HEAD AND NECK IMAGING VARIANTS

The McGraw-Hill Radiology Series

This innovative series offers indispensable workstation reference material for the practicing radiologist. Within this series is a full range of practical, clinically relevant works divided into three categories:

- **Patterns Books:** organized by modality, they provide a pattern-based approach to constructing practical differential diagnosis.
- **Variants Books:** structured by modality as well as anatomy, help decode appearances that are often misdiagnosed.
- **Case Books:** highlight classic case presentations by pathology.

HEAD AND NECK IMAGING VARIANTS

Achilles G. Karagianis, DO
Assistant Professor
Chief of Head and Neck Radiology
Department of Radiology
Northwestern Memorial Hospital
Northwestern University Feinberg School of Medicine

Mc Graw Hill Education

New York Chicago San Francisco Athens London Madrid Mexico City
Milan New Delhi Singapore Sydney Toronto

Head and Neck Imaging Variants

1 2 3 4 5 6 7 8 9 0 DSS/DSS 20 19 18 17 16

ISBN 978-0-07-180867-5
MHID 0-07-180867-1

Notice

Medicine is an ever-changing science. As new research and clinical experience broaden our knowledge, changes in treatment and drug therapy are required. The authors and the publisher of this work have checked with sources believed to be reliable in their efforts to provide information that is complete and generally in accord with the standards accepted at the time of publication. However, in view of the possibility of human error or changes in medical sciences, neither the authors nor the publisher nor any other party who has been involved in the preparation or publication of this work warrants that the information contained herein is in every respect accurate or complete, and they disclaim all responsibility for any errors or omissions or for the results obtained from use of the information contained in this work. Readers are encouraged to confirm the information contained herein with other sources. For example and in particular, readers are advised to check the product information sheet included in the package of each drug they plan to administer to be certain that the information contained in this work is accurate and that changes have not been made in the recommended dose or in the contraindications for administration. This recommendation is of particular importance in connection with new or infrequently used drugs.

This book was set in TradeGothic Light by Cenveo® Publisher Services.
The editors were Michael Weitz and Peter J. Boyle.
The production supervisor was Richard Ruzycka.
Project management was provided by Anupriya Tyagi, Cenveo Publisher Services.
The designer was Eve Siegel.
RR Donnelley/Shenzhen was printer and binder.

This book was printed on acid-free paper.

Library of Congress Cataloging-in-Publication Data

Head and neck imaging variants / editor, Achilles Karagianis.
p. ; cm.
Includes bibliographical references and index.
ISBN 978-0-07-180867-5 (hardcover : alk. paper)—ISBN 0-07-180867-1 (hardcover : alk. paper)
I. Karagianis, Achilles, editor, contributor.
[DNLM: 1. Head—pathology—Atlases. 2. Head—pathology—Case Reports. 3. Neck—pathology—Atlases. 4. Neck—pathology—Case Reports. 5. Diagnosis, Differential—Atlases. 6. Diagnosis, Differential—Case Reports. 7. Diagnostic Imaging—Atlases. 8. Diagnostic Imaging—Case Reports. 9. Head—radiography—Atlases. 10. Head—radiography—Case Reports. 11. Neck—radiography—Atlases. 12. Neck—radiography—Case Reports. WE 17]
RC936
617.5′10757—dc23

This book is dedicated to my late father, George Karagianis.
Thank you for showing me what true ambition means.
You will always be my inspiration.

CONTENTS

Chapter 2: Larynx, Hyoid, and Trachea 85

Christopher J. Therasse, Achilles G. Karagianis, Benjamin P. Liu

Chapter 3: Neck 213

Nishant D. Parekh, Christopher Reilly, Achilles G. Karagianis

Chapter 11: Calvarium, Scalp, and the Temporalis Musculature 1421

Noah Schwind, Achilles G. Karagianis

Chapter 12: Vascular 1539

Rishi Seth, Achilles G. Karagianis, Matthew T. Walker

CONTRIBUTORS

Tarek A. Hijaz, MD
Assistant Professor
Section of Neuroradiology
Department of Radiology
Northwestern Memorial Hospital
Northwestern University Feinberg School of Medicine
Chicago, Illinois
Chapter 9

Achilles G. Karagianis, DO
Assistant Professor
Chief of Head and Neck Radiology
Section of Neuroradiology
Department of Radiology
Northwestern Memorial Hospital
Northwestern University Feinberg School of Medicine
Chicago, Illinois
Chapters 1-12

Catherine Kim-Gavino, MD
Neuroradiologist
Medical Director
Premier Health Services
Chicago, Illinois
Chapter 4

Alexander W. Korutz, MD
Assistant Professor
Section of Neuroradiology
Department of Radiology
Northwestern Memorial Hospital
Northwestern University Feinberg School of Medicine
Chicago, Illinois
Chapter 5

Malisa S. Lester, MD
Assistant Professor
Section of Neuroradiology
Department of Radiology
Northwestern Memorial Hospital
Northwestern University Feinberg School of Medicine
Chicago, Illinois
Chapters 1 and 6

Vanessa A. Lewis, MD
Radiology Resident
Department of Radiology
Northwestern Memorial Hospital
Northwestern University Feinberg School of Medicine
Chicago, Illinois
Chapter 10

Benjamin P. Liu, MD
Assistant Professor
Section of Neuroradiology
Department of Radiology
Northwestern Memorial Hospital
Northwestern University Feinberg School of Medicine
Chicago, Illinois
Chapters 2 and 10

Erin N. McComb, MD
Assistant Professor
Section of Neuroradiology
Department of Radiology
Northwestern Memorial Hospital
Northwestern University Feinberg School of Medicine
Chicago, Illinois
Chapter 8

Nishant D. Parekh, MD
Clinical Instructor
Section of Thoracic Radiology
Department of Radiology
Northwestern Memorial Hospital
Northwestern University Feinberg School of Medicine
Chicago, Illinois
Chapter 3

Christopher Reilly, MD
Neuroradiologist
Radiologic Associates of Duluth
Grand Rapids, Minnesota
Chapter 3

Noah Schwind, MD
Interventional Radiologist
Department of Radiology
Saint Joseph's Medical Center
Joliet, Illinois
Chapter 11

Rishi Seth, MD
Section of Neuroradiology
Radiology Associates of North Texas
Fort Worth, Texas
Chapter 12

Kamran A. Shah, MD
Assistant Professor
Radiology Residency Program Director
Section of Neuroradiology
Department of Radiology
Detroit Medical Center
Wayne State University School of Medicine
Detroit, Michigan
Chapter 9

Christopher J. Therasse, MD
Clinical Instructor
Section of Neuroradiology
Department of Radiology
Northwestern Memorial Hospital
Northwestern University Feinberg School of Medicine
Chicago, Illinois
Chapter 2

Matthew T. Walker, MD
Professor
Chief of Neuroradiology
Department of Radiology
Northshore University Health Systems
University of Chicago Pritzker School of Medicine
Chicago, Illinois
Chapter 12

PREFACE

Sometimes the most challenging aspect of interpreting head and neck imaging is not in identifying the finding, but in determining whether the finding is truly abnormal or merely a variant. *Head and Neck Imaging Variants* aims to address this common dilemma. Imaging variants affecting all areas of head and neck imaging are addressed in this textbook, including selected vascular and calvarial variants. In addition, companion cases are included with almost all of the primary variant cases to help illustrate key differentiating imaging features. Because imaging of the posttreated head and neck may also simulate pathology, a large number of postsurgical and irradiated head and neck imaging cases are included.

An understanding of the important characteristics of a variant or disease process is vital to interpret images accurately. Thus, short discussions about the variant and relevant pathology are provided in this textbook. Similarly, the salient features of a surgical procedure are discussed to aid in interpreting the postsurgical head and neck.

Since imaging variants are normal findings and should not be resected or biopsied, pathologic confirmation was not possible in some cases. However, peer-reviewed literature is referenced for the vast majority of the variants, as well as for the companion cases. Because some of the variants presented in this text are quite rare and have a paucity of literature written about them, they are in essence case reports. In these instances, the author used his personal experience to label and characterize the variant.

Head and Neck Imaging Variants is written in an attempt to address common head and neck diagnostic imaging issues and pitfalls that face the radiologist on a daily basis. This book is geared for head and neck radiologists and general radiologists who interpret head and neck imaging. It is also ideal, particularly as a resource text, for residents and fellows who are learning head and neck imaging as well as for otolaryngologists.

Achilles G. Karagianis, DO

ACKNOWLEDGMENTS

I would first like to thank all the contributors who helped make this book possible. Thank you all for your hard work and dedication. I would also like to thank all the staff radiologists who trained me during my residency and fellowship. While there are too many to list, I would specifically like to acknowledge two by name. Dr. Henry Pribram was one of the staff neuroradiologists during my residency at the University of California, Irvine. Thank you, Dr. Pribram—especially for not accepting any of my "lazy answers" and for motivating me to become a better radiologist. Your teaching inspired me to pursue a career as an academic neuroradiologist. The other radiologist that I would like to thank is Dr. Hugh Curtin from the Massachusetts Eye and Ear Infirmary. Everyone in the head and neck radiology community already know of Dr. Curtin, but I would nevertheless be remiss in not acknowledging him. Dr. Curtin taught me just about everything I know in head and neck. He is the best radiologist that I have ever come across, and an even better human being.

On a personal level, I would like to thank my beautiful wife, Vivian, for her encouragement and unconditional love. I would have never completed this project without you. I would like to thank my mother, Kalliope, who in addition to my father, sacrificed so much so that their children would have every opportunity to succeed. Thank you for your wisdom and guidance throughout my life. I would also like to thank others in my family for their love and support over the years, including my brother, Eleftherios, my sister, Iphigenia, and my godparents, Vassilios and Maria Dionyssopoulos.

HEAD AND NECK IMAGING VARIANTS

CHAPTER 1

PHARYNX

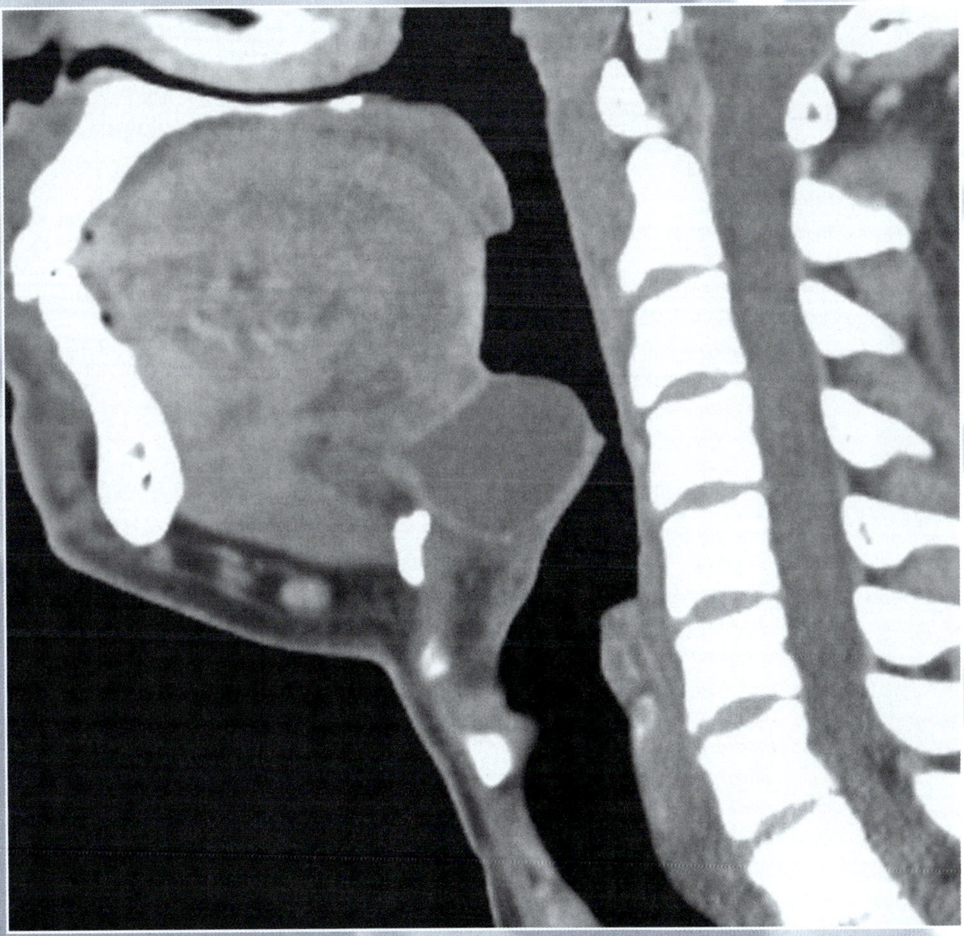

Malisa S. Lester, Achilles G. Karagianis

I. PHARYNX

1. Coapted fossa of Rosenmueller
    i. *Companion case*: Nasopharyngeal squamous cell carcinoma
2. Retention cyst in the fossa of Rosenmueller
    i. *Companion case*: Free fluid in the fossa of Rosenmueller
    ii. *Companion case*: Torus tubarius retention cysts
3. Eustachian tube cartilage mineralization
4. Hypertrophy of the Ostmann fat pad
    i. *Companion case*: Torus tubarius enlargement due to inflammation
    ii. *Companion case*: Denervation atrophy of the levator veli palatini muscle
5. Adenoid lymphoid hyperplasia
    i. *Companion case*: Nasopharyngeal squamous cell carcinoma
6. Tornwaldt cyst
7. Adenoid retention cyst
    i. *Companion case*: Sjögren syndrome affecting the nasopharynx minor salivary glands
8. Incidental adenoid diffusion restriction
    i. *Companion case*: Nasopharyngeal lymphoma
9. Tonsilloliths
    i. *Companion case*: Retained fish bone
    ii. *Companion case*: Displacement of a small tooth fracture fragment following intubation
    iii. *Companion case*: Displacement of an entire tooth
10. Palatine tonsil lymphoid hyperplasia
    i. *Companion case*: Unilateral palatine tonsil lymphoid hyperplasia due to a contralateral palatine tonsillectomy
    ii. *Companion case*: Vascular malformation involving a palatine tonsil
    iii. *Companion case*: Palatine tonsil squamous cell carcinoma
11. Air-filled palatine tonsil crypts
    i. *Companion case*: Fluid-filled palatine tonsil crypts
12. Palatine tonsil retention cyst
    i. *Companion case*: Palatine tonsil edema
    ii. *Companion case*: Palatine intratonsillar abscess
    iii. *Companion case*: Peritonsillar abscess
    iv. *Companion case*: Partially necrotic palatine tonsil squamous cell carcinoma
13. Lingual tonsil lymphoid hyperplasia
    i. *Companion case*: Base of tongue squamous cell carcinoma
14. Air-filled lingual tonsil crypts
15. Lingual tonsil retention cyst
    i. *Companion case*: Lingual tonsil edema
    ii. *Companion case*: Base of tongue squamous cell carcinoma
    iii. *Companion case*: Oropharyngeal wall retention cyst varying in size over time
    iv. *Companion case*: Vallecular retention cyst
16. Lingual thyroid
17. Coapted pyriform sinus
    i. *Companion case*: Pyriform sinus squamous cell carcinoma
    ii. *Companion case*: Retained oral contrast in the hypopharynx
18. Postcricoid region of the hypopharynx
    i. *Companion case*: Postcricoid region squamous cell carcinoma
    ii. *Companion case*: Impacted date seed at the cricopharyngeus muscle
19. Appearance of the pharynx during breath-hold or swallowing
    i. *Companion case*: Incidental soft palate abutment against the posterior pharyngeal wall
    ii. *Companion case*: Pharyngeal airway collapse related to an indwelling tracheostomy tube
    iii. *Companion case*: Large tumor compromising the pharyngeal airway
20. Denervation atrophy of the pharyngeal wall

CASE 1 Coapted fossa of Rosenmueller

The fossa of Rosenmueller, or lateral pharyngeal recess, is a mucosa-lined recess immediately posterior to the torus tubarius.

A coapted (ie, collapsed) fossa of Rosenmueller results from apposition of the torus tubarius with the ipsilateral posterior nasopharyngeal mucosa.

Differentiating this normal finding from a nasopharyngeal carcinoma can be difficult. With coaptation, the mucosal surfaces that are apposed to one another can usually be delineated, particularly with MRI. The submucosa should be intact and there should be no regional mass effect with coaptation. By contrast, if a mass is present, the mucosal surfaces will be disrupted and there will usually be mass effect.

COMPANION CASES

- **Nasopharyngeal squamous cell carcinoma.** Nasopharyngeal squamous cell carcinoma usually arises from within the fossa of Rosenmueller. Like other squamous cell carcinomas, this tumor is typically isointense on precontrast T1, iso- to hyperintense on T2, and diffusely enhances. Lymph nodes are present in 90% of patients at diagnosis and are usually bilateral and extensive, although the size of the primary tumor does not necessarily correlate with the extent of lymphadenopathy. The pharyngobasilar fascia, a tough fascia that encircles the nasopharyngeal mucosal space, tends to limit the extension of a nasopharyngeal carcinoma laterally, although aggressive tumors may directly breach the pharyngobasilar fascia, extend through the sinus of Morgagni (a space through which the Eustachian tube traverses), or it may directly invade the clivus. Because of the propensity of this tumor to involve the torus tubarius (and therefore obstruct or result in Eustachian tube dysfunction), the nasopharynx should be scrutinized in any patient who has a mastoid effusion, particularly when unilateral. In the United States, this tumor tends to affect males more than females, particularly in the sixth decade.Although a relatively uncommon cancer in the United States, it is more common in Asian Americans than non-Asian Americans, and it is extremely common in Asia (particularly southern China).

  It is important to evaluate for a pathologically enlarged node of Rouviere in every head and neck imaging study, particularly when there is a possible nasopharyngeal abnormality. The generally accepted size criterion for a pathologically enlarged node of Rouviere is 8 mm or larger when measured in greatest long axis dimension. Occasionally, young healthy patients can have measurements slightly greater than 8 mm and may simply represent a benign reactive lymph node. Conversely, in cases where a nasopharyngeal tumor is suspected, a node of Rouviere that is slightly less than 8 mm may be pathologic. As always, any lymph node that is significantly heterogeneous, regardless of size, should be considered abnormal.

Coapted fossa of Rosenmueller

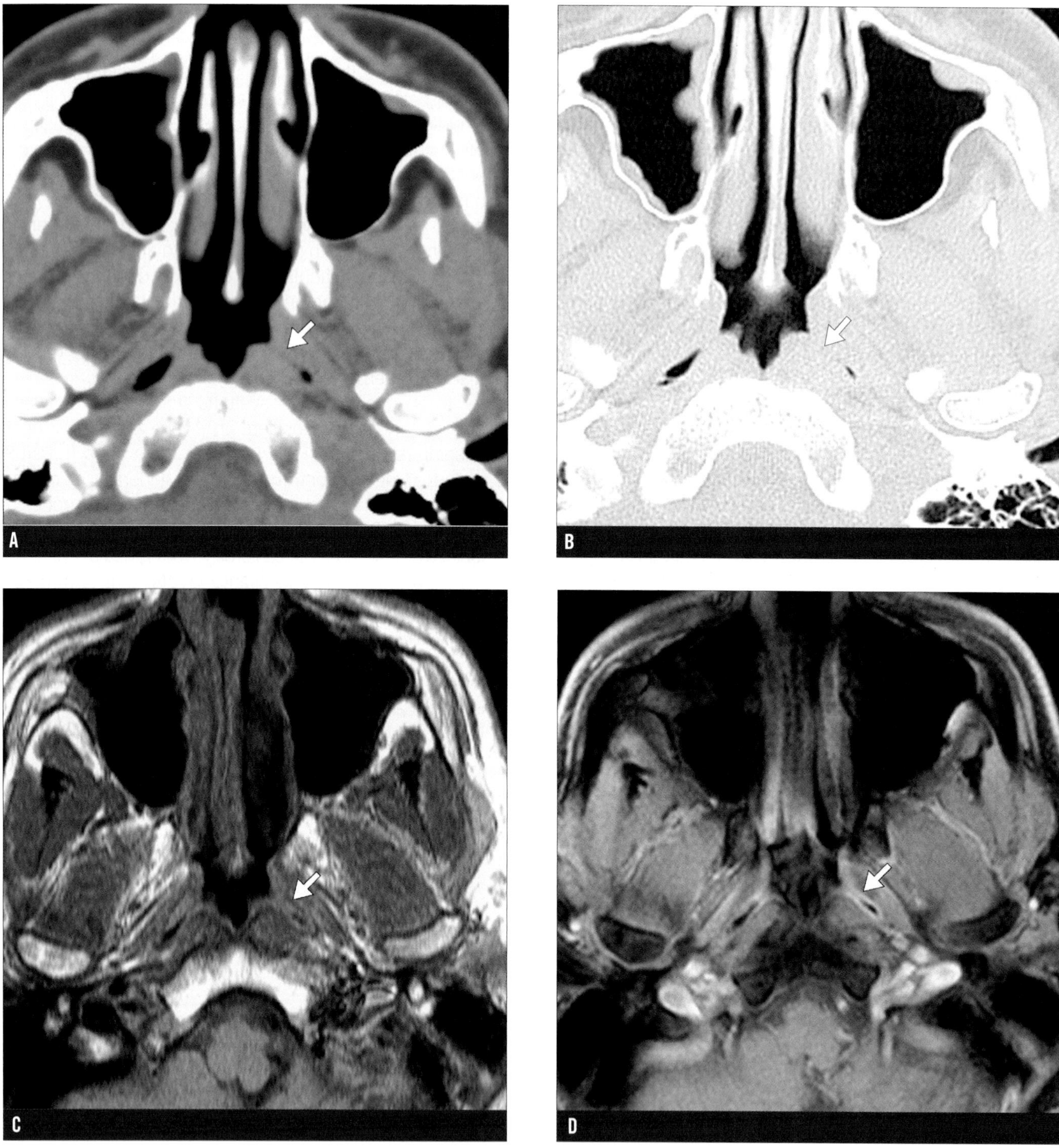

Unenhanced axial CT images through the level of the nasopharynx viewed with a soft tissue window (**A**) and wide window (**B**) demonstrating a partially coapted left fossa of Rosenmueller (arrows, **A**, **B**) with small amount of air deep in the fossa, a normal finding. Precontrast (**C**) and postcontrast (**D**) T1-weighted MR images of the same patient demonstrate normal smooth mucosal enhancement and normal submucosal architecture of the posterior nasopharynx (arrows, **C**, **D**).

Companion case: Nasopharyngeal squamous cell carcinoma

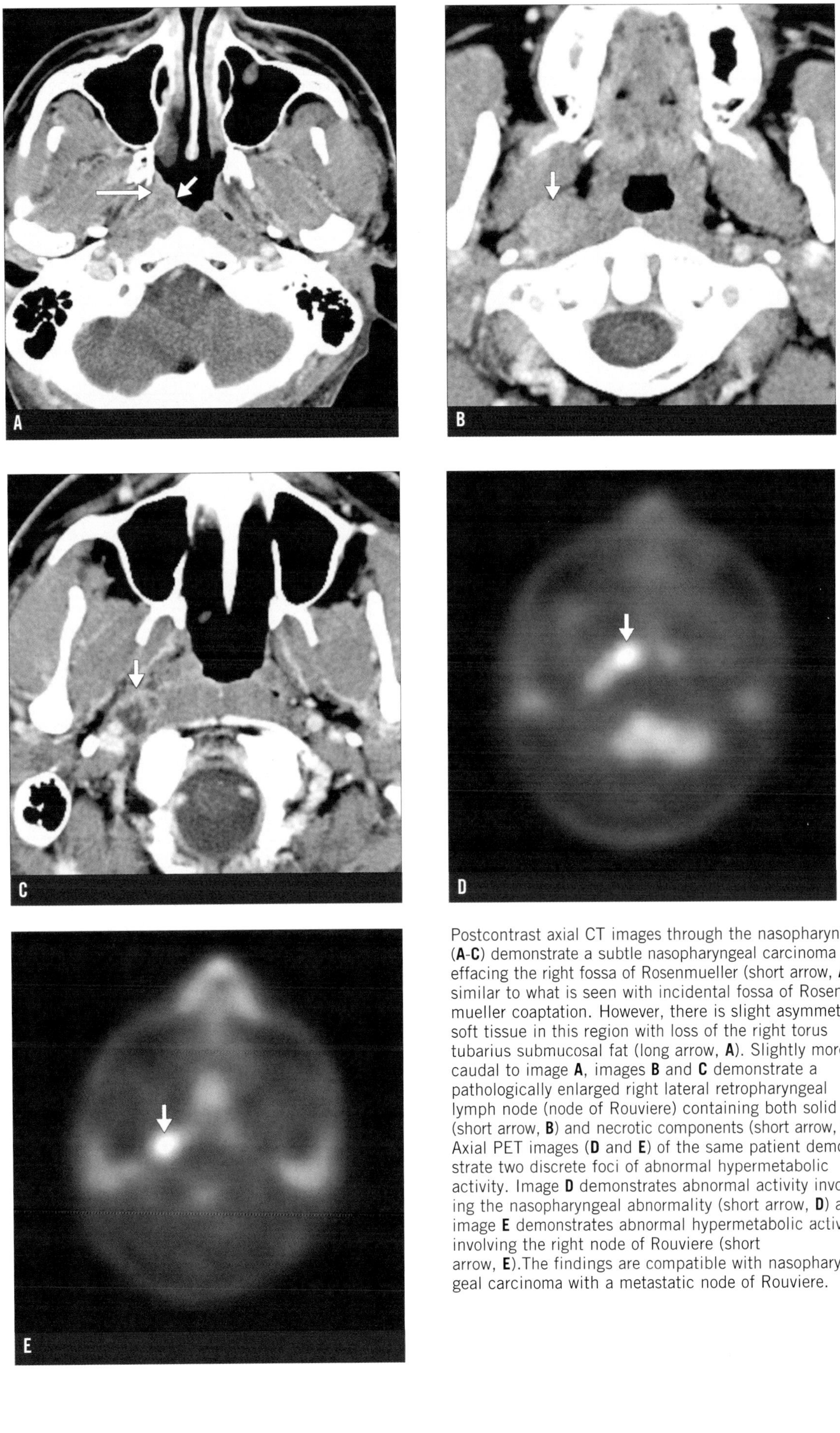

Postcontrast axial CT images through the nasopharynx (**A**-**C**) demonstrate a subtle nasopharyngeal carcinoma effacing the right fossa of Rosenmueller (short arrow, **A**), similar to what is seen with incidental fossa of Rosenmueller coaptation. However, there is slight asymmetric soft tissue in this region with loss of the right torus tubarius submucosal fat (long arrow, **A**). Slightly more caudal to image **A**, images **B** and **C** demonstrate a pathologically enlarged right lateral retropharyngeal lymph node (node of Rouviere) containing both solid (short arrow, **B**) and necrotic components (short arrow, **C**). Axial PET images (**D** and **E**) of the same patient demonstrate two discrete foci of abnormal hypermetabolic activity. Image **D** demonstrates abnormal activity involving the nasopharyngeal abnormality (short arrow, **D**) and image **E** demonstrates abnormal hypermetabolic activily involving the right node of Rouviere (short arrow, **E**).The findings are compatible with nasopharyngeal carcinoma with a metastatic node of Rouviere.

REFERENCES

Davis WL et al. Retropharyngeal space: evaluation of normal anatomy and diseases with CT and MR imaging. *Radiology.* 1990;174(1):59-64.

Lloyd SK et al. Cysts of the fossa of Rosenmuller: report of two cases. *Ear Nose Throat J.* August 2010;89(8):E19-E21.

Mancuso AA et al. Computed tomography of the nasopharynx: normal and variants of normal. *Radiology.* October 1980;137:113-121.

Silver AJ et al. Computed tomography of the nasopharynx and related spaces. Part I: normal anatomy. *Radiology.* June 1983;147:725-731.

Young KI et al. Nasopharyngeal carcinoma: posttreatment changes of imaging findings. *Am J Otolaryngol.* 2003;24(4):224-230.

CASE 2 Retention cyst in the fossa of Rosenmueller

Retention cysts are a common incidental and asymptomatic finding that may be found anywhere within the oral cavity and pharynx. There are two basic types of retention cysts: mucous and serous. A mucous retention cyst is more common and results from obstruction of a seromucinous gland. A serous retention cyst results from accumulation of fluid in the submucosal layer. Mucous and serous retention cysts are indistinguishable by imaging and appear as smooth, outwardly convex soft tissue masses. Depending on the location, or if the cyst becomes large enough, symptoms such as dysphagia may occur. Retention cysts generally have low attenuation values on CT imaging. On MRI, retention cysts are most often hypointense on T1 and hyperintense on T2, although their signal characteristics can be variable, depending on their protein content. Following intravenous contrast administration, a thin rim of enhancement may be observed on either CT or MRI, but retention cysts should not solidly enhance.

COMPANION CASE

- **Free fluid in the fossa of Rosenmueller.** Free fluid may also collect within the fossa of Rosenmueller. Free fluid may be indistinguishable from a retention cyst; however, free fluid may resolve on follow-up studies, whereas retention cysts generally persist. Additionally, a retention cyst may expand the fossa of Rosenmueller, while free fluid does not.
- **Torus tubarius retention cysts.**

Retention cyst in the fossa of Rosenmueller

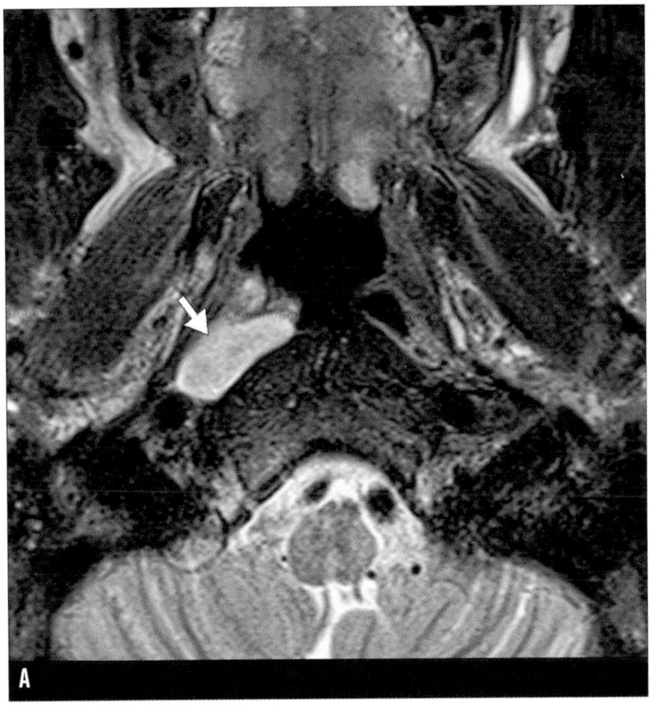

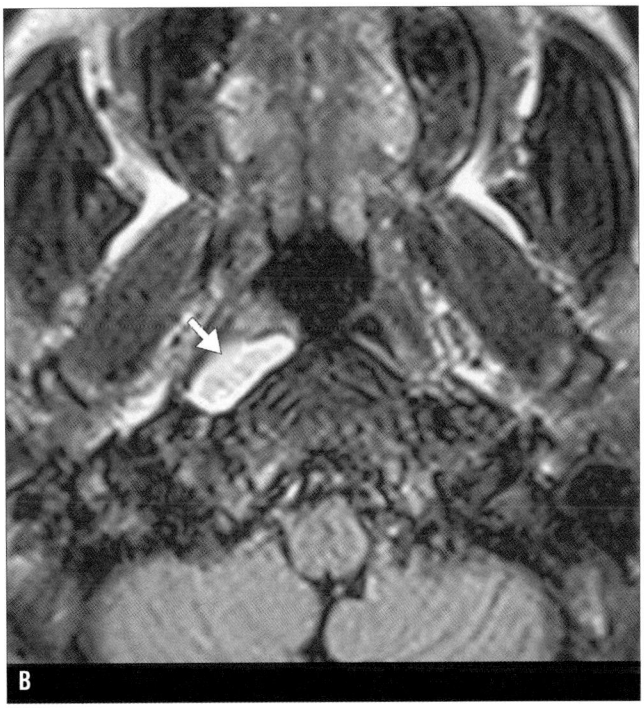

Axial T2 (**A**), axial FLAIR (**B**), axial T1 (**C**), sagittal T1 (**D**), and axial postcontrast MPRAGE (**E**) MR images. Images **A** and **B** demonstrate an oval, T2/FLAIR hyperintense finding within and expanding the right fossa of Rosenmueller (arrows, **A, B**). Images **C** and **D** demonstrate the finding to be markedly hyperintense on T1, compatible with proteinaceous content within the lesion (arrows, **C, D**). Image **E** does not demonstrate the lesion to enhance relative to the precontrast imaging (arrow, **E**). The lesion expands the right fossa of Rosenmueller, but the submucosa is normal. The findings are compatible with an incidental proteinaceous retention cyst and is of no clinical significance at this size.

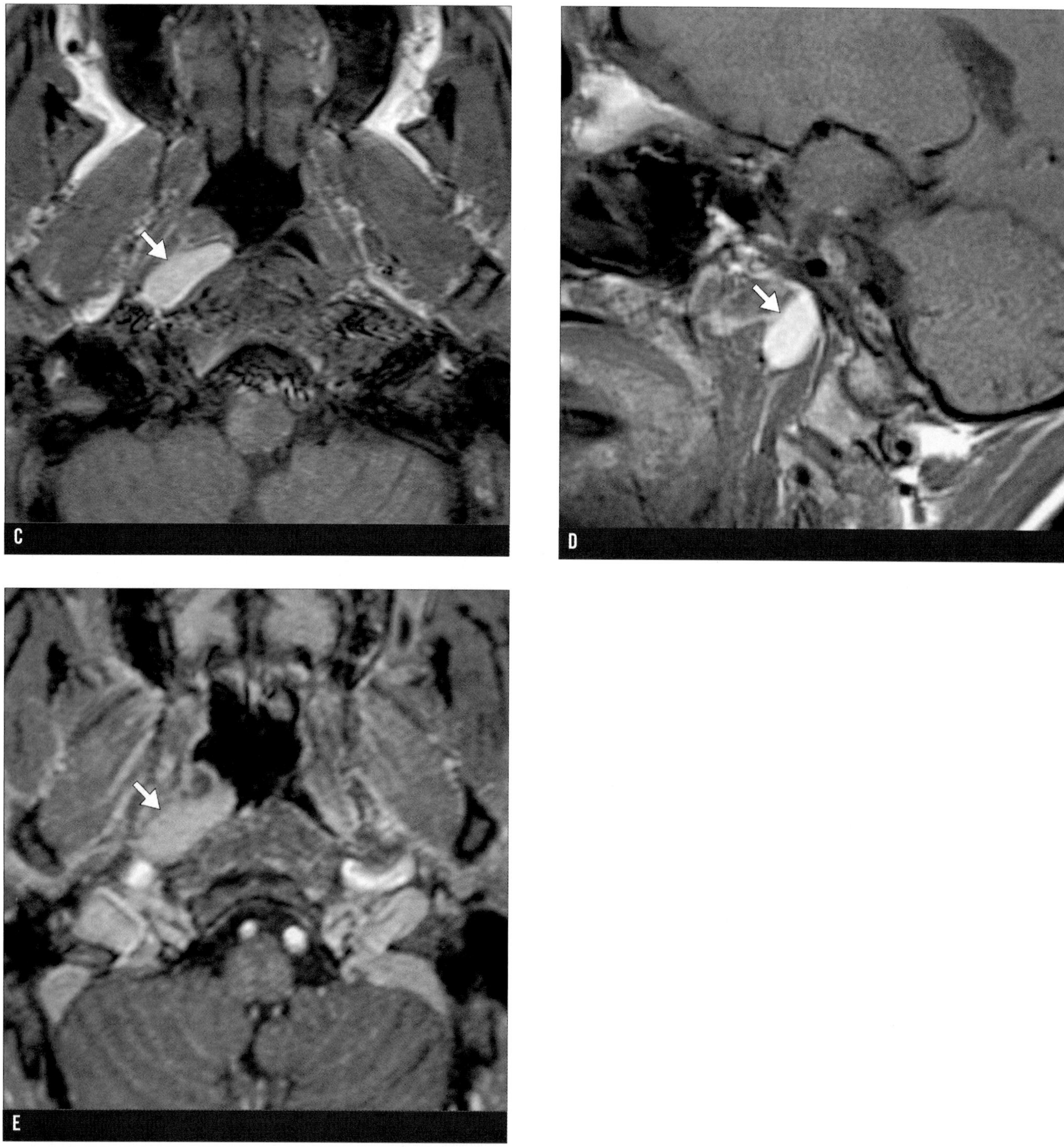
C
D
E

Retention cyst in the fossa of Rosenmueller

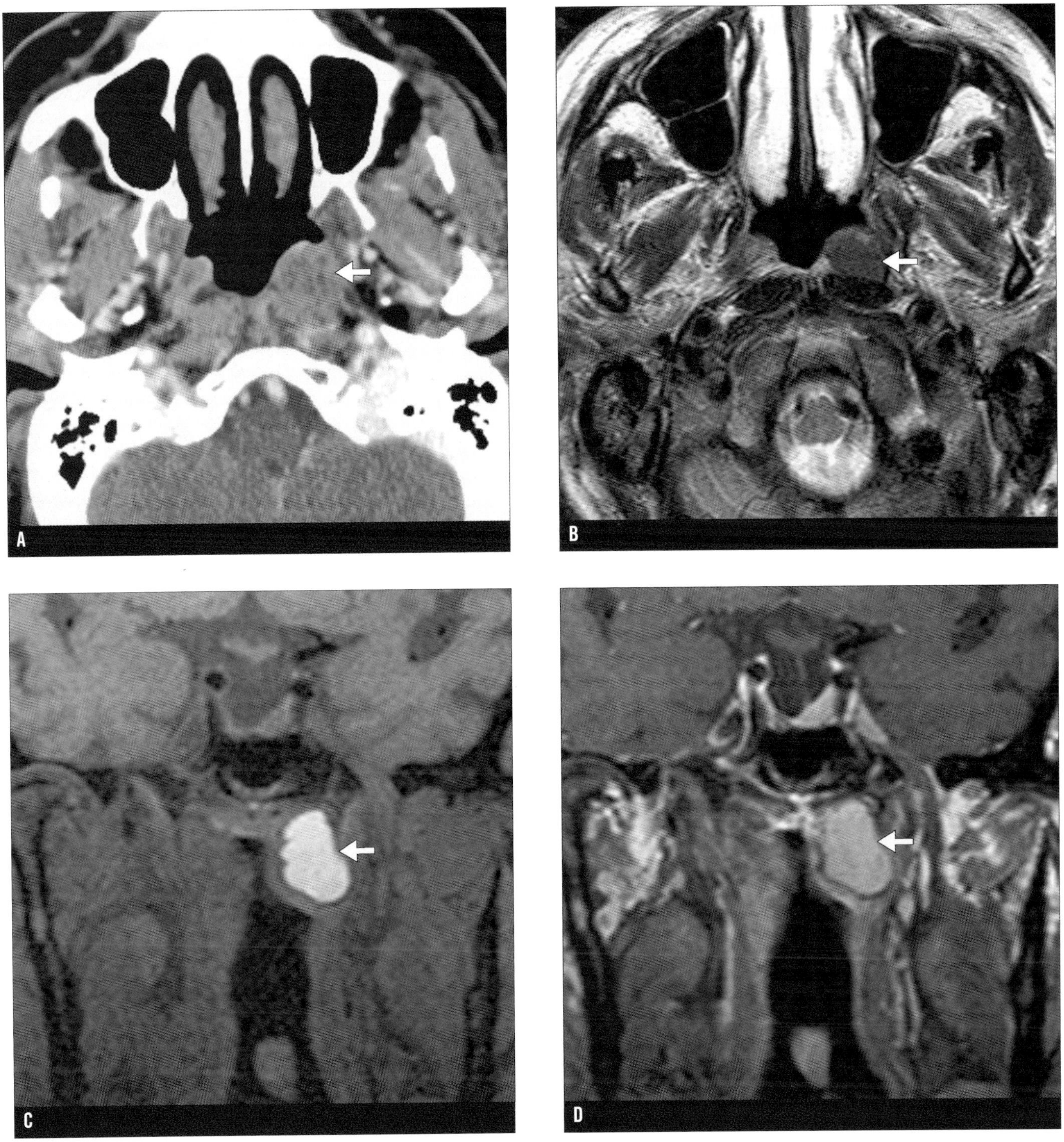

Different patient. A contrast-enhanced axial CT image through the nasopharynx (**A**) demonstrates a focal mass at the left fossa of Rosenmueller, concerning for a primary tumor at this location (arrow, **A**). However, axial T2 (**B**), fat-suppressed coronal T1 without contrast (**C**), and fat-suppressed coronal T1 with contrast (**D**) MR images obtained shortly before the CT study demonstrate a T2 hypointense, markedly intrinsically T1 hyperintense, nonenhancing oval lesion in the left fossa of Rosenmueller, compatible with an incidental retention cyst (arrows, **B**-**D**).

Free fluid in the fossa of Rosenmueller

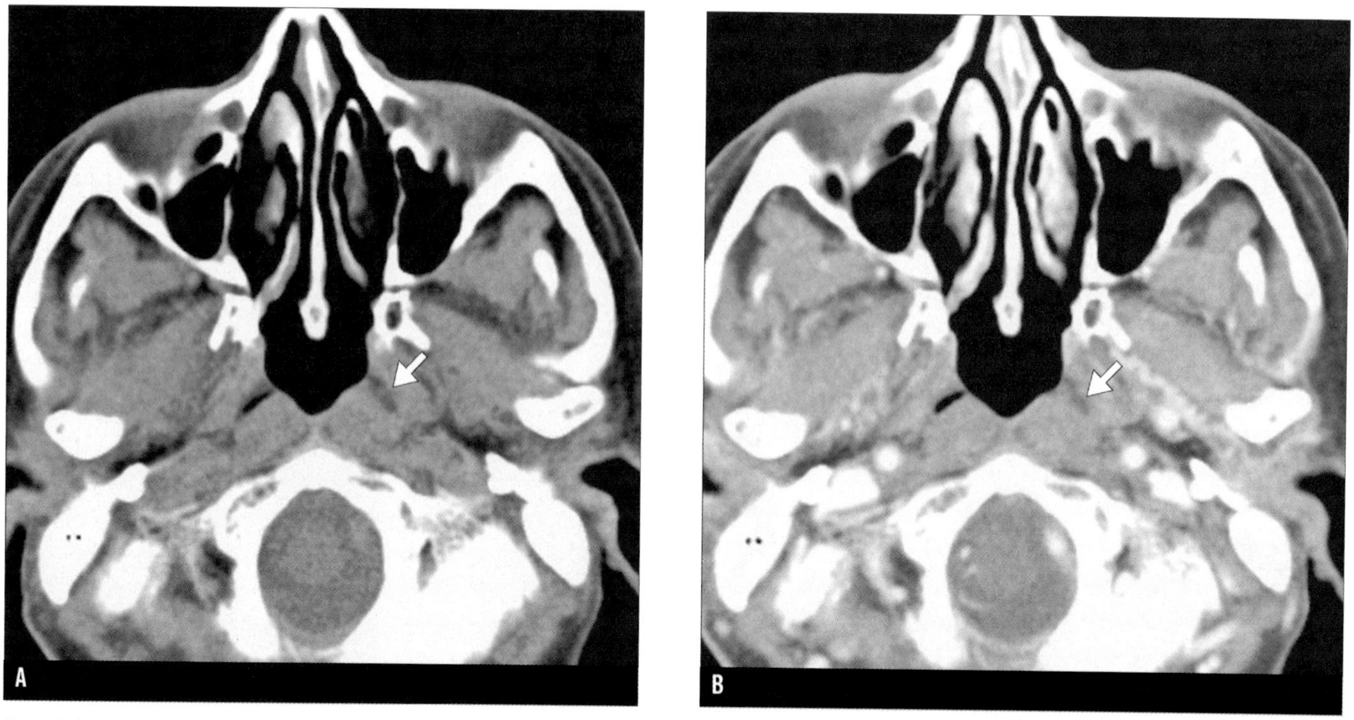

An axial precontrast CT image through the level of the nasopharynx (**A**) demonstrates an attenuated left fossa of Rosenmueller (arrow, **A**) compared to the contralateral side. An axial postcontrast CT image through the same level (**B**) does not demonstrate abnormal enhancement in the left fossa of Rosenmueller. The Hounsfield units within the left fossa of Rosenmueller measured fluid density. Thus, the attenuation of the fossa in this case was related to incidental fluid.

Torus tubarius retention cysts

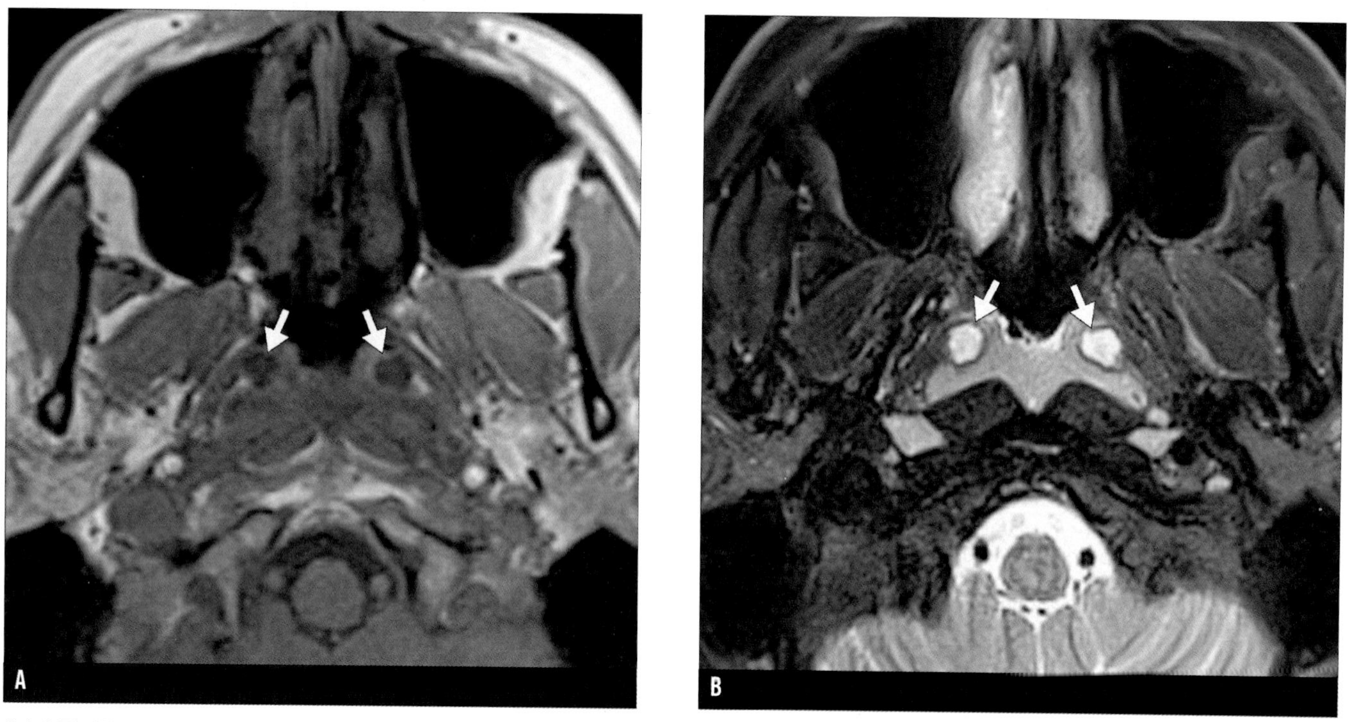

Axial T1 (**A**), axial T2 with fat saturation (**B**), and axial postcontrast T1 with fat saturation (**C**) demonstrate symmetric,T1 hypointense, T2 hyperintense, nonenhancing round foci within each torus tubarius most compatible with incidental retention cysts (arrows, **A-C**). These presumably occurred because of accumulation of mucous from obstructed seromucinous glands embedded within each torus tubarius.

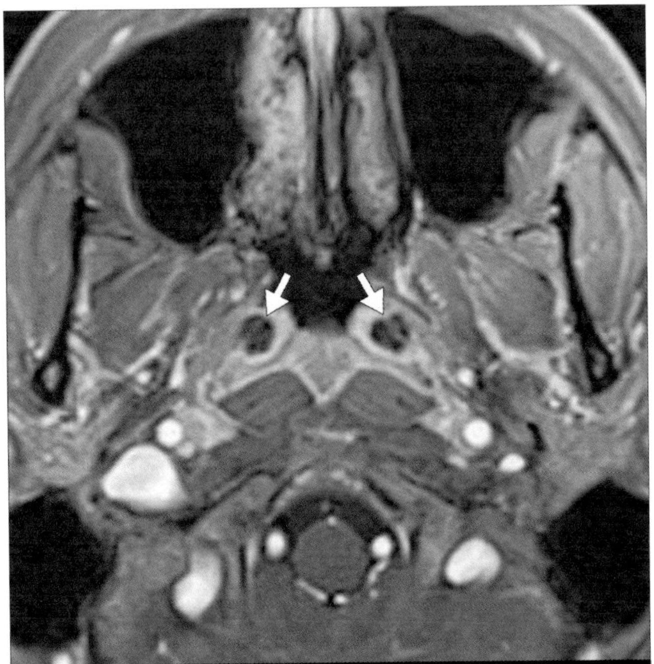

C

REFERENCES

Burgener F et al. *Differential diagnosis in computed tomography.* 2nd ed. New York, NY.: Thieme; 2012.

Lloyd SK et al. Cysts of the fossa of Rosenmuller: report of two cases. *Ear Nose Throat J.* Aug 2010;89(8):E19-E21.

Muro-Cacho C et al. Nasopharyngeal cysts. *Am J Otolaryngol.* 2000;21(2):108-111.

Pilch BZ. Head and neck surgical pathology. Philadelphia, PA:Lippincott Williams and Wilkins;2001.

Salem DB et al. Imaging of nasopharyngeal cysts and bursae. *Eur Radiol.* 2006;16:2249-2258.

CASE 3 Eustachian tube cartilage mineralization

Elastic cartilage surrounds a portion of the Eustachian tube and can mineralize, particularly in the torus tubarius. Mineralization of the Eustachian tube cartilage may be idiopathic, dystrophic (benign senescent mineralization), or present in the setting of hypercalcemic disease states, such as renal failure. Mineralization of the cartilage may cause Eustachian tube dysfunction, although it is an incidental finding in most patients, particularly the elderly when it almost always represents benign senescent mineralization. This finding may simulate a foreign body.

Eustachian tube cartilage mineralization

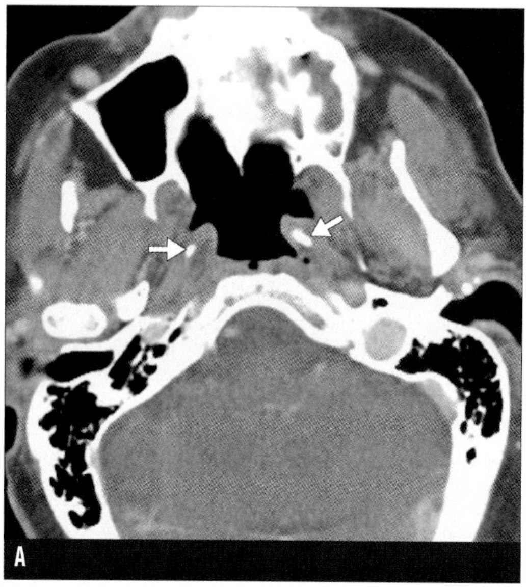

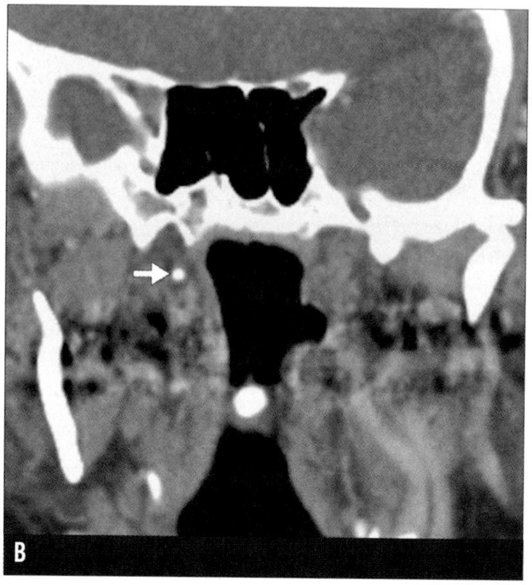

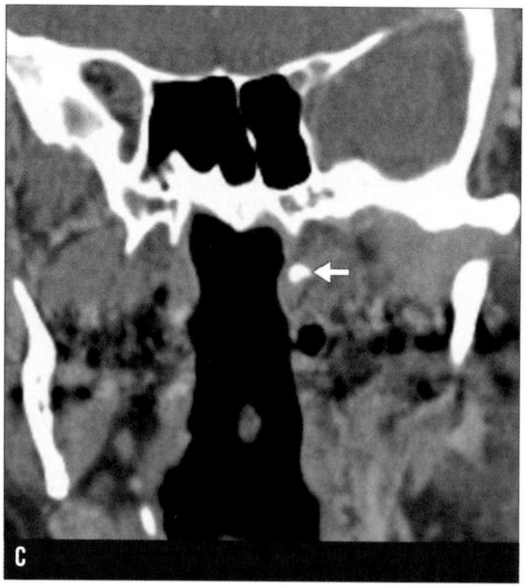

An axial postcontrast CT image through the nasopharynx (**A**) demonstrates mineralization of the Eustachian tube cartilage within each torus tubarius (arrows, **A**). Coronal reformatted postcontrast images through the pharynx (**B, C**) demonstrate the Eustachian tube mineralization in the coronal plane (arrows, **B, C**).

REFERENCES

Morshedi M, Mafee M. Calcification of the cartilaginous Eustachian tube. *Neuroradiology.* May 2012;54(5):525-527. Epub 2011 Sep 24.

Takasaki K et al. Ossification of Eustachian tube cartilage and Ostmann's fatty tissue in chronic renal failure. *Otolaryngol Head Neck Surg.* 2000;122:567-571.

The Eustachian tube orifice is located along the anterolateral aspect of the torus tubarius. The distal aspect of Eustachian tube is composed of cartilage and is surrounded by submucosal fat termed the Ostmann fat pad. The Ostmann fat pad lies between the Eustachian tube lumen and the tensor veli palatini muscle and may play a protective role by maintaining the Eustachian tube in a closed position. This fat pad may hypertrophy and result in enlargement of the torus tubarius. If the fatty hypertrophy encroaches upon the Eustachian tube orifice, then Eustachian tube dysfunction can occur.

COMPANION CASES

- **Torus tubarius enlargement due to inflammation.** A nasopharyngitis (ie, common cold) is most often due to a virus and may result in enlargement as well as enhancement of the torus tubarius.
- **Denervation atrophy of the levator veli palatini muscle.** This small muscle resides in the torus tubarius and is innervated by the pharyngeal plexus, primarily via the pharyngeal branch of CN X; therefore, injury to CN X can result in denervation atrophy of the levator veli palatini muscle. The function of the levator veli palatini muscle is to elevate the soft palate during deglutition and thus prevent food from entering the nasopharynx.

Hypertrophy of the Ostmann fat pad

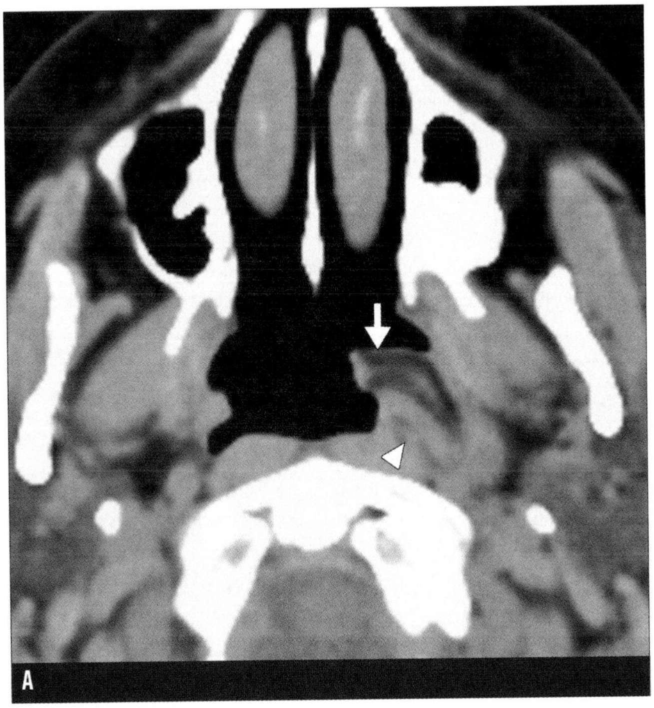

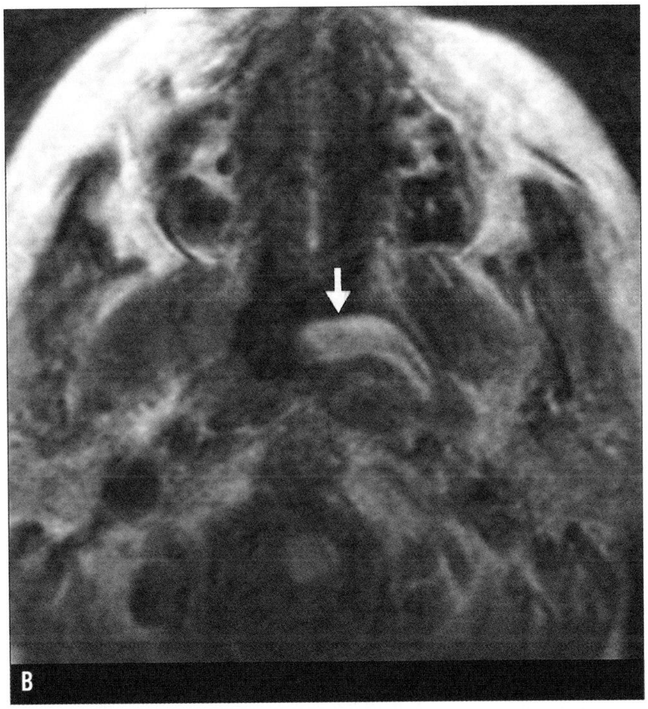

An axial noncontrast CT image (**A**) and an axial T1-weighted noncontrast MR image (**B**) through the level of the nasopharynx demonstrate the left torus tubarius to be significantly larger than the right and to protrude into the left aspect of the nasopharynx. The left torus tubarius contains a large amount of fat which represents a hypertrophied Ostmann fat pad (arrows, **A**, **B**). The hypertrophied left Ostmann fat pad also attenuates the left fossa of Rosenmueller (arrowhead, **A**). An axial CT image through the left mastoid and tympanic cavity (**C**) demonstrates an opacified left mastoid and left tympanic cavity (arrow, **C**), compatible with Eustachian tube dysfunction.

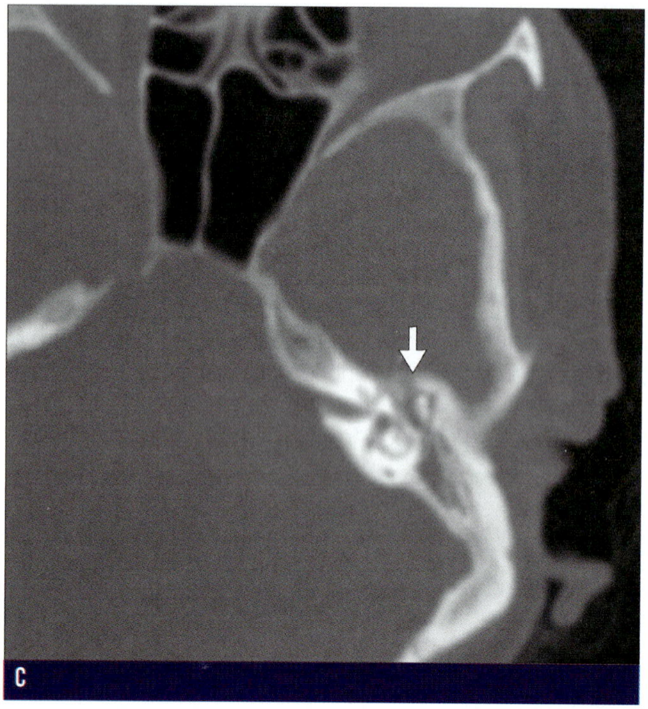

Companion case: Torus tubarius enlargement due to inflammation

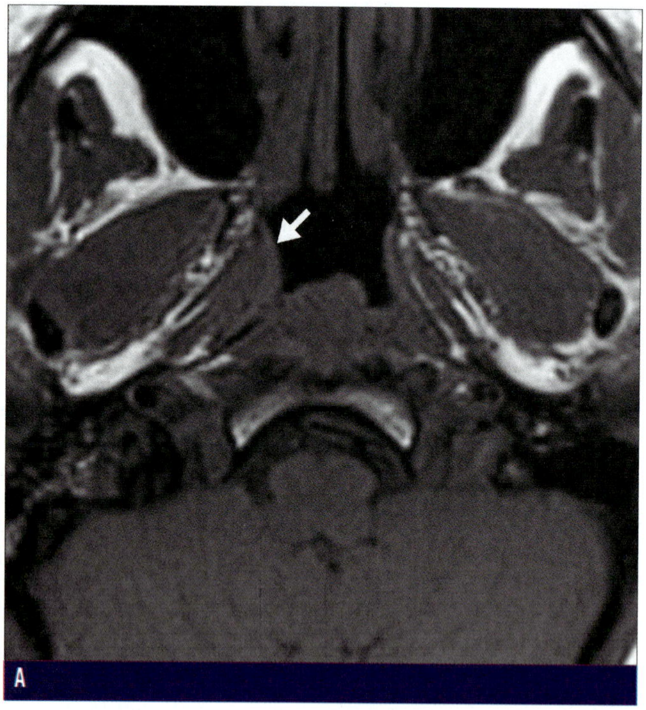

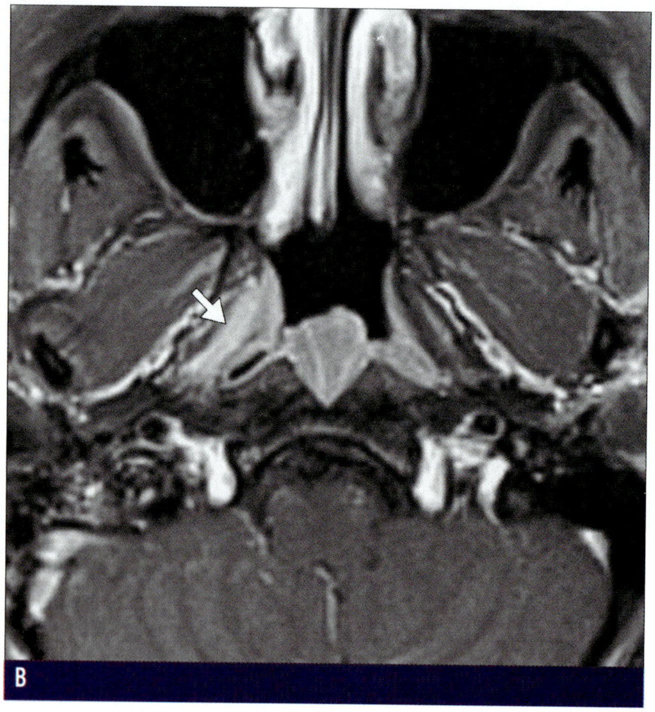

A 39-year-old woman with right hearing loss and right Eustachian tube dysfunction. Axial T1 (**A**), axial postcontrast T1 with fat saturation (**B**, **C**), and coronal postcontrast T1 without fat saturation (**D**) MR images. Image **A** demonstrates asymmetric enlargement in the region of the right torus tubarius with loss of the fat planes within and adjacent to the torus tubarius (arrow, **A**). Image **B** demonstrates enhancement in the region of the cartilaginous right Eustachian tube (arrow, **B**), whereas image **C** demonstrates asymmetric enlargement and enhancement of the right torus tubarius, consistent with edema (arrow, **C**). Image **D** demonstrates the Eustachian tube enhancement in the coronal plane (arrow, **D**). These findings do not represent a hypertrophied Ostmann fat pad, given the paucity of fat and the pronounced enhancement. While there is enhancement of the right torus tubarius, there is no discrete mass in the fossa of Rosenmueller to suggest nasopharyngeal carcinoma. Nevertheless, infiltrating squamous cell carcinoma of the Eustachian tube could have a similar appearance and follow-up clinically and/or with imaging to resolution for a finding such as this would be prudent.

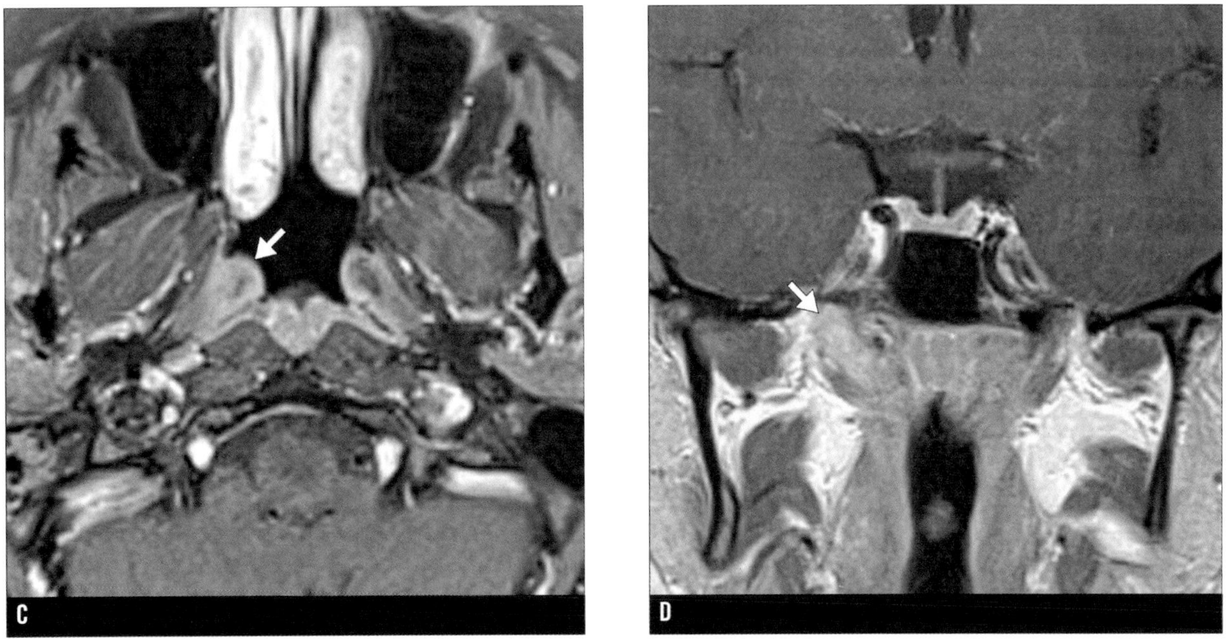

Companion case: Denervation atrophy of the levator veli palatini muscle

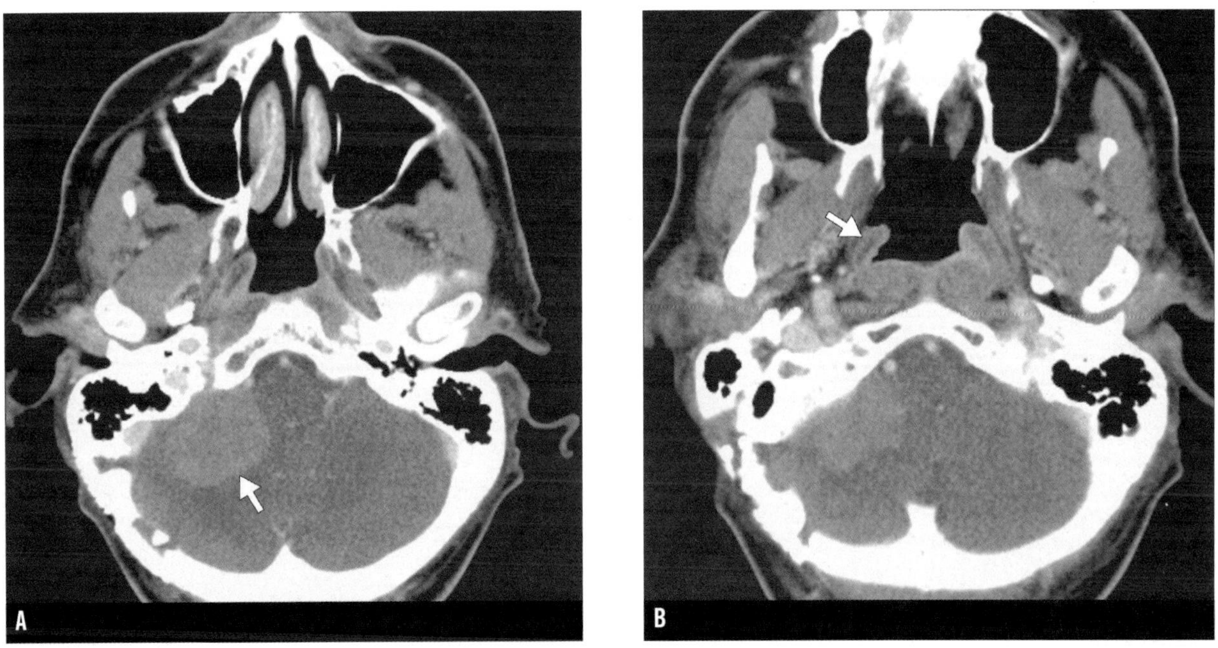

An axial postcontrast CT image through the posterior fossa (**A**) subtly demonstrates a large mass in the right aspect of the posterior fossa, which was pathologically proven non-Hodgkin lymphoma (arrow, **A**). An axial postcontrast CT image through nasopharynx (**B**) demonstrates atrophy and fatty infiltration of the right torus tubarius (arrow, **B**). This is related to denervation atrophy of the right levator palatini muscle due to injury of cranial nerve X by the mass. In contrast to hypertrophy of the Ostmann fat pad, this entity is associated with volume loss of the torus tubarius, whereas hypertrophy of the Ostmann fat pad is associated with enlargement of the torus tubarius and regional mass effect.

REFERENCES

Hayden MG et al. Cerebellopontine angle cyst compressing the vagus nerve: case report. *Neurosurgery*. June 2007;60(6):E1150.

Massey EW. Spinal Accessory Nerve Lesions. *Semin Neurol*. 2009;29(1):82-84.

Takasaki K et al. Ossification of Eustachian tube cartilage and Ostmann's fatty tissue in chronic renal failure. *Otolaryngol Head Neck Surg*. 2000;122:567-571.

CASE 5 Adenoid lymphoid hyperplasia

The Waldeyer ring (adenoids, palatine tonsils, and lingual tonsil) is normally large in children, adolescents, and young adults owing to lymphoid hyperplasia. However, while adenoid lymphoid hyperplasia is a benign entity, airway compromise, obstructive sleep apnea, and Eustachian tube dysfunction can be present in severe cases of adenoid lymphoid hyperplasia. Mild prominence of the adenoid tissue in children should not be misinterpreted as abnormal. In fact, if the adenoids are not prominent in children, then the child may be immunocompromised. Generally speaking, the maximum size of the adenoids occurs at approximately 5 years of age and involution of the adenoids begins around the time of puberty. While normal adenoid tissue may persist into the sixth decade, enlarged adenoids in older patients should be viewed with suspicion, particularly when asymmetric. When in doubt, enlarged adenoids in the older patients should be correlated with direct inspection to exclude a malignancy, such as nasopharyngeal carcinoma or lymphoma.

COMPANION CASE

Nasopharyngeal squamous cell carcinoma. Differentiating between a nasopharyngeal tumor (such as nasopharyngeal carcinoma, lymphoma, etc) from normal adenoids/lymphoid hyperplasia can be difficult. While lymphoid hyperplasia can simulate a neoplasm, lymphoid hyperplasia affecting the adenoids is typically a diffuse process rather than a focal asymmetric process, the latter more commonly identified with neoplasms. In addition, lymphoid hyperplasia often has a frond-like morphology, a feature that is not common with malignancy. Because of the propensity of a nasopharyngeal carcinoma to involve the torus tubarius (and therefore obstruct or result in dysfunction of the Eustachian tube), the nasopharynx should be scrutinized in any patient who has a mastoid effusion, particularly when the mastoid effusion is unilateral.

Adenoid lymphoid hyperplasia

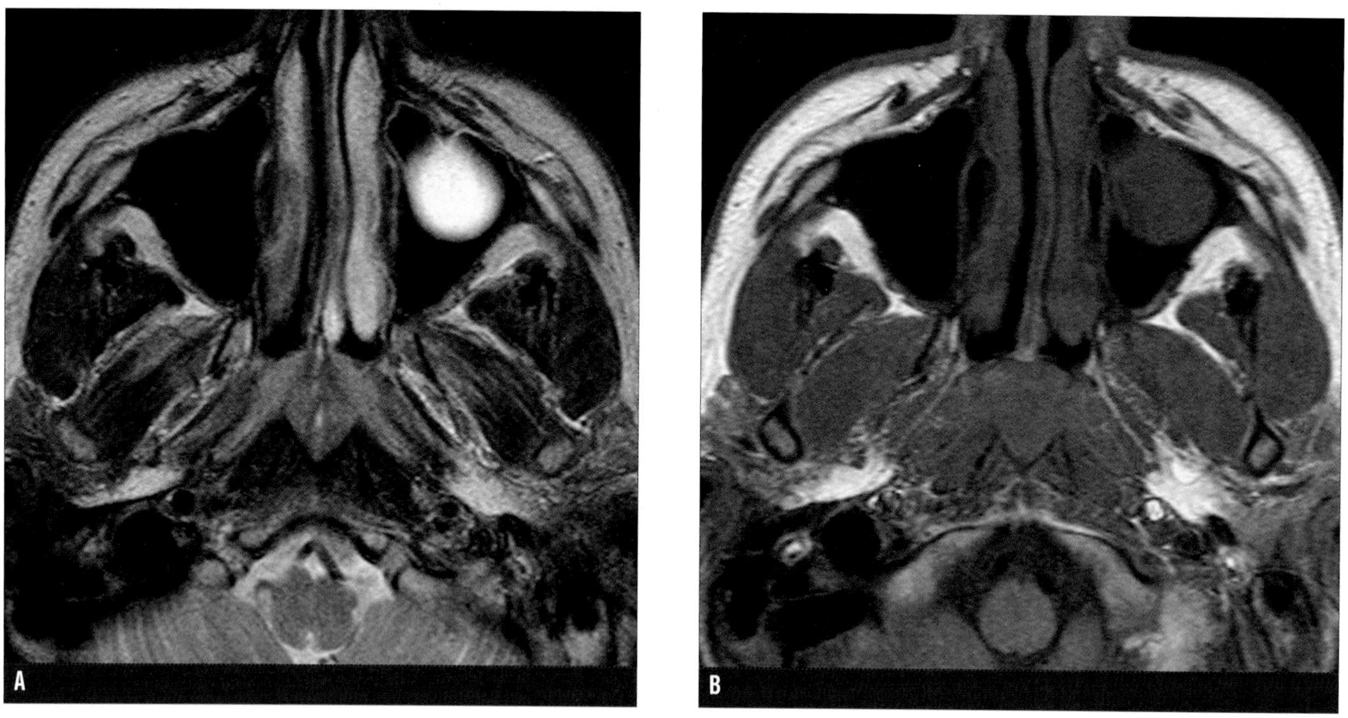

Axial T2 (**A**), axial precontrast T1 (**B**), and axial postcontrast T1 (**C**) MR images through the nasopharynx and a midline sagittal noncontrast T1-weighted MR image (**D**) demonstrate adenoid lymphoid hyperplasia in a healthy 14-year-old patient.

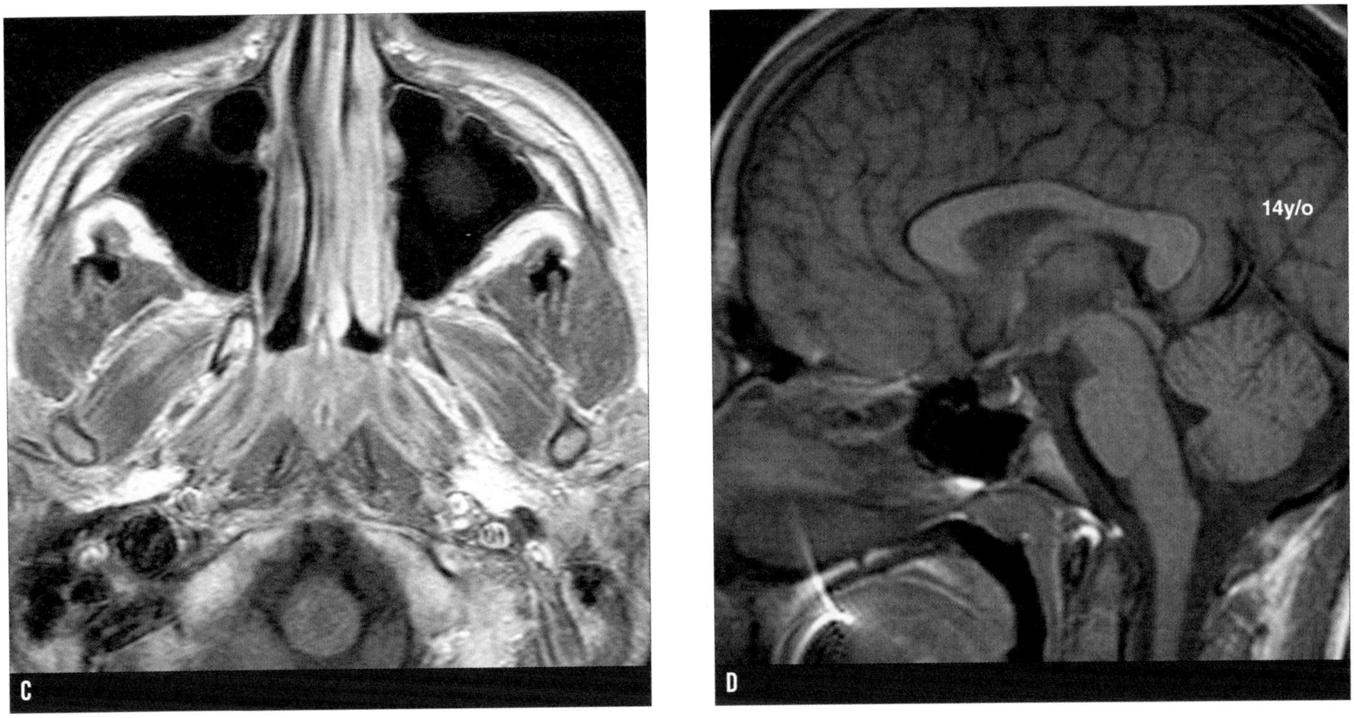

Adenoid lymphoid hyperplasia

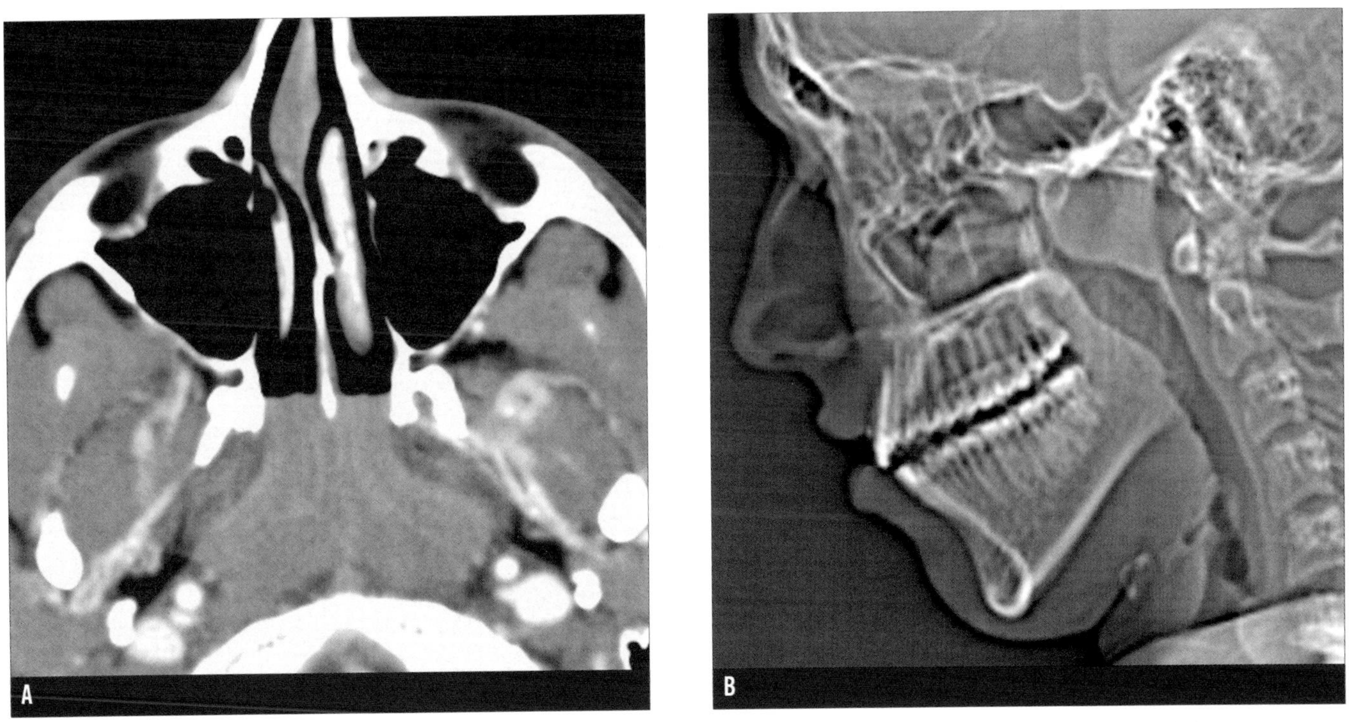

An axial postcontrast CT image obtained through the adenoids (**A**) and the sagittal scout image from the same CT study (**B**) demonstrate adenoid lymphoid hyperplasia in a healthy 17-year-old patient.

Adenoid lymphoid hyperplasia

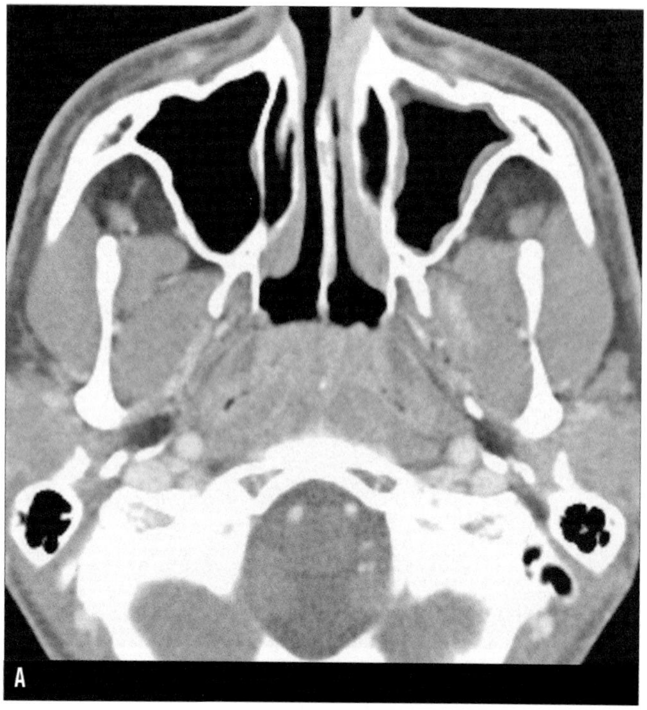

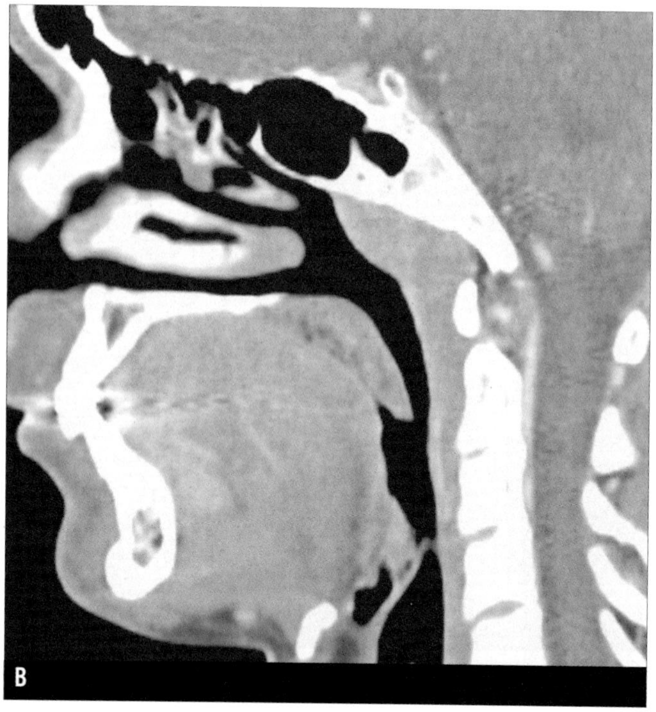

An axial postcontrast CT image through the nasopharynx (**A**) and a midline sagittal postcontrast reformatted CT image from the same study (**B**) demonstrate adenoid lymphoid hyperplasia in a healthy 19-year-old patient.

Companion case: Nasopharyngeal squamous cell carcinoma

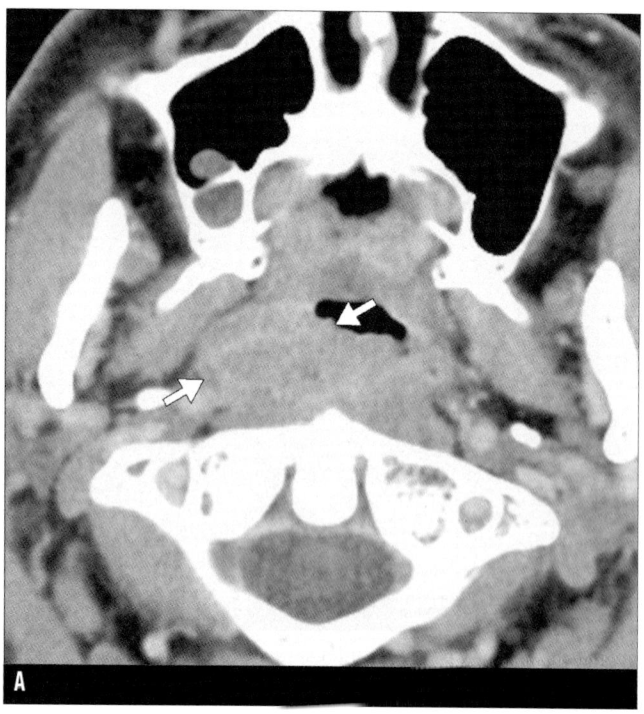

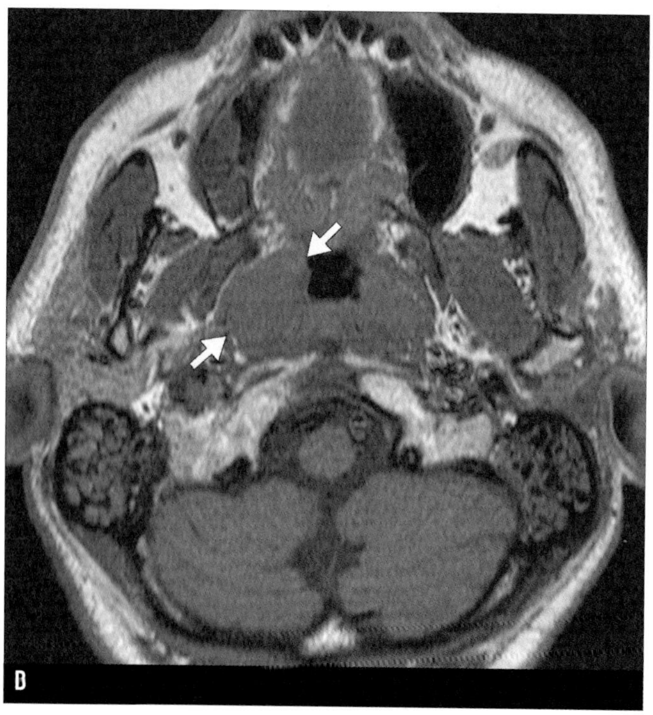

An axial postcontrast CT image through the nasopharynx (**A**) demonstrates a large nasopharyngeal mass primarily involving the right aspect of the nasopharynx (arrows, **A**). Axial noncontrast T1 (**B**), axial postcontrast T1 with fat saturation (**C**), and axial T2 (**D**) MR images demonstrate the same lesion on MRI, in this case representing nasopharyngeal carcinoma (arrows, **B-D**).

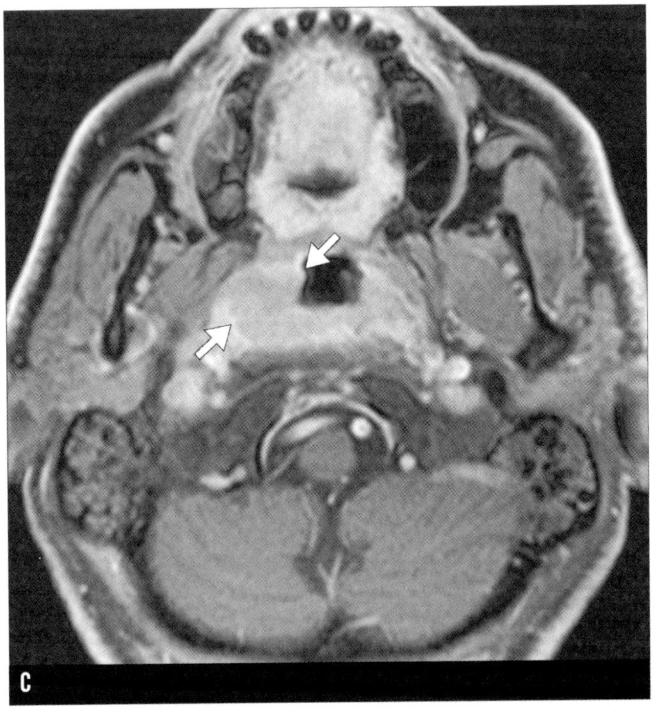

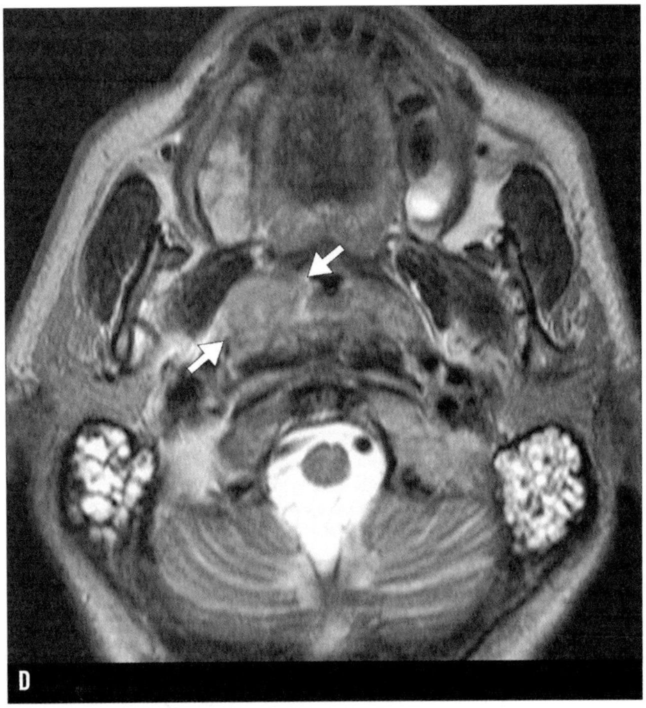

REFERENCES

Harley EH. Asymmetric tonsil size in children. *Arch Otolaryngo Head Neck Surg.* July 2002;128(7):767-769.

Som Peter M, Curtin Hugh D.. 4th ed. 2 vols. St. Louis, MO: Mosby; 2003.

Stambuk HE et al. Nasopharyngeal carcinoma: recognizing the radiographic features in children. *AJNR Am J Neuroradiol.* 2005;26(6):1575-1579.

Vogler RC et al. Age specific size of the adenoid pad on magnetic resonance imaging. *Clin Otolaryngol Allied Sci.* October 2000;(5):392-395.

CASE 6 Tornwaldt cyst

A Tornwaldt cyst is a benign notochordal remnant and represents the location where the embryologic notochord and endoderm of the primitive pharynx come into contact. It is a circumscribed structure most often located in the midline of the posterior nasopharyngeal soft tissues. A Tornwaldt cyst is a very common entity, present in approximately 5% of MRI studies that include the nasopharynx. The differential diagnosis of a Tornwaldt cyst includes a submucosal retention cyst, though a submucosal retention cyst is typically off-midline. Tornwaldt cysts may exhibit temporal variations in size, but they are normal variants and do not require biopsy. There are some reports of associated halitosis and Eustachian tube dysfunction (if large and obstructing the Eustachian tube orifice). The T1 and T2 signal characteristics vary based on a Tornwaldt cyst's proteinaceous content, although generally Tornwaldt cysts are T1 hypointense and T2 hyperintense. They do not centrally enhance, although they may have mild rim enhancement.

Tornwaldt cyst

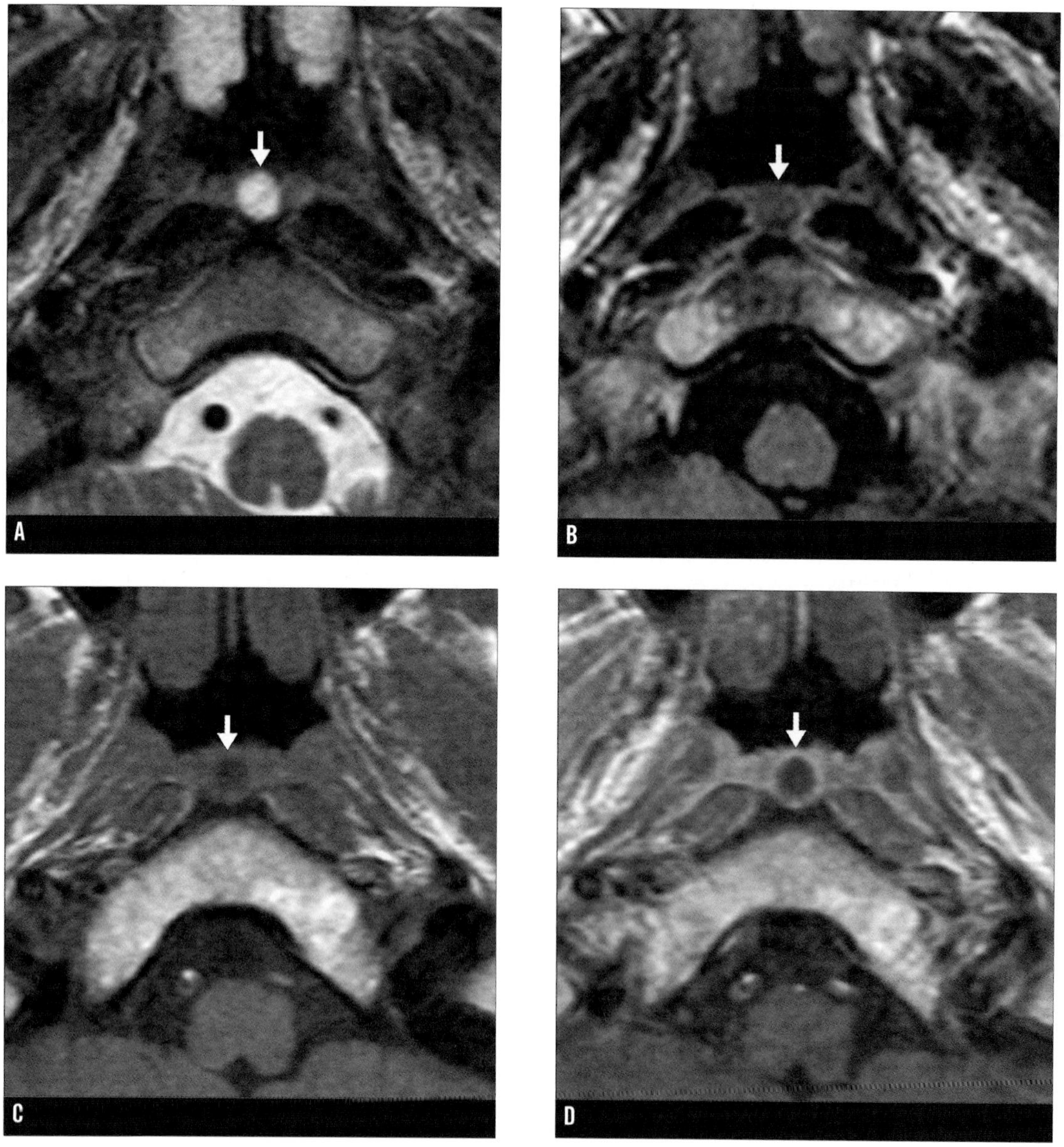

Axial T2 (**A**), axial FLAIR (**B**), noncontrast axial T1 (**C**), and postcontrast axial T1 (**D**) MR images through the level of the nasopharynx. There is a circumscribed, round lesion in the midline posterior nasopharyngeal soft tissues that is T2 hyperintense (arrow, **A**), relatively isointense on FLAIR (arrow, **B**), hypointense on precontrast T1 (arrow, **C**), and minimally enhances peripherally (arrow, **D**), compatible with a Tornwaldt cyst.

Enlarging Tornwaldt cyst

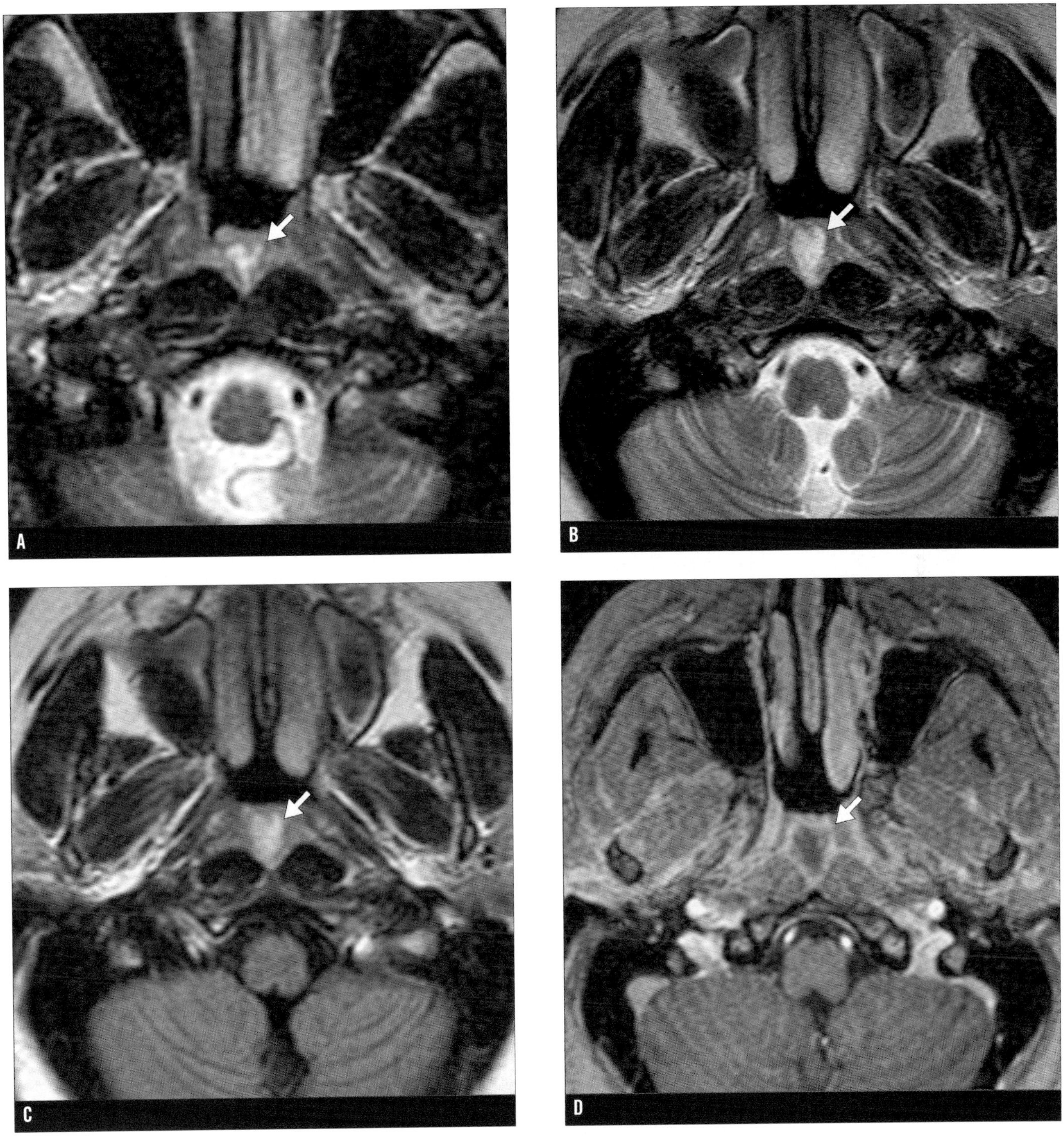

An axial T2-weighted MR image through the level of the nasopharynx obtained in July of 2007 (**A**) demonstrates a small focus of T2 hyperintense signal in the midline submucosa of the adenoids (arrow, **A**). Axial T2 (**B**), axial FLAIR (**C**), and axial postcontrast T1 (**D**) MR images through the nasopharynx obtained in March of 2008 demonstrate enlargement of the Tornwaldt cyst (arrows, **B-D**). There is mild rim enhancement demonstrated on image **D**, an incidental finding.

Proteinaceous Tornwaldt cyst

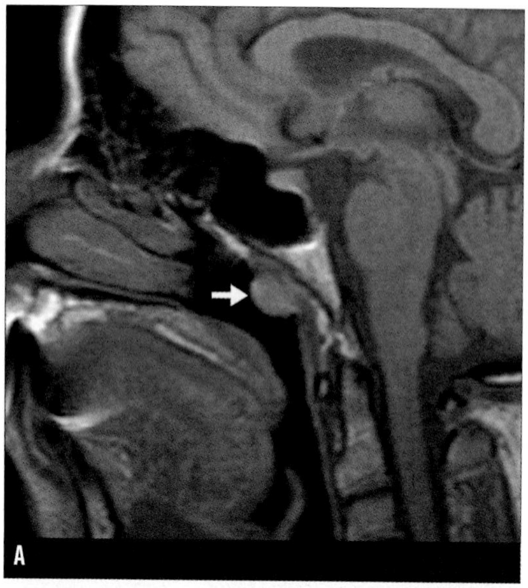

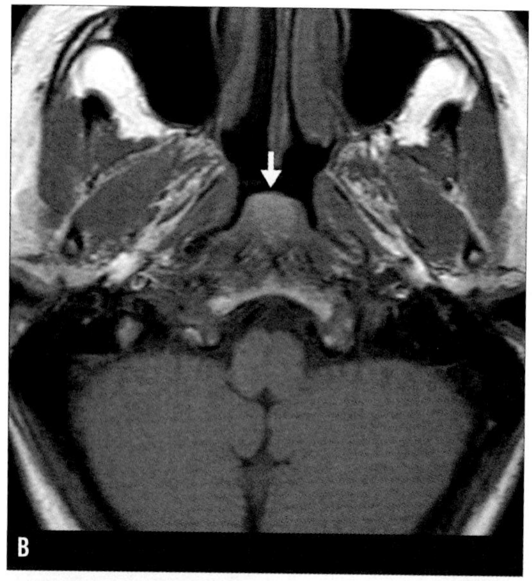

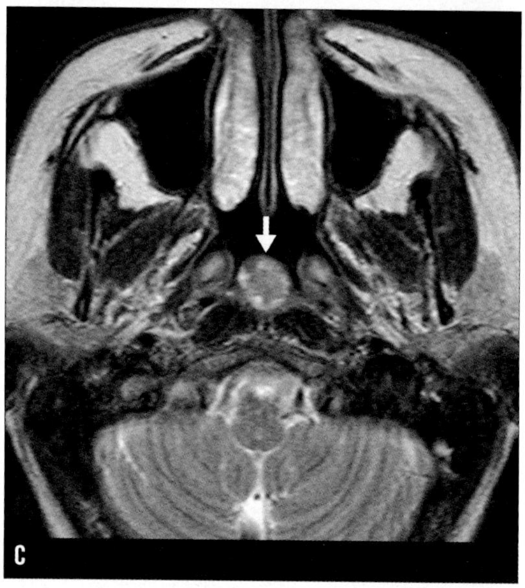

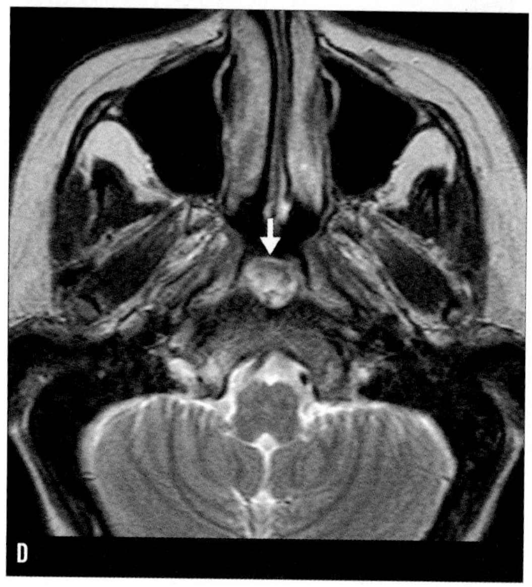

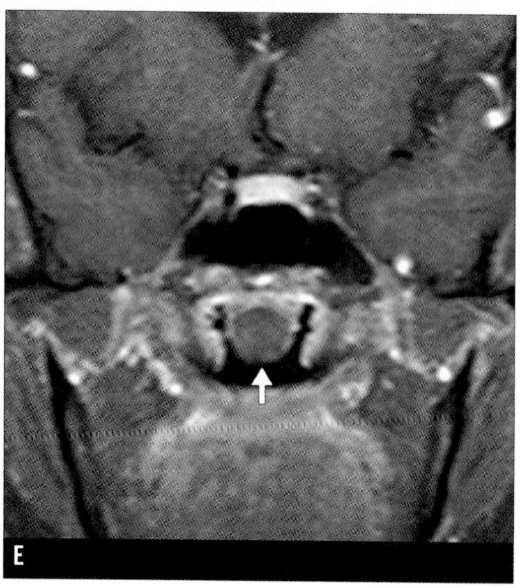

Unenhanced midline sagittal T1 (**A**), unenhanced axial T1 (**B**), axial T2 (**C, D**), and contrast-enhanced coronal T1 with fat suppression (**D**) MR images demonstrate a midline nasopharyngeal lesion compatible with a Tornwaldt cyst (arrows, **A-E**). Images **A** and **B** demonstrate mild T1 shortening within the Tornwaldt cyst, compatible with proteinaceous content. Images **C** and **D** demonstrate the Tornwaldt cyst to be heterogeneous on T2-weighted imaging, also compatible with proteinaceous content. Image **E** demonstrates expected lack of central enhancement of the Tornwaldt cyst.

Tornwaldt cyst

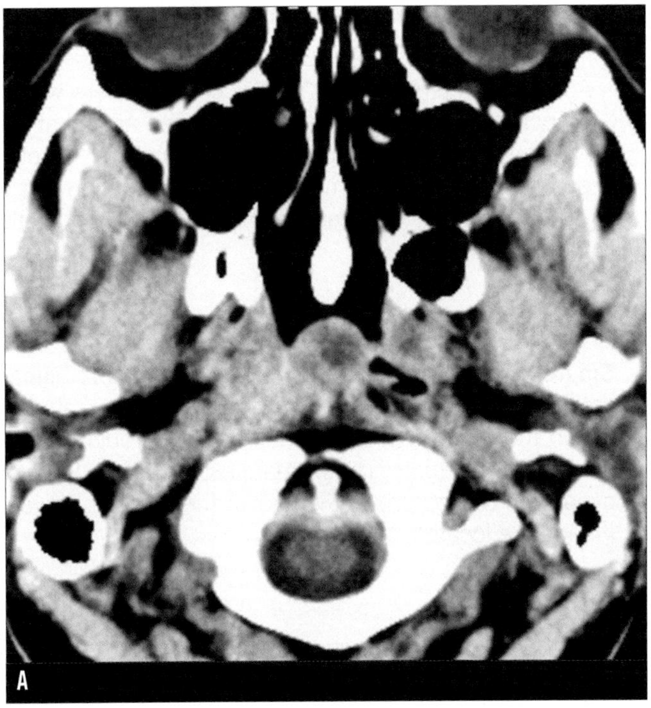

An axial CT image through the nasopharynx (**A**) demonstrates a hypoattenuating round lesion centered in the midline aspect of the adenoids, compatible with a typical Tornwaldt cyst.

REFERENCES

Ford WJ et al. Thornwaldt cyst: an incidental MR diagnosis. *AJNR Am J Neuroradiol.* 1987;8(5):922-923.

Lin JH et al. Huge Thornwaldt cyst: a case report. *Kaohsiung J Med Sci.* 2006;22:524–528.

Salem DB et al. Imaging of nasopharyngeal cysts and bursae. *Eur Radiol.* 2006;16:2249-2258.

CASE 7 Adenoid retention cyst

Retention cysts are a common incidental and asymptomatic finding that may be found anywhere within the oral cavity and pharynx. There are two basic types of retention cysts: mucous and serous. A mucous retention cyst is more common and results from obstruction of a seromucinous gland. A serous retention cyst results from accumulation of fluid in the submucosal layer. Mucous and serous retention cysts are indistinguishable by imaging and appear as smooth, outwardly convex soft tissue masses. Depending on the location, or if the cyst becomes large enough, symptoms such as dysphagia may occur. Retention cysts generally have low attenuation values on CT imaging. On MRI, retention cysts are most often hypointense on T1 and hyperintense on T2, although their signal characteristics can be variable, depending on their protein content. Following intravenous contrast administration, a thin rim of enhancement may be observed on either CT or MRI, but retention cysts should not solidly enhance.

Adenoidal retention cysts can occur anywhere within the adenoids. However, a midline cyst in the nasopharynx typically represents a Tornwaldt cyst, which is a notochordal remnant. Furthermore, adenoid retention cysts tend to be multiple, whereas a Tornwaldt cyst is a single lesion.

COMPANION CASES

- **Sjögren syndrome affecting the nasopharynx minor salivary glands.** Minor salivary glands are scattered within the mucosa and lymphoid tissue throughout the aerodigestive tract. Thus, manifestations of Sjögren syndrome can be present wherever these minor salivary glands are located.

Adenoid retention cysts

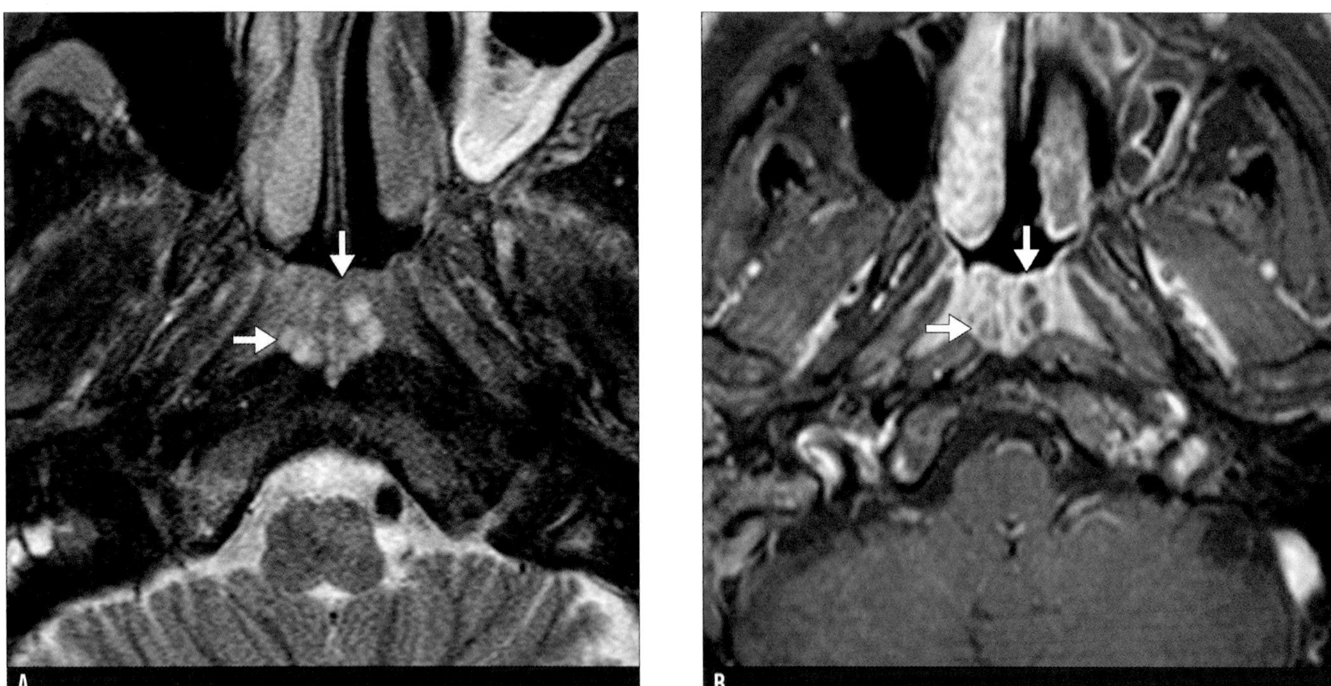

Axial T2 (**A**) and axial postcontrast T1 with fat saturation (**B**) demonstrate several T2 hyperintense, nonenhancing foci scattered within the adenoids, consistent with incidental adenoid retention cysts (arrows, **A, B**). An axial postcontrast CT image of the same patient (**C**) demonstrates a couple of these foci as hypoattenuating lesions (arrow, **C**). These imaging findings are typical of adenoid retention cysts and do not require biopsy or follow-up imaging.

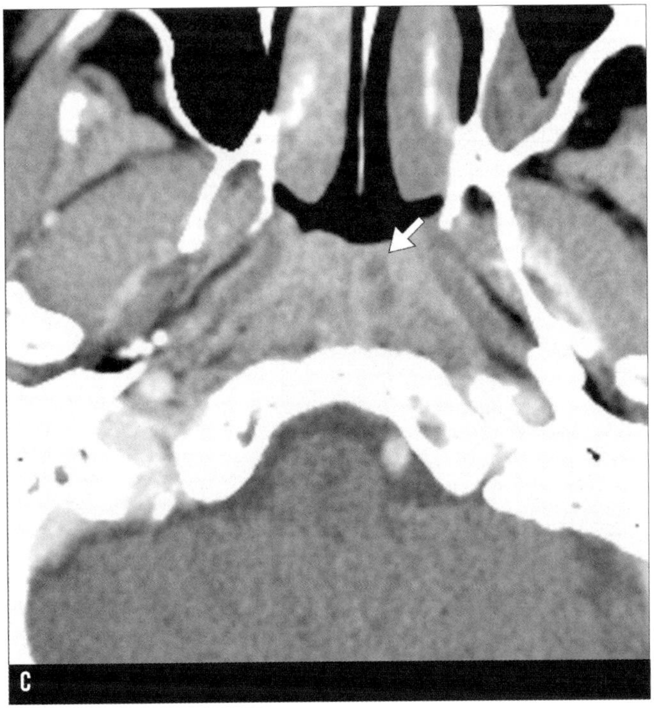

C

Adenoid retention cysts

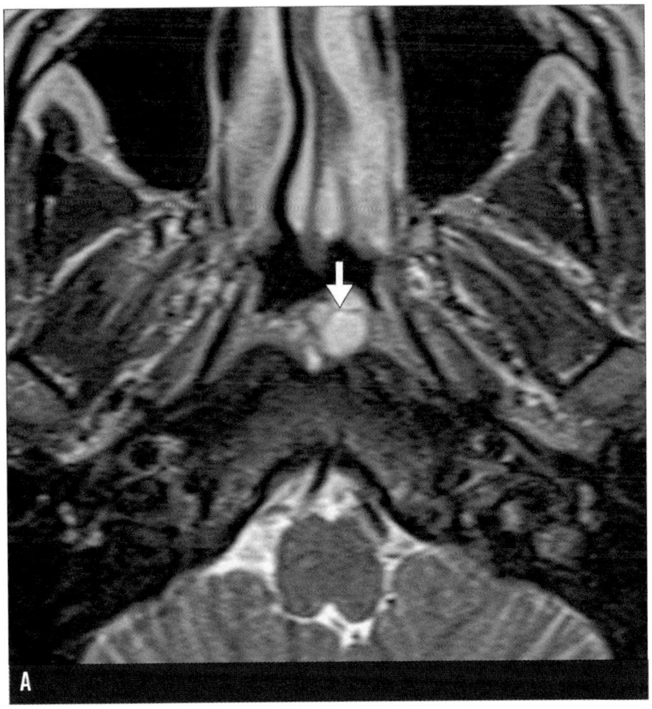

A

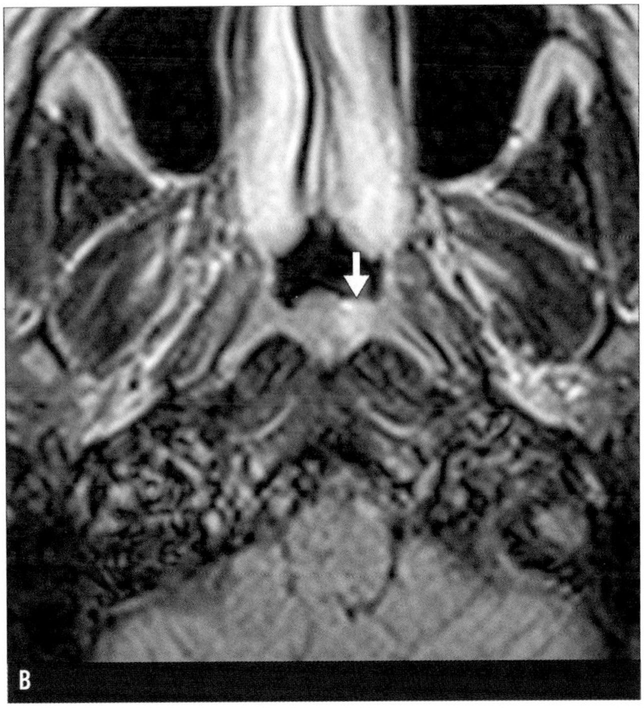

B

Different patient. Axial T2 (**A**), axial FLAIR (**B**), noncontrast axial T1 (**C**), and fat-suppressed postcontrast axial T1 (**D**) MR images through the nasopharynx demonstrate multiple T2 hyperintense, FLAIR hyperintense, and nonenhancing lesions in the adenoids, compatible with incidental adenoid retention cysts (arrows, **A-D**). The elevated FLAIR signal is reflective of proteinaceous content within the cysts.

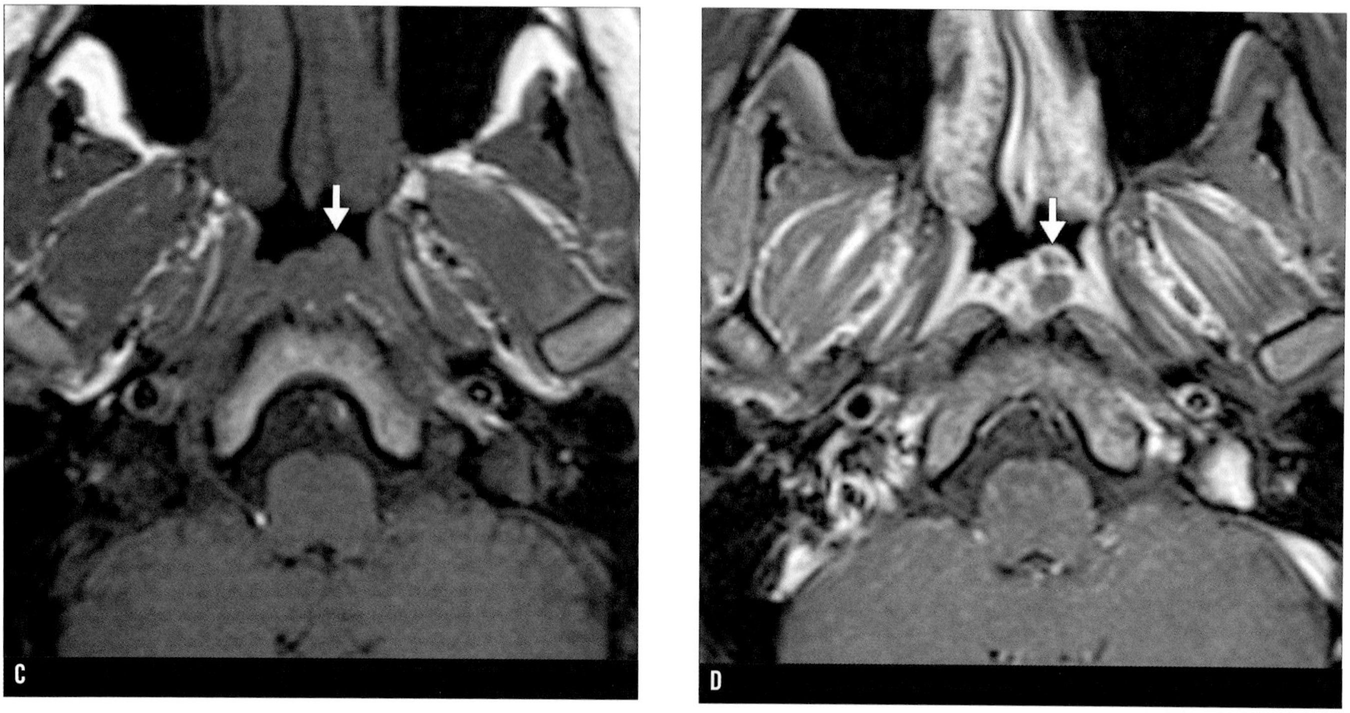

Adenoid retention cyst simulating a neoplasm on CT

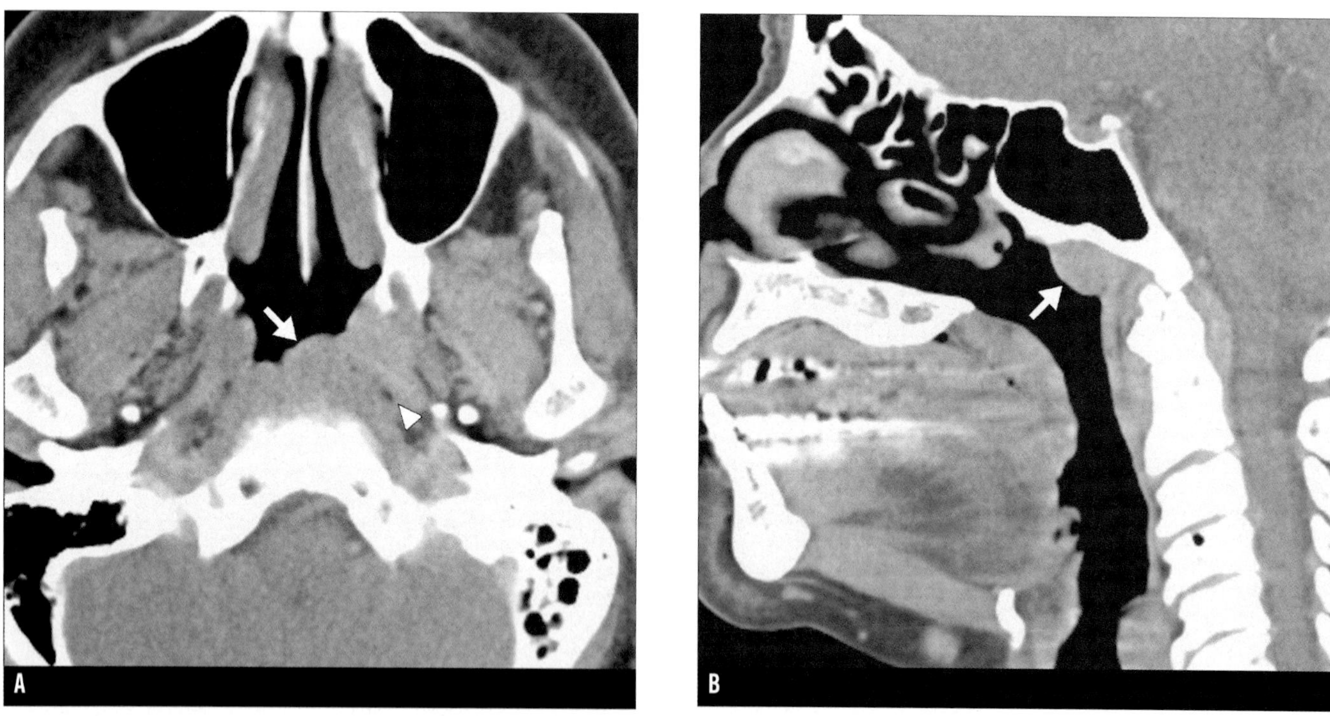

Contrast-enhanced axial (**A**) and sagittal reformatted (**B**) CT images through the nasopharynx demonstrate an asymmetric, rounded soft tissue lesion within the left aspect of the nasopharynx (arrows, **A, B**). The left fossa of Rosenmueller is minimally air-filled (arrowhead, **A**). Sagittal T1 (**C**), axial T1 (**D**), axial T2 (**E**), and postcontrast axial T1 with fat saturation (**F**) MR images demonstrate the lesion in question to be isointense on precontrast T1 (arrows, **C, D**), hypointense on T2 (arrow, **E**), and peripherally enhancing following contrast (arrow, **F**), compatible with an incidental proteinaceous adenoid retention cyst. It is difficult to exclude a neoplasm on the CT images, although the fossa of Rosenmueller is typically involved with nasopharyngeal cancer, which appears spared in this case.

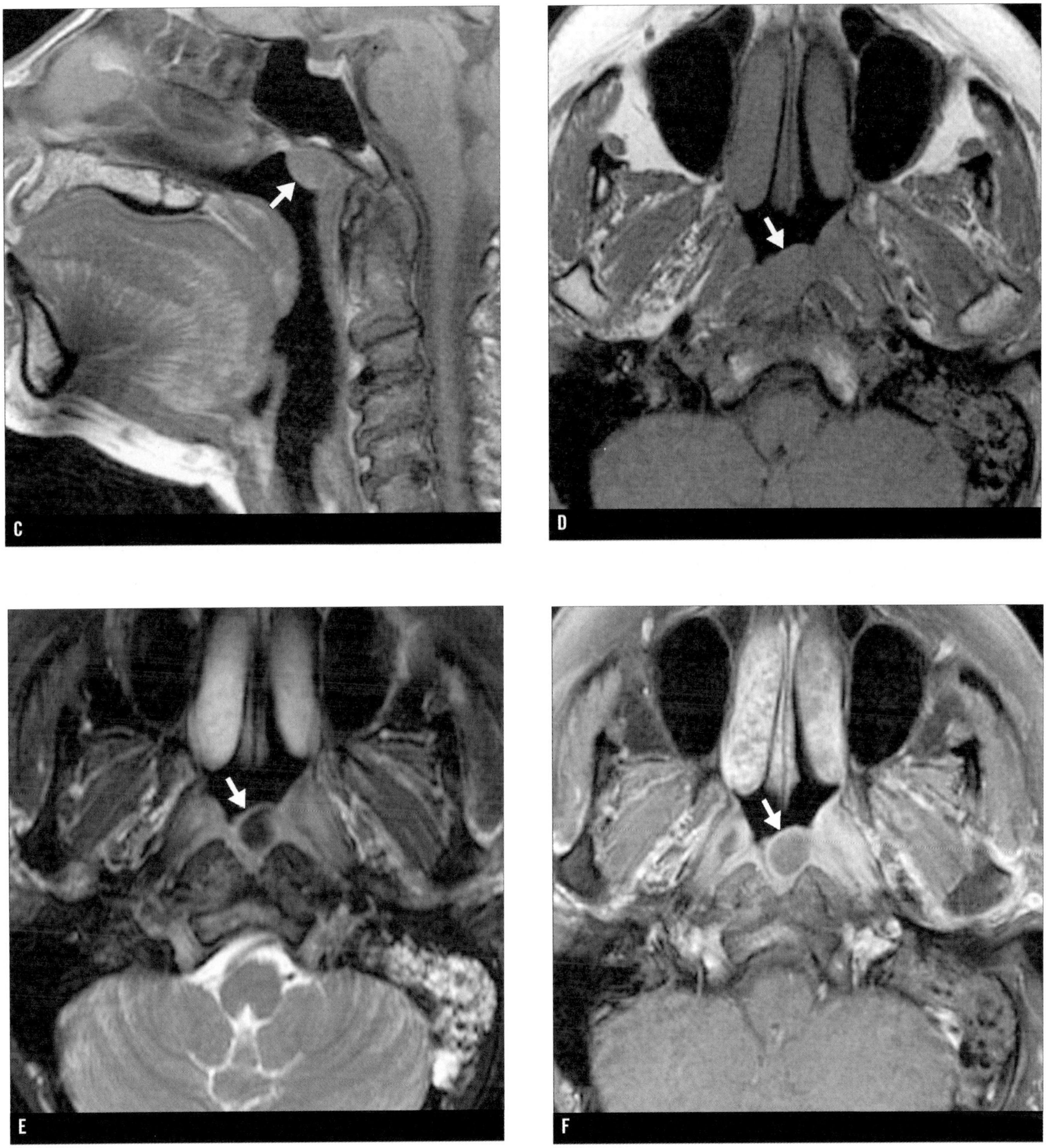
C
D
E
F

Companion case: Sjögren syndrome affecting the nasopharynx minor salivary glands

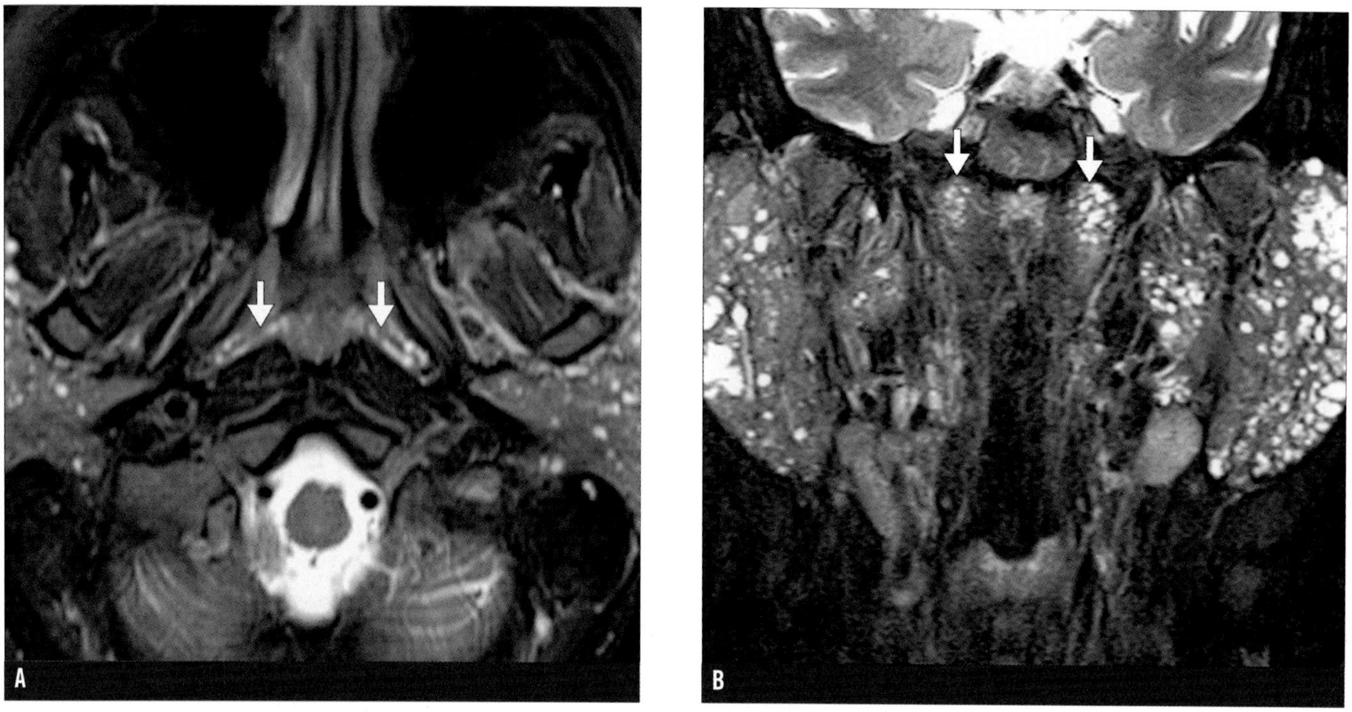

Axial (**A**) and coronal (**B**) T2-weighted MR imaging with fat suppression demonstrates innumerable, rounded, T2 hyperintense foci scattered throughout the bilateral parotid glands in a patient with known Sjögren syndrome. There is also evidence of similar findings in the adenoids (arrows, **A**, **B**). In the setting of Sjögren syndrome, these hyperintense foci represent abnormally dilated acini in the parotid glands and in minor salivary glands embedded within the adenoids.

REFERENCES

Lin JH et al. Huge Thornwaldt cyst: a case report. *Kaohsiung J Med Sci.* 2006;22:524-528.

Salem DB et al. Imaging of nasopharyngeal cysts and bursae. *Eur Radiol.* 2006;16:2249-2258.

CASE 8 Incidental adenoid diffusion restriction

While tumors of the adenoids with a high nuclear-to-cytoplasmic ratio (such as lymphoma) can restrict on diffusion-weighted imaging (DWI), the presence of diffusion restriction within the adenoids is a nonspecific finding and cannot be used to reliably differentiate between normal tissue and malignancy. Nevertheless, if there is clinical concern, then a biopsy of the adenoid tissue may be necessary.

COMPANION CASES

- **Nasopharyngeal lymphoma.** When lymphoma involves the pharynx, the most common site of involvement is the Waldeyer ring, in particular the palatine tonsil, followed by the adenoids. While primary nasopharyngeal lymphoma is overall less common than nasopharyngeal squamous cell carcinoma, differentiating between these two entities can be difficult. One source suggests favoring nasopharyngeal lymphoma over nasopharyngeal squamous cell carcinoma if the mass is homogeneous, diffusely enhanced, is symmetrically distributed within the nasopharynx, lacks regional invasion, and has low apparent diffusion coefficient (ADC) values on DWI. However, ultimately, a biopsy of the lesion would likely be necessary to differentiate these entities.

Incidental adenoid diffusion restriction

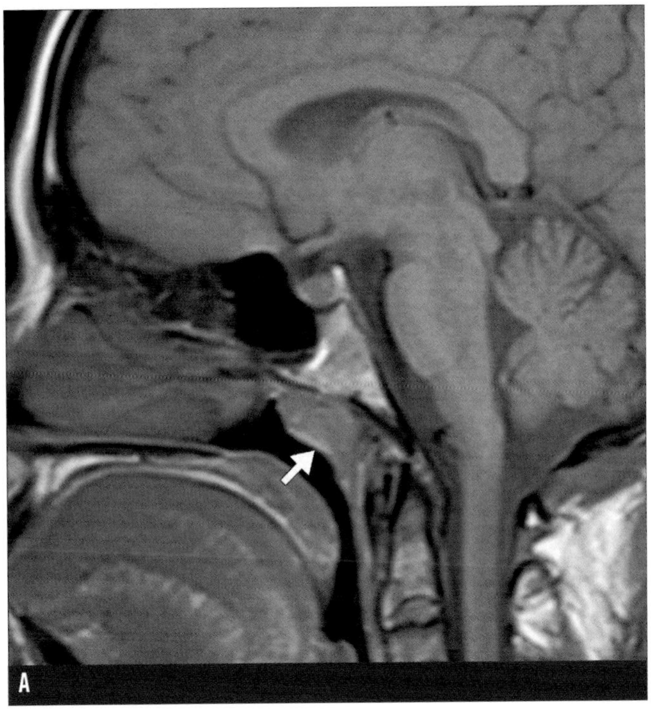

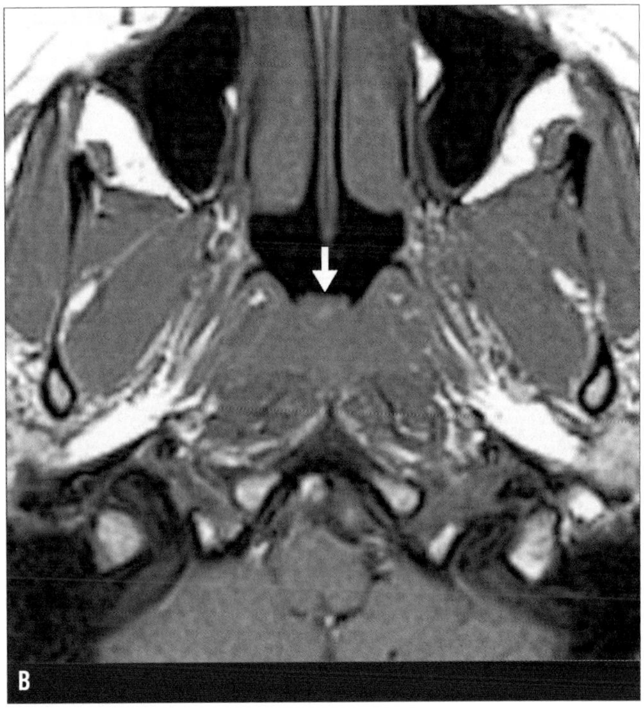

Midline sagittal T1 (**A**), axial T1 (**B**), postcontrast axial T1 with fat suppression (**C**), and axial T2 (**D**) MR images through the nasopharynx. Images **A** and **B** demonstrate enlarged adenoids in this 45-year-old patient (arrows, **A, B**). There is diffuse, homogeneous enhancement following contrast administration (arrow, **C**) and diffuse mildly hypointense signal on T2-weighted imaging (arrow, **D**). An axial DWI (**E**) and corresponding ADC map (**F**) demonstrate diffusion restriction involving the enlarged adenoid tissue. This patient had no history of cancer and the diffusion restriction in this case was incidental.

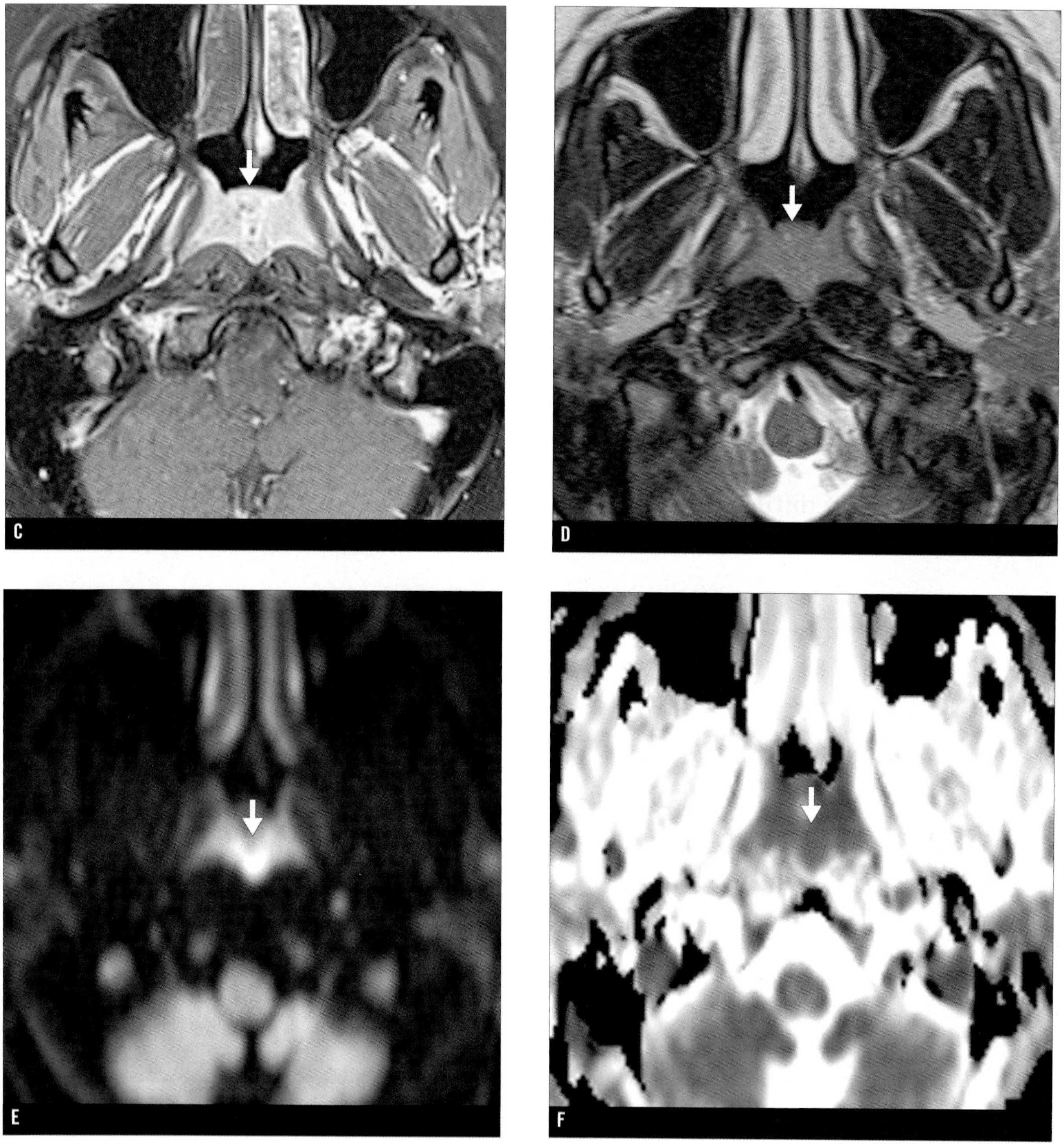
C
D
E
F

Companion case: Nasopharyngeal lymphoma

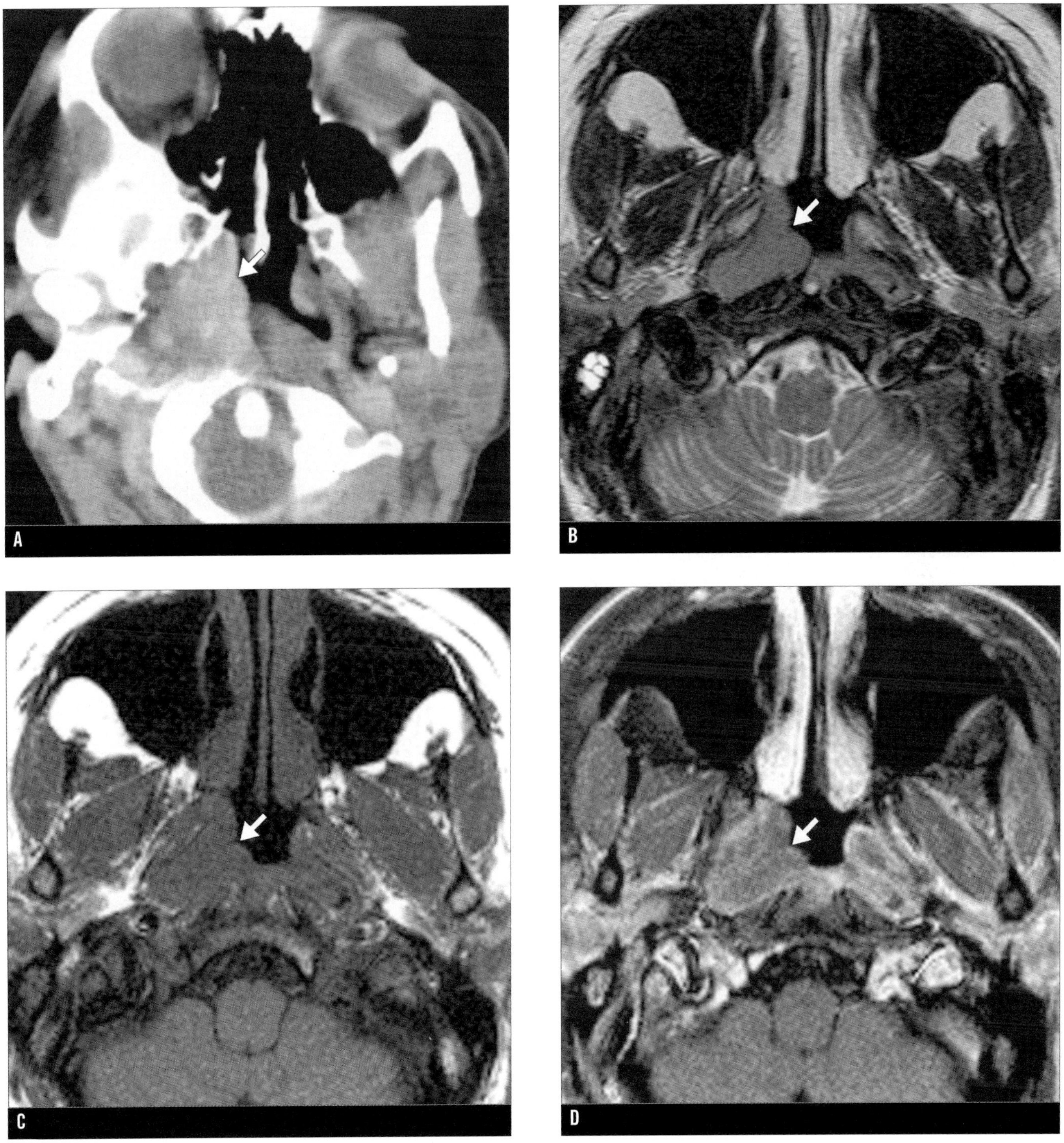

An axial postcontrast CT image (**A**) demonstrates a presumably enhancing mass in the right aspect of the nasopharynx (arrow, **A**). Axial T2 (**B**), unenhanced axial T1 (**C**) and postcontrast axial T1 with fat suppression (**D**) MR images demonstrate the mass to be T2 hypointense (arrow, **B**), T1 isointense (arrow, **C**), and relatively nonenhancing (arrow, **D**). Axial DWI (**E**) and the accompanying ADC map (**F**) demonstrate restricted diffusion within the lesion (arrows, **E, F**). Restricted diffusion may be present with both benign lymphoid hyperplasia and with malignancies. However, a unilateral mass in the nasopharynx, as is present in this case, should always be viewed with suspicion and investigated with direct inspection. An axial T2-weighted MR image (**G**) also demonstrates a right mastoid effusion because of Eustachian tube dysfunction and/or obstruction (arrow, **G**), a common finding in the setting of a nasopharyngeal tumor.

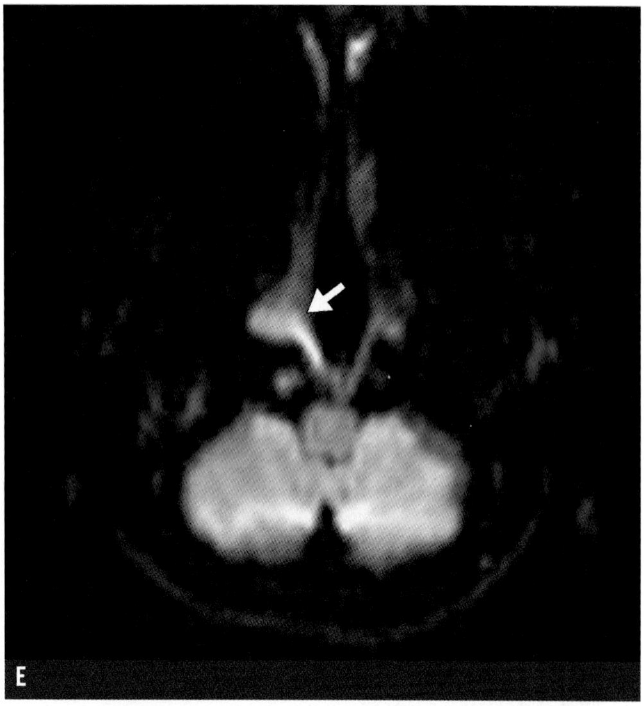

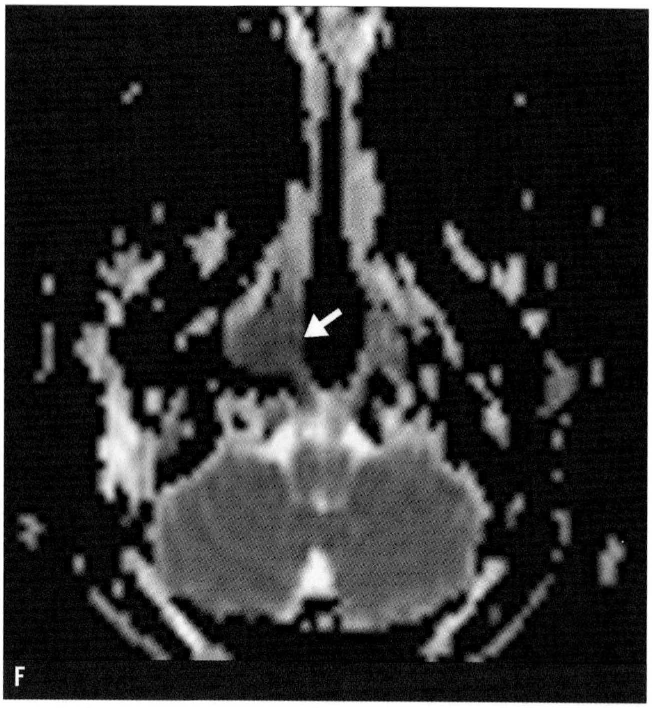

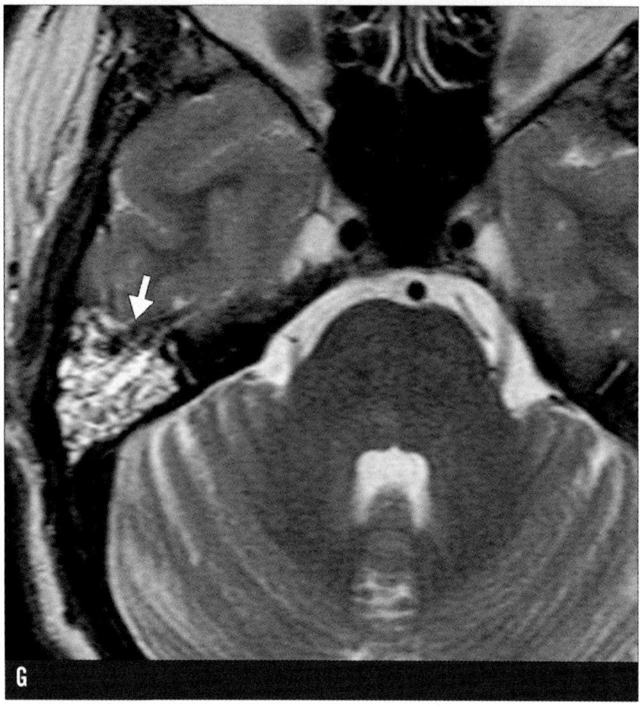

REFERENCES

Becker M et al. Imaging of the larynx and hypopharynx. *Eur J Radiol.* June 2008;66(3):460-470.

Cho KS, Kang DW, Kim HJ, Lee JK, Roh HJ. Differential diagnosis of primary nasopharyngeal lymphoma and nasopharyngeal carcinoma focusing on CT, MRI, and PET/CT. *Otolaryngol Head Neck Surg.* April 2012;146(4):574-578. Epub 2012 Jan 18.

Holzapfel K et al. Value of diffusion-weighted MR imaging in the differentiation between benign and malignant cervical lymph nodes. *Eur J Radiol.* 2009;72(3):381-387.

King AD et al. Malignant cervical lymphadenopathy: diagnostic accuracy of diffusion-weighted MR imaging. *Radiology.* 2007;245;806-813.

Maeda M et al. Usefulness of the apparent diffusion coefficient in line scan diffusion-weighted imaging for distinguishing between squamous cell carcinomas and malignant lymphomas of the head and neck. *AJNR Am J Neuroradiol.* 2005;26(5):1186-1192.

Misa S et al. Diagnostic ability of apparent diffusion coefficients for lymphomas and carcinomas in the pharynx. *European Radiology.* 2007;17(10):2631-2637.

CASE 9 Tonsilloliths

Tonsilloliths occur in the Waldeyer ring (adenoids, palatine tonsils, and lingual tonsil). They are most often punctate and are composed primarily of calcium and other minerals. Therefore, tonsilloliths are hyperdense on CT and plain radiographs. While the exact pathogenesis of these calcifications is not known, they are believed to result from a prior infection (such as from various fungi or bacteria). The incompletely resolved pus and debris from these infections are thought to serve as a nidus for stone formation. Tonsilloliths, particularly when small, are usually asymptomatic. Large tonsilloliths may cause symptoms, including chronic sore throat, odynophagia, or a globus sensation.

COMPANION CASES

- **Retained fish bone.**
- **Displacement of a small tooth fracture fragment following intubation**
- **Displacement of an entire tooth**

Adenoid tonsillolith

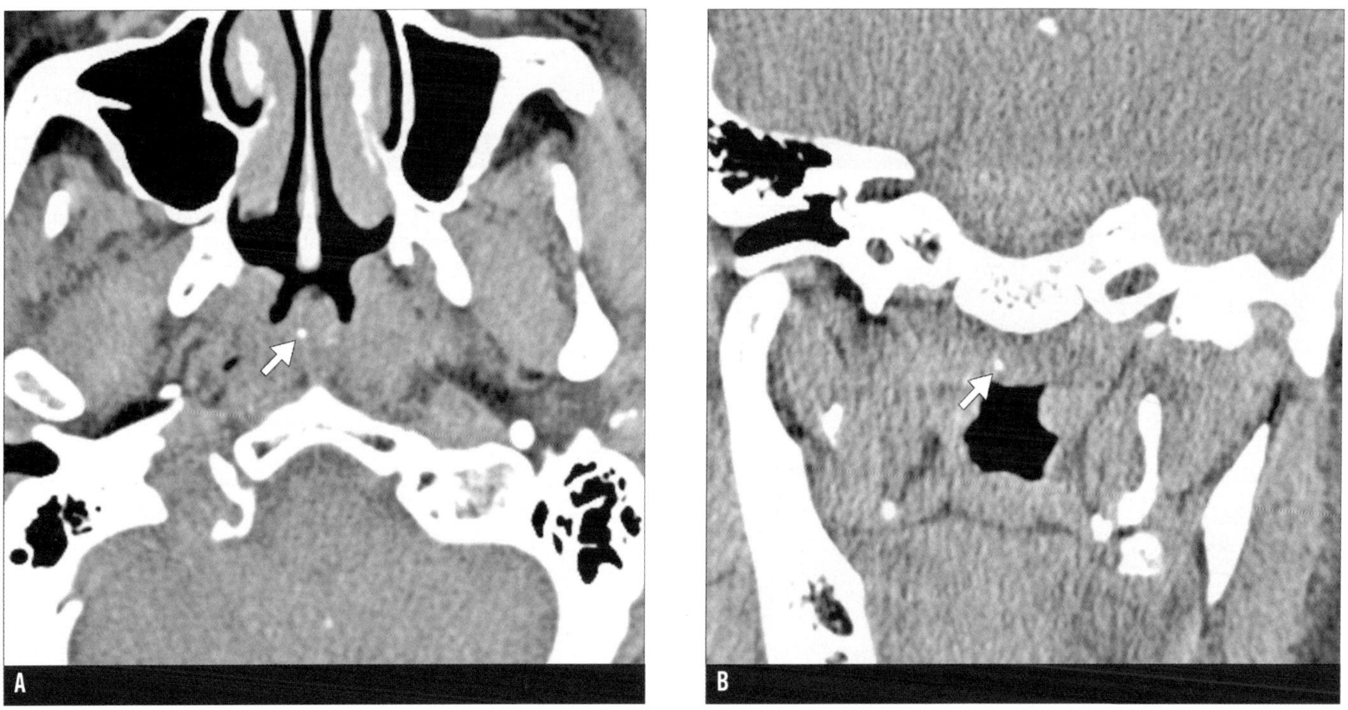

Axial (**A**) and coronal reformatted (**B**) unenhanced CT images through the nasopharynx demonstrate a punctate focus of mineralization compatible with an adenoidal tonsillolith (arrows, **A, B**).

Palatine tonsilloliths

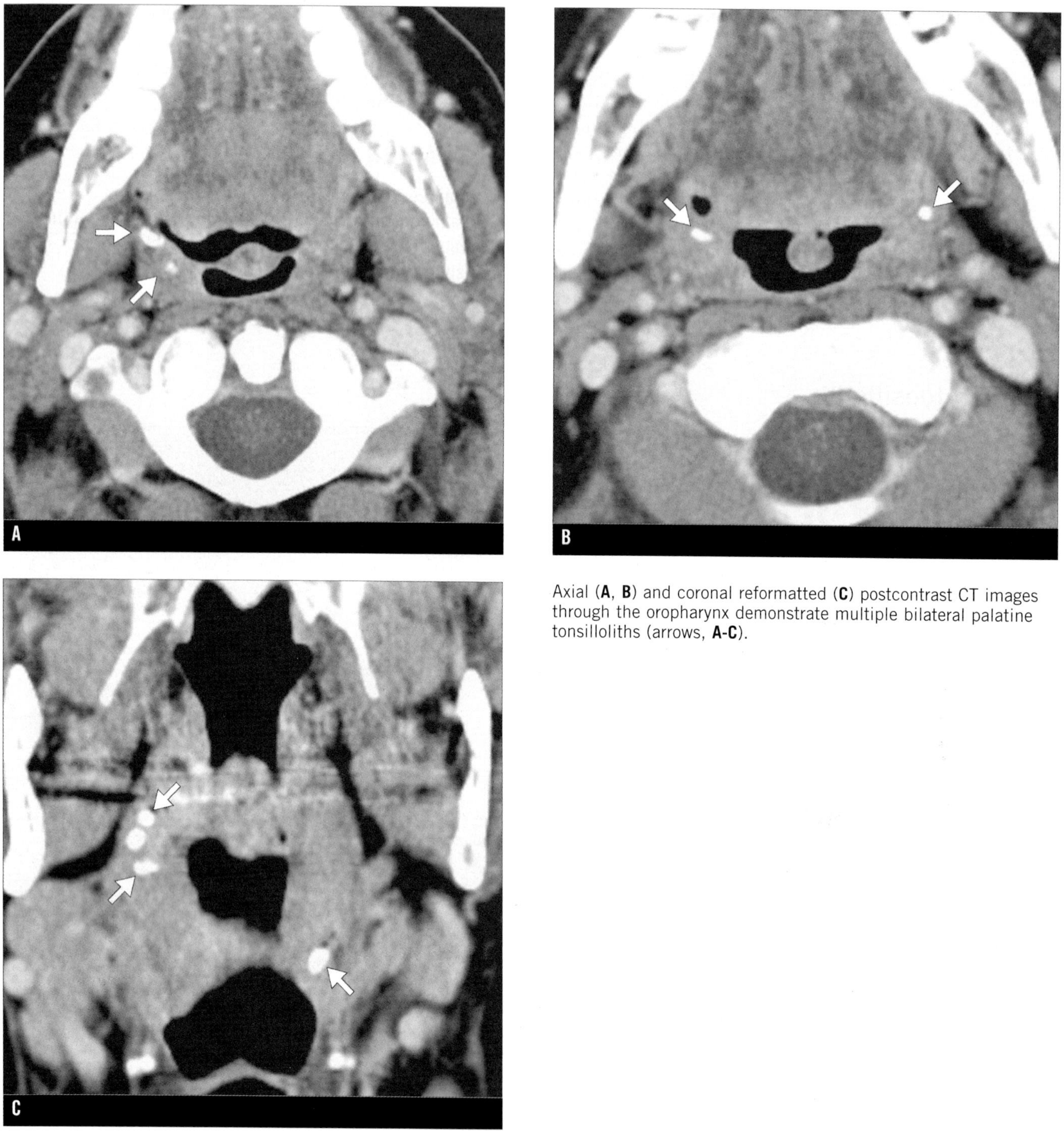

Axial (**A**, **B**) and coronal reformatted (**C**) postcontrast CT images through the oropharynx demonstrate multiple bilateral palatine tonsilloliths (arrows, **A-C**).

Lingual tonsilloliths

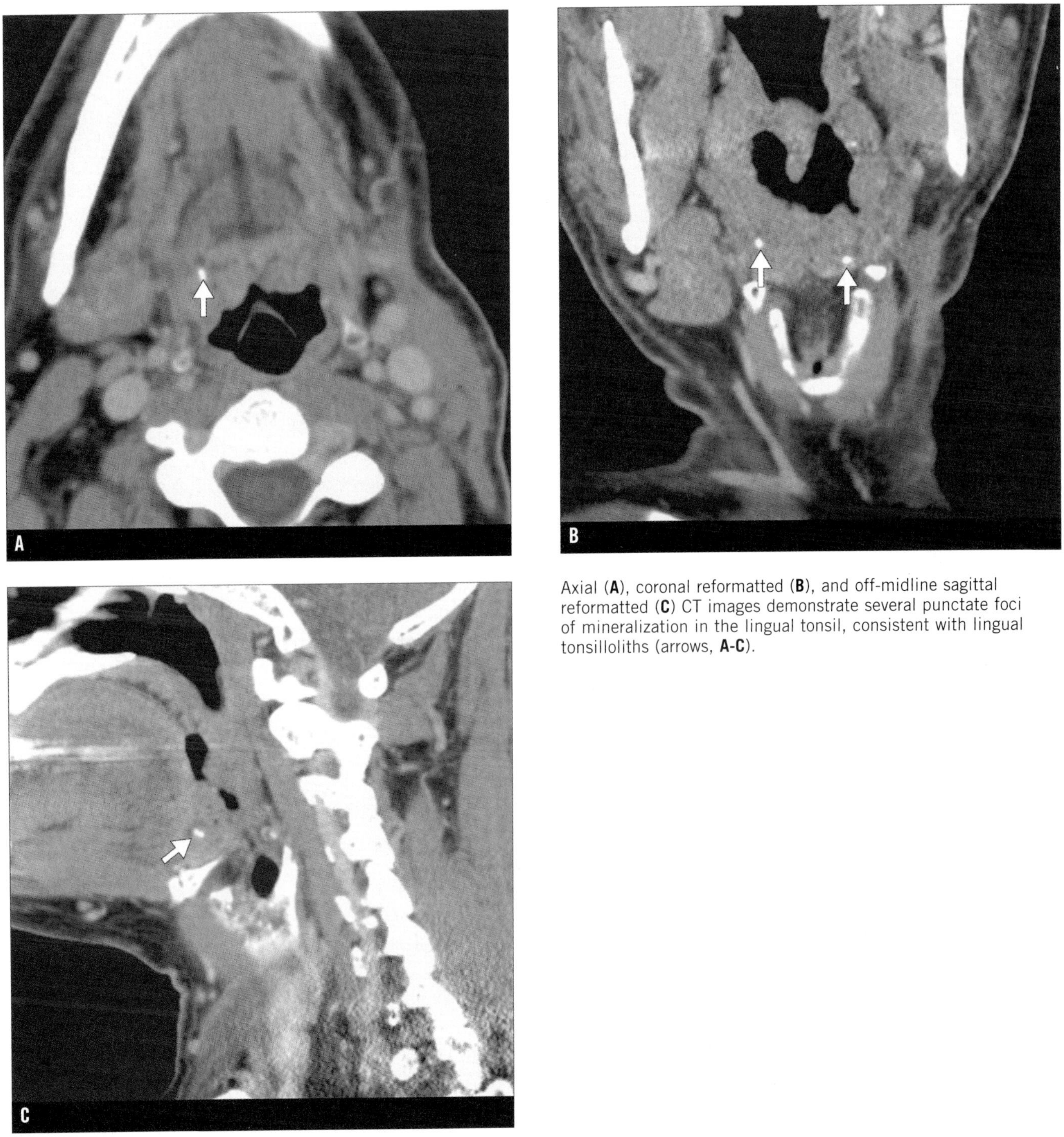

Axial (**A**), coronal reformatted (**B**), and off-midline sagittal reformatted (**C**) CT images demonstrate several punctate foci of mineralization in the lingual tonsil, consistent with lingual tonsilloliths (arrows, **A-C**).

Companion case: Retained fish bone

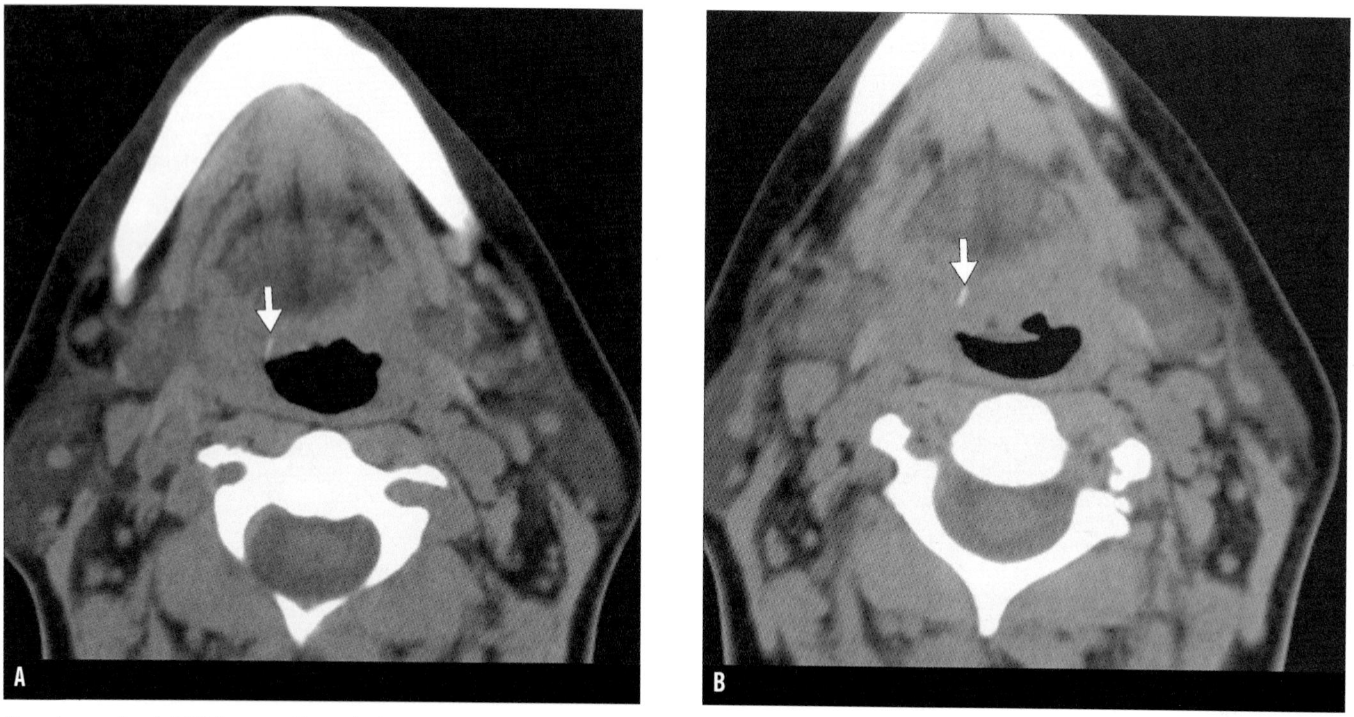

Unenhanced axial CT images through the oropharynx (**A, B**) demonstrate a linear, hyperdense focus within the right aspect of the lingual tonsils (arrows, **A, B**). This represented a retained fish bone.

Companion case: Displacement of a small tooth fracture fragment following intubation

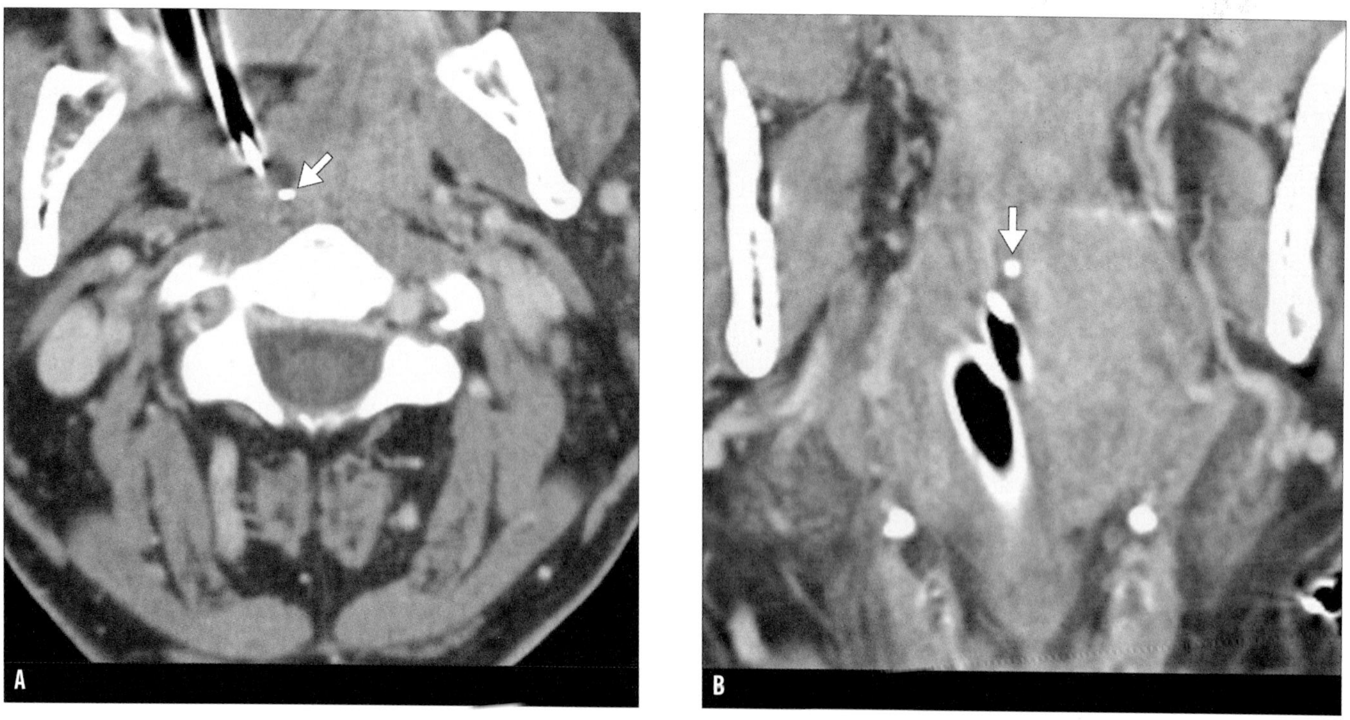

Axial postcontrast CT image through the oropharynx (**A**) demonstrates a punctate focus of mineralization (arrow, **A**) that could be misinterpreted as a lingual or palatine tonsillolith, except that it appears to be centered within the oropharyngeal airway. Coronal reformatted (**B**) and sagittal reformatted (**C**) postcontrast CT images also demonstrate this punctate focus of mineralization to be centered within the oropharyngeal airway (arrows, **B, C**). A coronal reformatted CT image viewed with a bone window through the midline maxillary teeth (**D**) demonstrate avulsion fractures of the maxillary left medial and lateral incisors arrowhead, **D**. The punctate focus of mineralization in the oropharyngeal airway represented a displaced portion of a tooth that was fractured during intubation or a previously fractured tooth that was displaced during intubation.

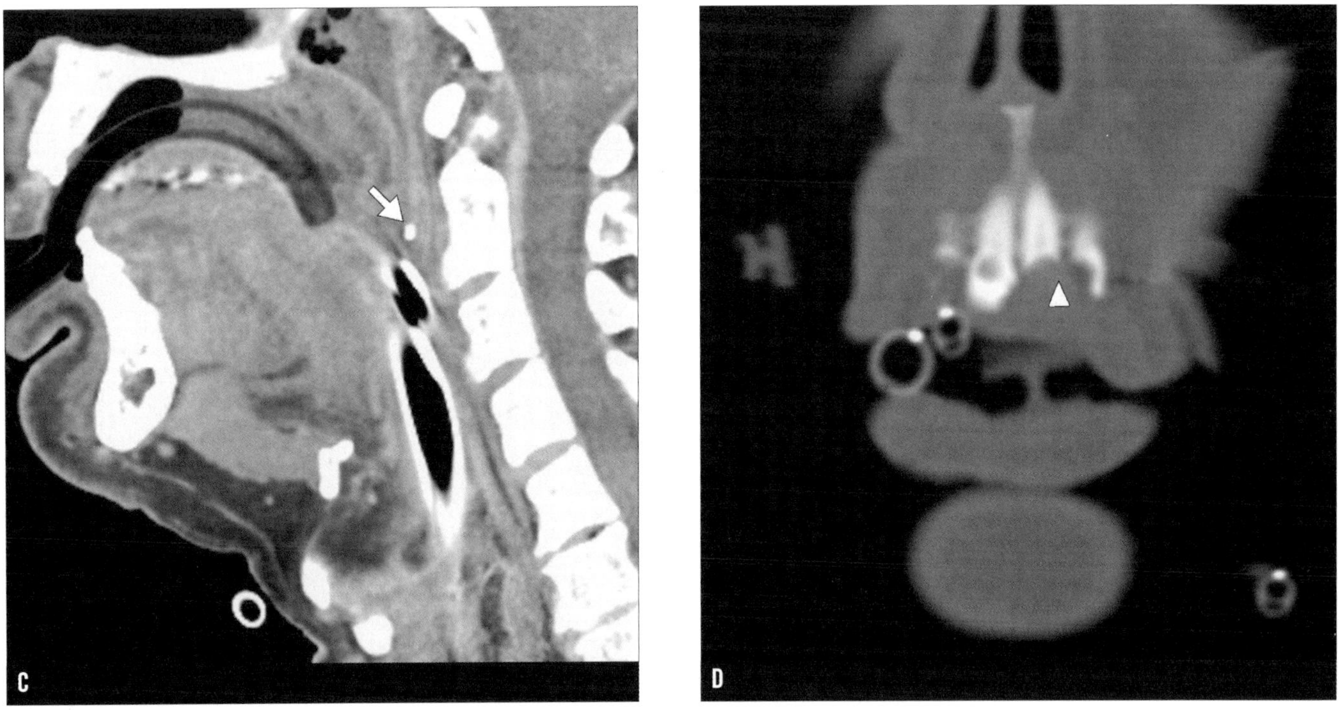

Companion case: Displacement of an entire tooth

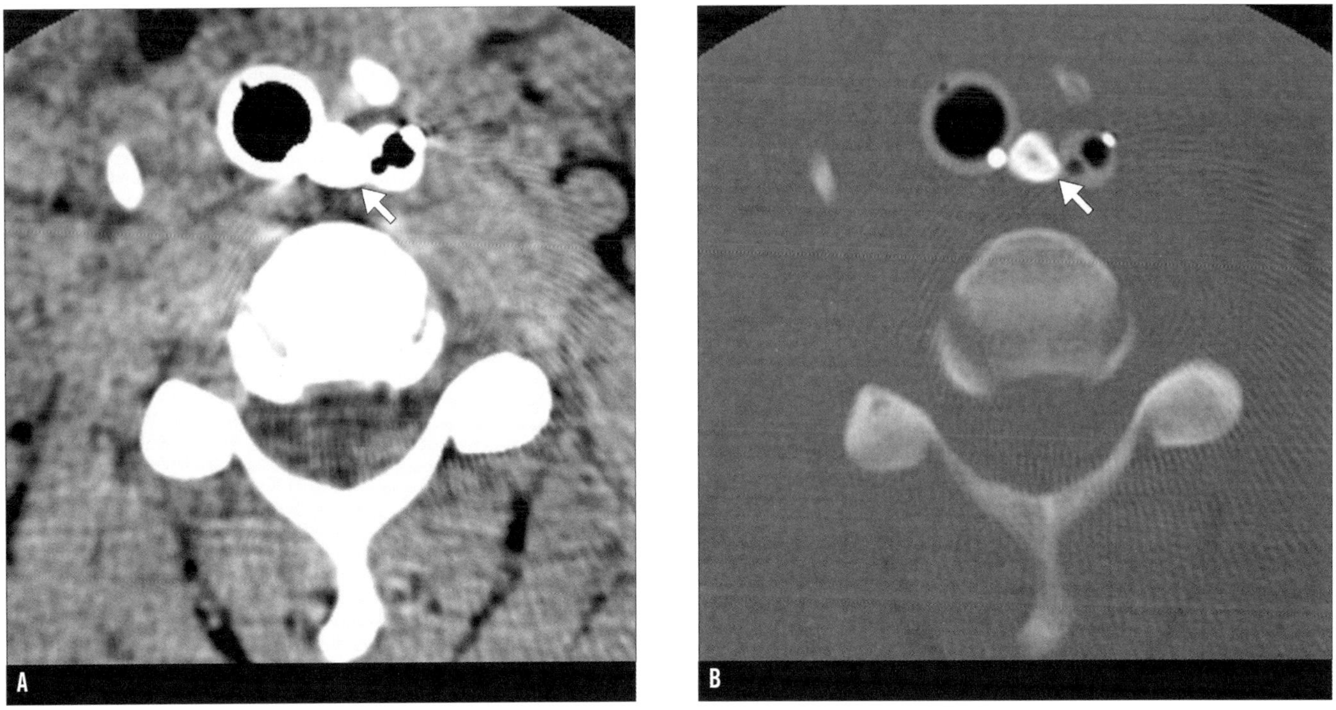

Different patient. Axial CT images viewed with a soft tissue algorithm (**A**) and a bone algorithm (**B**) demonstrate an osseous foreign body interposed between an endotracheal tube and a nasogastric tube (arrows, **A, B**). Sagittal reformatted (**C**) and coronal reformatted (**D**) CT images better demonstrate that the osseous abnormality represents an entire tooth lodged in the lower oropharynx (arrows, **C, D**). This tooth was most likely displaced during intubation.

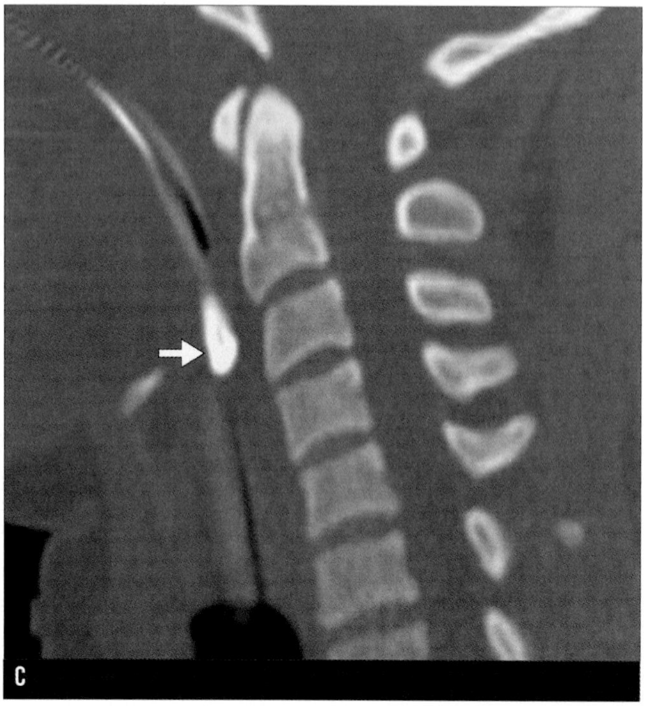

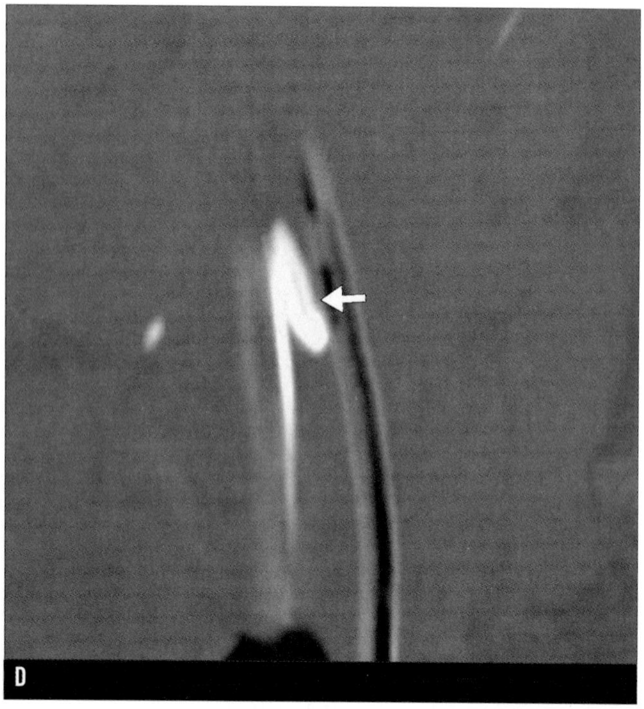

REFERENCES

De Moura M et al. Tonsillolith: a report of three clinical cases. *Med Oral Patol Oral Cir Buca.* 2007;12:E130-E133.

Donat F et al. Giant tonsillolith: report of a case. *Med Oral Patol Oral Cir Bucal.* 2005;10:239-242.

Sezer B et al. An unusual tonsillolith. *Oral Surg Oral Med Oral Pathol Oral Radiol Endod.* April 2003;95(4):471-473.

CASE 10 Palatine tonsil lymphoid hyperplasia

The Waldeyer ring (adenoids, palatine tonsils, and lingual tonsil is normally large in children, adolescents, and young adults due to lymphoid hyperplasia. Generally, the maximum size of the palatine tonsils occurs around the time of puberty. Mild, symmetric lymphoid hyperplasia should not be interpreted as abnormal in these age groups. However, with the recent increase incidence of squamous cell carcinoma (SCC) in the setting of human papilloma virus infection, one must more strongly consider the possibility of SCC in young adults, particularly when a unilaterally enlarged tonsil is identified, there is no history to suggest inflammation, or there is no history of a contralateral tonsillectomy to account for the asymmetry. Occasionally, enlargement of the Waldeyer ring can persist in older patients, with at least some lymphoid hyperplasia likely attributed to cigarette smoking. While palatine lymphoid hyperplasia is a benign entity, if severe lymphoid hyperplasia is present, then it can be associated with pharyngeal airway compromise and/or obstructive sleep apnea.

COMPANION CASE

- **Unilateral palatine tonsil lymphoid hyperplasia due to a contralateral palatine tonsillectomy.** If a patient undergoes a unilateral palatine tonsillectomy, then the contralateral intact palatine tonsil may undergo hypertrophy, simulating a tumor. Tonsil hypertrophy may occur if any of the tonsil tissues is not completely removed following a tonsillectomy.
- **Vascular malformation involving a palatine tonsil.** Vascular malformations of the head and neck are a diverse group of lesions and include arteriovenous malformation (AVM), venous malformation (VM), and lymphatic malformation (LM). Vascular malformations may be high-flow lesions (AVM), low-flow lesions (VM, LM), or a combination of both. Properly categorizing these lesions is important in order to determine proper treatment. Most vascular malformations are present at birth, although trauma can result in an AVM.

  VMs are essentially an abnormal collection of venous channels, fat, and degenerated muscle matrix. The veins in a VM can thrombose and form phleboliths, the latter suggesting this entity. LMs represent an abnormal collection of lymphatic vessels. LMs are subcategorized into macrocystic and microcystic forms. The macrocystic form, commonly referred to as a cystic hygroma, is composed of large cystic spaces containing proteinaceous fluid and lymphocytes that are interspersed with septa. The microcystic form contains 2 mm or smaller-sized cysts within a solid matrix.

  The hallmark of a vascular malformation is its transpatial nature (ie, often involving more than one compartment in the neck) and its softness to palpation. A vascular malformation may or may not be associated with mass effect. On MRI, both a VM and a macrocystic LM will be hyperintense on T2. Following contrast, a VM will contain patchy enhancement throughout the lesion, while a macrocystic LM will only enhance along its periphery and/or septa. A hemorrhagic fluid level may be identified in a macrocystic LM, frequently associated with an abrupt clinical enlargement and is strongly suggestive of LM when present. However, VMs and LMs frequently coexist in a lesion and are thus termed venolymphatic malformations when both are present. MRI is usually superior to CT in evaluating vascular malformations of the head and neck.
- **Palatine tonsil squamous cell carcinoma.** Generally speaking, if an older patient presents with a pathologically enlarged and/or necrotic, dominant unilateral level II lymph node, and there is no history of infection to explain the finding, then an ipsilateral palatine tonsil or base of tongue malignancy should be excluded. This is because the normal lymphatic drainage pattern of the base of tongue and palatine tonsil begins in the ipsilateral level II region. Thus, the threshold should be low for describing any subtle ipsilateral palatine tonsil or base of tongue asymmetry in this setting. Additionally, primary malignancies of the palatine tonsil or base of tongue may only be visible on delayed postcontrast imaging. Therefore, delayed postcontrast imaging should be considered if there is a clinical suspicion of a primary malignancy in these regions.

Palatine tonsil lymphoid hyperplasia

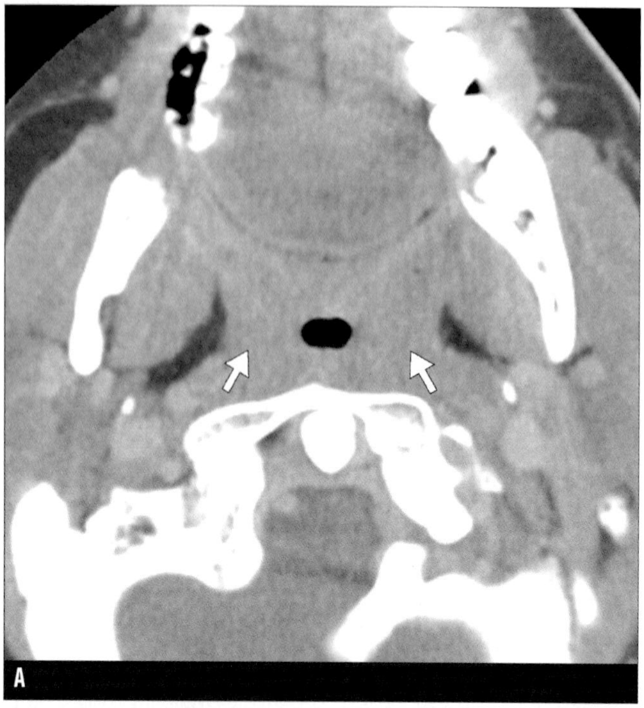

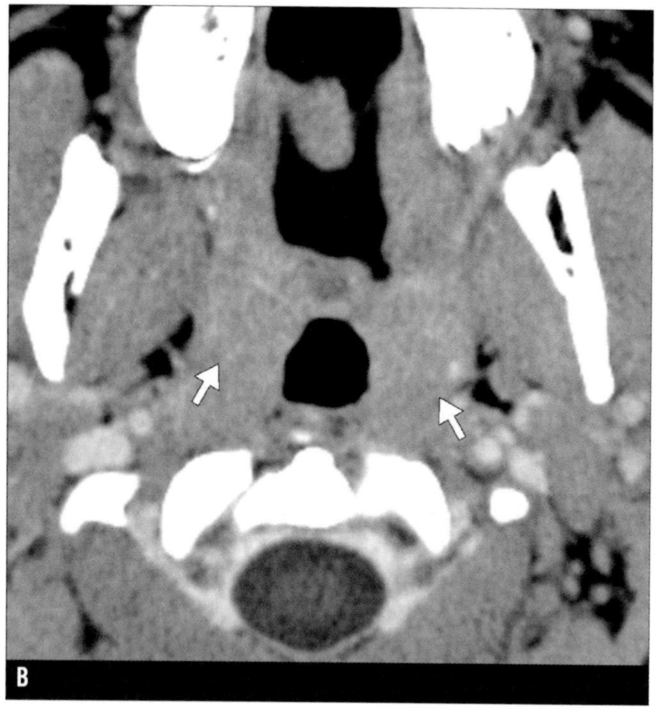

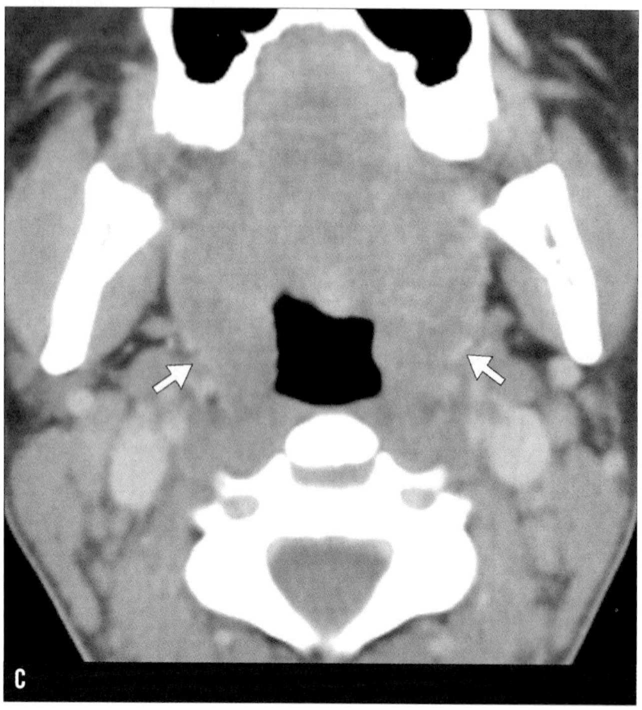

Axial postcontrast CT images from three different patients, ranging from 16 to 18 years of age. Each case demonstrates incidental lymphoid hyperplasia of the bilateral palatine tonsils in this age group (arrows, **A-C**).

Companion case: Unilateral palatine tonsil lymphoid hyperplasia due to a contralateral palatine tonsillectomy

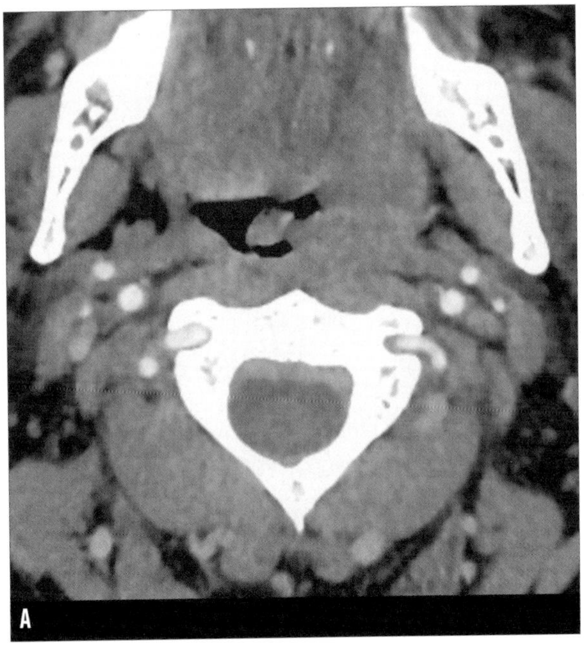

An axial CT image from a CTA **(A)** demonstrates asymmetric enlargement of the left palatine tonsil, likely due to compensatory lymphoid hyperplasia in this patient with a history of a right palatine tonsillectomy.

Companion case: Vascular malformation involving a palatine tonsil

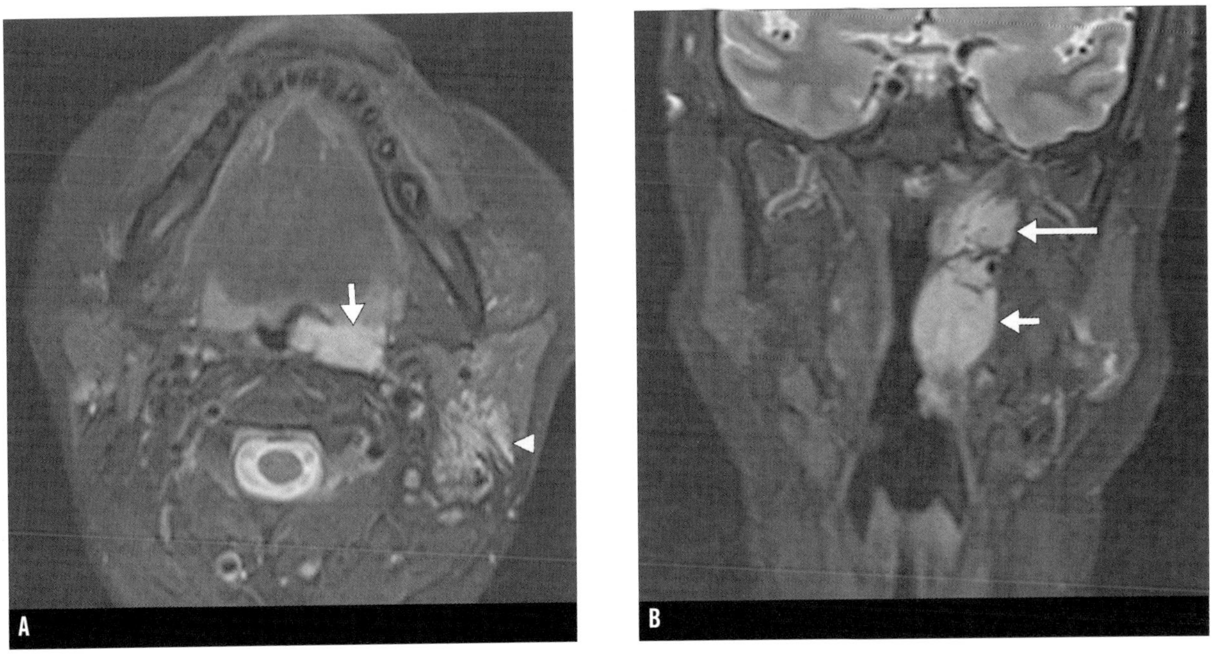

Axial (**A**) and coronal (**B**) T2 with fat suppression, axial T1 (**C**), and contrast-enhanced axial T1 with fat suppression (**D**) MR images demonstrate the left palatine tonsil to be diffusely T2 hyperintense and enhancing (short arrows, **A-D**). There is also a similar T2 hyperintense and enhancing lesion in the left parotid gland that appears infiltrating (arrowheads, **A, D**). The lesion also affects the left aspect of the nasopharynx, as demonstrated on image **B** (long arrow). The multifocality and imaging characteristics are compatible with a vascular malformation, likely venous or venolymphatic.

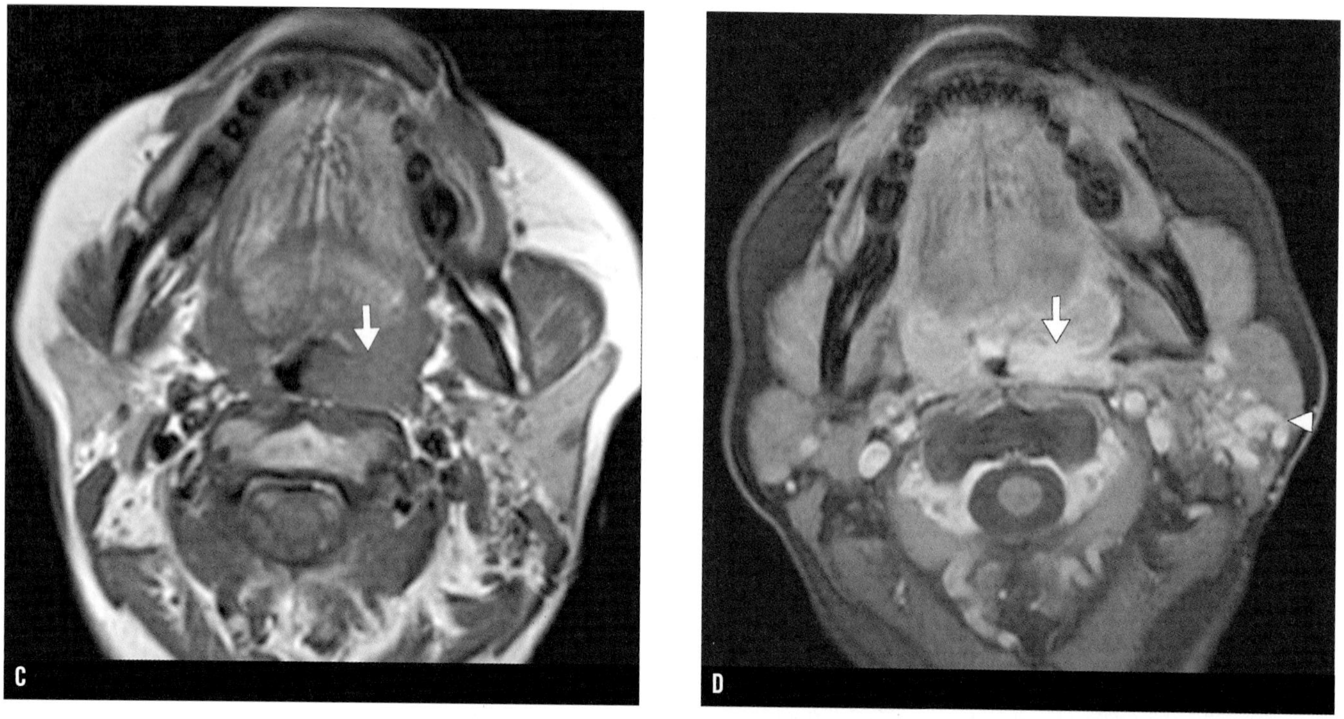

Companion case: Palatine tonsil squamous cell carcinoma

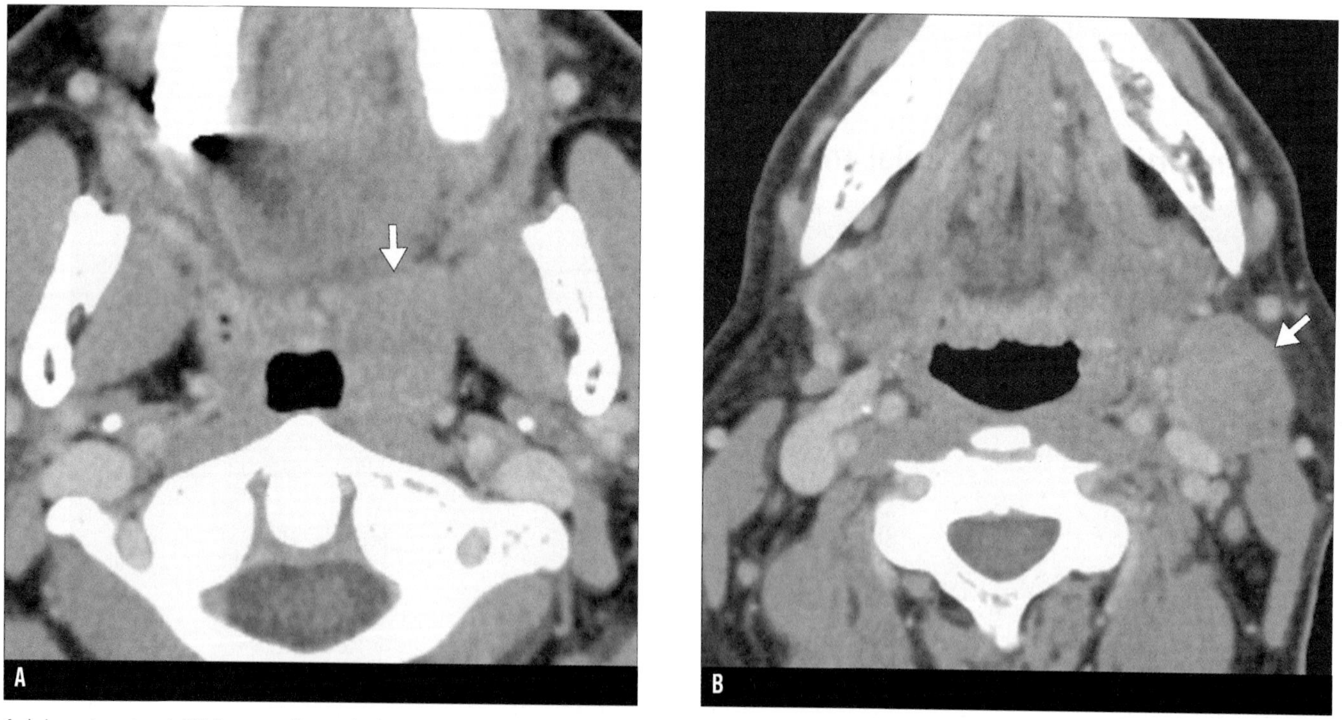

Axial postcontrast CT images through the oropharynx (**A**) and level II nodal station (**B**). Image **A** demonstrates an asymmetrically enlarged left palatine tonsil (arrow). Image **B** demonstrates a pathologically enlarged left level IIA lymph node (arrow). Together, these findings are compatible with a left palatine tonsil carcinoma, statistically a squamous cell carcinoma.

REFERENCES

Dubois J, Soulez G, Oliva VL, Berthiaume MJ, Lapierre C, Therasse E. Soft-tissue venous malformations in adult patients: imaging and therapeutic issues. *Radiographics*. 2001;21(6):1519-1531.

Flors L et al. MR imaging of soft-tissue vascular malformations: diagnosis, classification, and therapy follow-up. *Radiographics*. September-October 2011;31(5):1321-1340.

Nguyen NP, Ly BH, Betz M, Vinh-Hung V. Importance of age as a prognostic factor for tonsillar carcinoma. *Ann Surg Oncol*. 2010;17(10):2570-2577.

Peter M. Som and Hugh D. Curtin. 4th ed. 2 vols. St. Louis, MO: Mosby; 2003: 1467, 1470.

CASE 11 Air-filled palatine tonsil crypts

The palatine tonsils have invaginations, or crypts, extending from their surface into the substance of the lymphoid tissue. Air can be interposed between the crypts and is an incidental finding.

COMPANION CASE

- **Fluid-filled palatine tonsil crypts.**

Air-filled palatine tonsil crypts

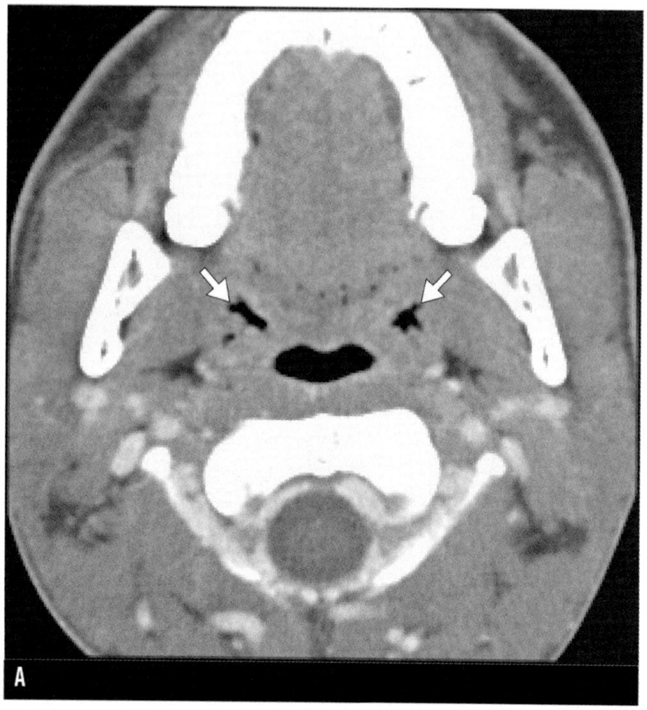

An axial postcontrast CT image through the palatine tonsils (**A**) demonstrates pockets of air in the bilateral palatine tonsils, compatible with incidental air-filled palatine tonsil crypts (arrows).

Companion case: Fluid-filled palatine tonsil crypts

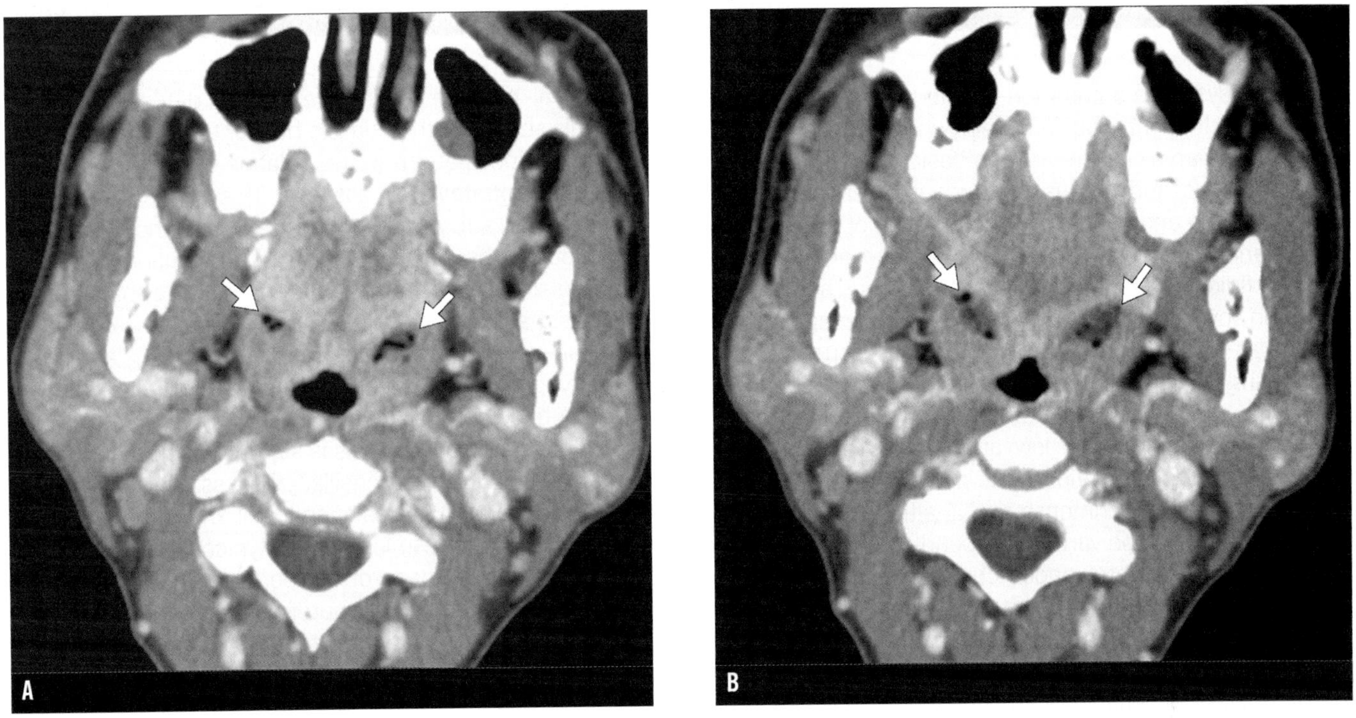

Contrast-enhanced axial CT images (**A**, **B**) demonstrate discrete, oval, and symmetric areas of hypoattenuation within the ventral aspect of both palatine tonsils, representing a combination of fluid and foci of air. The findings are compatible with partially fluid-filled palatine tonsil crypts (arrows, **A**, **B**).

REFERENCES

Lin JH et al. Huge Thornwaldt cyst: a case report. *Kaohsiung J Med Sci.* 2006;22:524-528.

Salem DB et al. Imaging of nasopharyngeal cysts and bursae. *Eur Radiol.* 2006;16:2249-2258.

CASE 12 Palatine tonsil retention cyst

Retention cysts are a common incidental and asymptomatic finding that may be found anywhere within the oral cavity and pharynx. There are two basic types of retention cysts: mucous and serous. A mucous retention cyst is more common and results from obstruction of a seromucinous gland. A serous retention cyst results from accumulation of fluid in the submucosal layer. Mucous and serous retention cysts are indistinguishable by imaging and appear as smooth, outwardly convex soft tissue masses. Depending on the location, or if the cyst becomes large enough, symptoms such as dysphagia may occur. Retention cysts generally have low attenuation values on CT imaging. On MRI, retention cysts are most often hypointense on T1 and hyperintense on T2, although their signal characteristics can be variable, depending on their protein content. Following intravenous contrast administration, a thin rim of enhancement may be observed on either CT or MRI, but retention cysts should not solidly enhance.

Differentiating this incidental finding from a palatine tonsil abscess on imaging can be difficult. The lack of a thick rim of enhancement, a nonenlarged/nonedematous tonsil, and the lack of surrounding inflammatory change can support the diagnosis of an incidental retention cyst and help exclude an abscess.

COMPANION CASES

- **Palatine tonsil edema.** This is often present in patients presenting with an uncomplicated pharyngitis. The bilateral palatine tonsils are usually diffusely enlarged in this setting, with a classic horizontal, linearly-oriented "tiger stripe" pattern in the palatine tonsils.
- **Palatine intratonsillar abscess.** This abscess is located within the substance of the palatine tonsil. This can sometimes be distinguished from a retention cyst by its irregular margins and thick peripheral enhancement. Additional imaging findings of a tonsillar abscess usually include surrounding inflammatory stranding and retropharyngeal fluid. These lesions are typically aspirated at the bedside.
- **Peritonsillar abscess.** This is significantly more common than a palatine intratonsillar abscess. This abscess is located lateral to the palatine tonsil and within the peritonsillar fossa. These lesions are typically treated with an incision and drainage of the peritonsillar fossa and the patient is placed on an appropriate antibiotic regimen.
- **Partially necrotic palatine tonsil squamous cell carcinoma.** Most squamous cell carcinomas of the oropharynx are solid soft tissue masses. However, occasionally an area of necrosis within the tumor may be identified, particularly with large tumors or those that are being treated.

Palatine tonsil retention cysts

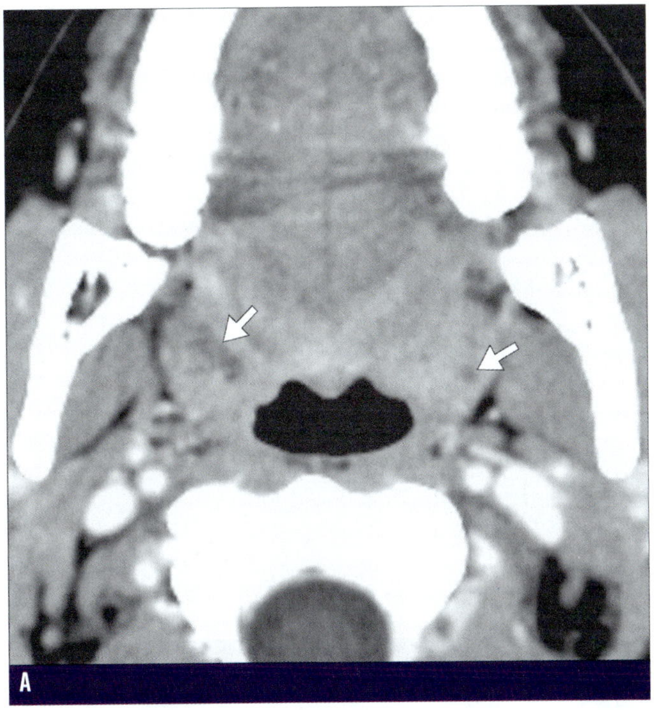

An axial postcontrast CT image through the level of the oropharynx (**A**) demonstrates incidental bilateral palatine tonsil retention cysts, right larger than left, in this asymptomatic patient (arrows).

Palatine tonsil retention cyst

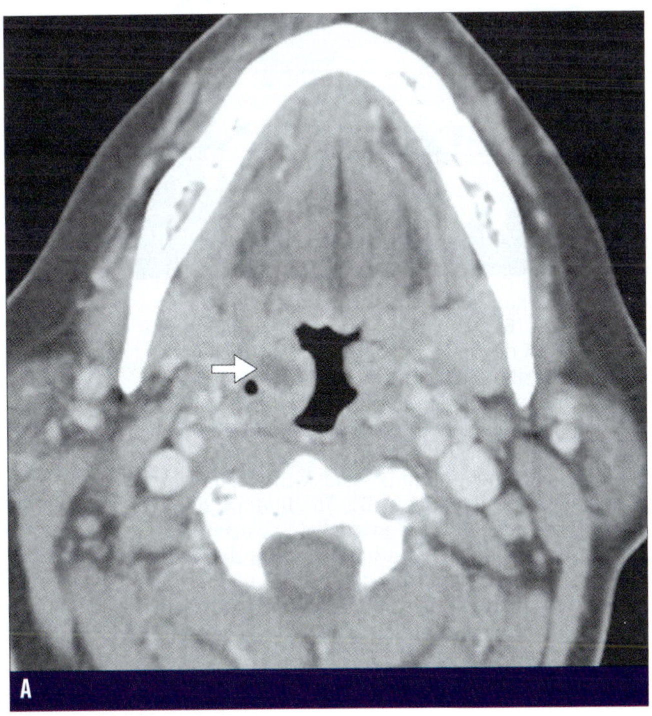

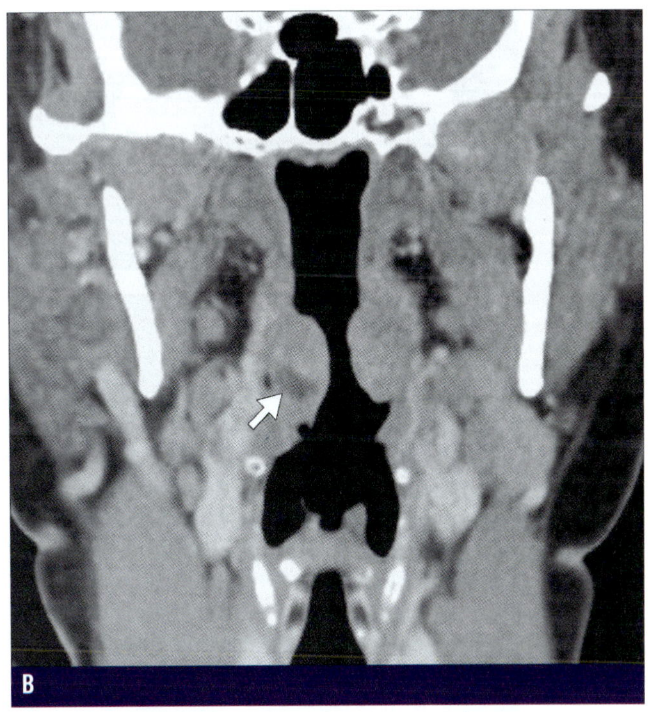

Different patient. Axial (**A**) and coronal reformatted (**B**) CT images demonstrate a nonenhancing, focal, hypoattenuating lesion within the right palatine tonsil (arrows, **A, B**). An axial T2-weighted MR image (**C**) demonstrates a focal area of T2-hyperintensity corresponding to the same lesion (arrow, **C**). Given the lack of surrounding inflammatory changes and the lack of significant peripheral enhancement, the lesion is most compatible with an incidental palatine tonsil retention cyst. Care should be taken not to confuse this finding with a tonsillar abscess.

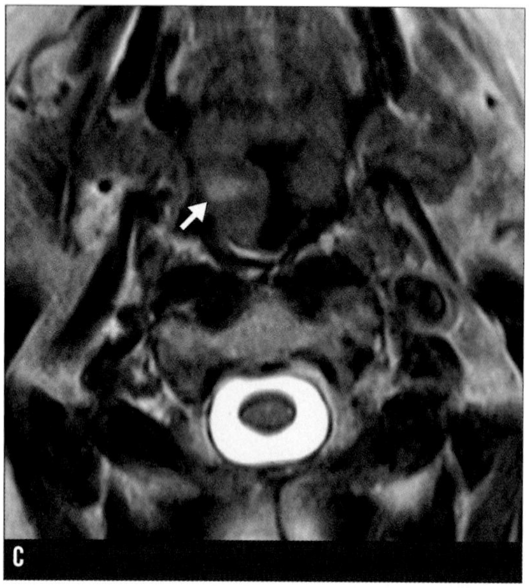

Companion case: Palatine tonsil edema

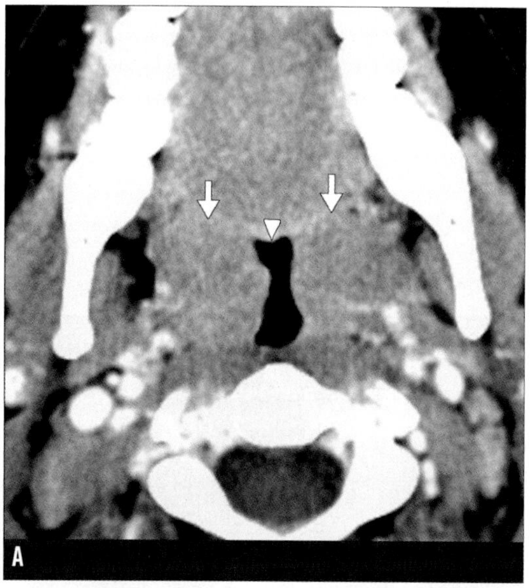

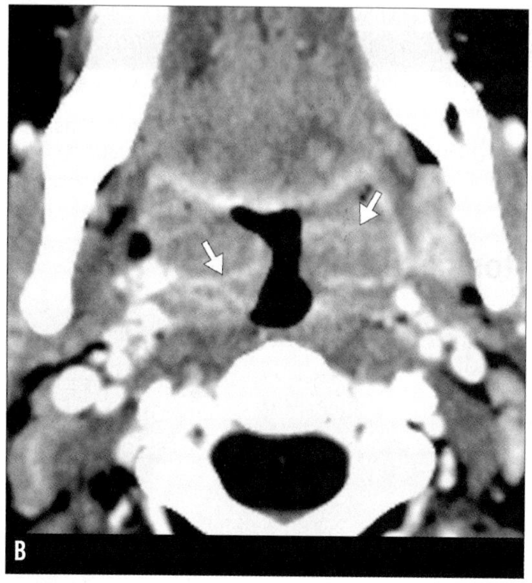

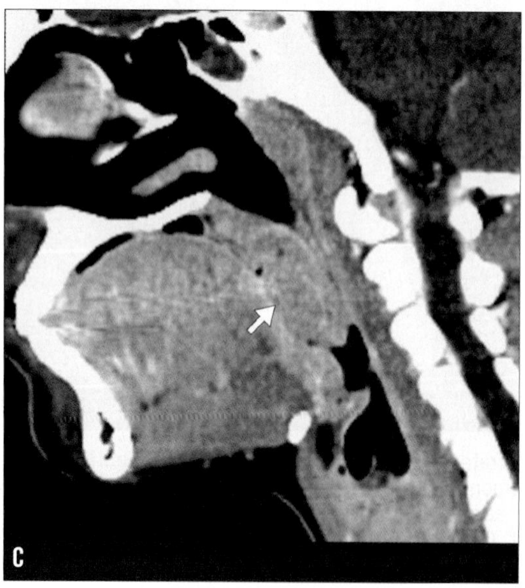

Axial immediate postcontrast (**A**) and axial delayed postcontrast (**B**) CT images through the palatine tonsils. Image **A** demonstrate symmetrically enlarged palatine tonsils (arrows, **A**) without a discrete focus of abnormal attenuation in either palatine tonsil. The oropharyngeal airway is narrowed (arrowhead, **A**). Image **B** demonstrates tranversely-oriented, linear enhancement often present with edema of the palatine tonsils (arrows, **B**). The findings on image **B** are occult on the immediate postcontrast image (**A**) and demonstrate the benefit of delayed postcontrast imaging in this setting. Off-midline sagittal reformatted postcontrast CT image (**C**) demonstrates an apparent mass involving the uvula or pharynx (arrow, **C**). This merely represents partial inclusion of the edematous palatine tonsil, and not a neoplasm.

Companion case: Palatine tonsil edema

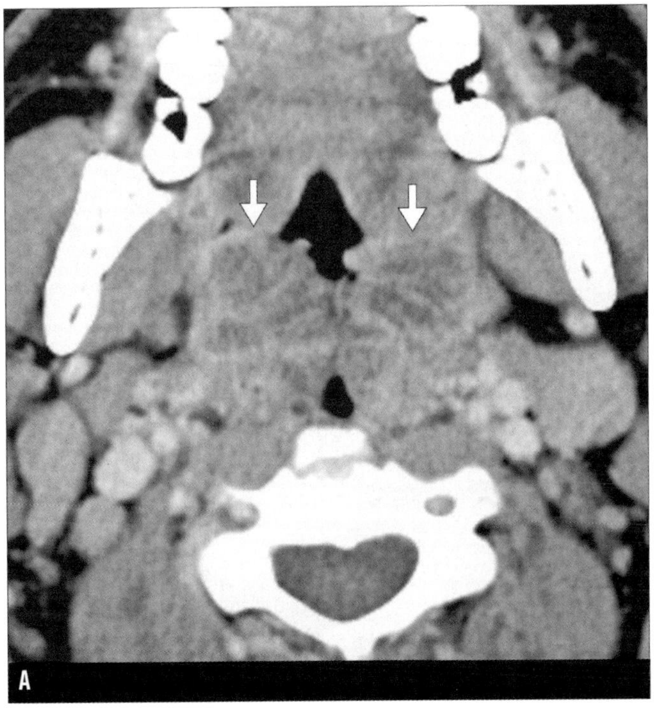

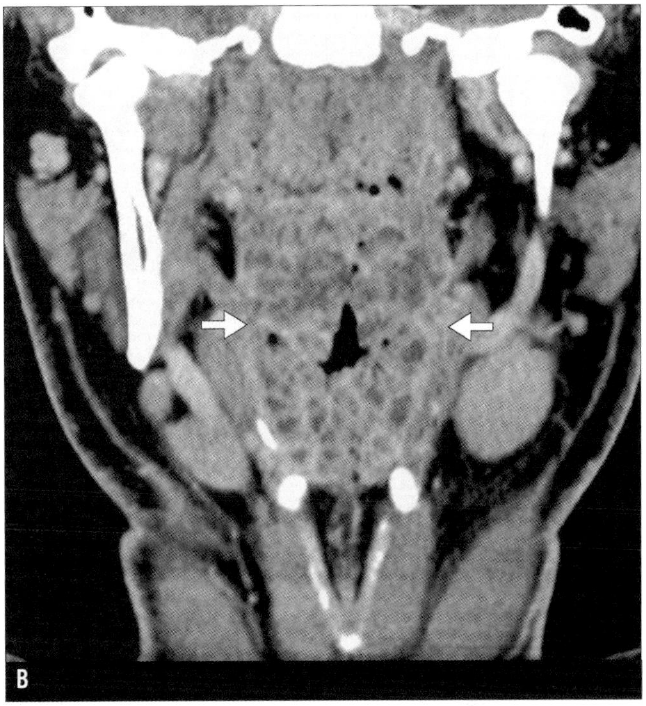

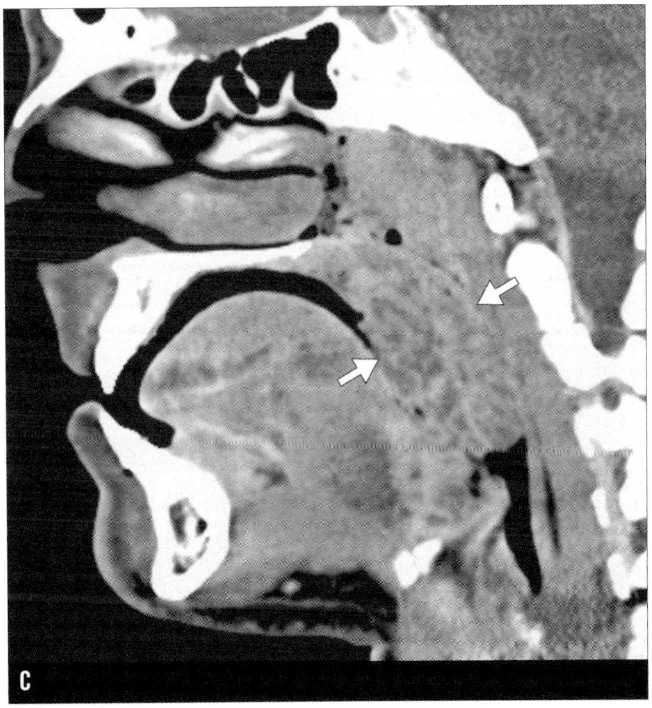

Different patient. An axial postcontrast CT image (**A**) demonstrates largely parallel-oriented, linear hyperattenuation and hypoattenuation in markedly enlarged bilateral palatine tonsils (arrows, **A**). Coronal (**B**) and sagittal (**C**) reformatted postcontrast CT images from the same study demonstrate numerous serpentine hyperattenuating areas outlining oval areas of hypoattenuation (arrows, **B**, **C**). The findings are most compatible with extensive palatine tonsillitis, particularly based on the axial image. Given the extensive edema, clinical evaluation of the airway was recommended.

Companion case: Palatine intratonsillar abscess

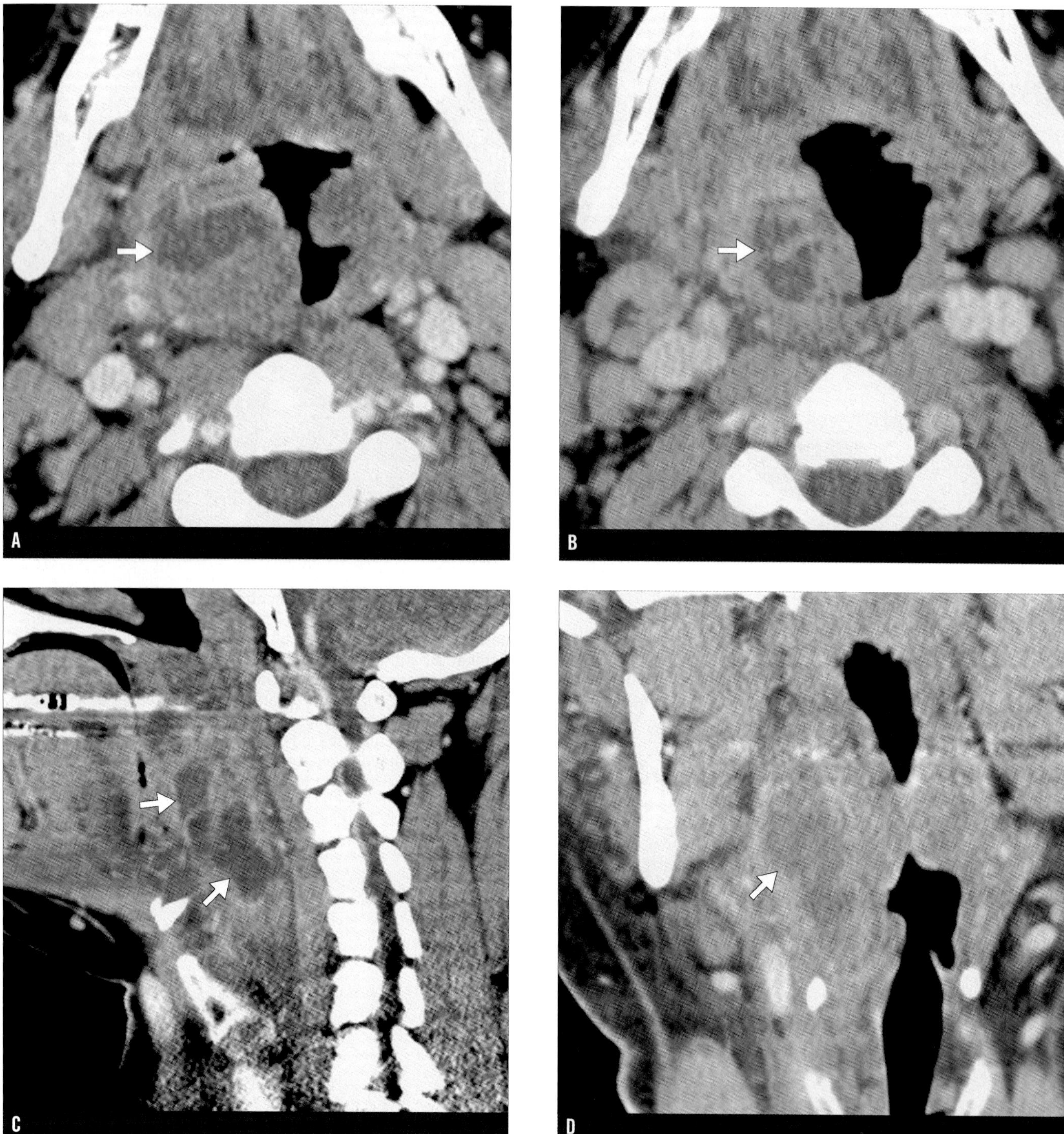

Axial (**A, B**), sagittal reformatted (**C**), and coronal reformatted (**D**) postcontrast CT images through the oropharynx demonstrate a peripherally enhancing, irregular, multiseptated fluid collection in the right palatine tonsil, consistent with an abscess (arrows, **A-D**). This is distinguished from a retention cyst by its irregular margins and thick peripheral enhancement, although the peripheral enhancement in this case is faint. Additional imaging findings related to a intratonsillar abscess may include surrounding inflammatory stranding and retropharyngeal fluid.

Companion case: Peritonsillar abscess

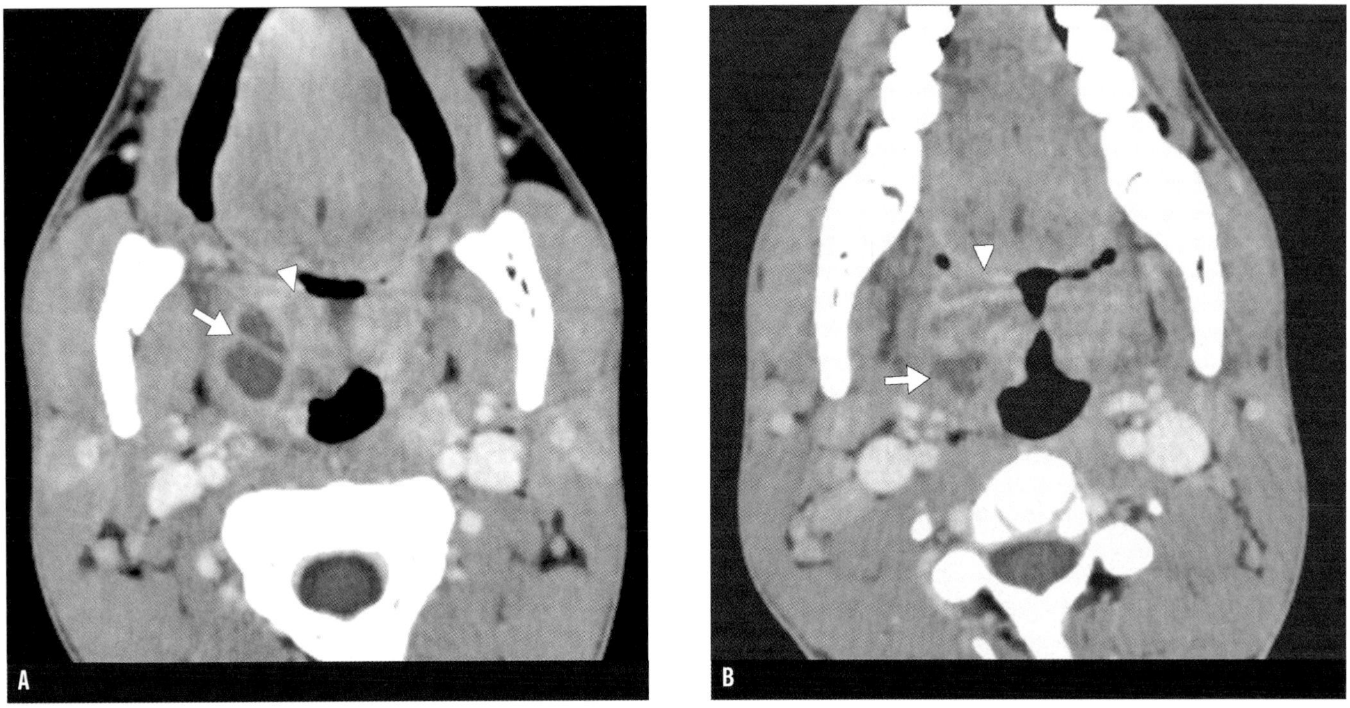

Postcontrast axial images through the oropharynx at slightly different levels (**A** and **B**) demonstrate a partially septated fluid collection in the right peritonsillar fossa, consistent with a right peritonsillar abscess (arrows, **A, B**). The right palatine tonsil is edematous and displaced medially (arrowheads, **A, B**).

Companion case: Partially necrotic palatine tonsil squamous cell carcinoma

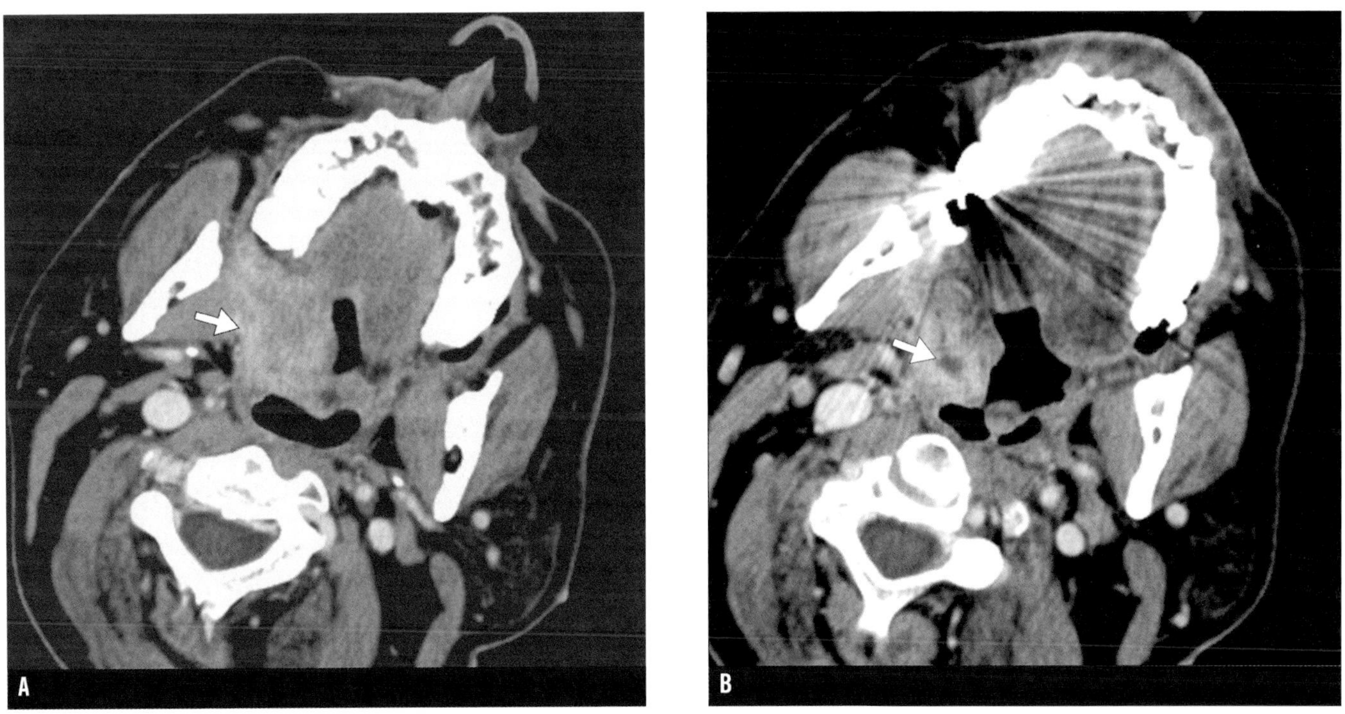

Contrast-enhanced axial CT images of the oropharynx (**A, B**) demonstrate a large right palatine tonsil squamous cell carcinoma, which is mostly composed of densely enhancing tumor (arrow, **A**), although a small focus of necrosis is identified (arrow, **B**).

REFERENCES

Gan EC, Ng YH, Hwang SY, Lu PK. Intratonsillar abscess: a rare cause for a common clinical presentation. *Ear Nose Throat J.* December 2008;87(12):E9.

Hsu CH, Lin YS, Lee JC. Intratonsillar abscess. *Otolaryngol Head Neck Surg.* December 2008;139(6):861-862.

Salem DB et al. Imaging of nasopharyngeal cysts and bursae. *Eur Radiol.* 2006;16:2249-2258.

CASE 13 Lingual tonsil lymphoid hyperplasia

The lingual tonsils form the anterior-inferior aspect of the Waldeyer ring and are located at the base of the tongue. While occasionally a diagnostic dilemma, normal lingual tonsil should maintain a frond-like morphology, rather than a solid, rounded morphology that is typically present with malignancies. If in doubt, direct inspection and/or follow-up imaging should be advised. While lingual tonsil lymphoid hyperplasia is a benign entity, marked enlargement can lead to oropharyngeal airway compromise.

COMPANION CASES

Base of tongue squamous cell carcinoma. Generally speaking, if an older patient presents with a pathologically enlarged and/or necrotic, dominant unilateral level II lymph node, and there is no history of infection to explain the finding, then an ipsilateral palatine tonsil or base of tongue malignancy should be excluded. This is because the normal lymphatic drainage pattern of the base of tongue and palatine tonsil begins in the ipsilateral level II region. Thus, the threshold should be low for describing any subtle ipsilateral palatine tonsil or base of tongue asymmetry in this setting. Additionally, primary malignancies of the palatine tonsil or base of tongue may only be visible on delayed postcontrast imaging. Therefore, delayed postcontrast imaging should be considered if there is a clinical suspicion of a primary malignancy in these regions.

Lingual tonsil lymphoid hyperplasia

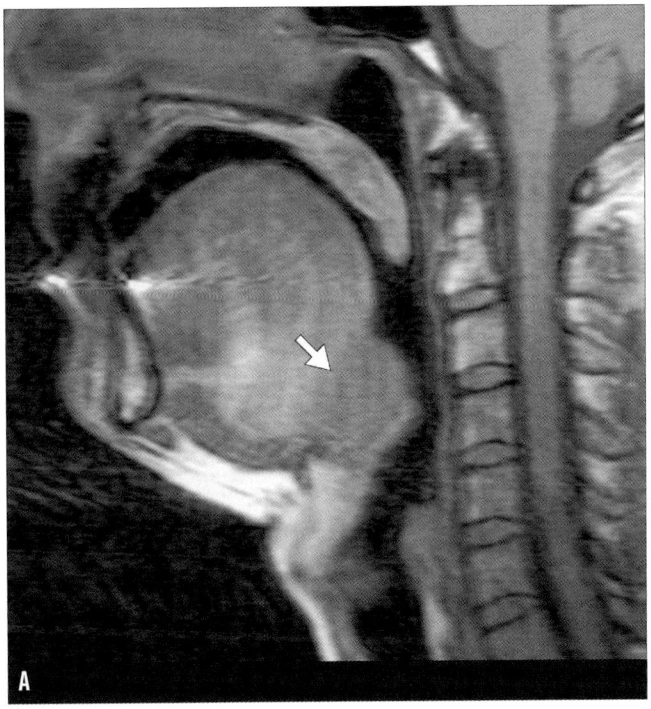

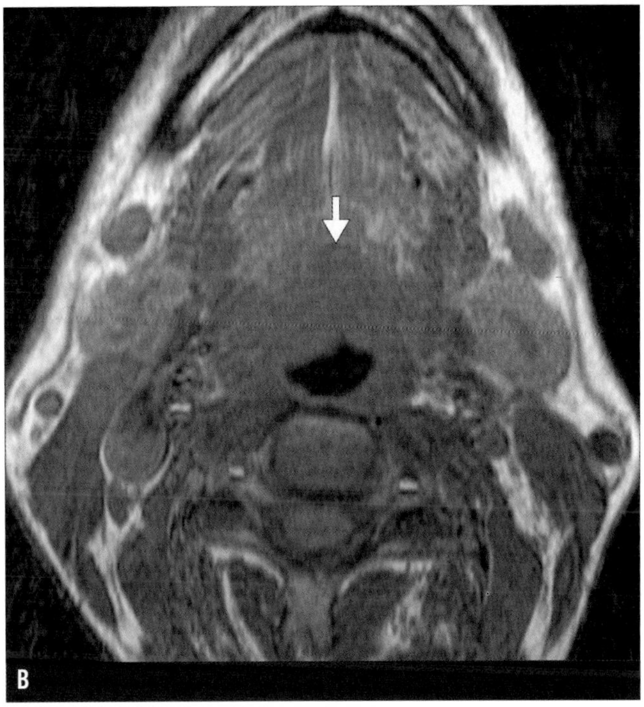

A 46-year-old man. Midline sagittal T1 (**A**), axial T1 (**B**), postcontrast sagittal T1 with fat saturation (**C**), and postcontrast axial T1 with fat saturation (**D**) MR images demonstrate mild enhancement of a diffusely enlarged lingual tonsil in this patient who is HIV positive (arrows, **A-D**). An axial T2-weighted MR image with fat suppression (**E**) demonstrates the enlarged lingual tonsil to be diffusely T2 hyperintense (arrow, **E**), typical of benign lingual tonsil. An axial postcontrast CT image of the same patient **(F)** demonstrates the CT correlate of lingual tonsillar hypertrophy (arrow, **F**).

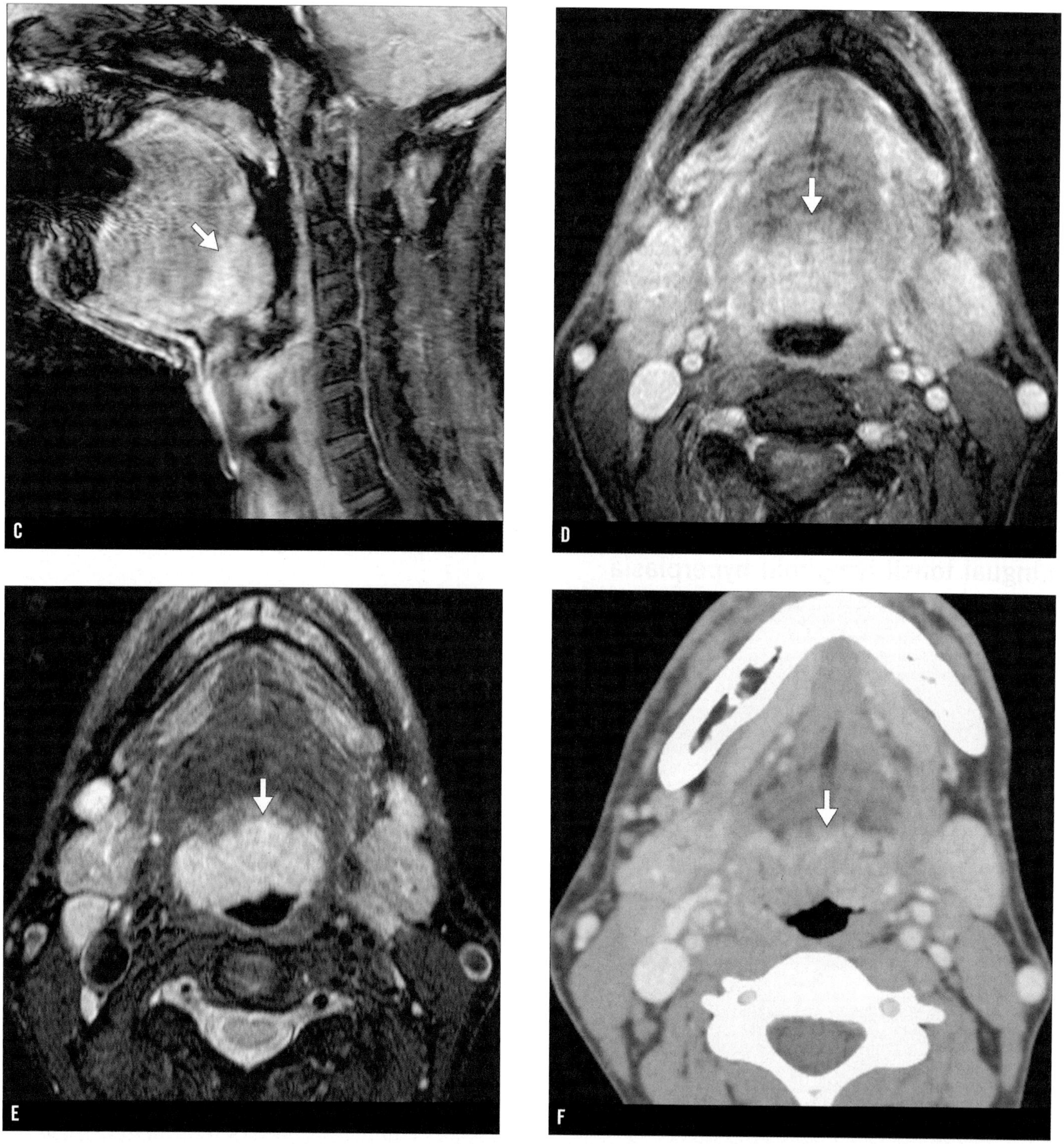
C
D
E
F

Lingual tonsil lymphoid hyperplasia

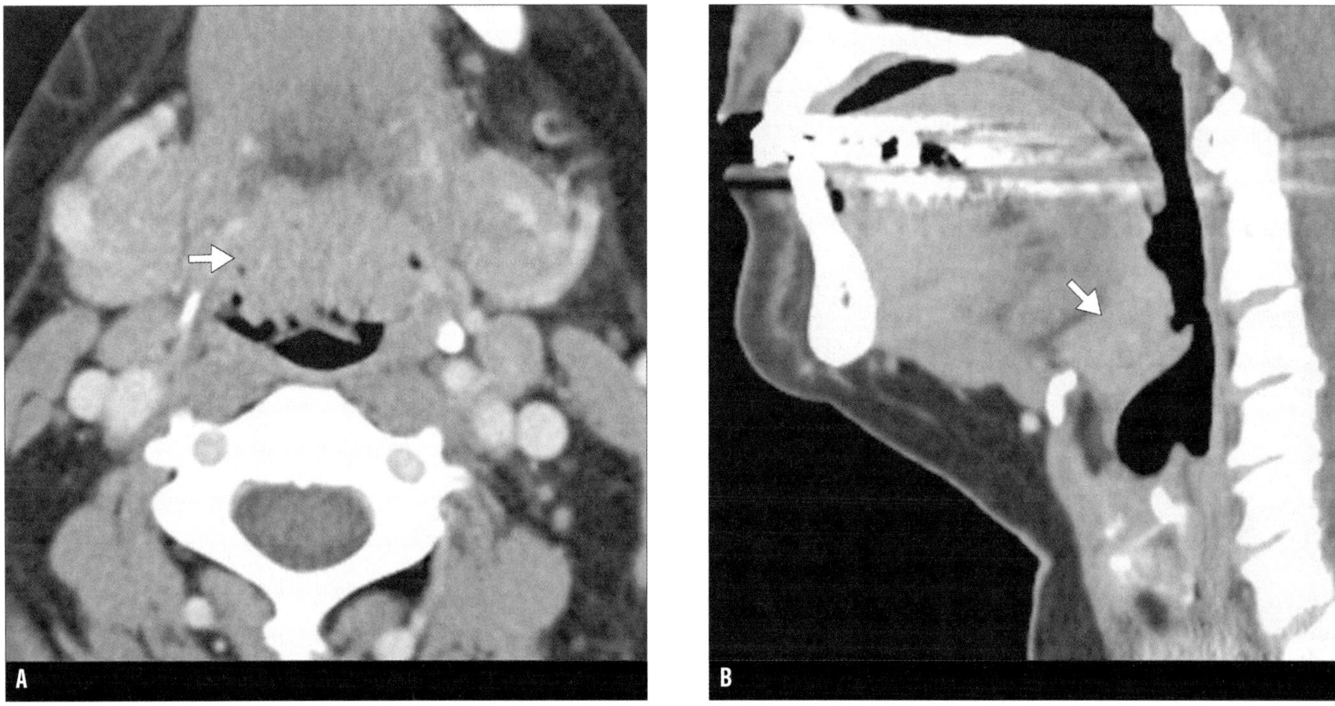

A 63-year-old woman. Axial (**A**) and sagittal reformatted (**B**) postcontrast CT images through the oropharynx demonstrate hypertrophied lingual tonsils occupying the majority of the vallecula (arrows, **A**, **B**). The lingual tonsillar tissue has a normal frond-like morphology with air extending into the crypts/crevices of the tonsil. This finding was completely stable compared to a CT scan obtained 9 years earlier, compatible with benignity.

Companion case: Base of tongue squamous cell carcinoma

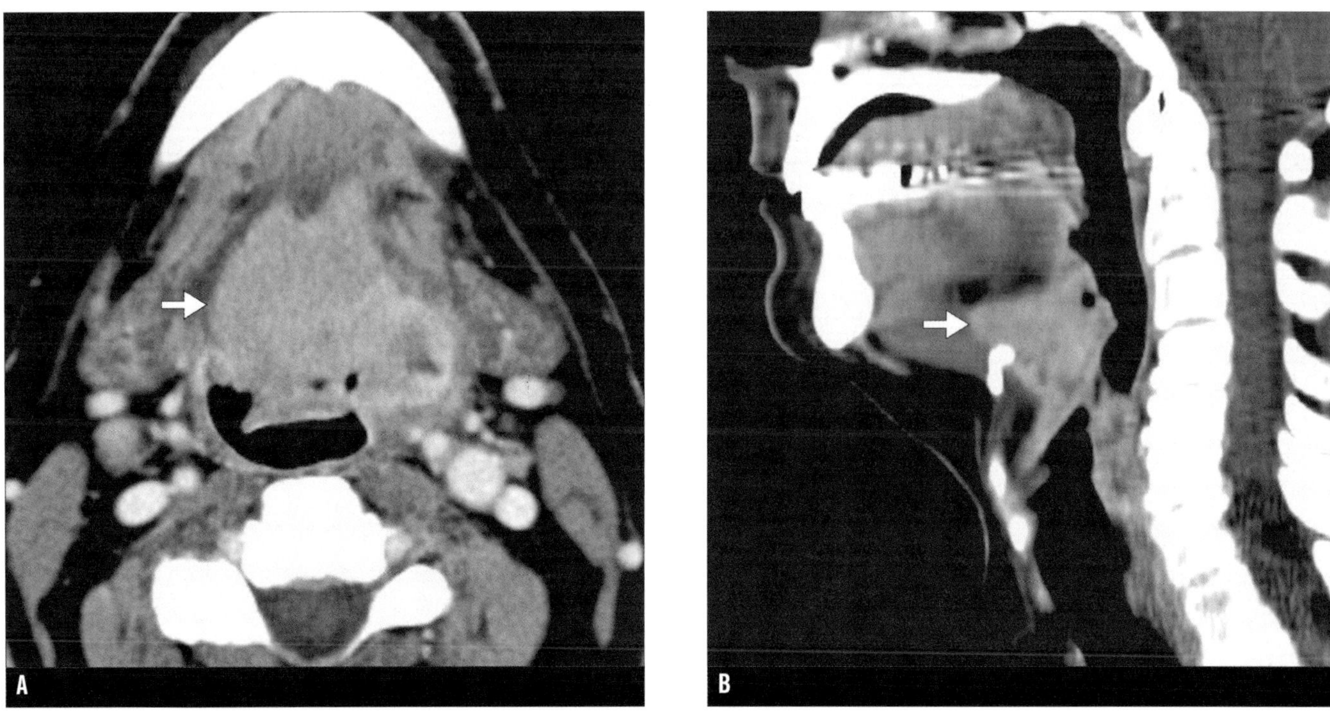

Axial (**A**) and sagittal reformatted (**B**) CT images performed with contrast demonstrate a large base of tongue mass consistent with squamous cell carcinoma (arrows, **A**, **B**). An axial postcontrast CT image through the supraglottic larynx (**C**) demonstrates the mass to extend into the left paraglottic fat, left aryepiglottic fold, and anterolaterally into the left strap muscles (arrow, **C**).

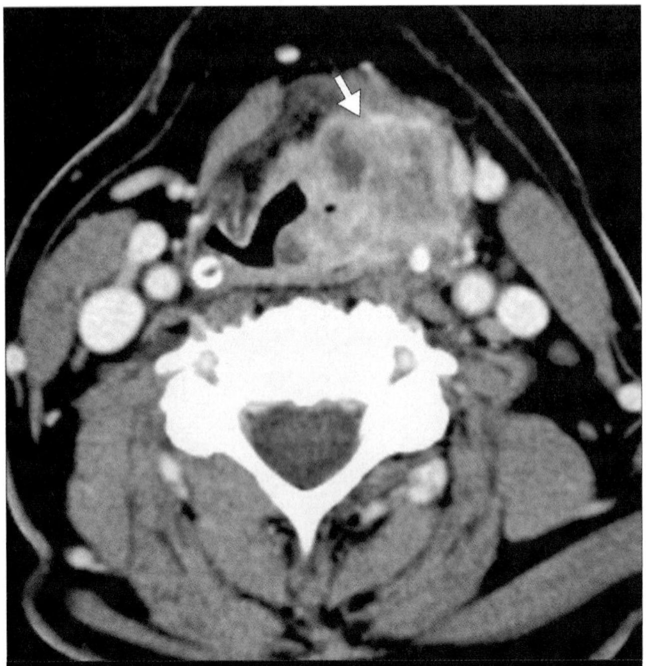

C

REFERENCES

Dillon WP et al. Magnetic Resonance Imaging of the nasopharynx. *Radiology.* 1984;152;731-738.

Fricke B et al. Comparison of lingual tonsil size as depicted on MR imaging between children with obstructive sleep apnea despite previous tonsillectomy and adenoidectomy and normal controls. *Pediatr Radiol.* 2006;36(6):518-523.

Friedman M et al. Measurements of adult lingual tonsil tissue in health and disease. *Otolaryngol Head Neck Surg.* 2010;142(4):520-525.

CASE 14 Air-filled lingual tonsil crypts

The palatine and lingual tonsils contain invaginations, or crypts, extending from their surface into the substance of the tissue. These crypts are usually potential spaces that are not visible by imaging. However, air or retention cysts can occasionally occupy the crypts and be visualized on imaging.

Air-filled lingual tonsil crypts

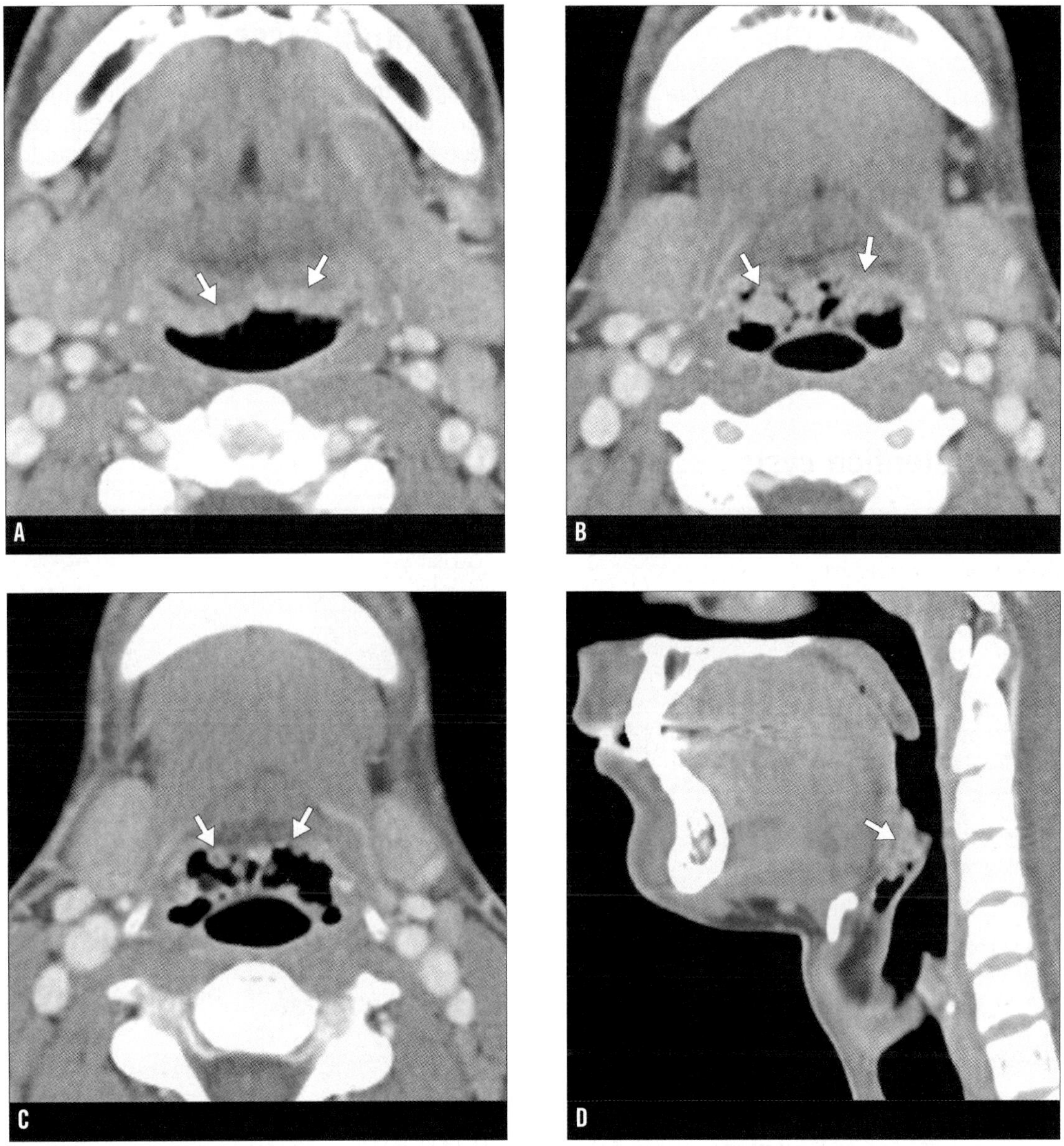

Sequential postcontrast axial CT images through the oropharynx (**A**-**C**). Image **A** demonstrates a typical, normal tongue base (arrows, **A**). Slightly inferior to image **A**, images **B** and **C** demonstrate a frond-like morphology of the lingual tonsil with air interdigitating within the crypts of the tonsil (arrows, **B**, **C**). A sagittal reformatted postcontrast CT image (**D**) also demonstrates the normal frond-like morphology of the lingual tonsil (arrow, **D**).

REFERENCES

Lin JH et al. Huge Thornwaldt cyst: a case report. *Kaohsiung J Med Sci.* 2006;22:524-528.

Salem DB et al. Imaging of nasopharyngeal cysts and bursae. *Eur Radiol.* 2006;16;2249-2258.

CASE 15 Lingual tonsil retention cyst

Retention cysts are a common incidental and asymptomatic finding that may be found anywhere within the oral cavity and pharynx. There are two basic types of retention cysts: mucous and serous. A mucous retention cyst is more common and results from obstruction of a seromucinous gland. A serous retention cyst results from accumulation of fluid in the submucosal layer. Mucous and serous retention cysts are indistinguishable by imaging and appear as smooth, outwardly convex soft tissue masses. Depending on the location, or if the cyst becomes large enough, symptoms such as dysphagia may occur. Retention cysts generally have low attenuation values on CT imaging. On MRI, retention cysts are most often hypointense on T1 and hyperintense on T2, although their signal characteristics can be variable, depending on their protein content. Following intravenous contrast administration, a thin rim of enhancement may be observed on either CT or MRI, but retention cysts should not solidly enhance.

Differentiating this incidental finding from a lingual tonsil abscess can be difficult on imaging. The lack of a thick rim of enhancement, a nonenlarged/nonedematous tonsil, and the lack of surrounding inflammatory change can support the diagnosis of an incidental retention cyst and help exclude an abscess.

COMPANION CASES

- **Lingual tonsil edema.** In this setting, the lingual tonsils are often enlarged and contain linear, parallel-oriented areas of enhancement within the lingual tonsil.
- **Base of tongue squamous cell carcinoma.** Please refer to the companion case from Case 13 for discussion.
- **Oropharyngeal wall retention cyst varying in size over time.**
- **Vallecular retention cyst.**

Lingual tonsil retention cysts

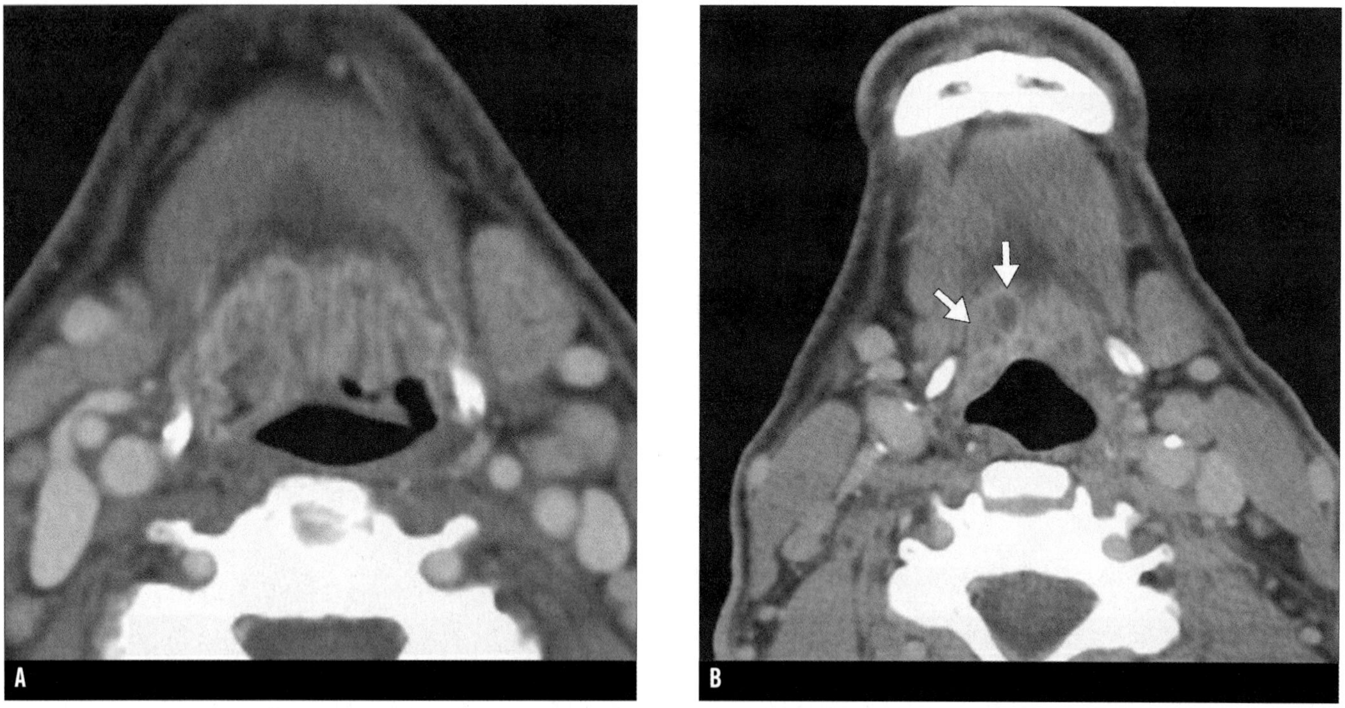

Sequential postcontrast axial CT images through the inferior oropharynx at the level of the lingual tonsils (**A-C**). Images **A** and **C** demonstrate normal lingual tonsil whereas image **B** demonstrates at least two discrete retention cysts with mild peripheral enhancement located in the right aspect of the tonsil (arrows, **B**).

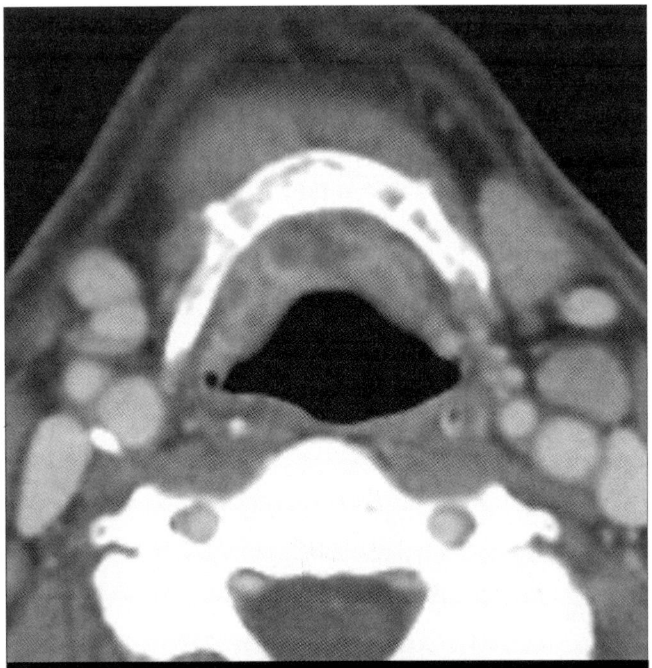

C

Lingual tonsil retention cyst

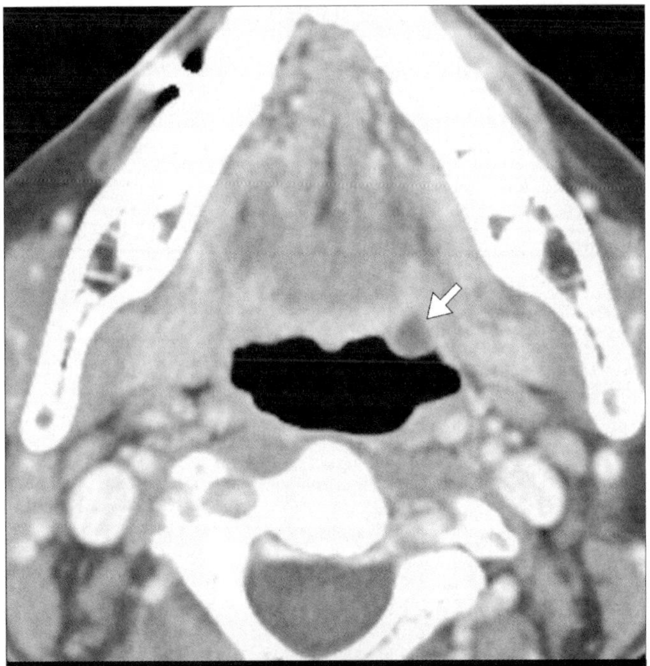

A

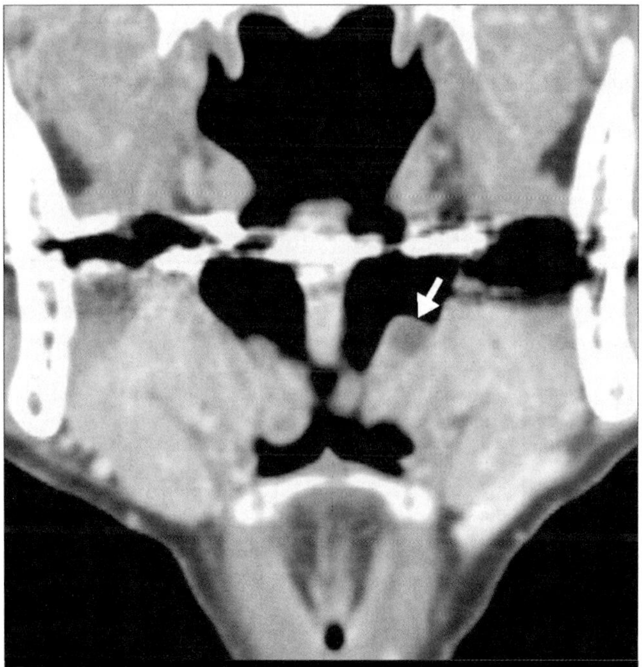

B

Different patient. Axial (**A**), coronal reformatted (**B**), and sagittal reformatted (**C**) postcontrast CT images through the oropharynx demonstrate a nonenhancing, round, circumscribed hypoattenuating lesion located at the left base of tongue, consistent with an incidental lingual tonsil retention cyst (arrows, **A-C**).

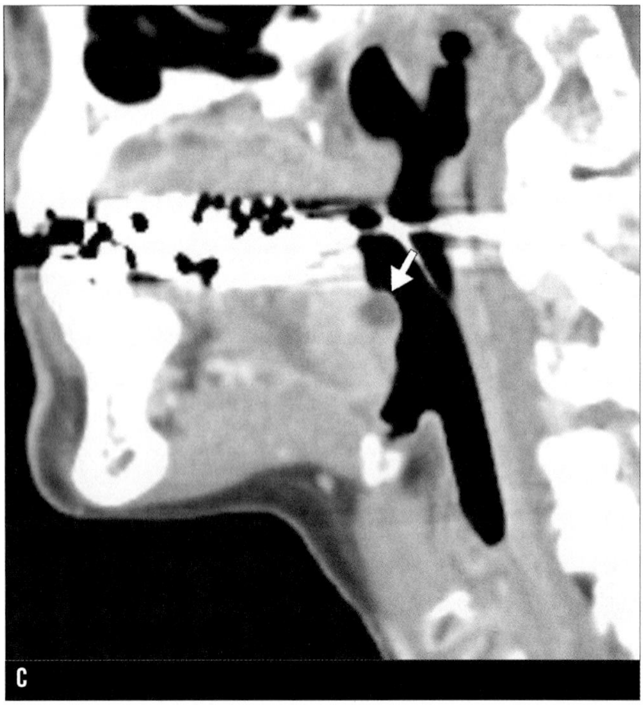

Lingual tonsil retention cyst

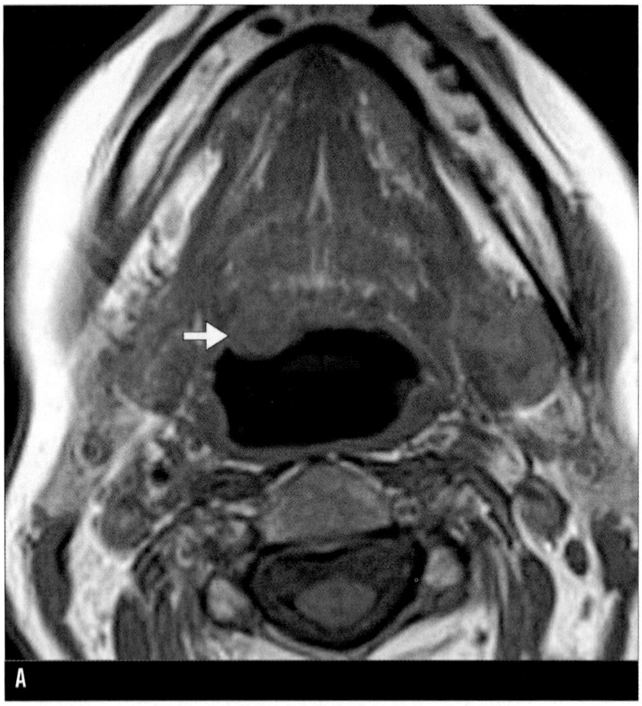

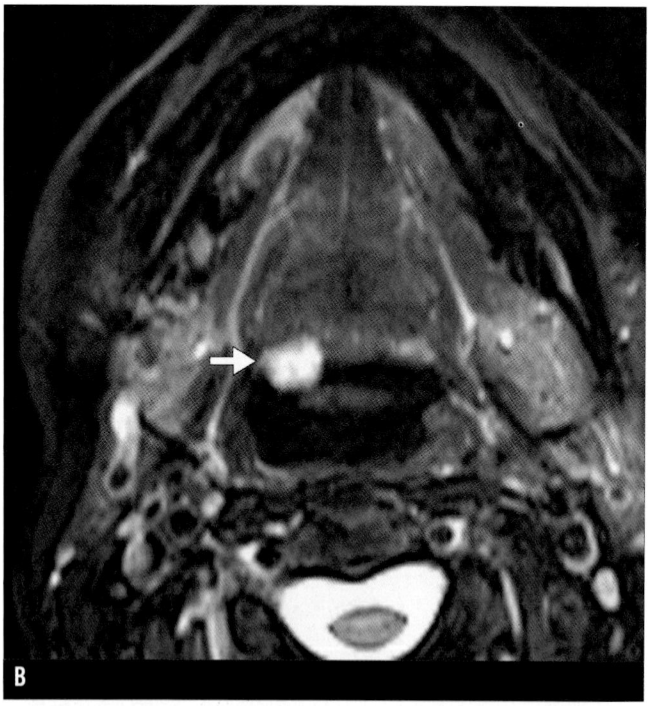

Different patient. Noncontrast axial T1 (**A**), axial T2 with fat saturation (**B**), and postcontrast axial T1 with fat saturation (**C**) MR images through the oropharynx demonstrate a nonenhancing, round, circumscribed hypoattenuating lesion at the right base of tongue, compatible with an incidental retention cyst (arrows, **A-C**).

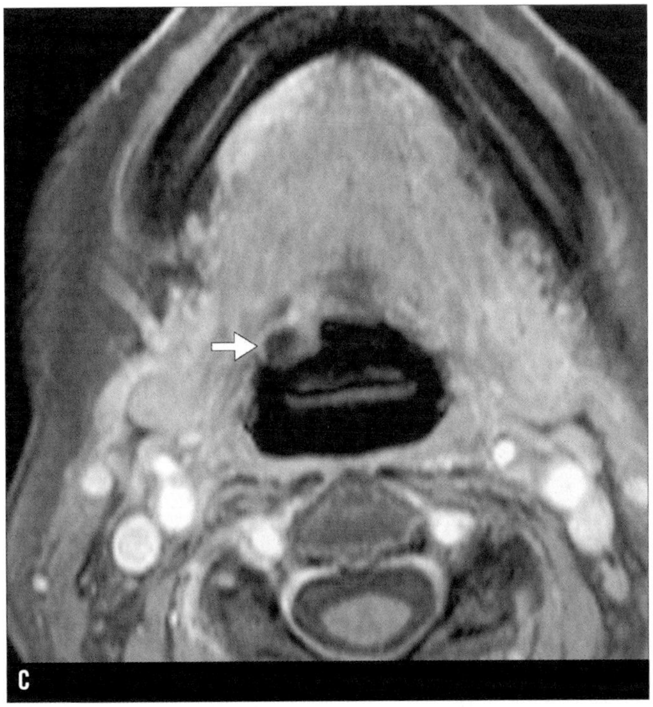

Companion case: Lingual tonsil edema

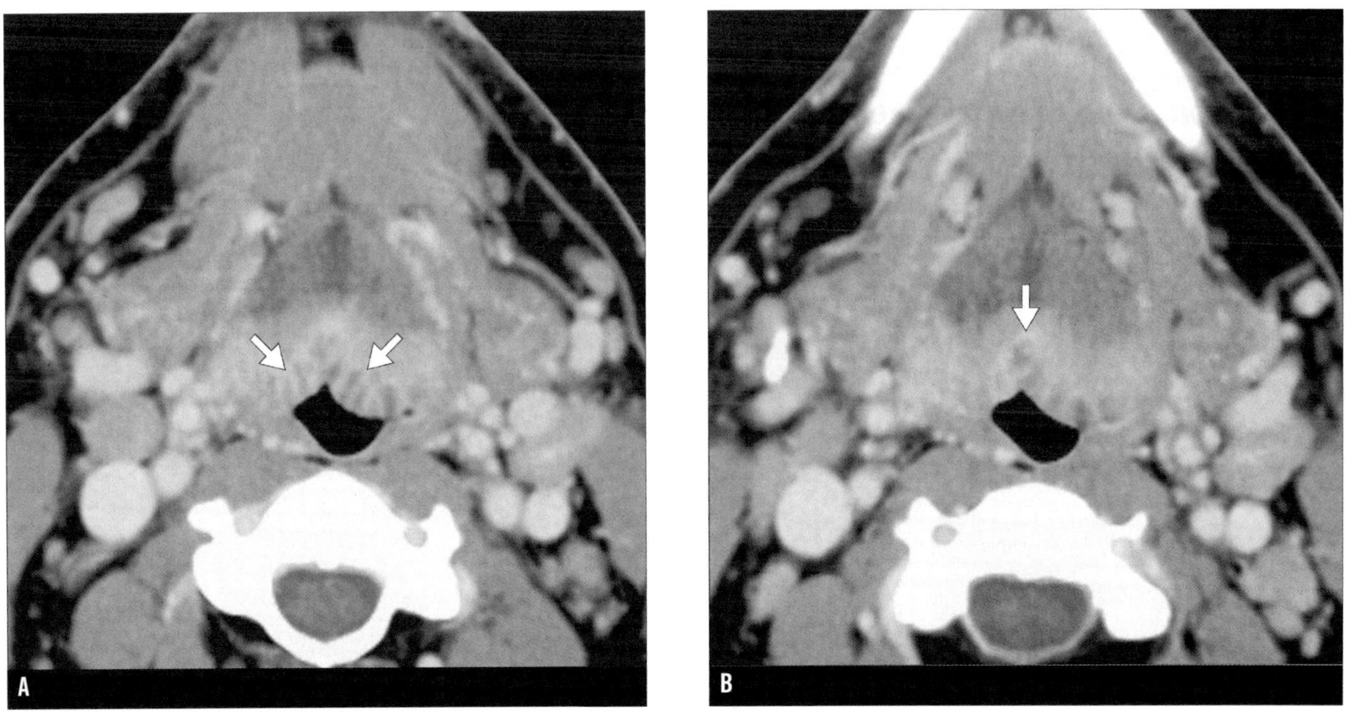

Patient presenting with clinical symptoms of pharyngitis. Postcontrast axial CT images through the lower oropharynx (**A** and **B**) demonstrate several hypoattenuating, parallel-oriented foci surrounded by mild inflammation, compatible with lingual tonsil edema. It is important to not mistake lingual edema/tonsillitis, as is present in this case, from a lingual tonsil abscess, as the former can be treated symptomatically whereas the latter is typically surgically drained. An attempt to aspirate the lingual tonsils with this imaging appearance will usually be unproductive and nondiagnostic. When in doubt, direct inspection and/or short-term imaging follow-up would be prudent.

Companion case: Base of tongue squamous cell carcinoma

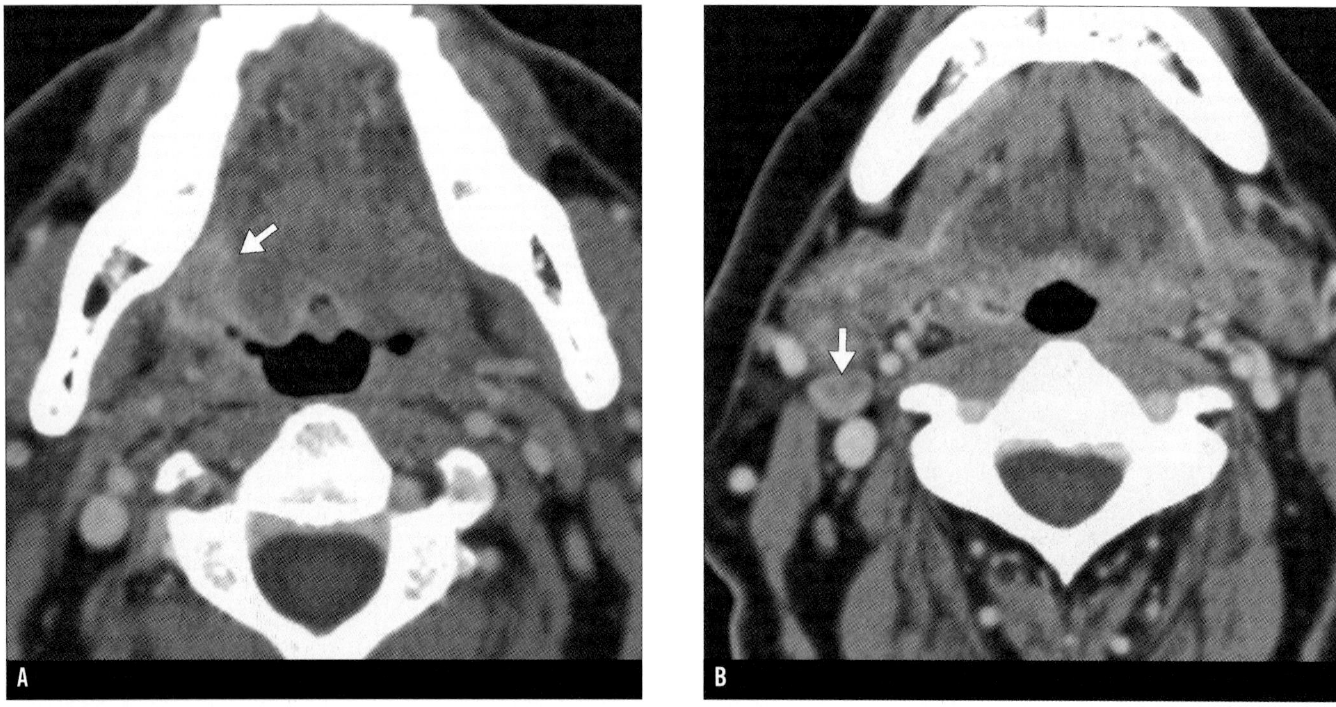

An axial postcontrast CT image through the base of tongue (**A**) and slightly lower through the base of tongue and level II nodal station (**B**). Image **A** demonstrates an irregularly enhancing mass at the right base of tongue with involvement of the lingual tonsil and right glossotonsillar sulcus (arrow, **A**). This was pathologically proven to be squamous cell carcinoma of tongue base. Image **B** demonstrates a nonenlarged, but heterogeneously enhancing, right level IIA lymph node that appears pathologic, given its enhancing characteristics, and represented a metastatic lymph node at pathology (arrow, **B**).

Companion case: Oropharyngeal wall retention cyst varying in size over time

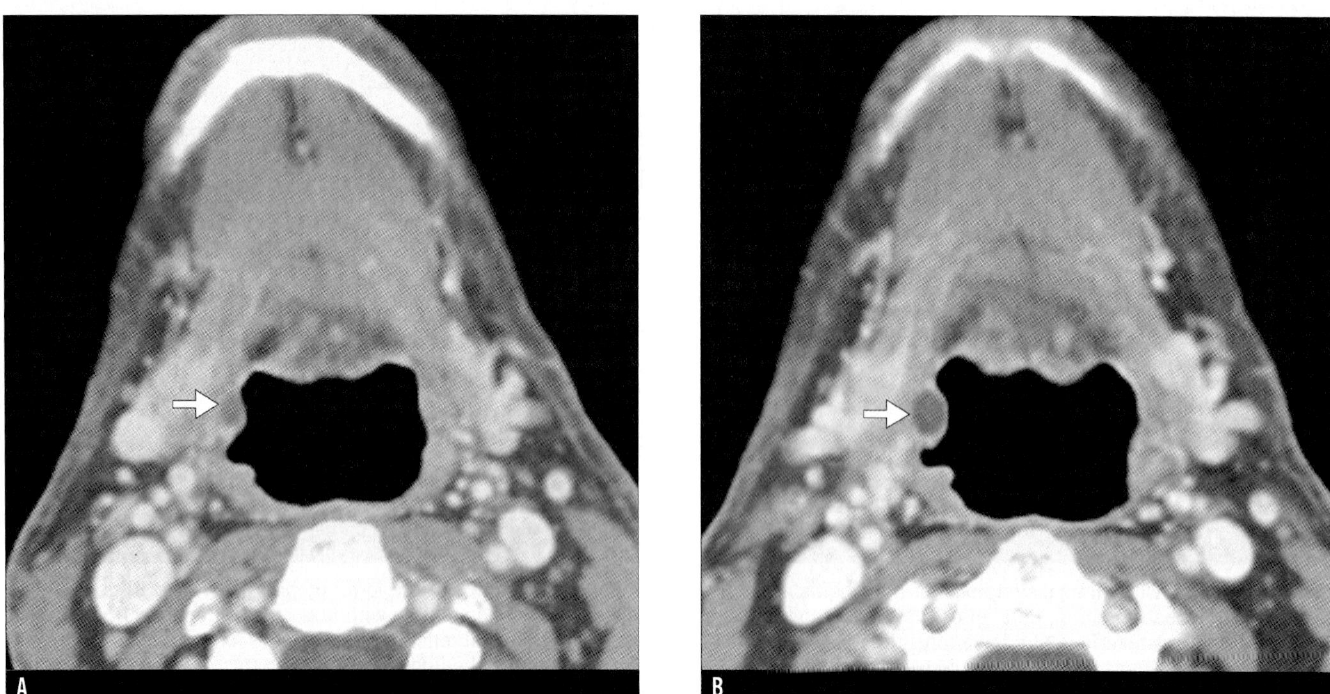

Axial postcontrast CT images through the oropharynx (**A**), 2 months after **A** (**B**), and 6 months after **B** (**C**) demonstrate a varying size of a circumscribed, fluid attenuating lesion embedded within the right aspect of the oropharyngeal wall (arrows, **A-C**). The imaging appearance of the finding is compatible with an incidental retention cyst. This case illustrates that retention cysts can vary in size over time and enlargement does not necessarily imply malignancy. Seromucinous glands are scattered throughout the upper respiratory tract mucosa; therefore, retention cysts may form anywhere along the upper respiratory tract mucosa.

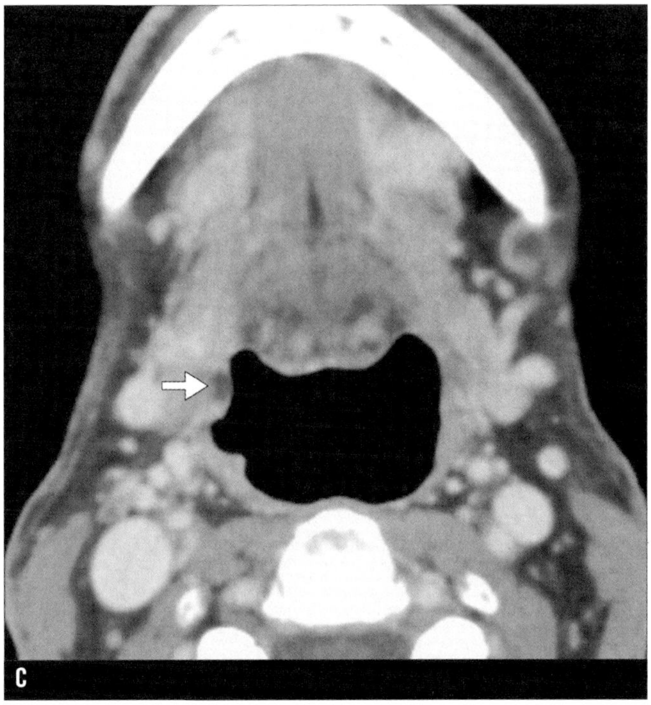

Companion case: Vallecular retention cyst

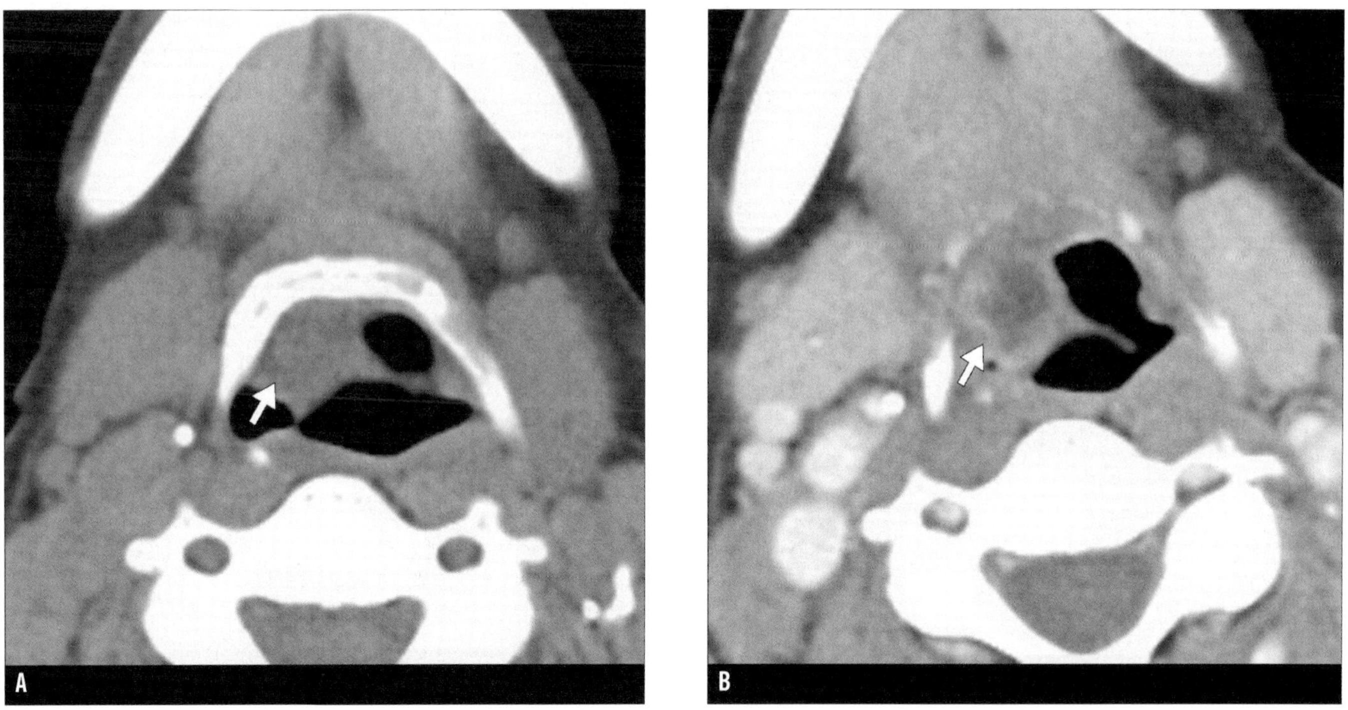

Noncontrast axial (**A**), postcontrast axial (**B**), and delayed postcontrast axial (**C**) CT images through the vallecula. Image **A** demonstrates nonspecific opacification of the right vallecula (arrow, **A**). Images **B** and **C** demonstrate a round, fluid-containing, peripherally enhancing lesion in the right vallecula, consistent with an incidental vallecular cyst (arrows, **B, C**).

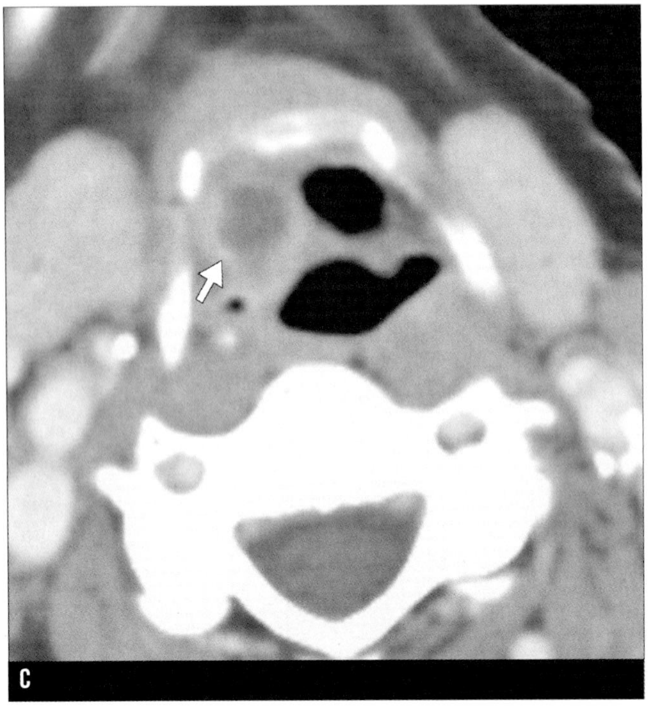

Companion case: Vallecular retention cyst

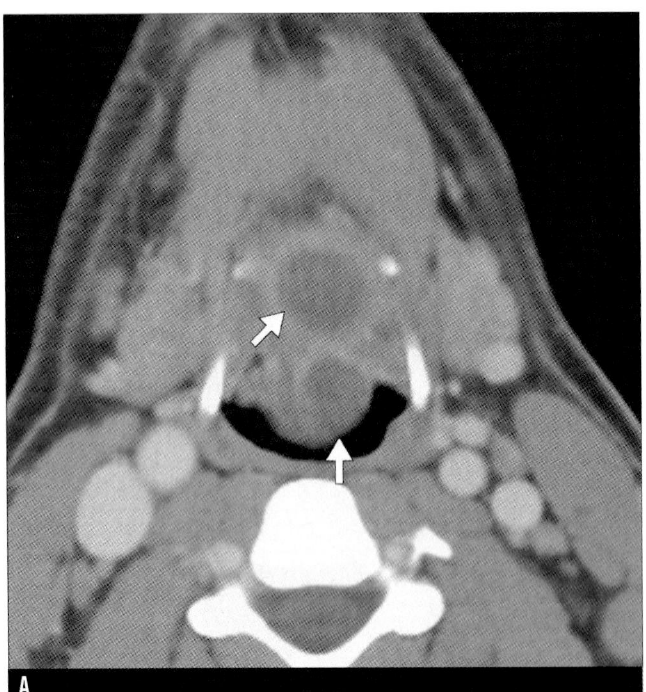

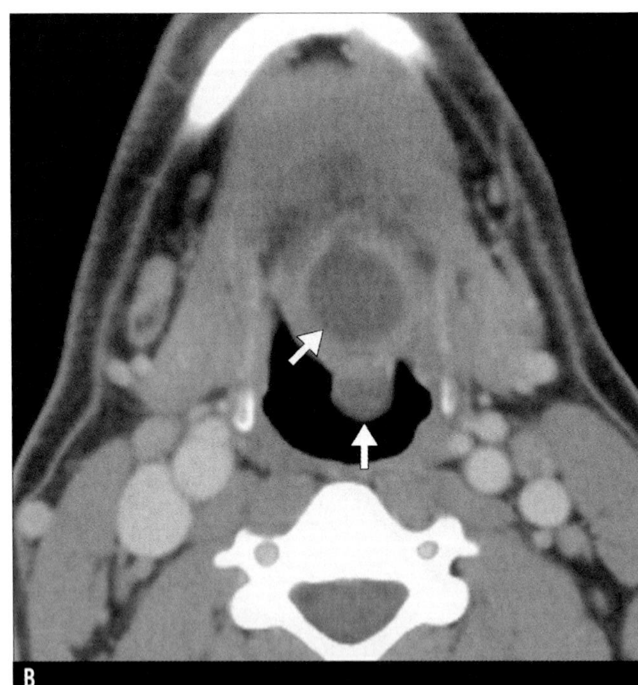

Different patient. Axial (**A** and **B**) and midline sagittal reformatted (**C**) postcontrast CT images through the lower oropharynx demonstrate a large, bilobed, circumscribed fluid density lesion located in the vallecula (arrows, **A**-**C**). The patient underwent surgical drainage soon after these images were obtained. The fluid that was aspirated was negative for malignancy. Follow-up axial (**D** and **E**) and midline sagittal reformatted (**F**) postcontrast CT images through the lower oropharynx obtained 1 month after images **A**-**C** demonstrate the lesion to be larger, despite drainage, and is now unilocular rather than bilobed (arrows, **D**-**F**). While a cystic neoplasm can be difficult to exclude in this case, the smooth, barely perceptible walls, circumscribed margin, lack of solid tissue associated with the cyst, and normal adjacent soft tissues support a benign etiology.

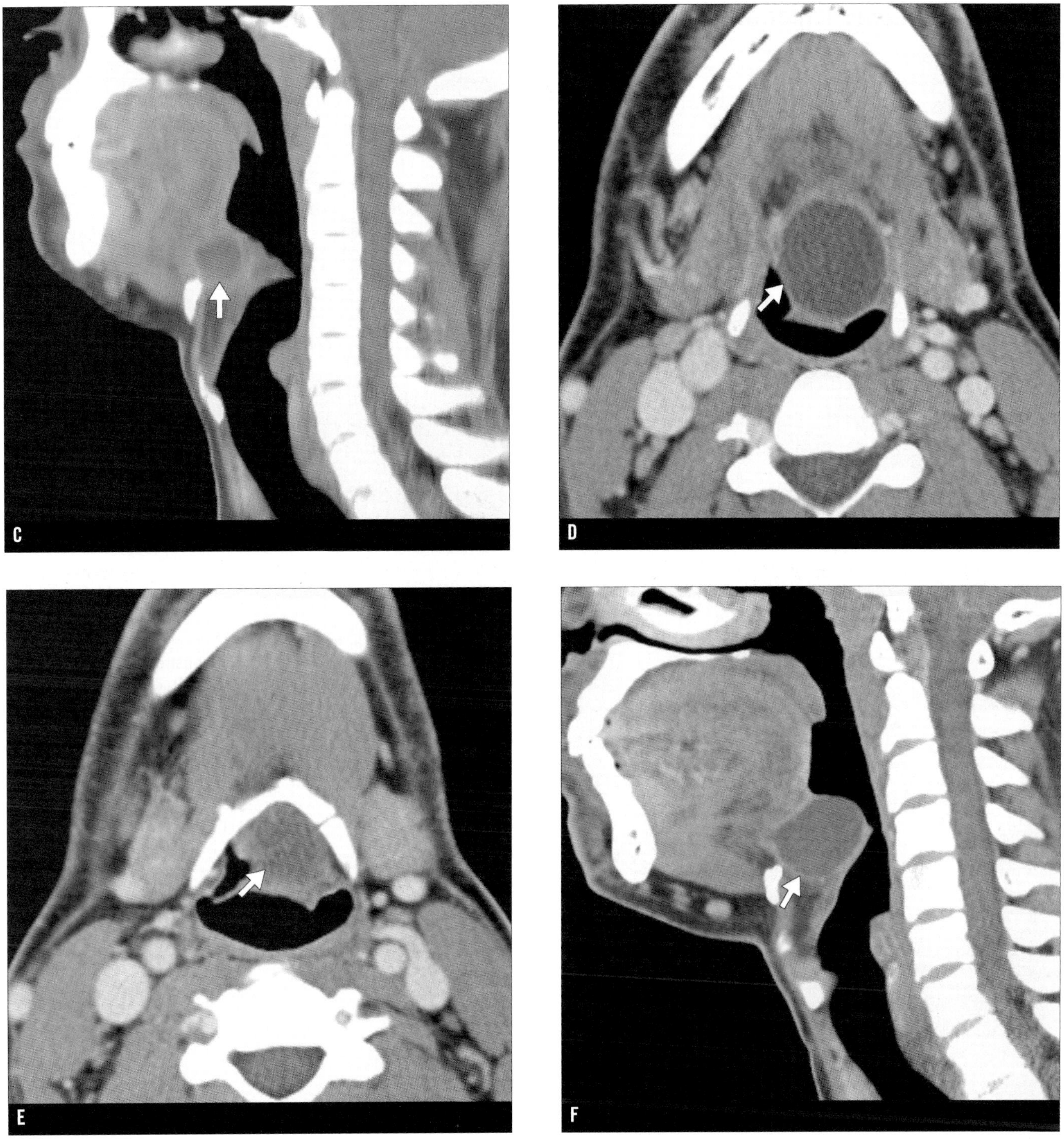
C
D
E
F

Companion case: Vallecular retention cyst with mineralization

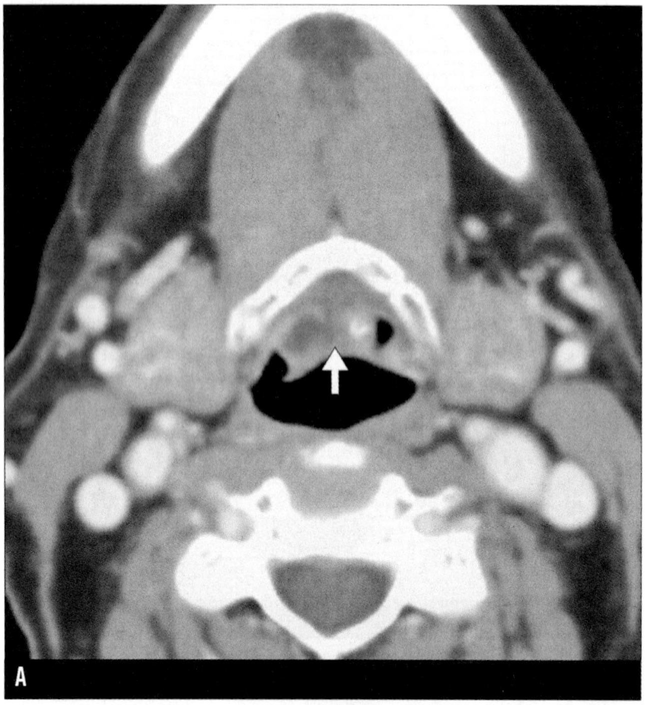

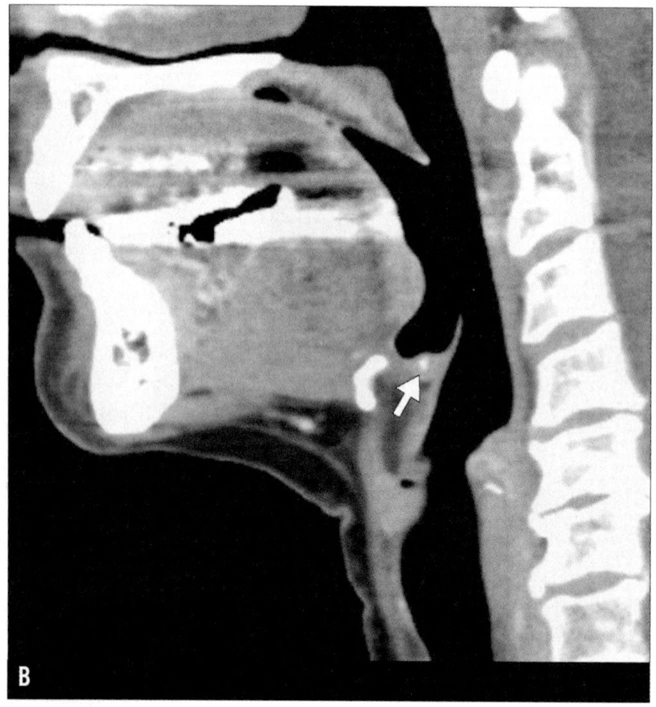

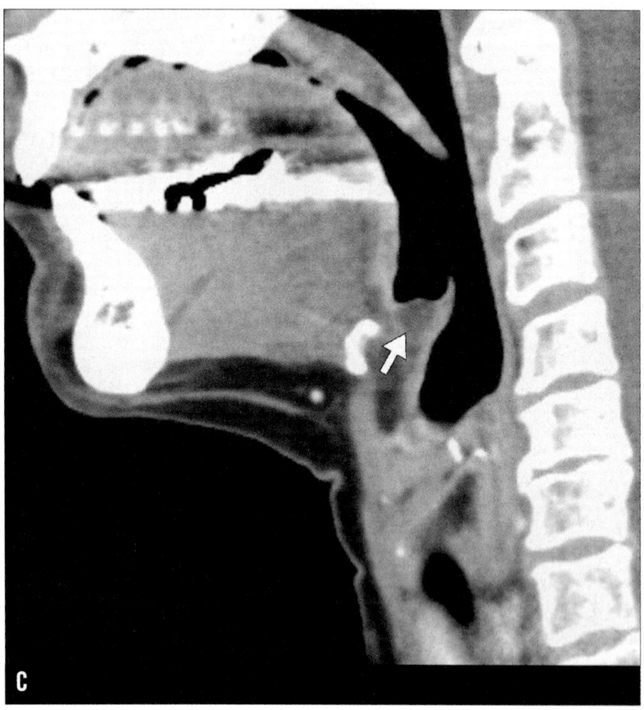

Axial (**A**) and sagittal reformatted (**B**, **C**) postcontrast CT images through the level of the oropharynx demonstrate a partially mineralized vallecular retention cyst (arrows, **A-C**).

REFERENCES

Grant PD et al. Pharyngeal dysphagia: what the radiologist needs to know. *Curr Probl Diagn Radiol.* 2009;38(1):17-32.

Lin JH et al. Huge Thornwaldt cyst: a case report. *Kaohsiung J Med Sci.* 2006;22:524-528.

Salem DB et al. Imaging of nasopharyngeal cysts and bursae. *Eur Radiol.* 2006;16:2249-2258.

Woodfield CA et al. Pharyngeal retention cysts: radiographic findings in seven patients. *AJR Am J Roentgenol.* 2005;184(3):793-796.

Lingual thyroid represents ectopically located thyroid tissue at the tongue base or floor of mouth, and it is the most common location for ectopic thyroid tissue. This developmental anomaly is related to failure of the thyroid gland to descend during early embryogenesis. Normally, the thyroid gland descends along the thyroglossal duct tract to reside in the lower anterior neck. However, if there is disruption of the normal descent, ectopic thyroid tissue can be found anywhere along this tract, usually from the foramen cecum at the tongue base to the level of the lower neck ventral to the trachea.

Ectopic thyroid tissue is many times more prevalent in females than males. Some patients with a lingual thyroid do not have a thyroid gland in the normal expected lower neck location. In cases where both are present, the lingual thyroid is usually smaller than 1 cm. If the lingual thyroid gland is the only functioning thyroid tissue, then its removal will lead to profound hypothyroidism and should be avoided in these cases, if possible. When large, lingual thyroid tissue may cause dysphagia, obstruct the airway, and result in a difficult intubation. While rare, reports of malignancy involving lingual thyroid tissue have been described.

Lingual thyroid tissue will image the same as the typical thyroid gland on CT and MRI. It will usually be hyperattenuating on precontrast CT imaging, just like normal thyroid.

Lingual thyroid

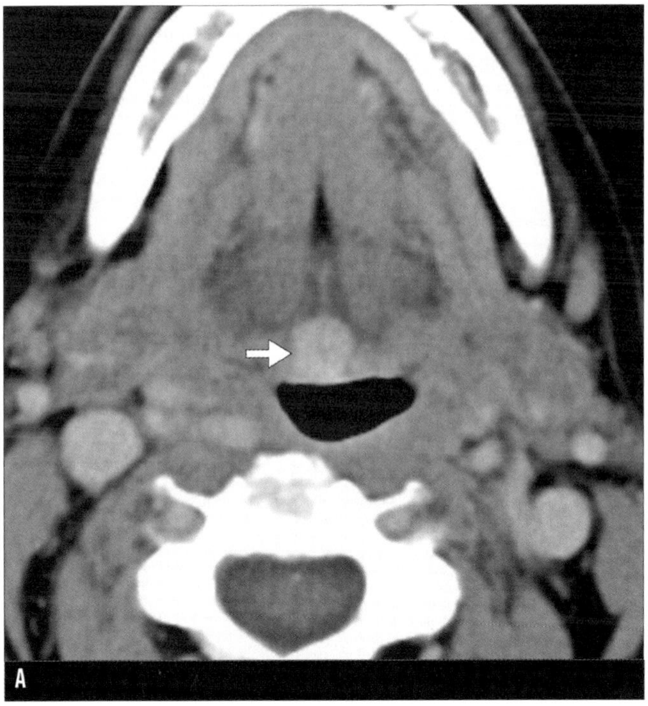

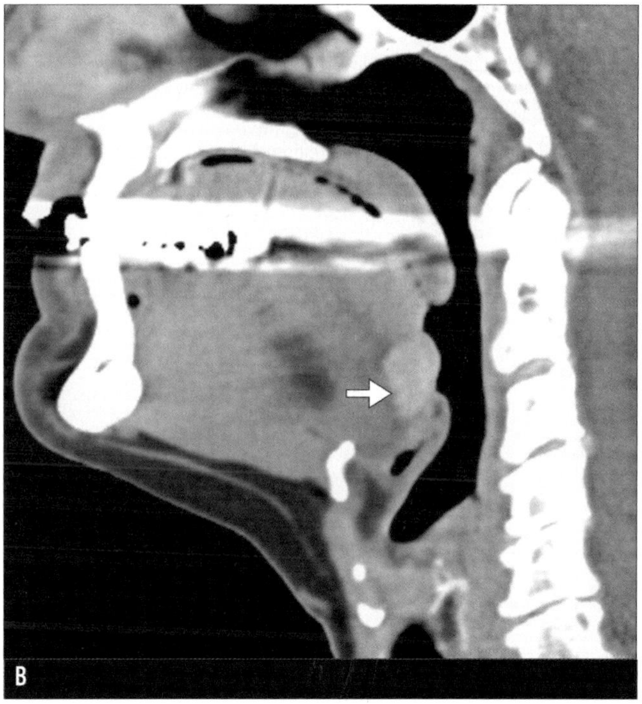

Axial (**A**), sagittal reformatted (**B**), and coronal reformatted (**C**) postcontrast CT images through the oral cavity demonstrate a small, oval, hyperdense finding at the base of the tongue near the midline (arrows, **A-C**). The location and density of the lesion is compatible with lingual thyroid. A postcontrast axial CT image through the lower neck (**D**) also demonstrates the presence of a normal thyroid gland (arrows, **D**), which may not be present when there is a lingual thyroid.

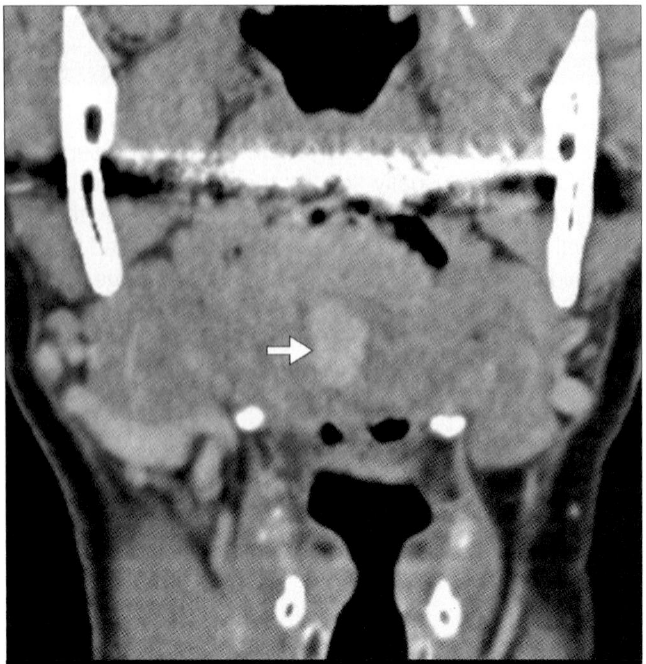
C

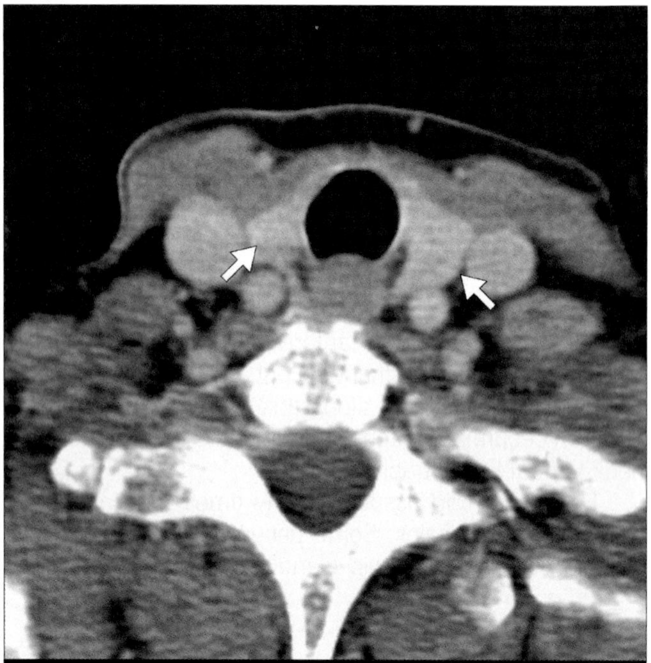
D

REFERENCES

El-Shafie OT, Hussain S, Sankhla D, Woodhouse N. Radioactive iodine-131 therapy in the management of ectopic thyroid tissue. *Sultan Qaboos Univ Med J.* 2014 Nov;14(4):e571-e574.

Massine RE et al. Lingual thyroid carcinoma: a case report and reviews of the literature. *Thyroid.* 2001;11(12):1191-1196.

Pisanu A, Deplano D, Uccheddu A, Cardu M. Unexpected and asymptomatic lingual thyroid as a cause of difficult intubation. *J Clin Anesth.* 2012 Aug;24(5):429-430.

CASE 17 Coapted pyriform sinus

The pyriform (or piriform) sinuses are air-filled recesses along the lateral aspects of the hypopharynx, bound ventrally by the posterior wall of the aryepiglottic fold and posteriorly by the posterior wall of the hypopharynx. Occasionally, asymmetry of the pyriform sinus may be present due to incidental coaptation of the aryepiglottic fold with the posterior wall of the hypopharynx.

Careful inspection of an asymmetric pyriform sinus is important in order to exclude the presence of a mass. Incidental coaptation of the pyriform sinus should not be associated with abnormal enhancement, the submucosal fat will be preserved, and the mucosal surfaces that are apposed are usually well-delineated. Conversely, tumors occupying the pyriform sinus generally enhance focally, obliterate the submucosal fat, and can have mass effect. If any of these findings that are typically present with tumors are identified, then direct inspection would be warranted. A PET scan can also be useful in this setting.

Coapted pyriform sinus

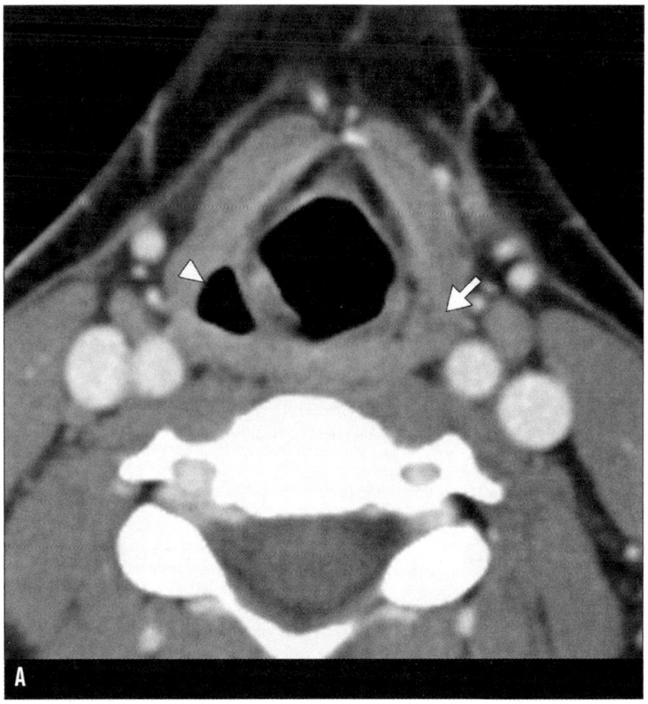

An axial postcontrast CT image through the level of the pyriform sinus (**A**) demonstrates asymmetric pyriform sinuses. The pyriform sinus on the right is air filled (arrowhead), whereas the pyriform sinus on the left is devoid of air (arrow). Careful inspection of the left pyriform sinus demonstrates preservation of the submucosal fat and lack of mass effect. The findings are consistent with incidental coaptation of the left pyriform sinus walls.

COMPANION CASES

- **Pyriform sinus squamous cell carcinoma.** Pyriform sinus squamous cell carcinomas tend to be very aggressive tumors with early metastasis and local spread. Owing to a large amount of lymphatic drainage from the hypopharynx, most patients have metastatic lymphadenopathy at presentation. Excessive alcohol and tobacco use are the primary risk factors for hypopharyngeal cancer.
- **Retained oral contrast in hypopharynx.** Oral contrast, frequently given for a CT abdomen and pelvis examination that is obtained concurrently with a CT neck, may be retained in the oral cavity and can be difficult to differentiate from an enhancing pharyngeal tumor. When in doubt, direct inspection or a follow-up CT neck study without oral contrast may be necessary.

Coapted pyriform sinus

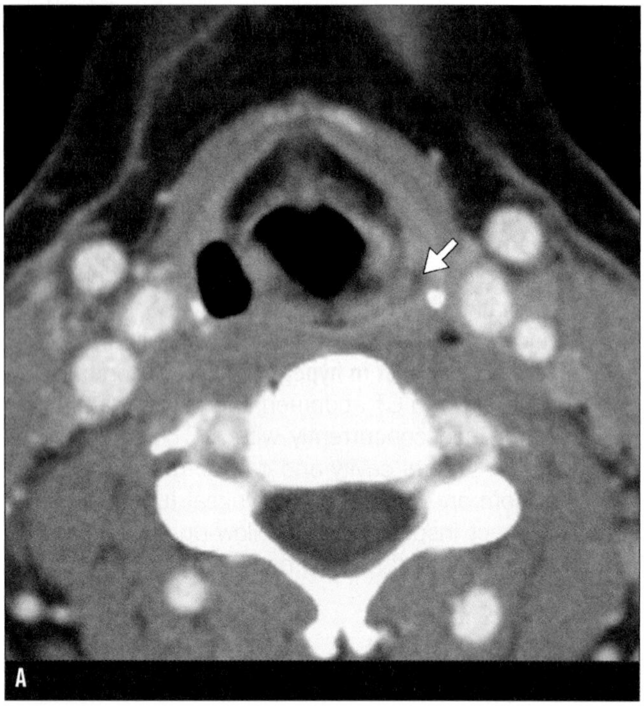

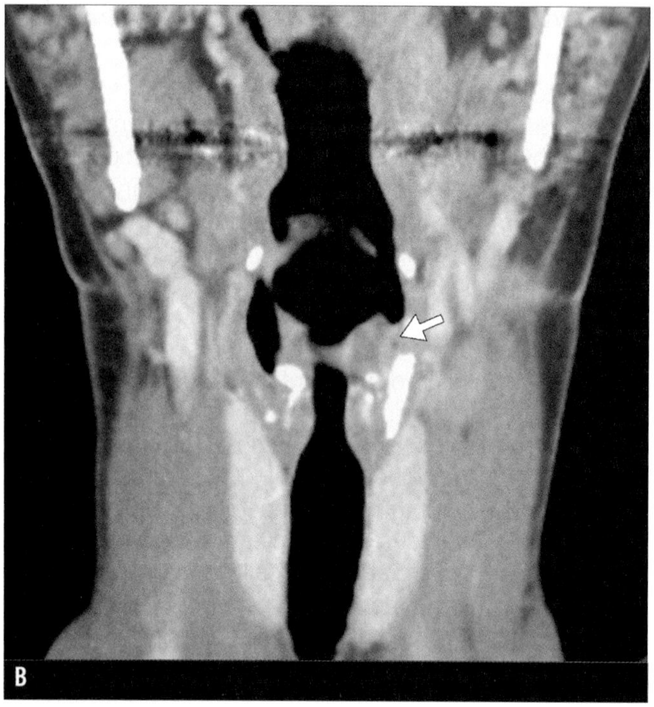

Different patient. An axial postcontrast CT image through the pyriform sinuses (**A**) demonstrates coaptation of the left pyriform sinus (arrow, **A**) with preservation of the submucosal fat and lack of mass effect. While there is enhancement of the hypopharyngeal mucosa, it is mild, smooth, and nonfocal, suggesting benignity, as was the case in this patient. A coronal reformatted postcontrast CT image through the level of the pyriform sinuses (**B**) also demonstrates coaptation of the left pyriform sinus (arrow, **B**).

Companion case: Pyriform sinus squamous cell carcinoma

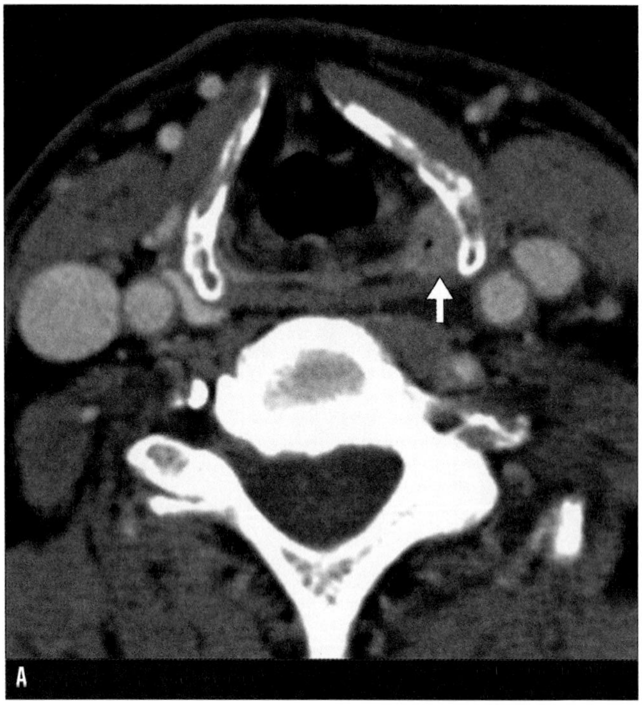

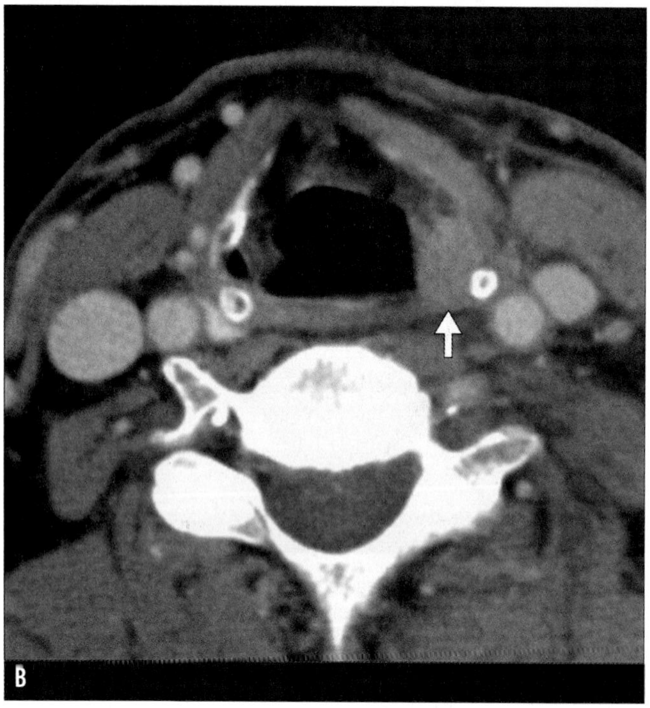

Axial postcontrast CT images through the pyriform sinuses (**A**, **B**) demonstrate asymmetric enhancement and mass effect within the left pyriform sinus, consistent with pyriform sinus carcinoma (arrows, **A**, **B**). The appearance of this finding can be differentiated from incidental coaptation of the pyriform sinuses by the greater degree of focal enhancement and the loss of the normal submucosal fat in this region. A postcontrast axial CT image through the level II nodal station (**C**) demonstrates extensive lymphadenopathy with extracapsular spread, strongly suggesting a malignant process (arrow, **C**).

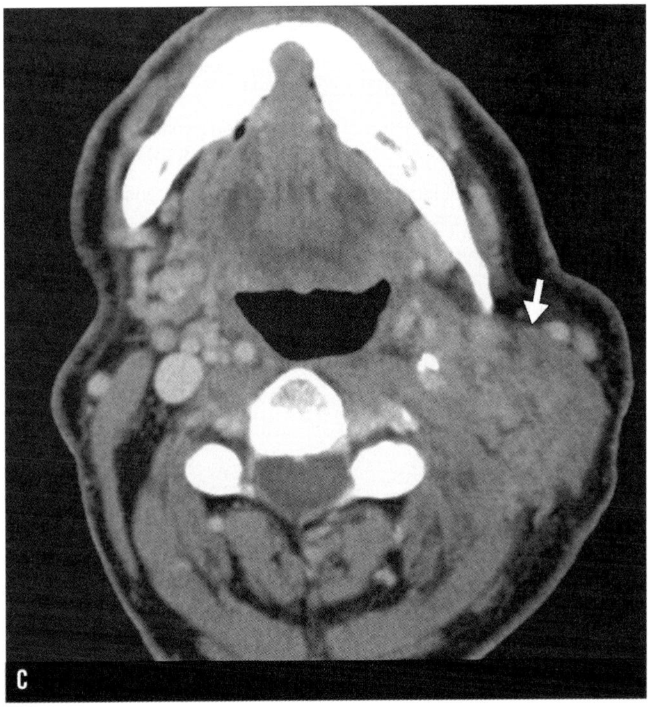

Companion case: Retained oral contrast in the hypopharynx

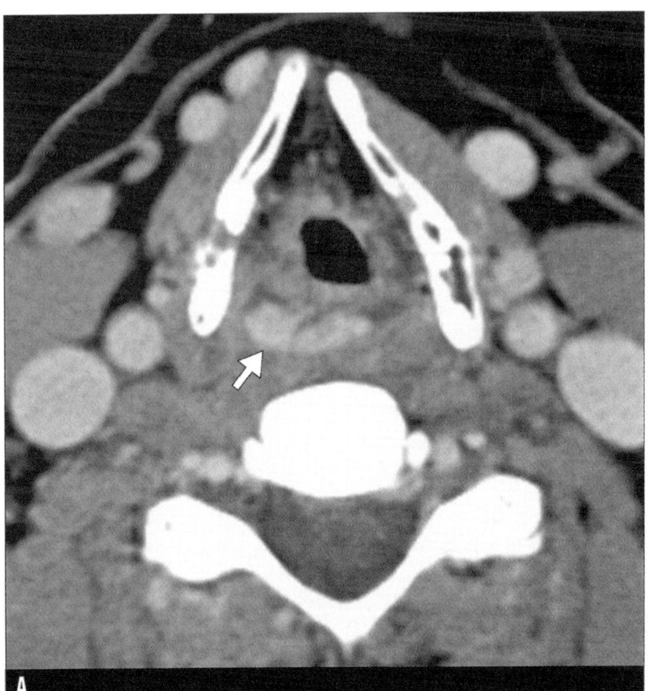

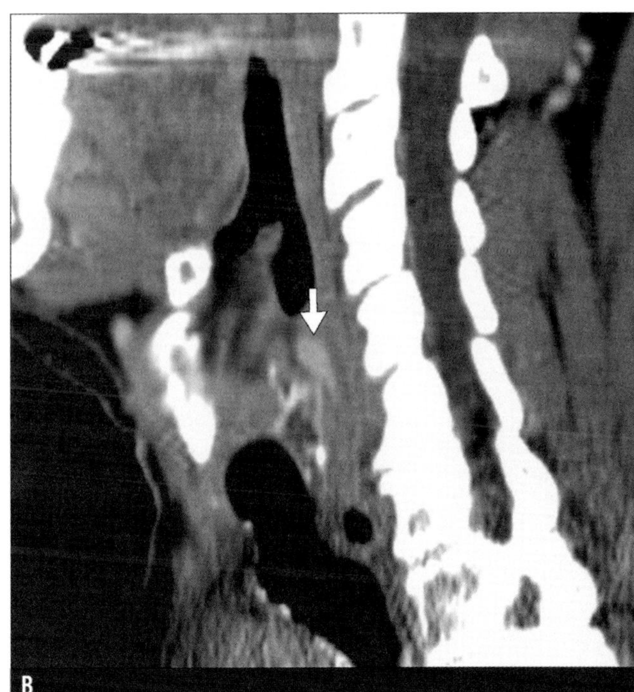

Contrast-enhanced axial (**A**) and sagittal reformatted (**B**) CT images demonstrate focal increased attenuation within the inferior aspect of the right piriform sinus (arrows, **A**, **B**). A contrast-enhanced axial CT image at the same level as image **A** obtained 2 months later (**C**) demonstrates complete resolution of the finding. The finding on images **A** and **B** was related to retained oral contrast that was given for a CT abdomen and pelvis examination which was obtained concurrently with the CT neck study.

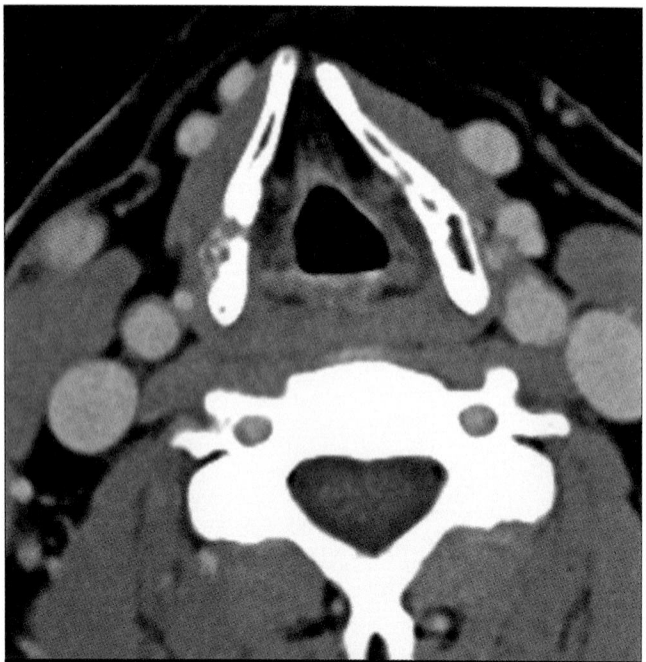

C

REFERENCES

Blot WJ et al. Smoking and drinking in relation to oral and pharyngeal cancer. *Cancer Res.* 1988;48(11):3282-3287.

Gamsu G et al. Ct in carcinoma of the larynx and pyriform sinus: value of phonation scans. *AJR Am J Roentgenol.* 1981;136(3):577-584

Hermans R. Staging of laryngeal and hypopharyngeal cancer: value of imaging studies. *Eur Radiol.* 2006;16(11):2386-2400.

Lell et al. Multiplanar functional imaging of the larynx and hypopharynx with multislice spiral CT. *Eur Radiol.* 2004;14(12):2198-2205.

Uzcudun AE et al. Clinical features of pharyngeal cancer: a retrospective study of 258 consecutive patients. *J Laryngol Otol.* 2001;115(2):112-118.

CASE 18 Postcricoid region of the hypopharynx

Tumors of the hypopharynx often grow in a submucosal fashion and are frequently advanced at presentation. Assessment of the adjacent fat and muscle planes of the hypopharynx, as well as the adjacent cartilage, is helpful in identifying these tumors. While complex, understanding the anatomy that comprises this region is vital to interpreting the hypopharynx on imaging.

The hypopharynx extends from the level of the hyoid bone to the cricopharyngeus sphincter (esophageal verge). Three regions comprise the hypopharynx: the pyriform (or piriform) sinuses, the postcricoid region, and the posterior hypopharyngeal wall. The pyriform sinus is a paired structure that is located superolaterally within the hypopharynx. Each pyriform sinus has the shape of an inverted pyramid, with its apex directed caudally. The aryepiglottic folds are an important anatomic landmark in this region, serving to subdivide the posteriorly located pyriform sinuses from the anteriorly located supraglottic larynx. Furthermore, the ventral wall of the aryepiglottic fold is considered a portion of the supraglottic larynx, whereas the posterior wall of the aryepiglottic fold is considered a portion of the pyriform sinus.

The postcricoid region represents the anterior wall of the hypopharynx. In the craniocaudal direction, the postcricoid region extends from the posterior aspect of the arytenoid cartilage to the cricopharyngeus sphincter. This craniocaudal length differs from the posterior hypopharyngeal wall, which extends more cephalad, namely from the oropharynx to the cricopharyngeus sphincter.

The anterior muscular layer of the postcricoid region hypopharynx is formed by the posterior cricoarytenoid muscles, which reside along the posterior margin of the cricoid and arytenoid cartilages. The posterior muscular layer of the hypopharynx is formed by the middle and inferior constrictor muscles. Thus, the layers of the hypopharynx on imaging from anterior to posterior at the level of the cricoid are as follows: the posterior cricoarytenoid muscles, submucosal fat, a stripe of soft tissue density (that sometimes enhances) representing coapted walls of the hypopharyngeal mucosa, additional submucosal fat, and the posterior hypopharyngeal muscular wall. The fat posterior to this posterior hypopharyngeal muscular wall represents the retropharyngeal fat.

The normal postcricoid portion of the hypopharynx is almost always collapsed during imaging. However, there are imaging criteria that aid in evaluating this region. The AP dimension of the postcricoid portion of the hypopharynx is fairly constant in size and should not measure greater than 10 mm. In addition, the postcricoid portion of the hypopharynx normally tapers as it descends toward the esophagus. While not always visible, identifying the normal muscles and intramural fat planes of the postcricoid region on axial imaging is also very helpful in determining whether pathology is present. These normal muscles and intramural fat planes are more likely to be identified on axial CT imaging rather than on axial MR imaging.

COMPANION CASE

- **Postcricoid region squamous cell carcinoma.**
- **Impacted date seed at the cricopharyngeus muscle.** Most esophageal foreign bodies in children become impacted at the cricopharyngeus muscle, whereas most esophageal foreign bodies in adults become impacted at the lower esophageal sphincter. The majority of foreign bodies will pass through the digestive system. However, if left untreated, a persistently lodged esophageal foreign body can be life threatening and result in esophageal perforation, fistulization, and empyema formation. The treatment for choice for a persistently lodged esophageal foreign body is endoscopic retrieval.

Postcricoid region of the hypopharynx

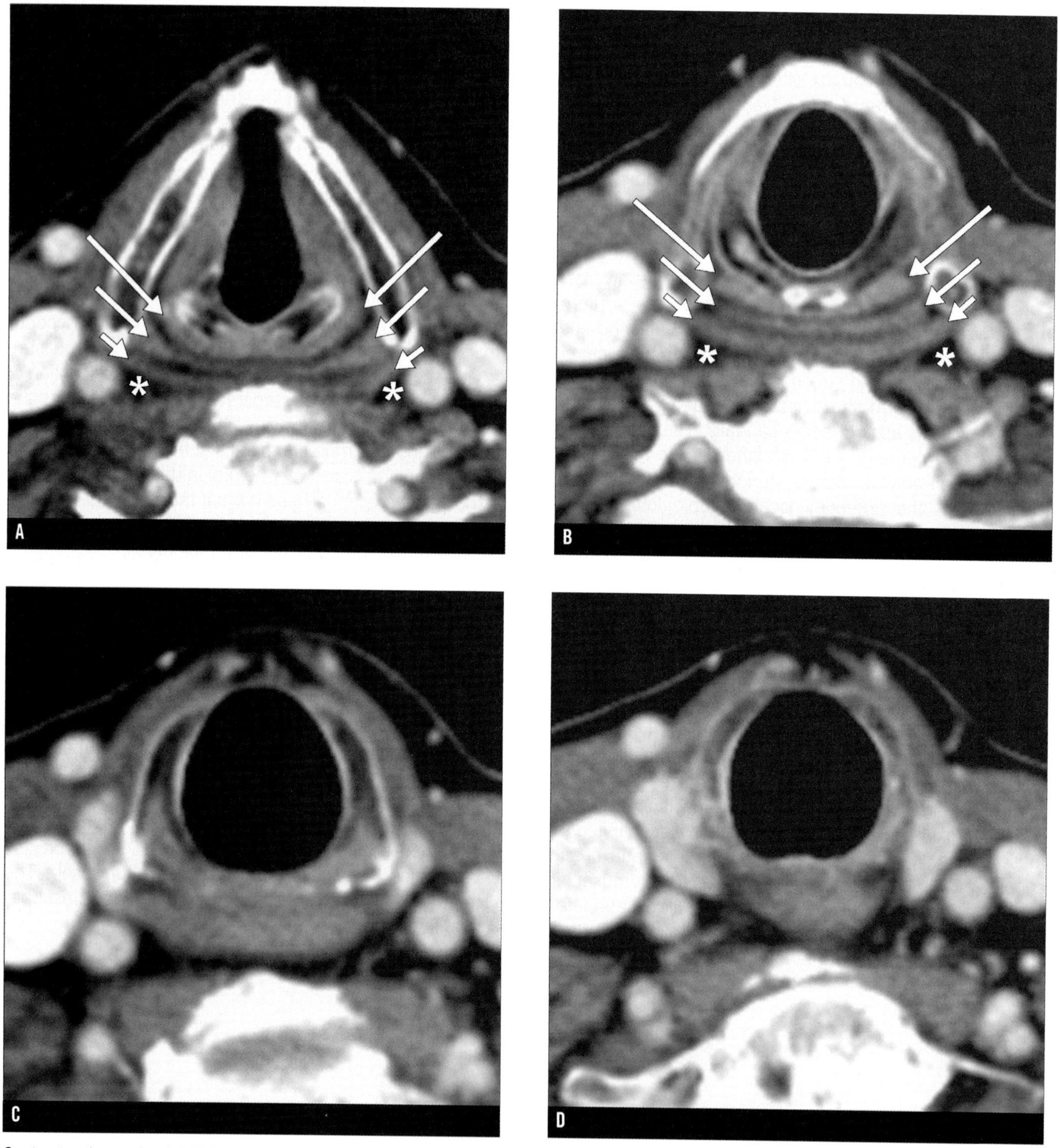

Contrast-enhanced axial (**A-D**) and sagittal reformatted (**E**) CT images through the postcricoid region demonstrate the normal hypopharyngeal anatomy at this level. The postcricoid region represents the anterior wall of the hypopharynx and is formed by the posterior cricoarytenoid muscles (long arrows, **A**, **B**, **E**). The normal collapsed mucosal surfaces of the hypopharynx are demarcated by the medium arrows (**A**, **B**, **E**). The posterior hypopharyngeal wall is demarcated by the short arrows (**A**, **B**, **E**). Interposed between the posterior cricoarytenoid muscle, apposed mucosa, and posterior hypopharyngeal wall are thin strips of fat, representing the submucosal fat layers. The retropharyngeal fat pad is also identified (asterisks, **A**, **B**). More caudal, the hypopharynx tapers in the transverse dimension as it approaches the cricopharyngeus sphincter and esophageal verge (**C**, **D**).

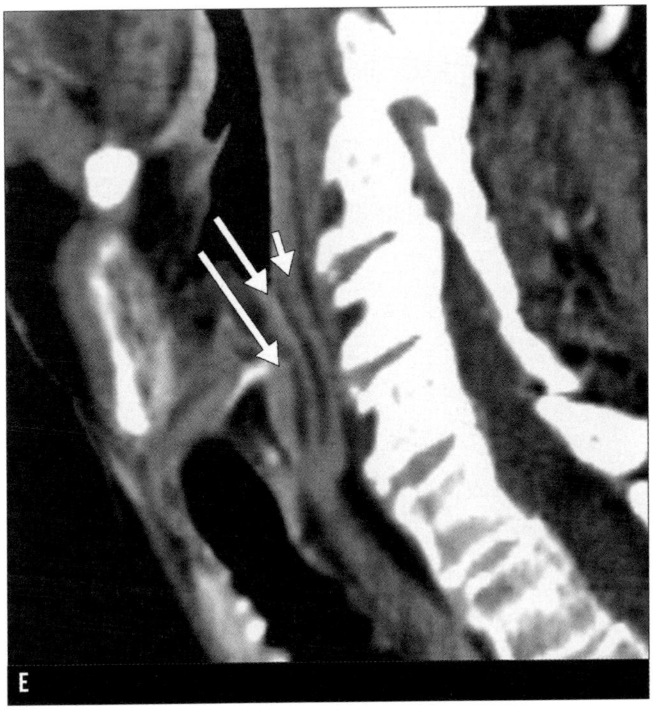

Companion case: Postcricoid region squamous cell carcinoma

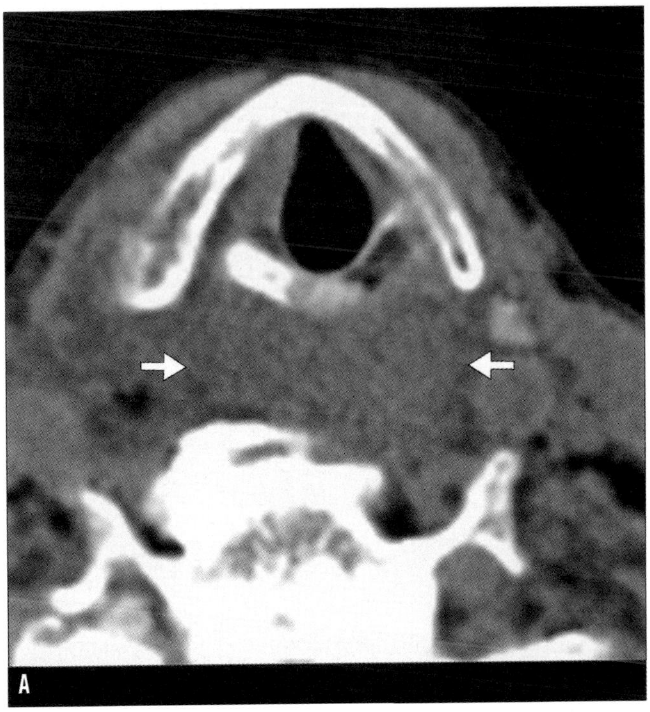

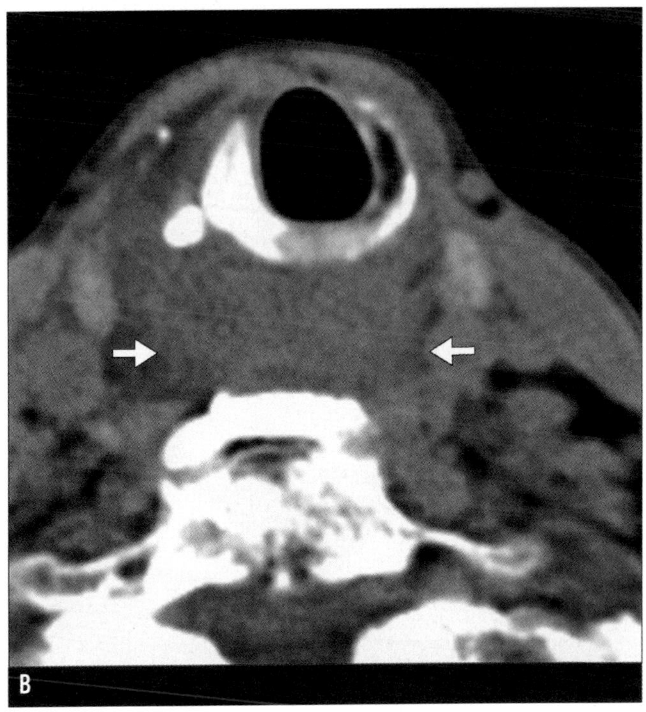

Contrast-enhanced axial (**A**, **B**) and sagittal reformatted (**C**) CT images through the postcricoid region of the hypopharynx demonstrate abnormal anterior-posterior thickening of this region (arrows, **A-C**), much larger than 1 cm or less that is present in normal patients. The muscle and fat planes are also grossly absent. An axial CT image viewed with a bone window (**D**) demonstrates overt sclerosis of right aspect of the cricoid cartilage (arrow, **D**), suggesting tumor infiltration, in this case related to squamous cell carcinoma.

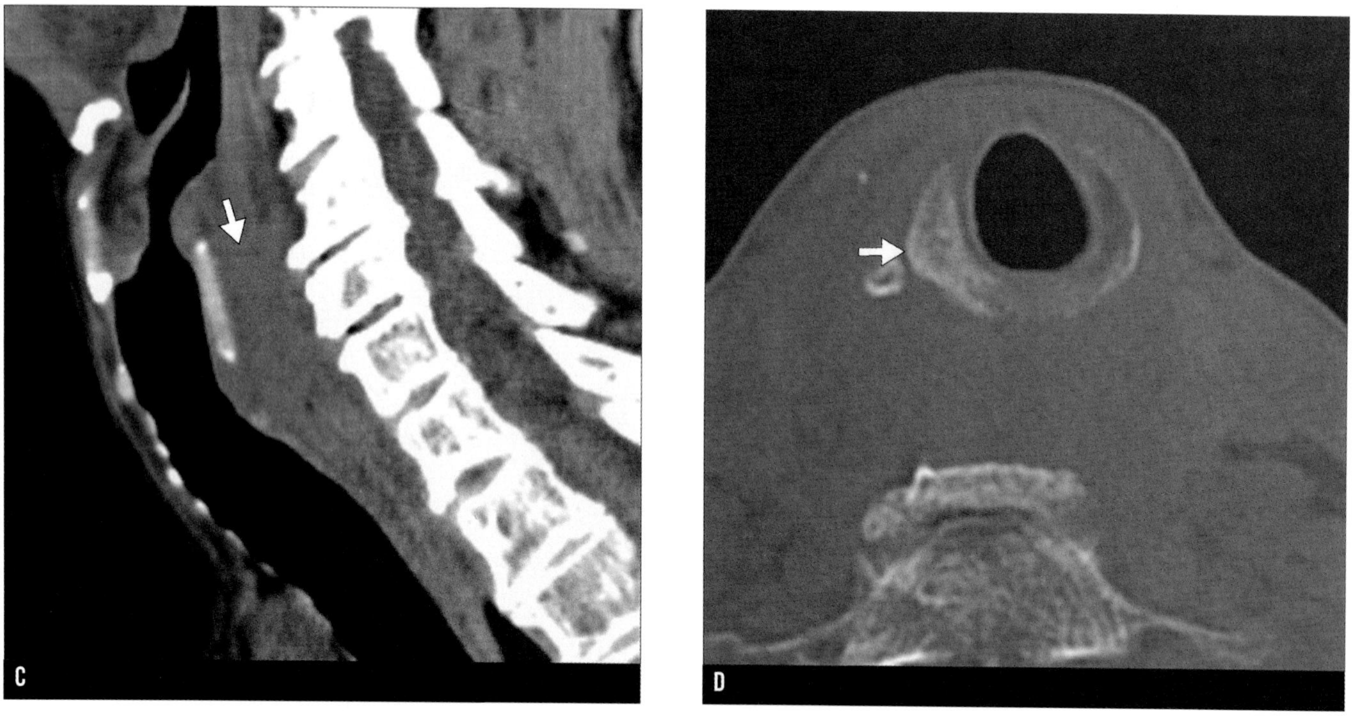

Companion case: Impacted date seed at the cricopharyngeus muscle

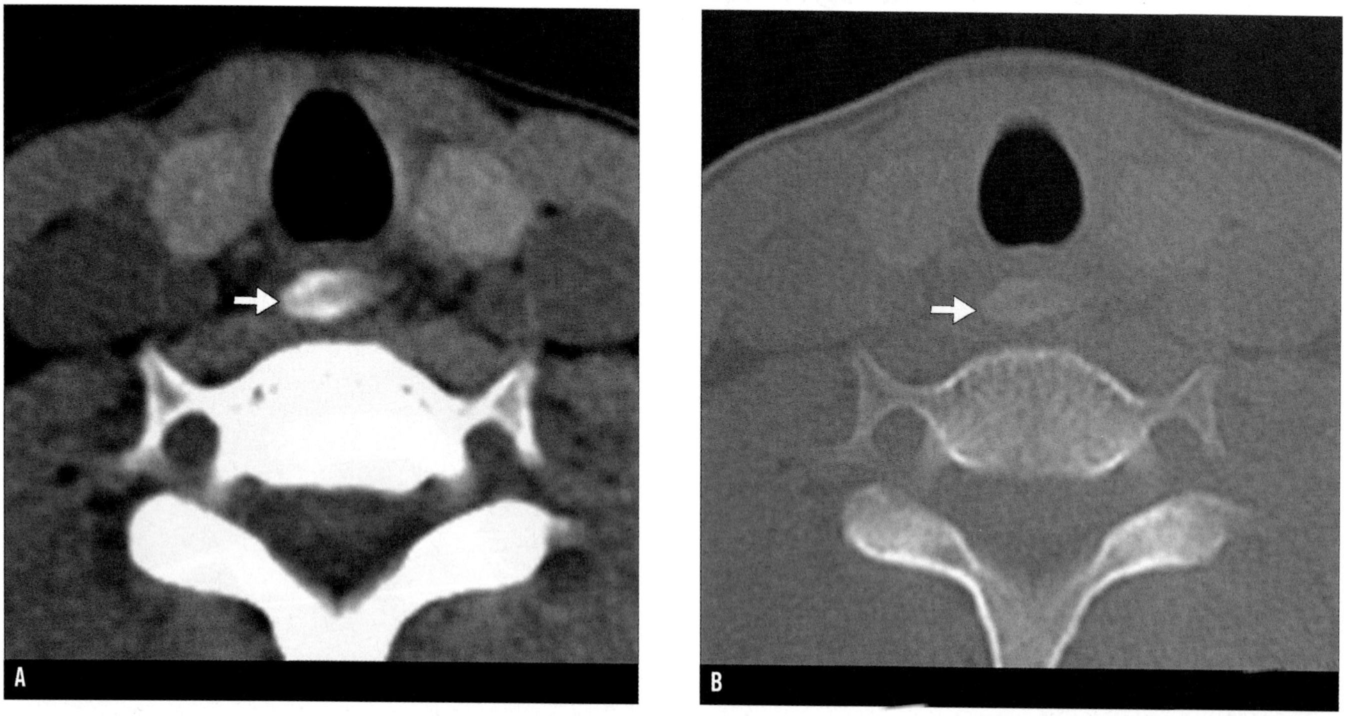

Unenhanced axial CT images viewed with a soft tissue window (**A**) and bone window (**B**) as well as coronal reformatted (**C**) and sagittal reformatted (**D**) CT images viewed with a soft tissue window demonstrate an elliptical, dense foreign body (arrows, **A-D**) that is obliquely oriented in the coronal plane (arrow, **C**) and located at the expected location of the cricopharyngeus muscle. This represented a date seed that was inadvertently swallowed in a 31-year-old patient. While most esophageal foreign bodies in adults become lodged at the lower esophageal sphincter, this foreign body likely lodged at the cricopharyngeus sphincter due to its large size. This was successfully removed via endoscopy.

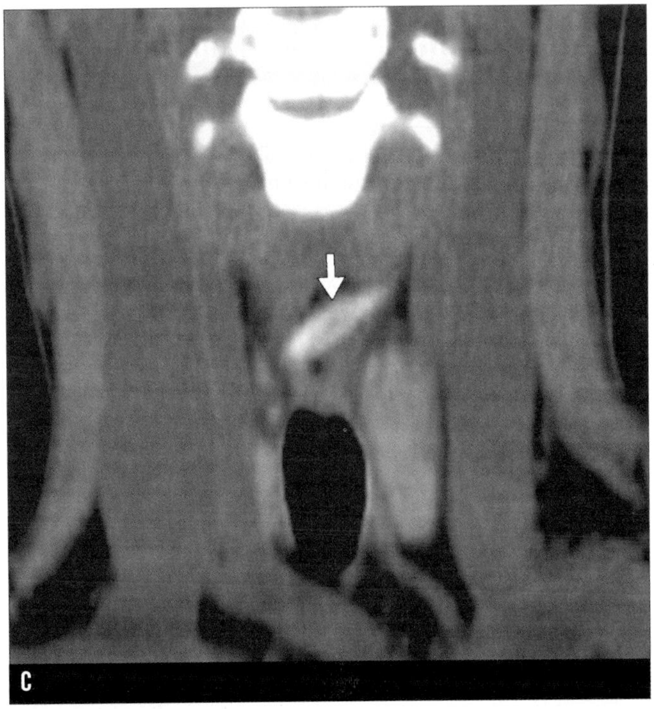

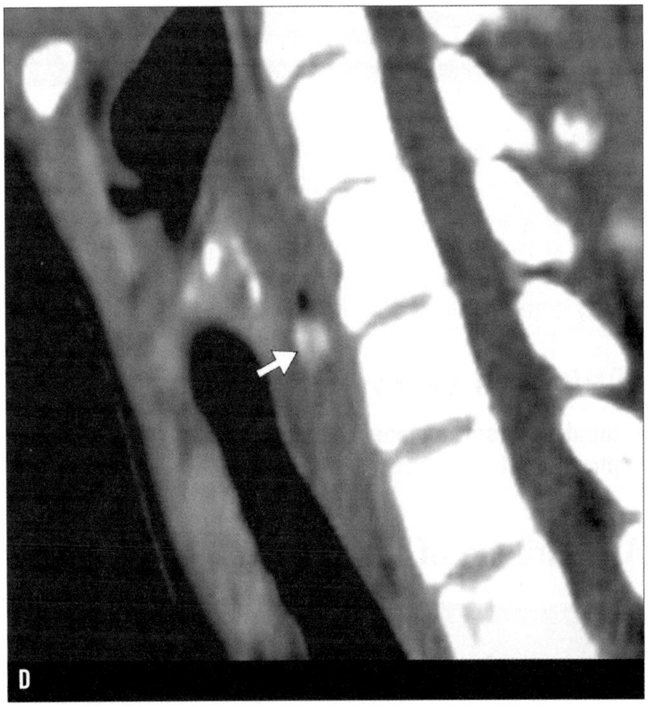

REFERENCES

Al-Qudah A, Daradkeh S, Abu-Khalaf M. Esophageal foreign bodies. *Eur J Cardiothorac Surg*. May 1998;13(5):494-498.

Hermans R (ed). Head and Neck Cancer Imaging, Medical Radiology. Diagnostic Imaging, DOI: 10.1007/174_2011_370, Springer-Verlag Berlin Heidelberg; 2012.

Schmalfuss IM, Mancuso AA, Tart RP. Postcricoid region and cervical esophagus: normal appearance at CT and MR imaging. *Radiology*. January 2000;214(1):237-246.

CASE 19 Appearance of the pharynx during breath-hold or swallowing

A CT examination performed while the patient is holding their breath or while in the act of swallowing can have a profound effect on the imaging appearance of the pharynx. The pharyngeal airway can significantly narrow during these actions, sometimes simulating a mass or spurious airway compromise.

COMPANION CASES

- **Incidental soft palate abutment against the posterior pharyngeal wall**. Occasionally, the soft palate and uvula may abut the oropharyngeal walls on imaging. This is a normal and typically transitory finding.
- **Pharyngeal airway collapse related to an indwelling tracheostomy tube.** Frequently, an indwelling tracheostomy tube will result in partial or complete collapse of the pharyngeal lumen. This pharyngeal collapse essentially precludes an accurate assessment of the pharynx.
- **Large tumor compromising the pharyngeal airway.**

Appearance of the pharynx during breath-hold

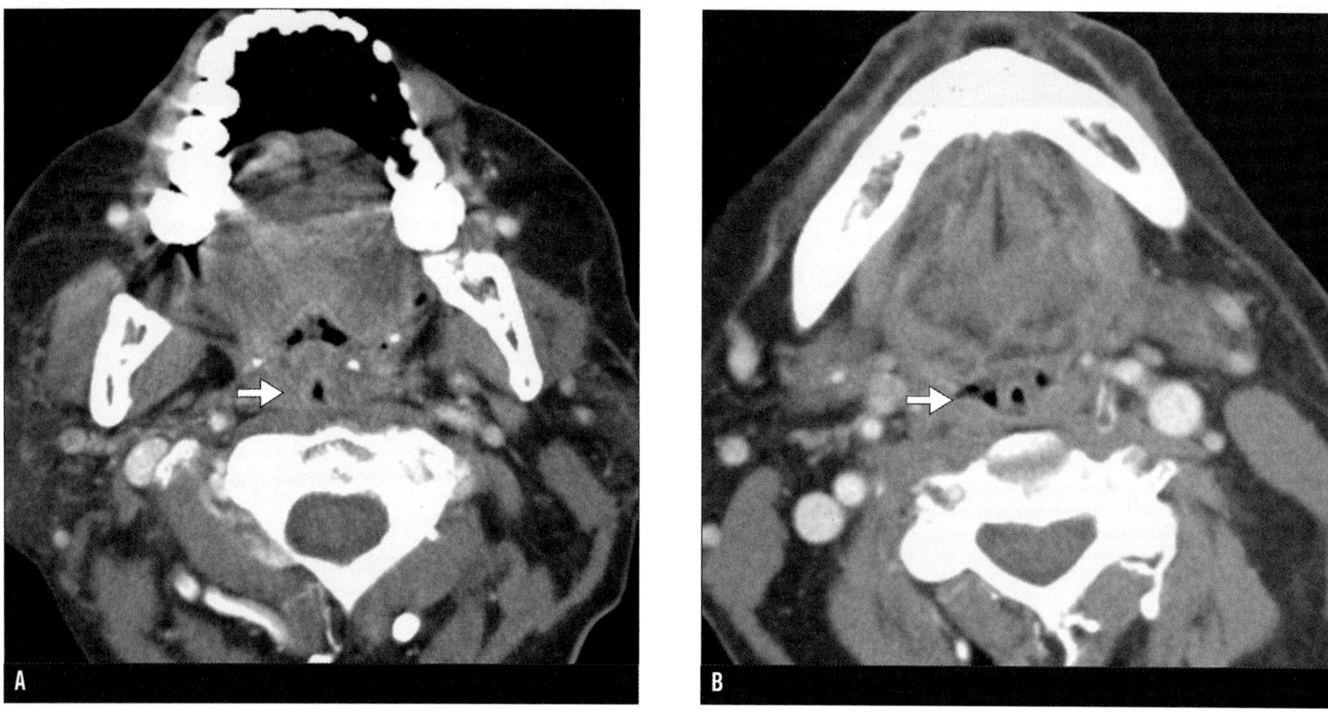

Postcontrast axial CT images through the upper oropharynx (**A**) and level of the epiglottis (**B**) demonstrate marked attenuation of the pharyngeal airway (arrows, **A, B**). Axial (**C**) and coronal reformatted (**D**) postcontrast CT images through the level of the true vocal cords demonstrate apposition of the true vocal cords, compatible with the patient's breath-hold during the scan (arrows, **C, D**). Delayed postcontrast axial imaging obtained through the oropharynx (**E**), epiglottis (**F**), and the aryepiglottic folds (**G**) approximately 2 minutes after images **A-D** were obtained demonstrate a normal pharyngeal airway, due to the cessation of the patient's breath-hold.

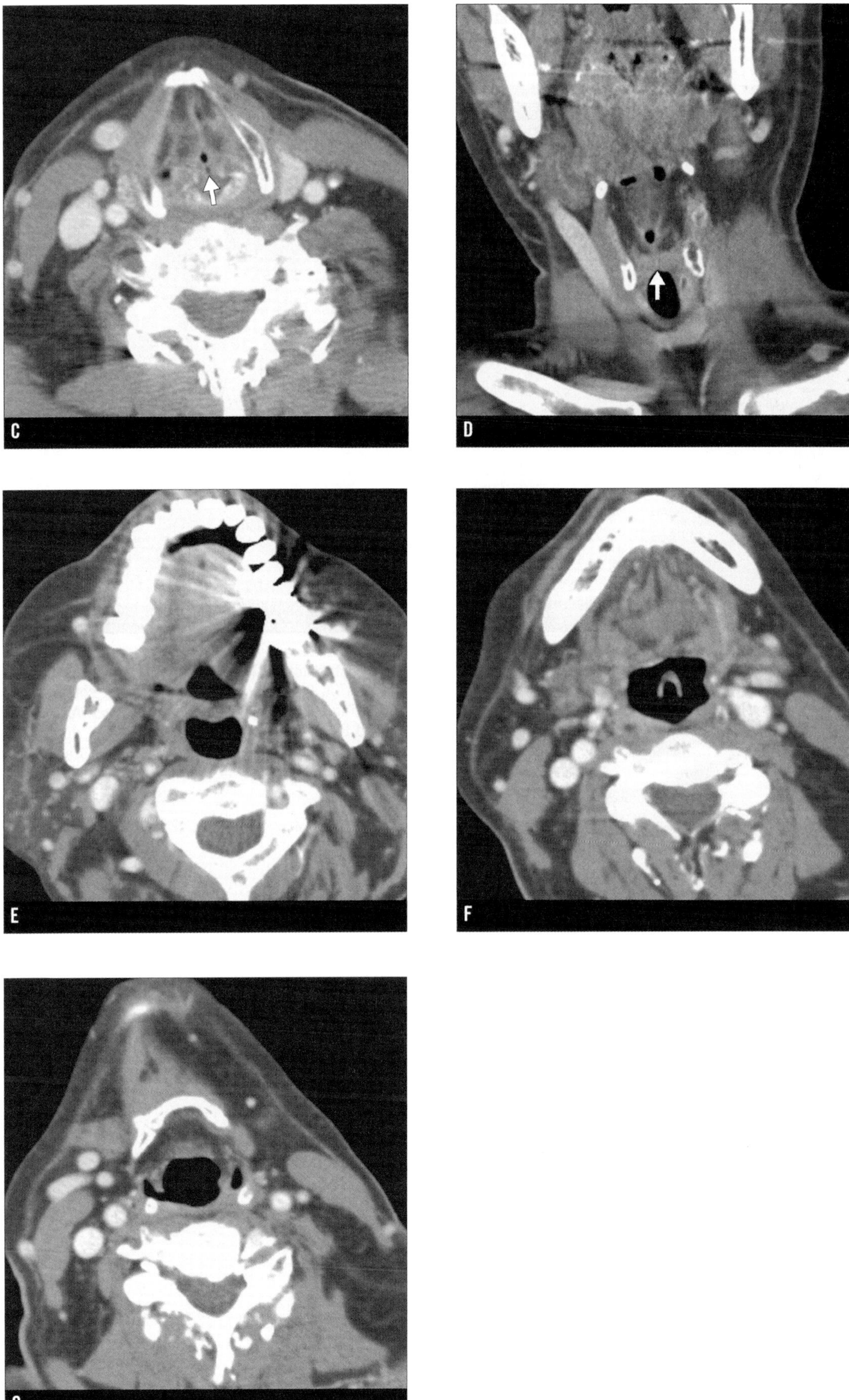
C
D
E
F
G

Companion case: Incidental soft palate abutment against the posterior pharyngeal wall

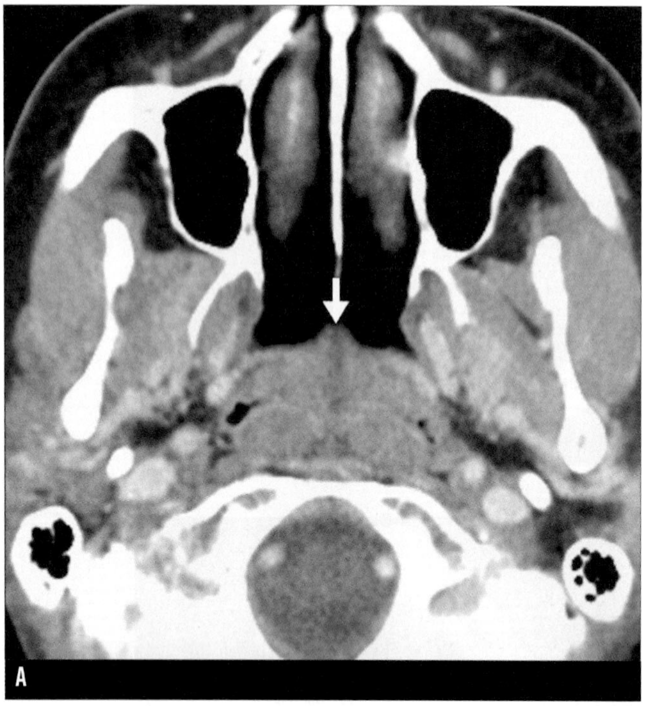

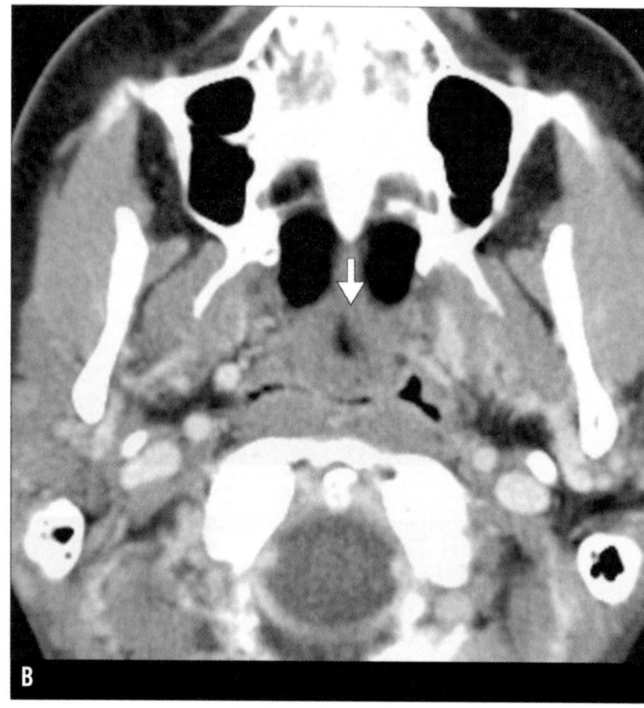

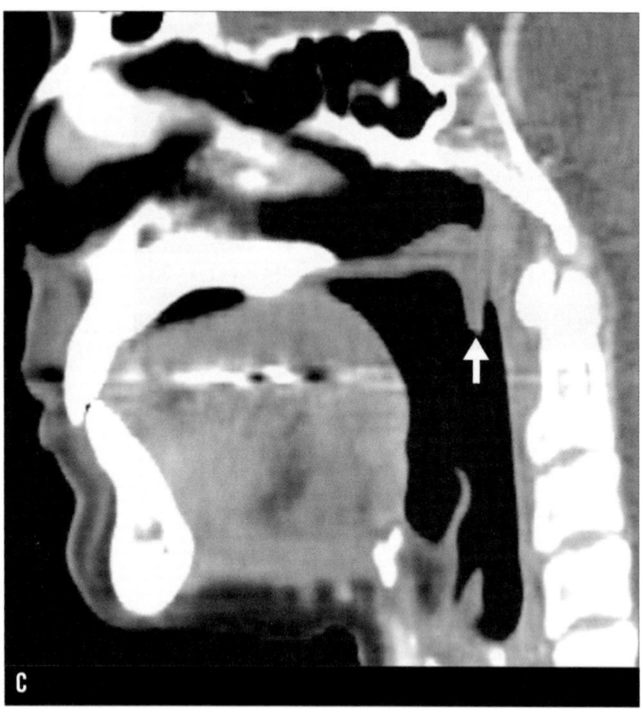

Axial postcontrast CT images through the nasopharynx–oropharynx junction (**A, B**) demonstrate an apparent soft tissue abnormally occupying the airway at this level (arrows, **A**, **B**). A sagittal reformatted CT image from the same study (**C**) demonstrates that the soft tissue merely represents abutment of the soft palate with the posterior pharyngeal wall (arrow, **C**).

Companion case: Pharyngeal airway collapse related to an indwelling tracheostomy tube

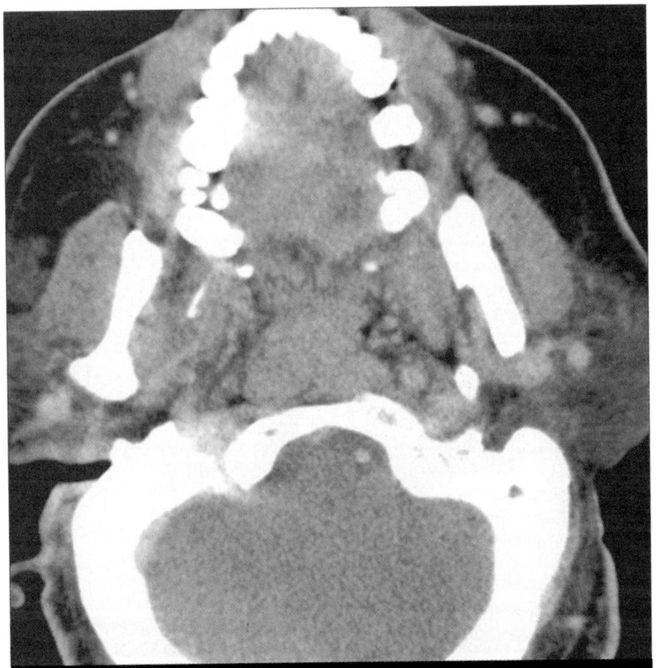

A

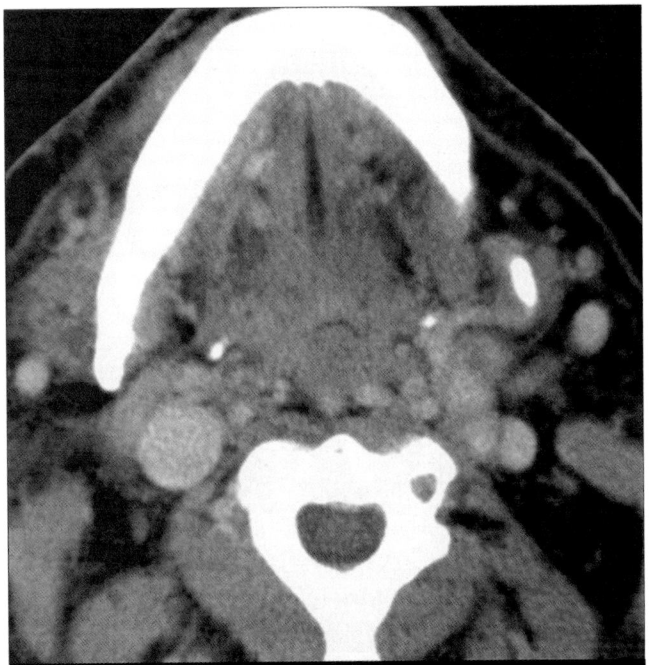

B

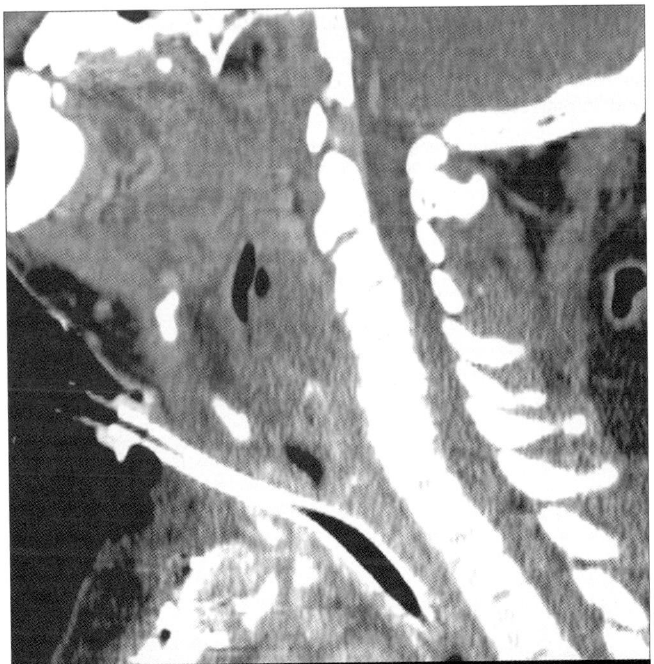

C

A contrast-enhanced axial CT image through the junction of the nasopharynx and oropharynx (**A**), a contrast-enhanced axial CT image through the oropharynx (**B**), and a contrast-enhanced sagittal reformatted CT image (**C**) demonstrate a large amount of soft tissue density occupying the upper pharynx, simulating the presence of a mass. However, this patient did not have a mass and the finding was simply related to pharyngeal collapse because of an indwelling tracheostomy tube demonstrated on image **C**. Nevertheless, the presence of a collapsed airway essentially precludes an accurate imaging assessment of the pharynx.

Companion case: Large tumor compromising the pharyngeal airway

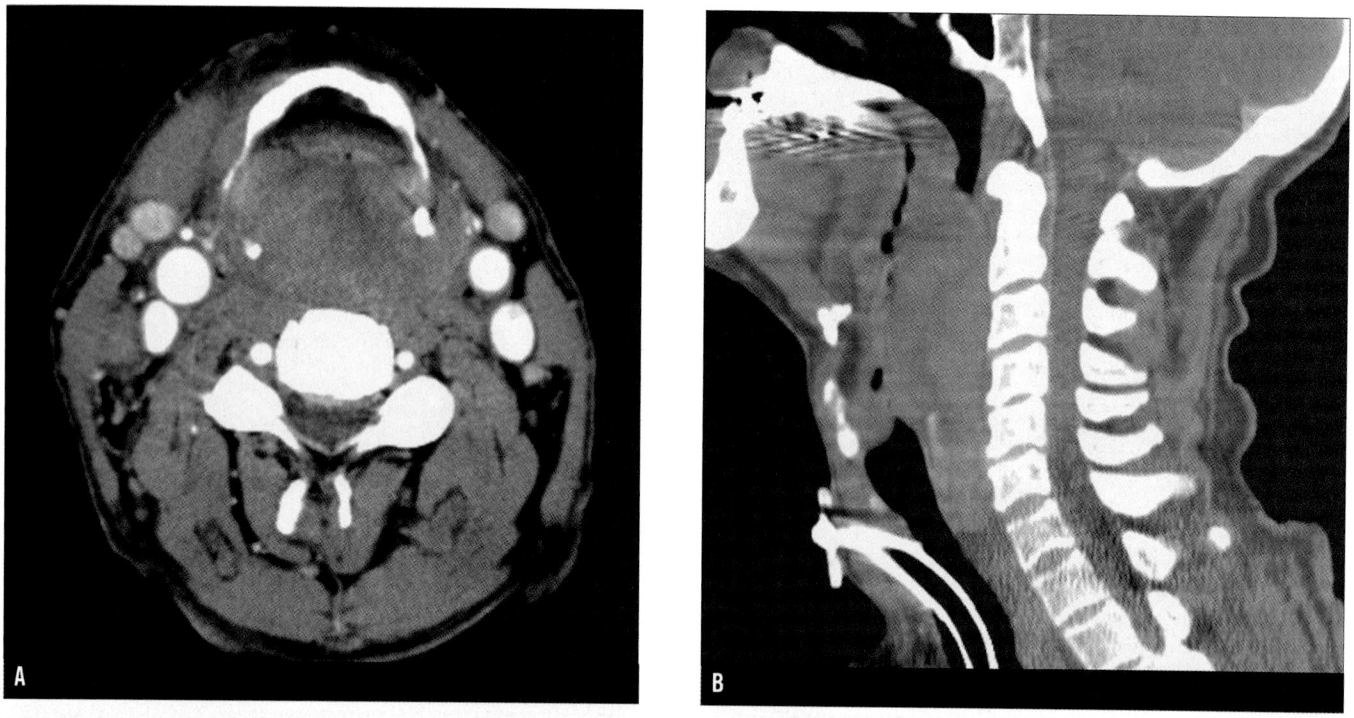

Contrast-enhanced axial (**A**) and sagittal reformatted (**B**) CT images demonstrate near-complete effacement of the oropharyngeal and hypopharyngeal airway due to a large tumor, in this case a squamous cell carcinoma. A tracheostomy tube is noted to be in place, which may also contribute to the pharyngeal airway narrowing. However, this case illustrates the difficulty in differentiating between incidental pharyngeal effacement because of an indwelling tracheostomy tube and pharyngeal effacement because of a tumor.

REFERENCES

Lell MM et al. Multiplanar functional imaging of the larynx and hypopharynx with multislice spiral CT. *Eur Radiol.* December 2004;14(2):2198-2205.

Massey EW. Spinal accessory nerve lesions. *Semin Neurol.* 2009;29(1):82-84.

Suojanen JN et al. Spiral CT in evaluation of head and neck lesions: work in progress. *Radiology.* 1992;183:281-283.

Wear et al. Evaluating "eee" phonation in multidetector CT of the larynx. *AJNR Am J Neuroradiol.* 2009;30(6):1102.

CASE 20 Denervation atrophy of the pharyngeal wall

Denervation atrophy of the pharyngeal wall can occur from a variety of causes. One such cause is a tumor at the skull base affecting the cranial nerve (CN) IX, CN X, and the cranial division of CN XI, all of which contribute to the pharyngeal nervous plexus. When present, other denervated muscles will also frequently be identified, including the thyroarytenoid muscle of the true vocal cord and posterior cricoarytenoid muscles (both innervated by the recurrent laryngeal nerve which originates from CN X), as well as the sternocleidomastoid and trapezius muscles (both innervated by CN XI).

Denervation atrophy of the pharyngeal wall

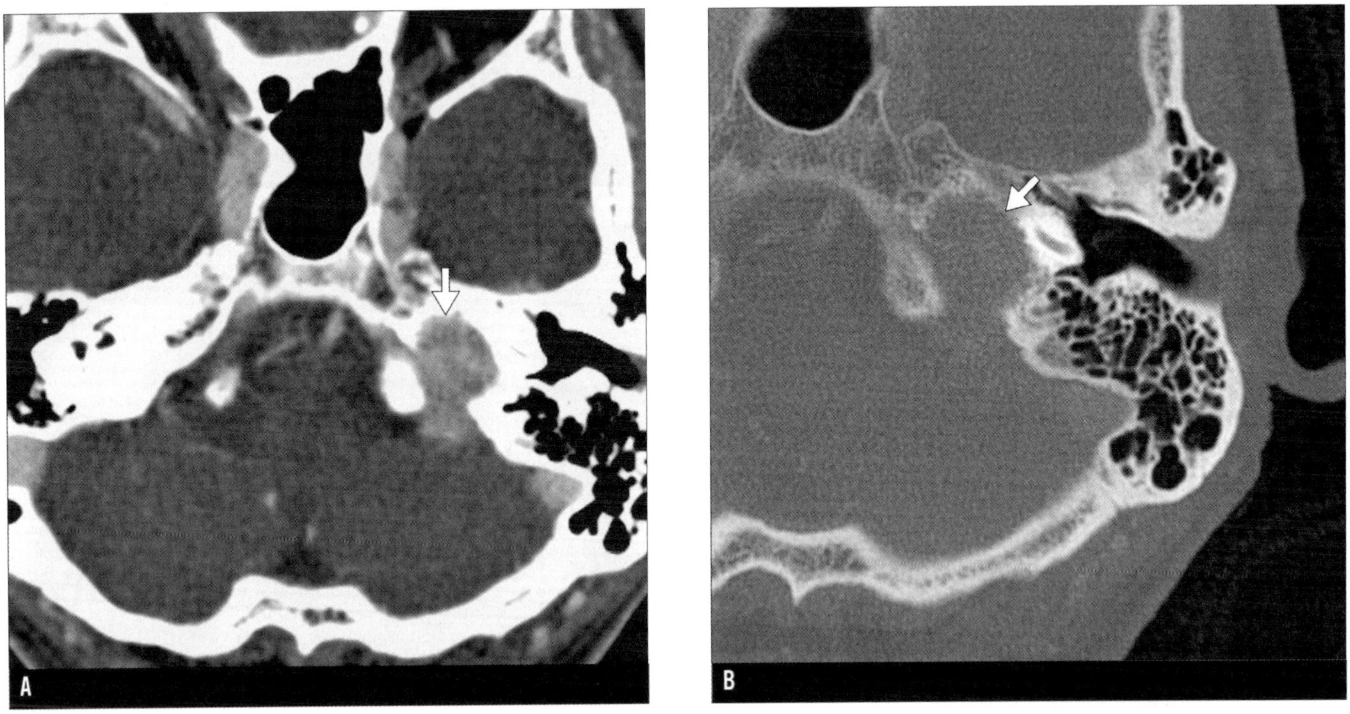

An axial CT image viewed with a soft tissue window (**A**) and bone window (**B**) through the jugular foramen demonstrates an enhancing mass in the left jugular foramen (arrow, **A**) associated with iregular osseous erosion of the left jugular foramen walls (arrow, **B**). Precontrast axial T1 (**C**) and fat-suppressed postcontrast axial T1 (**D**) MR images of the same patient demonstrate an irregular enhancing mass in the left jugular foramen with a "salt and pepper" enhancement pattern (arrows, **C, D**). The findings from the CT and MRI studies are compatible with a left glomus jugulare tumor. An axial postcontrast CT image (**E**) and an axial T2-weighted MR image (**F**) of the same patient demonstrate subtle denervation atrophy of the left pharyngeal wall constrictor muscles (arrows, **E, F**). This is a sequela of a left pharyngeal plexus injury (which is comprised of CN IX and X fibers) by the glomus jugulare tumor. When a jugular foramen mass is present, one should evaluate for denervation atrophy of all the muscles innervated by CN IX through CN XI, as some or all of these nerves may be involved by a tumor located in jugular foramen.

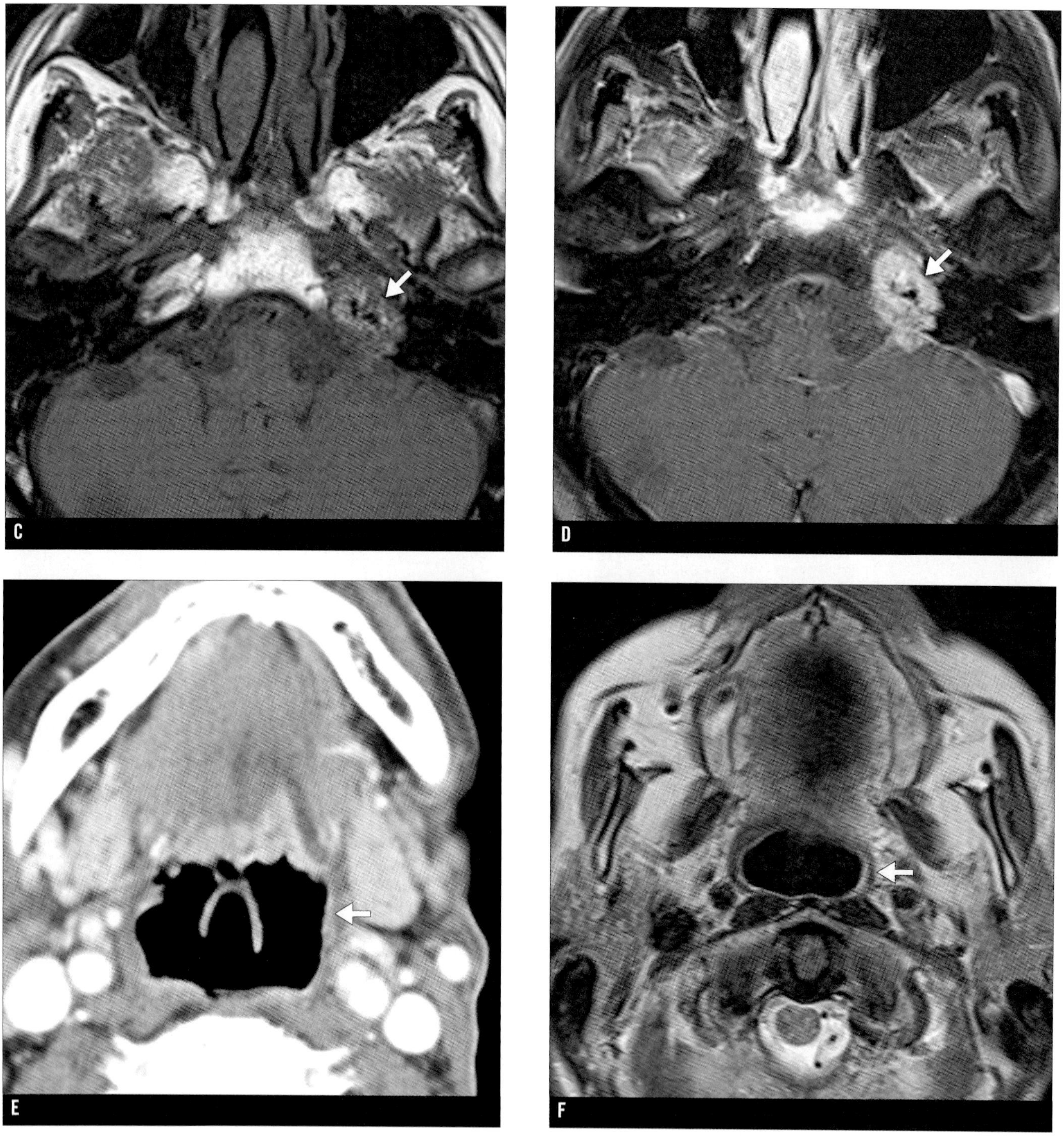

REFERENCE

Hayden MG et al. Cerebellopontine angle cyst compressing the vagus nerve: case report. *Neurosurgery*. June 2007;60(6):E1150

CHAPTER 2

LARYNX, HYOID, AND TRACHEA

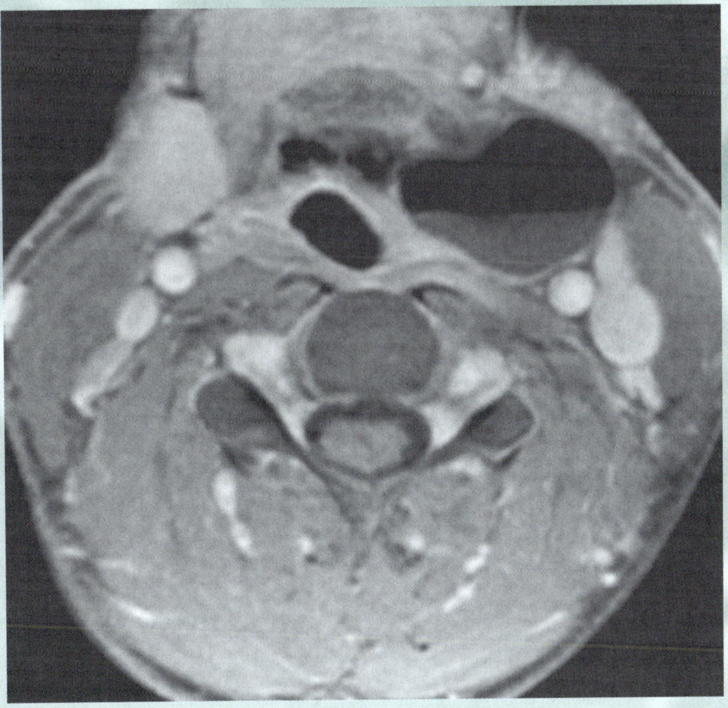

Christopher J. Therasse, Achilles G. Karagianis, Benjamin P. Liu

II. LARYNX, HYOID, AND TRACHEA

1. Variations of hyoid fusion
   i. *Companion case*: Hyoid body fracture
   ii. *Companion case*: Hyoid motion artifact due to swallowing
2. Thyrohyoid fusion anomalies
   Companion case: Mineralization of the triticeal cartilage
3. Variations of thyroid cartilage mineralization
   i. *Companion case*: Retained fish bone
   ii. *Companion case*: Multiple myeloma involving the thyroid cartilage
   iii. *Companion case*: Squamous cell carcinoma invading thyroid cartilage
   iv. *Companion case*: Radiation-induced chondronecrosis of the thyroid lamina
4. Thyroid cartilage pseudofracture
   i. *Companion case*: Acute thyroid cartilage fracture
   ii. *Companion case*: Thyroid cartilage fracture with healing
   iii. *Companion case*: Incidental focal angulation of thyroid lamina superior cornu
5. Variations of cricoid cartilage mineralization
   i. *Companion case*: Retained fish bone
   ii. *Companion case*: Cricoid cartilage chondrosarcoma
   iii. *Companion case*: Cricoid cartilage sclerosis due to squamous cell carcinoma invasion
   iv. *Companion case*: Radiation-induced chondronecrosis of the cricoid cartilage
6. Variations of arytenoid cartilage mineralization
   i. *Companion case*: Arytenoid cartilage sclerosis due to squamous cell carcinoma invasion
7. Mineralized epiglottis
   i. *Companion case*: Residual barium contrast layering along the epiglottis
8. Radiation-induced epiglottic edema
   i. *Companion case*: Acute epiglottitis
   ii. *Companion case*: Epiglottic squamous cell carcinoma
9. Thickened thyrohyoid membrane and median thyrohyoid ligament
   i. *Companion case*: Thyroglossal duct cyst
   ii. *Companion case*: Ectopic thyroid
10. Variations of the laryngeal ventricle
    i. *Companion case*: Abnormal enlargement of laryngeal ventricle due to true vocal cord paralysis
    ii. *Companion case*: Endotracheal tube cuff in supraglottic larynx
    iii. *Companion case*: Squamous cell carcinoma infiltrating the laryngeal ventricle
11. Laryngeal appendix
    i. *Companion case*: Air-filled internal laryngoceles
    ii. *Companion case*: Small fluid-filled laryngeal appendices/laryngoceles
    iii. *Companion case*: Large fluid-filled internal laryngocele
    iv. *Companion case:* Large fluid-filled internal and external laryngocele
    v. *Companion case*: Submucosal tumor invasion into paraglottic fat
12. Laryngeal apparatus rotation or slice selection resulting in an apparent true vocal cord abnormality
    i. *Companion case*: True vocal cord asymmetry due to denervation atrophy
    ii. *Companion case*: True vocal cord polyp
    iii. *Companion case*: True vocal cord squamous cell carcinoma
13. Closed glottis due to breath-hold
    i. *Companion case*: Closed glottis due to an indwelling tracheostomy tube
    ii. *Companion case*: Transglottic tumor
14. Characteristic findings of true vocal cord paralysis
    i. *Companion case*: Laryngeal tumor simulating true vocal cord paralysis
15. Injection laryngoplasty
    i. *Companion case*: Subglottic extrusion of Radiesse with calcium hydroxylapatite injectate
16. Medialization thyroplasty
17. MRI chemical shift artifact in the subglottic larynx simulating abnormal soft tissue
    i. *Companion case*: Subglottic granulation tissue
    ii. *Companion case*: Subglottic tumor extension
18. Posttreatment appearance of the larynx following radiation therapy
    i. *Companion case*: Posttreated larynx with recurrent tumor
    ii. *Companion case*: Posttreated larynx with superimposed tumor
19. Laryngectomies
    i. *Companion case*: Radiation necrosis and fistulization of a supraglottic laryngectomy
    ii. *Companion case*: Total laryngectomy with abscess formation 1 month following surgery
    iii. *Companion case*: Total laryngectomy with abscess resulting in a tracheo-pharyngo-cutaneous fistula
    iv. *Companion case*: Total laryngectomy with tumor recurrence
20. Tracheoesophageal puncture and prosthesis
    i. *Companion case*: Tracheal stoma closure with residual tracheal cartilage irregularity
    ii. *Companion case*: Granulation tissue and hemorrhage within the tracheostomy and subglottic airway
    iii. *Companion case*: Tracheal stoma recurrent tumor
21. Tracheal collapse during expiration
    i. *Companion case*: Thyroid carcinoma with tracheal wall invasion and luminal narrowing
22. Tracheal diverticulum
    i. *Companion case*: Apical lung herniation

CASE 1 Variations of hyoid fusion

The hyoid bone, situated in the anterior midline neck between the mandible and the larynx, is a horseshoe-shaped structure that serves to support the tongue and provides attachment sites to numerous muscles. The hyoid bone is an essential component in speaking and swallowing, and it is unique in that it does not articulate directly with any other bone but rather lies suspended in the mid neck by its ligamentous attachments.

Developed from cartilages of the second and third pharyngeal arches, the hyoid bone is composed of a central body and paired horn-like projections that are termed the greater and lesser cornua (also called greater and lesser horns, respectively). Ossification takes place both before and after birth via two centers in the body and one center in each cornu. The cornua are initially joined to the body via cartilaginous synchondroses and, in some patients, by osseous fusion later in life. The age at which this union occurs is highly variable. Moreover, there is considerable disparity in the frequency and extent of fusion among patients, resulting in several fusion variants such as unilateral fusion, bilateral fusion, and bilateral nonfusion.

COMPANION CASES

- **Hyoid body fracture.** The hyoid bone is relatively well protected from injury by virtue of its mobility as well as by surrounding soft tissue and osseous structures of the head and neck. Hyoid bone fractures account for only .002% of all fractures and are more common with increasing age, likely on the basis of more rigidity and decreased flexibility as the hyoid cartilage progressively ossifies. The majority of hyoid bone fractures are the result of direct trauma to the neck through manual strangulation, hanging, blunt trauma, or projectile injury. Identifying a hyoid bone fracture and/or a fracture of the laryngeal apparatus is important as fractures of these structures may give rise to airway compromise.
- **Hyoid motion artifact due to swallowing.** Swallowing during a CT scan will result in motion artifact of the hyoid bone, sometimes simulating duplication of the hyoid bone or conceivably a hyoid fracture. Evaluating the hyoid bone on reformatted imaging usually helps to elucidate motion artifact as the cause of the apparent finding.

Unilateral fusion of the hyoid body and greater cornua

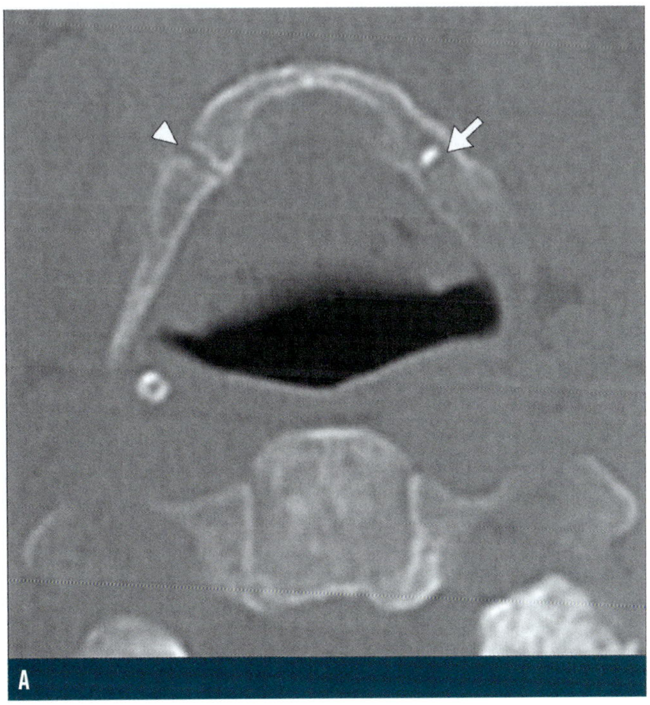

An axial CT image (**A**) demonstrates unilateral fusion of the articulation between the hyoid body and the left greater cornu (arrow) and lack of fusion on the contralateral side (arrowhead).

Bilateral fusion of the hyoid body and greater cornua

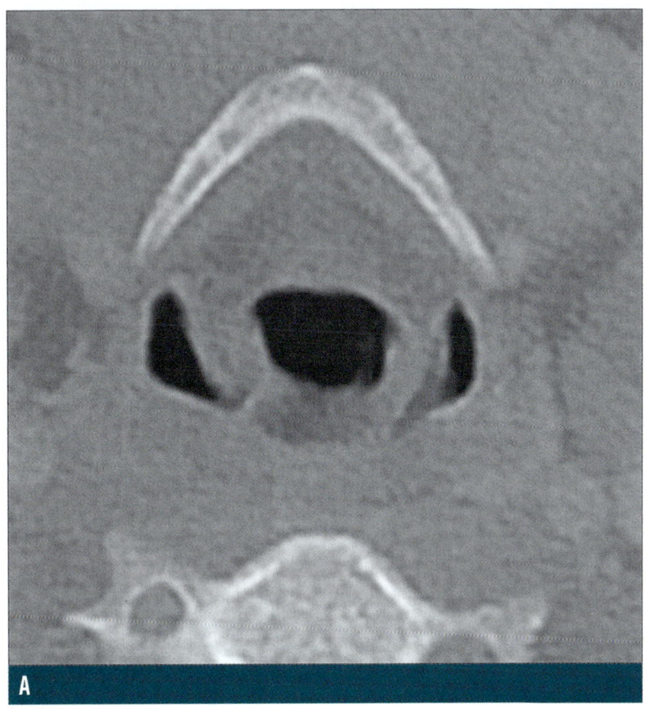

An axial CT image (**A**) demonstrates complete osseous fusion of the hyoid body with the bilateral greater cornua.

Bilateral nonfusion of the hyoid body and greater cornua

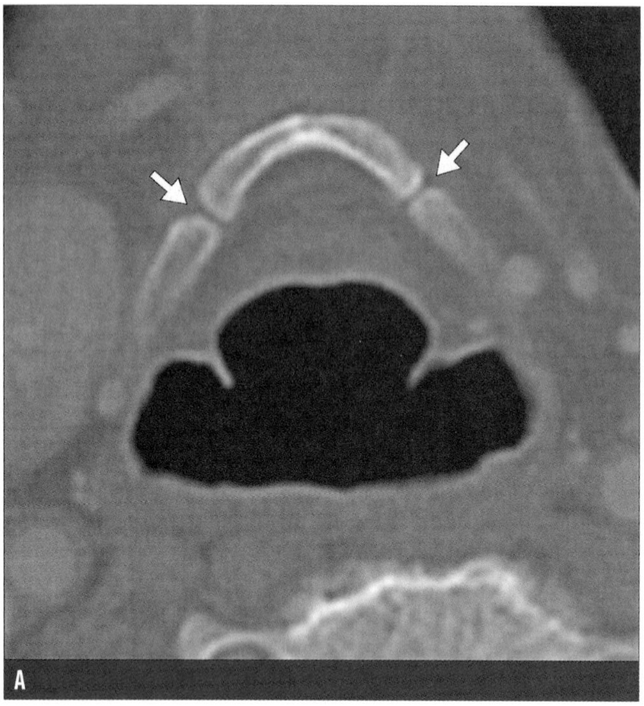

An axial CT image (**A**) demonstrates nonfusion of the articulations between the hyoid body and the greater cornua (arrows).

Focal angulation of hyoid greater cornu

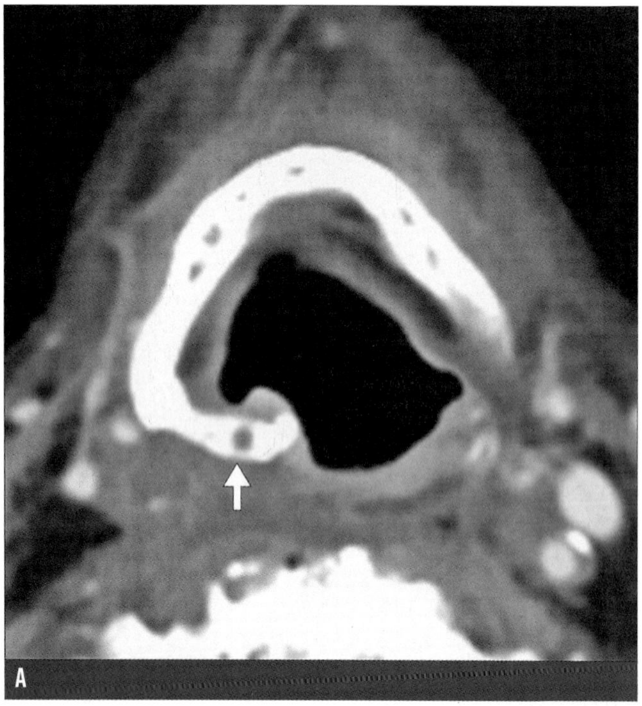

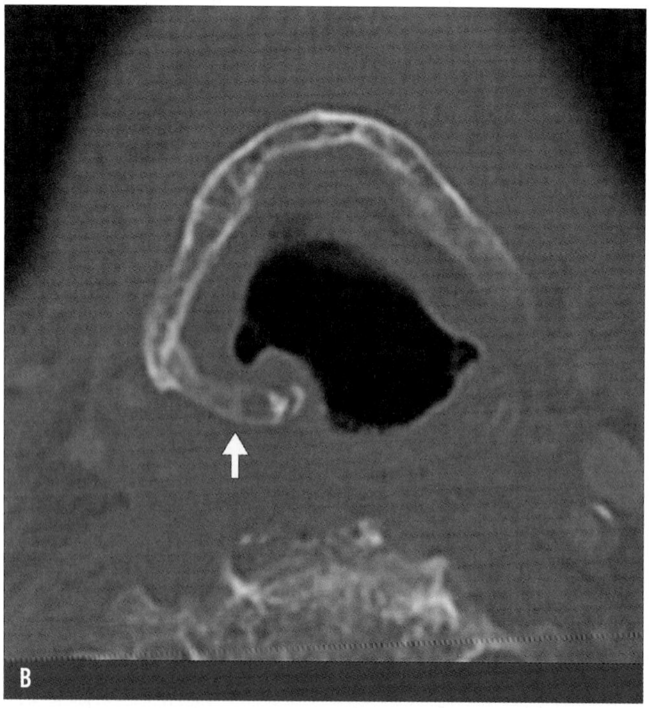

Contrast-enhanced axial CT images viewed with a soft tissue window (**A**) and bone window (**B**) demonstrate a focal, medially directed curvature of the right superior cornu of the hyoid (arrows, **A**, **B**), a normal variant.

Nonunion of hyoid lesser cornua

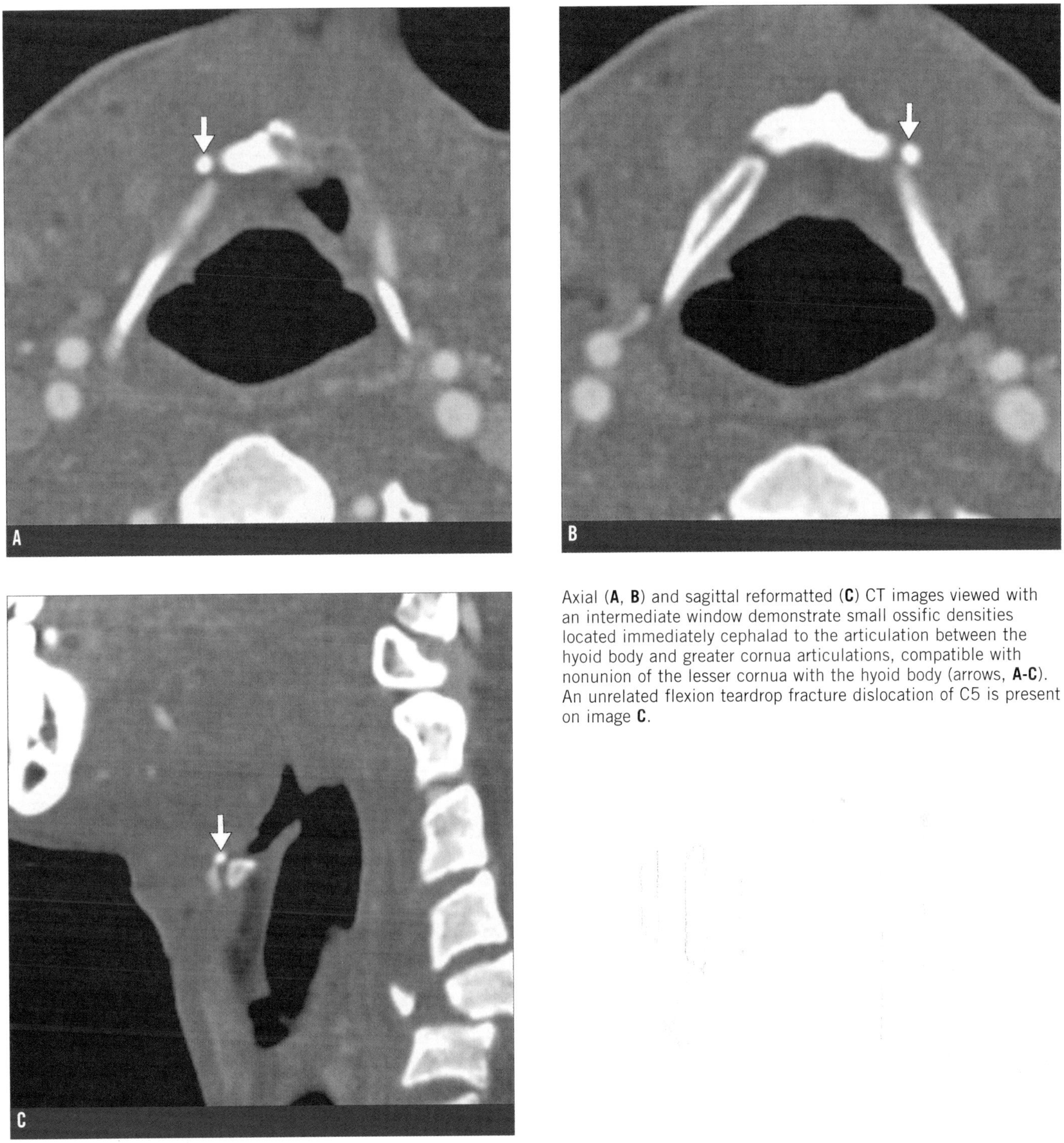

Axial (**A**, **B**) and sagittal reformatted (**C**) CT images viewed with an intermediate window demonstrate small ossific densities located immediately cephalad to the articulation between the hyoid body and greater cornua articulations, compatible with nonunion of the lesser cornua with the hyoid body (arrows, **A-C**). An unrelated flexion teardrop fracture dislocation of C5 is present on image **C**.

CASE 2 Thyrohyoid fusion anomalies

Deriving its name from the Greek alphabetic character upsilon (υ), the U-shaped hyoid bone serves to assist the complex motions of swallowing and vocalization. Situated at the midline within the ventral superior neck, the hyoid bone is held in position by paired stylohyoid ligaments above as well as the thyrohyoid membrane and thyrohyoid ligaments below. The hyoid bone serves as an attachment site for several muscles associated with the tongue, larynx, and pharynx, which contribute to additional stabilization and support for the hyoid.

The thyrohyoid membrane spans from the thyroid laminae to the hyoid bone. Specifically, it extends from the superior margin of the thyroid cartilage laminae and along the ventral margin of the thyroid cartilage superior cornua to the posterior-superior surface of the body and greater cornua of the hyoid bone. The paired, thickened, cord-like lateral thyrohyoid ligament is located along the posterolateral border of the thyrohyoid membrane and extends from the tip of the superior cornu of the thyroid lamina to the greater cornu of the hyoid bone. A small focus of cartilage, termed the triticeal cartilage (Latin *triticeus,* meaning grain of wheat), is embedded within the lateral thyrohyoid ligament. While the function of this cartilage is debated, it may aid in reinforcing the lateral thyrohyoid ligament.

Ossification of the lateral thyrohyoid ligament and/or the triticeal cartilage can result in various fusion anomalies between the posterior aspects of the hyoid greater cornua and the superior cornua of the thyroid laminae. These thyrohyoid fusion anomalies can represent a source of confusion for the radiologist and surgeon. Although the vast majority of these anomalies are asymptomatic and incidentally discovered on imaging or autopsy, there are scattered reports of symptoms related to thyrohyoid fusion anomalies.

COMPANION CASE

- **Mineralization of the triticeal cartilage.** Focal mineralization of the triticeal cartilage is not uncommon, occurring in 29% of males and 22% of females, and is most often an incidental finding. However, cases of dysphagia, cervicalgia, or globus sensation have been described. Moreover, the constellation of symptoms may mimic Eagle syndrome, which represents symptoms related to compression of regional structures by an elongated styloid process, ossified stylohyoid ligament, or ossified stylomandibular ligament. A focally mineralized or ossified triticeal cartilage may simulate a radiopaque foreign body, atherosclerosis, or fracture fragment on plain films or CT.

Various appearances of a thyrohyoid fusion anomaly

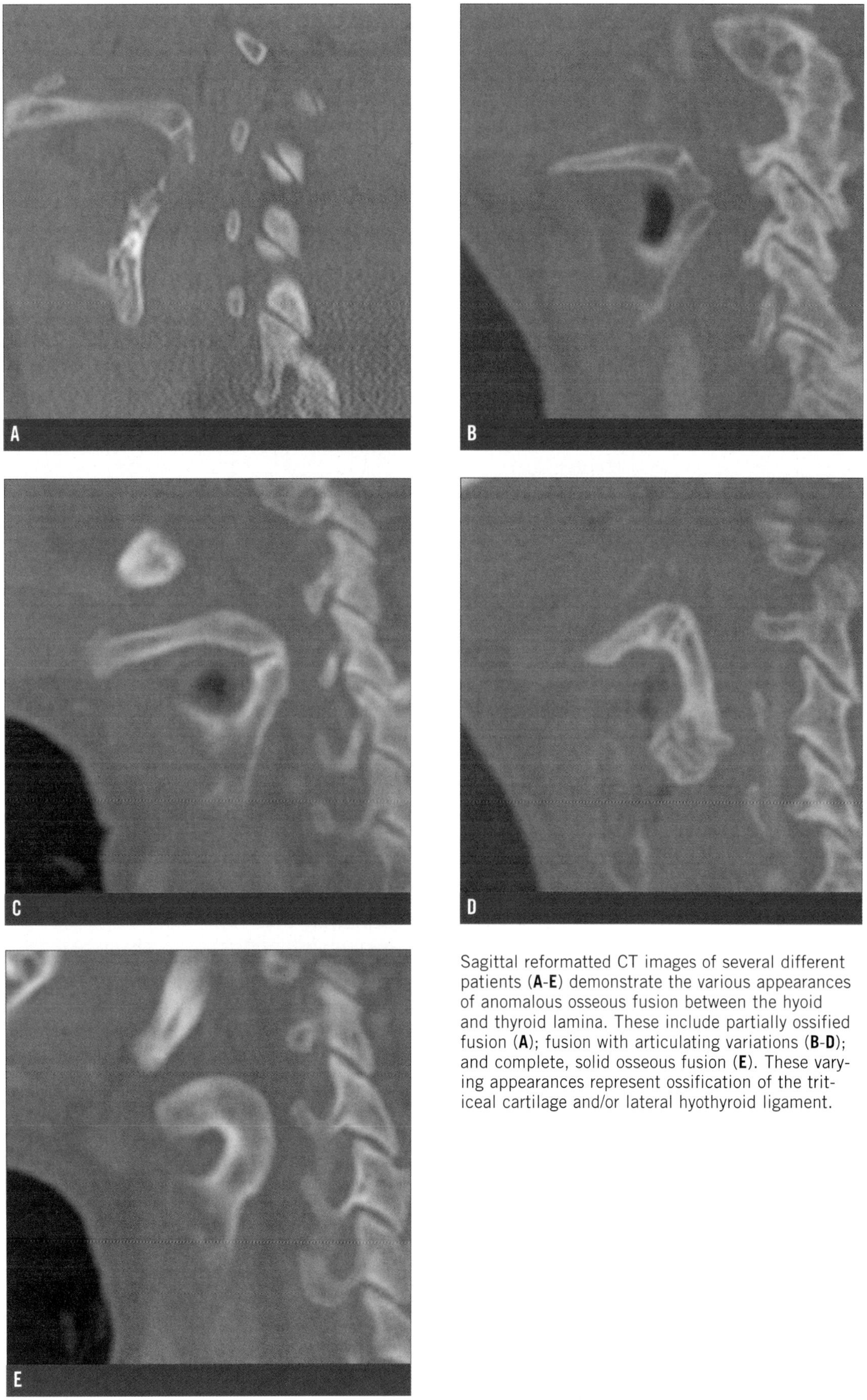

Sagittal reformatted CT images of several different patients (**A**-**E**) demonstrate the various appearances of anomalous osseous fusion between the hyoid and thyroid lamina. These include partially ossified fusion (**A**); fusion with articulating variations (**B**-**D**); and complete, solid osseous fusion (**E**). These varying appearances represent ossification of the triticeal cartilage and/or lateral hyothyroid ligament.

Unilateral thyrohyoid fusion resulting in a hyoid bone tilt

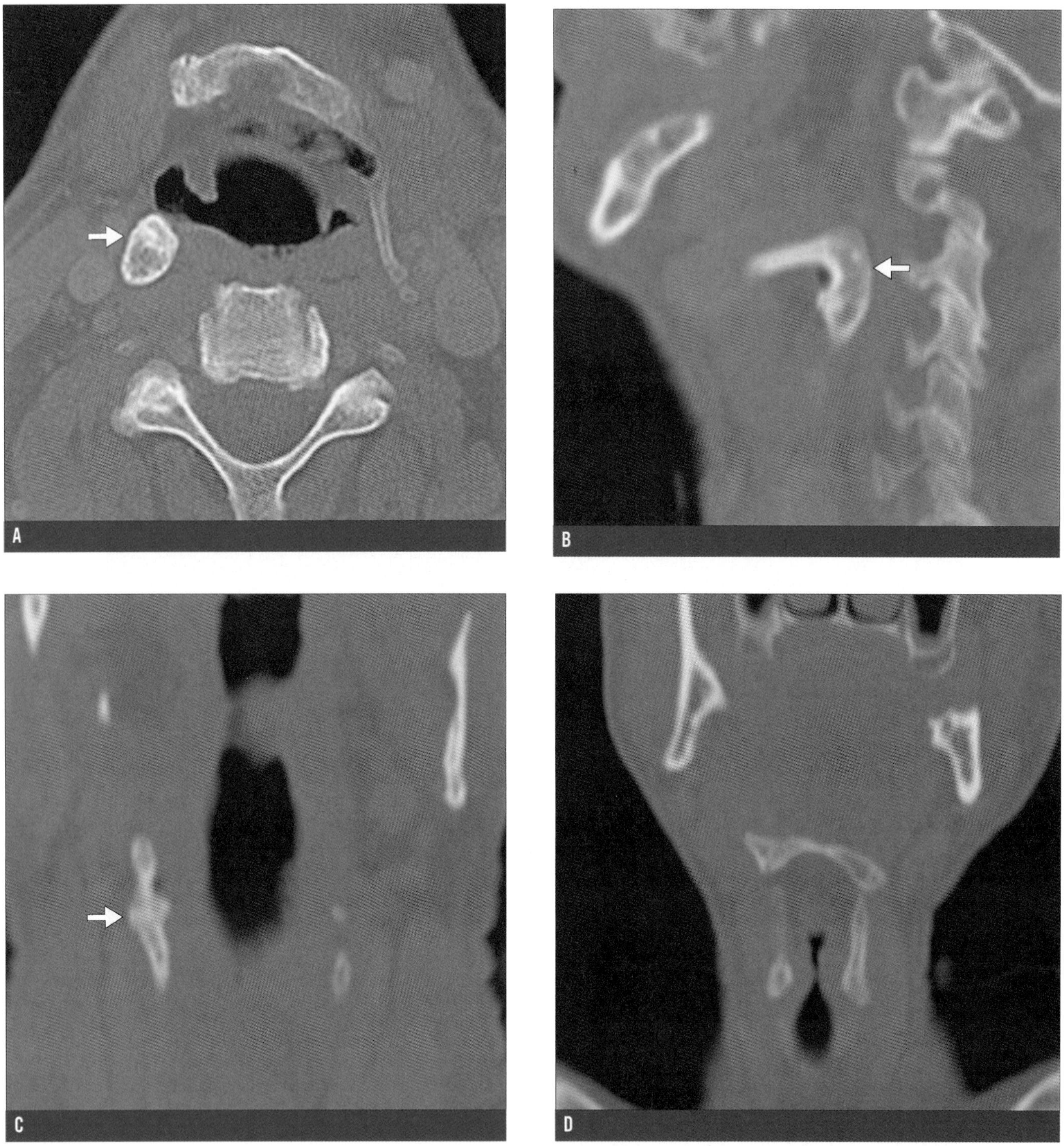

An axial CT image (**A**) and a sagittal reformatted CT image through the right aspects of the hyoid bone and thyroid lamina (**B**) demonstrate unilateral bulky osseous fusion between the posterior aspect of the right greater cornu of the hyoid bone and the right superior cornu of the thyroid lamina (arrows, **A**, **B**). This finding is also demonstrated on a coronal reformatted image (**C**, arrow). As a result of this asymmetric osseous fusion, the hyoid bone is tilted, with the right aspect significantly higher than the left, best appreciated on another coronal reformatted image (**D**).

Plain film appearance of near bilateral thyrohyoid osseous fusion

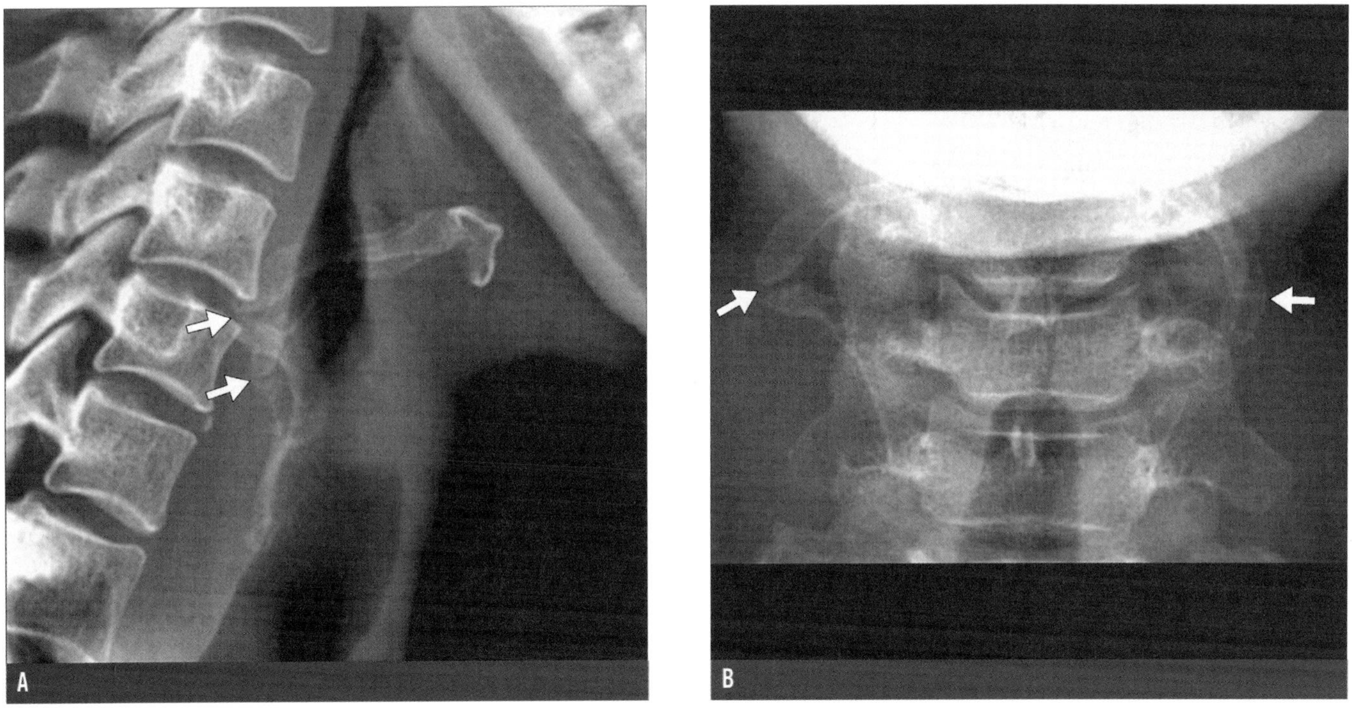

Lateral (**A**) and frontal (**B**) radiographs demonstrate near fusion between the bilateral greater cornua of the hyoid bone and superior cornua of the thyroid lamina with formation of bilateral articulations (arrows, **A**, **B**). This represents ossification of the bilateral triticeal and/or majority of the posterior thyrohyoid ligaments. This ossification, particularly when small and partially ossified, can simulate a radiopaque foreign body or fracture fragment on radiographs.

Companion case: Unilateral mineralization of the triticeal cartilage

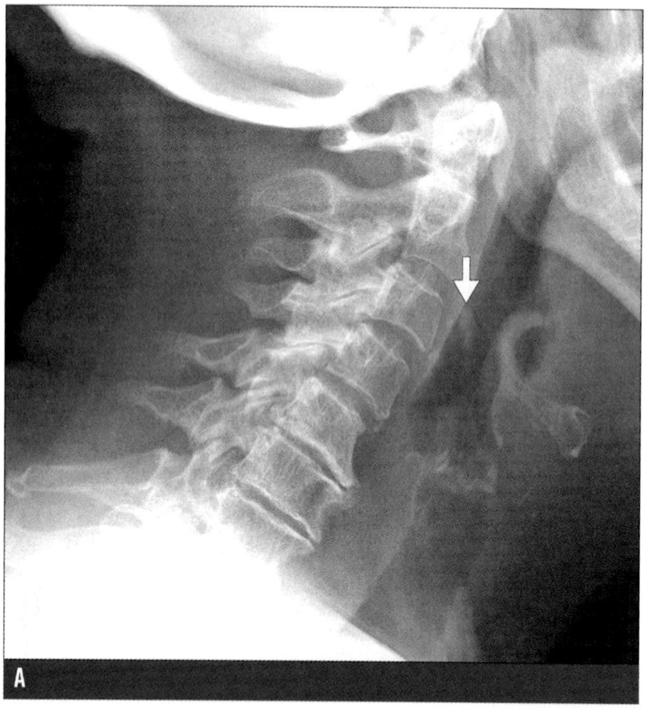

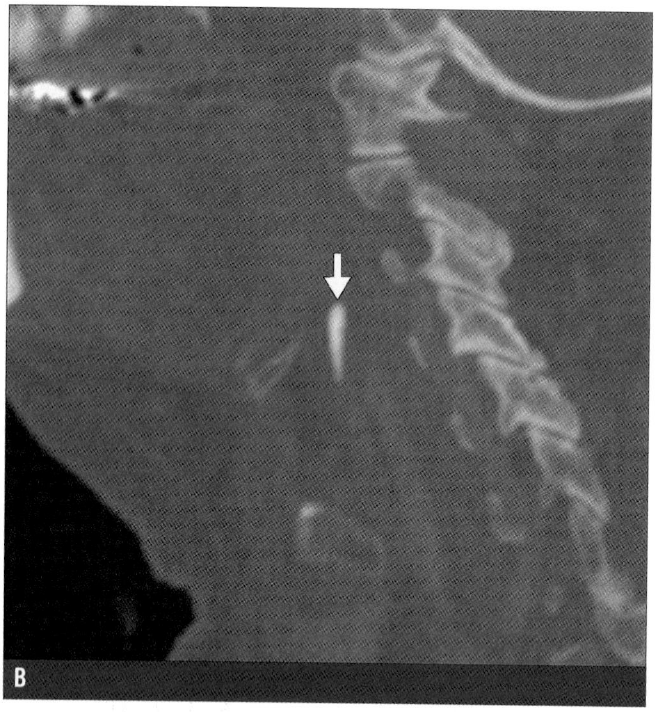

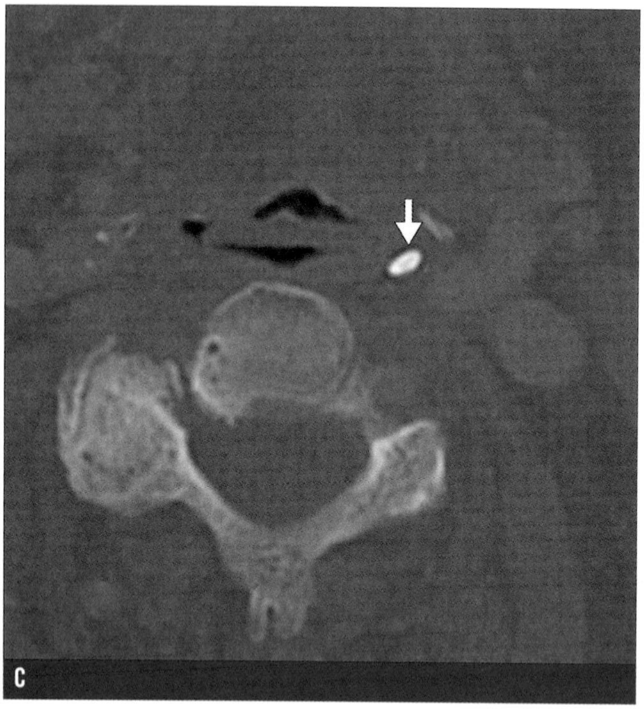

A lateral soft tissue neck radiograph (**A**) demonstrates a vertically oriented, linear hyperdensity that is suspicious for a foreign body (arrow). This finding was not appreciated on the frontal radiograph (not shown). Sagittal reformatted (**B**) and axial (**C**) CT images demonstrate the same finding to be located along the course of the left posterior thyrohyoid ligament and triticeal cartilage, compatible with incidental triticeal cartilage mineralization (arrows, **B**, **C**). A mineralized triticeal cartilage can simulate a displaced fracture fragment or a foreign body on CT or radiographs. This cartilage can vary from being radiographically occult to completely ossified.

Companion case: Bilateral mineralization of the triceal cartilages

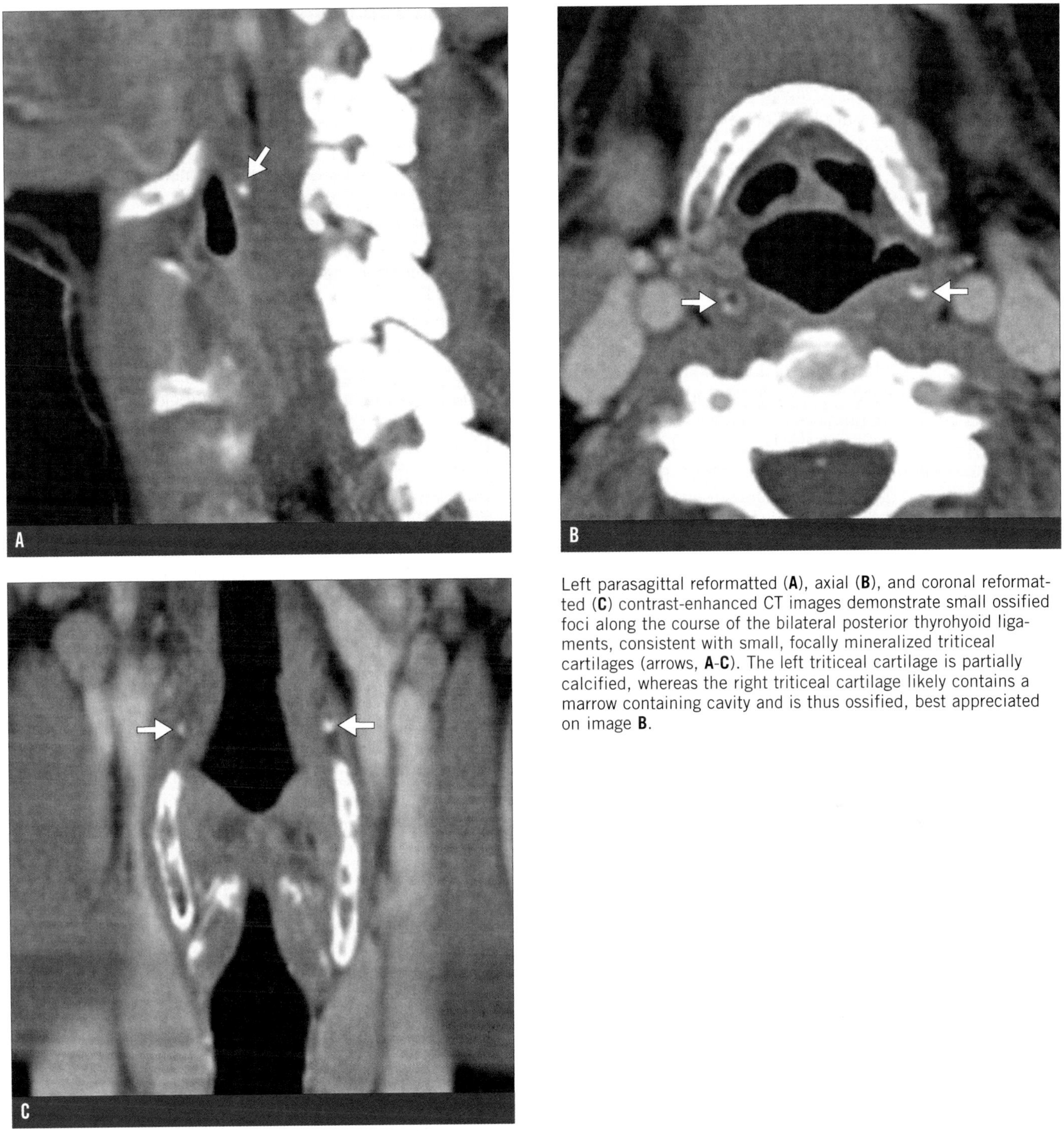

Left parasagittal reformatted (**A**), axial (**B**), and coronal reformatted (**C**) contrast-enhanced CT images demonstrate small ossified foci along the course of the bilateral posterior thyrohyoid ligaments, consistent with small, focally mineralized triticeal cartilages (arrows, **A**-**C**). The left triticeal cartilage is partially calcified, whereas the right triticeal cartilage likely contains a marrow containing cavity and is thus ossified, best appreciated on image **B**.

REFERENCES

Alsarraf R, Mathison S, Futran N. Symptomatic presentation of an enlarged, ossified triticeal cartilage. *Am J Otolaryngol.* 1998;19:339-341.

Drake RL, Gray H. *Gray's Atlas of Anatomy.* Philadelphia, PA: Churchill Livingstone; 2008.

Ilankovan V. An anomaly of the thyro-hyoid articulation. *J Laryngol Otol.* 1987;101:959-961.

Kopstein E. Hyoid syndrome. *Arch Otolaryngol.* 1975;101:484-485.

Murtagh RD, Caracciolo JT, Fernandez G. CT findings associated with Eagle syndrome. *AJNR Am J Neuroradiol.* 2001;22:1401-1402.

CASE 3 Variations of thyroid cartilage mineralization

The thyroid cartilage is composed of two laminae that fuse anteriorly to form the laryngeal prominence, commonly known as the "Adam's apple." Cephalad-directed projections along the posterior-superior margins of the thyroid laminae, termed the superior cornua, connect to the hyoid bone via the lateral thyrohyoid ligaments. The inferior cornua are located along the posterior-inferior aspects of the thyroid laminae and, in combination with the inferior margin of the thyroid laminae, serve as the superior attachment sites for the cricothyroid muscles, which function to tense the true vocal cords (TVCs) as well as manipulate vocal pitch.

Several studies have sought to establish patterns of mineralization involving the laryngeal cartilages. Hately, et al, described the mineralization process as beginning in the posterior-inferior third of the lamina and inferior cornu and progressing anteriorly along the inferior margin of the anterior two-thirds of the lamina. The superior cornua and anterior junctions of the two laminae generally mineralize much later.

While a general sequence of mineralization is accepted, variations are commonplace and likely owe to a combination of factors including nutrition, hormones, mechanical stresses, genetics, gender, and race. The normal thyroid cartilage may focally mineralize (and not contain a marrow cavity), ossify (and contain a marrow cavity), or be densely sclerotic. In addition, the degree and frequency of mineralization of the thyroid cartilage is often lower in females than in males, especially the anterior portions of the cartilage. Studies have also shown that African-American subjects may lack complete ossification, a pattern similar to all female subjects.

COMPANION CASES

- **Retained fish bone.** A swallowed fish bone can be retained in any portion of the pharynx and larynx. It will frequently appear as a discrete, linear focus, often with a nonanatomic angulation. It can simulate portions of the normal laryngeal apparatus, particularly the posterior margin of the thyroid laminae as well as the superior and inferior thyroid cornua.
- **Multiple myeloma involving the thyroid cartilage.** Multiple myeloma, an uncontrolled proliferation of monoclonal plasma cells resulting in a diffuse marrow replacement process, can occasionally manifest as a localized soft tissue mass arising from bone. Focal myelomatous involvement of the thyroid lamina is exceedingly rare. CT findings of thyroid lamina involvement include enlargement of the affected thyroid cartilage by soft tissue tumor and coarse calcifications. If large, the mass may compromise the laryngeal or upper tracheal airway.
- **Squamous cell carcinoma invading thyroid cartilage.** The vast majority of laryngeal cancers are squamous cell carcinomas, owing to the abundant squamous epithelium found throughout the larynx. Most cancers originate in the glottic larynx, followed by primary malignancies of the supraglottis and subglottis, in that order. While staging of laryngeal cancers is beyond the scope of this text, the American Joint Committee on Cancer has designated staging by the TNM classification. Invasion of the inner cortex of the thyroid cartilage by supraglottic or glottic tumors is considered a T3 lesion, whereas invasion through the thyroid cartilage constitutes at least a T4a lesion. Laryngeal cartilage invaded by tumor may be sclerotic or focally lytic on CT, which are appearances that may also be present with normal laryngeal cartilage. Therefore, it is imperative to evaluate for a mass if focal sclerosis or a suspicious focal lucency involving the laryngeal cartilage is encountered on CT. On MRI, tumor invading ossified laryngeal cartilage will generally lack normal marrow fat on non-fat-suppressed T1- and T2-weighted imaging, and it will abnormally enhance following contrast administration.
- **Radiation-induced chondronecrosis of the thyroid lamina.** Laryngeal edema, a well-known complication due to perichondritis and impairment of vascular and lymphatic channels, usually develops shortly following radiation treatment and tends to regress over time. A potentially devastating long-term complication of laryngeal radiation is chondronecrosis, which is characterized by demineralization, fragmentation, and collapse of the laryngeal skeleton with gas developing in the adjacent soft tissues. Chondronecrosis of the larynx is a generally irreversible process that may require laryngectomy due to the potential of life-threatening laryngeal instability.

Nonmineralized thyroid cartilage

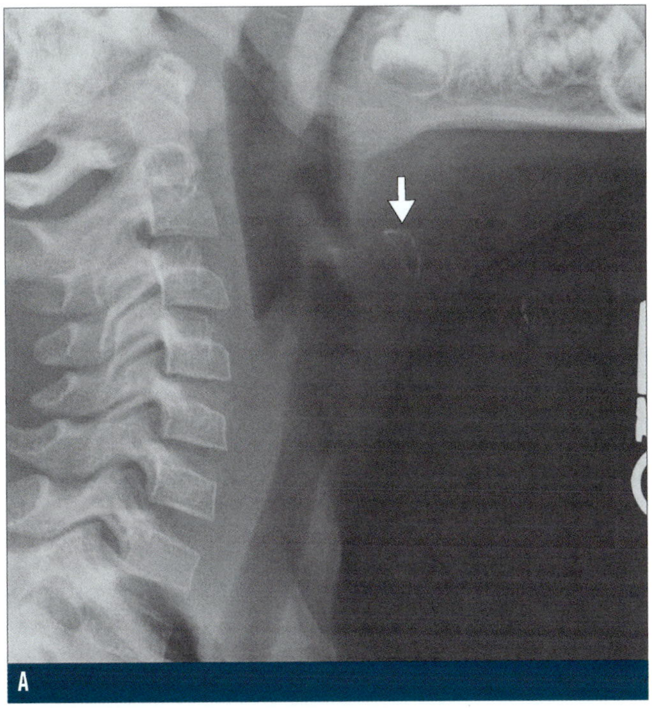

A lateral soft tissue neck radiograph of a 5-year-old boy (**A**) demonstrates a complete lack of thyroid lamina mineralization. The hyoid bone is at least partially ossified (arrow).

Nonmineralized thyroid cartilage

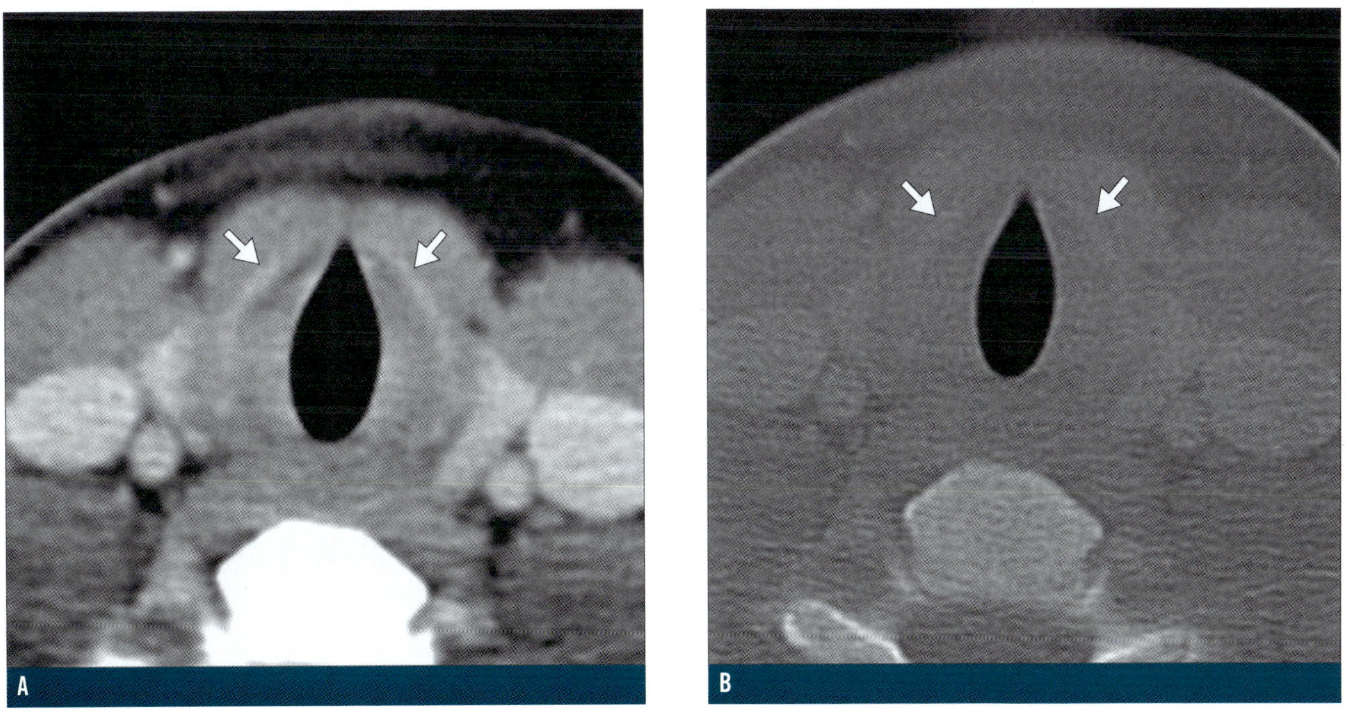

Different patient. Contrast-enhanced axial CT images viewed with a soft tissue window (**A**) and bone window (**B**) of a 19-year-old patient demonstrate faint visualization of the thyroid laminae cartilage, without evidence of mineralization (arrows, **A**, **B**).

Small amount of thyroid cartilage mineralization

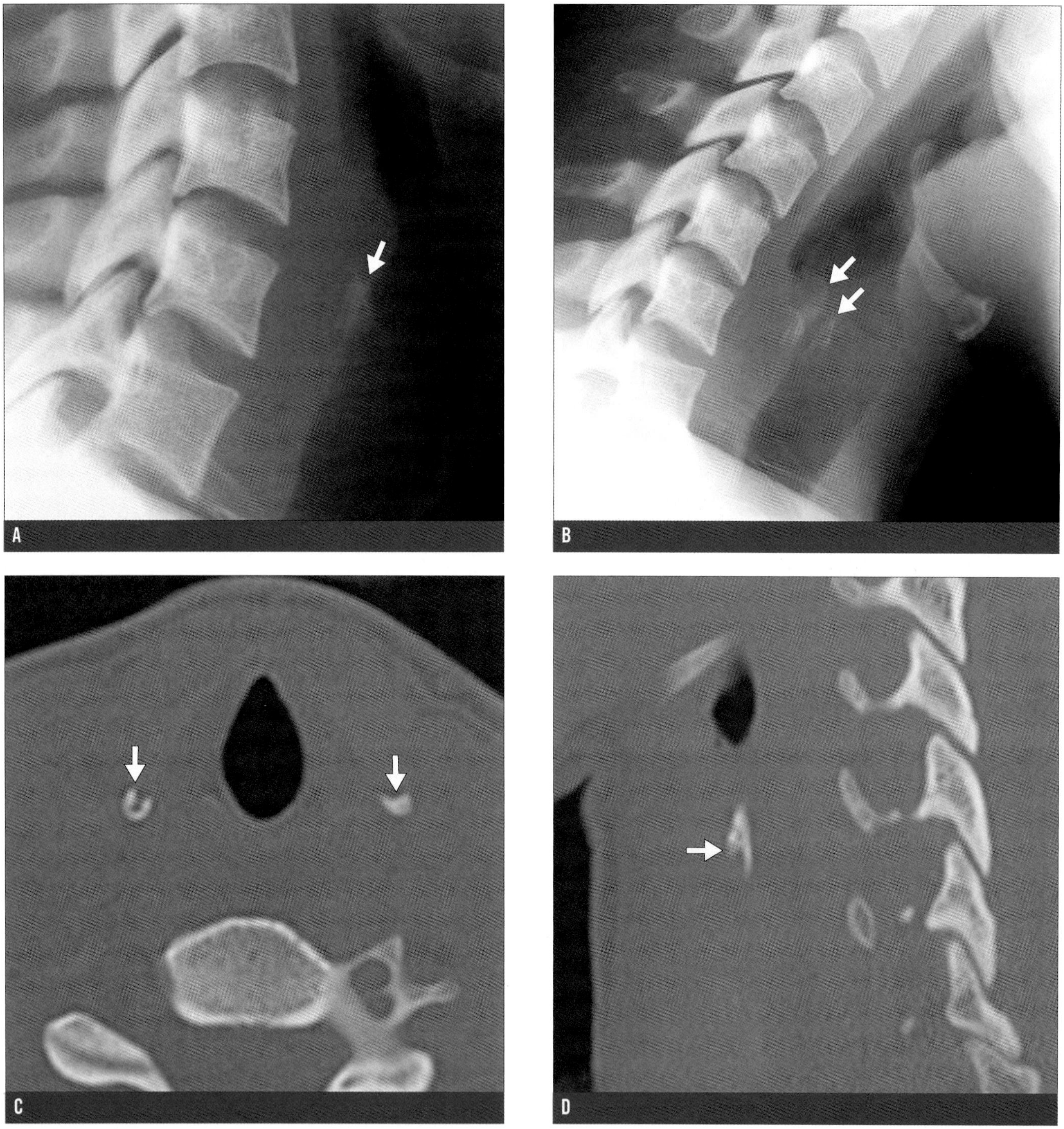

A lateral soft tissue neck radiograph of a 22-year-old-woman (**A**) demonstrates a focus of ossification along the posterior aspect of the upper airway which could be mistaken for a foreign body (arrow, **A**). A flexion lateral view from the same study (**B**) demonstrates the focus of mineralization to actually represent two foci (arrows, **B**). Axial (**C**) and sagittal (**D**) CT images of the same patient demonstrate the areas of mineralization on the plain films to represent normal early mineralization along the posterior aspects of the thyroid laminae (arrows, **C**, **D**).

Companion case: Retained fish bone

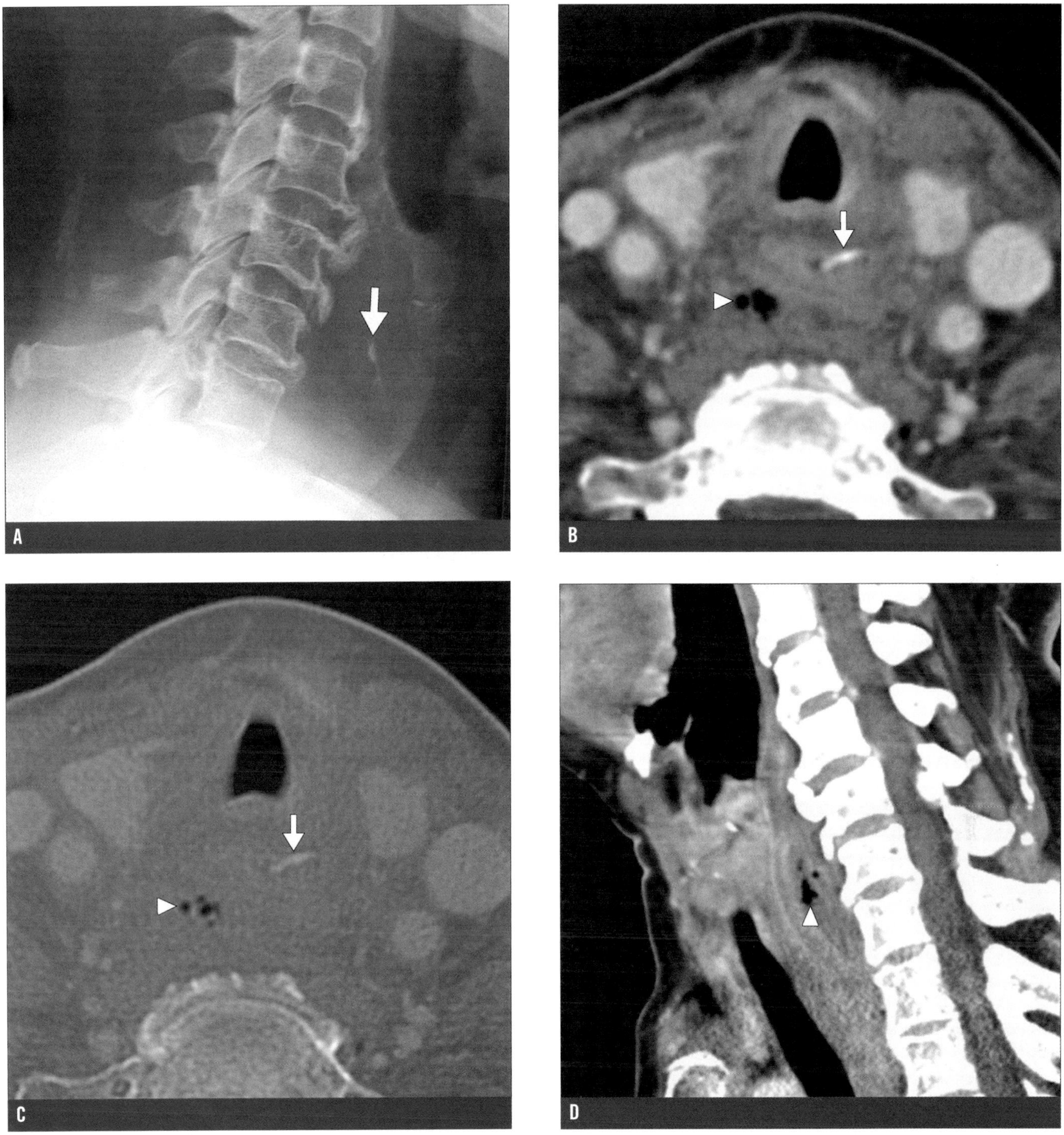

A lateral soft tissue neck radiograph of a 75-year-old-patient with a history of a fish bone ingestion **(A)** demonstrates a linear radiopaque density that is oriented vertically oblique (arrow, **A**), simulating thyroid cartilage mineralization. However, close inspection of the finding reveals that it resides posterior to the laryngeal apparatus, effectively excluding that the finding represents focal ossification of laryngeal cartilage. The prevertebral soft tissues are also abnormally thickened at this level. Contrast-enhanced axial CT images of the same patient viewed with a soft tissue window (**B**) and bone window (**C**) demonstrate the linear foreign body to reside primarily within the esophagus, compatible with an impacted fish bone (arrows, **B**, **C**). The tip of this fish bone has perforated the esophagus and free air is identified right posterolateral to the esophagus (arrowheads, **B**, **C**). A sagittal reformatted CT image viewed with a soft tissue window (**D**) best demonstrates the abnormal prevertebral edema in addition to the free air (arrowhead, **D**).

Moderate amount of thyroid cartilage ossification

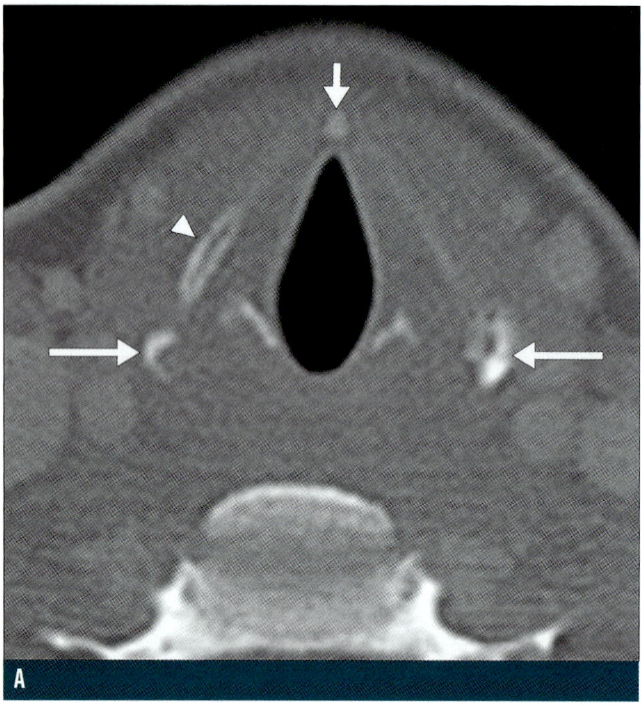

An axial CT image (**A**) demonstrates an intermediate stage of thyroid laminae ossification, with ossification along the posterior aspects of the thyroid laminae (long arrows), the mid right thyroid lamina (arrowhead), and at the apex of the thyroid laminae (short arrow).

Discontinuous ossification of the thyroid laminae

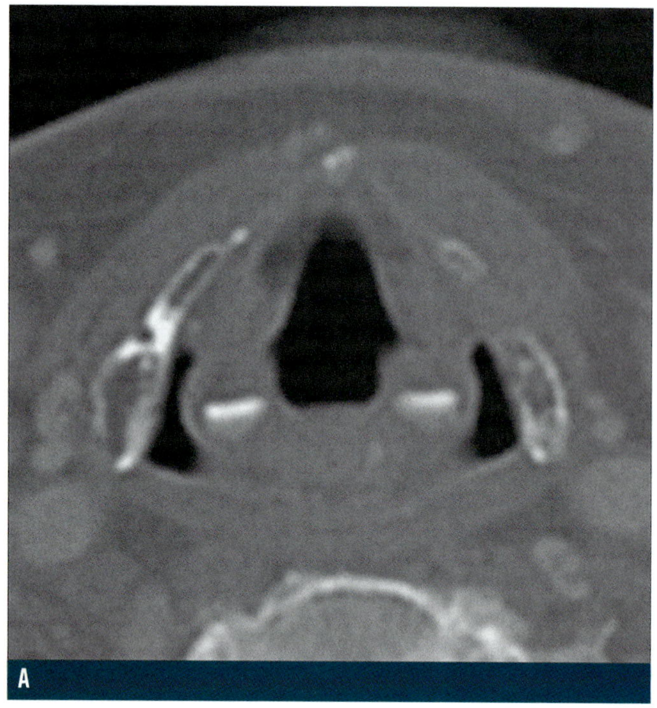

An axial CT image (**A**) demonstrates incidental discontinuous ossification of the bilateral thyroid laminae in this 80-year-old woman.

Fully ossified thyroid cartilage

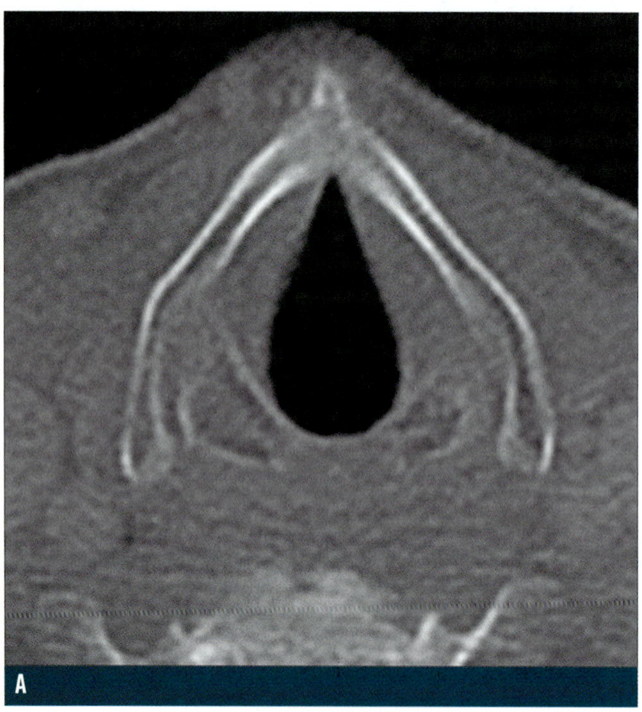

An axial CT image (**A**) demonstrates normal, diffuse, and symmetric ossification of the bilateral thyroid laminae.

Normal diffuse sclerosis of the thyroid laminae

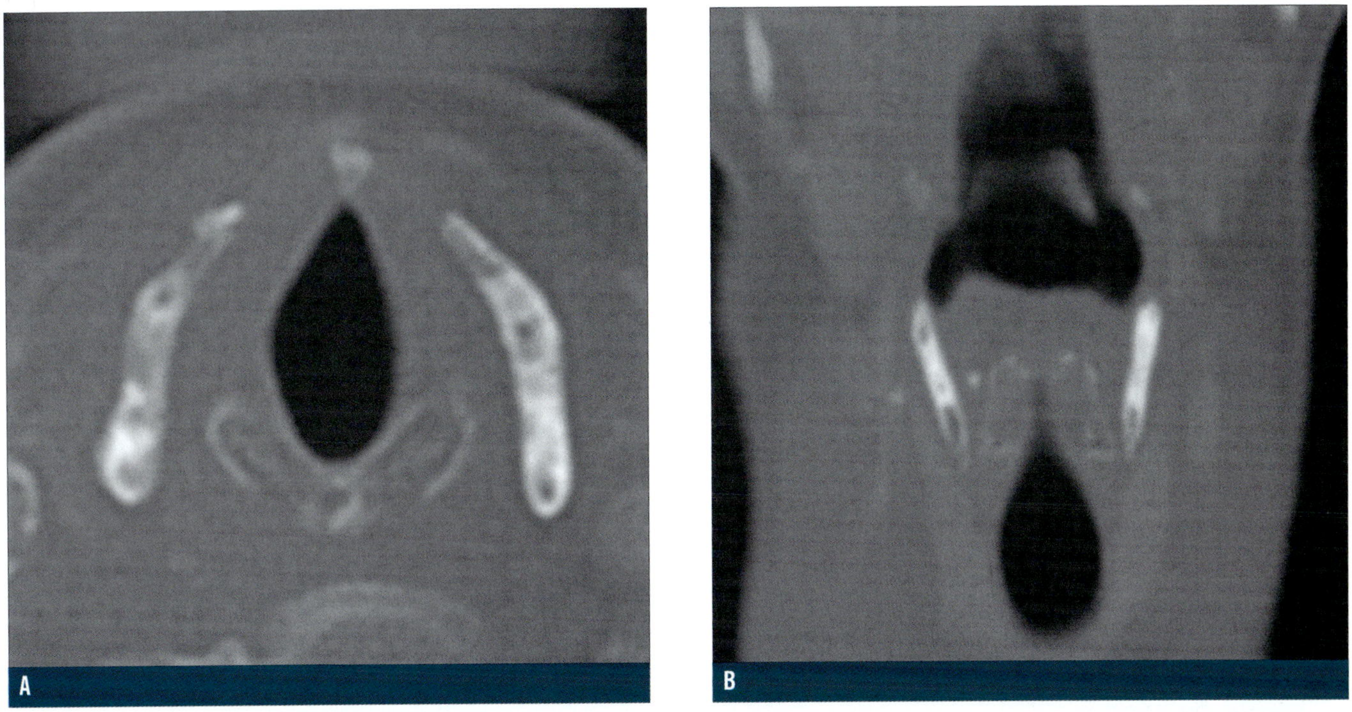

Axial (**A**) and coronal reformatted (**B**) CT images demonstrate diffusely sclerotic thyroid laminae. In this patient, this is a normal variation. However, if this appearance is encountered, then evaluation of the adjacent soft tissues, in particular the TVCs and supraglottic larynx, should be performed to exclude a cartilage invading lesion. Radiation may also result in thyroid laminae sclerosis and/or destruction.

Unilateral thyroid lamina focal marrow cavity

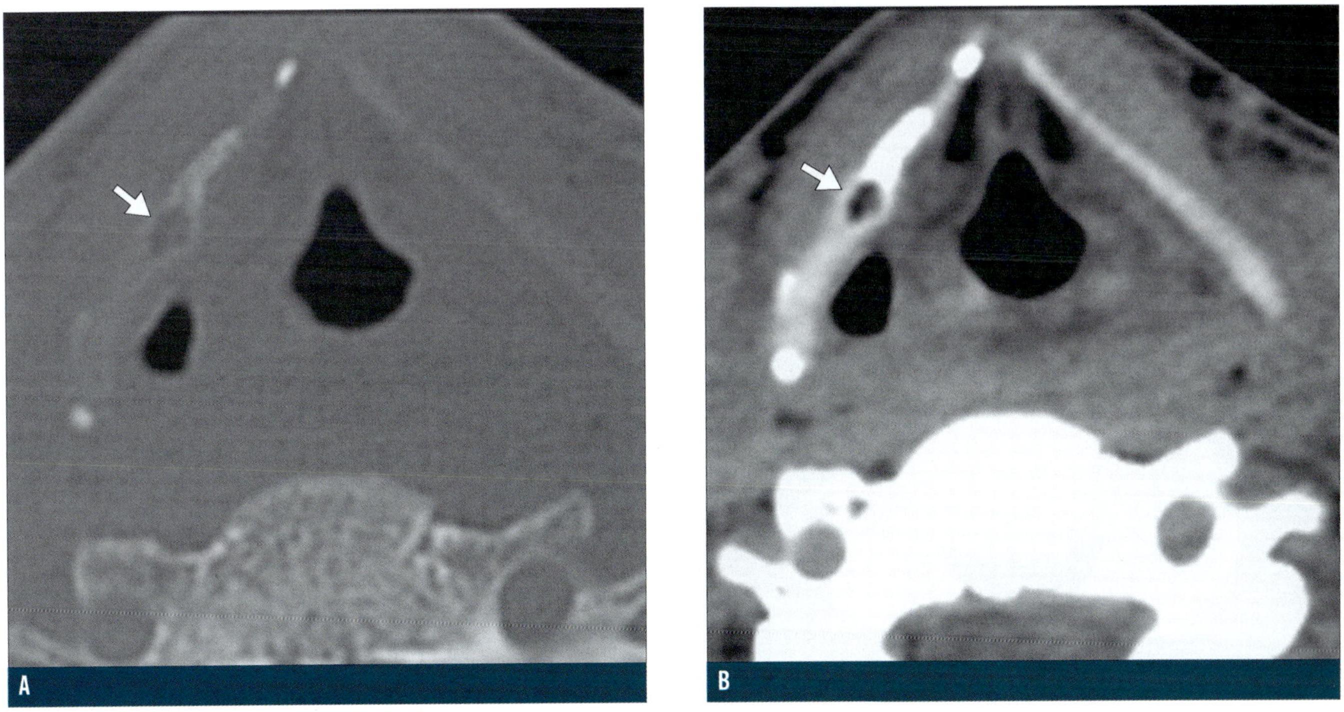

Axial CT images viewed with a bone window (**A**) and soft tissue window (**B**) demonstrate a focally dilated, marrow containing portion of the right thyroid lamina, a normal variant (arrows, **A**, **B**).

Focal marrow cavities of the thyroid laminae

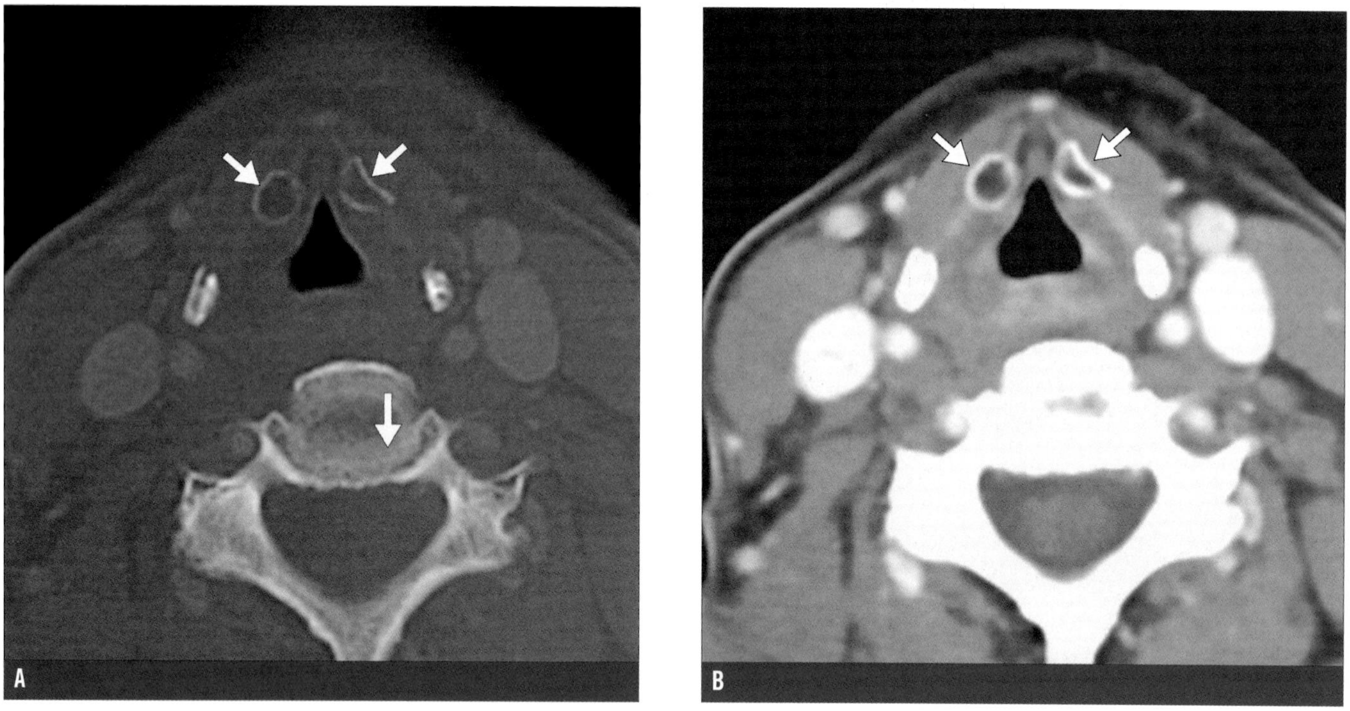

Axial CT images viewed with a bone window (**A**) and soft tissue window (**B**) demonstrate focally enlarged, marrow containing portions of the thyroid laminae (arrows, **A**, **B**). This is a normal variant.

Companion case: Multiple myeloma involving the thyroid cartilage

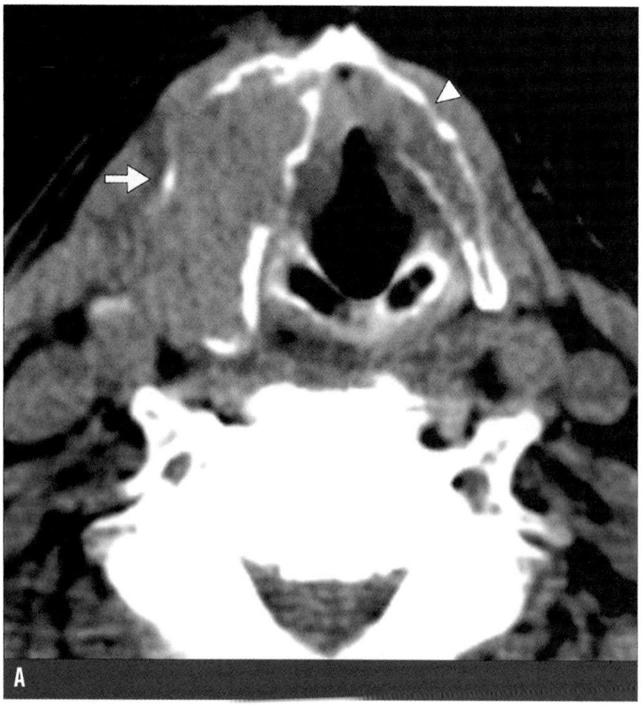

An unenhanced axial CT image (**A**) demonstrates a markedly expanded right thyroid lamina that contains soft tissue density (arrow). A mildly expanded left thyroid lamina is present as well, also containing abnormal soft tissue (arrowhead). Similar findings were present elsewhere in the body in this patient with multiple myeloma.

Companion case: Squamous cell carcinoma invading thyroid cartilage

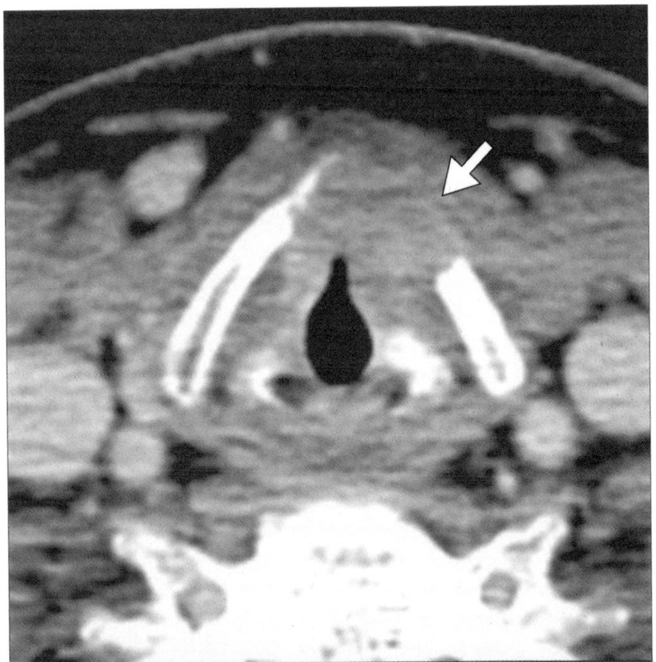

A

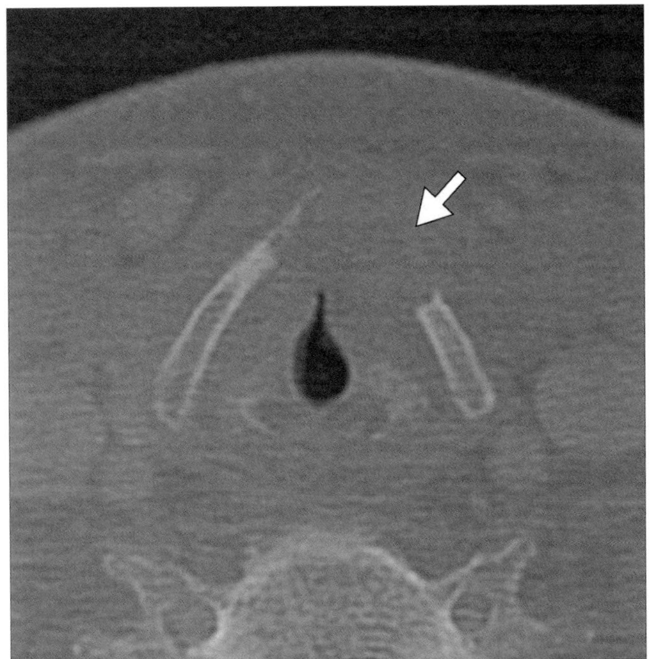

B

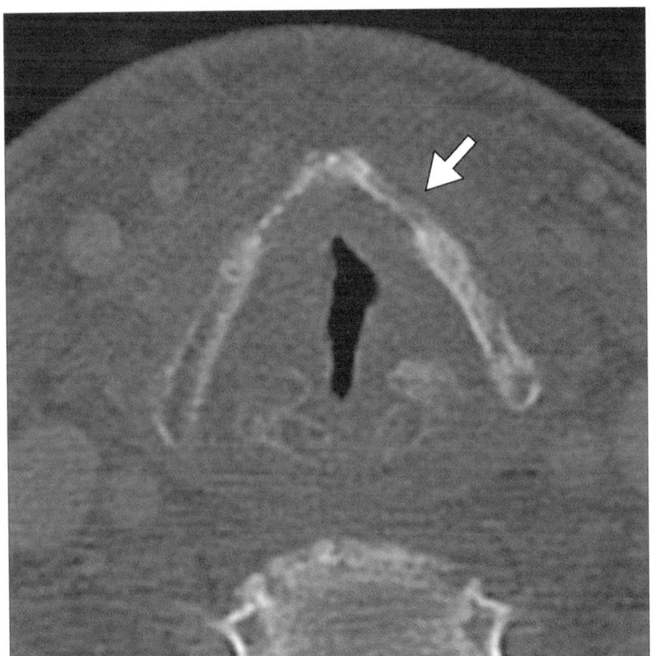

C

Contrast-enhanced axial CT images viewed with a soft tissue window (**A**) and bone window (**B**) demonstrate a left TVC tumor infiltrating and destroying the anterior aspect of the left thyroid lamina (arrows, **A**, **B**). An axial CT image viewed with a bone window obtained 1 year later (**C**) demonstrates marked improvement in the tumor and significant interval healing of the left thyroid lamina, which is now largely sclerotic (arrow, **C**).

Companion case: Squamous cell carcinoma invading thyroid cartilage

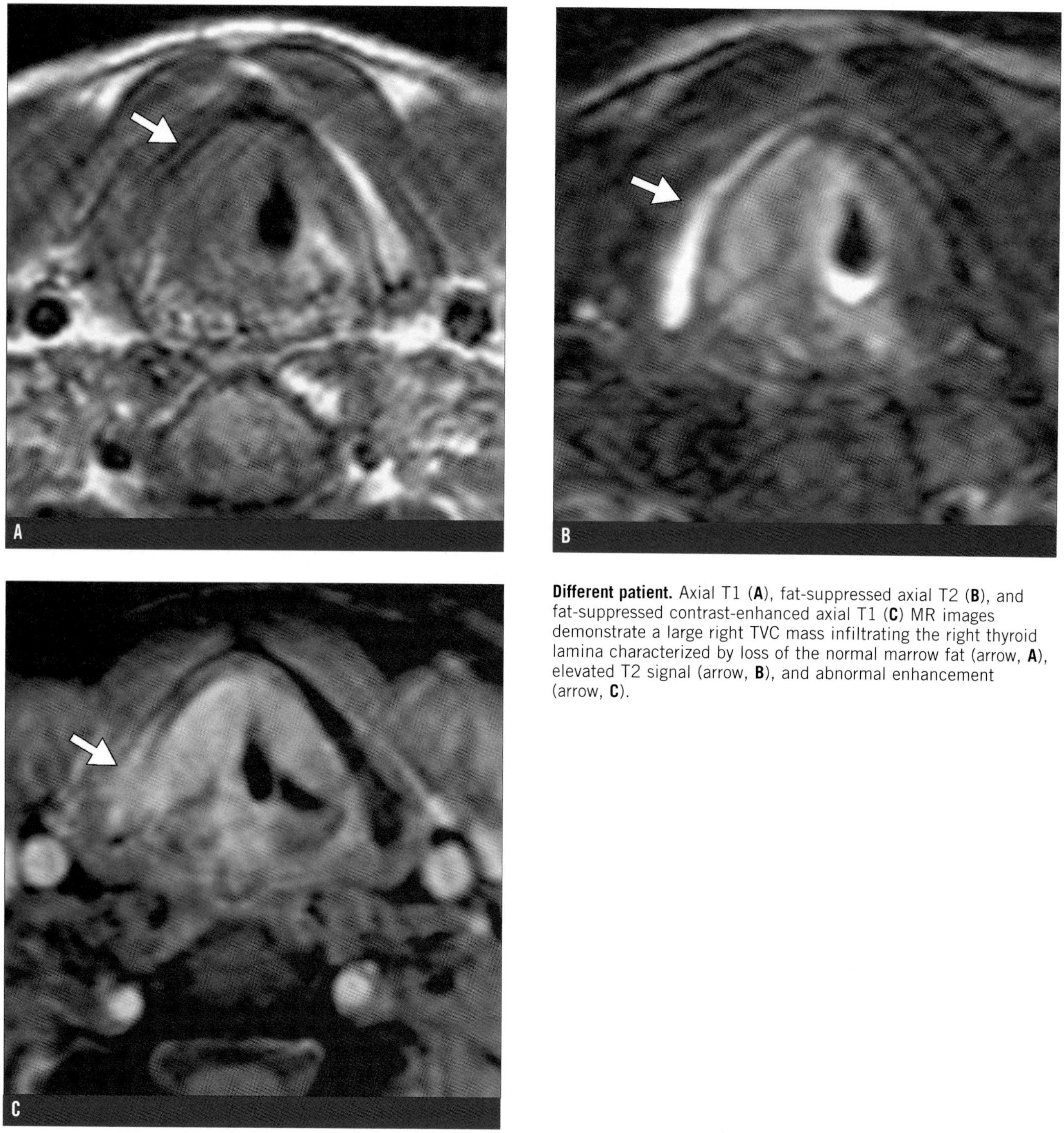

Different patient. Axial T1 (**A**), fat-suppressed axial T2 (**B**), and fat-suppressed contrast-enhanced axial T1 (**C**) MR images demonstrate a large right TVC mass infiltrating the right thyroid lamina characterized by loss of the normal marrow fat (arrow, **A**), elevated T2 signal (arrow, **B**), and abnormal enhancement (arrow, **C**).

Companion case: Radiation-induced chondronecrosis of the thyroid lamina

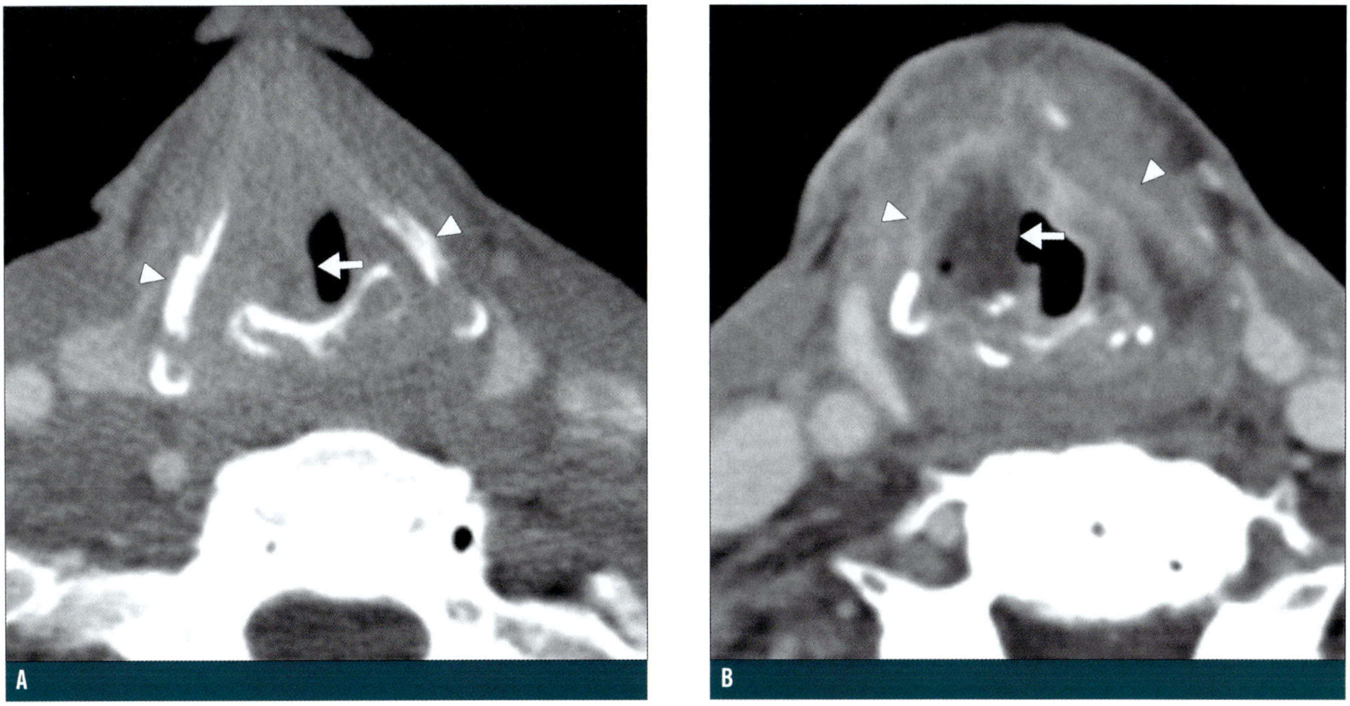

A contrast-enhanced axial CT image (**A**) demonstrates a right TVC mass (arrow, **A**) without overt destruction of either thyroid lamina (arrowheads, **A**), when allowing for incidental incomplete mineralization of the laminae. Approximately 1 year later and following radiation treatment, a contrast-enhanced axial CT image (**B**) demonstrates the tumor to be largely necrotic (arrow, **B**) and there is new demineralization of the thyroid laminae, compatible with chondronecrosis (arrowheads, **B**). While a portion of the right thyroid lamina chondronecrosis may have been due to interval direct invasion by the tumor, the left thyroid lamina was not affected by tumor and underwent chondronecrosis due to radiation treatment effect.

REFERENCES

de la Grandmaison GL, Banasr A, Durigon M. Age estimation using radiographic analysis of laryngeal cartilage. *Am J Forensic Med Pathol.* 2003;24:96-99.

Dispenza F, Sciandra D, Saraniti C. Thyroid cartilage involvement in patient affected by IgA multiple myeloma: case report. *Auris, Nasus, Larynx.* 2008;35:288-290.

Drake RL, Gray H.*Gray's Atlas of Anatomy.* 1st ed. Philadelphia, PA: Churchill Livingstone; 2008.

Fatterpekar GM, Mukherji SK, Rajgopalan P, Lin Y, Castillo M. Normal age-related signal change in the laryngeal cartilages. *Neuroradiology.* 2004;46:678-681.

Galline J, Marsot-Dupuch K, Bigel P, Lasjaunias P. Bilateral dystrophic ossification of the thyroid cartilage appearing as symmetrical laryngeal masses. *AJNR Am J Neuroradiol.* 2005;26:1339-1341.

Garvin HM. Ossification of laryngeal structures as indicators of age. *J Forensic Sci.* 2008;53:1023-7.

Hermans R[1], Pameijer FA, Mancuso AA, Parsons JT, Mendenhall WM. CT findings in chondroradionecrosis of the larynx. *AJNR Am J Neuroradiol.* 1998 Apr;19(4):711-718.

Marioni G, Marchese-Ragona R, Cartei G, Marchese F, Staffieri A. Current opinion in diagnosis and treatment of laryngeal carcinoma. *Cancer Treat Rev.* 2006;32:504-515.

Sosna J, Slasky BS, Paltiel O, Pizov G, Libson E. Multiple myeloma involving the thyroid cartilage: case report. *AJNR Am J Neuroradiol.* 2002;23:316-318.

CASE 4 Thyroid cartilage pseudofracture

Normal channels traversing the cartilage may be identified in the thyroid laminae. These cartilaginous channels represent tubes of vascularized mesenchyme and are believed to provide nourishment to the cartilage. Cartilaginous channels as well as normal asymmetric ossification of the cartilage can simulate a thyroid lamina fracture.

COMPANION CASES

- **Acute thyroid cartilage fracture**. Laryngeal fractures are uncommon, representing less than 1% of all blunt traumas. Etiologies include penetrating injuries, such as gunshot or stab wounds, or blunt trauma that may occur during motor vehicle collisions, sport injuries, strangulation, hanging, or assault. Iatrogenic injuries during surgical procedures or resuscitation attempts have also been described as a cause of laryngeal fracture.

  Specific injury patterns differ by location of the traumatic force. Supraglottic trauma commonly produces horizontal fractures of the thyroid laminae, whereas glottic forces may result in fractures near the attachment of the TVCs, resulting in dysphonia or aphonia. Subglottic forces may disrupt the cricothyroid joint via injury to the inferior cornu of the thyroid lamina.
- **Thyroid cartilage fracture with healing.** Like healing fractures elsewhere, healing fractures of the thyroid lamina are usually identified with areas of new bone formation along the margin of the fracture.
- **Incidental focal angulation of thyroid lamina superior cornu.** Occasionally, one may encounter a focal angulation of the thyroid lamina superior cornu. While trauma may result in this appearance, it is most often a normal variation and of no clinical significance.

Thyroid cartilage pseudofractures

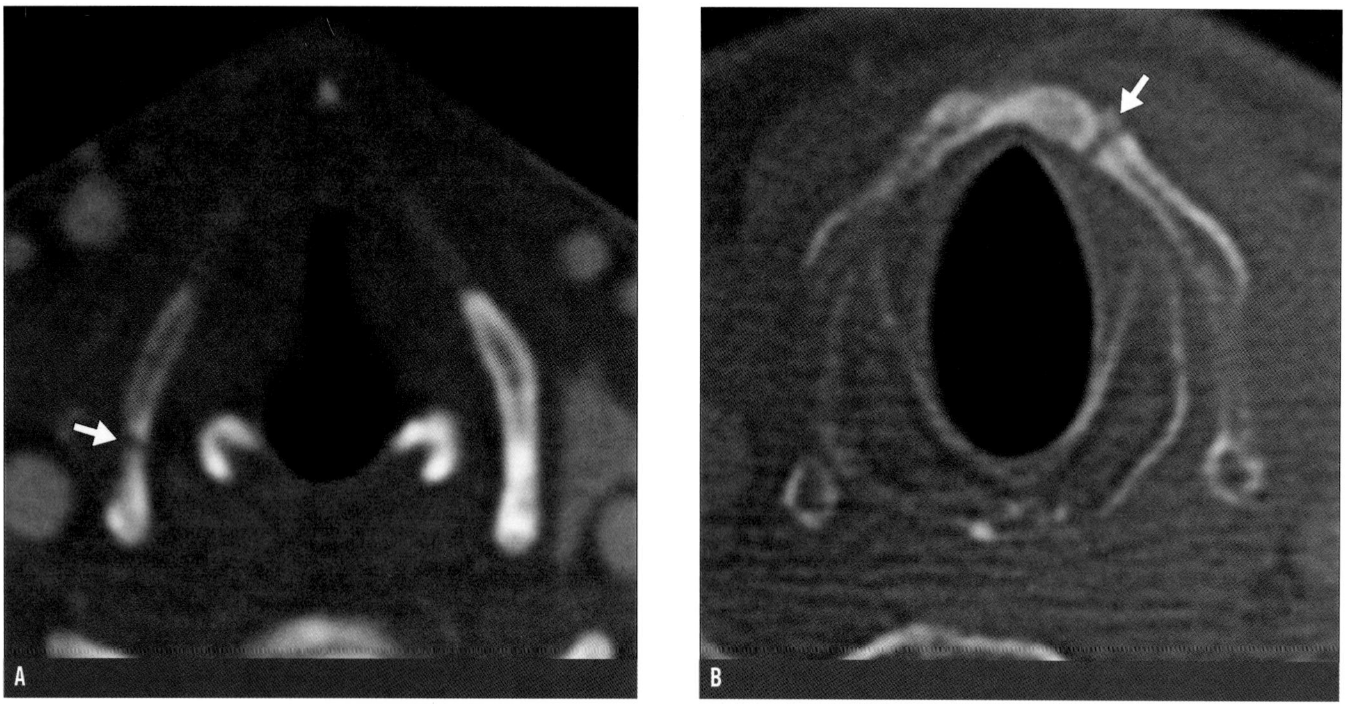

Axial CT images from three different patients ranging from 19 to 86 years of age (**A-C**) demonstrate corticated, linear lucencies through the thyroid lamina simulating fractures (arrows, **A-C**). These were incidental findings in all three patients and are compatible with incidental vascular channels within the thyroid laminae. However, fractures can have a similar appearance and these findings should be interpreted in conjunction with the clinical context.

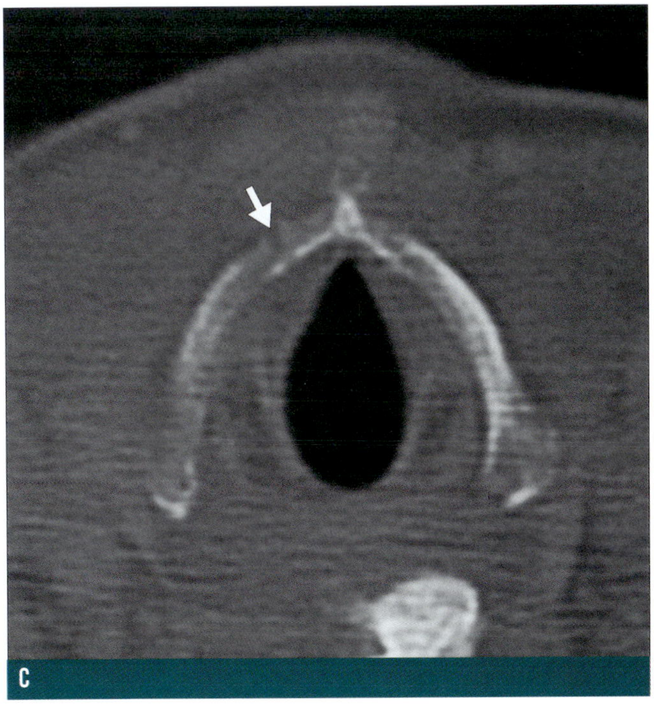

Companion case: Acute thyroid cartilage fracture

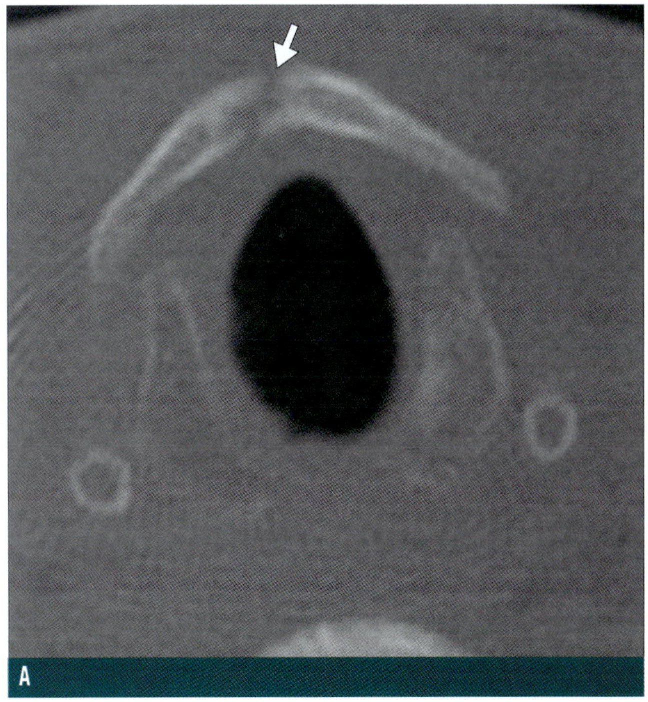

An axial CT image (**A**) demonstrates an acute fracture through the paramedian right thyroid lamina in this patient who experienced acute trauma to the thyroid lamina (arrow).

Companion case: Thyroid cartilage fracture with healing

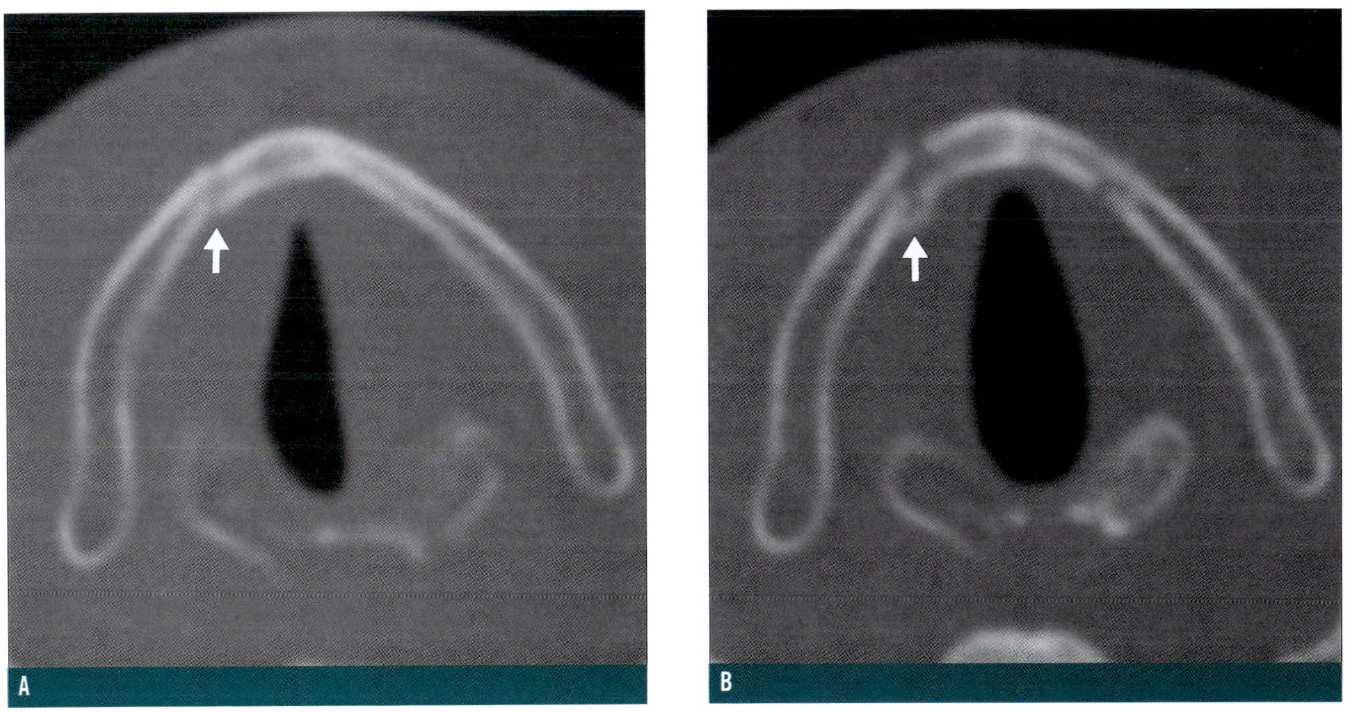

An axial CT image (**A**) demonstrates an acute fracture through the anterior aspect of the right thyroid lamina (arrow) in a 30-year-old patient who was struck in the neck with a hockey puck. One month later, an axial CT image (**B**) demonstrates interval new bone formation surrounding the fracture, compatible with interval healing (arrow).

Companion case: Incidental focal angulation of thyroid lamina superior cornu

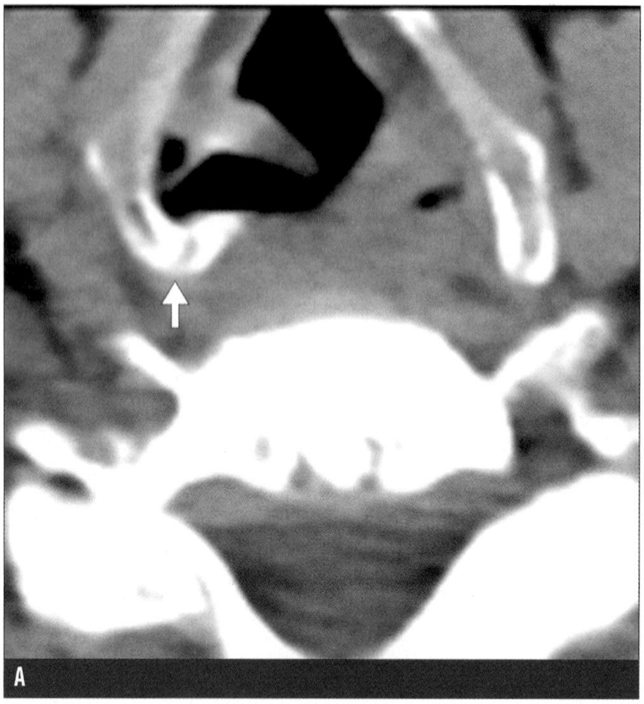

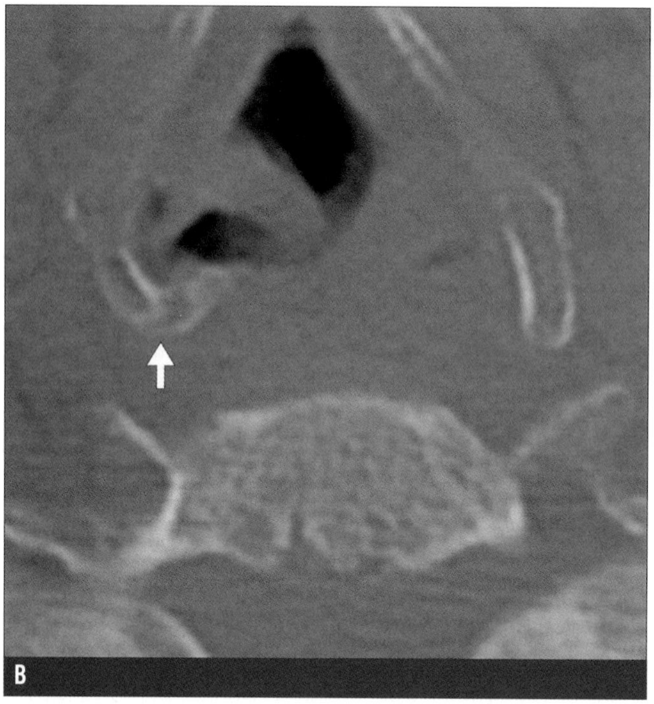

Axial CT images viewed with a soft tissue window (**A**) and bone window (**B**) demonstrate focal angulation of the right thyroid lamina superior cornu (arrows, **A**, **B**). This was a completely incidental finding.

REFERENCES

Claassen H, Kirsch T, Simons G. Cartilage canals in human thyroid cartilage characterized by immunolocalization of collagen types I, II, pro-III, IV and X. *Anat Embryol (Berl).* 1996;194:147-153.

de la Grandmaison GL, Banasr A, Durigon M. Age estimation using radiographic analysis of laryngeal cartilage. *Am J Forensic Med Pathol.* 2003;24:96-99.

Drake RL, Gray H. *Gray's Atlas of Anatomy.* 1st ed. Philadelphia, PA: Churchill Livingstone; 2008.

Fatterpekar GM, Mukherji SK, Rajgopalan P, Lin Y, Castillo M. Normal age-related signal change in the laryngeal cartilages. *Neuroradiology.* 2004;46:678-681.

Galline J, Marsot-Dupuch K, Bigel P, Lasjaunias P. Bilateral dystrophic ossification of the thyroid cartilage appearing as symmetrical laryngeal masses. *AJNR Am J Neuroradiol.* 2005;26:1339-1341.

Garvin HM. Ossification of laryngeal structures as indicators of age. *J Forensic Sci.* 2008;53:1023-1027.

Kim JP, Cho SJ, Son HY, Park JJ, Woo SH. Analysis of clinical feature and management of laryngeal fracture: recent 22 case review. *Yonsei Med J.* 2012;53:992-998.

Nerurkar N, Tandon S, Zodpe P, Bradoo R. Thyroid cartilage fracture: an unusual presentation. *Arch Otolaryngol Head Neck Surg.* 2005;131:262-265.

CASE 5 Variations of cricoid cartilage mineralization

The cricoid cartilage is located at the inferior aspect of the laryngeal apparatus, just caudal to the thyroid laminae. The cricoid cartilage is a complete ring of cartilage, often compared to a "signet ring," since it consists of a broad posterior lamina and a more slender arch circling anteriorly. The complete ring morphology of the cricoid is in contradistinction to the tracheal rings; the trachea has a membraneous posterior wall and therefore is composed of an incomplete ring of cartilage. The cricoid cartilage provides attachment sites for several muscles, ligaments, and cartilages involved in airway dynamics and vocalization.

Cricoid cartilage mineralization begins at nearly the same time as thyroid cartilage mineralization, commencing along the superior border of the posterior lamina followed by the remainder of the posterior lamina. The anterior arch is last to mineralize.

As with other cartilages of the larynx, variations of mineralization are commonplace and are likely because of a combination of factors, including nutrition, hormones, mechanical stresses, genetics, gender, and race. For instance, the degree and frequency of mineralization of the cricoid cartilage is often lower in females than in males, similar to thyroid cartilage mineralization. The normal cricoid cartilage can lack mineralization (particularly early in life), can ossify and contain a marrow cavity, or can be incidentally sclerotic.

COMPANION CASES

- **Retained fish bone.** A swallowed fish bone can be retained in any portion of the pharynx and larynx. It will frequently appear as a discrete, linear focus, often with a nonanatomic angulation. However, two regions of focal cricoid cartilage mineralization may simulate a foreign body on lateral radiographs. One is the superior margin of the cricoid lamina (which mineralizes early and may be the only portion of the signet ring that is calcified for a period of time), and the other is vertical mineralization along the posterior margin of the cricoid lamina.
- **Cricoid cartilage chondrosarcoma.** Chondrosarcoma is rarely encountered in the larynx and accounts for less than 1% of all laryngeal tumors; however, approximately three-fourths of these tumors arise from the cricoid cartilage. Laryngeal chondrosarcoma is a relatively low-grade, slow-growing neoplasm. While it poorly responds to chemotherapy and radiation, laryngeal chondrosarcoma is often successfully managed by local excision. The expected 5-year survival rate for patients with low-grade chondrosarcoma is greater than 70%. An important exception is the dedifferentiated chondrosarcoma, a highly aggressive malignancy with a mean patient survival of just 6 months.

  Imaging findings of laryngeal chondrosarcoma on CT include an expansile mass with areas of coarse or stippled calcification that are characteristic of a chondroid matrix. On MRI, a chondrosarcoma will be hypointense to isointense to muscle on T1, diffusely hyperintense on T2 (owing to the water content of the cartilage), and minimally enhance. Areas of matrix mineralization within the tumor will be hypointense on all pulse sequences. Dedifferentiated chondrosarcoma cannot be reliably distinguished from well-differentiated chondrosarcoma, or even a benign chondroma, by imaging alone.
- **Cricoid cartilage sclerosis due to squamous cell carcinoma invasion.** The vast majority of laryngeal cancers are squamous cell carcinomas, owing to the abundant squamous epithelium found throughout the larynx. Most cancers originate in the glottic larynx, followed by primary malignancies of the supraglottis and subglottis, in that order. While staging of laryngeal cancers is beyond the scope of this text, the American Joint Committee on Cancer has designated staging by the TNM classification. Subglottic tumors invading the cricoid or thyroid cartilage constitutes at least a T4a lesion by the TNM classification system. Laryngeal cartilage invaded by tumor may be sclerotic or focally lytic on CT, which are appearances that may also be present with normal laryngeal cartilage. Therefore, it is imperative to evaluate for a mass if focal sclerosis or a suspicious focal lucency involving the laryngeal cartilage is encountered on CT. On MRI, tumor invading ossified laryngeal cartilage will generally lack normal marrow fat on non-fat suppressed T1 and T2-weighted imaging, and it will abnormally enhance following contrast administration.

  Radiation-induced chondronecrosis of the cricoid cartilage. Laryngeal edema, a well-known complication due to perichondritis and impairment of vascular and lymphatic channels, usually develops shortly following radiation treatment and tends to regress over time. A potentially devastating long-term complication of laryngeal radiation is chondronecrosis, which is characterized by demineralization, fragmentation, and collapse of the laryngeal skeleton and/or gas bubbles within the adjacent soft tissues. Chondronecrosis of the larynx is a generally irreversible process that may require laryngectomy due to the potential for life-threatening laryngeal instability.

Nonmineralized cricoid cartilage

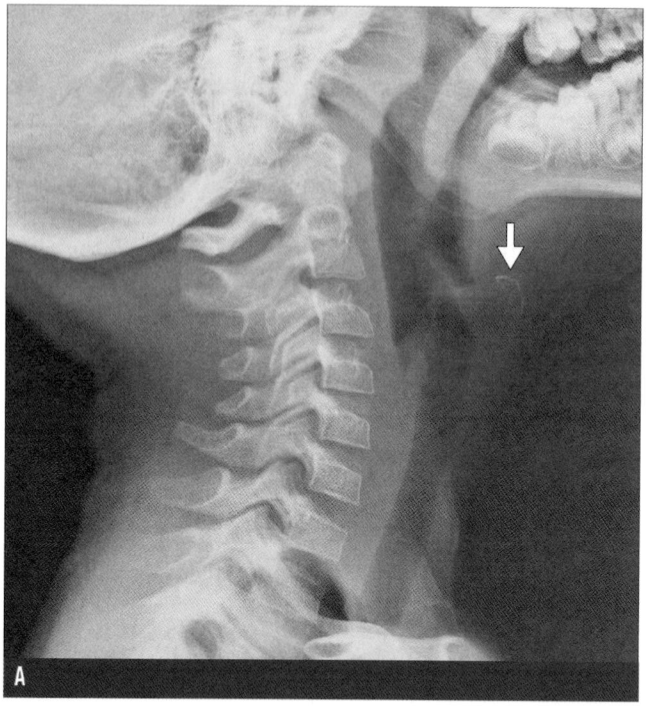

A lateral soft tissue neck radiograph of a 5-year-old boy (**A**) demonstrates a complete lack of cricoid cartilage mineralization. The hyoid bone is at least partially ossified (arrow).

Nonmineralized cricoid cartilage

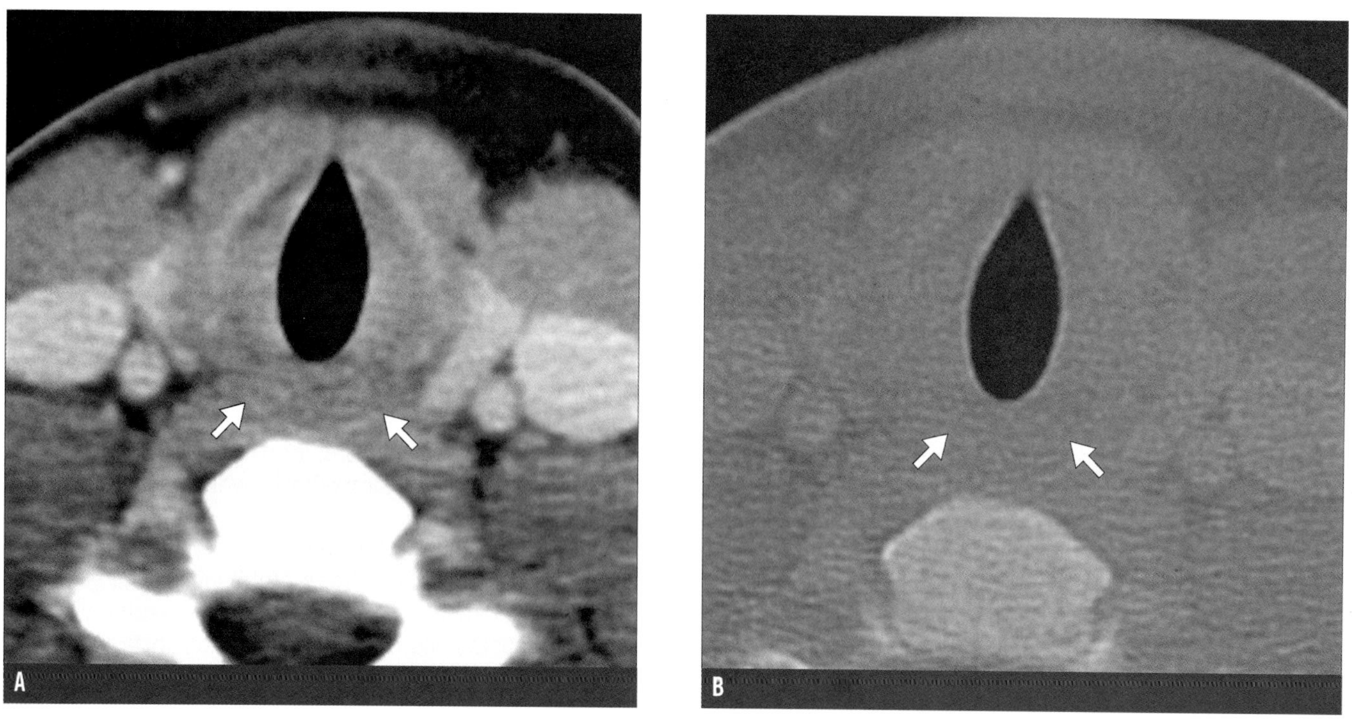

Different patient. Contrast-enhanced axial CT images viewed with a soft tissue window (**A**) and bone window (**B**) of a 19-year-old patient demonstrate absent mineralization at the expected location of the cricoid cartilage (arrows, **A**, **B**).

Small amount of cricoid cartilage mineralization

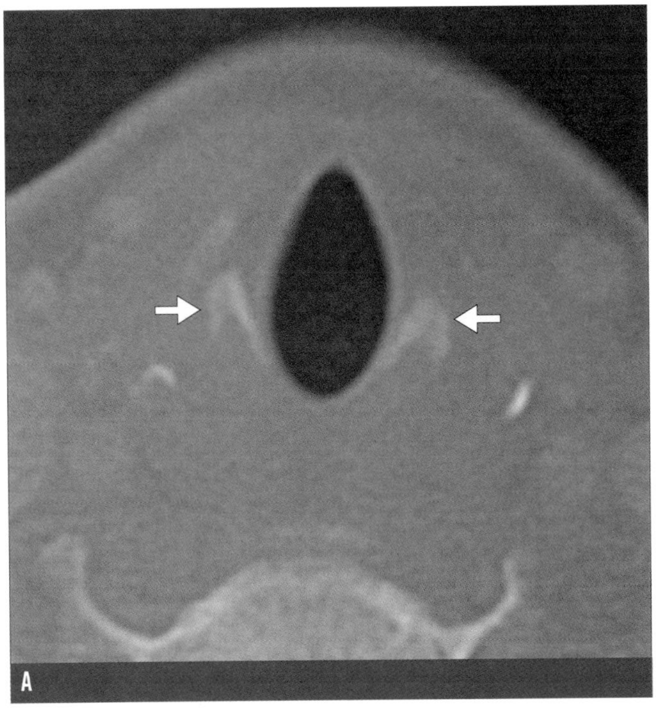

An axial CT image (**A**) demonstrates a small amount of cricoid cartilage mineralization in this 37-year-old female (arrows).

Moderate amount of cricoid cartilage ossification

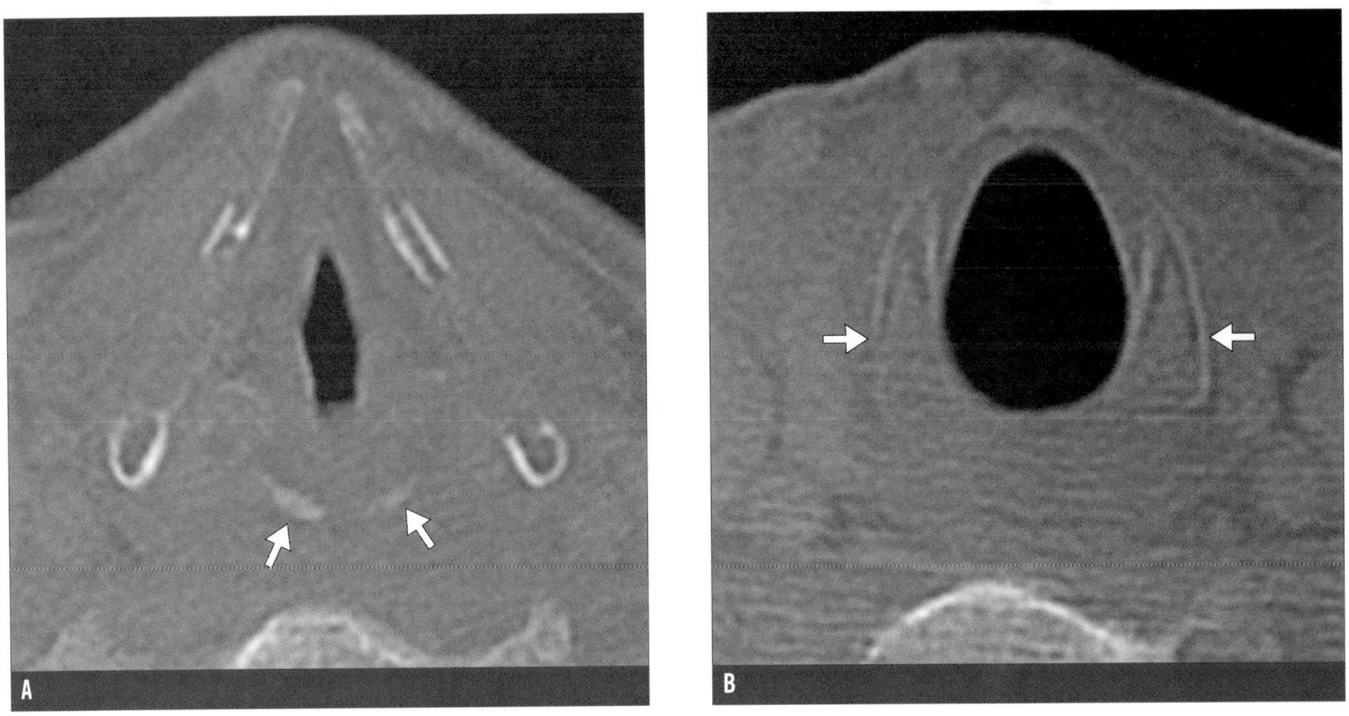

Axial CT images (**A**, **B**) demonstrate an overall moderate amount of cricoid cartilage ossification in this 60-year-old patient (arrows, **A**, **B**).

Fully ossified cricoid cartilage

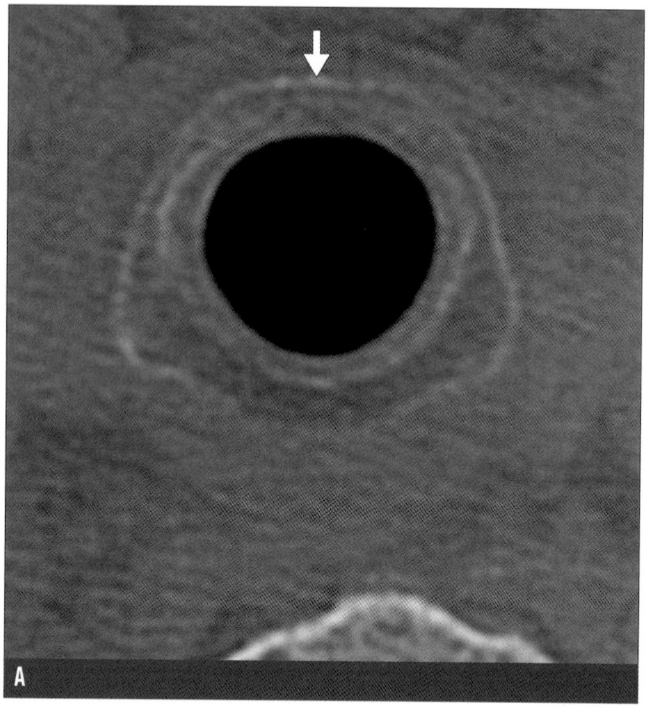

An axial CT image (**A**) demonstrates a fully ossified cricoid, including the anterior arch of the cricoid (arrow).

Focal mineralization of the cricoid cartilage

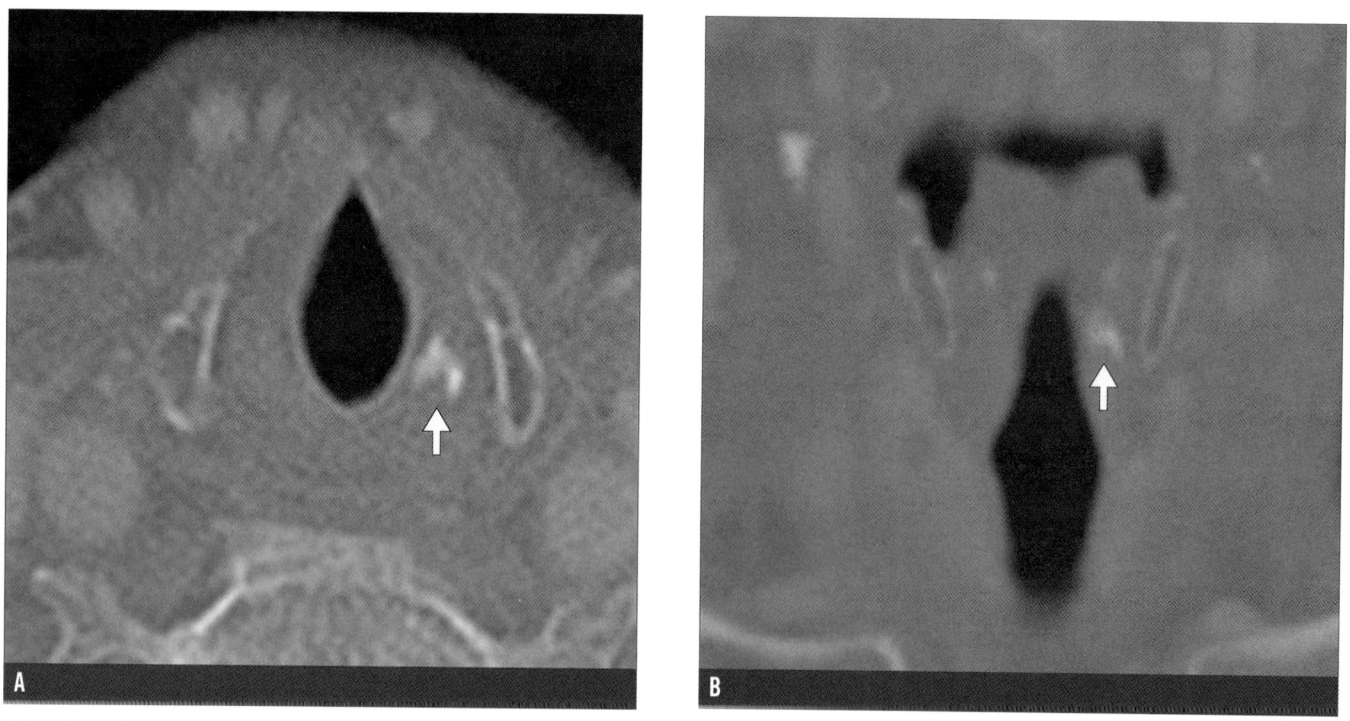

Axial (**A**) and coronal reformatted (**B**) CT images demonstrate a small focal area of ossification along the left aspect of the cricoid cartilage in this 85-year-old woman (arrows, **A**, **B**).

Focal mineralization of the cricoid cartilage

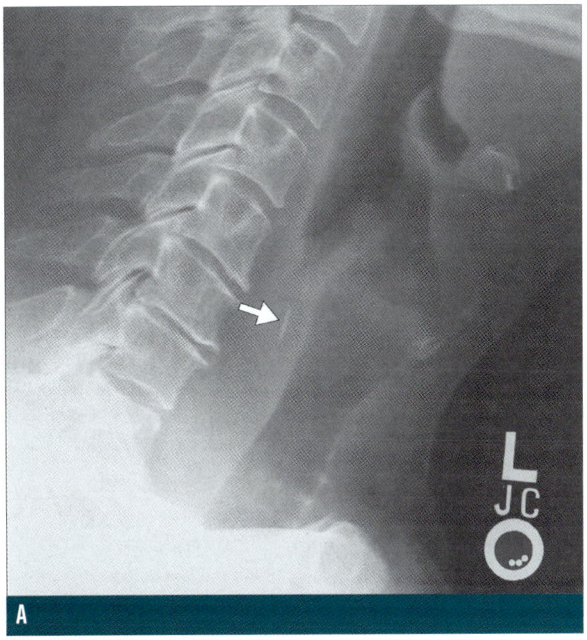

Different patient. A lateral soft tissue neck radiograph of a 54-year-old man with concern of a swallowed chicken bone impacted in the pharynx (**A**) demonstrates a vertically oriented focus of ossification anterior to C5-C6 (arrow). The patient underwent a direct laryngoscopy and cervical esophagoscopy, both of which were negative for a foreign body. The finding in this case represents normal, vertically oriented mineralization along the posterior margin of the cricoid cartilage.

Companion case: Retained fish bone

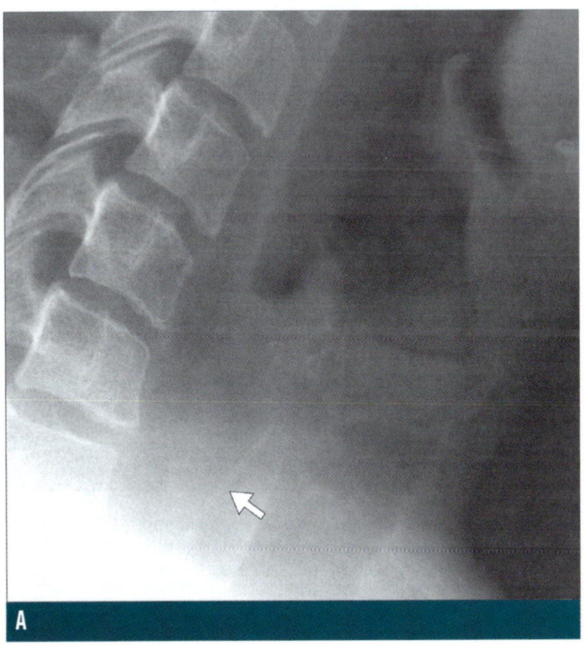

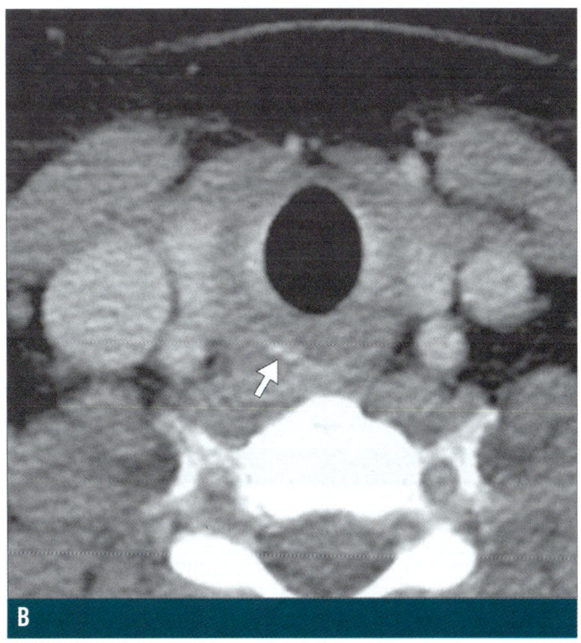

A lateral soft tissue neck radiograph (**A**) demonstrates a subtle, linear, vertically oblique oriented hyperdensity, located posterior to the trachea and inferior to the laryngeal apparatus (arrow, **A**). Contrast-enhanced axial (**B**) and coronal reformatted (**C**) CT images demonstrate the finding to be located in the proximal esophagus (arrows, **B**, **C**). Per the patient's history, this finding represented a retained fish bone.

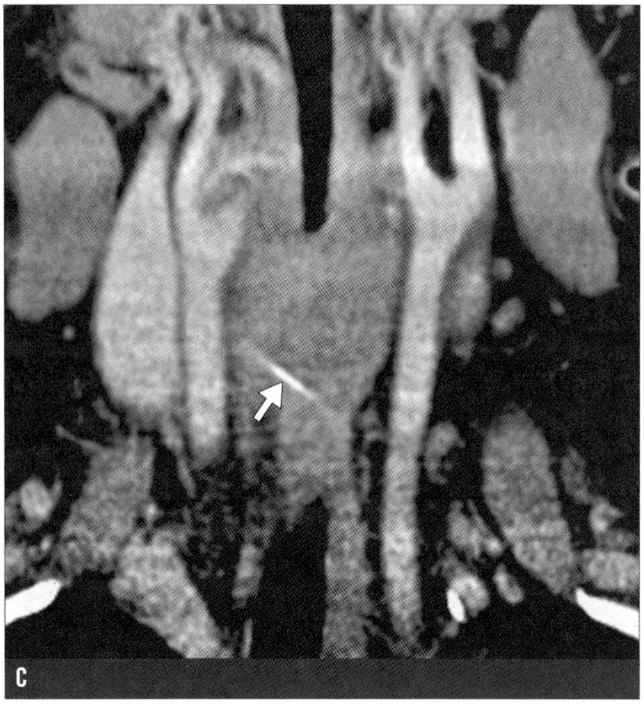

Companion case: Cricoid cartilage chondrosarcoma

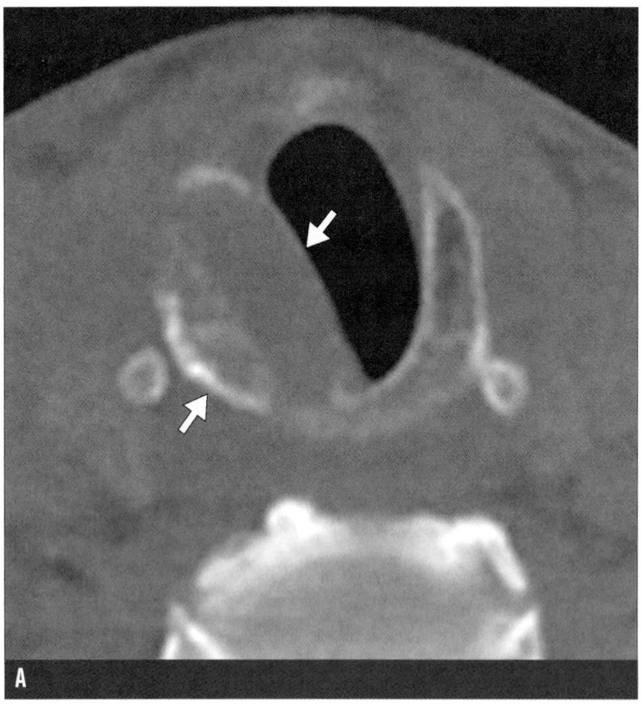

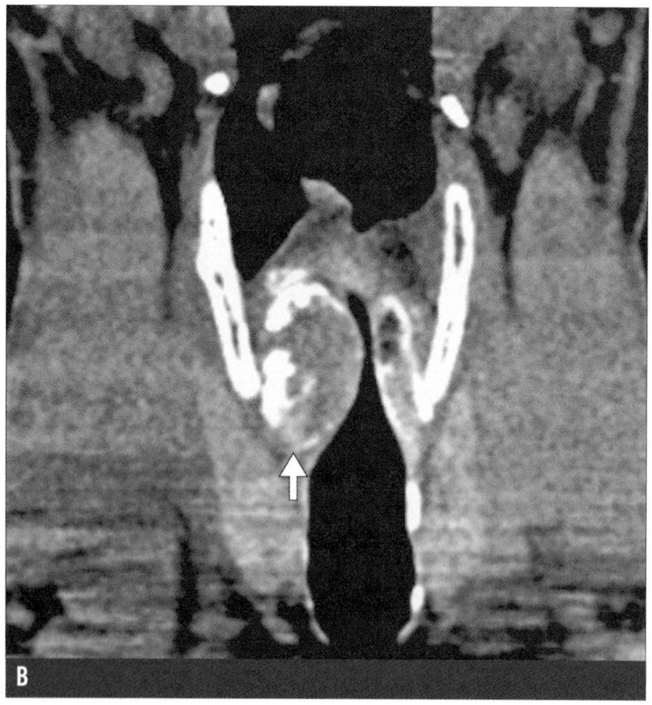

An unenhanced axial CT image viewed with a bone window (**A**) as well as a coronal reformatted CT image viewed with a soft tissue window (**B**) in a 51-year-old patient. The images demonstrate an abnormally expanded cricoid cartilage along its right posterolateral aspect that contains both soft tissue density and sclerosis (arrows, **A**, **B**). A cartilage matrix within the soft tissue component is subtly demonstrated on image **B**. Axial T1 (**C**), contrast-enhanced fat suppressed axial T1 (**D**), and fat suppressed axial T2 (**E**) MR images of the same patient demonstrate the mass to be T1 isointense (arrow, **C**), mildly enhancing (arrow, **D**), and T2 hyperintense (arrow, **E**). There is also loss of the normal marrow signal within an affected portion of the cricoid (arrowhead, **C**). The findings suggest a primary cricoid tumor, such as chondrosarcoma, which was confirmed at pathology.

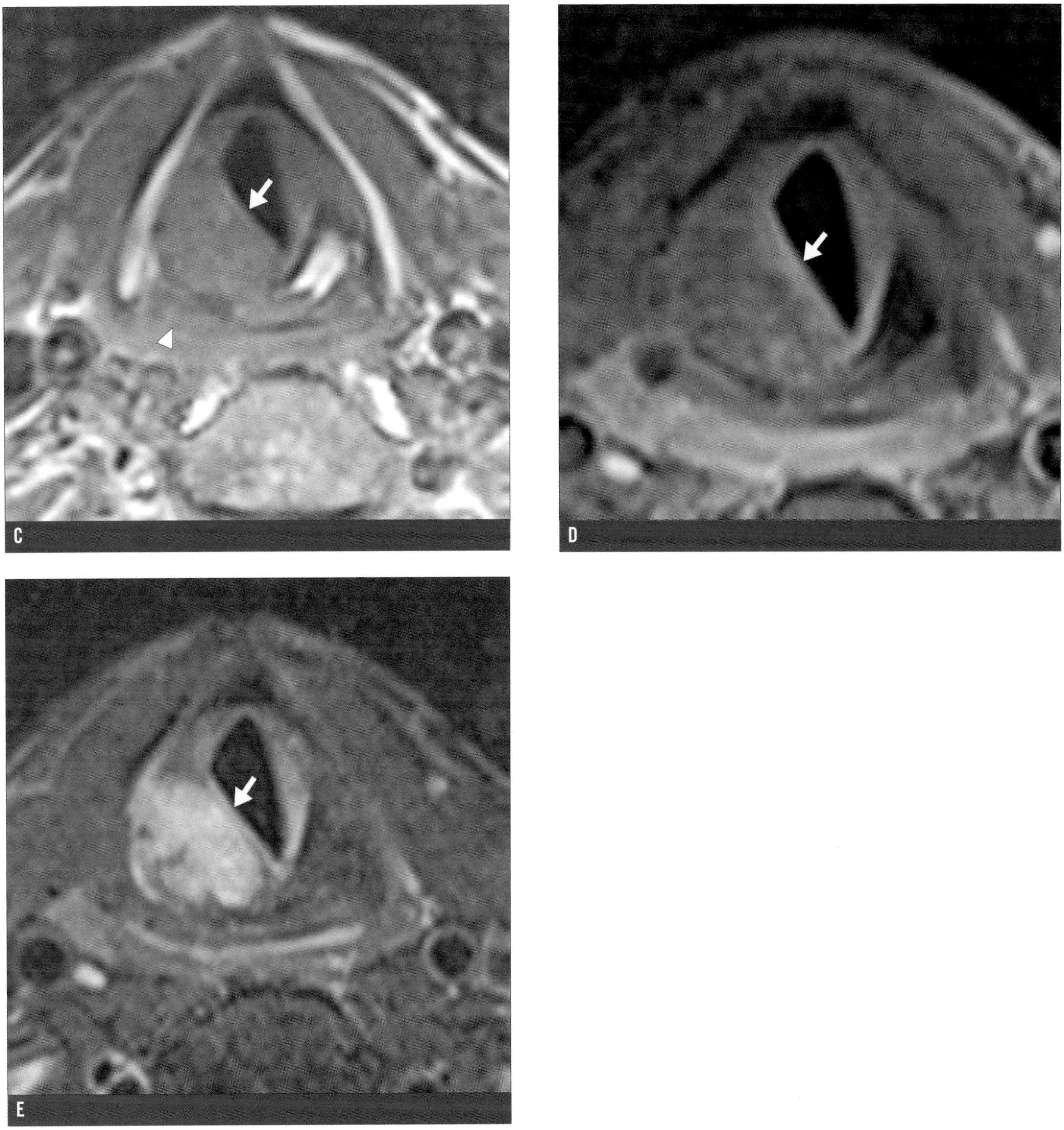
C
D
E

Companion case: Cricoid cartilage sclerosis due to squamous cell carcinoma invasion

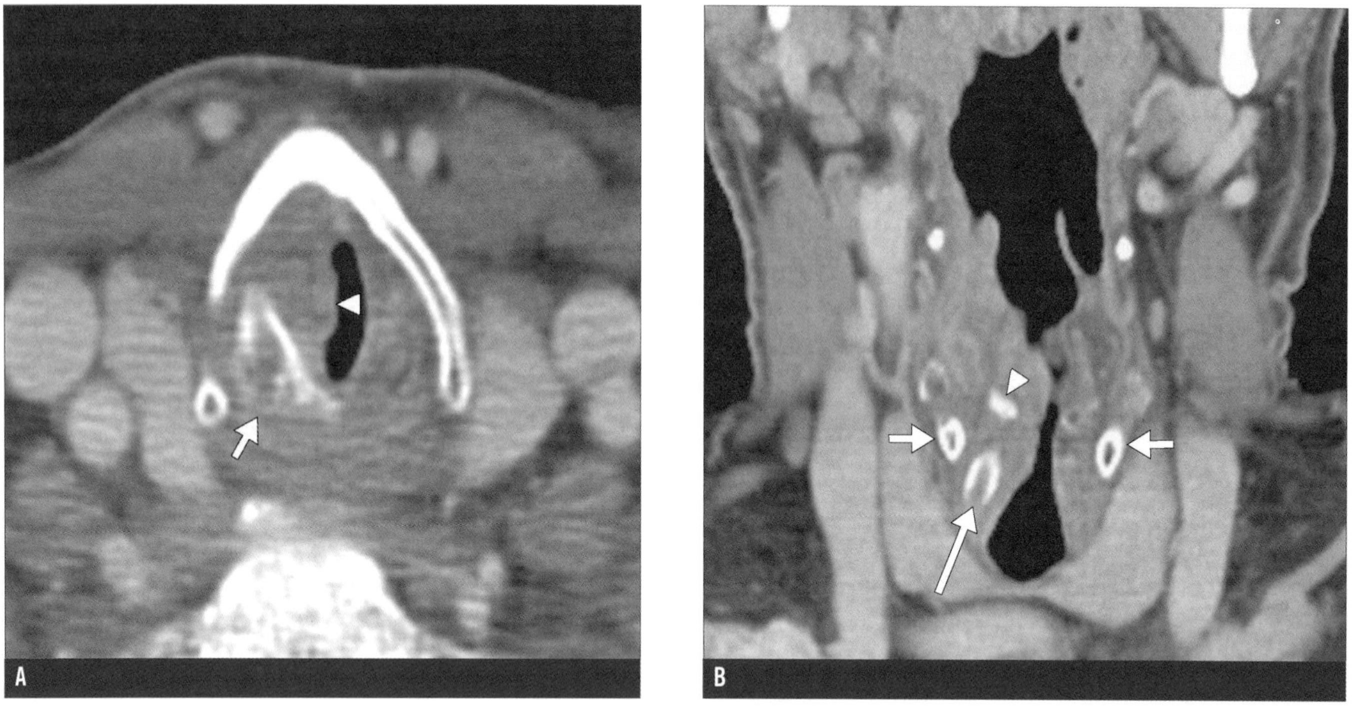

Contrast-enhanced axial CT image (**A**) demonstrates asymmetric sclerosis of the right aspect of the cricoid (short arrow, **A**) due to a squamous cell carcinoma of the right TVC that extends into the subglottic larynx (arrowhead, **A**). A coronal reformatted CT image (**B**) demonstrates the sclerotic portion of the cricoid (long arrow, **B**) as well as sclerosis of the right arytenoid cartilage (arrowhead, **B**). The sclerosis of these structures is compatible with tumor invasion, given the presence of an adjacent soft tissue mass. The thyroid laminae are also present on this image (short arrows, **B**).

Companion case: Radiation-induced chondronecrosis of the cricoid cartilage

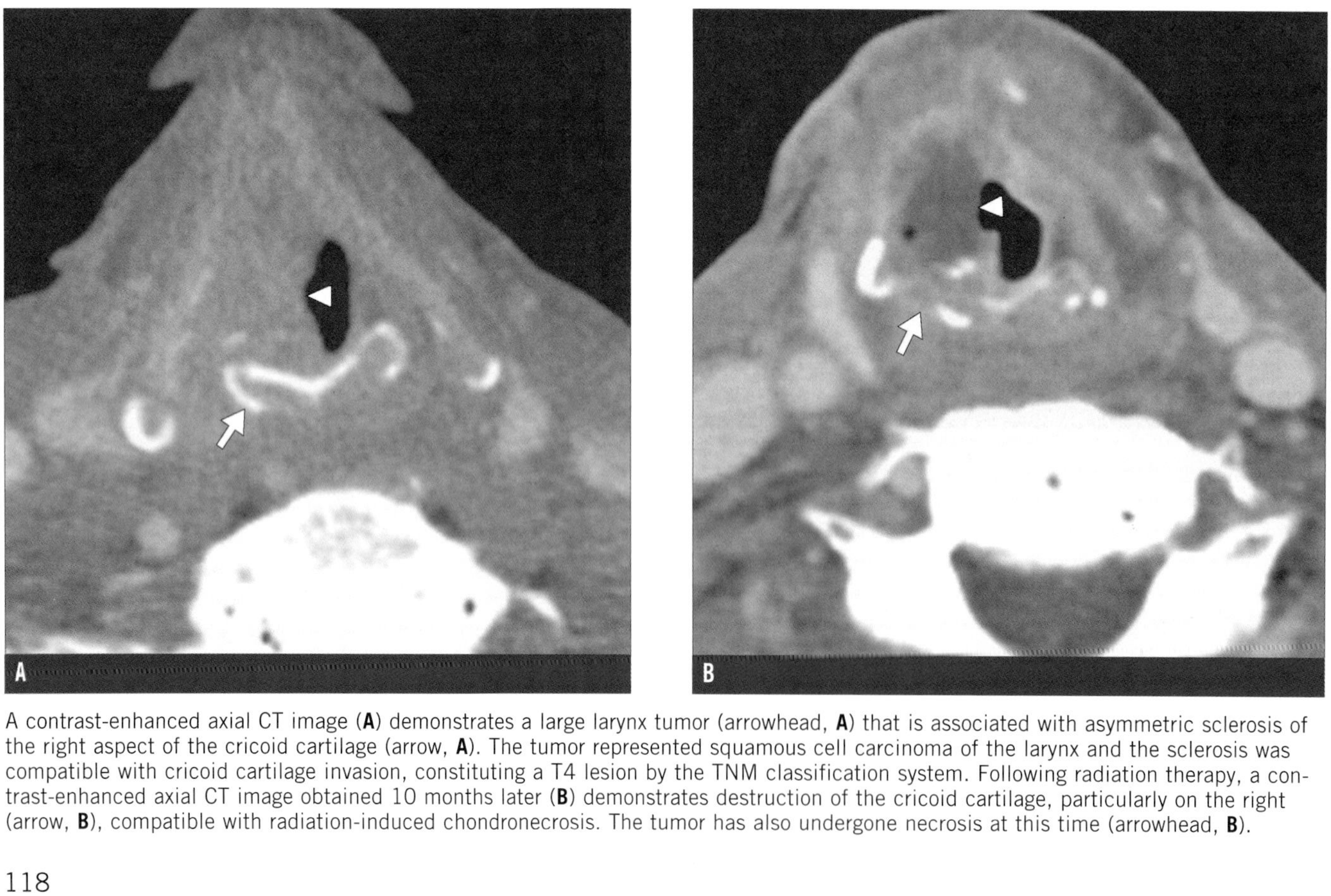

A contrast-enhanced axial CT image (**A**) demonstrates a large larynx tumor (arrowhead, **A**) that is associated with asymmetric sclerosis of the right aspect of the cricoid cartilage (arrow, **A**). The tumor represented squamous cell carcinoma of the larynx and the sclerosis was compatible with cricoid cartilage invasion, constituting a T4 lesion by the TNM classification system. Following radiation therapy, a contrast-enhanced axial CT image obtained 10 months later (**B**) demonstrates destruction of the cricoid cartilage, particularly on the right (arrow, **B**), compatible with radiation-induced chondronecrosis. The tumor has also undergone necrosis at this time (arrowhead, **B**).

REFERENCES

de la Grandmaison GL, Banasr A, Durigon M. Age estimation using radiographic analysis of laryngeal cartilage. *Am J Forensic Med Pathol.* 2003;24:96-99.

Drake RL, Gray H. *Gray's atlas of anatomy.* 1st ed. Philadelphia, PA: Churchill Livingstone; 2008.

Fatterpekar GM, Mukherji SK, Rajgopalan P, Lin Y, Castillo M. Normal age-related signal change in the laryngeal cartilages. *Neuroradiology.* 2004;46:678-681.

Garvin HM. Ossification of laryngeal structures as indicators of age. *J Forensic Sci.* 2008;53:1023-1027.

Hermans R[1], Pameijer FA, Mancuso AA, Parsons JT, Mendenhall WM. CT findings in chondroradionecrosis of the larynx. *AJNR Am J Neuroradiol.* 1998 Apr;19(4):711-718.

Marioni G, Marchese-Ragona R, Cartei G, Marchese F, Staffieri A. Current opinion in diagnosis and treatment of laryngeal carcinoma. *Cancer Treat Rev.* 2006;32:504-515.

Mupparapu M, Vuppalapati A. Ossification of laryngeal cartilages on lateral cephalometric radiographs. *Angle Orthod.* 2005;75:196-201.

Murphey MD1, Walker EA, Wilson AJ, Kransdorf MJ, Temple HT, Gannon FH. From the archives of the AFIP: imaging of primary chondrosarcoma: radiologic-pathologic correlation. *Radiographics.* 2003 Sep-Oct;23(5):1245-1278.

Sakai O, Curtin HD, Faquin WC, Fabian RL. Dedifferentiated chondrosarcoma of the larynx. *AJNR Am J Neuroradiol.* 2000;21:584-586.

CASE 6 Variations of arytenoid cartilage mineralization

Located superior to the cricoid cartilage, the arytenoid cartilages are paired, pyramidal-shaped hyaline cartilages to which the TVCs, vocal ligaments, and numerous skeletal muscles attach. Each cartilage consists of three surfaces (posterior, antero-lateral, medial), a base, and an apex. The base of each arytenoid articulates with the cricoid cartilage (cricoarytenoid joint), whereas small cartilaginous structures termed the corniculate cartilages are situated atop the arytenoid cartilages.

Like other portions of the laryngeal cartilage apparatus, ossification of the arytenoid cartilages undergoes progressive endochondral ossification with age. Also like other portions of the laryngeal cartilage apparatus, there is a relationship between the ossification patterns and the distribution of mechanical forces applied to the cartilages. Ossification of the arytenoid cartilages tends to initially occur along their lateral one-third (the site where the lateral and posterior cricoarytenoid muscles attach) and progresses toward the center of the cartilage with age. Studies have demonstrated an increased incidence of normal arytenoid sclerosis in women relative to men, and when unilateral, the left arytenoid cartilage is more affected than the right. Despite these trends, normal arytenoid mineralization, ossification, or sclerosis are common in both genders. If asymmetric arytenoid mineralization, or for that matter focal mineralization of any of the laryngeal cartilages is identified, then careful evaluation of the mucosal surfaces and submucosa of the larynx is warranted to exclude a tumor resulting in the focal mineralization. Conversely, the mere presence of asymmetric arytenoid cartilage mineralization should not be misinterpreted as tumor invasion if there is no history or evidence of tumor adjacent to the arytenoid cartilage.

COMPANION CASE

- **Arytenoid cartilage sclerosis due to squamous cell carcinoma invasion.** Squamous cell carcinoma is overwhelmingly the most common laryngeal malignancy and thus is the most common malignancy that can invade the arytenoid cartilage. CT criteria suggesting neoplastic arytenoid invasion include sclerosis, cartilage erosion/lysis, extralaryngeal tumor completely encasing the arytenoid, and obliteration of the medullary space.

Nonmineralized arytenoid cartilages

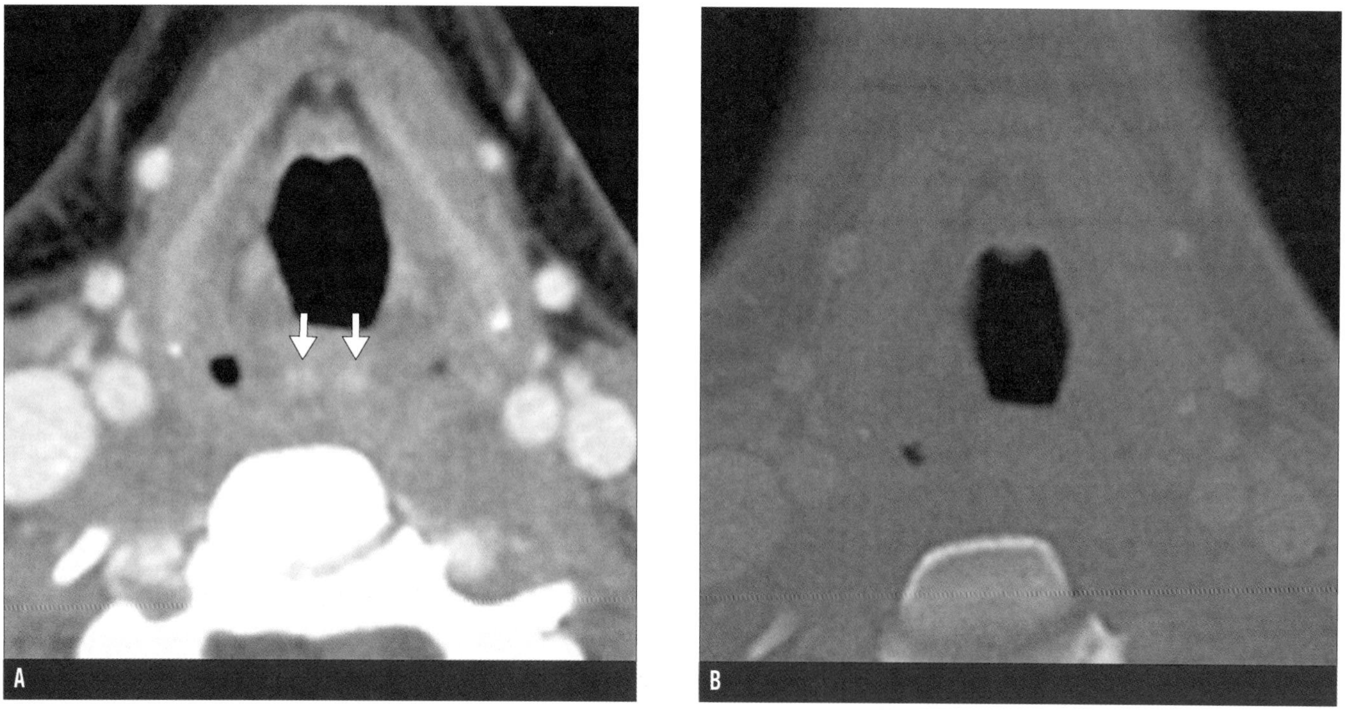

Contrast-enhanced axial CT images viewed with a soft tissue window (**A**) and bone window (**B**) demonstrate nonmineralized bilateral arytenoid cartilages in a 38-year-old female (arrows, **A**).

Ossification of both arytenoid cartilages

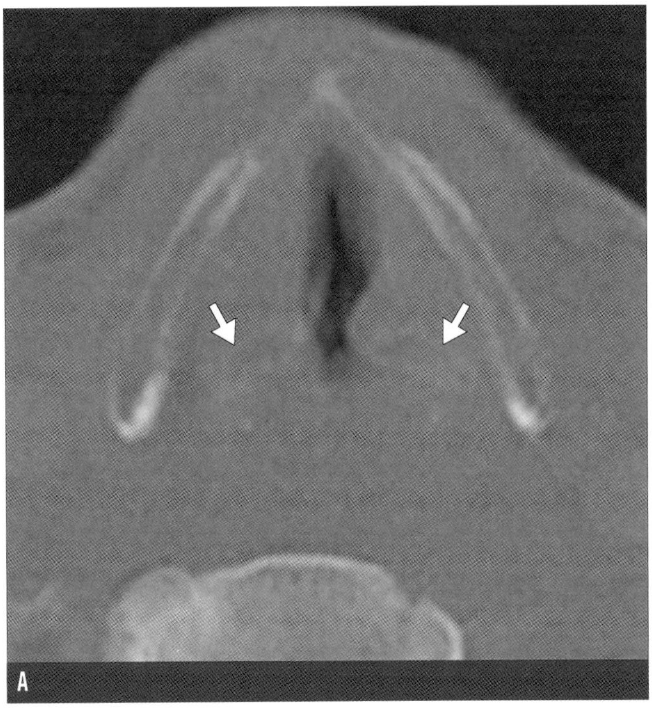
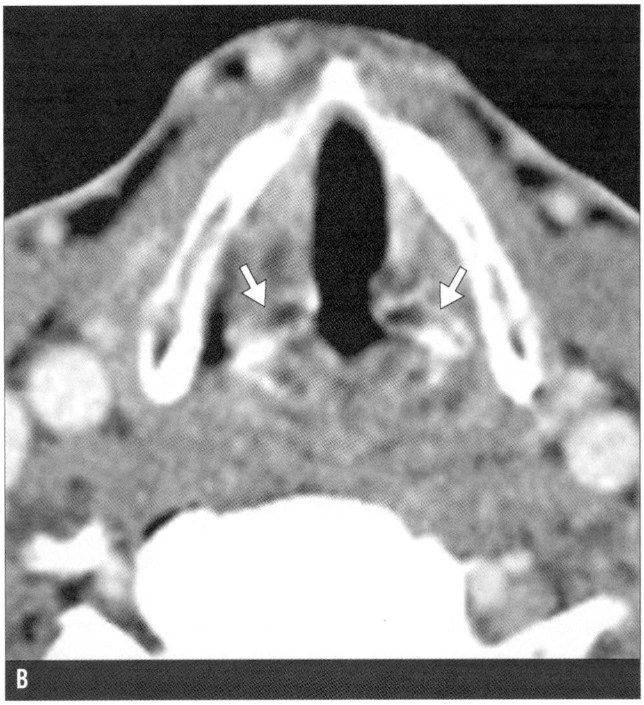

Contrast-enhanced axial CT images viewed with a bone window (**A**) and soft tissue window (**B**) demonstrate normal ossification of both arytenoid cartilages (arrows, **A**, **B**).

Unilateral arytenoid cartilage sclerosis

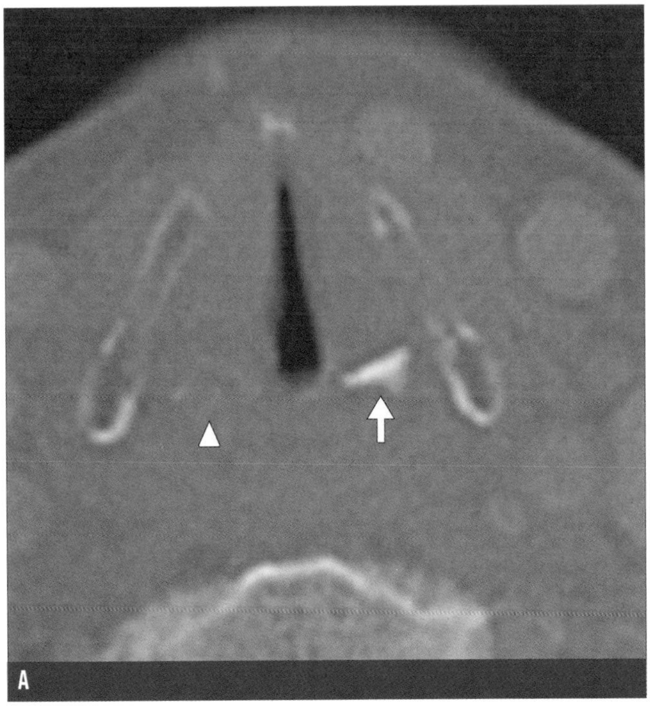
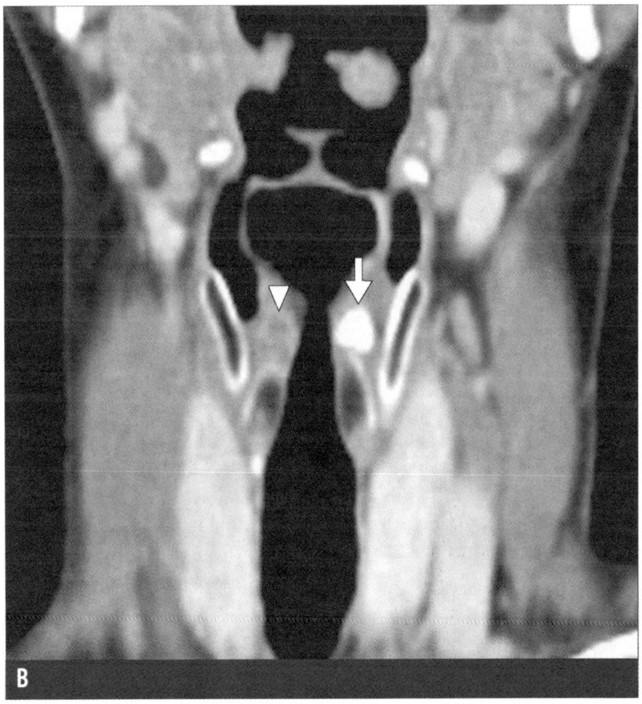

A contrast-enhanced axial CT image viewed with a bone window (**A**) and a coronal reformatted CT image viewed with a soft tissue window (**B**) demonstrate dense sclerosis of the left arytenoid cartilage (arrows, **A**, **B**), an incidental finding in this case. There is only mild mineralization of the right arytenoid cartilage (arrowheads, **A**, **B**).

Bilateral arytenoid cartilage sclerosis

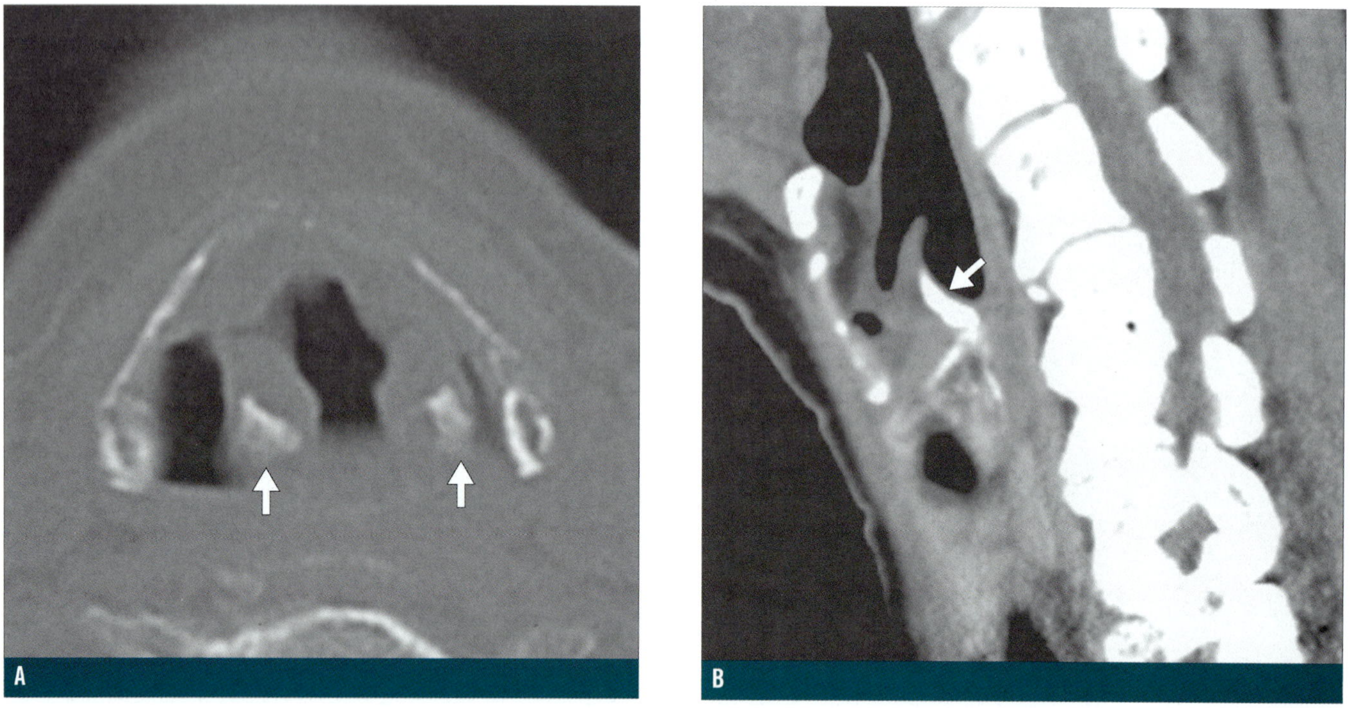

An axial CT image viewed with a bone window (**A**) demonstrates incidental dense sclerosis of both arytenoid cartilages (arrows, **A**). A coronal reformatted CT image viewed with a soft tissue window (**B**) demonstrates one of the sclerotic arytenoid cartilages in the sagittal plane (arrow, **B**).

Companion case: Arytenoid cartilage sclerosis due to squamous cell carcinoma invasion

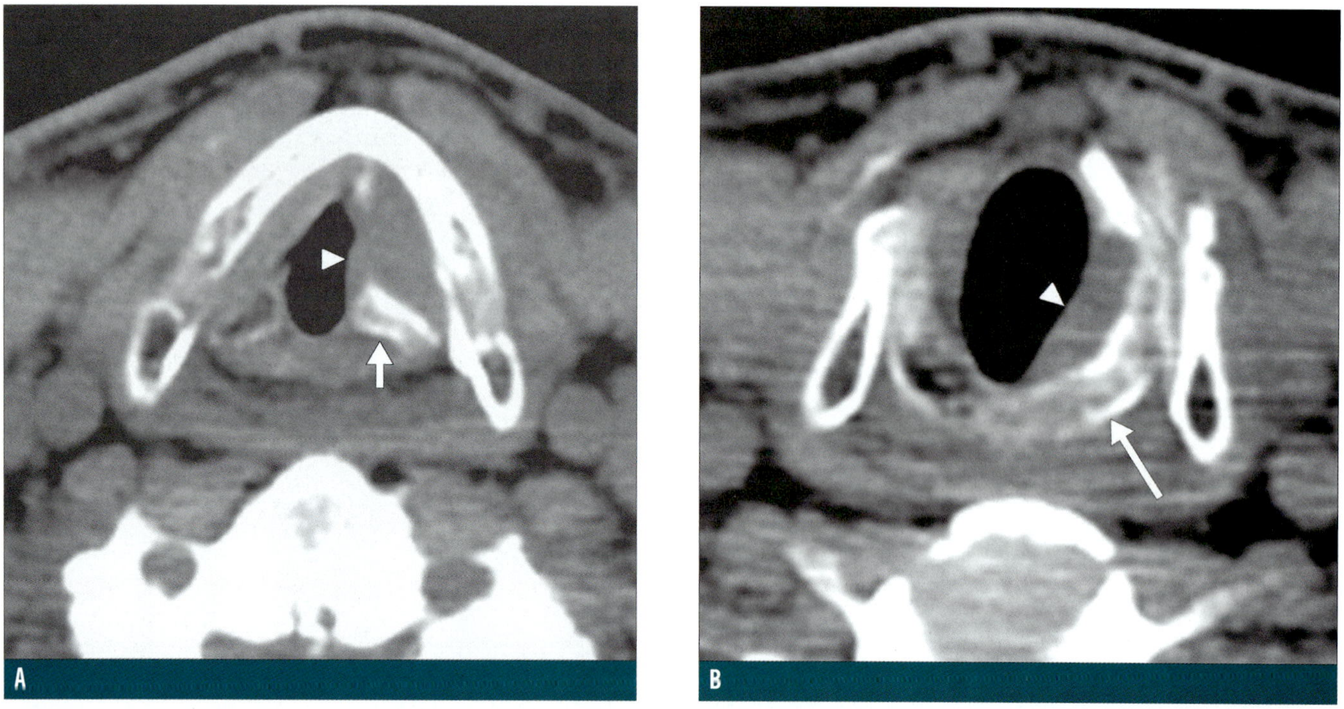

Noncontrast axial CT images (**A**, **B**) demonstrate a soft tissue mass, representing squamous cell carcinoma, arising from the left TVC (arrowhead, **A**) and extending into the subglottic larynx (arrowhead, **B**). There is focal sclerosis of the left arytenoid cartilage (short arrow, **A**) as well as the posterolateral left aspect of the cricoid cartilage (long arrow, **B**). Given the proximity of the malignancy and the focality of the areas of cartilaginous sclerosis, the areas of cartilaginous sclerosis are compatible with tumor infiltration and a T4 tumor grade by the TNM classification system.

REFERENCES

Becker M, Zbaren P, Casselman JW, Kohler R, Dulguerov P, Becker CD. Neoplastic invasion of laryngeal cartilage: reassessment of criteria for diagnosis at MR imaging. *Radiology.* 2008;249:551-559.

Becker M, Zbaren P, Laeng H, Stoupis C, Porcellini B, Vock P. Neoplastic invasion of the laryngeal cartilage: comparison of MR imaging and CT with histopathologic correlation. *Radiology.* 1995;194:661-669.

de la Grandmaison GL, Banasr A, Durigon M. Age estimation using radiographic analysis of laryngeal cartilage. *Am J Forensic Med Pathol.* 2003;24:96-99.

Drake RL, Gray H. *Gray's Atlas of Anatomy.* 1st ed. Philadelphia, PA: Churchill Livingstone; 2008.

Fatterpekar GM, Mukherji SK, Rajgopalan P, Lin Y, Castillo M. Normal age-related signal change in the laryngeal cartilages. *Neuroradiology.* 2004;46:678-681.

Garvin HM. Ossification of laryngeal structures as indicators of age. *J Forensic Sci.* 2008;53:1023-1027.

Hatley W, Samuel E, Evison G. The pattern of ossification in the laryngeal cartilages: a radiological study. *Bri J Radiol.* 1965;38:585-591.

Muñoz A, et al. Laryngeal carcinoma: sclerotic appearance of the cricoid and arytenoid cartilage—CT-pathologic correlation. *Radiology.* 1993;189:433-437.

Schmalfuss IM, Mancuso AA, Tart RP. Arytenoid cartilage sclerosis: normal variations and clinical significance. *AJNR Am J Neuroradiol.* 1998;19:719-722.

Zan E, Yousem DM, Aygun N. Asymmetric mineralization of the arytenoid cartilages in patients without laryngeal cancer. *AJNR Am J Neuroradiol.* 2011;32:1113-1118.

CASE 7 Mineralized epiglottis

The epiglottis, a cartilaginous projection attached to the entrance of the larynx, serves to cover the glottis during swallowing, preventing food from entering the trachea and instead directing it toward the posteriorly located esophagus. The epiglottis is vertically oriented during breathing and folds posteriorly to a horizontal position during deglutition. While the epiglottis is considered to represent a portion of the supraglottic larynx, some consider its ventral margin (ie, lingual surface), in addition to the vallecula, to represent a portion of the oropharynx. The epiglottis is subdivided into a suprahyoid portion (free upper margin) and an infrahyoid portion (lower fixed portion), which are subdivided by the hyoepiglottic ligament. The hyoepiglottic ligament attaches the ventral margin of the epiglottis to the superior margin of the hyoid body. Whereas the free upper margin has a leaf-like configuration, the inferior epiglottis tapers to a fixed short stalk, termed the petiole, to which the thyroepiglottic ligament joins. The thyroepiglottic ligament attaches the petiole to the inner margin of laryngeal prominence, just caudal to the superior thyroid notch. Additionally, the epiglottis is attached to the root of the tongue at the anterior midline via the median glossoepiglottic fold. Relationships to adjacent structures also include lateral attachments to the pharynx via the pharyngoepiglottic folds and inferior attachments to the arytenoid cartilages via the aryepiglottic folds.

The epiglottis is somewhat unique in that it is composed of elastic cartilage. This type of cartilage is found in only a few structures in the human body, including the external ear, eustachian tube, the vocal process of the arytenoid cartilage, and bronchiolar cartilages. In contrast to hyaline cartilage, mineralization of elastic cartilage has been described as rare and usually the sequela of granulomatous infection, trauma, or radiation therapy. However, it is likely that mineralization of the epiglottis is more common than previously reported. When present, it is most frequently encountered in elderly patients and likely represents senescent mineralization. It may also be identified in patient's with altered calcium and phosphorus metabolism, such as with end-stage renal failure. Epiglottic mineralization may involve any or all portions of the epiglottic leaflet and petiole. Occasionally, a focal area of epiglottic mineralization may simulate a foreign body such as a retained fish bone.

COMPANION CASE

- **Residual barium contrast layering along the epiglottis.** Barium coating of the epiglottis can be distinguished from epiglottic mineralization by evaluating the location of the increased attenuation. Specifically, barium will be located on the mucosal surface of the epiglottis, whereas mineralization will be within the substance of the epiglottis.

Mineralized epiglottis

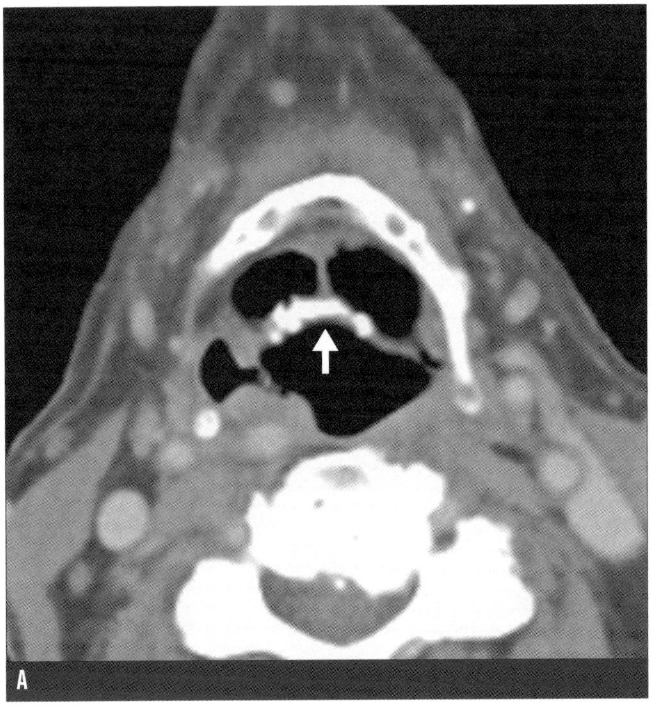

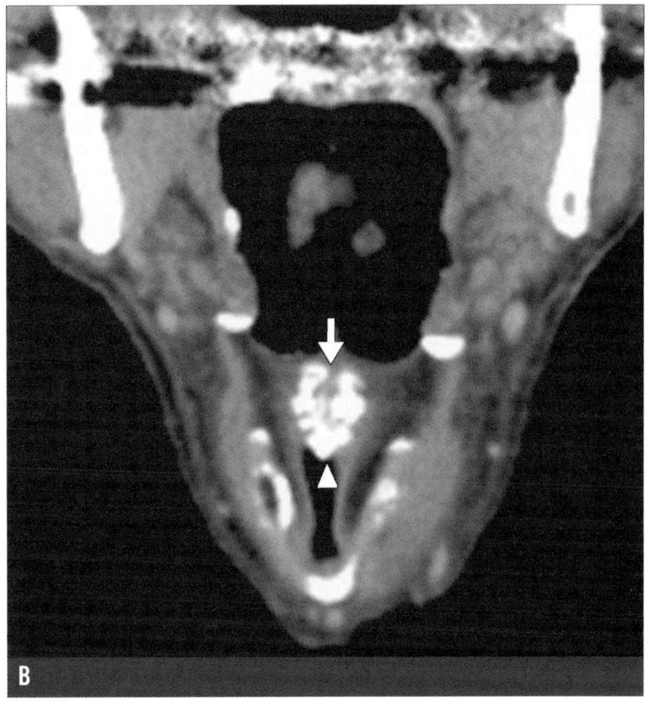

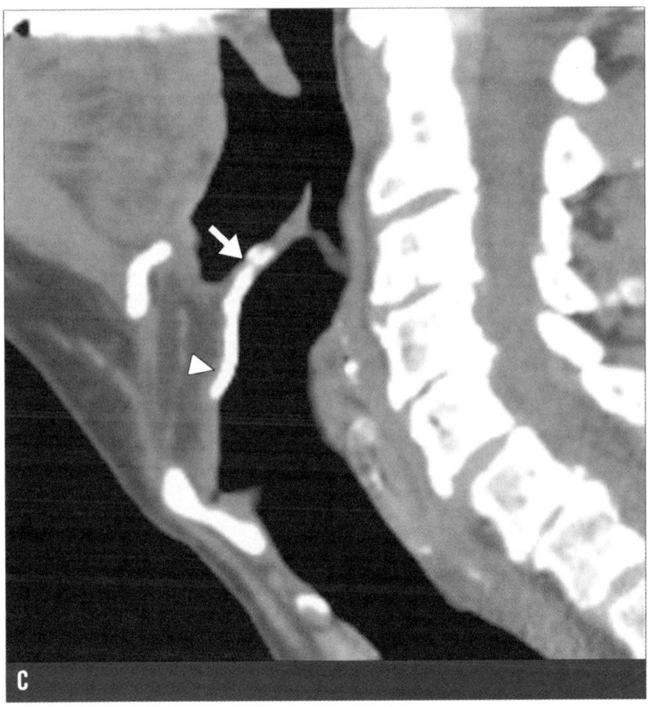

Contrast-enhanced axial (**A**), coronal reformatted (**B**), and sagittal reformatted (**C**) CT images demonstrate dense mineralization of a portion of the epiglottic leaflet (arrows, **A-C**) and the epiglottic petiole (arrowheads, **B**, **C**). This is an incidental, most likely senescent finding in this 88-year-old patient.

Focal mineralization of the epiglottic petiole

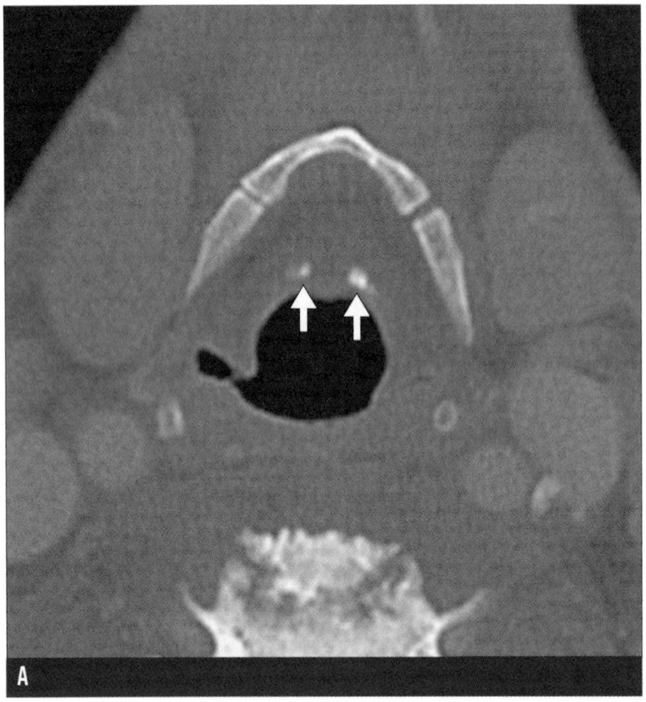

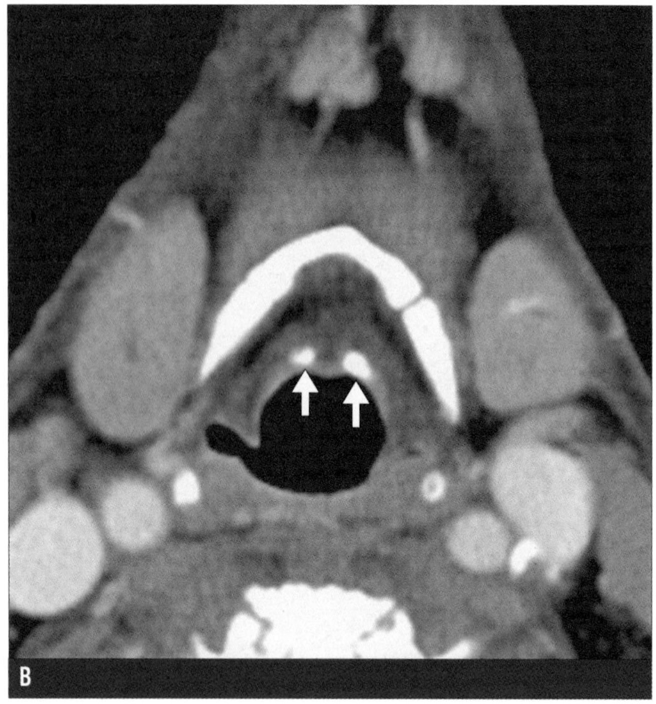

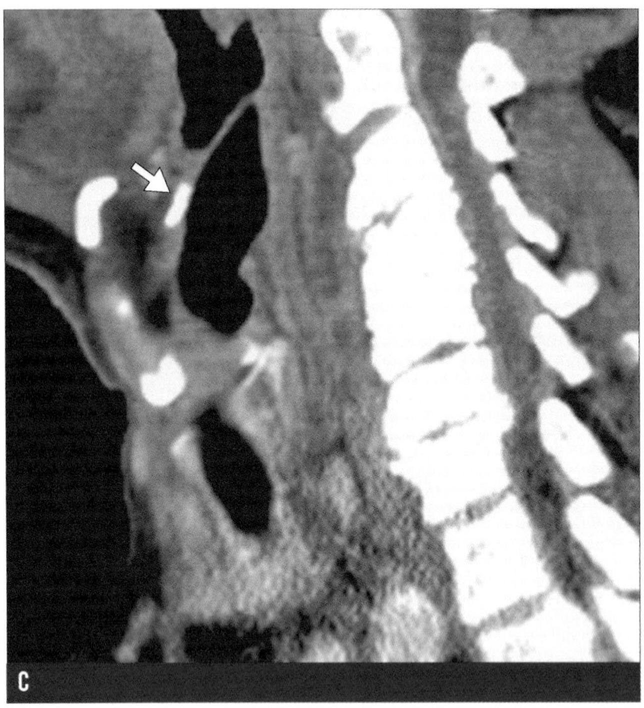

Contrast-enhanced axial CT images viewed with a bone (**A**) and soft tissue (**B**) window as well as a sagittal reformatted image viewed with a soft tissue window (**C**) demonstrate focal mineralization along the lateral margins of the epiglottic petiole (arrows, **A**-**C**). This was a 49-year-old patient with end-stage renal disease.

Companion case: Residual barium contrast layering along the epiglottis

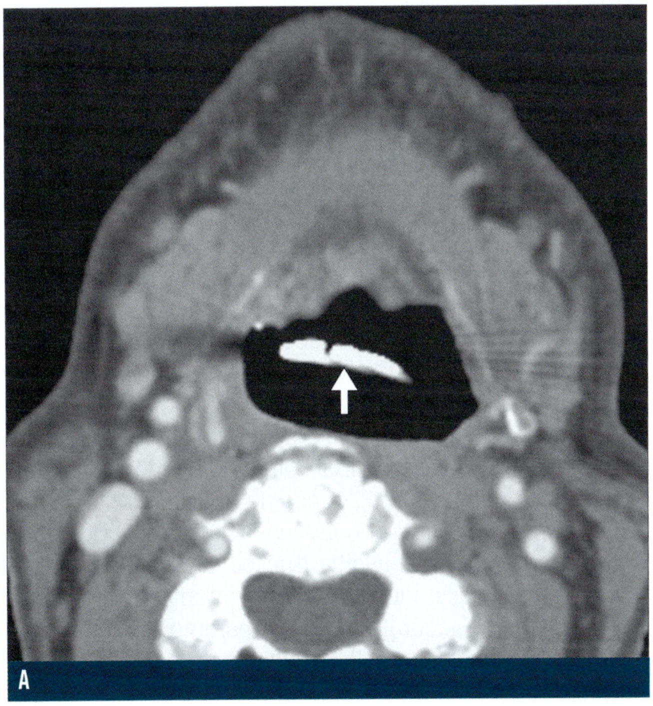

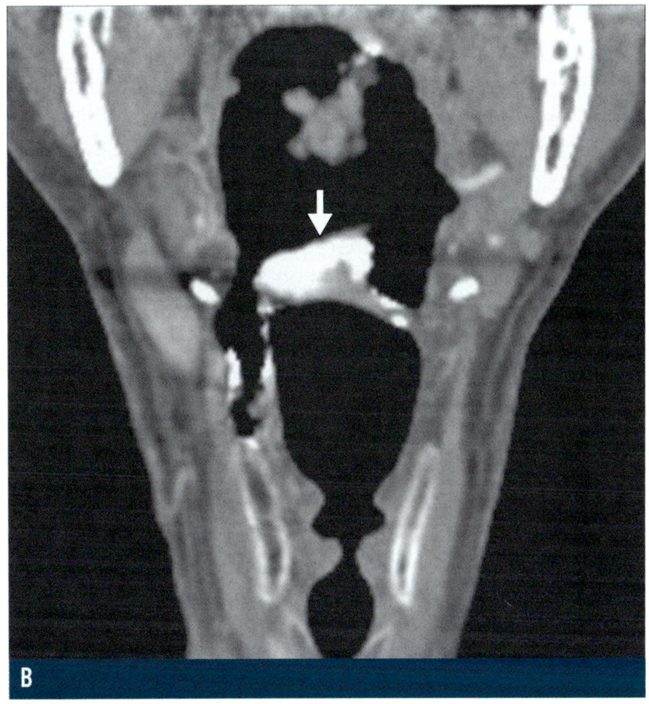

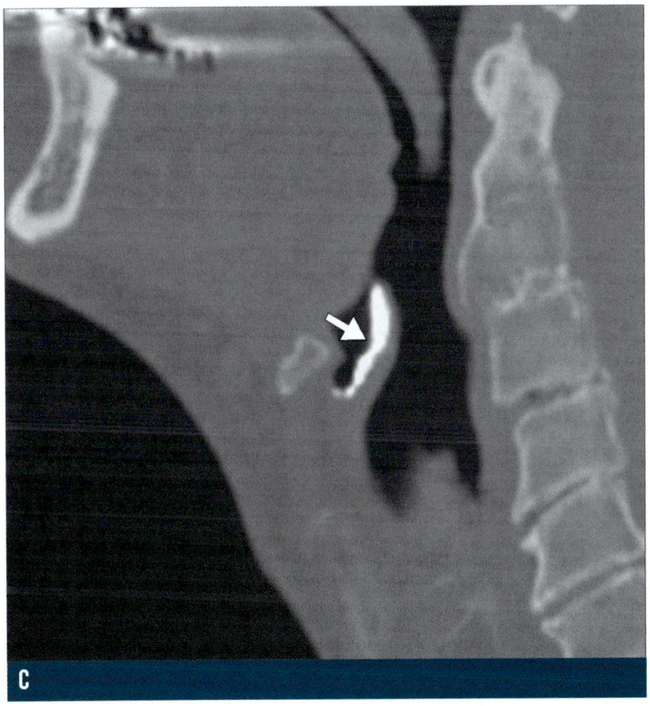

Contrast-enhanced axial (**A**) and coronal reformatted (**B**) CT images viewed with a soft tissue window as well as a sagittal reformatted CT image viewed with a bone window (**C**) demonstrate high density along the epiglottis (arrows, **A-C**). Image **C** best demonstrates that the finding is located along the ventral (ie, lingual) surface of the epiglottis, rather than within the substance of the epiglottis, as would be expected with epiglottic mineralization. This high density represented residual barium contrast from an immediately preceding esophagram study.

REFERENCES

Amis TC, O'Neill N, Somma ED, Wheatley JR. Epiglottic movements during breathing in humans. *J Physiol.* 1998;512:307-314.

Ardran GM. Calcification of the Epiglottis. *Bri J Radiol.* 1965;38:592-595.

Fernández-Rodríguez A, Benito-Orejas JI, Jiménez-Pérez AE, Morais-Pérez D. Calcification of the epiglottis. *Acta Otorrinolaringol Esp. May-June* 2009;60(3):215-216.

Kano M, Shimizu Y, Okayama K, Igari T, Kikuchi M. A morphometric study of age-related changes in adult human epiglottis using quantitative digital analysis of cartilage calcification. *Cells Tissues Organs.* 2005;180:126-137.

Som PM, Curtin HD. *Head and Neck Imaging.* 5th ed. St. Louis, MO: Elsevier Mosby; 2011.

CASE 8 Radiation-induced epiglottic edema

While radiation therapy is a useful adjunct treatment for many head and neck malignancies, there are clinically important acute and long-term complications that may occur following treatment. The laryngeal apparatus, which includes the epiglottis, will become diffusely edematous following radiation therapy, usually peaking at 6 to 24 weeks following completion of therapy. Laryngeal edema may persist for greater than 12 to 18 months, while chronic changes of atrophy and fibrosis may develop months or years after the edematous phase.

Laryngeal edema due to radiation therapy may simulate a tumor, particularly if one is not aware of prior radiation. Therefore, an accurate history and evaluation of other areas of edema that may have been in the radiation field are helpful in accurately evaluating this expected finding following radiation. If the primary tumor is remote from the larynx, then laryngeal edema following radiation is usually incidental and can be attributed to expected radiation effect. However, if the primary tumor arose from the larynx, then evaluation of residual or recurrent tumor following radiation treatment can be very challenging. In this setting, any new or persistent soft tissue density in the vicinity of the treated tumor should be viewed with suspicion. Short-term follow-up is usually necessary and can be aided with fluorodeoxyglucose (FDG) PET/CT in difficult cases. While the optimal time interval between completion of therapy and the first follow-up FDG-PET/CT has not been definitively established in the literature, a recommendation of 8 to 12 weeks following treatment is generally believed to balance the risks of imaging prematurely (and yielding a false positive result) against that of a delayed diagnosis.

COMPANION CASES

- **Acute epiglottitis.** Rarely encountered in modern practice given the success of widespread *Haemophilus influenzae* type b (Hib) vaccination, acute epiglottitis is a medical emergency often presenting with fever, difficulty swallowing, hoarseness, and drooling. While most commonly secondary to *Haemophilus* infection, additional etiologies include other bacterial pathogens, thermal injury from crack cocaine abuse, caustic injury, or trauma from foreign body ingestion. The appearance of an edematous epiglottis that occurs with epiglottitis can be virtually identical to an irradiated epiglottis. Therefore, an accurate history is paramount.
- **Epiglottic squamous cell carcinoma.** A supraglottic larynx malignancy is almost exclusively a squamous cell carcinoma (SCCA). The supraglottic larynx represents the second most common site of SCCA involvement of the laryngeal apparatus, second only to glottic SCCA. SCCA can usually be distinguished from edema secondary to radiation or infection by its density and focality; a SCCA is typically of soft tissue density and/or focally enhances, whereas edema is diffusely hypoattenuating.

Radiation-induced epiglottic edema

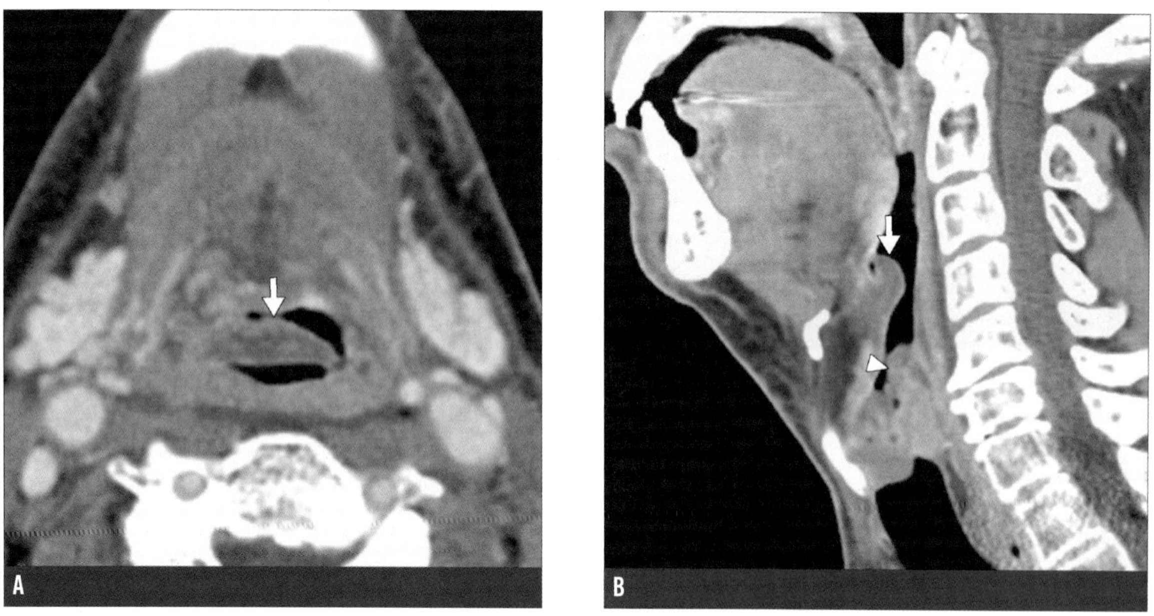

Contrast-enhanced axial (**A**) and sagittal reformatted (**B**) CT images demonstrate extensive thickening of the epiglottis (arrows, **A**, **B**) in this patient who received radiation for treatment of their base of tongue cancer. Additional radiation effect is identified involving other portions of the laryngeal apparatus (arrowhead, **B**).

Companion case: Acute epiglottitis

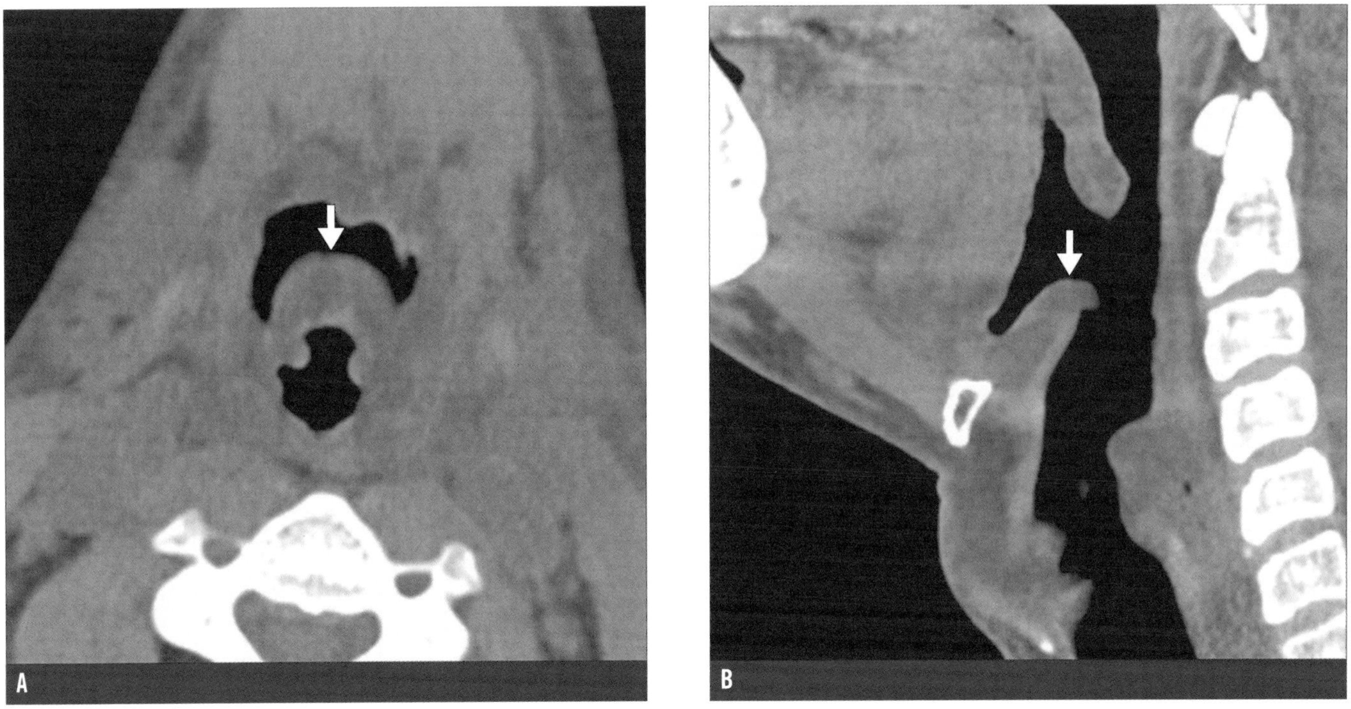

Unenhanced axial (**A**) and sagittal reformatted (**B**) CT images demonstrate diffuse thickening of the epiglottis (arrows, **A**, **B**) in this patient with a fever, white count, and a sore throat. The patient did not have a history of neck radiation. The findings are compatible with acute epiglottitis secondary to infection, which was confirmed clinically.

Companion case: Epiglottic squamous cell carcinoma

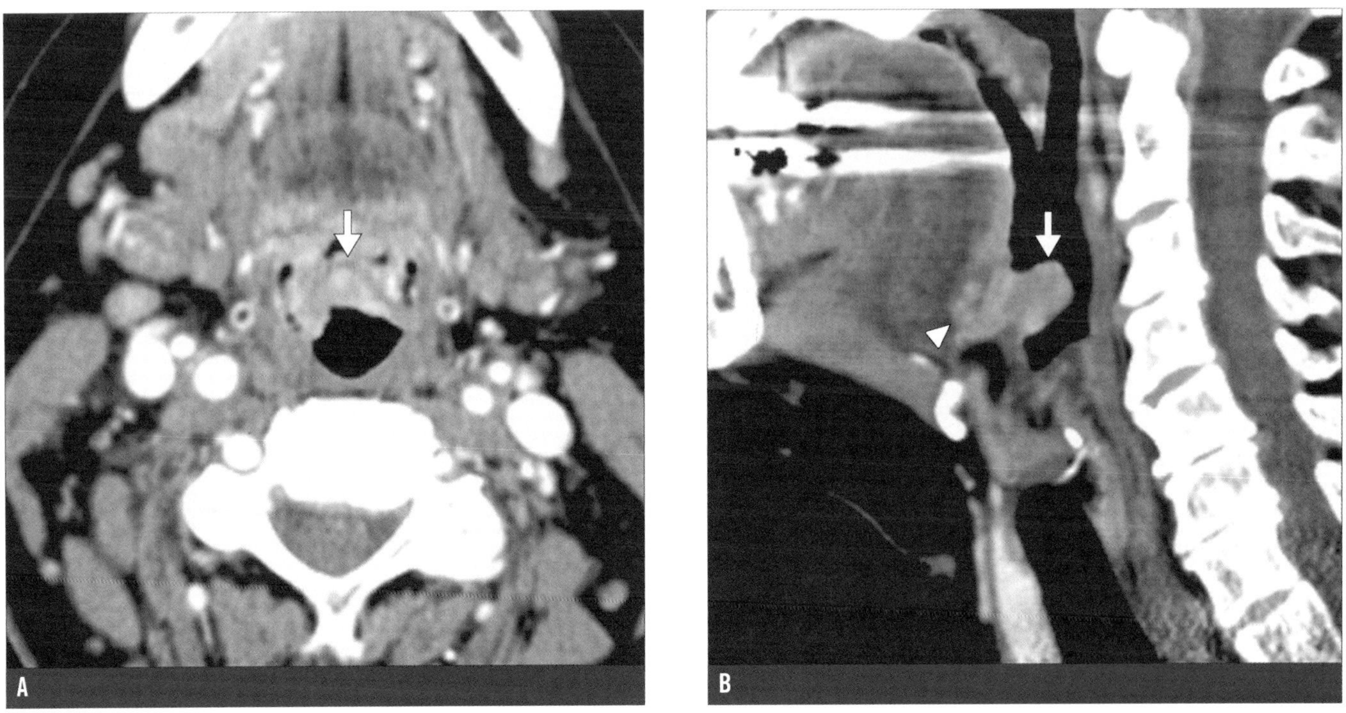

Contrast-enhanced axial (**A**) and sagittal reformatted (**B**) CT images demonstrate heterogeneously enhancing, abnormal thickening of the epiglottis in a 66-year-old woman (arrows, **A**, **B**). The soft tissue likely extends into the vallecula and base of tongue (arrowhead, **B**). The findings are compatible with a tumor of the epiglottis, most likely squamous cell carcinoma, which was confirmed at pathology.

REFERENCES

Bronstein AD, Nyberg DA, Schwartz AN, Shuman WP, Griffin BR. Soft-tissue changes after head and neck radiation: CT findings. *AJNR Am J Neuroradiol.* 1989;10:171-175.

Drake RL, Gray H. *Gray's atlas of anatomy.* 1st ed. Philadelphia, PA: Churchill Livingstone; 2008.

Fu KK, Woodhouse RJ, Quivey JM, Phillips TL, Dedo HH. The significance of laryngeal edema following radiotherapy of carcinoma of the vocal cord. *Cancer.* 1982;49:655-658.

Glastonbury CM, Parker EE, Hoang JK. The postradiation neck: evaluating response to treatment and recognizing complications. *AJR Am J Roentgenol.* 2010;195:W164-W171.

Hermans R, Pameijer FA, Mancuso AA, Parsons JT, Mendenhall WM. CT findings in chondroradionecrosis of the larynx. *AJNR Am J Neuroradiol.* 1998;19:711-718.

Kim SY, et al. The Feasibility of 18F-FDG PET scans 1 month after completing radiotherapy of squamous cell carcinoma of the head and neck. *J Nuc Med.* 2007;48:373-378.

King KG, Kositwattanarerk A, Genden E, Kao J, Som PM, Kostakoglu L. Cancers of the oral cavity and oropharynx: FDG PET with contrast-enhanced CT in the posttreatment setting. *Radiographics.* 2011;31:355-373.

Nomayr A, Lell M, Sweeney R, Bautz W, Lukas P. MRI appearance of radiation-induced changes of normal cervical tissues. *Eur Radiol.* 2001;11:1807-1817.

Yousefzadeh DK, Tewfik HH, Franken EA, Jr. Epiglottic enlargement following radiation treatment of head and neck tumors. *Pediatr Radiol.* 1981;10:165-168.

CASE 9 Thickened thyrohyoid membrane and median thyrohyoid ligament

The thyrohyoid membrane is a vertically oriented sheet of fibro-elastic tissue that spans between the thyroid cartilage and hyoid bone. Along the mid-lateral, thinner aspects of the membrane are small paired openings through which the superior laryngeal vessels and the internal branch of each superior laryngeal nerve enter the larynx. For further description of the thyrohyoid membrane anatomy, see Case 2 from this chapter.

The median (or middle) thyrohyoid ligament results in normal anatomic thickening at the midline of the thyrohyoid membrane. Occasionally, there may be incidental thickening of the thyrohyoid membrane and more pronounced incidental thickening of the median thyohyoid ligament. This may be due to patient positioning in the scanner, anatomic variation, or other incidental causes, and its appearance can simulate a mass on CT, such as an isoattenuating thyroglossal duct cyst. Usually, the thyrohyoid membrane and median thyroid ligament have a smooth, elongated shape in the craniocaudal dimension and a nonfocal, curvilinear morphology in the axial dimension, imaging features which aid in differentiating these normal structures from pathology. While thyroglossal duct cysts can be isodense to muscle on CT due to proteinaceous content, most thyroglossal duct cysts are hypoattenuating relative to muscle and can be differentiated from the isoattenuating thyrohyoid membrane and median thyrohyoid ligament. However, if it is still unclear whether the finding is abnormal by CT, then MRI can usually differentiate pathology from incidental thyrohyoid membrane and median thyrohyoid ligament thickening.

COMPANION CASES

- **Thyroglossal duct cyst.** The developing thyroid gland begins its descent at the foramen cecum of the tongue, located at the anterior midline tongue base. From there, the developing thyroid gland descends ventral to the hyoid body followed by a slightly cephalad course immediately posterior to the hyoid body. It then resumes its descent to its final resting place along the ventral-lateral aspect of the proximal trachea. During its descent, the developing thyroid gland is attached to the foramen cecum via the thyroglossal duct (TGD), which elongates as the thyroid descends the neck, only to involute by the eight fetal week. If any portion of a TGD fails to involute, then epithelial cells contained within the TGD can form a cyst.

  TGD cysts are the most common congenital neck mass. These lesions are painless, freely moveable masses that usually present clinically before the age of 20. Most TGD cysts are found at the level of the hyoid bone and may extend posterior to the hyoid body. If above the hyoid bone, then a TGD is typically midline. If a TGD cyst is located caudal to the hyoid bone, then it is typically off-midline. TGD cysts should be completely or partially embedded deep to the strap muscles. If not, then another etiology to explain the finding should be considered. Because of the increased risk of malignancy associated with TGD cysts (particularly papillary thyroid carcinoma), a TGD cyst and its tract are sometimes surgically removed with a Sistrunk procedure, which includes removing the hyoid body.
- **Ectopic thyroid.** In the course of thyroid development, rests of thyroid tissue along the course of the TGD may lead to the formation of ectopic thyroid tissue. The most common location is at the base of the tongue near the foramen cecum, but it can be found anywhere along the course of the TGD. Ectopic thyroid tissue may be the only thyroid tissue present or it may be present in conjunction with the normal thyroid gland. If the ectopic thyroid tissue is the only identifiable thyroid tissue present (ie, the normal thyroid gland is absent), then removal of the ectopic thyroid tissue will result in hypothyroidism. Due to its iodine content, normal thyroid gland and ectopic thyroid tissue are characteristically higher in attenuation relative to the muscle on unenhanced CT examinations, usually measuring between 70 and 120 Hounsfield units.

Thickened thyrohyoid membrane and median thyrohyoid ligament

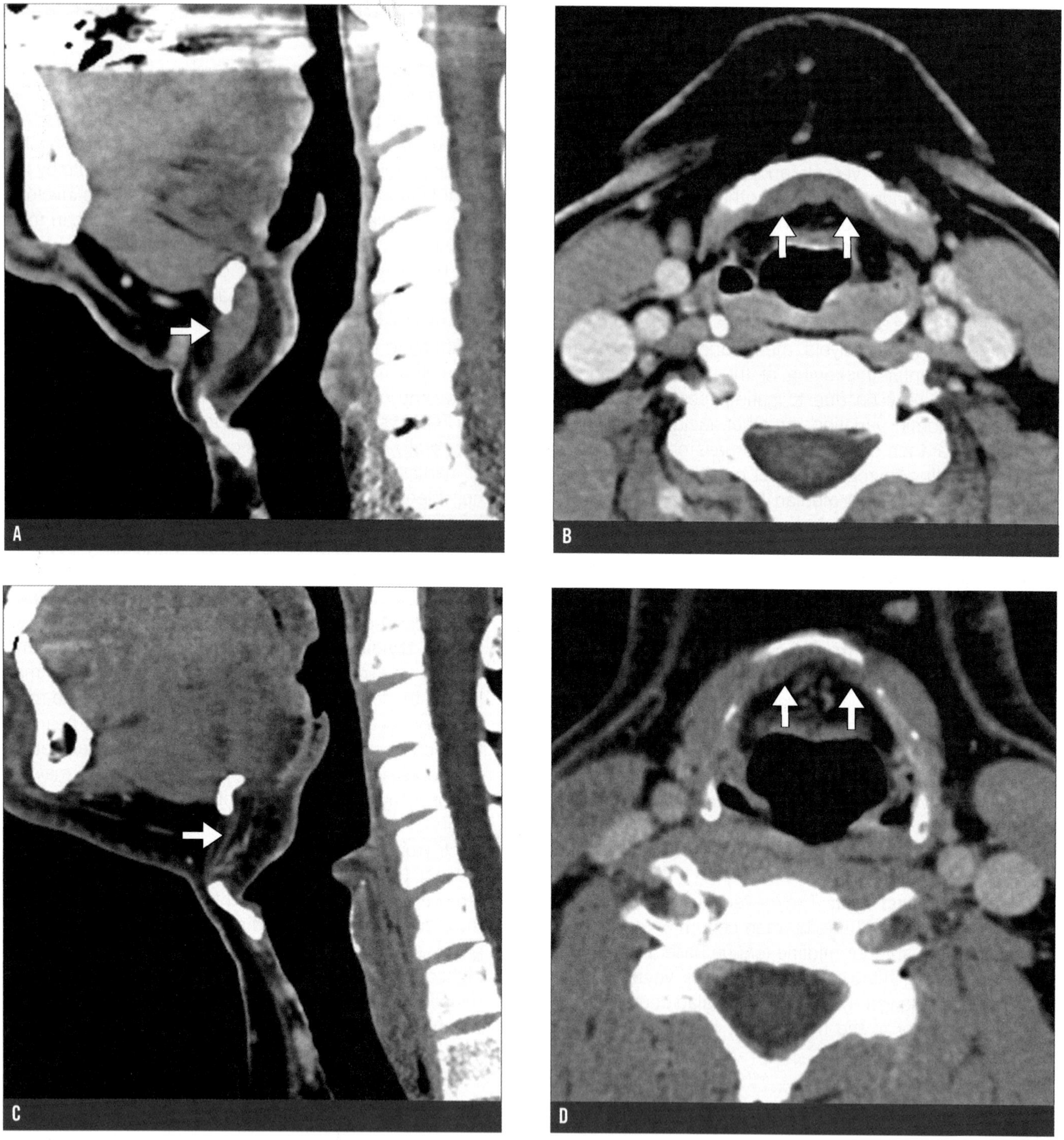

Sagittal reformatted (**A**) and axial (**B**) postcontrast CT images demonstrate thickened soft tissue between the superior aspect of the thyroid cartilage and the posterior margin of the hyoid body (arrows, **A**, **B**), possibly representing a thyroglossal duct cyst. However, the curvilinear morphology of the finding on image **B** is more compatible with a normal, incidentally thickened thyrohyoid membrane and median thyrohyoid ligament rather than a thyroglossal duct cyst, with the latter usually identified as a focal and round lesion in the axial plane. Sagittal reformatted (**C**) and axial (**D**) postcontrast CT images of a different patient demonstrate a more typical appearance of a normal thyrohyoid membrane and median thyrohyoid ligment (arrows, **C**, **D**).

Companion case: Thyroglossal duct cyst

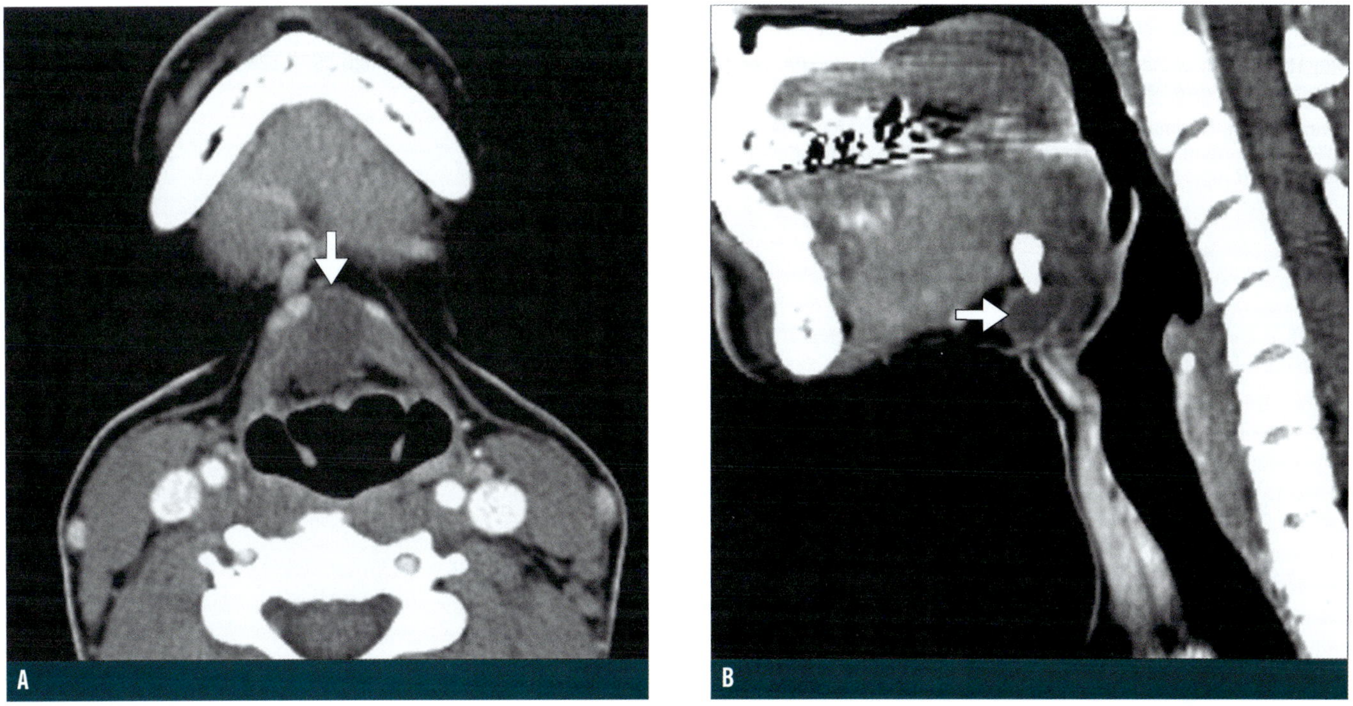

Axial (**A**) and sagittal reformatted (**B**) postcontrast CT images demonstrate a fluid density lesion (arrows, **A**, **B**) located deep to the strap muscles and which extends posterior to the hyoid bone. The findings are consistent with a thyroglossal duct cyst.

Companion case: Ectopic thyroid

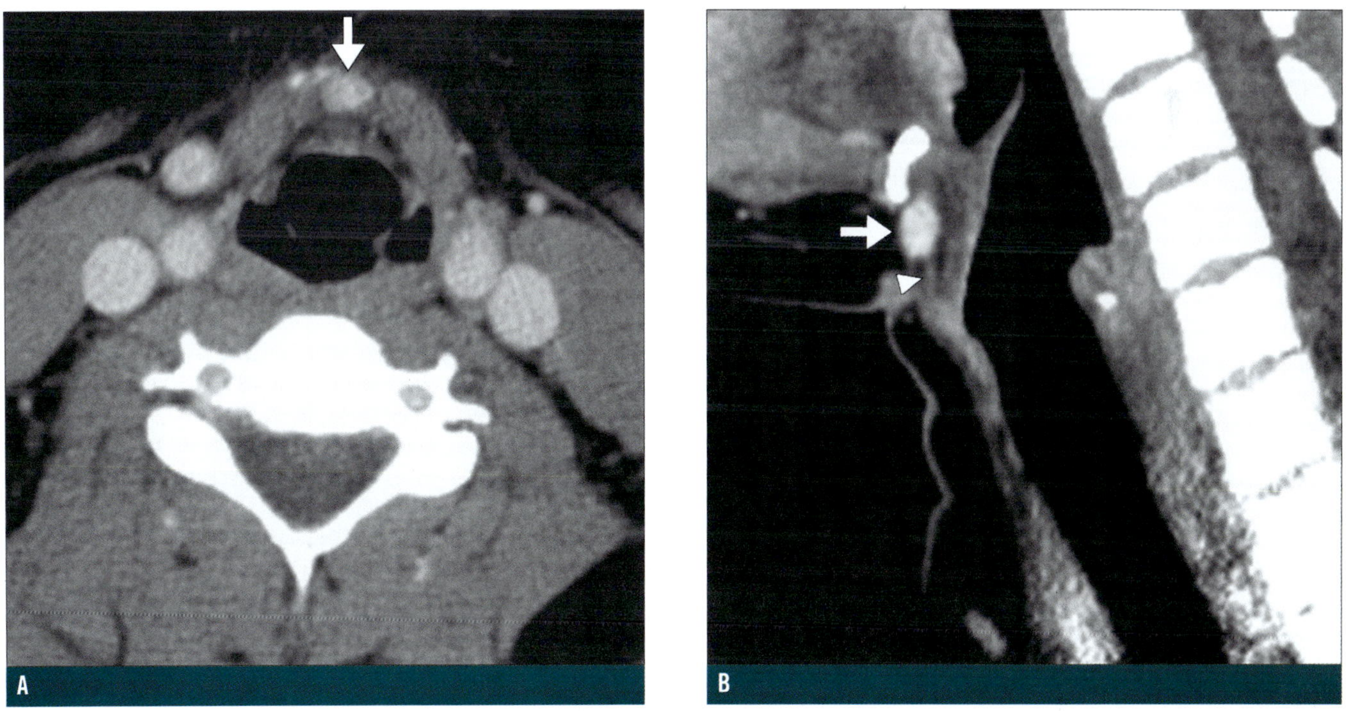

Axial (**A**) and sagittal reformatted (**B**) postcontrast CT images demonstrate a hyperdense nodule (arrows, **A**, **B**) deep to the strap muscles and immediately abutting the ventral aspect of the median thyrohyoid ligament (arrowhead, **B**). The location and density of the finding is compatible with ectopic thyroid tissue. Incidentally, if this ectopic thyroid tissue is normally functioning, then it would also be hyperattenuating on unenhanced CT imaging due to the presence of iodine. In addition to this ectopic thyroid tissue, the patient had a normal-sized thyroid gland at the expected anatomic position lower in the neck (not shown).

REFERENCES

Acierno SP, Waldhausen JHT. Congenital cervical cysts, sinuses and fistulae. *Otolaryngol Clin North Am.* 2007;40(1):161–176, vii–viii.

Gray H. *Anatomy of the Human Body.* 20th ed. Philadelphia, PA: Lea & Febiger; 1918. www.bartleby.com. Accessed December 12, 2012.

Silverman PM, Newman GE, Korobkin M, Workman JB, Moore AV, Coleman RE. Computed tomography in the evaluation of thyroid disease. *AJR Am J Roentgenol.* 1984;141:897-902.

Weber, AL, Randolph G, Aksoy FG. The thyroid and parathyroid glands: CT and MR imaging and correlation with pathology and clinical findings. *Radiol Clin North Am.* 2000;38(5):1105-1129.

Wolf BS, Nakagawa H, Yeh HC. Visualization of the thyroid gland with computed tomography. *Radiology.* 1977;123:368.

CASE 10 Variations of the laryngeal ventricle

Located between the false and true vocal cords (also called vocal folds), the laryngeal ventricle is a paired lateral depression lined by mucosa. Superolateral tubular extensions from the ventricles, termed laryngeal appendices (also called saccules), contain mucous glands that function to lubricate the TVCs.

The laryngeal ventricle is best evaluated on coronal imaging and is usually at least partially occupied with air, allowing clear delineation of the false vocal cord (FVC) above from the TVC below. However, the normal laryngeal ventricle can have various appearances, ranging from completely effaced to having a deep lateral depression. While laryngeal ventricle effacement may relate to normal anatomy or secretions occupying the ventricle, care should be taken to evaluate for a tumor in this region if laryngeal ventricle effacement is encountered on imaging.

COMPANION CASES

- **Abnormal enlargement of laryngeal ventricle due to true vocal cord paralysis.** Enlargement of the laryngeal ventricle is often present with an ipsilateral chronic TVC paralysis. While this may appear similar to a normal, asymmetrically prominent laryngeal ventricle, several additional findings are usually present with a TVC paralysis to aid in the proper diagnosis. For further discussion, see Case 14.
- **Endotracheal tube cuff in supraglottic larynx.** Normally when placing an endotracheal tube, the endotracheal tube is advanced so that the endotracheal tube cuff is inflated caudal to the TVCs. If the cuff is inadvertently insufflated cephalad to the TVCs, then there is a strong possibility that the endotracheal tube will become dislodged and airway protection will be lost. On imaging, a supraglottic location of an inflated endotracheal tube cuff can simulate grossly enlarged laryngeal ventricles in the coronal plane, though the morphology of the former has a wider and rounder contour compared to the latter.
- **Squamous cell carcinoma infiltrating the laryngeal ventricle.** The larynx is subdivided into three portions: the supraglottis, glottis, and subglottis. The laryngeal ventricle represents a portion of the supraglottic larynx along with the ventral wall of the aryepiglottic folds, arytenoid cartilages, FVCs, paraglottic fat, and preepiglottic fat. The epiglottis is also part of the supraglottic larynx, although some consider the ventral (also called lingual) surface of the epiglottis to be a part of the oropharynx. The boundary between the supraglottis and glottis is defined by a horizontal plane through the mid aspect of the laryngeal ventricle. Therefore, the superior half of the laryngeal ventricle resides in the supraglottis and the inferior half of the laryngeal ventricle resides in the glottis. The TVCs reside at the level of the glottis. The boundary between the glottis and subglottis is somewhat controversial, with some literature stating that it resides approximately 1 cm below the plane of the TVCs, others stating 5 mm below the free margin of the TVCs, whereas others stating that it resides along the undersurface of the TVCs. However, there is no debate with respect to the inferior border of the subglottis, which is considered to terminate at the inferior margin of the cricoid cartilage. Transglottic tumors represent laryngeal tumors that cross at least two of the three portions of the larynx, whether it be along the mucosa, submucosa/paraglottic fat, or both.

Widely patent laryngeal ventricles

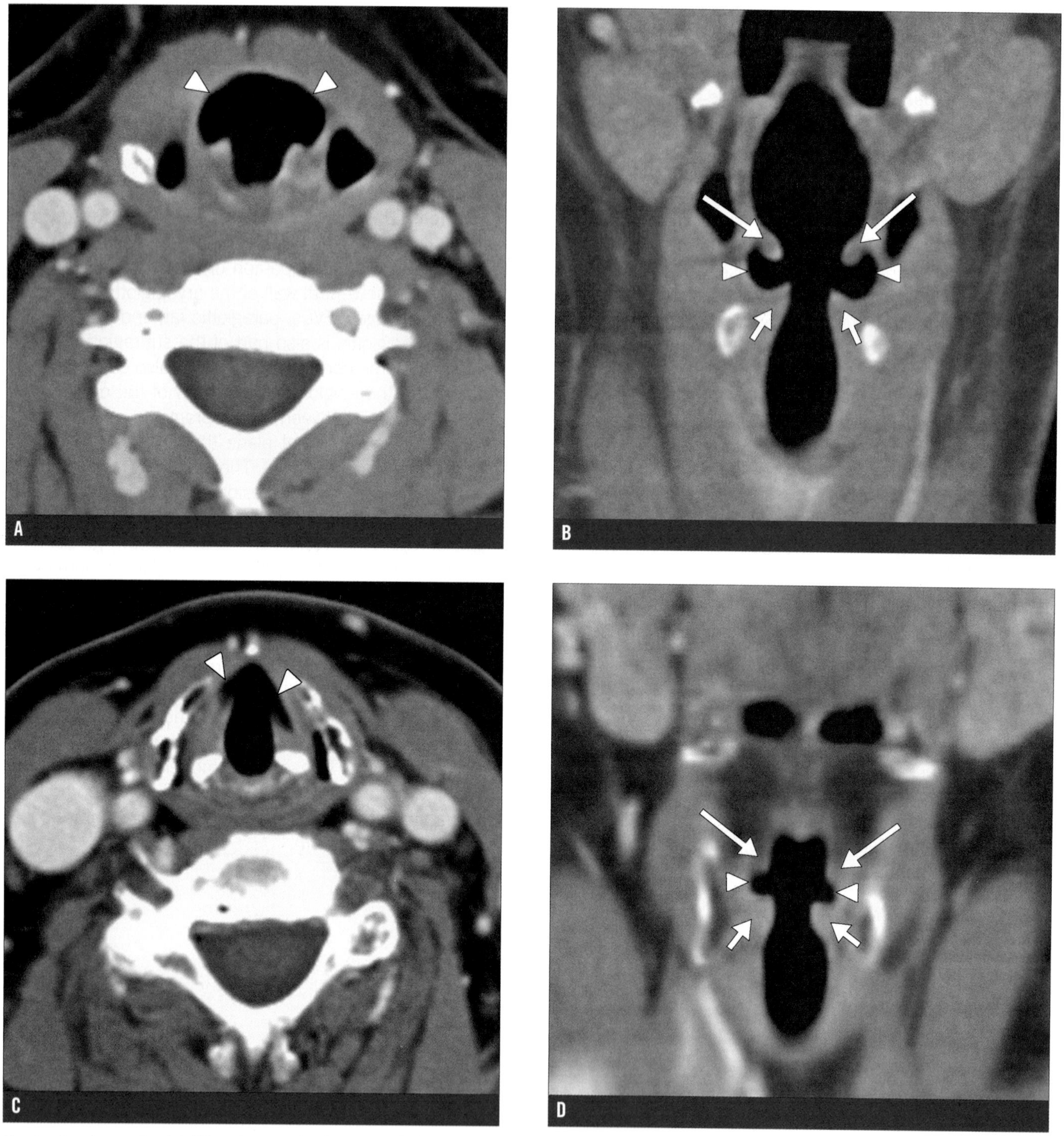

Contrast-enhanced axial (**A**) and coronal reformatted (**B**) CT images demonstrate widely patent laryngeal ventricles (arrowheads, **A**, **B**) which have an incidental curvature along their superolateral aspects when viewed on image **B**. Only a portion of the laryngeal ventricles are included on image **A**, due to slice selection. Contrast-enhanced axial (**C**) and coronal reformatted (**D**) CT images of a different patient demonstrate a slightly different but also normal appearance of the laryngeal ventricles, which are widely patent as well (arrowheads, **C**, **D**). The relationship of the laryngeal ventricle relative to the FVCs and TVCs is best appreciated on the coronal reformatted images. The FVCs (long arrows, **B**, **D**) are located cephalad to the laryngeal ventricles, whereas the TVCs (short arrows, **B**, **D**) are located caudal to the laryngeal ventricles.

Widely patent laryngeal ventricles in the lateral projection

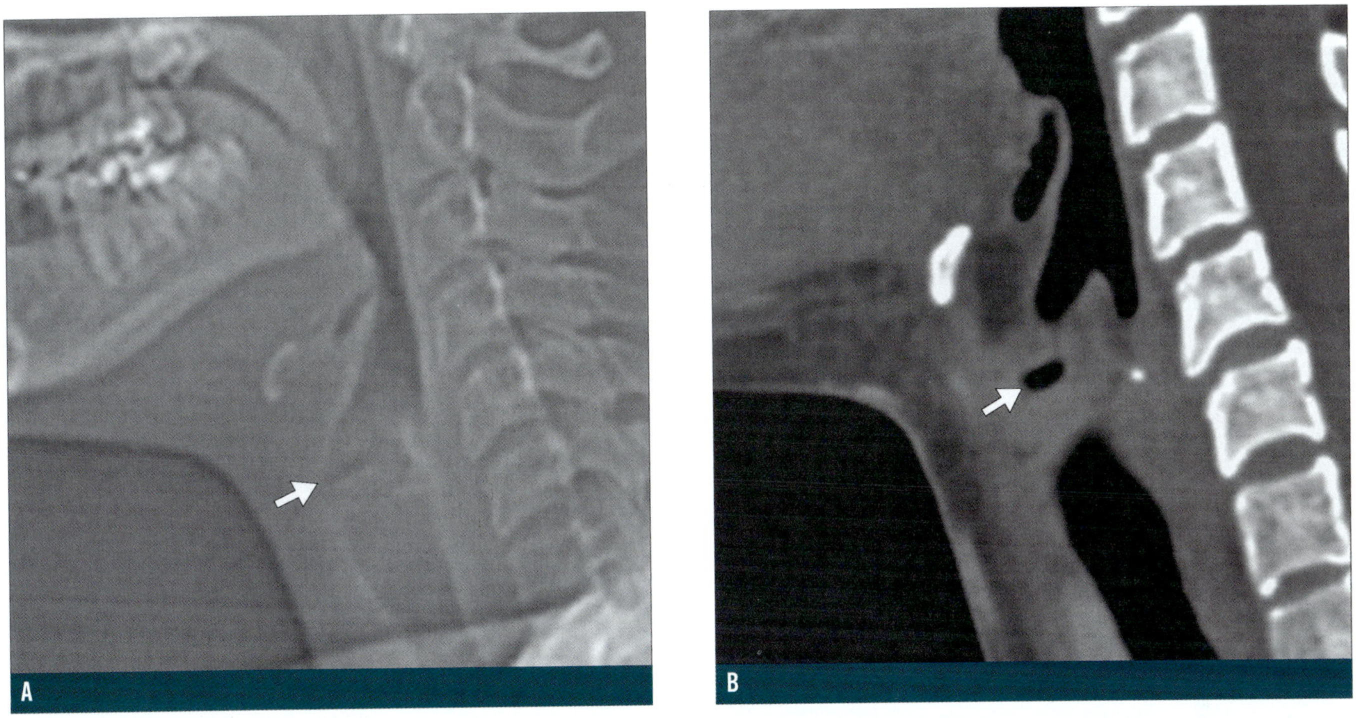

Different patient. A sagittal scout image from a CT (**A**) and a sagittal reformatted CT image from the same study (**B**) demonstrate the normal appearance of a widely patent laryngeal ventricle from a lateral perspective (arrows, **A, B**).

Shallow laryngeal ventricles

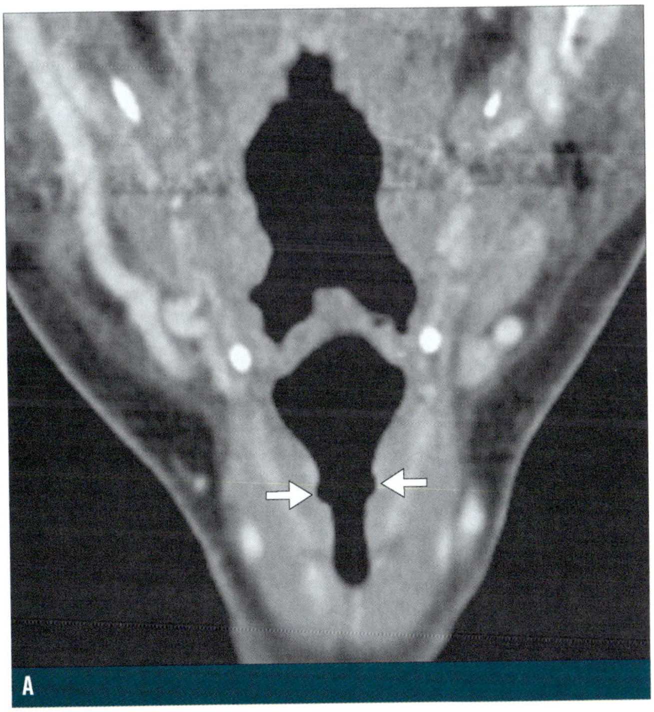

A contrast-enhanced coronal reformatted CT image (**A**) demonstrates a shallow appearance of the bilateral laryngeal ventricles (arrows), a normal variation.

Effaced laryngeal ventricles

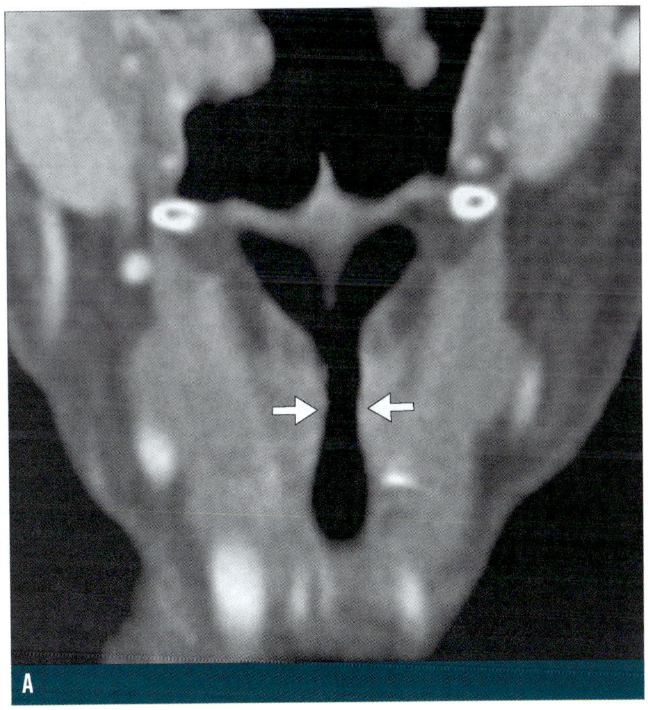

A contrast-enhanced coronal reformatted CT image (**A**) demonstrates complete effacement of the bilateral laryngeal ventricles (arrows), an incidental finding in this patient.

Companion case: Abnormal enlargement of laryngeal ventricle due to true vocal cord paralysis

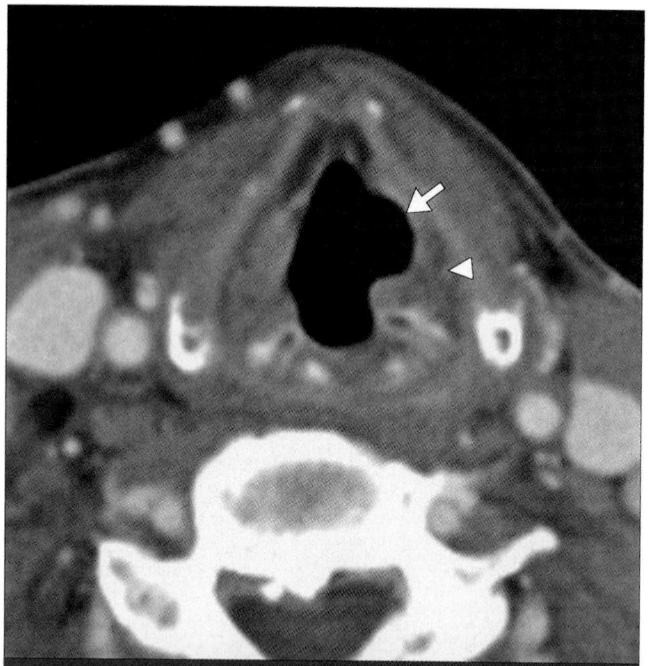

A

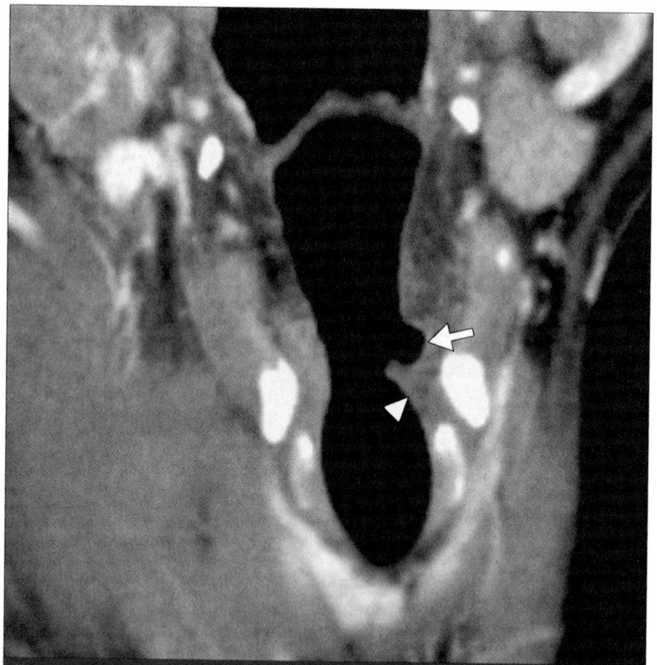

B

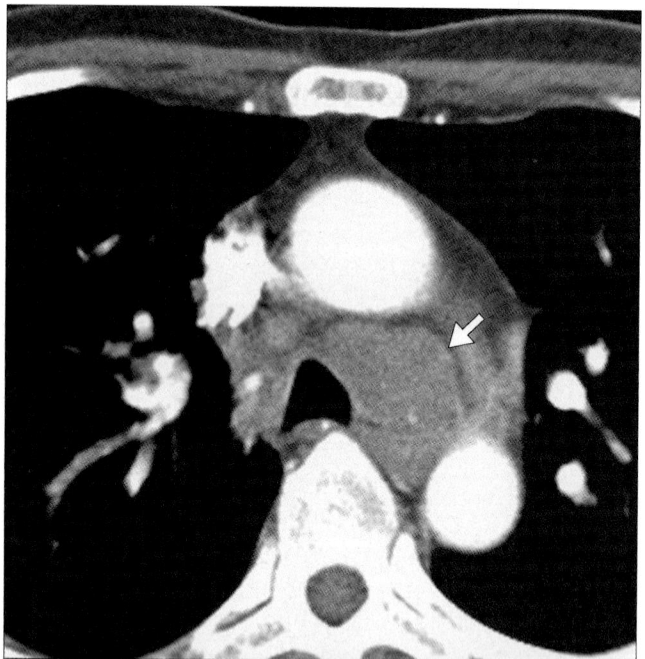

C

Contrast-enhanced axial (**A**) and coronal reformatted (**B**) CT images through the larynx demonstrate asymmetric enlargement of the left laryngeal ventricle (arrows, **A**, **B**) associated with fatty infiltration of the left TVC (arrowhead, **A**) as well as volume loss of the left TVC (arrowhead, **B**), compatible with a left TVC paralysis. An axial CT image from the same study through the superior mediastinum (**C**) demonstrates a large mass (arrow, **C**) at the aortopulmonary window, resulting in a left vagus nerve injury and the left TVC paralysis.

Companion case: Endotracheal tube cuff in supraglottic larynx

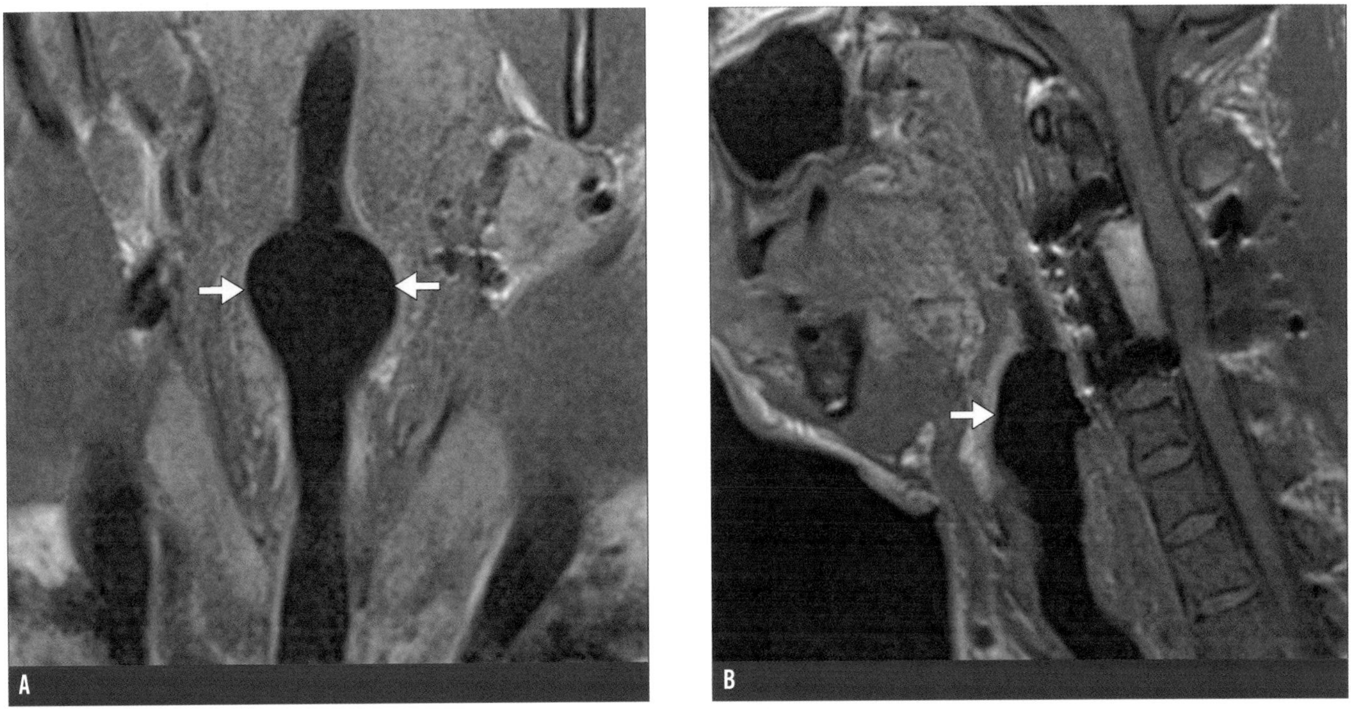

Coronal (**A**) and sagittal (**B**) T1-weighted MR images demonstrate abnormal positioning of an insufflated endotracheal tube cuff (arrows, **A**, **B**) located above the level of the TVCs. The finding could be confused with markedly enlarged bilateral laryngeal ventricles, although the morphology of the cuff is much rounder and wider than would be expected for normally prominent laryngeal ventricles. This endotracheal tube is at risk for dislodgement and subsequent loss of airway protection. Thus, this tube should be repositioned, with the cuff re-insufflated below the laryngeal apparatus.

Companion case: Squamous cell carcinoma infiltrating the laryngeal ventricle

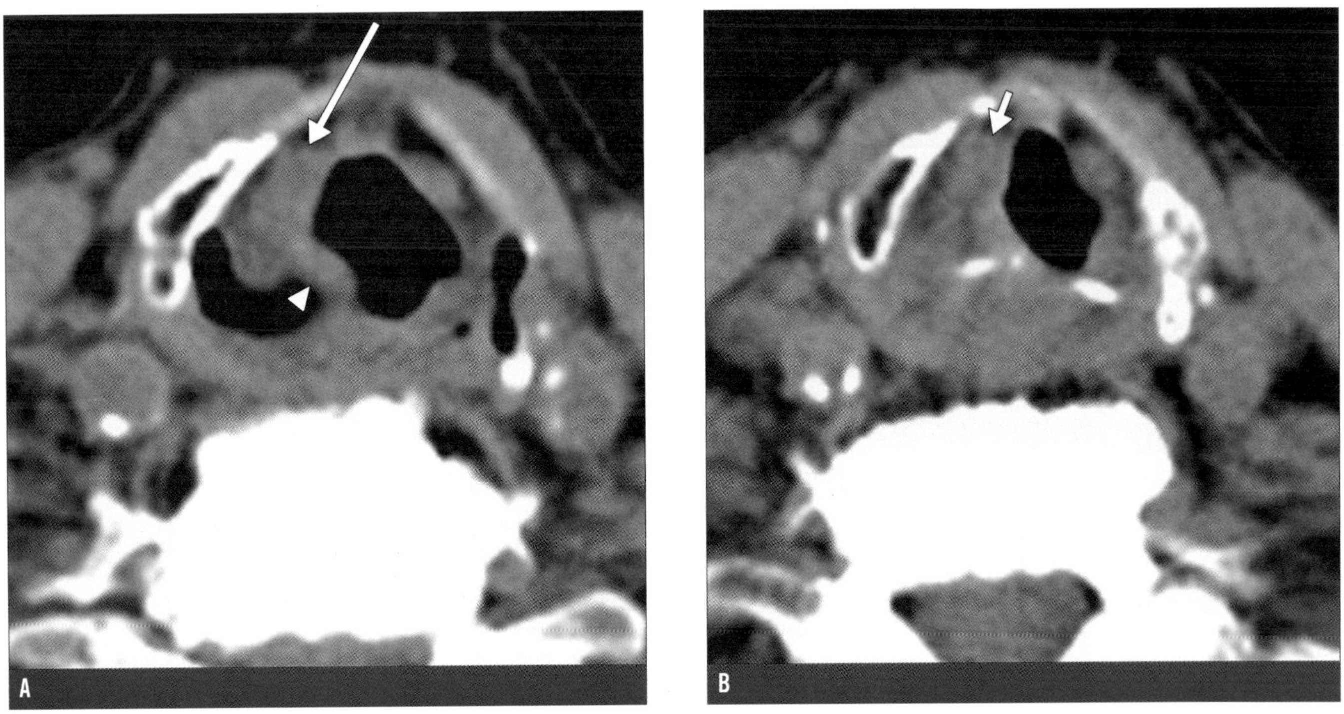

Unenhanced axial (**A-D**) and coronal reformatted (**E**) CT images through the larynx demonstrate a large right transglottic mass that extends from the right aryepiglottic fold (arrowhead, **A**) and paraglottic fat (long arrows, **A**, **E**), involves the right FVC (short arrow, **B**), both the right laryngeal ventricle and TVC (medium arrows, **C**, **E**), and the right aspect of the subglottic larynx (short arrows, **D**, **E**). As a reference, the left laryngeal ventricle is shown on image **E** and remains patent (arrowhead, **E**).

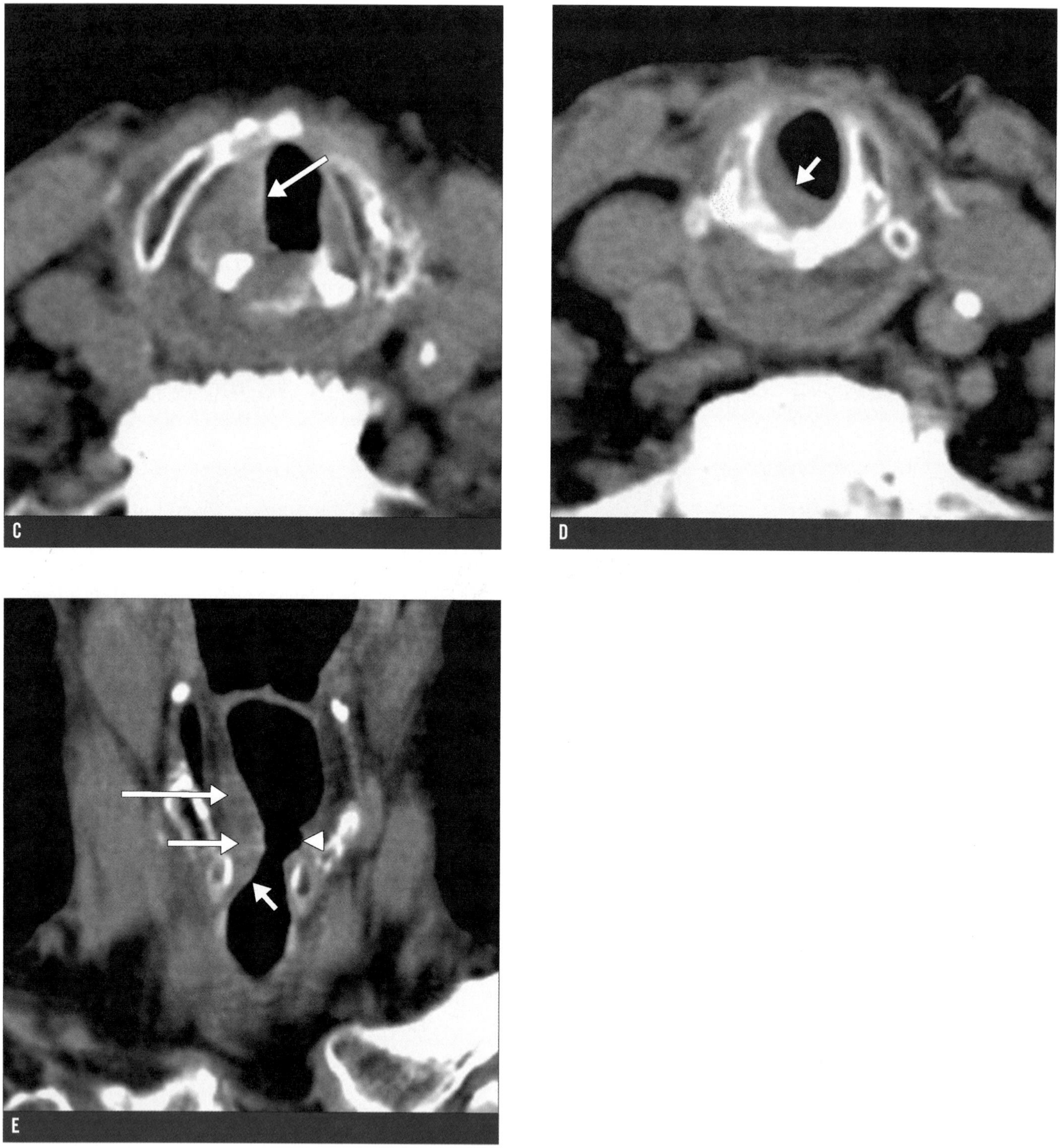

REFERENCES

American Society of Clinical Oncology, et al. American Society of Clinical Oncology clinical practice guideline for the use of larynx-preservation strategies in the treatment of laryngeal cancer. *J Clin Oncol.* 2006; 24:3693-3704.

Chin S-C, Edelstein S, Chen C-Y, Som PM. Using CT to localize side and level of vocal cord paralysis. *AJR Am J Roentgenol.* 2003; 180:1165-1170.

Drake RL, Gray H. *Gray's Atlas of Anatomy.* 1st ed. Philadelphia, PA: Churchill Livingstone; 2008.

Edge S, Byrd DR, Compton CC, Fritz AG, Greene FL, Trotti A. (eds.). *AJCC Cancer Staging Manual.* 7th ed. New York, NY: Springer; 2010.

Grundfast KM, Harley E. Vocal cord paralysis. *Otolaryngol Clin North Am.* 1989;22:569-597.

Kitzing P, Sonesson B. Shape and shift of the laryngeal ventricle during phonation. *Acta Otolaryngol.* 1967;63:479-488.

Romo LV, Curtin HD. Atrophy of the posterior cricoarytenoid muscle as an indicator of recurrent laryngeal nerve palsy. *AJNR Am J Neuroradiol.* 1999;20:467-471.

CASE 11 Laryngeal appendix

Situated within the paraglottic fat, the laryngeal appendix (also called saccule) is a mucosa-lined paired sac that is contiguous with, and extends superolaterally from, the ipsilateral laryngeal ventricle. Compression of the appendix from the surrounding laryngeal musculature results in expression of mucus that contributes to TVC lubrication.

On CT, normal collapsed laryngeal appendices are often identified as thin linear soft tissue density structures within both aspects of the paraglottic fat, each emanating from their respective laryngeal ventricles. Single or multiple foci of air are frequently detected along the course of the laryngeal appendix, which is an incidental finding. In cases of laryngeal carcinoma, knowledge of the normal laryngeal appendices is helpful in order to avoid misinterpreting these structures as areas of paraglottic tumor spread.

When a laryngeal appendix is abnormally enlarged, then the term laryngocele is used. Laryngoceles are classified, in part, by their location—internal, external, and mixed (combined). Internal laryngoceles are confined by the thyrohyoid membrane, whereas external laryngoceles are located outside the thyrohyoid membrane. The mixed type has features of both.

Laryngoceles are also classified as air-filled, fluid-filled, or infected (laryngopyocele). Chronically increased intralaryngeal pressures may result in the formation of an incidental air-filled laryngocele, as may be identified in chronic coughers, woodwind/brass instrumentalists, and glass blowers.

A fluid-filled laryngocele represents accumulation of mucous within an expanded laryngeal appendix. This may occur because of an obstruction of the laryngeal ventricle by a benign or malignant laryngeal process. Therefore, a fluid-filled laryngocele should prompt radiologic and clinical evaluation of the laryngeal ventricle to exlude an obstructing mass.

A laryngopyocele is uncommon. Clinical presentations may include a painful neck mass, hoarseness, or acute airway obstruction.

COMPANION CASES

- **Air-filled internal laryngoceles.**
- **Small fluid-filled laryngeal appendices/laryngoceles.**
- **Large fluid-filled internal laryngocele.**
- **Large fluid-filled internal and external laryngocele.**

- **Submucosal tumor invasion into paraglottic fat.** Most carcinomas arising from the larynx are at least partially located along the mucosal surface and are therefore commonly identified by the otolaryngologist during laryngoscopy. However, the otolaryngologist cannot usually determine whether there is submucosal spread of tumor into the paraglottic or pre-epiglottic fat, the presence of which can affect management and prognosis. However, identification of tumor spread into these areas can be assessed by the radiologist, either by CT or MRI. A thorough evaluation of tumor extension into these areas should be performed in every case of carcinoma affecting the laryngeal apparatus. Tumor involving the paraglottic or pre-epiglottic fat on imaging will usually be of soft tissue density/signal, infiltrative, and sometimes exert mass effect.

Normal laryngeal appendices

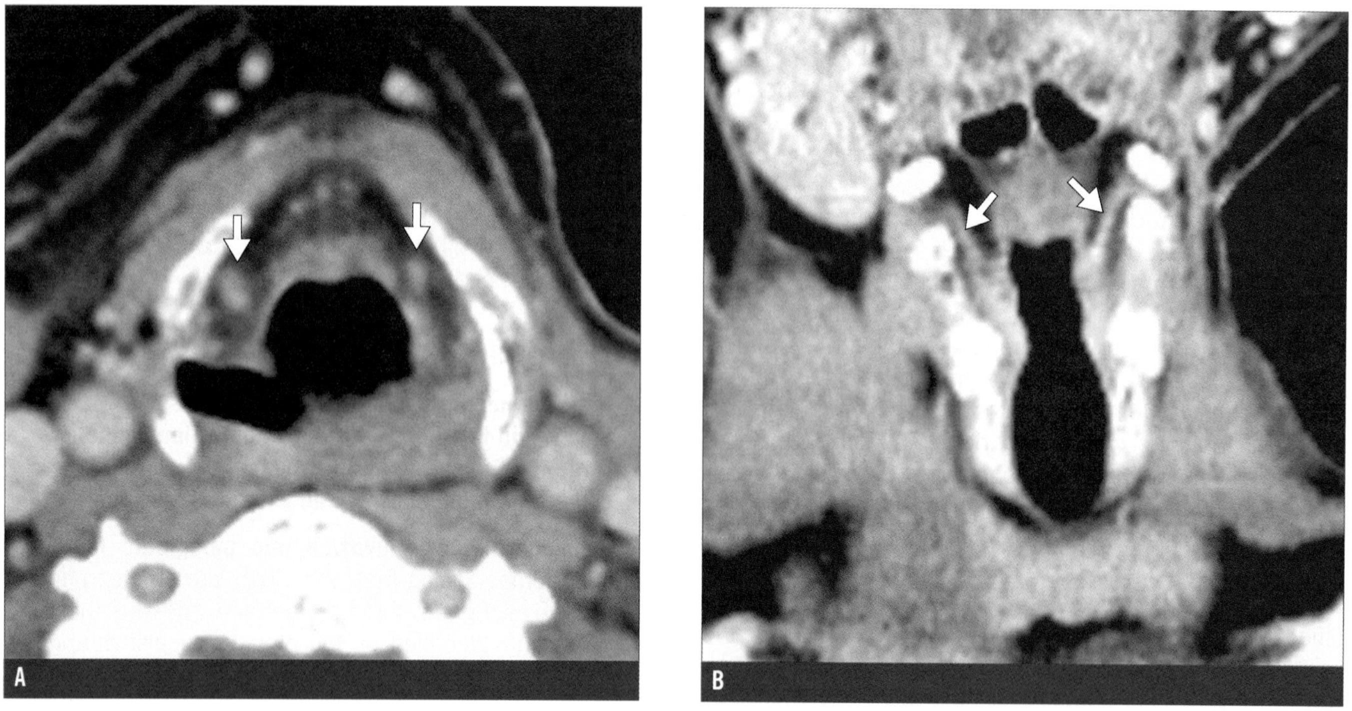

Contrast-enhanced axial (**A**) and coronal reformatted (**B**) CT images demonstrate paired soft tissue densities that are oval in the axial plane (arrows, **A**) and thin, vertically oriented in the coronal plane (arrows, **B**). These represent the normal laryngeal appendices.

Asymmetric laryngeal appendix

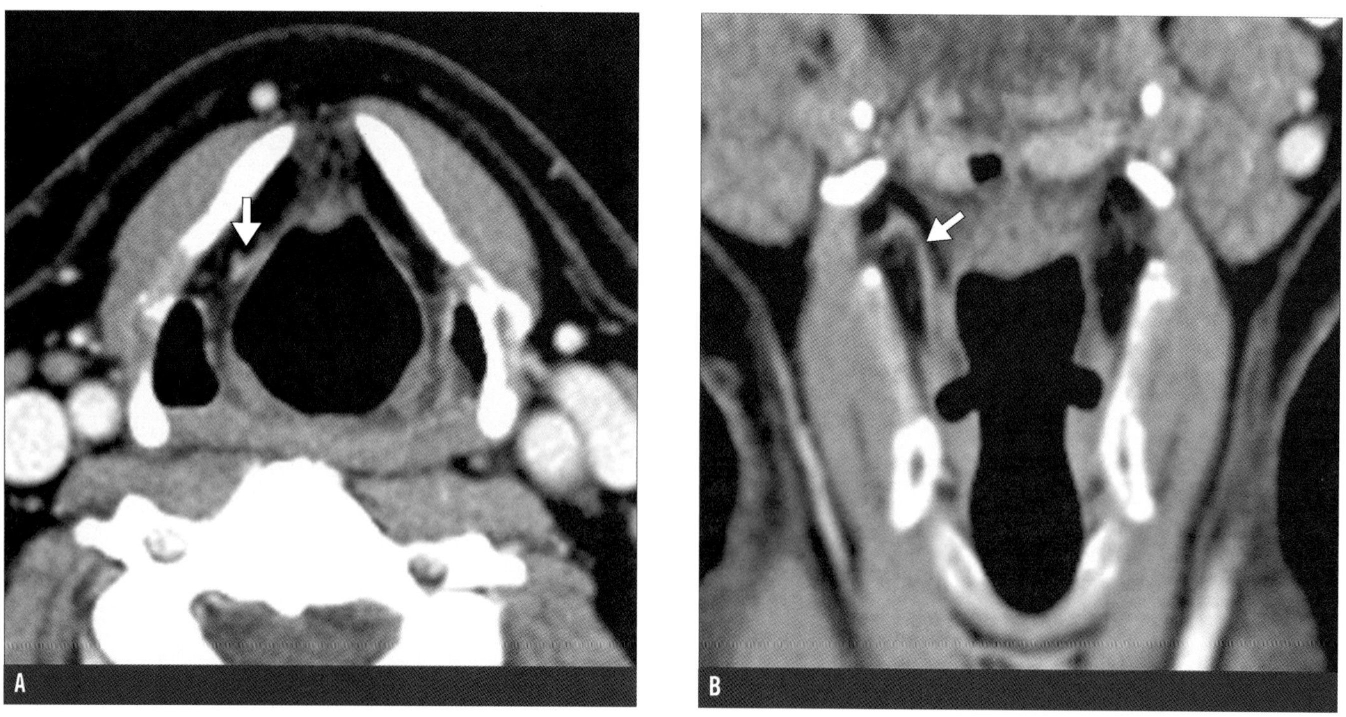

Contrast-enhanced axial (**A**) and coronal reformatted (**B**) CT images demonstrate an asymmetrically visualized right laryngeal appendix, a normal variant (arrows, **A**, **B**).

Air within proximal laryngeal appendix

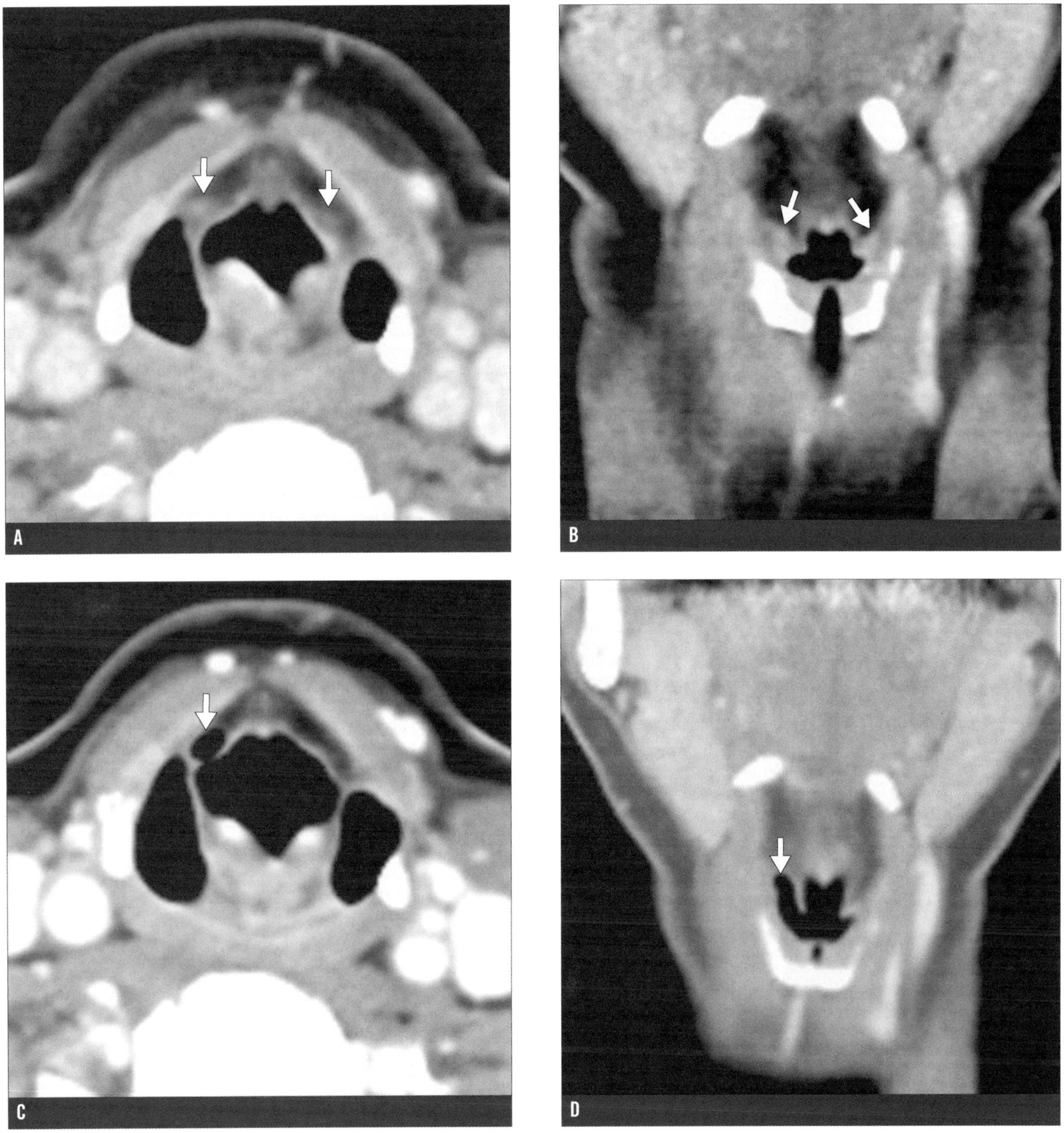

Contrast-enhanced axial (**A**) and coronal reformatted (**B**) CT images demonstrate the normal laryngeal appendices (arrows, **A**, **B**). Approximately 6 months later, axial (**C**) and coronal reformatted (**D**) contrast-enhanced CT images demonstrate a small amount of air extending from the right laryngeal ventricle into the proximal aspect of the right laryngeal appendix (arrows, **C**, **D**).The size of this air-filled laryngeal appendix is roughly the same as the laryngeal ventricles and could be considered incidental. Nevertheless, some might consider this a small, air-filled, internal laryngocele.

Companion case: Air-filled internal laryngoceles

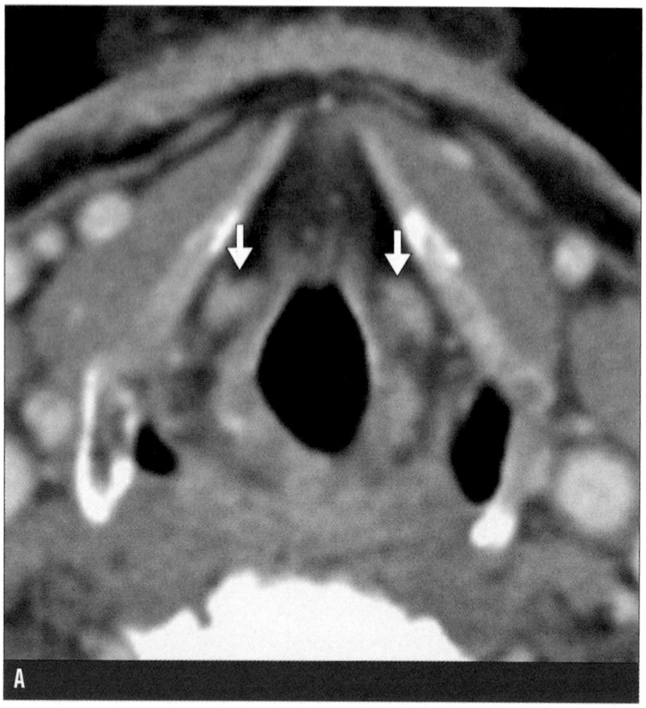

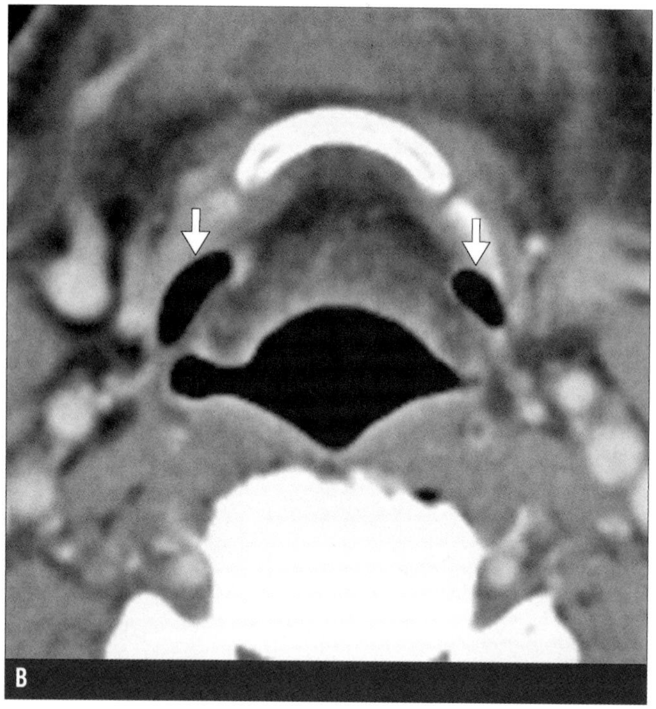

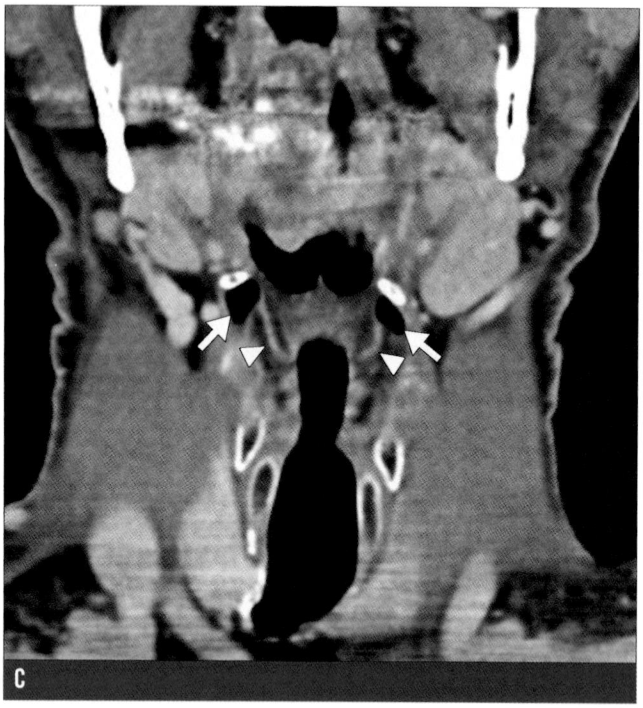

A contrast-enhanced axial CT image (**A**) demonstrates small foci of soft tissue density in the bilateral paraglottic fat that represent normal, collapsed laryngeal appendices (arrows, **A**). Slightly more cephalad, a contrast-enhanced axial CT image (**B**) demonstrates air within and mildly expanding the distal aspects of the laryngeal appendices, compatible with small, air-filled, internal laryngoceles (arrows, **B**). A contrast-enhanced coronal reformatted CT image (**C**) also demonstrates the normal, proximally collapsed bilateral laryngeal appendices (arrowheads, **C**) and the small, air-filled, distal laryngeal appendices, compatible with internal laryngoceles (arrows, **C**).

Companion case: Small fluid-filled laryngeal appendices/laryngoceles

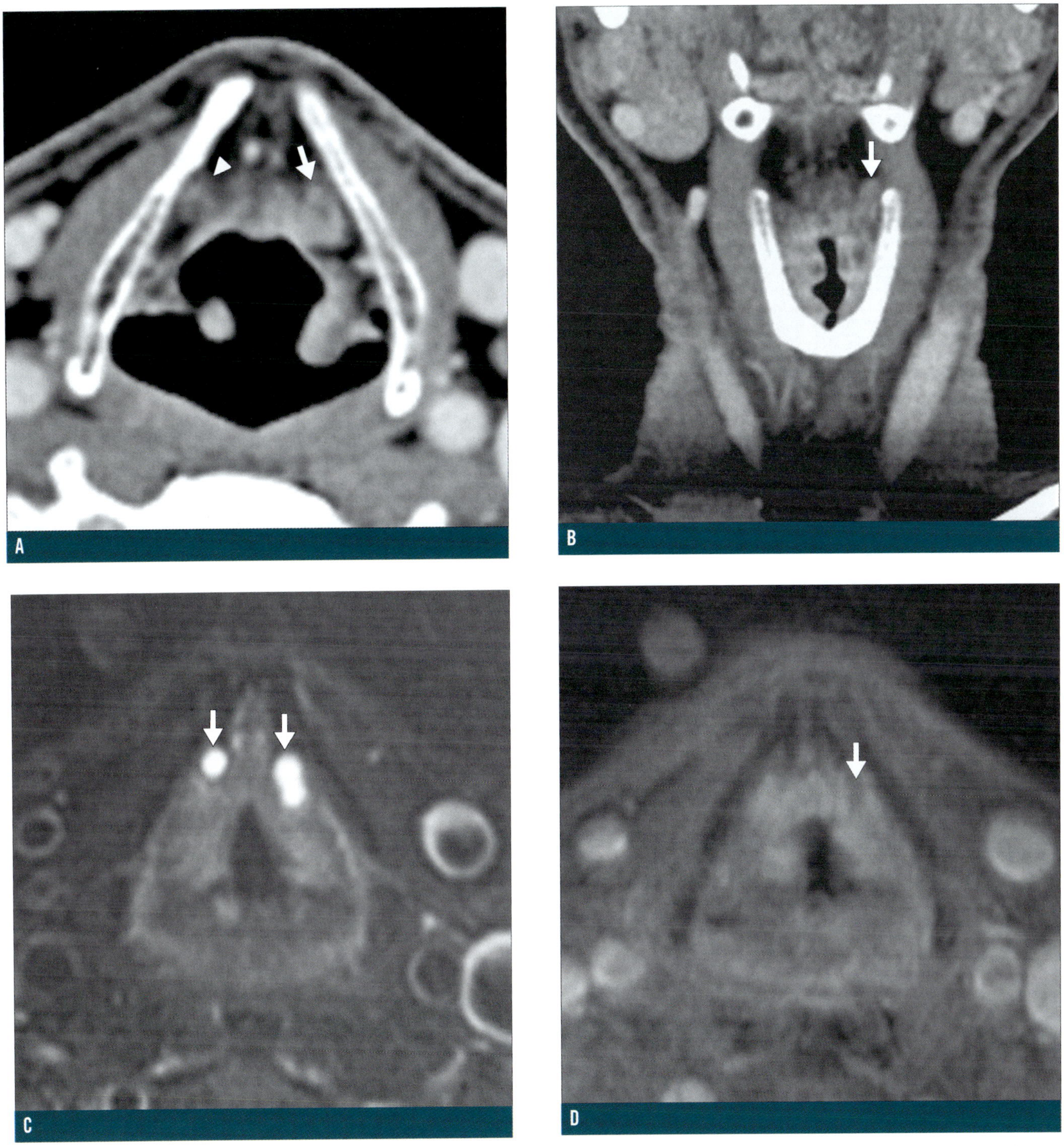

Contrast-enhanced axial (**A**) and coronal reformatted (**B**) CT images demonstrate asymmetric enlargement of the left laryngeal appendix (arrows, **A**, **B**) compared to the right (arrowhead, **A**). An axial fat-suppressed T2-weighted MR image (**C**) demonstrates the laryngeal appendices to be T2 hyperintense (arrows, **C**). A contrast-enhanced axial T1-weighted MR image without fat suppression (**D**) demonstrates the left laryngeal appendix to be nonenhancing (arrow, **D**). The right laryngeal appendix, while not clearly visualized, is also not overtly enhancing. The findings are most compatible with fluid-filled laryngeal appendices/laryngoceles, left larger than right.

Companion case: Large fluid-filled internal and external laryngocele

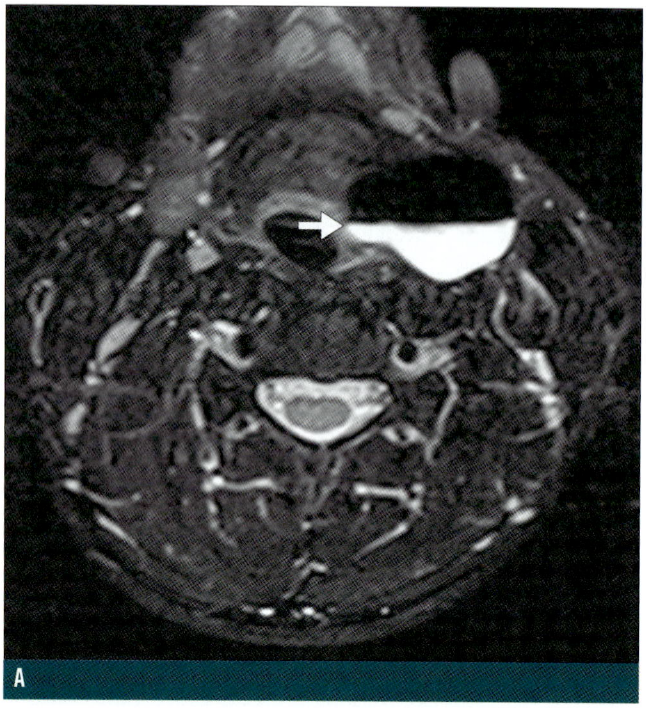

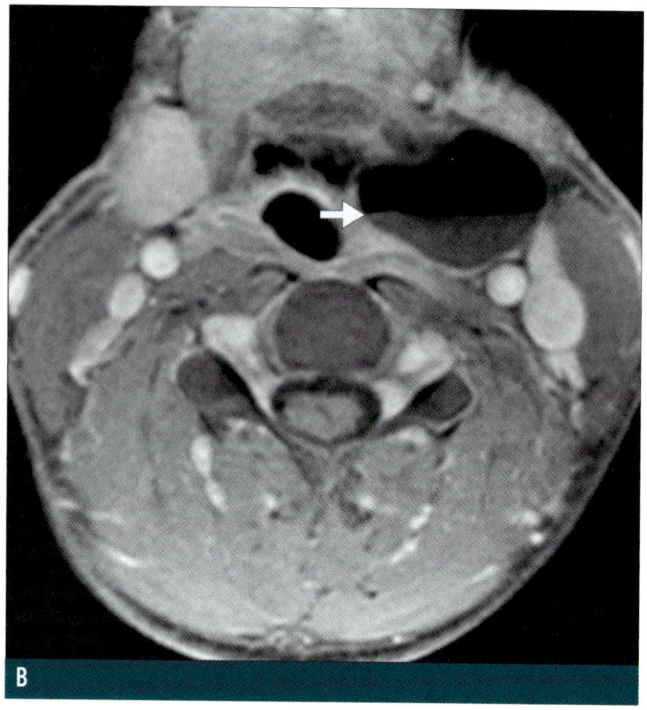

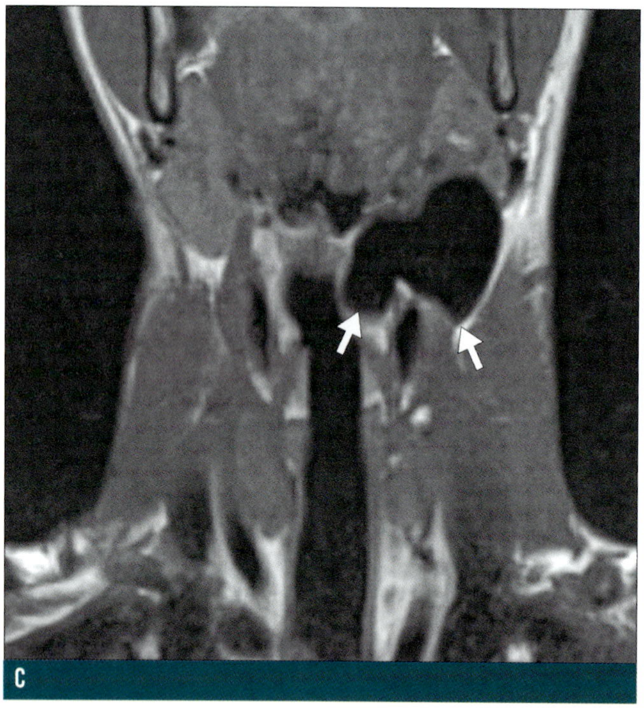

Different patient. Axial T2 with fat suppression (**A**), contrast-enhanced axial T1 with fat suppression (**B**), and coronal T1 (**C**) MR images demonstrate a large, nonenhancing lesion that contains a large fluid level spanning from the left paraglottic fat to the soft tissues left lateral to the laryngeal apparatus (arrows, **A-C**). The finding is compatible with a large, partially fluid-filled, internal and external (i.e. mixed) laryngocele.

Companion case: Submucosal tumor invasion into paraglottic fat

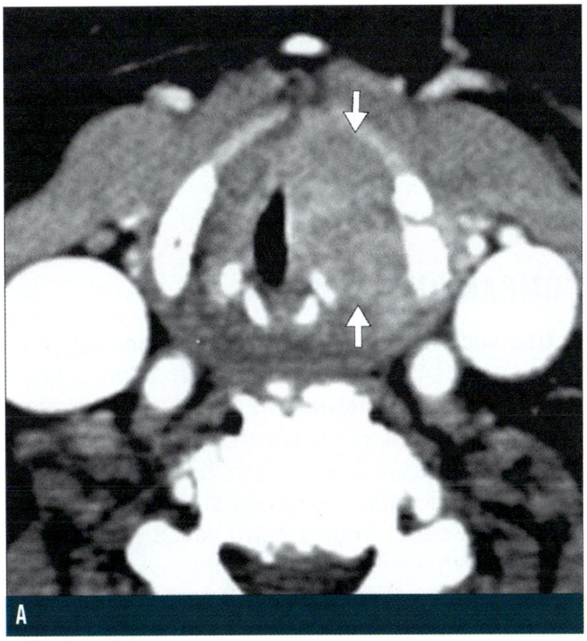

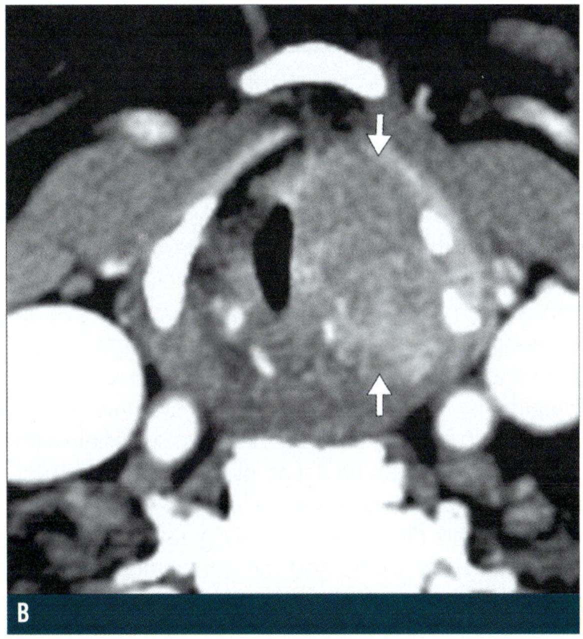

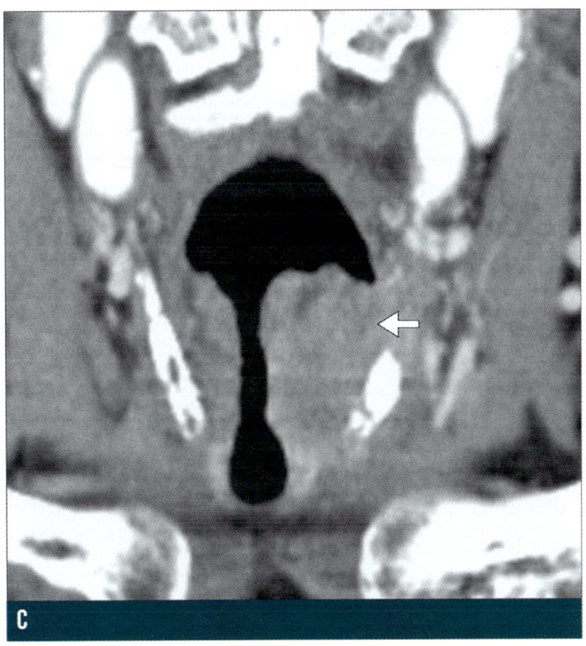

Contrast-enhanced axial CT images through the level of the TVCs (**A**) and slightly more cephalad through the level of the paraglottic fat (**B**) demonstrate a heterogeneously enhancing, large soft tissue density transglottic mass involving the left TVC (arrows, **A**) and the left paraglottic fat (arrows, **B**). A coronal reformatted image (**C**) also demonstrates bulky left paraglottic involvement (arrow, **C**). This lesion is differentiated from a fluid-filled laryngocele, in part, by its soft tissue density and heterogeneous enhancement. Other findings, such as cartilage invasion and lymphadenopathy were also present (not shown) and compatible with tumor.

REFERENCES

Bassett LW, Hanafee WN, Canalis RF. The appendix of the ventricle of the larynx. *Radiology*. 1976;120:571-574.

DeSanto LW. Laryngocele, laryngeal mucocele, large saccules, and laryngeal saccular cysts: a developmental spectrum. *Laryngoscope*. 1974;84:1291-1296.

Drake RL, Gray H. *Gray's Atlas of Anatomy*. 1st ed. Philadelphia, PA: Churchill Livingstone; 2008.

Dursun G, Ozgursoy OB, Beton S, Batikhan H. Current diagnosis and treatment of laryngocele in adults. *Otolaryngol Head Neck Surg*. 2007;136:211-215.

Fredrickson KL, D'Angelo AJ, Jr. Internal laryngopyocele presenting as acute airway obstruction. *Ear Nose Throat J*. 2007;86:104-106.

Frohlich S, O'Sullivan E. Repeated episodes of airway obstruction caused by a pyolaryngocele. *Eur J Emerg Med*. 2011;18:179-180.

Glazer HS, Mauro MA, Aronberg DJ, Lee JK, Johnston DE, Sagel SS. Computed tomography of laryngoceles. *AJR Am J Roentgenol*. 1983;140:549-552.

Micheau C, Luboinski B, Lanchi P, Cachin Y. Relationship between laryngoceles and laryngeal carcinomas. Laryngoscope. 1978;88:680-688.

Vasileiadis I, Kapetanakis S, Petousis A, Stavrianaki A, Fiska A, Karakostas E. Internal laryngopyocele as a cause of acute airway obstruction: an extremely rare case and review of the literature. *Acta Otorhinolaryngol Ital*. 2012;32:58-62.

CASE 12 Laryngeal apparatus rotation or slice selection resulting in an apparent true vocal cord abnormality

The TVCs are normally angulated with the anterior aspects of the TVCs, including the anterior commissure, slightly caudal in position relative to the posterior aspects of the TVCs and posterior commissure. As a result, straight axial imaging through the TVCs often results in partial volume averaging with the FVCs, laryngeal ventricles or subglottic larynx on a given axial image. This partial volume averaging can result in an apparent anatomic asymmetry and even simulate pathology of the TVCs. When dedicated TVC imaging is necessary, such as to evaluate a TVC malignancy, thin section imaging (1-2 mm) parallel to the TVCs is optimal. This can be accomplished by reconstructing the direct axial image data set parallel to the C4-C5 disc space, as this disc space usually parallels the TVCs. Evaluating the TVCs, FVCs, and the intervening laryngeal ventricles in the coronal plane is often very useful and complementary to evaluating these structures on angled axial images parallel to the TVCs.

Laryngeal apparatus rotation in the coronal plane is a common finding that may be identified incidentally, or the result of mass effect, such as with a thyroid goiter. The rotation will frequently result in asymmetry of the TVCs on axial imaging, sometimes simulating medialization of one TVC compared to the contralateral TVC, and thus raising the possibility of a TVC paralysis or tumor. When encountered with this scenario, the coronal reformatted images are extremely useful to assess whether the finding represents true pathology or is merely related to laryngeal apparatus rotation.

COMPANION CASES

- **True vocal cord asymmetry due to denervation atrophy.** See Case 14 for further discussion of this entity.
- **True vocal cord polyp.** TVC polyps may be very subtle and are sometimes easily missed on CT when viewed with a soft tissue window. A wide window, such as a lung window, will often outline any subtle contour abnormalities that result from a polyp which may otherwise be occult with a soft tissue window.
- **True vocal cord squamous cell carcinoma.** A TVC tumor will usually be associated with an increased volume of the TVC. Soft tissue that extends from the TVC to the subglottic larynx should be considered a tumor, until proven otherwise. Moreover, a clinical history of a paralyzed cord does not always equate to a TVC paralysis, as a TVC carcinoma can fix the TVC and result in an apparent "paralyzed" state. A TVC tumor usually enhances on CT and will usually be isointense on T1, variable on T2, and almost always enhance on MRI.

Normal study with thin section imaging parallel to true vocal cords

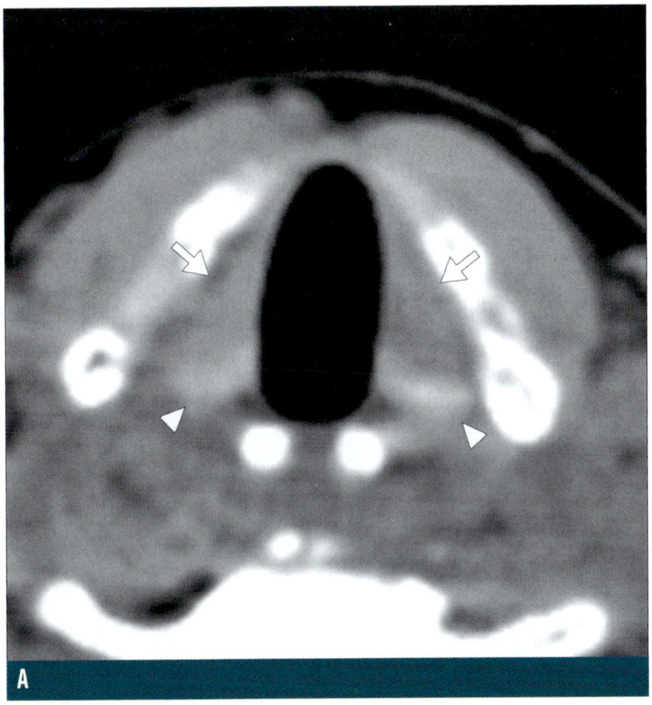

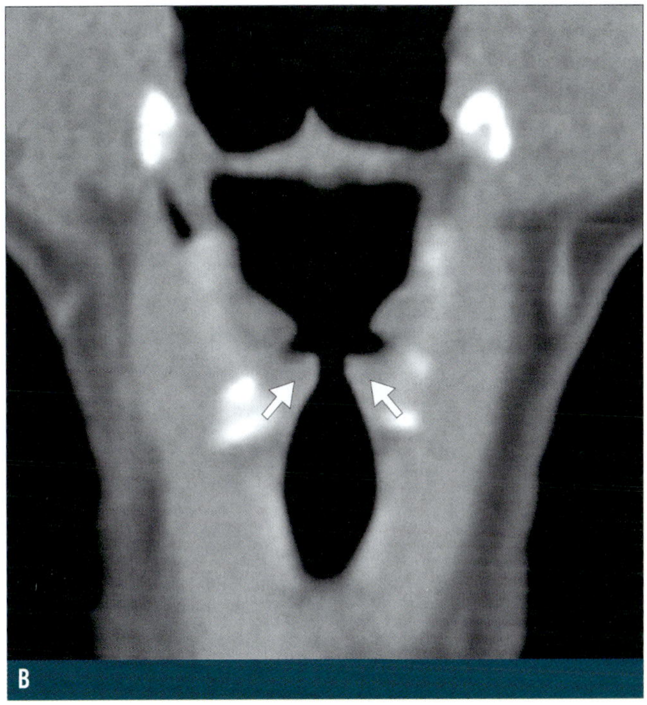

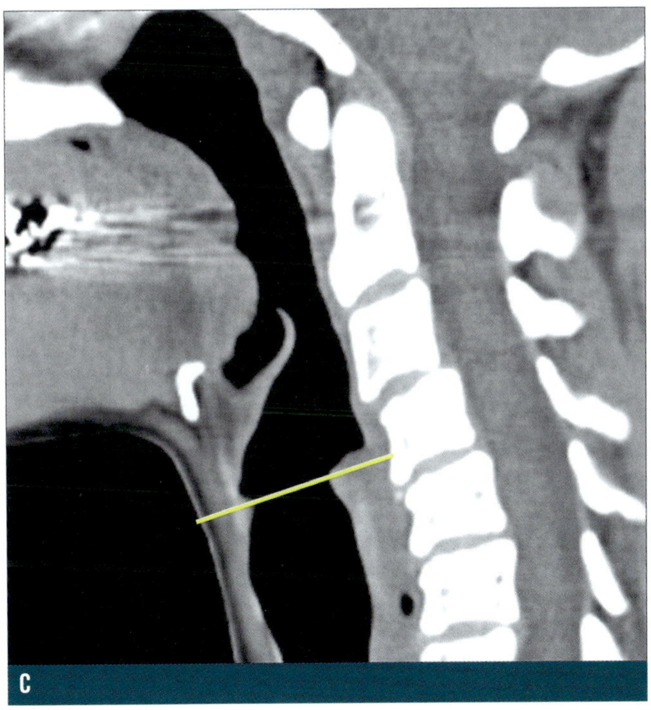

Unenhanced axial (**A**) and coronal reformatted (**B**) CT images demonstrate normal, symmetric TVCs (arrows, **A**, **B**). The location of the TVCs on axial imaging can usually be identified at the level of the cricoarytenoid articulations (arrowheads, **A**). In this case, a dedicated larynx protocol was performed with thin 1.5-mm images reconstructed from the initial straight 4-mm data set and angled parallel to the C4-C5 disc space, as demonstrated on a sagittal reformatted image (**C**, yellow angled line). The C4-C5 disc space is generally parallel to the plane of the TVCs and allows complete visualization of the entire length of the TVC. Conversely, straight axial images will only visualize a portion of the TVCs on any given image.

Volume averaging with the normal laryngeal ventricle

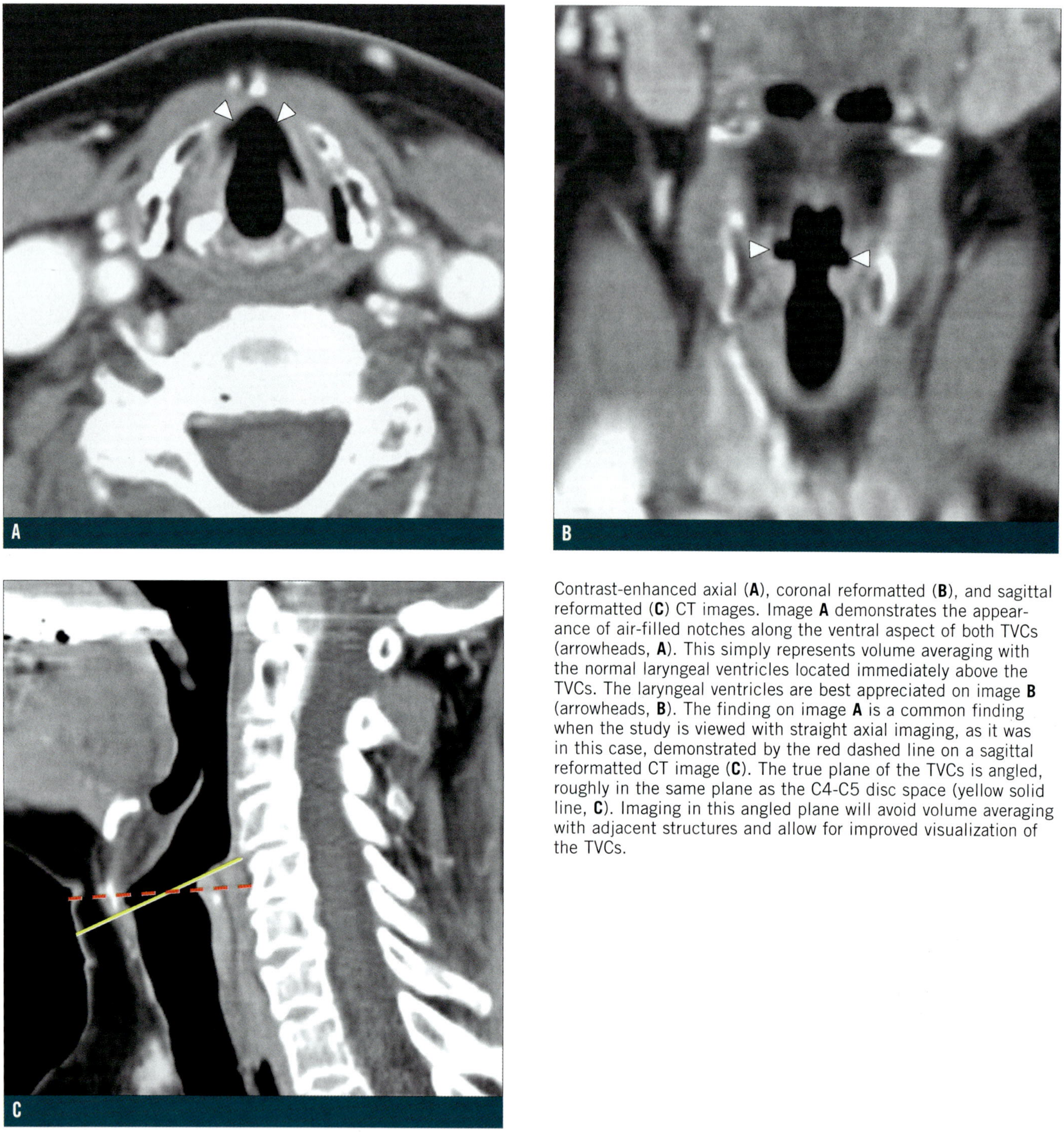

Contrast-enhanced axial (**A**), coronal reformatted (**B**), and sagittal reformatted (**C**) CT images. Image **A** demonstrates the appearance of air-filled notches along the ventral aspect of both TVCs (arrowheads, **A**). This simply represents volume averaging with the normal laryngeal ventricles located immediately above the TVCs. The laryngeal ventricles are best appreciated on image **B** (arrowheads, **B**). The finding on image **A** is a common finding when the study is viewed with straight axial imaging, as it was in this case, demonstrated by the red dashed line on a sagittal reformatted CT image (**C**). The true plane of the TVCs is angled, roughly in the same plane as the C4-C5 disc space (yellow solid line, **C**). Imaging in this angled plane will avoid volume averaging with adjacent structures and allow for improved visualization of the TVCs.

Laryngeal rotation simulating true vocal cord pathology

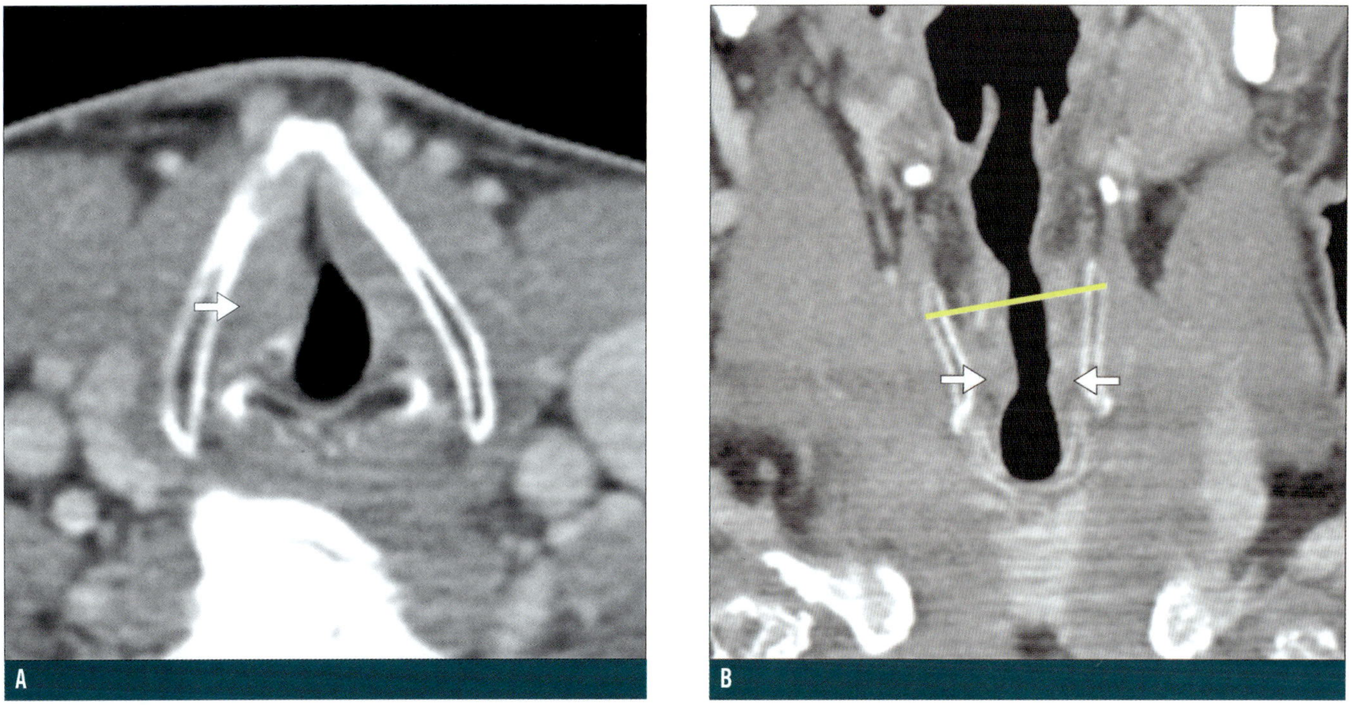

A contrast-enhanced axial CT image (**A**) demonstrates an apparent fullness of the right TVC (arrow, **A**) relative to the left. A coronal reformatted CT image from the same study (**B**) demonstrates a right lateral rotation of the laryngeal apparatus (yellow angled line) which accounts for the TVC asymmetry on axial imaging. The TVCs are completely symmetric and unremarkable on image **B** (arrows, **B**).

Laryngeal rotation simulating true vocal cord pathology

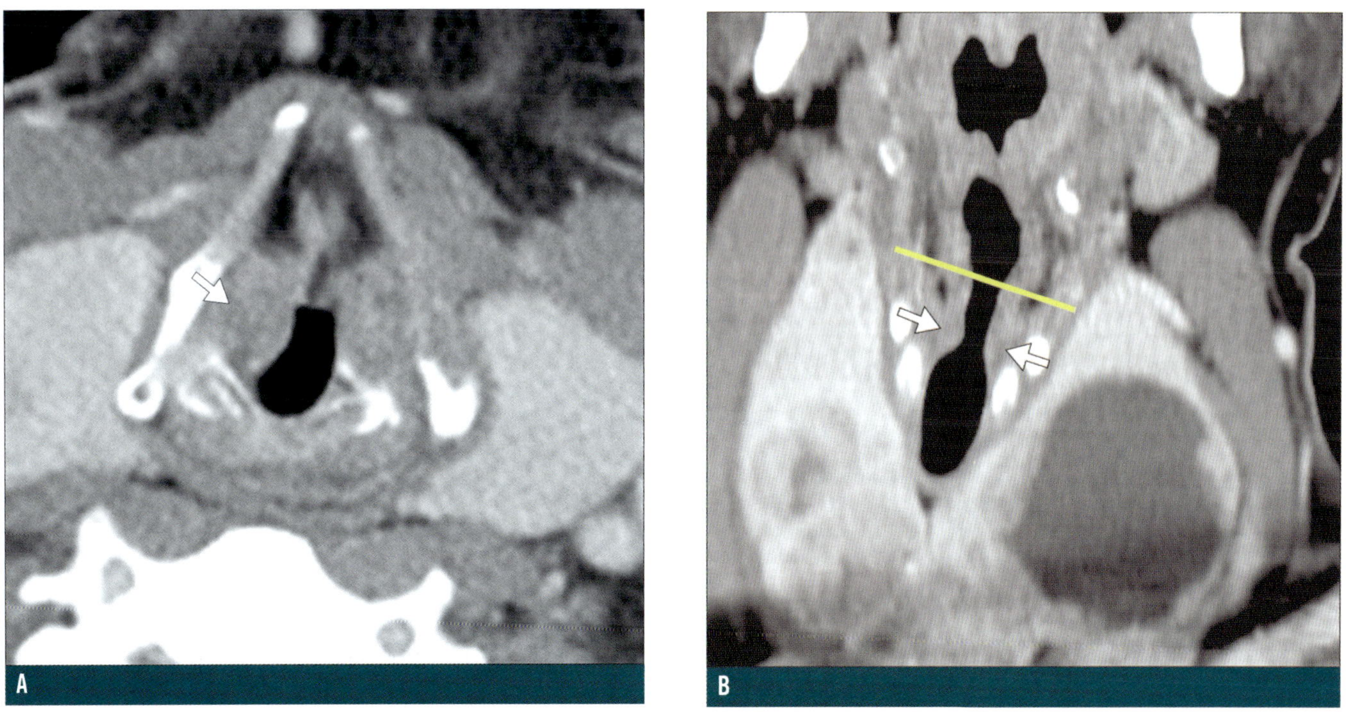

Different patient. A contrast-enhanced axial CT image (**A**) demonstrates apparent asymmetric fullness of the right TVC simulating a tumor (arrow, **A**). A coronal reformatted CT image from the same study (**B**) demonstrates marked rotation of the laryngeal apparatus (yellow angled line) due to a large multinodular thyroid goiter with completely symmetric and normal TVCs (arrows, **B**). Frequently, evaluating the TVCs with coronal reformatted imaging is helpful to determine whether incidental rotation of the laryngeal apparatus accounts for an asymmetric TVC finding on axial imaging and often allows for a more accurate assessment of any TVC asymmetry.

Companion case: True vocal cord asymmetry due to denervation atrophy

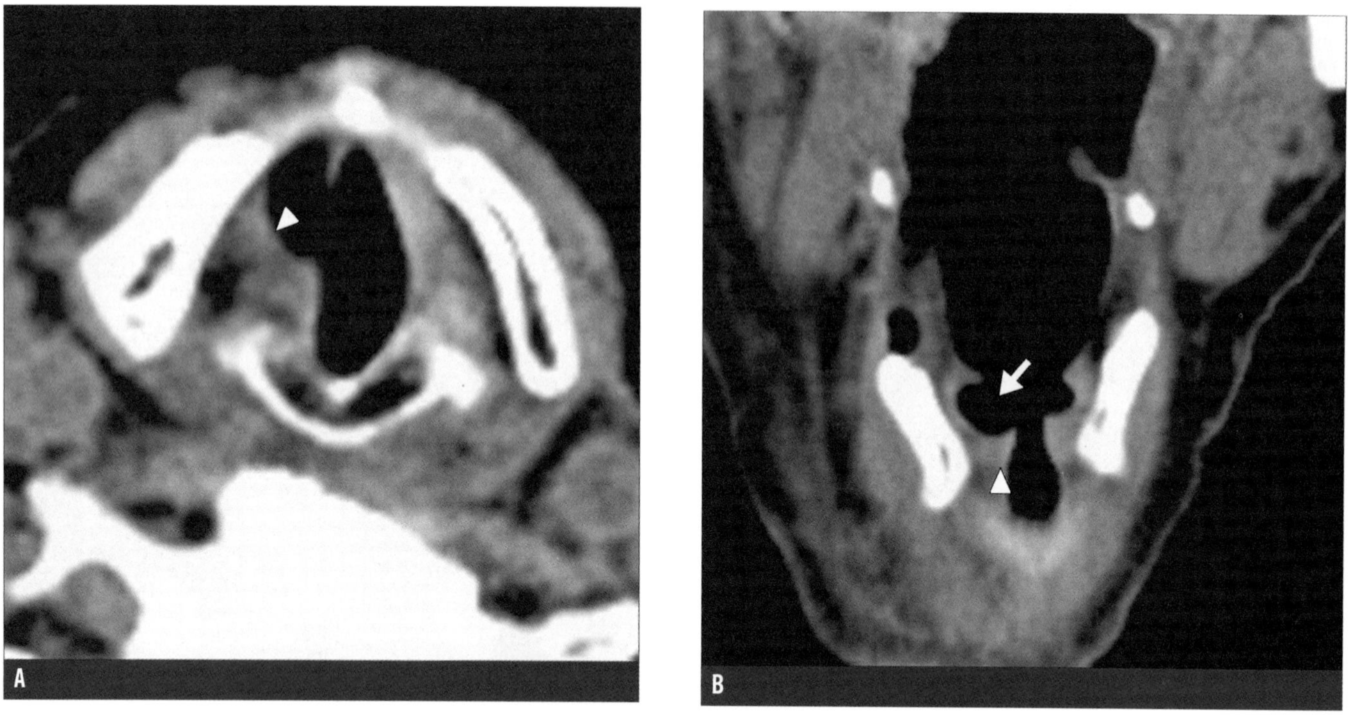

An unenhanced axial CT image (**A**) demonstrates diffuse abnormal fatty infiltration of the right TVC (arrowhead, **A**). A coronal reformatted CT image (**B**) demonstrates volume loss of the right TVC (arrowhead, **B**), although the fatty infiltration is not as well appreciated on this image. These findings are compatible with a TVC paralysis. Associated ipsilateral dilation of the right laryngeal ventricle is also present (arrow, **B**). Volume averaging with the enlarged laryngeal ventricle is present on image **A**, an abnormal finding in this case.

Companion case: True vocal cord polyp

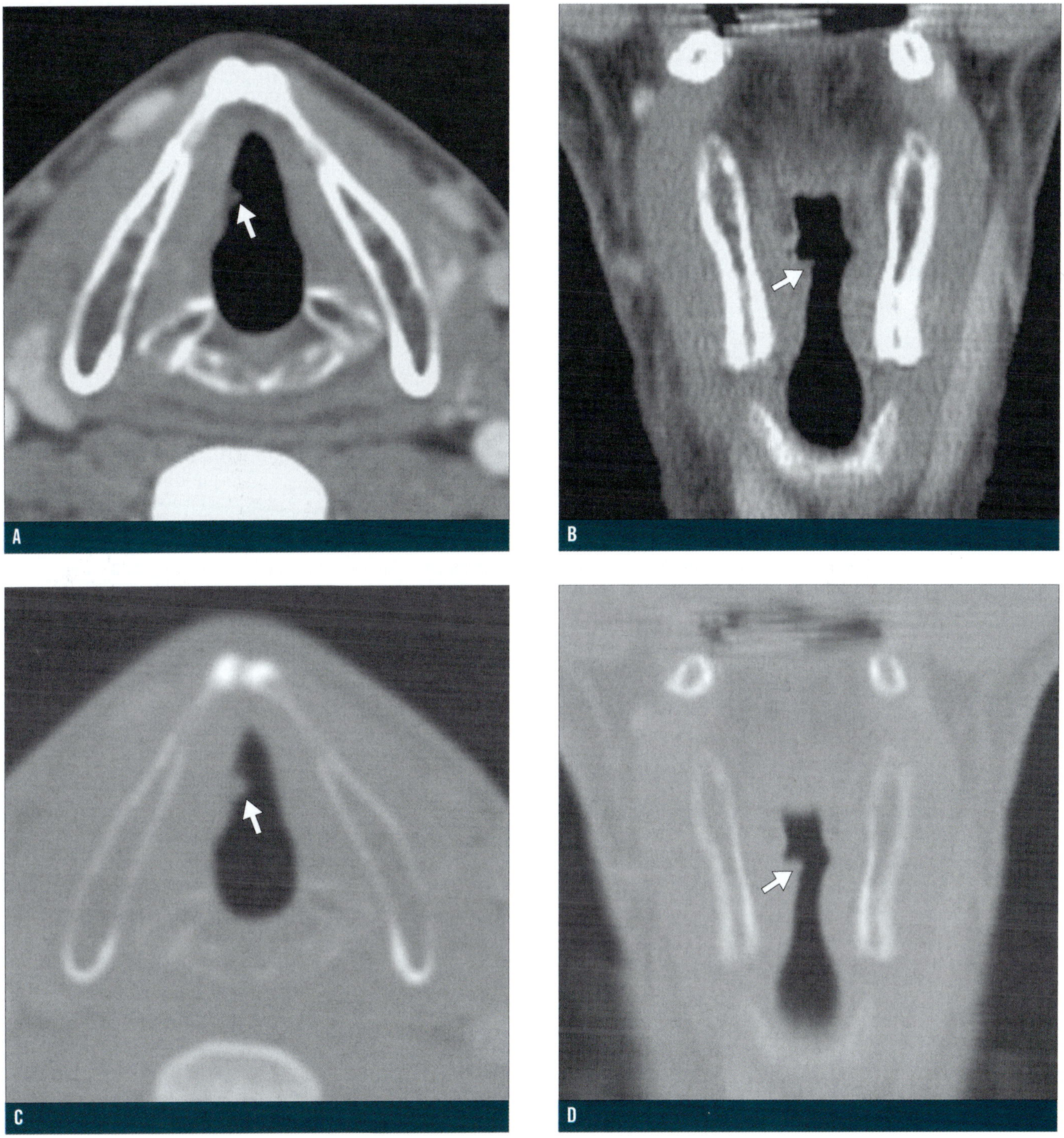

Contrast-enhanced axial (**A**) and coronal reformatted (**B**) CT images viewed with a soft tissue window demonstrate a very subtle irregularity along the medial margin of the right TVC that could be mistaken for mild, incidental asymmetry (arrows, **A**, **B**). However, the same images viewed with a wide window (**C**, **D**) more clearly demonstrate the contour abnormality and a clinically suspected TVC polyp. Using a wide window (such as a lung window) when evaluating the TVCs and trachea will often improve visualization of subtle contour irregularities that may be difficult to appreciate on soft tissue windows.

Companion case: True vocal cord squamous cell carcinoma

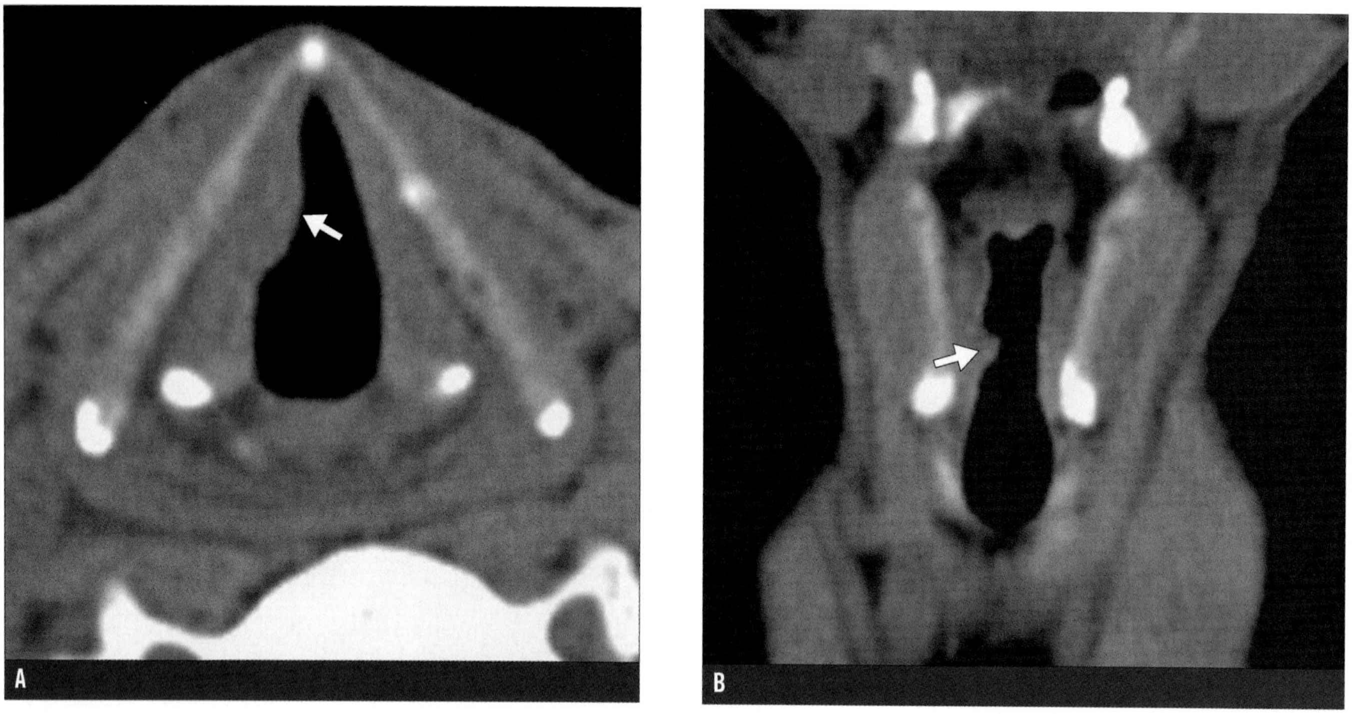

Unenhanced axial (**A**) and coronal reformatted (**B**) CT images demonstrate asymmetric fullness of the right TVC (arrows, **A**, **B**). The asymmetry in this case proved to be a true finding and represented invasive squamous cell carcinoma of the right TVC.

REFERENCES

Becker M, Burkhardt K, Dulguerov P, Allal A. Imaging of the larynx and hypopharynx. *Eur J Radiol.* 2008;66:460-479.

Chin S-C, Edelstein S, Chen C-Y, Som PM. Using CT to localize side and level of vocal cordparalysis. *AJR Am J Roentgenol.* 2003; 180:1165-1170.

Kumar VA, Lewin JS, Ginsberg LE. CT Assessment of Vocal Cord Medialization. *Am J Neuroradiol.* 2006;27:1643-1646.

Mafee M, Becker M. *Imaging of the Head and Neck.* Second edition. Georg Thieme Verlag; New York, 2005.

Paquette CM, Manos DC, Psooy BJ. Unilateral vocal cord paralysis: a review of CT findings, mediastinal causes, and the course of the recurrent laryngeal nerves. *Radiographics.* 2012;32:721-740.

Zinreich SJ. Imaging in laryngeal cancer: computed tomography, magnetic resonance imaging, positron emission tomography. *Otolaryng Clin North Am.* 2002;35:971-991, v.

CASE 13 Closed glottis due to breath-hold

Representing the voice-producing portion of the larynx, the glottis consists of two TVCs and the opening between the TVCs termed the rima glottidis. The rima glottidis is the narrowest part of the laryngeal cavity and changes shape and size with breathing and phonation.

Manipulation of the glottis occurs via a complex interplay between numerous sets of muscles, nearly all of which are innervated by the recurrent laryngeal nerve, a branch of the vagus nerve. The exception is the cricothyroid muscle, which is innervated by the external branch of the superior laryngeal nerve, although this is also a branch of the vagus nerve.

During normal inspiration, the TVCs separate and allow air entry into the lungs, while during expiration, the TVCs partially—but not fully—close. However, during phonation or breath-hold, the TVCs essentially completely close. A closed glottis due to breath-hold or phonation will typically be identified by CT and not MRI, due to the quick acquisition time of the former and the relatively long acquisition time of the latter. A closed glottis due to breath-hold or phonation can usually be identified by recognizing that both arytenoid cartilages are medially rotated and the TVCs are abutting one another. However, other entities can simulate this incidental finding, including a large transglottic tumor or diffuse laryngeal edema, such as from an anaphylactic reaction or radiation therapy.

If a closed glottis due to breath-hold is frequently encountered on imaging from a particular CT scanner, then inquiring whether the patient is inappropriately being instructed to hold their breath by the technician, or by the automated voice generated by the CT scanner, should be performed. A closed glottis due to phonation may result in superimposed motion artifact of the TVCs. Finally, when a closed glottis is encountered that is the result of breath-hold or phonation, then a detailed evaluation of the glottic larynx is limited and the study may need to be repeated if this area is of concern.

COMPANION CASES

- **Closed glottis due to an indwelling tracheostomy tube.** The glottis is usually closed and the pharynx is often collapsed when a tracheostomy tube is in place. A closed glottis and collapsed pharynx often preclude an accurate imaging evaluation of these structures.
- **Transglottic tumor.** Transglottic tumors represent laryngeal tumors that cross at least two of the three portions of the larynx (supraglottis, glottis, or subglottis), whether it be along the mucosa, submucosa/paraglottic fat, or both. Squamous cell carcinoma is overwhelmingly the most common histologic subtype of laryngeal cancer.

Closed glottis due to breath-hold

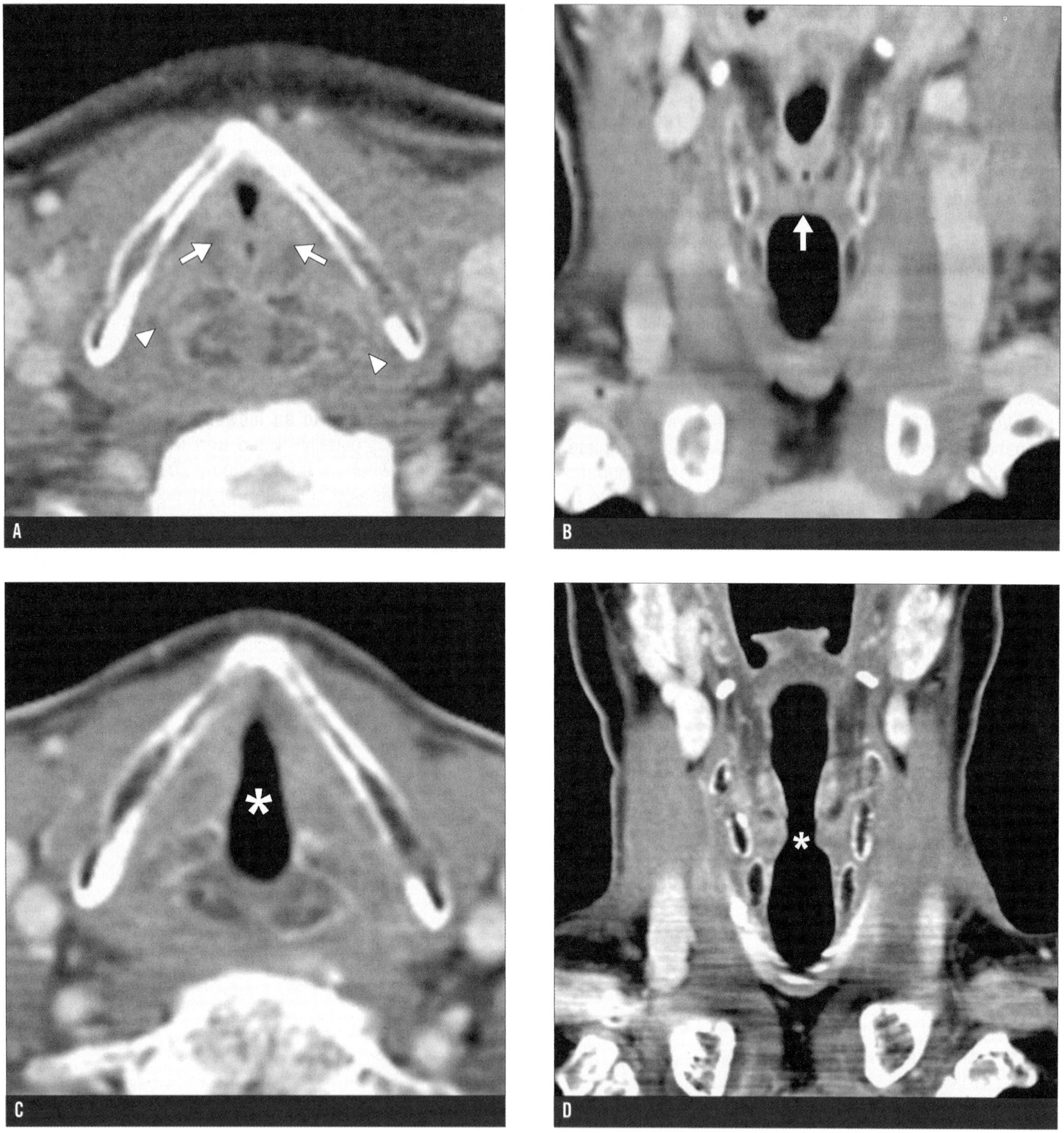

Contrast-enhanced axial (**A**) and coronal reformatted (**B**) CT images demonstrate apparent soft tissue fullness of the TVCs (arrows, **A**) and obliteration of the airway between the TVCs, known as the rima glottidis (arrow, **B**). Contrast-enhanced axial (**C**) and coronal reformatted (**D**) CT images from a follow-up study demonstrate a widely patent rima glottidis (asterisks, **C**, **D**). The findings on images **A** and **B** related to a breath-hold during the scan that resulted in apposition of the TVCs and closure of the rima glottidis. The arytenoid cartilages during breath-hold are medially rotated (arrowheads, **A**), an additional clue that the patient was holding their breath during the scan. Phonation during the scan will result in a similar finding, sometimes with superimposed motion artifact.

Companion case: Closed glottis due to an indwelling tracheostomy tube

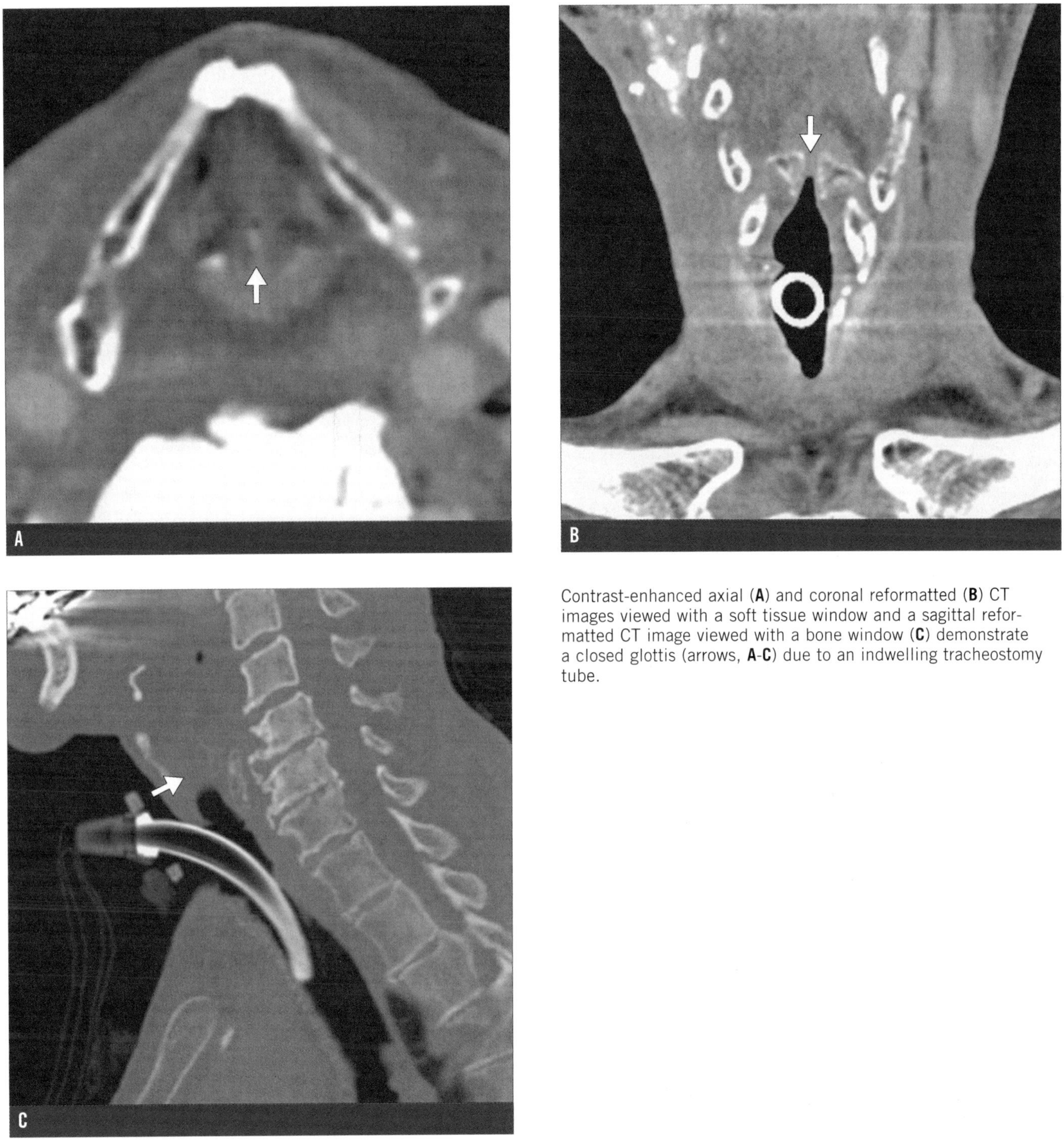

Contrast-enhanced axial (**A**) and coronal reformatted (**B**) CT images viewed with a soft tissue window and a sagittal reformatted CT image viewed with a bone window (**C**) demonstrate a closed glottis (arrows, **A**-**C**) due to an indwelling tracheostomy tube.

Companion case: Transglottic tumor

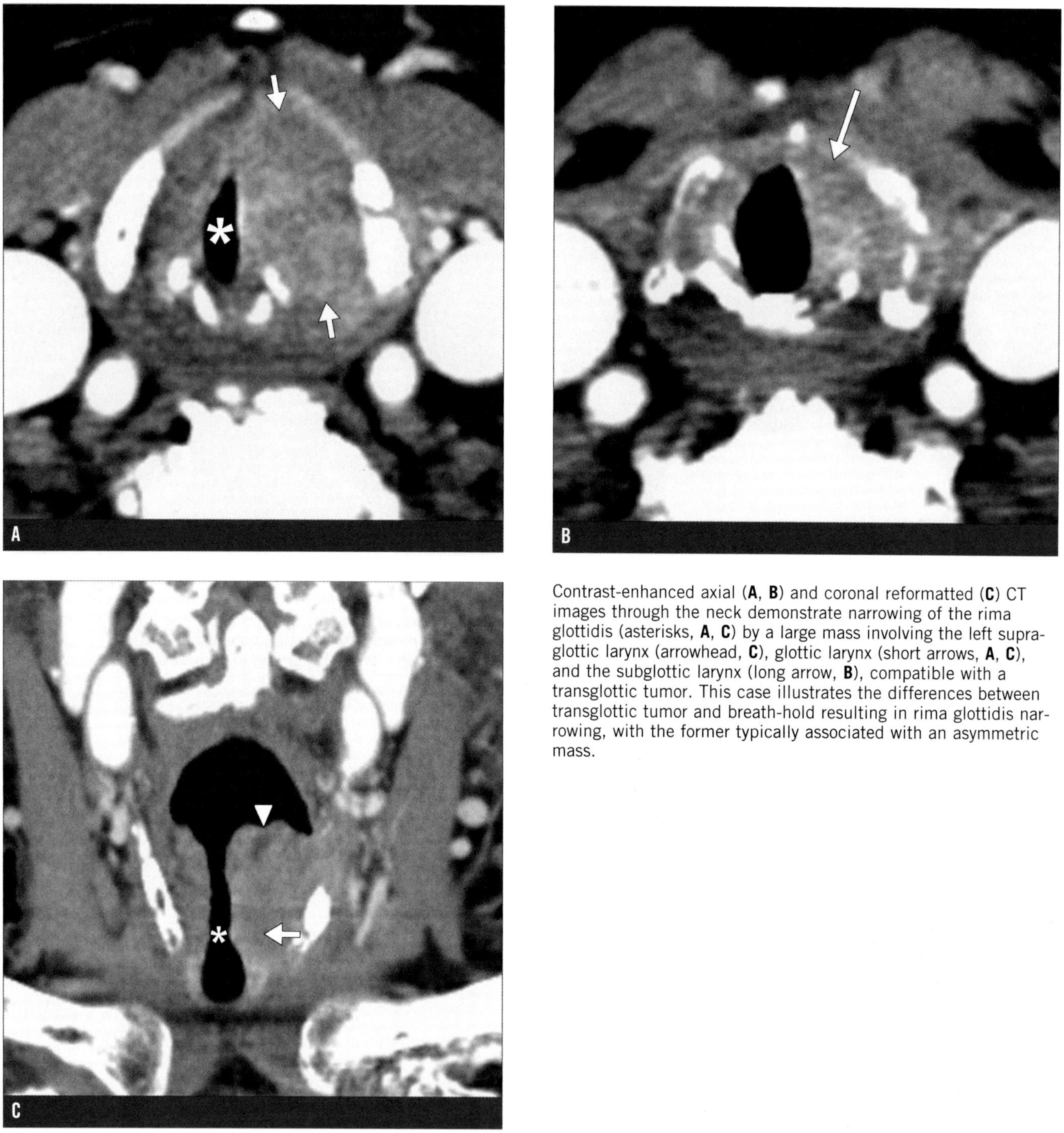

Contrast-enhanced axial (**A**, **B**) and coronal reformatted (**C**) CT images through the neck demonstrate narrowing of the rima glottidis (asterisks, **A**, **C**) by a large mass involving the left supraglottic larynx (arrowhead, **C**), glottic larynx (short arrows, **A**, **C**), and the subglottic larynx (long arrow, **B**), compatible with a transglottic tumor. This case illustrates the differences between transglottic tumor and breath-hold resulting in rima glottidis narrowing, with the former typically associated with an asymmetric mass.

REFERENCES

Barnes L. *Surgical Pathology of the Head and Neck.* New York, NY: Dekker; 1985:171-172.

Mendelsohn MS, Martin RE. Airway protection during breath-holding. *Ann Otol Rhino Laryngol.* 1993;102:941-944.

Noordzij JP, Ossoff RH. Anatomy and physiology of the larynx. *Otolaryngol Clin North Am.* 2006;39:1-10.

Shah RR, Lewin JS. Imaging of the infrahyoid neck. *Neuroimaging Clin N Am.* 1998;8:219-234.

CASE 14 Characteristic findings of true vocal cord paralysis

The etiologies of a true vocal cord paralysis (TVC) are varied and include iatrogenic causes from surgery or endotracheal intubation, noniatrogenic trauma, primary or metastatic neoplasms, and infectious/inflammatory processes. However, a cause of TVC paralysis is not always evident by imaging. If a cause of TVC paralysis is identified on imaging, it will usually reside along the course of the vagus nerve or recurrent laryngeal nerve. The vagus nerve travels posterior to the carotid artery within the carotid sheath as it descends within the neck. Each vagus nerve gives rise to a recurrent laryngeal nerve. On the left, the recurrent laryngeal nerve arises anterior to the aortic arch and wraps anterior to posterior along the undersurface of the arch within the aortopulmonary window. On the right, the vagus nerve gives rise to the right recurrent laryngeal nerve as it crosses anterior to the right subclavian artery. The recurrent laryngeal then courses caudal and ascends posterior to the right subclavian artery. Both recurrent laryngeal nerves continue to ascend along their respective tracheoesophageal grooves and divide into anterior and posterior rami at the level of the larynx to supply the laryngeal musculature.

The recurrent laryngeal nerves innervate all the muscles of the larynx, with the exception of the cricothyroid muscle, which is innervated by the external branch of the superior laryngeal artery (also a branch of the vagus nerve). In every case of TVC paralysis, it is critical to evaluate the course of the vagus nerve as well as the course of both recurrent laryngeal nerves in order to determine whether there is an imaging finding to explain a TVC paralysis.

Mimics and imaging pitfalls of a TVC paralysis can generally be avoided if one considers the hallmarks of TVC paralysis—laryngeal muscle denervation atrophy and shifing of the supraglottic structures because of regional volume loss. Several imaging findings at the level of the TCVs and aryepiglottic folds directly relate to this pathophysiology. The ipsilateral thyroarytenoid muscle, and often the ipsilateral posterior cricoarytenoid muscle, will be fatty infiltrated and atrophic with a chronic TVC paralysis, since both muscles are innervated by the recurrent laryngeal nerve. Additional ipsilateral findings may include dilation of the pyriform sinus, enlargement of the laryngeal ventricle, medialization of the TVC, medialization and thickening of the aryepiglottic fold, medial rotation of the arytenoid cartilage, and enlargement of the cricothyroid notch (space between the cricoid and thyroid cartilages on axial imaging).

Acute denervation is often accompanied by edema that results in enlargement of the affected muscle. Thus, with acute TVC paralysis, the affected TVC will be enlarged and diffusely mildly hypoattenuating (but not fat attenuating) on CT. On MRI, a TVC with acute denervation will be enlarged, T2 hyperintense, and enhance. Because there is considerable overlap in the appearance of an acutely paralyzed TVC and a TVC tumor, history in these cases is paramount.

Laryngeal FDG-uptake during a PET scan is symmetric and low level in the normal resting vocal apparatus. With vocalization at or near the time of FDG administration, a relatively increased amount of FDG-uptake will be present due to increased metabolic activity of the contracting muscles. However, with a unilateral TVC paralysis, there will be a paucity of metabolic activity in the paralyzed cord and asymmetric radiopharmaceutical uptake in the contralateral normal contracting TVC, a finding that may simulate tumor in the normal functioning TVC.

COMPANION CASE

- **Laryngeal tumor simulating true vocal cord paralysis.** An isolated, medialized TVC not accompanied by ancillary findings supporting acute or chronic denervation should not be assumed to represent a TVC paralysis. In fact, a TVC may be medialized or clinically "paralyzed" due to a tumor. A medialized TVC due to tumor will be characterized by increased volume of the TVC rather than volume loss of the TVC, as would be expected with chronic denervation. In addition, a tumor of the TVC on CT and MRI will be composed of soft tissue density and signal, respectively, as opposed to fat (as is present with chronic denervation) or edema (as is present with acute denervation). Unexplained subglottic soft tissue identified in conjunction with a medialized TVC should always be viewed with suspicion and is tumor until proven otherwise.

Chronic true vocal cord paralysis

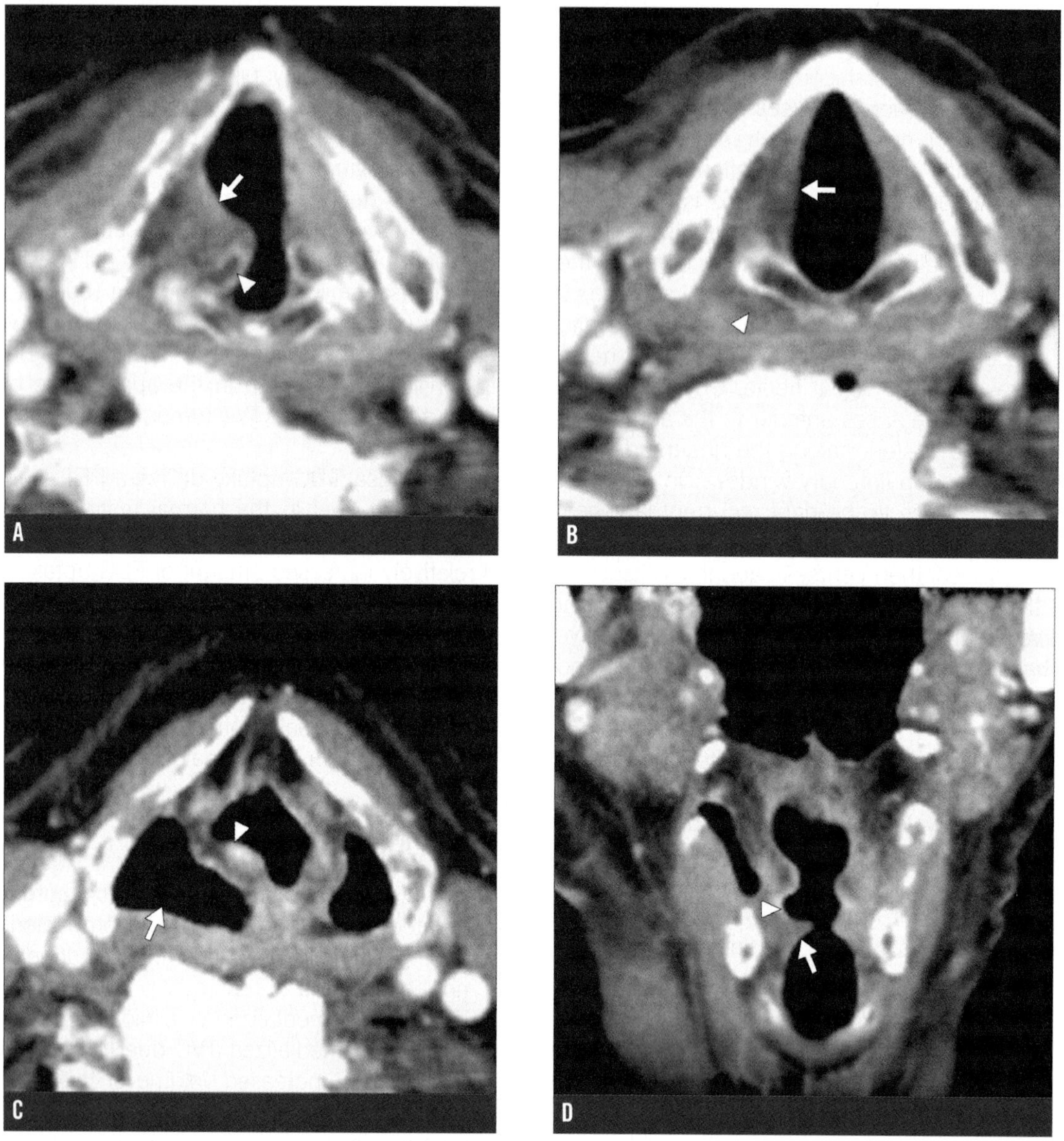

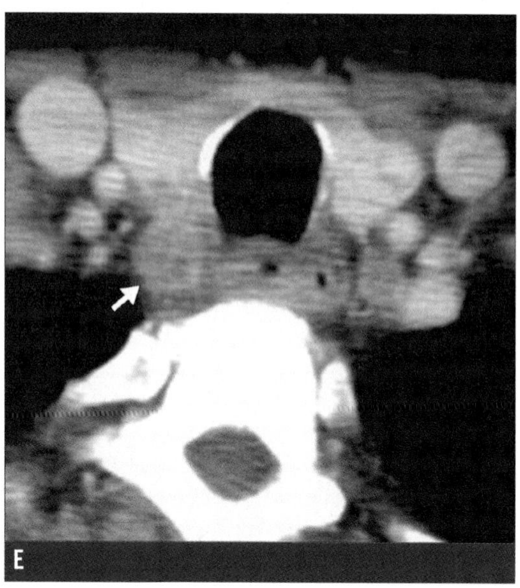

Contrast-enhanced axial (**A-C**) and coronal reformatted (**D**) CT images demonstrate classic findings of a right TVC paralysis. There is diffuse fatty infiltration and medialization of the right TVC (arrows, **A**, **B**), medial rotation of the right arytenoid cartilage (arrowhead, **A**), atrophy of the right posterior cricoarytenoid muscle (arrowhead, **B**), medialization of the ipsilateral aryepiglottic fold (arrowhead, **C**), enlargement of the ipsilateral pyriform sinus (arrow, **C**), volume loss of the right TVC (arrow, **D**), and dilation of the ipsilateral laryngeal ventricle (arrowhead, **D**). An axial CT image of the lower neck (**E**) demonstrates a right paraesophageal mass (arrow, **E**), likely infiltrating the right recurrent laryngeal nerve at the right tracheoesophageal groove and resulting in the TVC paralysis.

Chronic true vocal cord paralysis

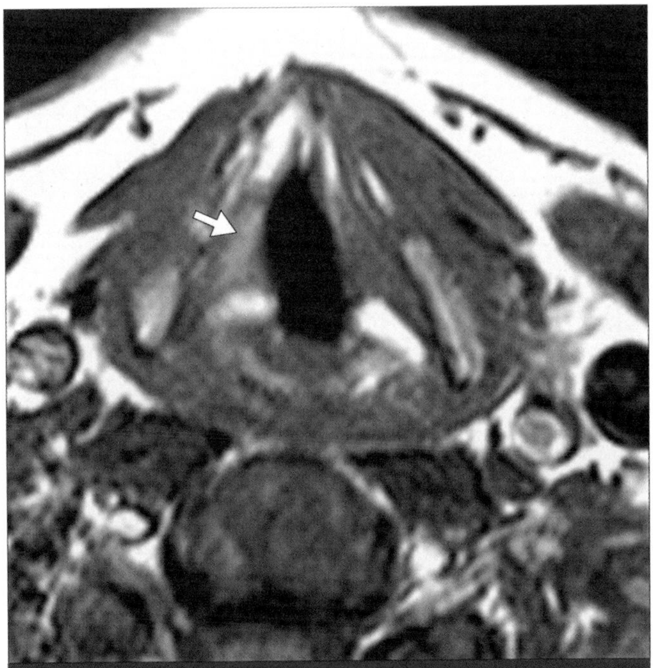

A

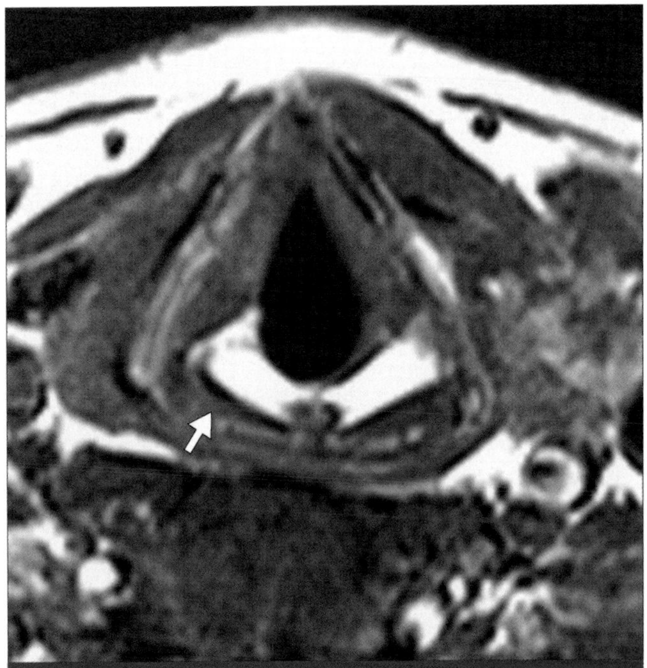

B

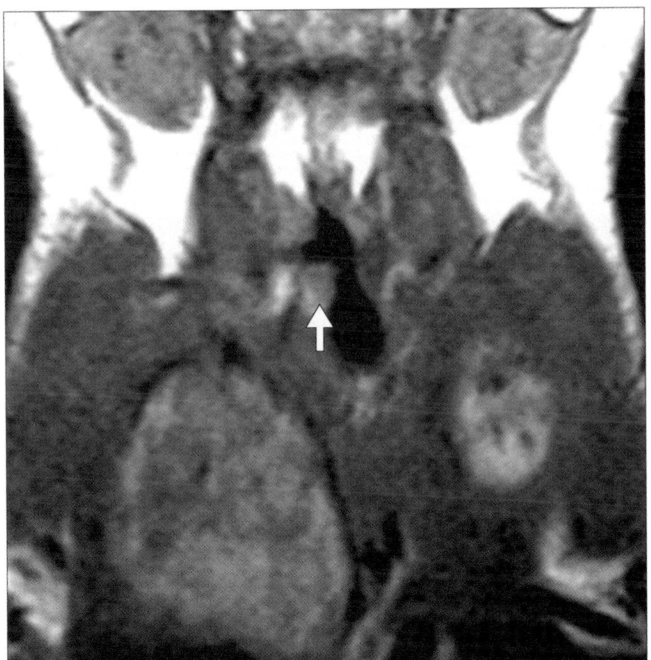

C

Different patient. Unenhanced axial T1 (**A**, **B**) and coronal T1 (**C**) MR images demonstrate fatty infiltration of the right TVC, compatible with TVC paralysis and denervation atrophy (arrows, **A**, **C**). While image **C** does not reflect this, right TVC volume loss was present, as is evident on image A (arrow, **A**). Image **B** demonstrates associated volume loss and denervation atrophy of the right posterior cricoarytenoid muscle (arrow, **B**).

Acute true vocal cord paralysis

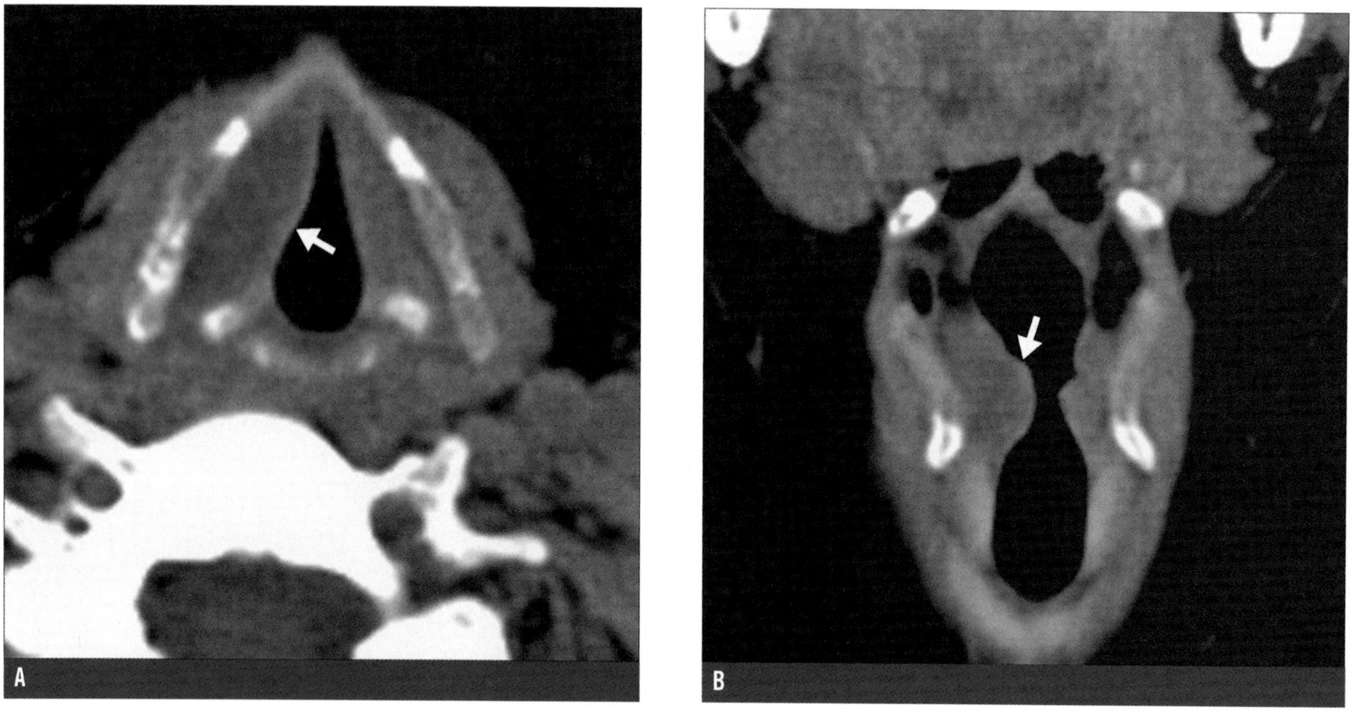

Unenhanced axial (**A**) and coronal reformatted (**B**) CT images demonstrate a diffusely enlarged and edematous right TVC (arrows, **A**, **B**) relative to the left. This patient developed acute hoarseness following a cardiac transplant that persisted for several days. The right TVC was demonstrated to be paralyzed during laryngoscopy on POD #4, the day this imaging was obtained. The findings are compatible with acute denervation atrophy of the right TVC and presumably the result of right recurrent laryngeal nerve injury during the cardiac transplant.

True vocal cord paralysis on PET

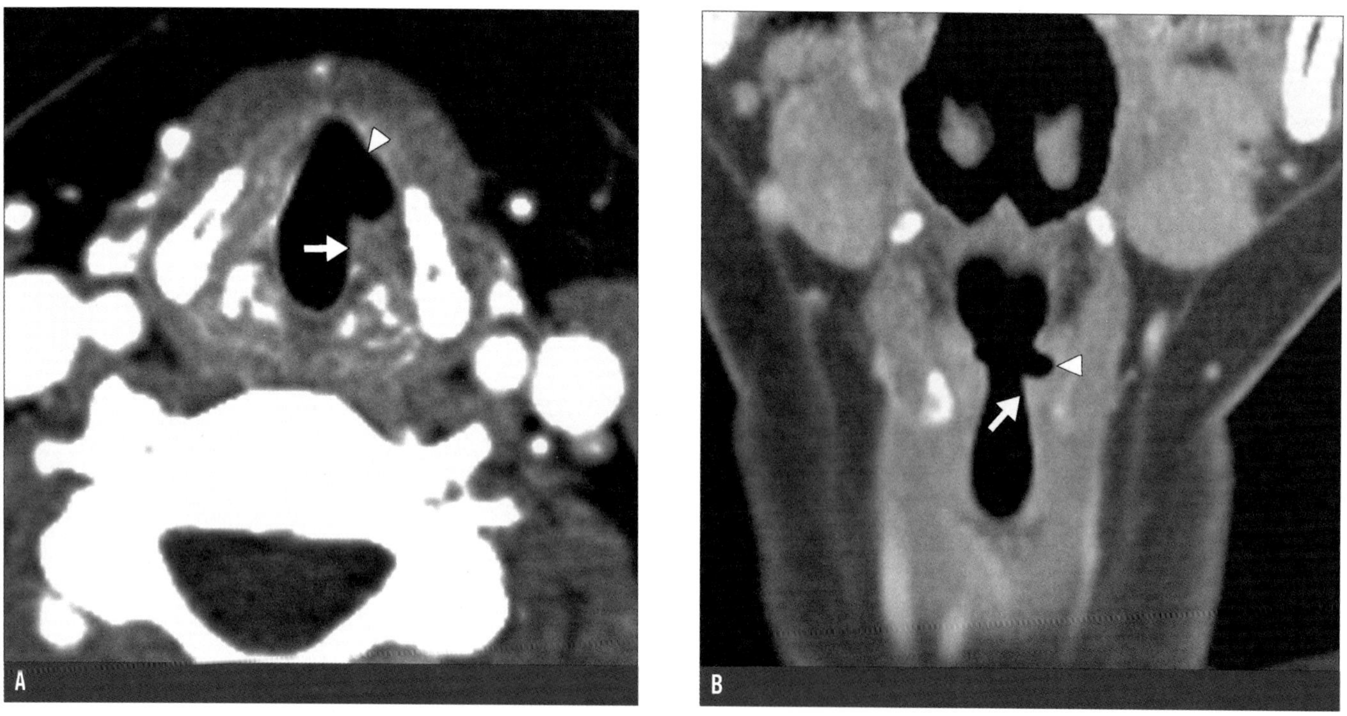

Contrast-enhanced axial (**A**) and coronal reformatted (**B**) CT images demonstrate findings compatible with a left TVC paralysis, including volume loss and fatty infiltration of the left TVC (arrows, **A**, **B**) and ipsilateral dilation of the left laryngeal ventricle (arrowheads, **A**, **B**). Axial (**C**) and coronal (**D**) FDG–PET images of the same patient demonstrate normal, expected metabolic activity of the right TVC (arrows, **C**, **D**) as well as expected lack of metabolic activity of the paralyzed left TVC. This asymmetry can simulate a mass involving the nonparalyzed TVC.

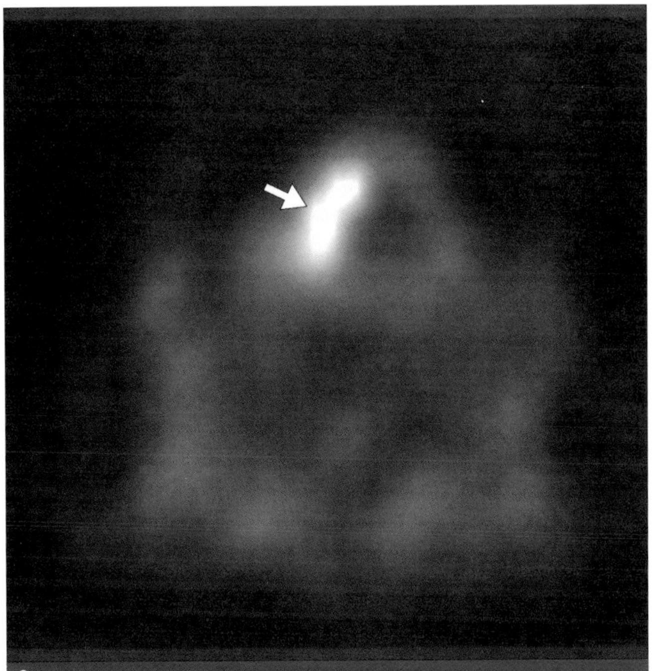

C

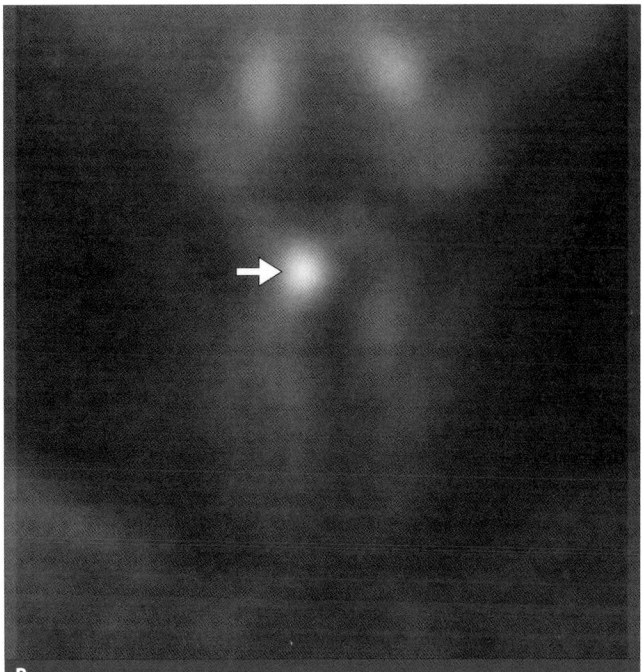

D

Companion case: Laryngeal tumor simulating true vocal cord paralysis

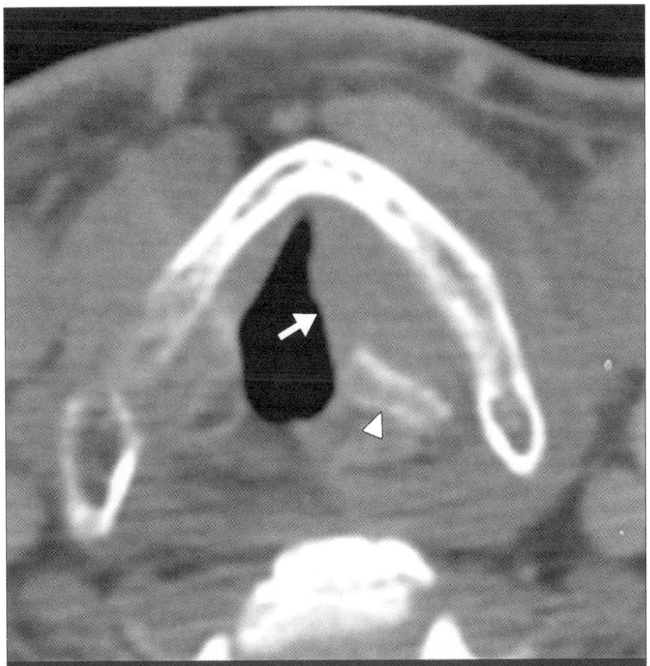

A

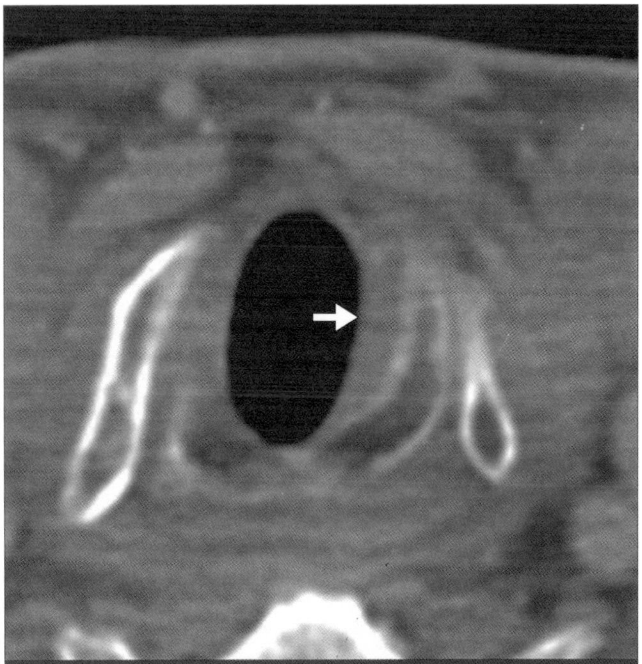

B

Contrast-enhanced axial CT images (**A**, **B**) demonstrate medialization of the left TVC (arrow, **A**) in this patient who presented with "TVC paralysis." A mass was not demonstrated at the initial laryngoscopy and the images were interpreted as findings compatible with TVC paralysis, given the medialization of the TVC. However, there is a small amount of abnormal soft tissue in the left subglottic larynx (arrow, **B**) as well as soft tissue density and fullness of the left TVC, rather than volume loss and fatty infiltration as would be expected with a chronic TVC paralysis. Moreover, there is asymmetric sclerosis of the left arytenoid cartilage (arrowhead, **A**) which in the setting of a suspected adjacent mass, raises the possibility of tumor infiltration of the cartilage. The constellation of findings are suspicious for a left TVC tumor with subglottic extension, which was eventually confirmed at pathology. In order to diagnose TVC paralysis, volume loss of the TVC as well as regional associated volume loss (ie, enlarged ipsilateral laryngeal ventricle, enlarged ipsilateral pyriform sinus, etc) should be present. In addition, soft tissue in the subglottic larynx should always be viewed with suspicion, particularly if associated with ipsilateral TVC fullness.

REFERENCES

Chin S-C, Edelstein S, Chen C-Y, Som PM. Using CT to localize side and level of vocal cord paralysis. *AJR Am J Roentgenol.* 2003;180:1165-1170.

Komissarova M, Wong KK, Piert M, Mukherji SK, Fig LM. Spectrum of 18F-FDG PET/CT findings in oncology-related recurrent laryngeal nerve palsy. *AJR Am J Roentgenol.* 2009;192:288-294.

Kostakoglu L, Wong JC, Barrington SF, Cronin BF, Dynes AM, Maisey MN. Speech-related visualization of laryngeal muscles with fluorine-18-FDG. *J Nucl Med.* 1996;37:1771-1773.

Kumar VA, Lewin JS, Ginsberg LE. CT assessment of vocal cord medialization. *AJNR Am J Neuroradiol.* 2006;27:1643-1646.

Myssiorek D. Recurrent laryngeal nerve paralysis: anatomy and etiology. *Otolaryngol Clin North Am.* 2004;37:25-44.

Nakamoto Y, Tatsumi M, Hammoud D, Cohade C, Osman MM, Wahl RL. Normal FDG distribution patterns in the head and neck: PET/CT evaluation. *Radiology.* 2005;234:879-885.

Paquette CM, Manos DC, Psooy BJ. Unilateral vocal cord paralysis: a review of CT findings, mediastinal causes, and the course of the recurrent laryngeal nerves. *Radiographics.* 2012;32:721-740.

Rosenthal LHS, Benninger MS, Deeb RH. Vocal fold immobility: a longitudinal analysis of etiology over 20 years. *Laryngoscope.* 2007;117:1864-1870.

Rubin AD, Sataloff RT. Vocal fold paresis and paralysis. *Otolaryngol Clin North Am.* 2007;40:1109-1131, viii-ix.

CASE 15 Injection laryngoplasty

Glottic insufficiency refers to a group of abnormalities that includes vocal cord paralysis, paresis, scar, and atrophy that result in incomplete closure of the glottis and the formation of a glottic gap. Glottic insufficiency may be characterized by hoarseness, increased phonatory effort, vocal fatigue, and reduction in vocal volume. A number of treatment options exist for patients with glottic insufficiency, including medical therapies (steroids, antiviral medications), voice therapy, injection augmentation (ie, injection laryngoplasty), thyroplasty, and other laryngeal framework surgery.

Injection laryngoplasty is a procedure that augments and medializes the abnormal TVC so that it may abut the contralateral TVC. In cases of presbylaryngis (thinning or aging of the TVCs), bilateral TVC paresis, unilateral TVC paralysis with contralateral bowing, and some neurologic conditions such as Parkinson disease, bilateral TVC medialization may be pursued. The injectable is typically placed deep within the lateral aspect of the thyroarytenoid/lateral cricoarytenoid muscle complex. Injection laryngoplasty is usually only performed for mild/moderate glottic insufficiency (up to 3 mm of a glottic gap during phonation); greater degrees of glottic insufficiency are more appropriately treated by other means or in conjunction with laryngoplasty. Direct laryngoscopy, with or without intubation, is usually performed during an injection laryngoplasty procedure. Direct laryngoscopy allows for visualization of the TVC during the injection and for monitoring any possible complications as they occur. Preferably, a laryngoplasty is performed in the awake patient. In addition to avoiding general anesthesia, the awake patient is able to phonate and allow for real-time feedback during the procedure. The injection can be performed in the office by several percutaneous routes, including directly through the thyroid lamina (preferably in noncalcified thyroid cartilage/young patients), through the thyrohyoid membrane, or traversing the cricothyroid membrane. The injectable may also be placed via oral or transnasal endoscopic approaches.

There are numerous products available for an injection laryngoplasty that are broadly categorized as temporary (lasting months) and permanent/long lasting (lasting years). Temporary materials include carboxymethylcellulose (Radiesse Voice Gel), collagen-based products, bovine gelatin (Gelfoam), and hyaluronic acid (Restylane). Temporary laryngoplasty injectables are generally reserved for patients whose glottic incompetence prognosis is unclear, such as those patients who present with an acute unilateral TVC paralysis from an unknown etiology. Permanent/long-lasting laryngoplasty materials include Radiesse with calcium hydroxylapatite and autologous fat.

- **Radiesse Voice Gel injection laryngoplasty.** Composed of water, glycerin, and sodium carboxymethylcellulose, Radiesse Voice Gel is an FDA-approved material for injection augmentation of the TVCs. This compound does not require additional preparation time as other available products and effectively medializes the paralyzed TVC for a period of 1 to 3 months. This substance is hypoattenuating on CT. Because denervation atrophy of the TVC is also hypoatttenuating on CT, Radiesse Voice Gel may not be readily identied on CT without a history of the procedure. On MRI, it is hyperintense on T2 and hypointense on T1.
- **Fat injection laryngoplasty.** Autologous fat laryngoplasty may last from 1 to 3 years. As expected, this injection will have fat density on CT and fat signal on MRI. Accurate history is important in order to avoid misinterpreting this postprocedure appearance as fatty infiltration of the TVC as a result of denervation atrophy.
- **Radiesse with calcium injection laryngoplasty hydroxylapatite.** This injectable is FDA approved and utilizes the same carboxymethylcellulose carrier as Radiesse Voice Gel but contains calcium hydroxylapatite; thus, it is used for permanent/long-lasting laryngoplasty. This material will be hyperattenuating on CT and T1 as well as T2 hypointense on MRI. It has been shown that Radiesse with calcium hydroxylapatite is very frequently FDG-PET avid, particularly within the first 18 months following the procedure.
- **Teflon injection laryngoplasty.** Teflon (paste of polytetrafluoroethylene) was the favored synthetic substrate from the 1960s to the early 1990s, until concern over long-term side effects led to a search for more desirable compounds. Today, Teflon is rarely used for injection laryngoplasty. Complications from Teflon injections that were identified included migration of particles, giant cell foreign body reaction with granuloma formation, and difficulty in removing Teflon at subsequent surgery. A Teflon granuloma has been shown to be FDG PET avid, although this is a nonspecific finding that may be seen with a normal injectable, such as Radiesse with calcium hydroxylapatite.

COMPANION CASE

- **Subglottic extrusion of Radiesse with calcium hydroxylapatite injectable.** Local tissue reactions, including mild postprocedural edema and TVC polyp formation, are the most common complications of injectable calcium hydroxylapatite. Superficial injection into the subepithelial space is a rare complication that may lead to over-medialization of the cord and undesirable voice outcomes. Because of the low viscosity of the calcium hydroxylapatite preparation (which is designed to allow passage through a 25-gauge needle) the compound can track through tissue planes and into unplanned locations during placement or postoperatively during phonation or with coughing. While rare, a foreign body reaction can ensue which can disrupt vocal mechanics, threaten airway patency, and require surgical correction.

Temporary injection laryngoplasty: Radiesse Voice Gel

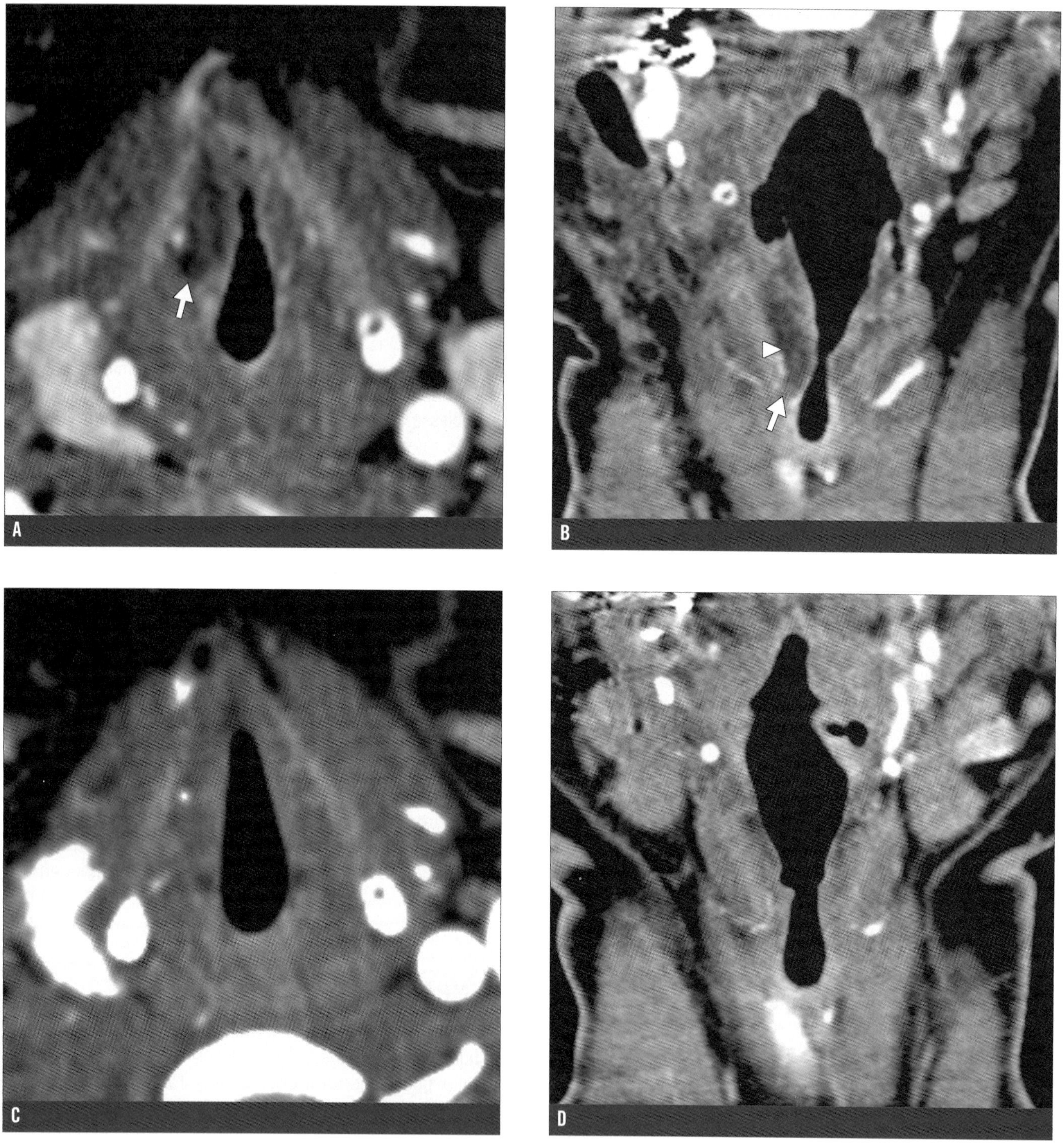

Contrast-enhanced axial (**A**) and coronal reformatted (**B**) CT images demonstrate low attenuation within the right TVC (arrows, **A**, **B**) as well as extending into the right supraglottic larynx (arrowhead, **B**). This finding represents Radiesse Voice Gel, an injectable used for temporary medialization of the TVC. Without history, this finding could be mistaken for right TVC edema or fatty infiltration, although the nonanatomic extension of the finding into the supraglottic larynx is evidence that this is related to an injectable. Contrast-enhanced axial (**C**) and coronal reformatted (**D**) CT images of the same patient obtained 6 months later demonstrate resolution of the right TVC and supraglottic extension of Radiesse Voice Gel.

Temporary injection laryngoplasty: Radiesse Voice Gel

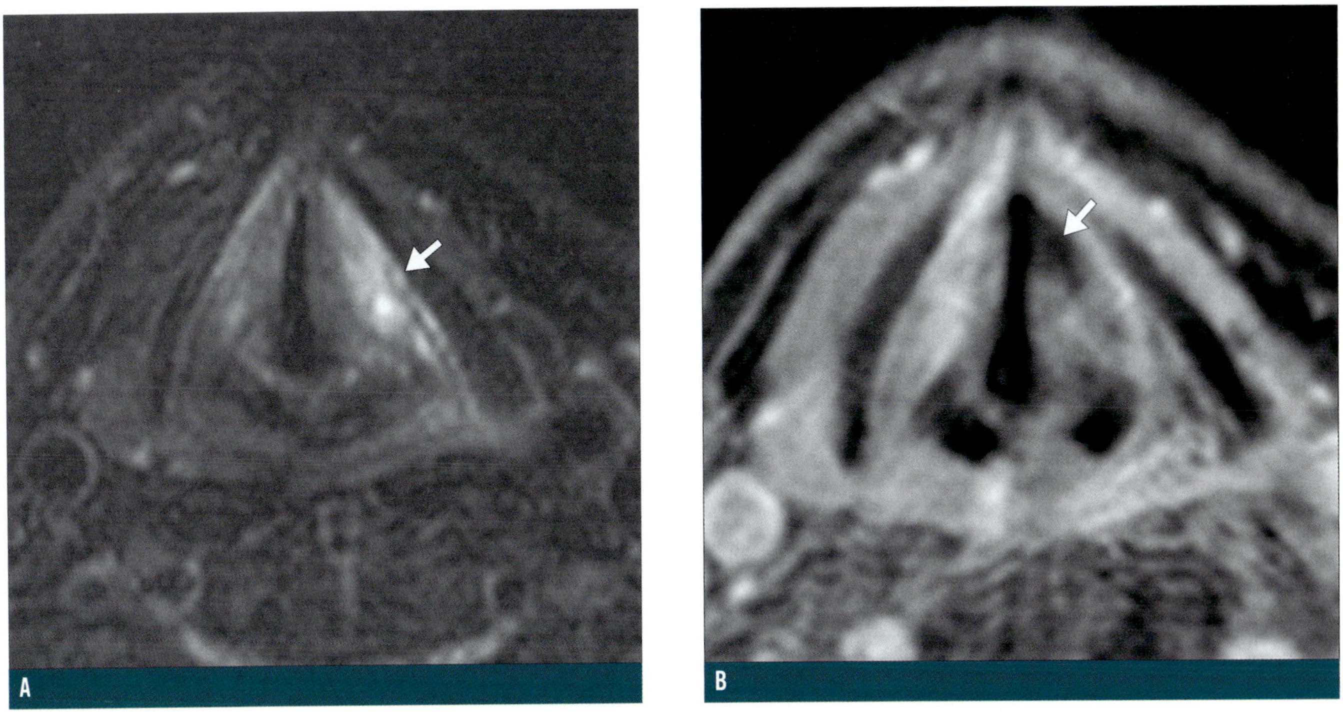

Different patient. Fat-suppressed axial T2 (**A**) and fat-suppressed contrast-enhanced axial T1 (**B**) MR images of a patient who had Radiesse Voice Gel injected into the left TVC. Image **A** demonstrates diffuse elevated T2 signal in the left TVC (arrow, **A**). Image **B** does not demonstrates any significant enhancement (arrow, **B**) when compared to the contralateral TVC and allowing for normal TVC enhancement.

Long-lasting injection laryngoplasty: Fat

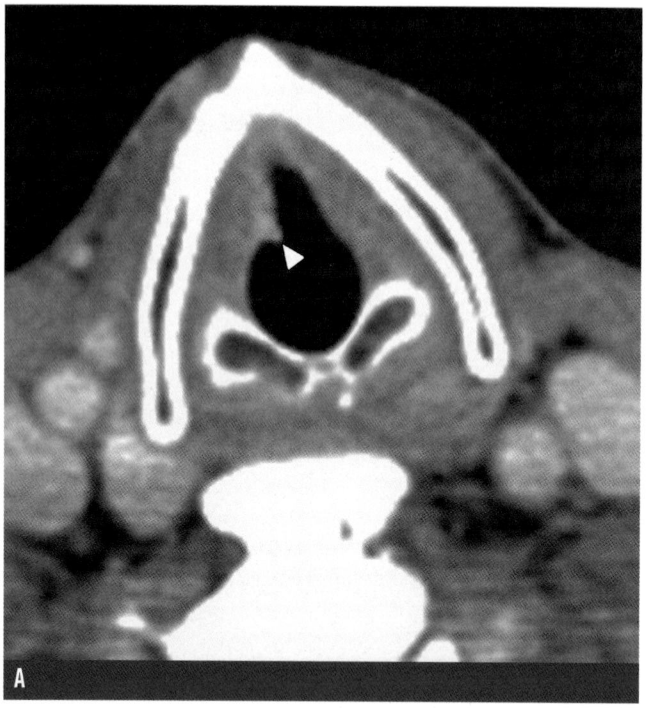

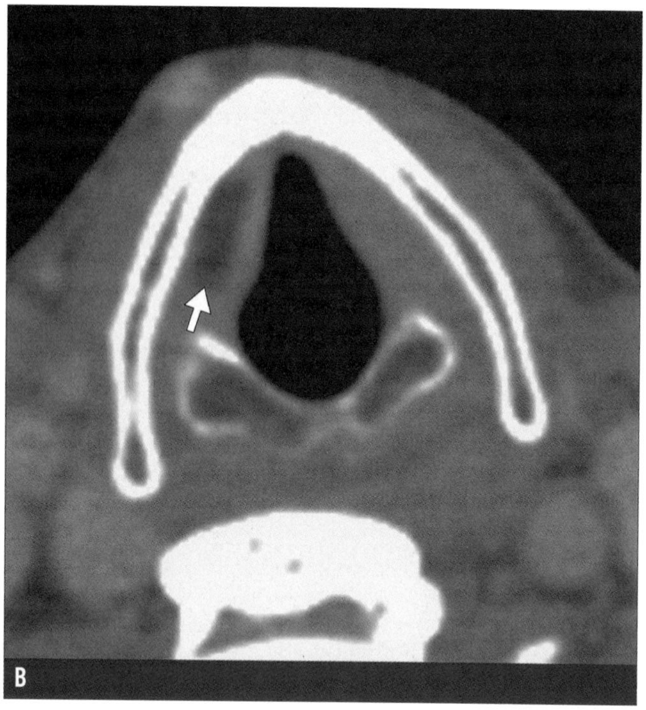

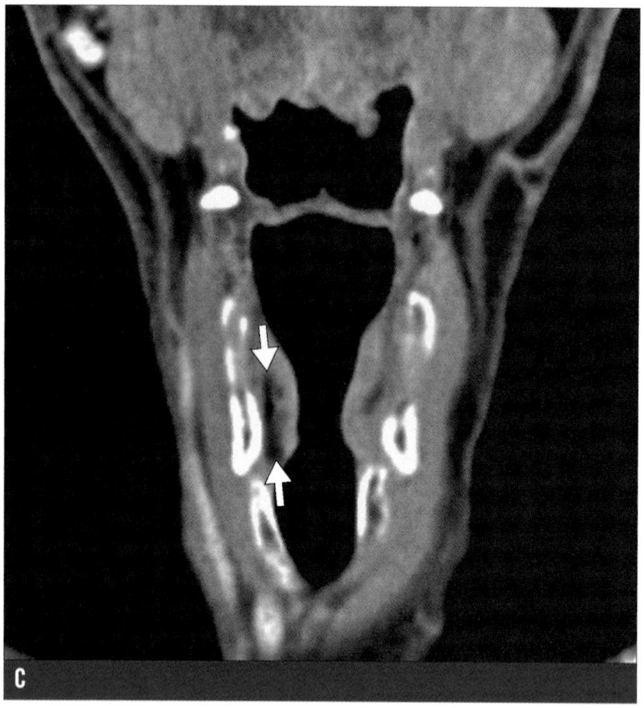

A contrast-enhanced axial CT image (**A**) demonstrates a small nodule arising from the right TVC, in this case representing a squamous cell carcinoma (arrowhead, **A**). Following treatment, the patient required right TVC augmentation. Fat was chosen to be the injectate, which was obtained from the patient's own periumbilical region. Following the fat injection laryngoplasty, contrast-enhanced axial (**B**) and coronal reformatted (**C**) CT images demonstrate the fat injectate infiltrating the right TVC (arrows, **B**, **C**).

Permanent/long-lasting unilateral injection laryngoplasty: Radiesse with calcium hydroxylapatite

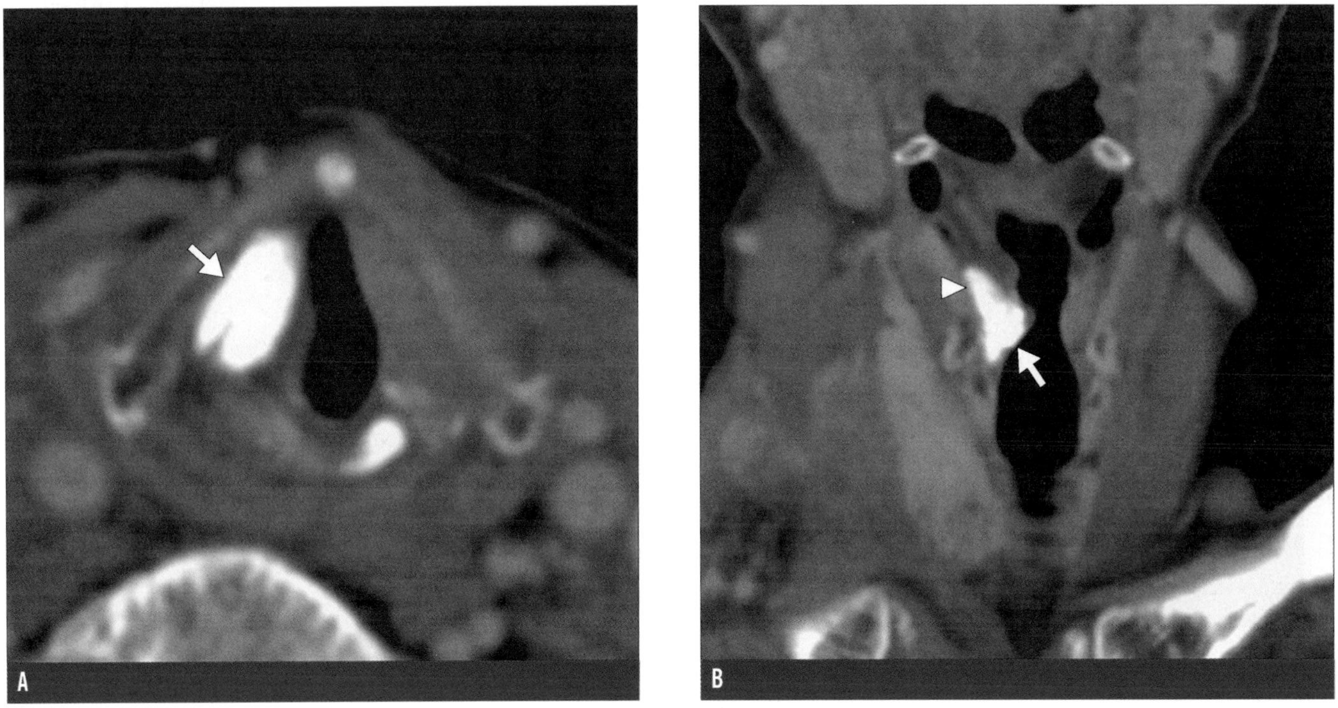

Contrast-enhanced axial (**A**) and coronal reformatted (**B**) CT images demonstrate increased attenuation in the right TVC (arrows, **A**, **B**) extending into the right supraglottic larynx (arrowhead, **B**) in this patient who received Radiesse with calcium hydroxylapatite, which is considered a permanent/long-lasting injectable.

Permanent/long-lasting bilateral injection laryngoplasty: Radiesse with calcium hydroxylapatite

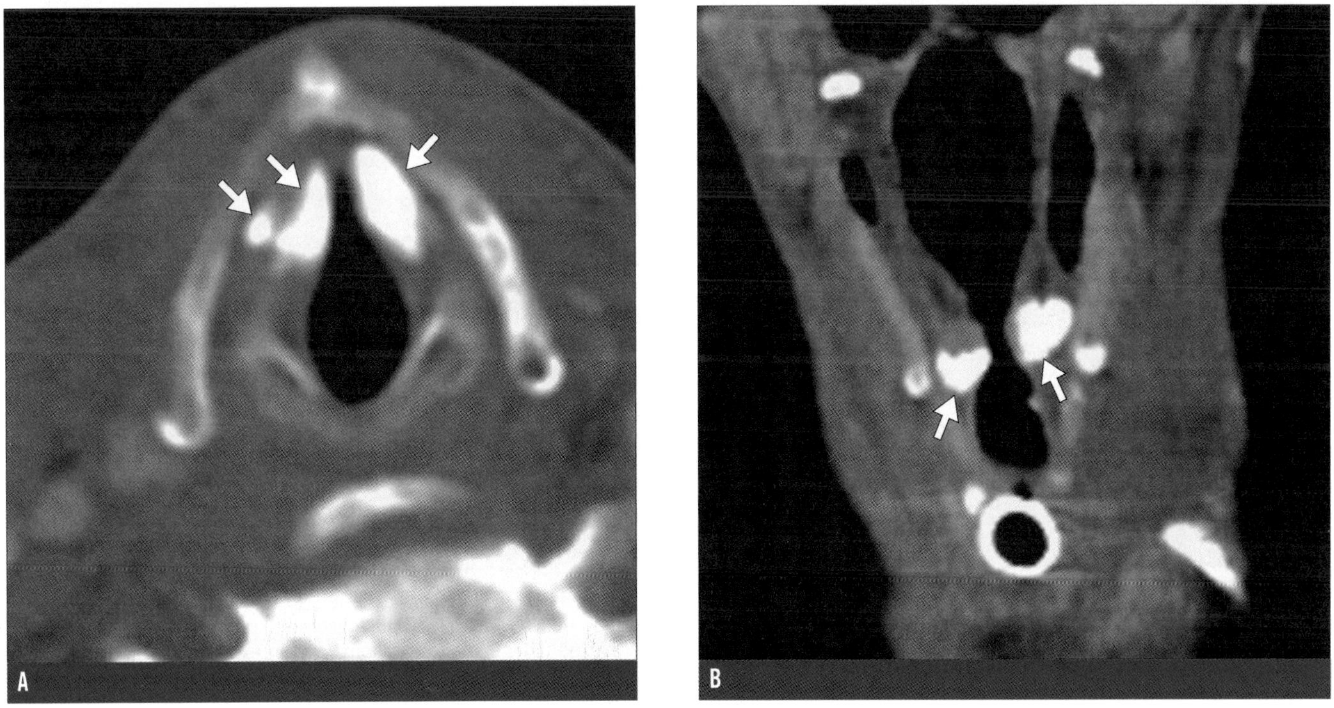

Contrast-enhanced axial (**A**) and coronal reformatted (**B**) CT images demonstrate increased attenuation in both TVCs, left greater than right, representing Radiesse with calcium hydroxylapatite (arrows, **A**, **B**). For this patient, the injectable was placed via a needle that traversed the thyroid lamina, though numerous other options are available for instillation of this material.

Permanent injection laryngoplasty: Teflon

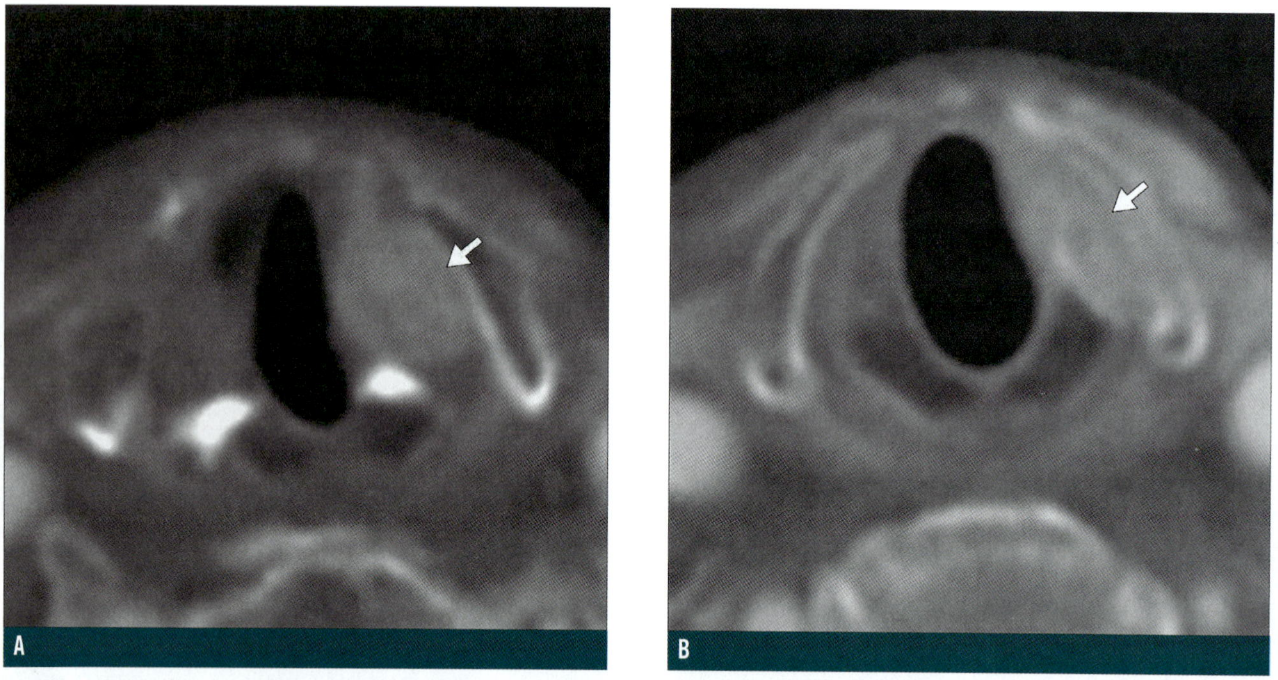

Contrast-enhanced axial CT images viewed with a bone window (**A**, **B**) demonstrate mildly increased attenuation centered in the left TVC and minimally in the subglottis (arrows, **A**, **B**). This increased attenuation represents Teflon that was injected into the TVC, a substance that is considered a permanent injectable. This substance is no longer routinely used due to its propensity to result in a foreign body reaction.

Permanent injection laryngoplasty: Teflon with FDG-PET avidity

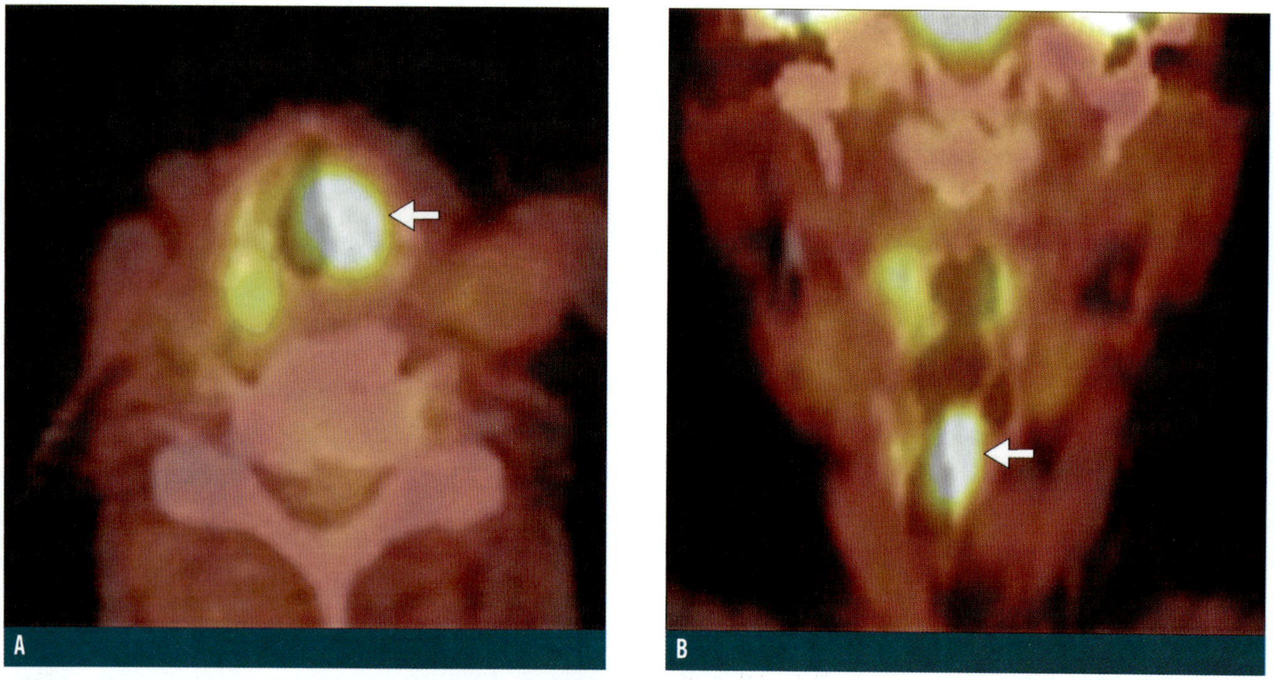

Axial (**A**) and coronal reformatted (**B**) PET-CT images demonstrate asymmetric FDG-PET avidity of the left TVC, which was described as a possible mass on the PET radiology report (arrows, **A**, **B**). On exam, the left TVC was fixed but a discrete, superficial left TVC mass was not appreciated. Contrast-enhanced axial (**C**) and coronal reformatted (**D**) CT images demonstrate an expansile, oval, mildly hyperattenuating finding centered in the left TVC (arrows, **C**, **D**). Axial T1 (**E**), fat suppressed axial T2 (**F**), and fat-suppressed contrast-enhanced coronal T1 (**G**) MR images demonstrate the finding to be isointense on T1 (arrow, **E**), hypointense relative to the contralateral TVC on T2 (arrow, **F**), and mildly enhancing (arrow, **G**). This patient had a history of a left TVC injection with Teflon. While the findings may represent a Teflon granuloma, this was not pathologically proven and the finding was stable on a follow-up FDG-PET/CT exam obtained over 4 years later. PET avidity is a nonspecific finding in the setting of an injection laryngoplasty and may be identified with a Teflon injection granuloma or with an uncomplicated Radiesse with calcium hydroxylapatite injection laryngoplasty.

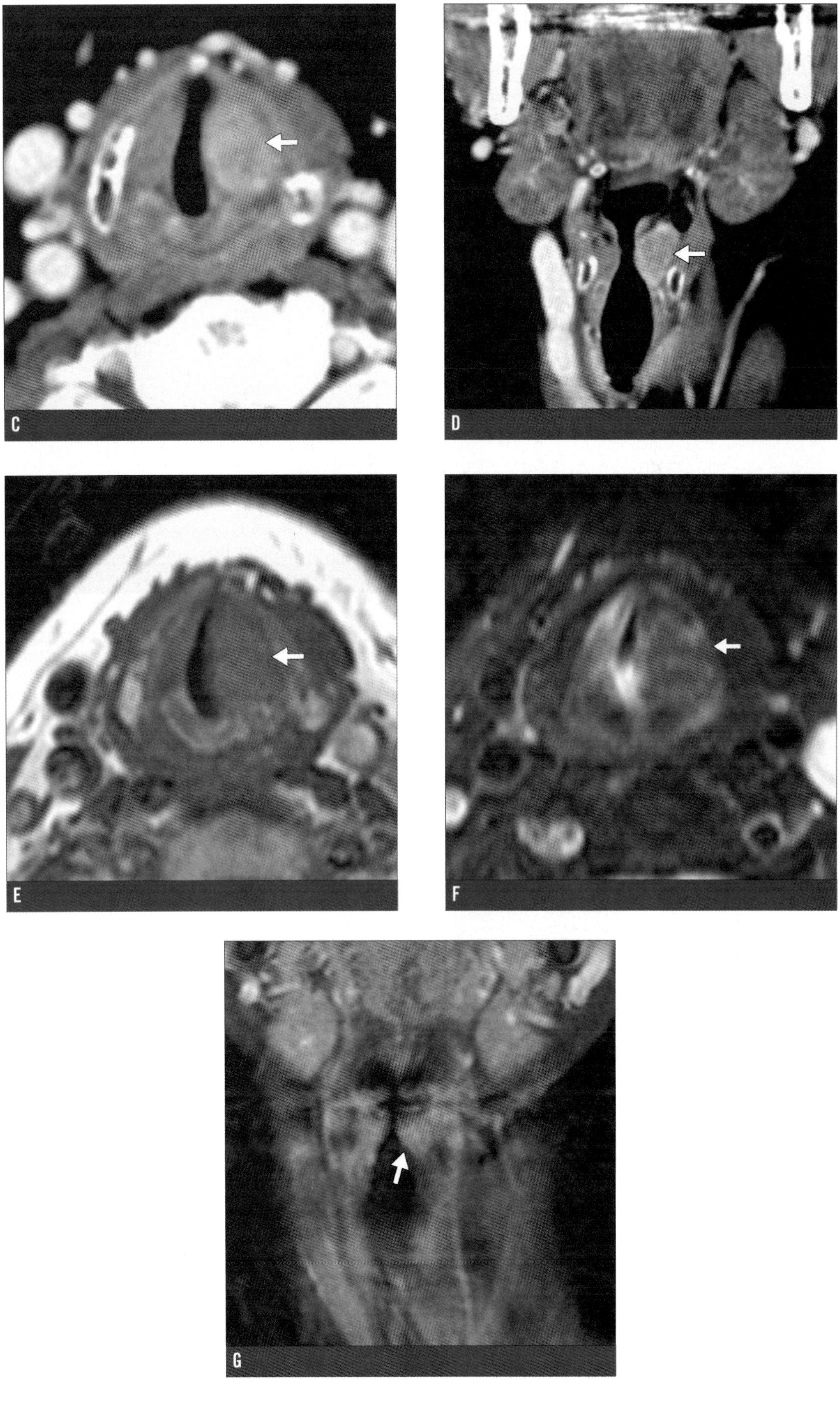
C
D
E
F
G

Companion case: Subglottic extrusion of Radiesse with calcium hydroxylapatite

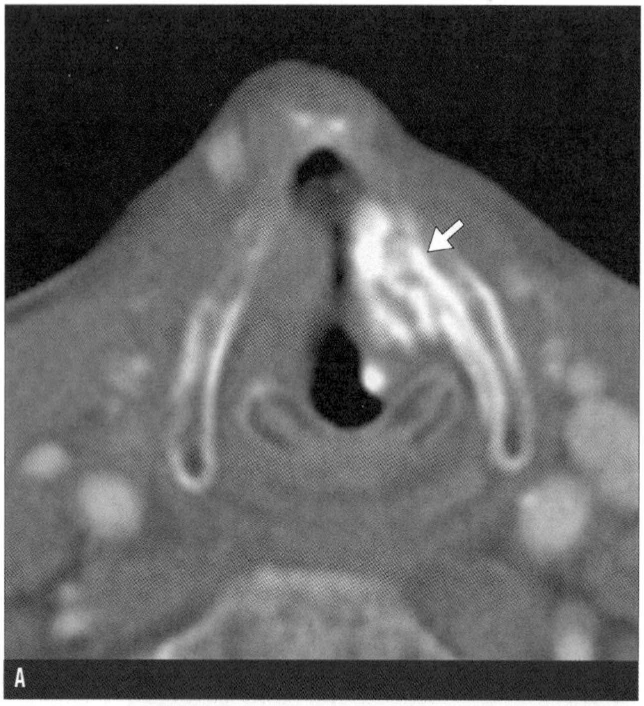

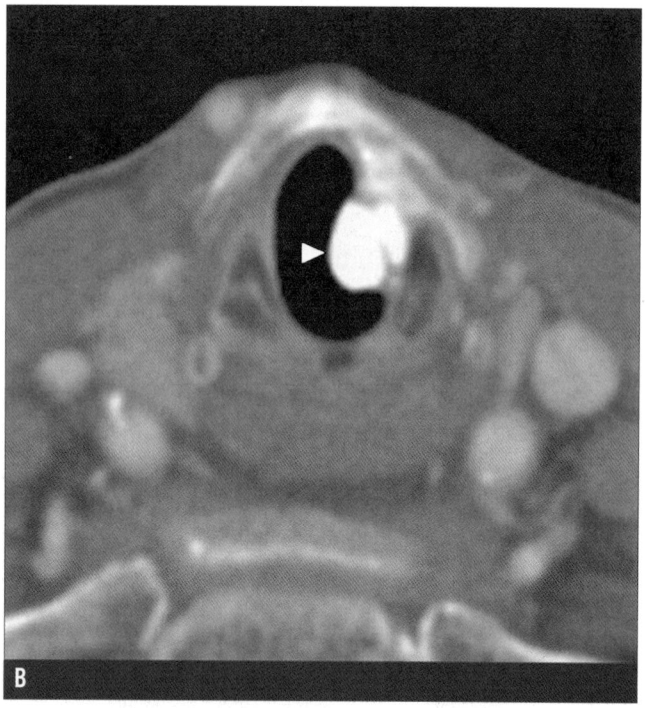

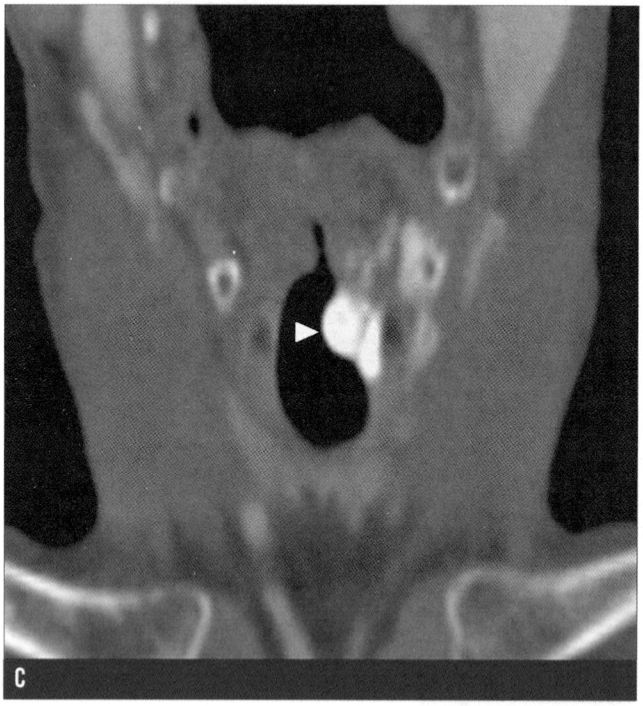

A contrast-enhanced axial CT image (**A**) demonstrates increased attenuation in the left TVC related to instillation of Radiesse with calcium hydroxylapatite (arrow, **A**). Axial (**B**) and coronal reformatted (**C**) CT images from the same study demonstrate inadvertent extrusion of the injectable into the left aspect of the subglottis (arrowheads, **B**, **C**).

REFERENCES

Chark DW[1], Boyd JW, Crumley RL. Vocal fold polyp resulting from calcium hydroxylapatite injection. *Laryngoscope.* 2010;120 (Suppl 4): S194. doi: 10.1002/lary.21661.

Chheda NN, Rosen CA, Belafsky PC, Simpson CB, Postma GN. Revision laryngeal surgery for the suboptimal injection of calcium hydroxylapatite. *Laryngoscope.* 2008;118(12):2260-2263.

DeFatta RA, Chowdhury FR, Sataloff RT. Complications of injection laryngoplasty using calcium hydroxylapatite. *J Voice.* 2012;26(5):614-618.

Harrigal C, Branstetter BF, Snyderman CH, Maroon J. Teflon granuloma in the nasopharynx: a potentially false-positive PET/CT finding. *Am J Neuroradiol.* 2005;26:417-420.

King JM, Simpson CB. Modern injection augmentation for glottic insufficiency. *Curr Opin Otolaryngology Head Neck Surg.* 2007;15:153-158.

Kwon T-K, Buckmire R. Injection laryngoplasty for management of unilateral vocal fold paralysis. *Curr Opin Otolaryngol Head Neck Surg.* 2004;12:538-542.

Kwon TK, An SY, Ahn JC, Kim KH, Sung MW. Calcium hydroxylapatite injection laryngoplasty for the treatment of presbylaryngis: long-term results. *Laryngoscope.* 2010;120(2):326-329. Montgomery thyroplasty implant system. Boston Medical products product insert/information.

Kwon TK, Lee JE, Cha WJ, Song CM, Sung MW, Kim KH. Serial computed tomographic and positron emission tomographic properties of injection material used for vocal fold augmentation. *Laryngoscope.* 2013 Oct;123(10):2491-2496.

Ondik MP, Kang J, Bayerl MG, Bruno M, Goldenberg D. Teflon laryngeal granuloma presenting as laryngeal cancer on combined positron emission tomography and computed tomography scanning. *J Laryngol Otol.* 2009;123:575-578.

Postma GN, Blalock PD, Koufman JA. Bilateral medialization laryngoplasty. *Laryngoscope.* 1998;108(10):1429-1434.

Rivera-Serrano CM, Smith LJ. Laryngeal teflon granuloma: endoscopy, laryngeal videostroboscopy, and CT imaging. *Ear Nose Throat J.* 2011 Mar;90(3):E25-E26.

Rosen CA[1], et al. Vocal fold augmentation with calcium hydroxylapatite: twelve-month report. *Laryngoscope.* 2009 May;119(5):1033-1041.

Truong MT, Erasmus JJ, Macapinlac HA, Podoloff DA. Teflon injection for vocal cord paralysis: false-positive finding on FDG PET-CT in a patient with non-small cell lung cancer. *AJR Am J Roentgenol.* 2004;182(6):1587-1589.

VoCoM prosthesis

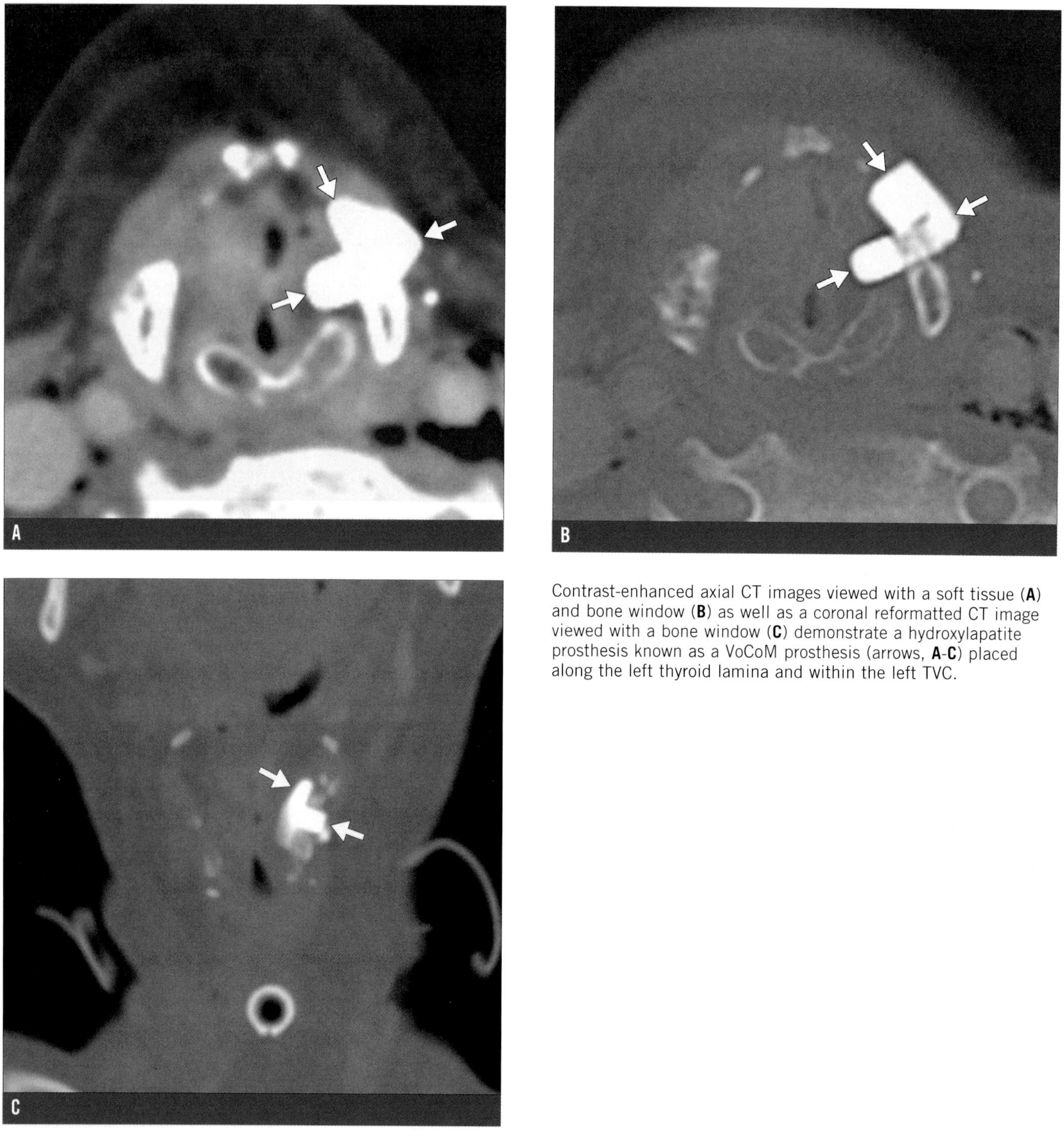

Contrast-enhanced axial CT images viewed with a soft tissue (**A**) and bone window (**B**) as well as a coronal reformatted CT image viewed with a bone window (**C**) demonstrate a hydroxylapatite prosthesis known as a VoCoM prosthesis (arrows, **A-C**) placed along the left thyroid lamina and within the left TVC.

REFERENCES

Hendricker RM, deSilva BW, Forrest LA. Gore-Tex medialization laryngoplasty for treatment of dysphagia. *Otolaryngol Head Neck Surg.* 2010;142(4):536-539.

Isshiki N.Progress in laryngeal framework surgery. *Acta Otolaryngol.* 2000 Mar;120(2):120-127.

Montgomery thyroplasty implant system. Boston Medical products product insert/information.

VoCom: The complete surgical system of implants and instruments that increases accuracy and decreases surgical time in vocal cord medialization. Gyrus ACMI product insert/information.

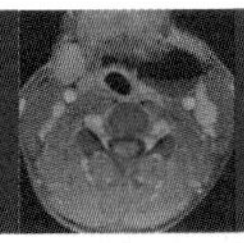

CASE 17 MRI chemical shift artifact in the subglottic larynx simulating abnormal soft tissue

There is considerable discrepancy in the literature with respect to the superior border of the subglottic larynx, with some literature stating that it resides approximately 1 cm below the plane of the TVCs, others stating 5 mm below the free margin of the TVCs, while others stating that it resides along the undersurface of the TVCs. However, there is no debate with respect to the inferior border of the subglottis, which is considered to terminate at the inferior margin of the cricoid cartilage.

Chemical shift artifact occurs because protons in fat resonate at 220 Hz downfield from protons in water. As a result of this difference in frequency, misregistration in the frequency encoding direction occurs, particularly on spin echo T1-weighted images without fat suppression. This artifact is linearly proportional to the MRI field strength. Chemical shift artifact will occur at the level of the subglottic larynx because of the cricoid marrow fat (if ossified) and/or the fat surrounding the cricoid. Since most MR imaging of the neck is performed with the frequency encoding direction from right to left, this artifact at the level of the cricoid is almost always identified along the left subglottic larynx. This can be particularly problematic if there is suspected or known tumor affecting the left TVC and the presence or absence of subglottic tumor affects management. If needed, swapping the phase and frequency encoding directions (ie, phase encoding performed from right to left and frequency encoding performed from anterior to posterior) should resolve the left subglottic chemical shift artifact. Additionally, chemical shift artifact should not be present on fat-suppressed images or with fast spin echo T2. If there is still a question as to the presence of a left subglottic abnormality, a CT examination should clarify the issue.

COMPANION CASES

- **Subglottic granulation tissue.** The subglottic larynx should be free of soft tissue within its lumen or along its walls. If soft tissue is present, then the finding is abnormal, though it may still be a benign finding. One such benign entity, granulation tissue, is often present in patients who have an indwelling tracheostomy tube. This finding is usually circumferential and smooth, though superimposed aerated debris may also be identified. Prior intubation may also result in granulation tissue or scar with subsequent stenosis of the subglottic larynx.
- **Subglottic tumor extension.** Primary malignancy arising from the subglottis is uncommon, accounting for less than 5% of all laryngeal malignancies. A primary TVC abnormality extending into the subglottic larynx is much more common than a primary tumor of the subglottis. Moreover, while there are various nonmalignant lesions that may affect the TVC and/or subglottis (amyloid, tuberculosis, etc), by far the most common etiology in the adult population that simultaneously affects both areas is squamous cell carcinoma. Thus, any lesion of the TVC that is associated with subglottic soft tissue should be considered squamous cell carcinoma until proven otherwise.

Companion case: Subglottic tumor extension

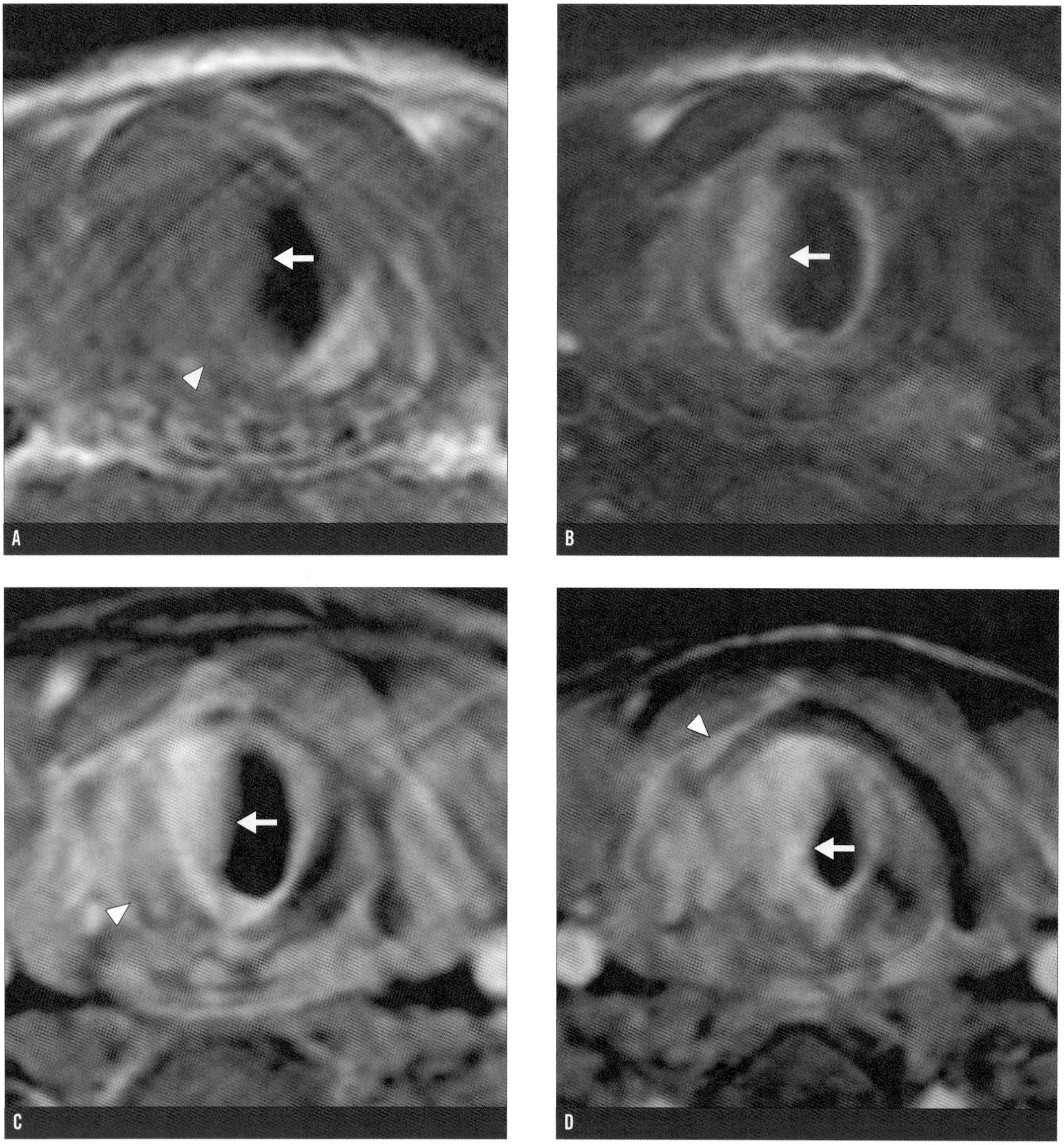

An axial T1-weighted MR image (**A**) demonstrates T1 isointense signal fullness in the right subglottic larynx (arrow, **A**). This does not represent incidental chemical shift artifact for a couple of reasons. First, the finding is on the right, whereas subglottic chemical shift artifact is on the left, assuming the frequency encoding direction was obtained from right to left. Second, there is loss of the normal marrow fat within the right aspect of the cricoid (arrowhead, **A**). Fat-suppressed axial T2 (**B**) and fat-suppressed contrast-enhanced axial T1 (**C**, **D**) MR images demonstrate further evidence that the finding on image **A** is abnormal. The finding in the subglottic larynx is hyperintense on T2 (arrow, **B**), enhances (arrow, **C**), and involves the right TVC (arrow, **D**). There is also abnormal enhancement of the cricoid cartilage (arrowhead, **C**) and right thyroid lamina with extension into the overlying strap muscles (arrowhead, **D**). Moreover, coronal T1 (**E**) and fat-suppressed contrast-enhanced coronal T1 (**F**) MR images demonstrate the lesion to represent a transglottic mass, extending from the right supraglottic larynx (long arrows, **E**, **F**), involving the TVC (arrowheads, **E**, **F**), and into the subglottic larynx (short arrows, **E**, **F**). This lesion represented a squamous cell carcinoma.

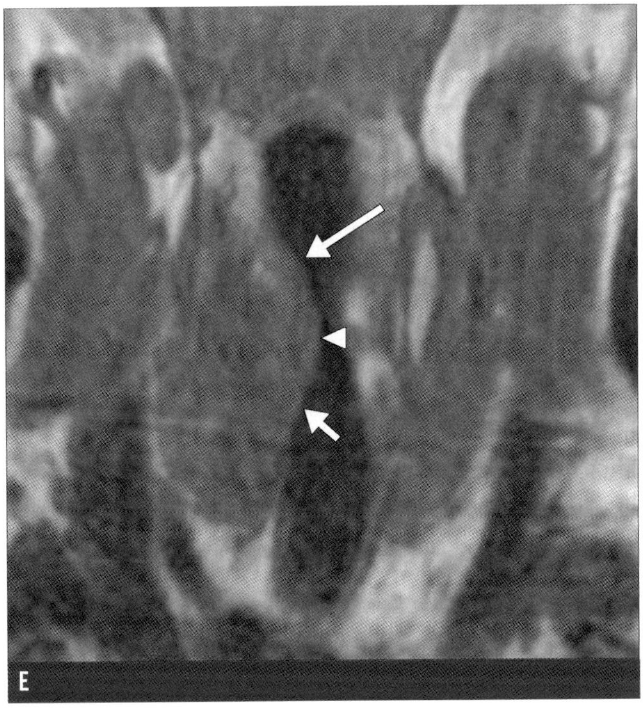

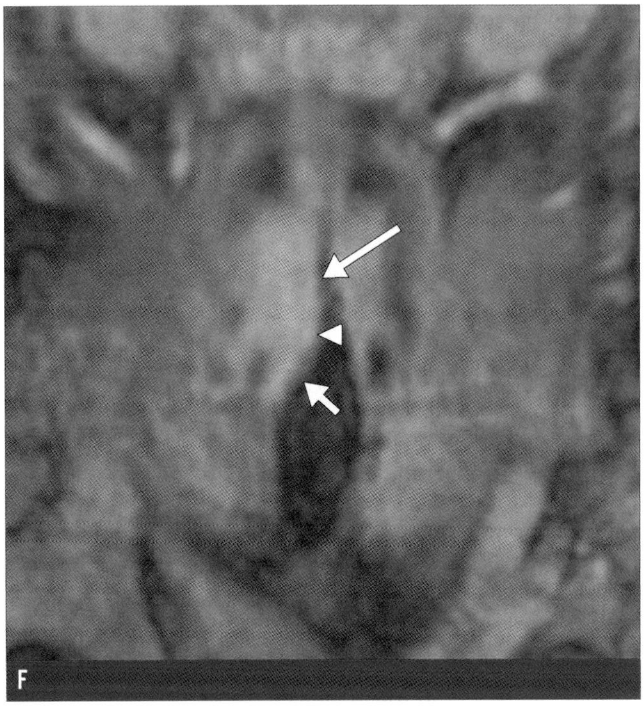

REFERENCES

Benning S, Technau-Ihling K, Fisch P, Fradis M, Schipper J, Maier W. Amyloid tumor of the larynx associated with plasma cell infiltration: differential diagnosis. *Ear Nose Throat J.* 2004;83:839-843.

Chiesa F, et al. Surgical treatment of laryngeal carcinoma with subglottis involvement. *Oncol Rep.* 2001;8:137-140.

Paisley S, et al. Results of radiotherapy for primary subglottic squamous cell carcinoma. *Int J Radiat Oncol Biol Phys.* 2002;52:1245-1250.

Prince JS, Duhamel DR, Levin DL, Harrell JH, Friedman PJ. Nonneoplastic lesions of the tracheobronchial wall: radiologic findings with bronchoscopic correlation. *Radiographics.* 2002;22 Spec No:S215-230.

Sakai F, Gamsu G, Dillon WP, Lynch DA, Gilbert TJ. MR imaging of the larynx at 1.5 T. *J Comput Assist Tomogr.* 1990;14:60-71.

Santoro R, Turelli M, Polli G. Primary carcinoma of the subglottic larynx. *Eur Arch Otorhinolaryngol.* 2000;257:548-551.

Yousem DM, Tufano RP. Laryngeal imaging. *Magn Reson Imaging Clin N Am.* 2002;10:451-465.

Zhuo J, Gullapalli RP. AAPM/RSNA physics tutorial for residents: MR artifacts, safety, and quality control. *Radiographics.* 2006;26:275-297.

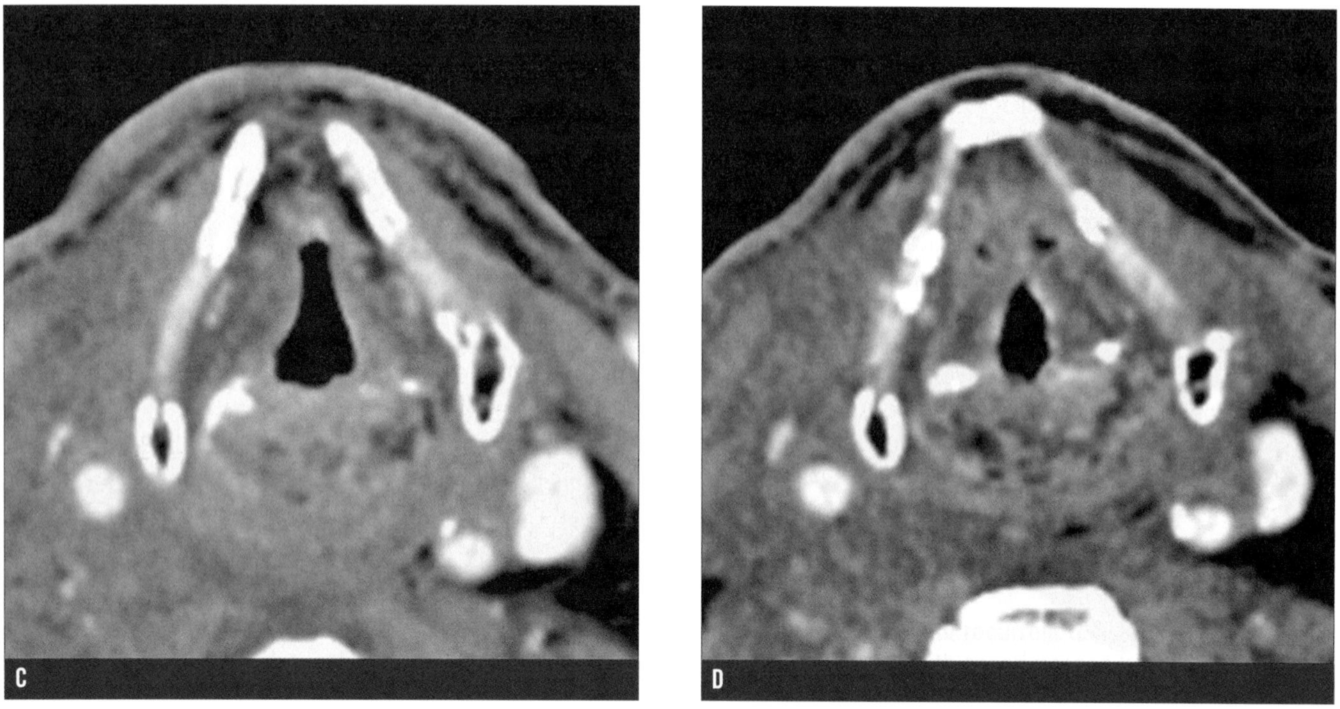

Companion case: Posttreated larynx with recurrent tumor

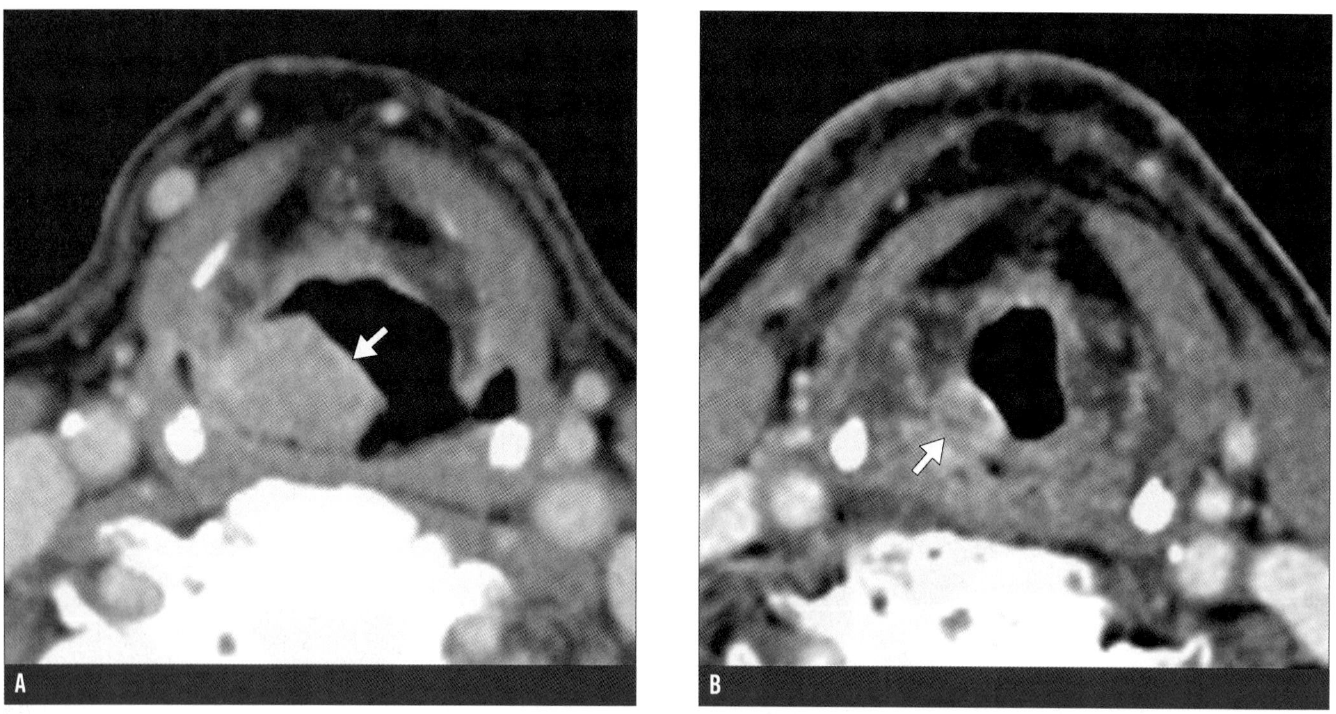

A contrast-enhanced axial CT image (**A**) demonstrates a focal mass centered along the ventral aspect of the right aryepiglottic fold, representing a supraglottic squamous cell carcinoma (arrow, **A**). Following radiation therapy, a contrast-enhanced axial CT image obtained 8 months later (**D**) demonstrates diffuse edematous change involving the supraglottic larynx and likely a small amount of residual tumor (arrow, **B**). A contrast-enhanced axial CT image obtained 11 months after the initial study (**C**) demonstrates diffuse edematous change, without focality, though the edematous tissues are slightly increased in attenuation diffusely (arrows, **C**). A contrast-enhanced axial CT image obtained 15 months after the initial study (**D**) now demonstrates an exophytic mass in the supraglottic larynx, compatible with tumor recurrence (arrow, **D**). This case illustrates the importance of close follow-up imaging.

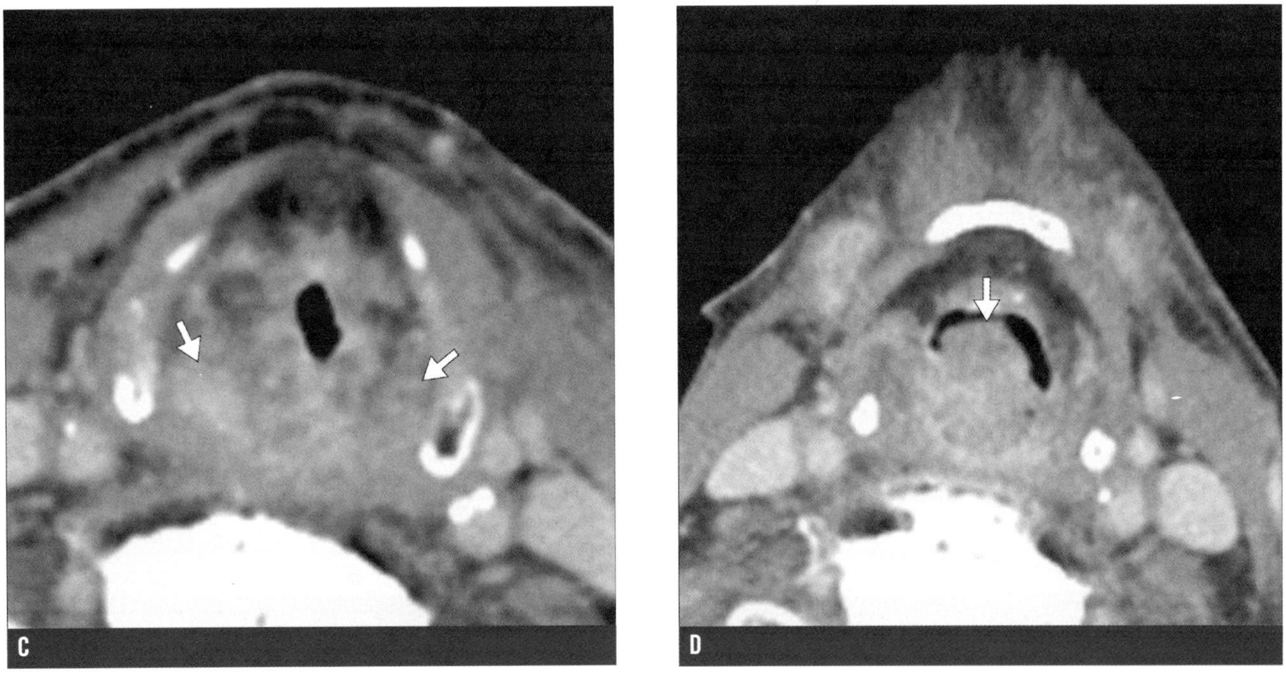

Companion case: Posttreated larynx with superimposed tumor

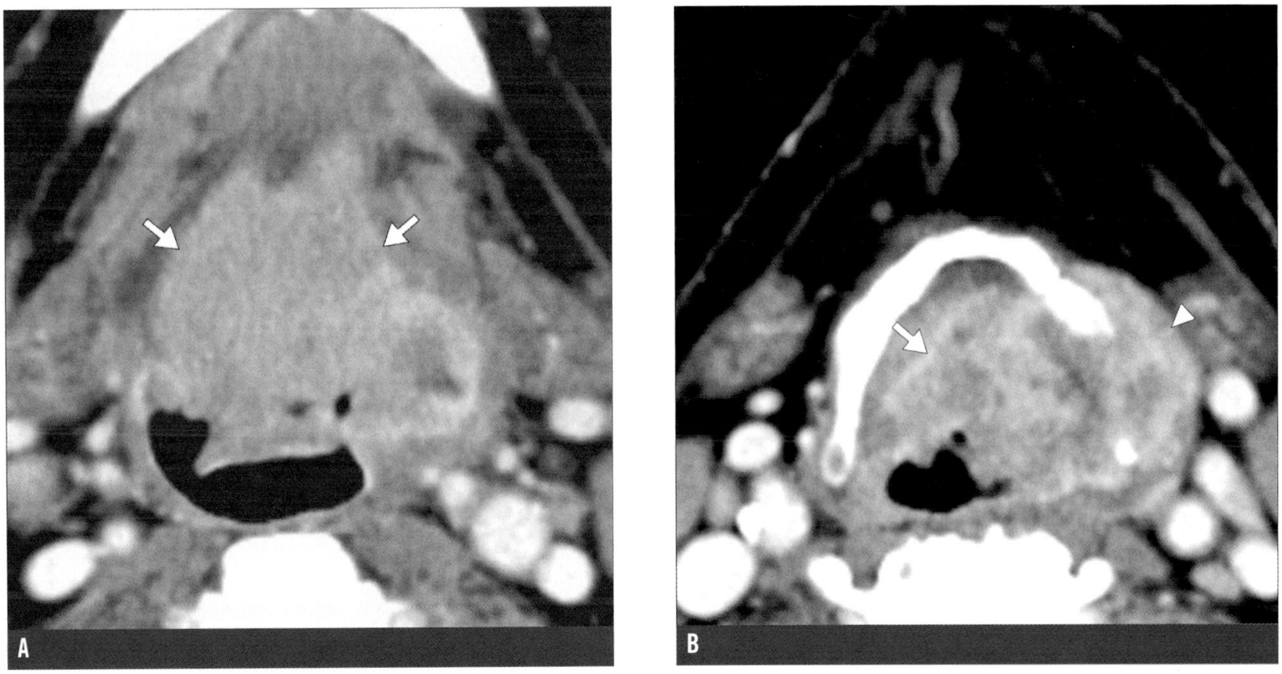

Contrast-enhanced axial CT images through the oropharynx (**A**) and supraglottic larynx (**B**) demonstrates a large base of tongue mass (arrows, **A**) that extends to involve the supraglottic larynx (arrow, **B**) and is associated with extra-laryngeal extension (arrowhead, **B**). Following radiation treatment, a contrast-enhanced axial CT image obtained 5 months after the initial study (**C**) demonstrates marked improvement of the mass at the supraglottic level, likely with residual tumor on the left (arrow, **C**). A contrast-enhanced axial CT image obtained 8 months after the initial study (**D**) demonstrates marked edematous change of the supraglottic larynx (asterisks, **D**). Slightly caudal to this level, an axial CT image from the same study (**E**) demonstrates diffuse edematous thickening of the supraglottic soft tissues, although the density of the thickening is more soft tissue than fluid (arrows, **E**). This was misinterpreted as likely treatment effect. No clear mass was identified by the otolaryngologist during visual inspection, but the clinical examination was reportedly difficult due to the extensive treatment effect. Two weeks later, an axial PET/CT image (**F**) demonstrates marked hypermetabolic activity in this region suggestive of tumor (arrows, **F**). This patient underwent a total laryngectomy shortly after the PET/CT scan and extensive, moderately differentiated invasive squamous cell carcinoma was present. This tumor likely reflected marked growth of an insufficiently radiated or radiation-resistant tumor. This case illustrates the need for careful evaluation for any residual or developing soft tissue that is present in the postradiated larynx on imaging, short term follow-up (particularly during the early stages of treatment), and the usefulness of PET imaging in difficult cases.

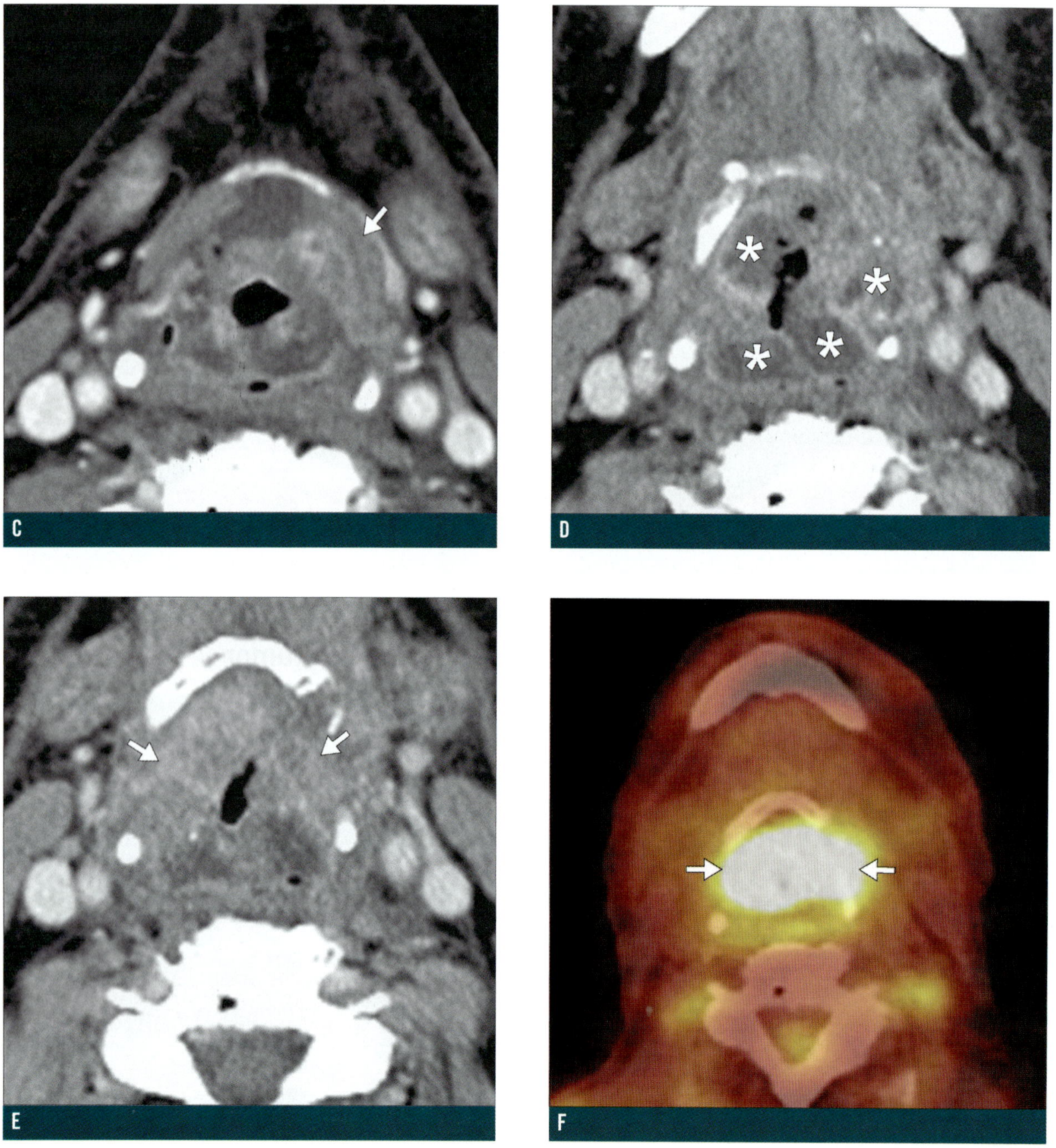

REFERENCES

Andrade RS, et al. Posttreatment assessment of response using FDG-PET/CT for patients treated with definitive radiation therapy for head and neck cancers. *Int J Radiat Oncol Biol Phys.* 2006;65(5): 1315-1322. Epub 2006 Jun 5.

Glastonbury CM, Parker EE, Hoang JK. The postradiation neck: evaluating response to treatment and recognizing complications. *AJR Am J Roentgenol.* 2010;195:W164-171.

Goerres GW, et al. Positron emission tomography in the early follow up of advanced head and neck cancer. *Arch Otolaryngol Head Neck Surg.* 2004;130(1):105-109; discussion 120-121.

Greven KM, et al. Serial positron emission tomography scans following radiation therapy of patients with head and neck cancer. *Head Neck.* 2001;23(11):942-946.

Kim SY, et al. The Feasibility of 18F-FDG PET scans 1 month after completing radiotherapy of squamous cell carcinoma of the head and neck. *J Nucl Med.* 2007;48:373-378.

King KG, Kositwattanarerk A, Genden E, Kao J, Som PM, Kostakoglu L. Cancers of the oral cavity and oropharynx: FDG PET with contrast-enhanced CT in the posttreatment setting. *Radiographics.* 2011;31:355-373.

Nam SY, et al. Early evaluation of the response to radiotherapy of patients with squamous cell carcinoma of the head and neck using 18FDG-PET. *Oral Oncol.* 2005;41(4):390-395.

Nomayr A, Lell M, Sweeney R, Bautz W, Lukas P. MRI appearance of radiation-induced changes of normal cervical tissues. *Eur Radiol.* 2001;11:1807-1817.

Wong RJ. Current status of FDG-PET for head and neck cancer. *J Surg Oncol.* 2008;97(8):649-652.

CASE 19 Laryngectomies

Accounting for approximately 12,500 new cases each year in the United States, laryngeal cancer is a generalized term referring to carcinoma of the supraglottic, glottic, or subglottic structures. Squamous cell carcinoma is by far the most common histologic subtype of laryngeal cancer, although there are numerous other histologies, including adenocarcinoma, chondrosarcoma, lymphoma, and plasmacytoma. Clinical behavior, treatment, and prognosis depend on several factors, including tumor location and tumor grade. Ultimately, the goal of treatment is to control or cure the patient of the tumor and, if feasible, preserve larynx function.

Partial or conservative laryngectomy aims to preserve a portion of the larynx in order to maintain phonation, respiration, and swallowing. Several conservative techniques have been developed, including endoscopic laser excision and cordectomy, vertical hemilaryngectomy (also called vertical partial laryngectomy), supraglottic laryngectomy (also called horizontal partial laryngectomy), and near-total laryngectomy. Ideally, tumors of the larynx should be excised with a 1 to 2 cm margin of normal tissue, although a slightly less than 1 cm tumor free margin is often sufficient.

- **Hemilaryngectomy.** A hemilaryngectomy involves surgery on the ipsilateral side of the laryngeal tumor with removal of a portion or all of the thyroid lamina, TVC, FVC, laryngeal ventricle, anterior commisure, arytenoid cartliage, and the mucosa of the aryepiglottic fold to the superior aspect of the cricoid cartilage. A small anterior portion of the contralateral TVC may also be resected. To perform a hemilaryngectomy, the tumor may involve the entire length of the affected TVC and anterior commissure, but it should not involve more than the anterior 1/3 of the contralateral TVC. A small amount of subglottic extension is acceptable, as a portion of the subglottis is often resected during this surgery. Ipsilateral arytenoid cartilage fixation by tumor, posterior commisure involvement, advanced transglottic tumor spread to involve the FVC, or extralaryngeal extension of tumor are contraindications of a vertical hemilaryngectomy.
- **Supraglottic laryngectomy.** A typical supraglottic laryngectomy involves removal of the epiglottis, FVCs, the laryngeal ventricles, upper 1/3 of the thyroid laminae, and the thyrohyoid membrane. The remaining lower portion of the thyroid laminae are retracted cephalad and attached to the hyoid via a procedure termed a thyrohyoidopexy. Laryngeal tumors that would be amenable to a suprahyoid laryngectomy include: tumor confined to the suprahyoid endolarynx without extension caudally to the level of the FVCs, freely mobile bilateral arytenoid cartilages, lack of oropharynx extension (therefore no extension to the lingual surface of the suprahyoid epiglottis), no cartilage invasion, no involvement of the postcricoid area, and no pyriform sinus involvement. Bilateral suprahyoid larynx involvement is acceptable. If the tumor is confined to the suprahyoid epiglottis and the pre-epiglottic fat is devoid of tumor, then an isolated epiglottidectomy may suffice.
- **Total laryngectomy.** Total or radical laryngectomy is a surgical option for patients with advanced disease, such as tumors that have penetrated through the laryngeal cartilages, have invaded into the extralaryngeal soft tissues of the neck, extensively involve the base of the tongue, or have circumferential submucosal involvement. A total laryngectomy may also be considered for those patients who have failed radiation therapy or conservative laryngectomy procedures; in these settings, the surgery may be termed a "salvage laryngectomy". Less common indications include radiation necrosis (chondroradionecrosis) or severe aspiration.

A total laryngectomy consists of removal of all laryngeal structures (epiglottis, aryepiglottic folds, true and FVCs, and subglottic larynx) as well as the supporting fibromuscular and osseous structures (hyoid bone, thyroid cartilage, arytenoid cartilages, cricoid cartilage, and a few proximal tracheal rings). Myocutaneous flaps, most commonly the pectoralis major flap, may be used to augment laryngopharyngeal repair in cases of extensive tumor involvement or salvage laryngectomy. If a pectoralis major flap is used, then the pedicle flap is reflected superiorly, tunneled beneath the superficial pectoralis major fascia but over the clavicle, and placed along the neck and/or used for the laryngopharyngeal repair. On imaging, the reflected pectoralis major flap will be identified as asymmetric muscle fullness along the upper chest on the side the flap was taken. Depending upon the timing of the imaging, a recently placed myocutaneous flap can appear to represent a large tumor, particularly soon after placement. Over time, these flaps will decrease in volume. Knowledge of prior myocutaneous flap placement is paramount in order to appropriately interpret these cases. See Chapter 3 for further discussion regarding neck reconstructions. One important imaging pitfall that may be identified with a total laryngectomy relates to repositioning of the thyroid gland during the procedure. Often, the thyroid gland is bisected at the thyroid isthmus and one or both lobes of the thyroid are positioned more laterally in the neck. The morphology of the repositioned thyroid lobe(s) is also commonly altered. These changes to the thyroid gland may simulate a metastatic lymph node or potentially an arterial aneurysm.

COMPANION CASES

Problems related to wound healing, from a minor dehiscence to frank laryngocutaneous fistula formation, are the most encountered complications following laryngectomy. Other less common complications include superficial flap necrosis, abscess formation, and wound hematoma. Evaluation for recurrent tumor can be very difficult following a laryngectomy, and when present, they often recur along surgical margins.

- Radiation necrosis and fistulization of a supraglottic laryngectomy
- Total laryngectomy with abscess formation 1 month following surgery
- Total laryngectomy with abscess resulting in a tracheo-pharyngo-cutaneous fistula
- Total laryngectomy with tumor recurrence

Hemilaryngectomy

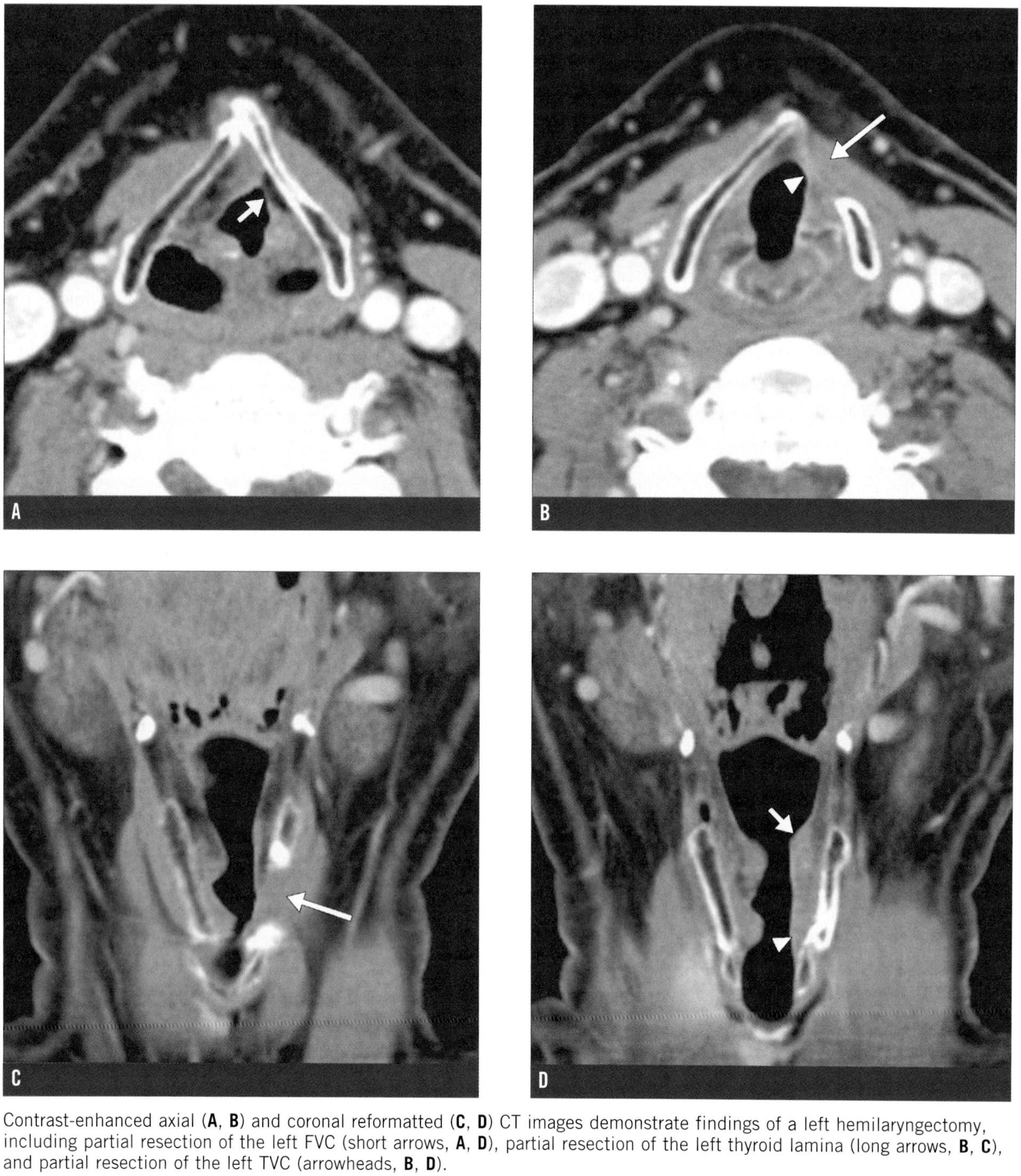

Contrast-enhanced axial (**A**, **B**) and coronal reformatted (**C**, **D**) CT images demonstrate findings of a left hemilaryngectomy, including partial resection of the left FVC (short arrows, **A**, **D**), partial resection of the left thyroid lamina (long arrows, **B**, **C**), and partial resection of the left TVC (arrowheads, **B**, **D**).

Supraglottic laryngectomy

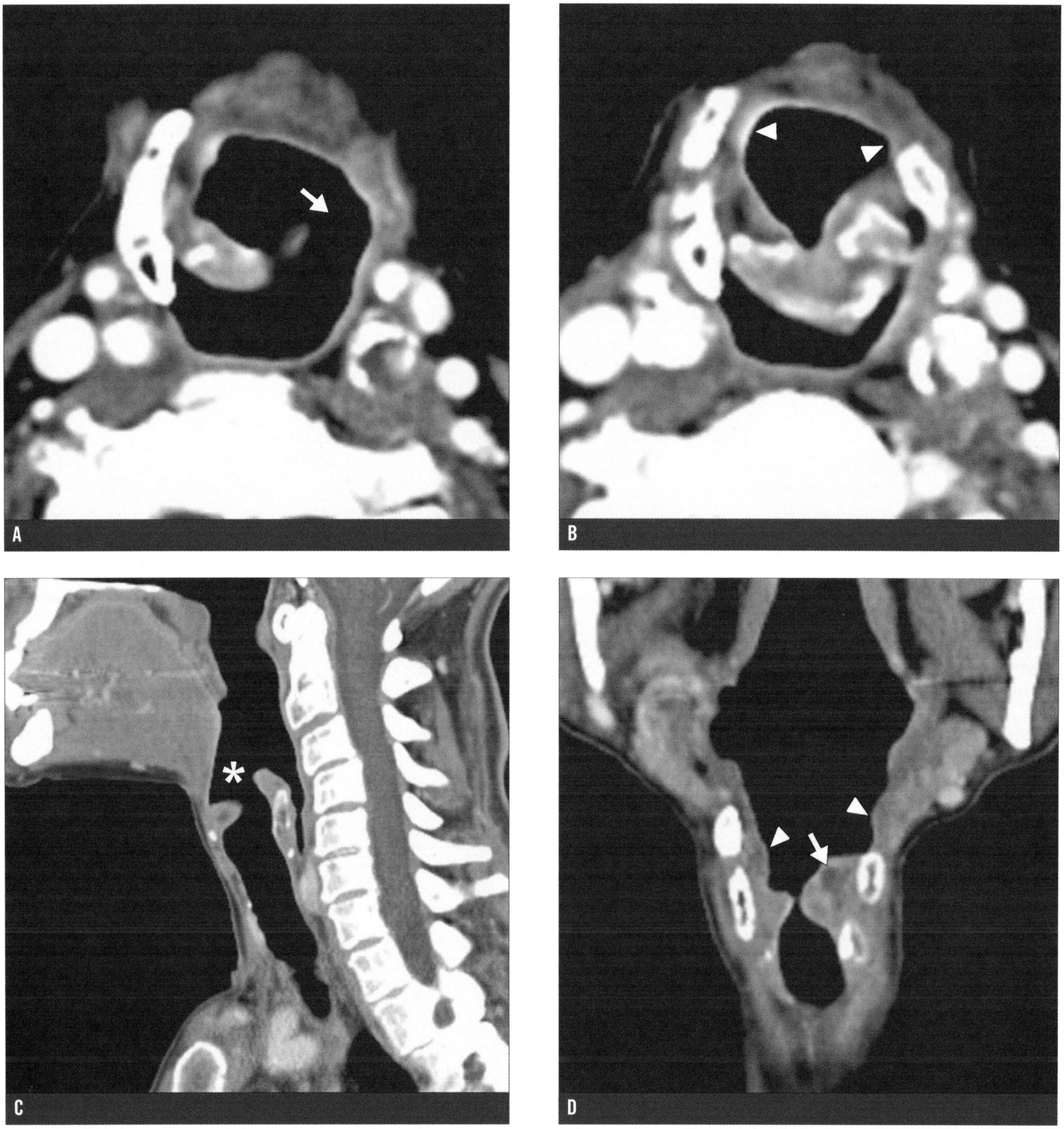

Contrast-enhanced axial CT images viewed from cephalad to caudad (**A**, **B**) as well as sagittal reformatted (**C**), and coronal reformatted (**D**) CT images demonstrate findings compatible with a supraglottic laryngectomy, including an epiglottectomy (asterisk, **C**), resection of the left aryepiglottic fold (arrow, **A**), and resection of the bilateral false vocal cords (arrowheads, **B**, **D**). The patient underwent a left TVC laryngoplasty with injection of Radiesse Voice Gel approximately 1 month prior to this study which accounts for the enlarged and heterogeneous left TVC appearance (arrow, **D**).

Supraglottic laryngectomy

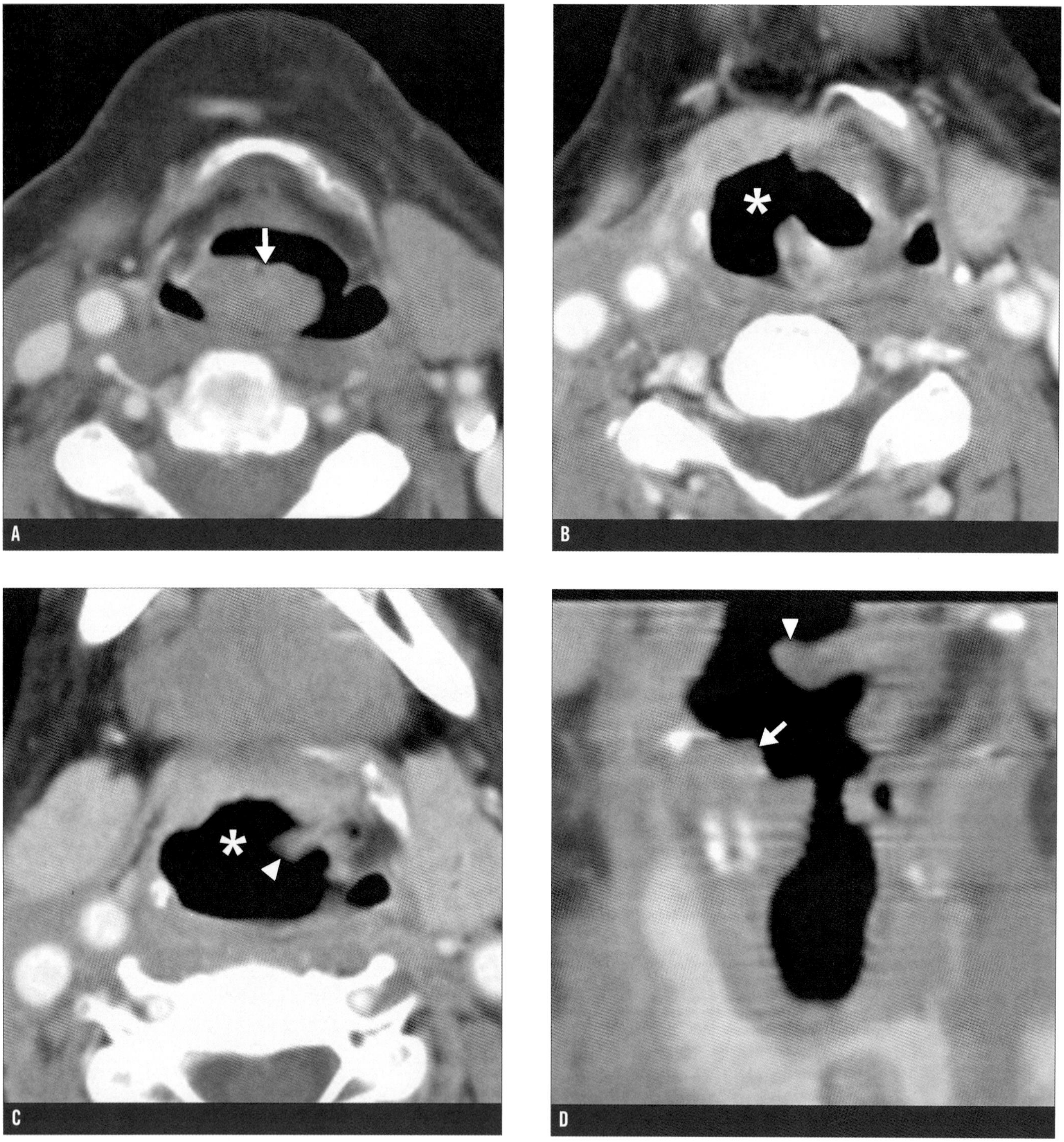

Different patient. A contrast-enhanced axial CT image through the aryepiglottic folds (**A**) demonstrates a mass along the right aryepiglottic fold representing squamous cell carcinoma (arrow, **A**). Contrast-enhanced axial CT images following a right supraglottic laryngectomy (**B**, **C**) demonstrate resection of the right aryepiglottic fold (asterisk, **B**) and a right hemiepiglottectomy (asterisk, **C**). Image **C** and a coronal reformatted CT image (**D**) demonstrate the residual left aspect of the epiglottis (arrowheads, **C**, **D**). Only a small portion of the right FVC was likely resected, best demonstrated on image **D** (arrow, **D**).

Total laryngectomy - 3 weeks following surgery

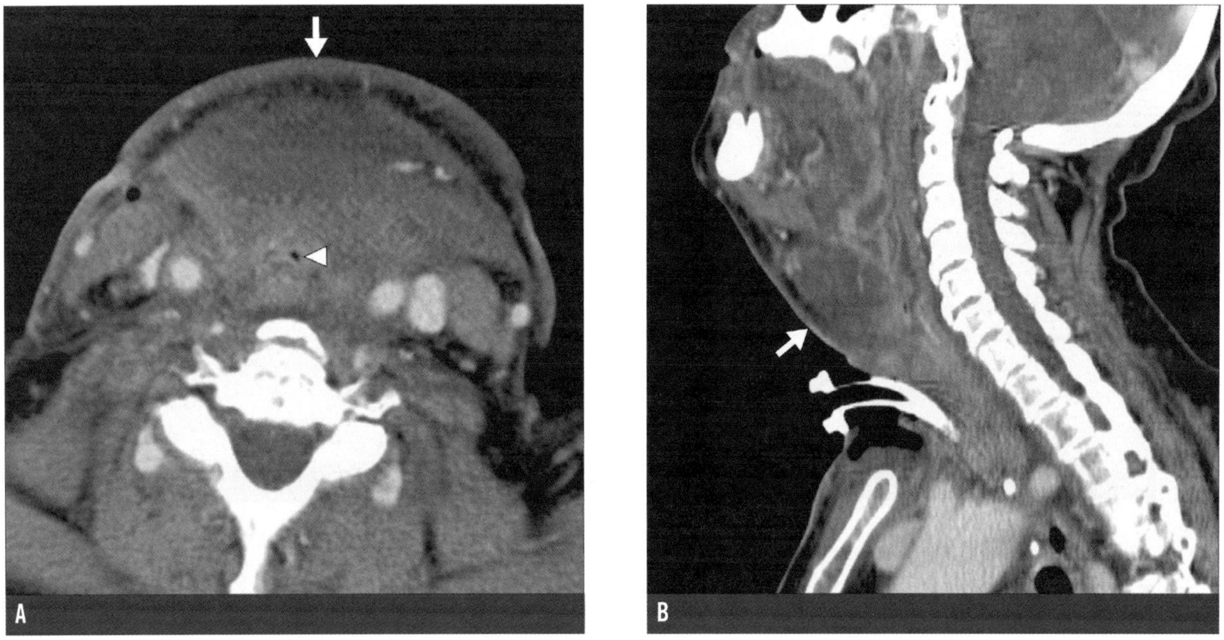

Contrast-enhanced axial (**A**) and sagittal reformatted (**B**) CT images demonstrate absence of the laryngeal apparatus and large, edematous soft tissue along the anterior neck, representing a large pectoralis major myocutaneous flap that was recently placed approximately 3 weeks prior to this scan (arrows, **A**, **B**). Without appropriate history, one could mistake this flap to represent a large tumor. A neopharynx is faintly visible on image **A** (arrowhead, **A**).

Total laryngectomy - 2 months following surgery

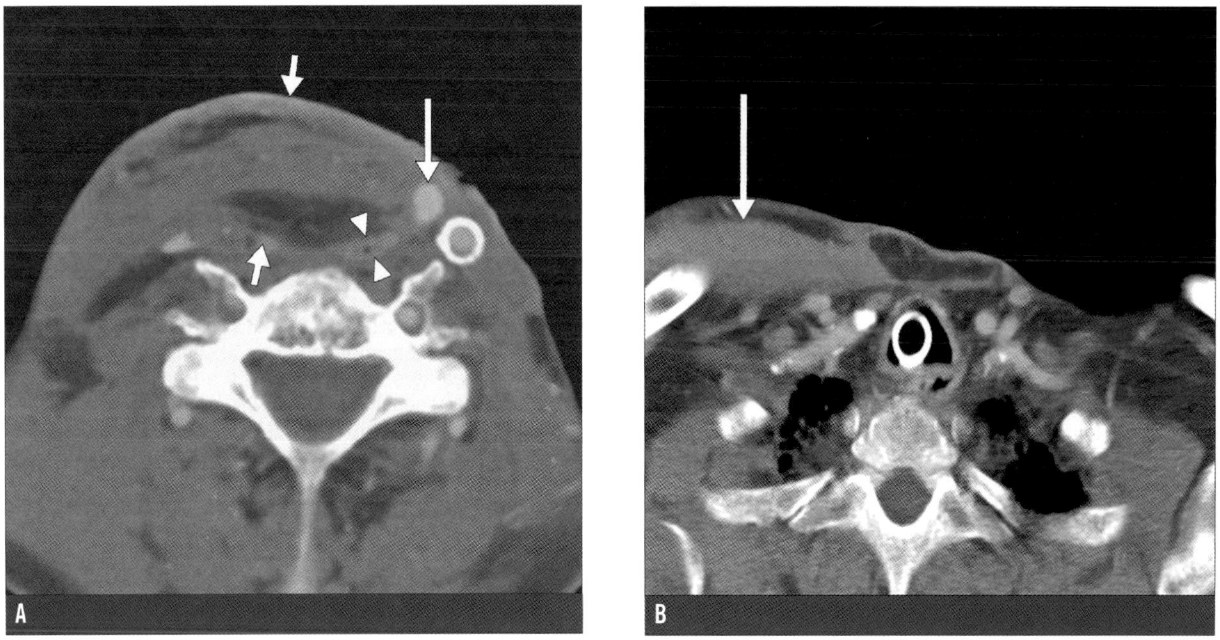

Contrast-enhanced axial (**A**, **B**), sagittal reformatted (**C**), and coronal reformatted (**D**) CT images demonstrate complete removal of the larynx, formation of a neopharynx (arrowheads, **A**, **C**), and placement of a pectoralis major myocutaneous flap (short arrows, **A**, **C**, **D**) that was performed approximately 2 months prior to this CT scan. In this patient, the neopharynx was partially reconstructed with the pectoralis major flap, which is composed of both muscle and fat. The flap origin is evident in the upper chest, where the right pectoralis major muscle is reflected superiorly (long arrow, **B**). An oval hyperdense focus in the left neck is also present, simulating a hyperdense suspicious lymph node (medium arrows, **A**, **D**). However, this represents a repositioned portion of the normal thyroid gland. There is frequently an unusual thyroid gland location and morphology following a total laryngectomy as the thyroid gland is often surgically altered and repositioned during this surgery.

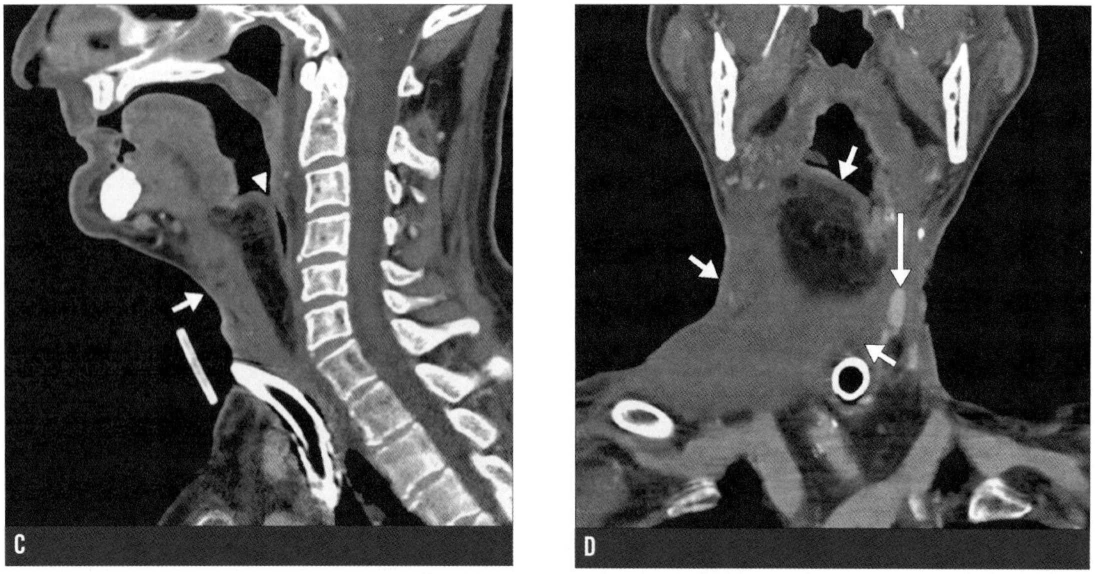

Total laryngectomy - several years following surgery

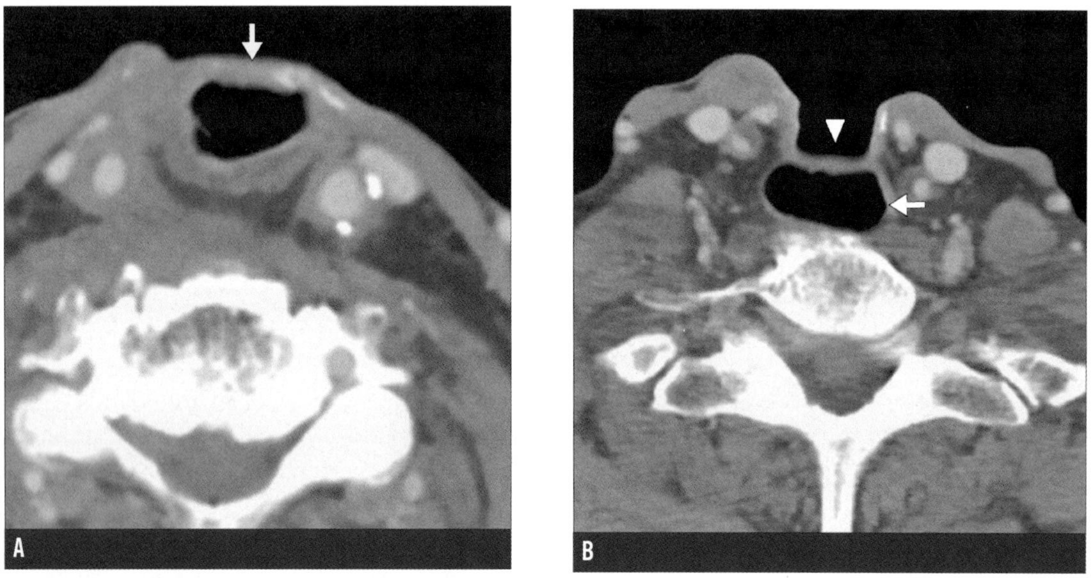

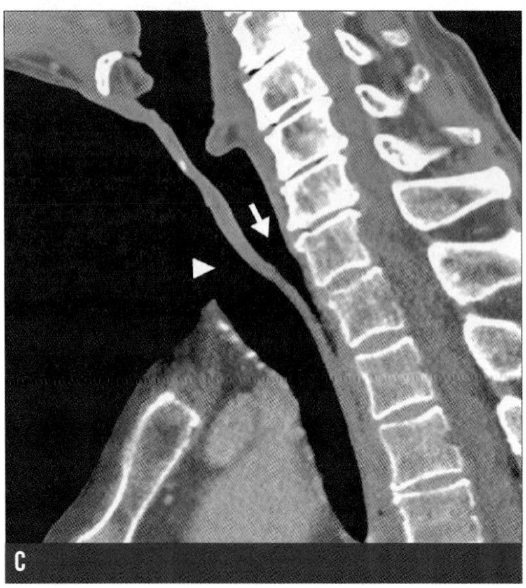

Contrast-enhanced axial (**A**, **B**) and sagittal reformatted (**C**) CT images demonstrate absence of the laryngeal apparatus, compatible with a total laryngectomy. The reconstructed pharynx (arrows, **A**-**C**) is a completely separate conduit from the trachea, as intended. The tracheal stoma is indicated by the arrowheads on images **B** and **C**.

Companion case: Radiation necrosis and fistulization of a supraglottic laryngectomy

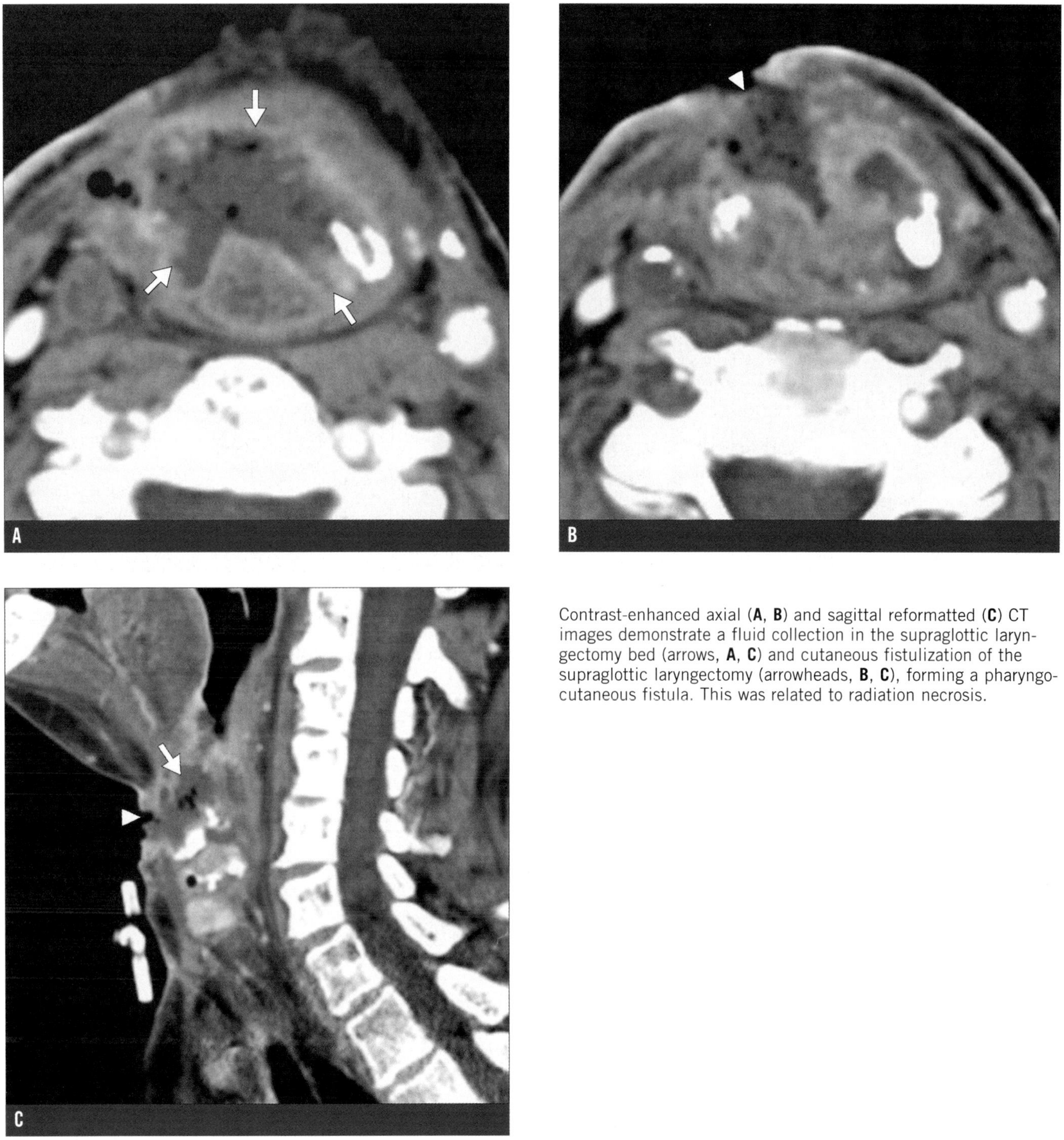

Contrast-enhanced axial (**A**, **B**) and sagittal reformatted (**C**) CT images demonstrate a fluid collection in the supraglottic laryngectomy bed (arrows, **A**, **C**) and cutaneous fistulization of the supraglottic laryngectomy (arrowheads, **B**, **C**), forming a pharyngocutaneous fistula. This was related to radiation necrosis.

Companion case: Total laryngectomy with abscess formation 1 month following surgery

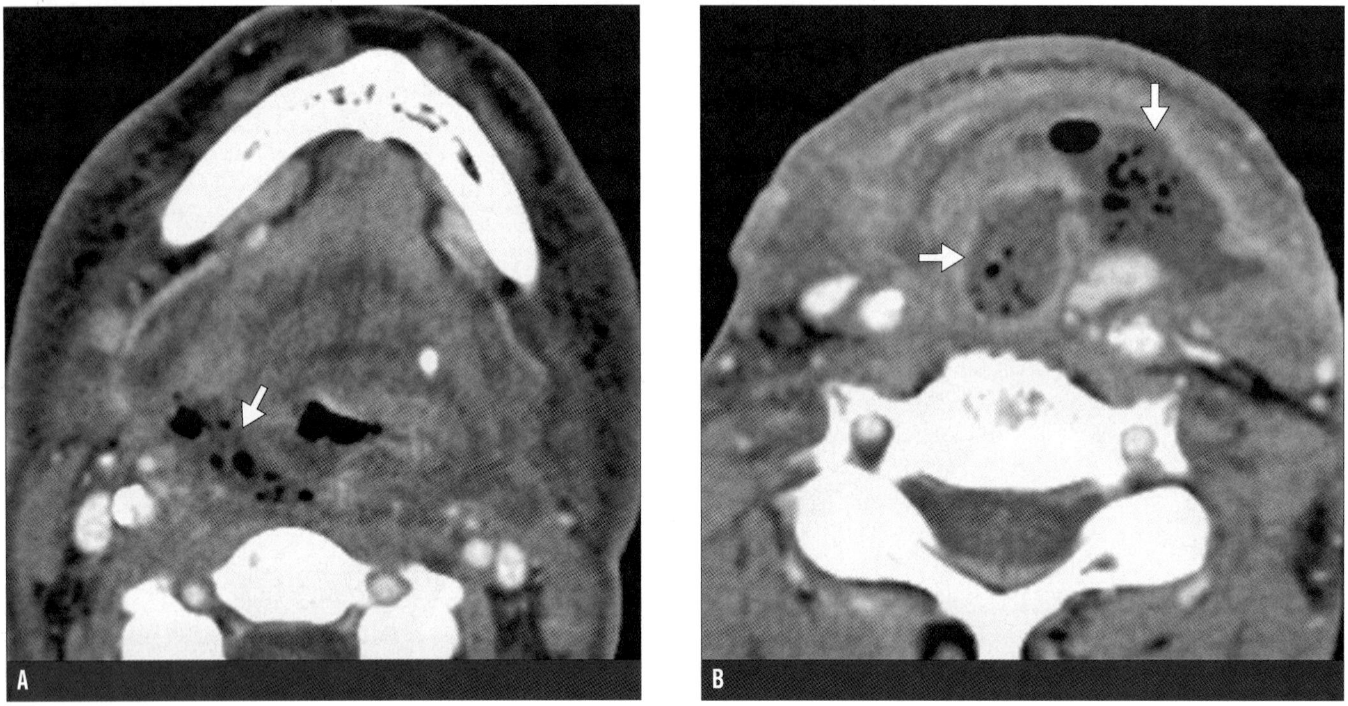

Contrast-enhanced axial CT images (**A**, **B**) demonstrate absence of the laryngeal apparatus, compatible with a total laryngectomy. This patient also underwent a limited hypopharyngectomy and placement of a left pectoralis myocutaneous flap. However, purulent drainage developed approximately 1 month following surgery and this CT neck was then performed. Evident on this imaging is a complex, partially aerated and likely peripherally enhancing fluid collection within the reconstruction with areas of fistulous communication (arrows, **A**, **B**). These findings represented a *staphylococcus aureus* abscess.

Companion case: Total laryngectomy with abscess resulting in a tracheo-pharyngo-cutaneous fistula

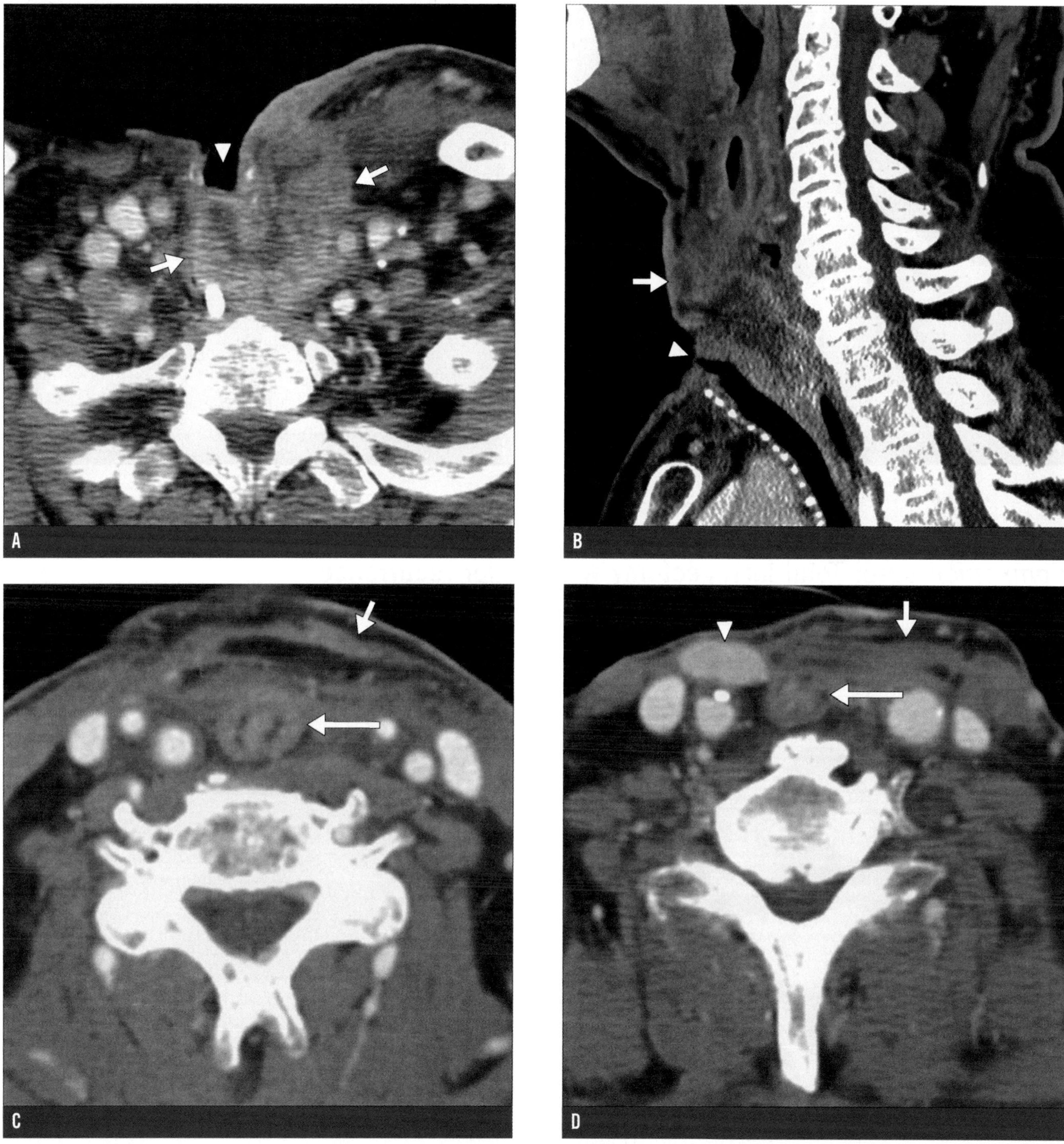

Different patient. Contrast-enhanced axial (**A**) and sagittal reformatted (**B**) CT images demonstrate absence of the laryngeal apparatus, compatible with a total laryngectomy. At and just above the tracheostomy stoma (arrowheads, **A**, **B**), a large, heterogeneous mass is present (short arrows, **A**, **B**), which was a new finding for this patient. While the findings could certainly represent a large tumor, in this case, the lesion was an abscess. Contrast-enhanced axial (**C**-**E**) and sagittal reformatted (**F**) CT images of the same patient following successful treatment of the abscess. These images better demonstrate the postsurgical appearance of the total laryngectomy, neopharynx (medium arrows, **C**, **D**), and pectoralis major flap (short arrows, **C**, **D**, **F**). The reflected, cephalad-directed pectoralis major muscle flap was taken from the left, as evidenced by asymmetric muscle fullness along the left anterior chest (arrowhead, **E**). While the acute inflammation related to the abscess had resolved, the patient developed a pharyngocutaneous fistula as a sequela of the infection, with communication between the neopharynx, trachea, and skin (long arrows, **E**, **F**). Due to this tracheo-pharyngo-cutaneous fistula, the patient was NPO and fed via tube feedings. Incidentally, residual thyroid tissue is present in the right lower neck simulating a vessel or abnormal lymph node (arrowhead, **D**). The thyroid gland is often repositioned and can have an unusual morphology following a laryngectomy.

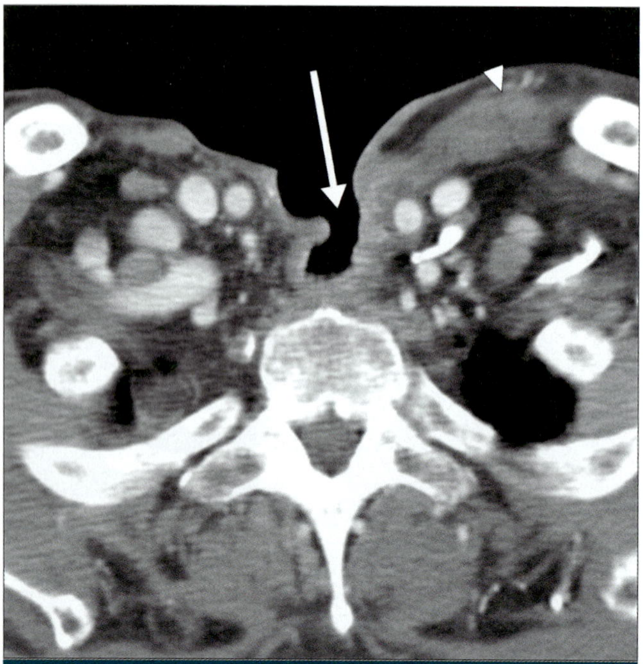

E

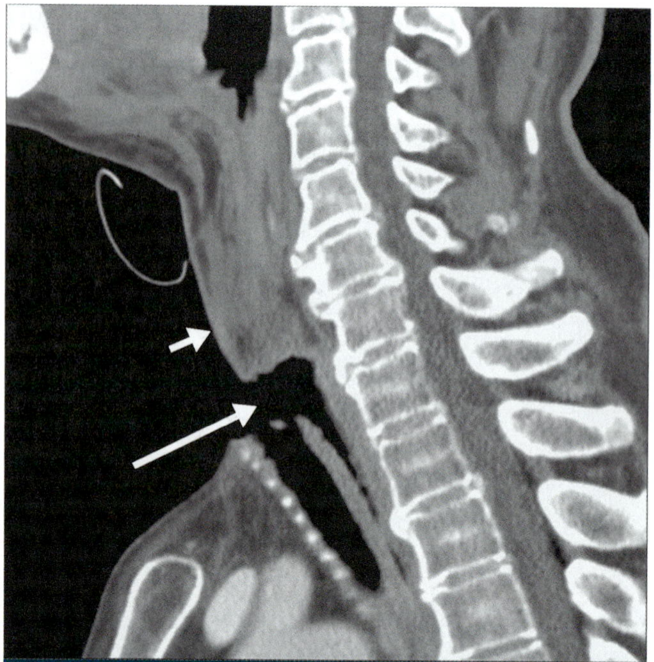

F

Companion case: Total laryngectomy with tumor recurrence

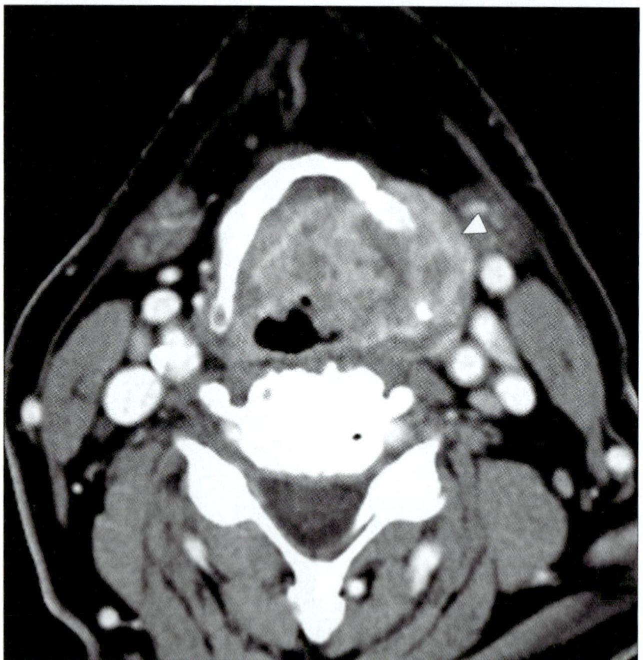

A

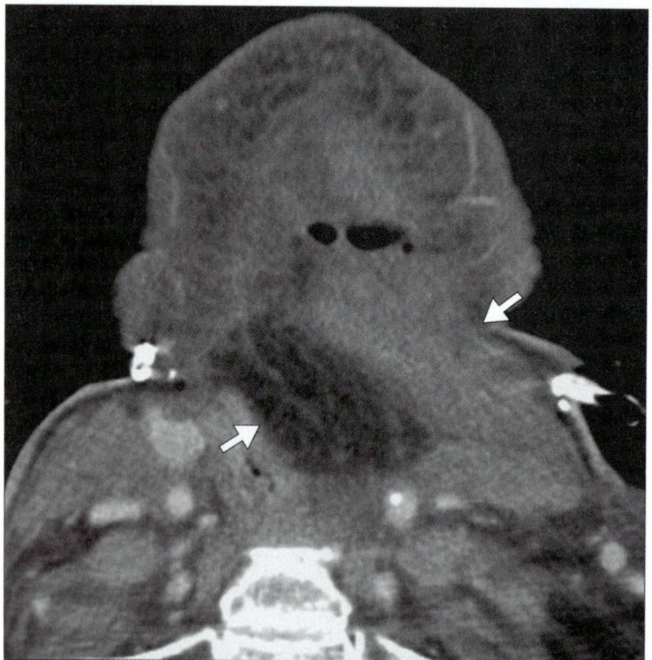

B

A contrast-enhanced axial CT image (**A**) demonstrates a large mass involving the supraglottic larynx with extralaryngeal extension (arrowhead, **A**). Contrast-enhanced axial CT images following surgery (**B**, **C**) demonstrate a total laryngectomy, tongue base resection, and a pectoralis flap closure (arrows, **B**, **C**). A pharyngoesophageal reconstruction utilizing the pectoralis major flap was also performed (arrowheads, **C**). However, a contrast-enhanced axial CT image obtained 6 months later (**D**) demonstrates tumor recurrence along the margins of the reconstruction and floor of mouth (arrows, **D**).

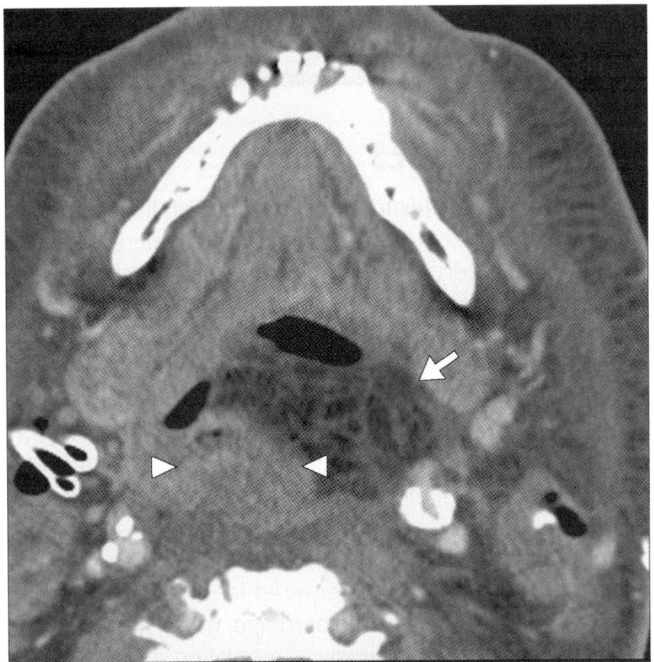

C

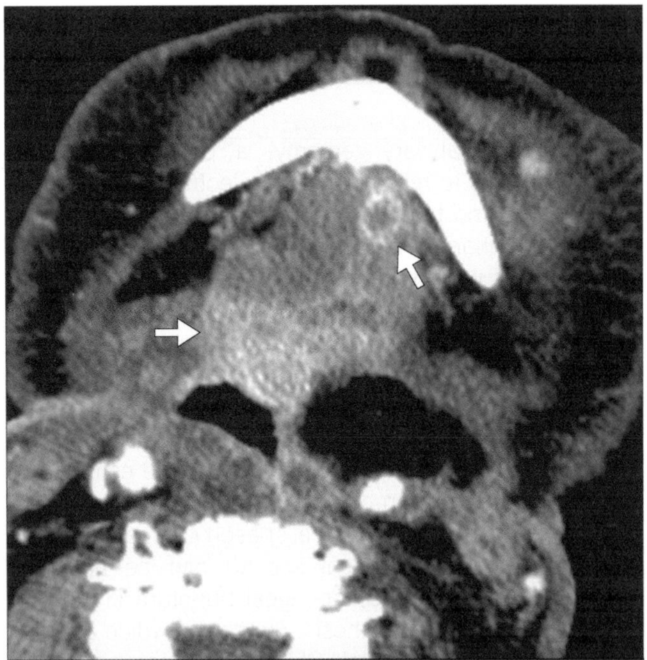

D

REFERENCES

Agrawal N, Goldenberg D. Primary and salvage total laryngectomy. *Otolaryngol Clin North Am.* 2008;41:771-780, vii.

American Society of Clinical Oncology, et al. American Society of Clinical Oncology clinical practice guideline for the use of larynx-preservation strategies in the treatment of laryngeal cancer. *J Clin Oncol.* 2006;24:3693-3704.

Bely-Toueg N, Halimi P, Laccourreye O, Laskri F, Brasnu D, Frija G. Normal laryngeal CT findings after supracricoid partial laryngectomy. *AJNR Am J Neuroradiol.* 2001;22:1872-1880.

Brasnu DF. Supracricoid partial laryngectomy with cricohyoidopexy in the management of laryngeal carcinoma. *World J Surg.* 2003; 27:817-823.

Clark JR, Gilbert R, Irish J, Brown D, Neligan P, Gullane PJ. Morbidity after flap reconstruction of hypopharyngeal defects. *Laryngoscope.* 2006;116(2):173-181.

Ferreiro-Arguelles C, et al. CT findings after laryngectomy. *Radiographics.* 2008;28:869-882; quiz 914.

Ganly I, et al. Analysis of postoperative complications of open partial laryngectomy. *Head Neck.* 2009;31(3):338-345.

Laramore GE, Coltrera MD. Organ preservation strategies in the treatment of laryngeal cancer. *Curr Treat Options Oncol.* 2003;4:15-25.

Sarra LD, Rodriguez JC, Garcia Valea M, Bitar J, Da Silva A. [Fistula following total laryngectomy. Retrospective study and bibliographical review]. *Acta Otorrinolaringol Esp.* 2009;60:186-189.

Weissman JL, Curtin HD, Johnson JT. Thyroid gland after total laryngectomy: CT appearance. *Radiology.* 1998 May;207(2):405-409.

CASE 20 Tracheoesophageal puncture and prosthesis

Following a total laryngectomy, a patient has three primary options to restore speech: electrolarynx, esophageal speech, and tracheoesophageal speech, all of which rely on vibrations induced along the pharynx and/or esophagus as well as the aid of natural anatomic resonators, namely the tongue, teeth, and lips. An electrolarynx is a handheld, battery-operated device that is held against the upper anterior neck which mechanically induces vibrations along the pharynx and esophagus. Esophageal speech is a learned form of speech that utilizes air flow in the pharynx and esophagus to vibrate the esophageal walls during exhalation. However, for a number of reasons, the success of esophageal speech is variable among patients. Tracheoesophageal speech can be achieved by performing a tracheoesophageal puncture (TEP) and placement of a TEP prosthesis. Successful voice acquisition occurs in approximately 95% of long-term users of a TEP prosthesis.

Because the trachea is effectively closed to the pharynx following a laryngectomy, a tracheal stoma is created to allow air to enter the lungs. However, in order for speech to be generated, a tracheostoma needs to be occluded by a finger or a with a one-way self-occluding valve that is placed over the stoma, the latter with the additional benefit of allowing patients to more easily express themselves with hand gestures. This one-way valve allows air to enter the trachea and lungs during inhalation but closes during exhalation. The TEP represents a horizontally oriented fistula between the trachea and esophagus that is performed roughly at the level of the third tracheal ring. The TEP provides a shunt for exhaled pulmonary air to enter the esophagus. A TEP prosthesis represents a small silicone tube that is placed within the TEP. The prosthesis contains a small valve which remains closed during swallowing, thereby excluding secretions and food debris from entering the trachea, but opens during exhalation, allowing pulmonic air to enter the esophagus and allow for tracheoesophageal speech.

COMPANION CASES

- **Tracheal stoma closure with residual tracheal cartilage irregularity.** Many tracheostomies, particularly those in place for a short duration, close within days of extubation. The term "persistent stoma" is utilized for those stomas persisting greater than 3 months following tracheostomy tube removal and range in size from small sinus tracts to full tube size defects. Etiologic factors for persistent tracheal stomas include prolonged tracheostomy tube placement with tract epithelialization, debilitated condition, severe metabolic derangements, chronic steroid use, and other comorbidities affecting wound healing. Surgical closure with tract debridement and muscle flap may be required for proper healing.
- **Granulation tissue and hemorrhage within the tracheostomy and subglottic airway.** Granulation tissue is often present along the tracheostomy and/or within the subglottic airway when there is an indwelling tracheostomy tube. It may also be present months or years after a tracheostomy tube has been removed. The granulation tissue is typically smooth in morphology and is most often present as a continuous rind of tissue. Occasionly, granulation in these areas may be identified as an incomplete rind of soft tissue; in this case tumor can be difficult to exclude in patients with a history of tumor in this region. Superimposed aerated debris, particularly with an indwelling tracheostomy tube, may also be identified, as is demonstrated in the case provided.
- **Tracheal stoma recurrent tumor.** Differentiating tumor from scar tissue adjacent to a tracheal stoma following a tumor resection can be extremely difficult. Enhancing tissue adjacent to the tracheal stoma should be viewed with suspicion, particularly if new. If soft tissue adjacent to a tracheal stoma is identified and no prior imaging is available, then short-term follow-up to document stability is warranted. When in doubt, a biopsy may be necessary.

Tracheoesophageal puncture (TEP) and prosthesis

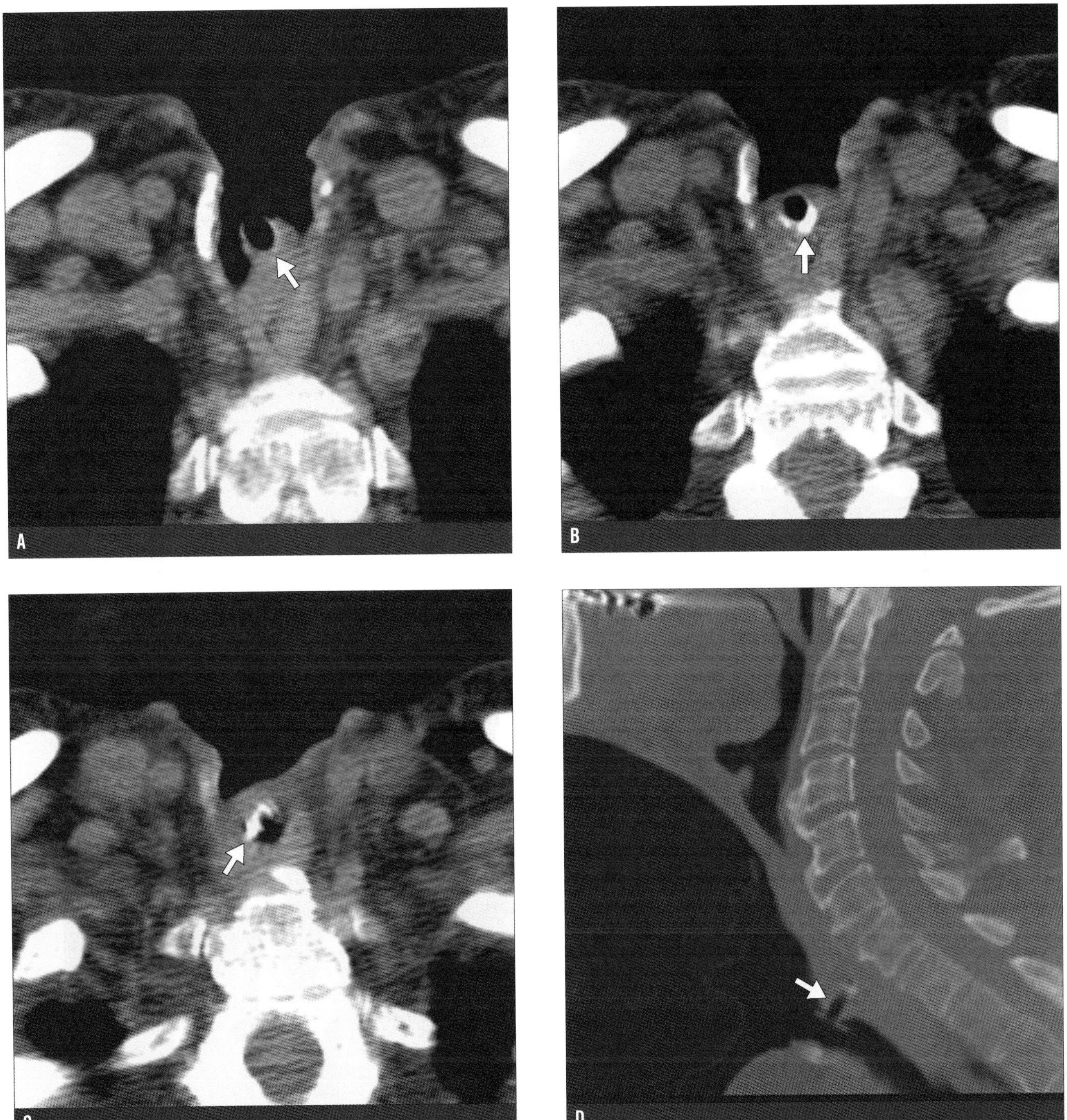

Unenhanced axial CT images viewed with a soft tissue window (**A-C**) and a sagittal reformatted CT image viewed with a bone window (**D**) demonstrate a total laryngectomy and a tubular device extending from the posterior wall of the trachea at the level of the tracheal stoma and into the esophagus, representing the TEP prosthesis (arrows, **A-D**). This prosthesis is placed through a surgically formed fistula between the trachea and the esophagus. A one-way valve over the tracheal stoma is not present in this case; the patient either removed the valve prior to this CT scan or uses their finger to occlude the stoma during tracheoesophageal speech.

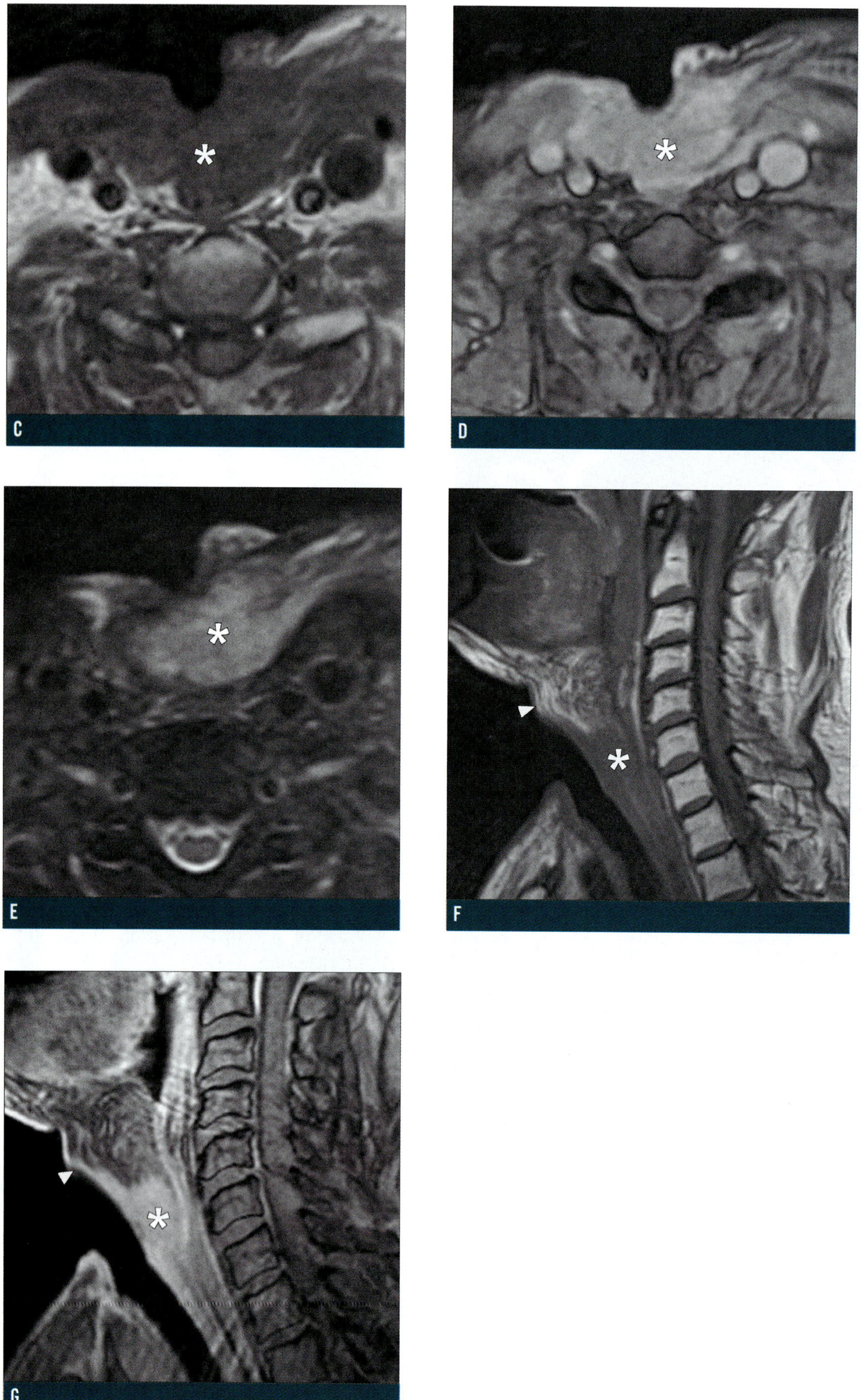

REFERENCES

American Speech-Language-Hearing Association. *Evaluation and treatment for tracheoesophageal puncture and prosthesis: technical report* [Technical Report]. 2004. Available from www.asha.org/policy.

Bishop JB, Bostwick J, Nahai F. Persistent tracheostomy stoma. *Am J Surg.*1980;140:709-710.

De Leyn P, et al. Tracheotomy: clinical review and guidelines. *Eur J Cardiothorac Surg.* 2007;32:412-421.

Doctor VS. In-office unsedated tracheoesophageal puncture. *Curr Opin Otolaryngol Head Neck Surg.* 2007;15:405-408.

Elmiyeh B, et al. Surgical voice restoration after total laryngectomy: an overview. *Indian J Cancer.* 2010;47:239-247.

Engels PT, Bagshaw SM, Meier M, Brindley PG. Tracheostomy: from insertion to decannulation. *Can J Surg.* 2009;52:427-433.

Pawar PV, Sayed SI, Kazi R, Jagade MV. Current status and future prospects in prosthetic voice rehabilitation following laryngectomy. *J Canc Res Therapeut.* 2008;4:186-191.

Stafford FW. Current indications and complications of tracheoesophageal puncture for voice restoration after laryngectomy. *Curr Opin Otolaryngol Head Neck Surg.* 2003;11:89-95.

Sue RD, Susanto I. Long-term complications of artificial airways. *Clin Chest Med.* 2003;24:457-471.

Composed of 16 to 20 horseshoe-shaped hyaline cartilage rings which support the anterior and lateral walls, the trachea is lined with mucus-producing ciliated pseudostratified columnar epithelial cells that serve to trap inhaled foreign particles and transport them upward toward the pharynx where they can be swallowed or expelled—a system collectively known as the mucociliary escalator. The posterior tracheal wall (known as the membranous portion of the trachea) is devoid of cartilage and is comprised of a thin membrane of smooth muscle and fibrous tissue. The membranous portion of the trachea contacts the ventral esophageal wall and is compliant during inspiration and expiration. This compliance also allows normal bulging of the esophagus into the trachea during deglutition and expiration.

Greater than 50% reduction in the cross-sectional area of the tracheal lumen during expiration has historically been considered diagnostic of tracheomalacia. However, recent studies of normal subjects have demonstrated a wide range of expiratory tracheal collapsibility and ventral bulging of the esophagus into the tracheal lumen, sometimes resulting in a greater than 50% decrease in the cross-sectional area of the tracheal lumen.

COMPANION CASE

- **Thyroid carcinoma with tracheal wall invasion and luminal narrowing.** Tracheal narrowing or invasion by thyroid cancer is associated with poorly differentiated tumors and reduced survival. It has been estimated that greater than 50% of all deaths from thyroid malignancy have been attributed to airway obstruction and bleeding, although the overall death rate of thyroid malignancy remains low because most thyroid malignancies are well-differentiated.

  Evaluating tracheal narrowiang and/or invasion by CT or MRI is best made by carefully evaluating for any asymmetric thickness and/or enhancement of the tracheal wall relative to the contralateral, normal side. In addition, reviewing the images with a CT lung window may increase the sensitivity of identifying subtle extension of tumor into the tracheal lumen.

Tracheal collapse during expiration

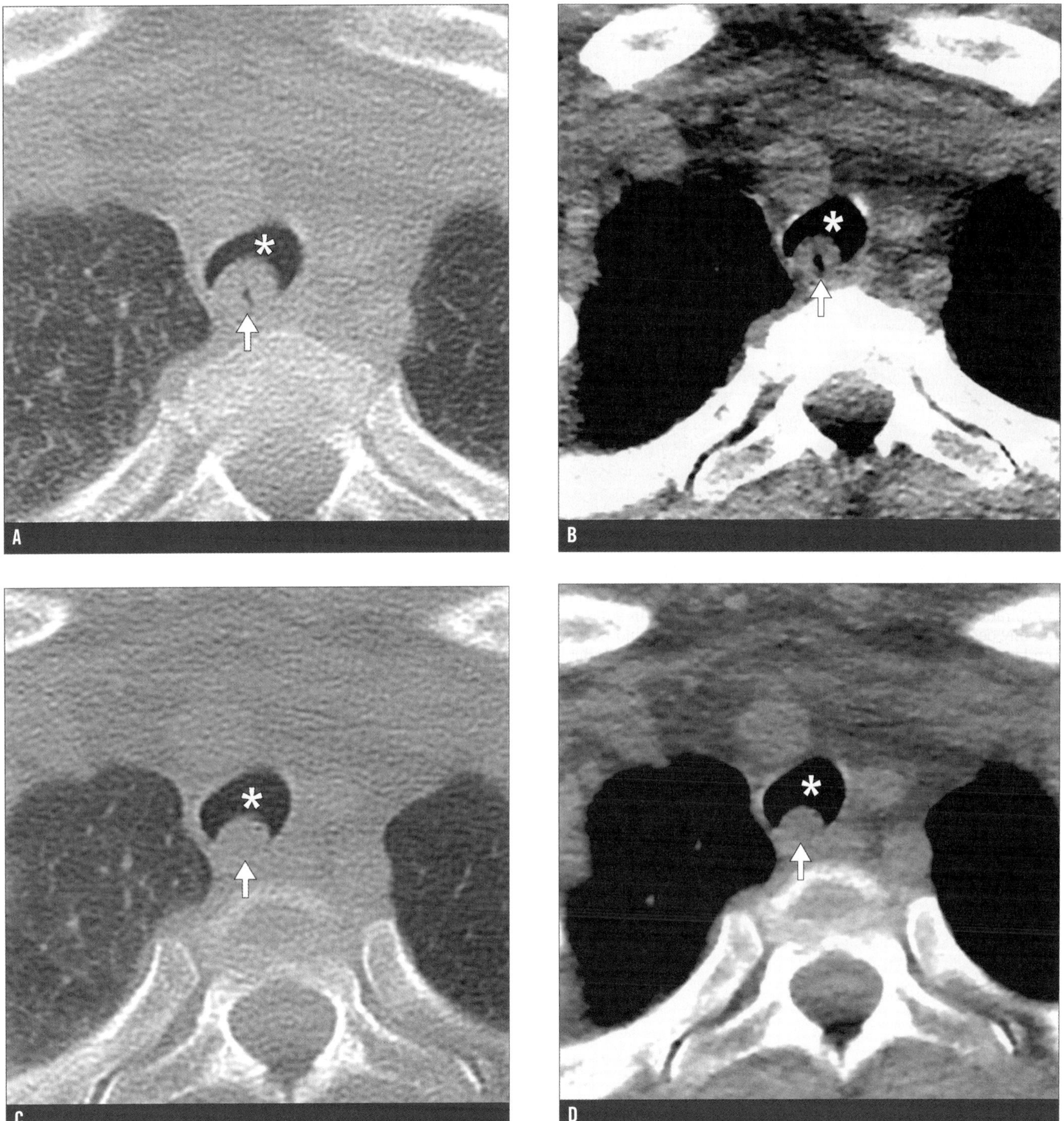

Unenhanced axial CT images viewed with a lung (**A**) and soft tissue (**B**) window demonstrate a ventrally bulging esophagus (arrows, **A**, **B**) and narrowing of the tracheal lumen (asterisks, **A**, **B**). The lungs on image **A** are ground glass in appearance, suggesting a poor inspiration. Approximately 3 weeks later, the same patient underwent another CT examination. Images from this study viewed at the same level and with the same windows as images **A** and **B** (**C**, **D**) demonstrate less ventral bulging of the esophagus (arrows, **C**, **D**) and a larger tracheal lumen (asterisks, **C**, **D**). There is improved lung aeration on image **C** relative to image **A**, illustrating the variability in tracheal lumen volume with varying respiratory effort. This patient had no history of symptoms referable to the trachea or esophagus during either scan.

Tracheal collapse during expiration

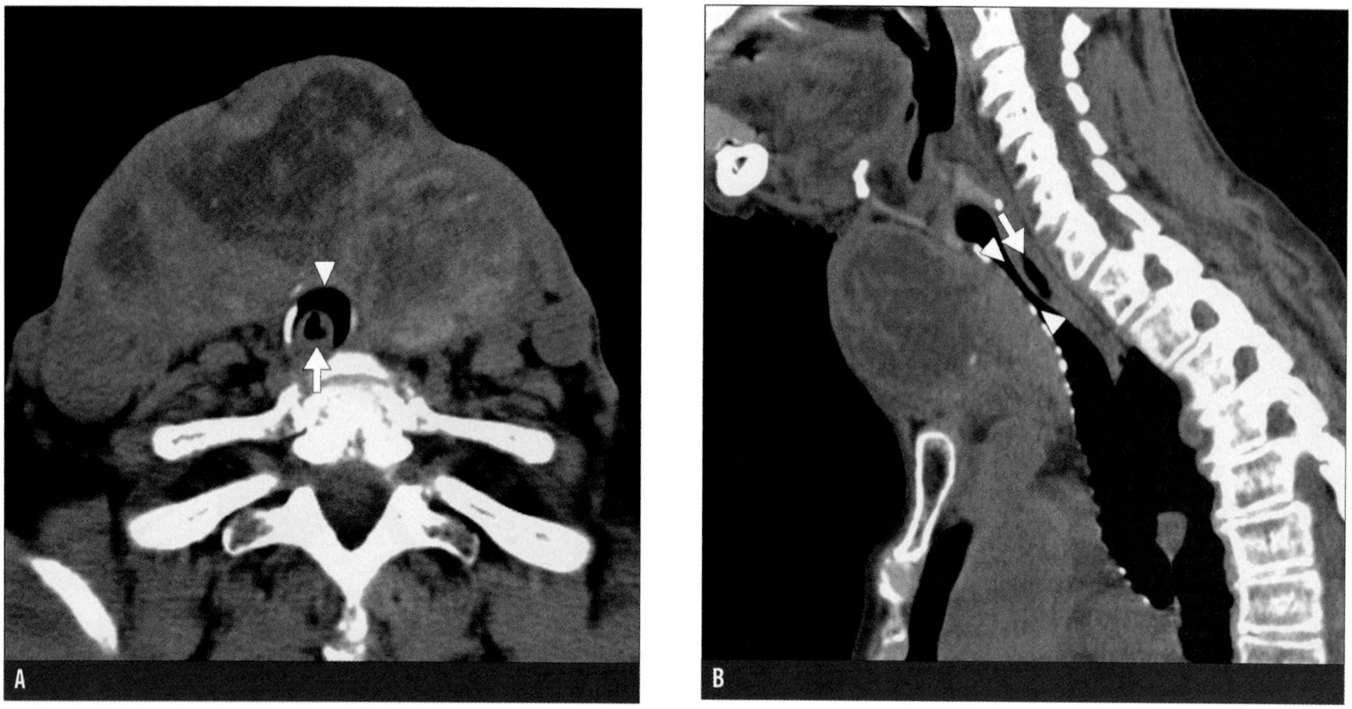

Different patient. Unenhanced axial (**A**) and sagittal reformatted (**B**) CT images demonstrate pronounced ventral bulging of the esophagus (arrows, **A**, **B**) into the trachea, resulting in pronounced narrowing of the tracheal lumen (arrowheads, **A**, **B**). This was presumably related to expiration during the scan. However, if presented with a case as pronounced as this, then correlation with pulmonary function tests and any pertinent symptoms referable to the finding would be advised. This patient did not have any symptoms pertinent to this finding. The large thyroid goiter is likely an unrelated issue, as the finding is related to the relative plasticity of the membranous portion of the trachea, which is not deformed by thyroid goiter.

Companion case: Thyroid carcinoma with tracheal wall invasion and luminal narrowing

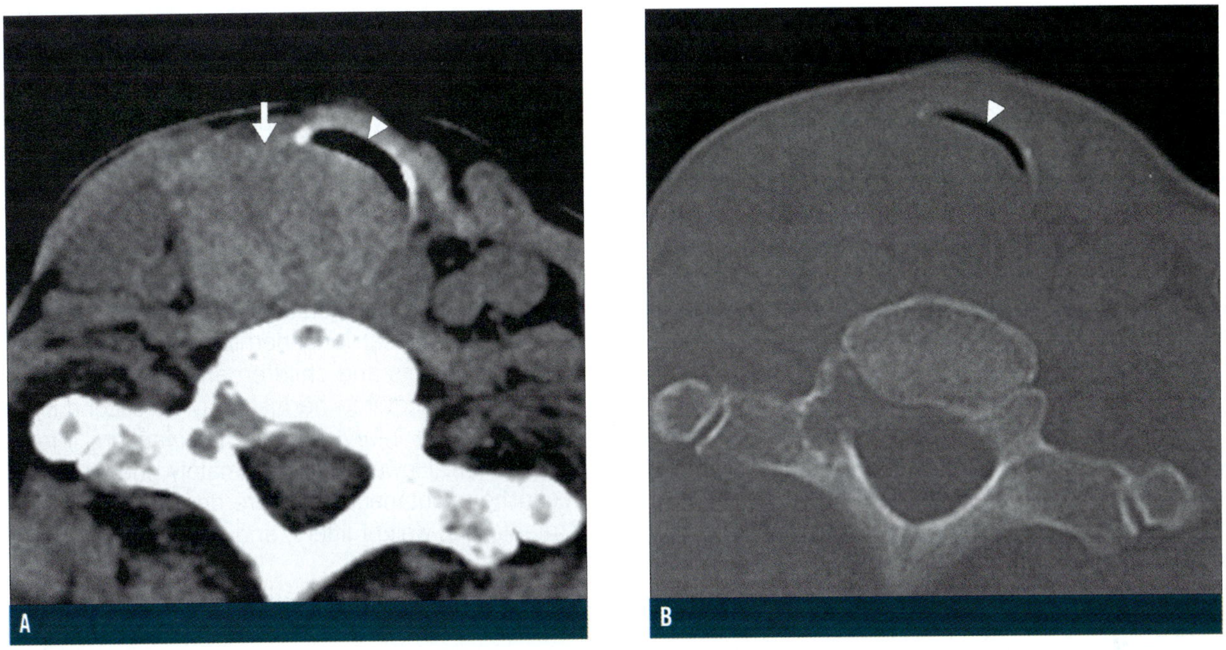

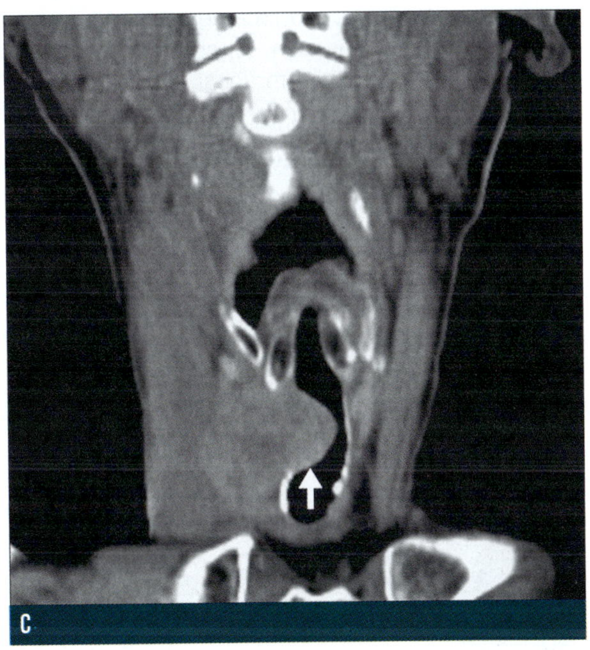

Unenhanced axial CT images viewed with a soft tissue window (**A**) and bone window (**B**) as well as a coronal reformatted CT image viewed with a soft tissue window (**C**) demonstrate a large mass arising from the thyroid gland (arrows, **A**, **C**) and invading the dorsolateral right tracheal wall, resulting in marked narrowing of the tracheal lumen (arrowheads, **A**, **B**). This thyroid lesion represented a thyroid carcinoma.

REFERENCES

Boiselle PM, et al. Tracheal collapsibility in healthy volunteers during forced expiration: assessment with multidetector CT. *Radiology.* 2009;252:255-262.

Carden KA, Boiselle PM, Waltz DA, Ernst A. Iracheomalacia and tracheobronchomalacia in children and adults: an in-depth review. *Chest.* 2005;127:984-1005.

Chung JH, Kanne JP, Gilman MD. CT of diffuse tracheal diseases. *AJR Am J Roentgenol.* 2011;196:W240-W246.

Gaissert HA, Burns J. The compromised airway: tumors, strictures, and tracheomalacia. *Surg Clin North Am.* 2010;90:1065-1089.

Javidan-Nejad C. MDCT of trachea and main bronchi. *Radiolog Clin North Am.* 2010;48:157-176.

Park CM, Goo JM, Lee HJ, Kim MA, Lee CH, Kang M-J. Tumors in the tracheobronchial tree: CT and FDG PET features1. *Radiographics.* 2009;29:55-71.

Seo YL, et al. Locally advanced thyroid cancer: can CT help in prediction of extrathyroidal invasion to adjacent structures? *AJR Am J Roentgenol.* 2010;195(3):W240-W244.

Webb EM, Elicker BM, Webb WR. Using CT to diagnose nonneoplastic tracheal abnormalities: appearance of the tracheal wall. *AJR Am J Roentgenol.* 2000;174:1315-1321.

CASE 22 Tracheal diverticulum

A tracheal diverticulum represents a unilocular or multilocular collection of air at the level of the thoracic inlet, characteristically located along the posterior-right aspect of the trachea. It can either be acquired or congenital and it occurs in approximately 2% to 3% of the population. A tracheal diverticulum may communicate directly with the tracheal lumen in up to 35% of cases and is usually best appreciated with a CT examination. The majority of diverticula are asymptomatic, incidentally noted structures on cross-sectional studies, although they may act as reservoirs for secretions and result in recurrent tracheobronchial infections.

The acquired form of a tracheal diverticulum is commonly attributed to bronchopulmonary disorders, such as chronic obstructive pulmonary disease (COPD). In COPD, the increased intraluminal pressure results in herniation of the mucous membrane through a weak point in the tracheal wall. The acquired tracheal diverticulum is typically larger and more variably located than congenital diverticula. The more aptly termed "pseudodiverticula" is used to describe these acquired diverticula, as their wall is formed solely by respiratory epithelium and lacks the smooth muscle and cartilage of the parent structure. By contrast, congenital tracheal diverticula possess complete tracheal anatomy. The etiology of congenital diverticula is debated, with several proposed theories including vestigial supernumerary lung, an aborted and abnormally high division of primary lung bud, or a defect in endodermal differentiation or tracheal cartilage formation.

COMPANION CASE

- **Apical lung herniation.** A rare condition, apical lung herniation may be congenital (~20%) or acquired (~80%). Congenital apical lung herniations are identified most often in infants and children and usually resolve spontaneously. Acquired hernias may be secondary to penetrating lung injury, surgical intervention, infection, or neoplasm. However, approximately one-fourth of cases can be spontaneous and are described in wind instrumentalists, weight lifters, and individuals with a chronic cough.

  An apical lung herniation is secondary to a defect in Sibson fascia, a continuation of endothoracic fascia over the apex of the lung. The defect is often large enough to prevent trapping and incarceration of lung, although these complications can infrequently occur. Surgical repair is often reserved for local mass effect symptoms such as dysphagia, hernia incarceration, or significant cosmetic deformity.

Tracheal diverticulum

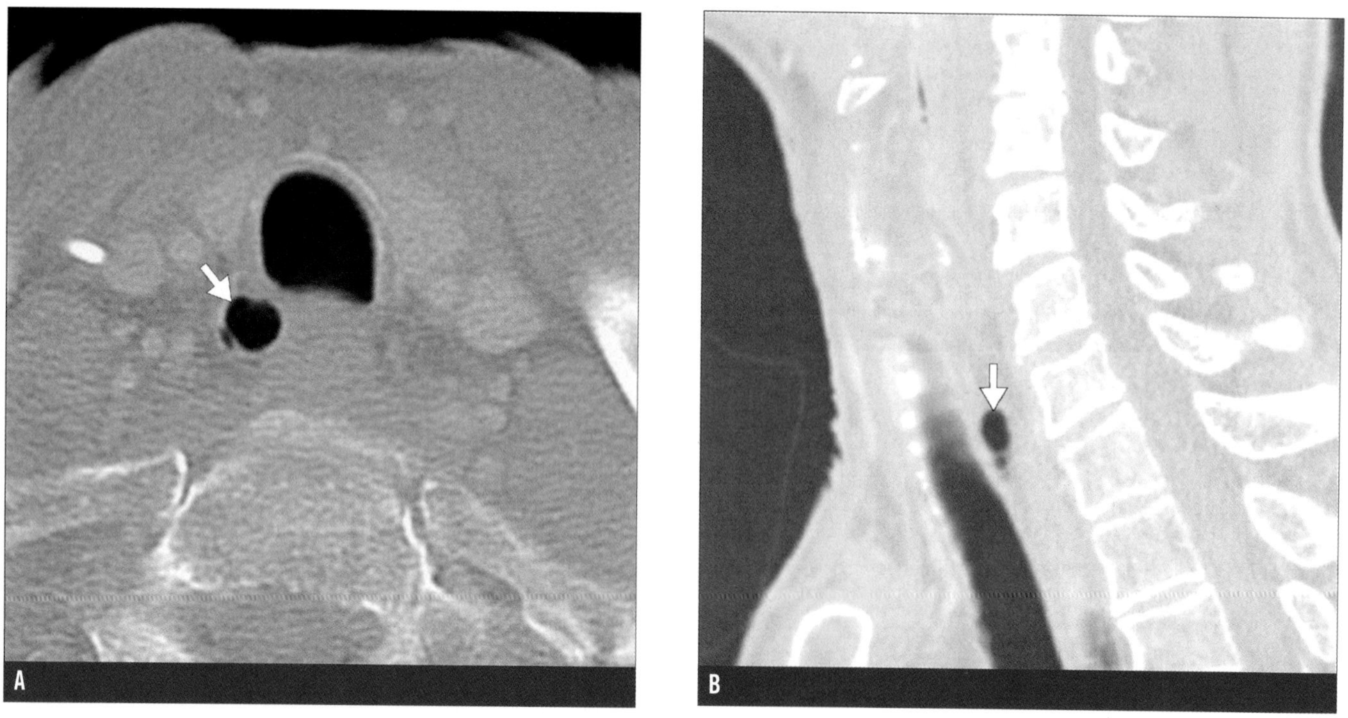

Axial (**A**) and sagittal reformatted (**B**) CT images demonstrate a small tracheal diverticulum along the right dorsolateral aspect of the trachea (arrows, **A**, **B**).

Tracheal diverticulum

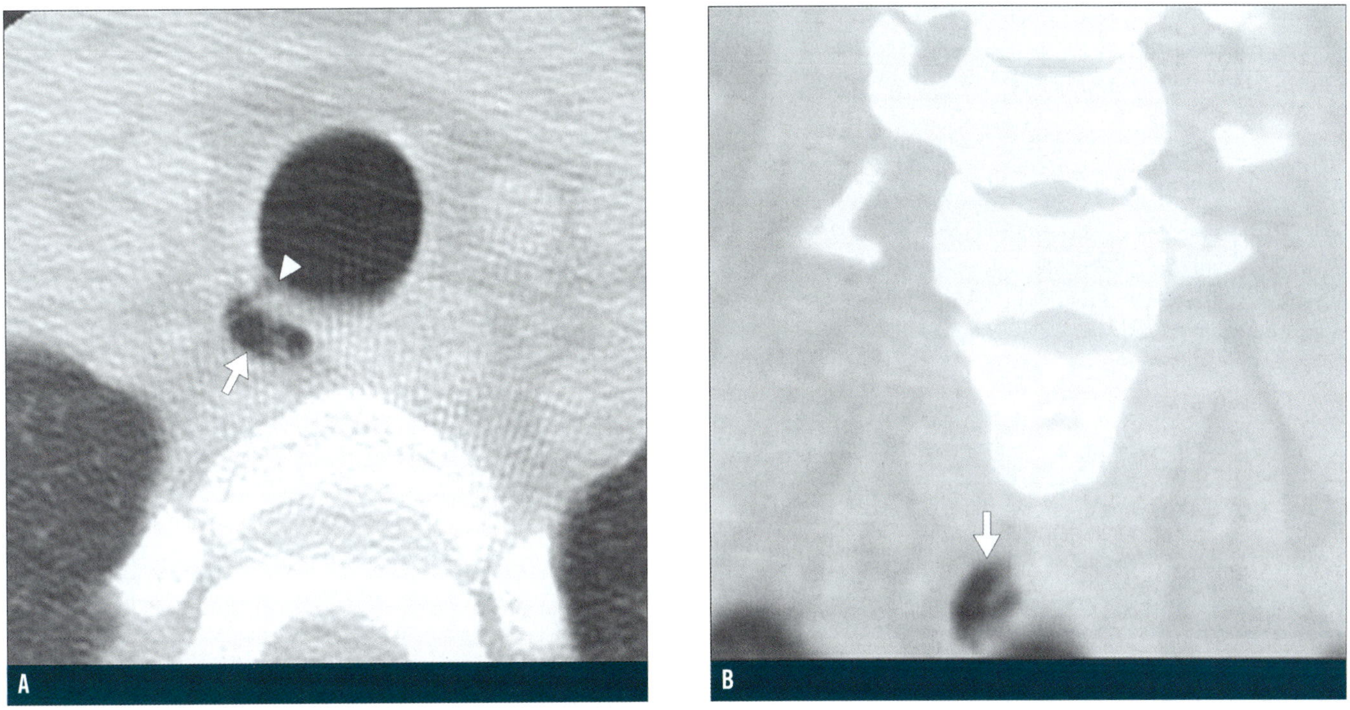

Different patient. Axial (**A**) and coronal reformatted (**B**) CT images demonstrate a small right dorsolateral tracheal diverticulum (arrows, **A**, **B**) with a small air-filled communication between the diverticulum and the trachea (arrowhead, **A**).

Companion case: Apical lung herniation

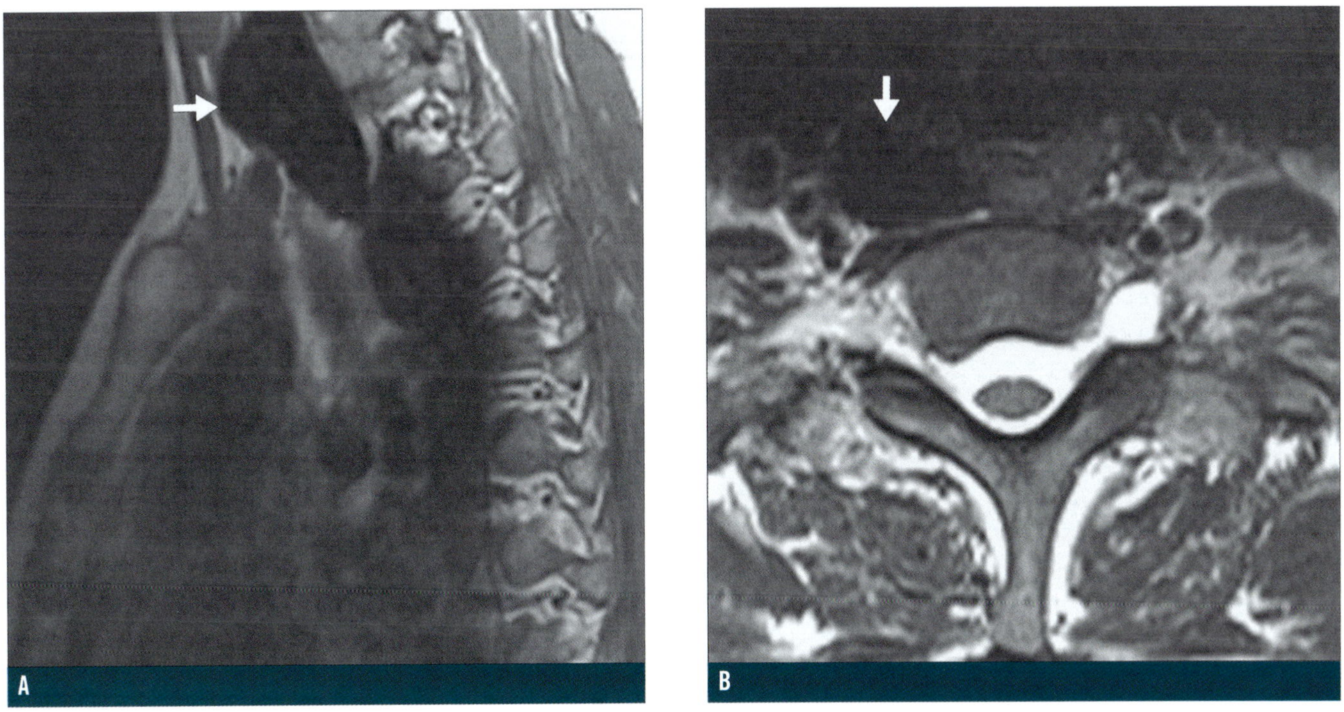

Sagittal T1 (**A**) and axial T2 (**B**, **C**) MR images demonstrate a large right apical lung herniation (arrows, **A**-**C**).

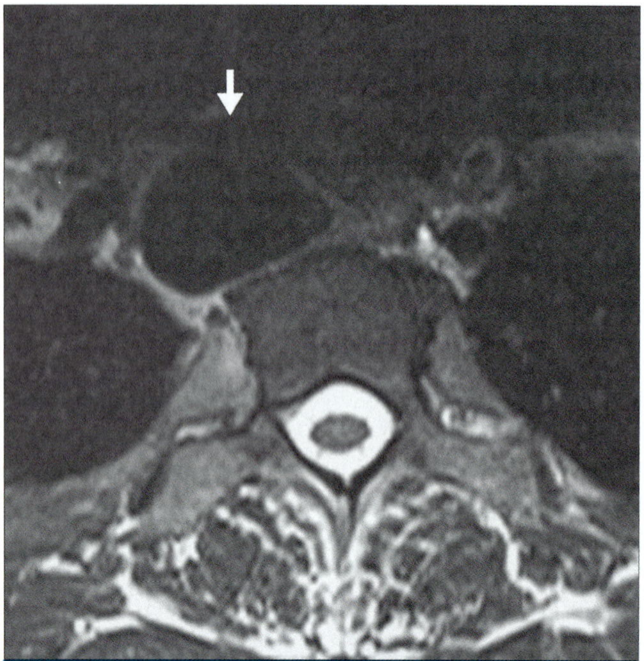

C

REFERENCES

Bhalla M, Leitman BS, Forcade C, Stern E, Naidich DP, McCauley DI. Lung hernia: radiographic features. *AJR Am J Roentgenol.* 1990;154:51-53.

Buterbaugh JE, Erly WK. Paratracheal air cysts: a common finding on routine CT examinations of the cervical spine and neck that may mimic pneumomediastinum in patients with traumatic injuries. *AJNR Am J Neuroradiol.* 2008;29:1218-1221.

Early EK, Bothwell MR. Congenital tracheal diverticulum. Otolaryngology - Head & Neck Surgery 2002;127:119-121.

Goo JM, et al. Right paratracheal air cysts in the thoracic inlet: clinical and radiologic significance. *AJR Am J Roentgenol.* 1999;173:65-70.

McAdams HP, Gordon DS, White CS. Apical lung hernia: radiologic findings in six cases. *AJR Am J Roentgenol.* 1996;167:927-930.

Ranu H, Jackson M. Apical lung herniation. Thorax 2011;66:740.

Soto-Hurtado EJ, Penuela-Ruiz L, Rivera-Sanchez I, Torres-Jimenez J. Tracheal diverticulum: a review of the literature. Lung 2006;184:303-

CHAPTER 3

NECK

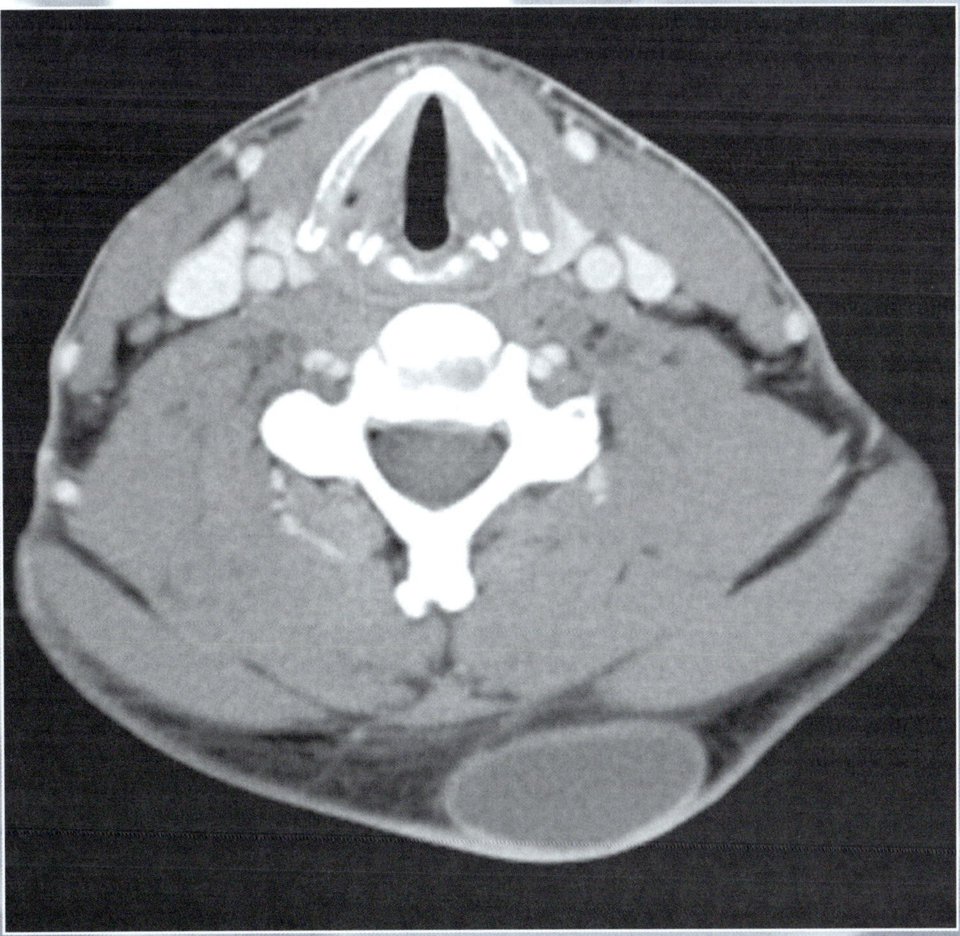

Nishant D. Parekh, Christopher Reilly,
Achilles G. Karagianis

III. NECK

1. Asymmetric strap muscles
   i. *Companion case*: Thyroglossal duct cyst with proteinaceous content
   ii. *Companion case*: Strap muscle lipoma
2. Epidermal inclusion cyst
   i. *Companion case*: Typical thyroglossal duct cyst
   ii. *Companion case*: Infected thyroglossal duct cyst
   iii. *Companion case*: Thyroglossal duct cyst containing thyroid carcinoma
   iv. *Companion case*: Metastatic lymph node (Delphian node)
3. Levator claviculae
   i. *Companion case*: Accessory muscle of the levator scapulae muscle
4. Unilateral third head of the sternocleidomastoid muscle
5. Sternocleidomastoid muscle hypertrophy
   i. *Companion case*: Sternocleidomastoid muscle myositis
   ii. *Companion case*: Sternocleidomastoid muscle *Staphylococcus aureus* abscess
   iii. *Companion case*: Sternocleidomastoid muscle hematoma
   iv. *Companion case*: Sternocleidomastoid muscle aggressive fibromatosis
   v. *Companion case*: Sternocleidomastoid muscle lymphoma
   vi. *Companion case*: Sternocleidomastoid muscle venolymphatic malformation
6. Disuse neck muscle atrophy from cervical scoliosis
   i. *Companion case*: Diffuse atrophy of the semispinalis capitis and splenius capitis muscles
7. Neck dissection types
   i. *Companion case*: Recurrent metatastic lymphadenopathy following a neck dissection
8. Neck reconstructions
9. Levator scapulae muscle hypertrophy following a neck dissection
   i. *Companion case*: Asymmetric levator scapulae muscle without surgery
   ii. *Companion case*: Levator scapulae muscle aggressive fibromatosis
   iii. *Companion case*: Levator scapulae muscle fibrosarcoma
10. Irradiated neck
    i. *Companion case*: Carotidynia
    ii. *Companion case*: Metastatic disease to the neck dermis and soft tissues
    iii. *Companion case*: Paraffinoma following mineral oil injection
11. Brown fat
    i. *Companion case*: Madelung disease
    ii. *Companion case*: Intramuscular neck lipoma
    iii. *Companion case*: Liposarcoma
    iv. *Companion case*: Epidermal inclusion cyst
12. Normal minimal fat in the neck
    i. *Companion case*: Cachexia
13. Incomplete fat suppression on MRI
14. Brachial plexus
    i. *Companion case*: Parsonage-Turner syndrome
15. Thoracic duct
    i. *Companion case*: Contrast reflux into the thoracic duct on CT
    ii. *Companion case*: Contrast reflux into the thoracic duct on MRI
    iii. *Companion case*: Change in the thoracic duct size during inspiration and expiration
    iv. *Companion case*: Cervical thoracic duct cyst
    v. *Companion case*: Metastatic lymphadenopathy from papillary thyroid carcinoma
    vi. *Companion case*: Chylous leak with the formation of a lymphocele and a chylous pleural effusion
16. Right lymphatic duct
    i. *Companion case*: Right lymphatic duct cyst
17. Venous valves and focal dilation of veins
    i. *Companion case*: Supraclavicular lymphadenopathy
    ii. *Companion case*: Iatrogenically injected air located in a focally dilated vein
    iii. *Companion case*: Internal jugular vein phlebectasia
18. Mixing of opacified and unopacified blood simulating internal jugular vein thrombus
    i. *Companion case*: Nonocclusive thrombus in the internal jugular vein
    ii. *Companion case*: Occlusive thrombus in the internal jugular vein
    iii. *Companion case*: Lemierre syndrome
19. Retropharyngeal lipoma
    i. *Companion case*: Retropharyngeal edema
    ii. *Companion case*: Retropharyngeal abscess
    iii. *Companion case*: Retropharyngeal lymphatic malformation
20. Large fatty hilum within a normal lymph node
    i. *Companion case*: Pathologic lymph node with a preserved fatty hilum
    ii. *Companion case*: Necrotic metastatic lymph node from papillary thyroid cancer
    iii. *Companion case*: Lymph node necrosis secondary to tuberculosis (scrofula)
21. Second branchial cleft cyst versus necrotic metastatic lymphadenopathy
22. Normal anterior rectus capitis muscles simulating nodes of Rouvière
    i. *Companion case*: Normal node of Rouvière
    ii. *Companion case*: Non-necrotic pathologic node of Rouvière
    iii. *Companion case*: Necrotic node of Rouvière
    iv. *Companion case*: Poststyloid parapharyngeal space schwannoma
23. Focal atrophy of the longus capitis muscle
    i. *Companion case*: Fatty infiltration of the longus capitis muscle
24. Longus colli tendon hydroxyapatite deposition
    i. *Companion case*: Acute calcific tendonitis of the longus colli muscle
    ii. *Companion case*: Enlarging longus colli tendon hydroxyapatite deposition
    iii. *Companion case*: C1 anterior vertebral osteophyte formation
    iv. *Companion case*: Retropharyngeal course of an atherosclerotic internal carotid artery

25. Asymptomatic marked ossification of the stylohyoid ligament
    i. *Companion case*: Symptomatic ossification of the stylohyoid ligament (Eagle syndrome)
    ii. *Companion case*: Eagle syndrome resulting in a chronic, nonocclusive internal jugular vein thrombus
    iii. *Companion case*: Normal intermediate tendon of the digastric muscle
26. Cervical rib
27. Ligamentum nuchae ossification
    i. *Companion case*: Acute cervical-thoracic junction spinous process fractures
    ii. *Companion case*: Chronic cervical spinous process avulsion fracture versus an ununited secondary ossification center
28. Vagal nerve stimulator
    i. *Companion case*: Occipital nerve stimulator

Mild asymmetry of the cervical musculature is common and is often either not noticed or not remarked upon. More severe asymmetry may present clinically as a palpable mass or may be misinterpreted as a significant lesion on imaging. One of the most common etiologies of muscle asymmetry is scoliosis, where the muscle asymmetry is the result of the deformity; however, muscle asymmetry may also play a role in forming the scoliosis. Other etiologies of muscle asymmetry include developmental variation, denervation atrophy (from trauma or tumor-related nerve damage), surgery, or asymmetric usage (golfing, carrying large shoulder bags, etc).

The strap muscles, also termed the infrahyoid muscles, function to depress the hyoid and larynx during speech and deglutition. They include the sternohyoid, sternothyroid, thyrohyoid, and omohyoid muscles. Apart from nerve damage resulting in atrophy of the strap muscles, no literature was found specifically pertaining to incidental asymmetry of the strap muscles. However, it is likely that many of the same causes of asymmetric muscle hypertrophy/atrophy that occur with other muscles of the neck are also applicable to the strap muscles. Moreover, incidental asymmetry related to normal variation likely accounts for some cases.

COMPANION CASES

- **Thyroglossal duct cyst with proteinaceous content.** TGD cysts may accumulate proteinaceous material because of prior infection or trauma. This proteinaceous material may render the lesion isodense to the surrounding muscle on CT and the only clue to its existence may be asymmetric apparent enlargement of the adjacent strap muscle. However, MRI will usually reveal the underlying TGD and its proteinaceous contents. For further discussion of TGD cysts, see the companion cases from Case 2.
- **Strap muscle lipoma.** Lipomas are benign, encapsulated, usually slow-growing tumors composed of fat. These tumors are painless and may occur at any age, but most commonly present in individuals aged between 40 and 60 years. Simple lipomas contain homogeneous fat attenuation on CT and homogeneous fat signal characteristics on all MRI pulse sequences. More complex lipomas, especially if there is fat necrosis or inflammatory change, may be difficult to distinguish from well-differentiated liposarcomas. However, certain findings within a fat-containing mass should favor a liposarcoma over a benign lipoma, including, thick septations, nodular and/or globular areas of nonadipose tissue, associated nonadipose masses, and nonadipose tissue comprising more than 25% of the lesion. Simple lipomas may be resected for cosmesis, with an overall recurrence rate of 1% to 2%; however, intramuscular lipomas, even when simple appearing on radiology studies or at pathology, have a much higher local recurrence rate (19%).

Asymmetric strap muscles

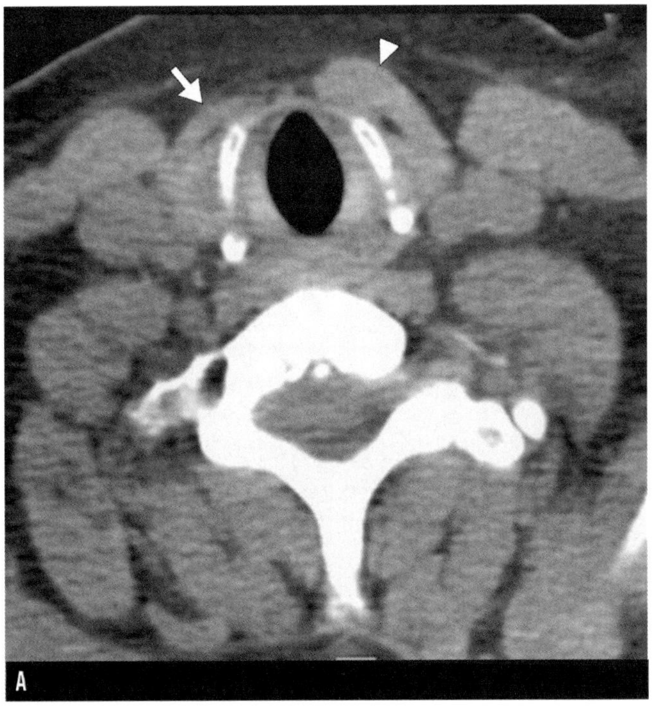

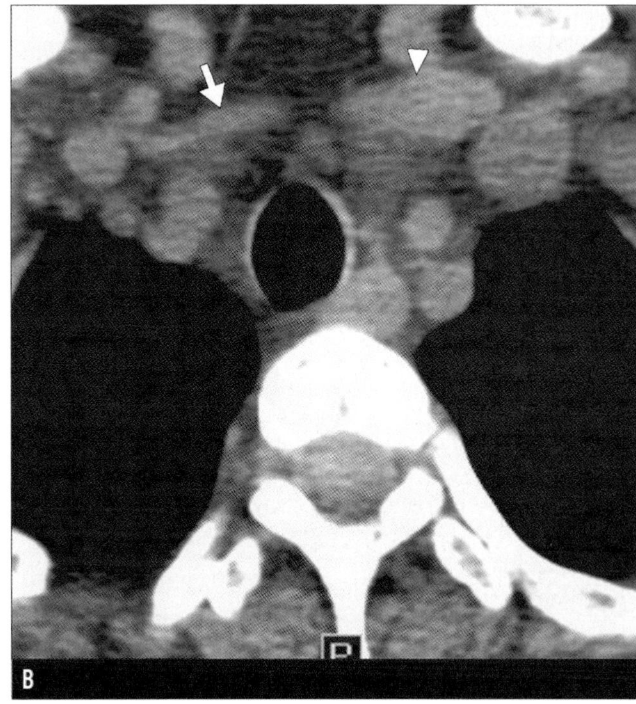

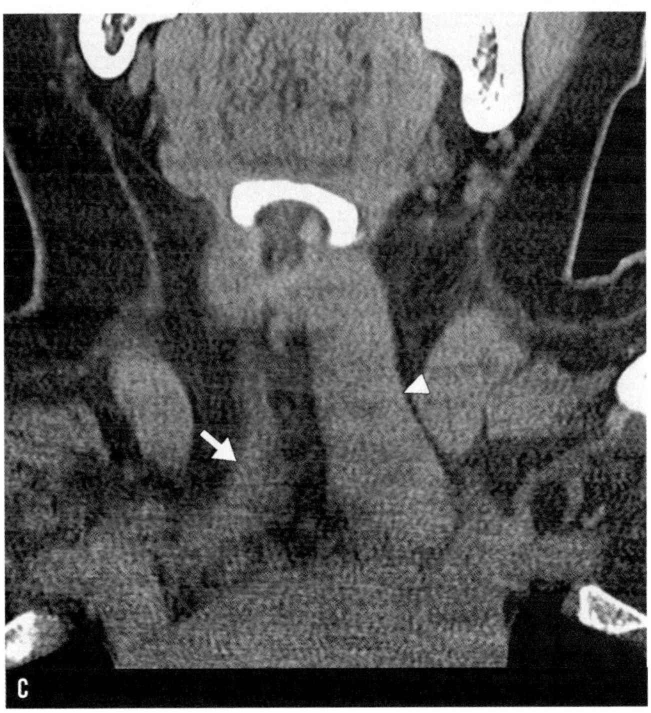

Unenhanced axial (**A**, **B**) and coronal reformatted (**C**) CT images demonstrate asymmetrically smaller right strap muscles (arrows, **A-C**) compared to the normal sized left strap muscles (arrowheads, **A-C**).

Epidermal inclusion cyst

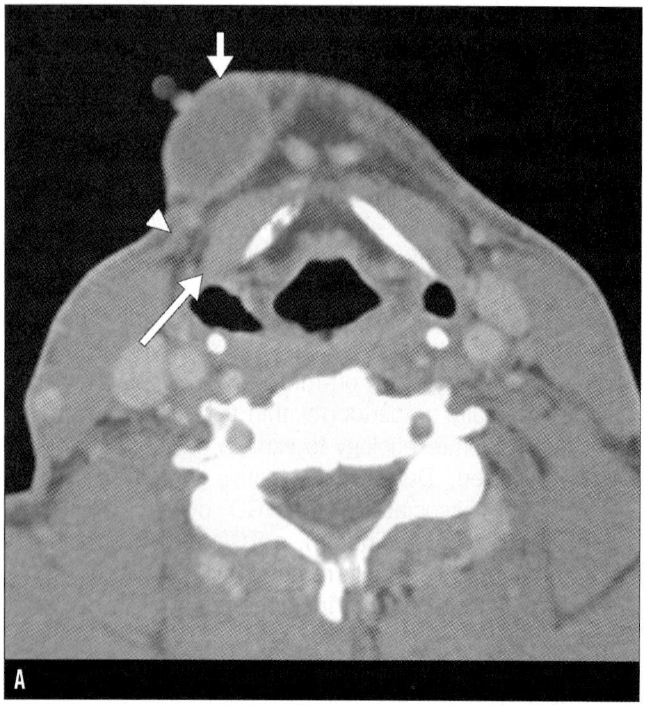

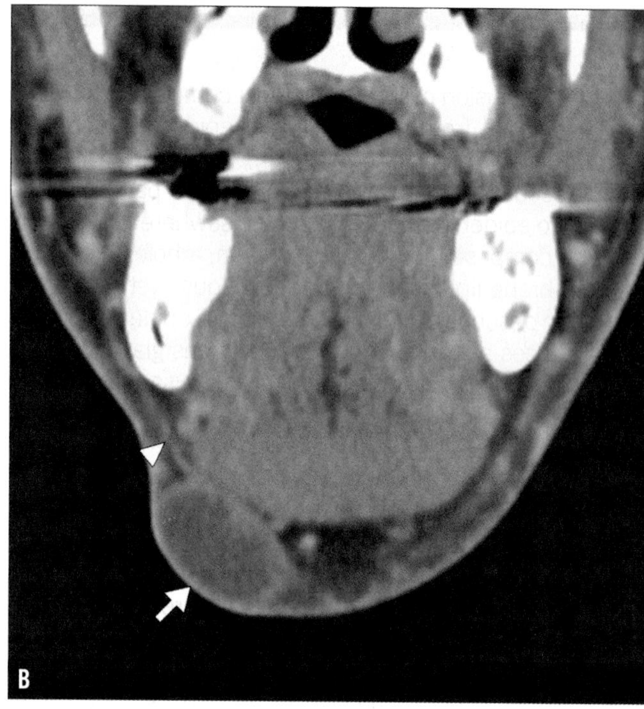

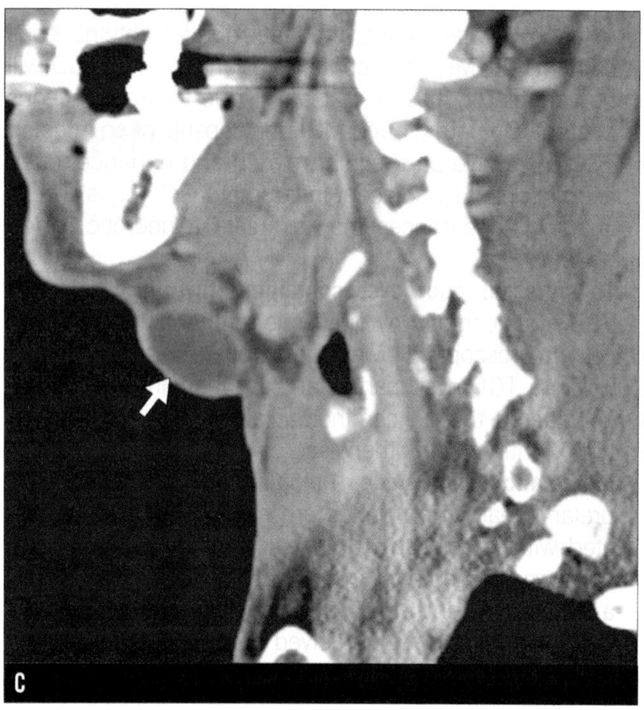

This patient presented with a history of a "slowly enlarging right submandibular mass." Axial (**A**), coronal reformatted (**B**), and sagittal reformatted (**C**) contrast-enhanced CT images through the neck demonstrate a thin-walled, fluid-attenuated, cystic appearing lesion located in the anterior neck subcutaneous soft tissues to the right of midline (short arrows, **A**-**C**). The lesion is superficial to the strap muscles (long arrow, **A**), superficial to the platysma muscle (arrowheads, **A**, **B**), and abuts the dermis. The superficial location of the lesion (in particular superficial to the strap muscles) would be highly atypical of a thyroglossal duct cyst, which are almost always at least partially embedded within the strap muscles. Given the location and dermal abutment, the lesion is most compatible with an epidermal inclusion cyst.

Companion case: Typical thyroglossal duct cyst

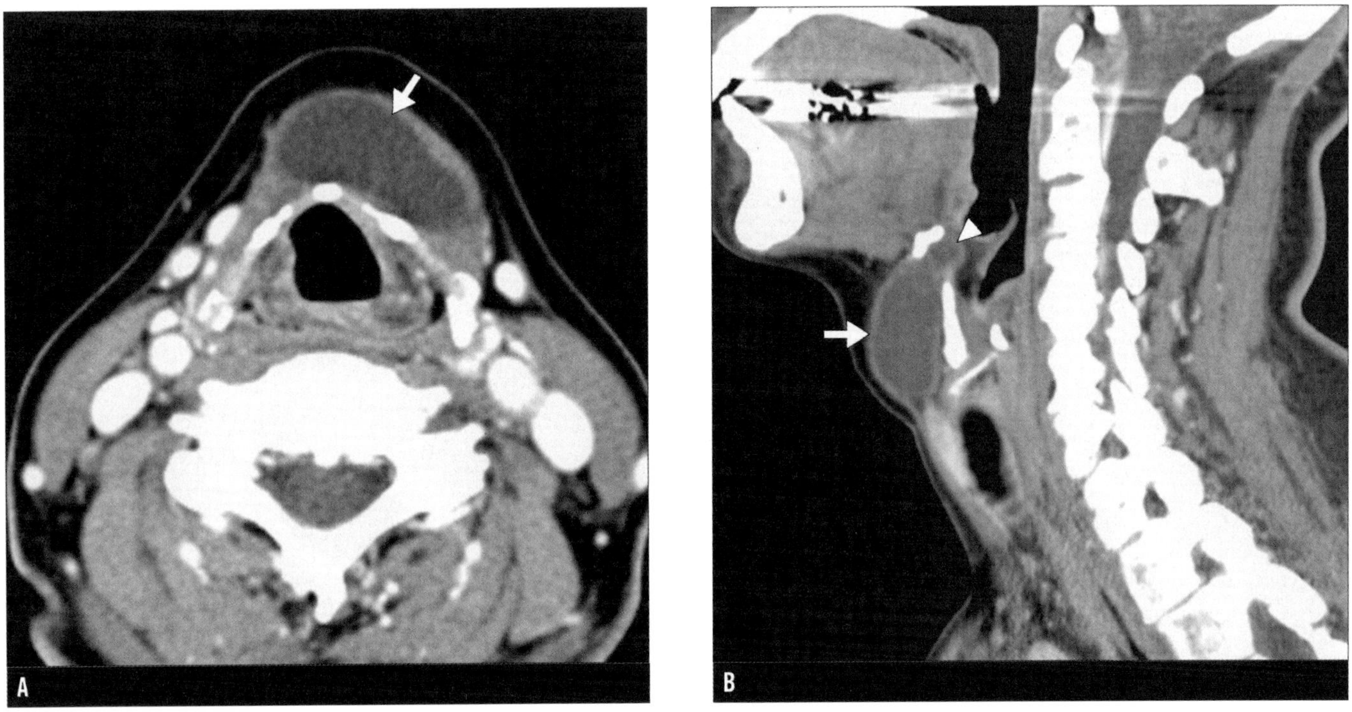

Contrast-enhanced axial (**A**) and sagittal reformatted (**B**) CT images demonstrate a large fluid-filled lesion (arrows, **A**, **B**) embedded deep to the strap muscles, with a small portion extending posterior to the body of the hyoid bone (arrowhead, **B**), compatible with a thyroglossal duct cyst. This lesion is differentiated from an epidermal inclusion cyst by its location, as discussed in the preceding case.

Companion case: Infected thyroglossal duct cyst

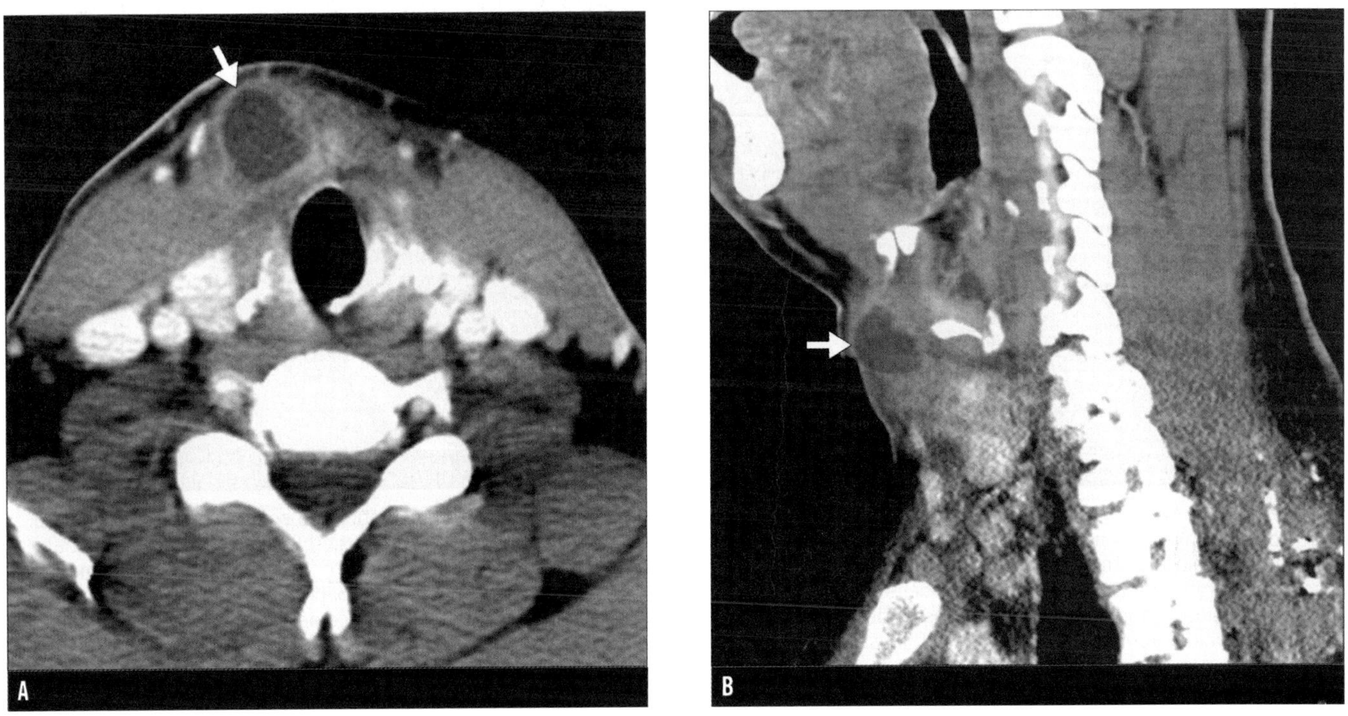

Axial (**A**) and sagittal reformatted (**B**) contrast-enhanced CT images demonstrate an oval, presumably peripherally enhancing lesion embedded within the right strap muscles (arrows, **A**, **B**). The finding is associated with surrounding inflammatory change. This finding represented an infected thyroglossal duct cyst.

Companion case: Thyroglossal duct cyst containing thyroid carcinoma

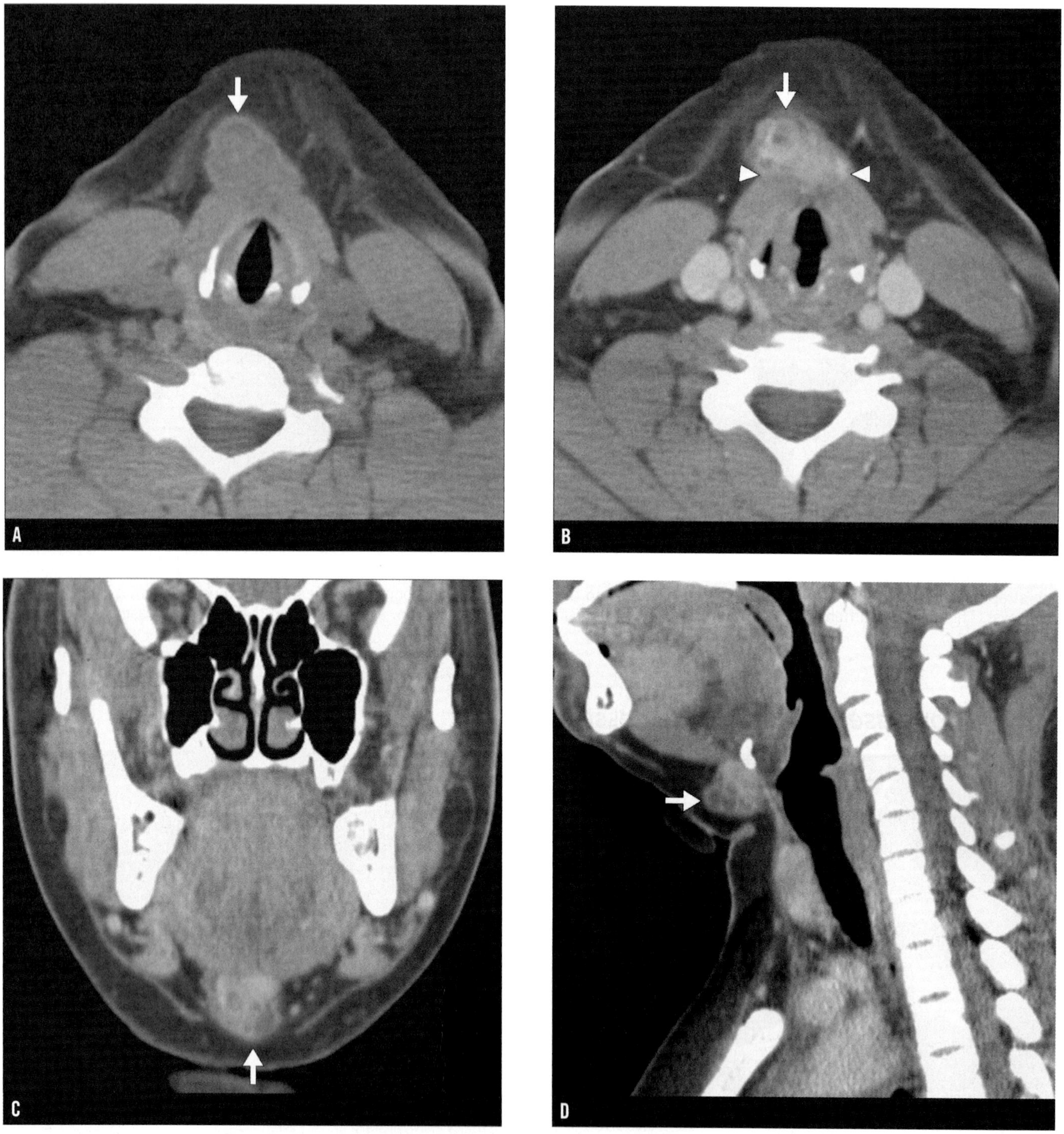

An unenhanced axial CT image through the level just caudal to the hyoid bone (**A**) demonstrates a lobulated soft tissue mass (arrow, **A**). A postcontrast axial CT image through the mass (**B**) demonstrate heterogeneous enhancement of the lesion (arrow, **B**), which is partially embedded within the strap muscles (arrowheads, **B**). Coronal reformatted (**C**) and sagittal reformatted (**D**) contrast-enhanced CT images also demonstrate the heterogeneous enhancement of the lesion (arrows, **C**, **D**). This lesion represented papillary thyroid carcinoma arising from a thyroglossal duct cyst. Any thyroglossal duct cyst that contains heterogeneous soft tissue enhancement is malignant (typically papillary thyroid carcinoma), until proven otherwise.

Companion case: Metastatic lymph node (Delphian node)

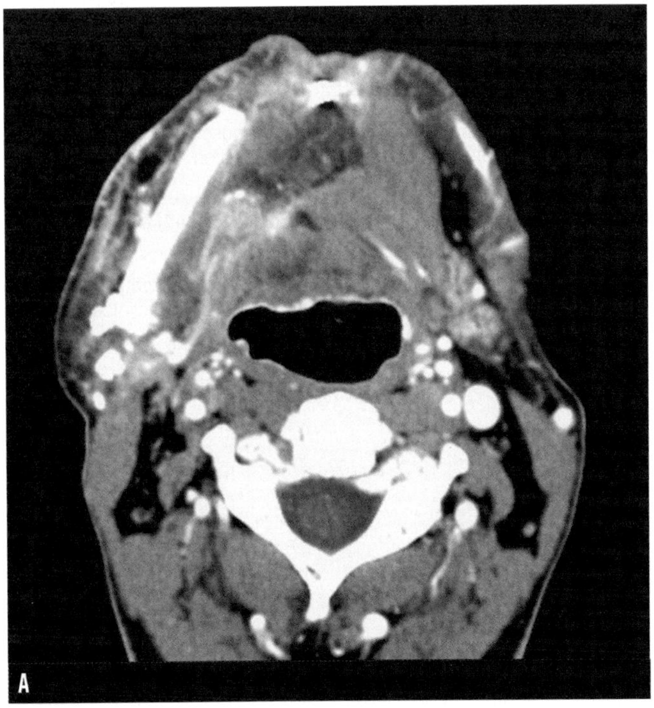

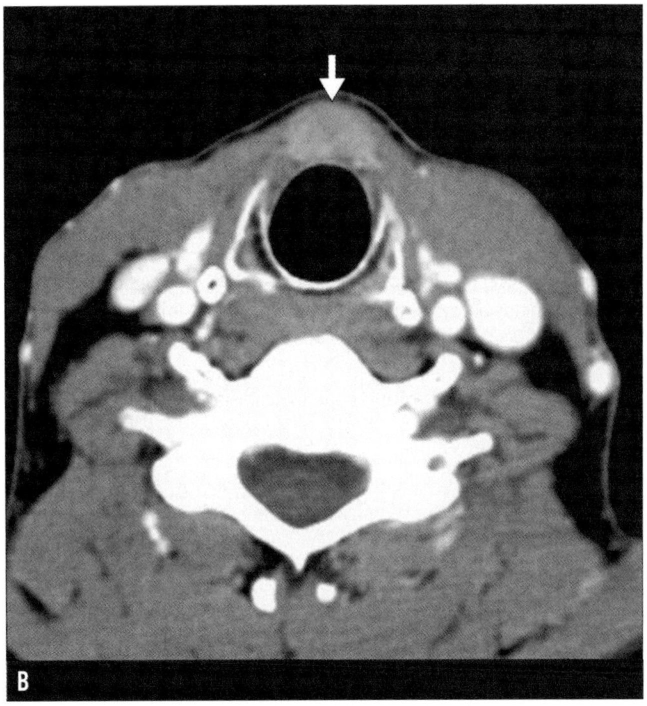

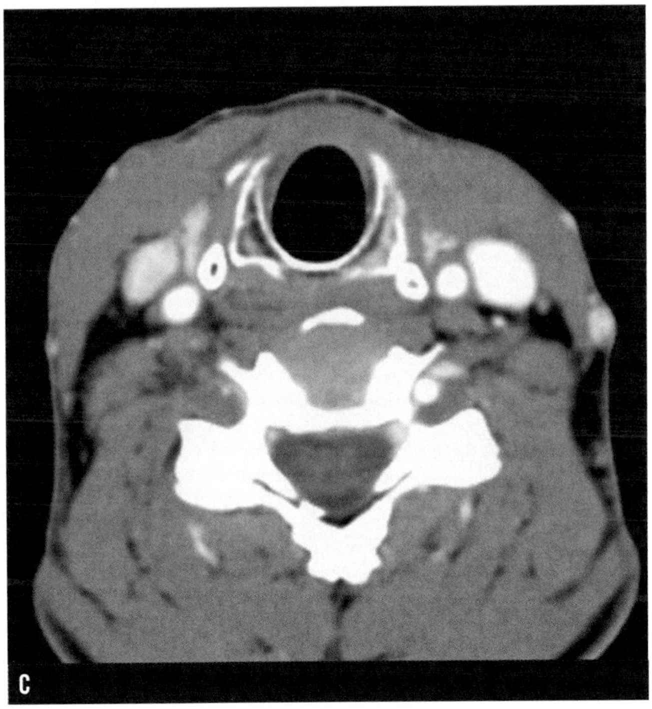

Axial postcontrast CT images through the oral cavity (**A**) and the subglottic level (**B**). Image **A** demonstrates marked postoperative changes at the level of the oral cavity in a patient being treated for oral cavity squamous cell carcinoma. Image **B** demonstrates an oval lesion immediately ventral to the subglottis (arrow, **B**), suspicious for a metastatic Delphian lymph node, given the clinical scenario. An axial postcontrast CT image at the same level as image **B** (**C**), obtained 5 months later after chemotherapy and radiation, demonstrates resolution of the Delphian lymph node.

REFERENCES

Acierno SP, Waldhausen JHT. Congenital cervical cysts, sinuses and fistulae. *Otolaryngol clin North Am.* 2007;40(1):161-176, vii-viii.

Golden BA, Zide MF. Cutaneous cysts of the head and neck. *J Oral Maxillofac Surg.* 2005;63(11):1613-1619.

Gross E and, Sichel JY. Congenital neck lesions. *Surg Clin North Am.* 2006;86(2):382-392.

Isaacs JD, Lundgren CI, Sidhu SB, Sywak MS, Edhouse PJ, Delbridge LW. The Delphian lymph node in thyroid cancer. *Ann Surg.* 2008;247(3):477-482.

Kim HK, Kim SM, Lee SH, Racadio JM, Shin MJ. Subcutaneous epidermal inclusion cysts: ultrasound (US) and MR imaging findings. *Skeletal Radiol.* 2011;40(11):1415–1419. Epub 2010 Dec 4.

Kim WW, Yang SI, Kim JH, Choi YS, Park Y-H, Kwon SK. Experience and analysis of Delphian lymph node metastasis in patients with papillary thyroid carcinoma. *World J Surg Oncol.* 2012;10(1):226.

Murono S, Hirota K, Kondo S, Wakisaka N, Furukawa M, Yoshizaki T. An extremely rare case of large Delphian node metastasis preceding primary laryngeal cancer. *Auris Nasus Larynx.* 2009;36(5):614-617.

Pandya K A, Radke F. Benign skin lesions: lipomas, epidermal inclusion cysts, muscle and nerve biopsies. *Surg clin North Am.* 2009;89(3):677-687.

Shpizner BA, Holliday RA. Levator scapulae muscle asymmetry presenting as a palpable neck mass: CT evaluation. *AJNR. Am J neuroradiol.* 1993;14(2):461-464.

Som PM and, Curtin HD. *Head and Neck Imaging.* 4th ed. St. Louis, MO: Mosby Inc.; 2003.

Weber, AL, Randolph G, Aksoy FG. The thyroid and parathyroid glands: CT and MR imaging and correlation with pathology and clinical findings. *Radiol Clin North Am.* 2000;38(5):1105-1129.

Weedon D, Strutton *G. Cysts and Sinuses in Skin Pathology.* 2nd ed. Edinburgh, Scotland: Churchill Livingstone; 2002.

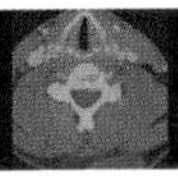

CASE 3 Levator claviculae

The levator claviculae muscle is a normal muscular variant present in 1% to 3% of the population that arises from the anterior aspect of the upper cervical vertebrae transverse processes and inserts upon the lateral half of the clavicle. It is a separate muscle that resides just lateral to the scalene muscles, medial to the sternocleidomastoid muscle and anterior or anterolateral to the levator scapulae muscle. On a single axial or sagittal image, it may appear to represent a normal or an abnormally enlarged cervical lymph node; however, evaluating this muscle on consecutive images allows for accurate characterization. Like other muscles of the neck, a levator claviculae muscle may undergo physiologic hypertrophy. In addition, because this variant is usually unilateral, this muscle may present clinically as an unexplained neck mass, with or without muscular hypertrophy.

COMPANION CASE

- **Accessory muscle of the levator scapulae muscle.** Normally, the levator scapulae muscle originates from the dorsal tubercles of the C1 to C4 transverse processes and inserts upon the superior medial aspect of the scapula, specifically between the triangular smooth surface of the scapula spine and the medial angle. As the name implies, the main function of the levator scapulae is to elevate the scapula, but it also assists in retraction and adduction of the scapula. There are rare reports of atypical origins and insertions of the levator scapulae muscle, including originating from the transverse processes of C5 to C7, or the skull, as well as inserting onto any of the following: first ten ribs, serratus anterior and serratus posterior muscles, trapezius muscle, scalene muscles, and rhomboideus major muscle. In the case provided, an accessory muscle arises from superior fibers of the left levator scapulae muscle, separates from the main levator scapulae muscle as it descends the neck, and inserts into the region of the superior muscle bundles of the left serratus anterior muscle rather than its typical insertion onto the scapula.

Levator claviculae

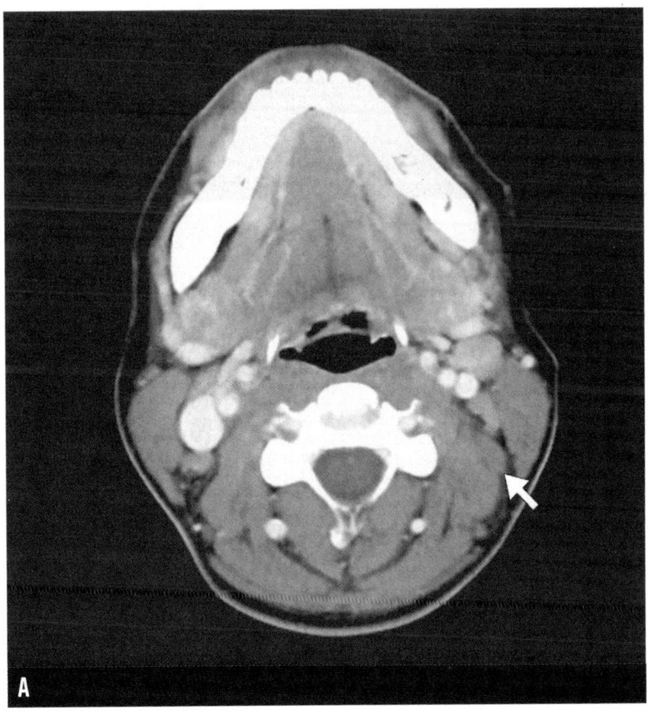

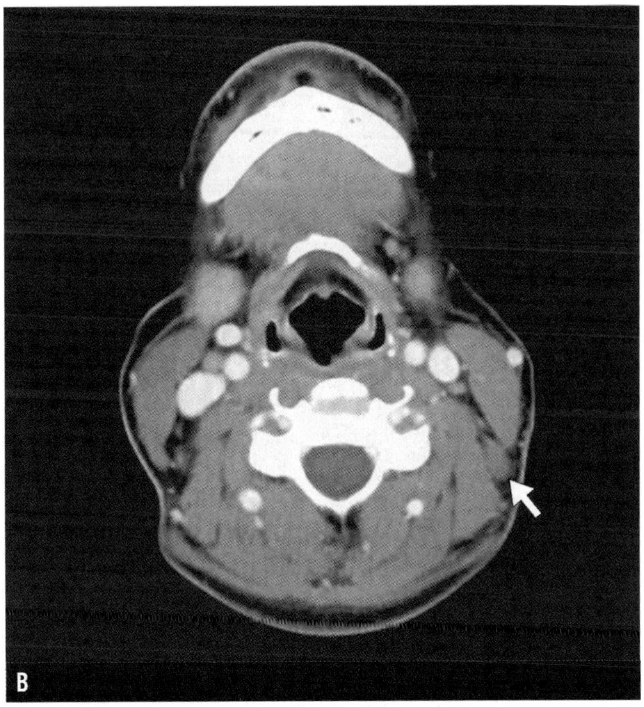

Axial (**A-D**), sagittal reformatted image through the left neck (**E**), sagittal reformatted through the right neck (**F**), and coronal reformatted (**G**) contrast-enhanced CT images. Several of these images demonstrate a typical levator clavicularis muscle on the left (arrows, **A-E**, **G**). The muscle simulates an abnormal lymph node when viewed separately on several of the provided images, such as images **B**, **C**, and **E**, although this should be easily distinguished from an abnormal lymph node when viewing consecutive images through the neck. Images **F** and **G** demonstrate the lack of a similar muscle in the right aspect of the neck.

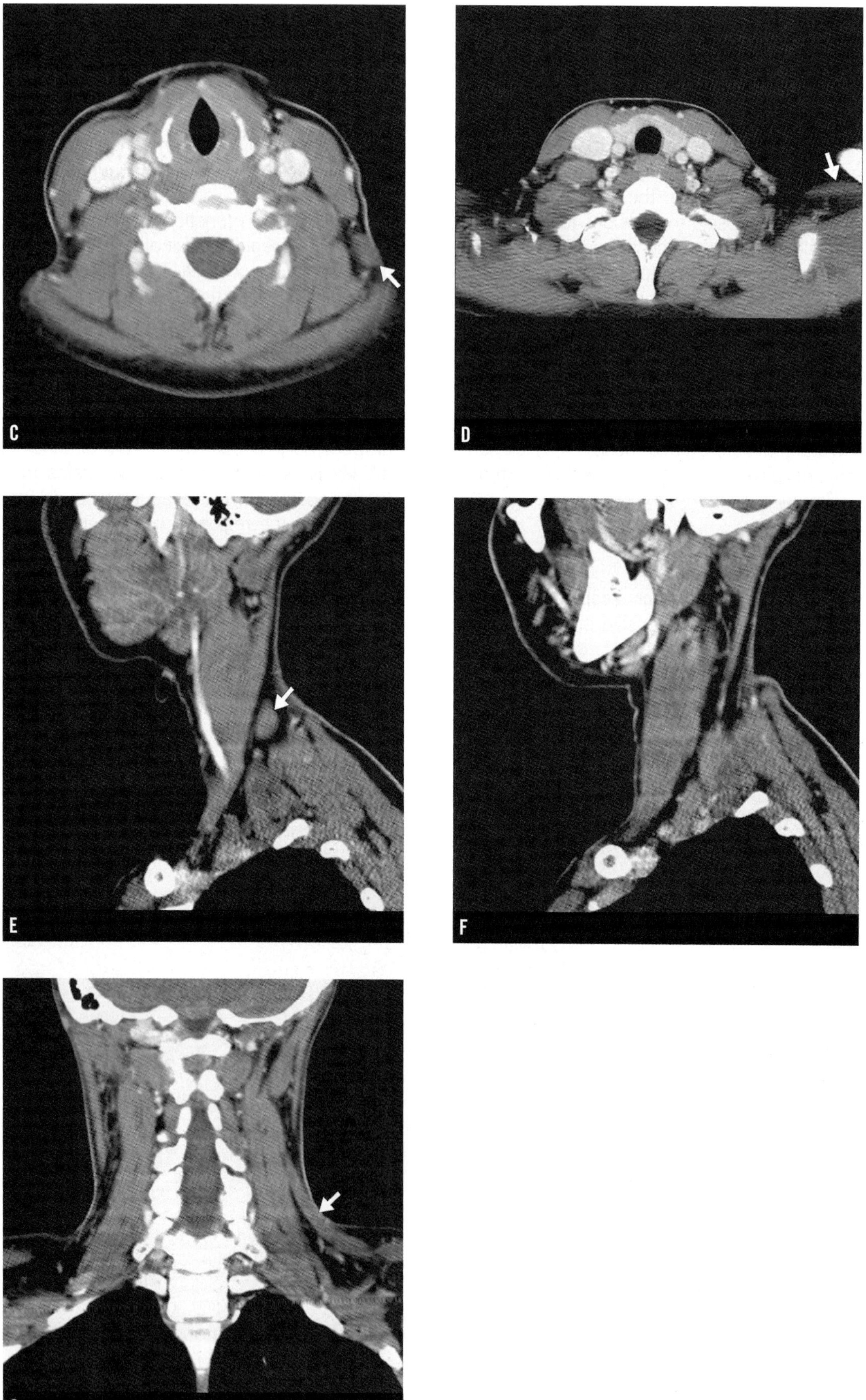
C
D
E
F
G

Companion case: Accessory muscle of the levator scapulae muscle

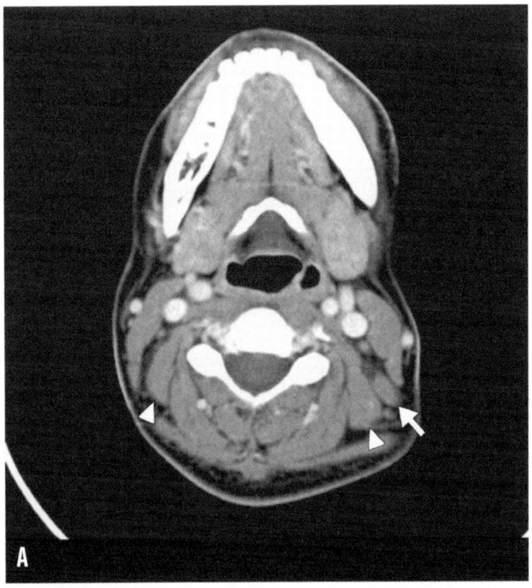

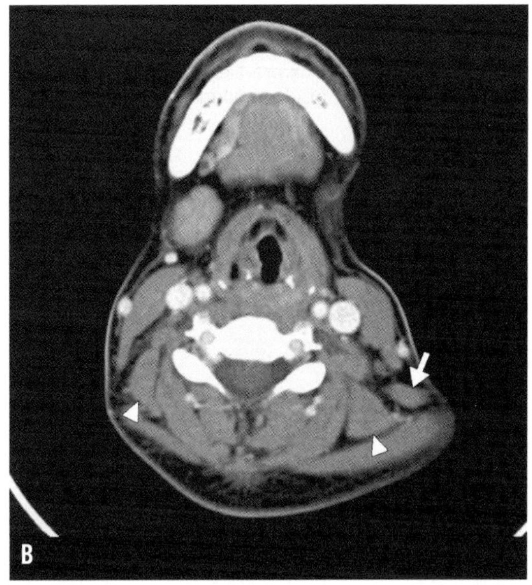

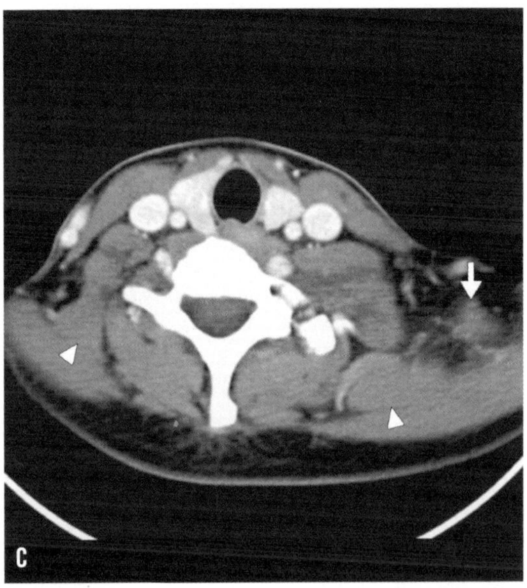

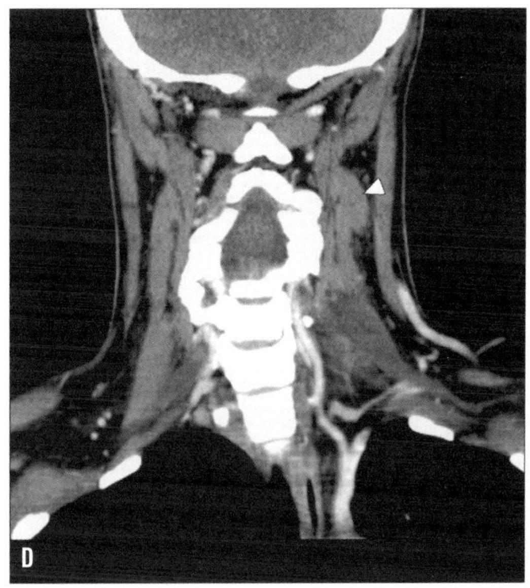

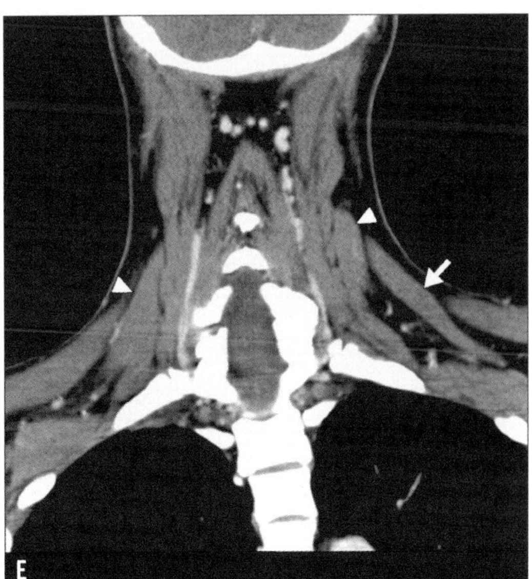

Contrast-enhanced axial (**A-C**) and a coronal reformatted (**D, E**) CT images through the neck. Images **A-C** and image **E** demonstrate an unusual accessory muscle (arrows, **A-C, E**) of the left levator scapulae muscle. This accessory muscle begins to separate from the normal left levator scapulae muscle superiorly in the neck (arrowhead, **D**) and then is more clearly defined as a separate muscle as it descends the neck. Image **C** demonstrates this accessory muscle (arrow) immediately prior to its merging with the superior muscle bundles of the left serratus anterior muscle (not shown). This is in contradistinction to the normal insertion of the levator scapulae muscle, which is the superior medial aspect of the ipsilateral scapula. In addition, this differs from the levator claviculae variant, which inserts onto the lateral half of the clavicle. The normal bilateral levator scapulae muscles are denoted as a reference (arrowheads, **A-C, E**).

REFERENCES

Gabriel Varjão Lima, et al. Unusual anatomical variation of the levator scapulae muscle. *Int. J. Morphol.* 2012;30(3):866-869.

Rubinstein D, Escott EJ, Hendrick LL. The prevalence and CT appearance of the levator claviculae muscle: a normal variant not to be mistaken for an abnormality. *AJNR Am J Neuroradiol.* 1999;20(4):583-586.

Rudisuli T. Demonstration of the musculus levator claviculae. *Surg Radiol Anat.* 1995;17:85-87

CASE 4 Unilateral third head of the sternocleidomastoid muscle

The sternocleidomastoid muscle (SCM) is a paired muscle located in the superficial, anterior neck and is the landmark that divides the neck into anterior and posterior cervical triangles. The SCM is typically composed of two heads, one head originating from the manubrium of the sternum and the other from the medial one-third of the clavicle. The sternal head is rounded in morphology, whereas the clavicular head is flattened in morphology. These muscles ascend obliquely and merge below the mid aspect of the neck, ultimately inserting via a tendon to the lateral aspect of the temporal bone mastoid process and via an aponeurosis to the lateral aspect of the occipital bone superior nuchal line. Symmetric contraction of the SCM results in neck flexion and head extension. Asymmetric contraction results in contralateral rotation of the head and lateral flexion of the ipsilateral neck.

Several variations of the SCM have been described. A relatively rare variant involves a developmental bifurcation of the clavicular head into medial and lateral components. The medial component originates from the medial one-third of the clavicle, whereas the lateral component originates from the middle one-third of the clavicle. This variant has been described as a "third head" or bipartite clavicular attachment and can be clinically important for head and neck surgeons preparing for a SCM flap reconstruction. It may also result in difficulty in attempting internal jugular vein access because of associated narrowing of the supraclavicular fossa by the variant. On axial imaging, it is often identified as a separate muscle along the posterior margin of the SCM at the level of the mid neck and as two separate muscles inserting onto the clavicle. Like other neck musculature, and in particular asymmetric muscular neck variants, viewing this variant on any given axial image may be confused with a normal or an abnormally enlarged lymph node. This can be avoided by viewing the variant on consecutive images. Asymmetric neck musculature variants may also simulate a neck mass or lymphadenopathy on clinical exam.

Unilateral third head of the sternocleidomastoid muscle

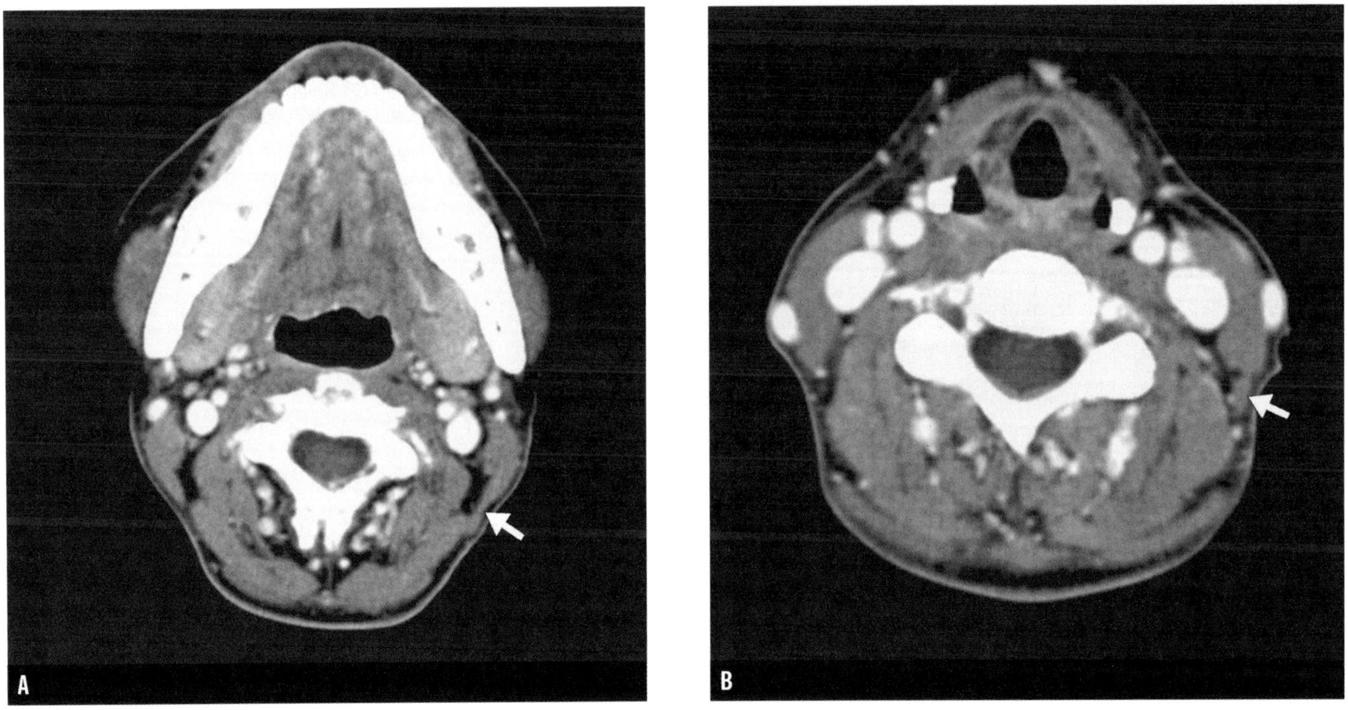

Axial postcontrast images from a CT neck (**A-D**) demonstrate a separate muscle along the posterior margin of the left SCM at the mid neck becoming two separate muscle bellies caudally in the neck, representing a bipartite clavicular head (also called "third" SCM head) (arrows, **A-D**). The asymmetric left SCM was palpated and thought to clinically represent lymphadenopathy, as denoted by a Vitamin E capsule on axial CT image **E** (arrow).

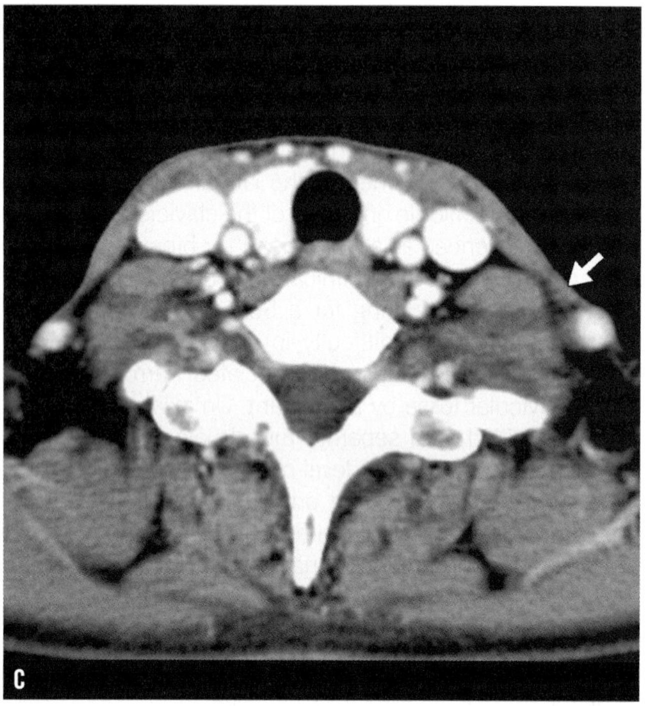

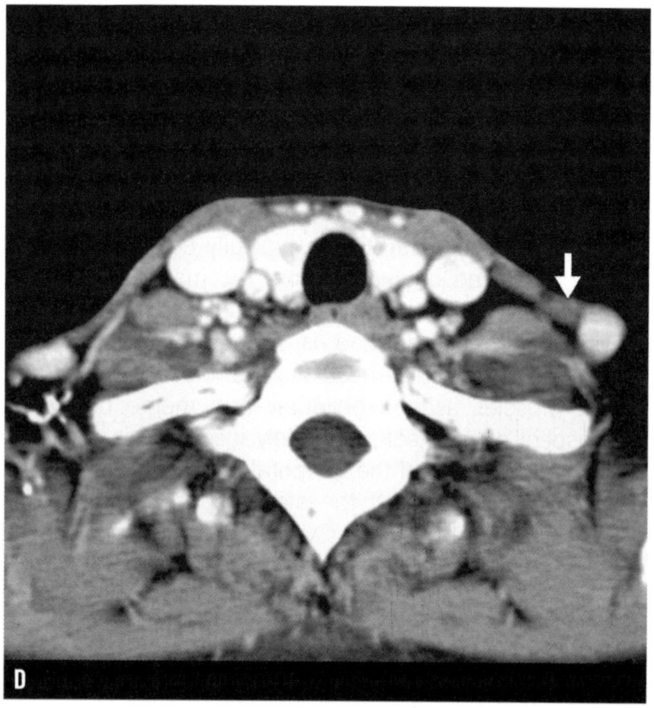

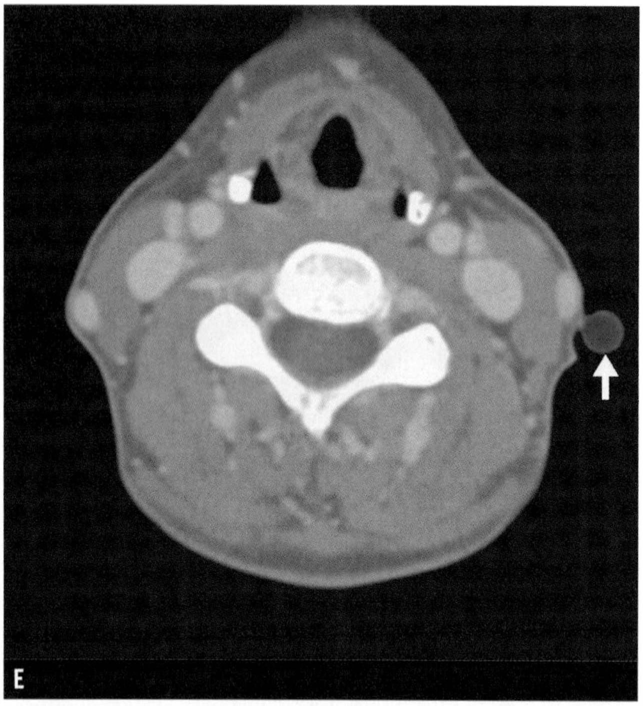

REFERENCES

Cherian SJ, Nayak S. A rare case of unilateral third head of sternocleidomastoid muscle. *Int. J. Morphol.* 2008; 26(1):99-101.

Coskun N, Yildirim FB, Ozkan O. Multiple muscular variations in the neck region–case study. *Folia morphol.* 2002;61(4):317-319.

Mehta V, et al. Bipartite clavicular attachment of the sternocleidomastoid muscle: a case report. *Anat Cell Biol.* 2012;45(1):66-69.

CASE 5 Sternocleidomastoid muscle hypertrophy

Incidental sternocleidomastoid muscle (SCM) hypertrophy may develop as a result of favoring one SCM over another during exercise or activity of daily living, in association with myotonic disorders (due to increased spontaneous activity), or idiopathically.

Apart from being asymmetrically enlarged, a hypertrophied SCM is otherwise normal in appearance on CT or MRI. If the SCM is enlarged, but there is attenuation or signal that deviates from normal muscle on CT or MRI, respectively, then an underlying cause of the muscle enlargement should be investigated. Also, it may be difficult to determine whether the SCM in question is hypertrophied or the contralateral SCM is atrophic. Assessment for ipsilateral trapezius muscle atrophy in the setting of suspected SCM atrophy is often helpful, since the SCM and trapezius muscle are both innervated by cranial nerve XI.

COMPANION CASES

- **Sternocleidomastoid muscle myositis.** Myositis represents an inflammation of muscle and can be due to several etiologies. Causes of diffuse myositis include various inflammatory conditions (eg, dermatomyositis, polymyositis, and systemic lupus erythematosis), illicit or iatrogenic drugs, bacterial infection, and viral infection. When isolated to a single muslce, a myositis may be the result of direct trauma or a focal bacterial infection.

  On unenhanced CT, muscles affected by myositis will be enlarged and hypoattenuating. On MRI, the affected muscles will be T1 isointense and T2 hyperintense. Myositis will enhance on both CT and MRI, but usually will enhance more avidly on MRI. In addition, inflammation of the surrounding fat will be identified on both CT and MRI.
- **Sternocleidomastoid muscle *Staphylococcus aureus* abscess.** An intramuscular abscess is usually the result of a bacterial infection, most commonly *Staphylococcus aureus,* and will often result in fever, swelling, and marked tenderness. The infection may be the result of a local bacterial infection or occur via hematogenous seeding from a remote site. On CT, an intramuscular abscess will be identified as an intramuscular fluid collection that peripherally enhances. On MRI, the abscess fluid is usually T1 iso- to hypointense and T2 hyperintense, and there will be peripheral enhancement following contrast. Restricted diffusion of the abscess fluid is also frequently evident on MRI. Surrounding inflammation is the rule with an acute abscess and will be identified on both CT and MRI; however, MRI will often demonstrate the extent of the infection to a better degree than will CT.
- **Sternocleidomastoid muscle hematoma.** An intramuscular hematoma is usually identified following penetrating or blunt trauma to the muscle and/or in patients receiving anticoagulant therapy. In the neck, a hematoma most commonly develops in the SCM and can occur following central line placement, a stab wound, or a seatbelt injury during a motor vehicle collision.

  The hematoma will result in masslike enlargement of the muscle. Acute hematomas may be isodense or mildly hyperdense to muscle on CT, usually with infiltrative changes of the adjacent fat. As the blood products begin to break down, the density and size of the hematoma will decrease. Chronic hematomas can occasionally become calcified (ie, myositis ossificans). On MRI, there is a variable pattern of signal on T1- and T2-weighted sequences based on the stage of blood product degradation. Intrinsic T1 shortening due to the presence of methemoglobin, or low T2 signal-intensity rims from deoxyhemoglobin or hemosiderin, may suggest the diagnosis of an intramuscular hematoma. An unexplained spontaneous intramuscular hemorrhage should be followed to resolution to exclude an underlying tumor as the source of the bleeding.
- **Sternocleidomastoid muscle aggressive fibromatosis.** Aggressive fibromatosis (AF) represents a benign, abnormal fibroblastic proliferation characterized by infiltrative growth and a high rate of local recurrence. AF affects females more often than males, and the most common clinical presentation is that of a painless, slowly growing mass arising in a patient during their 3rd or 4th decade. This entity may result in significant morbidity in the neck due to its potential to involve adjacent critical structures, such as vessels, nerves, and the airway. When AF is incompletely resected, radiation therapy is usually given for local control.

  On CT, aggressive fibromatosis may appear as an ill-defined soft tissue mass, but it may also be fairly innocuous and located entirely within muscle, its presence only suggested by an unexplained, slowly enlarging muscle in the neck. Attenuation on CT varies in proportion to the amount of collagen components, but it may be completely isodense to muscle. Contrast enhancement on CT may or may not be present. MRI is the imaging modality of choice to evaluate the presence and extent of disease. On T1, the lesion is typically isointense to slightly hyperintense to muscle. The T2 signal is highly variable and related to the proportion of collagen spindle cell and fibroblast content, although some of these tumors may be decidedly hypointense on T2. These lesions commonly enhance on MRI.
- **Sternocleidomastoid muscle lymphoma.** Though lymphoma can involve almost any type of tissue, intramuscular involvement is rare. Intramuscular lymphoma can present with localized pain and swelling, systemic symptoms of fever, diaphoresis, and weight loss. It can either be

indolent or rapidly progressive. On CT, the most common finding is that of muscle enlargement, usually with enhancement. Additional features that are supportive of the diagnosis include long segmental and/or multicompartmental involvement, subcutaneous stranding, skin thickening, and traversing vessels in the lesion. Many of these features are difficult to resolve by the relatively poor soft tissue resolution on CT and are more easily appreciated by MRI. On MRI, intramuscular lymphoma is generally isointense to mildly hyperintense on T1 relative to muscle, mildly hyperintense to muscle on T2, and enhances. Lymphoma should be considered in the differential diagnosis of unexplained, symptomatic muscle enlargement.

- **Sternocleidomastoid muscle venolymphatic malformation.** Vascular malformations of the head and neck are a diverse group of lesions and include arteriovenous malformation (AVM), venous malformation (VM), and lymphatic malformation (LM). Vascular malformations may be high-flow lesions (AVM), low-flow lesions (VM or LM), or mixed (a combination of VM and LM). Properly categorizing these lesions is important in order to determine appropriate treatment. Most vascular malformations are present at birth, although trauma can result in an AVM.

  VMs are an abnormal collection of venous channels, fat, and degenerated muscle matrix. The veins in a VM can thrombose and form phleboliths, the latter considered pathognomonic of this entity in the appropriate context. LMs represent an abnormal collection of lymphatic vessels. LMs are subcategorized into macrocystic and microcystic forms. The macrocystic form, commonly referred to as a cystic hygroma, is composed of large cystic spaces containing proteinaceous fluid and lymphocytes that are interspersed around septa. The microcystic form contains 2 mm or smaller-sized cysts within a solid matrix.

  The hallmark of a vascular malformation is its transpatial nature (ie, often involving more than one compartment in the neck) and its softness to palpation. A vascular malformation may or may not be associated with mass effect. MRI is usually superior to CT in evaluating vascular malformations of the head and neck. On MRI, both a VM and a macrocystic LM will be hyperintense on T2. Following contrast, a VM will undergo patchy enhancement on early postcontrast imaging that increases in extent on delayed postcontrast imaging, whereas a macrocystic LM will only enhance along its periphery and/or septa. A hemorrhagic fluid level may be identified in a macrocystic LM, frequently associated with an abrupt clinical enlargement and is strongly suggestive of a macrocystic LM when present. However, VMs and LMs often coexist in a lesion and are thus termed venolymphatic malformations (or mixed) when both are present.

Sternocleidomastoid muscle hypertrophy

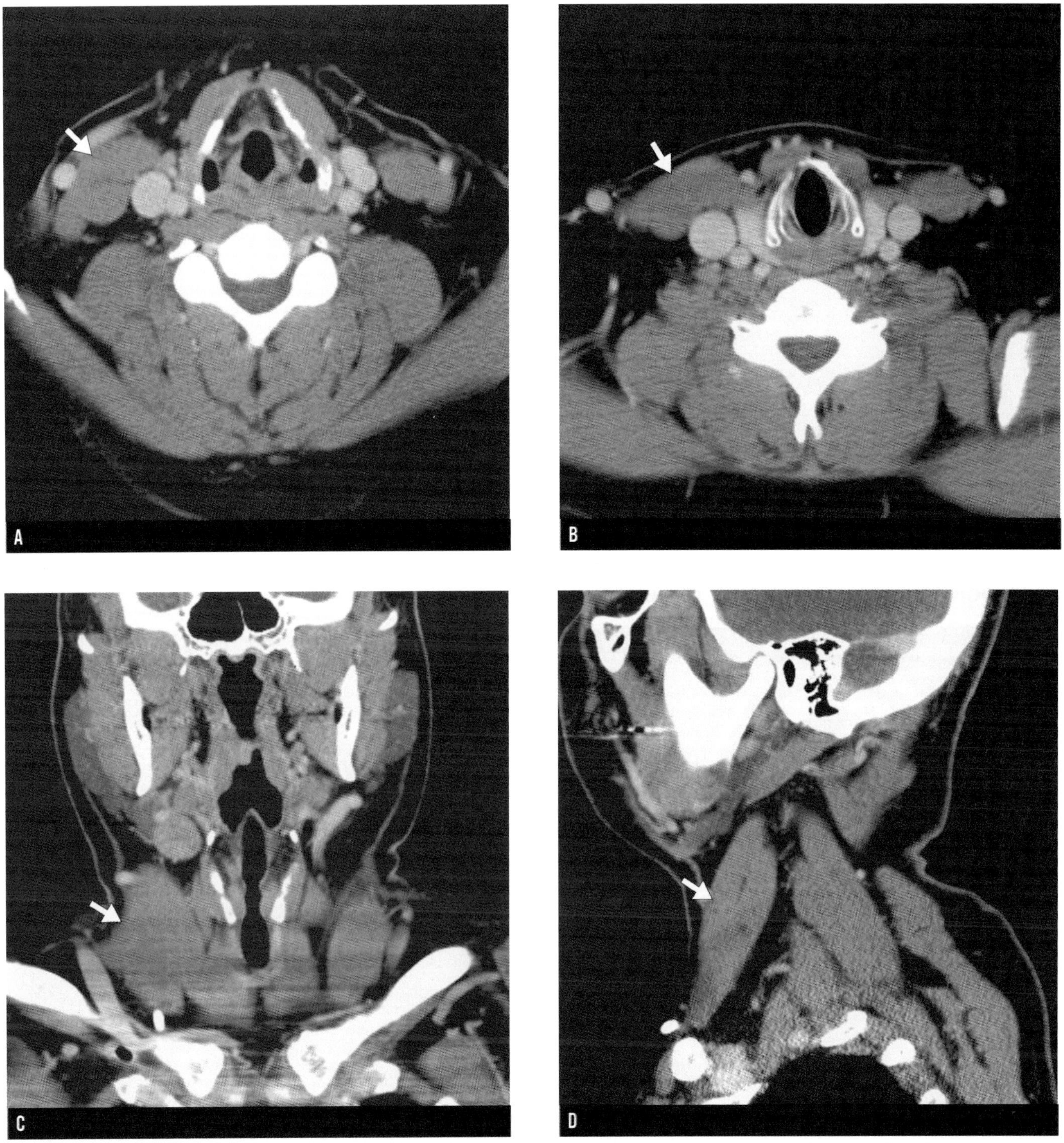

Contrast-enhanced axial (**A**, **B**) and coronal reformatted (**C**) CT images of the neck demonstrate asymmetric hypertrophy of the right sternocleidomastoid muscle (arrows, **A**-**C**). Sagittal reformatted CT images through the right (**D**) and left (**E**) aspects of the neck also demonstrate the asymmetric hypertrophy of the right SCM (arrow, **D**) relative to the left.

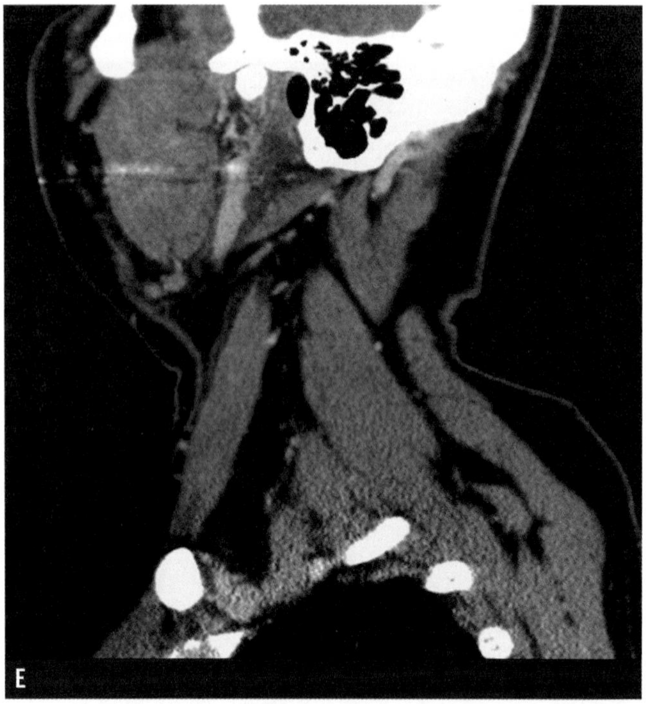

Sternocleidomastoid muscle hypertrophy

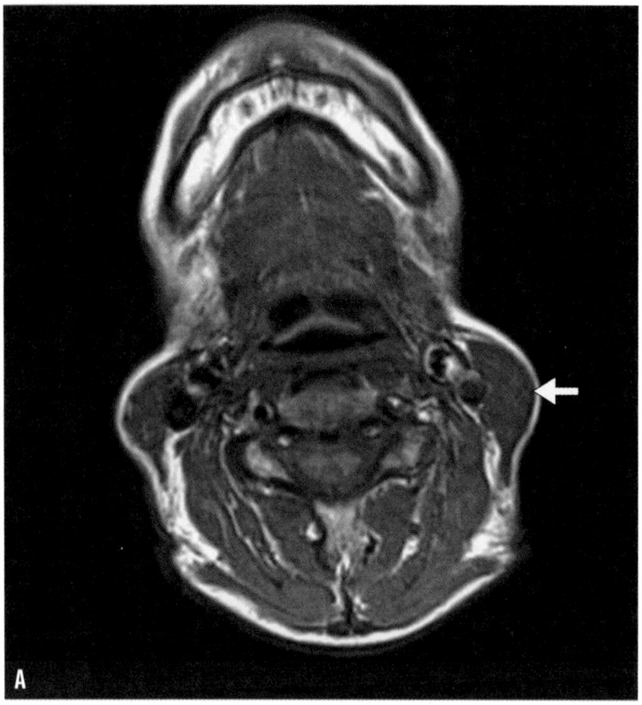

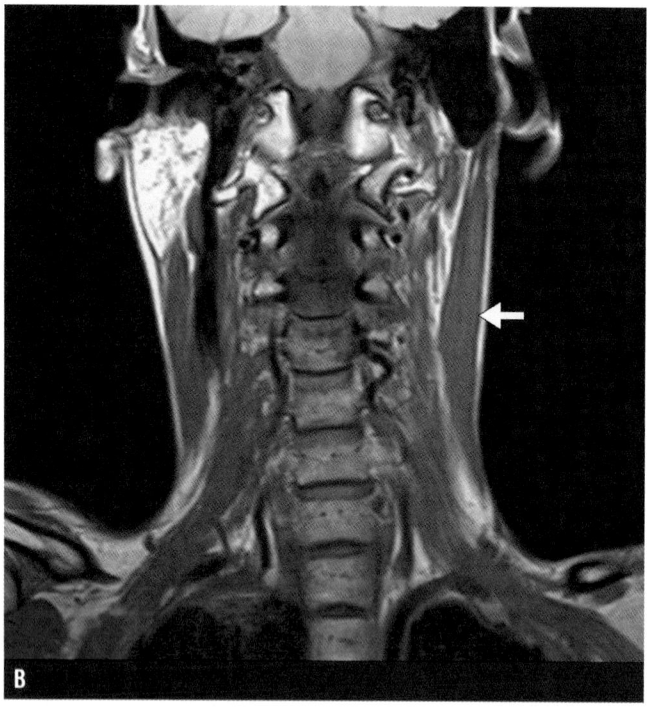

Different patient. Axial (**A**) and coronal (**B**) T1-weighted MR images of the neck demonstrate asymmetric hypertrophy of the left sternocleidomastoid muscle (arrows, **A**, **B**) relative to the right.

Companion case: Sternocleidomastoid muscle myositis

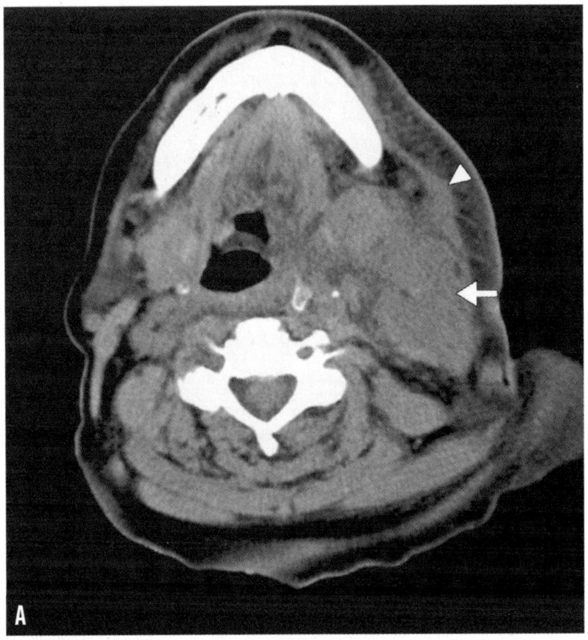

An unenhanced axial CT image through the neck (**A**) demonstrates asymmetric enlargement of the left sternocleidomastoid muscle (arrow), thickening of the left platysma muscle (arrowhead), and surrounding fat stranding as well as edema. The imaging findings in this case represented a myositis secondary to an infection. While edema and fat stranding as well as the platysma muscle thickening are often indicative of an acute inflammatory process, trauma can have an identical appearance.

Companion case: Sternocleidomastoid muscle *Staphylococcus aureus* abscess

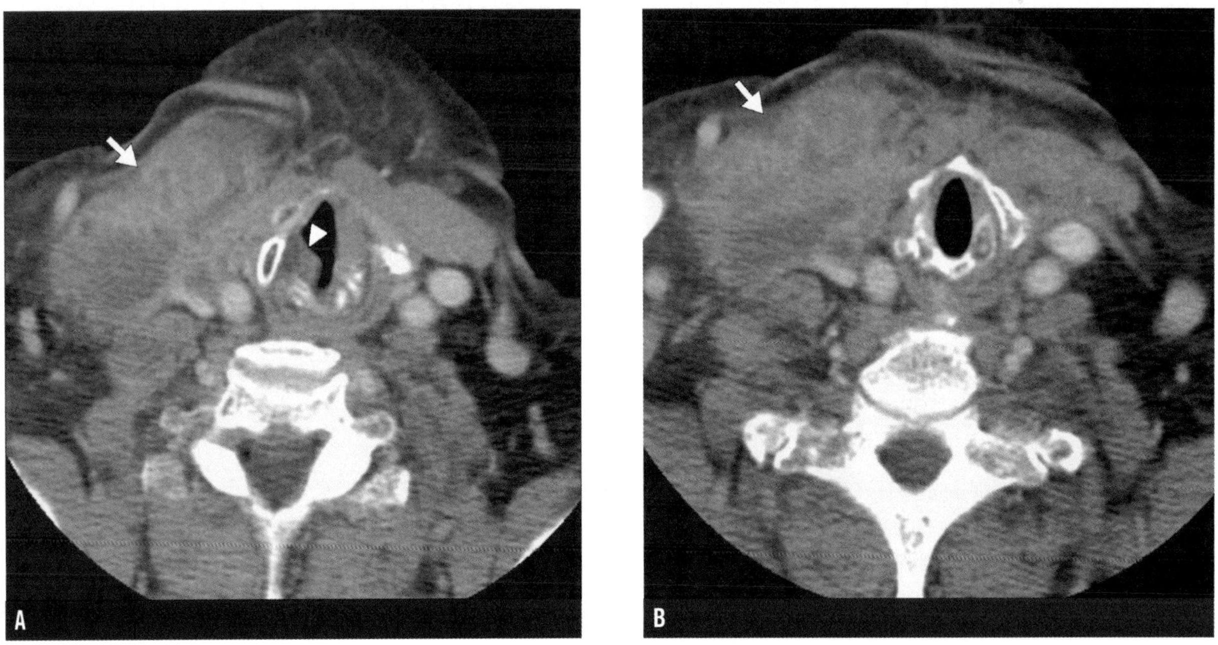

Postcontrast axial CT images of the neck (**A**, **B**) demonstrate a heterogeneously enhancing abnormality enlarging the right sternocleidomastoid muscle (arrows, **A**, **B**) with associated surrounding fat stranding. This was due to an abscess (*Staphylococcus aureus*), with aspiration of the lesion yielding green, purulent material. Incidentally noted is denervation atrophy of the right vocal cord (arrowhead, **A**), in this case possibly the result of remote prior thyroid surgery (not fully shown) and injury to the right recurrent laryngeal nerve.

Companion case: Sternocleidomastoid muscle hematoma

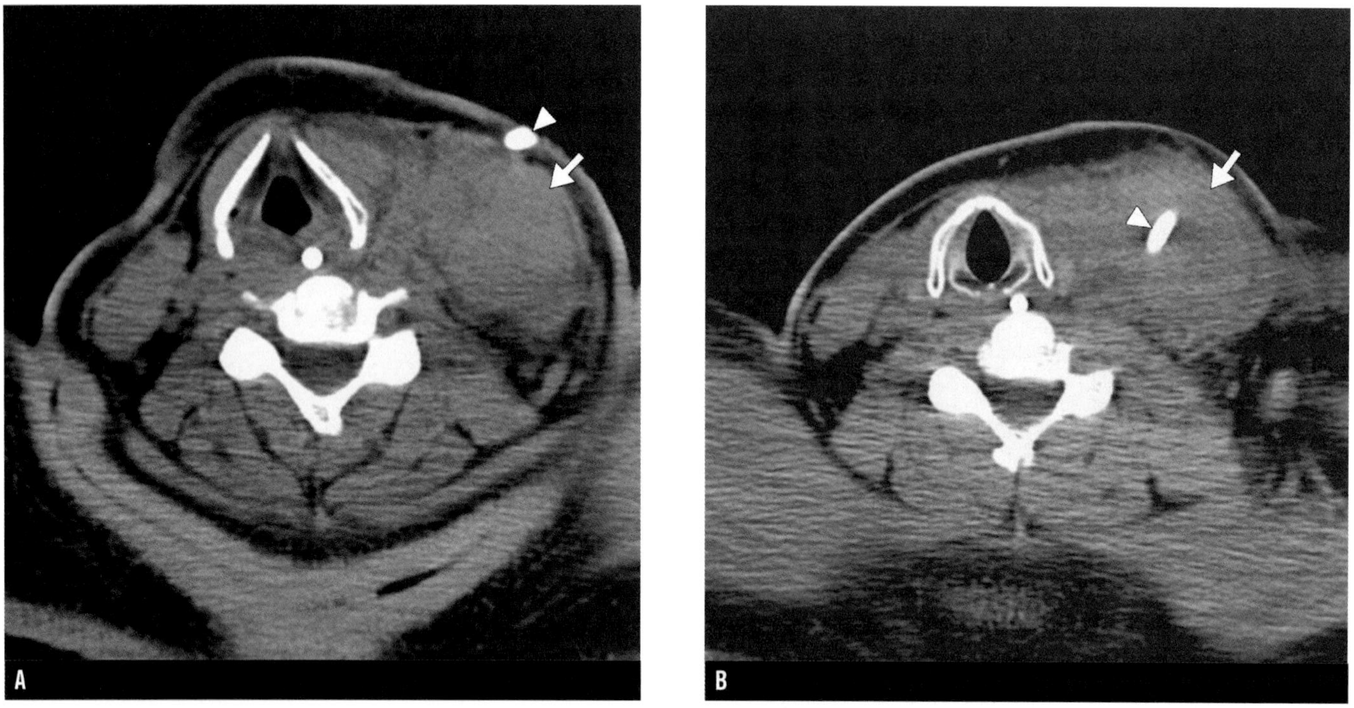

Unenhanced axial CT images of the neck (**A**, **B**) demonstrate an asymmetrically enlarged left sternocleidomastoid muscle (arrows, **A**, **B**) following an attempt at placing a left internal jugular vein line (arrowheads, **A**, **B**). Given the clinical scenario, the findings are compatible with hematoma formation within the left sternocleidomastoid muscle.

Companion case: Sternocleidomastoid muscle aggressive fibromatosis

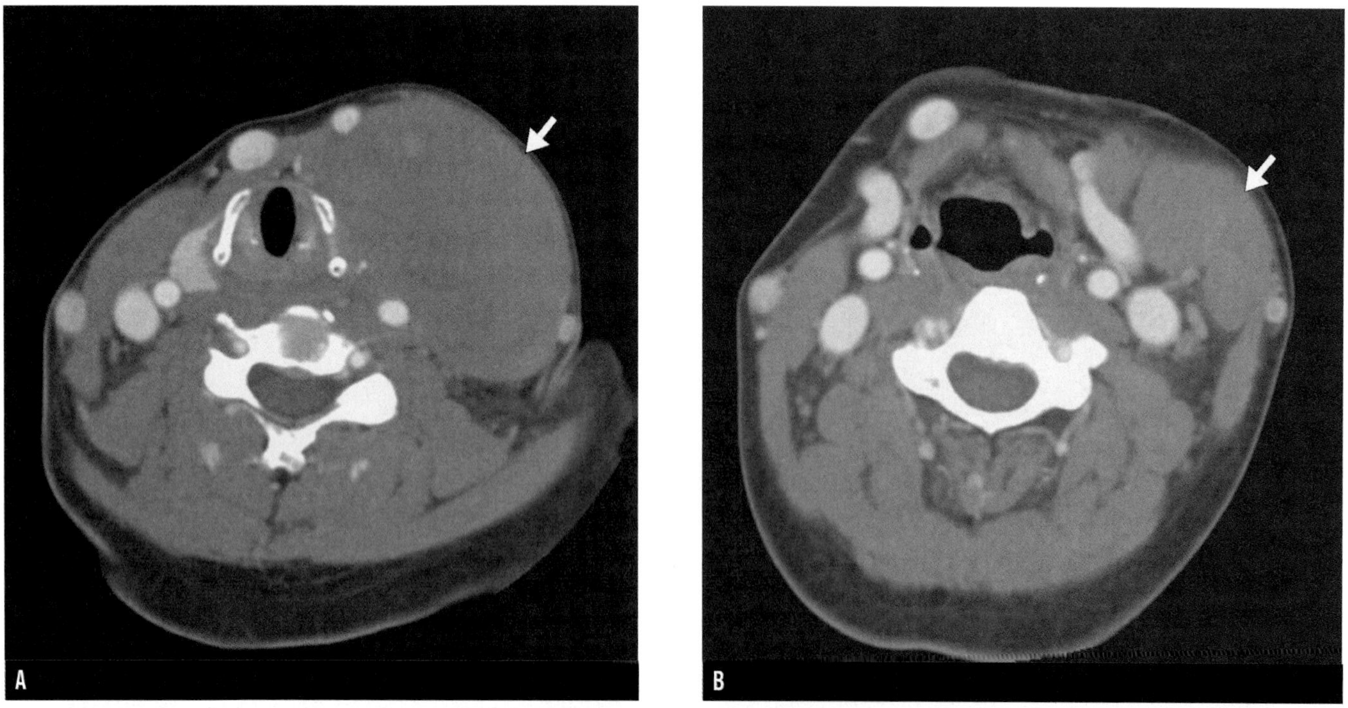

Postcontrast axial CT images from the same study (**A**, **B**) demonstrate a markedly enlarged left sternocleidomastoid muscle (arrows, **A**, **B**). This was a 36-year-old woman who presented with a slowly growing mass and difficulty with turning her head. Aggressive fibromatosis was demonstrated at pathology.

Companion case: Sternocleidomastoid muscle lymphoma

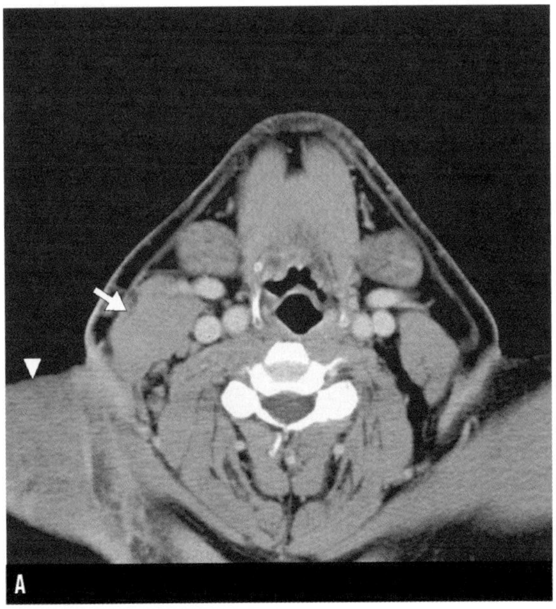

A postcontrast axial CT image (**A**) demonstrates asymmetric enlargement of the right sternocleidomastoid muscle (arrow), a non-specific imaging finding. In this case, lymphoma was demonstrated at pathology. Abnormal stranding and thickening of the right trapezius muscle is also partially visualized (arrowhead).

Companion case: Sternocleidomastoid muscle venolymphatic malformation

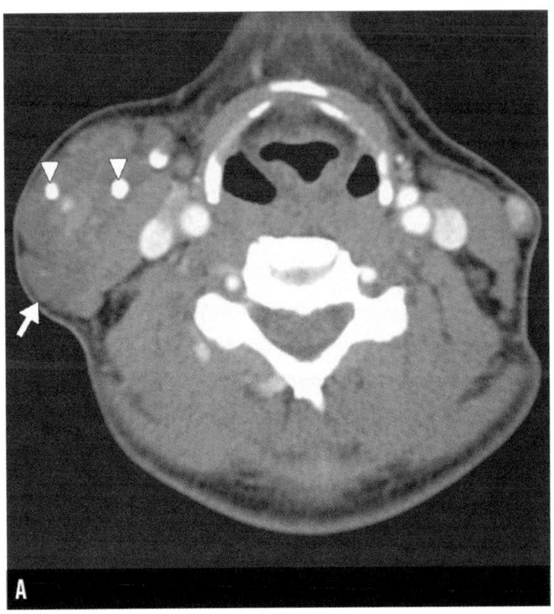

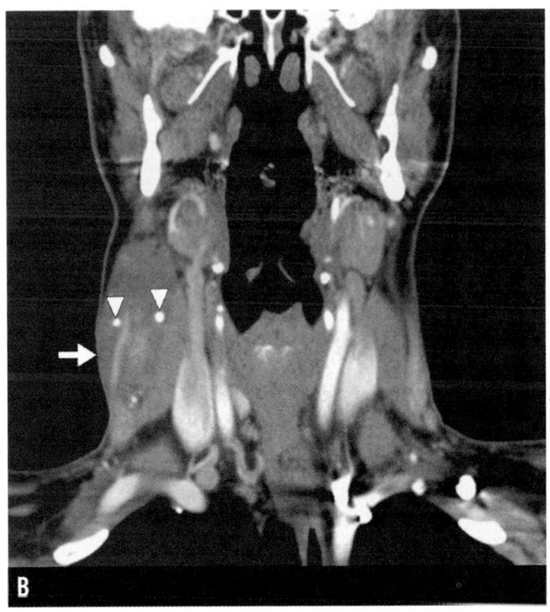

Contrast-enhanced axial (**A**) and coronal reformatted (**B**) CT images demonstrate asymmetric enlargement of the right sternocleidomastoid muscle (arrows, **A**, **B**). The right sternocleidomastoid muscle contains multiple calcifications suggestive of phleboliths (arrowheads, **A**, **B**) and heterogeneous, mild presumed enhancement. Fat-suppressed axial T2 (**C**), non-fat-suppressed axial T1 (D), and fat-suppressed postcontrast axial T1 (**E**) MR images of the same patient demonstrate the lesion to be mostly T2 hyperintense (arrow, **C**), contain patchy enhancement (arrow, **E**), and contain several small foci of hypointensity (arrowheads, **C**, **E**), the latter corresponding to the phleboliths demonstrated on CT. The enhancing component and phleboliths are compatible with a VM, whereas the nonenhancing component is compatible with a LM; thus, the lesion represents a venolymphatic malformation.

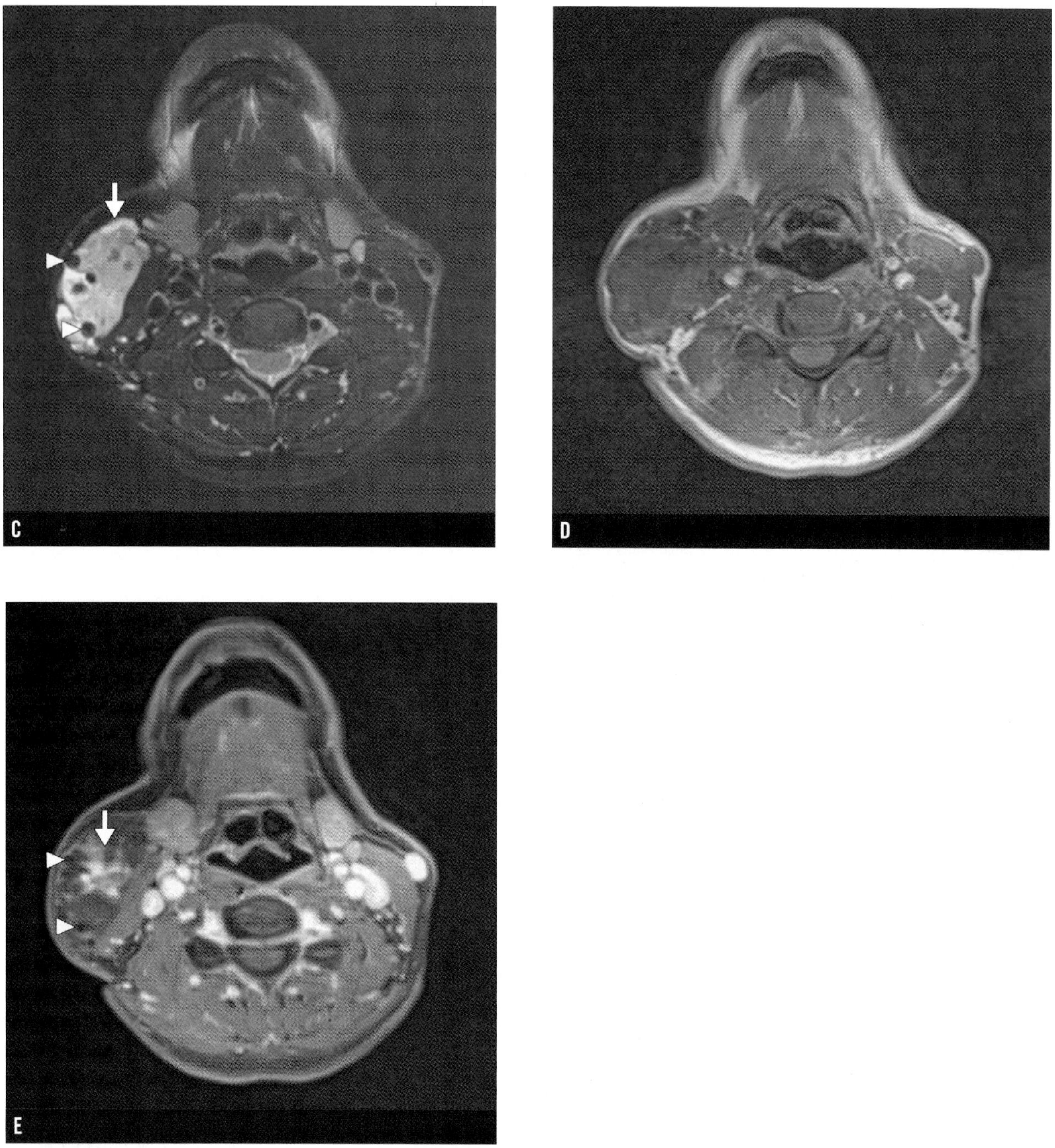

REFERENCES

Chun CW, et al. MRI features of skeletal muscle lymphoma. *Am J Roentgenol.* 2010;195:1355-1360.

Delman BN, Weissman JL, Som PM. Skin and soft tissue lesions. In: Som PM, Curtin HD, eds. *Head and Neck Imaging.* 5th ed. St Louis, Mo: Mosby; 2011: 2771-2822.

Donnelly LF, Adams DM, Bisset GS. Vascular malformations and hemangiomas: a practical approach in a multidisciplinary clinic. *Am J Roentgenol.* 2000;174:597-608.

Hein KD, Mulliken JB, Kozakewich HP, Upton J, Burrows PE. Venous malformations of skeletal muscle. *Plast Reconstr Surg.* 2002;110(7):1625-1635.

Koeller KK, Alamo L, Adair CF, Smirniotopoulos JG. Congenital Cystic masses of the neck: radiologic-pathologic correlation. *Radiographics.* 1999;19(1):121-146.

Lee JC, Thomas JM, Phillips S, Fisher C, Moskovic E. Aggressive fibromatosis: MRI features with pathologic correlation. *AJR Am J Roentgenol.* 2006;186(1):247-254.

May DA, Disler DG, Jones EA, Balkissoon AA, Manaster BJ. Abnormal signal intensity in skeletal muscle at MR imaging: patterns, pearls, and pitfalls. *Radiographics.* 2000;20:S295-S315.

McCafferty IJ, Jones RG. Imaging and management of vascular malformations. *Clin Radiol.* 2011;66(12):1208-1218. doi: 10.1016/j.crad.2011.06.014. Epub 2011 Sep 22. Review.

Neubauer H, et al. Diffusion-weighted MRI of abscess formations in children and young adults. *World J Pediatr.* 2012;8(3):229-234.

CASE 6 Disuse neck muscle atrophy from cervical scoliosis

Scoliosis involving any portion of the spine is defined as greater than 10° of spinal curvature in the coronal plane. Scoliosis is most commonly idiopathic, presents clinically during the adolescent growth spurt, and is more common in girls. Scoliosis related to congenital abnormalities (eg, hemivertibrae) is typically more severe. Syndromic scoliosis may be identified with Marfan syndrome, Down syndrome, and neurofibromatosis type 1, among others. In older patients, the most common cause of a scoliosis involving the cervical spine is degenerative facet disease progressing to ankylosis. Regardless of the cause of cervical scoliosis, the decreased range of cervical motion due to scoliosis, and the resultant altered muscular mechanics, often causes asymmetric atrophy and contralateral compensatory hypertrophy of the cervical musculature.

Disuse atrophy is a term that may be used to describe muscle(s) that become atrophic because of a long-term lack of use. Other causes of neck muscle atrophy include denervation atrophy related to tumor or prior surgery. Atrophy involving the posterior cervical musculature may be identified in up to 60% of patients who have undergone posterior surgical spinal fusion.

COMPANION CASE

- **Diffuse atrophy of the semispinalis capitis and splenius capitis muscles.** The semispinalis capitis and splenius capitis muscles are located in the posterior neck and function to extend the head. The splenius capitis muscle is located immediately deep to the trapezius muscle and immediately superficial to the semispinalis capitis muscle.

  Cervical muscle dysfunction has been theorized as a potential etiology of chronic headaches and/or neck pain, and a great deal of research has attempted to link neck muscle atrophy with symptoms. A subset of this research has focused on the extensor musculature of the neck, with multiple authors demonstrating decreased activation of the semispinalis capitis and multifidi muscles during electromyography and functional MRI in patients with chronic neck pain. While the etiology linking posterior cervical spinal musculature atrophy and chronic neck pain is unknown, some potential etiologies include prior injury (ie, whiplash), disuse related to pain, underlying nerve damage, and a focal inflammatory response.

Disuse neck muscle atrophy from cervical scoliosis

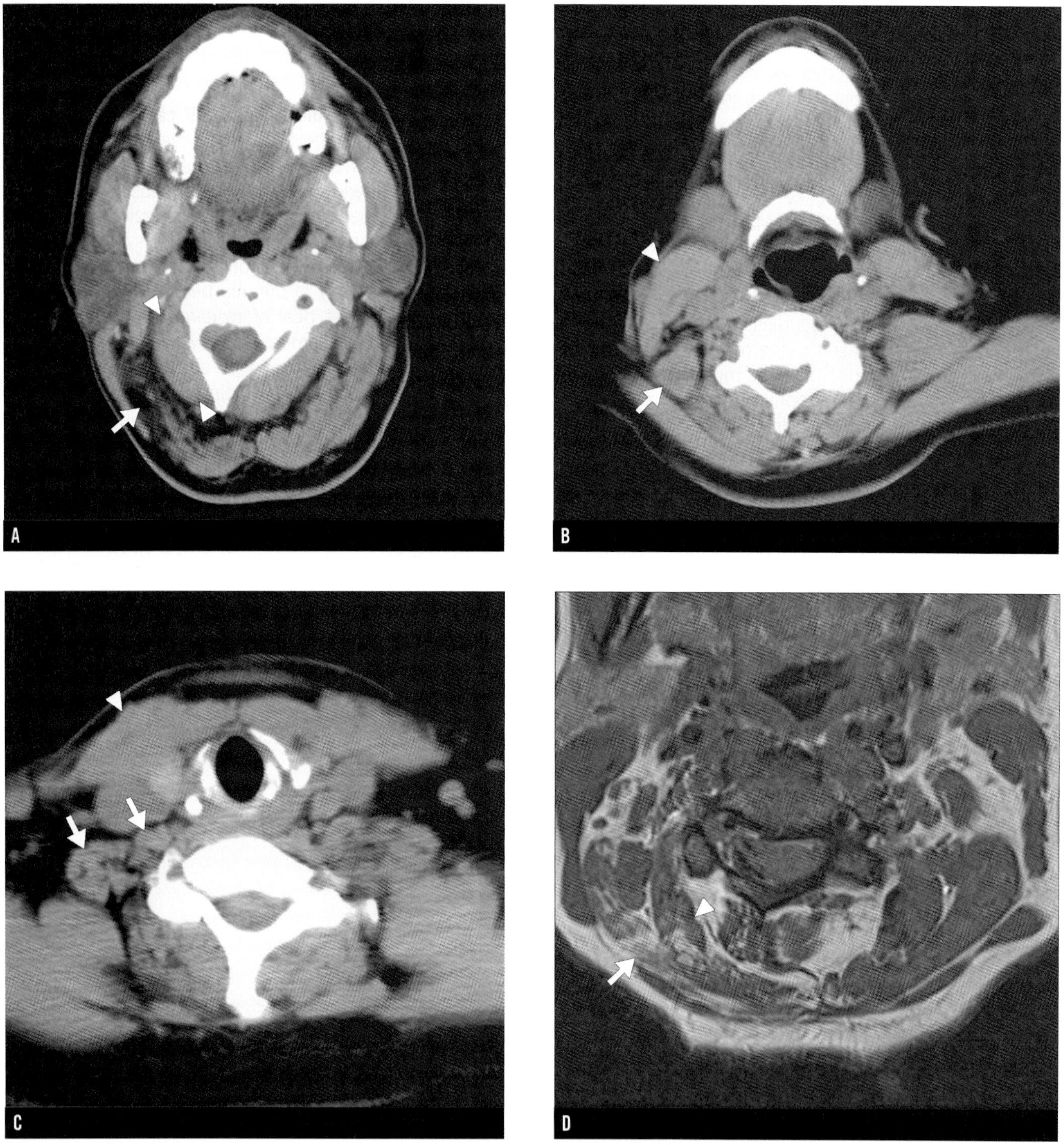

Unenhanced axial CT images (**A-C**) demonstrate hypoplasia/atrophy of the right obliquus capitis inferior muscles (arrowheads, **A**), the right semispinalis capitis and splenius capitis muscles (arrow, **A**), the right levator scapulae muscle (arrow, **B**), and the right scalene muscles (arrows, **C**). There is mild compensatory hypertrophy of the right sternocleidomastoid muscle (arrowheads, **B**, **C**). An axial T1-weighted MR image of the same patient (**D**) also demonstrates the right splenius capitis (arrow, **D**) and semispinalis capitis (arrowhead, **D**) muscle atrophy as seen on image **A**, although the muscles are better demonstrated on this MR image. Unenhanced coronal reformatted CT images viewed with a soft tissue window (**E**) and bone window (**F**) demonstrate a prominent dextroscoliosis of the cervical spine with fusion of several vertebrae (arrows, **F**). Muscle disuse related to the patient's scoliosis likely accounts for the right neck muscle atrophy.

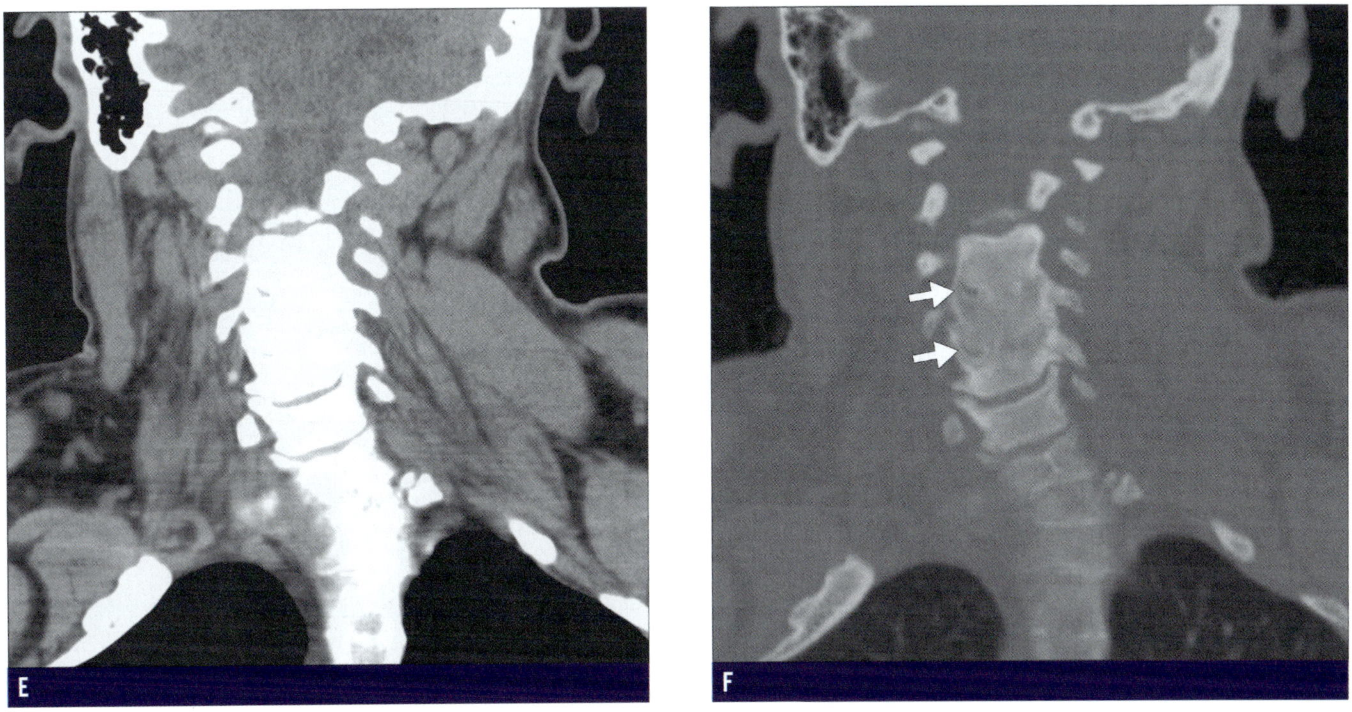

Companion case: Diffuse atrophy of the semispinalis capitis and splenius capitis muscles

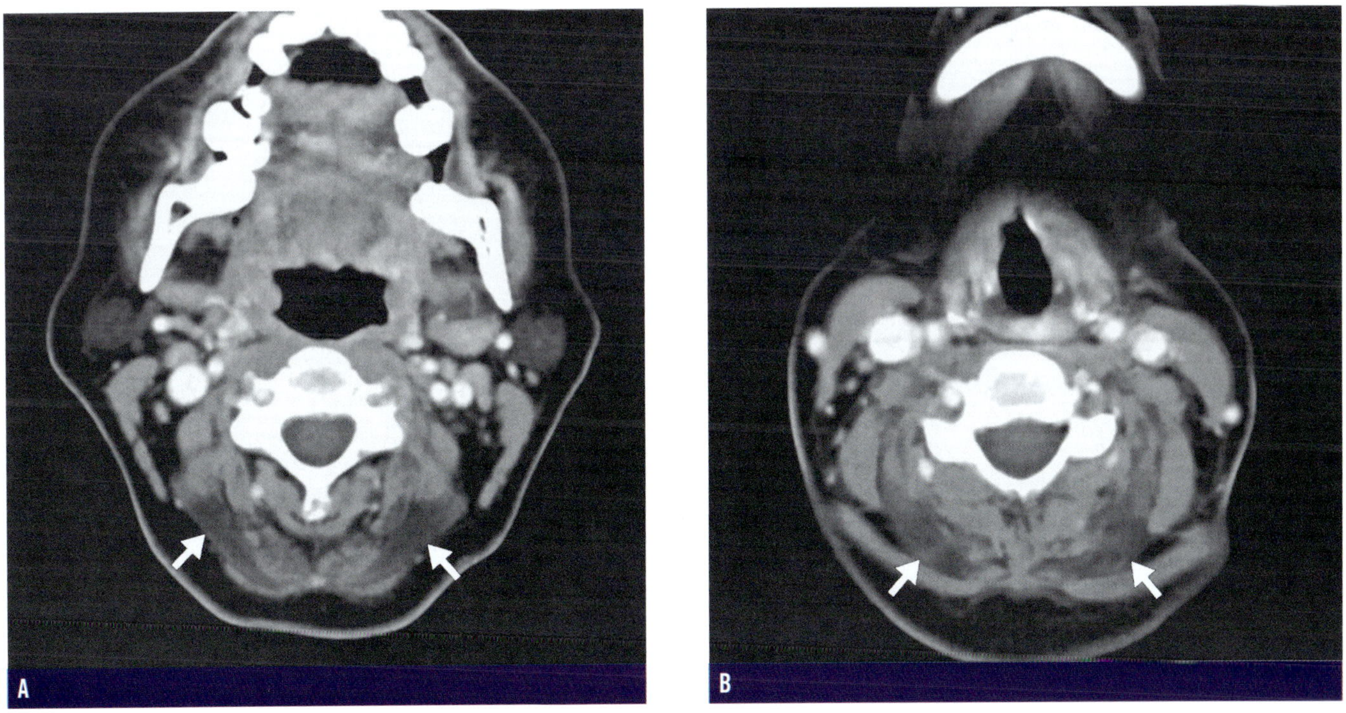

Contrast-enhanced axial (**A**, **B**), sagittal reformatted (**C**), and coronal reformatted (**D**) CT images through the neck demonstrate extensive atrophy isolated to the bilateral semispinalis and splenius capitis muscles (arrows, **A**-**D**). This patient complained of chronic headaches. Some authors have shown an association between chronic neck pain/headaches and neck extensor muscle atrophy.

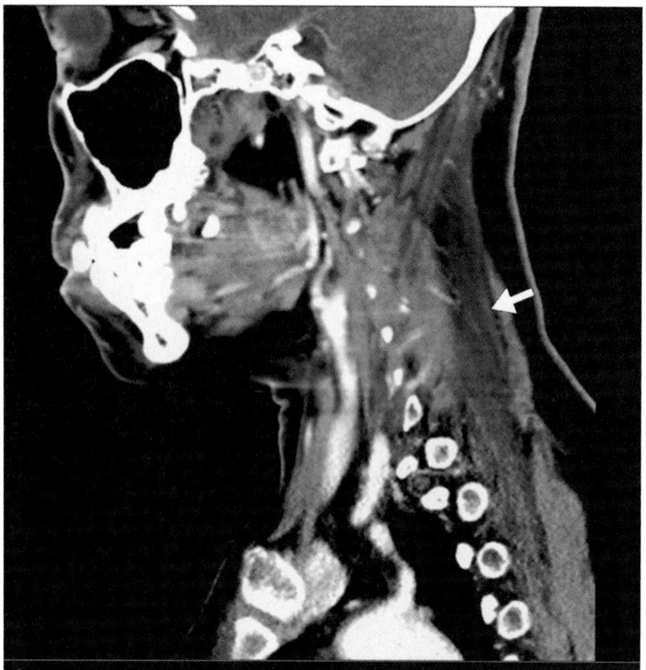

C

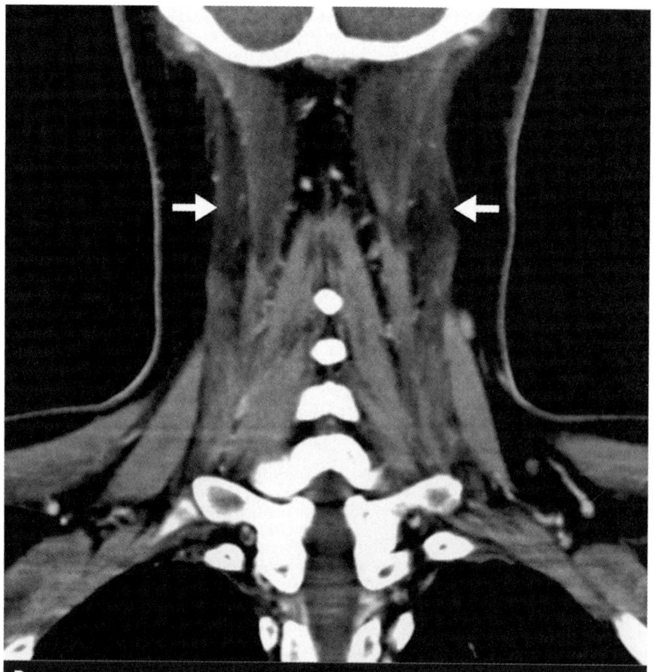

D

REFERENCES

Aebi M. The adult scoliosis. *Eur Spine J.* 2005;14(10):925-948.

Asher MA, Burton DC. Adolescent idiopathic scoliosis: natural history and long term treatment effects. *Scoliosis.* 2006;1(1):2.

Bogduk N, McGuirk B. Management of acute and chronic neck pain, an evidence-based approach. Edinburgh, Scotland: Elsevier; 2006.

O'Leary S, Falla D, Elliott JM, Jull G. Muscle dysfunction in cervical spine pain: implications for assessment and management. *J Orthop Sports Phys Ther.* 2009;39(5):324-333.

The radical neck dissection was first standardized in 1951 when Dr. Martin described what he believed to be the definitive surgical procedure to cure regional lymph node disease in head and neck cancer. The operation removed all structures from the platysma muscle to the prevertebral fascia, from the midline to the trapezius, roughly from the mandible to the clavicle. This early, standardized radical neck dissection only spared the carotid arteries, the phrenic, vagus, hypoglossal, and lingual nerves, as well as the brachial plexus. Today, a radical neck dissection is not as extensive and involves removal of the ipsilateral level I through V lymph nodes, sternocleidomastoid muscle, spinal accessory nerve, and internal jugular vein.

Modifications to the modern-day radical neck dissection have become commonplace. A modified radical neck dissection still includes removal of all the ipsilateral level I through V lymph nodes, but spares one or more non-lymphatic structures (ie, the sternocleidomastoid muscle, spinal accessory nerve, and internal jugular vein).

Since many head and neck malignancies have a predictable lymphatic drainage pattern, more targeted, limited neck dissections that remove only groups of lymph nodes are also a surgical option. Collectively termed selective neck dissections, these are the most common form of neck dissection in the United States. Selective neck dissection subtypes include: the supraomohyoid neck dissection for oral cavity carcinoma (nodal stations I-III and sometimes the submandibular gland for regional access), lateral/jugular chain neck dissection for oropharyngeal, some hypopharyngeal and some laryngeal carcinomas (nodal stations II-IV), and central/anterior neck dissection for carcinomas of the thyroid, cervical esophagus and trachea as well as advanced carcinomas of the piriform sinus, glottis, and subglottis (nodal station VI).

COMPANION CASE

- **Recurrent metastatic lymphadenopathy following a neck dissection.** Radiologic detection of recurrent metastatic carcinoma in the treated neck can be challenging, particularly in the absence of serial examinations or a prior baseline examination. The anatomy of the neck is often distorted and there may be a paucity of neck fat following a neck dissection and/or radiation. This results in potentially CT or MRI occult metastatic lymphadenopathy. Indeed, mild mass effect and/or ill-defined enhancement may be the only imaging findings of metastatic lymphadenopathy in these cases.

  In order to combat these challenges, an accurate and thorough history is vital to properly interpret the treated neck. Specifically, knowledge of the grade of tumor is important. A high grade malignancy increases the likelihood of metastatic disease, whereas a low grade carcinoma or previous carcinoma in situ is less likely to metastasize. Knowledge of the anatomic location of a previously present primary head and neck malignancy is also critical, not only for the detection of recurrent primary tumor, but also to evaluate for metastatic lymphadenopathy. As discussed previously, many primary head and neck malignancies have a predictable lymphatic drainage pattern; therefore, knowledge of the location of a previously present primary malignancy will often help in the radiologist's search pattern for metastatic lymphadenopathy. Certain primary malignancies are notorious for metastatic lymphadenopathy to the neck (eg, nasopharyngeal, oropharyngeal, supraglottic, and hypopharyngeal carcinomas), while others are less likely to metastasize to neck lymph nodes (eg, glottic, subglottic, and adenoid cystic carcinoma). Furthermore, some malignancies have a proclivity for bilateral metastatic lymphadenopathy to the neck (eg, nasopharyngeal carcinoma).

  It is also helpful to evaluate the precise location of previously present pathologic lymph nodes on imaging performed prior to treatment. While recurrent metastatic lymph nodes may occur anywhere in the treated neck, metastatic lymph nodes commonly recur at the site of prior lymphadenopathy. This is especially true if there was extracapsular spread of tumor from the lymph nodes prior to a neck dissection, or if the metastatic lymph nodes were subtotally resected.

  When metastatic lymphadenopathy is unable to be excluded with CT or MRI, or when it needs to be confirmed, then PET imaging is often useful. Viable tumors are typically hypermetabolic on PET imaging. However, because of expected soft tissue injury during surgery, PET imaging in the immediate postoperative period may result in a false-positive result. Therefore, common practice is to forgo PET imaging for the first 3 months following surgery.

Radical neck dissection

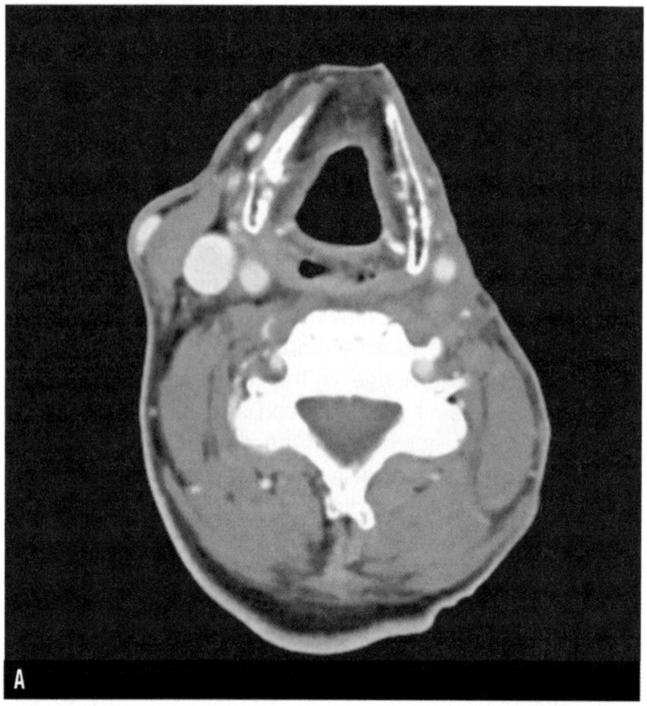

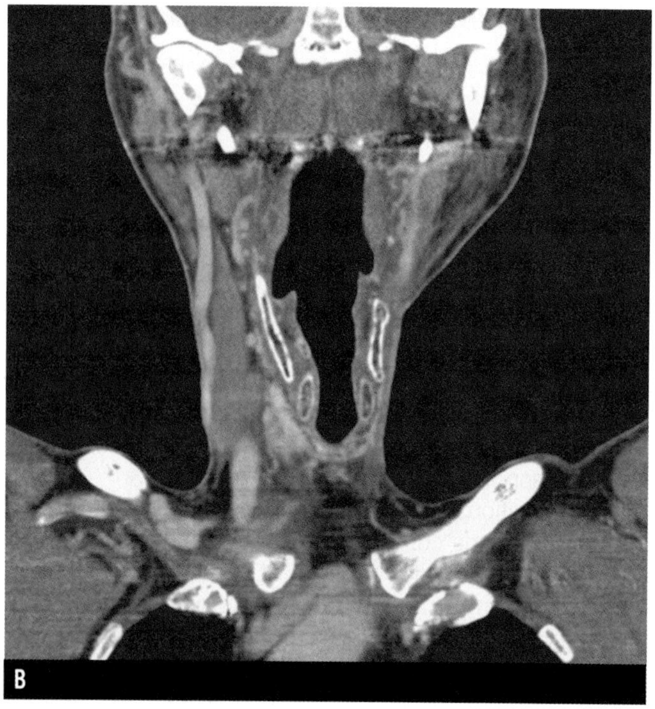

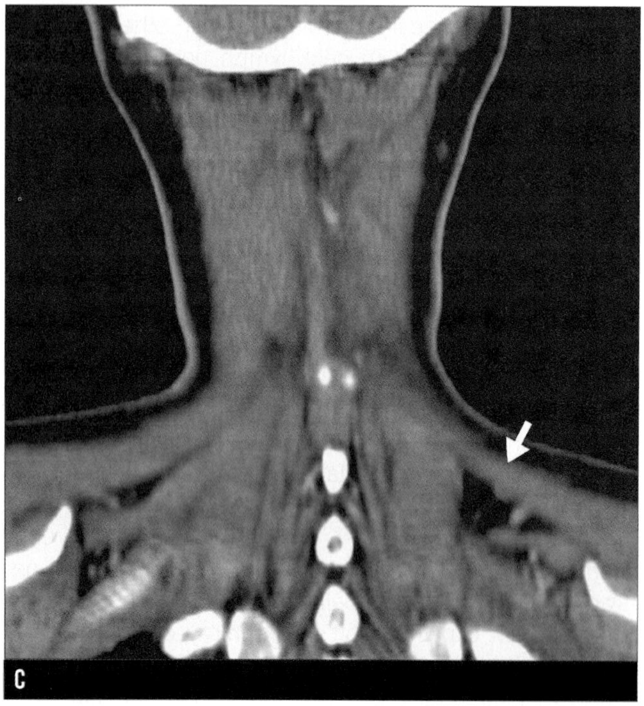

Contrast-enhanced axial (**A**) and coronal reformatted (**B**, **C**) CT images demonstrate a left radical neck dissection, with excision of the left sternocleidomastoid muscle (**A**, **B**), left internal jugular vein (**A**), and a left neck lymph node dissection. Atrophy of the left trapezius muscle (arrow, **C**) is evidence of left cranial nerve XI sacrifice.

Modified radical neck dissection

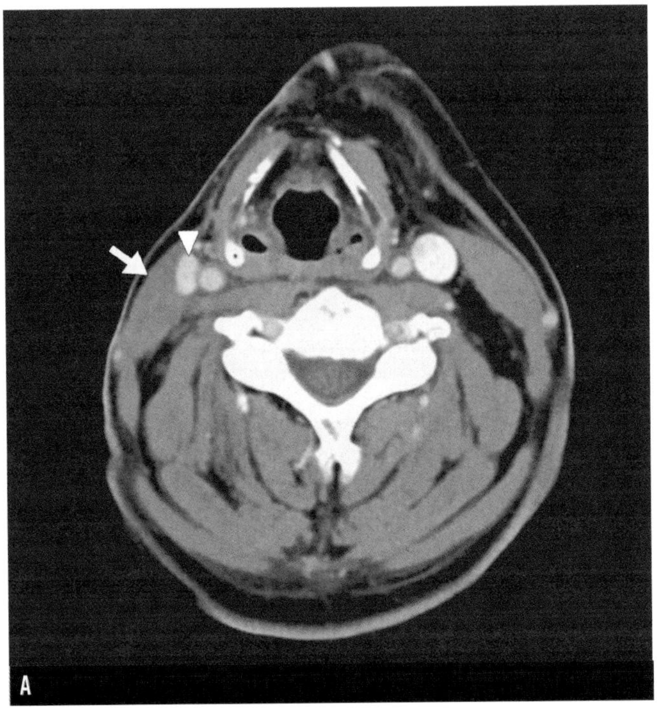

A

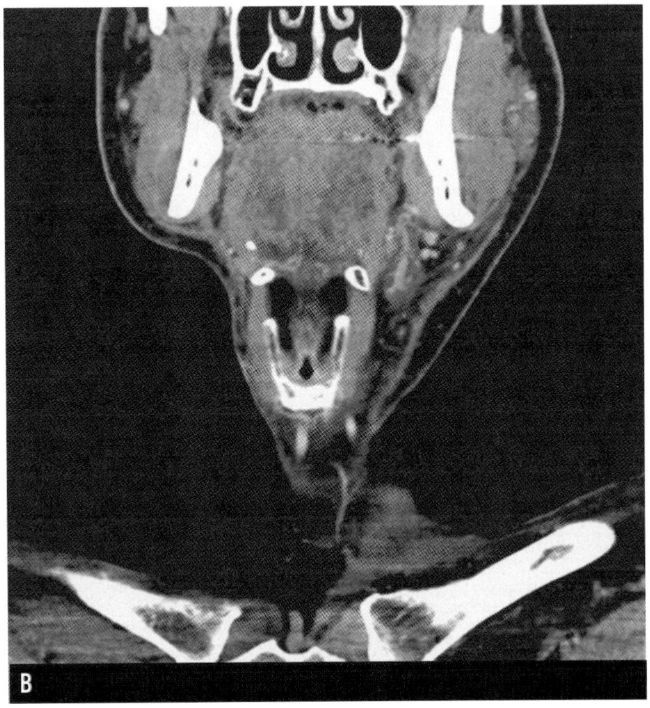

B

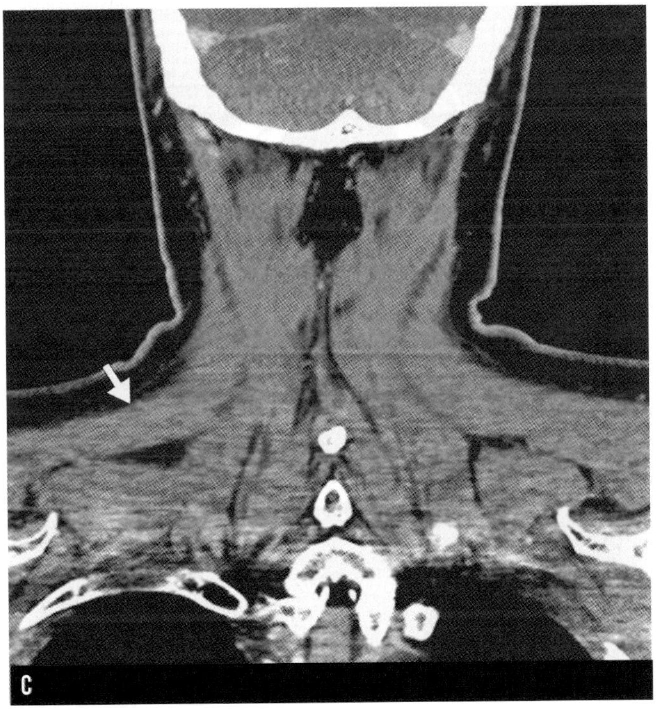

C

Contrast-enhanced axial (**A**) and coronal reformatted (**B**, **C**) CT images demonstrate a modified radical neck dissection. In this case, a right neck lymph node dissection was performed with preservation of the right SCM (arrow, **A**) and right internal jugular vein (arrowhead, **A**). Image **C** demonstrates atrophy of the right trapezius muscle (arrow, **C**), indicating that the right cranial nerve XI was sacrificed.

CASE 9 Levator scapulae muscle hypertrophy following a neck dissection

A neck dissection is typically performed to remove neck nodal metastasis. For a discussion regarding the main types of neck dissection that are performed today, please refer to Case 7 from this chapter.

Removal of the spinal accessory nerve during a radical or modified neck dissection will result in denervation atrophy of the ipsilateral sternocleidomastoid muscle and trapezius muscle. The patient may experience a postoperative shoulder drop because of denervation atrophy of the trapezius muscle. Most patients compensate for this loss of function by recruiting the ipsilateral levator scapulae muscle to elevate the scapula, often resulting in hypertrophy of the ipsilateral levator scapulae muscle. A potential imaging pitfall is mistaking this compensatory hypertrophy for a mass or recurrent neoplasm in the setting of head and neck malignancy. However, apart from hypertrophy of the muscle, the imaging characteristics of this entity are the same compared to normal muscle on CT and MRI.

COMPANION CASES

- **Asymmetric levator scapulae muscle without surgery.** Asymmetry of any muscle may be secondary to true hypertrophy or a normal developmental variant. As noted elsewhere in this chapter, muscle hypertrophy can be idiopathic or may develop as a result of unilateral preference during exercise, myotonic disorders (due to increased spontaneous activity), or scoliosis.
- **Levator scapulae muscle aggressive fibromatosis.** Aggressive fibromatosis (AF) represents a benign, abnormal fibroblastic proliferation characterized by infiltrative growth and high rate of local recurrence. AF affects females more often than males, and the most common clinical presentation is that of a painless, slowly growing mass arising in a patient during their 3rd or 4th decade. This entity may result in significant morbidity in the neck due to its potential to involve adjacent critical structures, such as vessels, nerves, and the airway. When AF is incompletely resected, radiation therapy is usually given for local control.

  On CT, aggressive fibromatosis may appear as an ill-defined soft tissue mass, but it may also be fairly innocuous and located entirely within muscle, its presence only suggested by an unexplained, slowly enlarging muscle in the neck. Attenuation on CT varies in proportion to the amount of collagen components, but it may be completely isodense to muscle. Contrast enhancement on CT may or may not be present. MRI is the imaging modality of choice to evaluate the presence and extent of disease. On T1, the lesion is typically isointense to slightly hyperintense to muscle. The T2 signal is highly variable and related to the proportion of collagen spindle cell and fibroblast content, although some of these tumors may be decidedly hypointense on T2. These lesions commonly enhance on MRI.
- **Levator scapulae muscle fibrosarcoma**. Fibrosarcoma is a relatively uncommon malignant tumor of fibroblasts that primarily affects adults between the fifth and seventh decades and has a slight predilection for males. While it can occur in the neck, the most commonly affected regions are the deep soft tissues of the extremities and trunk, often located intramuscularly. Clinically, these tumors usually present as a painless mass that slowly enlarges over several months.

  Owing to its superior soft tissue contrast resolution, MRI is the modality of choice to characterize, determine extent, and thus allow for more accurate preoperative planning of a fibrosarcoma. On MRI, fibrosarcomas are typically low to intermediate in signal intensity on T1. The literature is varied with respect to the T2 signal characteristics of a fibrosarcoma, ranging from hypointense to hyperintense. However, hypointense T2 signal may predominate with these tumors due to the presence of fibrous/collagen tissue, a high nuclear to cytoplasmic ratio, and mineralization.

  On CT, calcifications within the tumor and adjacent osseous erosion may be identified. Fibrosarcomas are often heterogeneous on CT, particularly if necrosis or hemorrhage within the tumor is present. However, the margin of a fibrosarcoma is often circumscribed due to the presence of a fibrous pseudocapsule. These lesions will enhance on postcontrast CT and MRI, often heterogeneously. Because of similar imaging characteristics, a malignant fibrous histiocytoma is in the imaging differential of a fibrosarcoma.

Levator scapulae muscle hypertrophy following a neck dissection

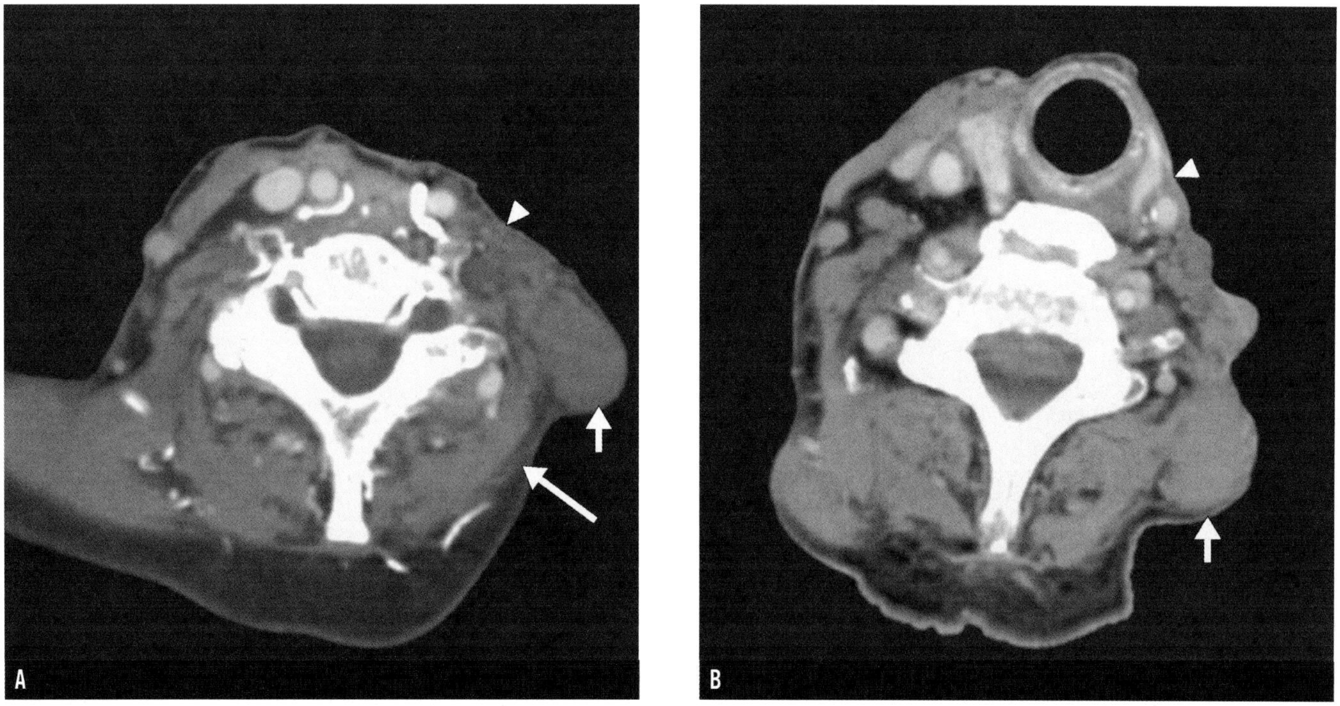

Postcontrast axial CT images of two different patients (**A**, **B**). In each case, the patient had undergone a radical neck dissection with resection of the left sternocleidomastoid muscle (arrowheads **A**, **B**) and left internal jugular vein. Also in both cases, the left levator scapulae muscle is hypertrophied (short arrows **A**, **B**). On image **A**, atrophy of the left trapezius muscle is also demonstrated (long arrow, **A**), a common sequela of a radical neck dissection related to sacrifice of the spinal accessory nerve.

Levator scapulae muscle hypertrophy following a neck dissection

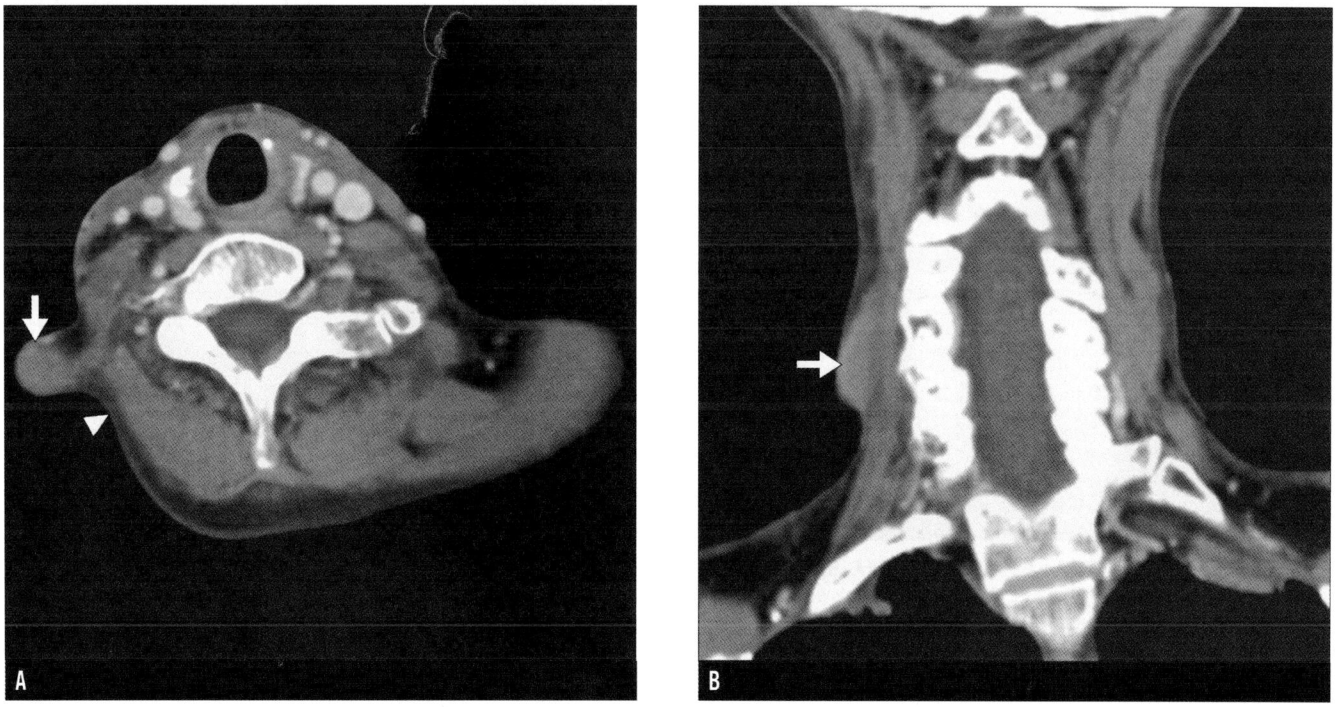

Different patient. Contrast-enhanced axial (**A**) and coronal reformatted (**B**) CT images demonstrate a right neck dissection with a focally enlarged and protuberant right levator scapulae muscle (arrows, **A**, **B**). An postcontrast axial CT image more cephalad than **A** (**C**) demonstrates atrophy of the right sternocleidomastoid muscle (arrow, **C**), compatible with muscle denervation from sacrifice of the ipsilateral spinal accessory nerve. In addition, images **A** and **C** demonstrate denervation atrophy of the right trapezius muscle (arrowheads **A**, **C**), also in keeping with sacrifice of the spinal accessory nerve.

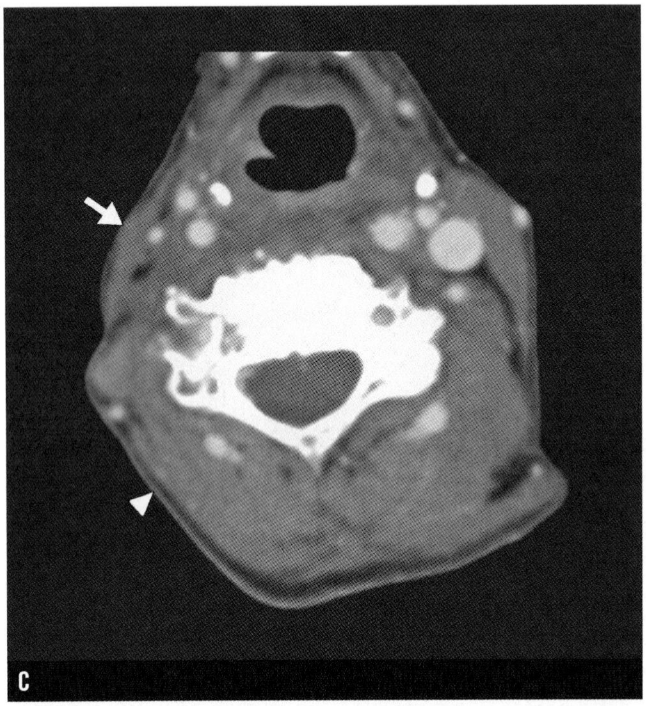

C

Companion case: Asymmetric levator scapulae muscle without surgery

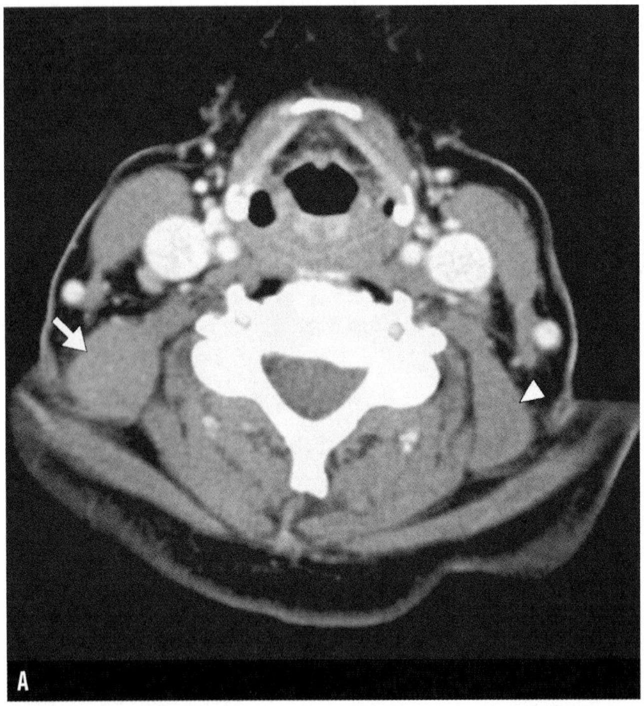

A

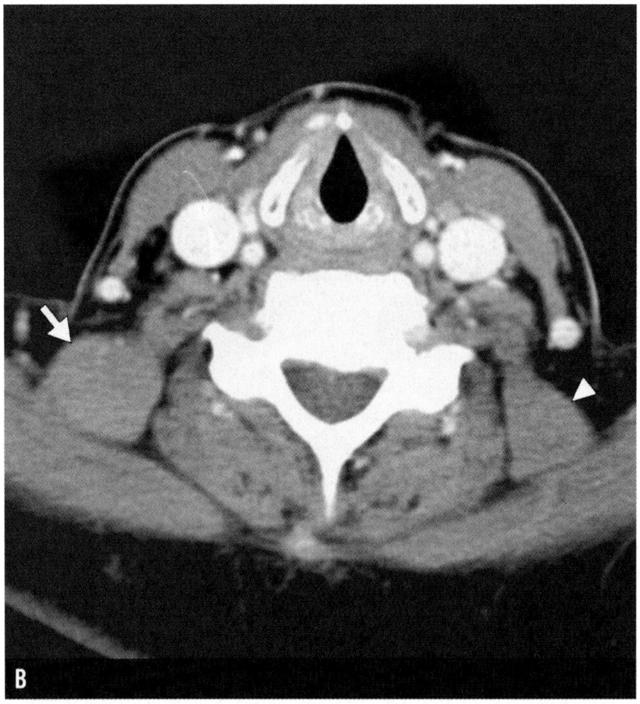

B

Contrast-enhanced axial CT images of the neck (**A**, **B**) demonstrate an asymmetrically larger right levator scapulae muscle (arrows, **A**, **B**) compared to the left (arrowheads, **A**, **B**) in a patient without prior neck surgery or other neck muscle asymmetry. The etiology of the muscle asymmetry was unclear; it may have been due to a cervical spondylosis (which was present in this patient but is not shown) resulting in overuse of the right and/or underuse of the left levator scapulae muscle.

Companion case: Levator scapulae muscle aggressive fibromatosis

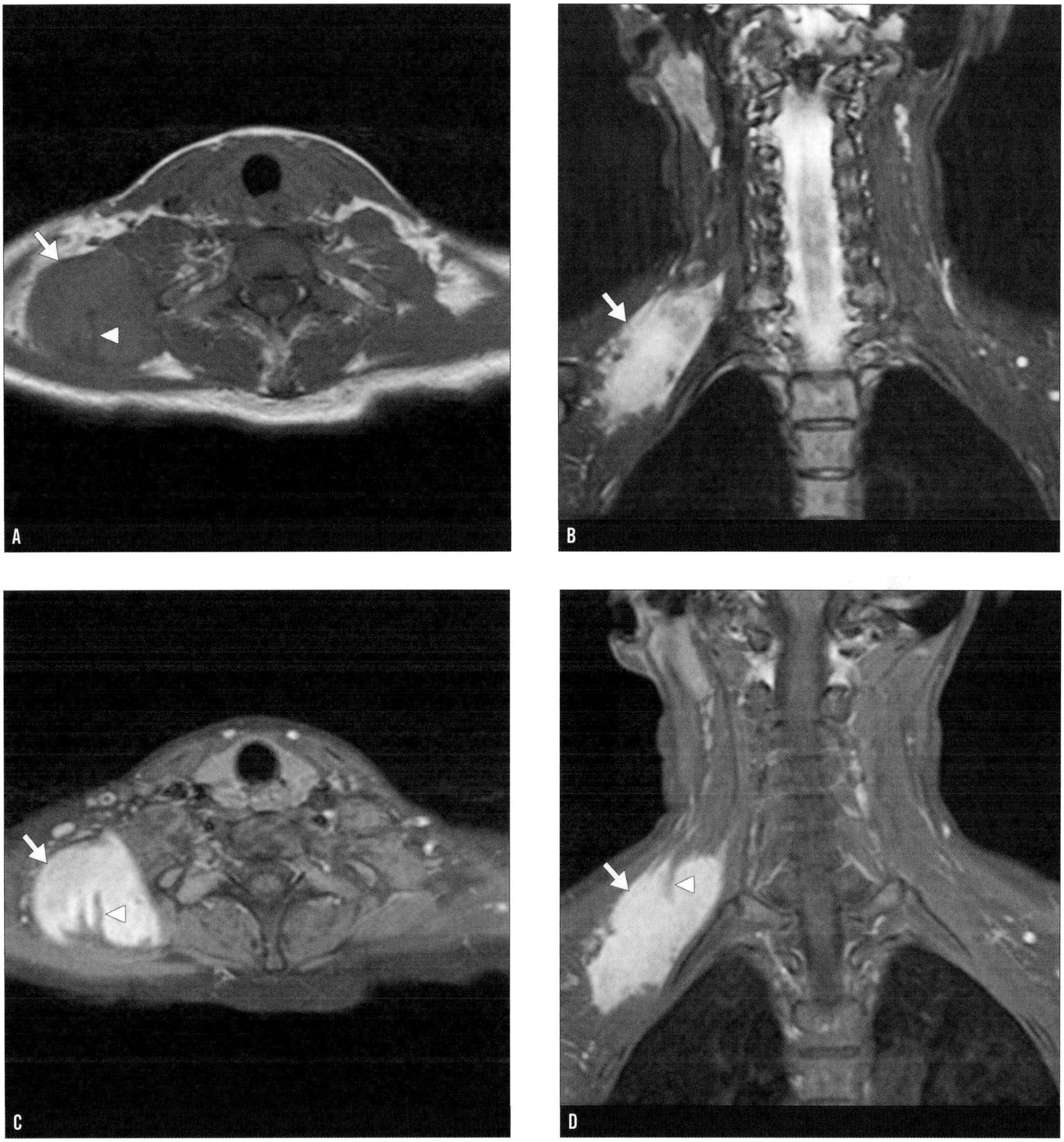

Axial T1 (**A**), fat-suppressed coronal T2 (**B**), postcontrast fat-suppressed axial T1 (**C**) and postcontrast fat-suppressed coronal T1 (**D**) MR images demonstrate a T1 isointense, T2 hyperintense, diffusely enhancing mass centered within the right levator scapulae muscle (arrows, **A-D**). The mass has mildly irregular margins and a couple muscle fibers are embedded within the lesion (arrowheads, **A**, **C**, and **D**). A biopsy of this mass was consistent with aggressive fibromatosis.

Companion case: Levator scapulae muscle fibrosarcoma

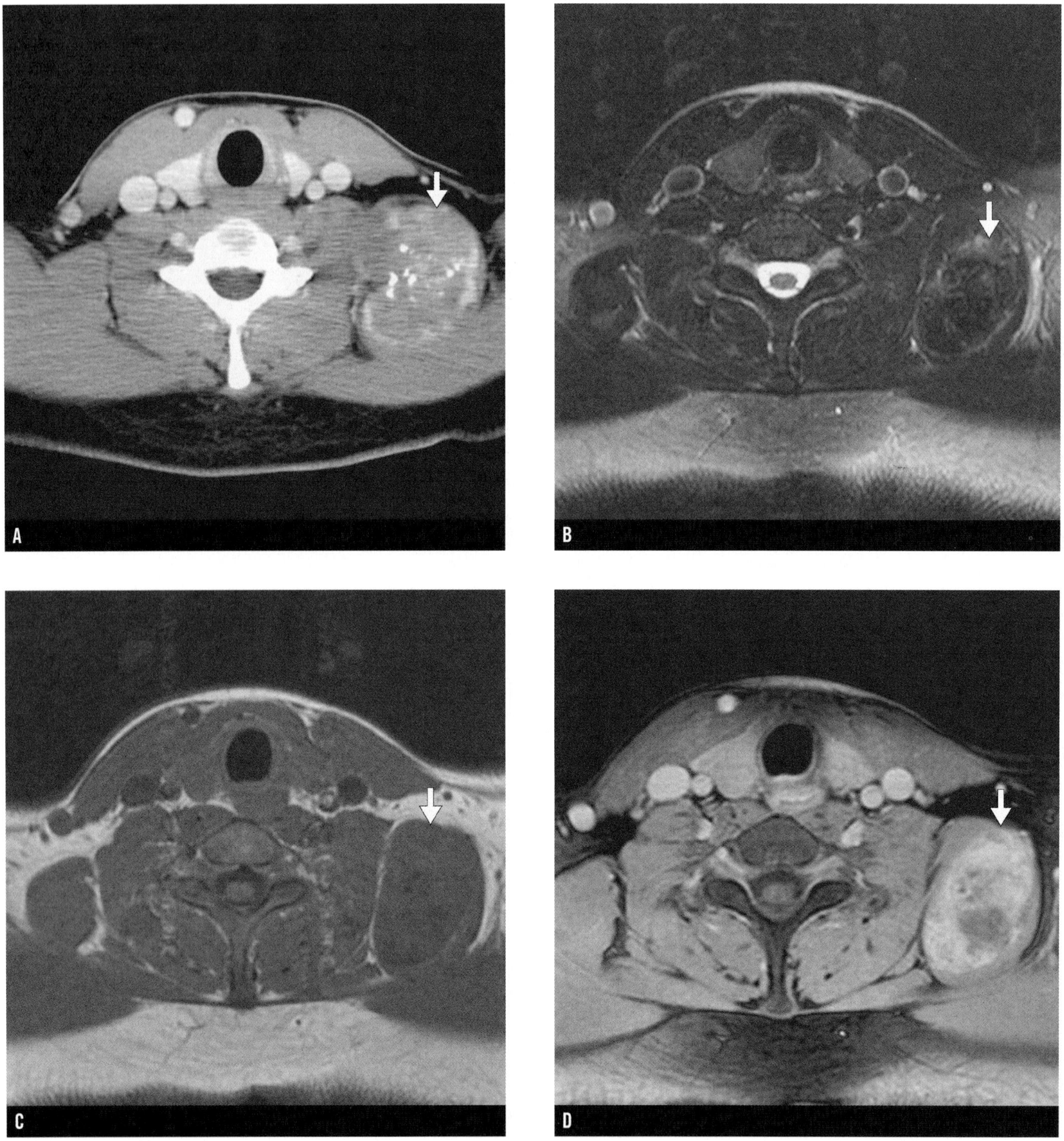

A contrast-enhanced axial CT image of the neck (**A**) demonstrates a large, heterogeneous, presumably enhancing and partially calcified mass occupying and expanding the left levator scapulae muscle (arrow, **A**). Axial T2 with fat suppression (**B**), axial T1 (**C**), and postcontrast axial T1 with fat suppression (**D**) MR images through the neck demonstrate the same mass as subtotally hypointense on T2 and heterogeneously enhancing following contrast administration (arrows, **B-D**). The calcification on CT, the hypointense signal on T2, and the enhancement, while nonspecific, are imaging findings that can be present with fibrosarcoma, which was pathologically demonstrated in this case.

REFERENCES

Borges A. Imaging of denervation in the head and neck. *Eur I Radiol.* 2010;74(2):378-390.

Hermans R. Posttreatment imaging in head and neck cancer. *Eur I Radiol.* 2008;66(3):501-511.

Kahn LB , Vigorita V. Fibrosarcoma of bone. In: Fletcher CDM et al, ed: *World Health Organization Classification of Tumours: Tumours of Soft Tissue and Bone. Lyon*, France: IARC Press; 2002: 289-290.

O'Connell TE, Castillo M, Mukherji SK. Fibrosarcoma arising in the maxillary sinus: CT and MR features. *J Comput Assist Tomogr.* Sep-Oct 1996;20(5):736-738.

Saito N, Nadgir RN, Nakahira M, et al. Posttreatment CT and MR imaging in head and neck cancer: what the radiologist needs to know. *Radiographics.* 2012;32(5):1261-1282.

Walker EA, Salesky JS, Fenton ME, Murphey MD. Magnetic resonance imaging of malignant soft tissue neoplasms in the adult. *Radiol Clin North Am.* 2011;49(6):1219-1234.

Radiation therapy, administered alone or in combination with chemotherapy and/or surgery, is one of the mainstays of head and neck cancer treatment. Distinguishing postradiation change from residual or recurrent tumor on imaging is often a challenging endeavor for the radiologist. Pretreatment imaging and baseline imaging following surgery and/or chemo-radiation are critical for the radiologist to accurately assess the imaging findings and to help differentiate posttreatment effect from residual/recurrent tumor.

Radiation therapy of the neck has improved over the years. Today's technology allows for a more focused tumor dose that minimizes normal tissue irradiation. 3D tumor mapping is often performed in conjunction with MRI or CT, resulting in more accurate dose mapping and beam intensity modulation. Chemotherapy is usually administered as an adjunct to radiation therapy. In addition to their primary therapeutic effect, chemotherapeutic agents often improve the effectiveness of radiation therapy and are thus termed radiation sensitizers.

Radiation at medically therapeutic doses (typically in the tens of Gy) results in direct tissue damage, with much of the antitumor effect the result of endothelial cell death within the microvascular bed supplying the tumor. This radiation damage manifests as interstitial edema, particularly in the acute to subacute stages. On imaging, interstitial edema most often manifests as skin thickening and stranding of the subcutaneous as well as deep fat planes. Delayed changes from radiation therapy include atrophy and fibrosis, often evolving years after therapy.

Enhancing and edematous pharyngeal walls as well as diffuse edematous thickening of the larynx are invariably present in the irradiated neck. This edema often results in a complicated imaging appearance, sometimes simulating a recurrent primary tumor, or a new primary tumor elsewhere in the pharynx or larynx. The symmetric, circumferential nature of the edema involving these structures usually allows for discrimination between posttreatment effect and recurrent tumor. However, any developing focal soft tissue density abnormality, particularly in the region of a previously treated primary tumor, should always be viewed with suspicion.

Atrophy of the submandibular glands and parotid glands invariably occurs if they are included in the field of radiation, usually developing within the first year of radiation and resulting in xerostomia. In addition to undergoing atrophy, the submandibular glands often hyperenhance, whereas the parotid glands may hyperenhance or undergo fatty infiltration. Hypothyroidism may also occur if the thyroid is included in the radiation field.

Neuropathy of the hypoglossal nerve, vagal nerve, or the brachial plexus may occur following radiation. When neuropathy occurs, it usually presents 2 to 4 years following treatment, although symptoms may be delayed up to 10 years following treatment.

COMPANION CASES

- **Carotidynia.** First described in 1927, carotidynia represents a self-limiting, atypical pain involving the neck associated with carotid artery sensitivity to pressure. The validity of this entity has been debated in the literature, although there does appear to be sufficient literature to support its existence. The cause of carotidynia is unknown, although some reports have described an apparent association between carotidynia and chemotherapy administration. While not recommended, prior biopsies of this entity have demonstrated focal inflammatory change without evidence of tumor. The imaging appearance is that of focal, ill-defined soft tissue surrounding the carotid bifurcation, with or without enhancement, and without carotid artery luminal compromise. Hypermetabolism on PET imaging isolated to the region of the carotid sheath in patients with carotidynia has also been described. Because carotidynia is self-limiting, symptomatic therapy with a course of nonsteroidal anti-inflammatory medications or a short course of steroids is often sufficient. Knowledge of this entity is important in order to properly interpret the imaging findings, and perhaps most importantly, avoid unnecessary biopsy. The imaging appearance of radiation therapy or a prior neck dissection can appear similar to carotidynia, except that in the case of carotidynia, the finding is isolated to the carotid bifurcation/sheath. Of course, history is also paramount in differentiating these entities.
- **Metastatic disease to the neck dermis and soft tissues.** Up to 5% to 10% of all cancer patients may develop metastasis to the dermis. While any malignancy may metastasize to the soft tissues, breast carcinoma is the most common culprit in women. Melanoma, followed by lung carcinoma, are the most frequently identified causes of metastasis to the soft tissues in men. Clinically, these metastatic lesions most often arise in patients older than 40 years of age and are usually multifocal, small, rubbery, or hard lesions. On imaging, the lesions are typically isointense relative to muscle on T1, iso- to mildly hyperintense to relative to muscle on T2, and typically enhance. Melanoma involving the dermis or soft tissues may also restrict on diffusion-weighted imaging.
- **Paraffinoma following mineral oil injection.** Injection of liquid paraffin (refined mineral oil) into various parts of the body has been documented for at least 100 years. While abandoned as a legitimate form of therapy, unqualified practitioners were known to be injecting these substances at least into the 1980s, primarily in

some Far East and Eastern European countries. Today, it is likely that most of the cases of injected paraffin are performed by the patients themselves. These injections are usually performed in an attempt to enlarge or change the shape of muscles or genitalia. In the realm of bodybuilding, targeted injection of mineral oils (so-called 'site enhancement') is prevalent and some products are even available commercially. The injected paraffin results in tissue damage which is sometimes extensive. The lesions formed have been termed parafffinomas or sclerosing lipogranulomas and are. A paraffinoma is characterized by oil cyst formation, muscle necrosis, foreign body giant cells, extensive surrounding granulomatous and fibrous tissue formation, vasculitis, and abscess formation. Paraffinomas may occur many years after injection. The clinical findings are generally irreversible, with cases of blindness, skin necrosis, emboli, acute pulmonary edema, and even death having been reported. On CT, extensive scarring with heterogeneous enhancement is usually evident. Round to oval areas of fat density may be identified on CT, wtih chronic lesions often containing coarse calcifications. The MRI appearance of a paraffinoma is variable and likely depends on the stage of the pathology. Some studies have demonstrated early changes related to liquid paraffin to be T1 hypo- to isointense, whereas other have demonstrated T1 shortening on unenhanced T1-weighted MR imaging. Early changes of liquid paraffin are usually hyperintense on T2. Later in the pathologic process, the paraffin presumably becomes semi-solid, resulting in hypointense T1 and T2 signal. The fibrous/granulomatous tissue surrounding the paraffin injections is usually hypo- to isointense on T1 and hypointense on T2, particularly later in the disease process when coarse calcifications may develop.

Chronic appearance of an irradiated neck

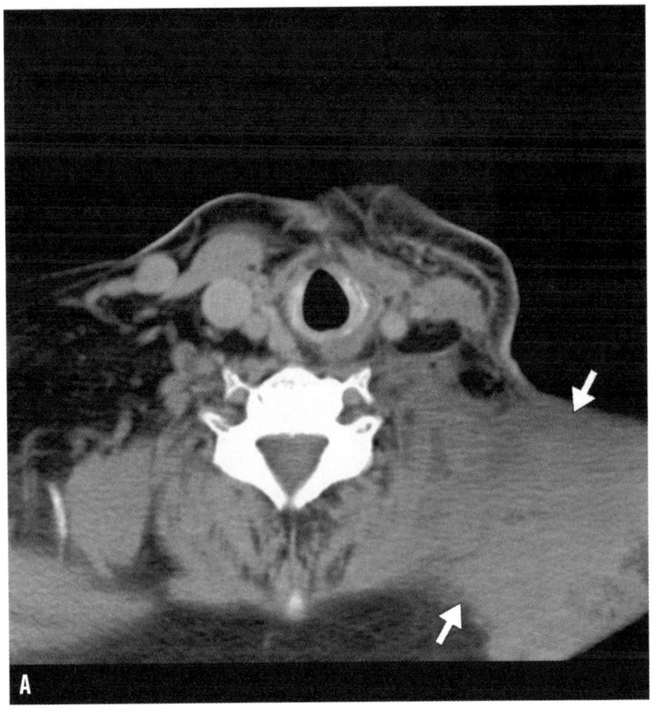

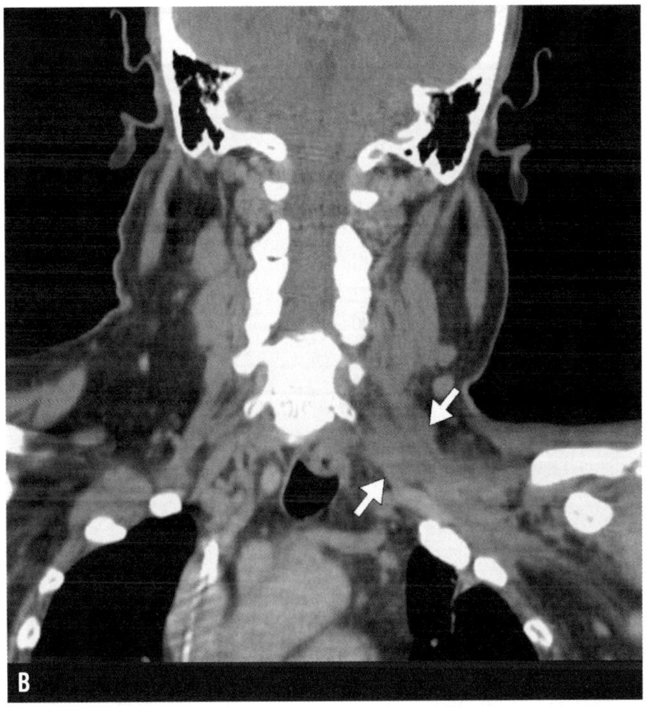

Axial (**A**) and coronal reformatted (**B**) contrast-enhanced CT images of the neck demonstrate marked radiation effect in the left lower neck following radiation treatment for breast cancer (arrows, **A**, **B**).

Evolving appearance of an irradiated neck

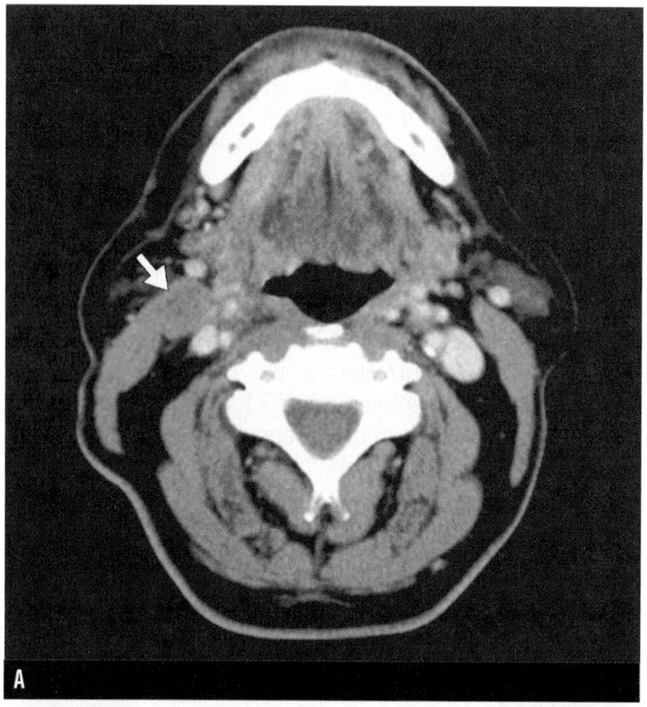

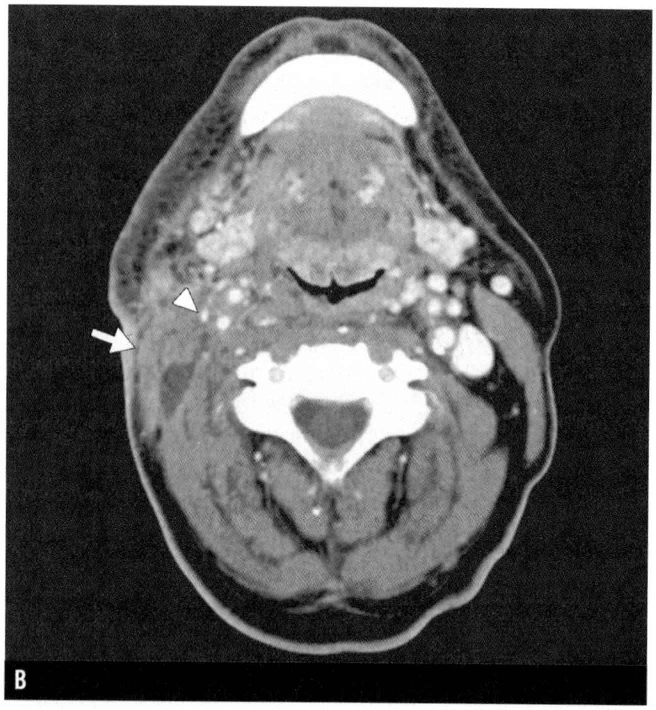

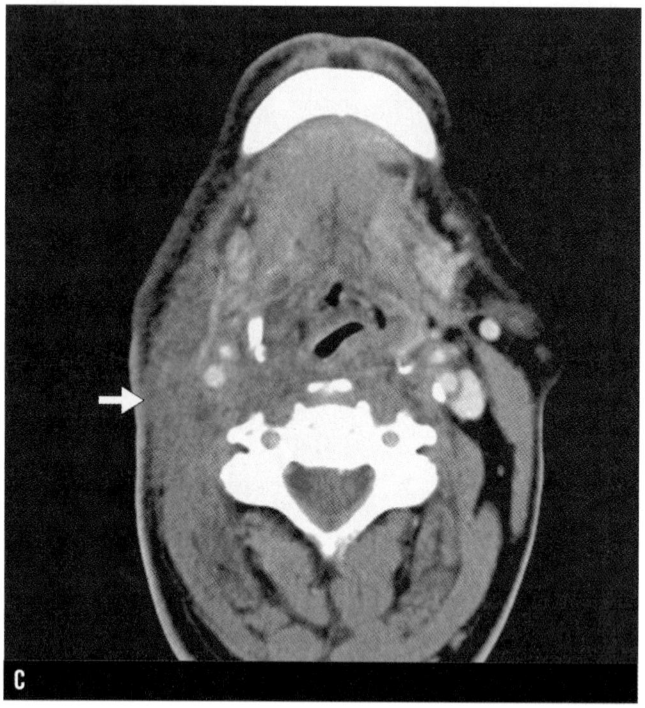

A postcontrast axial CT image of a patient who presented with a supraglottic squamous cell carcinoma (not shown) (**A**) demonstrates a pathologic lymph node in the right level IIA nodal station (arrow, **A**). A postcontrast axial CT image obtained 6 months later following a modified radical right neck dissection (**B**) demonstrates expected postoperative edema with preservation of the right sternocleidomastoid muscle (arrow, **B**) and right internal jugular vein, although the latter is markedly diminutive (arrowhead, **B**). Approximately 2 years later, a follow-up postcontrast axial CT image after radiation therapy (**C**) demonstrates marked scarring of the right sternocleidomastoid muscle and adjacent fat from radiation effect (arrow, **C**) as well as subsequent obliteration of the right internal jugular vein.

Companion case: Carotidynia

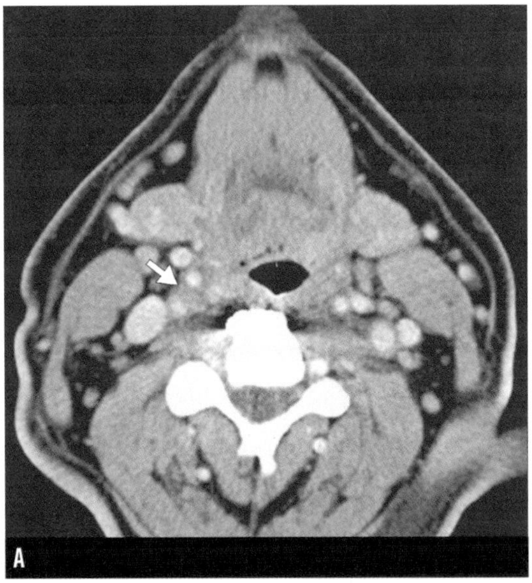

A contrast-enhanced axial CT image (**A**) demonstrates subtle soft tissue density in the right carotid sheath (arrow) in this patient with acute lymphocytic leukemia, acute right neck and right ear pain, chemotherapy administration, and no history of radiation. While presumptive, this patient's neck pain and imaging findings are compatible with carotidynia, possibly related to chemotherapy, which has been associated with carotidynia. The patient did not have a right temporal bone imaging abnormality (not shown) to account for the right ear pain. However, it is possible that the right ear pain was related to the carotidynia, as the inflammatory process surrounding the right carotid artery could have affected the immediately adjacent cranial nerve X and resulted in a referred ear pain via Arnold's nerve, a branch of cranial nerve X.

Companion case: Metastatic disease to the neck dermis and soft tissues

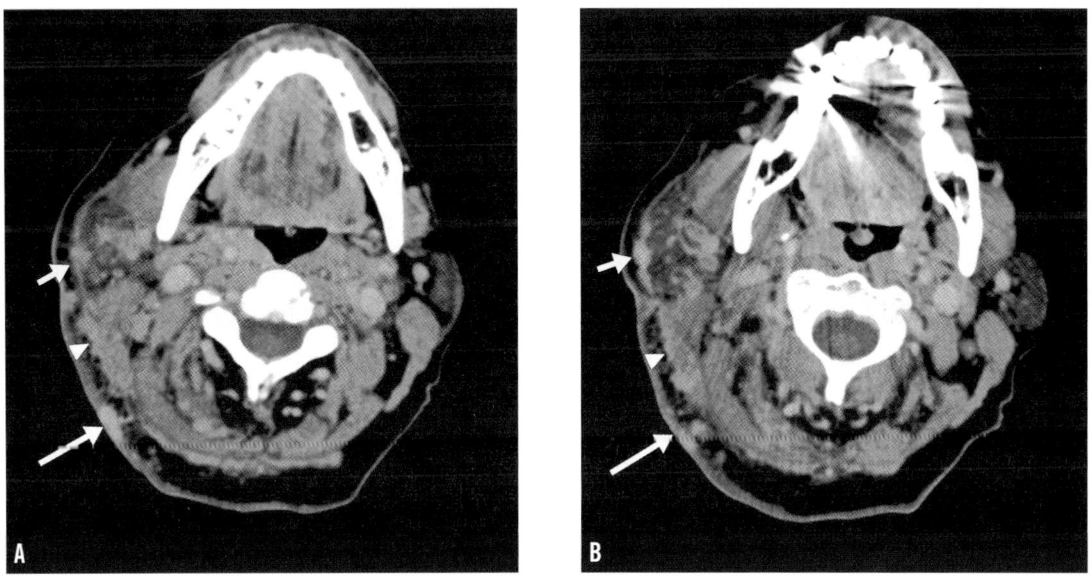

Axial (**A**, **B**) and coronal reformatted (**C**) contrast-enhanced CT images through the neck demonstrate ill-defined and nodular density involving the right neck dermis and subcutaneous tissues (long arrows, **A-C**), the right sternocleidomastoid muscle (arrowheads, **A**, **B**), and the right parotid capsule (short arrows, **A**, **B**). This represented metastatic disease from inflammatory breast carcinoma.

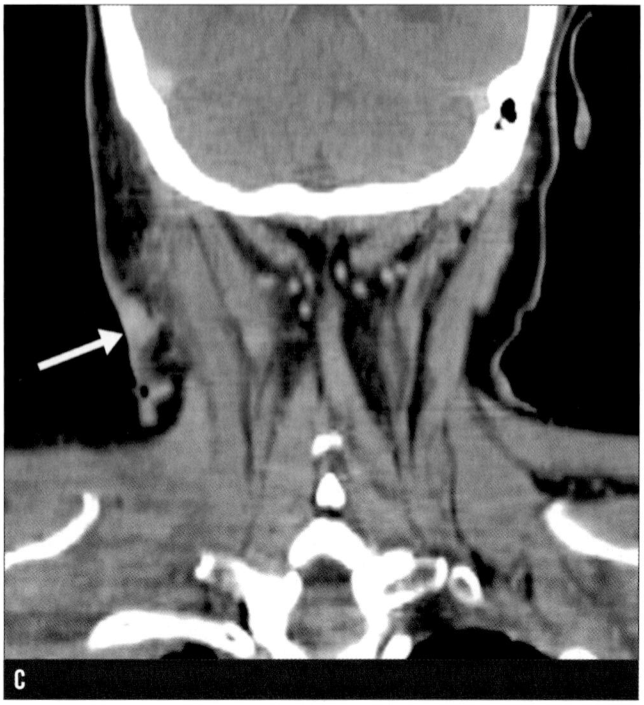

Companion case: Paraffinoma following mineral oil injection

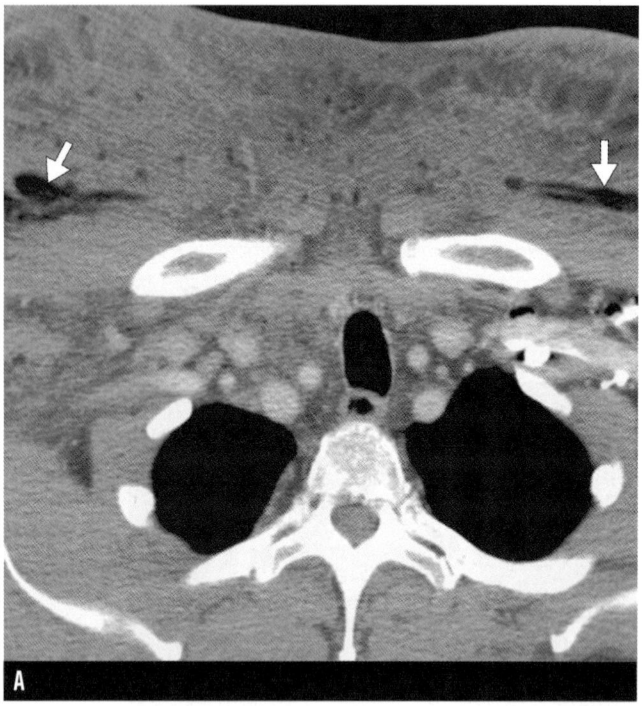

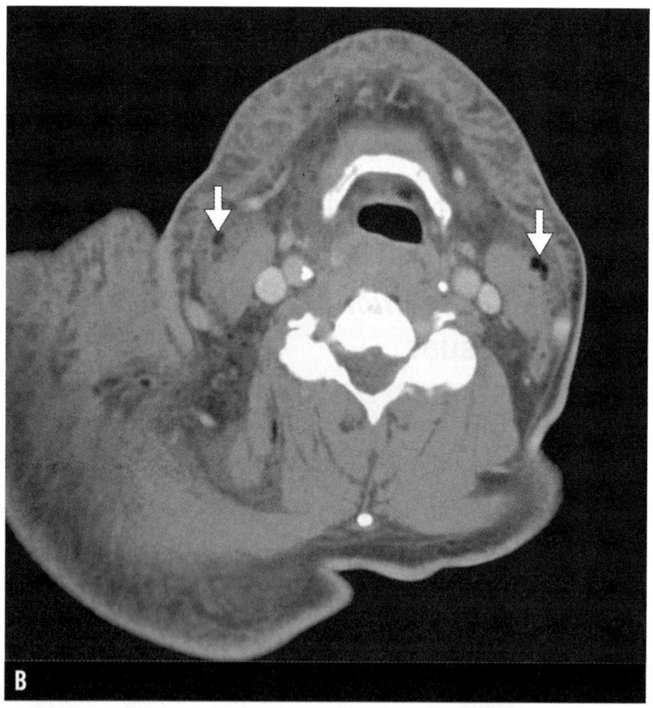

Postcontrast axial (**A**, **B**) and coronal reformatted (**C**) CT images of the neck demonstrate extensive edema and multifocal globular areas of fat density (arrows, **A-C**) scattered throughout the neck and visualized upper chest. The globular areas of fat density represent baby oil. This patient has gender identity disorder and self-injected baby oil in an attempt to change his sexual identity from a man to a woman. Unenhanced axial (**D**, **E**), coronal reformatted (**F**), and sagittal reformatted (**G**) CT images obtained nearly 1 year later demonstrate multifocal areas of calcified granuloma formation in the neck and upper chest (arrows, **D**, **F**, **G**) as well as in the retropharynx (arrowheads, **E**, **G**) as a result of the injected baby oil.

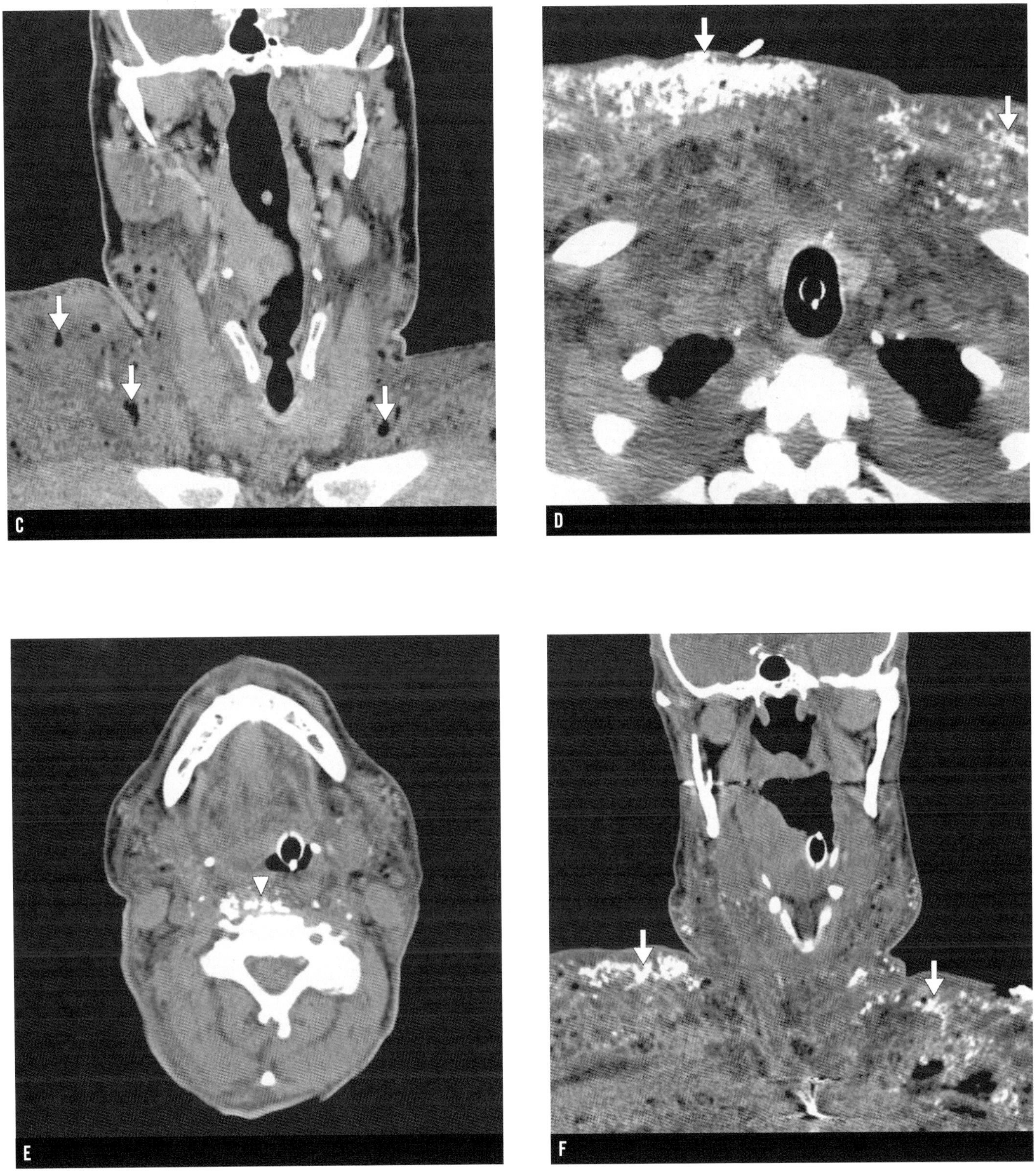
C
D
E
F

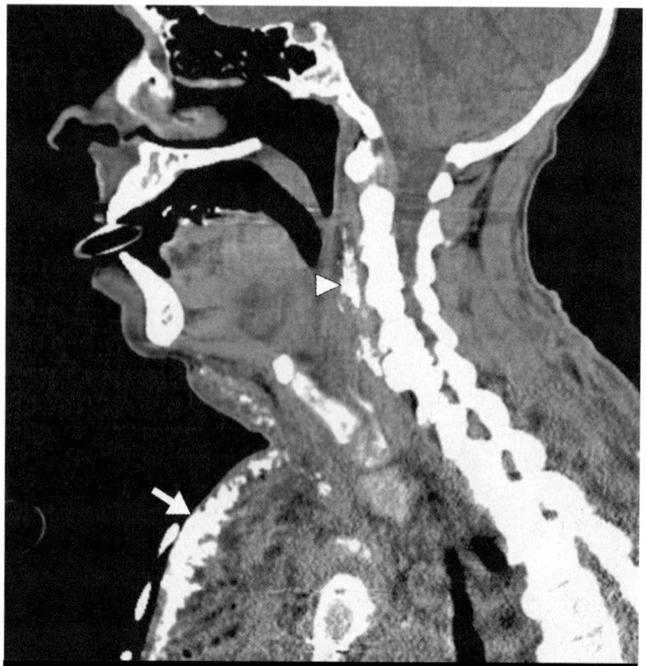
G

REFERENCES

Akkus E, et al. Paraffinoma and ulcer of the external genitalia after self-injection of vaseline. *J Sex Med.* 2006;3(1):170-172.

Banke IJ, et al. Irreversible muscle damage in bodybuilding due to long-term intramuscular oil injection. *Int J Sports Med.* 2012;33(10): 829-834. May 16, Epub 2012.

Beaman FD, et al. Superficial soft-tissue masses: analysis, diagnosis, and differential considerations. *Radiographics.* 2007;27(2):509-523.

Erguvan-Dogan B, et al. Direct injection of paraffin into the breast: mammographic, sonographic, and MRI features of early complications. *AJR Am J Roentgenol.* 2006;186(3):888-894.

Glastonbury CM, et al. The postradiation neck: evaluating response to treatment and recognizing complications. *AJR. Am J roentgenol.* 2010;195(2):W164-W171.

Gu DH, et al. CT features of foreign body granulomas after cosmetic paraffin injection into the cervicofacial area. *Diagn Interv Radiol.* 2010;16(2):125-128.

May DA, et al. Abnormal signal intensity in skeletal muscle at MR imaging: patterns, pearls, and pitfalls. *Radiographics.* 2000;20 Spec No:S295-S315.

Mukherji SK, et al. Evaluation of head and neck squamous cell carcinoma after treatment. *AJNR. Am J Neuroradiol.* 2003;24(9):1743-1746.

Rollins CE1, Reiber G, Guinee DG Jr, Lie JT. Disseminated Lipogranulomas and Sudden Death From Self-Administered Mineral Oil Injection. *Am J Forensic Med Pathol.* 1997;18(1):100-103.

CASE 11 Brown Fat

There are two types of fat found in mammals: brown and white. The main function of brown fat is to dissipate excess energy to create heat, whereas the main functions of white fat are to store energy as well as to insulate in order to retain heat. Brown fat contains a large number of modified mitochondria which contain iron; it is the iron in these mitochondria that gives brown fat its characteristic color. Brown fat is relatively abundant in newborns and helps compensate for their relative lack of sufficient skeletal muscle, which is the other major source of mammalian heat. The activity of brown fat remains high in children until they reach puberty.

Until the advent of PET imaging utilizing Fluorine-18 deoxyglucose (FDG), brown fat was thought to be nonfunctional in adults. However, up to 20% of adult patients will contain functional brown fat, which is more active in the winter months than in the summer months. Interestingly, a larger amount of brown fat activity will be demonstrated if PET imaging is performed in a cold room.

Brown fat in adults is predominantly found in the supraclavicular region and neck, and it is usually symmetric. While both brown fat and PET avid tumors have a standardized uptake value of greater than 2.5 (in the case of brown fat, roughly 4), the symmetry and characteristic location of brown fat helps differentiate brown fat from a PET avid tumor.

COMPANION CASES

- **Madelung disease.** Madelung disease is a rare lipodystrophy characterized by diffuse, symmetric, painless, unencapsulated, and irreversible lipomatosis. Common locations of Madelung disease include the face, neck, shoulders, upper trunk, arm, abdomen, and legs. It is male predominant (15:1) and a disease of middle age. The cause of this disease is unknown, but it has been associated with alcoholism in 60% to 90% of patients. Despite the reduced range of motion of the head and neck that may occur when this entity affects the neck, Madelung disease is most often asymptomatic and malignant transformation of this disease is extremely rare. The only effective therapy is surgical, either with dermolipectomy (removal of skin and fat) and/or suction-assisted lipectomy (removal of fat). Due to the presence of skin stretching that occurs as a result of the extensive lipomatosis, dermolipectomy is the preferred surgical option as it generally results in a greater degree of cosmesis.

  On imaging, the fat associated with Madelung disease is indistinguishable from normal fat except by its extent and associated pronounced mass effect on the surrounding musculature, vessels, and glands.
- **Intramuscular neck lipoma.** Lipomas are benign, encapsulated, usually slow-growing tumors composed of fat. These tumors may occur at any age but most commonly present as painless masses in individuals aged between 40 and 60 years. Simple lipomas contain homogeneous fat attenuation on CT and homogeneous fat signal characteristics on all MRI pulse sequences. Simple lipomas may be resected for cosmesis, with an overall recurrence rate of 1% to 2%; however, intramuscular lipomas, even when simple on radiology studies and at pathology, have a much higher local recurrence rate (19%).
- **Liposarcoma.** Liposarcomas are rare tumors occurring in 2.5 patients per million, although they are still the second most common soft-tissue sarcoma, after malignant fibrous histiocytoma. Five subtypes have been described: well-differentiated, dedifferentiated, myxoid, pleomorphic, and mixed type.

  A common challenge on cross-sectional imaging is to distinguish benign lipomas from well-differentiated liposarcomas. Kransdorf et al have described the following distinguishing factors that help favor a liposarcoma: large lesion size (>10 cm), thick septations (>2 mm), nodular/globular nonadipose tissue, associated nonadipose masses, and a total amount of nonadipose tissue comprising more than 25% of the lesion. Mild to moderate enhancement of the septations is also a reported finding that should raise the possibility of liposarcoma. Calcification associated with a lipomatous lesion is a nonspecific finding, though it is seen more often in liposarcomas relative to lipomas.
- **Epidermal inclusion cyst.** See Case 2 from this chapter for a full description.

Brown fat

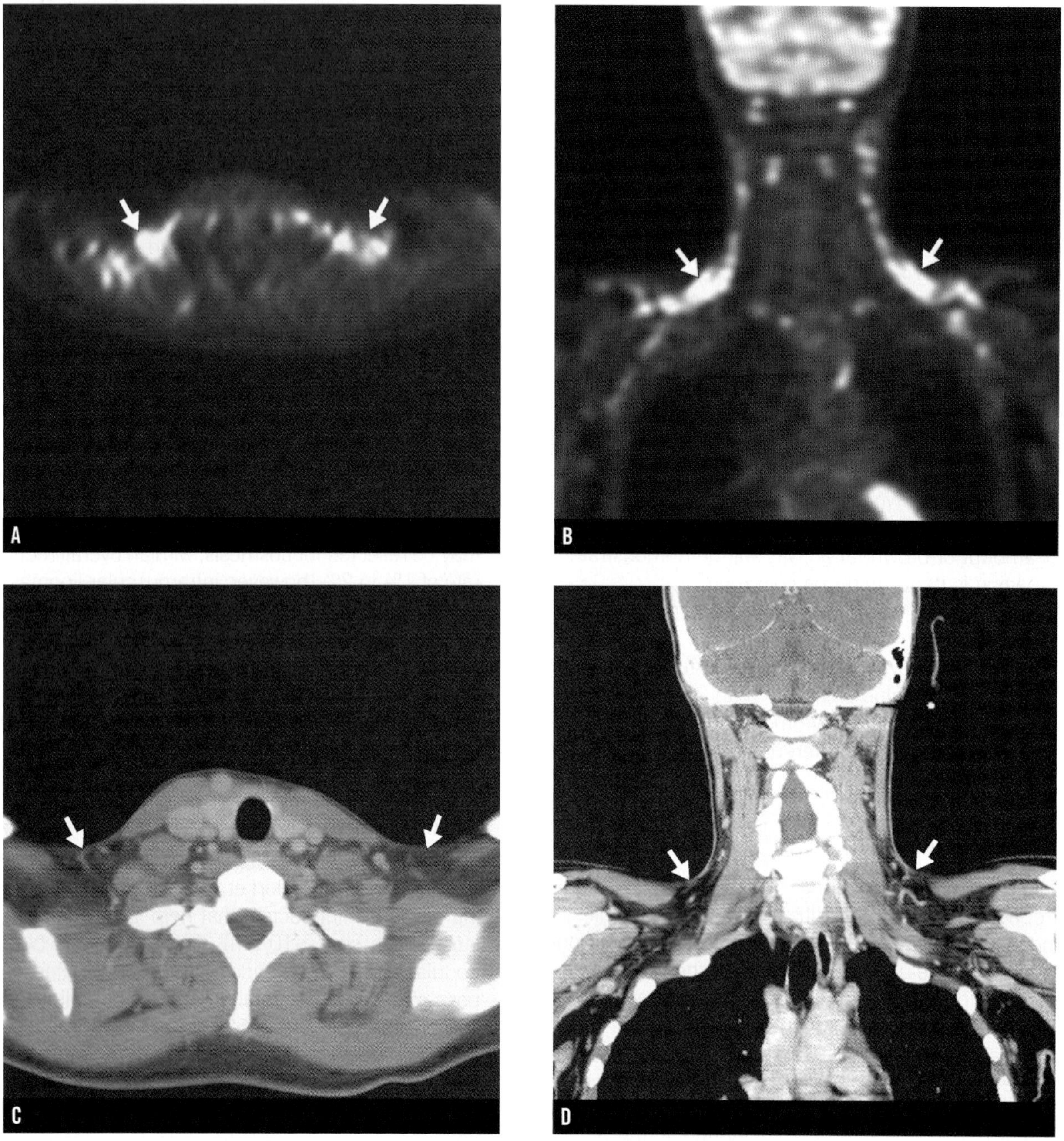

Axial (**A**) and coronal reformatted (**B**) PET images through the neck demonstrate increased metabolic activity in the bilateral aspects of the neck, particularly the supraclavicular regions (arrows, **A**, **B**). Axial (**C**) and coronal reformatted (**D**) postcontrast CT images of the neck at the same levels as image **A** and **B**, respectively, demonstrate that the increased activity on PET corresponds to normal fat (arrows, **C**, **D**). In conjunction with the PET findings, the fat in this case represents normal brown fat.

Companion case: Madelung disease

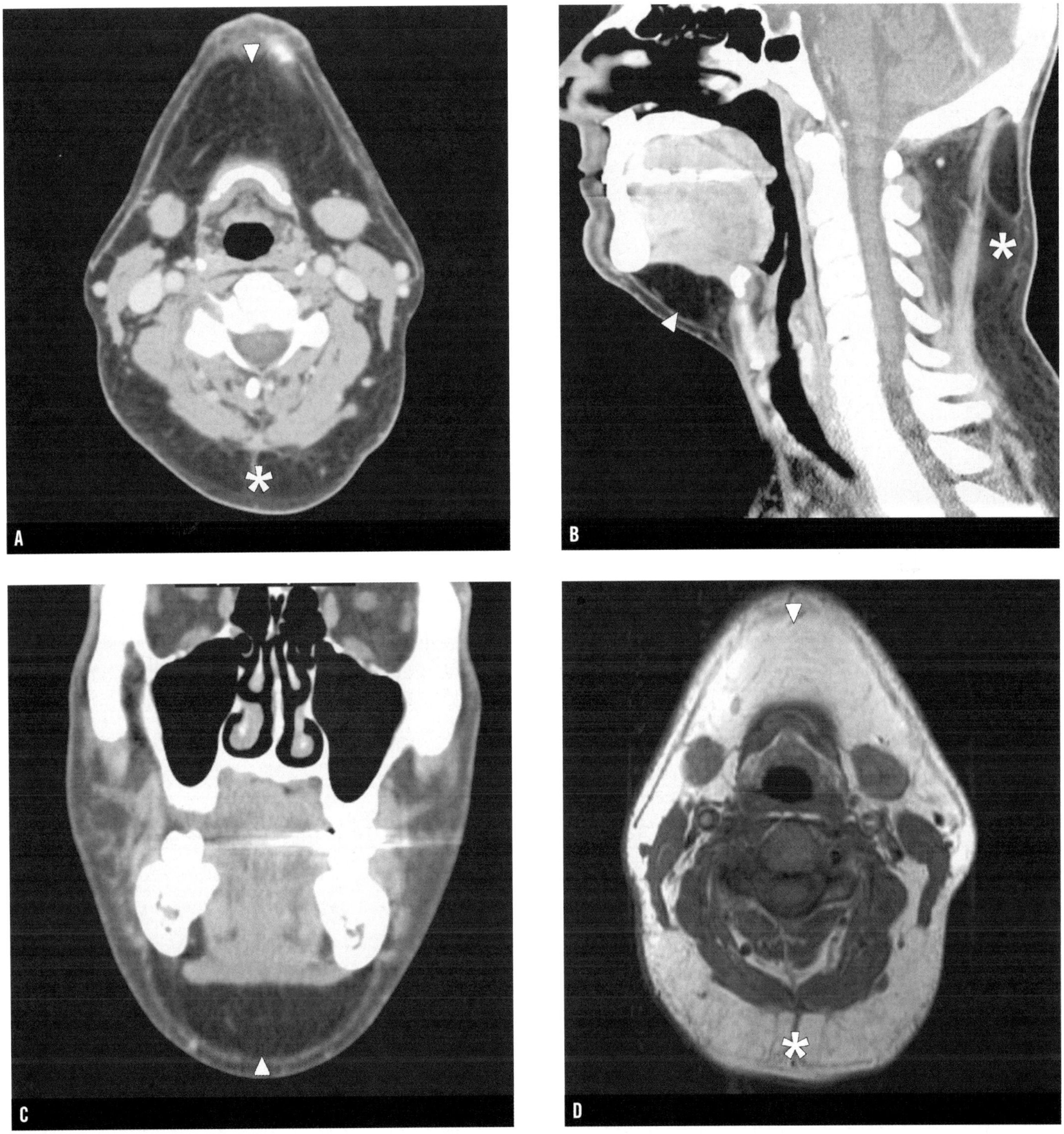

Postcontrast axial (**A**), sagittal reformatted (**B**), and coronal reformatted (**C**) CT images as well as an unenhanced axial T1-weighted MR image without fat suppression (**D**) demonstrate extensive fat deposition throughout the neck, in particular the posterior neck (asterisks, **A**, **B**, **D**) and submental regions (arrowheads, **A-D**). A postcontrast axial T1-weighted MR image with fat suppression (**E**) demonstrates expected fat suppression at the same locations. These findings are consistent with Madelung disease. The patient complained of disfiguring neck masses and was taken to surgery in an attempt to debulk the lipomas. This was achieved with variable success, as demonstrated on an axial T1-weighted MR image without fat suppression obtained following surgery (**F**).

Companion case: Intramuscular neck lipoma

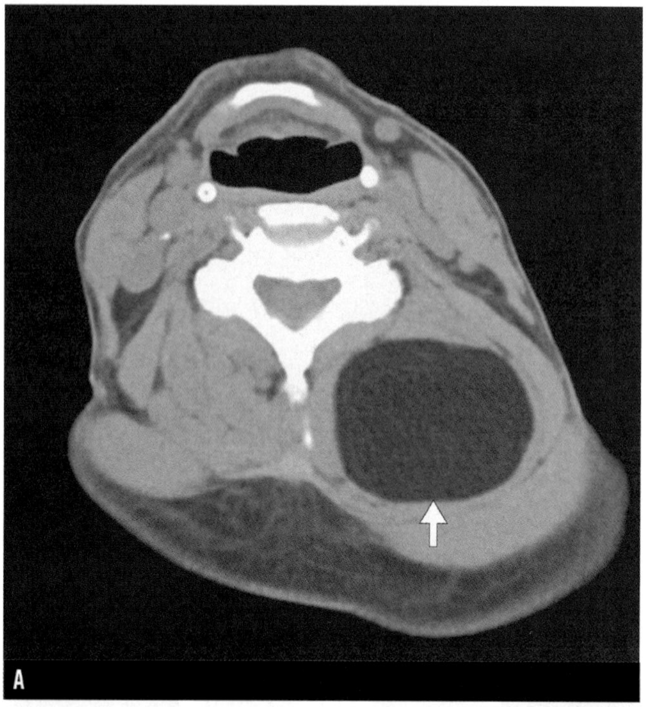

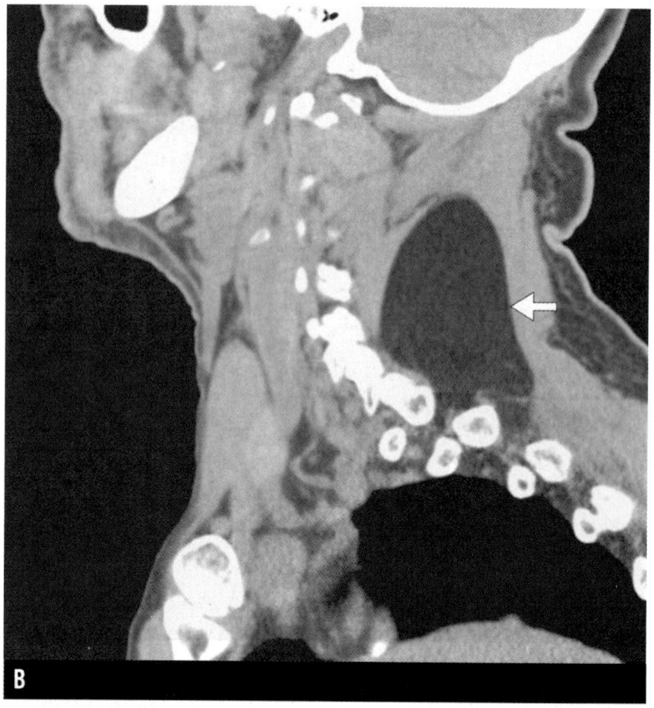

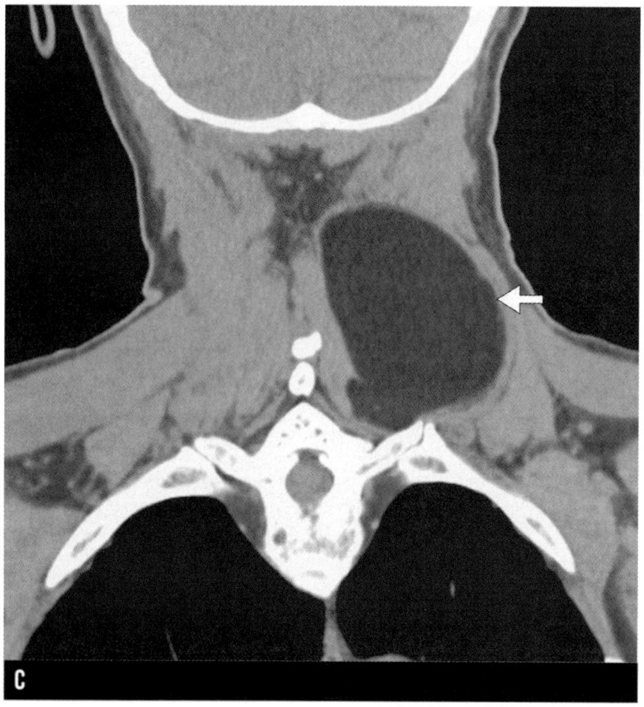

Axial (**A**), sagittal reformatted (**B**), and coronal reformatted (**C**) unenhanced CT images through the neck demonstrate a large, circumscribed, fat density mass embedded within the left posterior paraspinal muscles of the neck, compatible with a benign intramuscular lipoma (arrows, **A-C**).

Companion case: Liposarcoma

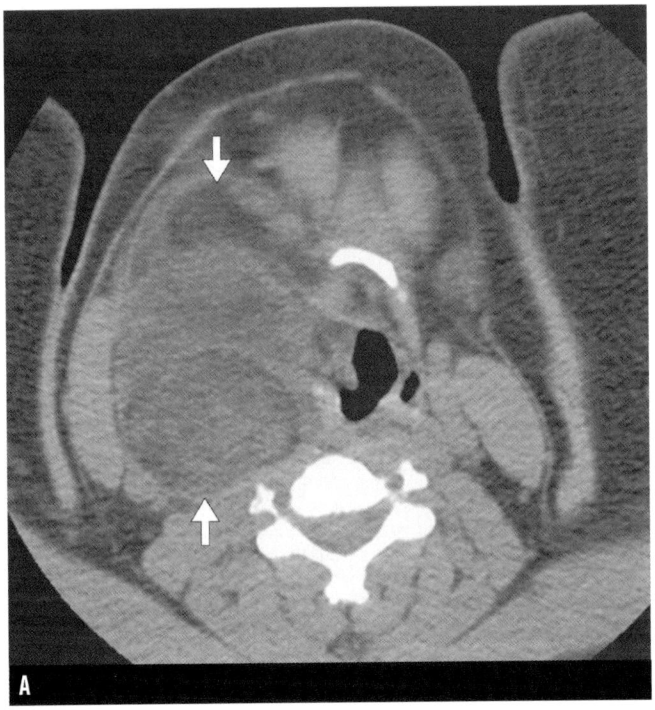

An unenhanced axial CT image through the neck (**A**) demonstrates a large, heterogeneous, partially fat-containing, soft tissue mass in the right aspect of the neck (arrows). This lesion was a liposarcoma at pathology.

Companion case: Epidermal inclusion cyst

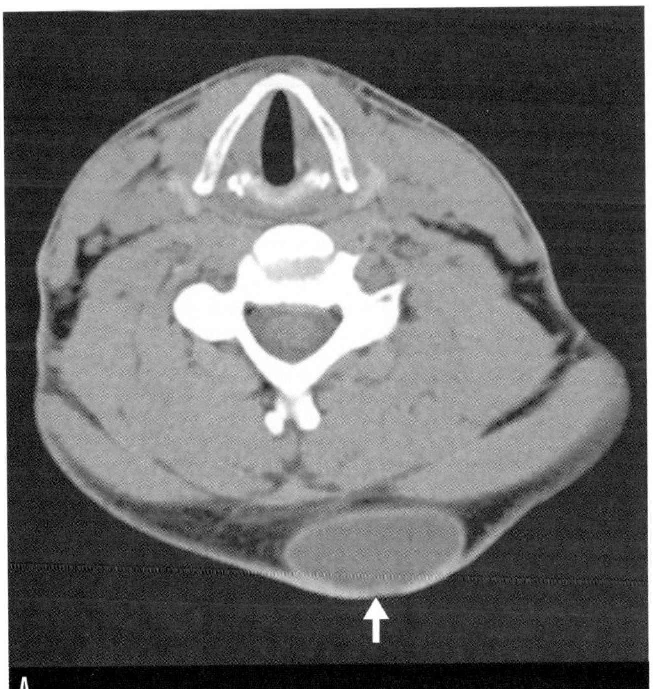

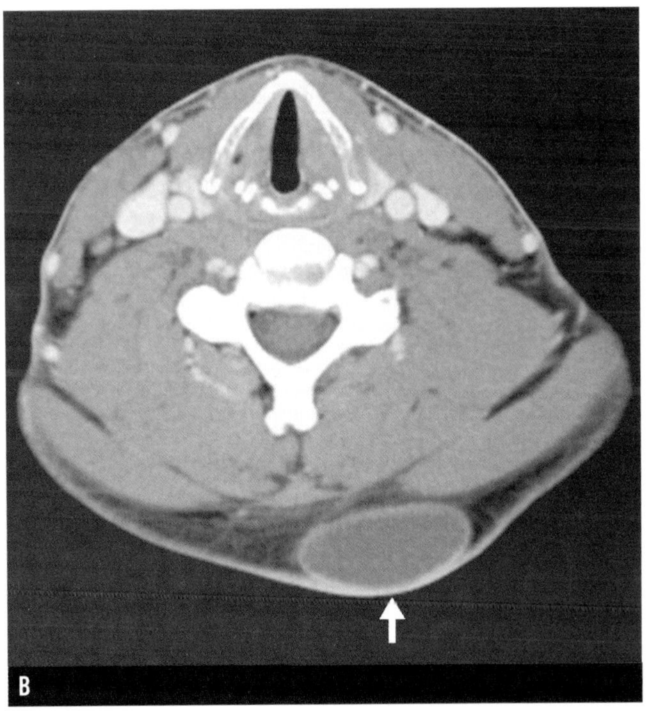

An axial noncontrast CT image (**A**) and contrast-enhanced axial (**B**), sagittal reformatted (**C**), and coronal reformatted (**D**) CT images of the neck demonstrate an ovoid, circumscribed, low density, nonenhancing mass in the subcutaneous tissues of the left posterior neck (arrows, **A-D**). The lesion is contiguous with the dermis and most consistent with an epidermal inclusion cyst.

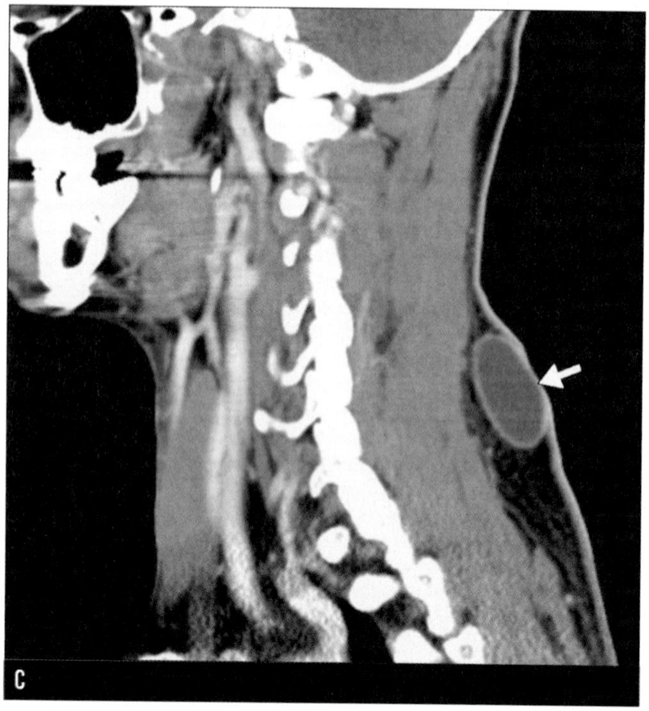

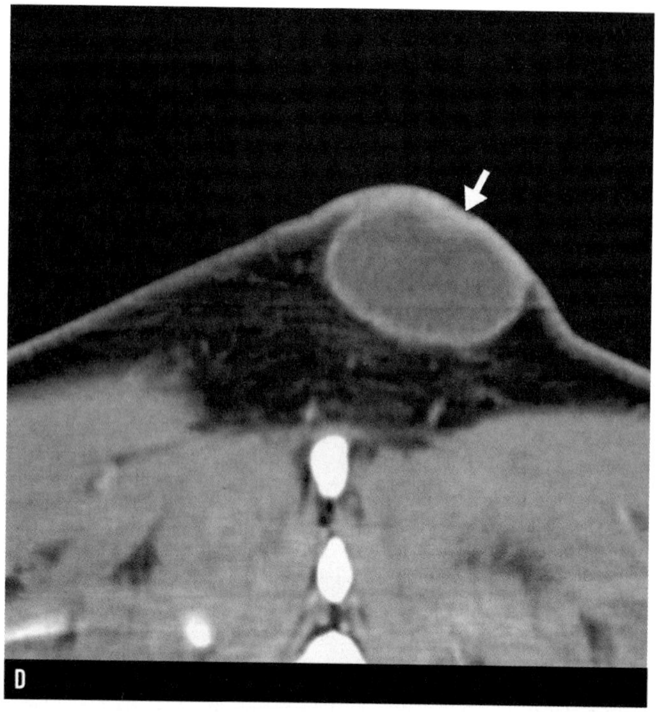

REFERENCES

Cypess AM, et al. Cold but not sympathomimetics activates human brown adipose tissue in vivo. *Proc Natl Acad Sci U S A.* 2012;109(25):10001-10005.

Daniels GH, et al. Brown Fat at PET/CT: correlation with patient characteristics. *Radiology.* 2012;263(3):836-842.

Kransdorf MJ, et al. Imaging of fatty tumors : distinction of lipoma and well-differentiated liposarcoma. *Radiology*;(1):99-104.

Landis MS, Etemad-Rezai R, Shetty K, Goldszmidt M. Case 143: Madelung disease. *Radiology.* 2009;250(3):951-954.

Murphey MD, et al. From the Archives of the AFIP Imaging of Musculoskeletal Liposarcoma with Radiologic-Pathologic correlation. *Radiographics.*2005;25:1371-1395.

Pandya KA, Radke F. Benign skin lesions: lipomas, epidermal inclusion cysts, muscle and nerve biopsies. *Surg Clin North Am.* 2009;89(3):677-687.

Pereira JM, Sirlin CB, Pinto PS, Casola G. CT and MR imaging of extrahepatic fatty masses of the abdomen and pelvis: techniques, diagnosis, differential diagnosis, and pitfalls. *Radiographics.* 2005; 25(1):69-85.

Ramos S, Pinheiro S, Diogo C, Cabral L, Cruzeiro C. Madelung disease: a not-so-rare disorder. *Ann Plast Surg.* 2010;64(1):122-124.

Virtanen KA, Nuutila P. Brown adipose tissue in humans. *Curr Opin Lipidol.* 2011;22(1):49-54.

Wang Y, Shi H. Dedifferentiated Liposarcoma of the Neck : CT findings. *AJNR Am J Neuroradiol.* 2012;33(1):E4-E6.

Zhang X, Li N, Xiao W. Madelung disease: manifestations of CT and MR imaging. *Oral Surg Oral Med Oral Pathol Oral Radiol Endod.* 2008;105(5):e57-e64.

CASE 12 Normal minimal fat in the neck

Normally, fat in the neck can be utilized as an intrinsic imaging contrast agent, with normal fat aiding in defining tissue planes. However, some patients, particularly athletes, may have a paucity of neck fat. As a result, there may be greater difficulty in localizing or identifying neck pathology in these patients, particularly abnormal lymph nodes.

COMPANION CASE

- **Cachexia.** Cachexia is the pathological loss of weight (as opposed to a desired loss of weight) and is frequently associated with muscle atrophy, anemia, fatigue, and weakness. Cachexia is commonly present in patients with malignancy, estimated to be present in 50% of all cancer patients and 80% of terminal cancer patients. The etiology of cachexia in cancer patients is multifactorial and relates to the hypermetabolic demands of the tumor, anorexia resulting from aggressive chemotherapy and/or radiation therapy, and overproduction of inflammatory cytokines. If loss of muscle and fat continues despite nutritional support, it is specifically termed "cancer cachexia." Additional causes of cachexia are numerous and include chronic infection (TB, AIDS), certain forms of drug abuse (most commonly amphetamines), COPD, and severe CHF. Imaging of cachectic patients will demonstrate diffuse loss of fat as well as diffuse muscle atrophy, the latter finding differentiating this entity from healthy patients with minimal neck fat.

Normal minimal fat in the neck

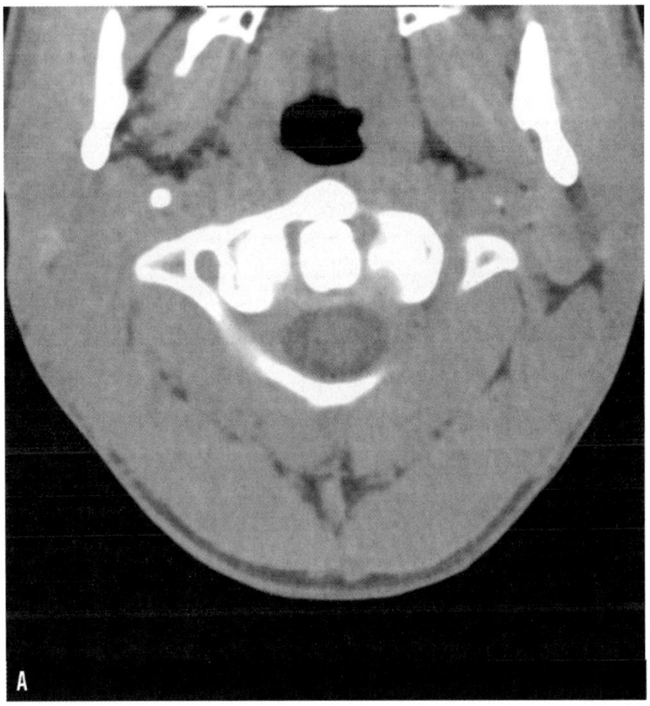

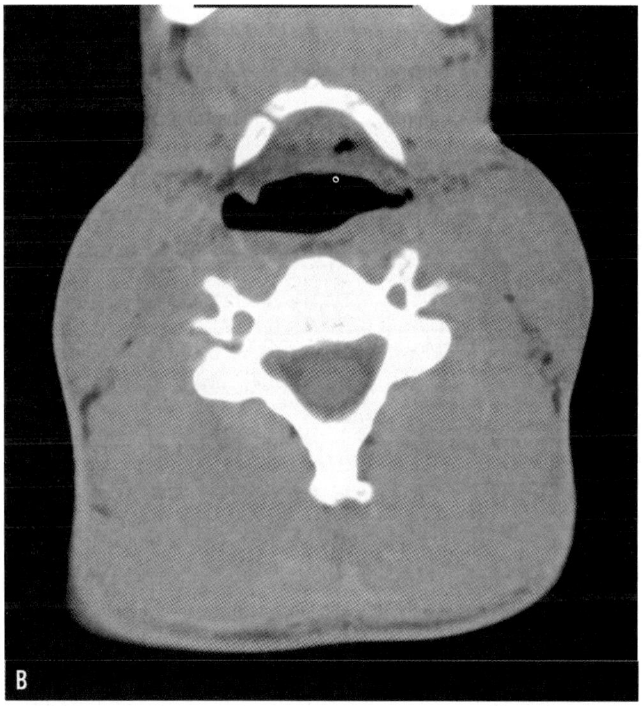

Axial (**A-C**) and coronal reformatted (**D**) CT images of the neck performed without contrast demonstrate a paucity of fat throughout the neck. This patient is a healthy 23-year-old patient, with normal neck muscle volume.

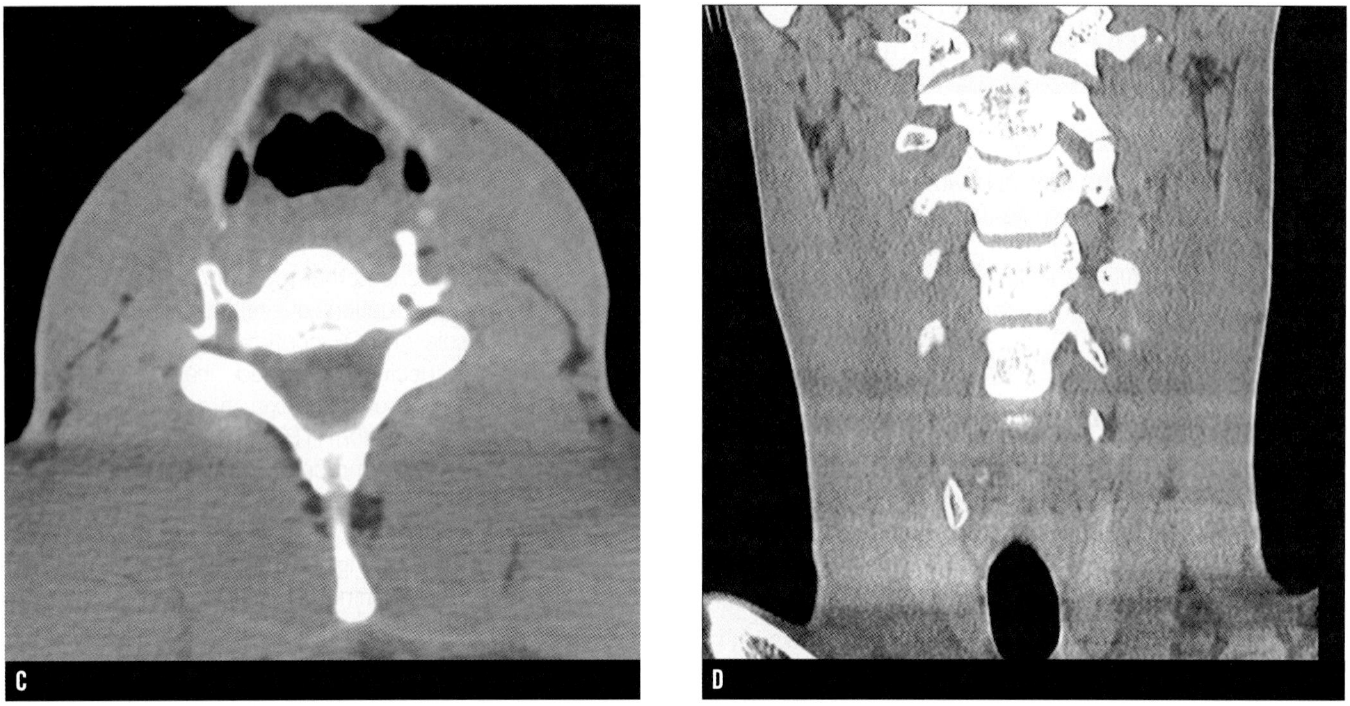

Companion case: Cachexia

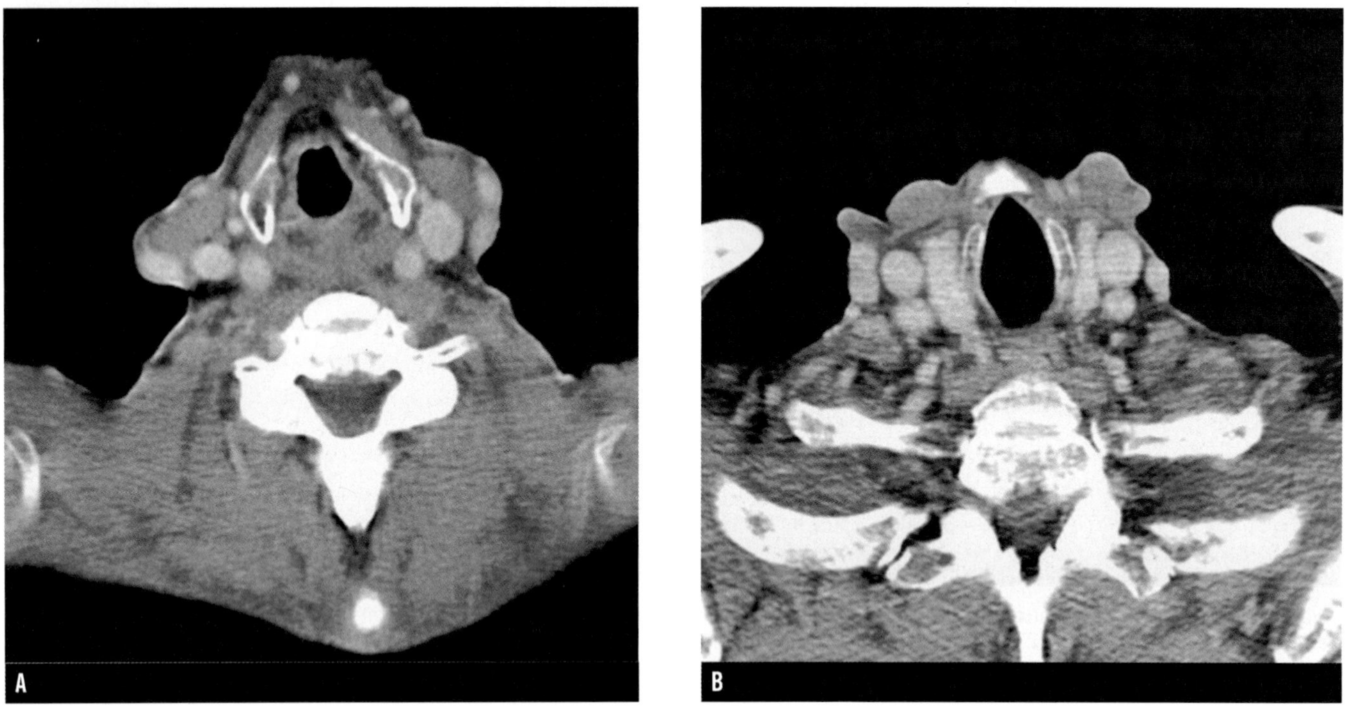

Axial postcontrast CT images through the neck (**A**, **B**) demonstrate diffuse loss of neck fat and muscle atrophy, compatible with cachexia. This patient was treated with chemotherapy and radiation for tonsillar squamous cell carcinoma.

Companion case: Cachexia

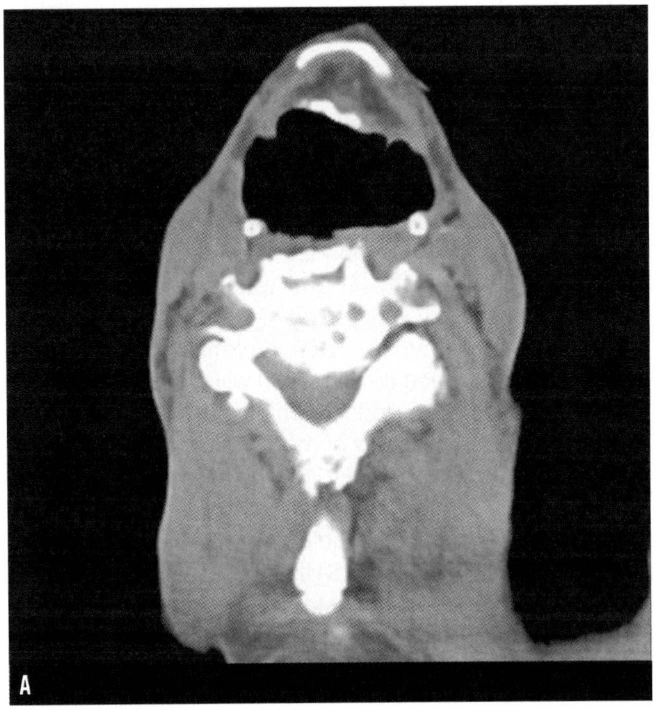

Different patient. An axial unenhanced CT image through the neck demonstrates marked loss of fat in the neck associated with diffuse muscle atrophy. This patient was newly diagnosed with base of tongue squamous cell carcinoma and metastatic disease to the lymph nodes (not shown).

REFERENCES

Fearon KCH, et al. Cancer cachexia. *Int J Cardiol.* 2002;85(1):73-81.

Freeman LM. The pathophysiology of cardiac cachexia. *Curr Opin Support Palliat Care.* 2009;3(4):276-281.

Tisdale MJ. Mechanisms of Cancer Cachexia. *Physiol Rev.* 2009;89(2):381-410.

Von Haehling S, et al. Cachexia as a major underestimated and unmet medical need: facts and numbers. *J Cachexia Sarcopenia Muscle.* 2010;1(1):1-5.

CASE 13 Incomplete fat suppression on MRI

Fat, along with water and gadolinium, is an essential source of signal on MR imaging. Fat is hyperintense on both T1 and T2 sequences, unless fat suppression (FS) techniques are applied. Unenhanced fat-suppressed T2 sequences are extremely useful for highlighting edema in bones and soft tissues. Contrast-enhanced T1-weighted imaging with FS is ideal for identifying enhancing lesions while suppressing potentially confounding neck and marrow fat.

Multiple FS techniques are available. Traditional spin-echo based, FS sequences utilize a presaturation pulse at a frequency specific to fat (at the given field strength of the magnet). This technique allows only signal from fat to be eliminated, and it can be applied to traditional T1 and T2 sequences with excellent signal preservation of nonfat containing tissues. The major disadvantage of this technique is that large areas of fat may not suppress if their precession frequency is shifted by a heterogeneous magnetic field. Metal will cause pronounced field heterogeneity and will often result in incomplete FS. Other causes include poor MRI magnet shimming and disparate interfaces, such as bone-air. A large enough frequency shift may occur in the setting of magnetic field heterogeneity such that water, instead of fat, is suppressed in some areas.

Short T1 (or short tau) inversion recovery (STIR) is an alternative technique that allows for subtraction of fat signal. This inversion recovery sequence is timed so that the rephasing pulse occurs when fat signal returns to baseline (ie, its null point). Both fat and water signal within fatty tissue is suppressed, which may result in improved tumor conspicuity. However, if fat is intermixed within tumor such that its relaxation time shifts, it will not fully suppress, potentially resulting in underestimation of tumoral fat. Furthermore, due to the timing of the pulse, some signal is lost from all tissues. This results in decreased signal-to-noise and is a disadvantage relative to FS sequences. However, STIR is not affected by field heterogeneity like conventional FS sequences; as a result, STIR is more efficient at suppressing fat than conventional FS sequences.

Knowledge of the causes of incomplete fat suppression and its appearance on MRI is essential in order to avoid image misinterpretation. Incomplete fat suppression should be suspected when there are geographic areas of increased signal that cross tissue planes.

Incomplete Fat Suppression On MRI

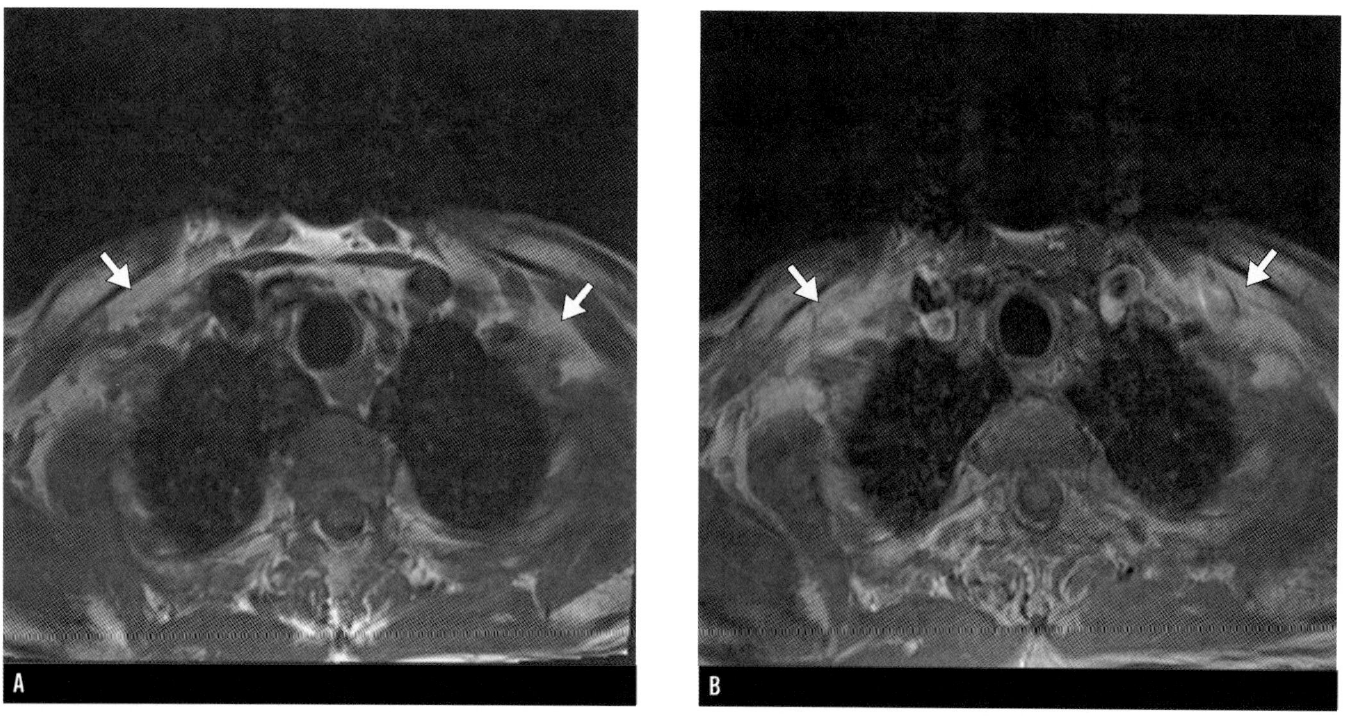

Axial T1 (**A**), axial postcontrast T1 with fat suppression (**B**), and axial T2 with fat suppession (**C**), as well as the same sequences in the coronal plane, respectively (**D-F**). Images **A** and **D** demonstrate normal fat in the bilateral supraclavicular regions (arrows, **A**, **D**). Images **B**, **C**, **E**, and **F** demonstrate incomplete fat suppression of the bilateral supraclavicular fat, simulating pathologic enhancement (arrows, **B**, **E**) and edema (arrows, **C**, **F**) in these regions.

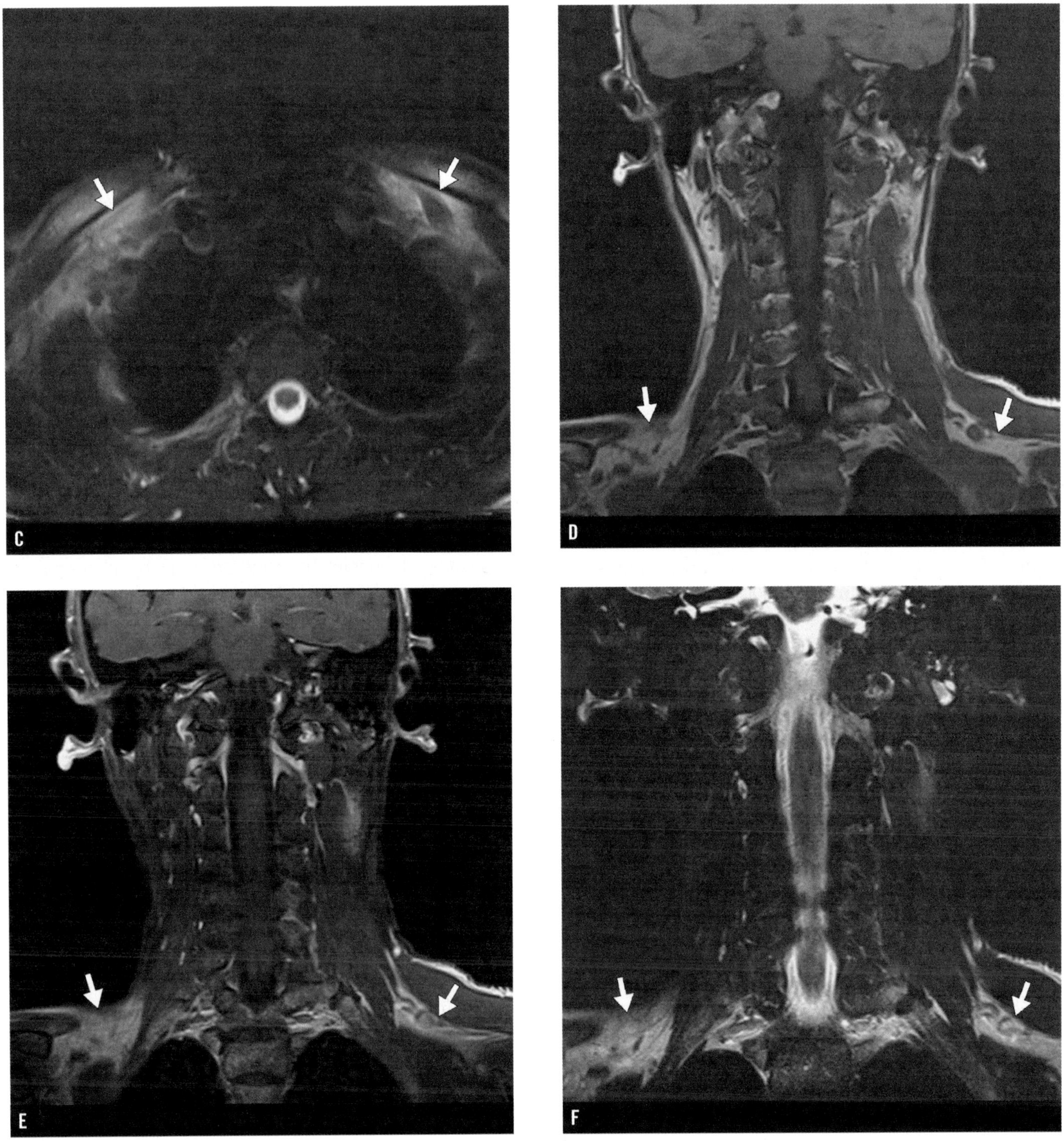

REFERENCES

Anne L, Herrick C. Pitfalls and encountered clinical artifacts in imaging of the spine1. 1998.1499 1521.

Beltran J, Johnson G. Fat suppression in MR imaging: techniques. *Radiographics.* 1998;18:373-382.

Bitar R, et al. MR pulse sequences: what every radiologist wants to know but is afraid to ask. *Radiographics.* 2006;26(2):513–537.

Taber KH1, Herrick RC, Weathers SW, Kumar AJ, Schomer DF, Hayman LA. Pitfalls and artifacts encountered in clinical MR imaging of the spine. *Radiographics.* 1998;18(6):1499-1521.

CASE 14 Brachial plexus

The brachial plexus is a complex weave of nerves composed of the C5 through T1 ventral rami. The nerves divide and merge, subdivided and named in the following order: roots, trunks, divisions, cords, and branches. The C5 through T1 roots exit at the C4-C5 through the T1-T2 levels. Proximally, the roots join to form the superior trunk (C5-C6), middle trunk (C7), and inferior trunk (C8-T1). Typically, the trunks pass between the anterior and middle scalene muscles, although a variable relationship relative to the scalene muscles has been described. The trunks separate into a total of six divisions, three anterior and three posterior, each with a superior, middle, and inferior division. The anterior divisions innervate the flexor muscles and the posterior divisions innervate the extensor muscles of the arm. These six divisions then merge to form three cords: a posterior cord, which is comprised of the three posterior divisions of trunks C5 to T1, a lateral cord, comprised of the anterior divisions of the upper and middle trunks of C5 to C7, and a medial cord, which represents a continuation of the anterior division of the lower trunk of C8 to T1.

The brachial plexus, although complex and difficult to image, is an increasingly important structure to delineate by imaging. This is particularly important in the setting of stereotactic radiosurgery, when avoiding the brachial plexus is ideal in order to prevent a brachial plexopathy. A brachial plexopathy typically occurs above 45Gy of absorbed radiation dose.

The normal brachial plexus is best identified with coronal MR imaging. It will appear low in signal and outlined by fat on T1. The brachial plexus will be hyperintense on fat suppressed T2 or STIR. Occasionally, the brachial plexus will also be identified on CT, often following fluid or near fluid attenuation as it traverses between the anterior and middle scalene muscles.

COMPANION CASE

- **Parsonage-Turner syndrome.** Parsonage-Turner syndrome (also called neuralgic amyotrophy, idiopathic brachial plexus neuritis, or acute brachial plexitis) is an idiopathic (possibly autoimmune) brachial neuritis that is characterized by a severe onset of acute shoulder pain that lasts a few days to a few weeks. This is often followed by weakness of the ipsilateral shoulder girdle muscles because of denervation atrophy. The condition affects men twice as often as women and usually resolves by 18 months, though up to 25% of patients can have a recurrence of this syndrome. The brachial neuritis of Parsonage-Turner typically affects the suprascapular nerve; less often it affects the axillary nerve and rarely does it involve the subscapular nerve. This syndrome may be misdiagnosed clinically as it can mimic other causes of neuropathy or shoulder pathology. Treatment is analgesics for pain and physical therapy for weakness.

  MR imaging findings of the brachial plexus with Parsonage-Turner syndrome include enlargement, enhancement, and a more pronounced amount of T2 hyperintensity of the affected brachial plexus than typically present. In the acute denervation phase, MR imaging of the shoulder usually demonstrates edema and/or enhancement of the muscles innervated by the suprascapular nerve, namely the infraspinatus and supraspinatus muscles. Chronically, the affected shoulder muscles may become atrophic and fatty infiltrated.

The normal brachial plexus on CT

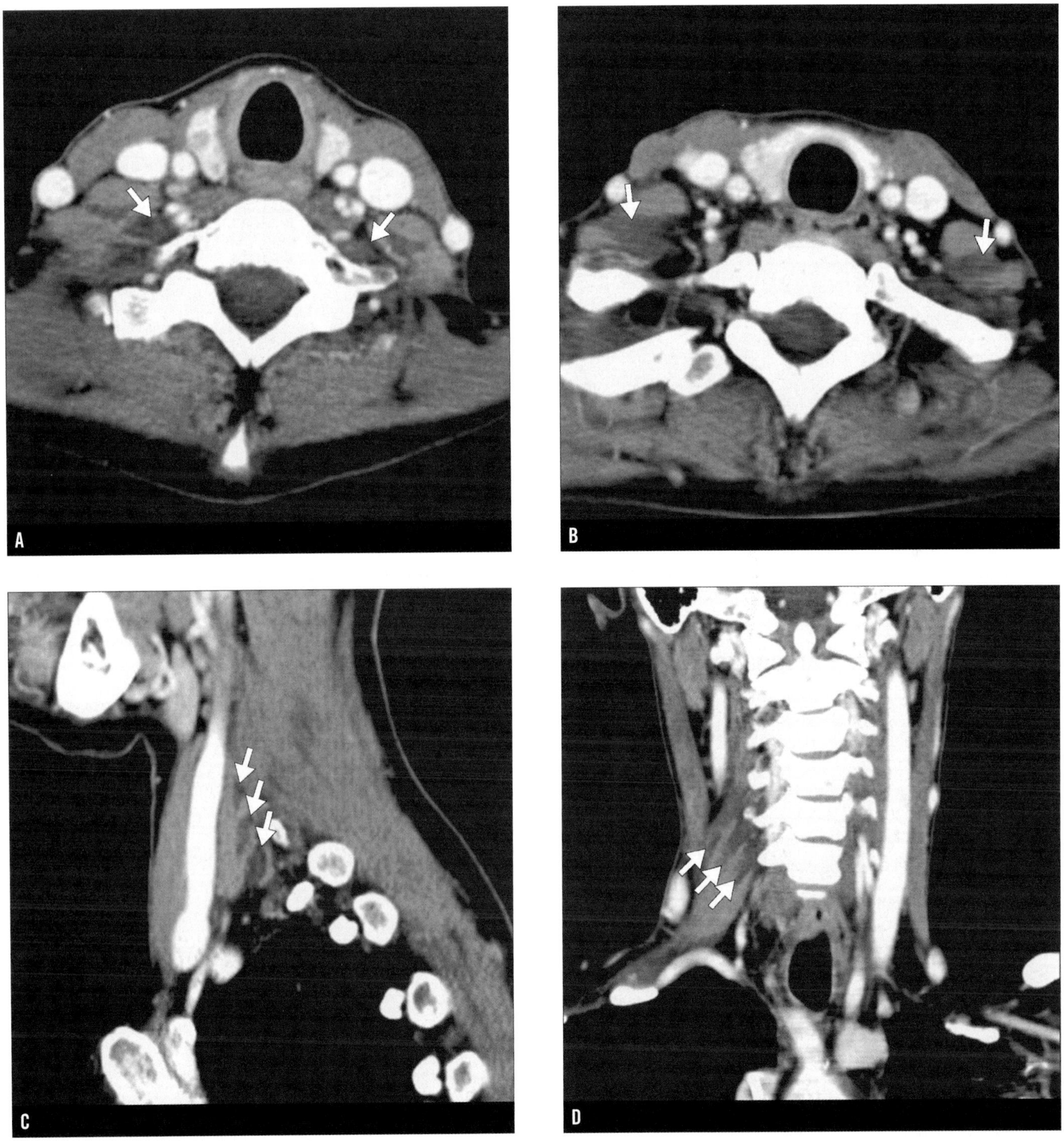

Axial (**A**, **B**), sagittal reformatted (**C**), and coronal reformatted (**D**) postcontrast CT images through the neck demonstrate normal hypoattenuating cervical roots of the brachial plexus (arrows, **A-D**). Image **B** best demonstrates the normal location of the brachial plexus interposed between the anterior and middle scalene muscles.

The normal brachial plexus on MRI

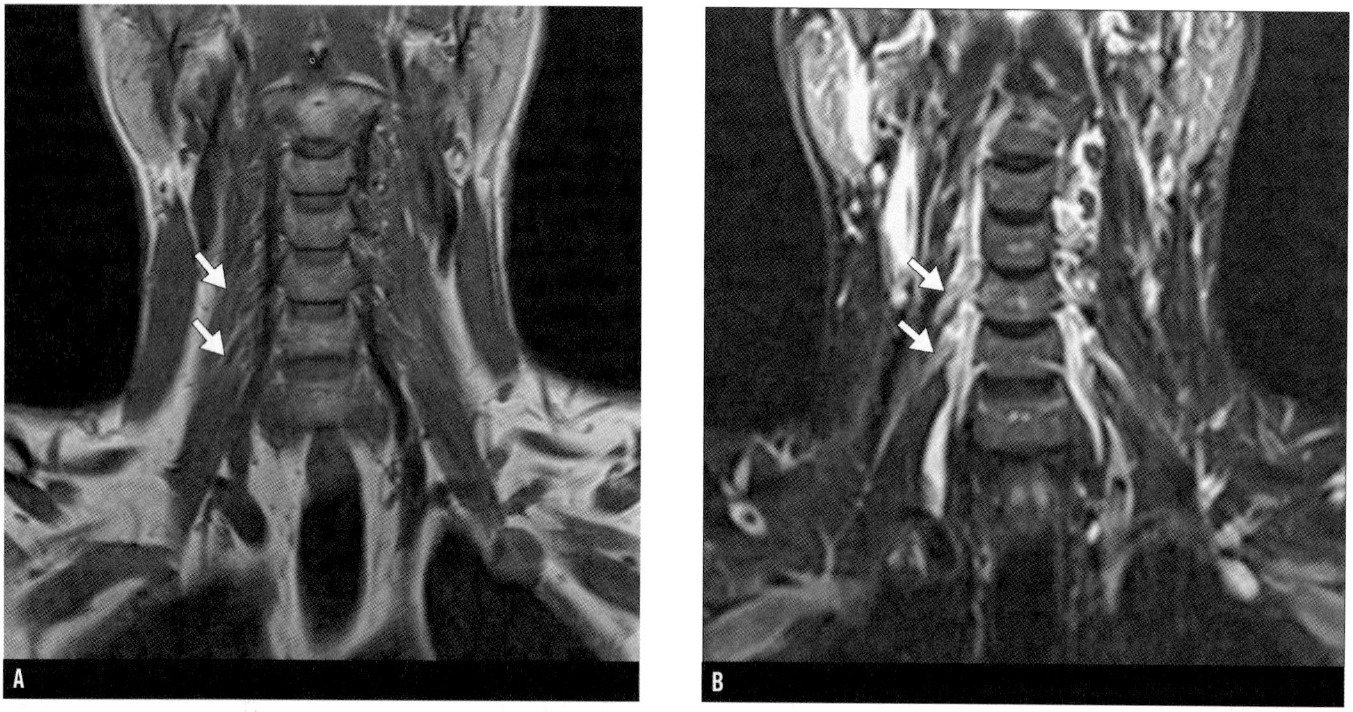

Different patient. Coronal T1 (**A**) and coronal STIR (**B**) MR images of the brachial plexus demonstrate some of the right cervical nerves contributing to a normal right brachial plexus (arrows, **A**, **B**).

Companion case: Parsonage-Turner syndrome

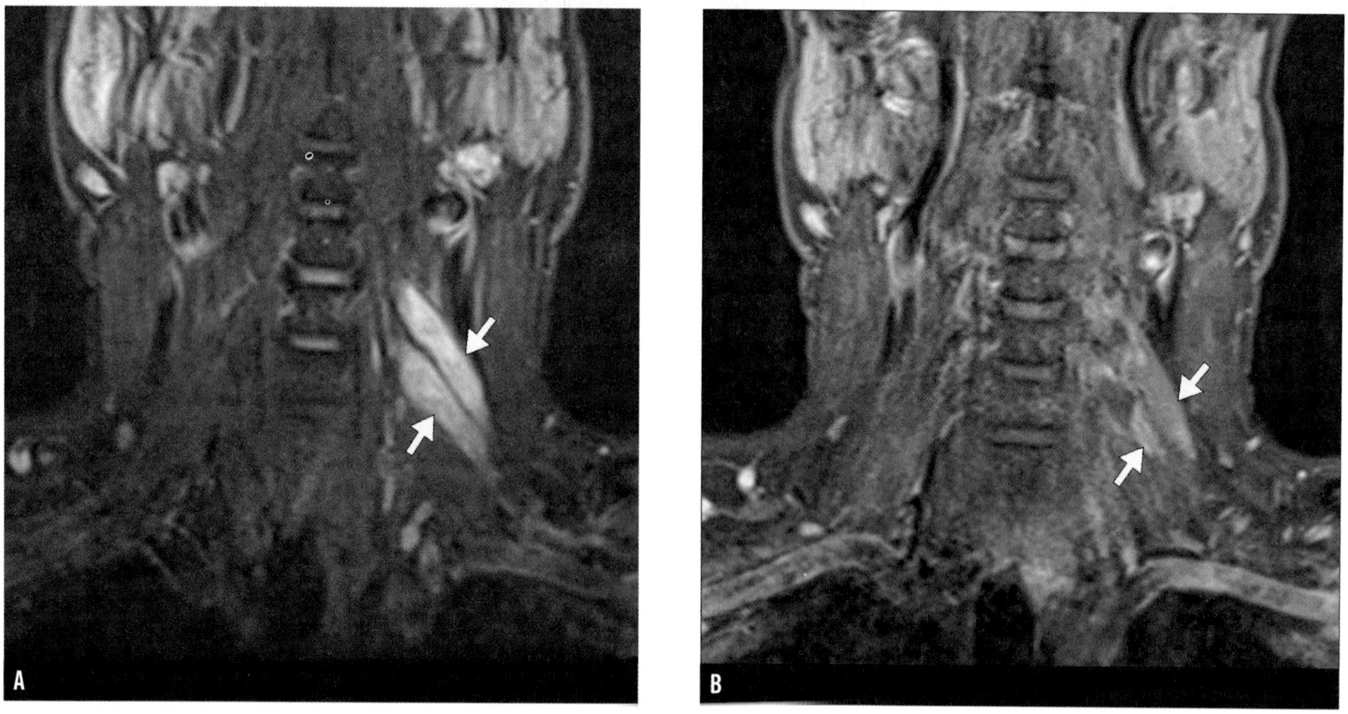

Coronal T2 (**A**), coronal postcontrast T1 with fat suppression (**B**), and axial postcontrast T1 with fat suppression (**C**) performed on a patient with acute left shoulder pain. The images demonstrate asymmetrically enlarged left C5 and C6 roots of the left brachial plexus which are abnormally T2 hyperintense (arrows, **A**) and abnormally enhancing (arrows, **B**, **C**). This patient had a clinical diagnosis of Parsonage-Turner syndrome.

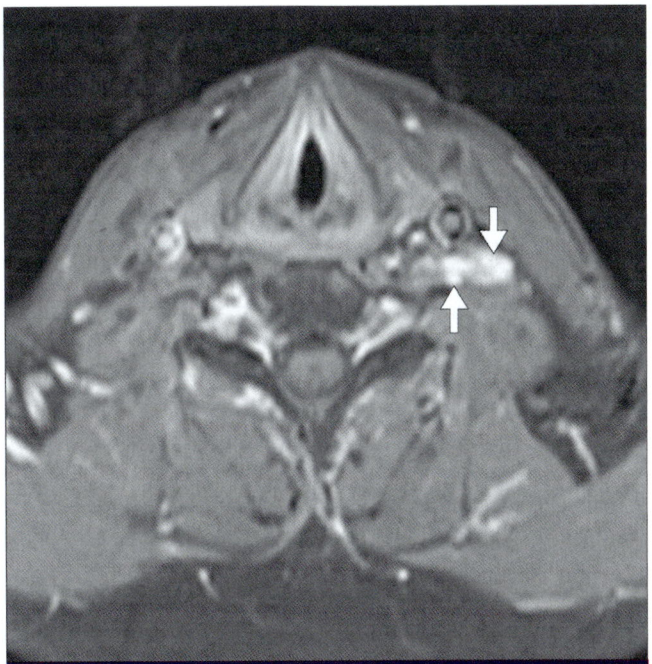

C

REFERENCES

Bowen BC, Verma A, Brandon AH, Fiedler JA. Radiation-induced brachial plexopathy: MR and clinical findings. *AJNR Am J Neuroradiol.* 1996;17(10):1932-1936.

Fathers E, Thrush D, Huson SM, Norman A. Radiation-induced brachial plexopathy in women treated for carcinoma of the breast. *Clin Rehabil.* 2002;16 (2):160-165.

Harry WG, Bennett JD, Guha SC. Scalene muscles and the brachial plexus: anatomical variations and their clinical significance. *Clin Anat.* 1997;10(4):250-252.

Helms CA, Martinez S, Speer KP. Acute brachial neuritis (Parsonage-Turner syndrome): MR imaging appearance—report of three cases. *Radiology.* 1998;207:255-259.

May DA, Disler DG, Jones EA, Balkissoon AA, Manaster BJ. Abnormal signal intensity in skeletal muscle at MR imaging: patterns, pearls, and pitfalls. *Radiographics.* 2000;20 Spec No:S295-S315.

Truong MT, Nadgir RN, Hirsch AE, Subramaniam RM, Wang JW, Wu R, Khandekar M, Nawaz AO, Sakai O. Brachial plexus contouring with CT and MR imaging in radiation therapy planning for head and neck cancer. *Radiographics.* 2010;30(4):1095-1103.

Xia P, Arnols HI, Ling CC. Three-dimensional con-formal radiation therapy and intensity-modulated radiation therapy. In: Leibel SA, Phillips TL, eds. *Textbook of Radiation Oncology.* Philadelphia, PA: Elsevier; 2004.

CASE 15 Thoracic duct

The thoracic duct is the common final trunk for many of the lymphatic channels. It has two primary roles: to carry 60% to 70% of ingested fat from the intestine to the circulatory system, and to carry lymph, which is made up of serous fluid, immunoglobulins, and lymphocytes. The thoracic duct measures approximately 38 cm to 45 cm in length in the adult patient and originates at the cisterna chyli, which is a patulous lymphatic sac located ventral to the second lumbar vertebra. The thoracic duct ascends in the medial right aspect of the thorax, typically crossing to the left of midline at the level of the aortic arch. The distal thoracic duct has a variable course, usually extending up to 3 cm cephalad to the clavicle; however, it can extend 5 cm or more cephalad to the clavicle prior to reversing its course to its venous termination. It normally extends posterior to the left internal jugular vein and most often terminates at or near the junction of the left internal jugular vein and left subclavian vein, although numerous variations of termination exist. The normal thoracic duct termination is focally enlarged and is termed the thoracic duct ampulla.

The thoracic duct generally follows fluid attenuation and signal on CT and MRI, respectively. Because of these imaging characteristics, a normal distal thoracic duct, especially its normally dilated ampullary portion, may be confused with a necrotic lymph node in the left supraclavicular region. Following the course of the thoracic duct from the left supraclavicular region and into the chest usually aids in differentiating this normal structure from pathology.

COMPANION CASES

- **Contrast reflux into the thoracic duct.** Normally, there are a couple of valves in the distal thoracic duct that prevent venous blood from refluxing into the thoracic duct. However, occasionally, venous contrast may reflux into the distal thoracic duct during a forceful contrast injection and can be visualized on either contrast-enhanced CT or MRI. This is an incidental finding.
- **Change in the thoracic duct size during inspiration and expiration.** There are many factors that influence the flow of lymph in the thoracic duct, one of which relates to respiration. During normal inspiration, negative intrathoracic pressure increases the amount of lymph flow into the intrathoracic portion of the thoracic duct, with numerous valves preventing significant backflow of lymph in the duct. During expiration, positive intrathoracic pressure promotes cephalad flow of lymph outside the chest and into the distal thoracic duct of the neck, which subsequently drains into the venous system. Therefore, during inspiration, the distal thoracic duct in the neck is small in caliber, and during expiration, the distal thoracic duct is enlarged in caliber. This change in size, which may be encountered if the patient has had a chest CT performed during inspiration and a neck CT performed during quiet respiration/expiration, may be a useful imaging finding in select cases where it is difficult to differentiate a normal distal thoracic duct from a necrotic lymph node.
- **Cervical thoracic duct cyst.** A cervical thoracic duct cyst represents a lymphocele of the neck arising from the distal thoracic duct or one of its adjacent tributaries. Resected specimens in the literature have shown the wall of these cysts to contain a thin endothelial lining and fibroconnective tissue but no epithelial lining. The lack of an epithelial lining differentiates a cervical thoracic duct cyst/lymphocele from a lymphangioma, which contains an epithelial lining. A cervical thoracic duct cyst most often presents as asymptomatic left supraclavicular fullness. However, symptoms of pain, pressure, dyspnea, dysphagia, and hoarseness from recurrent laryngeal injury have been described. While the etiology of a thoracic duct cyst is unknown, various theories have been proposed, including a congenital blind ending sac, a congenital weakness of the duct wall, or an acquired injury such as from prior trauma, inflammation, or infection. If asymptomatic, treatment is conservative. Surgery is advocated for symptomatic cases. As with the normal thoracic duct, a cervical thoracic duct cyst will be isodense and isointense to CSF on CT and MRI, respectively. Differentiating a cervical thoracic duct cyst from the normal ampulla of the thoracic duct can sometimes be difficult. However, a cervical thoracic duct cyst will be significantly larger and will have a saccular blind ending in the left lower neck, as opposed to a normal distal thoracic duct ampulla which can usually be traced to the thoracic duct.
- **Metastatic lymphadenopathy from papillary thyroid carcinoma.** Papillary thyroid carcinoma metastasizes to the cervical lymph nodes in 35% to 80% of patients. The metastatic lymphadenopathy from papillary thyroid carcinoma can have a myriad of appearances, ranging from completely or partially necrotic/cystic, solidly enhancing or containing a focal nodule of enhancement, or containing variable amounts of mineralization. Differentiating a cystic metastatic lesion in the left supraclavicular region (such as from papillary thyroid carcinoma) from a benign cervical thoracic duct cyst, or even a prominent ampulla of a normal thoracic duct, can be difficult. In indeterminate cases, fine needle aspiration of the finding may be necessary.
- **Chylous leak with the formation of a lymphocele and a chylous pleural effusion.** A chylous leak (fistula) generally occurs following trauma to a portion of the lymphatic system, especially the thoracic duct. Common traumatic causes include penetrating or blunt direct

injury, a fracture of the first rib, thoracic surgery, or during a neck dissection (occurring in 1%-2% of complete neck dissections). Most cases of chylous leaks are initially treated conservatively, including direct manual pressure and dietary restrictions. If this is not effective, then surgical repair with ligation of the injured duct(s) or an interventional procedure that embolizes the thoracic duct via percutaneous guided lymphangiogaphy can be performed. Briefly, this interventional procedure first requires a lymphangiogram, usually performed by accessing the lymphatic system of one or both feet. Once the cysterna chyli is visualized during the lymphangiogram, a needle followed by a catheter is placed percutaneously through the abdomen into the cysterna chyli to gain access to the thoracic duct. In order to avoid bowel perforation during this portion of the procedure, oral contrast is usually administered the night before the procedure to visualize the bowel. After the site of the chylous leak is fully imaged by fluoroscopy, coils and/or glue are placed into the thoracic duct to treat the chylous leak.

Normal thoracic duct

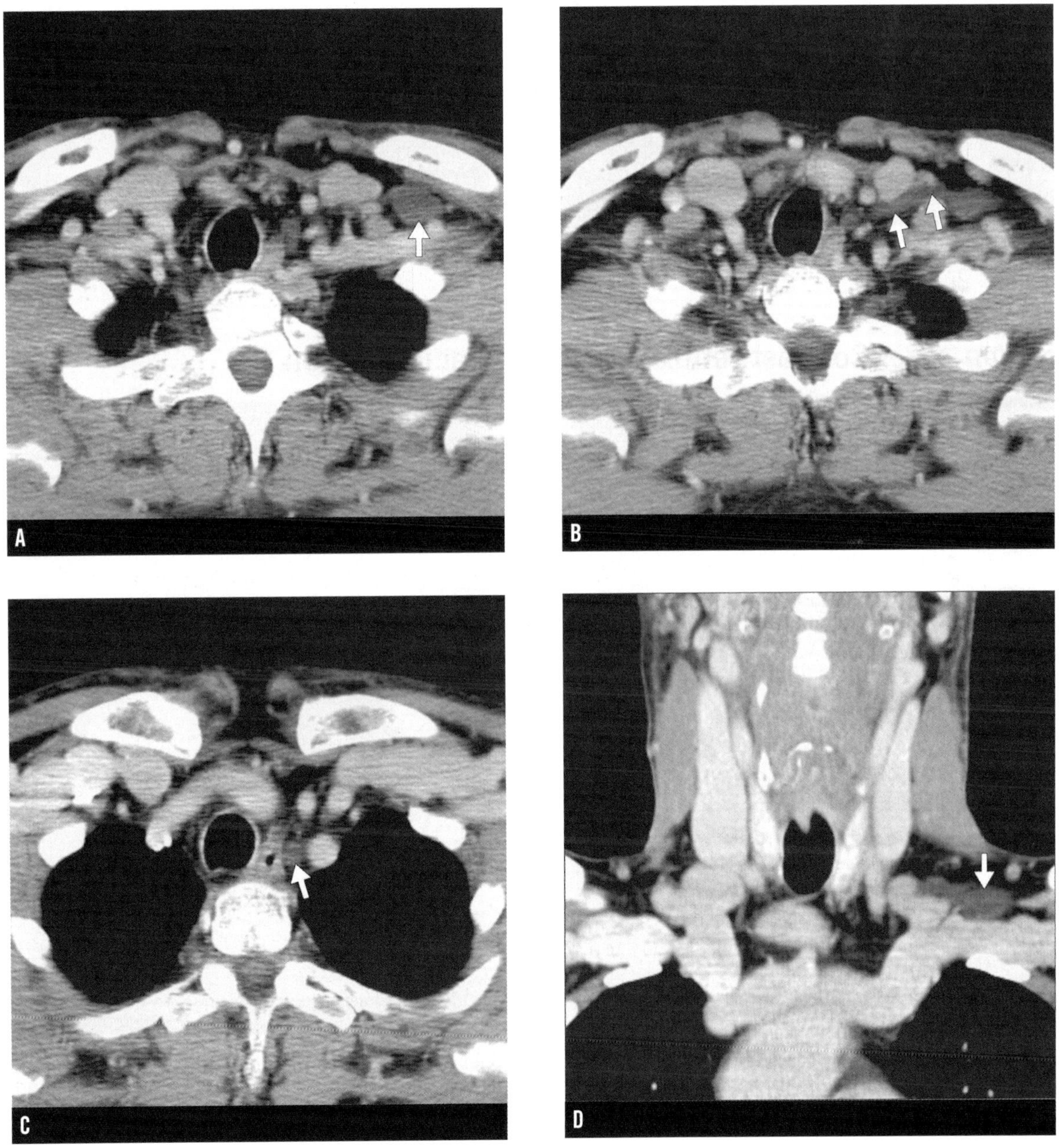

Postcontrast axial CT images through the neck from superior to inferior (**A-C**) and postcontrast coronal reformatted CT images through the neck from anterior to posterior (**D-F**) demonstrate a normal thoracic duct (arrows, **A-F**). A focally enlarged portion of the distal thoracic duct on images **A** and **D** could easily be confused with a necrotic lymph node. However, this focal prominence is in direct contiguity with the remainder of the thoracic duct and simply represents the normal thoracic duct ampulla.

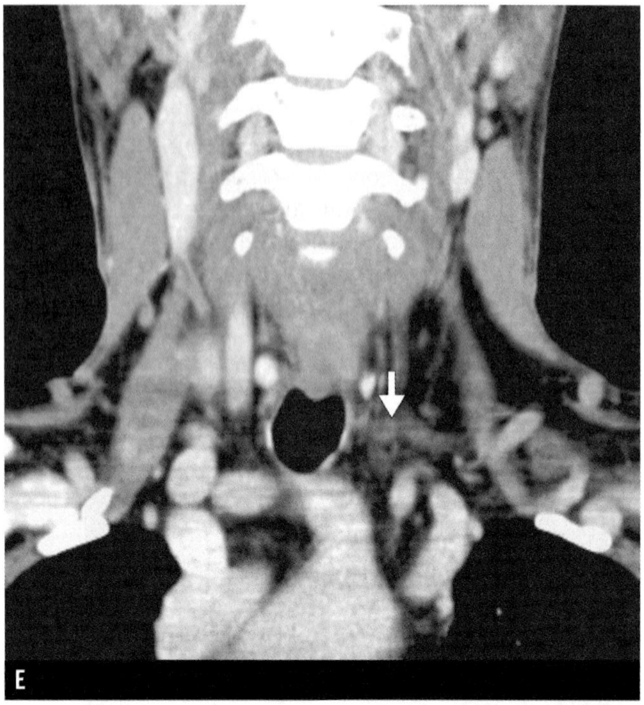

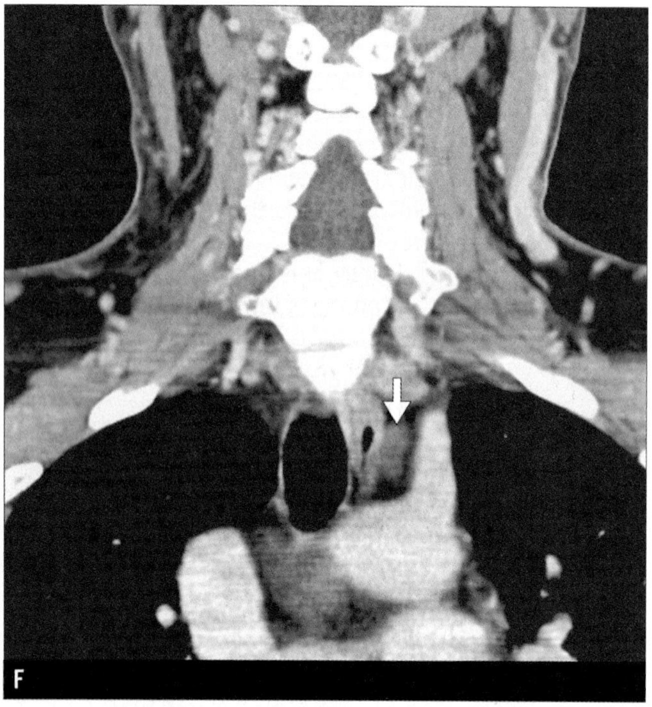

Companion case: Contrast reflux into the thoracic duct on CT

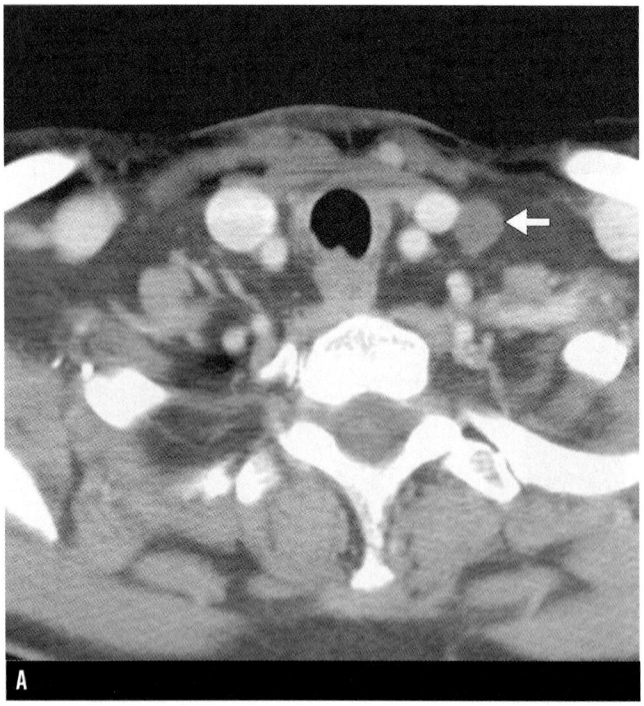

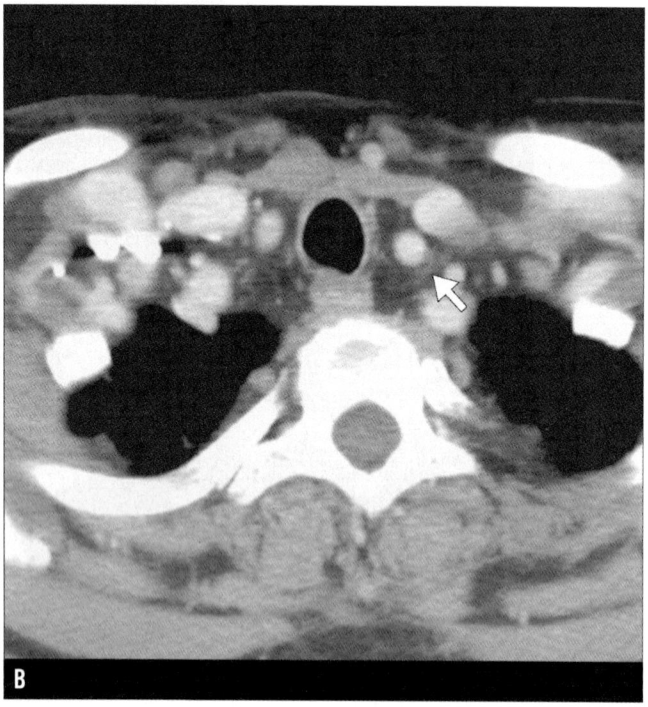

Contrast-enhanced axial CT images viewed from superior to inferior (**A**-**C**) demonstrate a circumscribed, oval hypodensity in the left supraclavicular region (arrow, **A**) that is contiguous with a small duct extending into the left aspect of the superior mediastinum (arrows, **B**, **C**), compatible with a normal thoracic duct. A coronal reformatted CT image from the same study (**D**) demonstrates normal focal dilation of the thoracic duct ampulla (arrow, **D**) terminating at the junction between the left internal jugular vein and the left subclavian vein. Contrast-enhanced axial (**E**, **F**) and coronal reformatted (**G**) CT images from a follow-up study of the same patient demonstrate pronounced contrast refluxing into ampulla of the thoracic duct (arrows, **E**-**G**).

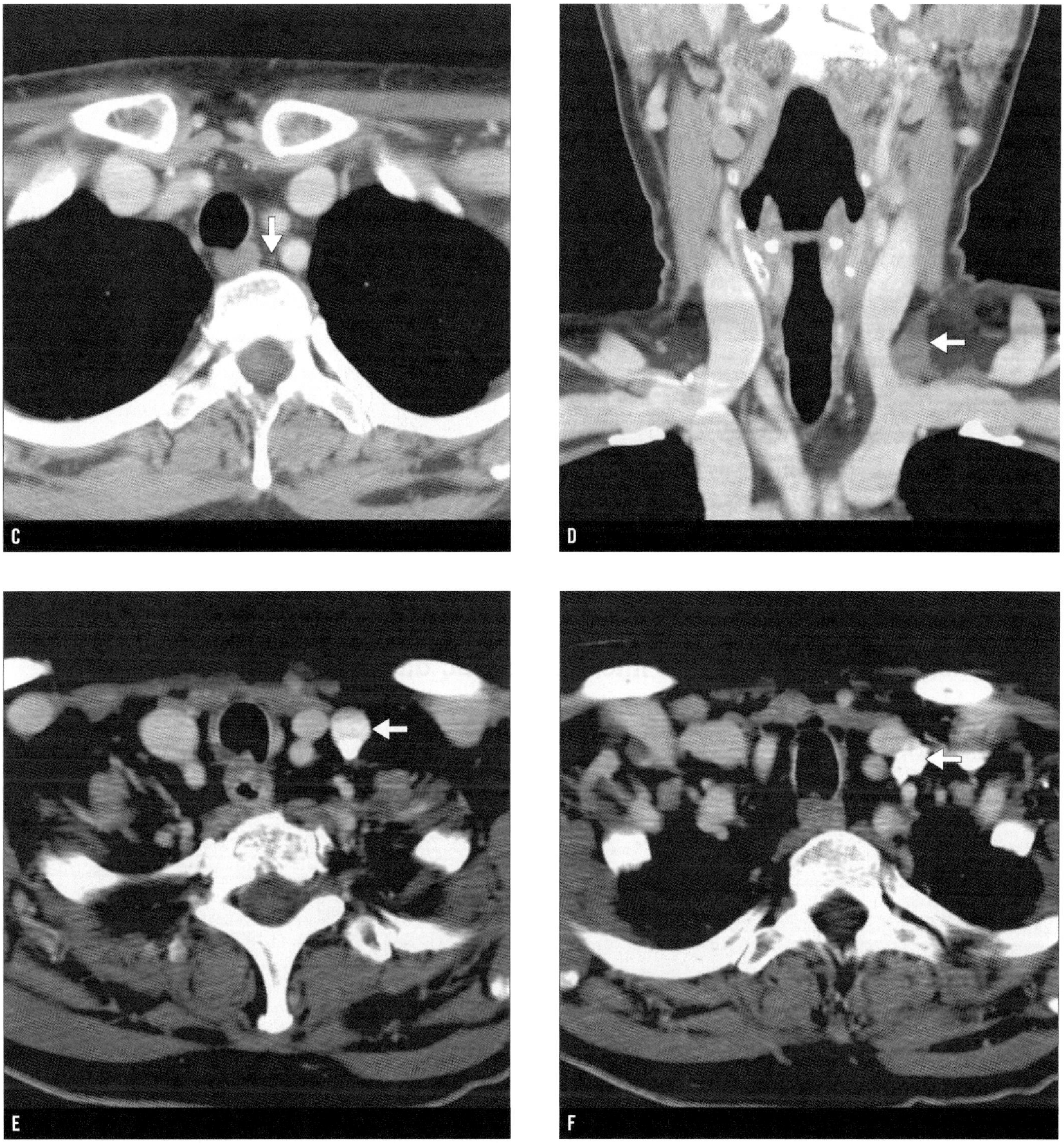

Companion case: Change in the thoracic duct size during inspiration and expiration

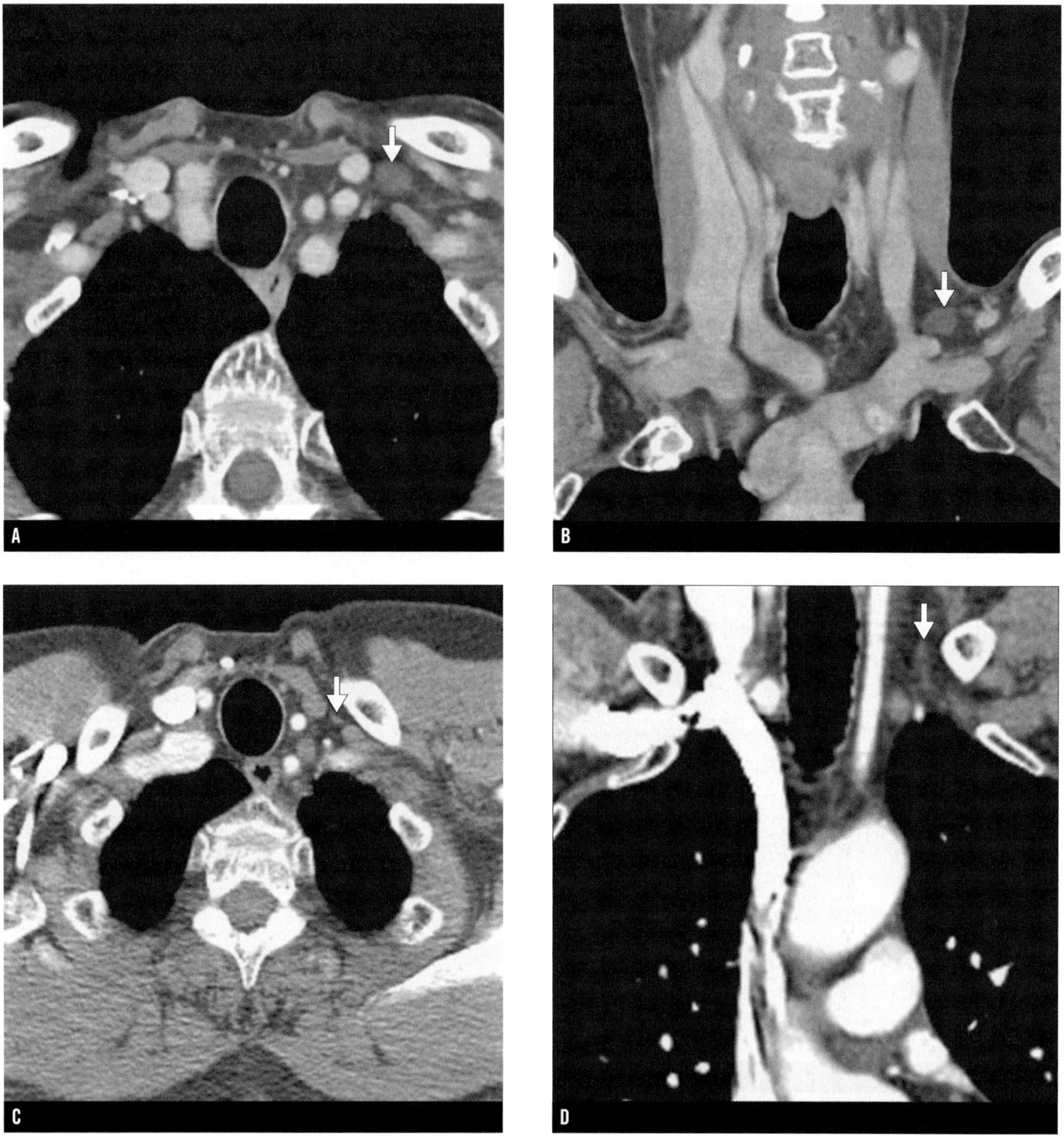

Contrast-enhanced axial (**A**) and coronal reformatted (**B**) CT images from a CT of the neck demonstrate normal dilation of the thoracic duct ampulla (arrows, **A**, **B**). Postcontrast axial (**C**) and coronal (**D**) CT images from a CT chest obtained on the same day and immediately preceding the neck CT demonstrate a decreased caliber of the distal thoracic duct (arrows, **C**, **D**). The relatively large distal thoracic duct on the CT neck occurs because it is obtained during quiet respiration, and the resultant relatively postitive lung pressure promotes lymph drainage from the chest into the distal thoracic duct. The small caliber of the distal thoracic duct during the CT chest occurs because it is obtained during inspiration and thus there is negative intrathoracic pressure. While negative intrathoracic pressure promotes flow of lymph in the intrathoracic portion of the thoracic duct, it does not promote flow of lymph into the neck.

Companion case: Cervical thoracic duct cyst

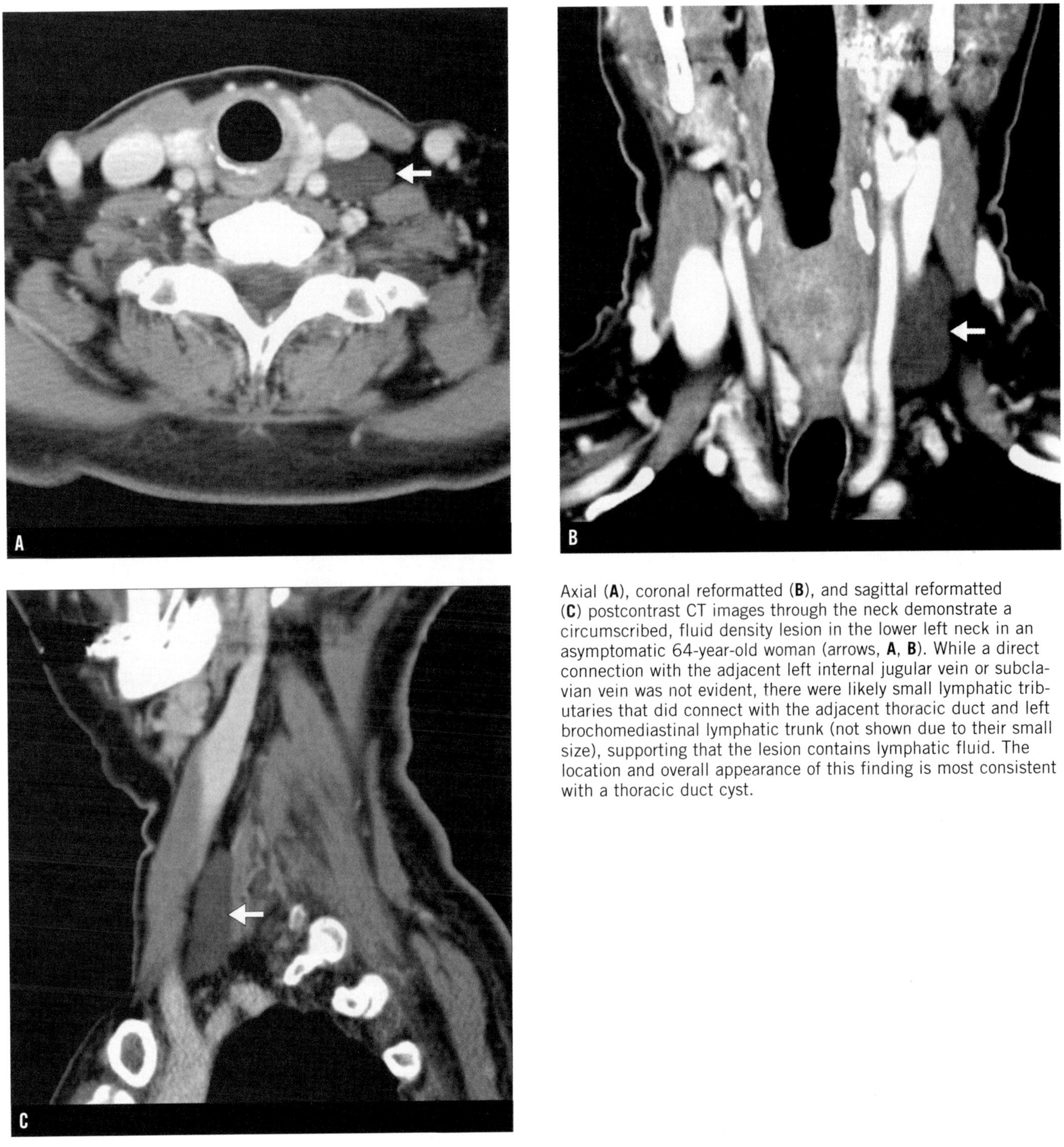

Axial (**A**), coronal reformatted (**B**), and sagittal reformatted (**C**) postcontrast CT images through the neck demonstrate a circumscribed, fluid density lesion in the lower left neck in an asymptomatic 64-year-old woman (arrows, **A**, **B**). While a direct connection with the adjacent left internal jugular vein or subclavian vein was not evident, there were likely small lymphatic tributaries that did connect with the adjacent thoracic duct and left brochomediastinal lymphatic trunk (not shown due to their small size), supporting that the lesion contains lymphatic fluid. The location and overall appearance of this finding is most consistent with a thoracic duct cyst.

Companion case: Metastatic lymphadenopathy from papillary thyroid carcinoma

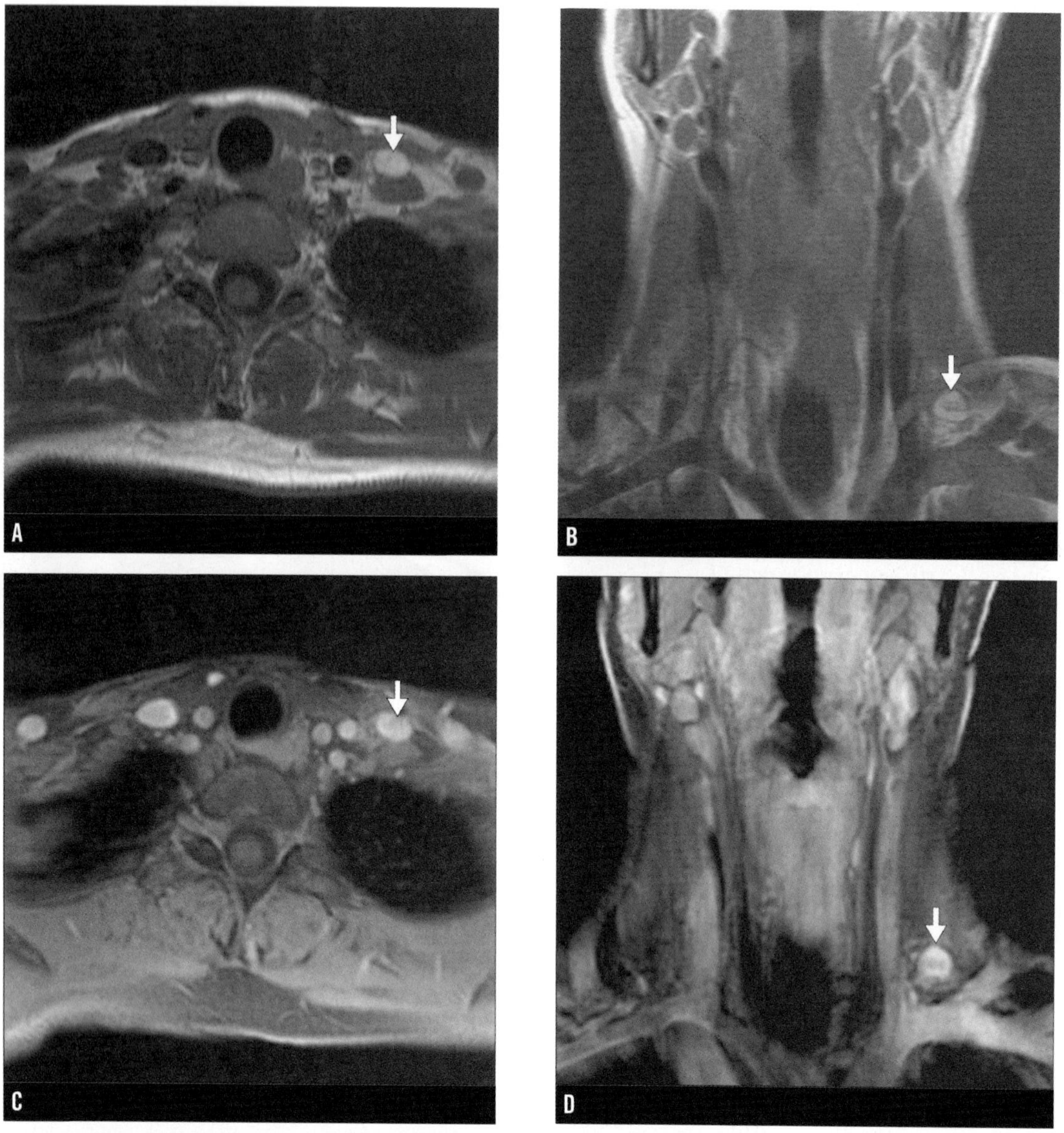

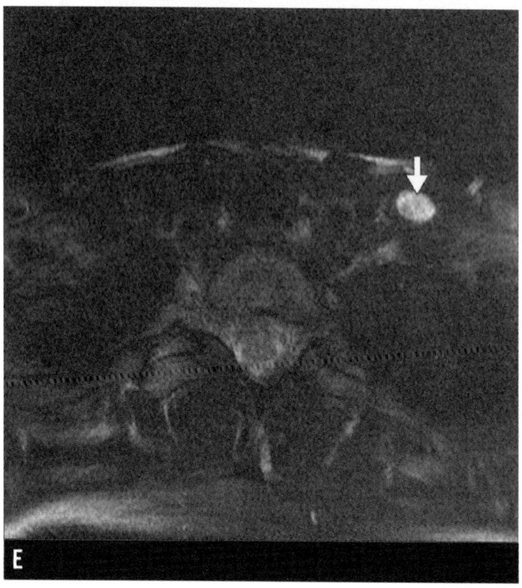

Axial (**A**) and coronal (**B**) unenhanced T1, axial (**C**) and coronal (**D**) postcontrast T1 with fat suppression, and axial T2 with fat suppression (**E**) MR images demonstrate an ovoid, enhancing, T2 hyperintense lesion (arrows, **A-E**) near the junction of the left internal jugular and left subclavian veins. While this is in a similar location as the normal thoracic duct termination, there is a lack of contiguity with left subclavian vein and/or left internal jugular vein and there is no evidence of a duct emanating from this finding into the superior mediastinum to suggest that this represents a portion of a normal thoracic duct. This finding was pathologically proven to represent a nodal metastasis in this 34-year-old woman with a history of papillary thyroid carcinoma.

Companion case: Chylous leak with the formation of a lymphocele and a chylous pleural effusion

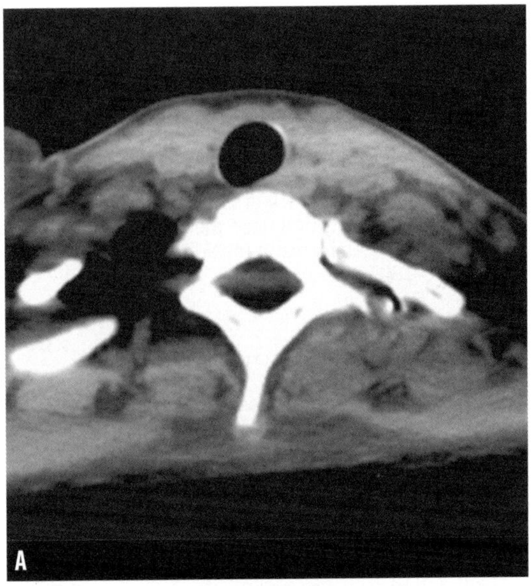

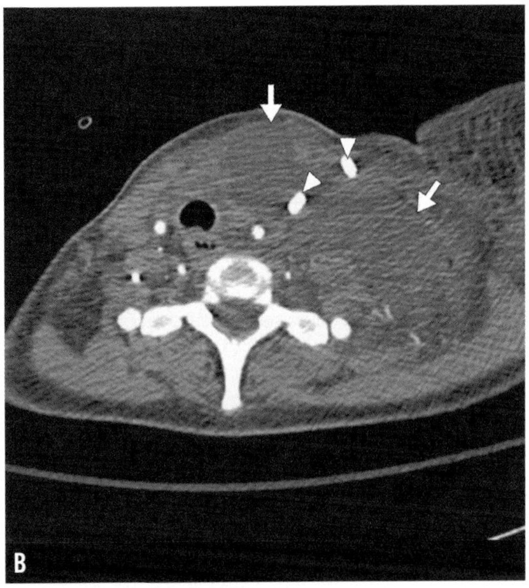

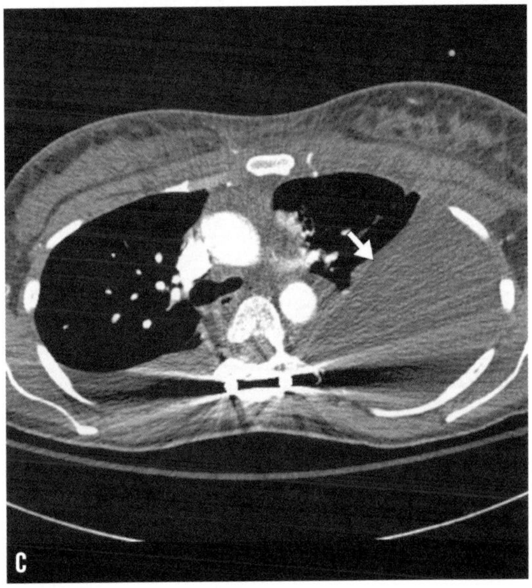

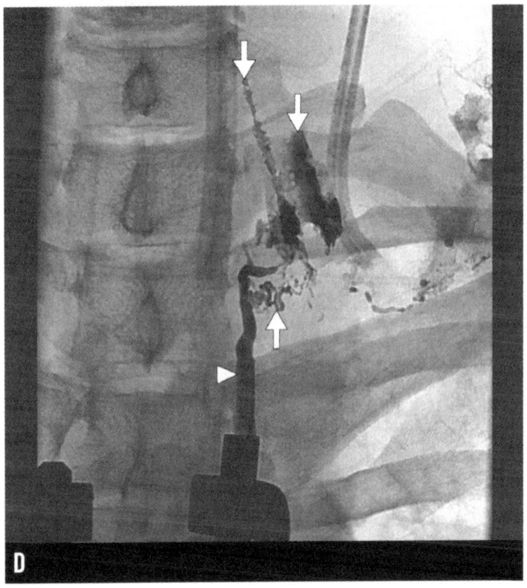

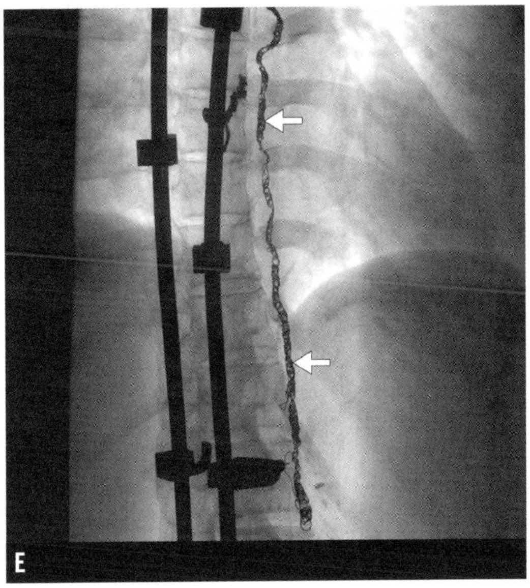

An unenhanced axial CT image through the lower neck prior to surgery (**A**) demonstrates a normal noncontrast appearance of the lower neck. Unenhanced axial CT images through the lower neck (**B**) and lungs (**C**) were obtained shortly following a left neck lymph node dissection for metastatic papillary thyroid carcinoma that was complicated by injury to the thoracic duct. Image **B** demonstrates a large, heterogeneous fluid collection in the lower left neck suspicious for a lymphocele, given the history (arrows, **B**). Image **C** demonstrates a large left pleural effusion, suspicious for a large left chylous pleural effusion (arrow, **C**), again given the history. A drain in the lower left neck is noted (arrowheads, **B**). An anterior to posterior (AP) image from a subsequently performed lymphangiogram (**D**) demonstrates a normal distal thoracic duct in the chest (arrowhead, **D**) and an injury to the distal-most aspect of the thoracic duct in the neck with evidence of extensive contrast extravasation (arrows, **D**). Following extensive coil embolization, an AP image (**E**) demonstrates therapeutic occlusion of the thoracic duct (arrows, **E**).

REFERENCES

Brauchle RW, Risin SA, Ghorbani RP, Pereira KD. Cervical Thoracic duct cysts: a case report and review of the literature. *Arch Otolaryngol Head Neck Surg.* 2003;129(5):581-583.

Greenfield, J and Gottlieb, M. Variations in the Terminal Portion of the Human Thoracic Duct. *AMA Arch Surg.* 1956;73(6):955-999.

Imhof H, Czerny C, Hörmann M, Krestan C. Tumors and tumor-like lesions of the neck: from childhood to adult. *Eur Radioll.* 2004;14 (Suppl 4):L155–L165.

Langford RJ, Daudia a T, Malins TJ. A morphological study of the thoracic duct at the jugulo-subclavian junction. *J Craniomaxillo Surg.* 1999;27(2):100-104.

Lecanu JB, Gallas D, Biacabe B, Bonfils P. Lymphocele of the thoracic duct presenting as a left supraclavicular mass: a case report and review of the literature. *Auris Nasus Larynx.* 2001;28(3):275-277.

Liu M-E, Branstetter BF, Whetstone J, Escott EJ. Normal CT appearance of the distal thoracic duct. *AJR. Am J Roentgenol.* 2006;187(6):1615-1620.

Moesgaard L, Baerentzen S, Mirz F. Cervical thoracic duct cyst: a differential diagnosis of left supraclavicular swelling. *Eur Arch Otorhinolaryngol.* 2007;264(7):797-799.

Scorza LB, Goldstein BJ, Mahraj RP. Modern management of chylous leak following head and neck surgery: a discussion of percutaneous lymphangiography-guided cannulation and embolization of the thoracic duct. *Otolaryngol Clin North Am.* 2008;41(6):1231-1240.

Wu L-M, et al. The accuracy of ultrasonography in the preoperative diagnosis of cervical lymph node metastasis in patients with papillary thyroid carcinoma: a meta-analysis. *Eur J Radiol.* 2012; 81(8):1798-1805.

CASE 16 Right lymphatic duct

The right lymphatic duct is the final common pathway of lymph drainage from the right aspect of the head and neck, right arm, right thorax, right lung, right heart, and a portion of the liver. The right jugular trunk, subclavian trunk, and bronchomediastinal trunk drain lymph from these areas and combine to form the right lymphatic duct; however, any or all of these major trunks may insert directly into the major veins near the right venous angle (ie, junction of the right internal jugular and subclavian veins). Unlike the thoracic duct, which usually measures up to 45 cm in the adult patient, the right thoracic duct is very small and only measures approximately 1.25 cm in length, most often terminating near right venous angle. Due to its small size, a right lymphatic duct may not able to be delineated on cross–sectional imaging. However, occasionally, it may be normally enlarged, particularly if there is a concomitantly hypoplastic thoracic duct.

COMPANION CASE

- **Right lymphatic duct cyst.** Like the cervical thoracic duct cyst, a right lymphatic duct cyst represents a lymphocele arising from the duct or one of its adjacent tributaries. Very little has been written about the right lymphatic duct cyst. However, it is likely that this entity shares the same characteristics and possible etiologies as the cervical thoracic duct cyst located in the left supraclavicular fossa. A right lymphatic duct cyst is usually an incidental finding, unless it is large enough to result in mass effect. On imaging, a right lymphatic duct cyst will be characterized as a circumscribed, blind ending fluid collection in the lower right neck that is isodense and isointense to CSF on CT and MRI, respectively. As is the case with a thoracic duct cyst, differentiating a right lower neck cystic metastatic lesion from an incidental right lymphatic duct cyst can be difficult. In indeterminate cases, fine needle aspiration may be necessary.

Right lymphatic duct

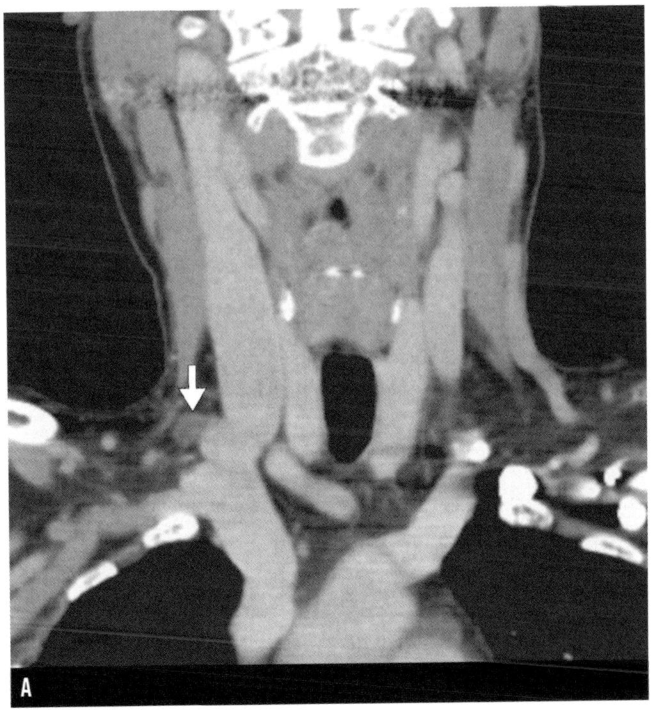

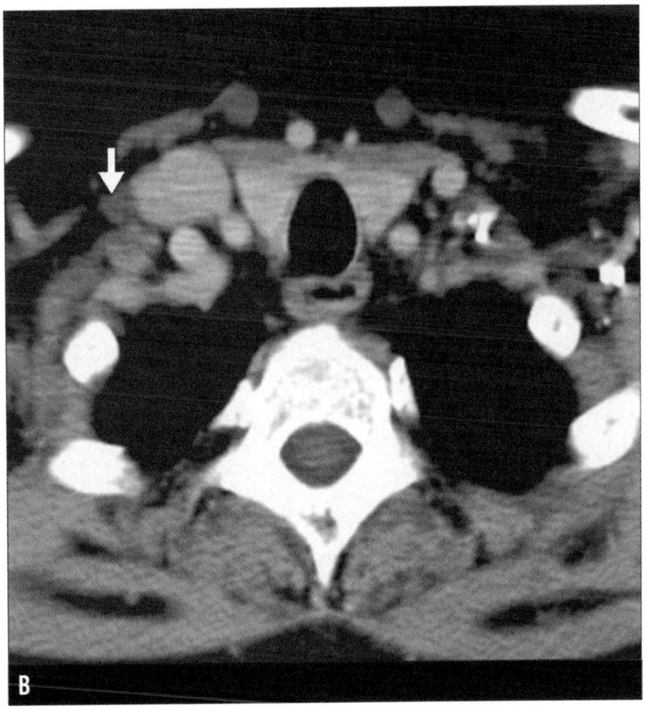

Postcontrast coronal reformatted CT image (**A**) and postcontrast axial CT images from inferior to superior (**B**-**E**) demonstrate a normal right lymphatic duct terminating in the distal right internal jugular vein (arrow, **A**) and extending slightly laterally (arrows, **B**, **C**). This continues cephalad and medially into the lower right neck as the jugular trunk (arrows, **D**, **E**).

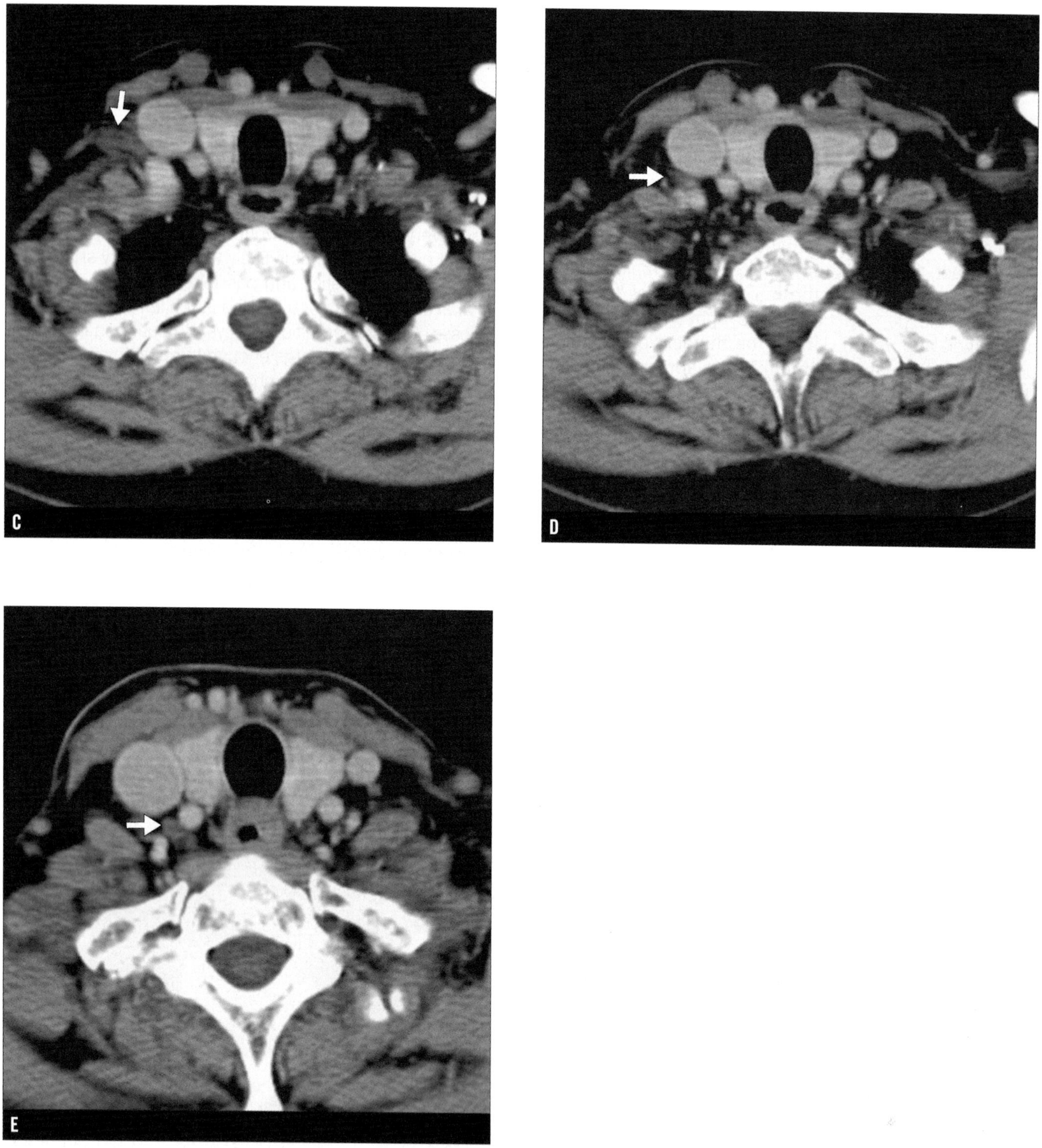
C
D
E

Right lymphatic duct

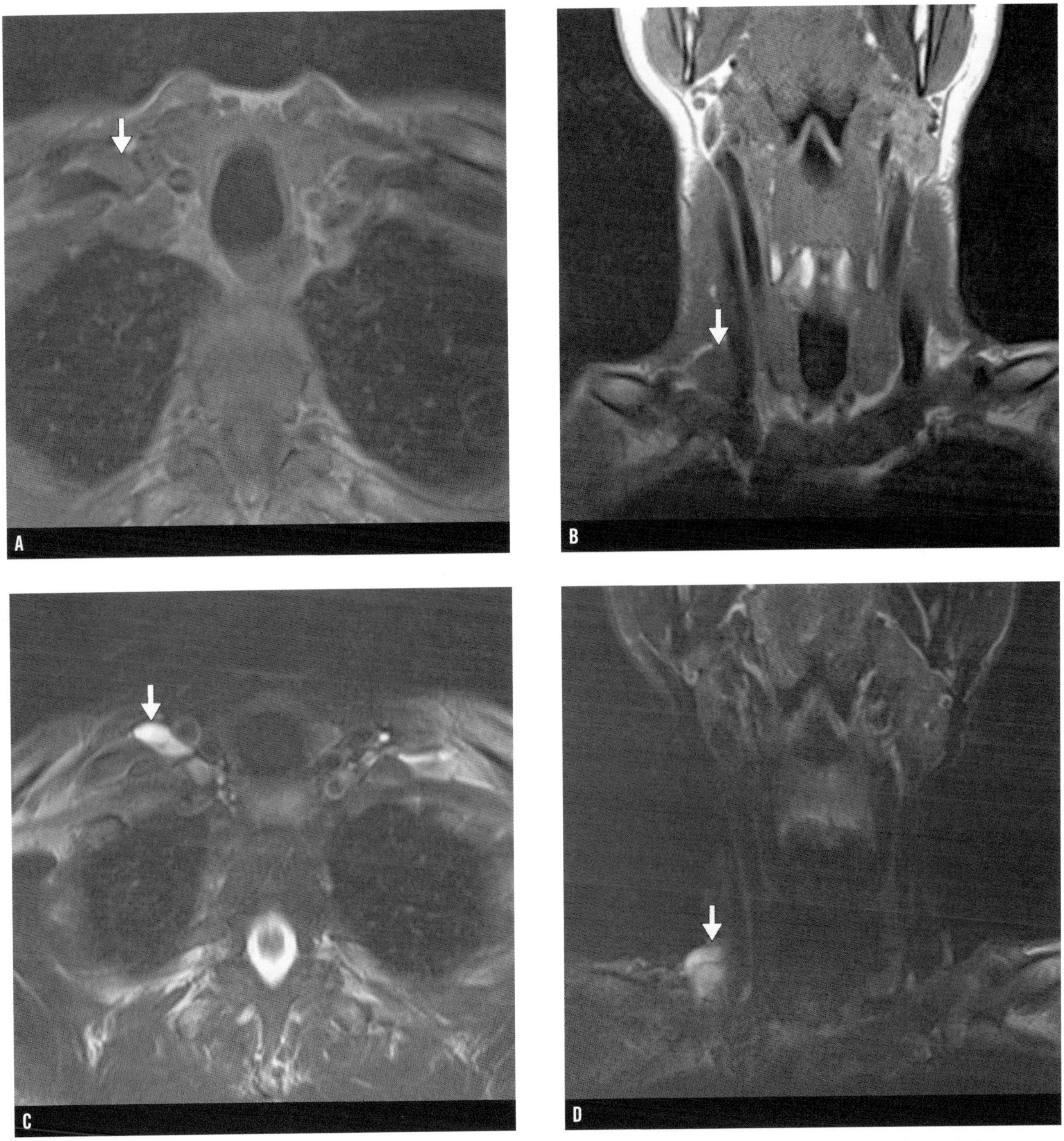

Different patient. Axial (**A**) and coronal (**B**) T1 as well as axial (**C**) and coronal (**D**) T2 with fat suppression MR images demonstrate a T1 isointense and T2 hyperintense structure at the junction between the right internal jugular vein and the right subclavian vein, compatible with the right lymphatic duct. Small T2 hyperintense tributaries were identified emanating from this structure (not shown), a finding which may be identified with a right lymphatic duct.

Companion case: Right lymphatic duct cyst

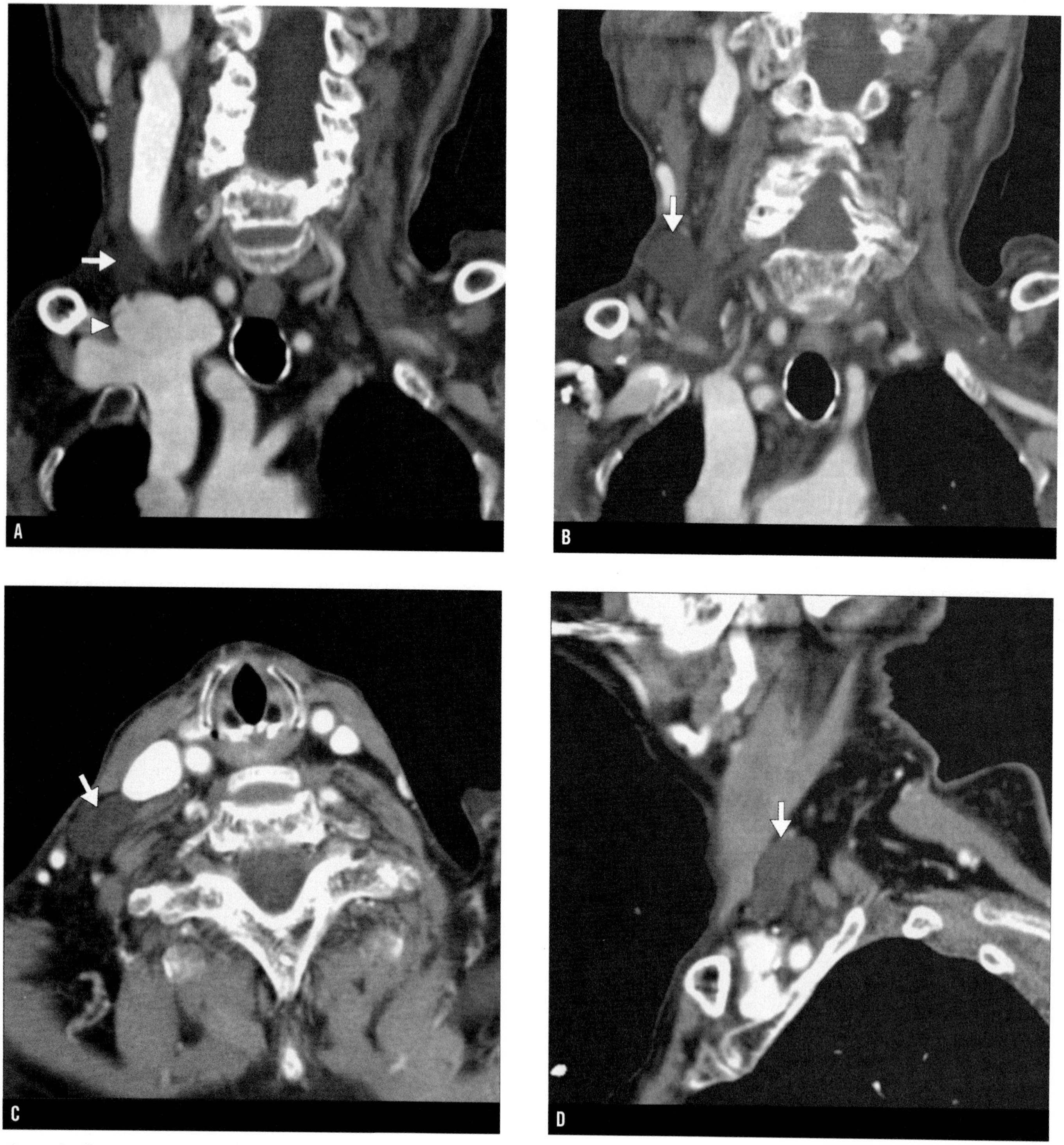

Coronal reformatted (**A**, **B**), axial (**C**), and sagittal reformatted (**D**) postcontrast CT images through the neck demonstrate a circumscribed, fluid density structure in the lower right neck (arrows, **A-D**), which communicates with a bulbous venous dilation at the junction between the right internal jugular vein and the right subclavian vein (arrowhead, **A**). Axial T2 (**E**) and postcontrast axial T1 (**F**) MR images through the neck demonstrate the same finding to be homogeneously T2 hyperintense and nonenhancing, respectively (arrows, **E**, **F**). A definable duct emanating from the fluid density structure was not evident on any of the additional images from the study, and therefore the finding was not consistent with a right lymphatic duct. Given its location, blind-ending morphology, and termination into the right venous angle, the constellation of findings is most consistent with a right lymphatic duct cyst.

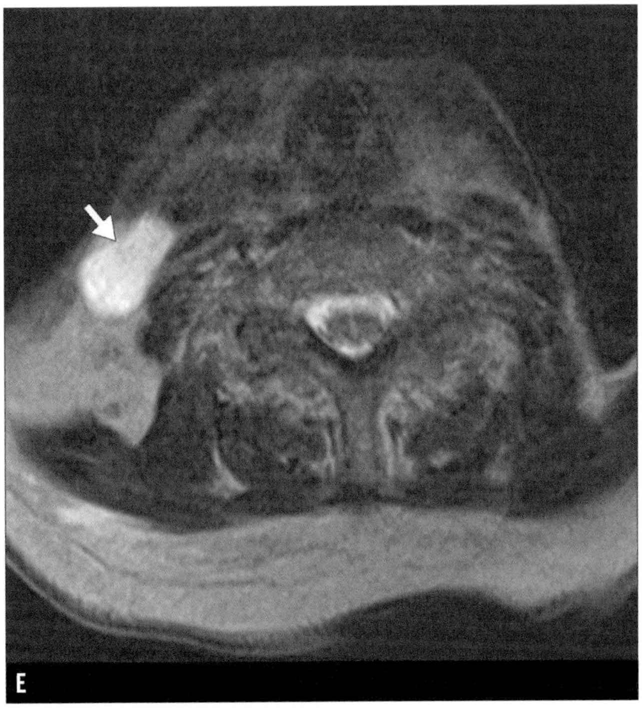

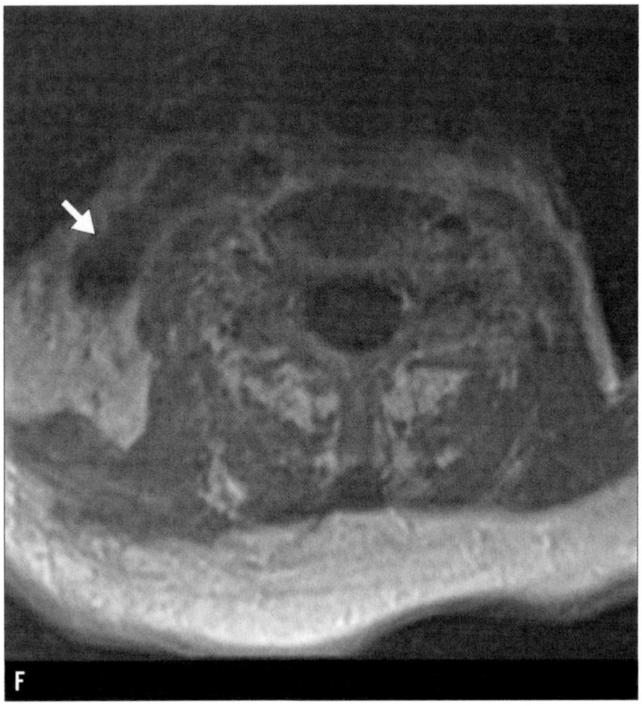

REFERENCES

Imhof H, Czerny C, Hörmann M, Krestan C. Tumors and tumor-like lesions of the neck: from childhood to adult. *Eur Radiol.* 2004;14 (Suppl 4):L155-L165.

Lecanu JB, Gallas D, Biacabe B, Bonfils P. Lymphocele of the thoracic duct presenting as a left supraclavicular mass: a case report and review of the literature. *Auris Nasus Larynx.* 2001;28(3):275-277.

Liu M-E, Branstetter BF, Whetstone J, Escott EJ. Normal CT appearance of the distal thoracic duct. *AJR Am J Roentgenology.* 2006;187(6):1615-1620.

Schünke M, Schulte E, Schumacher U, Ross LM, Lamperti ED. *Thieme Atlas of Anatomy: Neck and Internal Organs.* New York, NY: Thieme; 2006:370.

CASE 17 Venous valves and focal dilation of veins

Competent valves in veins function to prevent retrograde flow of venous blood as it returns to the heart. Relative to the flow of venous blood, the wall of the vein will often have a focal, tulip-shaped dilation immediately distal to the valves (ie, closer to the heart). This focal dilation is related to the distensibility of the vein and repetitive pooling of blood against closed valves. While most neck veins are valveless, valves in the neck will close during positive intrathoracic pressure (ie, expiration) and will open during negative intrathoracic pressure (ie, inspiration). Most of neck valves that have been described have a bicuspid morphology, although single cusp and tricuspid valves have also been reported. As it pertains to head and neck imaging, valves may be present in the internal jugular veins, bilateral subclavian veins, and uncommonly the left brachiocephalic vein, and each of these valves may be accompanied with focal dilation. These areas of focal dilation can be confused with soft tissue lesions, such as pathologic lymph nodes, particularly when unenhanced or poorly enhanced.

A few specific locations of normal venous dilation can be particularly problematic when interpreting CT or MRI neck imaging. These include the inferior jugular bulb, axillary vein, and subclavian vein.

The inferior bulb represents a focal dilation at the caudal termination of the internal jugular vein, just prior to its confluence with the ipsilateral subclavian vein. As an aside, the superior jugular bulb represents the commonly known jugular bulb located in the jugular fossa.

The axillary vein is a continuation of the basilic vein, beginning at the level of the lower margin of the teres major muscle and extending to the level of the lower border of the first rib, after which it becomes the subclavian vein. The subclavian vein lies upon its respective first rib, anterior to the anterior scalene muscle and posterior to clavicle. It joins with the ipsilateral internal jugular vein to form the innominate vein (also called brachiocephalic vein), which ultimately drains into the superior vena cava and right heart.

Depending on the side of the contrast injection, imaging immediately following a contrast injection can result in pronounced enhancement of the axillary, subclavian, and innominate veins on the side of the injection, but poor enhancement of the contralateral axillary, subclavian and innominate veins. The poorly enhanced veins may be similar in density to soft tissue and may be misinterpreted as a lesion, such as pathologically enlarged lymph nodes, particularly when there is normal focal dilation along the vein. In this setting, determining whether the attenuation of the finding is similar or different to other veins in the ipsilateral neck is helpful. In addition, reviewing the finding with coronal or sagittal reformatted imaging and determining whether the finding is contiguous with a vein is often useful. Occasionally, a small amount of contrast may be identified layering within the vein when viewed on the coronal or sagittal reformatted images, which essentially confirms that the finding represents a vein and not pathology.

COMPANION CASES

- **Supraclavicular lymphadenopathy.**
- **Iatrogenically injected air located in a focally dilated subclavian vein.** Iatrogenic injection of small volumes of venous air is not uncommon, most commonly occurring during intravenous catheter insertion.
- **Internal jugular vein phlebectasia.** Jugular vein phlebectasia refers to marked, fusiform dilation of the jugular vein, most commonly involving the right internal jugular vein. Most patients are pediatric patients that present with a nonpulsatile, nontender, soft neck mass which increases in size by maneuvers that elevate intrathoracic pressure, such as coughing, crying, and Valsava. Several internal jugular vein phlebectasia cases that have been resected demonstrate venous vessel wall pathology, including thinning of the venous wall, fibrosis, absence of the smooth muscle layer, and loss of elastic tissue, all of which likely play a role in the vessel enlargement. The imaging findings typically demonstrate marked enlargement of the right internal jugular vein, with no other complicating factors. Unless there is a cosmetic deformity or the rare symptom associated with this typically incidental entity, conservative management is the rule.

Inferior jugular bulb

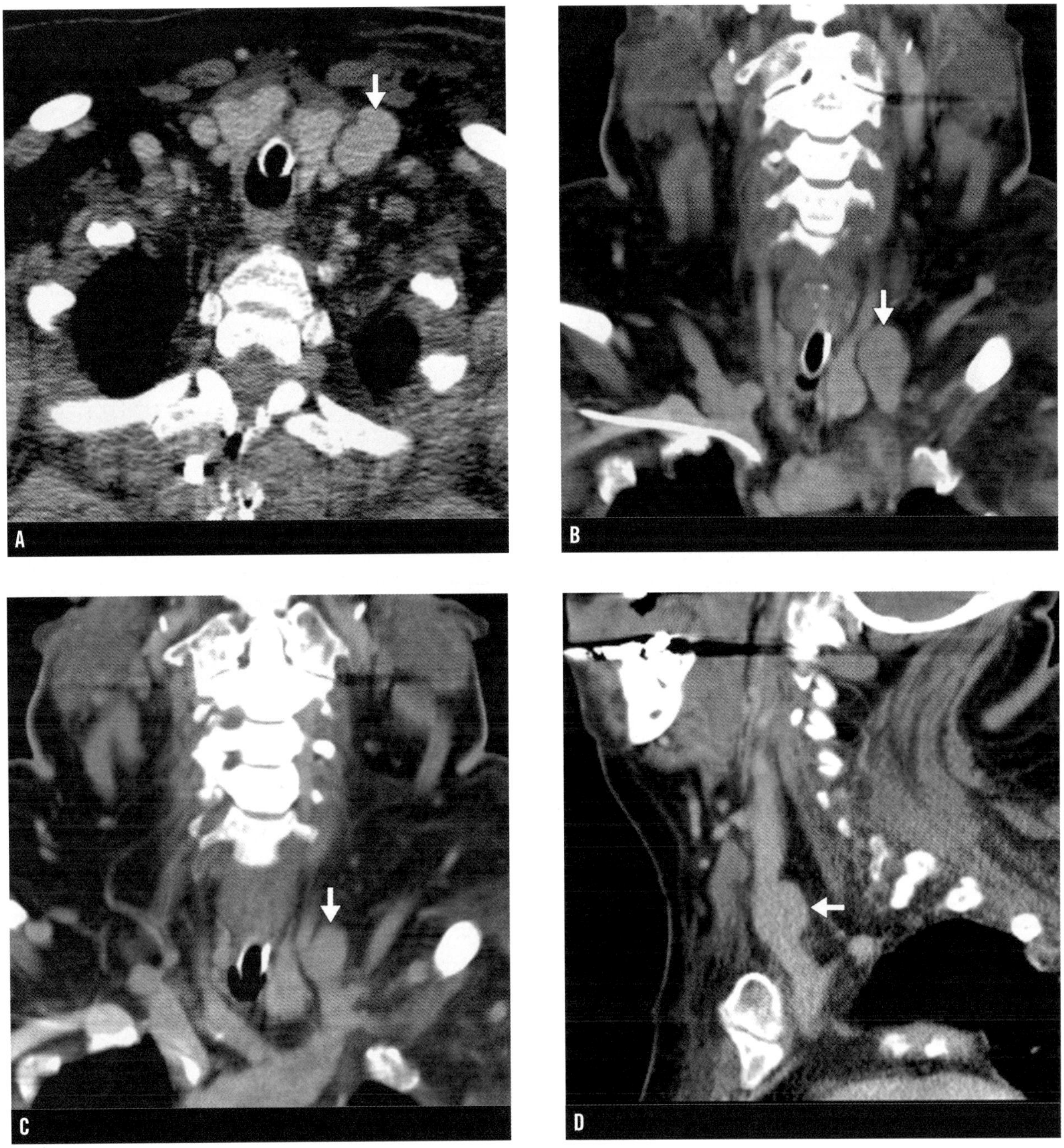

Axial (**A**), coronal reformatted (**B**, **C**), and sagittal reformatted (**D**) postcontrast CT images through the neck demonstrate a bulbous contour along the distal left internal jugular vein, compatible with a normal inferior jugular bulb (arrows, **A-D**).

Focal dilation of the subclavian vein

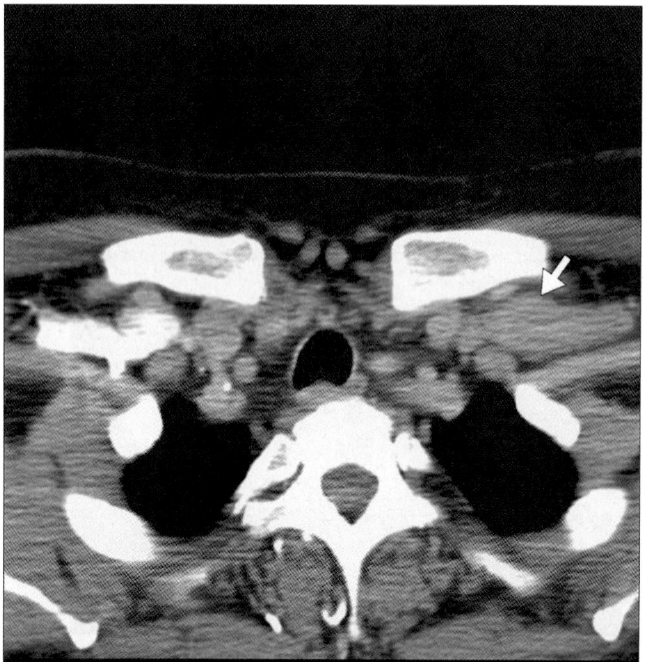

A

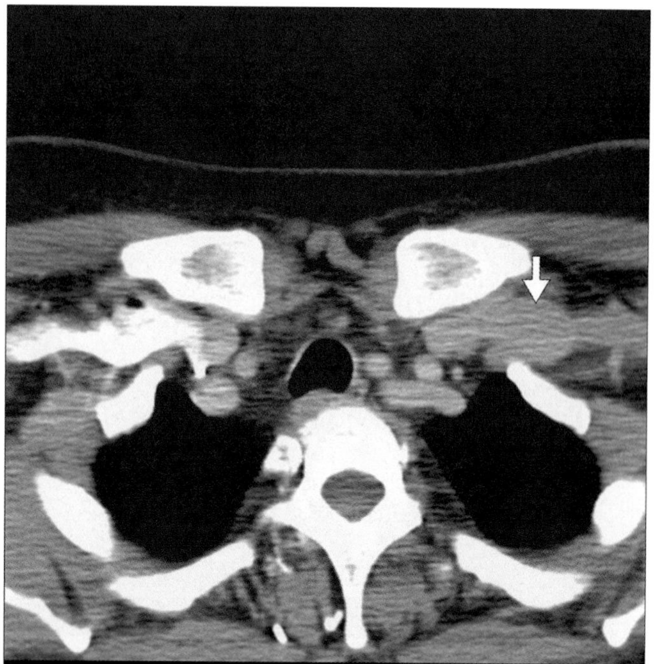

B

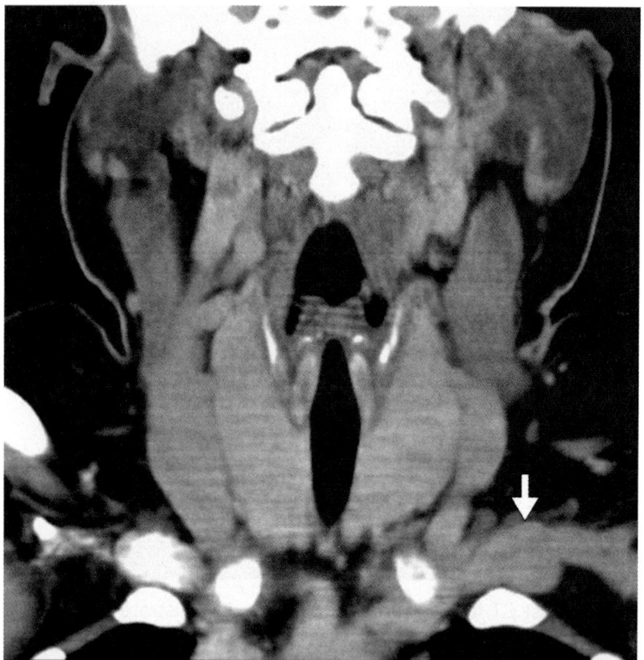

C

Axial (**A**, **B**) and coronal reformatted (**C**) postcontrast CT images demonstrate a normal bulbous contour along the left subclavian vein (arrows, **A-C**).

Normal focal dilations of the subclavian vein simulating pathologic lymph nodes

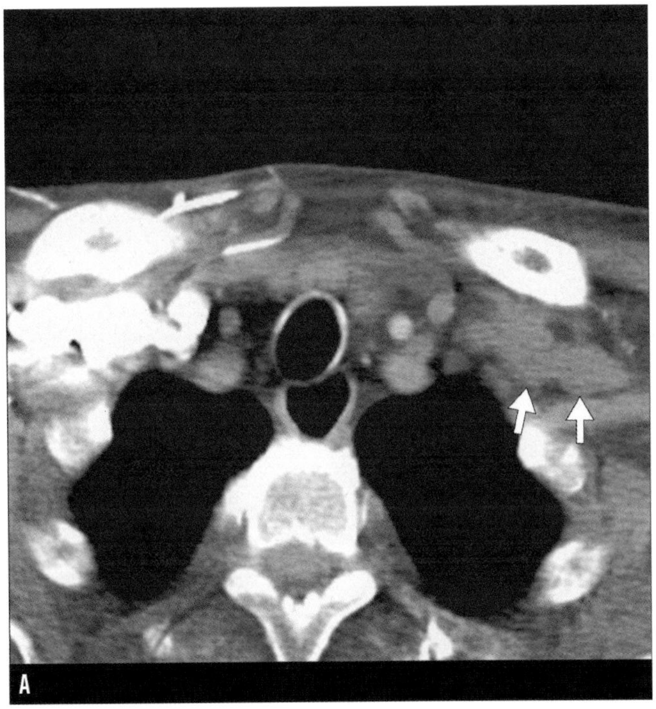

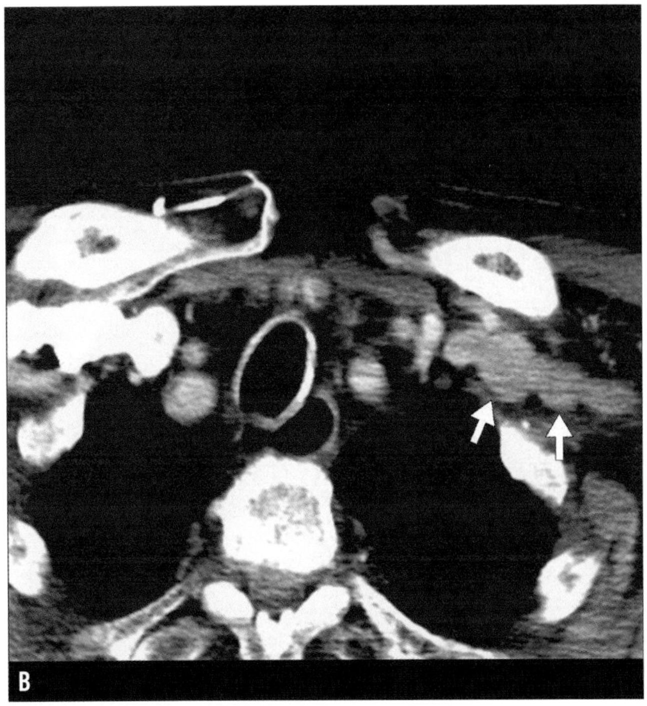

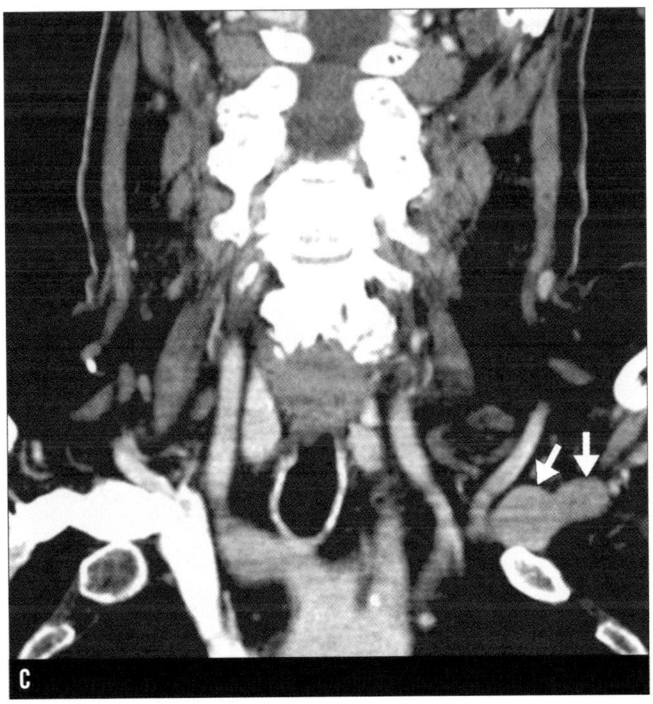

An axial postcontrast CT image through the lower neck obtained during a CT of the chest (**A**) demonstrates apparent soft tissue in the left supraclavicular region which was interpreted as lymphadenopathy (arrows, **A**). Axial (**B**) and coronal reformatted (**C**) postcontrast images from a CT of the neck obtained approximately 50 seconds following the CT of the chest demonstrate that the left supraclavicular finding simply represents the normal left subclavian vein, with the lobulations representing normal bulbous dilations of the vein related to valves (arrows, **B**, **C**). This patient was injected with contrast from the right antecubital vein, accounting for the delayed enhancement of the left subclavian vein between the CT chest and CT neck examinations.

Normal focal dilation of the axillary vein simulating a pathologic lymph node

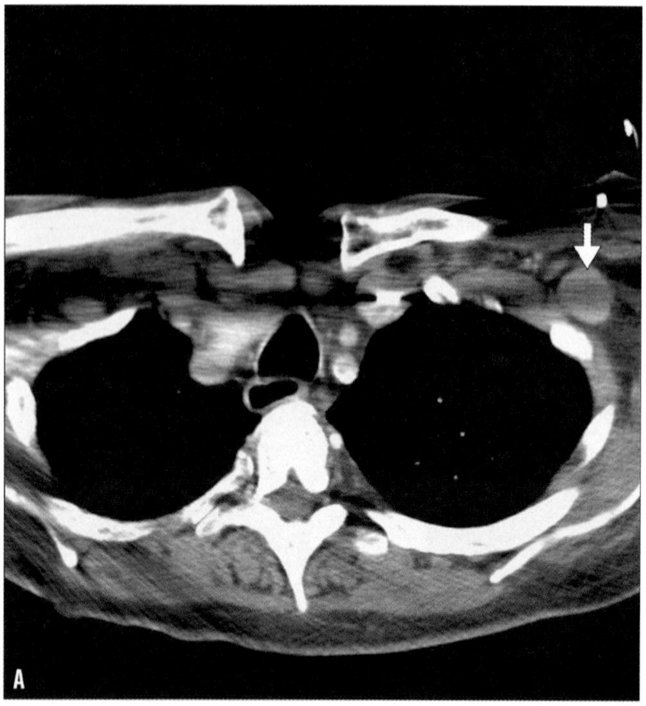

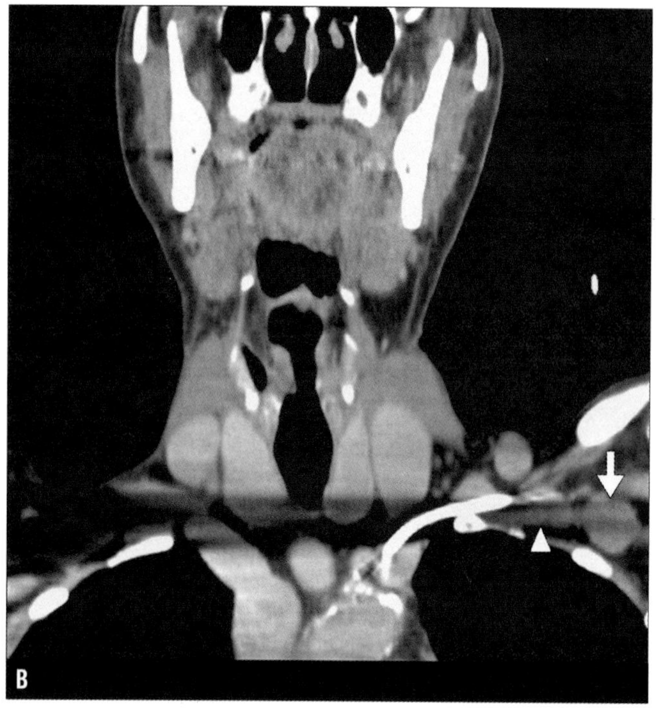

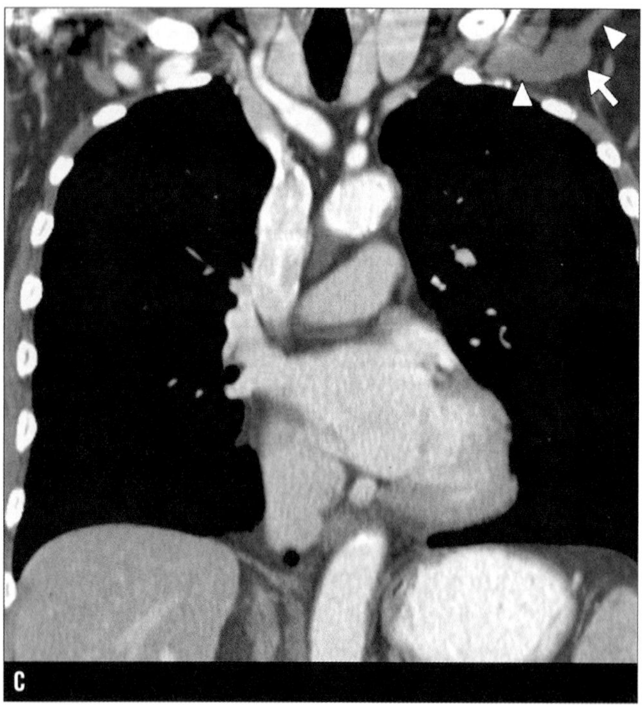

Different patient. Postcontrast axial (**A**) and coronal reformatted (**B**) CT images from a CT neck examination demonstrate a round, soft tissue density finding in the left axilla, which was interpreted as a pathologically enlarged lymph node in this patient with a history of chronic lymphocytic leukemia (arrow, **A**). Image **B** suggests that the finding is a continuation of the axillary vein (arrowhead, **B**), although this was not noticed during the interpretation. A postcontrast coronal reformatted CT image from a CT of the chest (**C**) performed in conjunction with the CT neck clearly demonstrates the bulbous finding (arrow, **C**) to be a continuation of the axillary vein (arrowheads, **C**) and to represent normal dilation of the vein rather than a pathologic lymph node.

Companion case: Supraclavicular lymphadenopathy

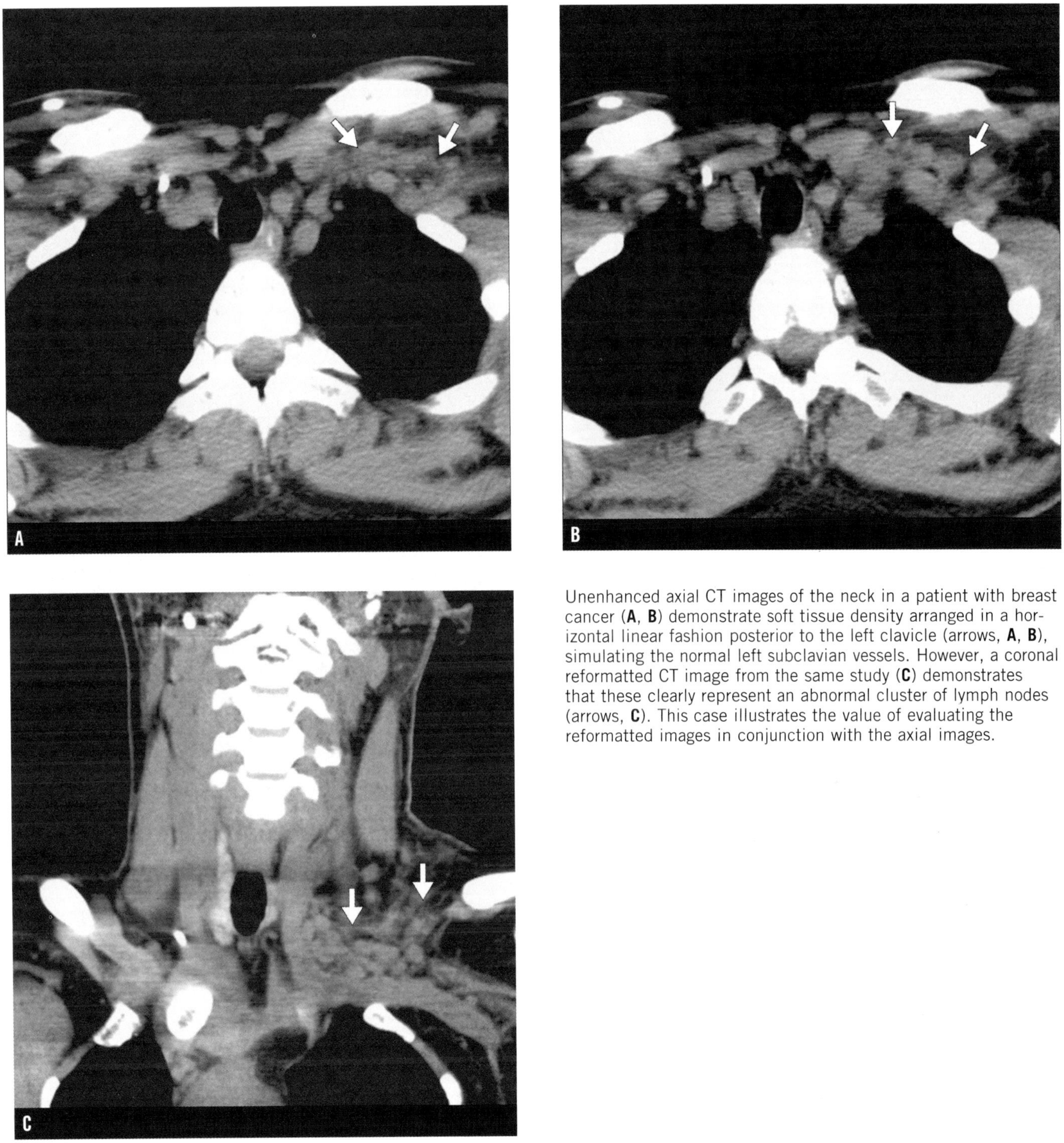

Unenhanced axial CT images of the neck in a patient with breast cancer (**A**, **B**) demonstrate soft tissue density arranged in a horizontal linear fashion posterior to the left clavicle (arrows, **A**, **B**), simulating the normal left subclavian vessels. However, a coronal reformatted CT image from the same study (**C**) demonstrates that these clearly represent an abnormal cluster of lymph nodes (arrows, **C**). This case illustrates the value of evaluating the reformatted images in conjunction with the axial images.

Companion case: Iatrogenically injected air located in a focally dilated subclavian vein

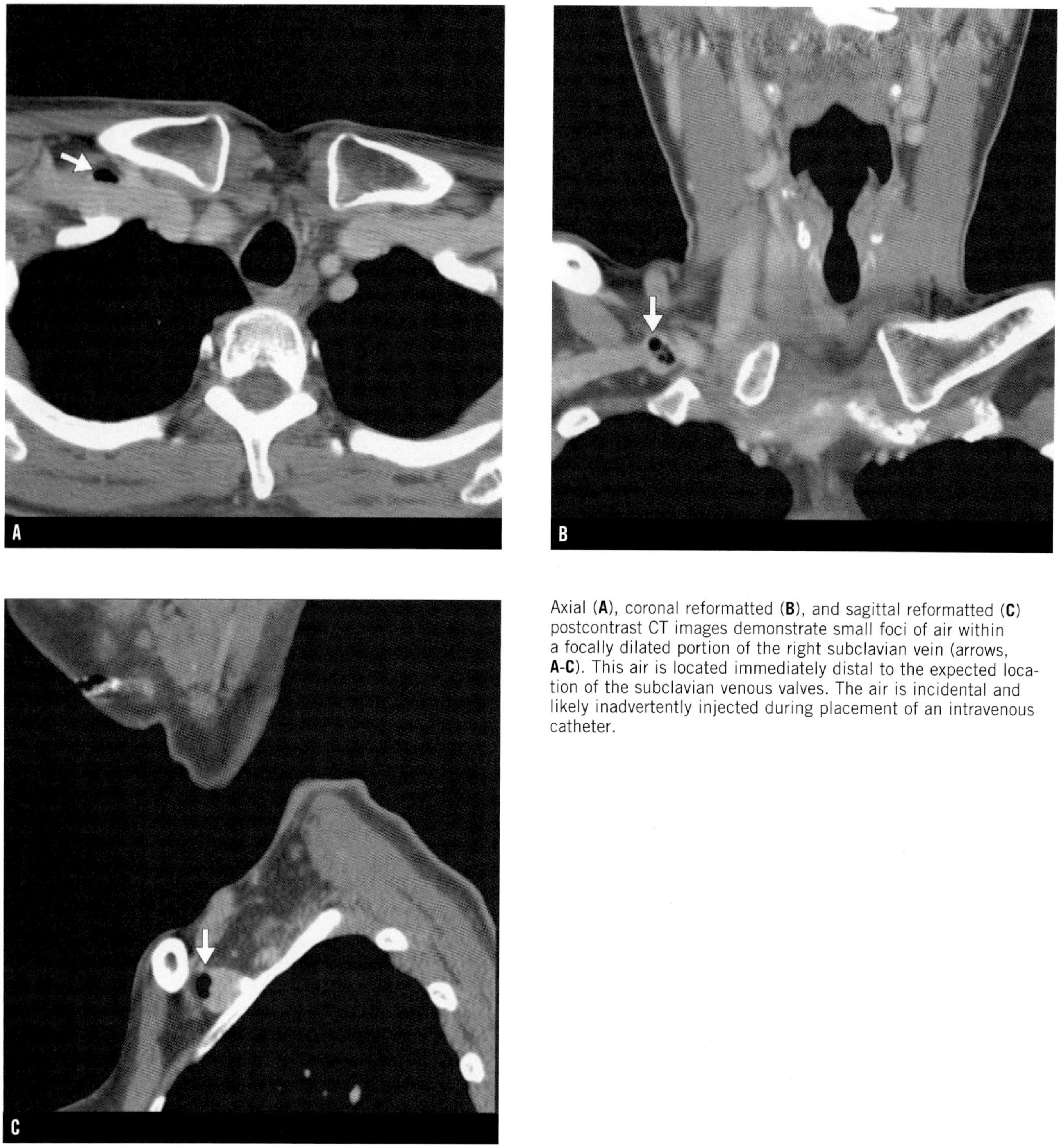

Axial (**A**), coronal reformatted (**B**), and sagittal reformatted (**C**) postcontrast CT images demonstrate small foci of air within a focally dilated portion of the right subclavian vein (arrows, **A-C**). This air is located immediately distal to the expected location of the subclavian venous valves. The air is incidental and likely inadvertently injected during placement of an intravenous catheter.

Companion case: Internal jugular vein phlebectasia

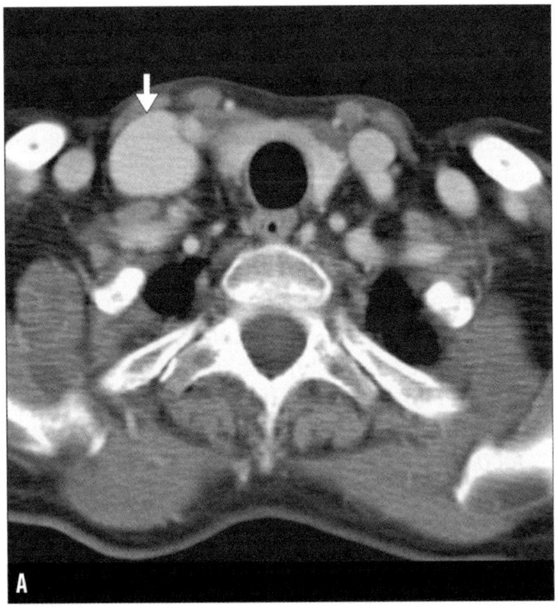

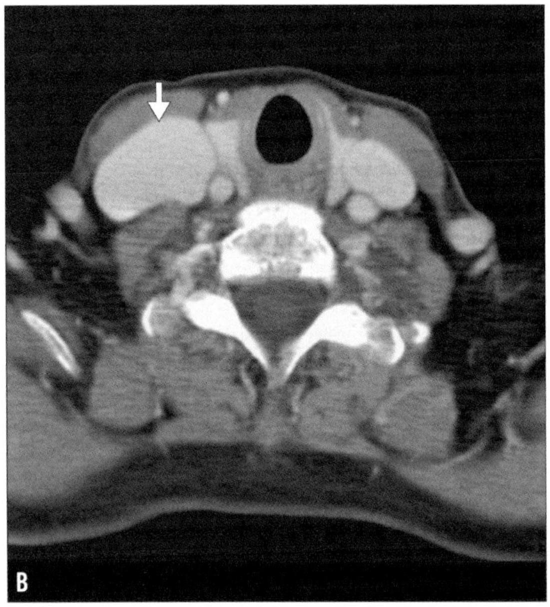

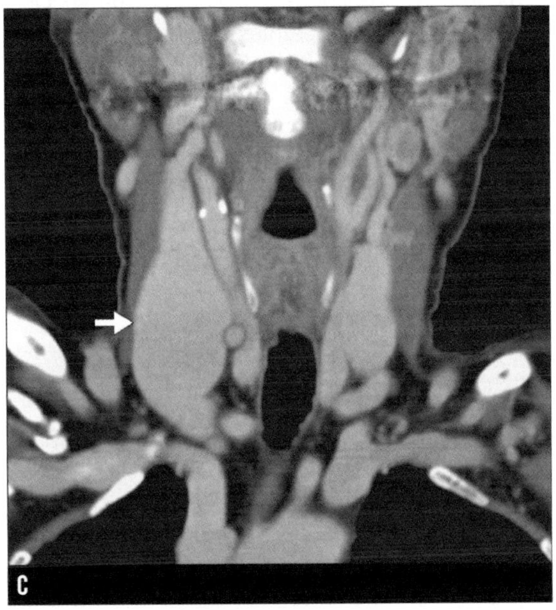

Axial (**A**, **B**) and coronal reformatted (**C**) postcontrast CT images through the neck demonstrate marked enlargement of the right internal jugular vein, compatible with right internal jugular vein phlebectasia (arrows, **A-C**).

REFERENCES

Aviram G, et al. Significance of reflux of contrast medium into the inferior vena cava on computerized tomographic pulmonary angiogram. *Am J Cardiol.* 2012;109(3):432-437.

Caramutti VM, Zaidman JC, Abud JA, Gabe ED. Azygos vein diverticulum. *Ann Thorac Surg.* 2000;70(2):665-666.

El Fakiri M-M, et al. Congenital internal jugular phlebectasia. *Eur Ann Otorhinolaryngol Head Neck Dis.* 2011;128(6):324-326.

Escott EJ, Branstetter BF. It's not a cervical lymph node, it's a vein: CT and MR imaging findings in the veins of the head and neck. *Radiographics.* 2006;26(5):1501-1515.

Ettekal Y, et al. Incidental vascular flaps on neck ultrasound. *J Cardiothorac Vasc Anesth.* 2013;27(1):199-200.

Gundlach U, Unlü C, Wüst AFJ, Voorwinde A. Unilateral jugular vein phlebectasia. *Vasc Endovascular Surg.* 2009;43(2):193-194.

Hung T, Campbell AI. Surgical repair of left internal jugular phlebectasia. *J Vasc Surg.* 2008;47(6):1337-1338.

Jianhong L, Xuewu J, Tingze H. Surgical treatment of jugular vein phlebectasia in children. *Am J Surg.* 2006;192(3):286-290.

Paleri V, Gopalakrishnan S. Jugular phlebectasia: theory of pathogenesis and review of literature. *Int J Pediatr Otorhinolaryngol.* 2001;57(2):155-159.

Som PM, Curtin HD, Mancuso AA. An imaging-based classification for the cervical nodes designed as an adjunct to recent clinically based nodal classifications. *Arch Otolaryngol Head Neck Surg.* 1999;125:388-396.

Som PM, Curtin HD, Mancuso AA. Imaging-based nodal classification for evaluation of neck metastatic adenopathy. *AJR Am J Roentgenol.* 2000;174:837-844.

Som PM. Lymph nodes of the neck. *Radiology.* 1987;165:593-600.

Valecchi D, et al. Internal jugular vein valves: an assessment of prevalence, morphology and competence by color Doppler echography in 240 healthy subjects. *Ital J Anat Embryol.* 2010;115(3):185-189.

CASE 18 Mixing of opacified and unopacified blood simulating internal jugular vein thrombus

The mixing of opacified blood with unopacified blood may create the false impression of thrombus in a vein. In the case of a neck CT, this is particularly true of the internal jugular vein. These "pseudoclots" typically have ill-defined margins and are only mildly hypoattenuating, as opposed to a true thrombus, which is usually well marginated and quite hypoattenuating. Occasionally, denser contrast may be identified layering dependently in the vein and support the presence of incidental mixing of contrast to explain the imaging appearance. Ultimately, problematic cases may require additional studies, such as ultrasonography or repeat CT imaging with a greater delay following contrast injection.

COMPANION CASES

- **Nonocclusive thrombus in the internal jugular vein.** A nonocclusive venous thrombus will typically appear as a rounded, homogeneous, hypoattenuating focus on CT that is eccentric or centrally located in a vein, with at least a portion surrounded by contrast.
- **Occlusive thrombus in the internal jugular vein.** An occlusive venous thrombus will occupy the entire diameter of the affected vein's lumen, often accompanied by upstream venous dilation, perivenous soft tissue edema, and opacification of dilated collateral veins. Chronic venous thrombi tend to have irregular margins and are associated with pronounced luminal narrowing. Occasionally, a venous thrombus can enhance on MRI, particularly a chronic thrombus.
- **Lemierre syndrome.** Lemierre syndrome is an uncommon but potentially life-threatening septic thrombophlebitis that results as a complication of an acute peritonsillar abscess in otherwise healthy patients. While the peritonsillar abscess is often initially caused by a *Streptococcus* bacterium, the abscess allows for abnormal growth of anaerobic bacteria that are part of the normal flora, namely the *Fusobacterium* genus of anaerobic bacteria (usually *Fusobacterium necrophorum*). The infection spreads to the ipsilateral parapharyngeal space as well as the ipsilateral carotid space. Occasionally, cranial IX-XI neuropathies may occur. The septic thrombophlebitis most often affects the internal jugular vein. The thrombophlebitis results in septicemia and septic embolization, with a predilection to the lungs. Given the propensity to develop septic emboli, imaging of the chest, abdomen, and pelvis is warranted in these cases.

Mixing of opacified and unopacified blood simulating bilateral internal jugular vein thrombi

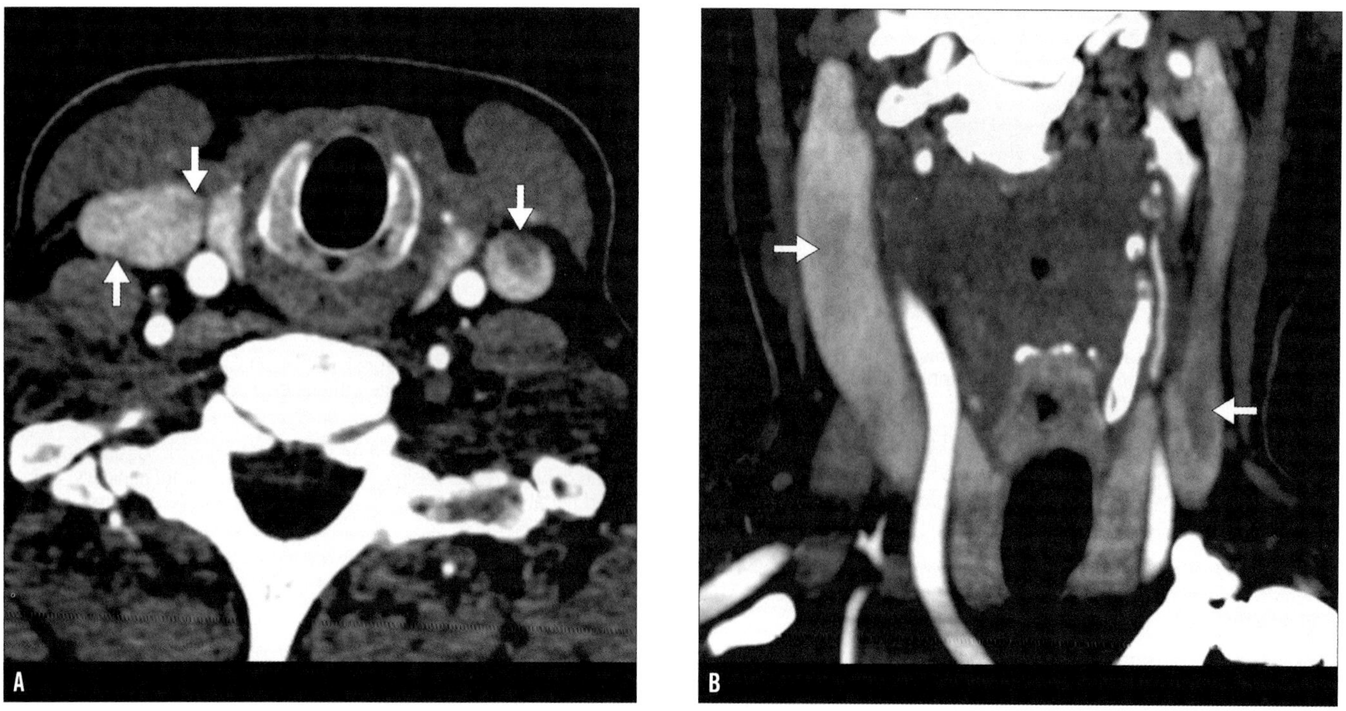

Axial (**A**) and coronal reformatted (**B**) postcontrast CT images through the neck demonstrate heterogeneous hypoattenuation within contrast opacified bilateral internal jugular veins (arrows, **A**, **B**). The heterogeneous hypoattenuation simulates nonocclusive venous thrombi. However, this simply represents unopacified blood intermixed with opacified blood within the internal jugular veins.

Companion case: Nonocclusive thrombus in the internal jugular vein

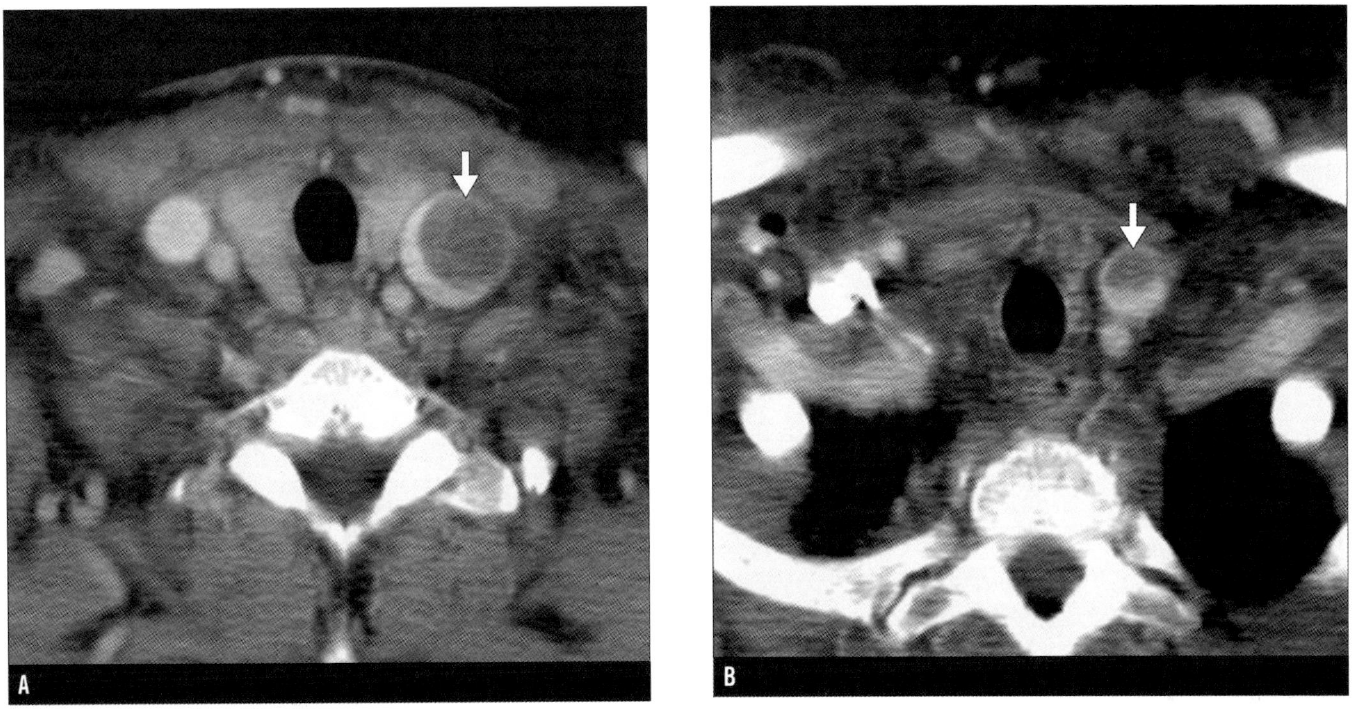

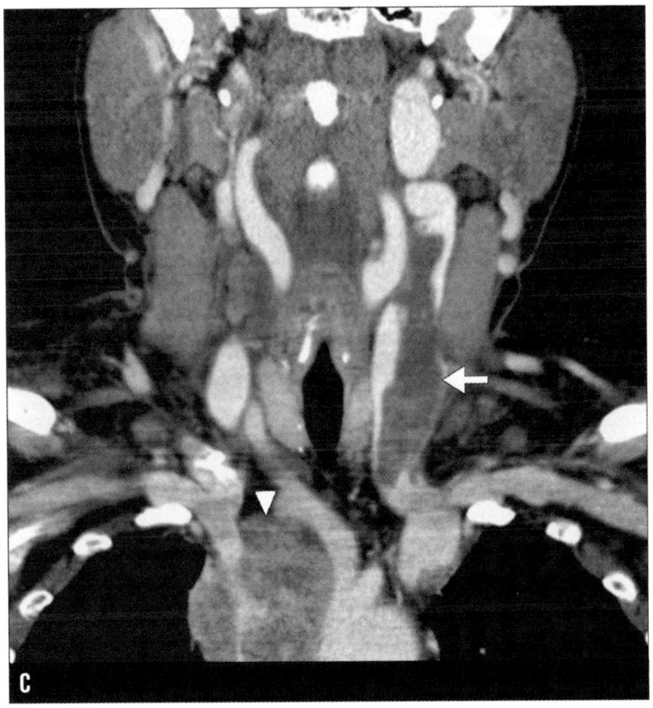

Axial (**A**, **B**) and coronal reformatted (**C**) postcontrast CT images through the neck demonstrate a large, nonocclusive thrombus in the left internal jugular vein (arrows, **A-C**). This patient has lung carcinoma, partially visualized on image **C** (arrowhead).

Companion case: Occlusive thrombus in the internal jugular vein

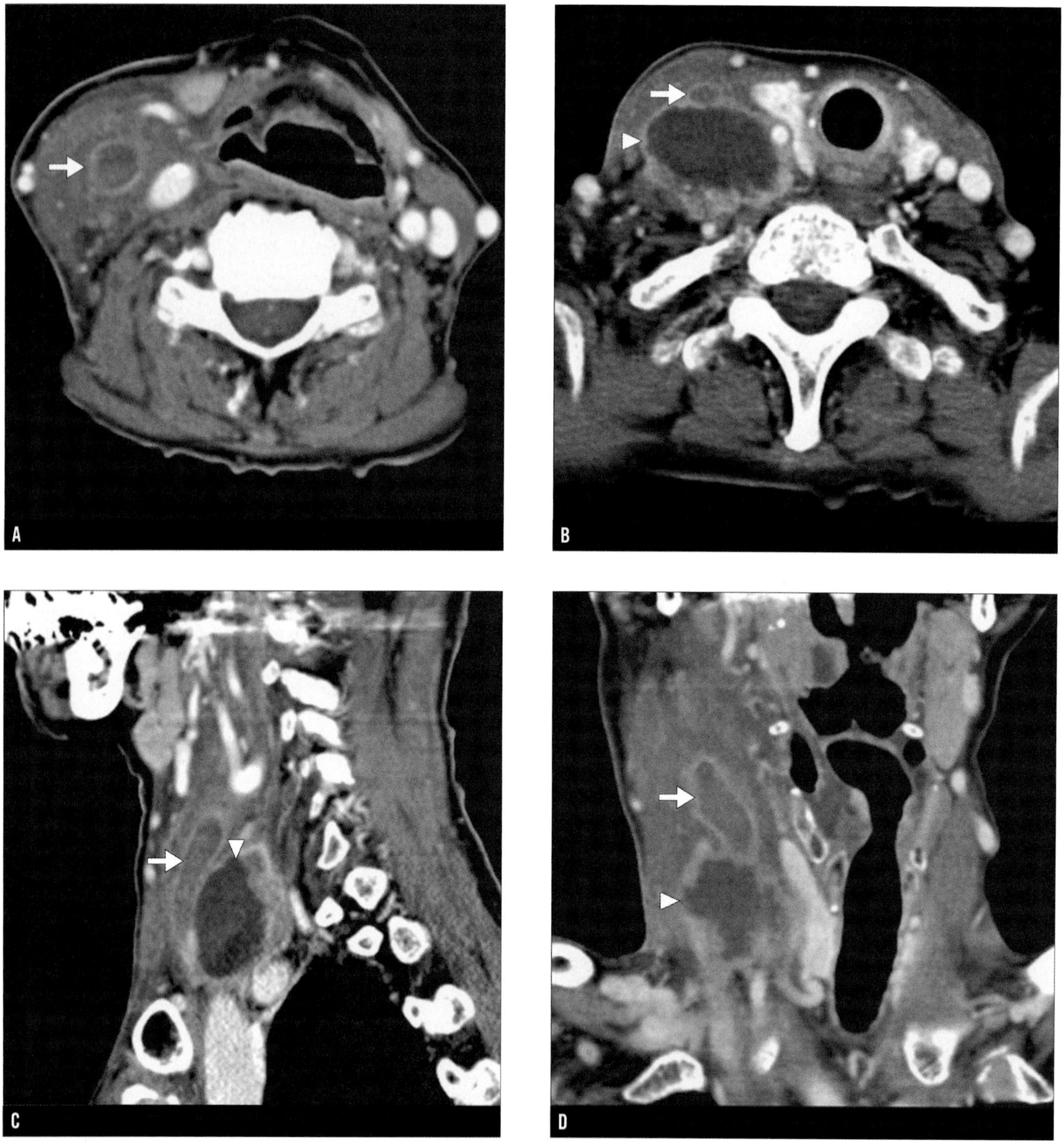

An axial postcontrast CT image (**A**) demonstrates a completely occluded right internal jugular vein (arrow, **A**). Axial (**B**), sagittal reformatted (**C**), and coronal reformatted (**D**) postcontrast CT images from the same study demonstrate a large necrotic mass (arrowheads, **B-D**) in the right lower neck resulting in occlusion of the right internal jugular vein (arrows, **B-D**). The right internal jugular vein is occluded with bland thrombus and/or tumor thrombus.

Companion case: Lemierre syndrome

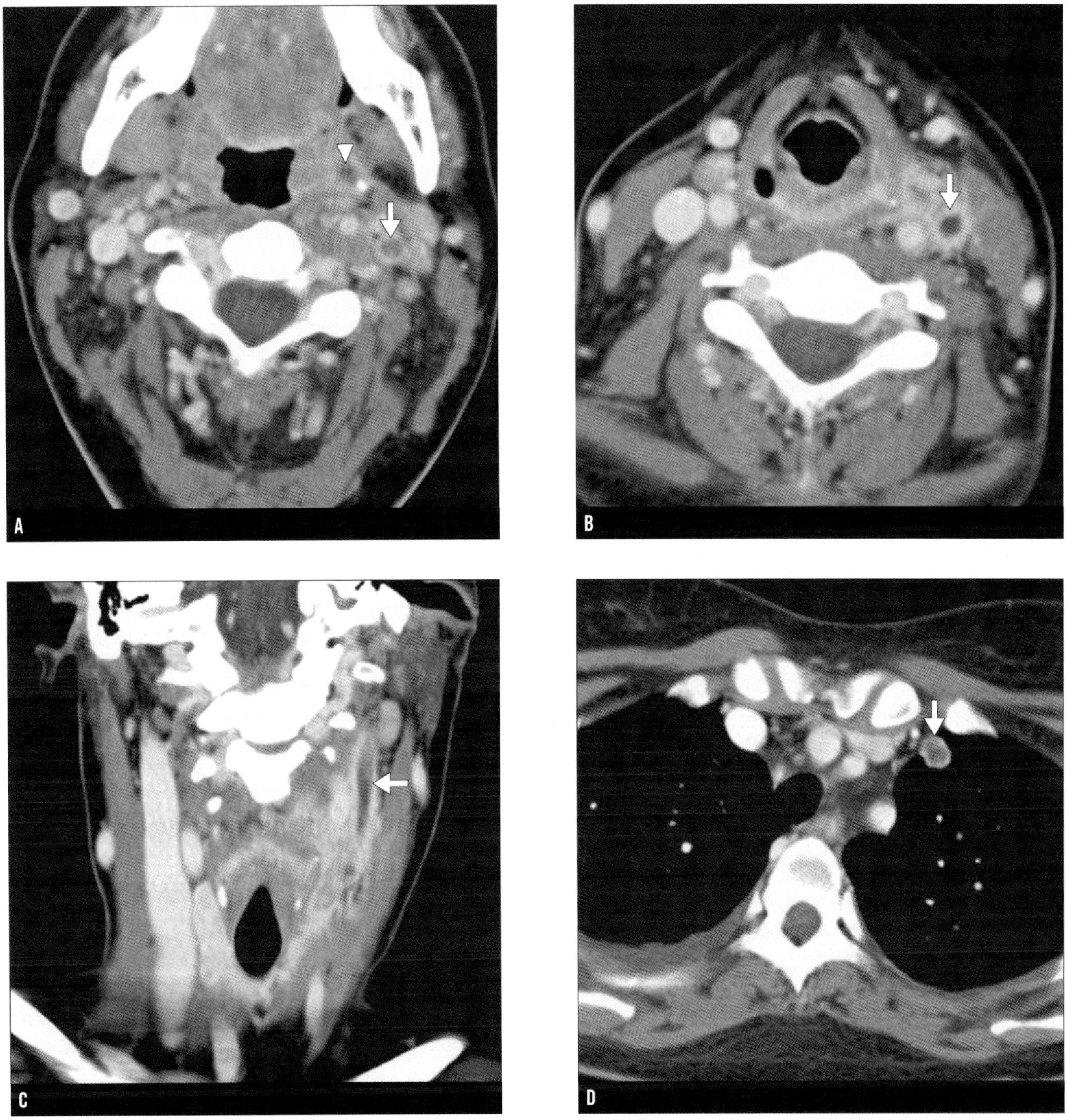

Axial (**A**, **B**) and coronal reformatted (**C**) postcontrast CT images through the neck demonstrate an occlusive thrombus in the left internal jugular vein (arrows, **A**-**C**) and a small left peritonsillar abscess (arrowhead, **A**). There is surrounding inflammatory change that is secondary to the peritonsillar abscess, occlusive venous thrombus, or both. An axial postcontrast CT image through the chest (**D**) demonstrates one of the patient's several septic emboli that occurred as a result of this entity (arrow, **D**).

REFERENCES

Ghaye B, Szapiro D, Willems V, Dondelinger RF. Pitfalls in CT venography of lower limbs and abdominal veins. *AJR Am J Roentgenol.* 2002;178(6):1465-1471.

Grenier PA, Beigelman C. Spiral computed tomographic scanning and magnetic resonance angiography for the diagnosis of pulmonary embolism. *Thorax.* 1998;53(Suppl 2):S25-S31.

Khosa F, Otero HJ, Prevedello LM, Rybicki FJ, Di Salvo DN. Imaging presentation of venous thrombosis in patients with cancer. *AJR Am J Roentgenol.* 2010;194(4):1099-1108.

Screaton NJ, Ravenel JG, Lehner PJ, Heitzman ER, Flower CDR. Lemierre syndrome : forgotten but not extinct—report of four cases. *Radiology.* 1999;213:369-374.

CASE 19 Retropharyngeal lipoma

The retropharyngeal space resides posterior to the pharynx and esophagus and anterior to the prevertebral musculature. The retropharyngeal space is a potential space, bound anteriorly by the visceral fascia, posteriorly by the prevertebral fascia (which is a portion of the deep layer of the deep cervical fascia), and laterally by the carotid spaces. A thin alar fascia, which is also a portion of the deep layer of the deep cervical fascia, subdivides the retropharyngeal space into two compartments: an anteriorly located true (or proper) retropharyngeal space and a posteriorly located danger space. This subdivision is unable to be delineated by imaging in normal patients but is sometimes able to be discerned in pathologic cases. The retropharyngeal space extends from the skull base to between T1 and T6, which represents the location where the alar fascia fuses with the visceral fascia. However, the danger space extends considerably more caudal, extending from the skull base, through the posterior mediastinum, and to the diaphragm. When an infection within the retropharyngeal space breaches the thin alar fascia, the infection may spread into the mediastinum via the danger space, hence the name "danger space." The danger space contains only loose areolar tissue and infection often spreads rapidly through this space.

Fat, lymph nodes, and small vessels normally occupy the suprahyoid retropharyngeal space, although only fat occupies the infrahyoid retropharyngeal space. Lipomas may be found within the retropharynx and represent benign, encapsulated, usually slow-growing tumors composed of fat. While small retropharyngeal lipomas are typically incidental, a large retropharyngeal lipoma can ventrally displace and compromise the pharynx, resulting in dyspnea, dysphagia or sleep apnea. A benign lipoma follows the same attenuation and signal characteristics of fat on CT and MRI, respectively.

COMPANION CASES

- **Retropharyngeal edema.** Retropharyngeal edema may result from numerous etiologies, including adjacent infection, inflammation (eg, calcific tendonitis longus colli), prior radiation, trauma, and tumor. Edema in the retropharynx on imaging will appear just as it does elsewhere in the body, and it can usually be demonstrated by the relative loss of fat attenuation or signal on CT or MRI, respectively. There should be no significant peripheral enhancement in cases of uncomplicated retropharyngeal edema. Retropharyngeal edema will resolve on its own when the offending cause is treated.
- **Retropharyngeal abscess.** In children, a retropharyngeal abscess is usually the result of a pharyngeal infection associated with a ruptured pyogenic lateral retropharyngeal lymph node (ie, node of Rouvière). In adults, a retropharyngeal abscess is usually the result of a spinal infection that has spread from the prevertebral space and into the retropharyngeal space. Due to the anatomy discussed above, a retropharyngeal abscess can spread into the danger space and subsequently into the mediastinum, resulting in a mediastinitis or mediastinal abscess. Additionally, infection can spread through fascia and into the adjacent neck soft tissues, resulting in a soft tissue neck abscess, venous thrombosis, or carotid artery pseudoaneurysm/rupture. The morphology of a retropharyngeal abscess is usually ovoid on axial imaging. It will most often have a rim of enhancement and may have significant mass effect that results in airway compromise. Due to the significant morbidity and mortality related to a retropharyngeal abscess, most require surgical drainage.
- **Retropharyngeal lymphatic malformation.** See case 5 for discussion regarding vascular malformations.

Retropharyngeal lipoma

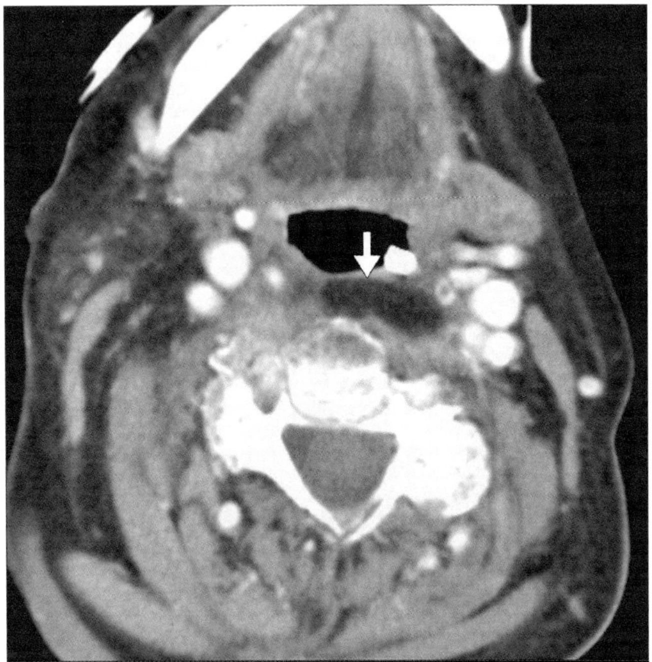

A

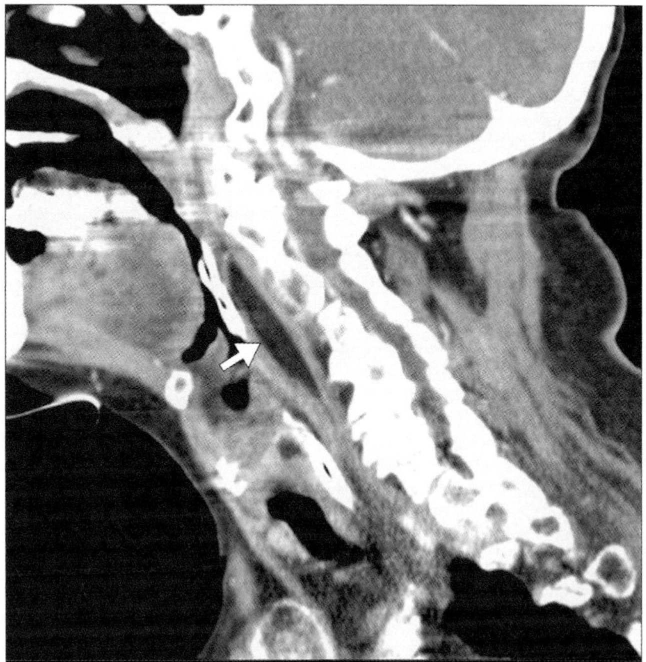

B

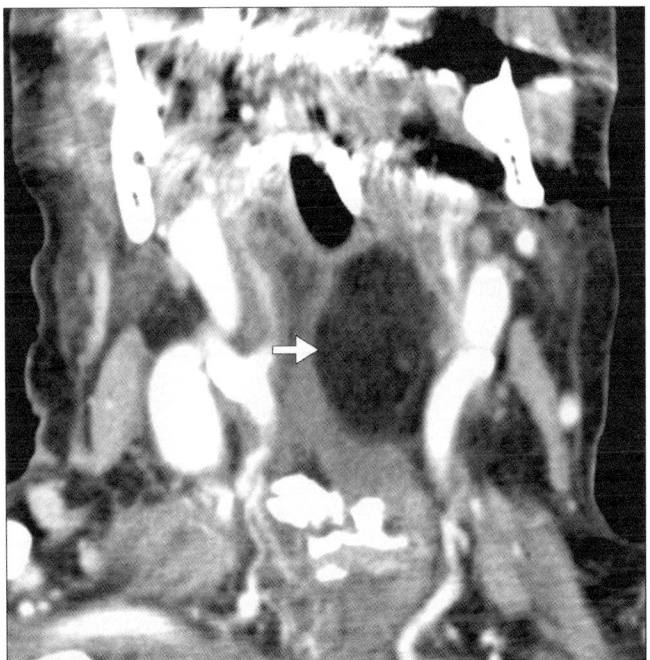

C

Axial (**A**), sagittal reformatted (**B**), and coronal reformatted (**C**) CT images demonstrate a circumscribed, fat-containing lesion in the left aspect of the retropharynx, compatible with a retropharyngeal lipoma (arrows, **A-C**).

Retropharyngeal lipoma

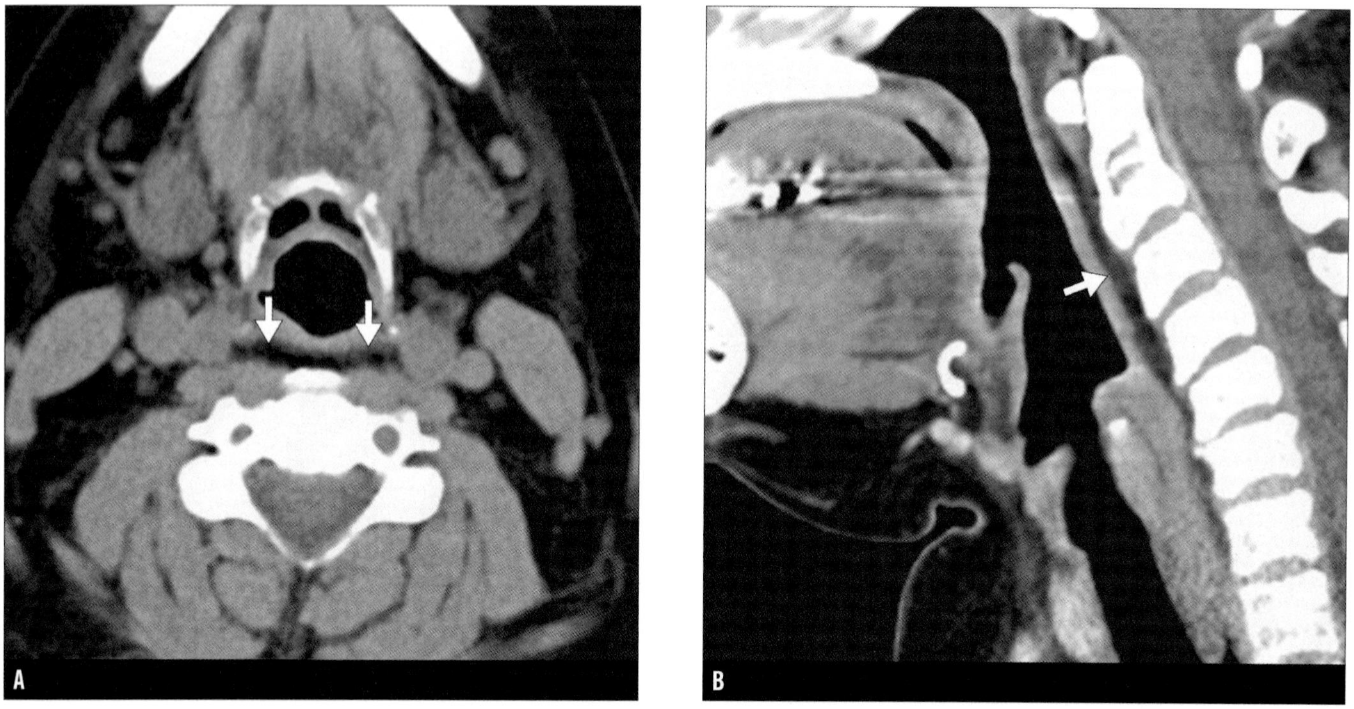

Different patient. Axial (**A**) and coronal reformatted (**B**) postcontrast CT images through the neck demonstrate fat extending through the entire transverse dimension of the retropharynx, compatible with a retropharyngeal lipoma (arrows, **A**, **B**).

Companion case: Retropharyngeal edema

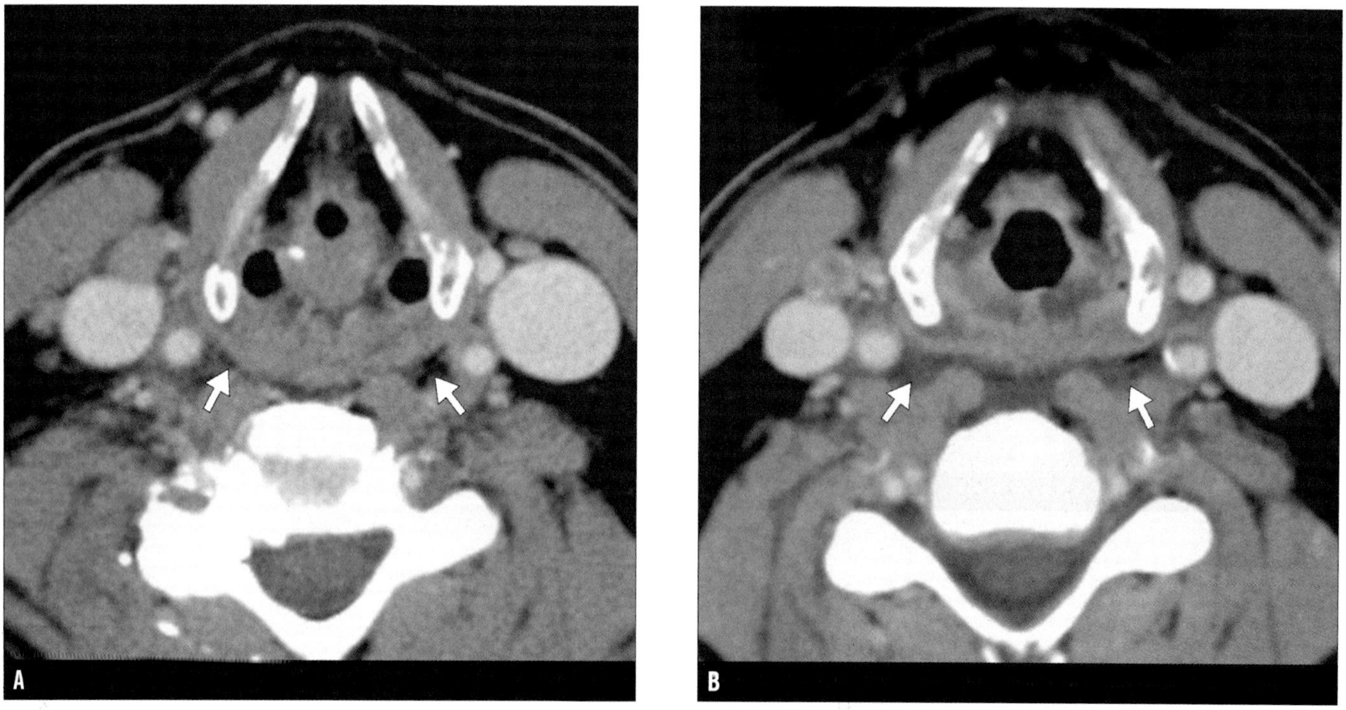

An axial postcontrast CT image (**A**) of a patient with newly diagnosed larynx carcinoma (not shown) demonstrates a normal thin amount of fat throughout the retropharynx (arrows, **A**) at the level of the hypopharynx. Following initiation of chemotherapy and radiation, a 3-month follow-up axial image from a postcontrast CT scan (**B**) demonstrates a small amount of new retropharyngeal edema (arrows, **B**). The lack of enhancement surrounding the fluid supports a reactive edema from the treatment rather than an infectious process. A 2-year follow-up axial image from a postcontrast CT scan (**C**) demonstrates marked progression of the retropharyngeal edema, again without significant enhancement (arrows, **C**), superimposed upon other posttreatment changes in the neck.

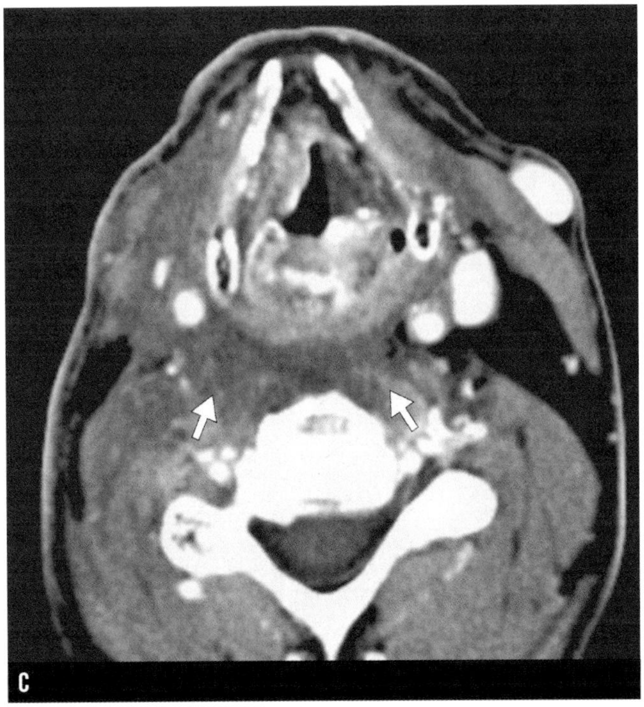

Companion case: Retropharyngeal abscess

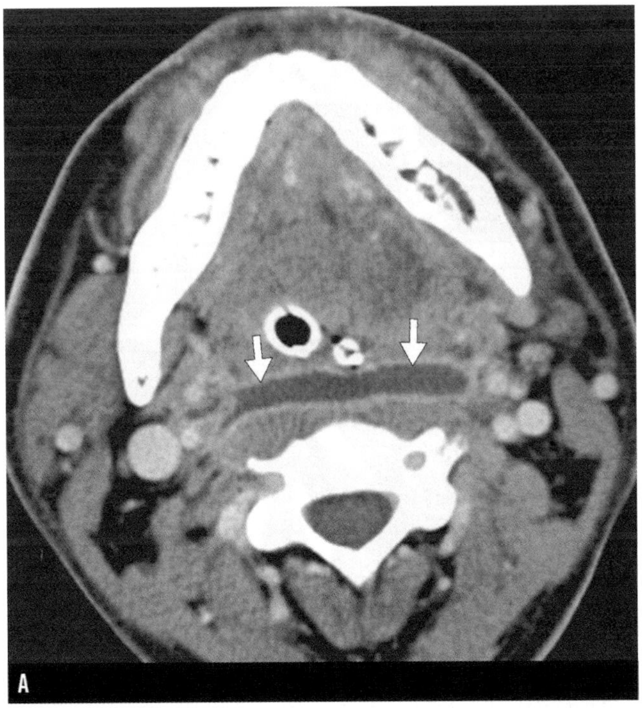

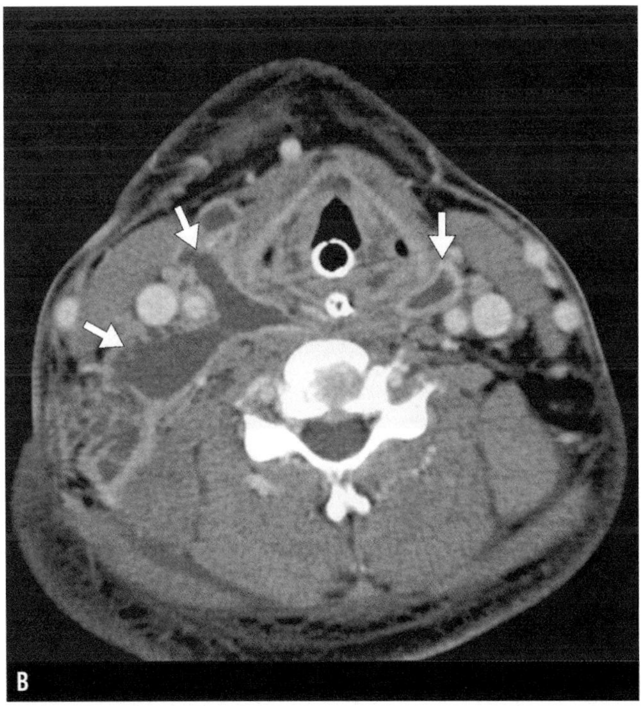

Axial (**A**, **B**), sagittal reformatted (**C**), and coronal reformatted (**D**) postcontrast CT images through the neck demonstrate a peripherally enhancing retropharyngeal fluid collection that extensively infiltrates the right aspect of the neck and to a lesser degree the left aspect of the neck (arrows, **A-D**). In addition to the extensive infiltration, the peripheral enhancement supports the diagnosis of a retropharyngeal abscess, as opposed to a sterile effusion which does not peripherally enhance.

Companion case: Pathologic lymph node with a preserved fatty hilum

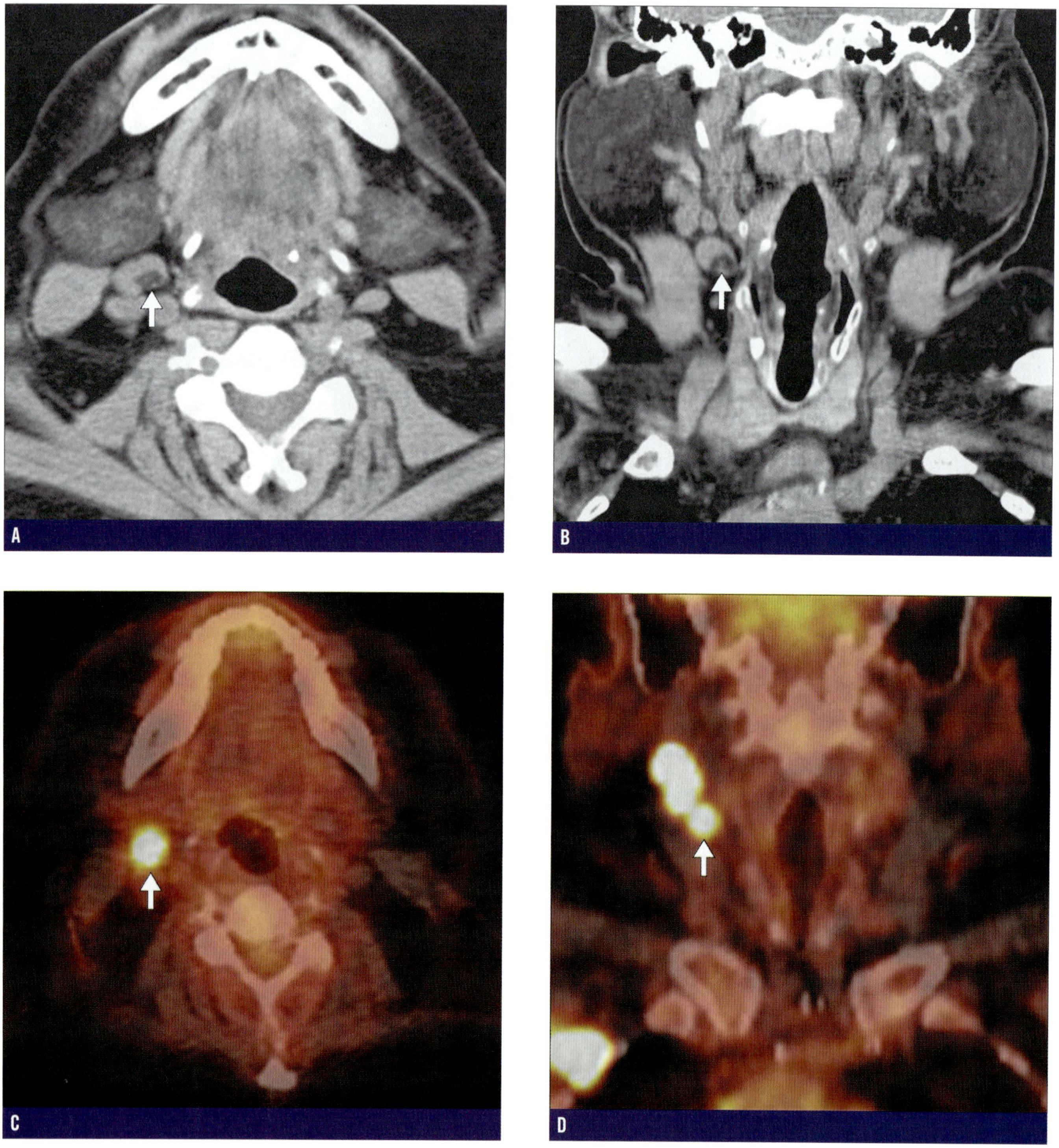

Axial (**A**) and coronal reformatted (**B**) unenhanced CT images of a patient with diffuse large B-cell lymphoma demonstrate a cluster of lymph nodes in the right level IIA nodal station, one of which contains a large fatty hilum (arrows, **A**, **B**). The presence of a fatty hilum typically suggests that a lymph node is benign. However, a PET scan obtained within a week of the CT examination demonstrates several abnormally hypermetabolic lymph nodes in the right IIA lymph nodal station, including the lymph node with a fatty hilum (arrows, **C**, **D**). This case illustrates that a fatty hilum, while usually a finding compatible with benignity, can still contain metastatic disease.

Companion case: Necrotic metastatic lymph node from papillary thyroid cancer

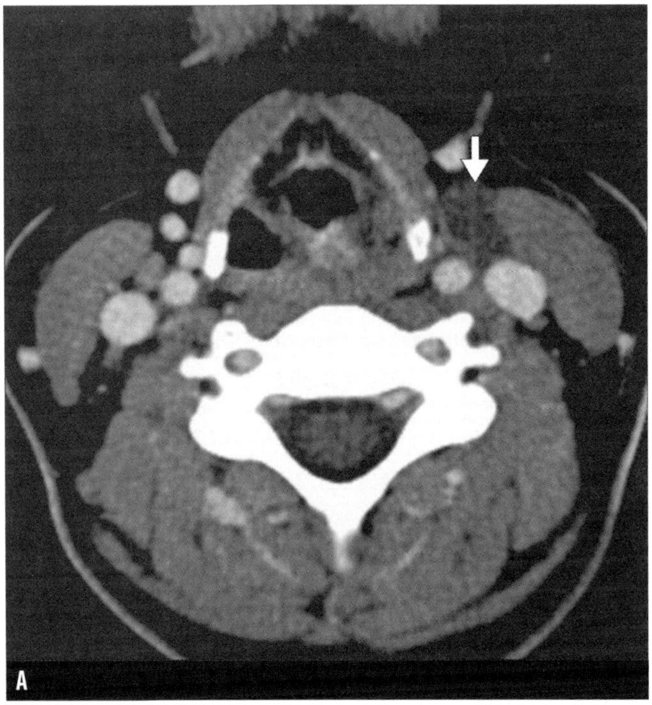

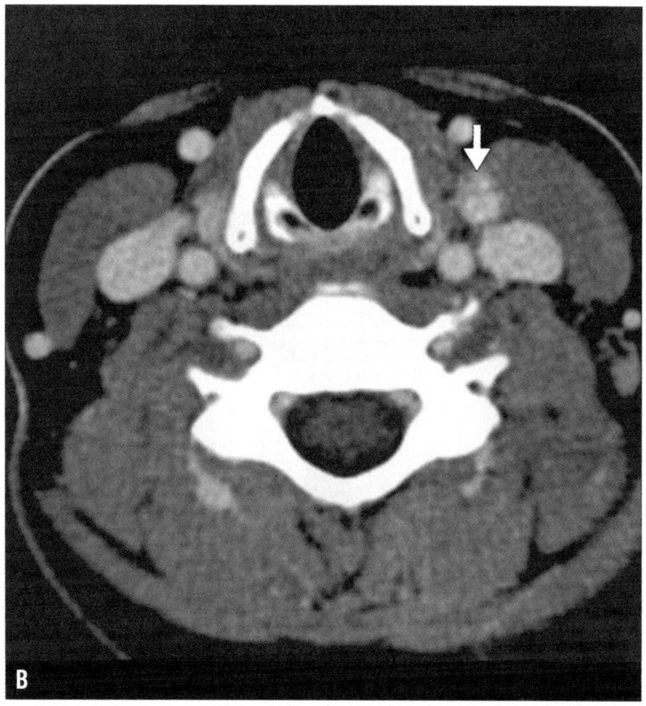

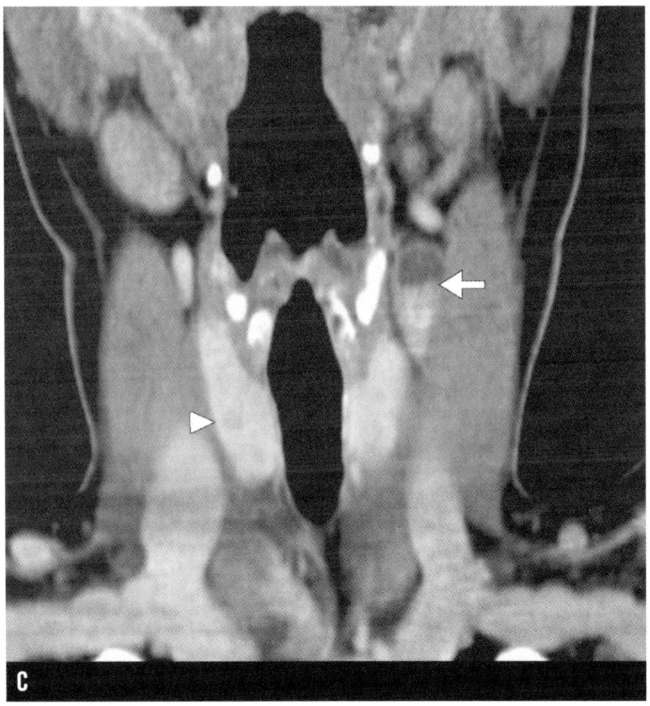

An axial postcontrast CT image through the neck (**A**) and an axial postcontrast CT image slightly caudal to this level (**B**) demonstrate a partially necrotic and partially presumably enhancing pathologic lymph node in the left level III nodal station (arrows, **A**, **B**). A coronal reformatted image from the same case (**C**) demonstrates the same finding in the coronal plane (arrow, **C**). The only identifiable thyroid finding in this case was a subtle subcentimeter focus of hypoattenuation in the right thyroid lobe (arrowhead, **C**), illustrating that a relatively unremarkable CT appearance of the thyroid gland does not exclude thyroid cancer, particularly in a young patient with a necrotic, unusually enhancing, or partially calcified lymph node in the neck.

Companion case: Lymph node necrosis secondary to tuberculosis (scrofula)

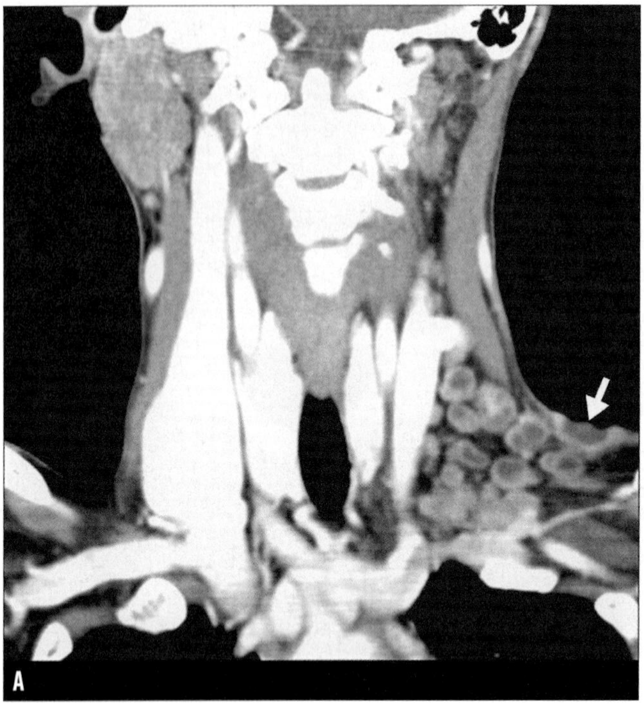

A coronal reformatted postcontrast CT image of the neck (**A**) demonstrates an abnormal cluster of numerous lymph nodes with central hypoattenuation in the left lower neck. The Hounsfield units of the hypoattenuation were of fluid density and therefore compatible with necrotic lymph nodes. One of the lymph nodes is associated with a cutaneous ulceration (arrow). This patient was purified protein derivative (PPD) positive and the findings are compatible with scrofula.

REFERENCES

Bellevre D, et al. Staging the axilla in breast cancer patients with ^{18}F-FDG PET: how small are the metastases that we can detect with new generation clinical PET systems? *Eur J Nucl Med Mol Imaging.* 2014;41(6):1103-1112.

Burrill J, Williams CJ, Bain G, Conder G, Hine AL, Misra RR.Tuberculosis: a radiologic review.*Radiographics.* 2007;27(5): 1255-1273.

Morris EA, Liberman L, Abramson AF. *Benign Lesions.* New York, NY: Springer;2005:140-163.

Norling R, Buron BM, Therkildsen MH, Henriksen BM, von Buchwald C, Nielsen MB. Staging of cervical lymph nodes in oral squamous cell carcinoma: adding ultrasound in clinically lymph nodenegative patients may improve diagnostic work-up. *PLoS One.* 2014;9(3):e90360.

Vaid S, Lee YY, Rawat S, Luthra A, Shah D, Ahuja AT. Tuberculosis in the head and neck – a forgotten differential diagnosis. *Clin Radiol.* 2010;65(1):73-81.

CASE 21 Second branchial cleft cyst versus necrotic metastatic lymphadenopathy

A branchial cleft cyst (BCC) is a benign congenital cystic remnant arising from the branchial apparatus.These are usually lined by stratified squamous epithelium, although respiratory epithelium occasionally lines some of these cysts. There are four types of BCC, with the second type by far the most common. A second BCC is usually located deep to the ventral aspect of the sternocleidomastoid muscle and lateral to the carotid space.

A necrotic level IIA metastatic lymph node (ie, jugulodigastric lymph node), most commonly from a squamous cell carcinoma (SCC) and less commonly from thyroid cancer, can be difficult to differentiate from a second BCC on imaging, although some generalizations can help differentiate these two entities. Since a BCC is congenital, they almost always present in patients less than 40 years of age, but usually much younger. Occasionally, they may be clinically occult until they become infected. By contrast, SCCs of the pharynx is a disease of older patients, usually between the fifth and seventh decades, although because of an increase in HPV-associated SCC, cancers of the pharynx are now being identified in younger patients. That said, as a general rule, any cystic lesion at the level IIA nodal station in a patient 40 years old or older should be considered a metastatic lymph node, until proven otherwise. Careful scrutiny of the ipsilateral palatine tonsil and/or tongue base should be performed in this scenario, given the high propensity of oropharyngeal cancer to metastasize to the level IIA nodal station. If available, the oropharynx should also be viewed with delayed postcontrast imaging, as delayed imaging can detect malignancies to a greater advantage compared to the more immediate postcontrast images.

An uninfected BCC has a thin, non-nodular wall, whereas an infected BCC usually has a thickened, irregular wall that diffusely enhances. On CT or MRI, BCCs can have variable density and signal characteristics, respectively, depending on the protein content of the cyst and/or whether it is infected. A necrotic metastatic lymph node will usually have some degree of enhancing nodularity along its walls.

While extracapsular spread (ECS) of tumor can appear similar to the fat stranding associated with an infected BCC, there are usually several imaging characteristics that help differentiate ECS of tumor from an infected BCC: there is usually more than one metastatic lymph node with ECS of tumor, the amount of fat stranding is usually more focal and less extensive with ECS of tumor, and there is milder thickening of the adjacent platysma muscle with ECS of tumor relative to an infected BCC, unless the platysma muscle frankly invaded by tumor. Furthermore, the clinical scenario of each entity is quite different and often aids in differentiating these two lesions.

PET imaging can be invaluable to evaluate primary malignancies of the pharynx and its metastatic disease, particularly if the primary tumor is not evident or there are indeterminate lymph nodes on MRI or CT. Just as with MRI and CT, assessment of the margin of the cystic lesion is important when evaluating these lesions on PET, as hypermetabolic activity along the margin of the lesion would favor a metastatic lesion over an uninfected BCC. While an infected BCC may be also hypermetabolic along its periphery, again the clinical scenario should help differentiate these two entities.

A primary malignancy arising from a BBC, termed a branchiogenic carcinoma, has been described in the literature, with much debate. Some argue that this is not a true diagnosis but rather a metastatic lymph node from an unknown primary. Nevertheless, this entity should be regarded only as a diagnosis of exclusion.

While a positive FNA of a suspected metastatic lymph node is useful, a negative FNA does not exclude malignancy, since there is a high rate of false negative results with an FNA. If there is persistent clinical concern despite a negative FNA, then an open biopsy and/or surgical removal of the lesion may be necessary.

Second branchial cleft cyst

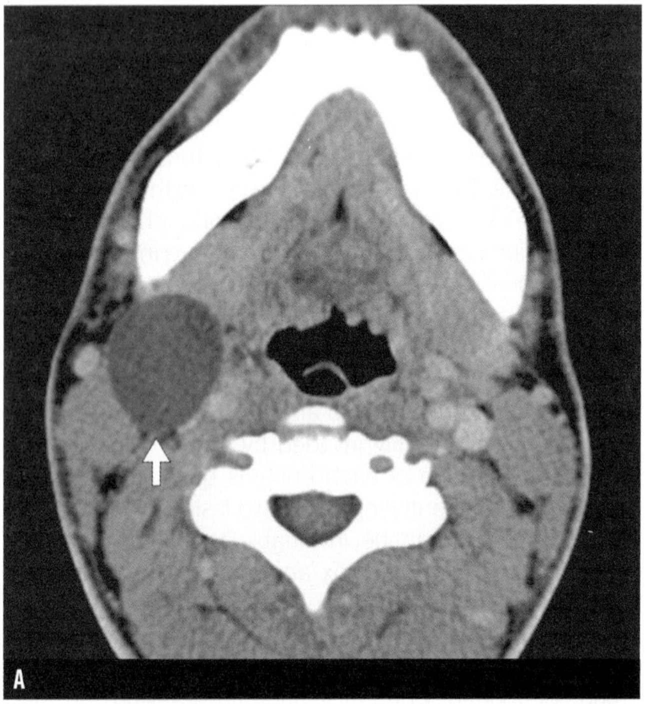

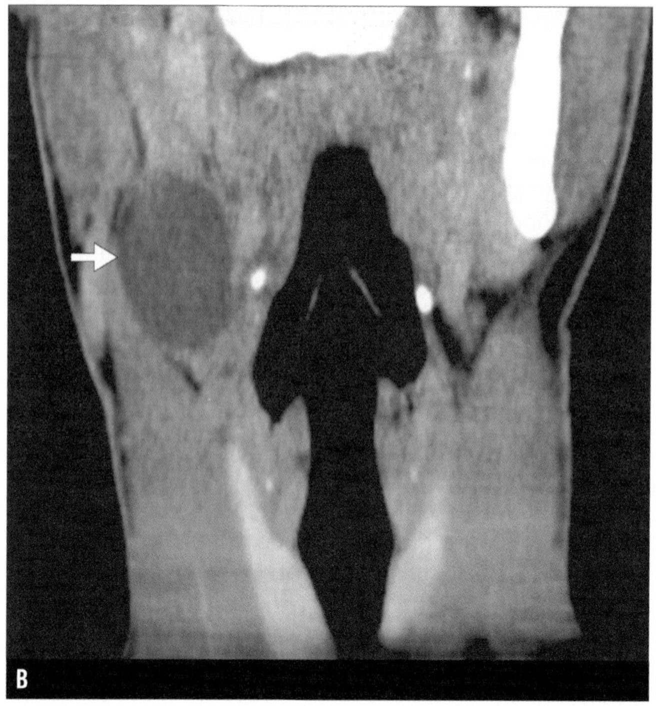

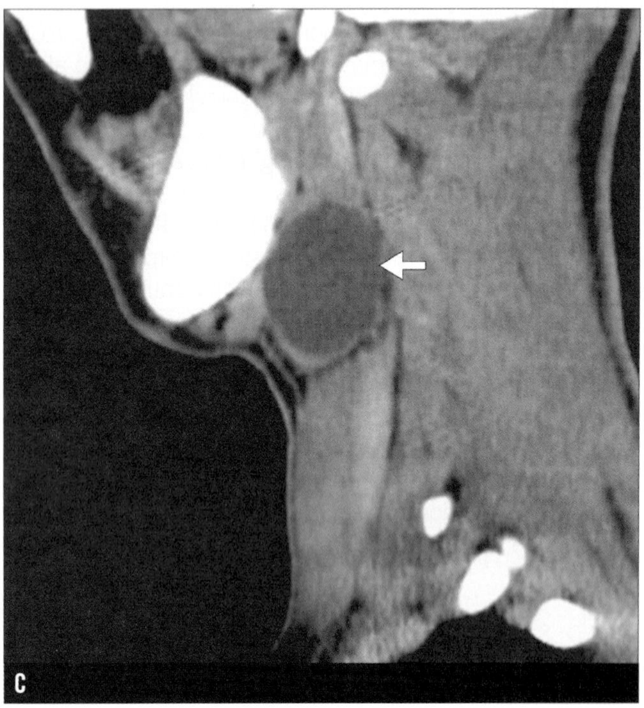

Axial (**A**), coronal reformatted (**B**), and sagittal reformatted (**C**) postcontrast CT images through the neck demonstrate an oval, circumscribed, nonenhancing, fluid attenuating lesion medial to the right sternocleidomastoid muscle in a 17-year-old patient (arrows, **A**-**C**). The location and imaging characteristics in a patient of this age are compatible with a second branchial cleft cyst, which was also demonstrated at pathology following resection.

Necrotic metastatic lymphadenopathy

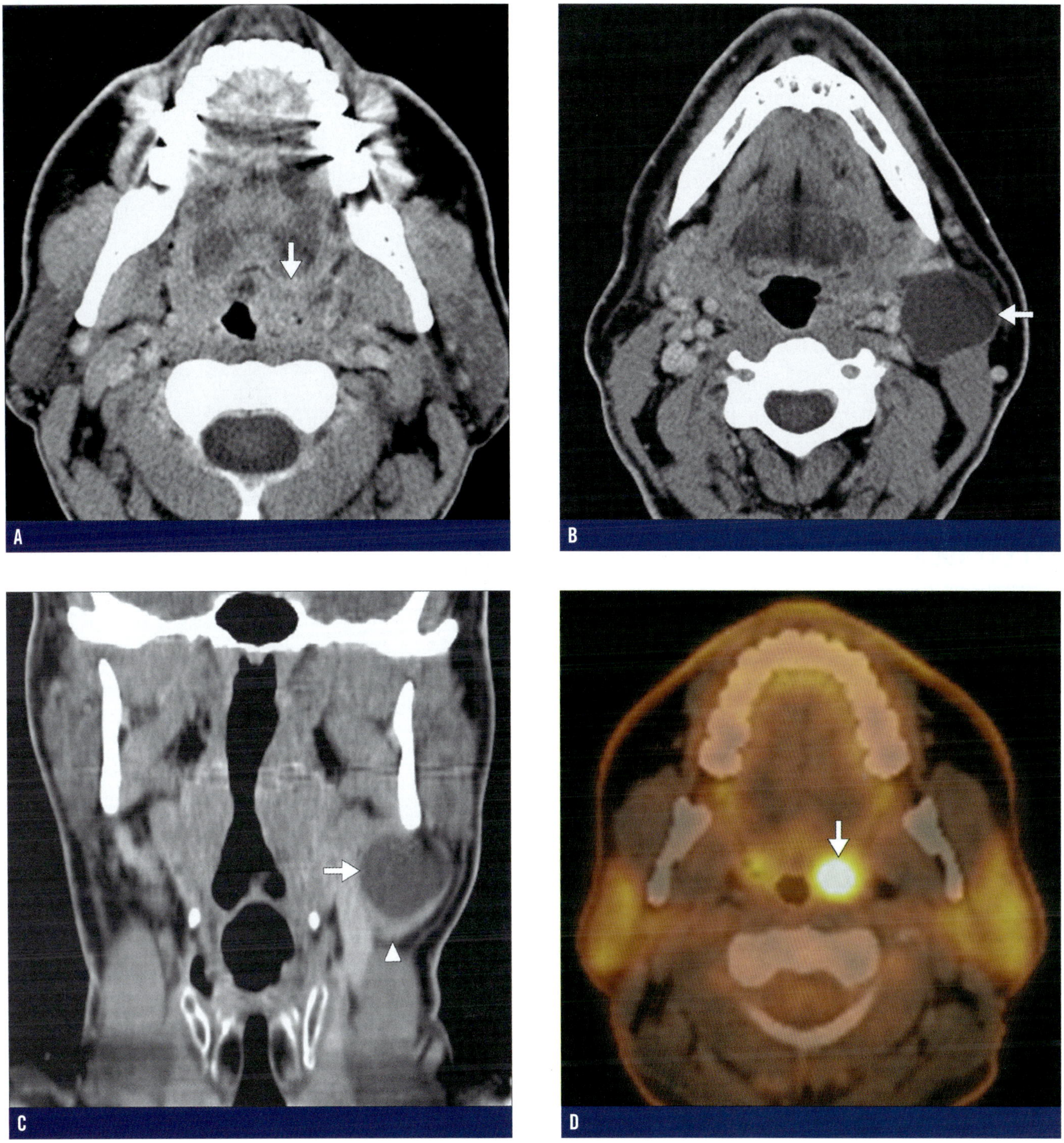

A contrast-enhanced axial CT image through the oropharynx (**A**) demonstrates mild asymmetric enlargement of the left palatine tonsil in a 49-year-old patient (arrow, **A**). Contrast-enhanced axial (**B**) and coronal reformatted (**C**) CT images from the same study demonstrate a fluid containing cystic lesion in the left neck, ventral to the left sternocleidomastoid muscle, simulating a branchial cleft cyst (arrows, **B**, **C**). However, image **C** demonstrates a thin rind of soft tissue along the undersurface of this finding (arrowhead, **C**), raising the possibility that the finding represents a necrotic lymph node, particularly given the left palatine tonsil finding. An axial PET CT image through the oropharynx (**D**) demonstrates pronounced hypermetabolic activity affecting the left palatine tonsil, compatible with tumor (arrow, **D**). Axial (**E**) and coronal reformatted (**F**) images from the same PET CT study demonstrate the left neck cystic lesion to be largely hypometabolic (arrows, **E**, **F**) except for subtle hypermetabolic areas along its periphery (arrowheads, **F**), consistent with a pathologic lymph node given the constellation of findings. This case illustrates that a cystic mass in the jugulodigastric region in a middle age or older patient (generally >40 years of age) should be considered malignant, rather than a benign cyst, until proven otherwise.

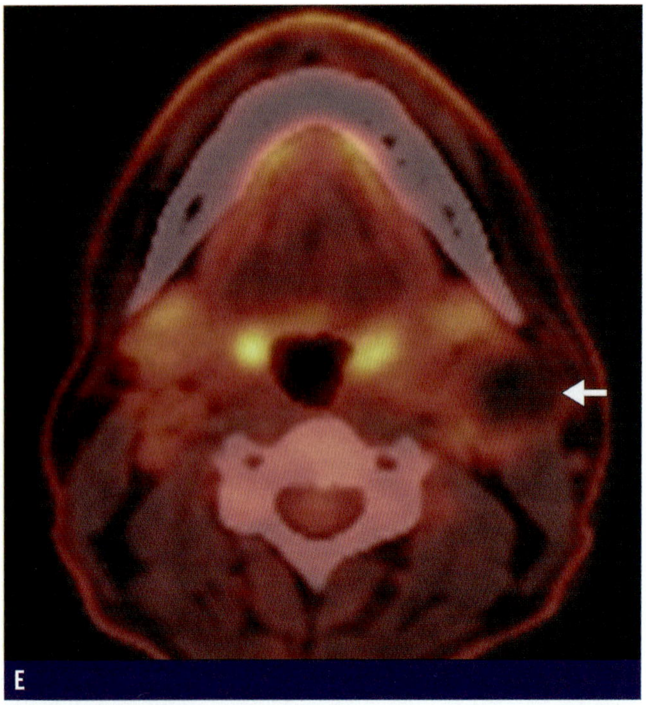

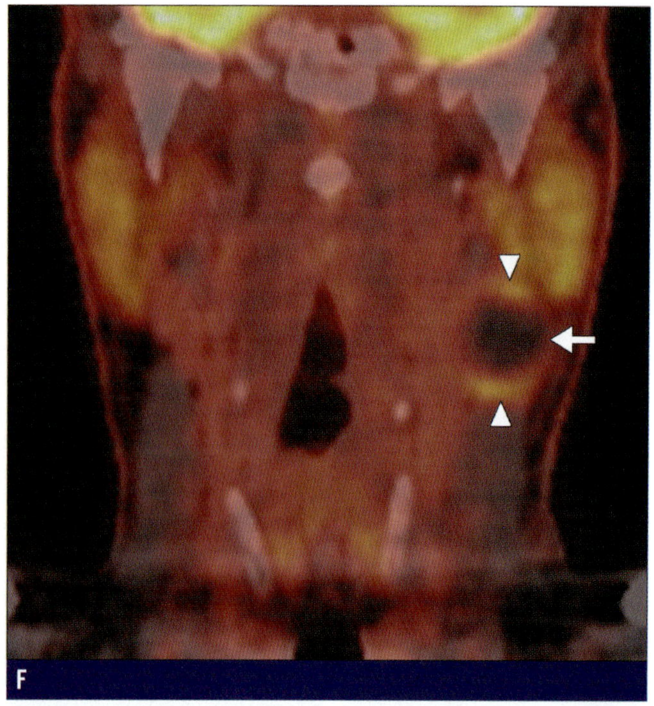

REFERENCES

Chi HS, Wang LF, Chiang FY, Kuo WR, Lee KW. Branchial cleft cyst as the initial impression of a metastatic thyroid papillary carcinoma: two case reports. *Kaohsiung J Med Sci.* 2007;23(12):634-638.

Devaney KO, et al. Squamous carcinoma arising in a branchial cleft cyst: have you ever treated one? Will you? *J Laryngol Otol.* 2008;122(6):547-550.

Pietarinen-Runtti P, Apajalahti S, Robinson S, Passador-Santos F, Leivo I, Mäkitie AA. Cystic neck lesions: clinical, radiological and differential diagnostic considerations. *Acta Otolaryngol.* 2010;130(2):300-304.

CASE 22 Normal anterior rectus capitis muscles simulating nodes of Rouvière

The anterior rectus capitis muscle is a short, thin, paired muscle that arises from the anterior margin of the C1 lateral mass and ascends superomedially to insert on each side of the basiocciput, just posterior to the longus capitis muscle. With the assistance of the longus capitis muscles, these muscles flex and rotate the head as well as return the head to neutral positioning following extension. The anterior rectus capitis muscles are innervated by C1 and C2.

The oval, circumscribed appearance of each anterior rectus capitis muscle on a single axial image can simulate abnormally enlarged retropharyngeal lymph nodes. However, evaluating the finding over several axial images, as well as the awareness of the normal location of this paired muscle, will allow one to appropriately differentiate these normal muscles from a potentially abnormal node of Rouvière.

COMPANION CASES

- **Normal node of Rouvière.** Both medial and lateral retropharyngeal lymph nodes exist, with the laterally located lymph nodes also referred to as the "nodes of Rouvière." In 1938, Dr. Rouvière established the anatomic locations of cervical lymph nodes and their drainage patterns according to surgical landmarks. The nodes of Rouvière are located anterior or just lateral to the longus colli muscle, medial to the carotid space, and typically posterior to the lateral aspect of the pharyngeal wall. Normal nodes of Rouvière are common in children and young adults, but are less commonly identified, or are very small, in older patients on imaging. While authors differ in the size criterion used for a normal node of Rouvière, most consider the largest axial dimension of 0.8 cm or less to be a normal size. However, in children and young adults who do not have a history of head and neck malignancy or an active infection, a node of Rouvière larger than 0.8 cm is often normal.
- **Non-necrotic pathologic node of Rouvière.** A circumscribed, enhancing lateral retropharyngeal space lesion should raise suspicion of a pathologic node of Rouvière, either arising from an infectious or metastatic etiology. Criteria for abnormal retropharyngeal nodes include a greatest axial dimension of larger than 0.8 cm (in the adult patient), abnormal nodular enhancement, and necrosis (focal or diffuse). Adjacent fat stranding may also be identified.
- **Necrotic node of Rouvière.** Focal or diffuse necrosis of a node of Rouvière is always abnormal. Common causes include a pyogenic infection of the upper pharynx and a metastatic lymph node, especially from a nasopharyngeal carcinoma. The margins of these nodes of Rouvière should be carefully inspected as both a suppurative lymph node from a pyogenic infection or a metastatic lymph node can result in extracapsular spread into the retropharyngeal space. In the case of a suppurative node of Rouvière with extracapsular spread, the infection may ultimately involve mediastinum via the danger space, a potentially life-threatening situation.
- **Poststyloid parapharyngeal space schwannoma.** Given their proximity, a tumor within the poststyloid parapharyngeal space may simulate a pathologic node of Rouvière, although the former will typically at least abut or sometimes reside between the internal carotid artery and internal jugular vein, whereas the latter does not. For further discussion regarding the parapharyngeal space, please refer to Chapter 7.

Normal anterior rectus capitis muscles

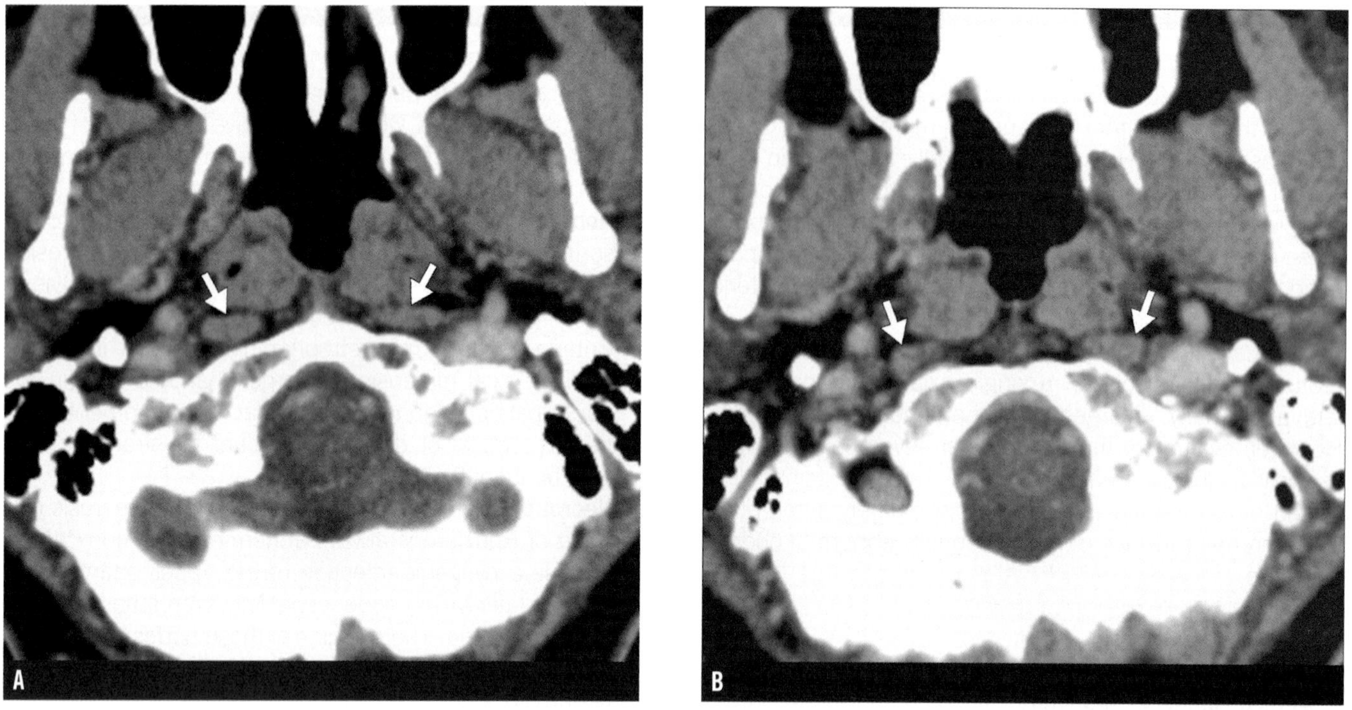

Postcontrast axial CT images through the level of the nasopharynx (**A**, **B**) demonstrate paired soft tissue densities (arrows, **A**, **B**) immediately anterior to the basiocciput. These findings represent the normal anterior rectus capitis muscles. These muscles can sometimes simulate abnormally enlarged retropharyngeal lymph nodes (also called nodes of Rouvière).

Companion case: Normal node of Rouvière

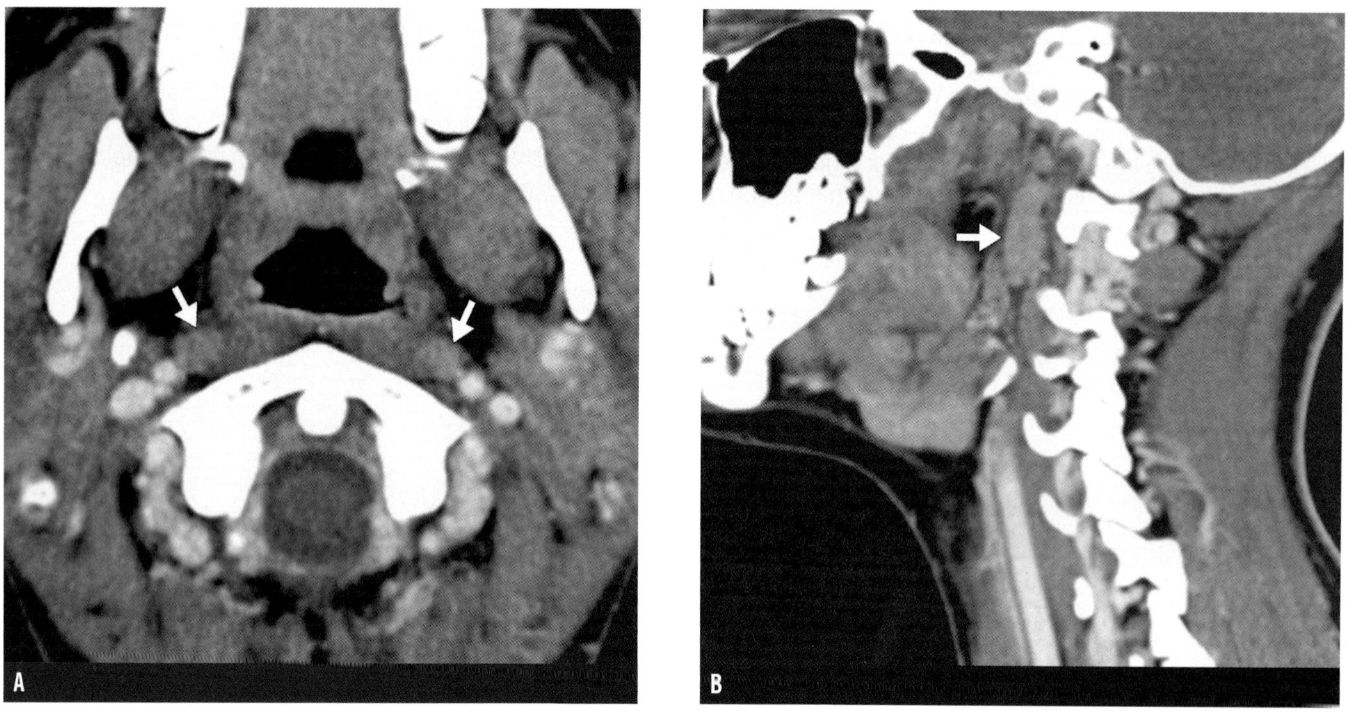

Axial (**A**) and sagittal reformatted (**B**) postcontrast CT images demonstrate prominent but normal nodes of Rouvière in a healthy 19-year-old patient (arrows, **A**, **B**).

Companion case: Normal node of Rouvière

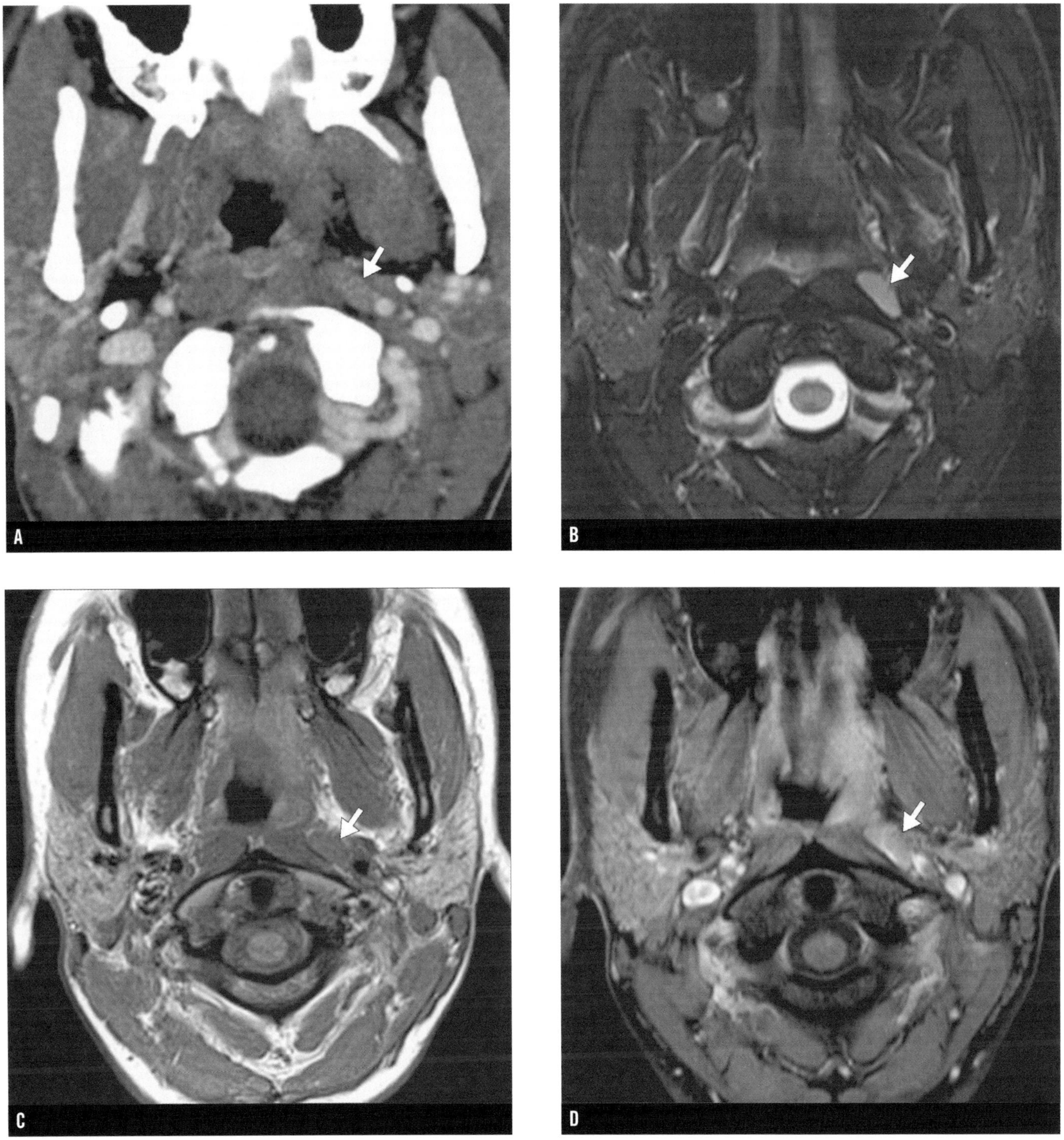

Different patient. A postcontrast axial CT image (**A**) as well as axial T2 with fat suppression (**B**), axial T1 (**C**), and postcontrast axial T1 with fat suppression (**D**) MR images through the nasopharynx demonstrate a prominent but normal left node of Rouvière in a healthy 24-year-old patient (arrows, **A-D**).

Companion case: Non-necrotic pathologic node of Rouvière

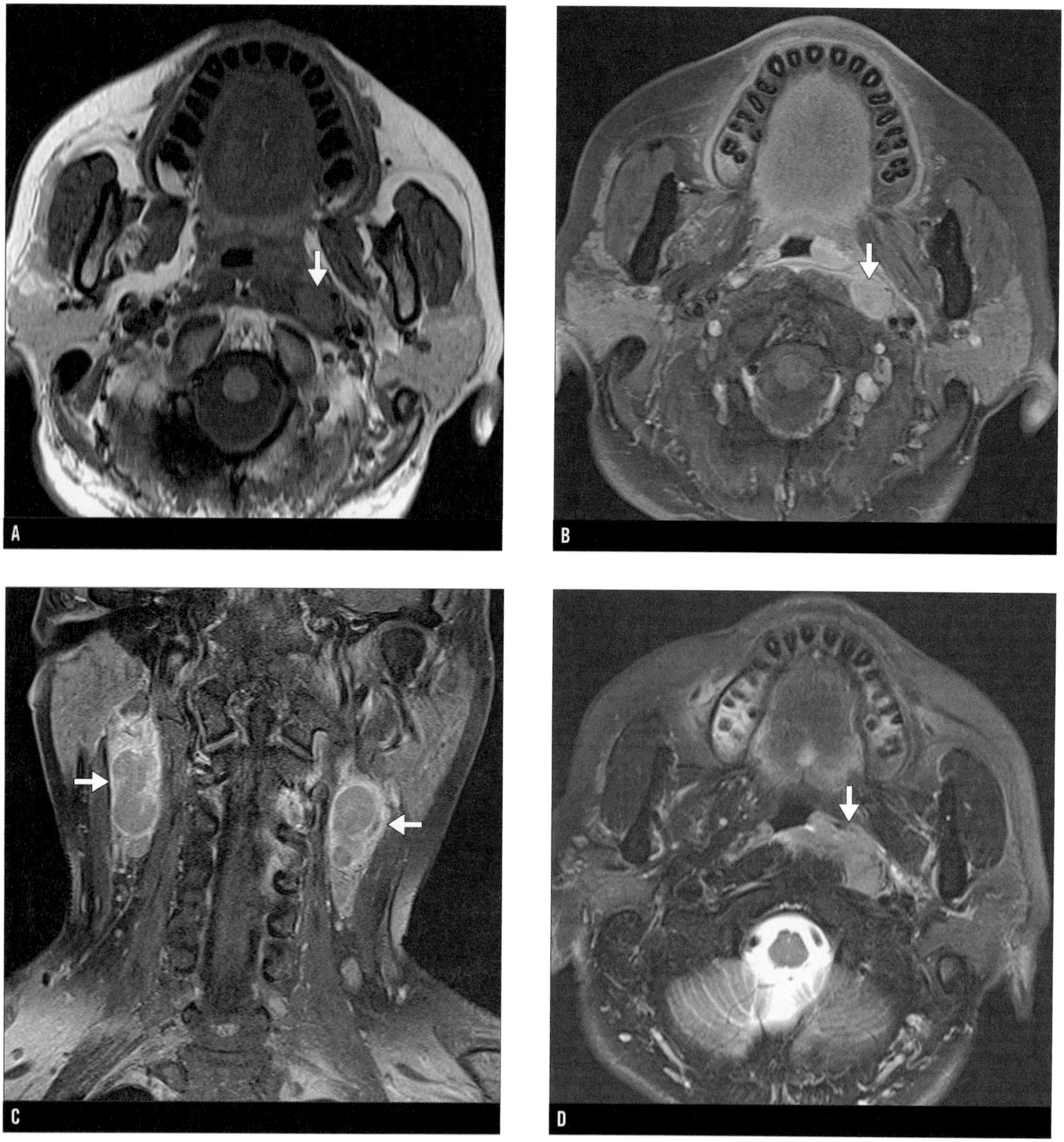

Axial T1 (**A**) and postcontrast axial T1 with fat suppression (**B**) MR images through the level of the nasopharynx demonstrate a pathologically enlarged, non-necrotic, left node of Rouvière (arrows, **A**, **B**). A postcontrast coronal T1-weighted MR image with fat suppression (**C**) demonstrates numerous additional pathologic lymph nodes in both sides of the neck (arrows, **C**). Axial T2 with fat suppression (**D**) and postcontrast axial T1 with fat suppression (**E**) demonstrate a left nasopharyngeal mass, compatible with nasopharyngeal carcinoma (arrows, **D**, **F**), which accounts for the pathologic lymph nodes. A postcontrast axial CT image of the same patient (**F**) demonstrates the CT appearance of the non-necrotic, pathologically enlarged left node of Rouvière (arrow, **F**).

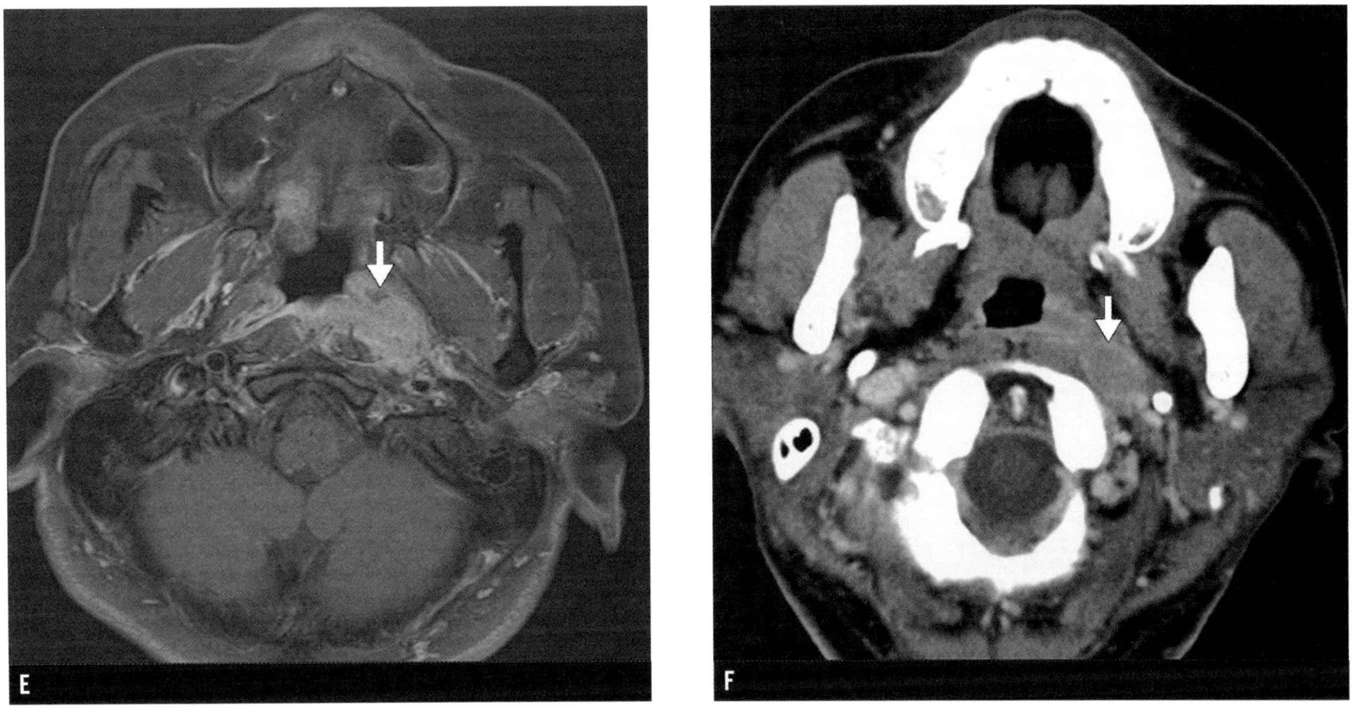

Companion case: Necrotic node of Rouvière

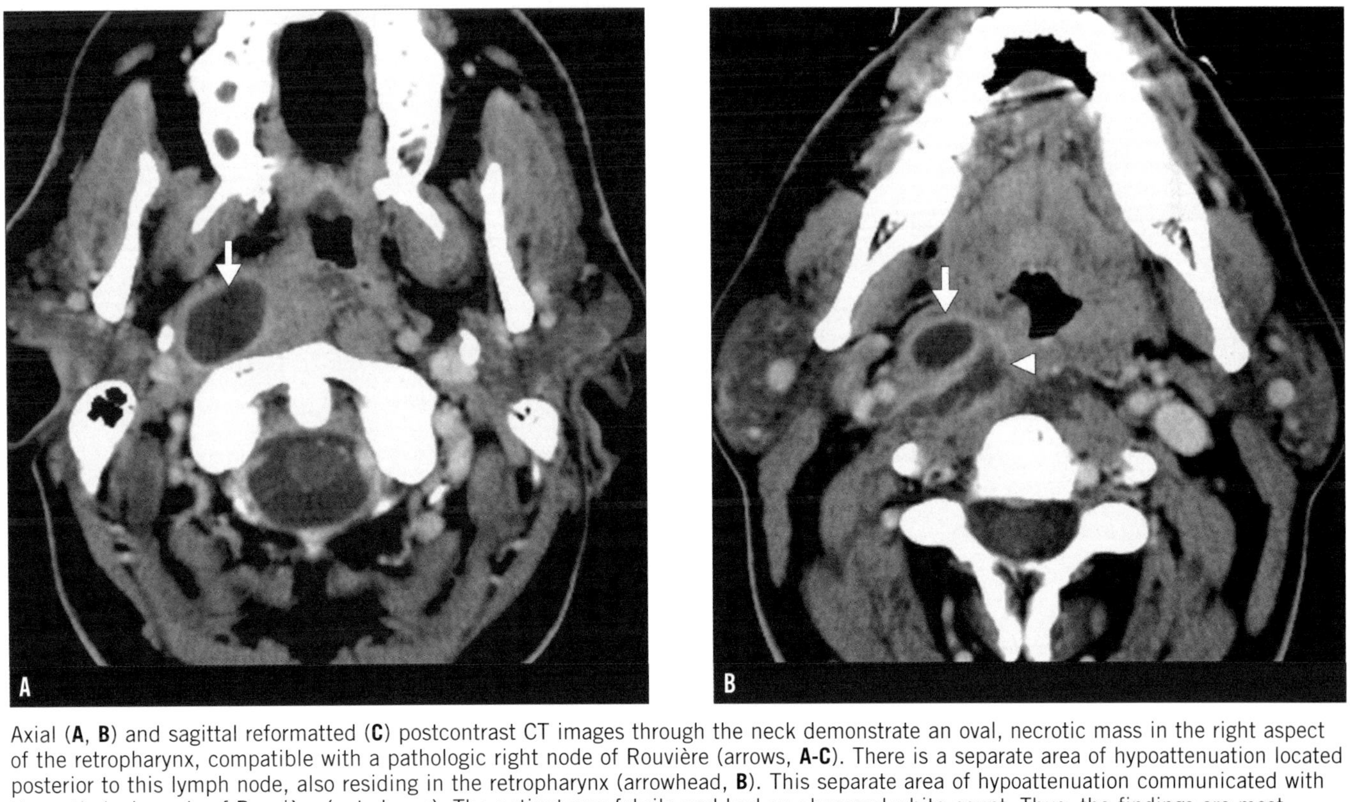

Axial (**A**, **B**) and sagittal reformatted (**C**) postcontrast CT images through the neck demonstrate an oval, necrotic mass in the right aspect of the retropharynx, compatible with a pathologic right node of Rouvière (arrows, **A-C**). There is a separate area of hypoattenuation located posterior to this lymph node, also residing in the retropharynx (arrowhead, **B**). This separate area of hypoattenuation communicated with the pathologic node of Rouvière (not shown). The patient was febrile and had an abnormal white count. Thus, the findings are most compatible with an abscess of the right node of Rouvière with extracapsular extension of the abscess into the retropharyngeal space. This patient developed a mediastinitis 2 days later that required emergent surgery.

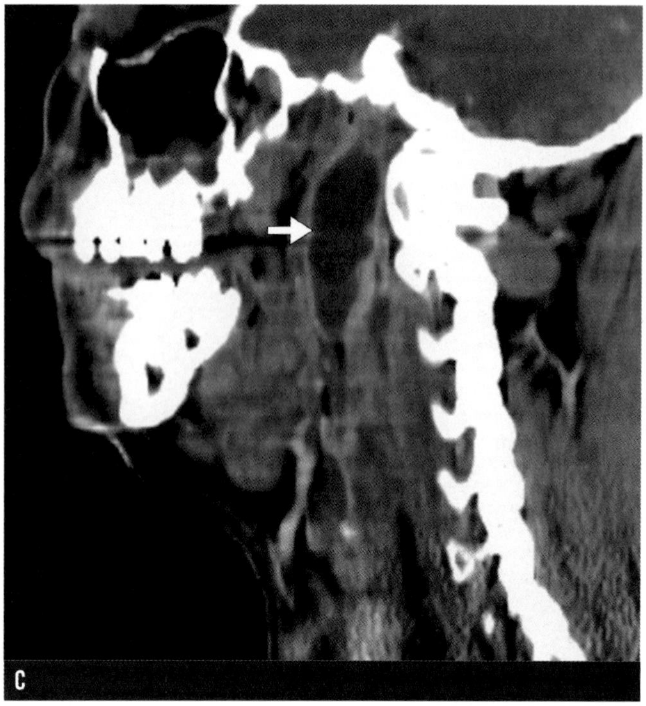

Companion case: Poststyloid parapharyngeal space schwannoma

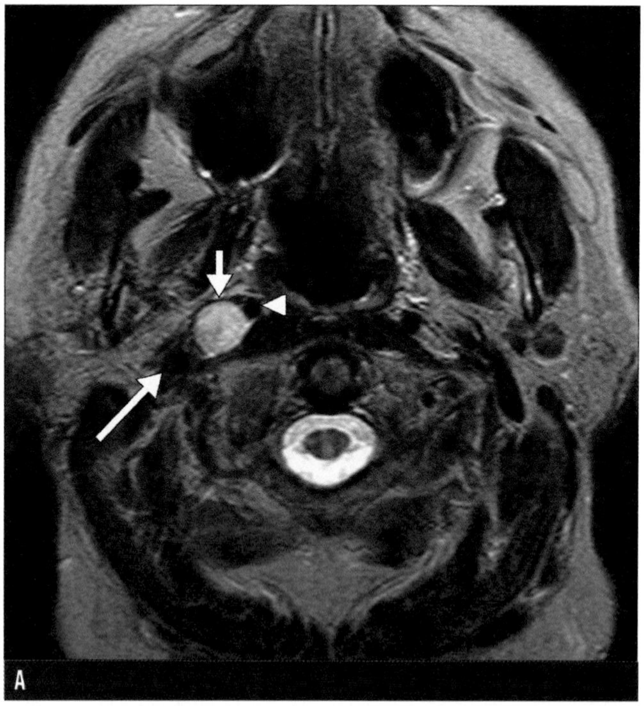

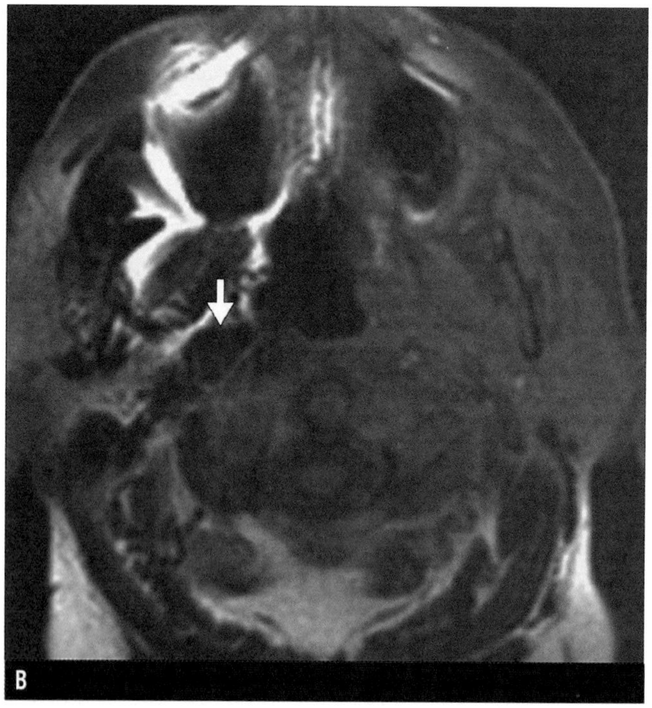

Axial T2 (**A**), unenhanced axial T1 with fat suppression (**B**), and contrast-enhanced axial MPRAGE (**C**) MR images as well as a contrast-enhanced axial CT image (**D**) demonstrate a mass in the right poststyloid parapharyngeal space (also called carotid space) (short arrows, **A**-**D**). This mass is interposed between the right cervical internal carotid artery, which is mildly displaced anteromedially (arrowheads, **A**, **C**, **D**), and the right internal jugular vein, which is situated posterolaterally (long arrows, **A**, **C**, **D**). This can be differentiated from a node of Rouvière by location; specifically, a node of Rouvière would be located in the retropharyngeal space and not centered in the poststyloid parapharyngeal space between these vessels. The mass is homogeneously hyperintense on T2, homogenously enhancing on T1, and mildly heterogeneously enhancing on CT. This was presumed to represent a schwannoma (either vagal or less likely sympathetic chain in origin) given its overall imaging characteristics. The imaging differential does include a paraganglioma, although the lack of a "salt and pepper" appearance (often present because of the increased vascularity of this tumor) makes this diagnosis less likely.

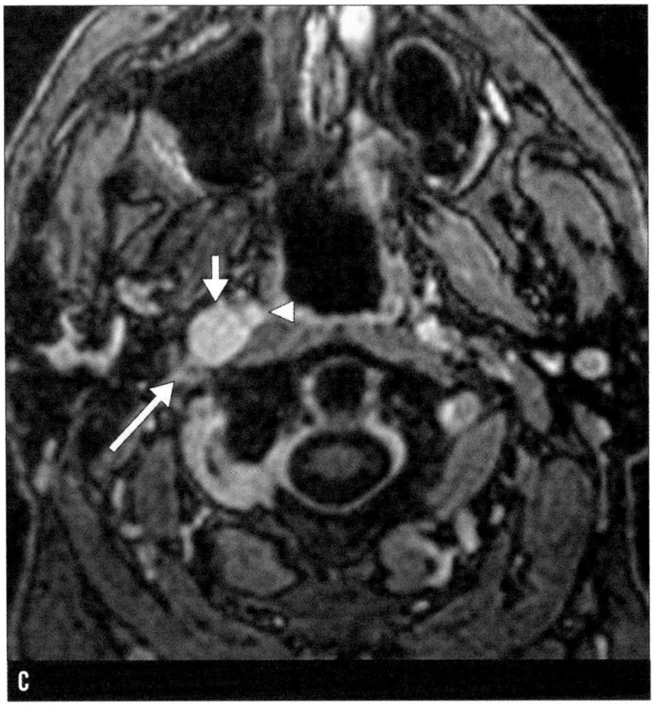

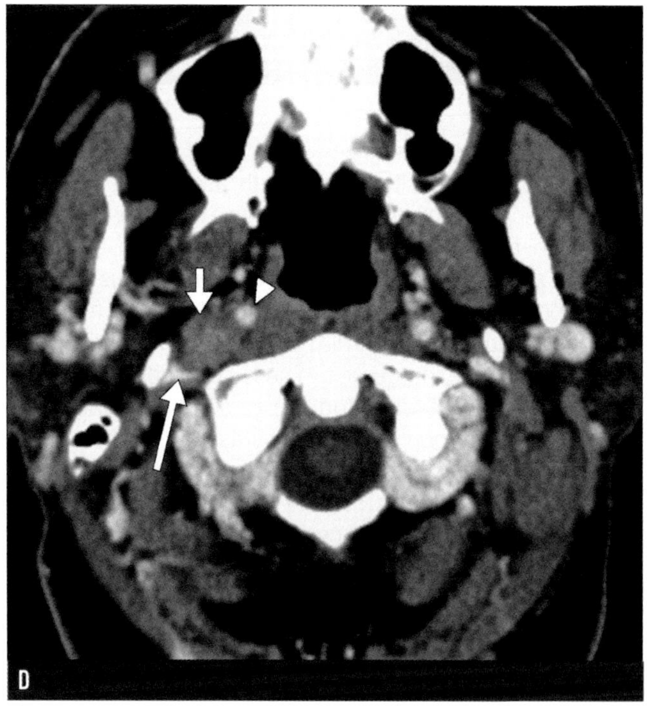

REFERENCES

Chong VF, Fan YF. Radiology of the retropharyngeal space. *Clinical radiology*. 2000;55(10):740-8.

Gupta A, Shah AD, Zhang Z, Phillips CD, Young RJ. Variability in the position of the retropharyngeal internal carotid artery. *Laryngoscope*. 2013;123(2):401-403.

Hoang JK, Eastwood JD, Iv BFB, Raduazo P, Glastonbury CM. Masses in the retropharyngeal space: key concepts on multiplanar CT and MR imaging. *Neurographics*. 2011;1(1):49–55.

Mancuso AA, Harnsberger HR, Muraki AS, Stevens MH. Computed tomography of cervical and retropharyngeal lymph nodes: normal anatomy, variants of normal, and applications in staging head and neck cancer. Part I: normal anatomy. *Radiology*. 1983;148(3):709-714.

Offiah CE, Hall E. Acute calcific tendinitis of the longus colli muscle: spectrum of CT appearances and anatomical correlation. *Br J Radiol*. 2009;82(978):e117-e121.

CASE 23 Focal atrophy of the longus capitis muscle

The longus capitis muscle is a paired muscle of the anterior superior capitis spine. With assistance from the anterior rectus capitus muscles, these muscles flex and rotate the head as well as return the head to a neutral position following extension. The longus capitis muscle is composed of four tendinous slips that arise from the anterior tubercles of the third through sixth cervical vertebrae transverse processes. These tendinous slips and muscle bundles traverse and merge superomedially, ultimately inserting upon the caudal parasagittal aspect of the basiocciput, just anterior to the anterior rectus capitis muscles. The longus capitis muscle is supplied by branches from the first through third cervical nerves.

Rarely, atrophy of one or both of these muscles may be encountered. Studies have suggested that deep cervical flexor muscle dysfunction may play a role in cervicalgia and cervicogenic headaches. However, the presence of longus capitis muscle atrophy is of unclear significance.

COMPANION CASES

- **Fatty infiltration of the longus capitis muscle.** Fatty infiltration of muscles is usually secondary to disuse atrophy or denervation atrophy. If atrophy and/or fatty infiltration of a cervical muscle is encountered, then evaluation of a potential etiology should be investigated. In the case of longus capitis muscle atrophy, this includes evaluation of a lesion along the first through third cervical nerves, such as from cervical degenerative changes or a mass.

Focal atrophy of the longus capitis muscle

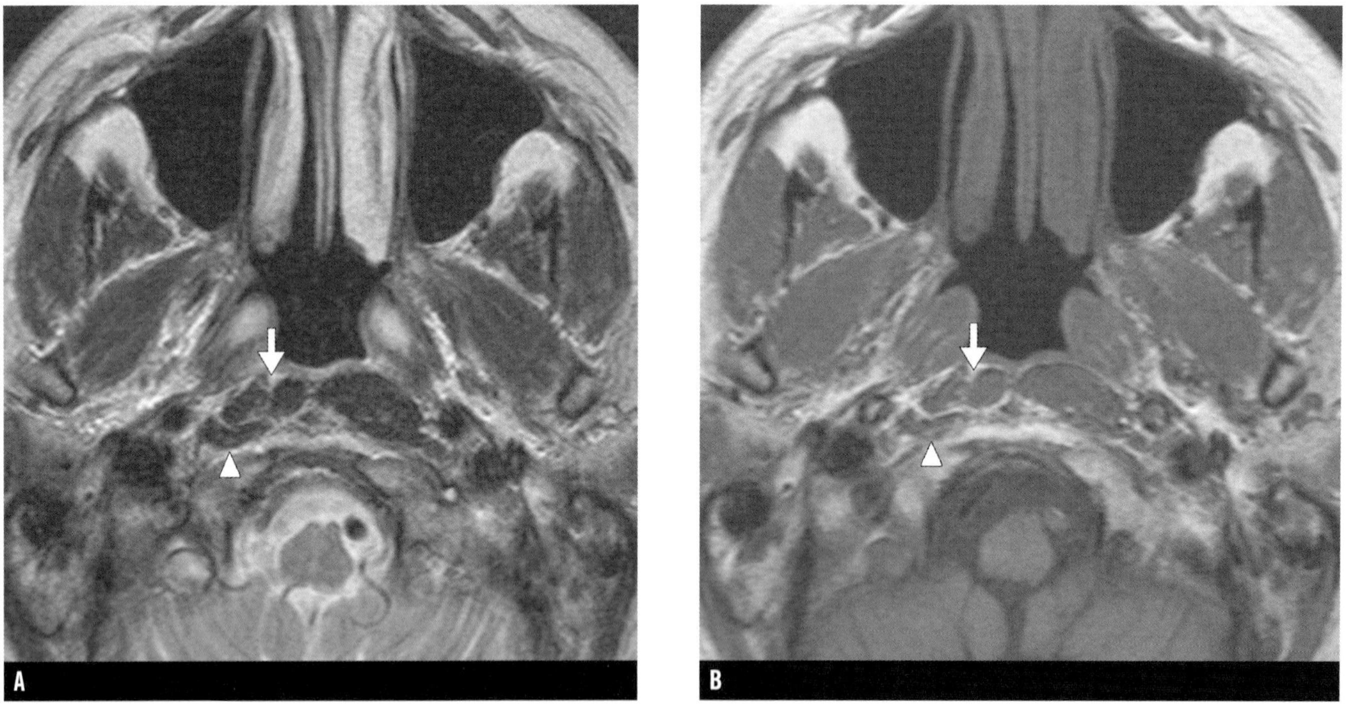

Axial T2 (**A**), axial T1 (**B**), and postcontrast axial T1 (**C**) MR images through the nasopharynx demonstrate focal atrophy of the right longus capitis muscle (arrows, **A-C**). This was an incidental finding. The normal right anterior rectus capitis muscle is present just posterior to this finding (arrowheads, **A-C**).

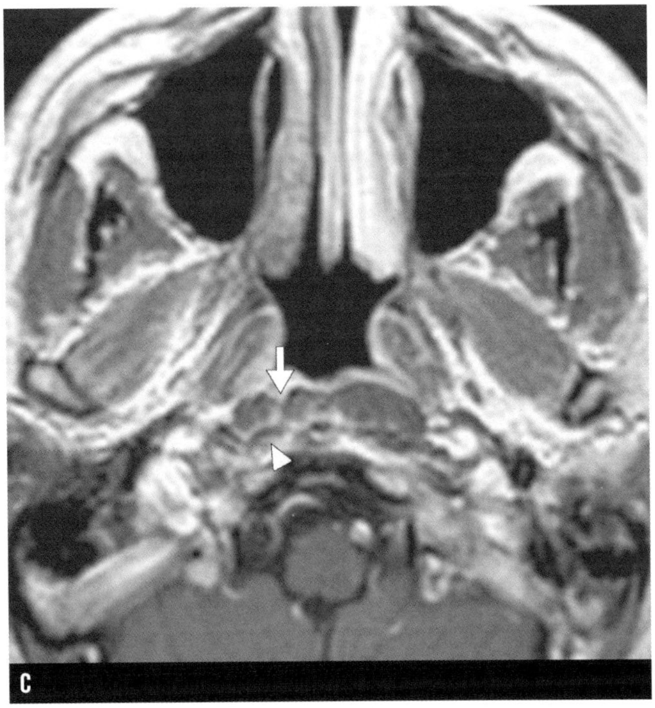

Fatty infiltration of the longus capitis muscle

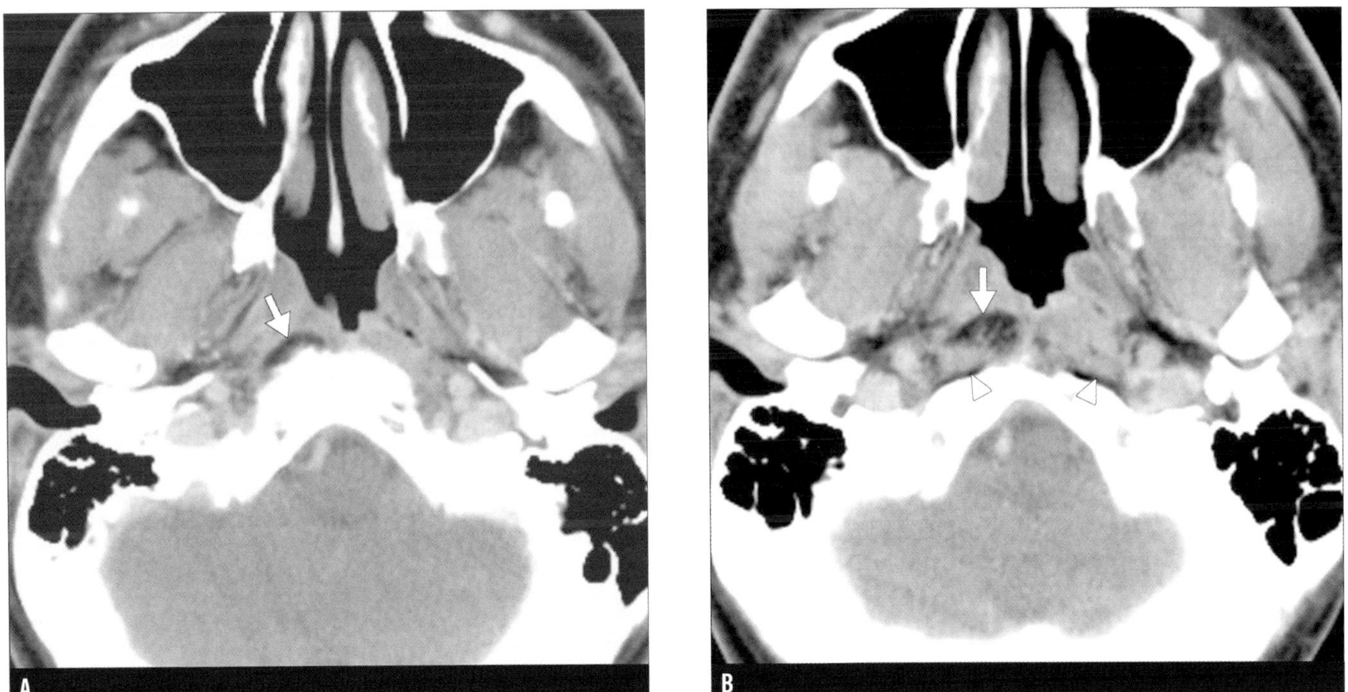

Postcontrast axial CT images through the nasopharynx (**A, B**) and oropharynx (**C**) as well as a sagittal reformatted CT image (**D**) demonstrate fatty infiltration along the superior aspect of the right longus capitis muscle (arrows, **A-D**). The etiology of this muscle's fatty infiltration was not able to be determined. As a reference, the normal anterior rectus capitis muscles (arrowheads, **B**) and longus colli muscles merging at the midline (arrowhead, **C**) are also shown. Both the longus capitis muscle and the anterior rectus capitis muscles insert upon the basiocciput, the former located anterior to the latter. By contrast, the longus colli muscles have several insertions, the most cephalad is located at the anterior tubercle of C1.

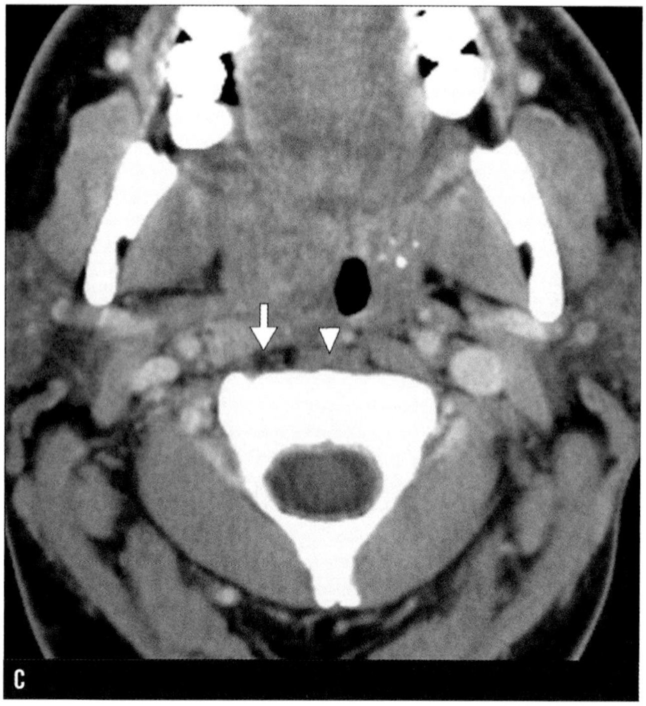

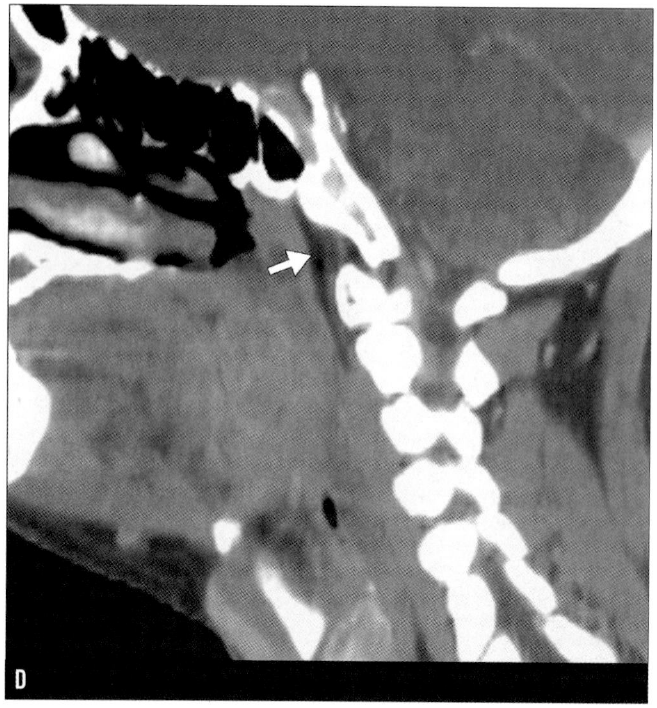

REFERENCES

Falla DL, Jull G, Hodges PW. Patients with neck pain demonstrate reduced electromyographic activity of the deep cervical flexor muscles during performance of the craniocervical flexion test. *Spine.* 2004;29(19):2108-2114.

Gray H. *Anatomy of the Human Body.* 1918. www.bartleby.com. Accessed December 2012.

Gray H. *Anatomy of the Human Body.* 20th ed. Philadelphia, PA: Lea & Febiger, 1918; www.bartleby.com. Accessed December 2012.

Jull G, Barrett C, Magee R, Ho P. Further clinical clarification of the muscle dysfunction in cervical headache. *Cephalalgia.* 1999;19:179-185.

Sakamoto Y. Spatial relationships between the morphologies and innervations of the scalene and anterior vertebral muscles. *Ann Anat.* 2012;194(4):381-388.

CASE 24 Longus colli tendon hydroxyapatite deposition

The longus colli muscle is a paired muscle located along the anterior aspect of the cervical and upper thoracic spine and constitutes the majority of the prevertebral space. The muscle has a complex configuration arising from three separate portions: a superior oblique, an inferior oblique, and a vertical (central) portion. The superior oblique portion arises from tendinous slips along the transverse processes of the C3 to C5 vertebrae and inserts upon the anterior tubercle of C1 at the midline. The inferior oblique portion arises from the ventral margin of the T1 to T3 vertebral bodies and inserts upon the anterior tubercles of the C5 and C6 transverse processes. The vertical portions arise from the ventral aspect of the C5 through T3 vertebral bodies and attach to the ventral aspect of the C2 to C4 vertebral bodies. Functionally, the longus colli muscle assists in flexion and rotation of the cervical spine, and its unilateral action leads to ipsilateral flexion. Because portions of the longus colli and longus capitis muscles are in close proximity and can be difficult to differentiate from one another on imaging, they are often referred to as the "longus colli-capitis complex."

Hydroxyapatite deposition disease (HADD) occurs when calcium hydroxyapatite crystals are deposited into tendons, bursae, or joint capsules. The mechanism of this deposition is unknown. However, it has been postulated to either represent a primary crystal deposition disease or to be the result of other disease processes, such as collagen vascular disorders, chronic kidney failure, or osteoarthritis. The most commonly affected site is the shoulder; however, deposition in the longus colli tendon is not uncommon. By CT or plain film radiography, these crystals appear as amorphous calcifications in the proximal fibers of the longus colli tendon, just inferior to the anterior arch of the atlas. HADD of the longus colli tendon has been primarily described in literature as it pertains to acute calcific tendinitis of the longus colli muscle. However, an asymptomatic *silent phase* of the disease has been described in the shoulder where the calcium deposits are completely contained within the tendon. Since HADD affecting the longus colli tendon is considered the same disease, it follows that one may also encounter these deposits incidentally in the longus colli tendon. The *mechanical phase* is considered the active, painful phase of the disease where aseptic inflammatory changes prevail. This results in the clinical entity termed acute calcific tendinitis of the longus colli muscle. During this phase, the deposits may increase in size and become less defined.

COMPANION CASES

- **Acute calcific tendinitis of the longus colli muscle.** Initially described by Hartley in 1964, this entity represents an acute inflammation of the superior oblique tendon fibers of the longus colli muscle because of the presence of calcium hydroxyapatite deposits. The classic clinical presentation is that of acute neck pain, stiffness, odynophagia, low-grade fever, and mild leukocytosis. Since many of these same symptoms can be identified with other clinical entities, namely a retropharyngeal abscess, acute calcific tendinitis of the longus colli muscle may be clinically misdiagnosed. CT, or sometimes plain film radiography, best demonstrates the hydroxyapatite crystals, frequently identified as amorphous calcifications in the prevertebral space located just caudal to the anterior arch of C1. On CT and MRI, there will be an associated prevertebral fluid effusion that is well defined and without peripheral enhancement. The lack of significant peripheral enhancement on either CT or MRI helps differentiate this entity from a retropharyngeal abscess. This is an important differentiation since a retropharyngeal abscess often requires surgical intervention, whereas acute calcific tendinitis of the longus coli is treated conservatively with nonsteroidal anti-inflammatory agents. The nonsteroidal anti-inflammatory agents often provide rapid symptomatic relief and usually lead to the dissolution of the hydroxyapatite deposits.
- **Enlarging longus colli tendon hydroxyapatite deposition.** This may represent an incidental finding at the onset of the *mechanical phase* of HADD, the sequela of a recent episode of acute calcific tendinitis, or simply a subclinical increase in the amount of calcium deposits.
- **C1 anterior vertebral osteophyte formation.** Osteoarthritis of the cervical spine most commonly affects the anterior aspect of the cervical spine, manifesting as anterior endplate osteophytes. This includes osteophytes that form along the anterior tubercle of the atlas. These C1 osteophytes can project inferiorly and mimic hydroxyapatite deposits. However, inferiorly projecting anterior C1 osteophytes are well corticated, may contain a marrow space, and are in contiguity with the C1 anterior tubercle, findings that are not identified with HADD.
- **Retropharyngeal course of an atherosclerotic internal carotid artery.** Atherosclerotic plaque can be calcified or noncalcified and usually occurs at areas of greatest shear force, such as at the bifurcation of the internal and external carotid arteries. When such calcified plaques are present along medialized cervical internal carotid arteries that course into the region of the retropharyngeal space, the calcified atherosclerosis may be mistaken for longus colli tendon calcification, particularly on sagittal reformatted CT imaging or lateral plain film radiography.

Longus colli tendon hydroxyapatite deposition

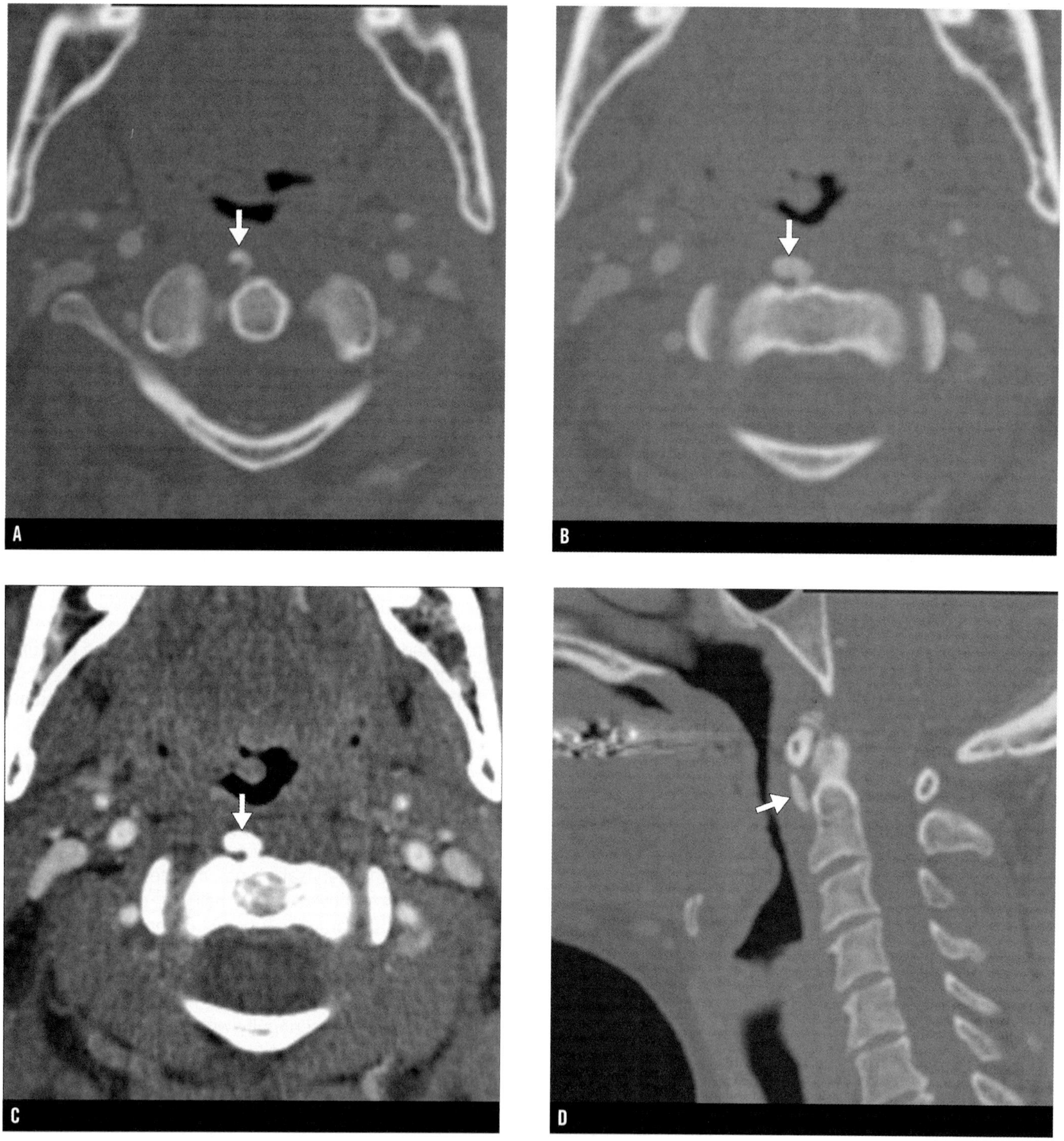

Postcontrast axial CT images viewed with a bone algorithm (**A**, **B**) and soft tissue algorithm (**C**) as well as a sagittal reformatted CT image viewed with a bone algorithm (**D**) demonstrate a focus of calcification in the region of the right longus colli tendon, most compatible with hydroxyapatite deposition (arrows, **A-D**). The lack of contiguity with the adjacent osseous structures favors that this represents hydroxyapatite deposition rather than osteophyte formation. There is no evidence of a retropharyngeal fluid collection. This patient was asymptomatic and the calcification presumably represented the silent phase of HADD. However, when this type of calcification is identified, one should evaluate for simple edema in the retropharynx to exclude acute calcific tendinitis of the longus colli muscle, particularly in patients who present with neck pain and odynophagia.

Companion case: Acute calcific tendinitis of the longus colli muscle

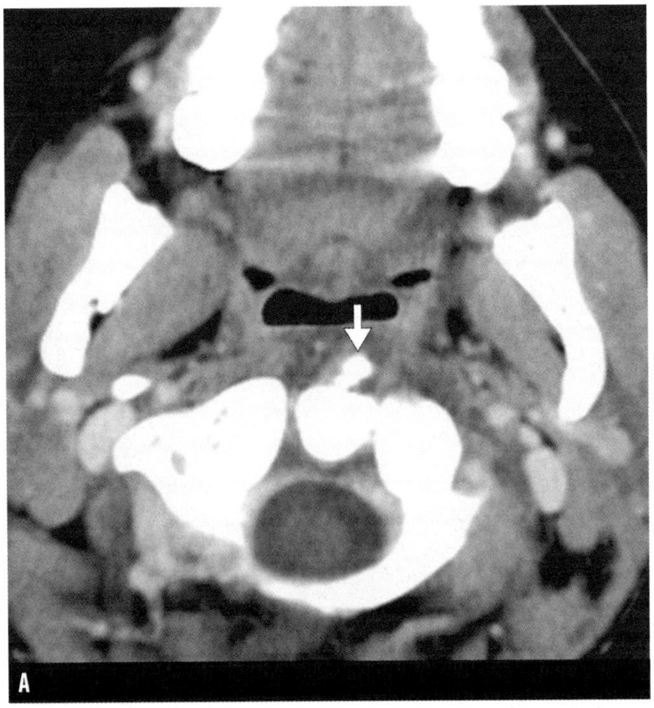

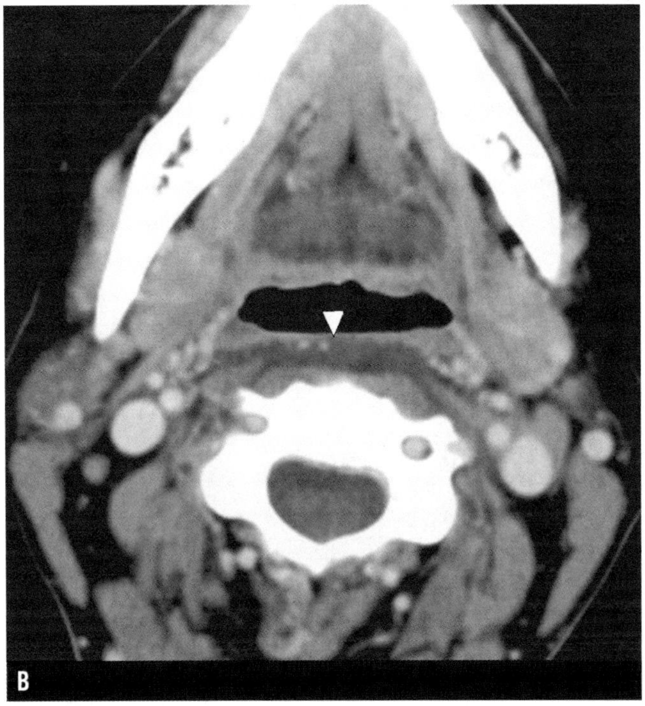

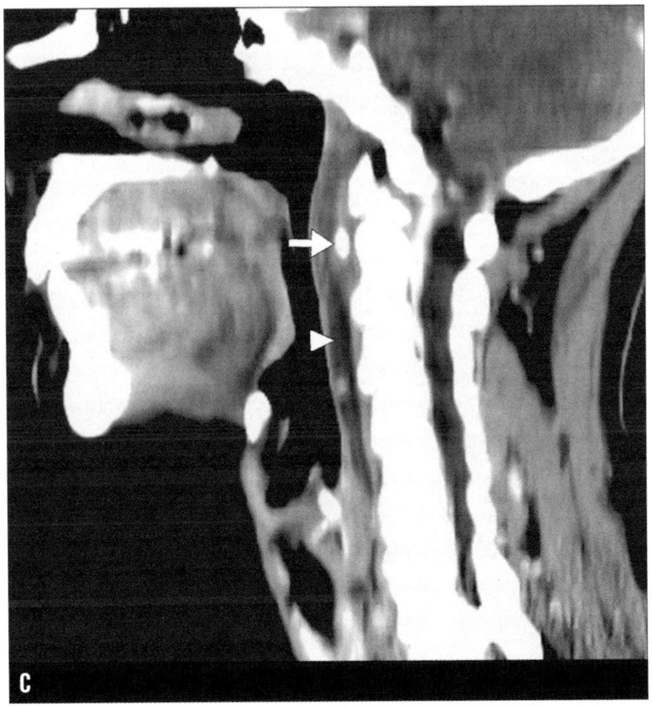

Axial (**A**, **B**) and coronal reformatted (**C**) postcontrast CT images demonstrate a focal area of calcification in the region of the longus colli tendon (arrows, **A**, **C**) and simple, nonenhancing fluid in the retropharynx (arrowheads, **B**, **C**). This patient presented with neck pain and odynophagia. The imaging findings and clinical presentation are compatible with acute calcific tendinitis of the longus colli muscle.

Companion case: Acute calcific tendinitis of the longus colli muscle with subsequent resolution

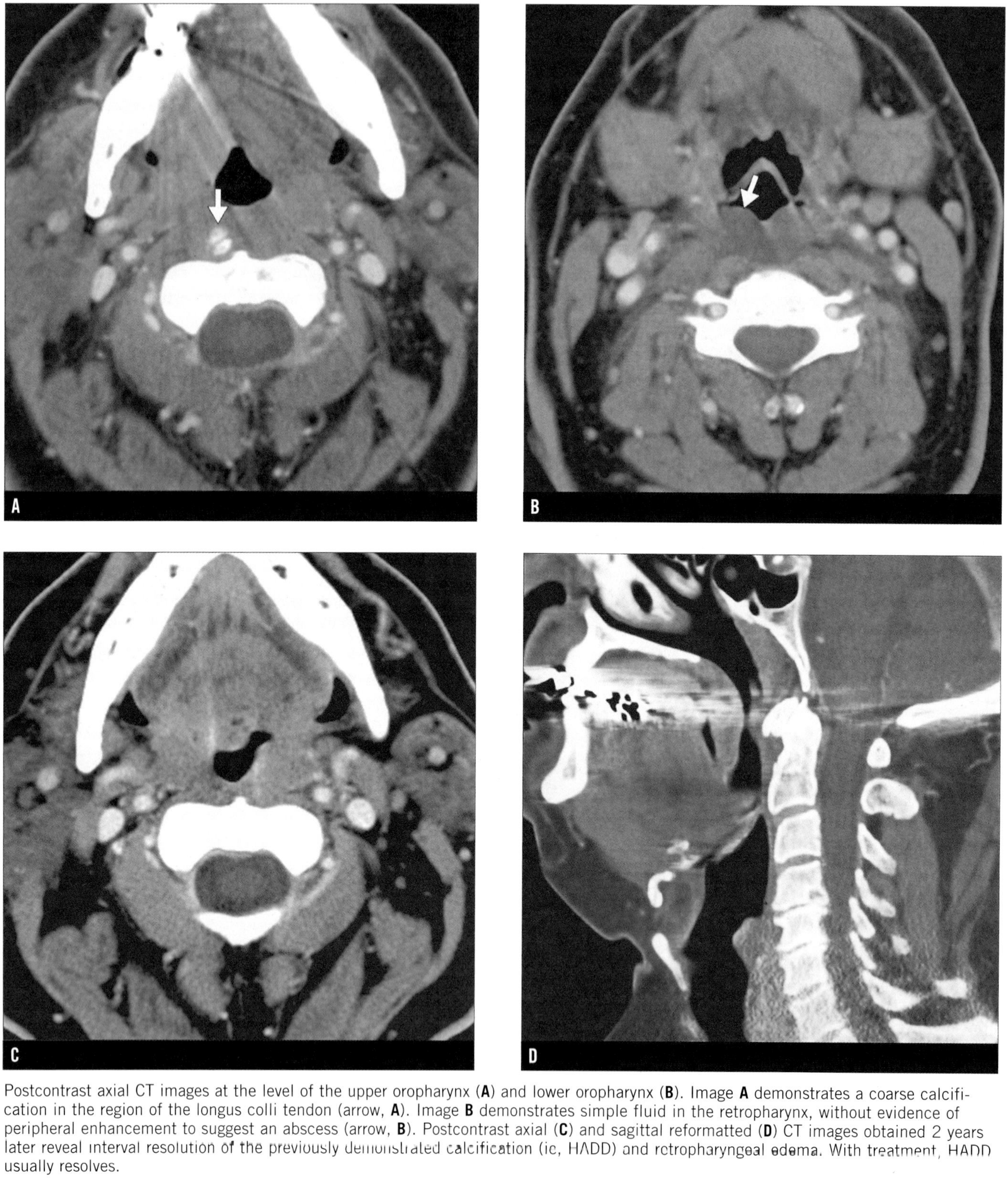

Postcontrast axial CT images at the level of the upper oropharynx (**A**) and lower oropharynx (**B**). Image **A** demonstrates a coarse calcification in the region of the longus colli tendon (arrow, **A**). Image **B** demonstrates simple fluid in the retropharynx, without evidence of peripheral enhancement to suggest an abscess (arrow, **B**). Postcontrast axial (**C**) and sagittal reformatted (**D**) CT images obtained 2 years later reveal interval resolution of the previously demonstrated calcification (ie, HADD) and retropharyngeal edema. With treatment, HADD usually resolves.

Companion case: Enlarging longus colli tendon hydroxyapatite deposition

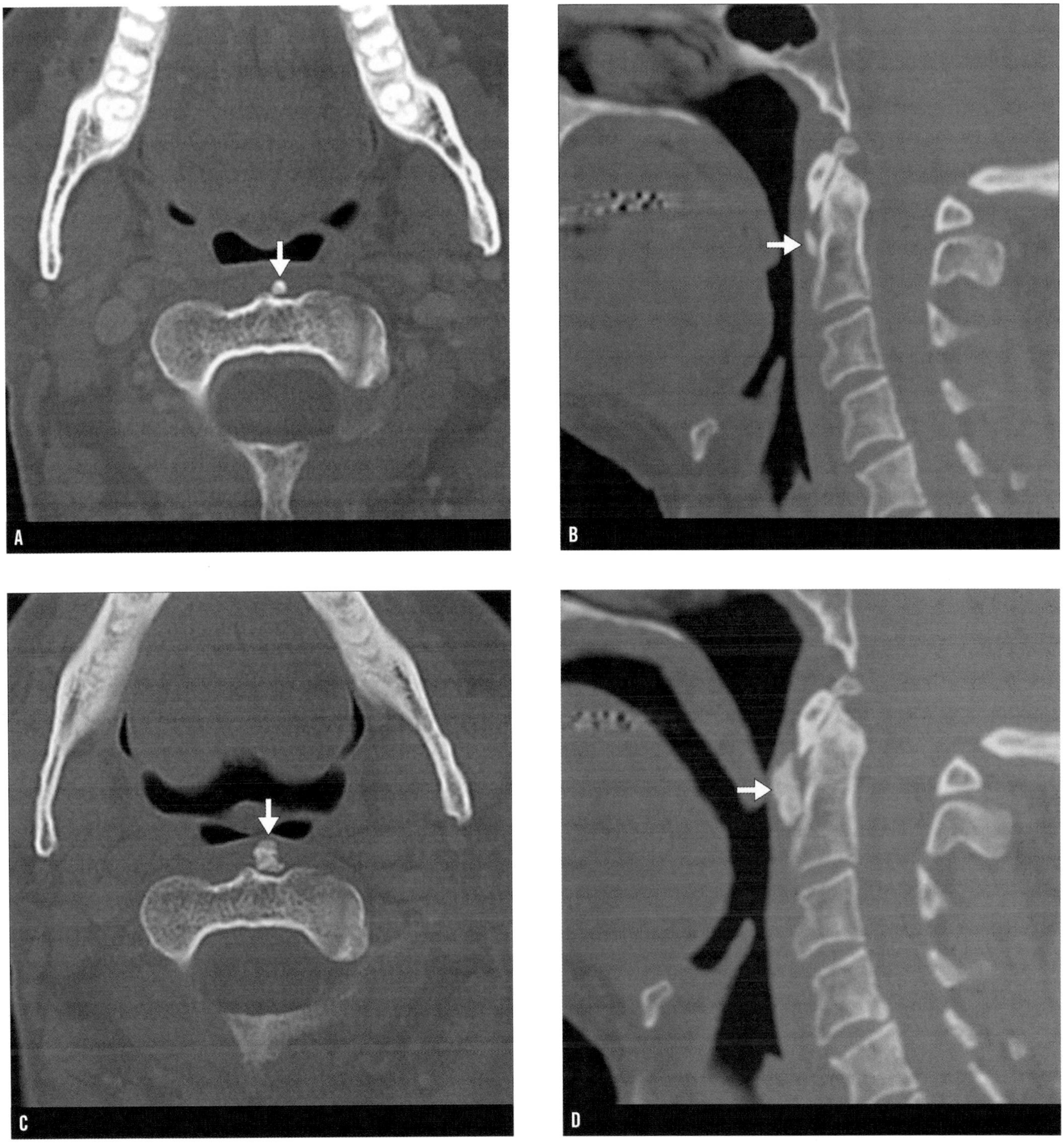

Axial (**A**) and sagittal reformatted (**B**) CT images demonstrate a small focus of calcification at the expected location of the longus colli tendon and distinctly separate from the anterior arch of C1, consistent with HADD (arrows, **A**, **B**). Four years later, axial (**C**) and coronal (**D**) CT images demonstrate significant enlargement of the mineralized focus, compatible with progressive HADD (arrows, **C**, **D**). There was no edema in the retropharynx (not shown) and there were no symptoms of odynophagia or neck pain to suggest acute calcific tendinitis of the longus colli. This HADD was presumably in the silent phase during both of these scans.

Companion case: C1 anterior vertebral osteophyte formation

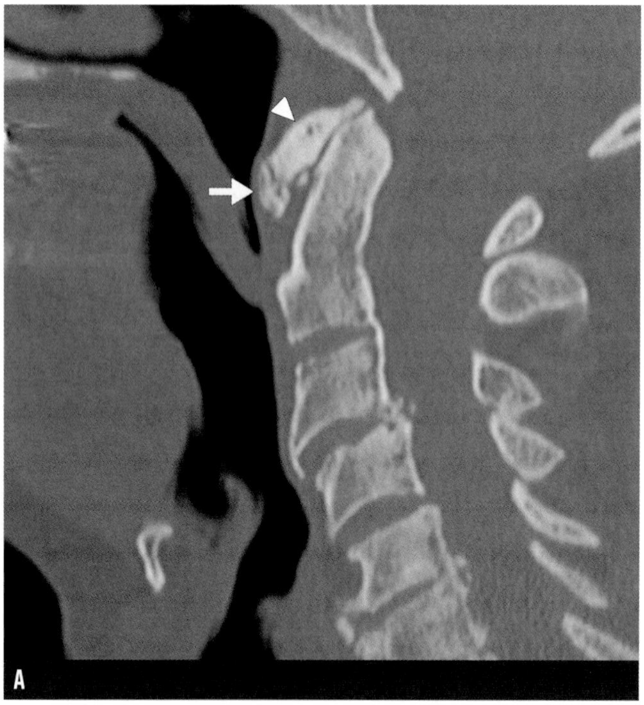

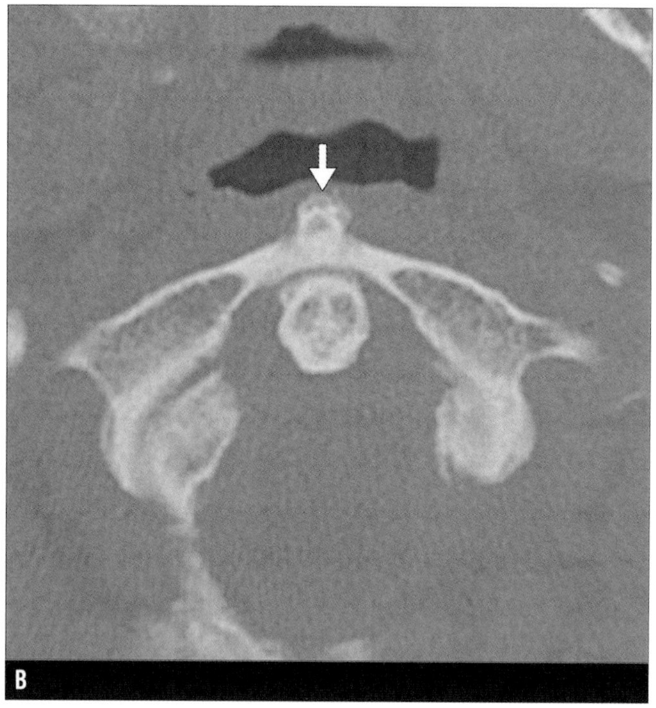

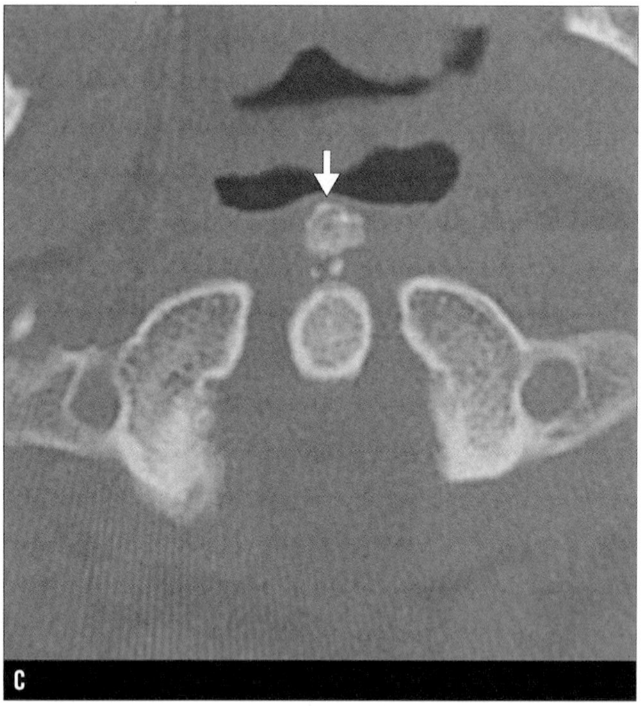

A sagittal reformatted CT image (**A**) and contiguous axial CT images (**B**, **C**) demonstrate a hypertrophic and degenerated anterior arch of C1 (arrowhead, **A**) associated with a caudally projecting osteophyte (arrows, **A**-**C**). The contiguity of the osseous finding with the C1 anterior arch and it's marrow containing matrix (best appreciated on image **C**) are helpful imaging features distinguishing this degenerative osteophyte from HADD.

Companion case: Retropharyngeal course of an atherosclerotic internal carotid artery

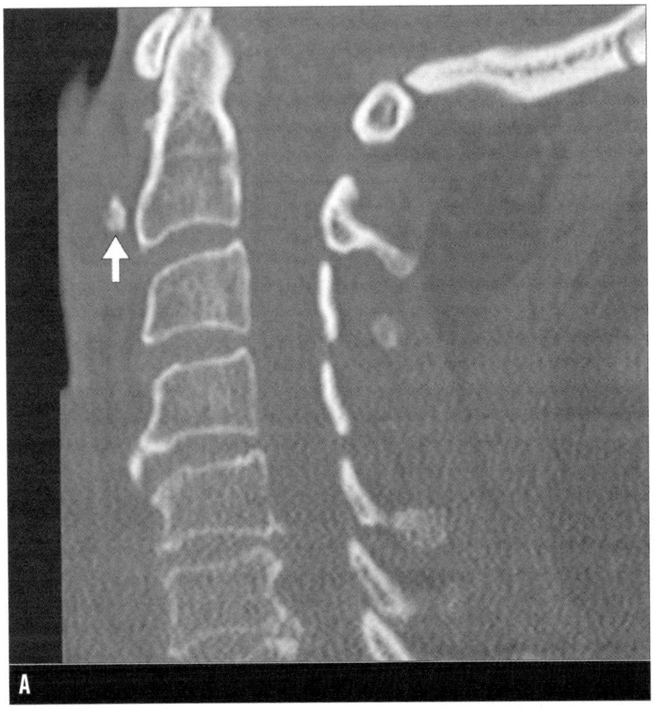

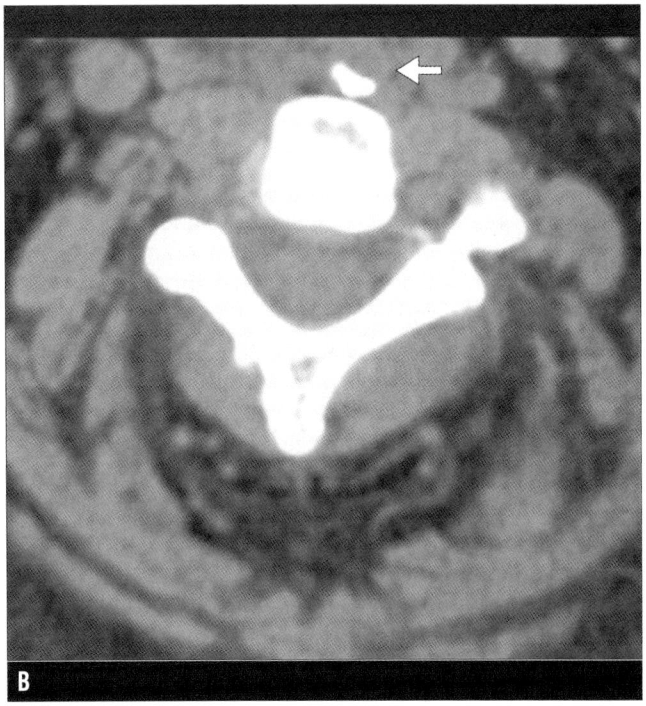

A sagittal reformatted unenhanced CT image through the neck viewed with a bone algorithm (**A**) demonstrates a focus of calcification that appears similar to hydroxyapatite deposition within the longus coli tendon, although it is located slightly more caudal than expected (arrow, **A**). An axial unenhanced CT image from the same case viewed with a soft tissue window (**B**) demonstrates that the finding is related to atherosclerosis from a retropharyngeal course of a subtly visualized left cervical internal carotid artery (arrow, **B**).

REFERENCES

Hayes CW, Conway WF. Calcium hydroxyapatite deposition disease. *Radiographics.* 1990;10(6):1031-1048.

Offiah CE, Hall E. Acute calcific tendinitis of the longus colli muscle: spectrum of CT appearances and anatomical correlation. *Br J Radiol.* 2009;82(978):e117-e121.

Resnick D. Degenerative diseases of the vertebral column. *Radiology.* 1985;156(1):3-14.

Siegal DS, Wu JS, Newman JS, Del Cura JL, Hochman MG. Calcific tendinitis: a pictorial review. *Can Assoc Radiol J.* 2009;60(5):263-272.

CASE 25 Asymptomatic marked ossification of the stylohyoid ligament

The stylohyoid ligament is a paired ligamentous band that arises from the tip of the temporal bone styloid process and extends to the lesser cornu of the hyoid bone. The stylohyoid ligament aids in regulating movement of the hyoid bone, mandible, pharynx, and tongue.

Occasionally, there may be ossification of the stylohyoid ligament in an asymptomatic patient. Moreover, an irregular, sclerotic appearing articulation may be identified between the styloid process and the ossified stylohyoid ligament, or between the lesser cornu of the hyoid bone and the ossified stylohyoid ligament, sometimes simulating a chronic fracture at either site. These findings can be explained embryologically. During normal fetal development, Reichert cartilage, which arises from the second pharyngeal arch, divides into four segments: tympanohyal, stylohyal, ceratohyal, and hypohyal. The tympanohyal portion gives rise to the upper, tympanic portion of the styloid process and the stapes of the ossicular chain. The stylohyal portion gives rise to the lower aspect of the styloid process. The stylohyal portion usually unites with the tympanohyal portion during puberty, giving rise to the adult styloid process. The hypohyal portion of Reichert cartilage gives rise to lesser cornu of the hyoid. Finally, the ceratohyal portion of Reichert cartilage usually deteriorates and gives rise to the stylohyoid ligament. However, the ceratohyal portion may ossify endochondrally and fuse with the styloid process and/or lesser cornu of the hyoid, resulting in ossification of the stylohyoid ligament. It is the junction between the ceratohyal portion (ie, ossified stylohyoid ligament) and the adult styloid process that results in a proximal irregular articulation that may simulate a chronic fracture. Similarly, it is the articulation between the ceratohyal portion and the hypohyal portion of Reichert cartilage that may simulate a chronic fracture near the hyoid bone.

COMPANION CASES

- **Symptomatic ossification of the stylohyoid ligament (Eagle syndrome).** Eagle syndrome, first described by Watt Eagle in 1937, represents a variety of symptoms related to compression of regional structures (including vascular structures) by an elongated styloid process, ossified stylohyoid ligament, or ossified stylomandibular ligament. The most common symptoms include recurrent throat pain, foreign body sensation, dysphagia, and facial pain. The diagnosis of Eagle syndrome is based on clinical symptoms and physical examination (either palpating the elongated styloid process via the tonsillar fossa or along the exterior of the neck) as well as imaging evidence (CT or radiographs). A styloid process greater than 3 cm in length may be considered elongated. However, it should be stressed that the mere presence of an elongated styloid process does not constitute Eagle syndrome, as many patients with an elongated styloid process are entirely asymptomatic.

  The treatment of a symptomatic ossified stylohyoid ligament is either surgical resection of the styloid process and ossified stylohyoid ligament or nonsurgical management, such as with nonsteroidal anti-inflammatory medications and steroid injections.
- **Eagle syndrome resulting in a chronic nonocclusive internal jugular vein thrombus.** There are reports of an elongated styloid process resulting in compression and dissection of the cervical internal carotid artery related to certain neck positioning, in some cases resulting in intracranial arterial occlusion. Moreover, some authors have suggested that compression of the internal jugular veins by elongated styloid processes may be a cause of intracranial hypertension. In the case presented herein, an elongated styloid process resulted in compression of the internal jugular vein and a chronic, nonocclusive thrombus. However, narrowing of the internal jugular vein by the styloid process is frequently identified on imaging and is often an incidental finding.
- **Normal intermediate tendon of the digastric muscle.** The digastric muscle has two bellies, an anterior and a posterior belly. Each belly is derived from different embryological origins and has different innervation. The anterior belly is derived from the first branchial arch and is innervated by the mylohyoid nerve, which is a branch of the trigeminal nerve. The posterior belly is derived from the second branchial arch and is supplied by the digastric branch of the facial nerve. The posterior belly of the digastric muscle originates from the mastoid notch and slopes antero-infero-medially toward the hyoid bone. The anterior belly of the digastric muscle originates from the digastric fossa, a small osseous depression located along the inner mandibular margin near the mandibular symphysis. The anterior belly is directed postero-infero-laterally, also toward the hyoid bone. The anterior and posterior bellies converge into a rounded tendon, named the intermediate tendon of the digastric muscle. A fibrous loop, which is attached to the junction of the body and greater cornu of the hyoid, encircles and supports the intermediate tendon. The intermediate tendon will often be identified on unenhanced CT. When identified, it will appear as a mildly hyperattenuating, linear structure located lateral to the hyoid bone and in line with the two bellies of the digastric muscle.

Asymptomatic marked ossification of the stylohyoid ligament

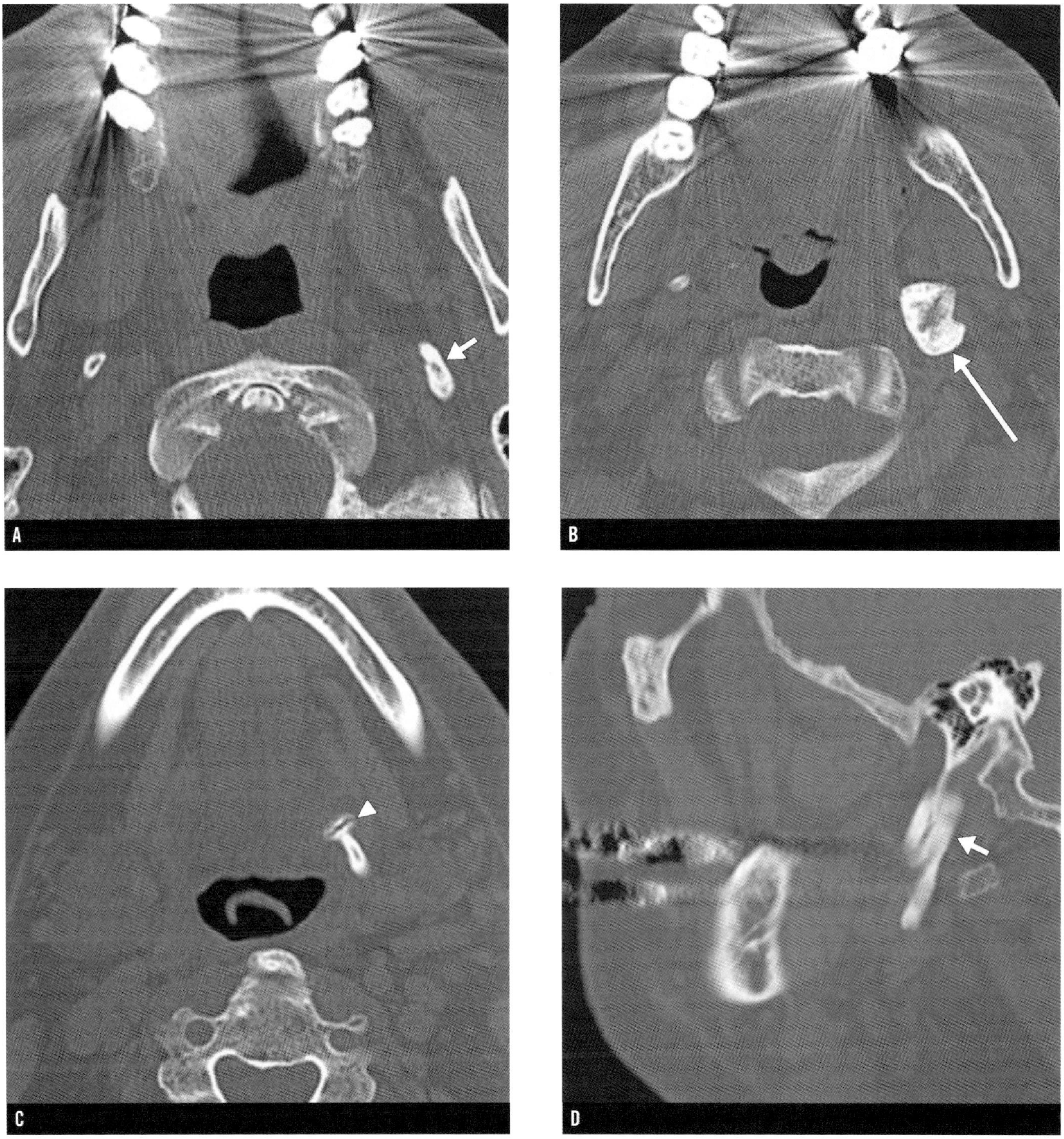

Axial CT images (superior to inferior, **A-C**) and sagittal reformatted CT images through the left stylohyoid ligament (lateral to medial, **D-G**). There is an enlarged left styloid process (short arrows, **A**, **D**) and extensive ossification of the left stylohyoid ligament (medium arrow, **F**). This patient did not have a history of symptoms related to this finding. A prominent sclerotic articulation is identified at either end of the stylohyoid ligament ossification. The proximal sclerotic articulation (long arrows, **B**, **E**) represents the junction between the stylohyal portion of the embryonic Reichert cartilage (which gives rise to the lower aspect of the styloid process) with the ceratohyal portion (which gives rise to the stylohyoid ligament). The distal articulation (arrowheads, **C**, **G**) represents the junction between the ceratohyal portion of the embryonic Reichert cartilage and the hypohyal portion (which gives rise to the lesser hyoid cornu).

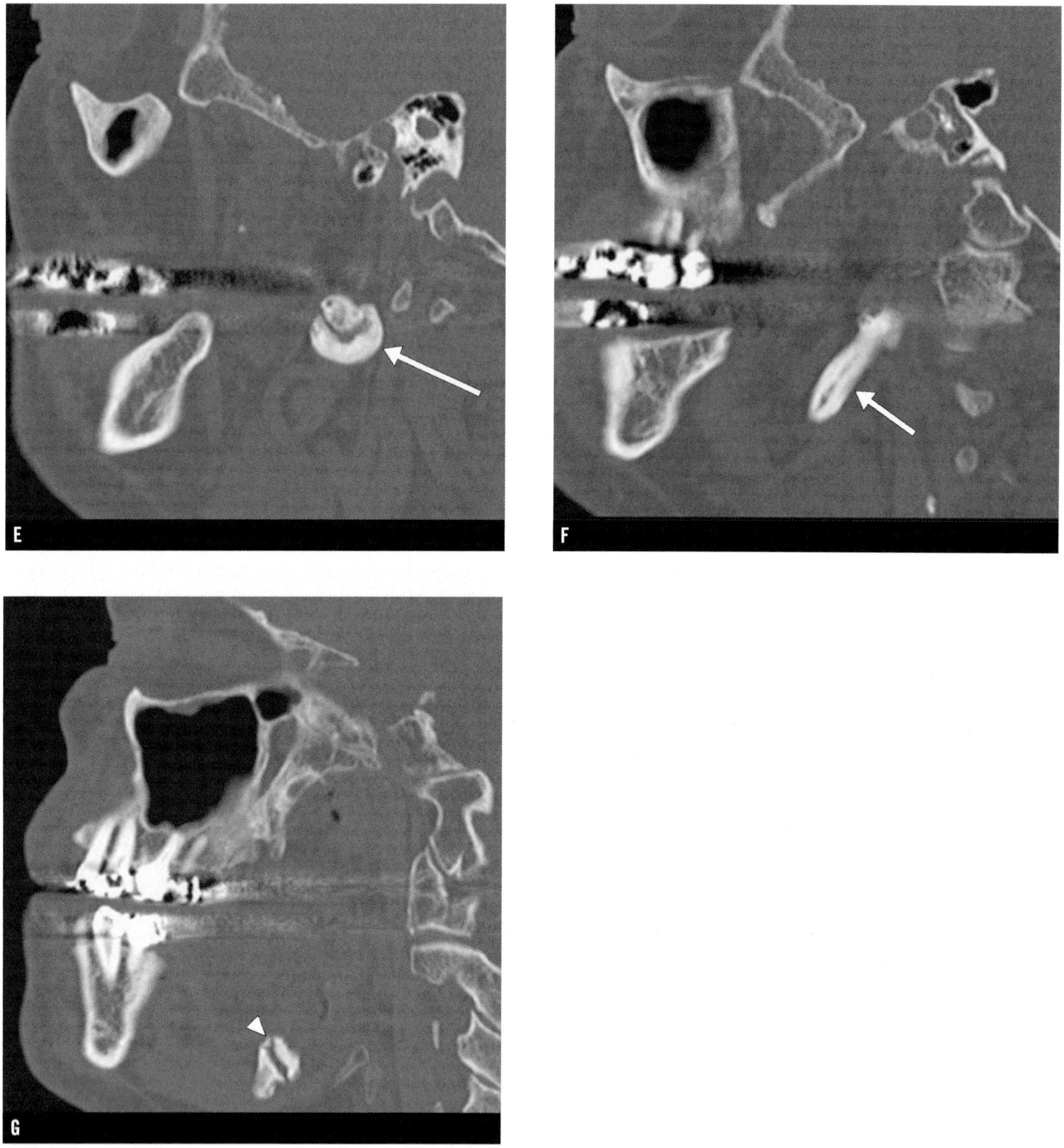
E
F
G

Companion case: Symptomatic ossification of the stylohyoid ligament (Eagle syndrome)

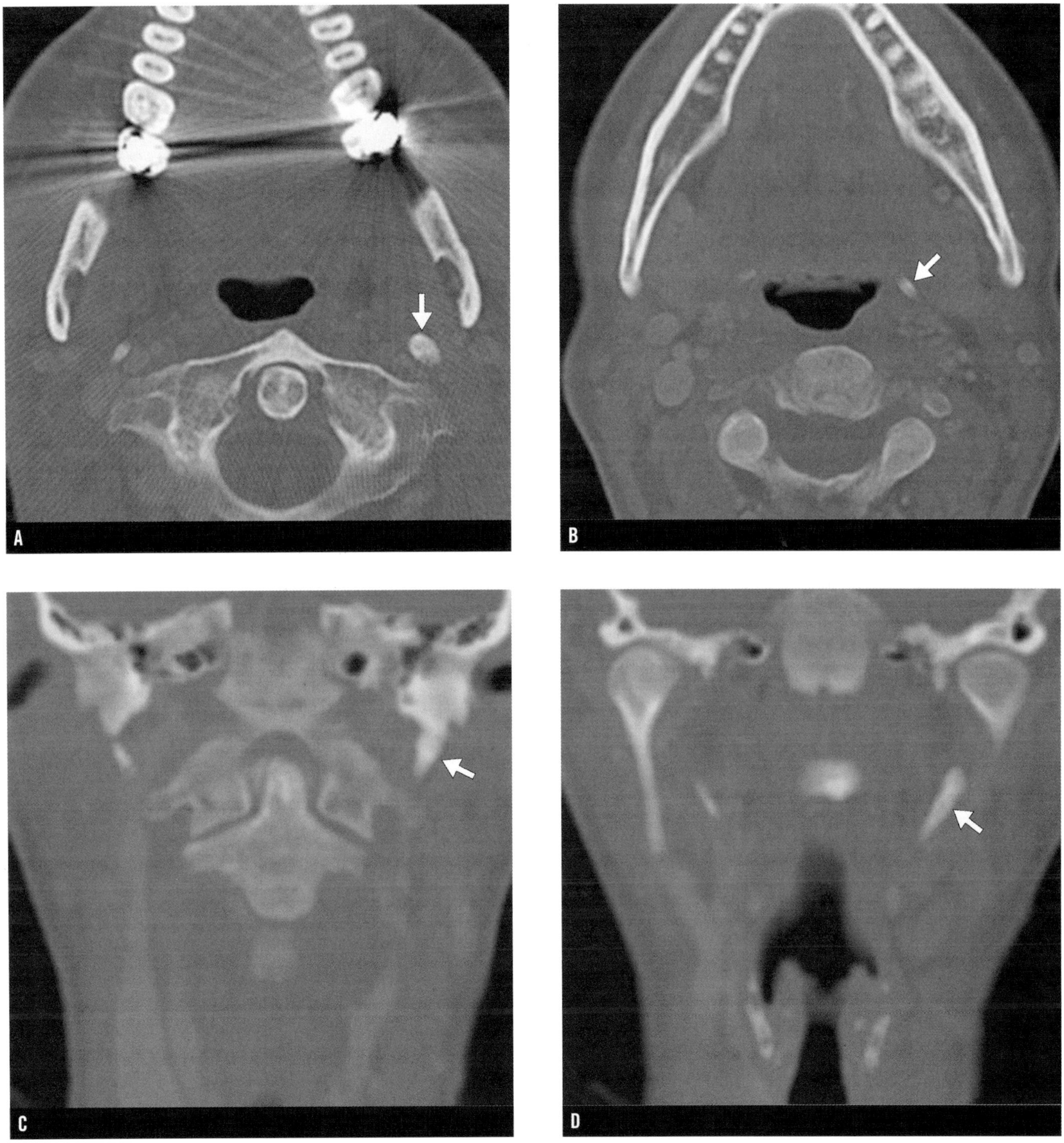

Axial (**A**, **B**) and coronal reformatted (**C**, **D**) CT images demonstrate ossification of the left stylohyoid ligament (arrows, **A-D**). This patient presented with a palpable left neck mass and a history of pain involving the left side of the face and throat as well as odynophagia. The ossified left stylohyoid ligament was surgically resected to treat these symptoms.

Companion case: Eagle syndrome resulting in a chronic nonocclusive internal jugular vein thrombus

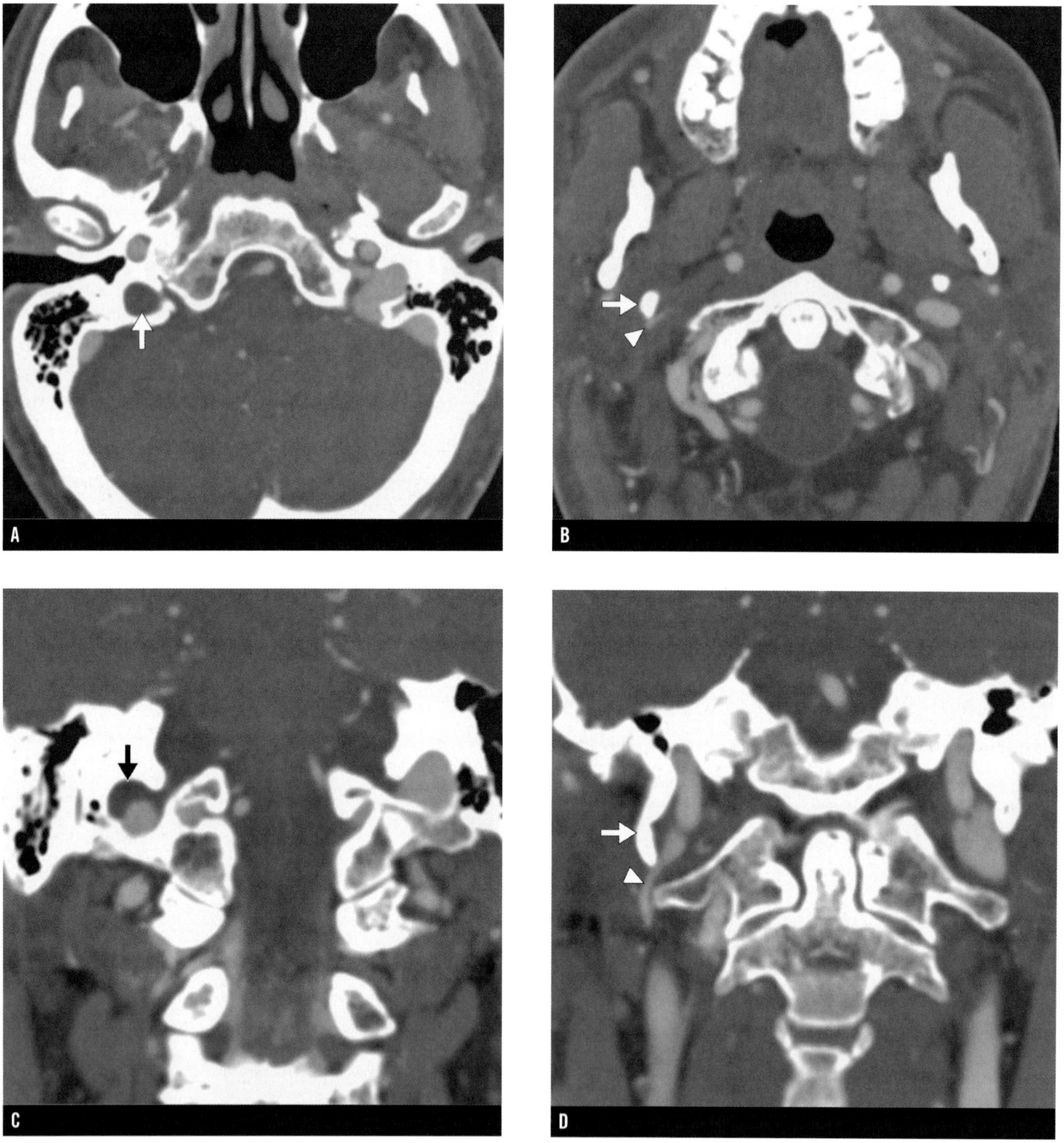

Axial (**A**, **B**) and coronal reformatted (**C**, **D**) postcontrast images from a CT venogram. Image **A** demonstrates lack of contrast in the right jugular bulb consistent with thrombus (arrow, **A**). Image **C** demonstrates that the thrombus is only partially occlusive and located within the superior aspect of the jugular bulb (arrow, **C**). Images **B** and **D** demonstrate a relatively normal-sized right styloid process (arrows, **B**, **D**). However, because of a medial angulation of the right styloid process, the adjacent right internal jugular vein is compressed against the adjacent right lateral mass of C1 (arrowheads, **B**, **D**). Coronal T2 (**E**) and sagittal postcontrast VIBE (**F**) MR images also demonstrate the nonocclusive thrombus in the superior aspect of the right jugular bulb (arrows, **E**, **F**), whereas a coronal 2D time-of-flight MRV MIP image (**G**) demonstrates the narrowing and deformity of the right internal jugular vein at the level of the styloid process and C1 lateral mass (arrow, **G**). While the right internal jugular vein is not completely compressed between the styloid process and the C1 lateral mass, it is likely that the narrowing was sufficient to result in relative stagnation of venous outflow and the formation of nonocclusive thrombus. The findings were stable for several years on follow-up imaging. Note that while narrowing of the internal jugular by the styloid process can result in thrombus formation, it is frequently identified as an incidental finding on imaging.

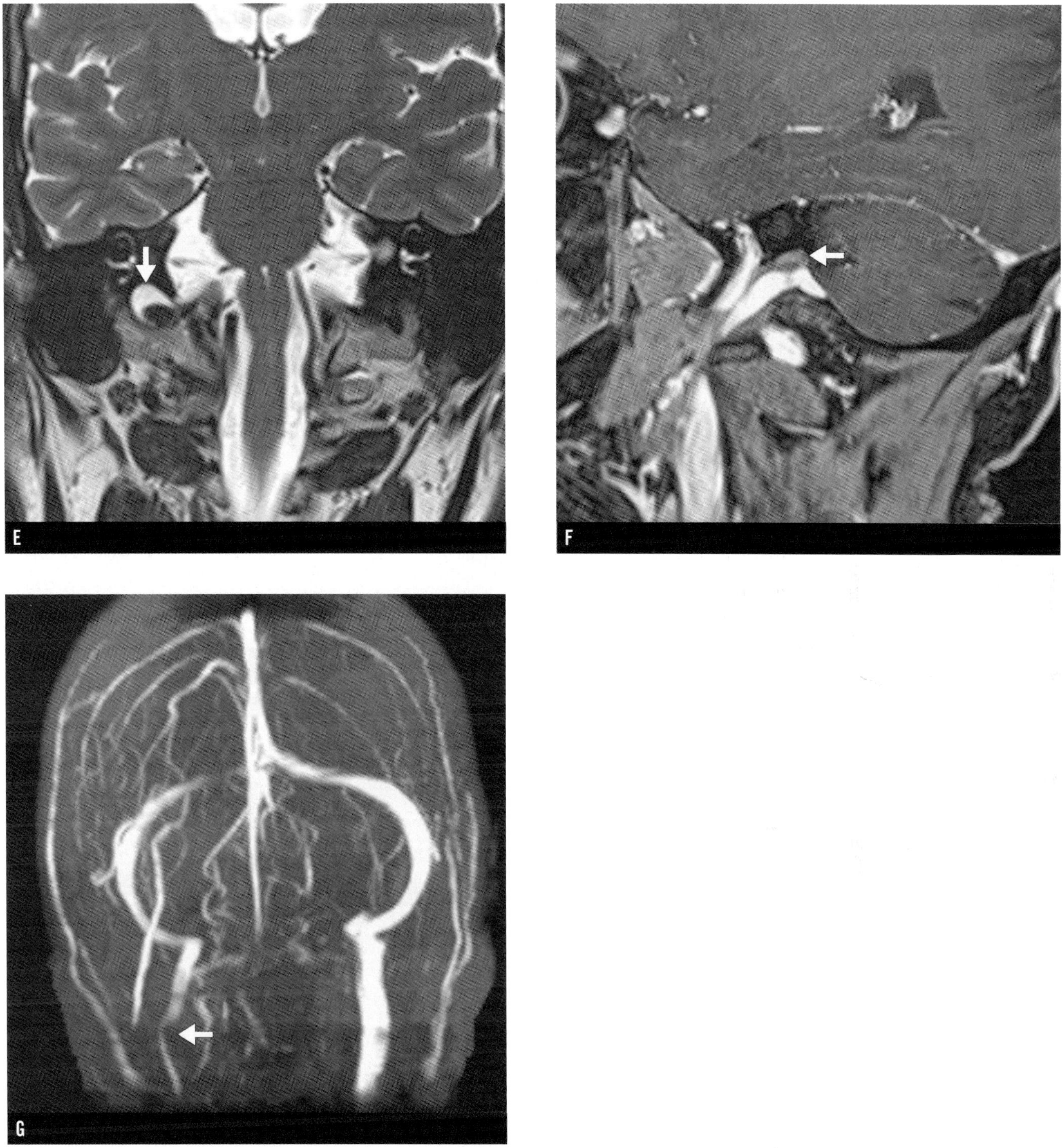
E
F
G

Companion case: Normal intermediate tendon of the digastric muscle

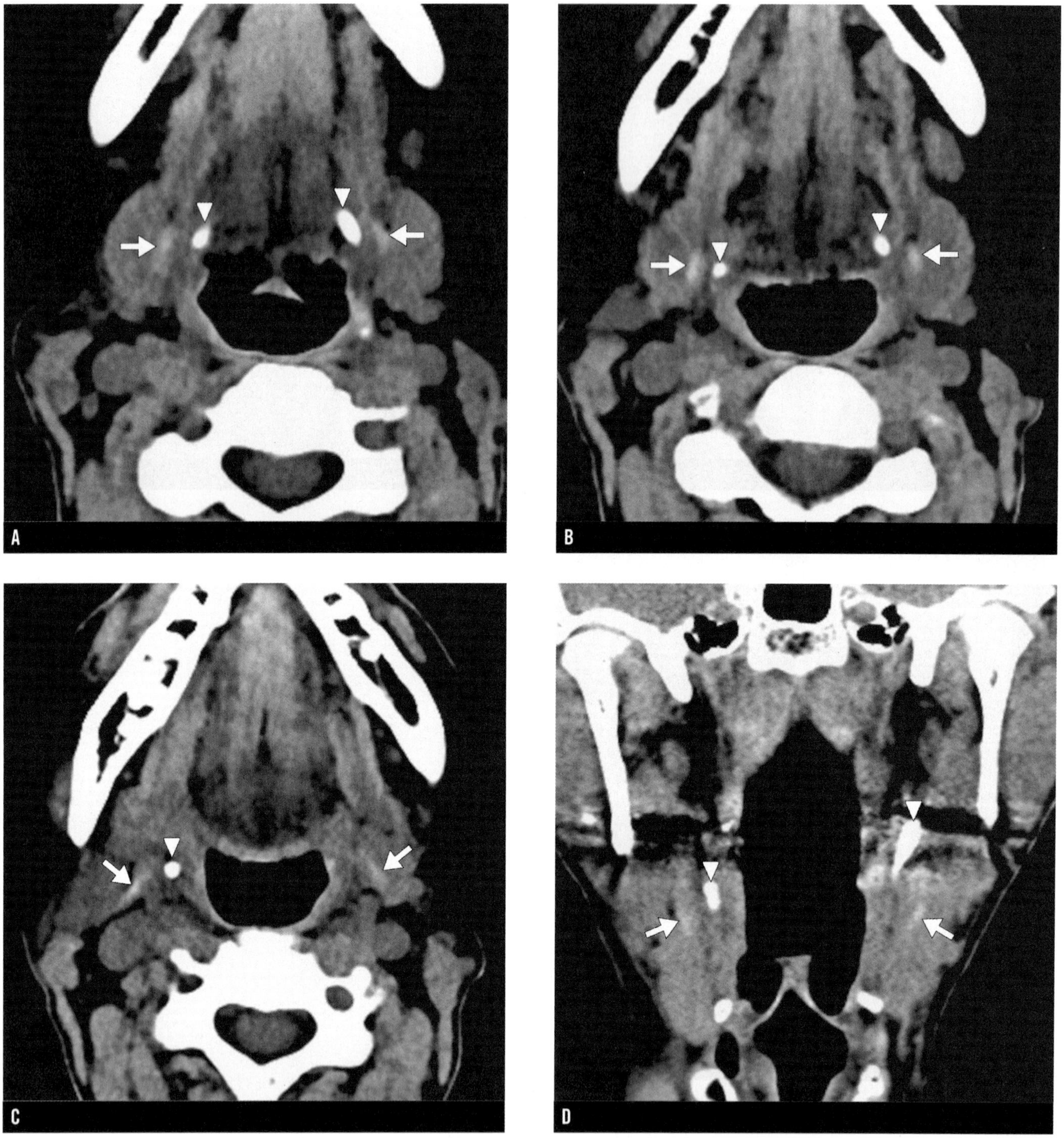

Unenhanced axial (**A-C**) and coronal reformatted (**D**) CT images demonstrate the normal bilateral intermediate tendons of the digastric muscles (arrows, **A-D**) adjacent to mostly ossified stylohoyoid ligaments, right greater than left (arrowheads, **A-D**).

REFERENCES

Dashti SR, et al. Styloidogenic jugular venous compression syndrome: diagnosis and treatment: case report. *Neurosurgery.* 2012;70(3):E795–E799.

De-Ary-Pires B, Ary-Pires R, Pires-Neto MA. The human digastric muscle: patterns and variations with clinical and surgical correlations. *Ann Anat.* 2003;185(5):471-479.

Ferrario VF, et al. Calcification of the stylohyoid ligament: incidence and morphoquantitative evaluations. *Oral Surg Oral Med Oral Pathol Oral Radiol Endod.* 1990;69:524-529.

Murtagh RD, Caracciolo JT, Fernandez G. Case Report CT Findings Associated with Eagle Syndrome. *AJNR Am J Neuroradiol.* 2001;22:1401-1402.

Omnell K, Gandhi C, Omnell M. Ossification of the human stylohyoid ligament: a longitudinal study. *Oral Surg Oral Med Oral Pathol Oral Radiol Endod.* 1998;85:226-232.

Ozgursoy OB, Kucuk B. Unique variation of digastric muscle: a confusing landmark for head and neck surgeons. *Acta Otolaryngol.* 2006;126(8):881-883.

Piagkou M, Anagnostopoulou S, Kouladouros K, Piagkos G. Eagle's syndrome: a review of the literature. *Clin Anat.* 2009;22(5):545-558.

Valerio CS, et al. Stylohyoid Syndrome. *J Craniofac Surg.* 2012;23(2):e138-e140.

Yavuz H, Caylakli F, Yildirim T, Ozluoglu LN. Angulation of the styloid process in Eagle's syndrome. *Eur Arch Otorhinolaryngol.* 2008;265:1393-1396.

that only 1.5% of PAs develop into CEPA if the tumor has been present for less than 5 years, although this increases to 9.5% if a PA has been present for more than 15 years. A CEPA can have a variable appearance, ranging from benign appearing to frankly malignant.

- **Adenoid cystic carcinoma.** Adenoid cystic carcinoma is a generally slow-growing mass that accounts for approximately 2% to 6% of all parotid gland tumors, most commonly occurring in patients who are in their fifth to sixth decade of life. This tumor has a high recurrence rate, particularly if high-grade, and it has a proclivity for perineural spread (50%-60%) which may result in facial paralysis or pain. Perineural spread may also "skip" along a nerve or nerves, which may be identified by imaging or pathologically. Additionally, while this tumor uncommonly metastasizes to lymph nodes, it will metastasize to bone, dura, and frequently to lung, sometimes resulting in slowly enlarging "cannonball" metastatic lung lesions. However, despite metastatic disease, many patients will have a prolonged survival. While a malignant salivary gland tumor, including an adenoid cystic carcinoma, may be indistinguishable from a benign tumor by CT or MR imaging, a salivary gland mass that has irregular margins should be considered malignant, until proven otherwise. In addition, while some benign tumors may have hypointense T2 signal (such as oncocytomas, Warthin tumors, occasionally PA, and others), a salivary gland mass that contains areas of hypointense T2 signal raises the possibility of malignancy, such as adenoid cystic carcinoma.
- **Adenocarcinoma.** Adenocarcinoma of the salivary glands represents a malignant tumor that arises from glandular elements. It accounts for approximately 3% of all parotid tumors. There are several types of adenocarcinoma, ranging from low-grade to high-grade. Some types include basal cell adenocarcinoma, cystadenocarcinoma, sebaceous adenocarcinoma, mucinous adenocarcinoma, and adenocarcinoma not otherwise specified. High-grade adenocarcinoma is typically aggressive, grows rapidly, and is painful. On MRI, an aggressive adenocarcinoma usually appears as an infiltrating mass that is T1 hypointense, T2 hypo- to isointense, and enhances. Metastatic disease is common with a high-grade adenocarcinoma.
- **Parotid sialocyst.** A parotid sialocyst (also called mucocele or retention cyst of the salivary gland) is a benign parotid cyst that usually develops from a postobstructive phenomenon, such as may occur with a sialolith or a postinflammatory stricture. Sialocysts represent true cysts because they are contained by an an epithelial lining. By contrast, a parotid sialocele represents an accumulation of saliva that typically occurs following trauma and does not represent a true cyst because it is only contained by a pseudocapsule. Sialocysts are painless, slowly enlarging lesions that do not recur if excised. Occasionally, hemorrhage may be present within a sialocyst. On MRI, the T1 and T2 signal characteristics vary and depend on the proteinaceous content of the sialocyst. On CT, a sialocyst is usually of fluid density, although again it may be complicated by proteinaceous fluid/hemorrhage. Following contrast, a sialocyst may peripherally enhance, but it will not centrally enhance.
- **First branchial cleft cyst.** The branchial apparatuses are divided into clefts, arches, and pouches. The first branchial cleft gives rise to the external auditory canal. The first branchial arch gives rise to the mandible, fifth cranial nerve, muscles of mastication, malleus, and incus. The first branchial pouch gives rise to the eustachian tube, tympanic cavity, and mastoid air cells.

  There are several classifications of first branchial cleft cysts that have been proposed by various authors, a couple of whom similarly subdivided them into Type I and Type II lesions. However, despite having described two types, the location and morphologic descriptions of the Type I and Type II lesions varied significantly between these authors. Perhaps the most currently accepted classification was described by Dr. Walter Work in 1972. In his classification, a Type I first branchial cleft cyst is ectodermal in origin and resides anterior, inferior, or posterior to the pinna, although most are located anterior. These cysts are contiguous with a tract that runs parallel to, and sometimes communicates with, the external auditory canal. A Type I first branchial cleft cyst is significantly less common than a Type II first branchial cleft cyst. A Type II first branchial cleft cyst contains both ectodermal and mesodermal elements and may extend from the angle of the mandible to near the membranous external auditory canal. They may be located in the subcutaneous soft tissues in this region, within the parotid, or in the parapharyngeal space. A Type II first branchial cleft cyst may be associated with a tract to the skin. Patients usually present earlier when a branchial cleft cyst is associated with a tract (typically in the first decade) and sometimes with purulent drainage. Complete surgical removal, rather than surgical drainage, is the treatment of choice for all branchial cleft cysts.
- **Periparotid varix.** A varix refers to a focal, abnormally dilated vein. It is differentiated from phlebectasia on imaging by its form; a varix is saccular whereas phlebectasia represents diffuse enlargement of the involved vein. Generally speaking, a varix is acquired.

Benign parotid lymph node (CT)

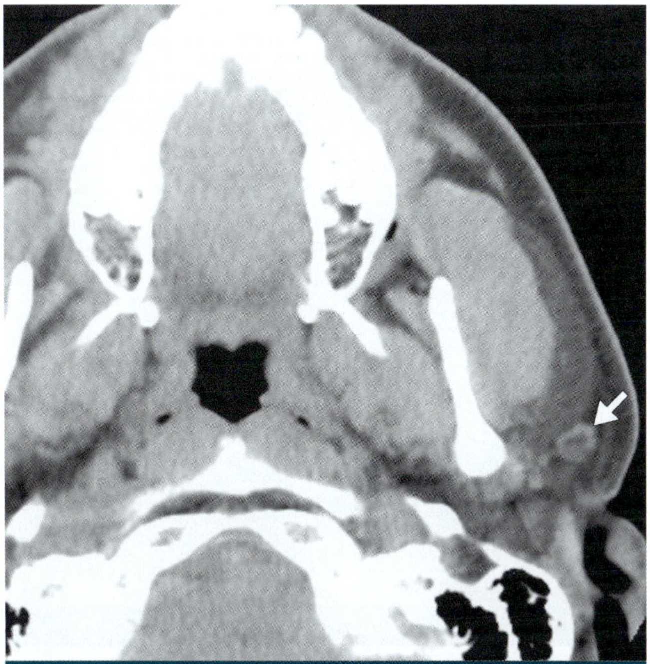

A

A postcontrast axial CT image through the level of the parotid glands (**A**) demonstrates a small lymph node in the left parotid gland which contains a fatty hilum, typical of a benign lymph node (arrow).

Benign parotid lymph node (MRI)

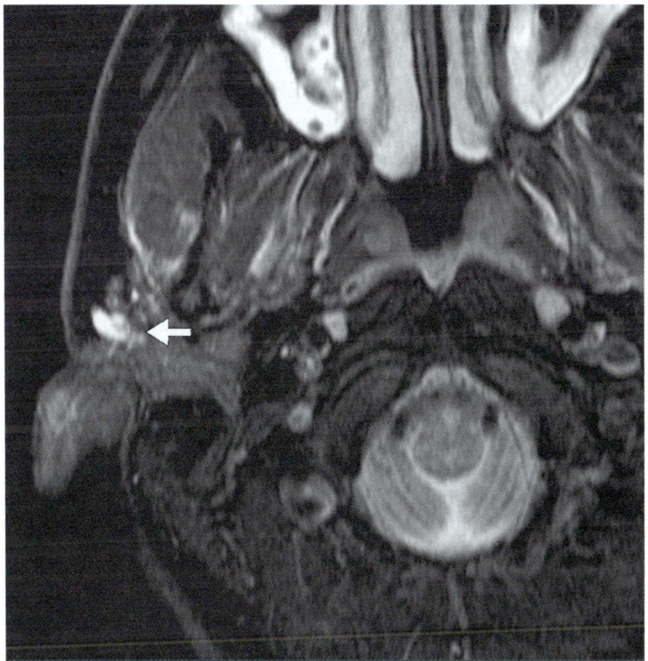

A

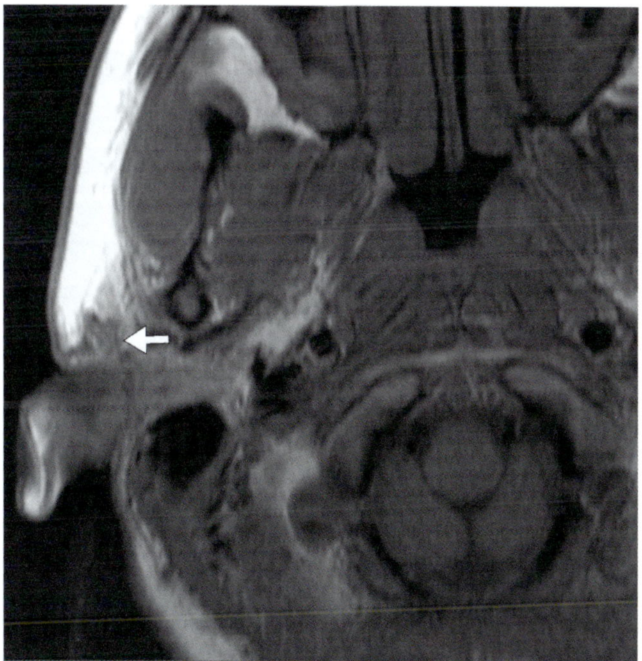

B

Different patient. Axial T2 with fat suppression (**A**), noncontrast axial T1 (**B**), noncontrast coronal T1 (**C**), and postcontrast coronal T1 with fat suppression (**D**) MR images demonstrate a small nodule that is T2 hyperintense, T1 isointense, and enhances located within the ventral superior margin of the right parotid gland (arrows, **A-D**). While nonspecific, given its relatively small size (particularly in the axial dimension), this was presumed to be a benign lymph node. However, if a finding such as this enlarges or is symptomatic for the patient, then a short-term follow-up or a biopsy of the finding may be warranted.

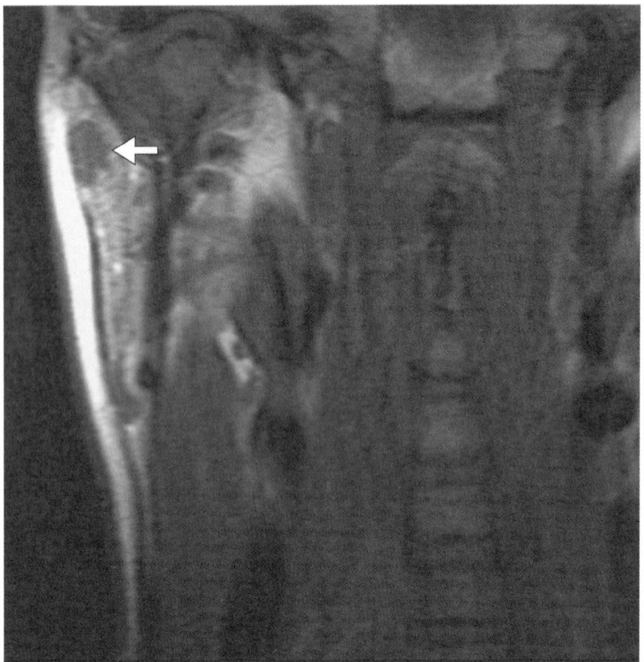

C

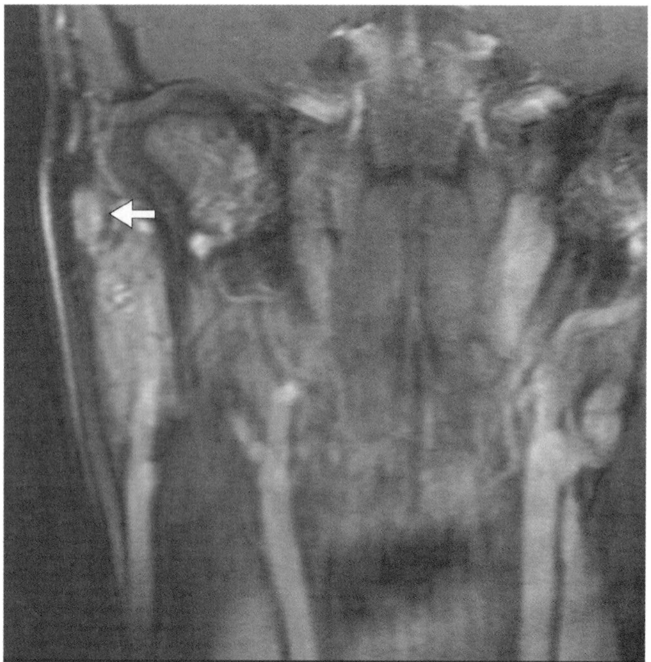

D

Companion case: Pathologic parotid lymph node

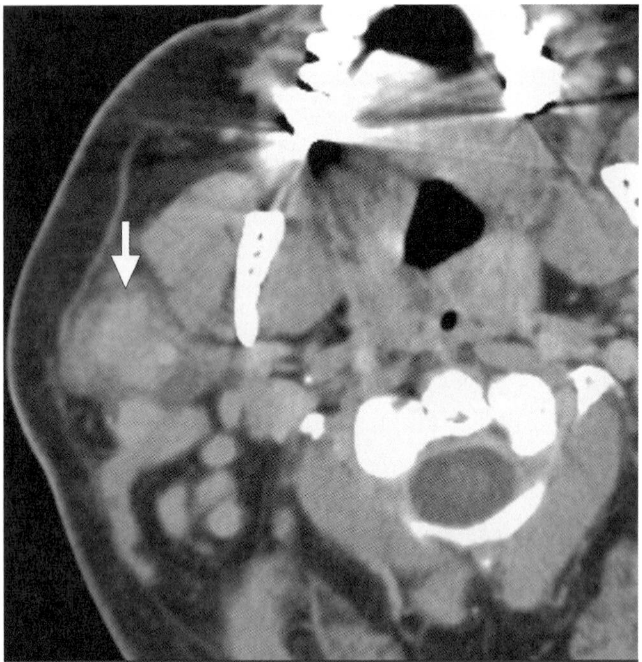

A

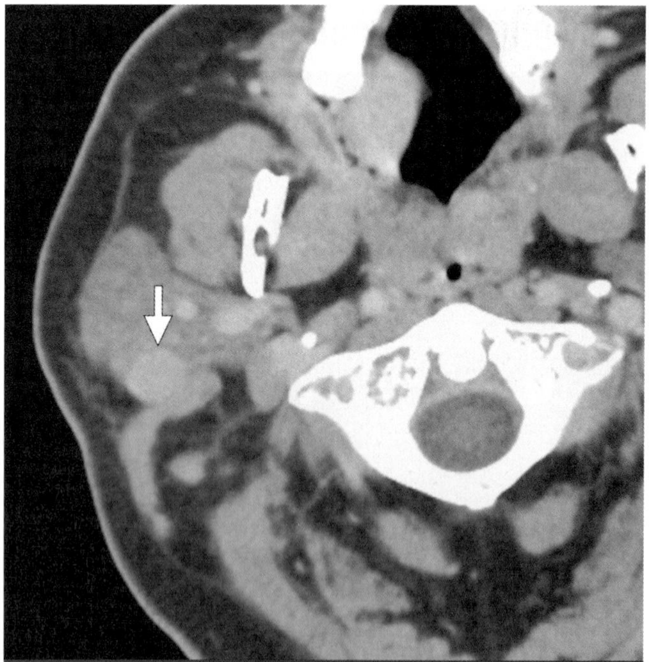

B

Postcontrast axial CT images through the level of the parotid glands (**A-C**) demonstrate a large soft tissue lesion in the right parotid gland (arrow, **A**) as well as mildly enlarged lymph nodes in the bilateral periparotid regions (arrows, **B, C**). This patient had a history of non-Hodgkin lymphoma and the lesion within the right parotid gland is consistent with a pathologic lymph node.

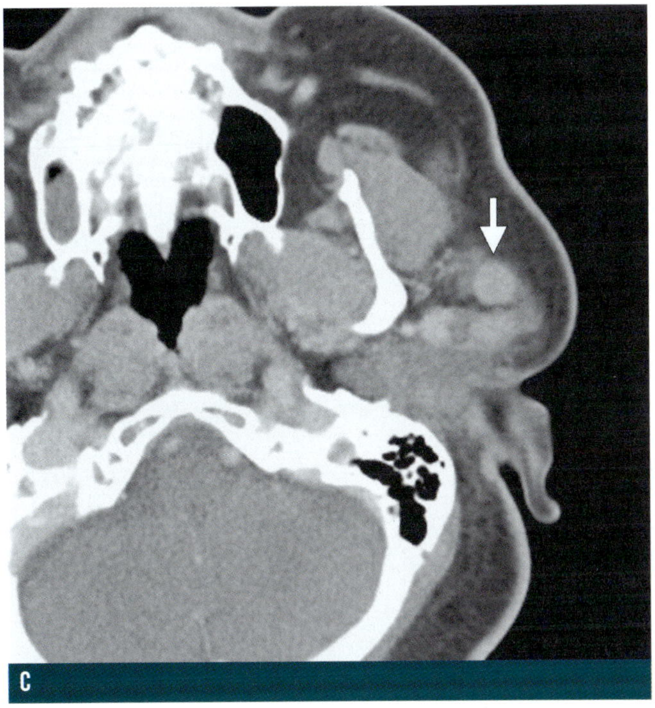

Companion case: Low-grade mucoepidermoid carcinoma

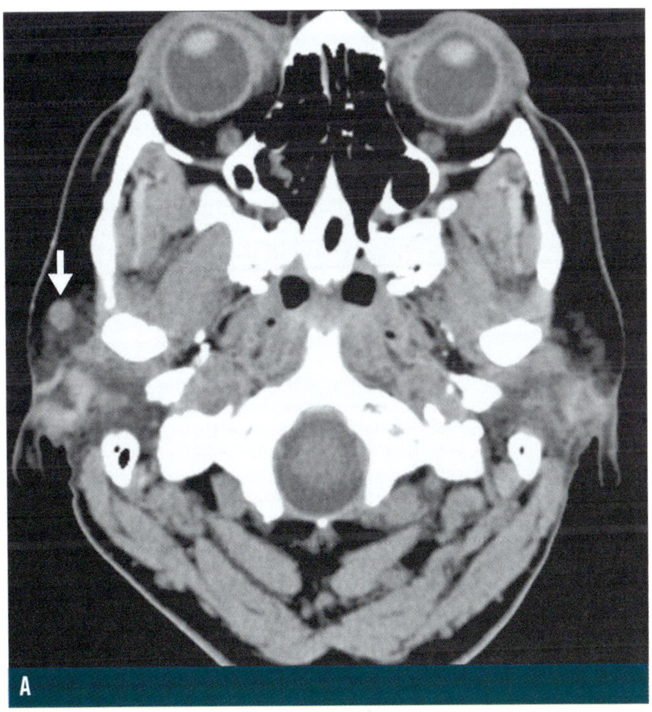

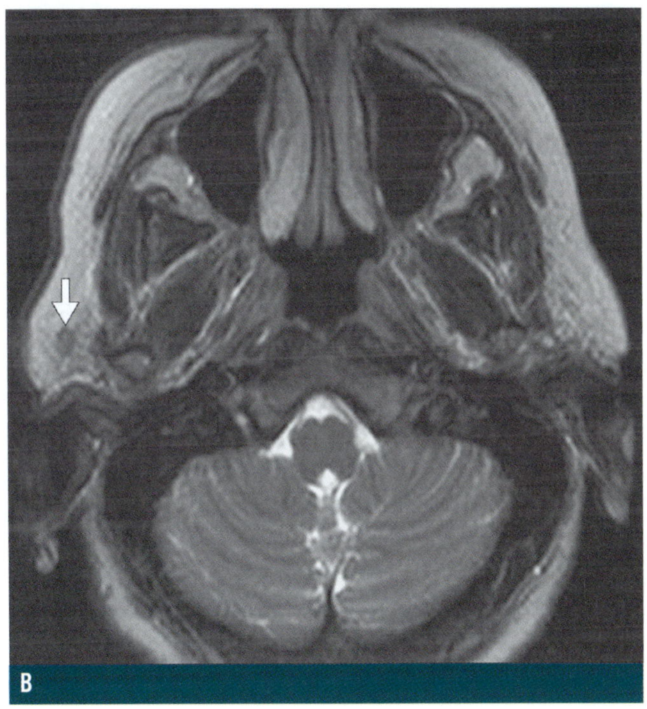

An unenhanced axial CT image at the level of the parotid glands (**A**) demonstrates a small, subcentimeter nodule within the ventral superficial aspect of the right parotid gland (arrow, **A**). Approximately 1 year later, axial T2 (**B**), coronal T1 (**C**), contrast-enhanced axial T1 with fat suppression (**D**), and contrast-enhanced coronal T1 with fat suppression (**E**) MR images demonstrate the same lesion to be unchanged in size, hypointense on T2 and T1 relative to the adjacent parotid gland, and enhance. Given the stability in size, this lesion was presumed to be benign. However, the patient had focal pain related to this finding and the lesion was surgically removed. The lesion represented a low-grade mucoepidermoid at pathology. In retrospect, the only finding on MRI that could have raised suspicion for malignancy was the hypointense T2 signal, which can be present with either benign or malignant parotid lesions. Nevertheless, if a parotid lesion is symptomatic, particularly if painful, then biopsy or removal of the lesion may be warranted.

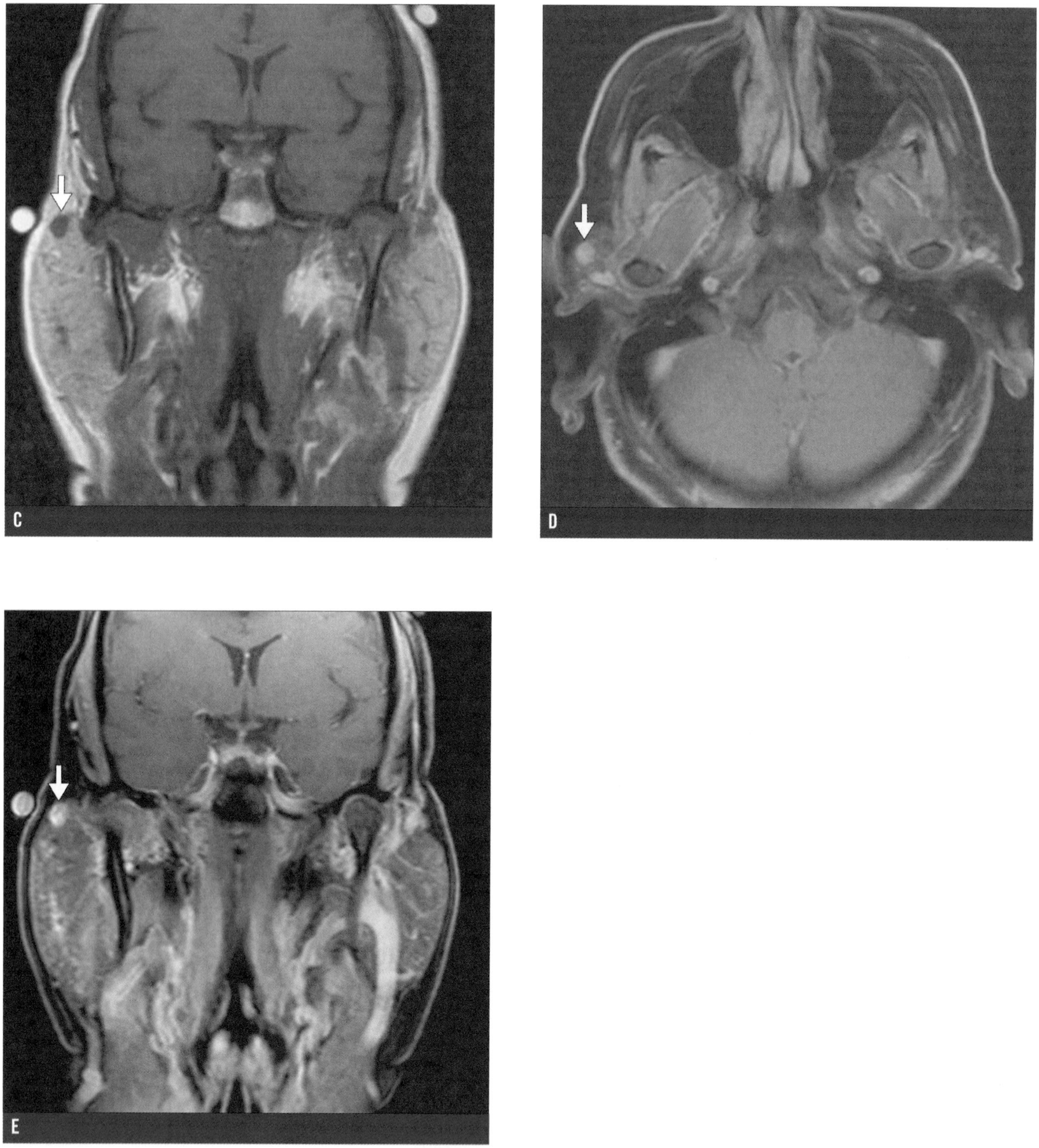
C
D
E

Companion case: High-grade mucoepidermoid carcinoma

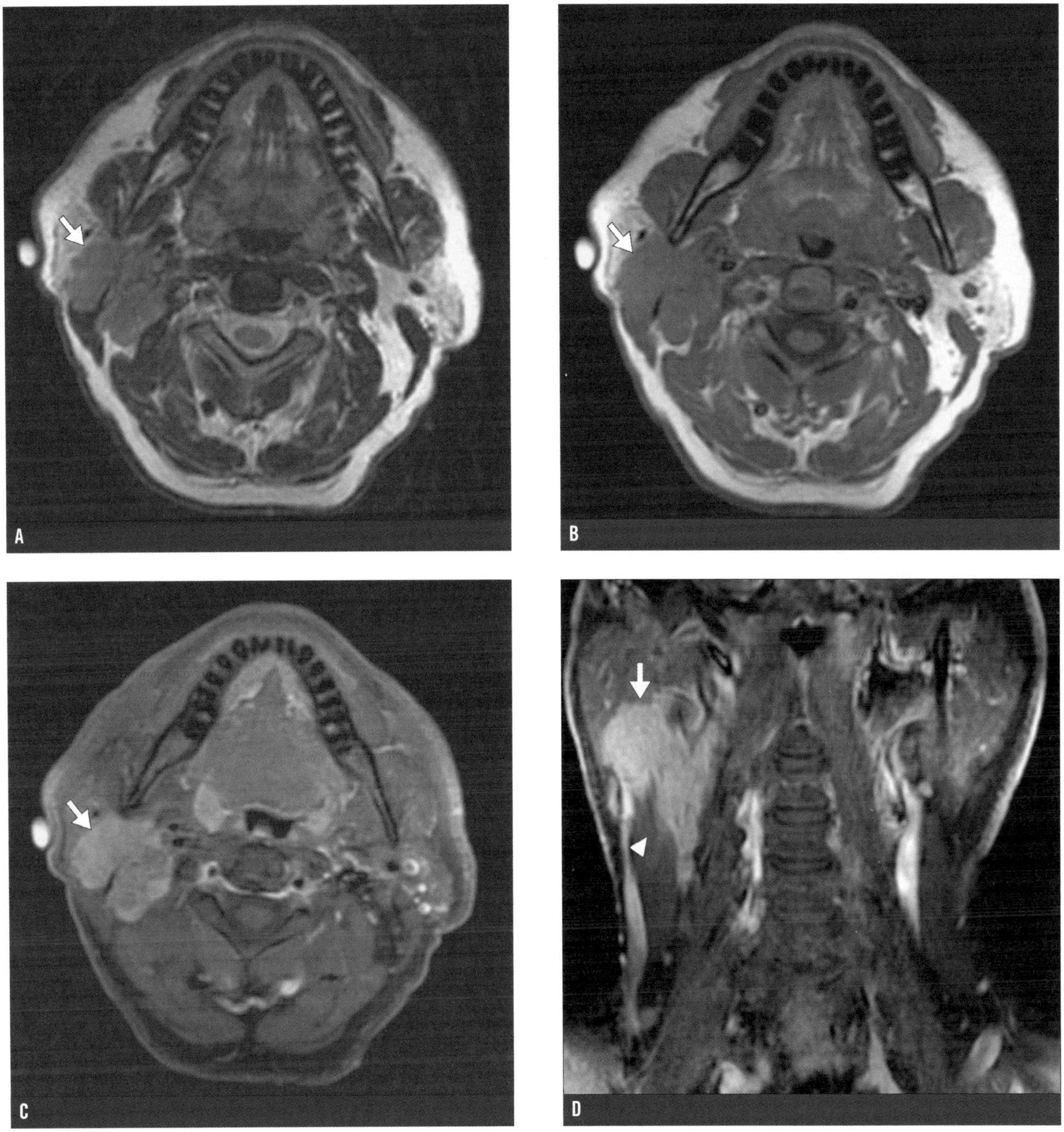

Axial T2 (**A**), axial T1 (**B**), contrast-enhanced axial T1 with fat suppression (**C**), and contrast-enhanced coronal T1 with fat suppression (**D**) MR images demonstrate a multilobulated, T2 and T1 hypointense (relative to adjacent parotid tissue), diffusely enhancing lesion located within the superficial and deep portions of the right parotid gland (arrows, **A-D**). Portions of the lesion are ill-defined (arrowhead, **D**). This lesion represented a high-grade mucoepidermoid carcinoma at pathology.

Companion case: Oncocytoma

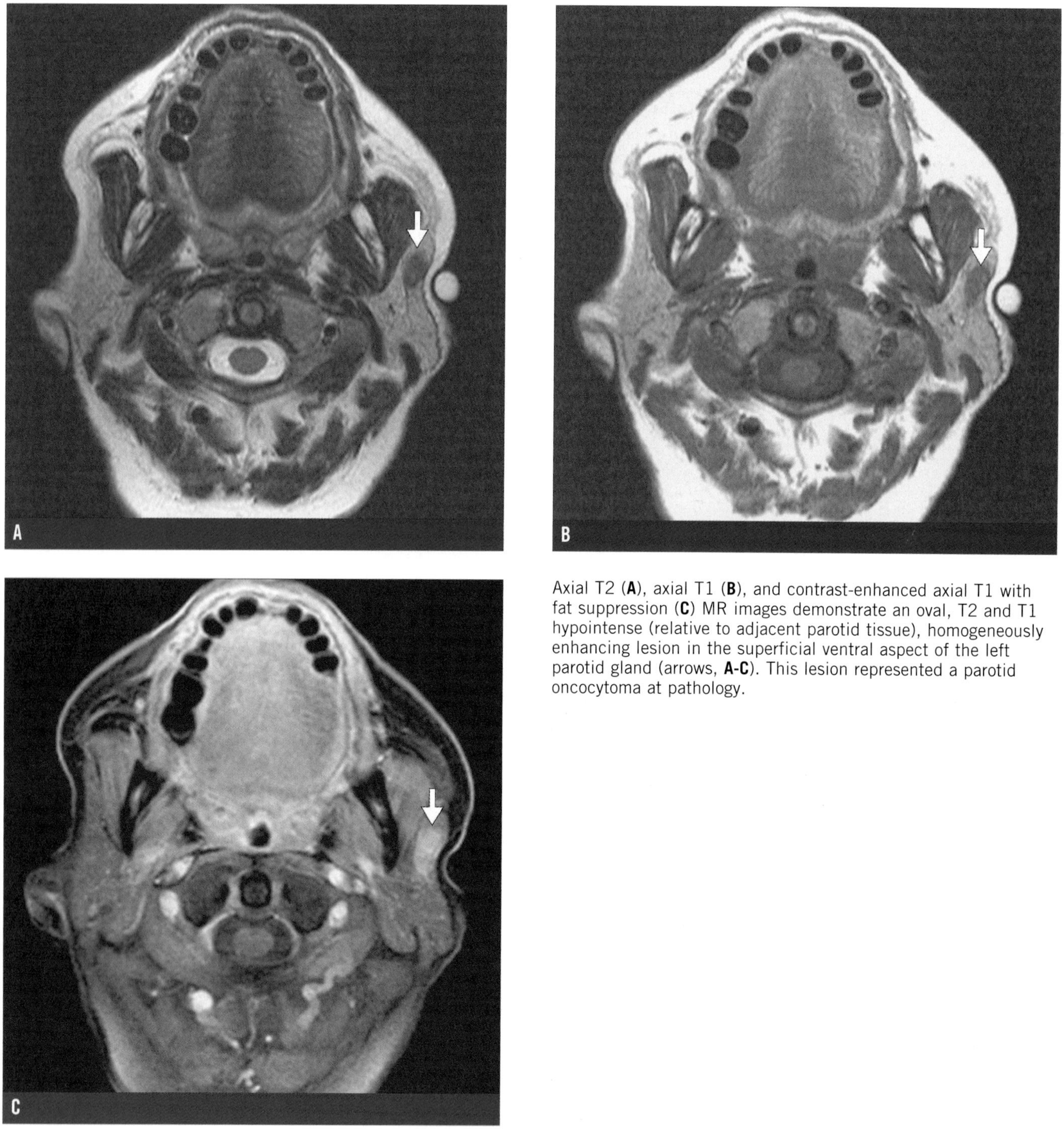

Axial T2 (**A**), axial T1 (**B**), and contrast-enhanced axial T1 with fat suppression (**C**) MR images demonstrate an oval, T2 and T1 hypointense (relative to adjacent parotid tissue), homogeneously enhancing lesion in the superficial ventral aspect of the left parotid gland (arrows, **A-C**). This lesion represented a parotid oncocytoma at pathology.

Companion case: Pleomorphic adenoma

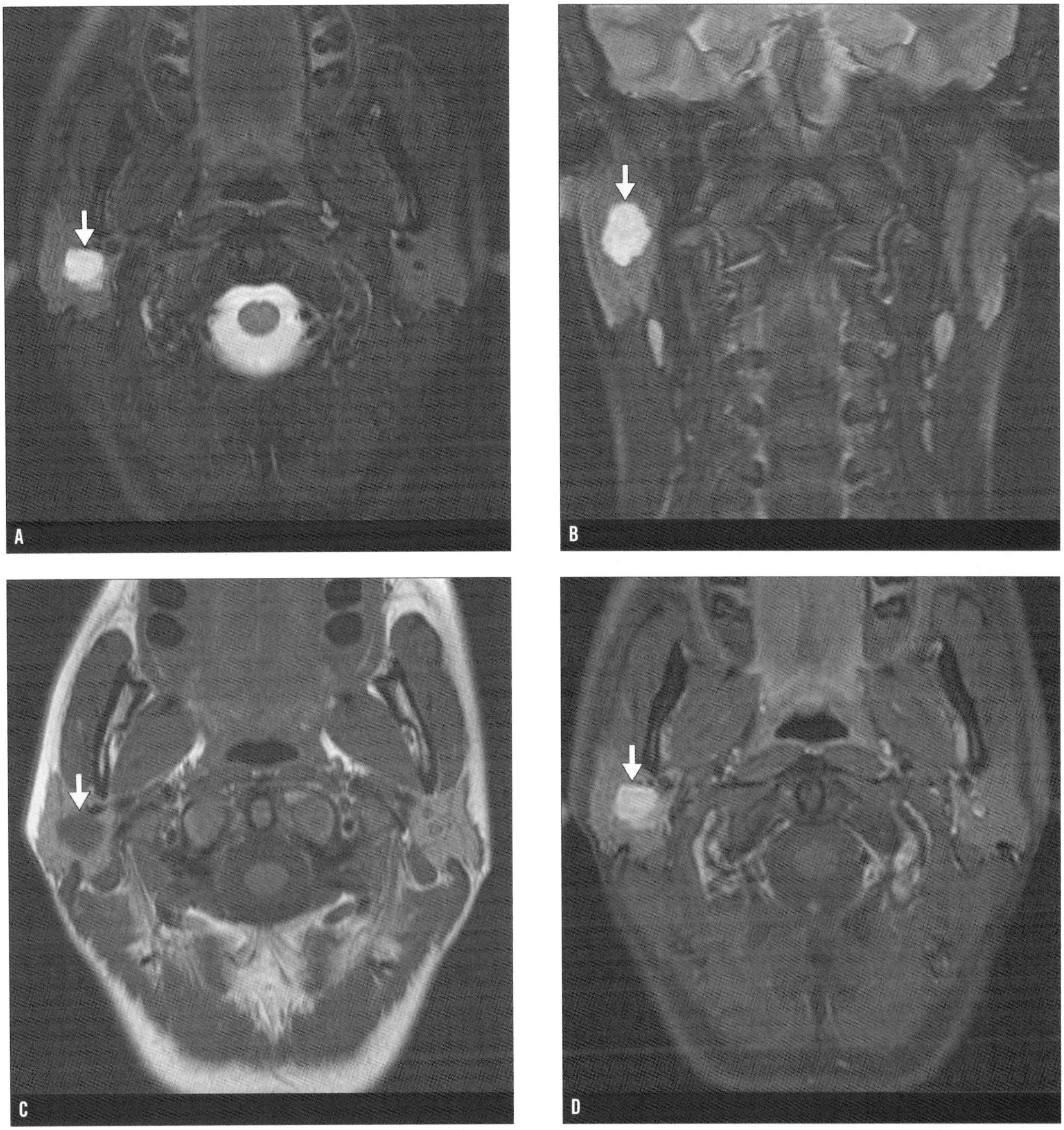

Axial T2 with fat suppression (**A**), coronal T2 with fat suppression (**B**), axial T1 (**C**), and contrast-enhanced axial T1 with fat suppression (**D**) MR images demonstrate a bosselated, diffusely T2 hyperintense, T1 hypointense (relative to adjacent parotid gland), and homogeneously enhancing lesion straddling the superficial and deep aspects of the right parotid gland (arrows, **A-D**). This represented a pleomorphic adenoma at pathology.

Companion case: Carcinoma ex pleomorphic adenoma

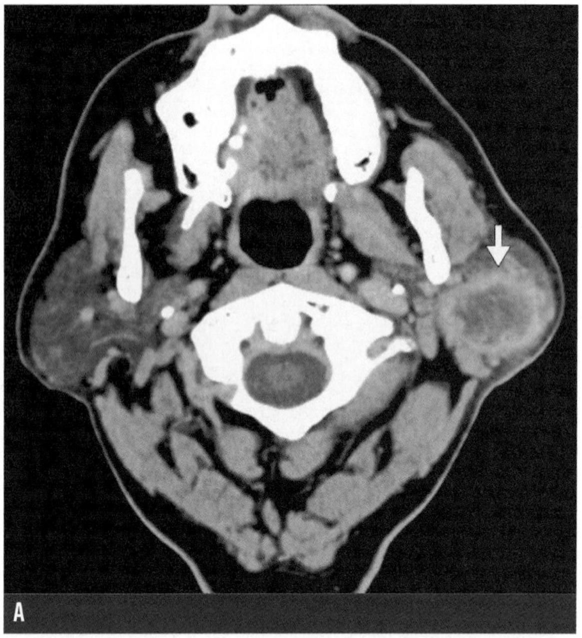

An unenhanced axial CT image (**A**) demonstrates a large, centrally necrotic mass with ill-defined margins located in the left parotid gland (arrow), in this case representing a carcinoma ex pleomorphic adenoma at pathology.

Companion case: Adenoid cystic carcinoma

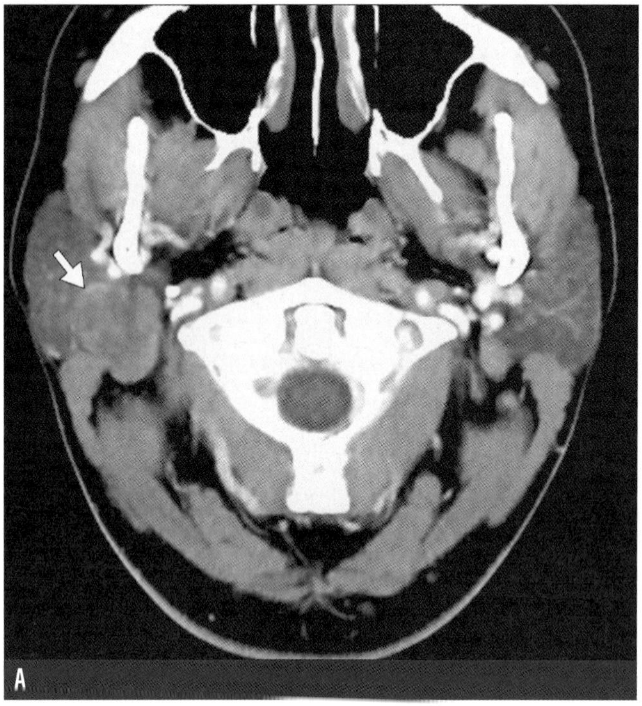

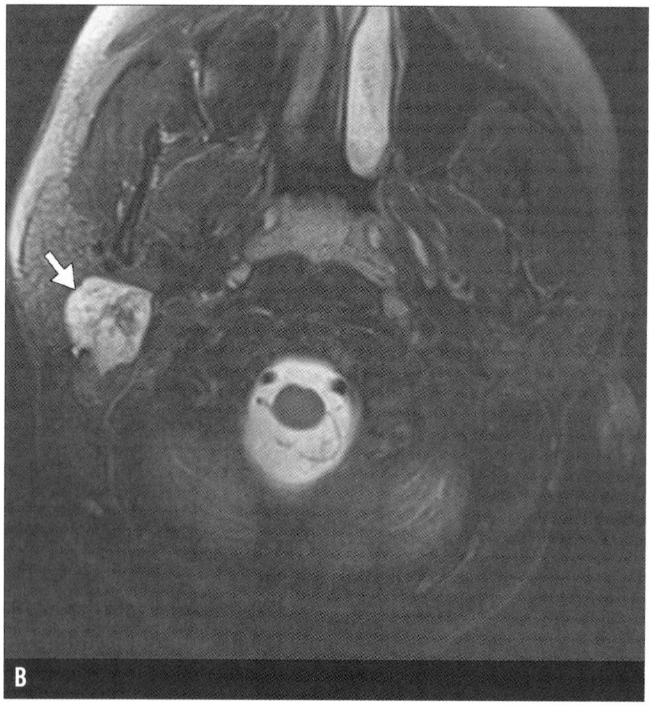

A contrast-enhanced axial CT image (**A**) demonstrates a circumscribed, heterogeneous mass centered in the deep aspect of the right parotid gland along the expected course of the right facial nerve. Fat-suppressed axial T2 (**B**), fat-suppressed coronal T2 (**C**), axial T1 (**D**), and contrast-enhanced axial T1 with fat suppression (**E**) MR images demonstrate the mass to be heterogeneous on T2, hypointense on T1 (relative to parotid gland), and heterogeneously enhancing (arrows, **A-E**). The focally hypointense T2 signal raises the possibility of, but is not specific for, malignancy. This was shown to represent adenoid cystic carcinoma at pathology. In addition, a contrast-enhanced axial T1-weighted MR image with fat suppression (**F**) demonstrates asymmetric enhancement of the right facial nerve mastoid segment, compatible with perineural spread (arrow, **F**). Perineural spread is a relatively common finding with adenoid cystic carcinoma.

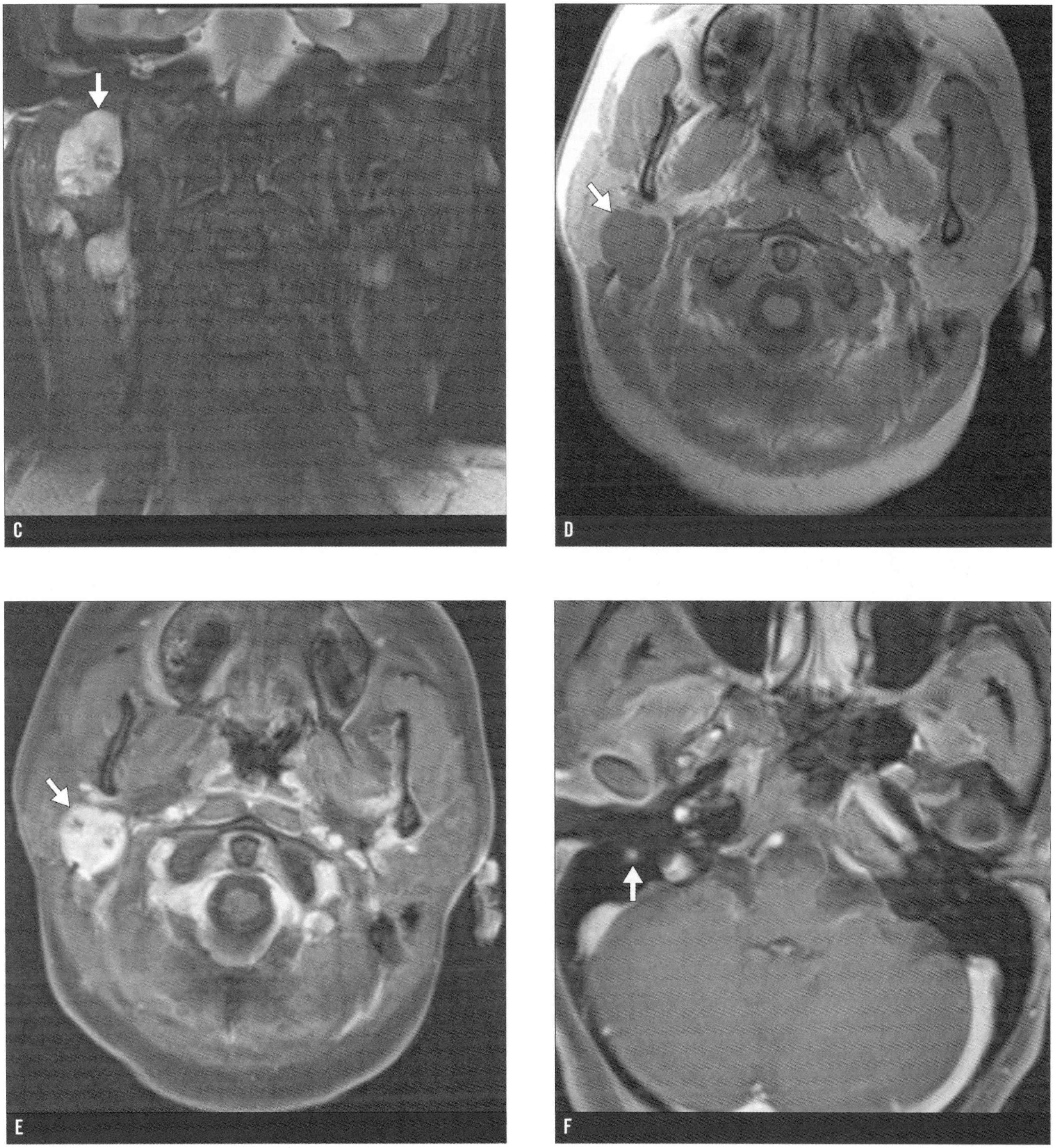
C
D
E
F

Companion case: Adenocarcinoma

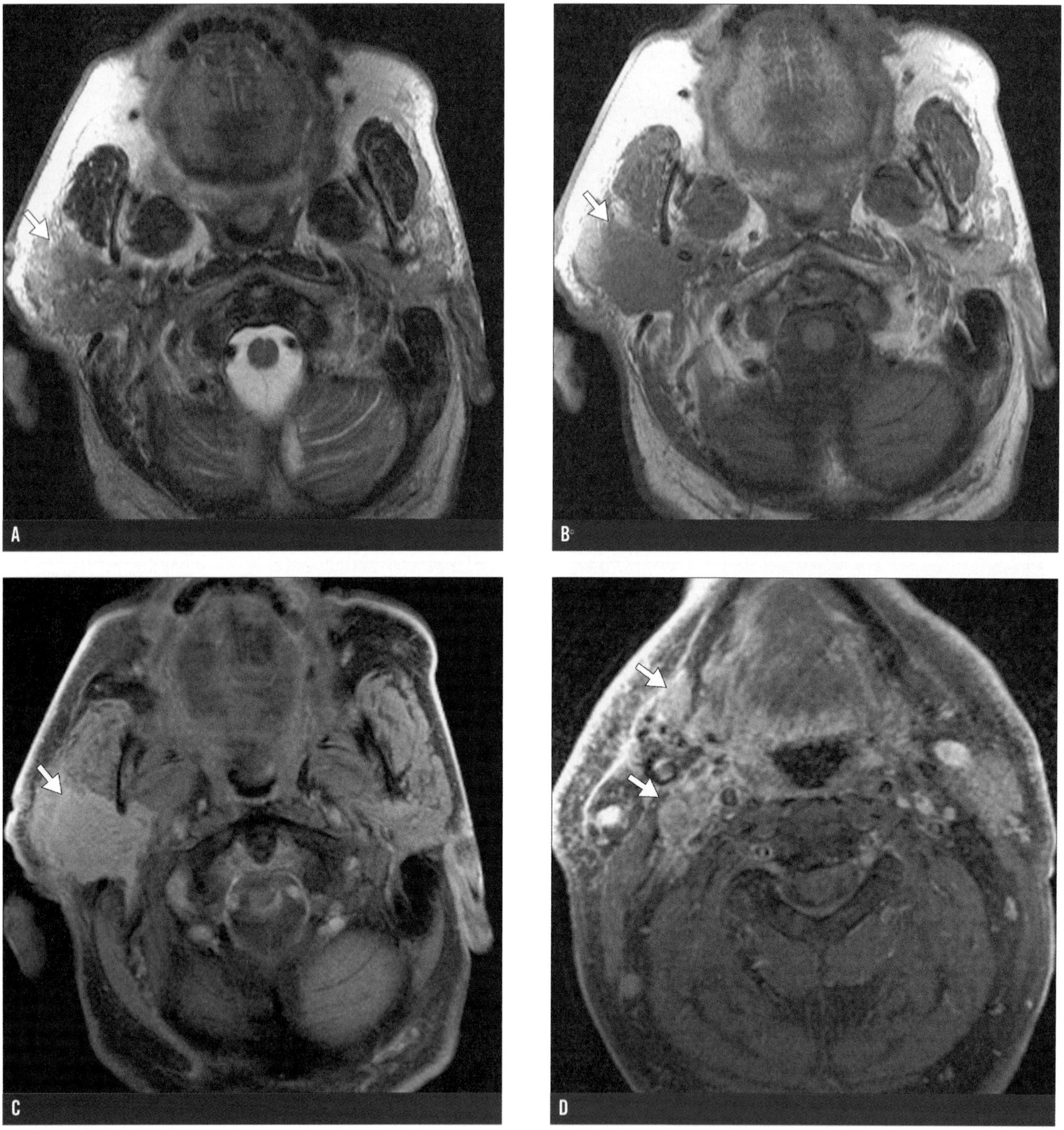

Axial T2 (**A**), axial T1 (**B**), and contrast-enhanced axial T1 with fat suppression (**C**) demonstrates a T2 and T1 hypointense (relative to the parotid gland), homogeneously enhancing right parotid mass that has ill-defined margins (arrows, **A-C**), representing an adenocarcinoma at pathology. A contrast-enhanced axial T1-weighted MR image with fat suppression (**D**) demonstrates ill-defined metastatic lymphadenopathy in the right upper neck (arrows, **D**).

Companion case: Parotid sialocyst

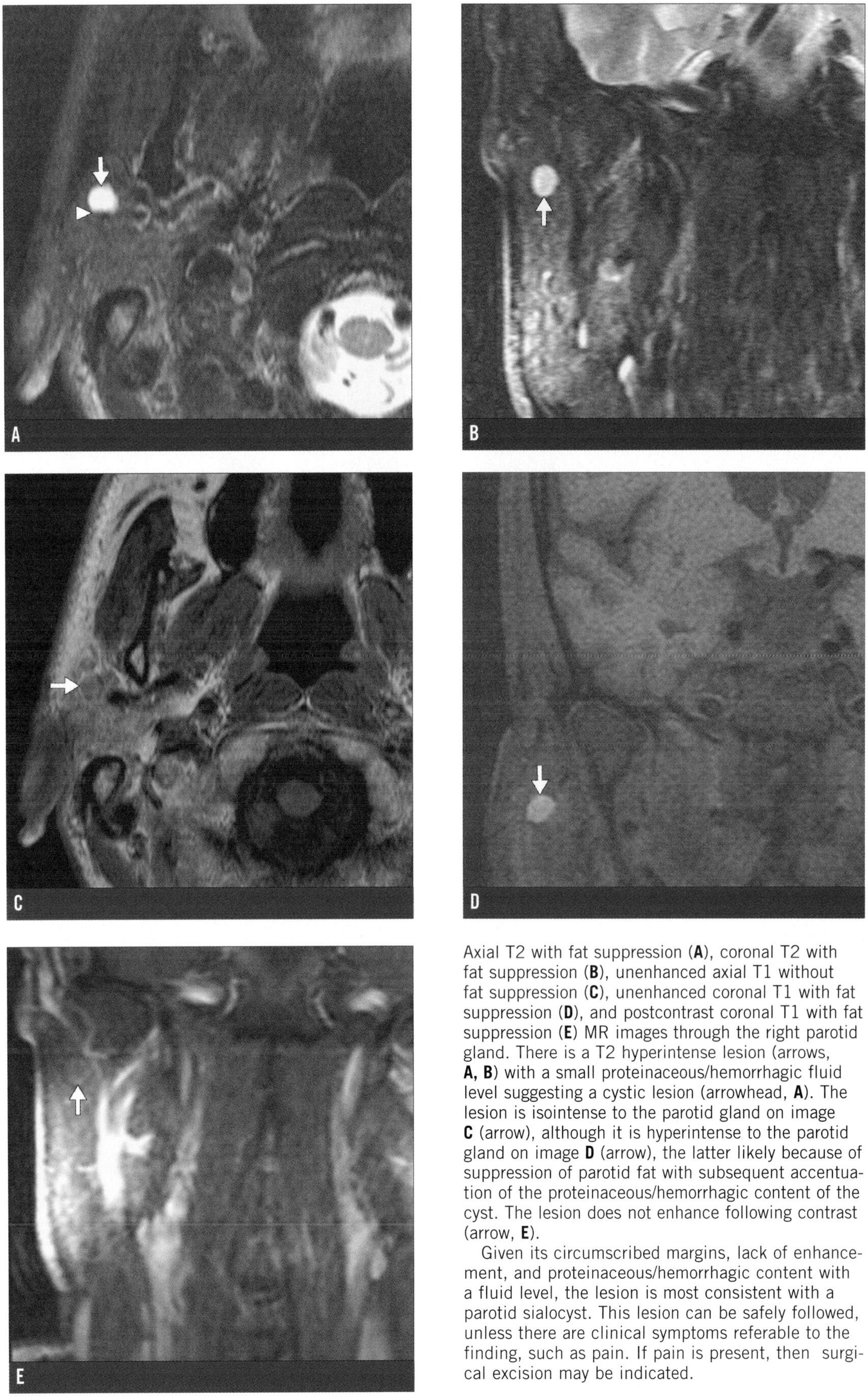

Axial T2 with fat suppression (**A**), coronal T2 with fat suppression (**B**), unenhanced axial T1 without fat suppression (**C**), unenhanced coronal T1 with fat suppression (**D**), and postcontrast coronal T1 with fat suppression (**E**) MR images through the right parotid gland. There is a T2 hyperintense lesion (arrows, **A, B**) with a small proteinaceous/hemorrhagic fluid level suggesting a cystic lesion (arrowhead, **A**). The lesion is isointense to the parotid gland on image **C** (arrow), although it is hyperintense to the parotid gland on image **D** (arrow), the latter likely because of suppression of parotid fat with subsequent accentuation of the proteinaceous/hemorrhagic content of the cyst. The lesion does not enhance following contrast (arrow, **E**).

Given its circumscribed margins, lack of enhancement, and proteinaceous/hemorrhagic content with a fluid level, the lesion is most consistent with a parotid sialocyst. This lesion can be safely followed, unless there are clinical symptoms referable to the finding, such as pain. If pain is present, then surgical excision may be indicated.

Companion case: First branchial cleft cyst

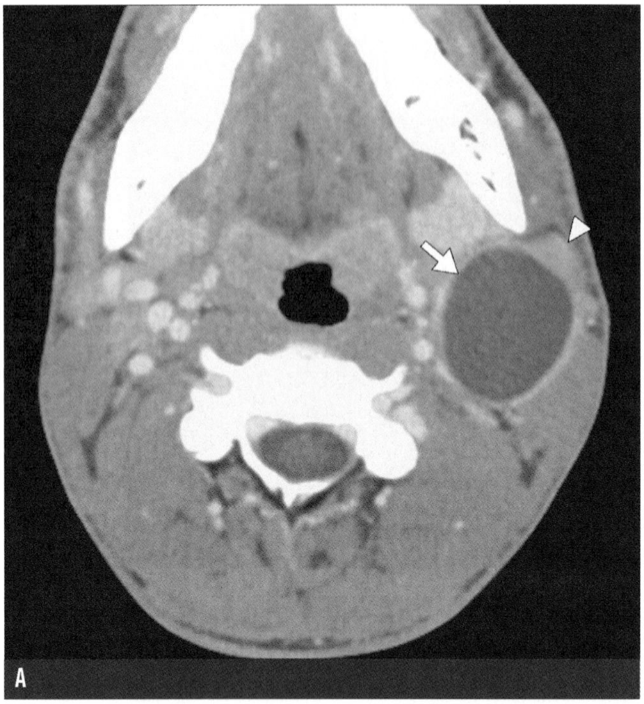

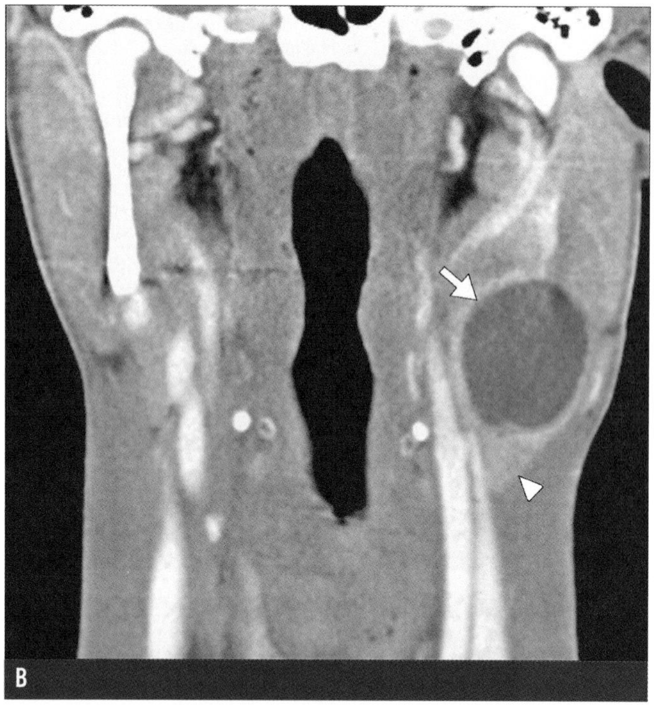

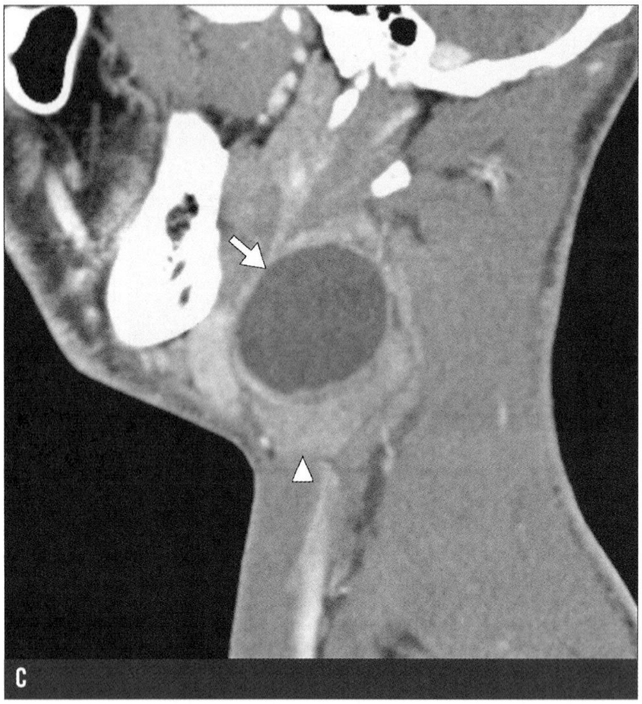

Axial (**A**), coronal reformatted (**B**), and sagittal reformatted (**C**) postcontrast CT images demonstrate a circumscribed, hypoattenuating mass in the left parotid gland of a 26-year-old patient, representing a Type II first branchial cleft cyst (arrows, **A-C**). The parotid tail surrounds the mass (arrowheads, **A-C**) and confirms the mass is intraparotid rather than periparotid in location.

Companion case: Periparotid varix

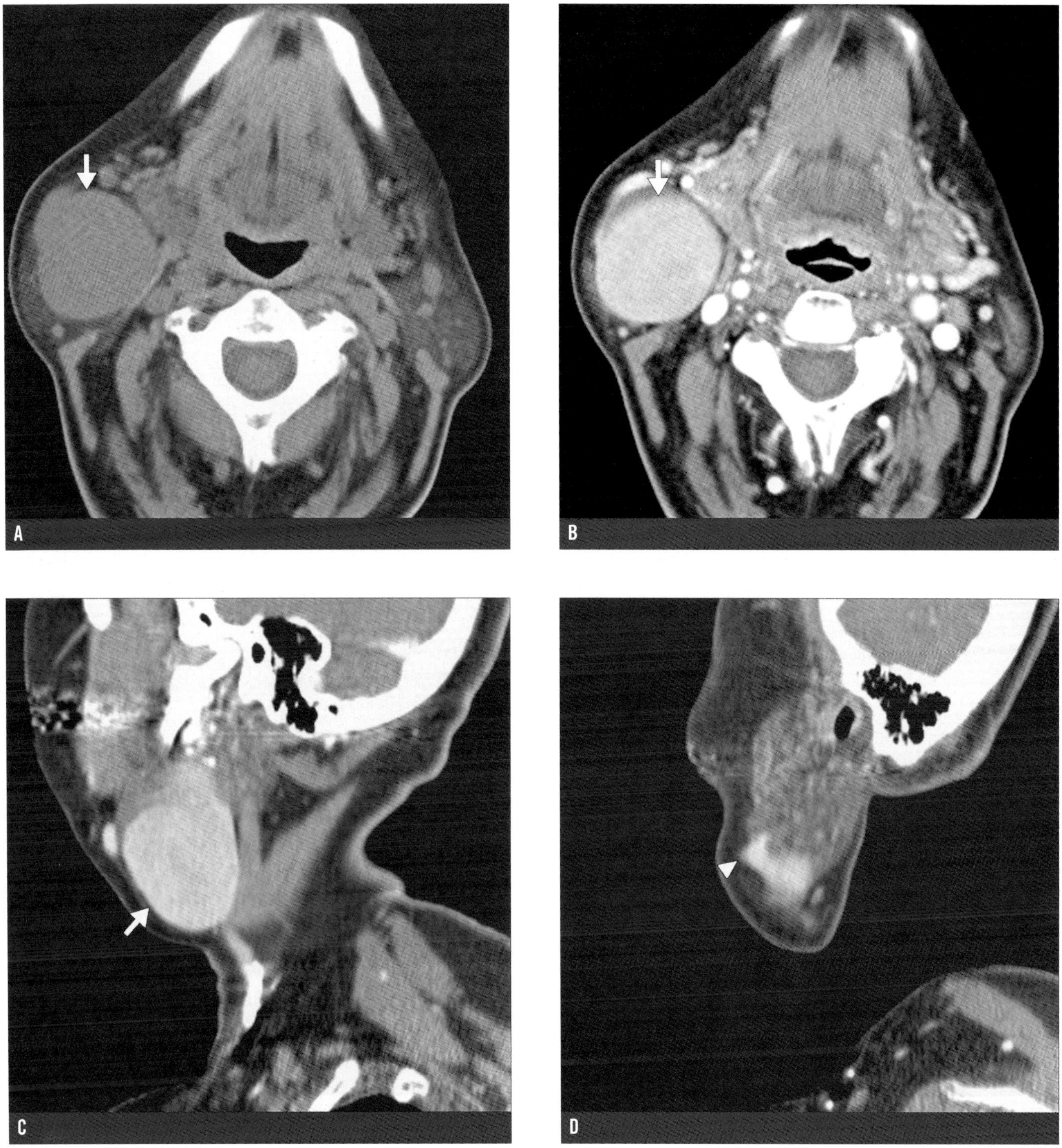

Precontrast axial (**A**), postcontrast axial (**B**), postcontrast right parasagittal reformatted (**C, D**), and postcontrast coronal reformatted (**E**) CT images. Image **A** demonstrates an isoattenuating mass (relative to muscle) adjacent to or within the right parotid tail (arrow, **A**). The postcontrast images demonstrate the large mass to densely enhance (arrows, **B, C, E**). Images **D** and **E** demonstrate a branch from the external jugular vein to extend directly into this lesion (arrowheads, **D, E**). Images **C** and **E** perhaps best demonstrate that the lesion causes mass effect on the right parotid gland and likely arises adjacent to the parotid tail. Real-time ultrasonography of the mass (**F, G**) demonstrates echogenic swirling within the lesion (arrows, **F, G**). Doppler imaging of the lesion (**H**) demonstrates venous flow within the lesion (arrow, **H**). This lesion was compressible on examination and is consistent with a periparotid venous varix. While tumors can be hyperenhancing on CT, in this case, the density of the enhancement on CT approaches that of the veins elsewhere in the neck. Additionally, tumors are generally firm lesions and not compressible. When a vascular lesion is suspected or cannot be accurately assessed by CT or MRI, then a Doppler ultrasound can be very useful in this setting.

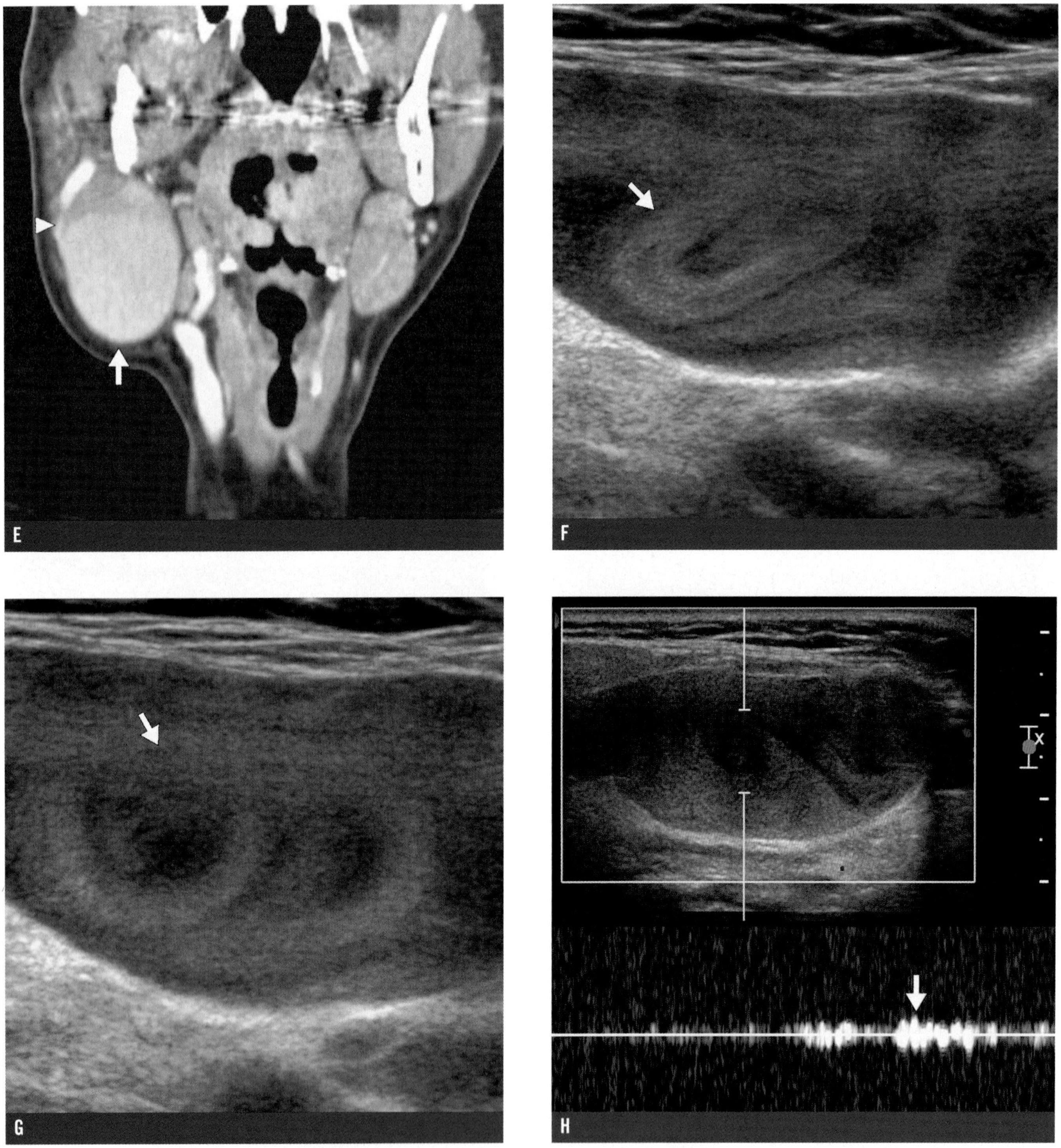
E
F
G
H

REFERENCES

Benson MT, Dalen K, Mancuso AA, Kerr HH, Cacciarelli AA, Mafee MF. Congenital anomalies of the branchial apparatus: embryology and pathologic anatomy. *Radiographics.* 1992;12(5):943-960.

Christe A, Waldherr C, Hallett R, Zbaeren P, Thoeny H. MR imaging of parotid tumors: typical lesion characteristics in MR imaging improve discrimination between benign and malignant disease. *AJNR Am J Neuroradiol.* 2011;32(7):1202-1207.

Godballe C, Schultz JH, Krogdahl A, Møller-Grøntved A, Johansen J. Parotid carcinoma: impact of clinical factors on prognosis in a histologically revised series. *Laryngoscope.* 2003;113(8):1411-1417.

Hamilton BE, Salzman KL, Wiggins RH 3rd, Harnsberger HR. Earring lesions of the parotid tail. *AJNR Am J Neuroradiol.* 2003;24(9):1757-1764.

Lev MH, Khanduja K, Morris PP, Curtin HD. Parotid pleomorphic adenomas: delayed CT enhancement. *AJNR Am J Neuroradiol.* 1998;19(10):1835-1839.

Moonis G, Patel P, Koshkareva Y, Newman J, Loevner LA. Imaging characteristics of recurrent pleomorphic adenoma of the parotid gland. *AJNR Am J Neuroradiol.* September 2007;28(8):1532-1536.

Mukherji SK, Tart RP, Slattery WH, Stringer SP, Benson MT, Mancuso AA. Evaluation of first branchial anomalies by CT and MR. *J Comput Assist Tomogr.* 1993;17(4):576-581.

Paleri V, Gopalakrishnan S. Jugular phlebectasia: theory of pathogenesis and review of literature. *Int J Pediatr Otorhinolaryngol.* 2001;57(2):155-159.

Patel ND, van Zante A, Eisele DW, Harnsberger HR, Glastonbury CM. Oncocytoma: the vanishing parotid mass. *AJNR Am J Neuroradiol.* 2011;32(9):1703-1706.

San Pedro EC, Lorberboym M, Machac J, Som P, Shugar J. Imaging of multiple bilateral parotid gland oncocytomas. *Clin Nucl Med.*1995;20(6):515-518.

Silvers AR, Som PM. Salivary glands. *Radiol Clin North Am.* 1998;36(5):941-966.

Stravropoulos SW, Mukherji SK, Mancuso AA. Recurrent parotid adenocarcinoma occurring within the cerebellopontine angle. *AJNR Am J Neuroradiol.* 1995;16(7):1529-1531.

Tan TJ, Tan TY. CT features of parotid gland oncocytomas: a study of 10 cases and literature review. *AJNR Am J Neuroradiol.* 2010;31(8):1413-1417.

Yousem DM, Kraut MA, Chalian AA. Major salivary gland imaging. *Radiology.* 2000;216(1):19-29.

CASE 2 Benign bilateral parotid lymph nodes

The presence of bilateral parotid lymph nodes is a common finding on imaging. As discussed in the preceding case, parotid lymph nodes that have circumscribed margins, are T2 hyperintense on MRI, contain a fatty hilum, and are less than 1 cm in size suggest benignity. There are numerous causes of bilateral parotid lymph node enlargement, including viral or bacterial infection, granulomatous disease, and metastatic disease, none of which may be able to be differentiated by imaging alone. In addition to bilateral parotid lymphadenopathy, specific entities enter the differential diagnosis when lesions affecting both parotid glands are encountered.

COMPANION CASES

- **Sjögren syndrome.** Sjögren syndrome is an autoimmune disorder in which lymphocytes infiltrate the salivary glands as well as the lacrimal glands and result in a sicca complex, manifested by dry eyes (xerophthalmia) and dry mouth (xerostomia). Sjögren syndrome commonly occurs in conjunction with a connective tissue disorder, most often rheumatoid arthritis. The lymphocytic infiltration initially results in glandular enlargement and premature fat deposition, but ultimately there is destruction of the glandular tissue and atrophy. On CT and MRI, variably sized fluid density and intensity foci, respectively, are usually scattered diffusely throughout both parotid glands, reflective of abnormally enlarged/destroyed acini. In addition, scattered calcifications are often present in the parotid glands with this entity. Sjögren syndrome is strongly associated with lymphoma, with some stating that the risk of developing lymphoma in patients with Sjögren syndrome increases by more than 4400% compared to the general population. Therefore, lymphoma should be suspected when an enlarging solid parotid lesion is identified in these patients. Sjögren syndrome and sarcoid involving the parotid glands may be indistinguishable on imaging, and sarcoid is also strongly associated with the development of lymphoma.
- **Benign lymphoepithelial lesions of HIV.** Benign lymphoepithelial lesions (BLELs) may occur sporadically or be the result of various pathologies, including recurrent parotitis of childhood. Furthermore, the term lymphoepithelial lesion has been used to describe the histopathological changes of Sjögren syndrome. However, BLELs are most commonly identified in the setting of HIV. While there may be imaging overlap between the Sjögren disease and BLELs of HIV, BLELs of HIV are generally more variably sized, larger, can enhance, may be solid, and are not associated with calcifications. Because BLELs of HIV can be solid, the term benign lymphoepithelial cysts of HIV has largely been replaced with the term BLELs. The etiology of BLELs of HIV is unclear although there are two theories. One theory describes lymphoid proliferation leading to ductal obstruction and acinar dilation, which in turn, leads to lesion formation. The other theory describes HIV-related lymphoproliferation within parotid lymph nodes that engulf a portion of adjacent parotid glandular epithelium and results in lesion formation. While BLELs are not invasive and do not have malignant potential, they may become large and disfiguring. Surgery is considered the gold standard for treating BLELs that are disfiguring.
- **Warthin tumors.** Also known as papillary cystadenoma lymphomatosum, a Warthin tumor represents the second most common benign parotid tumor, with pleomorphic adenoma being the most common. Warthin tumors are composed of a follicular stroma and an oncocytic epithelial component. These tumors are exclusive to the parotid or periparotid lymph nodes, with a propensity to involve the parotid tail. These tumors are most common in men between their fourth and seventh decades of life, Caucasians, and those who smoke tobacco; however, there are an increasing number of females with Warthin tumors, presumably because of an increasing number of female smokers. Multifocal tumors are common, and there are synchronous lesions in both parotid glands in 10% to 15% of cases. On CT, most Warthin tumors are circumscribed soft tissue masses. Cystic areas may be present, particularly with larger tumors. Pathologically enlarged periparotid lymph nodes that contain this tumor may have similar imaging characteristics as the parotid lesion(s) . On MRI, Warthin tumors are usually low, intermediate, or mixed in signal on T2. On T1, a focus or region of T1 shortening may be associated with the lesion(s), a finding that suggests a Warthin tumor in the appropriate clinical setting. However, T1 shortening, which likely represents proteinaceous content or hemorrhage within a cystic portion of the tumor, may also be identified in rarer parotid tumors, such as basal cell adenoma. Warthin tumors enhance early following contrast administration, but there is usually contrast washout from the tumor on delayed imaging. Both Warthin tumors and oncocytomas will exhibit intense and prolonged uptake with ^{99m}Tc-pertechnetate nuclear medicine imaging, an imaging characteristic that is unique for these tumors.
- **Bilateral parotid oncocytomas.** Please refer to Case 1 from this chapter for discussion.
- **Follicular lymphoma affecting both parotid glands.** Primary lymphoma of the parotid glands is rare. Most lymphomas affecting the parotid glands are related to systemic lymphoma, usually large B-cell lymphoma, although all forms of lymphoma have been reported.

Benign bilateral parotid lymph nodes

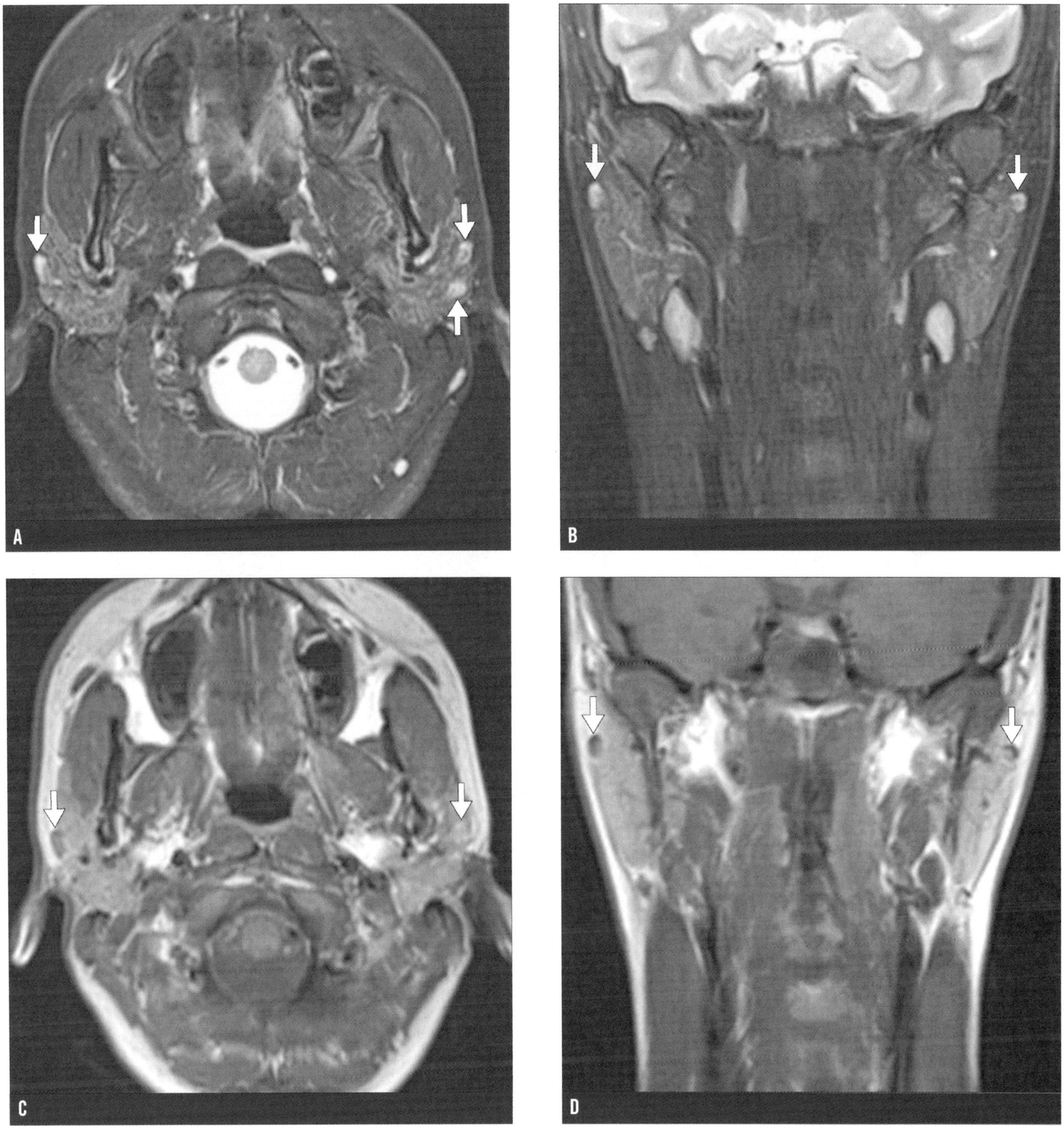

Fat-suppressed T2 in the axial (**A**) and coronal (**B**) planes, T1 in the axial (**C**) and coronal (**D**) planes, and contrast-enhanced axial T1 with fat suppression (**E**) MR images demonstrate several T2 hyperintense, enhancing nodules in the parotid glands, some of which contain fat, compatible with benign bilateral parotid lymph nodes (arrows, **A-E**).

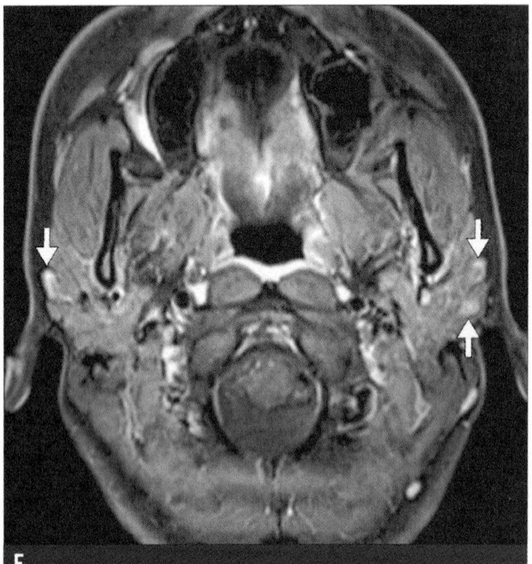

E

Companion case: Sjögren syndrome

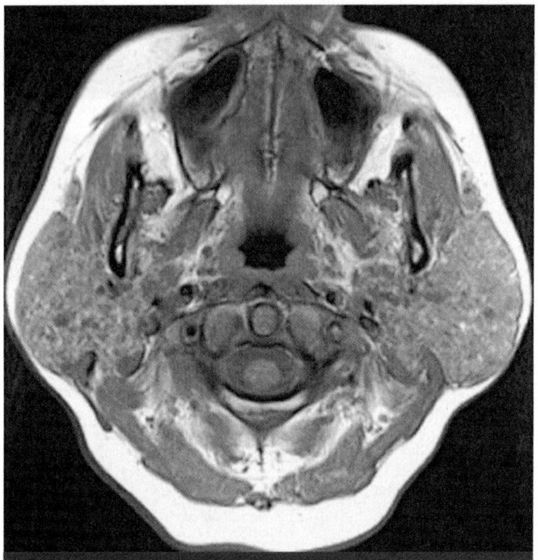

A

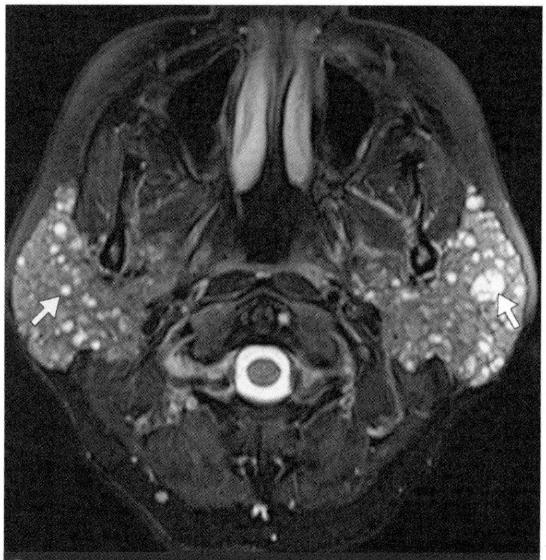

B

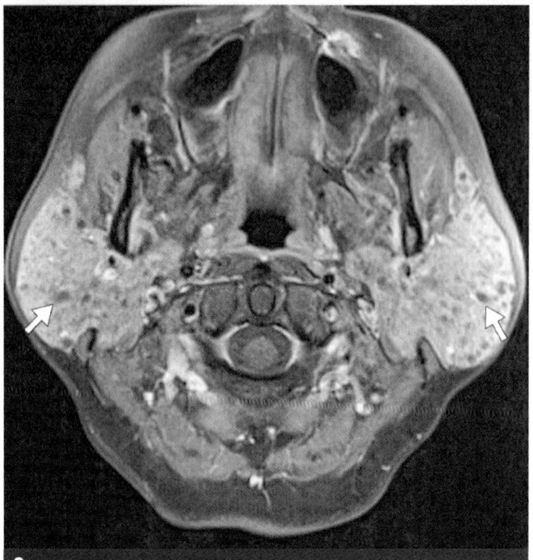

C

Axial T1 (**A**), fat-suppressed axial T2 (**B**), and fat-suppressed postcontrast axial T1 (**C**) MR images through the parotids glands. Images **B** and **C** best demonstrate innumerable, small foci throughout the parotid glands that are T2 hyperintense and nonenhancing, respectively, representing abnormally dilated acini, typical of Sjögren syndrome (arrows, **B**, **C**). The parotid glands are also diffusely enlarged, a finding that may be seen with Sjögren syndrome, depending on the stage of the disease.

Companion case: Benign lymphoepithelial lesions of HIV

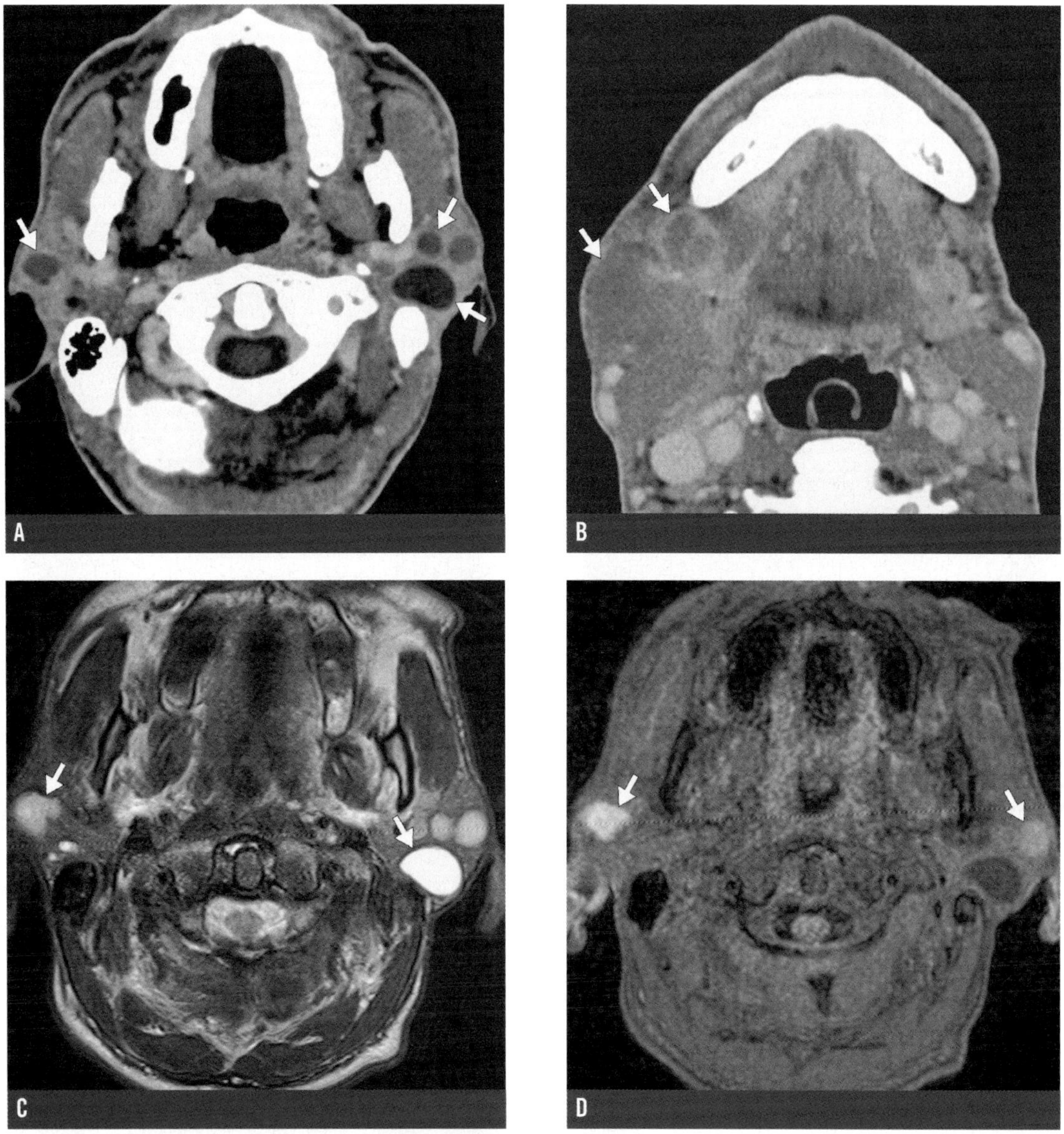

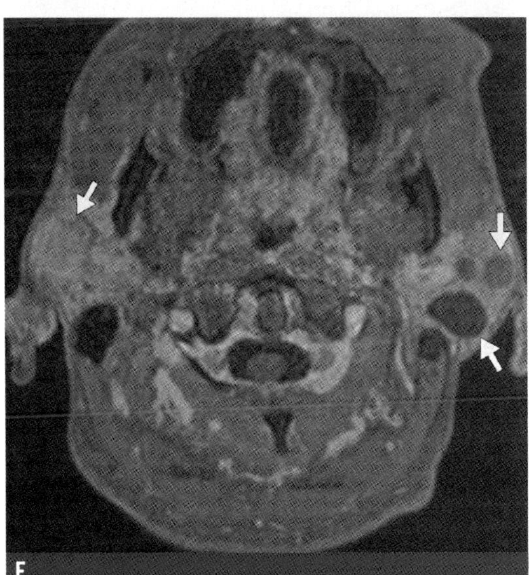

A postcontrast axial CT image through the parotid glands of an HIV patient (**A**) demonstrates several variably sized, round and oval circumscribed areas of varying hypoattenuation throughout the parotid glands, most compatible with benign lymphoepithelial lesions of HIV (arrows, **A**). A postcontrast axial CT image obtained through the level of the submandibular glands (**B**) demonstrates a large amount of lymphadenopathy in the right submandibular region in this patient with HIV-associated lymphoma (arrows, **B**). Axial T2 (**C**), precontrast axial MPRAGE (**D**), and postcontrast axial MPRAGE (**E**) MR images through the parotid glands of the same patient demonstrate the benign lymphoepithelial lesions to be hyperintense on T2 and contain varying amounts of proteinaceous content without enhancement (arrows, **C-E**). Images **D** and **E** were performed with the same technique. The intrinsically T1 hyperintense lesions on image **D** appear relatively less hyperintense on image **E** likely because of parotid gland enhancement. While not present in this case, benign lymphoepithelial lesions of HIV may be solid and can enhance.

Companion case: Follicular lymphoma affecting both parotid glands

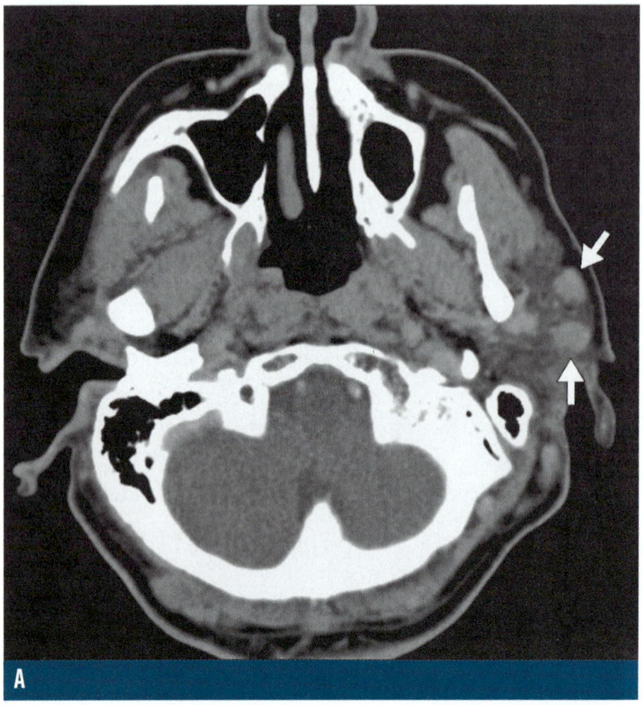

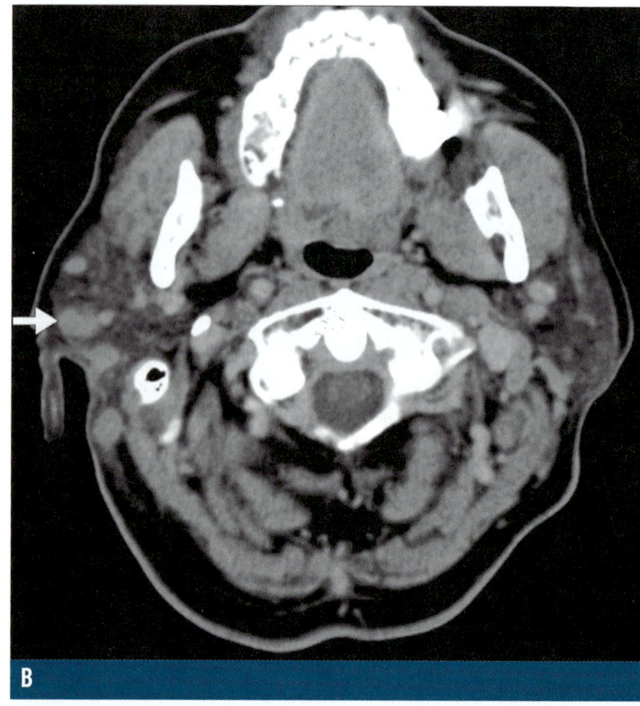

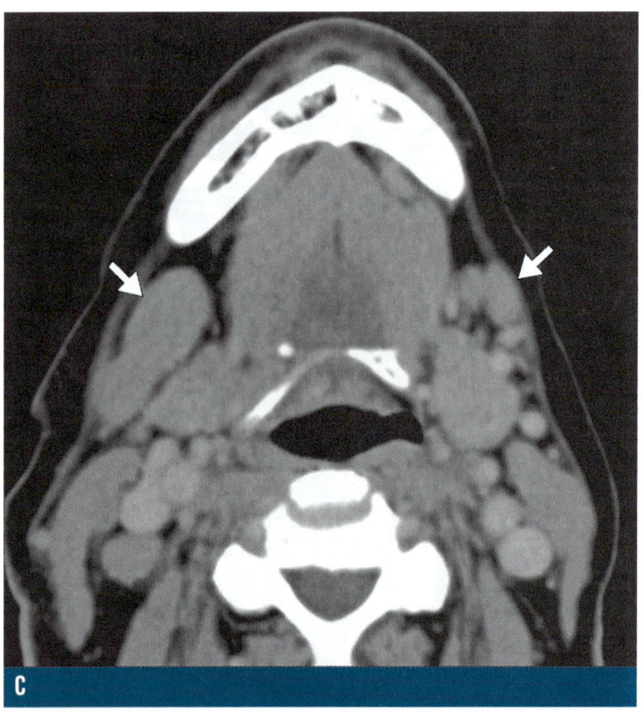

Contrast-enhanced axial CT images through the parotid glands (**A**, **B**) and submandibular region (**C**) demonstrate several soft tissue nodules in the parotid glands (arrows, **A**, **B**) as well as pathologically enlarged upper neck lymph nodes (arrows, **C**) in this patient with follicular lymphoma.

REFERENCES

Hamilton BE, Salzman KL, Wiggins RH 3rd, Harnsberger HR. Earring lesions of the parotid tail. *AJNR Am J Neuroradiol.* 2003;24(9):1757-1764.

O'Neill ID. New insights into the nature of Warthin's tumour. *J Oral Pathol Med.* 2009;38(1):145-149.

San Pedro EC1, Lorberboym M, Machac J, Som P, Shugar J. Imaging of multiple bilateral parotid gland oncocytomas. *Clin Nucl Med.*1995;20(6):515-518.

Silvers AR, Som PM. Salivary glands. *Radiol Clin North Am.* 1998;36(5):941-966.

Steehler MK, Steehler MW, Davison SP. Benign lymphoepithelial cysts of the parotid: long-term surgical results. *HIV AIDS (Auckl).* 2012;4:81-86.

Tan TJ, Tan TY. CT features of parotid gland oncocytomas: a study of 10 cases and literature review. *AJNR Am J Neuroradiol.* 2010;31(8):1413-1417.

Yousem DM, Kraut MA, Chalian AA. Major salivary gland imaging. *Radiology.* 2000;216(1):19-29.

CASE 3 Accessory parotid gland

An accessory parotid gland is located ventral to, and is separate from, the main parotid gland. It overlies the masseter muscle and is histologically as well as radiologically identical to the main parotid gland. This is a common entity, with most sources quoting an approximately 20% incidence. While neoplasms can arise in accessory parotid tissue, normal accessory parotid tissue may be palpated and mistaken for a mass during a clinical examination, particularly if it is asymmetrically enlarged relative to its contralateral counterpart.

COMPANION CASES

- **Enlarged accessory parotid glands with main parotid gland atrophy.** Most cases of accessory parotid tissue are associated with a normal accompanying main parotid gland. Occasionally, there is congenital absence or atrophy of the main parotid gland with normal or hypertrophied accessory parotid gland tissue, as is present in the case provided.
- **Tumor arising from an accessory parotid gland.** Because accessory parotid gland tissue represents the same tissue found in the main parotid gland, any process that arises from the main parotid gland can arise from an accessory parotid gland, including tumors.
- **Facial process of the parotid gland.** The facial process of the parotid gland is similarly located as accessory parotid gland tissue, but the facial process is directly contiguous with the main parotid gland, as opposed to the accessory parotid gland which is distinctly separate. Similar to accessory parotid gland tissue, the facial process of the parotid gland may also be mistaken for a mass during palpation.

Accessory parotid glands

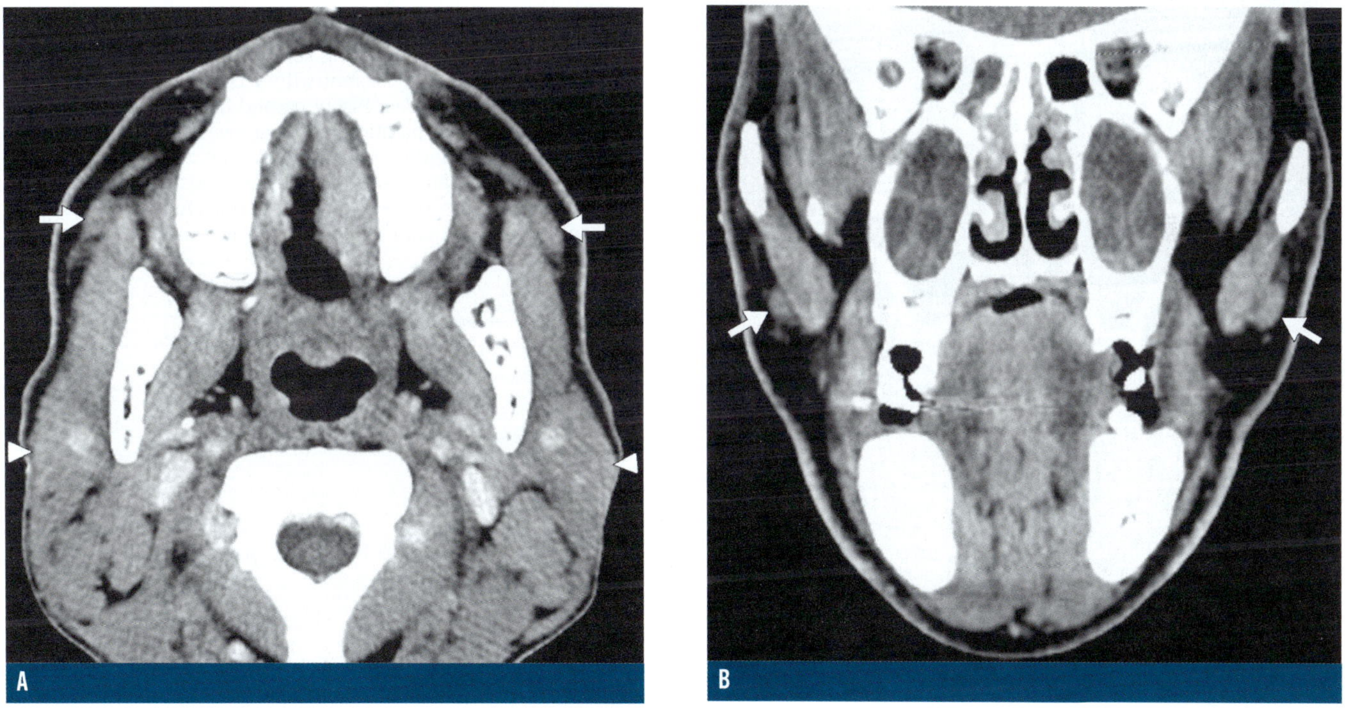

Axial (**A**) and coronal reformatted (**B**) contrast-enhanced CT images through the level of the parotid glands demonstrate bilateral accessory parotid tissue (arrows , **A**, **B**). Accessory parotid tissue is defined as anteriorly located parotid tissue that is separate from the main parotid glands, the latter denoted with arrowheads on image **A**.

Accessory parotid gland

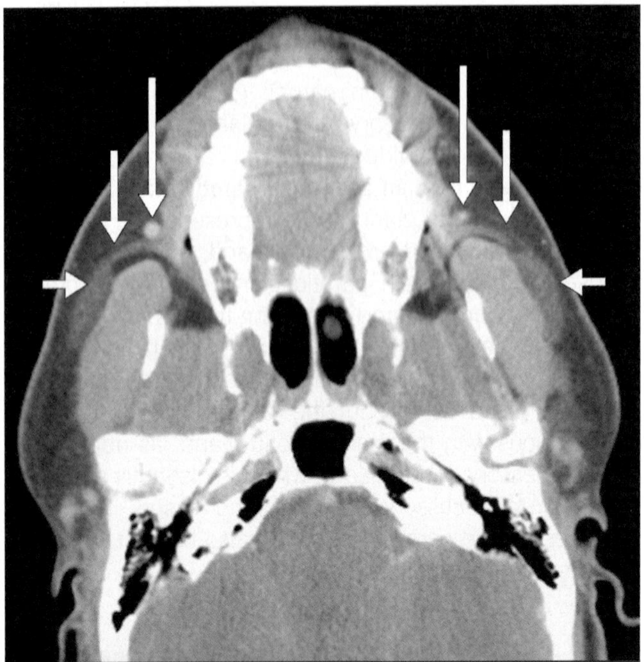

A

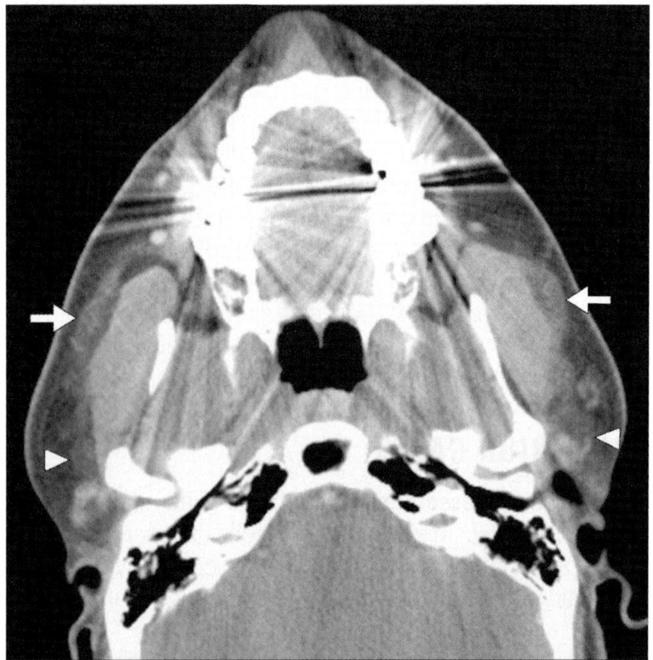

B

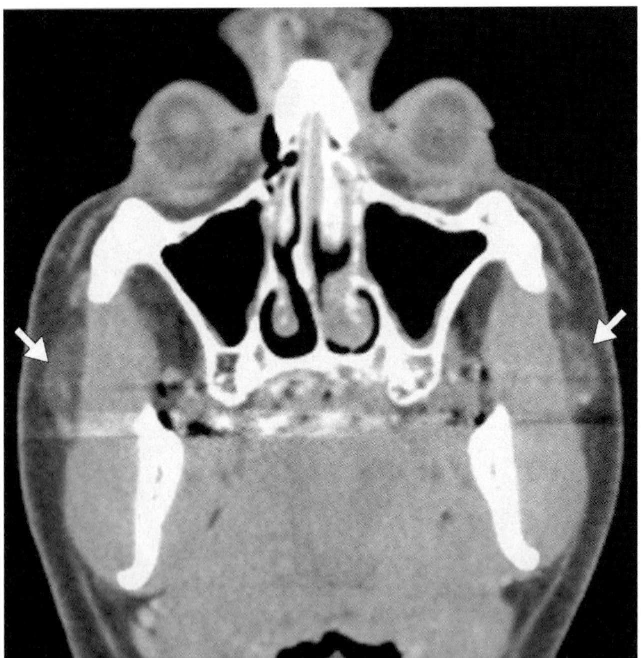

C

Different patient. Axial (**A**, **B**) and coronal reformatted (**C**) postcontrast CT images through the level of the parotid glands demonstrate symmetric hypoattenuating soft tissue overlying the masseter muscles, consistent with accessory parotid tissue (small arrows, **A-C**). The accessory parotid tissue is identical in density to the main parotid glands (arrowheads, **B**), which are only partially included on this image. The Stensen ducts (medium arrows, **A**) are identified and, as expected, are contiguous with the accessory parotid gland tissue. Anatomically, the Stensen ducts are located immediately posterior to the facial vein (long arrows, **A**).

Companion case: Enlarged accessory parotid glands with main parotid gland atrophy

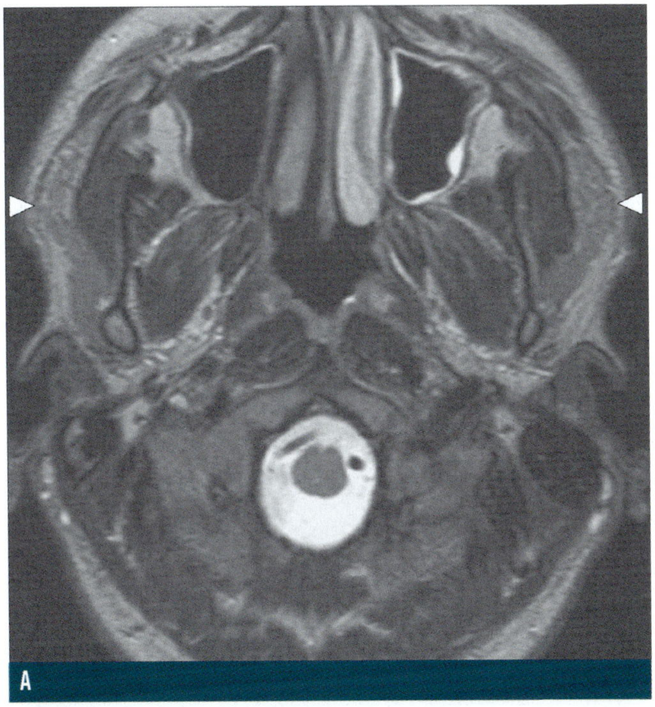

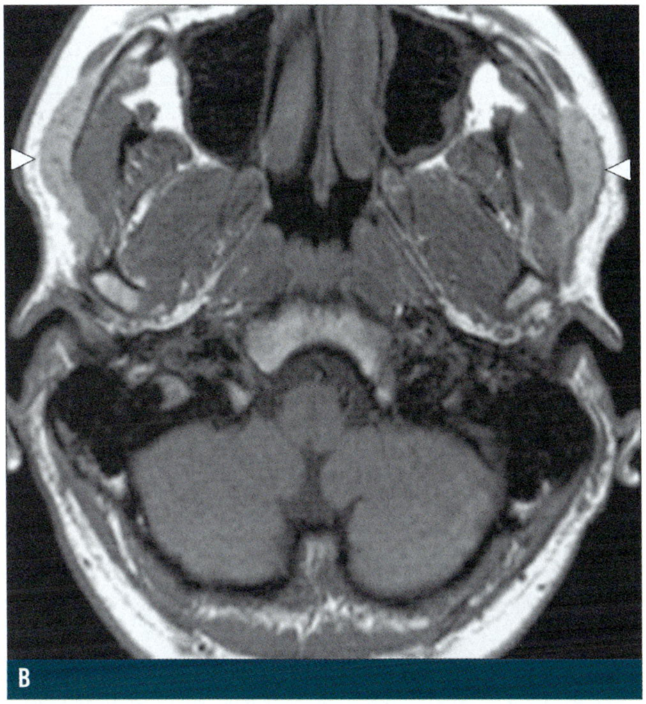

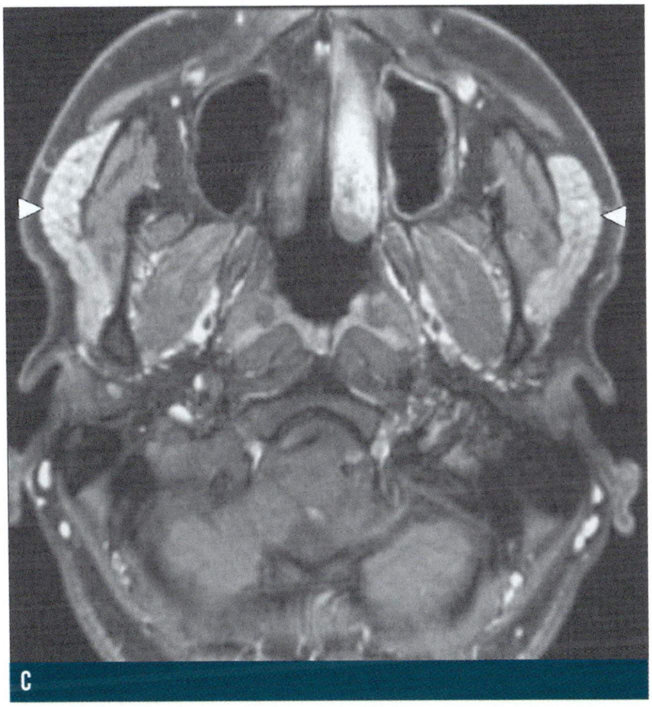

Axial T2 (**A**), axial T1 (**B**), and contrast-enhanced axial T1 with fat suppression (**C**) MR images demonstrate enlarged accessory parotid glands (arrowheads, **A-C**) that are associated with atrophy of the main parotid glands.

Companion case: Tumor arising from an accessory parotid gland

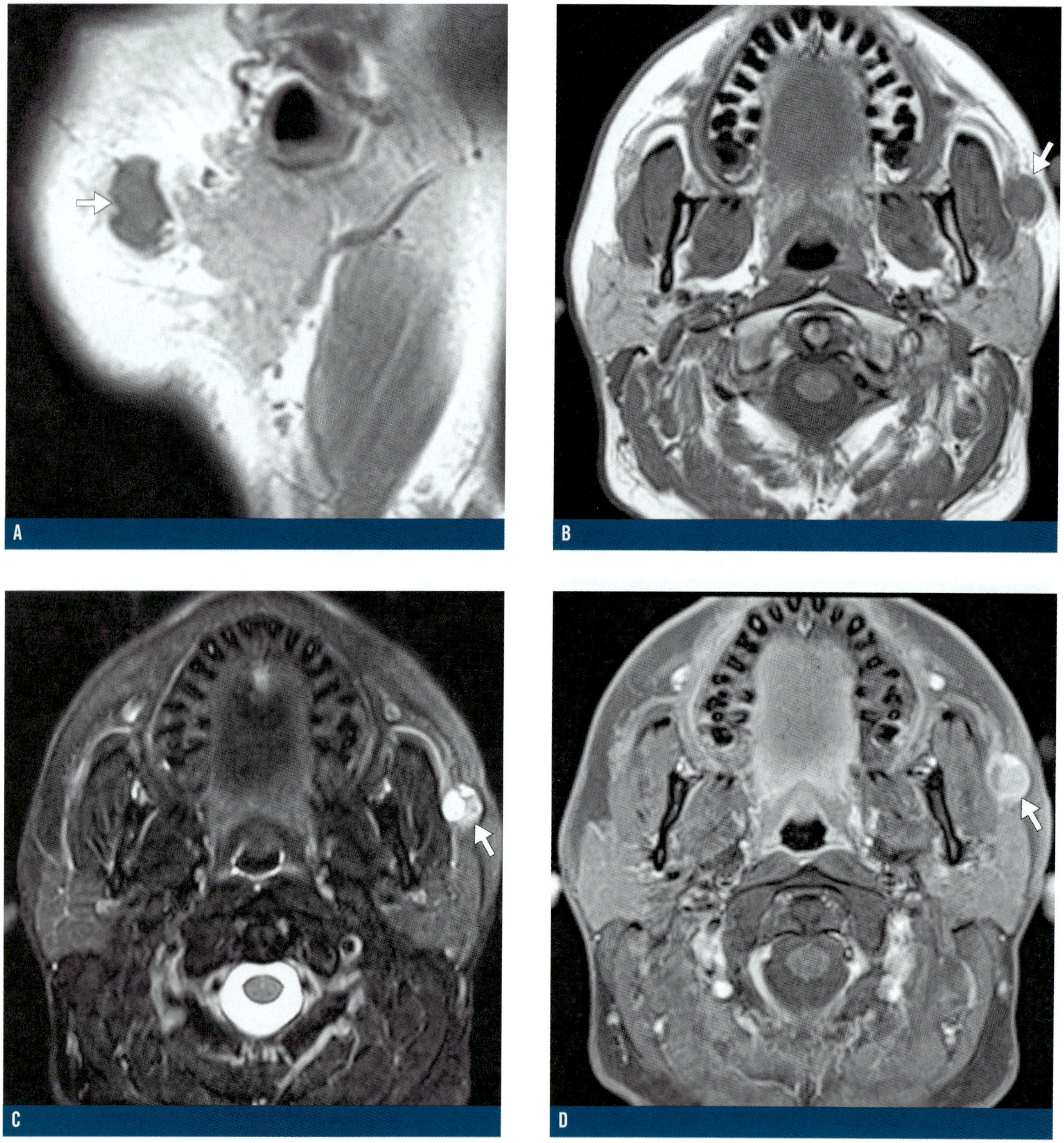

Sagittal T1 (**A**), axial T1 (**B**), axial T2 with fat suppression (**C**), and postcontrast axial T1 with fat suppression (**D**) MR images demonstrate an oval mass along the left Stensen duct (arrows, **A-D**). This lesion represented a mucoepidermoid carcinoma at pathology which arose from accessory left parotid gland tissue.

Companion case: Facial process of the parotid gland

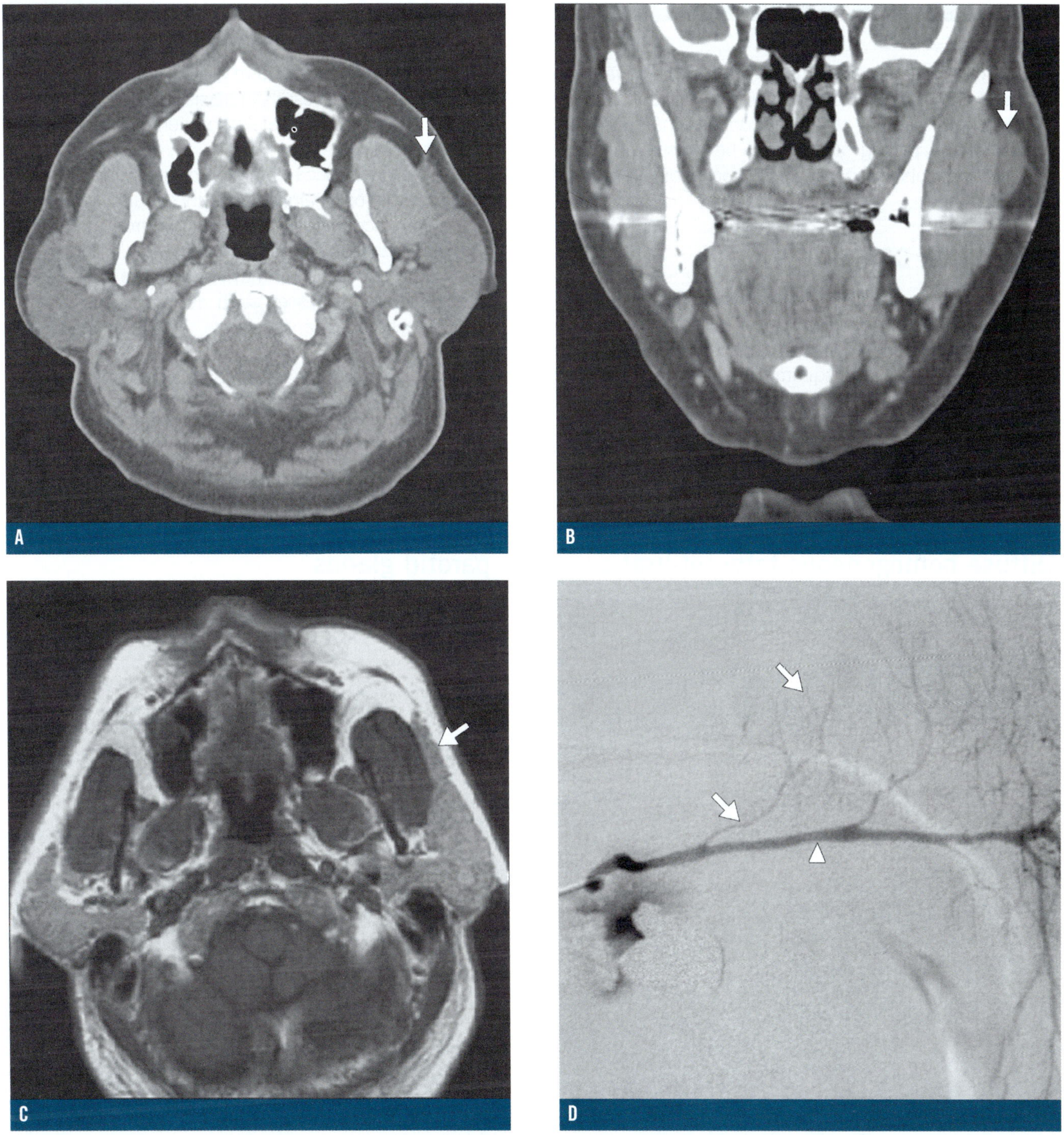

Axial (**A**) and coronal reformatted (**B**) unenhanced CT images through the parotid glands demonstrate asymmetric left parotid tissue that is directly contiguous with the main parotid gland and located immediately lateral to the left masseter muscle, compatible with a normal facial process of the left parotid gland (arrows, **A**, **B**). An axial T1-weighted MR image of the same patient (**C**) also demonstrates the asymmetric facial process of the left parotid gland (arrow, **C**). The facial process of the parotid gland can be palpable, particularly when unilateral, and may be mistaken clinically for a parotid mass. A lateral digitally subtracted left parotid sialography image of the same patient performed to evaluate left parotid symptoms (**D**) demonstrates a small duct and small branches within the facial process (arrows, **D**) emanating toward the left Stensen duct (arrowhead, **D**). As expected, the small duct and its branches within the facial process are normal.

REFERENCES

Currarino G, Votteler TP. Lesions of the accessory parotid gland in children. *Pediatr Radiol.* 2006;36:1-7.

Higley MJ, Walkiewicz TW, Miller JH, Curran JG, Towbin RB. Aplasia of the parotid glands with accessory parotid tissue. *Pediatr Radiol.* 2010;40:345-347.

CASE 4 Diffuse homogeneous fatty infiltration of the parotid gland

The parotid gland parenchyma normally contains fat, with a ratio of adipose to glandular tissue typically approaching 1:1. However, a larger ratio of fat deposition/fatty degeneration of the parotid glands may be present in obese patients, patients with chronic corticosteroid use, or in elderly patients.

COMPANION CASES

- **Stensen duct sialodocholithiasis resulting in parotid gland atrophy.** While the etiology of a sialolith is not completely understood, it likely begins with a nidus, such as from a focus of desquamated epithelium, bacteria and/or their degradation products, or a foreign body. Calcium-rich salts then form around the nidus. A sialolith, if obstructive, results in stasis of saliva, destruction of the acini, and ultimately parenchymal atrophy and fibrosis.
- **Sicca complex.** Sicca complex (or syndrome) refers to dry eyes (xerophthalmia) and dry mouth (xerostomia) that often accompanies Sjögren syndrome. However, not all patients with sicca symptoms have Sjögren syndrome. Sicca syndrome may also be present with other disease processes such as sarcoidosis, sialosis, viral infections, biliary cirrhosis, and graft-versus-host disease.
- **Sjögren syndrome. Please refer to Case 2 from this chapter for discussion.**

Diffuse homogeneous fatty infiltration of the parotid glands

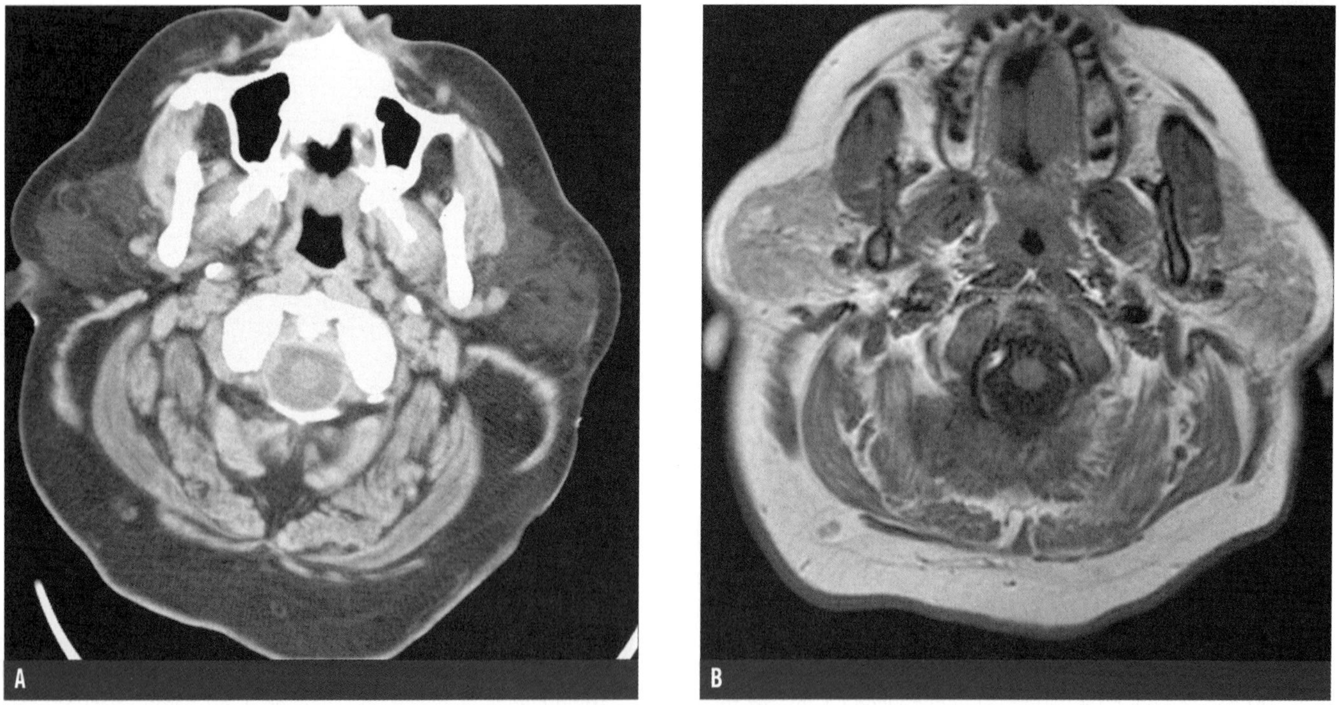

An unenhanced axial CT image (**A**) as well as unenhanced axial T1 (**B**) and axial T2 (**C**) MR images through the parotid glands demonstrate diffuse homogeneous fatty infiltration of the parotid glands. This 48-year-old patient is obese, likely accounting for the fatty infiltration of the parotid glands.

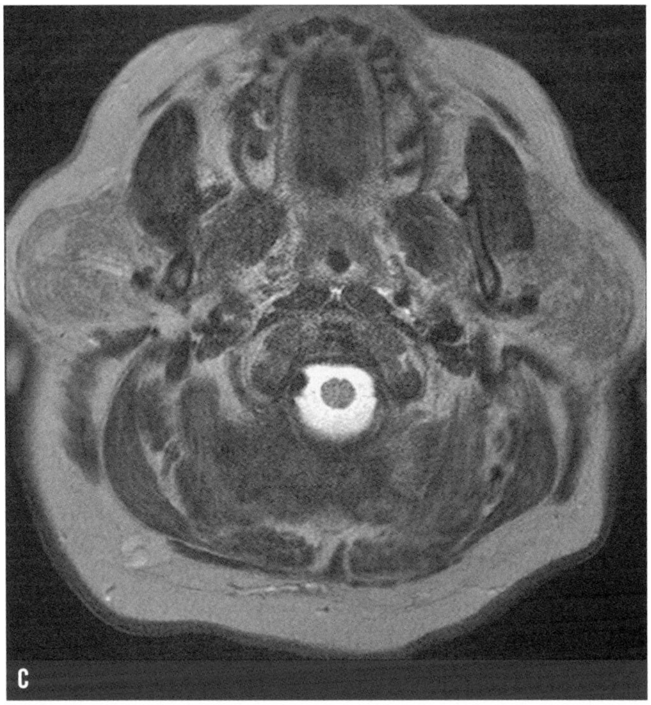

Companion case: Stensen duct sialodocholithiasis resulting in parotid gland atrophy

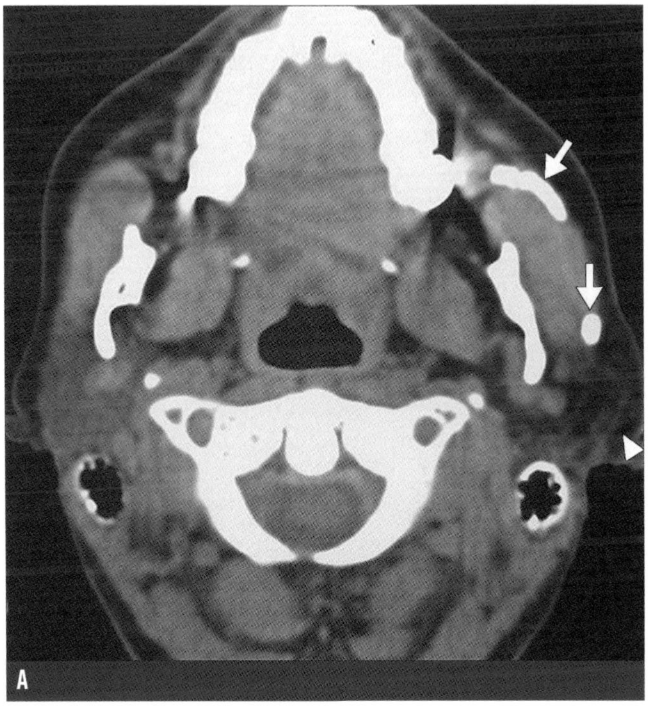

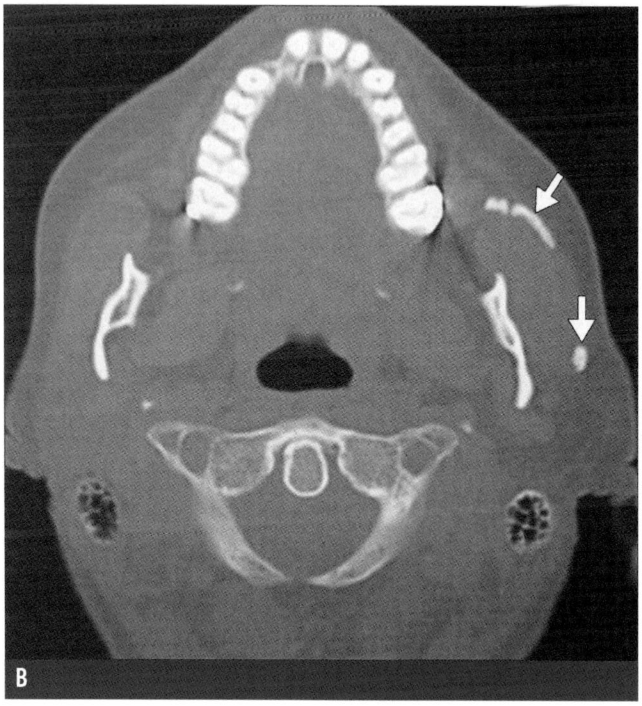

Unenhanced axial CT images viewed with a soft tissue window (**A**) and bone window (**B**) demonstrate a large amount of sialodocholithiasis in the left Stensen duct (arrows, **A**, **B**) resulting in atrophy and diffuse fatty infiltration of the left parotid gland (arrowhead, **A**).

Companion case: Sicca complex

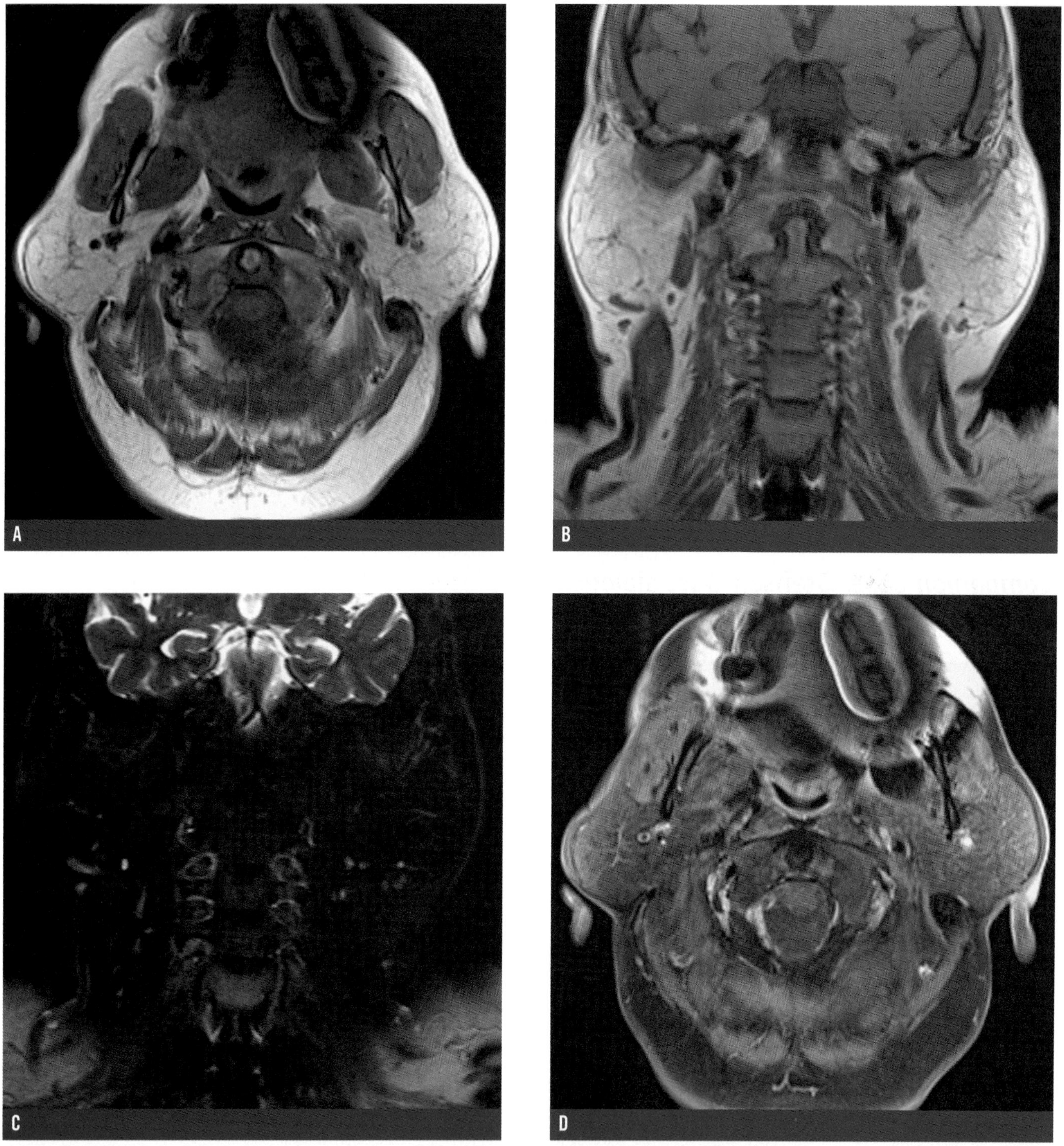

Axial T1 (**A**), coronal T1 (**B**), coronal T2 with fat suppression (**C**), and postcontrast axial T1 with fat suppression (**D**) MR images demonstrate diffuse fatty infiltration and enlargement of the parotid glands. This patient complained of xerostomia, which is a symptom associated with sicca complex.

Companion case: Sjögren syndrome

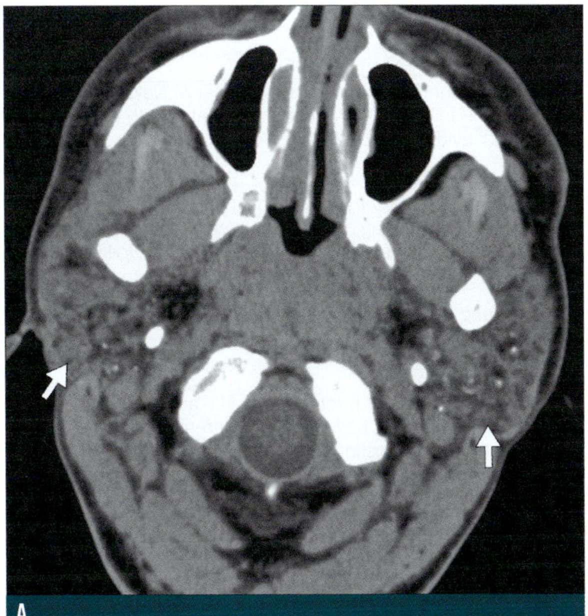

A

An unenhanced axial CT image (**A**) demonstrates marked heterogeneous fatty infiltration of the parotid glands with superimposed punctate foci of mineralization. The findings are consistent with an autoimmune disorder, such as Sjögren syndrome.

Companion case: Sjögren syndrome

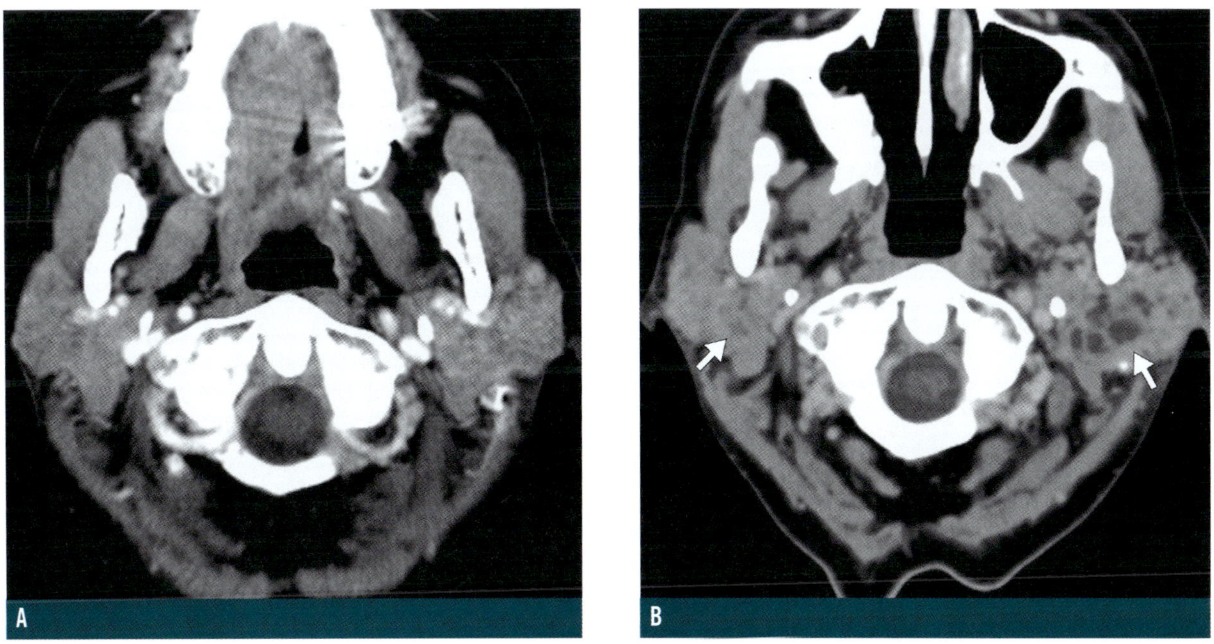

A B

Different patient. A postcontrast axial CT image of a patient who presents with left parotid tail swelling (**A**) demonstrates mildly enlarged parotid glands, left slightly larger than right, with equivocal punctate foci of hypoattenuation within the parotid glands. A postcontrast axial CT image obtained 8 years later than image **A** (**B**) demonstrates irregularly shaped hypoattenuating areas in the parotid glands, left significantly greater than right, suspicious for abnormally dilated acini (arrows, **B**). An axial T2-weighted MR image obtained 7 years after image **A** (**C**) better demonstrates findings consistent with abnormally dilated acini within the parotid glands (arrows, **C**). This patient had Sjögren syndrome clinically.

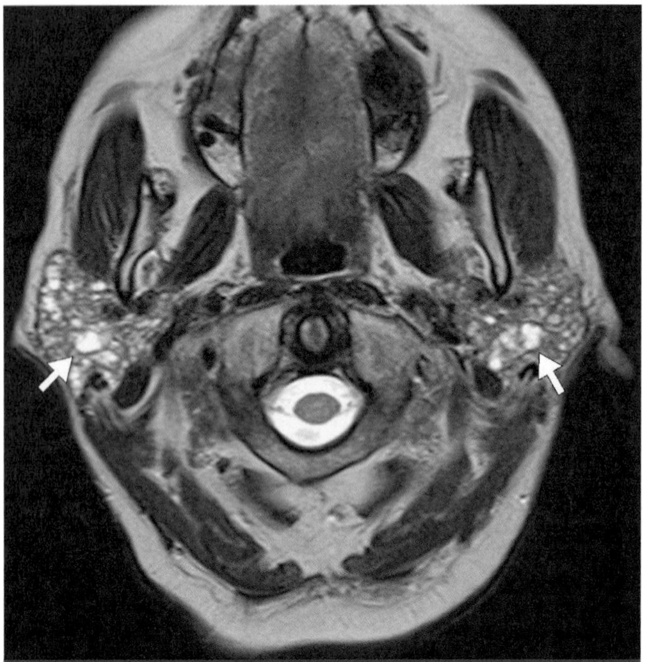

C

REFERENCES

Hamilton BE, Salzman KL, Wiggins RH 3rd, Harnsberger HR. Earring lesions of the parotid tail. *AJNR Am J Neuroradiol.* 2003;24(9):1757-1764.

Izumi M, Eguchi K, Nakamura H, Nagataki S, Nakamura T. Premature fat deposition in the salivary glands associated with Sjögren syndrome: MR and CT evidence. *AJNR Am J Neuroradiol.* May 1997;18:951-958.

Izumi M, Hida A, Takagi Y, Kawabe Y, Eguchi K, Nakamura T. MR imaging of the salivary glands in sicca syndrome: comparison of lipid profiles and imaging in patients with hyperlipidemia and patients with Sjögren's syndrome. *AJR Am J Roentgenol.* September 2000;175(3):829-834.

Sun Z, Zhang Z, Fu K, Zhao Y, Liu D, Ma X. Diagnostic accuracy of parotid CT for identifying Sjögren's syndrome. *Eur J Radiol.* 2012;81(10):2702-2709.

Takagi Y, Sumi M, Sumi T, Ichikawa Y, Nakamura T. MR microscopy of the parotid glands in patients with Sjogren's syndrome: quantitative MR diagnostic criteria. *AJNR Am J Neuroradiol. May* 2005;26(5):1207-1214.

Beriat GK, Akmansu SH, Kocatürk S, Ataoğlu O. Chronic Sclerosing Sialadenitis (Küttner tumour) of the Parotid Gland. *Malays J Med Sci.* 2010 Oct;17(4):57-61.

CASE 5 Focal fatty infiltration of the parotid gland

Occasionally, a geographic area of fatty infiltration within the parotid gland that is not associated with mass effect may be identified. This may be the result of numerous entities, such as a chronically obstructed/narrowed segmental duct, remote infection, or relatively greater focal involvement of a systemic process, such as sarcoid or Sjögren syndrome.

COMPANION CASES

- **Parotid lipoma.** Parotid lipomas represent an encapsulated collection of mature adipocytes that are slow-growing, asymptomatic, and freely mobile. Lipomas cannot be used for energy stores. As a result, while they can enlarge with weight gain, they do not decrease in size with weight loss. A parotid lipoma generally has some degree of mass effect whereas mass effect , as opposed to focal fatty infiltration of the parotid gland, which is not encapsulated and lacks mass effect.
- **Parotid sialocyst.** Please refer to Case 1 from this chapter for discussion.
- **Epidermal inclusion cyst adjacent to the parotid gland.** Epidermal inclusion cysts are the most common cutaneous cysts and occur from implantation of epidermal elements into the dermis and subcutaneous soft tissues. These cysts are pathologically identical to epidermoid cysts located elsewhere in the body and are composed of keratin, protein, cholesterol, and cell membrane lipids. The term sebaceous cyst should be avoided to describe this entity because an epidermal inclusion cyst does not arise from the sebaceous glands. Moreover, while sebaceous cysts do occur in the same locations as epidermal inclusion cysts, they are significantly less common. Epidermal inclusion cysts are benign lesions; however, there are rare reports of associated malignancies.

  Epidermal inclusion cysts are unilocular, circumscribed, and round to oval lesions that reside in the subcutaneous tissue and abut the dermis. They usually grow slowly over years or decades. They are fluid-attenuating on CT. On MRI, they are primarily iso- to hypoinon T1 relative to muscle (although they may contain small foci of mildly intrinsic T1 hyperintense signal), hyperintense on T2, and often restrict on diffusion-weighted imaging, similar to epidermoids elsewhere. A thin capsule surrounding these lesions is often appreciated on imaging. Epidermal inclusion cysts may mildly enhance along their periphery but they do not enhance centrally. Epidermal inclusion cysts may mineralize, particularly in the elderly.

Focal fatty infiltration of the parotid gland

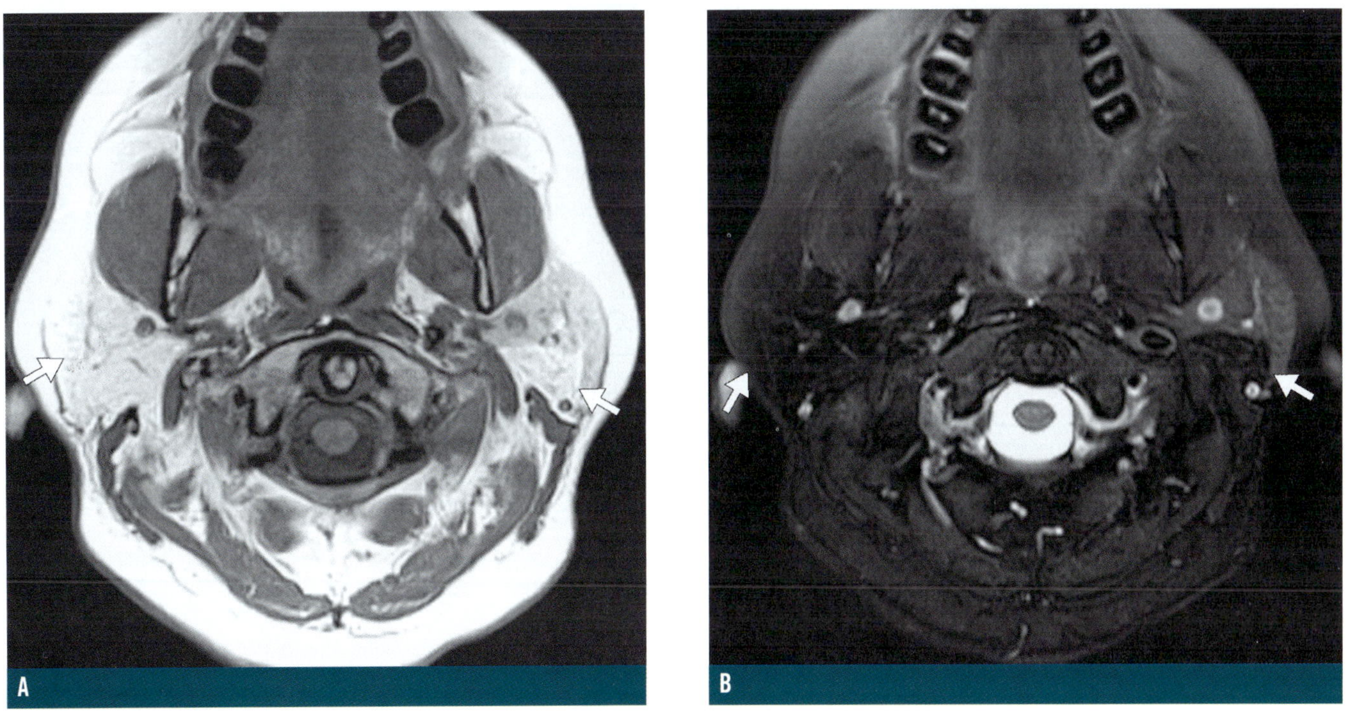

Axial T1 (**A**), fat-suppressed axial T2 (**B**), sagittal T1 through the right parotid gland (**C**) sagittal T1 through the left parotid gland (**D**), coronal T1 (**E**), and fat-suppressed postcontrast axial T1 (**F**) MR images demonstrate a diffusely fatty infiltrated right parotid gland and a focally fatty infiltrated left parotid gland along its posterior aspect (arrows, **A-F**). This patient did not have a diagnosis of Sjögren syndrome or complain of sicca symptoms.

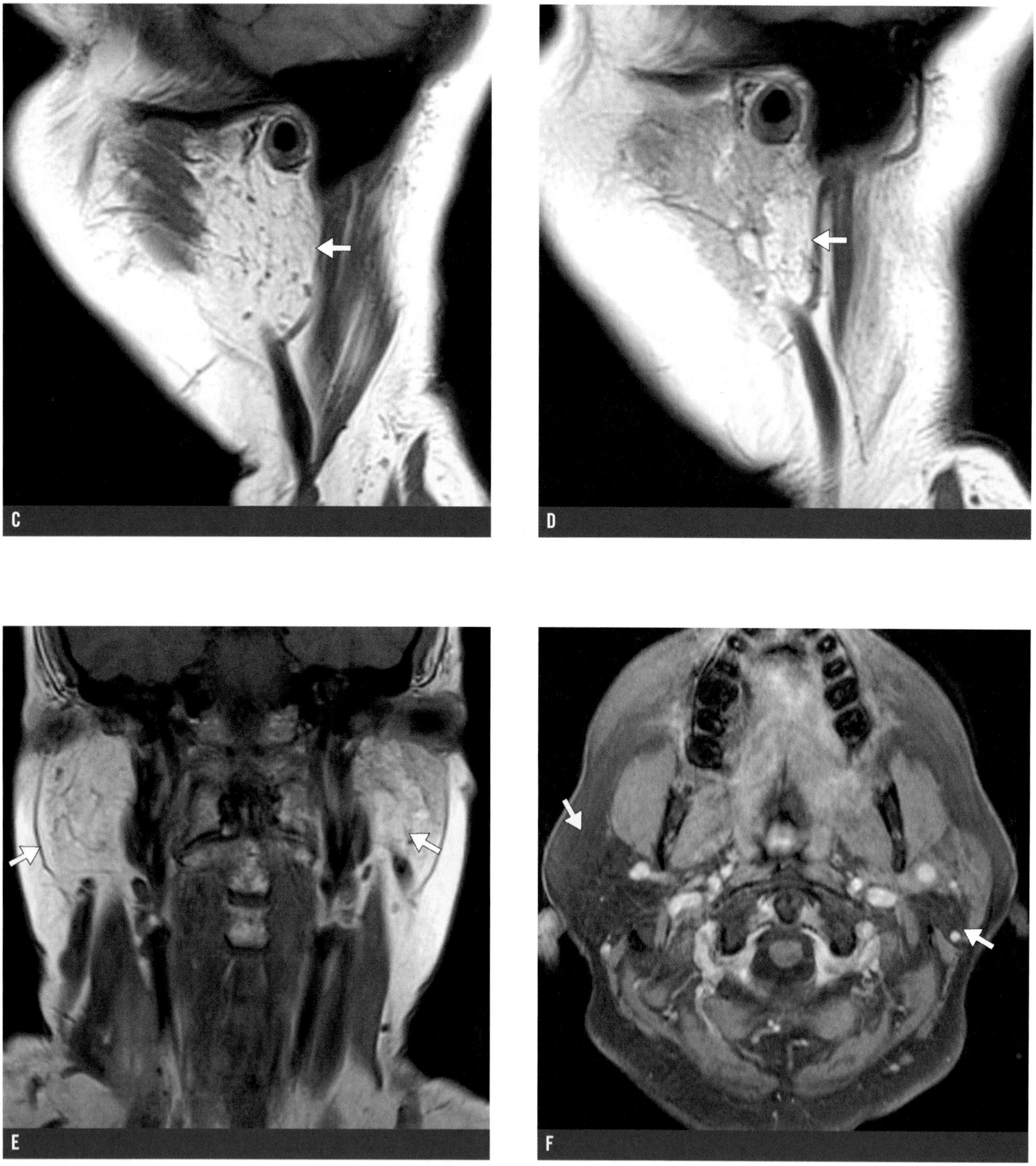
C
D
E
F

Companion case: Parotid lipoma

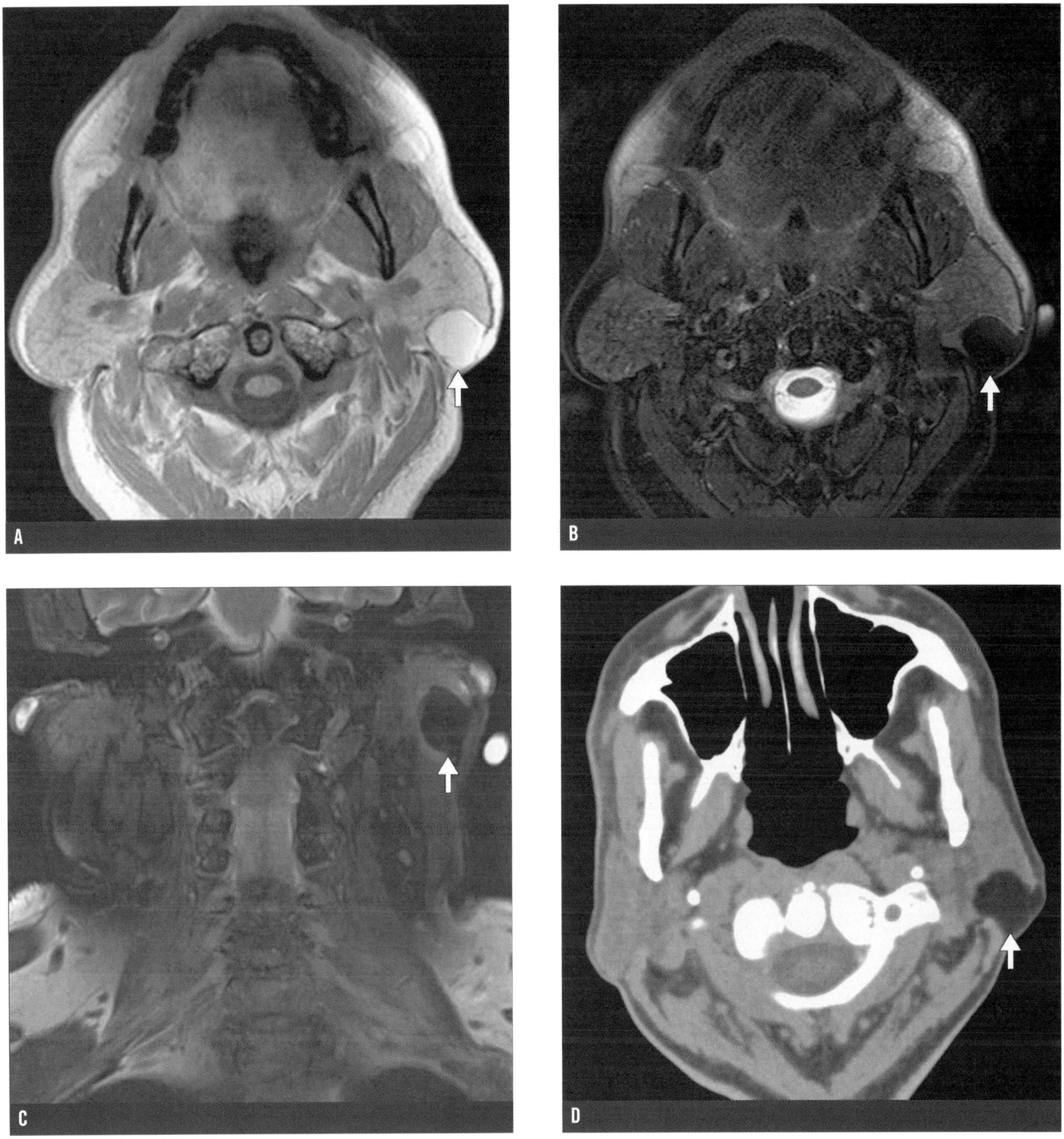

Axial T1 (**A**), axial T2 with fat suppression (**B**), and postcontrast coronal T1 with fat suppression (**C**) MR images as well as an unenhanced axial CT image (**D**) through the level of the parotid glands demonstrate a circumscribed, fat equivalent lesion within the dorsal aspect of the left parotid gland associated with mild regional mass effect, compatible with a parotid lipoma (arrows, **A-D**). This finding can be differentiated from focal fatty infiltration by the presence of mass effect; specifically, there is often mass effect from a lipoma and lack of mass effect related to focal fatty infiltration of the parotid gland. This finding was a palpable abnormality for the patient, as denoted by a Vitamin E capsule on images **B** and **C**.

Companion case: Parotid lipoma

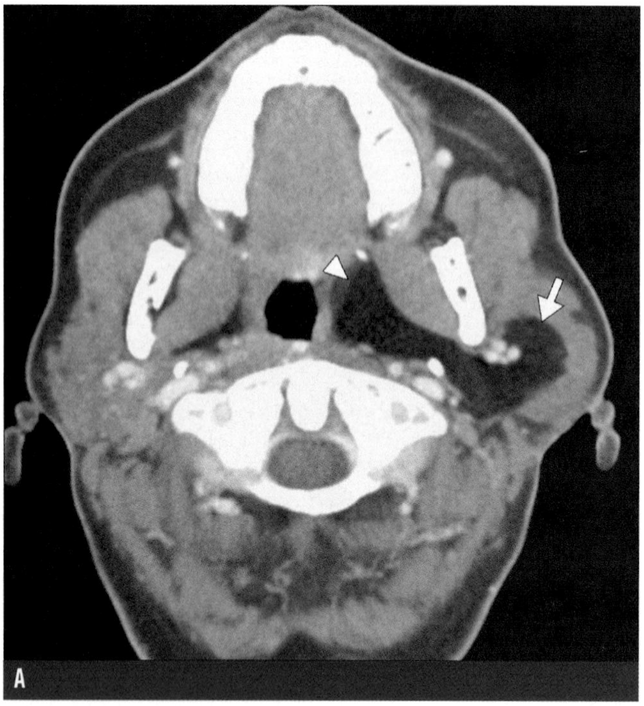

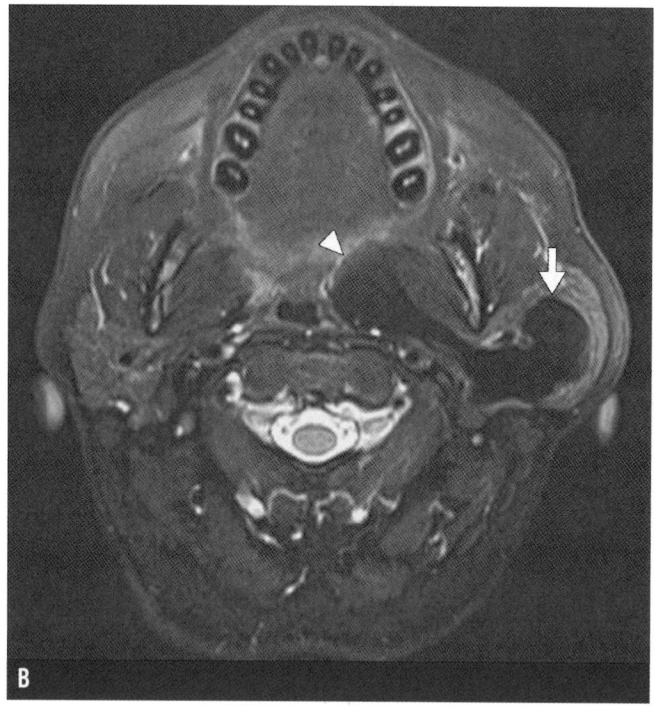

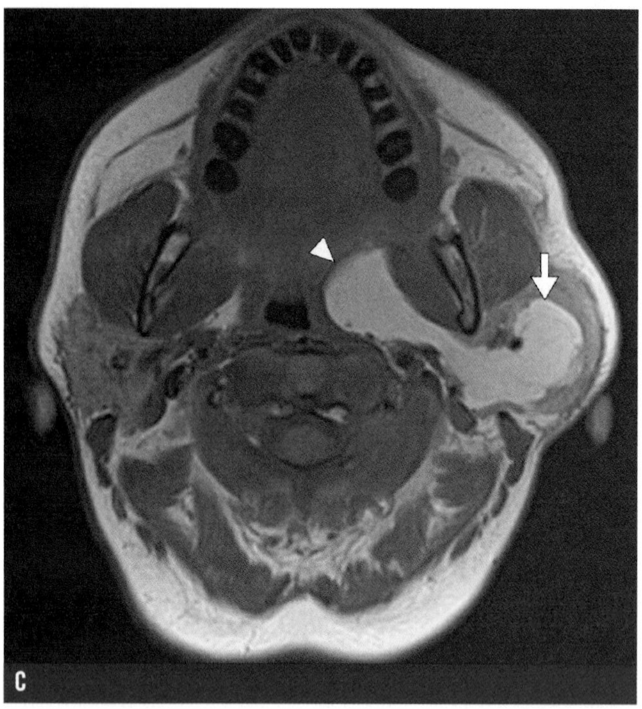

Different patient. A contrast-enhanced axial CT image (**A**) as well as axial T2 with fat suppression (**B**) and axial T1 without fat suppression (**C**) MR images demonstrate a large lipoma involving the superficial and deep aspects of the left parotid gland (arrows, **A-C**), extending through the stylomandibular tunnel and into the prestyloid left parapharyngeal space (arrowheads, **A-C**). The complete lesional suppression image **B** confirms that this represents a lipoma. Negative Hounsfield units within the lesion on the CT exam were also consistent with a lipoma.

Companion case: Parotid sialocyst

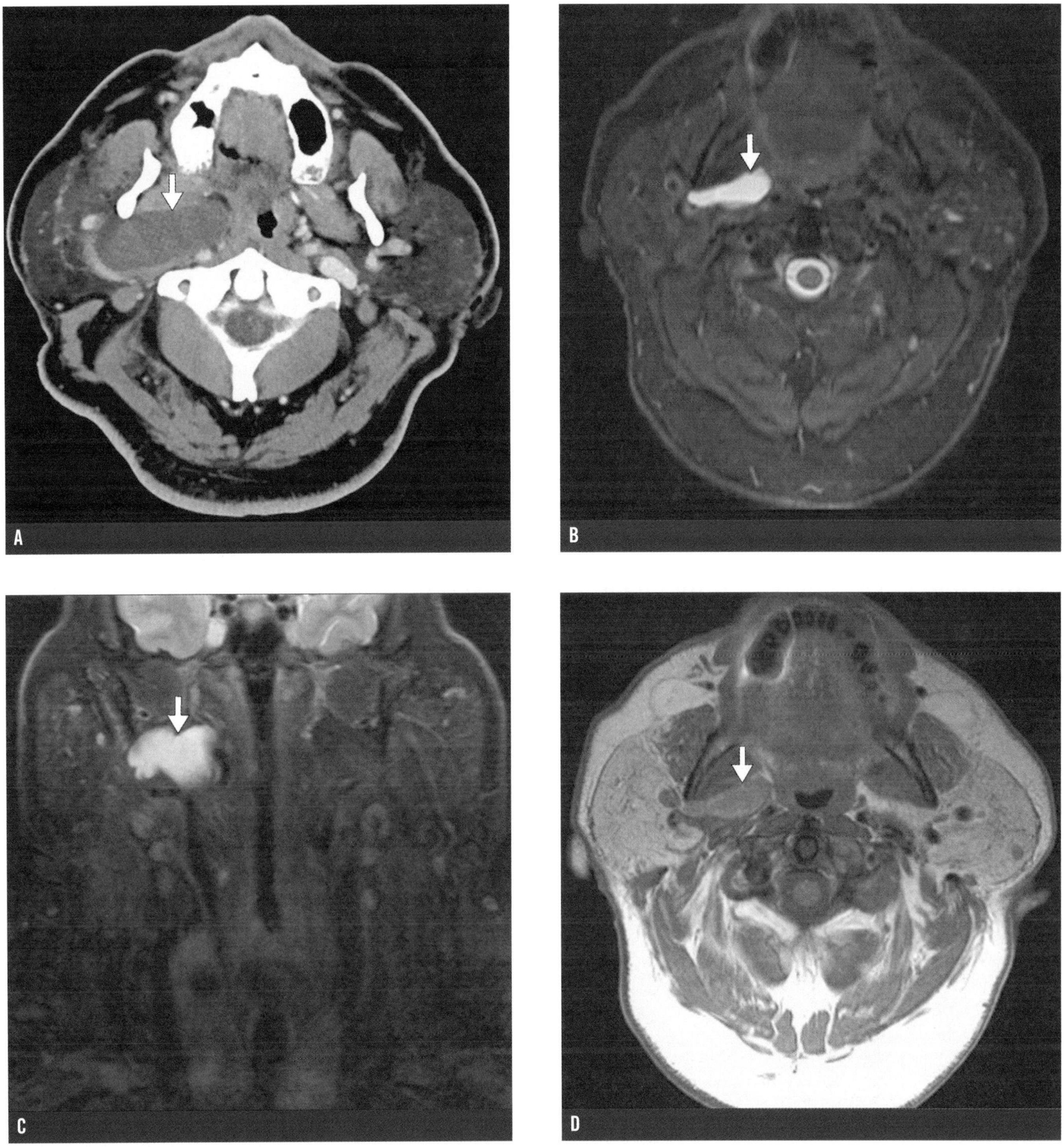

A contrast-enhanced axial CT image (**A**) demonstrates an elliptical-shaped, fluid density lesion centered within the right prestyloid parapharyngeal space (arrow, **A**) which abuts the deep aspect of the right parotid gland. Fat-suppressed axial T2 (**B**), fat-suppressed coronal T2 (**C**), axial T1 (**D**), and contrast-enhanced axial T1 with fat suppression (**E**) MR images following sampling of the lesion demonstrate the lesion to be smaller and T2 hyperintense, intrinsically T1 shortened to a mild degree, and minimally enhancing (arrows, **B-E**). The elevated signal on pre- and postcontrast T1-weighted imaging likely relates to the needle sampling. The fluid and tissue sample was shown to represent benign salivary fluid and tissue at pathology. This lesion could represent either a sialocyst (benign parotid cyst with a true epithelial capsule) or a sialocele (a collection of saliva typically following trauma and surrounded only by a pseudocapsule). However, this patient had no history of trauma and therefore the finding is most compatible with a sialocyst.

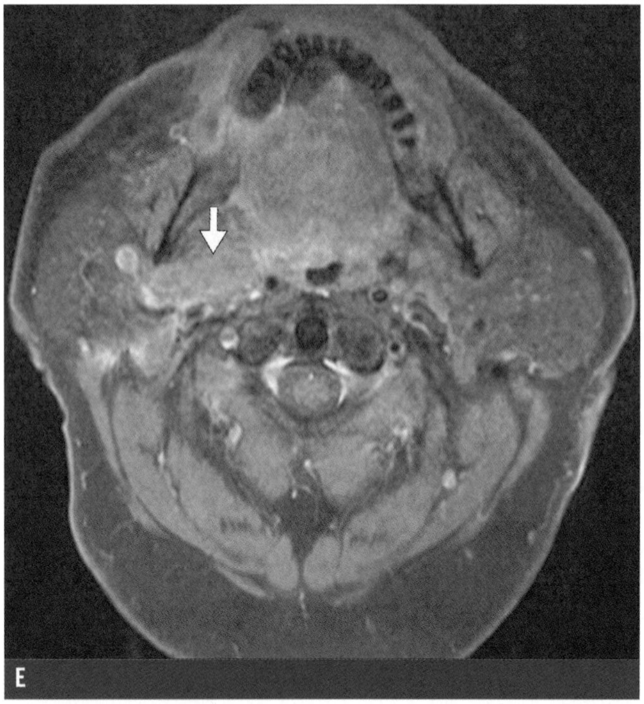

Companion case: Epidermal inclusion cyst adjacent to the parotid gland

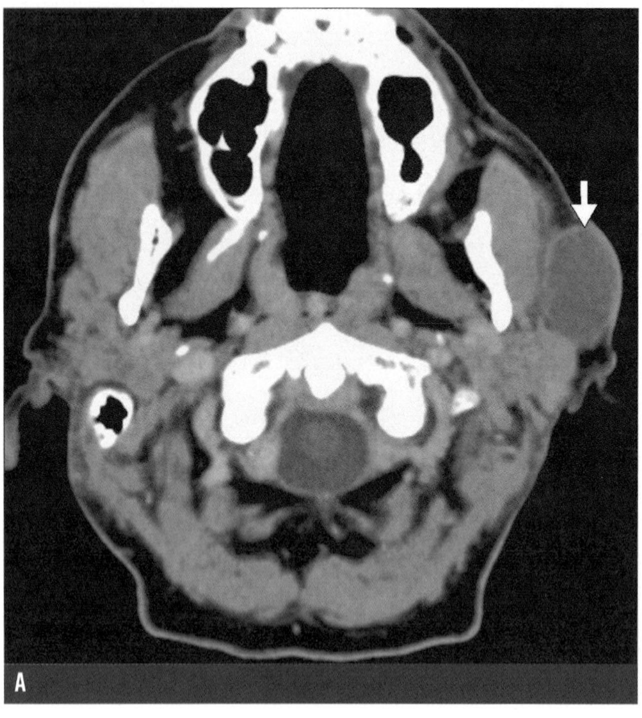

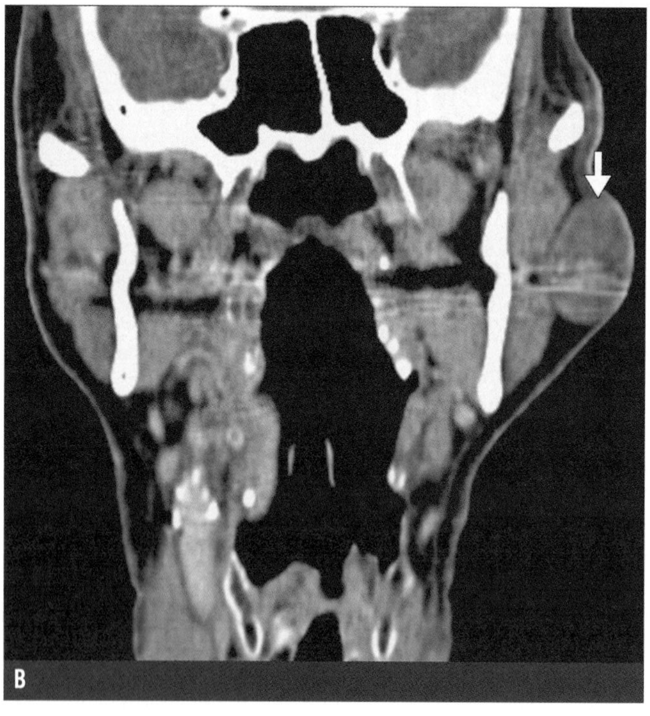

Axial (**A**) and coronal reformatted (**B**) contrast-enhanced CT images through the level of the parotid glands demonstrate a circumscribed, hypodense mass overlying the left masseter muscle that abuts the overlying dermis (arrows, **A**, **B**). Axial diffusion–weighted MR imaging (**C**) and its corresponding ADC map (**D**) demonstrate a portion of the lesion to restrict (arrows, **C**, **D**). The findings are most compatible with an epidermal inclusion cyst. While lymphoma can restrict on MRI, untreated lymphoma is typically isodense or mildly enhancing relative to muscle on CT, not hypoattenuating, as is present in this case.

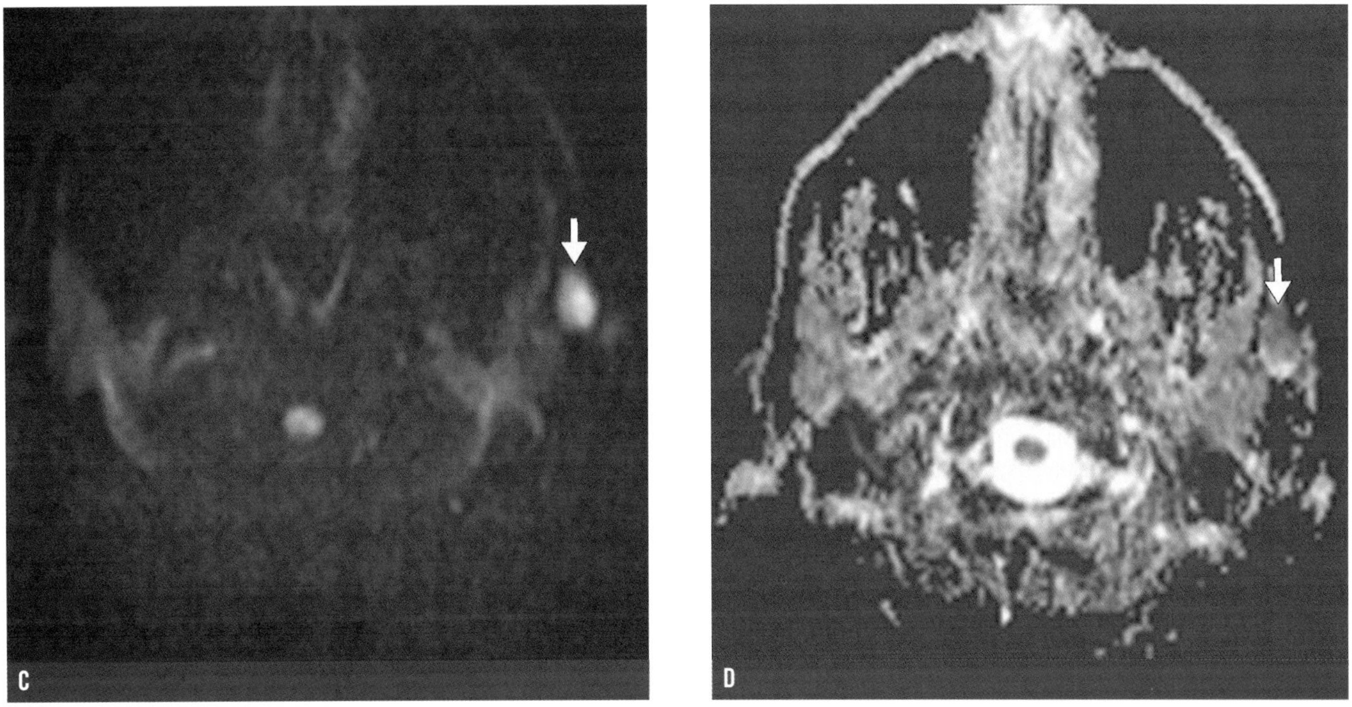

REFERENCES

Ansari MH. Superficial lobe parotid gland lipoma. *J Craniomaxillofac Surg*. 2006;34(1):47-49. Epub Dec 15, 2005.

Kim HK, Kim SM, Lee SH, Racadio JM, Shin MJ. Subcutaneous epidermal inclusion cysts: ultrasound (US) and MR imaging findings. *Skeletal Radiol*. 2011;40(11):1415-1419. Epub Dec 4, 2010.

Som PM, Curtin HD. *Head and Neck Imaging*. 4th ed. St. Louis, MO: Mosby Inc; 2003.

CASE 6 Parotid gland fatty infiltration simulating a contralateral parotid sialadenitis

Occasionally, a normal density parotid gland can appear "inflamed" on a contrast-enhanced CT examination if the contralateral parotid gland is diffusely fatty infiltrated. This misinterpretation can be avoided with the addition of unenhanced CT imaging through the parotid glands. The precontrast images will readily demonstrate the baseline differences between a potentially normal, denser parotid gland from the contralateral fatty infiltrated parotid gland. With the aid of these baseline images, it is easier to determine whether there is truly asymmetric enhancement of the parotid gland in question, or whether it just represents a normal, denser gland compared to the contralateral gland.

COMPANION CASE

- **Parotid sialadenitis.** Sialadenitis may be acute, arising from either a bacterial or viral etiology, or it may be chronic. When acute, it is usually the result of a bacterial infection, with *Staphylococcus aureus* the most common causative organism in the adult. Fever, chills, pain, erythema, and swelling often accompany an acute parotid sialadenitis. Purulent material may sometimes be expressed from the Stensen duct orifice when a parotid sialadenitis is bacterial in origin. Acute sialadenitis most commonly occurs when there is a decrease in salivary gland flow, such as may be present with chronic illnesses, dehydration, and medications, to name a few. Sialadenitis more commonly affects the parotid glands compared to the submandibular glands for several reasons. The submandibular gland produces a faster, more continuous flow of saliva compared to the parotid gland, and the Wharton duct orifice is smaller than the Stensen duct orifice; for both reasons, there is a decreased probability of retrograde spread of infection into the submandibular gland compared to the parotid gland. Furthermore, the saliva produced by the submandibular gland is more bacteriostatic relative to the saliva produced by the parotid gland. When a sialadenitis is bacterial in etiology, then treatment is primarily with antibiotics sensitive to the offending bacterial organism.

  When confronted with an imaging case of sialadenitis, particularly if unexplained or recurrent, it is imperative to evaluate for a sialolith, or more importantly, an obstructing tumor along the duct that may be the underlying cause of the sialadenitis. A tumor of the salivary duct is often best visualized with MRI and sometimes conventional sialography. However, if there is an acute bacterial parotid sialadenitis, then sialography should be deferred until the infection resolves so as to not promote retrograde spread of infection during the procedure. A tumor along a salivary duct may also be visualized by CT, although dental amalgam artifact can sometimes obscure the duct, particularly distally. That said, a sialolith is best visualized by CT.

Parotid gland fatty infiltration simulating a contralateral parotid sialadenitis

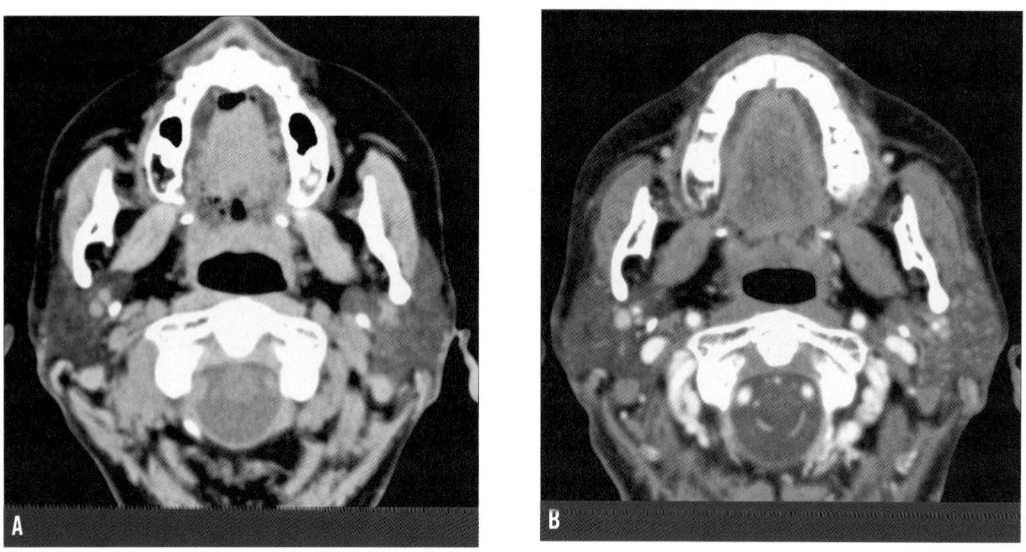

An unenhanced axial CT image through the level of the parotid glands (**A**) demonstrates diffuse fatty infiltration of the right parotid gland relative to the left. A postcontrast axial CT image (**B**) through the same level as image **A** demonstrates the same asymmetry between the parotid glands, again because of a greater amount of right parotid gland fatty infiltration. However, without the benefit of precontrast imaging, one could misinterpret that the left parotid gland is asymmetrically enhancing compared to the right,compatible with a mild left parotitis. Moreover, relative to image **A**, the left parotid gland does not significantly enhance, which would otherwise not be appreciated without the benefit of the unenhanced images. This patient did not have left parotid gland symptoms.

Companion case: Parotid sialadenitis

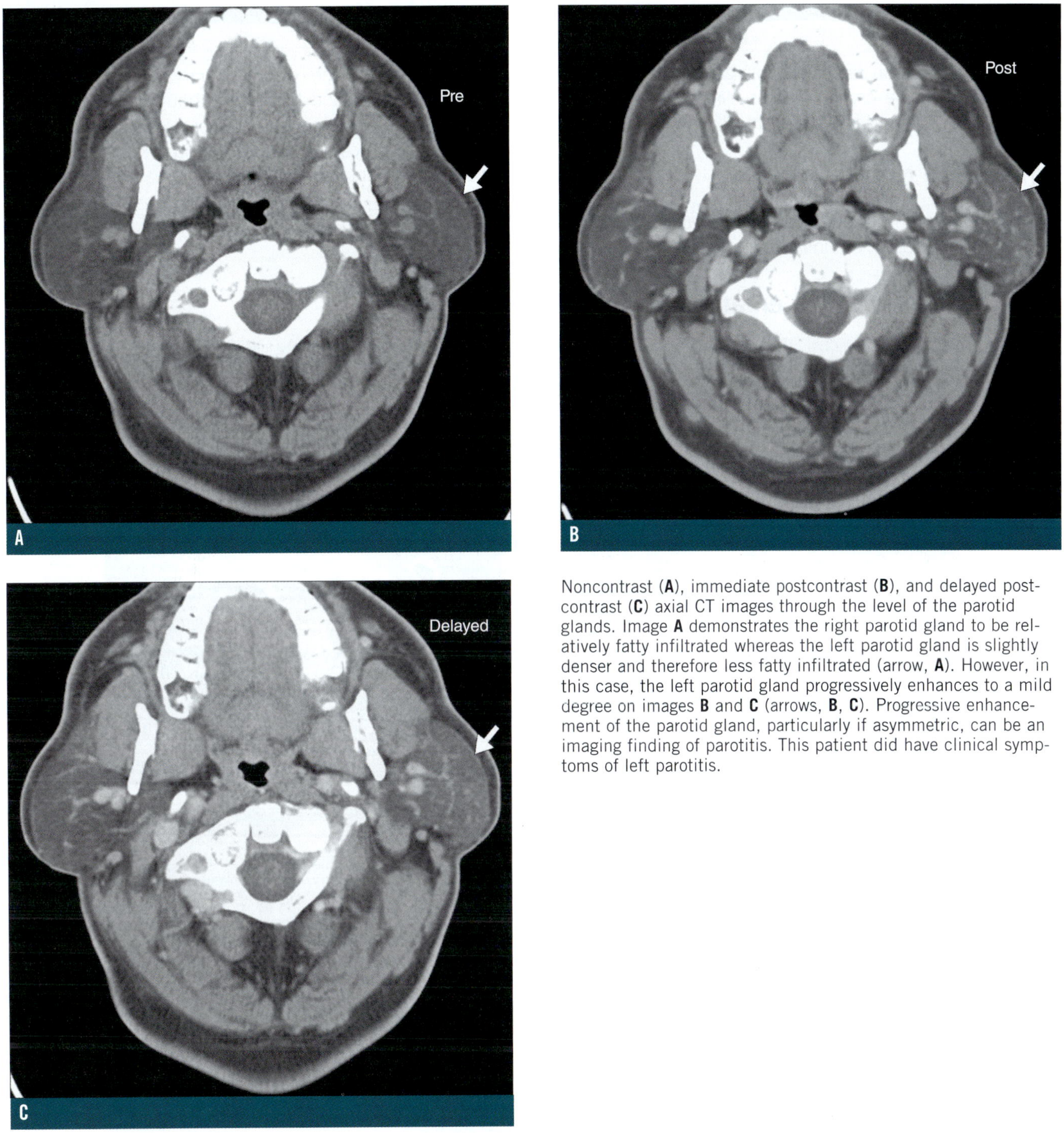

Noncontrast (**A**), immediate postcontrast (**B**), and delayed postcontrast (**C**) axial CT images through the level of the parotid glands. Image **A** demonstrates the right parotid gland to be relatively fatty infiltrated whereas the left parotid gland is slightly denser and therefore less fatty infiltrated (arrow, **A**). However, in this case, the left parotid gland progressively enhances to a mild degree on images **B** and **C** (arrows, **B**, **C**). Progressive enhancement of the parotid gland, particularly if asymmetric, can be an imaging finding of parotitis. This patient did have clinical symptoms of left parotitis.

REFERENCES

Ledesma-Montes C, et al. Giant sialolith: case report and review of the literature. *J Oral Maxillofac Surg.* 2007;65:128-130

Som PM, Curtin HD. *Head and Neck Imaging.* 5th ed. St. Louis, MO: Mosby Inc; 2011.

CASE 7 Parotid gland enlargement due to weight gain

Significant weight gain can cause enlargement of the parotid glands and simulate parotid masses clinically. The parotid glands will typically enlarge symmetrically in this setting.

COMPANION CASE

- **Sialosis.** Also known as sialadenosis, sialosis is defined as a non-neoplastic, noninflammatory, soft, and painless enlargement of the major salivary glands. Sialosis is typically diffuse and bilateral, although it can be asymmetric. There are several causes of sialosis, including alcoholic cirrhosis, diabetes mellitus, various medications, and malnutrition.

Parotid gland enlargement due to weight gain

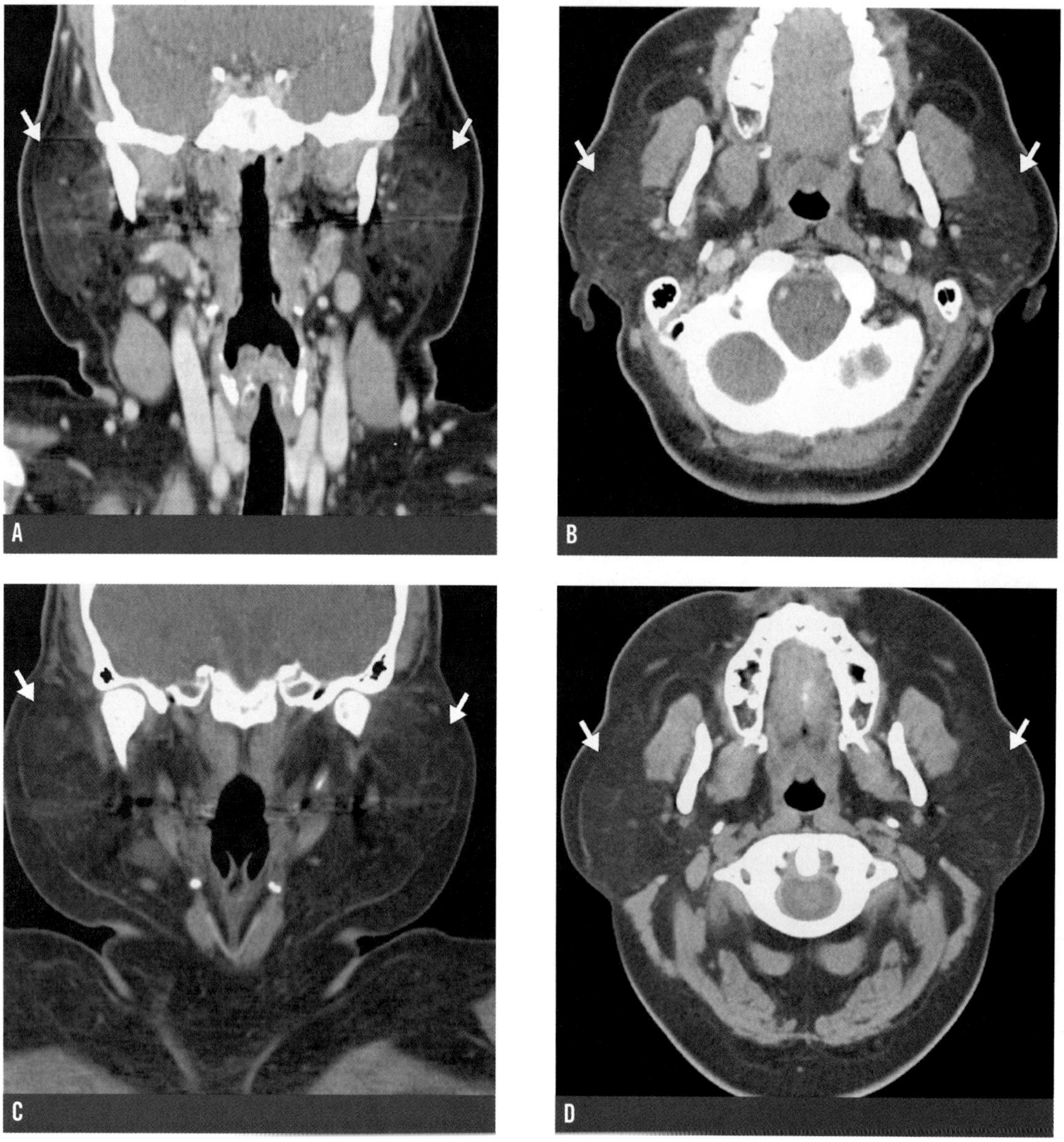

This patient complained of enlarging parotid glands. Coronal reformatted (**A**) and axial (**B**) postcontrast CT images demonstrate diffuse fatty infiltration of the parotid glands (arrows, **A**, **B**). Coronal reformatted (**C**) and axial (**D**) postcontrast CT images obtained 18 months after images **A** and **B** demonstrate enlargement of the parotid glands (arrows, **C**, **D**). This was because of weight gain with further fatty infiltration of the parotid glands rather than a mass or inflammation, as suspected clinically. A lateral scout CT image at the same time as images **A** and **B** (**E**) and a lateral scout image at the same time as images **C** and **D** (**F**) also demonstrate the weight gain.

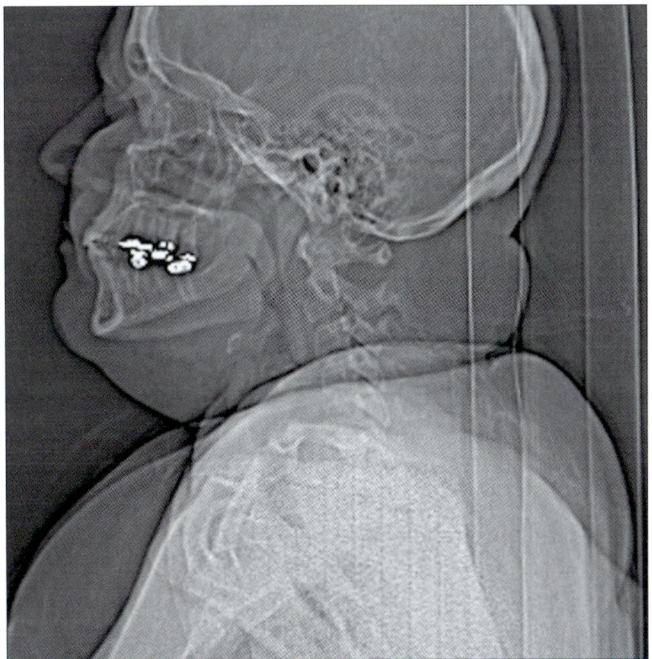

E

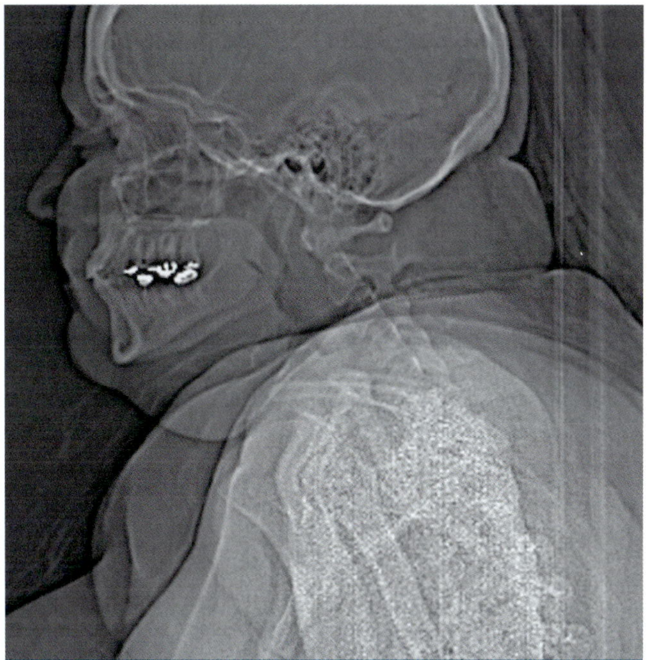

F

Companion case: Sialosis

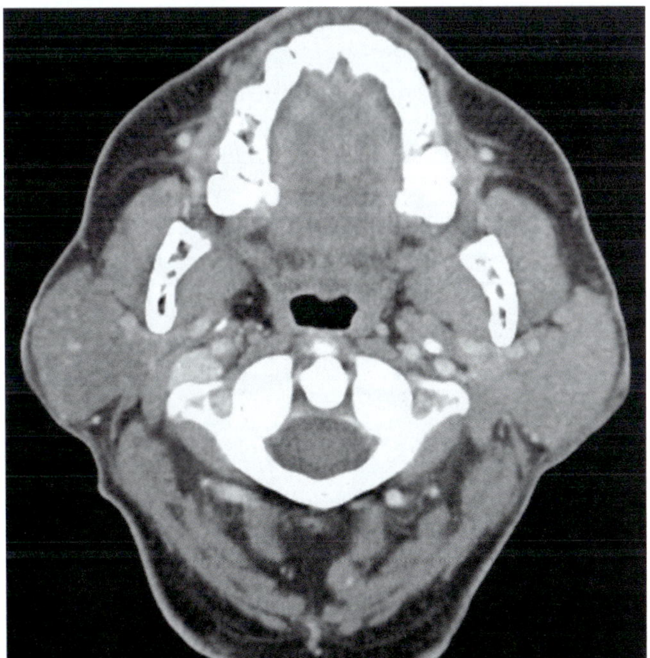

A

An axial CT image of the parotid glands (**A**) demonstrates diffuse bilateral parotid enlargement in this patient who complained of enlargement of the parotid glands but without clinical symptoms of sialadenitis. The enlarged parotid glands were entirely stable compared to a prior CT neck examination performed 7 years earlier (not shown). While nonspecific, given the clinical scenario and stability, the findings are consistent with sialosis.

REFERENCE

Rice DH. Noninflammatory, non-neoplastic disorders of the salivary glands. *Otolaryngol Clin North Am.* October 1999;32(5):835-843.

CASE 8 Volume averaging with the EAC simulating a parotid gland lesion

Because of the higher density of the normal external auditory canal (EAC) soft tissue and cartilage, volume averaging of the EAC with a normal parotid gland on CT may simulate a parotid mass. Usually, a mass can be excluded in this setting by viewing the coronal or sagittal reformatted CT images from the study.

COMPANION CASES

- **EAC adenocarcinoma.** A primary carcinoma of the EAC is relatively rare. Statistically, it is more common for a carcinoma to arise outside the EAC and subsequently invade the EAC than it is to have a primary carcinoma of the EAC. The most common malignancy of the EAC is squamous cell carcinoma, although adenoid cystic carcinoma, mucoepidermoid carcinoma, adenocarcinoma, and others may also arise from the EAC. On CT, a carcinoma of the EAC will present as a soft tissue mass, often with associated osseous erosion/destruction. On MRI, EAC carcinomas are usually isointense to muscle on T1, variable on T2, and enhance.
- **EAC mineralization simulating a parotid gland sialolith.** Occasionally, normal mineralization of the EAC can mimic a parotid sialolith on axial CT imaging because of the relative proximity of the EACs to the parotid glands. When possible, correlating with sagittal and/or coronal reformatted CT imaging is useful for differentiation.

Volume averaging with the external auditory canal simulating a parotid gland lesion

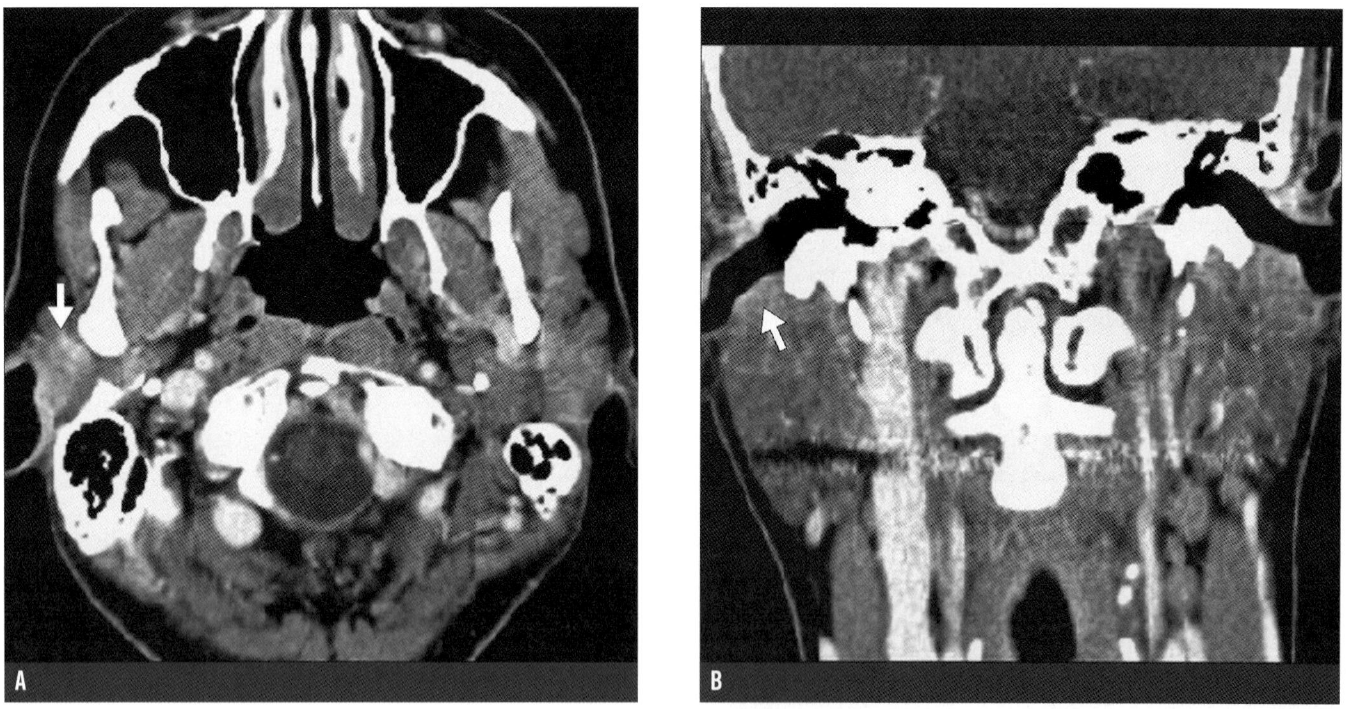

A postcontrast axial CT image (**A**) demonstrates apparent subtle asymmetric soft tissue at the superior aspect of the right parotid gland (arrow, **A**). However, a postcontrast coronal reformatted CT image (**B**) reveals that this merely represents volume averaging with the normal cartilaginous portion of the right external auditory canal rather than a focal mass (arrow, **B**).

Companion case: EAC adenocarcinoma

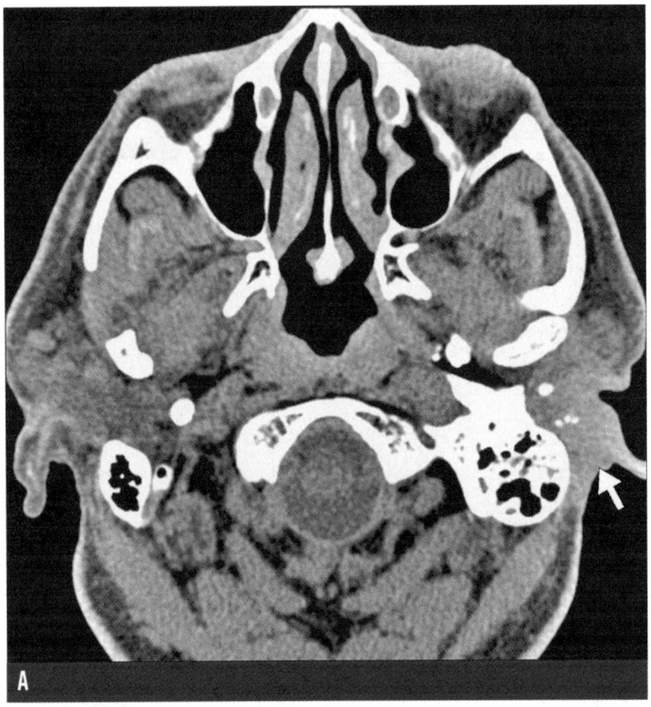

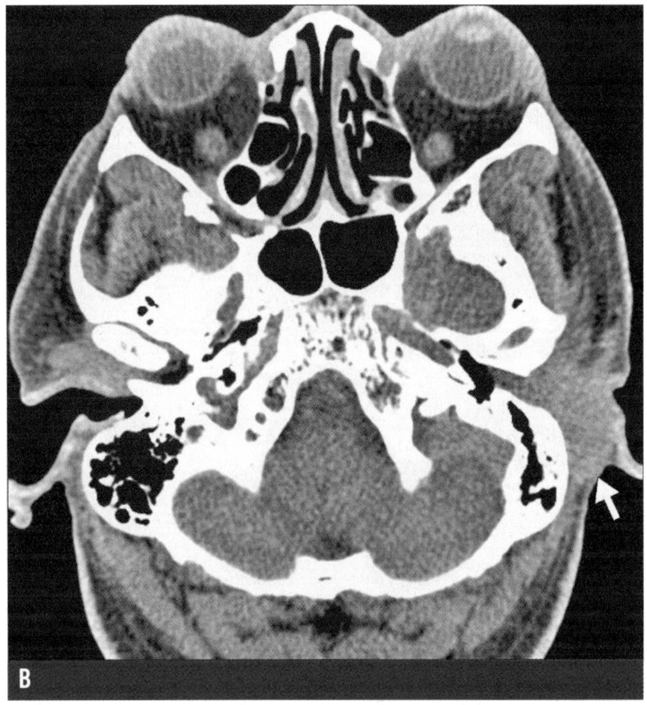

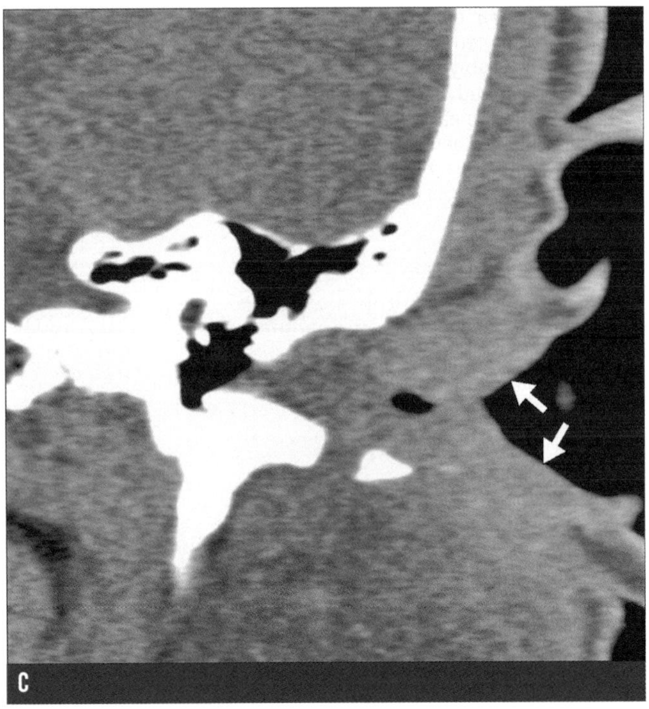

Axial (**A**, **B**) and coronal reformatted (**C**) unenhanced CT images through the temporal bones demonstrate a soft tissue mass along the left EAC (arrows, **A-C**). This lesion represented EAC adenocarcinoma at pathology. If available, coronal imaging is useful to determine whether an apparent mass in this region simply represents volume averaging with a normal EAC or if the finding represents a true EAC mass or parotid mass.

Companion case: EAC mineralization simulating a parotid gland sialolith

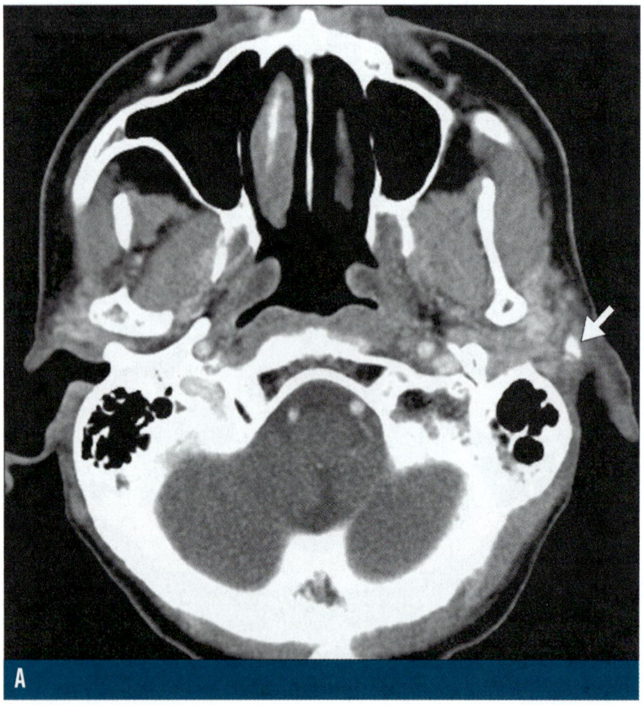

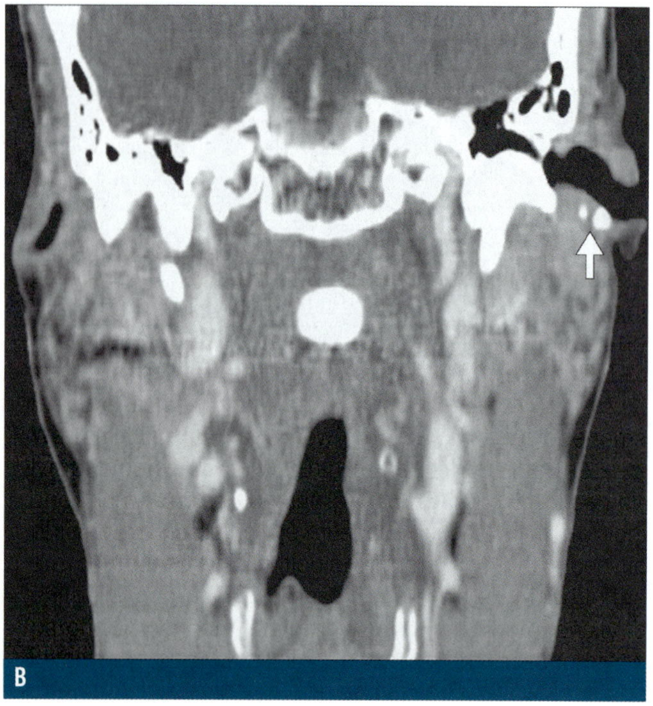

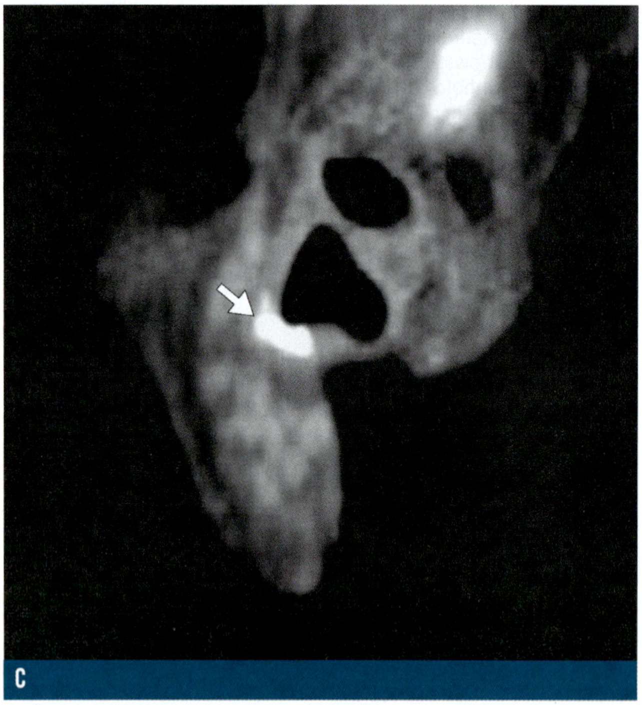

A contrast enhanced axial CT image through the superior aspect of the parotid glands (**A**) demonstrates a small focus of mineralization, possibly representing a left parotid sialolith (arrow, **A**). Coronal (**B**) and sagittal (**C**) reformatted contrast-enhanced CT images more clearly demonstrate that this finding represents incidental EAC mineralization (arrows, **B**, **C**).

REFERENCES

Chakeres DW, Kapila A, LaMasters D. Soft-tissue abnormalities of the external auditory canal: subject review of CT findings. *Radiology*. 1985;156:105-109.

Chatra PS. Lesions in the external auditory canal. *Indian J Radiol Imaging*. 2011;21(4):274-278.

Ong CK, Pua U, Chong VFH. Imaging of carcinoma of the external auditory canal: a pictorial essay. *Cancer Imaging*. 2008;8:191-198.

CASE 9 Parotidectomy

Parotidectomies are performed to resect benign or malignant tumors as well as chronic parotid gland infections that do not respond to medical therapy. When a tumor lies superficial to the facial nerve, a superficial parotidectomy is performed. When a tumor (particularly high-grade) resides deep to the facial nerve, a total parotidectomy is usually performed. A free fatty flap may be utilized to close the surgical wound.

COMPANION CASE

- **Pleomorphic adenoma seeding.** There are three histopathologic subtypes of pleomorphic adenoma: myxoid, classic, and cellular. The myxoid subtype is the most common and is responsible for the classic pronounced T2 hyperintense signal that is frequently present with pleomorphic adenomas. However, the myxoid variety is also the subtype that is most associated with a fragile, incomplete pseudocapsule and thus most prone to tumor seeding if incompletely resected during surgery. Therefore, during surgical extirpation, it is imperative that a pleomorphic adenoma is removed as a single, intact specimen to prevent tumor seeding into the operative bed. On MR imaging, pleomorphic adenoma tumor seeding will frequently appear as multiple T2 hyperintense, variably sized, enhancing nodules clustered in a grapelike manner within or adjacent to the operative bed. While growth of these recurrences is often slow, occasionally rapid growth may also be observed. Repeat surgery of these cases usually leads to poor results, as it is often extremely difficult to resect the entire volume of seeded tumor. It may also be difficult to preserve facial nerve function during repeat surgery.

  Fine needle aspiration of parotid neoplasms is usually reserved for those tumors that are believed to be malignant and when confirmation of malignancy is desired in order to appropriately plan the surgery. However, the need to biopsy a suspected benign pleomorphic adenoma is less clear. Biopsying a pleomorphic adenoma is generally believed to be unnecessary because most pleomorphic adenomas will be surgically removed irrespective of the biopsy results. It has been well documented that seeding of malignant parotid tumors as well as benign pleomorphic adenomas may occur during biopsy when using a large bore needle, particularly when performing multiple passes. However, even needles as small as a 22 gauge have been associated with pleomorphic adenoma tumor seeding. Therefore, regardless of whether biopsying a frankly malignant lesion or a benign pleomorphic adenoma, using a biopsy needle larger than a 25 gauge will increase the risk of tumor seeding and potentially irreversible consequences.

Parotidectomy

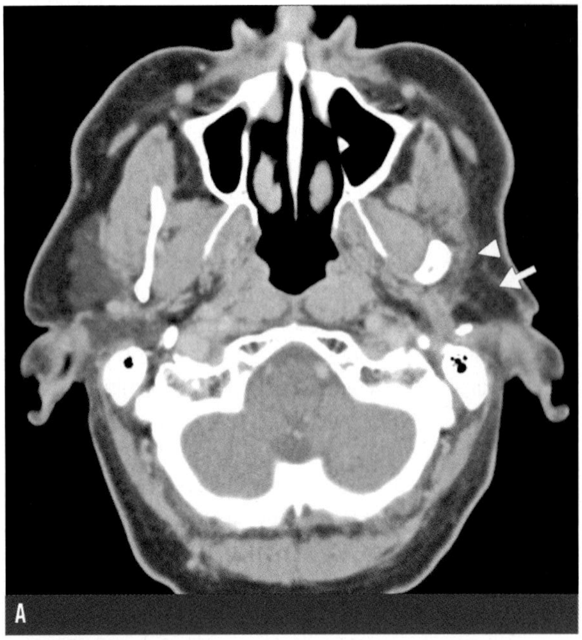

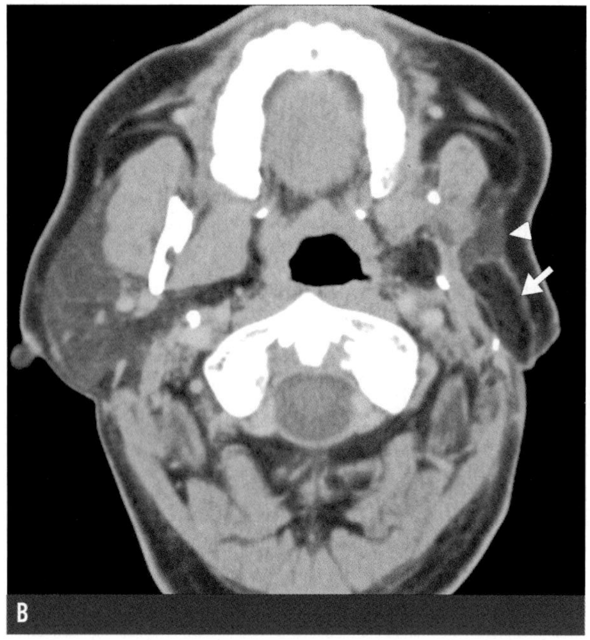

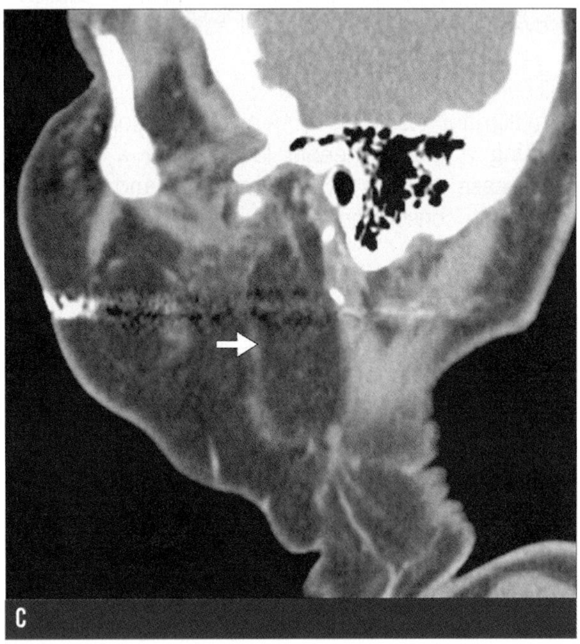

Postcontrast axial CT images through the parotid glands (**A**, **B**) demonstrate a subtotal left parotidectomy with a free fatty flap (arrows, **A**, **B**). A postcontrast sagittal reformatted CT image (**C**) demonstrates the same finding in the sagittal plane (arrow, **C**). A small amount of residual parotid tissue is present (arrowheads, **A**, **B**).

Companion case: Pleomorphic adenoma seeding

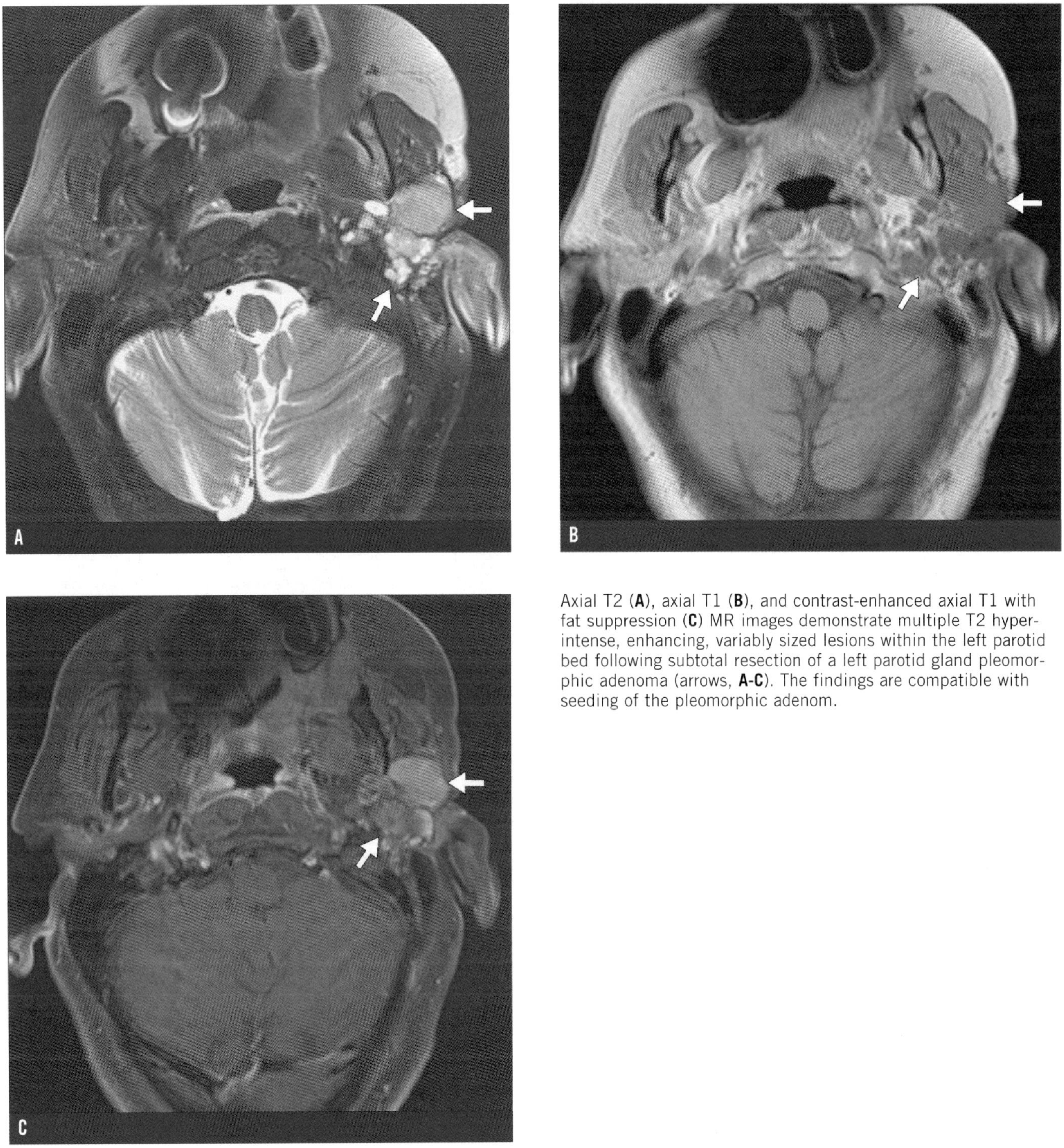

Axial T2 (**A**), axial T1 (**B**), and contrast-enhanced axial T1 with fat suppression (**C**) MR images demonstrate multiple T2 hyperintense, enhancing, variably sized lesions within the left parotid bed following subtotal resection of a left parotid gland pleomorphic adenoma (arrows, **A-C**). The findings are compatible with seeding of the pleomorphic adenom.

REFERENCES

Lev MH, Khanduja K, Morris PP, Curtin HD. Parotid pleomorphic adenomas: delayed CT enhancement. *AJNR Am J Neuroradiol.* 1998;19(10):1835-1839.

Moonis G, Patel P, Koshkareva Y, Newman J, Loevner LA. Imaging characteristics of recurrent pleomorphic adenoma of the parotid gland. *AJNR Am J Neuroradiol.* 2007;28(8):1532-1536.

Silvers AR, Som PM. Salivary glands. *Radiol Clin North Am.* 1998;36(5):941-966.

Supriya M, Denholm S, Palmer T. Seeding of tumor cells after fine needle aspiration cytology in benign parotid tumor: a case report and literature review. *Laryngoscope.* 2008;118(2):263-265.

CASE 10 Irradiated parotid and submandibular glands

Conventional radiation therapy for the treatment of head and neck malignancy is given in total doses of up to 70 Gy, usually administered over a 6- or 7-week period. This treatment can result in acute and chronic sequelae, including xerostomia, mucositis, hoarseness, and dysphagia, among others.

Some degree of xerostomia invariably occurs following radiation to the salivary glands. The consistency, volume, and pH of the saliva are altered by the radiation, resulting in a thicker saliva with an acidic pH. The changes in the saliva can result in oral discomfort/pain, dysphagia, dental caries, and oral infection. Xerostomia begins in the first week of radiation treatment and continues for several months after therapy. While some recovery of salivary gland function is possible following radiation therapy, radiation-induced xerostomia is typically irreversible and a chronic ailment for the patient.

On CT and MRI, irradiated glands become progressively atrophic and hyperenhancing over successive studies. Fatty infiltration, particularly of the parotid glands, may also occur.

Irradiated parotid glands

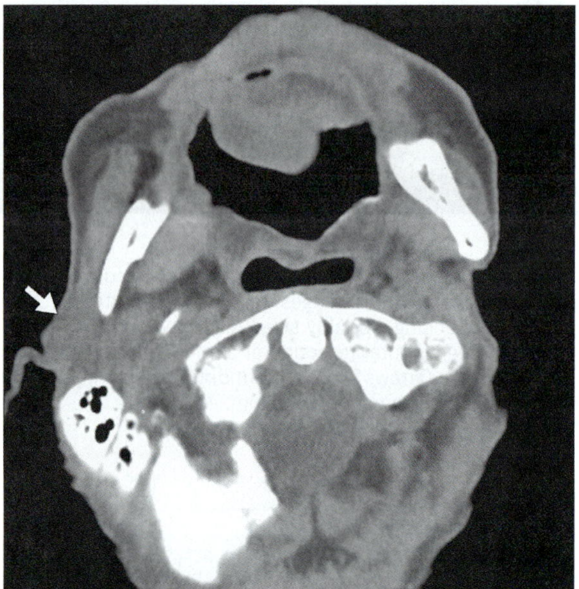

A

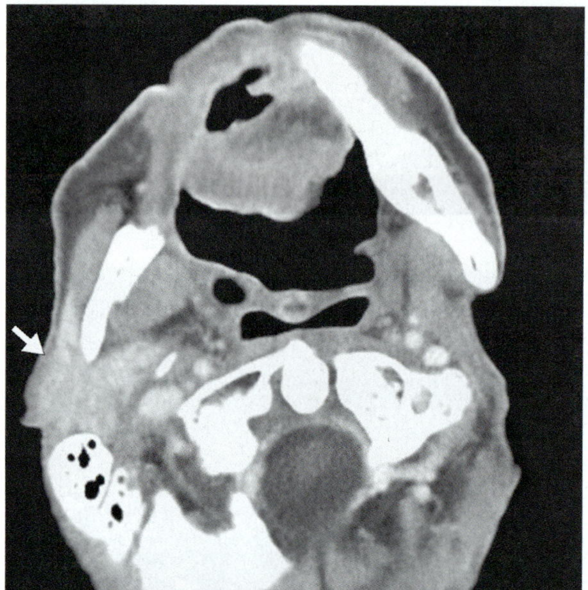

B

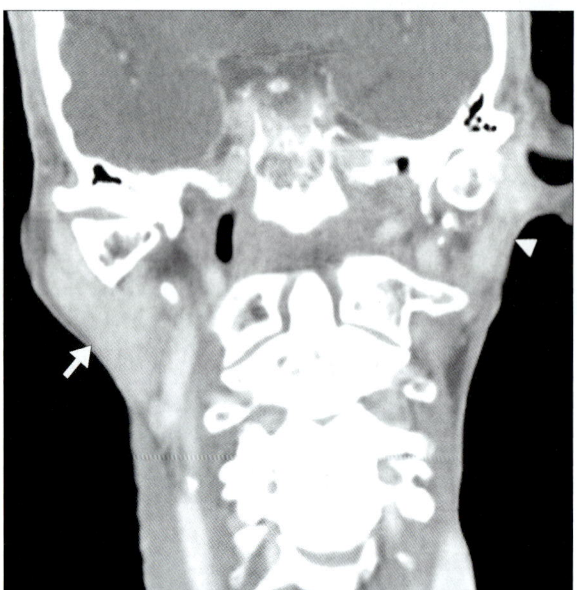

C

Noncontrast axial (**A**), postcontrast axial (**B**), and postcontrast coronal reformatted (**C**) CT images. Images **B** and **C** demonstrate dense enhancement of the right parotid gland (arrows, **B**, **C**) relative to image **A** in this patient with a history of radiation therapy for squamous cell cancer of the mandible. The left parotid gland is not in the same plane on the axial images although it is identified as densely enhancing on image **C** (arrowhead).

Irradiated parotid glands

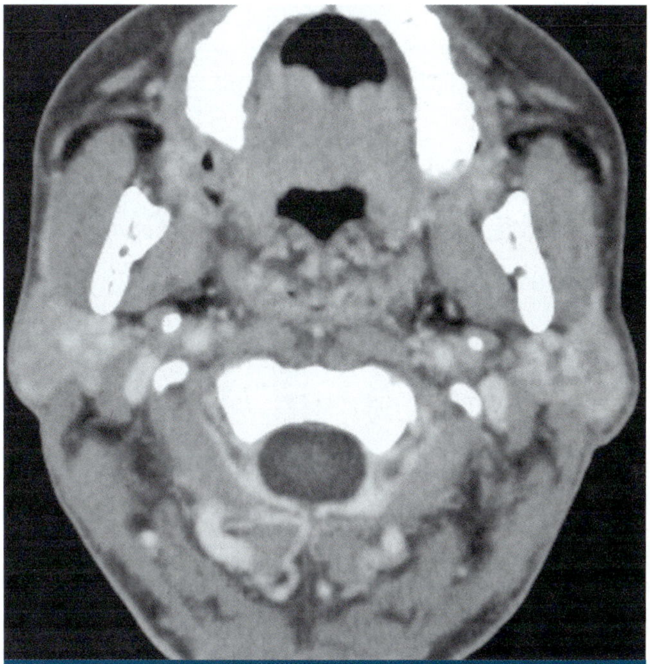

A

Different patient. A postcontrast axial CT image through the parotid glands (**A**) demonstrates dense and mild to moderately atrophic parotid glands, typical of postradiation effect.

Irradiated submandibular glands

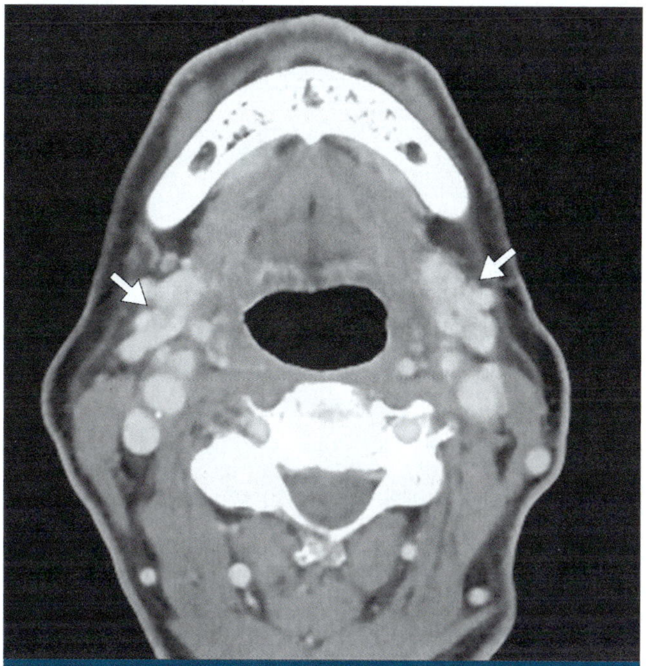

A

A postcontrast axial CT image through the level of the submandibular glands (**A**) demonstrates atrophic and densely enhancing submandibular glands (arrows), commonly present in the postradiation setting.

Irradiated submandibular glands

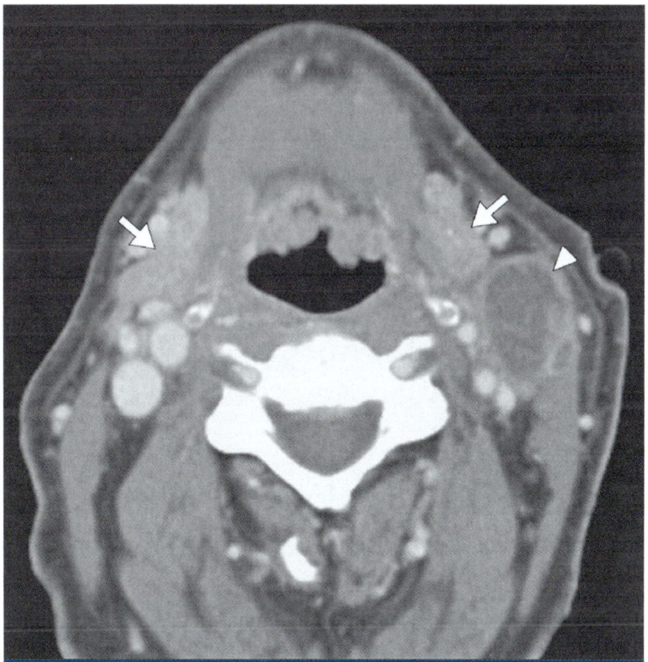

A

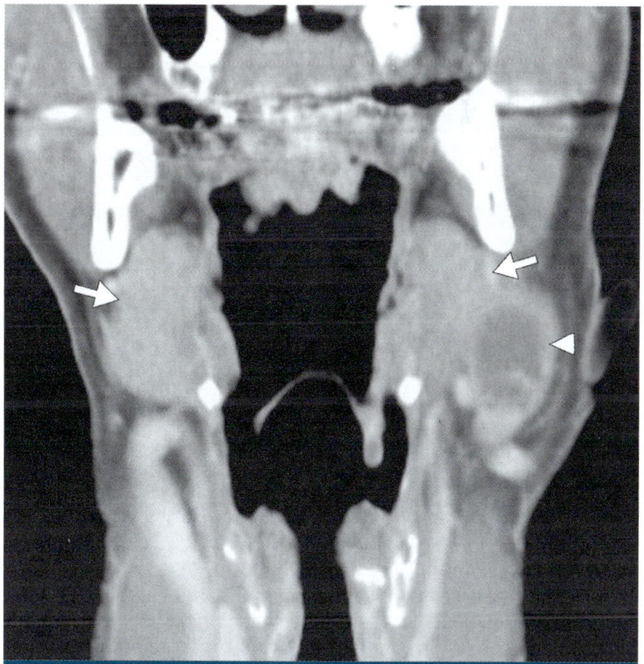

B

Different patient. Axial (**A**) and coronal reformatted (**B**) postcontrast CT images through the level of the submandibular glands demonstrate normal-sized submandibular glands (arrows, **A**, **B**), although the left submandibular gland is displaced anteromedially by a necrotic lymph node (arrowheads, **A**, **B**). Axial (**C**) and coronal reformatted (**D**) postcontrast CT images through the submandibular glands obtained 2 years later following radiation and chemotherapy. The submandibular glands are atrophic and densely enhancing (arrows, **C**, **D**), a common sequela following radiation treatment.

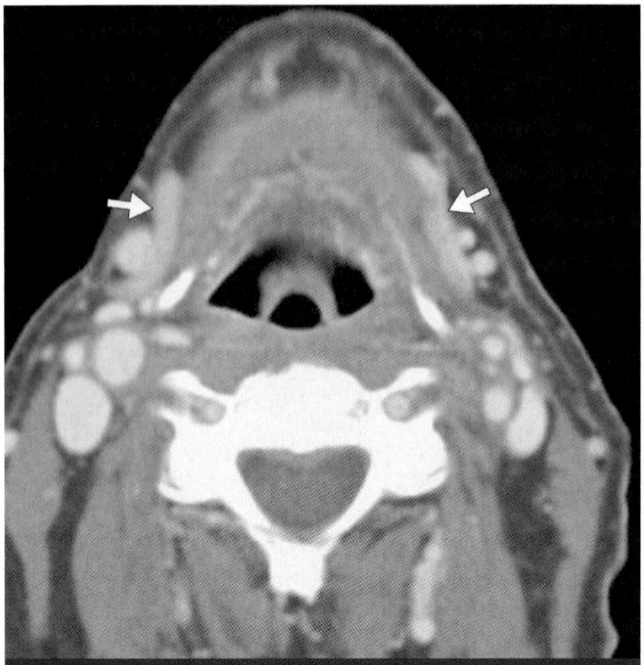

C

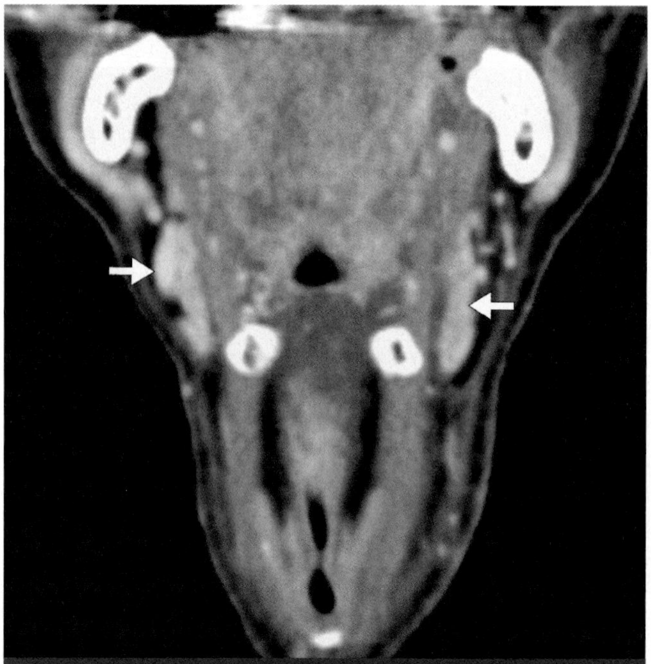

D

REFERENCE

Dirix P, Nuyts S, Van den Bogaert W. Radiation-induced xerostomia in patients with head and neck cancer: a literature review. *Cancer.* December 1, 2006;107(11):2525-2534.

CASE 11 Submandibular gland aplasia

Submandibular gland aplasia is a congenital entity that may be identified incidentally. This uncommon finding occurs as a result of disruption of submandibular gland development from the first and second branchial arches during embryogenesis. If unilateral, there is often compensatory hypertrophy of the contralateral submandibular gland. Furthermore, the sublingual glands, particularly the ipsilateral sublingual gland, may undergo compensatory hypertrophy in the setting of unilateral submandibular gland aplasia.

COMPANION CASES

- **Submandibular gland size asymmetry.** An asymmetrically smaller submandibular gland may be an abnormal finding, such as from unilateral chronic sialadenitis or the sequela of ipsilateral radiation. However, if the submandibular glands are asymmetric in size but are otherwise unremarkable (ie, normal symmetric attenuation and signal characteristics on CT and MRI, respectively), then submandibular gland size asymmetry can be considered a normal variant.
- **Diffuse fatty infiltration of the submandibular glands.** One or both submandibular glands can become fatty replaced and atrophic as a result of chronic sialadenitis. Fatty replacement of the submandibular glands may also occur in obese patients, although this is more commonly observed in the parotid glands. Diffusely fatty infiltrated submandibular glands often blend with adjacent neck fat and may appear aplastic on imaging.
- **Submandibular gland atrophy due to an obstructing sialolith.** In the acute setting, an obstructing sialolith can result in an acute sialadenitis or a gland abscess. A completely obstructing chronic sialolith can result in gland atrophy, whereas an incompletely obstructing sialolith can result in a mucocele within the gland.
- **Submandibular space lipoma.** A lipoma represents a focal, circumscribed collection of adipocytes that are often slow-growing, soft to palpation, mobile, and usually painless. Lipomas cannot be used for energy stores. As a result, while they can enlarge with weight gain, they do not decrease in size with weight loss.

Unilateral submandibular gland aplasia (MRI)

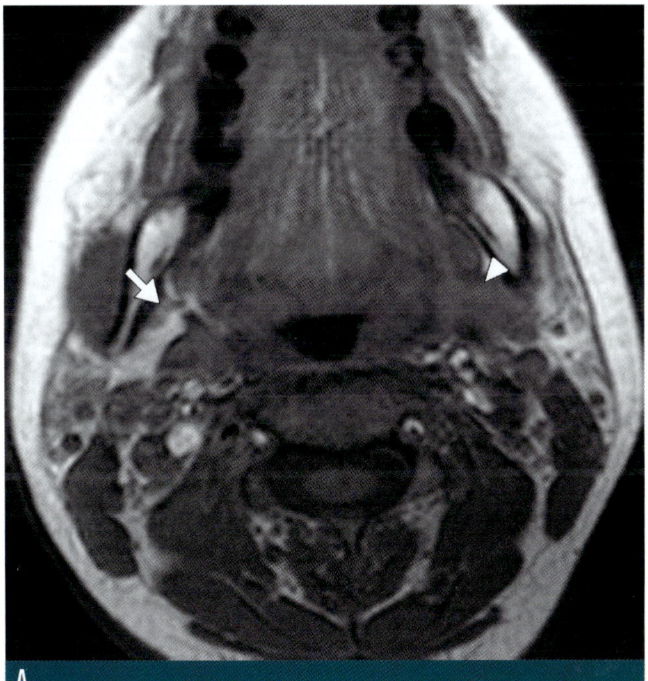
A

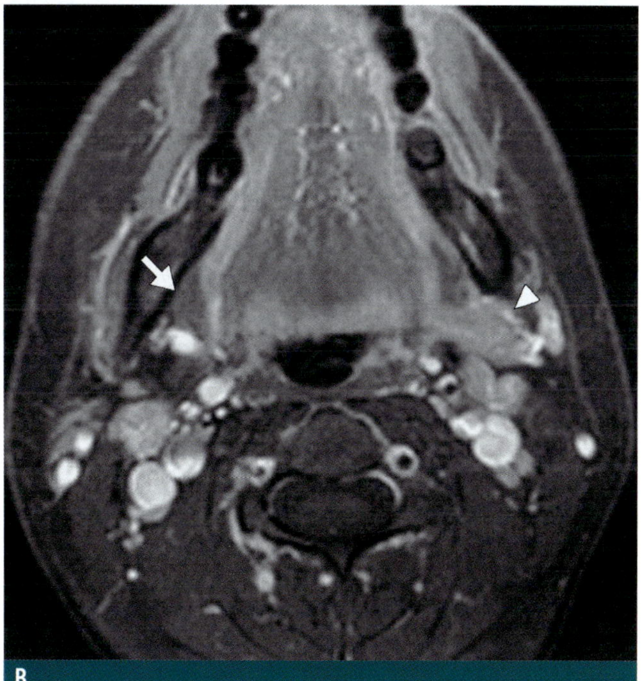
B

Axial unenhanced T1 (**A**), axial postcontrast T1 with fat suppression (**B**), axial T2 with fat suppression (**C**), and unenhanced coronal T1 (**D**) MR images through the level of the submandibular glands demonstrate congenital absence of the right submandibular gland (short arrows, **A-D**) and a small left submandibular gland (arrowheads, **A-D**). Incidentally noted are small lymph nodes in the right aspect of the submandibular space on image **D** (long arrow). An axial postcontrast T1-weighted MR image with fat suppression (**E**) demonstrates enlarged sublingual glands (short arrows, **E**), presumably representing compensatory hypertrophy because of the small left and the congenitally absent right submandibular glands.

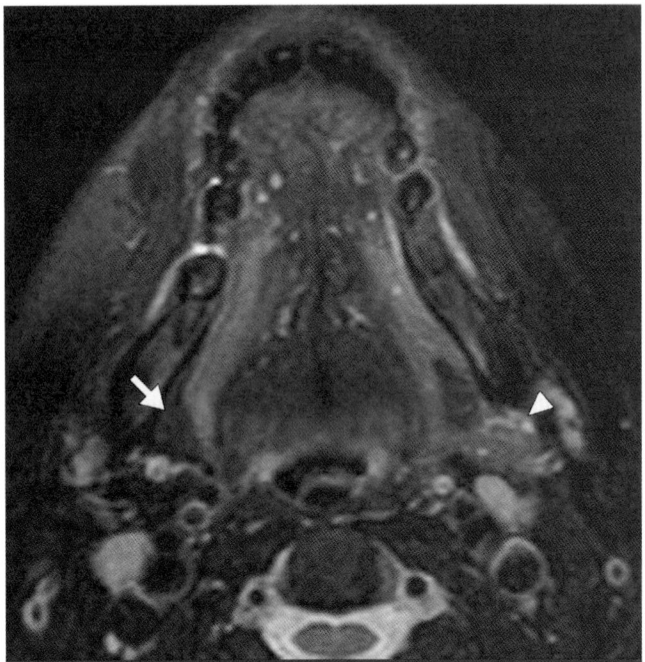

C

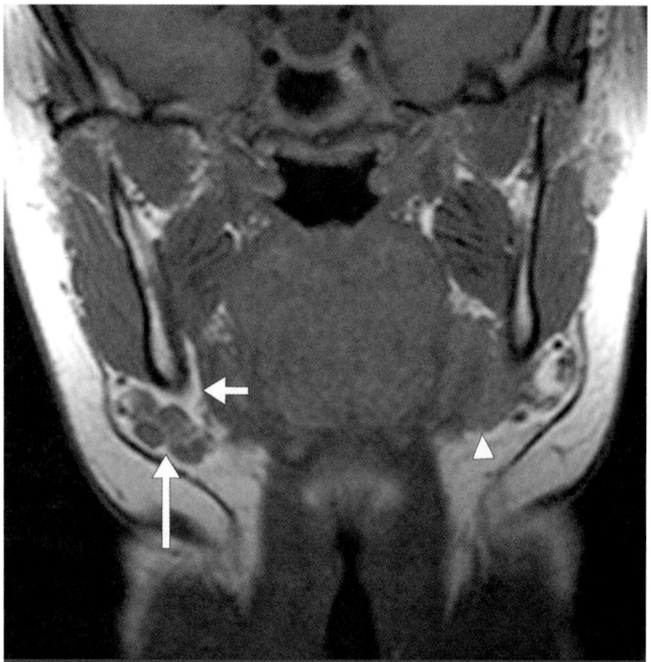

D

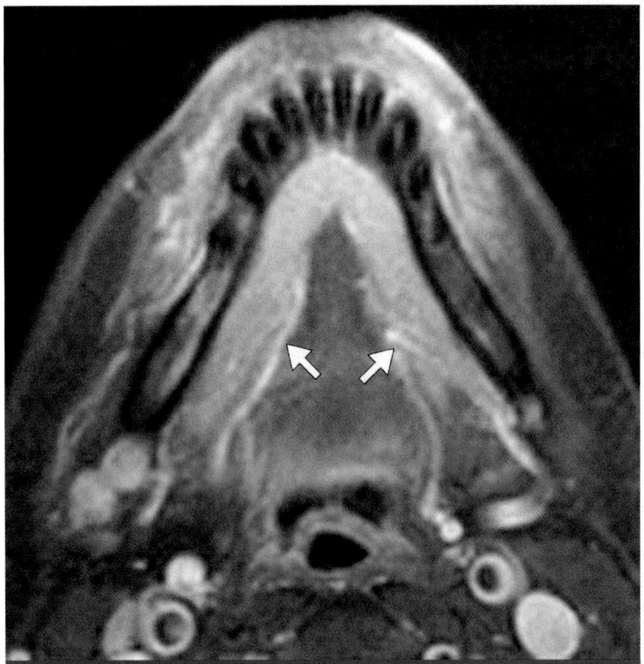

E

Unilateral submandibular gland aplasia (CT)

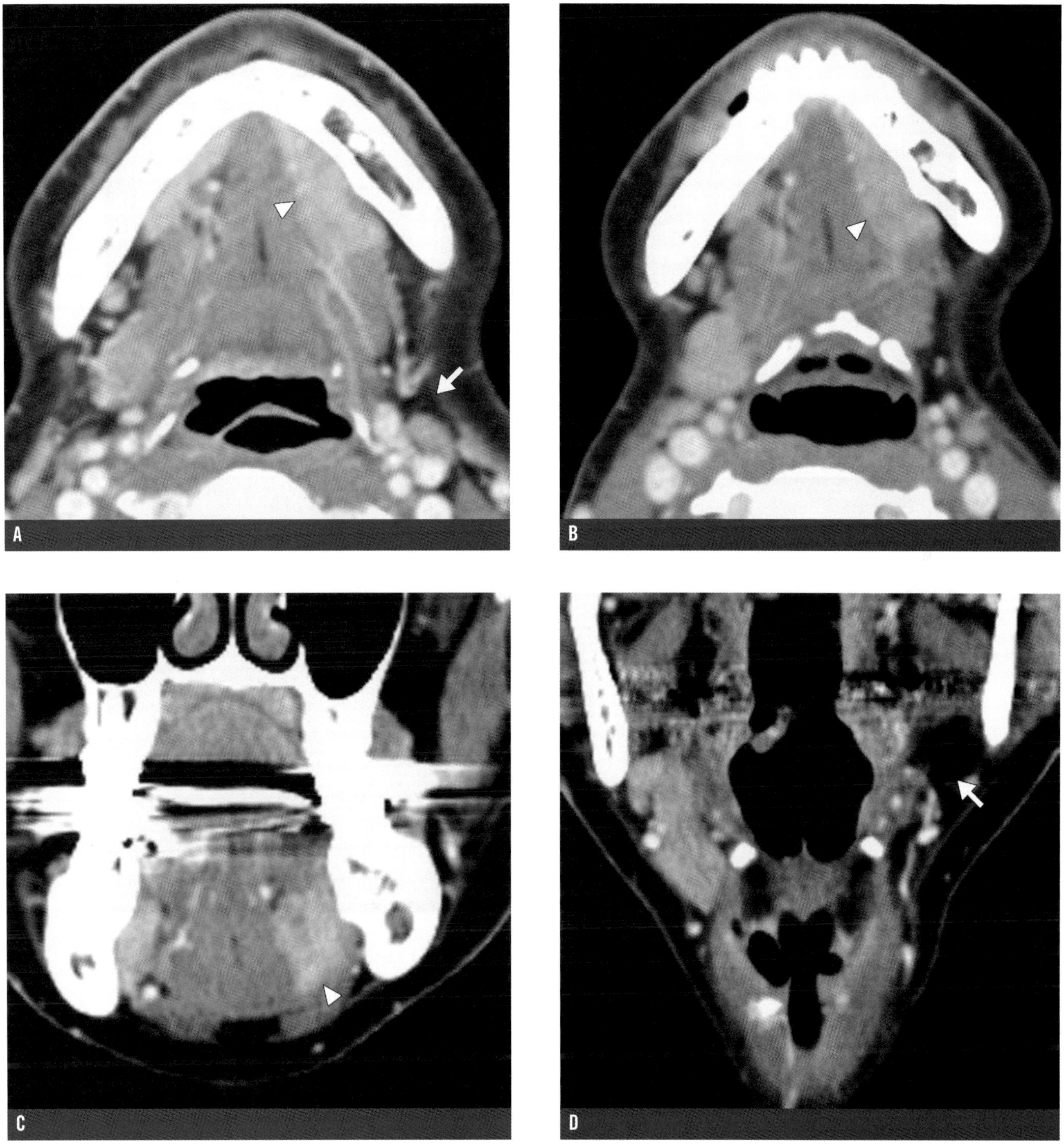

Different patient. Axial (**A**, **B**) and coronal reformatted (**C**, **D**) contrast-enhanced CT images demonstrate an aplastic left submandibular gland (arrows, **A**, **D**) and an asymmetrically enlarged left sublingual gland (arrowheads, **A**, **B**, **C**), presumably enlarged because of compensatory hypertrophy.

Bilateral submandibular gland aplasia

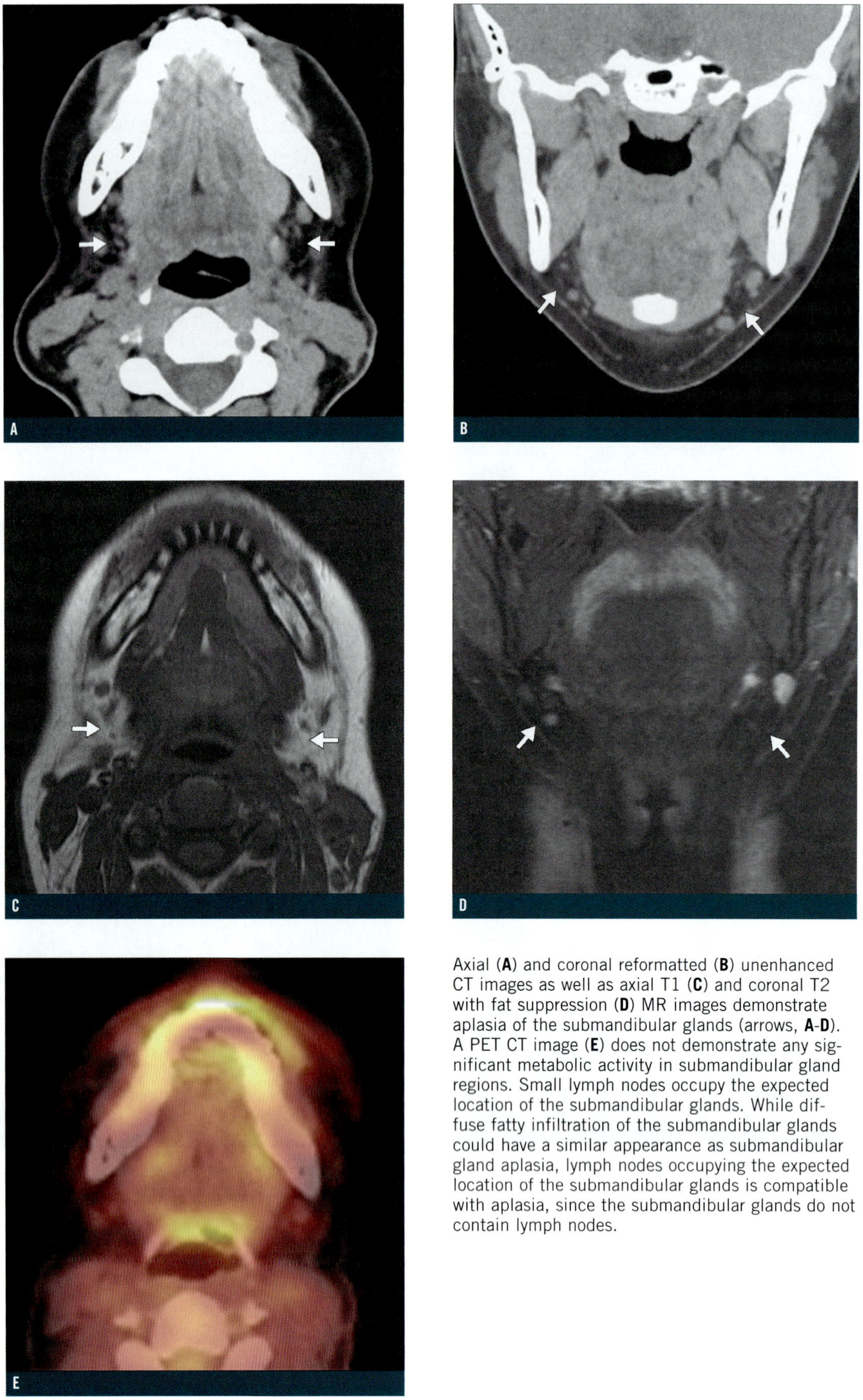

Axial (**A**) and coronal reformatted (**B**) unenhanced CT images as well as axial T1 (**C**) and coronal T2 with fat suppression (**D**) MR images demonstrate aplasia of the submandibular glands (arrows, **A**-**D**). A PET CT image (**E**) does not demonstrate any significant metabolic activity in submandibular gland regions. Small lymph nodes occupy the expected location of the submandibular glands. While diffuse fatty infiltration of the submandibular glands could have a similar appearance as submandibular gland aplasia, lymph nodes occupying the expected location of the submandibular glands is compatible with aplasia, since the submandibular glands do not contain lymph nodes.

Companion case: Submandibular gland size asymmetry

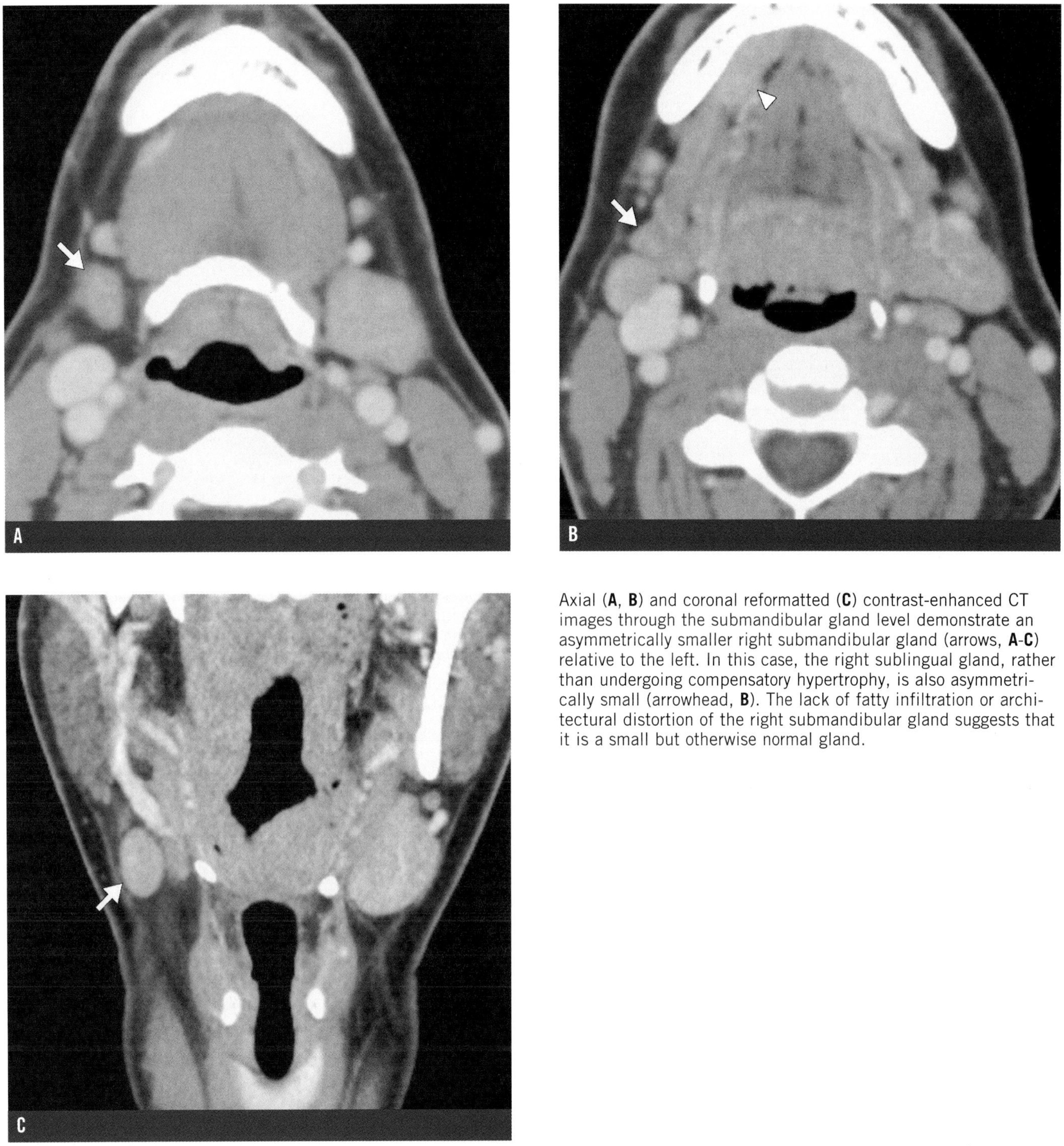

Axial (**A**, **B**) and coronal reformatted (**C**) contrast-enhanced CT images through the submandibular gland level demonstrate an asymmetrically smaller right submandibular gland (arrows, **A**-**C**) relative to the left. In this case, the right sublingual gland, rather than undergoing compensatory hypertrophy, is also asymmetrically small (arrowhead, **B**). The lack of fatty infiltration or architectural distortion of the right submandibular gland suggests that it is a small but otherwise normal gland.

Companion case: Diffuse fatty infiltration of the submandibular glands

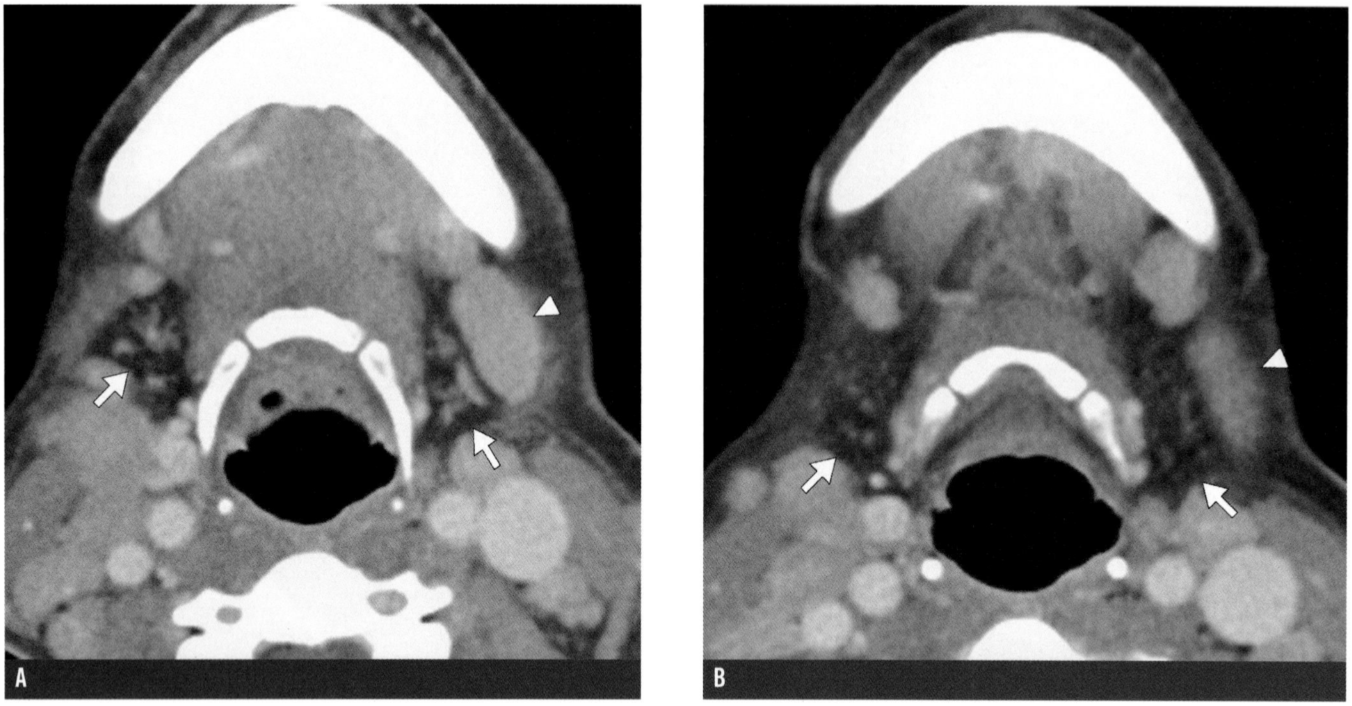

Postcontrast axial CT images through the level of the submandibular glands (**A**, **B**) demonstrate atrophic and diffusely fatty infiltrated submandibular glands (arrows, **A**, **B**). Small residual submandibular acinar and ductal elements surrounded by fat at the expected location of the submandibular glands are able to be visualized. A pathologically enlarged lymph node is present in the left submandibular space simulating a left submandibular gland (arrowheads, **A**, **B**). This patient had lymphoma which accounts for the pathologic lymph node. The lack of an identifiable branching ductal system within this lymph node helps differentiate this lymph node from the left submandibular gland.

Companion case: Diffuse fatty infiltration of one submandibular gland

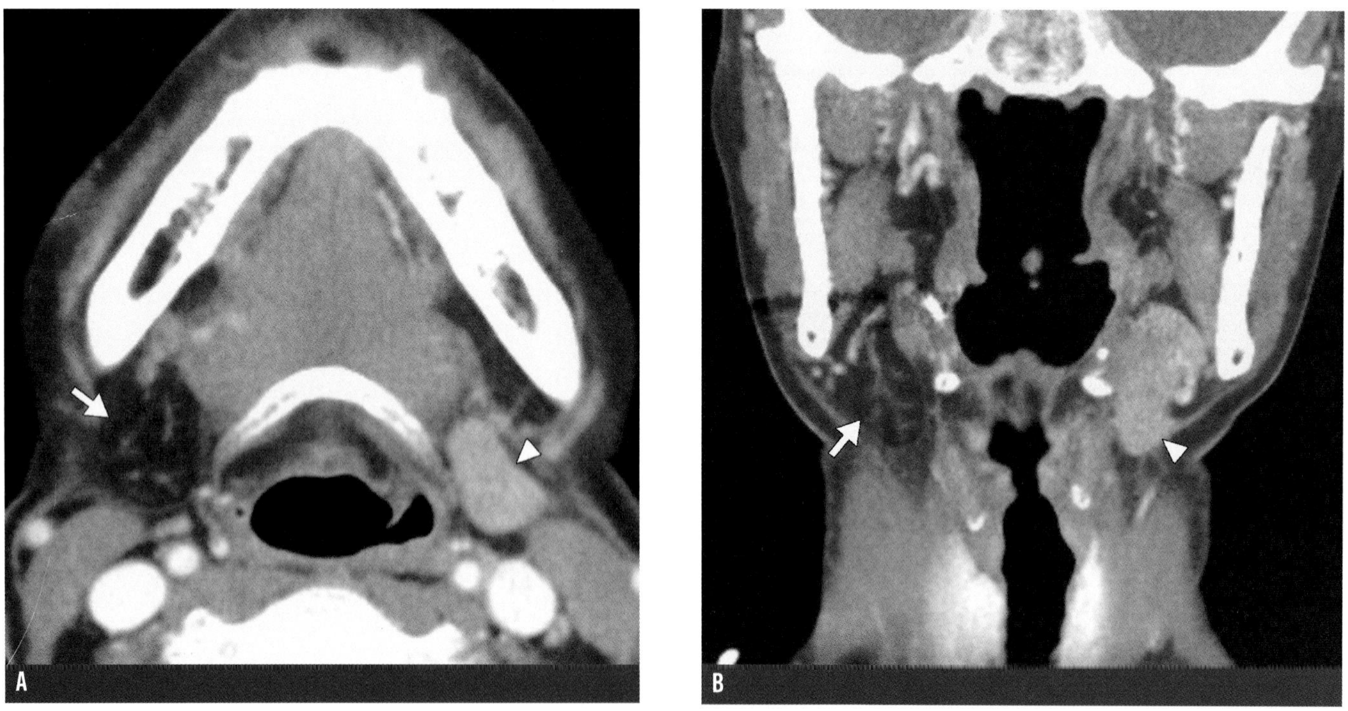

Axial (**A**) and coronal reformatted (**B**) contrast-enhanced CT images through the level of the submandibular glands demonstrate normal homogeneous parenchymal enhancement of the left submandibular gland (arrowheads, **A**, **B**) whereas fat completely replaces the right submandibular gland (arrows, **A**, **B**). Axial T1 (**C**), axial T2 with fat suppression (**D**), unenhanced coronal T1 (**E**), and contrast-enhanced coronal T1 with fat suppression (**F**) MR images of the same patient demonstrate primarily fat signal (arrows, **C**, **E**) and primarily fat suppression (arrows, **D**, **F**) at the expected location of the right submandibular gland. A normal MR appearance of the left submandibular gland is present (arrowheads, **C-F**).

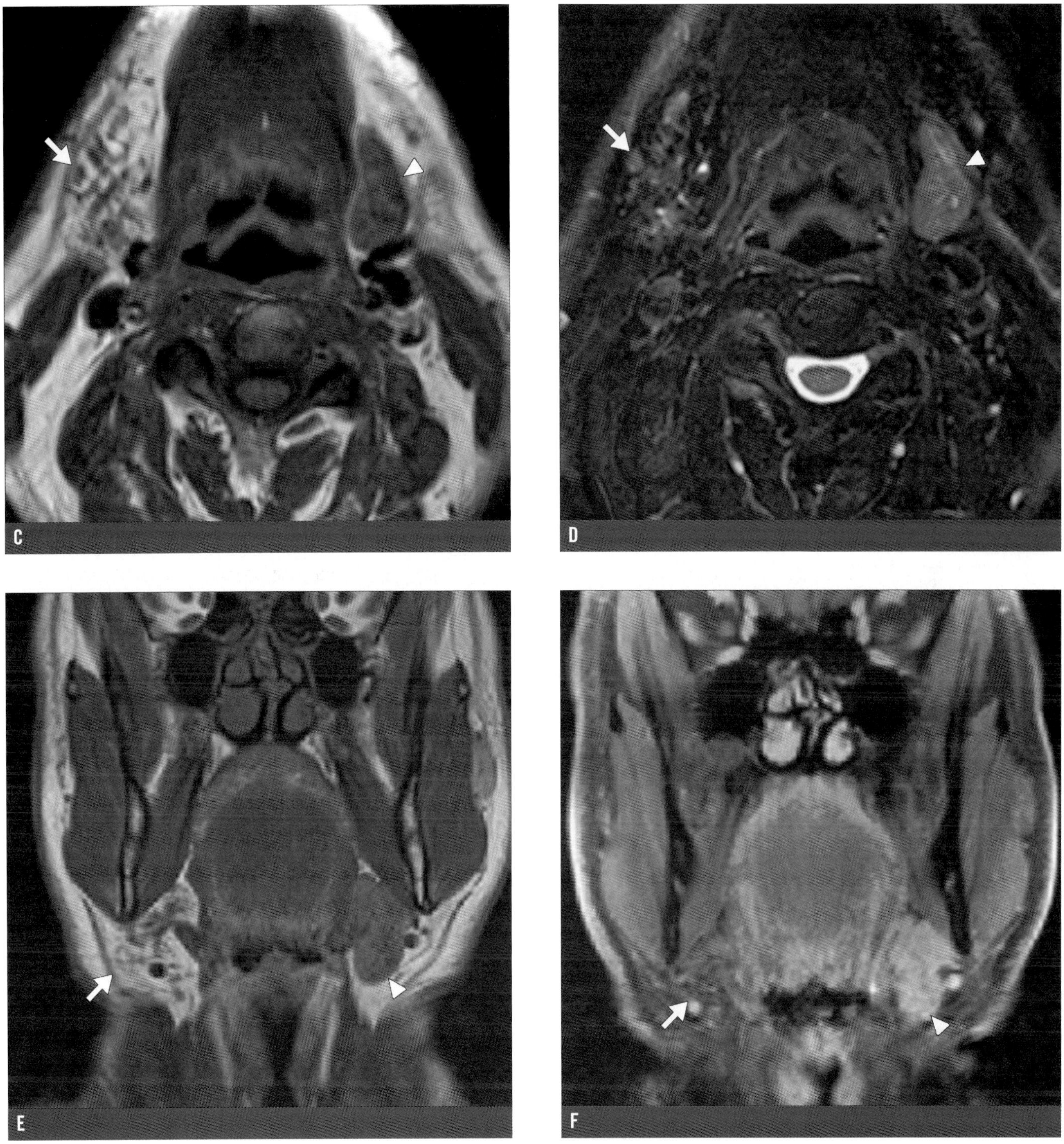
C
D
E
F

Companion case: Submandibular gland atrophy due to an obstructing sialolith

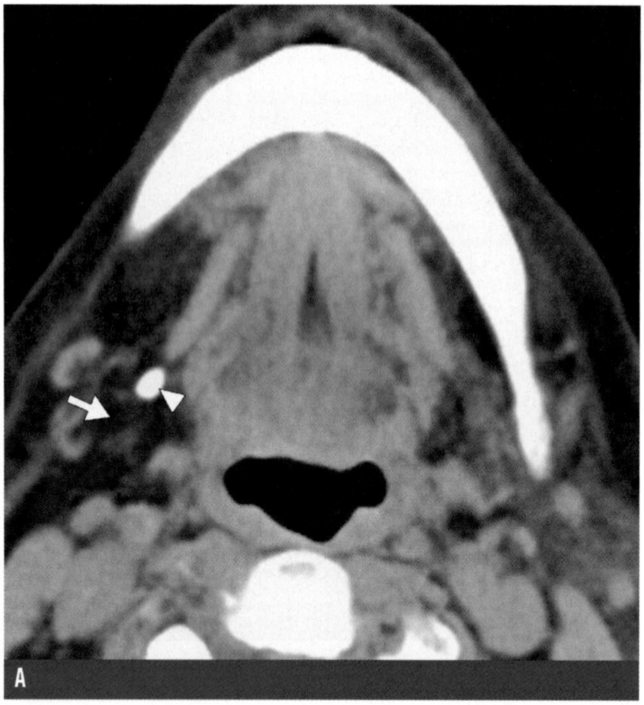

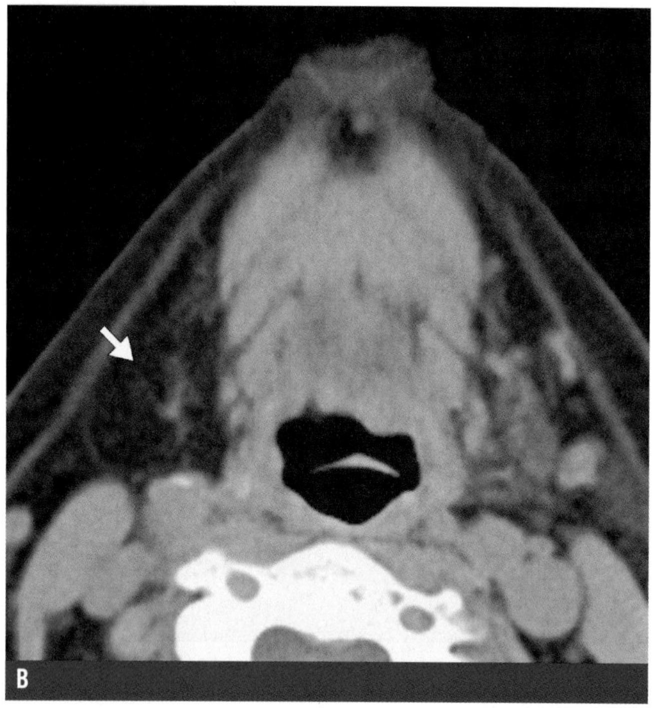

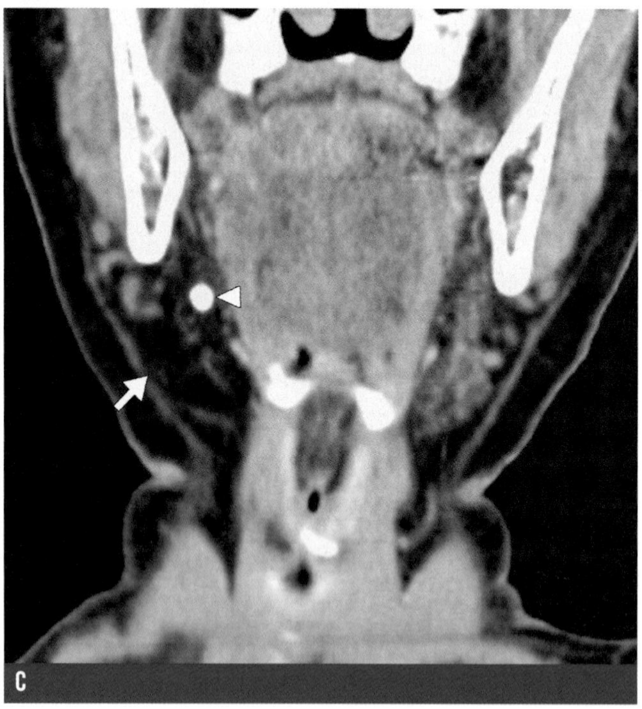

Axial (**A**, **B**) and coronal reformatted (**C**) contrast-enhanced CT images through the level of the submandibular glands demonstrate a diffusely fatty infiltrated right submandibular gland (arrows, **A-C**) due to chronic obstruction from a sialolith (arrowheads, **A**, **C**). When there is fatty infiltration and/or atrophy of a submandibular gland, one should inspect the course of the Wharton duct for a sialolith. Sialoliths are a common cause of submandibular gland atrophy and fatty infiltration.

Companion case: Submandibular space lipoma

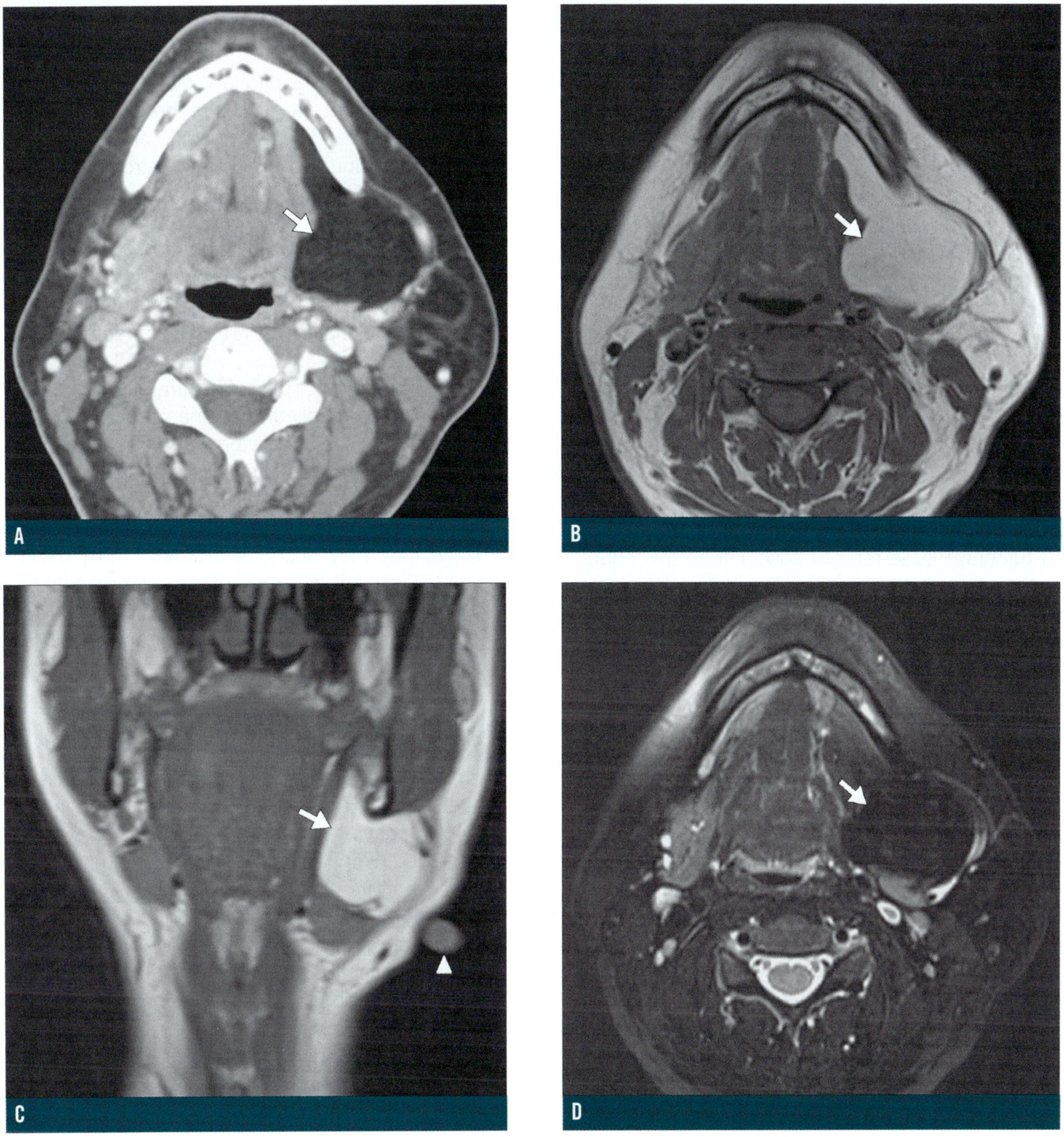

A postcontrast axial CT image (**A**) as well as axial T1 (**B**), coronal T1 (**C**), and axial T2 with fat suppression (**D**) MR images demonstrate a benign lipoma situated in the left aspect of the submandibular space (arrows, **A-D**) and located cephalad to the left submandibular gland. This mass fully suppresses on image **D**, verifying that the lesion is composed of fat and consistent with a lipoma. Negative Hounsfield units within the lesion on the CT were present and also consistent with a lipoma. This was mass-like to palpation, as denoted by a vitamin E capsule (arrowhead, **C**).

REFERENCES

Gupta N, Palacios E, Barry S. Unilateral submandibular gland aplasia: a rare phenomenon. *Ear Nose Throat J.* 2009;88(3):818-820.

Izumi M, Hida A, Takagi Y, Kawabe Y, Eguchi K, Nakamura T. MR Imaging of the salivary glands in sicca syndrome: comparison of lipid profiles and imaging in patients with hyperlipidemia and patients with Sjögren's syndrome. *AJR Am J Roentgenol.* 2000;175: 829-834.

Som PM, Curtin HD. *Head and Neck Imaging.* 4th ed. St. Louis, MO: Mosby Inc; 2003.

Srinivasan A, Moyer JS, Mukherji SK. Unilateral submandibular gland aplasia associated with ipsilateral sublingual gland hypertrophy. *AJNR Am J Neuroradiol.* 2006;27(10):2214-2216.

Sumi M, Izumi M, Yonetsu K, Nakamura T. The MR imaging assessment of submandibular gland sialoadenitis secondary to sialolithiasis: correlation with CT and histopathologic findings. *AJNR Am J Neuroradiol.* 1999;20:1737-1743.

CASE 12 Normal submandibular gland lobulation

It is not unusual for the submandibular gland to have normal lobulations. When imaged in the axial plane, these normal lobulations may simulate pathology, such as a focal submandibular gland tumor or a submandibular region pathologic lymph node. Viewing the apparent finding on sagittal or coronal imaging will usually allow one to differentiate normal submandibular gland lobulation from pathology.

COMPANION CASES

- **Submandibular gland benign epithelial cyst.** This represents a small benign cyst that contains an epithelial lining, usually the result of a focal ductal obstruction.
- **Submandibular gland pleomorphic adenoma.** A pleomorphic adenoma (also called benign mixed tumor) accounts for approximately 36% of all submandibular gland tumors. Please refer to Case 1 from this chapter for further discussion.
- **Submandibular gland carcinoma ex pleomorphic adenoma**. Please refer to Case 1 from this chapter for discussion.
- **Submandibular gland adenoid cystic carcinoma.** Adenoid cystic carcinoma only accounts for approximately 12% of all submandibular gland tumors, but it is the most common malignancy of the submandibular gland. This tumor has a proclivity for perineural spread (50%-60%), which when arising from the submandibular gland may affect the hypoglossal nerve, facial nerve, or trigeminal nerve. Please refer to Case 1 from this chapter for further discussion.
- **Submandibular gland Küttner tumor.** A misnomer, a Küttner tumor does not represent a neoplasm but rather a chronic sclerosing sialadenitis. It is believed to be part of a recently described IgG4-related disease spectrum, which includes several other head and neck entities, such as Mikulicz disease, Hashimoto thyroiditis, Riedel thyroiditis, orbital pseudotumor, and lymphocytic hypophysitis of the pituitary gland. Entities elsewhere in the body that are also considered part of the IgG4-related disease spectrum include autoimmune pancreatitis, sclerosing cholangitis, and retroperitoneal fibrosis, to name a few. Multi-organ involvement or elevated serum levels of IgG4 are very helpful in establishing the diagnosis, although not required. Histopathologically, the appearance of these lesions is similar, regardless of the organ, and are characterized by an abundance of IgG4-positive plasma cells and lymphocytes with associated organ fibrosis.

  A Küttner tumor may affect any of the salivary glands, but most commonly affects one or both of the submandibular glands. Patients present with a firm, mass-like submandibular gland, sometimes present for as little as a few weeks, although the presence of a firm mass for decades has also been described in some patients. While they may occur at any age, most patients that present with a Küttner tumor are older than 50 years. On imaging, the gland may be enlarged or atrophic, and the gland may be entirely abnormal or only focally involved. The abnormality is hypointense on T1, variable on T2 (typically hypointense but may be hyperintense on T2 with fat suppression), and enhances, often simulating a tumor. While differentiating this entity from a true tumor is not always possible, the identification of salivary gland ducts traversing through the signal abnormality is a helpful imaging finding and suggests a Küttner tumor rather than an epithelial neoplasm. Steroids are very effective in treating a Küttner tumor. Thus, if suspected clinically or with imaging, a trial of steroids should be considered prior to surgical intervention.
- **Lymphadenopathy simulating duplicated submandibular glands.** Occasionally, bulky lymphadenopathy adjacent to the submandibular glands may be mistaken for submandibular gland duplication, the latter an extremely rare entity.

Normal submandibular gland lobulation

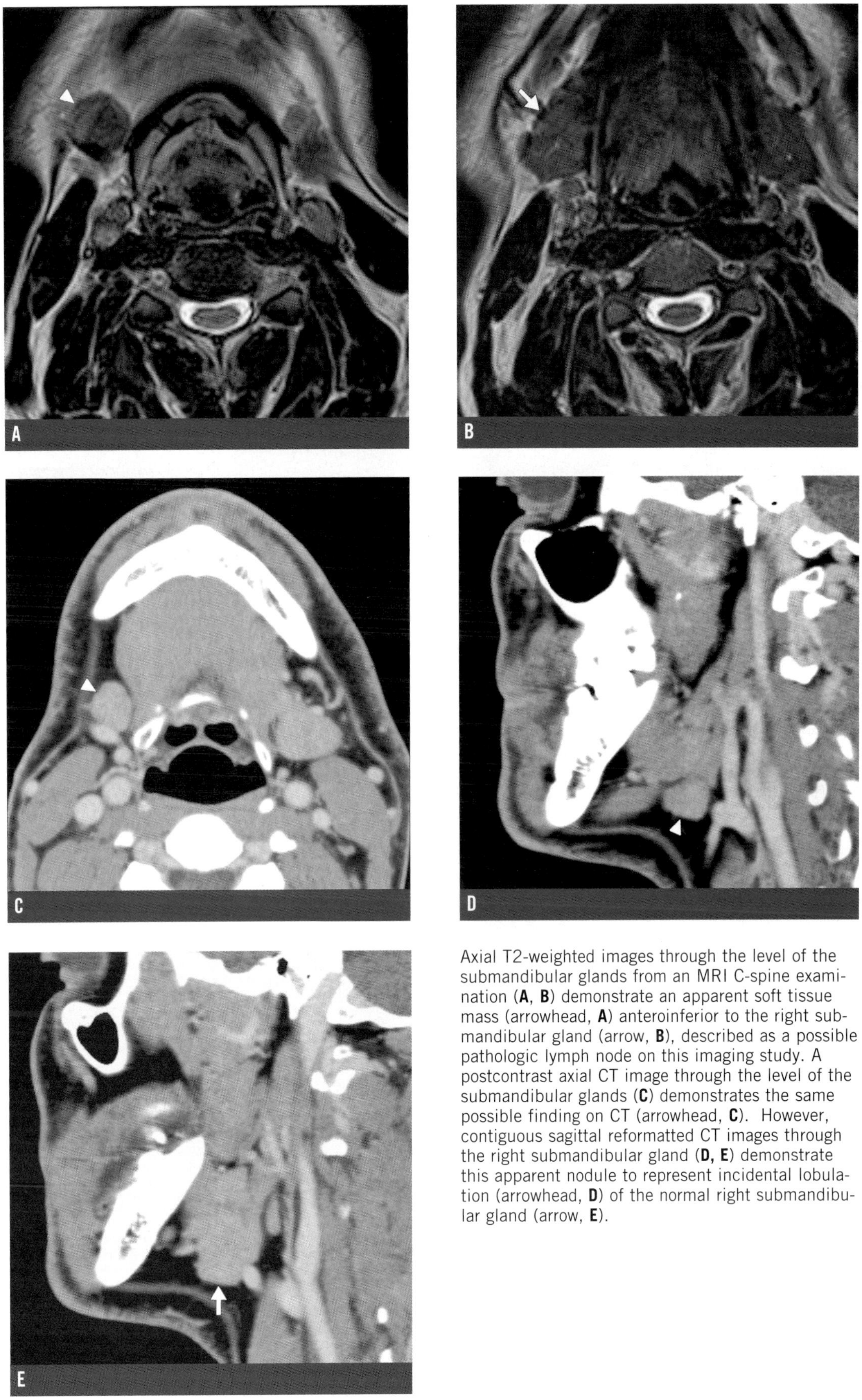

Axial T2-weighted images through the level of the submandibular glands from an MRI C-spine examination (**A**, **B**) demonstrate an apparent soft tissue mass (arrowhead, **A**) anteroinferior to the right submandibular gland (arrow, **B**), described as a possible pathologic lymph node on this imaging study. A postcontrast axial CT image through the level of the submandibular glands (**C**) demonstrates the same possible finding on CT (arrowhead, **C**). However, contiguous sagittal reformatted CT images through the right submandibular gland (**D, E**) demonstrate this apparent nodule to represent incidental lobulation (arrowhead, **D**) of the normal right submandibular gland (arrow, **E**).

Normal submandibular gland lobulation

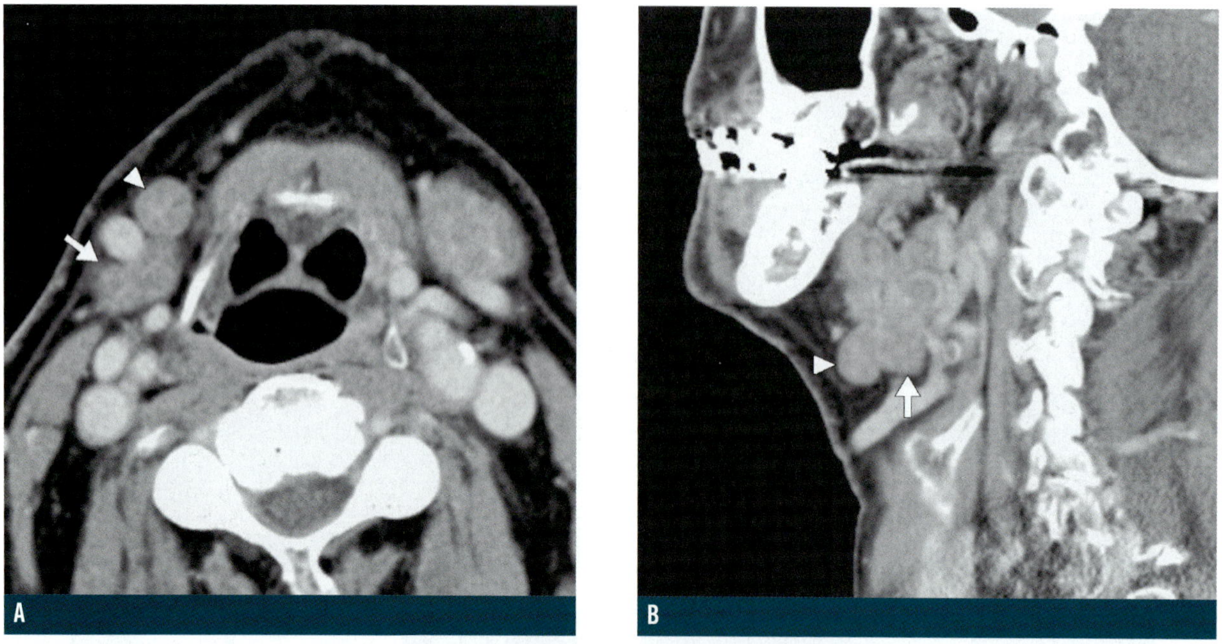

Different patient. A postcontrast axial CT image through the level of the submandibular glands (**A**) demonstrates a soft tissue nodule (arrowhead, **A**), possibly representing an abnormally enlarged lymph node, located at the same level as the right submandibular gland (arrow, **A**). However, the soft tissue nodule has the same attenuation as the adjacent submandibular gland, suggesting that it may represent a normal submandibular lobulation rather than an abnormally enlarged lymph node. A contrast-enhanced sagittal reformatted CT image from the same study (**B**) confirms that this nodule of soft tissue (arrowhead, **B**) is contiguous with the adjacent submandibular gland (arrow, **B**) and represents normal submandibular gland lobulation.

Companion case: Submandibular gland benign epithelial cyst

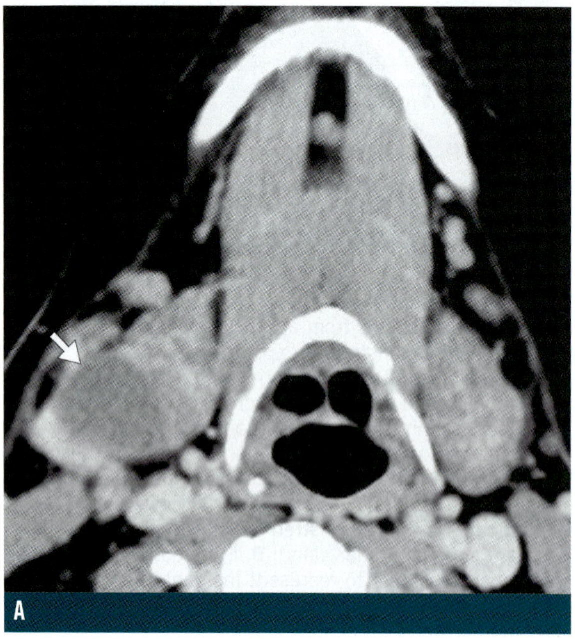

A postcontrast axial CT image through the submandibular glands (**A**) demonstrates a circumscribed, hypoattenuating oval lesion within the posterolateral aspect of the right submandibular gland (arrow). The Hounsfield units of this finding were consistent with simple fluid, which was present throughout much of the lesion. However, based solely on CT, a malignant lesion was not able to be excluded. This represented a benign epithelial cyst of the submandibular gland at pathology.

Companion case: Submandibular gland pleomorphic adenoma

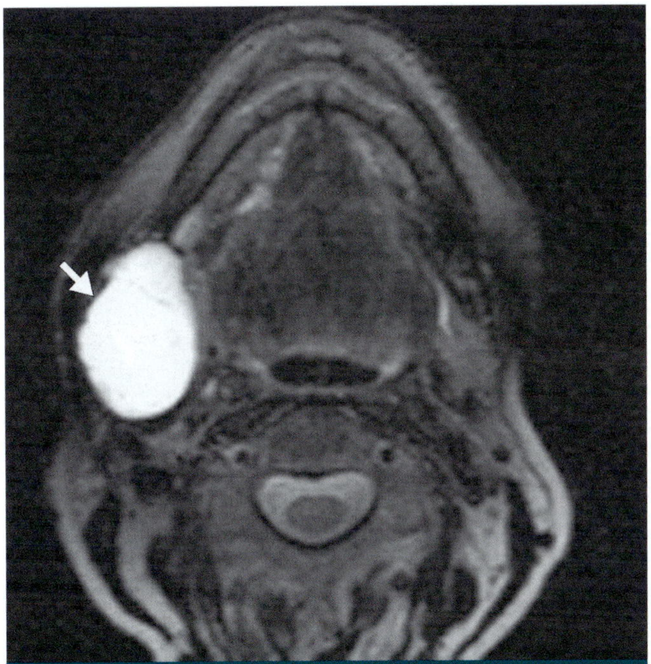

A

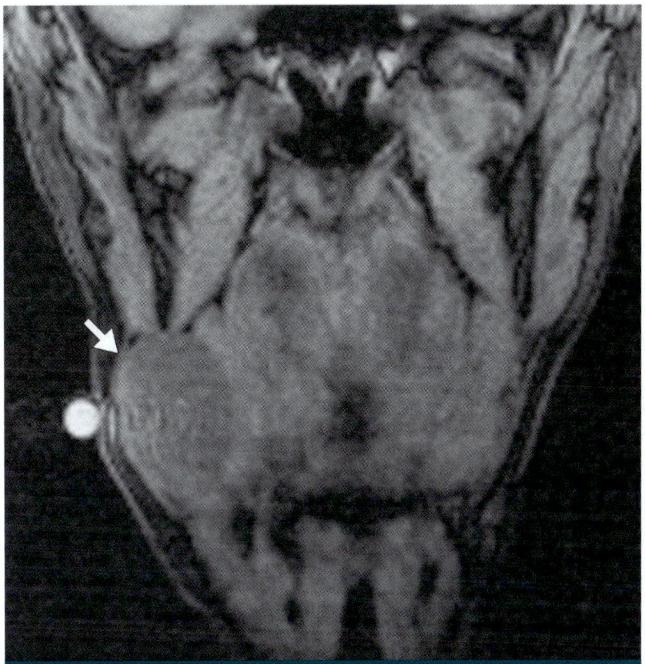

B

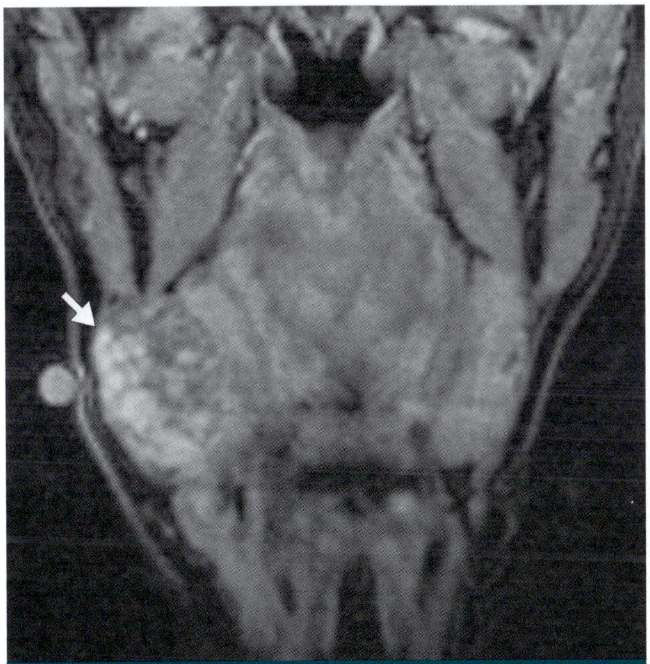

C

Axial T2 with fat suppression (**A**), unenhanced coronal T1 with fat suppression (**B**), and postcontrast coronal T1 with fat suppression (**C**) demonstrate an oval, diffusely and homogeneously T2 hyperintense, heterogeneously enhancing mass arising in the region of the right submandibular gland (arrows, **A-C**). Occasionally, determining whether a lesion arises from the submandibular gland or whether it represents a lesion separate from the submandibular gland is difficult. In this case, the location, signal characteristics (profoundly and homogeneously T2 hyperintense), and the presence of enhancement suggest a submandibular mass, most likely a pleomorphic adenoma, which was confirmed at pathology.

Companion case: Submandibular gland carcinoma ex pleomorphic adenoma

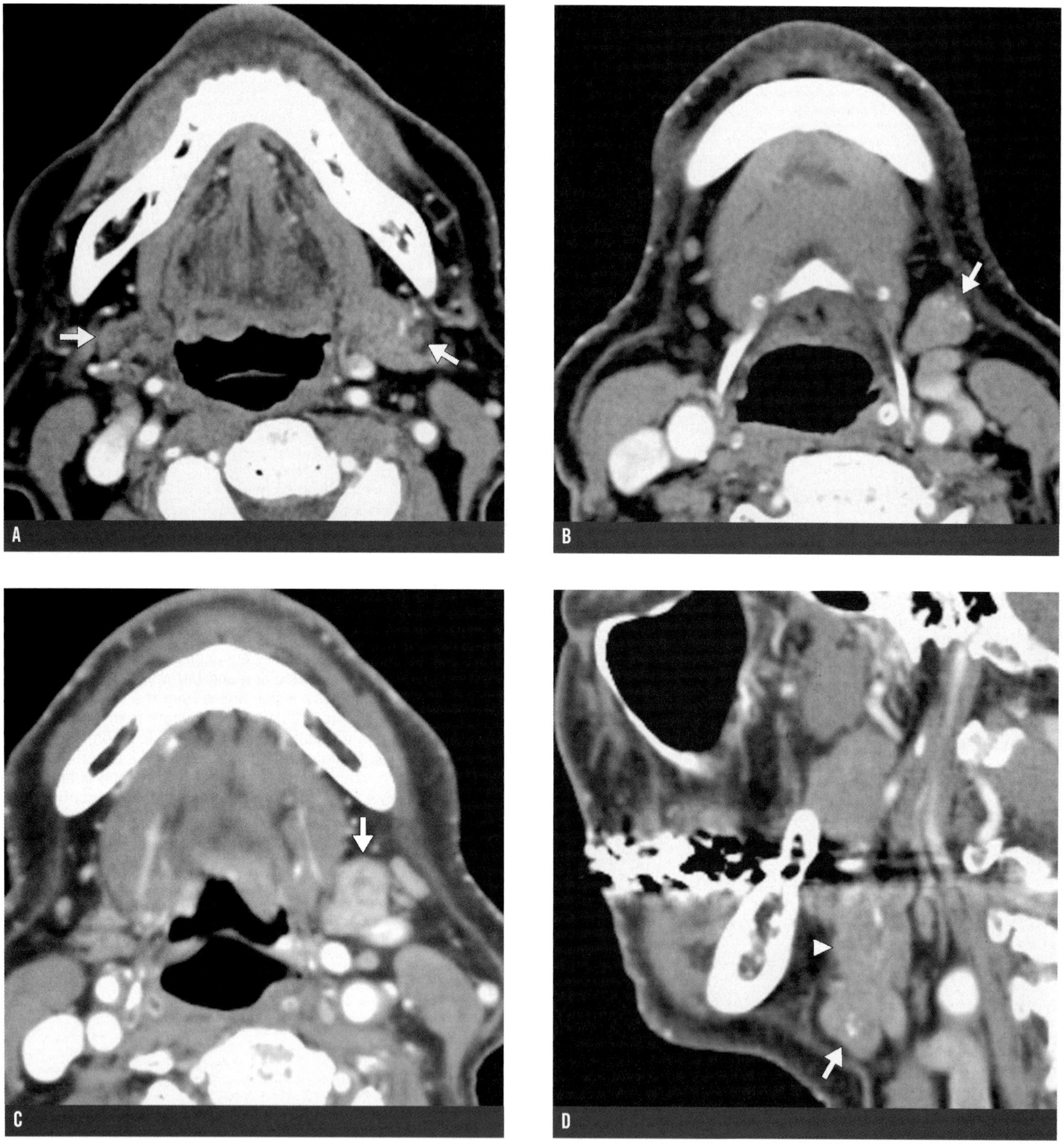

An axial postcontrast CT image through the level of the submandibular glands (**A**) demonstrates an asymmetrically larger left submandibular gland compared to the right (arrows, **A**). An axial postcontrast CT image slightly caudal to image **A** (**B**), demonstrates a lobulated lesion containing punctate calcifications projecting anteriorly, inferiorly, and laterally from the left submandibular gland (arrow, **B**). An axial delayed postcontrast CT image (**C**) demonstrates the lobulated finding to undergo mildly heterogeneous delayed enhancement (arrow, **C**). A postcontrast sagittal reformatted CT image (**D**) confirms that the lesion (arrow, **D**) arises from the left submandibular gland (arrowhead, **D**). The heterogeneous enhancement coupled with the focal punctate calcifications raises concern for a neoplasm. In this case, this lesion represented a carcinoma ex pleomorphic adenoma at pathology.

Companion case: Submandibular gland adenoid cystic carcinoma

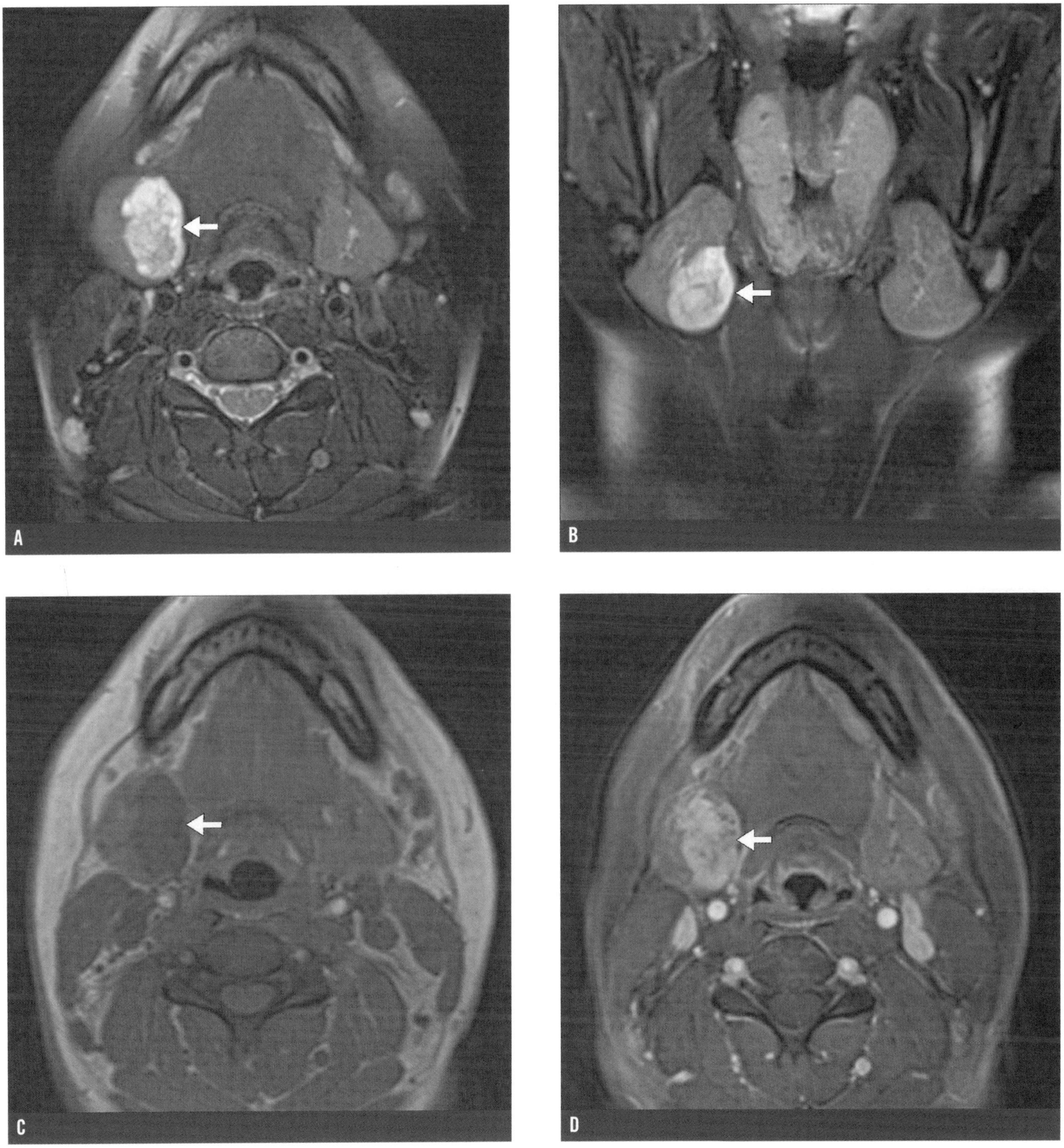

Axial T2 with fat suppression (**A**), coronal T2 with fat suppression (**B**), axial T1 (**C**), and contrast-enhanced axial T1 with fat suppression (**D**) MR images demonstrate a heterogeneously T2 hyperintense, heterogeneously enhancing mass involving the inferomedial aspect of the right submandibular gland (arrows. **A-D**), in this case representing an adenoid cystic carcinoma at pathology. The heterogeneous T2 signal within the lesion, while nonspecific, raises the possibility that the lesion may be malignant.

Companion case: Submandibular gland Küttner tumor

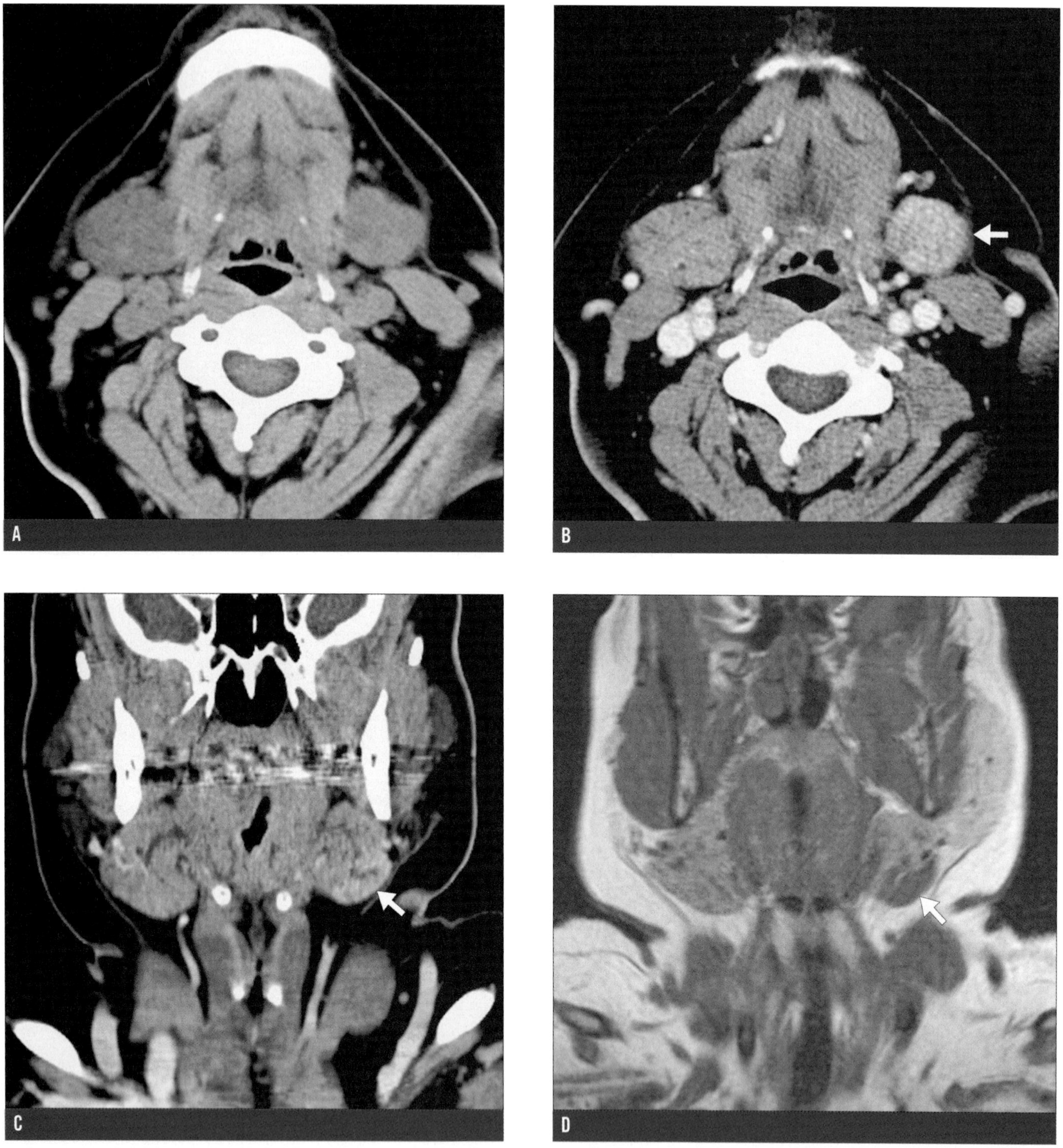

Unenhanced axial (**A**) as well as contrast-enhanced axial (**B**) and contrast-enhanced coronal reformatted (**C**) CT images through the level of the submandibular glands demonstrate an atrophic left submandibular gland that focally enhances along its inferior aspect (arrows, **B, C**). Coronal T1 (**D**), axial T1 (**E**), axial T2 with fat suppression (**F**), contrast-enhanced axial T1 with fat suppression (**G**), and contrast-enhanced coronal T1 with fat suppression (**H**) MR images demonstrate the inferior aspect of the left submandibular gland to be focally hypointense on T1, hyperintense on T2, and enhance (arrows, **D-H**). This 60-year-old female patient presented with a firm left submandibular gland mass. The gland was removed surgically, in part because tumor was raised as a possibility on imaging. However, the ducts within the gland in the area of abnormal signal and enhancement are preserved, a finding typically not present with a focal tumor. This represented chronic inflammation and fibrosis, consistent with Küttner tumor, with no evidence of tumor at pathology.

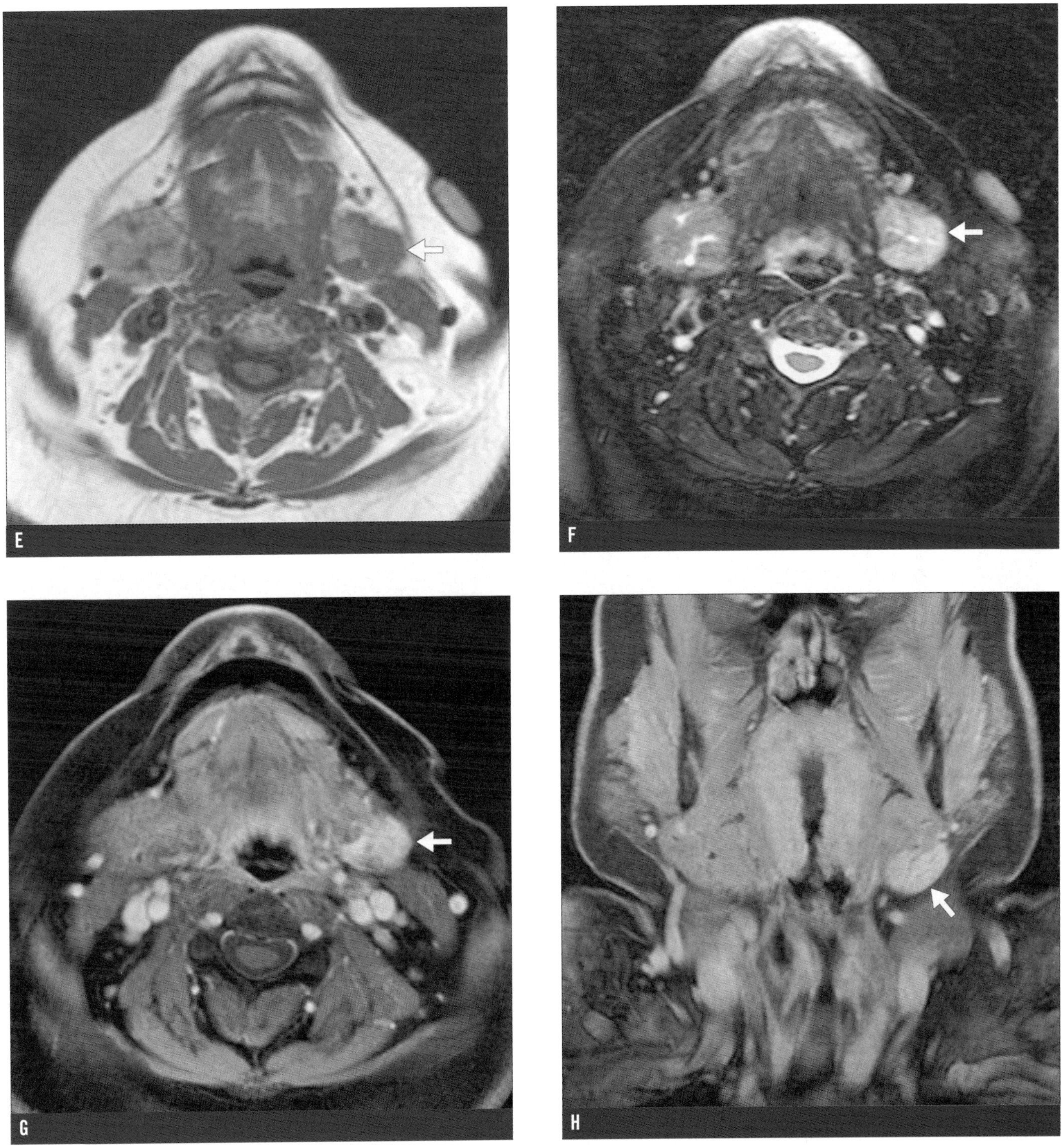
E
F
G
H

Companion case: Lymphadenopathy simulating duplicated submandibular glands

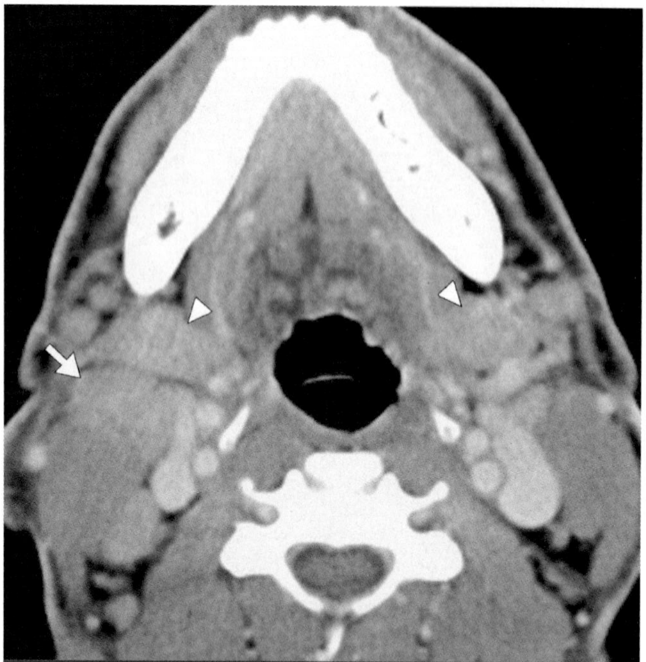

A

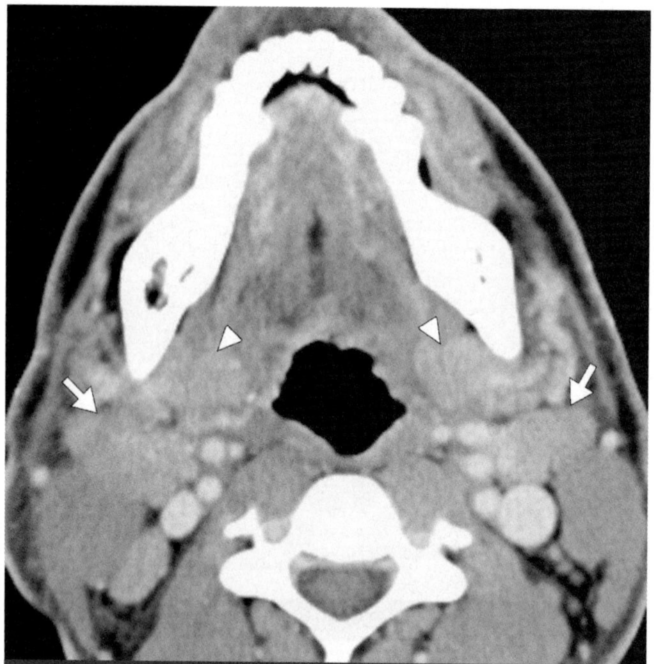

B

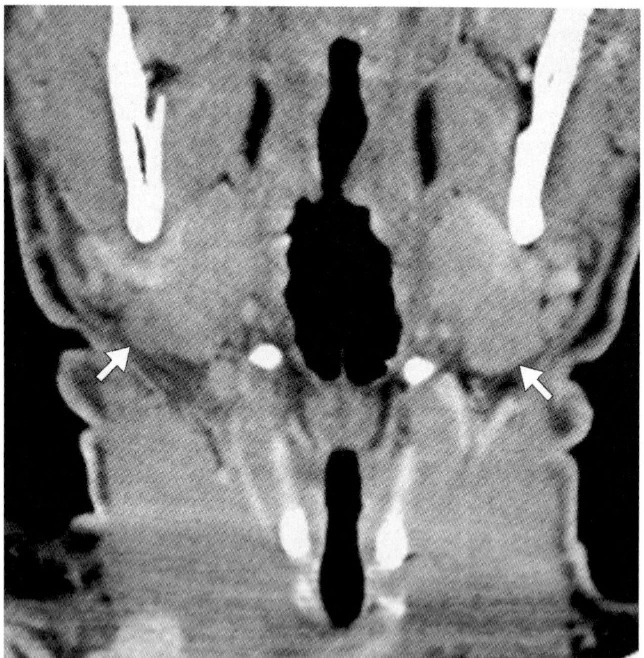

C

Axial (**A**, **B**) and coronal reformatted (**C**) contrast-enhanced CT images through the level of the submandibular glands in a patient with MRSA bacteremia and cervical lymphadenopathy. Markedly enlarged, homogeneously enhancing, oval shaped, bilateral level IIA lymph nodes (arrows, **A**-**C**) could be mistaken for salivary tissue. There are normal submandibular glands immediately anterior to these lymph nodes (arrowheads, **A**, **B**). Enlarged level IIA lymph nodes simulating duplicated submandibular glands are far more common than duplication of the submandibular glands, which is an extremely rare entity.

REFERENCES

Adeyemo WL, et al. Tumours of the submandibular salivary gland: a clinicopathologic review of cases over a 17-year period. *West Indian Med J.* 2009;58(4):388-391.

Browne RFJ, Golding SJ, Watt-Smith SR. The role of MRI in facial swelling due to presumed salivary gland disease. *Br J Radiol.* 2001;74:127-133.

Christe A, Waldherr C, Hallett R, Zbaeren P, Thoeny H. MR imaging of parotid tumors: typical lesion characteristics in MR imaging improve discrimination between benign and malignant disease. *AJNR Am J Neuroradiol.* 2011;32(7):1202-1207.

De Cocker LJ, D'Arco F, De Beule T, Tousseyn T, Blockmans D, Hermans R. IgG4-related systemic disease affecting the parotid and submandibular glands: magnetic resonance imaging features of IgG4-related chronic sclerosing sialadenitis and concomitant lymphadenitis. *Clin Imaging.* 2014;38(2):195-198.

Fujita A, Sakai O, Chapman MN, Sugimoto H. IgG4-related disease of the head and neck: CT and MRI imaging manifestations. *Radiographics.* 2012;32(7):1945-1958.

Kato H, Kanematsu M, Mizuta K, Ito Y, Hirose Y. Carcinoma ex pleomorphic adenoma of the parotid gland: radiologic-pathologic correlation with MR imaging including diffusion-weighted imaging. *AJNR Am J Neuroradiol.* 2008;29(5):865-867. Epub February 13, 2008.

Lev MH, Khanduja K, Morris PP, Curtin HD. Parotid pleomorphic adenomas: delayed CT enhancement. *AJNR Am J Neuroradiol.* 1998;19(10):1835-1839.

Lingam RK, Daghir AA, Nigar E, Abbas SA, Kumar M. Pleomorphic adenoma (benign mixed tumour) of the salivary glands: its diverse clinical, radiological, and histopathological presentation. *Br J Oral Maxillofac Surg.* 2011;49(1):14-20.

Moonis G, Patel P, Koshkareva Y, Newman J, Loevner LA. Imaging characteristics of recurrent pleomorphic adenoma of the parotid gland. *AJNR Am J Neuroradiol.* 2007;28(8):1532-1536.

Shi H, Wang P, Wang S, Yu Q. Pleomorphic adenoma with extensive ossified and calcified degeneration: unusual CT findings in one case. *AJNR Am J Neuroradiol.* 2008;29(4):737-738. Epub January 17, 2008.

Silvers AR, Som PM. Salivary glands. *Radiol Clin North Am.* 1998;36(5):941-966.

CASE 13 The submandibular ductal system

The submandibular duct, also known as the Wharton duct, drains the submandibular gland and measures approximately 5 to 6 cm in length. A small portion of the submandibular gland, known as the deep portion, extends cephalad from the submandibular space and over the free margin of the mylohyoid muscle. The Wharton duct arises from this portion of the submandibular gland and traverses anteromedially along the floor of the mouth in the sublingual space. Ultimately, each Wharton duct drains into its respective sublingual papilla (also called caruncle), each located immediately lateral to the tongue frenulum.

The normal intraluminal cross-sectional diameter of the Wharton duct is approximately 1 to 2 mm. The normal Wharton duct can sometimes be identified on cross-sectional imaging, usually best appreciated on coronal images. In the submandibular gland, the first- and second-order branches taper to an even smaller diameter. Nevertheless, normal intraglandular submandibular ductal branches may also be visualized on cross-sectional imaging and their identification does not necessarily imply pathology.

Determining whether the ducts are abnormally enlarged in one or both submandibular glands can be difficult, particularly since there are variations of normal among patients. Generally speaking, normal ducts in the submandibular gland should be no larger than the 1.5 mm in diameter. Symptoms referable to the submandibular glands are often helpful to determine whether the ductal prominence is abnormal. Any asymmetry of the intraglandular submandibular ducts should prompt evaluation for a sialolith, mass, or stricture. A conventional catheter sialogram or MR sialography may be necessary to identify a focal stricture.

In contradistinction to the normal intraglandular submandibular ductal system, visualization of the normal intraglandular parotid ductal system is usually not identified on cross-sectional imaging.

COMPANION CASES

- **Wharton duct sialolith resulting in abnormal submandibular ductal dilation.** A Wharton duct sialolith is a common cause of submandibular duct obstruction and dilation. Sialoliths may be identified on MRI and plain film radiography, but they are best visualized by CT. However, radiolucent sialoliths may be occult by CT and plain film radiography. The etiology of sialoliths is not entirely established, although most likely they arise from a nidus, such as from a focus of desquamated epithelium, bacteria and/or their degradation products, or a foreign body. Calcium-rich salts then form around the nidus. Sialoliths are more commonly associated with the Wharton duct rather than the Stensen duct for several reasons. The saliva produced by the submandibular gland is more alkaline, viscous, and contains more calcium as well as phosphorus, all of which promote the formation of a sialolith. In addition, the Wharton duct distal orifice is smaller than the Stensen duct distal orifice and therefore more likely to trap a sialolith. A sialolith, if obstructive, results in stasis of saliva, destruction of the acini, and parenchymal atrophy with fibrosis.

  Treatment of sialadenitis resulting from a sialolith is initially with oral hydration, sialogogues and gland massage. This treatment serves to provide symptomatic relief as well as promotes extrusion of the sialolith. Antibiotics are also administered if there is an associated active bacterial infection. If a sialolith is located near the ostium, it may be removed with dilation of the orifice. For other sialoliths, such as large, immobile sialoliths, or those located at the gland hilum, transoral removal via a floor of mouth incision has been shown to be effective with high patient satisfaction. Sialoendoscopy has also been shown to be highly effective, with success rates up to 95%. Sialoendoscopy uses a 1 to 2 mm diameter rigid scope that is placed into the duct. There is continuous instillation of saline to maintain duct luminal distension and to provide lubrication. Once the sialolith is visualized, it may be removed by a mini-grasper or a basket. Strictures may also be dilated during this procedure. If removal of a sialolith is not possible with these procedures, then the entire gland may need to be removed.
- **Anterior floor of mouth mass resulting in abnormal bilateral submandibular ductal dilation.** A floor of mouth mass can result in abnormal unilateral or bilateral submandibular ductal system dilation, depending on the location of the tumor. A tumor involving the floor of the mouth may not be readily identified on imaging because of several factors, including artifact from dental amalgam or because the mass is poorly enhancing. Furthermore, if there is obstruction of both submandibular ductal systems by a floor of mouth mass, then the symmetry of the ductal dilation may not alert the radiologist to search for an underlying cause. Thus, identifying submandibular ductal dilation on imaging, even when symmetric, should prompt careful scrutiny of the floor of mouth.
- **Blunt submandibular gland trauma.** Blunt trauma to the submandibular gland or sublingual gland without an accompanying mandibular fracture is rare, as these glands are generally well protected by the mandible. The most common causes of blunt injury to the submandibular glands are motor vehicle collisions, sports injuries, strangulation, and direct trauma during an altercation. The trauma may result in surrounding edema, hematoma, or a sialocele. On imaging, multiple clefts that often extend to the cortical surface of the gland will be visualized, and there are frequently ancillary signs of trauma, such as periglandular edema or hematoma formation.

Normal intraglandular submandibular ducts on CT

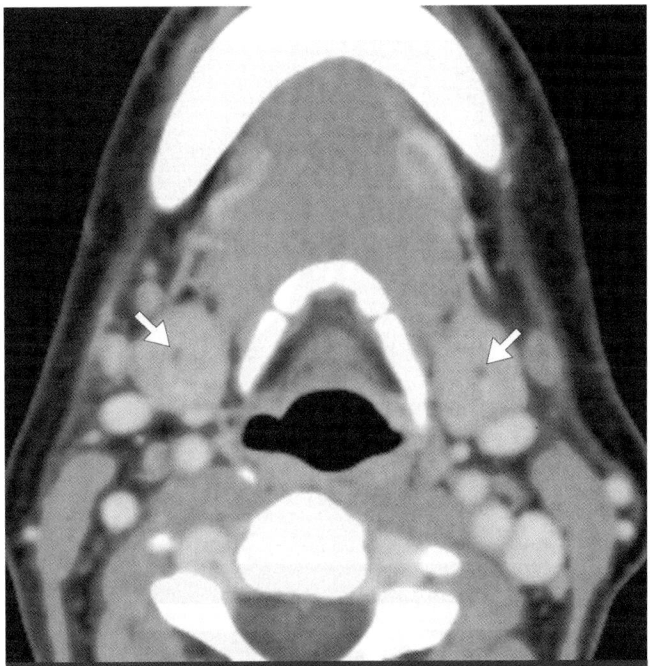

A

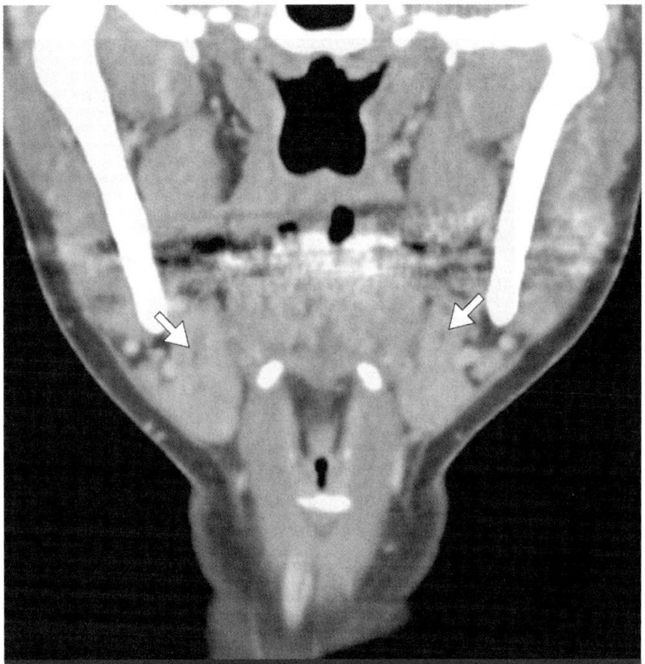

B

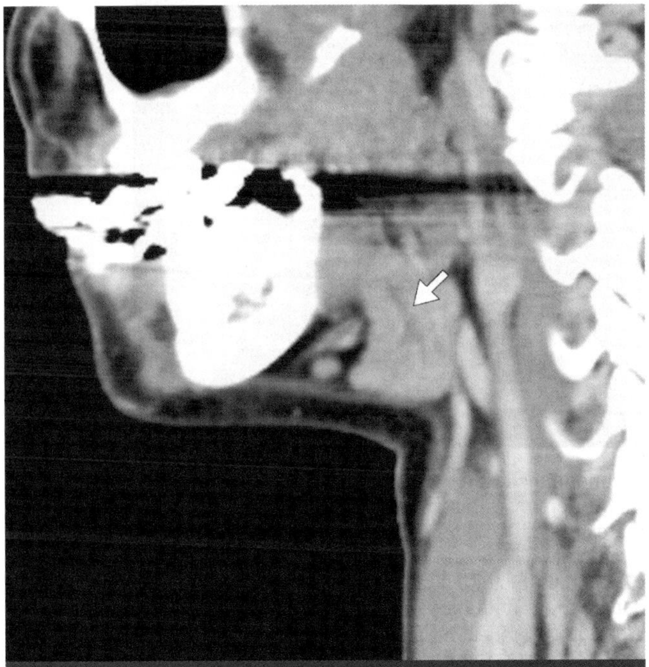

C

Axial (**A**), coronal reformatted (**B**), and sagittal reformatted (**C**) postcontrast CT images through the submandibular glands demonstrate conspicuous bilateral intraglandular submandibular ducts in an asymptomatic patient (arrows, **A-C**). There were no sialoliths or masses identified along the course of either Wharton duct. The bilateral, symmetric appearance of the ducts, absence of an obstructing sialolith/mass, and absence of symptoms in this patient are compatible with incidentally visualized and normal submandibular ducts.

CASE 14 Submandibular gland resection

Indications for a submandibular gland resection include chronic sialadenitis (usually secondary to sialodocolithiasis) and to remove a submandibular gland tumor. Occasionally, a submandibular gland is resected during a neck dissection in order to gain access to pathologic lymph nodes. The patient is usually asymptomatic following removal of one submandibular gland. Scar tissue or fat typically occupies the space vacated by the resected submandibular gland.

Submandibular gland resection

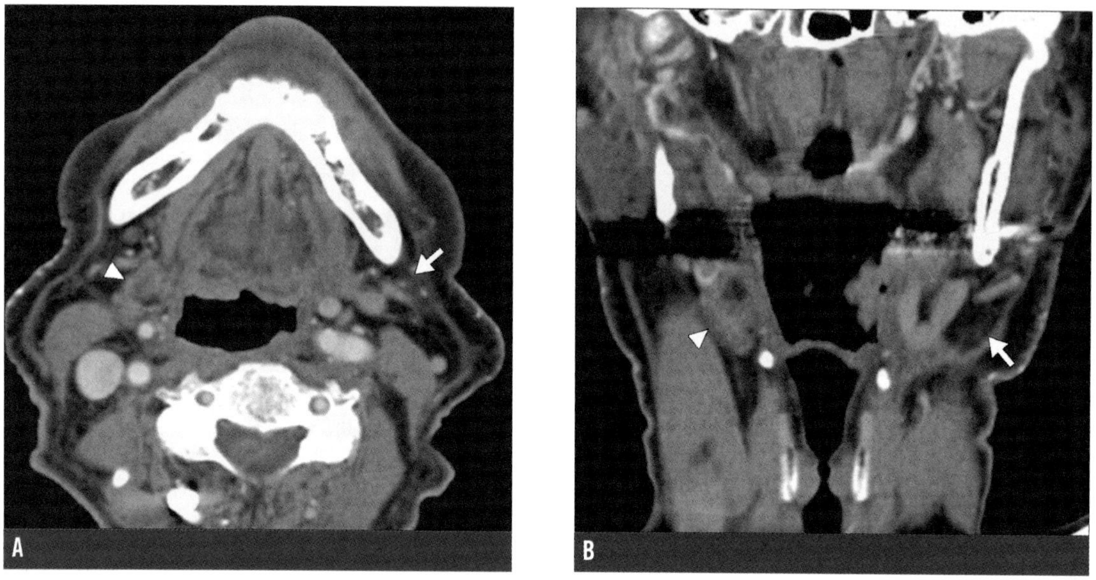

Axial (**A**) and coronal reformatted (**B**) contrast-enhanced CT images through the level of the submandibular glands demonstrate an atrophic right submandibular gland (arrowheads, **A**, **B**) and an absent left submandibular gland (arrows, **A**, **B**). The left submandibular gland was resected because it contained a carcinoma ex pleomorphic adenoma. Metallic surgical clips may or may not be utilized during a submandibular gland resection. In this case, no metallic surgical clips were used.

Submandibular gland resection

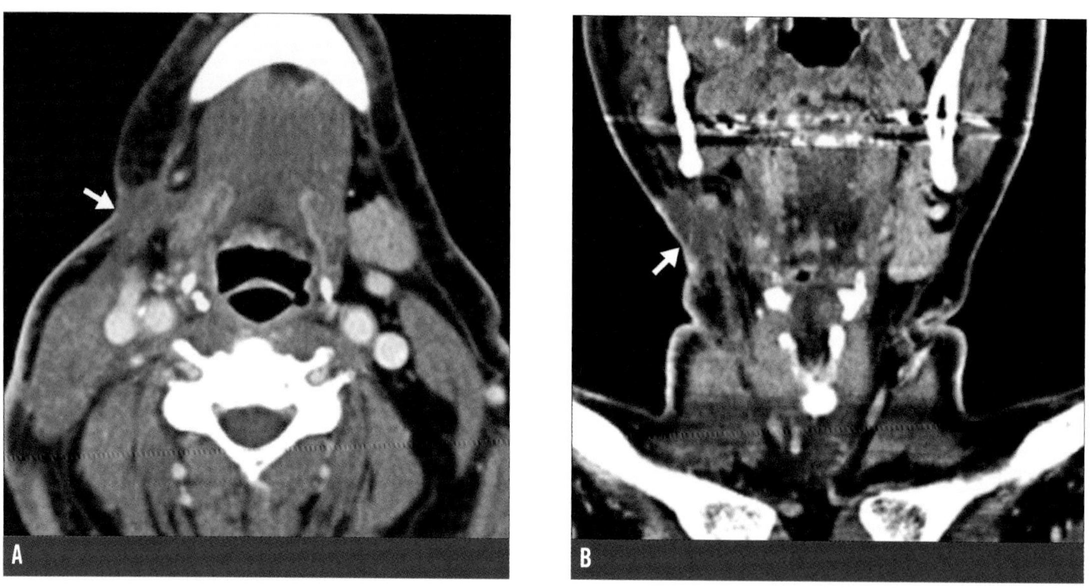

Different patient. Axial (**A**) and coronal reformatted (**B**) contrast-enhanced CT images through the level of the submandibular glands demonstrate surgical resection of the right submandibular gland with scar tissue in the resection bed (arrows, **A**, **B**).

CASE 15 Bartholin duct of the sublingual gland

There are approximately 20 individual ducts (named the ducts of Rivinus) that drain the sublingual gland. These ducts empty separately into the floor of the mouth along an elevated crest referred to as the sublingual fold. Occasionally, some of these ducts may form a single duct, termed the Bartholin duct, which drains a portion of the sublingual gland and joins with the ipsilateral Wharton duct. The development of a sialolith in a Wharton duct is not uncommon, but this rarely occurs in a Bartholin duct. However, if a Bartholin duct is present, a sialolith located distal to where the Bartholin duct joins the Wharton duct may result in sialadenitis affecting the ipsilateral sublingual and submandibular glands.

COMPANION CASES

- **Accessory submandibular duct.** Typically, ducts within the submandibular gland merge near the submandibular gland hilum to form the Wharton duct. Occasionally, an accessory submandibular duct draining a portion of the submandibular gland joins the Wharton duct after it exits the hilum. An accessory submandibular duct is differentiated from a Bartholin duct because a Bartholin duct, when present, drains the sublingual gland, not the submandibular gland.
- **Normal submandibular sialogram.** This case is provided to serve as a comparison for the Bartholin duct and accessory submandibular duct sialogram cases.

Bartholin duct of the sublingual gland

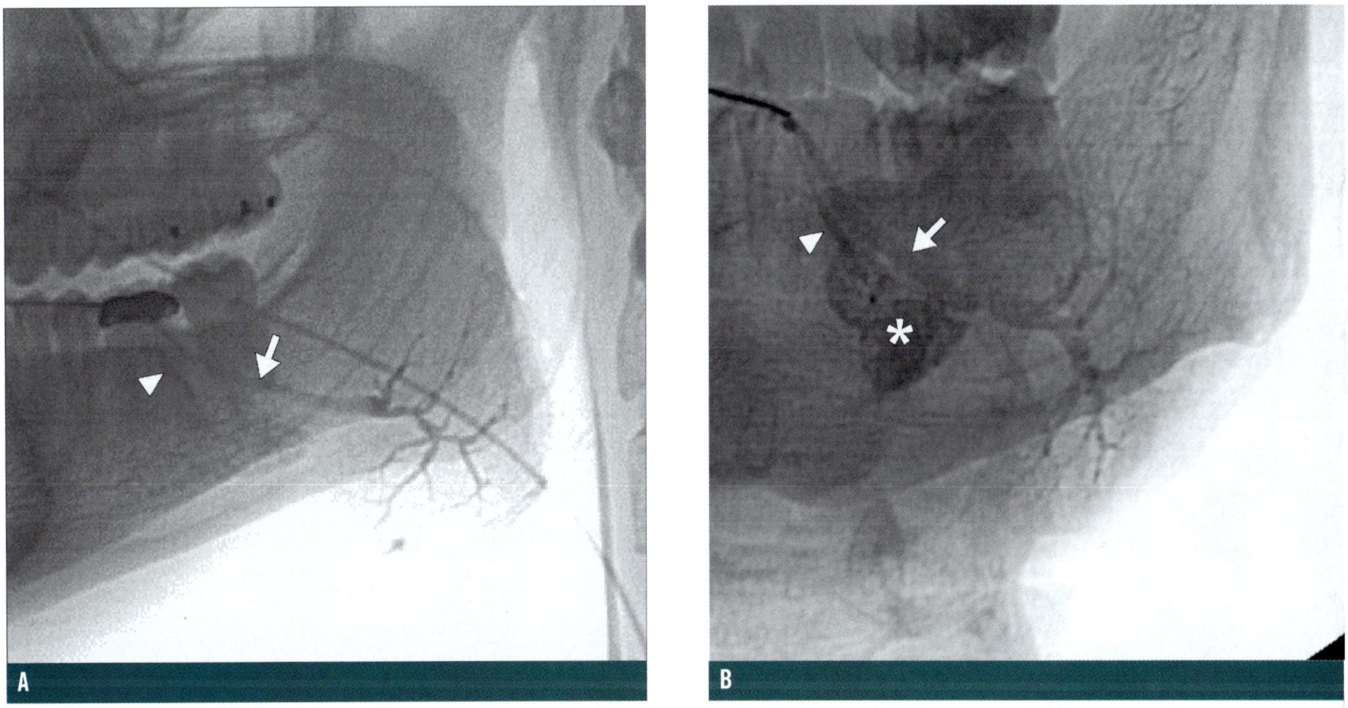

Lateral (**A**) and AP (**B**) fluoroscopic images from a left submandibular gland sialogram demonstrate a small duct consistent with a Bartholin duct (arrowheads, **A**, **B**) juxtaposed to the normal left Wharton duct (arrows, **A**, **B**). Image **B** demonstrates the normal union of the left Bartholin duct with the distal aspect of the left Wharton duct. Image **B** was obtained following a larger contrast bolus and reveals contrast opacifying the left sublingual gland (asterisk, **B**).

Presumed Bartholin duct of the sublingual gland

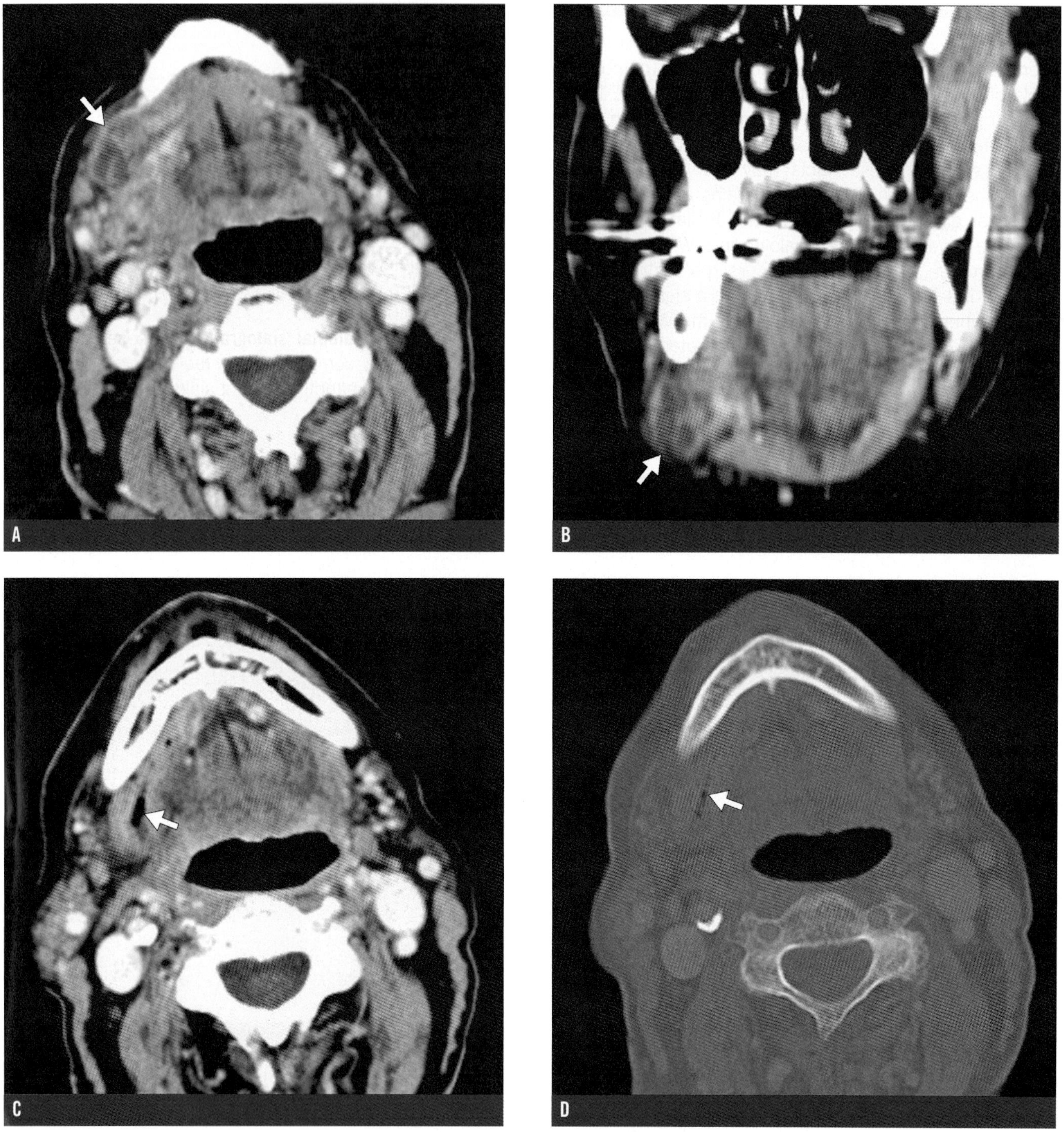

Different patient. Axial (**A**) and coronal reformatted (**B**) postcontrast CT images through the oral cavity demonstrate an enlarged and inflamed right sublingual gland herniating through a right mylohyoid defect, compatible with a boutonnière deformity (see Chapter 5 for discussion of boutonnière deformities). Postcontrast axial CT images through the right submandibular gland viewed with a soft tissue window (**C**) and bone window (**D**) demonstrate an edematous, hyperenhancing right submandibular gland with air in the right submandibular ductal system (arrows, **C**, **D**). The combination of an inflamed right sublingual gland and right submandibular gland suggests that a Bartholin duct exists between the right Wharton duct and the right sublingual gland. While speculative, the air within the right Wharton duct may have been related to a preexisting sialolith that had extruded prior to this examination.

Companion case: Accessory submandibular duct

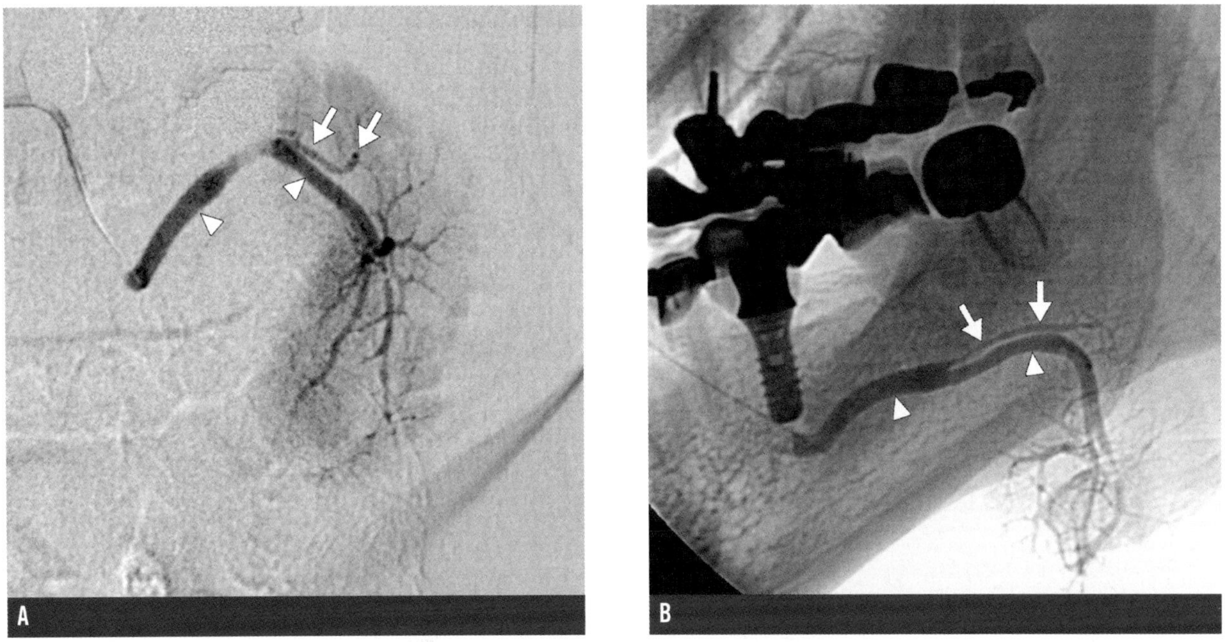

A digitally subtracted AP fluoroscopic image (**A**) and an unsubtracted lateral fluoroscopic image (**B**) from a left submandibular sialogram. There is an incidental small accessory submandibular duct (arrows, **A**, **B**) draining the superior aspect of the left submandibular gland. This accessory duct joins the Wharton duct (arrowheads, **A**, **B**) at its mid portion.

Companion case: Normal submandibular sialogram

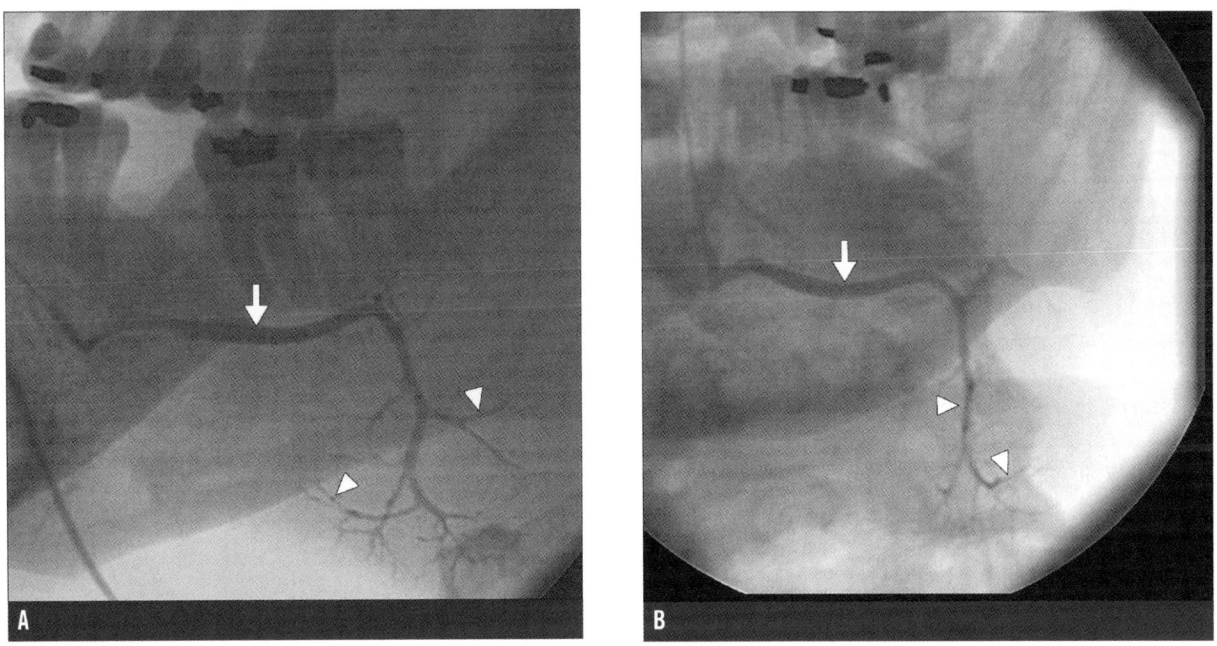

Lateral (**A**) and AP (**B**) fluoroscopic images from a right submandibular gland sialogram demonstrate a normal submandibular intraglandular ductal system (arrowheads, **A**, **B**) and a normal Wharton duct (arrows, **A**, **B**). Neither a Bartholin duct or an accessory submandibular duct are present in this case.

REFERENCES

Baurmash HD. Endoscopic technique for the diagnosis and treatment of obstructive salivary gland diseases. *J Oral Maxillofac Surg.* 1999;57:1401-1402.

Som PM, Curtin HD. *Head and Neck Imaging.* 4th ed. St. Louis, MO: Mosby Inc; 2003.

CASE 16 Sublingual gland aplasia

Similar to other salivary glands, the sublingual gland may be congenitally absent. Absence of a single sublingual gland is generally of no clinical significance. However, a normal or hypertrophied contralateral sublingual gland, or hypertrophy of the submandibular glands, may be occur in this setting and be mistaken for a salivary gland mass or sialadenitis. Fat occupies the location of the absent sublingual gland.

Sublingual gland aplasia

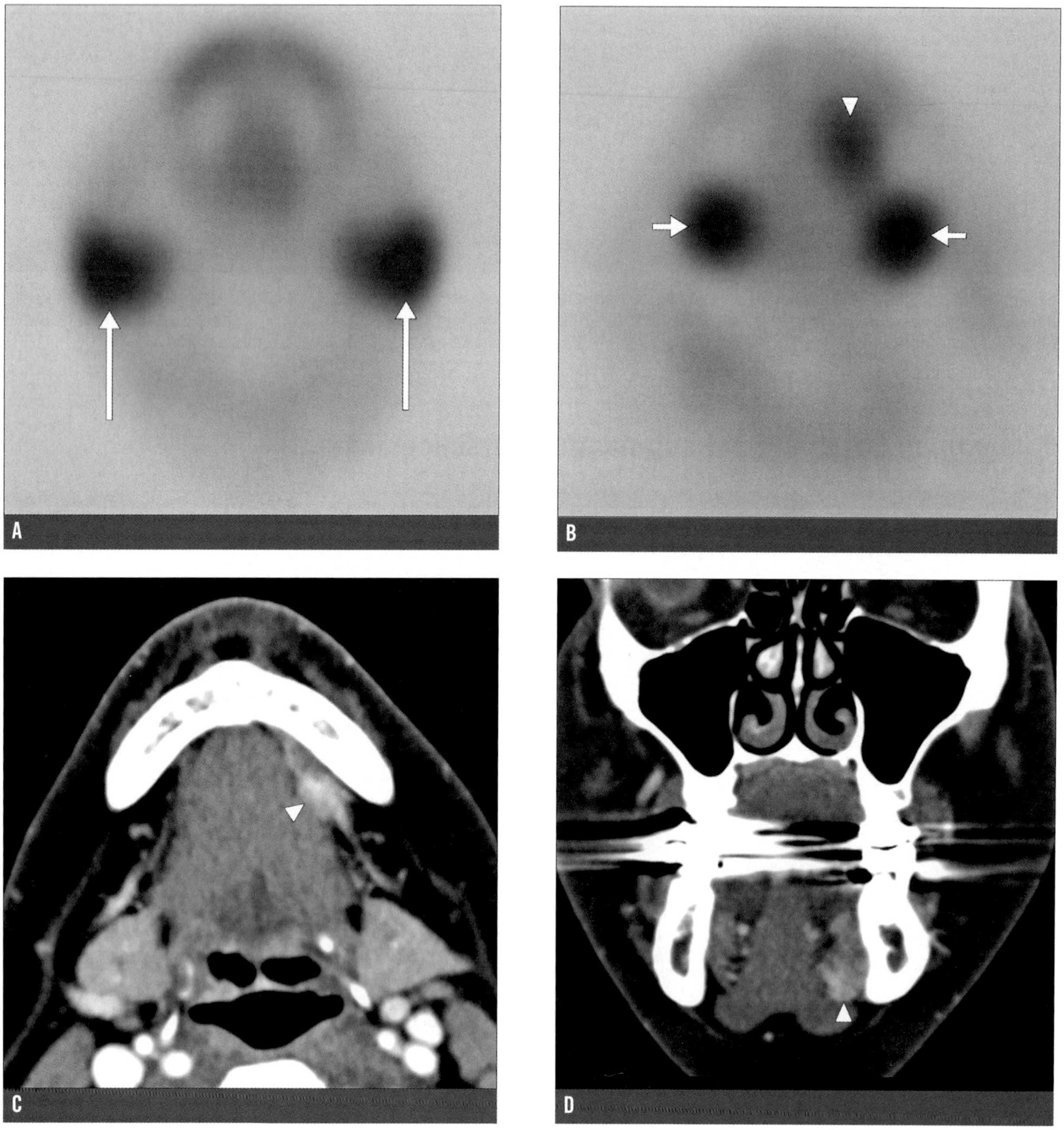

Axial images from a PET scan (**A**, **B**) demonstrate normal, symmetric metabolic activity within the parotid glands (long arrows, **A**) and the submandibular glands (short arrows, **B**). However, image **B** demonstrates asymmetric uptake within the left anterior floor of mouth (arrowhead, **B**) which was interpreted as a possible floor of mouth mass. Axial (**C**) and coronal reformatted (**D**) postcontrast CT images of the same patient demonstrate that the left floor of mouth uptake represents normal left sublingual gland (arrowheads, **C**, **D**) and is asymmetric because of the congenital absence of the right sublingual gland.

Embryologically, the major salivary glands develop from the first and second branchial arches. The mesenchyme divides the major salivary glands into lobules which ultimately form the glands. The sublingual glands form during the ninth week of gestation and are the last of the major salivary glands to form.

When one of the sublingual glands is hypertrophied, it may be accompanied by ipsilateral submandibular gland and/or contralateral sublingual gland hypoplasia or rarely aplasia. The hypertrophy of the gland is likely reflective of a compensatory hypertrophy. While this hypertrophy is incidental, it can present clinically as a palpable floor of mouth mass or may be mistaken for a tumor on imaging.

COMPANION CASES

- **Ranula**. A ranula is a mucous retention cyst that primarily arises from a sublingual gland, although the term has also been used when this lesion arises from a minor salivary gland. Two types of ranulas are described, the simple ranula and diving (also called plunging) ranula. The simple ranula is a cyst that contains an intact epithelial lining. A diving ranula is a ruptured cyst that does not contain an intact epithelial lining and can be viewed as a pseudocyst. While the distinction between these two types is only definitively made at pathology, a simple ranula resides entirely above the mylohyoid muscle and at least a portion of a the diving ranula extends below the mylohyoid.
- **Sublingual gland adenoid cystic carcinoma.** The smaller the major salivary gland affected, the greater the probability that a mass arising from that gland is malignant. Specifically, there is a 70% to 85% probability that a sublingual gland mass is malignant, an approximately 40% to 50% probability that a submandibular gland mass is malignant, and only a 20% to 30% probability that a parotid gland mass is malignant. Adenoid cystic carcinoma accounts for approximately 15% of all sublingual gland tumors and represents the most common malignancy of the sublingual gland. Please refer to Case 1 from this chapter for further discussion regarding adenoid cystic carcinoma.

Sublingual gland hypertrophy

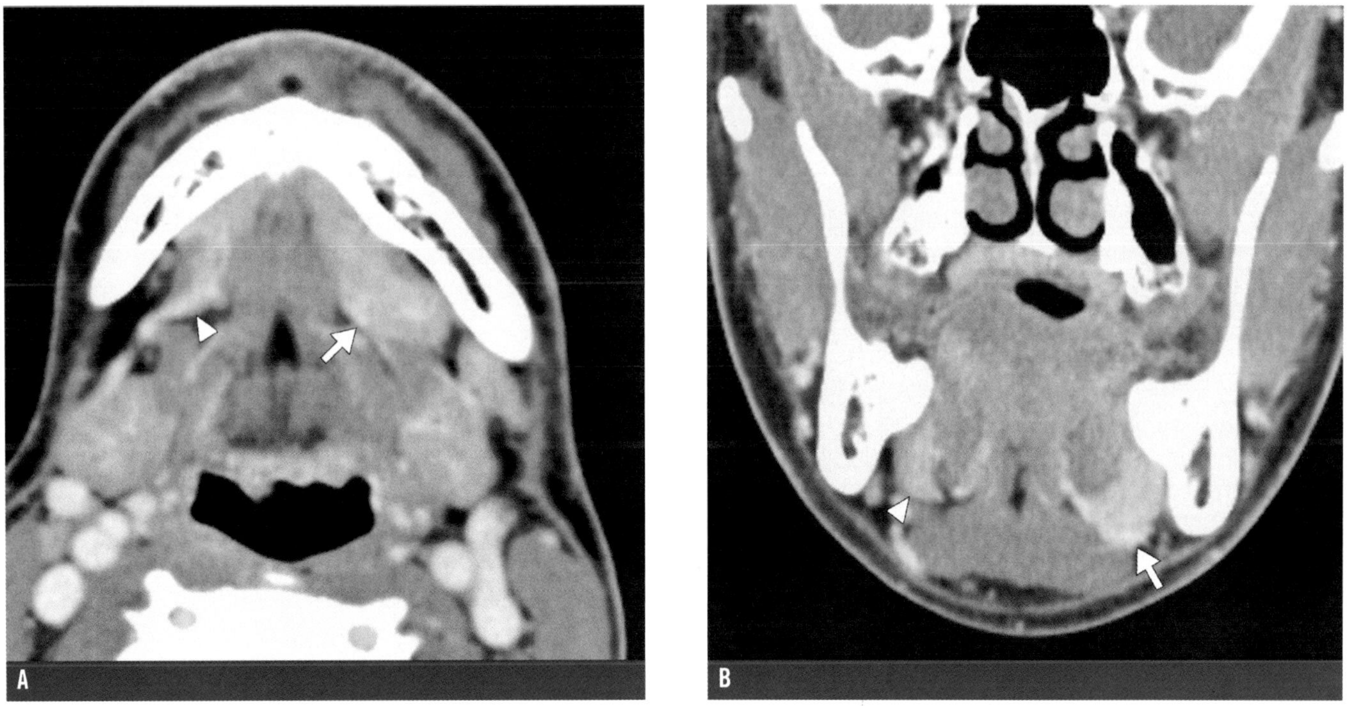

Axial (**A**) and coronal reformatted (**B**) contrast-enhanced CT images through the level of the sublingual glands demonstrate an incidental, asymmetrically enlarged left sublingual gland (arrows, **A**, **B**) relative to the right sublingual gland (arrowheads, **A**, **B**).

Sublingual gland hypertrophy

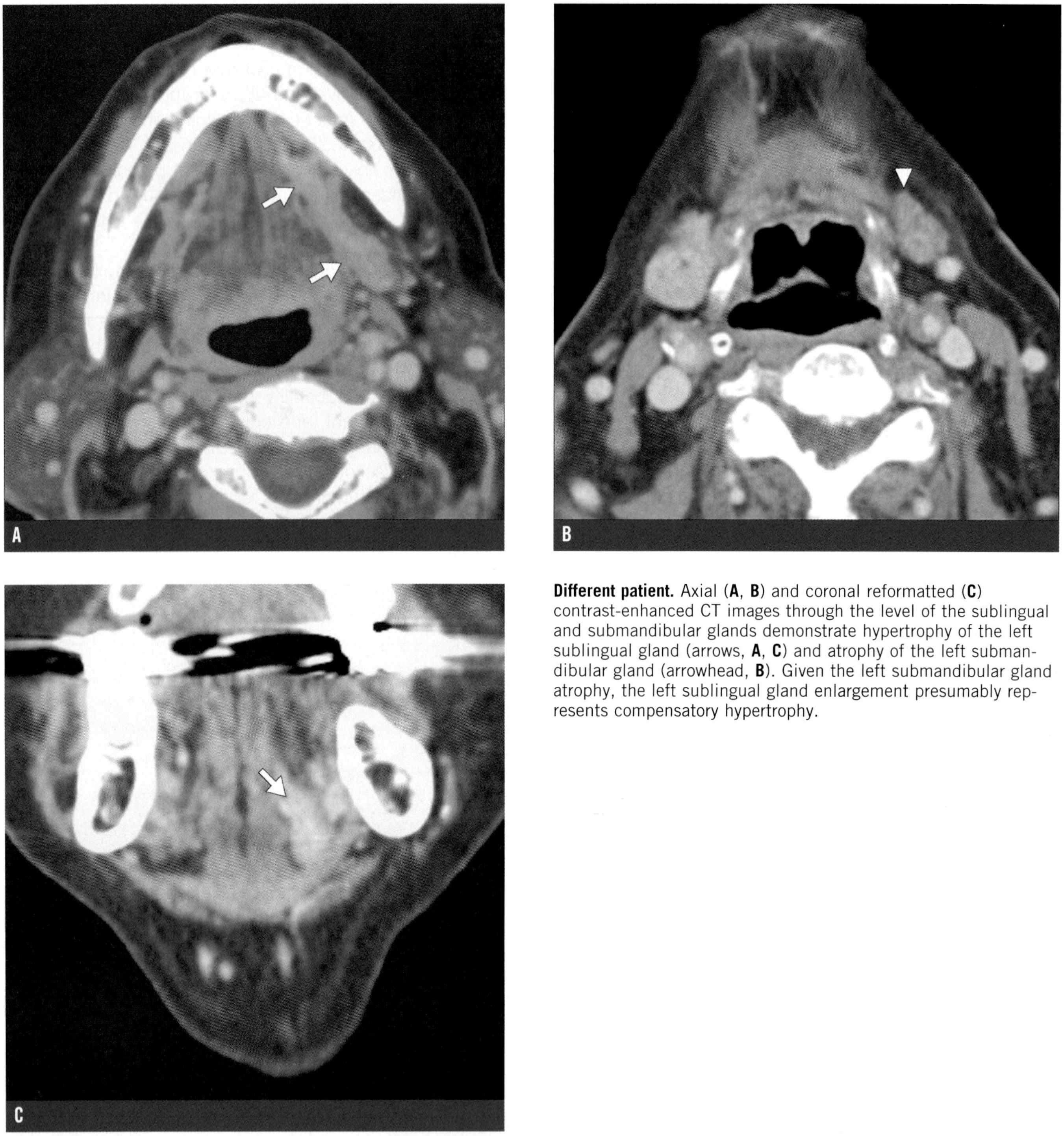

Different patient. Axial (**A**, **B**) and coronal reformatted (**C**) contrast-enhanced CT images through the level of the sublingual and submandibular glands demonstrate hypertrophy of the left sublingual gland (arrows, **A**, **C**) and atrophy of the left submandibular gland (arrowhead, **B**). Given the left submandibular gland atrophy, the left sublingual gland enlargement presumably represents compensatory hypertrophy.

Sublingual gland hypertrophy

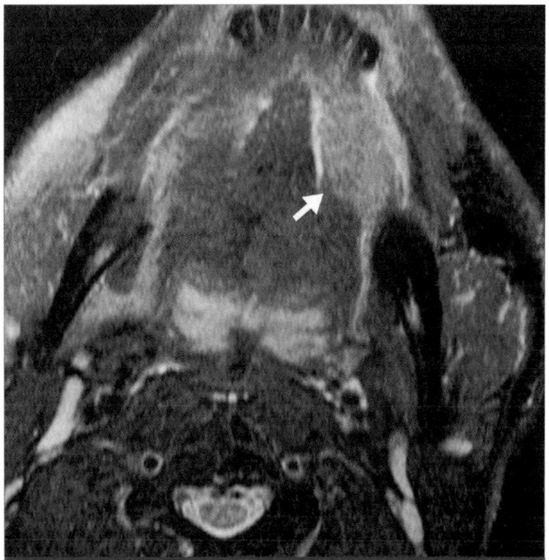

A

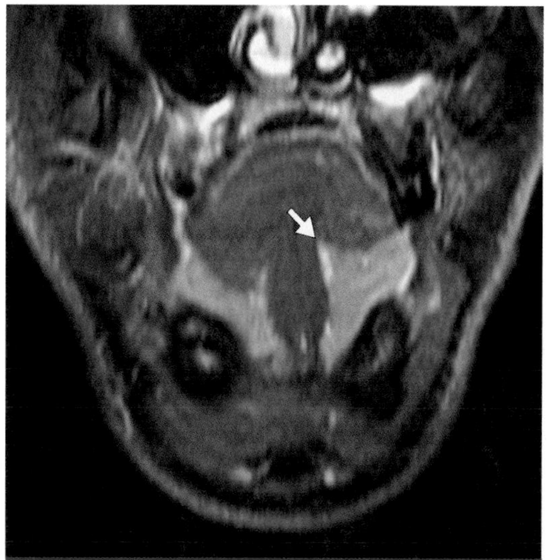

B

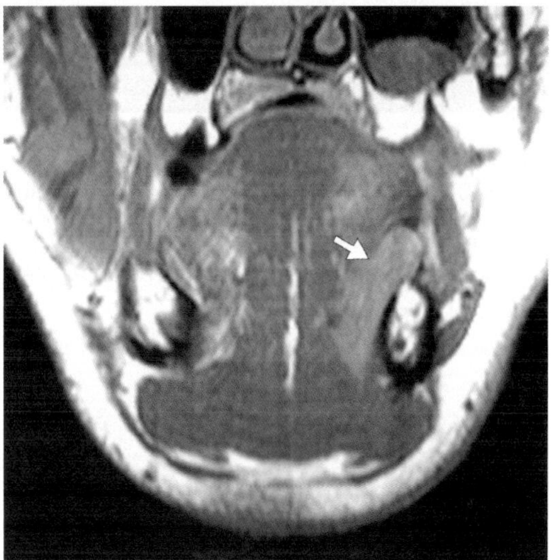

C

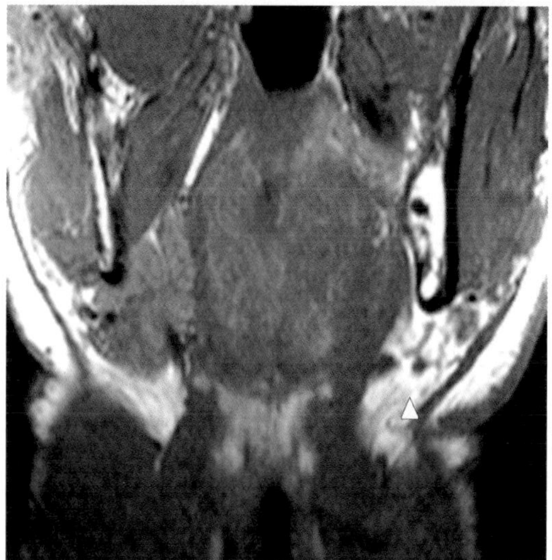

D

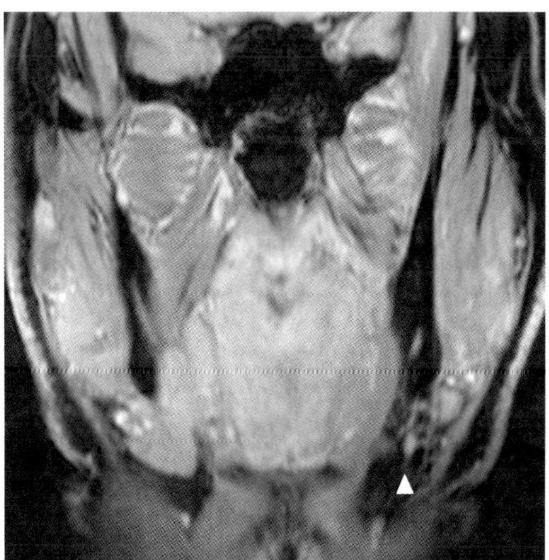

E

Different patient. Axial T2 with fat suppression (**A**) and coronal T2 with fat suppression (**B**) as well as coronal T1 (**C**) MR images through the sublingual glands demonstrate asymmetric hypertrophy of the left sublingual gland (arrows, **A-C**) compared to the right. Coronal T1 (**D**) and postcontrast coronal T1 with fat suppression (**E**) MR images through the submandibular glands demonstrate marked atrophy of the left submandibular gland (arrowheads, **D**, **E**). The left sublingual gland hypertrophy may represent compensatory enlargement secondary to the left submandibular gland atrophy.

Companion case: Ranula

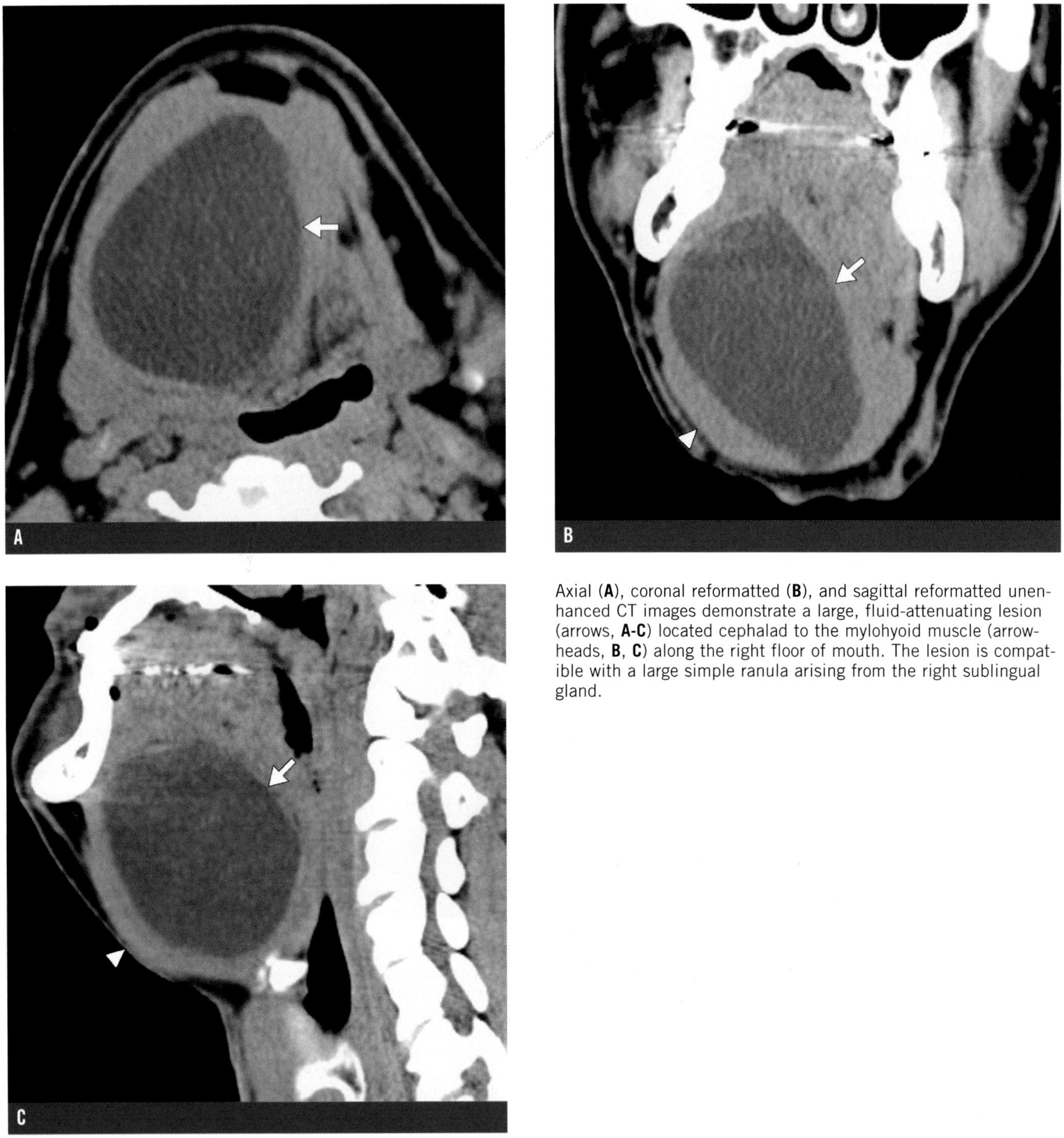

Axial (**A**), coronal reformatted (**B**), and sagittal reformatted unenhanced CT images demonstrate a large, fluid-attenuating lesion (arrows, **A-C**) located cephalad to the mylohyoid muscle (arrowheads, **B**, **C**) along the right floor of mouth. The lesion is compatible with a large simple ranula arising from the right sublingual gland.

Companion case: Sublingual gland adenoid cystic carcinoma

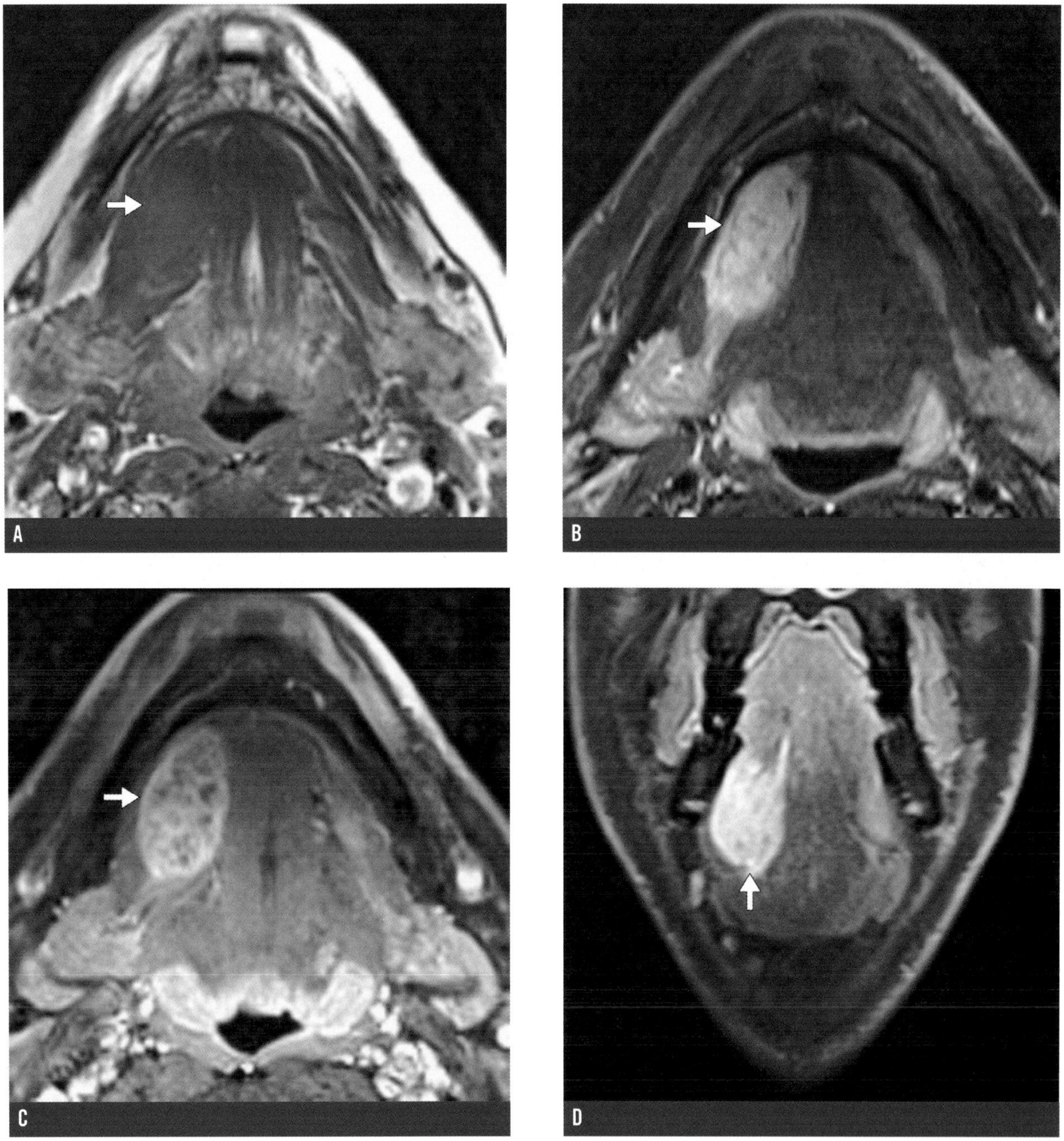

Axial T1 (**A**), axial T2 with fat suppression (**B**), contrast-enhanced axial T1 with fat suppression (**C**), and contrast-enhanced coronal T1 with fat suppression (**D**) MR images demonstrate a T2 hyperintense and enhancing mass involving the right sublingual gland (arrows, **A-D**). The heterogeneous appearance, particularly on image **C**, is more compatible with a mass rather than benign sublingual gland hyperplasia. Additionally, the anterior and posterior margins of this lesion are rounded which is more typical of a mass, rather than having tapered margins which is more commonly present with a normal sublingual gland, including those that are hypertrophied. This mass represented a sublingual gland adenoid cystic carcinoma at pathology.

REFERENCES

Macdonald AJ, Salzman KL, Harnsberger HR. Giant ranula of the neck: differentiation from cystic hygroma. AJNR Am J Neuroradiol. 2003;24(4):757-761.

Silvers AR, Som PM. Salivary glands. Radiol *Clin North Am.* September 1998;36(5):941-966.

Som PM and Curtin HD. Head and *Neck Imaging.* 4th ed. St. Louis, MO: Mosby Inc; 2003.

Srinivasan A, Moyer JS, Mukherji SK. Unilateral submandibular gland aplasia associated with ipsilateral sublingual gland hypertrophy. *AJNR Am J Neuroradiol.* November-December 2006;27(10): 2214-2216.

Yousem DM, Kraut MA, Chalian AA. Major salivary gland imaging. *Radiology.* July 2000;216(1):19-29.

CASE 18 Normal thyroid gland septa

The thyroid gland is surrounded by a thin capsule of connective tissue. This capsule extends into the substance of the gland where it forms numerous septa that surround lobules. These septa may be visualized on CT, particularly when the CT examination is performed without contrast.

COMPANION CASE

- **Air dissecting the thyroid gland septa.** Occasionally, penetrating injuries, such as from a knife wound, may result in air which dissects the thyroid gland septa, as is shown in the case provided. While this likely does not result in any permanent damage to the gland, the impact of dissecting air into the gland is not known given the paucity of literature discussing this topic.

Normal thyroid gland septa

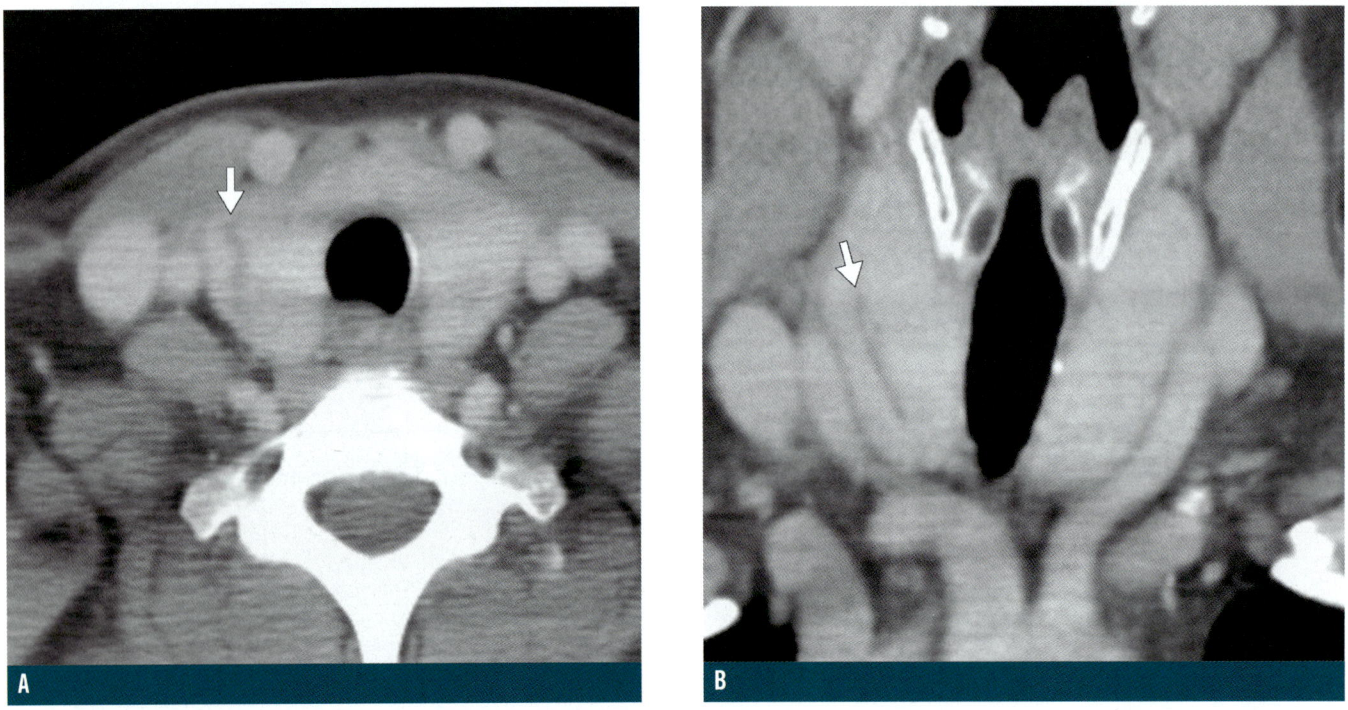

Axial (**A**) and coronal reformatted (**B**) contrast-enhanced CT images demonstrate a linear focus of hypoattenuation within the right thyroid lobe directed in AP and CC directions (arrows, **A**, **B**). This finding represents an incidentally thick but normal thyroid septum.

Normal thyroid gland septa

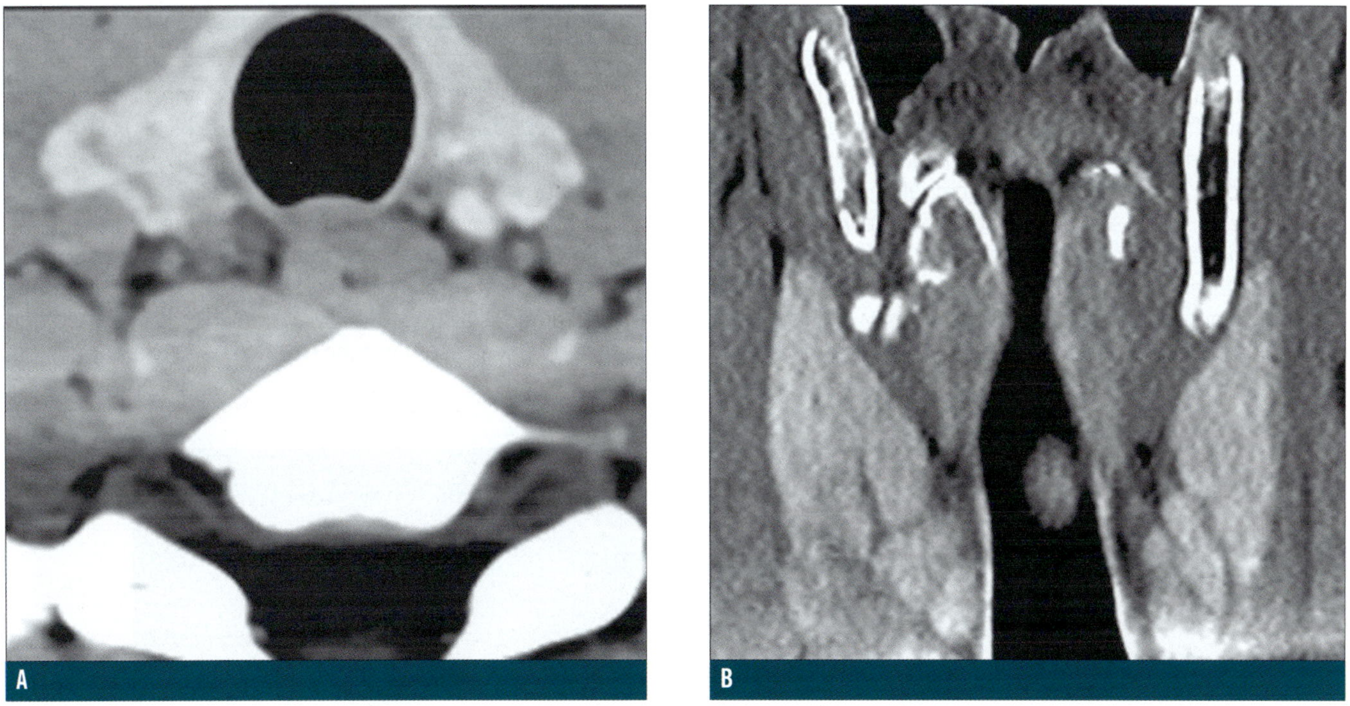

Different patient. Axial (**A**) and coronal reformatted (**B**) unenhanced CT images demonstrate pronounced incidental septa throughout the thyroid lobes.

Companion case: Air dissecting the thyroid gland septa

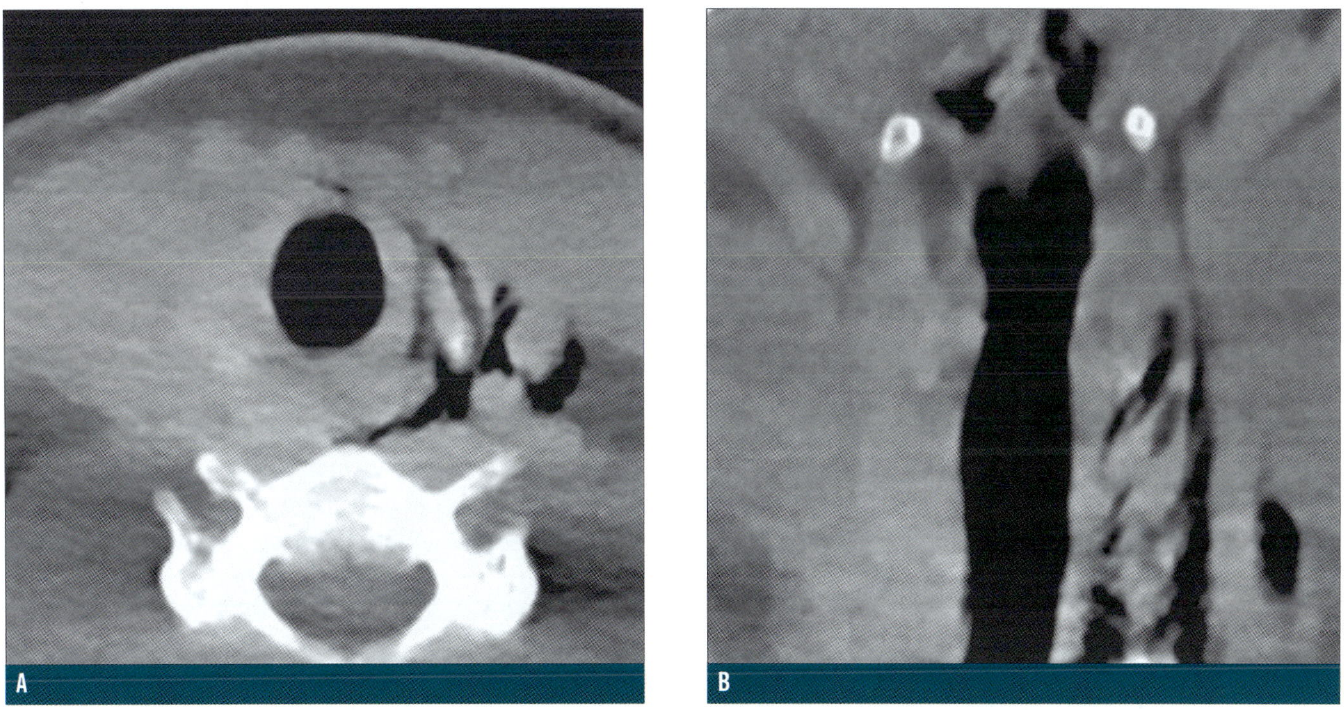

Axial (**A**) and coronal reformatted (**B**) unenhanced CT images of a patient who was stabbed in the neck shortly before this imaging study demonstrate air dissecting the left thyroid lobe septa. This resolved on a follow-up CT study performed 1 day later (not shown).

REFERENCE

Gray H. *Anatomy of the Human Body.* Philadelphia, PA: Lea & Febiger; 1918; Bartleby.com, 2000.

CASE 19 Thyroid gland pyramidal lobe

The pyramidal lobe is a vestigial remnant of thyroid tissue which arises from the caudal end of the thyroglossal duct tract. This normal variant often resides at the midline and is attached to the isthmus, but it may also be attached to either thyroid lobe. Various shapes of a pyramidal lobe have been described, including pyramid, string, nodule, and an inverted Y shape. Often, the pyramidal lobe thyroid tissue is nonfunctioning; therefore, it may not be seen on scintigraphic imaging. However, the pyramidal lobe tissue may become activated if functioning thyroid tissue is removed. In this scenario, elevated levels of thyroid-stimulating hormone may result in pyramidal lobe hypertrophy.

If a total thyroidectomy is planned, then the surgeon should be made aware of the presence of a pyramidal lobe preoperatively in order to ensure that the entire thyroid gland is removed. A pyramidal lobe is common and reported to be present in more than 50% of the population.

Thyroid gland pyramidal lobe

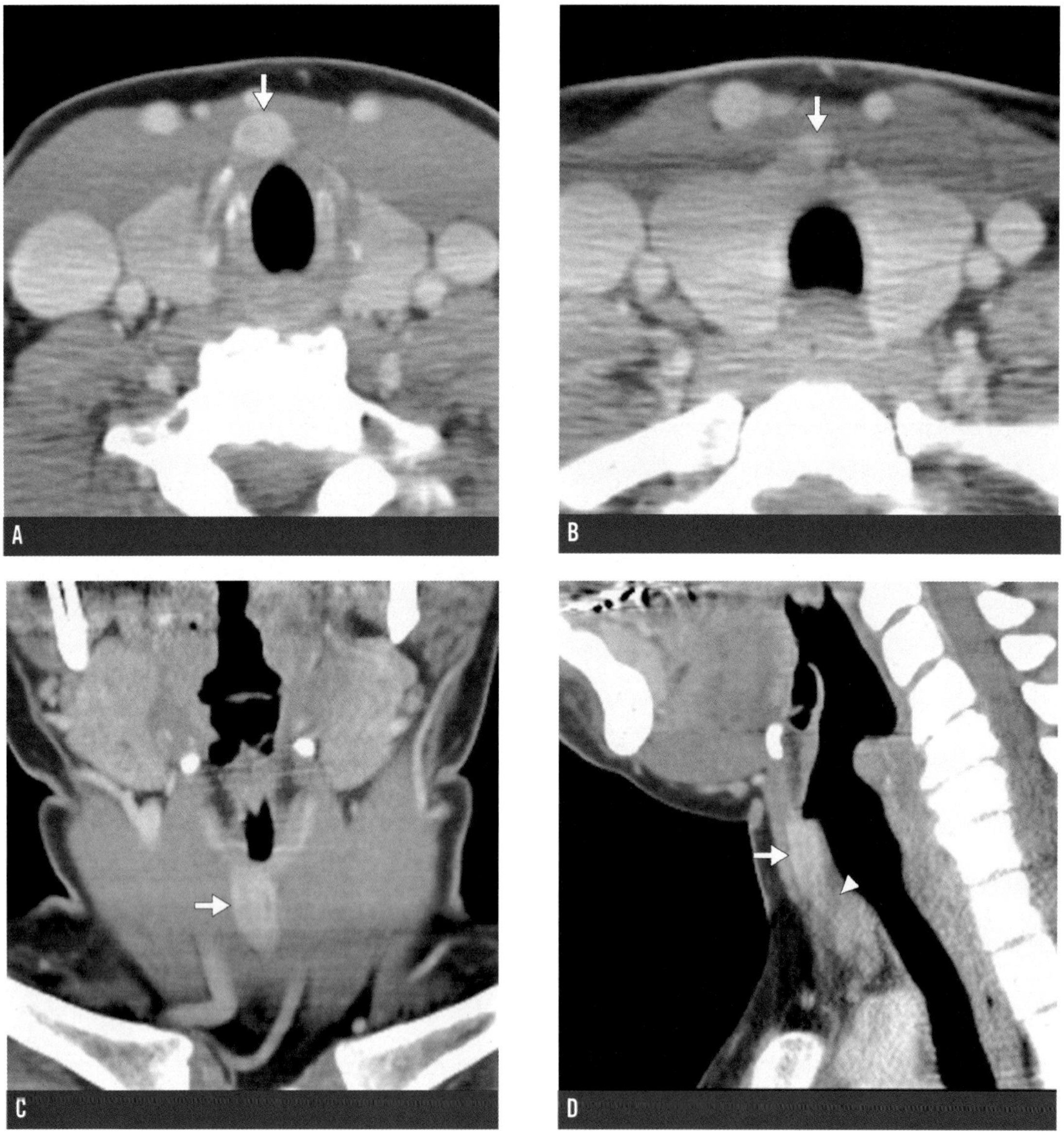

A contrast-enhanced axial CT image through the level of the thyroid gland (**A**) demonstrates oval-shaped, hyperdense soft tissue anterior to the trachea at the midline (arrow, **A**). The hyperdense soft tissue is the same density as the adjacent thyroid lobes. A contrast-enhanced axial CT image immediately caudal to image **A** (**B**) demonstrates that the hyperdense soft tissue is contiguous with the thyroid isthmus and compatible with a pyramidal lobe (arrow, **B**). Coronal reformatted (**C**) and sagittal reformatted (**D**) contrast-enhanced CT images from the same study also demonstrate the pyramidal lobe (arrows, **C**, **D**). The caudal margin of the pyramidal lobe is contiguous with the thyroid gland via a subtle small stalk (arrowhead, **D**).

Thyroid gland pyramidal lobe

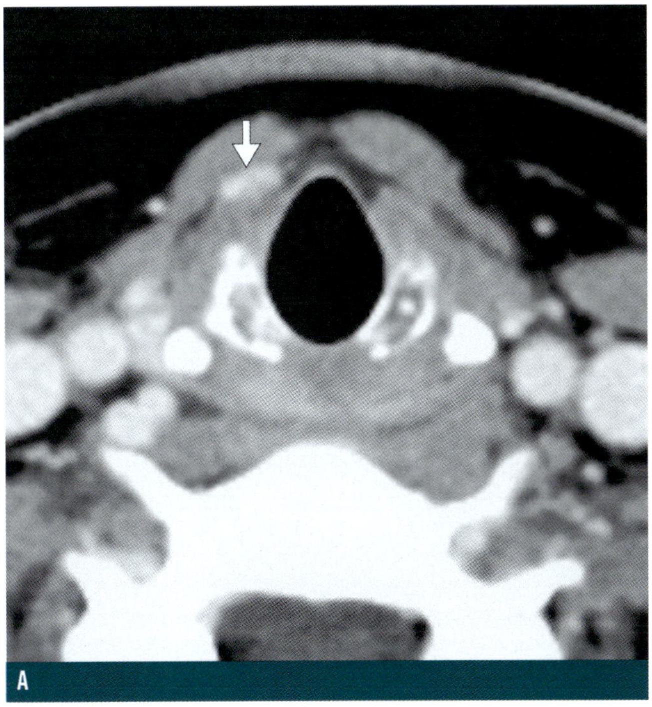

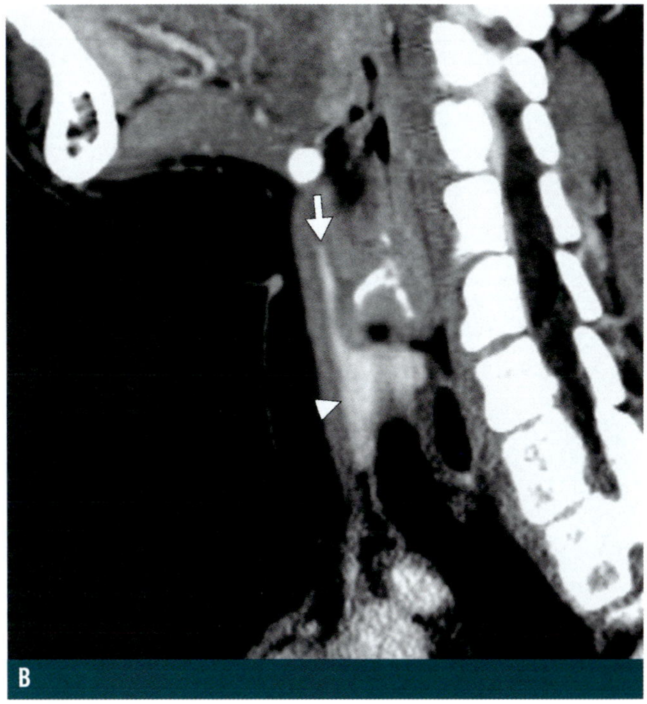

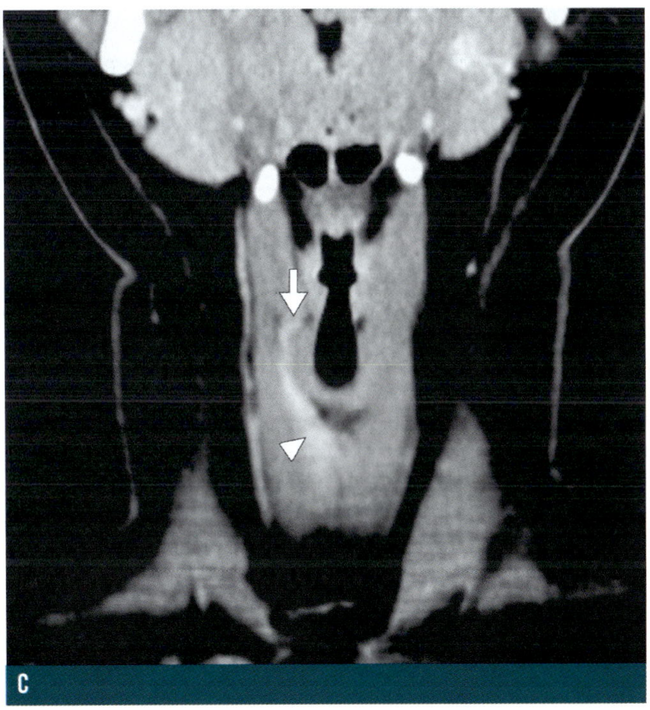

Different patient. Axial (**A**), sagittal reformatted (**B**), and coronal reformatted (**C**) contrast-enhanced CT images through the level of the thyroid. Image **A** demonstrates a small focus of hyperdense soft tissue to the right of midline and anterior to the trachea (arrow, **A**). Images **B** and **C** demonstrate the hyperdense tissue to be linear in morphology (arrows, **B**, **C**) and contiguous with the adjacent thyroid gland (arrowheads, **B**, **C**), compatible with an eccentrically located pyramidal lobe.

Thyroid gland pyramidal lobe

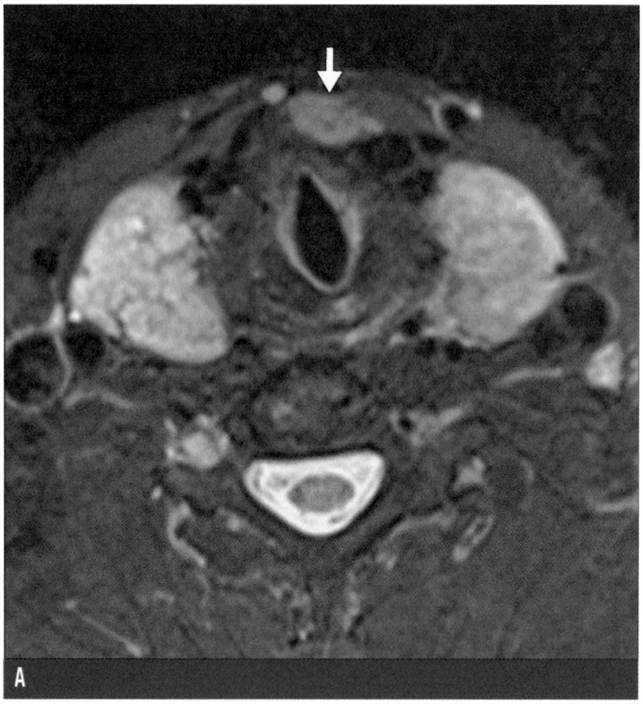

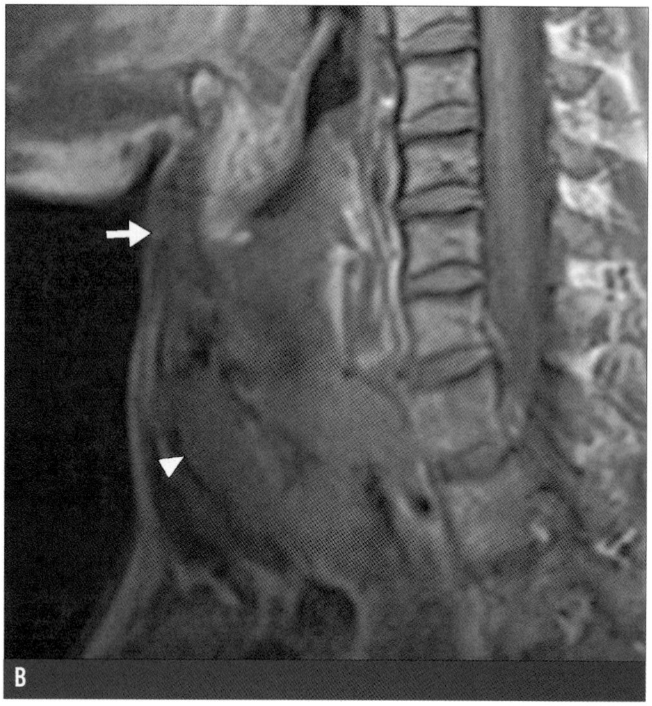

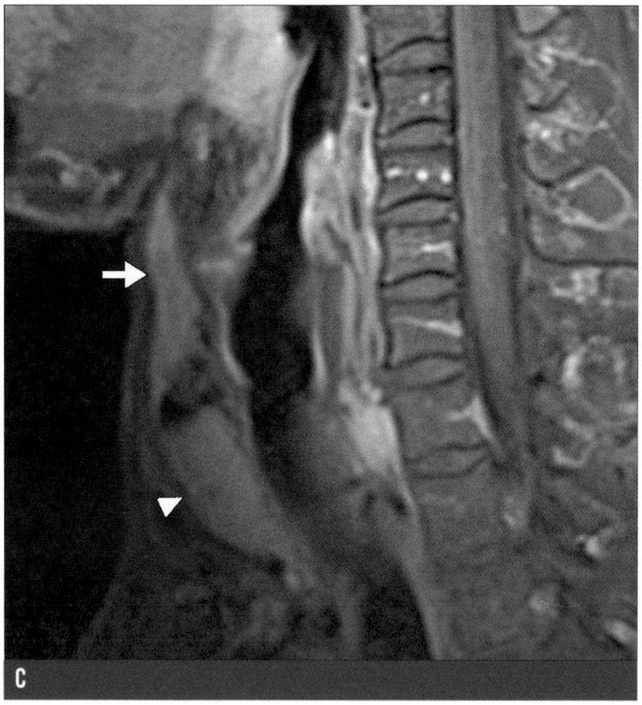

Different patient. Fat-suppressed axial T2 (**A**), sagittal T1 (**B**), and contrast-enhanced fat-suppressed sagittal T1 (**C**) MR images demonstrate the MRI appearance of a pyramidal lobe (arrows, **A-C**) emanating from the remainder of the thyroid gland (arrowheads, **B**, **C**).

REFERENCES

Braun EM, Windisch G, Wolf G, Hausleitner L, Anderhuber F. The pyramidal lobe: clinical anatomy and its importance in thyroid surgery. *Surg Radiol Anat.* 2007;29:21-27.

Izenstark JL, Forsaith AL, Horwitz NH. The pyramidal lobe in thyroid imaging. *J Nucl Med.* 1969;10(8):519-524.

CASE 20 Zuckerkandl tubercle (posteriorly directed pedunculated thyroid tissue)

A Zuckerkandl tubercle (ZT) represents a normal posteriorly directed protuberance of the thyroid gland that arises from the posterolateral aspect of the thyroid lobe. Statistically, a ZT more commonly arises from the right lobe of the thyroid compared to the left. There are several normal variations of a ZT, including posteriorly projected fullness of one or both thyroid lobes, focal posterior penduncluated thyroid tissue with a discrete intervening stalk, and a focal retroesophageal course. The ipsilateral common carotid artery may or may not abut the lateral margin of the intervening stalk with the posterior pedunculated variety. A ZT may serve as a landmark for the surgeon, as the recurrent laryngeal nerve consistently resides in the tracheoesophageal groove immediately medial to a ZT. A ZT is also often located adjacent to the ipsilateral superior parathyroid gland.

COMPANION CASES

- **Zuckerkandl tubercle thyroid nodule with vocal cord paralysis.** While a ZT is a normal finding, because it represents thyroid tissue, it is subject to the same pathology as the remainder of the thyroid gland. Given the proximity of a ZT to the tracheoesophageal groove, and thus the recurrent laryngeal nerve, a lesion involving a ZT may result in ipsilateral vocal cord paralysis.
- **Parathyroid adenoma.** The current radiotracer of choice for parathyroid scintigraphy is ^{99m}Tc-sestamibi. The range of sensitivity for detecting a parathyroid adenoma with ^{99m}Tc-sestamibi parathyroid scintigraphy has been reported to be between 50%-90% and is most sensitive if performed with single-photon emission computed tomography (SPECT). There is also improved localization of a parathyroid adenoma with the addition of SPECT. False positives most commonly arise from radiotracer accumulation within thyroid adenomas, but this may also occur with thyroiditis, thyroid carcinoma, and regional pathologic lymph nodes.

  A relatively new CT technique, described as a "4D CT technique," may also be used to diagnose a parathyroid adenoma. The efficacy of this technique is based on the principal that a parathyroid adenoma rapidly enhances and rapidly "washes out" to a greater degree than surrounding lymph nodes following the administration of contrast. This technique was initially described as imaging the parathyroid gland with thin section 1.25-mm slices viewed in three planes (sagittal, axial, and coronal) with the "fourth" dimension acquired from perfusion data related to precontrast, arterial, and venous (late phase) imaging. Modifications of this technique that entail significantly less radiation have since been described. The sensitivity of this technique to diagnose parathyroid adenomas is quite high, with at least one report describing up to 95% sensitivity.
- **Thyroid lobe extending posterior to the hypopharynx.** Both normal and goitrous thyroid tissue may project a considerable distance from the expected confines of the normal thyroid gland. However, these extensions of thyroid tissue are typically confined by fascia that form the visceral compartment (also called visceral space) of the neck. When viewed from a lateral perspective, the visceral compartment can be likened to a 3-D lower case lambda (λ). Anatomically, the lower limbs of the λ begin where a fold of fascia drapes over the inferior thyroidal artery. The anterior lower limb of the λ represents the pretracheal space. The pretracheal space of the visceral compartment houses the thyroid gland, parathyroid glands, trachea (despite its name "pretracheal"), recurrent laryngeal nerves, larynx, and portions of the sympathetic trunks. The posterior lower limb of the λ represents the lower retrovisceral space (also called retroesophageal space) of the visceral compartment. The pretracheal space communicates with the anterior mediastinum, whereas the retrovisceral space communicates with the posterior mediastinum. The retrovisceral space also extends cephalad and posterior to the pharynx and is known as the retropharyngeal space. The retropharyngeal space represents the upper limb of the λ. Thus, thyroid tissue may extend into the anterior mediastinum, posterior mediastinum, retroesophageal space, and the retropharyngeal space.

Zuckerkandl tubercle

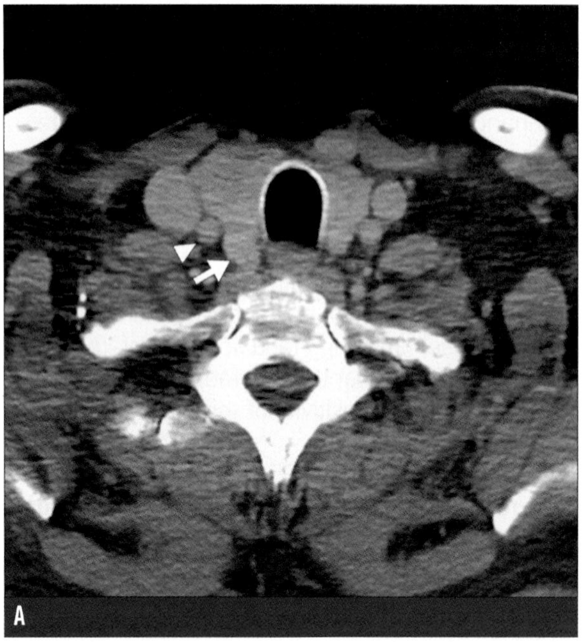

A contrast-enhanced axial CT image through the level of the thyroid gland (**A**) demonstrates posteriorly directed, pedunculated thyroid tissue arising from the right thyroid lobe, consistent with a right Zuckerkandl tubercle (arrow). In this case, the right common carotid artery (arrowhead) abuts the lateral aspect of the Zuckerkandl tubercle stalk.

Zuckerkandl tubercle

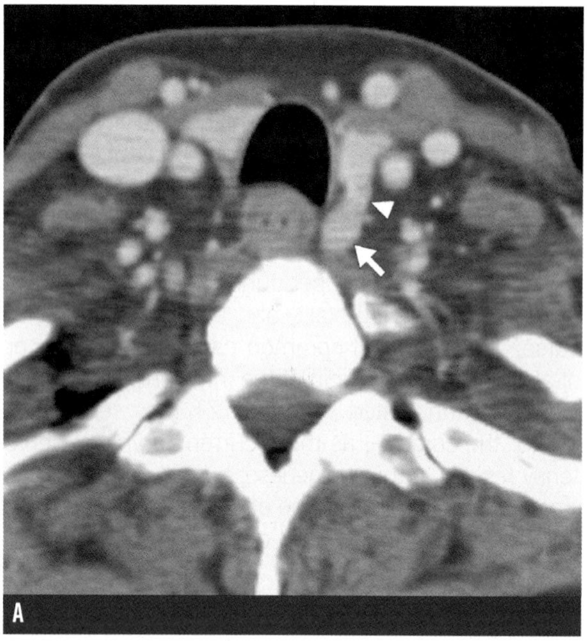

Different patient. A contrast-enhanced axial CT image through the level of the thyroid gland (**A**) demonstrates posteriorly pedunculated thyroid tissue (arrow) arising from the posterior aspect of the left thyroid lobe via an intervening stalk (arrowhead). This is compatible with a left Zuckerkandl tubercle.

Companion case: Zuckerkandl tubercle thyroid nodule with vocal cord paralysis

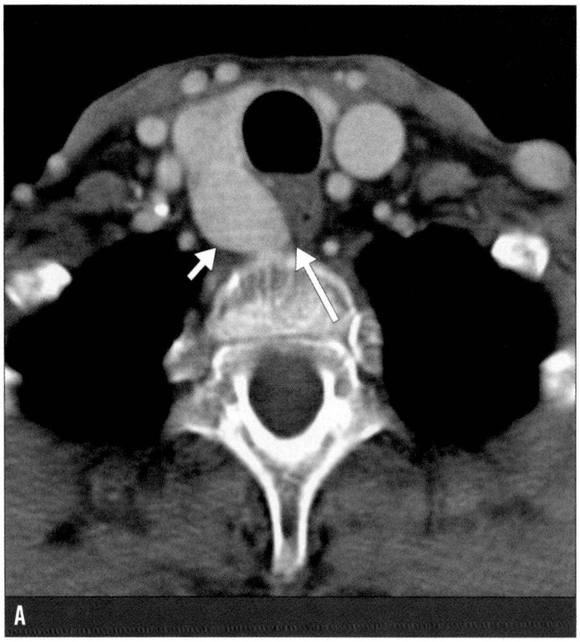

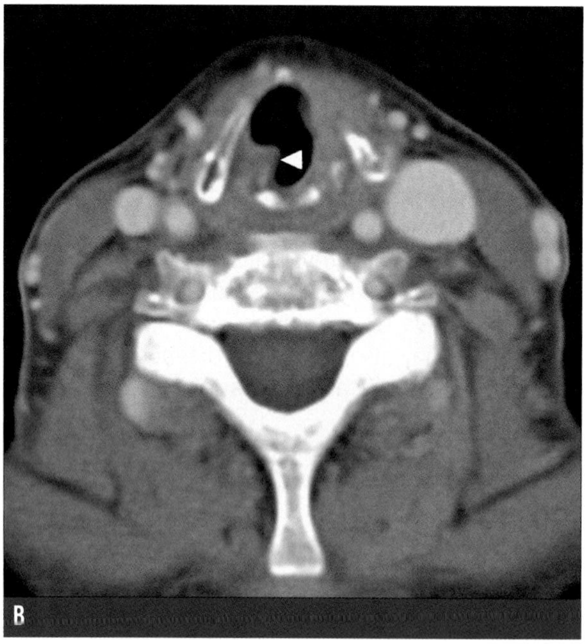

A contrast-enhanced axial CT image through the level of the thyroid gland (**A**) demonstrates a small to moderate-sized nodule projecting posteriorly from the right thyroid lobe, consistent with a thyroid nodule involving a right Zuckerkandl tubercle (short arrow, **A**). In this case, the nodule extends deeply into the right tracheoesophageal groove (long arrow, **A**) and results in mass effect upon the right aspect of the esophagus. Contrast-enhanced axial (**B**) and coronal reformatted (**C**) CT images through the larynx demonstrate fatty infiltration and volume loss of the right true vocal cord, compatible with a vocal cord paralysis (arrowheads, **B**, **C**), likely due to impingement of the right recurrent laryngeal nerve in the tracheoesophageal groove by the right Zuckerkandl tubercle thyroid nodule.

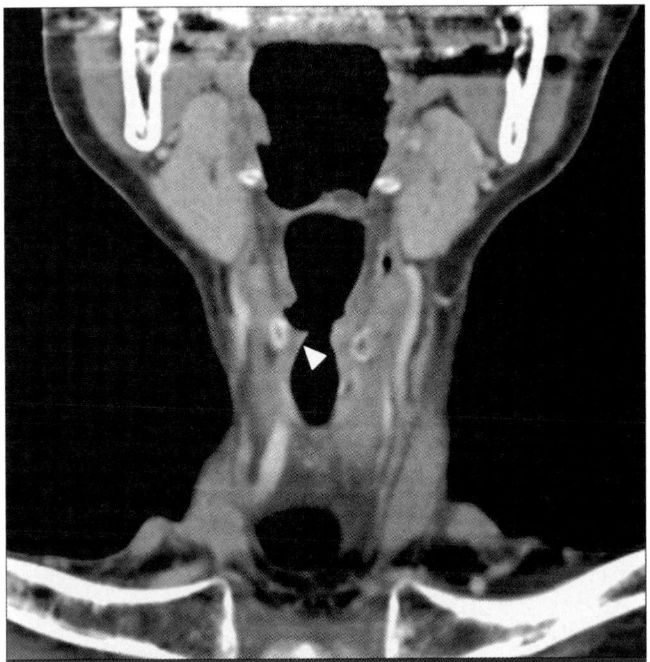

C

Companion case: Parathyroid adenoma

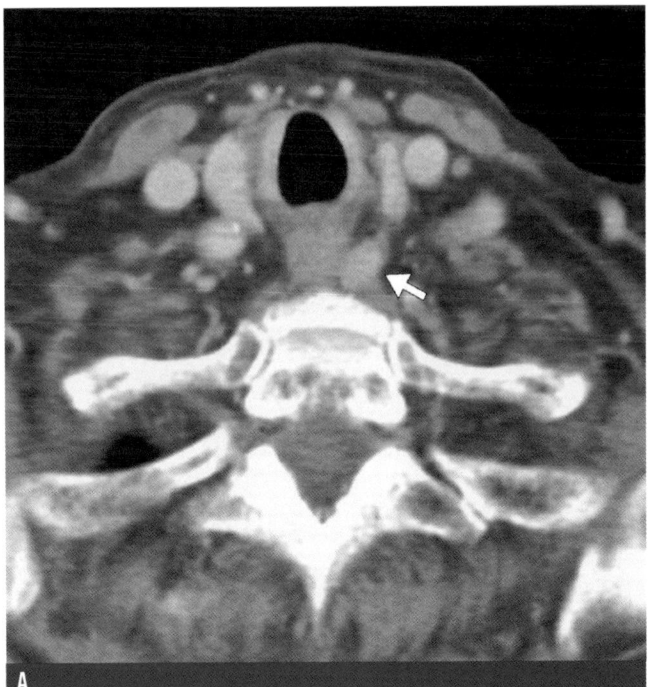

A

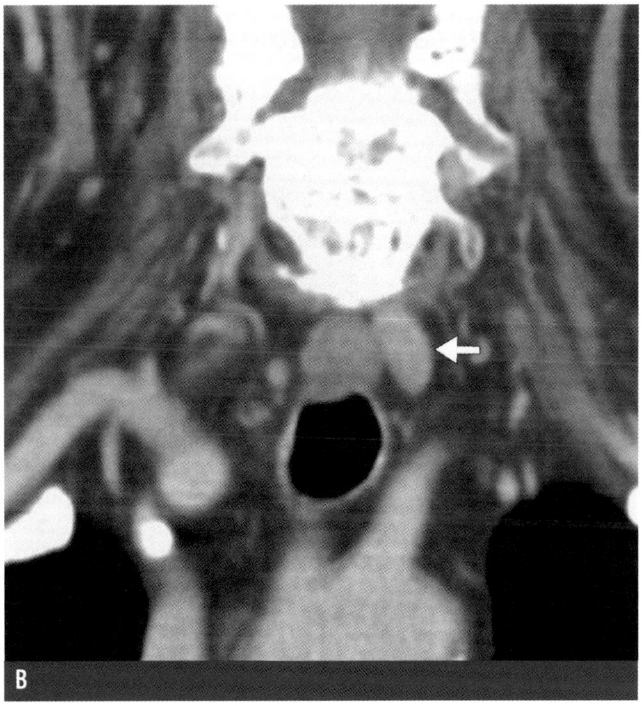

B

Axial (**A**), coronal reformatted (**B**), and sagittal reformatted (**C**) contrast-enhanced CT images demonstrate an oval soft tissue lesion located posterior to the left thyroid lobe (arrows, **A-C**). This finding was not contiguous with the thyroid gland on any of the images. An axial SPECT image with attenuation correction from a ^{99m}Tc-sestamibi parathyroid scan (**D**) demonstrates increased tracer uptake posterior to the left thyroid lobe corresponding to the finding demonstrated on CT (arrow, **D**). This patient had a 10-year history of hypercalcemia and elevated parathyroid hormone levels. The clinical history and imaging findings are compatible with a parathyroid adenoma.

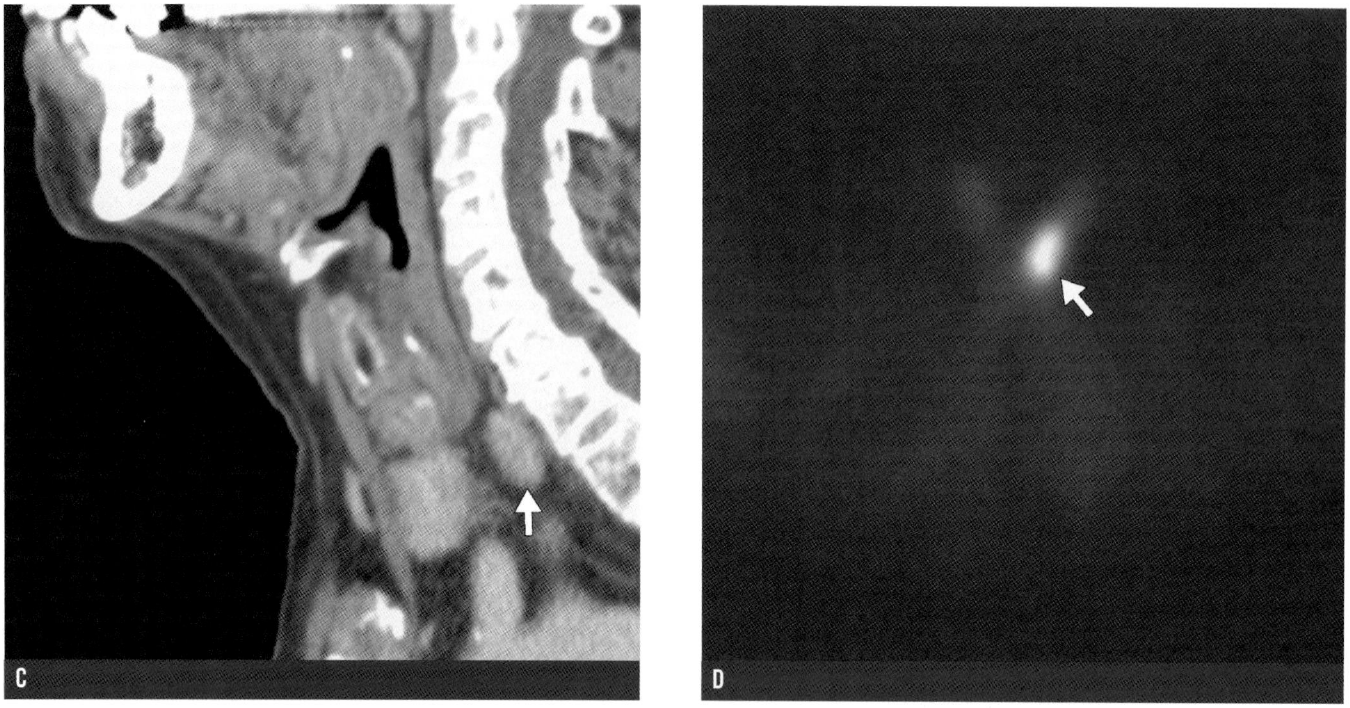

Companion case: Thyroid lobe extending posterior to the hypopharynx

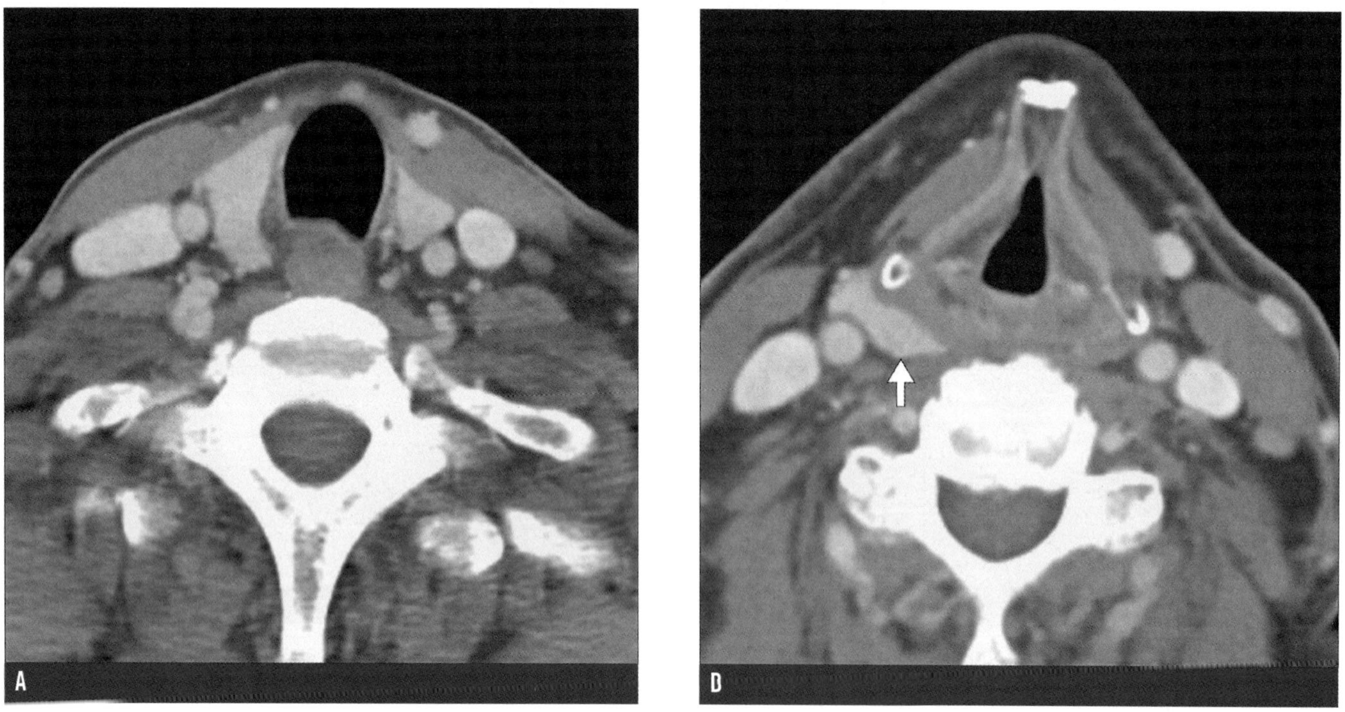

Contrast-enhanced axial CT images (**A-C**) and a contrast-enhanced sagittal reformatted CT image (**D**) of a patient without thyroid or pharyngeal symptoms. These images demonstrate incidental linear extension of the right lobe of the thyroid posterior to the right aspect of the hypopharynx (arrows, **B-D**). This extension of thyroid tissue resides in the retropharyngeal space of the visceral compartment.

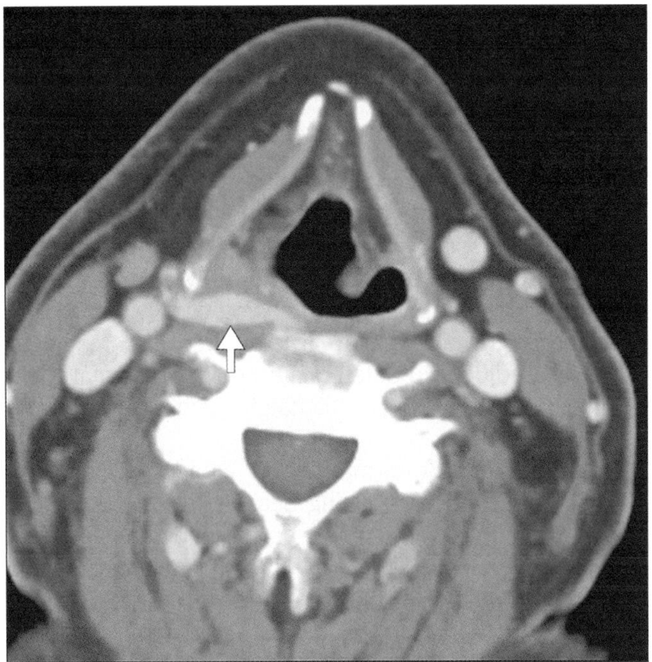

C

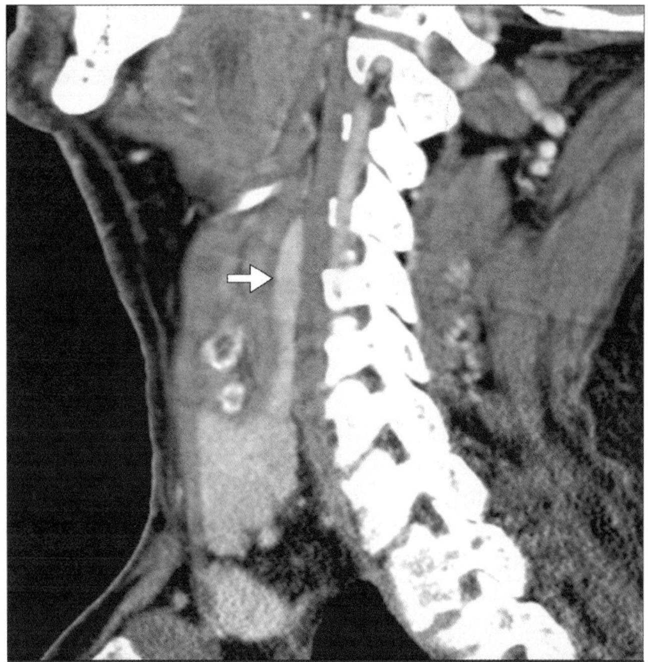

D

REFERENCES

Chien D, Jacene H. Imaging of parathyroid glands. *Otolaryngol Clin North Am.* 2010;43(2):399-415.

Chin SC, Rice H, Som PM. Spread of goiters outside the thyroid bed: a review of 190 cases and an analysis of the incidence of the various extensions. *Arch Otolaryngol Head Neck Surg.* 2003;129(11):1198-1202.

Lee TC, Selvarajan SK, Curtin H, Mukundan S. Zuckerkandl tubercle of the thyroid: a common imaging finding that may mimic pathology. *AJNR Am J Neuroradiol.* 2012;33(6):1134-1138.

Mehanna R, Murphy MS, Sheahan P. Thyroid tubercle of zuckerkandl is more consistently present and larger on the right: a prospective series. *Eur Thyroid J.* 2014;3(1):38-42.

CASE 21 Strap muscles simulating a thyroid nodule

Occasionally, the normal strap muscles may indent the ventral aspect of the thyroid gland and simulate a thyroid nodule on CT, particularly on axial imaging. Usually, sagittal and coronal reformatted CT images can help differentiate a normal strap muscle simulating a thyroid nodule from a true thyroid nodule.

COMPANION CASES

- **Thyroid nodule.** Most thyroid nodules represent follicular nodules and are benign. While a CT examination can depict most thyroid nodules, occasionally a thyroid nodule can be occult on CT when it enhances to the same degree as the adjacent normal iodine-containing thyroid tissue. Additionally, a well-depicted thyroid nodule on one CT examination may be occult on a follow-up CT examination of the same patient. This likely occurs due to differences in the timing of the contrast bolus relative to when the images are obtained. Furthermore, widespread malignancy within the thyroid gland may be CT occult. Thus, care should be taken to ascribe normalcy to the thyroid gland when there is a high clinical suspicion of thyroid malignancy or when suspicious lymph nodes suggesting thyroid malignancy (eg, partially calcified, containing a nodule of enhancement, etc) are present. While CT is useful to evaluate for substernal extension of a thyroid nodule/goiter prior to a thyroidectomy, thyroid ultrasonography is the imaging study of choice to evaluate a thyroid nodule. Thyroid ultrasound imaging is a useful adjunct to differentiate benign from malignant thyroid lesions although, ultimately, pathology is needed for the diagnosis.
- **Hypothyroidism.** A normal thyroid gland is hyperdense on unenhanced CT imaging because of its iodine content. In the case of thyroid gland atrophy and resultant chronic hypothyroidism, the thyroid gland on CT may be difficult to delineate due to its diminutive size and lack of iodine content, frequently resulting in an isodense and inconspicuous thyroid gland relative to the adjacent strap muscles. In some cases of acute thyroiditis, the thyroid gland may also be hypoattenuating because of the release of iodine, although in this setting the thyroid gland is often enlarged.

Strap muscles simulating a thyroid nodule

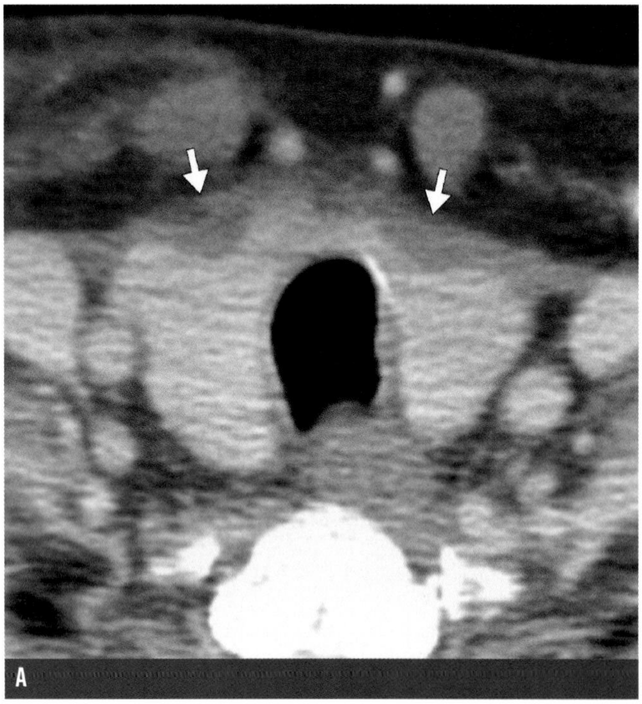

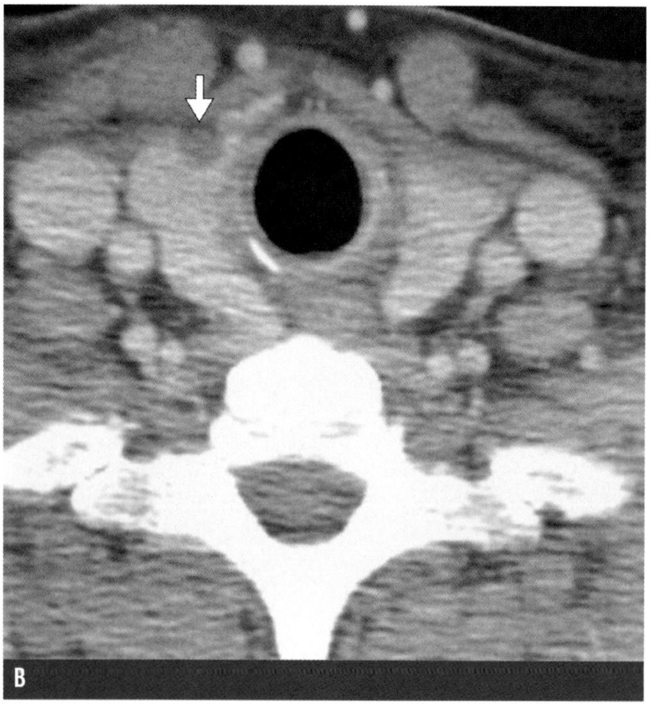

Axial (**A**, **B**) and coronal reformatted (**C**) contrast-enhanced CT images through the thyroid lobes as well as a contrast-enhanced sagittal reformatted CT image through the right thyroid lobe (**D**). Image **A** demonstrates the strap muscles mildly deforming and indenting the ventral margins of the thyroid lobes (arrows, **A**). Image **B** is located slightly cephalad to image **A** and demonstrates a focal hypodensity along the ventral margin of the right thyroid lobe (arrow, **B**), suggestive of a right thyroid nodule. However, images **C** and **D** do not demonstrate a right lobe thyroid nodule. The apparent finding on image **B** simply represents a focal incidental indentation along the ventral margin of the right thyroid lobe by the right strap musculature.

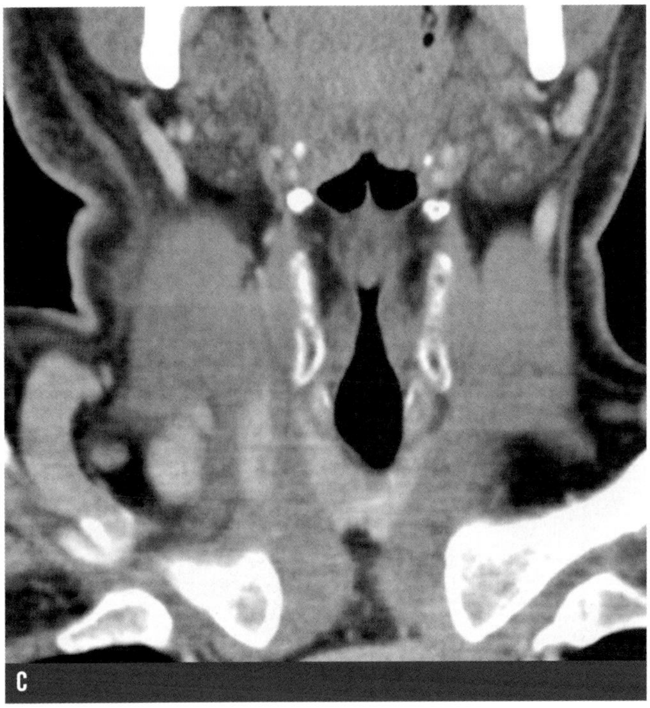

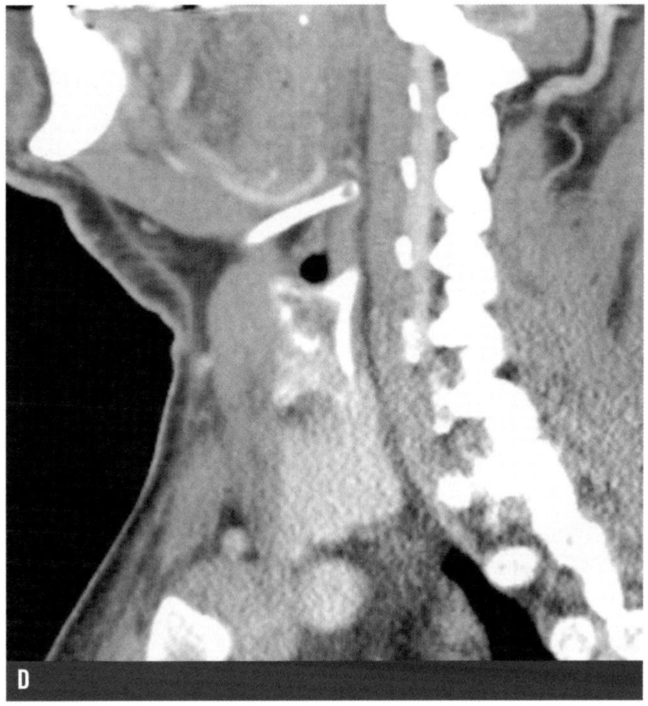

Companion case: Thyroid nodules

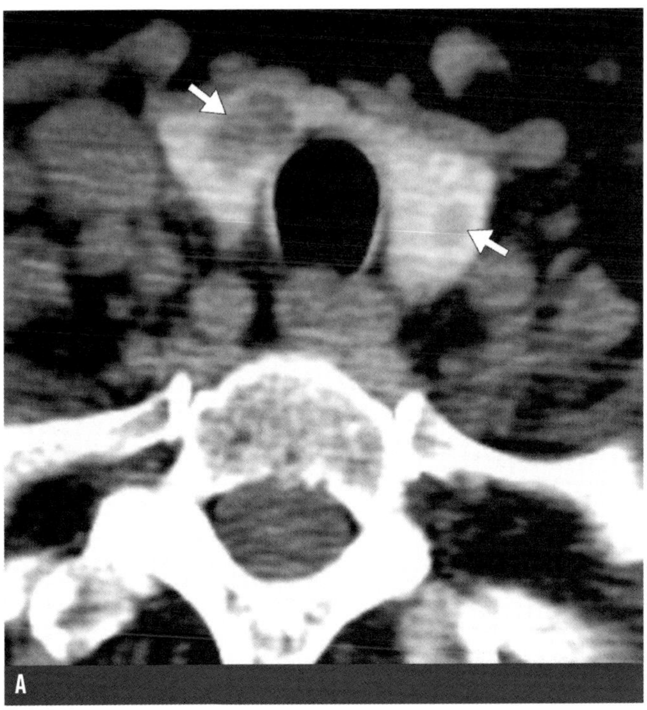

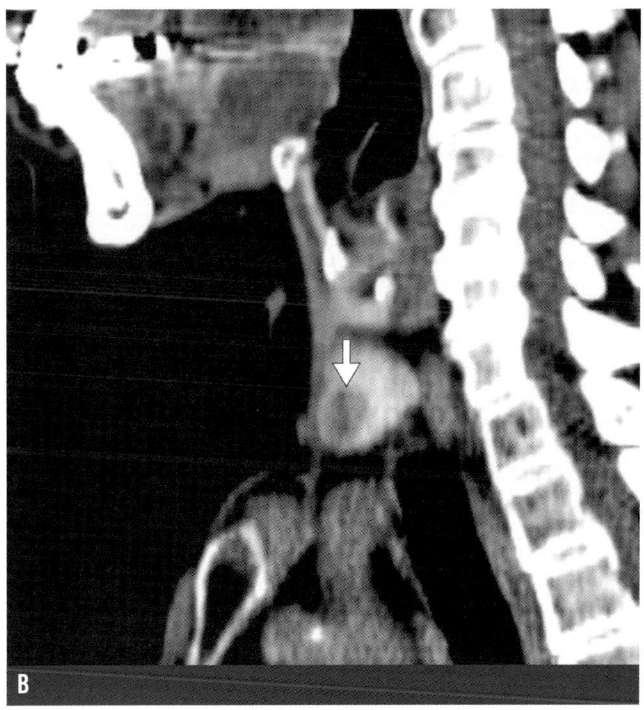

Axial (**A**) and sagittal reformatted (**B**) unenhanced CT images demonstrate typical thyroid nodules in the thyroid lobes (arrows, **A**, **B**). The thyroid nodules are well delineated on this study, despite the lack of intravenous contrast, because iodine content within normal portions of the thyroid gland silhouette the thyroid nodules.

Companion case: Hypothyroidism

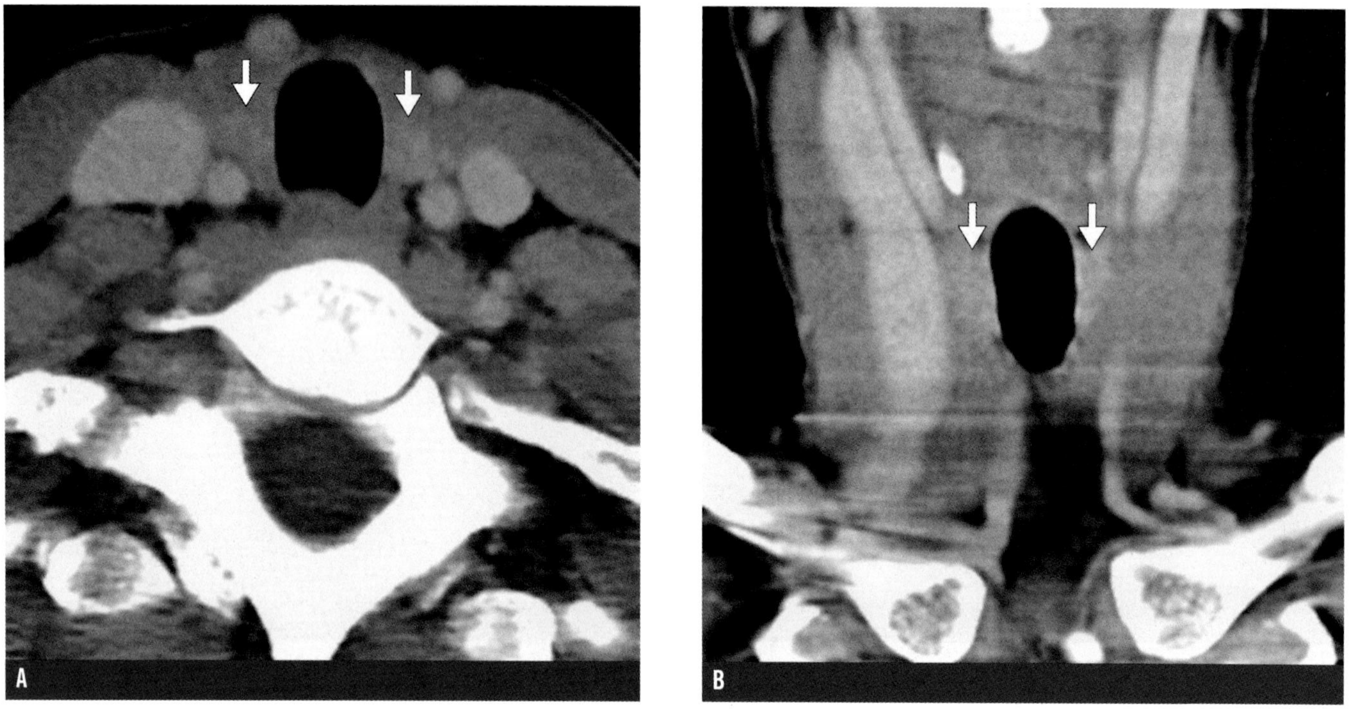

Axial (**A**) and coronal reformatted (**B**) postcontrast CT images demonstrate a small, barely perceptible thyroid gland (arrows, **A**, **B**) that is nearly isodense to adjacent musculature. The poor visualization of the thyroid gland can be explained by the lack of iodine content within the thyroid. This patient was clinically hypothyroid.

REFERENCE

Bomeli SR, LeBeau SO, Ferris RL. Evaluation of a thyroid nodule. *Otolaryngol Clin North Am.* 2010;43(2):229-238, vii.

CASE 22 Thyroidectomy bed

A thyroidectomy is a surgical procedure that involves removing all or a portion of the thyroid gland. This surgery is most commonly performed to remove a thyroid malignancy, a hyperactive thyroid, thyroid goiter, or to improve regional mass effect related to an enlarged thyroid gland from various causes.

Following a thyroidectomy, the thyroid bed is usually comprised of fat, may or may not contain metallic clips, and may contain lymph nodes. Thyroid malignancies have a propensity to metastasize to regional lymph nodes. Therefore, if a thyroidectomy was performed to resect a thyroid malignancy, then the lymph nodes within the thyroidectomy bed, regardless of size, should be closely monitored for any change. Additionally, thyroid malignancies, in particular papillary thyroid carcinoma, are notorious for resulting in a wide spectrum of pathologic lymph node appearances, including purely solid to cystic, nodular enhancing, and mineralized lymph nodes.

Thyroidectomy bed

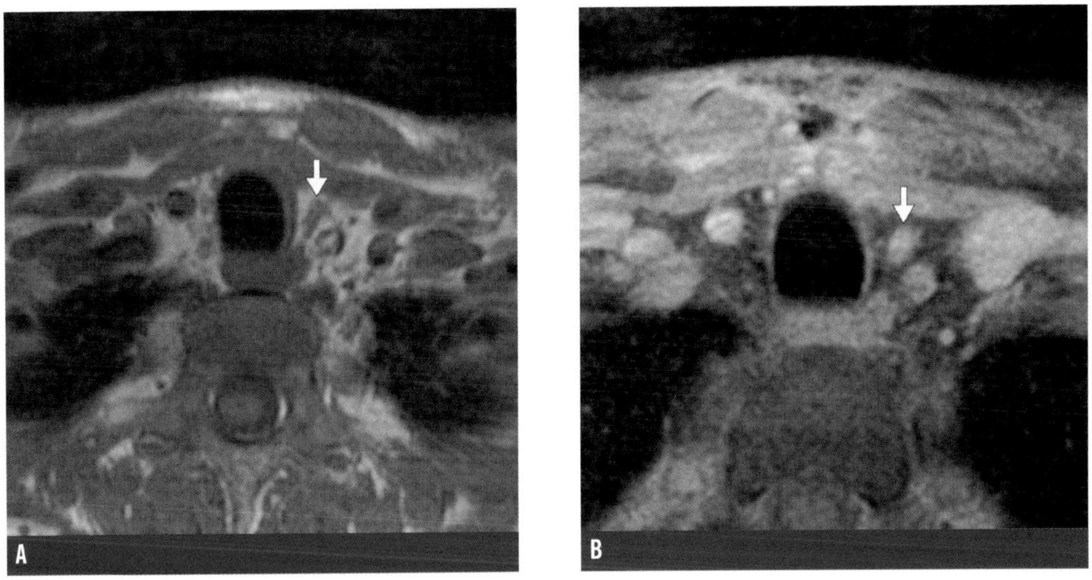

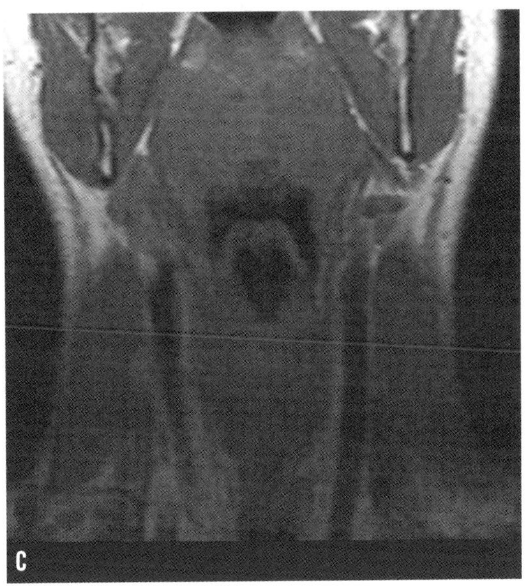

Unenhanced axial T1 (**A**), postcontrast axial T1 (**B**), and unenhanced coronal T1 (**C**) MR images through the lower neck demonstrate absence of the thyroid gland. The thyroid bed is largely occcupied with fat, although a small nonspecific soft tissue nodule is present in the left aspect of the thyroid bed (arrows, **A**, **B**). This small nodule may represent a non-pathologic lymph node. However, if this finding is identified in a patient with a history of prior thyroid carcinoma, then short-term follow-up studies and clinical assessment (such as evaluating for abnormal thyroglobulin levels) are necessary to ensure that this nodule is not a metastatic normal-sized lymph node.

Thyroidectomy bed

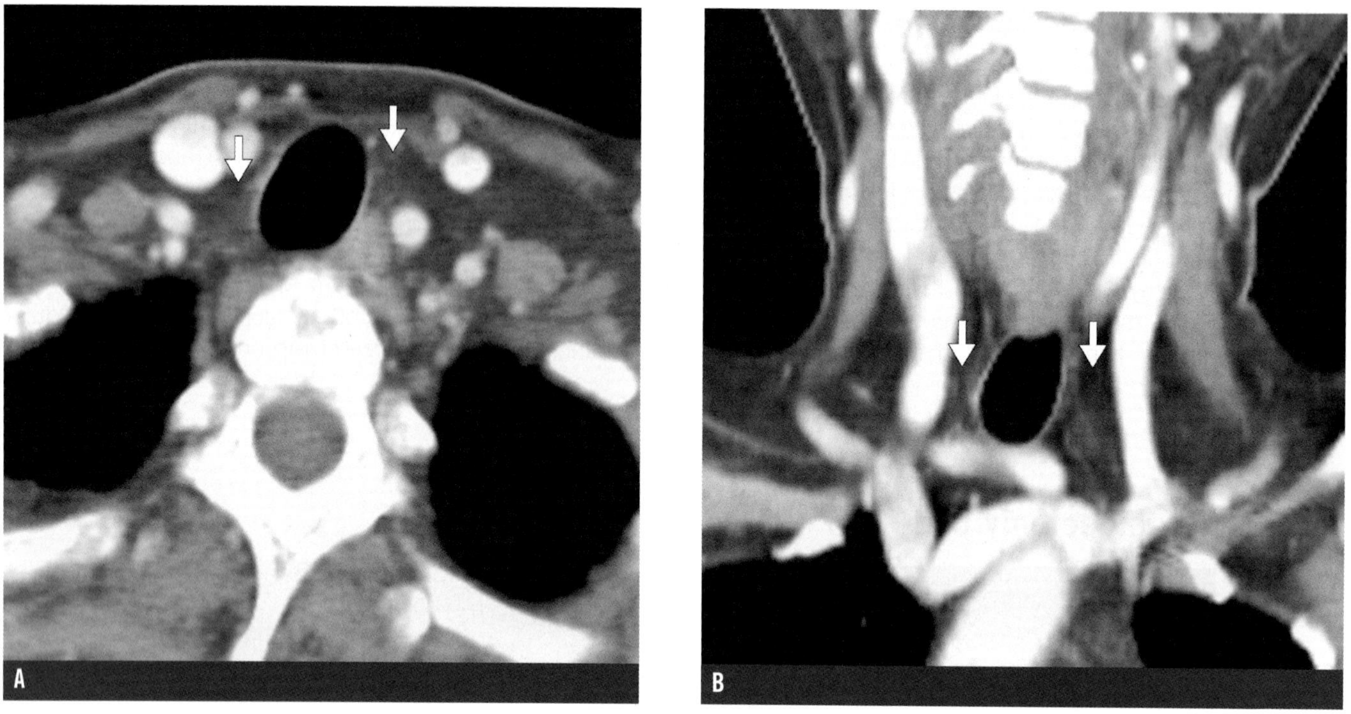

Different patient. Axial (**A**) and coronal reformatted (**B**) contrast-enhanced CT images through the lower neck demonstrate absence of the normal thyroid gland with fat occupying the thyroid bed (arrows, **A**, **B**).

REFERENCES

Lombardi D, Nicolai P, Antonelli AR, Maroldi R, Farina D, Shaha AR. Parapharyngeal lymph node metastasis: an unusual presentation of papillary thyroid carcinoma. *Head Neck.* 2004;26(2):190-196.

Verge J, et al. Cervical cystic lymph node metastasis as first manifestation of occult papillary thyroid carcinoma: report of seven cases. *Head Neck.* 1999;21:370-374.

CASE 23 Repositioning of residual thyroid gland following a laryngectomy

A laryngectomy is most commonly performed to remove the laryngeal apparatus in the setting of advanced carcinoma of the larynx. During a total laryngectomy, the thyroid gland is often disrupted, usually in the form of an ipsilateral hemithyroidectomy and/or isthmectomy. The residual portions of the thyroid gland are repositioned during the neck dissection to provide access to the larynx.

The fascial layers and surrounding musculature which normally contribute to the shape of the thyroid gland are also disrupted during a laryngectomy. As a result, the shape of the residual thyroid gland may vary following a laryngectomy. Because of the atypical location and unusual shape of the postoperative thyroid gland, the thyroid gland may simulate residual tumor, a mass, a lymph node, or even an abnormal vascular structure, such as a pseudoaneurysm.

Repositioning of residual thyroid gland following a laryngectomy

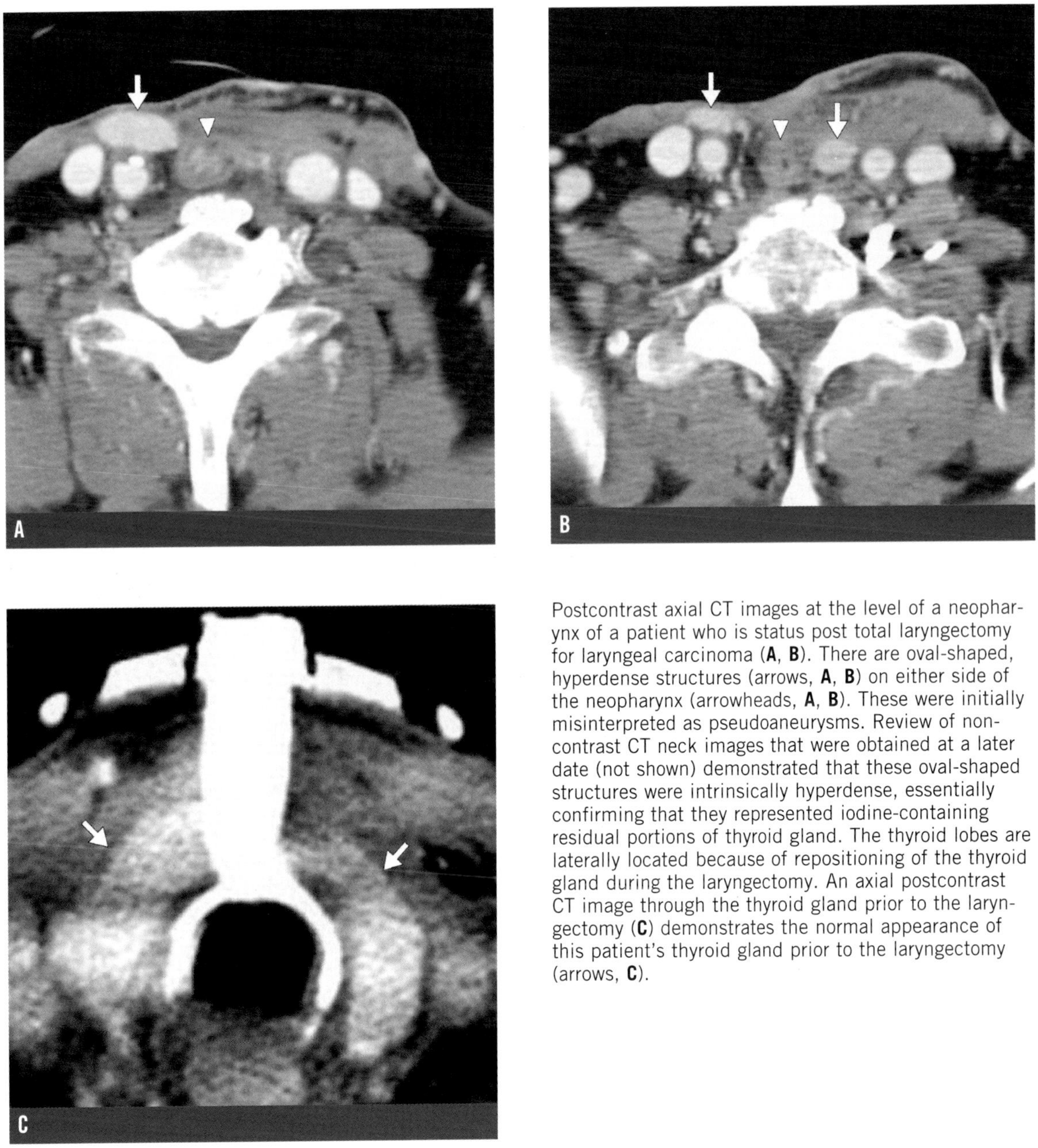

Postcontrast axial CT images at the level of a neopharynx of a patient who is status post total laryngectomy for laryngeal carcinoma (**A**, **B**). There are oval-shaped, hyperdense structures (arrows, **A**, **B**) on either side of the neopharynx (arrowheads, **A**, **B**). These were initially misinterpreted as pseudoaneurysms. Review of noncontrast CT neck images that were obtained at a later date (not shown) demonstrated that these oval-shaped structures were intrinsically hyperdense, essentially confirming that they represented iodine-containing residual portions of thyroid gland. The thyroid lobes are laterally located because of repositioning of the thyroid gland during the laryngectomy. An axial postcontrast CT image through the thyroid gland prior to the laryngectomy (**C**) demonstrates the normal appearance of this patient's thyroid gland prior to the laryngectomy (arrows, **C**).

Repositioning of residual thyroid gland following a laryngectomy

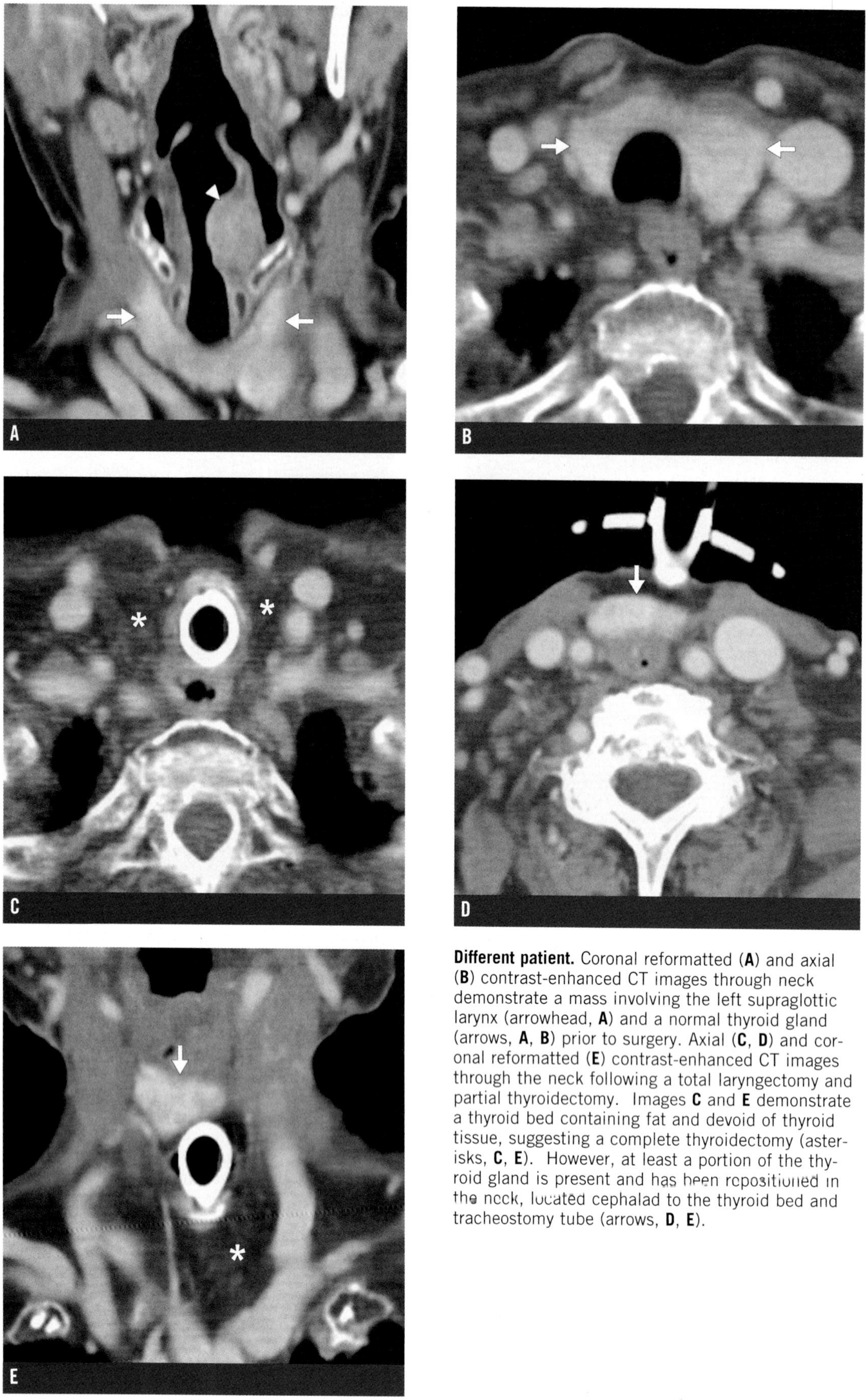

Different patient. Coronal reformatted (**A**) and axial (**B**) contrast-enhanced CT images through neck demonstrate a mass involving the left supraglottic larynx (arrowhead, **A**) and a normal thyroid gland (arrows, **A**, **B**) prior to surgery. Axial (**C**, **D**) and coronal reformatted (**E**) contrast-enhanced CT images through the neck following a total laryngectomy and partial thyroidectomy. Images **C** and **E** demonstrate a thyroid bed containing fat and devoid of thyroid tissue, suggesting a complete thyroidectomy (asterisks, **C**, **E**). However, at least a portion of the thyroid gland is present and has been repositioned in the neck, located cephalad to the thyroid bed and tracheostomy tube (arrows, **D**, **E**).

REFERENCES

Mendelson AA, Al-Khatib TA, Julien M, Payne RJ, Black MJ, Hier MP. Thyroid gland management in total laryngectomy: meta-analysis and surgical recommendations. *Otolaryngol Head Neck Surg.* 2009;140(3):298-305.

Weissman JL, Curtin HD, Johnson JT. Thyroid gland after total laryngectomy: CT appearance. *Radiology.* 1998;207:405-409.

Embryologically, the thymus develops from the third pharyngeal pouches during the sixth week of gestation. During the eighth week of gestation, the thymic primordium joins at the midline, attaches to the pericardium as it begins its caudal descent into the mediastinum. By the ninth week of gestation, the thymus reaches its final destination in the anterior mediastinum.

The function of the thymus is to transform hematopoietic precursors (thymocytes) into T cells, most of which are produced during childhood. The thymus grows during infancy and childhood and may be quite large when imaging these age groups. By adolescence, the thymus decreases in size and begins to be replaced by fat. However, it is not unusual to appreciate residual thymic tissue in the teen-aged or young adult patient. In this patient population, the thymus is most commonly triangular in shape, may have an inverted V morphology, and is located in the anterior-superior mediastinum. Normal thymus should not be associated with mass effect.

COMPANION CASES

- **Thymic cyst.** A thymic cyst is a branchial cleft remnant that may occur anywhere along the descent of the developing thymus, from the angle of the mandible to the superior mediastinum, although they are most commonly found in the superior mediastinum. When a thymic cyst is present in the neck, the term cervical thymic cyst is used. If a thymic cyst is present but normal thymic tissue is not identified in a child or young adult, then surgery to remove a thymic cyst should be at least temporarily avoided. This is because a thymic cyst may contain the only functioning thymic tissue for the patient. Mediastinal thymic cysts have been reported to be associated with myasthenia gravis.
- **Change in pericardial recess volume during inspiration and expiration.** The normal pericardial cavity may contain up to 25 mL of fluid. The pericardial recesses are extensions of the pericardial cavity and can simulate disease on imaging. In particular, the superior aortic pericardial recess may simulate a necrotic superior mediastinal mass (such as a necrotic lymph node) or a thymic cyst on imaging. However, redistribution of fluid within the pericardial recesses occurs during inspiration and expiration, and this fluid redistribution can aid in appropriately identifying the finding as a pericardial recess. Specifically, the superior aortic pericardial recess typically decreases in volume during an inspiratory effort and increases in volume during an expiratory effort. While literature explaining why this occurs is scant, this might be explained by the following: The pericardium is a relatively rigid structure and the pressure within the pericardial sac directly correlates with the intrathoracic pressure. During inspiration, the negative intrathoracic pressure results in decreased pericardial sac pressure as well as increased systemic venous return, subsequently resulting in enlargement of the right heart. The enlarged right heart attenuates and redistributes the superior aortic pericardial recess fluid. Conversely, during expiration, there is less venous return and thus less volume of blood in the right heart. This results in a greater accumulation of pericardial fluid in the superior aortic pericardial recess.

Normal thymic tissue

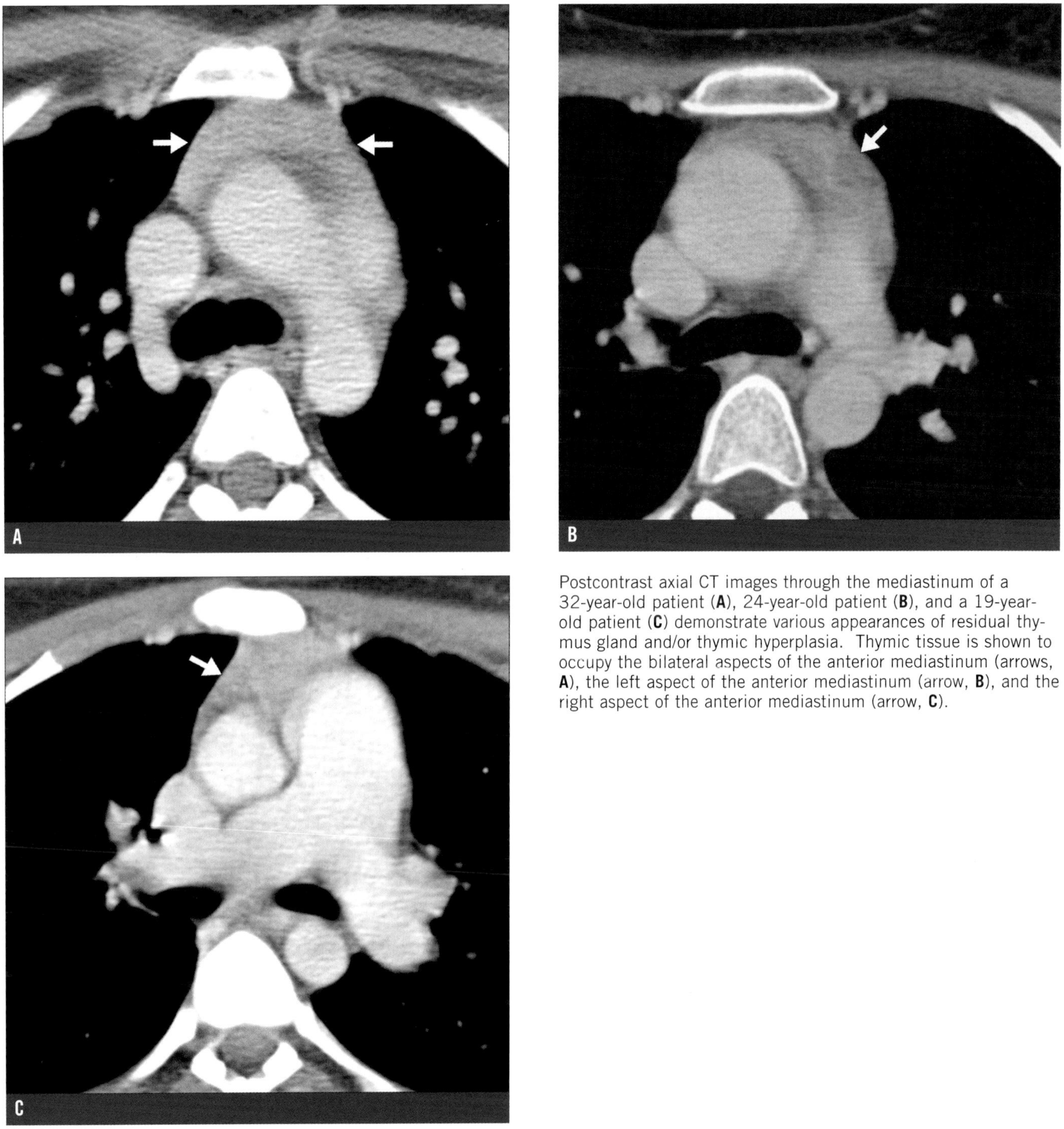

Postcontrast axial CT images through the mediastinum of a 32-year-old patient (**A**), 24-year-old patient (**B**), and a 19-year-old patient (**C**) demonstrate various appearances of residual thymus gland and/or thymic hyperplasia. Thymic tissue is shown to occupy the bilateral aspects of the anterior mediastinum (arrows, **A**), the left aspect of the anterior mediastinum (arrow, **B**), and the right aspect of the anterior mediastinum (arrow, **C**).

Residual thymic tissue

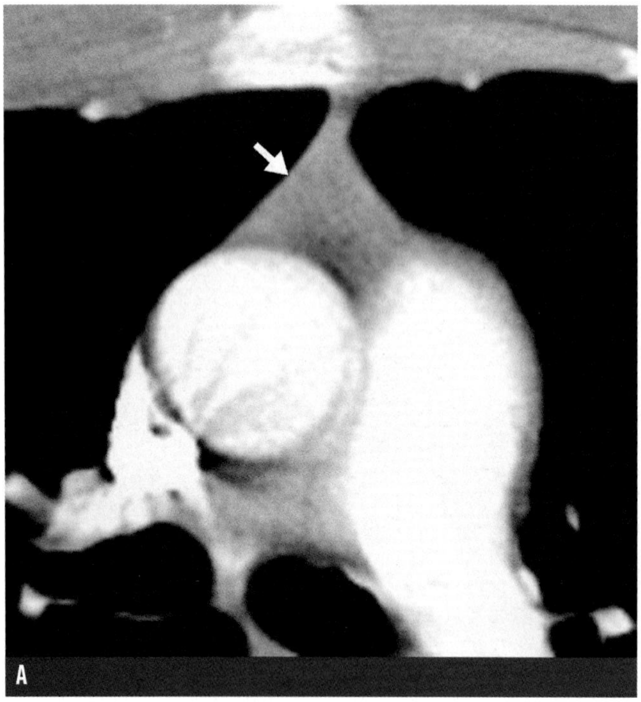

A postcontrast axial CT image through the superior mediastinum of a 27-year-old patient (**A**) demonstrates prominent, triangle-shaped soft tissue in the anterior aspect of the superior mediastinum, compatible with normal residual thymic tissue (arrow).

Companion case: Thymic cyst

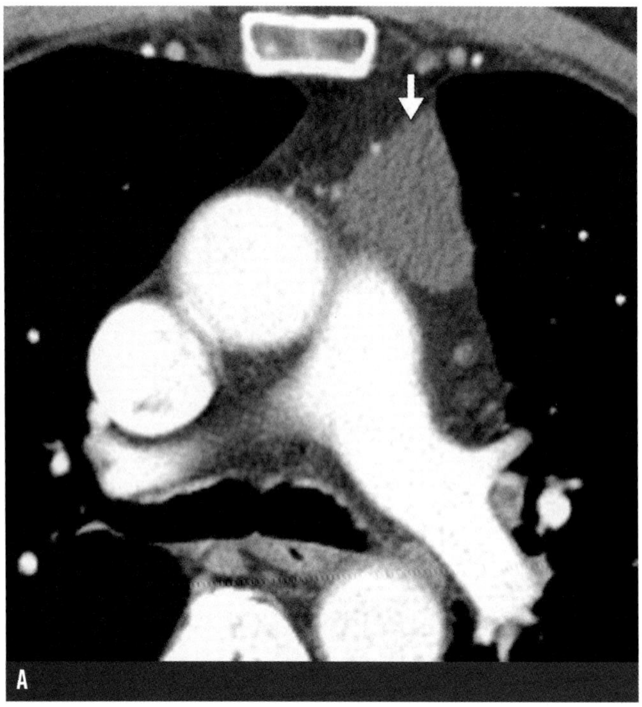

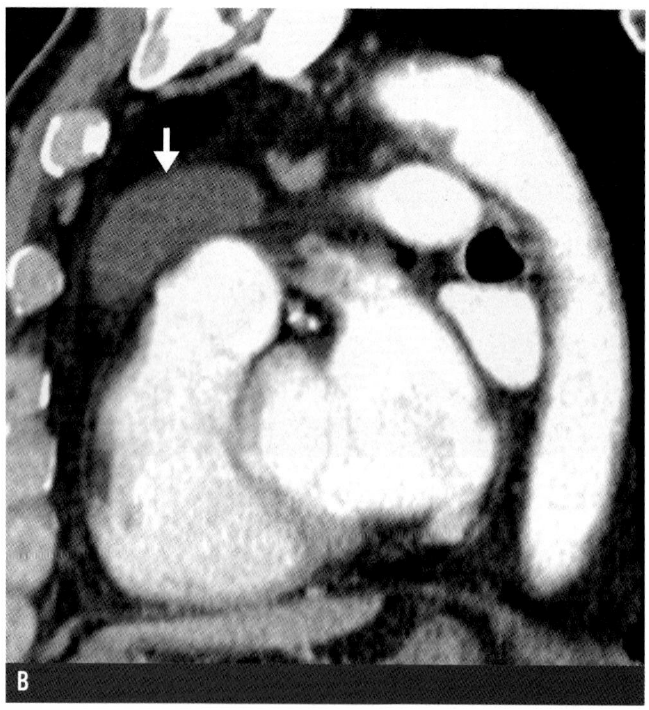

Axial (**A**), sagittal reformatted (**B**), and coronal reformatted (**C**) contrast-enhanced CT images demonstrate a circumscribed, fluid-attenuating structure within the anterior mediastinum that most likely represents a benign thymic cyst (arrows, **A-C**).

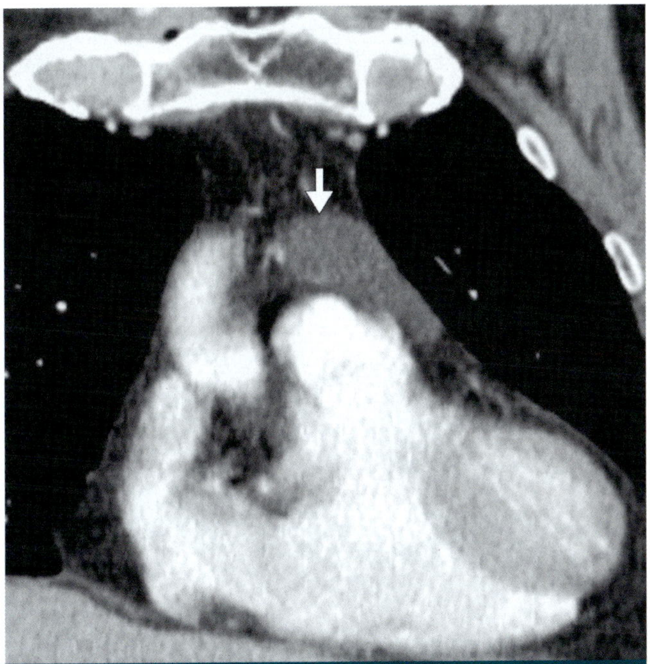

C

Companion case: Change in pericardial recess volume during inspiration and expiration

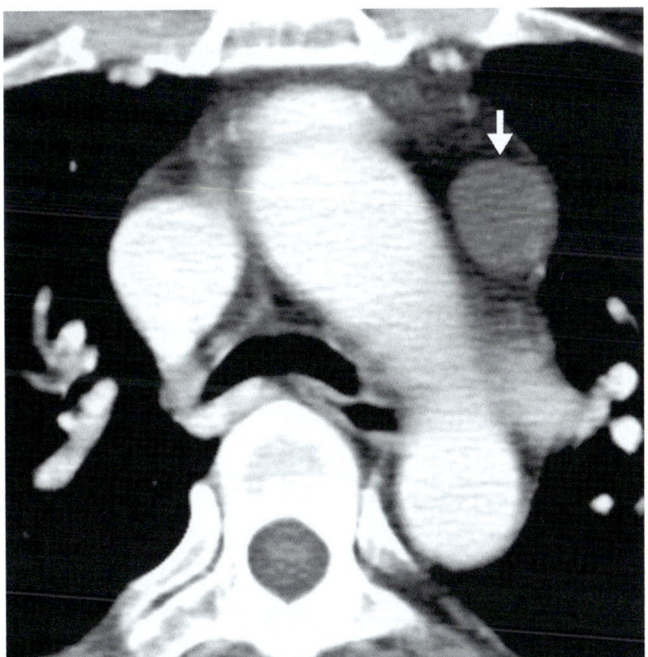

A

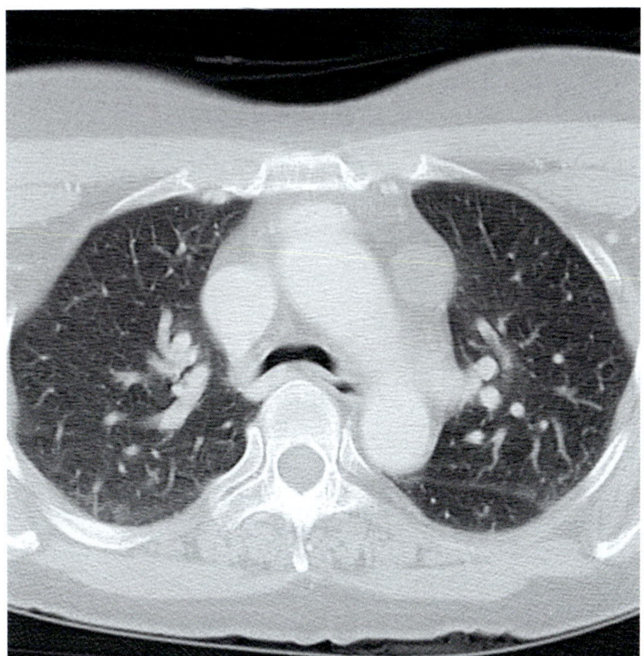

B

A postcontrast axial CT image through the mediastinum from a neck CT of a patient with papillary thyroid carcinoma (**A**) demonstrates a fluid density structure in the prevascular space of the mediastinum (arrow, **A**). The differential diagnosis for this finding includes a metastatic necrotic lymph node from papillary thyroid carcinoma, thymic cyst, or the anterior portion of the superior aortic pericardial recess, among others. An axial CT image viewed with a lung window from the same study and at the same level as image **A** (**B**) demonstrates a relatively poor inspiratory effort. An axial CT image through the mediastinum obtained from a CT of the chest (**C**) performed minutes after the neck CT demonstrates the finding in the prevascular space of the mediastinum to be much smaller in volume (arrow, **C**). The lung window from this chest CT (**D**) demonstrates a much improved inspiratory effort relative to image **B** from the neck CT. The change in volume of the finding effectively confirms that this represents an incidental superior aortic pericardial recess, because other entities (such as thymic cyst, tumor, or a pathologic lymph node) would not be expected to change in volume during inspiration and expiration.

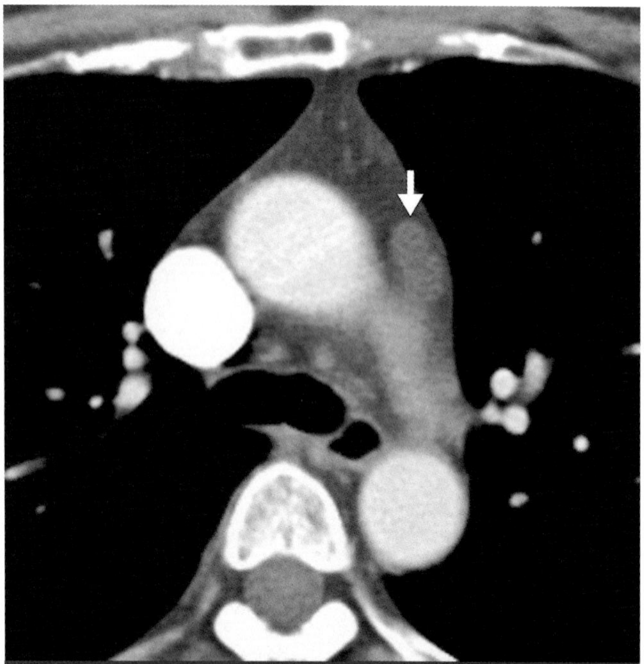

C

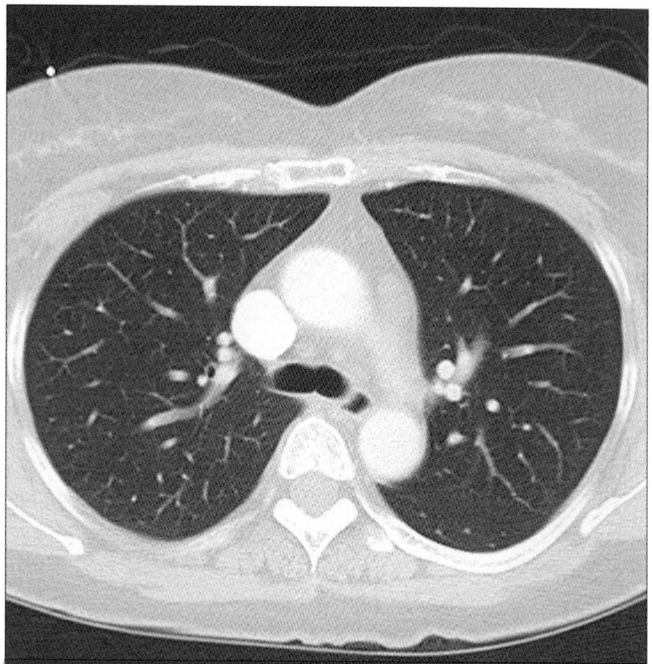

D

REFERENCES

Aribandi M. High-riding superior pericardial recess: temporal change can help distinguish from mediastinal pathology. *South Med J.* 2007;100(4):407-408.

Baron RL, Lee JK, Sagel SS, Peterson RR. Computed tomography of the normal thymus. *Radiology.* 1982;142:121.

Gawande RS, et al. Differentiation of normal thymus from anterior mediastinal lymphoma and lymphoma recurrence at pediatric PET/CT. *Radiology.* 2012;262(2):613-622. Epub December 12, 2011.

Michalopoulos N, et al. Cervical thymic cysts in adults. *Thyroid.* 2011;21(9):987-992. Epub May 19, 2011.

Som PM, et al. Parenchymal cysts of the lower neck. *Radiology.* 1985;157(2):399-406.

Yarom N, Zissin R, Apter S, Hertz M, Rahimi-Levene N, Gayerlnt G. Rebound thymic enlargement on CT in adults. *Int J Clin Pract.* 2007;61(4):562-568.

CASE 25 Rebound thymus

Thymic rebound (also called thymic hyperplasia) occurs after a significant illness or physical stress, such as following chemotherapy, severe burns, or steroid treatment. While a benign entity, a rebound thymus can simulate an anterior mediastinal mass. Thymic rebound may occur months after the illness/stress and persist for several years. Clinical history is important in these cases to help differentiate incidental thymic rebound from a tumor.

COMPANION CASE

- **Mediastinal lymphoma.** A tumor of the anterior mediastinum can be difficult to distinguish from an incidentally enlarged thymus gland or rebound thymus. Tumors of the anterior mediastinum may result in regional mass effect or may be heterogeneous on imaging, although some tumors (eg, lymphoma) may be entirely homogeneous. The clinical history or other areas of lymphadenopathy are often helpful to differentiate mediastinal lymphoma from a benign thymus gland. If the diagnosis is still in question, a PET CT may help differentiate these entities. Generally speaking, mediastinal lymphoma in the adult patient will have a greater standardized uptake value (SUV) than residual/rebound thymus, with one study determining an SUV of 3.4 or greater suggestive of mediastinal lymphoma. However, patients younger than 13 years of age may have normal thymus glands with SUVs significantly greater than 3.4 because of the greater physiologic activity of the thymus in these patients. While some have stated that the thymus ceases to be physiologically active beginning at 13 years of age, others have shown PET activity in normal thymus glands of patients older than 13.

Rebound thymus

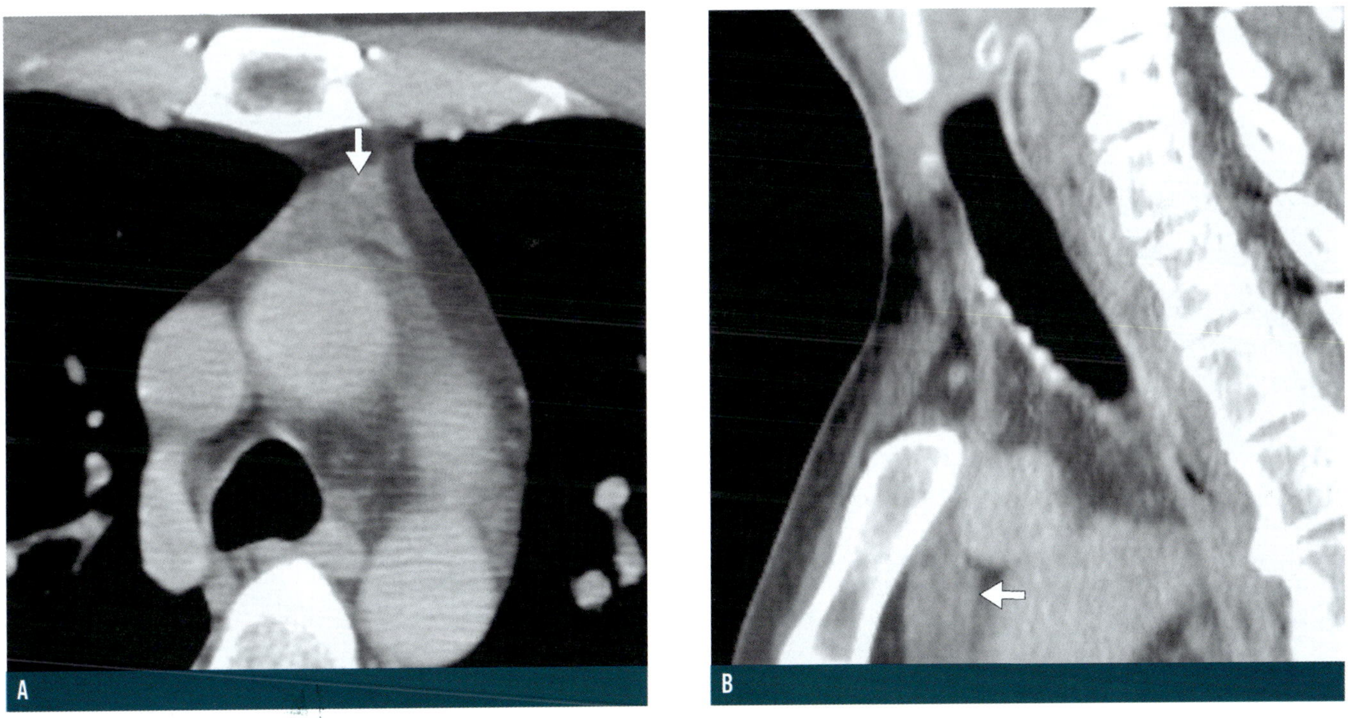

Axial (**A**), sagittal reformatted (**B**), and coronal reformatted (**C**) contrast-enhanced CT images through the lower neck and superior mediastinum of a 44-year-old patient following treatment of a tongue malignancy. These images demonstrate prominent, triangular-shaped soft tissue in the anterior aspect of the superior mediastinum, consistent with thymus gland (arrows, **A-C**). This thymus gland is enlarged for a patient of this age, most compatible with rebound thymus following cancer treatment.

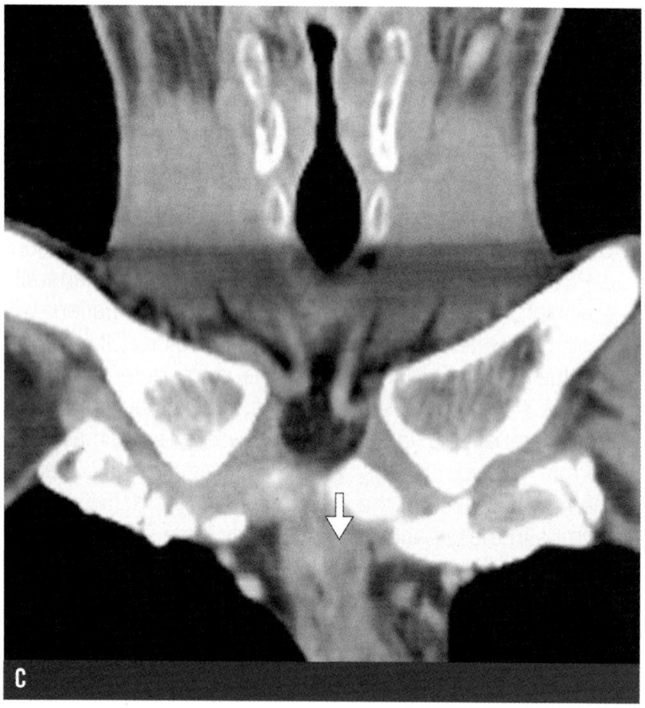

Rebound thymus

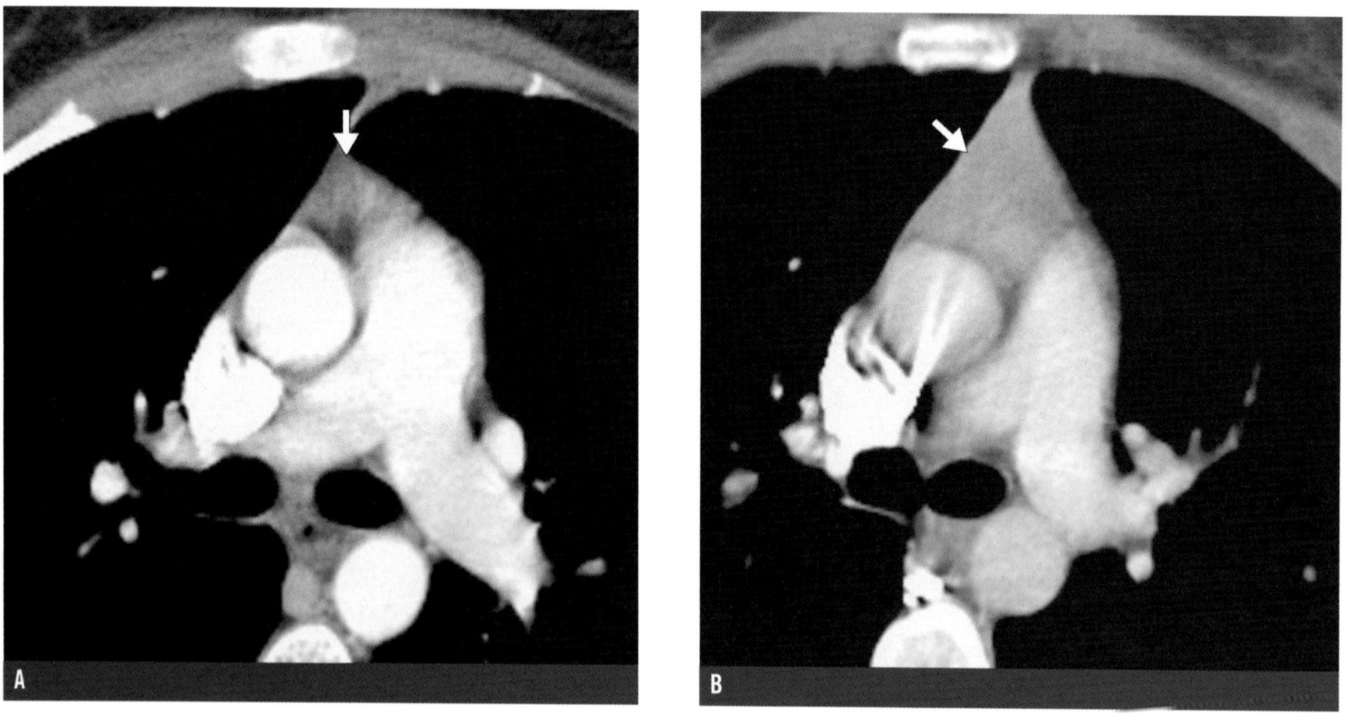

Different patient. A postcontrast axial CT image through the superior mediastinum when the patient was 29-year-old (**A**) demonstrates a small amount of triangle-shaped soft tissue in the anterior aspect of the superior mediastinum, compatible with normal residual thymic tissue (arrow, **A**). A postcontrast axial CT image obtained 4 years later (**B**) demonstrates interval enlargement of the thymic tissue with maintenance of its normal triangular-shape (arrow, **B**). This patient received chemotherapy during the interval and the findings are compatible with rebound thymus.

Companion case: Mediastinal lymphoma

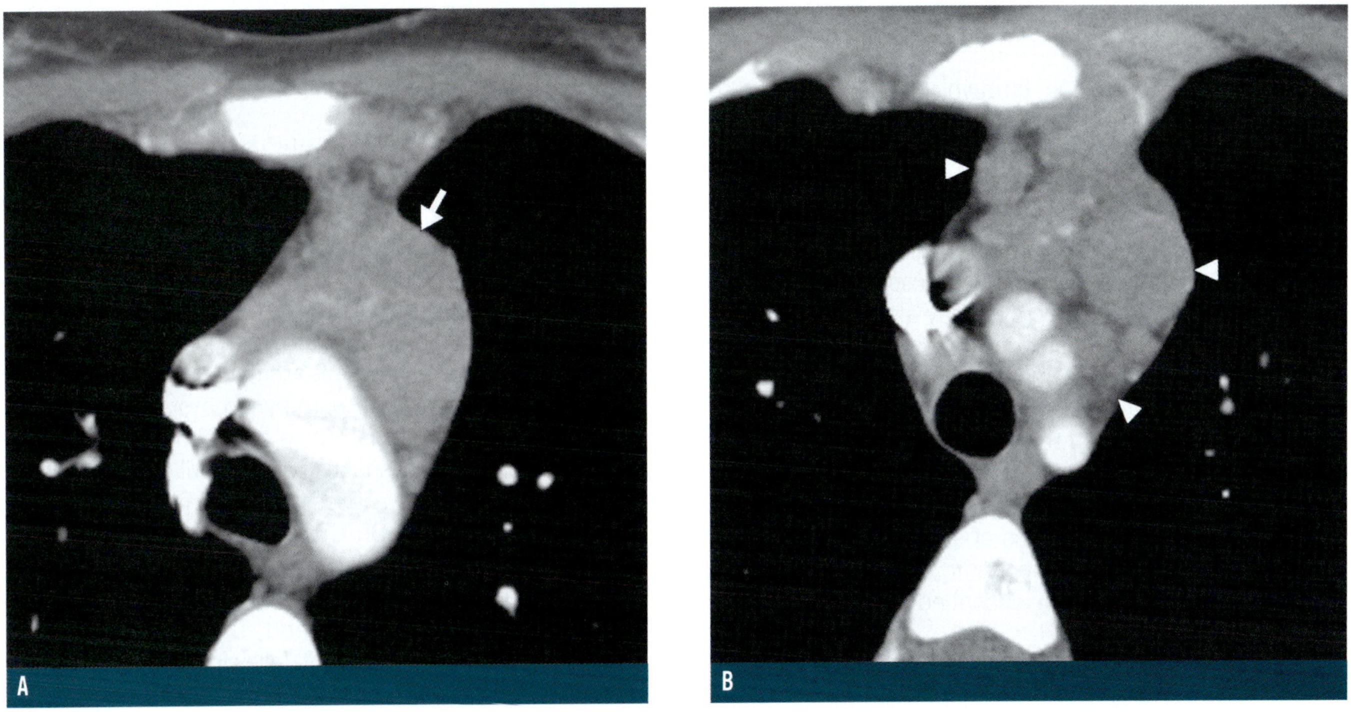

A postcontrast axial CT image through the superior mediastinum (**A**) demonstrates prominent soft tissue in the anterior mediastinum of a 24-year-old patient (arrow, **A**). The finding lacks angulated borders that are usually identified with residual or rebound thymus. A postcontrast axial image slightly more caudal than image **A** (**B**) demonstrates an abnormally large number of lymph nodes adjacent to the dominant finding (arrowheads, **B**). This patient had a history of Hodgkin lymphoma, and the findings are compatible with this diagnosis.

REFERENCES

Baron RL, Lee JK, Sagel SS, Peterson RR. Computed tomography of the normal thymus. *Radiology.* 1982;142:121.

Jerushalmi J, Frenkel A, Bar-Shalom R, Khoury J, Israel O. Physiologic thymic uptake of 18F-FDG in children and young adults: a PET/CT evaluation of incidence, patterns, and relationship to treatment. *J Nucl Med.* 2009;50(6):849-853.

Yarom N, Zissin R, Apter S, Hertz M, Rahimi-Levene N, Gayer G. Rebound thymic enlargement on CT in adults. *Int J Clin Pract.* 2007;61(4):562-568.

Any disruption during the embryological transit of the developing thymus can result in deposition of thymic tissue rests. Therefore, anomalies of the thymus gland may be present from the angle of the mandible to the mediastinum. A cervical thymus, if present, will follow the same imaging characteristics as normal thymic tissue located in the mediastinum, assuming it is composed of normal thymic tissue. A cervical thymic cyst may also develop in the neck, most commonly arising in the left neck and usually paralleling the sternocleidomastoid muscle.

Because 80% to 90% of discovered cervical thymus cases are asymptomatic, the true incidence of a cervical thymus is unknown. When large in size, mass effect from an ectopic thymus may compress or displace structures in the neck and cause symptoms of stridor, dysphagia, and hoarseness. Rarely, but importantly, thymic neoplasms (eg, thymoma), have been described to arise from an ectopic thymus.

If surgery to remove cervical thymic tissue is contemplated in a child or adolescent patient, then the presence of normal mediastinal thymus must be confirmed prior to resection. If normal mediastinal thymus is not present, then the cervical thymus may be the only functioning thymic tissue. Thus, removal of the cervical thymus in this setting should be avoided because it would likely result in deleterious effects to the developing immune system.

COMPANION CASE

- **Parathyroid cyst.** Parathyroid cysts are uncommon lesions that are frequently confused with thyroid cysts clinically and by imaging. Most parathyroid cysts are nonfunctional and asymptomatic. Occasionally, a parathyroid cyst may be functional and secrete parathyroid hormone (PTH), in which case it is treated the same as a hyperfunctioning parathyroid gland. Parathyroid cysts may occur anywhere from the mandible to the mediastinum, and large parathyroid cysts may result in compressive symptoms. While aspiration of a parathyroid cyst may decrease its size, most will recur following aspiration, frequently necessitating surgical removal for definitive treatment. On CT, parathyroid cysts manifest as a nonenhancing cystic mass, often arising from an inferior parathyroid gland. On MRI, parathyroid cysts follow fluid signal on T1- and T2-weighted imaging, and they lack enhancement following contrast administration. The diagnosis of a parathyroid cyst can be confirmed by fine-needle aspiration and assessing for an elevated C-terminal PTH level in the aspirate. Additionally, fluid from a parathyroid cyst is usually colorless and can be differentiated from a thyroid cyst, which is typically cloudy and hemorrhagic.

Cervical (ectopic) thymus

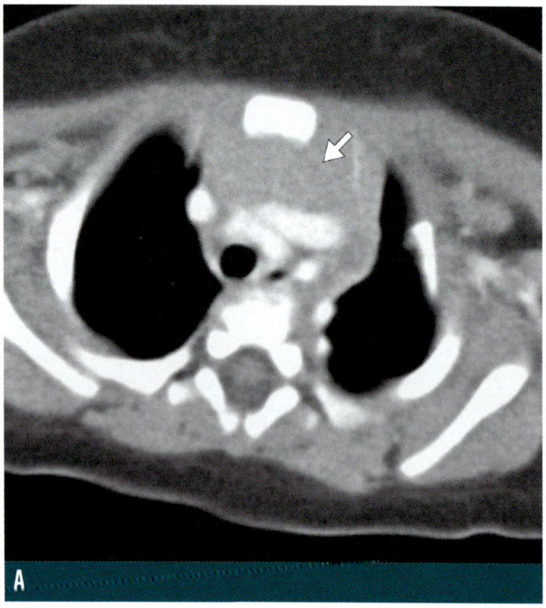

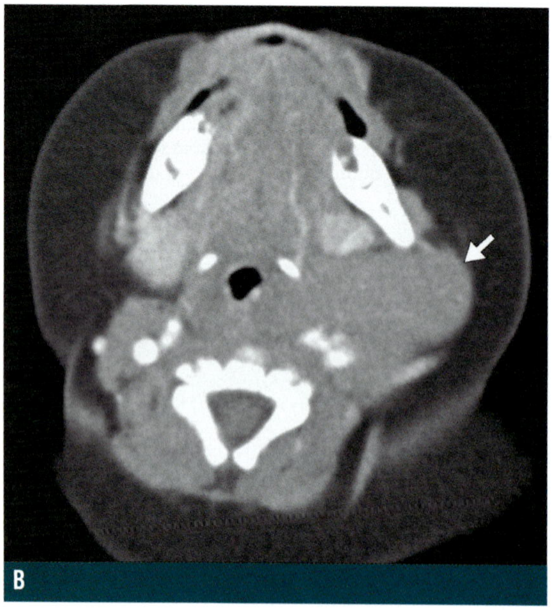

(Case courtesy of Alice Yao, MD, and Maura Ryan, MD, Children's Memorial Hospital, Chicago, IL). A postcontrast axial CT image through the superior mediastinum (**A**) demonstrates normal thymus in an infant (arrow, **A**). A postcontrast axial CT image obtained through the level of the oropharynx (**B**) demonstrates a mass in the left submandibular space (arrow, **B**). A Doppler ultrasound obtained in the transverse plane through the left submandibular region mass (**C**) does not demonstrate the mass to be hypervascular (arrow, **C**). Coronal T2 (**D**), noncontrast coronal T1 (**E**), and postcontrast coronal T1 with fat suppression (**F**) demonstrate the left submandibular region mass (arrows, **D-F**) to be isointense to the normal thymus (arrowheads, **D-F**) on all three pulse sequences. This finding represented a cervical thymus. (Case courtesy of Alice Yao, MD and Maura Ryan, MD.)

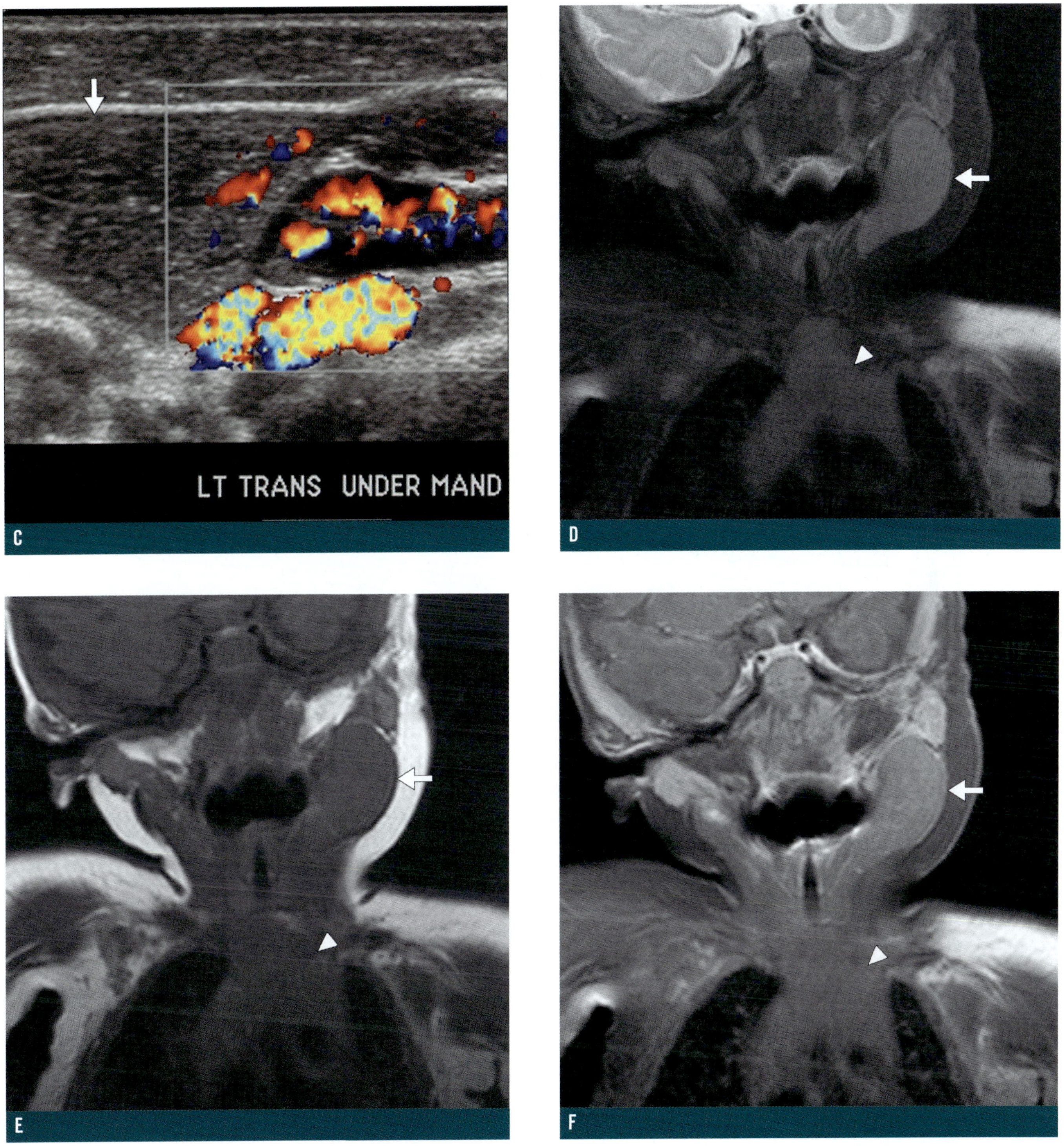
LT TRANS UNDER MAND
C
D
E
F

Companion case: Parathyroid cyst

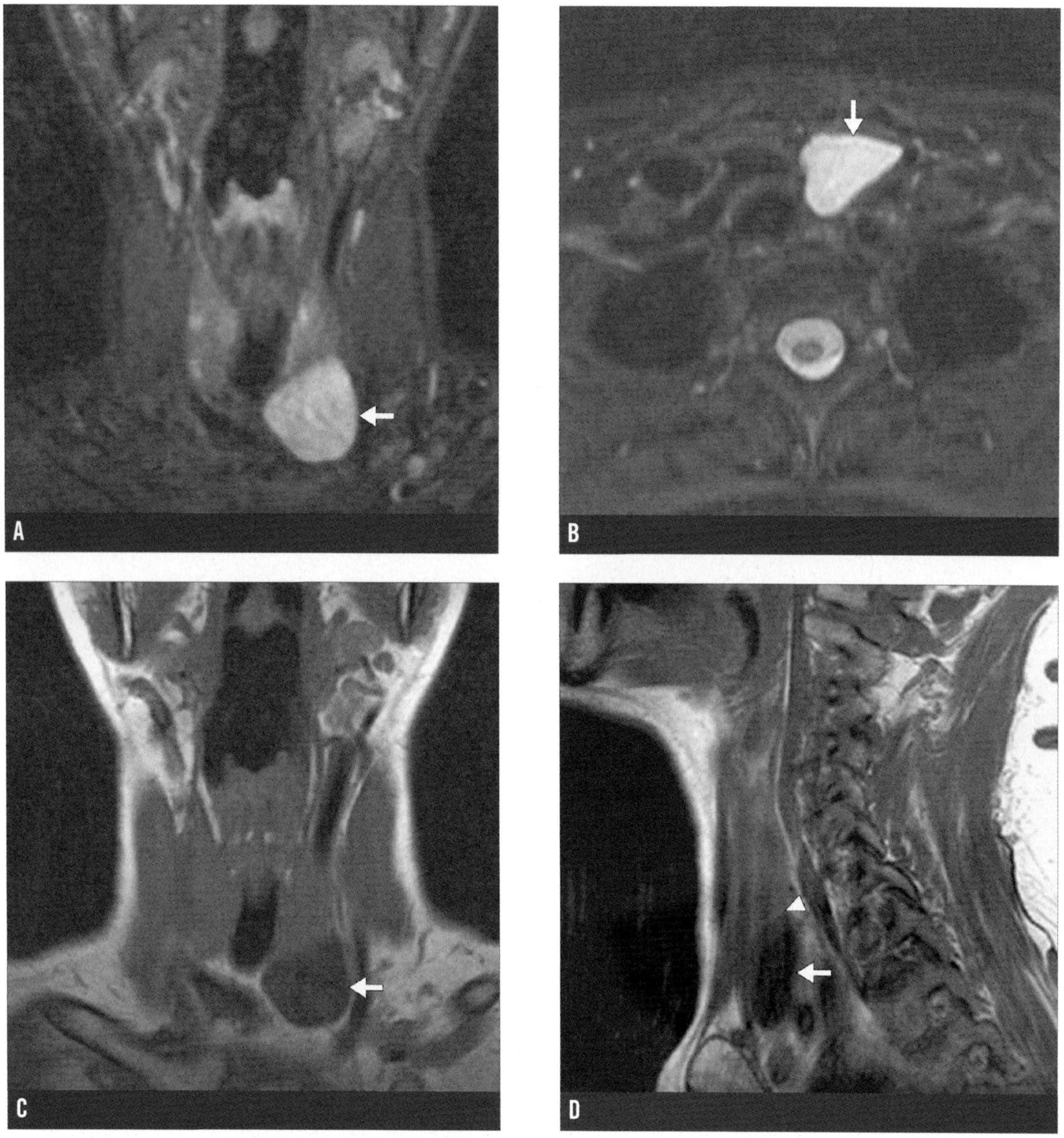

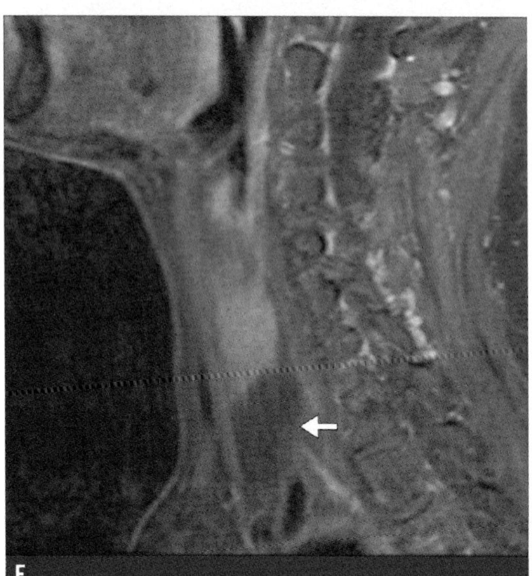

Coronal T2 with fat suppression (**A**), axial T2 with fat suppression (**B**), coronal T1 (**C**), and sagittal T1 (**D**) MR images demonstrate a circumscribed, T1 hypointense, T2 hyperintense lesion along the caudal aspect of the left thyroid lobe inferior pole (arrows, **A-D**). However, image **D** demonstrates a subtle fat plane between the thyroid gland and the lesion (arrowhead, **D**), suggesting that the finding does not arise from the thyroid gland. A contrast-enhanced sagittal T1 fat-suppressed MR image (**E**) does not demonstrate any lesional enhancement. This finding represented a nonfunctioning parathyroid cyst. However, by imaging, other entities are possible, including a cervical thymic cyst and a foregut duplication cyst.

REFERENCES

Herman TE, Siegel MJ. Cervical ectopic thymus. *J Perinatol.* 2009;29:173-174.

Jung JI, Kim HH, Park SH, Lee YS. Malignant ectopic thymoma in the neck: a case report. *AJNR Am J Neuroradiol.* 1999;20:1747-1749.

Pontikides N, et al. Diagnostic and therapeutic review of cystic parathyroid lesions. Hormones (Athens). 2012;11(4):410-418.

Saggese D, Ceroni Compadretti G, Cartaroni C. Cervical ectopic thymus: a case report and review of the literature. *Int J Pediatr Otorhinolaryngol.* 2002;66(1):77-80.

Som PM, Curtin HD. *Head and Neck Imaging.* 4th ed. St. Louis, MO: Mosby Inc; 2003.

Ujiki MB, Nayar R, Sturgeon C, Angelos P. Parathyroid cyst: often mistaken for a thyroid cyst. *World J Surg.* 2007;31(1):60-64.

Zielke AM, Swischuk LE, Hernandez JA. Ectopic cervical thymic tissue: can imaging obviate biopsy and surgical removal. *Pediatr Radiol.* 2007;37:1174-1177.

CHAPTER 5

THE ORAL CAVITY, TMJ, AND REGIONAL MUSCULATURE

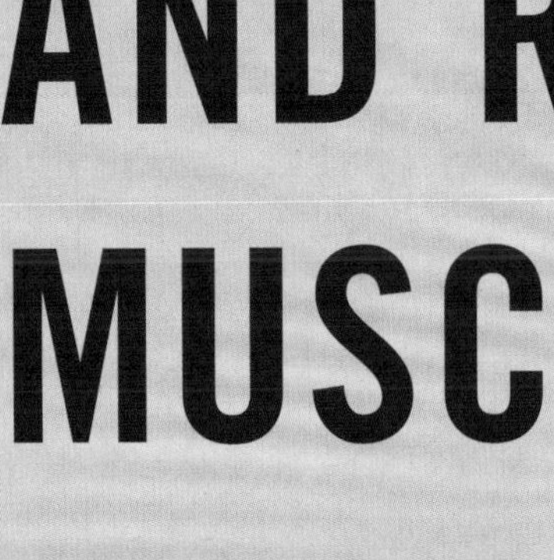

Alexander W. Korutz, Achilles G. Karagianis

V. The Oral Cavity, TMJ, and Regional Musculature

1. Normal nasopalatine canal and foramen
    i. *Companion case*: Nasopalatine duct cyst: Large, bilobulated, eccentrically located, and partially air-filled patterns
    ii. *Companion case*: Squamous cell carcinoma of the palate
2. Radicular cyst
    i. *Companion case*: Periapical abscess
    ii. *Companion case*: Dental abscess following a tooth extraction
    iii. *Companion case*: Odontogenic sinusitis
    iv. *Companion case*: Dentigerous cyst
    v. *Companion case*: Residual cyst
    vi. *Companion case*: Keratocystic odontogenic tumor
    vii. *Companion case*: Basal cell nevus syndrome
    viii. *Companion case*: Ameloblastoma
    ix. *Companion case*: Lymphoma of the mandible
    x. *Companion case*: Multiple myeloma
    xi. *Companion case*: Stafne cyst
3. Torus palatinus, Torus mandibularis, and Torus maxillaris
    i. *Companion case*: Mandibular osteoma
    ii. *Companion case*: Mandibular osteosarcoma
    iii. *Companion case*: Buccal alveolus venous malformation
    iv. *Companion case*: Chewing gum mimicking a torus palatinus
4. Supernumerary teeth
    i. *Companion case*: Unerupted teeth in a child
5. Dilaceration
6. Bifid or cleft morphology of the mandibular condyle
    i. *Companion case*: Mandibular condyle hypoplasia
    ii. *Companion case*: Motion artifact
7. Benign masticatory muscle hypertrophy
    i. *Companion case*: Benign masticatory muscle hypertrophy with hemimandibular hyperplasia
    ii. *Companion case*: Hemimandibular hyperplasia with dental malocclusion
    iii. *Companion case*: Leiomyosarcoma of the mandible
8. Pseudosubluxation of the temporomandibular joint
    i. *Companion case*: Anterior TMJ dislocation
    ii. *Companion case*: Malocclusion from tooth loss leading to ipsilateral TMJ subluxation
9. Enostosis
    i. *Companion case*: Fibrous dysplasia
    ii. *Companion case*: Cemento-osseous dysplasia
    iii. *Companion case*: Cementoblastoma
    iv. *Companion case*: Odontoma
10. Genial tubercle
    i. *Companion case*: Genial tubercle mimicking a Wharton duct sialolith
    ii. *Companion case*: Distal Wharton duct sialolith
11. Dental implants and restorations
    i. *Companion case*: Soft tissue abscess associated with an infected dental implant
    ii. *Companion case*: MRI artifact from dental restoration and dental braces
    iii. *Companion case*: CT streak artifact from normal dental enamel
12. Dentures
13. Macroglossia related to an edentulous state
    i. *Companion case*: Angioedema-induced macroglossia
    ii. *Companion case*: Vascular malformation of the tongue
    iii. *Companion case*: Squamous cell carcinoma of the tongue
14. Denervation atrophy of the tongue
    i. *Companion case*: Squamous cell carcinoma of the oral tongue
    ii. *Companion case*: Squamous cell carcinoma of the tongue base
15. Denervation atrophy of the floor of mouth musculature
16. Anomalies of the anterior bellies of the digastric muscles
17. Mylohyoid muscle defect (boutonnière deformity)
    i. *Companion case*: Ranula extending through a boutonnière deformity
18. Intraoral comestible foreign bodies
    i. *Companion case*: Wharton duct sialolith
    ii. *Companion case*: Retained oral contrast
19. Piercings
20. Oropharyngeal airway device and bite blocks
21. Palatal sutures mimicking a fracture
    i. *Companion case*: Palate fracture
    ii. *Companion case*: Cleft palate
22. Orthognathic surgery: Le Fort I and bilateral sagittal split osteotomies
23. Orthognathic surgery: Genioglossus advancement surgery
24. Midline mandibular osteotomy
    i. *Companion case*: Lingual foramen and canal
25. Chin augmentation
26. Normal presymphyseal fat pad
    i. *Companion case*: Chin abscess
27. Mandibular fixation following trauma
28. Fibular strut graft
29. Palatal obturator
30. Myocutaneous flap floor of mouth and oral tongue reconstruction
    i. *Companion case*: Tongue deviation simulating a partial glossectomy
    ii. *Companion case*: Ludwig angina
    iii. *Companion case*: Retromolar trigone squamous cell carcinoma
    iv. *Companion case*: Schwannoma of the oral cavity

CASE 1 Normal nasopalatine canal and foramen

The nasopalatine canal is located in the anterior midline palate and transmits the nasopalatine nerve, a branch of the maxillary division of the trigeminal nerve, as well as branches of the maxillary artery and vein. Superiorly, the nasopalatine canal opens into the floor of the nasal cavity via one or two foramina of Stensen. In some patients, up to four additional foramina, termed the foramina of Scarpa, are present within the floor of the nasal cavity. Inferiorly, the foramina of Stensen and/or Scarpa typically coalesce into a single canal that opens into the oral cavity via the nasopalatine foramen, also referred to as the incisive foramen. The nasopalatine canal is variable in width, usually measuring between 2 and 6 mm. Nasopalatine canal widths measuring between 6 and 10 mm may be considered normal, assuming there are no aggressive features, such as osseous destruction. However, when a canal diameter measures wider than 10 mm, a pathologic process could be present. Studies have shown that the nasopalatine canal can increase in size with both age and tooth loss, the former of which is thought to be due to age-related bone resorption.

COMPANION CASES

- **Nasopalatine duct cyst: Large, bilobulated, eccentrically located, and partially air-filled patterns.** Nasopalatine duct cysts, also referred to as incisive canal or nasopalatine cysts, are the most common nonodontogenic cysts. The cysts are thought to arise from epithelial remnants of the nasopalatine duct and, as such, are lined by stratified squamous epithelium with varying combinations of pseudostratified columnar, simple columnar, and simple cuboidal epithelial components. These cysts are usually asymptomatic; however, some patients may experience symptoms including burning or numbness from compression of the adjacent neurovascular bundle, swelling of the hard palate, drainage, and superinfection. The cysts are variable in size and can be quite large. In some patients, a nasopalatine duct cyst may communicate with the oral and/or nasal cavities, which may be on imaging suspected when air or debris is identified within the cyst.

  The cysts are normally located at or near the midline, have a thin sclerotic rim of cortical bone, and are round, ovoid or heart-shaped in configuration. Variant appearances include a bilobed shape or eccentric positioning within the hard palate. When the cyst is positioned more posteriorly within the palate, the more specific term, median palatal cyst, may be used.
- **Squamous cell carcinoma of the palate**. Squamous cell carcinoma (SCC) is the most common malignancy of the oral cavity. On CT, SCC usually manifests as a homogeneous soft tissue mass that may be associated with localized osseous destruction. On MRI, these tumors are typically iso- to hypointense on T1-weighted imaging. On T2-weighted imaging, SCC is variable in signal, but often T2 iso- to hyperintense relative to muscle. Smaller SCCs of the palate are usually homogeneously enhancing, whereas larger SCCs of the palate are usually heterogeneously enhancing, often due to necrosis. A helpful imaging finding to help distinguish tumors from benign cystic lesions of the maxilla is the presence of an associated soft tissue lesion/mass eroding the osseous margins of the lytic lesion. As is the case with other malignant tumors of the hard palate, examination for perineural spread of tumor is critical in cases of palate SCC, particularly along the greater and lesser palatine foramina as well as along the nasopalatine canal.

Normal nasopalatine canal

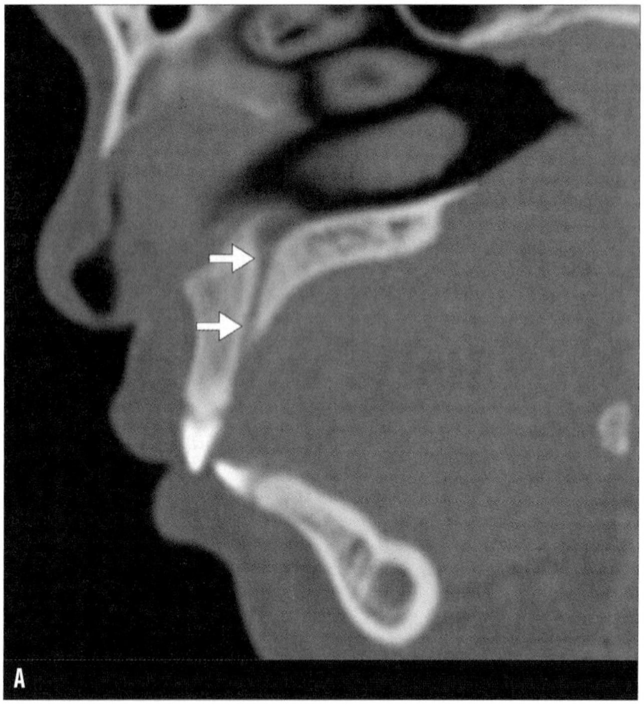

A sagittal reformatted CT image through the midline palate viewed with a bone window (**A**) demonstrates a normal nasopalatine canal (also called incisive canal) (arrows). Its inferior opening into the oral cavity is the nasopalatine foramen (also called incisive foramen).

Normal nasopalatine canal

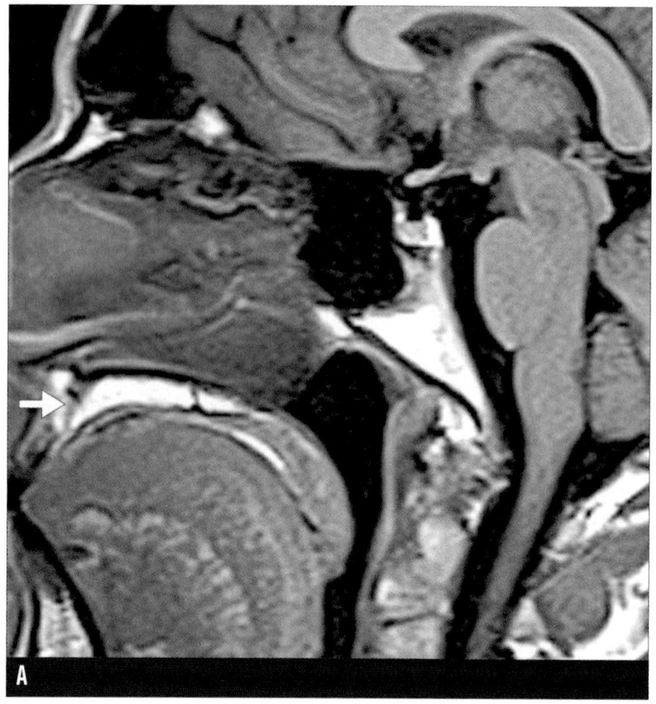

Different patient. A sagittal T1 MR image through the midline palate (**A**) demonstrates a normal nasopalatine canal (arrows).

Normal nasopalatine foramen with Stensen and Scarpa foramina

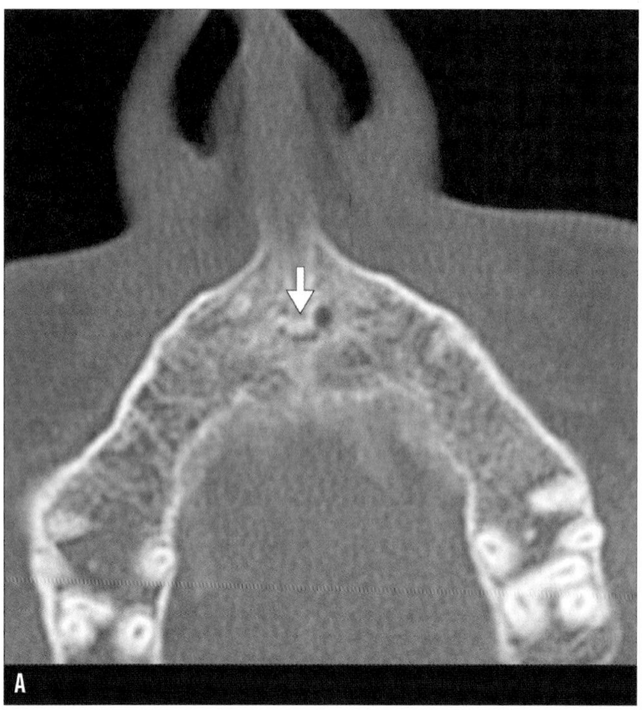

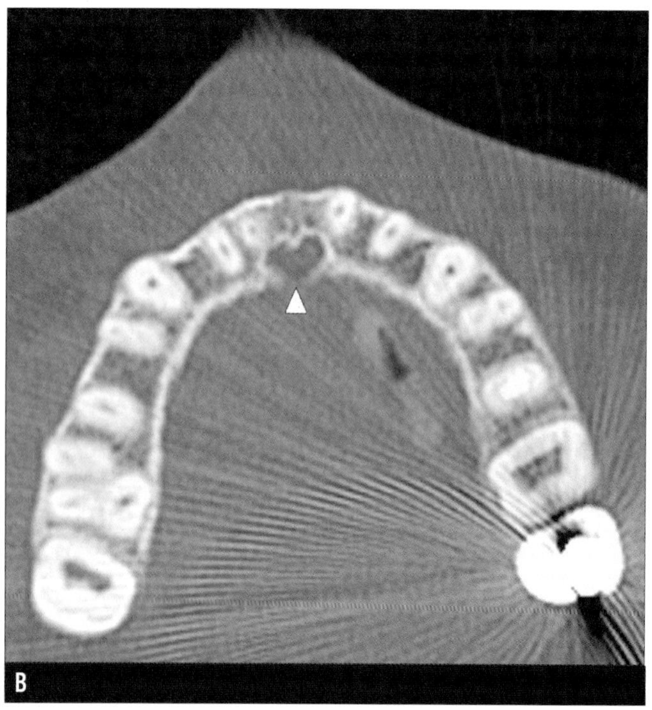

Axial CT images (**A**, **B**) demonstrate several small foramina of Stensen and Scarpa near the floor of the nasal cavity (arrow, **A**) and a single, normal, heart-shaped nasopalatine foramen at the level of the oral cavity (arrowhead, **B**).

Companion case: Large nasopalatine duct cyst

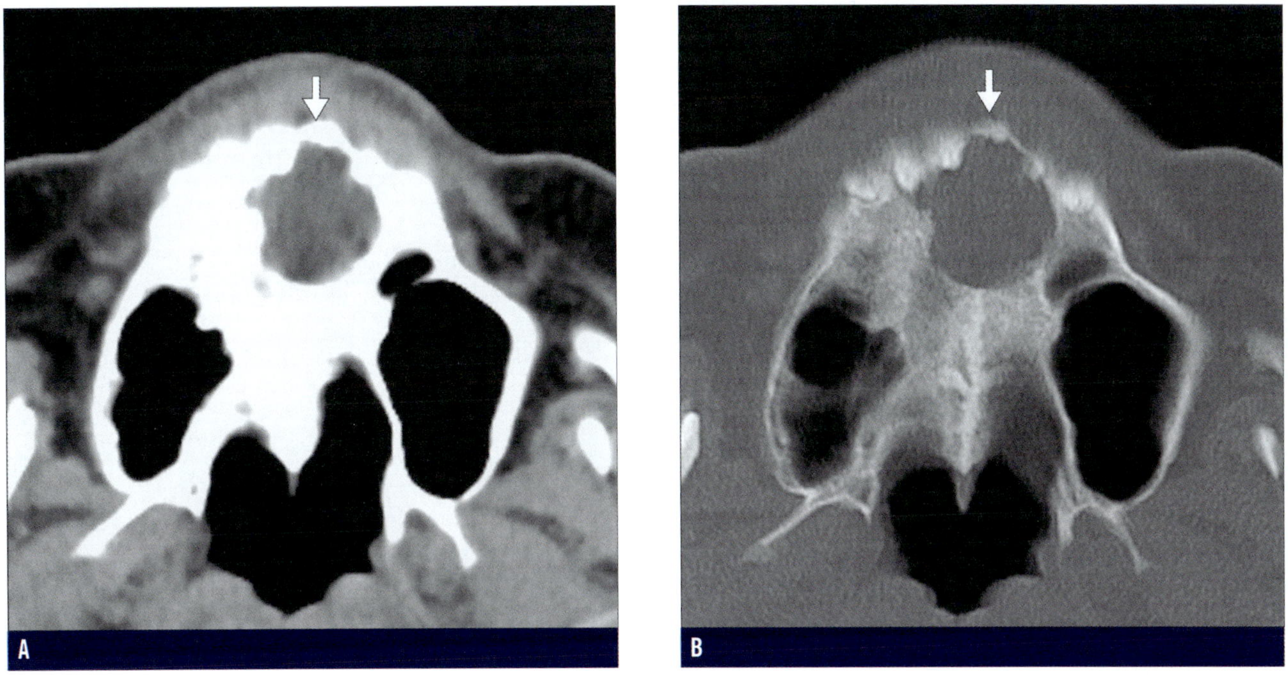

Unenhanced axial CT images viewed with a soft tissue window (**A**) and a bone window (**B**) through the anterior maxilla. Image **A** demonstrates an expansile lesion centered in the nasopalatine canal, which measured 25 mm in greatest axial dimension. The contents of the lesion are slightly lower in attenuation than muscle, suggesting fluid. The premaxillary soft tissues are unremarkable. Image **B** demonstrates marked expansion of the nasopalatine canal, though the wall of the lesion is fairly smooth and is intact. This patient was completely asymptomatic from this finding. The constellation of findings is most consistent with an enlarged nasopalatine duct cyst, an incidental finding. However, if the patient was symptomatic from this finding, then other etiologies would need to be considered, such as a tumor, and would warrant further evaluation with either contrast-enhanced CT or MRI.

Companion case: Bilobulated nasopalatine duct cyst

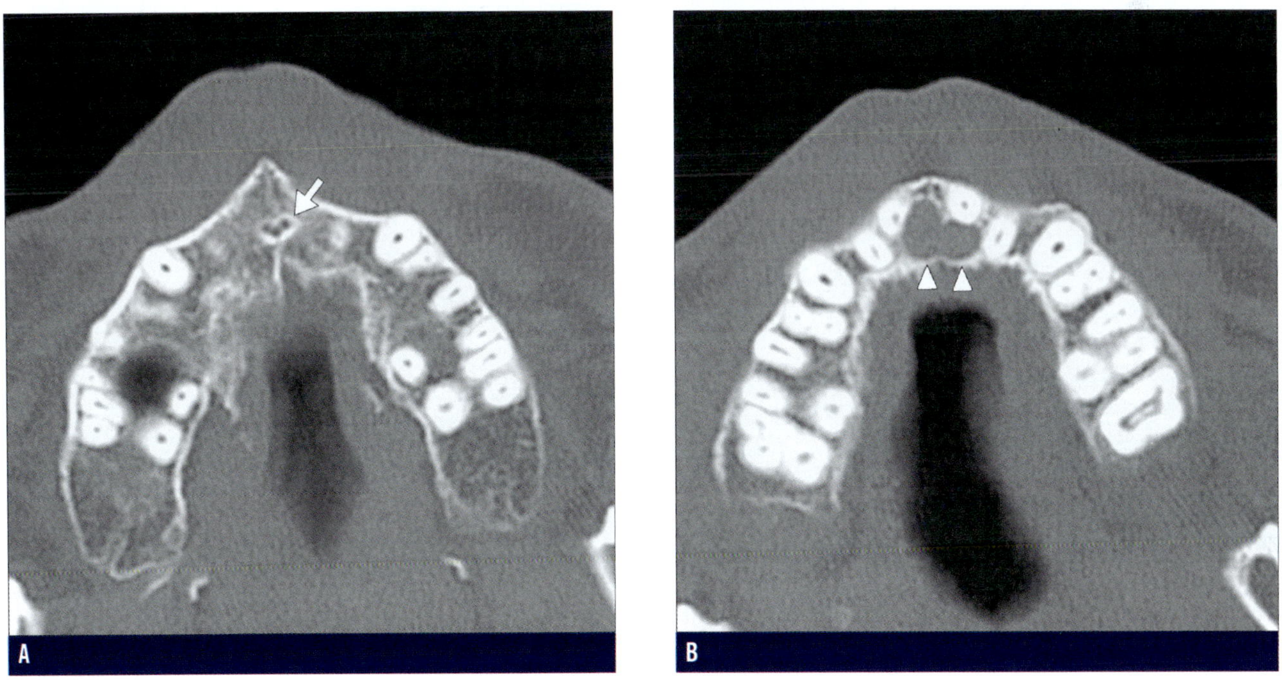

An axial CT image (**A**) demonstrates the midline nasopalatine foramina (arrow, **A**). A slightly more caudal axial image (**B**) as well as sagittal reformatted (**C**) and coronal reformatted (**D**) CT images demonstrate a 12 mm wide, bilobulate, expansile, lucent area consistent with a nasopalatine duct cyst (arrowheads, **B-D**). The lesion is located inferior to and contiguous with the nasopalatine canal (arrow, **C**).

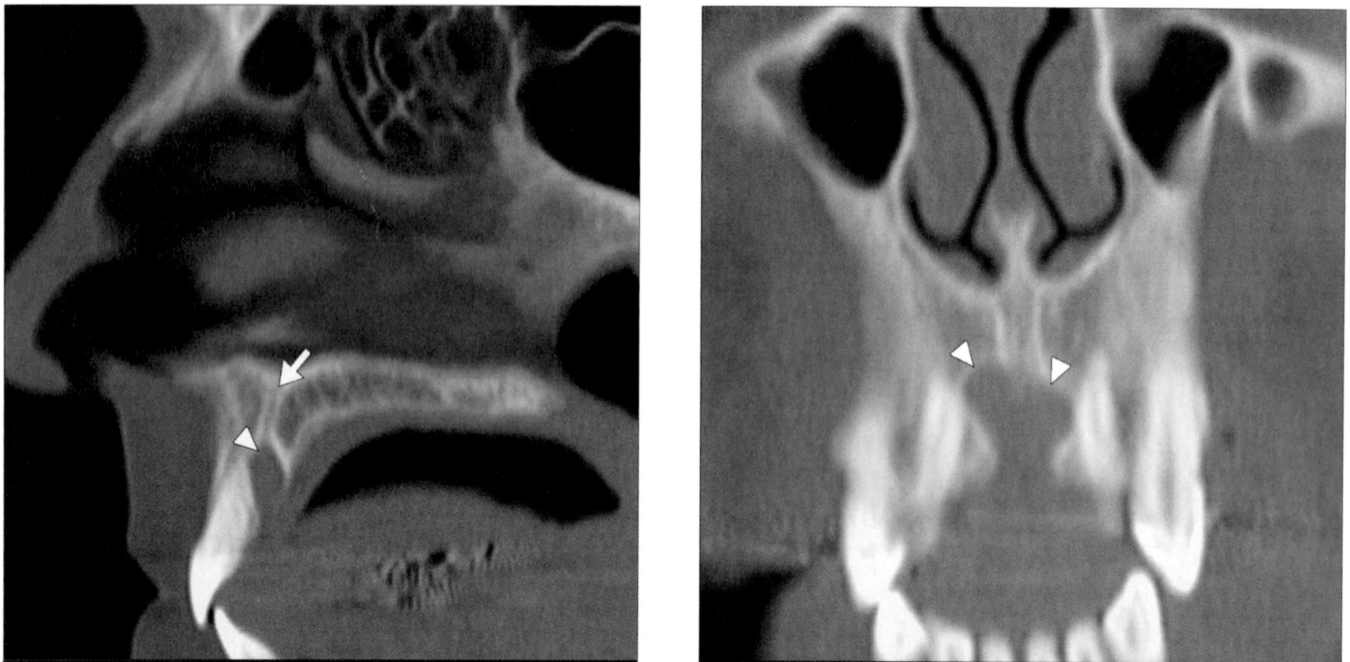

C **D**

Companion case: Eccentrically located nasopalatine duct cyst

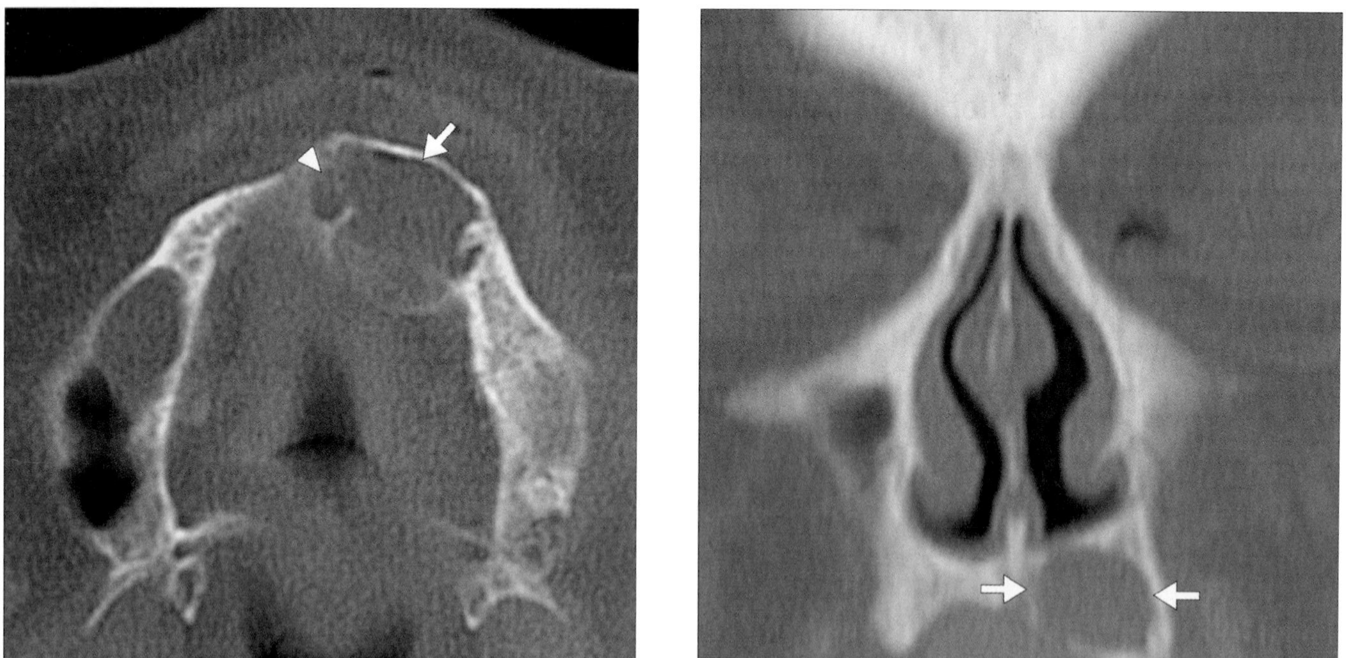

A **B**

Axial (**A**), coronal reformatted (**B**), and sagittal reformatted (**C**) CT images through the anterior maxillary alveolus viewed with a bone window demonstrate an expansile, lucent lesion (arrows, **A**-**C**) eccentrically located with respect to the nasopalatine canal (arrowhead, **A**). An axial CT image viewed with a soft tissue window at the same level as image **A** (**D**) demonstrates soft tissue/fluid occupying the expansile lucent lesion, most compatible with an eccentrically located nasopalatine duct cyst (arrow, **D**). Sagittal unenhanced T1 (**E**), axial T2 (**F**), and postcontrast axial T1 (**G**) MR images through the anterior maxillary alveolus demonstrates the same lesion on MRI. The lesion is slightly intrinsically hyperintense on T1 (arrow, **E**), isointense relative to muscle on T2 (arrows, **F**), and does not enhance on postcontrast T1-weighted imaging (arrows, **G**). The MRI findings are compatible with a benign proteinaceous cyst.

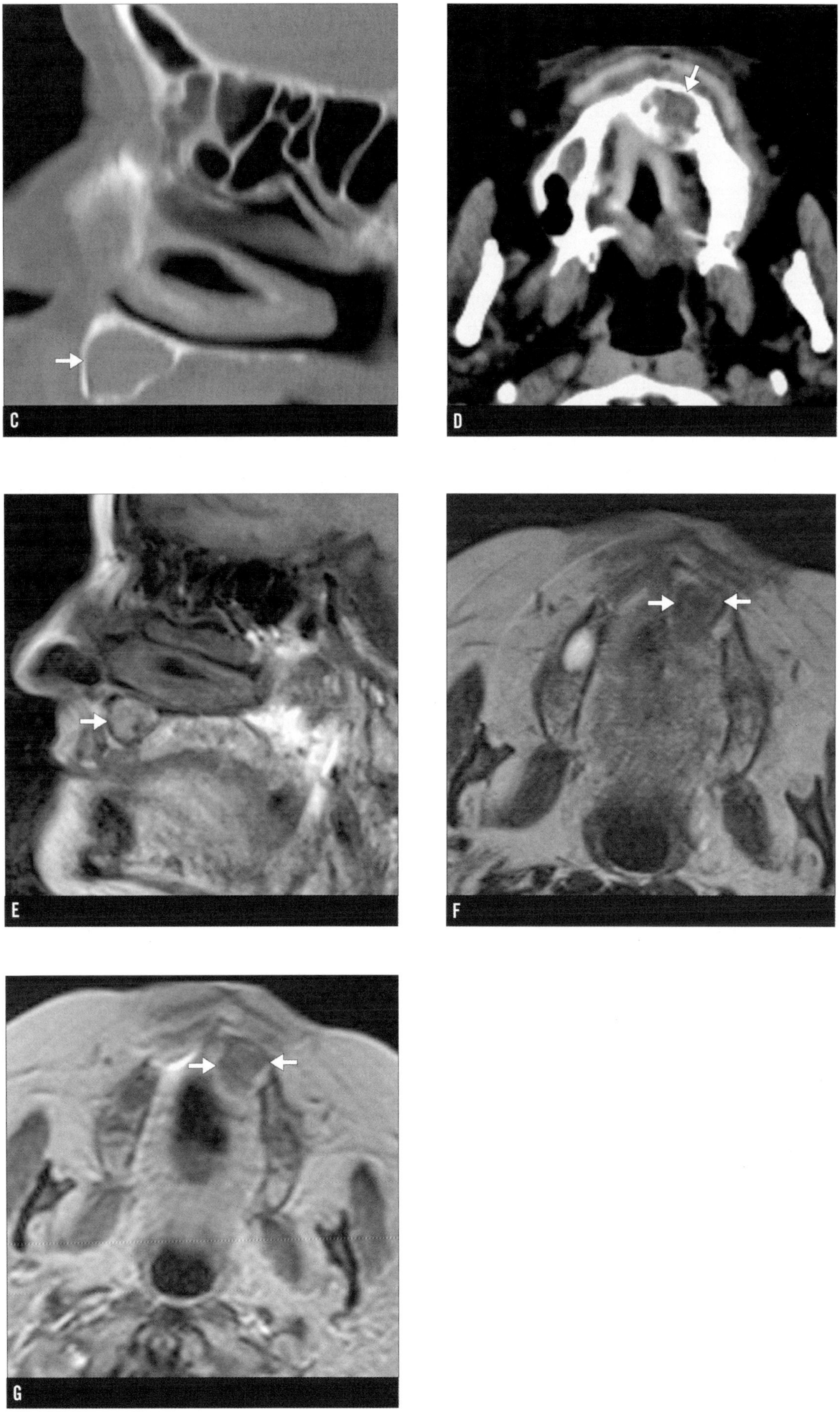
C
D
E
F
G

Companion case: Partially air-filled nasopalatine duct cyst

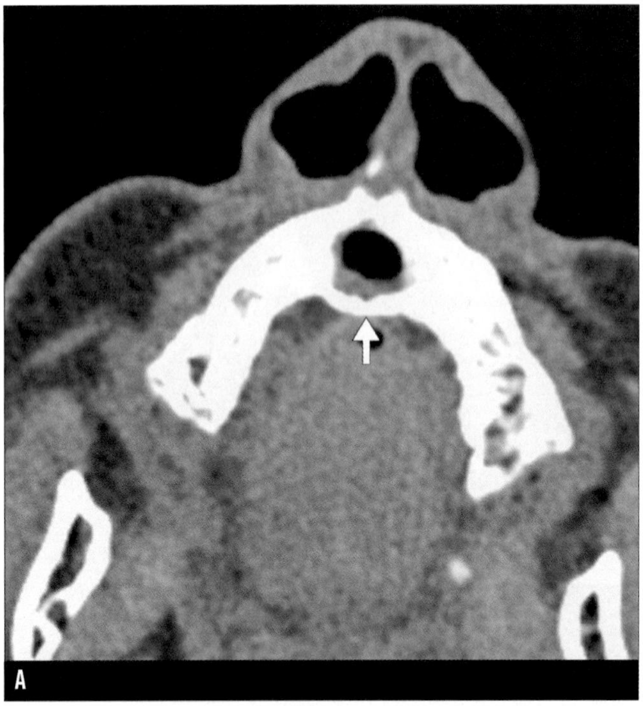

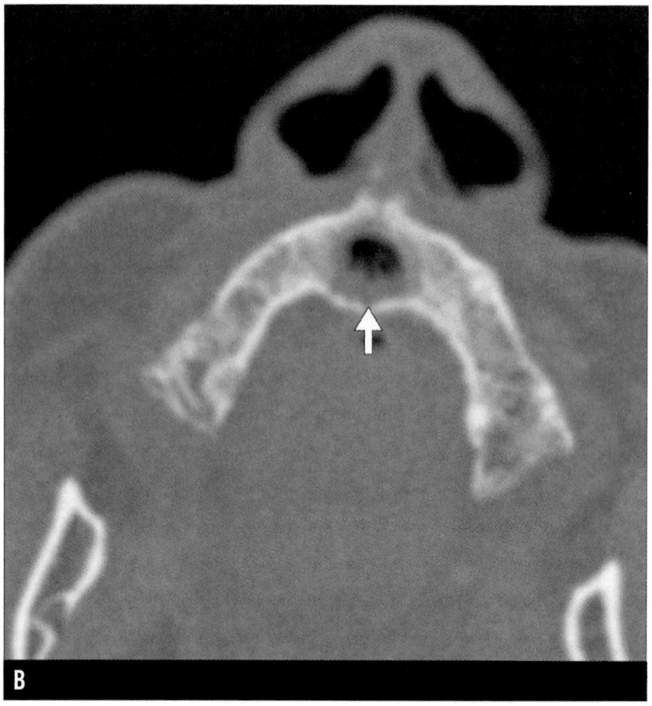

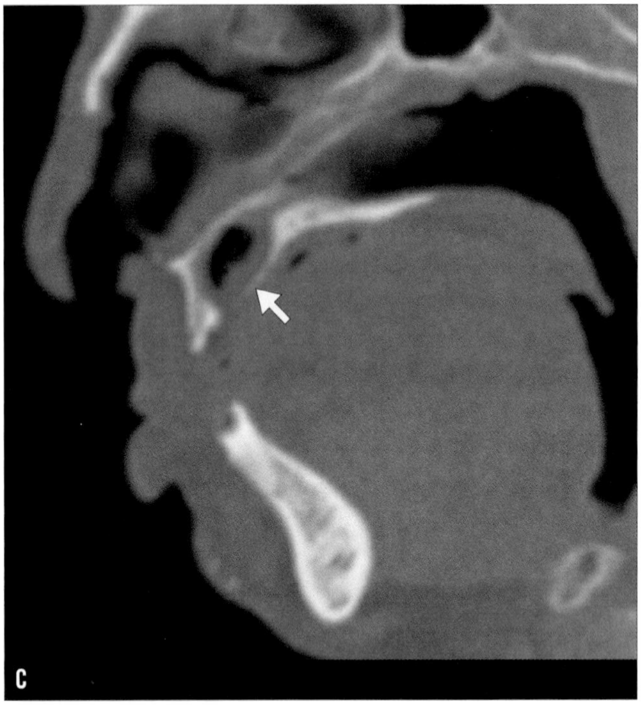

Axial CT images viewed with a soft tissue window (**A**) and bone window (**B**) as well as a sagittal reformatted CT image viewed with a bone window (**C**) demonstrate a nasopalatine duct cyst which is occupied with mucosa/debris and air (arrows, **A-C**). This is likely due to a communication between the nasopalatine duct cyst and the adjacent oral and/or nasal cavities.

Companion case: Squamous cell carcinoma of the palate

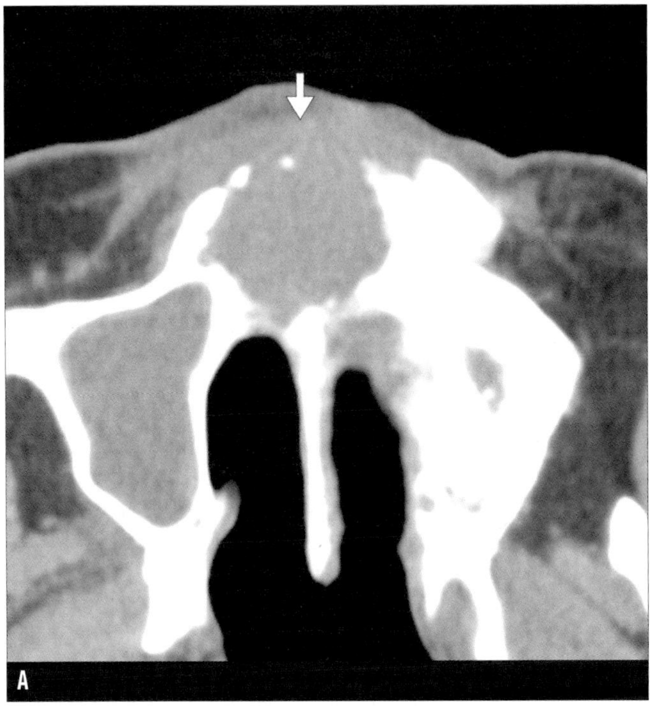

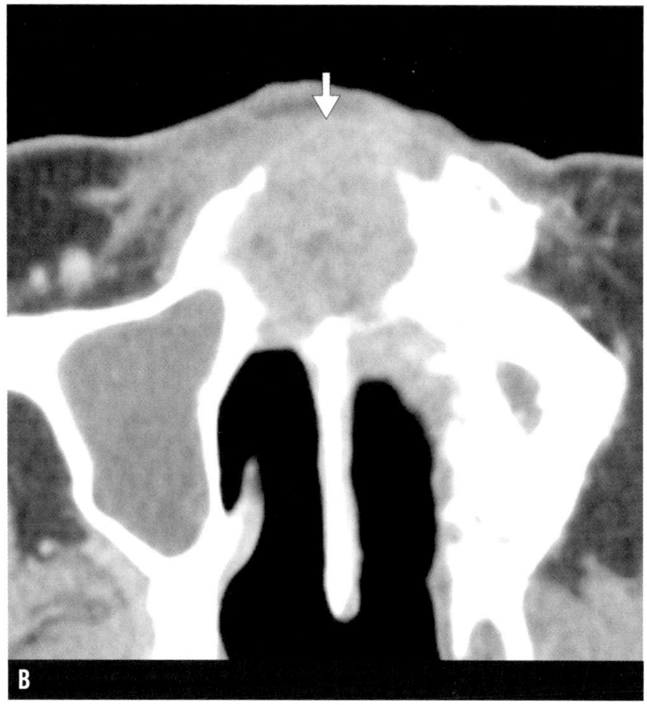

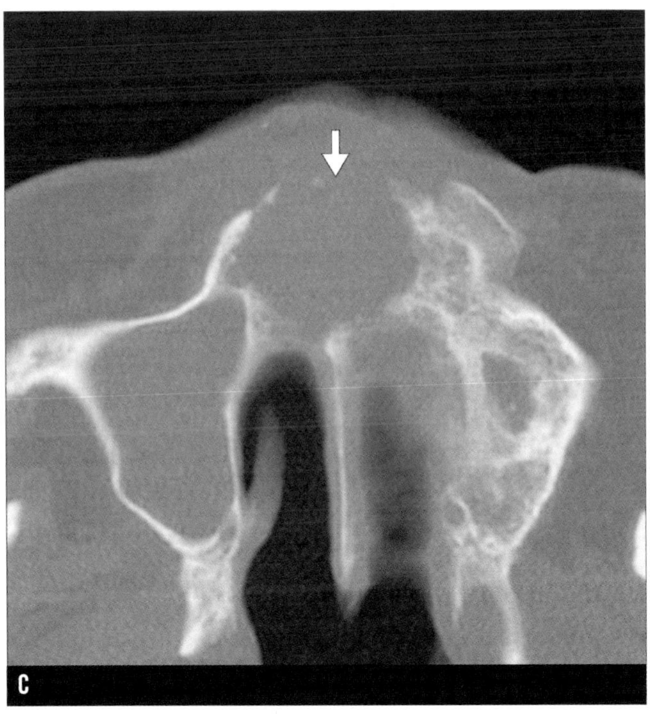

Axial pre- and postcontrast CT images (**A** and **B**, respectively) viewed with a soft tissue window demonstrate an enhancing, soft tissue mass within the ventral midline aspect of the hard palate with premaxillary soft tissue extension of the lesion (arrows, **A**, **B**). An axial CT image viewed with a bone window (**C**) best demonstrates associated osseous destruction, primarily along the ventral aspect of this lesion (arrow, **C**). This lesion was a pathologically proven squamous cell carcinoma. The osseous destruction, enhancement, and premaxillary soft tissue extension helps differentiate this case from a benign nasopalatine duct cyst.

REFERENCES

Beil CM, Keberle M. Oral and oropharyngeal tumors. *Eur J Radiol.* 2008;66(3):448-459.

Francoli JE, Marques NA, Aytes LB, Escoda CG. Nasopalatine duct cyst: report of 22 cases and review of the literature. *Med Oral Patol Oral Cir Bucal.* 2008;13(7):E438-E443.

Liang X, et al. Macro- and micro-anatomical, histological and computed tomography scan characterization of the nasopalatine canal. *J Clin Periodontol.* 2009;36:598-603.

Mraiwa N, et al. The nasopalatine canal revisited using 2D and 3D CT imaging. dentomaxillofacial. *Radiol.* 2004;33:396-402.

Swanson KS, Kaugars GE, Gunsolley JC. Nasopalatine duct cyst: an analysis of 334 cases. *J Oral Maxillofacial Surg.* 1991;49(3):268-271.

CASE 2 Radicular cyst

A radicular cyst (also called periapical cyst, periodontal cyst, or dental cyst) results when a periapical abscess or granuloma trigger the proliferation of epithelial rests located within the periodontal ligament, termed the epithelial rests of Malassez. It is these rests of Malassez that help form the radicular cysts. Like periapical granulomas, radicular cysts are often asymptomatic, though both types of cysts may enlarge over time.

On imaging, radicular cysts, periapical abscesses, and periapical granulomas all appear as a radiolucent lesions surrounding the root apex of the diseased tooth and generally cannot be differentiated by imaging alone. The exception is when there is a fluid collection in the adjacent perialveolar soft tissues, in which case an abscess can be favored. In some instances, the roots of the involved tooth will be resorbed, particularly when a periapical abscess is present. A radicular cyst is typically not treated.

COMPANION CASES

- **Periapical abscess.** When a dental caries extends to involve the pulp chamber of a tooth, the infection can violate the root apex of a tooth and spread into the adjacent alveolar process of the maxilla/mandible. During the acute infectious phase, this is termed a periapical abscess. If the infectious process extends through the cortex of the involved alveolar process of the maxilla/mandible, it may lead to spread of infection into the adjacent soft tissues or maxillary sinus, the latter of which is termed an odontogenic sinusitis. Patients with a dental abscess frequently complain of an exquisitely painful tooth. A periapical abscess may be treated with a root canal procedure or tooth extraction. A periapical granuloma differs from a periapical abscess in that it represents a low-grade inflammatory process that extends through the root apex of a tooth and results in the formation of granulation tissue.
- **Dental abscess following a tooth extraction.** Soft tissue infections may occur following a tooth extraction, particularly if the tooth extracted was a carious tooth. These infections usually involve the buccal space but may extend elsewhere in the neck if the abscess is large. On CT, an abscess will manifest as a peripherally enhancing fluid collection. On MRI, an abscess is often centrally T1 hypointense, centrally T2 hyperintense, and peripherally enhances following contrast administration. After identifying a soft tissue infection in this region, it is important to evaluate the mandible and/or maxilla for an extracted tooth socket (usually recently extracted), an indwelling carious tooth, or a tooth with periodontal/periapical lucency (particularly one associated with a focal cortical osseous defect) that could account for the abscess.
- **Odontogenic sinusitis.** This entity occurs when a dental abscess and/or periodontal disease along the maxillary alveolus perforates into the maxillary sinus lumen or when there is a breach in the maxillary sinus floor following a dental extraction. The maxillary sinus lumen may be partially or completely opacified, may contain a fluid level, and the inflammatory process may spread through the ostiomeatal unit to involve other paranasal sinuses. The patient may complain of headaches, tenderness over the affected maxillary sinus, and dental pain. Evaluation of any opacified maxillary sinus should include a survey of the maxillary teeth in order to identify this dental complication. The treatment of odontogenic sinusitis includes medical treatment of the sinus infection and dental surgical intervention.
- **Dentigerous cyst**. Dentigerous cysts are the second most common odontogenic cyst, second only to periapical cysts related to infection/inflammation. A dentigerous cyst forms as a result of fluid that accumulates between the follicular epithelium and the crown of an unerupted tooth. A unique characteristic of a dentigerous cyst is that it surrounds the dental crown and its margins merge at the cementoenamel junction. The cementoenamel junction represents the "neck" of the tooth, where the cementum (which covers the tooth roots) and the enamel (which covers the tooth crown) meet one another. A dentigerous cyst can slowly increase in size, potentially displacing adjacent teeth or eroding into the maxillary sinus. While dentigerous cysts are typically asymptomatic, facial pain, swelling, headache, and sinus obstruction have all been described. On radiography and CT, a dentigerous cyst is typically unilocular with defined, sclerotic borders that surround the crown of an unerupted tooth. On MRI, these cysts can appear iso- to hypointense on T1 and hyperintense on T2-weighted imaging. Some cysts will have thin peripheral enhancement. If an enhancing nodular component is identified, then other diagnoses should be considered.
- **Residual cyst.** The term residual cyst refers to an odontogenic cyst that remains after extraction of a tooth, regardless of whether the cyst is inflammatory or developmental in nature. Inflammatory cysts include a periapical abscess, periapical granuloma, and radicular cyst. Examples of developmental cysts include dentigerous cysts and keratocystic odontogenic tumors, among several others.
- **Keratocystic odontogenic tumor**. Formerly known as an odontogenic keratocyst, a keratocystic odontogenic tumor (KOT) is believed to arise from odontogenic epithelium, such as the dental lamina. A KOT is a cystic mass that most commonly occurs within the body or ramus of the mandible. On radiography and CT, a KOT

may be associated with an impacted tooth and varies in appearance, ranging from a unilocular, lucent lesion which has smooth, corticated margins, to a multilocular lesion which is associated with cortical thinning, tooth displacement, and root resorption. On MRI, a KOT is often T2 hyperintense, but its T2 signal characteristics may vary. A KOT is typically iso- to hyperintense on T1-weighted images, depending on the cyst contents. Postcontrast MR images will demonstrate a thin wall that may peripherally enhance. Because of the varying imaging appearance of a KOT, a prospective diagnosis of a KOT is often quite difficult. When a KOT has a benign appearance, it may be indistinguishable from a radicular or dentigerous cyst. When a KOT has an aggressive appearance, it may be indistinguishable from an ameloblastoma; however, an enhancing nodule is not typically present with a KOT, whereas one is commonly present with an ameloblastoma. KOTs are treated by complete resection because they will frequently recur if they are only treated with curettage.

- **Basal cell nevus syndrome.** Multiple KOTs are associated with basal cell nevus syndrome (Gorlin-Goltz syndrome). This syndrome is associated with multiple basal cell carcinomas, multiple mandibular KOTs, rib anomalies, intracranial calcifications, spinal kyphoscoliosis, and facial anomalies.
- **Ameloblastoma.** Ameloblastomas are benign cystic neoplasms that originate from the dental follicular epithelium. Most of these tumors arise within the ramus and posterior body of the mandible. Frequently, an ameloblastoma will be associated with the crown of an impacted tooth and contain a solid enhancing component. Approximately 50% of ameloblastomas originate from the epithelial lining of a dentigerous cyst, otherwise known as a mural ameloblastoma. While ameloblastomas are slow-growing lesions, they may exhibit locally aggressive behavior, including extension of a soft tissue component into the adjacent soft tissues. These lesions can vary in appearance, ranging from a unilocular, well-corticated cystic lesion to a multilocular, expansile lesion containing multiple internal septa. On CT, these lesions may contain both cystic and solid components, the latter often enhancing following contrast administration. On MRI, the cystic component is typically T1 hypointense and T2 hyperintense. On postcontrast MR images, the solid component will avidly enhance. An ameloblastoma may also have a thick enhancing wall or enhancing septa. These tumors are treated with a wide local excision.
- **Lymphoma of the mandible.** Osseous lymphoma, typically representing the Non-Hodgkin variety, most frequently occurs as a secondary process in a patient with primary nodal lymphoma, rather than presenting as a primary lesion. Imaging features of osseous lymphoma are protean and include lesions that are focally lytic, permeative, and with varying degrees of sclerosis. Periosteal reaction may be present, with imaging frequently revealing a lamellated appearance with or without cortical breakthrough. On MRI, lymphoma typically appears hypointense on T1-weighted images and enhances. On T2-weighted sequences, lymphoma can range in signal from hypointense to hyperintense. Lymphoma will often restrict on diffusion-weighted sequences due to its hypercellularity.
- **Multiple myeloma.** Multiple myeloma (MM) is a hematologic malignancy characterized by a monoclonal proliferation of plasma cells within the bone marrow. On radiographs and CT, MM characteristically presents as lytic, punched-out lesions which are not associated with significant periosteal new bone formation. Diffuse disease may only manifest as diffuse osteopenia without a focal lesion on radiographs. On MRI, MM may have a myriad of imaging appearances, ranging from a focal lesion, a variegated (salt and pepper) abnormally, to diffuse disease. MM is characteristically T1 hypointense, STIR hyperintense, and enhancing.
- **Stafne cyst.** A Stafne cyst (also called lingual salivary gland inclusion defect or static bone cavity) is a benign, incidental, focal scalloping along the lingual cortex of the posterior mandible, most commonly at the junction of the body and angle of the mandible. The osseous defect is usually occupied by a portion of the submandibular gland as well as fat and most likely represents a benign remodeling by the submandibular gland. On CT or radiography, a Stafne cyst is an ovoid lucency located along the inferior lingual margin of the mandible, just anterior to the angle.

Radicular cyst

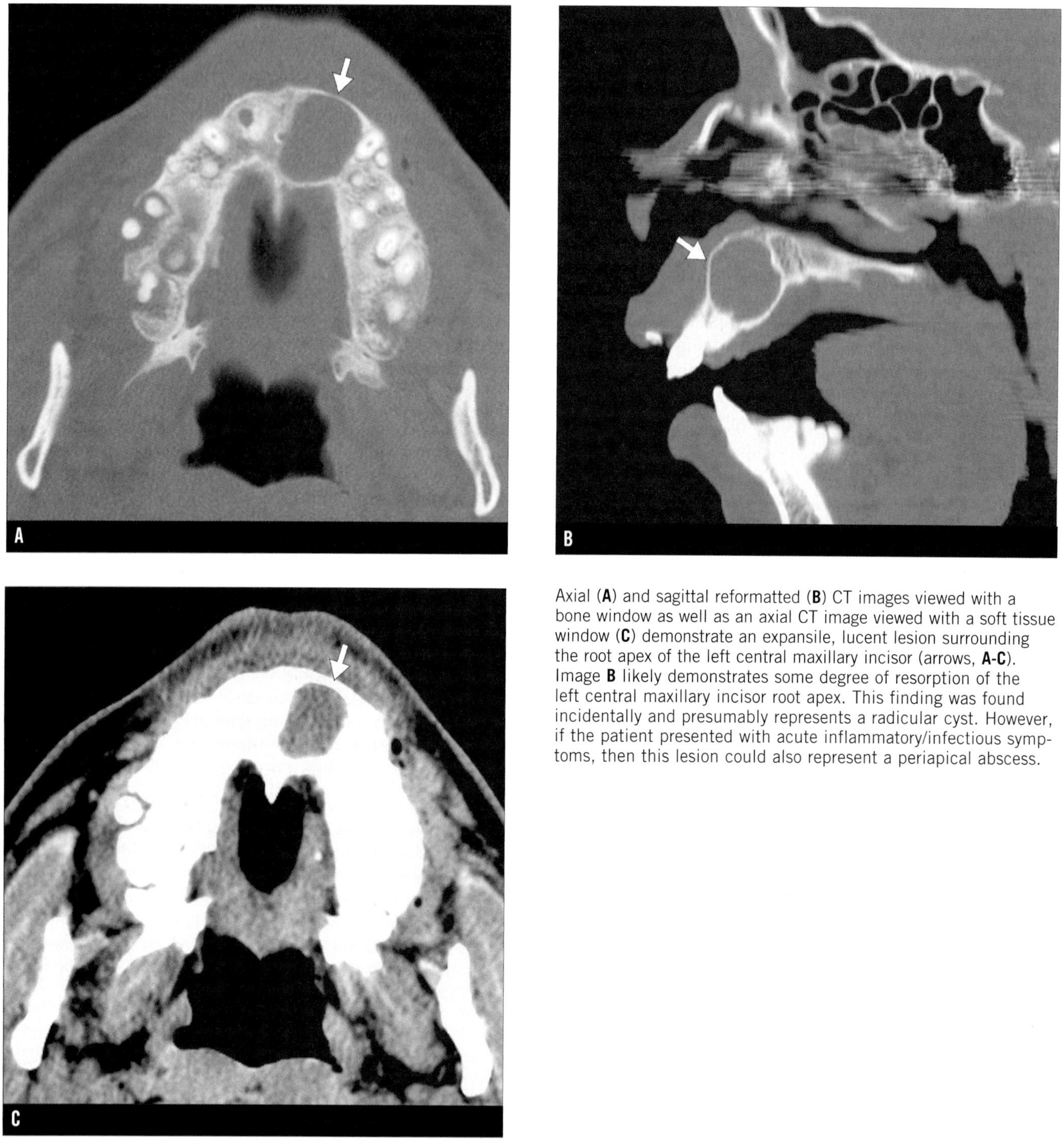

Axial (**A**) and sagittal reformatted (**B**) CT images viewed with a bone window as well as an axial CT image viewed with a soft tissue window (**C**) demonstrate an expansile, lucent lesion surrounding the root apex of the left central maxillary incisor (arrows, **A-C**). Image **B** likely demonstrates some degree of resorption of the left central maxillary incisor root apex. This finding was found incidentally and presumably represents a radicular cyst. However, if the patient presented with acute inflammatory/infectious symptoms, then this lesion could also represent a periapical abscess.

Radicular cyst

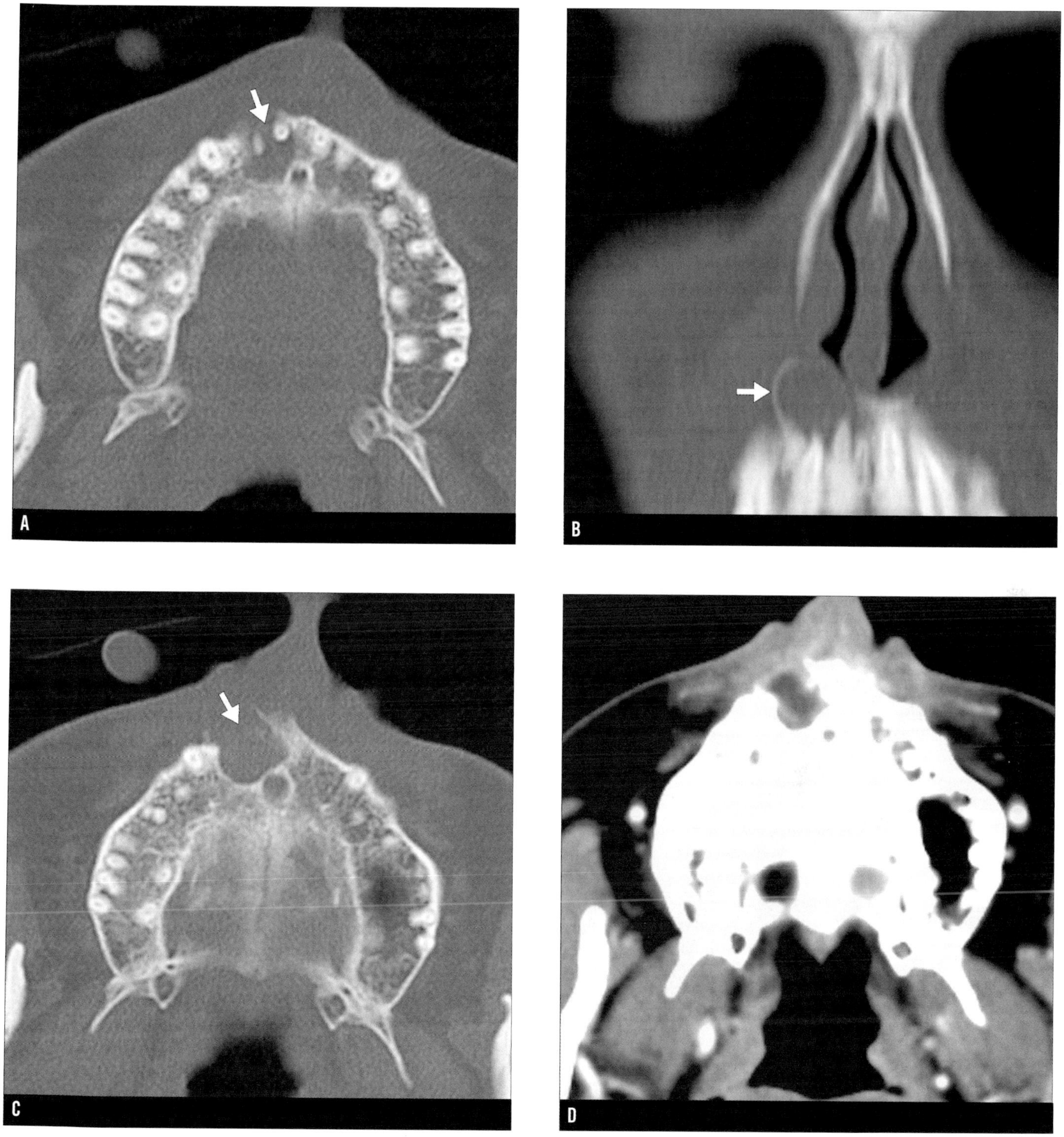

Different patient. This patient presented with a painless, palpable lump caudal to the right nasal ala. Axial (**A**) and coronal reformatted (**B**) CT images viewed with a bone window demonstrate a typical appearance of a radicular cyst (arrow, **A**, **B**), in this case surrounding the root apices of the medial and lateral right maxillary incisors. An axial CT image viewed with a bone window (**C**) demonstrates dehiscence along the ventral wall of the cyst with slight ventral bulging of the residual ventral wall, likely accounting for the palpable lump (arrow, **C**). While an axial postcontrast CT image viewed with a soft tissue window (**D**) does demonstrate apparent subtle peripheral enhancement along the margin of the lucency, there is no significant enhancement in the surrounding soft tissues, as is commonly identified with a periapical abscess. However, the clinical history is paramount in cases such as these in order to differentiate an incidental radicular cyst from a periapical abscess.

Companion case: Chewing gum mimicking a torus palatinus

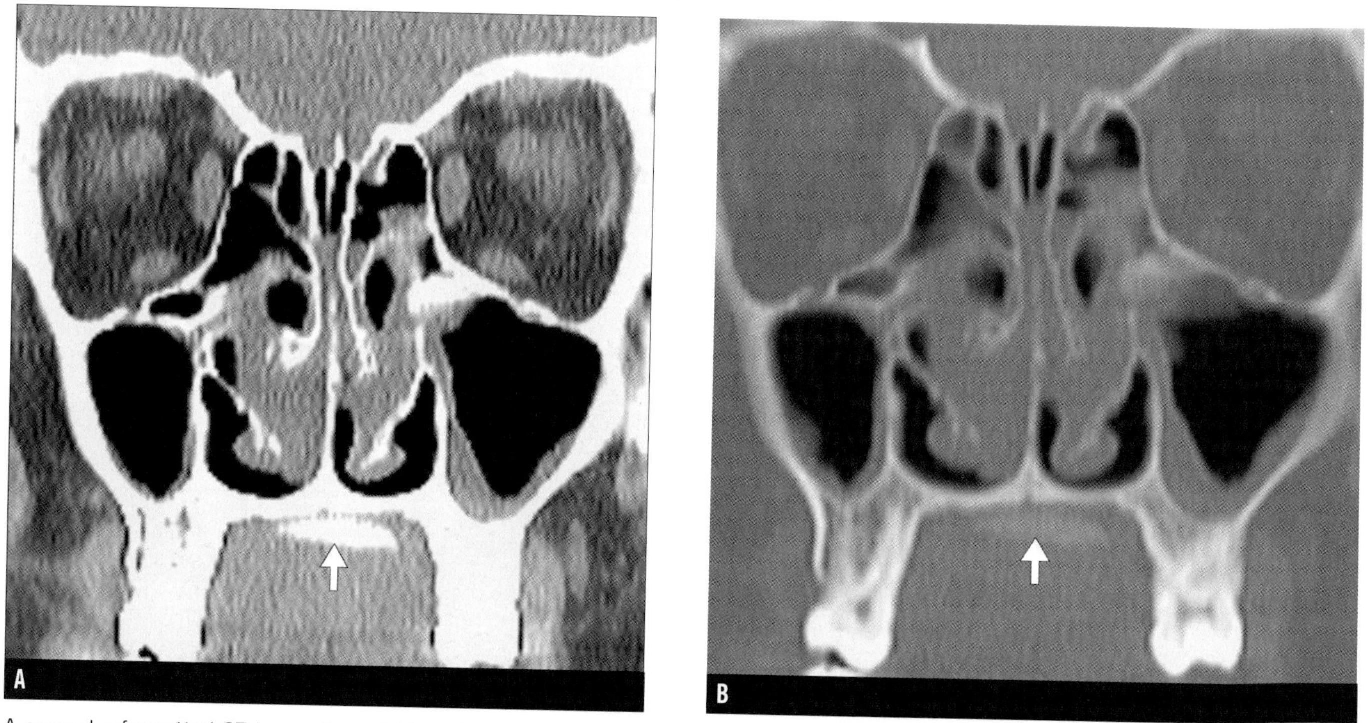

A coronal reformatted CT image through the mid hard palate viewed with a soft tissue window (**A**) and the same image viewed with a bone window (**B**). These images demonstrate a high-density finding located immediately subjacent, but separate from, the hard palate (arrows, **A**, **B**). The density of the finding on image **B** is considerably less than that of bone. The finding is compatible with a comestible foreign body, likely chewing gum. Comestibles often mimic tori.

REFERENCES

Flis CM, Connor SE. Imaging of head and neck venous malformations. *Eur Radiol.* 2005;15(10):2185-2193.

Garcia-Garcia AS, et al. Current Status of the Torus Palatinus and Torus Mandibularis. *Med Oral Patol Oral Cir Bucal.* 2010;15 (2):e353-e360.

Jainkittivong A, Apinhasmit W, Swasdison S. Prevalence and clinical characteristics of oral tori in 1,520 Chulalongkorn University Dental School patients. *Surg Radiol Anat.* 2007;29:125-131.

Johann AC, et al. Peripheral osteoma of the mandible: case report and review of the literature. *J CranioMaxillofac Surg.* 2005;33(4):276-281.

Lee YY, et al. Craniofacial osteosarcomas: plain film, CT, and MR findings in 46 Cases. *AJR Am J Roentgenol.* 1988;150(6):1397-1402.

McCafferty IJ, Jones RG. Imaging and management of vascular malformations. *Clin Radiol.* 2011;66(12):1208-1218. Doi: 10.1016/j.crad.2011.06.014. Epub Sep 2011. Review.

McDermott M, Branstetter BF, Escott EJ. What's in your mouth? The CT appearance of comestible intraoral foreign bodies. *AJNR Am J Neuroradiol.* 2008;29(8):1552-1555.

CASE 4 Supernumerary teeth

Supernumerary teeth refer to an excess of the normal 32 teeth in the adult and may occur with both primary and permanent dentition. Supernumerary teeth are present in up to 4% of adults and are more common in men by a 2:1 margin. However, supernumerary teeth, while often incidental, have been associated with abnormal conditions, such as Gardner syndrome, Fabry-Anderson syndrome, Ehlers-Danlos syndrome, cleft lip and palate, and cleidocranial dysplasia. In people who have supernumerary teeth, one supernumerary tooth is present in 75% to 86% of cases, two supernumerary teeth are present in 12% to 25% of cases, and three or more supernumerary teeth are present in only 1%.

The mesiodens is the most common supernumerary tooth, occurring in the anterior maxilla, adjacent to the central incisors. The mesiodens represents between one-third to two-thirds of all cases of supernumerary teeth. The remaining supernumerary teeth include the distomolar (also known as a distodens) which is located posterior to the third molar, the paramolar which is located adjacent to the molar teeth (except when located posterior to the third molar), the premolar (also known as a peridens) which is located in the premolar region, and the lateral incisor and canine supernumerary teeth, both of which occur in close proximity to the teeth of the same names.

Supernumerary teeth may extend into the nasal cavity or maxillary sinus and are frequently referred to as ectopic supernumerary teeth in these instances. Supernumerary teeth can also result in retention, delayed eruption, or displacement of the primary teeth as well as the formation of a dentigerous cyst. When a supernumerary tooth has a size and shape similar to that of a normal tooth, it may be termed a supplemental tooth.

COMPANION CASE

- **Unerupted teeth in a child.** The dental follicle is a structure that surrounds the crown of an unerupted tooth and is necessary for tooth eruption. On radiographs, the dental follicle appears as a radiolucent halo. The dental follicle is surrounded by a thin rim of compact bone that surrounds the roots of the teeth, known as the lamina dura. The lamina dura serves as the point of attachment for the periodontal ligament.

  The follicle surrounding unerupted teeth can vary in thickness, particularly in the case of maxillary canines, which can be surrounded by normal large follicular spaces that can mimic pathologic processes, such as a dentigerous cyst. Should a tooth become impacted, particularly over the span of multiple years, the normal follicle will often diminish is size or become absent on imaging. Some children may develop one or more prominent follicular spaces in the absence of pathology. In this circumstance, it may be helpful to apply the following rule: a pathologic process should be considered if the pericoronal halo is 2.5 mm or greater in thickness and there is evidence of irregularity of the surrounding rim of cortical bone. This general rule can be applied to all teeth, except the maxillary canines, which, as discussed above, can be normally associated with larger follicular spaces.

Supernumerary teeth and a supplemental tooth

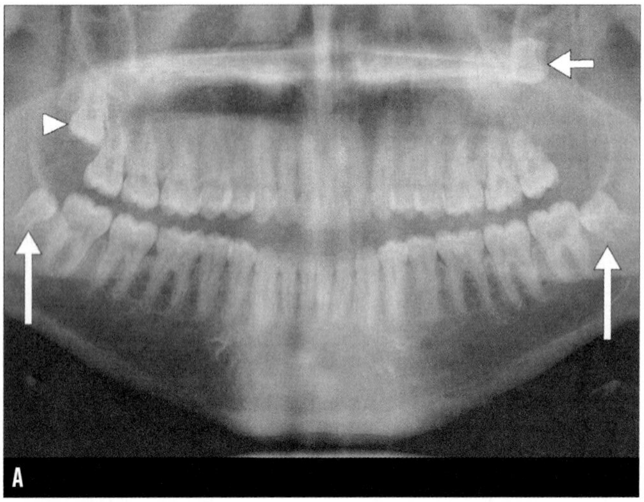

A single panorex image (**A**) demonstrates a total of 36 teeth with four supernumerary teeth. One of the supernumerary teeth is present in the left maxillary sinus floor and is compatible with a distomolar (short arrow). The supernumerary teeth located lateral (clinically posterior) to the third mandibular molars are smaller than the adjacent molars and are also considered distomolars (long arrows). However, the tooth lateral (clinically posterior) to the right third maxillary molar is essentially the same size and shape as the adjacent molar tooth and therefore can be termed a supplemental tooth (arrowhead).

Mesiodens supernumerary tooth with an A-P orientation

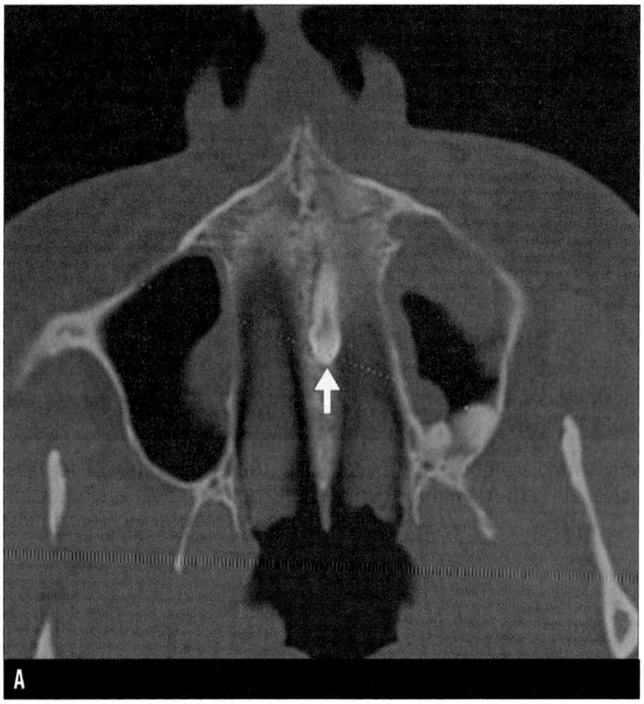

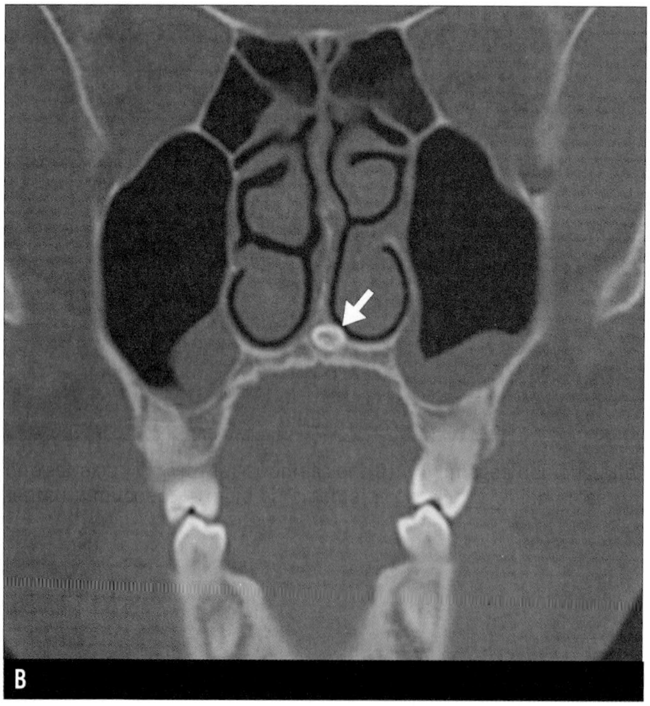

Axial (**A**) and coronal reformatted (**B**) CT images demonstrate a tooth in the midline of the hard palate, oriented anterior-posterior, compatible with a mesiodens (arrows, **A**, **B**).

Mesiodens supernumerary teeth with a vertical orientation

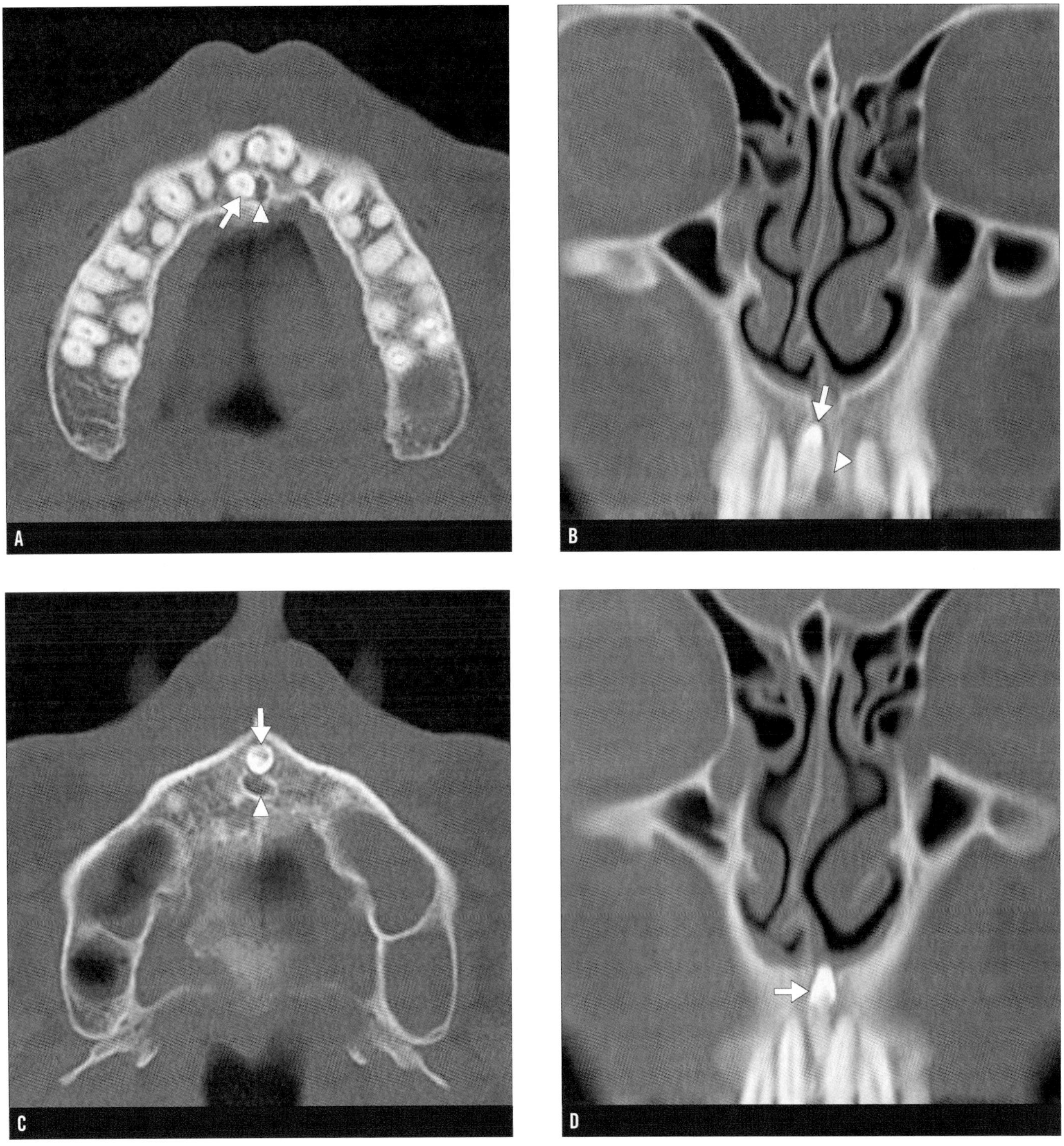

Axial (**A**) and coronal reformatted (**B**) CT images demonstrate a small, vertically oriented, supernumerary tooth (arrows, **A**, **B**) immediately posterior to the right maxillary central incisor and to the right of the nasopalatine canal (arrowheads, **A**, **B**). Notice the supernumerary tooth is inverted, as the enamel along its crown is directed superiorly. Axial (**C**) and coronal reformatted (**D**) CT images demonstrate a second small supernumerary tooth (arrows, **C**, **D**), also vertically oriented and inverted, situated between the maxillary central incisors and immediately anterior to the nasopalatine canal (arrowhead, **C**). Both of these teeth are compatible with supernumerary mesiodens teeth.

Mesiodens supernumerary tooth with an oblique orientation

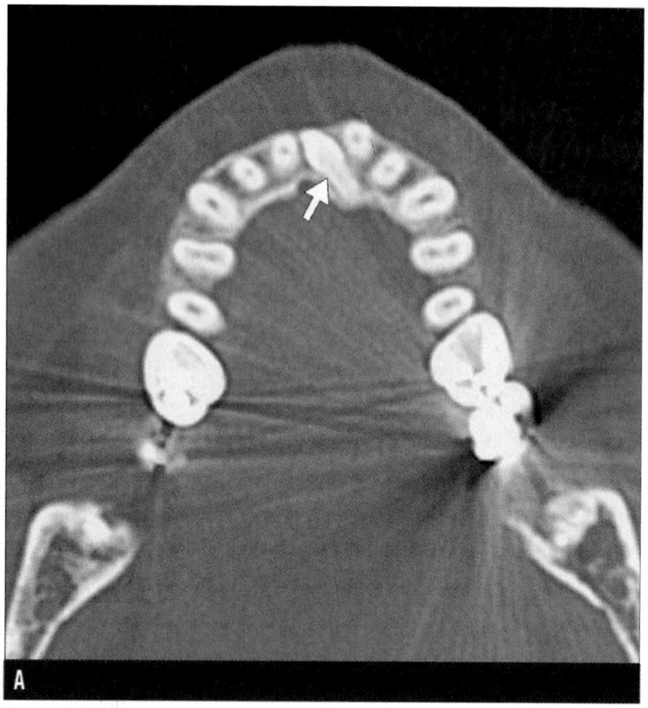

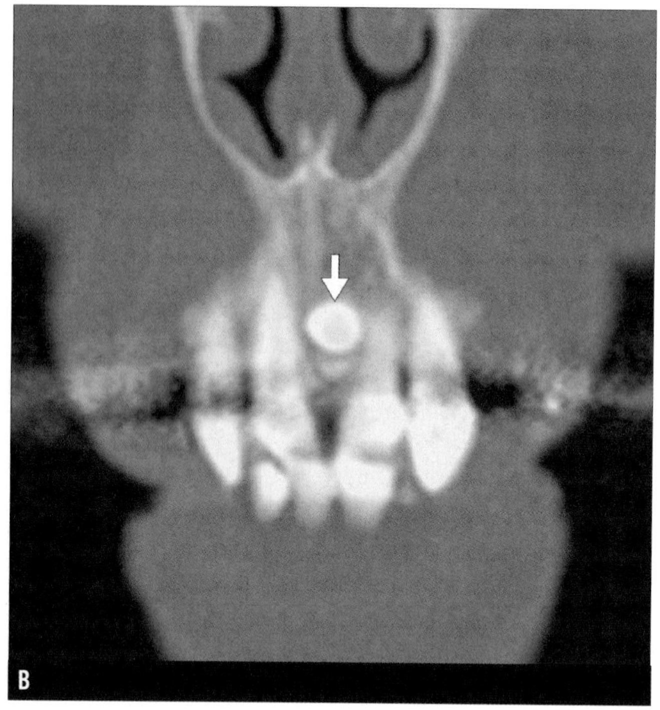

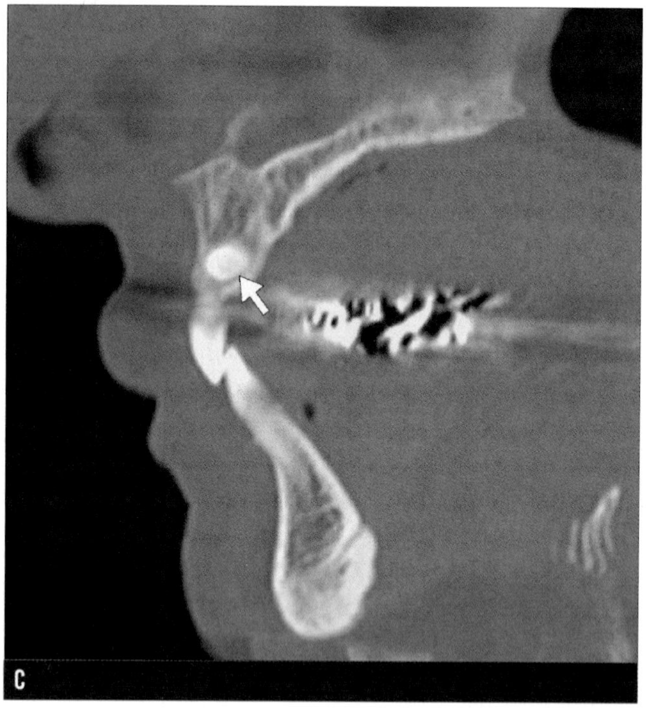

Axial (**A**), coronal reformatted (**B**), and sagittal reformatted (**C**) CT images demonstrate an obliquely oriented supernumerary tooth in the maxillary alveolus interposed between the maxillary central incisors, consistent with a mesiodens (arrows, **A-C**).

Canine supernumerary tooth associated with a retained primary tooth

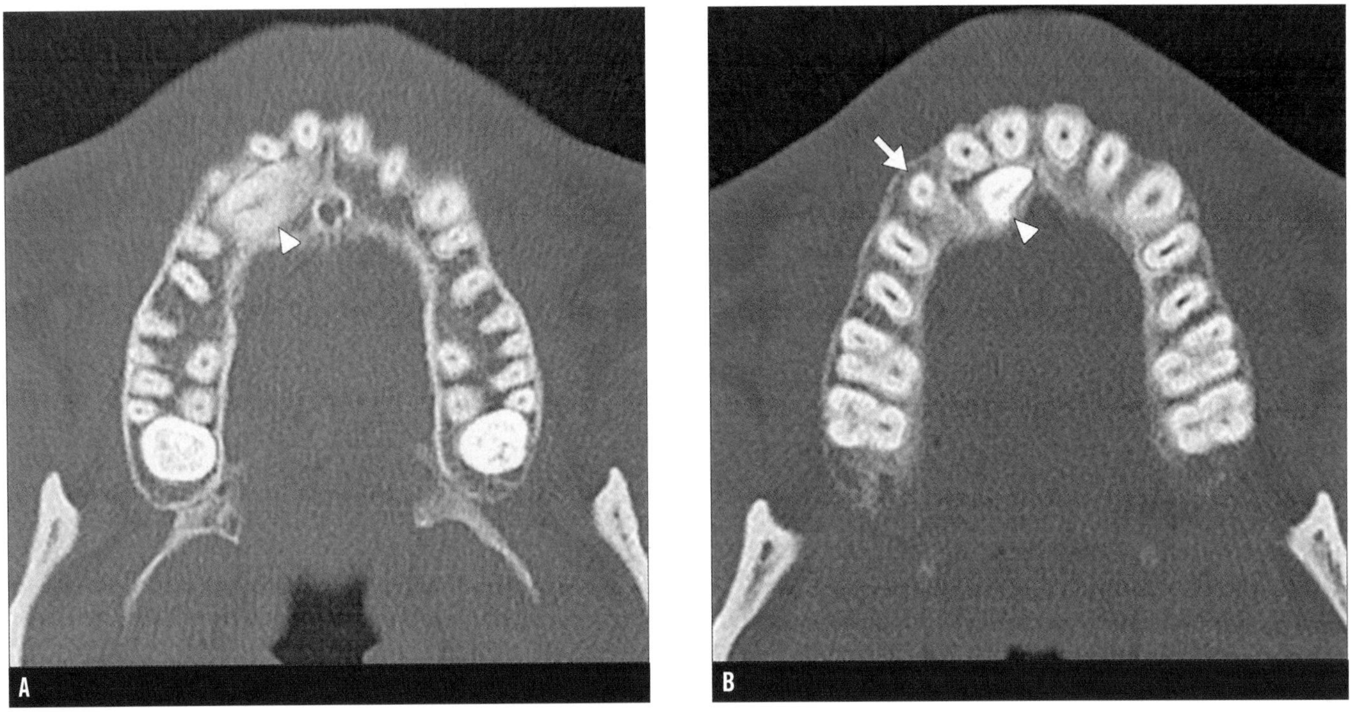

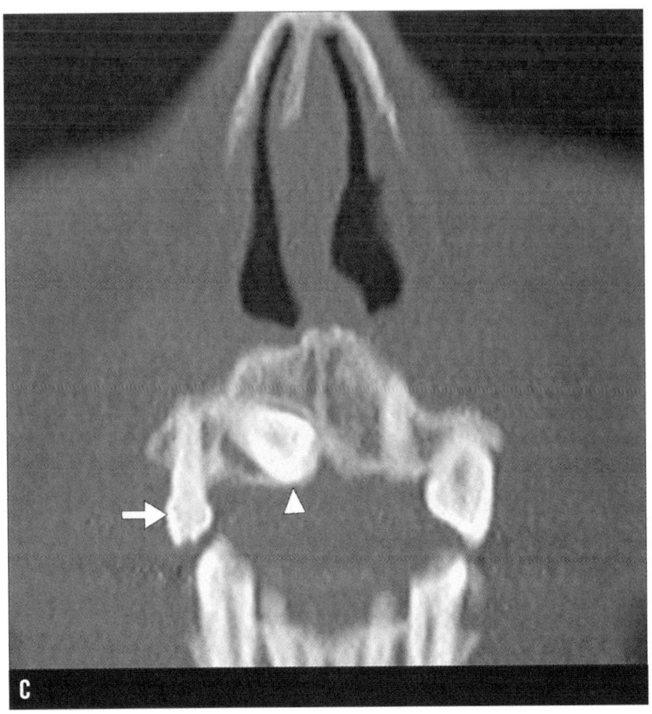

Axial (**A**, **B**) and coronal reformatted (**C**) CT images demonstrate an obliquely oriented supernumerary tooth adjacent to a right maxillary canine, compatible with a canine supernumerary tooth (arrowheads, **A-C**). The right maxillary canine tooth is diminutive, likely representing the residual primary tooth (arrows, **B**, **C**). Supernumerary teeth can be associated with retention, delayed eruption, or displacement of primary teeth.

Paramolar supernumerary teeth

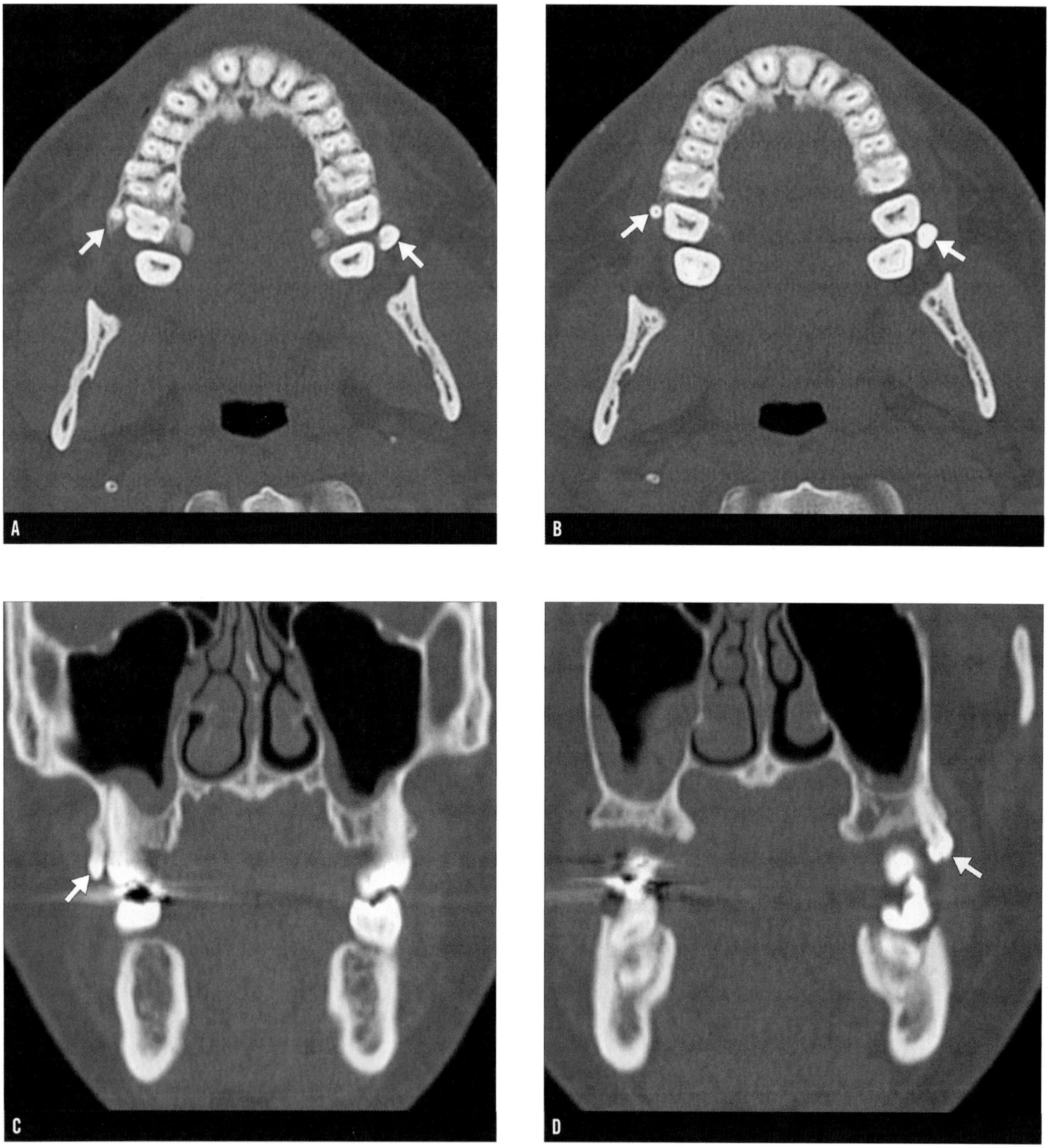

Axial (**A**, **B**) and coronal reformatted (**C**, **D**) CT images demonstrate small supernumerary teeth lateral to the bilateral molar teeth, consistent with bilateral paramolar teeth (arrows, **A-D**).

Paramolar supernumerary tooth

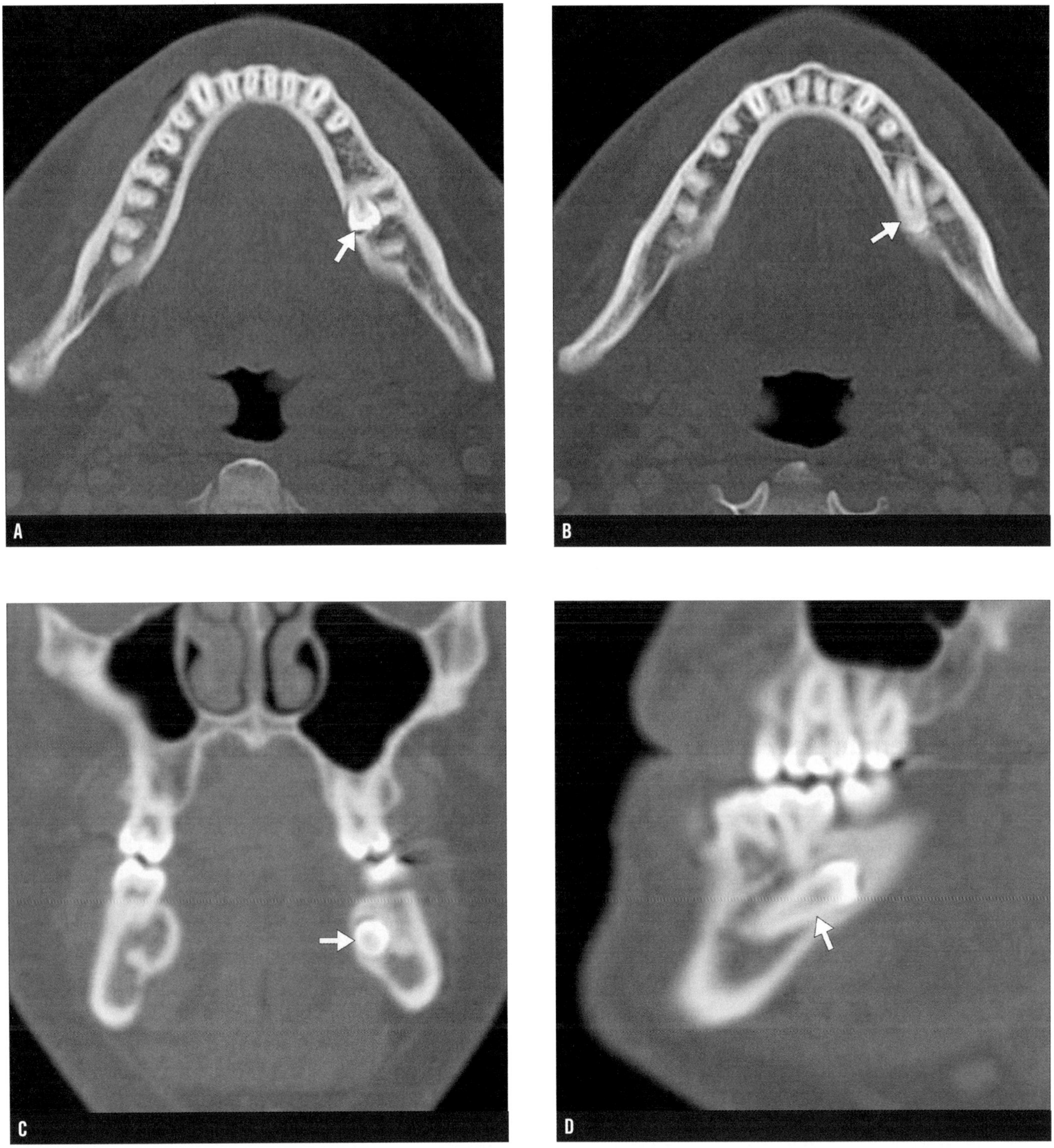

Axial (**A**, **B**), coronal reformatted (**C**), and sagittal reformatted (**D**) CT images through the mandible demonstrate an obliquely oriented supernumerary tooth in the left hemimandible (arrows, **A-D**), located caudal to the left mandibular molars. This tooth is consistent with a mandibular paramolar.

Ectopic supernumerary tooth in the maxillary sinus

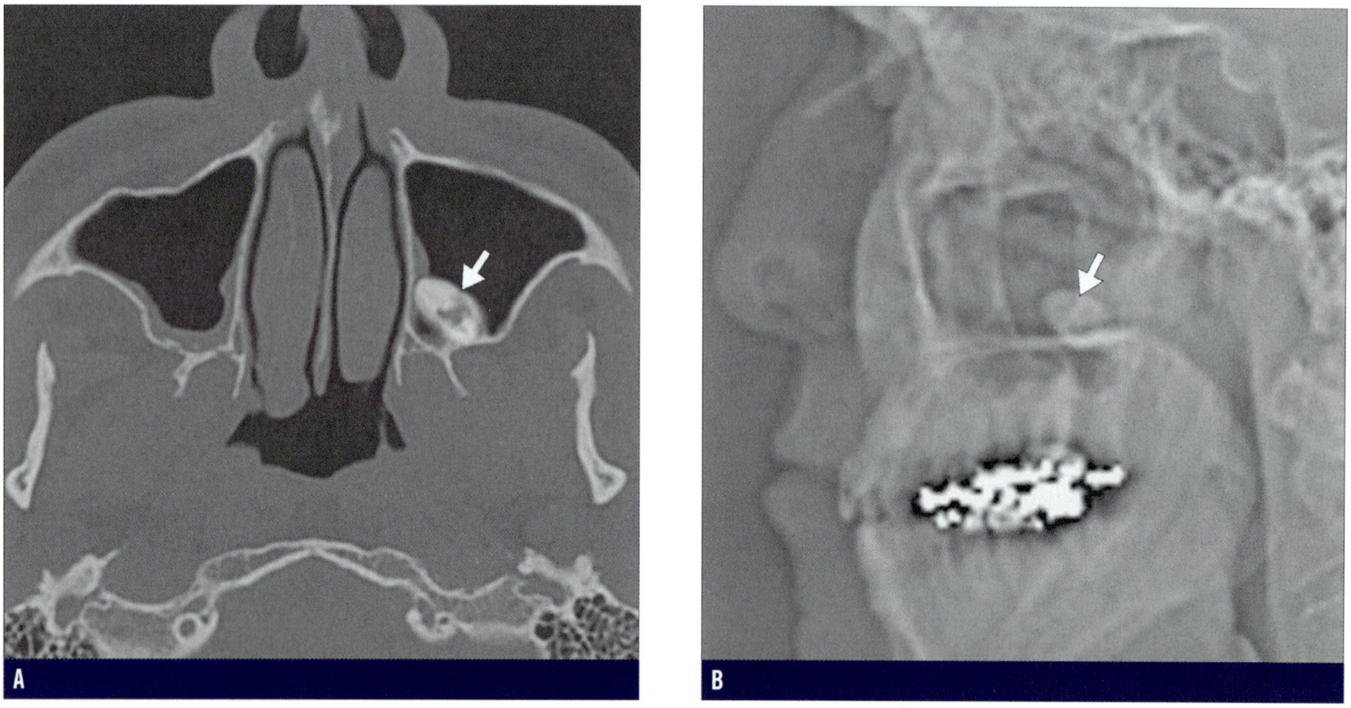

An axial CT image viewed with a bone window (**A**) demonstrates an ectopic supernumerary tooth within the posterior-inferior aspect of the left maxillary sinus lumen (arrow, **A**). The tooth is also appreciated on the lateral scout image **B** (arrow, **B**).

Ectopic supernumerary tooth embedded in the maxillary sinus wall

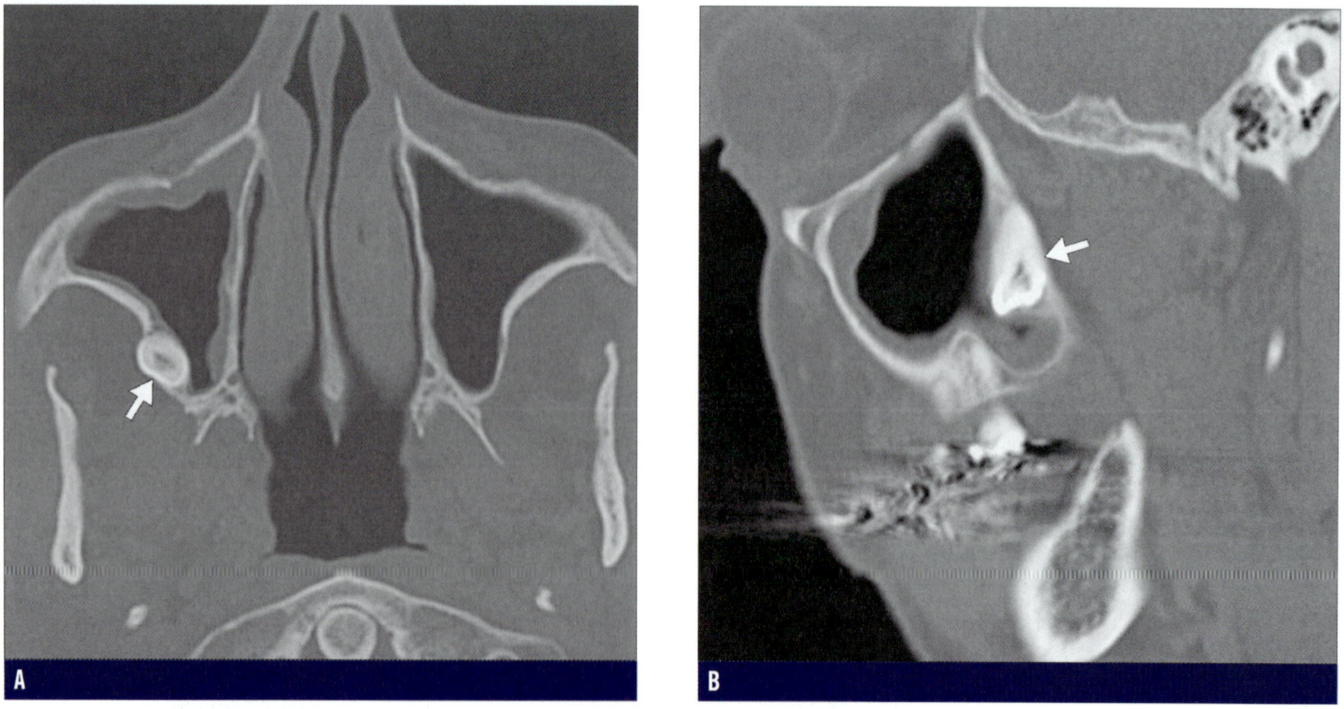

Axial (**A**), sagittal reformatted (**B**), and coronal reformatted (**C**) CT images demonstrate an ectopic supernumerary tooth within the wall of the right maxillary sinus (arrows, **A-C**).

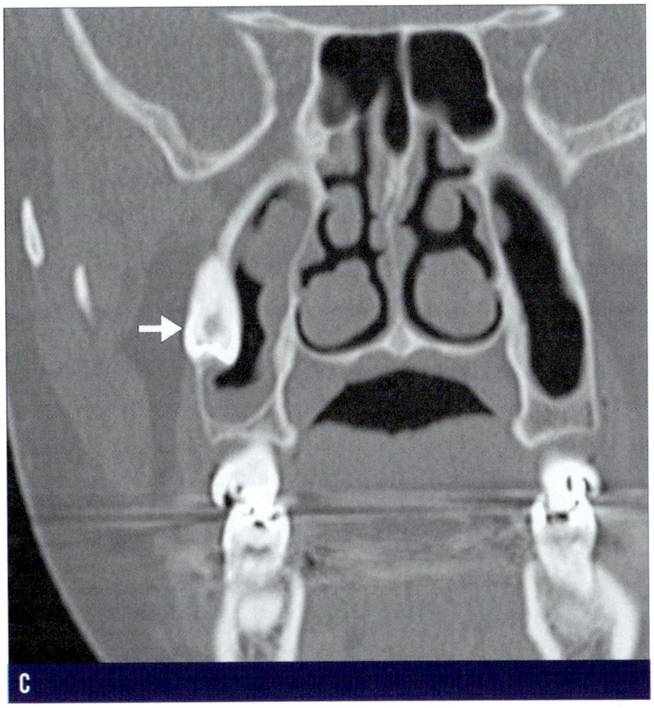

Ectopic supernumerary tooth with roots projecting into the maxillary sinus lumen

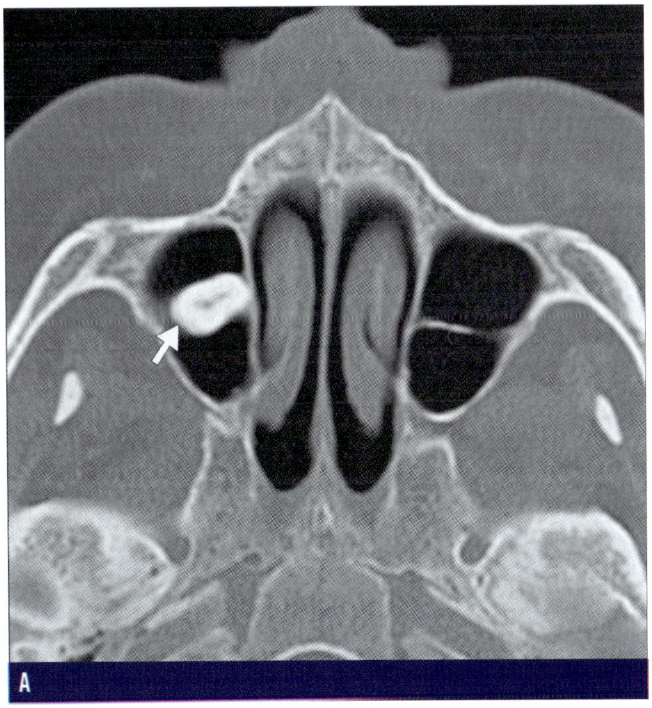

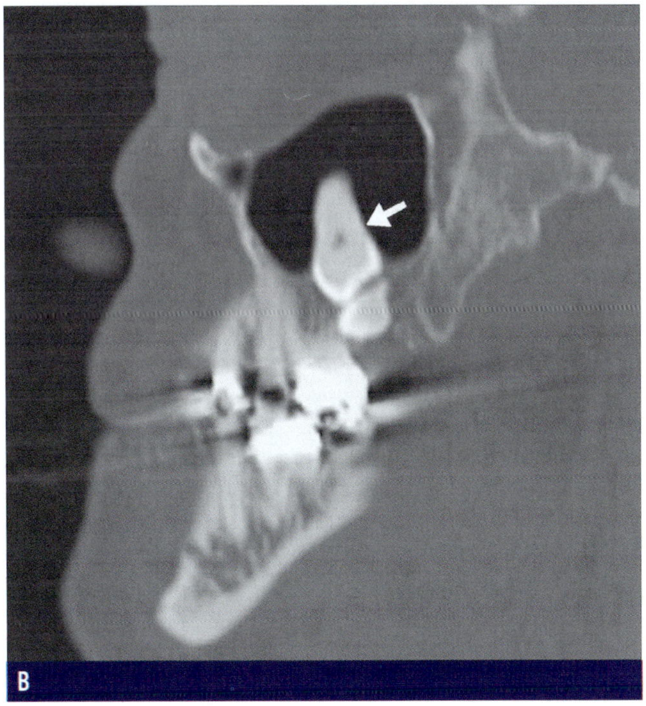

Axial (**A**), sagittal reformatted (**B**), and coronal reformatted (**C**) CT images demonstrate the roots of an ecotopic supernumerary tooth projecting into the lumen of the right maxillary sinus (arrows, **A-C**).

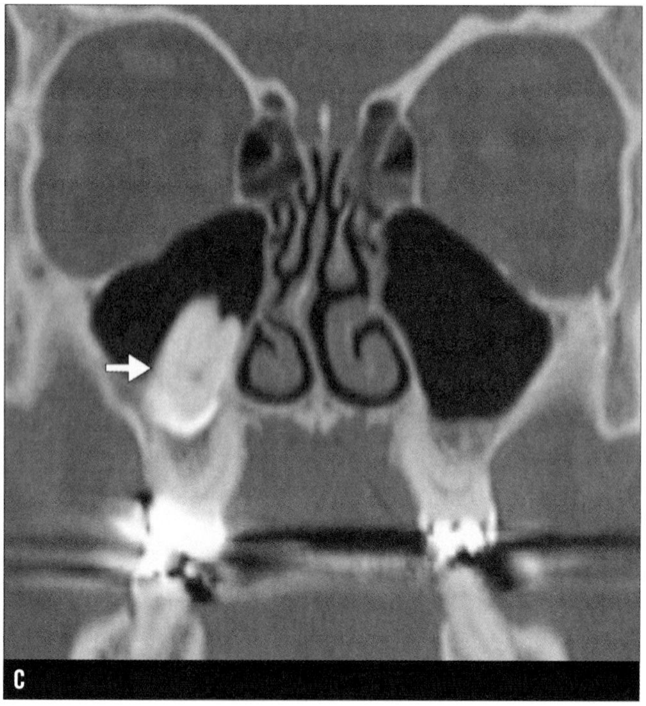

C

Companion case: Unerupted teeth in a child

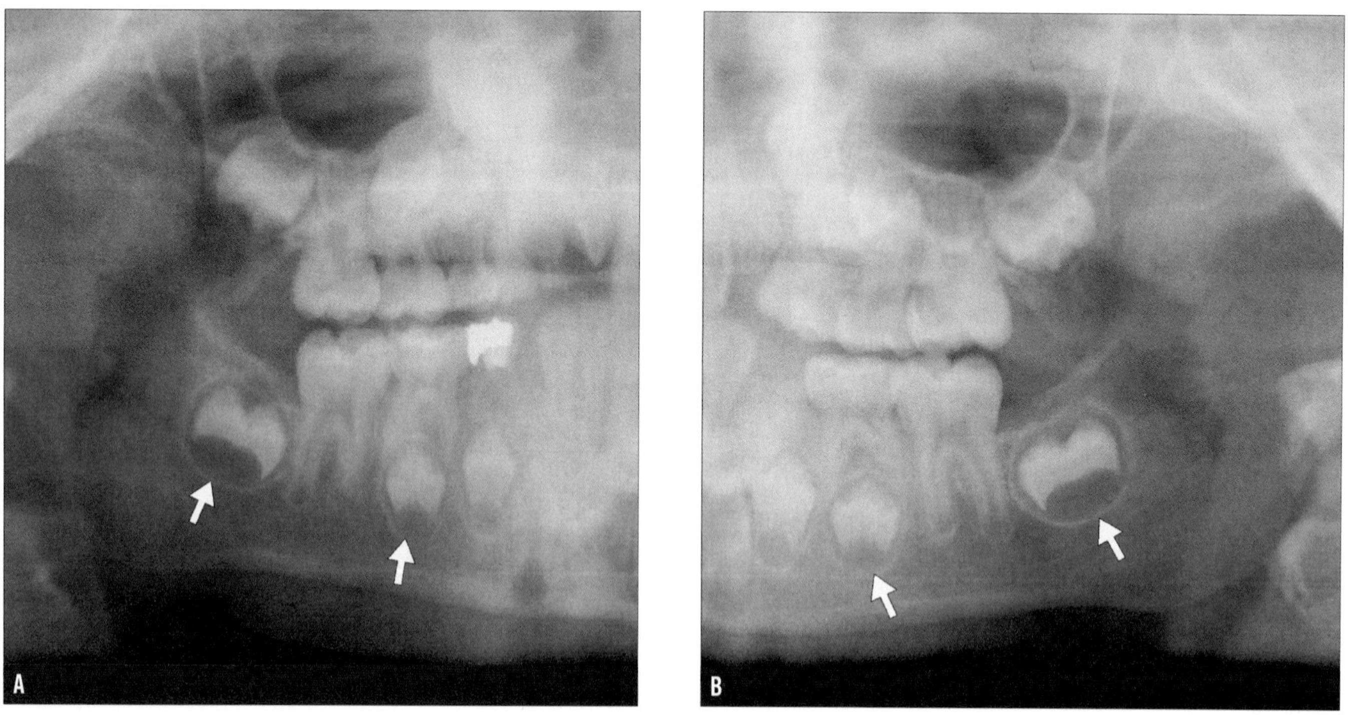

A B

Magnified images from a panorex radiograph of an 8 year old patient (**A**, **B**) demonstrate multiple developing, unerupted teeth. Many of these unerupted teeth are associated with prominent, but not pathologically enlarged, follicular spaces (arrows, **A**, **B**).

REFERENCES

Celikoglu M, Kamak H, Oktay H. Prevalence and characteristics of supernumerary teeth in a non-syndrome Turkish population: associated pathologies and proposed treatment. *Med Oral Patol Oral Cir Bucal.* 2010;15(4):e575-e578.

Fernandez Montenegro P, Valmaseda Castellon E, Berini Aytes L, Gay Escoda C. Restrospective study of 145 supernumerary teeth. *Med Oral Patol Oral Cir Buccal.* 2006;11(4):e339-e344.

Ramanojam S, Halli R, Hebbale M, Bhardwaj S. Ectopic tooth in maxillary sinus: Case series. *Ann Maxillofac Surg.* 2013;3(1):89-92.

Russell KA, Folwarczna MA. Mesiodens—diagnosis and management of a common supernumerary tooth. *J Can Dent Assoc.* 2003;69(6):362-366.

Saleem T, Khalid U, Hameed A, Ghaffar S. Supernumerary, ectopic tooth in the maxillary antrum presenting with recurrent haemoptysis. *Head Face Med.* 2010;6:26.

Santos AP, Ammari MM, Moliterno LF, Junior JC. First report of bilateral supernumerary teeth associated with bony primary and permanent maxillary canines. *J Oral Sci.* 2009;51(1):145-150.

CASE 5 Dilaceration

Dilaceration refers to deviation or bending of a tooth from a minimum angle of 20° to 90°, depending on the literature cited. Dilaceration may occur anywhere along the course of the tooth, from the crown to the root. Two theories exist for the etiology of this anomaly. The first theory suggests that trauma to the primary teeth damages the adjacent developing permanent tooth germ within the maxilla or mandible. The second suggests that the anomaly results primarily from ectopic development of the tooth bud. Identification of a dilacerated tooth is critical prior to endodontal intervention or extraction because it can lead to failure of endodontal therapy or prolonged/arduous tooth extraction. Most cases are not clinically evident, but dilacerations can clinically manifest as a deformed crown or a missing tooth if dilaceration prevents normal tooth eruption.

Dilaceration

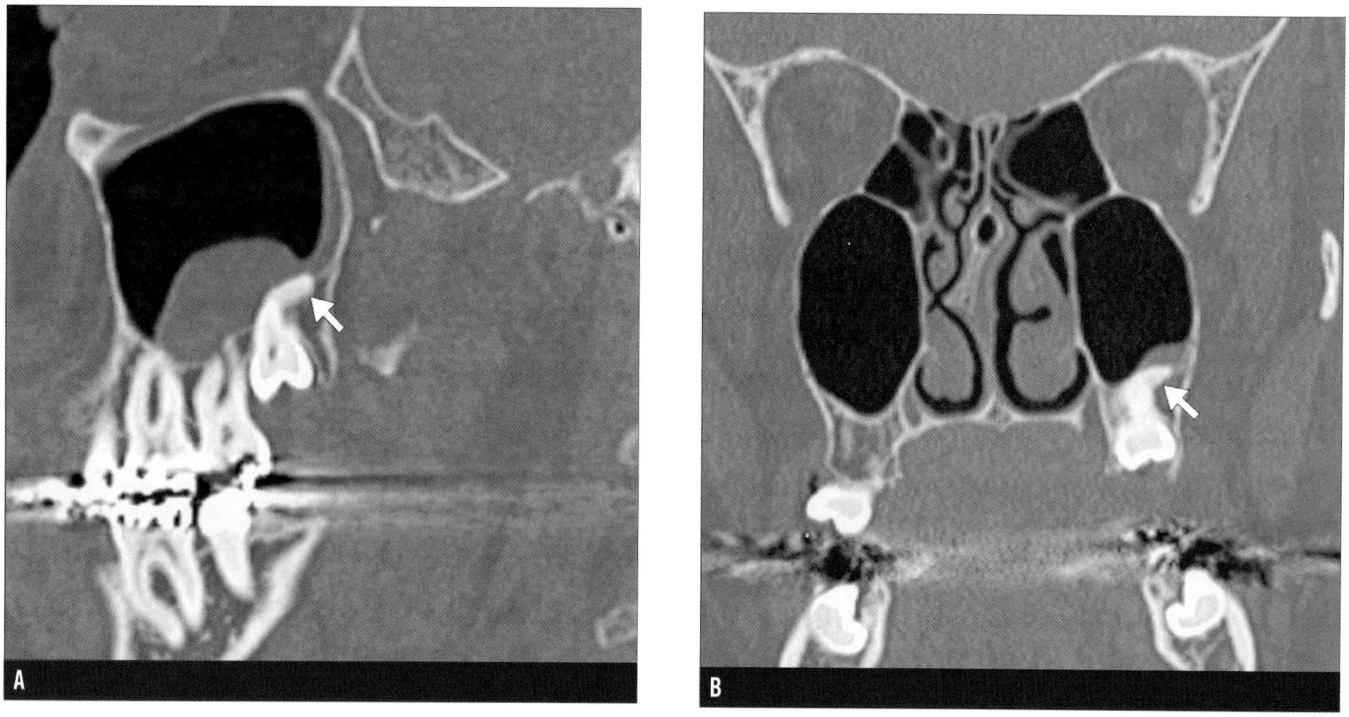

Sagittal reformatted (**A**) and coronal reformatted (**B**) CT images demonstrate pronounced posterior angulation involving the root of a left maxillary molar tooth, compatible with a dilacerated tooth root (arrows, **A**, **B**).

Dilaceration

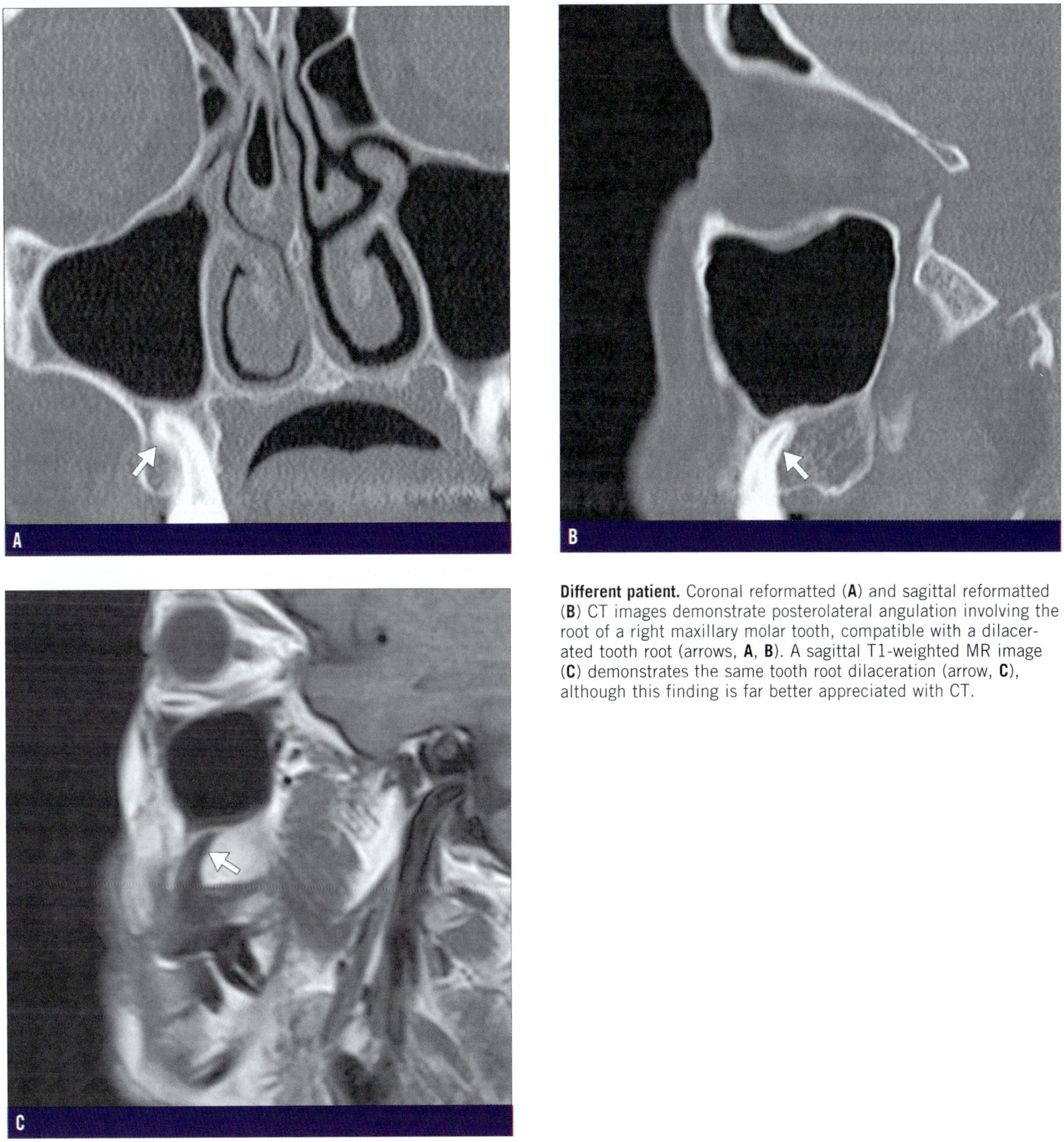

Different patient. Coronal reformatted (**A**) and sagittal reformatted (**B**) CT images demonstrate posterolateral angulation involving the root of a right maxillary molar tooth, compatible with a dilacerated tooth root (arrows, **A**, **B**). A sagittal T1-weighted MR image (**C**) demonstrates the same tooth root dilaceration (arrow, **C**), although this finding is far better appreciated with CT.

REFERENCES

Chohayeb AA. Dilaceration of permanent upper lateral incisors: frequency, direction, and endodontic treatment implications. *Oral Surg Oral Med Oral Pathol.* 1983;55(5):519-520.

Malcic A, et al. Prevalence of root dilaceration in adult dental patients in Croatia. *Oral Surg Oral Med Oral Pathol Oral Radiol Endod.* 2006;102(1):104-109

Miloglu O, et al. The prevalence of root dilacerations in a Turkish population. *Med Oral Patol Oral Cir Bucal.* 2010;15(3):e441-e444.

CASE 6 Bifid or cleft morphology of the mandibular condyle

The bifid mandibular condyle is a rare anomaly in which there is duplication of the articular heads with an interposed groove. Up to four separate condylar heads have been described in the literature, although a bifid condyle is most commonly unilateral. In the typical case of a bifid mandibular condyle, the duplicated mandibular heads are positioned in either the anterior-posterior or medial-lateral planes. Some authors use the terms mandibular condylar notch or cleft to describe grooves oriented in the sagittal plane, particularly when the intercondylar groove is shallow. Limited population studies among various ethnic groups have described this anomaly as occurring in up to 0.5% of individuals.

Two major theories to explain the etiology of this anomaly have been proposed. The first suggests that prior birth trauma or mandibular condyle fracture predisposes to the development of this anomaly. The second suggests that interruption of the blood supply to the condyle or the formation of fibrovascular septa during embryologic development leads to its development. Additional anecdotal causes of the bifid mandibular condyle include teratogenic drug use, infection, radiation exposure, or a genetic predisposition. In most cases, bifid condyles are asymptomatic; however, some patients report swelling, temporomandibular joint (TMJ) clicking, or TMJ pain. Uncommonly, the bifid mandibular condyle is associated with TMJ ankylosis.

COMPANION CASES

- **Mandibular condyle hypoplasia.** Aplasia and hypoplasia refer to nondevelopment or underdevelopment of the mandibular condyle, respectively. Aplasia of the mandibular condyle is a congenital condition, whereas hypoplasia of the mandibular condyle may be either congenital or acquired. Congenital aplasia or congenital hypoplasia usually occurs as part of a systemic condition that results in maldevelopment of the first and second branchial arches, such as mandibulofacial dysostosis (Treacher Collins syndrome). Acquired hypoplasia may be due to trauma, infection, irradiation, toxic agents, or rheumatoid arthritis. Aplasia or hypoplasia, when bilateral, can lead to the underdevelopment of the mandible and subsequent micrognathia.
- **Motion artifact**. Motion artifact is a common imaging pitfall that can mimic a variety of pathologic processes and anatomic variants. In the case of mandibular condyle motion artifact, motion artifact may involve the skull base and mandible (due to head movement), or it may be isolated to the mandible (due to speaking).

Bifid mandibular condyle

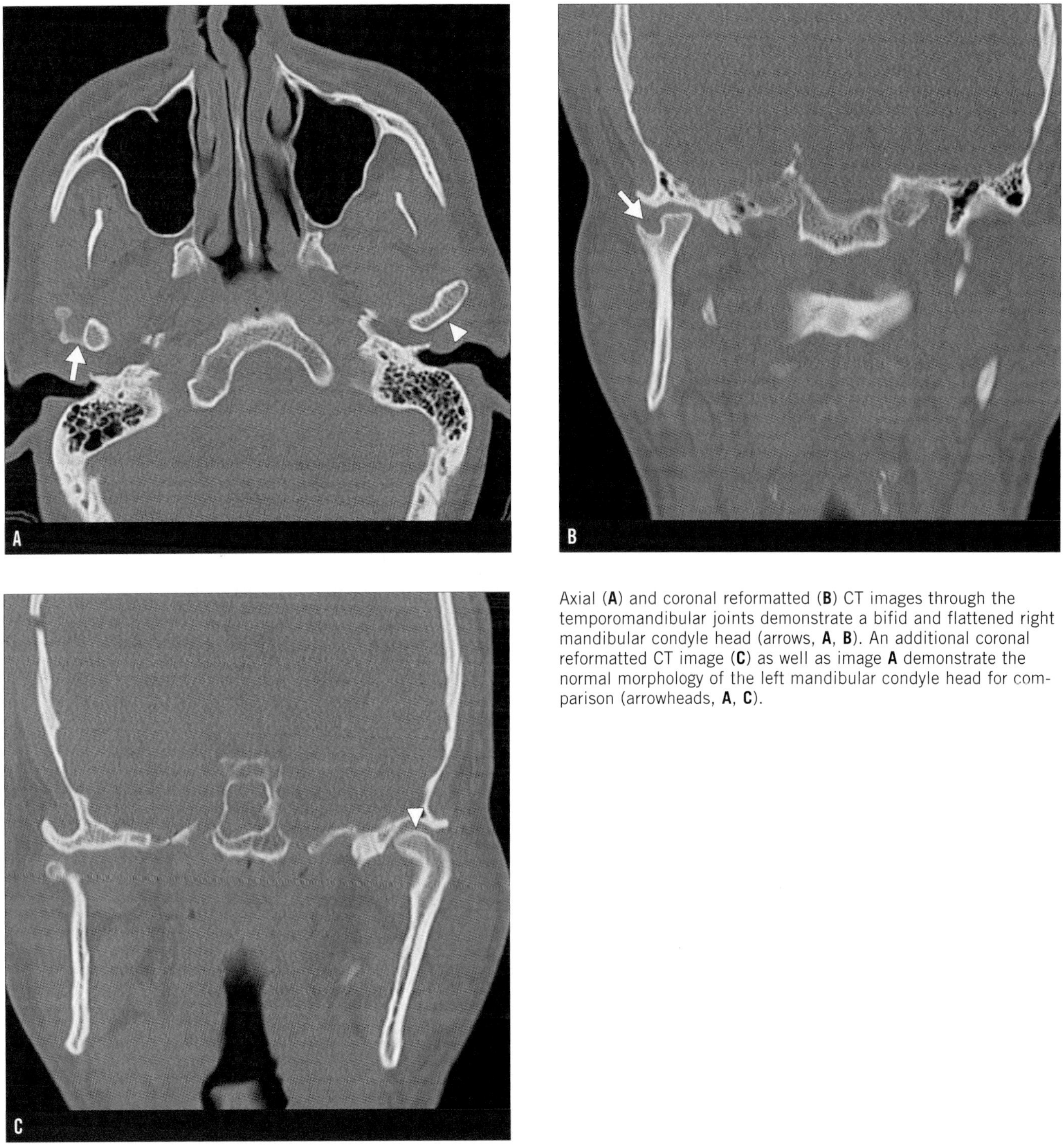

Axial (**A**) and coronal reformatted (**B**) CT images through the temporomandibular joints demonstrate a bifid and flattened right mandibular condyle head (arrows, **A**, **B**). An additional coronal reformatted CT image (**C**) as well as image **A** demonstrate the normal morphology of the left mandibular condyle head for comparison (arrowheads, **A**, **C**).

Mandibular condyle cleft

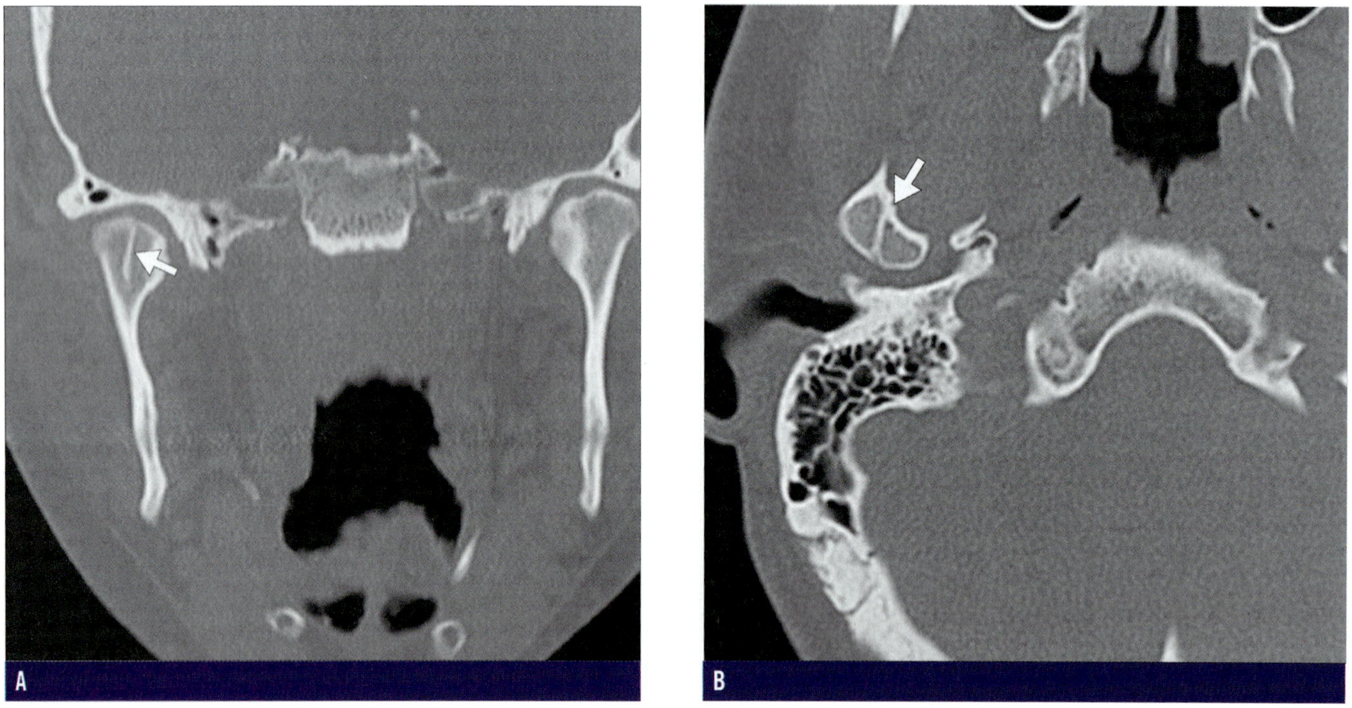

Coronal reformatted (**A**) and axial (**B**) CT images through the mandibular condyles demonstrate a vertically oriented right mandibular condyle cleft (arrows, **A**, **B**).

Companion case: Mandibular condyle hypoplasia

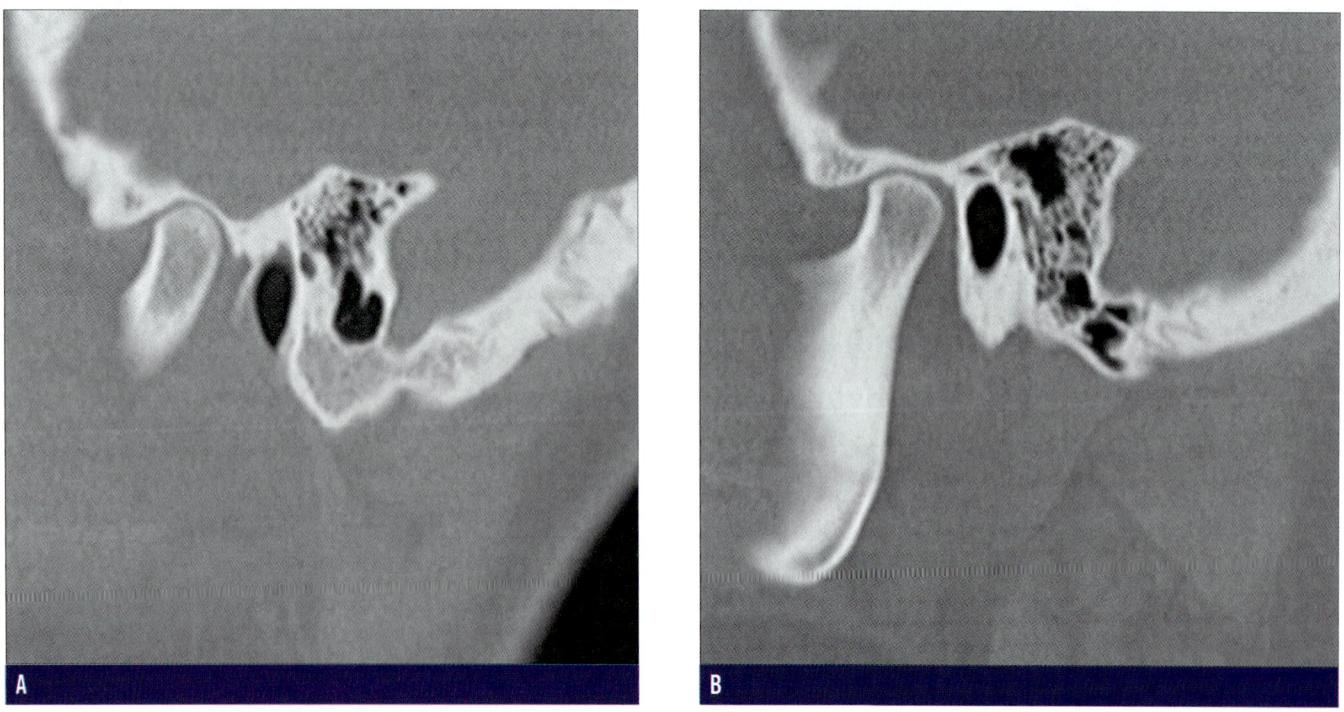

Sagittal reformatted CT images of the right TMJ (**A**) and left TMJ (**B**), as well as axial (**C**) and coronal reformatted (**D**) CT images through the TMJs . While the left mandibular condyle is slightly larger in the AP dimension on image **B**, the left mandibular condyle is clearly smaller in the transverse dimension and in overall volume on images **C** and **D** (arrows, **C**, **D**). A correspondingly hypoplastic left condylar fossa is also evident (**D**).

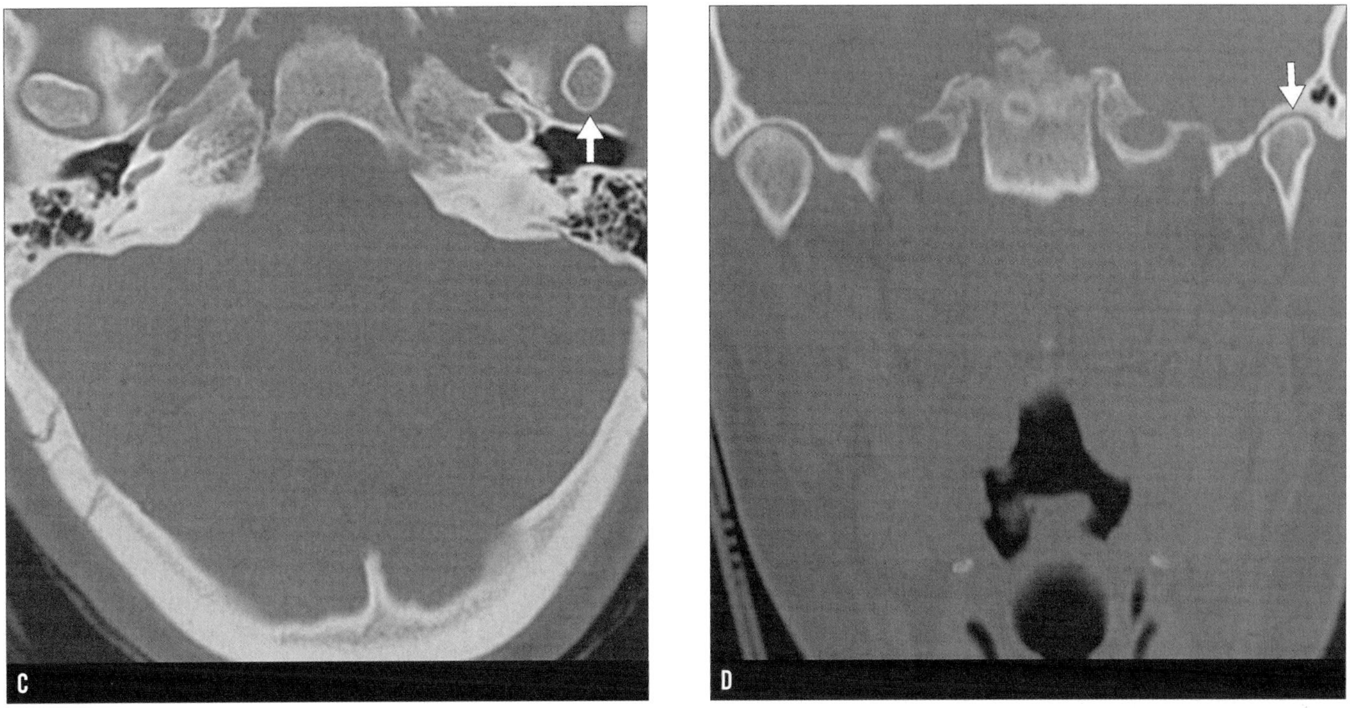

Companion case: Motion artifact

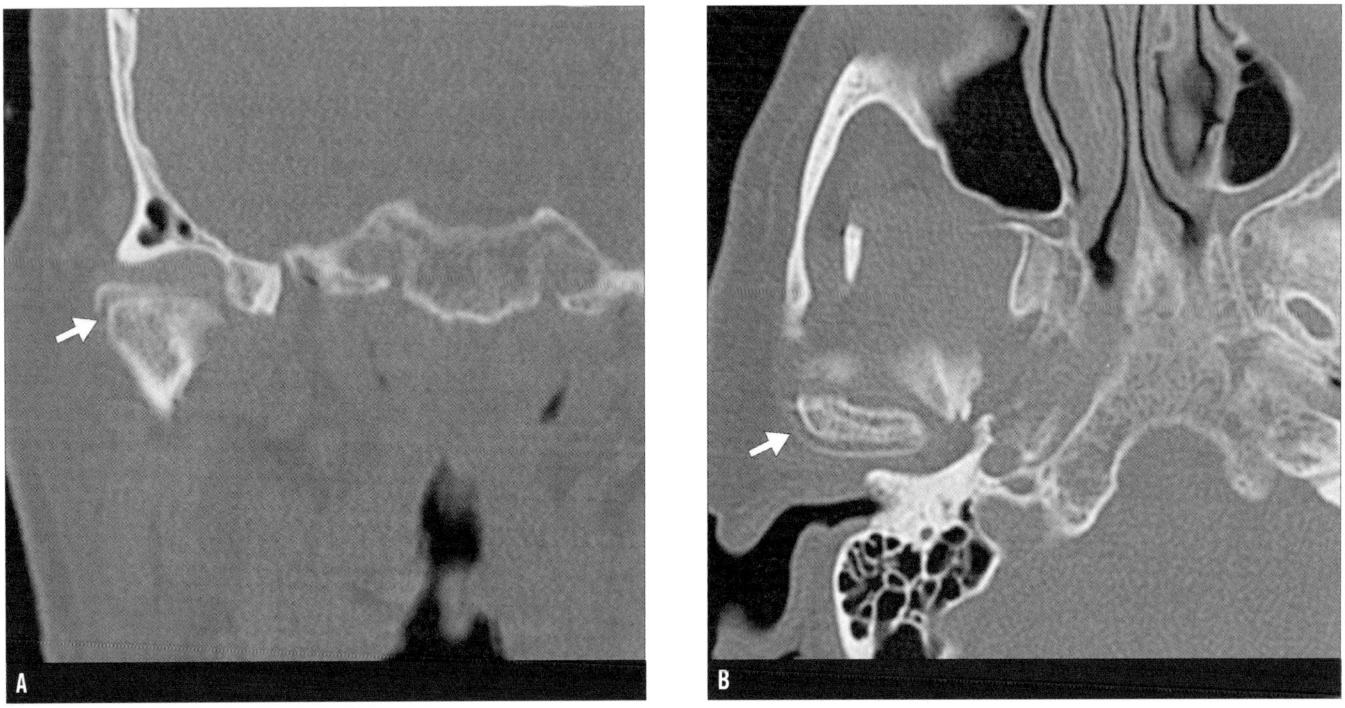

Coronal reformatted (**A**), axial (**B**), and sagittal reformatted (**C**) CT images through the right mandibular condyle demonstrate an apparent cleft within the right mandibular condyle (arrows, **A-C**). However, when evaluating all the images from this CT examination, it was clearly apparent that the finding simply represented motion artifact during the acquisition related to jaw movement.

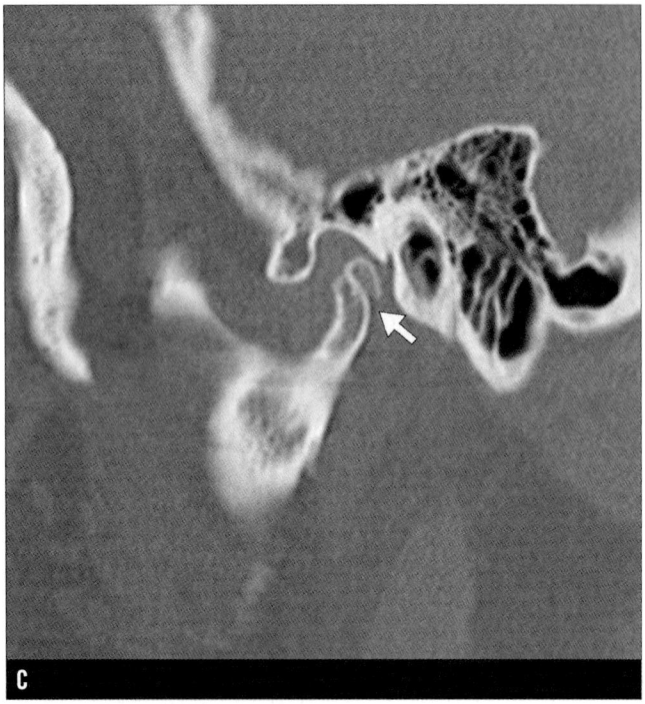

REFERENCES

Dennison J, Mahoney P, Herbison P, Dias G. The false and the true bifid condyles. *Homo.* 2008;59(2):149-159.

Faisal M, Ali I, Pai US, Bannerjee K. Bifid mandibular condyle: Report of two cases of varied etiology. *Nat Maxillofac Surg.* 2010; 1(1):78–80.

Kaneyama K, Segami N, Hatta T. Congenital deformities and developmental abnormalities of the mandibular condyle in the temporomandibular joint. *Congenit Anom (Kyoto).* 2008;48(3):118-125.

Lopez-Lopez, J, Ayuso-Montero R, Salas EJ, Rosello-Llabres X. Bifid condyle: review of the literature of the last 10 Years and report of two cases. *Cranio.* 2010;28(2):136-140.

Shriki J, et al. Bifid mandibular condyle: CT and MR imaging appearance in two patients: case report and review of the literature. *AJNR Am J Neuroradial.* 2005;26(7):1865-1868.

CASE 7 Benign masticatory muscle hypertrophy

There are four muscles of mastication: the masseter, temporalis, medial pterygoid, and lateral pterygoid muscles. The masseter and temporalis muscles, in particular, can hypertrophy, either in a unilateral or bilateral fashion. Temporalis muscle hypertrophy is discussed separately in Chapter 11. Multiple etiologies have been proposed for masticatory hypertrophy and include bruxism (ie, teeth grinding, such as during sleep or due to stress/anxiety), various temporomandibular joint disorders, and excessive gum chewing. Unilateral masticatory muscle hypertrophy can occur in those who have a tendency to chew or clench on only one side of their mouth. Occasionally, masticatory muscle hypertrophy can result in enlargement of the ipsilateral mandibular angle, likely the result of a stress response at the attachment site of the masseter muscle. Masticatory muscle hypertrophy is usually asymptomatic, but on occasion patients can experience facial pain or discomfort. On imaging, the hypertrophied muscle is asymmetrically larger than the contralateral side, but should otherwise be uniform in appearance, without evidence of a focal intramuscular mass.

COMPANION CASES

- **Benign masticatory muscle hypertrophy with hemimandibular hyperplasia.** Hemimandibular hyperplasia refers to uniform enlargement of one half of the mandible, including its condyle, with the enlarged portion of the hemimandible terminating at midline. The finding often results in displacement of the chin to the contralateral side and dental malocclusion. Hemimandibular hyperplasia occurs when a condylar growth center is hyperactive relative to the contralateral side. Proposed inciting factors for this entity include abnormal loading (ie, benign masticatory muscle hypertrophy due to bruxism, etc), trauma, infection, hormonal influences, hypervascularity, neoplasia, and heredity.
- **Leiomyosarcoma of the mandible**. Leiomyosarcoma is a malignant tumor that arises from smooth muscle. The average age of presentation is the late 30s. Often a patient with a leiomyosarcoma of the mandible will present with a painful mass. On imaging, a leiomyosarcoma is often an aggressive, destructive lesion associated with a soft tissue mass. Images obtained following contrast administration will demonstrate enhancement which is frequently heterogeneous.

Benign masticatory muscle hypertrophy

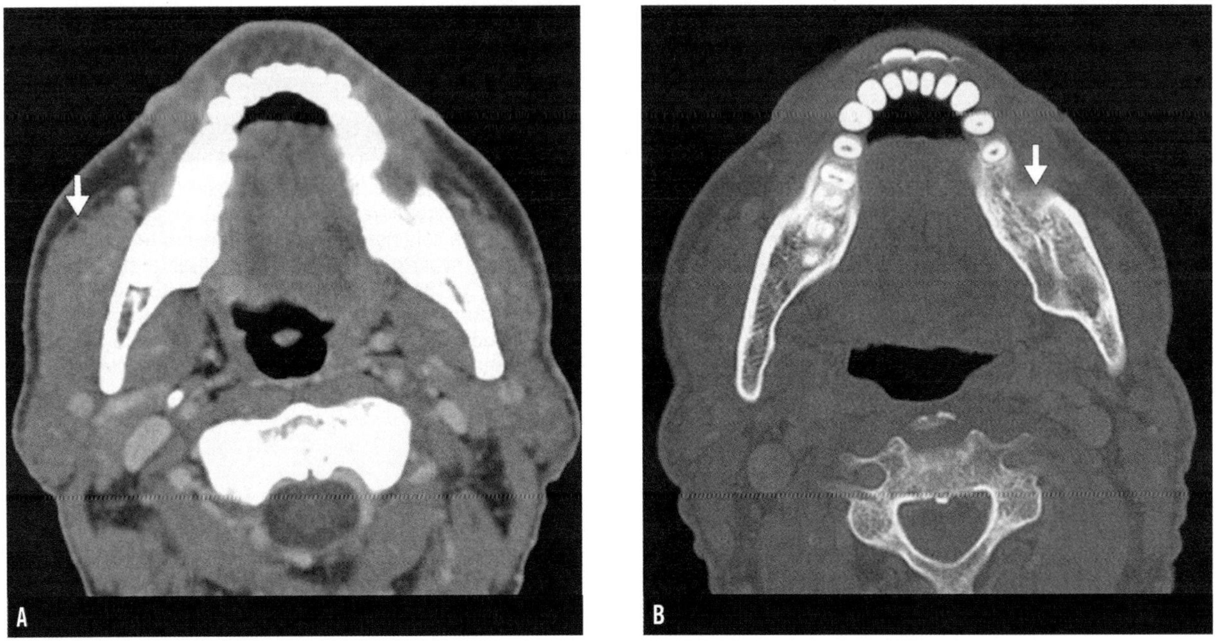

An axial CT image viewed with a soft tissue window (**A**) demonstrates asymmetric hypertrophy of the right masseter muscle (arrow, **A**). An axial CT image viewed with a bone window (**B**) demonstrates an old, healed fracture involving the left hemimandible (arrow, **B**). The right masseter hypertrophy presumably occurred due to a compensatory phenomenon following the left hemimandibular fracture.

Companion case: Benign masticatory muscle hypertrophy with hemimandibular hyperplasia

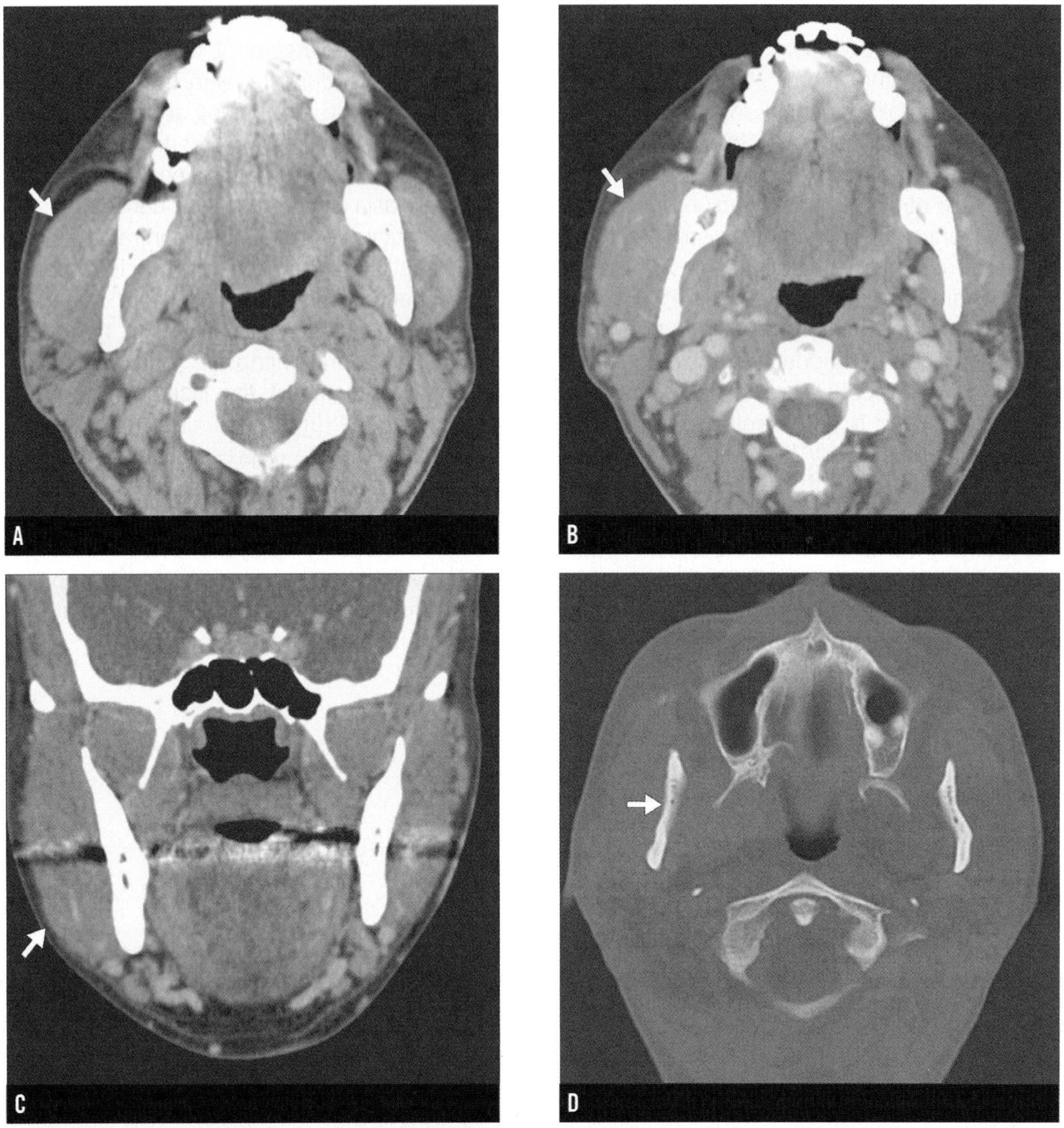

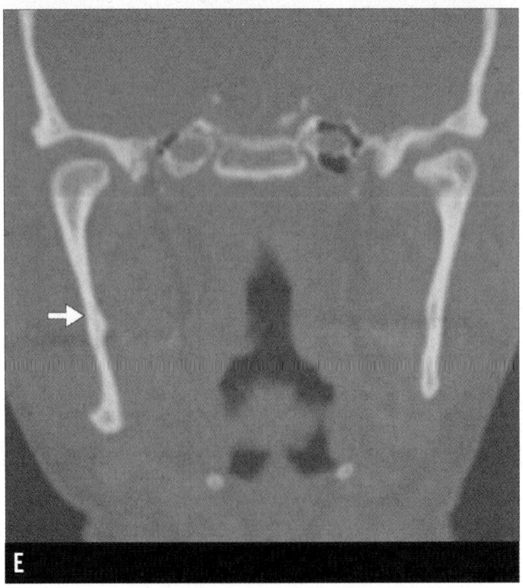

Unenhanced axial (**A**), postcontrast axial (**B**), and postcontrast coronal reformatted (**C**) CT images viewed with a soft tissue window demonstrate asymmetric hypertrophy of the right masseter muscle relative to the left (arrows, **A-C**). Axial (**D**) and coronal reformatted (**E**) CT images viewed with a bone window demonstrate the right hemimandible enlargement associated with the masseter muscle hypertrophy (arrows, **D**, **E**).

Companion case: Hemimandibular hyperplasia with dental malocclusion

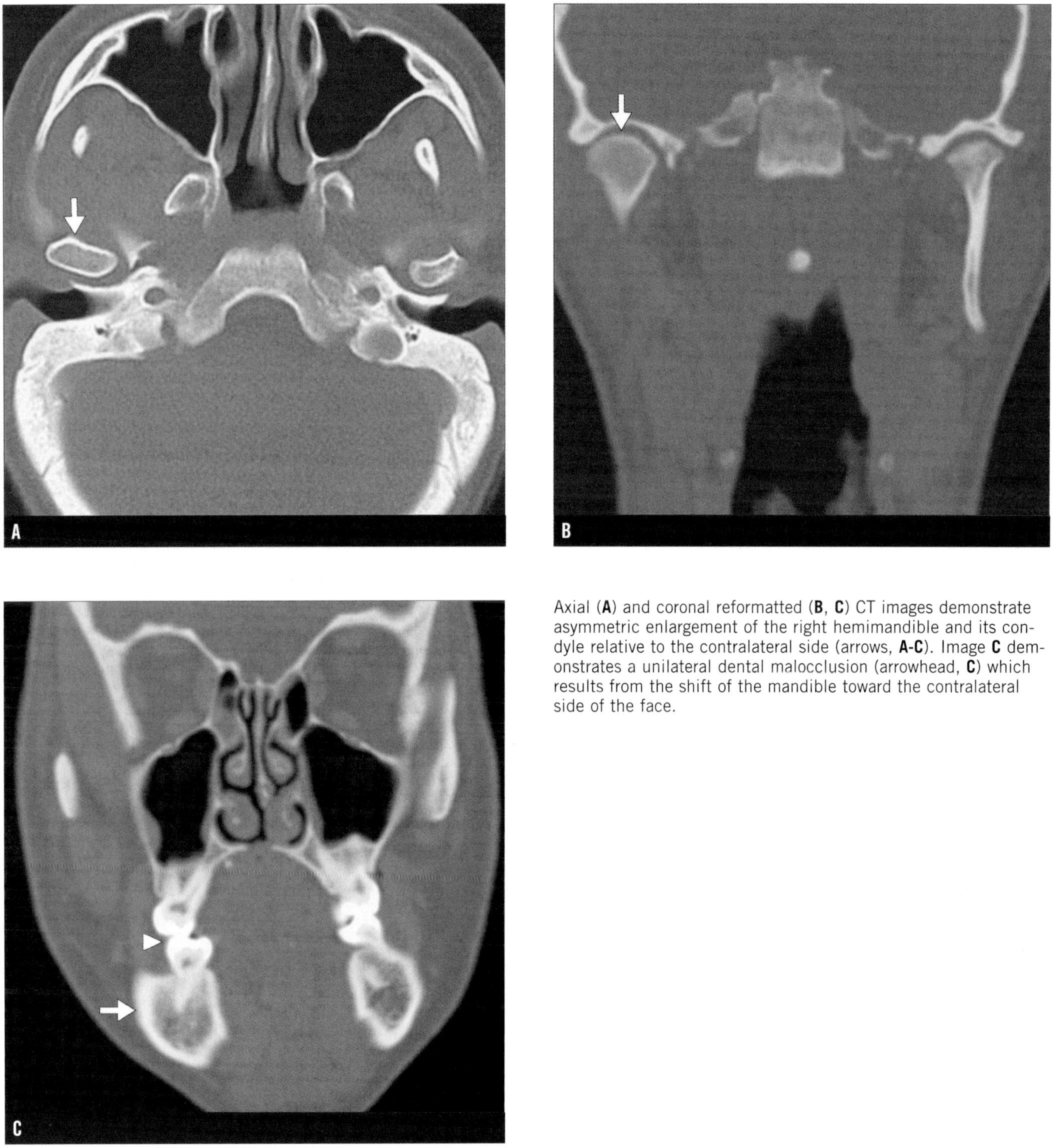

Axial (**A**) and coronal reformatted (**B**, **C**) CT images demonstrate asymmetric enlargement of the right hemimandible and its condyle relative to the contralateral side (arrows, **A-C**). Image **C** demonstrates a unilateral dental malocclusion (arrowhead, **C**) which results from the shift of the mandible toward the contralateral side of the face.

Companion case: Leiomyosarcoma of the mandible

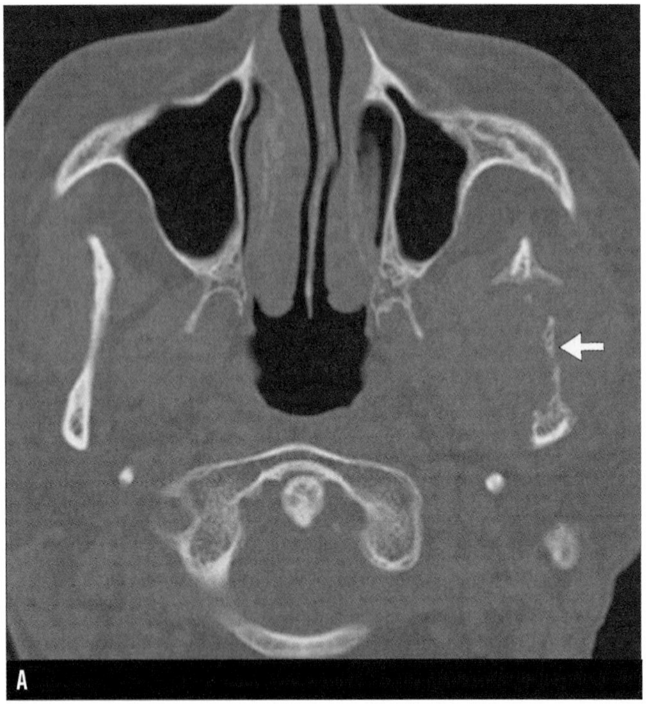

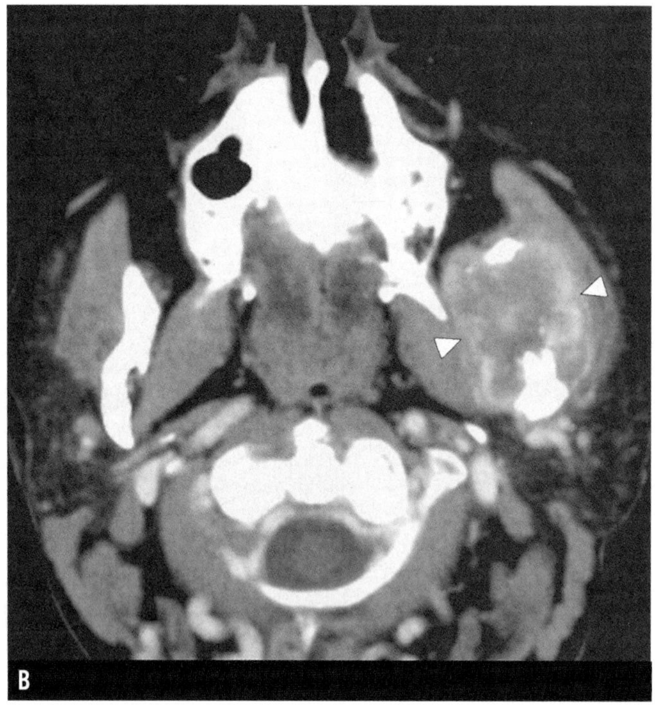

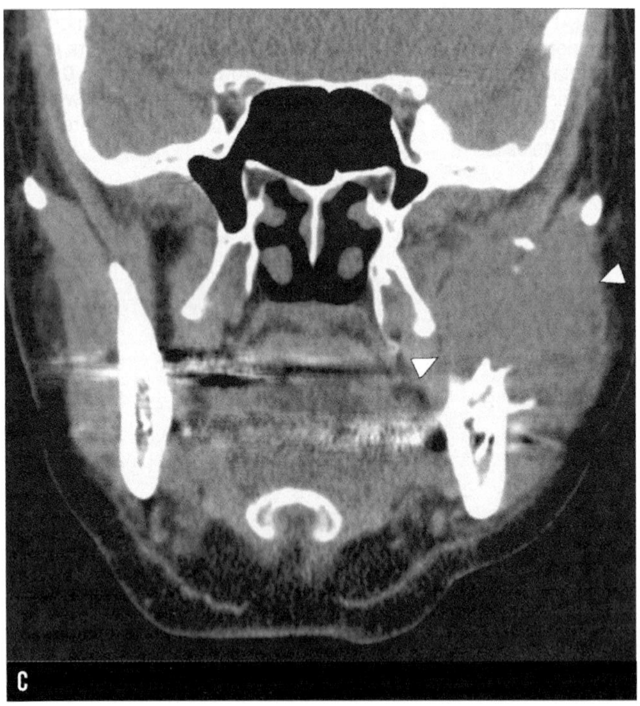

An axial CT image viewed with a bone window (**A**) demonstrates osseous destruction of the left hemimandible (arrow, **A**). Post-contrast axial (**B**) and noncontrast coronal reformatted (**C**) CT images viewed with a soft tissue window demonstrate a large, heterogeneously enhancing soft tissue mass surrounding the left hemimandible (arrowheads, **B**, **C**). The osseous destruction and heterogeneous enhancement differentiate this pathologic finding from benign masticator muscle hypertrophy.

REFERENCES

Bas B, Ozan B, Muglali M, Celebi N. Treatment of masseteric hypertrophy with botulinum toxin: a report of two cases. *Med Oral Patol Oral Cir Bucal.* 2010;15(4):e649-e652.

Braun IF, et al. Computed tomography of benign masseteric hypertrophy. *J Comput Assist Tomogr.* 1985;9(1):167-170.

Kaneyama K, Segami N, Hatta T. Congenital deformities and development abnormalities of the mandibular condyle in the temporomandibular joint. *Cogen Anom (Kyoto).* 2008;48(3):118-125.

Obwegeser HL, Makek MS. Hemimandibular hyperplasia—hemimandibular elongation. *J Maxillofac Surg.* 1986;14(4):183-208.

Rege IC, et al. High-grade primary leiomyosarcoma in the mandible: diagnosis and treatment. *Head Neck.* 2013; 35(2):E44-48.

Riefkohl R, Georgiade GS, Georgiade NG. Masseter Muscle Hypertrophy. *Ann Plast Surg.* 1984;12(6):528-532.

CASE 8 Pseudosubluxation of the temporomandibular joint

The temporomandibular joint (TMJ) is comprised of a fibrocartilage-covered mandibular condyle, the glenoid fossa (also called condylar fossa), the anterior articular eminence of the temporal bone, the meniscus, supporting musculature, ligaments, and a joint capsule. The joint capsule surrounding the TMJ is redundant and accommodates anterior translation of the mandibular condyle and meniscus that occurs with normal mouth opening. With normal open mouth positioning, the mandibular condyle may be positioned at the level of, or just anterior to, the articular eminence. The maximal degree of normal condylar translation can vary among individuals, typically ranging between 5 and 20 mm. Therefore, if a patient is imaged with their mouth open, normal anterior condyle translation may result in a subluxed appearance of the mandibular condyles on imaging.

COMPANION CASES

- **Anterior TMJ dislocation**. The TMJ may dislocate in various directions, including anteriorly, posteriorly, superiorly, medially, and laterally, each the result of a different mechanism. An anterior TMJ dislocation is the most common type and is discussed here. In an anterior TMJ dislocation, the normal sequence of jaw movement from an open mouth position to a closed position occurs in the wrong order. During normal mouth closure, the lateral pterygoid muscle, which attaches to the condyle and functions to protrude as well as depress the mandible, relaxes first, followed by contraction of the masseter and temporalis muscles, which function to elevate the mandible. This normal sequence of events allows for normal return of the condyle into the condylar fossa. With an anterior TMJ dislocation, the masseter and temporalis muscles contract prior to lateral pterygoid muscle relaxation. The combination of superior tension by the contracted masseter and temporalis muscles on the mandible as well as anterior and caudal traction by the contracted lateral pterygoid muscle on the condyle results in the anterior TMJ dislocation. Subsequent muscle spasm/trismus locks the condyle in place. An anterior dislocation may be unilateral or bilateral. The patient with bilateral TMJ dislocation will be unable to close their mouth.

  Anterior dislocations may occur as the result of trauma, yawning, laughing, taking large bites during eating, and undergoing intraoral procedures. Predisposing conditions that may contribute to a TMJ dislocation include being under the influence of medications which reduce muscular tone (ie, during intubation), a shallow articular eminence, or conditions which lead to joint laxity, such as a seizure disorder or Ehlers-Danlos syndrome.

  Distinguishing an anterior TMJ dislocation from a TMJ pseudosubluxation can be difficult and requires careful review of the images. Pseudosubluxation is an extremely common finding on CT because of the increased number of patients who are scanned with their mouth open. Compared to pseudosubluxation, an anteriorly dislocated mandibular condyle tends to be anteriorly-superiorly positioned relative to the inferior margin of the articular eminence, with the superior positioning a result of the constant upward force generated by the masseter and temporalis muscles. While the mandibular condyle may be located anterior to the articular eminence during a pseudosubluxation, it is generally not located superior to the level of the articular eminence. In addition, history supporting a TMJ dislocation should be present with a true anterior dislocation, such as the inability to close the patient's mouth following an inciting event. If the entire mandible is not included in the field of view on the axial or reconstructed images of a CT examination, then the scout lateral view from a CT examination is often helpful to evaluate the position of the mandible. However, in the case of pseudosubluxation, the patient may move their mandible between the acquisition of the scout and axial images.
- **Malocclusion from tooth loss leading to ipsilateral TMJ subluxation.** Dental malocclusion from various causes, including tooth loss, can result in unequal masticator muscle tension and subsequent TMJ subluxation.

Pseudosubluxation of the temporomandibular joint

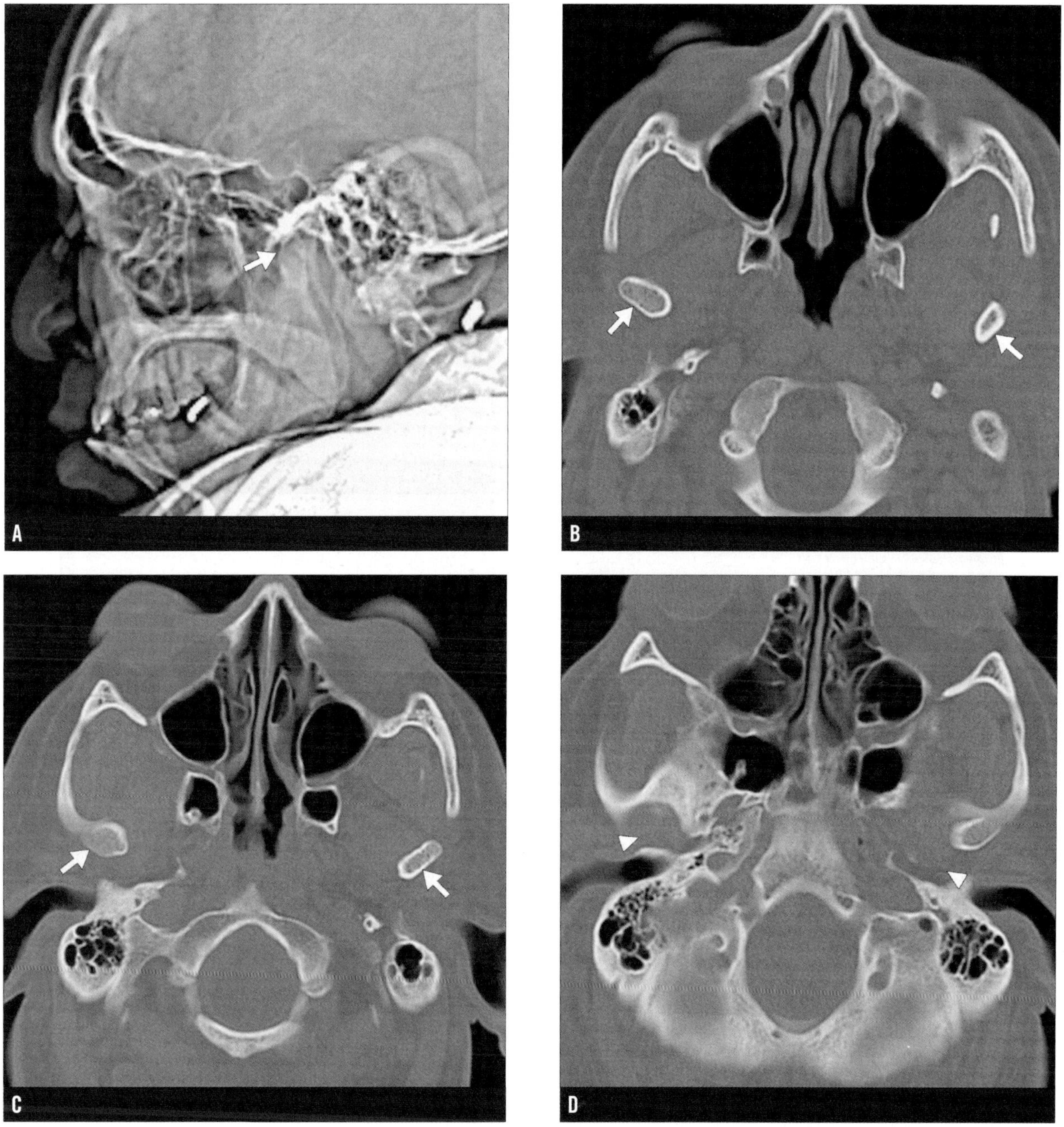

A lateral scout image from a facial bone CT (**A**) and axial CT images obtained through the TMJs (**B**-**D**). Image **A** is mildly rotated but demonstrates dental occlusion and the mandibular condyles fairly well seated in the glenoid fossae at the time the scout image was obtained (arrow, **A**). Images **B**-**D** demonstrate the mandibular condyles (arrows, **B**, **C**) to be anteriorly positioned relative to the glenoid fossae (arrowheads, **D**) during axial scanning. The patient opened their mouth during axial imaging resulting in normal anterior translation of the condylar heads relative to their respective articular eminences. This is not pathologic subluxation of the TMJs but rather normal TMJ movement. Similar findings are frequently identified in intubated patients who also have their mouth opened to accommodate the endotracheal tube.

Companion case: Fibrous dysplasia

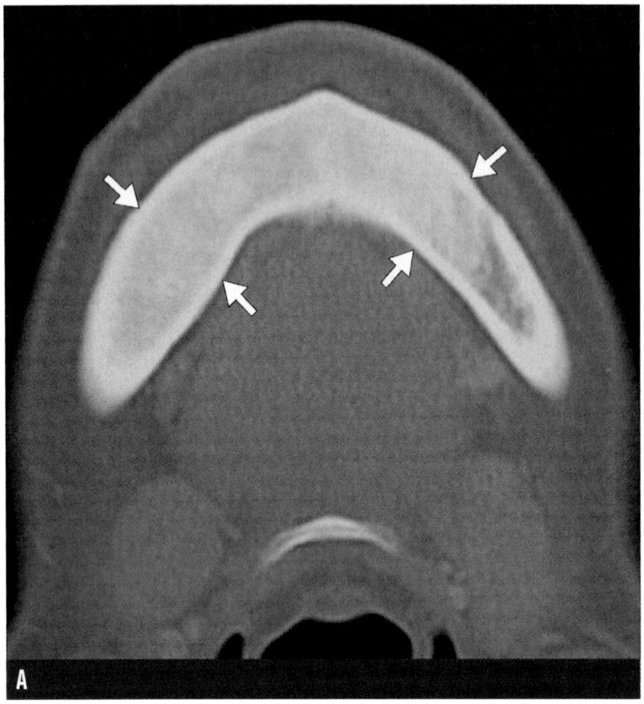

An axial CT image (**A**) demonstrates an expansile, sclerotic, ground-glass lesion involving the mandibular symphysis and the right greater than left hemimandibular body, compatible with fibrous dysplasia (arrows).

Companion case: Florid cemento-osseous dysplasia

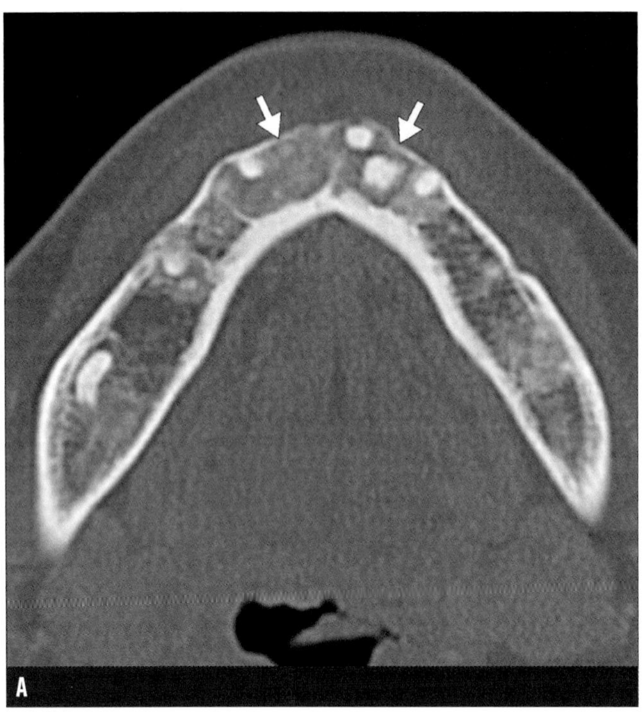

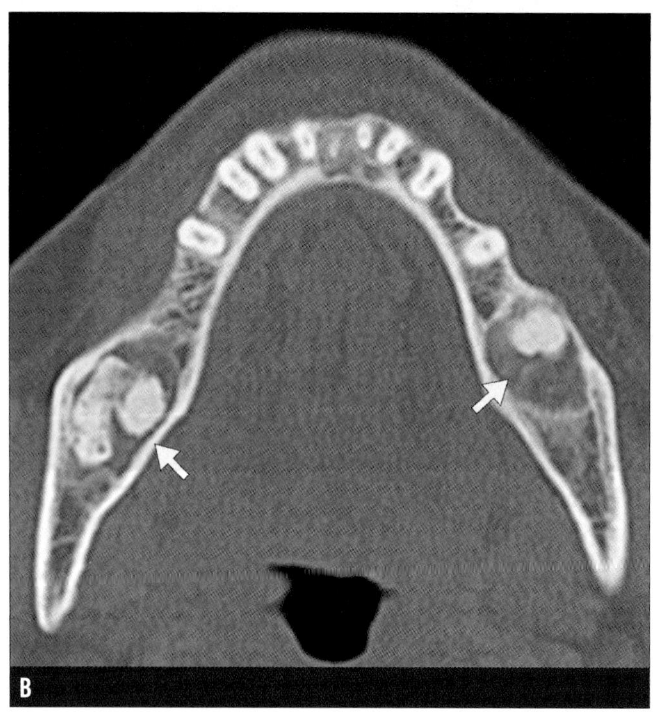

Axial (**A**, **B**), coronal reformatted (**C**), and sagittal reformatted (**D**, **E**) CT images demonstrate multiple heterogeneous, mixed lucent and sclerotic lesions surrounding the roots of multiple mandibular teeth, associated with mild expansion of the mandibular alveolus (arrows, **A-E**). These findings are typical for florid cemento-osseous dysplasia.

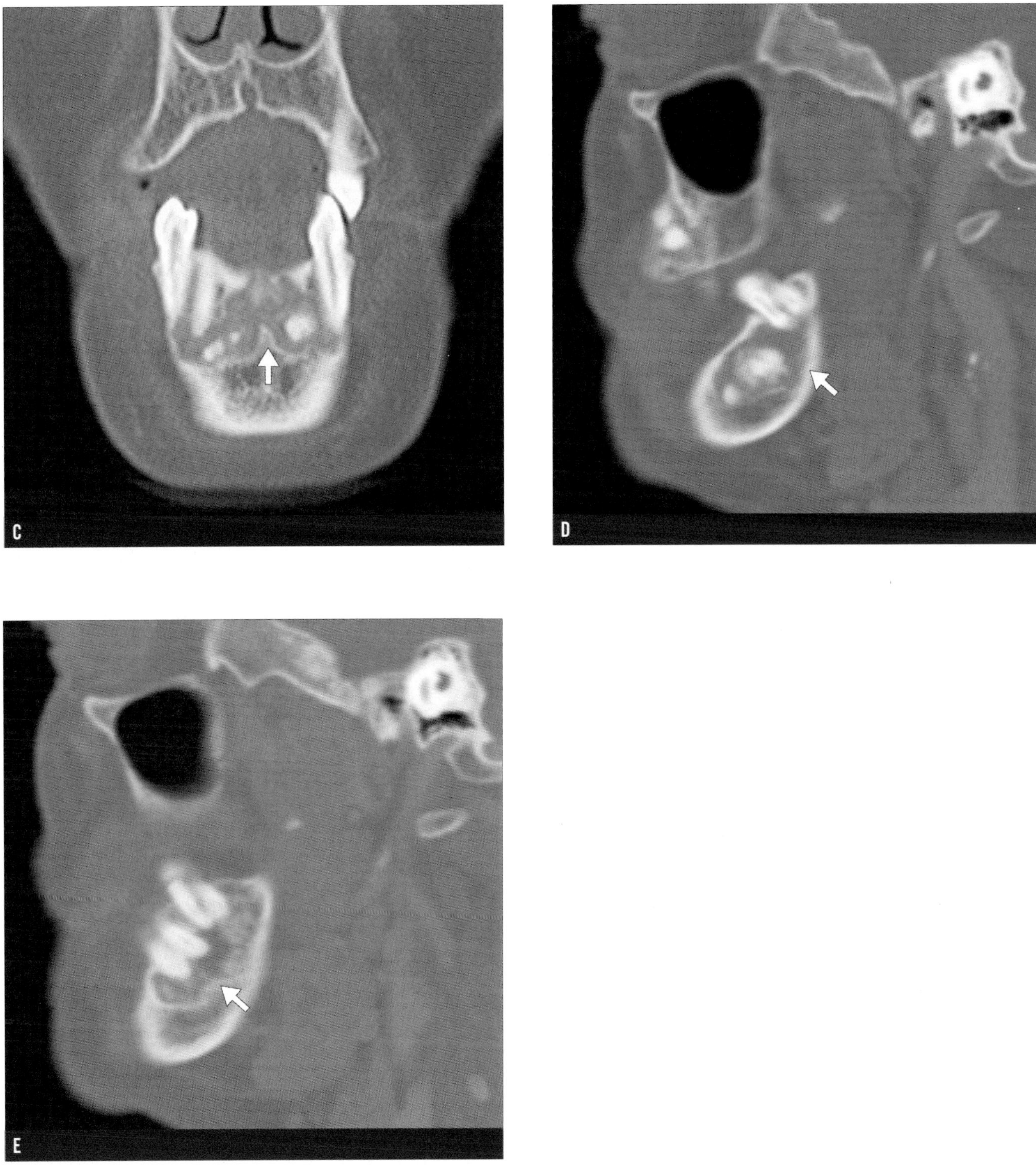
C
D
E

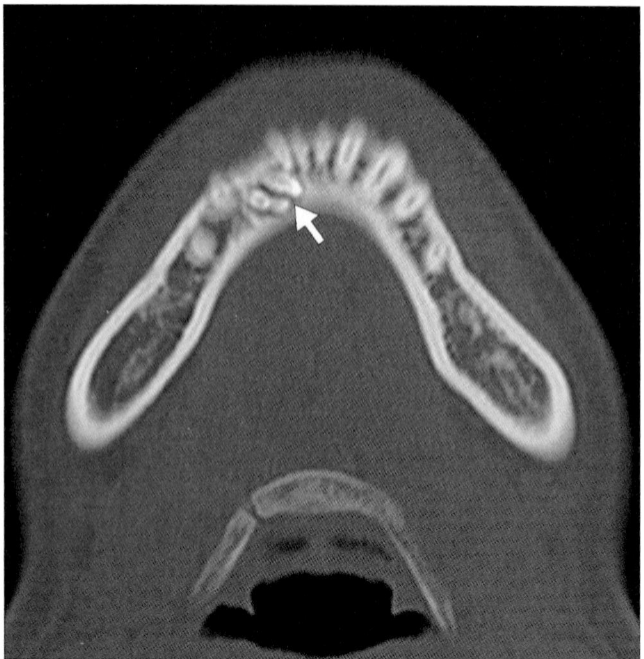

C

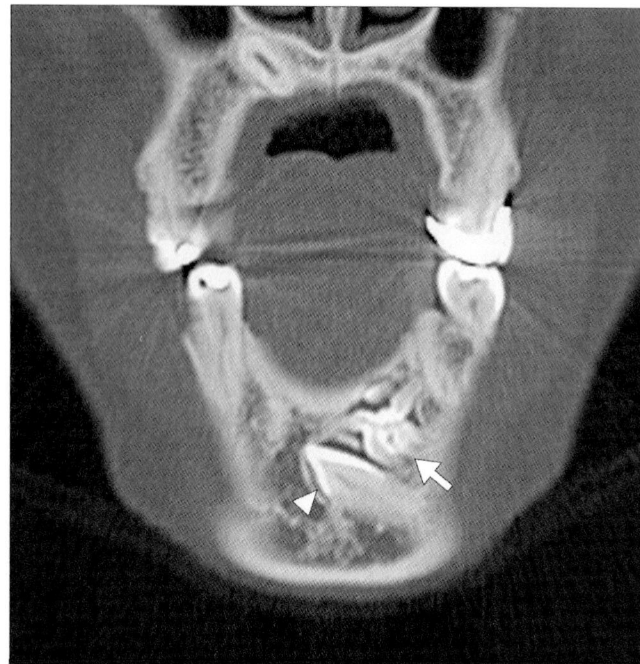

D

Companion case: Compound odontoma

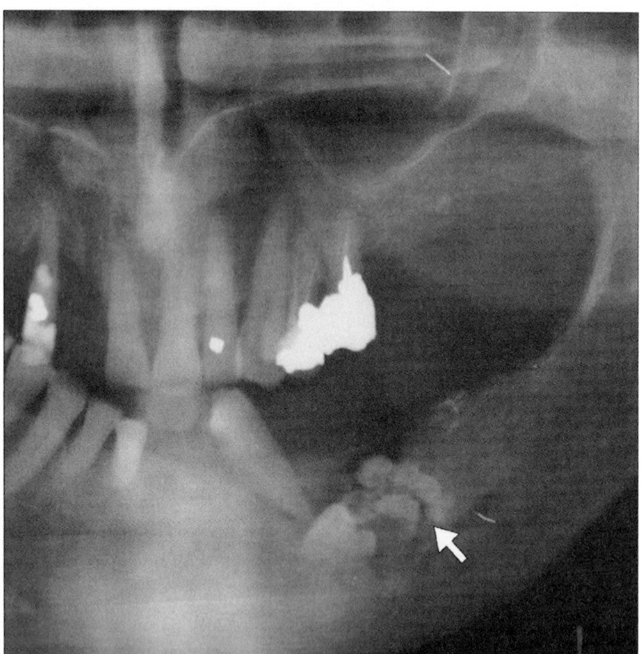

A

Different patient. A magnified panorex image (**A**) demonstrates a multilobulated, sclerotic lesion within the mandible composed of dental elements, consistent with a compound odontoma (arrow).

REFERENCES

Costa FW, et al. Maxillary cementoblastoma in a child. *J Craniofac Surg.* 2011;22(5):1910-1913.

Dunfee BL, Sakai O, Pistey R, Gohel A. Radiologic and pathologic characteristics of benign and malignant lesions of the mandible. *Radiographics.* 2006;26(6):1751-1768.

Eversole R, Su L, ElMofty S. Benign fibro-osseous lesions of the craniofacial complex. A Review. *Head Neck Pathol.* 2008;2(3):177-202.

Gould CF, et al. Bone tumor mimics: avoiding misdiagnosis. *Curr Probl Diagn Radiol.* 2007;36(3):124-141.

Kransdorf MJ, Moser RP, Gilkey FW. Fibrous dysplasia. *Radiographics.* 1990;10(3):519-537.

Wood NK, Kuc IM. Pericoronal radiolucencies. In: Wood NK, Goaz PW, eds. *Differential diagnosis of oral and maxillofacial lesions.* St. Louis, MO: Mosby Elsevier; 1997:279-295.

CASE 10 Genial tubercle

The genial tubercle is a small osseous projection located along the midline lingual aspect of the mandibular symphysis. The genial tubercle is most often a paired osseous projection, with an upside-down V-shaped morphology in the axial plane, although occasionally it may manifest as only a single osseous projection. The genial tubercle serves as the origin of the genioglossus and geniohyoid muscles. The genioglossus is a fan-shaped muscle that inserts in a radial fashion on the base of the tongue and provides anterior traction for tongue advancement. The geniohyoid muscle is a paired muscle that inserts upon the anterior aspect of the hyoid bone body. In combination with other floor of mouth muscles and the tongue, the geniohyoid elevates and pulls the hyoid bone anteriorly during deglutition.

A genial tubercle fracture can occur following trauma, denture placement, or as a spontaneous event in a person with a demineralized mandible. Identification of genial tubercle disruption is important, as loss of the anterior attachment of the genioglossus muscle with resultant loss of anterior traction on the tongue can result in compromise of the oropharyngeal airway.

COMPANION CASES

- **Genial tubercle mimicking a Wharton duct sialolith.** When evaluating the floor of mouth in the coronal plane on CT, a prominent genial tubercle may mimic a distal Wharton duct sialolith. This misinterpretation can easily be avoided by cross-referencing the finding on the axial images.
- **Distal Wharton duct sialolith**. The submandibular gland duct, otherwise known as the Wharton duct, measures approximately 5 cm in length. Following its exit from the submandibular hilum, the Wharton duct ascends posterior to the free margin of the mylohyoid and traverses anteriorly within the sublingual space, above the mylohyoid muscle. Each duct drains via its respective sublingual papilla, which are located on each side of the lingual frenulum. A sialolith within a Wharton duct may be confused with a prominent genial tubercle if the sialolith is located at or near the distal Wharton duct orifice. On CT, a radiopaque sialolith will appear as a calcified focus along the expected course of the Wharton duct. On T1 and T2-weighted MR images, a sialolith will appear as a hypointense focus.

Genial tubercle

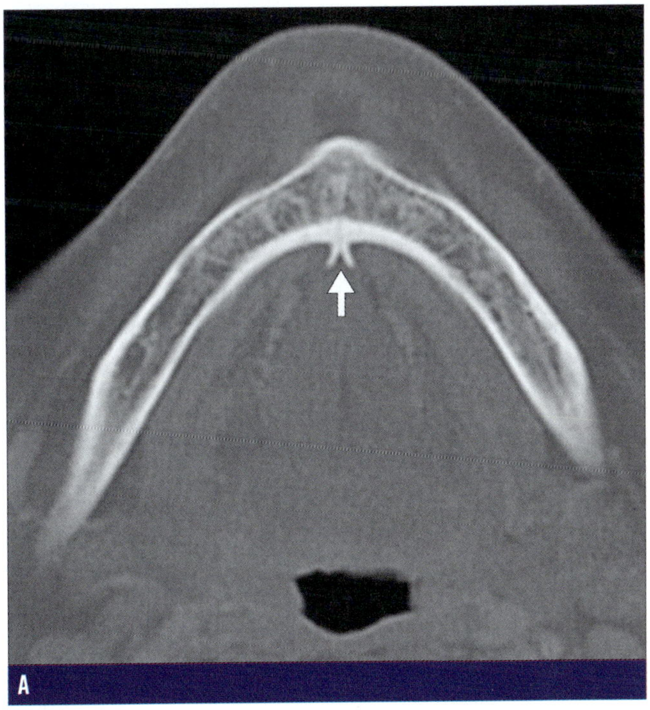

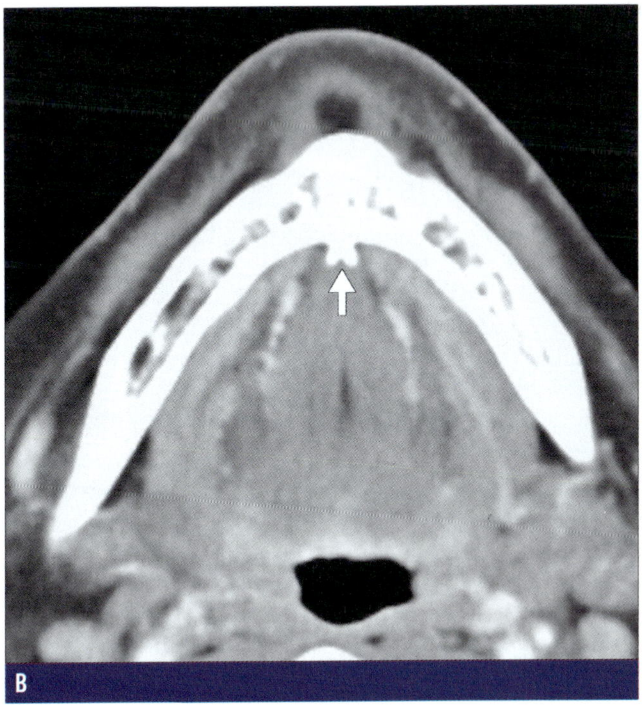

Axial CT images viewed with a bone window (**A**) and soft tissue window (**B**) as well as sagittal reformatted CT images viewed with a bone window (**C**) and soft tissue window (**D**) demonstrate a prominent but normal genial tubercle (arrows, **A-D**).

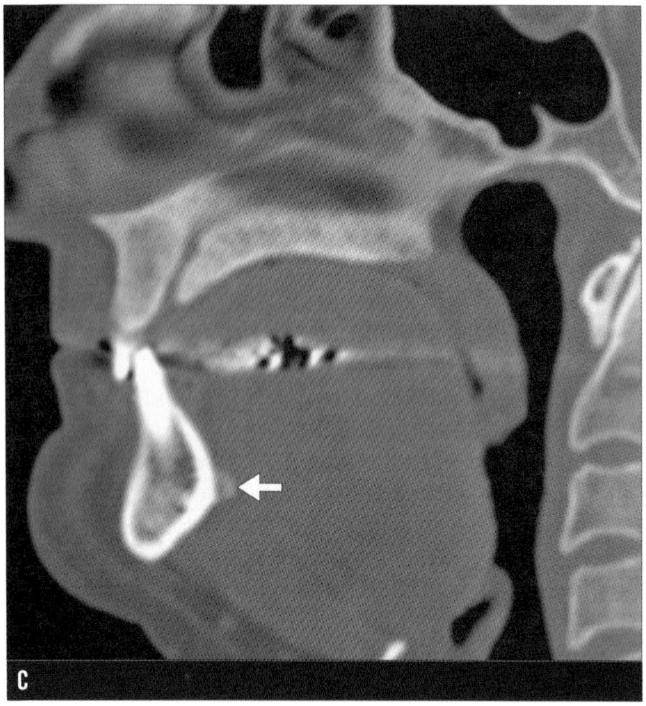

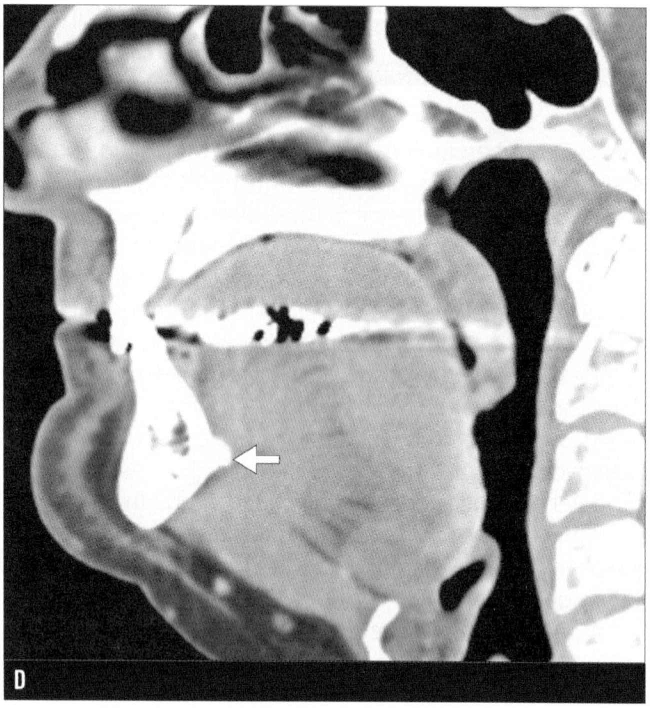

Genial tubercle

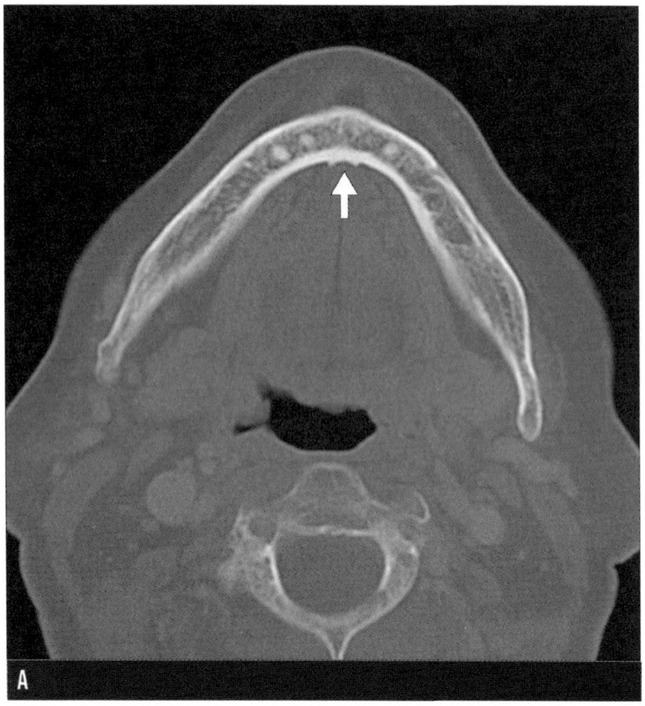

Different patient. A single axial CT image (**A**) demonstrates a flat and diminutive but normal genial tubercle (arrow).

Genial tubercle with a single osseous projection

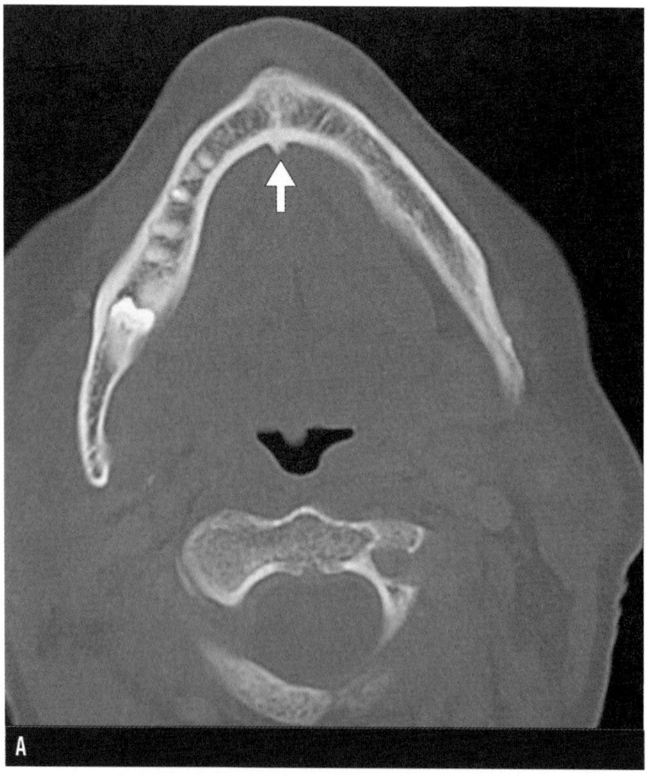

An axial CT image (**A**) demonstrates a genial tubercle with only one osseous projection, rather than paired osseous projections, as is more commonly present.

Companion case: Genial tubercle mimicking a Wharton duct sialolith

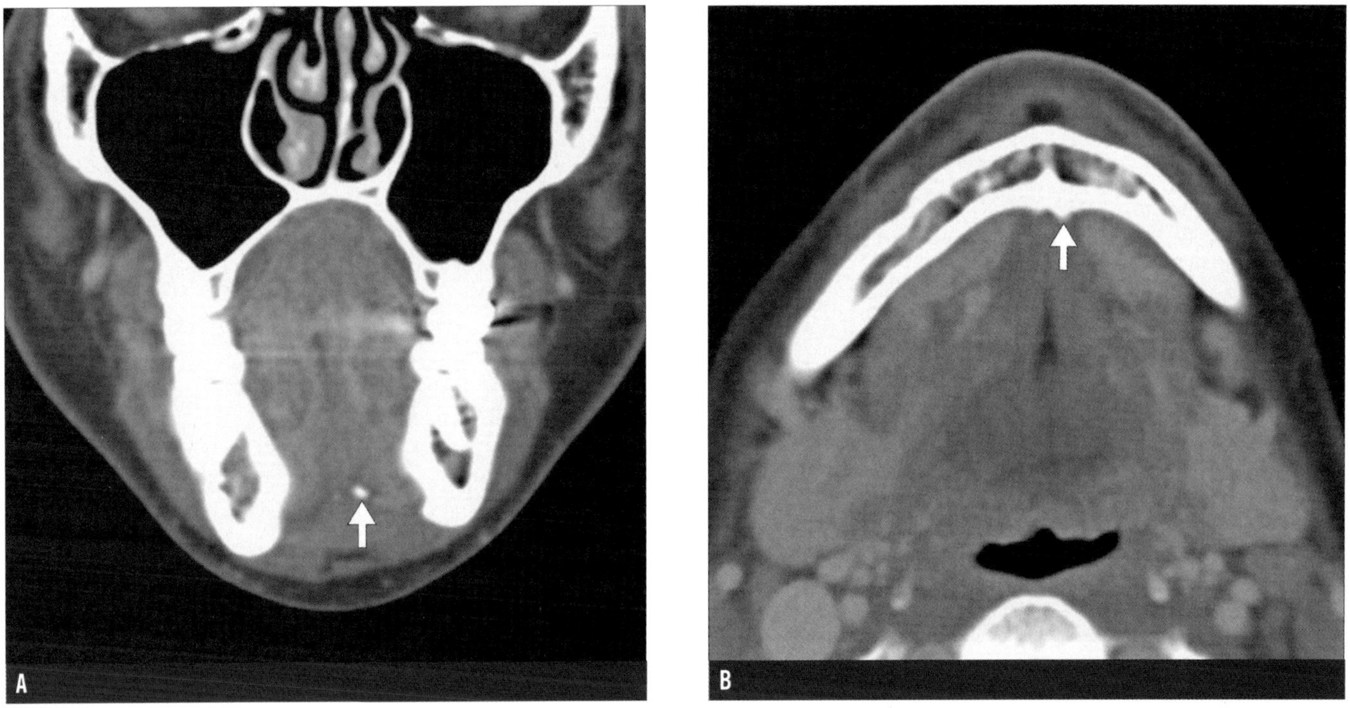

A coronal reformatted CT image (**A**) demonstrates an apparent left Wharton duct stone (arrow, **A**). An axial CT image (**B**) reveals that this structure represents a normal, asymmetrically prominent genial tuberosseous projection and not a Wharton duct sialolith (arrow, **B**).

Companion case: Distal Wharton duct sialolith

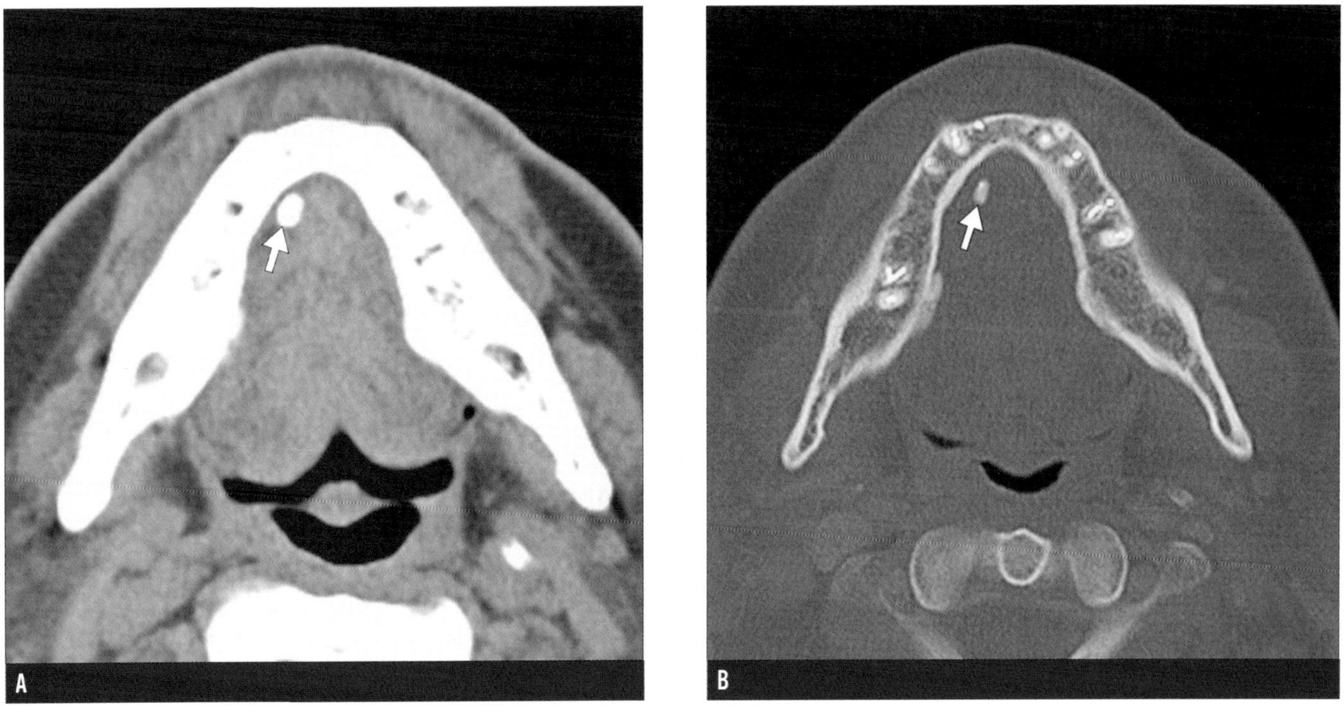

An axial CT image viewed with a soft tissue window (**A**) and axial CT images viewed with a bone window (**B**-**D**) demonstrate a sialolith in the distal aspect of the right Wharton duct (arrows, **A**, **B**) and a larger sialolith in the right submandibular gland hilum (arrows, **C**, **D**). In most cases, a distal Wharton duct sialolith is easily distinguishable from a genial tubercle (arrowhead, **D**).

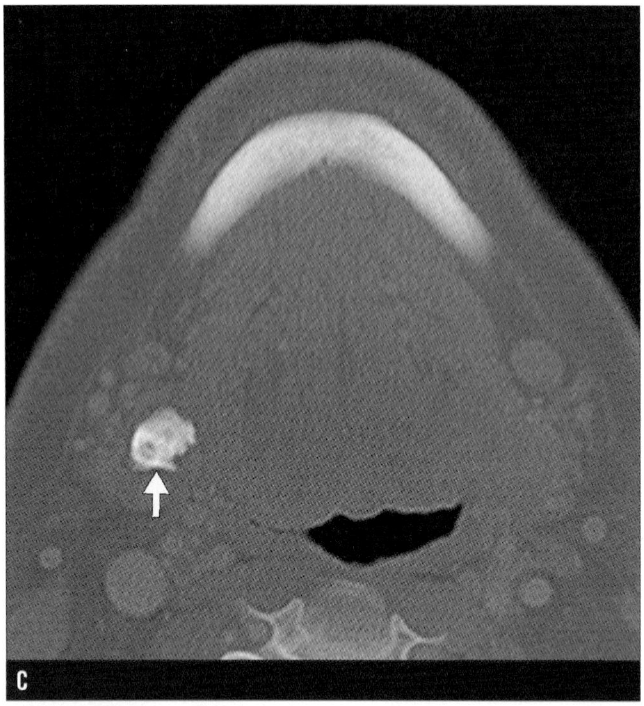

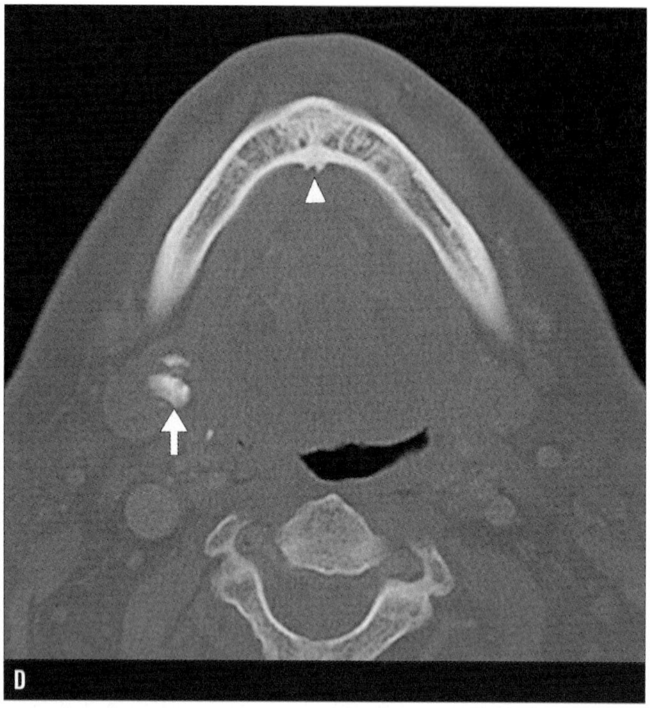

REFERENCES

Hennessee J, Miller FR. Anatomic analysis of the genial bone advancement trephine system's effectiveness at capturing the genial tubercle and its muscular attachments. *Otolaryngol Head Neck Surg.* 2005;133(2):229-233.

Hueman EM, et al. Accuracy of cone beam computed tomography in determining the location of the genial tubercle. *Otolaryngol Head Neck Surg.* 2007;137(1):115-118.

Jager L, et al. Sialolithiasis: MR sialography of the submandibular duct: an alternative to conventional sialography and US? *Radiology.* 2000;216(3):665-671.

Mintz SM, Ettinger AC, Geist JR, Geist RY. Anatomic relationship of the genial tubercles to the dentition as determined by cross-sectional tomography. *J Oral Maxillofac Surg.* 1995;53(11):1324-1326.

Ryan JM, Ross D, Obeid G. Genial tubercle fracture: a case report and review of the literature. *J Oral Maxillofac Surg.* 2010;68(9):2338-2341.

- **Dental implants**. Dental implants are a permanent solution to replace missing teeth. The modern day dental implant is an osteointegrated type that is typically constructed from titanium and drilled directly into the maxillary or mandibular bone. If the maxillary alveolus is deficient and cannot adequately anchor a dental implant fixture, then bone graft material is often placed along the floor of the maxillary sinus to aid in osseous integration of the fixture. This procedure is termed a maxillary sinus lift or maxillary sinus augmentation. When the fixture has incorporated with the adjacent bone (typically after a period of 4-9 months), the remainder of the implant, including the prosthetic tooth, is attached to the fixture. For further discussion regarding maxillary sinus lifts, please refer to Chapter 6.
- **Dental crowns.** A dental crown, also known as a dental cap, is used to "cap" a damaged or decaying tooth. Dental crowns may be used when a tooth is damaged so greatly that there isn't enough residual tooth that can be adequately repaired with dental amalgam. They may also be placed atop a fractured tooth in order to stabilize the fracture or used as integral portions of a dental bridge. Multiple different materials may be used to construct a crown, including various metals (eg, gold) and porcelain (a ceramic material). Porcelain crowns may be made entirely of porcelain, or its surface may be made of porcelain and the portion deep to the crown surface, termed the substructure, may be constructed with metal or other ceramics (eg, zirconium oxide). While a tooth crown made entirely of porcelain has a similar appearance on imaging to that of normal tooth enamel, those porcelain dental crowns with a metallic or other type of ceramic substructure will have an imaging appearance dependent on the material used.
- **Dental bridges.** Dental bridges are used to bridge a gap between one or more missing teeth. Dental bridges are constructed of two or more dental crowns and one or more intervening false teeth that are termed pontics. The dental crowns are anchored atop the remaining teeth or dental implants, referred to as abutment teeth, which serve to anchor the bridge. The abutment teeth are modified and frequently reduced in size to accommodate the dental crowns. Bridges are most commonly composed of porcelain for aesthetic purposes, although they may also be composed of alloys, silver, gold, or a combination of these materials. A dental bridge may be fixed or removable, the latter more commonly known as a removable partial denture. A fixed dental bridge is glued into place and cannot be removed by the patient. Dental bridges aim to restore dental functionality and improve oral health.
- **Dental amalgam.** Dental amalgam (also called dental fillings) refers to material composed of two or more metals which is used to fill defects within teeth, most commonly for the treatment of dental caries. The two most common metals used in dental amalgam are mercury and silver; however, small quantities of copper, tin, and zinc are also included to prevent corrosion. The metals used in dental amalgam are extremely dense and very radiopaque on radiographic imaging. Newer compounds used for teeth restoration include composite acrylic resins and glass ionomer cement, among others. The composite acrylic resins are naturally radiolucent. Therefore, in order to be visible on radiographs, radiopaque material must be added prior to their application. On imaging, composite acrylic resins are intermediate in attenuation, between that of dental amalgam and regular dental enamel.
- **Root canal**. The neurovascular bundle enters the tooth root apex via the apical foramen. The bundle then travels through the root canal and enters the pulp chamber. In endodontal disease, bacteria from dental caries enter the pulp chamber from above (typically from the crown). If a large enough infection forms, the infection can extend through the apical foramen into the bone of the maxilla or mandible. Once the infectious process has spread outside the tooth, a periapical abscess may develop. By contrast, periodontal disease occurs when bacteria from gingivitis attack the ligament which affixes the tooth roots to the tooth socket (termed the periodontal ligament). In periodontal disease, bone resorption occurs around the roots of the teeth.

  The root canal procedure is used to treat endodontal disease. In this procedure, the pulp cavity and root canal are drilled and its contents are removed. The pulp cavity and root canal are then injected with material termed gutta-percha. A dental crown may be placed at the end of the procedure. On imaging, a tooth treated with a root canal procedure has radiopaque gutta-percha occupying the normally radiolucent pulp chamber and root canal.

COMPANION CASES

- **Soft tissue abscess associated with an infected dental implant.** Dental implants may be utilized to replace a devitalized tooth resulting from chronic endodontal or periodontal disease. The oral cavity in these patients is colonized with bacteria from normal oral flora as well as from their underlying dental disease. Despite the best efforts by the treating clinician, bacteria may remain within the bone or gingiva after placement of an implant and serve as a nidus for a postprocedural infection. Peri-implant osteitis (also called peri-implantitis) is an inflammatory process that involves both the soft tissues and bone surrounding the implant. On radiography or

CT imaging, peri-implant osteitis will be radiolucent along a portion or the entire osseous margin of the implant.

- **MRI artifact from dental restoration and dental braces**. Metal can result in MR image distortion, signal loss, and signal "pile-up." Signal loss can result from two principal mechanisms. The first mechanism is when the metal object results in local differences in atomic spins, which leads to spin–spin dephasing and loss of the MRI signal. The second occurs when the metal object alters the frequency of atomic spins within a voxel such that those protons localize to a different voxel, creating a region of signal loss. The voxel which acquires the signal from the additional protons will have an increase in signal, otherwise known as signal "pile-up."

  In addition to signal loss and image distortion, metal may also cause difficulties with normal fat or cerebrospinal fluid suppression. Fat suppression MR imaging relies on the different resonant frequencies between the protons in water and fat. At 1.5T, fat resonance is 220 Hz lower than that of water. Since the resonant frequencies of protons in fat and water are different, fat can be selectively "excluded" from images to obtain the desired fat suppression. However, the resonant frequencies of protons near metal implants can be altered as much as 80 kHz, preventing fat from being adequately saturated. On FLAIR, metallic substances create magnetic field heterogeneity which may lead to incomplete nulling of CSF signal, potentially mimicking pathologic processes such as subarachnoid hemorrhage or meningitis.
- **CT streak artifact from normal dental enamel**. The density of normal dental enamel is higher than that of normal cortical bone. As a result, mild streak artifact may be present in a patient with normal dental enamel and without a history of prior dental intervention.

Dental implants and dental crowns

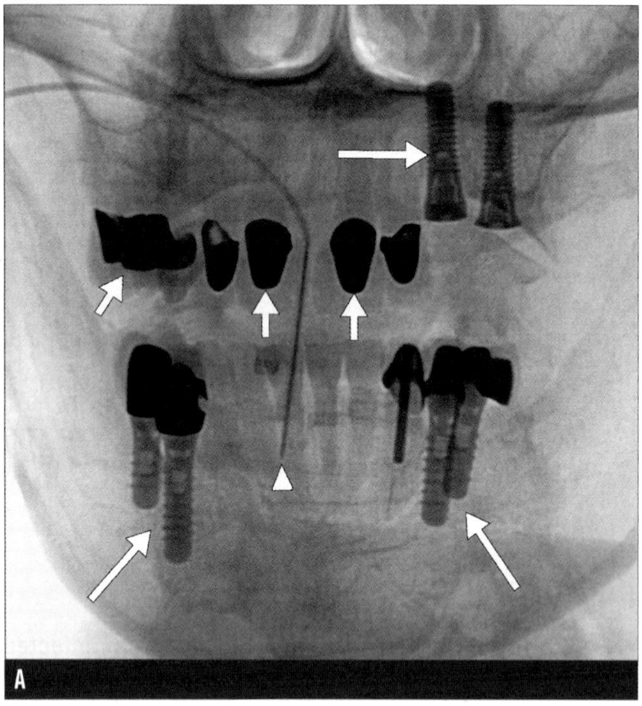

A frontal scout radiograph prior to a sialogram (**A**) demonstrates multiple threaded osteointegrated dental implants (long arrows) and multiple dental crowns (short arrows). A Rabinov sialography needle is also present on the image (arrowhead).

Dental crowns, dental amalgam, and a root canal

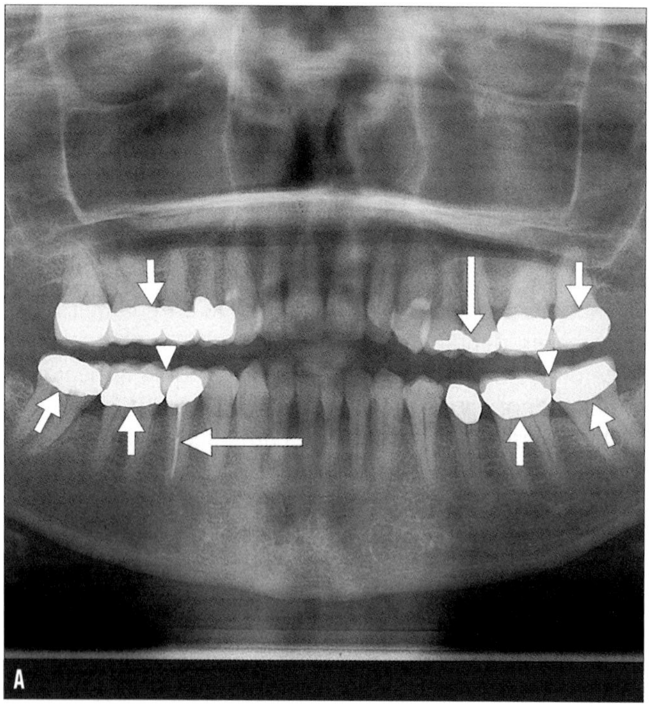

A panorex image (**A**) demonstrates multiple dental crowns, only some of which are denoted by small arrows. The high-density portion of the crowns represents a metallic substructure, whereas a small amount of less dense material along the cephalad aspect of the crowns represents ceramic material, presumably porcelain (arrowheads). This patient also has had a root canal procedure (long arrow) and placement of dental amalgam (medium arrow).

Dental bridge, dental crowns, and dental amalgam

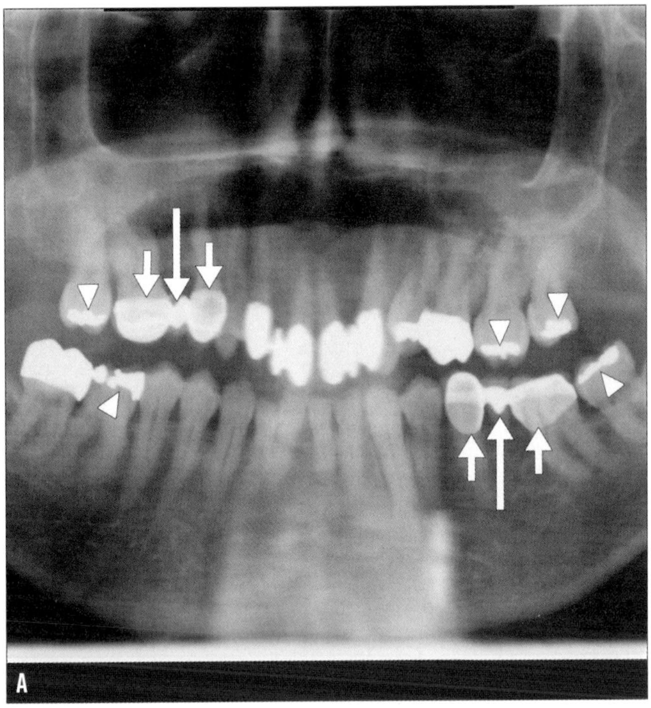

A panorex image (**A**) demonstrates right maxillary and left mandibular dental bridges (long arrows) which are affixed to existing teeth with dental crowns (small arrows). Several additional dental crowns as well as dental amalgam are present (arrowheads).

Dental amalgam

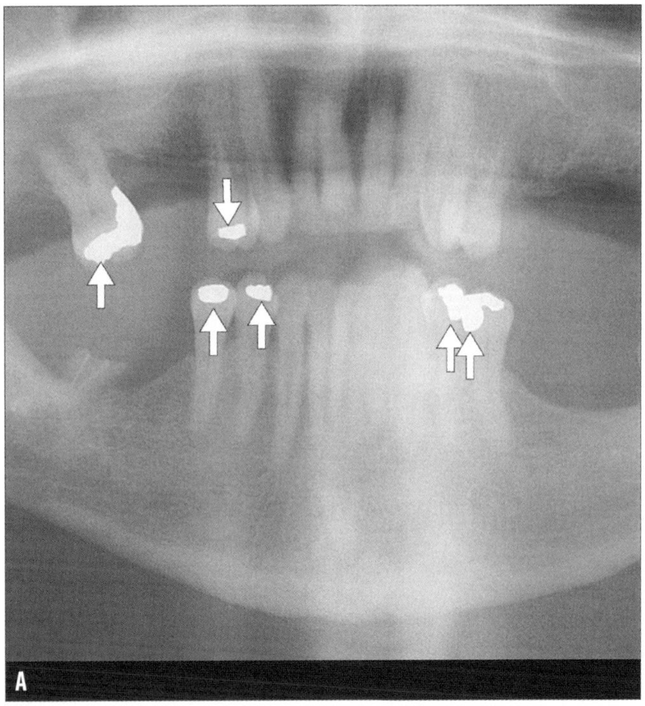

A panorex (**A**) image demonstrates dental amalgam overlying the crowns of several maxillary and mandibular teeth (arrows).

Root canals

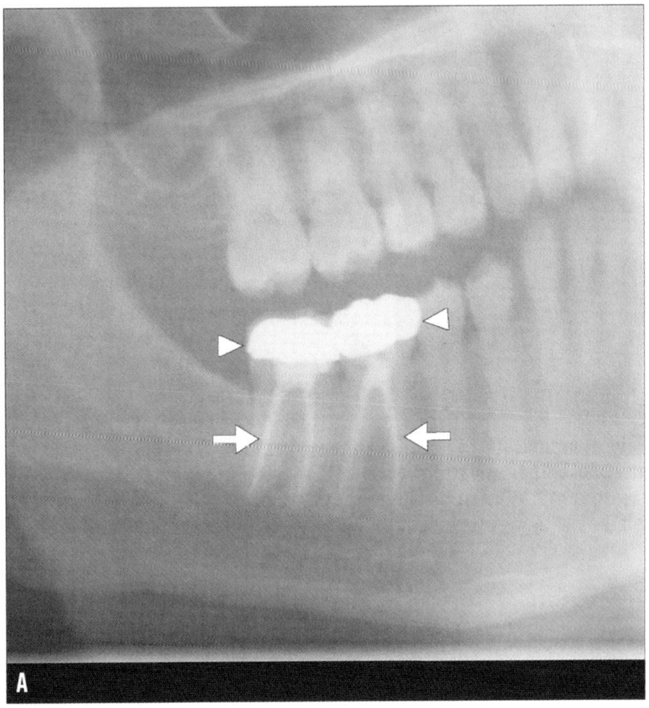

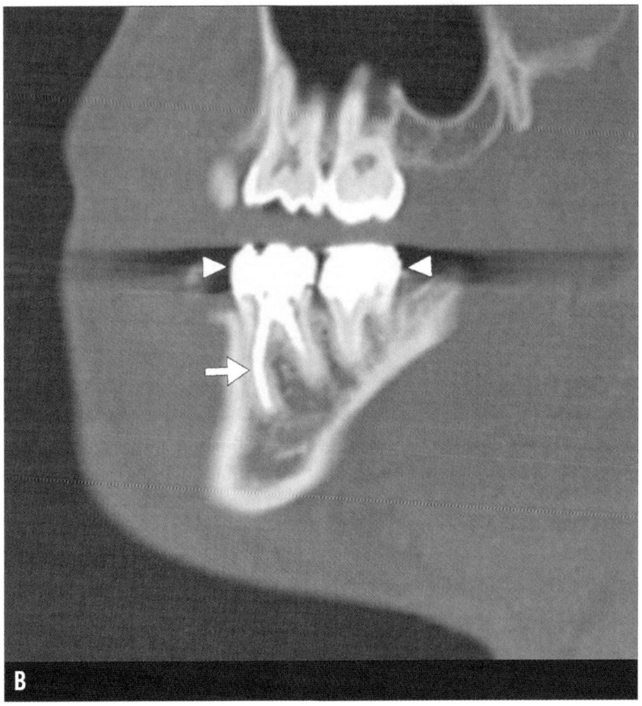

A cropped panorex image (**A**) and a sagittal reformatted CT imaged (**B**) demonstrate gutta-percha material related to a root canal procedure (arrows, **A**, **B**). Dental crowns are also present (arrowheads, **A**, **B**).

Companion case: Soft tissue abscess associated with an infected dental implant

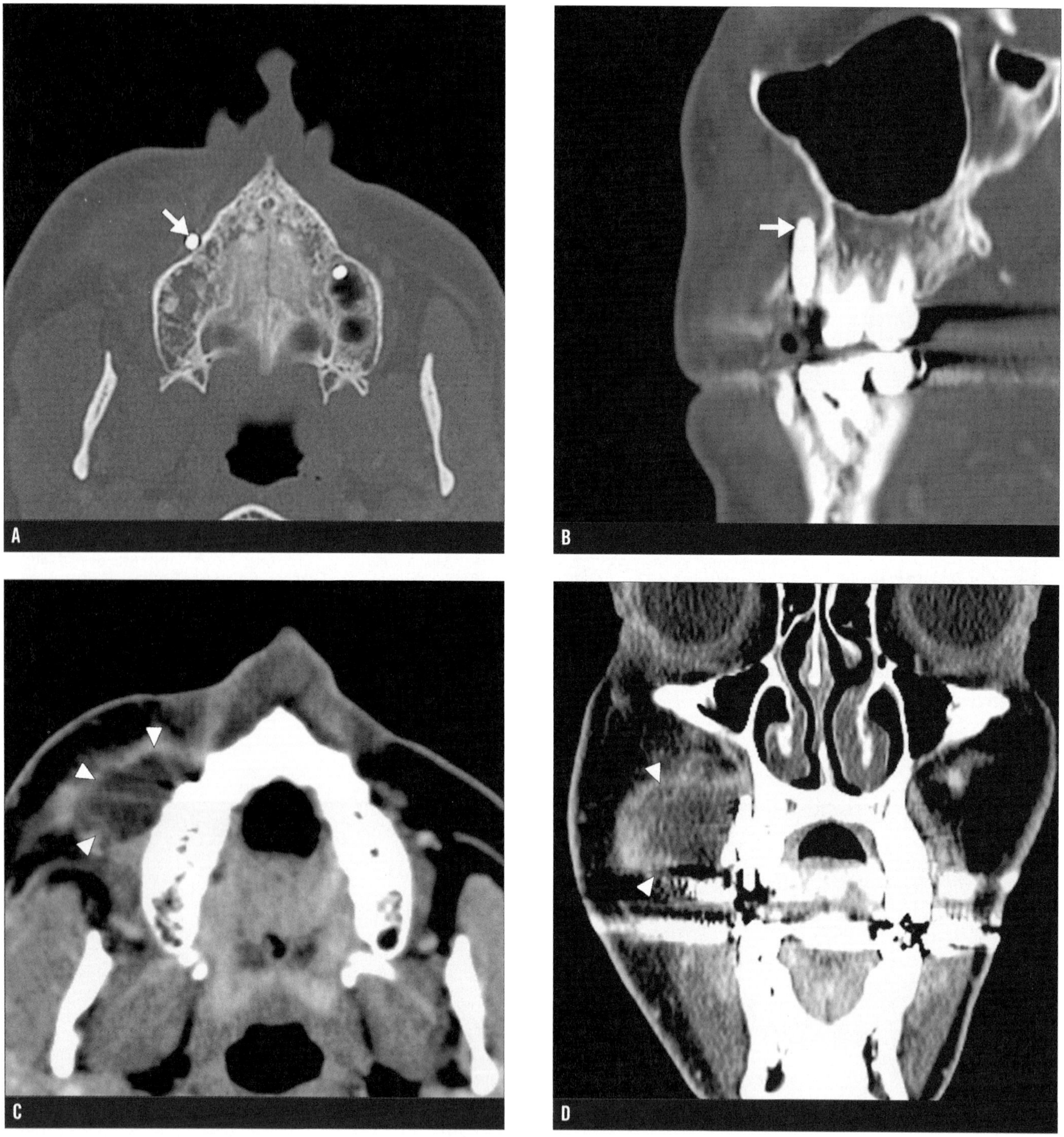

Axial (**A**) and sagittal reformatted (**B**) CT images viewed with a bone window demonstrate the cranial-most portion of a dental implant to protrude outside the confines of the maxillary alveolus and into the perialveolar soft tissues (arrows, **A**, **B**). Postcontrast axial (**C**) and coronal reformatted (**D**) CT images viewed with a soft tissue window demonstrate a mildly peripherally enhancing fluid collection within the right premaxillary soft tissues (arrowheads, **C**, **D**). These findings are consistent with a soft tissue abscess related to an infected dental implant.

Companion case: MRI artifact from dental restoration

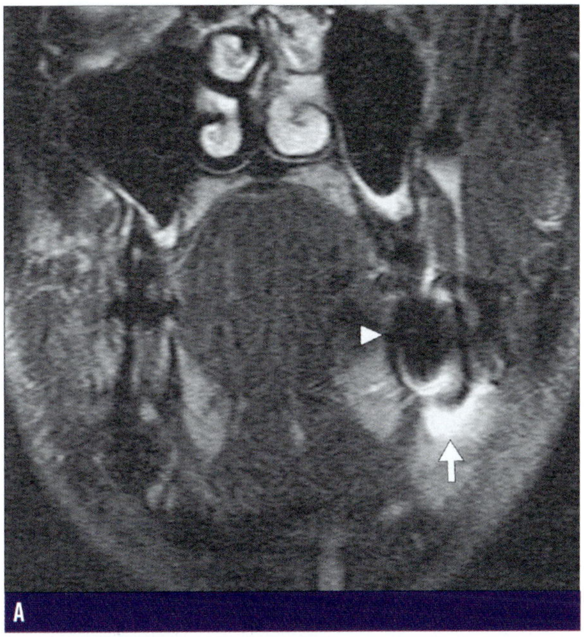

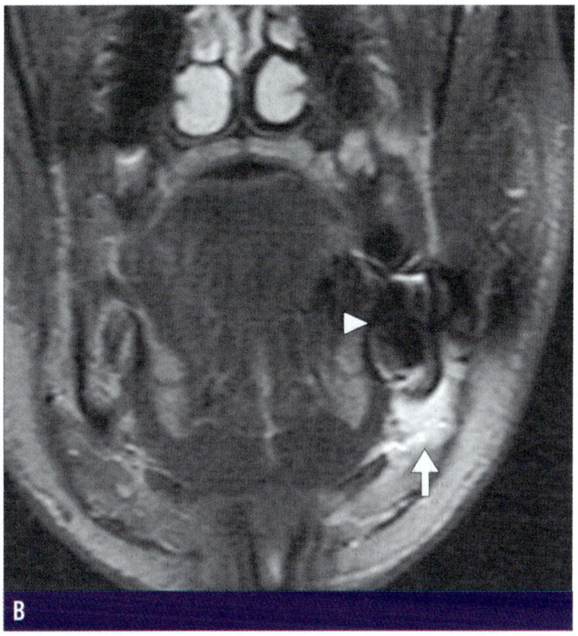

A coronal T2-weighted MR image with fat suppression (**A**) and the same MRI sequence from the same patient 6 months later (**B**) demonstrate stable hypointense signal along the left hemimandibular alveolus (arrowheads, **A**, **B**) and stable associated high T2 signal located primarily caudal to the left hemimandible (arrows, **A**, **B**), both of which are related to a dental restoration. While the elevated T2 signal on image **A** appears similar to edema, the stability of the finding for 6 months essentially confirms that the finding is artifactual. The T2 signal loss is due metal within the dental restoration that leads to local spin–spin dephasing as well as an alteration of the atomic spin frequency within a voxel, such that those protons localize to a different voxel. The elevated T2 signal relates to signal "pile up" that occurs from these displaced protons.

Companion case: MRI artifact from dental braces

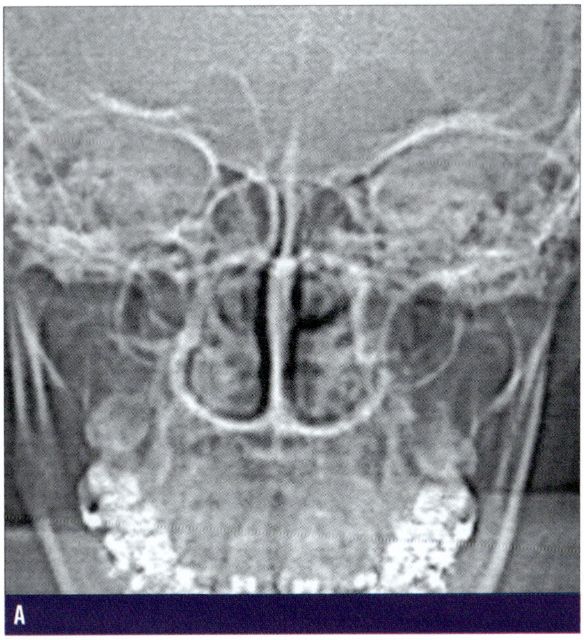

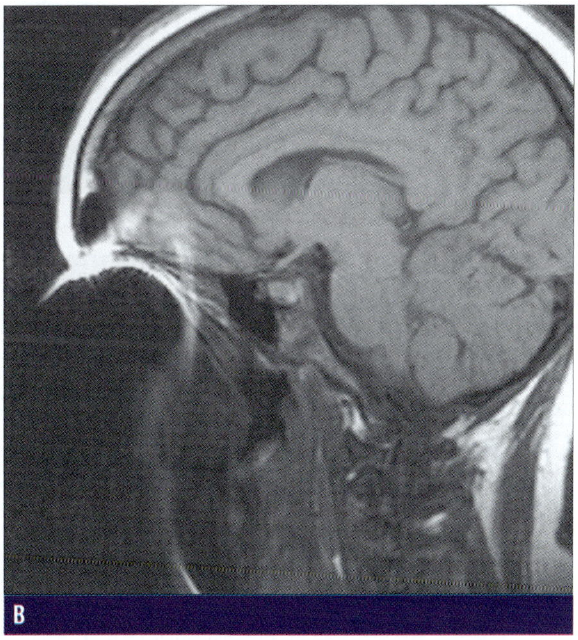

A scout image from a CT examination (**A**) demonstrates partially imaged dental braces. A concurrent sagittal T1-weighted MR image (**B**) demonstrates extensive metallic artifact resulting in nonvisualization of the entire face. A subsequent sagittal T1-weighted MR image performed following removal of the braces (**C**) demonstrates complete resolution of the metallic artifact. Axial T1 (**D**), axial T2 (**E**), axial DWI (**F**), and axial FLAIR (**G**) MR images of the same patient prior to removal of the dental braces also demonstrate extensive artifact. Image **G** demonstrates artifactually increased signal within multiple frontal lobe sulci, simulating an abnormal process in the subarachnoid space. This is due to field distortion and incomplete suppression of CSF from the dental braces. "Marching artifact," frequently identified with dental braces, is also present on image G and overlies temporal lobes, so named because it appears to "march" posteriorly on successive images.

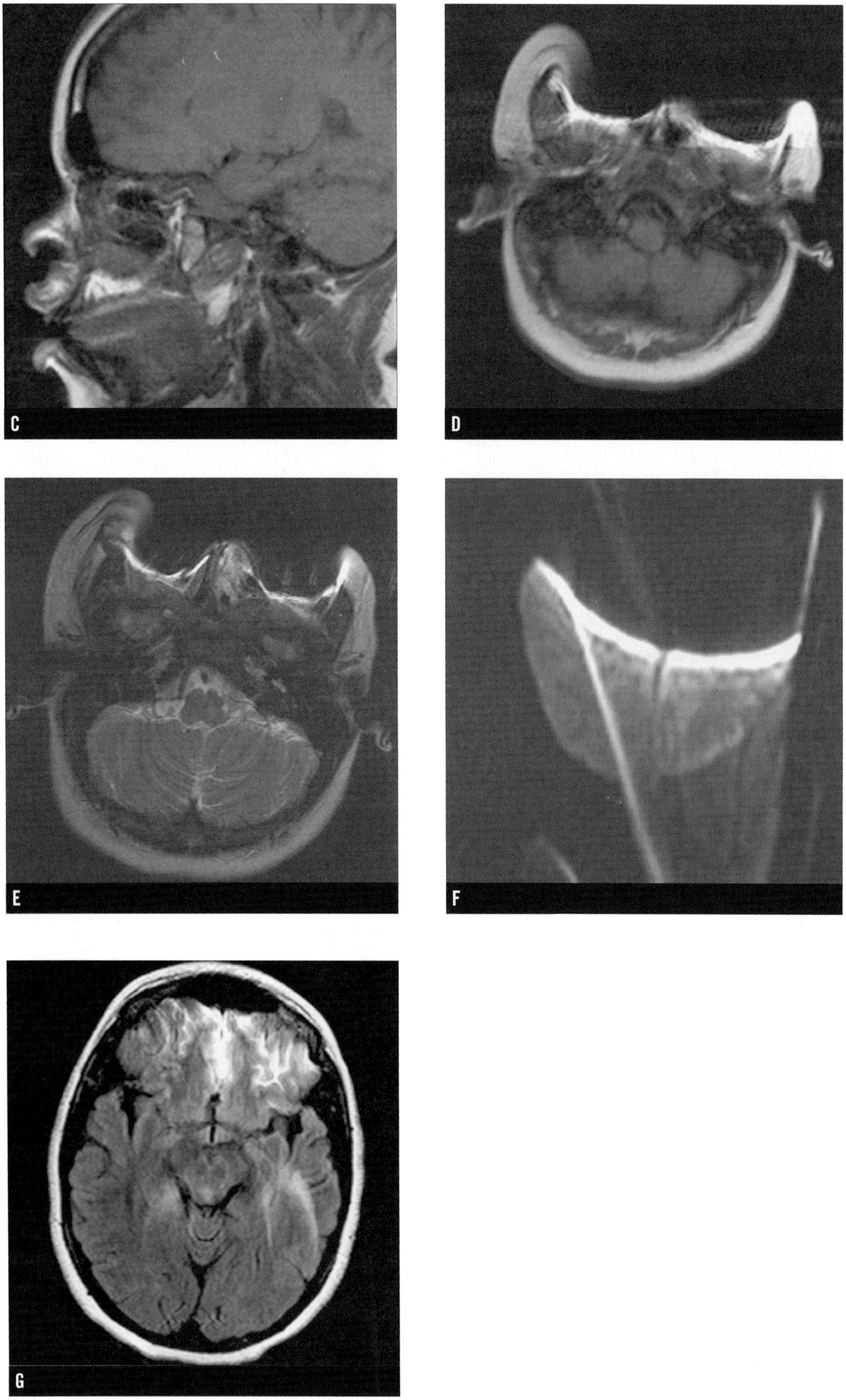
C
D
E
F
G

Companion case: CT streak artifact from normal dental enamel

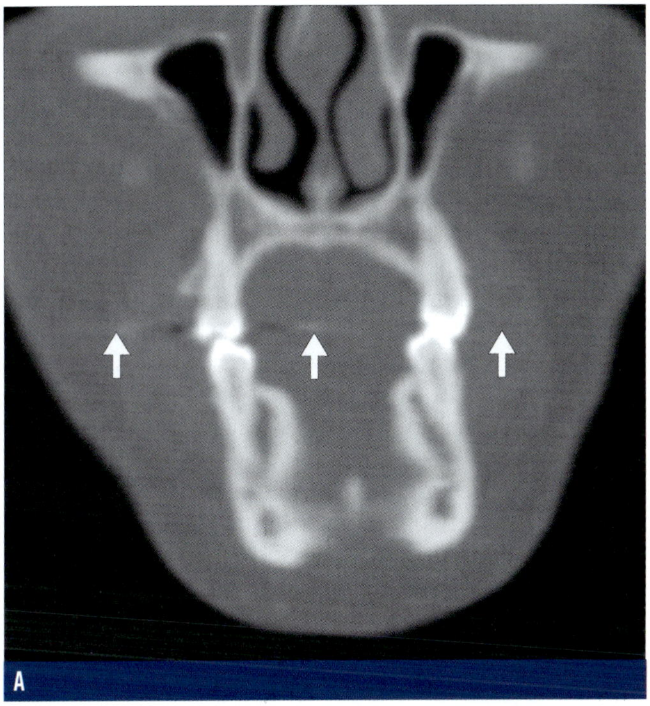

A single coronal reformatted CT image (**A**) demonstrates mild streak artifact from normal dental enamel (arrows).

REFERENCES

Abrahams JJ, Dental CT. Imaging: a look at the jaw. *Radiology.* 2001;219(2):334-345.

Bowen Antolin A, Pascua Garcia MT, Nasimi A. Infections in implantology: from prophylaxis to treatment. *Med Oral Patol Oral Cir Bucal.* 2007;12(4):E323-E330.

DelBalso AM, Greiner FG, Licata M. Role of diagnostic imaging in evaluation of the dental implant patient. *Radiographics.* 1994;14(4):699-719.

Hargreaves BA, et al. Metal-induced artifacts in MRI. *AJR Am J Roentgenol.* 2011;197(3):547-555.

Hunter TB, et al. Medical devices of the head, neck, and spine. *Radiographics.* 2004;24(1):257-285.

Manly RS, Hodge HC, Ange LE. Density and refractive index studies of dental hard tissues: II density distribution curves. *J Dental Res.* 1939;18(3):203-211.

Sconzo, J. The complete mandibular subperiosteal implant: an overview of its evolution. *J Oral Implantol.* 1998;24(1):14-15.

Stuckey SL, Goh TD, Heffernan T, Rowan D. Hyperintensity in the subarachnoid space on FLAIR MRI. *AJR Am J Roentgenol.* 2007;189(4):913-921.

CASE 12 Dentures

Dentures may replace some or all of the teeth in the oral cavity, referred to as partial and complete dentures, respectively. In addition, both partial and complete dentures may be removable or they may be fixed in place.

There are two main components of dentures, the dental base and the denture teeth. The purpose of the dental base is to provide a substrate for the dental teeth, cover the dental alveolus, and to help provide a normal facial contour. The dental base is typically constructed with a polymer resin (ie, polymethyl methacrylate, a form of plastic), metal (such as chromium), or a combination of both. A plastic dental base is most commonly used since it is easily molded and lighter in weight relative to a metallic dental base. A metallic dental base usually provides a more accurate fit for the patient and provides the additional benefit of transferring heat from fluids and foods to the palate, allowing for a more enjoyable eating experience.

Denture teeth are usually composed of either porcelain (a form of ceramic) or acrylic (a plastic). Porcelain dental teeth are usually more aesthetically pleasing and harder than plastic teeth, but they are paradoxically more likely to fracture compared to plastic teeth. Porcelain teeth will also erode opposing natural teeth with repeated contact. In addition, if porcelain teeth articulate with one another, they may result in an undesirable clicking sound during contact. Relative to porcelain denture teeth, plastic denture teeth are softer, easier to adjust, less likely to fracture, and do not erode natural teeth upon contact.

Plastic denture teeth readily bond chemically with a plastic denture base and give rise to a plastic tooth-plastic base denture combination. However, anteriorly placed porcelain denture teeth are affixed to the plastic denture base with metallic retentive pins. Posteriorly placed porcelain denture teeth are only placed when they oppose other denture teeth (either porcelain or plastic) and are usually affixed by acrylic resin to the plastic denture base. The acrylic resin extends into and fuses with small holes that are constructed along the gingival surface of the porcelain teeth, termed diatoric retentive holes.

With a well-seated plastic denture base, a thin layer of saliva provides enough traction to maintain an adequate seal between the denture base and the mucosa along the alveolar ridge and hard palate. However, over time, gaps between a plastic denture base and the mucosal surface may develop, often resulting in instability of the denture. The best method to correct this scenario is by adding a thin layer of plastic to a plastic denture base by a process termed relining. If this option is not used, numerous over the counter denture adhesive products are available in the form of a paste, powder, or adhesive strips.

Plastic denture base and porcelain teeth

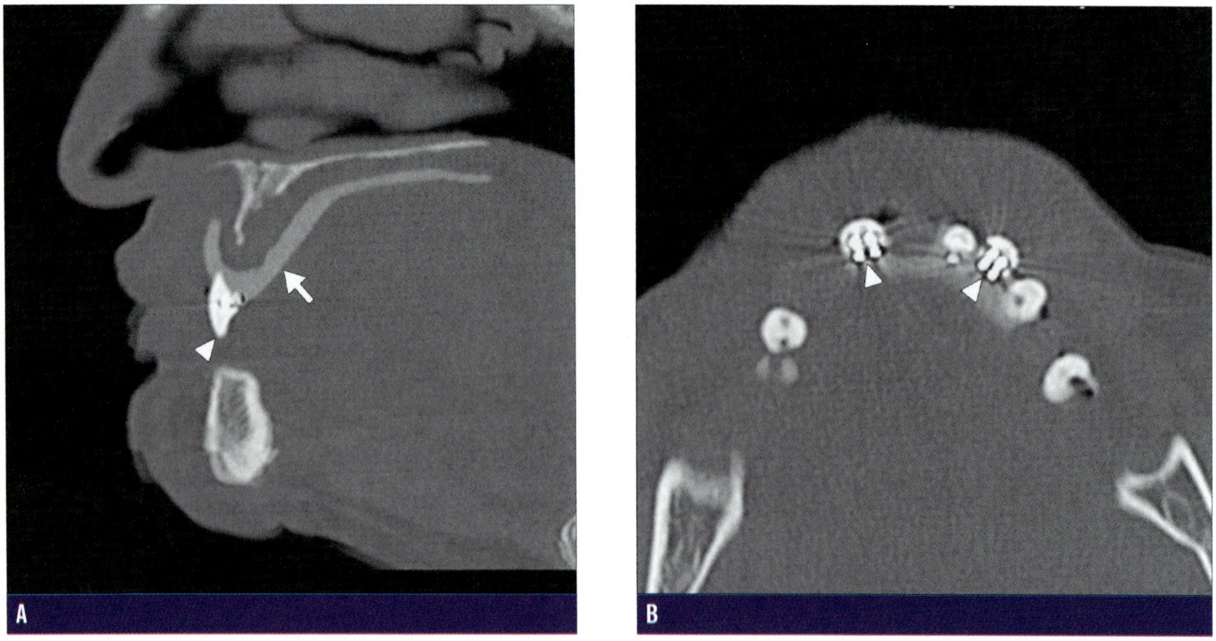

A sagittal reformatted CT image (**A**) demonstrates a removable denture along the maxilla. The linear, mildly high-density structure conforming to the hard palate and maxillary alveolus represents the denture base (arrow, **A**), whereas the arrowhead on image **A** denotes one of the denture teeth. The denture base is constructed of plastic. The tooth density is between that of metal and plastic; thus, it is most consistent with a porcelain tooth. An axial CT image of the same patient (**B**) confirms that the teeth are made of porcelain, as evidenced by the presence of retentive pins affixing the teeth to the plastic denture base (arrowheads, **B**).

Plastic denture base and porcelain teeth

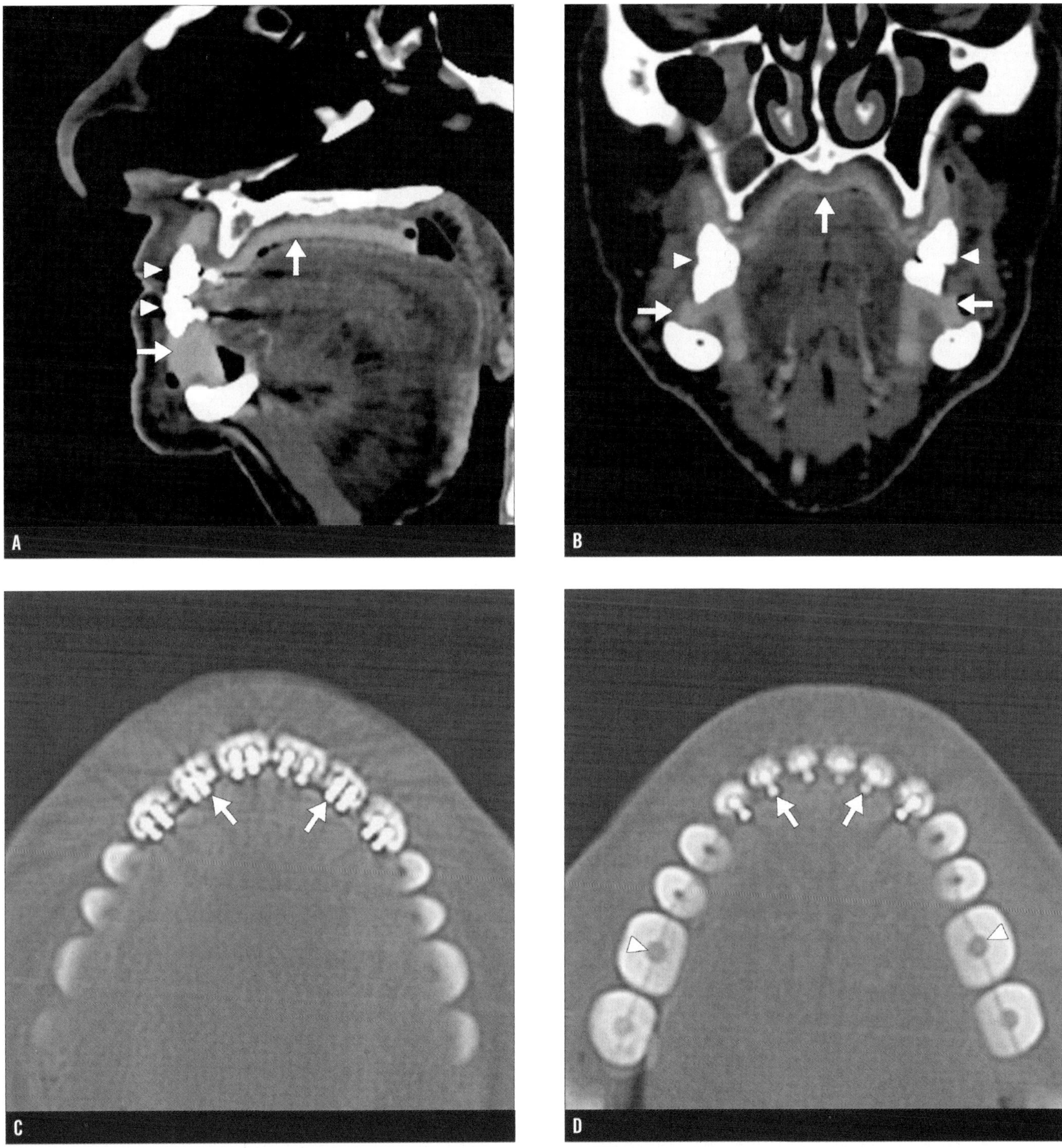

Different patient. Sagittal reformatted (**A**) and coronal reformatted (**B**) CT images viewed with a soft tissue window demonstrate plastic denture bases (arrows, **A**, **B**) and denture teeth (arrowheads, **A**, **B**) along the maxilla and mandible. Axial CT images viewed with a bone window (**C**, **D**) demonstrate the bilateral medial and lateral incisors as well as the bilateral canine denture teeth to contain retentive pins (arrows, **C**, **D**), which affix these teeth to the plastic denture base. Holes within the premolar and molar teeth (a couple annotated by arrowheads, **D**) represent diatoric retentive holes. Acrylic resin is placed into, and fuses with, the diatoric retentive holes as well as with the dental base, thereby fixating these molar and premolar teeth to the dental base. These represent porcelain teeth, given their density as well as the presence of retentive pin fixation and diatoric retentive holes.

Metallic-plastic combination dental base

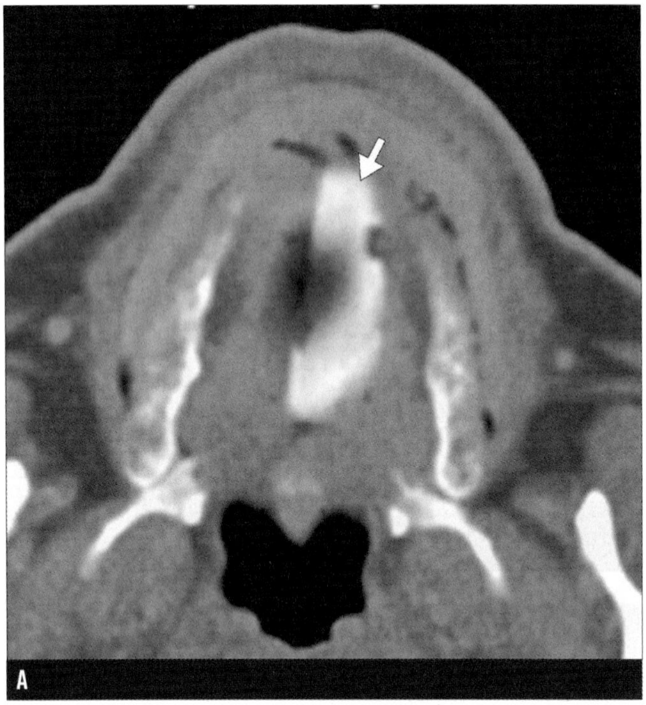

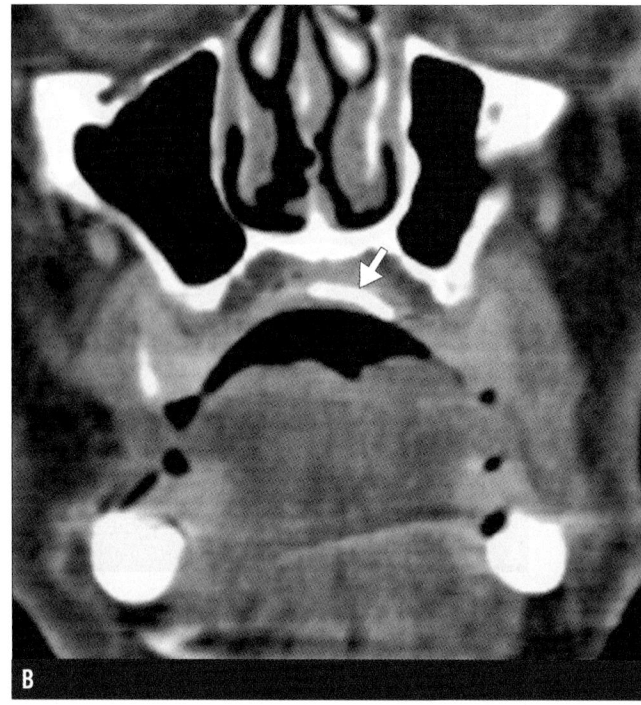

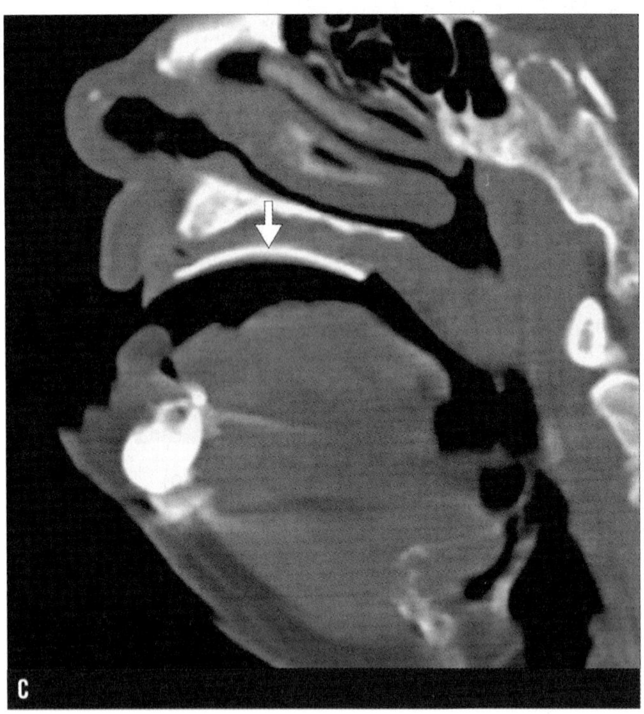

Axial (**A**), coronal reformatted (**B**), and sagittal reformatted (**C**) CT images demonstrate a thin, rectangular, high-density structure located within the left paramedian aspect of a maxillary denture dental base (arrows, **A-C**). This is consistent with metal that was used to construct a metallic-plastic combination dental base.

REFERENCES

Beaumont AJ. An overview of esthetics with removable partial dentures. *Quintessence Intl.* 2002;33(10):747-755.

Haidary A, Leider JS, Silbergleit R. Unsuspected swallowing of a partial denture. *AJNR Am J Neuroradiol.* 2007;28(9):1734-1735.

McCord JF, Grey NJ, Winstanley RB, Johnson A. A clinical overview of removable prostheses: I. Factors to consider in planning a removable partial denture. *Dent Update.* 2002;29(8):376-381.

Mericske-Stern RD, Taylor TD, Beiser U. Management of the edentulous patient. *Clin Oral Implants Res.* 2000;11(1):108-125.

Nallaswamy D. *Textbook of Prosthodontics.* Jaypee Brothers Publishers, 2008.

Rahn AO, Ivanhoe JR, Plummer KD. *Textbook of Complete Dentures.* 6th ed. People's Medical Publishing House, USA.

Zhao K, et al. Laboratory evaluation of a new denture adhesive. *Dent Mater.* 2004;20(5):419-424.

CASE 13 Macroglossia related to an edentulous state

Macroglossia can be congenital or acquired. One of the acquired forms of macroglossia may be identified in a chronically edentulous patient. Mastication is the primary role of the teeth, which function to crush and grind food, thereby increasing the surface area of food so that it is more amenable to degradation by enzymes. However, without teeth, the tongue plays a greater role in the breakdown of food, sometimes resulting in compensatory tongue hypertrophy and macroglossia. Macroglossia related to an edentulous state may regress if the patient is able to wear dentures.

Macroglossia may also result from numerous other causes, including secondary to angioedema, glossitis, venous and/or lymphatic malformations, various benign and malignant tumors, acromegaly, amyloidosis, and Beckwith-Wiedemann syndrome, among others. Reports of acute and life-threatening acquired macroglossia following oral cavity/oropharynx surgery, posterior fossa surgery, and immediately following extubation have also been reported.

No discrete size calculation defines macroglossia. Instead, the diagnosis and treatment of this condition are guided by clinical factors, including the presence of airway compromise, sleep apnea, dental malocclusion, and difficulties with swallowing or speaking.

COMPANION CASES

- **Angioedema-induced macroglossia.** Angioedema may be allergic or nonallergic in etiology. It is an edema that can affect numerous sites, including various portions of the head and neck, extremities, viscera, and genitalia. When involving the head and neck, life-threatening airway compromise may occur that necessitates emergent securing of the airway. Numerous medications have been implicated in causing angioedema, with angiotensin-converting enzyme (ACE) inhibitors the most common culprit, estimated to be responsible for 30% to 40% of all cases of angioedema in the United States emergency departments.
- **Vascular malformation of the tongue.** Vascular malformations are generally subdivided into low-flow lesions (ie, venous malformation, lymphatic malformation, and mixed malformation) and high flow lesions, such as an arteriovenous malformation (AVM). Properly categorizing these lesions is important in order to determine appropriate treatment. Most vascular malformations are present at birth, although some lesions, such as an AVM, may result from trauma.

  Venous malformations (VM) are essentially an abnormal collection of venous channels, fat, and degenerated muscle matrix. The venous components in a VM can thrombose and form phleboliths, the latter considered pathognomonic of this entity in the appropriate context. Lymphatic malformations (LM) represent an abnormal collection of lymphatic vessels. LMs are subcategorized into macrocystic and microcystic forms. The macrocystic form, commonly referred to as a cystic hygroma, is composed of large cystic spaces containing proteinaceous fluid and lymphocytes that are interspersed around septa. The microcystic form contains 2 mm or smaller sized cysts within a solid matrix. A mixed lesion refers to a low flow vascular lesion that contains both venous and lymphatic components (also called venolymphatic malformation).

  The hallmark of a vascular malformation is its transpatial nature (ie, often involving more than one compartment in the neck) and softness to palpation. A vascular malformation may or may not be associated with mass effect. On MRI, both a VM and a macrocystic LM will be hyperintense on T2. Following contrast, a VM will contain patchy enhancement throughout the lesion whereas a macrocystic LM will only enhance along its periphery and/or along its septa. When a hemorrhagic fluid level within a loculated fluid collection is associated with abrupt clinical enlargement, then the diagnosis of a macrocystic LM should be suspected. MRI is usually superior to CT at evaluating vascular malformations of the head and neck.
- **Squamous cell carcinoma of the tongue.** Similar to other regions of the head and neck, the most common malignant tumor affecting the tongue is squamous cell carcinoma (SCC), followed by a variety of tumors arising from the minor salivary glands. When examining the tongue on imaging, it is important to evaluate for distortion of the intrinsic and extrinsic tongue muscles (in particular the fat within the substance and between these muscles) as well as the lingual septum. The lingual septum is a fibrofatty structure that is present along the midline of the tongue and divides the tongue into two halves. If the normal appearance of any of these structures is disrupted, the tongue should be closely scrutinized for a pathologic process. On imaging, the appearance of SCC may range from a small enhancing mass to a large infiltrating tumor with regions of necrosis and adjacent mandibular erosion/destruction. A SCC of the tongue is typically iso- to hypointense on T1-weighted images, iso- to hyperintense on T2-weighted images, and enhances. Imaging findings of necrosis may be evident, particularly when the tumor is large.

Macroglossia related to an edentulous state

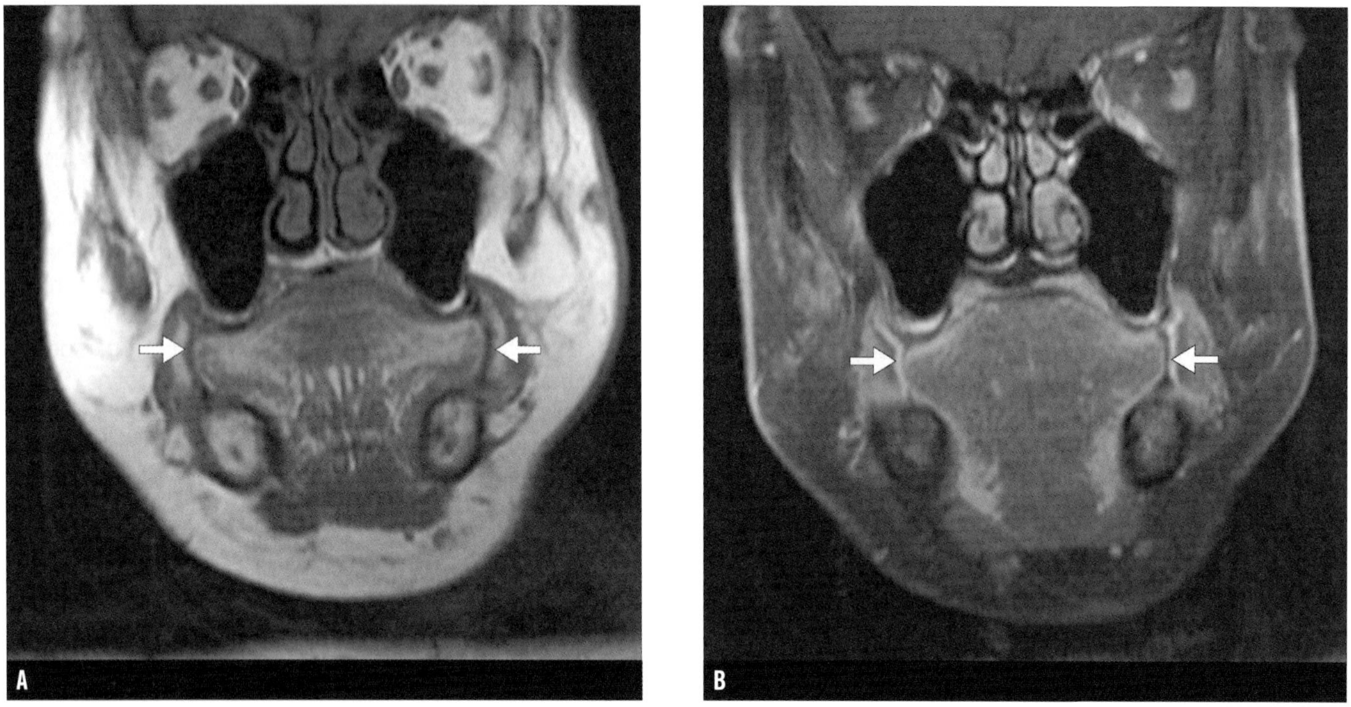

Coronal T1 (**A**) and postcontrast coronal T1 with fat suppression (**B**) MR images in an edentulous patient demonstrate diffuse enlargement of the tongue that extends lateral to bilateral alveolar ridges, suggestive of macroglossia (arrows, **A**, **B**).

Companion case: Angioedema-induced macroglossia

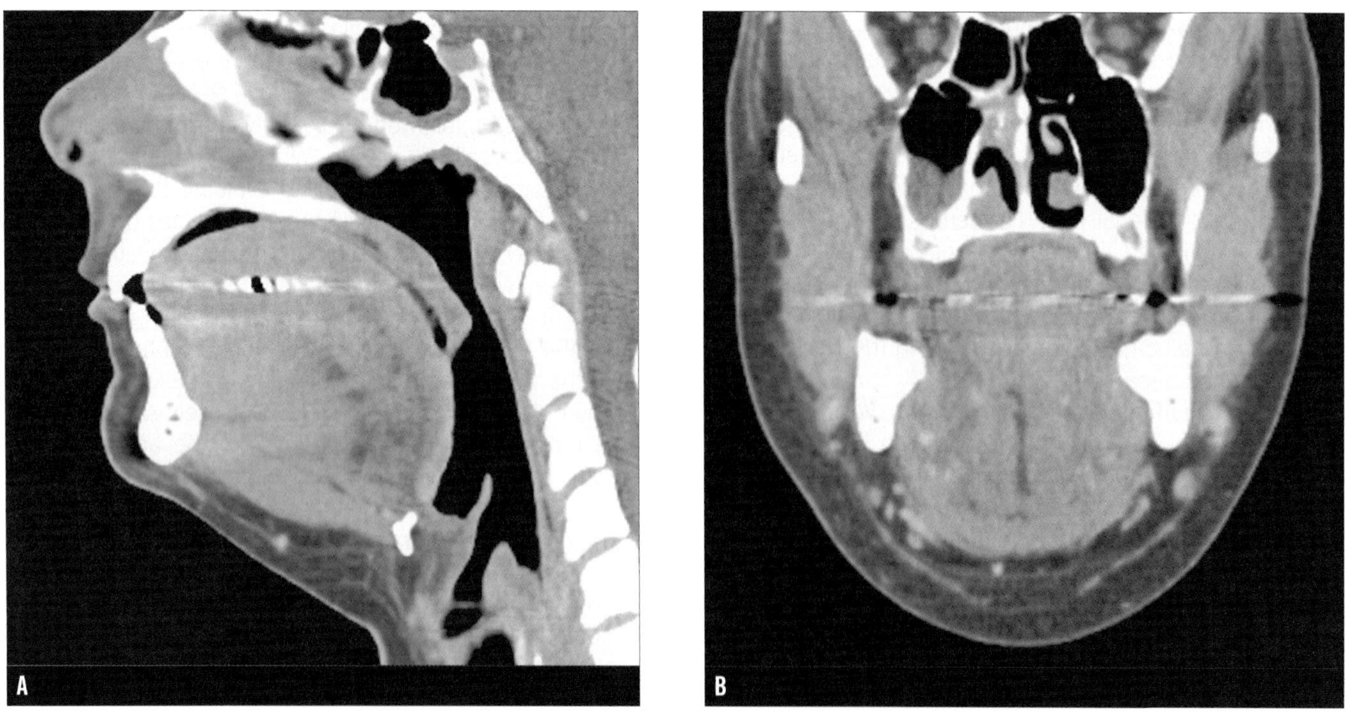

Sagittal reformatted (**A**) and coronal reformatted (**B**) contrast-enhanced CT images demonstrate diffuse prominence of the tongue without focal imaging findings. This patient had abrupt onset of marked macroglossia and facial edema clinically. After a complete workup, the macroglossia and facial edema was deemed the result of idiopathic angioedema, and completely resolved after steroids were administered to the patient.

Companion case: Vascular malformation of the tongue

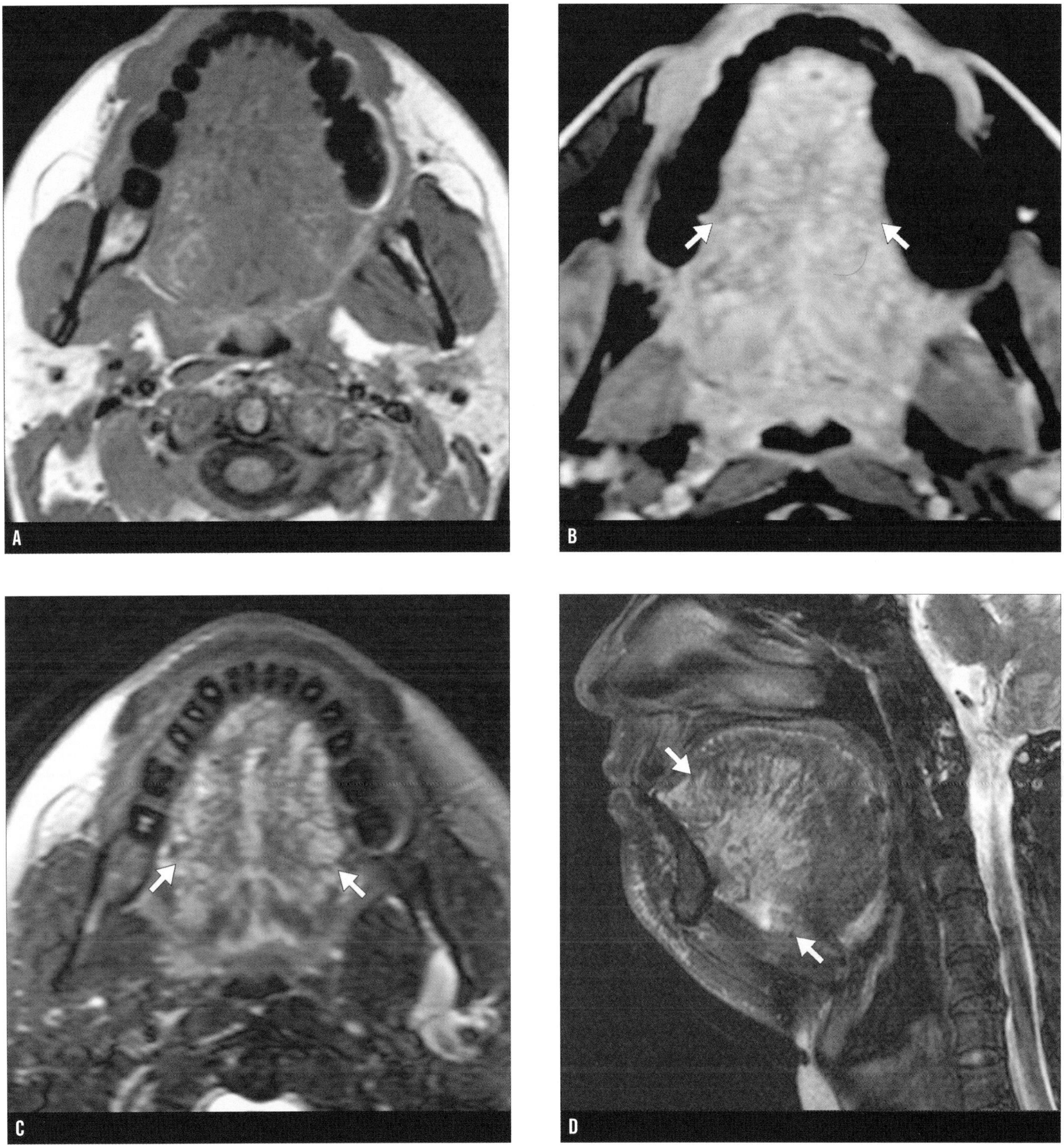

Axial T1 (**A**), postcontrast axial T1 with fat suppression (**B**), axial T2 with fat suppression (**C**), and sagittal T2 with fat suppression (**D**) MR images. Image **A** is unremarkable. However, image **B** demonstrates diffuse abnormal enhancement (arrows, **B**), whereas images **C** and **D** demonstrate heterogeneous increased T2 signal within a significant portion of the tongue (arrows, **C**, **D**). The findings, while nonspecific, represented a vascular malformation of the tongue in this patient with a history of macroglossia that was soft to palpation.

Companion case: Squamous cell carcinoma of the tongue

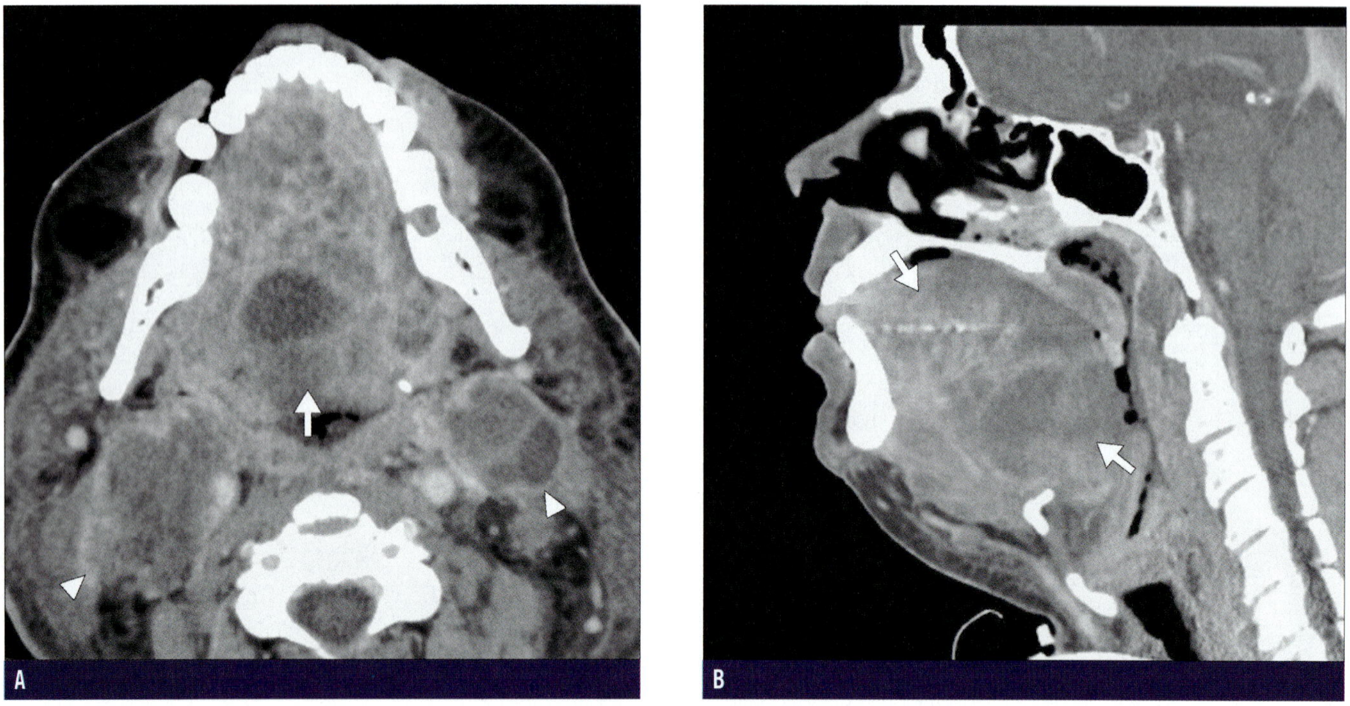

Axial (**A**) and sagittal reformatted (**B**) contrast-enhanced CT images demonstrate a diffusely enlarged tongue that is heterogeneous and contains multiple regions of low attenuation, compatible with areas of necrosis (arrows, **A**, **B**). Necrotic, bilateral level II lymph nodes are also present (arrowheads, **A**). This tongue lesion represented squamous cell carcinoma at pathology.

REFERENCES

Beil CM, Keberle M. Oral and oropharyngeal tumors. *Euro J Radiol.* 2008;66(3):448-459.

Chernoff R. Geriatric Nutrition: The Health Professional's Handbook. Sudbury, MA: Jones & Bartlett Learning; 2006.

El Hassani Y, Narata AP, Pereira VM, Schaller C. A reminder for a very rare entity: massive tongue swelling after posterior fossa surgery. *J Neurol Surg A Cent Eur Neurosurg.* 2012;73(3):171-174. Epub May 9, 2012.

Junghaenel S, et al. Massive macroglossia after palatoplasty: case report and review of the literature. *Eur J Pediatr.* 2012;171(3):433-437.

Lewis LM. Angioedema: etiology, pathophysiology, current and emerging therapies. *J Emerg Med.* 2013 45(5):789-796.

Perkins JA. Overview of macroglossia and its treatment. *Curr Opin Otolaryngol Head Neck Surg.* 2009;17(6):460-465.

Toyama S, Hoya K, Matsuoka K, Numai T, Shimoyama M. Massive macroglossia developing fast and immediately after endotracheal extubation. *Acta Anaesthesiol Scand.* 2012;56(2):256-259. doi: 10.1111/j.1399-6576.2011.02575.x. Epub November 21, 2011.

Wolford LM, Cottrell DA. Diagnosis of macroglossia and indications for reduction glossectomy. *Am J Orthod Dentofacial Orthop.* 1996;110(2):170-177.

CASE 14 Denervation atrophy of the tongue

The hypoglossal nerve innervates both the intrinsic muscles of the tongue (those muscles that lie entirely within the tongue) as well as four paired extrinsic tongue muscles (those muscles that attach the tongue to another structure). The extrinsic tongue muscles are the genioglossus, hyoglossus, styloglossus, and palatoglossus muscles. The hypoglossal nerve exits the preolivary sulcus of the medulla via multiple rootlets, traverses the premedullary cistern and enters the hypoglossal canal. After exiting the hypoglossal canal, the nerve travels caudally within the carotid space to the level of the hyoid bone, at which point the nerve turns slightly cranially and courses anteriorly in the sublingual space. A pathologic process that occurs along any portion of the course of this nerve may result in nerve dysfunction and denervation atrophy of the tongue. A unilateral tongue denervation atrophy will respect the midline and will usually involve the majority, if not all, of the oral hemitongue.

On CT, denervation injury is most commonly identified in the chronic stage, when the affected muscles undergo fatty atrophy and volume loss. In the setting of chronic tongue denervation atrophy, the affected side of the tongue base may partially prolapse posteriorly into the oropharynx due to loss of the normal anterior tongue traction provided by the tongue muscles. A prolapsed tongue following denervation atrophy may simulate a mass at the base of the tongue on imaging. On MRI, denervation injury has different appearances depending upon the phase of the denervation injury. In the acute/subacute phase, the involved muscle will be edematous and thus iso- to hypointense signal on T1, hyperintense signal on T2, and usually enhance. Care should be taken not to misinterpret the enhancement that occurs during this phase as tumor or infection. In the chronic phase, the affected tongue on MRI will contain intrinsic hyperintense T1 signal related to fatty infiltration and have associated volume loss.

COMPANION CASES

- **Squamous cell carcinoma of the oral tongue.** Squamous cell carcinoma (SCC) of the oral tongue usually enhances and may only involve one half of the tongue, similar to acute denervation atrophy. However, a SCC does not typically involve and conform to the entire affected hemitongue, as is often present with acute denervation atrophy. In addition, a SCC of the oral tongue may breach the midline lingual septum, a finding that is not present with acute unilateral tongue denervation.
- **Squamous cell carcinoma of the tongue base.** A SCC of the tongue base is considered a tumor of the oropharynx. This tumor may may prolapse into the oropharyngeal airway in a similar fashion to what is seen with chronic denervation atrophy of the tongue. However, the tongue with chronic denervation atrophy is usually fatty infiltrated and nonenhancing, as opposed to a SCC which enhances on CT and usually iso- to hypointense on T1-weighted imaging iso- to hyperintense on T2-weighted imaging, and enhances on MRI following contrast administration.

Chronic denervation atrophy of the tongue

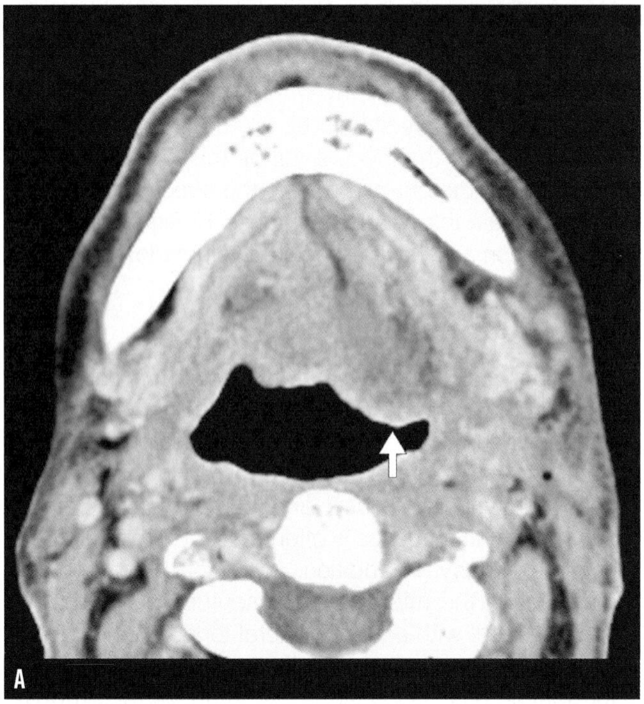

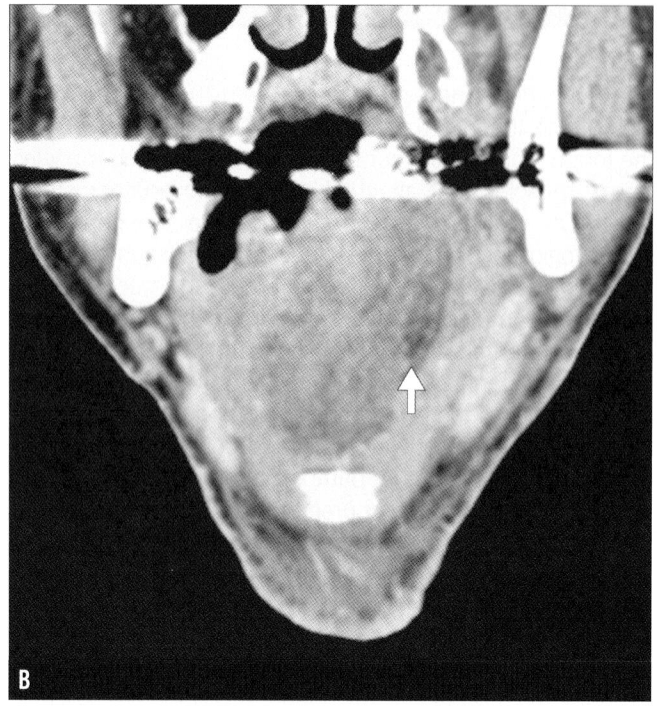

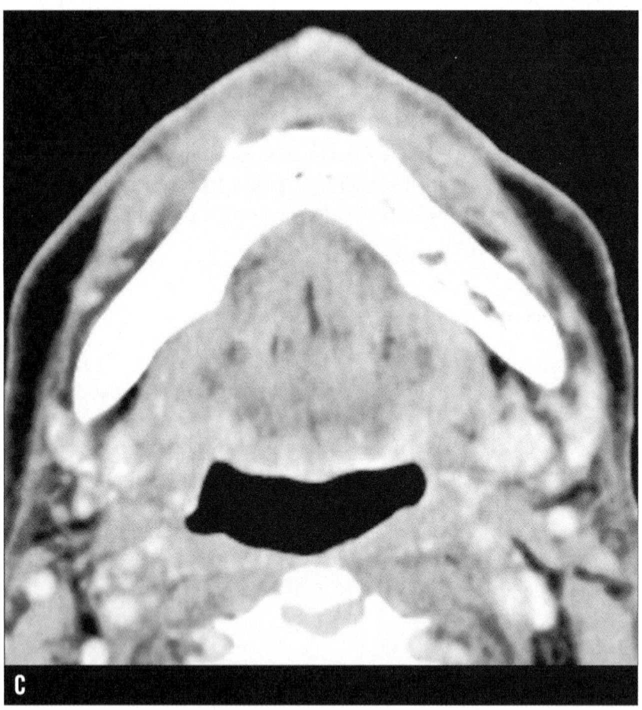

This patient had a history of a prior left neck tumor resection and radiation for metastatic squamous cell carcinoma related to an unknown primary. Postcontrast axial (**A**) and coronal reformatted (**B**) CT images demonstrate fatty infiltration of the left hemi-tongue (arrow, **B**) with partial prolapse of the left tongue base into the oropharynx (arrow, **A**), compatible with chronic denervation atrophy of the tongue. A postcontrast axial CT image of the same patient prior to surgery and radiation (**C**) demonstrates a normal appearance of the tongue.

Chronic denervation atrophy of the tongue

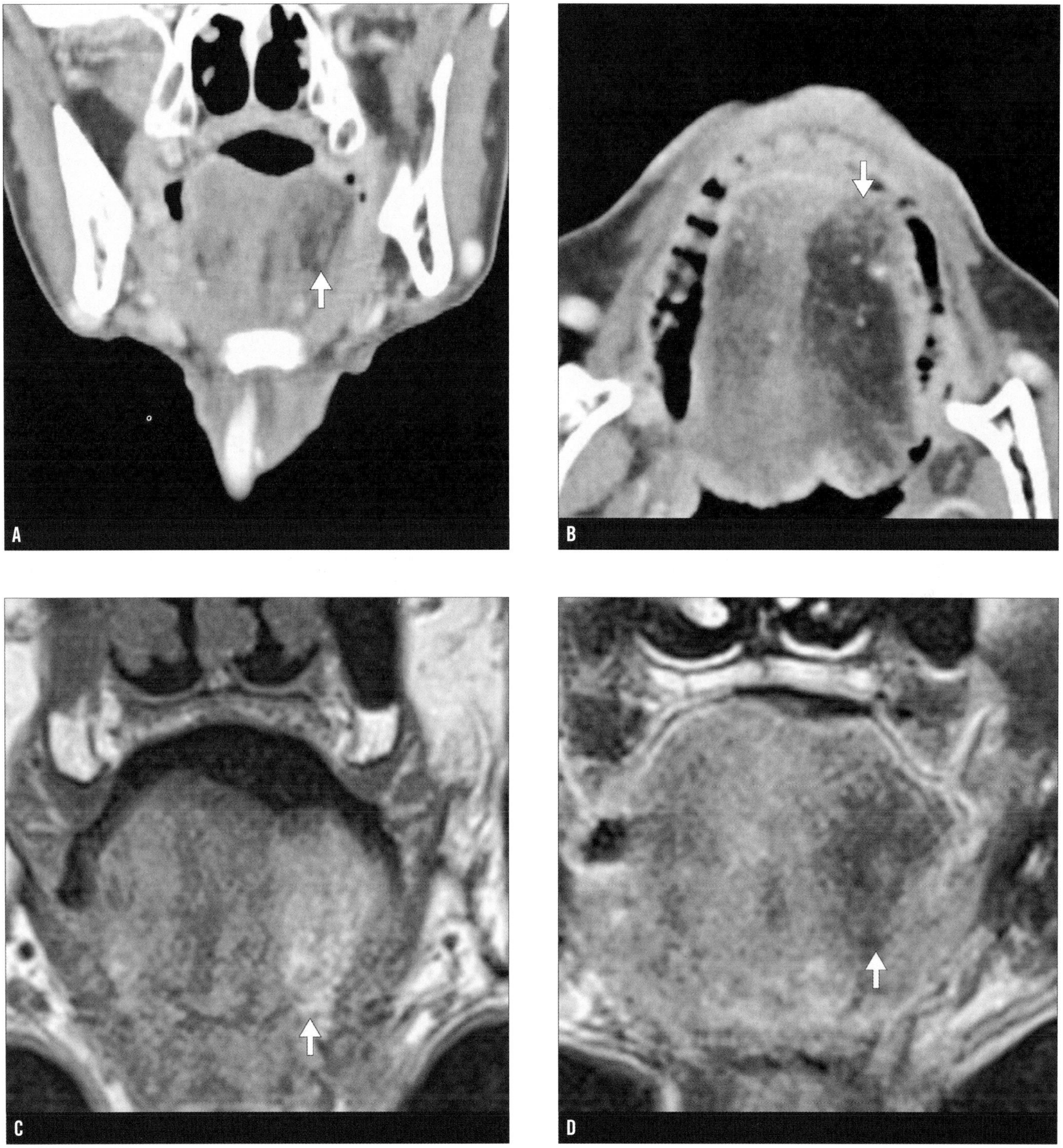

Different patient. Coronal reformatted (**A**) and axial (**B**) contrast-enhanced CT images viewed with a soft tissue window demonstrate asymmetric fatty infiltration of the left hemitongue, compatible with chronic left hemitongue denervation atrophy (arrows, **A**, **B**). Unenhanced coronal T1 without fat suppression (**C**) and contrast-enhanced coronal T1 with fat suppression (**D**) MR images demonstrate hyperintense T1 signal in the left hemitongue on image **C** (arrow, **C**) that fully suppresses on image **D** (arrow, **D**), also consistent with left hemitongue denervation atrophy. An unenhanced axial T1-weighted MR image through the jugular foramina (**E**) demonstrates an isointense (to muscle) lesion in the left jugular foramen (arrow, **E**). Fat-suppressed, contrast-enhanced axial T1-weighted MR images through the jugular foramina (**F**) and hypoglossal canals (**G**) demonstrate an enhancing lesion in the left jugular foramen (arrow, **F**) that also involves the left hypoglossal canal (arrow, **G**). The mass contains hypointense foci, suggestive of flow voids. A magnified axial CT image of the left jugular foramen viewed with a bone window (**H**) demonstrates irregular/erosive osseous margins (arrow, **H**). The findings at the skull base are consistent with a glomus jugulare tumor that also affects the left hypoglossal canal and nerve, which resulted in the chronic left hemitongue denervation atrophy. This patient also had multiple other locations of chronic denervation atrophy (associated with left CN X and XI), which are not shown.

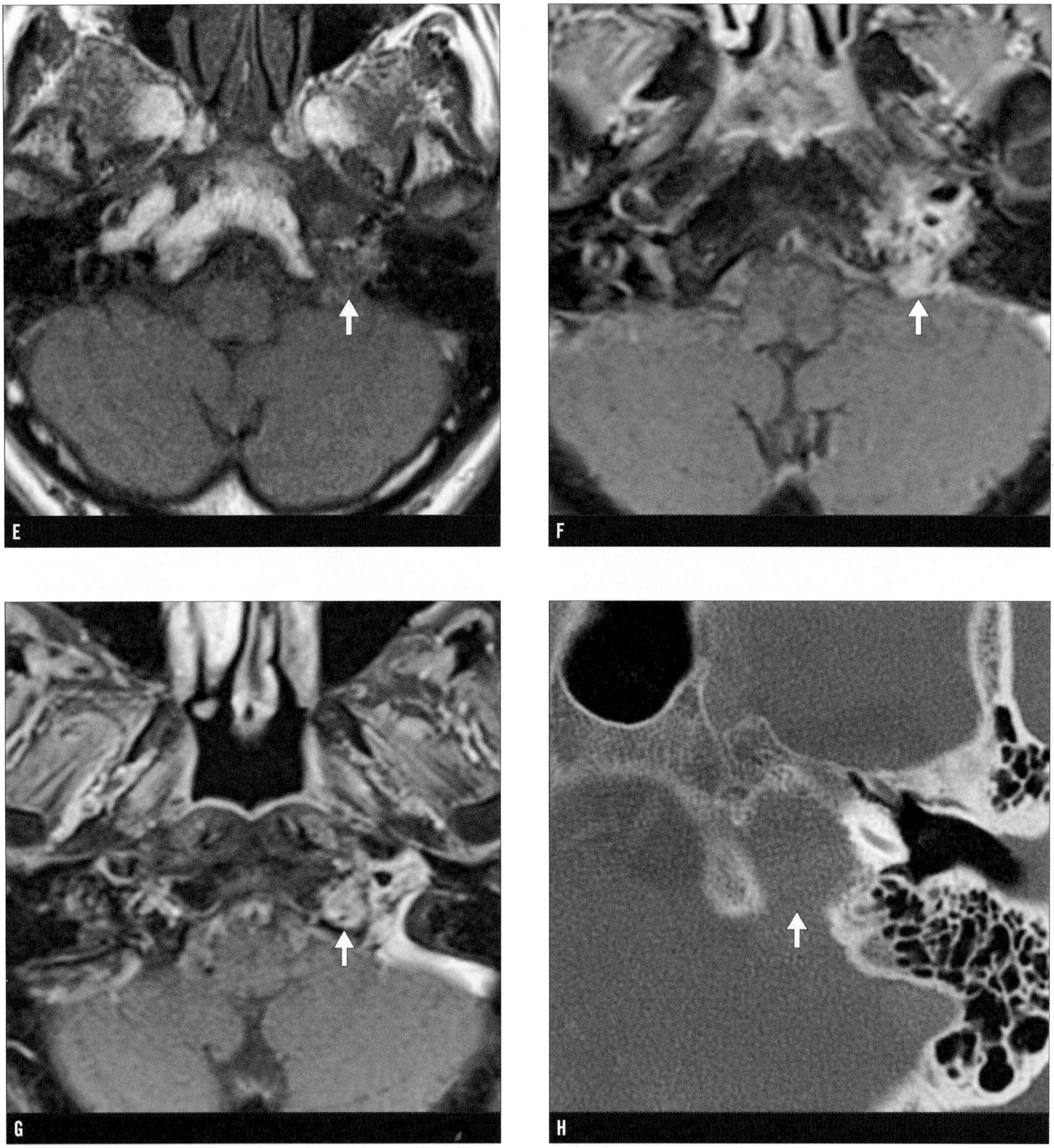
E
F
G
H

Acute denervation atrophy of the tongue

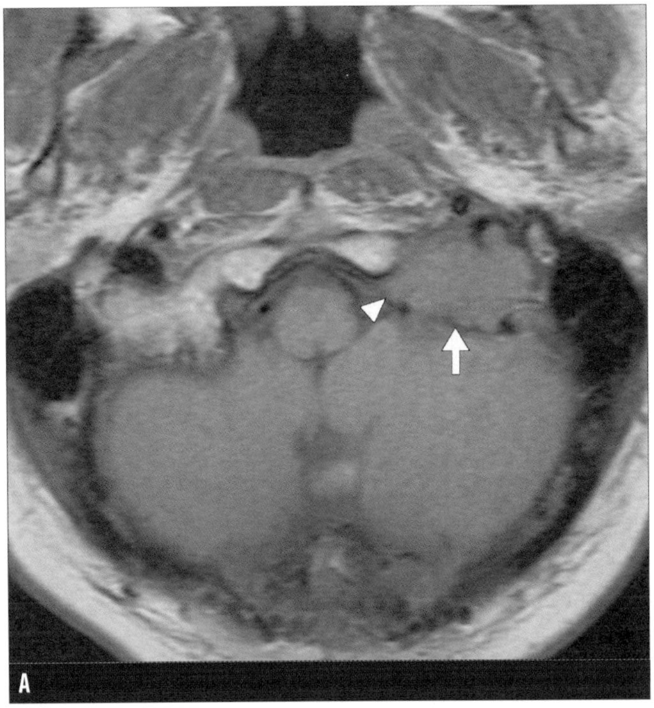

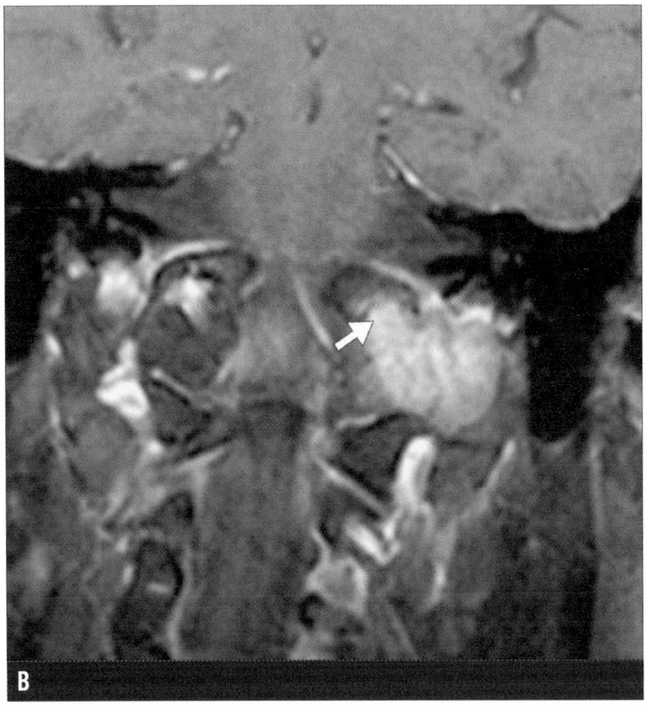

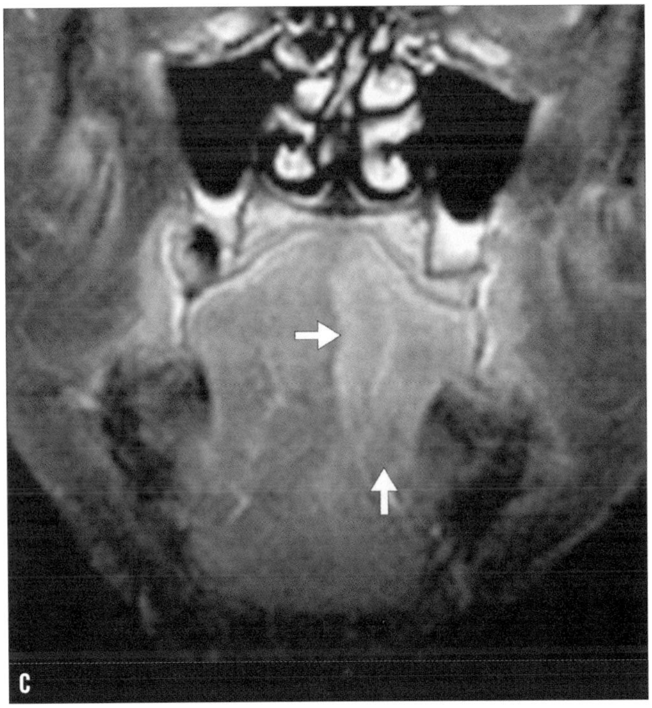

An axial T1-weighted MR image through the level of the hypoglossal canals (**A**) as well as fat-suppressed, postcontrast coronal T1-weighted MR images through the hypoglossal canals (**B**) and through the oral tongue (**C**) in a patient with small cell lung cancer and known metastatic disease. Image **A** demonstrates a mass at the left basiocciput (arrow, **A**) that involves the left hypoglossal canal (arrowhead, **A**). Image **B** demonstrates the mass to abnormally enhance and also demonstrates involvement of the left hypoglossal canal (arrow, **B**). Image **C** demonstrates robust enhancement of the left hemitongue (arrows, **C**) (relative to unenhanced T1-weighted imaging which is not shown). The constellation of findings is compatible with acute denervation atrophy of the tongue secondary to a metastatic lesion involving the left hypoglossal canal. The tongue enhancement in this setting can simulate a primary tumor of the tongue. A lesion involving the ipsilateral hypoglossal canal should be excluded in the setting of hemitongue enhancement or hemitongue atrophy, which may be the result of acute and chronic denervation atrophy, respectively.

Companion case: Squamous cell carcinoma of the oral tongue

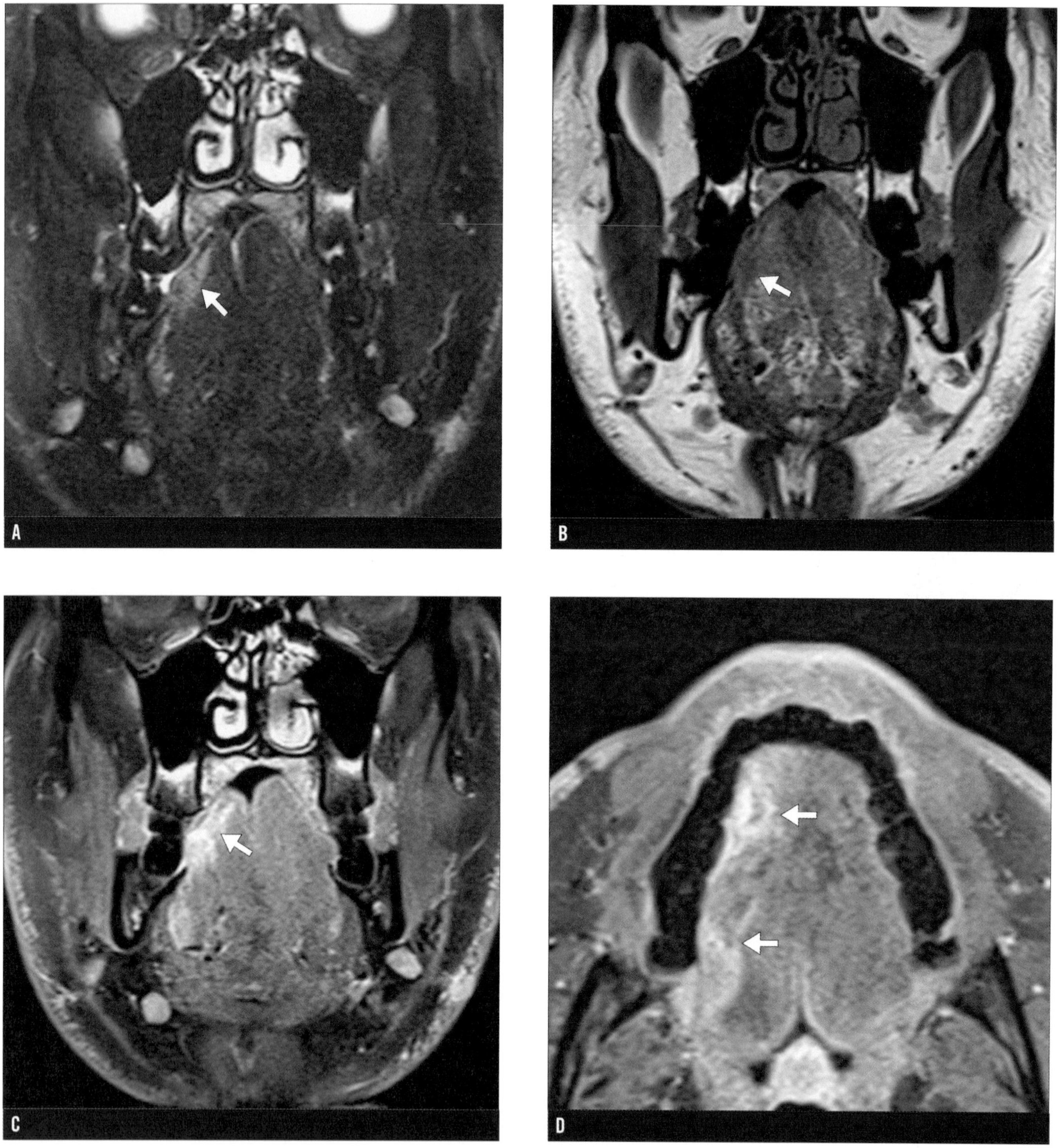

Coronal T2 with fat suppression (**A**), coronal T1 (**B**), postcontrast coronal T1 with fat suppression (**C**), and postcontrast axial T1 with fat suppression (**D**) MR images demonstrate a focal T2 hyperintense (arrow, **A**), subtly T1 hypointense (arrow, **B**), enhancing (arrows, **C**, **D**) lesion in the right hemitongue. This lesion involves a relatively small portion of the right hemitongue, in contradistinction to the signal abnormality related to denervation atrophy, which usually involves the entire hemitongue on the affected side.

Companion case: Squamous cell carcinoma of the tongue base

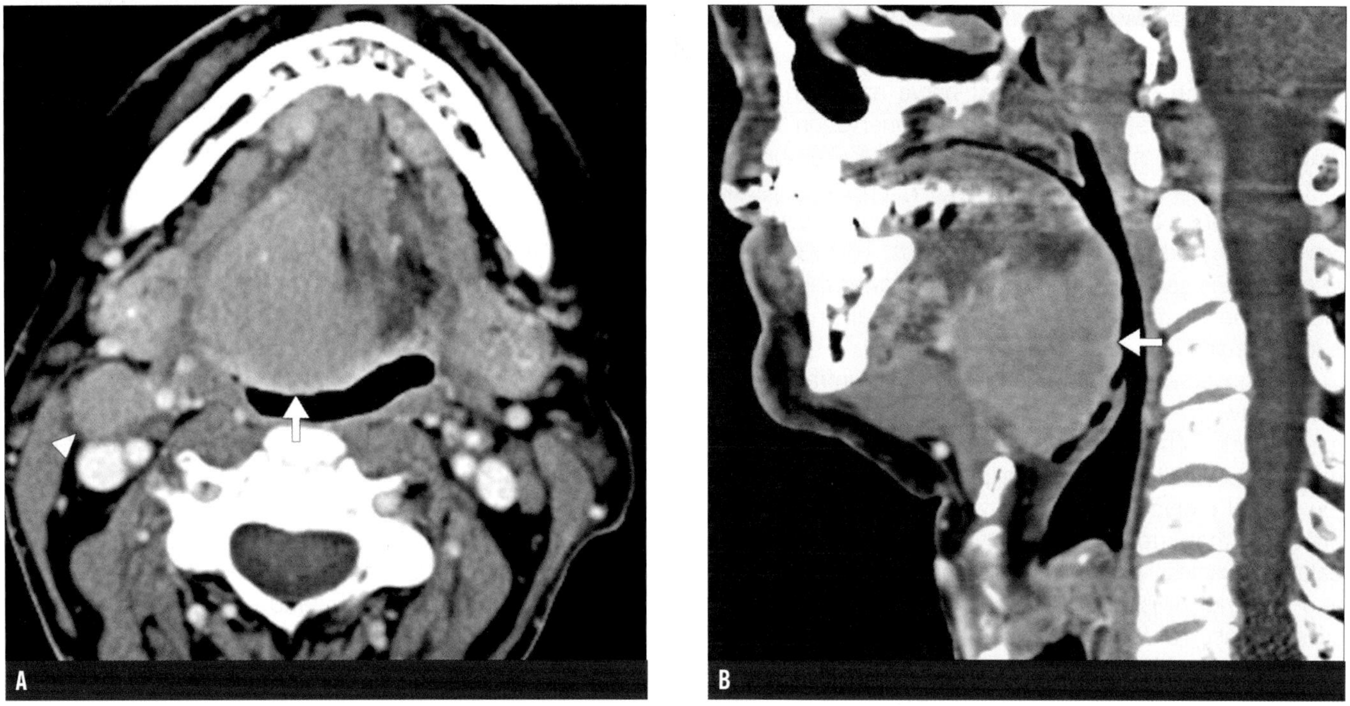

Axial (**A**) and coronal reformatted (**B**) postcontrast CT images demonstrate a large mass involving the right tongue base extending into the root of the tongue, compatible with a tumor, in this case representing a squamous cell carcinoma (arrows, **A**, **B**). While this lesion prolapses into the oropharynx similarly to what may be identified with tongue denervation atrophy, the increased density of the mass as well as mass effect upon the surrounding structures helps differentiate this lesion from base of tongue prolapse secondary to tongue denervation atrophy. In addition, a pathologic lymph node is identified in the right level IIA nodal station, compatible with metastatic disease (arrowhead, **A**).

REFERENCES

Beil CM, Keberle M. Oral and oropharyngeal tumors. *Euro J Radiol.* 2008;66(3):448-459.

El Hassani Y, Narata AP, Pereira VM, Schaller C. A reminder for a very rare entity: massive tongue swelling after posterior fossa surgery. *J Neurol Surg A Cent Eur Neurosurg.* 2012;73(3):171-174. Epub May 9, 2012.

Murakami R, et al. CT and MR findings of denervated tongue after radical neck dissection. *AJNR Am J Neuroradiol.* 1997;18(4):747-750.

Russo CP, Smoker WR, Weissman JL. MR appearance of trigeminal and hypoglossal motor denervation. *AJNR Am J Neuroradiol.* 1997;18(7):1375-1383.

CASE 15 Denervation atrophy of the floor of mouth musculature

The V3 branch of the trigeminal nerve has both motor and sensory fibers. It provides motor innervation for the four muscles of mastication (the masseter, temporalis, medial pterygoid, and lateral pterygoid muscles) as well as the anterior belly of the digastric, mylohyoid, tensor veli palatini, and tensor tympani muscles. The V3 branch also provides sensory innervation to the lower third of the face via the inferior alveolar, auriculotemporal, lingual, and buccal nerves.

V3 traverses the foramen ovale and infratemporal fossa, between the tensor veli palatini and the lateral pterygoid muscle. The main trunk of the nerve gives rise to the medial pterygoid nerve, which provides motor supply to the medial pterygoid muscle as well as gives rise to small branches that supply the tensor tympani and tensor veli palatini muscles. The main trunk then divides into anterior and posterior divisions. The anterior division gives rise to several muscular branches which innervate the remaining muscles of mastication. The posterior division gives rise to several sensory nerves and the lingual nerve, which has both sensory and motor fibers. The mylohyoid nerve arises from the inferior alveolar nerve and innervates the mylohyoid muscle and the anterior belly of the digastric muscle. Any pathologic process that occurs along the course of the V3 nerve may result in nerve dysfunction and denervation atrophy of the affected muscle group.

On CT, denervation injury is most commonly identified in the chronic stage, when the affected muscles undergo fatty atrophy. On MRI, denervation injury has different appearances depending upon the phase of the injury. In the acute/subacute phase, the involved muscle will be edematous and be iso- to hypointense signal on T1, hyperintense on T2, and enhance. Care should be taken not to misinterpret the enhancement that occurs during this phase as tumor or infection. In the chronic phase, the muscles affected will atrophy and contain intrinsic hyperintense T1 signal related to fatty infiltration.

Denervation atrophy of the floor of mouth musculature

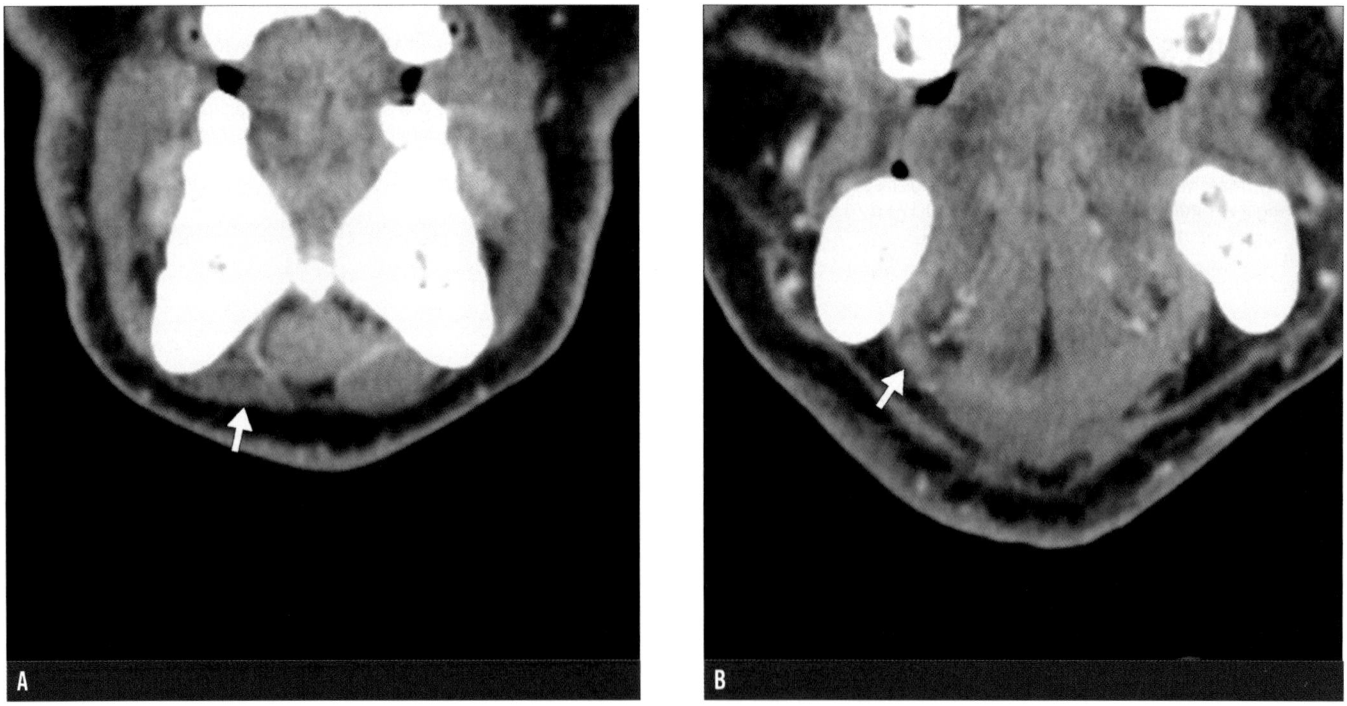

Postcontrast coronal reformatted CT images obtained through the floor of mouth (**A**, **B**) demonstrate fatty atrophy of the anterior belly of the right digastric muscle (arrow, **A**) and volume loss of the right mylohyoid muscle (arrow, **B**). This patient had a history of larynx cancer and a total laryngectomy (not shown), chemotherapy, and radiation. The therapy presumably resulted in the CN V, V3 denervation of the right floor of mouth.

Denervation atrophy of the floor of mouth musculature

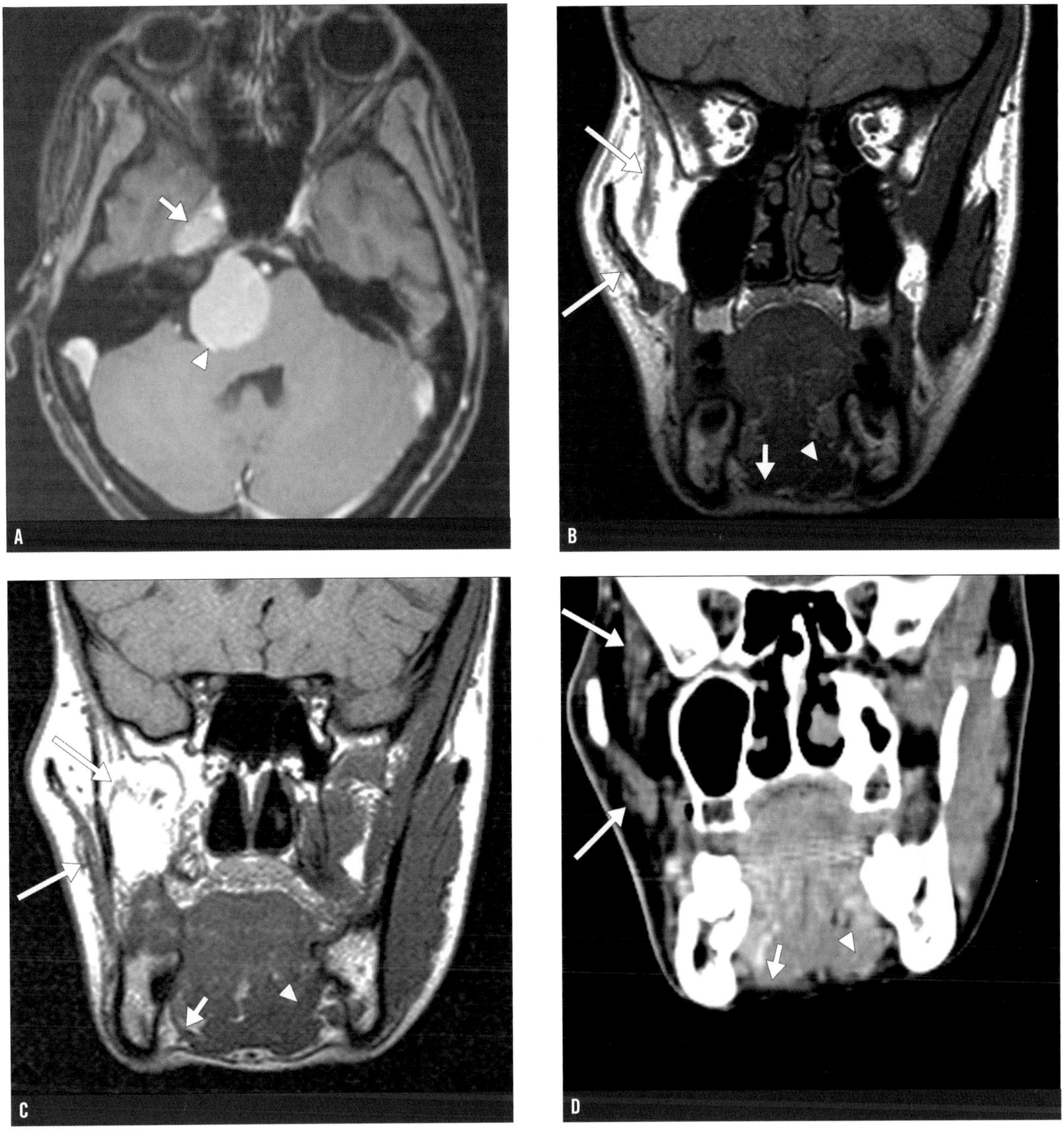

A postcontrast axial MPRAGE MR image (**A**) demonstrates a large mass anterior to, and resulting in marked mass effect upon, the right ventral aspect of the pons (arrowhead, **A**). The mass is located along the expected course of the right trigeminal nerve cisternal segment. Tumor also occupies the right Meckel cave (short arrow, **A**). This lesion represented a CN V primary melanoma at pathology. An unenhanced coronal T1-weighted MR image (**B**) demonstrates denervation atrophy of the right anterior belly of the digastric muscle (short arrow, **B**) relative to the normal sized anterior belly of the left digastric muscle (arrowhead, **B**). An unenhanced coronal T1-weighted MR image slightly more posterior to image **B** (**C**) demonstrates denervation atrophy of the right mylohyoid muscle (short arrow, **C**) relative to the normal left mylohyoid muscle (arrowhead, **C**). Postcontrast coronal reformatted CT of the same patient (**D**) also subtly demonstrates the right anterior belly digastric muscle denervation atrophy (short arrow, **D**) relative to the normal left anterior belly of the digastric muscle (arrowhead, **D**). A postcontrast axial CT image through the masticator space (**E**) as well as images **B**, **C**, and **D** demonstrate marked denervation atrophy of the right muscles of mastication (long arrows, **B-E**).

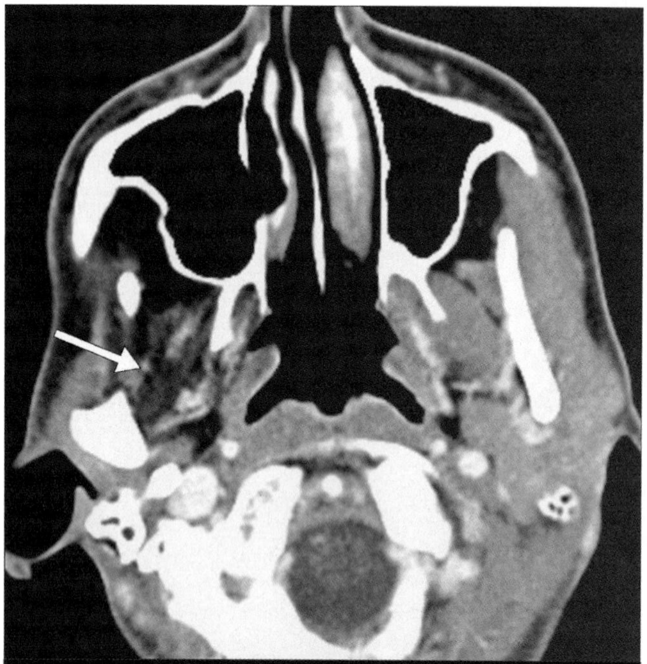
E

REFERENCES

Larsson SG. Hemiatrophy of the tongue and floor of the mouth demonstrated by computed tomography. *J Comp Assist Tomogr.* 1985;9(5):914-918.

Russo CP, Smoker WR, Weissman JL. MR appearance of trigeminal and hypoglossal motor denervation. *AJNR Am J Neuroradiol.* 1997;18(7):1375-1383.

CASE 16 Anomalies of the anterior bellies of the digastric muscles

The anterior bellies of the digastric muscles mark the lateral boundary of the submental triangle. Multiple anomalies of the anterior belly of the digastric muscles have been described in the literature. Most commonly, the one or both of the anterior bellies of the digastric muscles are duplicated. A second variant is a unilateral accessory anterior belly digastric muscle that obliquely crosses the midline and inserts onto the contralateral aspect of the mandible. Another variant that has been described is a hypoplastic anterior belly of the digastric muscle which courses medially and blends with the mylohyoid muscle. With this last variant, a normal sized digastric muscle will not be identified on the affected side.

Obliquely oriented anterior belly of the digastric muscle

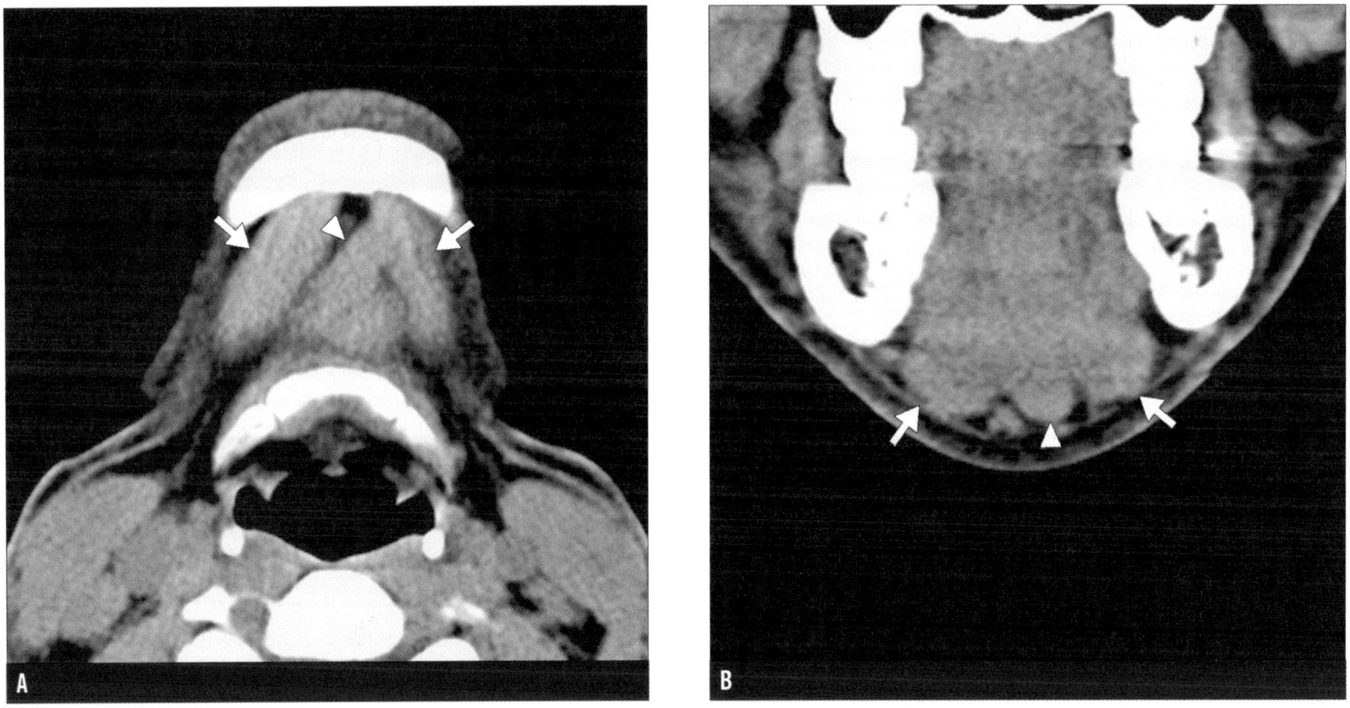

Axial (**A**) and coronal reformatted (**B**) unenhanced CT images through the oral cavity demonstrate an accessory anterior belly digastric muscle that is oriented obliquely along the floor of mouth (arrowheads, **A**, **B**). The typical bilateral configuration of the anterior belly of the digastric muscles is also present (arrows, **A**, **B**).

Unilateral hypoplasia of the anterior belly of the digastric muscle

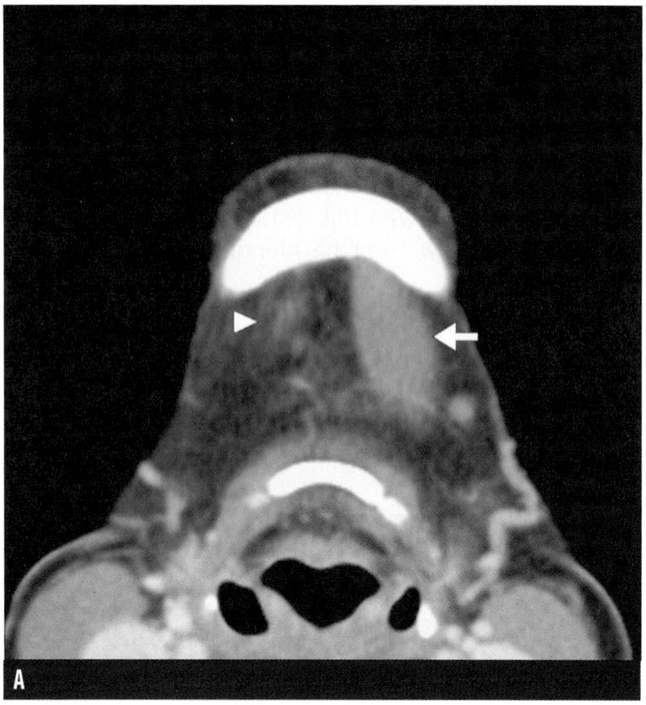

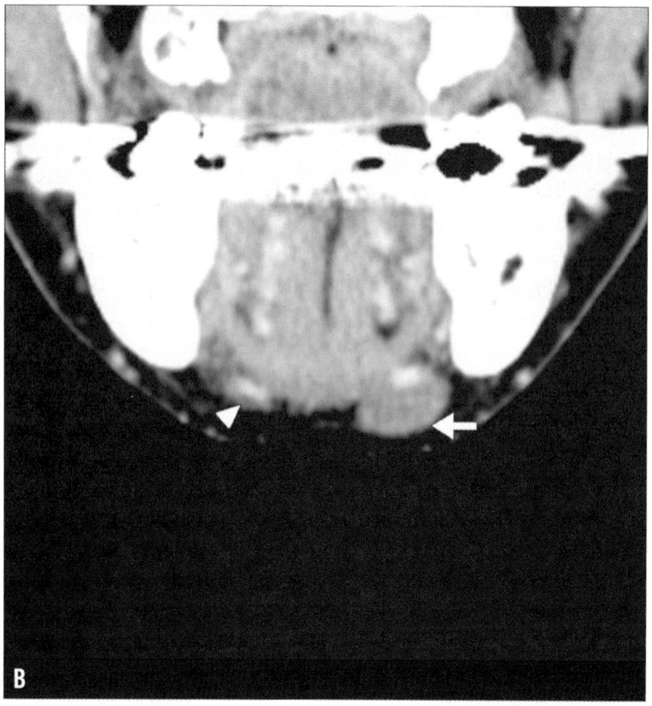

Axial (**A**) and coronal (**B**) unenhanced CT images through the submental triangle demonstrate a normal anterior belly of the left digastric muscle (arrows, **A**, **B**). The anterior belly of the right digastric muscle is markedly hypoplastic (arrowheads, **A**, **B**). The right mylohyoid muscle as well as the right muscles of mastication (not fully shown) were normal in volume, suggesting that the hypoplasia of the anterior belly of the right digastric muscle is a normal variant, rather than the result of a proximal injury to mylohyoid nerve arising from CN V, V3 division.

Unilateral merging of the anterior belly of the digastric muscle with the mylohyoid muscle

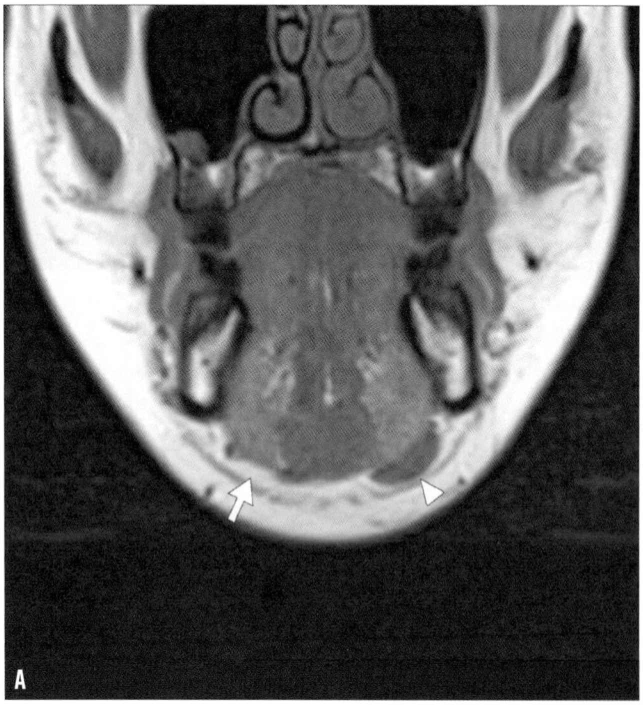

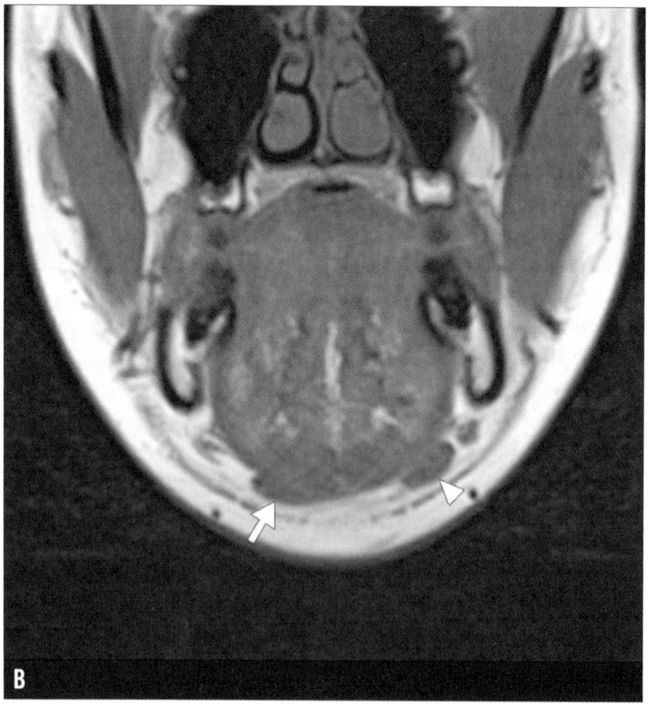

Sequential unenhanced coronal T1-weighted MR images viewed from anterior to posterior (**A**-**C**) and a single axial T1-weighted MR image (**D**) demonstrate a normal appearing anterior belly of the left digastric muscle (arrowheads, **A**-**D**). On the right, an anterior belly of the digastric muscle is not identified in its normal expected location (arrows, **A** and **D**). Instead, there is a diminutive anterior belly of the right digastric muscle which is located more medial than normal (arrow, **B**) and which partially merges with the muscle fibers of the mylohyoid muscle (arrow, **C**).

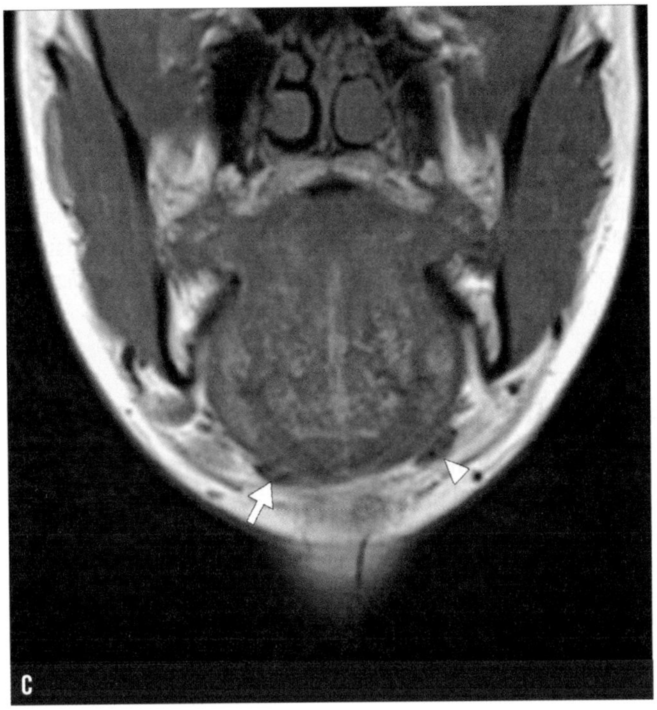

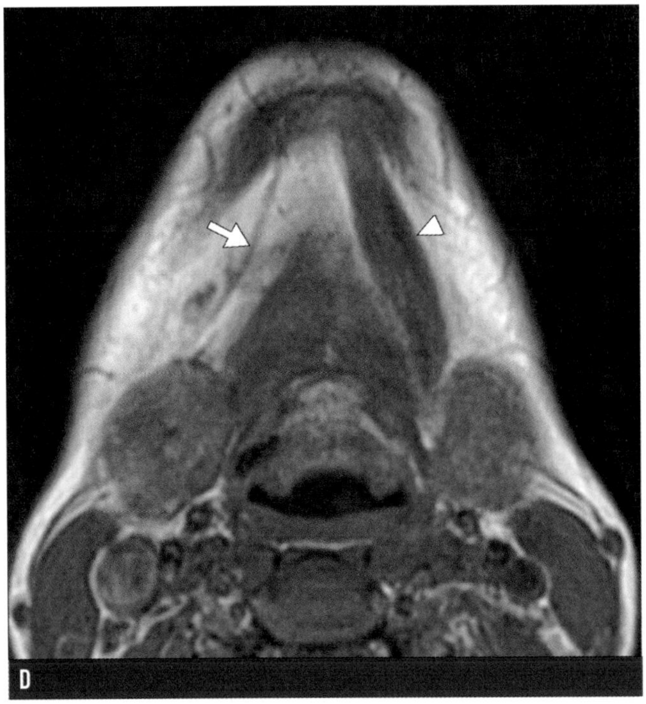

REFERENCES

Larsson SG, Lufkin RB. Anomalies of digastric muscles: CT and MR demonstration. *J Comput Assist Tomogr.* 1987;11(3):422-425.

Ozgur Z, Govsa F, Ozgur T. The cause of the difference in the submental region: aberrant muscle bundles of the anterior belly of the digastric muscle. *J Craniofac Surg.* 2007;18(4):875-881.

CASE 17 Mylohyoid muscle defect (boutonnière deformity)

The mylohyoid muscles are paired, sheet-like muscles that help form the floor of the mouth and serve as the primary boundary between the sublingual and submandibular spaces. The muscles arise from the mylohyoid line of the mandible, which is located along the lingual surface of the mandible. The muscle fibers course posteromedially, with the medial aspects of each muscle inserting onto a fibrous median raphe and the posteromedial aspects of each muscle inserting directly upon the hyoid body. The remainder of the posterior margin of each mylohyoid muscle represents a "free margin." A small portion of each submandibular gland extends cephalad and slightly anterior to this free margin, allowing each Wharton duct to traverse within the sublingual space.

A focal deficiency of the mylohyoid muscle is termed a boutonnière deformity. A boutonnière deformity is a common finding, with one series identifying this defect in 72% of cadavers. This deformity is most often an incidental finding but it can serve as a conduit for the spread of tumor or infection between the sublingual and submandibular spaces. In addition, a boutonnière deformity often allows the sublingual gland (historically referred to as a bouton), fat, or blood vessels to herniate from the sublingual space into the submandibular space. A boutonnière deformity is most frequently identified along the anterolateral two-thirds of the muscle belly. Herniated sublingual gland, fat, or vessels, if present, may range in size from a few millimeters to a few centimeters. A herniated sublingual gland through a boutonnière deformity may be mistaken for an enhancing mass or a pathologically enlarged lymph node in the submandibular space. Helpful imaging characteristics to avoid this interpretation pitfall include: similar attenuation or signal characteristics compared to other salivary tissue in the neck, identification of a narrow waist near the mid aspect of the suspected herniated sublingual gland at the level of the muscle defect, and visualization of fat or blood vessels that may also be herniating through the defect.

COMPANION CASE

- **Ranula extending through a boutonnière deformity**. A ranula is a sublingual or minor salivary gland mucous retention cyst or mucocele which usually results from prior salivary gland trauma or inflammation. On CT, a ranula is usually fluid attenuating and may enhance peripherally but does not enhance centrally. On MRI, a ranula is usually hyperintense on T2-weighted and iso- to hypointense on T1-weighed imaging, although its signal depends on the amount of proteinaceous content.

  A ranula may be classified into simple and plunging (also called diving) types. A simple ranula is a unilocular cystic lesion centered within the lateral aspect of the sublingual space. A plunging ranula typically occurs when a simple ranula ruptures posteriorly into the submandibular space over the posterior free margin of the mylohyoid muscle. However, infrequently, a simple ranula may extend through a boutonnière deformity (if present) and into the ipsilateral anterior aspect of the submandibular space. In this uncommon form of a ranula, a narrow waist along the ranula at the site of the mylohyoid defect is often visualized.

Unilateral boutonnière deformity with sublingual gland herniation

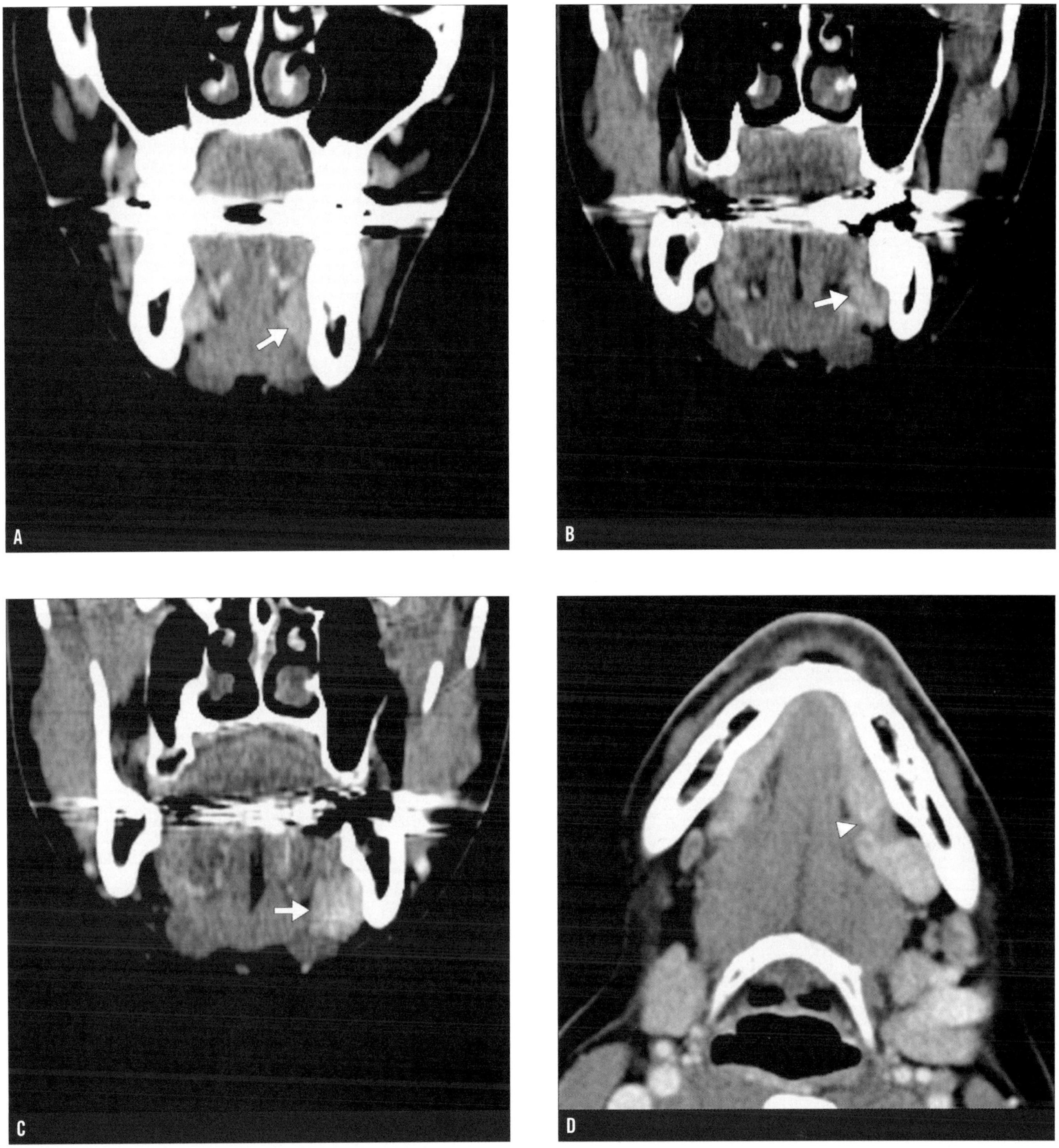

Sequential contrast-enhanced coronal reformatted CT images (**A-C**) demonstrate the left sublingual gland herniating through a left mylohyoid muscle defect (boutonnière deformity) (arrows, **A-C**). A contrast-enhanced axial CT image (**D**) demonstrates focal waisting of the left sublingual gland at the level of the left mylohyoid muscle, an imaging finding often identified with sublingual gland herniation through a boutonnière deformity (arrowhead, **D**).

Unilateral boutonnière deformity with sublingual gland herniation

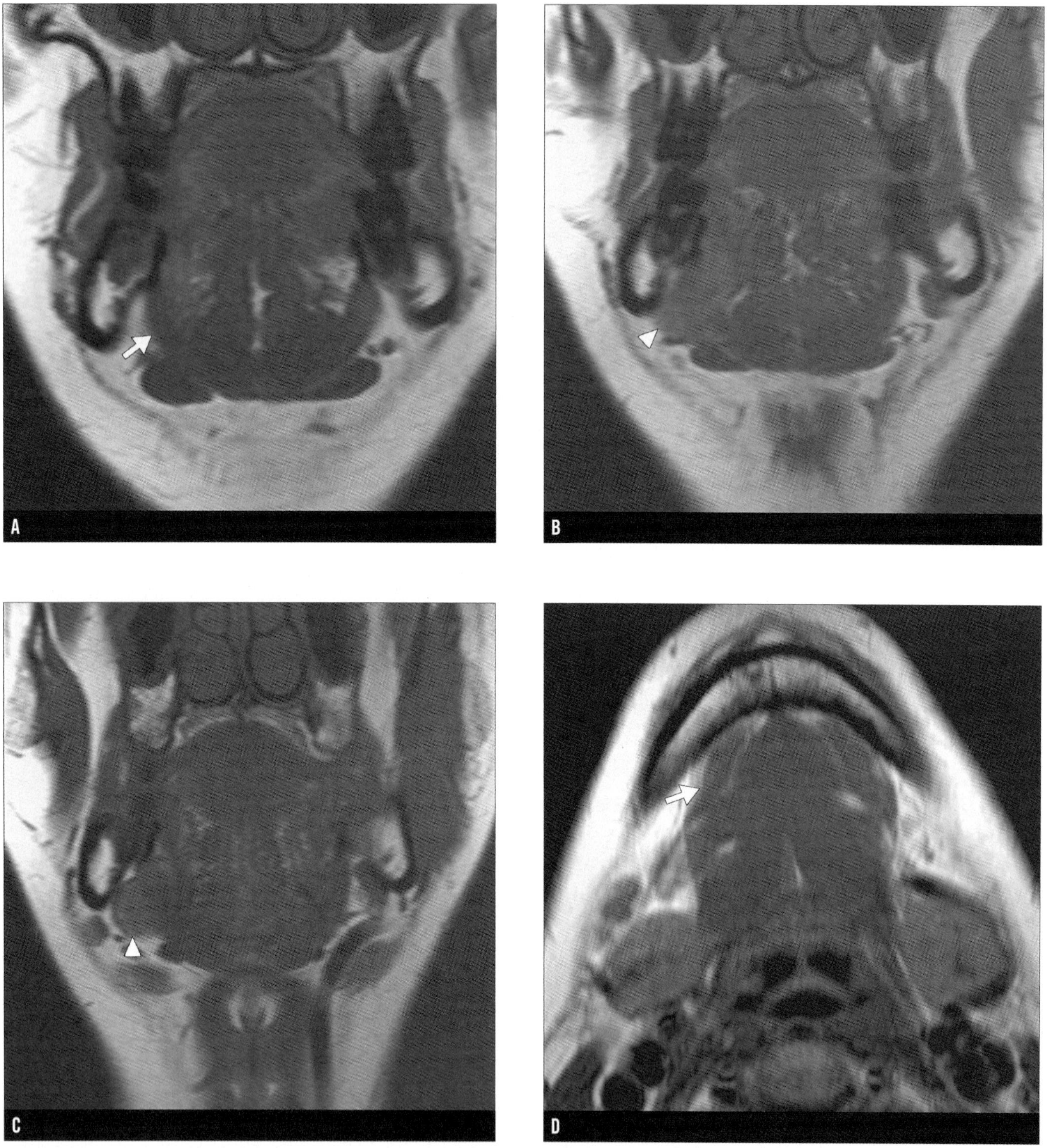

Different patient. Sequential coronal (**A-C**) and axial (**D-F**) unenhanced T1-weighted MR images through the floor of the mouth. Images **A** and **D** demonstrate the intact portion of the right mylohyoid muscle (arrows, **A**, **D**). Images **B**, **C**, **E**, and **F** demonstrate the right sublingual gland herniating through a right boutonnière deformity (arrowheads, **B**, **C**, **E**, **F**).

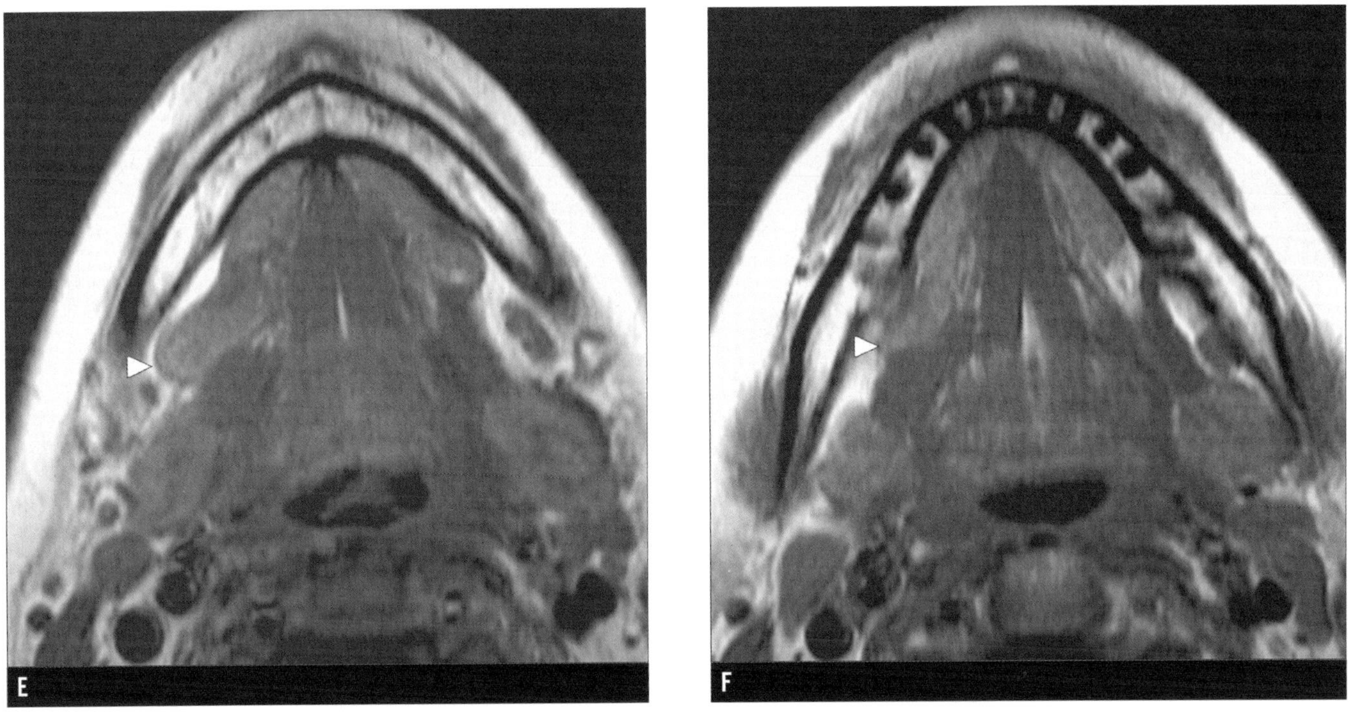

Bilateral boutonnière deformities with bilateral sublingual gland herniation

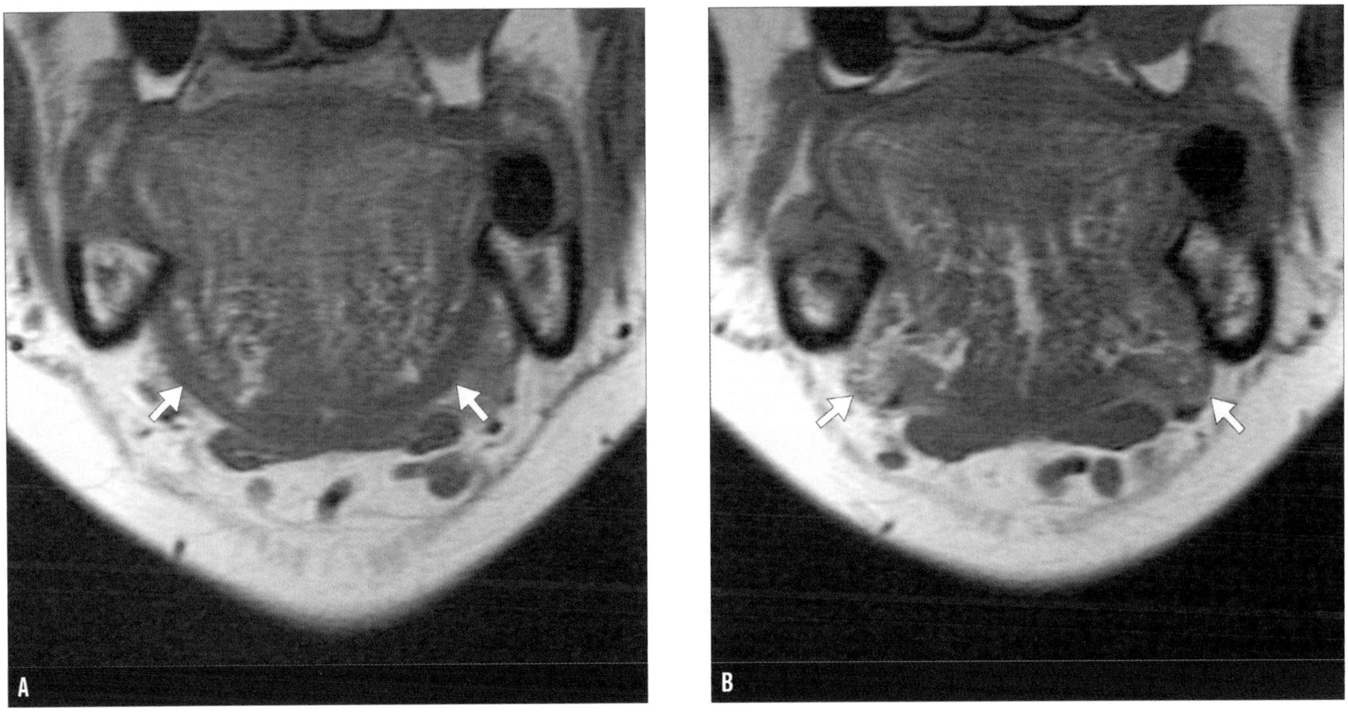

Noncontrast coronal T1 (**A**, **B**), fat-suppressed coronal T2 (**C**, **D**), noncontrast axial T1 (**E**), and fat-suppressed axial T2 (**F**) MR images obtained through the oral cavity. Images **A** and **C** demonstrate the intact portions of the bilateral mylohyoid muscles (arrows, **A**, **C**). More anterior, images **B** and **D** demonstrate the deficient portions of the bilateral mylohyoid muscle where there is herniation of both sublingual glands through boutonnière deformities (arrows, **B**, **D**). Images **E** and **F** also demonstrate the intact portion of the bilateral mylohyoid muscles posteriorly (arrows, **E**, **F**) and the deficient portion of the bilateral mylohyoid muscles with sublingual gland herniation more anterior (arrowheads, **E**, **F**).

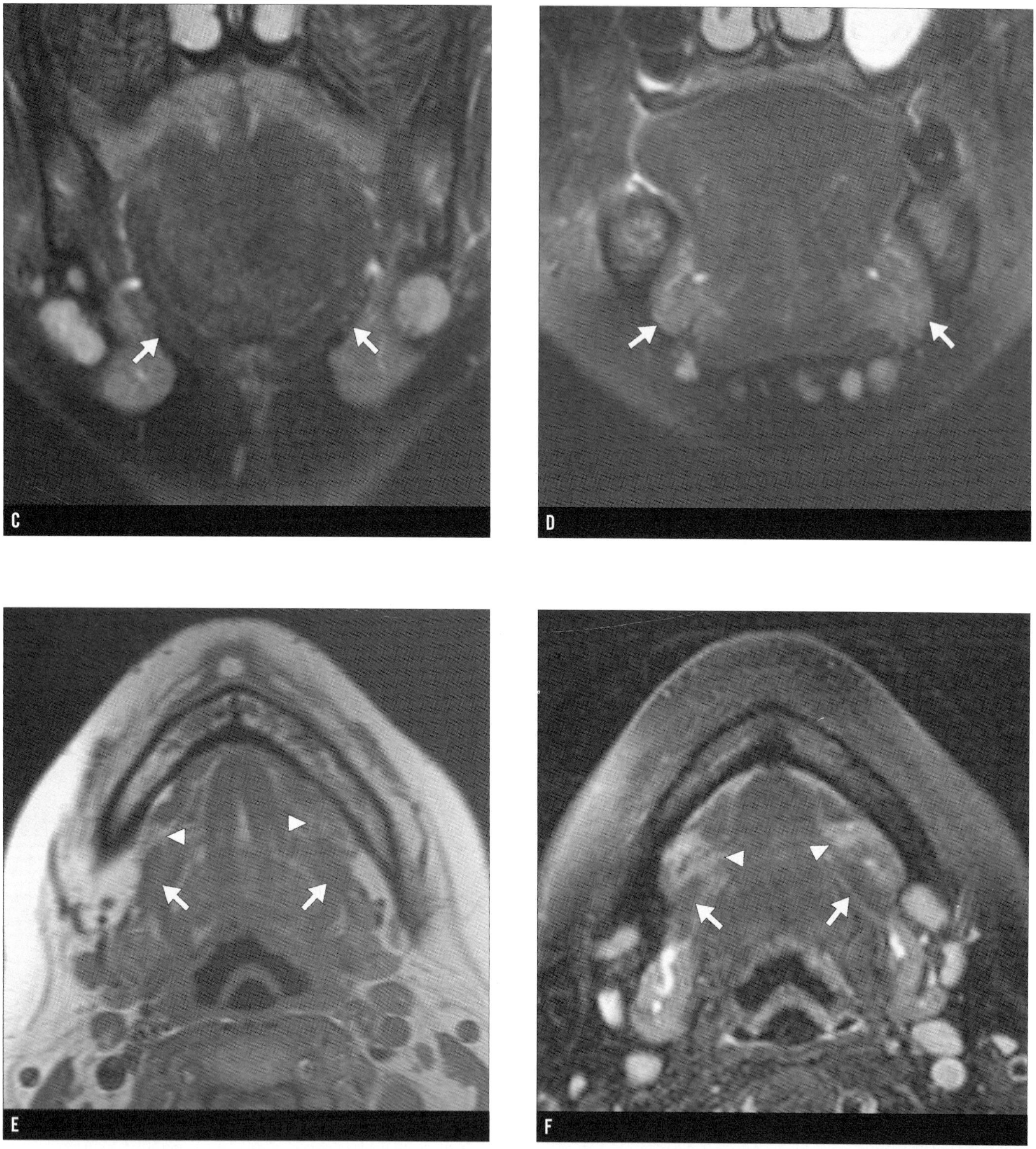
C
D
E
F

Companion case: Ranula extending through a boutonnière deformity

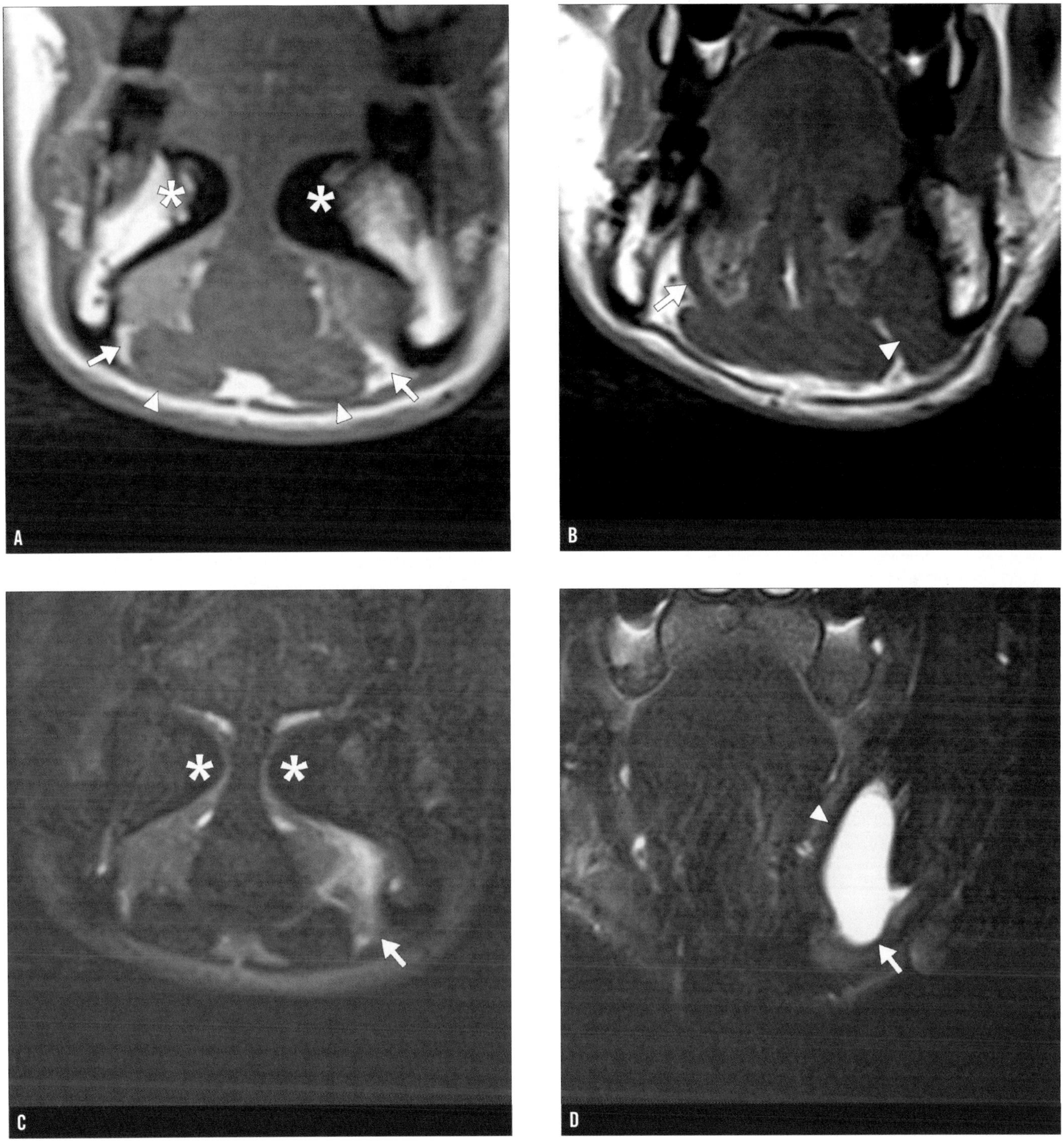

Noncontrast coronal T1 (**A**, **B**), coronal T2 with fat suppression (**C**, **D**), postcontrast coronal T1 with fat suppression (**E**-**G**), and axial T2 with fat suppression (**H**) MR images through the oral cavity. Image **A** demonstrates deficiency of both mylohyoid muscles along the ventral aspect of the oral cavity floor (arrows, **A**). The normal anterior bellies of the digastric muscles are delineated (arrowheads, **A**). More posterior, image **B** demonstrates the intact portion of the right mylohyoid muscle (arrow, **B**), whereas the left mylohyoid muscle is not seen. In expected location of the left mylohyoid muscle is an asymmetric lesion that is not the same signal as would be expected for normal sublingual gland extending into the left aspect of the submandibular space (arrowhead, **B**). Image **C** demonstrates T2 prolongation traversing the deficient left mylohyoid muscle (arrow, **C**). More posterior, image **D** demonstrates continuation of the T2 hyperintense lesion in the left aspect of the submandibular space (arrow, **D**), which displaces the intact portion of the left mylohyoid muscle superomedially (arrowhead, **D**). Image **E** demonstrates a linear, small amount of nonenhancing fluid (arrow, **E**). This nonenhancing fluid continues posterior into the left aspect of the submandibular space, as demonstrated on images **F** and **G** (arrows, **F**, **G**). Image **H** demonstrates the T2 hyperintense lesion in the axial plane (arrow, **H**). This case illustrates a ranula extending from the left sublingual gland, herniating through a left boutonnière deformity, and extending into the left aspect of the submandibular space. Incidentally, large bilateral tori mandibularis interna are present (asterisks, **A**, **C**, **E**).

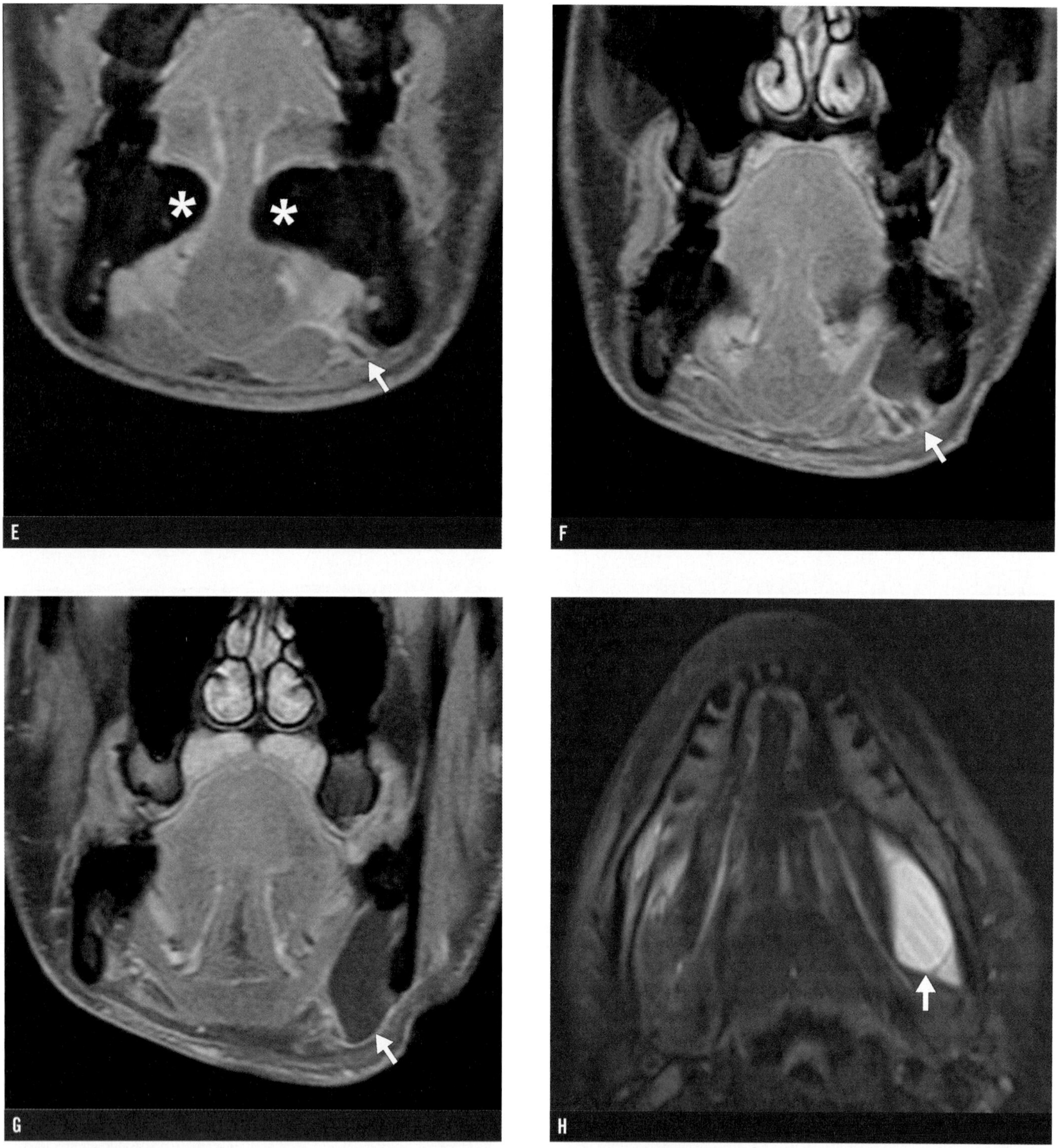

REFERENCES

Gaughran GR. Mylohyoid boutonniere and sublingual bouton. *J Anat.* 1963;97(4):565-568.

LaPorte SJ, Juttla JK, Lingam RK. Imaging of the floor of the mouth and the sublingual space. *Radiographics.* 2011;31(5):1215-1230.

White DK, et al. Accessory salivary tissue in the mylohyoid boutonniere: a clinical and radiologic pseudolesion in the oral cavity. *AJNR Am J Neuroradiol.* 2001;22(2):406-412.

CASE 18 Intraoral comestible foreign bodies

Comestible foreign bodies (food material) can have a confusing appearance on imaging and may mimic a variety of pathologic processes. Hard foreign bodies, such as hard candies or lozenges, tend to be higher in attenuation (300-475 Hounsfield units), have smooth borders, and maintain their oval or round shape. Soft foreign bodies, such as chewing gum, may be more difficult to recognize, particularly because they tend to be lower in attenuation (100-400 Hounsfield units) and their soft consistency allows them to be easily molded to the adjacent mucosal surfaces. On contrast-enhanced CT imaging, the inherent elevated attenuation of these foreign bodies and their location along a mucosal surface of the oral cavity can lead to misinterpreting these incidental findings as enhancing mucosal lesions, particularly if precontrast imaging is unavailable. Because soft foreign bodies can be easily chewed and manipulated within the mouth, they are typically irregular in shape and contain small locules of air within their interstices.

COMPANION CASES

- **Wharton duct sialolith**. There are paired submandibular gland ducts, also know as Wharton ducts, which measure approximately 5 cm in length. Each duct extends superiorly and medially into the sublingual space, above the mylohyoid muscle. The duct drains via its ipsilateral sublingual papilla which is located adjacent to the lingual frenulum. On CT, a sialolith will appear as a calcified structure along the expected course of the Wharton duct. On MRI, a sialolith will appear as a hypointense focus.
- **Retained oral contrast.** If a head and neck CT examination is being performed in conjunction with an abdomen CT examination, oral contrast being utilized for the CT of the abdomen may be retained in the oral cavity. On CT, the appearance of oral contrast will depend on whether the administered contrast is iodine-based water soluble contrast (less dense) or a barium agent (denser). In addition, the density on imaging will also vary based on the specific concentration of the contrast agent as well as the amount of oral secretions diluting the contrast material. Irrespective of these conditions, oral contrast will appear on CT as radiodense material lining the mucosal surfaces or pooling within the oral cavity. Unenhanced imaging is helpful in distinguishing retained oral contrast from an enhancing mucosal lesion.

Comestible foreign body: Chewing gum

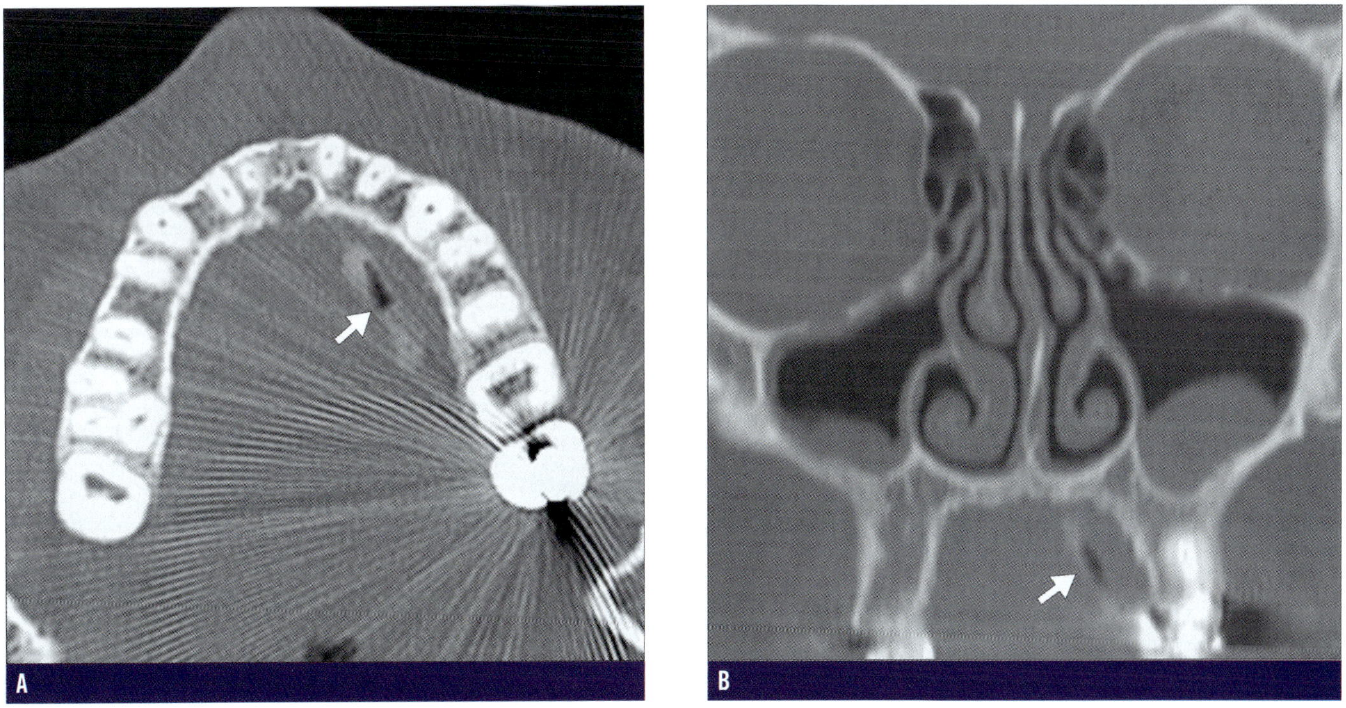

Unenhanced axial (**A**) and coronal reformatted (**B**) CT images demonstrate a comestible foreign body within the anterior left aspect of the oral cavity (arrows, **A**, **B**). The irregular morphology and a discrete focus of air in the interstices of the foreign body are compatible with chewing gum.

Comestible foreign body: Chewing gum

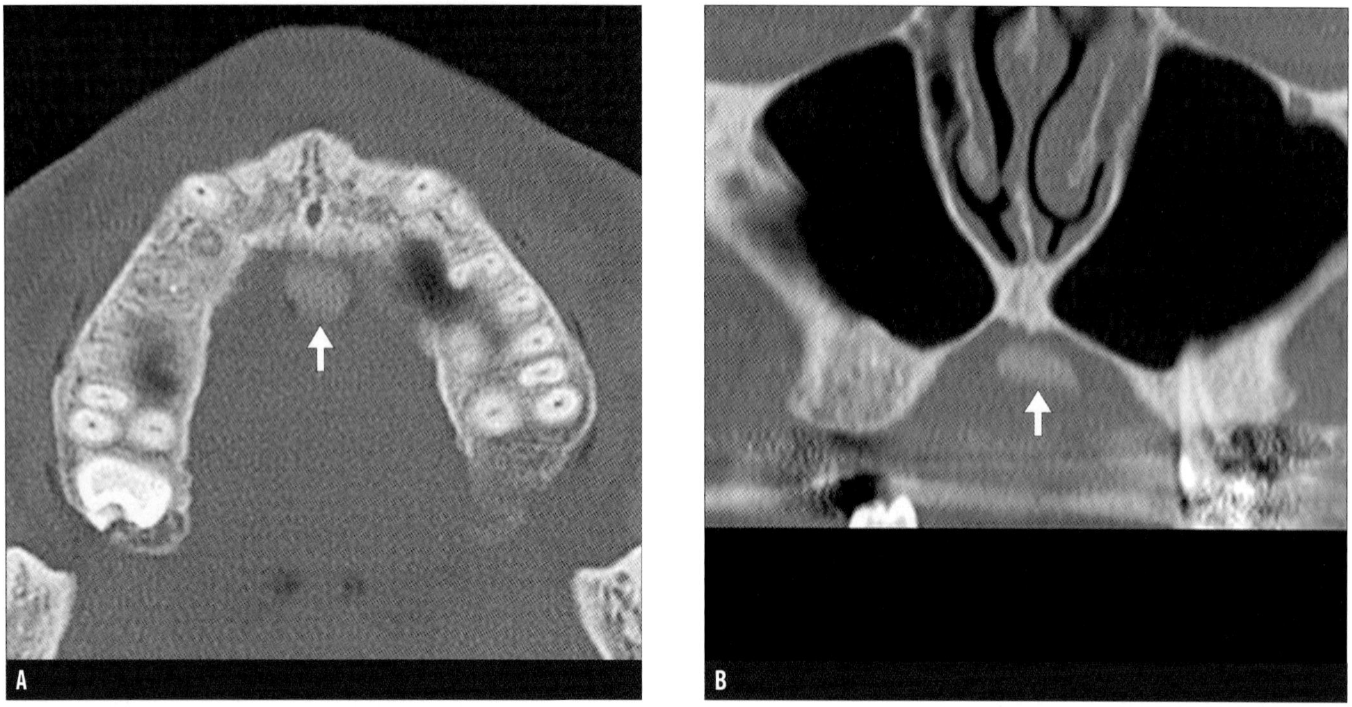

Different patient. Axial (**A**) and coronal reformatted (**B**) CT images demonstrate a foreign body in the anterior-superior aspect of the oral cavity, abutting the undersurface of the hard palate (arrows, **A**, **B**). The attenuation and flat morphology partially molding to the shape of the hard palate are compatible with chewing gum.

Comestible foreign body: Chewing gum

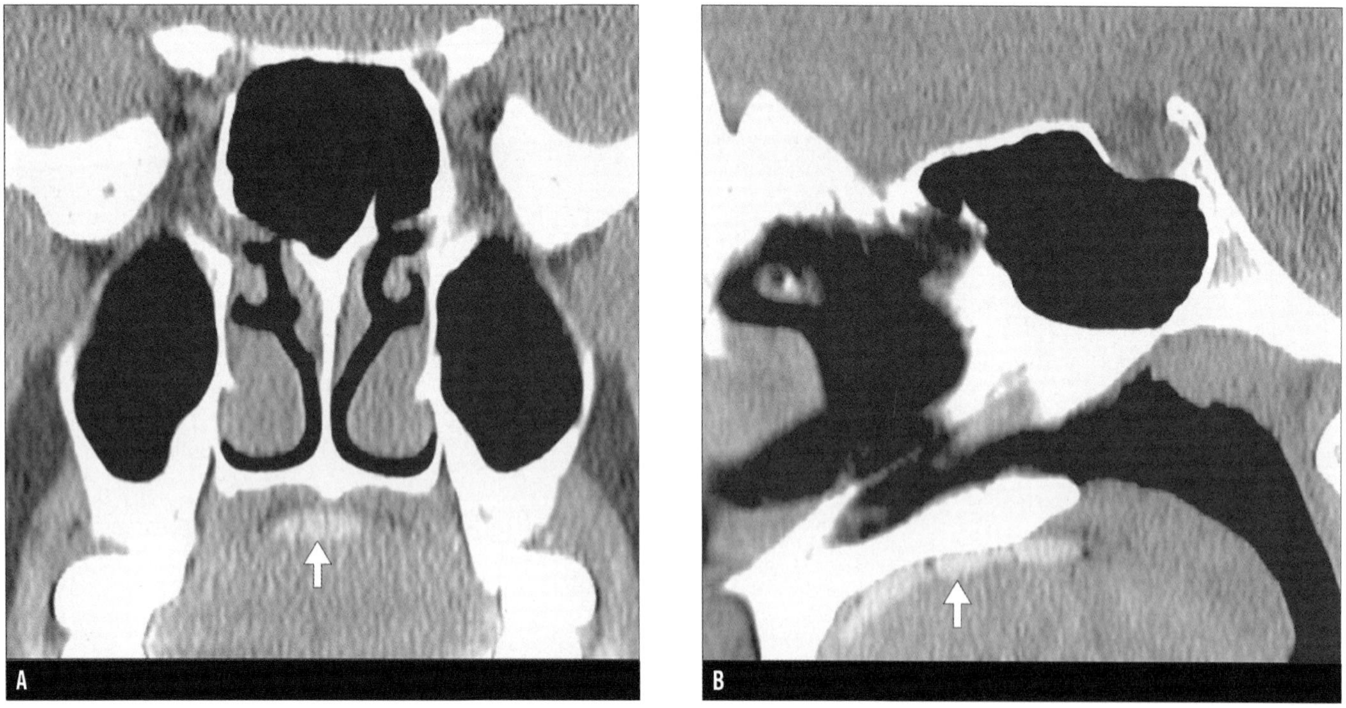

Different patient. Coronal reformatted (**A**) and sagittal reformatted (**B**) CT images demonstrate a linear high-density focus located subjacent and conforming to the shape of the hard palate, compatible with chewing gum (arrows, **A**, **B**).

Comestible foreign body: Hard candy

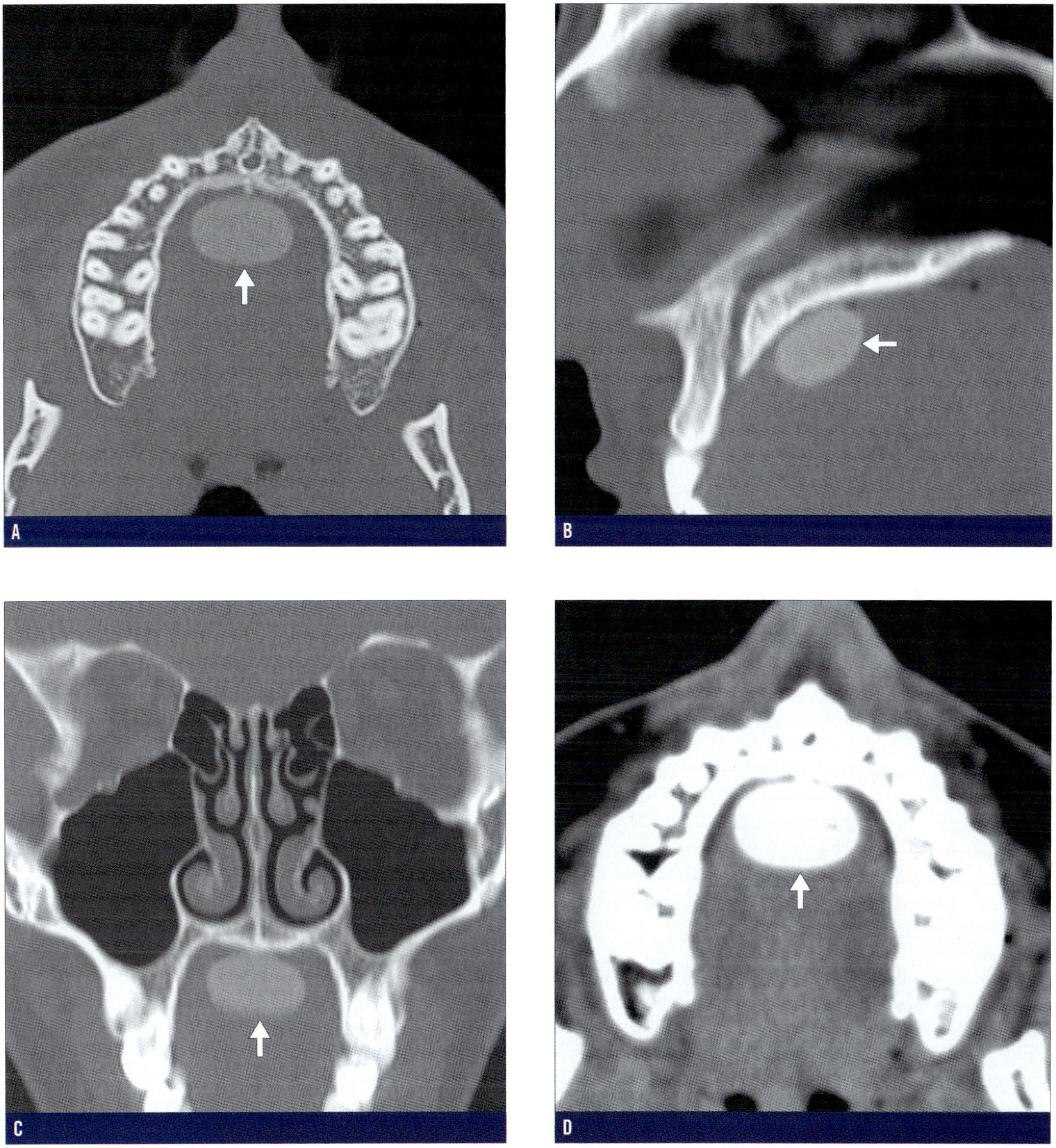

Axial (**A**), sagittal reformatted (**B**), and coronal reformatted (**C**) CT images viewed with a bone window as well as a corresponding axial postcontrast CT image viewed with a soft tissue window (**D**) through the oral cavity. These images demonstrate an oval, circumscribed, hyperattenuating density within the oral cavity, adjacent to the hard palate (arrows, **A-D**). The density of this foreign body is less than that of the osseous structures. These imaging findings are typical of hard candy.

Comestible foreign body: Hard candy

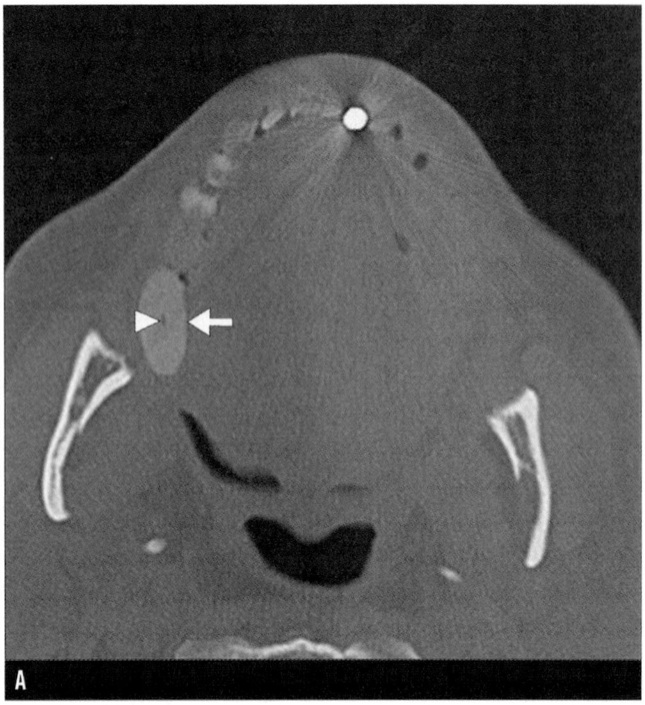

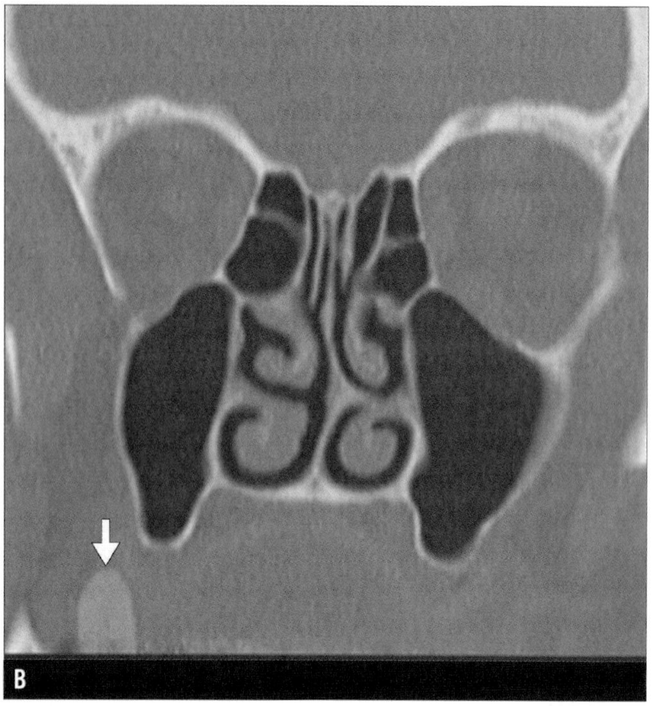

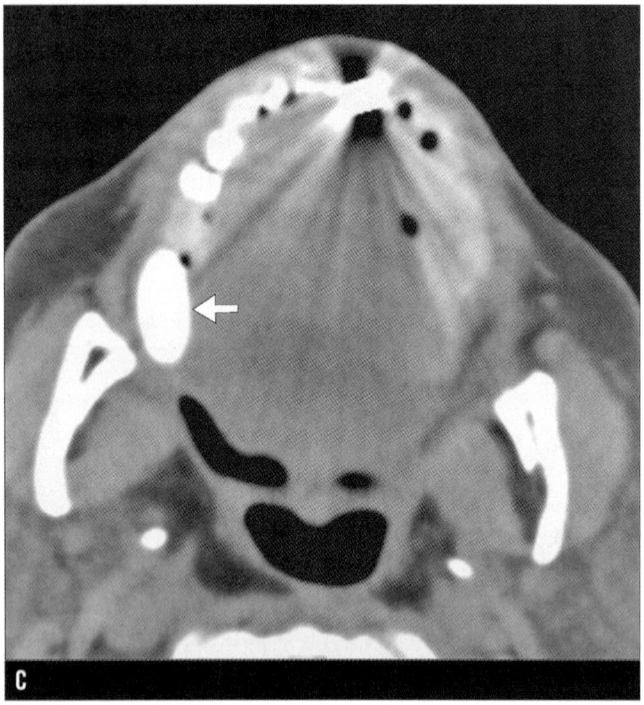

Different patient. Axial (**A**) and coronal reformatted (**B**) CT images viewed with a bone window as well as an unenhanced axial image viewed with a soft tissue window (**C**) demonstrate a dense, oval, circumscribed foreign body located in the right lateral aspect of the oral cavity (arrows , **A-C**). This foreign body contains a small lucent center (arrowhead, **A**). These imaging findings are consistent with hard candy.

Comestible foreign body: Hard candy

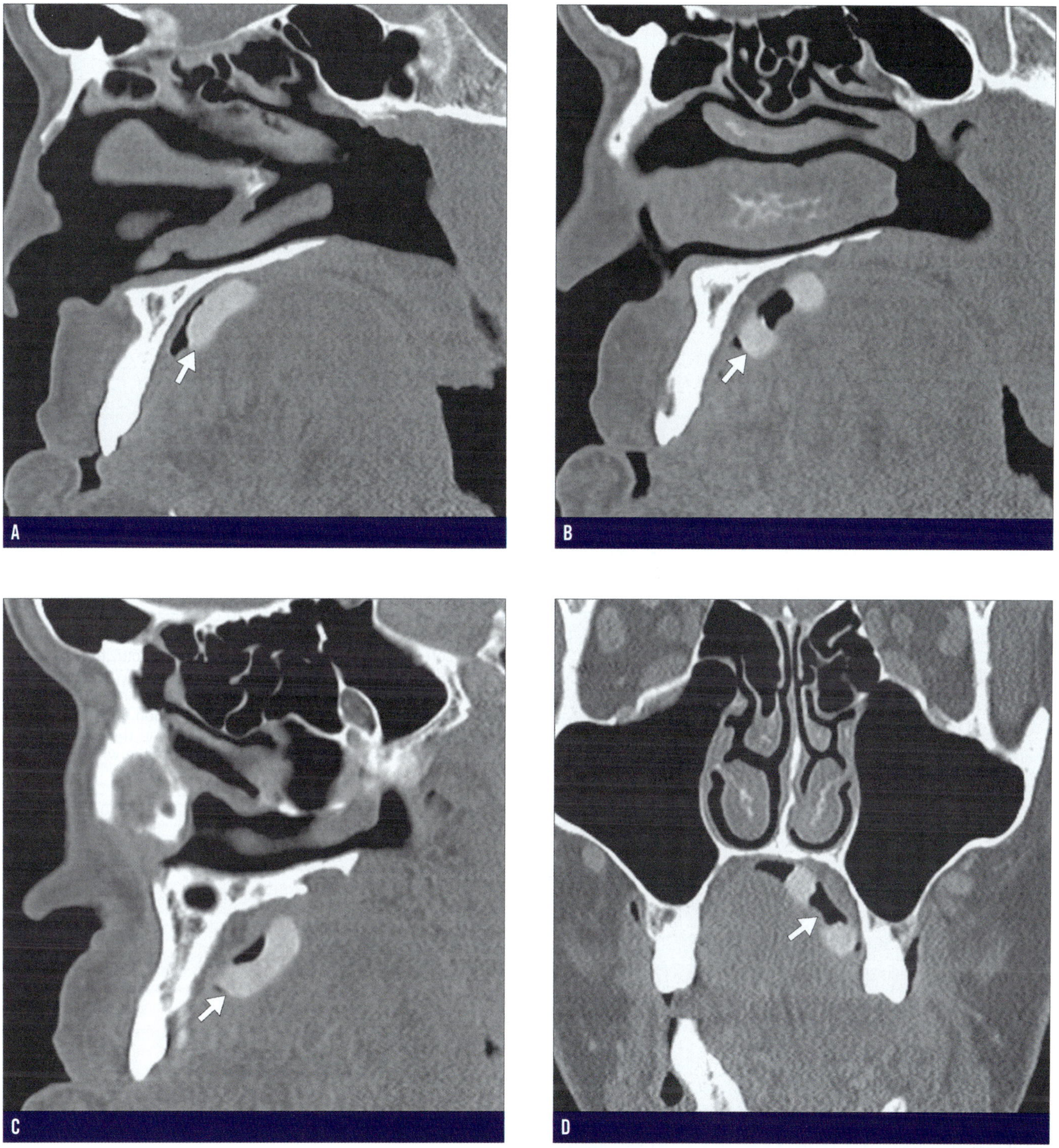

Different patient. Unenhanced sagittal reformatted (**A-C**) and coronal reformatted (**D**) CT images demonstrate a ring-shaped foreign body within the left aspect of the oral cavity, likely representing a Life Savers candy (arrows, **A-D**).

Companion case: Wharton duct sialolith (CT)

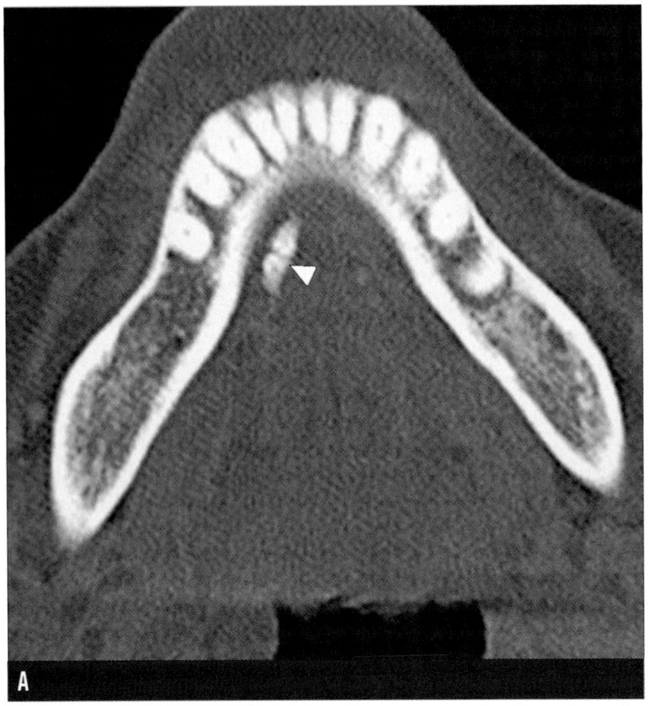

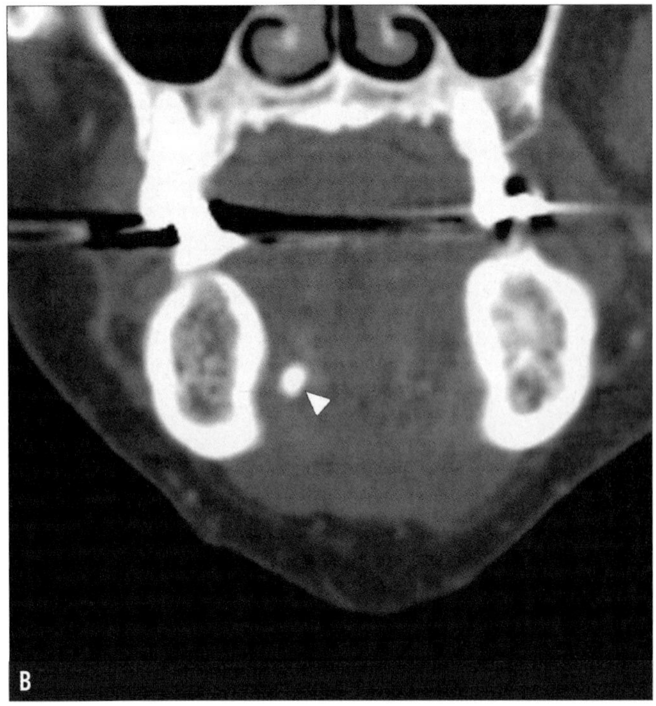

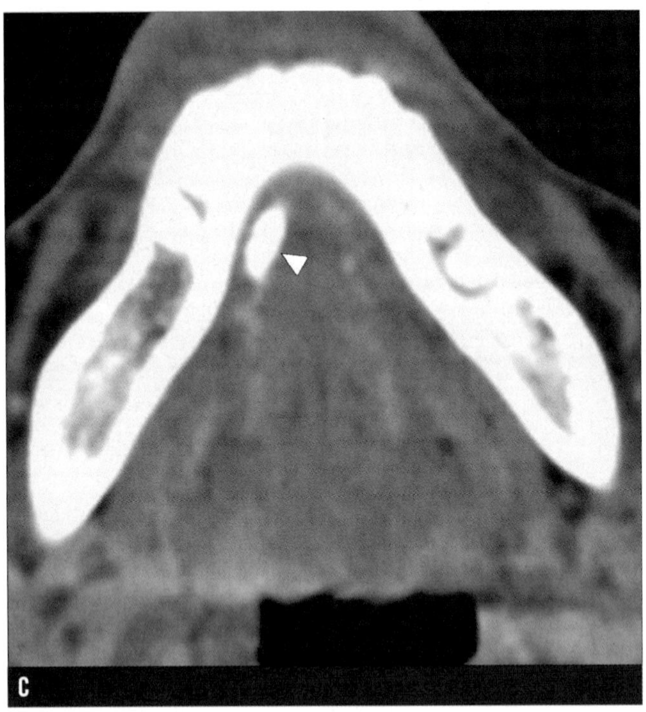

Axial (**A**) and coronal reformatted (**B**) CT images viewed with an intermediate window and a corresponding axial CT image viewed with a soft tissue window (**C**) demonstrate an ovoid, high-density abnormality along the course of the right Wharton duct (arrowheads, **A-C**). The density of the finding is similar to bone and compatible with calcium. Given the location along the expected location of the right Wharton duct and the calcific density of the finding, the finding is most compatible with a right Wharton duct sialolith.

Companion case: Wharton duct sialolith (MRI)

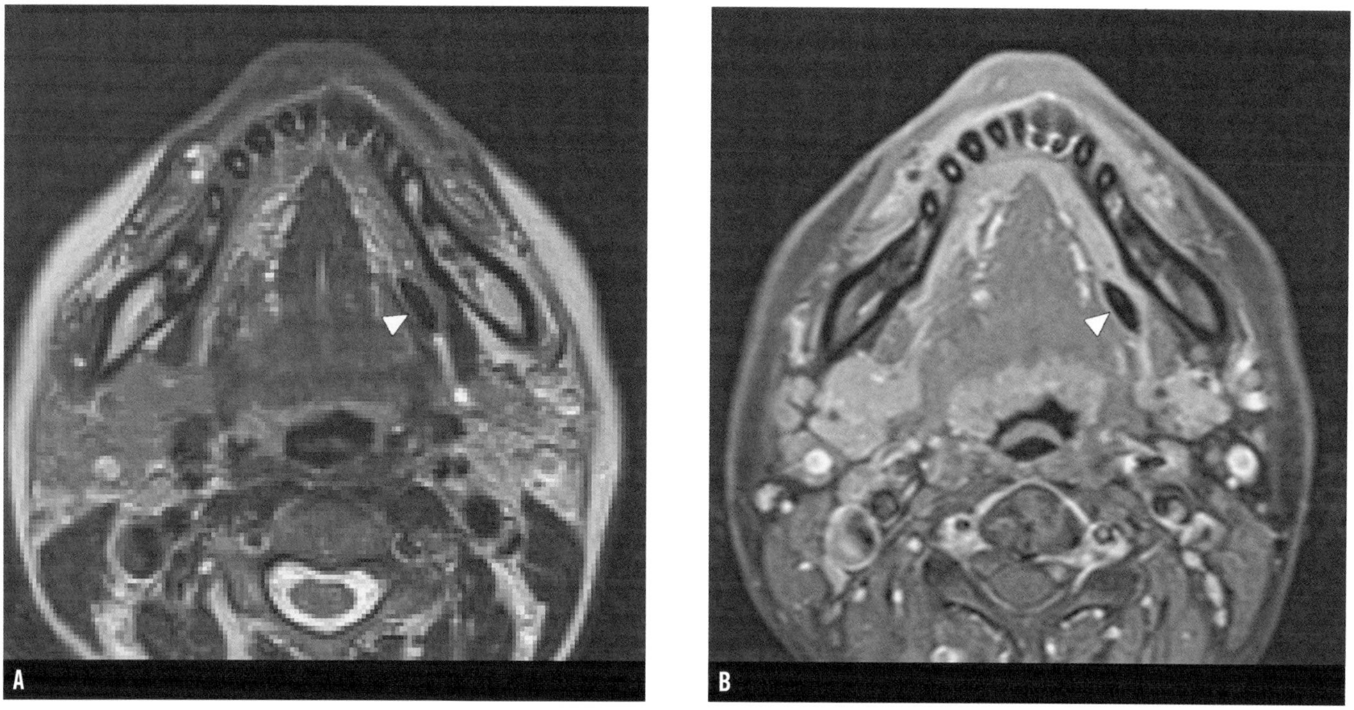

Axial T2 (**A**) and postcontrast axial T1 with fat suppression (**B**) MR images demonstrate an ovoid, hypointense focus along the expected course of the left Wharton duct, most compatible with a left Wharton duct sialolith (arrowheads, **A**, **B**).

Companion case: Obstructing Wharton duct sialolith

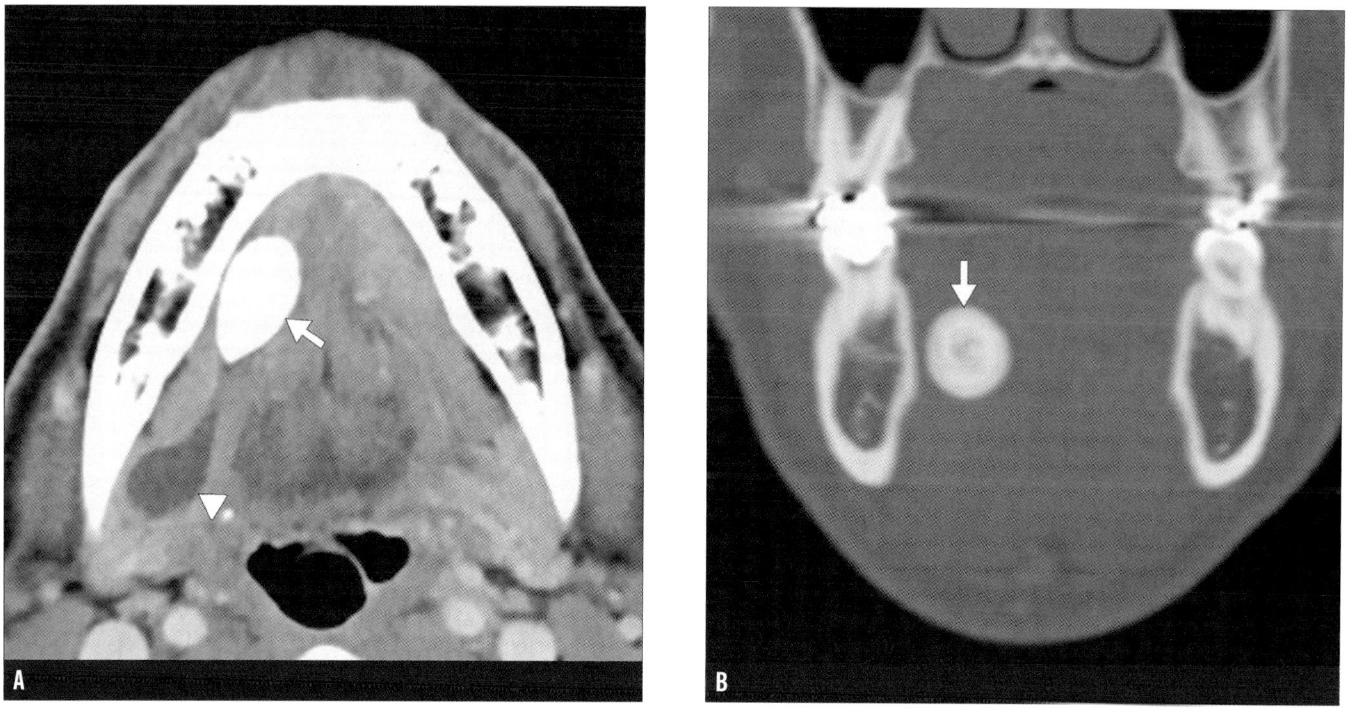

A postcontrast axial CT image through the oral cavity viewed with a soft tissue window (**A**) demonstrates a large, oval, high-density lesion within the right lower aspect of the oral cavity (arrow, **A**). An abnormally enlarged right Wharton duct is present posterior to the finding (arrowhead, **A**). The constellation of findings is compatible with a large, obstructing, right Wharton duct sialolith. Coronal reformatted (**B**) and sagittal reformatted (**C**) CT images from the same study viewed with a bone window demonstrate the large sialolith to contain multiple, oval, concentric lucencies and scleroses, consistent with lamination (arrows, **B**, **C**). A sagittal T1-weighted image from an MRI of the brain obtained 4 years prior to the CT (**D**) also demonstrates the large sialolith (arrow, **D**).

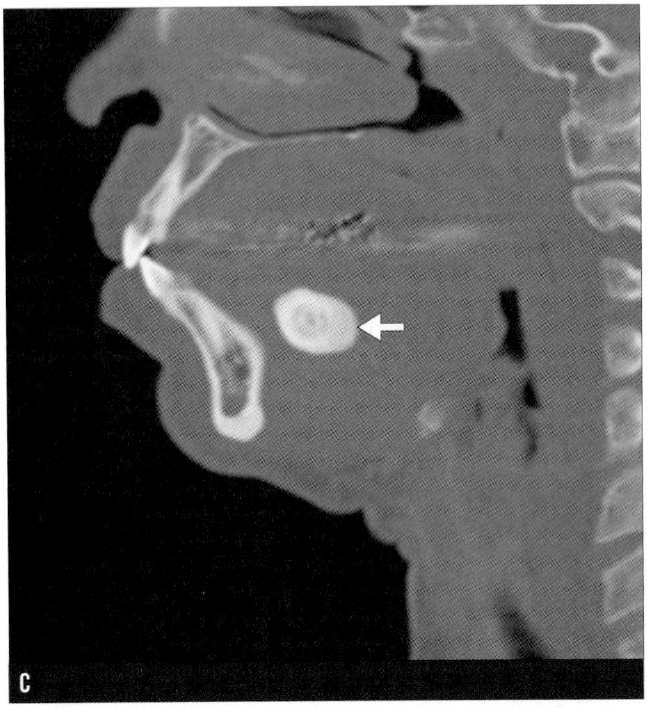

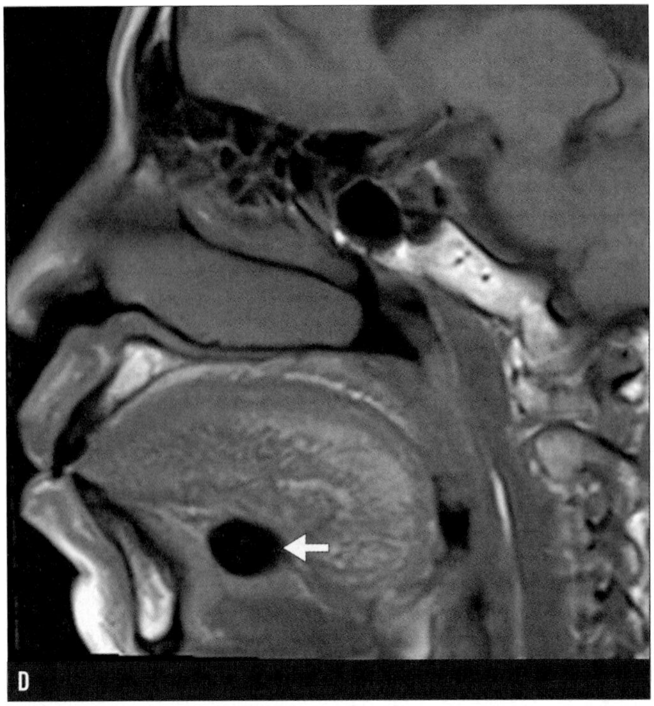

Companion case: Retained oral contrast

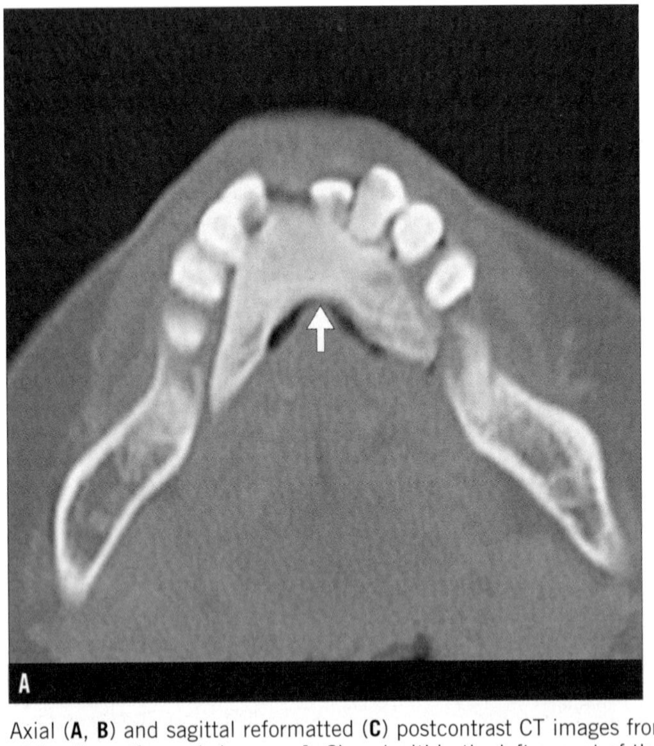

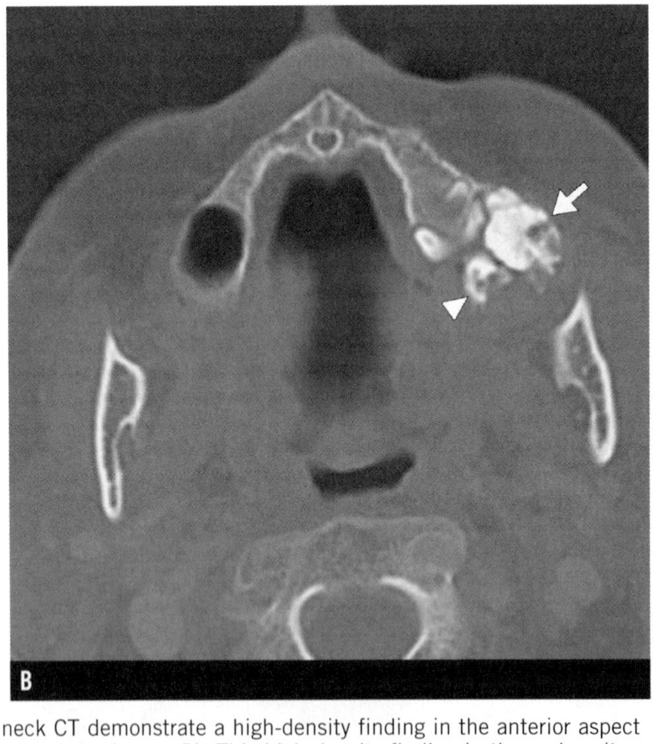

Axial (**A**, **B**) and sagittal reformatted (**C**) postcontrast CT images from a neck CT demonstrate a high-density finding in the anterior aspect of the floor of mouth (arrows, **A**, **C**) and within the left aspect of the buccal cavity (arrow, **B**). This high-density finding in the oral cavity was misinterpreted as some form of oral prosthesis, although the patient had no history of such a device. This patient was largely non-verbal and very ill during this scan, but was nevertheless given oral contrast for a CT abdomen examination that was to be performed in conjunction with this CT neck examination. Approximately 1 year later, a repeat CT neck was performed. Comparable imaging through the same levels as **A**-**C** (**D**-**F**) demonstrate resolution of the high density in the oral cavity, compatible in retrospect with oral contrast that was not swallowed on the prior examination. A partially imaged single remaining tooth, and not residual contrast, is incidentally noted on images **B** and **E** (arrowheads).

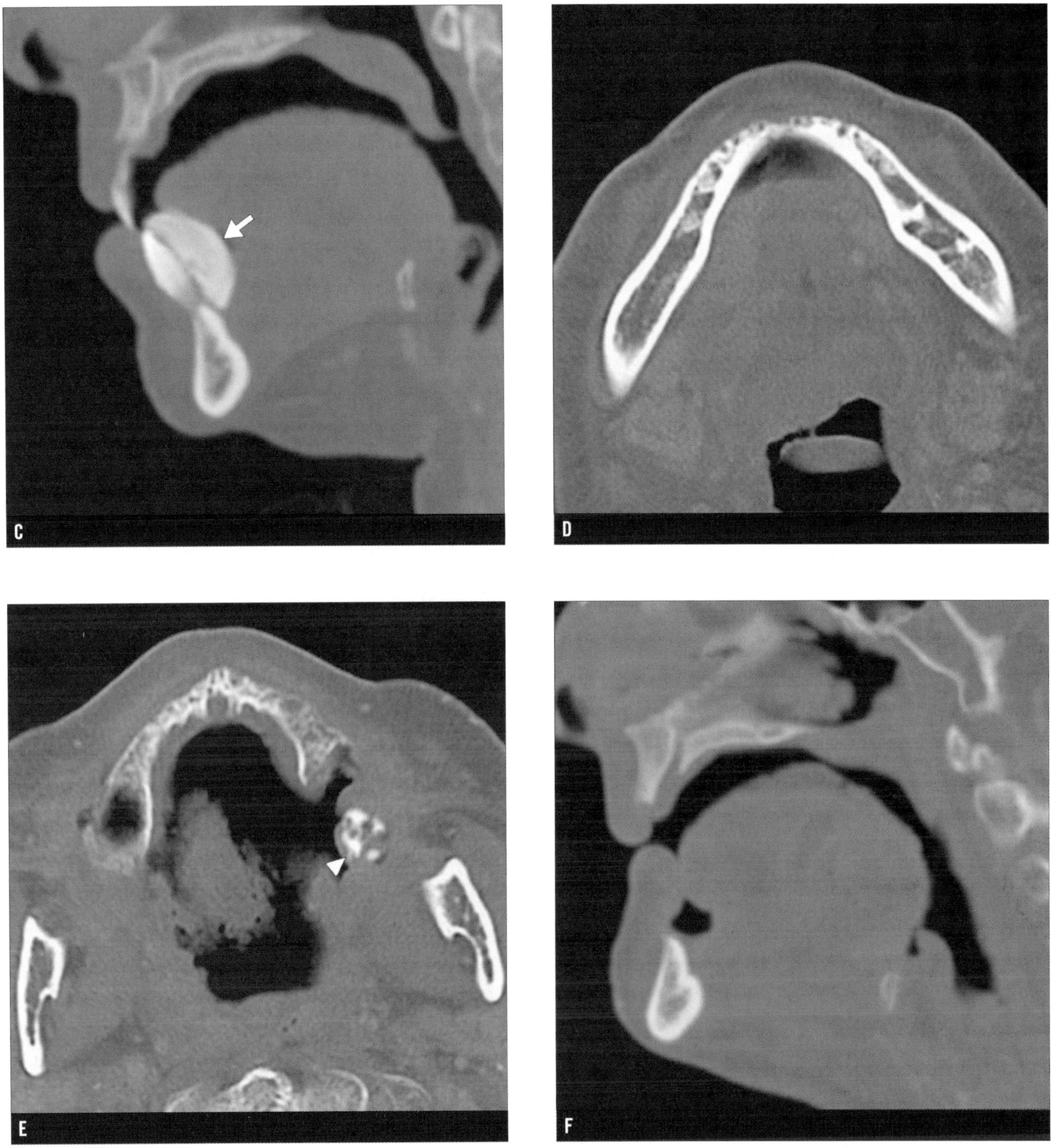

REFERENCES

Jager L, et al. Sialolithiasis:MR sialography of the submandibular duct: an alternative to conventional sialography and US? *Radiology*. 2000;216(3):665-671.

McDermott M, Branstetter BF, Escott EJ. What's in your mouth? The CT appearance of comestible intraoral foreign bodies. *AJNR Am J Neuroradiol.* 2008;29(8):1552-1555.

Towbin AJ. The CT appearance of intraoral chewing gum. *Pediatr. Radiol.* 2008;38(12):1350-1352.

CASE 19 Piercings

Oral piercings are becoming increasingly popular in today's society. The most common oral piercings include the tongue, labiomental groove, lip, and cheek. Jewelry used for piercing is most commonly made from metals such as stainless steel or titanium, but may also be made from synthetic materials, such as polytetrafluoroethylene (PTFE), nylon, or plastics. On imaging, it is important to be aware of potential complications that may occur in a patient with an oral piercing, including an associated soft tissue infection, hematoma, or a dental fracture.

Lip piercing

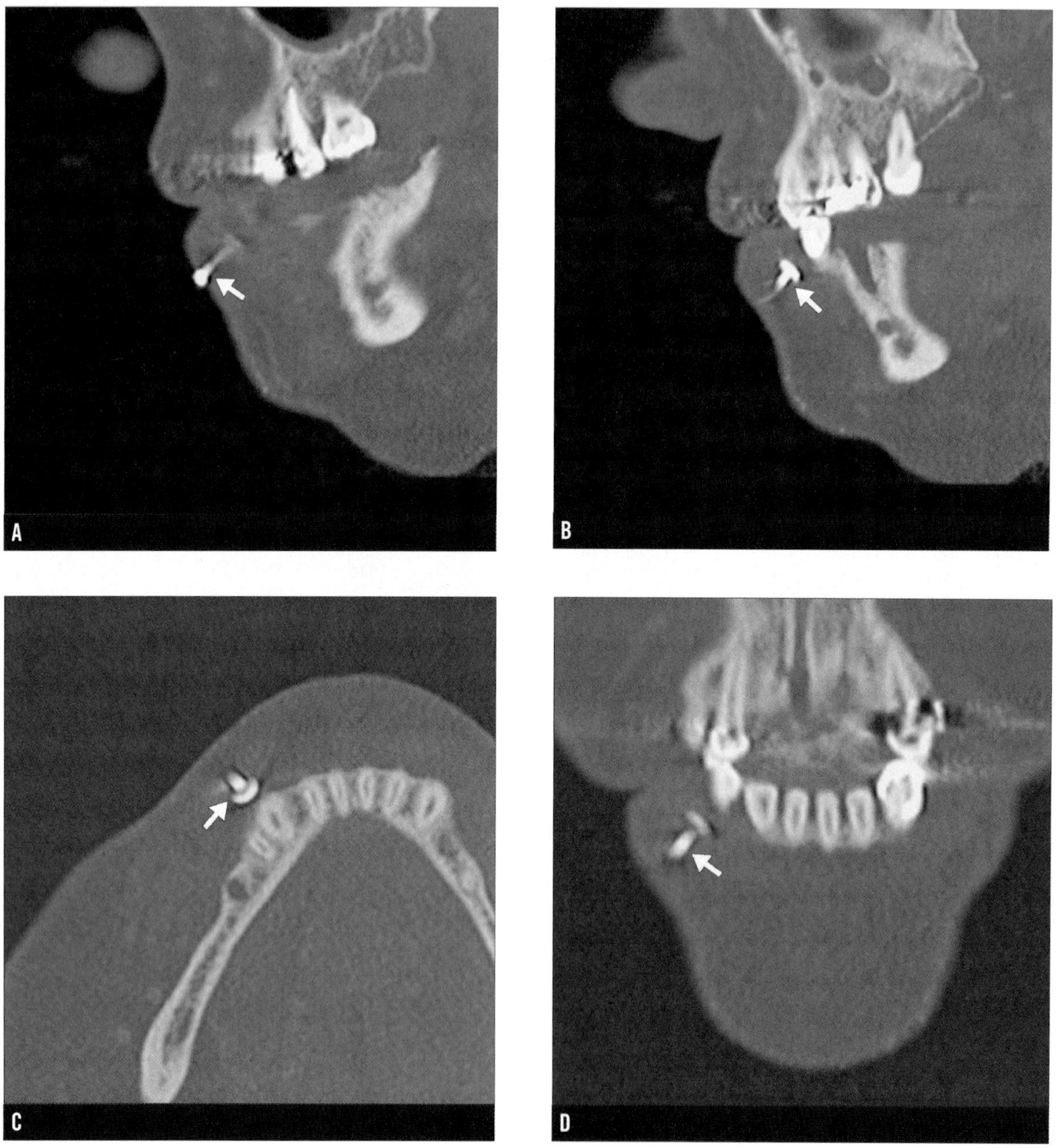

Sagittal reformatted (**A**, **B**), axial (**C**), and coronal reformatted (**D**) CT images demonstrate a metallic piercing along the right aspect of the lower lip (arrows, **A-D**).

Tongue piercing

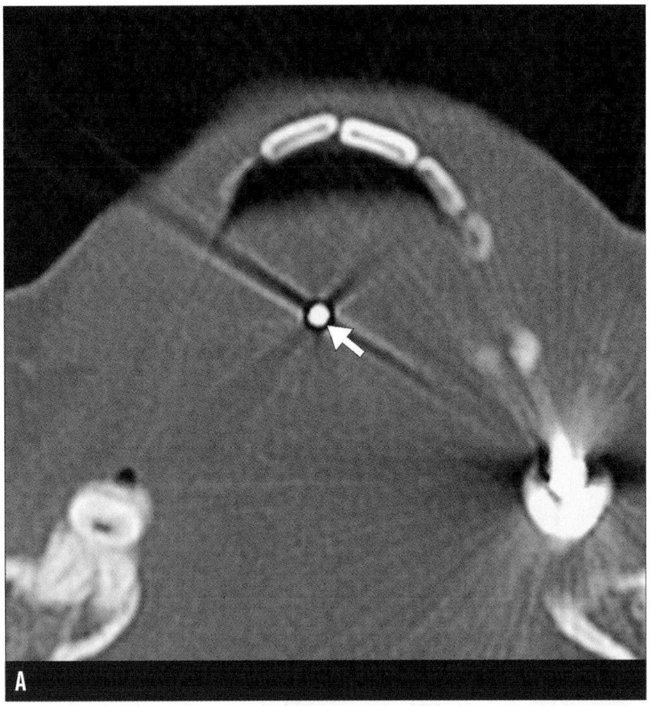

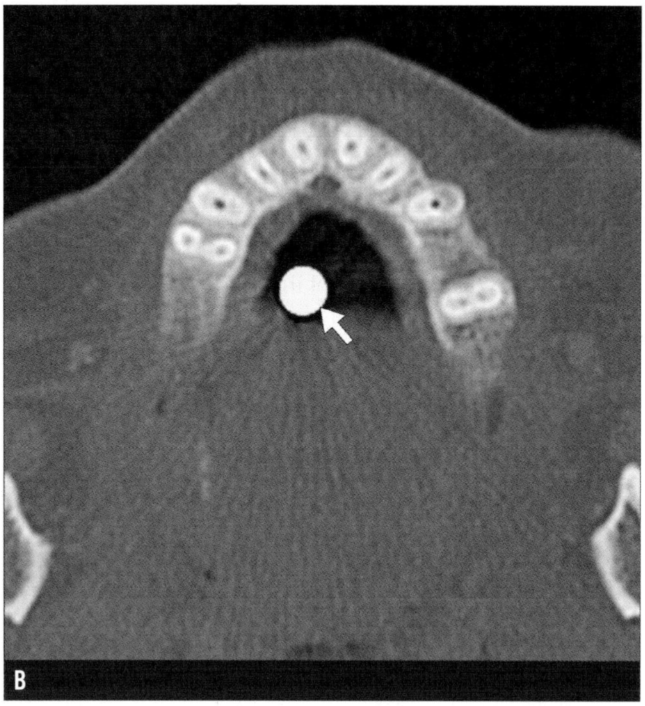

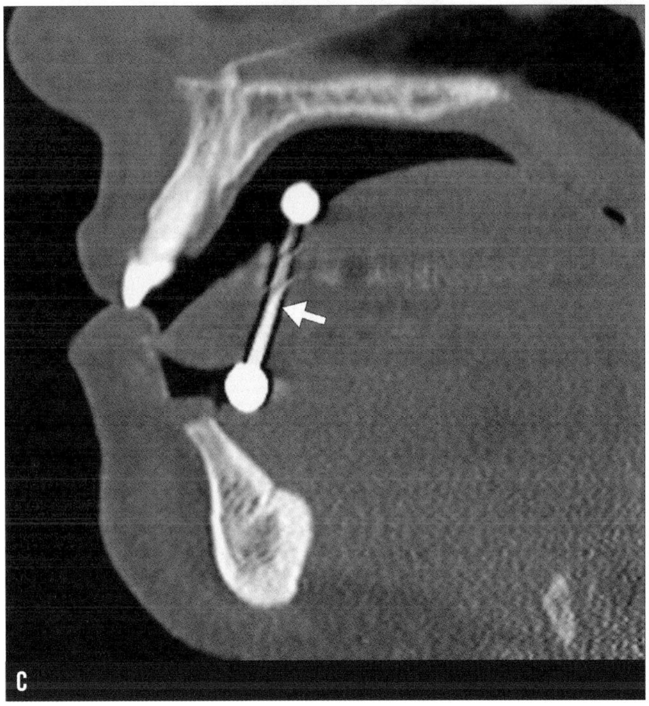

Axial (**A**, **B**) and sagittal reformatted (**C**) CT images demonstrate a tongue piercing through the anterior aspect of the oral tongue (arrows, **A-C**).

REFERENCES

Inchingolo F, et al. Oral piercing and oral diseases: a short time retrospective study. *Int J Med Sci.* 2011;8(8):649-652.

Ziebolz D, et al. Long-term effects of tongue piercing—a case control study. *Clin Oral Invest.* 2012;16(1):231-237.

CASE 20 Oropharyngeal airway device and bite blocks

In addition to endotracheal and enteric tubes, there are several other intraoral objects that may be used in the hospital or acute setting. Two of the most commonly encountered are the plastic oropharyngeal airway device and bite block. The oropharyngeal airway is a curved plastic device that parallels the contour of the tongue. It functions to prevent posterior displacement of the tongue and subsequent oropharyngeal airway compromise. Bite blocks are placed between the teeth to prevent chewing of an endotracheal and/or orogastric tube as well as to prevent biting of the tongue. Gauze bite blocks are created by rolling gauze into a tubular-shaped structure. A tongue depressor or other rigid structure may be used within a gauze bite block to add strength. A gauze bite block is typically low in attenuation and usually contains air which insinuates between the gauze fibers. Other objects, such as a syringe, may also be used as a bite block.

Oropharyngeal airway device

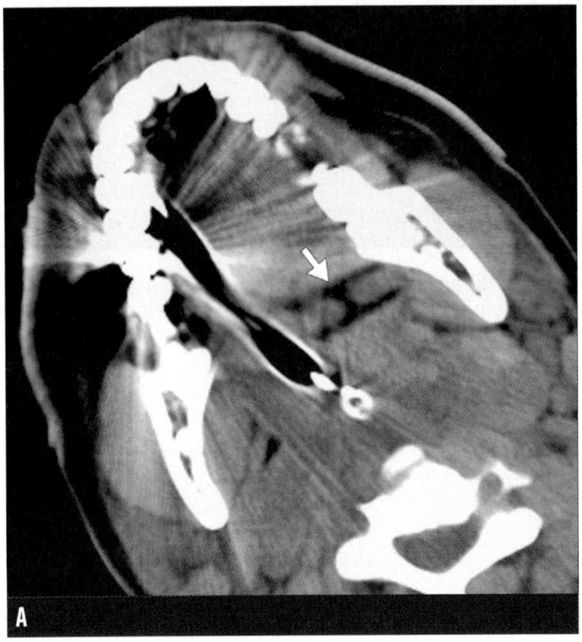

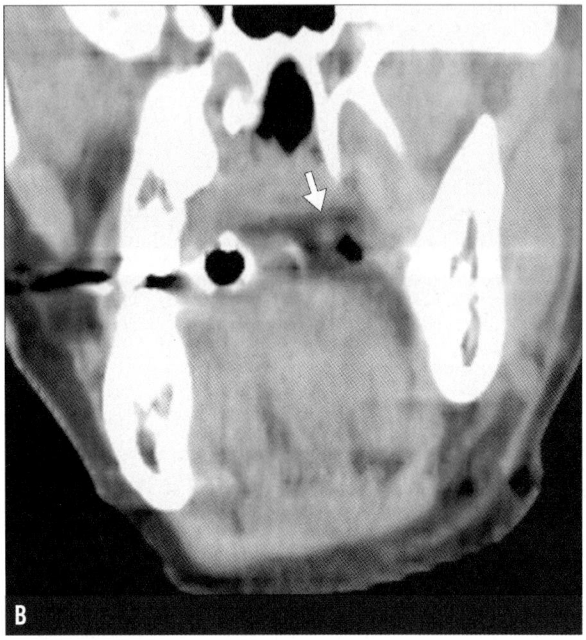

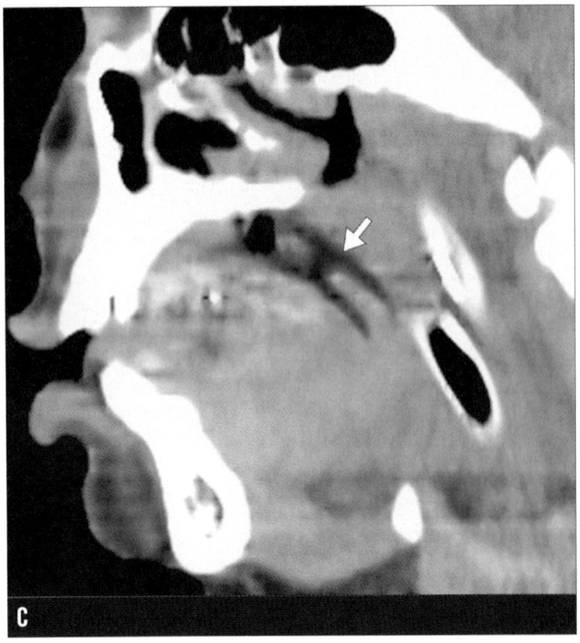

Axial (**A**), coronal reformatted (**B**), and sagittal reformatted (**C**) unenhanced CT images demonstrate an intubated patient with a polyethylene oropharyngeal airway device located in the oral cavity (arrows, **A-C**).

Gauze bite block

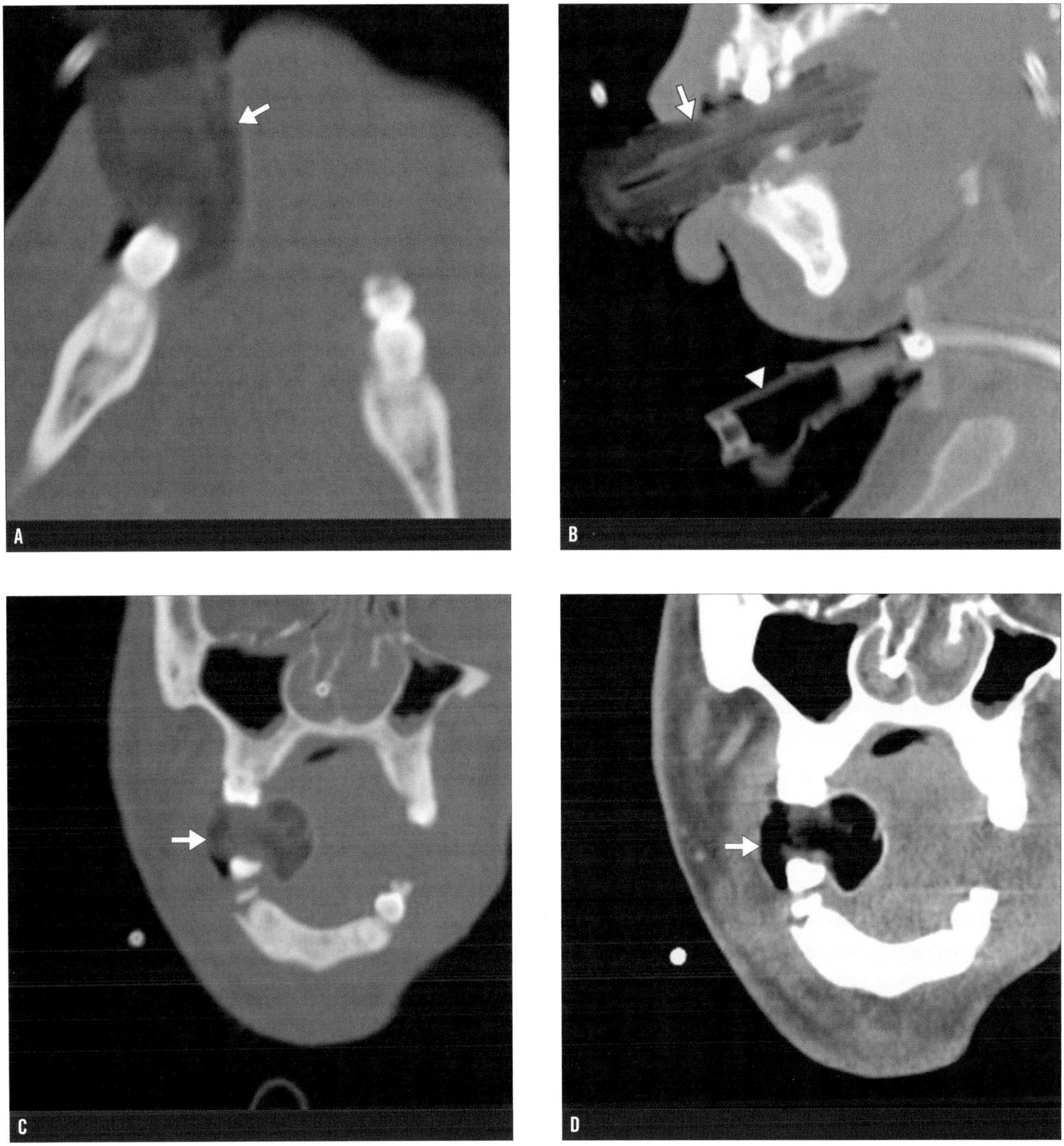

Axial (**A**), sagittal reformatted (**B**), and coronal reformatted (**C**) CT images viewed with a bone window demonstrates a bite block (arrows, **A-C**), which was created by the clinician by wrapping gauze around a flat, firm structure. A coronal reformatted CT image viewed with a soft tissue window (**D**) best demonstrates the air within the interstices of the gauze bite block (arrow, **D**). This patient has a tracheostomy tube also in place (arrowhead, **B**).

Syringe bite block

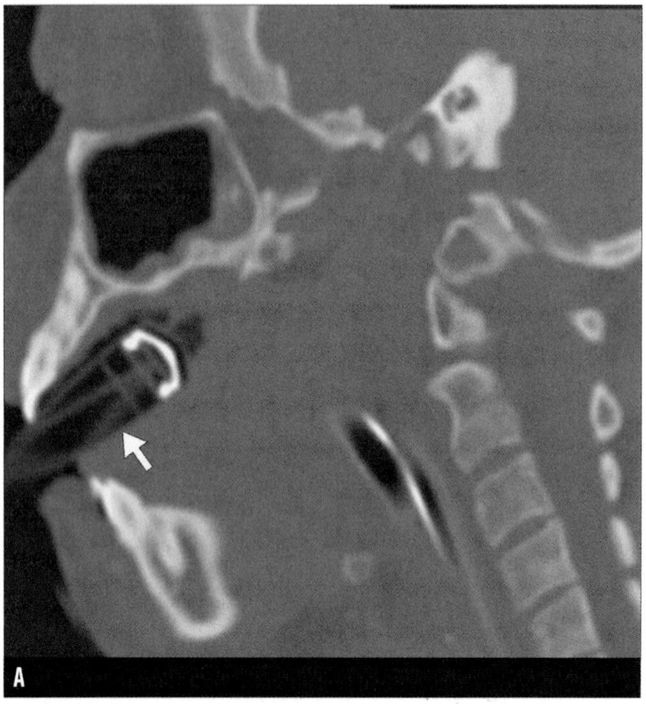

A single sagittal reformatted CT image (**A**) demonstrates a syringe being used as a bite block (arrow).

REFERENCES

Keller C, Sparr HJ, Brimacombe JR. Laryngeal mask bite blocks—rolled gauze versus Guedel airway. *Acta Anaesthesiol Scand.* 1997;41(9):1171-1174.

Kojima Y, Ina H, Yokuta S. Double gauze bite block for orotracheally intubated patients. *J Anesth.* 2005;19(3):271-272.

CASE 21 Palatal sutures mimicking a fracture

The hard palate is comprised of two palatal processes of the maxilla, and just posterior to them, two horizontal plates of the palatine bones. These bones are fused to each other and to the maxilla by several sutures. The palatal processes of the maxilla are fused at the midline by an anterior to posterior (AP) directed suture termed the mid-palatal suture (also called median palatal or intermaxillary suture), whereas the horizontal plates of the palatine bones are fused at the midline by an AP directed interpalatine suture. The transverse palatine suture (also called palatomaxillary suture) joins the posterior margin of the palatal processes of the maxilla and the anterior margins of the horizontal plates of the palatine bones. The ventral margins of the palatal processes of the maxilla are attached to the premaxilla by the premaxillary suture, located immediately posterior to the level of the nasopalatine canal.

Fusion of the mid-palatal suture is rarely complete before the third decade of life. If visible, the sutures of the hard palate can be usually differentiated from palatal fractures by their typical location as well as by their corticated margins.

COMPANION CASES

- **Palate fracture**. Fractures of the palate may occur in many orientations, including sagittal/parasagittal, transverse, oblique, and palato-alveolar. Palato-alveolar fractures occur at the junction of the hard palate and alveolar ridge, and they may occur at any location along the maxillary alveolar ridge. While most palatal fractures are readily identifiable, some palatal fractures may simulate the normal palatal sutures. For example, a sagittal directed fracture may simulate the mid-palatal or interpalatine sutures, a transverse fracture may simulate the transverse palatine suture, and an anteriorly located, transversely oriented palato-alveolar fracture may simulate the premaxillary suture.
- **Cleft palate**. A cleft lip and palate may be unilateral or bilateral, and may be characterized as an isolated cleft lip or a combined cleft lip and palate. A cleft palate may be further characterized as complete or incomplete. As the name implies, an isolated cleft lip only involves the lip. A combined cleft lip and palate extends from the lip through the maxillary alveolus, most commonly between the lateral incisor and the cuspid tooth. The cleft then extends posteriorly along the midline of the palate. A cleft palate may involve the anterior (primary) palate, the posterior (secondary) palate, or both. The primary and secondary palates are subdivided by the nearly transversely oriented premaxillary suture located near level of the incisive foramen. In a complete cleft palate, the defect extends through both the primary and secondary palates. In an incomplete cleft palate, the cleft involves only the posterior palate and potentially up to, but not anterior to, the premaxillary suture. Cleft palates may result in velopharyngeal insufficiency, an entity that results in a hypernasal voice, speech problems, and nasal regurgitation of food.

Mid-palatal, interpalatine, and transverse palatine sutures

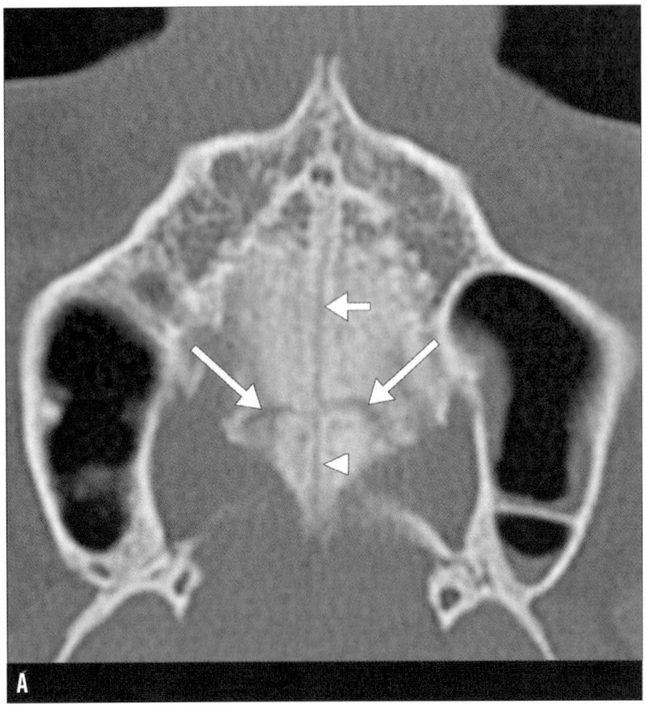

A single axial CT image (**A**) demonstrates the transverse palatine suture (long arrows). The mid-palatal suture (short arrow) and interpalatine suture (arrowhead) are also visible. These sutures can be differentiated from fractures by their typical location and corticated margins.

Mid-palatal, interpalatine, and transverse palatine sutures

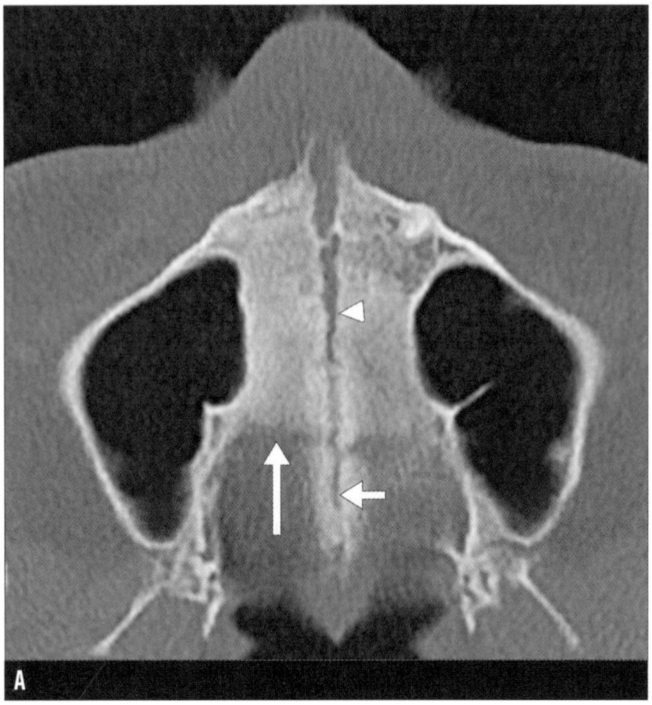

Different patient. A single axial CT image (**A**) demonstrates a fairly wide but normal mid-palatal suture (arrowhead) and interpalatine suture (short arrow). The transverse palatine suture is only faintly visible on this image (long arrow).

Premaxillary suture

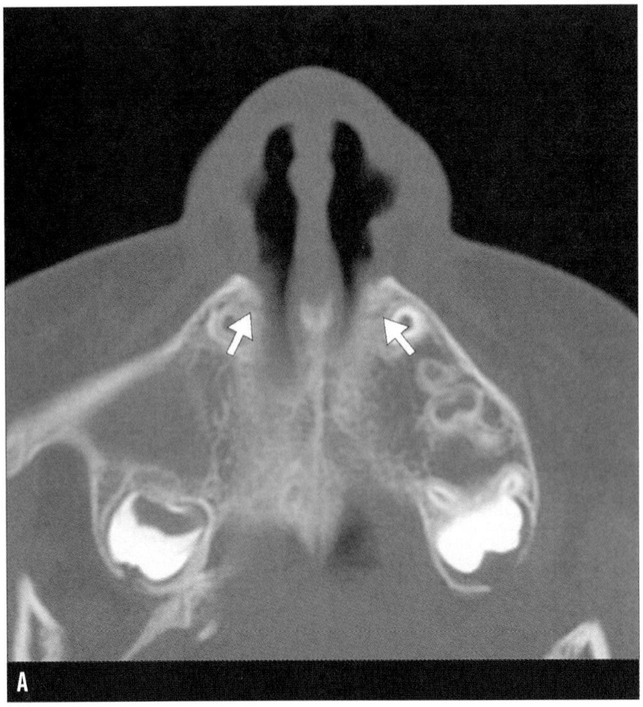

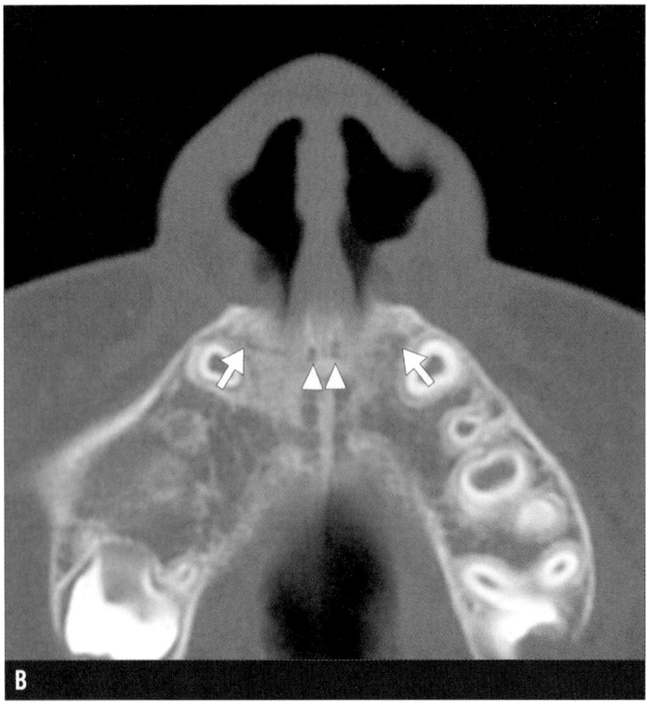

Axial CT images (**A, B**) demonstrate a subtle, normal premaxillary suture (arrows, **A**, **B**). This suture extends into the region two foramina of Stensen near the midline (arrowheads), which are the openings for the nasopalatine foramen.

Premaxillary suture

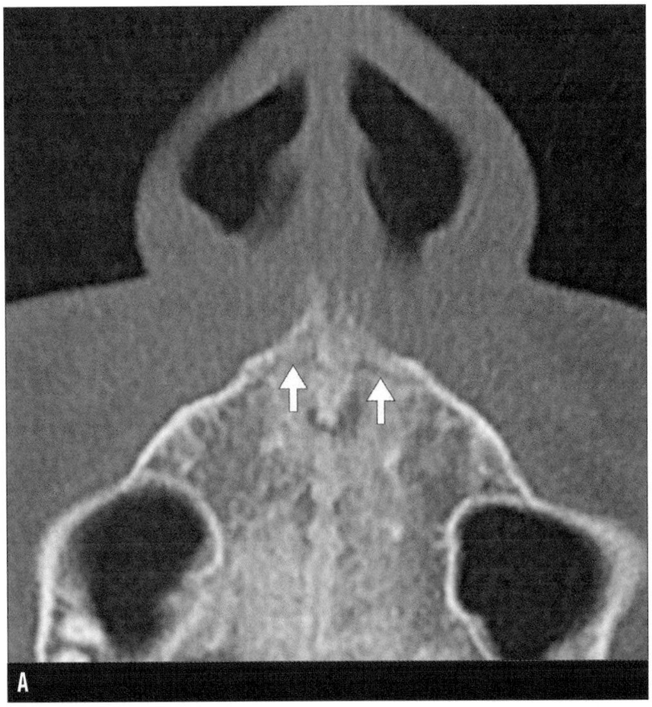

Different patient. An axial CT image (**A**) demonstrates a typical, normal premaxillary suture (arrows).

Companion case: Palato-alveolar fracture

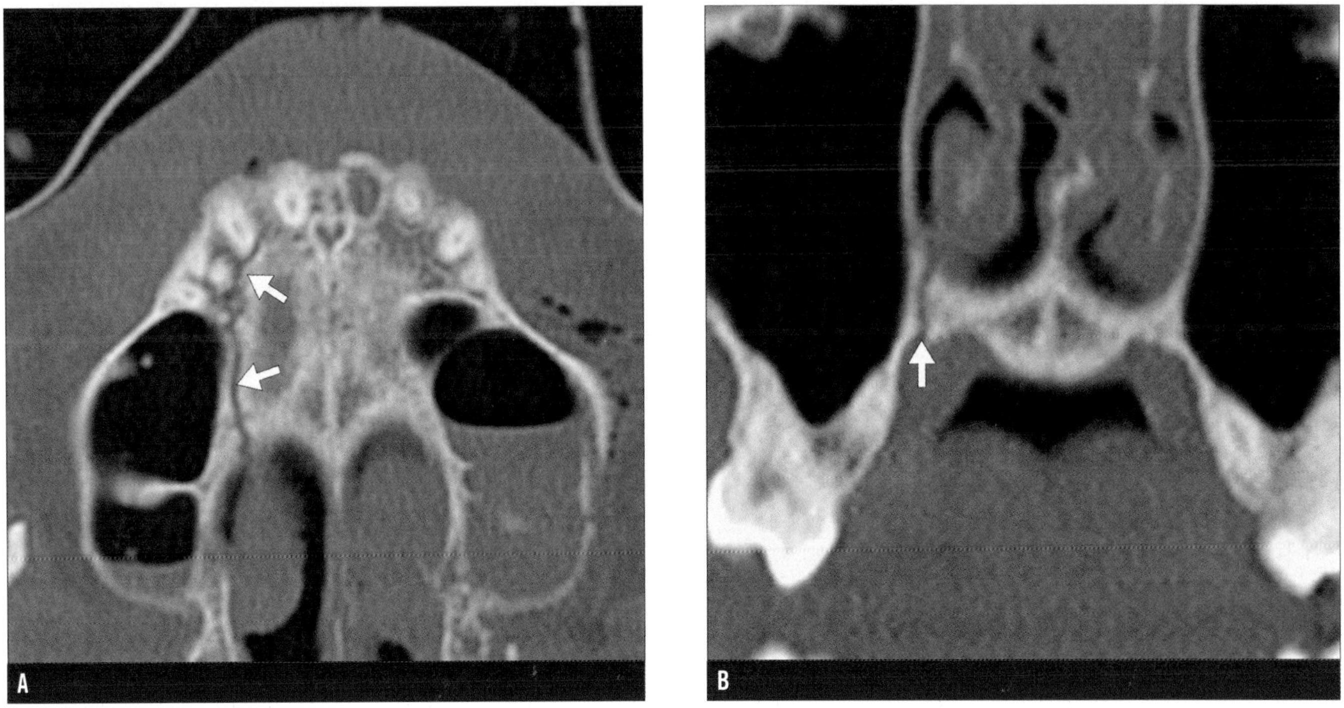

Axial (**A**) and coronal reformatted (**B**) CT images demonstrate a fracture through the hard palate and alveolar ridge, compatible with a palato-alveolar fracture (arrows, **A**, **B**).

Companion case: Transverse palate fracture

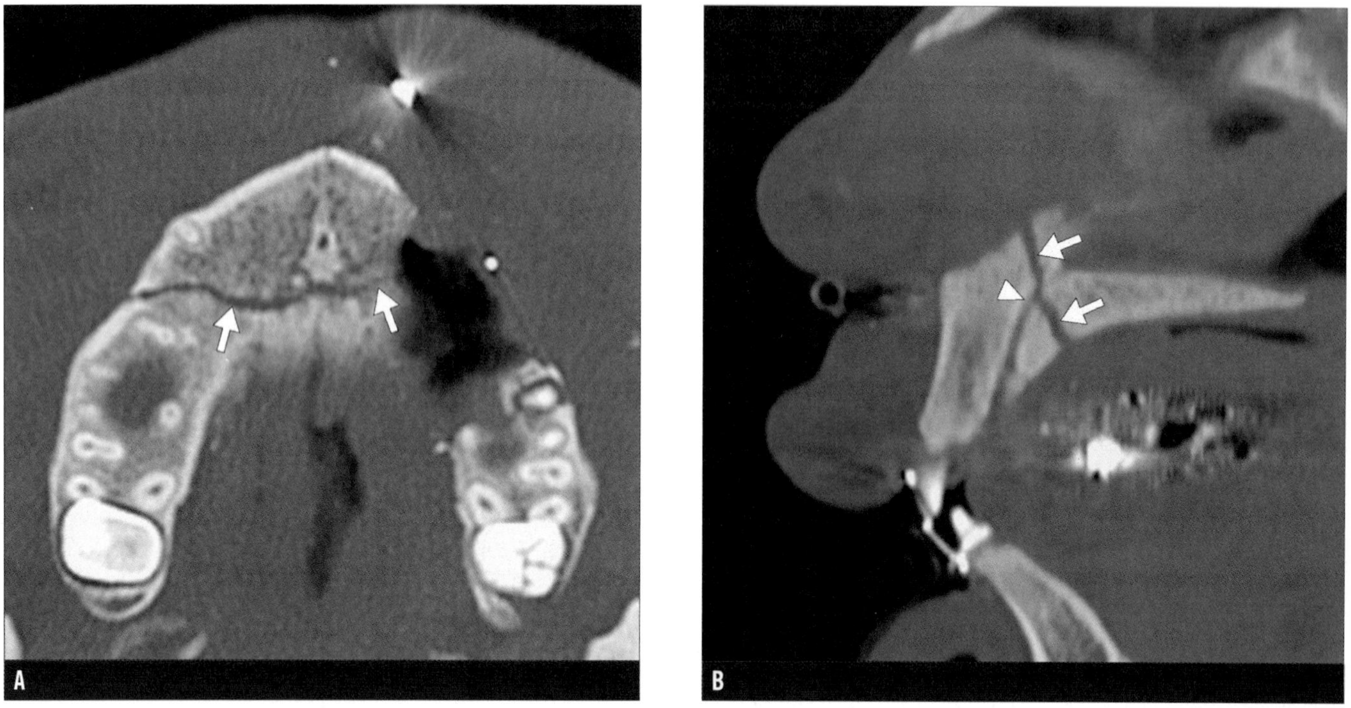

Axial (**A**) and sagittal reformatted (**B**) CT images demonstrate an acute transverse fracture through the anterior aspect of the hard palate (arrows, **A**, **B**). This fracture is similar in orientation to the normal premaxillary suture, although the margins of this finding are not corticated and the lucency extends to the cortex, typical of an acute fracture. The fracture line traverses the superior aspect of the nasopalatine canal (arrowhead, **B**) and therefore may involve the nasopalatine nerve.

Companion case: Complete cleft palate

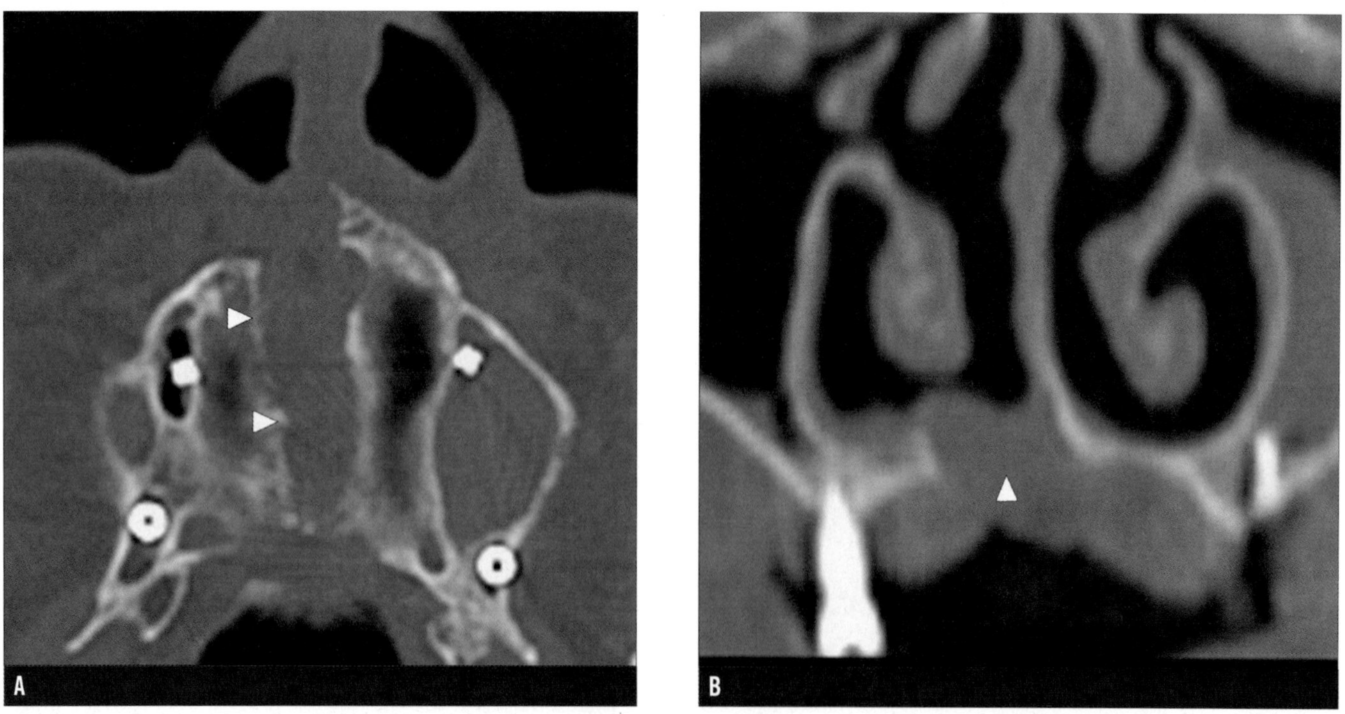

Axial (**A**) and coronal reformatted (**B**) CT images demonstrate a wide osseous defect through the maxillary alveolus and midline hard palate involving both the primary and secondary palates, compatible with a complete cleft palate (arrowheads, **A**, **B**).

Companion case: Incomplete (posterior) cleft palate

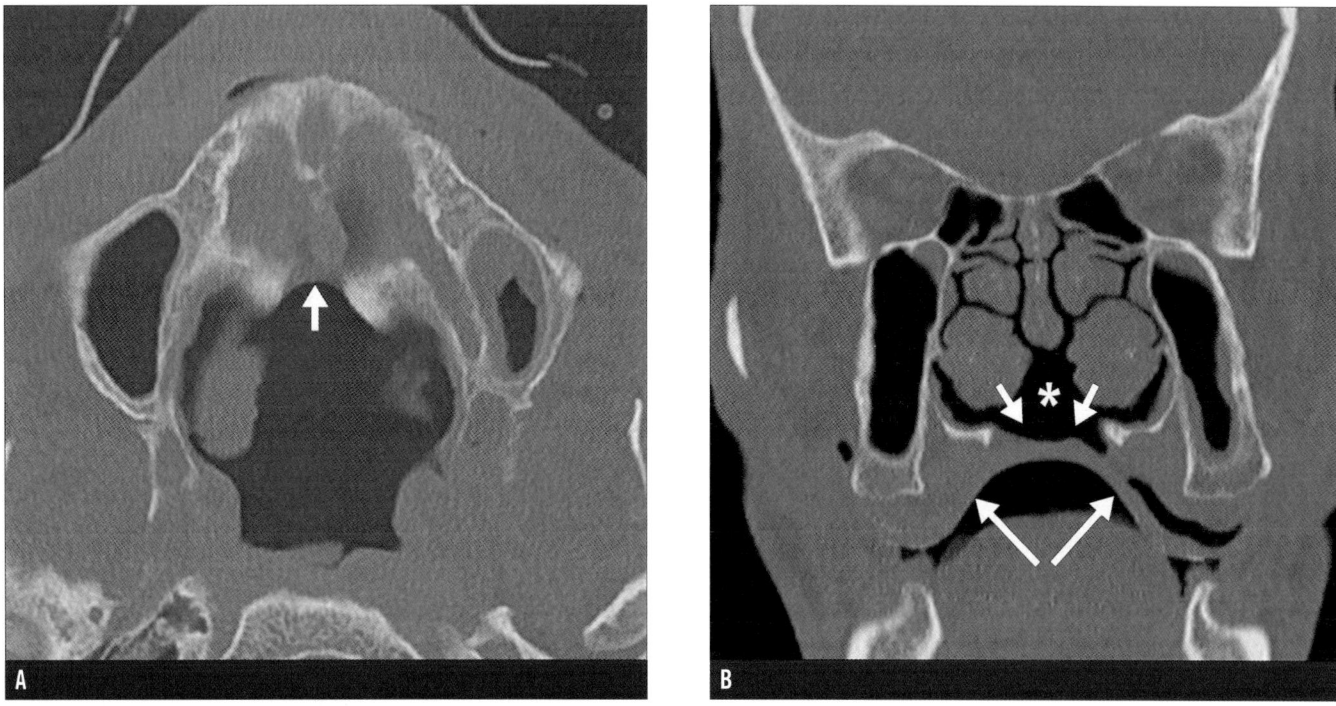

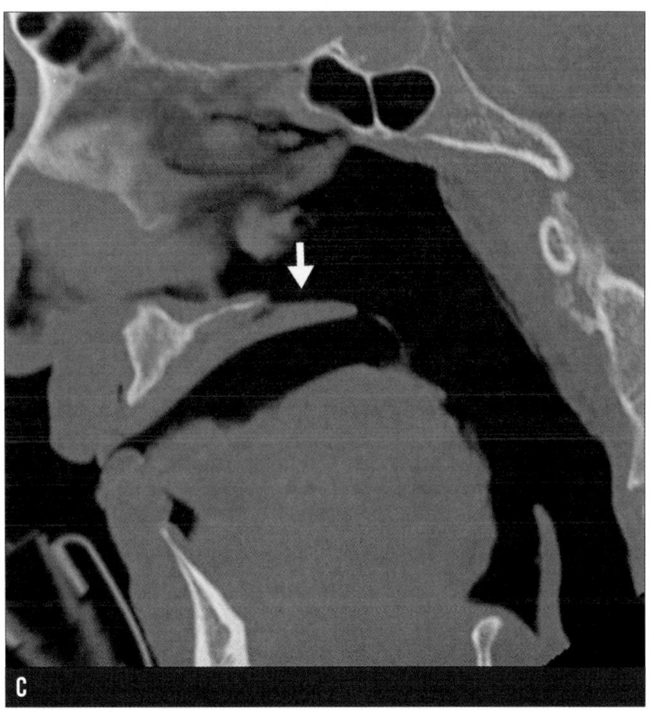

Axial (**A**), coronal reformatted (**B**), and sagittal reformatted (**C**) CT images demonstrate a wide defect involving the posterior aspect of the cleft palate (small arrows, **A-C**) as well as an associated deficiency of the nasal septum vomer (asterisk, **B**). Than anterior-most aspect of the hard palate (primary palate) is intact, and thus the finding is consistent with an incomplete, or posterior, cleft palate. A dental base from dentures (long arrows, **B**) effectively acts as palatal obturator, aiding in preventing nasal regurgitation of food.

REFERENCES

Baxter DJ, Shroff MM. Developmental maxillofacial anomalies. *Semin Ultrasound CT MRI.* 2011;32(6):555-568.

Lantham RA. The development, structure and growth pattern of the human mid-palatal suture. *J Anat.* 1971;108:31-41.

Pollock RA. The search for the ideal fixation of palatal fractures: innovative experience with a mini-locking plate. *Craniomaxillofac Trauma Reconstr.* 2008;1(1):15-24.

Skrzat J, Holiat D, Walocha J. A morphometrical study of the human palatine sutures. *Folia Morphol.* 2003;62(2):123-127.

CASE 22 Orthognathic surgery: Le Fort I and bilateral sagittal split osteotomies

There have been many surgical advancements over the years for the treatment of maxillary-mandibular size discrepancies, specifically, those patients who have maxillary or mandibular prognathia (jaw protrustion) or retrognathia (jaw retrusion). These procedures include the Le Fort I osteotomy, bilateral sagittal split osteotomy, and the horizontal sliding genioplasty. Any or a combination of these procedures may be performed for aesthetic purposes in order to correct a particular facial abnormality. During a Le Fort I osteotomy, the maxilla is mobilized via a horizontal osteotomy. The mobilized maxilla is then advanced anteriorly or retruded, as needed, and then plated in place. A Le Fort I osteotomy may also be paired with vertical maxillary osteotomies in order to enlarge or contract the maxilla in the craniocaudal dimension.

The bilateral sagittal split osteotomy (also called lateral mandibular osteotomy or ramus osteotomy) is a procedure that may be utilized to protrude or retrude the mandible. This paired osteotomy is made in an oblique fashion from anterior to posterior anywhere along the rami or bodies of the mandible, with careful attention made to avoid disrupting the adjacent mandibular canal and subsequent neurovascular injury. Various osteotomy shapes may be utilized, with some of the more complex osteotomy shapes performed in order to improve healing or to decrease movement of the mandible across the osteotomy line. Occasionally, bilateral sagittal split osteotomies are paired with a midline mandibular osteotomy to improve a maxillary-mandibular size discrepancy and to ensure that any concurrent dental occlusive abnormality is also corrected. The bilateral sagittal split osteotomy may also be paired with a chin advancement procedure (eg, horizontal sliding genioplasty) to create a more aesthetically pleasing facial profile. Bilateral sagittal split osteotomies may also be performed to treat obstructive sleep apnea. In this setting, the anterior retraction of the anterior mandible afforded by this procedure enlarges a narrowed oropharyngeal airway.

Le Fort I and bilateral sagittal split osteotomies

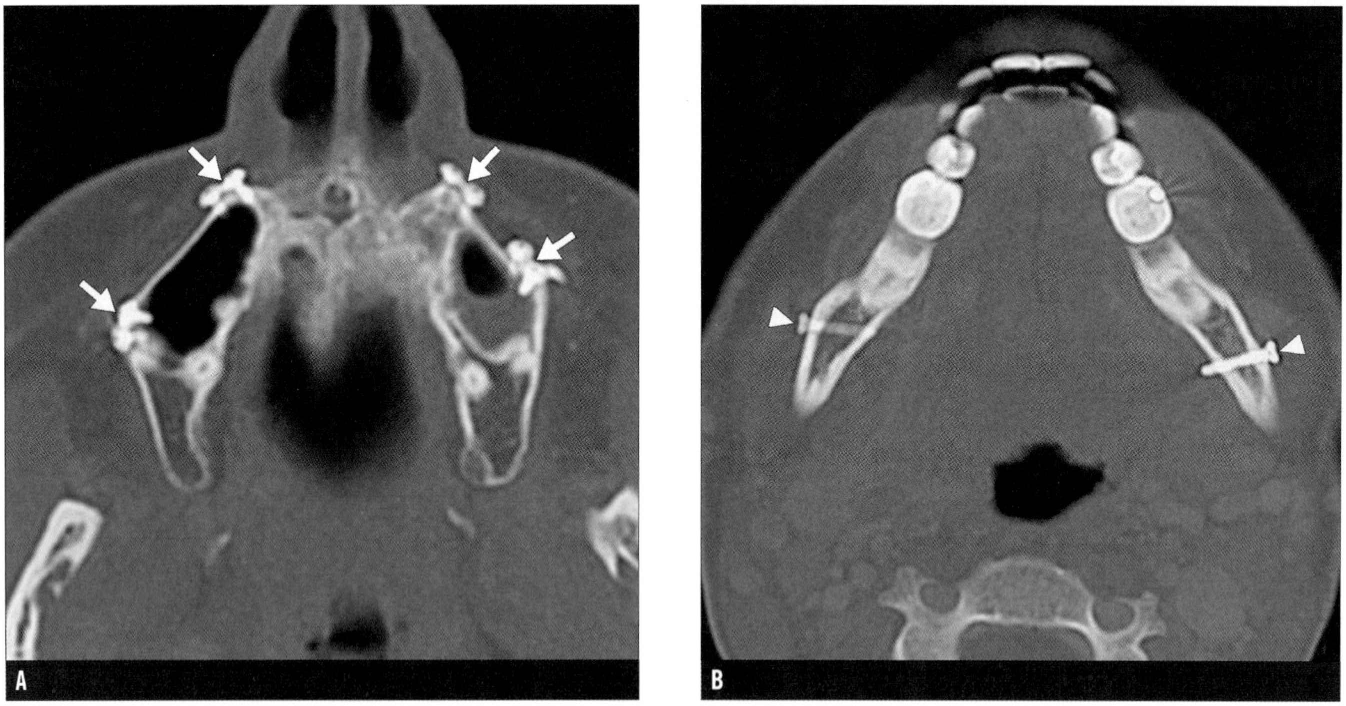

Axial (**A**,**B**), coronal reformatted (**C**), and sagittal reformatted (**D**, **E**) CT images demonstrate multiple plate and screws in the ventral maxilla, related to a Le Fort I osteotomy (arrows, **A**, **E**). There are also screws located along the rami and bodies of the mandible related to bilateral sagittal split osteotomies (arrowheads, **B**, **C**, **D**).

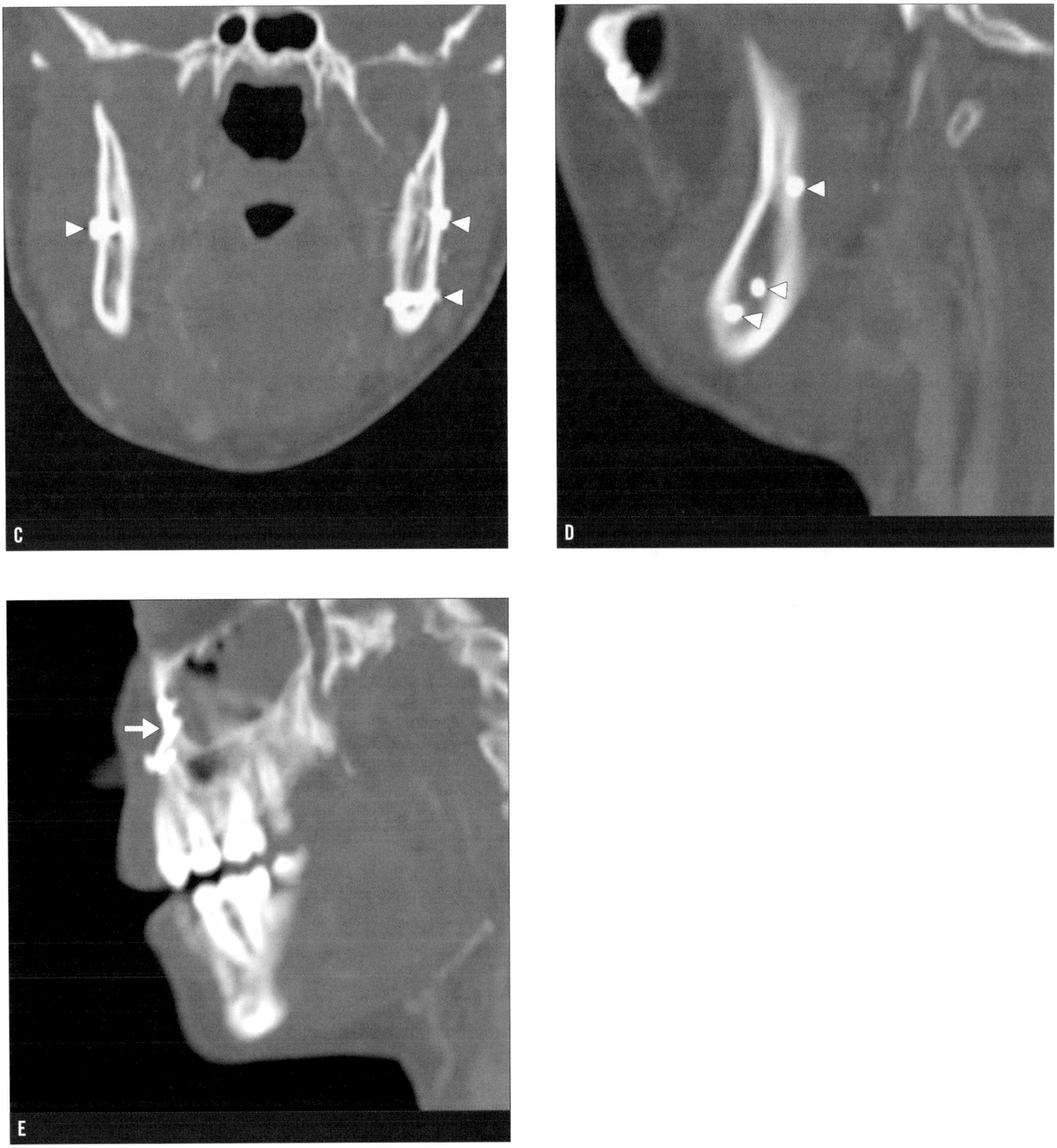
C
D
E

Le Fort I and bilateral sagittal split osteotomies

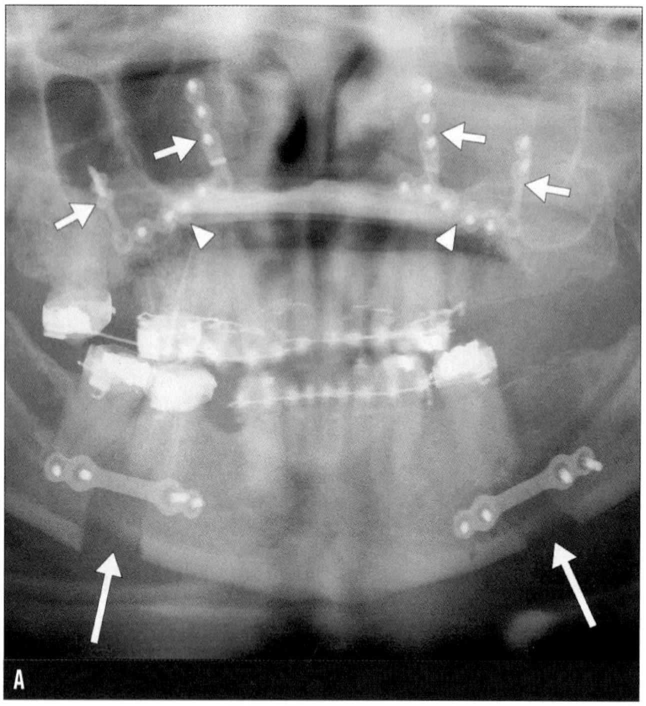

Different patient. A single panorex image (**A**) demonstrates surgical plates and screws along both aspects of the maxilla related to a prior Le Fort I osteotomy as well as bilateral vertical osteotomies that were performed to "constrict" the maxilla. The vertically oriented plates and screws (arrows) affix the Le Fort I osteotomy, whereas the horizontally oriented plate and screws (arrowheads) affix the vertical osteotomies. There are also surgical plates and screws that affix bilateral sagittal split osteotomies (long arrows).

REFERENCES

Anghinoni ML, et al. Midline mandibular osteotomy in an asymmetric patient. *Angle Orthod.* 2009;79(5):1008-1014.

Costello BJ, Posnick JC. The role of maxillofacial osteotomies in the treatment of obstructive sleep apnea. *Curr Opin Otolaryngol Head Neck Surg.* 2003;11(4):267-274.

Dowling PA, et al. LeFort I maxillary advancement: 3-year stability and risk factors for relapse. *Am J Orthod Dentofacial Orthop.* 2005;128(5):560-567.

Prinsell JR. Maxillomandibular advancement surgery in a site-specific treatment approach for obstructive sleep apnea in 50 consecutive patients. *Chest.* 1999;116(6):1519-1529.

Takahashi H, et al. Three lateral osteotomy designs for bilateral sagittal split osteotomy: biomechanical evaluation with three-dimensional finite element analysis. *Head Face Med.* 2010;6(4):1-10.

CASE 23 Orthognathic surgery: Genioglossus advancement surgery

Multiple subtypes of obstructive sleep apnea (OSA) have been described, each named based on the site of primary airway narrowing. For patients with the retrolingual subtype of OSA, genioglossus advancement surgery has been used for correction of this abnormality. The genial tubercle is a small osseous prominence or prominences along the lingual margin of the midline mandible which serves as the osseous site of origin for the genioglossus and geniohyoid muscles. Genioglossus advancement surgery may be performed to treat OSA. One type of genioglossus advancement surgery entails forming an osteotomy along the anterior mandible which encircles the genial tubercle. Various osteotomy shapes have been used, including elliptical, rectangular, and circular. After performing the osteotomy, the osteotomy flap is advanced anteriorly, rotated, and plated in place. By advancing the genial tubercle, there is resultant advancement of the genioglossus muscles and enlargement of the retrolingual airway.

Various other types of mandibular osteotomies have also been used to treat sleep apnea. The bilateral sagittal split osteotomy is one such surgical technique that may be performed to treat sleep apnea, in addition to being utilized for orthognathic procedures. The bilateral sagittal split osteotomy is more fully discussed in the preceding case.

Genioglossus advancement surgery: Elliptical osteotomy type

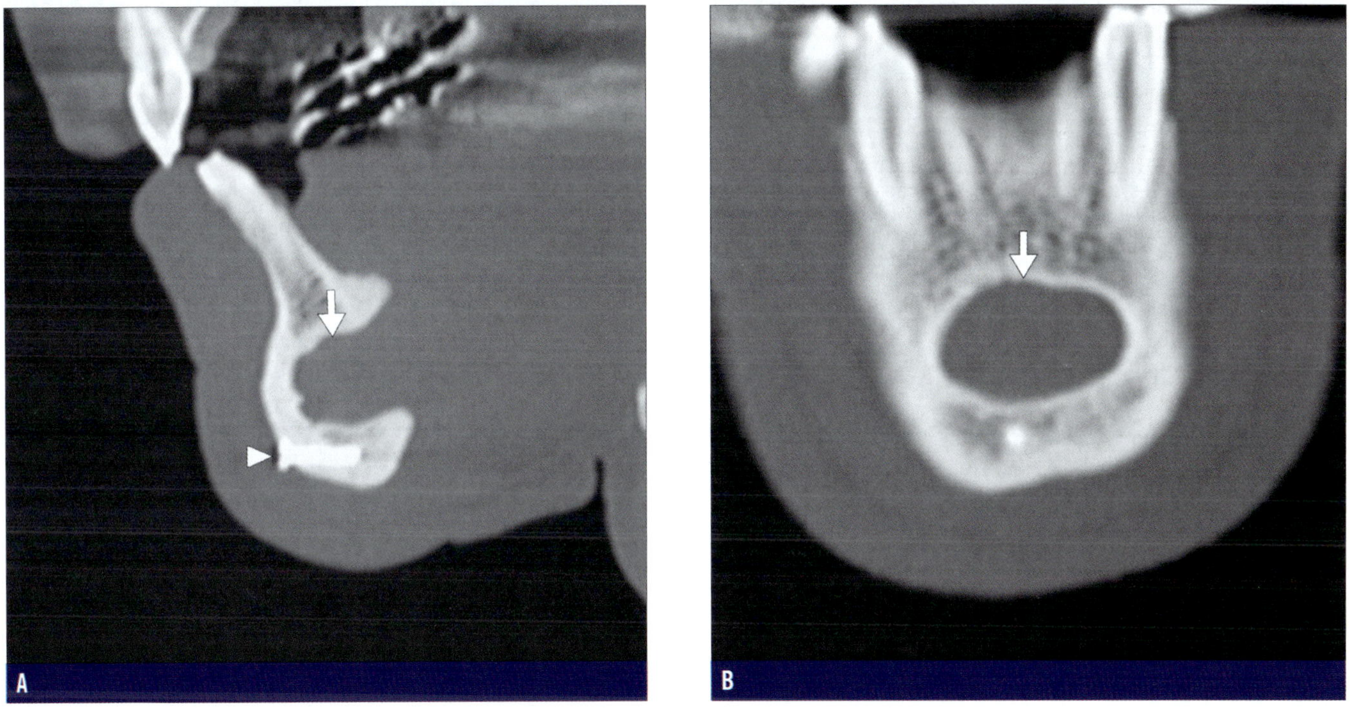

Sagittal reformatted (**A**), coronal reformatted (**B**), and axial (**C**, **D**) CT images demonstrate a well-defined, oval, surgical defect involving the symphysis of the mandible (arrows, **A**, **B**, **D**) with placement of a screw (arrowheads, **A**, **C**) in the symphysis just caudal to the surgical defect. These findings are consistent with genioglossus advancement surgery performed for obstructive sleep apnea. Because of the shape of the osteotomy, this form of genioglossus advancement surgery is termed the elliptical osteotomy type.

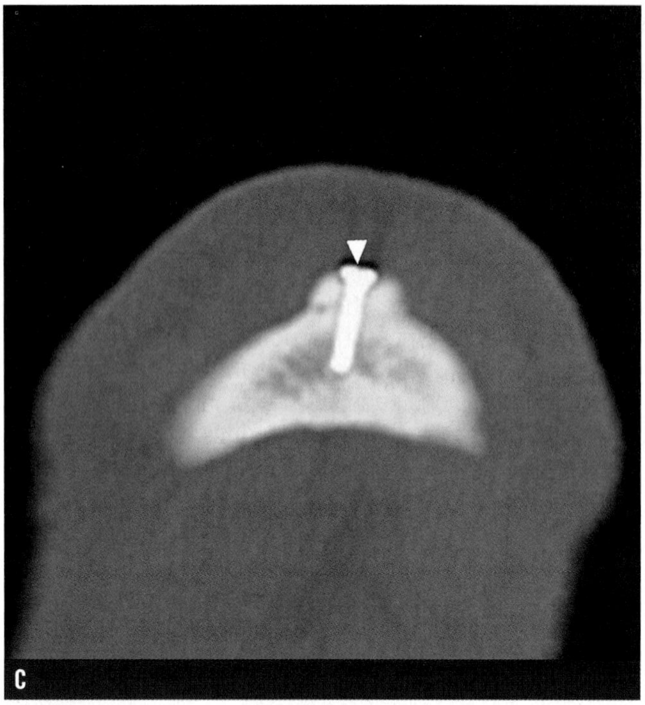

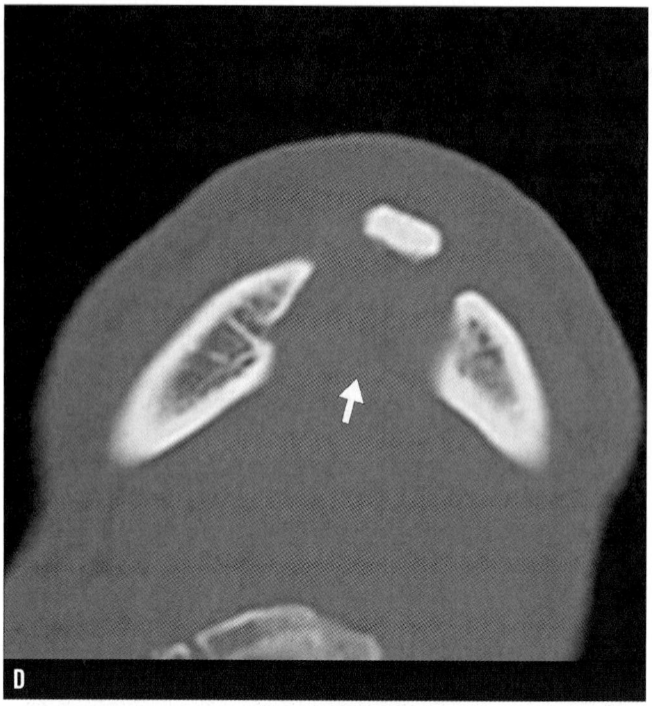

REFERENCES

Hennessee J, Miller FR. Anatomic analysis of the genial bone advancement trephine system's effectiveness at capturing the genial tubercle and its muscular attachments. *Otolaryngol Head Neck Surg.* 2005;133(2): 229-233.

Hueman EM, et al. Accuracy of cone beam computed tomography in determining the location of the genial tubercle. *Otolaryngol Head Neck Surg.* 2007;137(1):115-118.

Meslemani D, Jones LR. Skeletal surgery in sleep apnea. *Curr Opin Otolaryngol Head Neck Surg.* 2011;19(4):307-311.

CASE 24 Midline mandibular osteotomy

A midline mandibular osteotomy is frequently performed when a wide surgical exposure is needed, such as to resect tumors that are located within the deep aspects of the oral cavity and oropharynx or for tumors located in the parapharyngeal space. It may also be performed to improve dental occlusal harmony, often in conjunction with Lefort I and bilateral sagittal split osteotomies. As the name implies, a mandibular split osteotomy entails splitting the mandible in half via a midline osteotomy. The mandible may be widely distracted when performed to improve surgical exposure for a tumor resection. When performed to improve dental occlusion, the mandible may be widened in the transverse dimension (by distracting the bisected mandible), or narrowed in the transverse dimension (by resecting mandibular bone and teeth). Ultimately, the two halves of the mandible are reconnected with surgical plate and screws.

COMPANION CASE

- **Lingual foramen and canal**. The lingual foramen and canal are located at the midline of the mandible (also called symphysis or mentum) and directed anteroposteriorly, with the lingual foramen situated along the lingual surface of the symphysis and the canal often traversing the lingual cortex into a portion of the mandibular symphisis diploic space. The lingual foramen and canal can be single or multiple, with up to four separate canals described in the literature. When solitary, the foramen is typically positioned at or above the level of the genial tubercle. When multiple, one foramen is located superior to the genial tubercle, whereas the additional foramina are typically located inferior to the genial tubercle.

  There is debate in the literature regarding the contents of these canals. A solitary canal (or the canal located superior to the genial tubercle when multiple canals are present) likely transmits small branches of the lingual artery and nerve. When multiple lingual canals are present, the canal or canals located inferior to the genial tubercle likely transmit branches of either the lingual or submental arteries as well as branches of the mylohoid nerve. There have been reports of life-threatening emergencies as a result of arterial injury with subsequent formation of a large floor of mouth hematoma following placement of a dental implant in the region of the lingual foramen.

Midline mandibular osteotomy

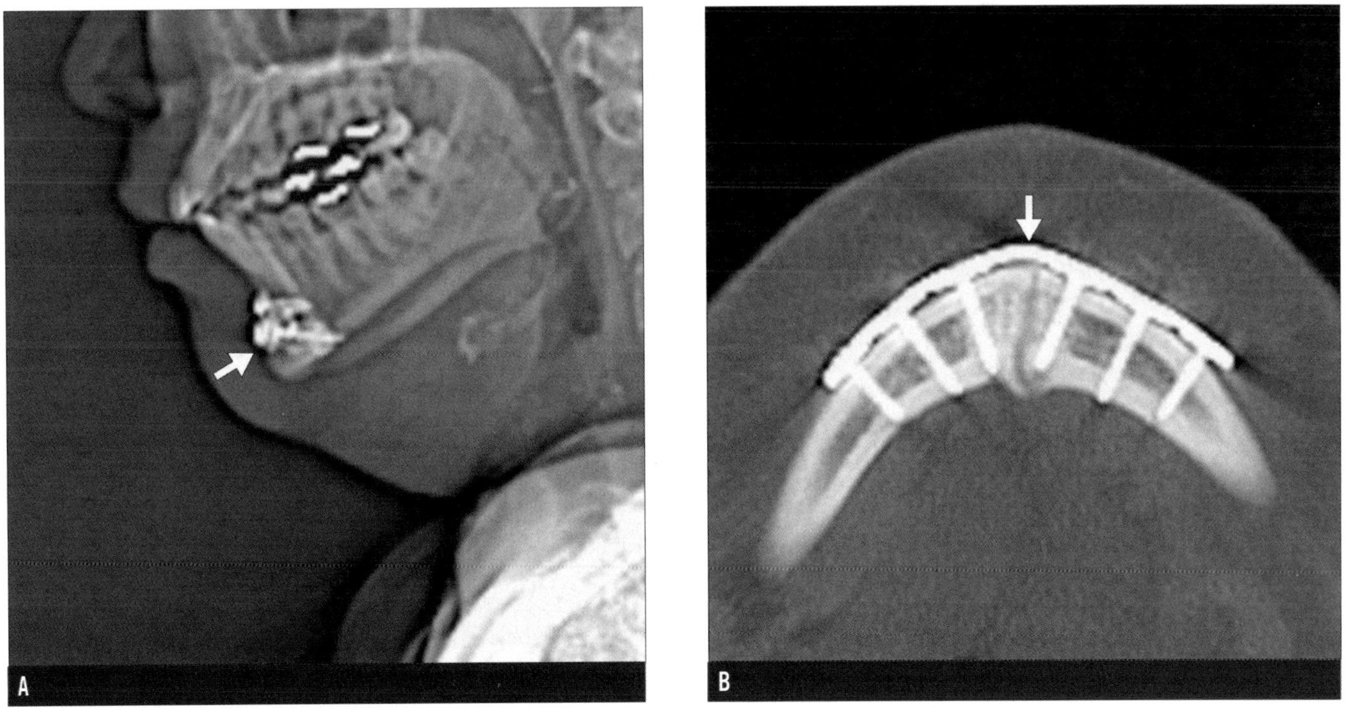

A lateral scout image (**A**) as well as axial (**B**, **C**) CT images demonstrate metallic surgical hardware related to a prior midline mandibular osteotomy (arrows, **A-C**). Image **C** demonstrates a small amount of new bone formation related to osseous healing along the lingual cortex of the midline osteotomy (arrowhead, **C**).

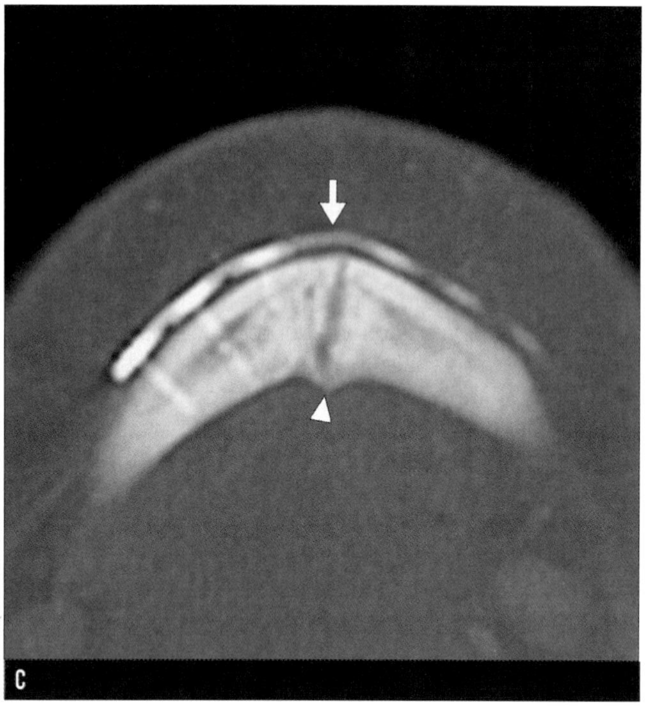

Companion case: Lingual foramen and canal

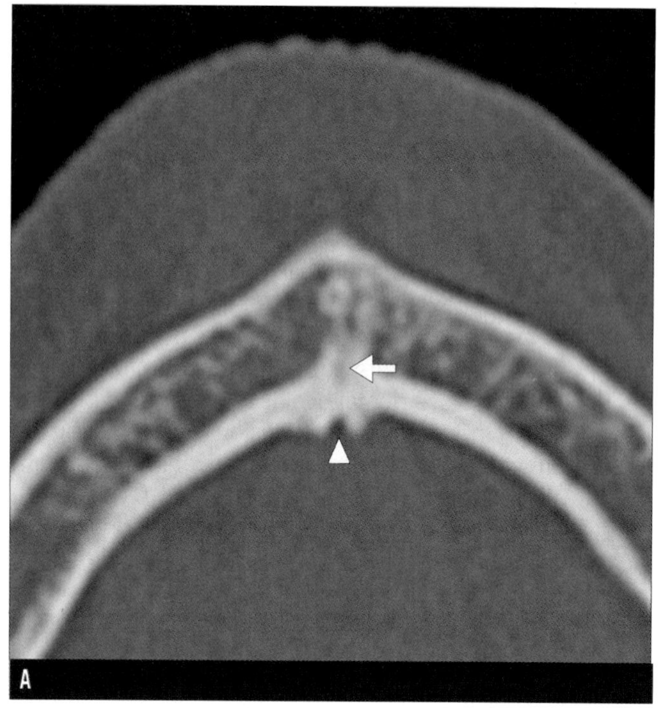

An axial CT image (**A**) demonstrates a normal-appearing lingual foramen (arrowhead) located between paired osseous projections of the genial tubercle. The lingual canal is identified extending into the diploic space of the mandibular symphysis (arrow).

Companion case: Two lingual foramina and canals

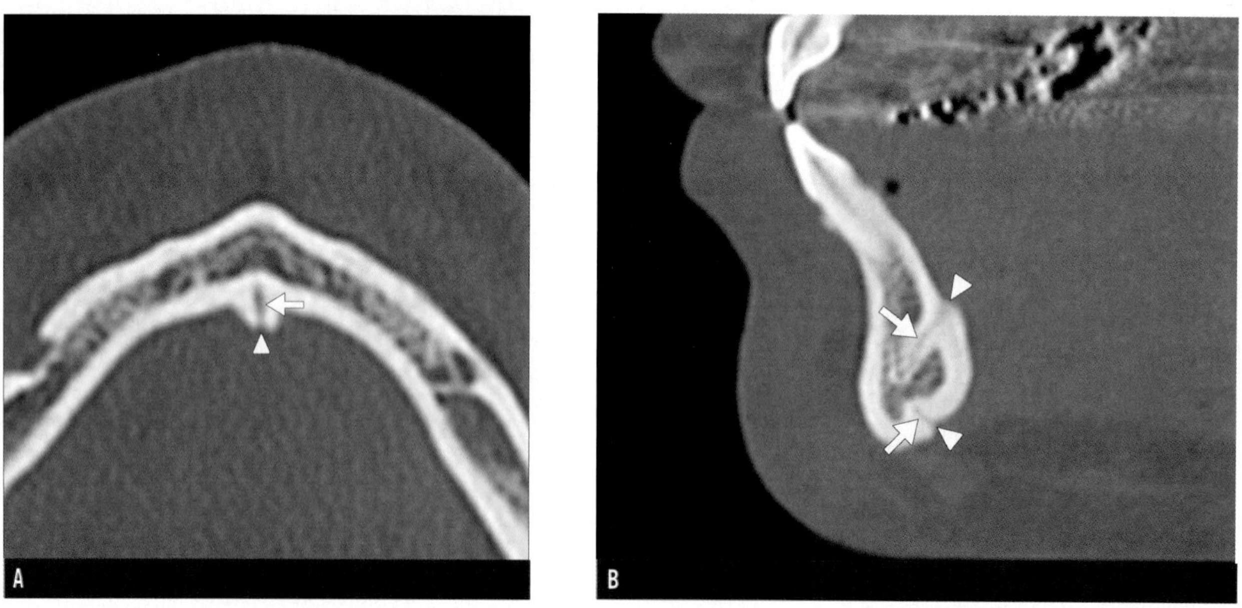

An axial CT image through the superior aspect of the mandibular symphysis (**A**) demonstrates a typical lingual foramen (arrowhead, **A**) and lingual canal (arrow, **A**). A sagittal reformatted CT image through the mandibular symphysis (**B**) demonstrates two separate lingual foramina (arrowheads, **B**) and lingual canals (arrows, **B**), one located at the superior aspect and the other at the inferior aspect of the mandibular symphysis.

REFERENCES

Brusati R, Sesenna E, Mannucci N, Gamoletti R. The midline mandibular osteotomy-ostectomy in the correction of dentofacial deformities. *Int J Adult Orthodon Orthognath Surg.* 1987;2(1):37-50.

Gahleitner A, et al. Lingual vascular canals of the mandible: evaluation with dental CT. *Radiology.* July 2001;220(1):186-189.

Liang X, Jacobs R, Lambrichts I, Vandewalle G. Lingual foramina on the mandibular midline revisited: a macroanatomical study. *Clin Anat.* 2007;20(3):246-251.

McDonnell D, Reza Nouri, Todd ME. The mandibular lingual foramen: a consistent arterial foramen in the middle of the mandible. *J Anat.* 1994;184:363-369.

Rosano G, et al. Anatomic assessment of the anterior mandible and relative hemorrhage risk in implant dentistry: a cadaveric study. *Clin Oral Implants Res.* 2009;20(8):791-795.

Uglesic V, Knezevic P, Kosutic D, Jokic D. Lag screw fixation for straight midline mandibulotomy: four-year experience. *Ann Plast Surg.* 2004;52(4):349-353.

CASE 25 Chin augmentation

Chin augmentation procedures (also called mentoplasty or genioplasty) are surgical procedures that are performed to reshape the contour of the chin. Many different techniques exist for chin augmentation, including implanting bone graft material or implanting synthetic materials such as polytetrafluoroethylene, high-density polyethylene, silicone, and polyester fiber mesh. Other procedures, such as the horizontal sliding genioplasty, may also be performed. The horizontal sliding genioplasty is a procedure that creates a horizontal osteotomy through the caudal aspect of the mandibular mentum. The freed portion of the mandibular mentum is then advanced forward and secured into place with a surgical plate and screws. This procedure can also be used for the treatment of obstructive sleep apnea or may be paired with an orthognathic procedure to enhance the chin profile.

The postoperative imaging appearance of these procedures is highly variable. The appearance of implanted materials on CT depends on the material used. A silicone chin implant tends to have smooth margins and is mildly hyperattenuating, usually between that of muscle and bone. In the case of the horizontal sliding genioplasty, the postsurgical deformity of the mandible is fixed in place with a surgical plate.

Chin augmentation: Synthetic chin implant

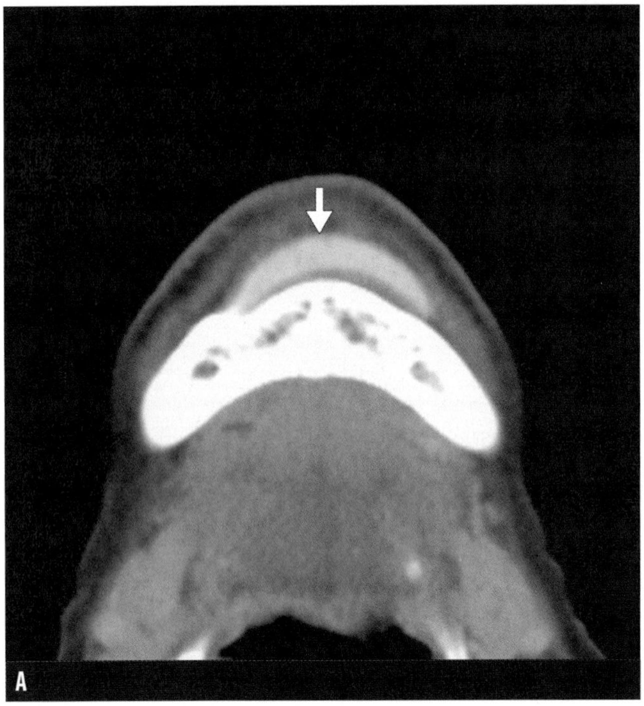

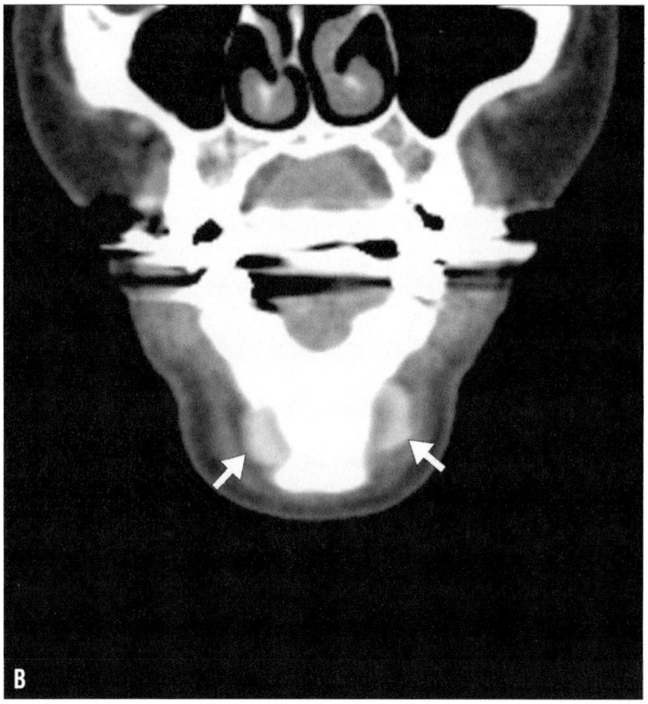

Axial (**A**), coronal reformatted (**B**, **C**), and sagittal reformatted (**D**) CT images demonstrate a foreign body that is closely apposed to the ventral cortex of the mandibular symphysis (arrows, **A-D**). It has a crescent shape, smooth margins, and is of high density, although it is less dense than the adjacent bone. This finding represents a synthetic chin implant.

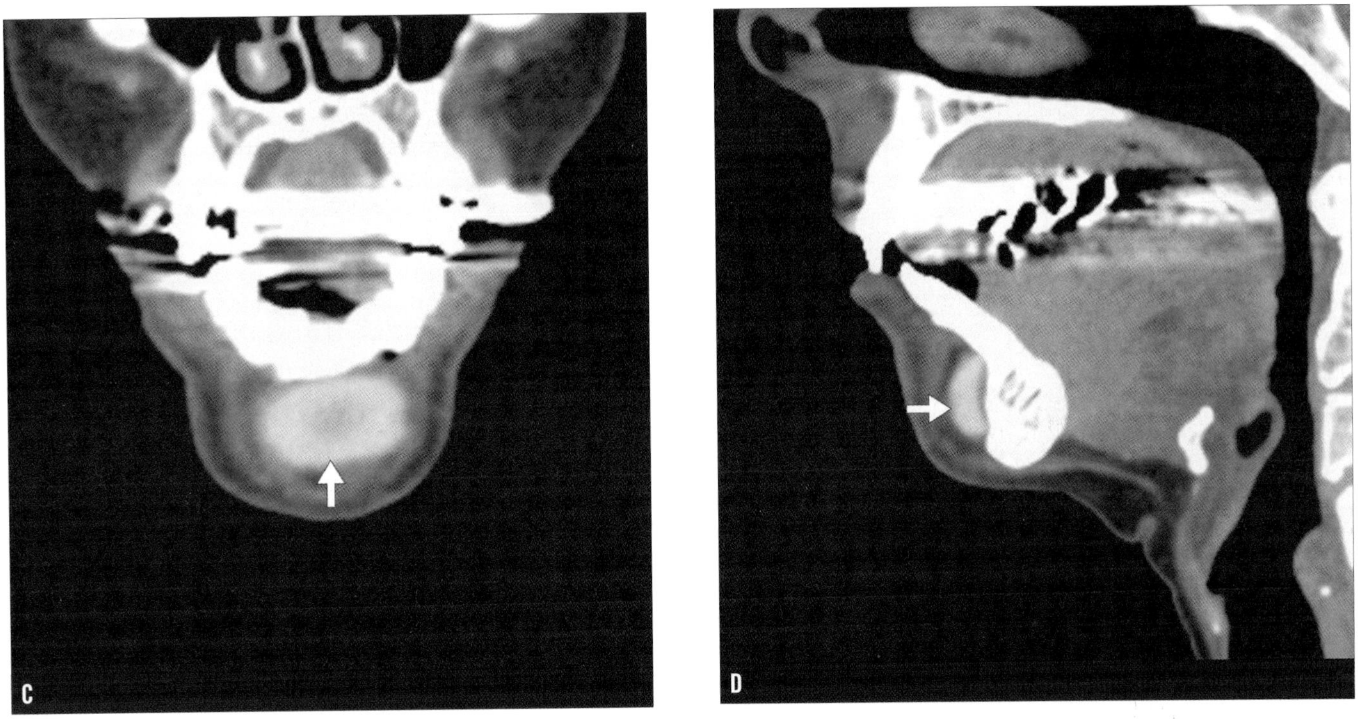

Chin augmentation: Synthetic chin implant

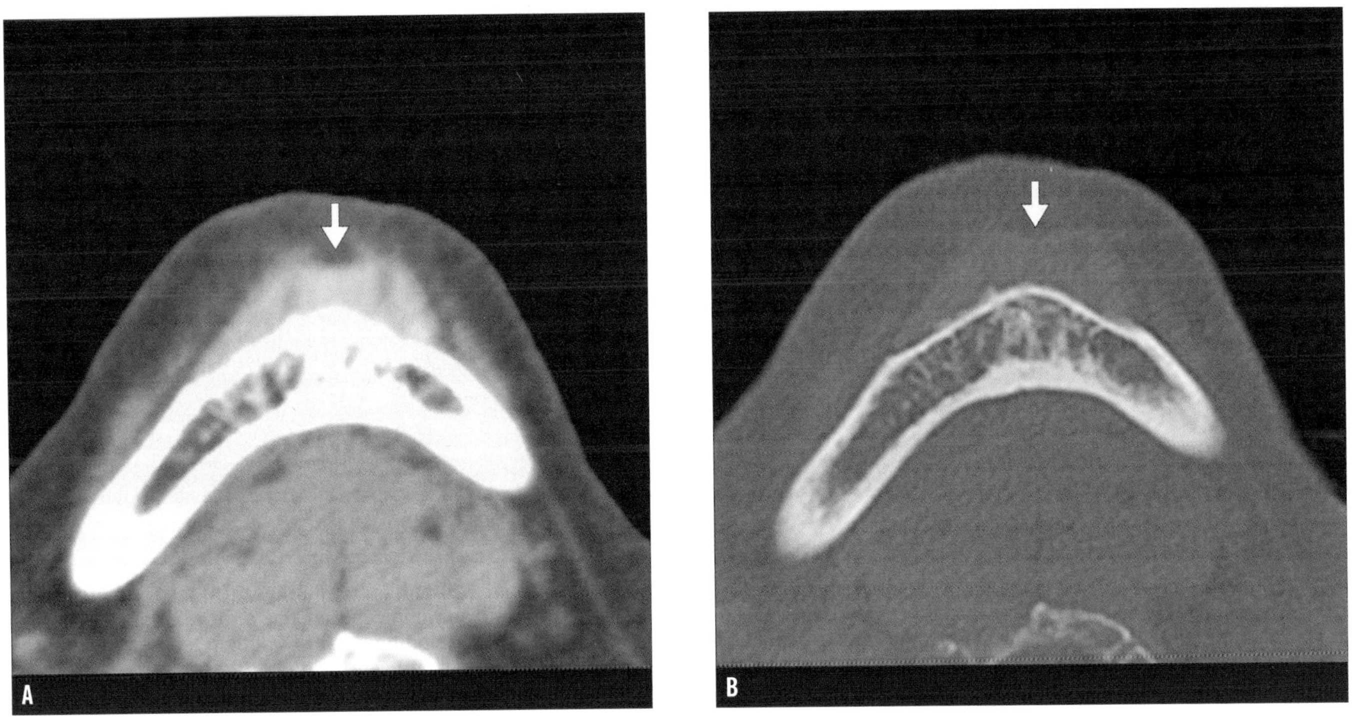

Different patient. An axial CT image viewed with an intermediate window (**A**) as well as axial (**B**), coronal reformatted (**C**, **D**), and sagittal reformatted (**E**) CT images viewed with a bone window demonstrate an intermediate-density foreign body closely apposed the outer cortex of the mandibular symphysis, compatible with a synthetic chin implant (arrows, **A-E**). Small holes in the implant, presumably used for implant fixation, are identified on image **C**. A sagittal scout image from the same study (**F**) also subtly demonstrates the chin implant (arrow, **F**).

CASE 27 Mandibular fixation following trauma

Mandibular fractures are most frequently encountered in young males and are usually the result of motor vehicle collisions, physical altercations, or gunshot wounds. In decreasing order of frequency, fractures of the mandible involve the condyle, body, angle, symphysis, alveolar ridge, ramus, and coronoid process. Treatment may be achieved by either an open surgery (surgically exposing and treating the fracture) or via a closed surgery (treating the fracture without surgical exposure).

Open reduction and internal fixation is the most frequently performed surgery to repair a mandibular fracture and involves the use of surgical plates, lag screws, or wires. A maxillomandibular fixation (MMF) is frequently performed in conjunction with either an open or closed reduction in order to create greater mandibular stability in the postoperative period. An MMF temporarily fixes the maxilla to the mandible. Various methods and materials exist for a MMF, including maxillary and mandibular arch bars, ivy loops, and suspension screws.

Arch bars are metallic bars that are affixed to the maxillary and mandibular teeth via thin wires, which are wrapped around individual teeth (also called circumdental wires). The arch bars along the maxilla and mandible are then attached to each other with wires or elastic bands.

Ivy loop placement is similar to arch bar placement, except that the MMF is created by wrapping individual metal wires in a figure-of-eight fashion around two posterior teeth in all four quadrants of the maxilla and mandible. Ivy loops along the maxilla and mandible are also connected with wires or elastic bands.

A third method of MMF requires placement of a total of four suspension screws into the maxilla and mandible which are then locked together with wires. Typically, screws are placed on each side just lateral to pyriform aperture and two screws are placed medial to the mental foramina.

Maxillomandibular fixation: Closed reduction with arch bars

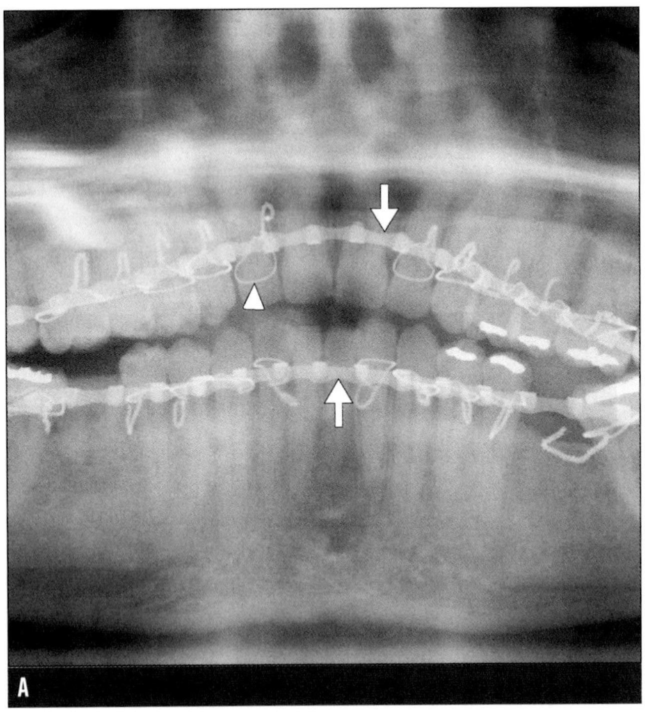

A single panorex image (**A**) of a patient following a gunshot injury to the mandible resulting in multiple fractures (not shown). The patient was treated with a closed reduction of the fractures and placement of arch bars (arrows) for maxillomandibular fixation. The arrowhead denotes one of the circumdental wires utilized to attach the arch bars to the teeth. For this patient, the arch bars on the maxilla and mandible were connected with elastic bands which are not visible.

Maxillomandibular fixation: Open reduction with surgical plate fixation

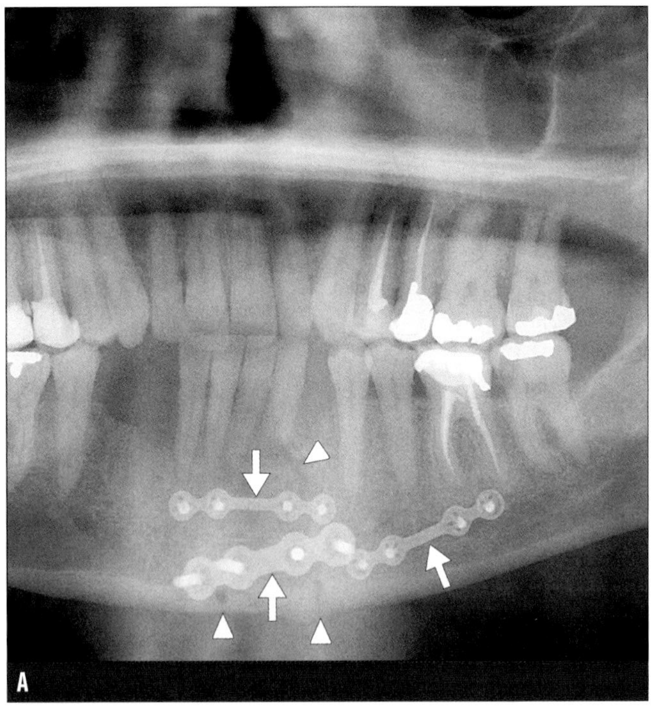

A magnified portion of a panorex image (**A**) demonstrates prior open reduction and internal fixation of comminuted left parasymphyseal and mandibular body fractures with three surgical plates and multiple surgical screws (arrows). A couple fracture lines are faintly visible (arrowheads).

Maxillomandibular fixation: Open reduction with surgical plate fixation and arch bars

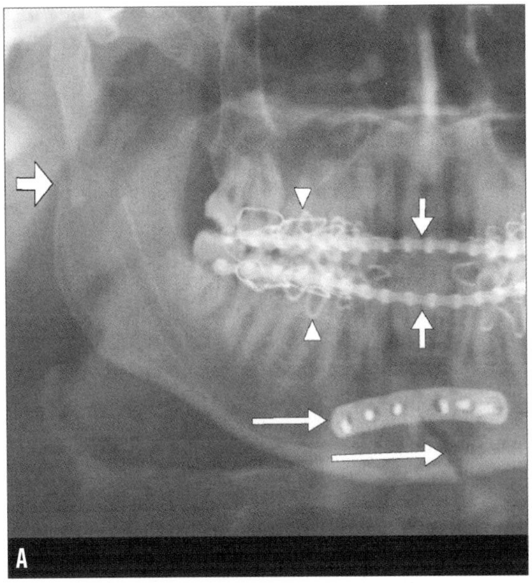

A magnified portion of a single panorex image (**A**) demonstrates prior open reduction and internal fixation of a symphyseal fracture (long arrow) with a surgical plate and screws (medium arrow). A displaced right mandibular ramus fracture is present as well (thick arrow). The mandible has been secured to the maxilla with arch bars (short arrows), consistent with maxillomandibular fixation. Multiple circumdental wires securing the arch bars to the teeth are also evident (arrowheads).

Maxillomandibular fixation: Open reduction with surgical plate fixation, suspension screws, and ivy loop fixation

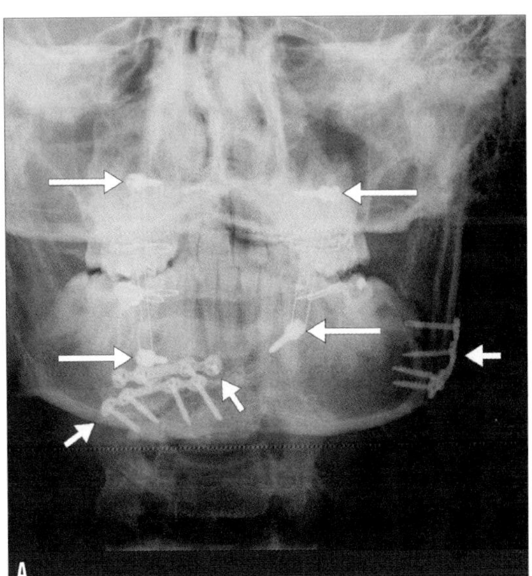

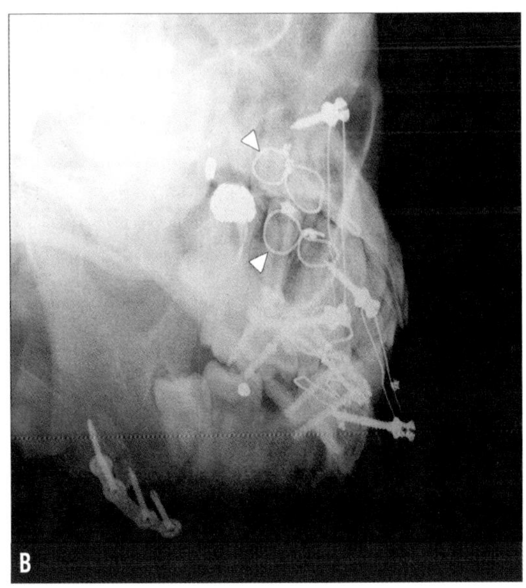

Frontal (**A**) and oblique (**B**) radiographs of the mandible demonstrate findings related to prior internal fixation of the mandible with surgical plates (short arrows, **A**). A maxillomandibular fixation has been achieved with suspension screws and wires (long arrows, **A**), and ivy loops (arrowheads, **B**).

REFERENCES

Ellis E, Muniz O, Anand K. Treatment considerations for comminuted mandibular fractures. *J Oral Maxillofac Surg.* 2003;61(8):861-870.

Stacey DH, et al. Management of mandible fractures. *Plast Reconstr Surg.* 2006;117(3):48e-60e.

Villarreal PM, et al. Mandibular condyle fractures: determinant of treatment and outcome. *J Oral Maxillofac Surg.* 2004;62(2):155-163.

Multiple osseous donor sites exist for mandibular reconstructive surgery, including the fibula, rib, ilium, radius, scapula, and metatarsal. The fibula is most frequently used because it is a site that is easily accessed and carries relatively low morbidity at the harvesting site relative to the other donor sites. The fibula may be grafted as a single piece or as a "double barrel" (ie, two stacked fibular grafts parallel to one another). The double barrel approach provides a greater height of the reconstructed mandible and often an improved dental occlusion relative to a single piece fibular strut graft.

Fibular strut graft with separate pieces of fibula

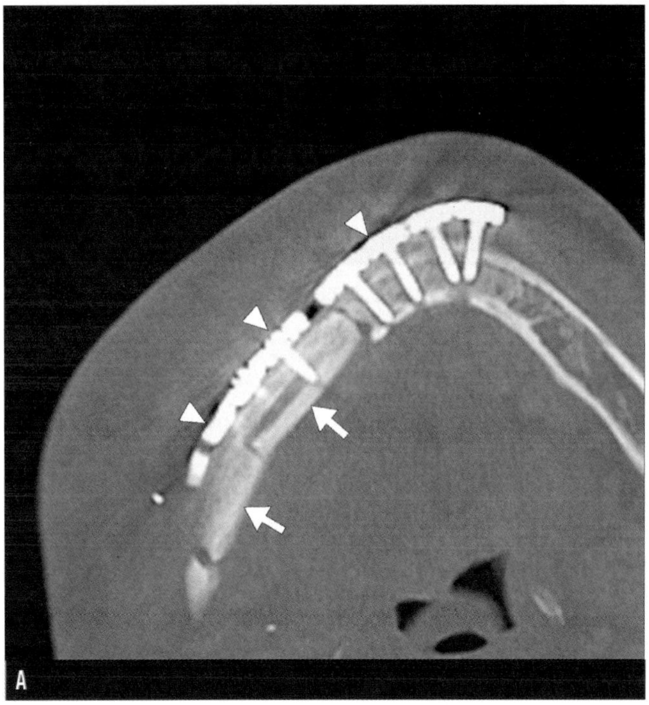

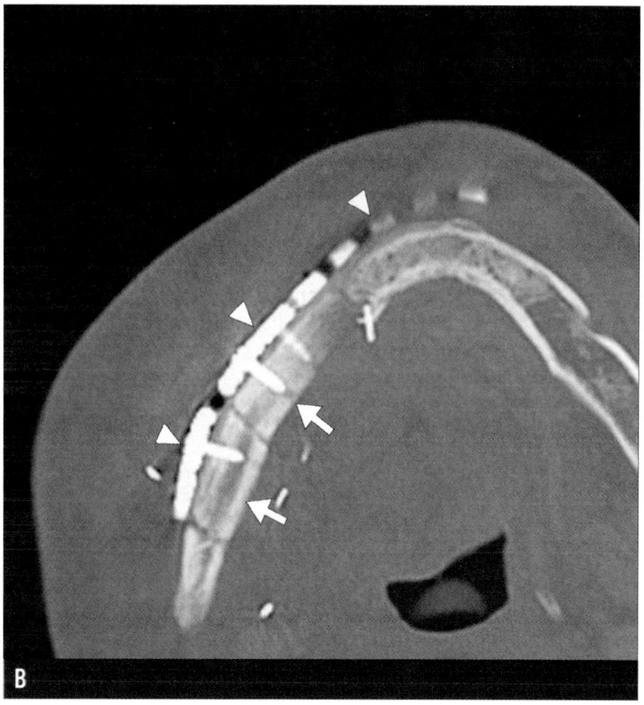

Sequential axial CT images from cranial (**A**) to caudal (**B**) demonstrate a fibular strut graft which was constructed from separate pieces of fibula (arrows, **A**, **B**) and fixed in place with surgical plate and screws (arrowheads, **A**, **B**).

Fibular strut graft with a single piece of fibula

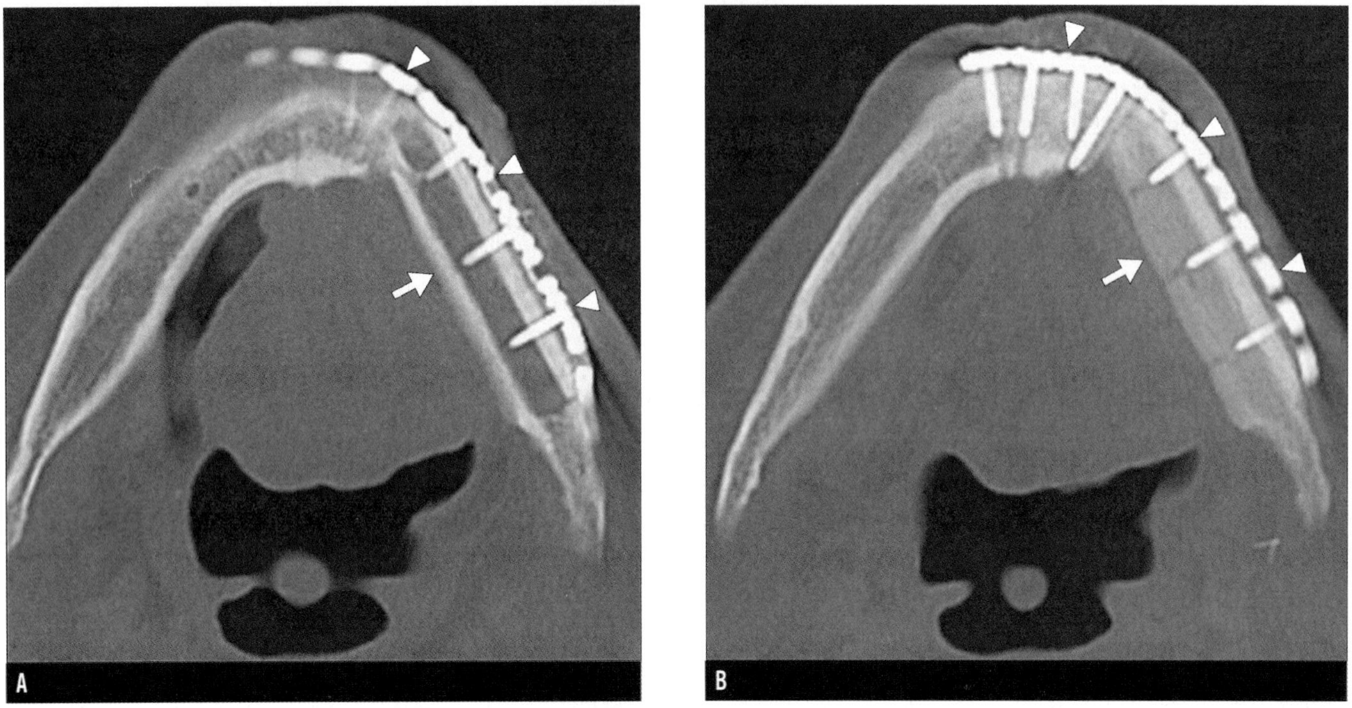

Sequential axial CT images from cranial (**A**) to caudal (**B**) demonstrate a fibular strut graft composed of one piece of fibula (arrows, **A**, **B**), which is fixed in place with surgical plate and screws (arrowheads, **A**, **B**).

REFERENCES

Bahr W, Stoll P, Wachter R. Use of the "double barrel" free vascularized fibula in mandibular reconstruction. *J Oral Maxillofac Surg.* 1998;56(1): 38-44.

Hidalgo DA. Fibula free flap: A new method of mandible reconstruction. *Plast Reconstr Surg.* 1989;84(1):71-79.

CASE 29 Palatal obturator

Defects of the palate may be congenital or they may be acquired as a result of prior surgery or trauma. A palatal obturator is a device that can be used to close a palatal defect between the oral and nasal cavities. Obturators may be constructed from metal, acrylic resins, polymethyl methacrylate, or silicone. The imaging appearance of an obturator prosthesis depends on the materials from which it is constructed. On CT, nonmetallic materials can appear homogeneously hyperattenuating or isoattenuating. Small foci of air may be present within the obturator if small locules of air are incorporated into the material as it is mixed and molded. In the absence of precontrast imaging, it is important to not confuse hyperattenuating obturators for enhancing lesions. Similarly, it is important to not confuse obturators that contain internal foci of air with an infectious process.

Synthetic palatal obturator

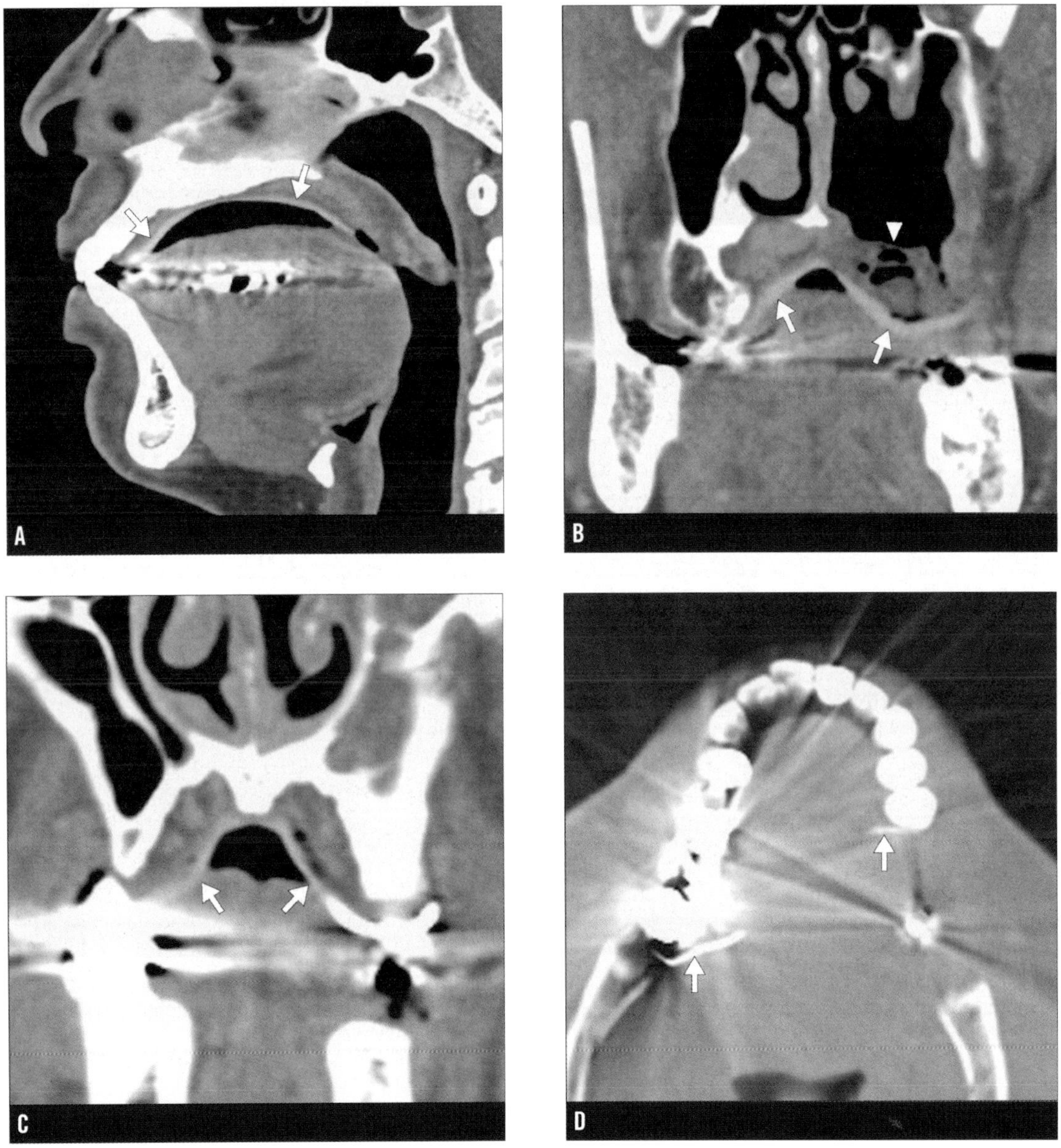

Sagittal reformatted (**A**) and coronal reformatted (**B**, **C**) postcontrast CT images viewed with an intermediate window demonstrate a palatal obturator (arrows, **A-C**). The patient had a left hard hemipalatectomy for resection of an adenoid cystic carcinoma of the hard palate. Debris is present cephalad to the hemipalatectomy (arrowhead, **B**). An axial CT image through the oral cavity viewed with a bone window (**D**) demonstrates wires affixing the obturator in place (arrows, **D**).

Metallic palatal obturator

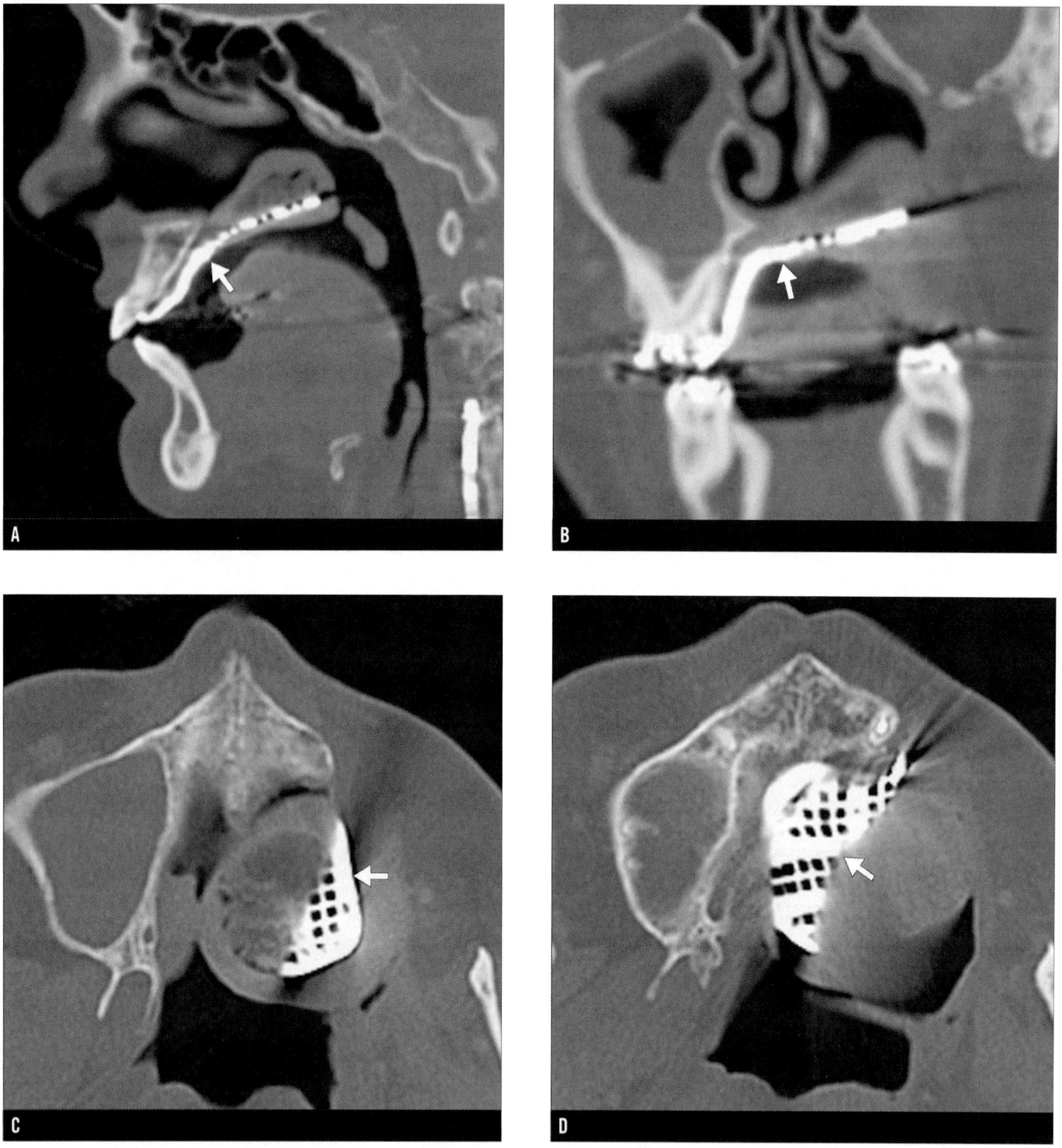

Sagittal reformatted (**A**), coronal reformatted (**B**), and multiple sequential axial CT images from superior to inferior (**C**-**E**) demonstrate a metallic palatal obturator (arrows, **A**-**E**) in a patient with a prior history of a left hemipalatectomy. An additional axial image further inferior (**F**) demonstrates multiple wires affixing the obturator to the maxillary teeth (arrowheads, **F**).

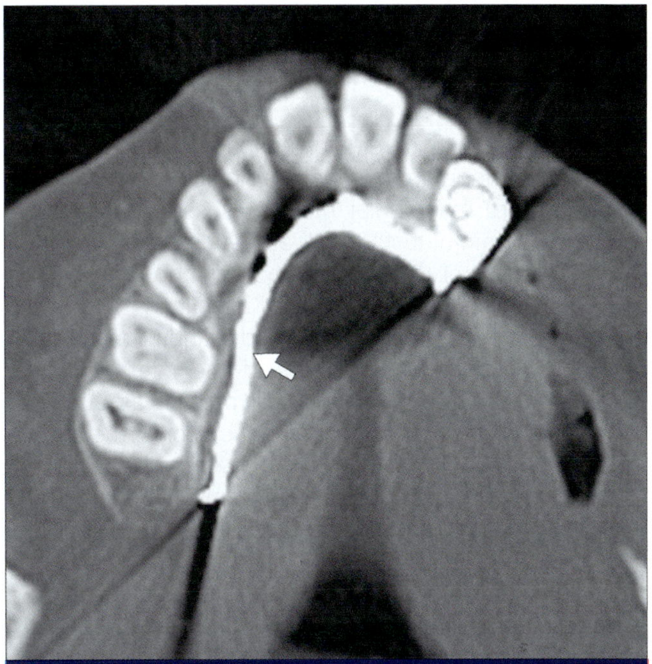

E

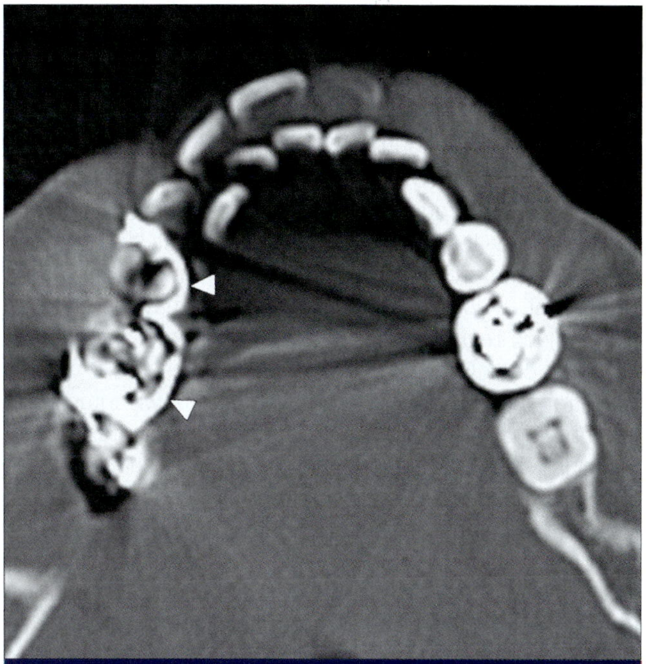

F

REFERENCES

Goiato MC, et al. Patient satisfaction with maxillofacial prosthesis. Literature review. *J. Plast Reconstr Aesthet Surg.* 2009;62(2):175-180.

Keyf F. Obturator prostheses for hemimaxillectomy patients. *J Oral Rehabil.* 2001;28(9):821-829.

Kumar VA, Hofstede TM, Ginsberg LE. CT imaging features of obturator prostheses in patients following palatectomy or maxillectomy. *AJNR Am J Neuroradiol.* 2011;32(10):1926-1929.

Rilo B, da Silva JL, Martinez-Insua A, Santana U. A titanium and visible light-polymerized resin obturator. *J Prosthet Dent.* 2002;87(4):407-409.

CASE 30 Myocutaneous flap floor of mouth and tongue reconstruction

Multiple floor of mouth reconstruction techniques exist following an oral cavity malignancy resection, including skin grafts, loco-regional flaps, and free flaps. Skin grafts are reserved to treat superficial mucosal defects that result following resection of a tumor. When a larger defect is present, a loco-regional or free flap may be utilized. During loco-regional flap surgery, the tissue flap and its vascular pedicle are obtained locally. This tissue flap is then transposed into the oral cavity and sewn into place. Loco-regional flaps include a pectoralis major musculocutaneous, deltopectoral, nasolabial, sternocleidomastoid, and platysma muscle flaps. In contradistinction to a loco-regional flap, a free flap and its pedicle are harvested from a remote site and then transplanted to the resection bed within the head and neck. Free flaps include the radial forearm, fibular, rectus abdominus myocutaneous, vastus lateralis and anterolateral thigh muslce flaps. In the cases of a radial forearm or fibular free flap, a portion of the radius or fibula bone, respectively, may also be harvested and used to repair a destroyed or resected portion of the mandible.

A mobile tongue reconstruction is usually performed with an anterolateral thigh free flap. One technique for this type of reconstruction, termed the "cathedral triptych" technique, is performed by folding and suturing a portion of the anterolateral thigh free flap to form the tongue shape. The neotongue is formed at the thigh site, and the flap and neotongue are then transferred to the oral cavity defect where a microanastamosis is performed. The best perforating vascular pedicle is included in the reconstruction, as is the lateral femoral cutaneous nerve, the latter allowing for resensitization of the newly formed tongue via the lingual nerve following transfer. This technique yields sufficient neotongue volume to allow for dental, palatal, and lip contact. A mobile tongue reconstruction can restore a near normal mobile tongue shape and improve functional results with improved deglutition and oral clearance compared to not performing a neotongue reconstruction.

COMPANION CASES

- **Tongue deviation simulating a partial glossectomy.** Occasionally, a patient may move their tongue during a CT scan and simulate a tongue abnormality or prior surgery, such as a partial glossectomy. Inspecting the entire tongue in three planes can aid in determining whether the tongue is fully intact or whether there is a true focal defect.
- **Ludwig angina.** Ludwig angina is a potentially life-threatening cellulitic infection that involves the floor of the mouth and often the submandibular space soft tissues. The vast majority of cases of Ludwig angina result from local spread of an odontogenic infection, most commonly from periapical infections of the second or third mandibular molars. Presenting symptoms include a painful tooth, neck and submandibular swelling, elevation of the tongue, and stridor. Complications of this process include spread of infection into the deep fascial spaces of the neck or mediastinum, mandibular osteomyelitis, and thrombosis of the internal jugular vein. On CT, Ludwig angina will present as an ill-defined enhancing lesion involving the floor of the mouth. There is often associated skin thickening, edema and stranding of the subcutaneous fat, muscle edema, and generalized loss of the normal fat planes of the submandibular space. If severe, a soft tissue abscess or soft tissue emphysema may be present.
- **Retromolar trigone squamous cell carcinoma**. The retromolar trigone is a small, mucosal covered, triangular-shaped region that overlies the anterior surface of the ascending mandibular ramus, located just posterior to the third mandibular molar. Because of its location, a tumor of the retromolar trigone may spread to involve several different structures and compartments of the head and neck, including the buccinator muscle and buccal space, masticator space, tongue, oropharynx, maxilla, and mandible. The pterygomandibular raphe (PMR), a ligamentous band that attaches the posterior margin of the buccinator muscle to the anterior margin of the superior pharyngeal constrictor muscle, is located in close proximity to the retromolar trigone. The PMR can serve as a conduit for cephalo-caudal spread of tumor, specifically superiorly to the attachment of the PMR along the medial pterygoid plate hamulus and inferiorly to the posterior margin of the mylohyoid muscle.

  Like other mucosa-lined areas of the head and neck, the most common malignancy affecting the retromolar trigone is squamous cell carcinoma (SCC). On CT, SCC tends to present as a homogeneous soft tissue mass which may be associated with localized osseous destruction. On MRI, these tumors are typically iso- to hypointense on T1-weighted imaging and iso- to hyperintense on T2-weighted imaging. SCC typically enhances avidly, with small tumors usually homogeneous and large tumors often heterogeneous in their enhancement pattern.
- **Schwannoma of the oral cavity**. A schwannoma is a benign nerve sheath tumor that originates from Schwann cells. In the oral cavity, the tongue is the most common location of a schwannoma. Less common locations in the oral cavity include the palate, floor of mouth, buccal mucosa, lips, and mandible. Schwannomas are usually solitary lesions, but they can be multiple in patients with neurofibromatosis.

On imaging, schwannomas are usually circumscribed round or oval lesions. These lesions tend to be iso- to hypoattenuating on precontrast CT images and variably enhance. On MRI, schwannomas are usually T1 isointense and T2 hyperintense. Following gadolinium administration, schwannomas classically avidly enhance, although they may contain nonenhancing cystic components.

Total glossectomy with a myocutaneous flap floor of mouth reconstruction

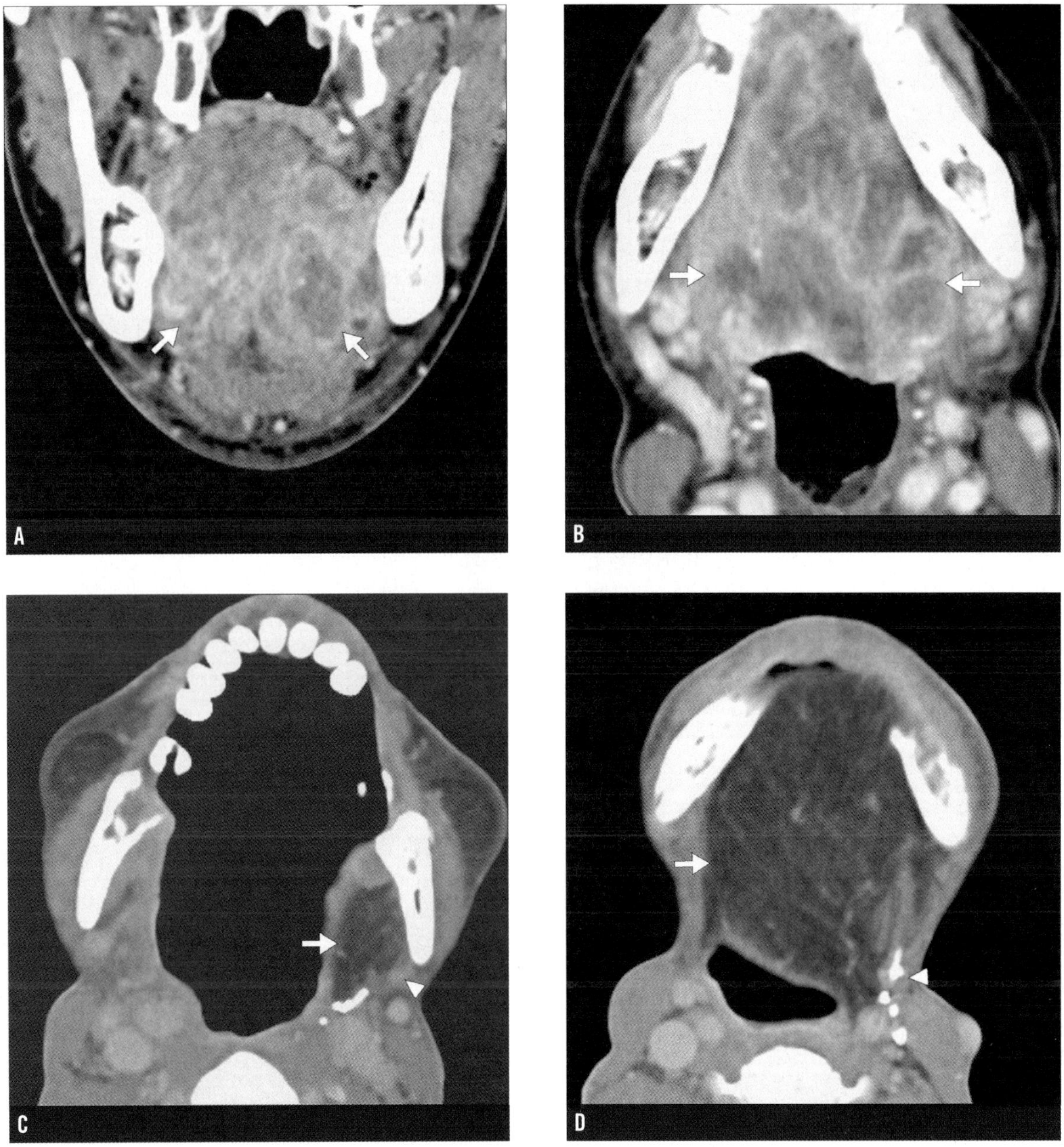

Coronal reformatted (**A**) and axial (**B**) contrast-enhanced CT images demonstrate a heterogeneously enhancing mass occupying almost the entire tongue (arrows , **A**, **B**). This was pathologically proven to represent a squamous cell carcinoma. Axial (**C**, **D**), sagittal reformatted (**E**), and coronal reformatted (**F**) contrast-enhanced CT images were obtained following a total glossectomy and floor of mouth reconstruction utilizing a myocutaneous flap, in this case an anterolateral thigh myocutaneous free flap. A large amount of fat is present within the free flap (arrows, **C-F**). The arrowhead on image **C** denotes the vascular pedicle, whereas the arrowhead on image **D** denotes the suture material used for the anastomosis.

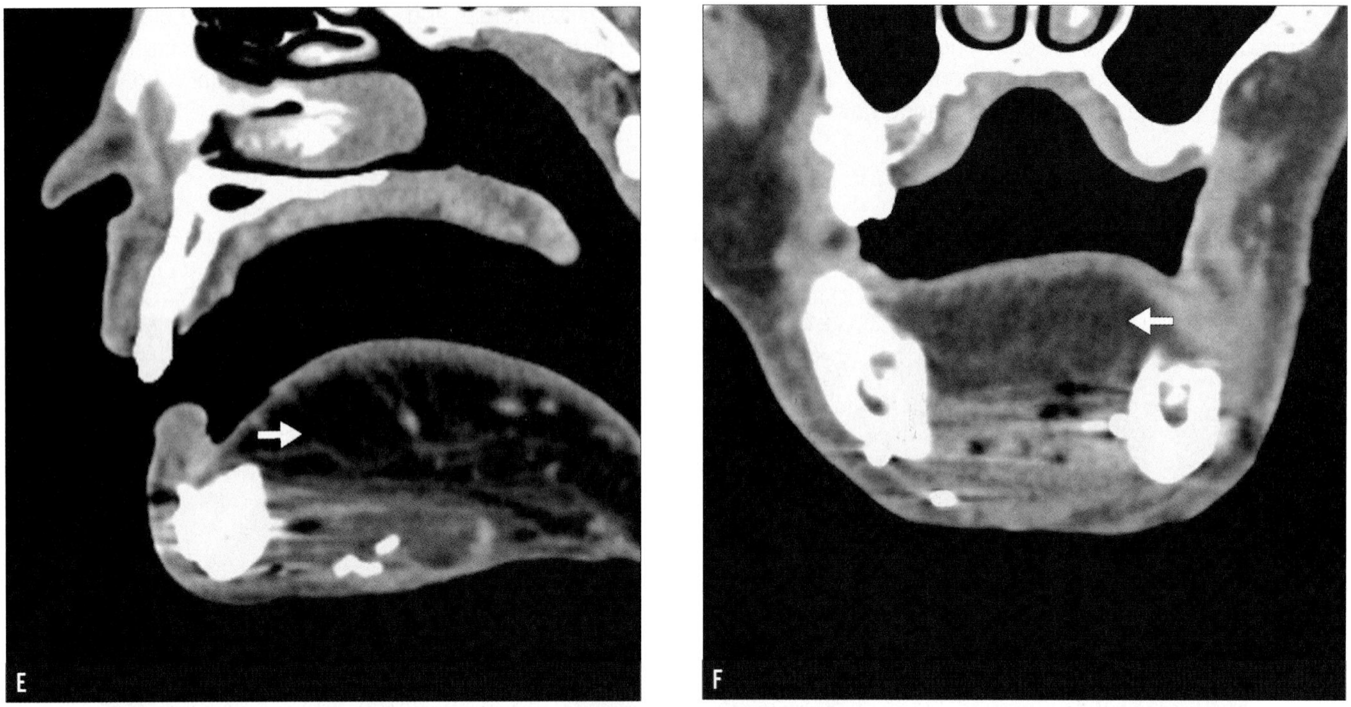

Partial glossectomy with a myocutaneous flap floor of mouth reconstruction

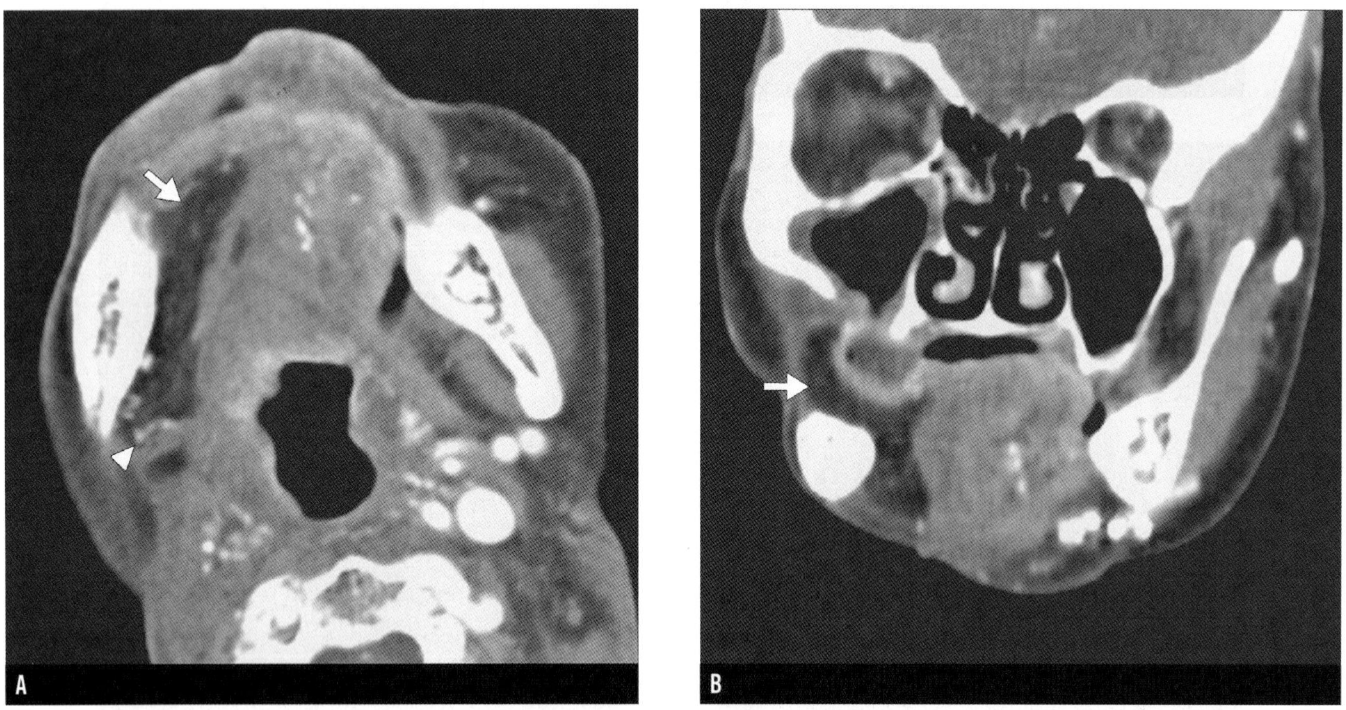

Axial (**A**) and coronal reformatted (**B**) contrast-enhanced CT images demonstrate surgical changes related to a prior a partial right glossectomy and loco-regional myocutaneous flap reconstruction of floor of mouth (arrows, **A**, **B**). In this case, a pectoralis major myocutaneous flap was utilized. The arrowhead on image **A** denotes the vascular pedicle of the flap.

Evolution of an osteocutaneous fibular free flap utilized for a floor of mouth reconstruction

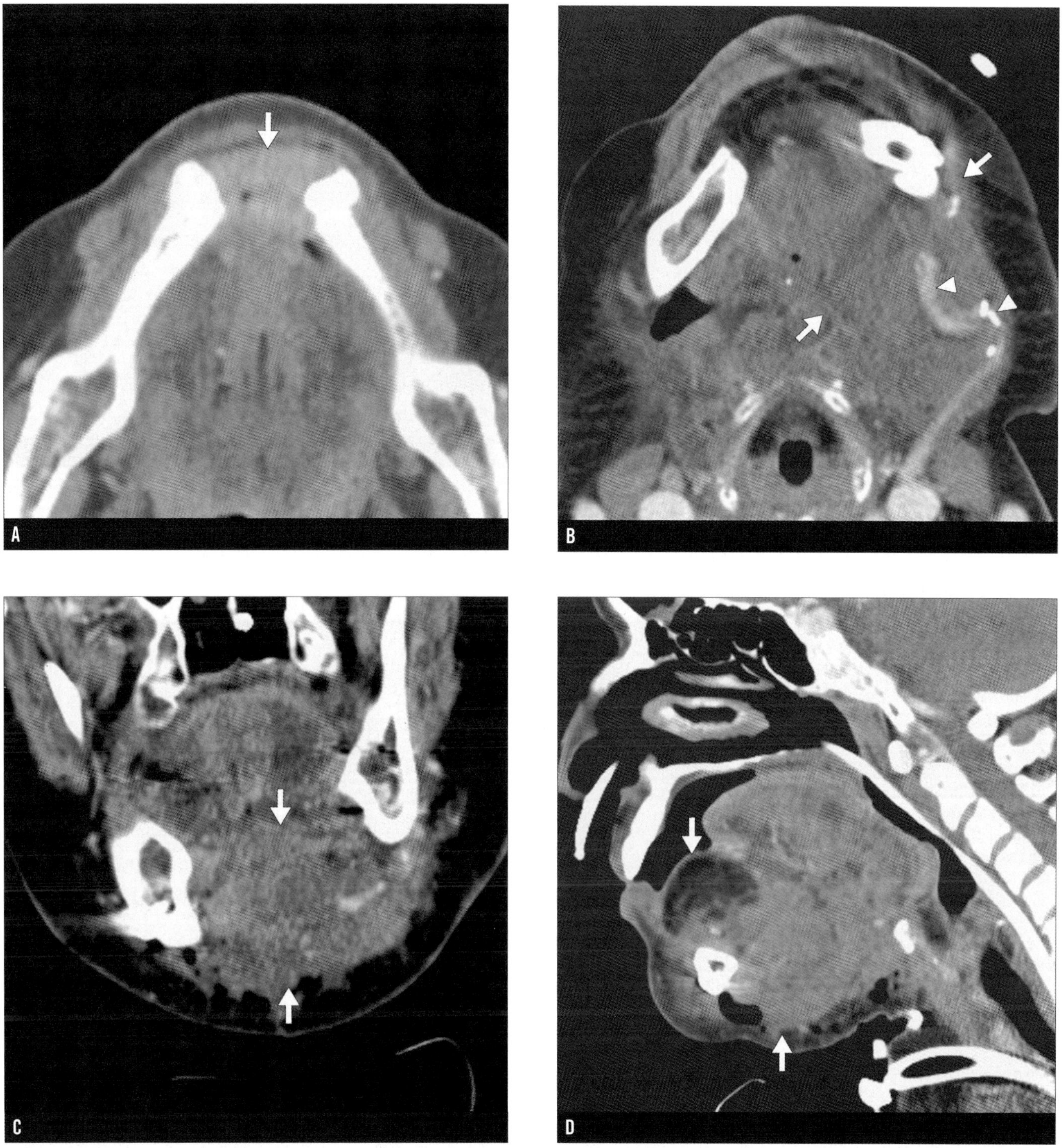

A postcontrast axial CT image through the oral cavity (**A**) demonstrates a focal mass along the mentum of the mandible, in this case representing an alveolar ridge squamous cell carcinoma (arrow, **A**). The patient underwent a composite resection of the tumor with placement of an osteocutaneous fibula free flap and a mandibular reconstruction. Axial (**B**), coronal reformatted (**C**), and sagittal reformatted (**D**) postcontrast CT images were obtained less than 1 week following the tumor resection and reconstruction. Images **B**-**D** demonstrate a large amount of new soft tissue along the floor of mouth which represents the new fibular free flap; this fibular free flap could be mistaken for a large mass without adequate history. The fibular free flap vascular pedicle and its anastomosis are shown on image **B** (arrowheads). Axial (**E**) and coronal reformatted (**F**) postcontrast CT images obtained 1.5 years later demonstrate expected evolution and volume loss of the fibular free flap. Image **E** demonstrates persistent enhancement of the vascular pedicle (arrowhead, **E**).

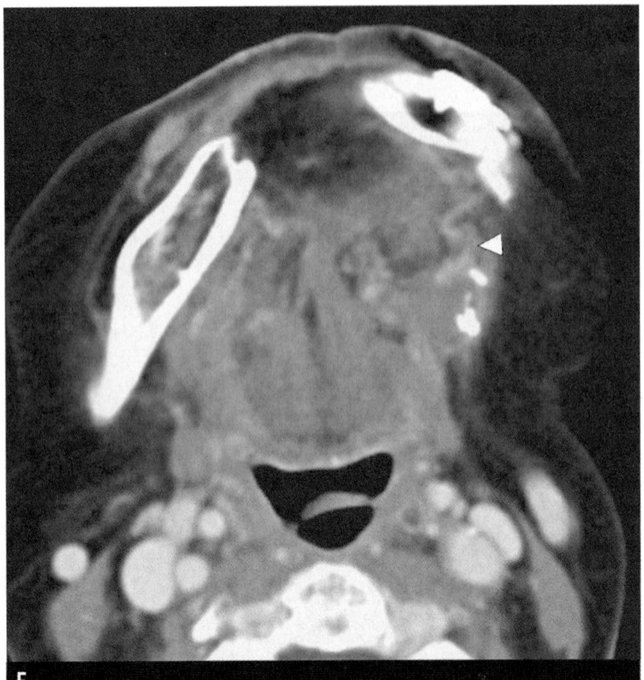

E

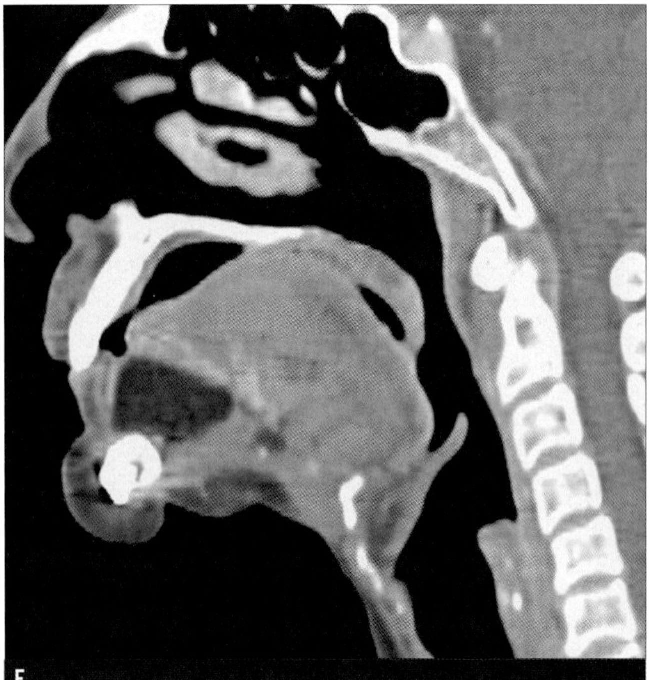

F

Total glossectomy with a myocutaneous free flap and total mobile tongue reconstruction

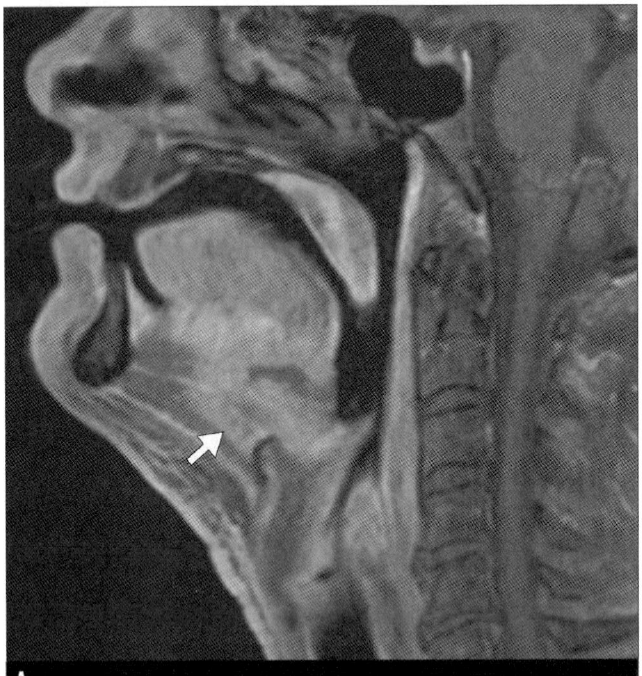

A

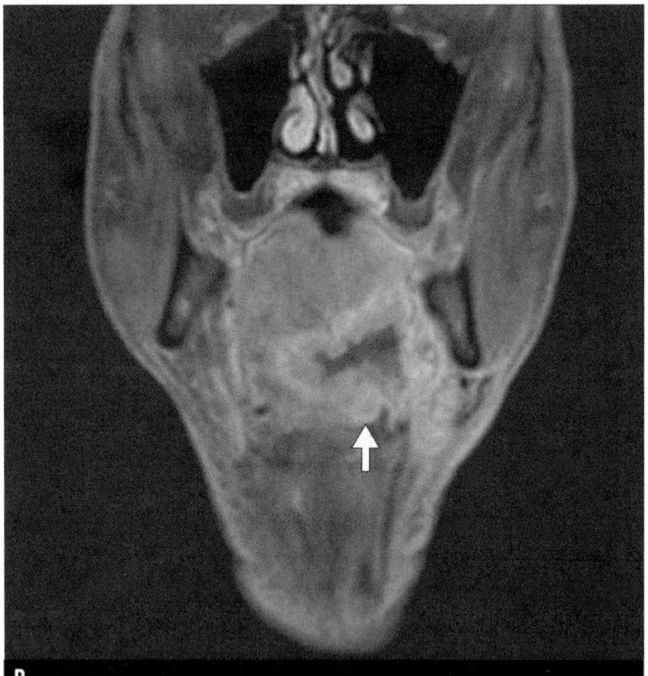

B

Postcontrast sagittal (**A**) and coronal (**B**) fat suppressed T1-weighted MR images demonstrate a peripherally enhancing necrotic tongue root mass relative to unenhanced imaging (not shown), pathologically shown to represent squamous cell carcinoma with perineural invasion (arrows, **A**, **B**). The patient underwent a total glossectomy and mobile tongue reconstruction with an anterolateral thigh and vastus lateralis free flap. Unenhanced sagittal (**C**) and coronal (**D**) T1-weighted MR images as well as contrast-enhanced sagittal (**E**) and coronal (**F**) fat-suppressed T1-weighted MR images demonstrate the results of the surgery approximately 1 month after the operation. The tumor has been removed following the glossectomy and the mobile tongue reconstruction results in a near-normal tongue morphology. In addition to being more aesthetically pleasing, a mobile tongue reconstruction improves deglutition and oral clearance compared to not performing a mobile tongue reconstruction.

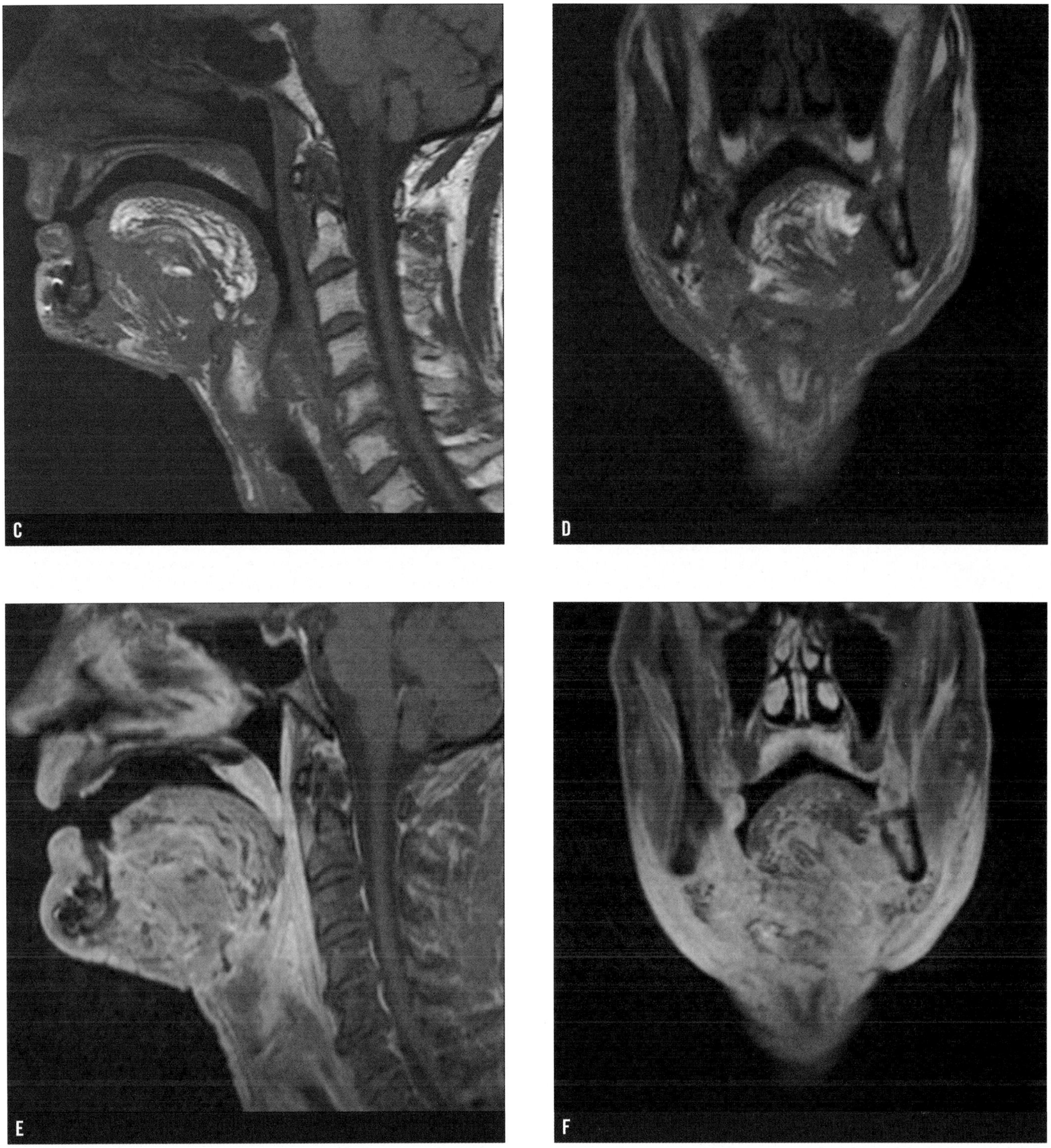

Companion case: Tongue deviation simulating a partial glossectomy

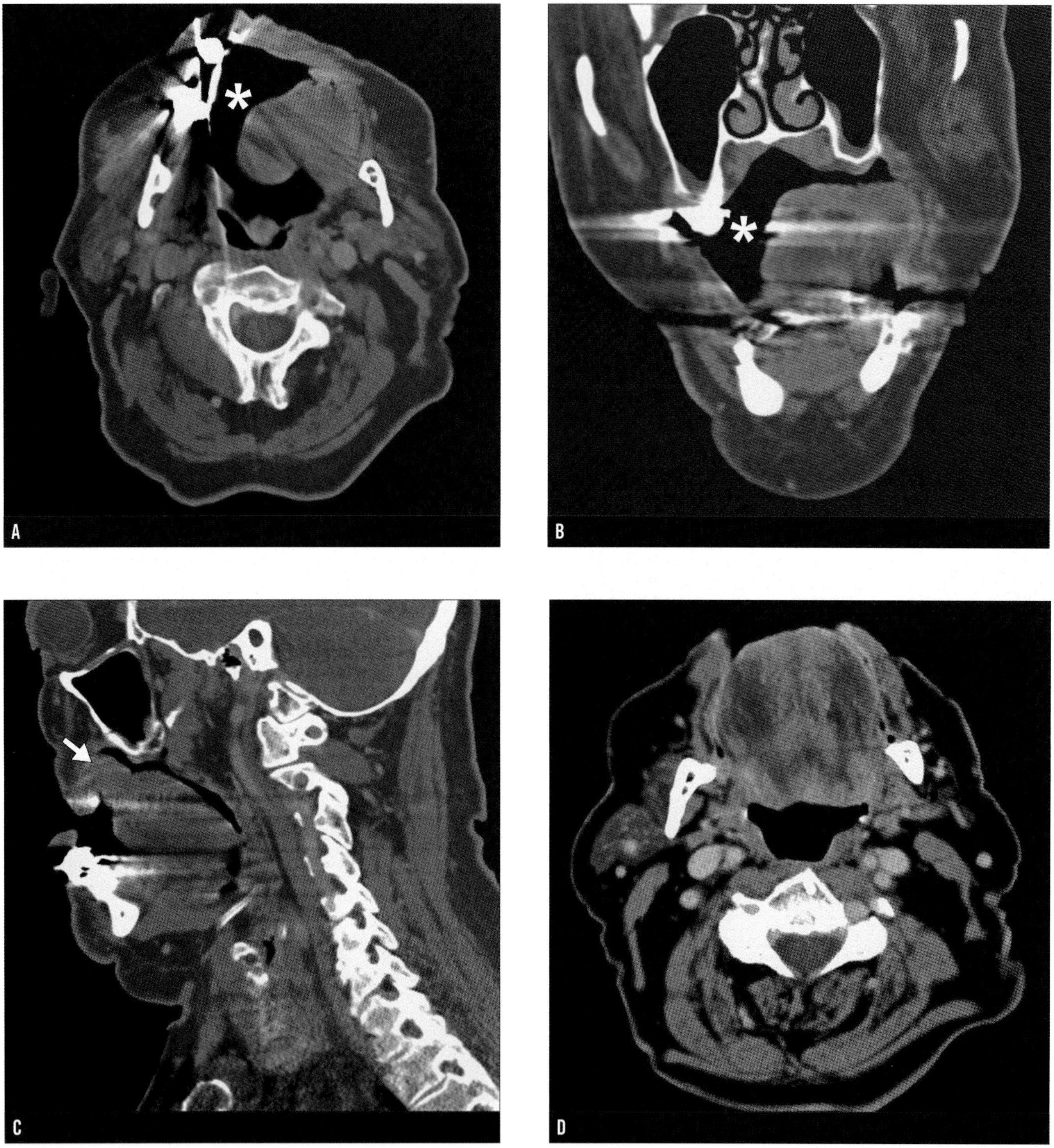

Postcontrast axial (**A**) and coronal reformatted (**B**) CT images demonstrate an apparent defect along the right aspect of the oral tongue, suggesting a partial right glossectomy (asterisks, **A**, **B**). A postcontrast left parasagittal reformatted CT image from the same imaging study (**C**) demonstrates that the tip of the tongue is touching the left anterior buccal surface of the upper lip (arrow, **C**), perhaps in an effort to clean away debris in the oral cavity. A delayed postcontrast axial CT image from the same imaging study demonstrates a normal position and volume of the tongue, verifying that the appearance of the tongue on images **A** and **B** was related to tongue positioning and not a true finding.

Companion case: Ludwig angina

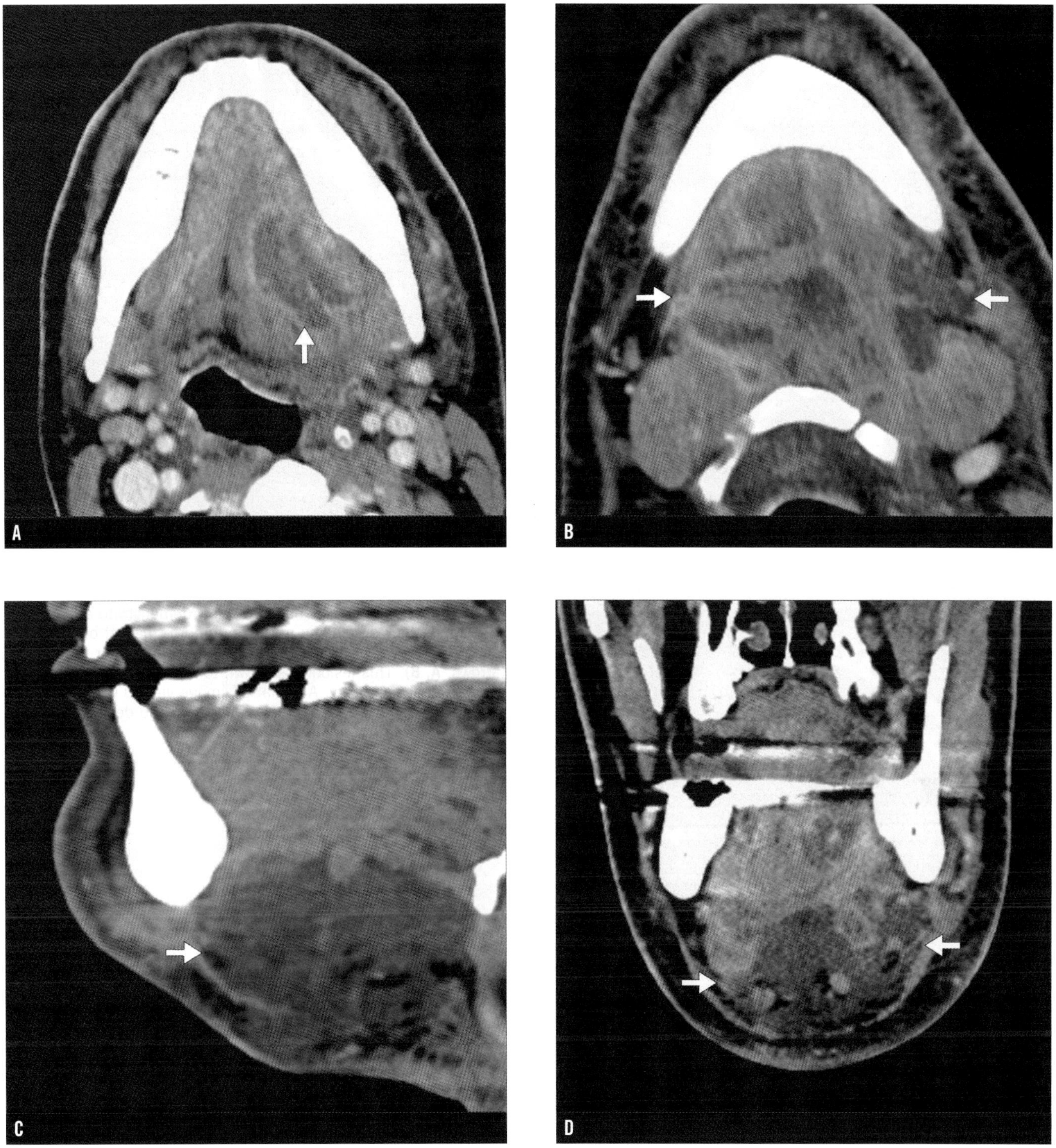

Axial (**A**, **B**), sagittal reformatted (**C**), and coronal reformatted (**D**) contrast-enhanced CT images demonstrate extensive edema, fat-stranding, and loss of the normal fat planes within the floor of the mouth (arrows, **A-D**). This patient had a recent extraction of ADA tooth number 18 with clinical findings of edema in the submental region associated with odynophagia, trismus, and car pain. The history and imaging findings are consistent with Ludwig angina. The heterogeneity and mild peripheral enhancement of the finding suggests a developing abscess.

VI. PARANASAL SINUSES AND NASAL CAVITY

CASE 1 Aplastic frontal sinuses

The frontal sinuses are usually not fully developed until after puberty and their development is quite variable among patients. The frontal sinuses may develop asymmetrically, may be diminutive, or may be aplastic. Aplasia is uncommon, reportedly found in approximately 3% to 5% of cases in several published

Aplastic right frontal sinus

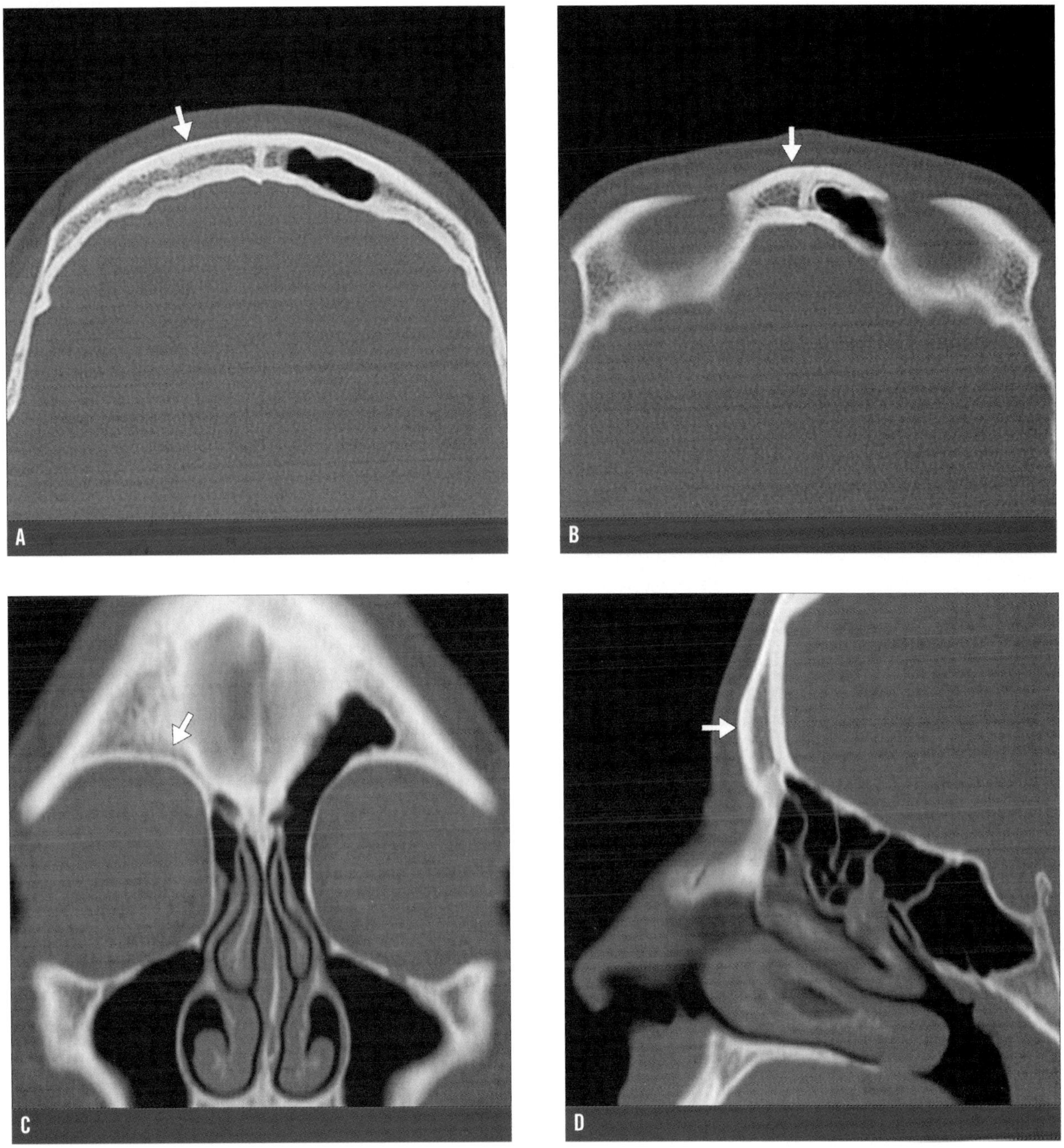

Axial (**A**, **B**), coronal reformatted (**C**), and sagittal reformatted (**D**) CT images demonstrate aplasia of the right frontal sinus (arrows, **A-D**).

Aplastic frontal sinuses

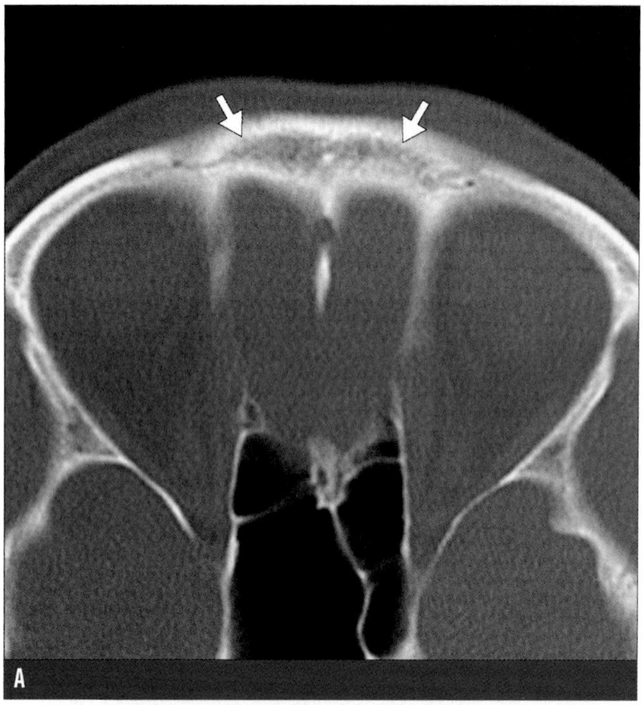

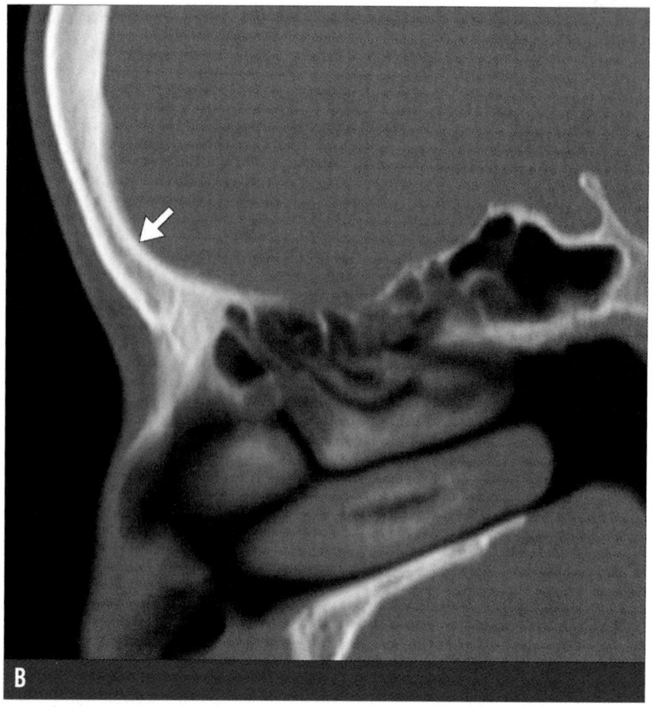

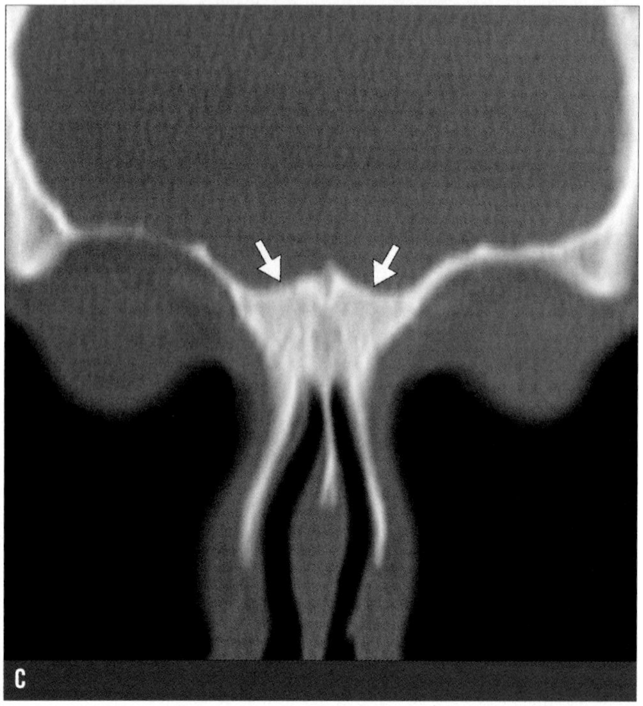

Axial (**A**), sagittal reformatted (**B**), and coronal reformatted (**C**) CT images demonstrate aplasia of the frontal sinuses (arrows, **A-C**).

REFERENCES

Beale TJ, Madani G, Morley SJ. Imaging of the paranasal sinuses and nasal cavity: normal anatomy and clinically relevant anatomical variants. Semin Ultrasound CT MR. 2009 Feb;30(1):2-16.

Orlandi, RR, Wiggins RH 3rd. Radiological sinonasal findings in adults with cystic fibrosis. *Am J Rhinol Allergy.* May-June 2009;23(3):307-311.

Kountakis E, et al. *The Frontal Sinus.* 1st ed. Verlag Berlin Heidelberg, Germany: Springer; 2005.

CASE 2 Dominant frontal sinus extending across midline

One frontal sinus is often larger than the other. Occasionally, the larger frontal sinus may extend across midline and sometimes may be the only frontal sinus present. When a single frontal sinus is present, the sidedness of the sinus can be determined by the side where its draining frontal recess (also called frontoethmoidal recess) is located.

Dominant left frontal sinus extending across midline

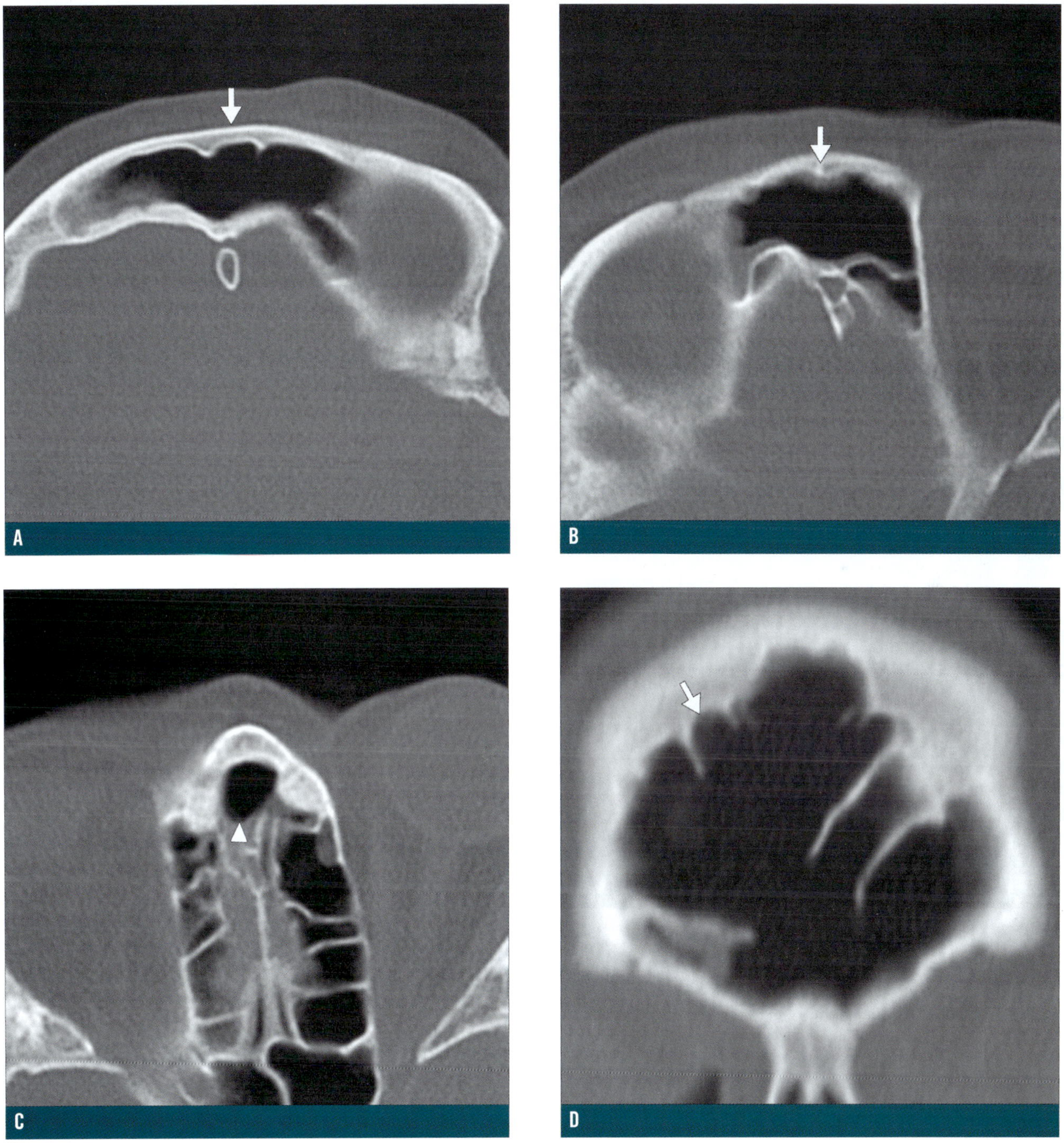

Axial (**A-C**), coronal reformatted (**D-F**), and sagittal reformatted (**G**) CT images through the paranasal sinuses. There is a dominant, heavily pneumatized single frontal sinus (arrows, **A**, **B**, **D**, **E**). A single left frontal recess (arrowheads, **C**, **F**, **G**) serves as the outflow tract for this sinus. Therefore, the sinus is best described as a large left frontal sinus that extends across the midline. There was no native right frontal sinus in this patient.

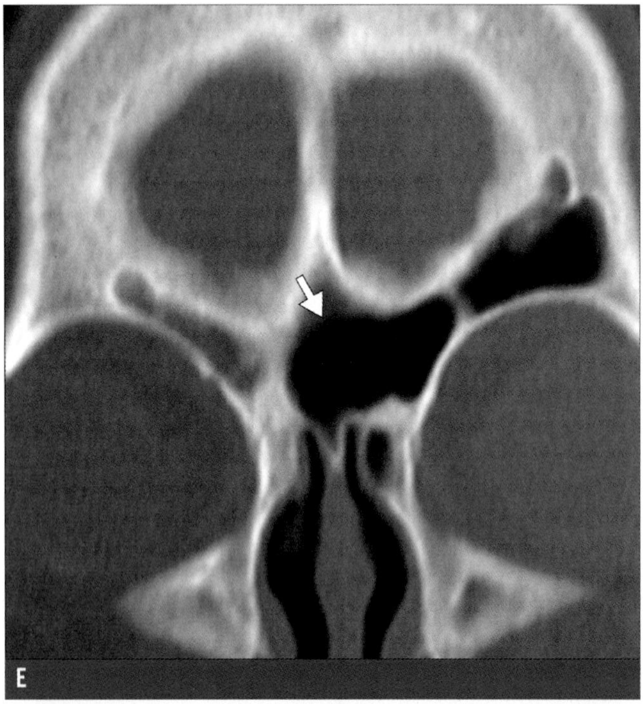

E

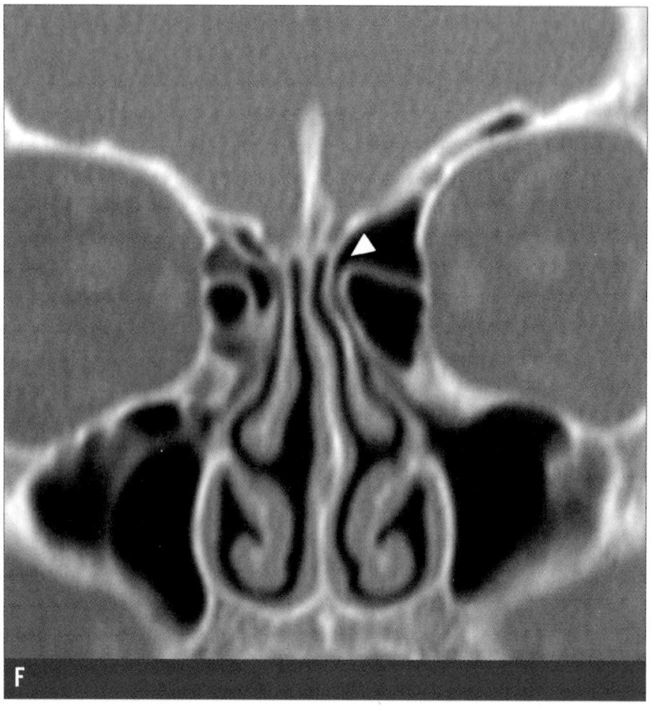

F

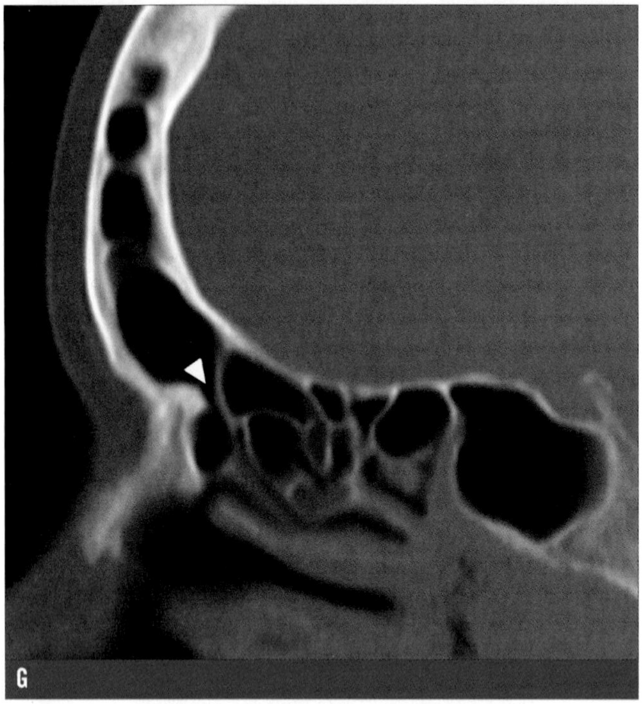

G

REFERENCE

David M, Saxena R. Use of frontal sinus and nasal septum patterns as an aid in personal identification: a digital radiographic pilot study. *J Forensic Dent Sci.* 2010;2(2):77-80.

CASE 3 Frontal sinus hypersinus

A hypersinus is defined as an enlarged, aerated sinus that remains confined to the normal native bone boundaries and maintains normal bone wall thickness. This is considered a clinically asymptomatic variant.

COMPANION CASES

- **Frontal sinus pneumosinus dilatans.** Pneumosinus dilatans (PD) is defined as an abnormally expansile, aerated sinus that extends beyond the normal confines of the native bone. The sinus involved with PD usually has a normal wall thickness. However, PD can be associated with a meningioma, which may induce sinus wall hyperostosis.

  The etiology of PD remains unknown. While PD is usually idiopathic, it has been described in association with many conditions, including:

  Meningioma
  McCune-Albright syndrome
  Fibrous dysplasia
  Arachnoid cyst
  Brain tumors
  Prolonged CSF shunting
  Cerebral hemiatrophy infantile meningoencephalitis
  von Recklinghausen disease
  Acromegaly
- **Frontal sinus and ethmoid air cell pneumosinus dilatans with fibrous dysplasia.** With fibrous dysplasia, normal bone is replaced by fibrous tissue which consists of spindle cell bundles and immature woven bone. This process results in expansion of the affected bone. It may affect a single site (monostotic) or multiple sites (polyostotic). The most common CT appearance of fibrous dysplasia is a ground-glass (sclerotic) pattern. However, fibrous dysplasia can less commonly appear as a heterogeneously sclerotic and lucent lesion (Pagetoid form) or as a cystic lesion (cystic form). On MRI, fibrous dysplasia has a nonspecific appearance and may mimic other osseous lesions, including malignant entities. Thus, any suspicious osseous lesion on MRI should be interpreted in combination with CT, or when appropriate, radiographs. Typically, fibrous dysplasia is low-to-intermediate in T1 signal and enhances on MRI. The T2 signal characteristics are variable and depend on the ratio of mineralized matrix to fibrous tissue.
- **Frontal sinus pneumocele.** Like pneumosinus dilatans, a sinus pneumocele is an enlarged paranasal sinus that extends beyond the normal confines of the native bone. However, at least a portion of the walls of a sinus pneumocele are thinned or sometimes dehiscent, unlike the walls of pneumosinus dilatans which are normal or thickened. The etiology of a pneumocele is unknown, although a one-way ball-valve mechanism has been proposed, characterized by air entering but not escaping the affected sinus. The source of the proposed one-way ball-valve mechanism may be from developmental, posttraumatic, inflammatory, or neoplastic etiologies. Most pneumoceles are asymptomatic, although a dull pain or pressure with atmospheric changes, as well as with nose blowing, have been reported. Rarely, pneumocephalus may occur because of a fistulous communication between the affected sinus and the intracranial compartment. While there is no standardized treatment for a pneumocele, successful treatment has been reported by surgical enlargement of the outflow tract with preservation of the mucosa of the outflow tract and affected sinus.

Frontal sinus hypersinus

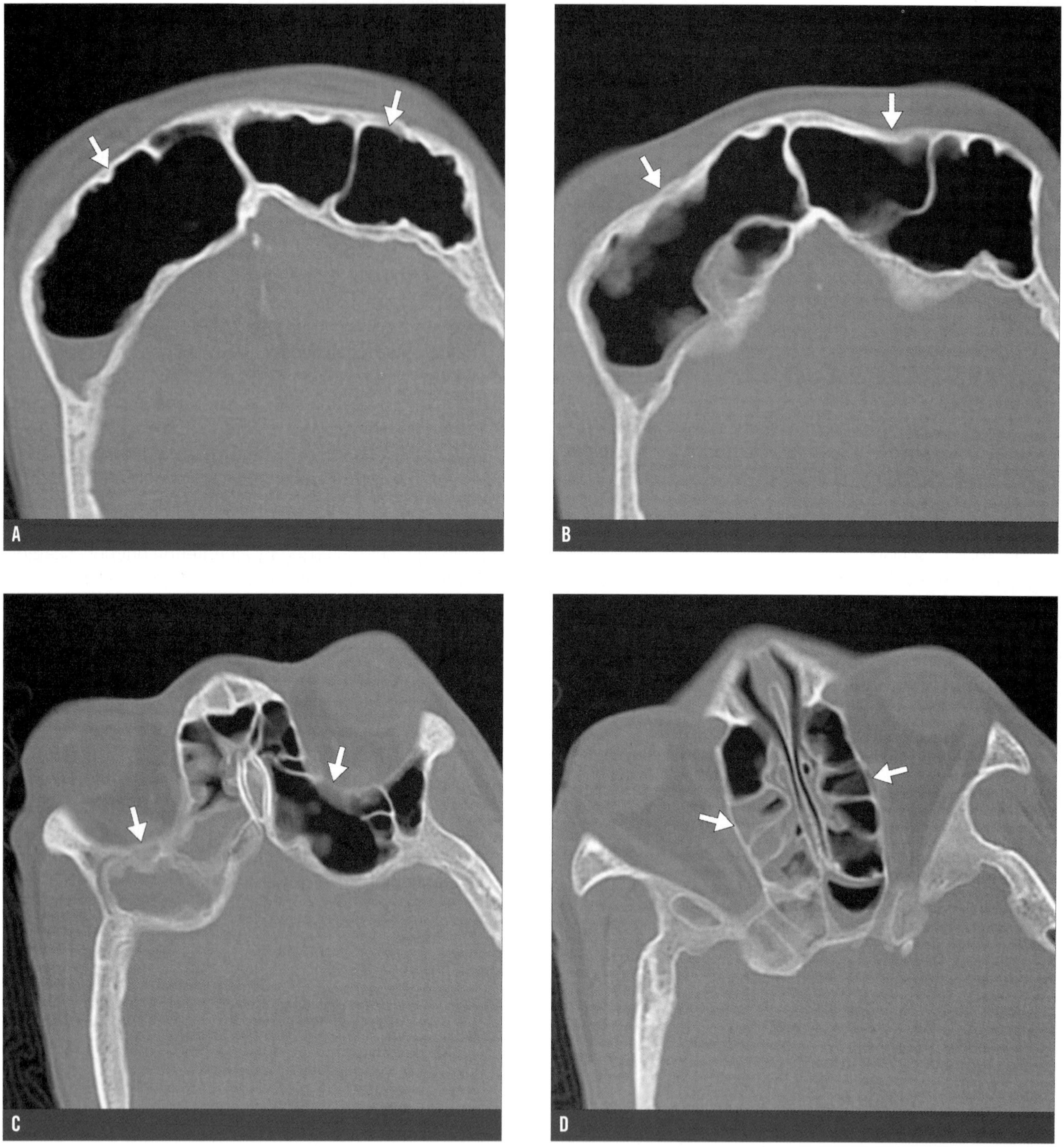

Axial CT images through the frontal sinuses (**A, B**), the supraorbital ethmoid air cells (**C**), and the ethmoid air cells (**D**) demonstrate hypersinus of the frontal sinuses (arrows, **A, B**) and of the supraorbital ethmoid air cells (arrows, **C**). The right supraorbital ethmoid air cell is opacified. The ethmoid air cells (arrows, **D**) are unremarkable in size but mostly opacified on the right.

Companion case: Frontal sinus pneumosinus dilatans

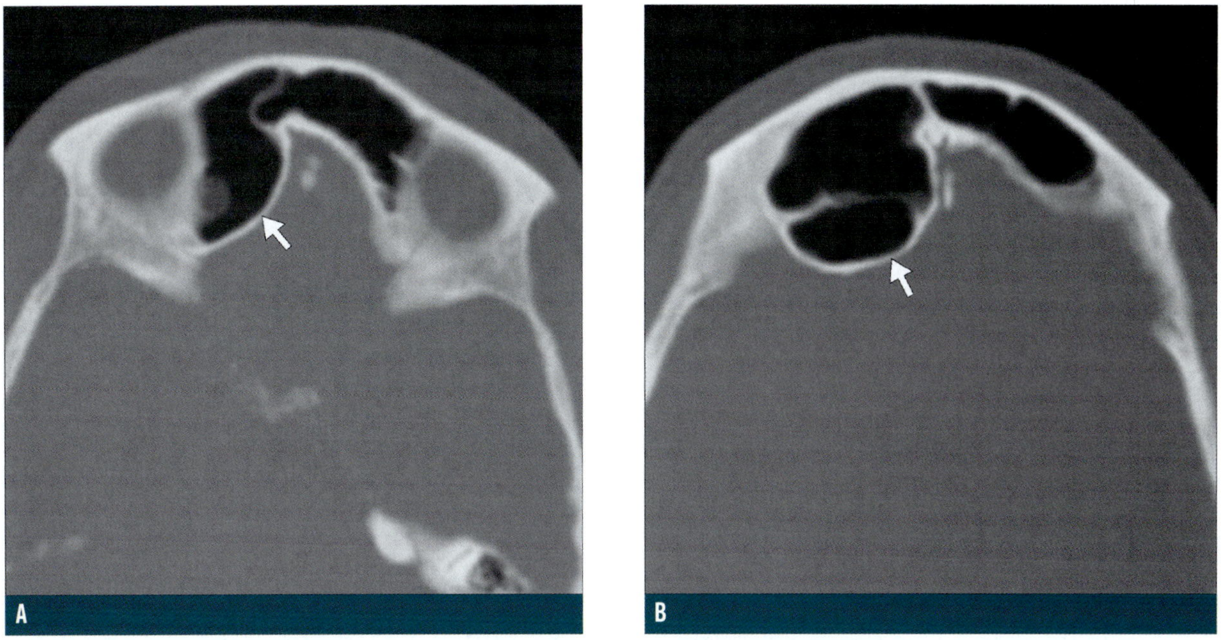

Axial CT images through the frontal sinuses (**A, B**) demonstrate an expansile right frontal sinus that extends outside the confines of the normal frontal sinus and has normal sinus wall thickness, compatible with pneumosinus dilatans (arrows, **A, B**).

Companion case: Frontal sinus and ethmoid air cell pneumosinus dilatans with fibrous dysplasia

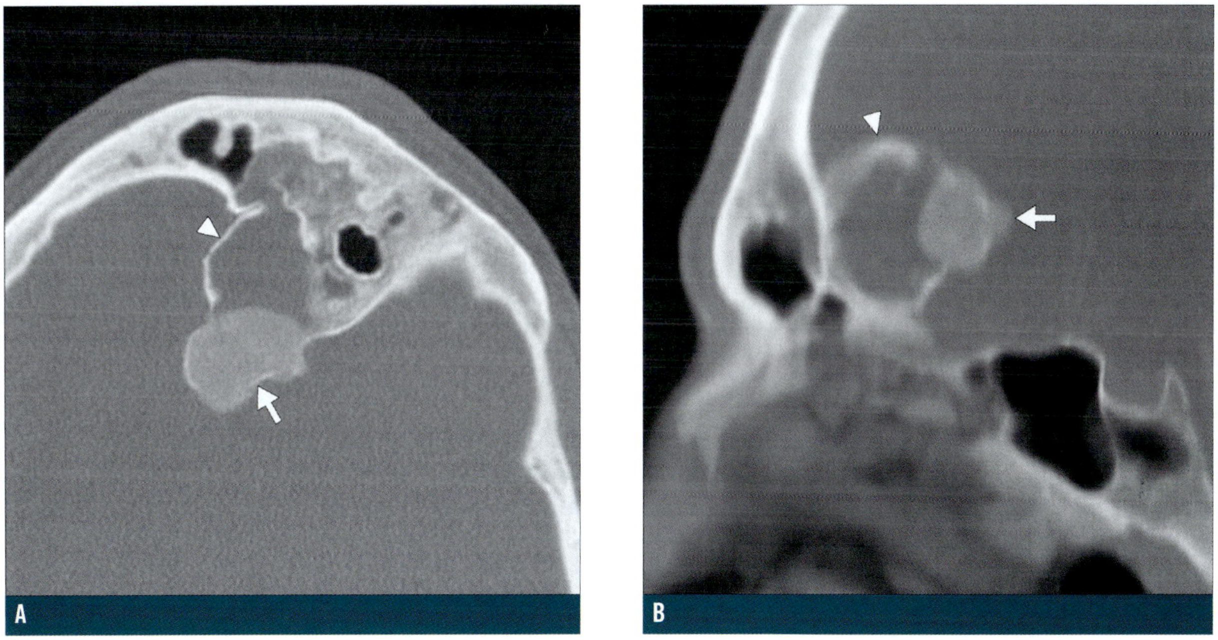

Axial (**A**), sagittal reformatted (**B**), and coronal reformatted (**C**) CT images through the anterior cranial fossa demonstrate an expansile, mixed-density area of new bone formation which contains focally lucent areas (arrowheads, **A-C**) and areas of ground-glass bone formation (arrows, **A, B**). The ground-glass portion is compatible with fibrous dysplasia. The lucent area may represent a cystic area of fibrous dysplasia or an opacified portion of pneumosinus dilatans. Axial (**D**) and sagittal reformatted (**E**) CT images of the same patient demonstrate aerated pneumosinus dilatans of the left frontal sinus and adjacent left ethmoid air cells (arrows, **D, E**) with the area of fibrous dysplasia along their cephalad aspects. Sagittal T1 (**F**), axial T1 (**G**), axial T2 (**H**), coronal T2 (**I**), and axial postcontrast MPRAGE (**J**) MR images of the same patient demonstrate nonenhancing, T1 hypointense, and T2 hyperintense signal (arrowheads, **F-J**) corresponding to the prominent lucent area of bone demonstrated on images **A-C**. There is nonenhancing, T1 hyperintense, and T2 hypointense signal (arrows, **F, G, H, J**) corresponding to the ground-glass area of fibrous dysplasia demonstrated on CT.

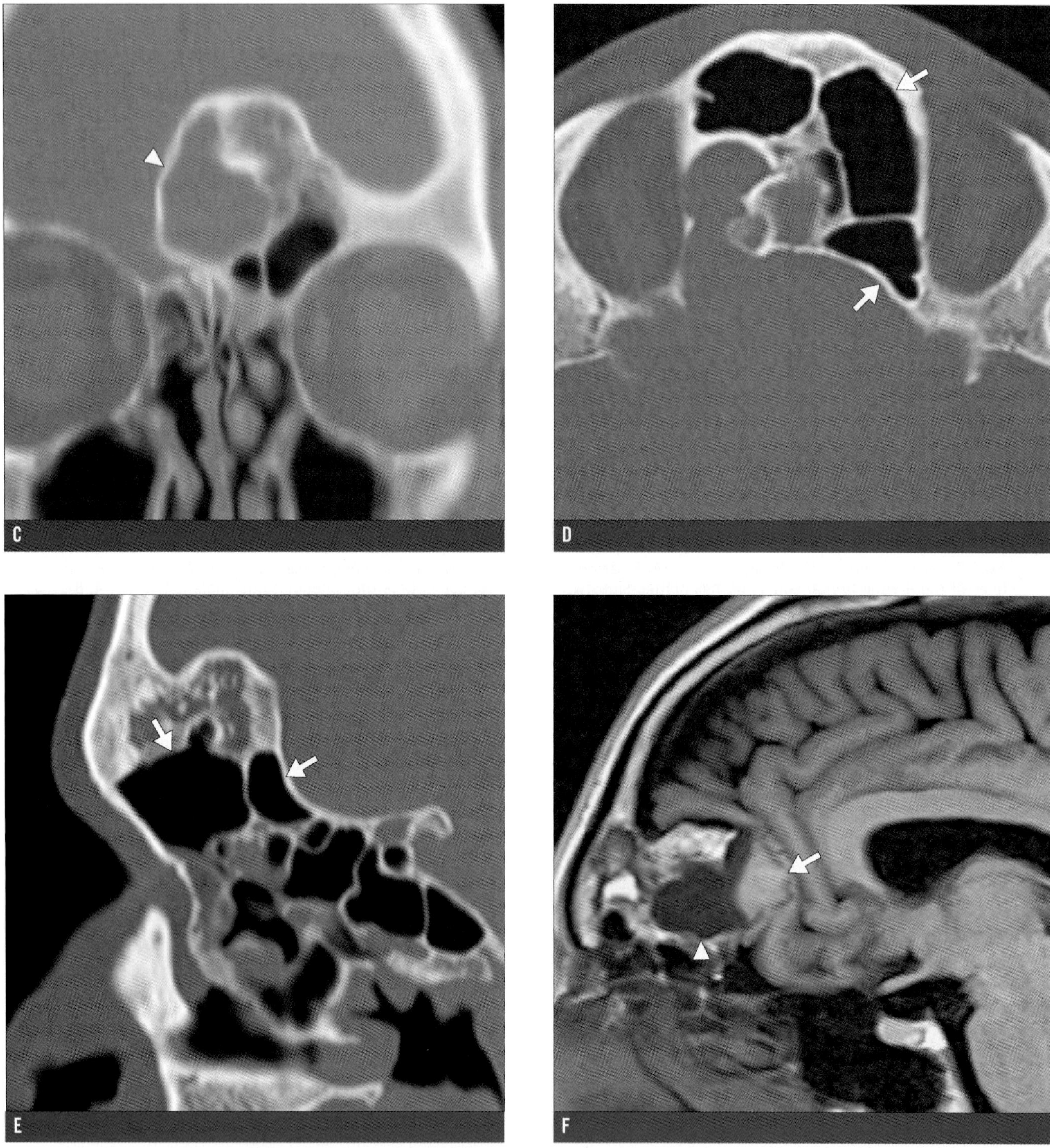
C
D
E
F

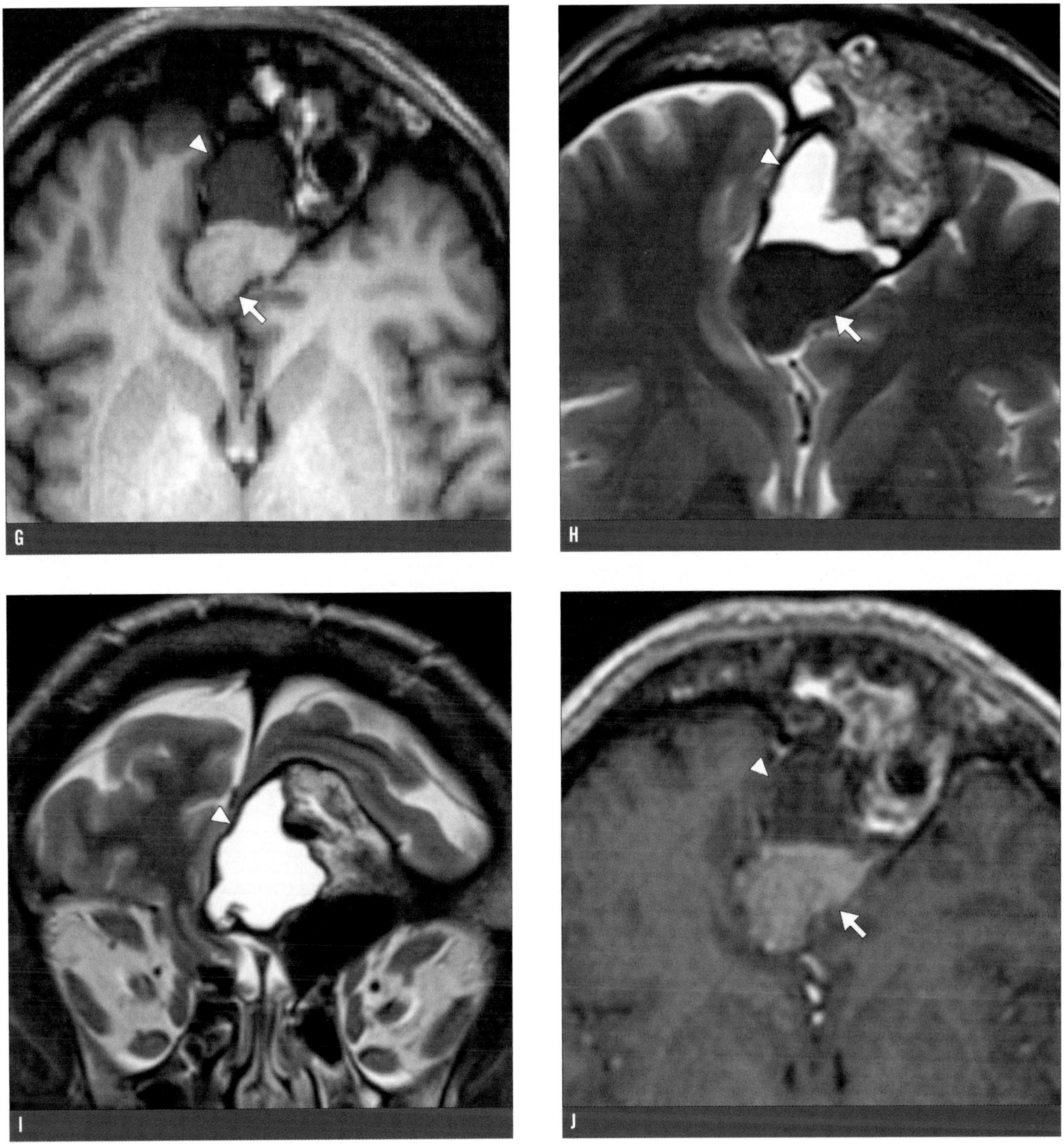

Companion case: Frontal sinus pneumocele

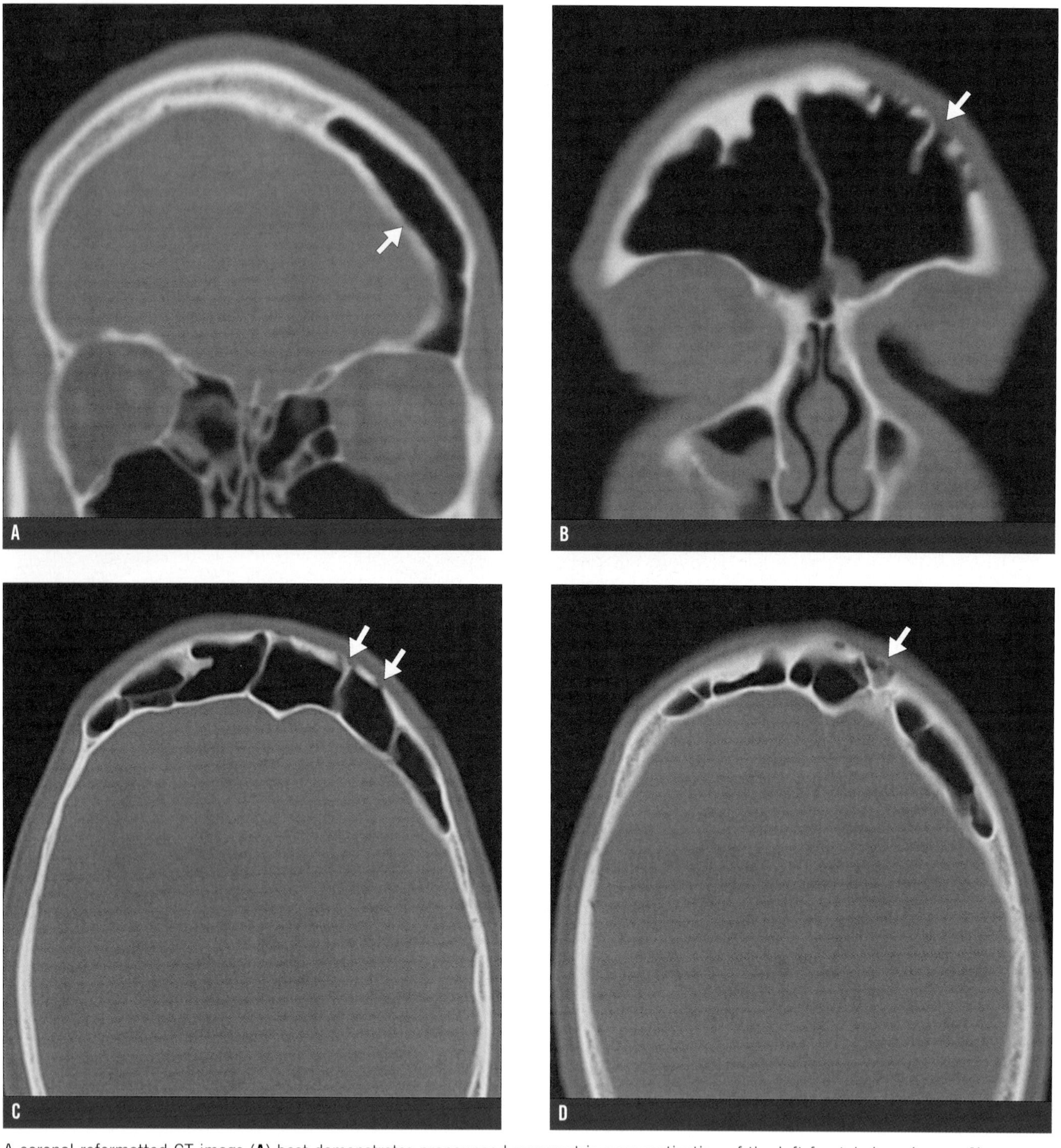

A coronal reformatted CT image (**A**) best demonstrates pronounced asymmetric pneumatization of the left frontal sinus (arrow, **A**). Coronal reformatted (**B**) and axial (**C**, **D**) CT images demonstrate pronounced thinning of the left frontal sinus anterior table (arrows, **B**-**D**). The expansion and wall thinning of the sinus are compatible with a pneumocele.

REFERENCES

Abdel-Aal AK, Abayazeed AH, Raghuram K, Curé JK. Pneumocele of the frontal sinus producing orbital roof defect: case report and review of literature. *Am J Otolaryngol.* 2010;31(3):202-204.

Acar M, Yucel A, Degirmenci B, Yilmaz MD, Albayrak R. Pneumocele vs. pneumosinus dilatans: review of the literature with a case of frontal sinuspneumocele. *Tohoku J Exp Med.* 2004;202(4): 295-297. Review.

Dhillon RS, Williams DC. Pneumosinus dilatans. *J Laryngol Otol.* 1987;101:828-832.

Flint PW, Haughey BH, Niparko JK, Richardson MA, Lund VJ, Robbins KT, Lesperance MM, Thomas JR, *Cummings Otolaryngology: Head and Neck Surgery.* 5th ed. St. Louis, MO: Mosby; 2010.

Park CY, Kim KS. Spontaneous pneumocephalus associated with pneumocele of the frontal sinus. *Cephalalgia.* 2010;30(11):1400-1402.

Schmalfuss IM, Camp M. Skull base: pseudolesion or true lesion? *Eur Radiol.* 2008;18:1232-1243.

CASE 4 Interfrontal sinus septal cell

An interfrontal sinus septal cell is defined as an air cell that results from pneumatization of a midline or paramedian bony septum located between the frontal sinuses. It can drain into its own separate recess or into either of the native frontal recesses.

COMPANION CASE

- **Interfrontal sinus septal cell mucocele.** If an interfrontal sinus septal cell does not have a patent outflow tract, either developmentally or otherwise, then the cell is "isolated". In these circumstances, the interfrontal sinus septal cell will be frequently opacified. Over time, this opacified cell may develop a mucocele and expand, sometimes obstructing one or both frontal recesses.

Interfrontal sinus septal cell draining via its own recess

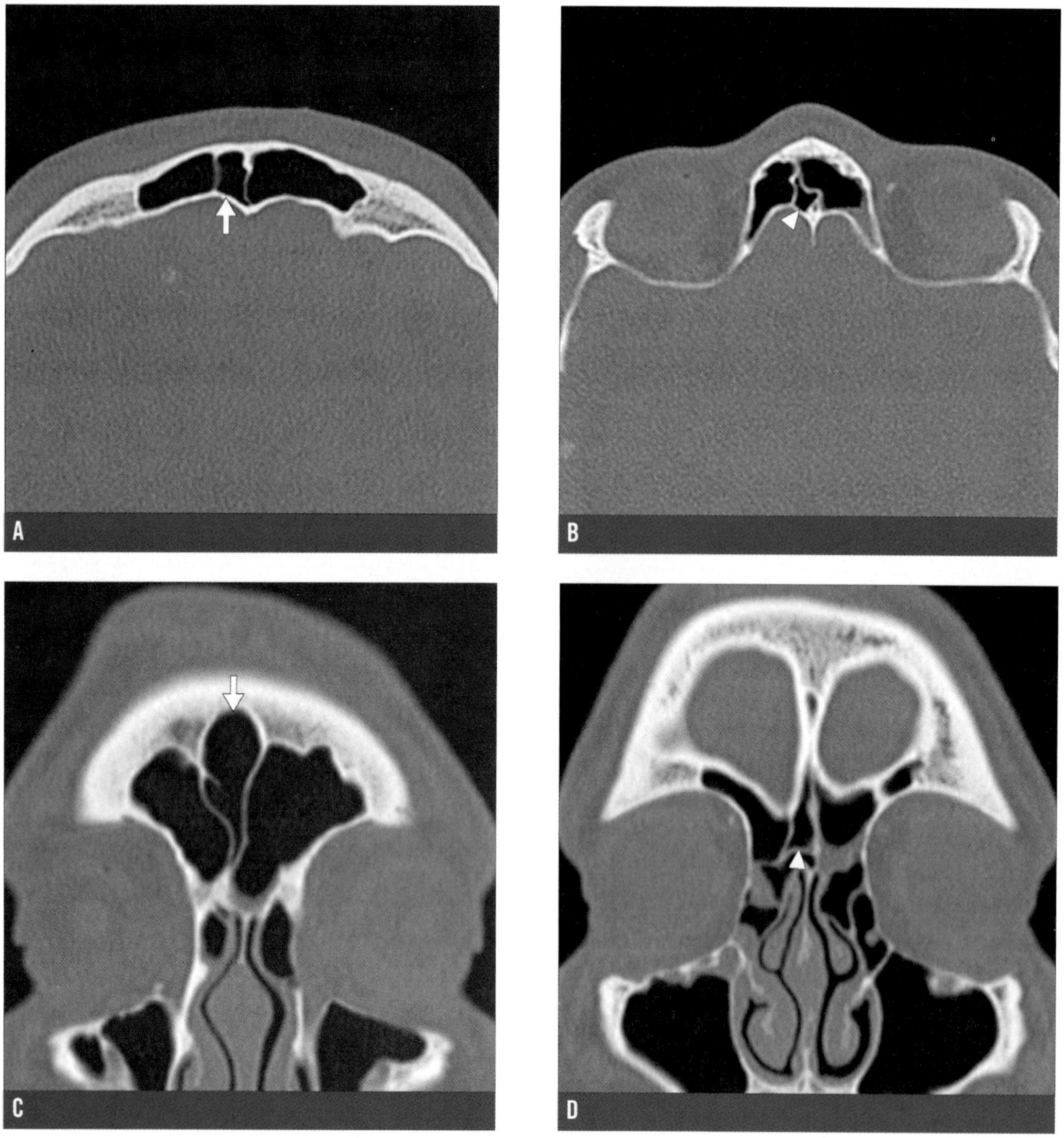

Axial CT images (**A, B**) demonstrate an interfrontal sinus septal cell (arrow, **A**) with its own separate outflow tract (arrowhead, **B**). Coronal reformatted CT images (**C-E**) also demonstrate the interfrontal sinus septal cell (arrow, **C**) and its own separate outflow tract (arrowheads, **D, E**).

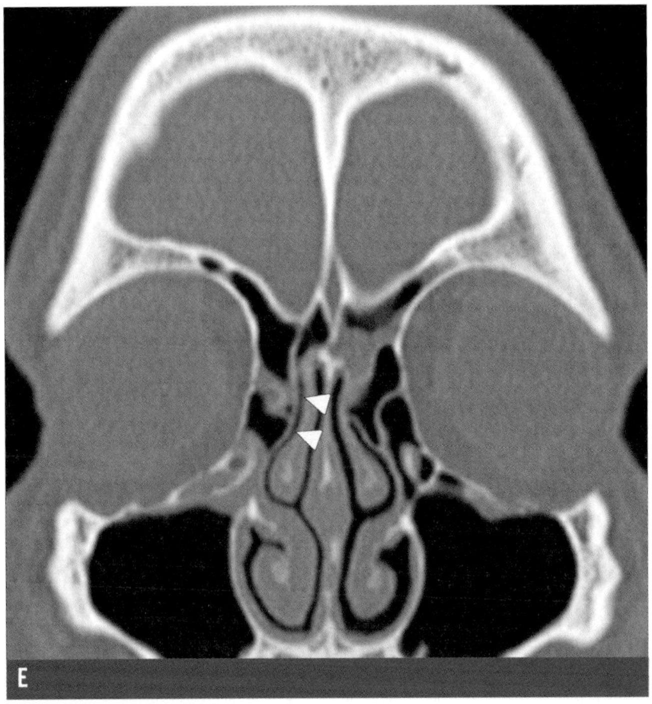

Interfrontal sinus septal cell draining via a frontal recess

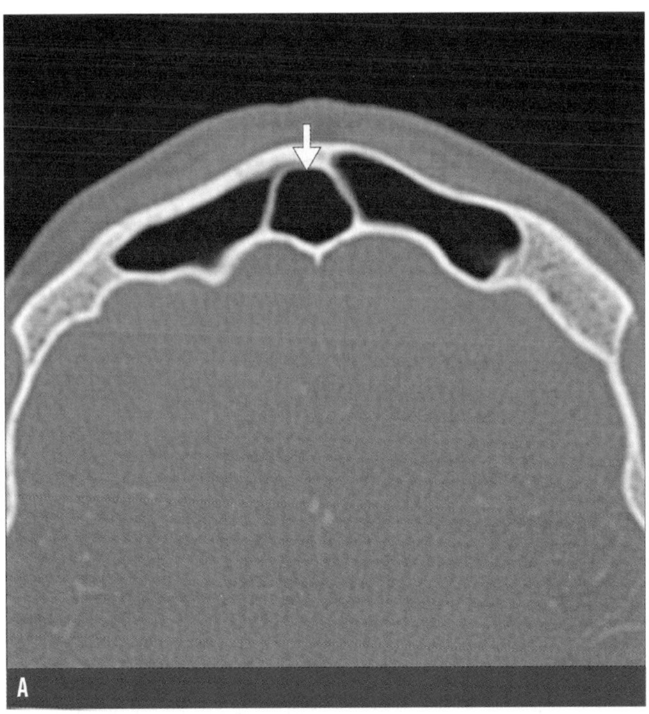

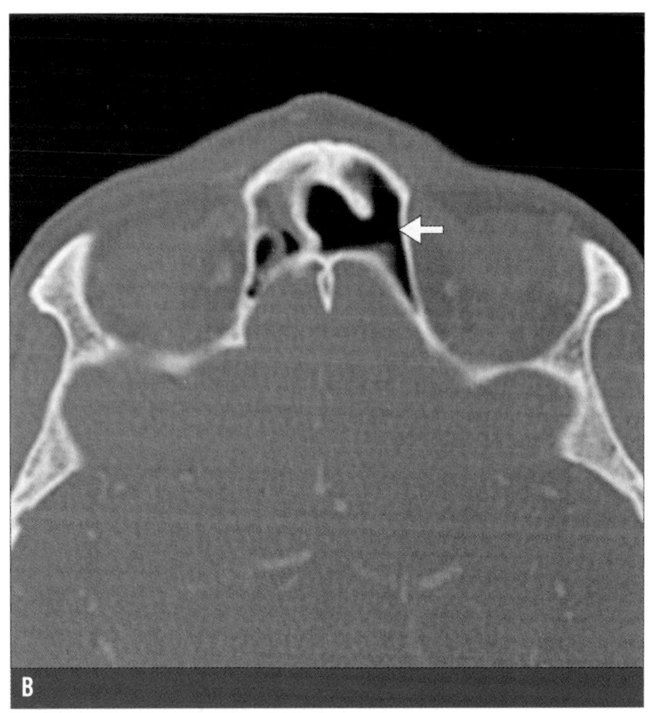

Axial (**A, B**) and coronal reformatted (**C, D**) CT images demonstrate an interfrontal sinus septal cell (arrows, **A, C**) that communicates with the left frontal recess (arrows, **B, D**).

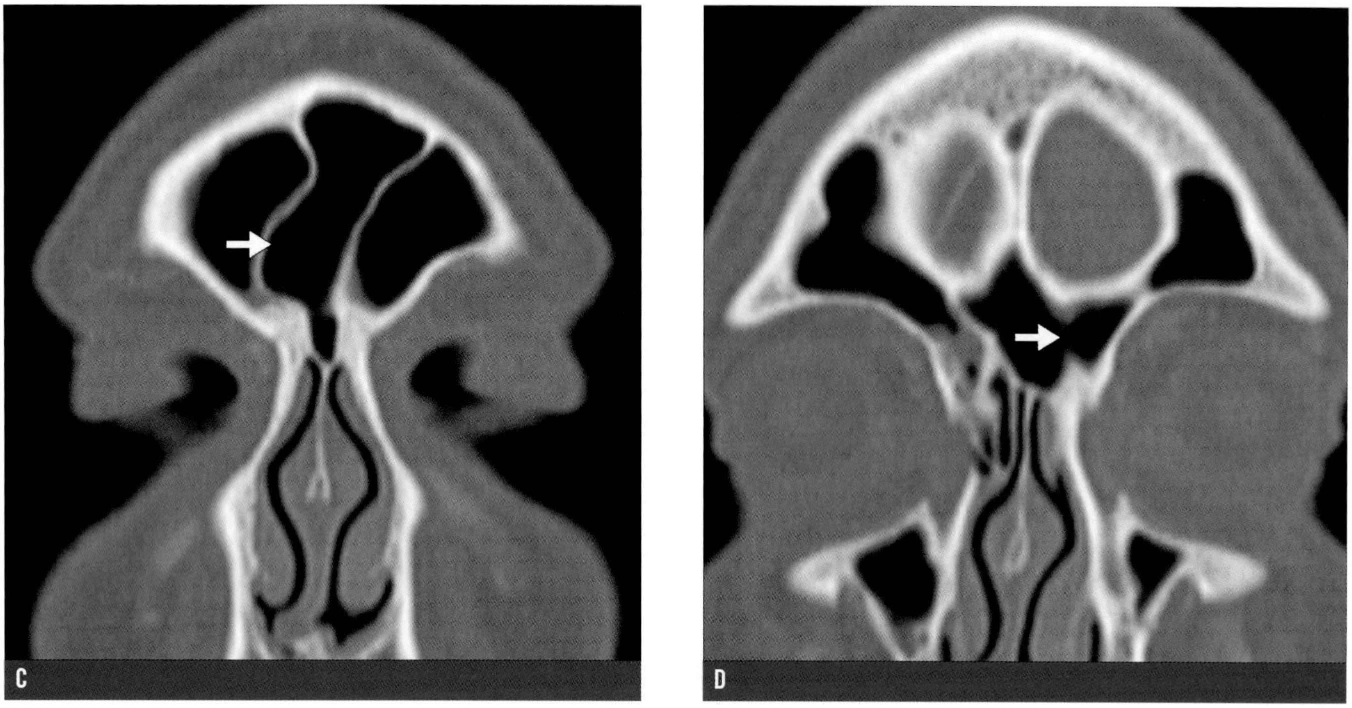

Opacified and isolated interfrontal sinus septa cell

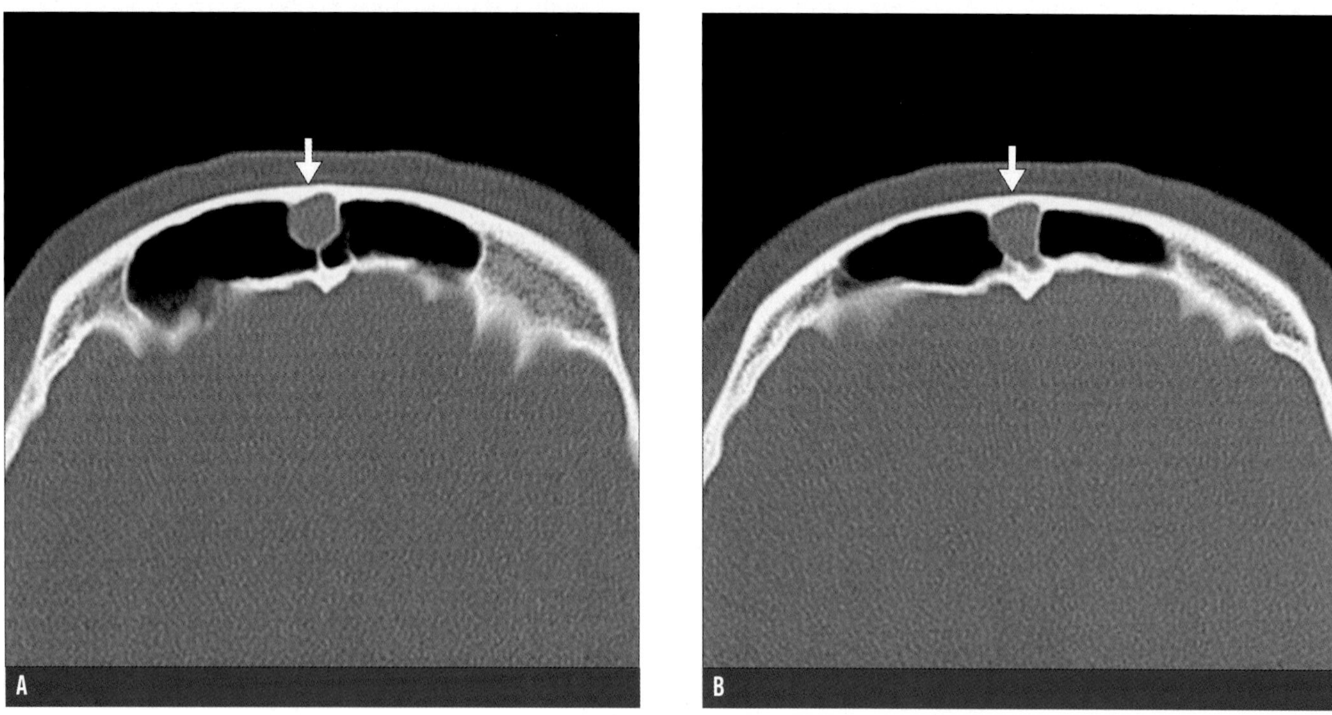

Axial (**A, B**), coronal reformatted (**C**), and sagittal reformatted (**D**) CT images demonstrate an opacified interfrontal sinus septal cell (arrows, **A-D**). The interfrontal sinus septal cell is isolated from the remaining paranasal sinuses as it does not contain its own outflow tract or drain into either frontal recess. Mild sclerosis along the superior margin of this interfrontal sinus septal cell suggests an element of chronic sinus disease (arrowhead, **C**).

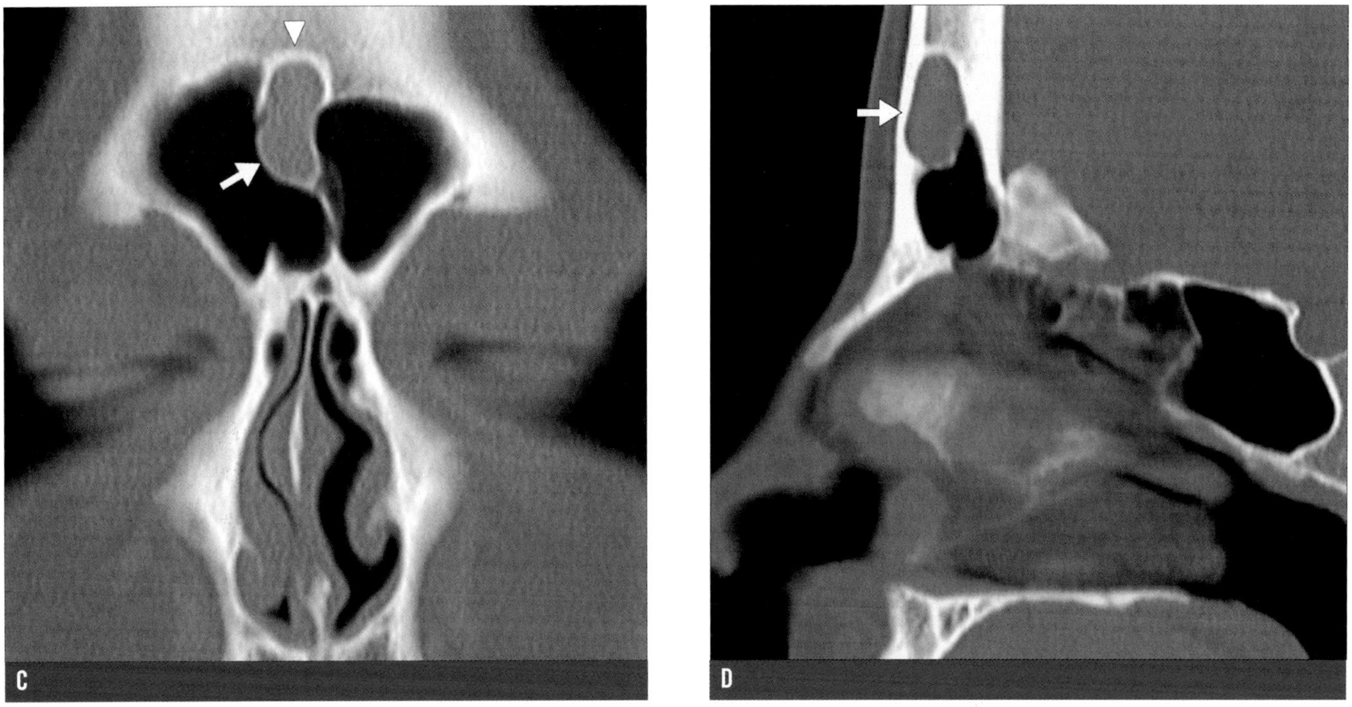

Companion case: Interfrontal sinus septal cell mucocele

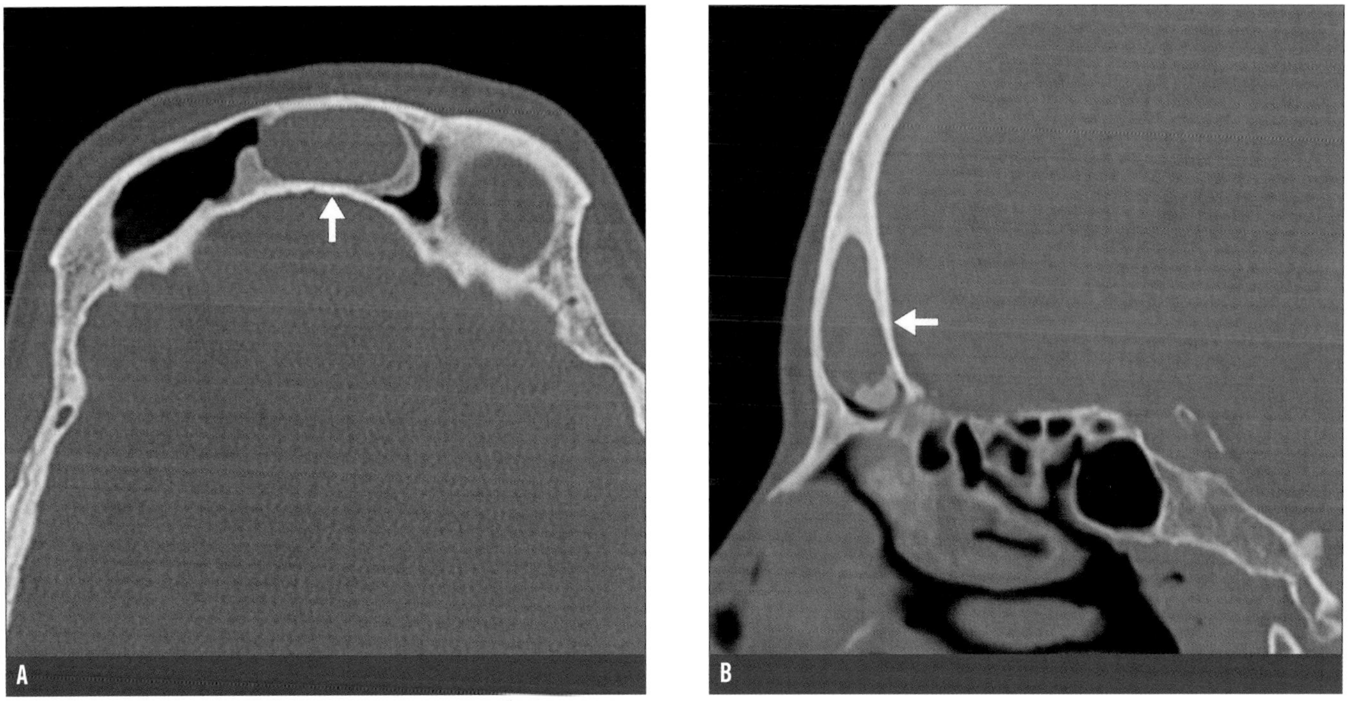

Axial (**A**), sagittal reformatted (**B**), and coronal reformatted (**C, D**) CT images demonstrate a completely opacified and expansile interfrontal sinus septal cell, compatible with a mucocele (arrows, **A-D**). Portions of the interfrontal sinus septal cell walls are thickened, compatible with a chronic process.

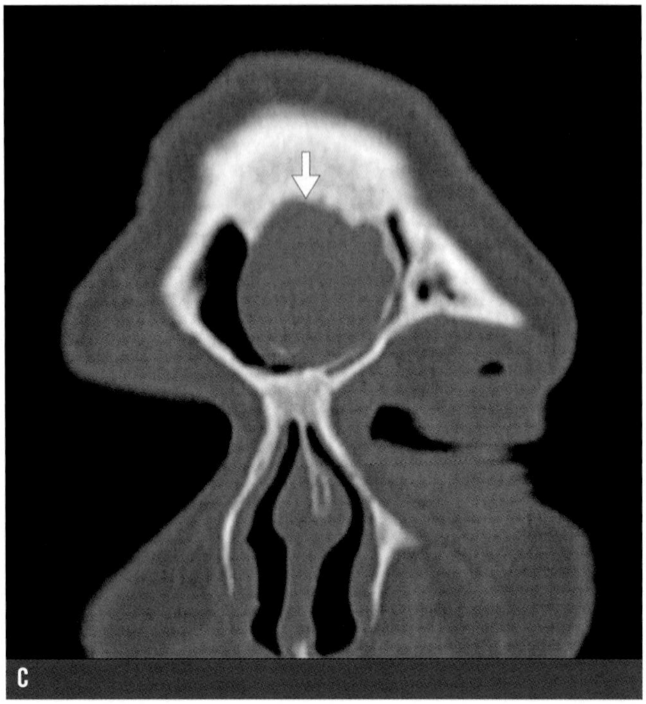

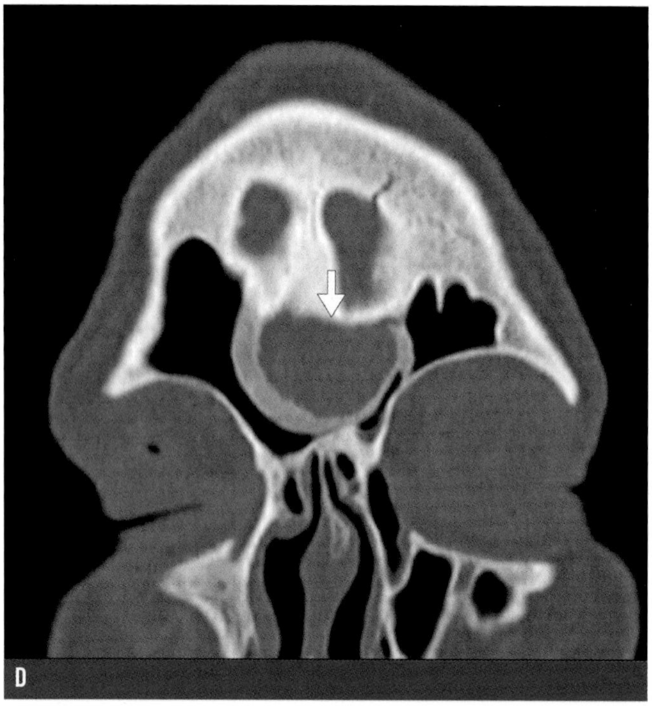

REFERENCE

Som PM, Lawson W. Interfrontal sinus septal cell: a cause of obstructing inflammation and mucoceles. *AJNR Am J Neuroradiol.* 2008;29:1369-1371.

CASE 5 Frontal bulla

A frontal bulla is as an anterior ethmoid air cell that extends cephalad into the posterior aspect of the frontal recess and into the frontal sinus. It resides posterior to an agger nasi cell (if present) and anterosuperior to the ethmoid bulla. Moreover, to constitute a frontal bulla, the posterior wall of a frontal bulla shares a wall with the anterior skull base, and its anterior wall is a free partition within the frontal sinus. If large, or when strategically located, a frontal bulla may impair drainage of a frontal sinus/recess.

COMPANION CASES

- **Suprabullar air cell.** Like a frontal bulla, this represents an air cell that is located anterosuperior to the ethmoid bulla. However, unlike a frontal bulla, the suprabullar air cell does not extend into the frontal sinus. The superior wall of the suprabullar air represents the anterior cranial fossa skull base.

Frontal bulla narrowing the ipsilateral frontal recess

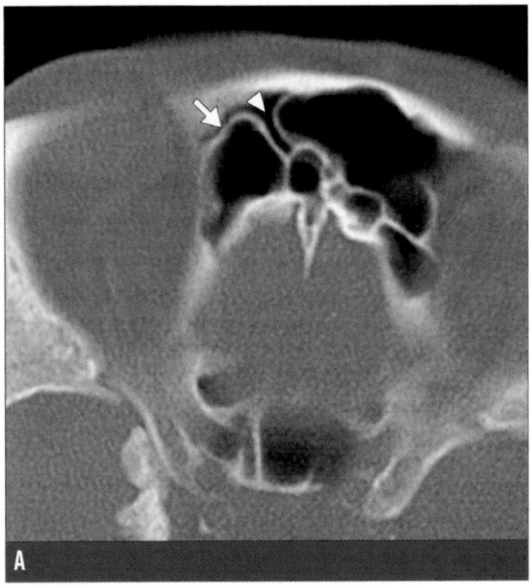

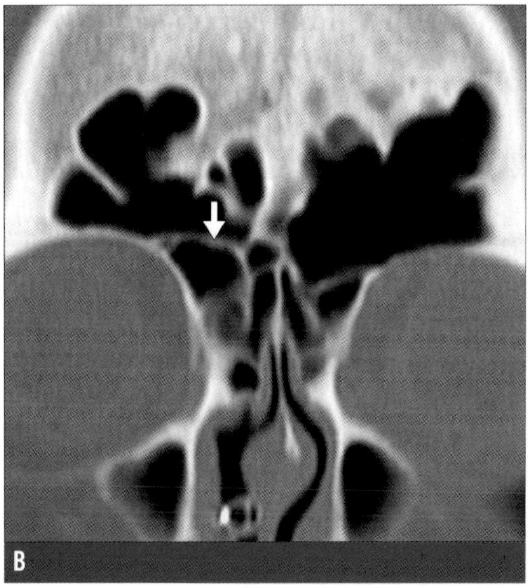

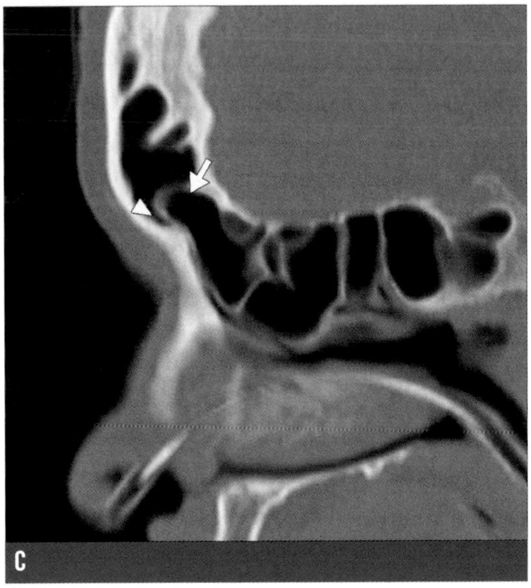

Axial **(A)**, coronal reformatted (**B**), and sagittal reformatted (**C**) CT images demonstrate a moderate-sized right frontal bulla (arrows, **A-C**) extending into the right frontal sinus and narrowing the right frontal recess (arrowheads, **A, C**).

Frontal bulla partially obstructing the ipsilateral frontal recess

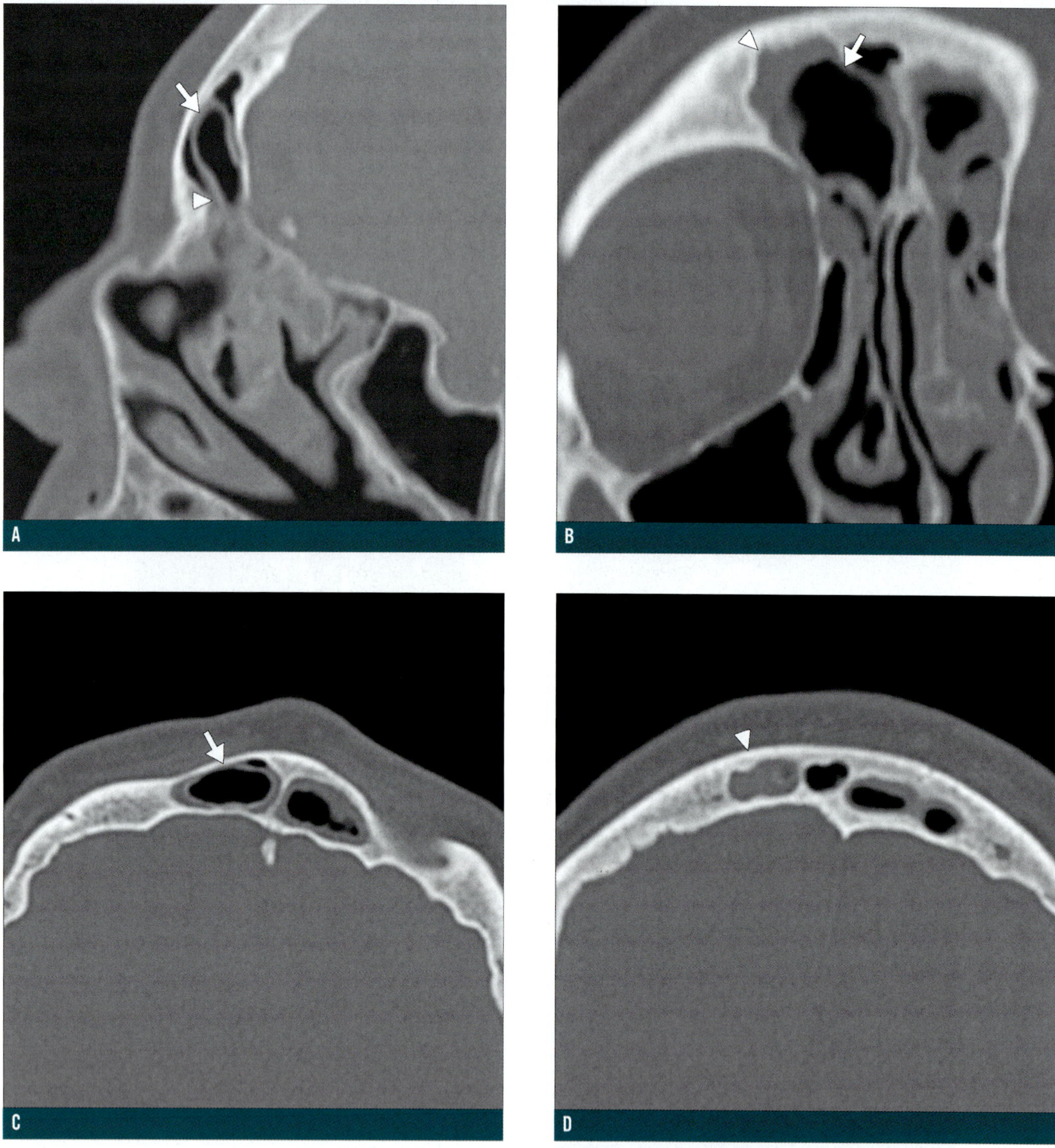

Sagittal reformatted (**A**), coronal reformatted (**B**), and axial (**C, D**) CT images demonstrate a large right frontal bulla (arrows, **A-C**) narrowing the right frontal recess (arrowhead, **A**) and associated with partial opacification of the right frontal sinus (arrowheads, **B, D**).

Companion case: Suprabullar air cell

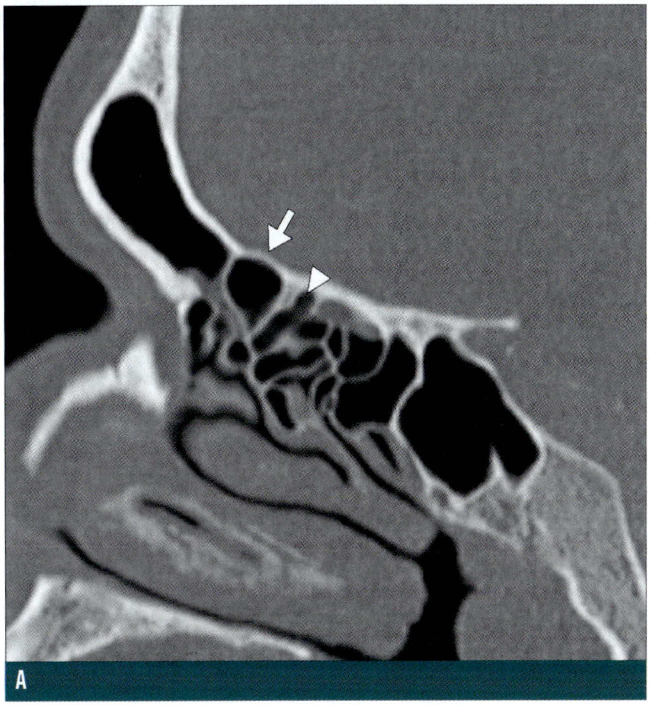

A sagittal reformatted CT image **(A)** demonstrates a suprabullar air cell (arrow) located immediately anterosuperior to the ethmoid bulla (arrowhead).

REFERENCE

Lee WT, Kuhn FA, Citardi MJ. 3D computed tomographic analysis of frontal recess anatomy in patients without frontal sinusitis. *Otolaryngol Head Neck Surg.* 2004;131(3):164-173.

CASE 6 Frontal cells

Frontal cells are ethmoid air cells that extend cephalad into the frontal recess or frontal sinus. However, unlike a frontal bulla, the posterior wall of a frontal cell represents a distinct partition between the frontal cell and the frontal recess/sinus , whereas for a frontal bulla, its ventral wall represents a free partition in the frontal recess/sinus. If a frontal cell extends into the frontal sinus, then the anterior wall of the frontal cell represents the anterior wall of the frontal sinus. Additionally, all frontal cells, when present, reside superior to the agger nasi air cell, as opposed to a frontal bulla, which resides posterior to the agger nasi cell. Please refer to the immediately preceding case for further discussion regarding a frontal bulla. If large, or when strategically located, a frontal cell or frontal bulla may obstruct a frontal sinus/recess.

Frontal air cells were classified into four types by Bent and Kuhn in 1994.

Type I—A single air cell located superior to the agger nasi cell that does not extend into the frontal sinus and its posterior wall is a free partition in the frontal recess
Type II—A tier of two or more air cells located superior to the agger nasi cell and their posterior walls are free partitions in the frontal sinus/recess
Type III—A single large air cell located superior to the agger nasi cell that extends superiorly into the frontal sinus lumen and its posterior wall is a free partition in the frontal sinus/recess
Type IV—A single air cell contained entirely within the frontal sinus and its posterior wall is a free partition in the frontal sinus

Type I frontal cell

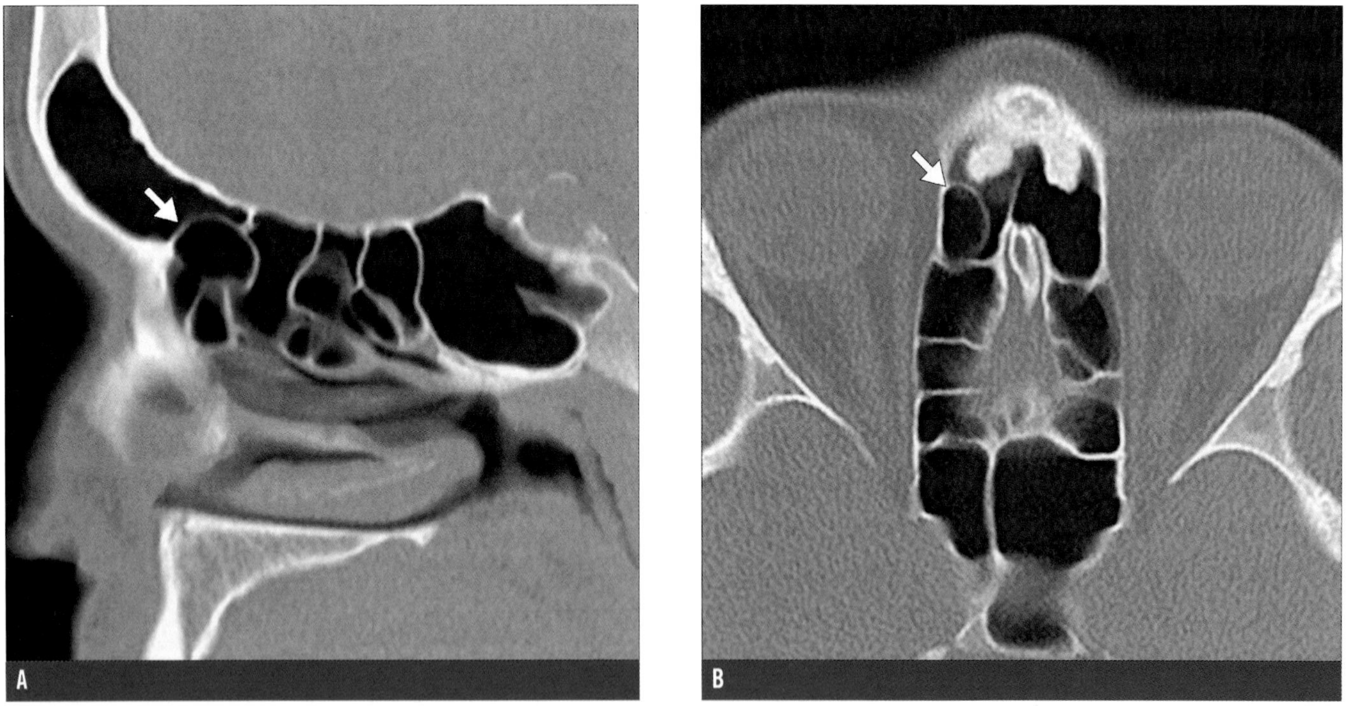

Sagittal reformatted (**A**) and axial (**B**) CT images demonstrate a type I frontal cell (arrows, **A**, **B**).

Type II frontal cell

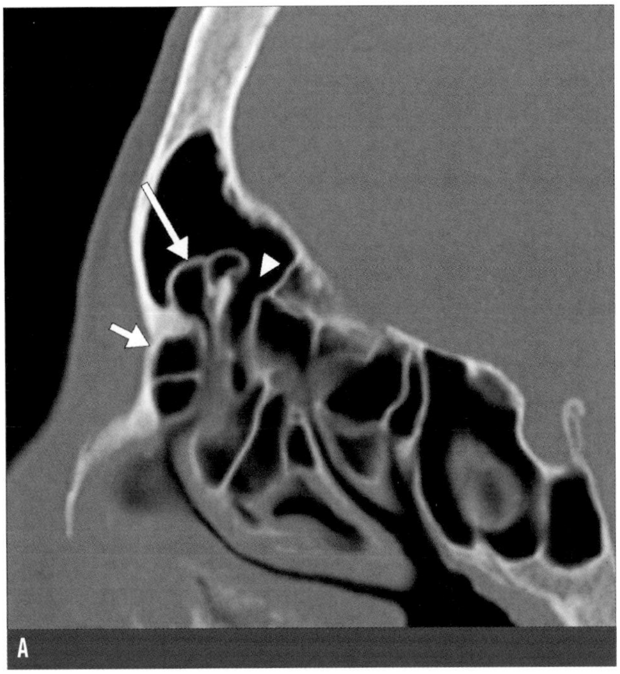

A sagittal reformatted CT image through the frontal sinus and frontal recess **(A)** demonstrates multiple tiered air cells (long arrow) located above an agger nasi air cell (short arrow). These multiple tiered air cells extend cephalad into the frontal sinus and recess, compatible with type II frontal cells. The frontal recess is patent in this case (arrowhead).

Type III frontal cell

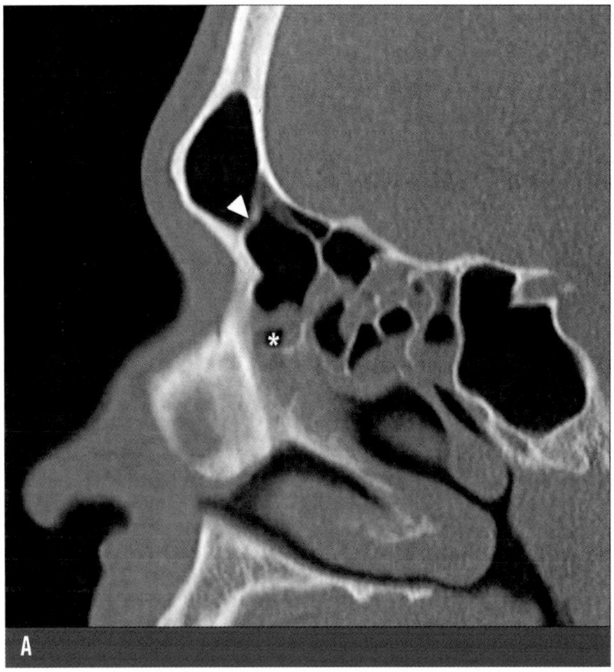

A sagittal reformatted CT image (**A**) demonstrates a single air cell that traverses the frontal recess as well as extends into the frontal sinus (arrowhead). This air cell is located cephalad to an agger nasi cell (asterisk) and its posterior wall represents a free partition in the frontal recess and frontal sinus. The combination findings is compatible with a Type III frontal cell.

Type IV frontal cell

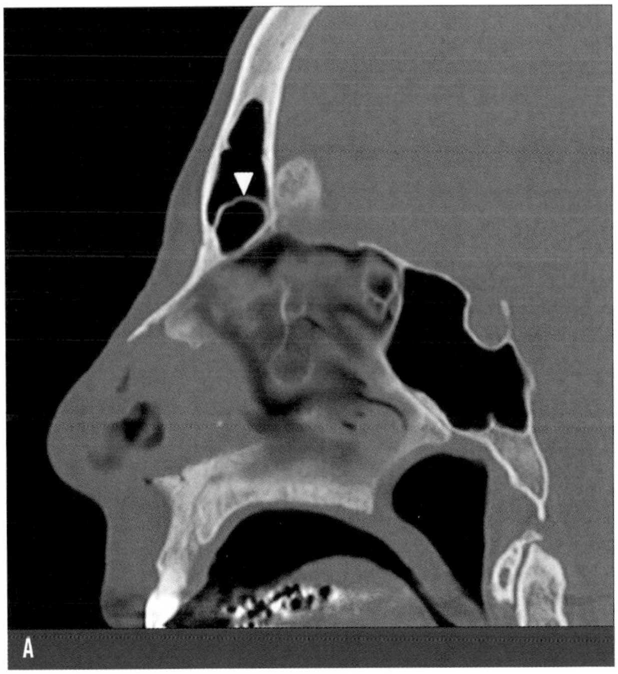

A sagittal reformatted CT image **(A)** demonstrates an isolated air cell in a frontal sinus (arrowhead) in which its anterior-inferior margin is the anterior wall of the frontal sinus and its posterior wall represents a free partition in the frontal sinus. These findings are consistent with a type IV frontal cell.

REFERENCES

Bent JP, Cuilty-Siller C, Kuhn FA. The frontal cell as a cause of frontal sinus obstruction. *Am J Rhinol.* 1994;8(4):185-191.

Huang BY[1], Lloyd KM, DelGaudio JM, Jablonowski E, Hudgins PA. Failed endoscopic sinus surgery: spectrum of CT findings in the frontal recess. *Radiographics.* 2009;29(1):177-195.

Lee WT, Kuhn FA, Citardi MJ. 3D computed tomographic analysis of frontal recess anatomy in patients without frontal sinusitis. *Otolaryngol Head Neck Surg.* 2004;131(3):164-173.

Navarro JAC. *The Nasal Cavity and Paranasal Sinuses: Surgical Anatomy.* New York, NY: Springer-Verlag Berlin Heidelberg; 1997.

Yildirim A. Is it more reasonable to categorize frontal cells on the basis of their location rather than on their type? *Ear Nose Throat J.* 2010; 89(9):E19.

CASE 7 Frontal sinusotomies

A frontal sinusotomy is a surgical procedure performed to treat chronic inflammatory frontal sinus disease that is refractory to medical treatment. To understand the indications of a frontal sinusotomy, as well as to determine whether there has been a sufficient resection, it is imperative to understand the complex anatomy of the frontal sinus outflow tract.

The frontal sinus outflow tract represents a combination of the funnel-shaped inferior portion of the frontal sinus (also called frontal infundibulum), frontal sinus ostium, and frontal recess. The frontal sinus ostium represents the opening between the frontal sinus and frontal recess and is located at the level of the frontal sinus floor, demarcated by the nasofrontal process (also called frontal beak). The walls of the frontal recess are not inherent to the recess but are rather derived from the walls of several regional air cells, collectively termed frontal recess air cells. Many of these frontal recess air cells are only variably present and include the frontal cell, frontal bulla, agger nasi air cell, supraorbital ethmoid air cell, suprabullar air cell, and interfrontal sinus air cell.

The borders of the frontal recess are as follows:

- Anterior, inferior, and a portion of the lateral boundary are formed by the agger nasi bone or air cell.
- Lateral boundary is formed by the lamina papyracea.
- Medial boundary is formed by the most anterior-superior aspect of the middle turbinate and the lateral wall of the olfactory fossa.
- Posterior boundary is formed by the ethmoid bulla and, if present, the suprabullar air cell.
- Superior boundary is formed by the fovea ethmoidalis.

The size and configuration of the frontal recess air cells often dictate the caliber and relative patency of the frontal sinus outflow tract. The frontal recess air cells need to be adequately resected if they represent the cause of a frontal sinus outflow obstruction. The frontal sinus outflow tract, including its postoperative appearance, is best appreciated with sagittal reformatted CT imaging.

There are several types of frontal sinusotomies, first described by Wolfgang Draf in the early 1990s. These are endoscopic surgeries that are performed if the frontal sinus disease does not improve with classic ostiomeatal complex surgery. The Draf procedures may be performed in a progressive three-stage approach if the preceding surgery fails to provide relief. There have been modifications to these procedures over the years and the Draf nomenclature has been replaced with other terminology by some authors. However, generally speaking, these procedures are as follows, from least to most extensive:

- Endoscopic frontal recess approach (Draf type I)—This surgery completely removes the anterior ethmoid cells, uncinate process, and any obstructing air cells, such as frontal cells. However, the mucosa of the frontal recess and frontal ostium is left intact.
- Extended frontal sinusotomy (Draf type II)—The floor of the frontal sinus is resected, from the level of nasal septum medially to the lamina papyracea laterally. The anterior face of the frontal recess is also resected. When viewed in the coronal plane, a Draf I and Draf II procedure will appear similar; the two procedures are best differentiated by sagittal reformatted CT imaging, with at least a portion of the frontal sinus floor intact with a Draf I procedure but the frontal sinus floor completely absent with a Draf II procedure.
- Endoscopic modified Lothrop (Draf type III)—This surgery is performed for severe refractory frontal sinusitis. It involves removal of the inferior aspect of the interfrontal septum, the superior portion of the nasal septum, and the floor of both frontal sinuses laterally to the level of the orbit. The lamina papyracea and posterior walls of the frontal sinuses are left intact.

COMPANION CASE

- **Trephination.** Trephination is a surgical procedure that is performed from an external approach. It entails an incision made superior to the brow with careful attention made to avoid injury to the supratrochlear and supraorbital neurovascular bundles. The anterior wall of the abnormal frontal sinus is drilled. The frontal sinus disease may be removed and the sinus irrigated from this approach. This procedure, in conjunction with an endoscopic approach, may be performed to gain access to the frontal sinus and allow for placement of a frontal recess stent. It may also be performed to allow for greater access to the anterior skull base, such as to aid in an anterior skull base CSF leak repair. Correlation with imaging is necessary to accurately localize the frontal sinuses prior to a trephination procedure.
- **Osteoplastic flap procedure with frontal sinus obliteration.** This procedure is performed in cases when endoscopic treatment fails, for resection of large frontal tumors, or in cases of severe facial fractures involving the anterior paranasal sinus drainage pathways that are damaged beyond repair. They may also be performed to treat far lateral frontal sinus or supraorbital ethmoid air cell mucocele formation that is not amenable to an endoscopic approach. The procedure begins with osteotomies. The frontal sinus mucosa is then removed and replaced with an autologous fat graft and soft tissue, followed by replacement of the bony flap. The imaging appearance of the frontal sinus obliteration depends on the tissues placed, although at least a portion of the obliteration almost always includes fat.

Frontal sinusotomy via an endoscopic frontal recess approach (Draf type I)

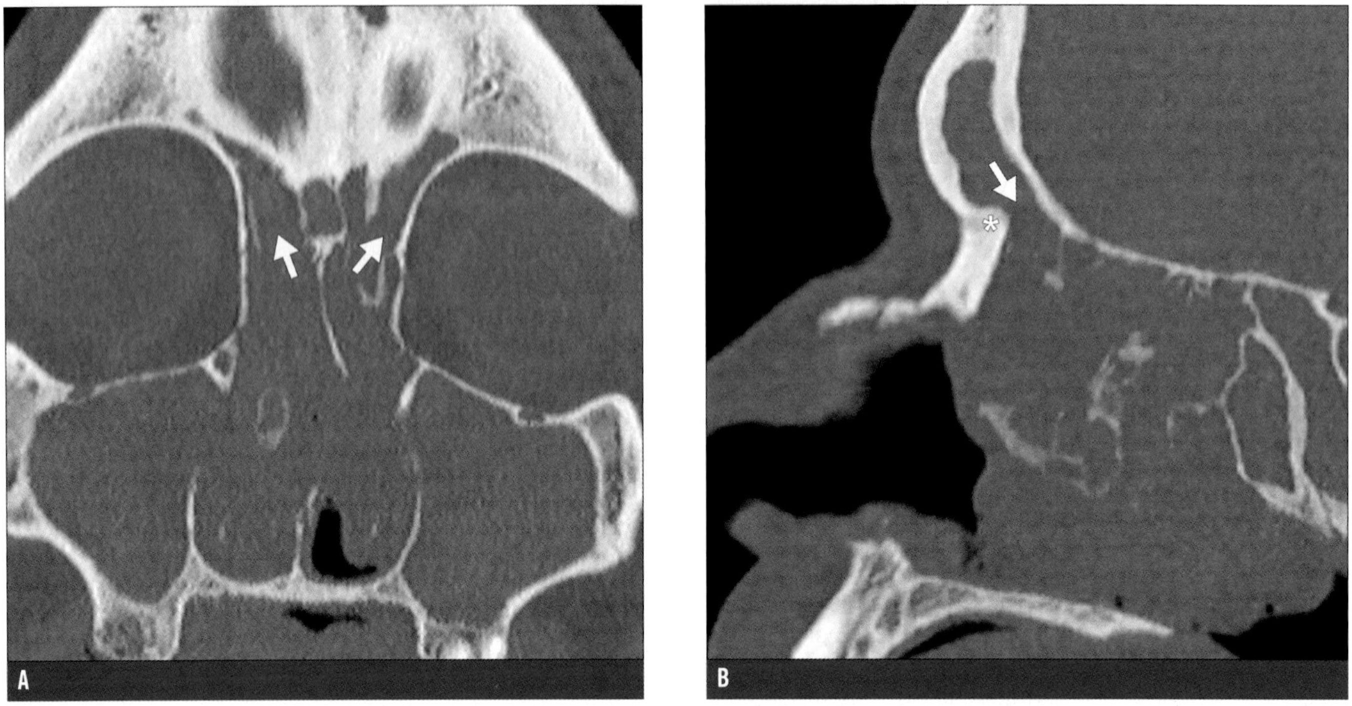

A coronal reformatted CT image (**A**) demonstrates bilateral frontal sinusotomies (arrows, **A**). A right parasagittal CT image (**B**) demonstrates the right frontal sinusotomy (arrow, **B**) with an intact frontal sinus floor, as evidenced by a fully intact nasofrontal process or frontal beak (asterisk, **B**). These findings constitute an endoscopic frontal recess approach, or Draf I frontal sinusotomy.

Extended frontal sinusotomy (Draf type II)

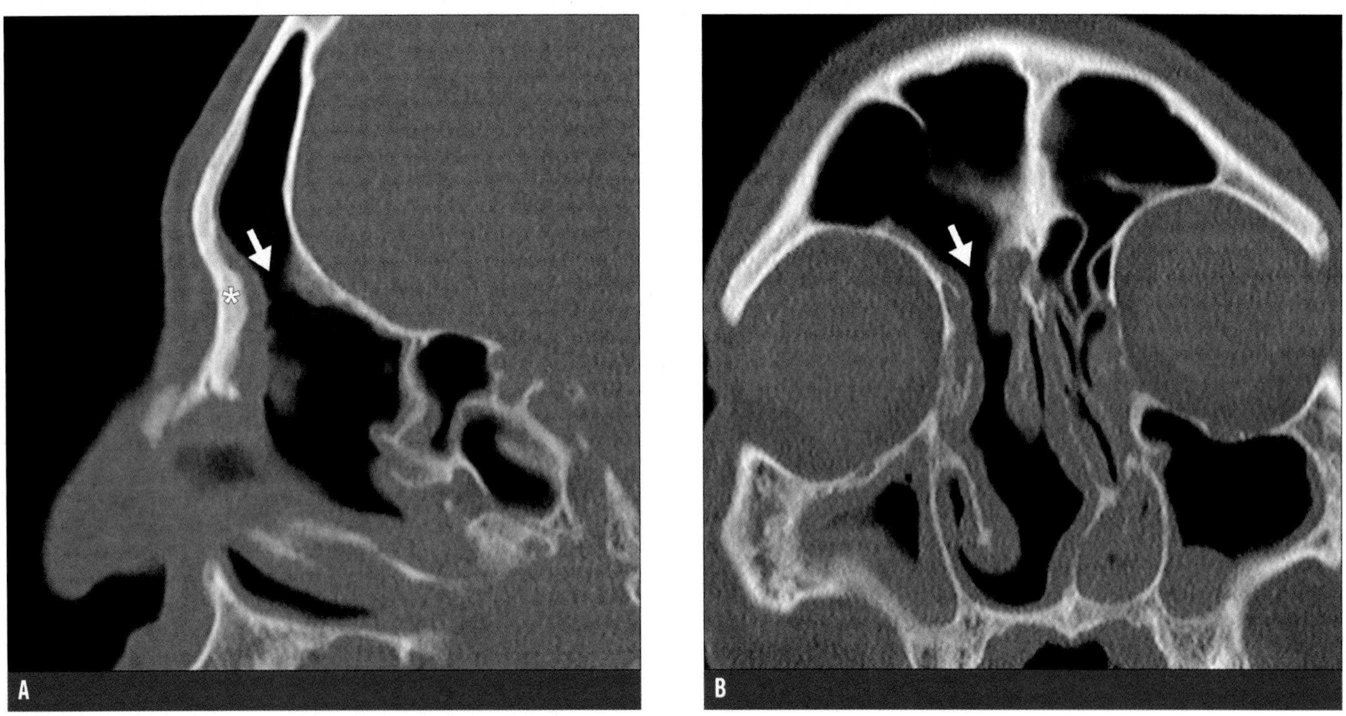

Right parasagittal (**A**) and coronal reformatted (**B**) CT images demonstrates a right frontal sinusotomy (arrows, **A, B**). The lack of a right frontal sinus floor, as evidenced by a blunted nasofrontal process (asterisk, **A**) as well as an intact nasal septum (appreciated on image **B**) constitute an extended frontal sinusotomy, or Draf II frontal sinusotomy.

Frontal sinusotomy via an endoscopic modified Lothrop approach (Draf type III)

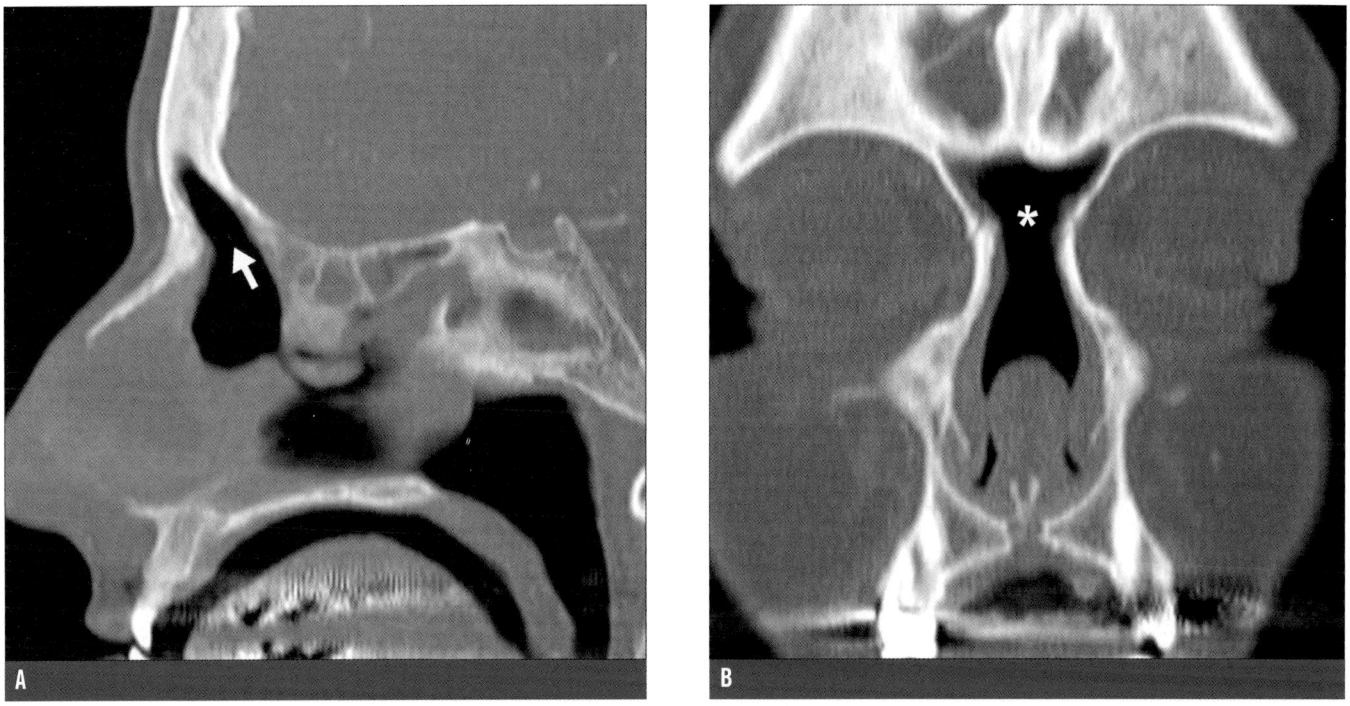

A right parasagittal reformatted CT image (**A**) demonstrates a right frontal sinusotomy (arrow, **A**) in this patient with severe refractory frontal sinusitis. A coronal reformatted CT image (**B**) demonstrates absence of the superior aspect of the osseous nasal septum (asterisk, **B**), characteristic of a modified Lothrop procedure, or Draf type III frontal sinusotomy.

Companion case: Trephination

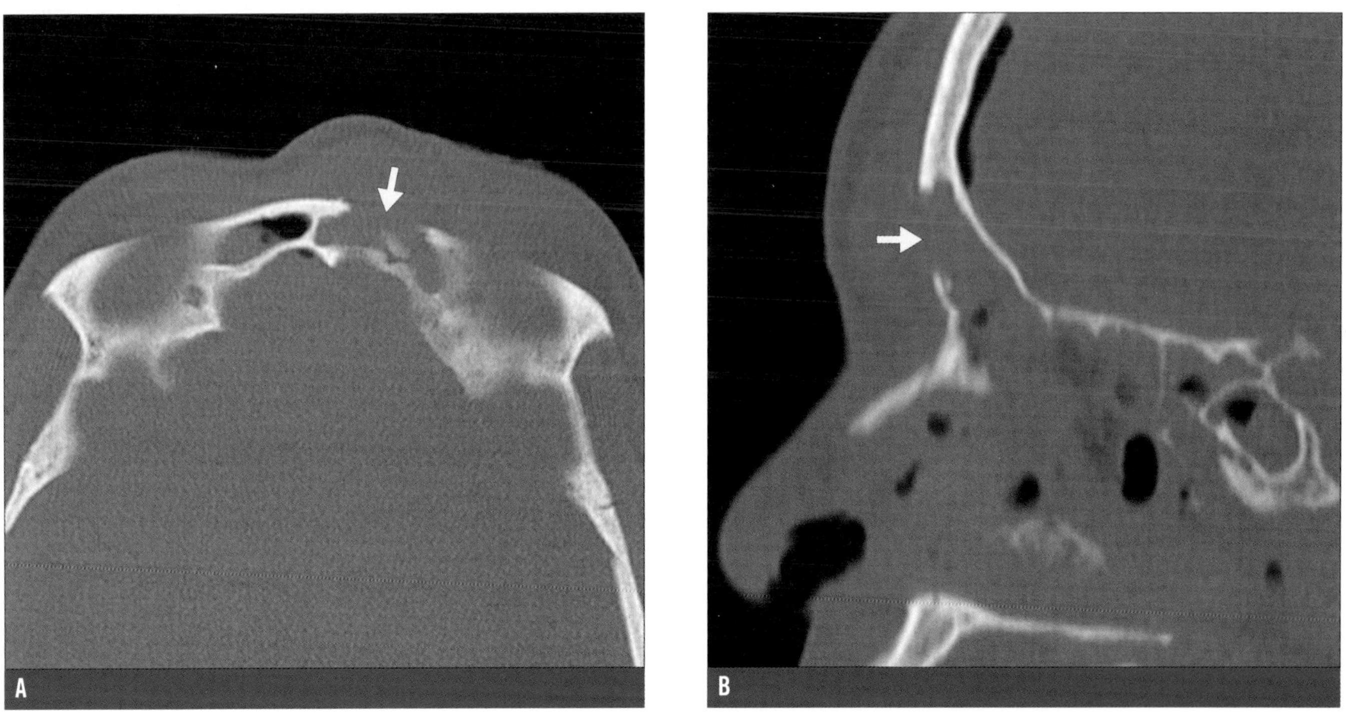

Axial (**A**) and left parasagittal reformatted (**B**) CT images demonstrate an osseous defect involving the anterior wall of the left frontal sinus, consistent with a left frontal sinus trephination surgery (arrows, **A**, **B**). In this patient, this was performed to access and treat an anterior cranial fossa CSF leak (not shown).

Companion case: Osteoplastic flap procedure with frontal sinus obliteration

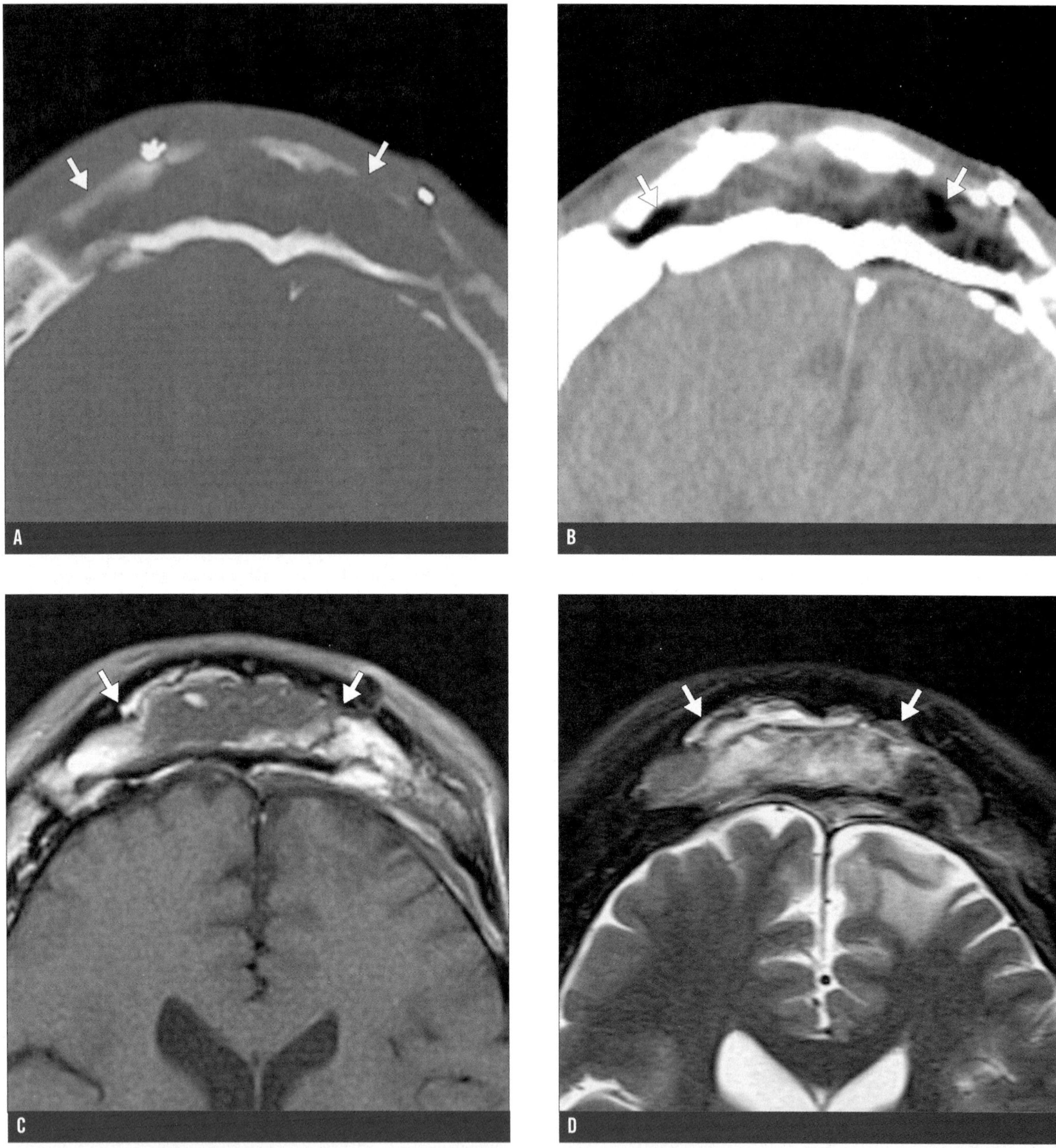

Axial CT images viewed with a bone window (**A**) and soft tissue window (**B**) demonstrate postoperative changes involving both frontal sinuses with soft tissue/granulation tissue and fat packing in both frontal sinuses (arrows, **A**, **B**), compatible with an osteoplastic flap procedure and frontal sinus obliteration. Axial T1 (**C**), axial T2 (**D**), and axial (**E**) as well as sagittal (**F**) fat-suppressed postcontrast T1-weighted MR images demonstrate the same postoperative changes on MRI (arrows, **C-F**).

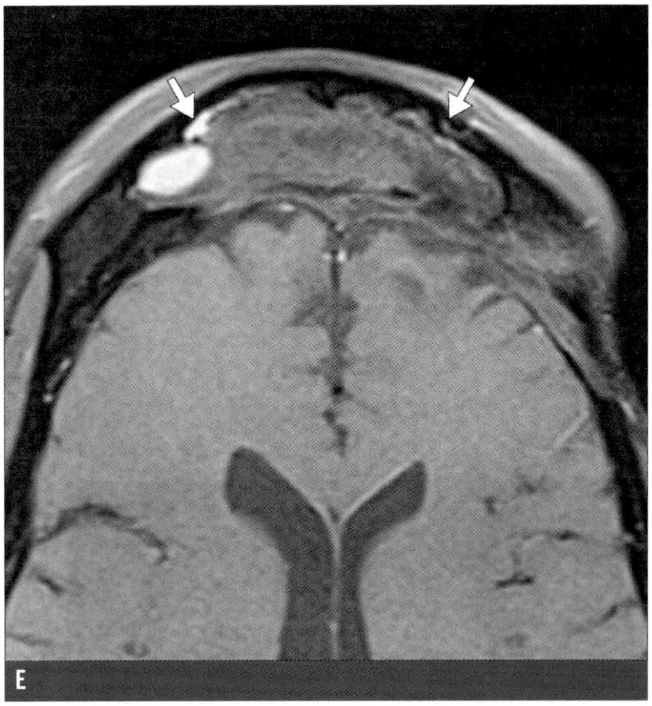

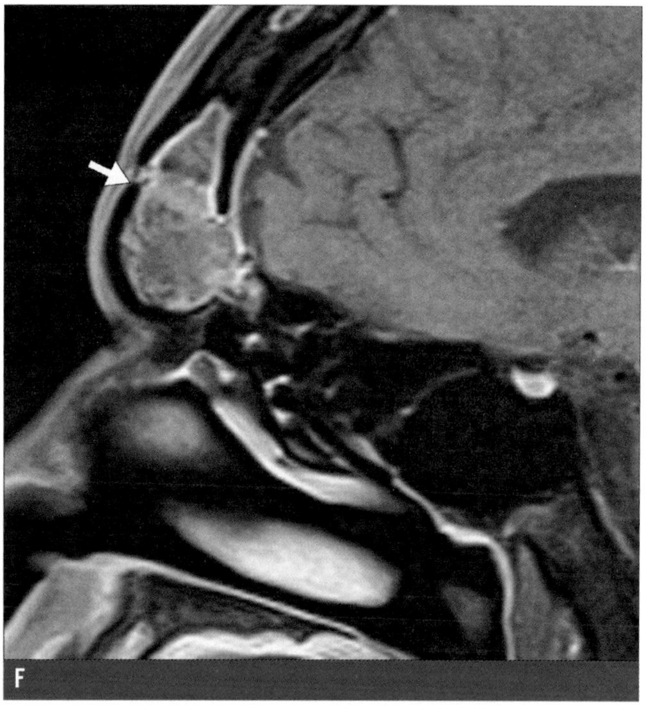

REFERENCES

Beale TJ, Madani G, Morley SJ. Imaging of the paranasal sinuses and nasal cavity: normal anatomy and clinically relevant anatomical variants. *Semin Ultrasound CT MR*. 2009;30(1):2-16.

Benoit CM, Duncavage JA. Combined external and endoscopic sinusotomy with stent placement: a retrospective review. *Laryngoscope*. 2001;111:1246-1249.

Huang BY, Lloyd KM, DelGaudio JM, Jablonowski E, Hudgins PA. Failed endoscopic sinus surgery: spectrum of CT findings in the frontal recess. *Radiographics*. 2009;29(1):177-195.

Weber R, Draf W, Kratzsch B, Hosemann W, Schaefer SD. Modern concepts of frontal sinus surgery. *Laryngoscope*. 2001;111(1):137-146.

CASE 8 Frontal sinusotomy stent

Synechia or mineralization may develop within a frontal sinusotomy following surgery. These changes may result in obstruction of the frontal sinusotomy and subsequent frontal sinus mucocele formation. If the patient is at high risk for developing synechia and/or mineralization, then a frontal sinusotomy stent may be placed to allow for postoperative patency. A variety of stent materials may be used, including silicone. These stents are typically removed in the office approximately 4 weeks following surgery. However, if a stent is placed to correct a postoperative stenosis, then the stent may need to remain in place for 6 to 12 months following surgery.

Frontal sinusotomy stent

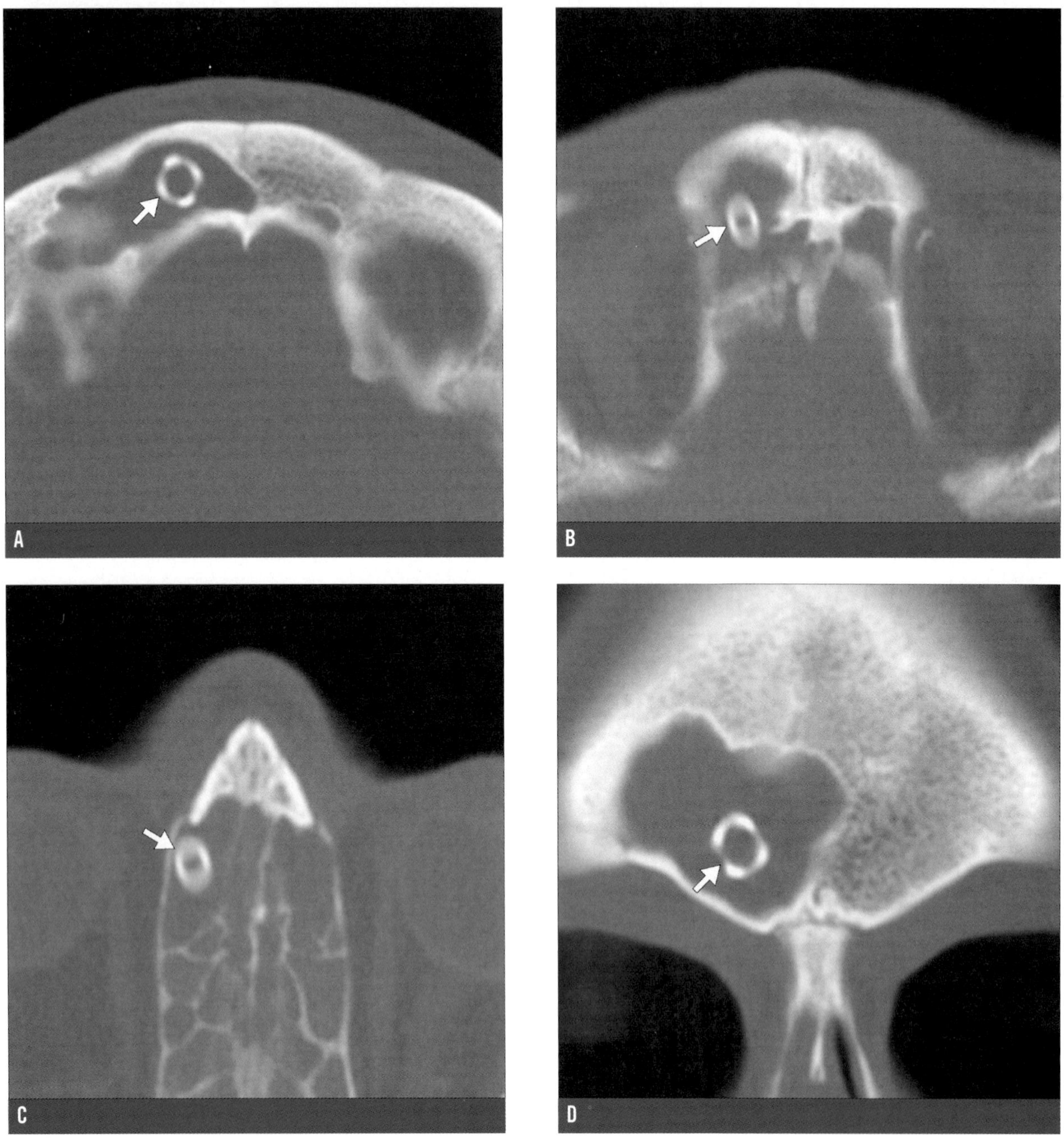

Axial (**A-C**) and coronal reformatted (**D-F**) CT images demonstrate a stent traversing from the frontal sinus to the ethmoid air cells (arrows, **A-F**).

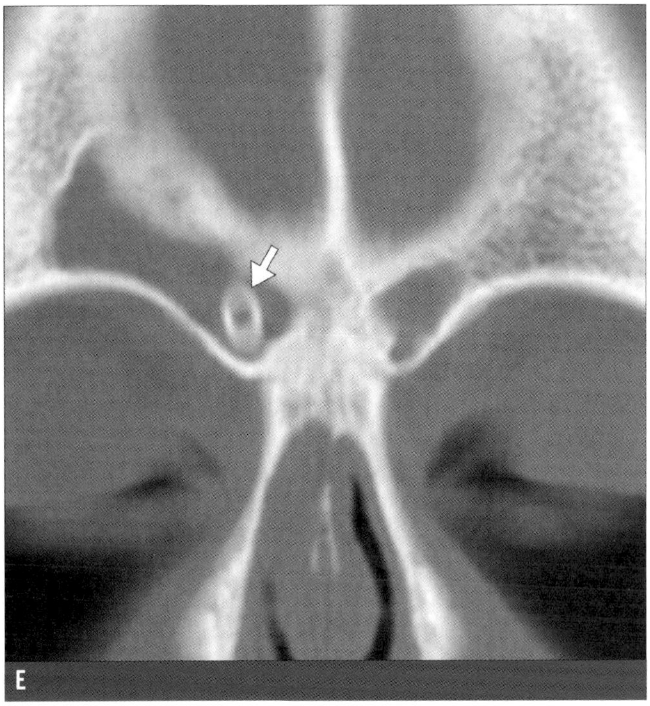

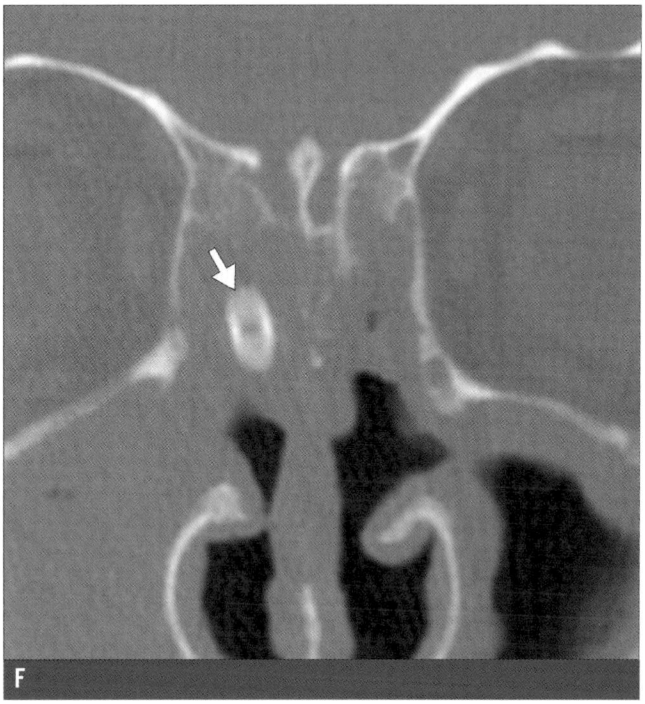

REFERENCES

Benoit CM, Duncavage JA. Combined external and endoscopic sinusotomy with stent placement: a retrospective review. *Laryngoscope.* 2001;111:1246-1249.

Freeman SB, Blom ED. Frontal sinus stents. *Laryngoscope.* 2000;110(7):1179-1182.

CASE 9 Supraorbital ethmoid air cell

A supraorbital ethmoid air cell is an ethmoid air cell that extends into the supraorbital plate of the frontal bone and resides posterior to the frontal sinus. They usually arise from anterior ethmoid air cells, although occasionally they arise from posterior ethmoid air cells. The recess that drains a supraorbital ethmoid air cell resides posterior to the frontal recess, with an osseous septum often separating the two recesses. Because supraorbital ethmoid air cells may appear to represent a frontal sinus in the coronal plane, these cells are usually best identified on axial or sagittal reformatted imaging.

COMPANION CASES

- **Supraorbital ethmoid air cell mucocele.** Mucoceles are benign, mucous-filled, encapsulated, and epithelial-lined lesions of the paranasal sinuses that result from an obstruction of the sinus ostium or outflow tract. Persistent physiologic mucus secretion by the epithelial lining within the obstructed sinus results in expansile osseous remodeling of the affected sinus and occasional dehiscence, potentially extending into the orbital and intracranial compartments. Precipitating factors include trauma, chronic sinusitis, neoplasm, or postoperative complications that result in an outflow obstruction. The frontal sinuses and ethmoidal air cells are the most common sites of sinus mucocele formation. Occasionally, a supraorbital ethmoid mucocele may occur, often following sinus surgery and secondary to lateralization of a middle turbinate remnant with synechiae that obstruct the supraorbital ethmoid outflow tract. When superinfected, a mucocele may be referred to as a mucopyocele.
- **Differentiating a supraorbital ethmoid air cell mucocele from a frontal sinus mucocele.** The frontal sinus drains into the frontal sinus recess, whereas a supraorbital ethmoid air cell drains posterior to the frontal recess. Thus, determining whether a mucocele is located in the frontal sinus or supraorbital ethmoid air cell is crucial in order to widen the appropriate outflow tract during surgery. Furthermore, preoperative identification of a supraorbital air cells is important because they may be mistaken for the true frontal ostium endoscopically. Treatment options of a mucocele depend on the location of the mucocele. Most mucoceles can be treated endoscopically, although occasionally a frontal craniotomy with osteoplastic flap and frontal sinus obliteration may be necessary to treat far lateral frontal sinus mucoceles or supraorbital mucoceles that cannot be reached by endoscopy alone.

Supraorbital ethmoid air cell

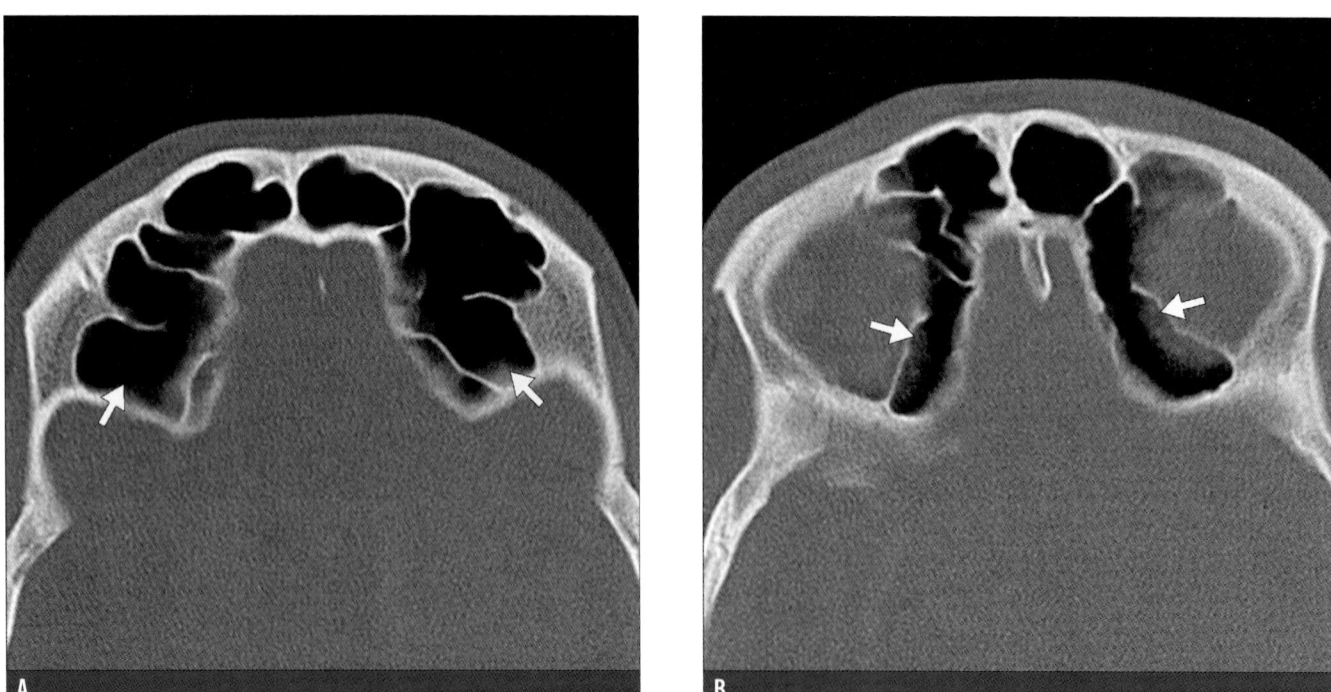

Axial (**A, B**) and coronal reformatted (**C**) CT images demonstrate large bilateral supraorbital ethmoid air cells (arrows, **A-C**).

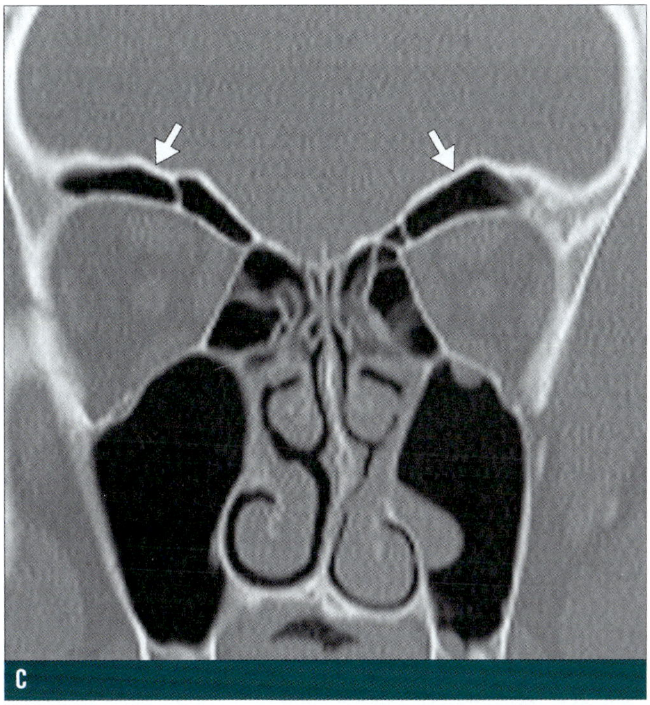

Supraorbital ethmoid air cell

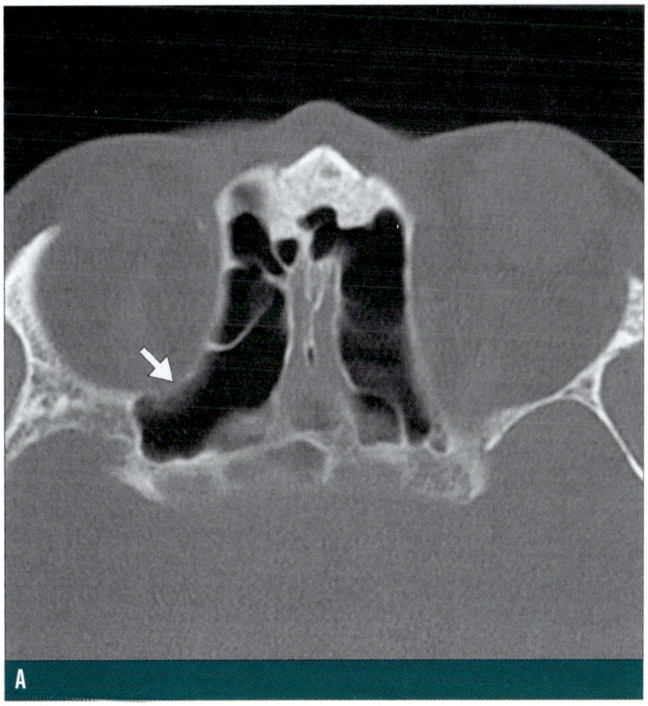

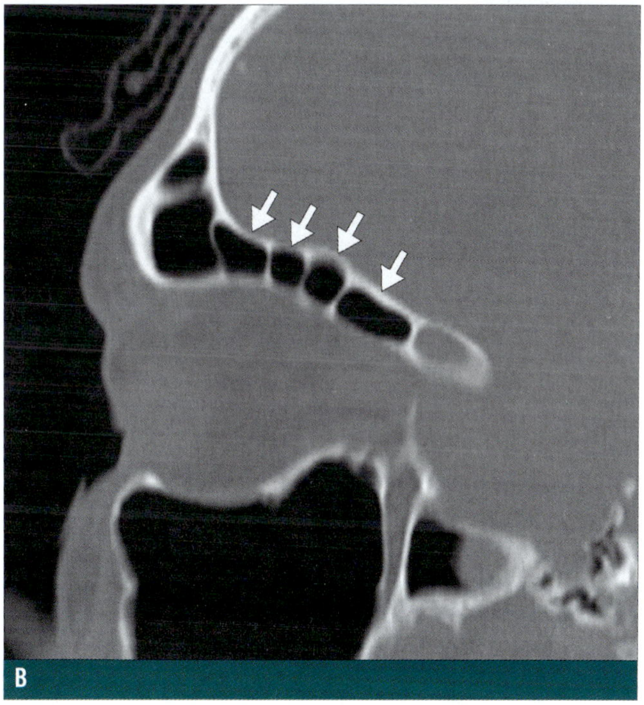

Different patient. Axial (**A**) and right parasagittal reformatted (**B**) CT images. Image **A** demonstrates extension of a posterior ethmoid air cell above the orbit, compatible with a supraorbital ethmoid air cell (arrow, **A**). Image **B** demonstrates that this supraorbital ethmoid air cell contains multiple setpa (arrows, **B**).

Supraorbital ethmoid air cell (MRI)

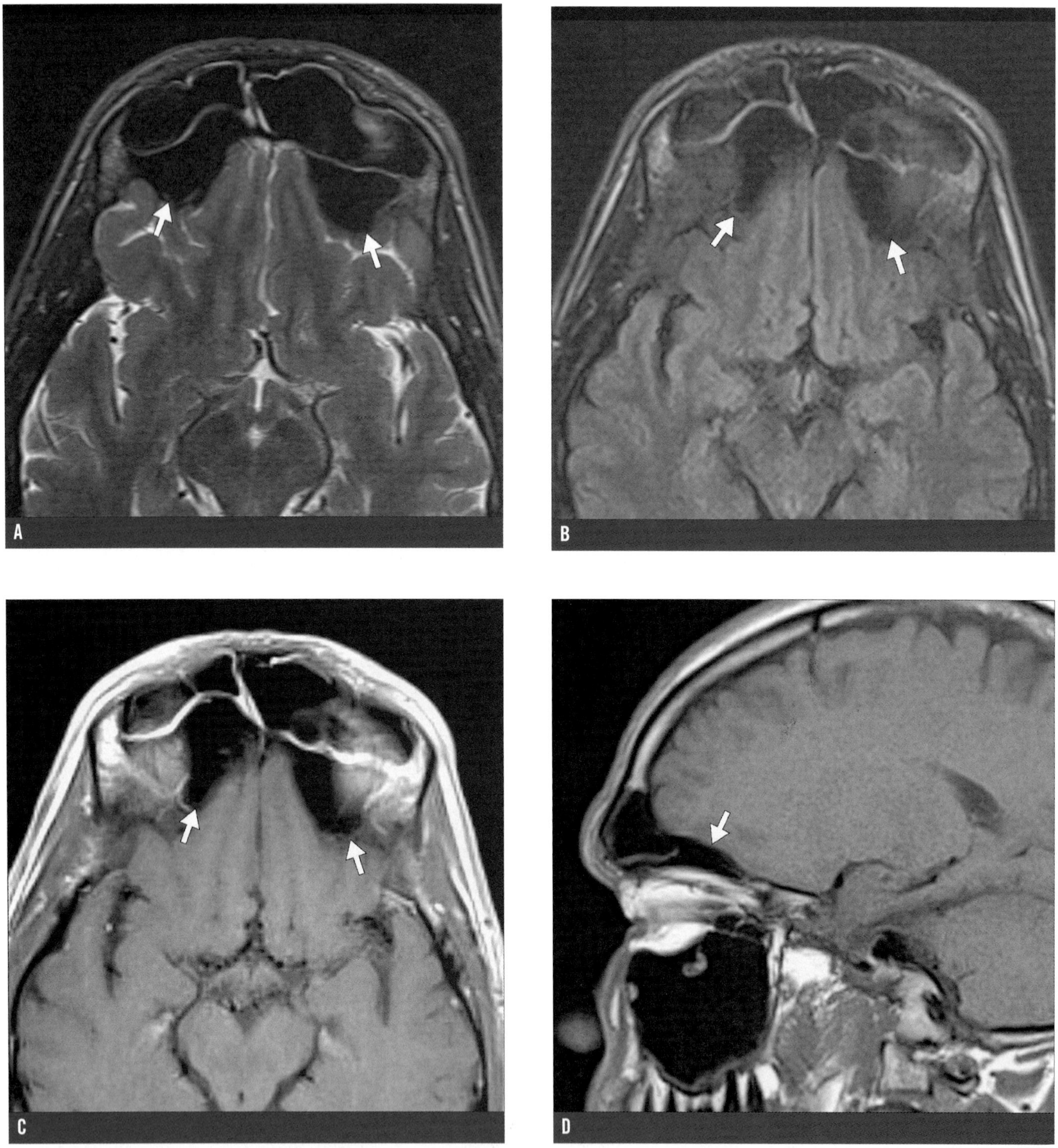

Different patient. A different patient. Axial T2 (**A**), axial FLAIR (**B**), and axial postcontrast T1 (**C**) MR images demonstrate bilateral supraorbital air cells (arrows, **A-C**). A sagittal T1-weighted MR image (**D**) subtlety demonstrates one of the supraorbital air cells (arrow, **D**).

Supraorbital ethmoid air cell simulating a lesion on MRI

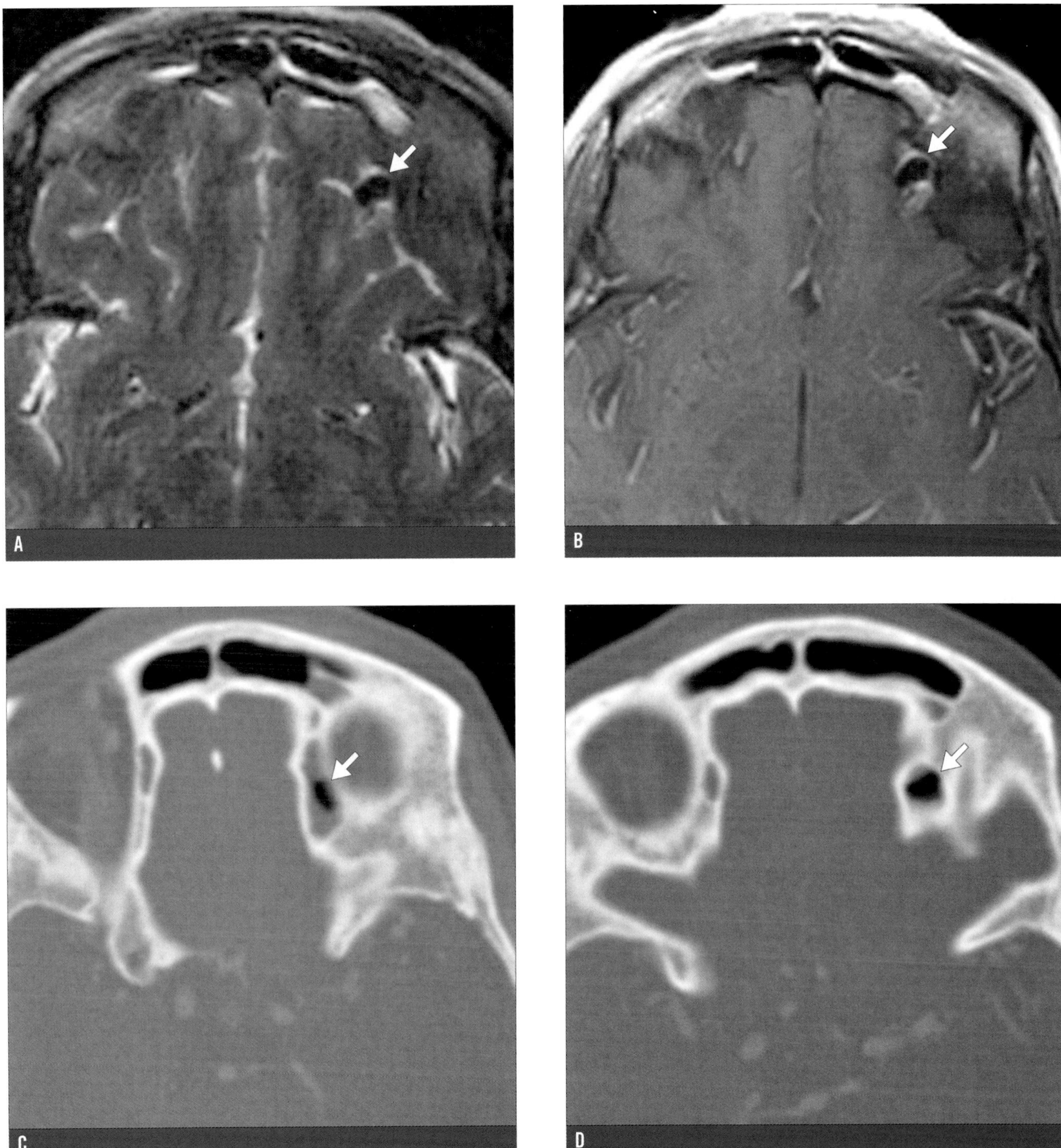

Axial T2 (**A**) and postcontrast axial T1 (**B**) MR images as well as axial CT images (**C, D**) through the supraorbital region. Images **A** and **B** demonstrate a nonspecific, hypointense, nonenhancing apparent lesion in the left frontal region (arrows, **A**, **B**). Images **C** and **D** demonstrate this lesion to simply represent an incidental, partially opacified left supraorbital ethmoid air cell (arrows, **C**, **D**).

Companion case: Supraorbital ethmoid air cell mucocele

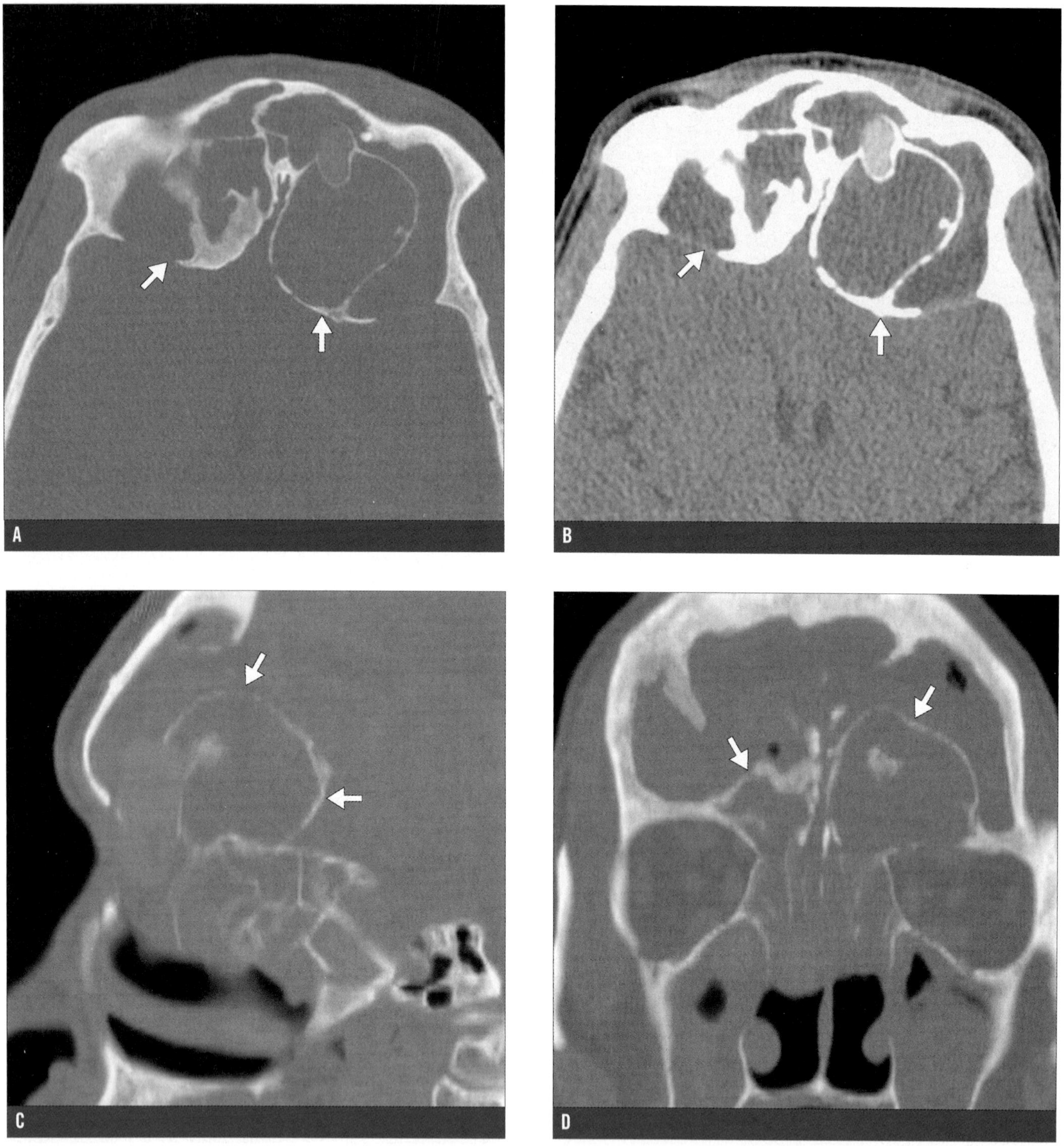

Unenhanced axial CT images viewed with a bone window (**A**) and soft tissue window (**B**) as well as sagittal reformatted (**C**) and coronal reformatted (**D**) CT images viewed with bone window demonstrate opacified and markedly expansile supraorbital ethmoid air cells compatible with mucoceles that extend intracranially (arrows, **A-D**). Axial and coronal T2 with fat suppression (**E, F**), axial T1 (**G**), and postcontrast coronal T1 with fat suppression (**H**) MR images demonstrate the same mucoceles on MRI (arrows, **E-H**). In this case, the hypointense areas on MRI represented new areas of sinus aeration which was confirmed on a follow-up CT (not shown). However, sinus aeration on MRI cannot be accurately assessed because densely inspissated secretions and/or fungal disease may result in "pseudoaeration" of the sinuses due to the lack of water content in these entities.

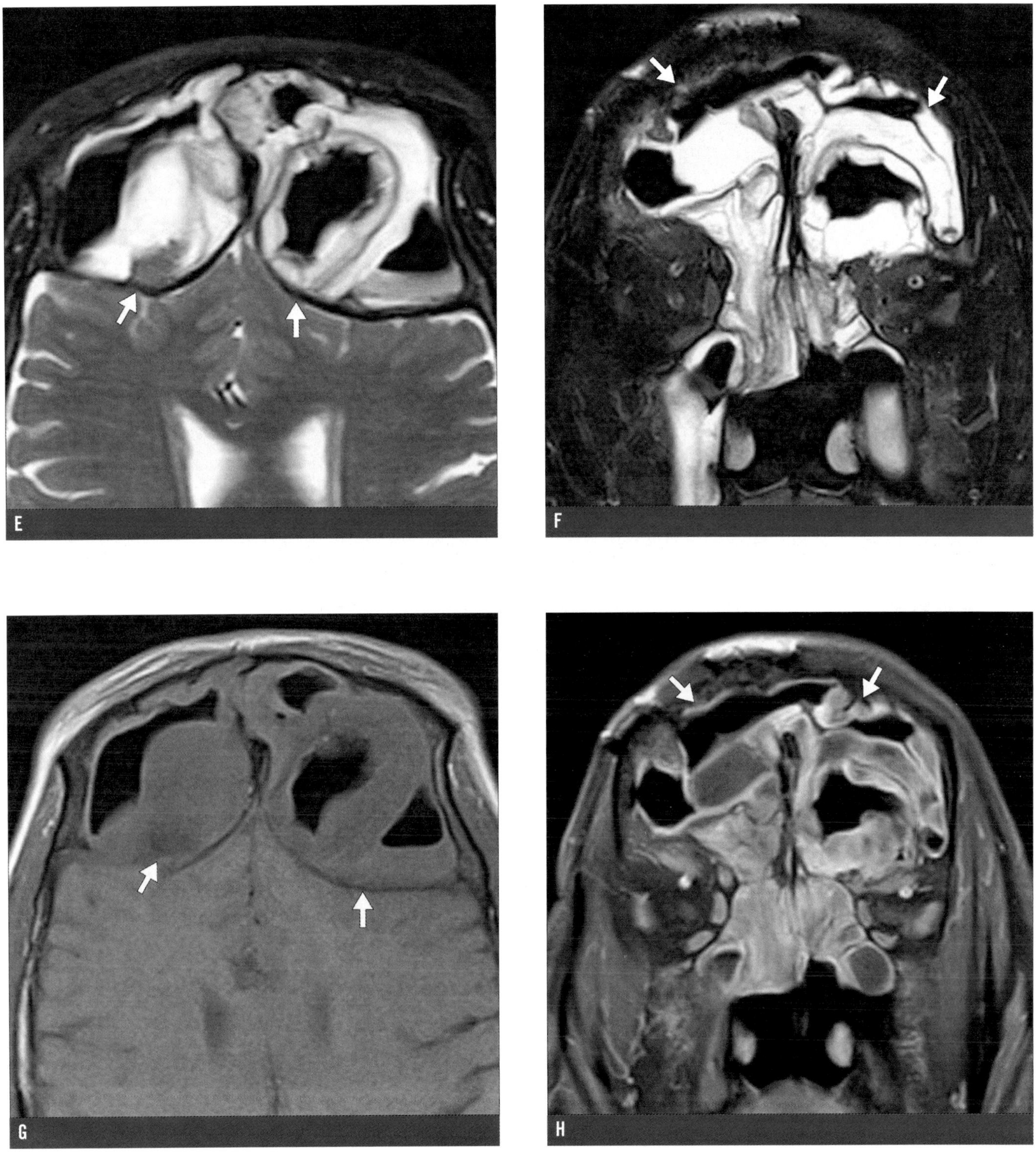
E
F
G
H

Companion case: Differentiating a supraorbital ethmoid air cell mucocele from a frontal sinus mucocele

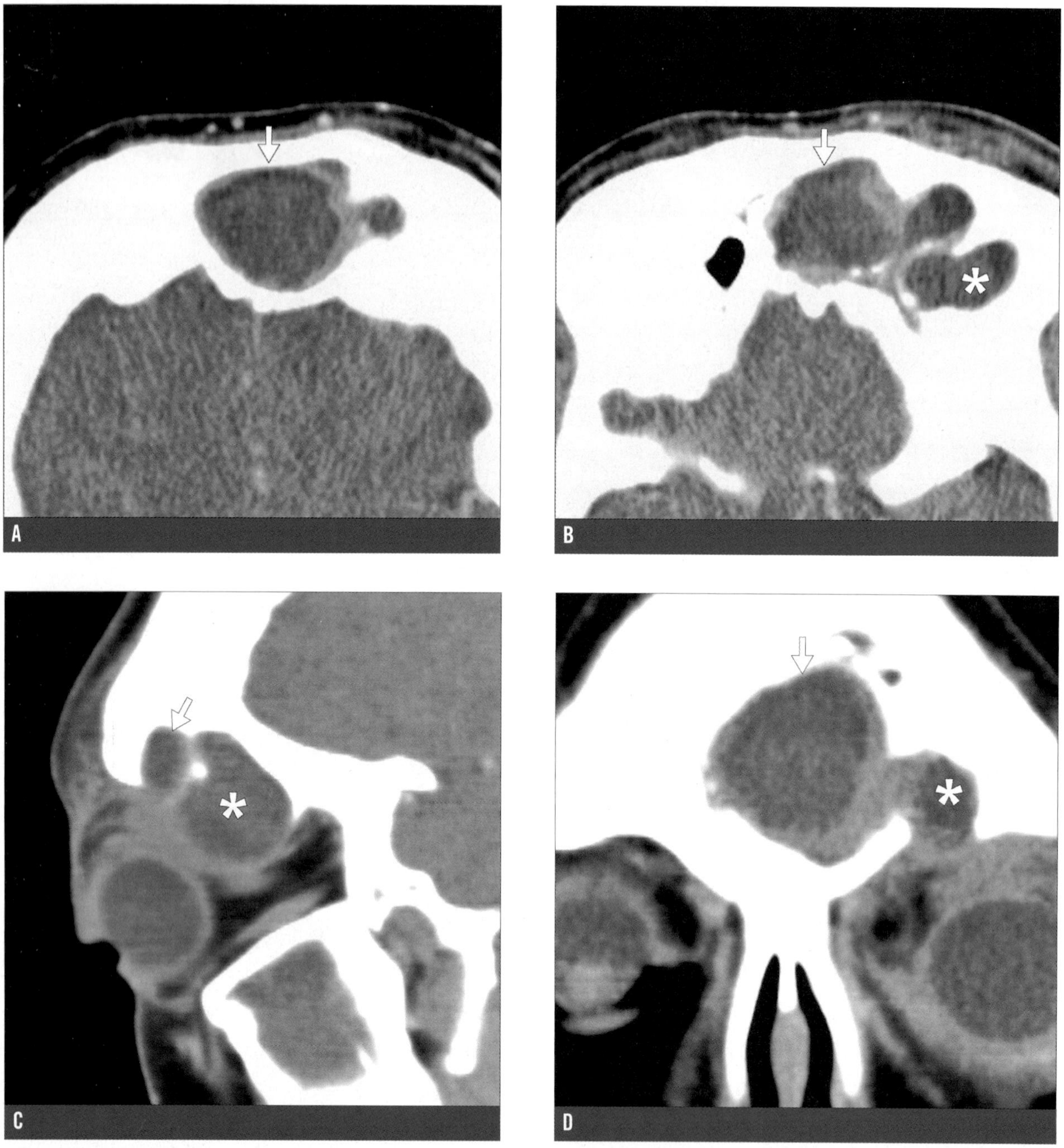

Unenhanced axial (**A, B**), sagittal reformatted (**C**), and coronal reformatted (**D**) CT images demonstrate a completely opacified, expansile left frontal sinus, compatible with a left frontal sinus mucocele (arrows, **A-D**). An additional coronal reformatted CT image (**E**) as well as images **B-D** also demonstrate a completely opacified, expansile left supraorbital ethmoid air cell, compatible with a left supraorbital ethmoid air cell mucocele (asterisks, **B-E**). Caudal displacement of the left globe (ie, hypoglobus) is present on images **C** and **D**, whereas an axial CT image through the orbits (**F**) demonstrates mild-to-moderate left globe proptosis. The patient underwent functional endoscopic sinus surgery that only addressed the left frontal sinus outflow tract and therefore only the left frontal sinus mucocele. A follow-up CT examination 3 years later with unenhanced axial (**G, H, K**), sagittal reformatted (**I**), and coronal reformatted (**J**) CT images demonstrate significant interval enlargement of the left supraorbital ethmoid mucocele (asterisks, **G-J**) and an interval decrease in size of the left frontal sinus mucocele that is now more aerated (arrows, **G, J**). The degree of mass effect from the larger supraorbital ethmoid air cell mucocele upon the superior aspect of the left orbit has significantly progressed (**I, J**), as has the degree of proptosis (**K**). This case illustrates the importance of precisely identifying where a mucocele and its corresponding obstructed outflow tract are located. In this patient, the coexisting supraorbital ethmoid mucocele was not treated. This was because it was not identified as a mucocele that was separate from the frontal sinus mucocele and that each mucocele had separate obstructed outflow tracts. As as result, the patient was incompletely treated and the supraorbital mucocele significantly grew following surgery.

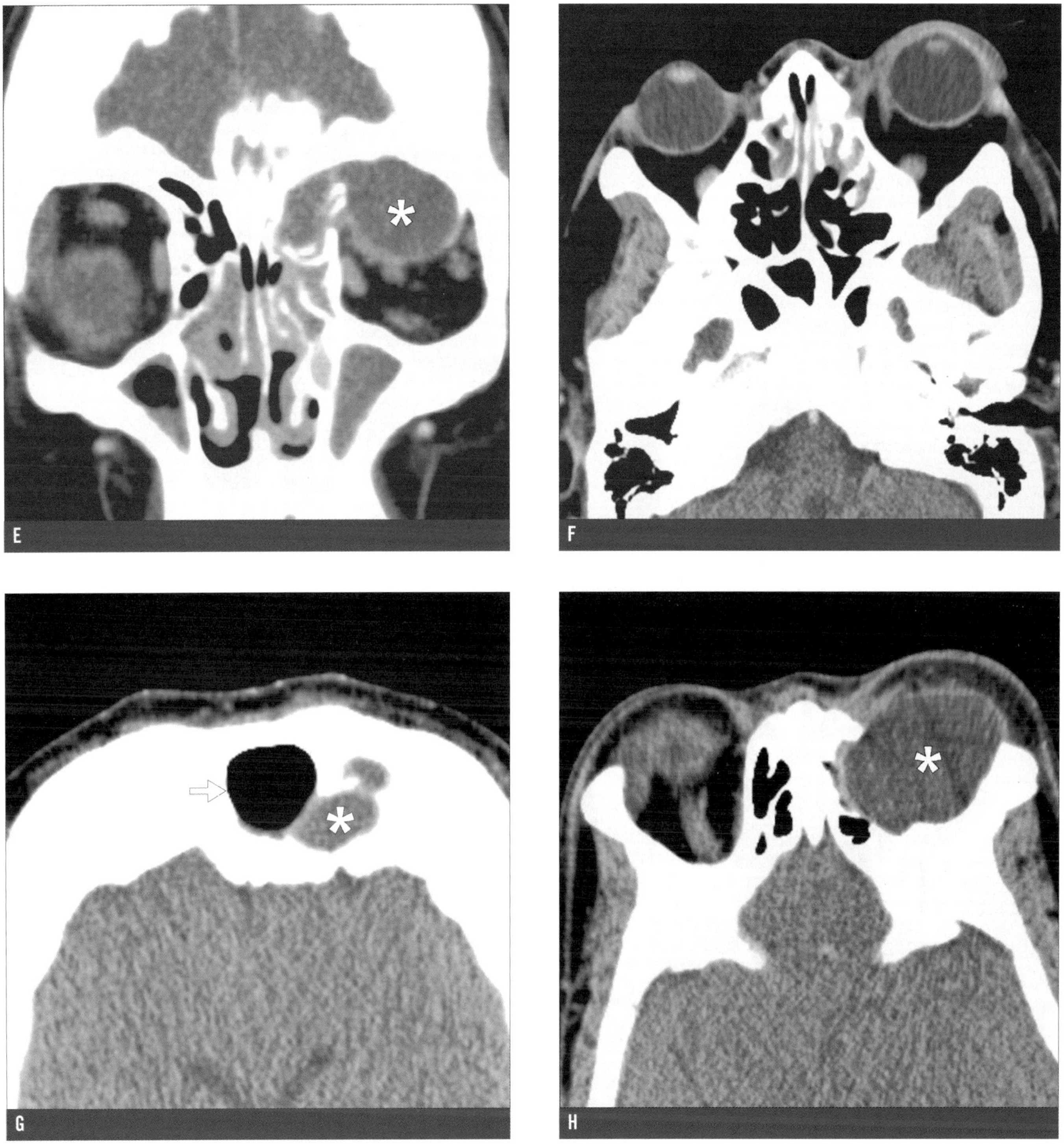
E
F
G
H

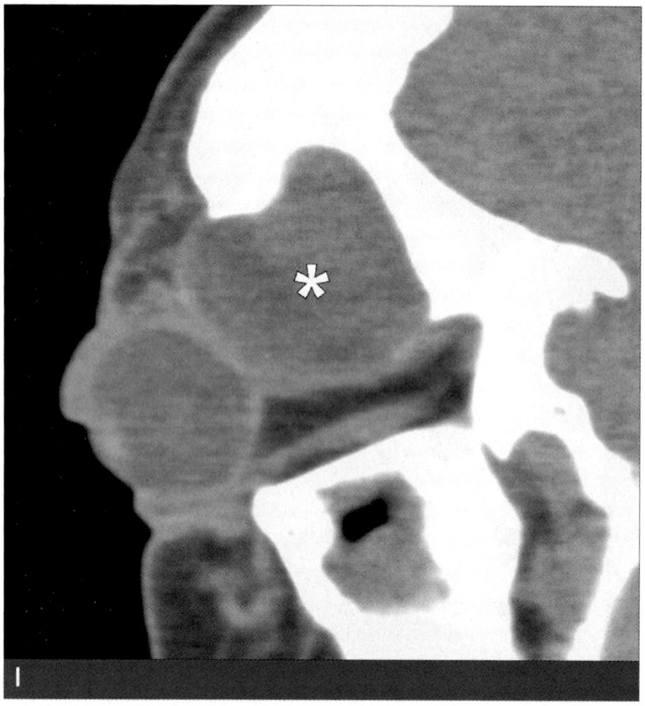

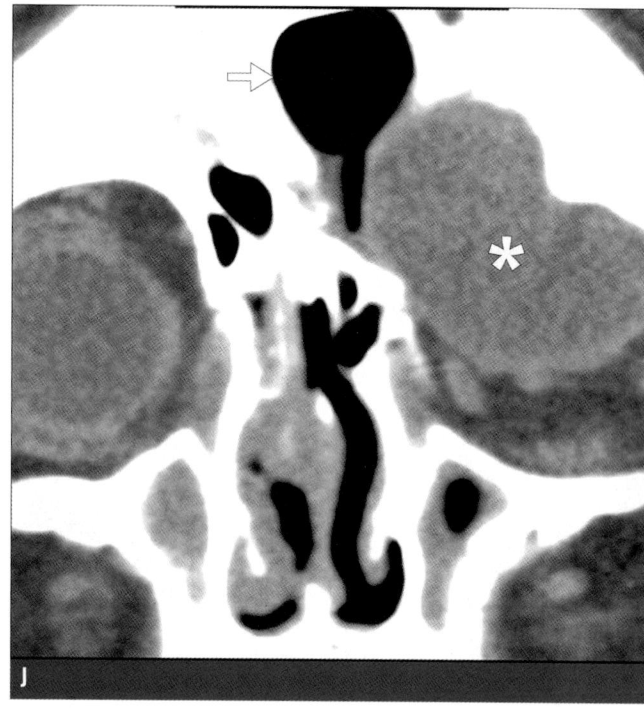

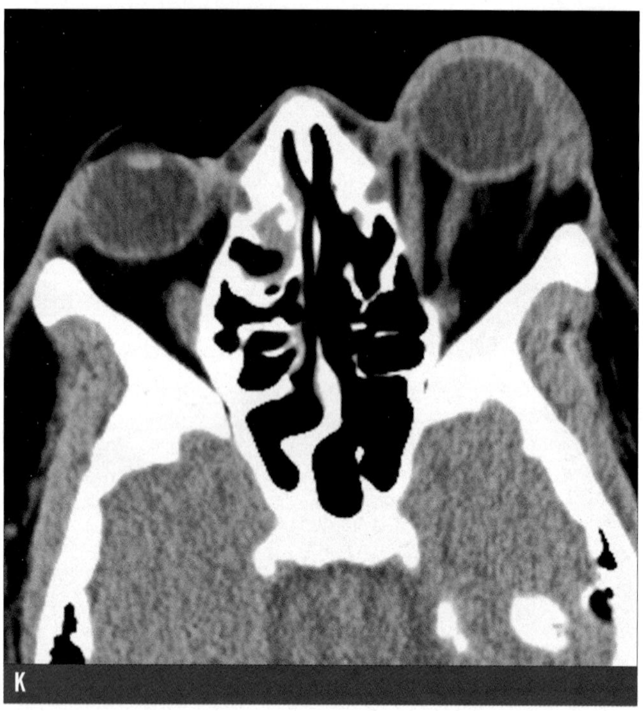

REFERENCES

Beale TJ, et al. Imaging of the paranasal sinuses and nasal cavity: normal anatomy and clinically relevant anatomical variants. *Semin Ultrasound CT MR.* 2009;30(1):2-16.

Chiu AG, Vaughan WC. Management of the lateral frontal sinus lesion and the supraorbital cell mucocele. *Am J Rhinol.* 2004;18(2):83-86.

Herndon M, et al. Presentation and management of extensive fronto-orbital-ethmoid mucoceles. *Am J Otolaryngol.* 2007;28:145-147.

Lanzieri CF, et al. Use of gadolinium-enhanced MR imaging for differentiating mucoceles from neoplasms in the paranasal sinuses. *Radiology.* 1991;178:425-428.

Lee WT, Kuhn FA, Citardi MJ. 3D computed tomographic analysis of frontal recess anatomy in patients without frontal sinusitis. *Otolaryngol Head Neck Surg.* 2004;131(3):164-173.

Man LX[1], McLean CC, Pierce ML, Fakhri S.Laryngoscope. Endoscopic trans(naso)orbital management of supraorbital mucoceles with biliary T-tube stenting. 2013;123(2):326-330.

Rao VM, El-Noueam KI. Sinonasal imaging: anatomy and pathology. *Radiol Clin North Am.* 1998;36:921-939.

Zhang L, et al. Computed tomographic and endoscopic analysis of supraorbital ethmoid cells. *Otolaryngol Head Neck Surg.* 2007; 137(4):562-568.

CASE 10 Haller cell

Haller cells, sometimes referred to as infraorbital ethmoid cells, are anterior ethmoid air cells that extend inferomedial to the orbital floor and into the superomedial aspect of the maxillary sinus lumen. While most often incidental, Haller cells can narrow or obstruct the infundibulum and/or the primary maxillary sinus ostium if they encroach upon these structures.

COMPANION CASE

- **Obstructed infundibulum due to a Haller cell.**

Haller cells

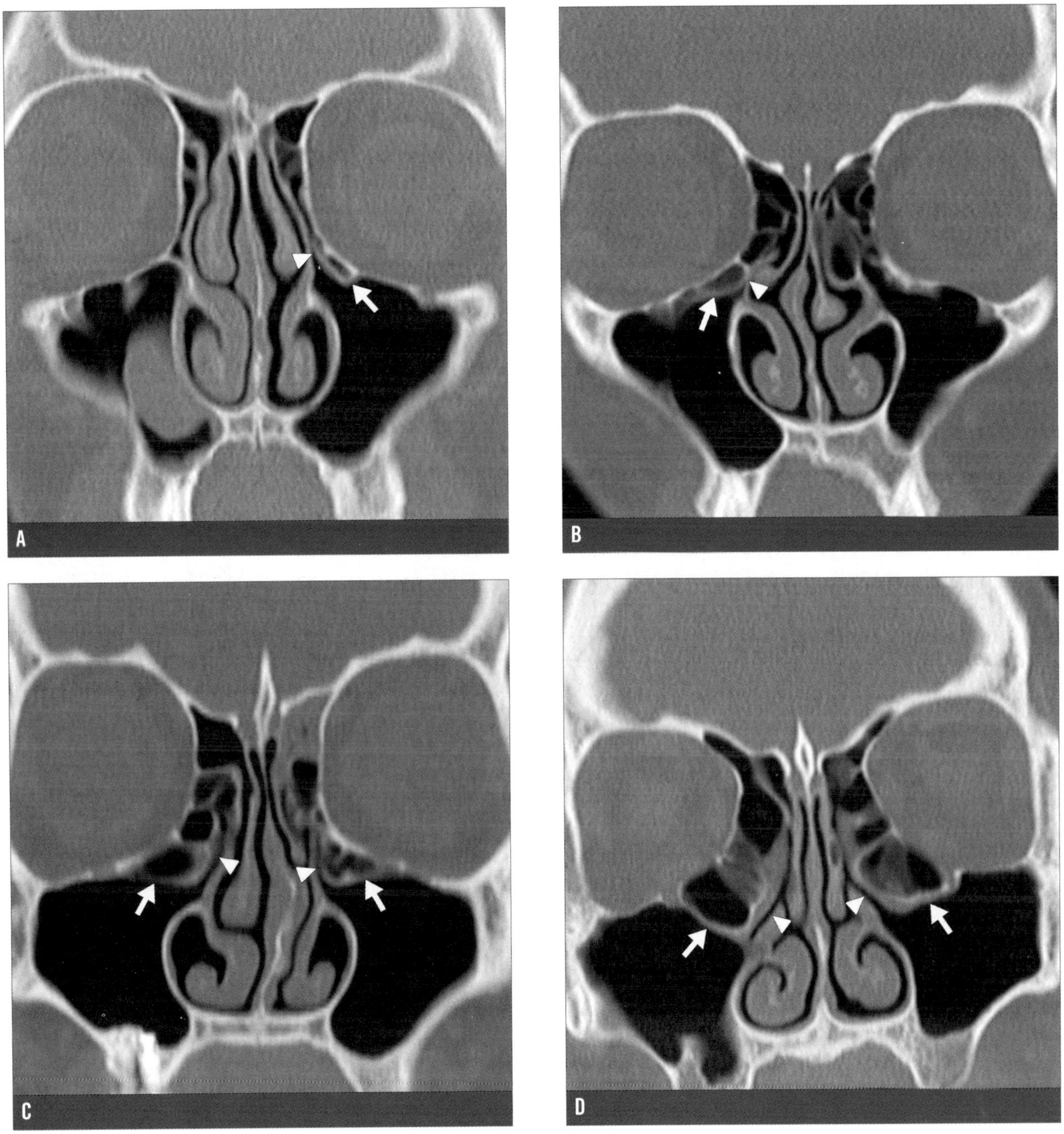

Coronal reformatted CT images of 4 different patients demonstrating Haller cells (**A-D**). Each case demonstrates various sizes of Haller cells (arrows, **A-D**) and varying degrees of infundibular narrowing (arrowheads, **A-D**), some with no significant narrowing and one case with apparent obstruction (arrowhead, **B**). However, evaluating the entire infundibulum in the coronal plane is necessary in order to assess for a patent air channel. A sagittal reformatted image from the same patient as image **D** (**E**) demonstrates a Haller cell in the sagittal plane (arrow, **E**).

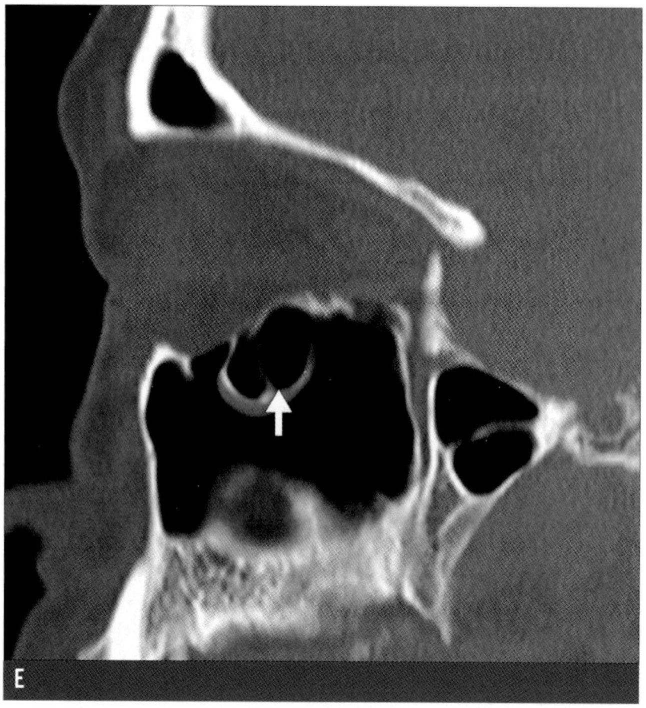

Companion case: Obstructed infundibulum due to a Haller cell

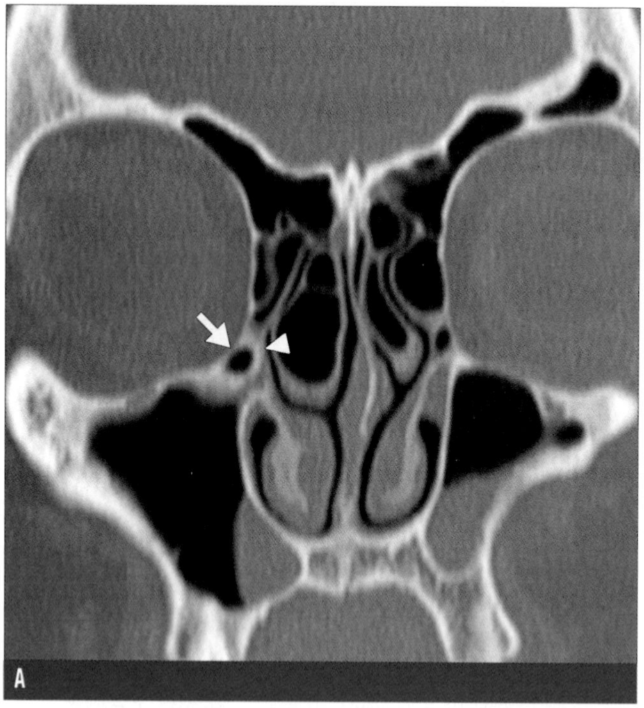

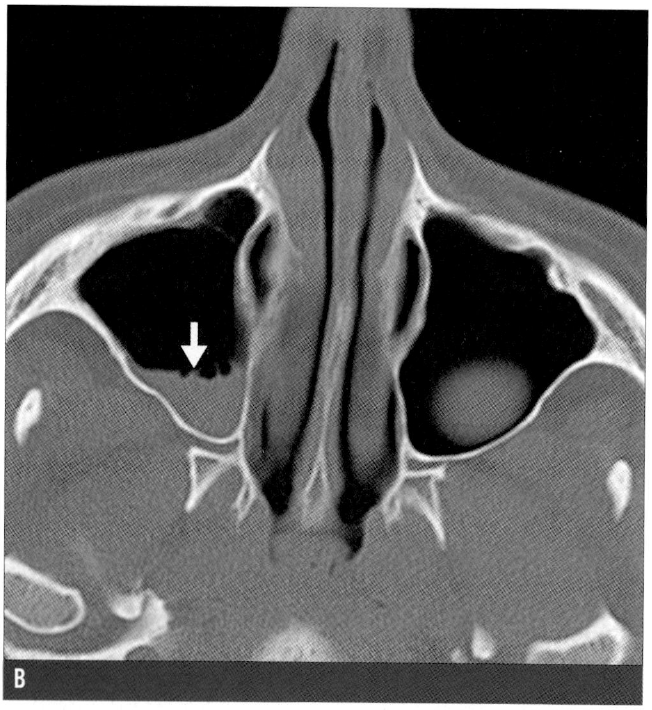

A coronal reformatted CT image through the right ostiomeatal unit (**A**) demonstrates a relatively small right Haller cell (arrow, **A**) obstructing the right infundibulum (arrowhead, **A**). An axial CT image through the maxillary sinuses (**B**) demonstrates an air fluid level in the right maxillary sinus (arrow. **B**), compatible with postobstructive sinusitis. A coronal reformatted CT image through the left ostiomeatal unit (**C**) demonstrates a patent left infundibulum for comparison purposes (arrow, **C**).

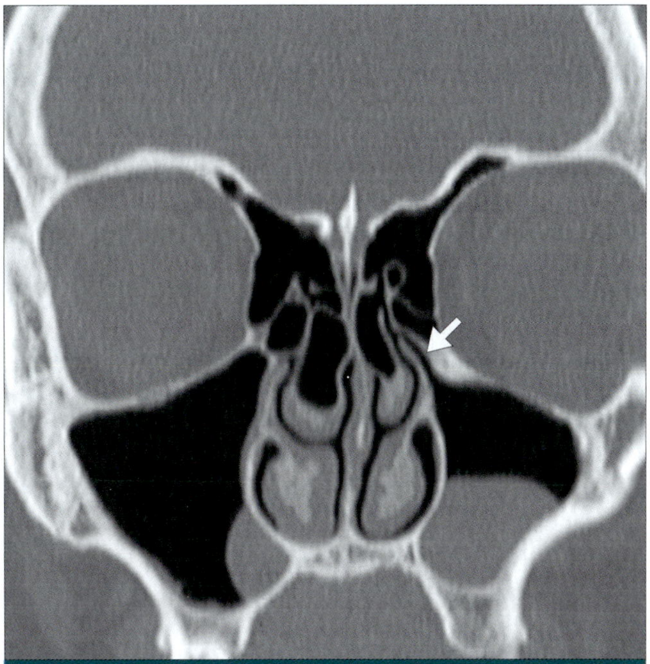

C

REFERENCES

Arslan H, et al. Anatomic variations of the paranasal sinuses: CT examination for endoscopic sinus surgery. *Auris Nasus Larynx.* 1999;26:39-48.

Beale TJ, et al. Imaging of the paranasal sinuses and nasal cavity: normal anatomy and clinically relevant anatomical variants. *Semin Ultrasound CT MR.* 2009;30(1):2-16.

Kantarci M, et al. Remarkable anatomic variations in paranasal sinus region and their clinical importance. *Eur J Radiology.* 2004;50:296-302.

Perez-Pinas I, et al. Anatomical variations in the human paranasal sinus region studied by CT. *J Anat.* 2000;197:221-227.

The Onodi cell, also known as a sphenoethmoidal air cell, is a posteriormost located ethmoid air cell in which its posterolateral wall shares a common wall with the optic canal. Usually, an Onodi cell resides cephalad to the sphenoid sinus and is sometimes best identified with coronal CT imaging. Identifying an Onodi cell prior to surgery is important to avoid inadvertent breach of the optic canal and/or superior orbital fissure during surgery to the ethmoid air cells. Additionally, an aggressive Onodi cell infection (ie, invasive fungal sinusitis), or a mucocele in an Onodi cell, may result in mechanical compression of the optic nerve and clinically present as optic nerve pathology.

A helpful imaging finding to determine the presence of an Onodi cell is to track the course of the sphenoethmoidal recesses. If the sphenoethmoidal recess communicates with the air cell in question, then the air cell is consistent with the sphenoid sinus. However, if the sphenoethmoidal recess does not communicate with the air cell in question, then the air cell is consistent with an Onodi cell.

COMPANION CASE

- **Pneumosinus dilatans of an Onodi cell.** Pneumosinus dilatans (PD) is defined as an abnormally expansile, aerated sinus that extends beyond the normal confines of the native bone. The sinus involved with PD usually has a normal wall thickness. However, PD can be associated with a meningioma, which may induce sinus wall hyperostosis.

  The etiology of PD remains unknown. While PD is usually idiopathic, it has been described in association with many conditions, including:
  - Meningioma
  - McCune-Albright syndrome
  - Fibrous dysplasia
  - Arachnoid cyst
  - Brain tumors
  - Prolonged CSF shunting
  - Cerebral hemiatrophy infantile meningoencephalitis
  - von Recklinghausen disease
  - Acromegaly

Onodi cell

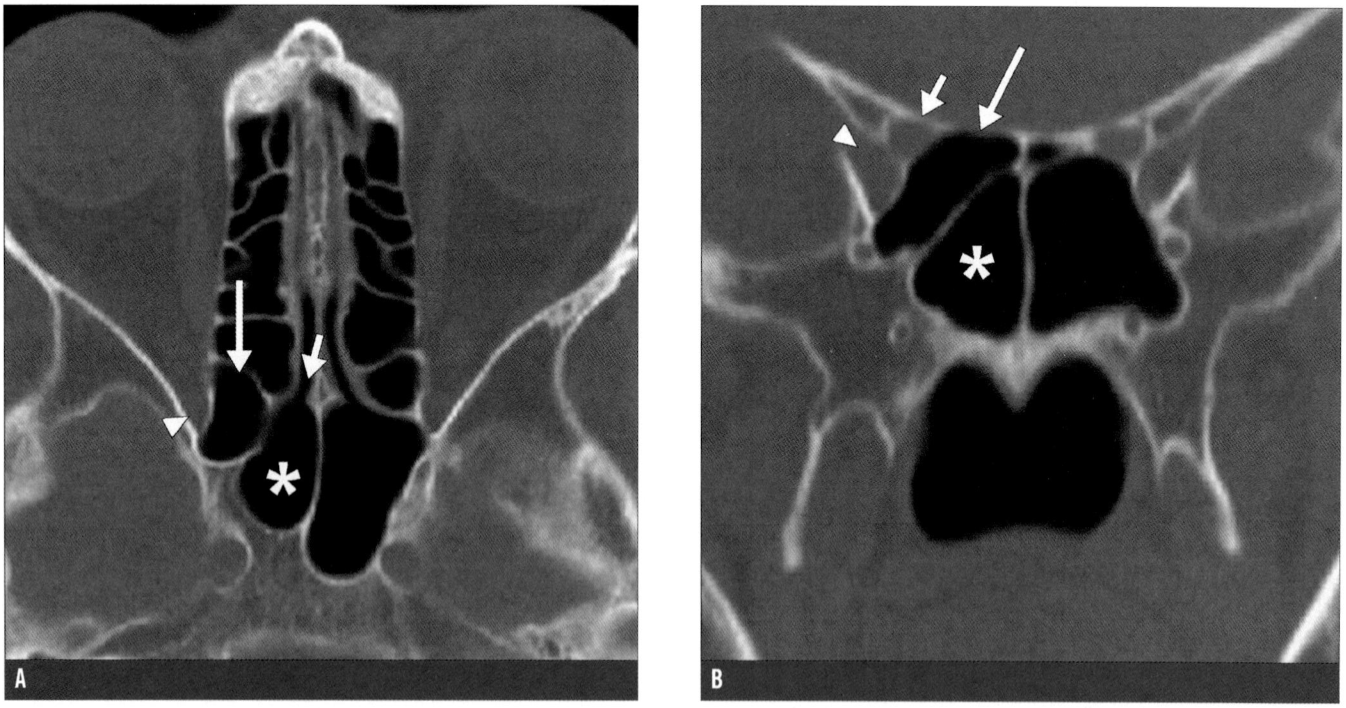

Axial (**A**) and coronal reformatted (**B**) CT images demonstrate a right Onodi air cell. Image **A** demonstrates a posterior-most right ethmoid air cell (long arrow, **A**) that is located lateral to the right aspect of the sphenoid sinus (asterisk, **A**). The sphenoid sinus is differentiated from the right Onodi cell on this image by the right sphenoethmoidal recess (short arrow, **A**), which communicates directly with the right aspect of the sphenoid sinus, but not the Onodi cell. Image **B** demonstrates the typical location of an Onodi cell (long arrow, **B**) as it extends cephalad to the right aspect of the sphenoid sinus (asterisk, **B**) and shares a common wall with the right optic canal (short arrow, **B**). In this case, the Onodi cell also shares a wall with the right superior orbital fissure (arrowheads, **A**, **B**).

Companion case: Pneumosinus dilatans of an Onodi cell

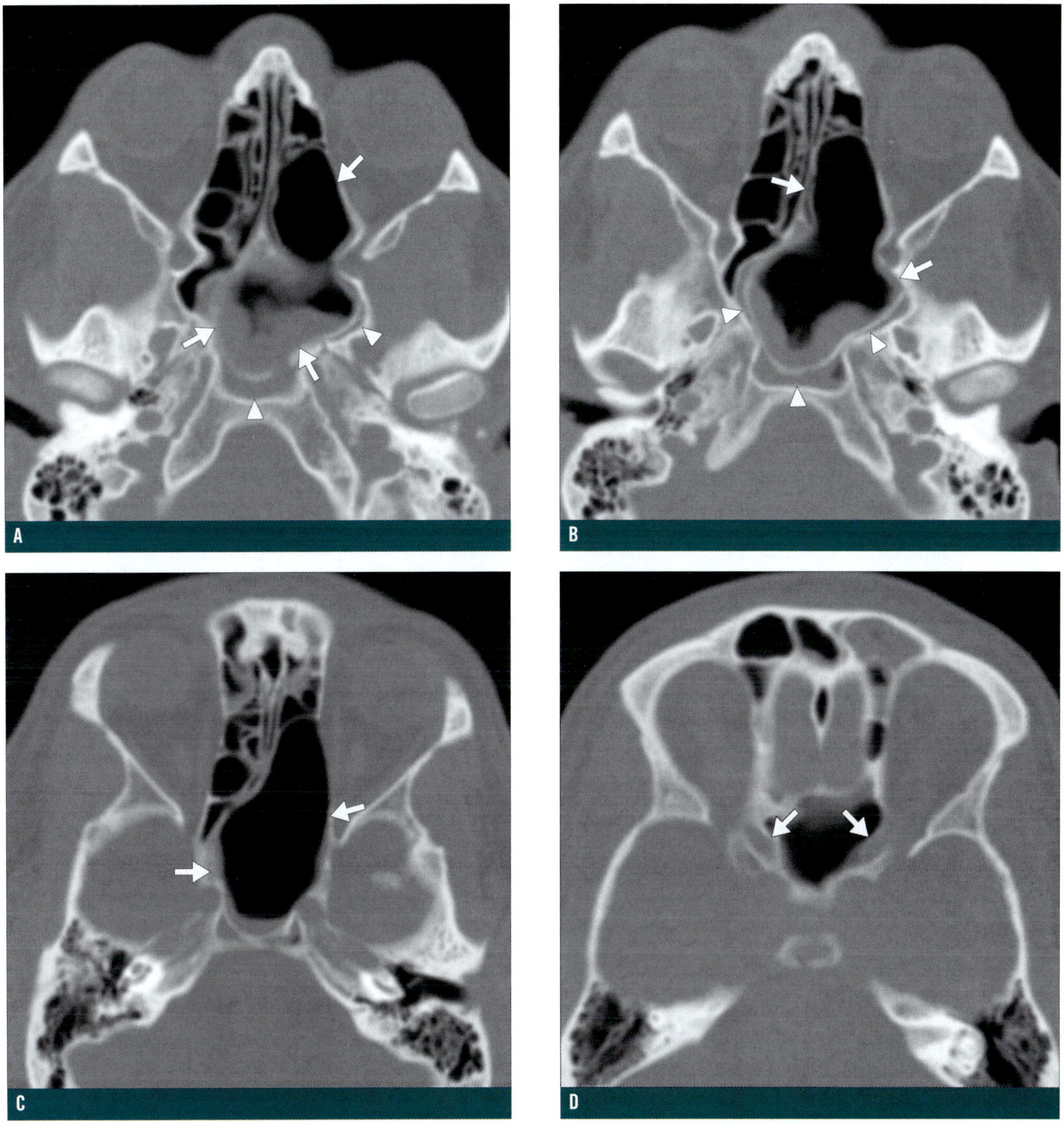

Axial CT images (**A**-**C**) demonstrate a large, expansile air cell (arrows, **A**-**C**) occupying the posterior left ethmoid air cells and markedly attenuating the left sphenoid sinus lumen. Only a small portion of the left aspect of the sphenoid sinus is visible (arrowheads, **A**, **B**). This large air cell is larger than the native "mother bone" and therefore consistent with pneumosinus dilatans. An additional axial image (**D**) demonstrates that the air cell shares a common wall with the optic canals (arrows, **D**). Therefore, this air cell is consistent with pneumosinus dilatans of an Onodi cell.

REFERENCES

Arslan H, et al. Anatomic variations of the paranasal sinuses: CT examination for endoscopic sinus surgery. *Auris Nasus Larynx.* 1999;26:39-48.

Kantarci M, et al. Remarkable anatomic variations in paranasal sinus region and their clinical importance. *Eur J Rad.* 2004;50:296-302.

Meloni F, et al. Anatomic variations of surgical importance in ethmoid labyrinth and sphenoid sinus. a study of radiological anatomy. *Surg Radiol Anat.* 1992;14:65-70.

Perez-Pinas I, et al. Anatomical variations in the human paranasal sinus region studied by CT. *J Anat.* 2000;197:221-227.

Schmalfuss IM, Camp M. Skull base: pseudolesion or true lesion? *Eur Radiol.* 2008;18:1232-1243.

CASE 12 Ethmomaxillary sinus

An ethmomaxillary sinus is defined as an expansile posterior ethmoid air cell that extends into the posterior-superior aspect of the maxillary sinus and drains into the superior meatus. While its presence may not be a predisposing factor for paranasal sinus disease, it may result in disorientation during an endoscopic procedure.

Ethmomaxillary sinuses

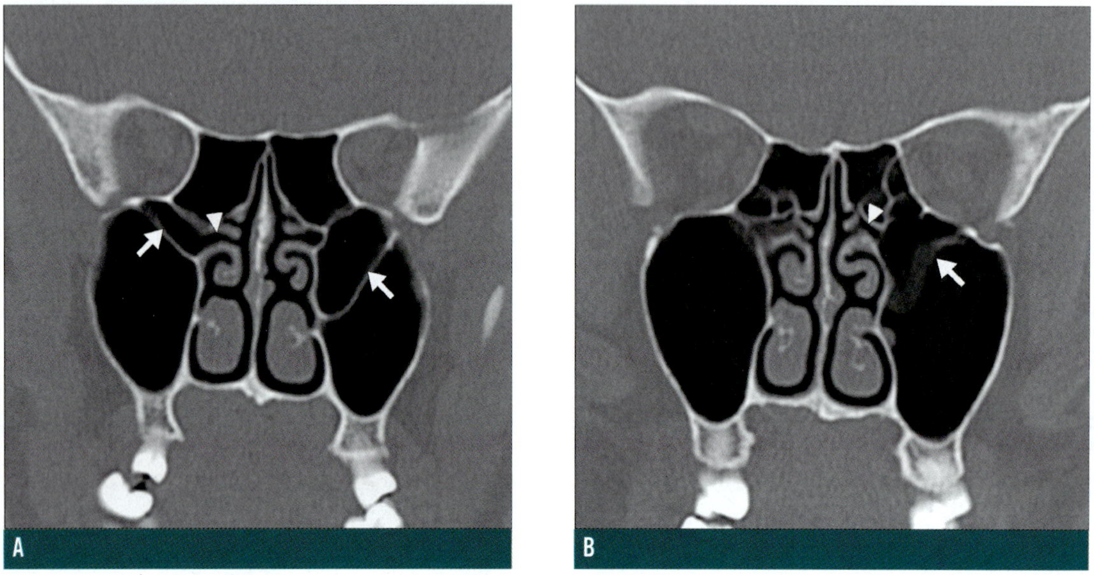

Coronal reformatted CT images (**A**, **B**) demonstrate bilateral ethmomaxillary sinuses within the posterior-superior aspects of both maxillary sinuses (arrows, **A**, **B**). Each ethmomaxillary air sinus drains into its respective superior meatus (arrowheads **A**, **B**).

Ethmomaxillary sinuses

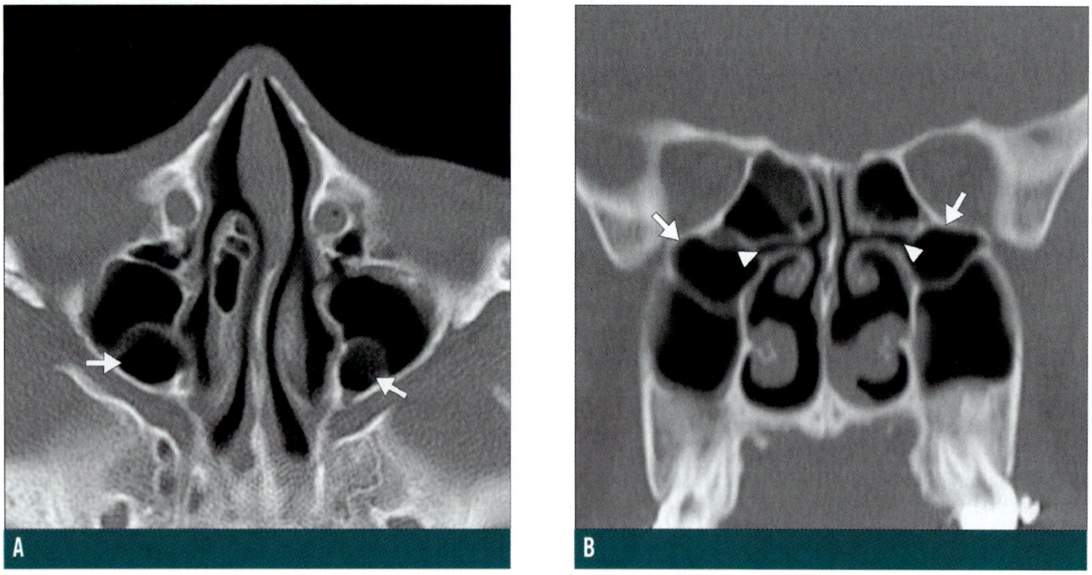

Different patient. Axial (**A**) and coronal reformatted (**B**) CT images demonstrate bilateral ethmomaxillary sinuses within the posterosuperior aspect of each maxillary sinus (arrows, **A**, **B**). Each ethmomaxillary sinus drains via its respective superior meatus (arrowheads, **B**).

REFERENCES

Chrcanovic B, Freire-Maia B. Maxillary sinus aplasia. *Oral Maxillofac Surg.* 2010;14(3):187-191.

Sirikci A, et al. Ethmomaxillary sinus: a particular anatomic variation of the paranasal sinuses. *Eur Radiol.* 2004;14(2):281-285.

CASE 13 Agger nasi air cell

The agger nasi is a mound of bone that represents the intranasal, posterior extension of the frontal process of the maxilla. It is pneumatized in the vast majority of individuals, and when pneumatized, it is termed an agger nasi air cell. An agger nasi air cell represents the most anteriorly located ethmoid air cell and its walls form part of the anterior, inferior, and a portion of the lateral boundary of the frontal recess. An agger nasi air cell is considered an extramural ethmoid air cell because it extends outside the confines of the ethmoid bone. Often, an agger nasi air cell will extend anterior to the level of the nasolacrimal canal and into the frontal process of the maxilla. Given the close relationship of this air cell to the lacrimal bone and nasolacrimal canal, epiphora (excessive tearing) may occur in patients with sinus disease (eg, mucoceles, etc) that affects an agger nasi cell.

COMPANION CASE

- **Obstructed frontal recess due to an agger nasi cell.** Most agger nasi air cells are incidental. However, if extensively pneumatized, an agger nasi air cell may primarily narrow the frontal recess or it may displace the attachment of the middle turbinate superomedially and secondarily narrow the frontal recess.

Agger nasi air cells

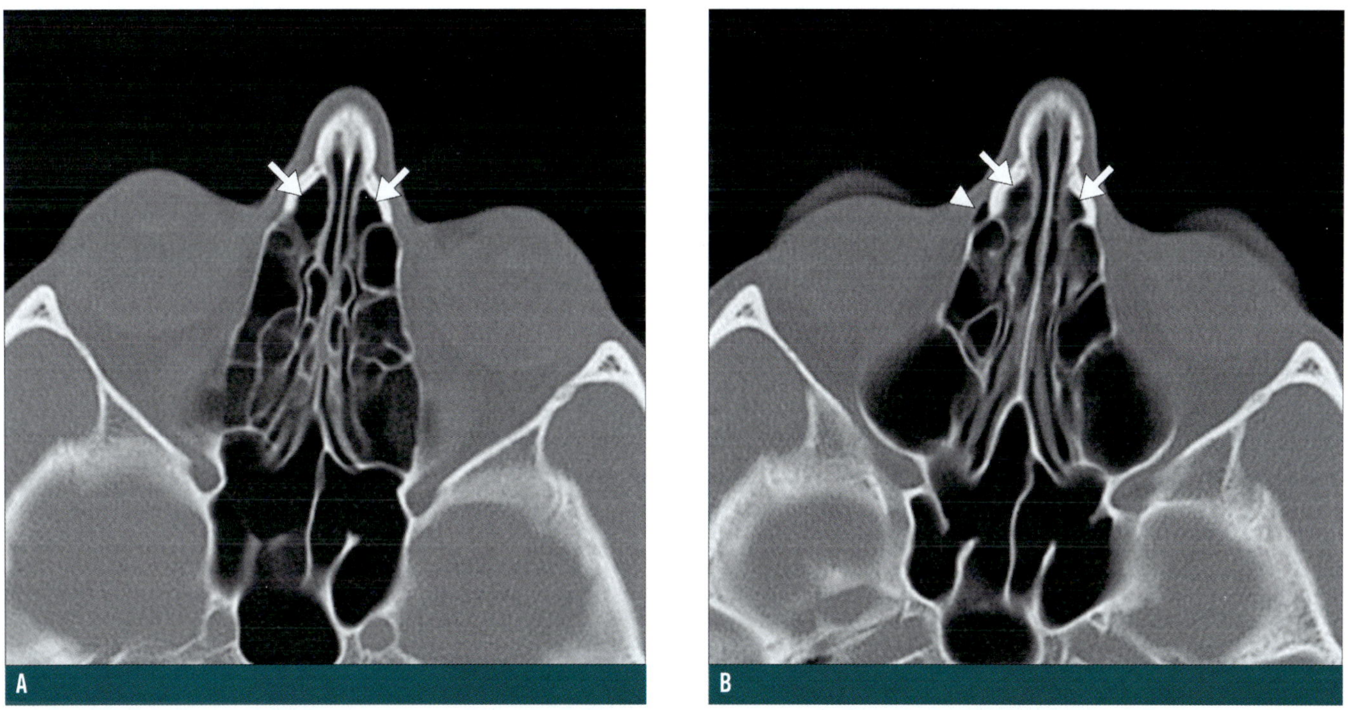

Axial (**A, B**) and coronal reformatted (**C, D**) CT images demonstrate bilateral agger nasi air cells (arrows, **A-D**). These air cells are anterior-most ethmoid air cells that are located ventral to the nasolacrimal canals or frontal recesses. The location of the right nasolacrimal canal is denoted by arrowheads on images **B** and **C**.

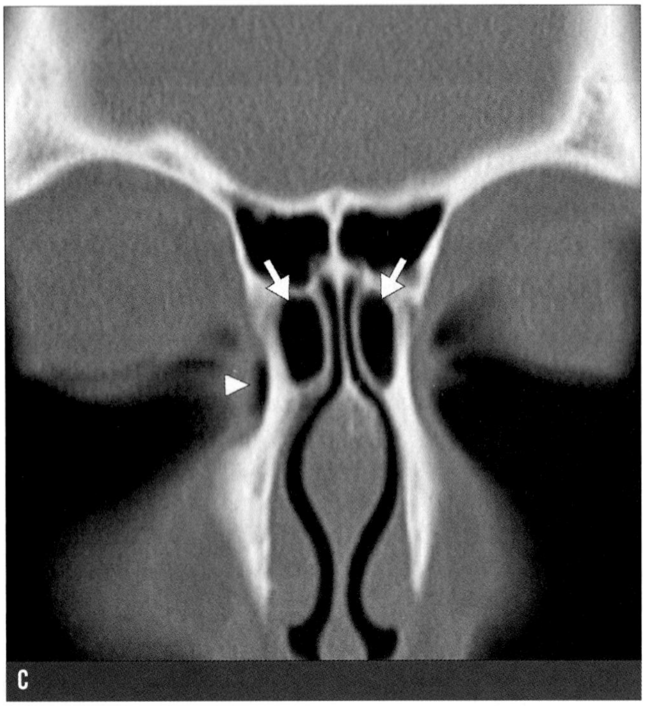

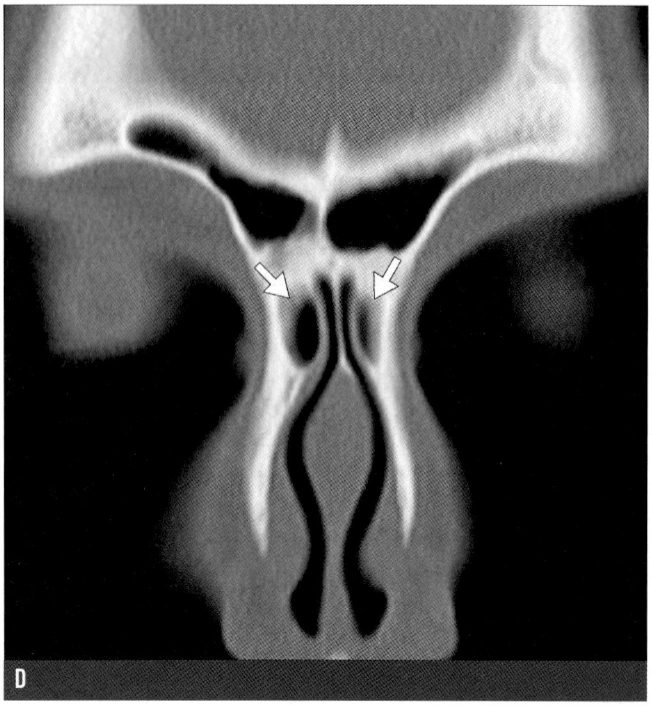

Agger nasi air cells

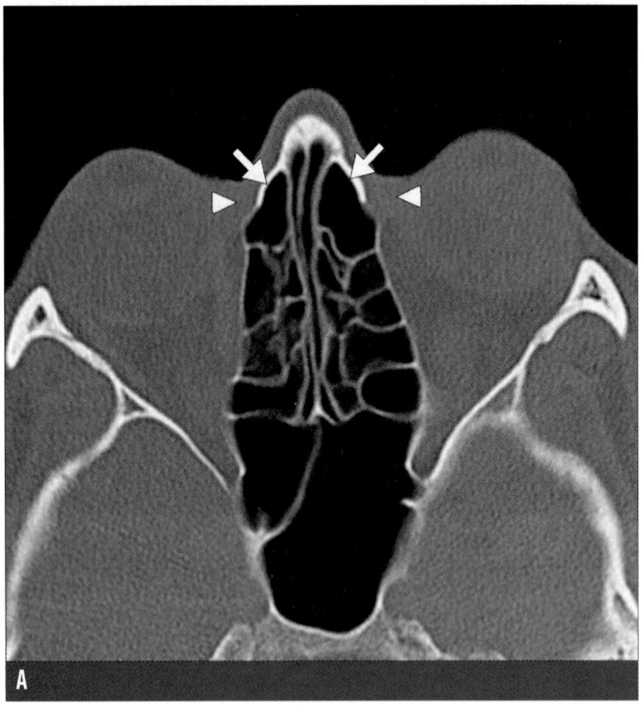

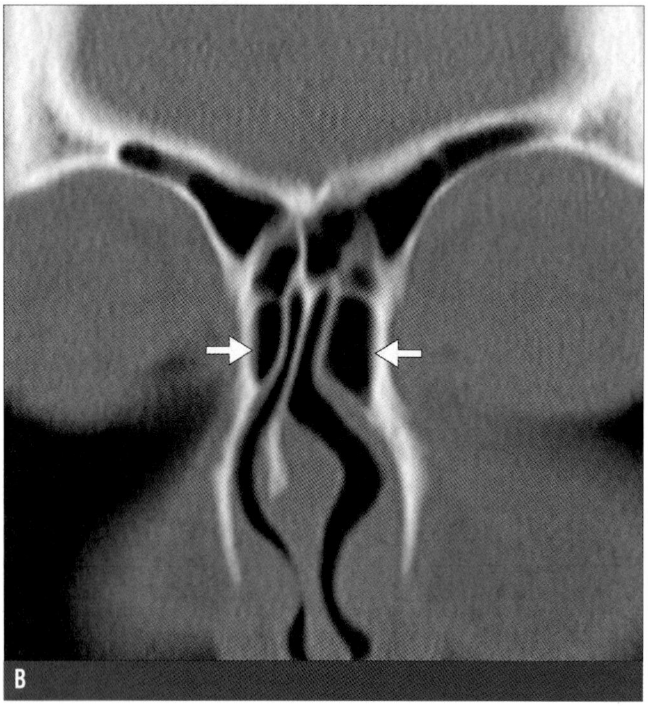

Different patient. Axial (**A**), coronal reformatted (**B**), and sagittal reformatted (**C**) CT images demonstrate anteriorly positioned ethmoid airs cells at the level of, and ventral to, the nasolacrimal ducts (arrowheads, **A**), compatible with agger nasi air cells (arrows, **A-C**).

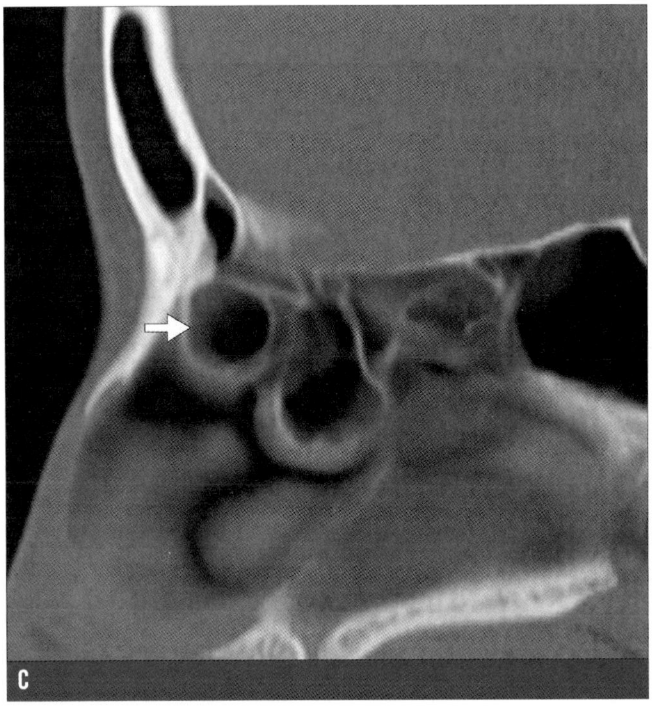

Companion case: Obstructed frontal recess due to an agger nasi cell

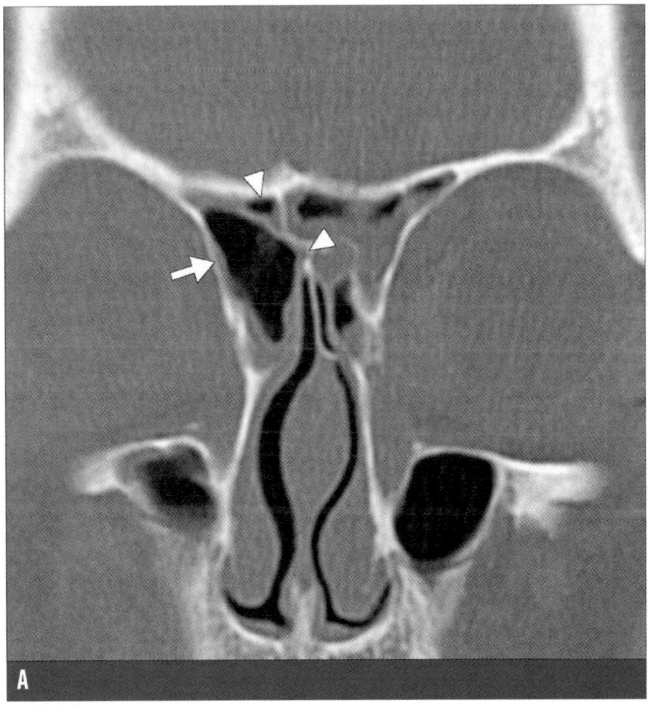

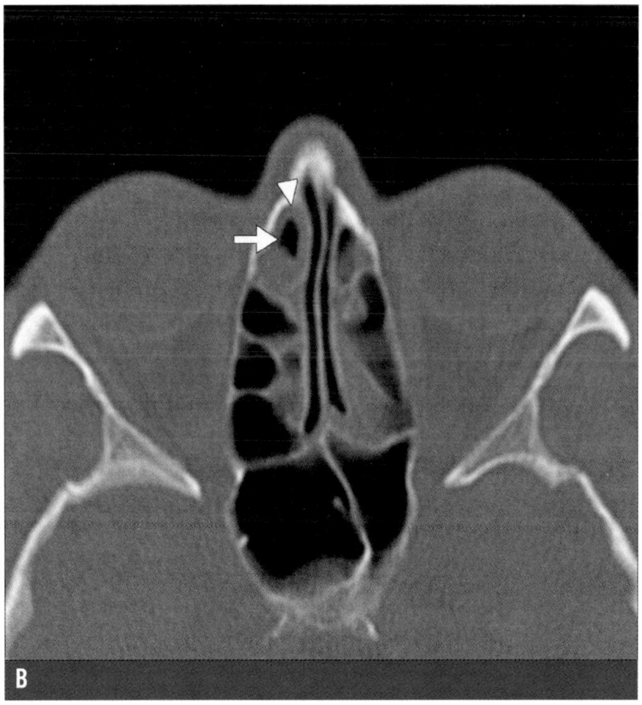

A coronal reformatted CT image through the frontal recesses (**A**) demonstrates a large right agger nasi cell (arrow, **A**) that obstructs the right frontal recess (arrowheads, **A**). An axial CT image through the inferior aspect of the agger nasi cell (**B**) also demonstrates that the agger nasi cell (arrow, **B**) subtotally occupies and obstructs the mucosal-lined right frontal recess (arrowhead, **B**). An axial CT image through the frontal sinus (**C**) demonstrates postobstructive sinus disease within the right frontal sinus (arrow, **C**).

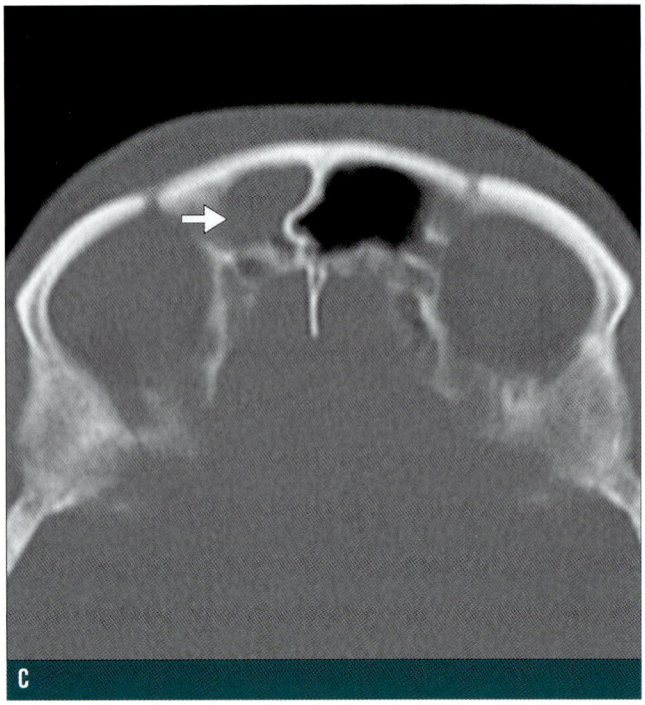

REFERENCES

Beale TJ, et al. Imaging of the paranasal sinuses and nasal cavity: normal anatomy and clinically relevant anatomical variants. *Semin Ultrasound CT MR*. 2009;30(1):2-16.

Daniels DL, et al. The frontal sinus drainage pathway and related structures. *AJNR Am J Neuroradiol*. 2003;24(8):1618-1627.

Huang BY, Lloyd KM, DelGaudio JM, Jablonowski E, Hudgins PA. Failed endoscopic sinus surgery: spectrum of CT findings in the frontal recess. *Radiographics*. 2009;29(1):177-195.

Kantarci M, et al. Remarkable anatomic variations in paranasal sinus region and their clinical importance. *Eur J Radiol*. 2004;50:296-302.

Perez-Pinas I, et al. Anatomical variations in the human paranasal sinus region studied by CT. *J Anat*. 2000;197:221-227.

CASE 14 Intraethmoidal lipoma

A lipoma of the ethmoid air cells is a rarely encountered entity. It represents an intraosseous lipoma that may be entirely composed of adipose tissue, or it may contain a combination of adipose tissue, bone, osteoblasts, and hematopoietic marrow. Lipomas may also undergo changes due to ischemia or trauma which may lead to infarction, hemorrhage, and ultimately mineralization. Its CT and MRI appearance depends upon its histologic components; an ethmoid air cell lipoma composed purely of adipose tissue will follow fat attenuation or fat signal on CT and all MRI pulse sequences, respectively. However, the presence of hemorrhage and/or mineralization may complicate its imaging appearance, in which case it could be mistaken for numerous other entities, such as fibrous dysplasia, enchondroma, chondrosarcoma, and osteoblastoma. A lipoma of the ethmoid air cells is a benign entity that is typically asymptomatic and requires no surgical treatment, unless it results in a sinus obstruction.

Intraethmoidal lipoma

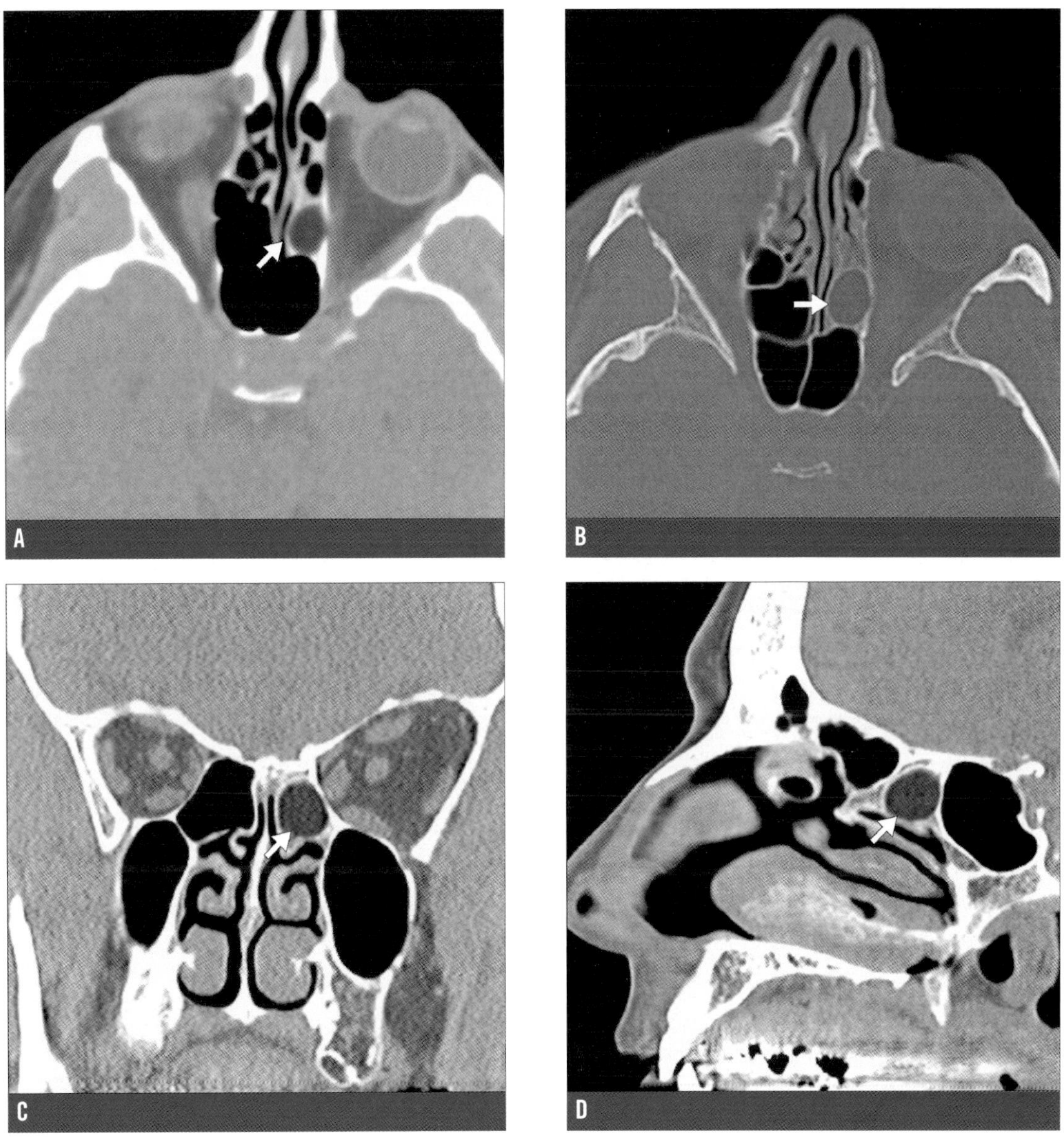

An axial CT image viewed with a soft tissue window (**A**), an axial CT image viewed with a bone window (**B**), and coronal reformatted (**C**) as well as sagittal reformatted (**D**) CT images viewed with an intermediate window demonstrate a fat equivalent lesion in the left posterior ethmoids, consistent with an intraethmoidal lipoma (arrows, **A-D**). A primary intraethmoidal lipoma is rare. Fat herniation into the ethmoid air cells following a lamina papyracea is far more common than an intraethmoidal lipoma. Posttraumatic changes were not present in this case.

REFERENCES

Abdalla W, et al. Intraosseous lipoma of the left frontoethmoidal sinuses and nasal cavity. *AJNR Am J Neuroradiol.* 2007;28(4):615-617.

Elsurer C, Hancı D, Cakir A, Dal T. Isolated intraosseous lipoma of the ethmoid sinus. *J Craniomaxillofac Surg.* 2013;41(8):718-720.

Fu YS, Perzin KH. Non-epithelial tumors of the nasal cavity, paranasal sinuses and nasopharynx: a clinicopathologic study. VIII. Adiopose tissue tumors (lipoma and liposarcoma). *Cancer.* 1977;40(3): 1312-1317.

Gupta N, et al. Fine needle aspiration cytology in lesions of the nose, nasal cavity and paranasal sinuses. *Acta Cytologica.* 2011;55:135-141.

Schwentner I, Schmutzhard J, Krugmann J, Sprinzl GM. Lipoma of the paranasal sinus: a rare but noticeable entity. *J Otolaryngol Head Neck Surg.* 2008;37(5):E133-E134

Uysal A, et al. Maxillary sinus lipoma: an unanticipated diagnosis. *J Craniofac Surg.* 2007;18(5):1153-1155.

CASE 15 Paranasal sinus osteoma

Paranasal sinus osteomas are benign, slow-growing hamartomatous tumors that arise from the membranous bone of the paranasal sinuses. While they are usually incidental, patients may experience local pain or headaches with osteomas. Paranasal osteomas are most frequently found in the frontal sinuses, frontal recesses, and ethmoid air cells. If they cause obstruction of sinus drainage, they will predispose patients to sinus infection and mucocele formation, although this is relatively infrequent. Multiple osteomas may be seen in patients with Gardner syndrome.

COMPANION CASE

- **Paranasal sinus fibrous dysplasia.** With fibrous dysplasia, normal bone is replaced by fibrous tissue which consists of spindle cell bundles and immature woven bone. This process results in expansion of the affected bone. It may affect a single site (monostotic) or multiple sites (polyostotic). The most common CT appearance of fibrous dysplasia is a ground-glass (sclerotic) pattern. However, fibrous dysplasia can less commonly appear as a heterogeneously sclerotic and lucent lesion (Pagetoid form) or as cystic lesion (cystic form). On MRI, fibrous dysplasia has a nonspecific appearance and may mimic other osseous lesions, including malignant entities. Thus, any suspicious primary osseous lesion on MRI should be interpreted in combination with CT, or when appropriate, radiographs. Typically, fibrous dysplasia is low-to-intermediate in T1 signal and enhances on MRI. The T2 signal characteristics are variable and depend on the ratio of mineralized matrix to fibrous tissue.

Ethmoid air cell osteoma

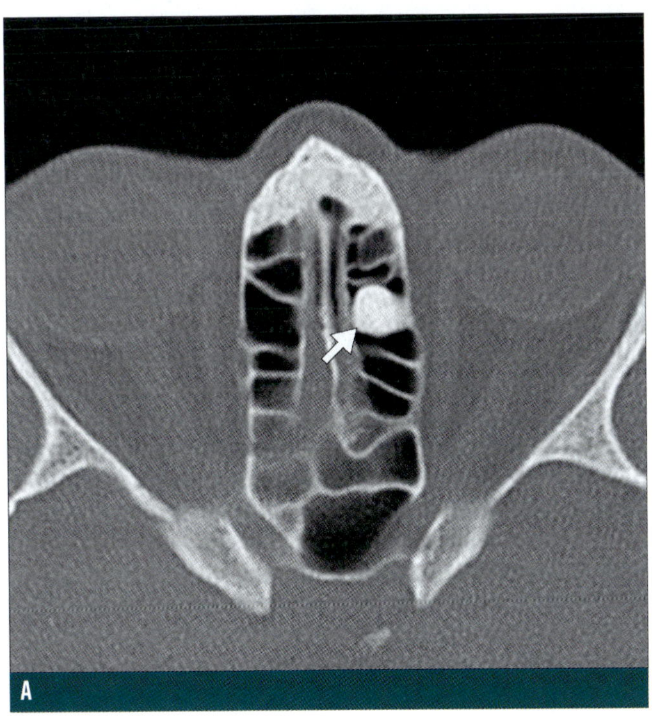

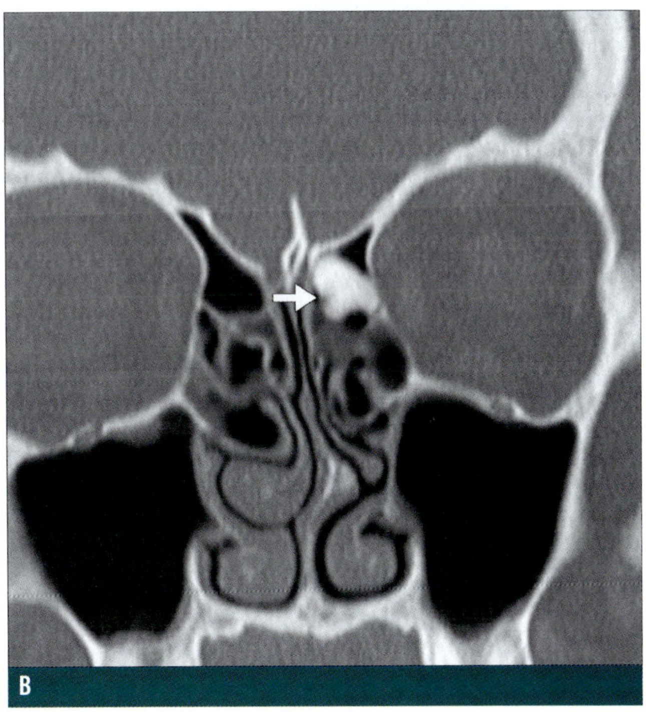

Axial (**A**), coronal reformatted (**B**), and sagittal reformatted (**C**) CT images demonstrate an osteoma within the left anterior ethmoid air cells (arrows, **A-C**).

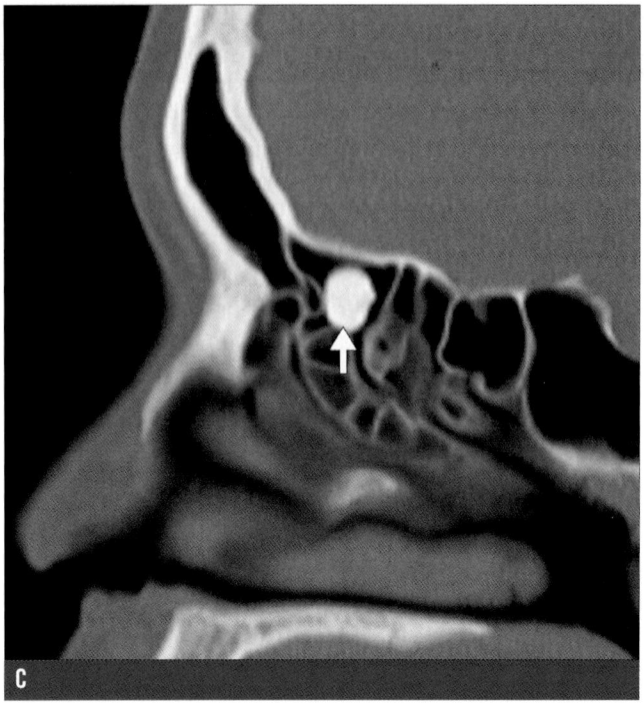

Frontal recess osteoma

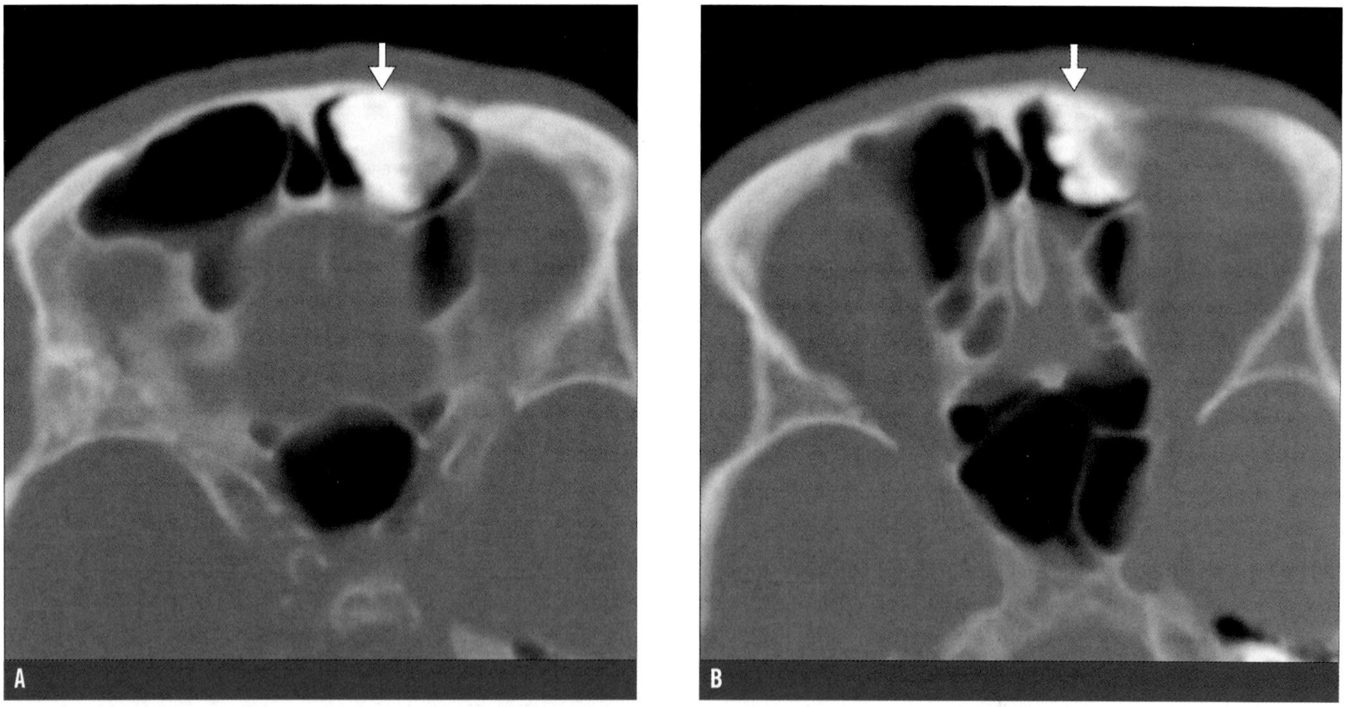

Axial CT images through the frontal recesses (**A**, **B**) demonstrate a large, densely ossified mass centered within the left frontal recess (arrows, **A**, **B**). This lesion is compatible with a benign osteoma.

Progressively enlarging frontal recess osteoma

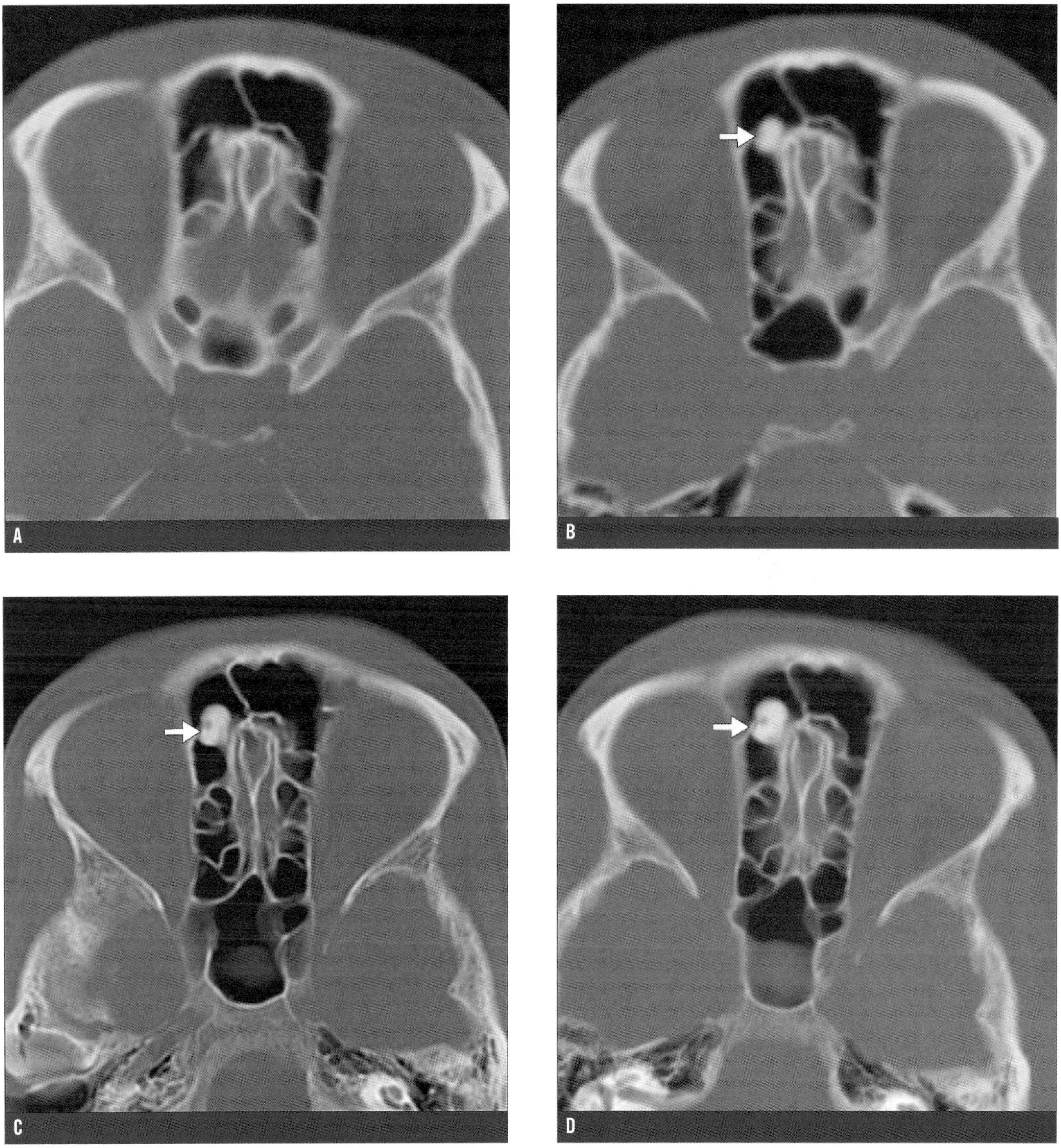

Axial CT images through the level of the frontal recesses obtained over a 6-year span (**A-D**) demonstrate a progressively enlarging osteoma within the right frontal recess (arrows, **A-D**).

Companion case: Ethmoid air cell fibrous dysplasia

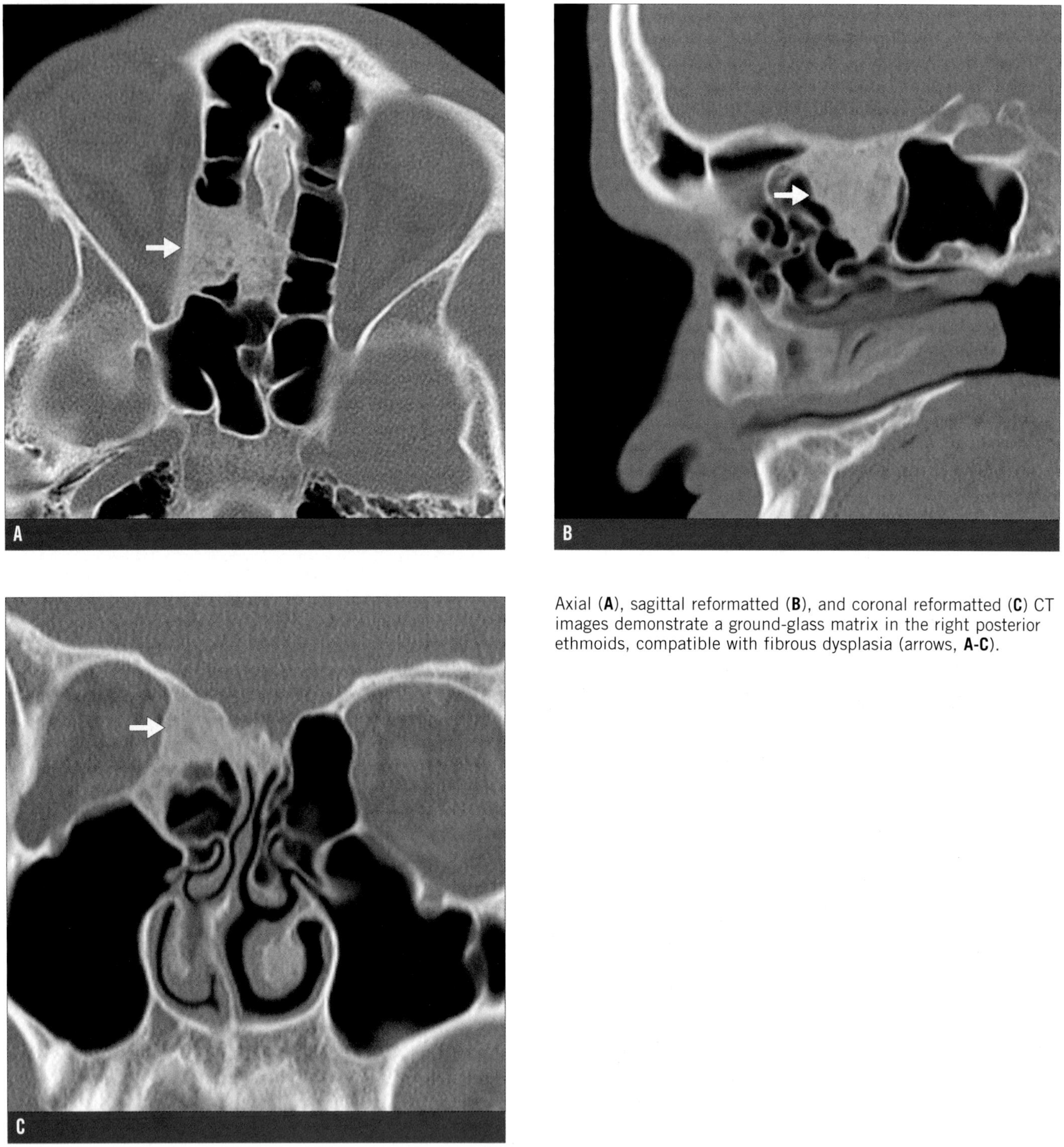

Axial (**A**), sagittal reformatted (**B**), and coronal reformatted (**C**) CT images demonstrate a ground-glass matrix in the right posterior ethmoids, compatible with fibrous dysplasia (arrows, **A-C**).

Companion case: Frontal recess fibrous dysplasia

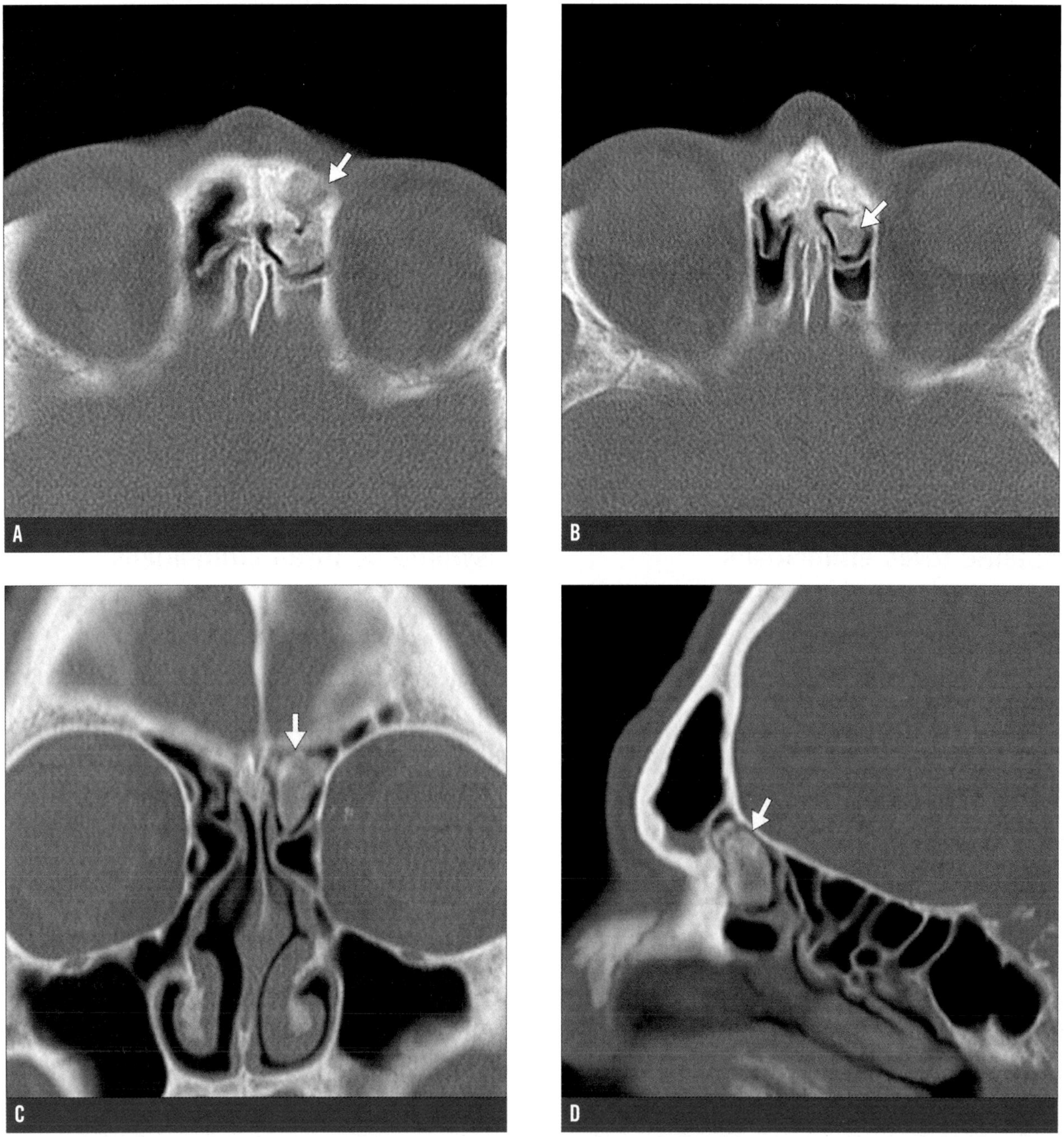

Axial (**A**, **B**), coronal reformatted (**C**), and sagittal reformatted (**D**) CT images through the level of the frontal recesses demonstrate an osseous lesion with a ground-glass matrix occupying the majority of the left frontal frontal recess, compatible with fibrous dysplasia (arrows, **A-D**).

REFERENCES

Camilleri AE. Craniofacial fibrous dysplasia. *J Laryngol Otol.* 1991;105:662-666.

Clauser L, Marchetti C, Piccione M, Bertoni F. Craniofacial fibrous dysplasia and Ollier's disease: combined transfrontal and transfacial resection using the nasal-cheek flap. *J Craniofac Surg.* 1996;7(2):140-144.

Cruz AAV, Constanzi M, Attie de Castro FA, Carlos dos Santos AC. Apical involvement with fibrous dysplasia: implications for vision. *Ophthal Plast Reconstr Surg.* 2007;23(6):450-454.

Demirdover C, Sahin B, Ozkan HS, Durmus EU, Oztan HY. Isolated fibrous dysplasia of the zygomatic bone. *J Craniofac Surg.* 2010;21:1583-1584.

MacDonald-Jankowski DS. Fibro-osseous lesions of the face and jaws. Clin *Radiol.* 2004;59:11-25.

Yücel A, Acar M, Haktanır A, Albayrak R, Değirmenci B. Orbital extension of a large frontal sinus osteoma associated with fibrous dysplasia. *Eur J Gen Med.* 2004;1(4):74-77.

CASE 16 Asymmetric fovea ethmoidalis

The fovea ethmodalis, or roof of the ethmoid air cells, is very commonly asymmetric. One fovea ethmoidalis is often more caudal or has a steeper slope than the other. This is a normal, incidental finding but awareness to its presence is important due to its surgical implications, as discussed below.

COMPANION CASE

- **Surgical injury of the fovea ethmoidalis.** The fovea ethmoidalis is the superior limit of dissection during functional endoscopic sinus surgery (FESS). An asymmetrically low-lying or steep slope of the fovea ethmodalis may be problematic during FESS. Specifically, these scenarios increase the chance of inadvertent breech of the more caudally positioned or steeper sloped fovea ethmodalis by the unsuspecting surgeon. Complications that may occur if the fovea ethmoidalis is disrupted include herniation of the brain and/or meninges into the superior nasal cavity or ethmoids, brain damage, hemorrhage, CSF leak, arterio-venous fistula, and recurrent meningitis.

Asymmetric fovea ethmoidalis

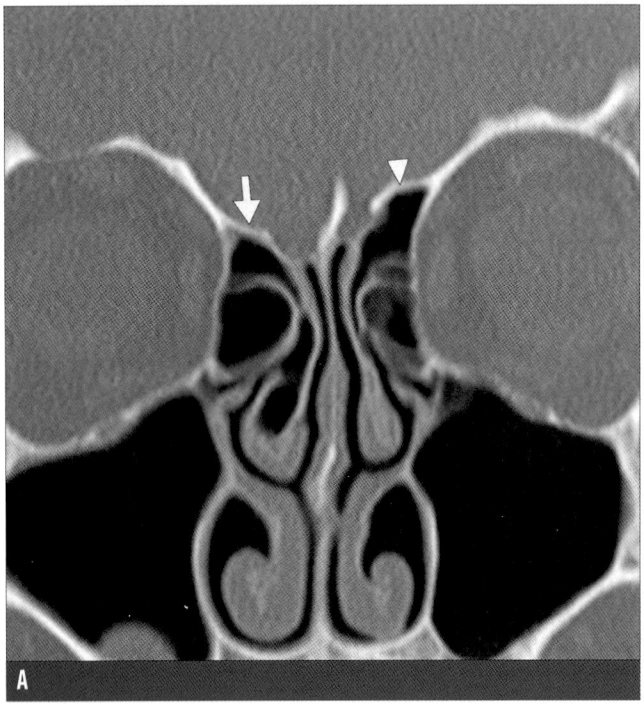

A coronal reformatted CT image (**A**) demonstrates the right fovea ethmoidalis (arrow) to be more caudal in position compared to the left fovea ethmoidalis (arrowhead).

Asymmetric fovea ethmoidalis

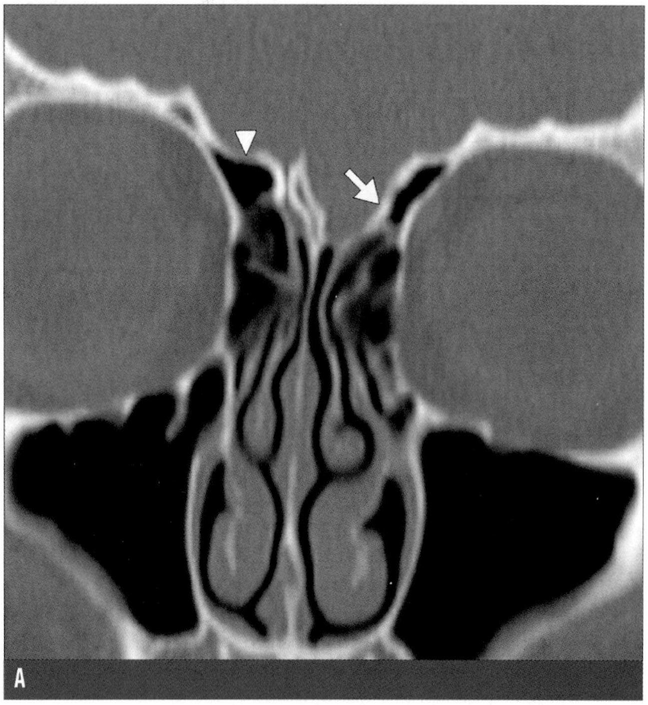

Different patient. A coronal reformatted CT image (**A**) demonstrates the left fovea ethmoidalis (arrow) to be more caudally positioned and to have a greater slope than the right fovea ethmoidalis (arrowhead).

Companion case: Surgical injury of the fovea ethmoidalis

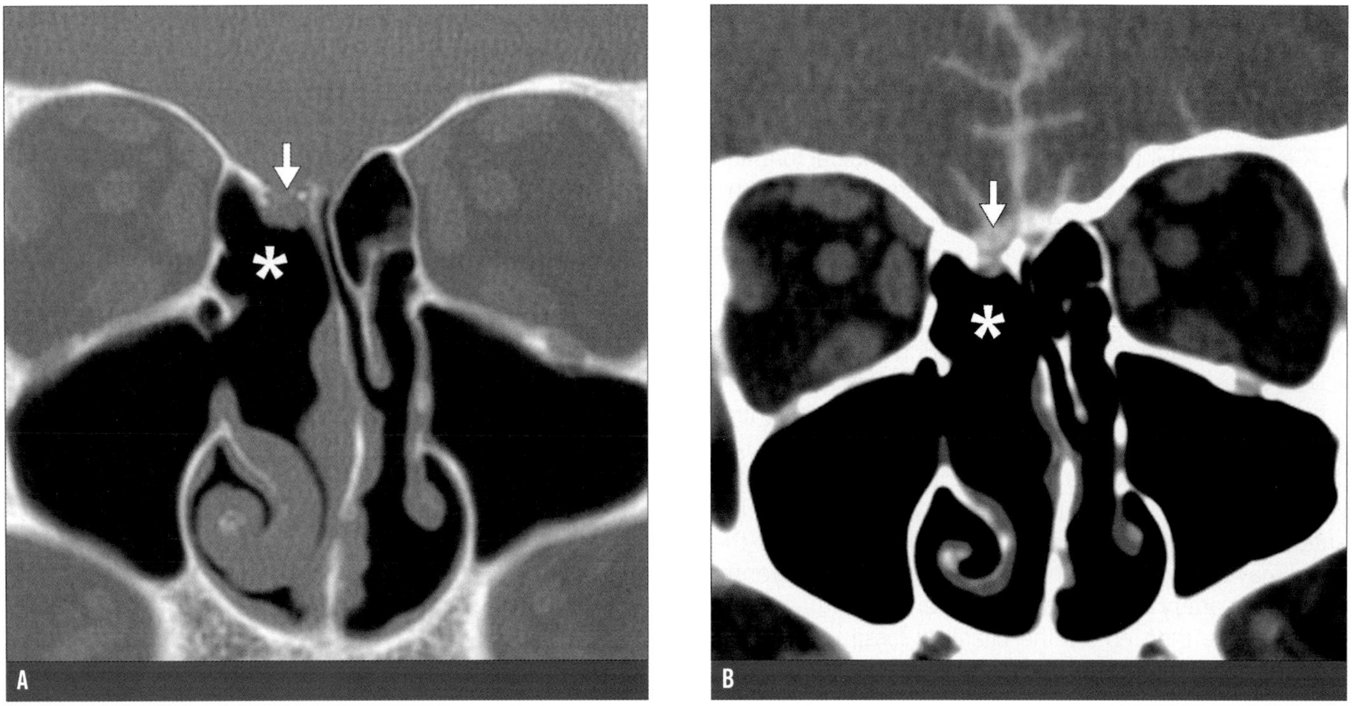

A coronal CT image viewed with a bone window (**A**) and a coronal CT image viewed with a soft tissue window (**B**) obtained following intrathecal contrast demonstrate a right fovea ethmoidalis defect (arrows, **A**, **B**). A small cephalocele is present within the defect, best appreciated on image **B**. This was a surgical complication of a right internal ethmoidectomy performed during functional endoscopic sinus surgery (FESS) (asterisks, **A**, **B**).

REFERENCES

Bayram M, et al. Important anatomic variations of the sinonasal anatomy in light of endoscopic surgery: a pictorial review. *Eur Radiol.* 2001;11(10):1991-1997.

Meloni F, et al. Anatomic variations of surgical importance in ethmoid labyrinth and sphenoid sinus. A study of radiological anatomy. *Surg Radiol Anat.* 1992;14:65-70.

Nouraei SA, et al. Variations in paranasal sinus anatomy: implications for the pathophysiology of chronic rhinosinusitis and safety of endoscopic sinus surgery. *J Otolaryngol Head Neck Surg.* 2009;38(1):32-37.

CASE 17 Anterior ethmoidal artery canal

The anterior ethmoidal artery (AEA) typically arises from the distal one-third of the intraorbital ophthalmic artery. The AEA exits the orbit through the anterior ethmoidal foramen and then the anterior ethmoidal canal, the latter representing a medially directed, pyramidal-shaped notch located along the superior aspect of the lamina papyracea. The anterior ethmoidal canal serves as a surgical landmark and demarcates the posterior edge of the frontal recess. The anterior ethmoidal canal is avoided during functional endoscopic sinus surgery in order to prevent injury to the AEA. If breached, the anterior ethmoidal artery can retract intraorbitally and result in uncontrolled intraorbital hemorrhage.

After exiting the orbit, the AEA enters the ethmoid labyrinth. The AEA may be surrounded by an extension of the anterior ethmoidal canal into the ethmoid labyrinth, or the canal may be absent or dehiscent in the ethmoid labyrinth, leaving the artery unprotected by bone.

The AEA then enters the olfactory fossa of the skull base through the lateral lamella of the cribriform plate via a structure termed the ethmoidal groove (also called ethmoidal sulcus).

From the anterior skull base, the AEA has several branches, including several nasal branches which traverse caudally back through the anterior skull base to anastomose with the nasal branches of the sphenopalatine artery, subsequently forming the Kiesselbach plexus.

An anterior ethmoidal canal may sometimes simulate a lamina papyracea fracture, although this can usually be differentiated from a fracture by its typical morphology and location.

COMPANION CASE

- **Lamina papyracea fracture.** This is a very common fracture following significant orbital trauma. Occasionally, a lamina papyracea fracture may extend into the anterior ethmoidal canal and result in AEA injury with subsequent hemorrhage in the orbit.

Anterior ethmoidal canals

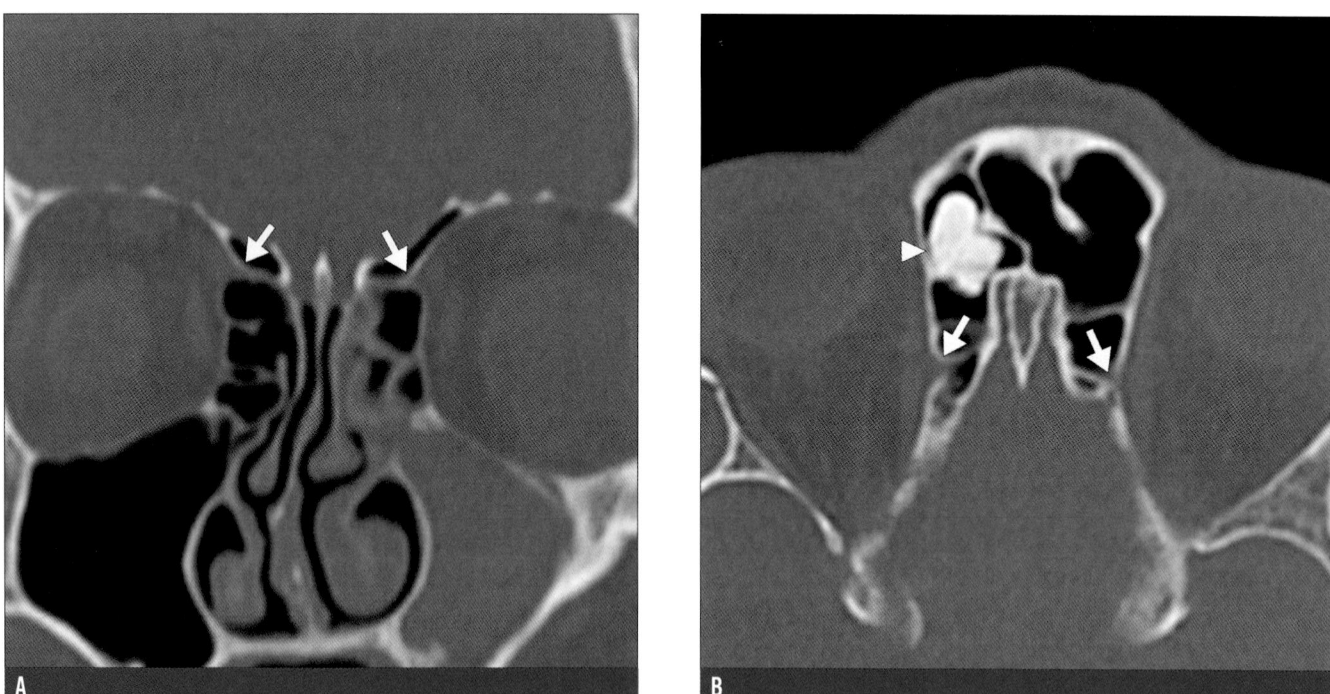

Coronal reformatted (**A**) and axial (**B**) CT images viewed with a bone window demonstrate bilateral anterior ethmoidal canals (arrows, **A, B**). The anterior ethmoidal foramen is located at the entrance site of each canal. An incidental right anterior ethmoid osteoma is demonstrated on image **B** (arrowhead).

Anterior ethmoidal canals

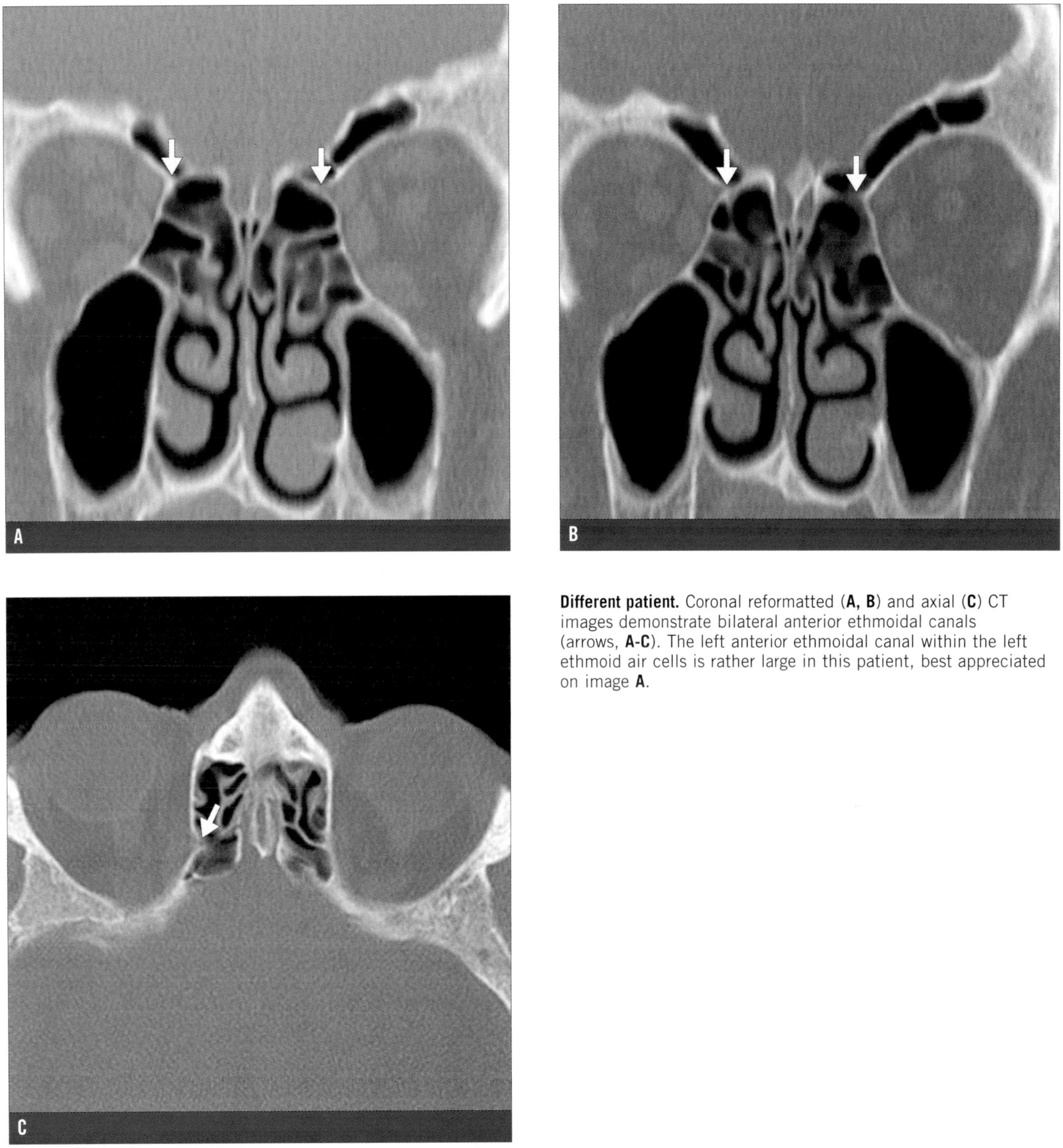

Different patient. Coronal reformatted (**A, B**) and axial (**C**) CT images demonstrate bilateral anterior ethmoidal canals (arrows, **A-C**). The left anterior ethmoidal canal within the left ethmoid air cells is rather large in this patient, best appreciated on image **A**.

Companion case: Lamina papyracea fractures

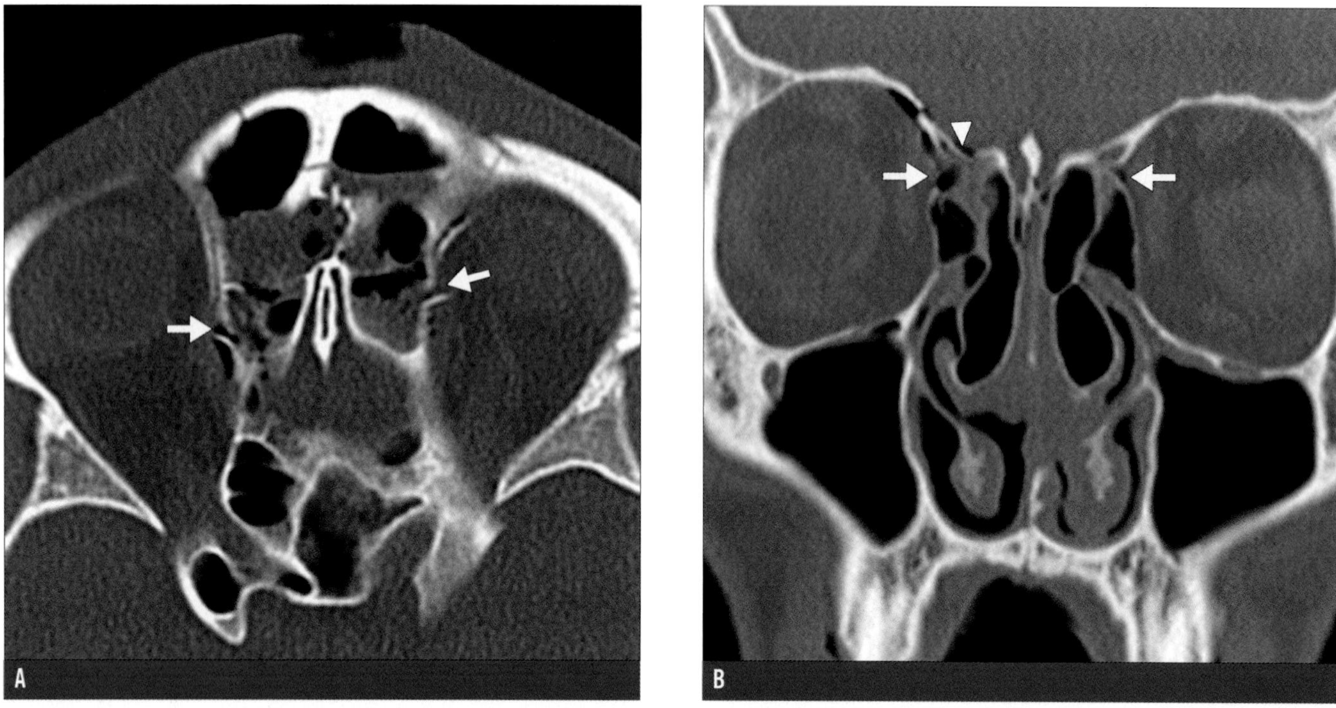

Axial (**A**) and coronal reformatted (**B**) CT images demonstrate bilateral lamina papyracea fractures that involve the bilateral anterior ethmoidal canals (arrows, **A**, **B**) and the right fovea ethmoidalis (arrowhead, **B**). The step-off at the fracture sites and the adjacent extraconal and intracranial air confirm the presence of acute fractures. This patient did not have significant intraorbital hemorrhage (not shown), but disruption of the anterior ethmoidal artery may result in extensive intraorbital hemorrhage.

REFERENCES

Cankal F, et al. Evaluation of the anterior and posterior ethmoidal canal by computed tomography. *Clin Radiol.* November 2004;59(11):1034-1040.

Meloni F, et al. Anatomic variations of surgical importance in ethmoid labyrinth and sphenoid sinus. A study of radiological anatomy. *Surg Radiol Anat.* 1992;14:65-70.

Moon HJ, et al. Surgical anatomy of the anterior ethmoidal canal in ethmoid roof. *Laryngoscope.* 2001;111:900-904.

CASE 18 Internal ethmoidectomy

An ethmoidectomy is a surgical procedure that resects portions or all the ethmoid septa and is performed to treat sinus mucosal disease that involves the ethmoid air cells. An internal ethmoidectomy is a surgical procedure performed during a functional endoscopic sinus surgery (FESS), whereas an external ethmoidectomy is performed from an external approach.

Today, FESS has replaced the external approach to treat ethmoid air cell mucosal disease. However, an external ethmoidectomy approach may be used to ligate the ethmoidal artery (in cases of epistaxis), drain an orbital abscess, reduce a fracture, expose the optic nerve, remove a large osteoma, or to gain wide exposure for removal of a regional tumor.

Partial internal ethmoidectomy

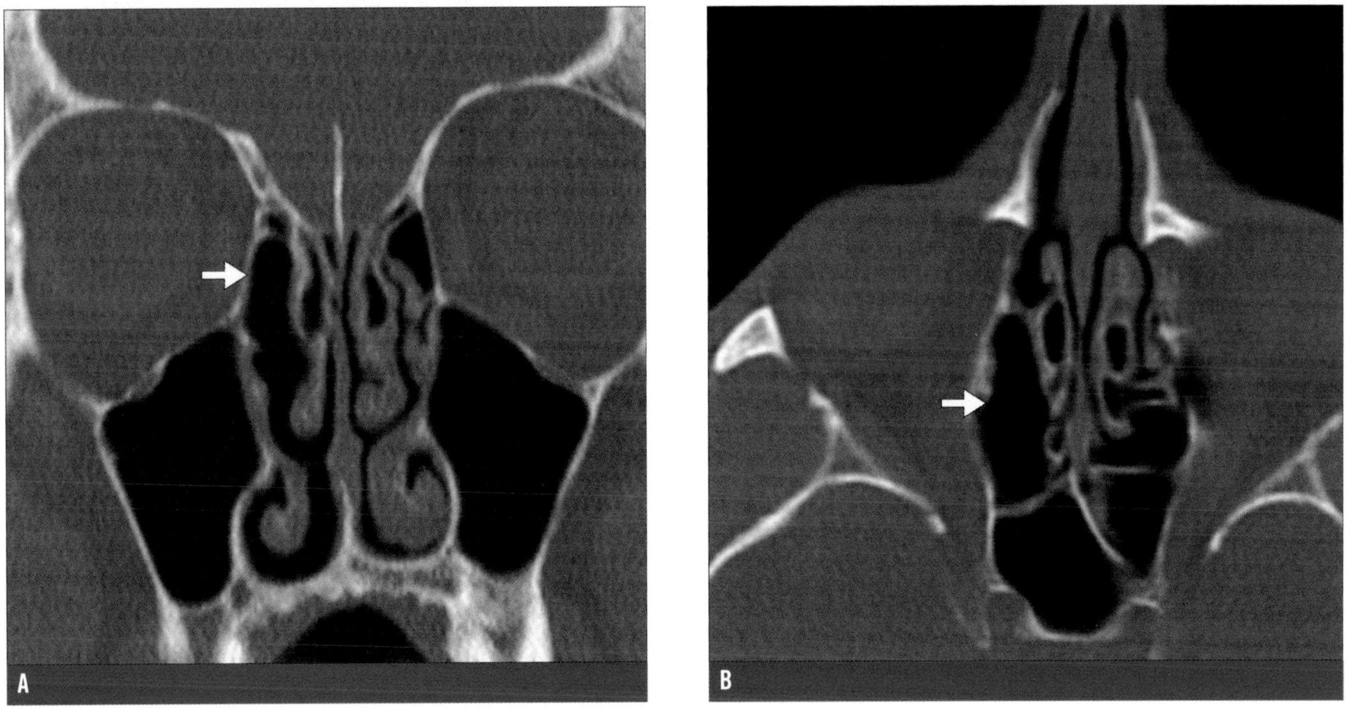

Coronal reformatted (**A**) and axial (**B**) CT images demonstrate typical postoperative changes from a partial right internal ethmoidectomy (arrows, **A**, **B**).

Complete internal ethmoidectomies

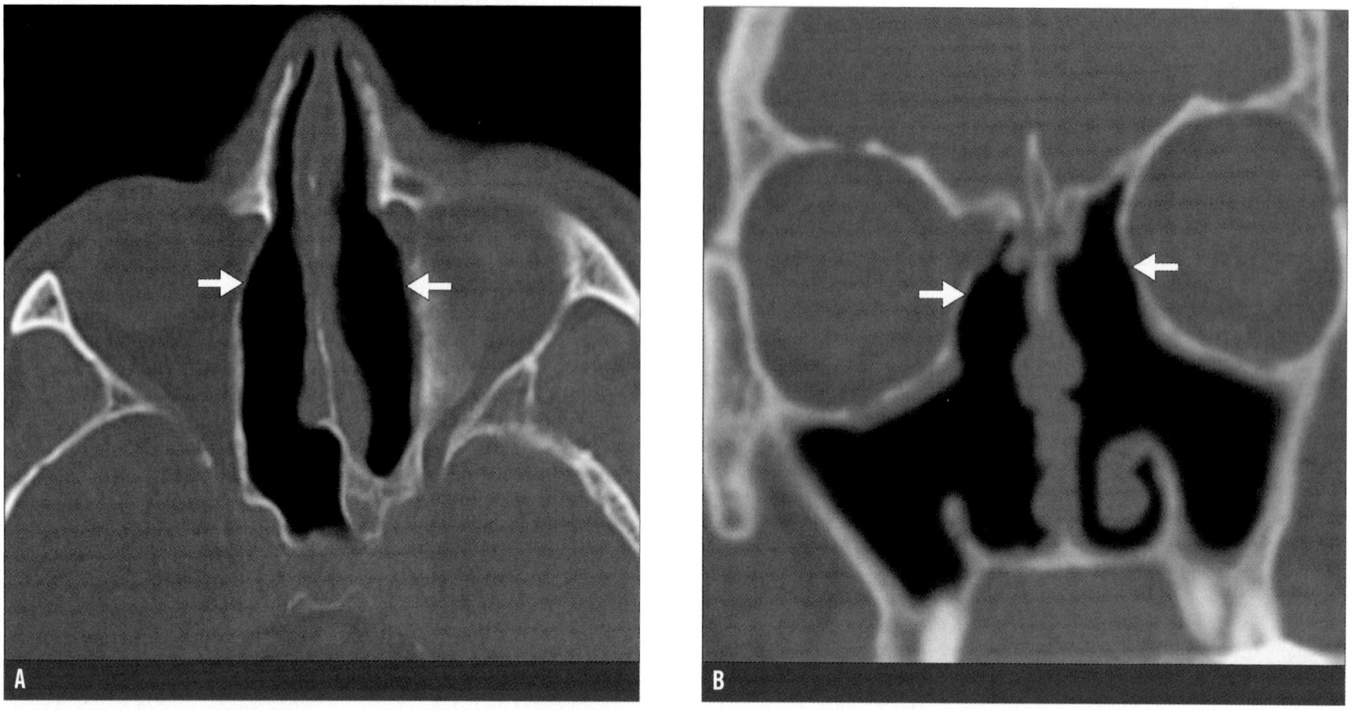

Axial (**A**) and coronal reformatted (**B**) CT images demonstrate complete bilateral internal ethmoidectomies (arrows, **A**, **B**), among other postsurgical sinus changes.

REFERENCES

Kountakis S E, et al. Revision Sinus Surgery. Berlin-Heidelberg, Germany: Springer; 2008.

Myers EN. *Operative Otolaryngology.* 2nd ed. Philadelphia, PA: Saunders; 2008.

CASE 19 Hypoplastic sphenoid sinus

Hypoplasia on either side of the sphenoid sinus is along the spectrum of pneumatization variants. See Chapter 7 for a full discussion regarding arrested pneumatization of the skull base (ie, sphenoid sinus).

COMPANION CASE

- **Cystic fibrosis-related sphenoid sinus hypoplasia.** Hypoplasia of the paranasal sinuses is a common finding in patients with cystic fibrosis, although the pathogenesis of hypoplasia is not fully understood. High-viscosity mucus with impaired mucociliary transport and superimposed inflammatory sinus disease occurring during sinus development are proposed etiologies.

Hypoplastic sphenoid sinus

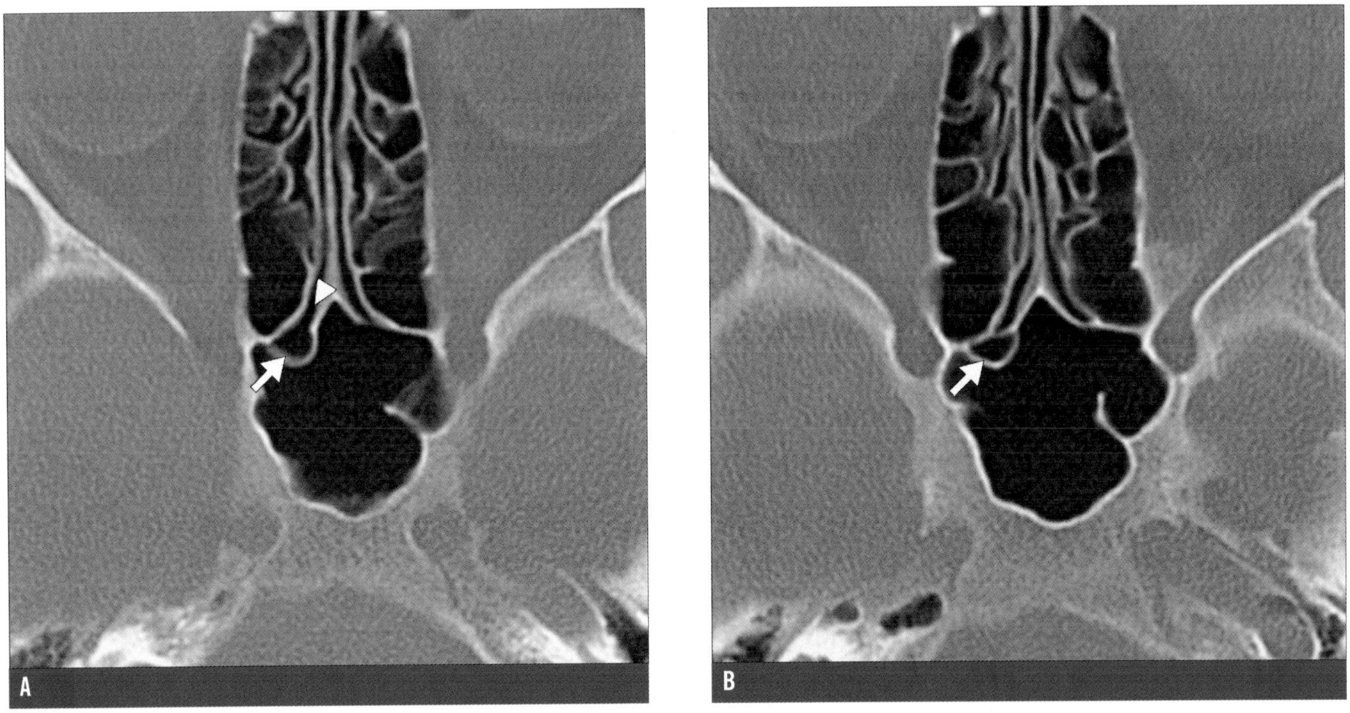

Axial CT images (**A, B**) demonstrate a hypoplastic right aspect of the sphenoid sinus (arrows, **A**, **B**). The right sphenoethmoidal recess (arrowhead, **A**) directly communicates with the right aspect of the sphenoid sinus. The direct communication with the right sphenoethmoidal recess indicates that this represents a hypoplastic sphenoid sinus rather than a posteriorly located ethmoid air cell.

Companion case: Cystic fibrosis-related sphenoid sinus hypoplasia

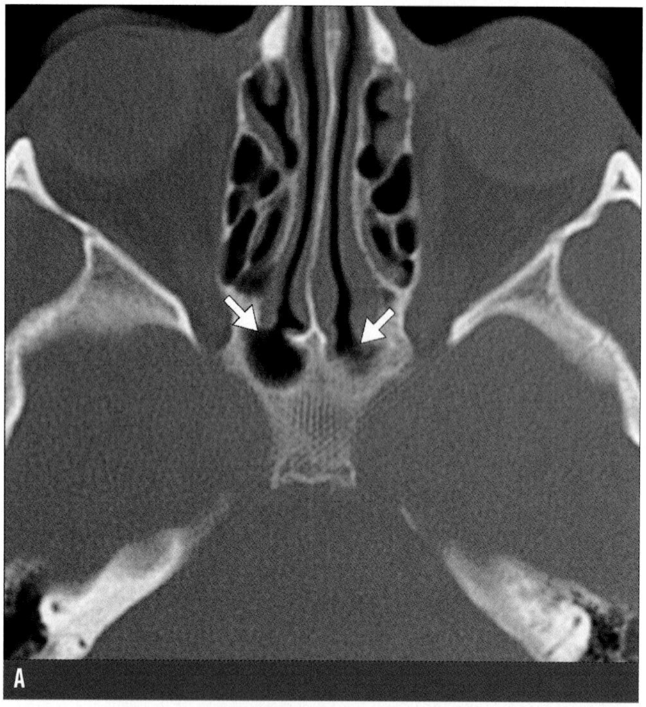

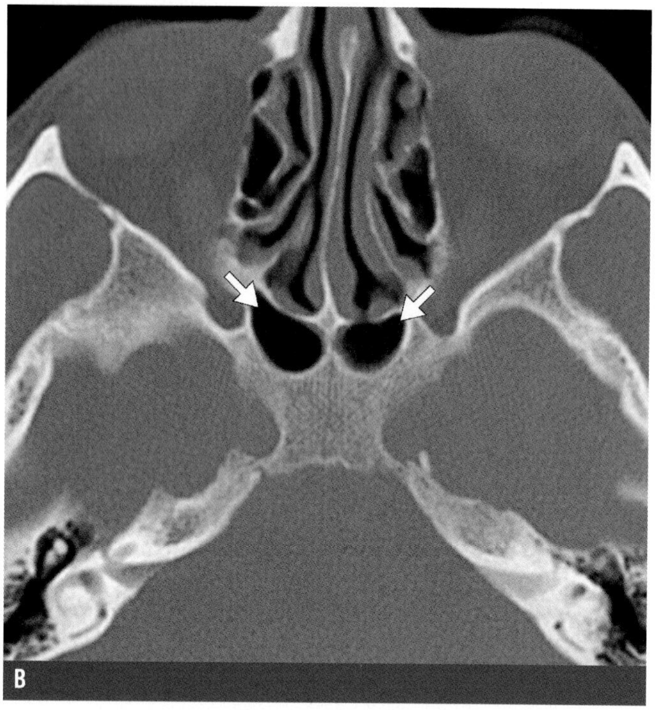

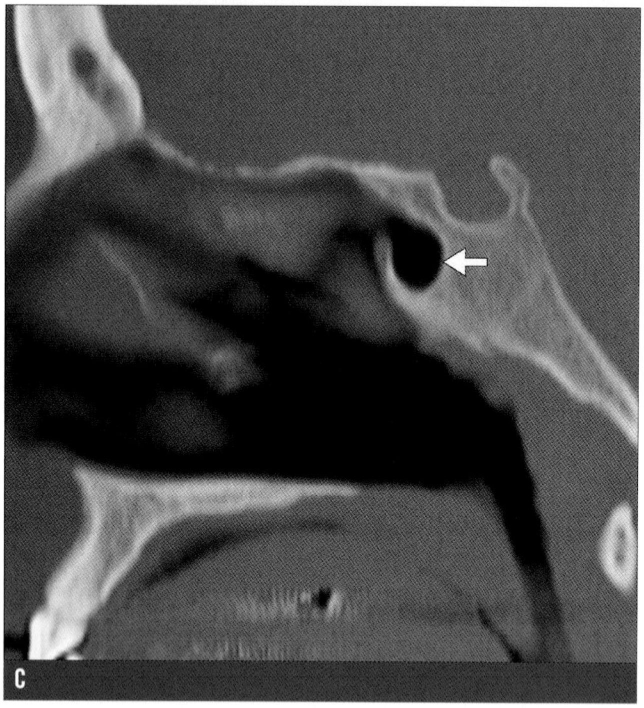

Axial (**A**, **B**) and sagittal reformatted (**C**) CT images in a patient with cystic fibrosis demonstrate hypoplasia of the sphenoid sinus (arrows, **A-C**), a common finding with this disease.

REFERENCES

Eggesbø HB, et al. CT Characterization of inflammatory paranasal sinus disease in cystic fibrosis. *Acta Radiol.* 2002;43:21-28.

Eggesbø HB, et al. Proposal of a CT scoring system of the paranasal sinuses in the diagnosis of cystic fibrosis. *Eur Radiol.* 2003;13:1451-1460.

Haktanir A, et al. Combined sphenoid and frontal sinus aplasia accompanied by bilateral maxillary and ethmoid sinus hypoplasia. *Br J Radiol.* 2005;78:1053-1056.

Jenkins JR. *Atlas of Neuroradiologic Embryology, Anatomy, and Variants.* Philadelphia, PA: Lippincott, Williams, and Wilkins; 2000.

Orlandi, RR, Wiggins RH 3rd. Radiological sinonasal findings in adults with cystic fibrosis. *Am J Rhinol Allergy.* 2009;23(3):307-311.

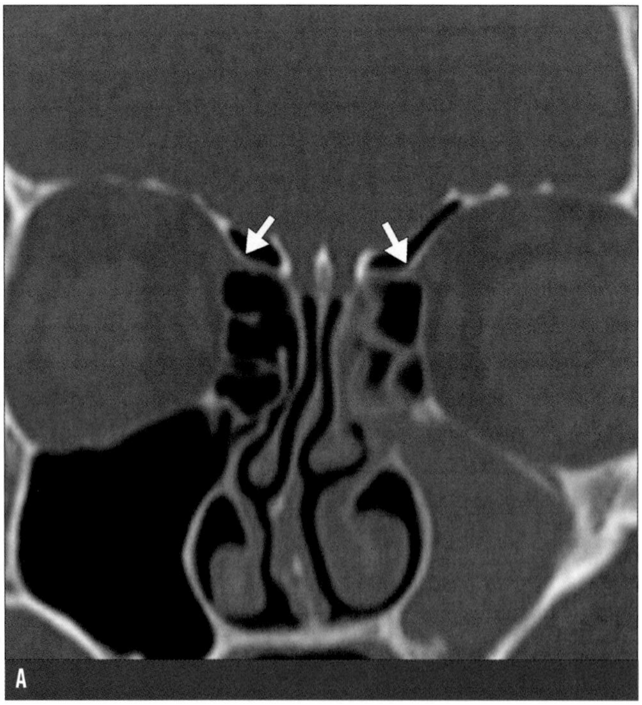

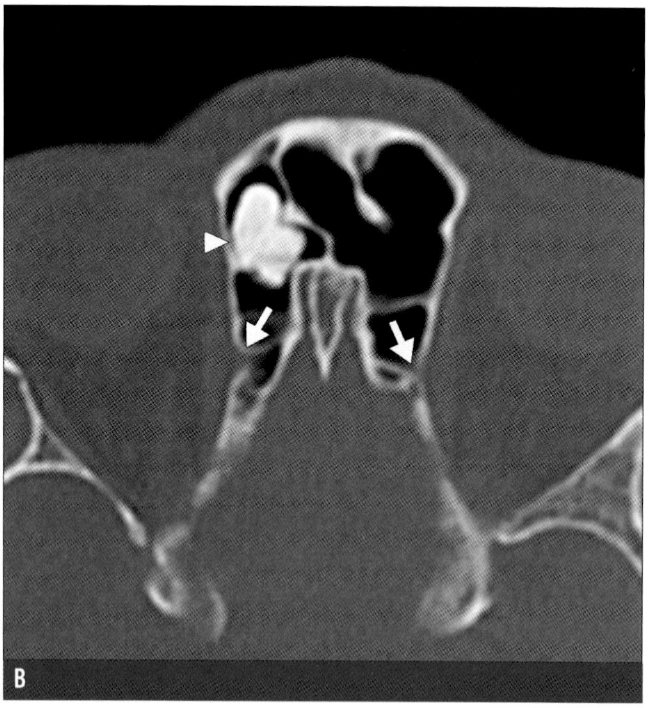

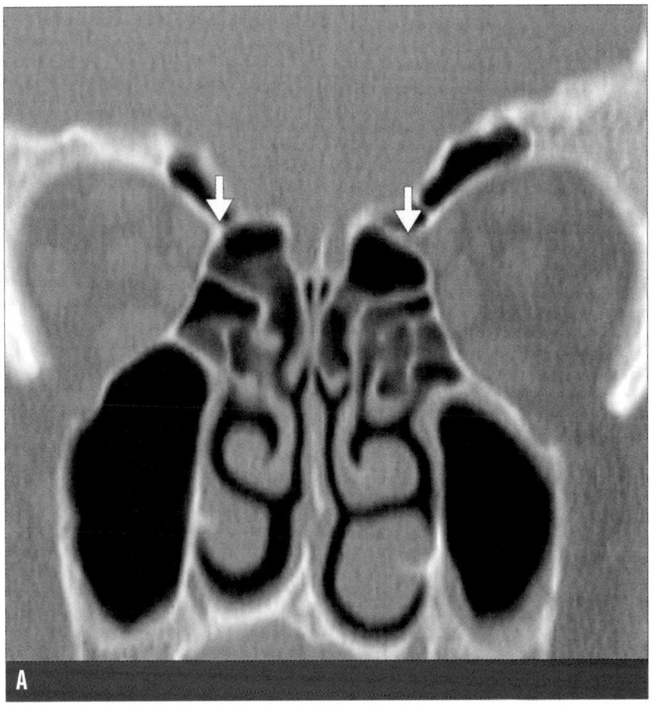

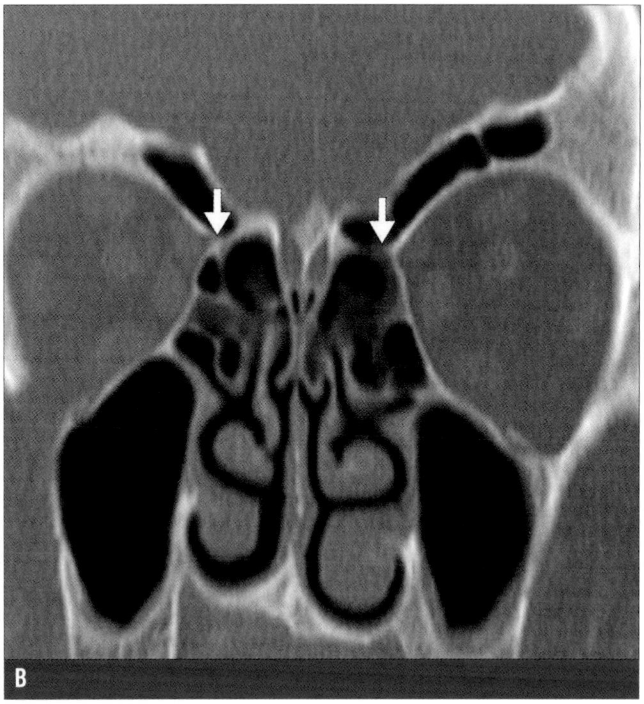

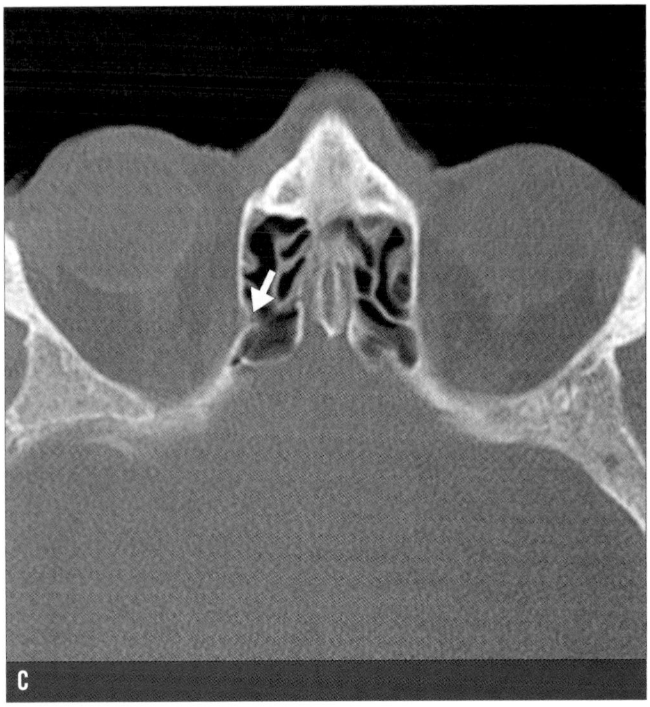

A maxillary sinus lift (or augmentation) is a procedure that is performed for patients requiring dental implants but who have an insufficient osseous alveolar ridge to stabilize the dental implant. A maxillary sinus lift entails placing bone graft material along the maxillary sinus floor in order to increase the height of the maxillary alveolus and provide support for the dental implant.

A wide variety of materials may be used for the bone graft, including autogenous bone (typically from an iliac crest donor site), Surgicel, freeze dried bone, and hydroxyapatite.

After the bone graft material is placed, typically 4 to 9 months (depending on the material used) are needed for the bone graft material to integrate with the native maxillary alveolus and to provide adequate support for the dental implant. Therefore, there may or may not be a dental implant in the area of the bone graft material at the time of imaging.

If the interpreting radiologist is unaware of this procedure, the bone graft material along the maxillary sinus floor could be misinterpreted as fibrous dysplasia, an osteoma, or other bone-forming tumor.

COMPANION CASES

- **Maxillary sinus osteoma.** Paranasal sinus osteomas are benign, slow-growing tumors arising from the membranous bone of the paranasal sinuses. While they are usually incidental, patients may have local pain or headaches associated with osteomas. If they cause obstruction of sinus drainage, they can predispose patients to sinus infection and mucocele formation, although this is relatively infrequent. Multiple osteomas may be seen in patients with Gardner syndrome.
- **Antrolith.** An antrolith is a term that is used to describe a stone in the maxillary antrum. While a stone in the nasal cavity (termed rhinolith) can occur from endogenous causes (pus, fungus, etc) or from exogenous causes (ie, various foreign bodies), an antrolith typically only occurs from endogenous causes because of its location relative to the outside environment.

Maxillary sinus lifts without dental implants

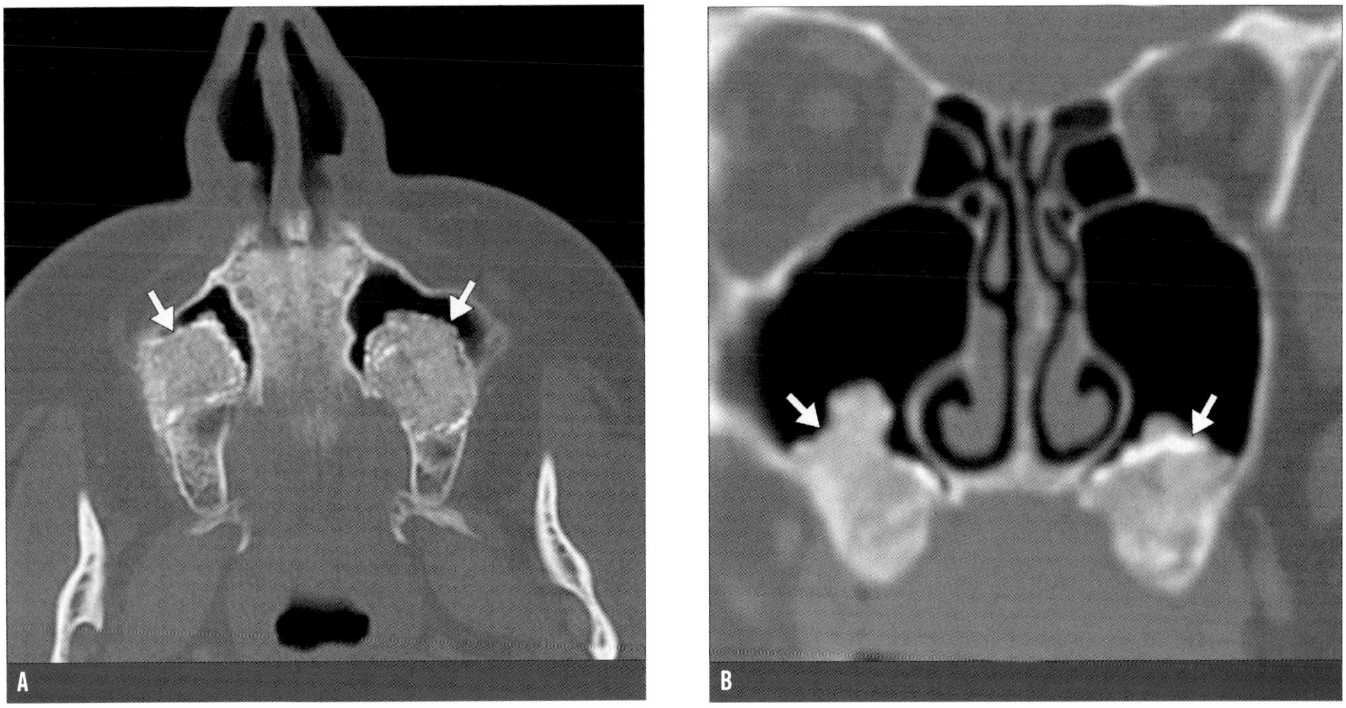

Axial (**A**) and coronal reformatted (**B**) CT images through the maxillary sinuses demonstrate bone graft material along the floors of both maxillary sinuses that has fully integrated with the maxillary alveolus, compatible with healed sinus lifts (arrows, **A**, **B**). Dental implants have not yet been placed in this patient at the time of imaging.

Normal evolution of a maxillary sinus lift without dental implants

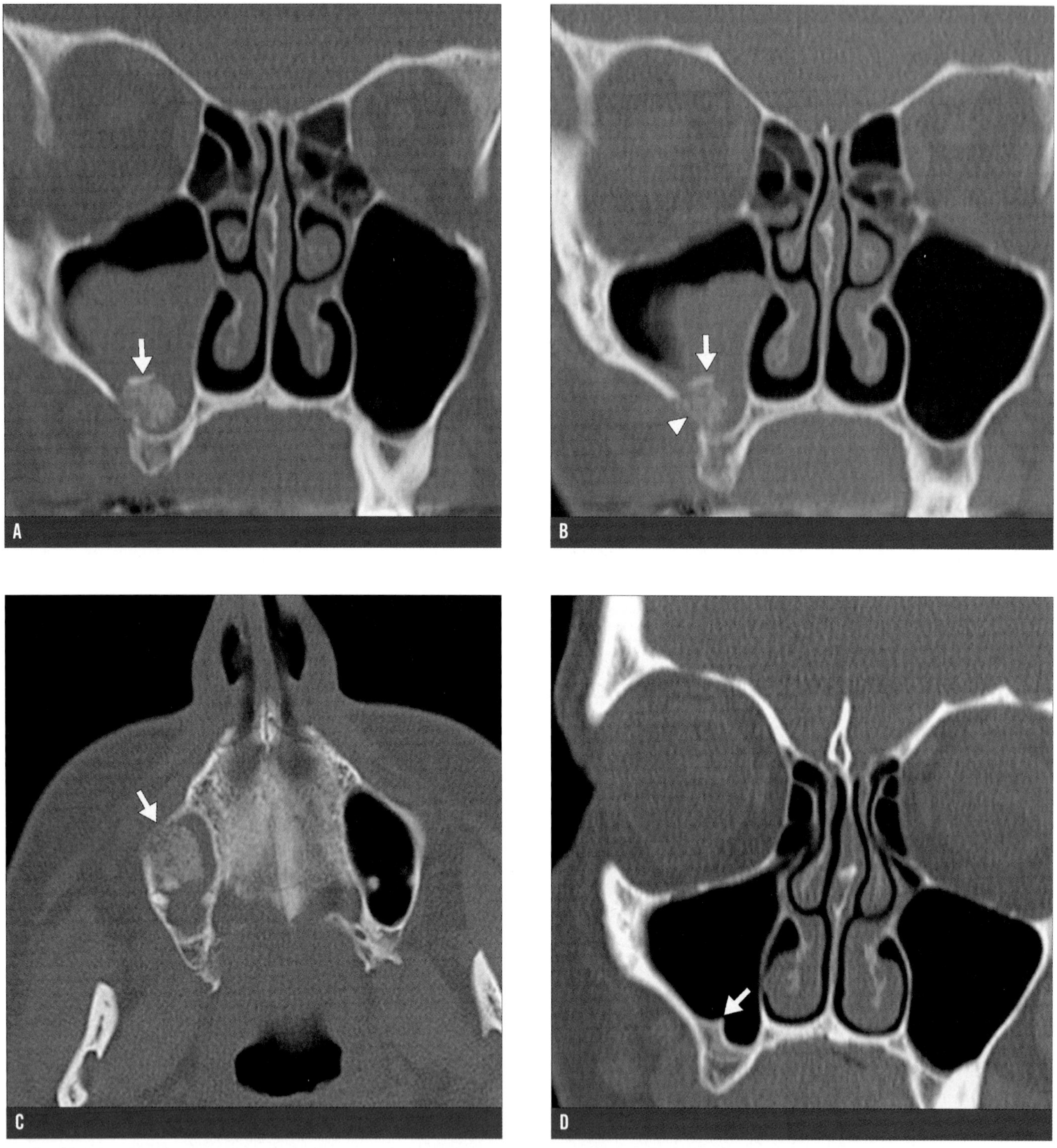

Coronal reformatted (**A, B**) and axial (**C**) CT images through the maxillary sinuses demonstrate ill-defined bone graft material along the floor of the right maxillary sinus which has not yet integrated with the maxillary alveolus (arrows, **A-C**). A right maxillary sinus floor defect is present (arrowhead, **B**), presumably representing the maxillary antrum entrance site for placement of the bone graft material. A coronal reformatted CT image obtained 16 months later (**D**) demonstrates the bone graft material to be fully integrated with the maxillary alveolus (arrow, **D**).

Maxillary sinus lifts with a dental implant

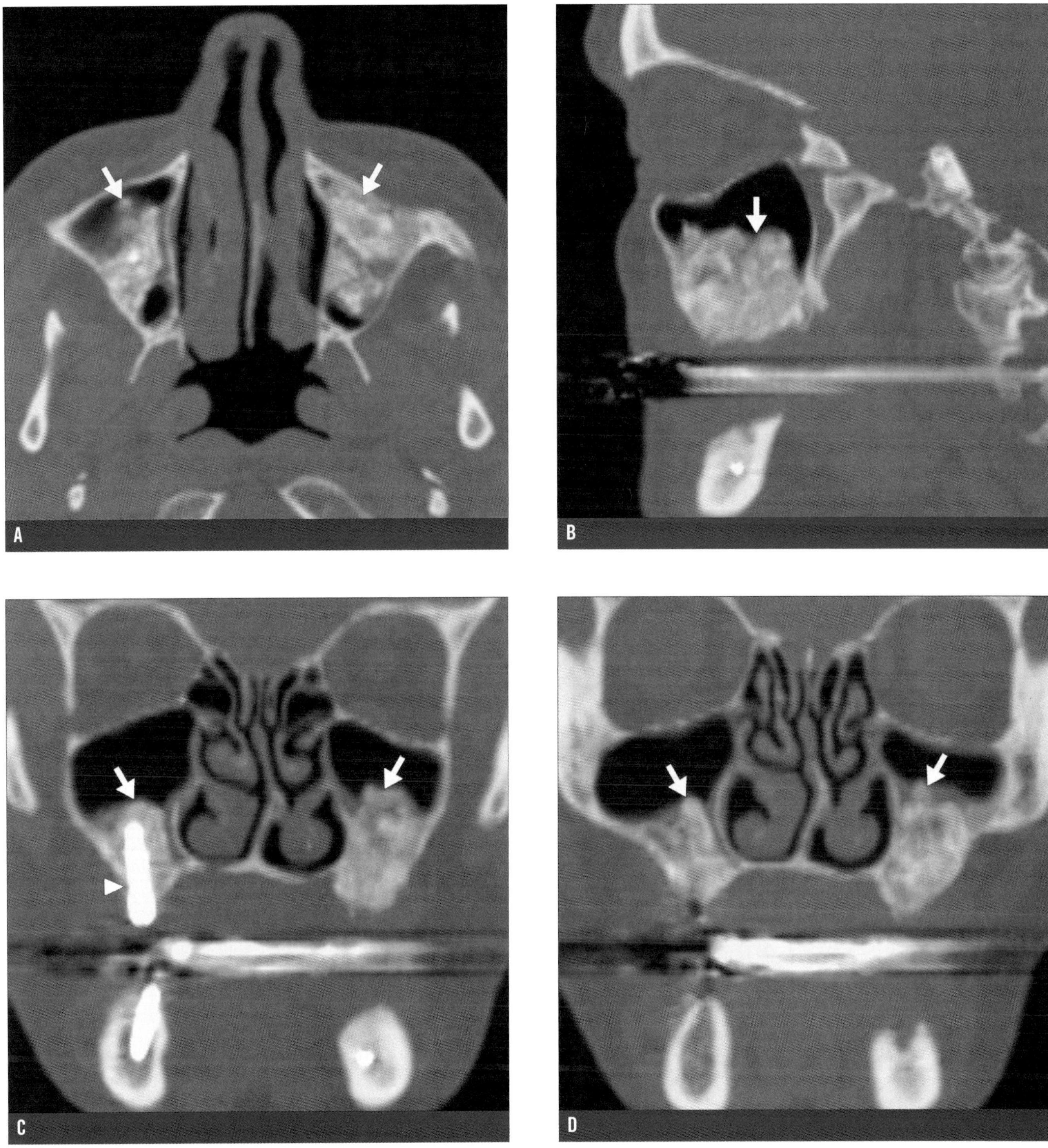

Axial (**A**), sagittal reformatted (**B**), and coronal reformatted (**C, D**) CT images through the maxillary sinuses demonstrate a large amount of bone graft along the floors of the maxillary sinuses (arrows, **A-D**), compatible with large bilateral sinus lifts. A dental implant within the right maxillary sinus lift is present (arrowhead, **C**).

Companion case: Maxillary sinus osteoma

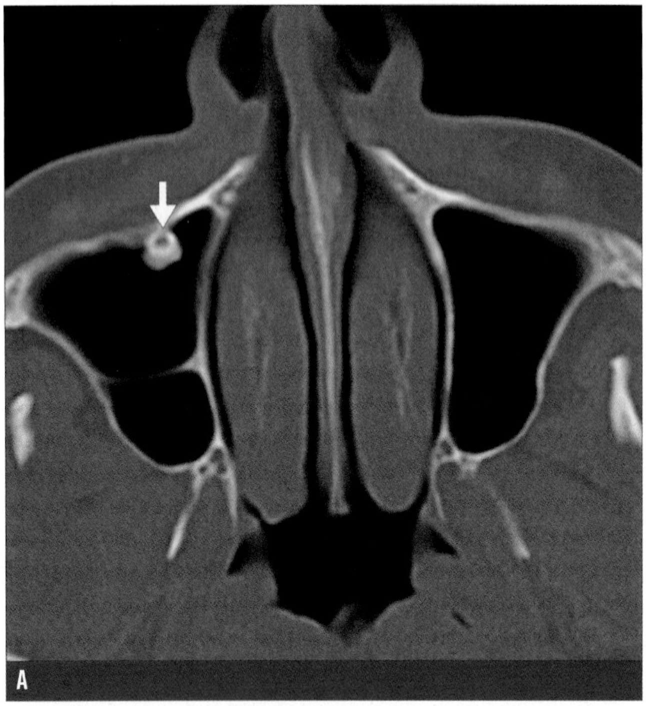

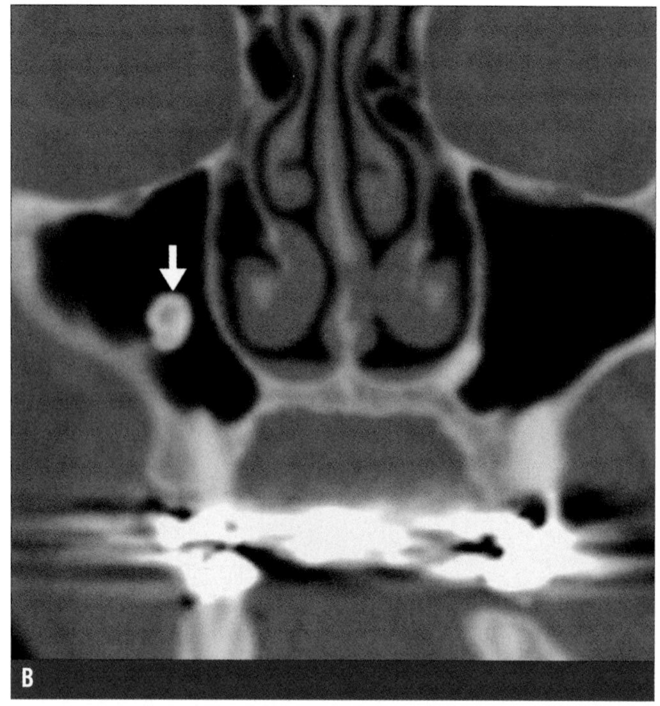

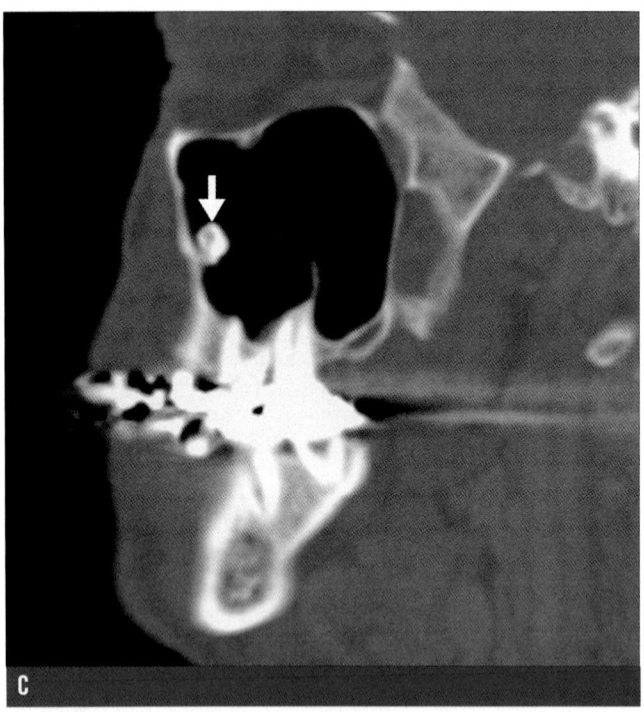

Axial (**A**), coronal reformatted (**B**), and sagittal reformatted (**C**) CT images demonstrate a small pedunculated ossified density arising from the inner table of the right maxillary sinus wall and projecting into the maxillary sinus lumen, compatible with a maxillary sinus osteoma (arrows, **A-C**).

Companion case: Antrolith

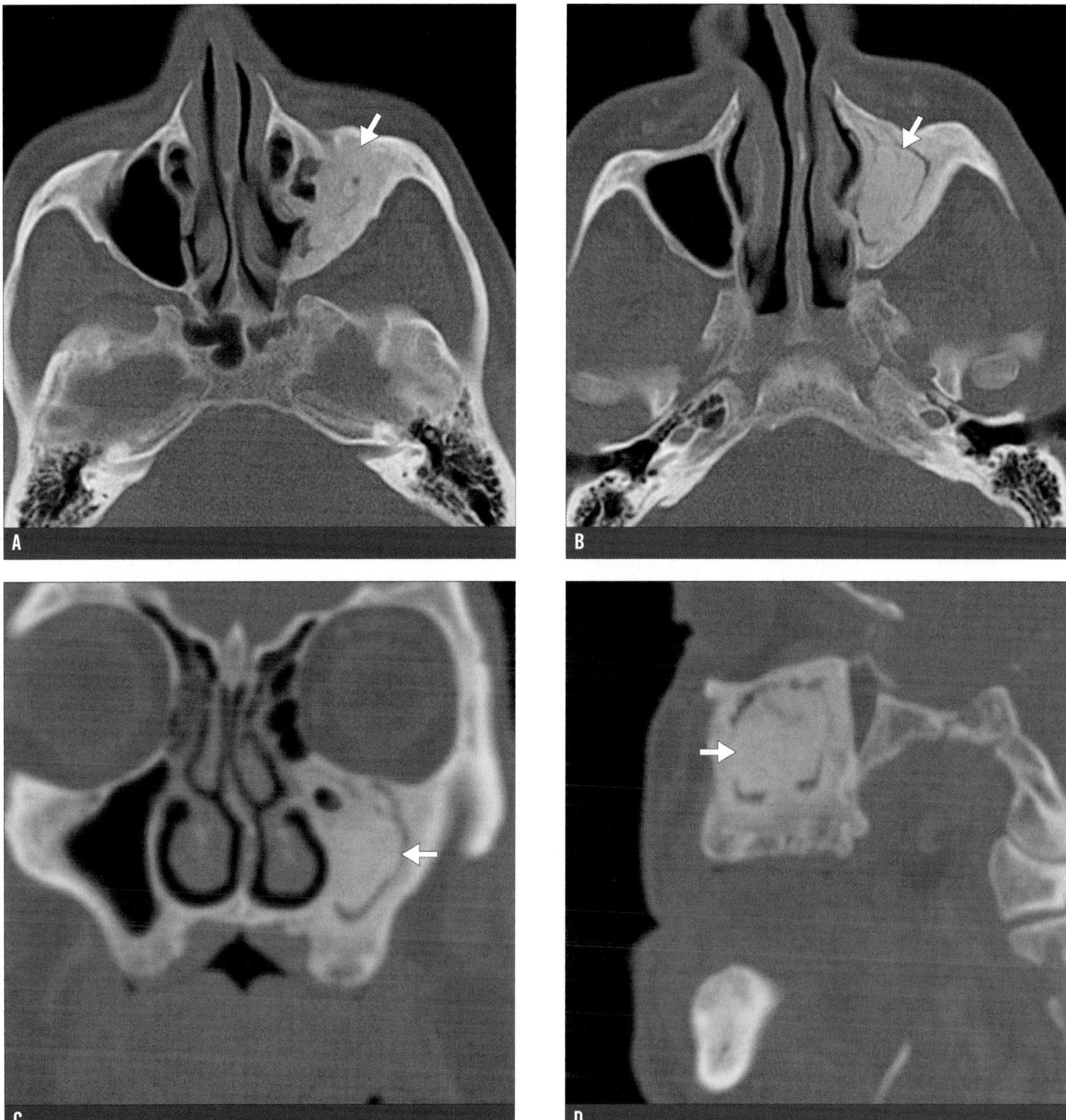

Axial (**A, B**), coronal reformatted (**C**), and sagittal reformatted (**D**) CT images demonstrate a large osseous abnormality subtotally occupying the left maxillary sinus, compatible with a large antrolith (arrows, **A-D**). The antrolith is likely the result of chronic inspissated sinus disease that has mineralized/ossified, supported by the presence of sclerotic left maxillary sinus walls which are often present with chronic maxillary sinus disease.

REFERENCES

Abrahams JJ, et al. Sinus lift procedure of the maxilla in patients with inadequate bone for dental implants: radiographic appearance. *AJR Am J Roentgenol.* 2000;174:1289-1292.

Edmond M, et al. A large atypical osteoma of the maxillary sinus: a report of a case and management challenges. *Eur Arch Otorhinolaryngol.* 2011;268(2):315-318. Epub December 4, 2010.

Gray CF, et al. Magnetic resonance imaging assessment of a sinus lift operation using reoxidised cellulose (Surgicel) as graft material. *Clin Oral Impl Res.* 2001;12:526-530.

Maroldi R, et al. Paranasal sinus imaging. *Eur J Radiol.* 2008;66(3):372-386.

Price HI, et al. CT of benign disease of the paranasal sinus. *Radiographics.* 1983;3(1):107-140.

CASE 27 Variant course of the infraorbital canal

The infraorbital canal typically has a course along the orbital floor. However, variations in its course have been described, including a course through the anterosuperior aspect of the maxillary sinus lumen. Rarely, the infraorbital canal may extend along the lateral wall of the maxillary sinus. Identifying a variant course of the infraorbital canal is important to prevent iatrogenic injury of the infraorbital nerve during sinus surgery, particularly if a Caldwell-Luc approach is utilized. While functional endoscopic sinus surgery has supplanted a Caldwell-Luc approach for treatment of sinus inflammatory disease, a Caldwell-Luc procedure is sometimes utilized for resection of neoplasms, orbital floor repair, and ligation of the internal maxillary artery.

Variant course of the infraorbital canal through the maxillary sinus lumen

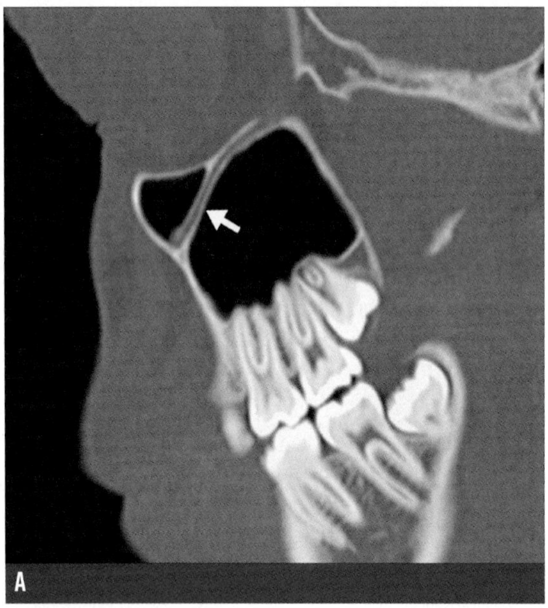

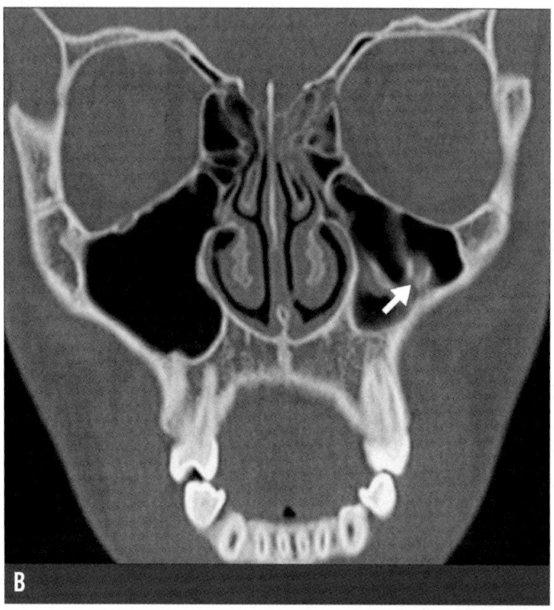

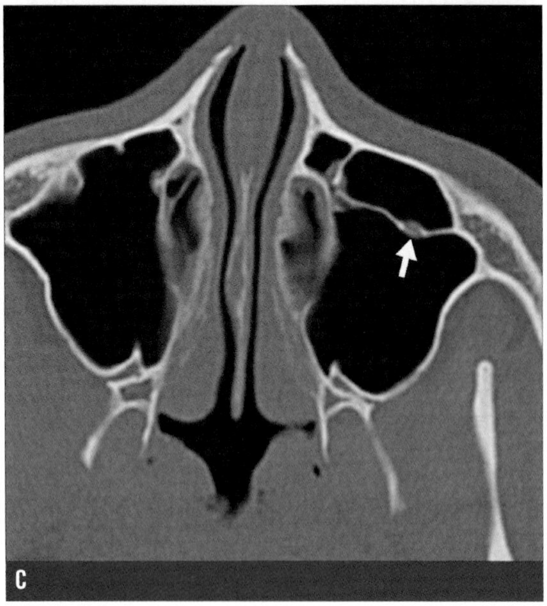

Sagittal (**A**), coronal (**B**), and axial (**C**) CT images demonstrate the left infraorbital canal extending through the anterosuperior aspect of the left maxillary sinus lumen (arrows, **A-C**).

Variant course of the infraorbital canal along the maxillary sinus lateral wall

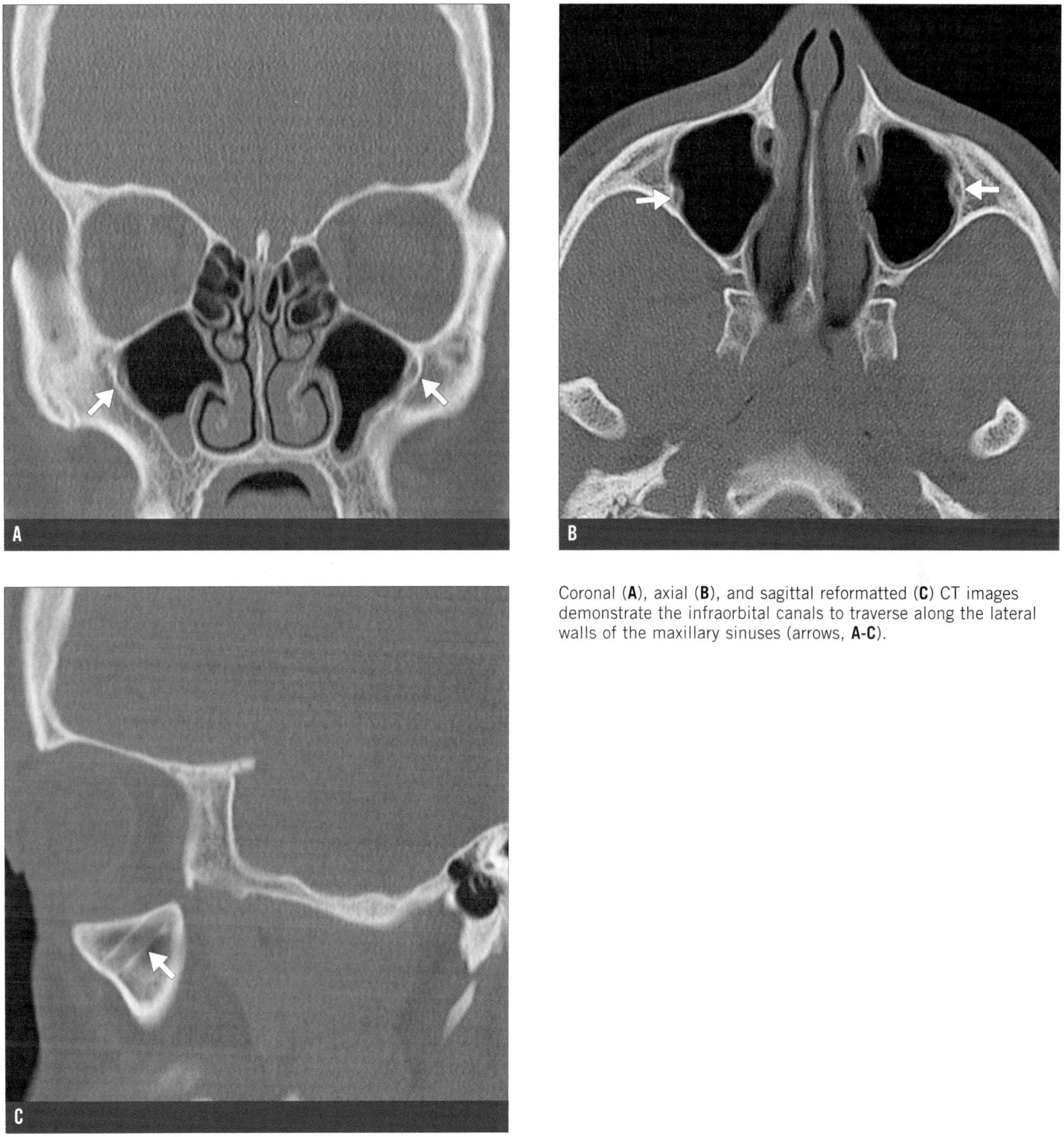

Coronal (**A**), axial (**B**), and sagittal reformatted (**C**) CT images demonstrate the infraorbital canals to traverse along the lateral walls of the maxillary sinuses (arrows, **A-C**).

REFERENCES

Chandra RK, Kennedy DW. Surgical implications of an unusual anomaly of the infraorbital nerve. *Ear Nose Throat J.* 2004:83(11);766-767.

Mailleux P, et al. Ectopic infraorbital nerve in a maxillary sinus septum: another potentially dangerous variant for sinus surgery. *JBR-BTR.* 2010;93(6):308-309.

Whittet HB. Infraorbital nerve dehiscence: the anatomic cause of maxillary sinus "vacuum headache"? *Otolaryngol Head Neck Surg.* 1992;107(1):21-28.

CASE 28 Secondary maxillary sinus ostium

The main drainage pathway for the maxillary sinus is the primary maxillary sinus ostium, which leads directly into the infundibulum and subsequently the middle meatus of the ostiomeatal unit. A secondary maxillary sinus ostium is an accessory air channel located along the medial wall of the maxillary sinus, near its mid aspect. A secondary maxillary sinus ostium serves as an additional drainage pathway between the maxillary sinus and the middle meatus. Other names given to a secondary maxillary ostium include a posterior fontanelle or an accessory maxillary ostium.

A secondary maxillary sinus ostium may simulate a surgical defect, such as a small maxillary antrostomy. Furthermore, a maxillary antrostomy may widen a preexisting secondary maxillary sinus ostium. However, typically, if the medial maxillary wall defect is attributable to surgery, then there is usually evidence of other sinus surgery, such as uncinectomies or ethmoidectomies.

Unilateral secondary maxillary sinus ostium

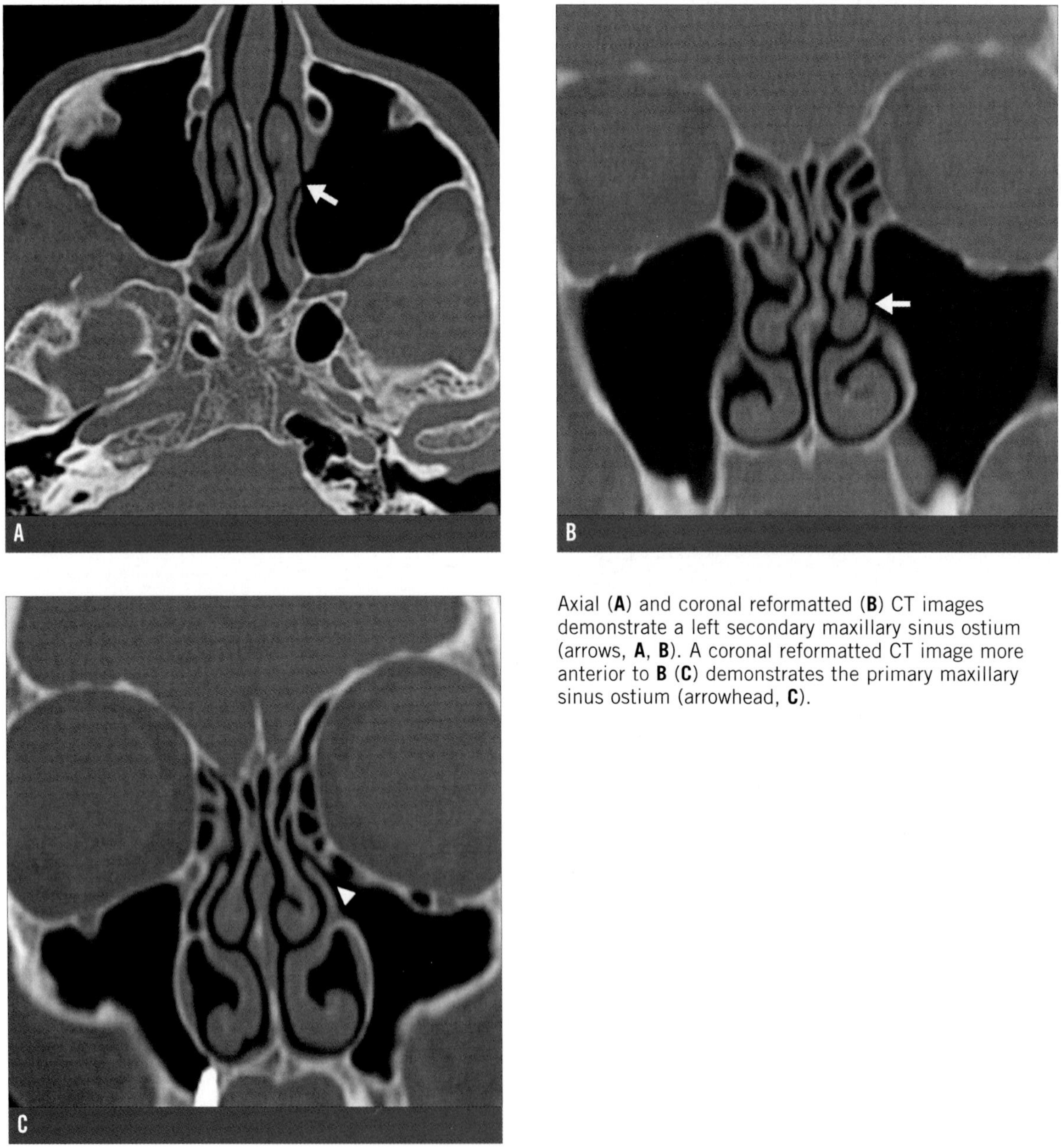

Axial (**A**) and coronal reformatted (**B**) CT images demonstrate a left secondary maxillary sinus ostium (arrows, **A**, **B**). A coronal reformatted CT image more anterior to **B** (**C**) demonstrates the primary maxillary sinus ostium (arrowhead, **C**).

CASE 26 Maxillary sinus lift

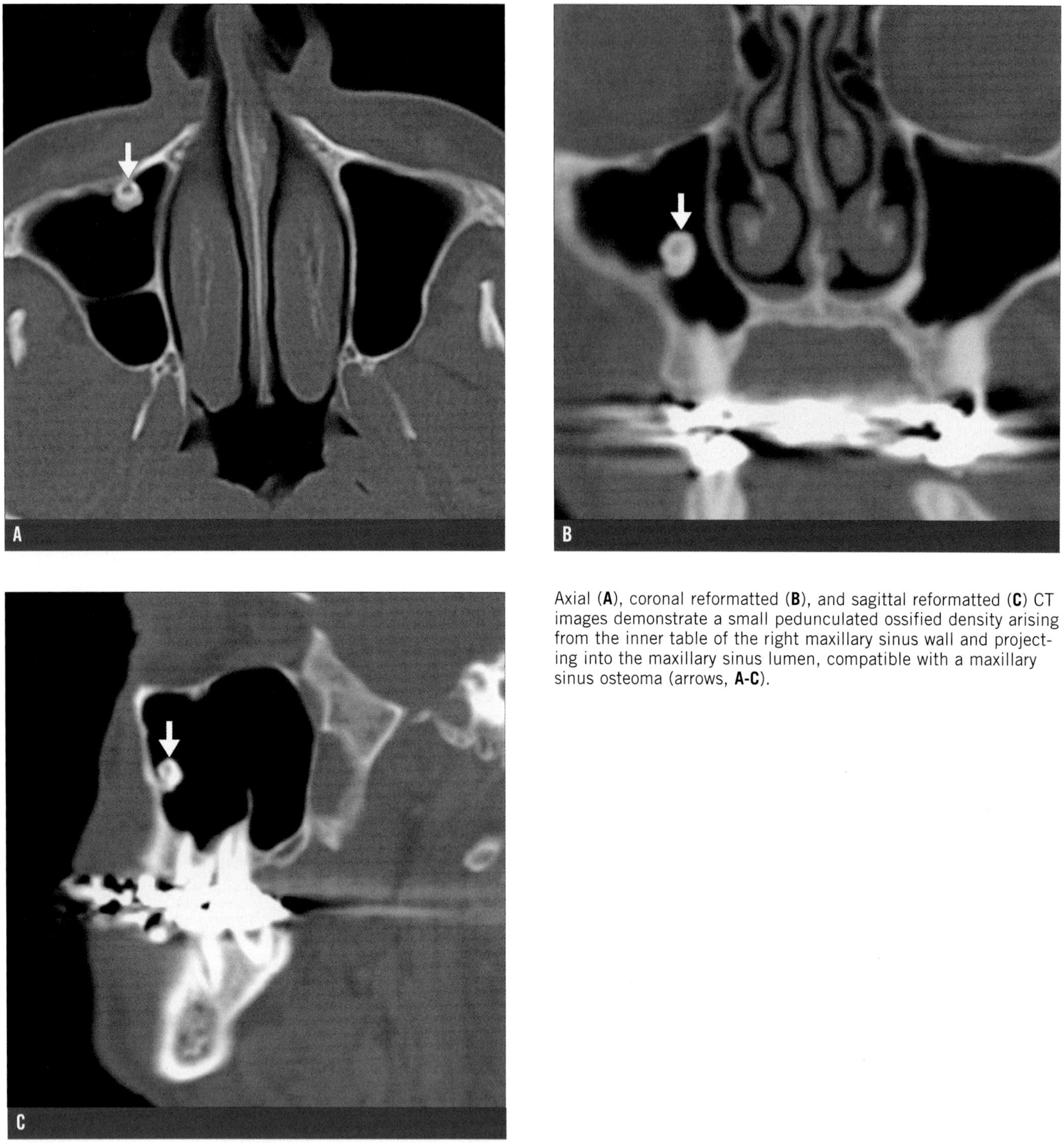

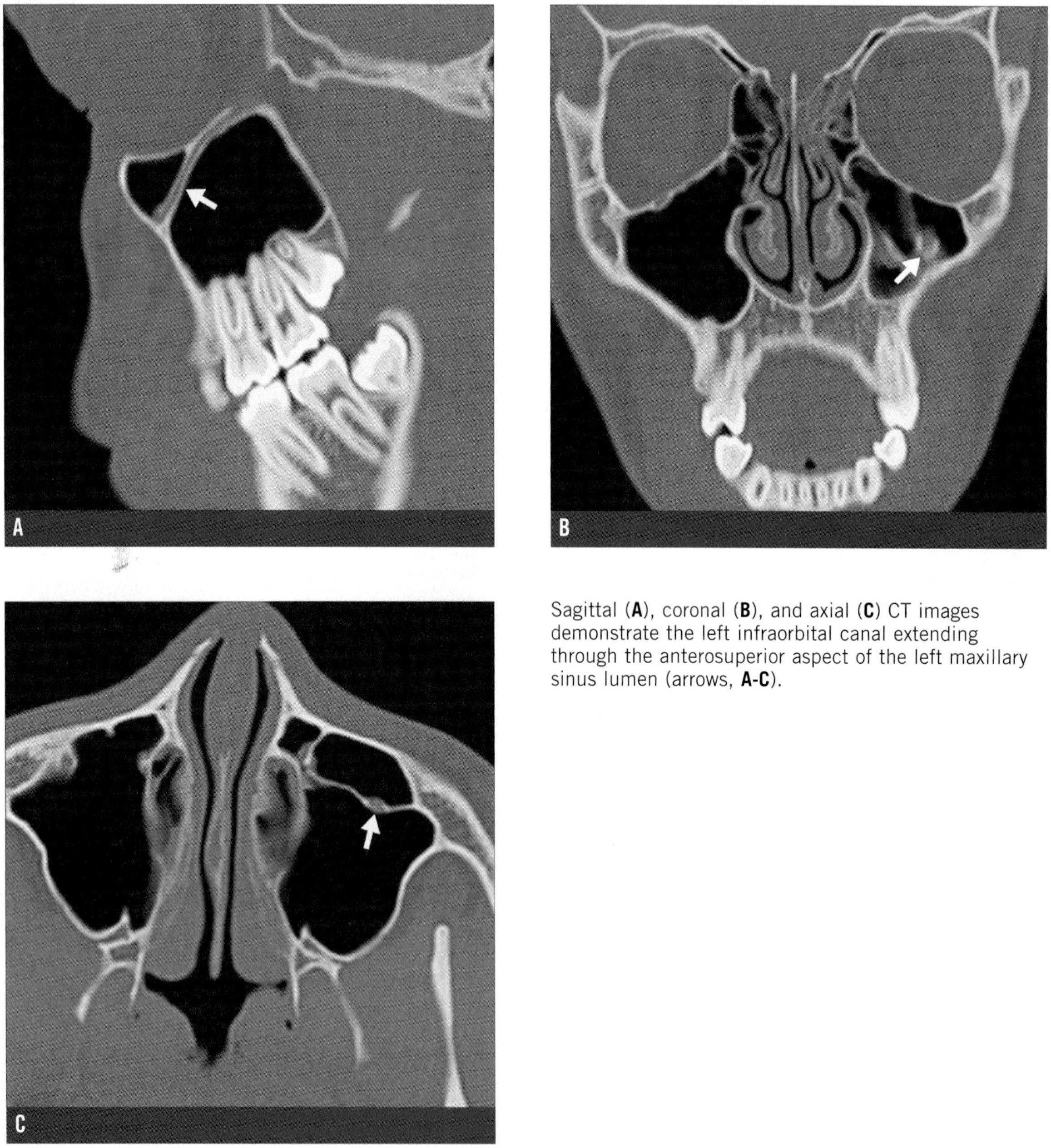

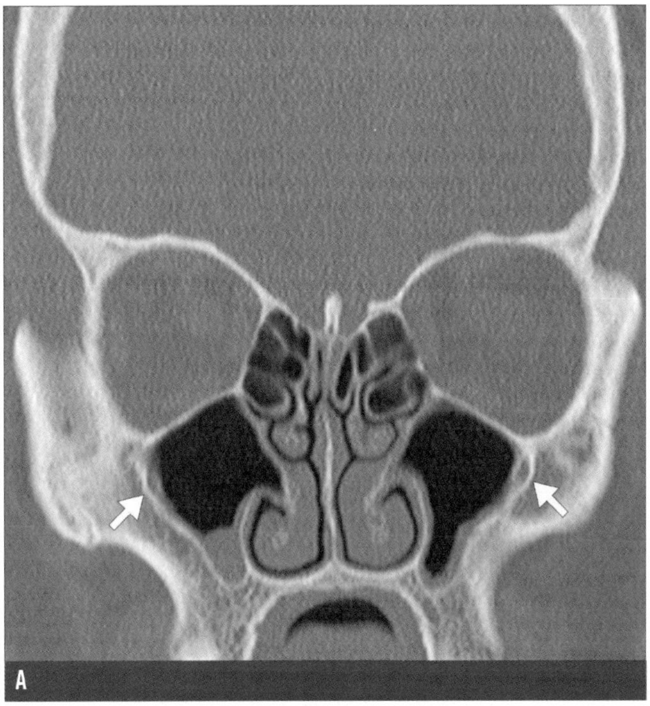

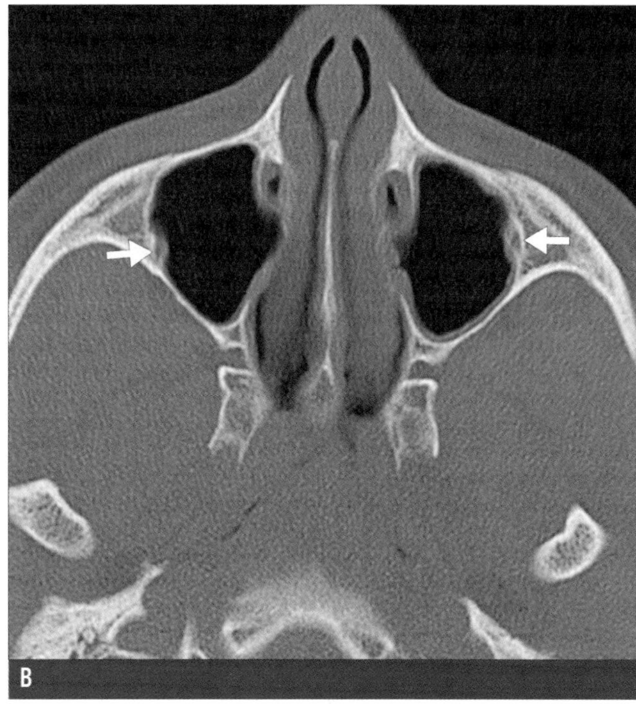

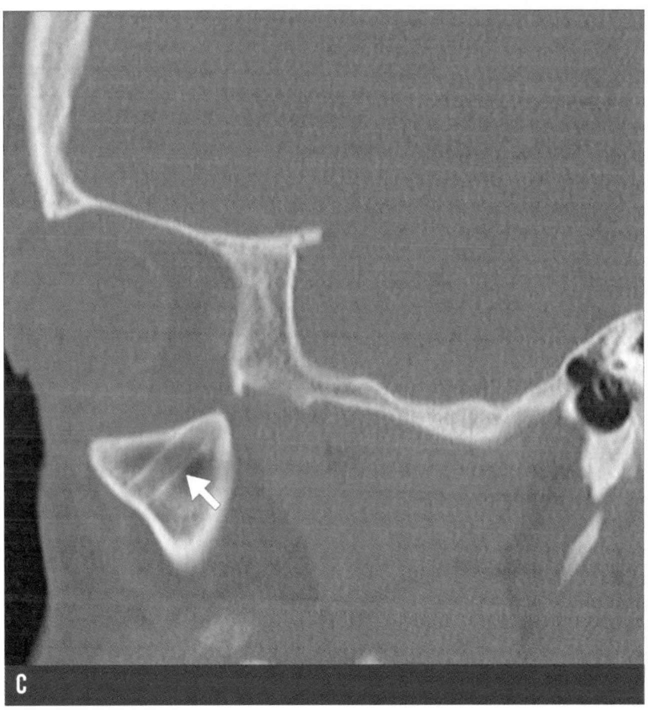

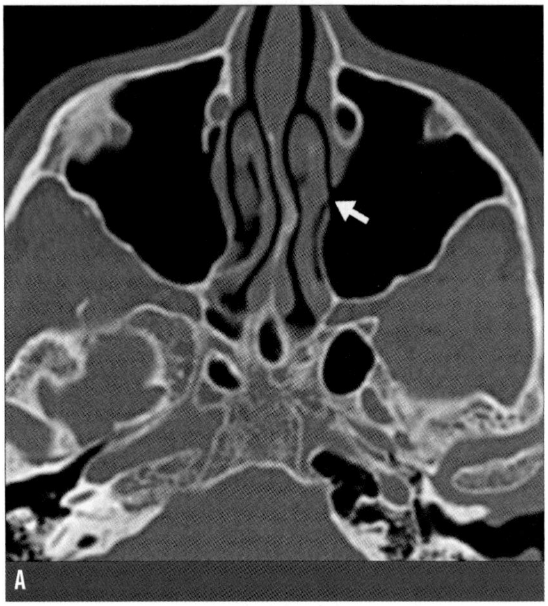

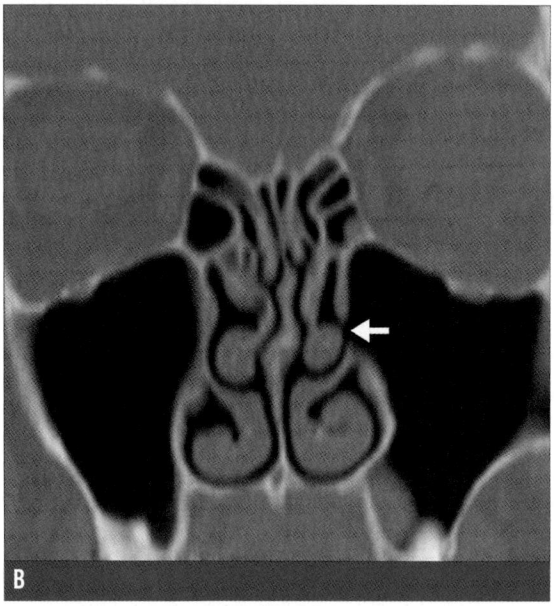

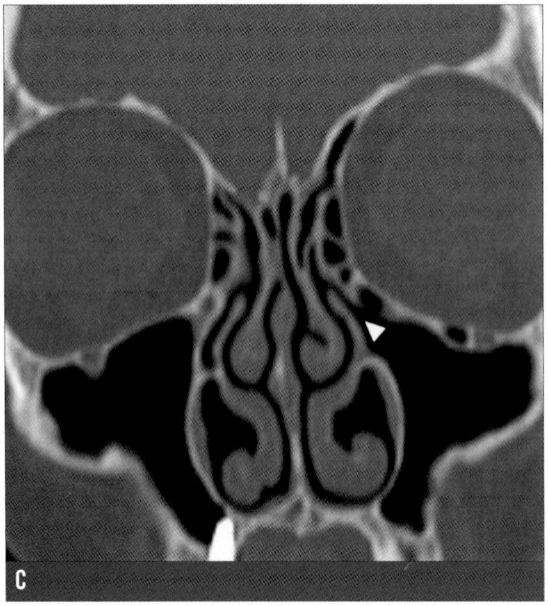

Bilateral secondary maxillary sinus ostia

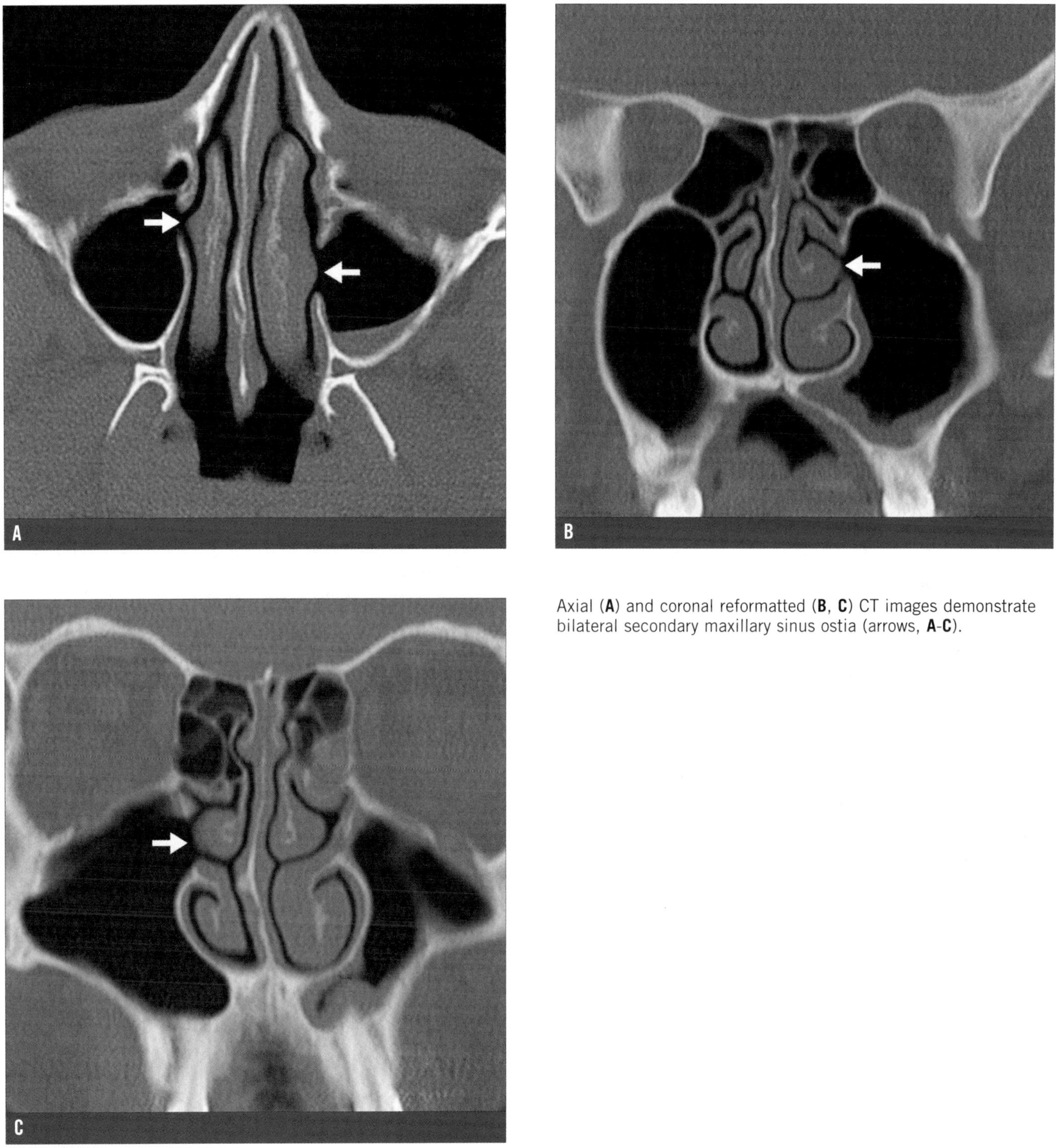

Axial (**A**) and coronal reformatted (**B**, **C**) CT images demonstrate bilateral secondary maxillary sinus ostia (arrows, **A**-**C**).

REFERENCES

Beale TJ, et al. Imaging of the paranasal sinuses and nasal cavity: normal anatomy and clinically relevant anatomical variants. *Semin Ultrasound CT MR*. 2009;30(1):2-16.

Earwaker J. Anatomic variants in sinonasal CT. *Radiographics*. 1993;13(2):381-415.

CASE 29 Maxillary sinus antrostomy

An uncinectomy with formation of a maxillary sinus antrostomy performed during functional endoscopic sinus surgery is the surgical treatment of choice for chronic maxillary sinus disease that is refractory to medical treatment. These sites are surgically targeted because the normal physiological pattern of mucous clearance by the maxillary sinus cilia occurs in a centripetal fashion toward the primary maxillary sinus ostium, which represents the entrance site of the ostiomeatal unit.

During this surgery, an endoscopic septoplasty (if needed) is performed first. This is then followed by an uncinectomy, which forms the antrostomy and allows for surgical enlargement of the primary maxillary sinus ostium.

Maxillary sinus antrostomies

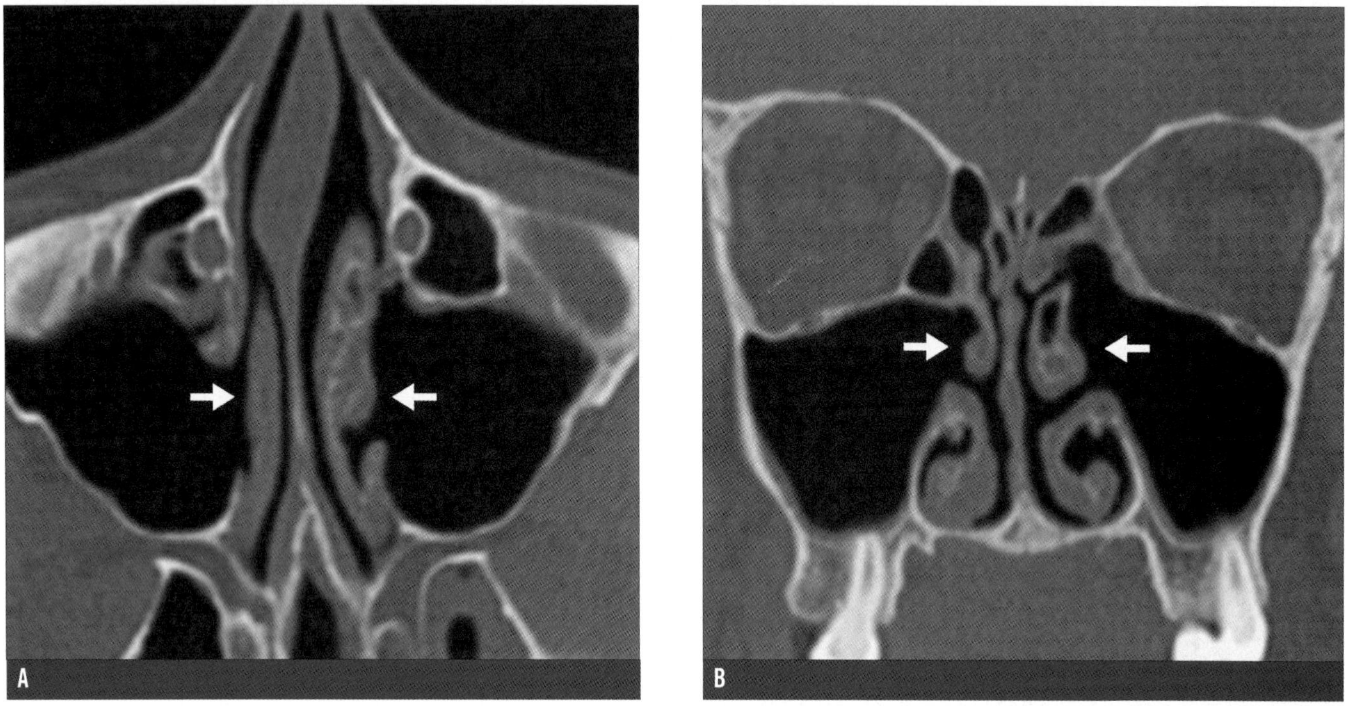

Axial (**A**) and coronal reformatted (**B**) CT images through the maxillary sinuses demonstrate surgical removal of the bilateral uncinate processes with formation of bilateral maxillary sinus antrostomies (arrows, **A, B**).

Maxillary sinus antrostomies

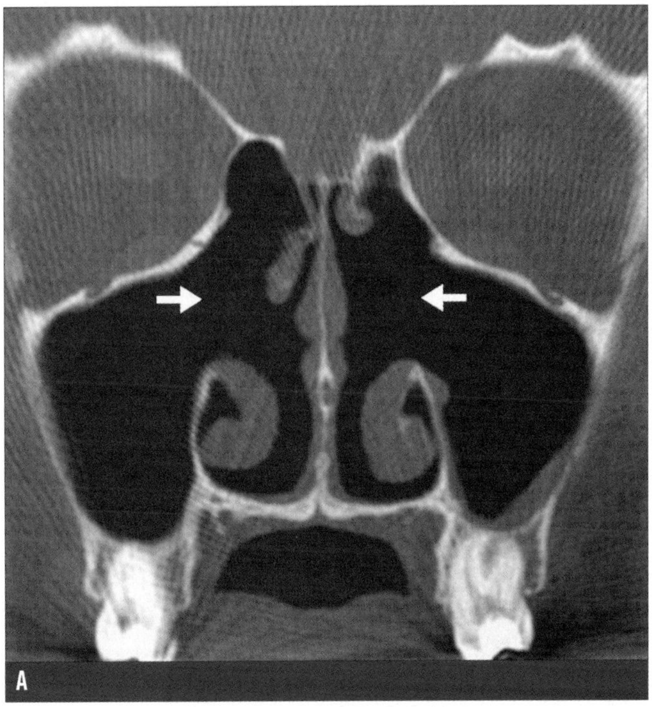

Different patient. A coronal reformatted CT image (**A**) demonstrates large uncinectomies with formation of large bilateral maxillary antrostomies (arrows). Internal ethmoidectomies, a left middle turbinectomy, and a right middle turbinate head reduction have also been performed.

REFERENCE

Luong A, Marple BF. Sinus surgery: indications and techniques. *Clin Rev Allergy Immunol.* 2006;30:217-222.

CASE 30 Caldwell-Luc surgery

Until the mid 1980s, the Caldwell-Luc procedure was the primary surgical procedure for treating maxillary sinus disease that was refractory to medical treatment. Since then, it has been supplanted by functional endoscopic sinus surgery (FESS).

The Caldwell-Luc procedure involves an inferior meatal antrostomy (ie, nasoantral window) and maxillotomy via an incision above the canine fossa. The belief was that inflammatory sinus disease would preferentially exit the inferior meatal antrostomy into the nasal cavity due to gravity. However, this procedure often failed in treating maxillary sinus inflammatory disease. This is because the normal physiologic mucociliary flow is centripetal toward the primary maxillary sinus ostium and infundibulum, rather than gravity dependent.

Currently, the main indication for a Caldwell-Luc procedure is to access tumors that involve, or are adjacent to, the maxillary sinus. Other indications include improved access to allow for ligation of an abnormal internal maxillary artery or for orbital floor repairs.

Caldwell-Luc surgery

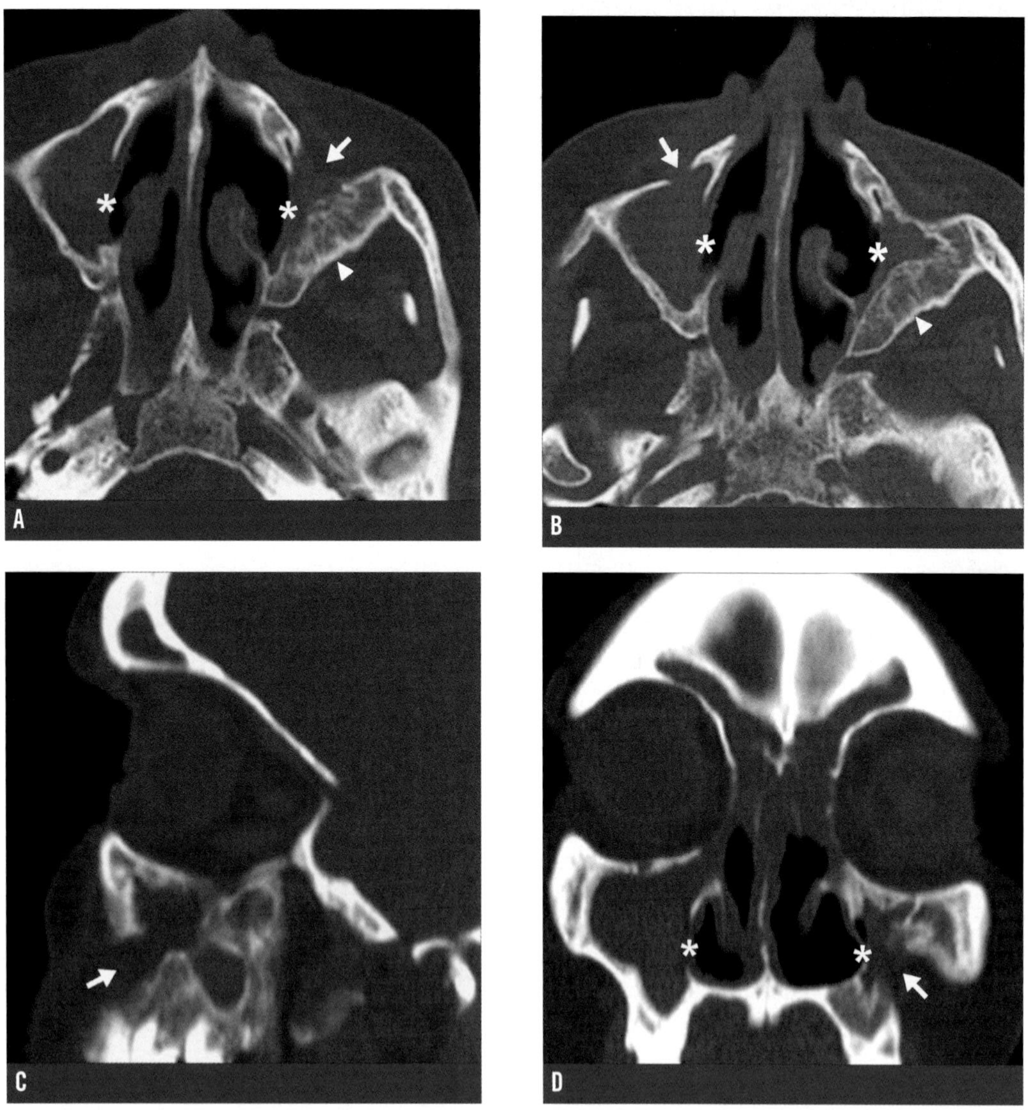

Axial (**A, B**), sagittal reformatted (**C**), and coronal reformatted (**D**) CT images demonstrate typical changes of a bilateral Caldwell-Luc surgery. There are osseous defects involving the anterior walls of the maxillary sinuses representing maxillotomies formed during the Caldwell-Luc surgery (arrows, **A, B**). The left maxillotomy is also shown on images **C** and **D** in the sagittal and coronal planes, respectively (arrows, **C, D**). Nasoantral windows formed during the Caldwell-Luc surgery are present bilaterally (asterisks, **A, B, D**). This is marked chronic hyperostotic bone formation, particularly involving the left maxillary sinus posterolateral wall (arrowheads, **A, B**), a common unintended sequela of this surgery.

REFERENCES

Chandra RK, Kennedy DW. Surgical implications of an unusual anomaly of the infraorbital nerve. *Ear Nose Throat J.* 2004:83(11);766-767.

Kim E, Duncavage JA. Prevention and management of complications in maxillary sinus surgery. *Otolaryngol Clin N Am.* 2010;43:865-873.

Luong A, Marple BF. Sinus surgery: indications and techniques. *Clin Rev Allergy Immunol.* 2006;30:217-222.

Tichenor WS, et al. Nasal and sinus endoscopy for medical management resistant rhinosinusitis, including postsurgical patients. *J Allergy Clin Immun.* 2008;121(4):917-927.

CASE 31 Horizontal orientation of the uncinate process

Several uncinate process variants have been described. These include deviation (such as horizontal orientation), hypertrophy, and pneumatization. While most of these uncinate process variations are incidental, they can result in an anatomic outflow obstruction of the ostiomeatal unit. A horizontal orientation of an uncinate process is often associated with an ipsilaterally enlarged ethmoid bulla.

Horizontal orientation of the uncinate processes

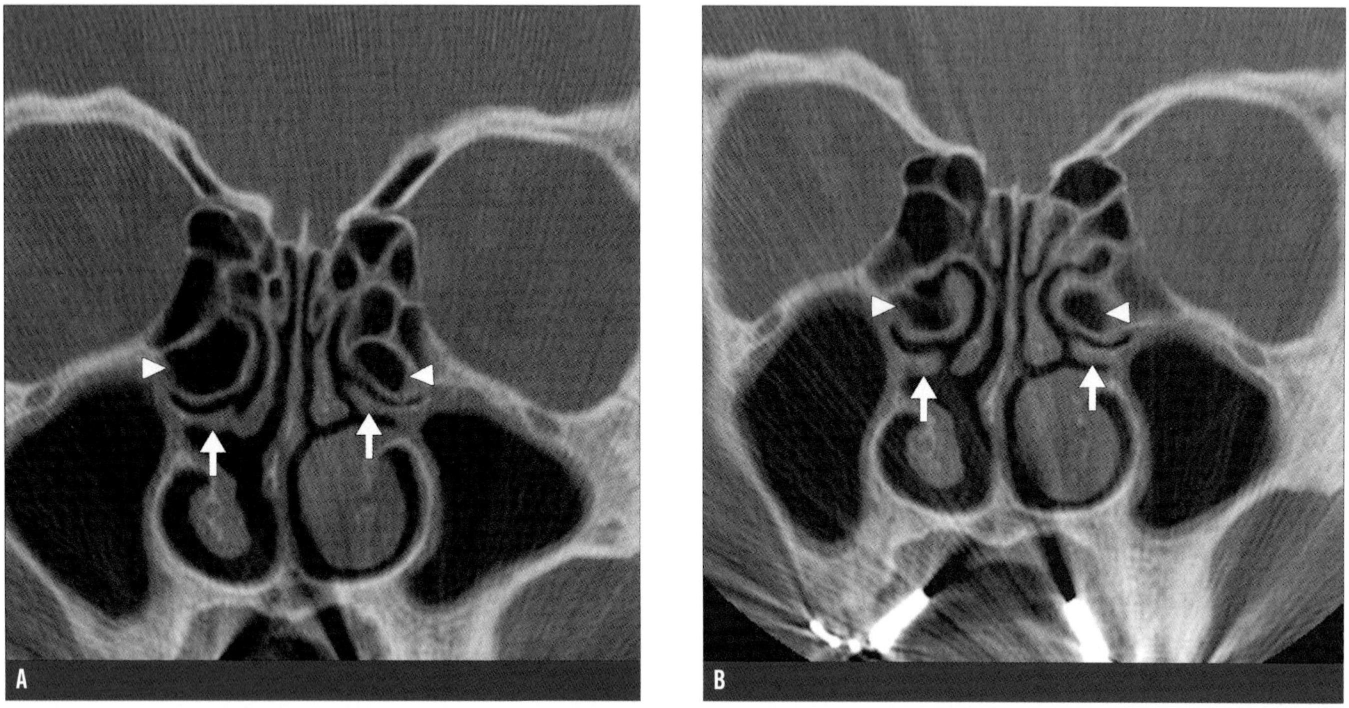

Coronal reformatted CT images (**A, B**) demonstrate horizontally oriented bilateral uncinate processes (arrows, **A, B**). Mildly enlarged ethmoid bullae are also present (arrowheads, **A, B**).

REFERENCES

Beale TJ, et al. Imaging of the paranasal sinuses and nasal cavity: normal anatomy and clinically relevant anatomical variants. *Semin Ultrasound CT MR.* 2009;30(1):2-16.

Earwaker J. Anatomic variants in sinonasal CT. *Radiographics.* 1993;13(2):381-415.

Isobe M, et al. Variations of the uncinate process of the lateral nasal wall with clinical implications. *Clin Anat.* 1998;11:295-303.

Kantarci M, et al. Remarkable anatomic variations in paranasal sinus and their clinical importance. *Eur J Radiol.* 2004;50:296-302.

Miranda CMNR, et al. Anatomical variations of paranasal sinuses at multislice computed tomography: what to look for. *Radiol Bras.* 2011;44(4):256-262.

Perez-Pinas I, et al. Anatomical variations in the human paranasal sinus region studied by CT. *J Anat.* 2000;197:221-227.

CASE 32 Pneumatized uncinate process

Pneumatization of an uncinate process may also be referred to as an uncinate bulla. This is a relatively uncommon variant in which pneumatization extends into the uncinate process, typically from an adjacent agger nasi air cell. If large, a pneumatized uncinate process may contact the middle turbinate neck and result in infundibular narrowing and obstruction of the ostiomeatal complex.

Bilateral pneumatized uncinate processes

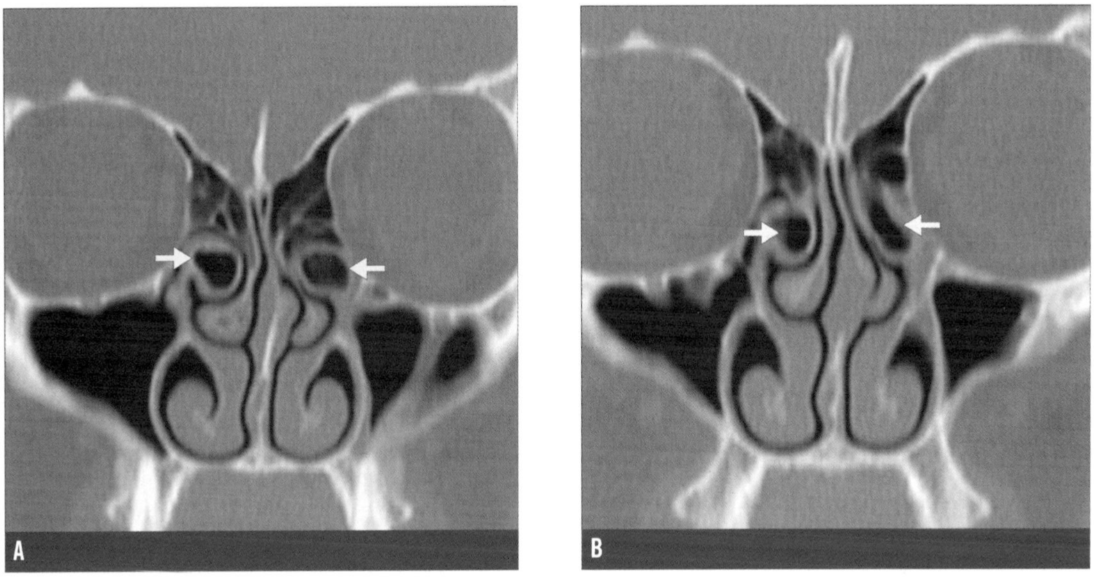

Coronal reformatted CT images (**A, B**) demonstrate pneumatization of the uncinate processes (arrows, **A**, **B**).

Unilateral pneumatized uncinate process

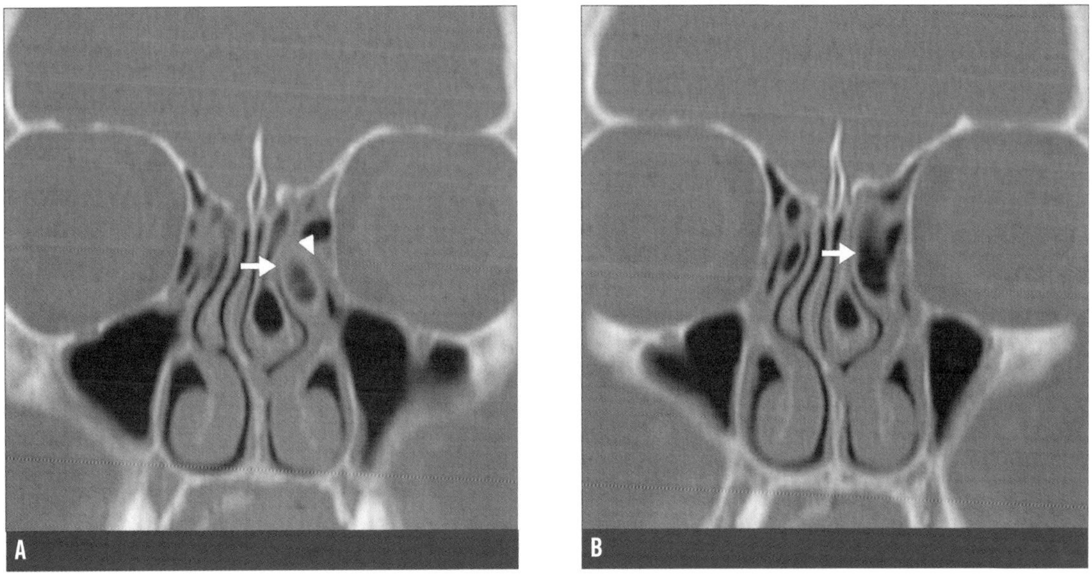

Coronal reformatted CT images (**A-D**). Images **A** and **B** demonstrate a pneumatized left uncinate process (arrow, **A**) that extends ventrally and communicates with a prominent left agger nasi air cell (arrows, **B-D**). The left infundibulum (arrowhead, **A**) is narrowed by the pneumatized left uncinate process. A small right agger nasi air cell that is not associated with a pneumatized uncinate process is also present (arrowhead, **D**).

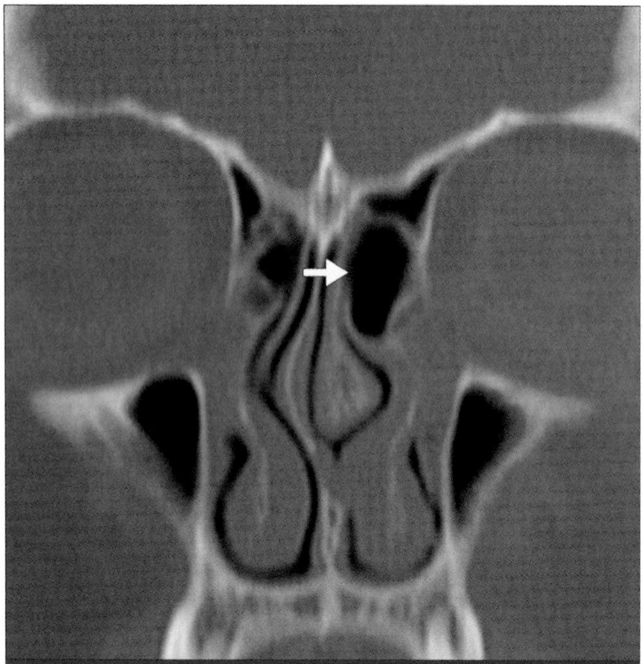

C

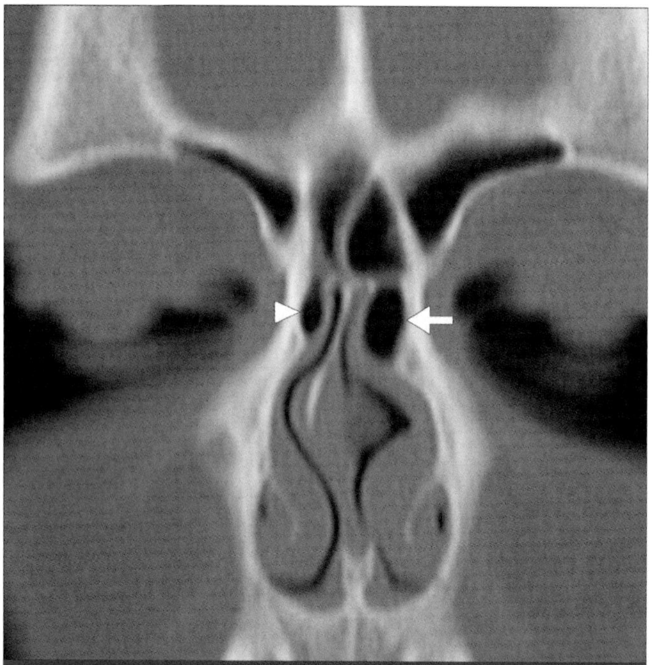

D

REFERENCES

Isobe M, et al. Variations of the uncinate process of the lateral nasal wall with clinical implications. *Clin Anat.* 1998;11:295-303.

Kantarci M, et al. Remarkable anatomic variations in paranasal sinus and their clinical importance. *Eur J Radiol.* 2004;50:296-302.

Kennedy D. *Diseases of the Sinuses: Diagnosis and Management.* Hamilton, ON: BC Decker; 2001.

Miranda CMNR, et al. Anatomical variations of paranasal sinuses at multislice computed tomography: what to look for. *Radiol Bras.* 2011;44(4):256-262.

Perez PI, et al. Anatomical variations in the human paranasal sinus region studied by CT. *J Anat.* 2000;197:221-227.

CASE 33 Recessus terminalis

A recessus terminalis is present when the tip of the uncinate process terminates at the medial wall of the orbit, caudal to the frontal recess ostium. When this variant is present, the frontal sinus drains directly into the middle meatus.

COMPANION CASES

There are two other positions of uncinate process termination that have been described. One is cephalad extension of the uncinate process that attaches to the fovea ethmoidalis, and the other is a medial deviation of the uncinate process that terminates at the lateral wall of the middle turbinate neck. In both of these other uncinate positions, the frontal sinus directly drains into the infundibulum and then the middle meatus.

- ***Companion case*: Uncinate process attachment to the anterior skull base.**
- ***Companion case*: Recessus terminalis and uncinate process attachment to a middle turbinate concha bullosa neck.**

Recessus terminalis

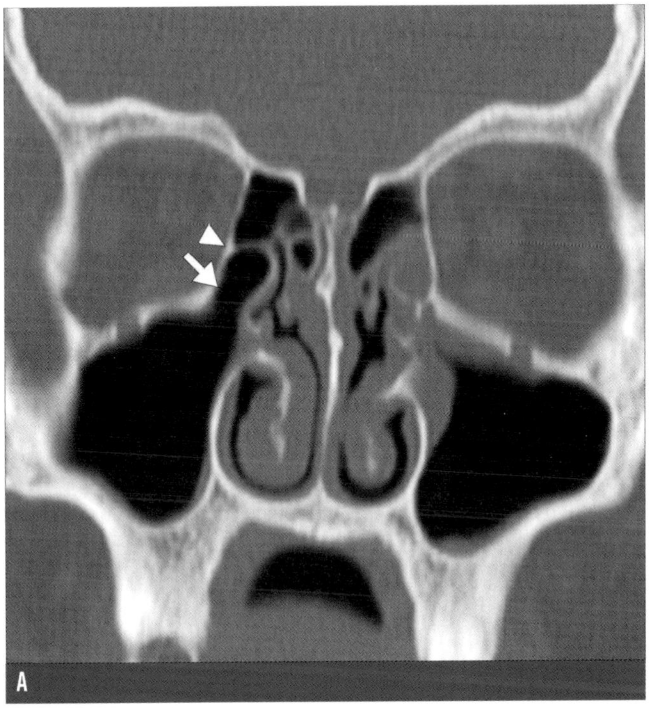

A coronal reformatted CT image (**A**) demonstrates the tip of the right uncinate process to terminate at the right lamina papyracea (arrowhead), forming a right recessus terminalis (arrow).

Companion case: Uncinate process attachment to the anterior skull base

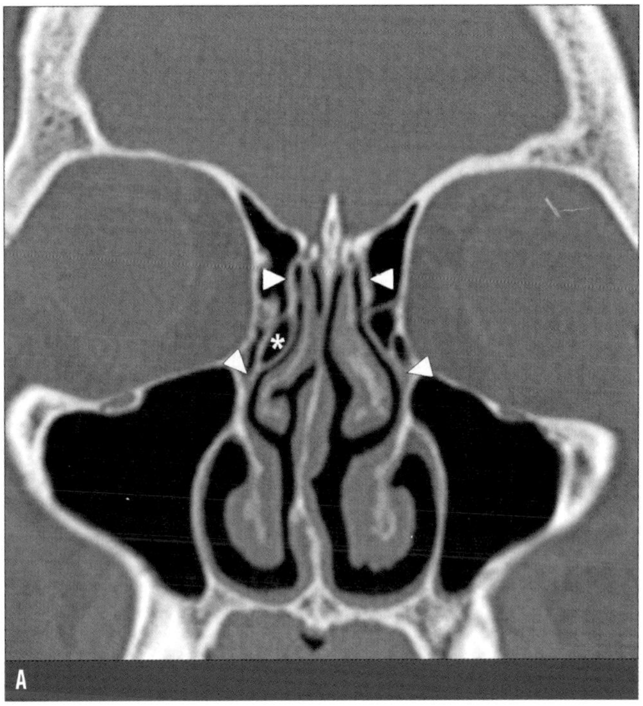

A coronal reformatted CT image (**A**) demonstrates cephalad extension of the uncinate processes (arrowheads) which ultimately attach to the lateral lamellae. In this scenario, the frontal recesses drain into the infundibula (not clearly shown on this image). Incidental note is made of right uncinate process pneumatization, a normal variant (asterisk).

Companion case: Recessus terminalis and uncinate process attachment to a middle turbinate concha bullosa neck

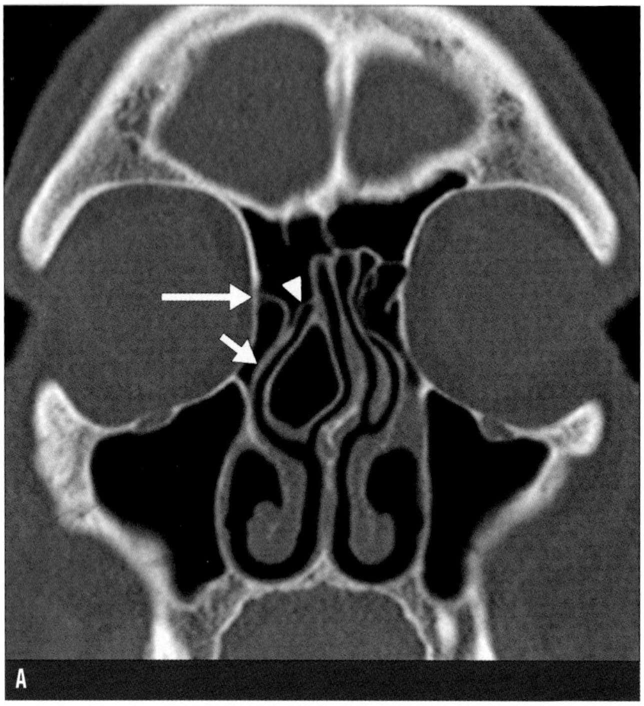

A coronal reformatted CT image (**A**) demonstrates two distal attachment sites of the right uncinate process (short arrow). One attachment site is to the right lamina papyracea, compatible with a recessus terminalis (long arrow). The other attachment site is to the lateral aspect of a right middle turbinate concha bullosa neck (arrowhead). Given the duality of the uncinate process distal attachment sites, the right frontal recess drainage for this patient presumably represents a combination of direct drainage into the right infundibulum and into the right middle meatus.

REFERENCES

Daniels DL, et al. The frontal sinus drainage pathway and related structures. *AJNR Am J Neuroradiol.* 2003;24(8):1618-1627.

Lee WT, Kuhn FA, Citardi MJ. 3D computed tomographic analysis of frontal recess anatomy in patients without frontal sinusitis. *Otolaryngol Head Neck Surg.* 2004;131(3):164-173.

CASE 34 Enlarged ethmoid bulla

An ethmoid bulla is defined as an anterior-inferior ethmoid air cell that is located directly superior and posterior to the infundibulum and hiatus semilunaris.

While most often incidental, an excessively pneumatized ethmoid bulla may encroach upon the ostiomeatal unit and result in an anatomic outflow obstruction.

Enlarged ethmoid bullae

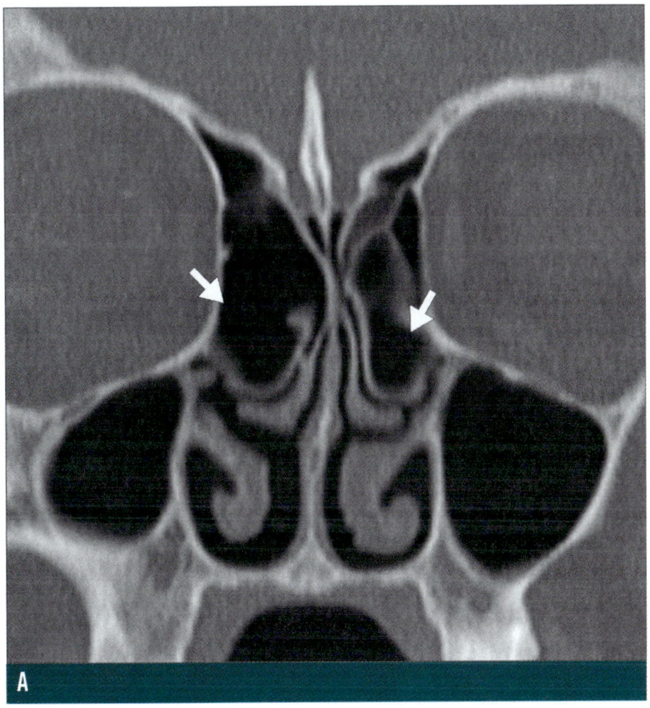

A coronal reformatted CT image through the ethmoid air cells (**A**) demonstrates enlarged ethmoid bullae, right larger than left (arrows).

REFERENCES

Kennedy DW, et al. *Diseases of the Sinuses: Diagnosis and Management.* Part 611. Hamilton, ON: BC Decker; 2001.

Perez PI, et al. Anatomical variations in the human paranasal sinus region studied by CT. *J Anat.* 2000;197:221-227.

CASE 35 Superior concha bullosa

The term concha bullosa literally translates to an "air-filled turbinate." A pneumatized superior nasal turbinate is therefore termed a superior concha bullosa. However, the term superior concha bullosa should be reserved for pneumatization that involves the head of the superior turbinate, which is often enlarged in this setting, rather than when the pneumatization solely involves the neck of the superior turbinate. A superior concha bullosa is most often an incidental finding. However, as with any unusual or excessive air cell pneumatization, a large concha bullosa could result in an obstruction of an adjacent outflow tract. In the case of a large superior concha bullosa, the superior meatus can be obstructed.

Bilateral superior conchae bullosa

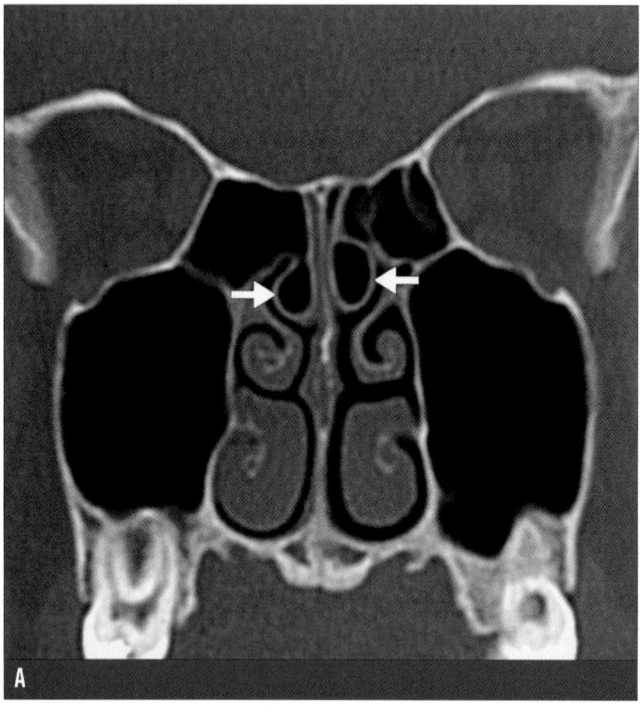

A coronal reformatted CT image (**A**) demonstrates pneumatization of the bilateral superior turbinate heads, compatible with superior conchae bullosa (arrows).

REFERENCES

Kantarci M, et al. Remarkable anatomic variations in paranasal sinus region and their clinical importance. *Eur J Radiol.* 2004;50:296-302.

Sarna A, et al. Coronal imaging of the osteomeatal unit: anatomy of 24 variants. *J Comp Assist Tomogr.* 2002;26(1):153-157.

CASE 36 Middle concha bullosa

A pneumatized middle turbinate head is termed a middle concha bullosa. If pneumatization is isolated to the middle turbinate neck, then it is more appropriately referred to as a "lamellar concha" or "interlamellar cell of Grünwald." If large enough, a middle concha bullosa may result in an anatomic obstruction of the ostiomeatal unit, most commonly of the middle meatus. There is a strong association between a middle concha bullosa and contralateral deviation of the nasal septum. The associated nasal septal deviation is likely the result of a developmental phenomenon and not related to mass effect from the concha bullosa.

Middle concha bullosa

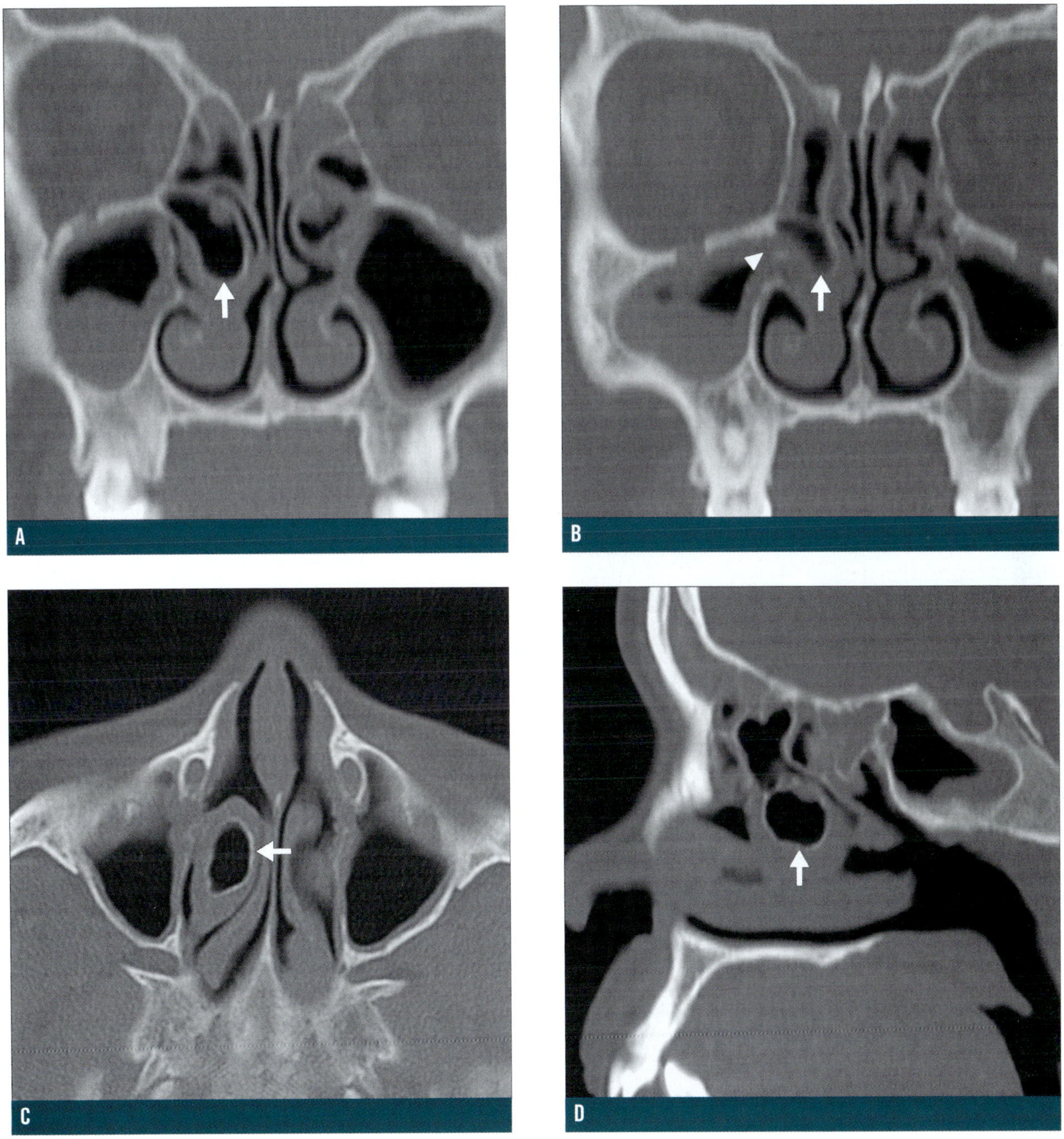

Coronal reformatted CT images (**A, B**) demonstrate a large right middle concha bullosa (arrows, **A**, **B**). The right middle concha bullosa is associated with compromise of the right ostiomeatal unit infundibulum (arrowhead, **B**). Axial (**C**) and sagittal reformatted (**D**) CT images demonstrate the same concha bullosa in different planes (arrows, **C**, **D**).

Middle concha bullosa

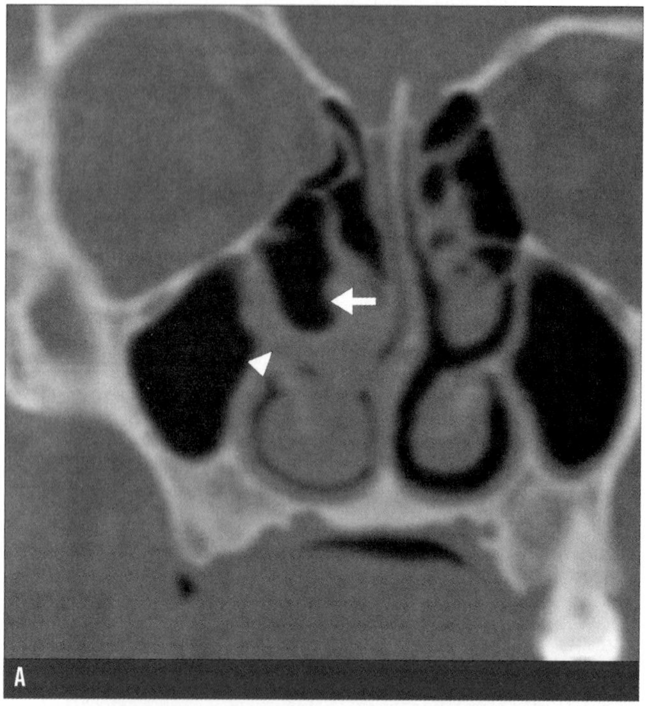

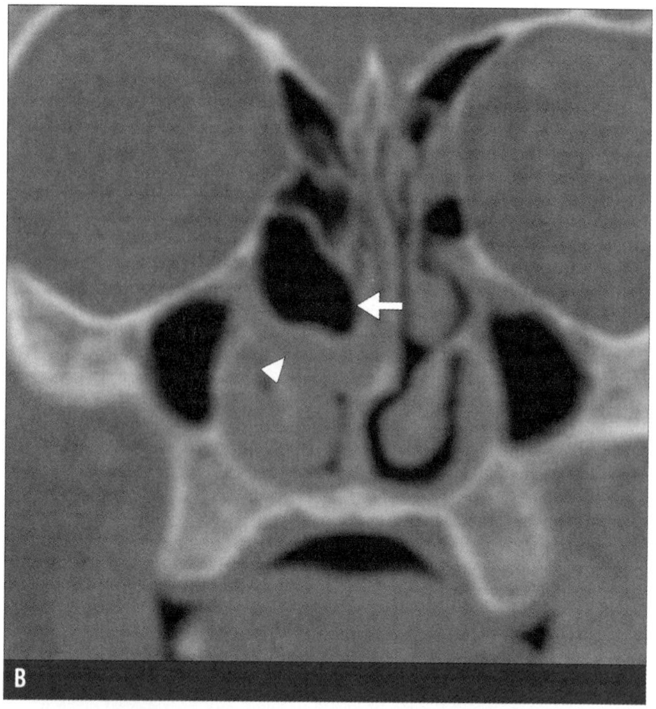

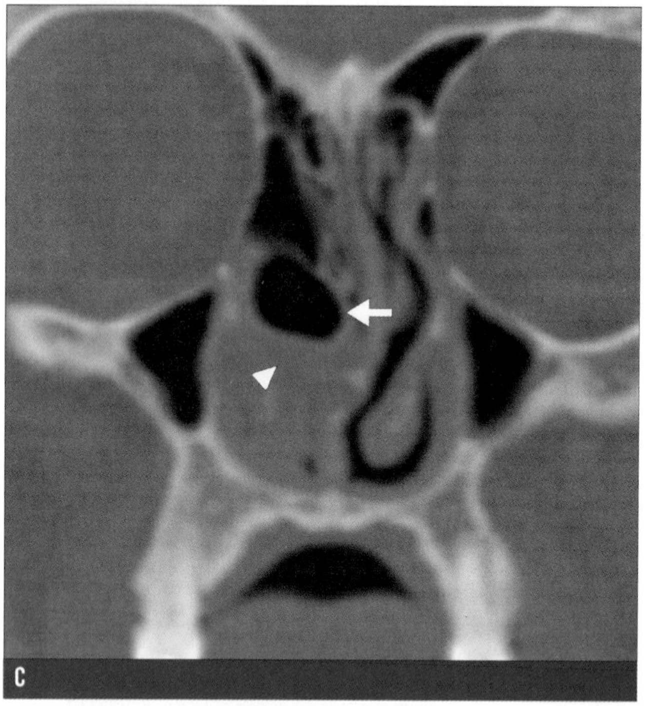

Different patient. Coronal reformatted CT images (**A-C**) demonstrate a large right middle concha bullosa (arrows, **A-C**). The right middle concha bullosa is associated with compromise of the right ostiomeatal complex middle meatus (arrowheads, **A-C**).

Middle concha bullosa

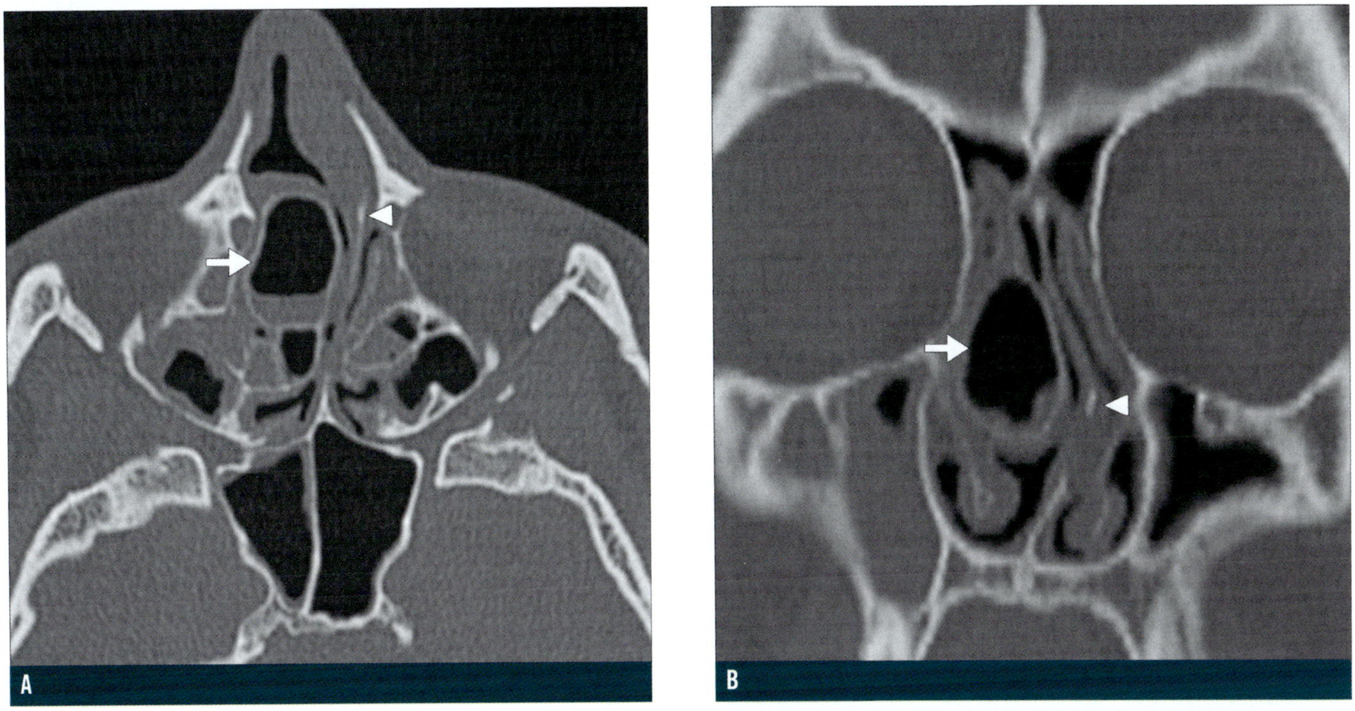

Different patient. Axial (**A**) and coronal reformatted (**B**) CT images demonstrate a large right middle concha bullosa (arrows, **A, B**) which contains mucosal thickening and possibly fluid. There is a moderate to severe associated leftward nasal septal deviation (arrowheads, **A, B**). A contralateral nasal septal deviation is often present in conjunction with a large middle concha bullosa.

REFERENCES

Kantarci M, et al. Remarkable anatomic variations in paranasal sinus and their clinical importance. *Eur J Radiol.* 2004;50:296-302.

Perez PI, et al. Anatomical variations in the human paranasal sinus region studied by CT. *J Anat.* 2000;197:221-227.

Sarna A, et al. Coronal imaging of the osteomeatal unit: anatomy of 24 variants. *J Comp Assist Tomogr.* 2002;26(1):153-157.

Stallman JS, Lobo JN, Som PM. The incidence of concha bullosa and its relationship to nasal septal deviation and paranasal sinus disease. *AJNR Am J Neuroradiol.* 2004:25(9);1613-1618.

CASE 37 Paradoxical middle nasal turbinate

A nasal turbinate is considered paradoxical if there is reversal of the curvature at the junction of the turbinate head and neck, from its typical medial convexity to a lateral convexity. The head of a paradoxical nasal turbinate is thus directed medially. A paradoxical curvature may be partial or complete. A paradoxical configuration is most often associated with a middle nasal turbinate, but it may involve any nasal turbinate. It is typically an incidental finding; however, rarely, a paradoxical nasal turbinate can result in compromise of its ipsilateral meatus.

Paradoxical middle nasal turbinate

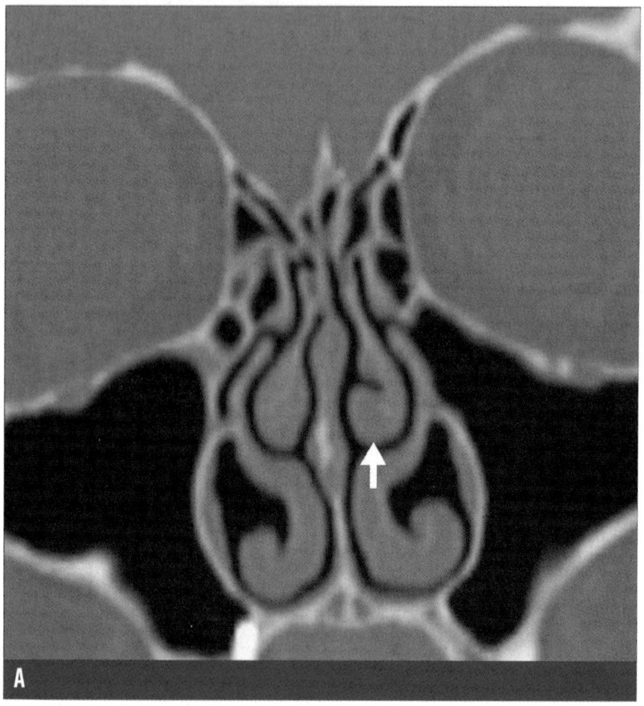

A coronal CT image through the nasal cavity and maxillary sinuses (**A**) demonstrates a paradoxical left middle nasal turbinate (arrow). The head of the left middle nasal turbinate is directed medially, rather than its typical lateral direction, as is present with both inferior nasal turbinates.

REFERENCES

Beale TJ, et al. Imaging of the paranasal sinuses and nasal cavity: normal anatomy and clinically relevant anatomical variants. *Semin Ultrasound CT MR.* 2009;30(1):2-16.

Ozcan KM, et al. Anatomical variations of nasal turbinates. *J Craniofac Surg.* 2008;19(6):1678-1682.

Perez-Pinas I, et al. Anatomical variations in the human paranasal sinus region studied by CT. *J Anat.* 2000;197:221-227.

Sarna A, et al. Coronal imaging of the osteomeatal unit: anatomy of 24 variants. *J Comp Assist Tomogr.* 2002;26(1):153-157.

CASE 38 Secondary middle nasal turbinate

A secondary middle nasal turbinate represents a fully duplicated middle turbinate with its own turbinate neck. It is defined as an osseous projection that is covered by mucosa and may arise from several locations, inlcuding the lateral wall of the middle meatus, lateral wall of the ethmoid bulla, or from the wall of the lamina papyracea. If a secondary middle nasal turbinate arises from the wall of the lamina papyracea, then resection of a secondary nasal turbinate can result in an inadvertent fracture of the lamina papyracea. This entity is not typically associated with obstruction of the ostiomeatal complex.

COMPANION CASE

- **Accessory middle nasal turbinate.** An accessory middle nasal turbinate is formed directly from a medially curved uncinate process, simulating a secondary middle nasal turbinate. However, this entity differs from a secondary middle nasal turbinate because it represents an extension of the uncinate process, rather than a fully duplicated nasal turbinate.
- **Bifid middle nasal tubinates.** When the middle nasal turbinate head is partially divided into two portions, it is termed a bifid middle nasal turbinate. A bifid middle nasal turbinate is usually of no clinical significance.

Secondary middle nasal turbinate

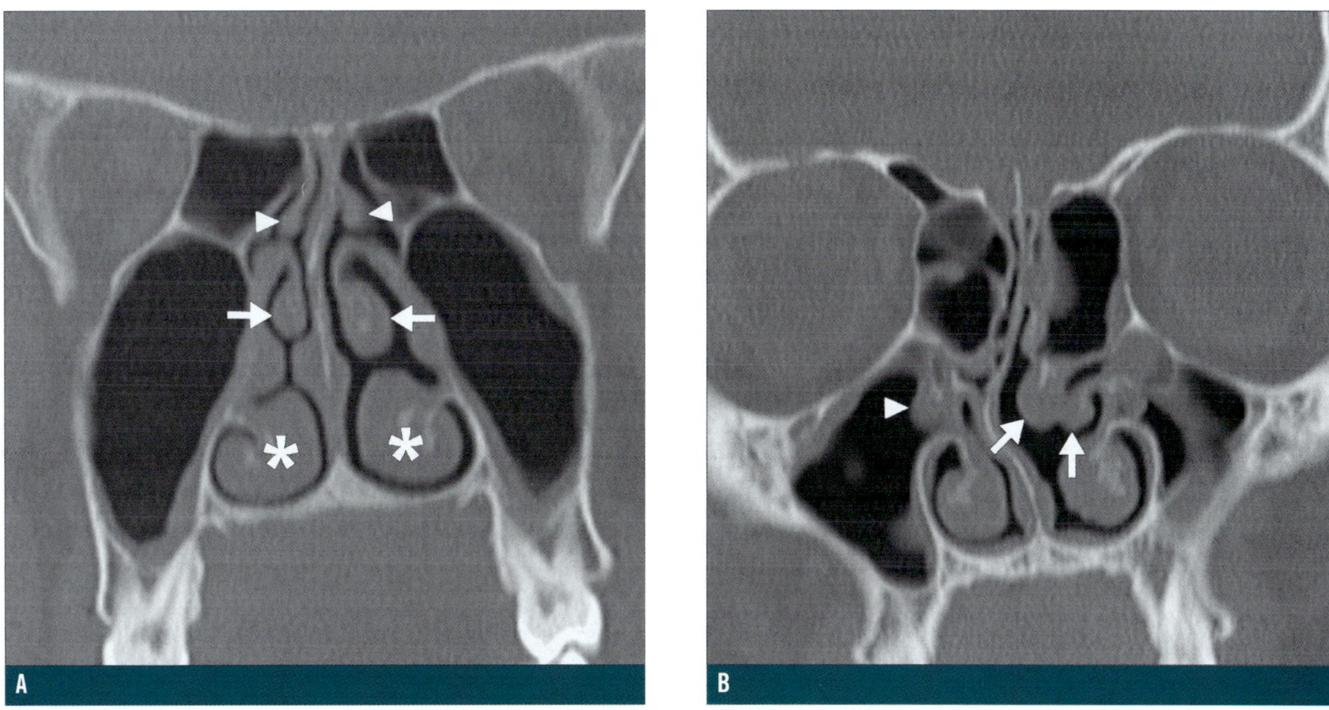

Coronal reformatted CT images obtained at the mid to posterior aspect of the nasal cavity (**A**) and the mid to anterior aspect of the nasal cavity (**B**). Image **A** demonstrates normal paired superior nasal turbinates (arrowheads), middle nasal turbinates (arrows), and inferior nasal turbinates (asterisks). Image **B** demonstrates two left secondary middle nasal turbinates (arrows) and one right secondary middle nasal turbinate (arrowhead). These do not represent polyps as there is evidence of a cartilaginous superstructure within the tissue, compatible with normal conchal cartilage. An axial image (**C**) demonstrates the two left secondary middle nasal turbinates in the axial plane (arrows).

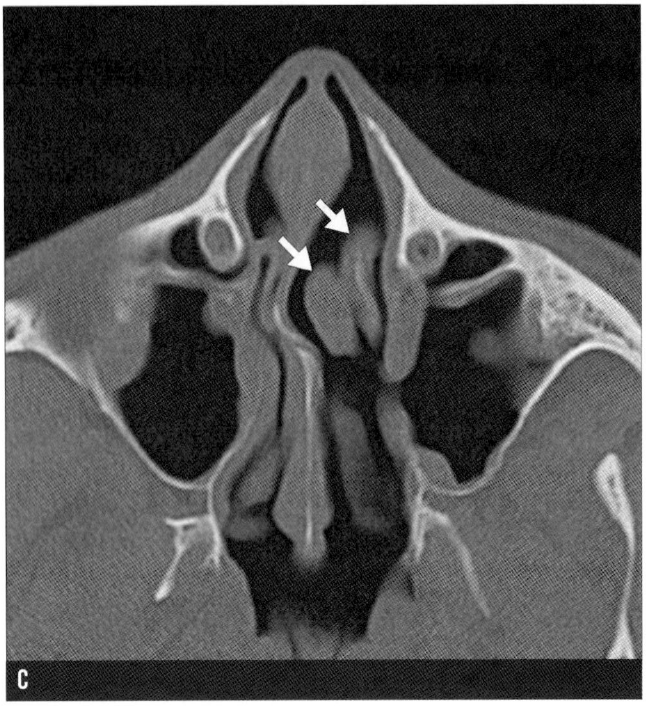

Companion case: Accessory middle nasal turbinate

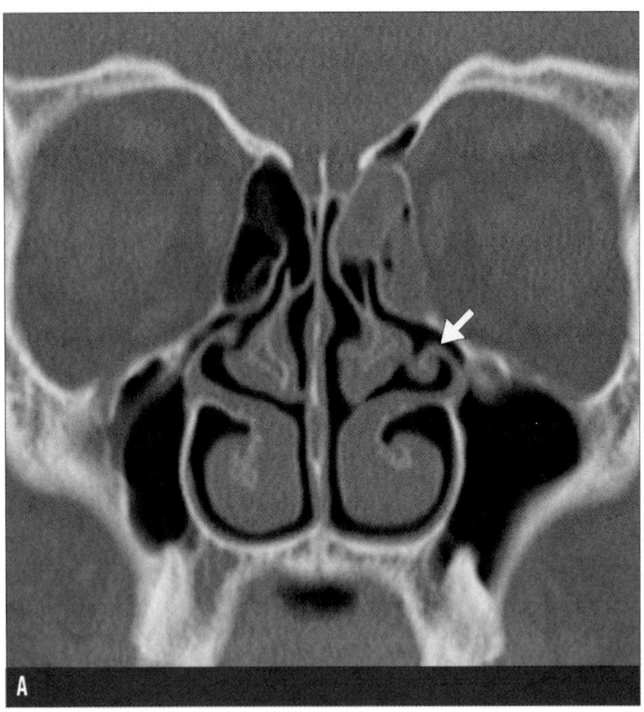

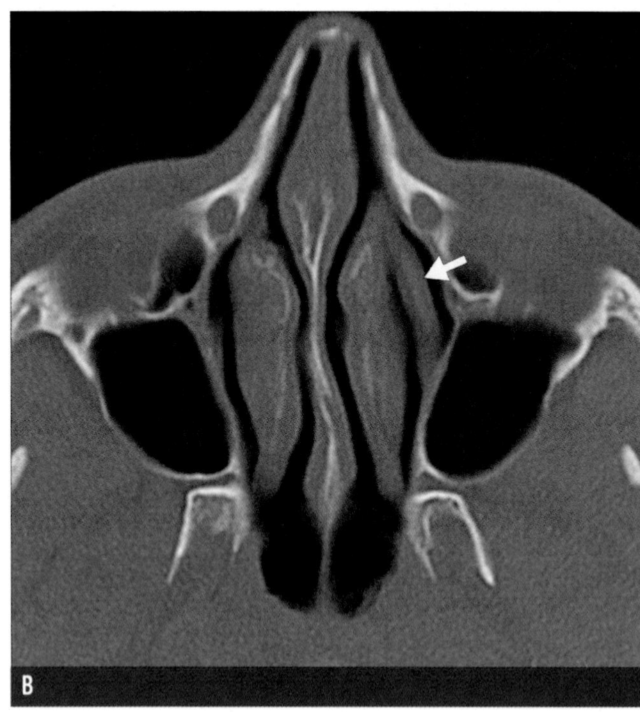

Coronal reformatted (**A**) and axial (**B**) CT images demonstrate an accessory left middle nasal turbinate (arrows, **A**, **B**). An accessory middle nasal turbinate arises from the uncinate process, whereas a secondary nasal turbinate has its own separate turbinate neck and does not represent an extension of the uncinate process.

Companion case: Bifid middle nasal turbinates

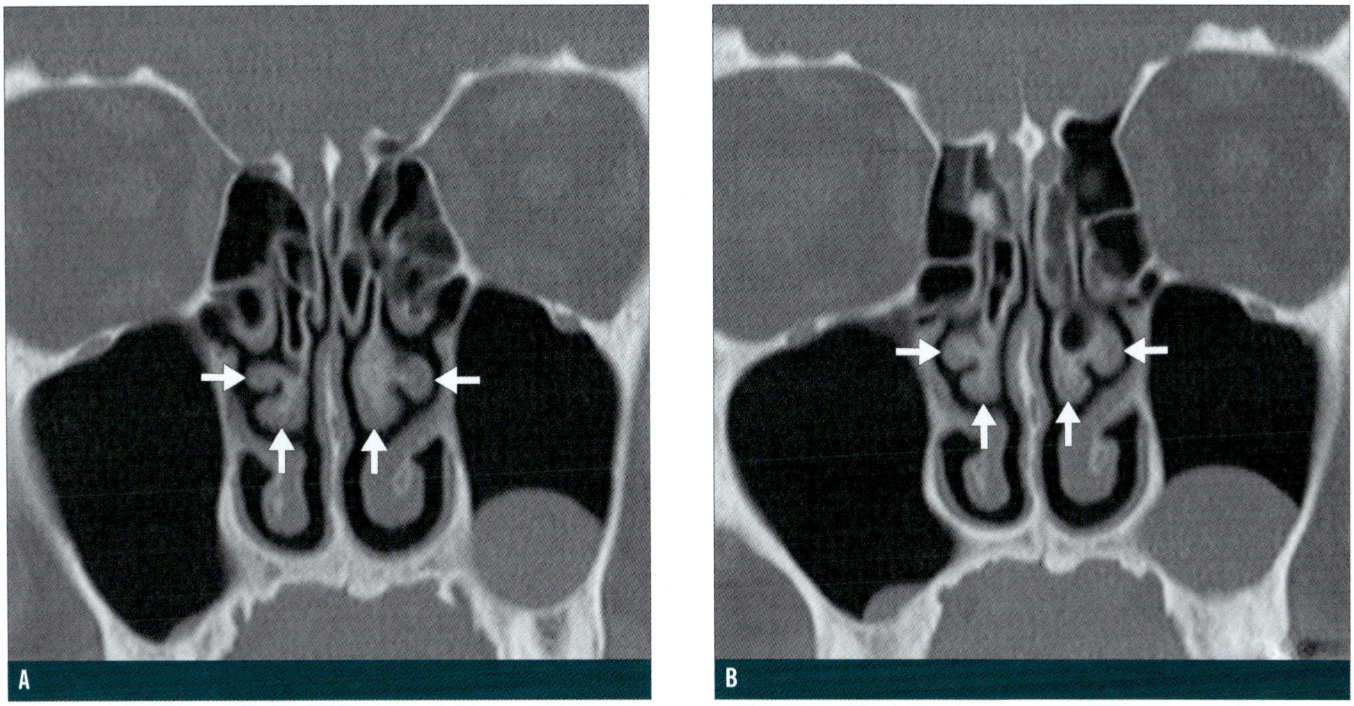

Coronal reformatted CT images through the nasal cavity (**A, B**) demonstrate an incidental bifid configuration of both middle nasal turbinate heads (arrows, **A, B**).

REFERENCES

El-Shazly AE, et al. Anatomical variations of the lateral nasal wall: the secondary and accessory middle turbinates. *Clinl Anal.* 2012;25:340-346.

Eweiss A. Trifurcate middle turbinate; an unusual anatomical variation. *Rhinology.* 2008;46(3):246-248.

Khanobthamchai K, Shankar L, Hawke M, Bingham B. The secondary middle turbinate. *J Otolaryngol.* 1991;20:412-413.

Ozcan KM, et al. Anatomical variations of nasal turbinates. *J Craniofac Surg.* 2008;19(6):1678-1682.

CASE 39 Nasal cycle

Changes in the nasal mucosal volume occur cyclically and alternate sides, each cycle ranging from 1 to 6 hours. This normal process is termed the nasal cycle. The mucosal volume changes related to the nasal cycle may be observed on CT or MRI, and it may involve the mucosa of the nasal turbinates, nasal septum, nasal cavity walls, nasolacrimal ducts, and ethmoidal air cells. Because of the normal nasal cycle, asymmetrically enlarged nasal turbinates, particularly when unilateral, are almost always an incidental finding. Application of a topical vasoconstrictor will interrupt the nasal cycle.

The nasal cycle may not be seen in all individuals and can become less pronounced with age.

Nasal cycle

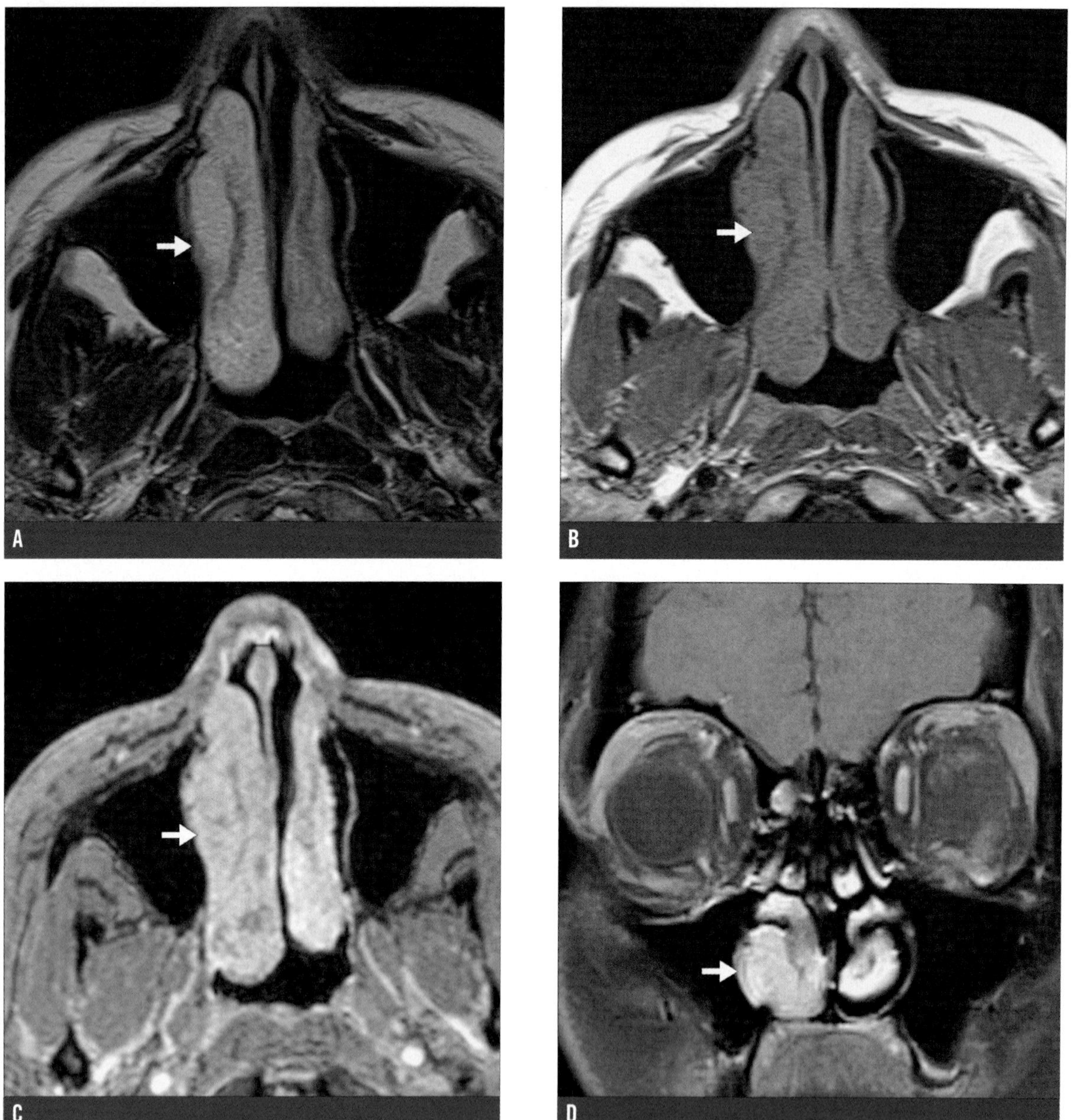

Axial T2 (**A**), unenhanced axial T1 (**B**), postcontrast axial MPRAGE (**C**), and postcontrast fat-saturated coronal T1 (**D**) MR images demonstrate asymmetric enlargement of the right inferior nasal turbinate (arrows, **A-D**). Axial T2 (**E**), unenhanced axial T1 (**F**), postcontrast axial MPRAGE (**G**), and postcontrast fat-saturated coronal T1 (**H**) MR images performed for a 4-month follow-up study demonstrate asymmetric enlargement of the left inferior nasal turbinate (arrows, **E-H**). This case illustrates the normal nasal cycle. A normal nasal cycle occurs every 1 to 6 hours and alternates sides during each cycle.

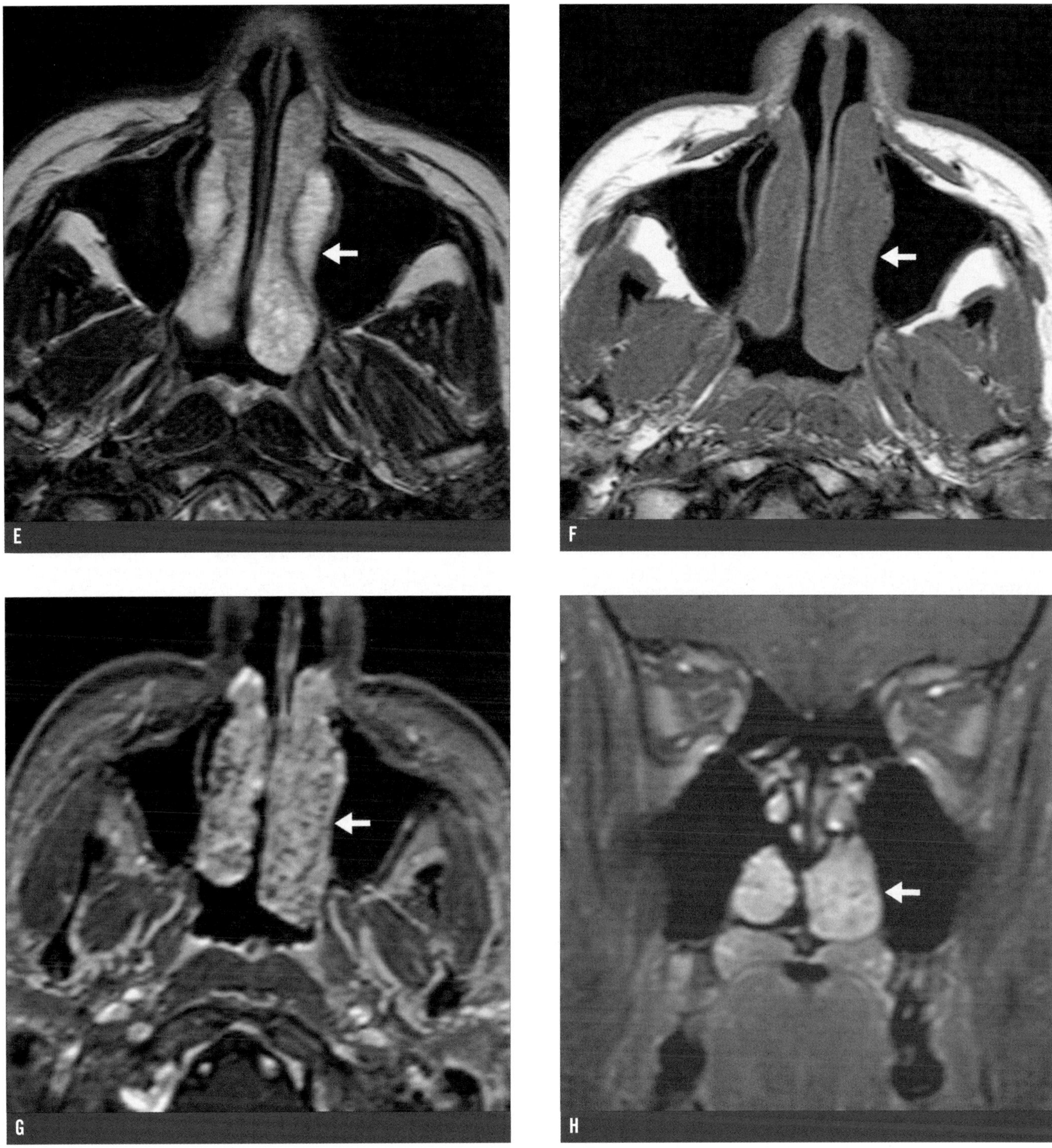
E
F
G
H

Nasal cycle

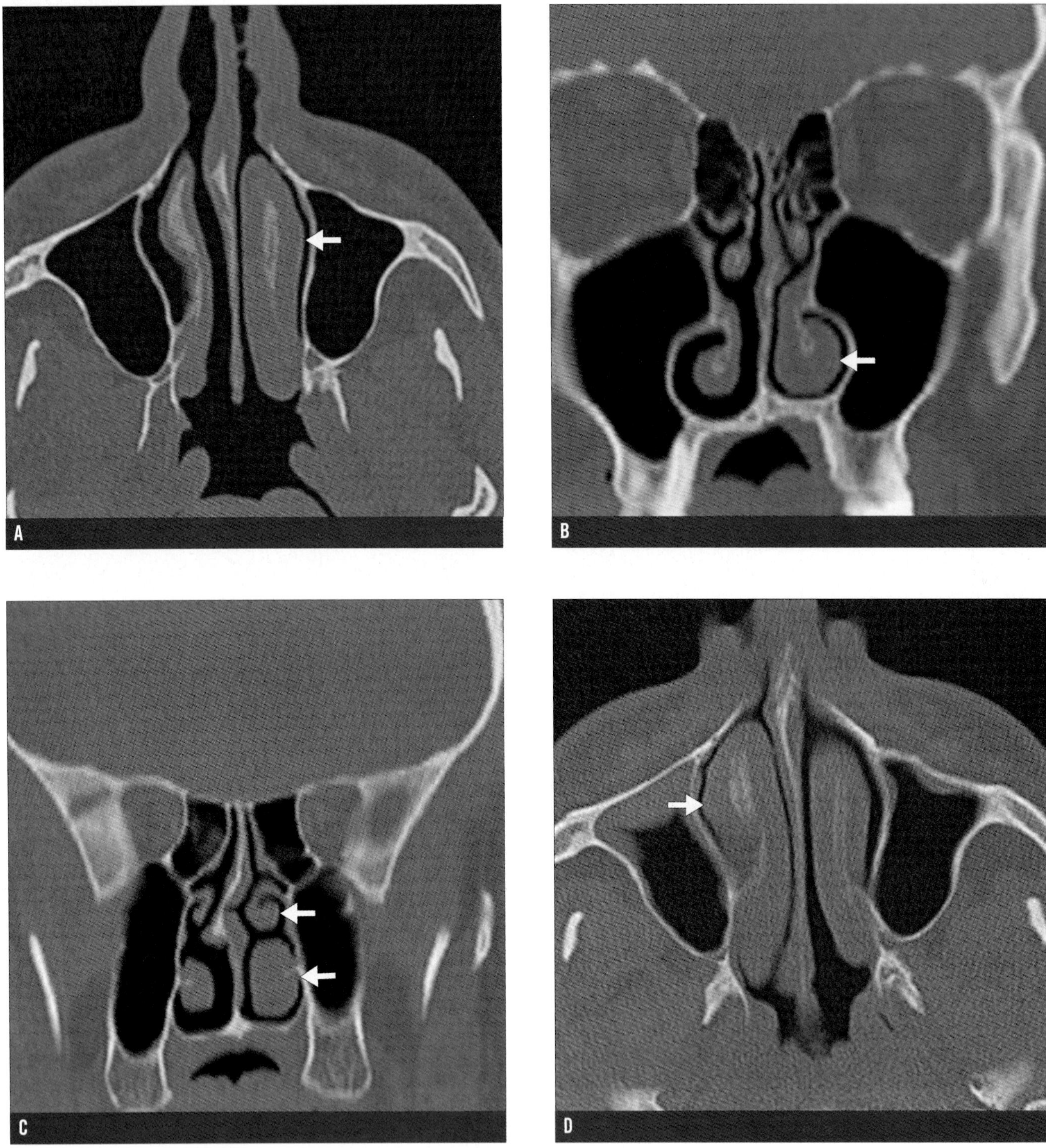

Different patient. Axial (**A**) and coronal reformatted (**B, C**) CT images through the nasal cavity demonstrate left nasal turbinate enlargement (arrows, **A-C**). Axial (**D**) and coronal reformatted (**E, F**) CT images of the same patient from a study performed 5 years later now demonstrate right nasal turbinate enlargement (arrows, **D-F**).

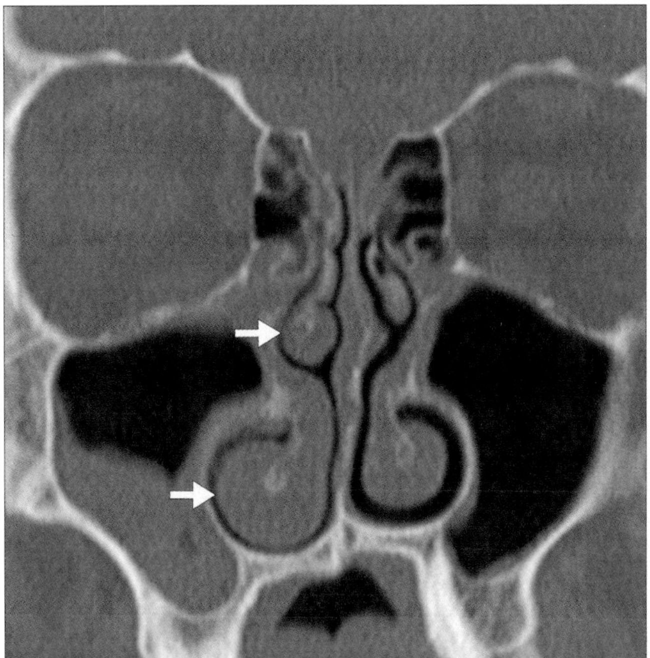

E

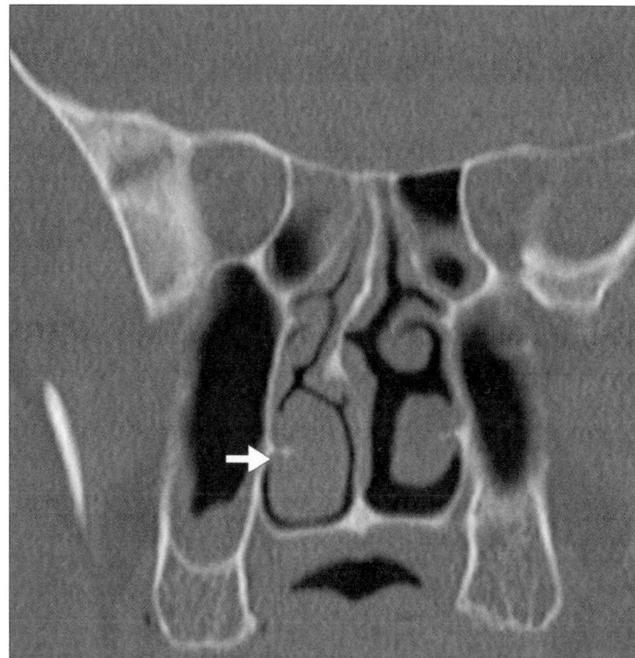

F

REFERENCES

Eggesbø HB. Radiological imaging of inflammatory lesions in the nasal cavity and paranasal sinuses. *Eur Radiol.* 2006;16:872-888.

Rak KM, et al. Paranasal sinuses on MR images of the brain: significance of mucosal thickening. *AJR Am J Roentgenol.* 1991;156: 381-384.

Zinreich SJ, et al. MR imaging of normal nasal cycle: comparison with sinus pathology. *J Comp Assist Tomogr.* 1988;12(6):1014-1019.

CASE 40 Nasal turbinate hypertrophy

Nasal turbinate hypertrophy that is not related to the normal nasal cycle may occur with allergic rhinitis or vasomotor (nonallergic) rhinitis. In these cases, the nasal turbinate enlargement is usually bilateral and due to inflammation. Occasionally, nasal turbinate hypertrophy may involve only one nasal turbinate and be associated with a nasal septal defect, regional osseous remodeling, or extend through the nasal choana into the nasopharynx. In this setting, the enlarged nasal turbinate is likely developmentally enlarged, although care should be taken to ensure that there are no findings to suggest a tumor, such as cartilaginous tumor matrix on CT or abnormal mucosal signal on MRI. A tumor arising from a nasal turbinate will most often contain different T2 signal and enhance differently than will turbinates that are uninvolved by tumor. However, with nasal turbinate hypertrophy, the enlarged turbinate will be of the same T2 signal and enhance the same as the remaining turbinates.

COMPANION CASE

- **Fungal disease of the nasal turbinates ("Black turbinate" sign).** Invasive fungal sinusitis is a life-threatening infection that has a proclivity for immunocompromised or poorly controlled diabetic patients. It is usually caused by *Mucor*, *Rhizopus*, or *Absidia* fungal species. The spores from these fungi invade the sinus and/or turbinate mucosa of susceptible patients and then germinate, forming angioinvasive hyphae. These angioinvasive hyphae result in infarction and gangrene of the involved tissue. The devitalized, gangrenous sinus/turbinate mucosa will not enhance on MRI and will often be hypointense on T2. These nasal turbinate findings on MRI have been described as the "black turbinate" sign. Prompt recognition and appropriate therapy is of paramount importance to effectively treat invasive fungal sinusitis.

Nasal turbinate hypertrophy

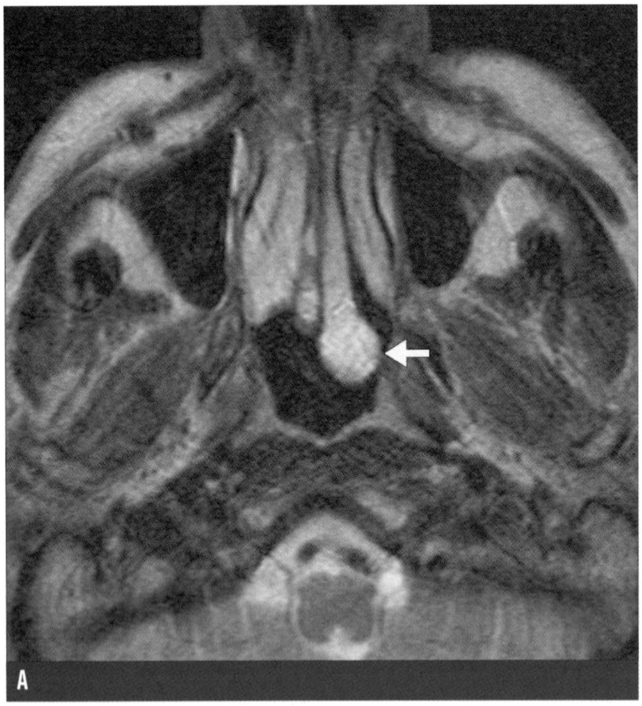

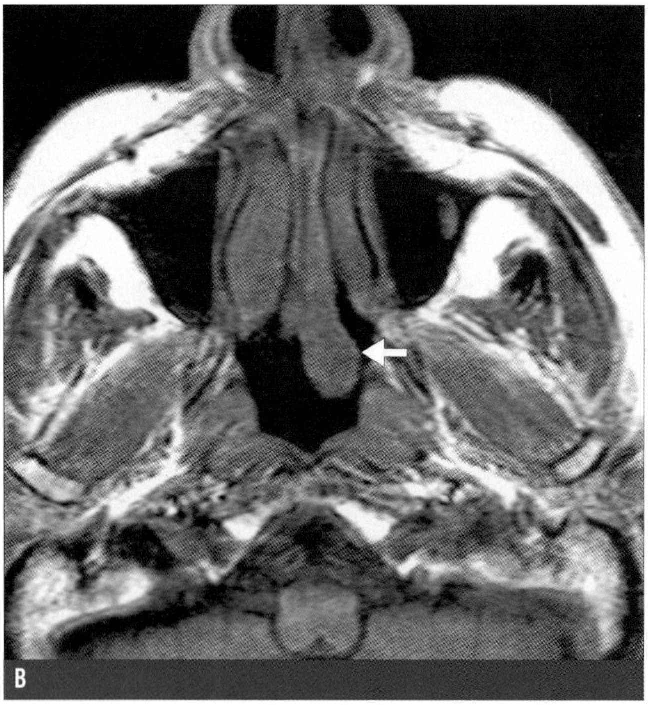

Axial T2 (**A**), noncontrast axial T1 (**B**), and postcontrast axial T1 (**C**) MR images demonstrate a bulbous posterior aspect of the left inferior nasal turbinate (arrows, **A-C**). The pre- and postcontrast MRI signal of this finding follows the same signal as the remaining nasal turbinates. This represents incidental nasal turbinate hypertrophy and is not pathologic.

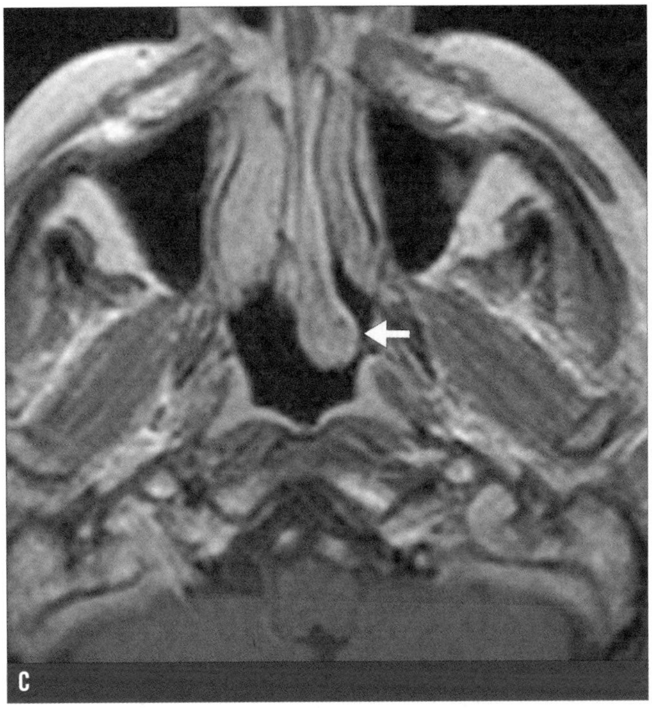

Developmental nasal turbinate hypertrophy

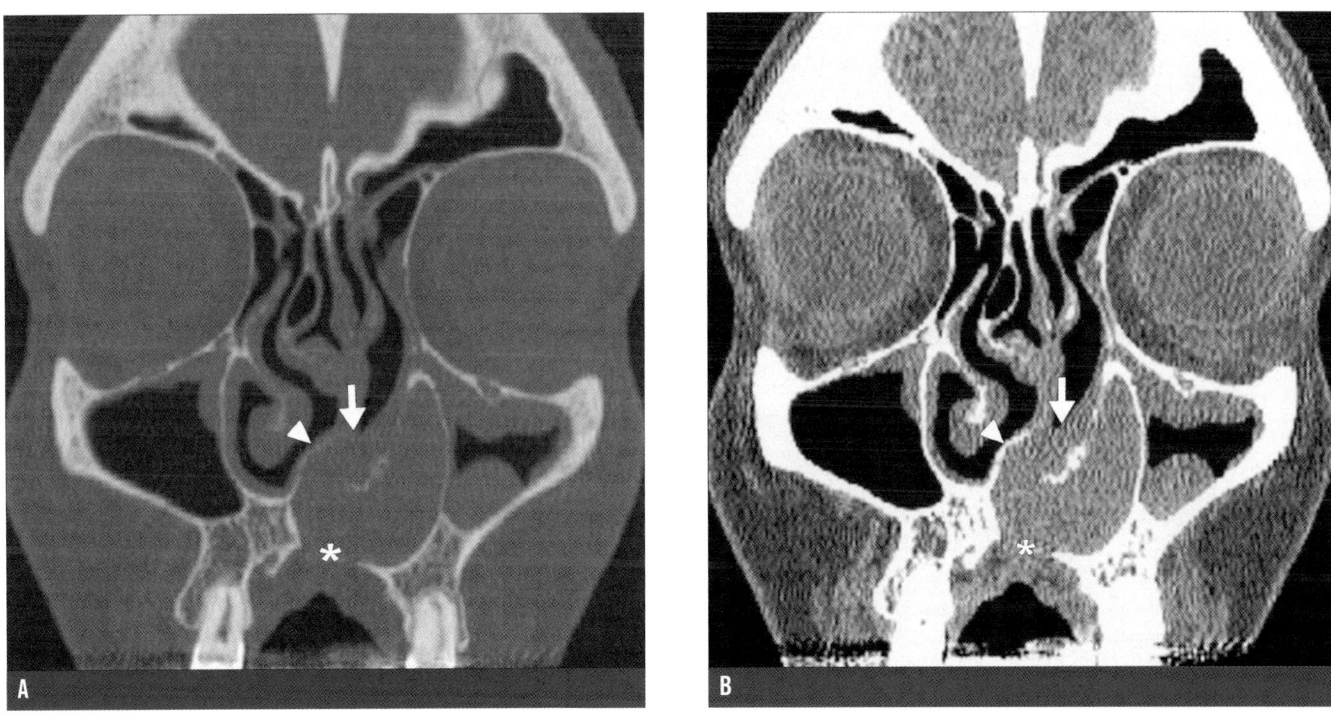

Coronal reformatted CT images viewed with a bone window (**A**) and intermediate window (**B**) demonstrates a large left inferior nasal turbinate (arrows, **A, B**). These images also demonstrate a chronic deformity of the osseous nasal septum (arrowheads, **A, B**) and focal osseous loss of the hard palate (asterisks, **A, B**), suggestive of a developmental anomaly. An axial CT image viewed with a soft tissue window (**C**) demonstrates the large left inferior nasal turbinate to extend from the posterior aspect of the nasal vestibule (arrowhead, **C**) to the nasopharynx (asterisk, **C**). Axial T1 (**D**), postcontrast axial T1 with fat suppression (**E**), axial T2 with fat suppression (**F**), and unenhanced sagittal T1 (**G**) MR images obtained 18 months prior to the CT also demonstrate marked hypertrophy of the left inferior nasal turbinate (arrows, **D-G**). This marked nasal turbinate hypertrophy has the same signal characteristics as the contralateral inferior nasal turbinate compatible with benignity.

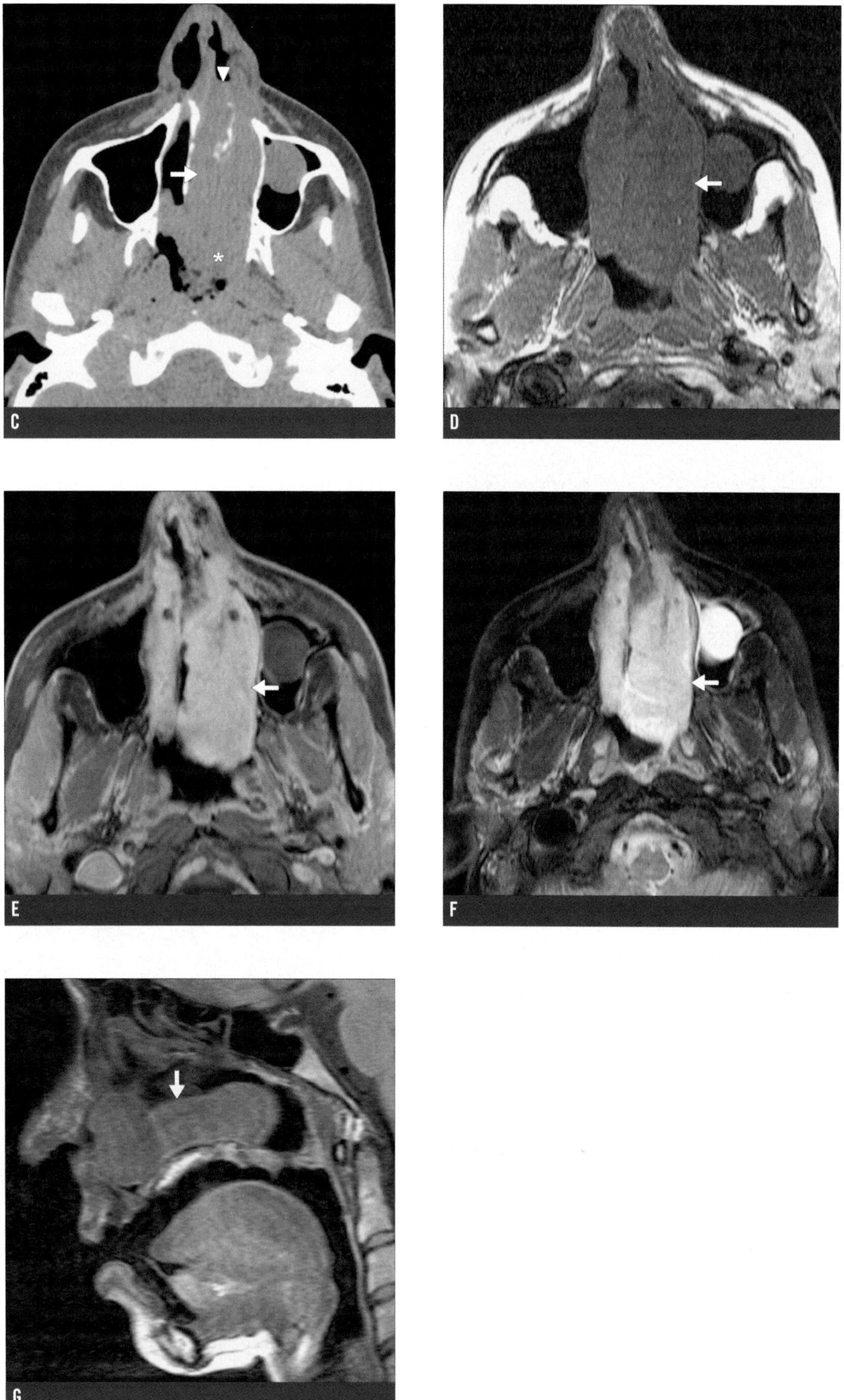
C
D
E
F
G

Companion case: Fungal disease of the nasal turbinates ("Black turbinate" sign)

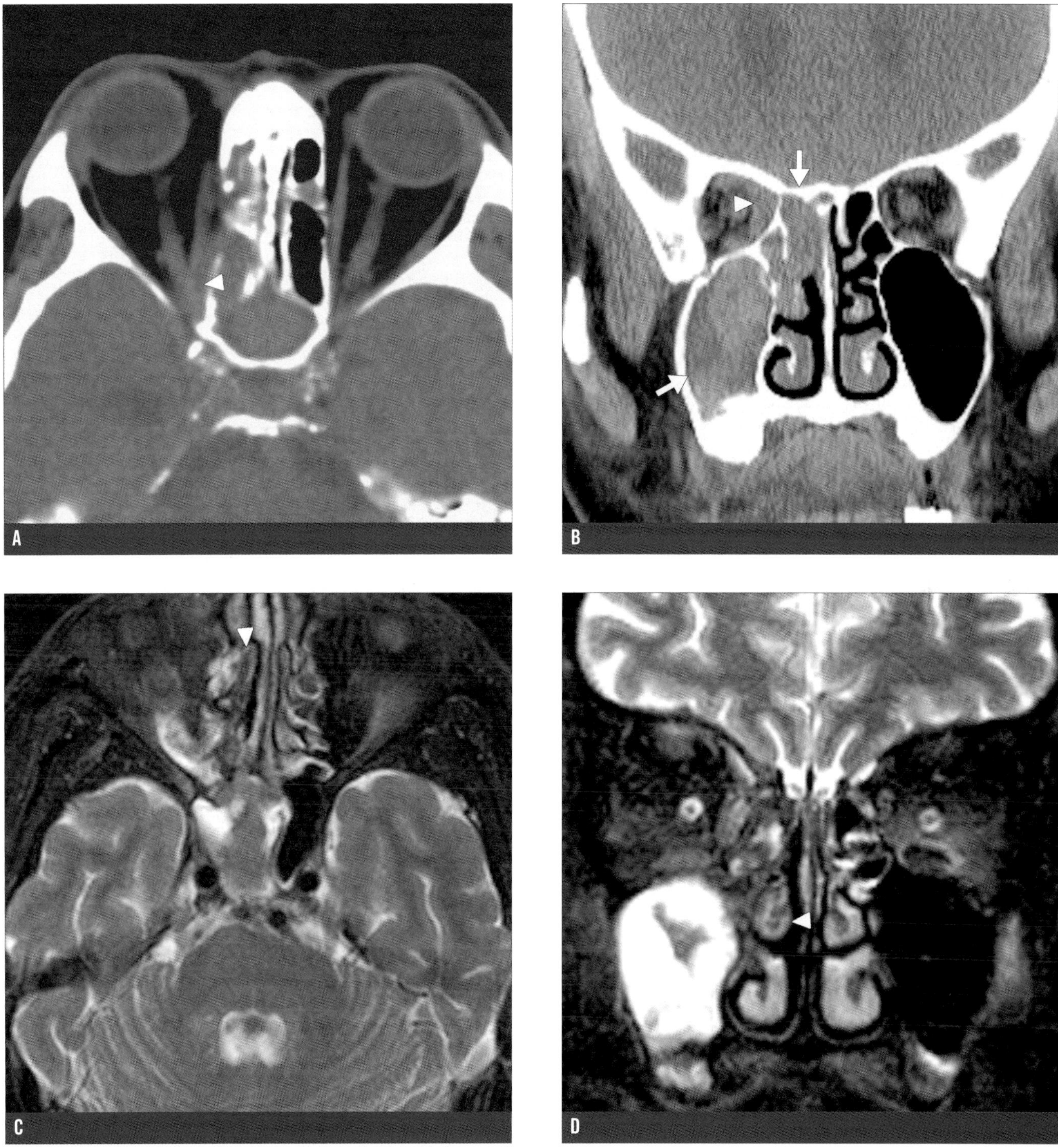

Unenhanced axial (**A**) and coronal reformatted (**B**) CT images of the paranasal sinuses demonstrate extensive opacification of the right maxillary sinus and right ethmoid air cells (arrows, **B**) with associated abnormal extension of the finding into the posteromedial aspect of the right orbit (arrowheads, **A, B**). The findings are nonspecific based on these images, although they do suggest an aggressive abnormality, such as an invasive tumor or infection. T2 fat-suppressed MR images in the axial (**C**) and coronal (**D**) planes demonstrate subtle abnormal hypointense T2 signal involving the right middle nasal turbinate (arrowheads, **C, D**) as well as scattered hypointense T2 signal within several of the visualized sinuses. The finding affecting the right middle nasal turbinate is compatible with a "black turbinate sign" of invasive fungal sinusitis, in the appropriate clinical setting, which was pathologically confirmed in this patient. A postcontrast axial T1-weighted MR image with fat suppression (**E**) demonstrates subtle hypoenhancement of the right middle nasal turbinate (arrow, **E**). Nonenhancement or hypoenhancement of the affected nasal turbinate may be identified with the invasive fungal sinusitis because of the angioinvasive nature of the fungus and resultant devitalization of the mucosa.

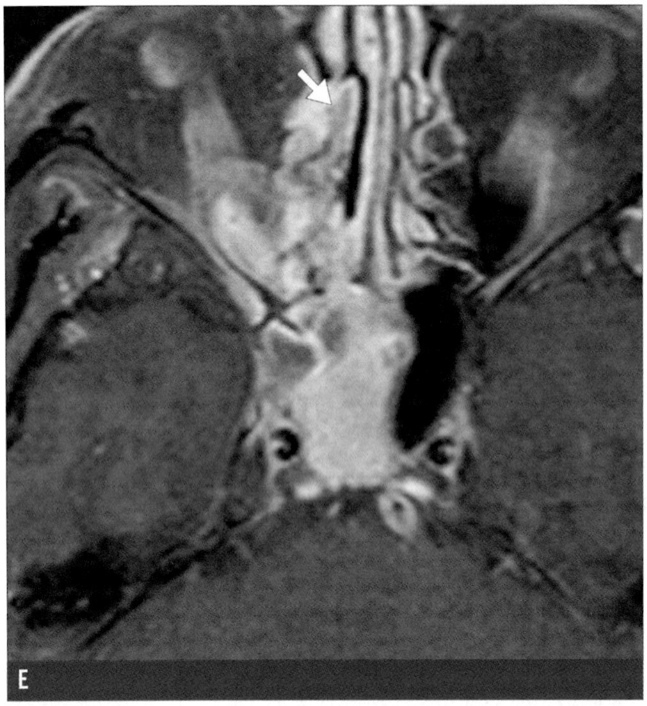

REFERENCES

Akoğlu E, et al. Evaluation of the turbinate hypertrophy by computed tomography in patients with deviated nasal septum. *Otolaryngol Head Neck Surg.* 2007;136(3):380-384.

Eggesbø HB. Radiological imaging of inflammatory lesions in the nasal cavity and paranasal sinuses. *Eur Radiol.* 2006;16(4):872–888. Epub January 4, 2006.

Lee JH. Congenital vomeral bone defect: report of two cases and a review of the literature. *Acta Otolaryngol.* 2006;126(11):1229-1231.

Safder S, Carpenter JS, Roberts TD, Bailey N. The "Black Turbinate" sign: an early MR imaging finding of nasal mucormycosis. *AJNR Am J Neuroradiol.* 2010;31(4):771-774. Epub November 26, 2009.

Scheithauer MO. Surgery of the turbinates and "empty nose" syndrome. *GMS Curr Top Otorhinolaryngol Head Neck Surg.* 2010;9.

CASE 41 Nasal turbinate head reduction

A nasal turbinate head reduction is a surgical procedure that removes a portion of a nasal turbinate head. It is the primary surgical therapy to treat patients who have refractory allergic rhinitis or chronic rhinosinusitis. This procedure serves to enlarge the nasal airway and allows the nasal fossa to accommodate nasal turbinate swelling that occurs as a result of sinus inflammation. Currently, there are a variety of techniques that may be employed to surgically reduce nasal turbinate tissue, including an outfracture, submucosal resection, laser vaporization, radiofrequency ablation, and coblation.

COMPANION CASES

- **Nasal turbinectomy.** This refers to resection of the head as well as the neck of the nasal turbinate, as opposed to a nasal turbinate head reduction, which involves resection of only the nasal turbinate head.
- **Nasal turbinate cleft simulating a surgical defect.** Occasionally, an incidental, anatomic variant cleft within a nasal turbinate may simulate a surgical defect, such as partial resection of a nasal turbinate neck.
- **Empty nose syndrome.** The nasal turbinates are important structures that function to humidify, filtrate, and warm the air. Therefore, a radical nasal turbinectomy should be avoided because it can result in an entity termed empty nose syndrome (ENS). Despite an enlarged nasal cavity airspace afforded by a radical nasal turbinectomy, clear paranasal sinuses and a clear nasal cavity in patients with ENS will be associated with a paradoxical sensation of nasal congestion because of a lack of adequate air humidification. Additional symptoms of ENS include crusting and dryness of the nasal cavity, facial pain, and headache.

Nasal turbinate head reduction

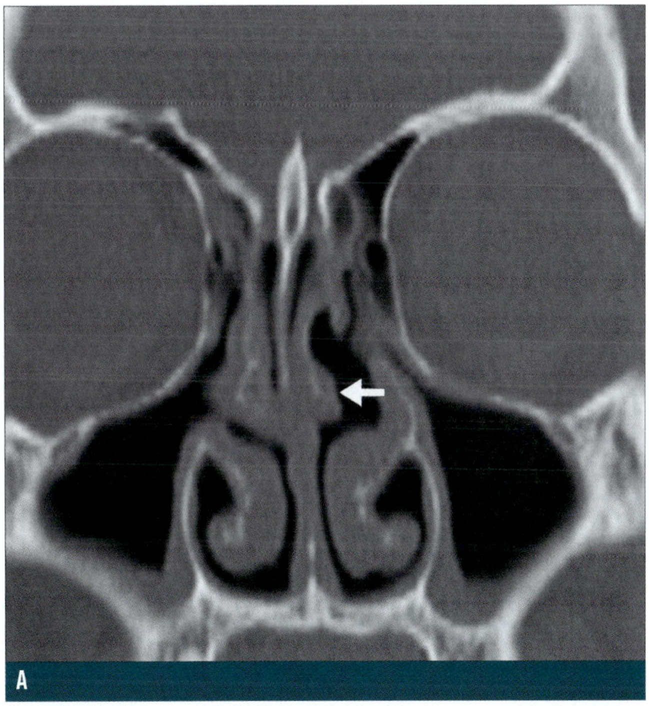

A coronal reformatted CT image (**A**) demonstrates a typical nasal turbinate head reduction, in this case involving the left middle nasal turbinate head (arrow).

Companion case: Nasal turbinectomies

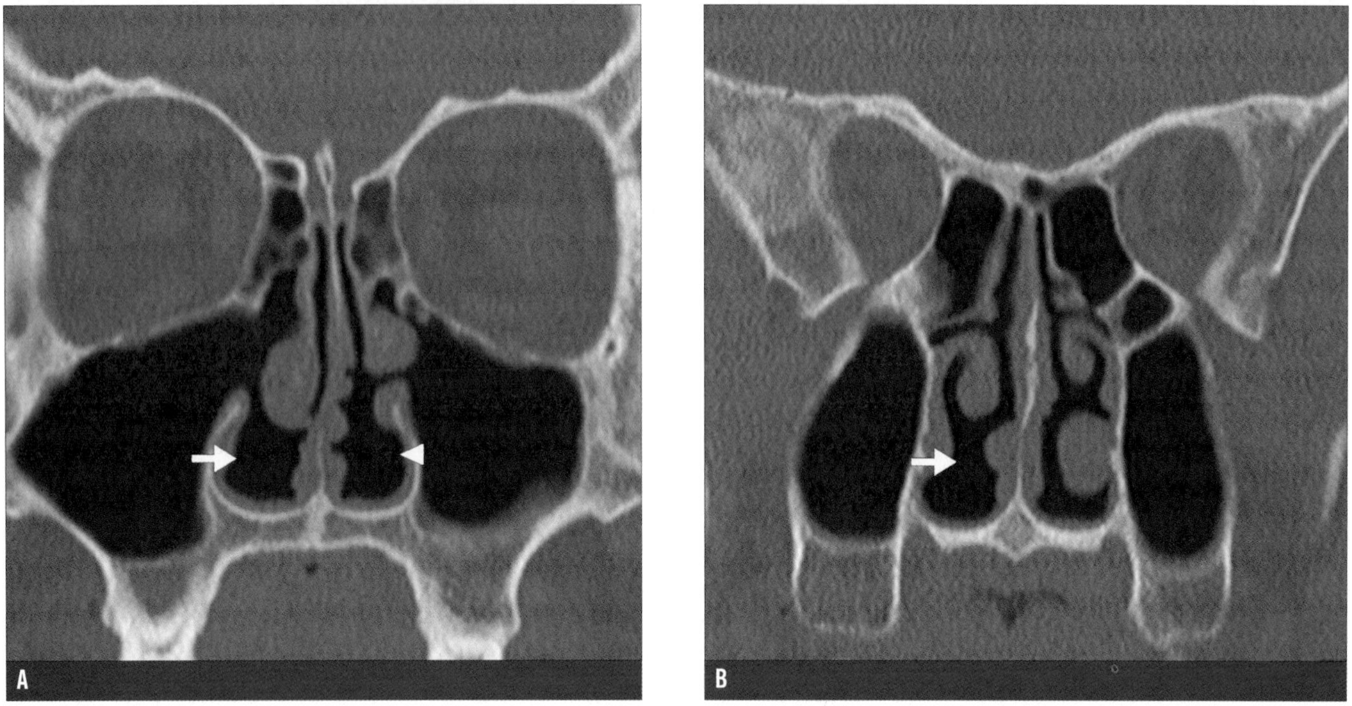

Coronal reformatted CT images (**A**, **B**) demonstrate a total right inferior nasal turbinectomy (arrows, **A**, **B**) and a partial left inferior nasal turbinectomy (arrowhead, **A**).

Companion case: Nasal turbinate cleft simulating a surgical defect

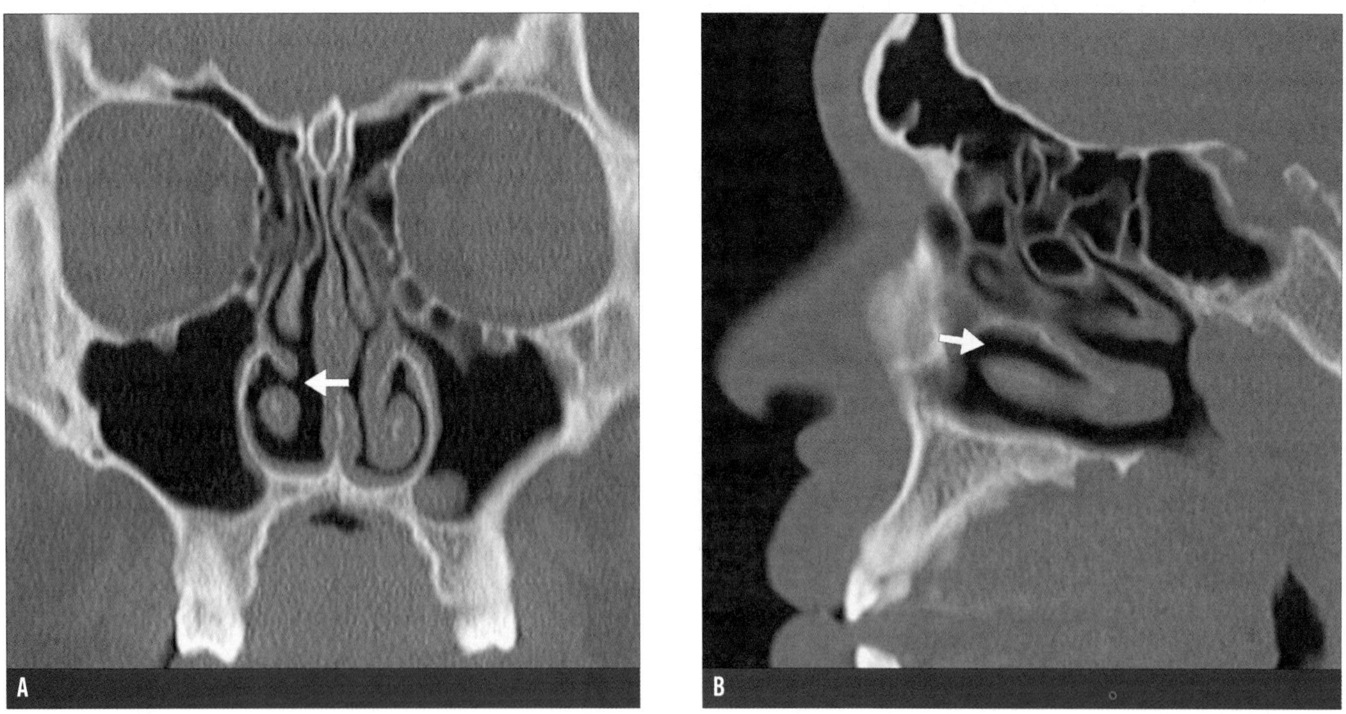

A coronal reformatted CT image through the nasal cavity (**A**) demonstrates an apparent defect in the neck of the right inferior nasal turbinate (arrow, **A**). A sagittal reformatted CT image from the same study (**B**) demonstrates a cleft through the neck of the right inferior nasal turbinate (arrow, **B**) accounting for the finding demonstrated on image **A**. This patient did not have a history of prior nasal turbinate surgery.

Companion case: Empty nose syndrome

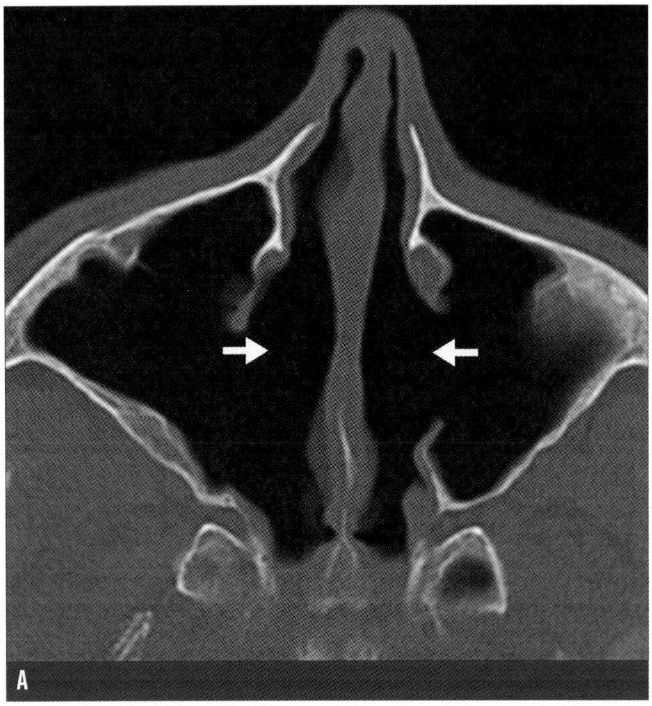

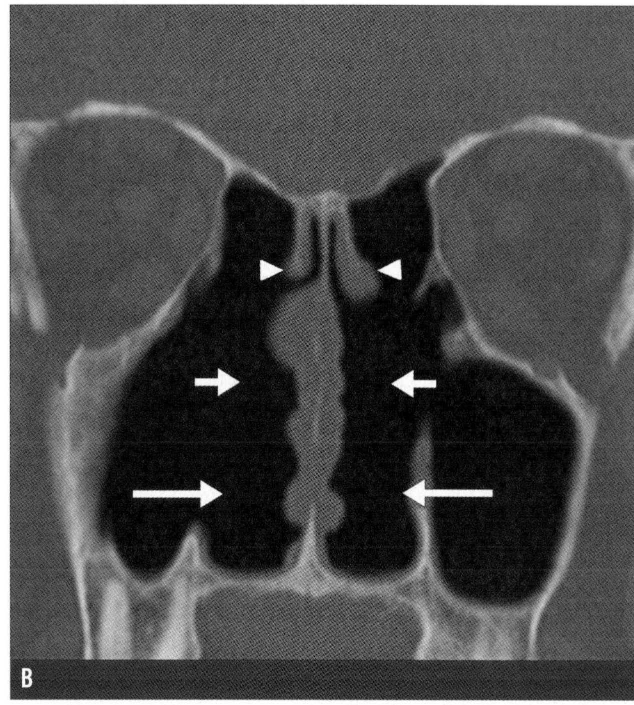

An axial CT image (**A**) demonstrates absent nasal turbinates at the level of the maxillary sinuses (short arrows, **A**). A coronal reformatted CT image (**B**) demonstrates absent bilateral middle nasal turbinates (short arrows, **B**) and inferior nasal turbinates (long arrows, **B**). The bilateral superior nasal turbinates are still present (arrowheads, **B**). The nasal turbinates function to humidify air and thus the lack of nasal turbinates may result in a paradoxical congested sensation, despite the absence of nasal cavity and paranasal sinus mucosal disease. This is a clinical diagnosis and should be suspected if the patient experiences persistent congestion following advanced nasal turbinate resection, which was present in this case.

REFERENCES

Chhabra N, Houser SM. The surgical management of allergic rhinitis. *Otolaryngol Clin N Am.* 2011;44:779-795.

Jang YJ, et al. Empty nose syndrome. *Laryngoscope.* 2011;121(6):1308-1312.

Scheithauer MO. Surgery of the turbinates and “empty nose” syndrome. *GMS Curr Top Otorhinolaryngol Head Neck Surg.* 2010;9.

Deviation of the nasal septum is an extremely common finding and often incidental. However, if pronounced, a nasoseptal deviation can narrow an adjacent nasal meatus and result in an outflow obstruction.

A nasoseptal spur often accompanies a nasoseptal deviation. Occasionally, a nasoseptal deviation and spur can be associated with deformity of an adjacent nasal turbinate. Some authors have proposed that this scenario may result in a "contact point" headache. These are thought to occur as a result of referred headaches from stimulation of the trigeminal nerves (specifically V1 and V2) that innervate the nasal cavity mucosa. Some have shown that these referred headaches can resolve following surgical removal of the nasoseptal spur and a septoplasty. However, a nasal turbinate deformity associated with a nasoseptal deviation and spur is not a primary indication for surgery. In fact, some authors have disputed "contact point" headaches altogether. Other potential causes for a patient's headache should always be considered prior to performing a septoplasty to specifically treat this symptom.

Nasoseptal deviation and spur

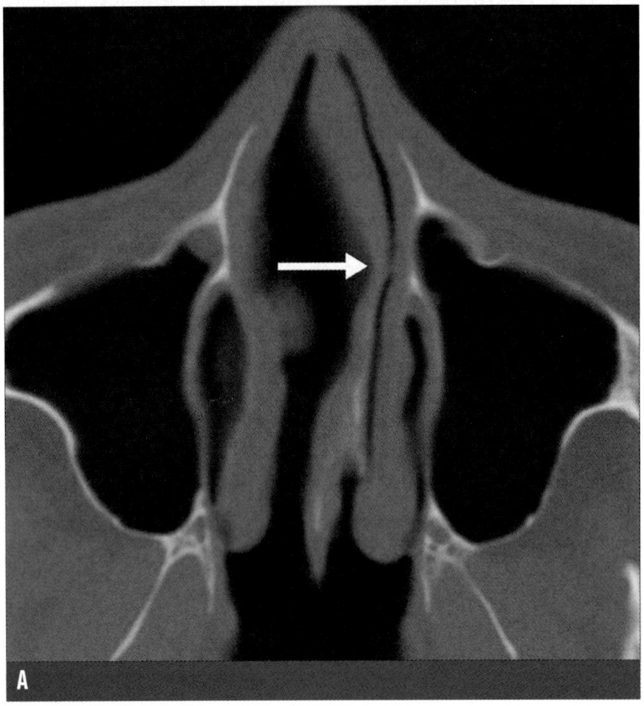

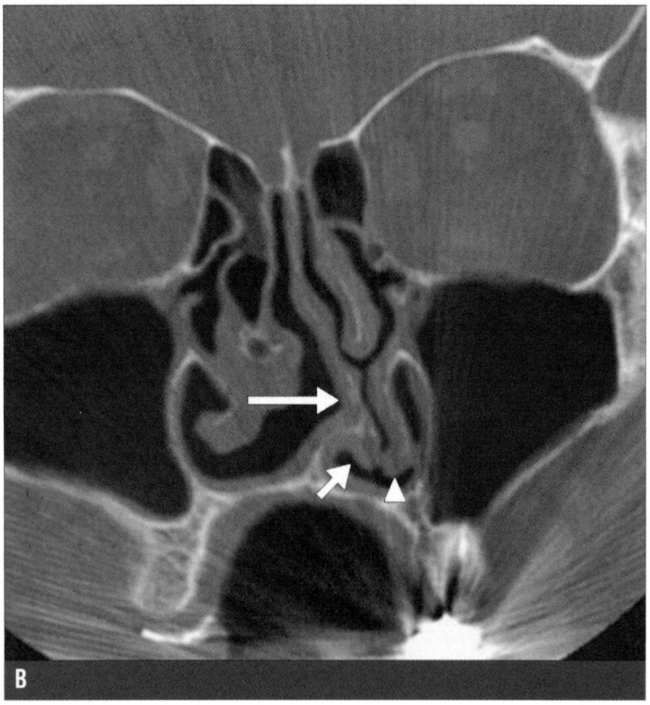

Axial (**A**) and coronal reformatted (**B**) CT images demonstrate severe leftward nasoseptal deviation (long arrows, **A**, **B**) and a small nasal spur (short arrow, **B**). As a result of the nasoseptal deviation and spur, there is pronounced narrowing of the left aspect of the nasal cavity, in particular the left inferior nasal meatus. There is also an associated mild deformity of the left inferior nasal turbinate head (arrowhead, **B**).

Nasoseptal deviation and spur

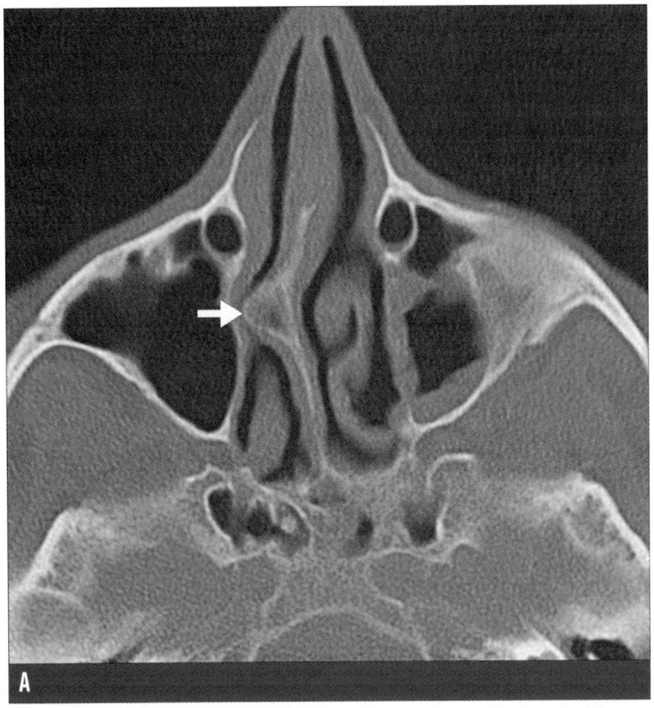

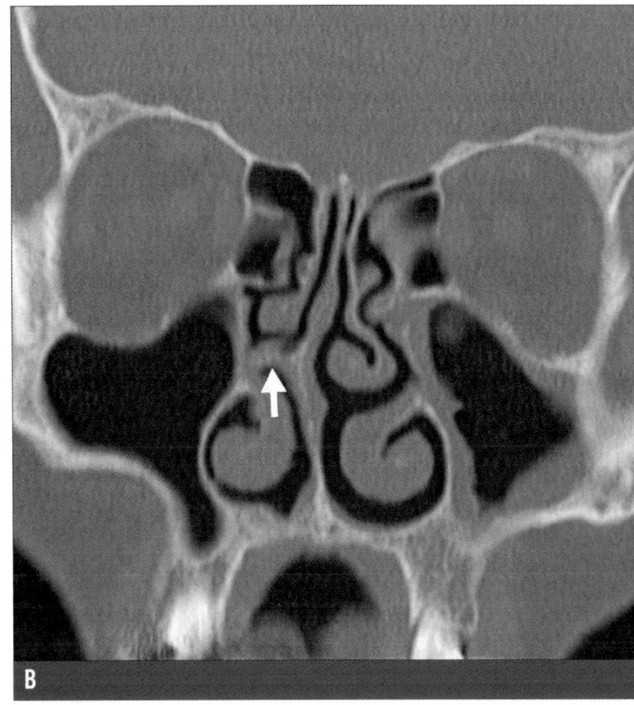

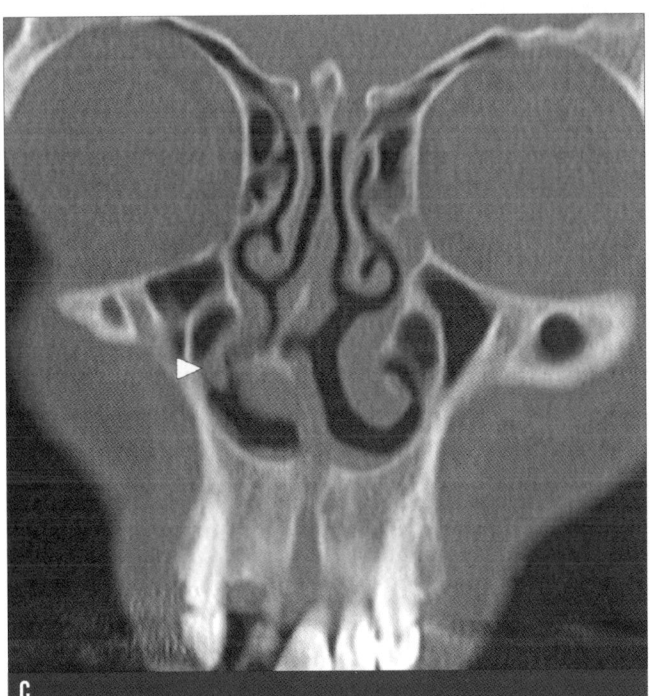

Different patient. Axial (**A**) as well as coronal reformatted (**B**, **C**) CT images demonstrate a moderate rightward-directed nasoseptal deviation and large spur (arrows, **A**, **B**) that is associated with deformity of the right inferior nasal turbinate head (arrowhead, **C**).

REFERENCES

Abu-Bakra M, Jones NS. Prevalence of nasal mucosal contact points in patients with facial pain compared with patients without facial pain. *J Laryngol Otol.* 2001;115(8):629-632.

Parsons DS, Batra PS. Functional endoscopic sinus surgical outcomes for contact point headaches. *Laryngoscope.* 1998;108(5):696-702.

Perez-Pinas I, et al. Anatomical variations in the human paranasal sinus region studied by CT. *J Anat.* 2000;197:221-227.

CASE 43 Nasoseptal retention cyst

Nasoseptal retention cysts likely result from an obstruction of a mucous or serous gland embedded within the nasal septal mucosa, much like other retention cysts found elsewhere in the paranasal sinuses. Other authors have proposed that these occur following surgery, perhaps because of entrapment of nasal mucosa into the submucosal space following surgery. Regardless of the cause, the signal characteristics of a nasoseptal retention cyst vary on MRI and may be hypointense or hyperintense on T1 and T2, depending on the protein content of the cyst. While a retention cyst may peripherally enhance, retention cysts should never solidly enhance on MRI. The morphology of a nasoseptal retention cyst is typically oval in shape, smooth, and nonaggressive appearing. On CT, nasoseptal retention cysts are typically of the same density as the nasal mucosa and may therefore be relatively occult on CT, though a contour deformity is usually evident. These lesions are nonspecific on CT and could represent any number of entities. Melanoma is in the differential of an intrinsically T1 hyperintense nasal septal lesion. However, nasoseptal melanoma would be expected to at least partially enhance and often invades adjacent structures, neither of which are features of a nasoseptal retention cyst. If the benignity of a nasoseptal lesion is in question on imaging, then direct inspection is indicated.

Nasoseptal retention cyst

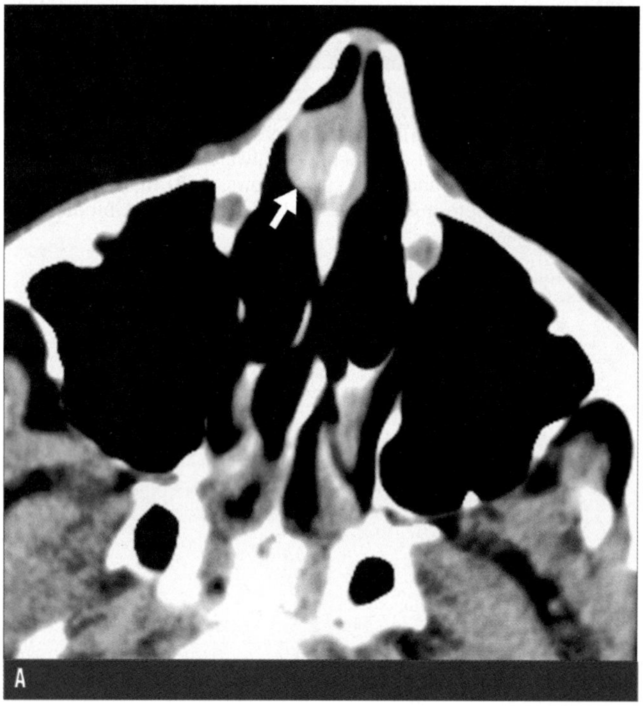

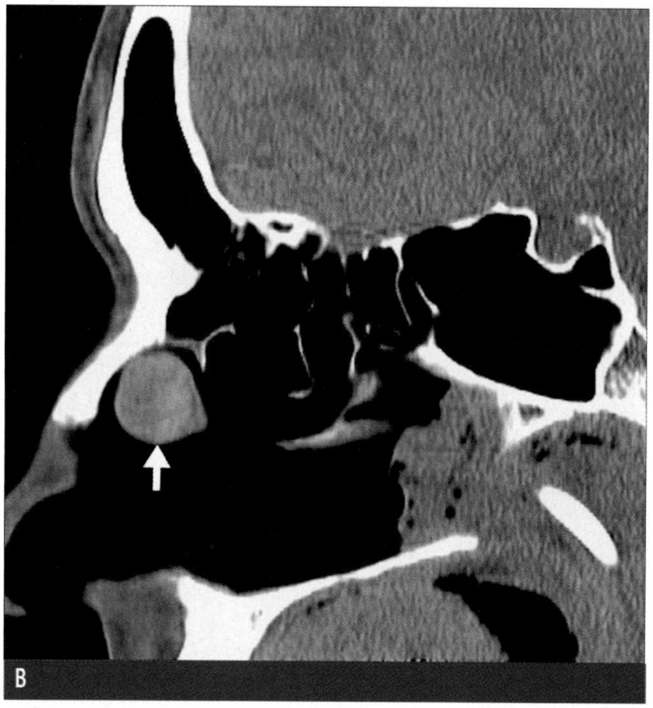

Axial (**A**), sagittal reformatted (**B**), and coronal reformatted (**C**) unenhanced CT images through the nasal cavity. The images demonstrate a soft tissue mass along the anterior right aspect of the nasal septum (arrows, **A-C**). Based on this CT examination, the lesion is nonspecific and could represent any number of benign and malignant entities. Axial T1 (**D**), sagittal T1 (**E**), axial T2 (**F**), and postcontrast fat-suppressed coronal T1 (**G**) MR images demonstrate the lesion to be hyperintense on precontrast T1 (arrows, **D, E**), hypointense on T2 (arrow, **F**), and not significantly enhance (arrow, **G**). The findings are compatible with an incidental nasoseptal retention cyst with proteinaceous content.

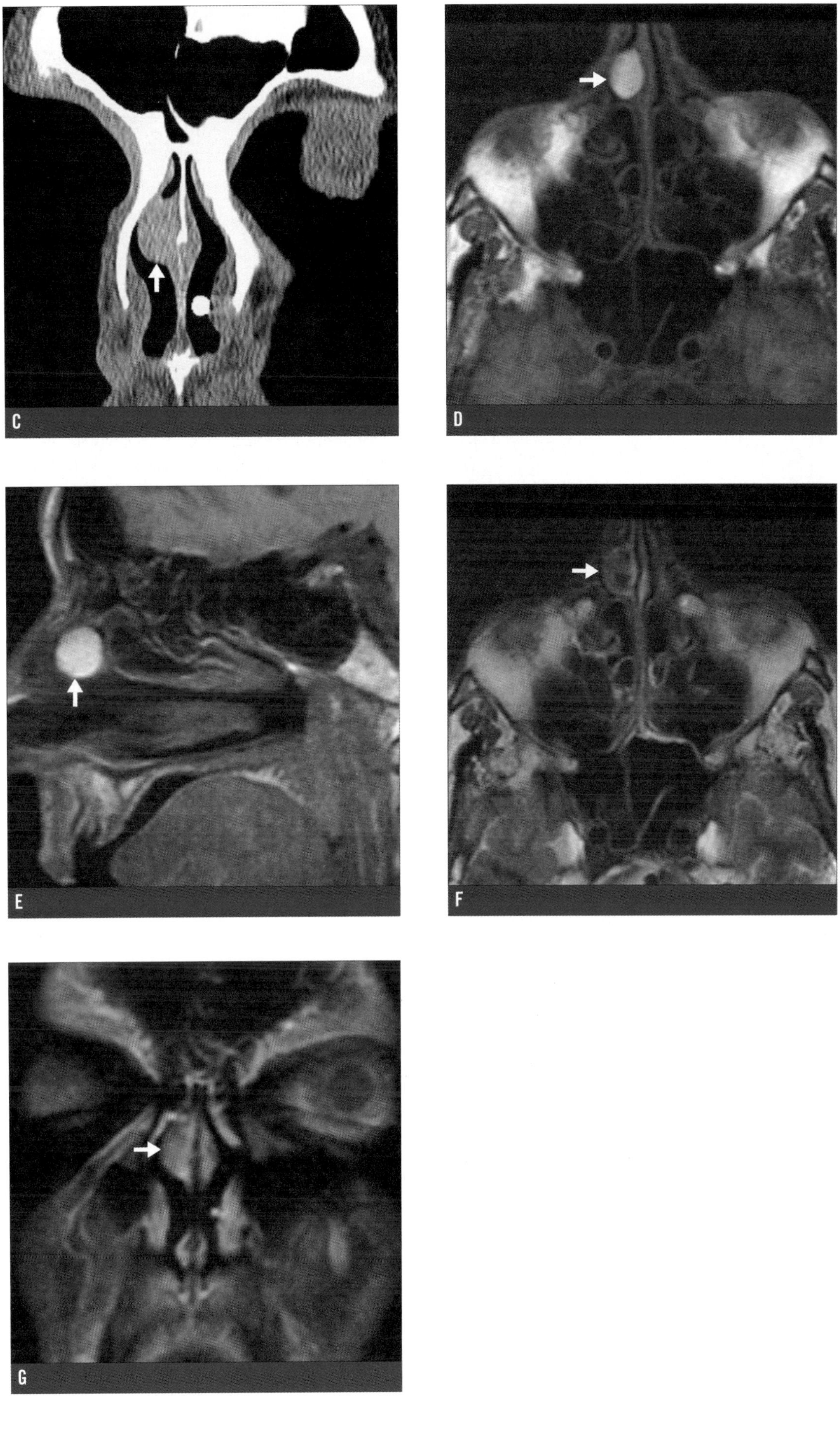
C
D
E
F
G

Nasoseptal retention cyst

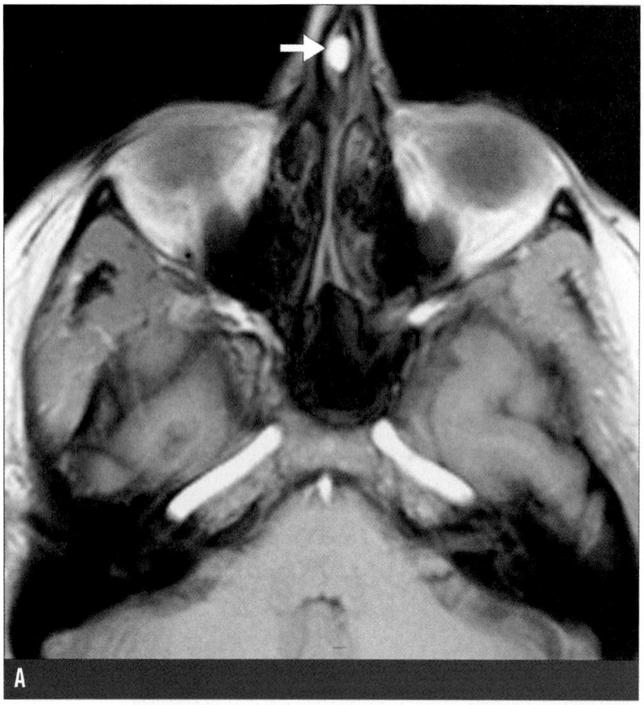

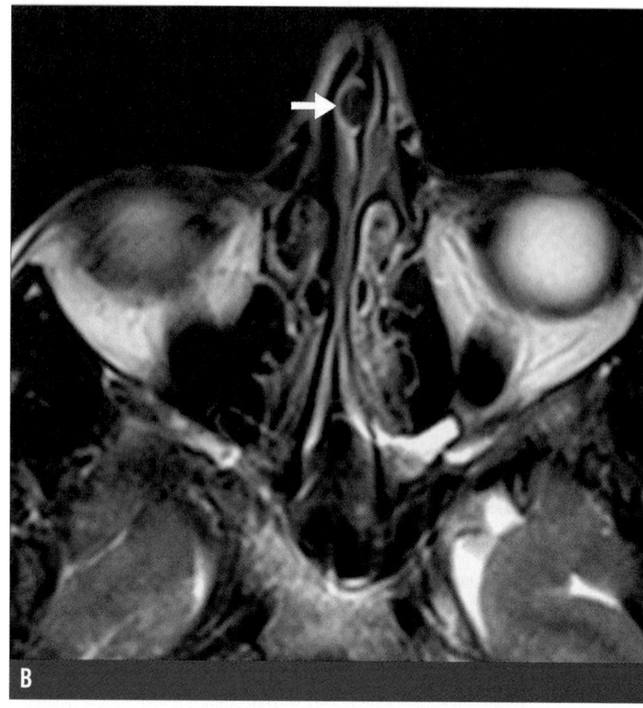

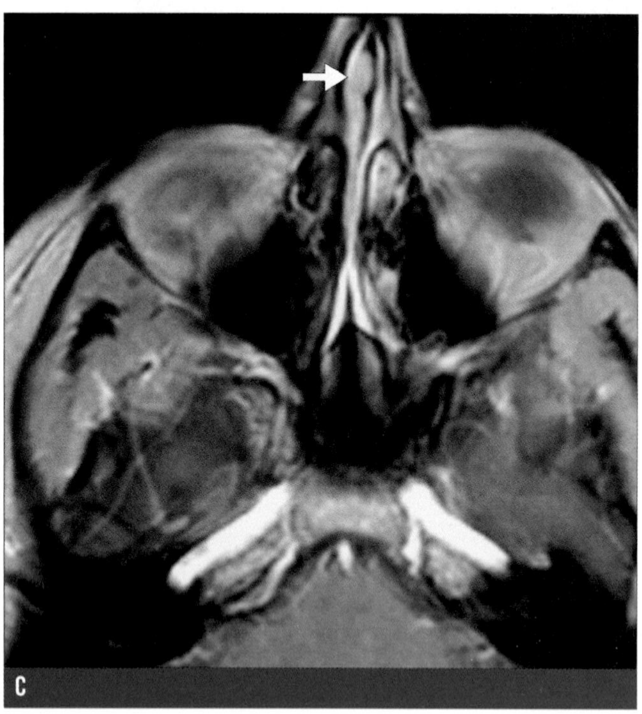

Different patient. Axial T1 (**A**), axial T2 (**B**), and postcontrast axial T1 (**C**) MR images through the nasal cavity demonstrate a small focus of T1 hyperintensity likely along the cartilaginous nasal septum, compatible with an incidental proteinaceous nasoseptal retention cyst (arrows, **A-C**).

REFERENCE

Leong AC, Sharp HR. Nasal septal cyst: a rare phenomenon. *Auris Nasus Larynx.* February 2009;36(1):96-99. Epub July 2008.

CASE 44 Septoplasty

A septoplasty is a surgical procedure that is performed in order to straighten the nasal septum and improve nasal cavity airflow. A septoplasty can be performed as an open procedure or endoscopically. During this surgery, mucoperichondrial and/or mucoperiosteal flaps are raised from the nasal septum. The deviated cartilage and/or bone are then selectively removed in order to straighten the nasal septum. Generally, the amount of cartilage and bone that is removed should be limited because excessive removal may predispose to a cosmetic nasal deformity.

Common indications for a septoplasty include symptomatic developmental or posttraumatic nasoseptal deviation. A septoplasty is frequently performed in combination with other sinus surgery during functional endoscopic sinus surgery, such as internal ethmoidectomies and uncinectomies.

A septoplasty can be suspected on CT imaging if there are partially or completely absent nasoseptal bones (ie, perpendicular plate of the ethmoid and vomer) or when the nasal septum is unusually straight.

COMPANION CASE

- **Septoplasty with a nasoseptal perforation.** Devascularization of the nasoseptal mucosa during a septoplasty, such as with the use of excessive electrocautery, can predispose to nasoseptal perforations.

Septoplasty

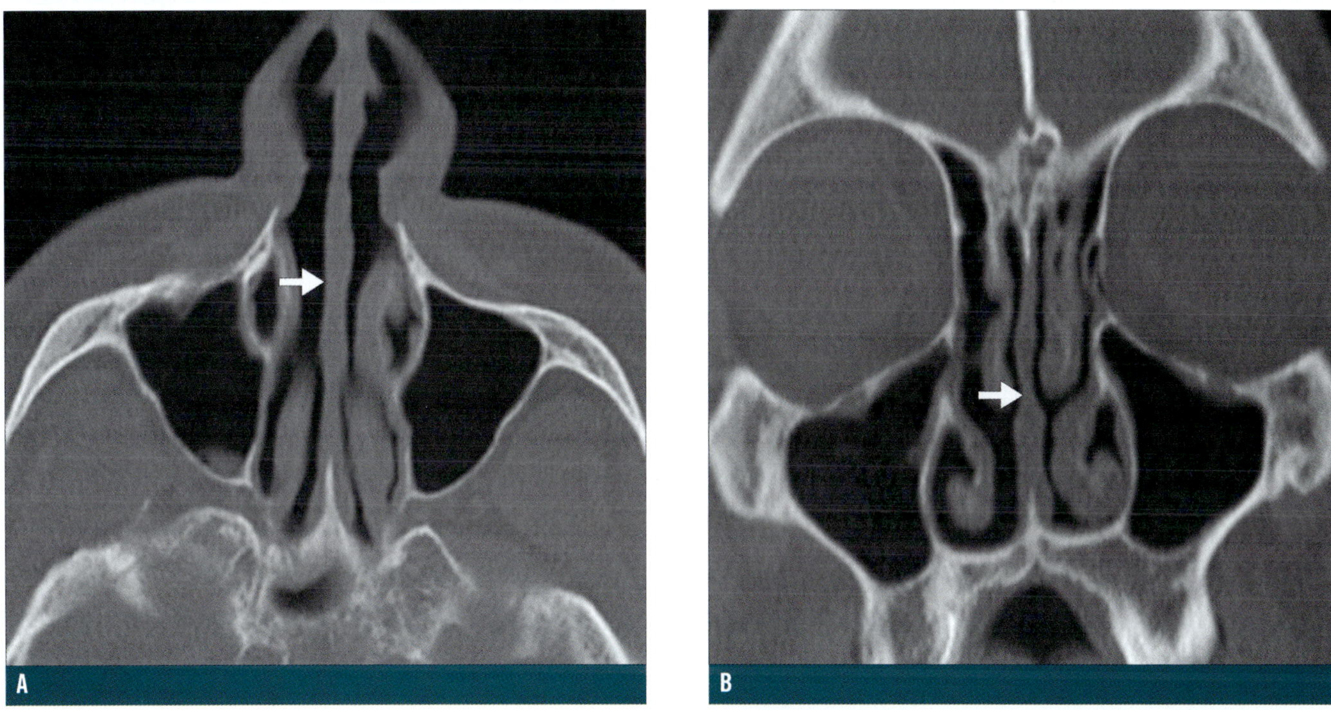

Axial (**A**) and coronal reformatted (**B**) CT images through the paranasal sinuses demonstrate a mostly absent osseous nasal a straightened nasal septum with most of its bones absent (arrows, **A, B**), compatible with a prior septoplasty.

Companion case: Septoplasty with a nasoseptal perforation

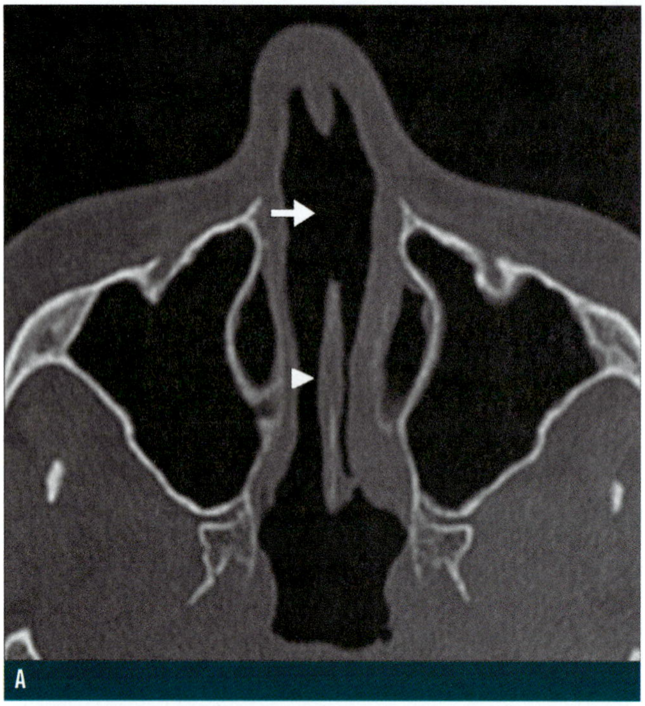

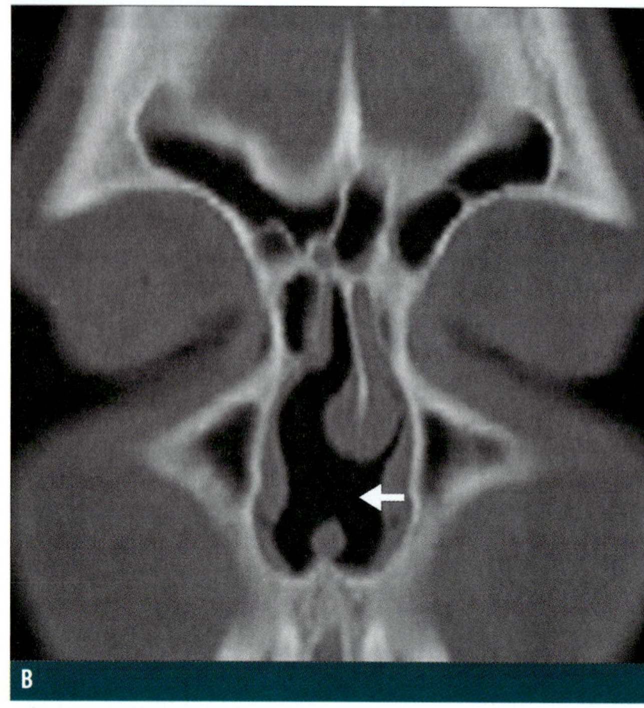

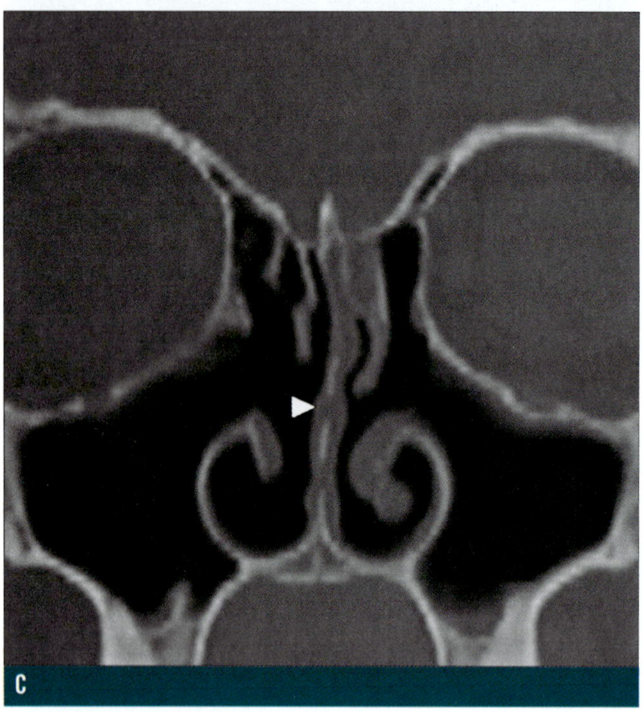

Axial (**A**) and coronal reformatted (**B**) CT images through the nasal cavity demonstrate a large nasoseptal perforation (arrows, **A**, **B**). An additional coronal reformatted CT image (**C**) as well as image A demonstrate septoplasty changes, as evidenced by straightening of the nasal septum with osseous discontinuity (arrowheads, **A**, **C**).

REFERENCES

Ketcham AS, Han JK. Complications and management of septoplasty. *Otolaryngol Clin N Am.* 2010;43:897-904.

Weber R, Hochapfel WD. Packing and stents in endonasal surgery. *Rhinology.* 2000;38:49-62.

CASE 45 Nasal cavity stents

Nasal stents are surgical products that are typically inserted on each side of the nasal septum at the conclusion of nasoseptal surgery. Nasal stents are intended to keep wound surfaces separated in order to prevent stenosis and adhesions as well as to aid in wound healing. These surgical products can be made from various materials, including silicone (Silastic), polyethylene, and polyurethane.

COMPANION CASES

- **Nasal breathing tubes.** These surgical products share the same benefits as nasal stents but also improve the patency of the nasal airway because of their hollow chambers.
- **Nasal balloon.** A nasal balloon is used to control nasal epistaxis. These devices may have lubricated fabric to ease placement. Once placed, air is injected in the balloon in order to tamponade the bleeding source. An external cuff connected to the balloon is used to monitor the pressure.
- **Nasal packing.** Nasal packing is placed in the nasal cavity in order to control epistaxis from various causes, including following a septoplasty. Nasal packing may also serve to stabilize the nasal septum, prevent synechiae formation, and prevent restenosis. Several types of nasal packing products have been used, including latex rubber packed with foam, gauze, cellulose, a colloidal suspension of irradiated polyethylene oxide and water, and gelfoam.

  Nasal packing provides the ideal medium for bacterial growth and increases the risk of toxic shock syndrome following a septoplasty. The risk of toxic shock syndrome following a septoplasty is estimated to be under 0.02%, although it is fatal in 10% of patients who contract it. Therefore, nasal packing should be removed as soon as it is deemed to no longer provide additional benefit.
- **Rhinolith.** Rhinoliths are relatively rare masses that can arise from endogenous causes (pus, fungus, etc) or from exogenous causes (ie, various foreign bodies). Rhinoliths may increase in size over time and patients may present with nasal obstruction, purulent rhinorrhea, epistaxis, headache, and halitosis.

Nasal stents

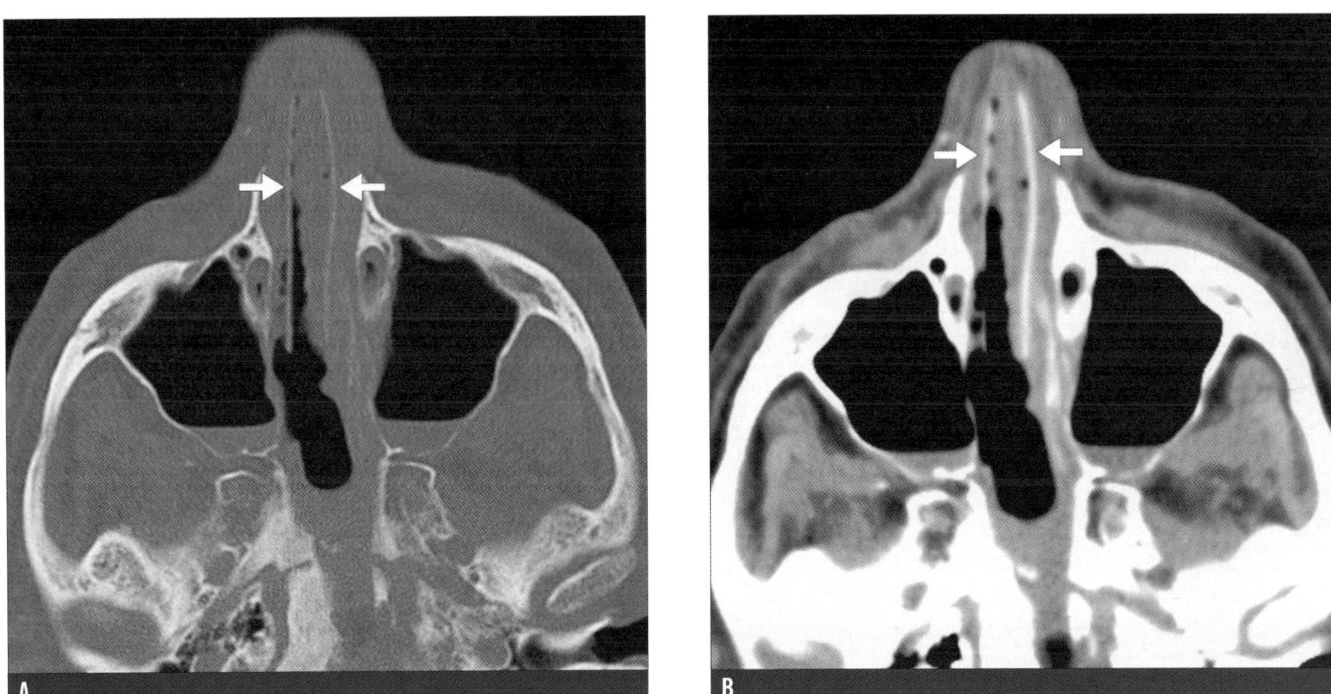

Axial CT images viewed with a bone window (**A**) and soft tissue window (**B**) as well as coronal reformatted CT images viewed with a bone window (**C**, **D**) demonstrate linear hyperdense surgical prostheses in the bilateral aspects of the nasal cavity representing Silastic stents (arrows, **A-D**). These were placed at the conclusion of septoplasty surgery to help prevent the formation of synechiae/stenosis as well as to promote healing.

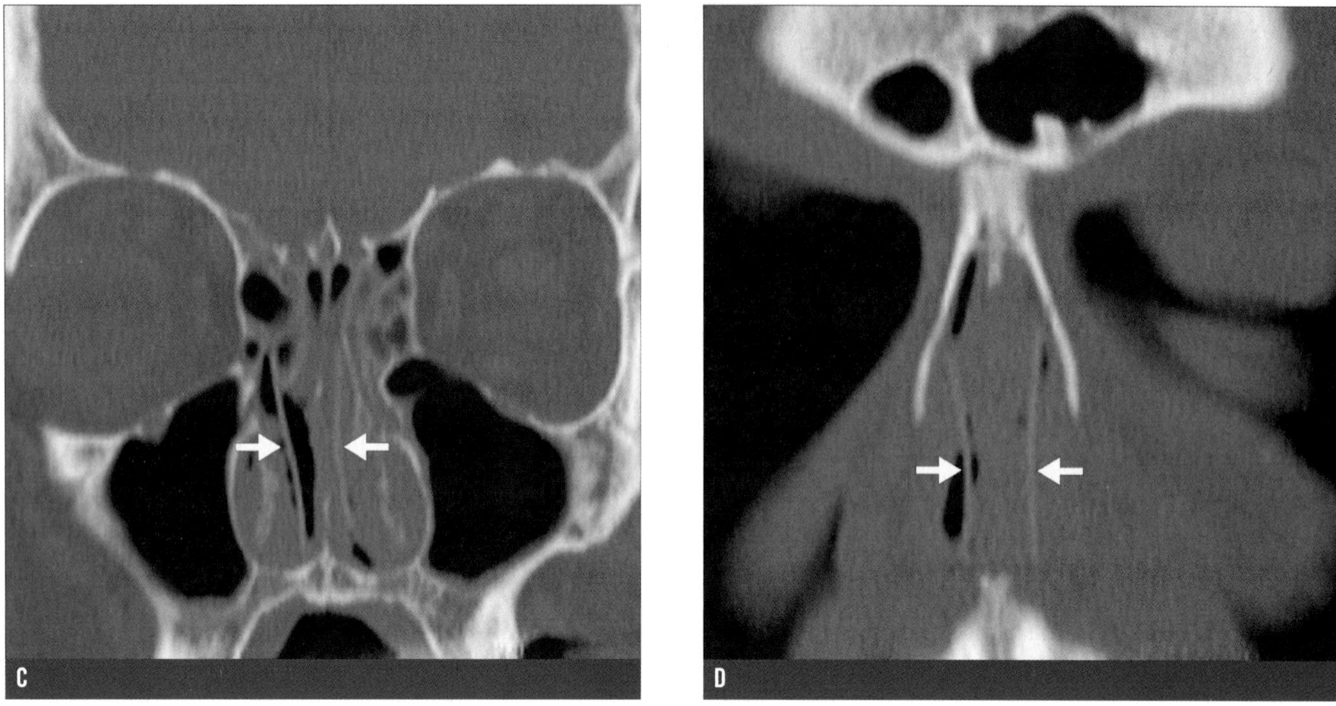

Companion case: Nasal breathing tubes

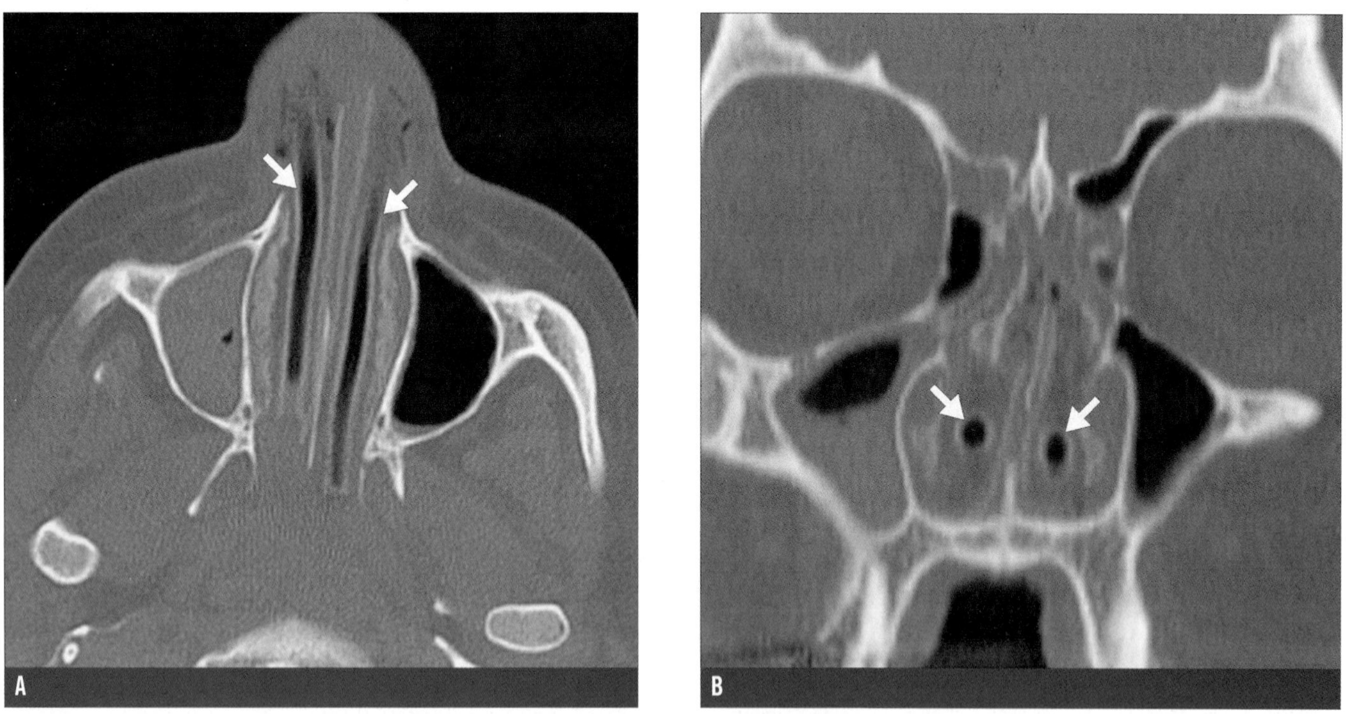

Axial (**A**), coronal reformatted (**B**), and sagittal reformatted (**C**) CT images demonstrate nasal breathing tubes in the bilateral aspects of the nasal cavity (arrows, **A-C**). These were placed to help prevent the formation of synechiae/stenosis and to aid in breathing following surgery.

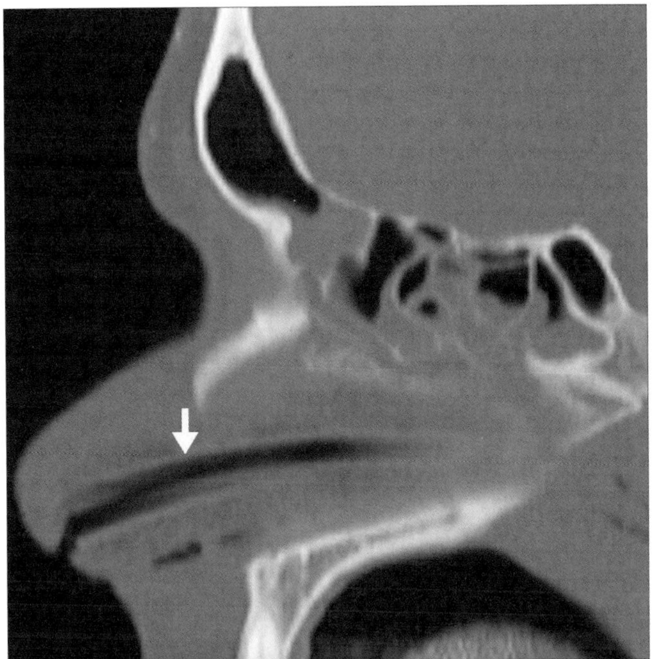

C

Companion case: Nasal balloon

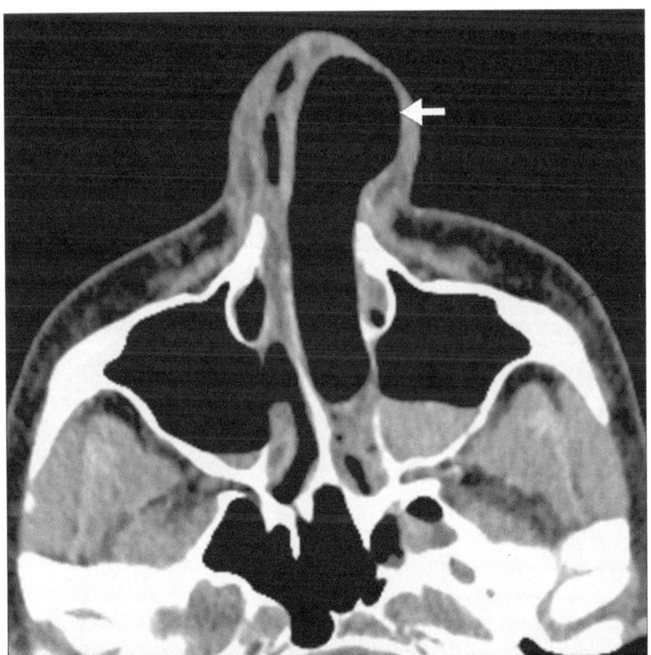

A

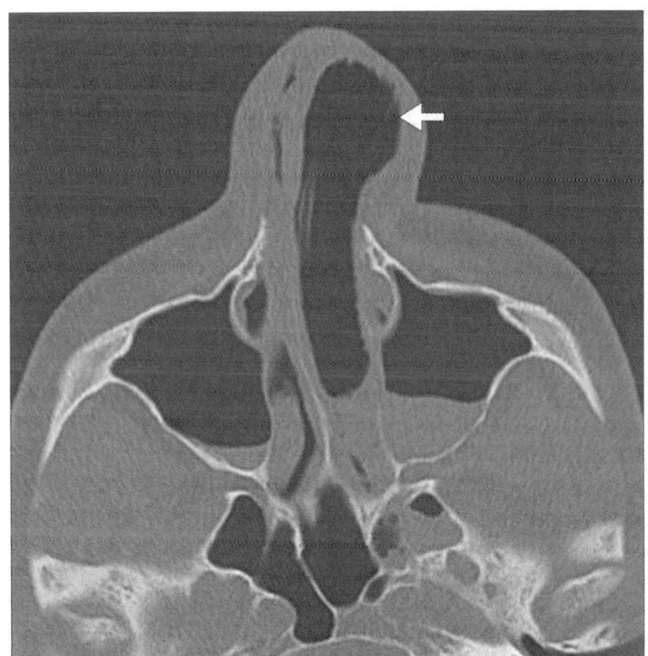

B

Axial CT images viewed with a soft tissue window (**A**) and bone window (**B**) as well as coronal reformatted (**C**) and sagittal reformatted (**D**) CT images viewed with a bone window demonstrate expansion of the left nasal vestibule and left aspect of the nasal cavity with a nasal balloon (arrows, **A-D**). The nasal balloon was placed to control epistaxis. An associated catheter can be identified within the balloon.

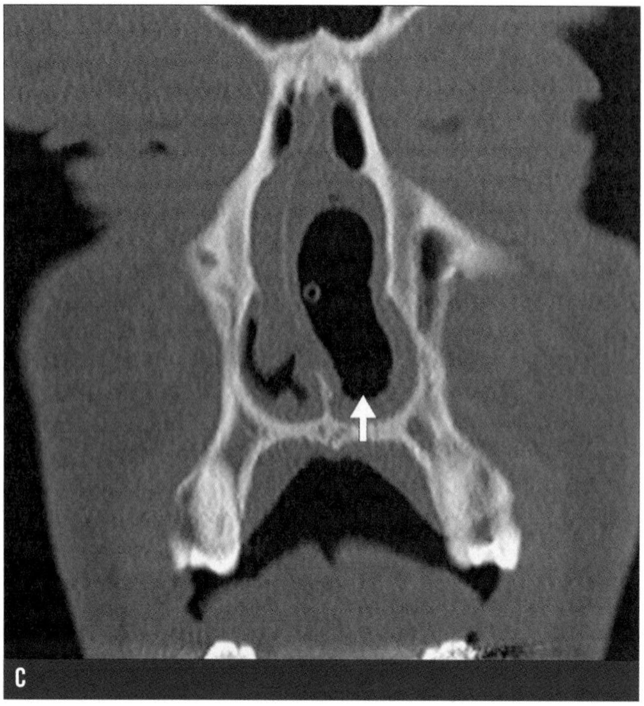

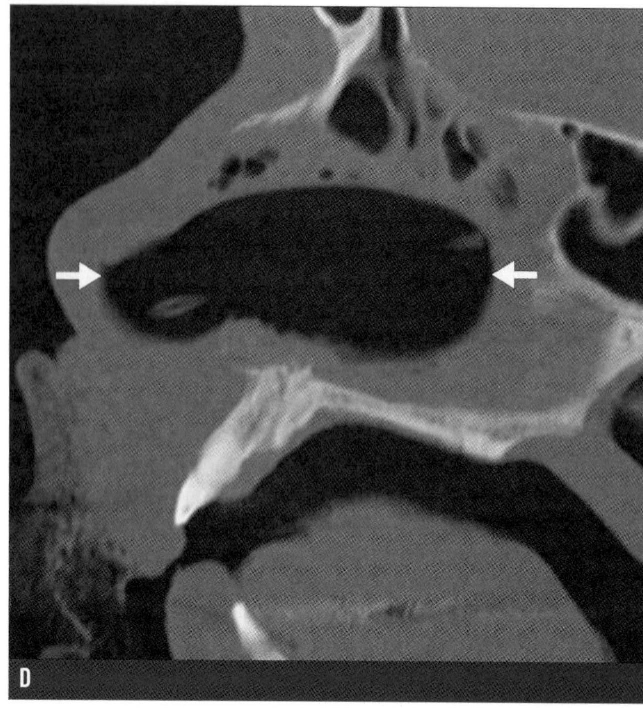

Companion case: Nasal packing

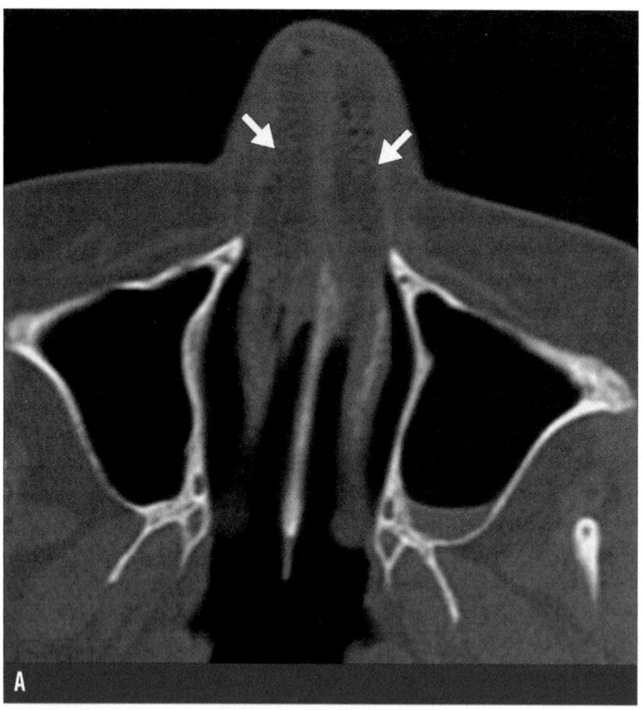

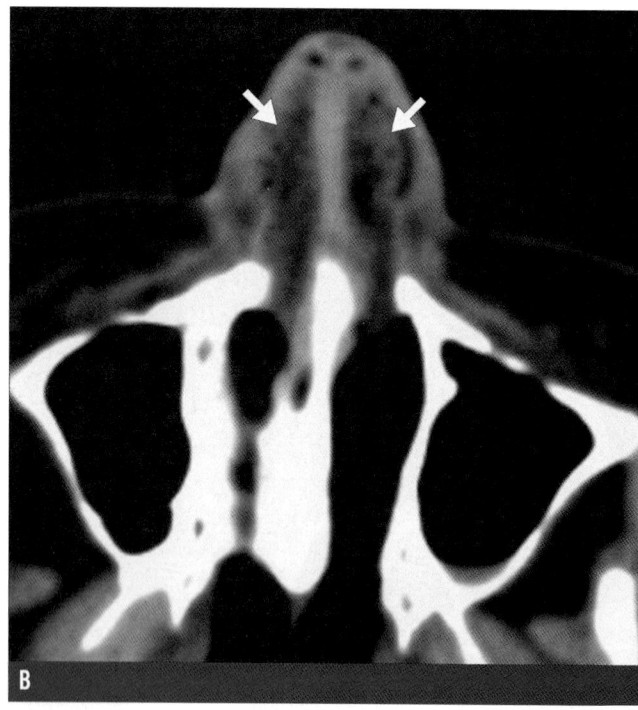

Axial CT images viewed with a bone window **(A)** and soft tissue window **(B)** as well as a coronal reformatted CT image viewed with a bone window **(C)** demonstrate opacification of the nasal vestibules with packing material (arrows, **A-C**). There are small foci of air interspersed within this nasal packing which is often identified with gauze or other similar nasal packing materials used for hemostasis.

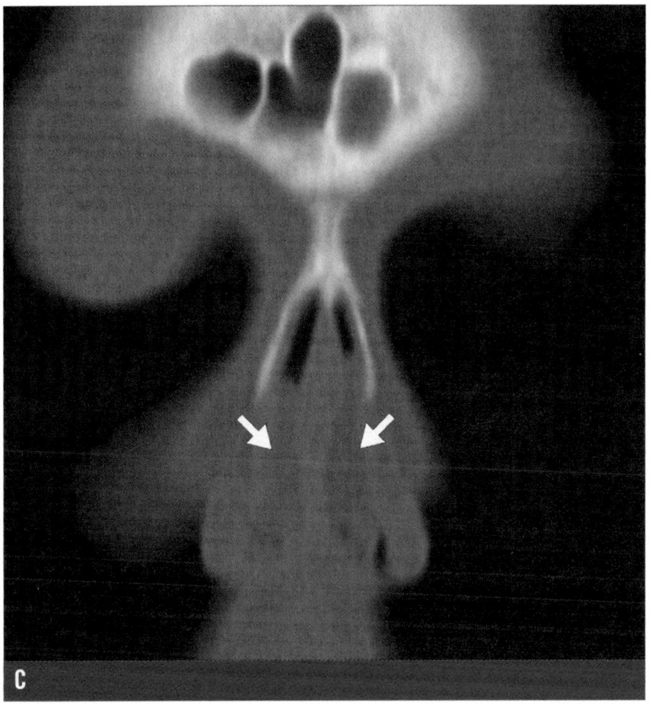

Companion case: Nasal packing

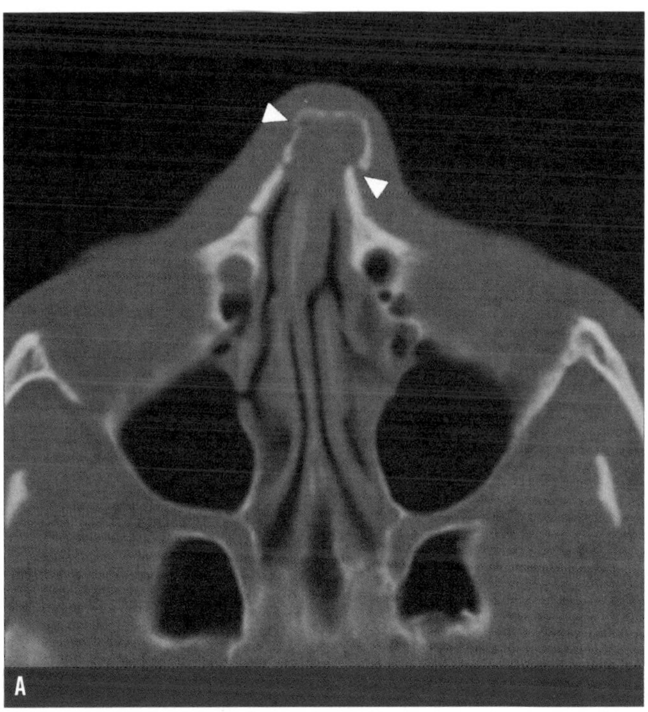

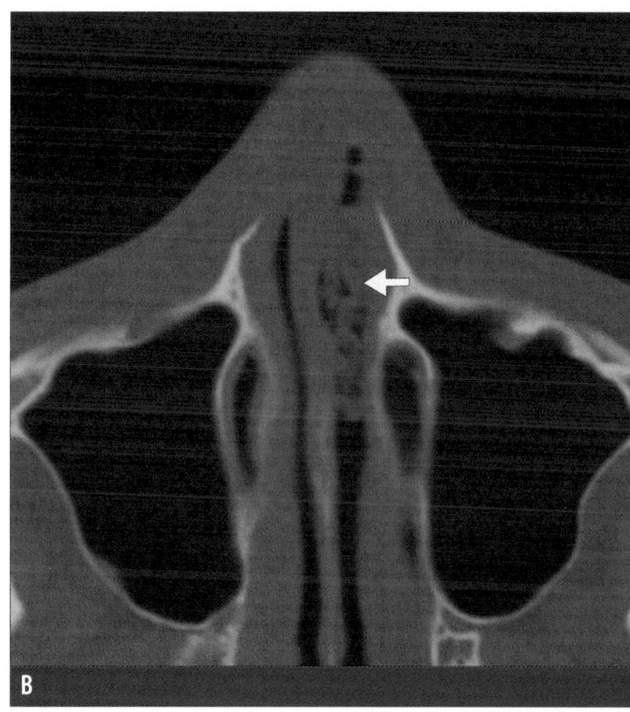

Different patient. Axial (**A-C**), coronal reformatted (**D**), and sagittal reformatted (**E**) CT images demonstrate fractures of the nasal bones (arrowheads, **A, D, E**) and a lobulated foreign body located in the left aspect of the nasal cavity and nasal vestibule (arrows, **B-E**). This foreign body contains small interspersed air pockets and is consistent with nasal packing used for hemostasis.

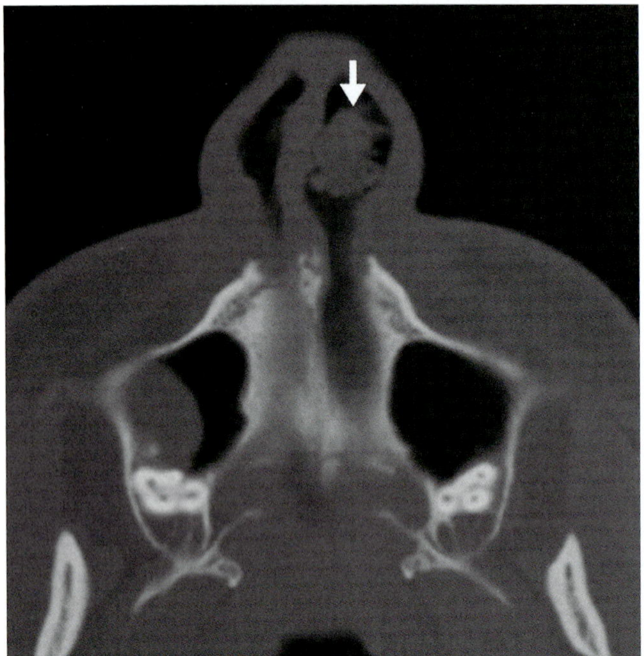

C

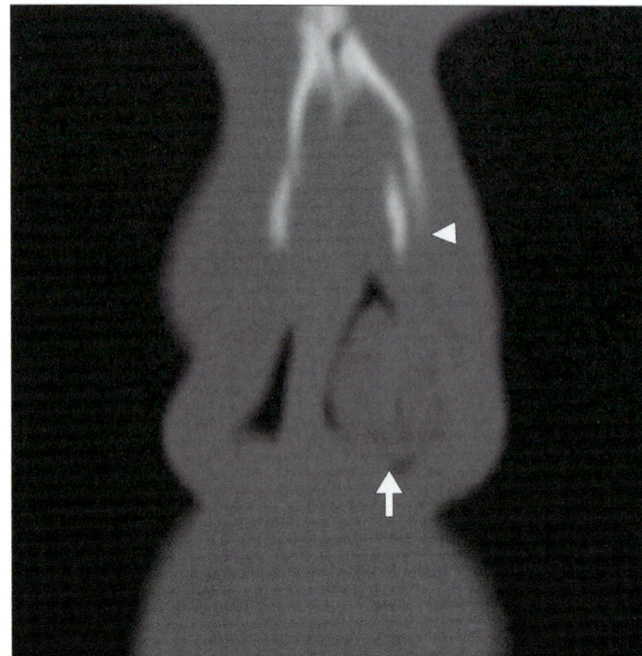

D

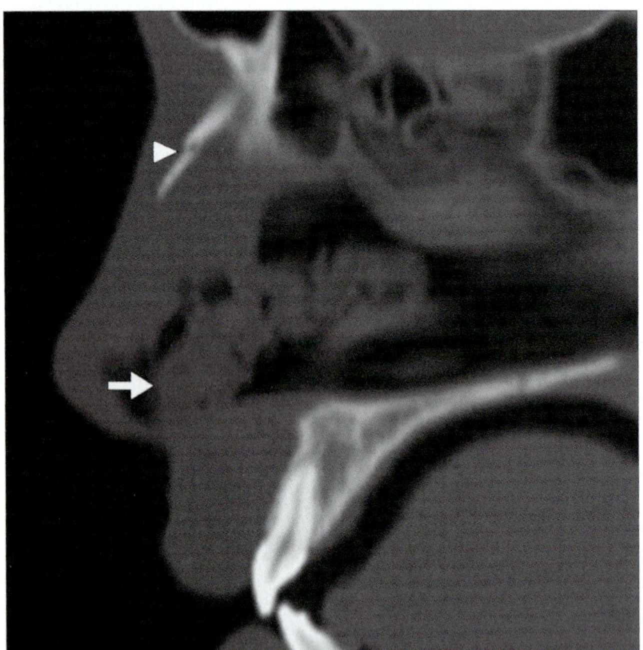

E

Companion case: Rhinolith

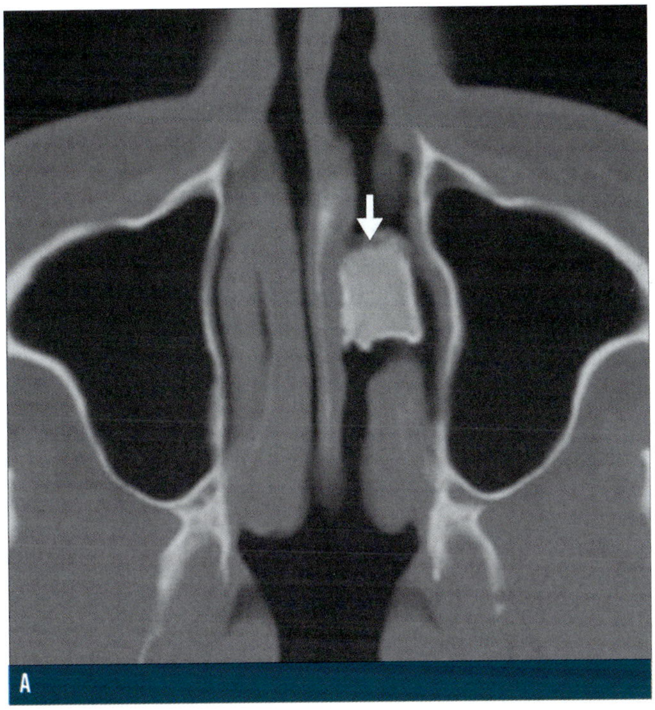

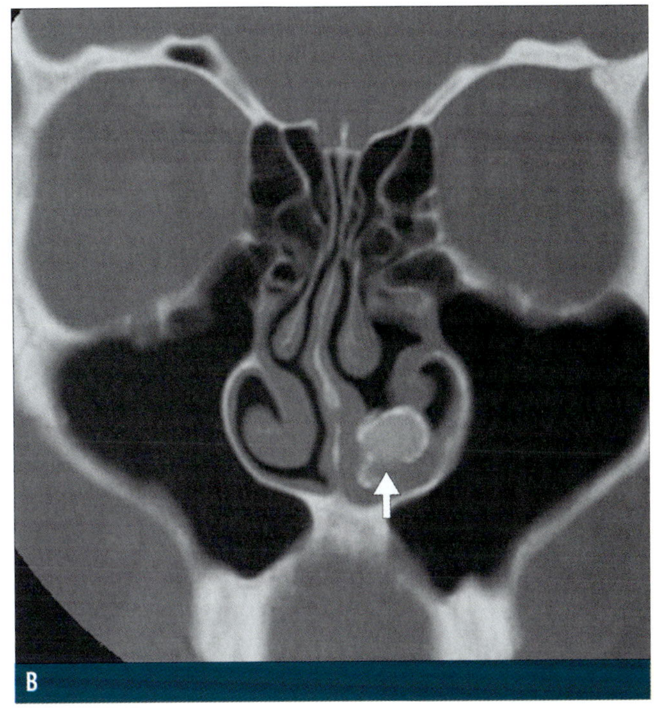

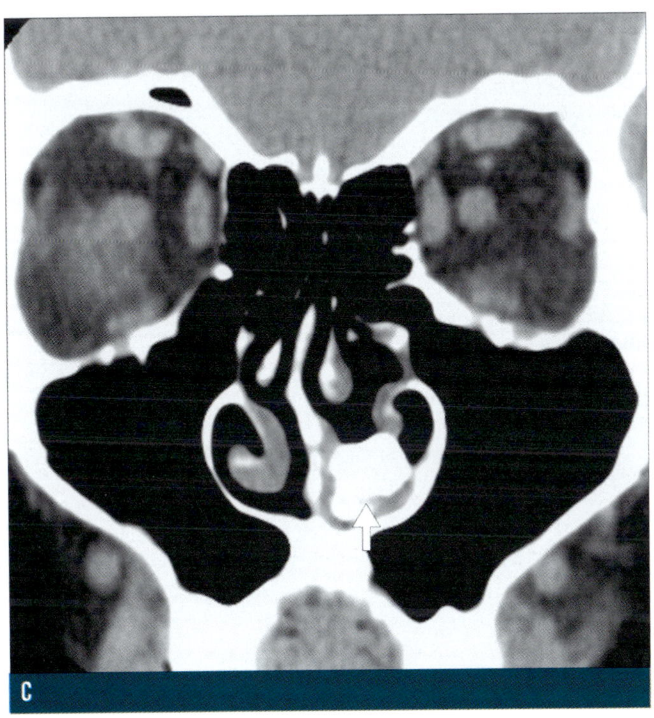

Axial (**A**) and coronal reformatted (**B**) CT images viewed with a bone window as well as a coronal reformatted CT image viewed with a soft tissue window (**C**) obtained through the nasal cavity. The images demonstrate an ossified mass (arrows, **A-C**) that is distinct from the nasal septum and left inferior turbinate. This was a mineralized foreign body at surgery. At pathology, it was described as a foreign body (polarizable) with bacterial colonization, calcium encrustation, and an admixture of respiratory epithelium with acute inflammatory cells. The imaging and pathology are consistent with a rhinolith.

REFERENCES

Brehmer D. The rhinolith-a possible differential diagnosis of a unilateral nasal obstruction. *Case Rep Med.* 2010;2010:845671.

Ketcham AS, Han JK. Complications and management of septoplasty. *Otolaryngol Clin N Am.* 2010;43:897-904.

Orhan K, et al. Rhinolithiasis: an uncommon entity of the nasal cavity. *Oral Surg Oral Med Oral Pathol Oral Radiol Endod.* 2006;101(2):e28-e32.

Ozdemir S, et al. Rhinolithiasis: review of 21 cases. *Am J Rhinol Allergy.* 2010;24(6):136-139.

Weber R, Hochaptel WD. Packing and stents in endonasal surgery. *Rhinology.* 2000;38:49-62.

CHAPTER 7

SKULL BASE AND INFRATEMPORAL FOSSA

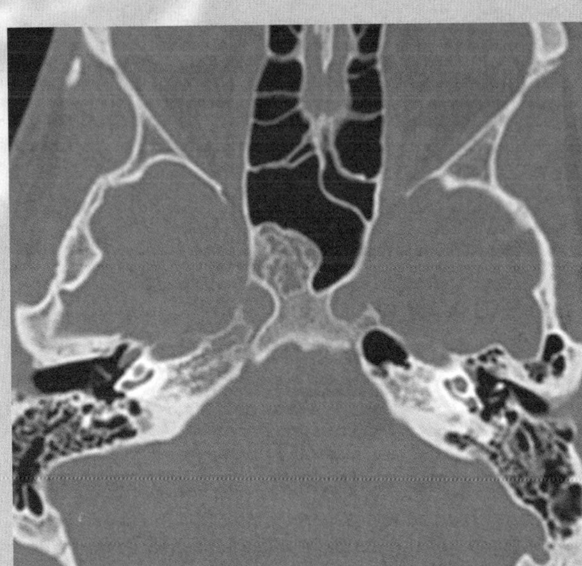

Achilles G. Karagianis

VII. SKULL BASE AND INFRATEMPORAL FOSSA

1. Spheno-occipital synchondrosis
2. Canalis basilaris medianus
3. Ecchordosis physaliphora
  i. *Companion case*: Classic clival chordoma
  ii. *Companion case*: Poorly differentiated clival chordoma
  iii. *Companion case*: Petroclival synchondrosis chondrosarcoma
4. Clival lipoma
5. Arrested pneumatization of the skull base
  i. *Companion case*: Fibrous dysplasia
  ii. *Companion case*: Skull base metastatic disease
6. Anterior clinoid process pneumatization simulating an aneurysm
7. Asymmetric sphenoid sinus pneumatization simulating a lesion on MRI
  i. *Companion case*: Intraosseous meningioma
8. Asymmetric sphenoid sinus pneumatization deforming the sella turcica
  i. *Companion case*: Pneumatization of the dorsum sella
9. Interclinoid bar
10. Occipital bone air cell
  i. *Companion case*: Fluid-filled occipital bone air cell
11. Crista galli pneumatization
  i. *Companion case*: Ossified crista galli
  ii. *Companion case*: Crista galli pneumosinus dilatans with an associated meningioma
12. Normal ethmoidal grooves
  i. *Companion case*: Anterior skull base fracture
  ii. *Companion case*: Anterior ethmoidal artery fistula
  iii. *Companion case*: Posterior ethmoidal canals
13. Orbital roof diploic veins
  i. *Companion case*: Anterior skull base fracture
14. Arachnoid granulations
  i. *Companion case*: Middle cranial fossa arachnoid cysts with adjacent osseous remodeling
  ii. *Companion case*: Brain herniation into the transverse dural venous sinus
  iii. *Companion case*: Middle cranial fossa meningocele
  iv. *Companion case*: Encephalocele and CSF leak associated with idiopathic intracranial hypertension
15. Meckel cave cephalocele
  i. *Companion case*: Intrasellar cephalocele herniating into the clivus
  ii. *Companion case*: Hypoplastic Meckel cave
16. Incidental asymmetric enlargement of the foramen ovale
  i. *Companion case*: Foramen ovale meningocele
  ii. *Companion case*: Foramen rotundum meningocele
17. Foramen Vesalius
18. Foramen spinosum
  i. *Companion case*: Absent and hypoplastic foramina spinosum
  ii. *Companion case*: Bifurcated foramen spinosum
19. Canaliculus innominatus
20. Iatrogenic venous air at the skull base
21. Iophendylate (Pantopaque) contrast at the skull base
22. Lateral pterygoid plate foramen simulating a fracture
23. Normal pterygoid venous plexus
  i. *Companion case*: Internal maxillary veins draining the pterygoid venous plexuses
  ii. *Companion case*: Venous plexuses surrounding the temporomandibular joints
24. The parapharyngeal space and normal pharyngeal venous plexus
  i. *Companion case*: Air in the pharyngeal venous plexus
  ii. *Companion case*: Prestyloid parapharyngeal space pleomorphic adenoma
  iii. *Companion case*: Poststyloid parapharyngeal space glomus vagale
25. CN V, V3 denervation atrophy
26. Normal pterygopalatine fossa enhancement
27. Postoperative pterygopalatine fossa appearance
  i. *Companion case*: Perineural spread along the pterygopalatine fossae
28. MRI susceptibility artifact in the retromaxillary fat pad and pterygopalatine fossa
29. Normal CN III in the cavernous sinus
  i. *Companion case:* Abnormal enhancement of CN III
30. Normal enhancing venous plexuses of the CN V, V2 and V3 divisions as well as of the Meckel cave
  i. *Companion case*: Asymmetrically enlarged but normal Meckel cave enhancing venous plexus
  ii. *Companion case*: Presumed schwannoma of the CN V, V2 division and pterygopalatine fossa
  iii. *Companion case*: Presumed CN V, V3 division schwannoma
  iv. Perineural spread of tumor along the CN V, V2 and V3 divisions as well as the vidian nerve
  V. *Companion case*: Meckel cave schwannoma or meningioma
  VI. *Companion case*: Meckel cave "white" epidermoid
31. Meckel cave CN V rootlets
  i. *Companion case*: Pathologically enhancing Meckel cave rootlets
32. Normal sensory and motor roots of the CN V cisternal segment
33. The jugular foramen and pars nervosa
  i. *Companion case*: Nonocclusive distal sigmoid venous sinus and jugular bulb thrombus
  ii. *Companion case*: CN IX-XI complex schwannoma
  iii. *Companion case*: CT occult glomus jugulare tumor
34. Normal spinal accessory nerve root
  i. *Companion case*: Presumed spinal accessory nerve schwannoma
35. Normal hypoglossal canal enhancement
  i. *Companion case*: Asymmetrically enlarged anterior condylar vein
  ii. *Companion case*: CN XII meningioma
  iii. *Companion case*: CN XII schwannoma
36. Mastoid emissary veins
  i. *Companion case*: Mildly enlarged mastoid emissary vein in Crouzon syndrome
  ii. *Companion case*: Acquired occipital bone vascular channels related to an arteriovenous fistula
37. Posterior condylar canal and vein
38. Petrosquamosal sinus
39. Occipital sinus
40. Air-tissue interface artifact on 3T MRI

CASE 1 Spheno-occipital synchondrosis

A synchondrosis is a cartilaginous joint between two bones which allows for growth until the cartilage ossifies. The spheno-occipital synchondrosis is located between the sphenoid and occipital bones, residing approximately in the middle of the clivus. The age at which the spheno-occipital synchondrosis fuses varies among studies and may vary among ancestry. In a study by Bassed, et al analyzing the spheno-occipital synchondrosis in the Australian population, fusion was well underway by the age of 15 and essentially fused by 17. According to this study, females showed a greater degree of fusion than males at age 15, but completely fused at essentially the same age. The synchondrosis fuses from cephalad to caudad and a scar in the clivus can be seen up to the age of 25.

Spheno-occipital synchondrosis

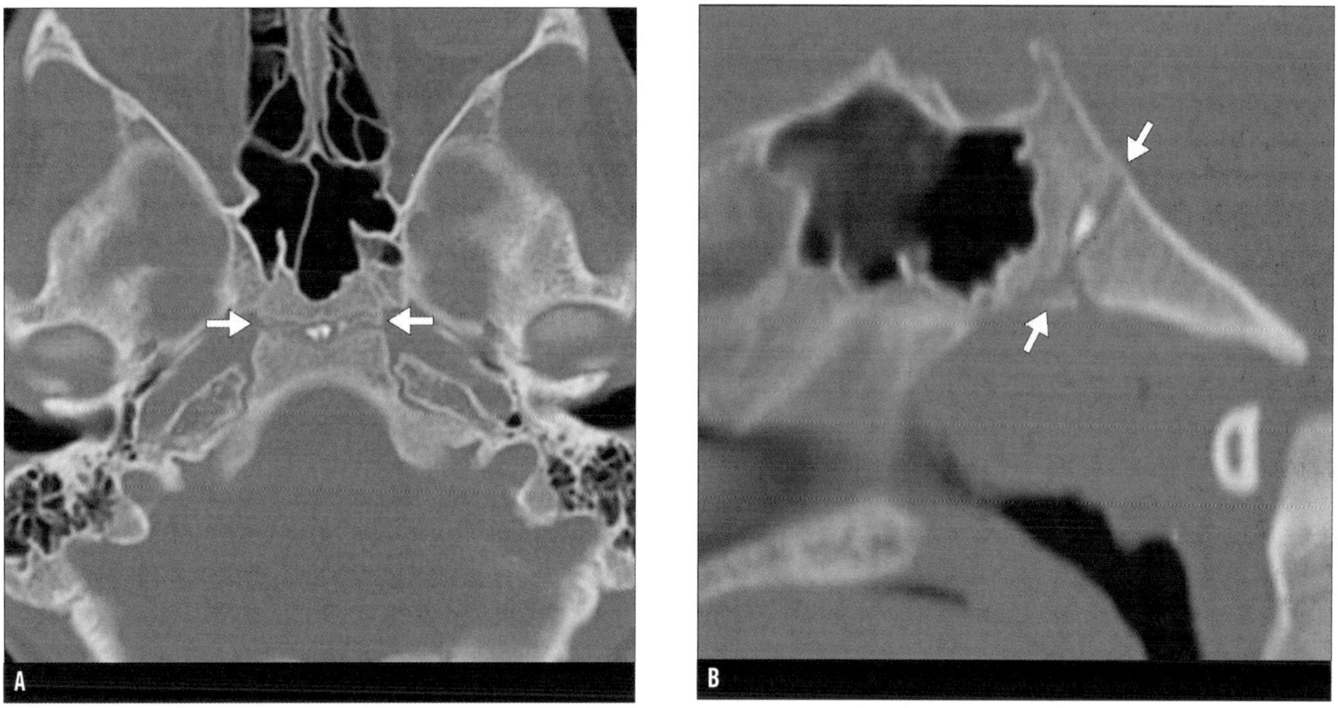

Axial (**A**) and sagittal reformatted (**B**) CT images demonstrate the normal spheno-occipital synchondrosis in a 14-year-old (arrows). The high density within the synchondrosis likely reflects early ossification and partial fusion of the synchondrosis.

REFERENCES

Bassed RB, Briggs C, Drummer OH. Analysis of time of closure of the spheno-occipital synchondrosis using computed tomography. *Forensic Sci Int*. 2010;200(1-3):161-164. Epub May 2010.

S Standring, ed. *Grays Anatomy: The Anatomical Basis of Clinical Practice*. 39th ed. Edinburgh: Elsevier Churchill Livingstone; 2005.

CASE 2 Canalis basilaris medianus

The canalis basilaris medianus (CBM) is characterized as a well-defined osseous channel that is located primarily at the midline of the basiocciput. A total of six types of CBM have been described, three complete and three incomplete.

The complete forms are as follows:

- Superior: A cleft along the posterior margin of the clivus that forms a small ossicle
- Inferior: A cleft extending through the entire inferior aspect of the clivus from anterior to posterior
- Bifurcated: Same as the inferior form, but also forming a separate small ossicle along its posterior margin

The incomplete forms are as follows:

- Superior basiocciput recess: An incomplete notch along the posterior margin of the clivus.
- Inferior basiocciput recess: An incomplete notch along the ventral margin of the clivus. Other literature describes this form of CBM as the fossa navicularis magna.
- Long channel in the basiocciput and posterior sphenoid: A vertically oriented channel extending the length of the sphenoid body and basiocciput.

The incomplete forms of CBM are considered anatomic variants and almost always of no clinical significance. One case of clival osteomyelitis has been described in the setting of a pharyngeal abscess that spread into the clivus via a fossa navicularis magna (inferior basiocciput recess type). In addition, rare descriptions of meningitis have been reported with the complete forms of CBM, in particular those which allow for a communication between the intracranial compartment and the nasopharynx.

There are two theories describing the etiology of a CBM, one describing that it represents the cephalad aspect of a notochordal remnant, and the other describing that it represents a vascular channel for the basivertebral vein. However, the general consensus seems to favor a notochordal remnant etiology.

A craniopharyngeal canal, while having a similar morphology and involving the same region, can be distinguished from a CBM. In contradistinction to a CBM, a craniopharyngeal canal extends from the floor of the sella to the level of the nasopharynx. There have been reports of cephalocele and pituitary gland herniation through a large, patent craniopharyngeal canal.

Incomplete CBM: Inferior basiocciput recess type (fossa navicularis magna)

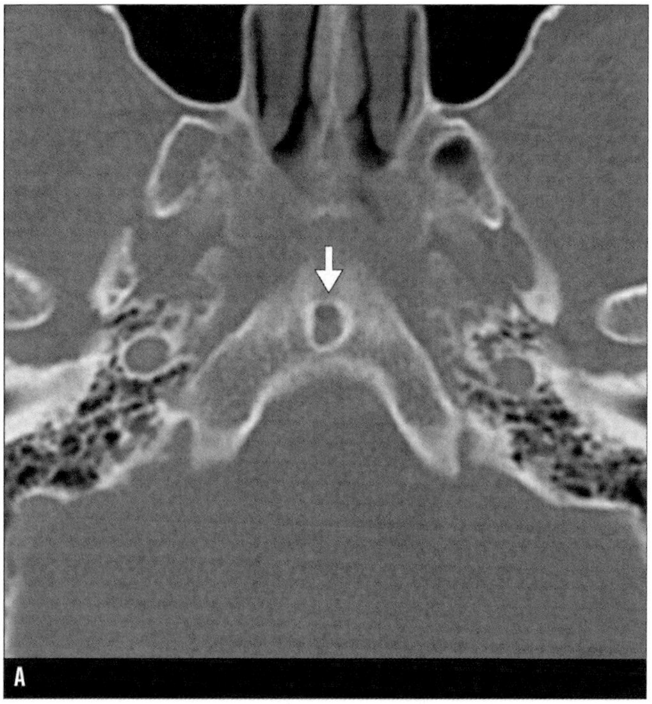

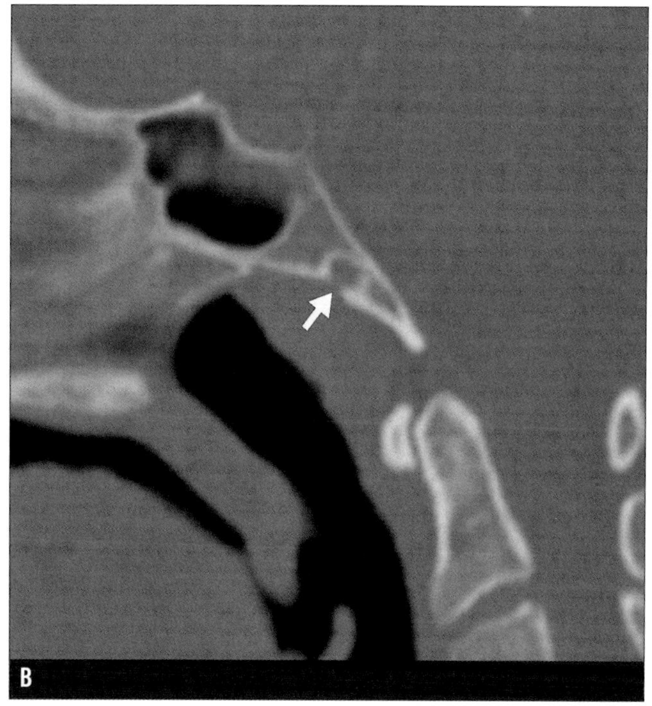

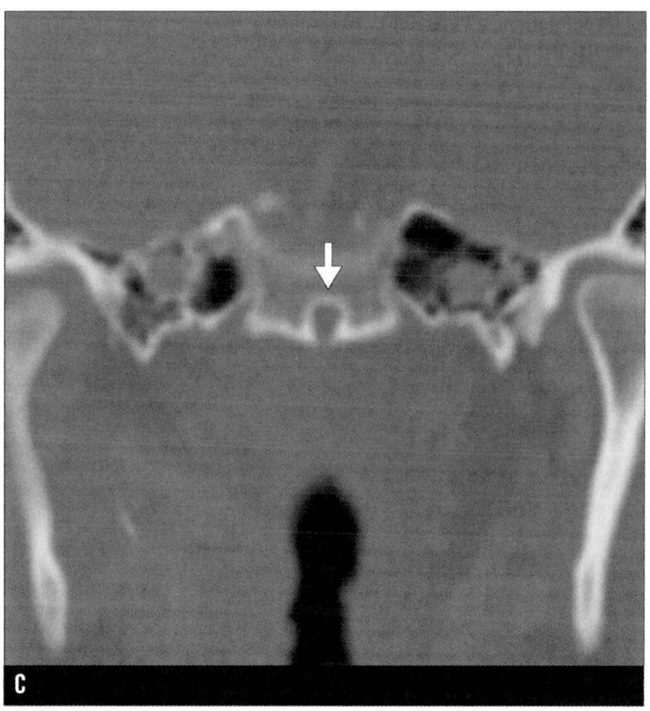

Axial (**A**), sagittal reformatted (**B**), and coronal reformatted (**C**) CT images demonstrate a well-defined osseous notch with sclerotic margins along the ventral basioccipital portion of the clivus, consistent with the inferior basiocciput recess type of an incomplete canalis basilaris medianus (arrows, **A**-**C**).

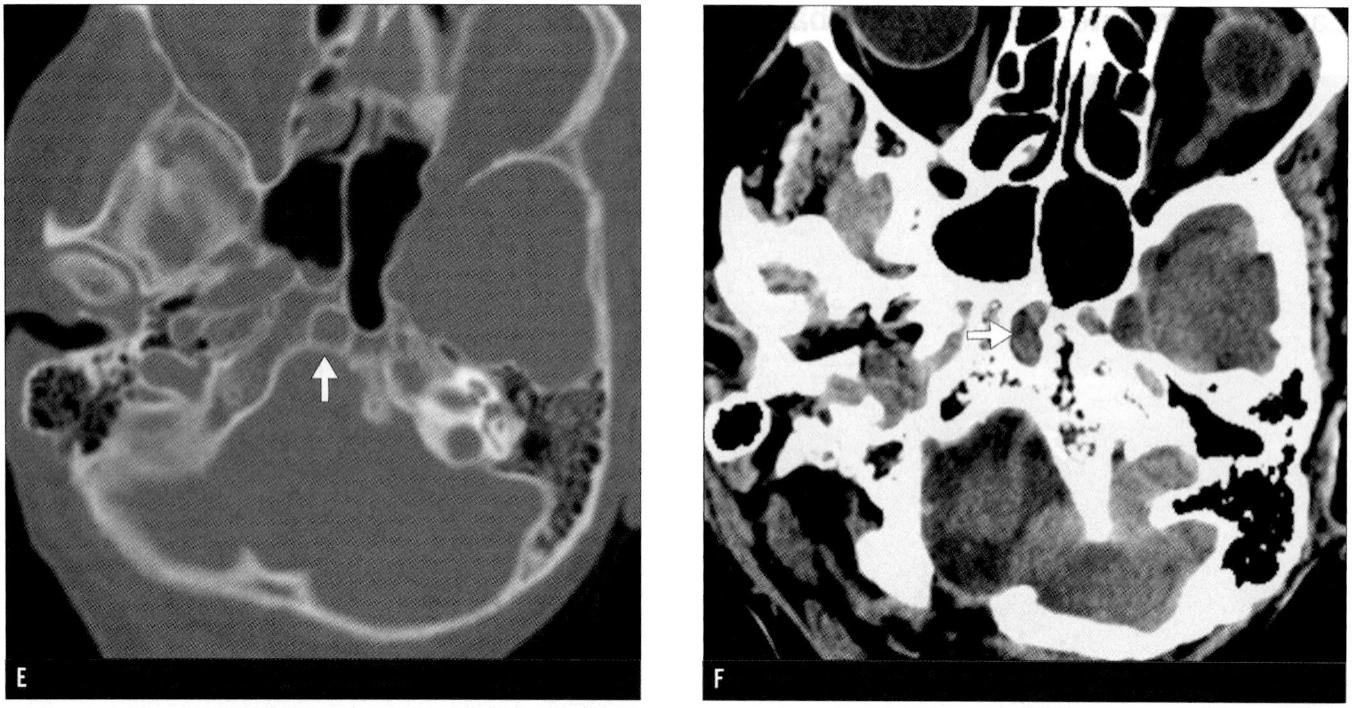

Incomplete CBM: Superior basiocciput recess type

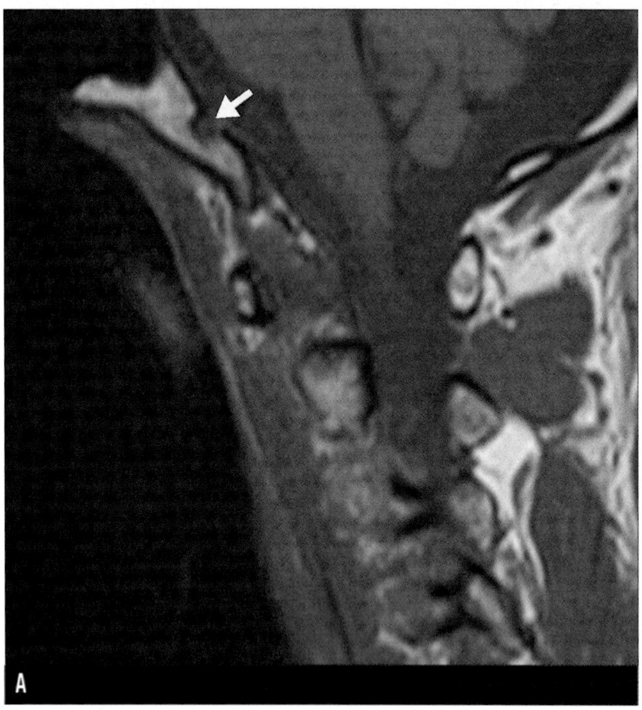

A sagittal T1-weighted MR image (**A**) demonstrates a discrete osseous notch along the posterior basioccipital aspect of the clivus (arrow), compatible with the superior basiocciput recess type of an incomplete canalis basilaris medianus.

Incomplete CBM: Long channel in basiocciput

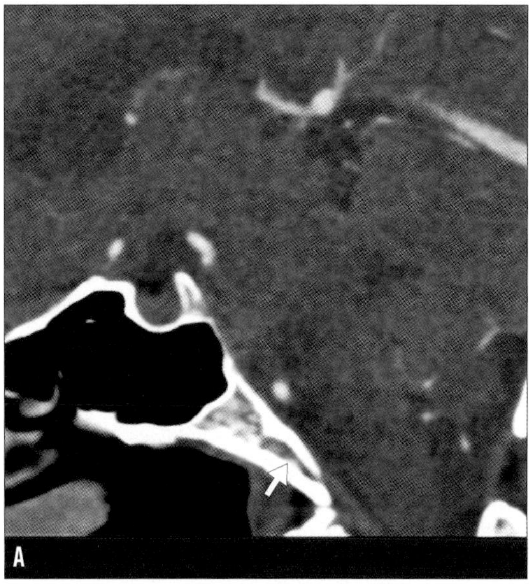

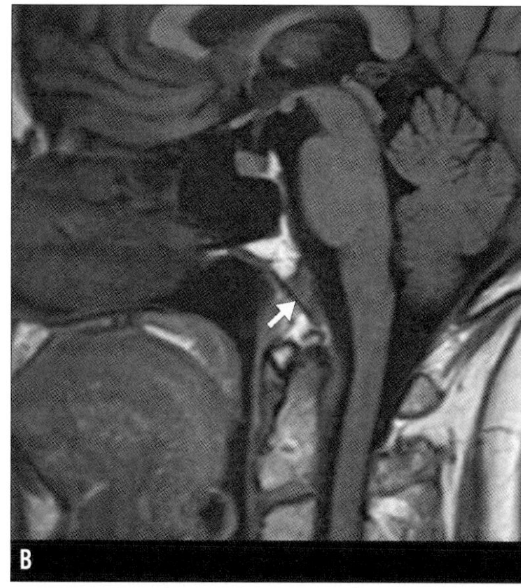

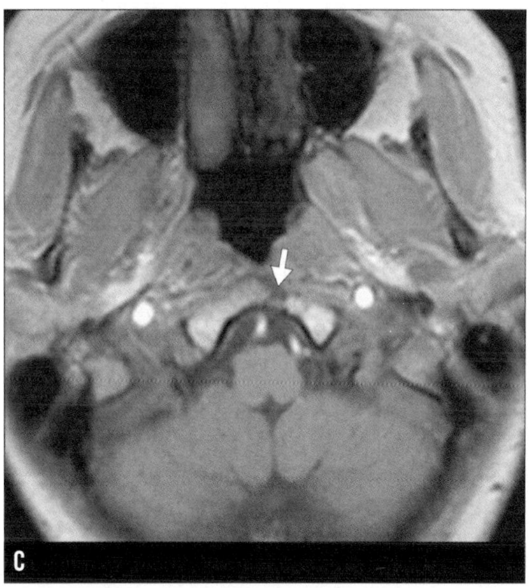

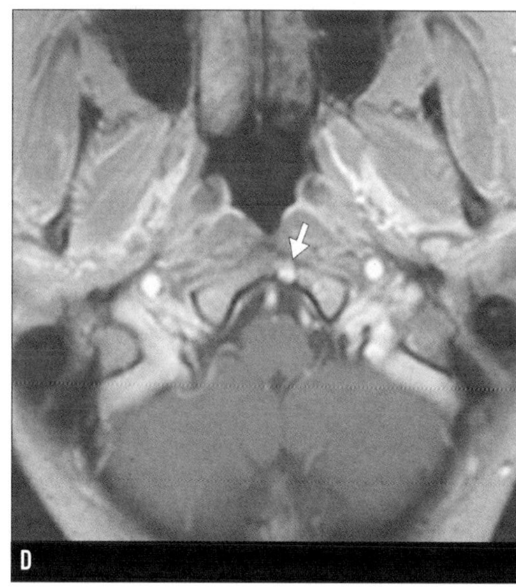

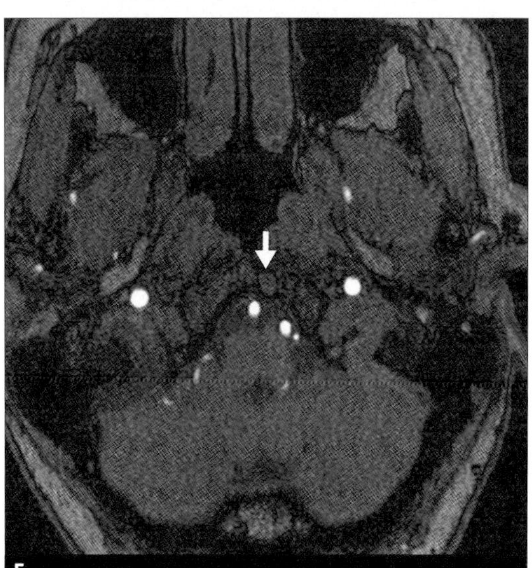

A postcontrast sagittal reformatted CT image (**A**) demonstrates a subtle channel extending along the length of the basioccipital portion of the clivus, compatible with a canalis basilaris medianus (arrow, **A**). Unenhanced sagittal T1 (**B**), unenhanced axial T1 (**C**), and contrast-enhanced axial T1 (**D**) MR images demonstrate the same finding on MRI (arrows, **B**-**D**). Image **D** demonstrates an enhancing vessel within the canalis medianus basilaris (arrow, **D**). An axial time-of-flight MRA source image (**E**) does not demonstrate arterial flow-related signal within this vessel, verifying that the enhancing vessel in the basiocciput is venous (arrow, **E**). At least in this case, the canalis basilaris is vascular in etiology, rather than a notochordal remnant etiology.

REFERENCES

Currarino G. Canalis basilaris medianus and related defects of the basiocciput. *AJNR Am J Neuroradiol.* 1988;9:208-211.

Jacquemin C, Bosley TM, al Saleh M, Mullaney P. Canalis basilaris medianus: MRI. *Neuroradiology.* 2000;42(2):121-123.

Prabhu SP, Zinkus T, Cheng AG, Rahbar R. Clival osteomyelitis resulting from spread of infection through the fossa navicularis magna in a child. *Pediatr Radiol.* 2009;39(9):995-998.

Schick B, Prescher A, Hofmann E, Steigerwald C, Draf W. Two occult skull base malformations causing recurrent meningitis in a child: a case report. *Eur Arch Otorhinolaryngol.* 2003;260(9):518-521. Epub May 2003.

CASE 3 Ecchordosis physaliphora

During development of the axial skeleton, the notochord becomes incorporated into the spine and contributes to the formation of the intervertebral disc nucleus pulposus. However, at the clival and sacral regions, the incorporation of the notochord into the spine is more variable, often resulting in notochordal variants in each of these areas. The notochord has a sinuous course in the clivus, extending to the clival surface three times. They are, from inferior to superior the posterior clivus, pharyngeal surface, and dorsum sella. Notochordal remnants can be identified in each of these locations, including the Tornwlaldt cyst (along the pharyngeal surface), most believe the canalis basilaris medianus (along the ventral and/or posterior clivus), and the ecchordosis physaliphora (EP) (posterior to the dorsum sella/clivus).

While EP may be identified anywhere along the spinal axis, it is most frequently identified at the midline immediately posterior to the clivus and dorsum sella. EP is a gelatinous excrescence, and it may be intradural or extradural. If intradural, a thin stalk may be identified extending toward the clivus. EP is found in up to 2% of autopsies.

On MRI, EP is T1 hypointense and T2 hyperintense, often appearing as a grape-like collection of small foci. EP does not enhance, in contradistinction to a chordoma, which variably enhances. While there may be mild irregularity along the dorsal clivus, there is no clival destruction with EP, also a differentiating feature compared to a chordoma, which usually destroys the adjacent clivus. However, it should be noted that small biopsy samples of EP may not be able to be distinguished from a chordoma on histology or immunohistochemistry. EP is usually asymptomatic, although cases of hemorrhage and cranial nerve palsies have been described.

COMPANION CASE

- **Classic clival chordoma.** Chordomas are slow-growing tumors that arise from undifferentiated notochordal remnants located within the axial skeleton. While historically considered more common in the sacrum, recent medical literature suggests that chordomas are nearly equally distributed among the clivus, spine, and sacrum. These tumors are uncommon in patients younger than 40 years, and when arising in the clivus, patients commonly present with cranial nerve palsies. Histologically, chordomas are characterized by cells with large, clear vacuoles, termed physaliferous cells (from the Greek word meaning *bubble-bearing*). While most are considered low-grade neoplasms, these tumors are locally aggressive, invasive, relatively radioresistant, and have a high recurrence rate. Five percent of chordomas are metastatic at presentation, with up to 65% metastatic in advanced cases. However, interestingly, the presence of local recurrence is considered to be more predictive of poorer survival than metastatic disease. Additionally, the most important factor determining cure relates to the amount of tumor removed at the initial resection. On imaging, a chordoma will expand the bone of origin and frequently invade adjacent structures. A clival chordoma frequently deforms the ventral pons and may encase the basilar artery. On CT, osseous destruction will often result in scattered bone fragments within the lesion. On MRI, a classic clival chordoma is most often T1 hypointense, T2 hyperintense (due to the increased fluid content in physaliferous cells), and variably enhances, from no enhancement to marked enhancement.
- **Poorly differentiated clival chordoma.** While most clival chordomas are low grade, occasionally poorly differentiated clival chordomas may occur. An MR imaging finding that may help differentiate a classic clival chordoma from a poorly differentiated clival chordoma relates to their T2 signal characteristics; a classic clival chordoma is diffusely T2 hyperintense, whereas a poorly differentiated clival chordoma may be T2 hypointense.
- **Petroclival synchondrosis chondrosarcoma.** A chondrosarcoma, graded from low to high, is a tumor that contains atypical chondrocytes and enlarged hyperchromatic nuclei interspersed within a cartilaginous matrix. Discerning between a chondrosarcoma and a classic chordoma can be difficult on imaging, with both often being markedly T2 hyperintense and variably enhancing. Perhaps the most reliable imaging characteristic differentiating these two entities relates to their location. A clival chordoma tends to be located at the midline, whereas a skull base chondrosarcoma usually occurs at the petroclival synchondrosis where there is a relative abundance of cartilage. Recent literature also suggests that there are significant apparent diffusion coefficient (ADC) differences between a clival chordoma (poorly differentiated clival chordoma more so than a classic clival chordoma) and a petroclival junction chondrosarcoma, with a chordoma having significantly lower ADC values compared to a chondrosarcoma.

Ecchordosis physaliphora

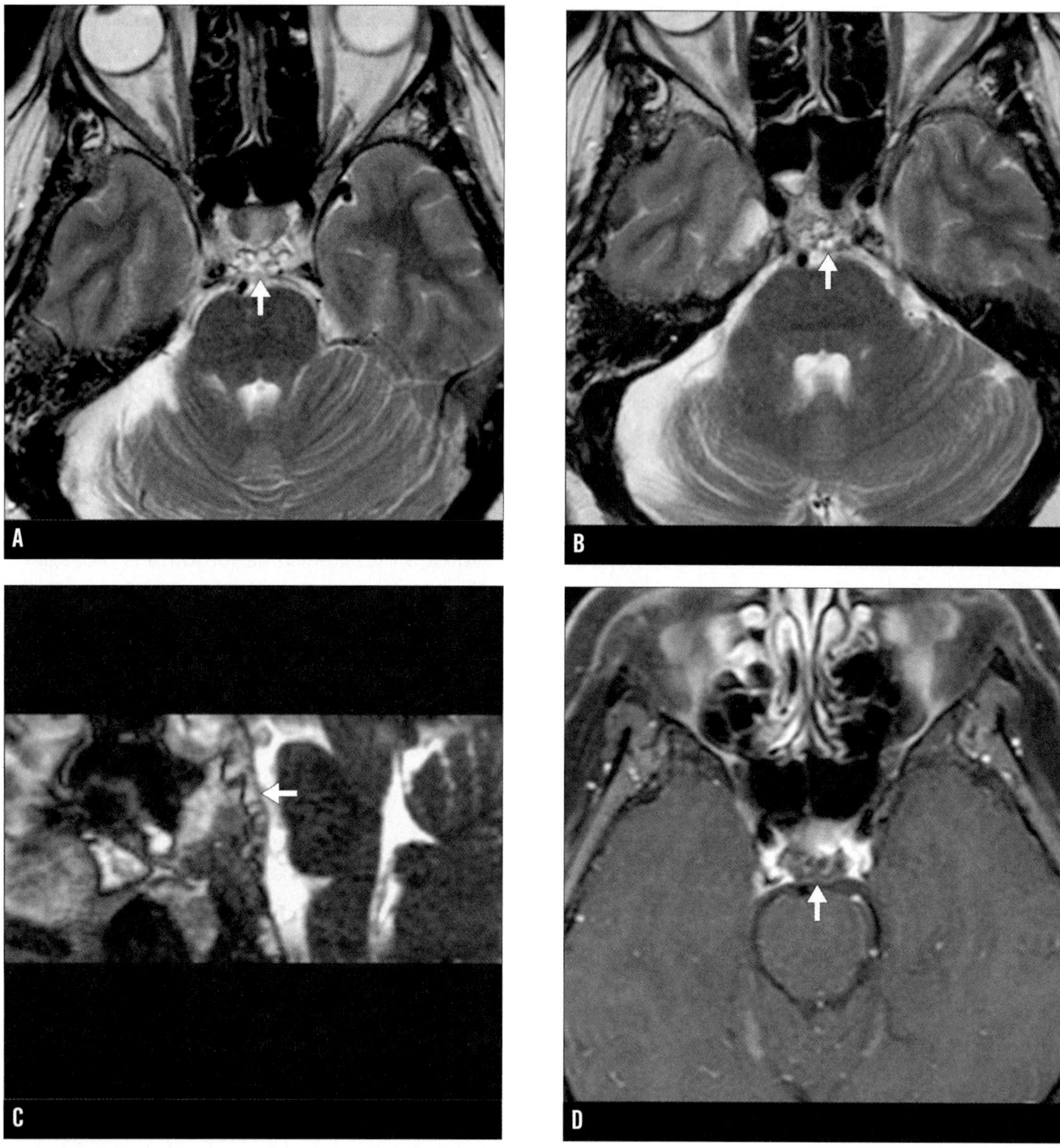

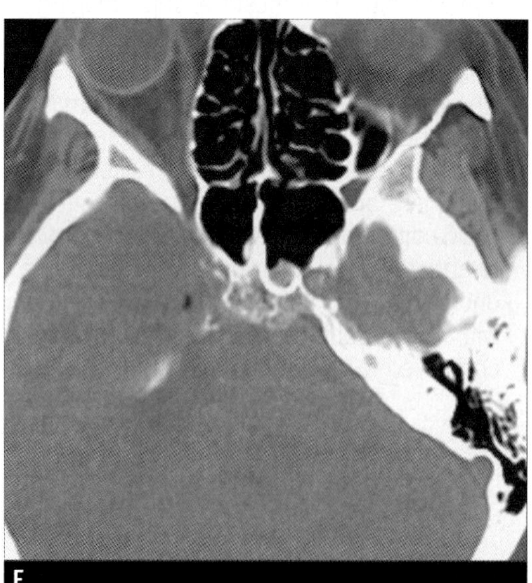

Axial T2 (**A, B**), sagittal reconstructed constructed interference in the steady state (CISS) (**C**), and contrast-enhanced fat-suppressed axial T1 (**D**) MR images demonstrate an extradural, grape-like cluster of T2 hyperintense, nonenhancing foci immediately dorsal to the clivus and dorsum sella (arrows, **A-D**). Image **C** demonstrates an undulating contour of the dorsal clivus and dorsum sella, although the bone appears grossly intact. An axial CT image viewed with an intermediate window (**E**) confirms the lack of bone destruction and the presence of normal marrow fat.

Companion case: Classic clival chordoma

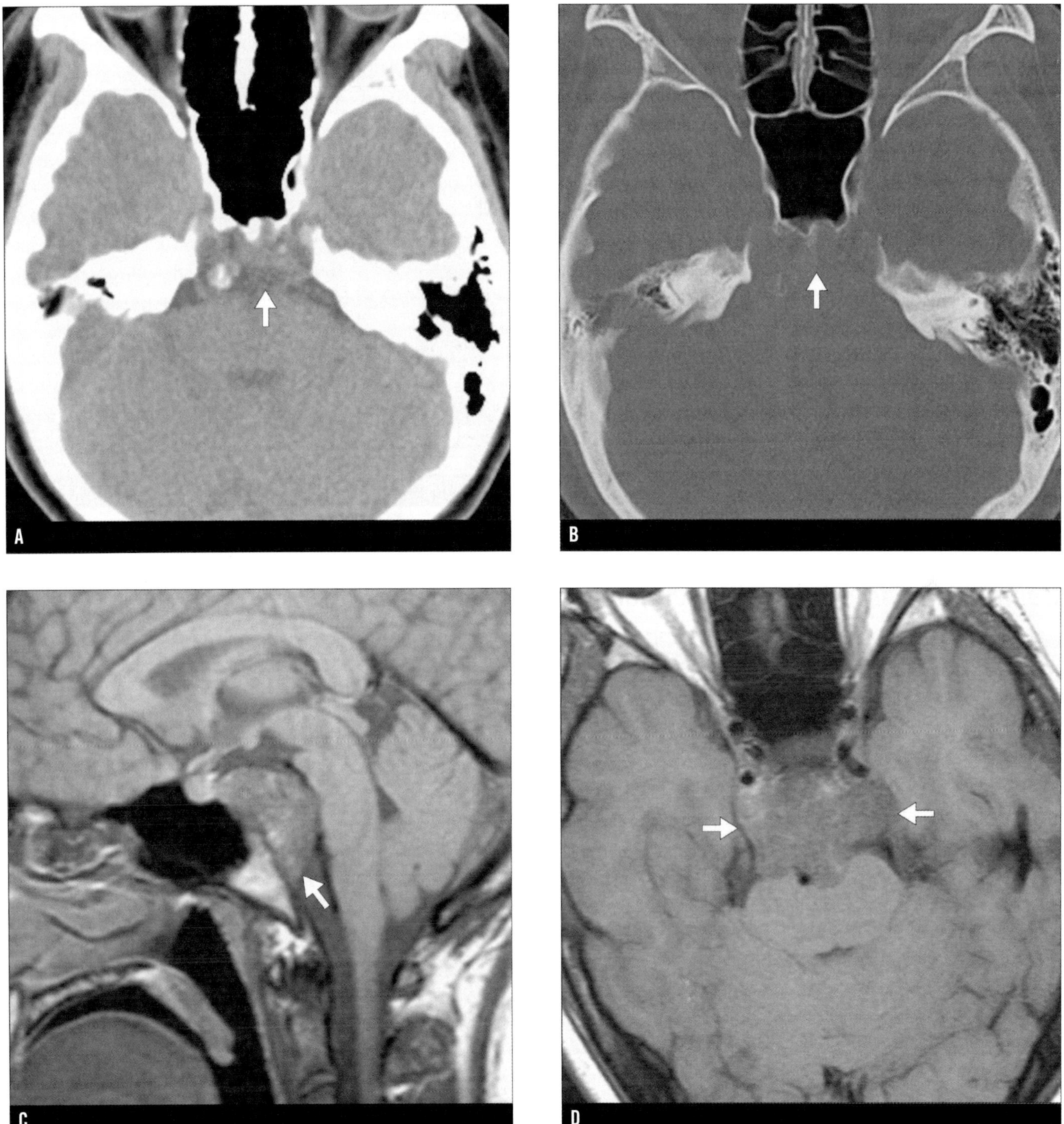

Axial CT images through the clivus viewed with a soft tissue window (**A**) and bone window (**B**) demonstrate a dorsally projecting soft tissue mass (arrow, **A**) arising from the clivus associated with osseous erosion of the clivus (arrow, **B**). Unenhanced sagittal T1 (**C**), unenhanced axial T1 (**D**), axial T2 (**E**), and postcontrast axial MPRAGE (**F**) MR images of the same patient. The exophytic lesion arising from the clivus is mildly heterogeneous on precontrast T1 (arrows, **C, D**), profoundly hyperintense on T2 (arrows, **E**), and contains trace enhancement (arrows, **F**). The erosive nature on CT, exophytic appearance, minimal enhancement, and the pronounced T2 hyperintensity are most compatible with a chordoma.

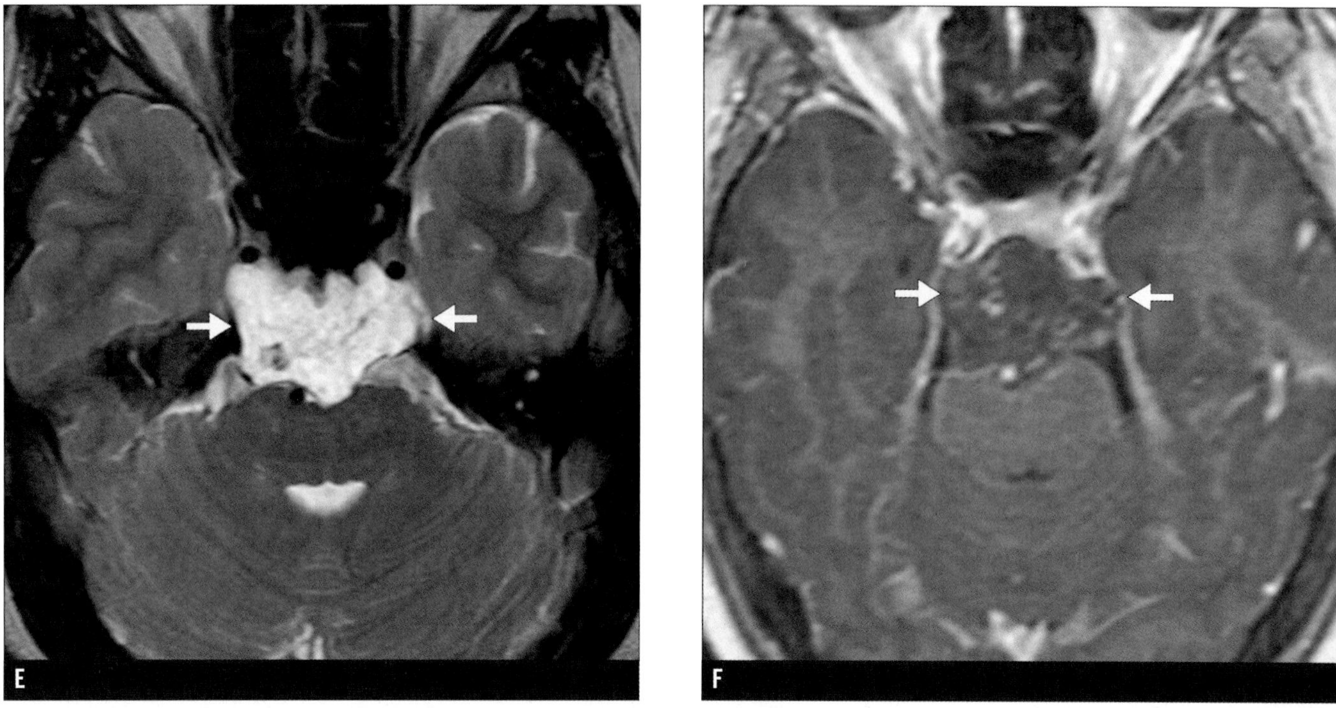

Companion case: Poorly differentiated clival chordoma

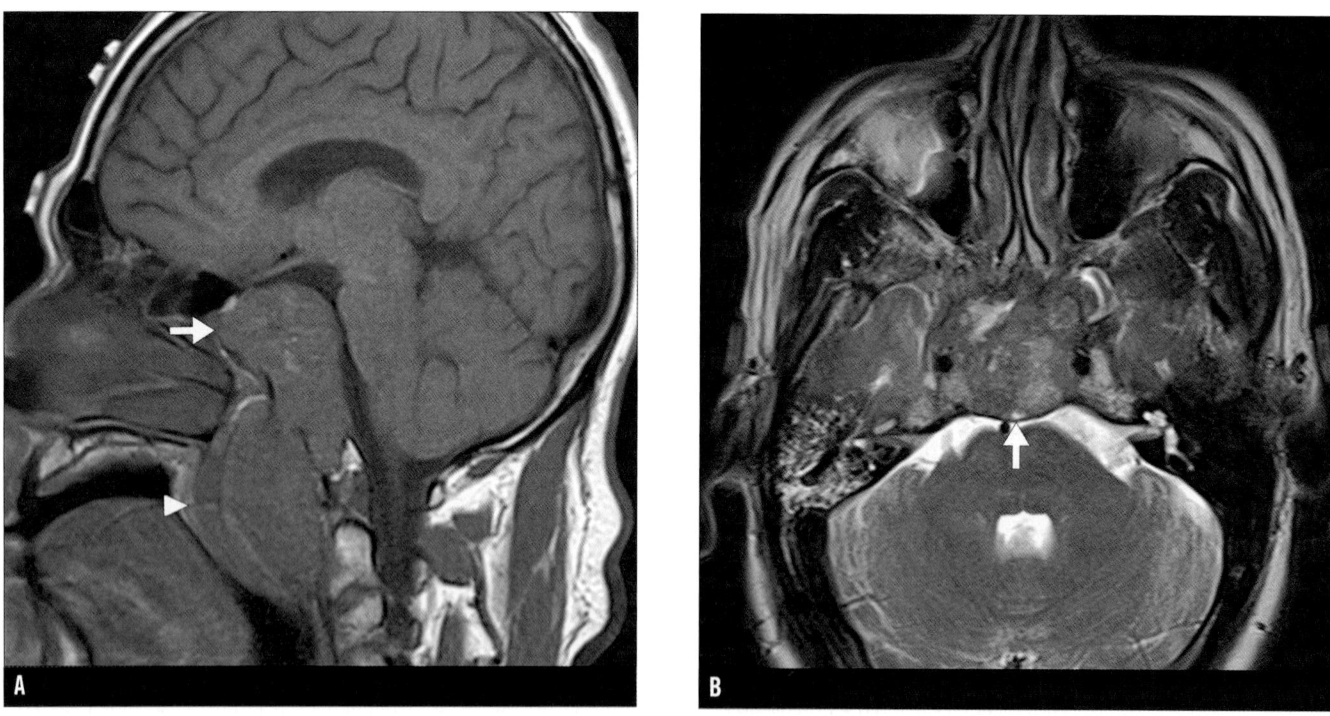

Sagittal T1 (**A**), axial T2 (**B**), and contrast-enhanced axial MPRAGE (**C**) MR images demonstrate a large, T1 hypointense, T2 hypointense, enhancing mass involving the clivus (arrows, **A-C**), This large mass also has a large prevertebral/retropharyngeal component (arrowhead, **A**). Axial DWI (**D**) and its corresponding ADC map (**E**) demonstrate significant restricted diffusion within the tumor (arrows, **D, E**). This mass could represent a variety of primary tumors or a large metastatic lesion. This tumor represented a poorly differentiated chordoma at pathology, which is supported by its clival location, hypointense T2 signal, and restricted diffusion.

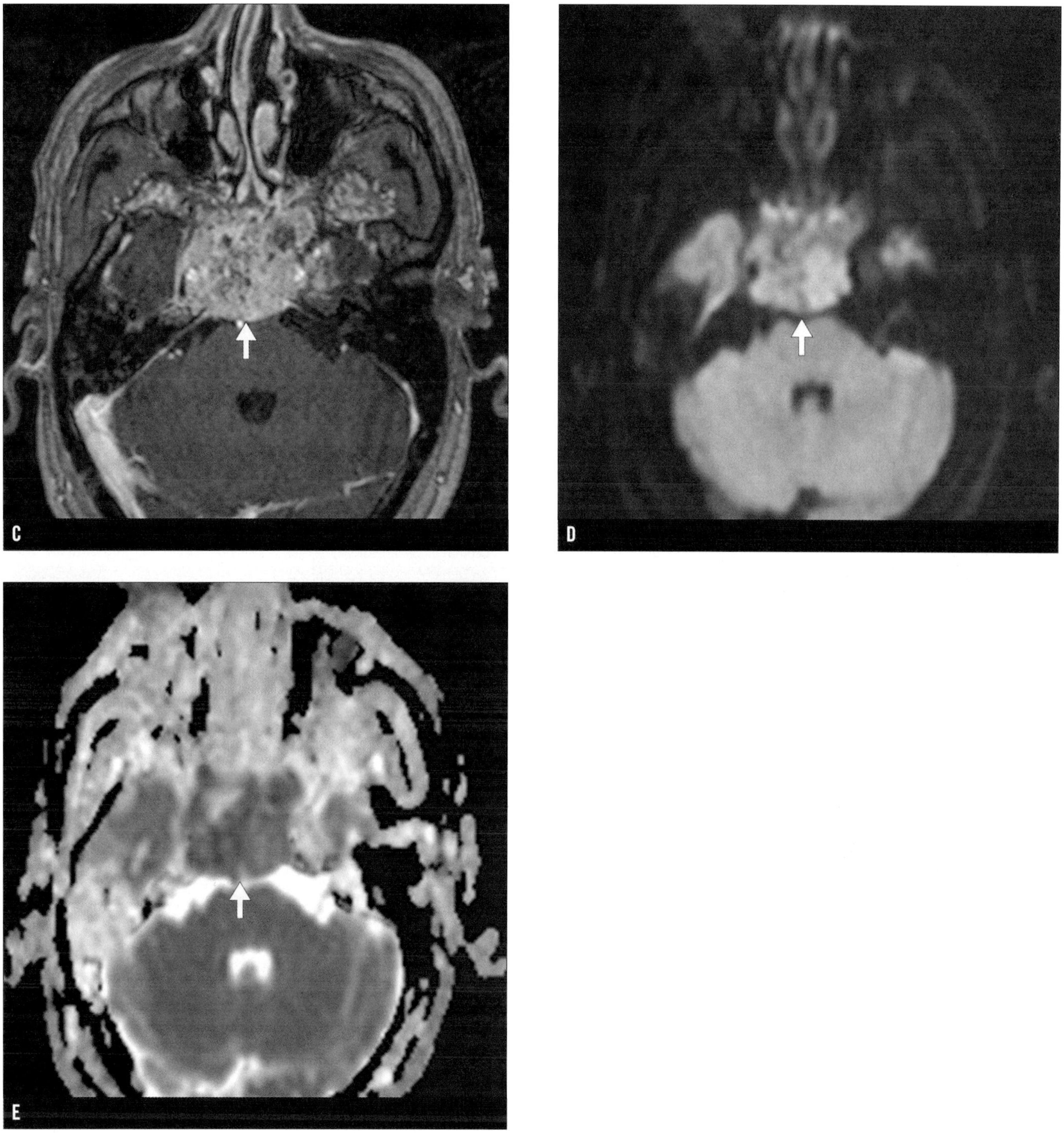
C
D
E

Companion case: Petroclival synchondrosis chondrosarcoma

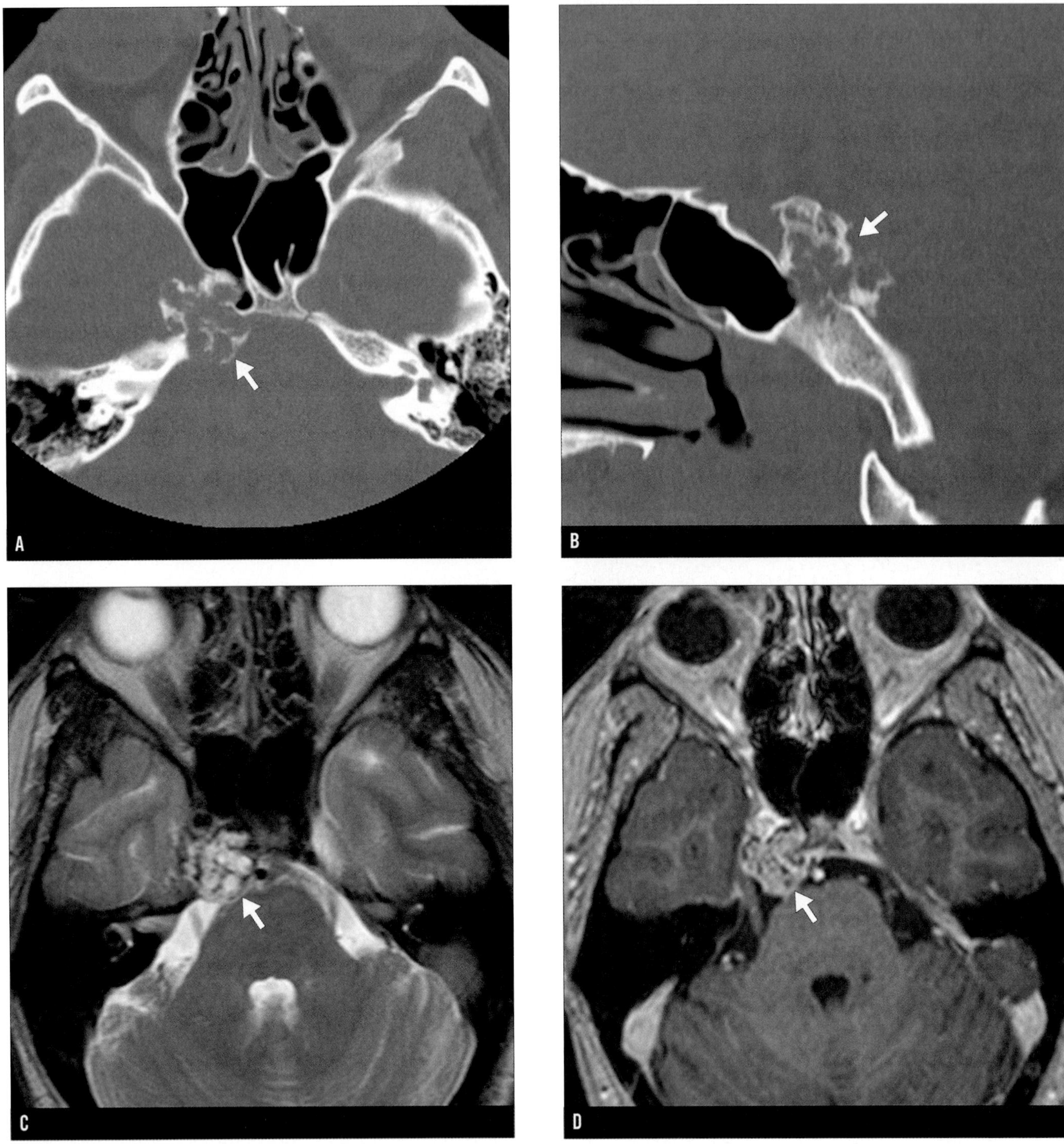

Axial (**A**) and sagittal reformatted (**B**) CT images demonstrate a bubbly, expansile, lytic mass with a chondroid matrix involving the right petroclival synchondrosis (arrows, **A, B**). Axial T2 (**C**) and contrast-enhanced axial MPRAGE (**D**) MR images demonstrate the lesion to be T2 hyperintense (arrow, **C**) and enhancing (arrow, **D**) relative to precontrast T1-weighted imaging (not shown). The location of the lesion at the petroclival synchondrosis and its signal characteristics are suggestive of a chondrosarcoma. Furthermore, axial DWI (**E**) and its corresponding ADC map (**F**) do not demonstrate significant diffusion restriction, also in keeping with a chondrosarcoma (arrows, **E**, **F**). This was a low-grade chondrosarcoma at pathology.

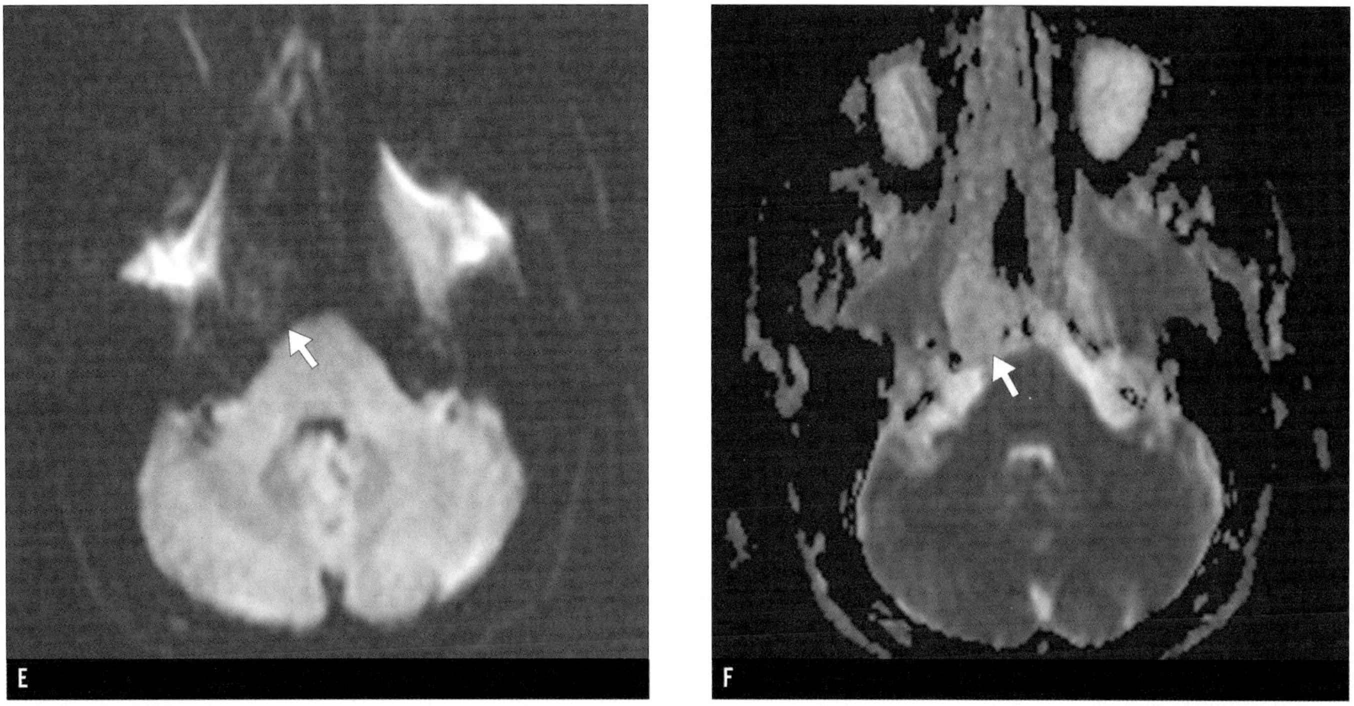

REFERENCES

Mehnert F, Beschorner R, Küker W, Hahn U, Nägele T. Retroclival ecchordosis physaliphora: MR imaging and review of the literature. *AJNR Am J Neuroradiol.* 2004;25(10):1851-1855. Review.

Ng SH, Ko SF, Wan YL, Tang LM, Ho YS. Cervical ecchordosis physaliphora: CT and MR features. *Br J Radiol.* 1998;71(843):329-331.

Walcott BP, Nahed BV, Mohyeldin A, Coumans JV, Kahle KT, Ferreira MJ. Chordoma: current concepts, management, and future directions. *Lancet Oncol.* 2012;13(2):e69-e76.

Yeom KW, et al. Diffusion-weighted MRI: distinction of skull base chordoma from chondrosarcoma. *AJNR Am J Neuroradiol.* 2013;34(5):1056-1061

CASE 4 Clival lipoma

Intraosseous lipomas are a proliferation of mature lipocytes within the marrow. A benign lipoma confined to the sphenoid bone or elsewhere in the skull base should be left alone. Rarely, a clival lipoma can extend into the sella turcica and result in mass effect upon the optic chiasm, resulting in hypopituitarism and visual disturbance, respectively. When confined to the clivus, a clival lipoma and incidental marrow fat within the clivus are in the same spectrum.

Clival lipoma

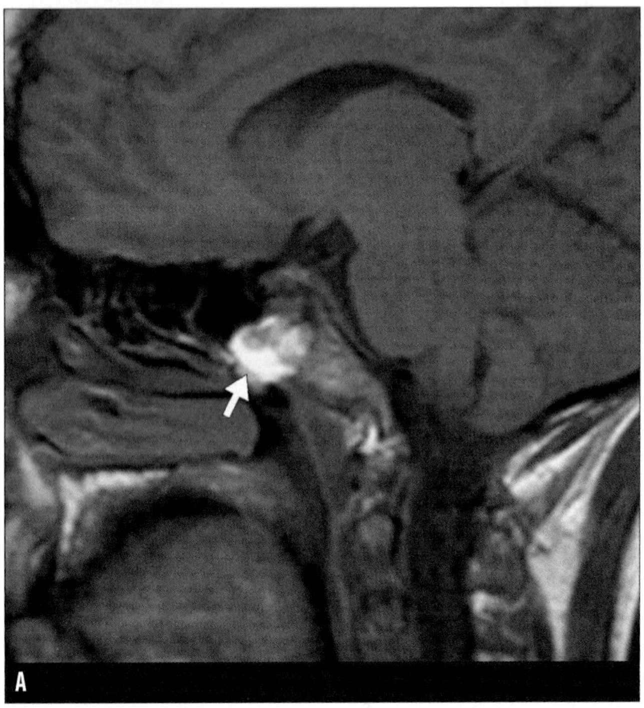

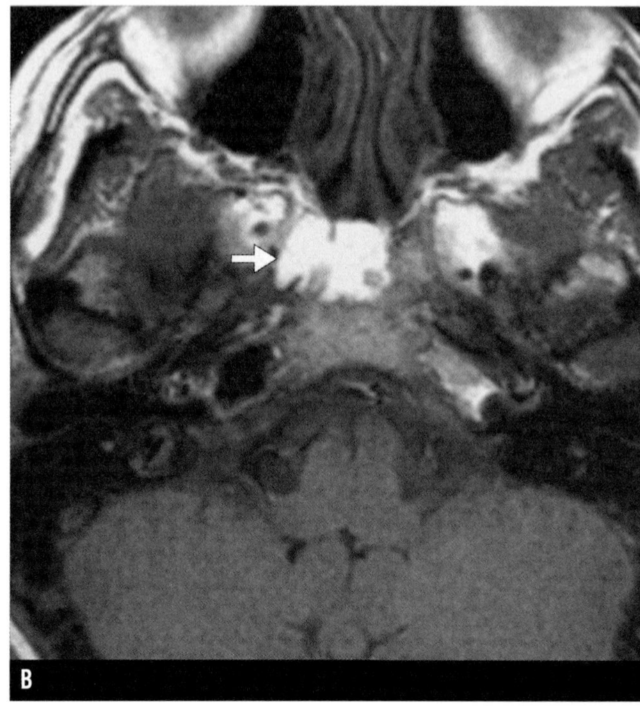

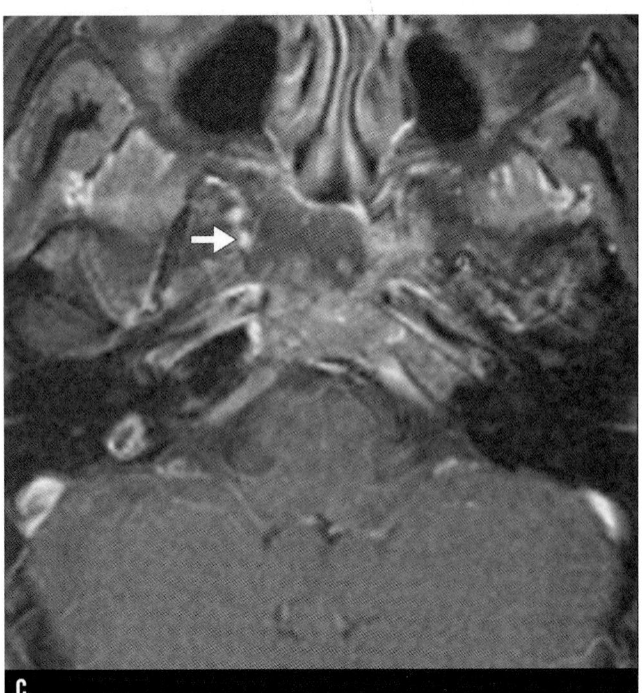

Sagittal (**A**) and axial (**B**) unenhanced T1-weighted MR images without fat suppression and a postcontrast coronal T1-weighted MR image with fat suppression (**C**). Images **A** and **B** demonstrate a relatively round, discrete, T1 hyperintense lesion located in the right aspect of the sphenoid body (arrows, **A**, **B**). Image **C** demonstrates the lesion to be hypointense with fat suppression (arrow, **C**), confirming the presence of a clival lipoma.

Clival lipoma (normal clival marrow fat)

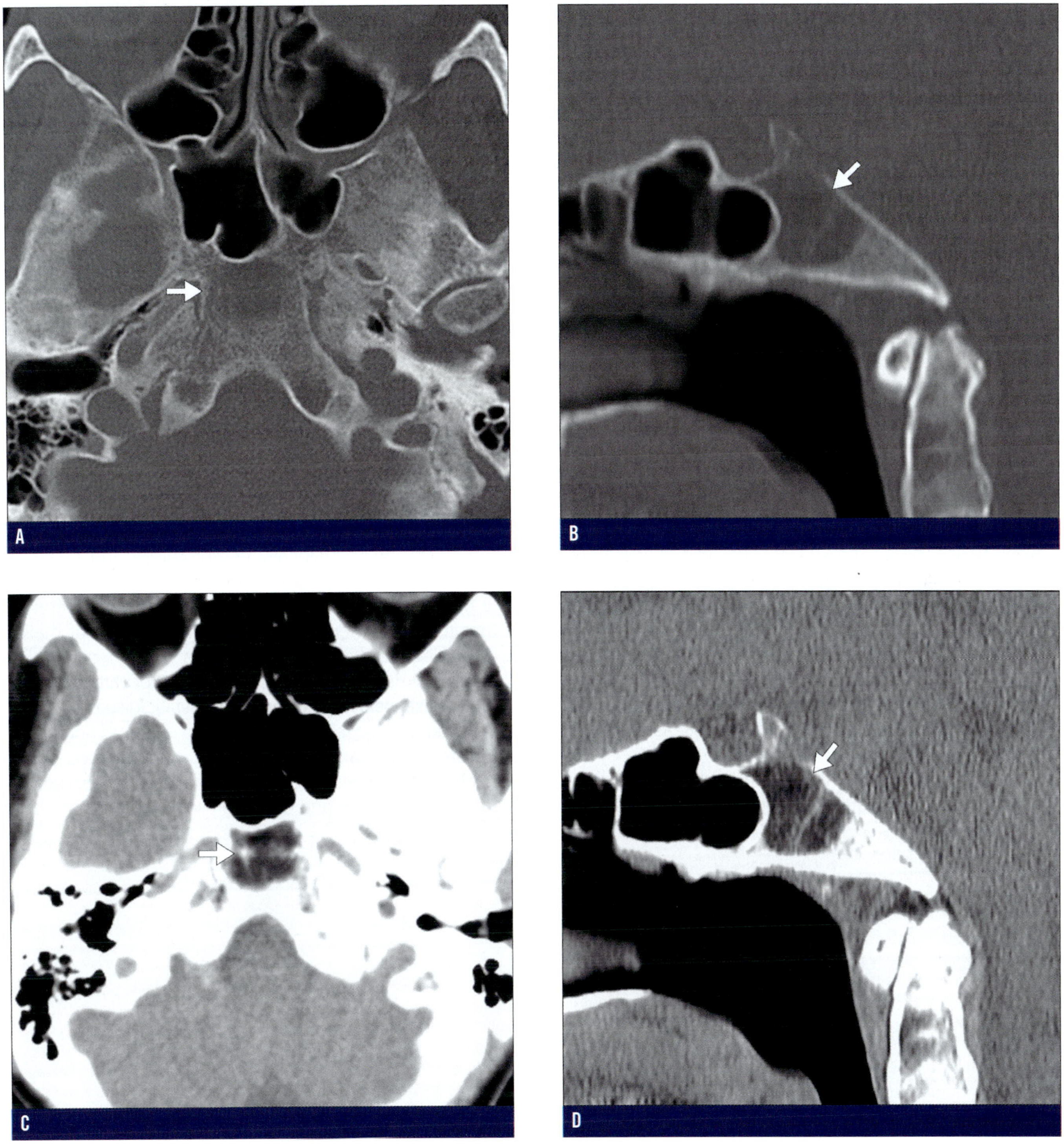

Different patient. Axial (**A**) and sagittal reformatted (**B**) CT images viewed with a bone window demonstrate lucency within the clivus that could be misinterpreted as a lytic lesion, possibly a lytic metastasis (arrows, **A**, **B**). However, these same images viewed with a soft tissue window (**C**, **D**) demonstrate fat attenuation within the finding, compatible with a clival lipoma or normal clival marrow fat (arrows, **C**, **D**). If it is unclear whether a lucency in bone relates to fat or a lytic mass, then MR imaging to include a fat suppression sequence should clarify the finding.

REFERENCES

Lanisnik, B Didanovic, V. Sphenoclival intraosseus lipoma: case report and literature review. *Skull base.* 2007;17(3):211-214.

MacFarlane, M, Soule, S, Hunt, P. Intraosseous lipoma of the body of the sphenoid bone. *J Clin Neurosci.* 2005;12(1):105-108.

CASE 5 Arrested pneumatization of the skull base

Arrested pneumatization of the skull base is a benign developmental variant which can be mistaken for a pathologic process because of its heterogeneous appearance. Most of the normal sphenoid sinus pneumatization occurs between 1 and 5 years, although the full size of a pneumatized sphenoid occurs between 12 and 14 years. For some unknown reason, the sphenoid sinus may not become fully pneumatized in some individuals and is thus "arrested." This benign entity is located within the sphenoid bone, contains fat, is nonexpansile, contains sclerotic defined margins, and does not violate the adjacent foramina.

COMPANION CASES

- **Fibrous dysplasia.**

  Fibrous dysplasia (FD) is a developmental disorder resulting in an abnormal proliferation of fibroblasts that replaces the normal bone with immature, structurally weak bone. There is no known cause of FD, and it may be monostotic (affecting a single site) or polyostotic (affecting more than one site). Craniofacial involvement occurs in 30% of monostotic forms and 50% of polyostotic forms of disease. While FD is classified as nonneoplastic, it often expands the affected bone and can be locally aggressive. Most cases of FD do not progress after adolescence, although occasionally the lesion may grow during adulthood.

  Three patterns of FD have been described, depending on the ratio of osseous and fibrous tissue. These are: sclerotic, cystic, and pagetoid (or mixed) patterns. The classic CT appearance of the sclerotic variety is a diffusely ground-glass lesion that has a thin cortex and expands the involved bone. With the cystic form of FD, there are one or more lucent areas and the margins may be quite sclerotic. Soft tissue density is often identified within the cystic areas on CT. The pagetoid form is a combination of the sclerotic and cystic forms. While FD is generally hypointense on T1, it varies greatly in its signal characteristics on T2, and it often enhances. FD is particularly notorious for mimicking a malignancy on MRI and is a common reason why any unusual appearing osseous lesion on MRI should also be evaluated with CT or plain film radiography.

  FD may mimic arrested pneumatization of the skull base on imaging. However, in contradistinction to arrested pneumatization of the skull base, FD does not typically contain fat and is most often expansile. Since FD often expands the bone, the foramina of the skull base may be occasionally compromised and result in cranial nerve compression. Treatment of FD is surgical if there is a cosmetic deformity, intractable pain, cranial nerve impingement, or if there is a suspicion of malignant degeneration. In the absence of such issues, FD can be simply monitored clinically and/or with imaging.
- **Skull base metastatic disease.** Metastatic disease, as well as other skull base entities such as chordomas and chondrosarcomas, can be differentiated from arrested pneumatization of the skull base because they are destructive, may be expansile, and do not preserve regional fat.

Arrested pneumatization of the skull base

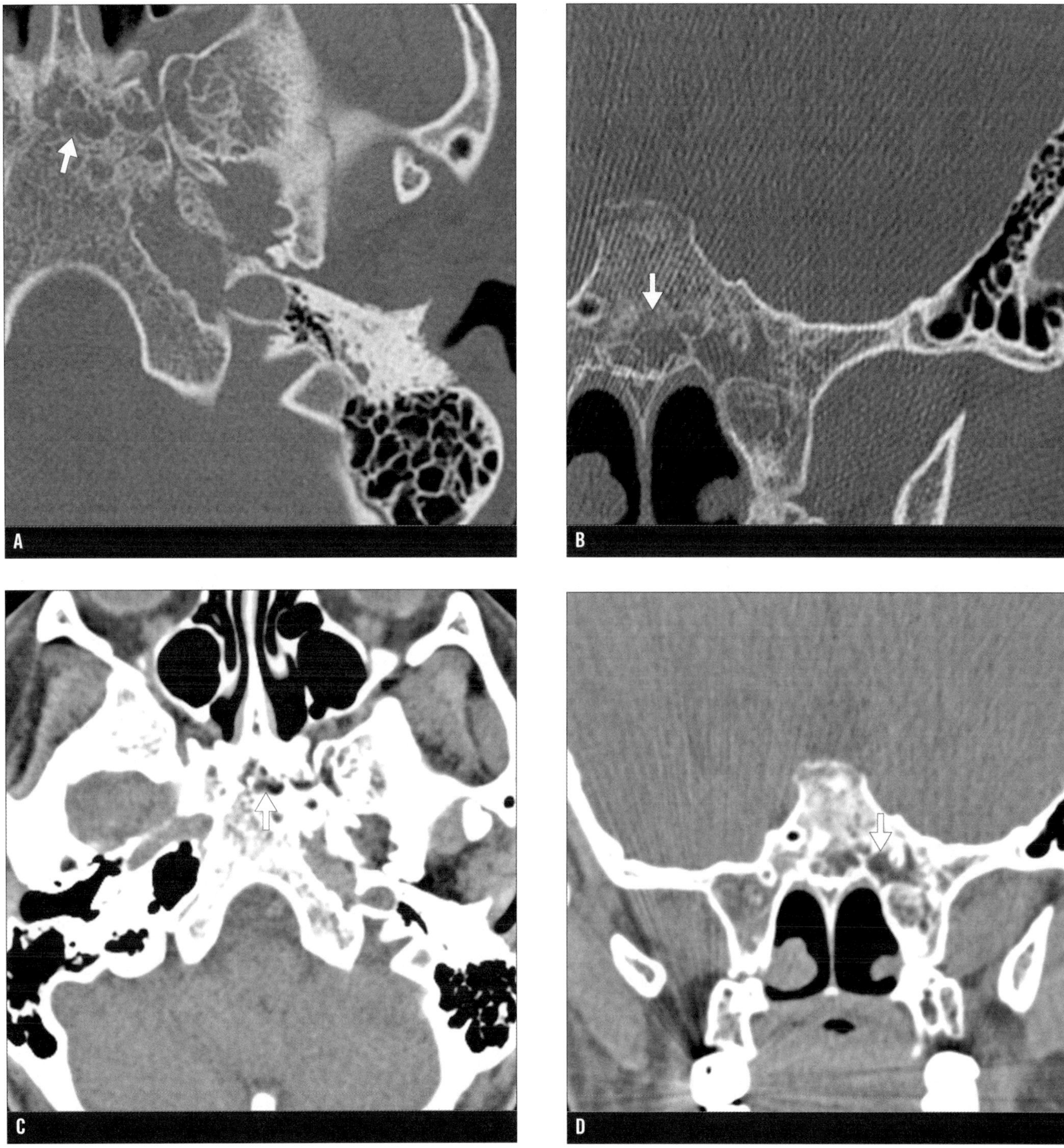

Axial (**A**) and direct coronal (**B**) CT images viewed with a bone window demonstrate several discrete lucent areas with defined borders interspersed within the left aspect of the sphenoid body (arrows **A, B**). The same images as **A** and **B** but viewed with a soft tissue window (**C** and **D**, respectively) demonstrate fat attenuation within the lucent areas, compatible with normal fat containing marrow and incidental arrested pneumatization of the skull base (arrows, **C, D**).

Arrested pneumatization of the skull base

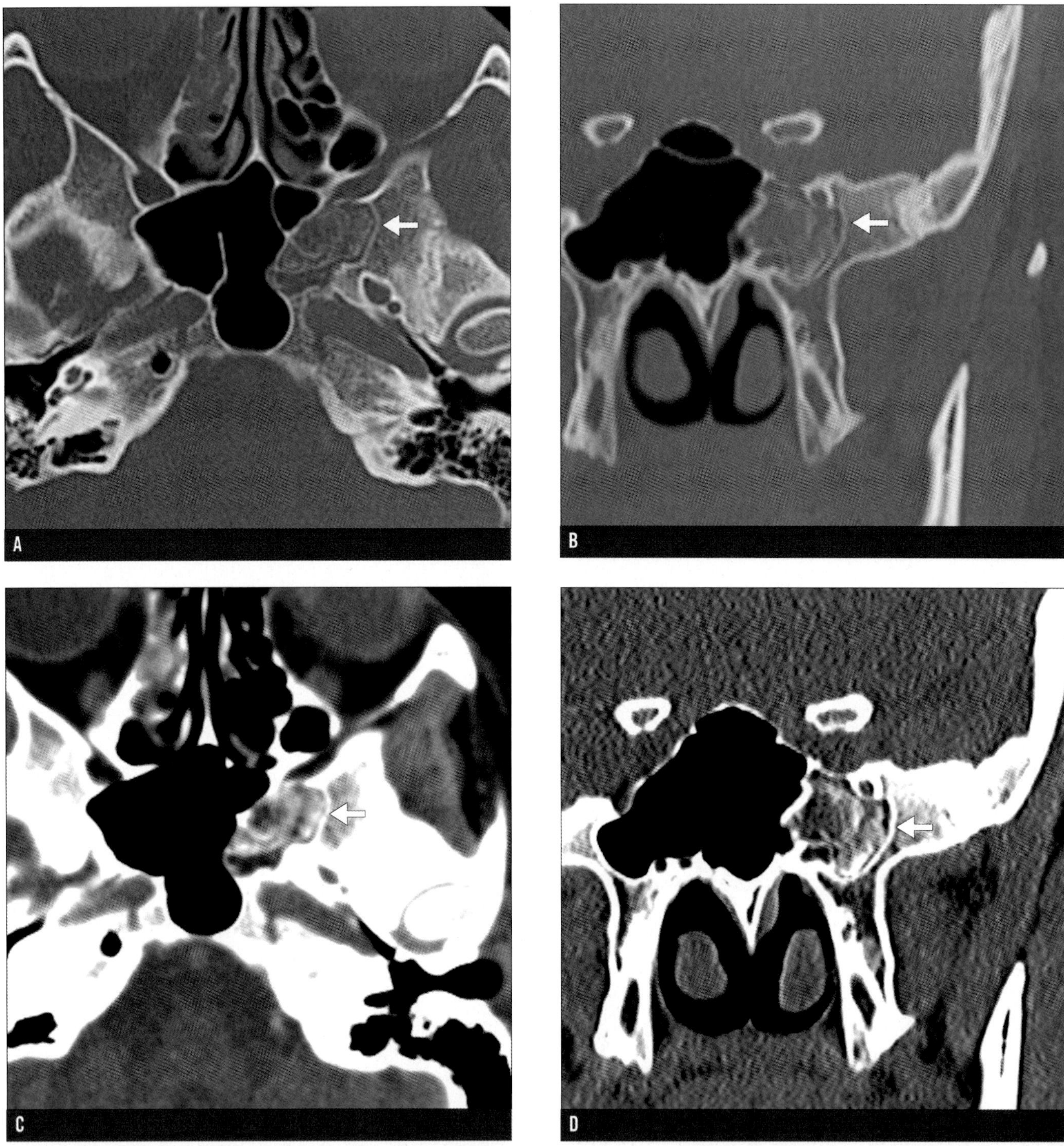

Different patient. Axial (**A**) and coronal reformatted (**B**) CT images viewed with a bone window demonstrate a lucent, circumscribed lesion with a bone matrix located immediately left lateral to the pneumatized sphenoid sinus (arrows, **A**, **B**). The same images as **A** and **B**, but viewed with a soft tissue window (**C** and **D**, respectively), demonstrate the lesion to contain fat attenuation, compatible with fatty marrow and incidental arrested pneumatization of the skull base (arrows, **C**, **D**).

Arrested pneumatization of the skull base

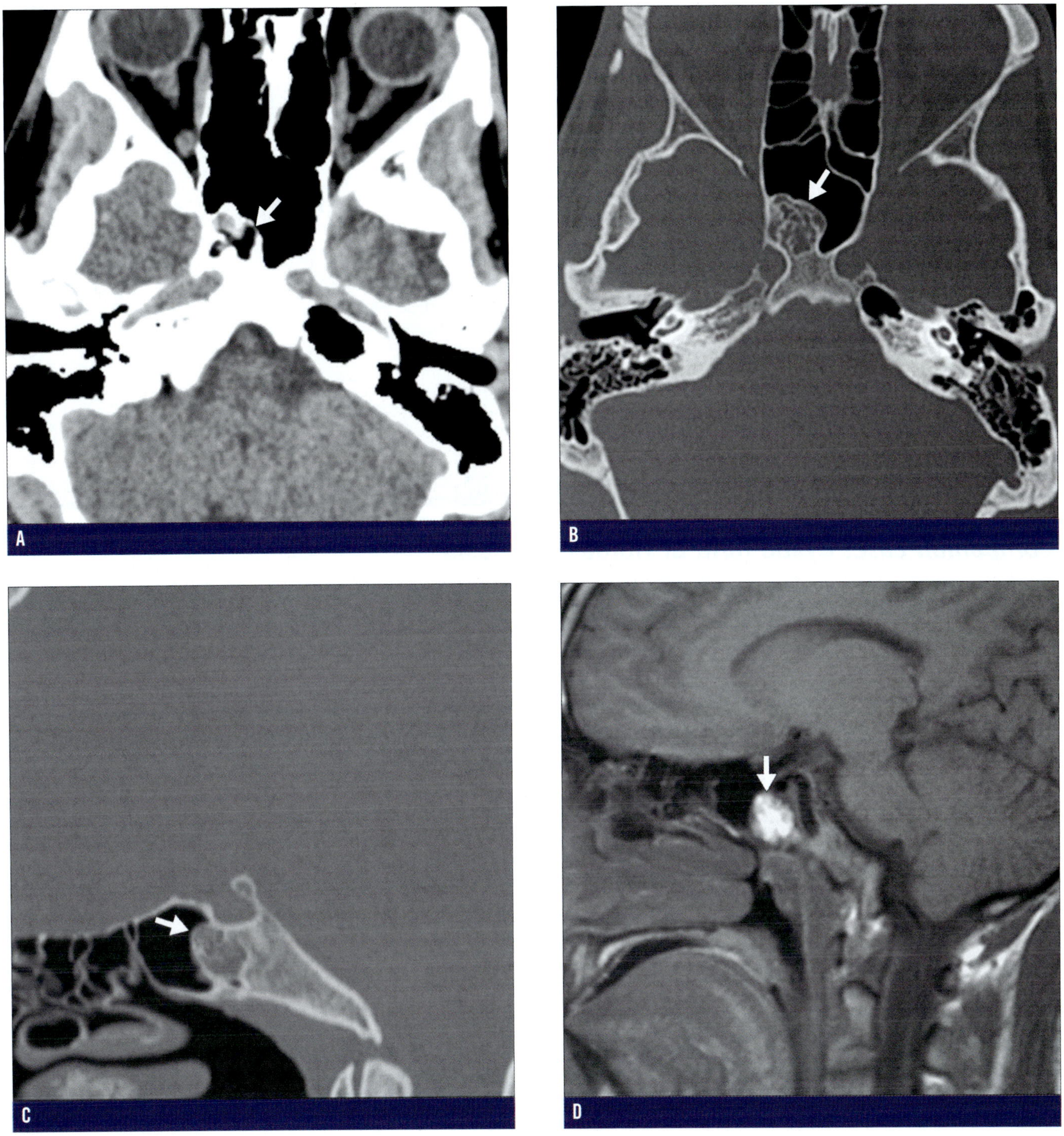

Different patient. An axial CT image through the sphenoid sinus viewed with a soft tissue window (**A**) as well as axial (**B**) and sagittal reformatted (**C**) CT images viewed with a bone window. These images demonstrate a round, exophytic, heterogeneous osseous finding arising from the right posterior wall of the sphenoid sinus and projecting into the sphenoid sinus lumen (arrows, **A-C**). While the finding is exophytic, it contains hypoattenuation suggestive of fat, as demonstrated on image **A** (arrow). Sagittal T1 (**D**), axial T1 (**E**), and axial T2 (**F**) MR images demonstrate fat equivalent signal on all pulse sequences. In combination with the CT images, the findings are consistent with benignity and incidental arrested pneumatization of the skull base. Surgery had been planned on this patient based on an initial interpretation that described this finding as a skull base mass. Fortunately, surgery was avoided once this lesion was correctly interpreted as an incidental finding.

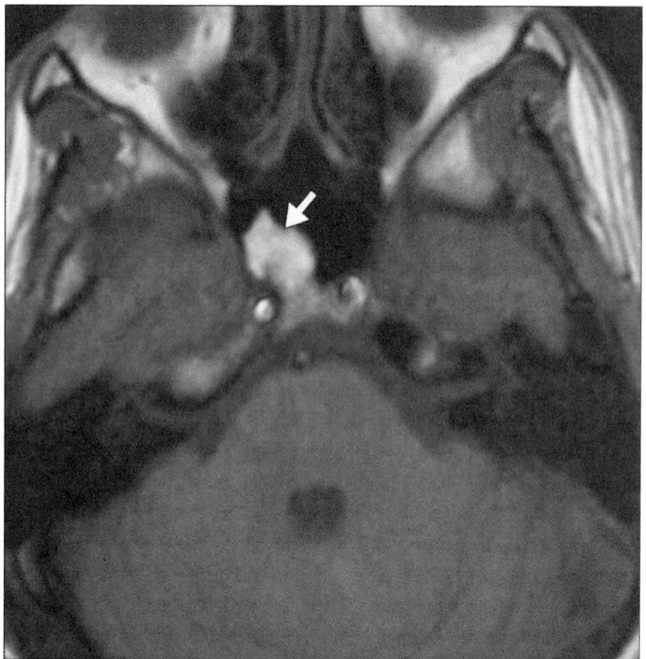

E

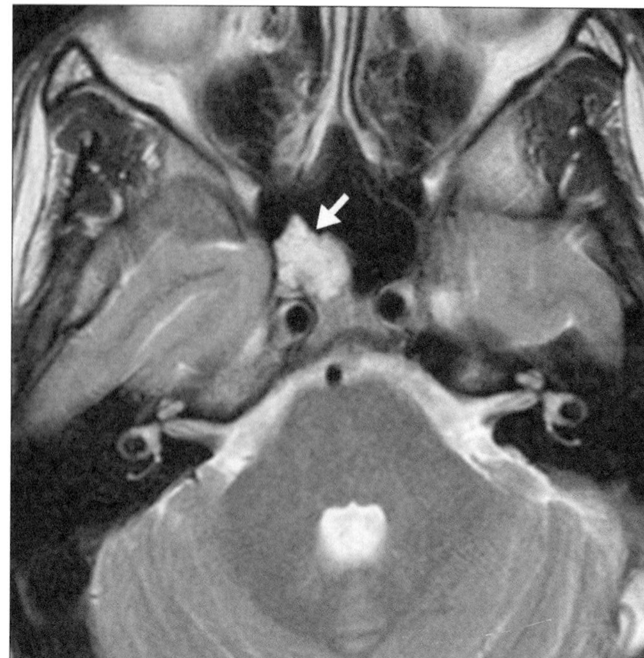

F

Companion case: Cystic form of fibrous dysplasia

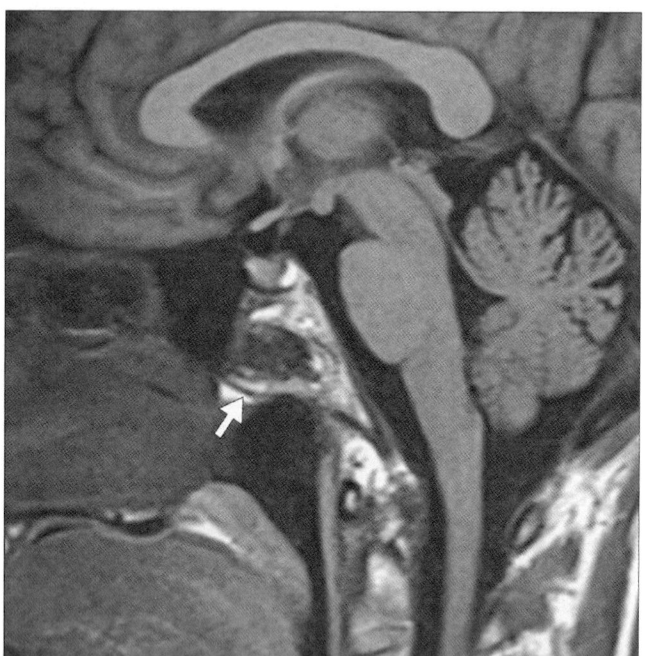

A

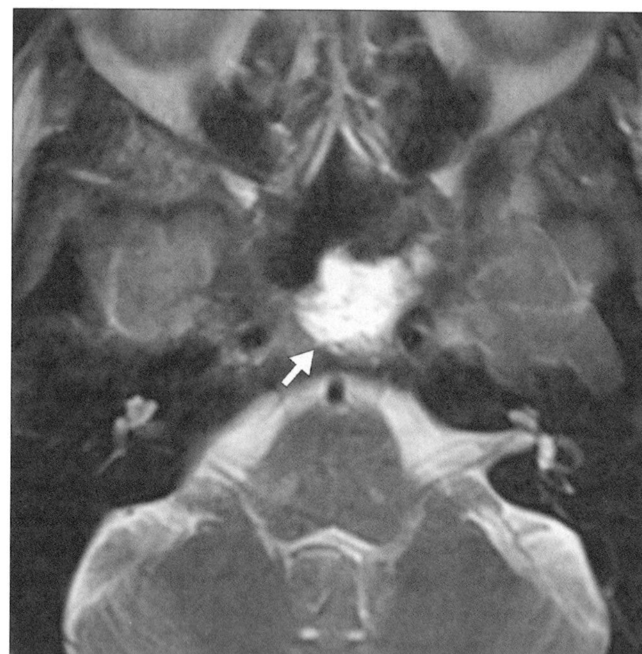

B

Sagittal T1 (**A**), axial T2 (**B**), unenhanced axial T1 (**C**), and postcontrast axial T1 (**D**) MR images through the skull base. There is a lesion in the left aspect of the sphenoid body that contains T1 hypointensity (arrow, **A**), predominantly T2 hyperintensity (arrow, **B**), speckled intrinsic T1 shortening (arrow, **C**), and minimally enhances (**D**). The MR imaging appearance can be confusing and could easily be mistaken for a malignancy, although the speckled T1 shortening is generally a sign of benignity. An axial CT image of the same patient viewed with a bone window (**E**) demonstrates an expansile, lucent lesion with sclerotic margins involving the body and left greater wing of the sphenoid, fairly characteristic of the cystic form of fibrous dysplasia (arrows, **E**). The same image viewed with a soft tissue window (**F**) demonstrates soft tissue attenuation within the lesion (arrow, **F**). The imaging findings affecting the skull base were stable over several years. A coronal reformatted CT image through the sphenoid bone and mandible (**G**) demonstrates destruction of the left vidian canal (arrow, **G**), with the normal right vidian canal annotated for reference (arrowhead, **G**). An additional expansile, ground-glass lesion involving the left hemimandible is also present on image **G**.

The constellation of imaging findings is compatible with polyostotic fibrous dysplasia, with a cystic pattern involving the sphenoid and a sclerotic pattern involving the mandible. This case demonstrates the benefit of CT imaging for osseous lesions and the rather complex MRI appearance of fibrous dysplasia. In general, fibrous dysplasia will be more confidently diagnosed with CT.

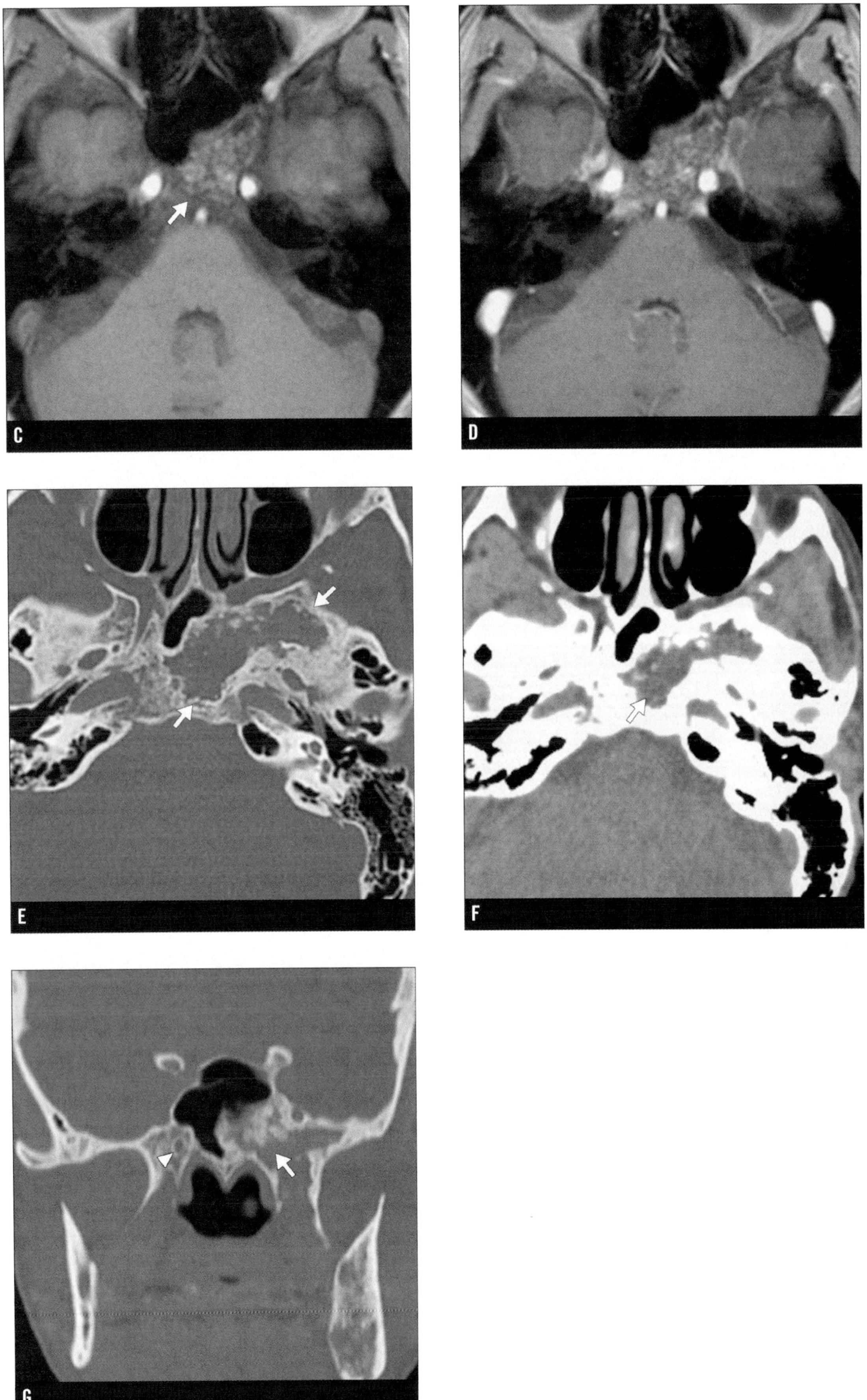
C
D
E
F
G

Companion case: Pagetoid (mixed) form of fibrous dysplasia

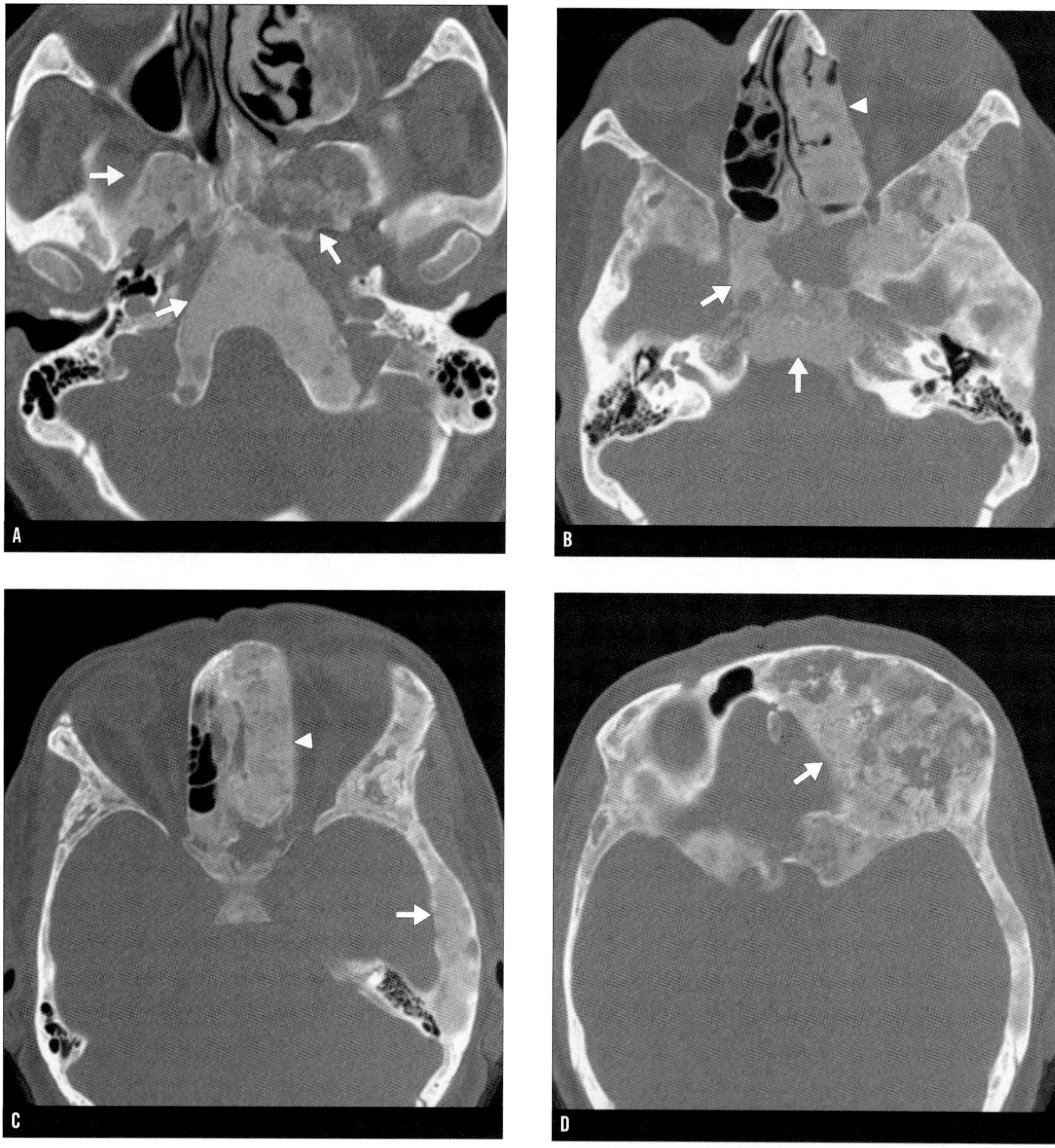

Several axial images extending from the central skull base through the roof of the orbits viewed with a bone window (**A-D**) demonstrate a pronounced, partially ground glass, partially cystic, expansile abnormality involving the central skull base (arrows, **A, B**), the left ethmoid air cells (arrowheads, **B, C**), squamosal portion of the left temporal bone (arrow, **C**), and the roof of the left orbit (arrow, **D**). Axial CT images through the same levels as images **B** and **D** but viewed with a soft tissue window (**E, F**) demonstrate soft tissue attenuation within the lytic portions of the abnormality. The ground-glass, lytic, and, expansile nature of the abnormality is consistent with the pagetoid (mixed) form of fibrous dysplasia.

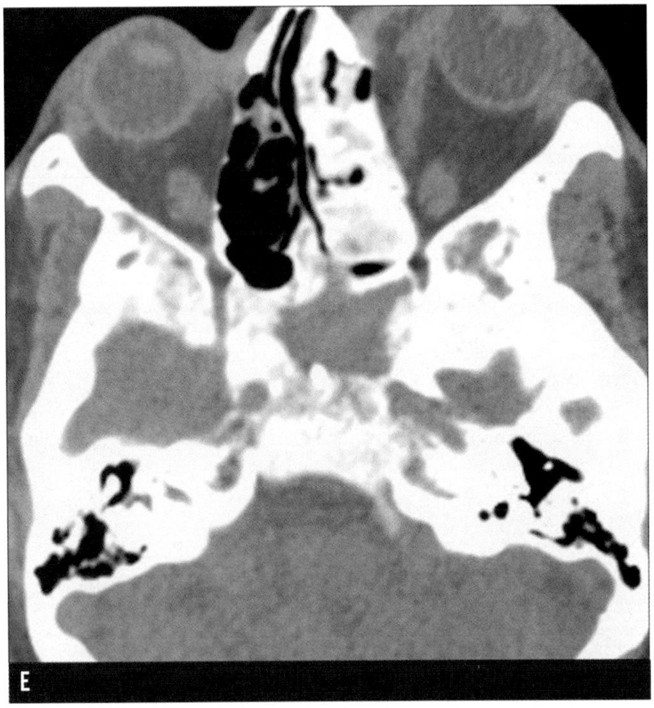

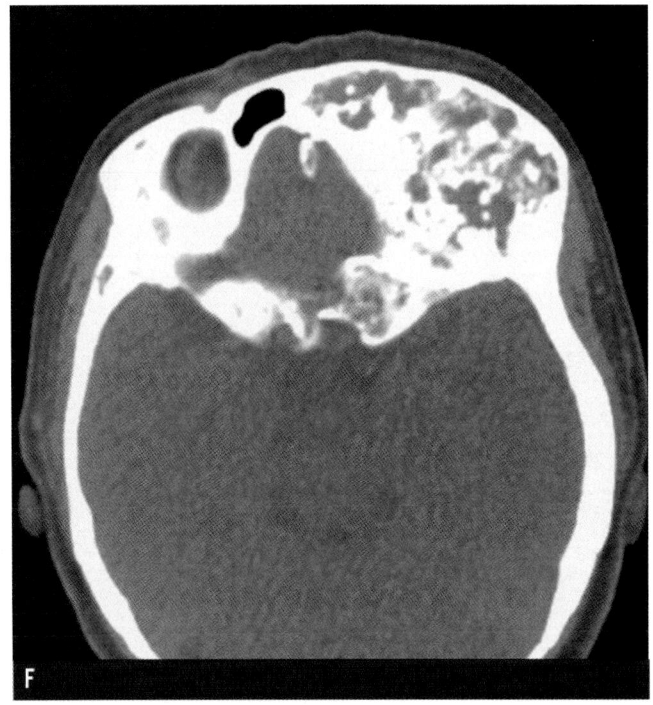

Companion case: Sclerotic (ground-glass) form of fibrous dysplasia

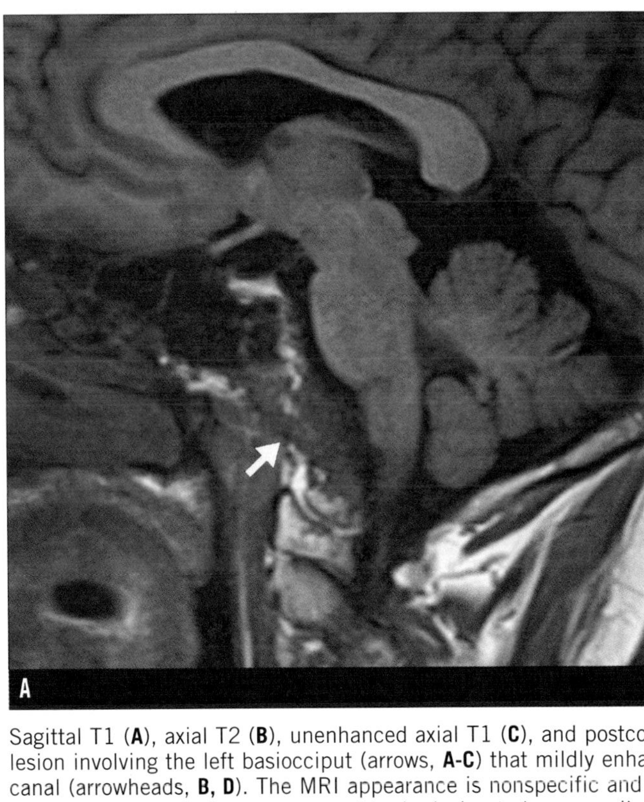

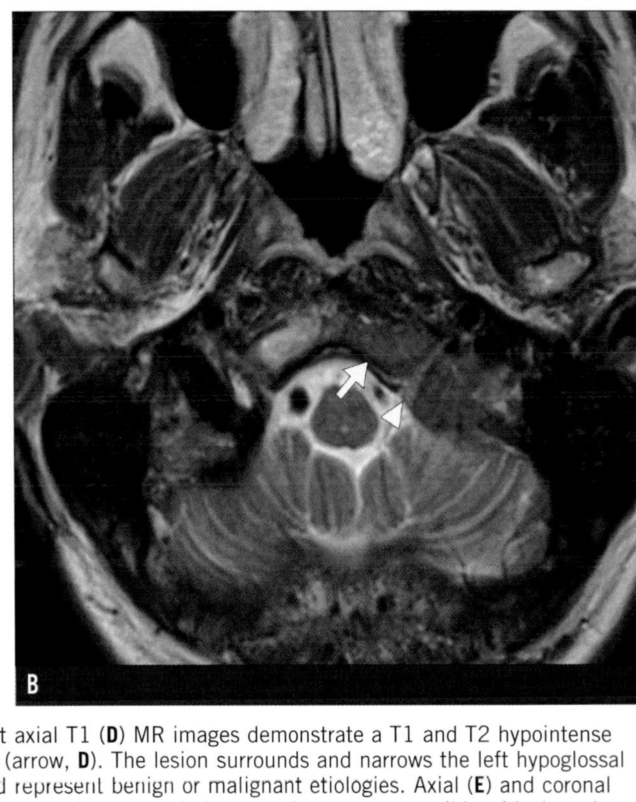

Sagittal T1 (**A**), axial T2 (**B**), unenhanced axial T1 (**C**), and postcontrast axial T1 (**D**) MR images demonstrate a T1 and T2 hypointense lesion involving the left basiocciput (arrows, **A-C**) that mildly enhances (arrow, **D**). The lesion surrounds and narrows the left hypoglossal canal (arrowheads, **B, D**). The MRI appearance is nonspecific and could represent benign or malignant etiologies. Axial (**E**) and coronal reformatted (**F**) CT images demonstrate the lesion to be expansile and to contain a ground-glass matrix, most compatible with the sclerotic form of fibrous dysplasia and not malignancy (arrows, **E**, **F**). However, it would likely be prudent to do imaging follow-up to document stability and to exclude malignancy when confronted with a case such as this. While the left hypoglossal canal is narrowed by the fibrous dysplasia, the patient did not have any clinical symptoms referable to the tongue.

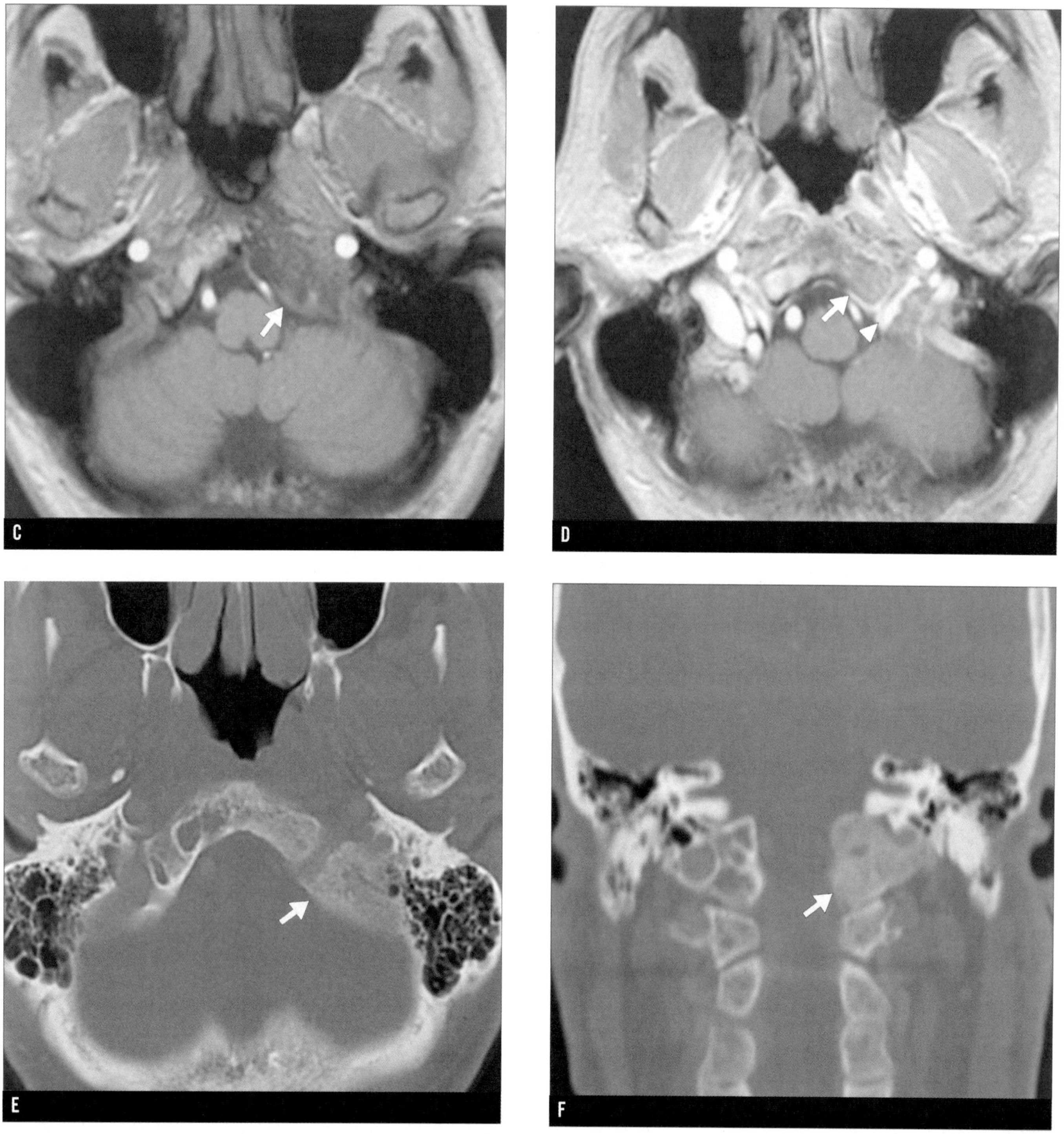

C
D
E
F

Companion case: Skull base metastatic disease

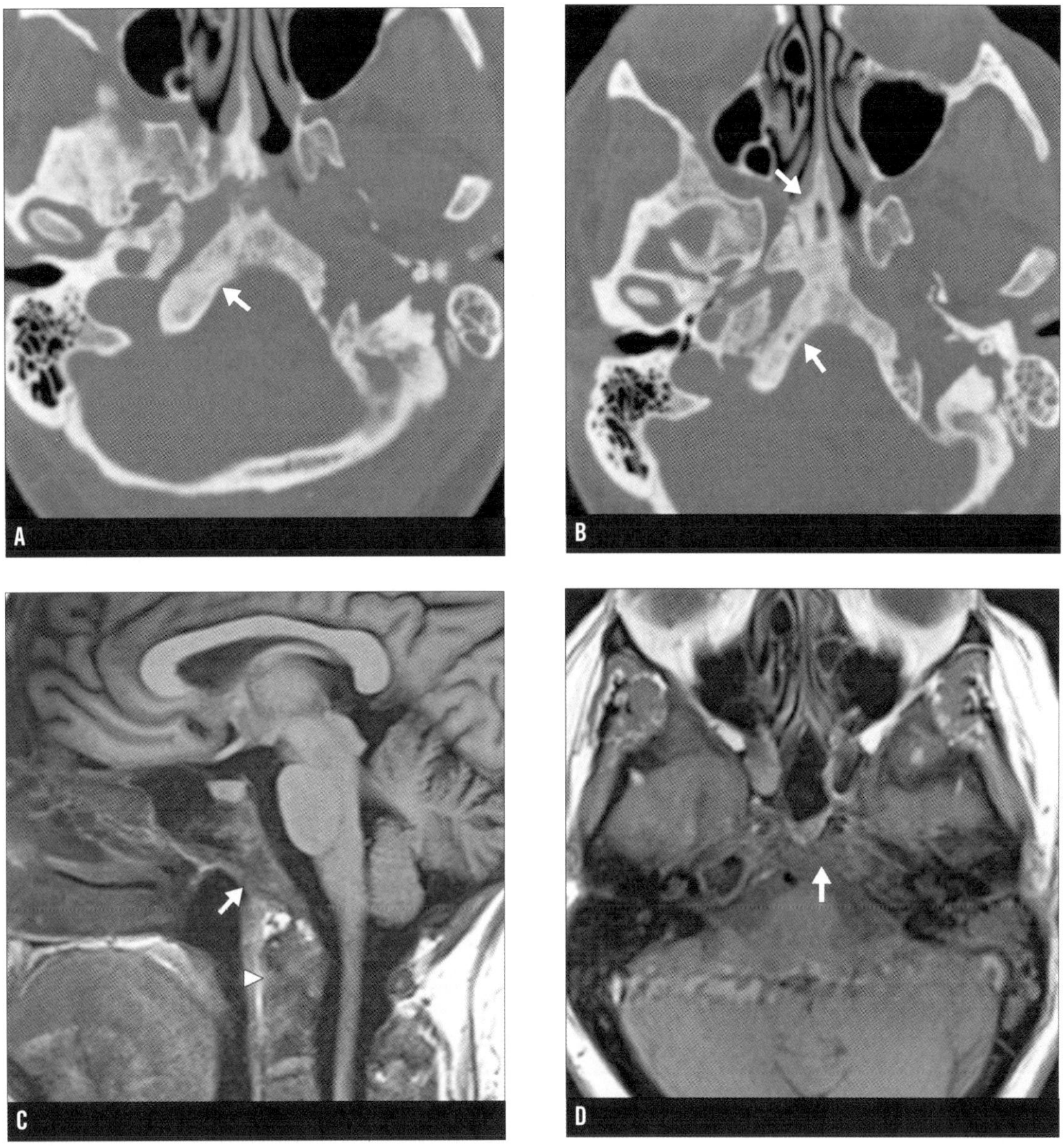

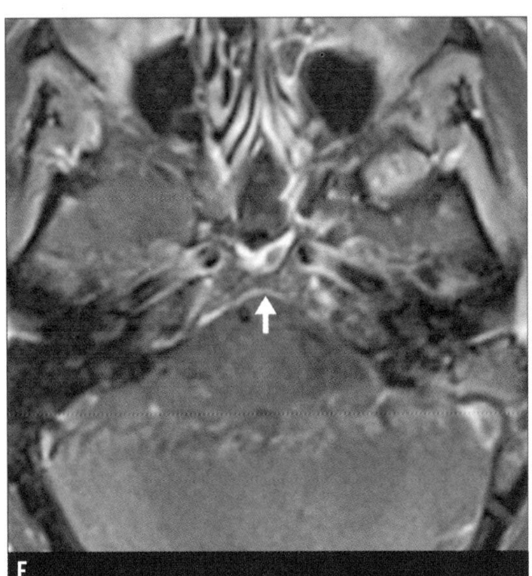

History of breast cancer. Axial CT images viewed with a bone window obtained through the skull base (**A, B**) demonstrate a sclerotic lesion involving the central skull base (arrows, **A, B**). There is no evidence of osseous expansion, best demonstrated on image **B**. While metastatic disease may certainly result in osseous expansion, the lack of expansion effectively excludes a fibro-osseous lesion. Unenhanced sagittal T1 (**C**), unenhanced axial T1 (**D**), and postcontrast axial T1 with fat suppression (**E**) MR images demonstrate a minimally enhancing, T1 hypointense lesion involving the skull base (arrows, **C-E**). There is also abnormal precontrast T1-weighted signal in the cervical spine (arrowhead, **C**). Given the history of breast cancer, the findings are compatible with osteoblastic metastatic disease. Minimal or lack of enhancement can be seen with osteoblastic metastasis.

REFERENCES

Adada B, Al-Mefty O: Fibrous dysplasia of the clivus. *Neurosurgery.* 2003:52;318-322; discussion 323.

Aoki S, Dillon WP, Barkovich AJ, Norman D. Marrow conversion before pneumatization of the sphenoid sinus: assessment with MR imaging. *Radiology.* 1989; 172:373-375.

Kim E. Fibrous dysplasia of the clivus. *J Korean Neurosurg Soc.* 2010;48(5):441-444. Epub November 2010.

Scuderi AJ, Harnsberger HR, Boyer RS. Pneumatization of the paranasal sinuses: normal features of importance to the accurate interpretation of CT scans and MR images. *AJR Am J Roentgenol.* 1993;160:1101-1104.

Sirvanci M, Karaman K, Onat L, Duran C, Ulusoy OL. Monostotic fibrous dysplasia of the clivus: MRI and CT findings. *Neuroradiology.* 2002;44:847-850.

Welker KM, DeLone DR, Lane JI, Gilbertson JR. Arrested pneumatization of the skull base: imaging characteristics. *AJR Am J Roentgenol.* 2008;190:1691-1696.

CASE 6 Anterior clinoid process pneumatization simulating an aneurysm

Pneumatization of the anterior clinoid process is a common variant, demonstrated as being present in 4.6% of cases in one study and 14.7% in another study. While an incidental finding and readily identifiable on CT, anterior clinoid process pneumatization may simulate an aneurysm on MR imaging of the brain. Susceptibility artifact on a gradient-recalled echo (GRE) sequence related to air within anterior clinoid process pneumatization may aid in differentiating this incidental finding from an aneurysm. However, when in doubt, a CT study to rule in a pneumatized anterior clinoid process, or alternatively, a CTA or MRA to rule out an aneurysm, may be necessary. A pneumatized anterior clinoid process almost always communicates with the paranasal sinuses, typically the sphenoid sinus or posterior ethmoid air cells. Thus, a breach of a pneumatized anterior clinoid process during surgery may result in CSF rhinorrhea, and its presence should be relayed to the surgeon prior to surgery in this region.

Anterior clinoid process pneumatization simulating an aneurysm

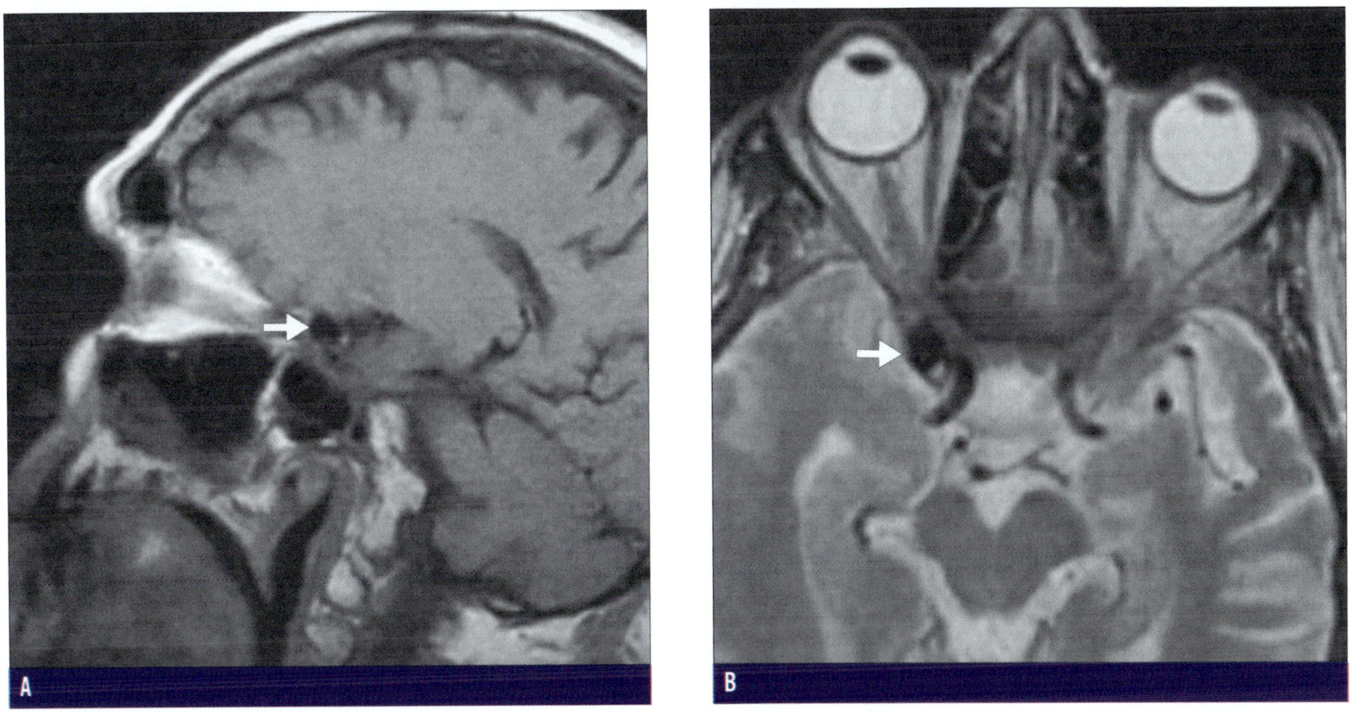

Sagittal T1 (**A**), axial T2 (**B**), and axial proton density (**C**) MR images demonstrate a prominent apparent flow void in the right paraclinoid region, raising the possibility of a right paraclinoid aneurysm (arrows, **A-C**). An axial CT image viewed with a bone window through the same level as images **B** and **C** (**D**) demonstrates that the apparent flow void on MRI simply represents a pneumatized anterior clinoid process and not an aneurysm (arrow, **D**).

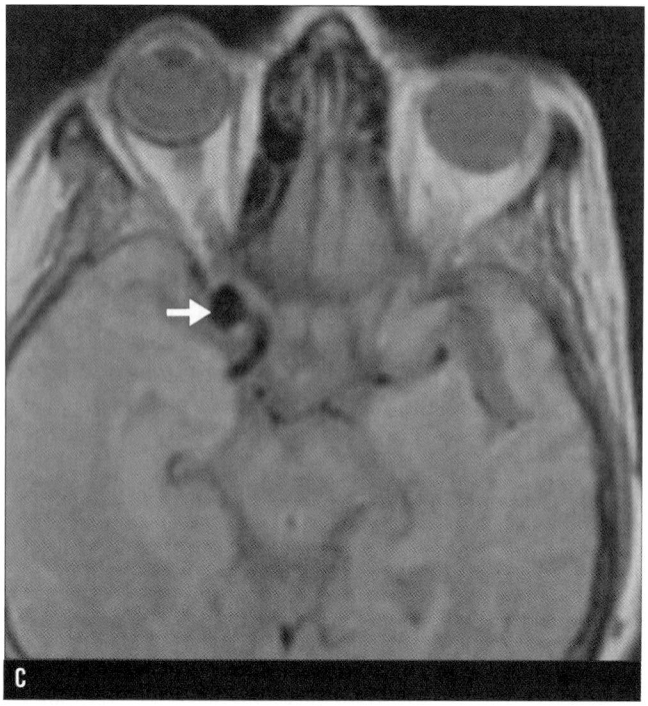

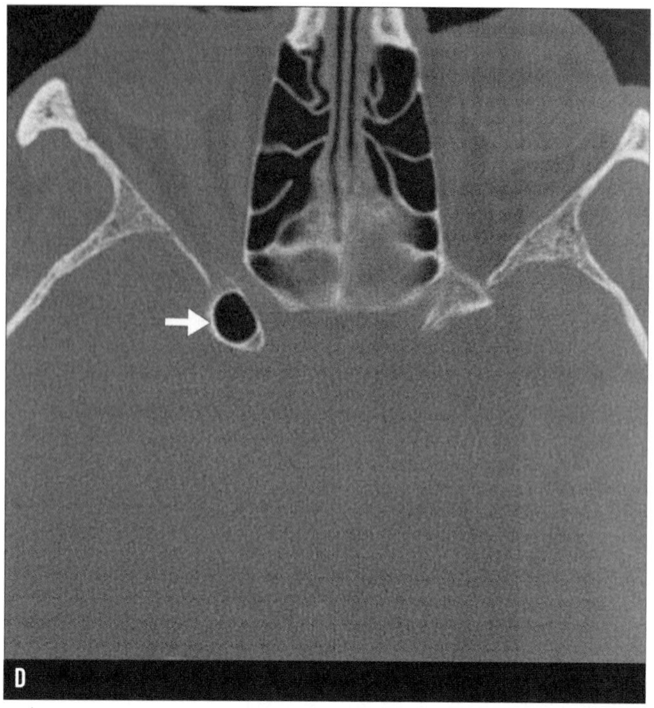

Anterior clinoid process pneumatization simulating an aneurysm adjacent to a true aneurysm

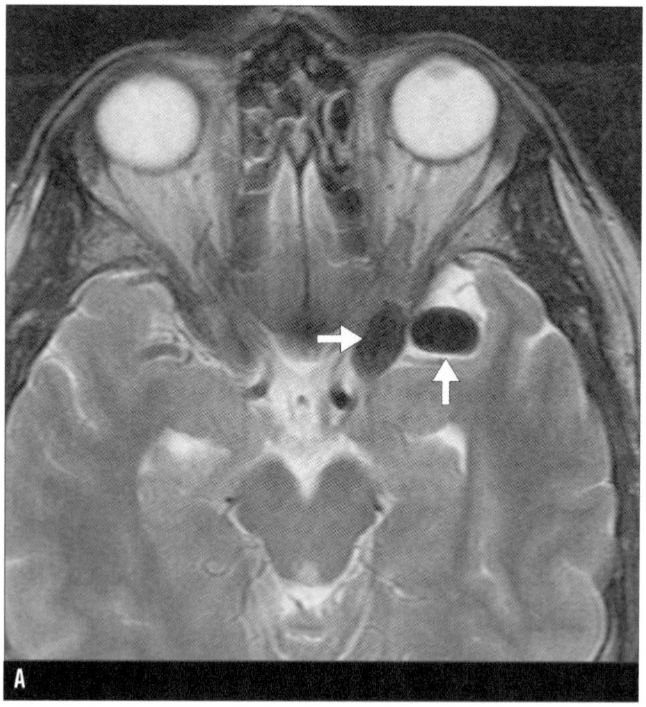

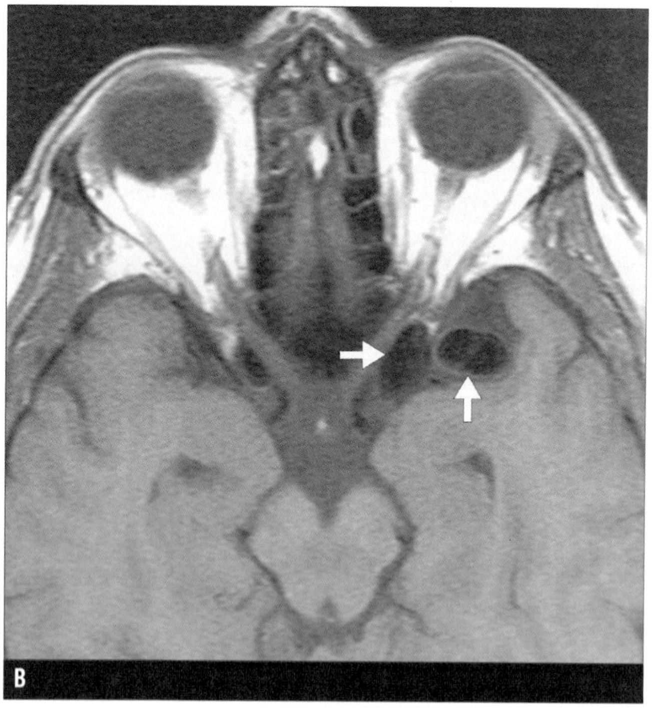

Different patient. Axial T2 (**A**) and axial T1 (**B**) MR images demonstrate two oval, circumscribed hypointense structures nearly perpendicular to one another in the left paraclinoid region (arrows, **A**, **B**). An axial postcontrast T1-weighted MR image (**C**) through the same level demonstrates the more lateral oval finding to enhance (arrow, **C**). An axial source image from a time of flight MRA through this level (**D**) demonstrates flow-related signal through the more lateral oval finding (arrow, **D**). Axial (**E**) and coronal reformatted (**F**) postcontrast images from a CTA demonstrate the more lateral oval finding to represent an aneurysm (arrows, **E**, **F**), and the more medial apparent lesion to simply represent a pneumatized left anterior clinoid process (arrowheads, **E**, **F**). To a lesser degree, there is also pneumatization of the right anterior clinoid process.

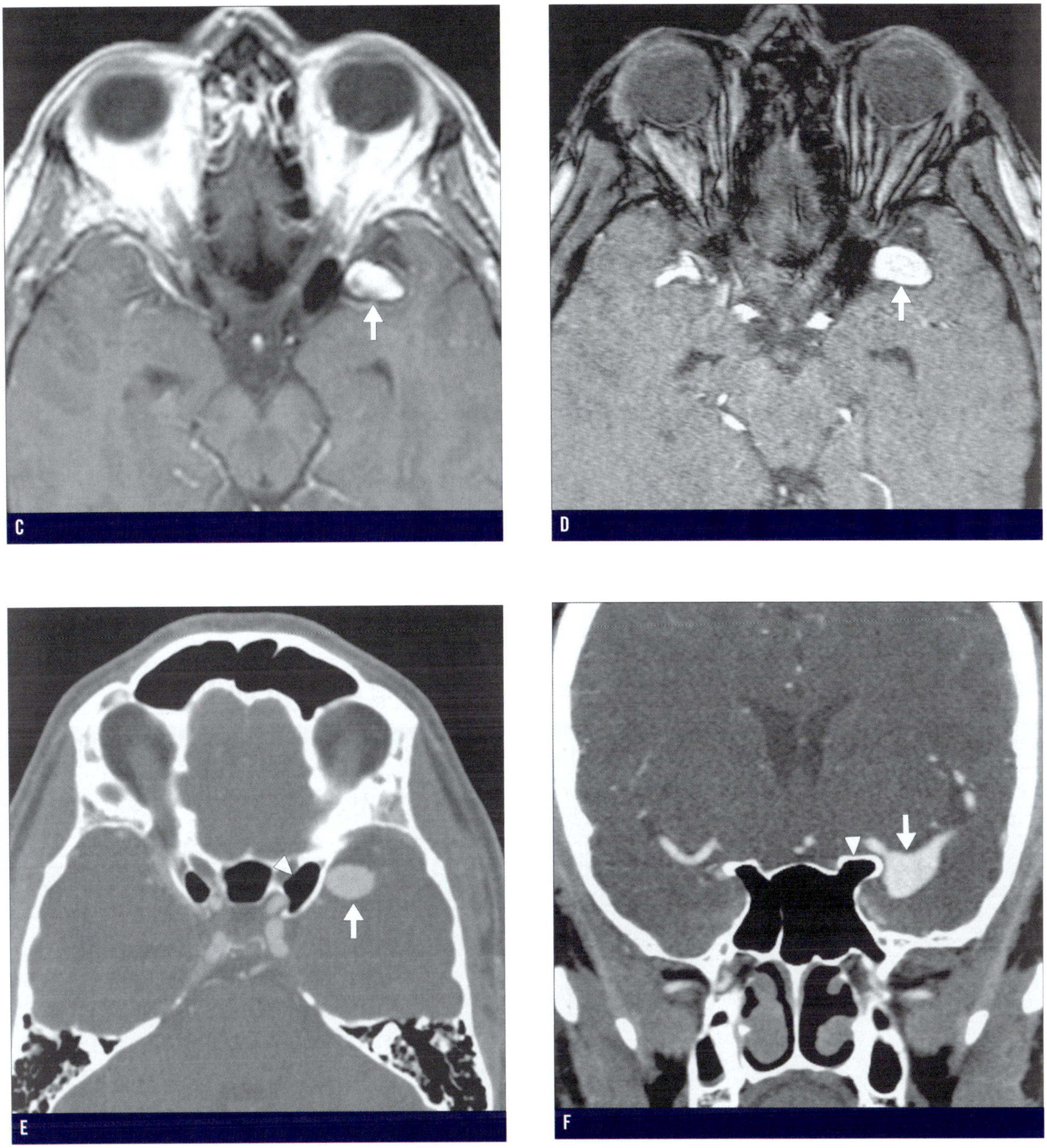

REFERENCES

Gean, AD, et al. A pneumatized anterior clinoid mimicking an aneurysm on MR imaging. Report of two cases. *J Neurosurg.* 1989;71:128-132.

Mikami T, et al. Anatomical variations in pneumatization of the anterior clinoid process. *J Neurosurg.* 2007;106:170-174.

CASE 7 Asymmetric sphenoid sinus pneumatization simulating a lesion on MRI

Various portions of the sphenoid bone may pneumatize and asymmetrically enlarge the sphenoid sinus, often yielding confusing imaging findings on MRI. An asymmetrically pneumatized sphenoid sinus on MRI may simulate an ipsilateral sclerotic lesion or, because of the asymmetry, a mass affecting the contralateral nonpneumatized portion of the sphenoid. Sphenoid sinus pneumatization may extend into the lateral/pterygoid recesses of the sphenoid, greater and lesser wings of the sphenoid, clivus, anterior and posterior clinoid processes, and the optic strut, among other areas. Recognizing certain patterns of sphenoid sinus pneumatization may aid surgical entry into the sphenoid sinus and impact a surgeon's approach to lesions within or adjacent to the sphenoid sinus. Conversely, the lack of awareness of asymmetric sphenoid sinus pneumatization during surgery may result in injury to critical structures, such as the carotid canal or optic nerve.

COMPANION CASE

- **Intraosseous meningioma.** Intraosseous meningiomas may involve the calvarium or skull base. These tumors are hypothesized to arise from arachnoid rests or cap cells that have undergone abnormal migration during embryogenesis, often arising near sutures. Most intraosseous meningiomas are osteoblastic and induce hyperostosis. Occasionally, lytic intraosseous meningiomas may occur, which tend to be more aggressive. On CT, most intraosseous meningiomas will result in thickening and sclerosis of the diploic space as well as the inner and outer calvarial tables. On MRI, intraosseous meningiomas tend to be T1 hypointense, T2 hypointense and heterogeneously enhance. Compared to CT, MRI is more sensitive in detecting the presence of an extraosseous soft tissue component, which is usually more homogeneously enhancing relative to the intraosseous component.

Asymmetric sphenoid sinus pneumatization simulating a lesion on MRI

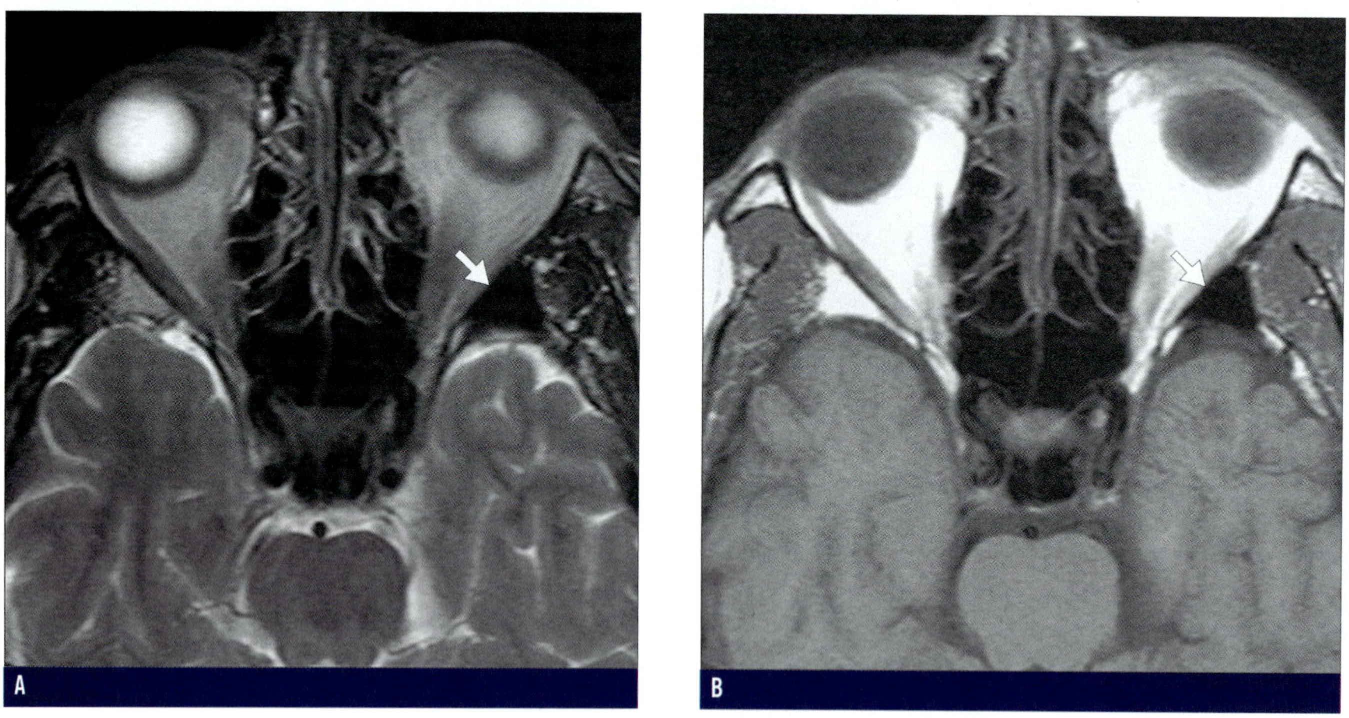

Axial T2 (**A**), unenhanced axial T1 (**B**), and postcontrast axial T1 (**C**) MR images through the greater wings of the sphenoid demonstrate hypointense signal in the left greater wing of the sphenoid on all three sequences (arrows, **A-C**). Based on MRI, this finding is nonspecific and could represent incidental pneumatization of the left greater wing of the sphenoid or a densely sclerotic mass. Axial CT images through the sphenoid sinus (**D**, **E**) demonstrate incidental asymmetric pneumatization of the left greater wing of the sphenoid corresponding to the finding on MRI (arrows, **D**, **E**).

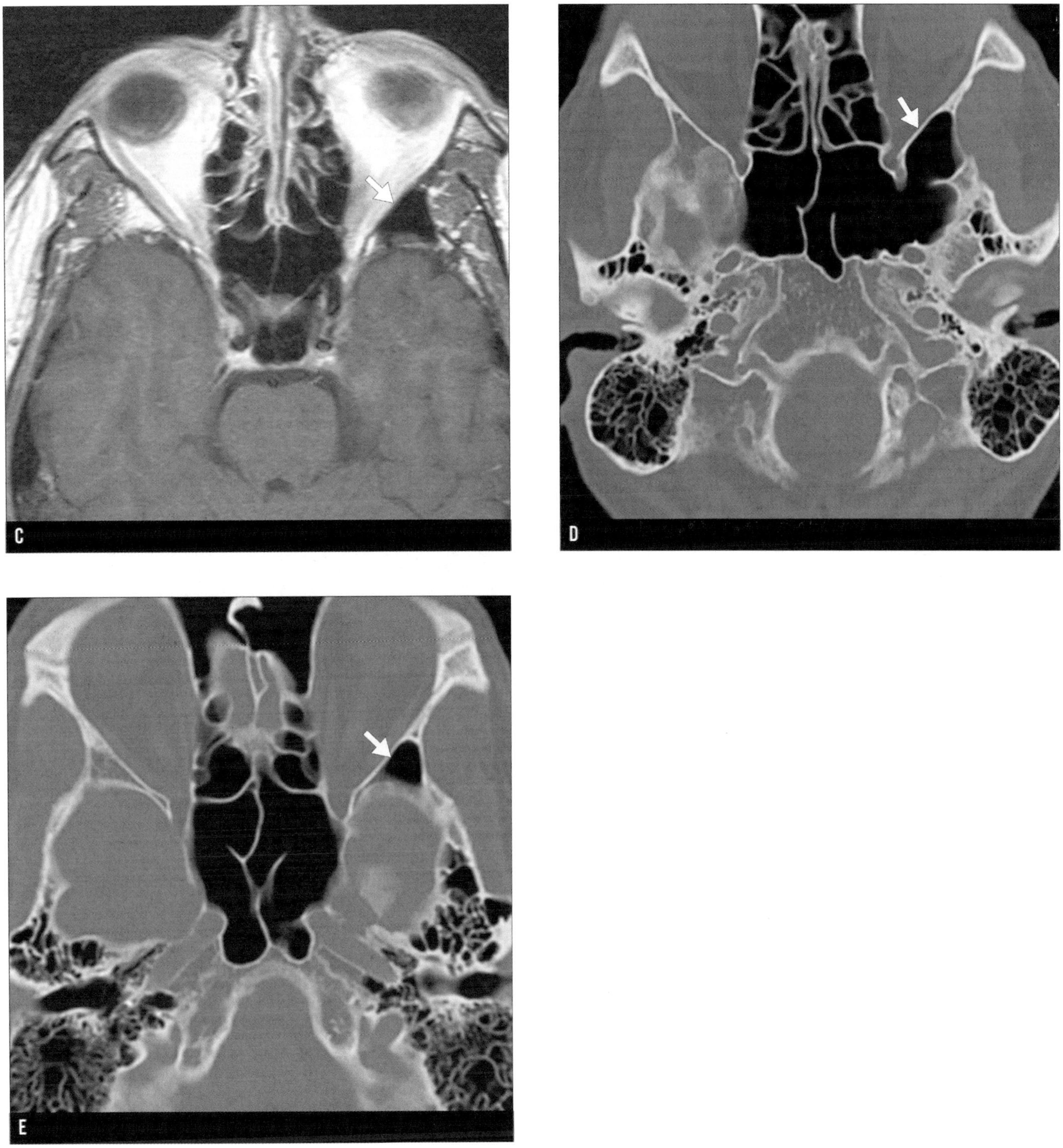

Companion case: Intraosseous meningioma

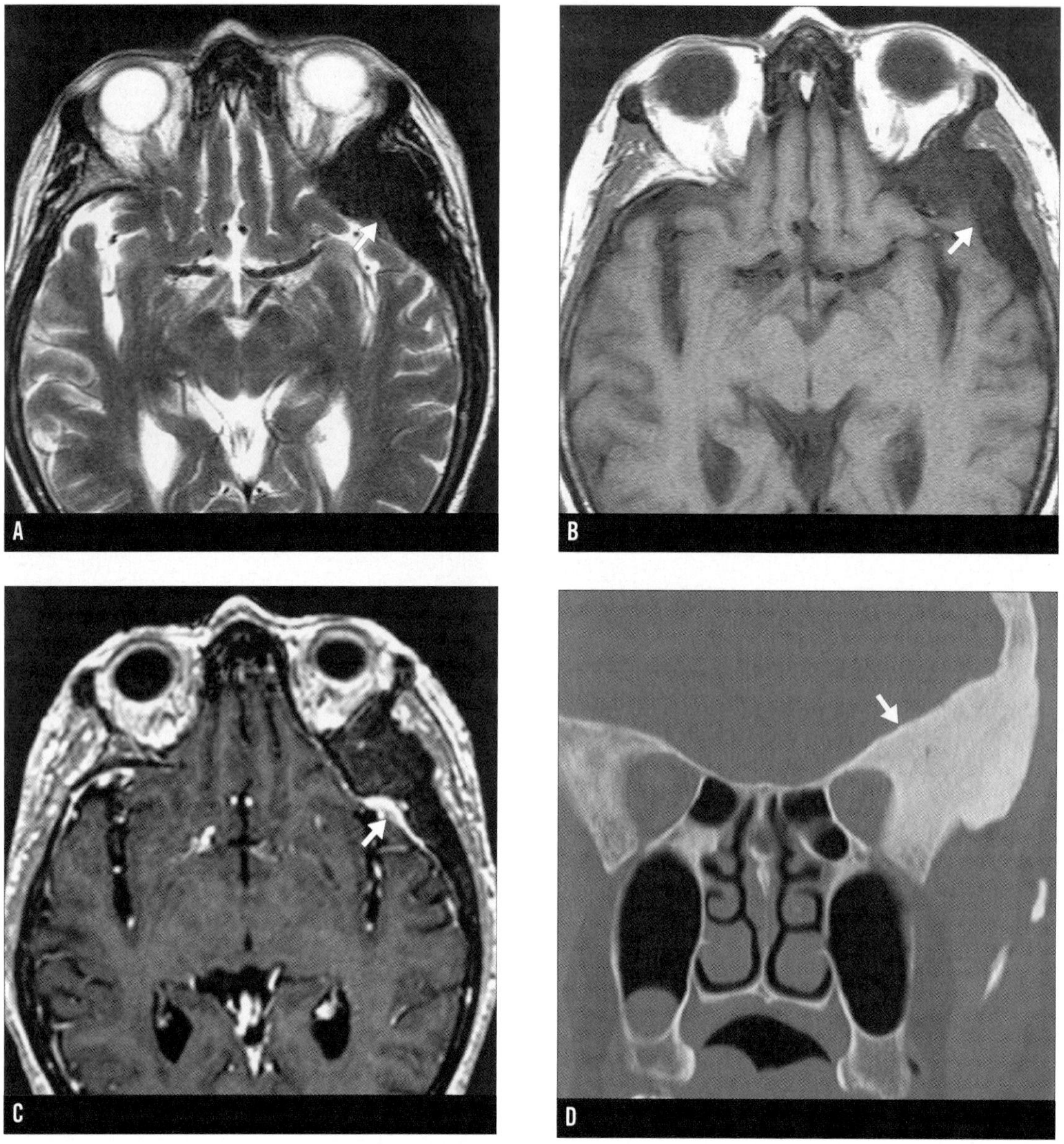

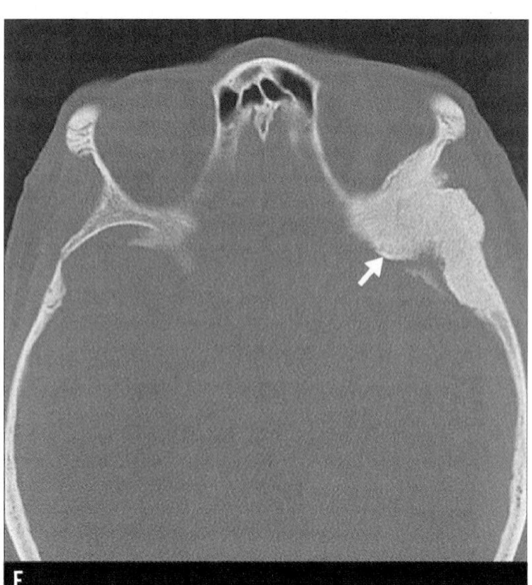

Axial T2 (**A**) and unenhanced axial T1 (**B**) MR images through the lower brain demonstrate a T2 and T1 hypointense, expansile lesion centered in the left greater wing of sphenoid and involving the lateral wall of the orbit (arrows, **A**, **B**). A postcontrast axial MPRAGE MR image through the same level (**C**) demonstrates pachymeningeal thickening and enhancement (arrow, **C**), although the osseous portion of the lesion does not enhance. Axial (**D**) and coronal reformatted (**E**) CT images demonstrate the lesion to be markedly thickened and diffusely sclerotic (arrows, **D**, **E**). The findings are consistent with an intraosseous meningioma.

REFERENCES

Lee HY, et al. Intraosseous meningioma: CT and MR Appearance. *J Comput Assist Tomogr.* 1992;16(6):1000-1001.

SË irikci A, Bayazõt YA, Bayram M, Mumbuç S, Güngör K, Kanlõkama M. Variations of sphenoid and related structures. *Eur Radiol.* 2000;10:844-848.

Wang J, Bidari S, Inoue K, Yang H, Rhoton A. Extensions of the sphenoid sinus: a new classification, *Neurosurgery.* 2010;66(4):797-816.

CASE 8 Asymmetric sphenoid sinus pneumatization deforming the sella turcica

As discussed in preceding cases within this chapter, the sphenoid sinus pneumatizes to a varying degree and sometimes asymmetrically. If the asymmetric pneumatization is in the region of the sella turcica, then the pneumatization may deform the sella turcica, occasionally simulating a pituitary abnormality on MRI.

COMPANION CASE

- **Pneumatization of the dorsum sella.** While incidental, this finding almost always communicates with the sphenoid sinus, and inadvertent breach of a pneumatized dorsum sella during surgery may result in a CSF leak.

Asymmetric sphenoid sinus pneumatization deforming the sella turcica

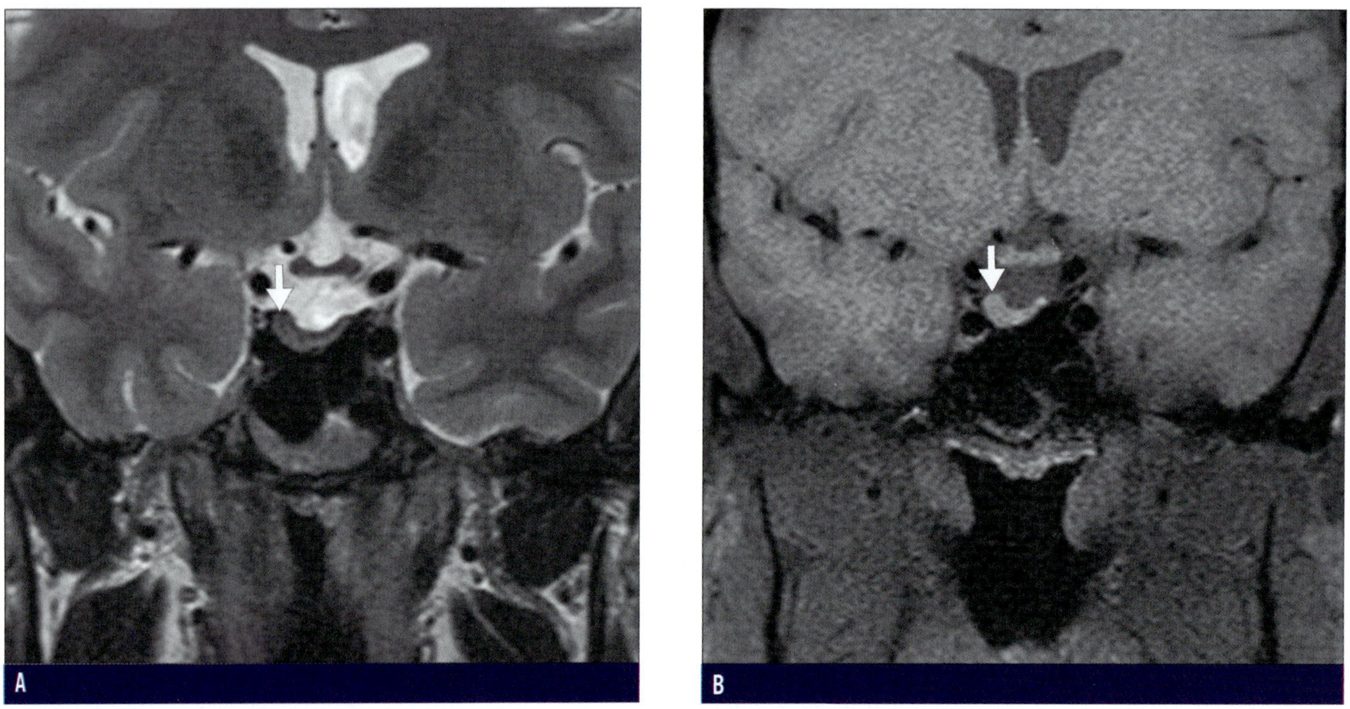

Coronal T2 (**A**), precontrast coronal T1 with fat suppression (**B**), and postcontrast coronal T1 with fat suppression (**C**) MR images demonstrate asymmetry of the pituitary gland, with the right aspect larger than the left, raising the possibility of a right-sided pituitary gland lesion (arrows, **A-C**). Axial CT images through the sella turcica viewed with a soft tissue window (**D**) and a bone window (**E**) as well as a coronal reformatted CT image viewed with an intermediate window (**F**) demonstrate an asymmetrically larger degree of pneumatization within the sphenoid sinus along the left aspect of the sella turcica (arrows, **D**, **E**) that results in deformity of the left aspect of the sella turcica (arrow, **F**). This accounts for the relatively larger, but normal, right aspect of the pituitary gland demonstrated on MRI.

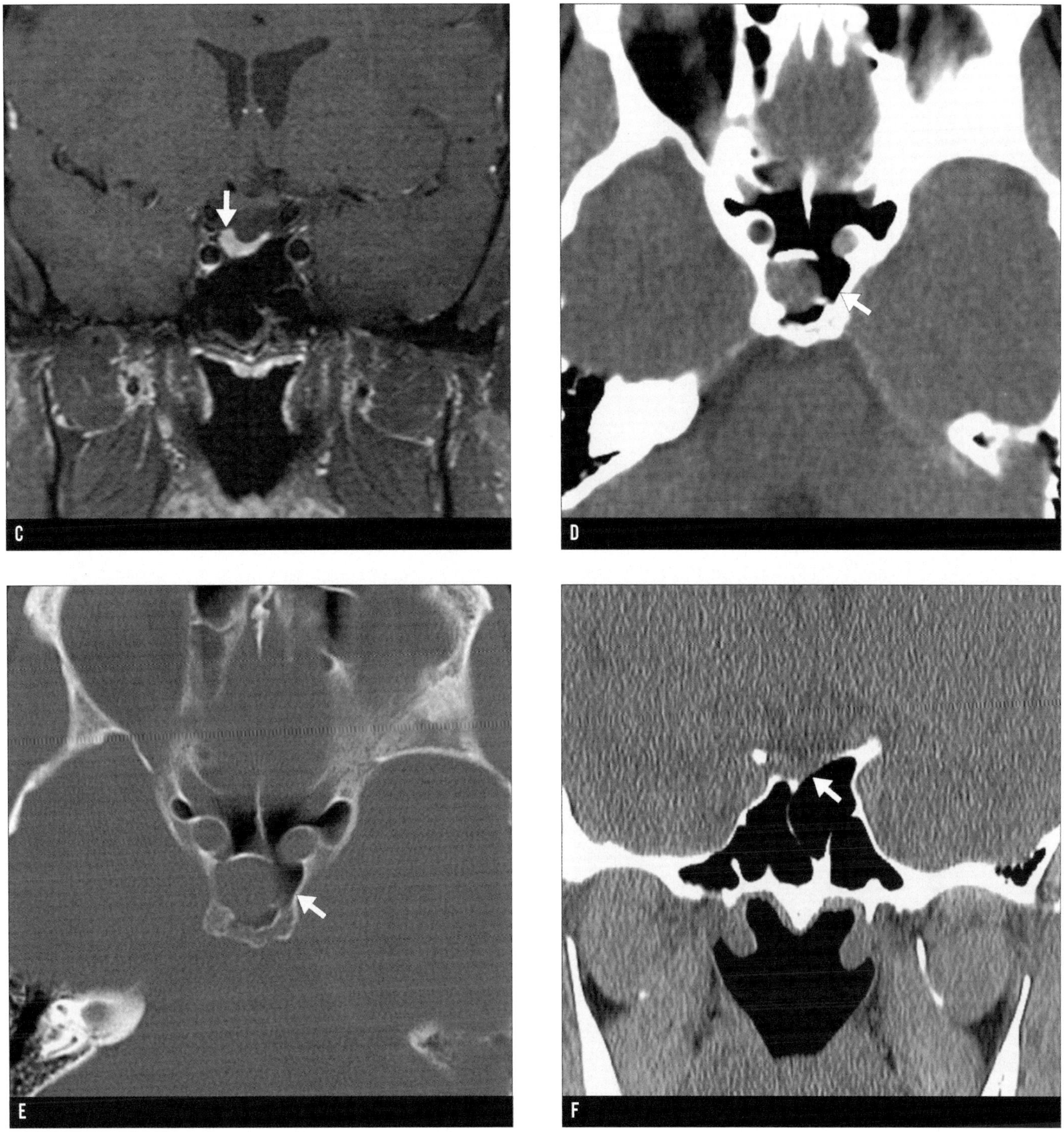
C
D
E
F

Companion case: Pneumatization of the dorsum sella

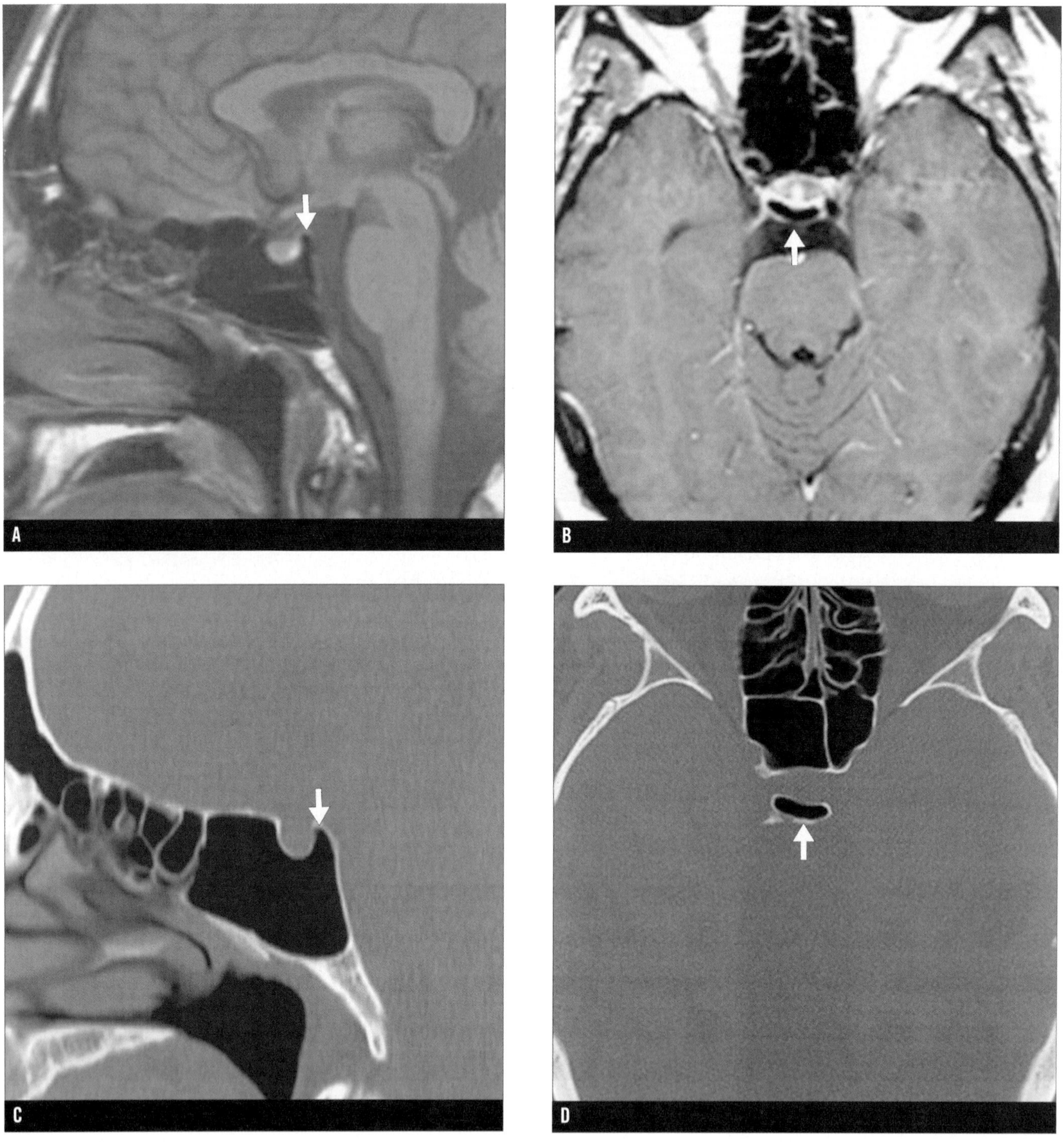

Sagittal T1 (**A**) and postcontrast axial T1 (**B**) MR images demonstrate hypointense T1 signal posterior to the pituitary gland (arrows, **A**, **B**). While the finding is certainly suggestive of incidental pneumatization of the dorsum sella on image **A**, the finding could be confused with pathology if only assessed on image **B**. Sagittal reformatted (**C**) and axial (**D**) CT images confirm the presence of incidental pneumatization of the dorsum sella (arrows, **C**, **D**), which is fully contiguous with the sphenoid sinus.

REFERENCE

Hamid O, El Fiky L, Hassan O, Kotb A, El Fiky S. Anatomic variations of the sphenoid sinus and their impact on trans-sphenoid pituitary surgery. *Skull Base*. 2008;18(1):9-15.

CASE 9 Interclinoid bar

Interclinoid bars are important to recognize, both for their surgical implications and for their propensity to simulate pathology on imaging, particularly on MRI. Various etiologies have been proposed to explain the formation of interclinoid bars, although they likely result from ossification of normally present ligaments at these locations—specifically, the pterygospinous, interclinoid, and caroticoclinoid ligaments.

There are four types of interclinoid bars that have been described by Archana et al, often forming foramina beneath the bars. These interclinoid bars may be complete, incomplete (approaching but not contacting), or minimally contacting one another. The infrequently discussed middle clinoid processes referred to below represent small paired osseous eminences along the lateral margins of the anterior sella turcica wall.

- Type I is a bridge between the anterior and middle clinoid processes, forming an anterior interclinoid (also called caroticoclinoid) foramen beneath the bar. A portion of the intracranial carotid artery passes through the anterior clinoid foramen.
- Type II is a bridge between the anterior, middle, and posterior clinoid processes. This forms an anterior interclinoid foramen anteriorly and a posterior interclinoid foramen posteriorly beneath the bar. The lateral portion of the posterior intercavernous sinus traverses through the posterior interclinoid foramen.
- Type III is a bridge between the anterior and posterior clinoid processes (also called "sella turcica bridge"), forming a large, common interclinoid foramen beneath the bar. A portion of the intracranial carotid artery traverses through the anterior aspect of this foramen, whereas the lateral portion of the posterior intercavernous sinus traverses through the posterior aspect of this foramen.
- Type IV is a bridge between the middle and posterior clinoid processes, forming a posterior interclinoid foramen beneath the bar.

Removal of an anterior clinoid process is often necessary to gain access and to properly visualize lesions in this region, such as clinoidal segment aneurysms, carotid-cavernous fistulas, and regional meningiomas. Similarly, the presence of an interclinoid bar will frequently need to be removed to gain access to these types of lesions. Also, several cranial nerves are in this vicinity, such as cranial nerves II and III. These cranial nerves may be injured during resection of an anterior clinoid process and are possibly at even more risk for injury if an interclinoid bar is present.

On MRI, interclinoid bars may simulate a pituitary adenoma (due to volume averaging with the interclinoid bar marrow space), result in midline shift of the pituitary gland, or result in a dysmorphic pituitary gland shape.

Interclinoid bar

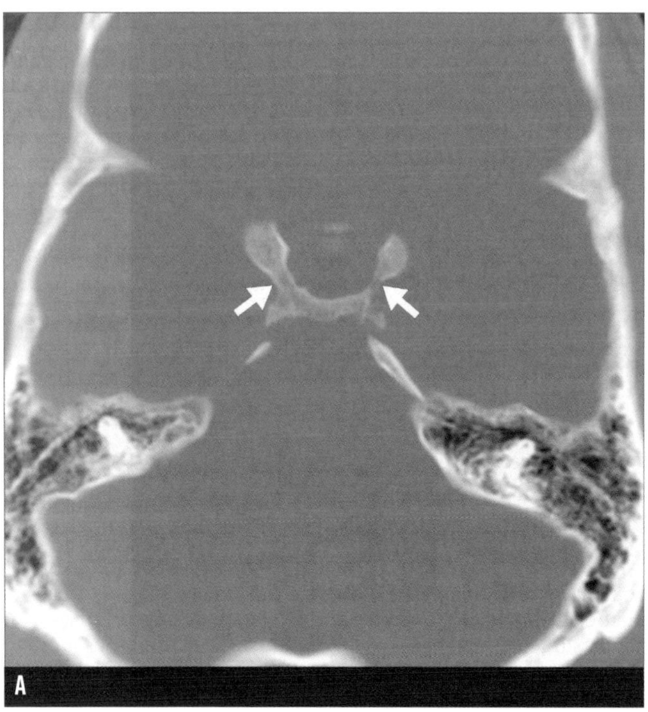

An axial CT image (**A**) demonstrates typical bilateral interclinoid bars, right larger than left (arrows). These likely represent Type III interclinoid bars given that the osseous bridges extend between the anterior and posterior clinoid processes. The middle clinoid processes cannot be visualized on this image, but if they are contributing to the bars, then these would constitute Type II interclinoid bars.

Interclinoid bar simulating a pituitary mass on MRI

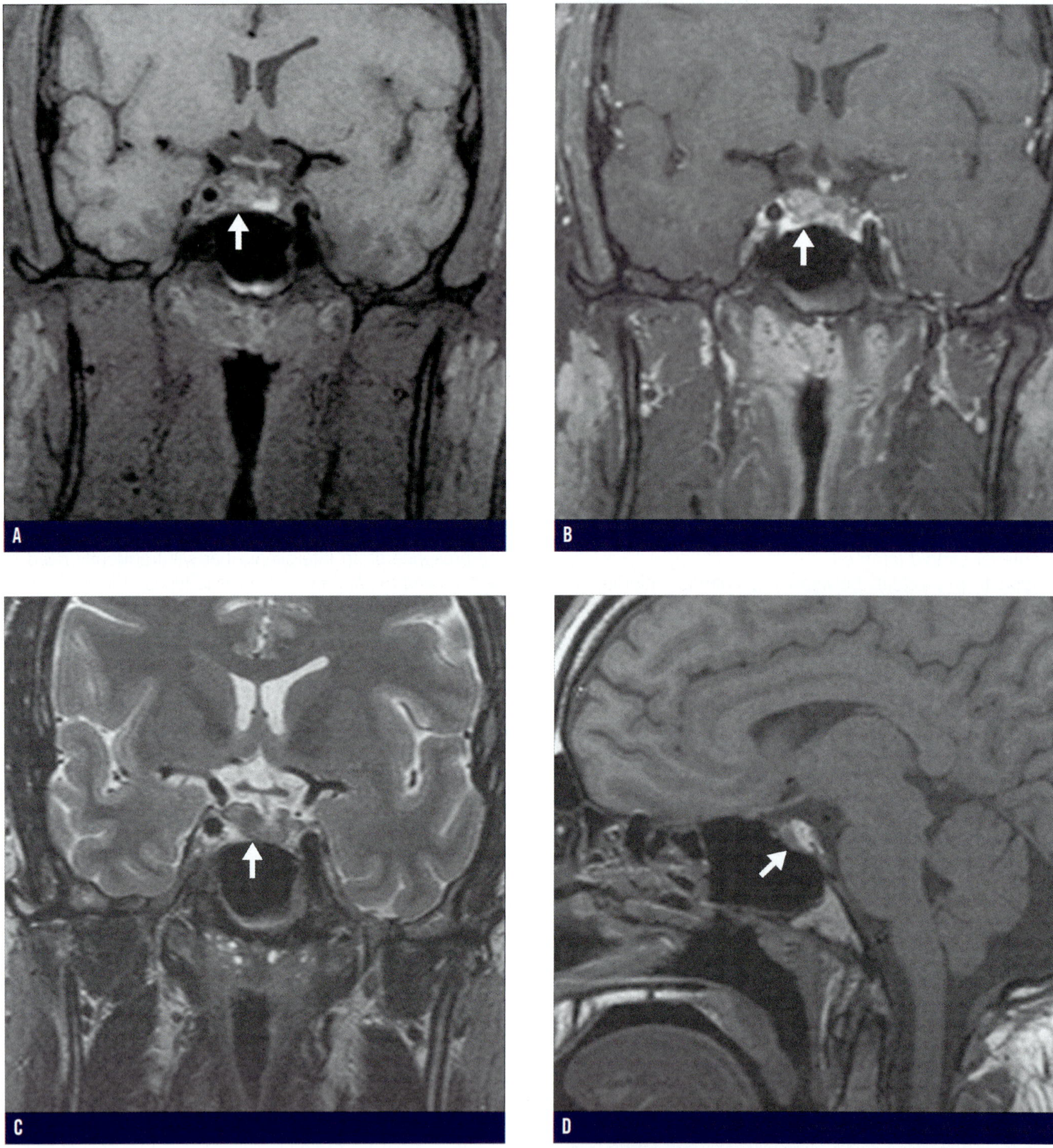

Unenhanced coronal T1 with fat suppression (**A**), contrast-enhanced coronal T1 with fat suppression (**B**), and coronal T2 (**C**) MR images through the sella turcica. There is an apparent lesion within the right aspect of the sella turcica (arrows, **A**-**C**). An unenhanced sagittal T1-weighted MR image through the right aspect of the sella turcica (**D**) demonstrates an unusually small right aspect of the sella turcica (arrow, **D**). An axial CT image through the level of the dorsum sella (**E**) demonstrates a complete or near complete Type III right interclinoid bar (arrow, **E**). A sagittal reformatted CT image just to the right of the sella turcica (**F**) also demonstrates a portion of the right interclinoid bar (arrow, **F**). A coronal CT image through the dorsum sella (**G**) best demonstrates that the apparent MRI finding of a pituitary mass merely represented volume averaging with the marrow of the interclinoid bar (arrow, **G**).

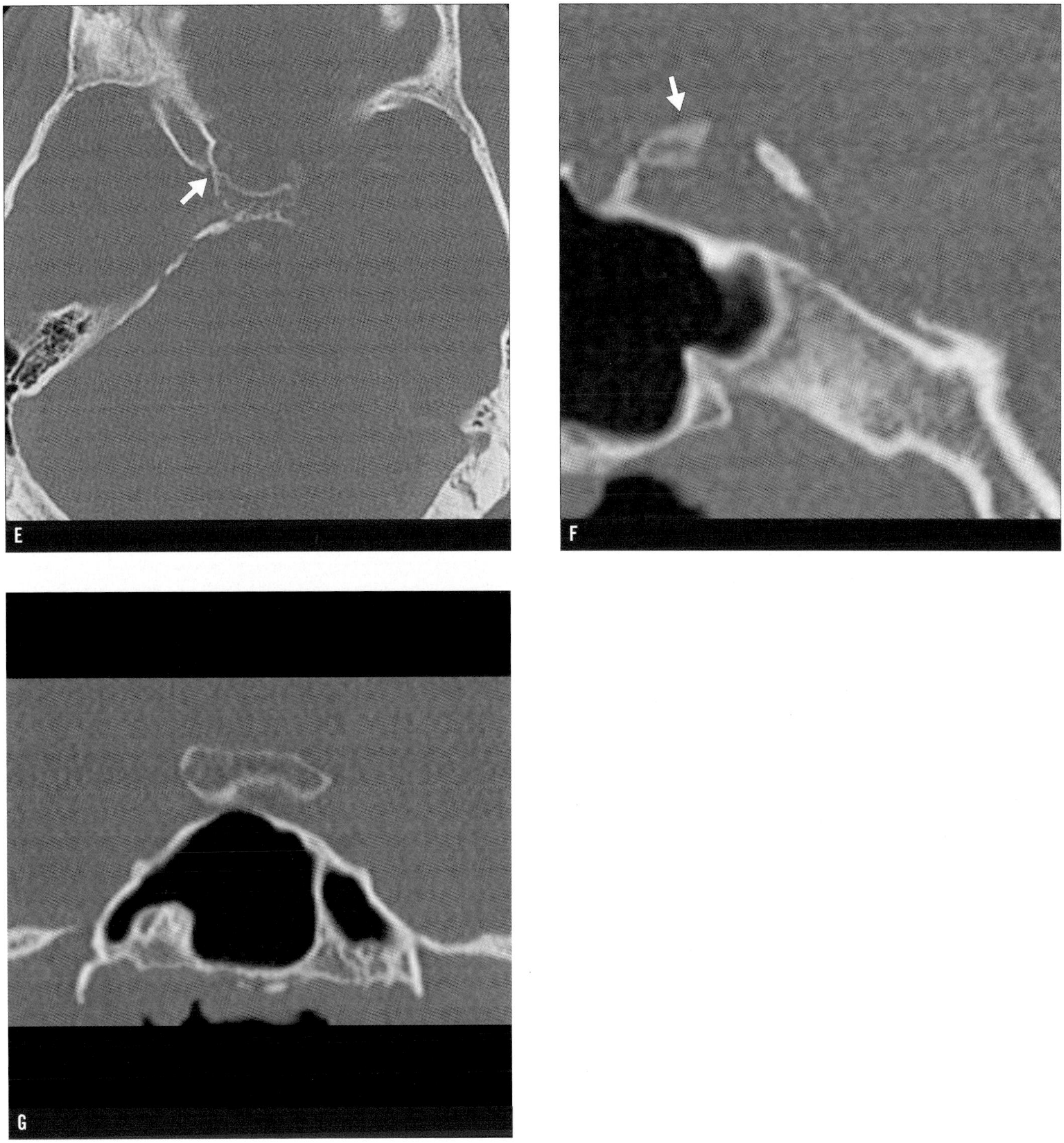
E
F
G

Incomplete interclinoid bar resulting in pituitary gland shift

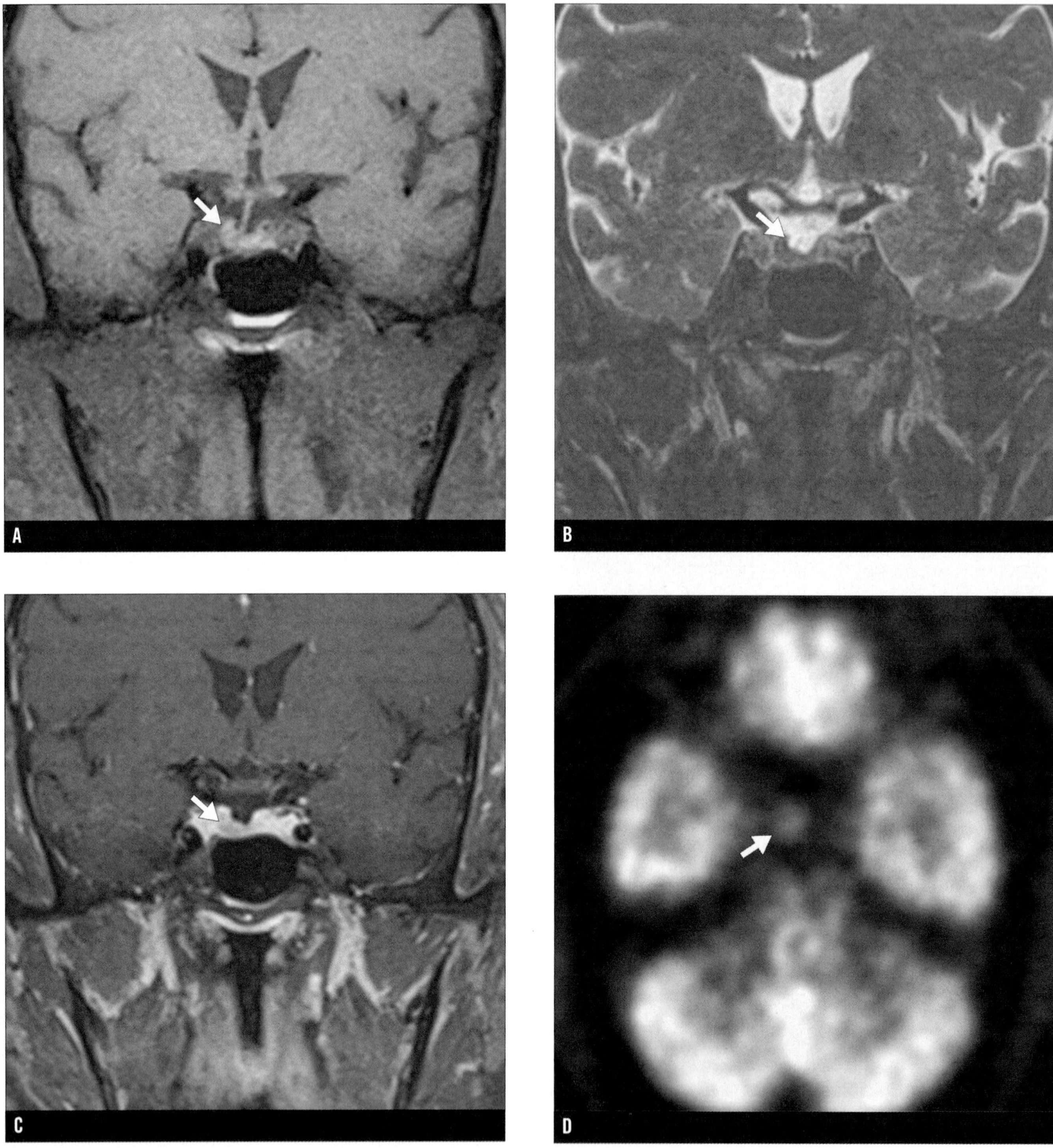

Coronal T1 with fat suppression (**A**), coronal T2 (**B**), and postcontrast coronal T1 with fat suppression (**C**) MR images demonstrate a rightward shift of the pituitary gland and infundibulum (arrows, **A-C**) without an apparent intrasellar mass. Axial (**D**) and coronal (**E**) PET images through the brain from a PET CT also demonstrate the rightward pituitary gland shift (arrows, **D, E**). Axial CT images from the PET CT (**F, G**) explain the finding. There is asymmetric enlargement of the left posterior clinoid process (arrows, **F, G**) approaching but not fusing with the left anterior clinoid process, thus representing an incomplete Type III interclinoid bar. The result is an asymmetrically smaller left aspect of the sella turcica with rightward shift of the pituitary gland and infundibulum.

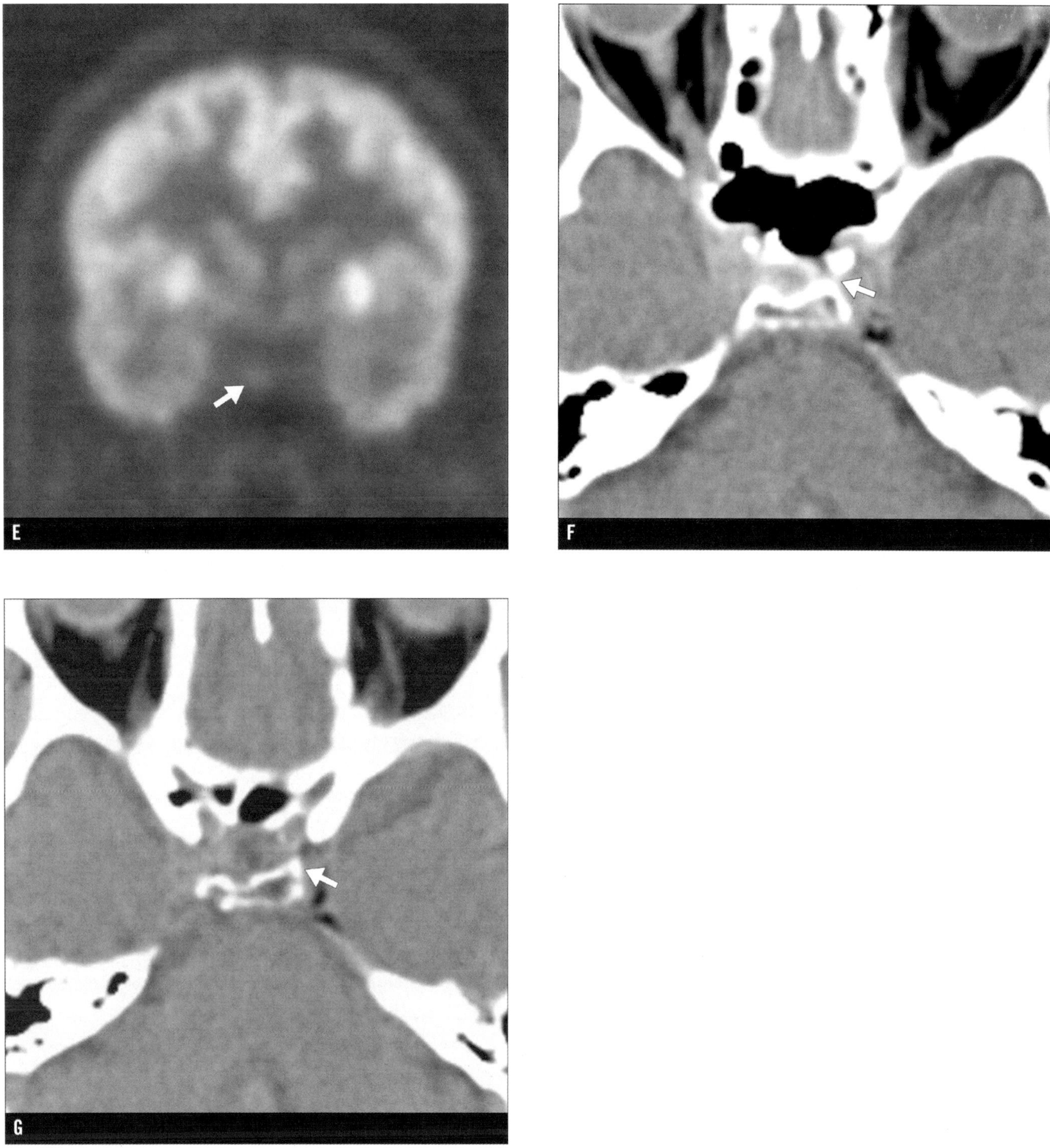

REFERENCES

Archana R, Anita R, Jyoti C, Punita M, Rakesh D. Incidence of osseous interclinoid bars in Indian population. *Surg Radiol Anat.* 2010;32(4):383-387. Epub October 2009.

Ray B, Gupta N. Caroticoclinoid foramen with interclinoid osseous bar. *Clin Anat.* 2006;19(8):732-733.

Williams PL, Bannister LH, Martin MM. *Gray's Anatomy.* 38th ed. London: Churchill Livingstone; 1995.

CASE 10 Occipital bone air cell

Normal pneumatization of the temporal bone begins in the weeks just prior to birth, progressing throughout childhood and into puberty. Pneumatization of the temporal bone can be divided into four regions: mastoid, middle ear, perilabyrinthine, and petrous apex. However, other areas within or surrounding the temporal bones may also pneumatize and are termed accessory sites of pneumatization. These accessory sites include the occipital bone, zygomatic process, squamosal temporal bone, and styloid process. While pneumatization of these accessory sites may be considered normal variants, occasionally excessive pneumatization of these structures, in particular the occipital bone, may result in a fistulous communication and the formation of a pneumatocele. A pneumatocele represents a separate, abnormal collection of air; in the temporal-occipital region, a pneumatocele may develop in the adjacent soft tissues or in the intracranial compartment, the latter representing pneumocephalus, typically extradural in location. Pneumatoceles of this region may occur following minor trauma or during an abrupt pressure change, such as with a Valsalva maneuver or during deep sea diving. The etiology of occipital bone pneumatization is likely the result of extension of pneumatization from the adjacent mastoid via a partially patent occipitomastoid synchondrosis, which remains partially patent during the teenage years or early adulthood.

COMPANION CASE

- **Fluid-filled occipital bone air cell.** Like mastoid opacification, a fluid-filled occipital bone air cell may be symptomatic or completely asymptomatic. However, it is important to properly identify this usually incidental finding from a more aggressive finding, such as a mass.

Occipital bone air cell

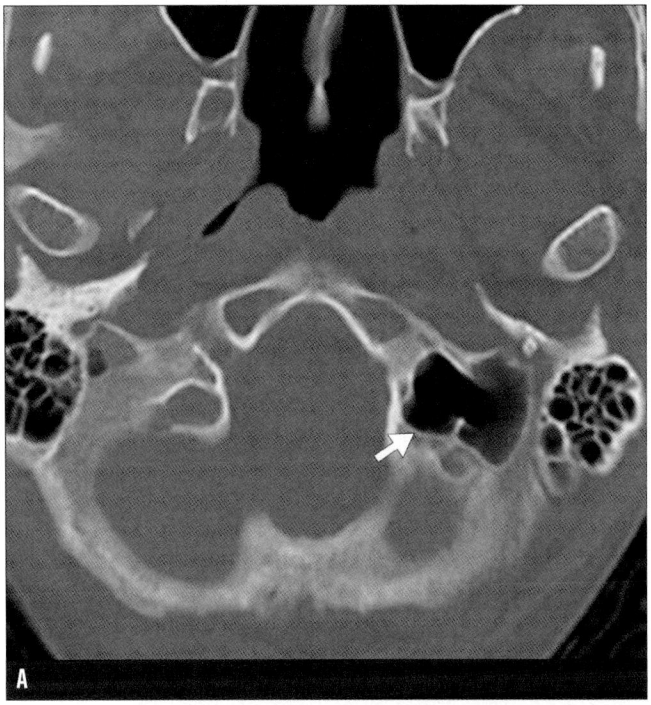

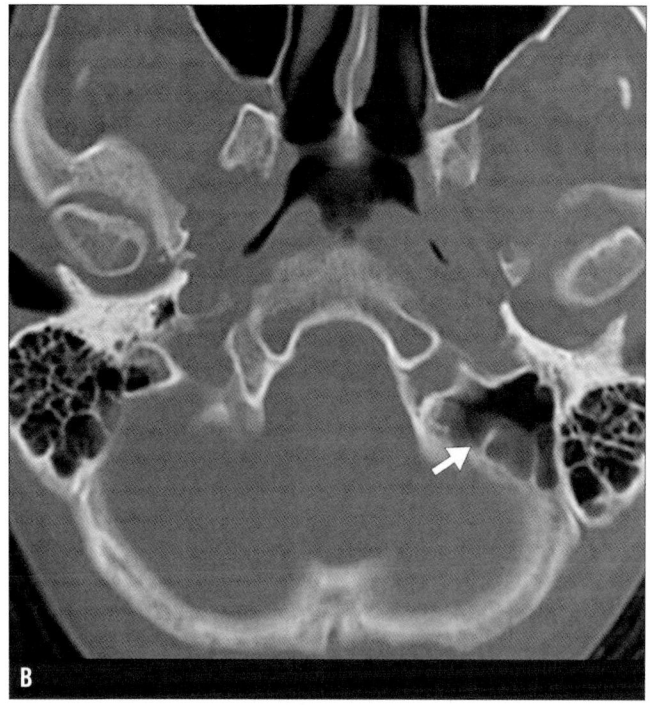

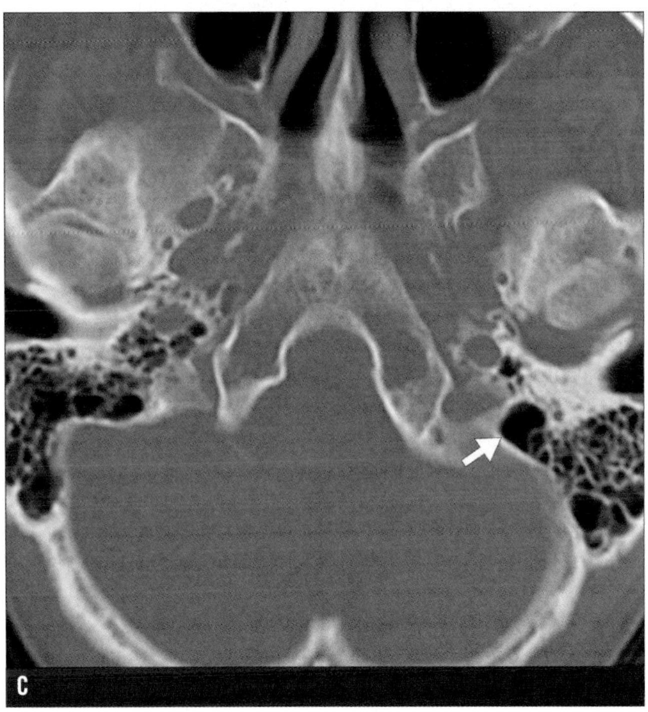

Axial CT images (**A**-**C**) demonstrate incidental pneumatization of the left aspect of the occipital bone (arrows, **A**-**C**).

Companion case: Fluid-filled occipital bone air cell

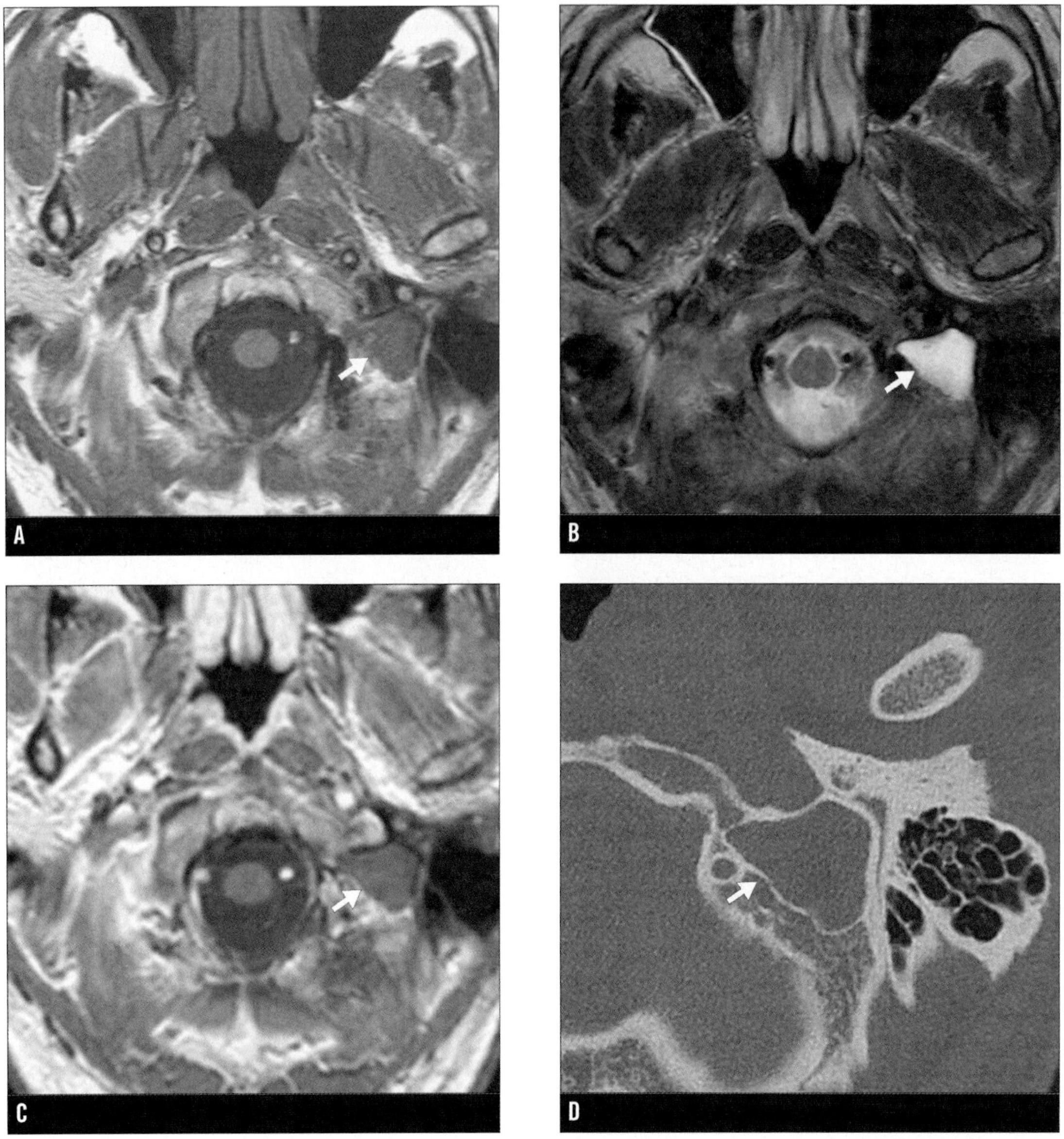

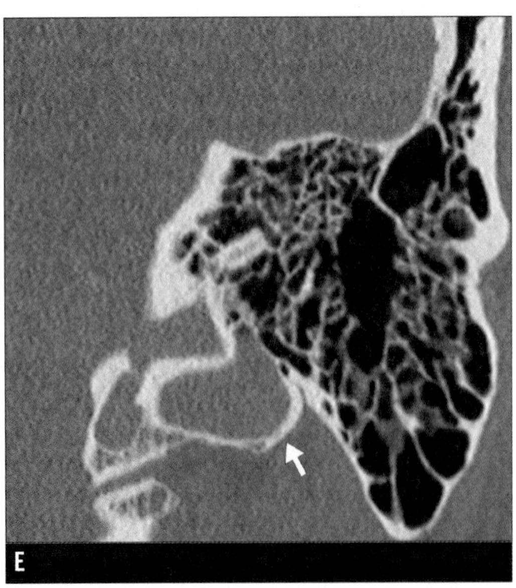

Unenhanced axial T1 (**A**), axial T2 (**B**), and contrast-enhanced axial T1 (**C**) MR images of the left temporal bone demonstrate a region of signal abnormality in the left aspect of the occipital bone. This region contains isointense T1 signal (arrow, **A**), hyperintense T2 signal (arrow, **B**), and does not enhance (arrow, **C**). Noncontrast axial (**D**) and coronal reformatted (**E**) CT images of the left temporal bone from the same patient demonstrate a circumscribed, opacified air cell in the left aspect of the occipital bone (arrows, **D**, **E**) corresponding to the area of signal abnormality on the MR images. There is no evidence of osseous erosion or destruction. The imaging findings are consistent with a fluid-filled, pneumatized air cell in the left aspect of the occipital bone.

REFERENCES

Moss M, Biggs M, Fagan P, Forer M, Davis M, Roche J. Complications of occipital bone pneumatization. *Australas Radiol.* 2004;48(2):259-263.

Petritsch B, Goltz JP, Hahn D, Wendel F. Extensive craniocervical bone pneumatization. *Diagn Interv Radiol.* 2011;17(4):308-310.

Rebol J, Munda A, Tos M. Hyperpneumatization of the temporal, occipital, and parietal bones. *Eur Arch Otorhinolaryngol.* 2004;261(8): 445-448. Epub December 2003.

CASE 11 Crista galli pneumatization

An aerated crista galli may communicate with the adjacent paranasal sinuses, most commonly one of the frontal sinuses, via a diverticular-like extension. Therefore, an aerated crista galli is subject to the same pathology that affects the paranasal sinuses (ie, sinusitis, mucoceles, etc).

COMPANION CASES

- **Ossified crista galli**. When the crista galli is ossified, its marrow cavity often results in fat attenuation and signal on CT and MRI, respectively. Alternatively, a sclerotic crista galli will be hyperattenuating on CT and lack signal on all MRI pulse sequences.
- **Crista galli pneumosinus dilatans with an associated meningioma.** Pneumosinus dilatans (PD) is defined as an abnormally expanded, aerated sinus that extends beyond the normal confines of the native bone. The sinus involved with PD usually has a normal wall thickness. However, PD can be associated with a meningioma, which may induce sinus wall hyperostosis.

  The etiology of PD remains unknown. While PD is idiopathic, it has been described in association with many conditions, including:

  Meningioma
  McCune-Albright syndrome
  Fibrous dysplasia
  Arachnoid cyst
  Brain tumors
  Prolonged CSF shunting
  Cerebral hemiatrophy infantile meningoencephalitis
  von Recklinghausen disease
  Acromegaly

Crista galli pneumatization

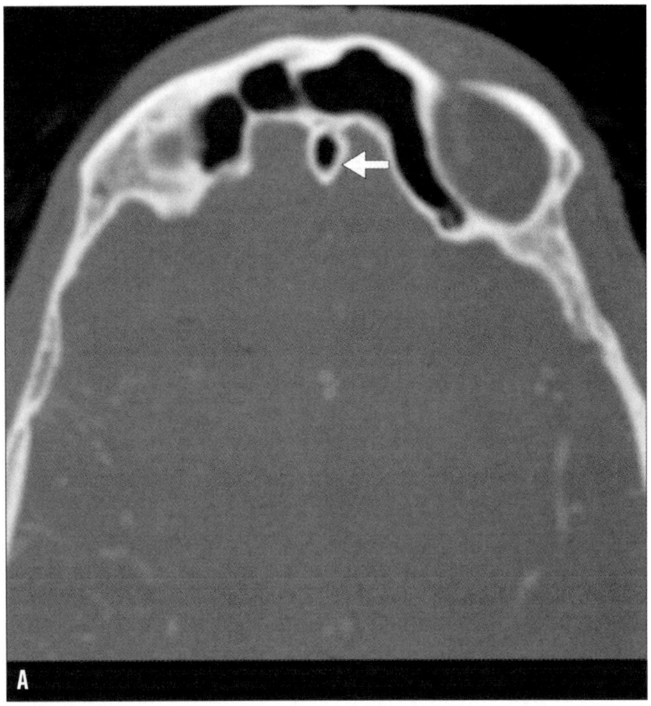

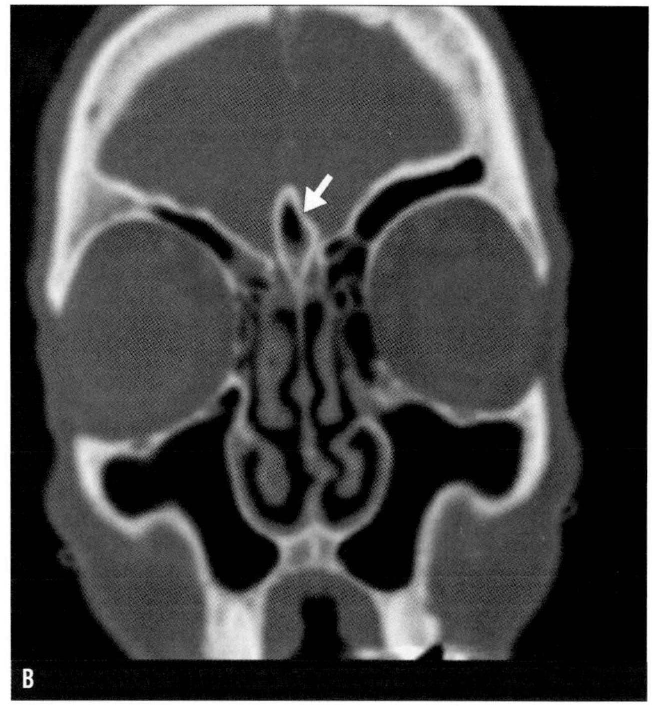

Axial (**A**), coronal reformatted (**B**), and sagittal reformatted (**C**) CT images obtained through the anterior skull base demonstrate a pneumatized crista galli (arrows, **A**-**C**) directly communicating with a frontal sinus (arrowhead, **C**).

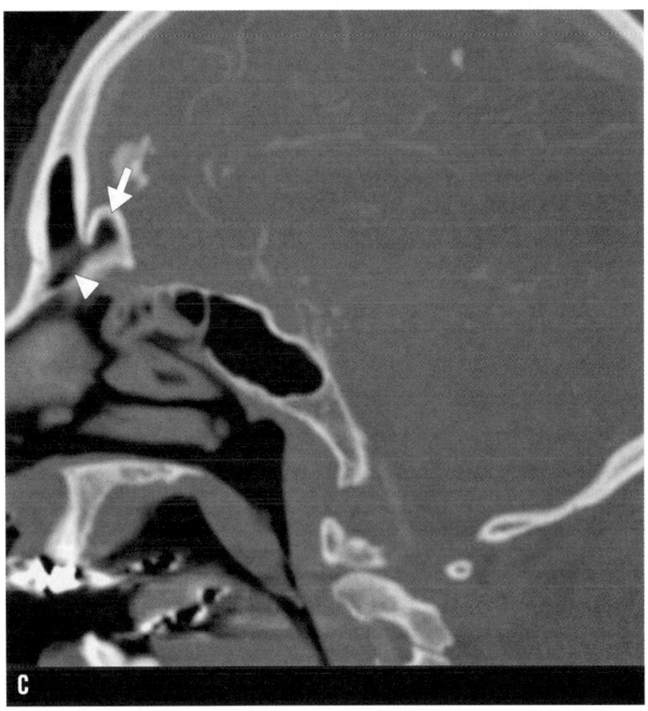

Companion case: Ossified crista galli

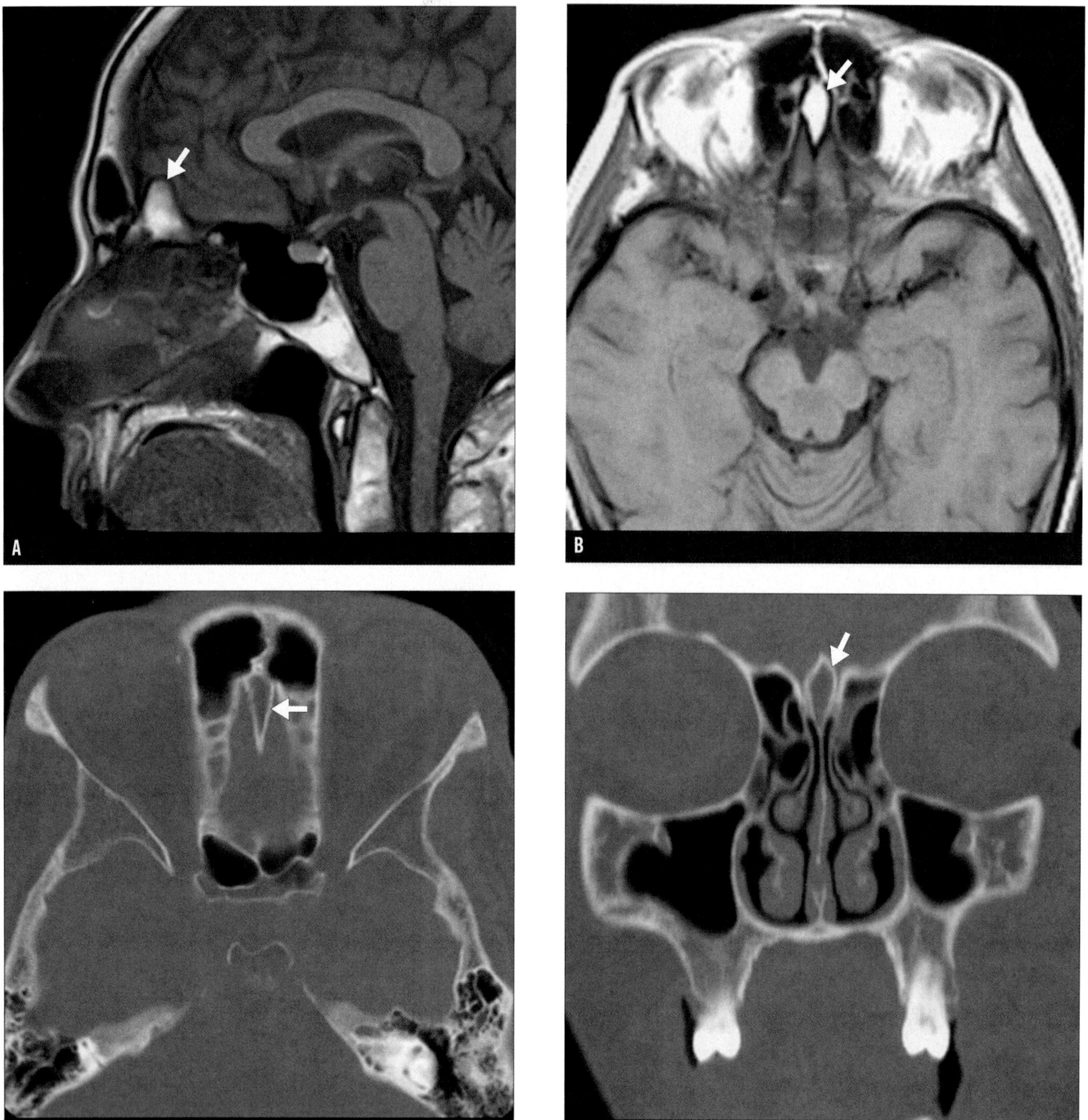

Sagittal T1 (**A**) and axial T1 (**B**) MR images through the anterior skull base demonstrate normal fatty marrow in an ossified crista galli (arrows, **A**, **B**). Axial (**C**) and coronal reformatted (**D**) CT images of a different patient obtained through the anterior skull base demonstrate normal marrow containing bone in an ossified crista galli (arrows, **C**, **D**).

Companion case: Crista galli pneumosinus dilatans with an associated meningioma

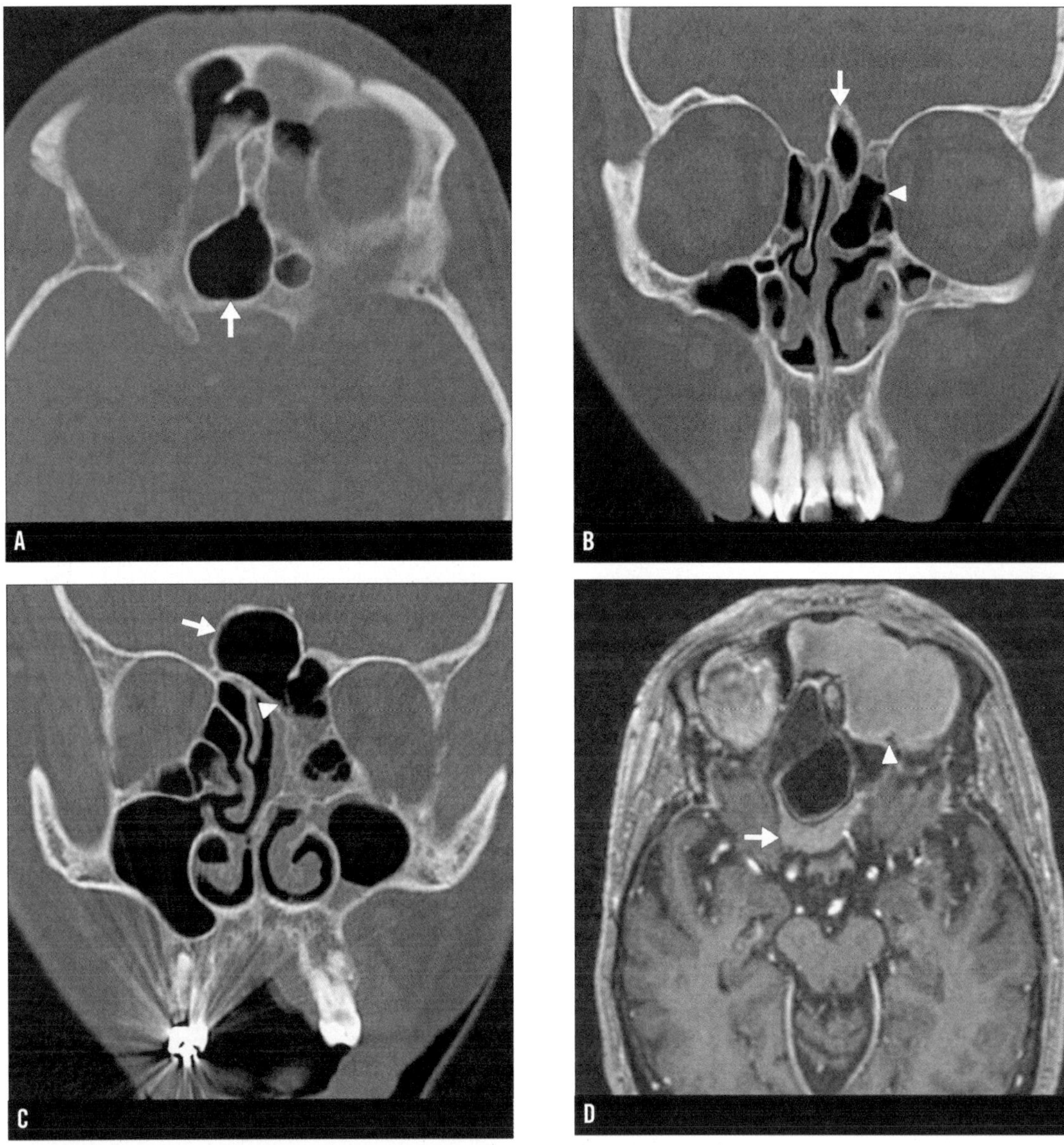

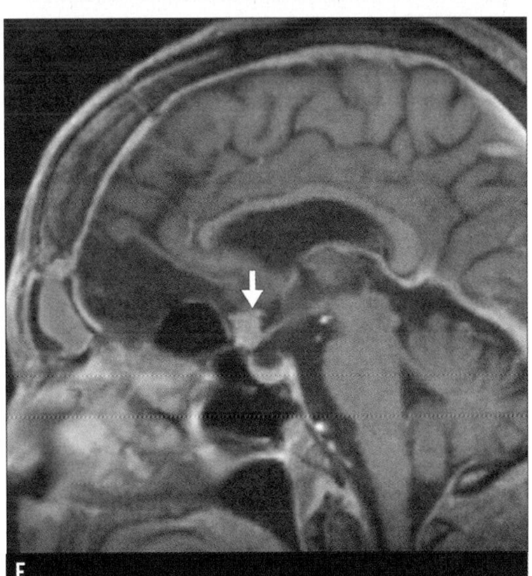

Axial (**A**) and coronal reformatted (**B**, **C**) CT images through the anterior skull base demonstrate a markedly expanded and pneumatized crista galli (arrows, **A**-**C**) which extends to involve the left ethmoid air cells (arrowheads, **B**, **C**), compatible with pneumosinus dilatans. Axial (**D**) and sagittal reformatted (**E**) MPRAGE MR images obtained several years later demonstrate a meningioma along the posterior margin of the pneumosinus dilatans (arrows, **D**, **E**). The patient also developed a large left frontal mucocele (arrowhead, **D**) because of a left frontal recess outflow obstruction.

REFERENCES

Dhillon RS, Williams DC. Pneumosinus dilatans. *J Laryngol Otol.* 1987;101:828-832

Flint PW, et al, eds. *Cummings Otolaryngology: Head and Neck Surgery.* 5th ed. Philadelphia, PA: Mosby Elsevier; 2010.

Hajiioannou J, et al. Evaluation of anatomical variation of the Crista Galli using computed tomography. *Clinical Anatomy.* 2010; 23:370-373.

Schmalfuss IM, and Camp M. Skull base: pseudolesion or true lesion? *Eur Radiol.* 2008;18:1232-1243.

Som PM, et al. Crista Galli pneumatization is an extension of the adjacent frontal sinuses. *AJNR Am J Neuroradiol.* 2008;30:31-33.

CASE 12 Normal ethmoidal grooves

The anterior ethmoidal artery (AEA) typically arises from the distal one-third of the intraorbital ophthalmic artery. The AEA exits the orbit through the anterior ethmoidal foramen and then anterior ethmoidal canal, the latter representing a medially directed, pyramidal-shaped notch located along the superior aspect of the lamina papyracea. After exiting the orbit, the AEA enters the ethmoid labyrinth and then the olfactory fossa of the anterior skull base through the ethmoidal groove (also called ethmoidal sulcus). The ethmoidal groove is a small notch-like osseous channel located within the lateral lamella of the anterior skull base. This normal ethmoidal groove can sometimes simulate a skull base fracture. The groove is present bilaterally and is variably identified on CT, usually dependent on the slice thickness and quality of the study.

COMPANION CASES

- **Anterior skull base fracture.** Identifying the normal expected location of the ethmoidal groove along the lateral lamella on CT usually helps differentiate an anterior skull base fracture from the normal ethmoidal groove.
- **Anterior ethmoidal artery fistula.** Given the anatomic course of the anterior ethmoidal arteries, an anterior ethmoidal artery fistula may be suspected if an intracranial tangle of vessels near the midline of the anterior skull base is identified on imaging. Iatrogenic injury or trauma to the lateral lamella of the anterior skull base can result in an AEA tear and result in an arteriovenous fistula. This fistula has a higher risk of hemorrhage than most other fistulae and thus warrants treatment. Its arterial supply is often bilateral, and its venous drainage is typically via cortical veins along the frontal lobes.
- **Posterior ethmoidal canals.** A posterior ethmoidal artery (PEA) has a more variable origin compared to an AEA. While the PEA typically arises from the proximal one-third of the intraorbital ophthalmic artery, it may also arise from the AEA or from the middle meningeal artery. The PEA exits the posterior-superior-medial aspect of the orbit via the posterior ethmoidal foramen and continues into the posterior ethmoidal canal, both of which are located a few millimeters anterior to the sphenoid sinus, and then enters the skull base. As opposed to the AEA, the PEA does not typically traverse the ethmoid labyrinth.

Normal ethmoidal grooves

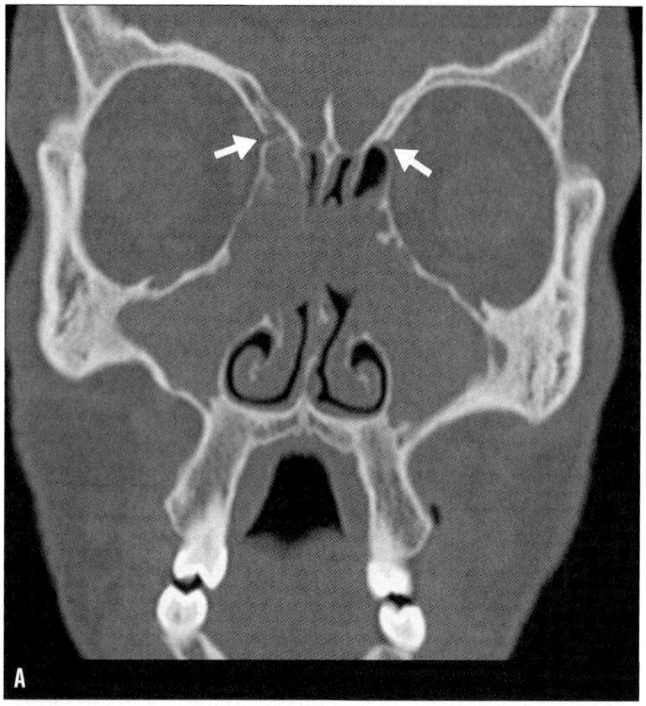

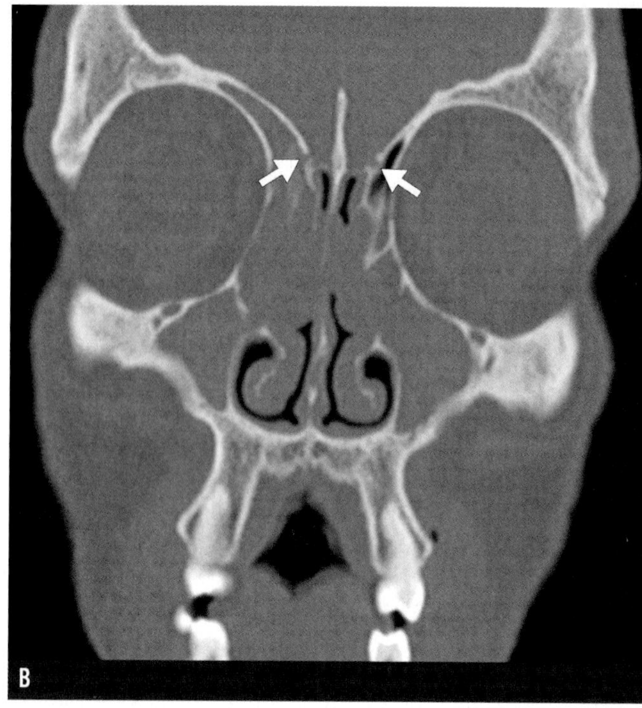

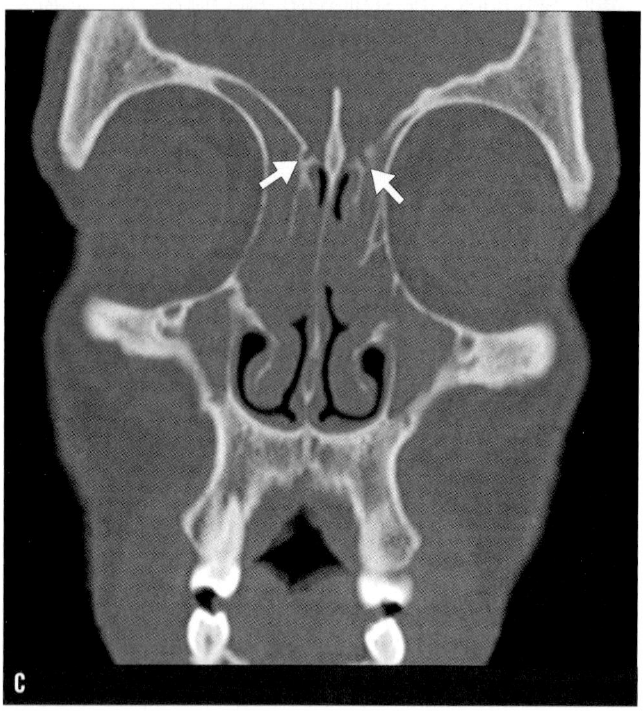

Coronal reformatted CT images from anterior to posterior (**A**-**C**). Image **A** demonstrates the normal anterior ethmoidal canals through which the anterior ethmoidal arteries traverse (arrows, **A**). The anterior ethmoidal arteries then exit the orbit, traverse the ethmoid labyrinth, and enter the skull base via the ethmoidal grooves along the lateral lamellae of the cribriform plate (arrows, **B**, **C**). The ethmoidal grooves are normal anatomic structures that may mimic skull base fractures.

Normal ethmoidal grooves

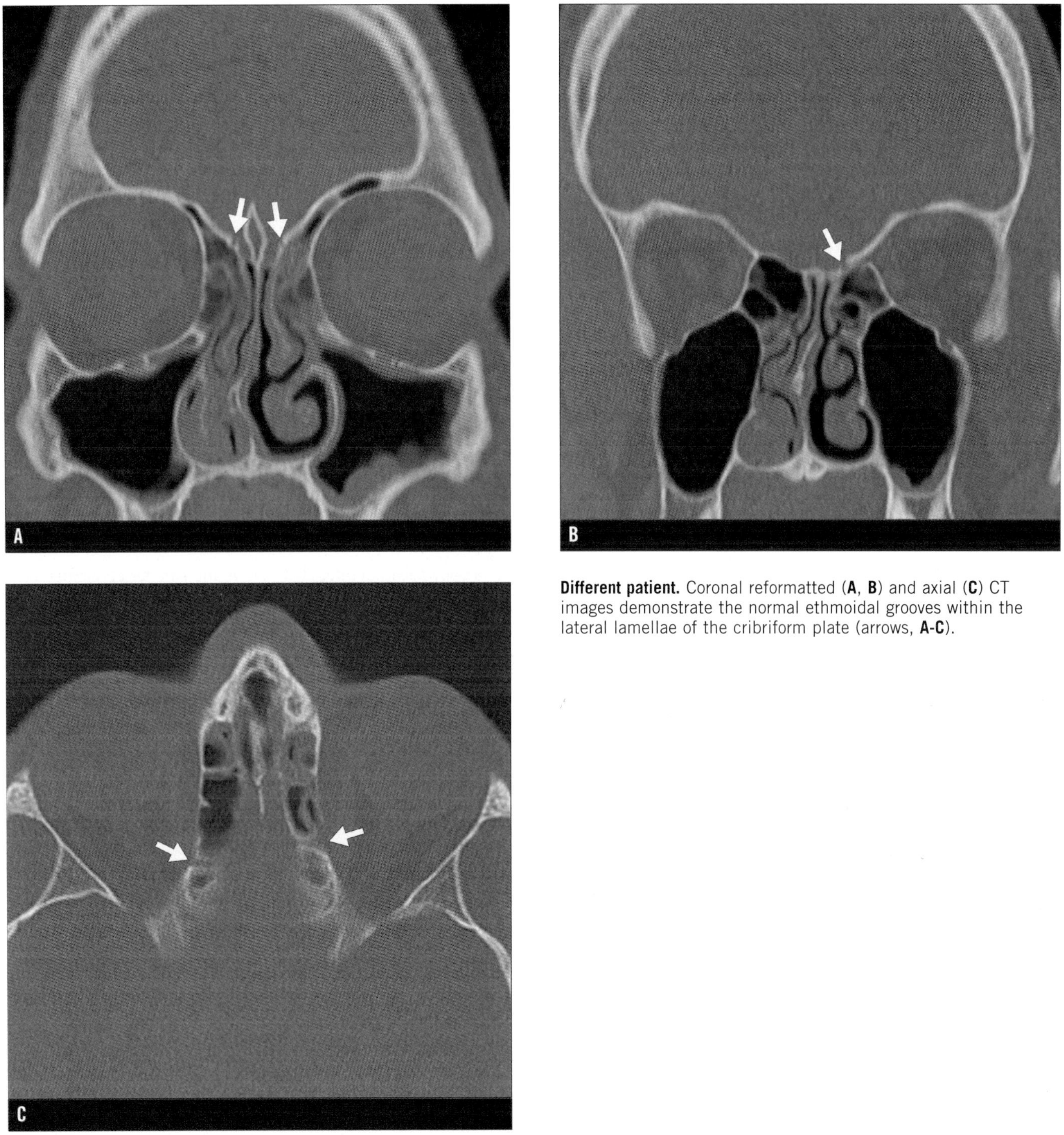

Different patient. Coronal reformatted (**A**, **B**) and axial (**C**) CT images demonstrate the normal ethmoidal grooves within the lateral lamellae of the cribriform plate (arrows, **A-C**).

Companion case: Anterior skull base fracture

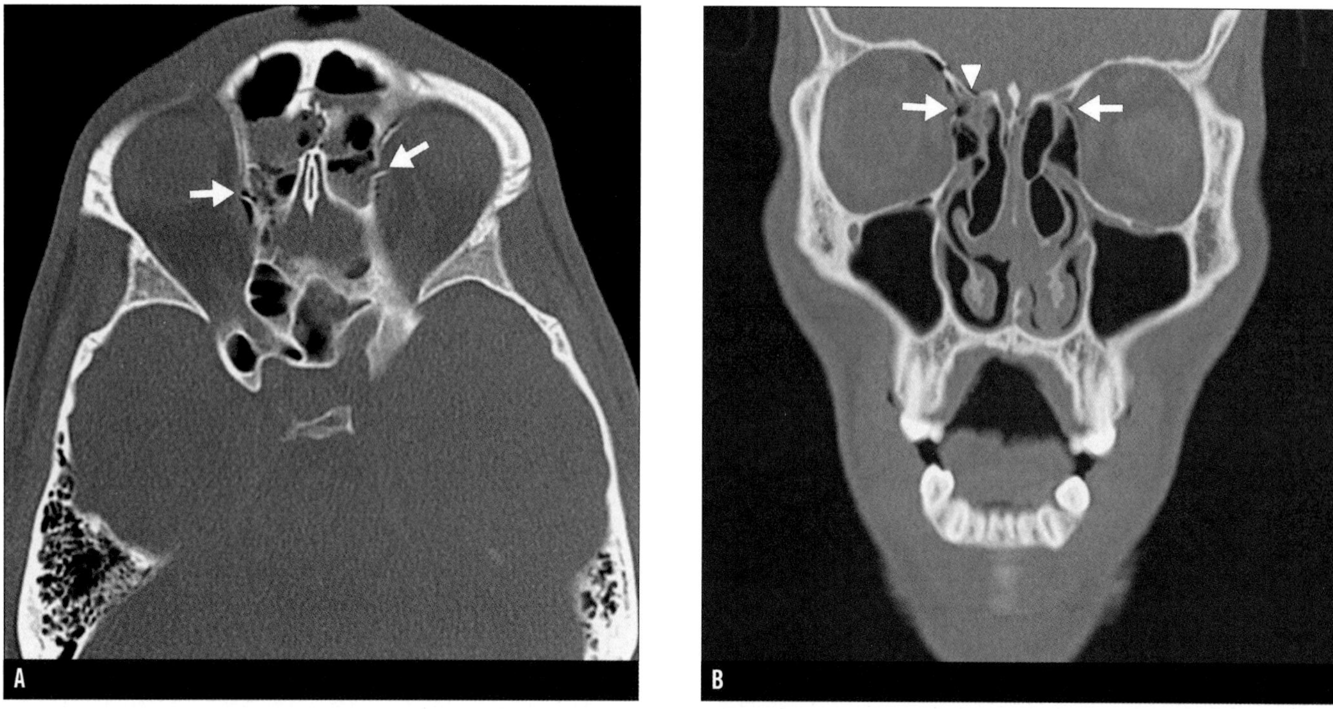

Axial (**A**) and coronal reformatted (**B**) CT images demonstrate bilateral lamina papyracea fractures that involve the anterior ethmoidal canals (arrows, **A, B**) and the anterior skull base at the right fovea ethmoidalis (arrowhead, **B**). The offset at the fracture sites and the adjacent abnormally located pockets of air confirm the presence of acute fractures.

Companion case: Anterior ethmoidal artery fistula

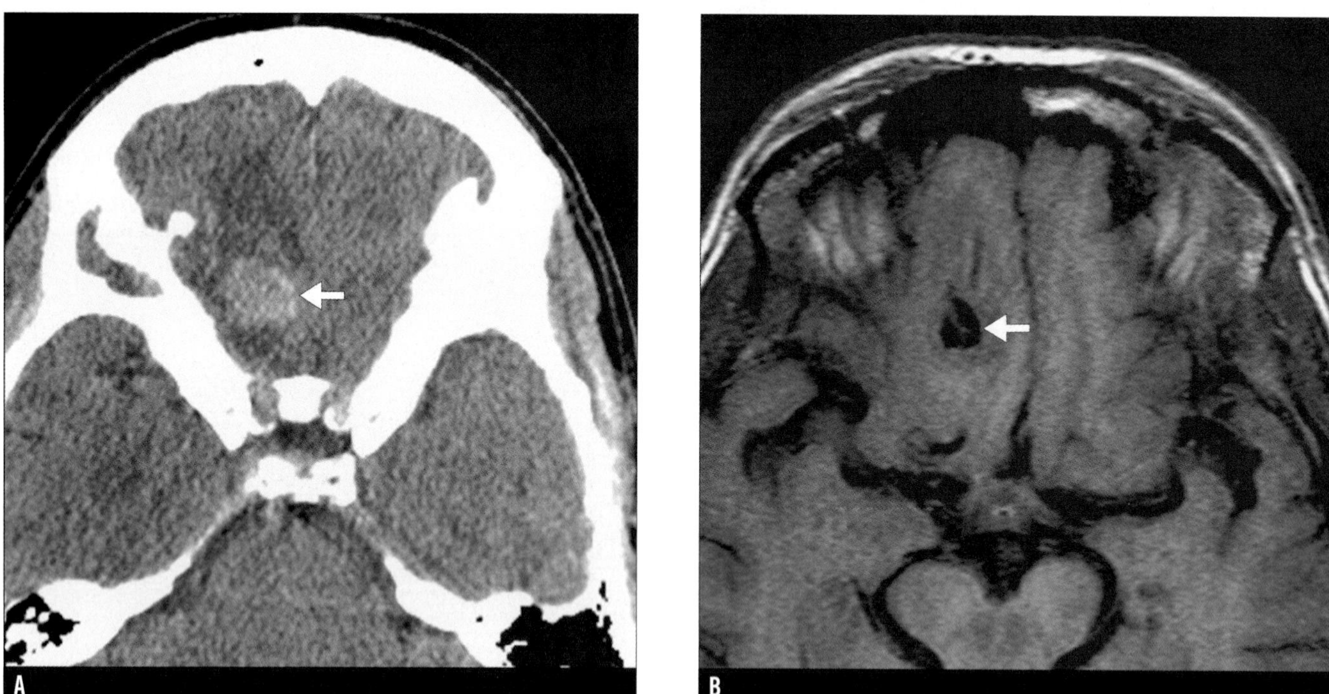

An unenhanced axial CT image (**A**) demonstrates a focal area of apparent hemorrhage in the inferior aspect of the right frontal lobe (arrow, **A**). Axial T1 (**B**), axial FLAIR (**C**), and postcontrast axial T1 (**D**) MR images demonstrate the finding to be hypointense on T1 (arrow, **B**), hypointense on FLAIR (arrow, **C**), and enhance (arrow, **D**). Image **C** also best demonstrates edema surrounding the finding. A lateral view (**E**) and transorbital view (**F**) from a catheter angiogram of the same patient demonstrate early cortical venous filling (arrowheads, **E**, **F**) arising directly from the right anterior ethmoidal artery (short arrows, **E**, **F**), consistent with an anterior ethmodial artery fistula. The right ophthalmic artery, which gives rise to the right anterior ethmodial artery, is also depicted (long arrows, **E**, **F**). An anterior ethmoidal artery fistula may arise sporadically or following trauma.

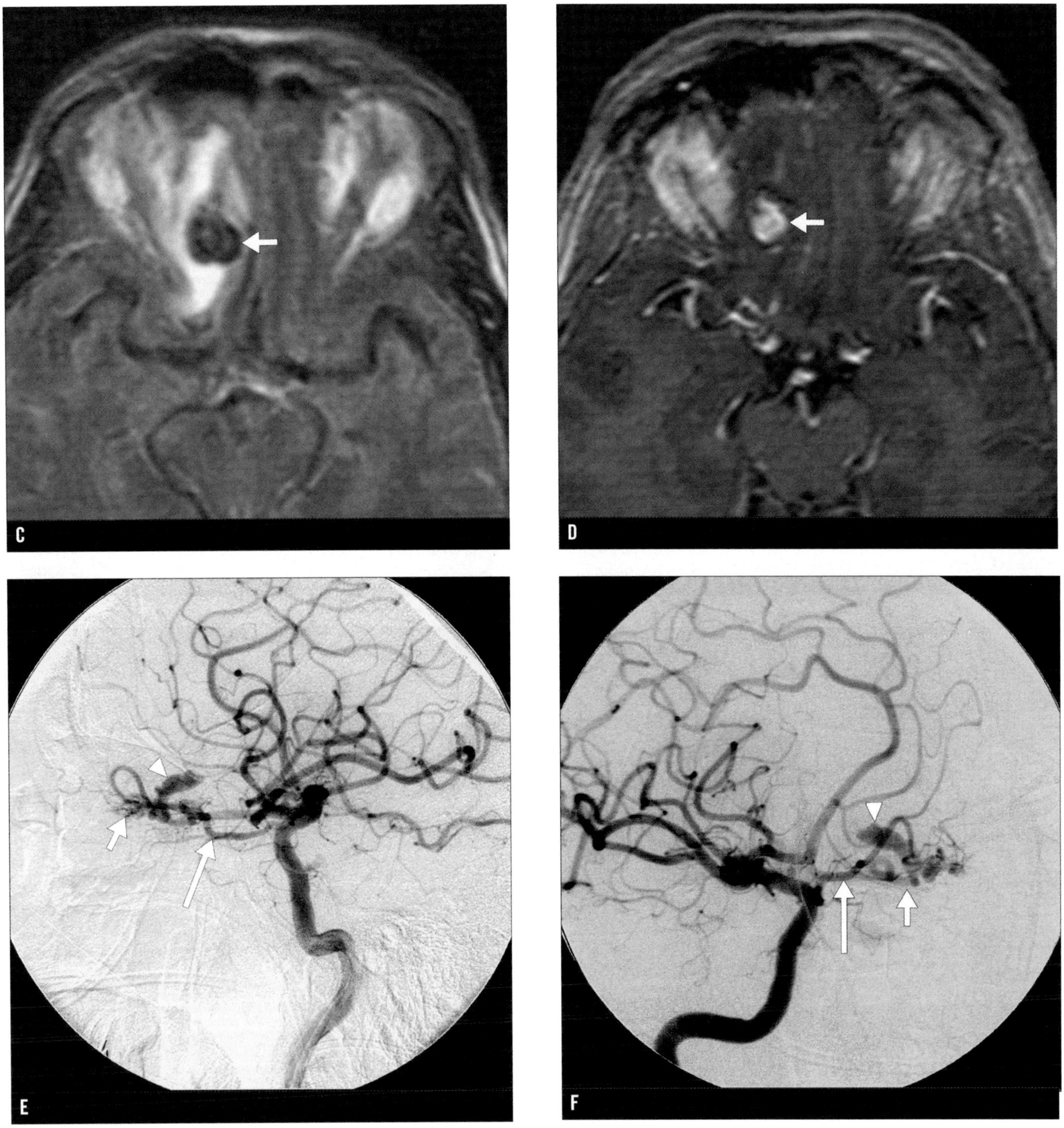
C
D
E
F

Companion case: Posterior ethmoidal canals

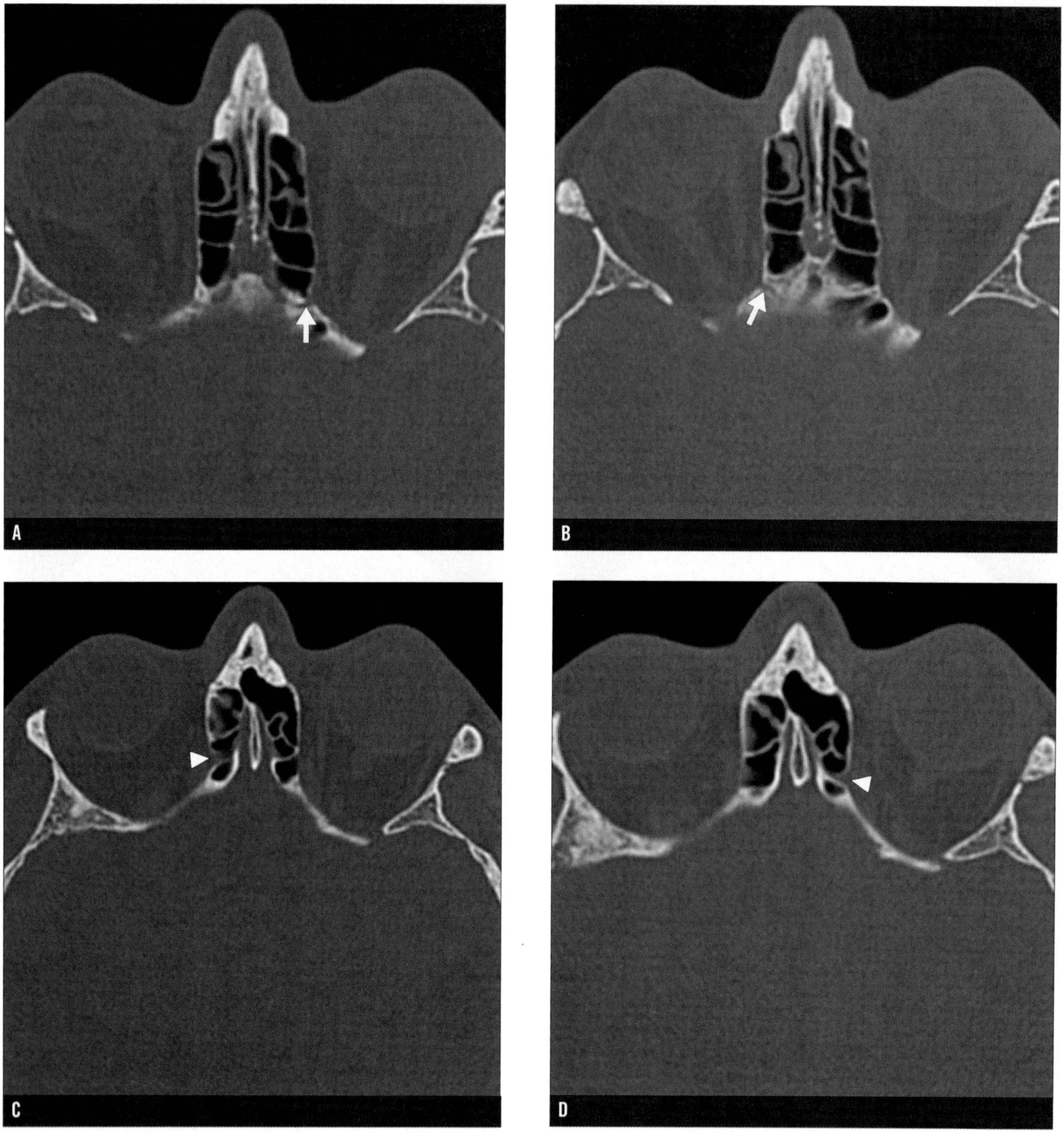

Axial CT images through the ethmoid air cells (**A, B**) demonstrate the posterior ethmoidal canals (arrows, **A, B**). As a reference, additional axial CT images (**C, D**) demonstrate the anterior ethmoidal canals in this patient (arrowheads, **C, D**). Coronal reformatted CT images from the same study (**E, F**) demonstrate the posterior ethmoidal canals (arrows, **E**) and anterior ethmoidal canals (arrowheads, **F**). The foramina of the anterior and posterior ethmoidal canals are located at their entrance sites. The anterior ethmoidal arteries traverse the ethmoid labyrinth prior to entering the skull base, whereas the posterior ethmoidal arteries enter the skull base directly, just a few millimeters anterior to the ventral wall of the sphenoid sinus. As is the case with the ethmoidal grooves at the lateral lamellae, the posterior ethmoidal canals are normal anatomic structures that may mimic skull base fractures.

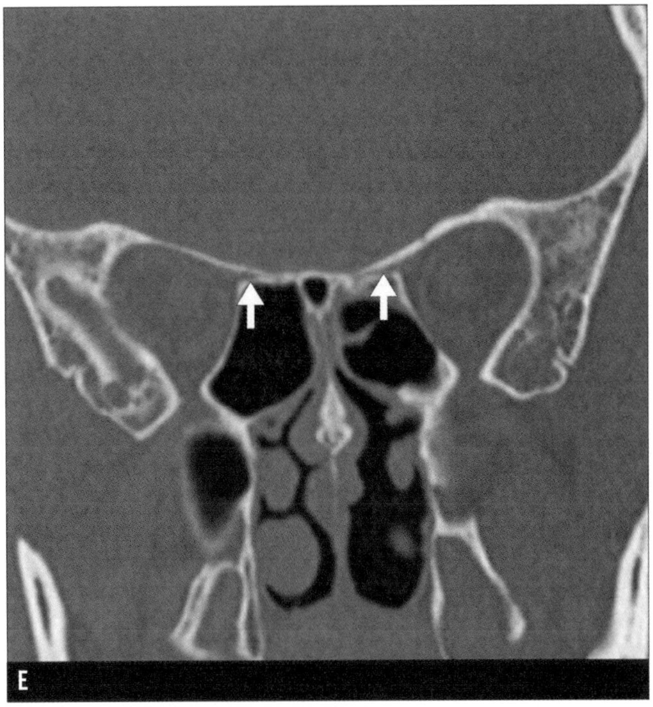

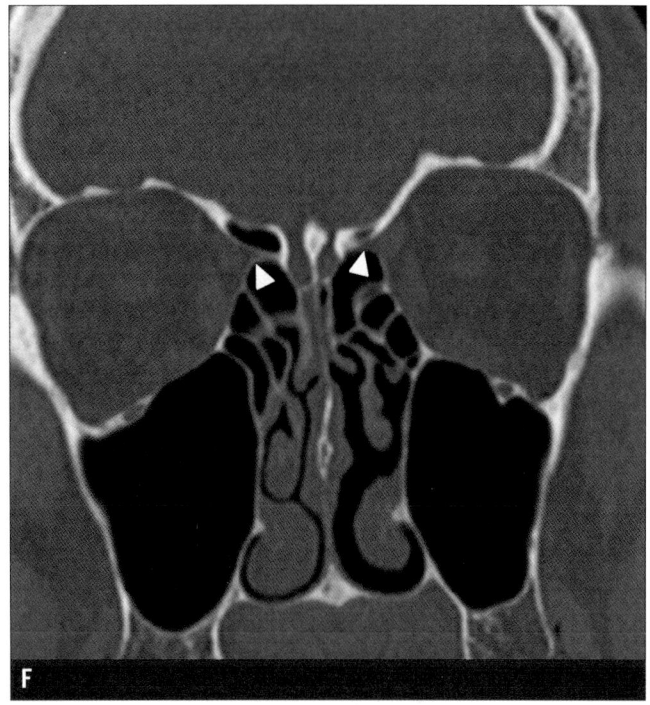

REFERENCES

Cankal F, et al. Evaluation of the anterior and posterior ethmoidal canal by computed tomography. *Clin radiol.* 2004;(59)11:1034-1040.

Meloni F, et al. Anatomic variations of surgical importance in ethmoid labyrinth and sphenoid sinus. A study of radiological anatomy. *Surg Radiol Anat.* 1992;14:65-70.

Moon HJ, et al. Surgical anatomy of the anterior ethmoidal canal in ethmoid roof. *Laryngoscope.* 2001;111:900-904.

Patterson R, et al. *Patterson's Allergic Diseases.* 7th ed. Baltimore, MD: Lippincott Williams & Wilkins; 2009

Ros de San Pedro J, et al. Bilateral ethmoidal dural arteriovenous fistula: unexpected surgical diagnosis. *Clin Neurol Neurosurg.* 2010;112:903-908.

CASE 13 Orbital roof diploic veins

The veins within the osseous diploic space are valveless and are therefore bidirectional. Calvarial diploic veins communicate with both the intracranial and extracranial compartments. Intracranially, they communicate with the dural venous sinuses and pachymeningeal veins along the inner table of the calvarium. Extracranially, they communicate with extracalvarial veins via emissary veins. The diploic vein anatomy is variable among individuals, although most of the diploic veins are concentrated in the high frontal, parietal, and occipital bones.

Diploic veins along the orbital roof may be confused with skull base fractures. The normal orbital roof diploic veins are typically wavy, ill-defined, and branching lucencies. Coronal and sagittal reformatted CT imaging helps to localize these normal lucencies within in the diploic space as well as exclude extension of the lucencies to the cortical surface, as would be expected with a fracture.

COMPANION CASE

- **Anterior skull base fracture.** Anterior skull base fractures that involve the orbital roof are non-corticated, discrete lucencies, often accompanied by regional trauma or other fractures on CT imaging. On coronal and sagittal reformatted CT imaging, an anterior skull base fracture will extend to the cortical surface, as opposed to orbital roof diploic veins which are isolated to the diploic space.

Orbital roof diploic veins

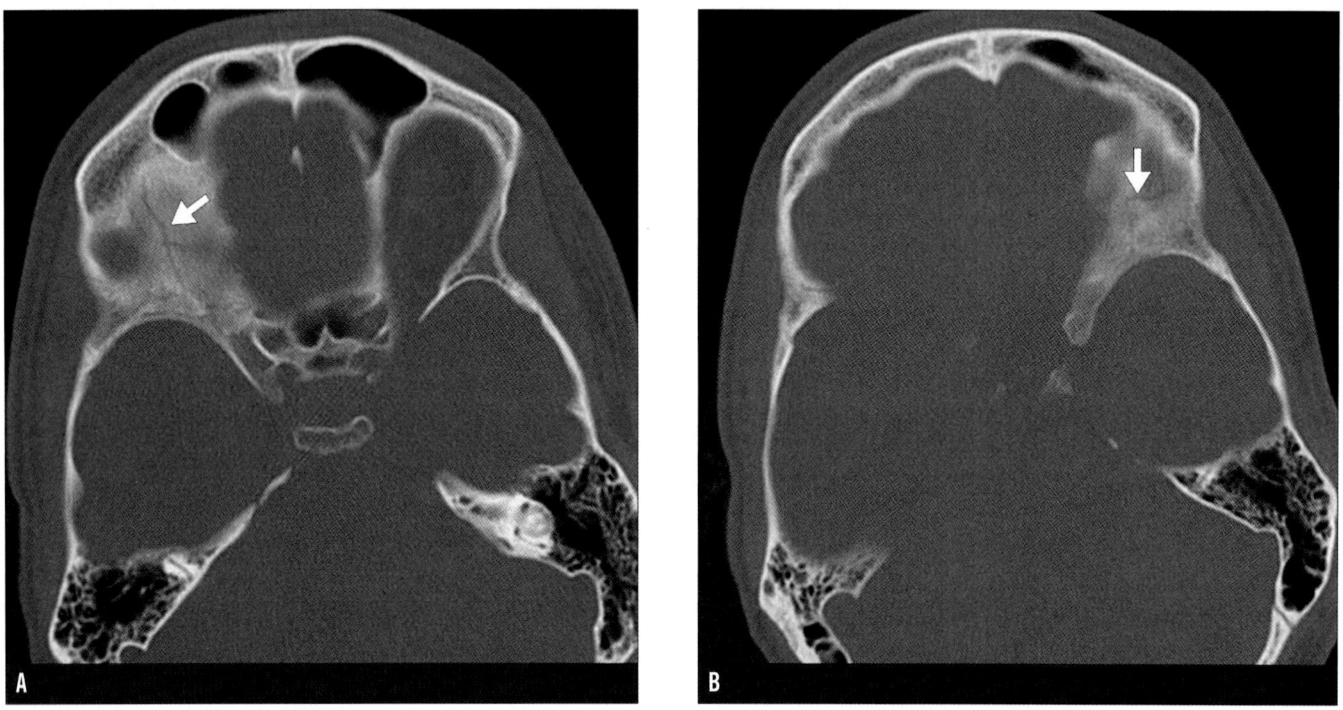

Axial CT images through the roof of the right orbit (**A**) and left orbit (**B**) demonstrate wavy, branching linear lucencies in the roof of both orbits which could be mistaken for fractures (arrows, **A**, **B**). Coronal reformatted (**C**, **D**) and left parasagittal reformatted (**E**) CT images through the orbits demonstrate these lucencies as discrete, well-corticated channels isolated within the diploic space, compatible with normal diploic veins (arrows, **C**-**E**).

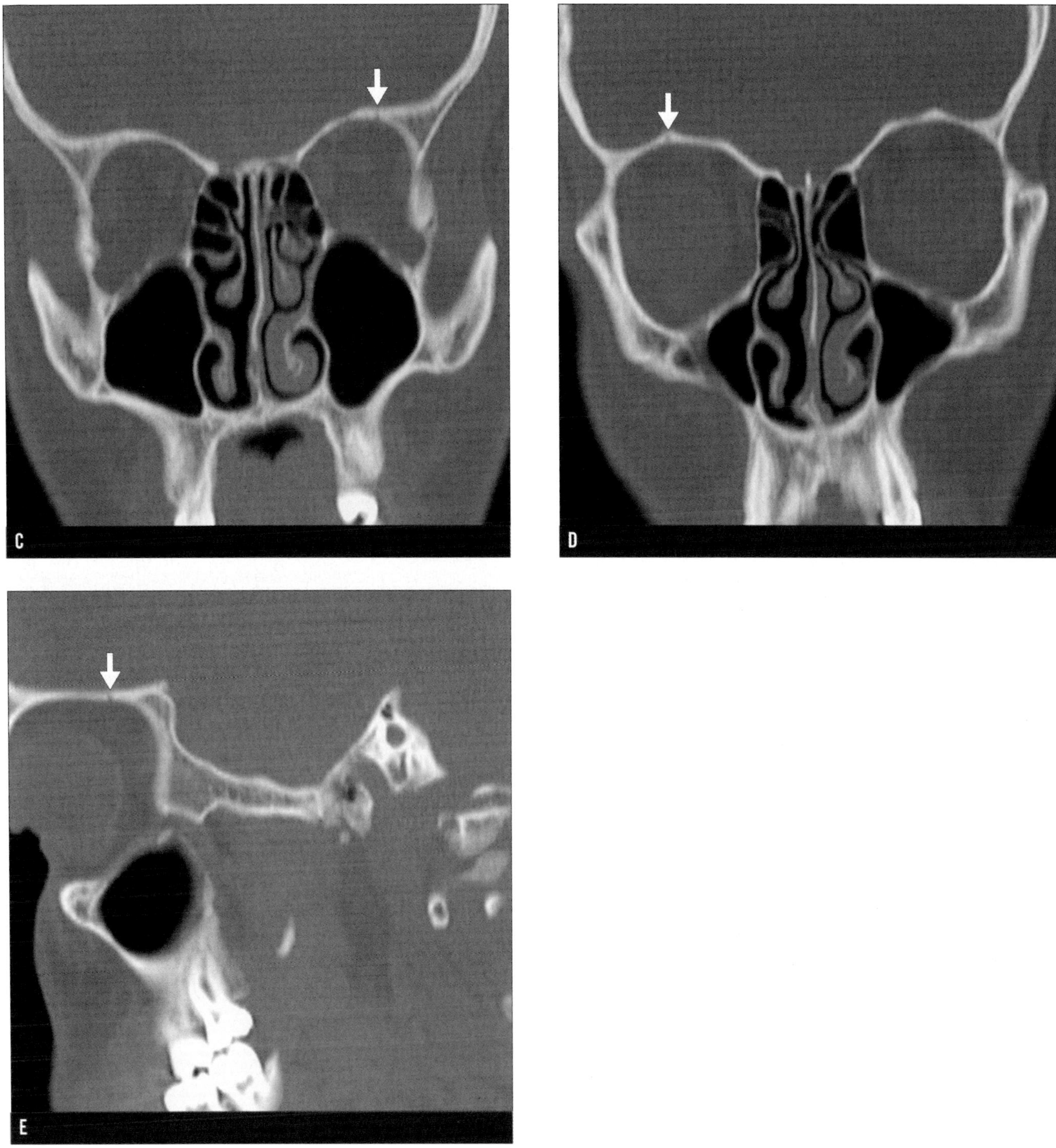
C
D
E

Companion case: Anterior skull base fracture

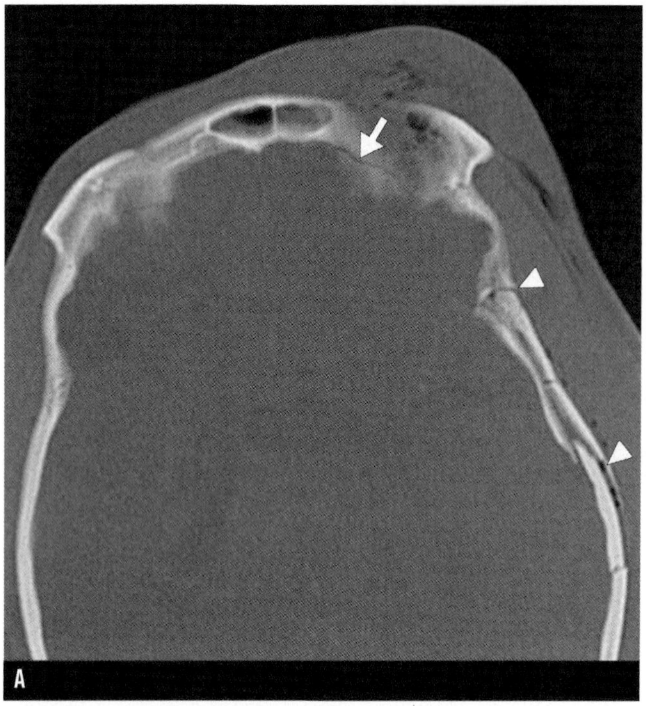

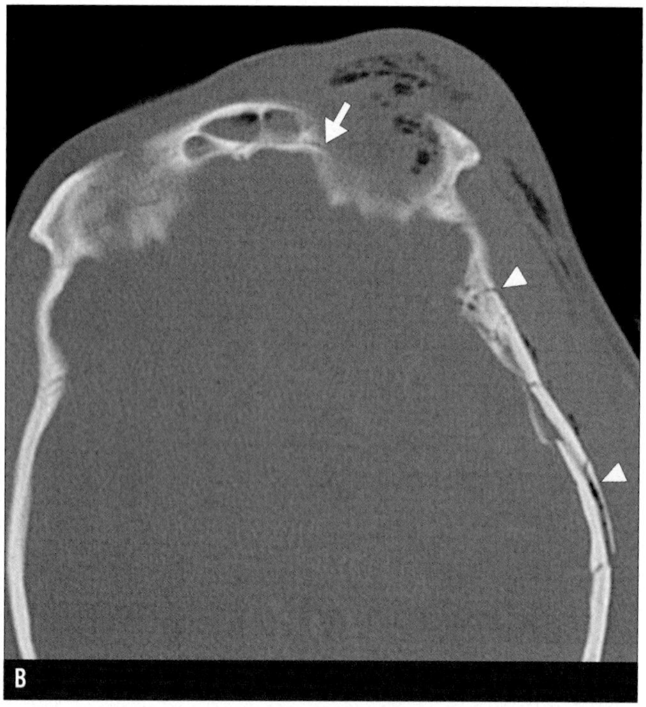

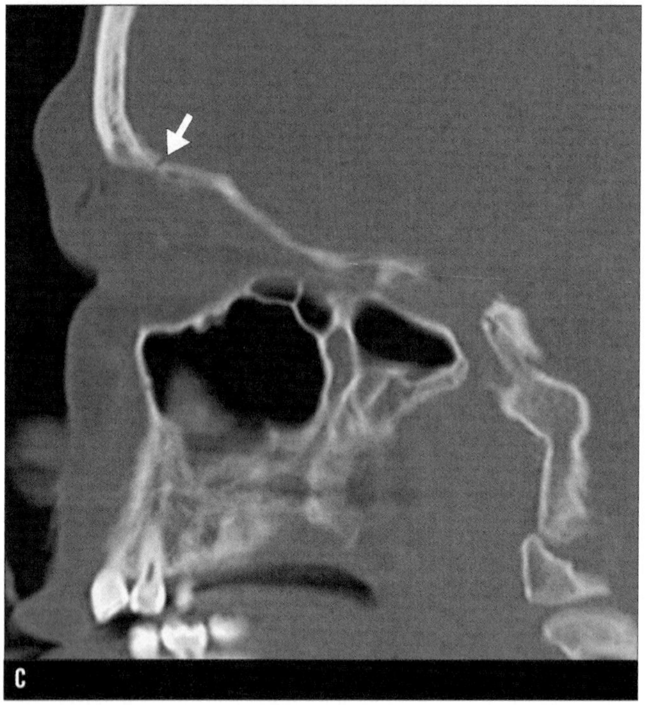

Axial CT images through the roofs of the orbits and squamosal potions of the temporal bones (**A**, **B**) as well as a sagittal reformatted CT image through the left orbit (**C**) demonstrate fractures through the roof of the left orbit (arrows, **A**-**C**) and primarily the squamosal portion of the left temporal bone (arrowheads **A**, **B**). While this case demonstrates imaging findings that are obvious for acute fractures, including overt subcutaneous emphysema and soft tissue swelling, image **C** demonstrates the lucency to extend to the cortex. This can be a helpful imaging finding when it is difficult to differentiate between a skull base fracture and normal orbital roof diploic veins on axial CT images.

REFERENCE

Jivraj K, Bhargava R, Aronyk K, Quateen A, Walji A. Diploic venous anatomy studied in-vivo by MRI. *Clin Anat.* 2009;22(3):296-301.

CASE 14 Arachnoid granulations

Arachnoid granulations (also called **Pacchionian granulations**) are meningothelial-lined herniations of the arachnoid membrane that protrude through the dura mater and usually extend into the venous sinuses or venous lacunae on the surface of the brain. They are functionally and histologically similar to arachnoid villi and allow for filtration as well as resorption of cerebrospinal fluid (CSF) into the venous circulation.

When arachnoid granulations affect the skull base, they often appear as lytic abnormalities on CT, sometimes simulating metastatic disease or a bubbly primary bone tumor. The contents of an arachnoid granulation are CSF equivalent, unless an arachnoid granulation is large (>1 cm), in which case it may not be CSF equivalent. When a less than 1 cm focal skull base lucency or fluid signal focus involving the skull base is encountered on CT or MRI, respectively, then it is helpful to determine whether the finding is CSF equivalent and whether it communicates with the adjacent subarachnoid space; if the finding satisfies both of these imaging criteria, then the finding is highly likely to represent an arachnoid granulation. An arachnoid granulation that does not overlie a pneumatized air cell is most often incidental. However, if it overlies a pneumatized air cell, such as a paranasal sinus, and the intervening bone is sufficiently thinned and/or dehiscent, then the patient is at risk for a CSF leak from arachnoid granulation rupture.

COMPANION CASES

- **Middle cranial fossa arachnoid cysts with adjacent osseous remodeling.** An arachnoid cyst represents a benign, CSF-containing congenital lesion located within the arachnoid. The wall of an arachnoid cyst is composed of flattened arachnoid cells without a glial membrane or epithelial lining. Arachnoid cysts are smooth lesions that are most often unilocular and frequently have mass effect. If large enough, the calvarium and brain are often molded by an arachnoid cyst, and removal of the cyst does not result in reversal of the molded calvarial or brain contour. Most arachnoid cysts are supratentorial, and of those, most are located in the middle cranial fossa. While the etiology of an arachnoid cyst is unknown, one theory suggests that there is arachnoid separation and/or a diverticulum during development that fills with CSF. These lesions do not enhance and almost always follow CSF attenuation and signal on CT and MRI, respectively. Rarely, proteinaceous debris or hemorrhage may develop within an arachnoid cyst, particularly following trauma.

  Differentiating an arachnoid cyst from a giant arachnoid granulation (>1cm) can be difficult. When large, arachnoid cysts will be associated with mass effect upon the subjacent brain, whereas a giant arachnoid granulation typically does not result in mass effect. Additionally, veins do not traverse an arachnoid cyst (since it represents a contained cyst), whereas veins will traverse an arachnoid granulation.
- **Brain herniation into the transverse dural venous sinus.** Brain herniation through the dura and into a dural venous sinus is a recently recognized entity that is likely incidental and asymptomatic, although its clinical significance is not definitively known. The herniated portion of the brain results in an apparent filling defect in the affected dural venous sinus, similar to what can be identified with an arachnoid granulation. While some consider this entity distinct from an arachnoid granulation, it is certainly plausible that this entity represents brain that has herniated into a large arachnoid granulation, which in turn, has herniated into the dural venous sinus. This entity does not represent an encephalocele because an encephalocele requires herniation outside the confines of the cranium, which is not present with this entity. Brain herniation into a dural venous sinus is best delineated by MRI, and it will simply be characterized by brain equivalent signal in the dural sinus. Frequently, brain sulci will be identified along the herniated brain, best appreciated with thin section T2-weighted or CISS sequences.
- **Middle cranial fossa meningocele.** A cephalocele is a generic term that is used when the intracranial meninges and/or brain herniate outside the expected confines of the cranium. The term cranial meningocele is used when the intracranial meninges and CSF, but not brain, herniate outside the cranium, whereas the term encephalocele is used when brain also herniates through the defect. As expected, a meningocele will follow CSF attenuation and signal on CT and MRI, respectively. A giant arachnoid granulation and a focal meningocele involving the cranium are likely within the same imaging spectrum, although histologically the former herniates through the dura.
- **Encephalocele and CSF leak associated with idiopathic intracranial hypertension.** If there is no clear etiology for a CSF leak, such as from trauma, neoplasm, or a congenital abnormality, then a CSF leak is considered to be spontaneous. Some authors believe that arachnoid villi/granulations enlarge because of increasing CSF volume and intracranial pressure. This theory is supported by clinical and imaging findings in patients who have idiopathic intracranial hypertension (IIH), also known as pseudotumor cerebri. Patients with IIH are typically woman, obese, and often have numerous symptoms, including headaches, diplopia, and vision loss. The CSF opening pressure in patients with IIH is abnormally elevated and their symptoms improve with drainage of CSF. Imaging findings in patients with IIH include

multiple arachnoid granulations of the skull, a partially empty sella, and dilated optic nerve sheath complexes. If the arachnoid granulations are strategically located over a pneumatized air cell (ie. the paranasal sinuses or temporal bones), they can rupture and result in spontaneous CSF leaks. If a CSF leak due to an arachnoid granulation is present, then a focal osseous defect along the undersurface of an arachnoid granulation will be identified immediately cephalad to the affected pneumatized air cell, usually best demonstrated by CT. An encephalocele, if present, may predispose the patient to seizures, headaches, and meningitis.

Occipital bone arachnoid granulations

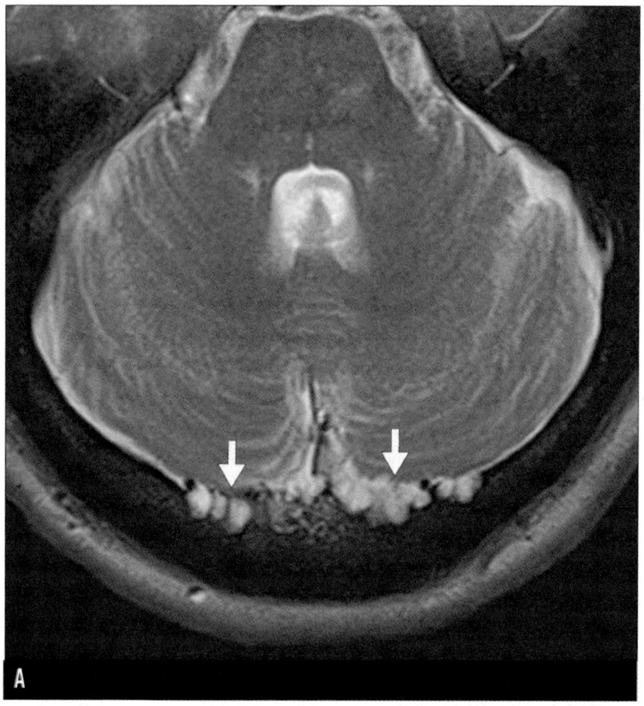

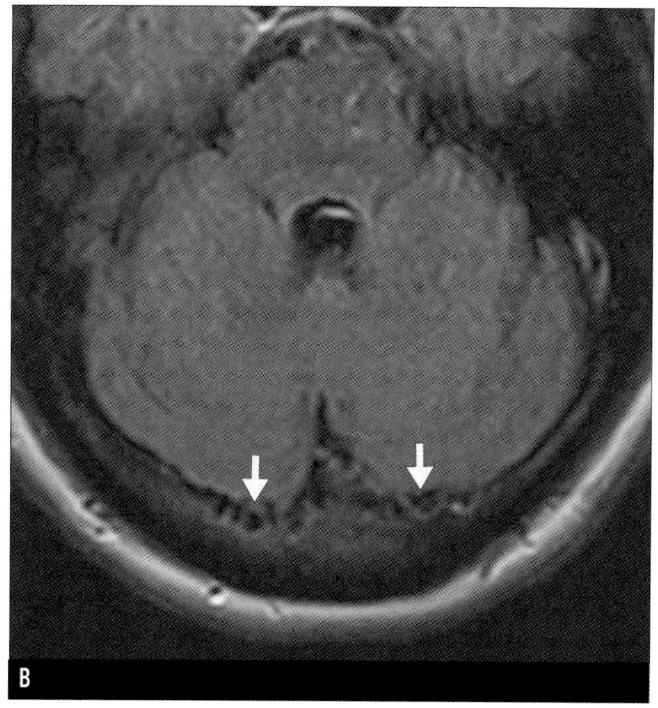

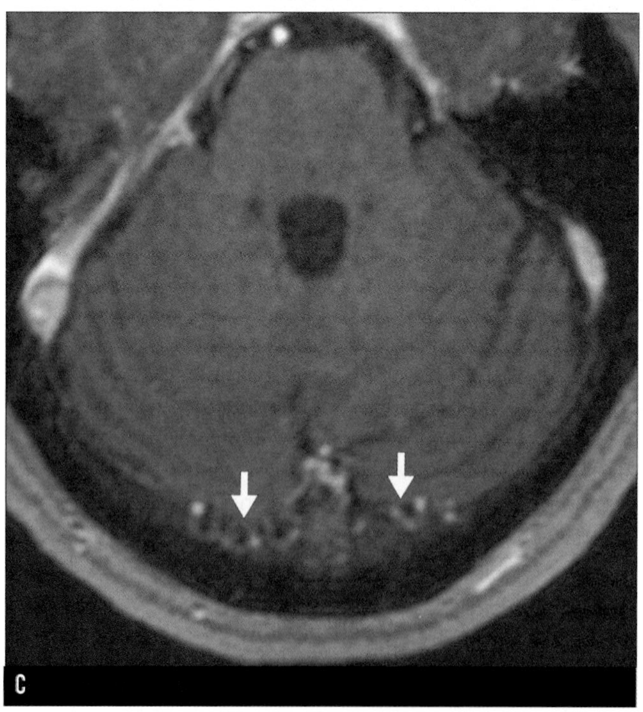

Axial T2 (**A**), axial FLAIR (**B**), and postcontrast axial T1 (**C**) MR images through the posterior fossa demonstrate multiple T2 hyperintense foci along the inner table of the occipital calvarium (arrows, **A**), which suppress on FLAIR (arrows, **B**) and do not enhance centrally following gadolinium administration (arrows, **C**). The findings are compatible with incidental arachnoid granulations.

Occipital bone arachnoid granulations

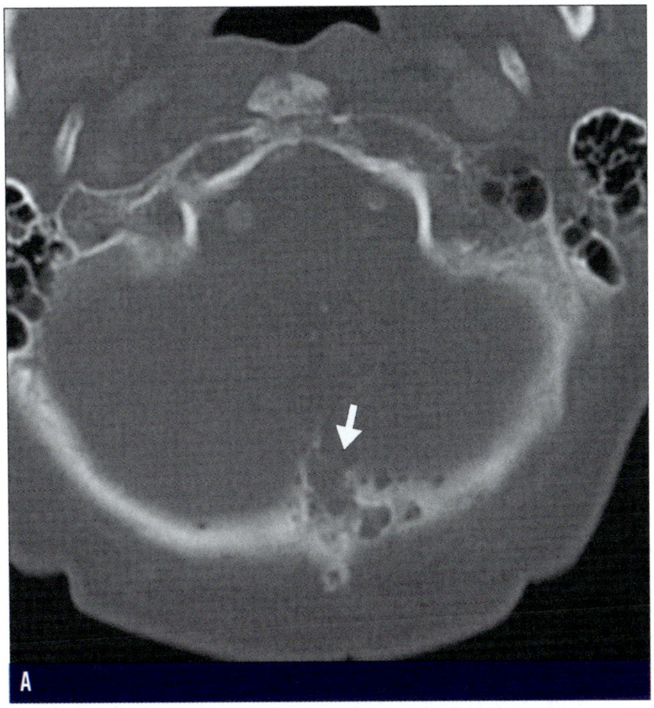

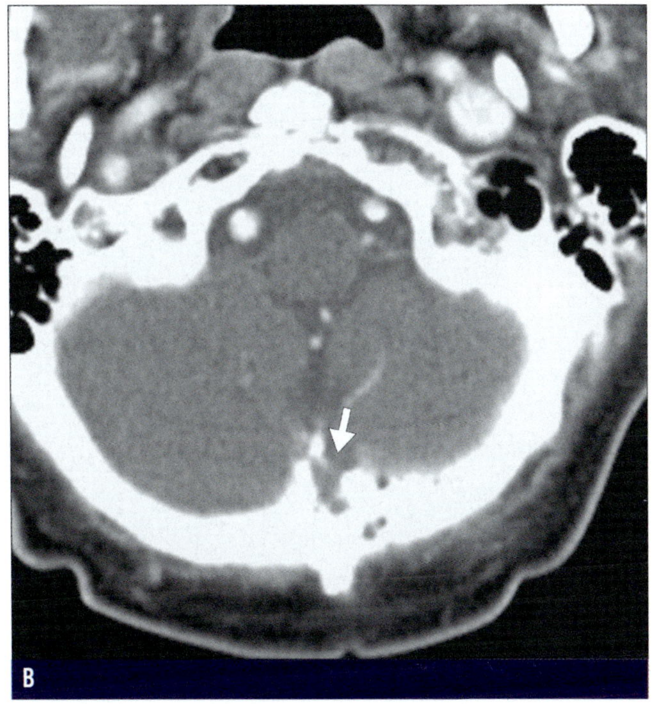

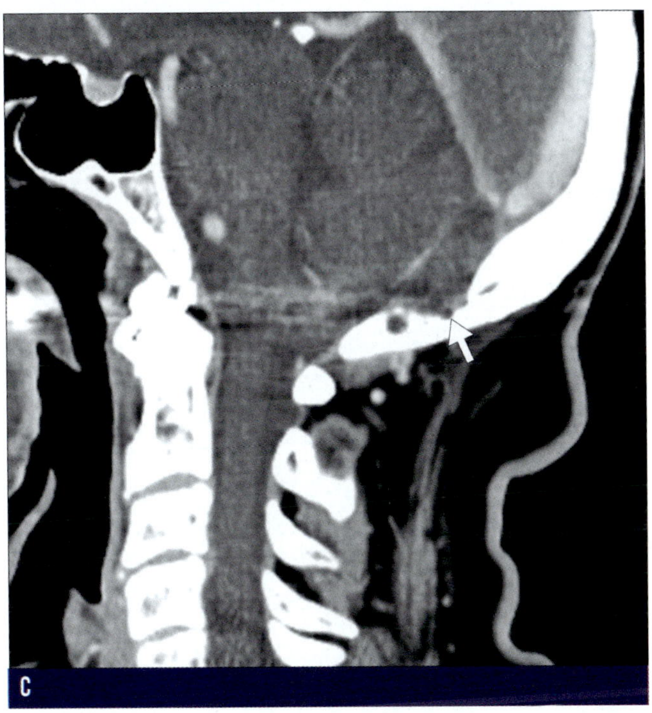

Different patient. Axial postcontrast CT images viewed with a bone window (**A**) and soft tissue window (**B**) as well as a sagittal reformatted CT image viewed with a soft tissue window (**C**). These images demonstrate multiple lytic foci along the inner table of the midline posterior fossa which do not enhance and are CSF equivalent (arrows, **A**-**C**). Image **C** best demonstrates that these lucencies communicate with the CSF, compatible with incidental arachnoid granulations.

Greater wing of the sphenoid arachnoid granulations

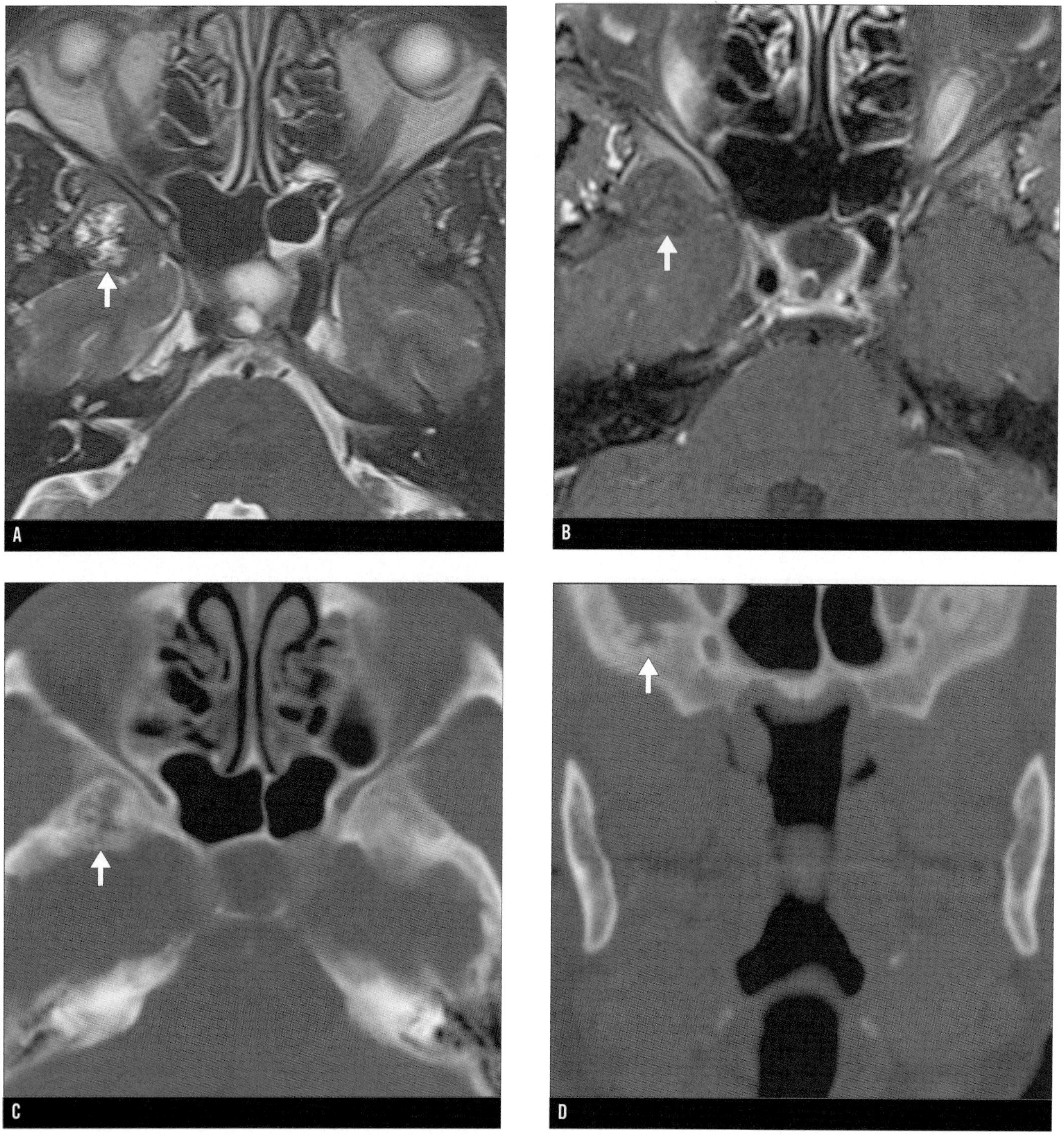

Axial T2 (**A**) and postcontrast axial T1 with fat suppression (**B**) MR images demonstrate a cluster of T2 hyperintense foci that do not enhance located in the right greater wing of the sphenoid (arrows, **A, B**). This is nonspecific based on MRI. However, axial (**C**) and coronal reformatted (**D**) CT images demonstrate benign-appearing lucencies (arrow, **C**) which communicate with the subarachnoid space (arrow, **D**). The findings are consistent with incidental arachnoid granulations.

Greater wing of the sphenoid arachnoid granulations

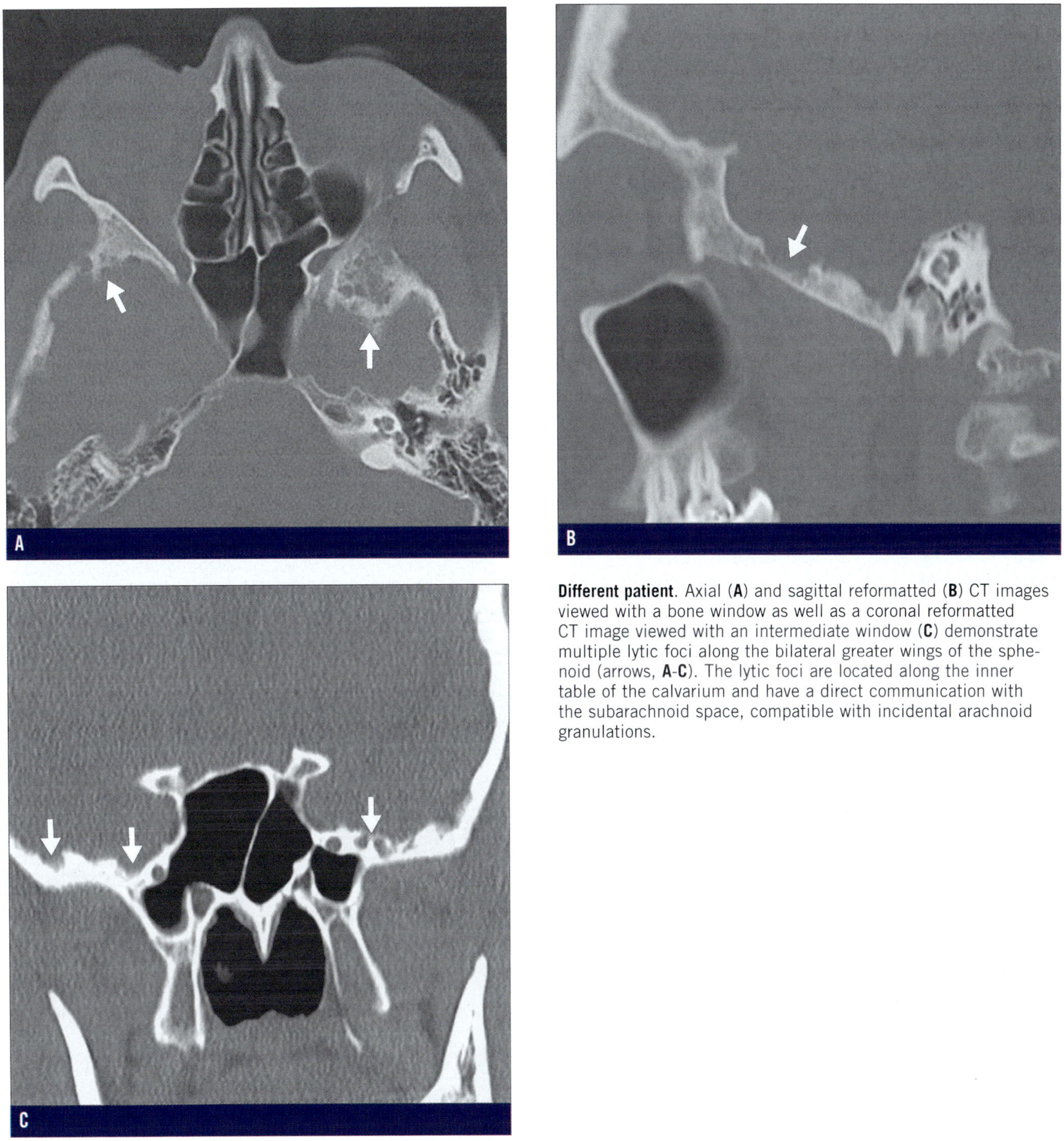

Different patient. Axial (**A**) and sagittal reformatted (**B**) CT images viewed with a bone window as well as a coronal reformatted CT image viewed with an intermediate window (**C**) demonstrate multiple lytic foci along the bilateral greater wings of the sphenoid (arrows, **A**-**C**). The lytic foci are located along the inner table of the calvarium and have a direct communication with the subarachnoid space, compatible with incidental arachnoid granulations.

Companion case: Middle cranial fossa arachnoid cysts with adjacent osseous remodeling

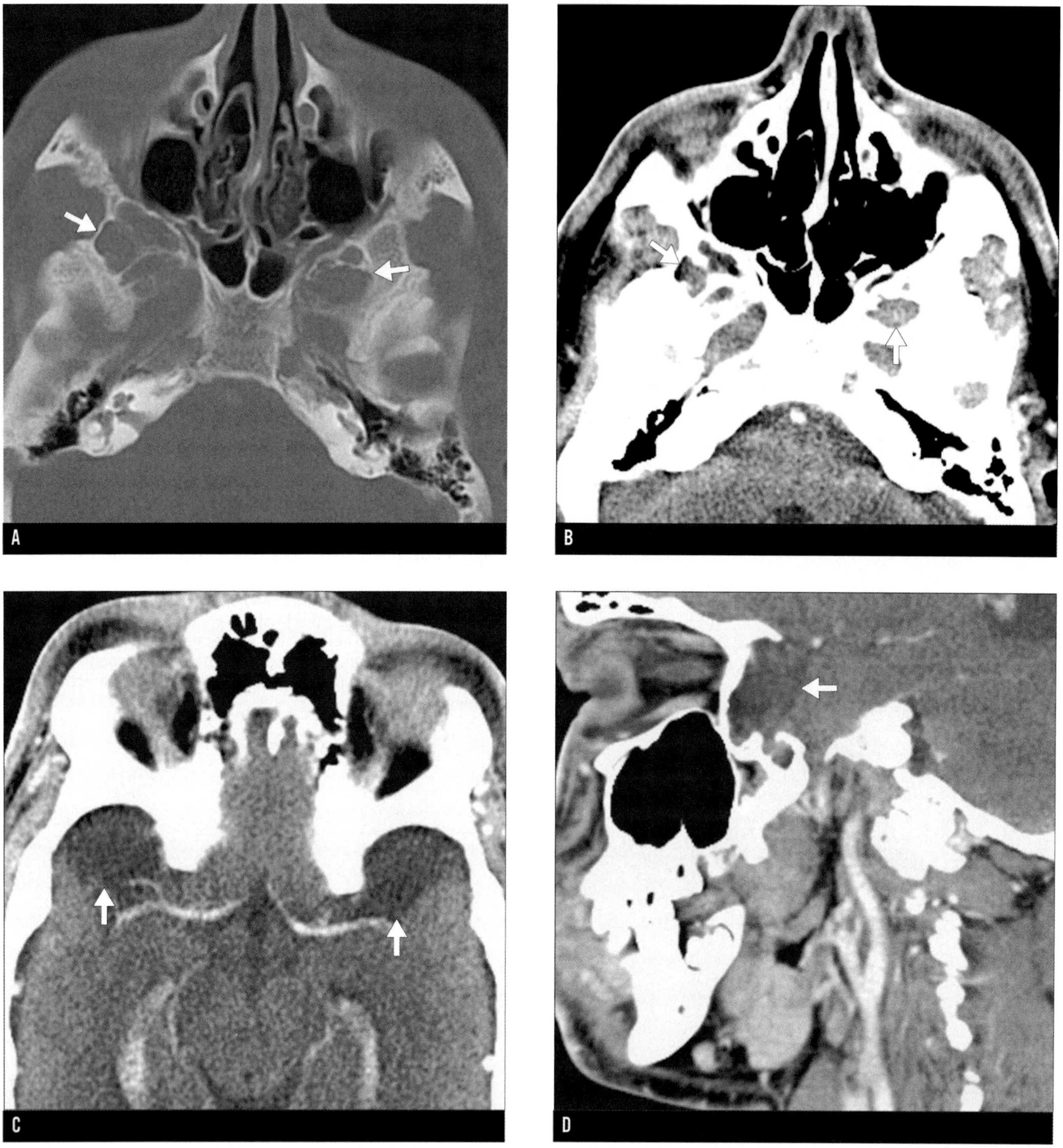

Axial CT images viewed with a bone window (**A**) and soft tissue window (**B**) demonstrate fairly large lucencies along the floors of the middle cranial fossae (arrows, **A**, **B**). These are larger than typical arachnoid granulations, which normally measure less than 1 cm. Axial (**C**) and sagittal reformatted (**D**) CT images viewed with a soft tissue window demonstrate arachnoid cysts in the middle cranial fossae, which are associated with mass effect upon the adjacent temporal lobes (arrows, **C**, **D**). These arachnoid cysts extend into, and result in, the middle cranial fossae lucencies. This patient has Hurler syndrome, which, along with other mucopolysaccharidoses, are often associated intracranial arachnoid cysts.

Companion case: Brain herniation into the transverse dural venous sinus

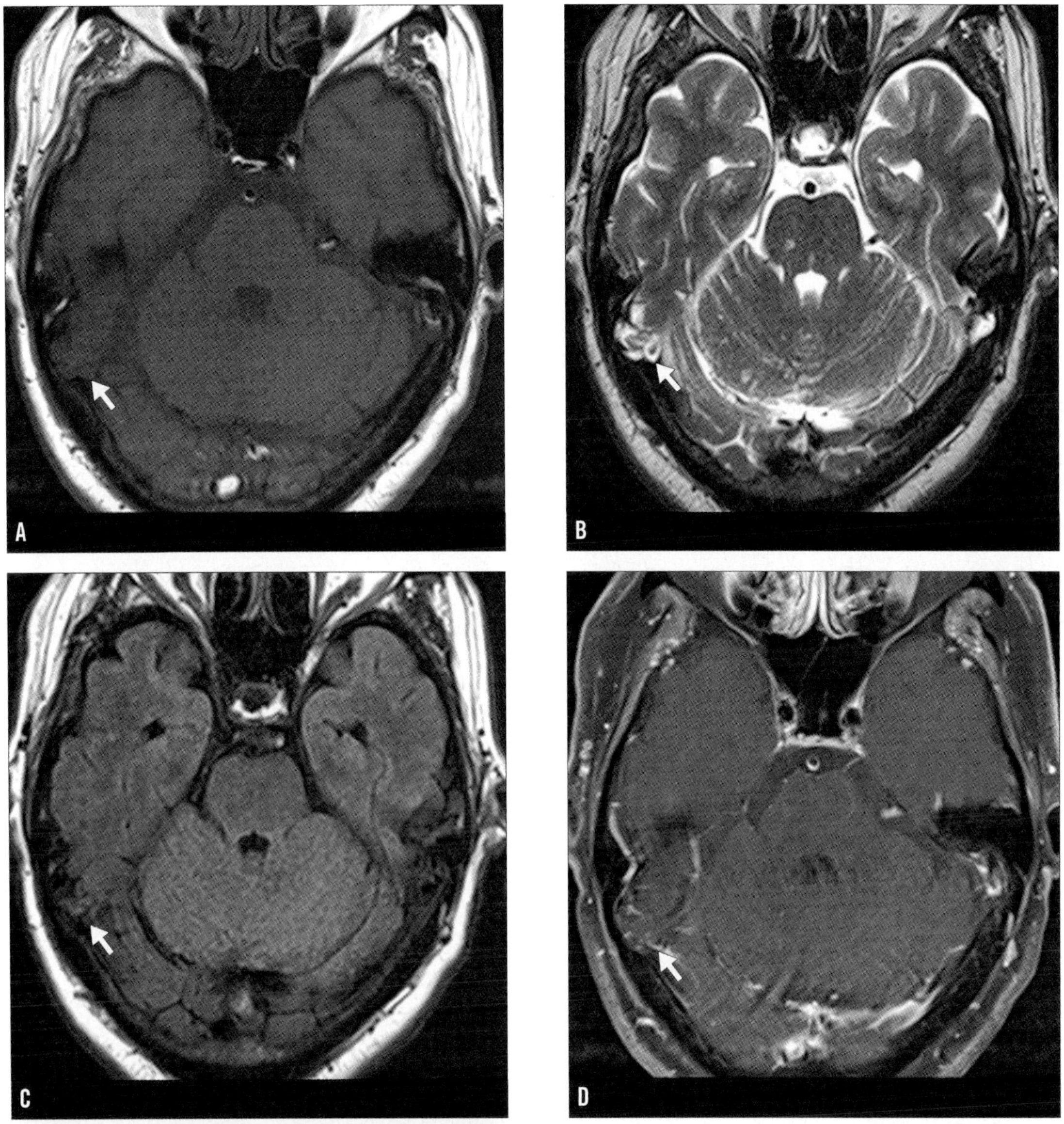

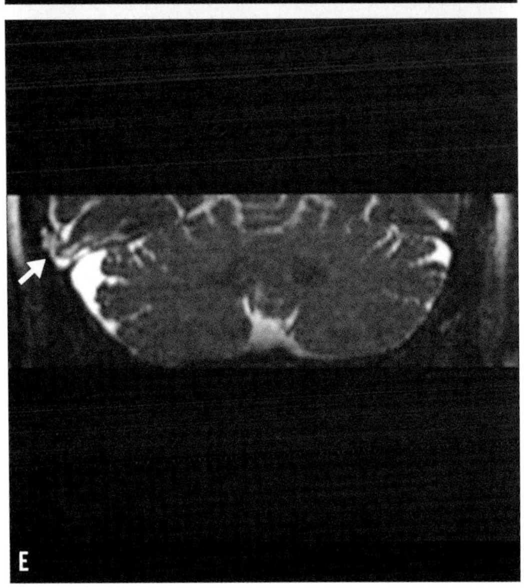

Axial T1 (**A**), axial T2 (**B**), axial FLAIR (**C**), contrast-enhanced axial T1 with fat suppression (**D**), and coronal reformatted CISS (**E**) MR images demonstrate typical features of brain herniation into a dural venous sinus, in this case the posterior aspect of the right temporal lobe into the right transverse venous sinus (arrows, **A-E**). Herniated sulci, helping confirm the presence of herniated brain, are best identified on images **B** and **E**.

Companion case: Middle cranial fossa meningocele

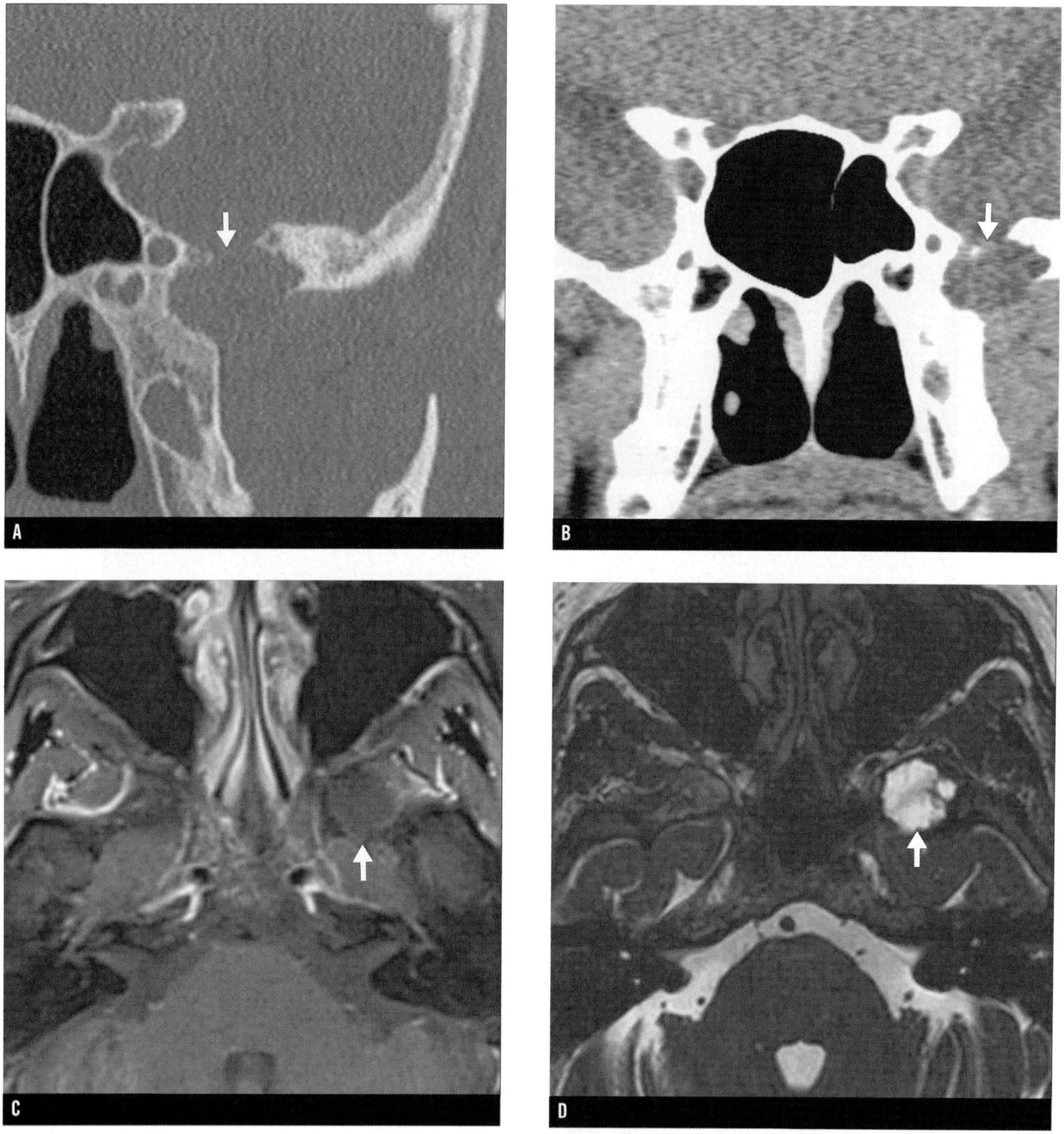

Coronal reformatted CT images through the left middle cranial fossa viewed with a bone window (**A**) and soft tissue window (**B**) demonstrate a moderate-sized, circumscribed, lucent lesion along the left middle cranial fossa floor (arrows, **A**, **B**), which communicates with the subarachnoid space (best demonstrated on image **B**). MR imaging of the same patient with fat-suppressed postcontrast axial T1 (**C**), axial CISS (**D**), and coronal reformatted CISS (**E**) demonstrate a CSF equivalent lesion in the left middle cranial fossa floor communicating with the overlying subarachnoid space and extending into the left infratemporal fossa (arrows, **C**-**E**). Axial diffusion-weighted MR imaging through this level (**F**) does not demonstrate restricted diffusion within the lesion, effectively excluding an epidermoid.

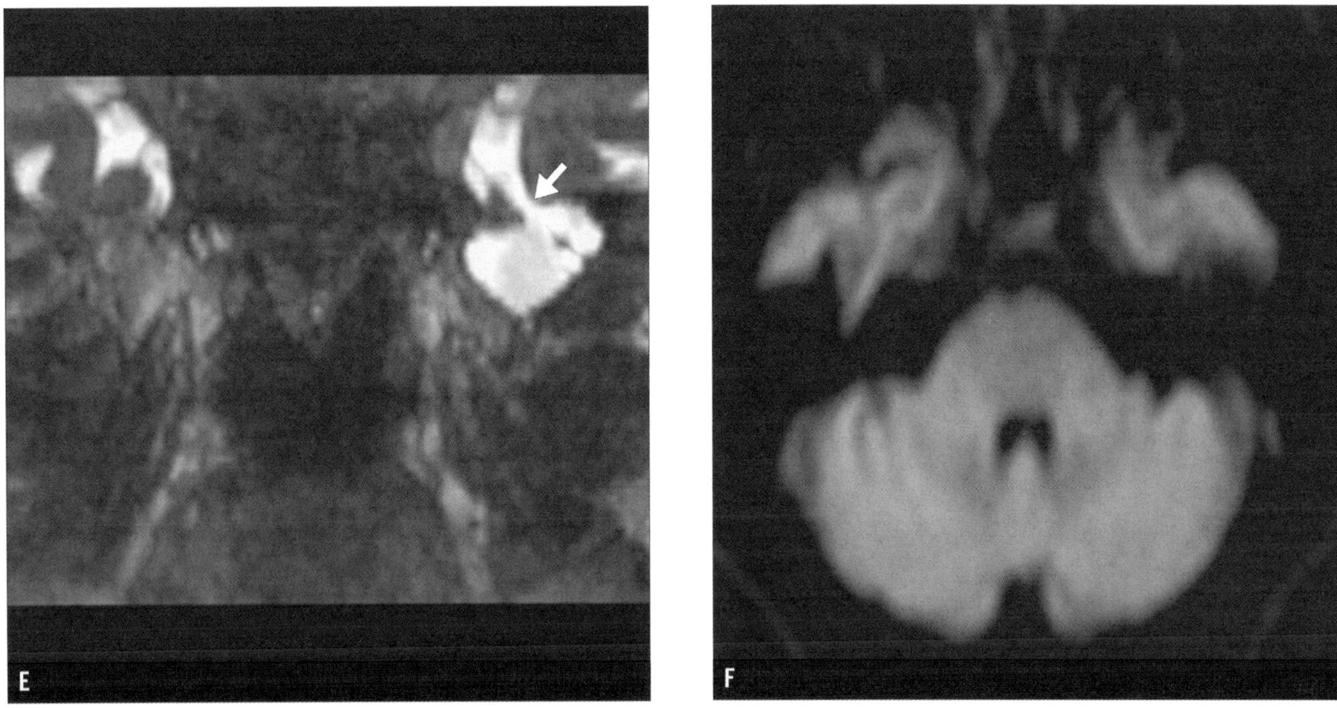

Companion case: Encephalocele and CSF leak associated with idiopathic intracranial hypertension

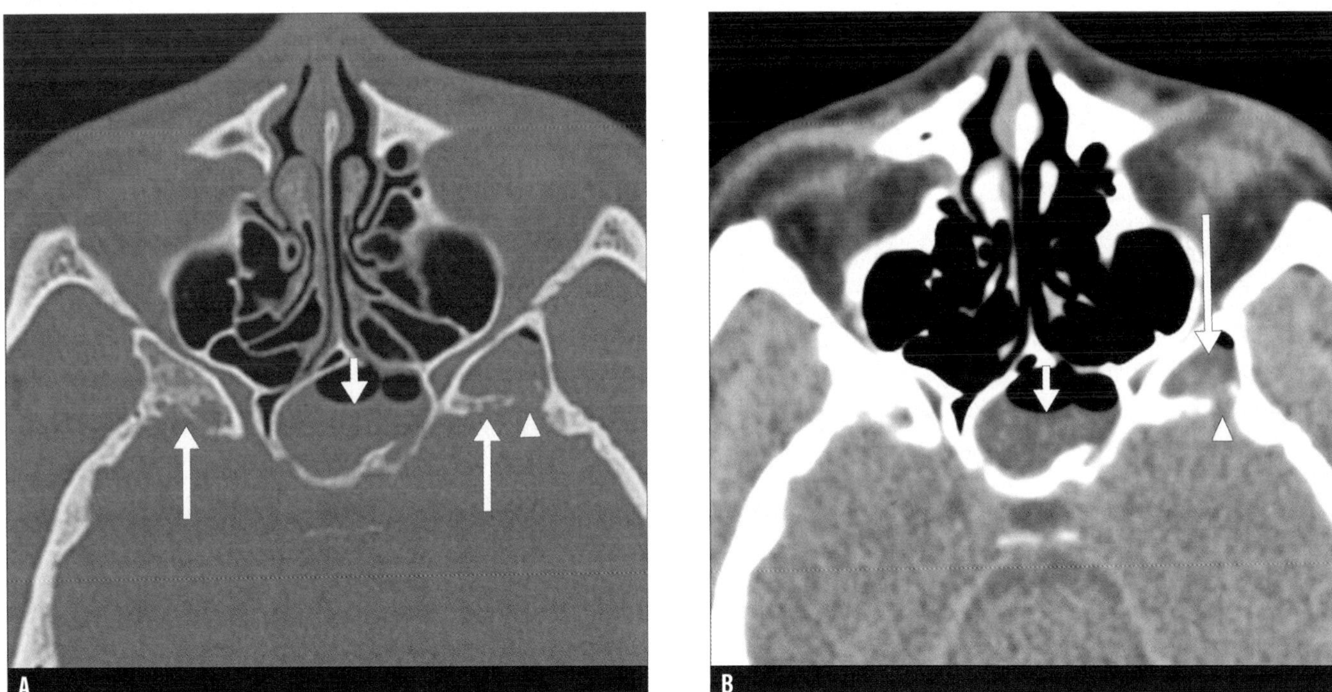

Axial CT images viewed with a bone window (**A**) and soft tissue window (**B**) demonstrate fluid attenuation in the sphenoid sinus (short arrows, **A, B**) as well as possible soft tissue density in a large, pneumatized left pterygoid recess of the sphenoid sinus (long arrow, **B**) in this patient with a known CSF leak and idiopathic intracranial hypertension. A small osseous defect is demonstrated along the posterior wall of the left pterygoid recess (arrowheads, **A, B**). Small arachnoid granulations are also present along the greater wings of the sphenoid (medium arrows, **A**). Sagittal reformatted CT images through the left pterygoid recess (**C, D**) also demonstrate the osseous defect (short arrow, **C**) and immediately adjacent arachnoid granulations (arrowhead, **D**). Sagittal T1 (**E**), axial T2 (**F**), and unenhanced axial T1 (**G**) MR images demonstrate an associated encephalocele extending through the defect (arrowhead, **E**). and into the pneumatized left pterygoid recess (short arrows, **E-G**) While most cases of arachnoid granulations are incidental, in this case, arachnoid granulations likely contributed to the osseous defect, CSF leak, and encephalocele.

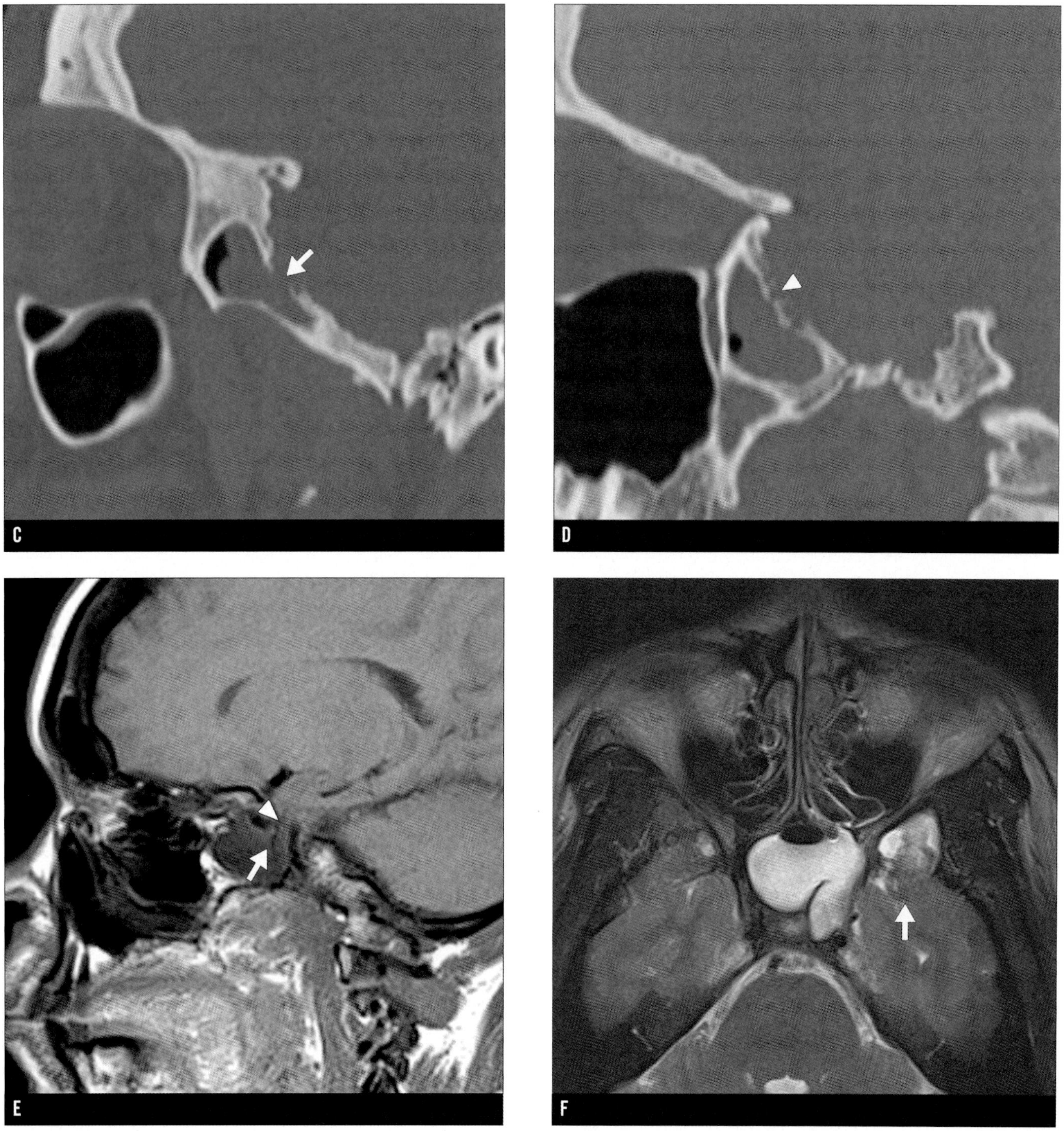
C
D
E
F

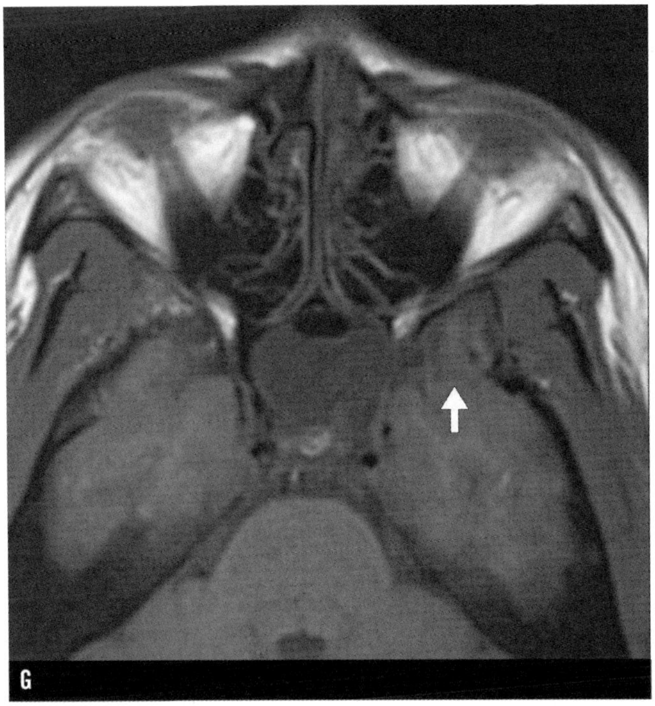

REFERENCES

Battal B, Castillo M.Brain herniations into the dural venous sinuses or calvarium: MRI of a recently recognized entity. *Neuroradiol J.* 2014;27(1):55-62.

Chen F, Deng XF, Liu B, Zou LN, Wang DB, Han H. Arachnoid granulations of middle cranial fossa: a population study between cadaveric dissection and in vivo computed tomography examination. *Surg Radiol Anat.* 2011;33(3):215-221. Epub October 2010.

Goddard JC, Meyer T, Nguyen S, Lambert PR. New considerations in the cause of spontaneous cerebrospinal fluid otorrhea. *Otol Neurotol.* 2010;31(6):940-945.

Trimble CR, Harnsberger HR, Castillo M, Brant-Zawadzki M, Osborn AG. "Giant" arachnoid granulations just like CSF?: NOT!! *AJNR Am J Neuroradiol.* 2010;31(9):1724-1728. Epub June 2010.

CASE 15 Meckel cave cephalocele

Focal expansion of a Meckel cave related to an increase in CSF volume has been termed a cephalocele, meningocele, or an arachnoid cyst. The more generic term cephalocele, rather than meningocele or arachnoid cyst, has been proposed because it is often difficult by imaging to differentiate between a meningocele and an arachnoid cyst. However, a Meckel cave cephalocele could be considered a misnomer. As discussed in the previous case, to be considered a cephalocele, the intracranial contents should herniate outside the confines of the cranium, which typically does not occur with this entity. Nevertheless, in keeping with the predominant current literature, the term Meckel cave cephalocele will be used hererin. A Meckel cave cephalocele is CSF equivalent on all imaging studies and can be unilateral or bilateral. If a Meckel cave cephalocele herniates into the adjacent petrous apex, then the term petrous apex cephalocele is used (which is further described in Chapter 8). Meckel cave cephaloceles are most often incidental findings. Thus, they are usually "do not touch" findings. However, occasionally, they may be associated with meningitis and CSF leaks as well as cranial nerve palsies. Surgical intervention should only be performed if there is sufficient clinical evidence that the patient's symptoms arise from the finding.

COMPANION CASES

- **Intrasellar cephalocele herniating into the clivus.** This is analogous to a Meckel cave cephalocele and petrous apex cephalocele, except in this case there is direct herniation of CSF from the sella into the sphenoid potion of the clivus.
- **Hypoplastic Meckel cave.** It is more common to identify a Meckel cave cephalocele than it is to identify Meckel cave hypoplasia. There are at least a couple reports in the literature describing hypoplasia of the gasserian ganglion in a Meckel cave in combination with hypoplasia of the ipsilateral trigeminal nerve cisternal segment. If the hypoplasia is symptomatic, then the patient may present with facial anesthesia which may result in painless corneal erosions or ulcerations. However, given the paucity of literature, the significance of Meckel cave hypoplasia is unclear.

Meckel cave cephalocele

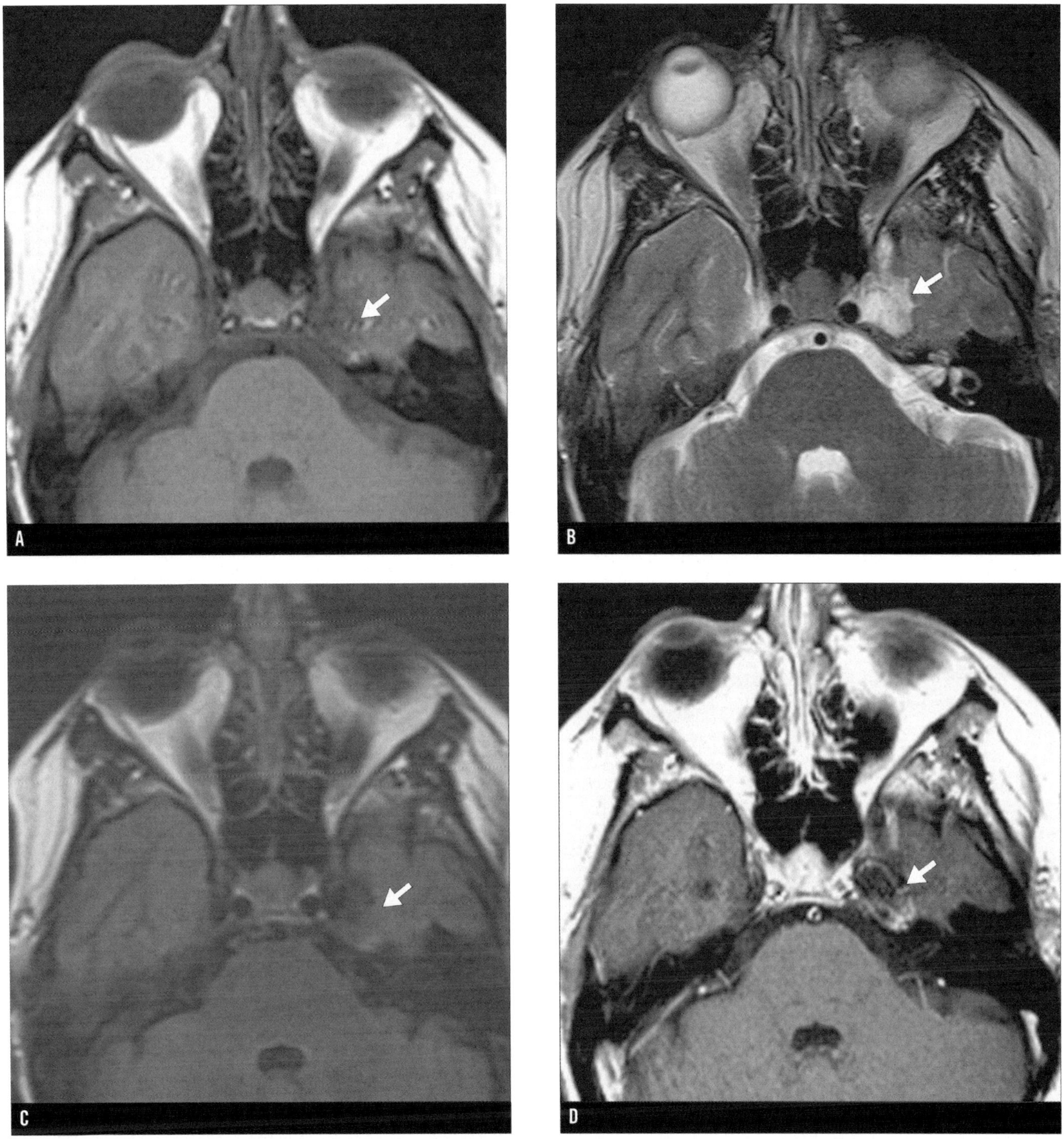

Unenhanced axial T1 (**A**), axial T2 (**B**), axial FLAIR (**C**), and postcontrast axial T1 (**D**) MR images through the mid-skull base demonstrate a CSF equivalent, nonenhancing, expansile lesion in the left Meckel cave (arrows, **A-D**). The finding does not extend into the left petrous apex and therefore is more appropriately characterized as a Meckel cave cephalocele, rather than a petrous apex cephalocele.

Companion case: Intrasellar cephalocele herniating into the clivus

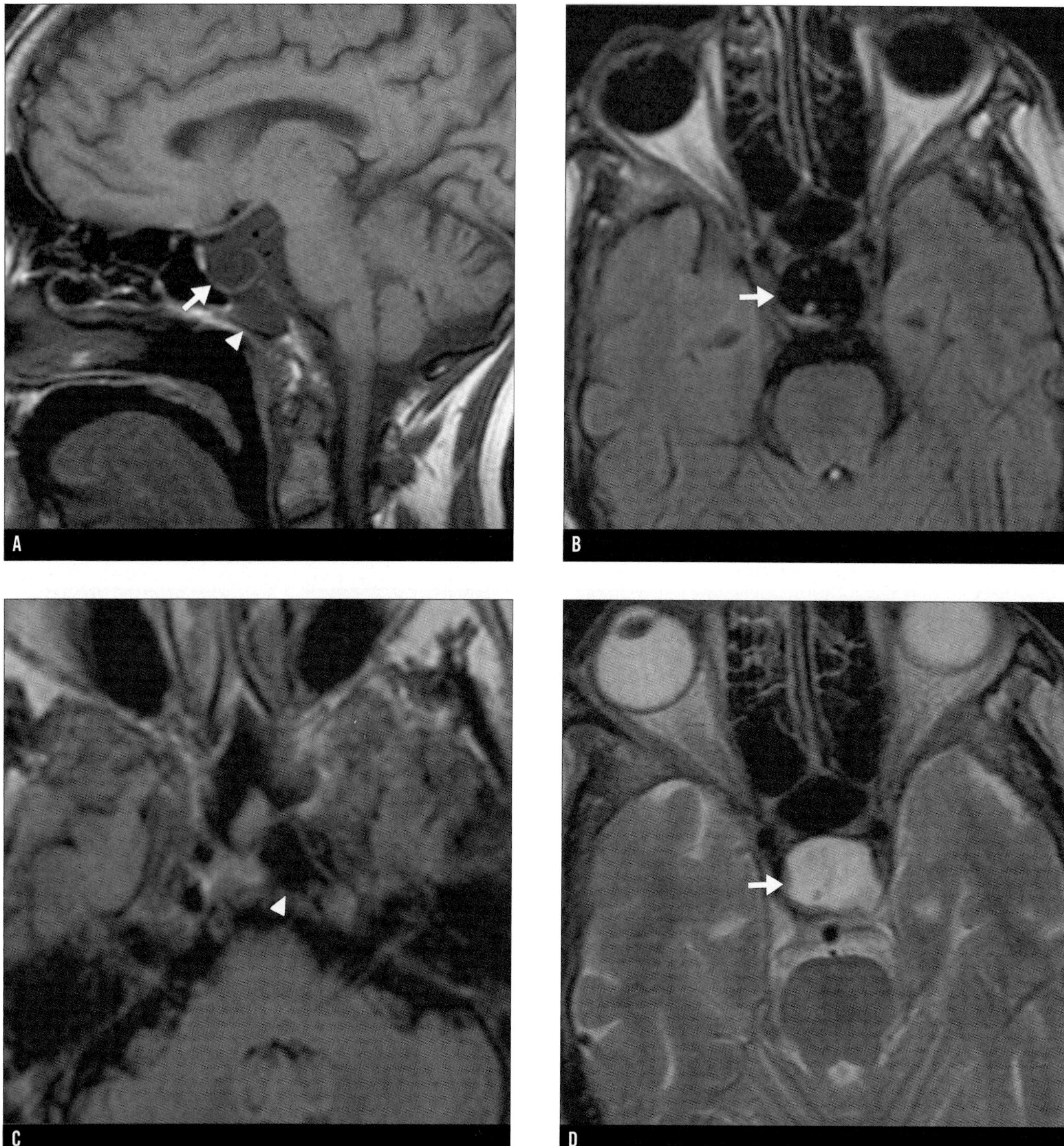

Sagittal unenhanced T1 (**A**), axial FLAIR (**B**, **C**), axial T2 (**D**, **E**), and postcontrast axial T1 (**F**, **G**) MR images demonstrate a nonenhancing, CSF equivalent lesion expanding and occupying the sella turcica (arrows, **A**, **B**, **D**, **F**) as well as herniating into the left aspect of the sphenoid portion of the clivus (arrowheads, **A**, **C**, **E**, **G**). This is similar in appearance to a petrous apex cephalocele and Meckel cave meningocele, with the exception of the intrasellar and clival location of the finding, suggesting that these entities likely reside in the same spectrum. Instead of a cephalocele, some might consider this an arachnoid cyst in the sella herniating into the clivus.

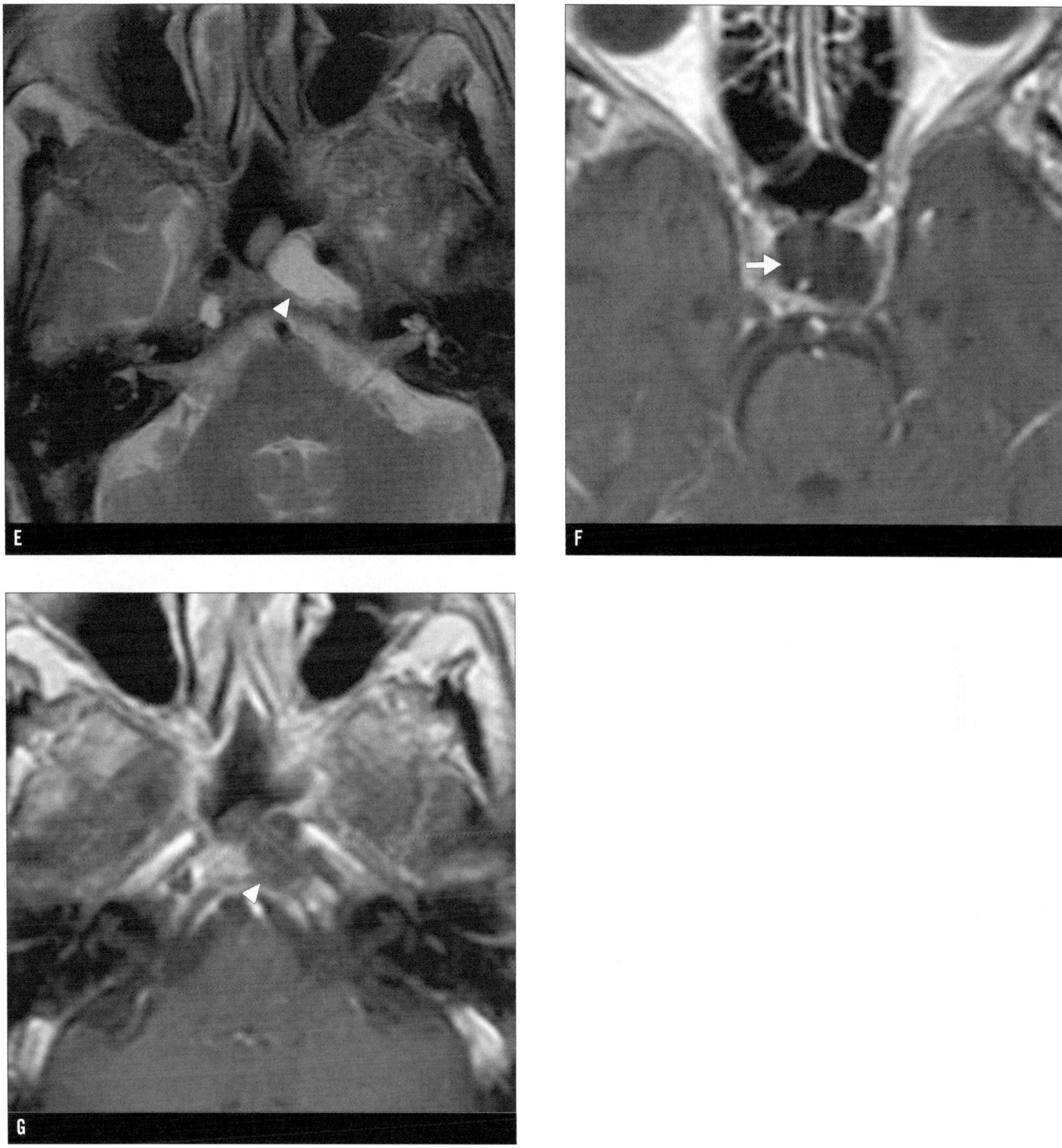

Companion case: Hypoplastic Meckel cave

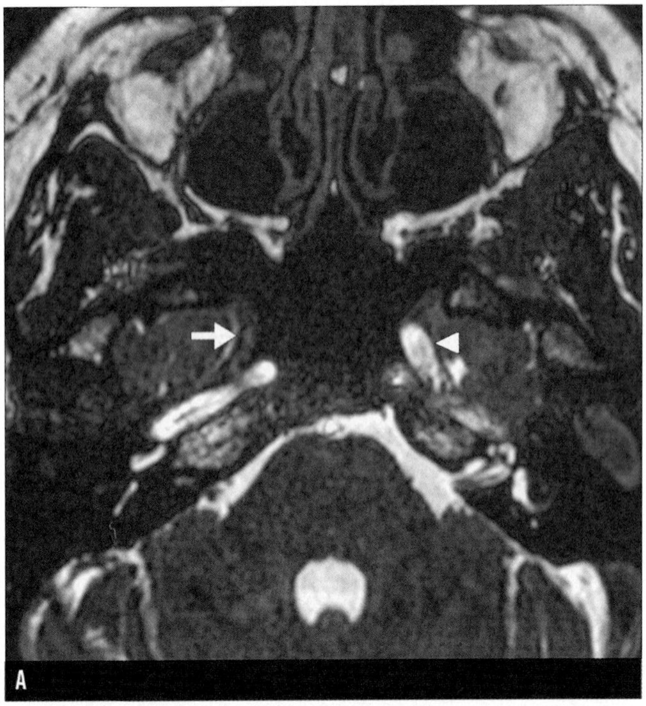

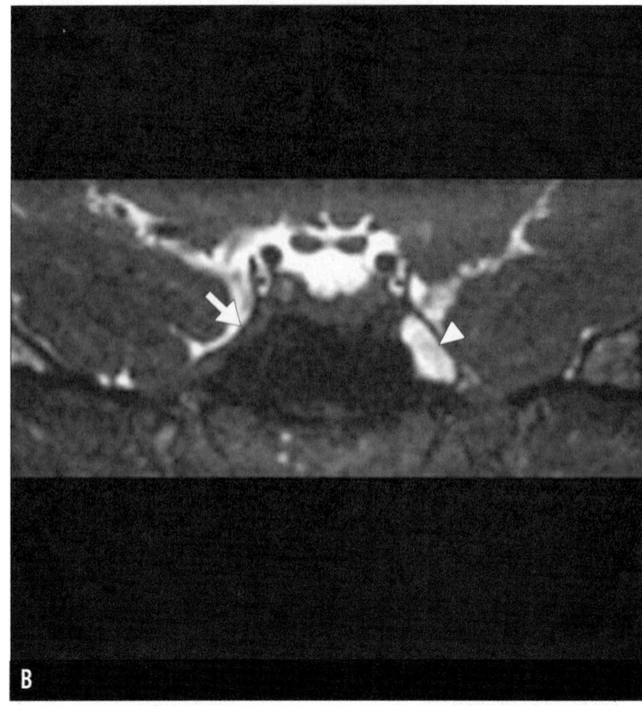

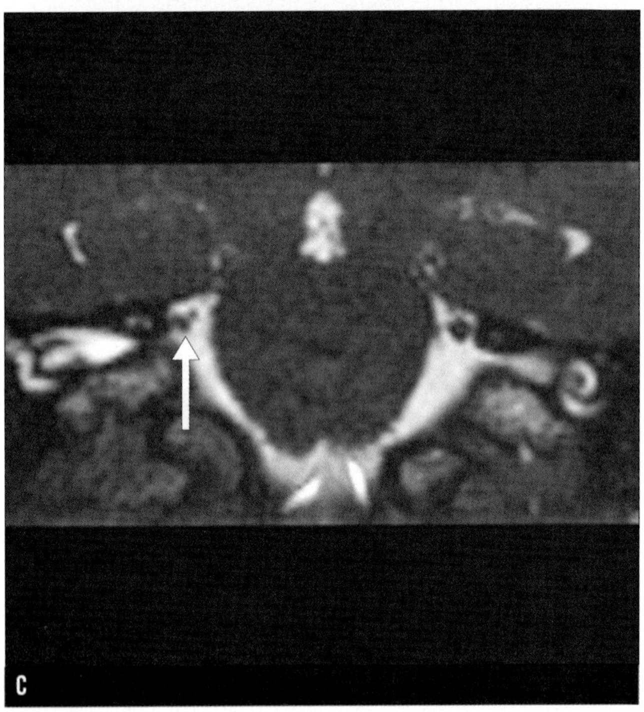

Axial CISS (**A**) and coronal reformatted CISS (**B**) MR images demonstrate a markedly hypoplastic right Meckel cave (short arrows, **A**, **B**) and a normal-sized left Meckel cave (arrowheads, **A**, **B**). A coronal reformatted CISS MR image through the cerebellopontine cistern (**C**) demonstrates a hypoplastic right trigeminal nerve cisternal segment (long arrow, **C**), suggesting that perhaps the right gasserian ganglion is also developmentally hypoplastic. This patient did have right trigeminal nerve symptomatology.

REFERENCES

Jacob M, Gujar S, Trobe J, Gandhi D. Spontaneous resolution of a Meckel's cave arachnoid cyst causing sixth cranial nerve palsy. *J Neuroophthalmol.* 2008;28(3):186-191.

Milne AD, Chui L, Mishra AV, Maxner CE. Unilateral hypoplasia of the trigeminal ganglion. *Can J Ophthalmol.* 2005;40(6):772-774.

Moore KR, Fischbein NJ, Harnsberger HR, Shelton C, Glastonbury CM, White DK, Dillon WP. Petrous apex cephaloceles. *AJNR Am J Neuroradiol.* 2001;22(10):1867-1871.

Schick B, Draf W, Kahle G, Weber R, Wallenfang T.Occult malformations of the skull base. *Arch Otolaryngol Head Neck Surg.* 1997;123(1):77-80.

CASE 16 Incidental asymmetric enlargement of the foramen ovale

Occasionally, incidental asymmetry of the skull base foramina and/or canals may be identified, particularly of the foramen ovale, where one study demonstrated a normal intrasubject foramen ovale mean difference of 0.5 mm. In this same study, there were less intrasubject right to left differences identified when evaluating the normal facial nerve canal, foramen rotundum, and pterygoid canal (ie, vidian canal) compared to the foramen ovale. Therefore, while asymmetry of the skull base foramina/canals may be normal in any given patient, in general, a foramen ovale that is larger by 0.5 mm or greater compared to its contralateral counterpart should be fully evaluated to exclude the possibility of a space occupying lesion (eg, mass, perineural tumor spread, cephalocele, etc). For other skull base foramina/canals, a discrepancy in size of 0.5 mm or less may require further investigation.

COMPANION CASES

- **Foramen ovale meningocele**. A foramen ovale meningocele represents CSF and meninges protruding through the foramen ovale. While a foramen ovale meningocele can be asymptomatic, it may also be associated with a CSF leak. Additionally, one should evaluate the contents of the meningocele for the presence of brain tissue; if present, then the term foramen ovale encephalocele should be used instead of meningocele.
- **Foramen rotundum meningocele.** Same as above, except that the meningocele extends through the foramen rotundum.

Incidental asymmetric enlargement of the foramen ovale

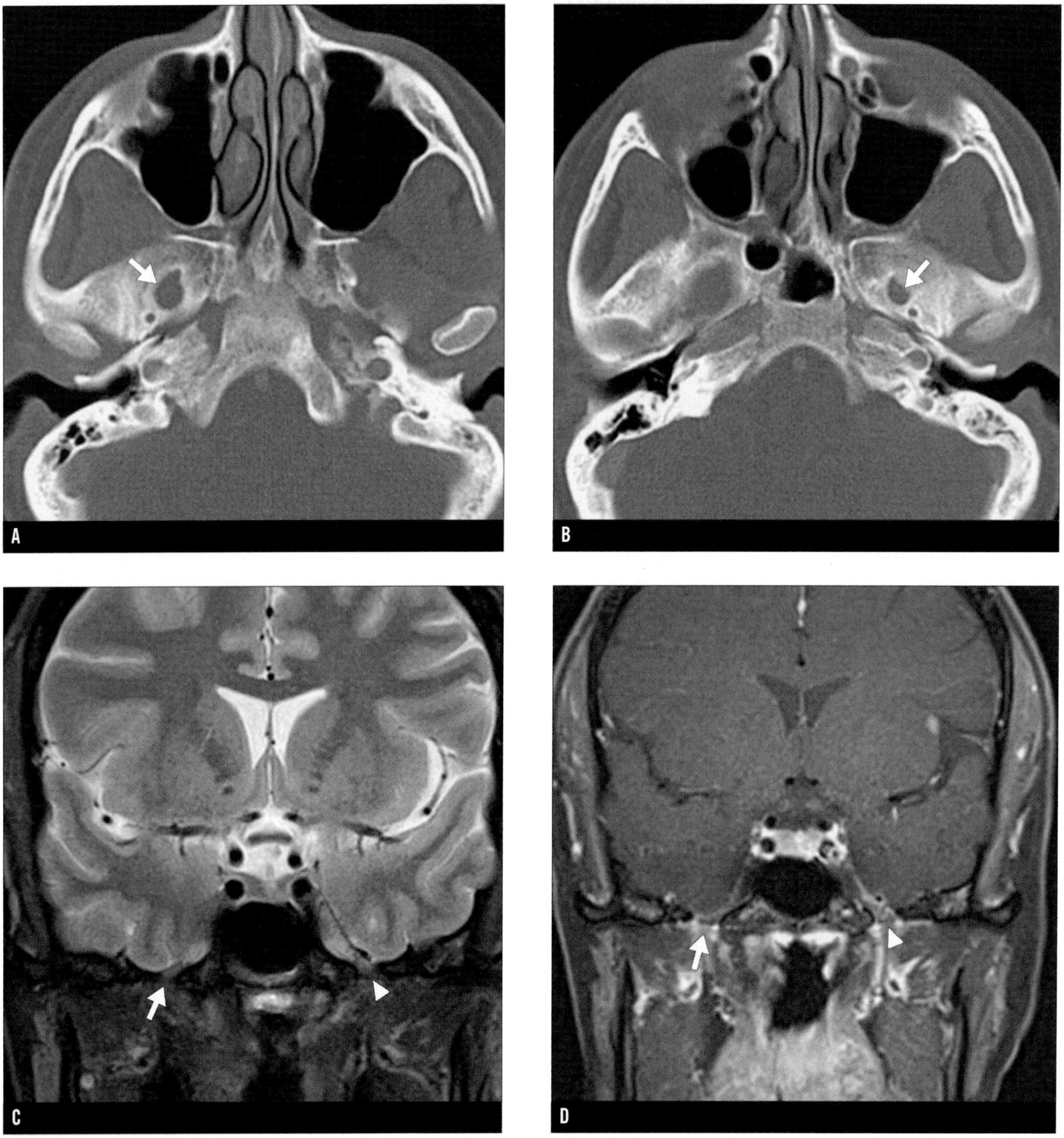

Axial CT images through the skull base from the same study demonstrate an asymmetrically larger right foramen ovale (arrow, **A**) relative to the left (arrow, **B**). Fat-suppressed coronal T2 (**C**) and fat-suppressed contrast-enhanced coronal T1 (**D**) MR images of the same patient do not demonstrate a mass within the right foramen ovale (arrows, **C**, **D**). For reference, the left foramen ovale is denoted by arrowheads on images **C** and **D**.

Companion case: Foramen ovale meningocele

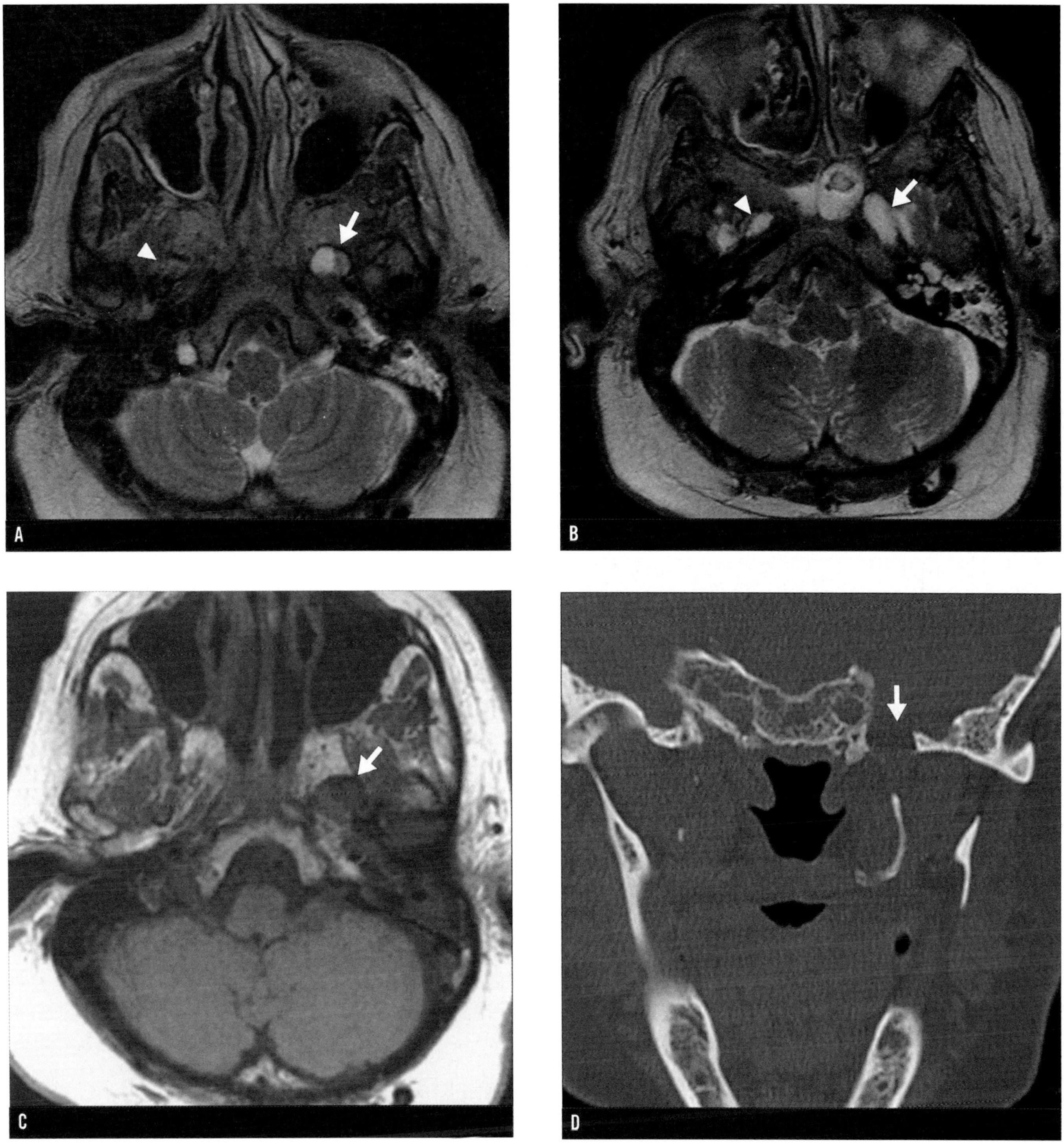

Axial T2 (**A**, **B**) and unenhanced axial T1 (**C**) MR images through the mid-skull base demonstrate asymmetric enlargement of the left foramen ovale (arrows, **A**, **C**) as well as asymmetric enlargement of the left Meckel cave (arrow, **B**). The right foramen ovale and Meckel cave are normal in size (arrowheads **A**, **B**, respectively). Postcontrast MR images (not shown) were of poor quality but did not demonstrate enhancement within the left Meckel cave or left foramen ovale. Direct coronal CT images through the mid skull base viewed with a bone window (**D**, **E**) also demonstrate the asymmetrically enlarged left foramen ovale (arrow, **D**) relative to the right (arrow, **E**). A coronal reformatted CT image viewed with a soft tissue window (**F**) demonstrates CSF equivalent density in the left foramen ovale (arrow, **F**). Following the injection of intrathecal contrast for a CT cisternogram, a coronal CT image through the left foramen ovale viewed with a soft tissue window (**G**) demonstrates contrast bulging through the left foramen ovale, consistent with a foramen ovale meningocele (arrow, **G**). This patient had multiple CSF leaks and arachnoid granulations (not shown). Benign idiopathic intracranial hypertension was clinically suspected in this patient.

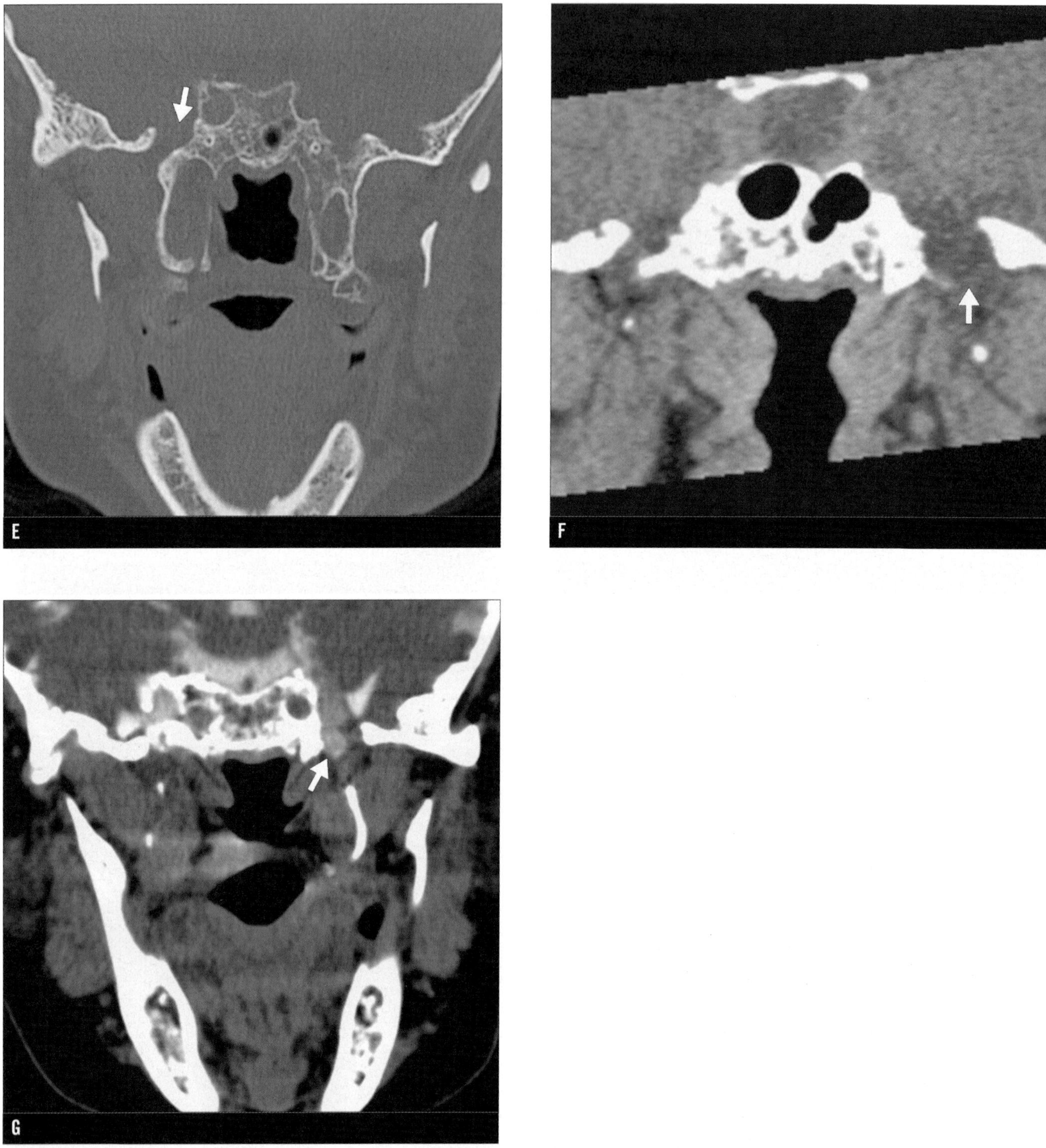

Companion case: Foramen rotundum meningocele

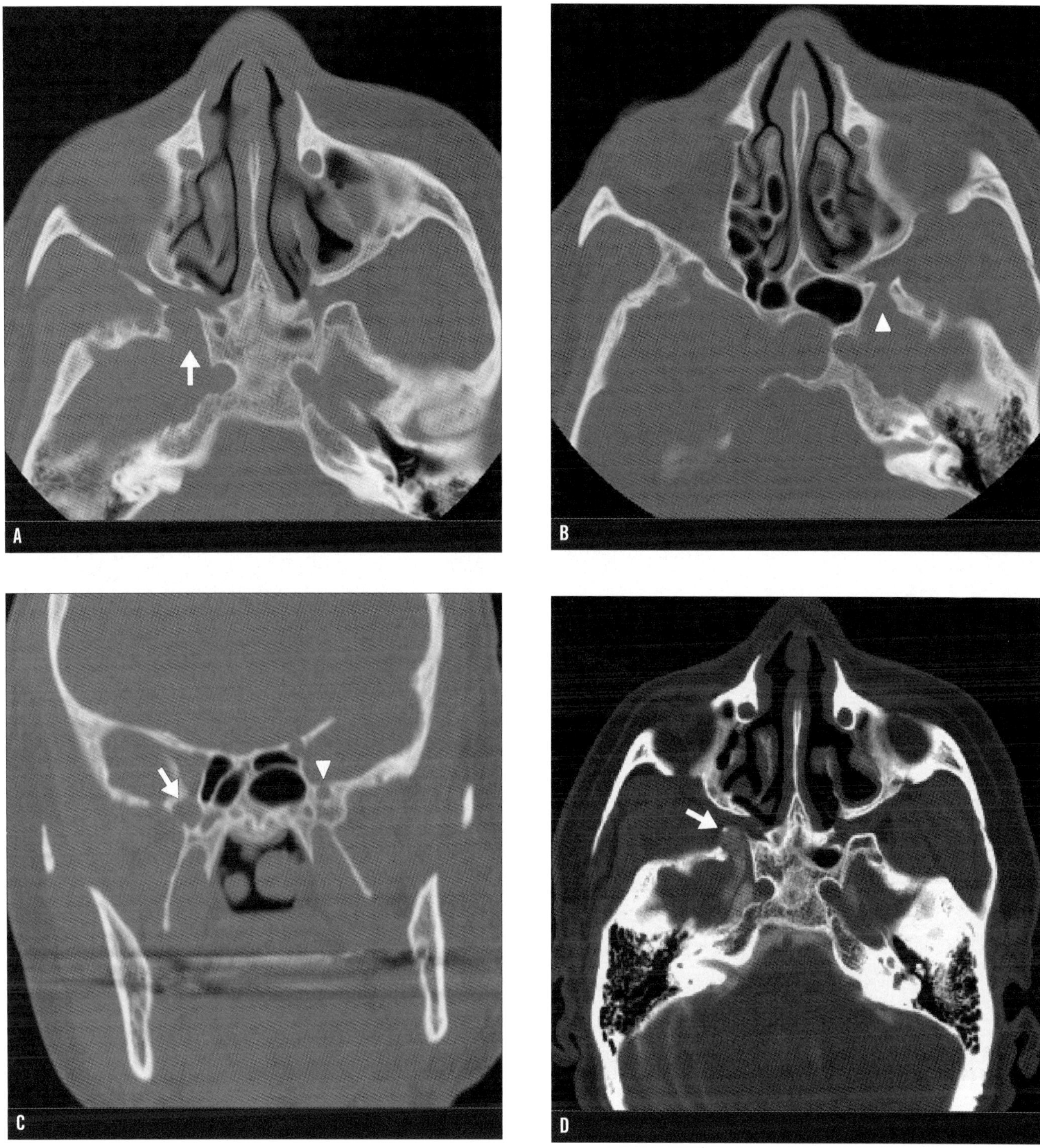

A patient with a suspected CSF leak. Axial (**A**, **B**) and coronal reformatted (**C**) CT images viewed with a bone window demonstrate an asymmetrically enlarged right foramen rotundum (arrows, **A**, **C**) compared to the left foramen rotundum (arrowheads, **B**, **C**). Axial (**D**) and coronal reformatted (**E**) CT images viewed with an intermediate window and following intrathecal administration of contrast for a CT cisternogram demonstrate contrast opacifying the enlarged right foramen rotundum (arrows, **D**, **E**), compatible with a foramen rotundum meningocele. T2-weighted MR images in the axial plane (**F**) and coronal plane (**G**) of the same patient demonstrate T2 hyperintense signal in the expanded right foramen rotundum (arrows, **F**, **G**). A coronal CT image from the cisternogram viewed with an intermediate window (**H**) demonstrates a right fovea ethmoidalis defect resulting in a CSF leak (arrow, **H**). The combination of a fovea ethmoidalis defect with a CSF leak and a foramen rotundum cephalocele suggests the possibility of an underlying benign idiopathic intracranial hypertension.

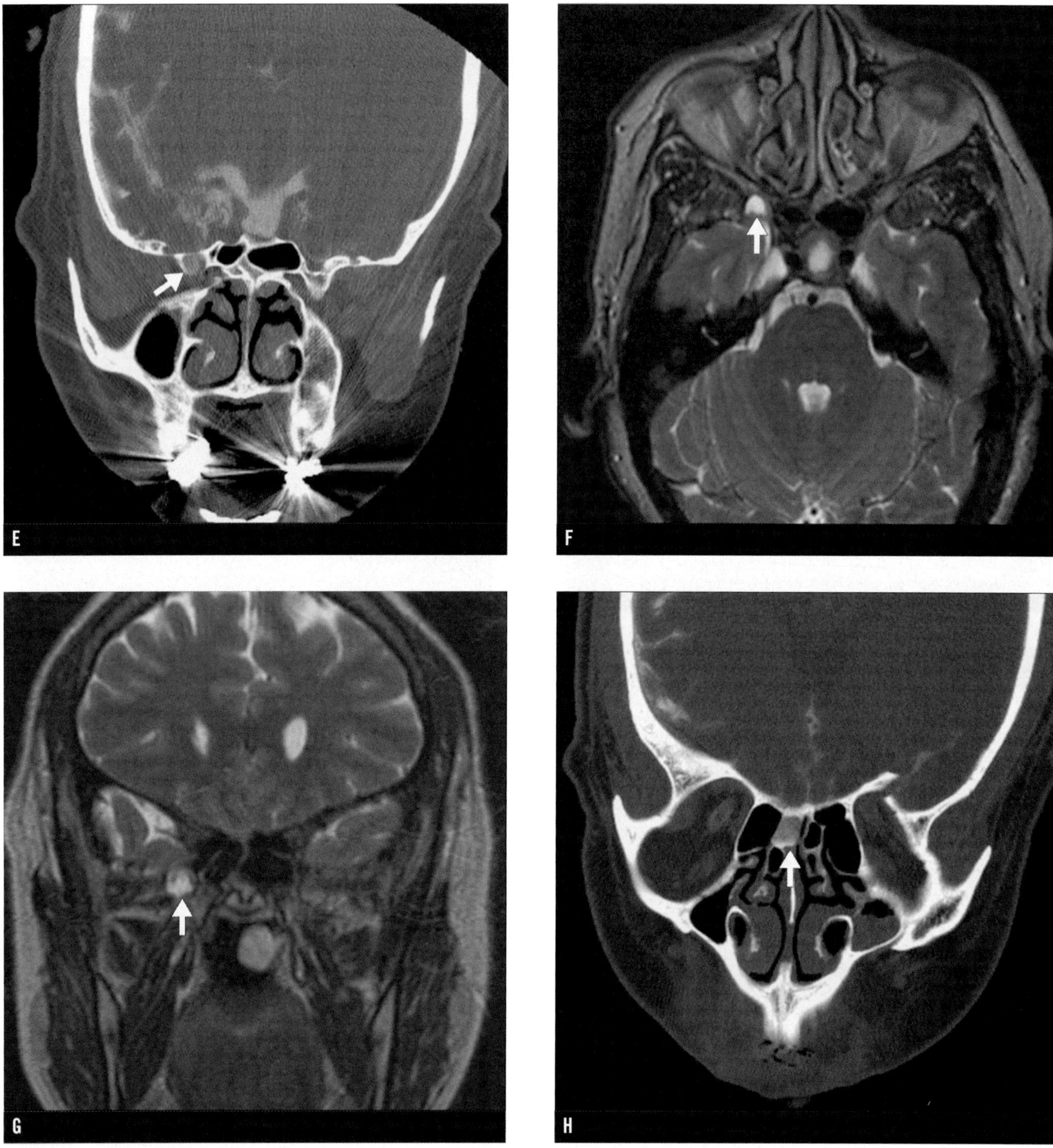

REFERENCES

Mylanus EA, et al. Transalar sphenoidal encephalocele and respiratory distress in a neonate: a case report. *Pediatrics.* 1999;103(1):E12.

Sepahdari AR, Mong S. Skull base CT: normative values for size and symmetry of the facial nerve canal, foramen ovale, pterygoid canal, and foramen rotundum. *Surg Radiol Anat.* 2013;35(1):19-24.

Schick B, Draf W, Kahle G, Weber R, Wallenfang T. Occult malformations of the skull base. *Arch Otolaryngol Head Neck Surg.* 1997;123(1):77-80.

CASE 17 Foramen Vesalius

The foramen Vesalius (also called the sphenoid emissary foramen) is a variably present foramen located immediately anteromedial to the foramen ovale. The foramen Vesalius transmits emissary veins which connect the cavernous sinus to the pterygoid venous plexus. If this structure is not present, the emissary vein which would normally traverse the foramen Vesalius most likely passes through the foramen ovale.

Foramen Vesalius

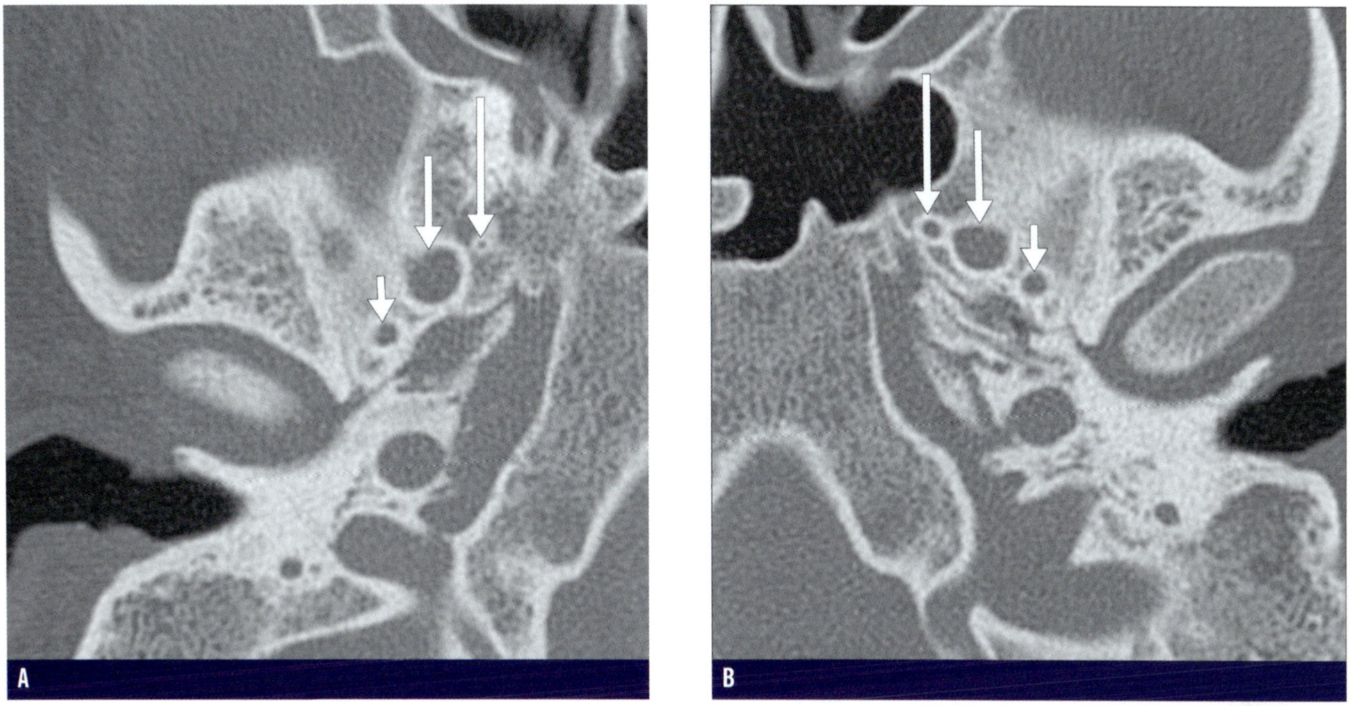

Axial CT images through the right (**A**) and left (**B**) temporal bones demonstrate the normal foramen Vesalius (long arrows, **A**, **B**), with the left being incidentally larger than the right. The foramina ovale (medium arrows, **A**, **B**) and foramina spinosum (short arrows, **A**, **B**) are denoted for reference.

REFERENCE

Ginsberg LE, Pruett SW, Chen MY, Elster AD. Skull-base foramina of the middle cranial fossa: reassessment of normal variation with high-resolution CT. *AJNR Am J Neuroradiol.* 1994;15(2):283-291.

CASE 18 Foramen spinosum

The foramen spinosum is traversed by the middle meningeal artery, middle meningeal veins, and a recurrent branch of the mandibular nerve. The foramen spinosum is located posterolateral to the foramen ovale and its size varies among individuals. The foramen spinosum is usually round or oval in shape and has a diameter of 1 to 4 mm (average 2 mm), absent in less than 1% of cases, and may be duplicated.

If the foramen spinosum is absent, then one should consider the presence of a persistent stapedial artery. A persistent stapedial artery is a rare congenital vascular anomaly that may be incidental or could present clinically as a middle ear mass with pulsatile tinnitus. While the foramen spinosum is absent when a persistent stapedial artery is present, not every case of an absent foramen spinosum is associated with a persistent stapedial artery. See Chapter 8 for further discussion regarding the persistent stapedial artery.

COMPANION CASES

- **Absent and hypoplastic foramina spinosum.** A hypoplastic foramen spinosum is considered within the realm of normal and is of no clinical significance. However, as discussed above, an absent foramen spinosum, while sometimes also incidental, raises the possibility of a persistent stapedial artery.
- **Bifurcated foramen spinosum.** This variant is believed to relate to an early bifurcation of the middle meningeal artery and is an incidental finding.

Foramen spinosum

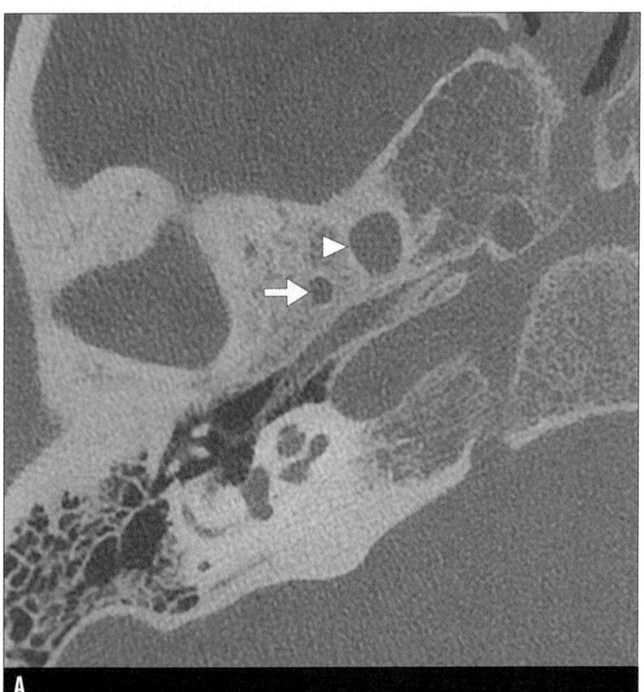

An axial CT image (**A**) demonstrates a normal right foramen spinosum (arrow). A normal right foramen ovale is denoted for reference (arrowhead).

Companion case: Absent and hypoplastic foramina spinosum

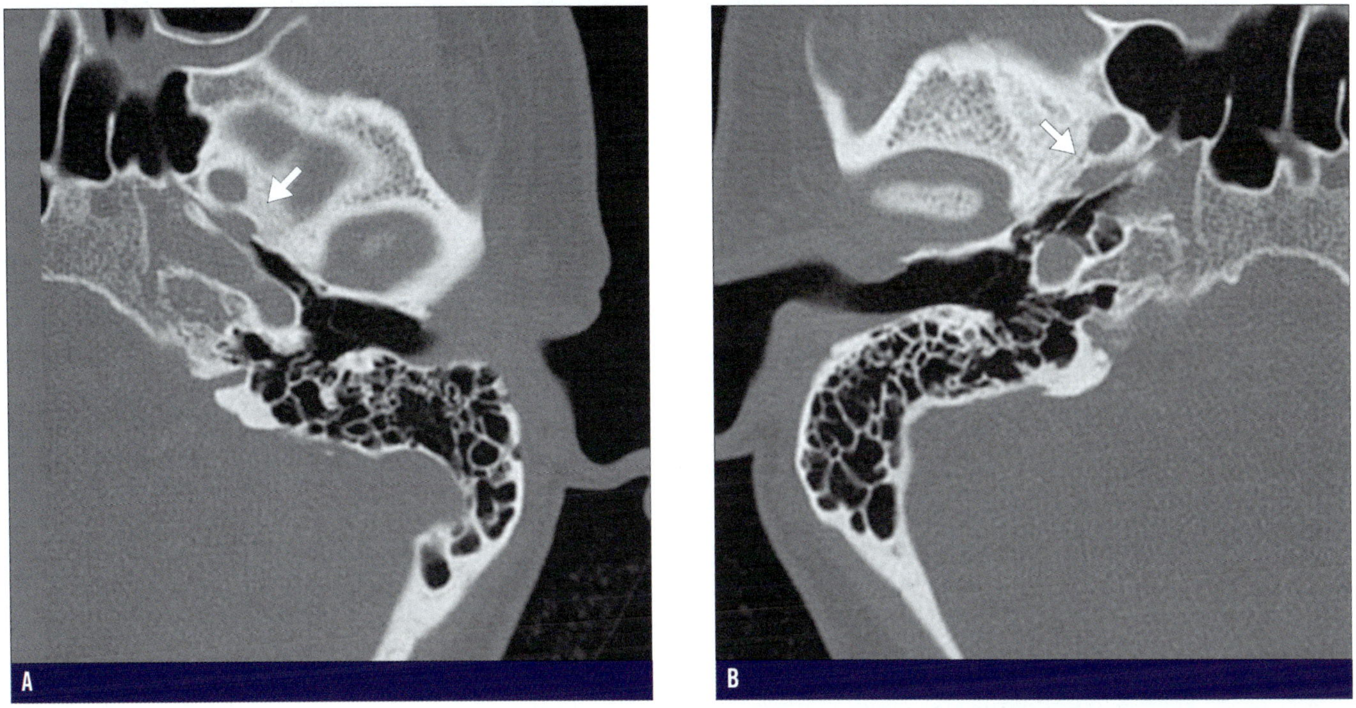

An axial CT image through the left mid-skull base (**A**) demonstrates absence of the left foramen spinosum. The arrow on image **A** indicates the expected location of the left foramen spinosum. An axial CT image through the right mid-skull base of the same patient (**B**) demonstrates a hypoplastic right foramen spinosum (arrow, **B**).

Companion case: Bifurcated foramen spinosum

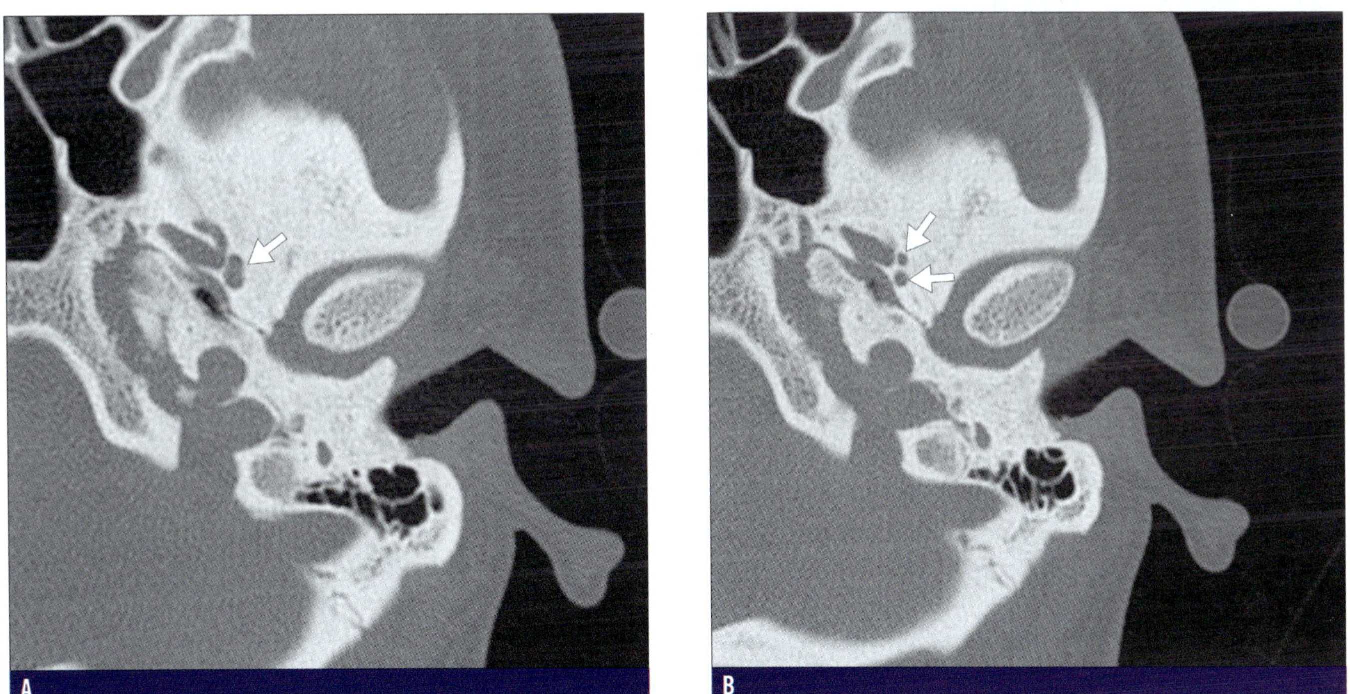

Axial CT images through the left mid-skull base (**A**, **B**) demonstrate an asymmetrically prominent left foramen spinosum (arrow, **A**) that subsequently bifurcates (arrows, **B**).

REFERENCES

Krayenbühl N, Isolan GR, Al-Mefty O. The foramen spinosum: a landmark in middle fossa surgery. *Neurosurg Rev.* 2008;31:397-402

Richard Silbergleit, et al. The persistent stapedial artery. *AJNR Am J Neuroradiol.* 2000; 21:572-577.

Schmalfuss H, Camp M. Skull base: pseudolesion or true lesion? *Eur Radiol.* 2008;18:1232-1243.

CASE 19 Canaliculus innominatus

The canaliculus innominatus (also called Arnold canal) is a very small canal situated medial to the foramen spinosum. This canal transmits the lesser superficial petrosal nerve, which is a small nerve originating from the tympanic branch of CN IX that provides parasympathetic innervation to the parotid gland. This canal is infrequently seen, with one study demonstrating its presence in 16% of cases. If it is not present, then the lesser superficial petrosal nerve traverses the foramen ovale.

Canaliculus innominatus

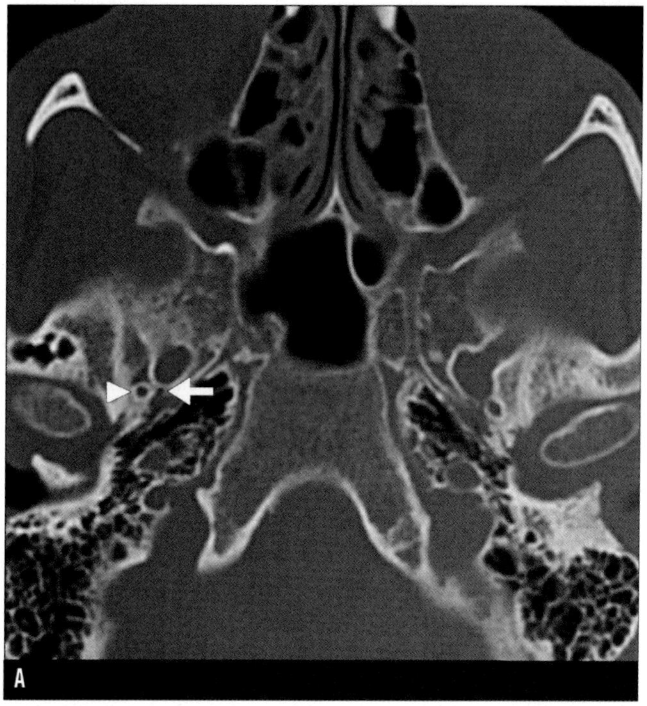

A single axial image through the skull base (**A**) demonstrates a very small foramen representing the canaliculus innominatus (arrow), located immediately medial to the right foramen spinosum (arrowhead).

REFERENCE

Ginsberg LE, Pruett SW, Chen MY, Elster AD. Skull-base foramina of the middle cranial fossa: reassessment of normal variation with high-resolution CT. *AJNR Am J Neuroradiol.* 1994;15(2):283-291.

CASE 20 Iatrogenic venous air at the skull base

Air identified in the veins of the head and neck most commonly occurs during initiation of intravenous cannulation and is the result of inadvertent injection of air. Air has been described in several veins of the head and neck, including the subclavian veins, internal jugular veins, scalp veins, infratemporal fossa, carotid canal, dural venous sinuses, and the superior ophthalmic veins. Generally speaking, there is no long-term sequela if the amount of air injected is small.

Iatrogenic venous air at the skull base

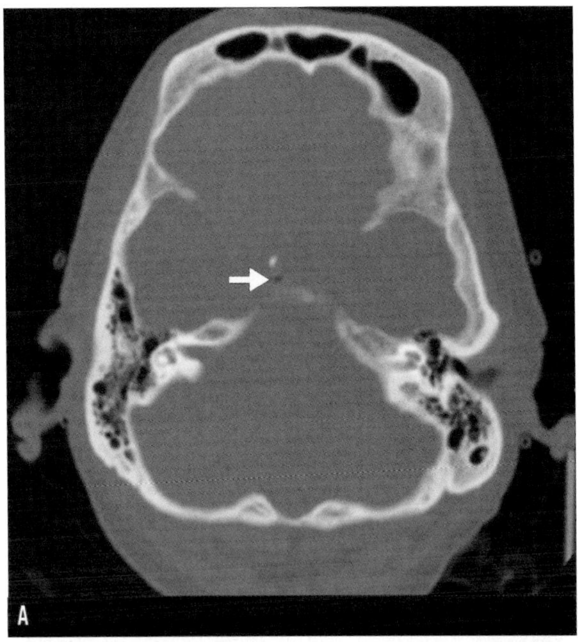

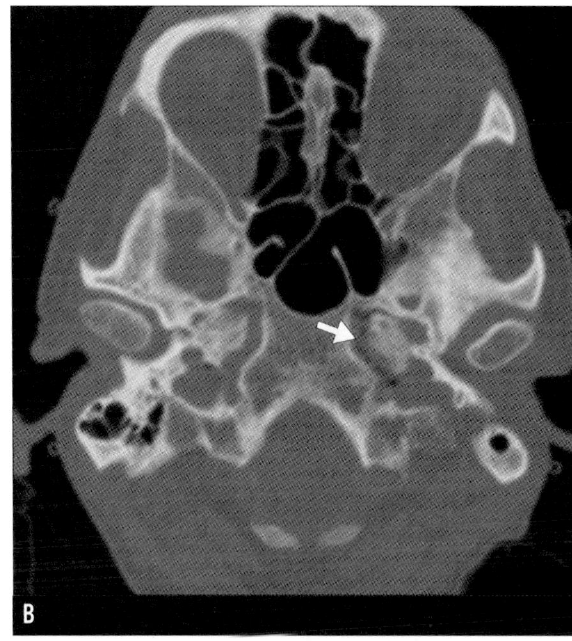

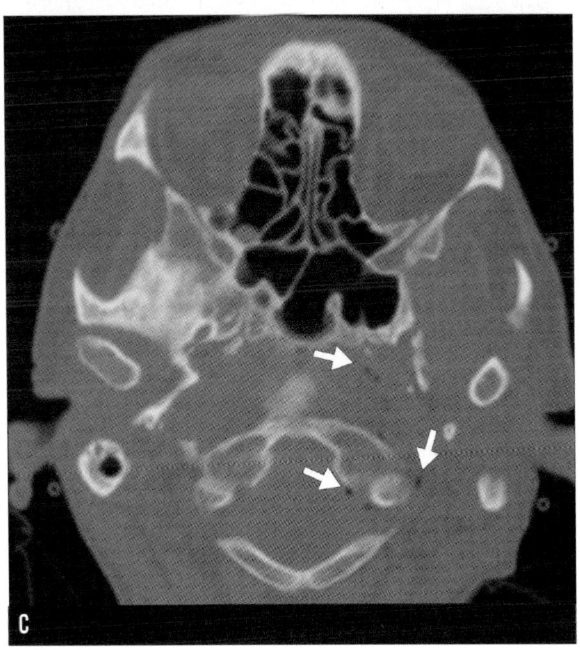

Axial CT images through the sella (**A**), mid-skull base (**B**), and the C1 vertebra (**C**) demonstrate scattered foci of air including in the sella (arrow, **A**), within the petro-occipital synchondrosis (arrow, **B**), and in the prevertebral soft tissues as well as in the venous plexus surrounding the left occipital condyle and left lateral mass of C1 (arrows, **C**). This air was incidental and the patient was not symptomatic from these findings.

REFERENCES

Bodkin PA, et al. Air in the cavernous sinus may be due to venous cannulation. *Br J Neurosurg.* 2010;24(3):309-310.

Rubinstein D, Dangleis K, Damiano TR. Venous air emboli identified on head and neck CT scans. *J Comp Assist Tomogr.* 1996;20(4):559-562.

CASE 21 Iophendylate (Pantopaque) contrast at the skull base

Iophendylate (Pantopaque) is an oil-based intrathecal contrast agent that was introduced in 1941 and used for nearly three decades. This agent has been subsequently replaced with water-soluble contrast agents. However, due to its lipid-soluble state and extremely slow rate of resorption, residual Pantopaque will often be demonstrated in patients who have received this agent years and even decades after its administration. The agent is typically more hyperdense than intravenous contrast used for CT and is similar in density to intravenous contrast used for conventional angiography. On MRI, the agent has similar imaging characteristics as fat and is hyperintense on precontrast T1-weighted imaging, hyperintense on T2-weighted imaging, and does not enhance.

Pantopaque can simulate an aneurysm on MRI, particularly on precontrast T1-weighted imaging, as both Pantopaque and methemoglobin in thrombosed aneurysms will be hyperintense on this sequence. If differentiating Pantopaque from an aneurysm cannot be made on an MRI/MRA or on a cerebral angiogram, then a noncontrast CT should help differentiate an aneurysm from Pantopaque material. Alternatively, a fat-suppression sequence typically suppresses Pantopaque but will not alter the appearance of methemoglobin within an aneurysm.

Iophendylate (Pantopaque) contrast at the skull base

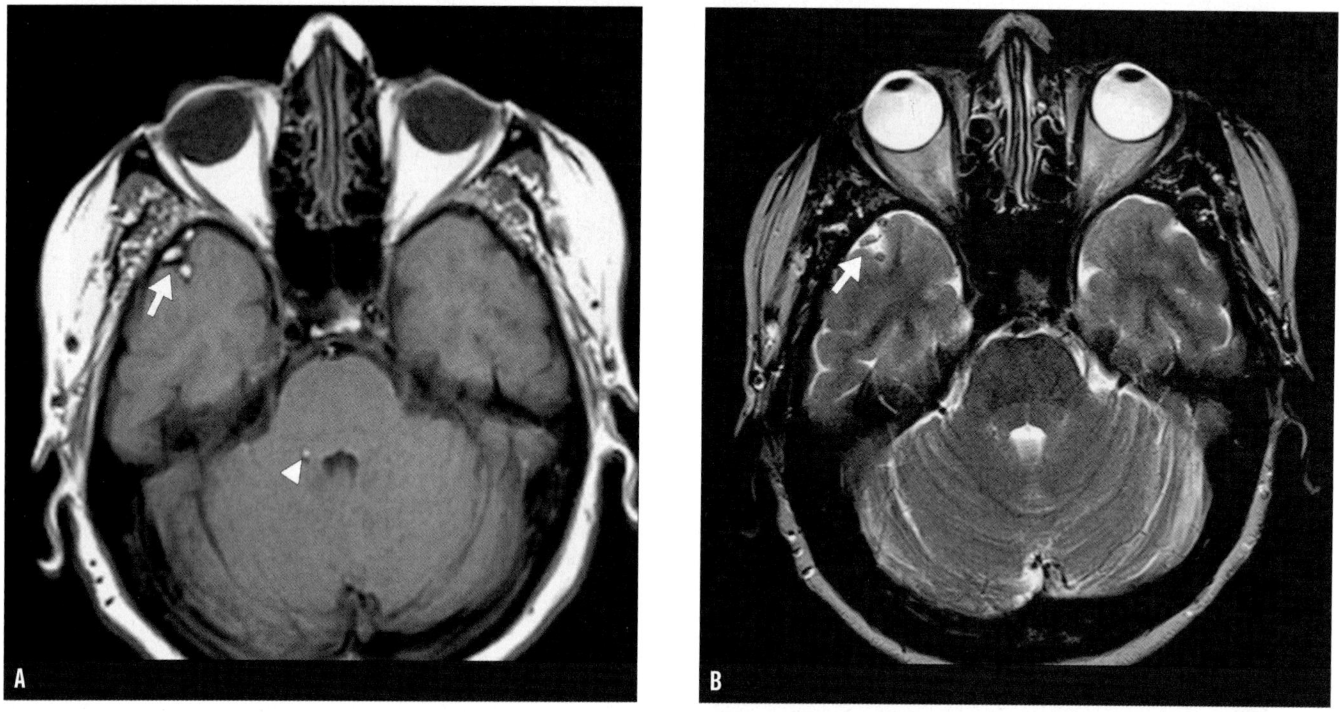

This patient had a remote history of a myelogram performed with Pantopaque. Unenhanced axial T1 (**A**), axial T2 (**B**), axial GRE (**C**), and postcontrast axial T1 (**D**) MR images demonstrate several nonspecific foci of signal abnormality in the anterior aspect of the right middle cranial fossa (arrows **A-D**) and just lateral to the right brachium conjunctivum (arrowheads, **A**, **C**, **D**). The findings are hyperintense on T1, hypointense on T2 and GRE, and do not enhance following contrast. Several axial CT images of the same patient obtained through the middle cranial fossa and temporal bones (**E-H**) demonstrate numerous punctate hyperdense foci scattered throughout the subarachnoid space, compatible with Pantopaque material. Residual Pantopaque material is demonstrated in the olfactory grooves (arrowhead, **E**), scattered in the middle cranial fossae (arrows, **E**, **F**), the cavernous sinus (arrowheads, **F**, **G**), and in the internal auditory canals (arrows, **H**). The findings on CT are pathognomonic of prior intrathecal Pantopaque contrast administration (or other oil-based contrast agent).

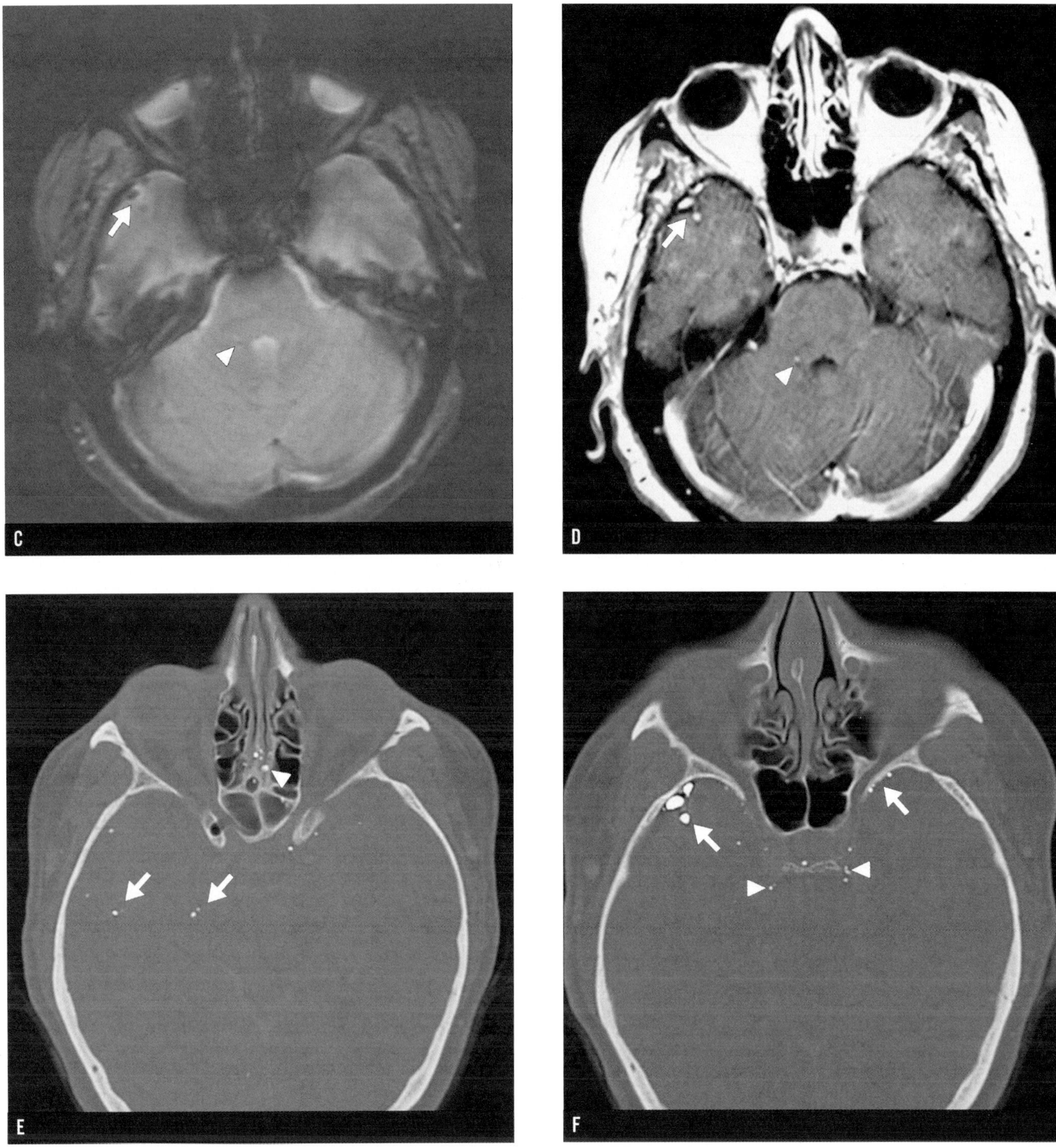
C
D
E
F

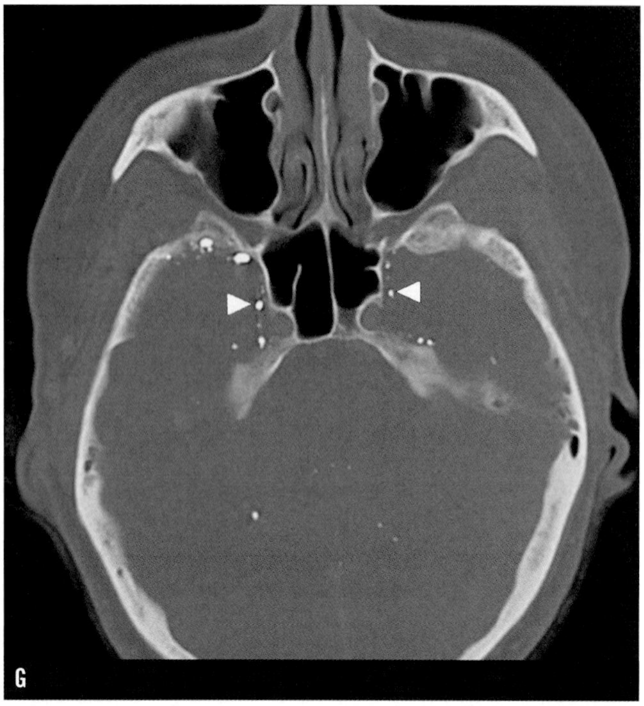

G

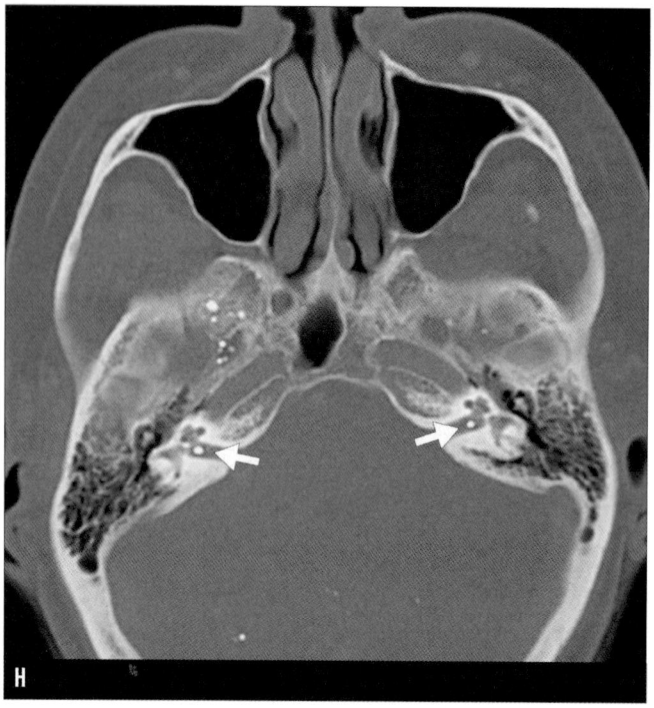

H

REFERENCE

Lidov MW, Silvers AR, Mosesson RE, Stollman AL, Som PM. Pantopaque simulating thrombosed intracranial aneurysms on MRI. *J Comput Assist Tomogr.* 1996;20(2):225-227.

CASE 22 Lateral pterygoid plate foramen simulating a fracture

This case demonstrates the need to evaluate possible fractures on CT in various planes to exclude a normal finding simulating a fracture. In the case provided an unusual foramen in the lateral pterygoid plate simulated a fracture on axial imaging, but was well-delineated as a foramen on the sagittal reformatted images.

Lateral pterygoid plate foramen simulating a fracture

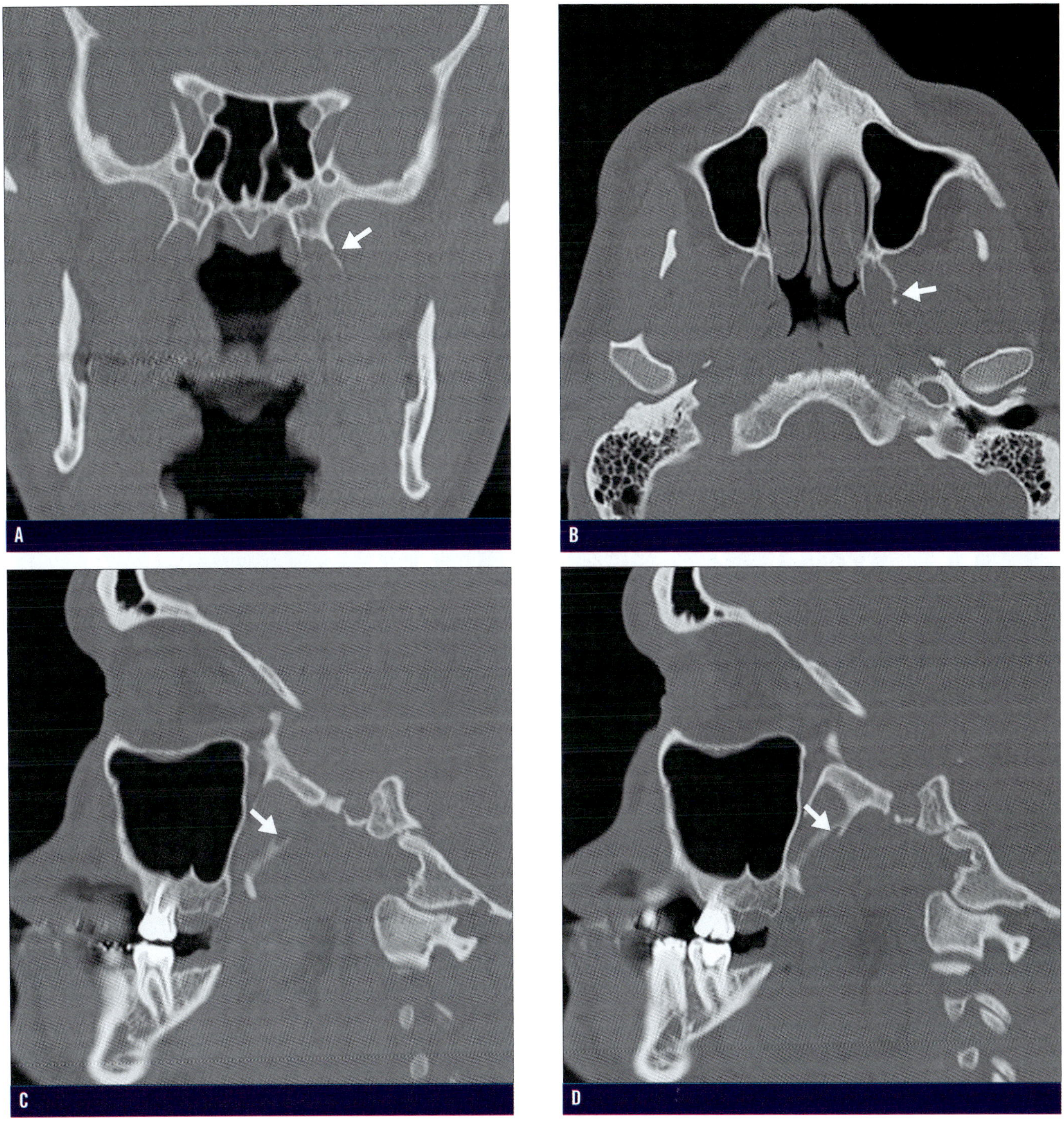

Coronal reformatted (**A**) and axial (**B**) CT images through the pterygoid plates demonstrate an apparent fracture through the left lateral pterygoid plate (arrows, **A**, **B**). However, two contiguous sagittal reformatted CT images through the left lateral pterygoid plate (**C**, **D**) demonstrate that this apparent fracture simply represents an incidental, normal variant foramen (arrows, **C**, **D**).

CASE 23 Normal pterygoid venous plexus

The pterygoid venous plexus is a normal paired plexus of valveless veins located along the pterygoid musculature. It drains a multitude of veins, including the infraorbital vein, middle meningeal vein, masseteric vein, anterior and posterior deep temporal veins, descending palatine vein, sphenopalatine vein, and alveolar veins. The pterygoid venous plexus also drains the cavernous sinus via venous branches extending through the foramen ovale, foramen Vesalius, and foramen lacerum. In addition, the pterygoid venous plexus anastomoses with the anterior facial vein; therefore, the pterygoid venous plexus may serve as a conduit for facial infections to spread to the cavernous sinus and result in a cavernous sinus thrombophlebitis. The pterygoid venous plexus is normally drained by its ipsilateral internal maxillary vein.

COMPANION CASES

- **Internal maxillary veins draining the pterygoid venous plexuses.** The internal maxillary vein arises from the pterygoid venous plexus and joins the superficial temporal vein to form the retromandibular vein. The retromandibular vein is one of the tributaries that forms the external jugular vein.
- **Venous plexuses surrounding the temporomandibular joints.** Rather than typical, discrete bilateral retromandibular veins, the case provided represents variant venous plexuses that likely supplant the bilateral retromandibular veins.

Asymmetric normal pterygoid venous plexuses

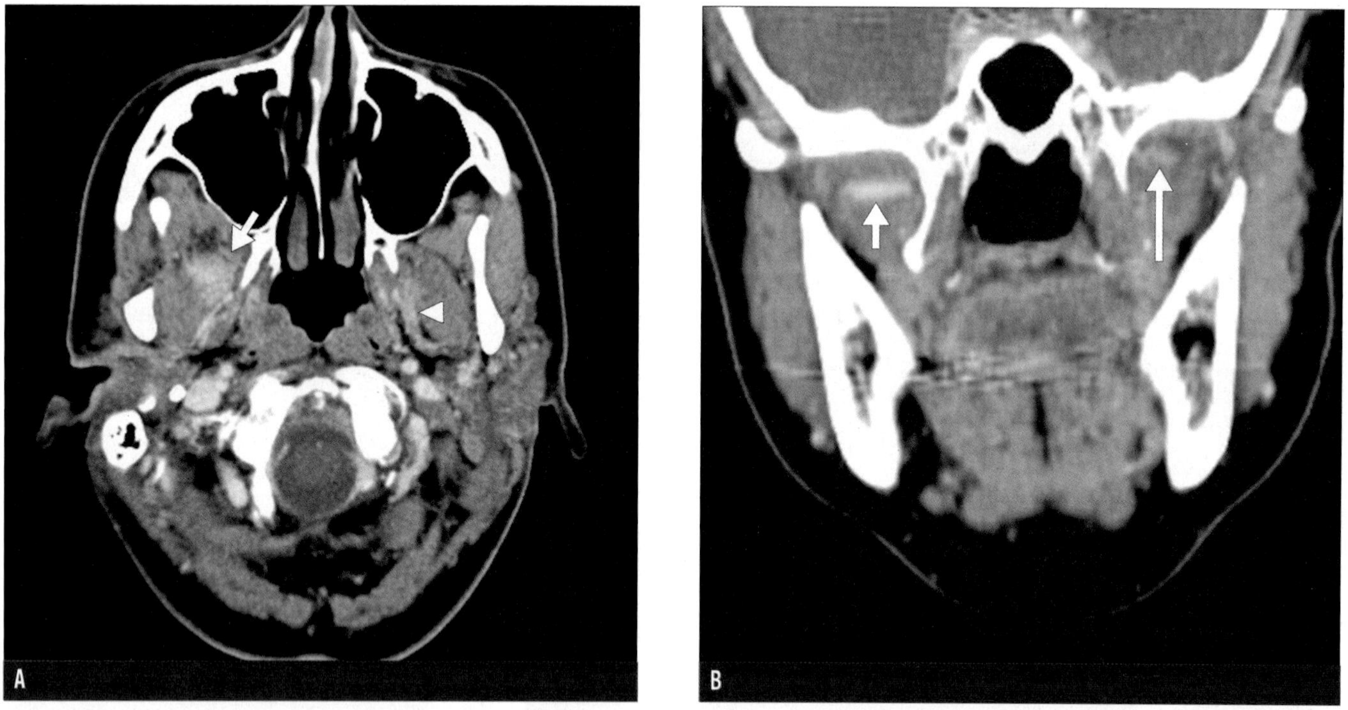

Postcontrast axial (**A**) and postcontrast coronal reformatted (**B**) CT images demonstrate focal asymmetric enhancement along the right lateral pterygoid muscle that is ill-defined on axial imaging (small arrow, **A**) and linear as well as more discrete on coronal reformatted imaging (small arrow, **B**). This is a normal appearance of a pterygoid venous plexus. An asymmetrically small left pterygoid venous plexus is identified (long arrow, **B**). The dominant left venous plexus in this region is located in the left parapharyngeal space and is more appropriately termed a parapharyngeal venous plexus (arrowhead, **A**).

Normal pterygoid venous plexuses

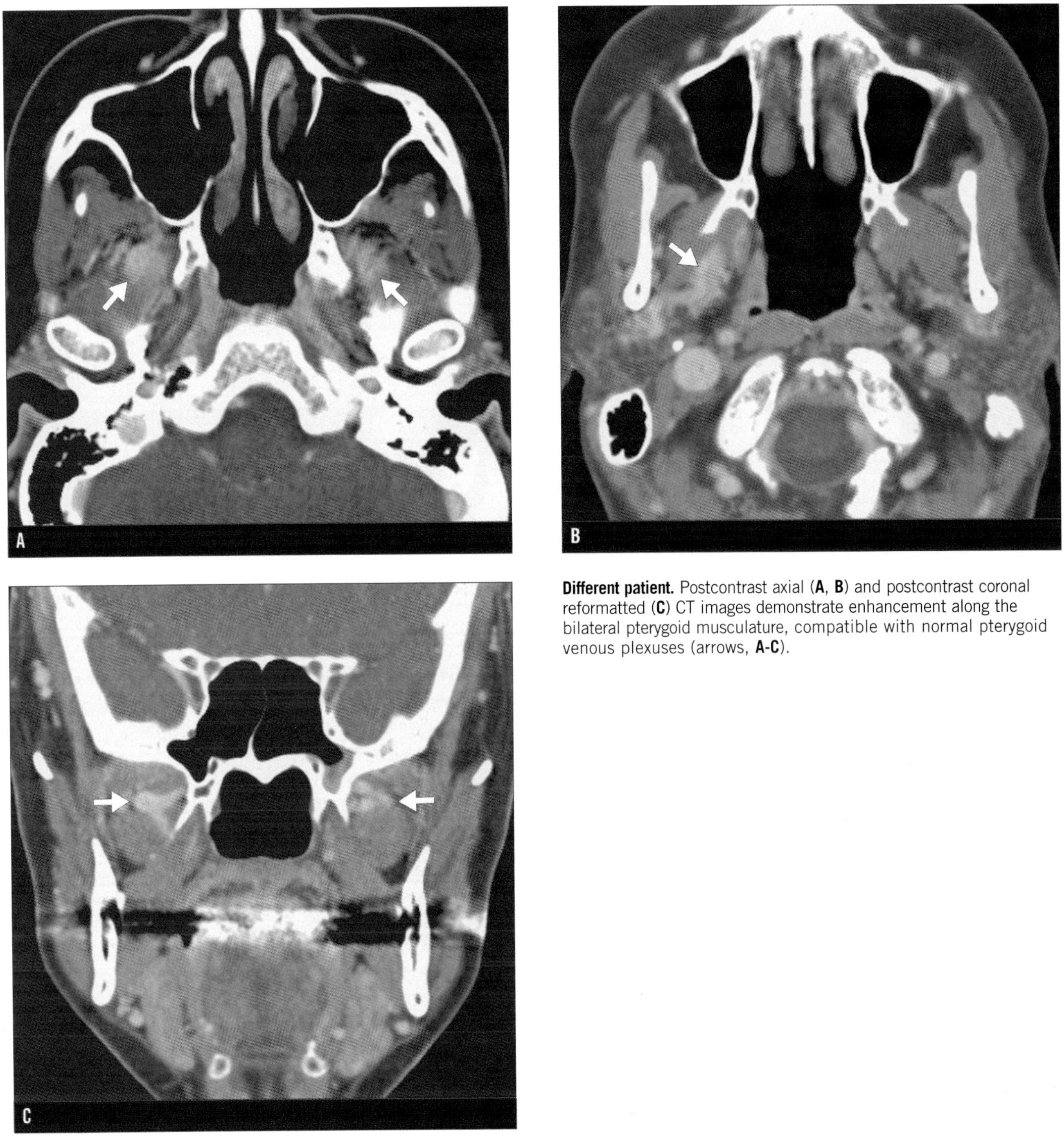

Different patient. Postcontrast axial (**A**, **B**) and postcontrast coronal reformatted (**C**) CT images demonstrate enhancement along the bilateral pterygoid musculature, compatible with normal pterygoid venous plexuses (arrows, **A-C**).

Normal pterygoid venous plexuses

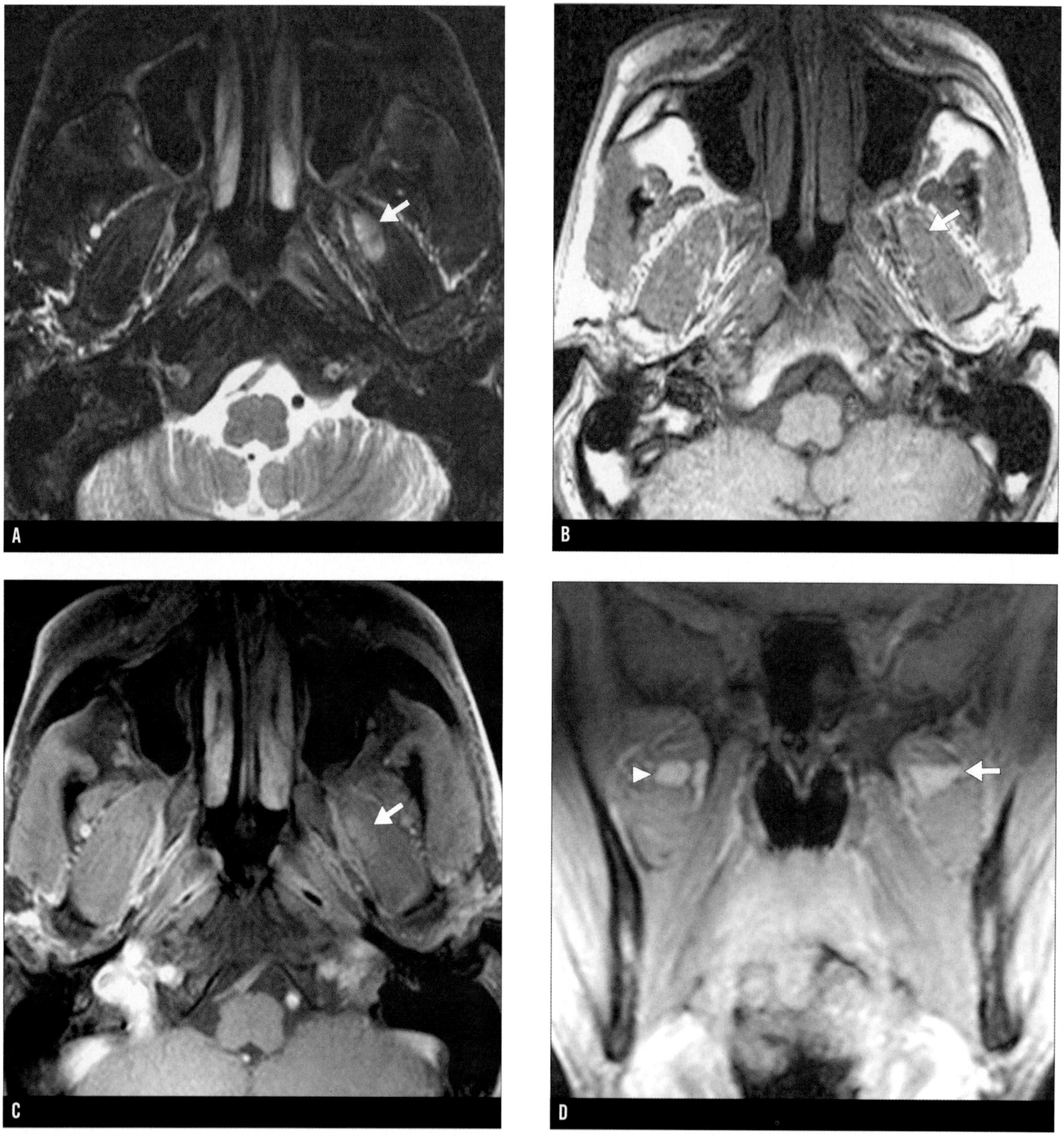

Different patient. Axial T2 (**A**), unenhanced axial T1 (**B**), postcontrast axial T1 with fat suppression (**C**), and postcontrast coronal T1 with fat suppression (**D**) MR images were obtained through the infratemporal fossa. Image **A** demonstrates a discrete oval area of T2 prolongation along the left lateral pterygoid muscle (arrow, **A**). Images **B** and **C** demonstrate this apparent lesion to be relatively occult with only minimal enhancement (arrows, **B**, **C**). This area more robustly enhances on image **D** (arrow, **D**). A similar but smaller focus of enhancement is present within the contralateral pterygoid musculature on image **D** (arrowhead, **D**). These findings are consistent with normal bilateral pterygoid venous plexuses.

Internal maxillary veins draining the pterygoid venous plexuses

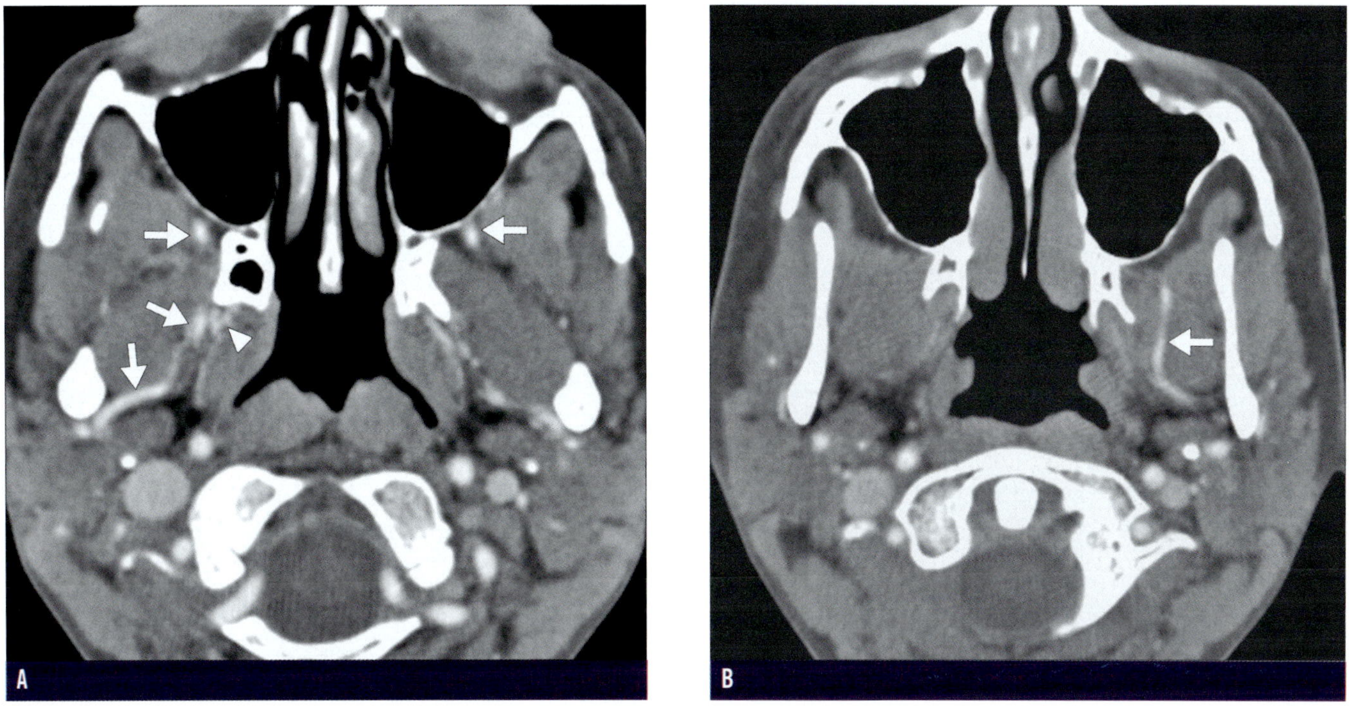

Postcontrast axial CT images (**A, B**) demonstrate enhancing vessels along the pterygoid musculature that represent the normal bilateral internal maxillary veins (arrows, **A, B**). These vessels drain the pterygoid venous plexuses and join the superficial temporal veins to form the retromandibular veins. A small portion of the right pterygoid venous plexus is identified on image **A** (arrowhead, **A**).

Venous plexuses surrounding the temporomandibular joints

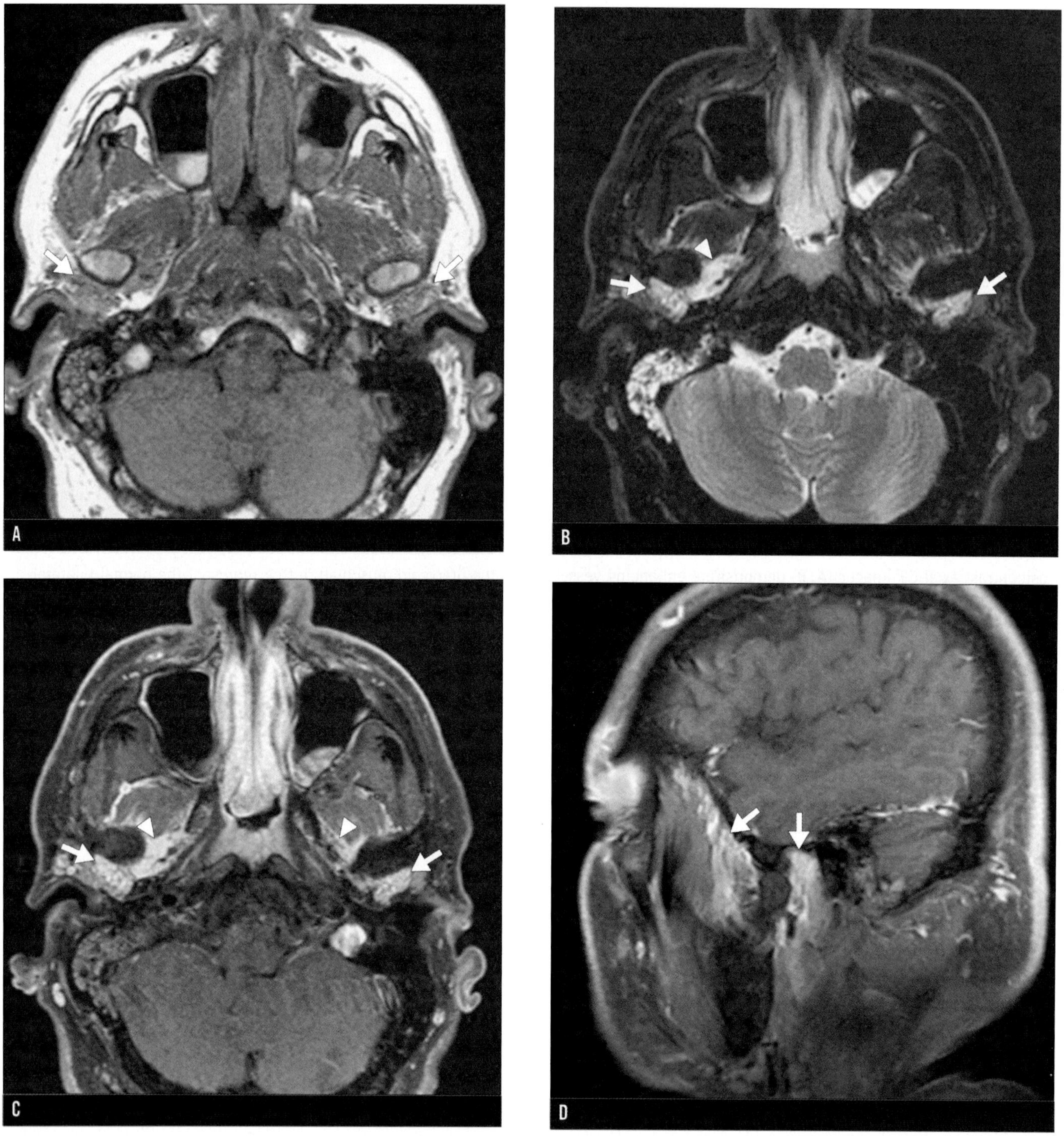

Axial T1 (**A**), axial T2 with fat suppression (**B**), postcontrast axial T1 with fat suppression (**C**) and postcontrast coronal T1 with fat suppression (**D**) MR images demonstrate pronounced normal venous plexuses surrounding the temporomandibular joints (arrows, **A-D**) which communicate with the pterygoid venous plexuses (arrowheads, **B, C**). The normal retromandibular veins were not identified in this patient and were likely supplanted by these temporomandibular venous plexuses.

REFERENCE

Henry G. *Anatomy of the Human Body.* 20th ed. Philadelphia, PA: Lea & Febiger; 1918; Bartleby.com, 2000. Published May 2000 by Bartleby.com; © 2000 Copyright Bartleby.com, Inc. (Terms of Use).

CASE 24 The parapharyngeal space and normal pharyngeal venous plexus

The parapharyngeal space is shaped like an inverted pyramid, with the base of the pyramid located at the skull base and the apex at the greater cornu of the hyoid. While there are technically three anatomic compartments comprising the parapharyngeal space, most subdivide the parapharyngeal space into two spaces: the prestyloid and poststyloid parapharyngeal spaces. The prestyloid parapharyngeal space is subdivided from the poststyloid parapharyngeal space by an obliquely oriented fascia termed the tensor-vascular-styloid fascia. The tensor-vascular-styloid fascia extends from the styloid process and traverses anteromedially to insert upon the inferior aspect of the tensor veli palatini. By imaging, differentiating the prestyloid from the poststyloid parapharyngeal space is best made by locating the styloid process; a lesion centered anterior to the styloid process is considered prestyloid, whereas a lesion centered posterior to the styloid process is considered poststyloid.

The prestyloid parapharyngeal space contains fat, the internal maxillary and ascending pharyngeal arteries, V3 branches of CN V, sympathetic chain, deep aspect of the parotid gland, and minor salivary gland tissue. It also includes the pharyngeal venous plexus. This plexus is comprised of unnamed tributaries that drain the adjacent pharyngeal wall. The pharyngeal plexus connects with the pterygoid venous plexus and drains into the internal jugular vein.

The poststyloid parapharyngeal space, also referred to by some as the carotid space, contains the carotid artery, internal jugular vein, glomus bodies, CN IX-XII, lymph nodes, and fat.

COMPANION CASES

- **Air in the pharyngeal venous plexus.** Occasionally, air may be identified in head and neck veins, including the pharyngeal venous plexus. Usually, this is related to inadvertent injection of air during the initiation of intravenous access. Air in veins may also be the result of external trauma, such as from a knife wound.
- **Prestyloid parapharyngeal space pleomorphic adenoma.** A pleomorphic adenoma (also called benign mixed tumor) is the most common tumor of the salivary glands and is also the most common tumor arising in the parapharyngeal space. On CT, these tumors may be relatively occult in the early phase following contrast administration; thus, delayed imaging is frequently helpful in identifying these tumors. On MRI, these tumors are usually isointense on T1, diffusely hyperintense on T2, have circumscribed bosselated margins, and enhance homogeneously or heterogeneously.
- **Poststyloid parapharyngeal space glomus vagale.** A glomus tumor arises from paraganglia tissue. The paraganglia are specialized organs that are located throughout the body, including the adrenal glands. In the head and neck, glomus tumors may arise from the carotid body, inferior ganglion of the vagus nerve, cervical portion of the vagus nerve (glomus vagale), jugular bulb (glomus jugulare), and the middle ear (glomus tympanicum). Most extra-adrenal paragangliomas are nonfunctioning. On MRI, paragangliomas are T1 isointense and T2 hyperintense relative to muscle. These tumors are highly vascular and therefore avidly enhance on CT and MRI. Moreover, on MRI, flow voids are often appreciated on T1 or T2-weighted imaging (so-called "salt and pepper" appearance). MRA will demonstrate increased vascularity and catheter angiography will demonstrate rapid arterial to venous shunting within these tumors.

Companion case: Air in the pharyngeal venous plexus

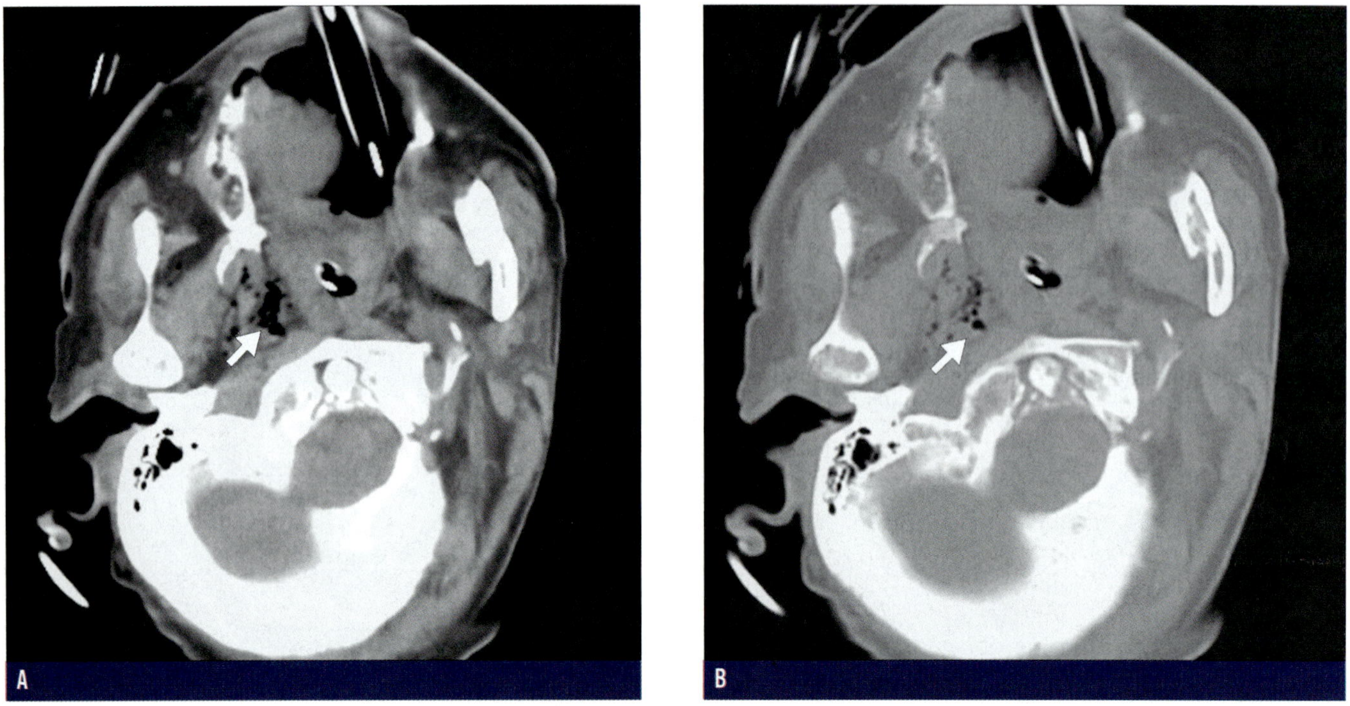

Axial CT images viewed with a soft tissue window (**A**) and an intermediate window (**B**) demonstrate air within the right pharyngeal venous plexus (arrows, **A, B**). The etiology of the air was unclear but it was presumably related to inadvertent injection of air during the initiation of venous access.

Companion case: Prestyloid parapharyngeal space pleomorphic adenoma

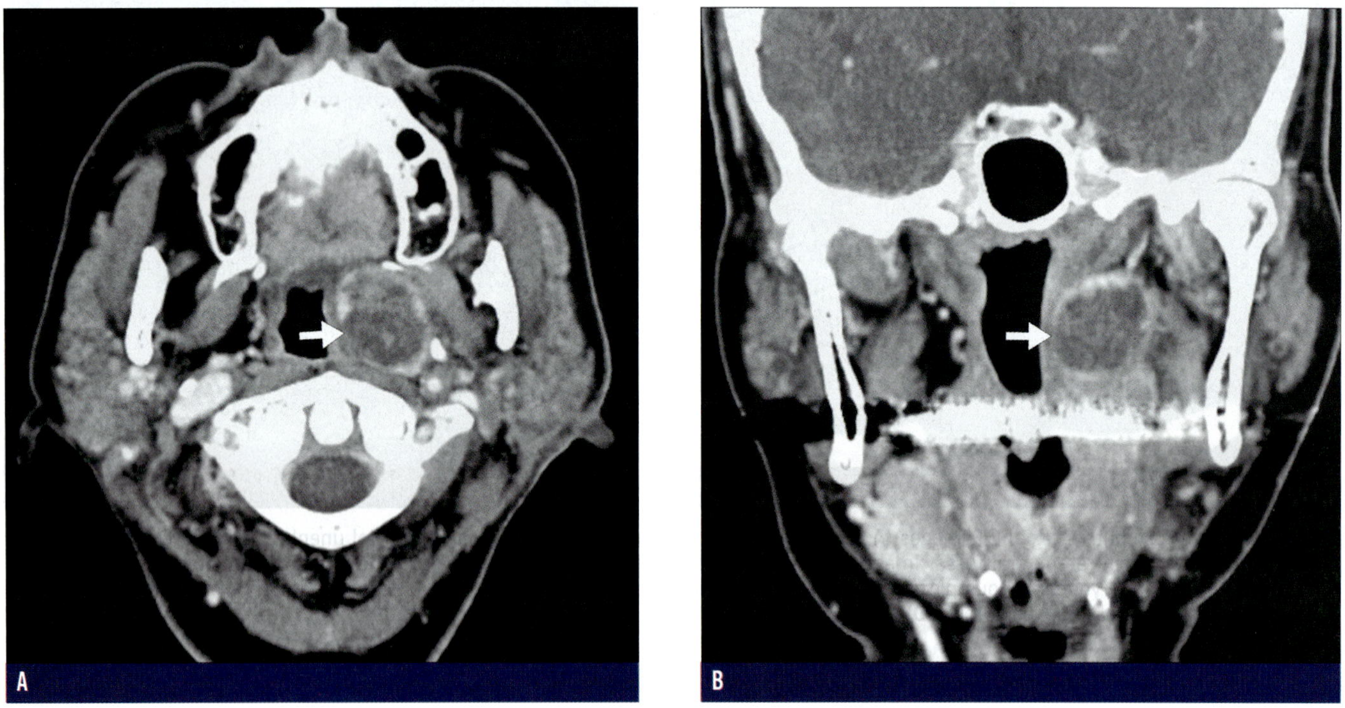

Axial (**A**) and coronal reformatted (**B**) postcontrast CT images through the parapharyngeal spaces demonstrate a heterogeneous mass in the left prestyloid parapharyngeal space which represented a pleomorphic adenoma at pathology (arrows, **A, B**). In this case, it is likely that the lesion arose from minor salivary gland rest tissue within the prestyloid parapharyngeal space since it appears separate from the parotid gland. This particular lesion has mass effect and is circumscribed, findings that are not present with a normal pharyngeal venous plexus.

Companion case: Poststyloid parapharyngeal space glomus vagale

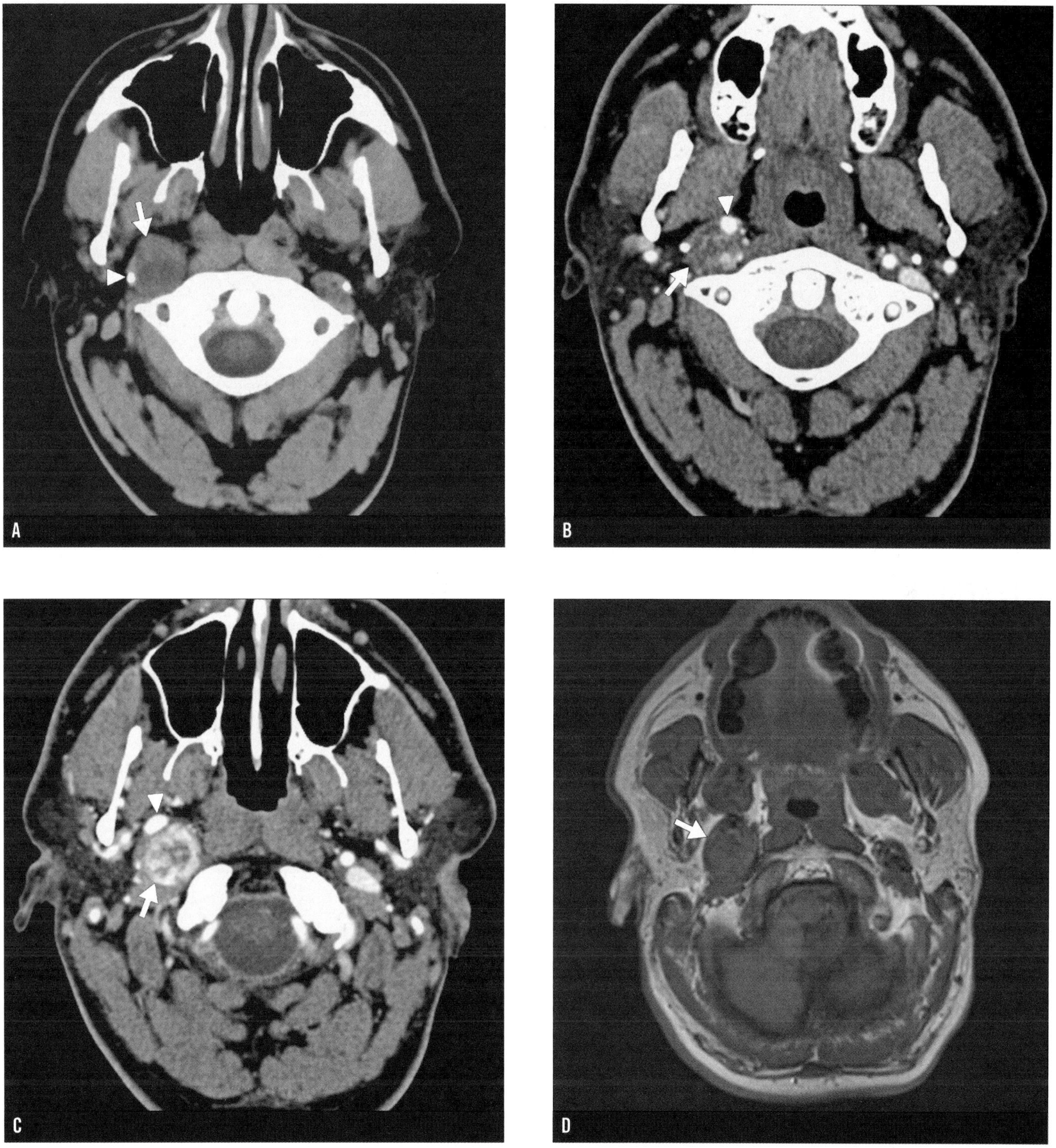

An unenhanced axial CT image (**A**) demonstrates a round, hypoattenuating mass (arrow, **A**). This mass is located medial to the styloid process (arrowhead, **A**). While it is difficult to determine whether this lesion arises anterior or posterior to the styloid process on the basis of this single image, the mass does appear to extrinsically compress the posterior aspect of the prestyloid parapharyngeal space and does not appear to arise from the prestyloid parapharyngeal space. Contrast-enhanced axial CT images from a CTA (**B, C**) demonstrate the lesion to heterogeneously enhance (arrows, **B, C**) and ventrally displace the right internal carotid artery (arrowheads, **B, C**), clear evidence that the lesion is located in the poststyloid parapharyngeal space. Axial T1 (**D**), contrast-enhanced axial T1 with fat suppression (**E**), and fat-suppressed axial T2 (**F**) MR images of the same patient demonstrate the lesion to avidly enhance and to be mildly heterogeneous on precontrast T1 and T2. The constellation of findings on CT and MRI is compatible with a glomus vagale.

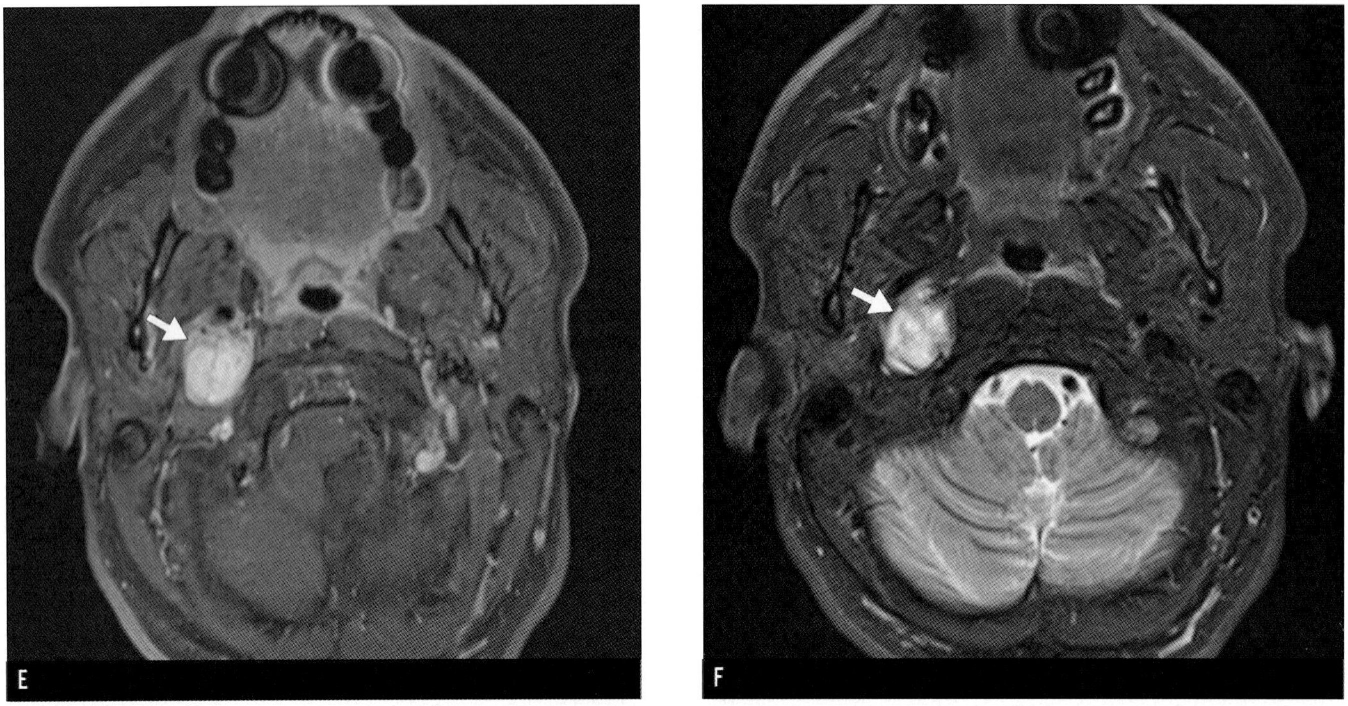

REFERENCES

Henry G. *Anatomy of the human body.* 20th ed. Published May 2000 by Bartleby.com; © 2000 Copyright Bartleby.com, Inc.

Lingam RK, Daghir AA, Nigar E, Abbas SA, Kumar M. Pleomorphic adenoma (benign mixed tumour) of the salivary glands: its diverse clinical, radiological, and histopathological presentation. *Br J Oral Maxillofac Surg.* 2011;49(1):14-20.

Mafee MF, Raofi B, Kumar A, Muscato C. Glomus faciale, glomus jugulare, glomus tympanicum, glomus vagale, carotid body tumors, and simulating lesions. Role of MR imaging. *Radiol Clin North Am.* 2000;38(5):1059-1076.

Shin JH, Lee HK, Kim SY, Choi CG, Suh DC. Imaging of parapharyngeal space lesions. *AJR Am J Roentgenol.* 2001;177(6):1465-1470.

CASE 25 CN V, V3 denervation atrophy

The V3 (mandibular) division of cranial nerve (CN) V innervates the muscles of mastication, which include the masseter, temporalis, medial pterygoid, and lateral pterygoid muscles. CN V, V3 denervation atrophy may occur following injury or when a lesion involves any portion of the nerve course, including at the brainstem nuclei level, Meckel cave, or along a portion of the V3 nerve.

While CT may detect denervation atrophy, particularly the chronic stage, MRI is superior at demonstrating the evolutionary changes of denervation atrophy, from acute to chronic.

After injury, a typical MRI denervation pattern ensues as follows:

Acute phase: The muscles enhance, are hyperintense on T2, and are enlarged from edema. Most authors consider acute denervation to occur anytime within 1 month of injury, although MR imaging may only detect changes as early as 2 weeks following the injury.

Subacute phase: The muscles continue to enhance and are hyperintense on T2. Some areas of T1 hyperintensity within the affected muscle are present, consistent with fatty atrophy. The muscle is typically no longer enlarged at this point. Most authors consider this phase to last anywhere between 1 month and 12 to 20 months.

Early or mild chronic phase: The muscles continue to undergo mild fatty atrophy. There is no enhancement, T2 prolongation, or appreciable volume loss involving the affected muscles during this phase. Most authors consider the early or mild chronic phase to occur after 12 to 20 months.

Long-standing chronic phase: Extensive volume loss and fatty infiltration of the denervated muscle is present. There is no enhancement or T2 prolongation involving the affected muscles during this phase.

Several studies have shown an increase in relative blood flow to denervated muscle compared to normal muscle. Thus, the MRI enhancement pattern of denervated muscle during the acute and subacute stages is likely in part due to this increase in relative blood flow. Additionally, there is likely accumulation of gadolinium within the extracellular space of denervated muscle that contributes to the enhancement pattern. One should be careful not to misinterpret the acute and subacute denervation atrophy phase of enhancement on MRI as tumor or an inflammatory process involving the muscle. With chronic denervation, care should be taken not to confuse the normal, unaffected side as abnormal.

Acute to subacute CN V, V3 denervation atrophy

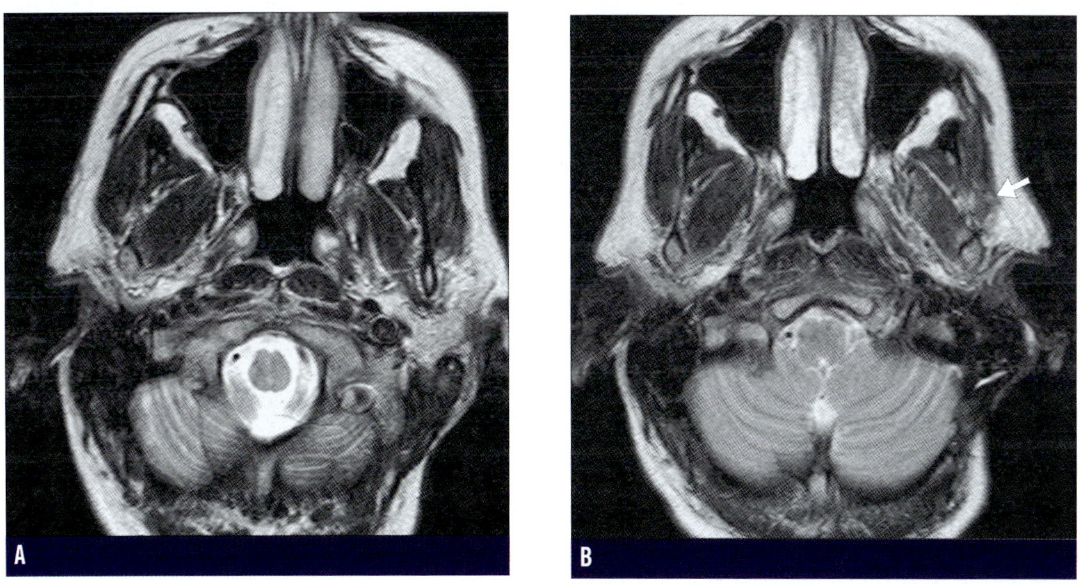

Axial T2 (**A-C**) and postcontrast axial MPRAGE (**D-F**) MR images demonstrate expected evolutionary changes that occur with CN V, V3 denervation atrophy. Images **A** and **D** were obtained at the same time and demonstrate symmetric muscles of mastication. Shortly thereafter, images **B** and **E** were obtained. Image **B** demonstrates mild asymmetric volume loss and subtle T2 prolongation of the left muscles of mastication (arrow, **B**), whereas image **E** demonstrates mild asymmetric enhancement of the left muscles of mastication (arrow, **E**). A couple of months later, images **C** and **F** were obtained. Image **C** demonstrates further volume loss and T2 prolongation (arrow, **C**), whereas image **F** demonstrates progressive enhancement of the left muscles of mastication (arrow, **F**). A postcontrast axial MPRAGE MR image through the Meckel caves (**G**) demonstrates that these findings were related to a mass involving the left Meckel cave (arrow, **G**), in this case due to a breast metastasis.

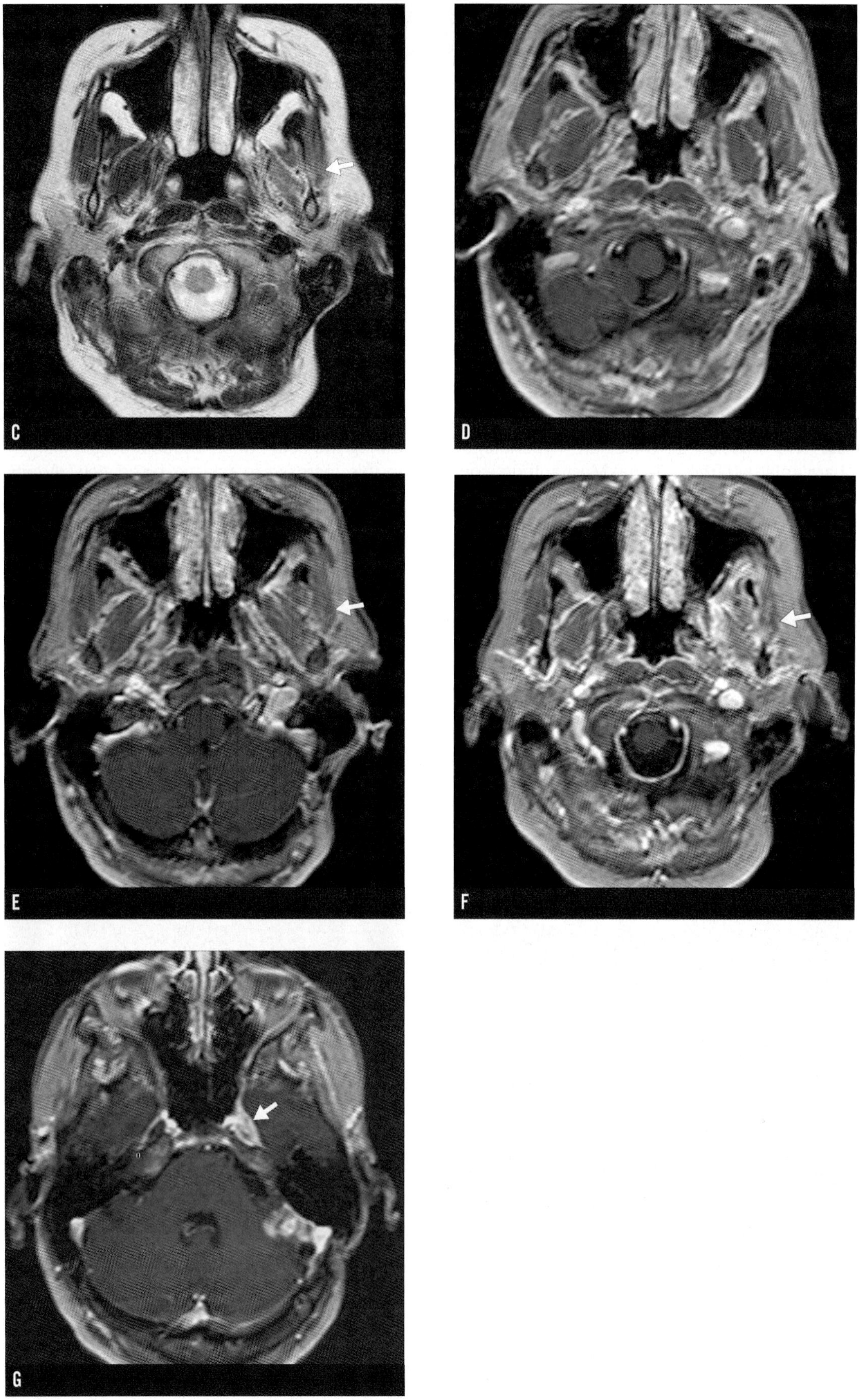
C
D
E
F
G

Subacute to chronic CN V, V3 denervation atrophy

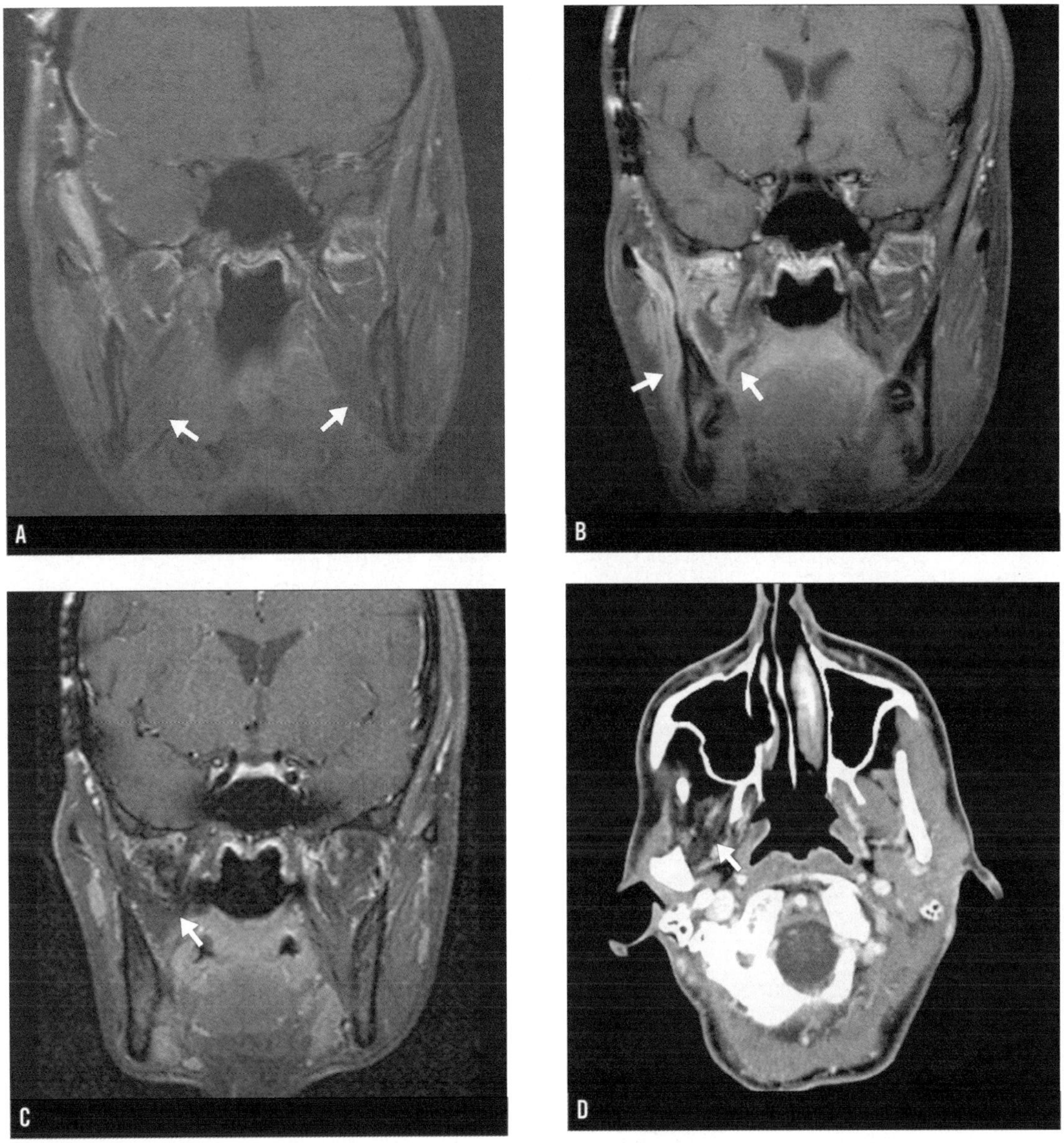

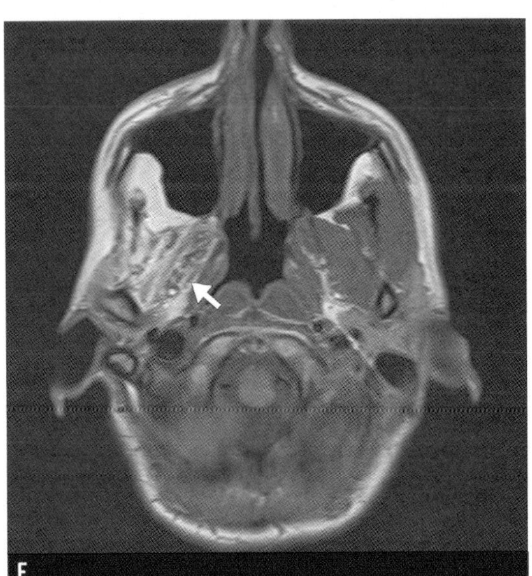

A postcontrast coronal T1-weighted MR image with fat suppression (**A**) demonstrates relatively symmetric muscles of mastication (arrows, **A**). A postcontrast coronal T1-weighted MR image with fat suppression taken nearly 1 year later demonstrates asymmetric enhancement of the right muscles of mastication relative to the left, compatible with subacute CN V, V3 denervation atrophy (arrows, **B**). A postcontrast coronal T1-weighted MR image with fat suppression taken 4 years after image **B** (**C**) demonstrates decreased signal consistent with suppressed fat as well as volume loss of the right muscles of mastication, compatible with chronic CN V, V3 denervation injury (arrow, **C**). A postcontrast axial CT image (**D**) and an unenhanced axial T1-weighted MR image (**E**) taken approximately 2 years later than image **C** also demonstrate the fatty infiltration and atrophy of the right muscles of mastication (arrows, **D**, **E**). The CN V, V3 denervation atrophy in this case was due to a melanoma metastasis to the right Meckel cave (not shown).

Chronic CN V, V3 denervation atrophy

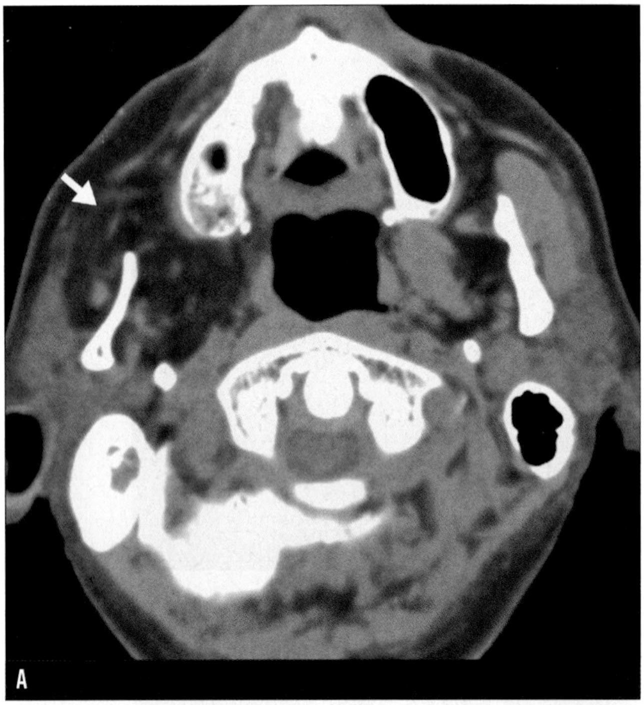

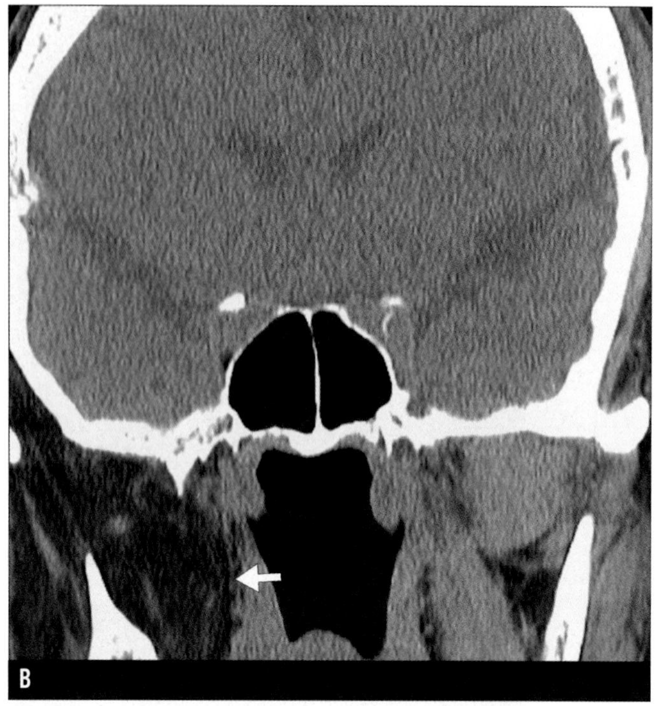

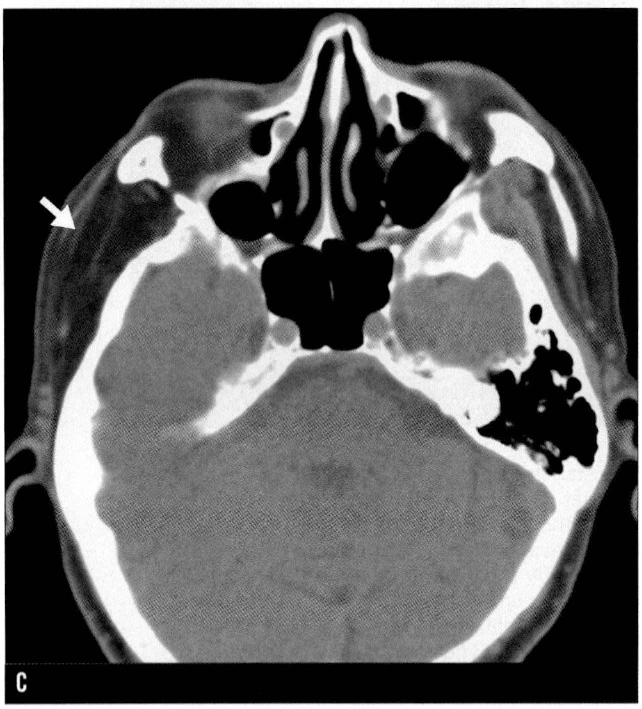

Axial (**A**, **C**) and coronal reformatted (**B**) unenhanced CT images demonstrate extensive volume loss and fatty infiltration of the right muscles of mastication, compatible with long-standing chronic CN V, V3 denervation atrophy (arrows, **A**-**C**). The cause of the denervation atrophy was unknown in this case.

REFERENCES

Davis SB, Mathews VP, Willaims DW 3rd. Masticator muscle enhancement in subacute denervation atrophy. *AJNR Am J Neuroradiol.* 1995;16:1292-1294.

Fischbein NJ, Kaplan MJ, Jackler RK, Dillon WP. MR Imaging in two cases of subacute denervation change in the muscles of facial expression. *AJNR Am J Neuroradiol.* 2001;22:880-884.

CASE 26 Normal pterygopalatine fossa enhancement

The pterygopalatine fossa is located immediately posterior to the maxillary sinus and contains the pterygopalatine ganglion, V2 division of CN V, terminal branches of the internal maxillary artery, and small veins. Due to the presence of normal vasculature within the pterygopalatine fossa, a small amount of enhancement in the pterygopalatine fossa is normal and should not be confused with pathology, particularly if the fat planes in the fossa are preserved.

Normal pterygopalatine fossa enhancement

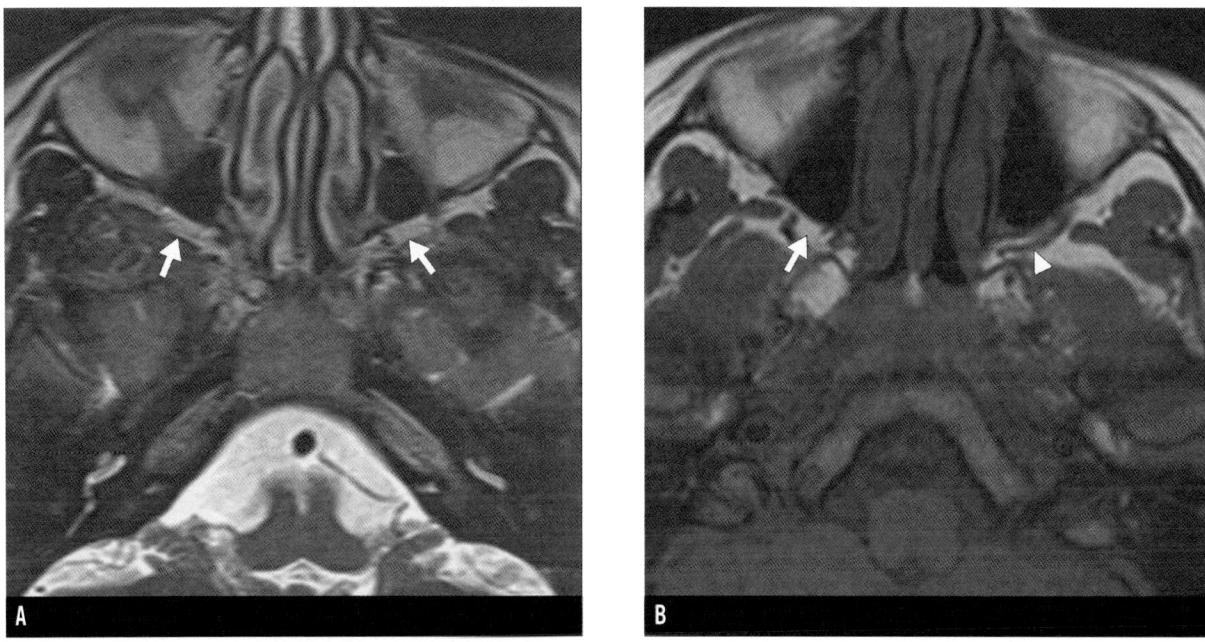

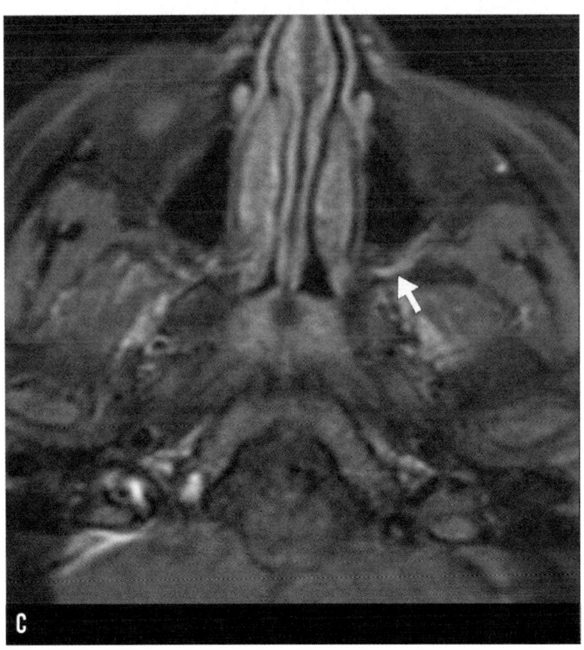

Axial T2 (**A**), unenhanced axial T1 (**B**), and postcontrast axial T1 with fat suppression (**C**) MR images. Images **A** and **B** demonstrate a normal pterygopalatine fossa with predominantly fat signal (arrows, **A**, **B**). A linear area of hypointense signal in the left pterygopalatine fossa (arrowhead, **B**) which enhances (arrow, **C**) is compatible with a normal traversing vessel.

REFERENCES

Chan LL, Chong J, Gillenwater AM, Ginsberg LE. The pterygopalatine fossa: postoperative MR imaging appearance. *AJNR Am J Neuroradiol.* 2000;21(7):1315-1319.

Curtin HD, Williams R. Computed tomographic anatomy of the pterygopalatine fossa. *Radiographics.* 1985;5:429-440.

CASE 27 Postoperative pterygopalatine fossa appearance

The pterygopalatine fossa may be violated during maxillectomies performed to remove maxillary sinus tumors or during infratemporal fossa tumor resections. Following surgery to this area, the normal fat planes and vessels in the pterygopalatine fossa are replaced by soft tissue attenuation and signal on CT and MRI, respectively. Moreover, the pterygopalatine fossa will consistently enhance on MRI following surgery, often mimicking perineural spread of tumor. Care should be taken to not mistake this common postoperative appearance for pathology, assuming that this finding has been stable over serial exams. A baseline MRI study should always be obtained after the pterygopalatine fossa has been violated following surgery. Serial follow-up imaging would then be necessary to assess for changes which that would suggest the presence of perineural spread of tumor, if this is of clinical concern.

COMPANION CASE

- **Perineural spread along the pterygopalatine fossae**

Postoperative pterygopalatine fossa appearance

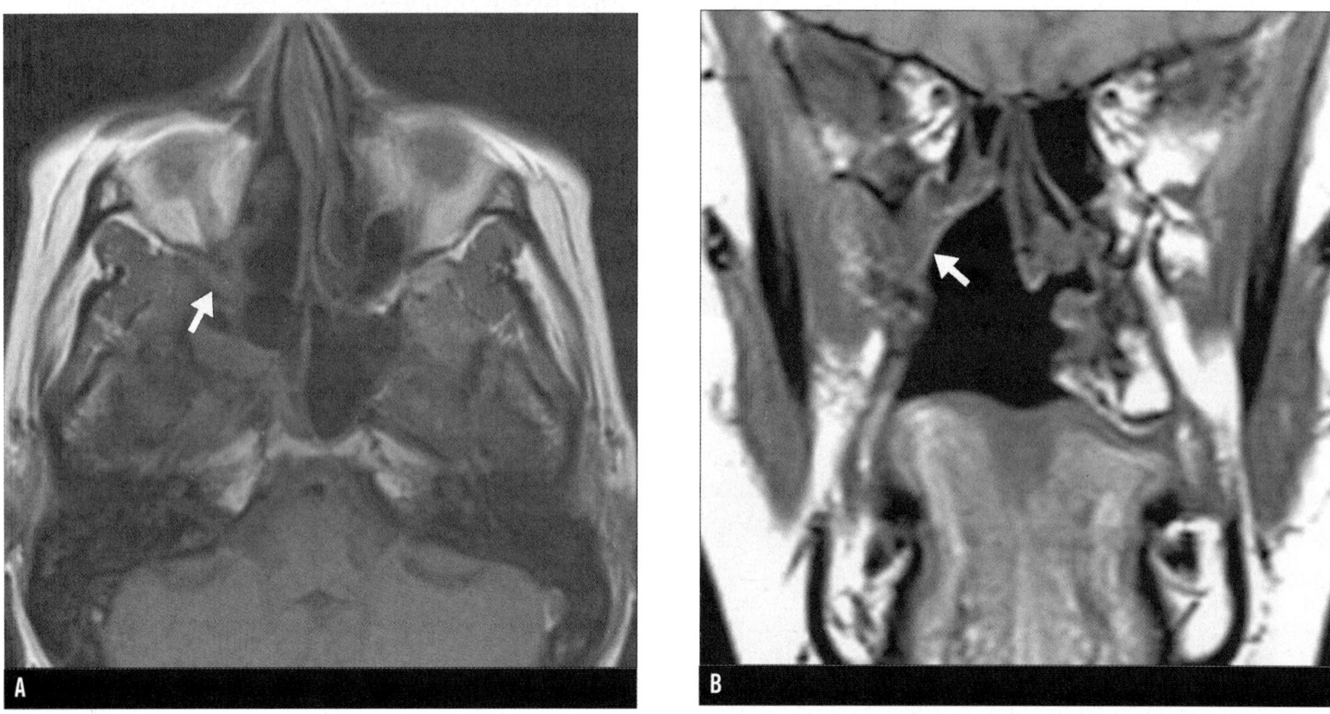

Status post right maxillary sinus surgery. Unenhanced axial T1 (**A**), unenhanced coronal T1 (**B**), axial T2 with fat suppression (**C**), and postcontrast axial T1 with fat suppression (**D**) MR images. There is isointense T1 signal relative to muscle in the right pterygopalatine fossa (arrows, **A, B**) with corresponding mildly hyperintense T2 signal (arrow, **C**) and enhancement (arrow, **D**). These are expected imaging findings if the pterygopalatine fossa has been violated during surgery. However, follow-up imaging of such a case is necessary to document stability and exclude perineural spread of tumor, if this is of concern.

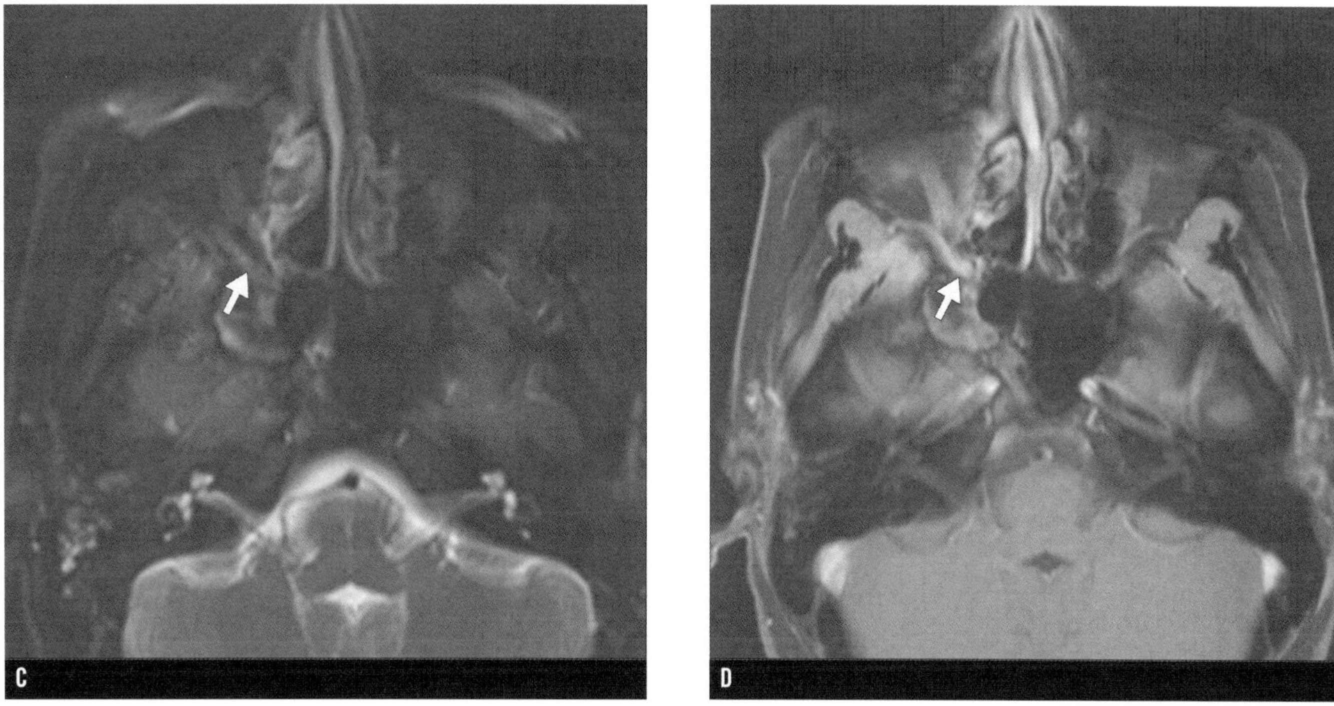

Companion case: Perineural spread along the pterygopalatine fossae

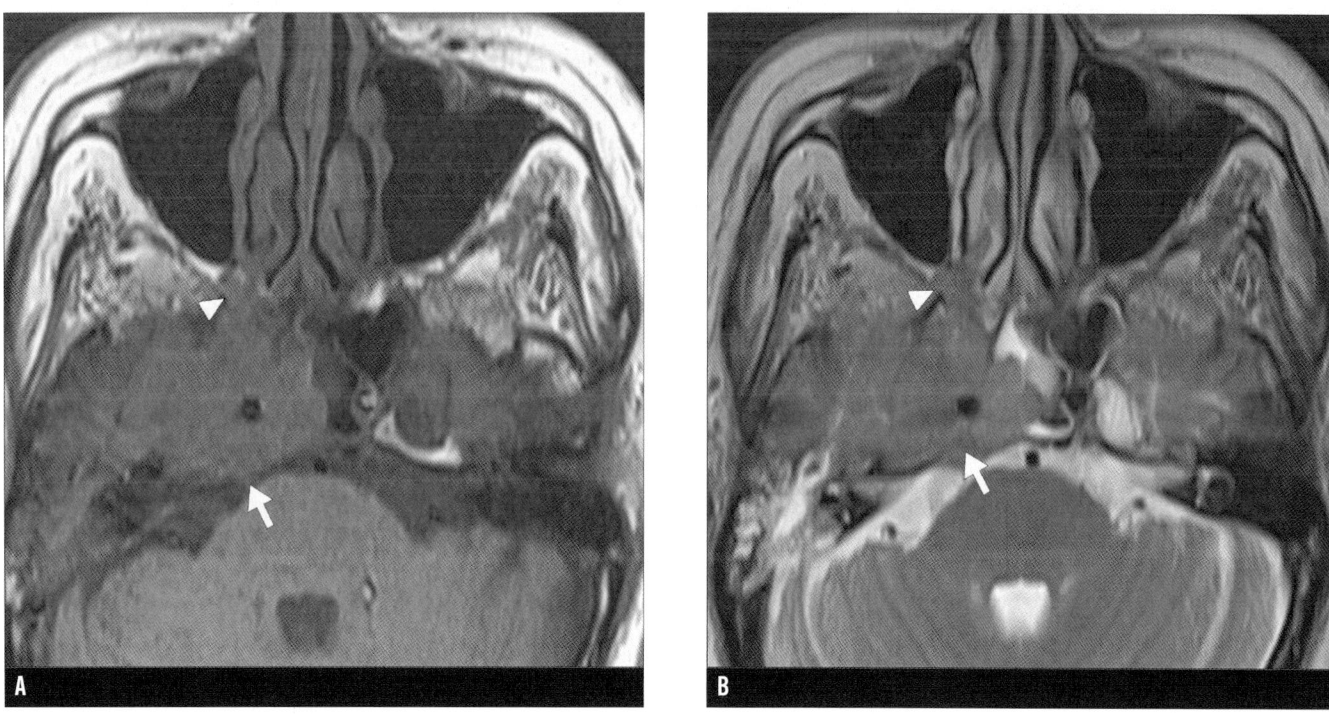

History of nasopharyngeal carcinoma. Unenhanced axial T1 (**A**), axial T2 (**B**), and postcontrast axial T1 with fat suppression (**C**) MR images demonstrate a large mass involving the right cavernous sinus and Meckel cave (arrows, **A-C**) with encasement of the right cavernous carotid artery as well as minimal extension of tumor into the right pterygopalatine fossa suggesting perineural spread (arrowheads, **A-C**). The same patient 4 years later with unenhanced axial T1 (**D**), axial T2 with fat suppression (**E**), and postcontrast axial T1 with fat suppression (**F**) MR images. These images demonstrate progression of enhancing tumor into the right pterygopalatine fossa (arrows, **D-F**) and new enhancing tumor extending into the left pterygopalatine fossa (arrowheads, **D-F**), compatible with progressive perineural spread of tumor.

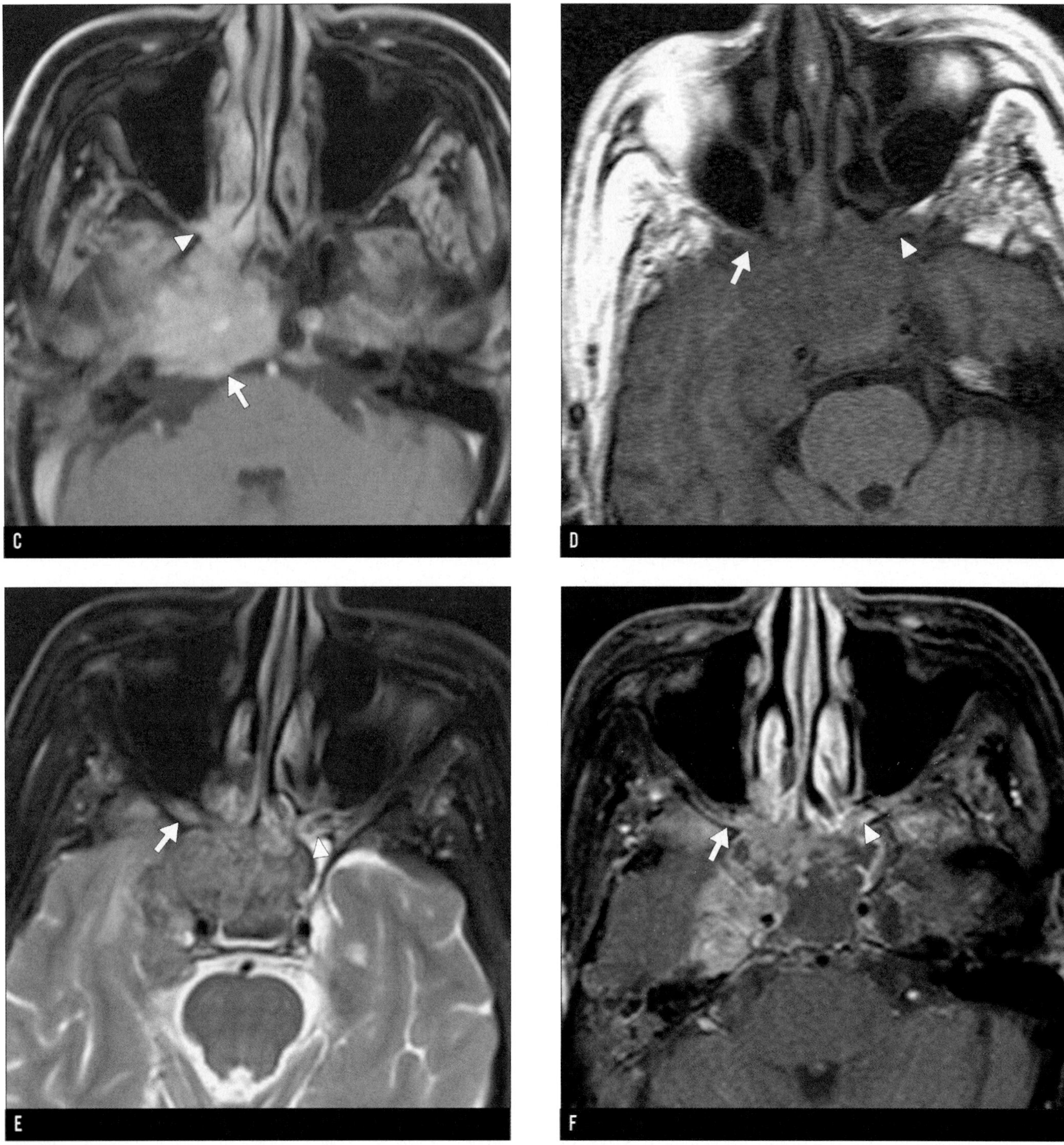

REFERENCE

Chan LL, Chong J, Gillenwater AM, Ginsberg LE. The pterygopalatine fossa: postoperative MR imaging appearance. *AJNR Am J Neuroradiol.* 2000;21(7):1315-1319.

CASE 28 MRI susceptibility artifact in the retromaxillary fat pad and pterygopalatine fossa

Artifact from dental amalgam is more pronounced on CT than on MRI. Nevertheless, dental amalgam can result in significant field heterogeneity and susceptibility artifact on MRI. Ferromagnetic dental amalgam results in this artifact by creating its own magnetic field and in effect altering the precessional frequencies of protons in the adjacent soft tissues, resulting in poor or no signal from this tissue. Additionally, largely nonmetallic materials used in dentistry, such as some ceramics and coloring agents in composites, can also result in artifact on CT and MRI due to small amounts of ferromagnetic substances contained within these materials.

MRI susceptibility artifact from dental amalgam may simulate disease in several regional locations, including the pterygopalatine fossa and retromaxillary fat pad. Susceptibility artifact is significantly more pronounced on a fat-suppressed pulse sequence and is much less prominent on a spin echo T1-weighted sequence. Moreover, if a sizeable lesion is truly present on the fat-suppressed sequence, then it will usually be visible on the unenhanced fat-suppressed sequence with a spin echo T1-weighted sequence. Therefore, one should confirm an apparent finding on a fat-suppressed sequence with a spin echo T1-weighted sequence. Additionally, if dental amalgam is suspected to account for a spurious asymmetric finding on fat-suppressed MR imaging, then there is usually evidence of an asymmetric degree of dental amalgam susceptibility artifact on a sagittal and/or coronal sequence.

MRI susceptibility artifact in the retromaxillary fat pad

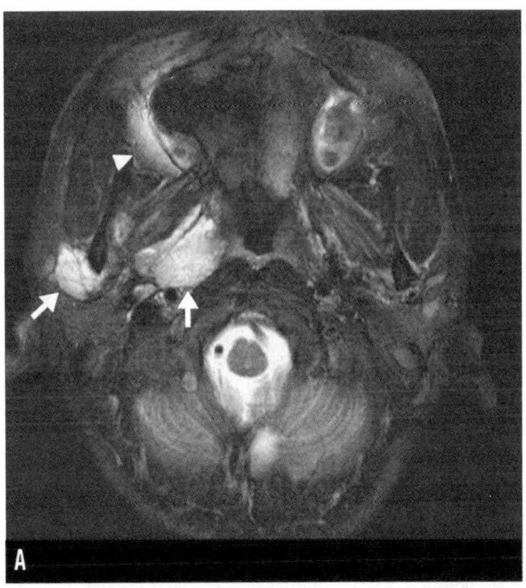

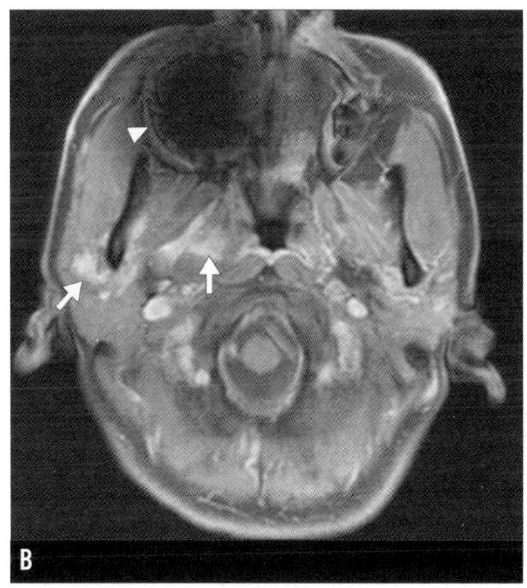

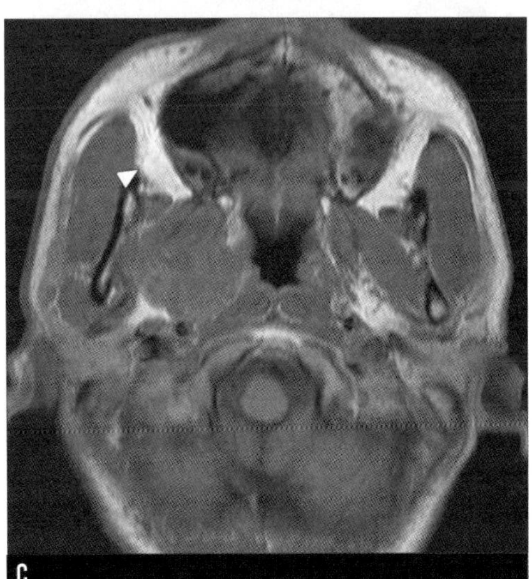

Axial T2 with fat suppression (**A**), postcontrast axial T1 with fat suppression, and noncontrast axial T1 without fat suppression (**C**) MR images. There is asymmetric increased T2 signal in the right retromaxillary fat pad (arrowhead, **A**). This area is obscured by dental amalgam artifact on image **B** (arrowhead, **B**), but image **C** demonstrates normal fat signal in this region (arrowhead, **C**), effectively excluding a lesion in the right retromaxillary fat pad. The finding on image **A** was related to susceptibility artifact from dental amalgam. However, this patient did have a facial vascular malformation in the right parapharyngeal space and adjacent to the right temporomandibular joint that is T2 hyperintense (arrows, **A**) and enhances (arrows, **B**).

MRI susceptibility artifact in the retromaxillary fat pad and pterygopalatine fossa from dental amalgam

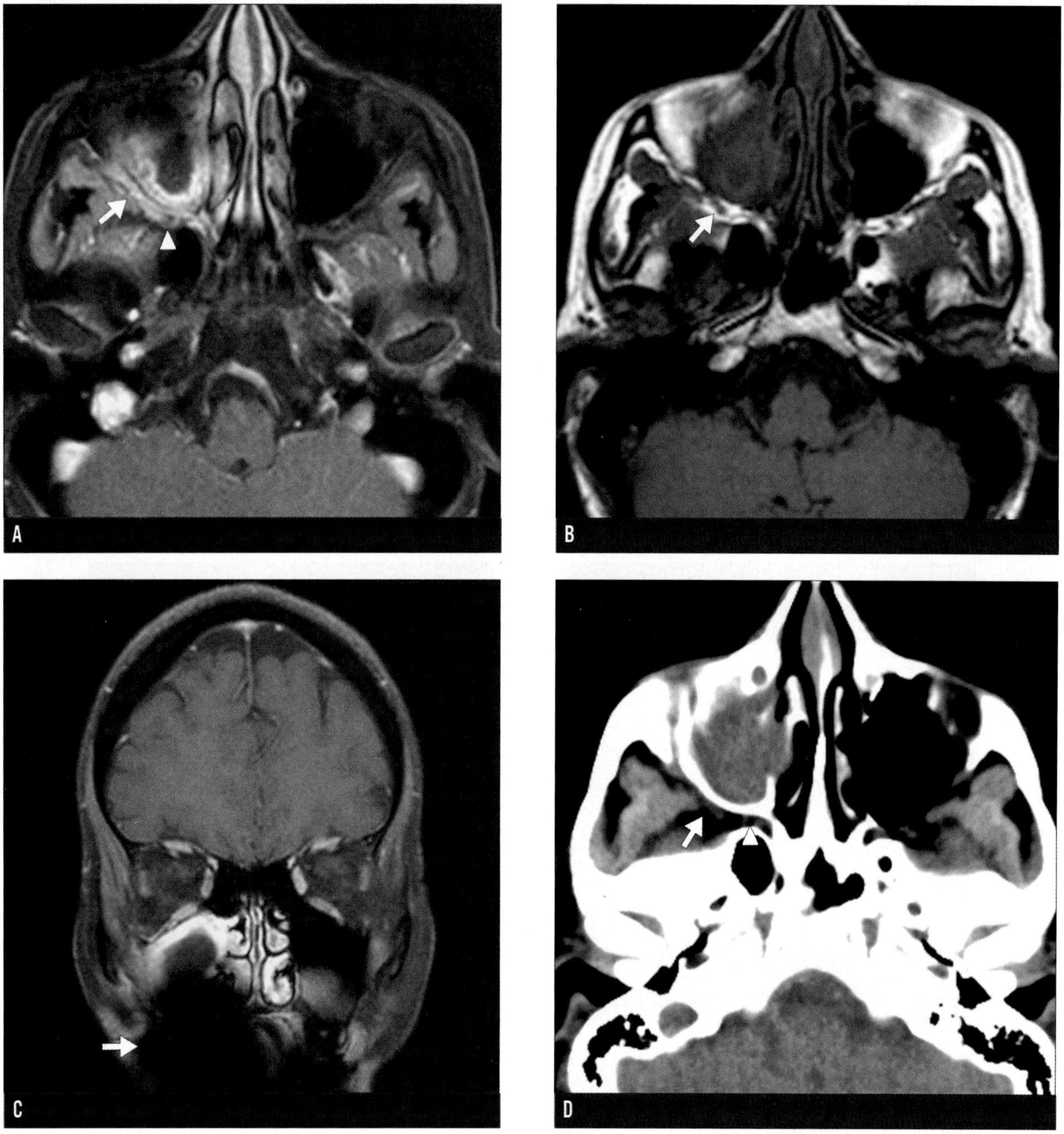

Postcontrast axial T1 with fat suppression (**A**), unenhanced axial T1 without fat suppression (**B**), and postcontrast coronal T1 with fat suppression (**C**) MR images through the level of the maxillary sinuses. Image **A** demonstrates advanced right maxillary sinus disease as well as increased signal in the right retromaxillary fat pad (arrow, **A**) and right pterygopalatine fossa (arrowhead, **A**). Given the extensive right maxillary sinus findings, one could interpret the findings in the right retromaxillary fat pad and pterygopalatine fossa as a lesion infiltrating these areas. However, image **B** demonstrates normal fat and a normal traversing vein in this region without a discrete abnormality (arrow, **B**). Image **C** demonstrates right greater than left dental amalgam artifact (arrow, **C**) accounting for the signal abnormality on image **A**. An axial CT image obtained shortly prior to the MRI (**D**) also demonstrates normal fat in the right retromaxillary space (arrow, **D**) and right pterygopalatine fossa (arrowhead, **D**).

REFERENCE

Klinke T, et al. Artifacts in magnetic resonance imaging and computed tomography caused by dental materials. *PLoS One*. 2012;7(2):e31766.

CASE 29 Normal CN III in the cavernous sinus

After exiting the brainstem at the level of the interpeduncular cistern, CN III (oculomotor nerve) traverses between the superior cerebellar artery and posterior cerebral artery and then enters the superolateral margin of the cavernous sinus wall through what is termed the porus (Latin for 'opening'). CN III then enters a cuff of dura-arachnoid within the cavernous sinus, known as the oculomotor cistern, where it is typically circumferentially surrounded by CSF. The oculomotor cistern is a horizontally oriented cistern that extends from the porus and tapers caudal to the anterior clinoid process tip. This cistern has surgical importance, as it allows for access and mobilization of CN III for lesions in and around the cavernous sinus.

The cavernous sinus portion of the CN III is typically best delineated on high resolution, thin section coronal T2-weighted and postcontrast coronal T1-weighted MR imaging (preferably with fat suppression). On coronal T2-weighted imaging, the cavernous sinus portion of the nerve is identified as a round focus that is isointense to brain and frequently surrounded by CSF. On postcontrast coronal T1-weighted imaging, the nerve is also demonstrated as a round focus that is isointense to brain, but it is hypointense to the adjacent hyperenhancing pituitary gland. Within the orbit, CN III subdivides into superior and inferior branches. The superior branch supplies the superior rectus and levator palpebrae muscles, whereas the inferior branch supplies the inferior and medial rectus muscles as well as the inferior oblique muscle.

COMPANION CASE

- **Abnormal enhancement of CN III.** Evaluating the entire course of a cranial nerve, from its nucleus to its end organ, is critical to fully evaluate a cranial nerve palsy on imaging. With respect to CN III, this includes the midbrain and region of the Edinger-Westphal nucleus as well as the cisternal, cavernous sinus, and intraorbital portions of CN III. At the level of the cavernous sinus, abnormal enhancement of the nerve can be quite subtle but should be excluded in cases of CN III palsy.

Normal CN III in the cavernous sinus

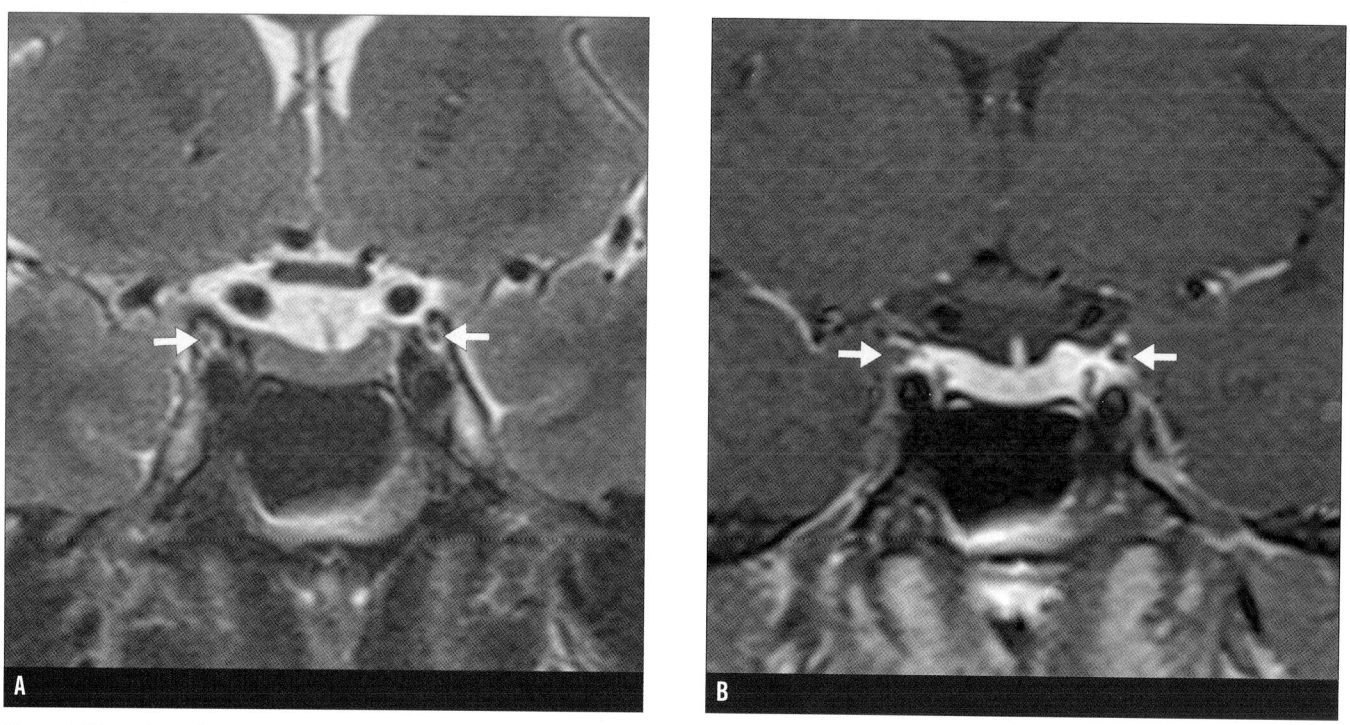

Coronal T2 without fat suppression (**A**) and postcontrast coronal T1 with fat suppression (**B**) MR images through the cavernous sinus demonstrate normal bilateral oculomotor nerves traversing within the superolateral walls of the cavernous sinus (arrows, **A**, **B**). On image **A**, the nerves are isointense in signal relative to brain, in this case surrounded by relatively prominent CSF in the oculomotor nerve cisterns. On image **B**, the oculomotor nerves and cisterns are isointense to slightly hypointense to brain but are silhouetted by densely enhancing cavernous sinus and pituitary gland.

Companion case: Abnormal enhancement of CN III

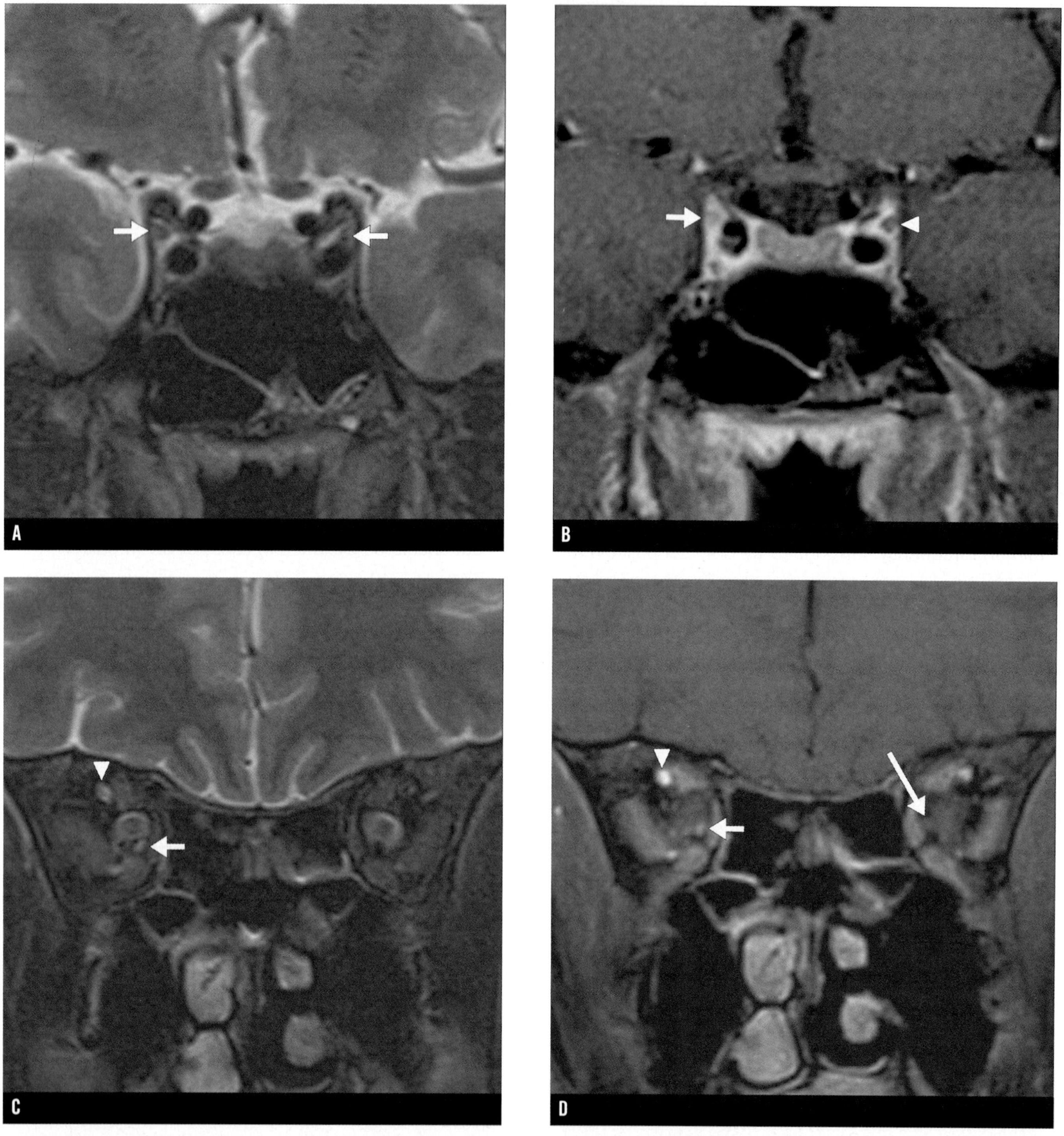

Coronal T2 with fat suppression (**A**) and postcontrast coronal T1 with fat suppression (**B**) MR images through the cavernous sinus. Image **A** demonstrates normal-sized and symmetric oculomotor nerves (short arrows, **A**). However, image **B** demonstrates asymmetric enhancement of the right oculomotor nerve (short arrow, **B**) and a normal nonenhancing left oculomotor nerve (arrowhead, **B**). Coronal T2 with fat suppression (**C**) and postcontrast coronal T1 with fat suppression (**D**) MR images through the orbits demonstrate abnormal T2 prolongation and enhancement of the inferior branch of the right oculomotor nerve that supplies the right medial rectus muscle (short arrows, **C**, **D**). These findings were related to perineural spread of tumor from Burkitt lymphoma. The normal right superior ophthalmic vein (arrowheads, **C**, **D**) and the normal inferior branch of the left oculomotor nerve innervating the left medial rectus muscle (long arrow, **D**) are depicted for reference.

REFERENCES

Everton KL, Rassner UA, Osborn AG, Harnsberger HR. The oculomotor cistern: anatomy and high-resolution imaging. *AJNR Am J Neuroradiol.* 2008;29(7):1344-1348.

Leblanc A. *Encephalo-Peripheral Nervous System: Vascularisation, Anatomy, Imaging.* Berlin: Springer; 2001.

CASE 30 Normal enhancing venous plexuses of the CN V, V2 and V3 divisions as well as of the Meckel cave

The gasserian ganglion resides within the anterior and inferolateral aspects of the Meckel cave and has a small semilunar configuration in the coronal plane. This ganglion, and a normal enhancing venous plexus located immediately cephalad to it, are often demonstrated on contrast-enhanced coronal T1-weighted MRI. Similarly, there are normal enhancing venous plexuses that surround the second (V2) and third (V3) divisions of CN V. Occasionally, incidental asymmetric enlargement of any of these venous plexuses may occur, sometimes simulating pathology.

COMPANION CASES

- **Asymmetrically enlarged but normal Meckel cave venous plexus.** The presence of asymmetric iso- to hypointense T2 signal with associated asymmetric enhancement in the Meckel cave certainly raises concern for a mass, such as a schwannoma or meningioma. However, if the finding is semilunar in configuration on coronal MRI and the finding is located in the inferolateral aspect of the Meckel cave, then a normal Meckel cave venous plexus is a consideration, particularly if the patient is asymptomatic and does not have a known systemic illness. Regardless, a finding such as this should be followed with serial imaging in order to exclude tumor.
- **Presumed schwannoma of the CN V, V2 division and pterygopalatine fossa.** Differentiating a V2 schwannoma from a normal V2 venous plexus is best made by identifying asymmetric enlargement of the nerve in addition to enhancement, both of which are typically present with a schwannoma. If the finding affects the foramen rotundum, then smooth enlargement of the foramen is typically present with a schwannoma.
- **Presumed CN V, V3 division schwannoma.** As discussed above, mass effect is typically present with a schwannoma and not present with a normal venous plexus. A schwannoma affecting the V3 division and extending through the foramen ovale will typically result in smooth enlargement of the foramen.
- **Perineural spread of tumor along the CN V, V2 and V3 divisions as well as the vidian nerve.** Evaluating for perineural spread of tumor can be challenging, particularly if the patient has had radiation to the area of interest. Radiation to the affected area may result in a radiation-induced neuritis that will often enhance indefinitely. The most reliable imaging finding to assess for perineural spread of tumor is progression of enhancement, sometimes accompanied by enlargement of the affected nerve. Therefore, baseline and follow-up MR imaging is essential to accurately assess for perineural spread. Enlargement of the foramen surrounding perineural spread of tumor may also be identified, usually best appreciated by CT.
- **Meckel cave schwannoma or meningioma.** Differentiating a schwannoma from a meningioma in the Meckel cave is not always possible by imaging. If the mass is contiguous with the cisternal segment of the trigeminal nerve, or contiguous with one or several divisions of CN V, then a schwannoma may be favored over a meningioma.
- **Meckel cave "white" epidermoid.** So called "white" epidermoids represent proteinaceous containing epidermoid cysts and are rare. The imaging appearance of these white epidermoids reflects their proteinaceous content and will therefore be hyperintense on T1 (hence the term "white"), hypointense on T2, and may be hyperattenuating on CT. Additionally, white epidermoids may not restrict on diffusion weighted imaging and may not be hyperintense on FLAIR (again, depending on their proteinaceous content), as is common with typical epidermoids.

Normal CN V, V2 division enhancing venous plexuses

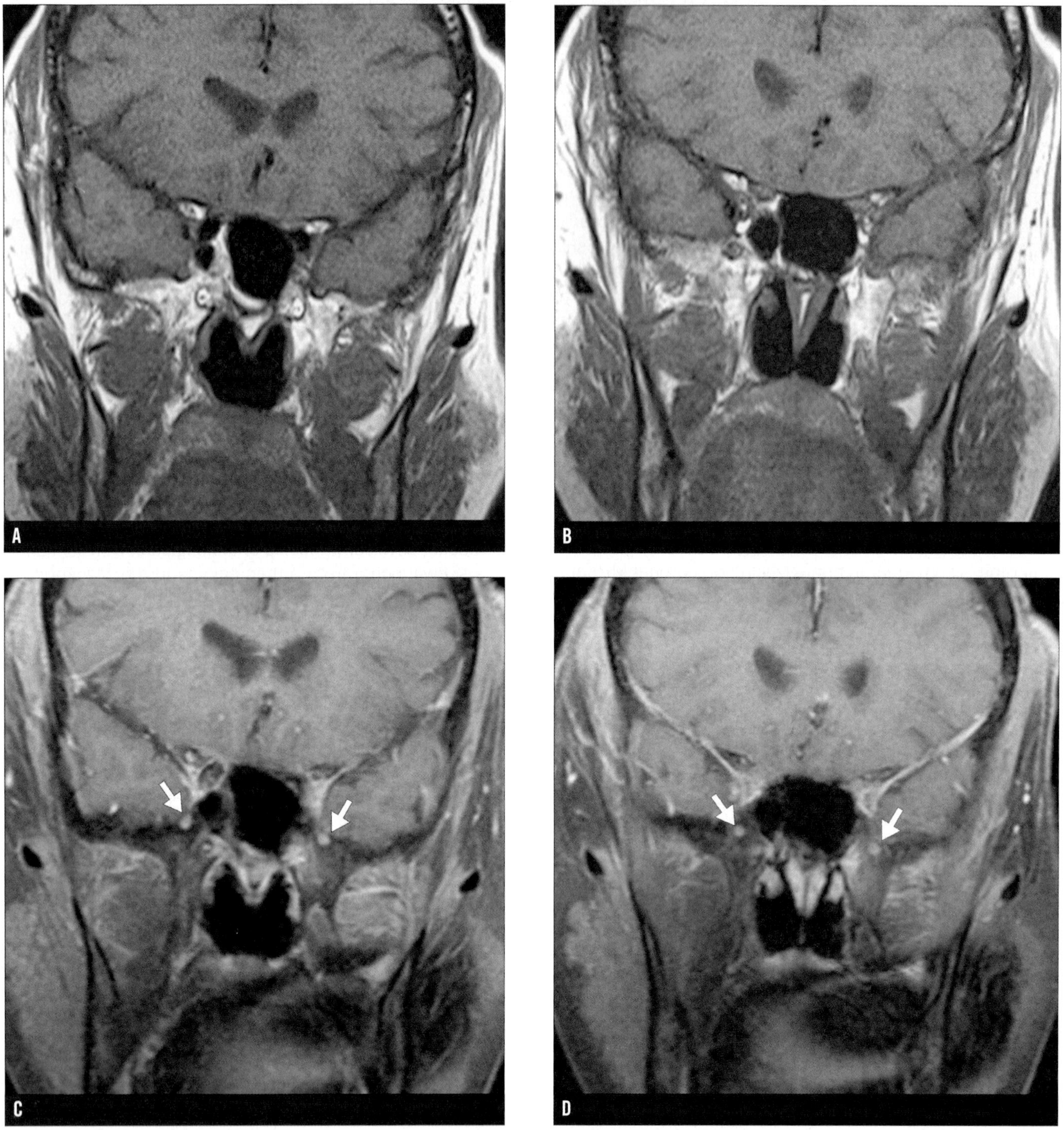

Unenhanced coronal T1-weighted MR images without fat suppression through the mid-skull base (**A**, **B**) and postcontrast coronal T1-weighted MR images with fat suppression through the same levels as **A** and **B** (**C**, **D**). Images **C** and **D** demonstrate symmetric enhancement of the V2 portions of both trigeminal nerves due to normal venous plexuses (arrows, **C**, **D**). This patient was asymptomatic and had no history of malignancy.

Normal CN V, V3 division enhancing venous plexuses

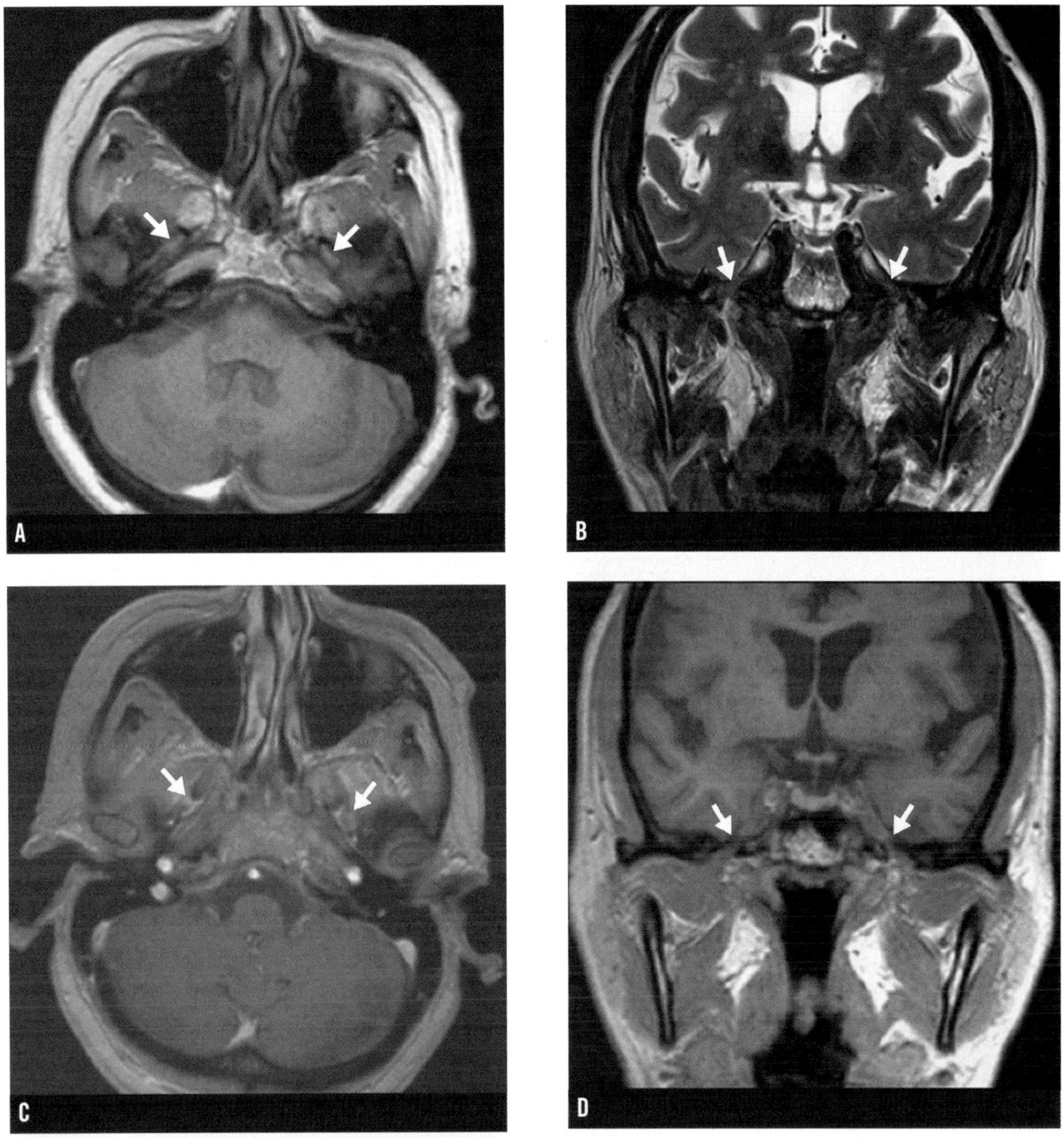

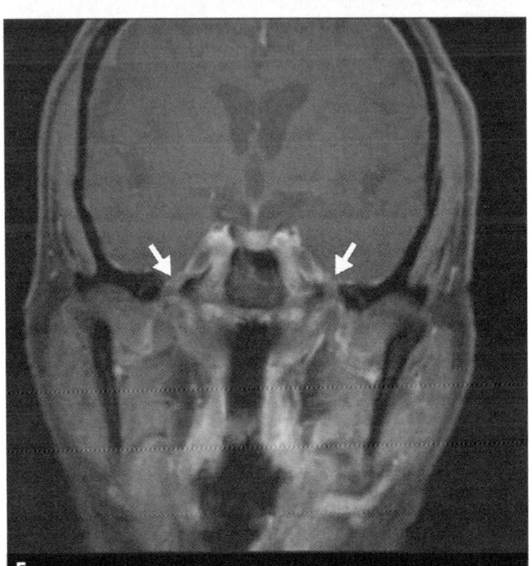

Unenhanced axial T1 (**A**), coronal T2 (**B**), postcontrast axial T1 with fat suppression (**C**), unenhanced coronal T1 (**D**), and coronal postcontrast T1 with fat suppression (**E**) MR images demonstrate normal precontrast T1 and T2 signal characteristics (arrows, **A, B, D**) and normal expected enhancement (arrows, **C, E**) of the V3 division of CN V. This is related to a normal venous plexus surrounding the V3 division, similar to what is normally present within the Meckel cave and along the V2 division of CN V.

Normal Meckel cave enhancing venous plexuses

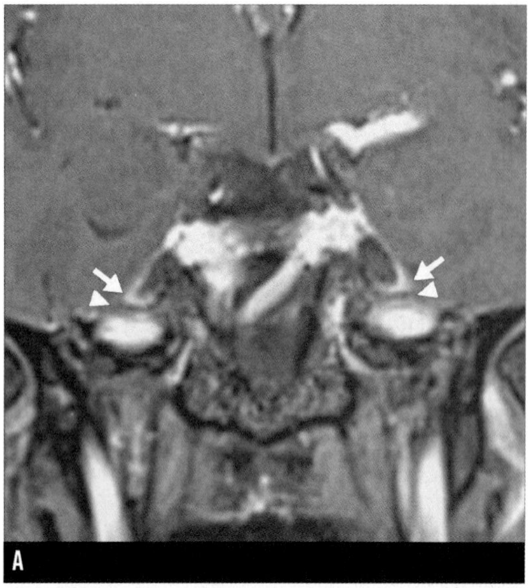

A postcontrast coronal T1-weighted fat-suppressed MR image (**A**) demonstrates symmetric, semilunar enhancing structures in the inferolateral aspects of both Meckel caves (arrows). These represent normal venous plexuses in the Meckel caves. The gasserian ganglia are located caudal to each venous plexus and each is demonstrated as a small nonenhancing focus (arrowheads). This patient did not have any CN V symptomatology.

Asymmetrically enlarged but normal Meckel cave enhancing venous plexus

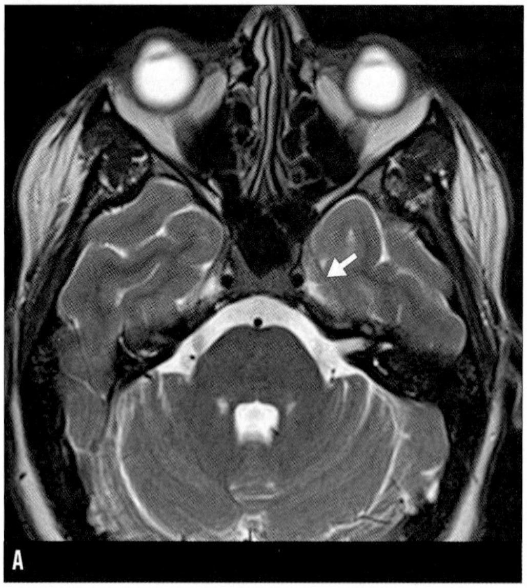

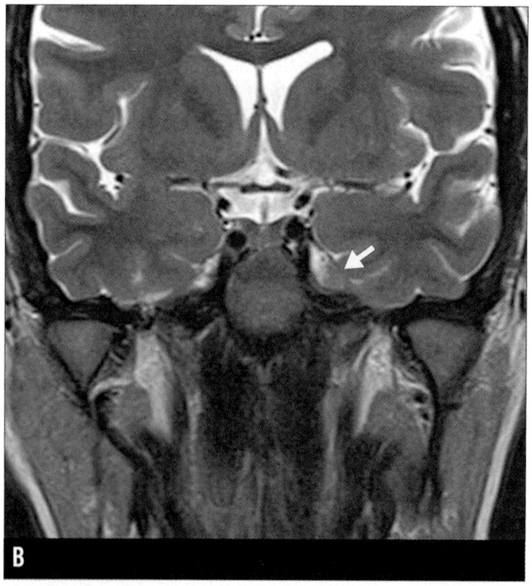

Axial T2 (**A**), coronal T2 (**B**), contrast-enhanced axial T1 with fat suppression (**C**), and contrast-enhanced coronal T1 with fat suppression (**D**) MR images demonstrate asymmetric soft tissue thickening and enhancement within the left Meckel cave (arrows, **A**-**D**). This was initially described as pathologic and concerning for perineural spread of tumor. However, the finding was entirely stable for 8 months and the patient did not have CN V symptomatology or a history of systemic illness. Furthermore, the finding has a normal semilunar configuration (best demonstrated on image **D**), typical of a normal Meckel cave venous plexus.

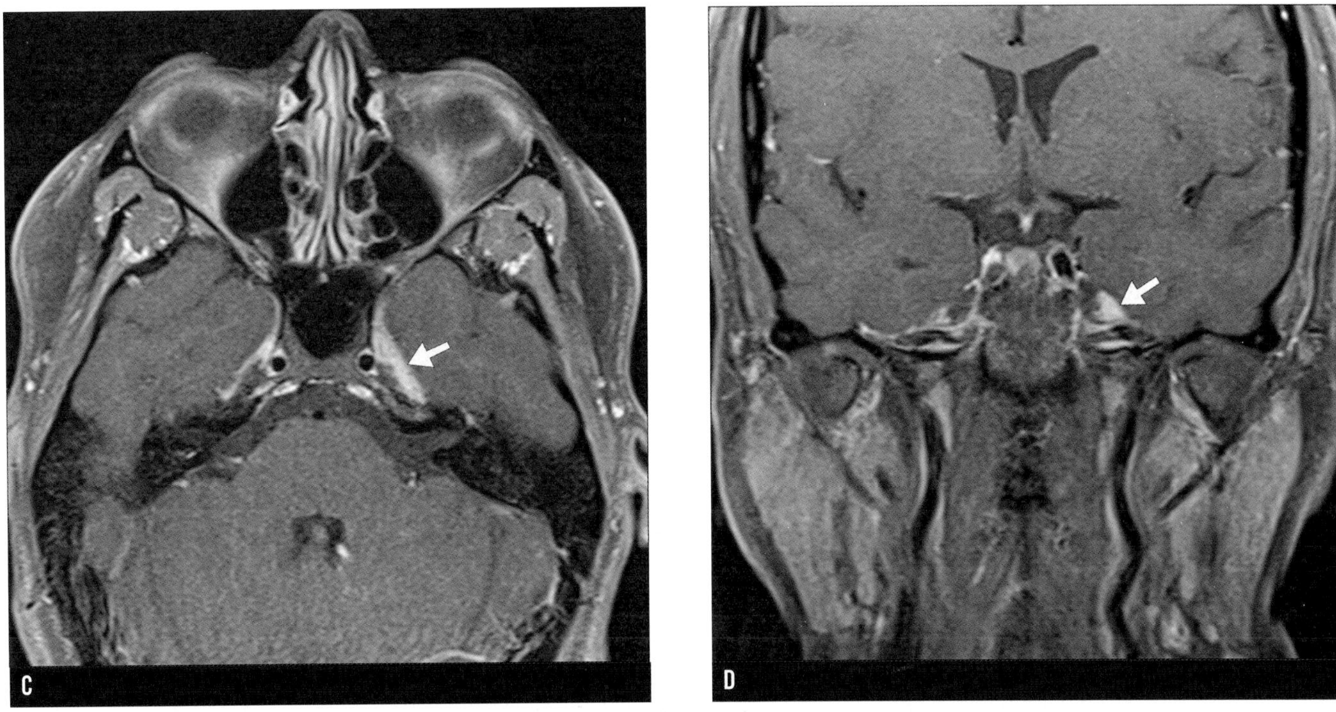

Companion case: Presumed schwannoma of the CN V, V2 division and pterygopalatine fossa

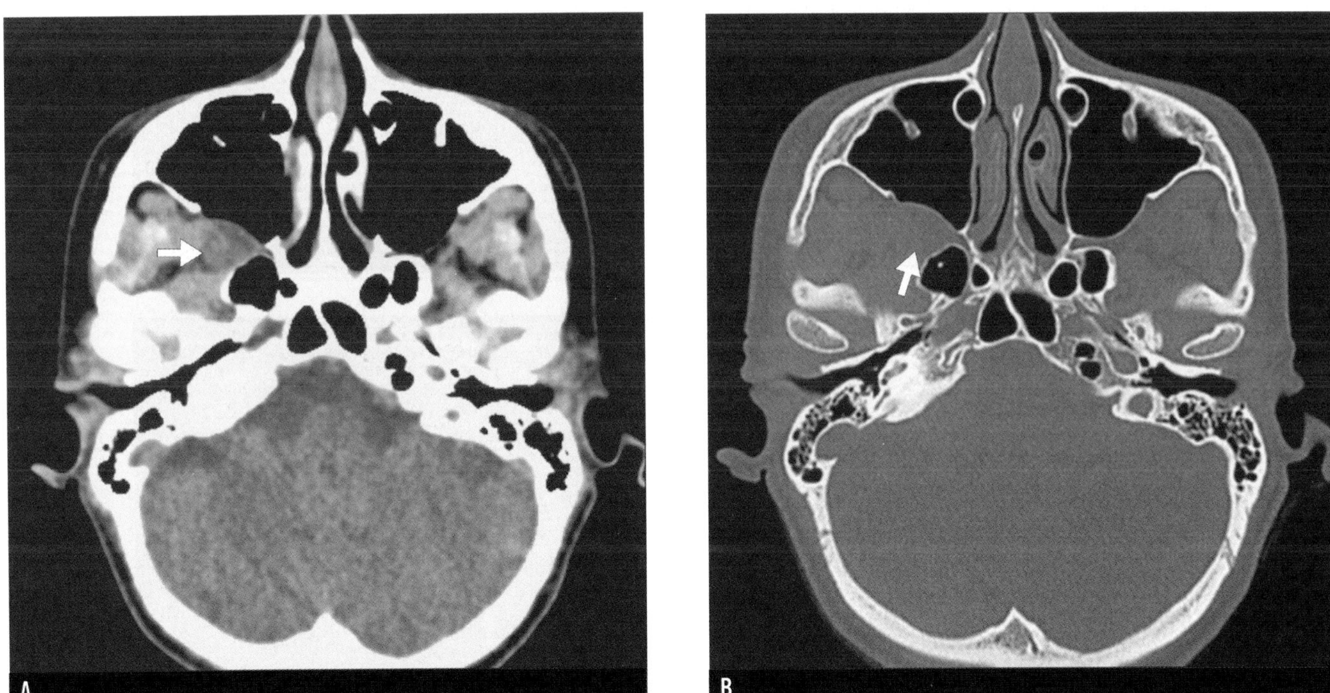

Unenhanced axial CT images through the level of the pterygopalatine fossa viewed with a soft tissue window (**A**) and bone window (**B**) demonstrate a mass within and expanding the right pterygopalatine fossa (arrows, **A**, **B**). Axial (**C**) and coronal reformatted (**D**) CT images viewed with a bone window demonstrate abnormal expansion of the right foramen rotundum (arrows, **C**, **D**). The normal left foramen rotundum is denoted for reference (arrowheads, **C**, **D**). Unenhanced axial T1 (**E**), axial T2 (**F**), and postcontrast axial T1 with fat suppression (**G**) MR images as well as a postcontrast coronal reformatted time of flight MRA image (**H**) demonstrate T1 and T2 isointense, enhancing mass in the right foramen rotundum (arrows, **E**-**H**) that also involves the right pterygopalatine fossa. The normal left foramen rotundum is demonstrated on image **H** (arrowhead, **H**). While not pathologically proven, the finding presumably represents a schwannoma.

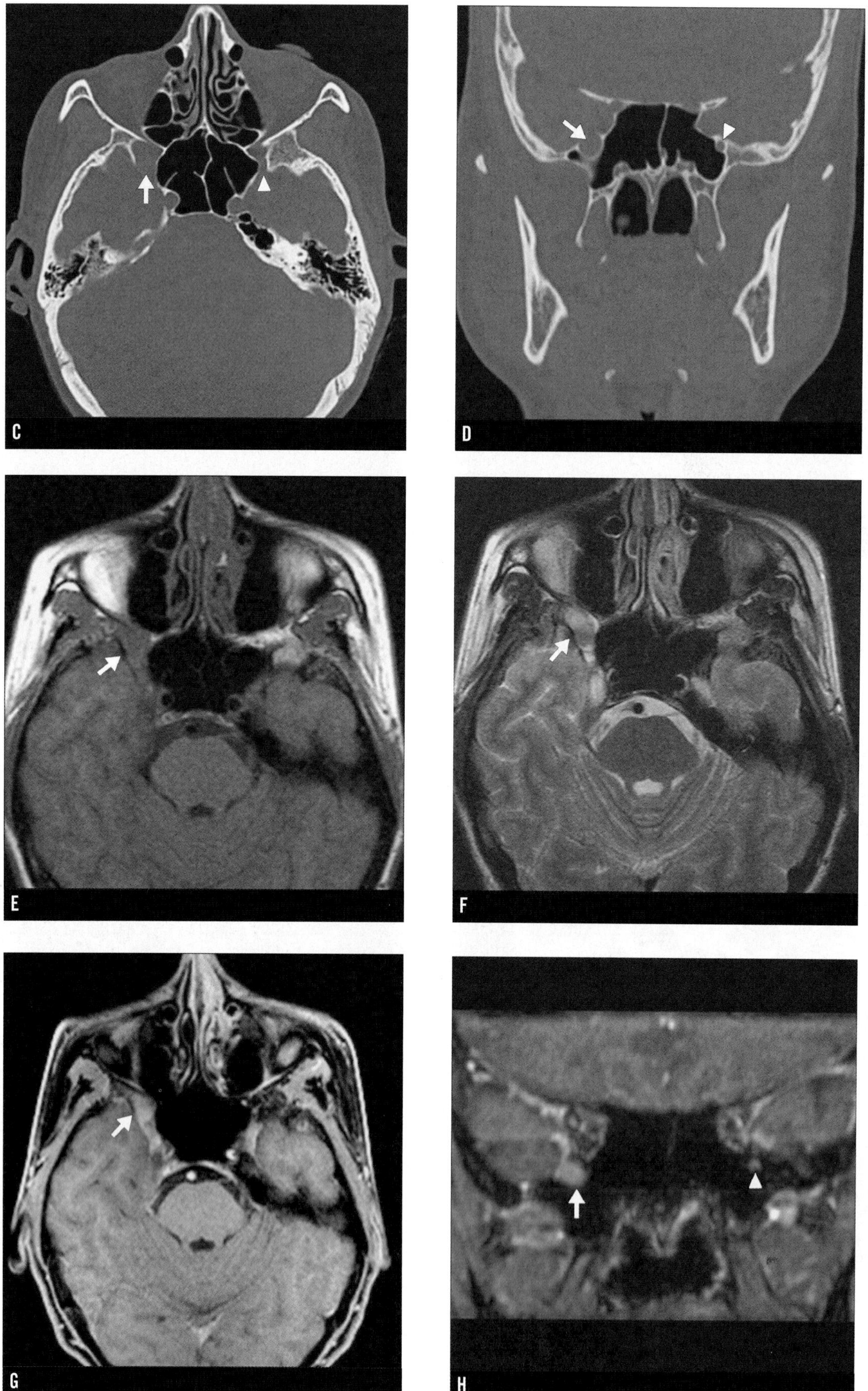
C
D
E
F
G
H

Companion case: Presumed CN V, V3 division schwannoma

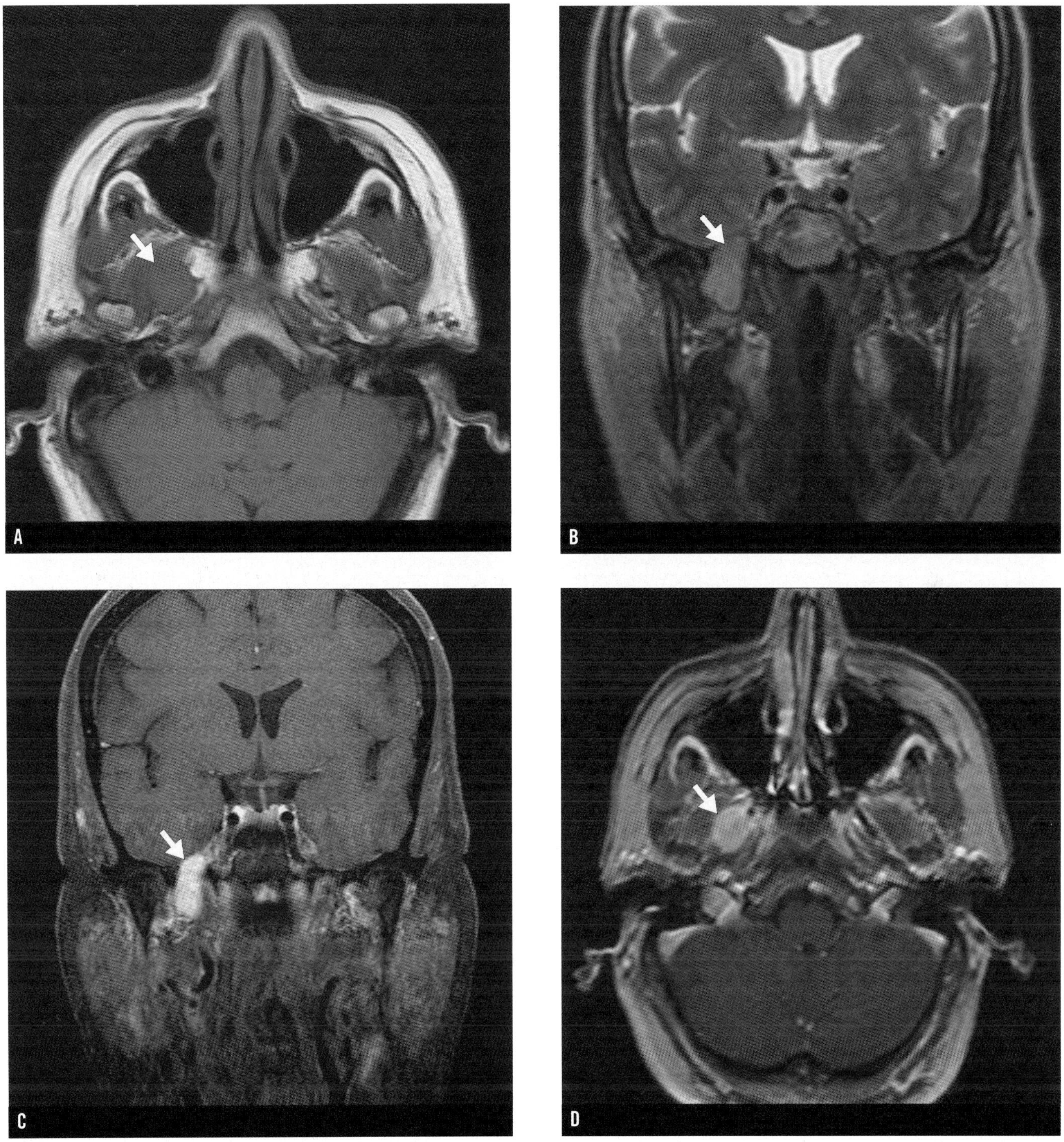

Unenhanced axial T1 (**A**), coronal T2 (**B**), postcontrast coronal T1 with fat suppression (**C**), and postcontrast axial MPRAGE (**D**) MR images demonstrate a homogeneously enhancing, mildly T2 hyperintense mass expanding the right foramen ovale and extending into the infratemporal fossa, most likely representing a schwannoma (arrows, **A**-**D**).

Perineural spread of tumor along the CN V, V2 and V3 divisions as well as the vidian nerve

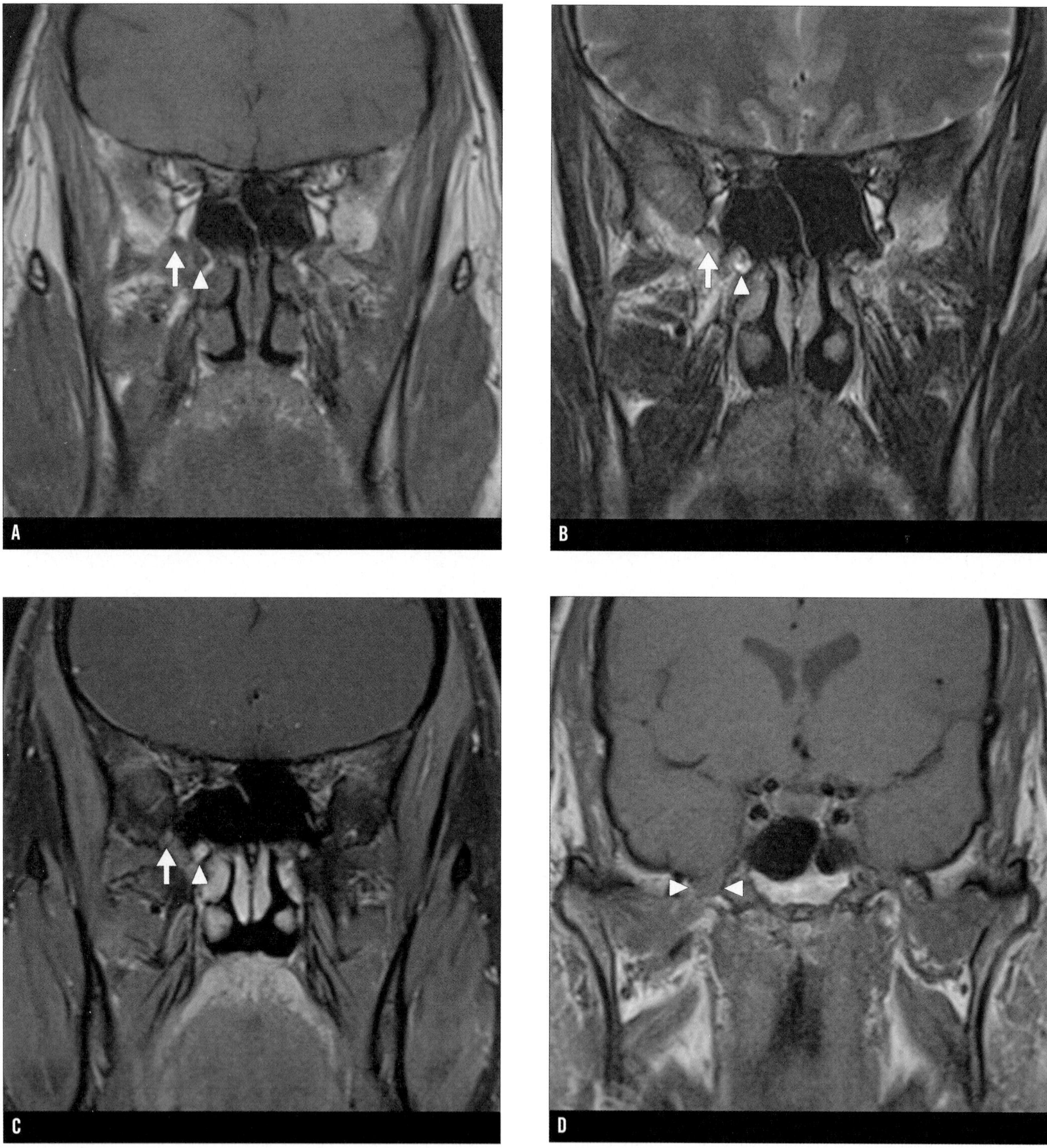

Coronal T1 (**A**), coronal T2 (**B**), and postcontrast coronal T1 with fat suppression (**C**) MR images through the level of the foramina rotundum and vidian canals. These images demonstrate T1 isointense and slightly T2 hyperintense signal as well as asymmetric enhancement of the CN V, V2 division in the right foramen rotundum (arrows, **A**-**C**) and of the vidian nerve in the right vidian canal (arrowheads, **A**-**C**). The right vidian nerve and canal are also asymmetrically larger. Coronal T1 (**D**), coronal T2 (**E**), and postcontrast coronal T1 with fat suppression (**F**) through the level of the foramina ovale demonstrate asymmetric enlargement with T1 isointense signal, T2 hyperintense signal, and enhancement along the right CN V, V3 segment (arrowheads, **D**-**F**). These findings were related to perineural spread of melanoma.

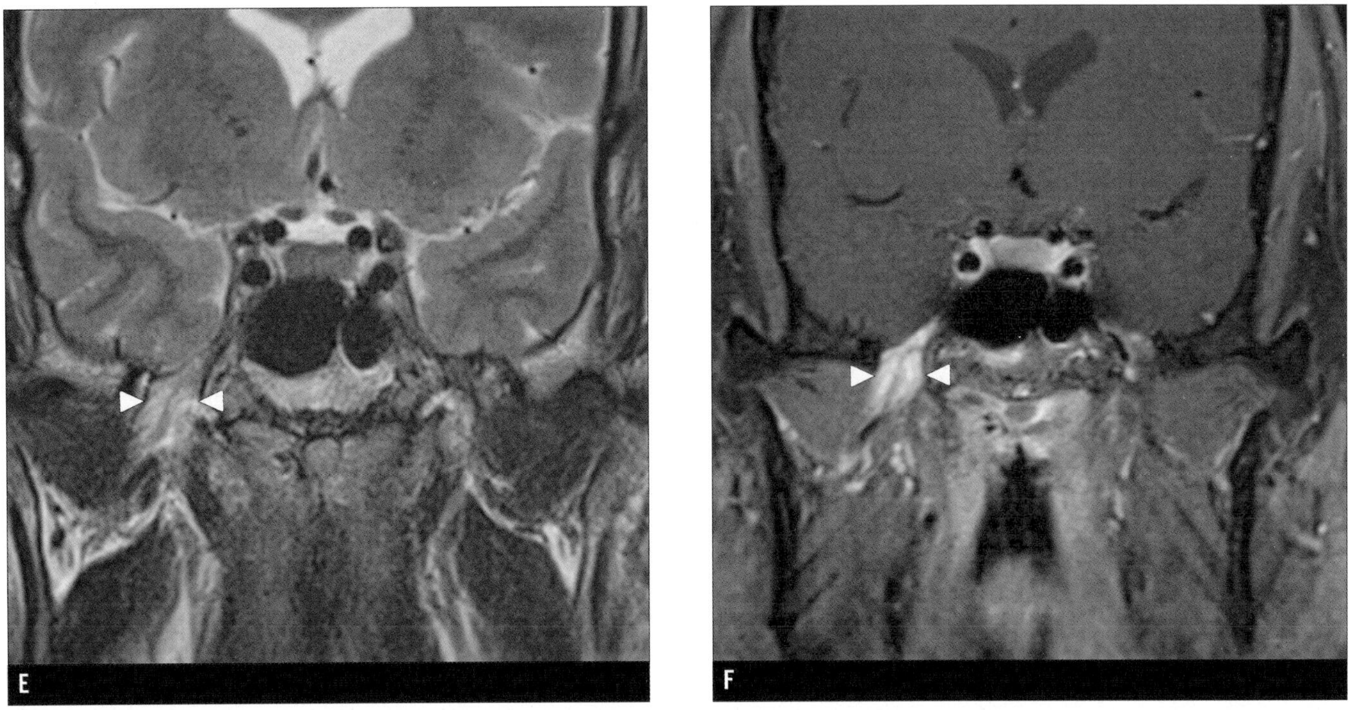
E
F

Companion case: Meckel cave schwannoma or meningioma

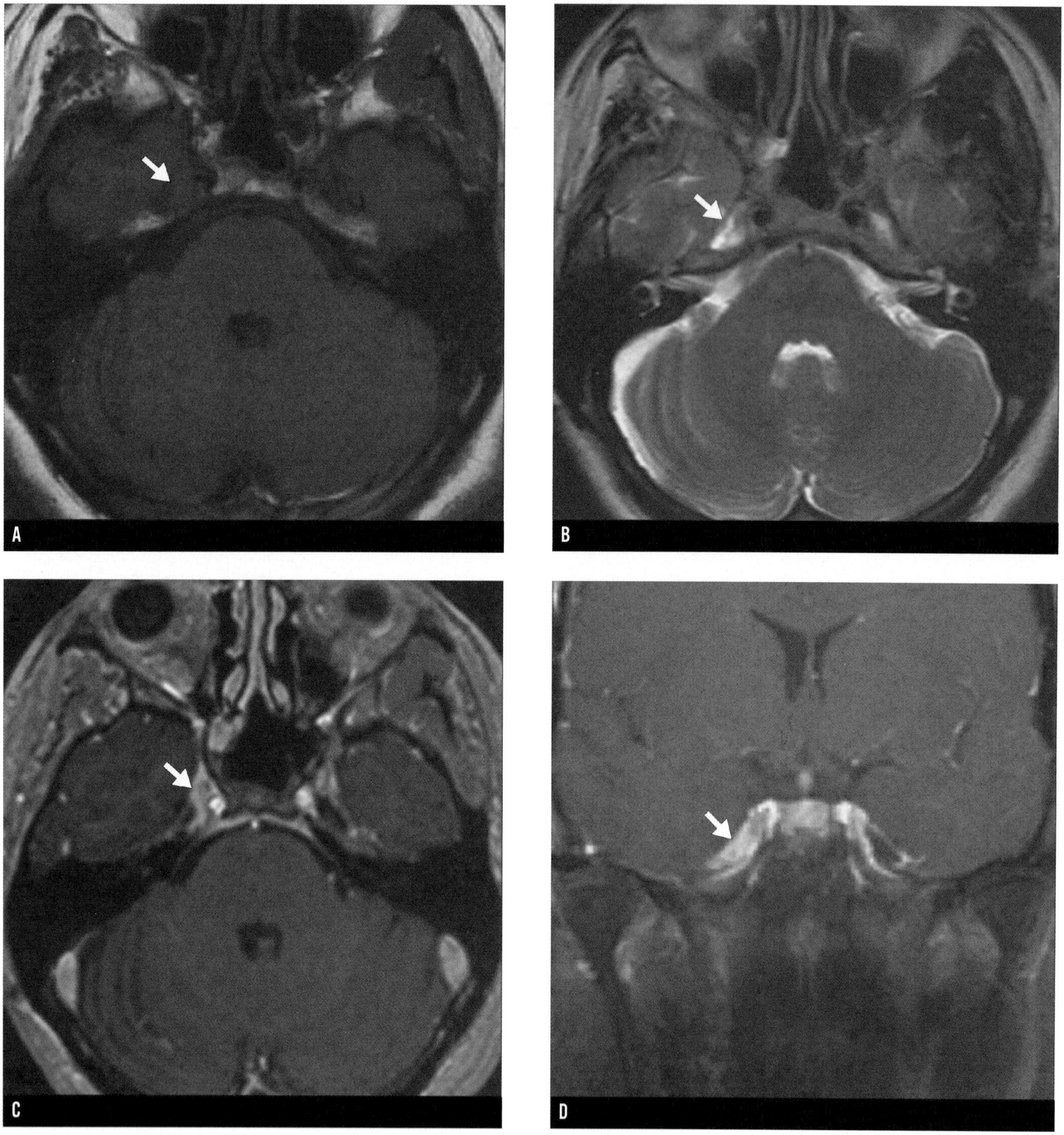

Unenhanced axial T1 (**A**), axial T2 (**B**), postcontrast axial MPRAGE (**C**), and postcontrast coronal T1 with fat suppression (**D**) MR images demonstrate a homogeneously enhancing, T2 hyperintense lesion centered within the right Meckel cave, consistent with either a schwannoma or meningioma (arrows, **A**-**D**). This is in contradistinction to a normal Meckel cave venous plexus, which is smaller, semilunar, and has a characteristic location, as discussed in the text.

Companion case: Meckel cave "white" epidermoid

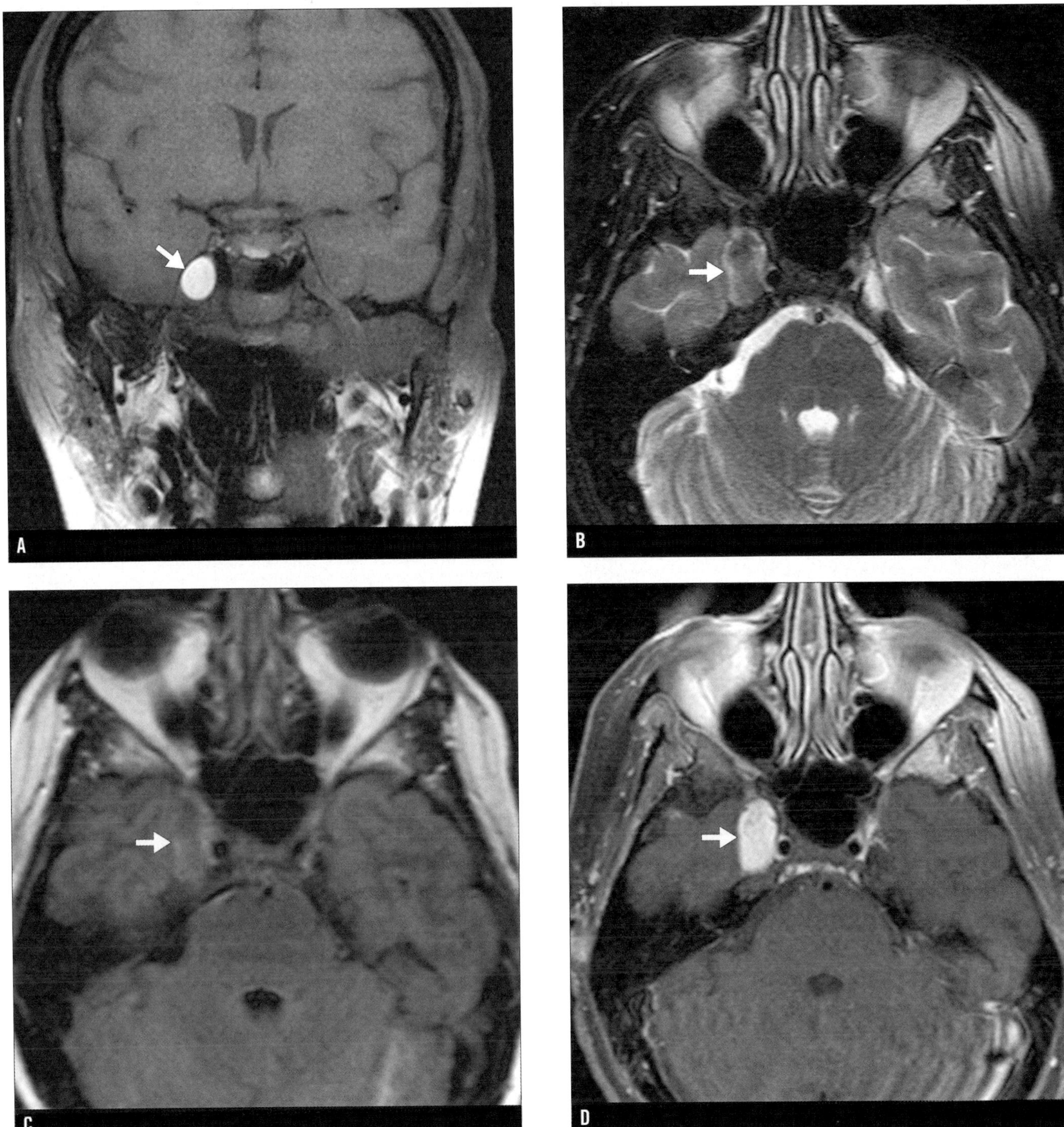

Unenhanced coronal T1 with fat suppression (**A**), axial T2 (**B**), axial FLAIR (**C**), and contrast-enhanced axial T1 with fat suppression (**D**) demonstrate an intrinsically T1 hyperintense, T2 isointense, minimally FLAIR hyperintense, unenhancing lesion located in the right Meckel cave (arrows, **A-D**). The lesion does not suppress on fat saturation imaging, effectively excluding a lipoma. The finding was a benign epidermoid tumor at pathology. The atypical "white" appearance on T1-weighted imaging is due to elevated proteinaceous content within the tumor.

REFERENCES

Puranik A, Sankhe S, Goel N, Mahore A. Cerebral shading sign in a giant intraparenchymal white epidermoid. *Neurol India*. 2012;60(2):265-266.

Williams LS, et al. MR imaging of the trigeminal ganglion, nerve, and the perineural vascular plexus: normal appearance and variants with correlation to cadaver specimens. *AJNR Am J Neuroradiol*. 2003;24(7):1317-1323.

On MRI, CN V enters the porus trigeminus (the opening of the Meckel cave) primarily as a single dominant nerve. However, occasionally, small CN V rootlets are distinctly demonstrated within the Meckel cave on MRI (best appreciated on thin section T2/CISS imaging) and are an incidental, normal finding. The CN V neural rootlets course anteriorly in the Meckel cave to form the gasserian ganglion.

COMPANION CASE

- **Pathologically enhancing Meckel cave rootlets.** Asymmetric enhancement of the Meckel cave rootlets should be viewed with suspicion and may be due to a variety of pathology, such as perineural spread of tumor or a neuritis. When encountered, follow-up imaging and correlation with the patient's history are usually necessary.

Meckel cave CN V rootlets

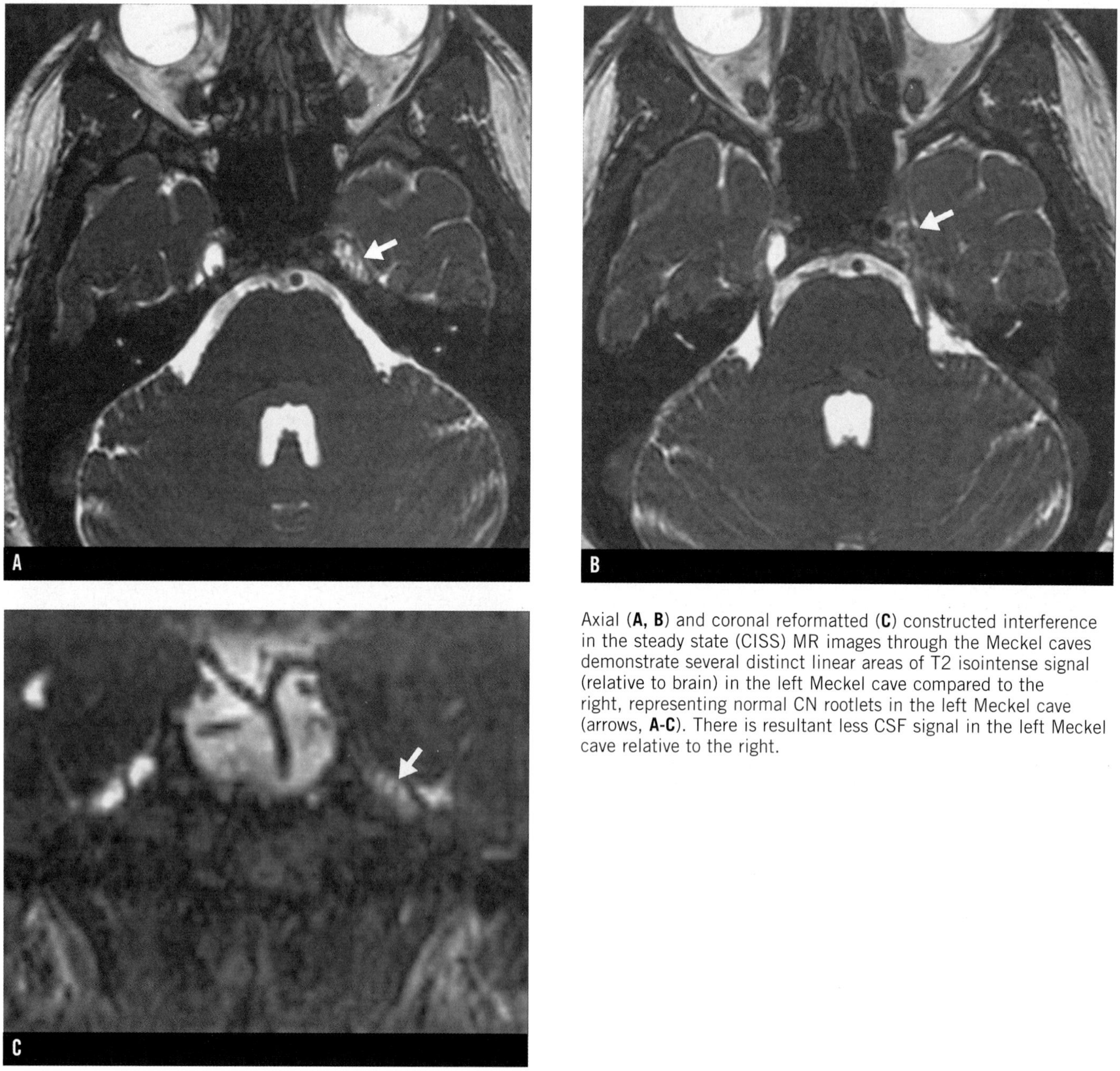

Axial (**A, B**) and coronal reformatted (**C**) constructed interference in the steady state (CISS) MR images through the Meckel caves demonstrate several distinct linear areas of T2 isointense signal (relative to brain) in the left Meckel cave compared to the right, representing normal CN rootlets in the left Meckel cave (arrows, **A-C**). There is resultant less CSF signal in the left Meckel cave relative to the right.

Companion case: Pathologically enhancing Meckel cave rootlets

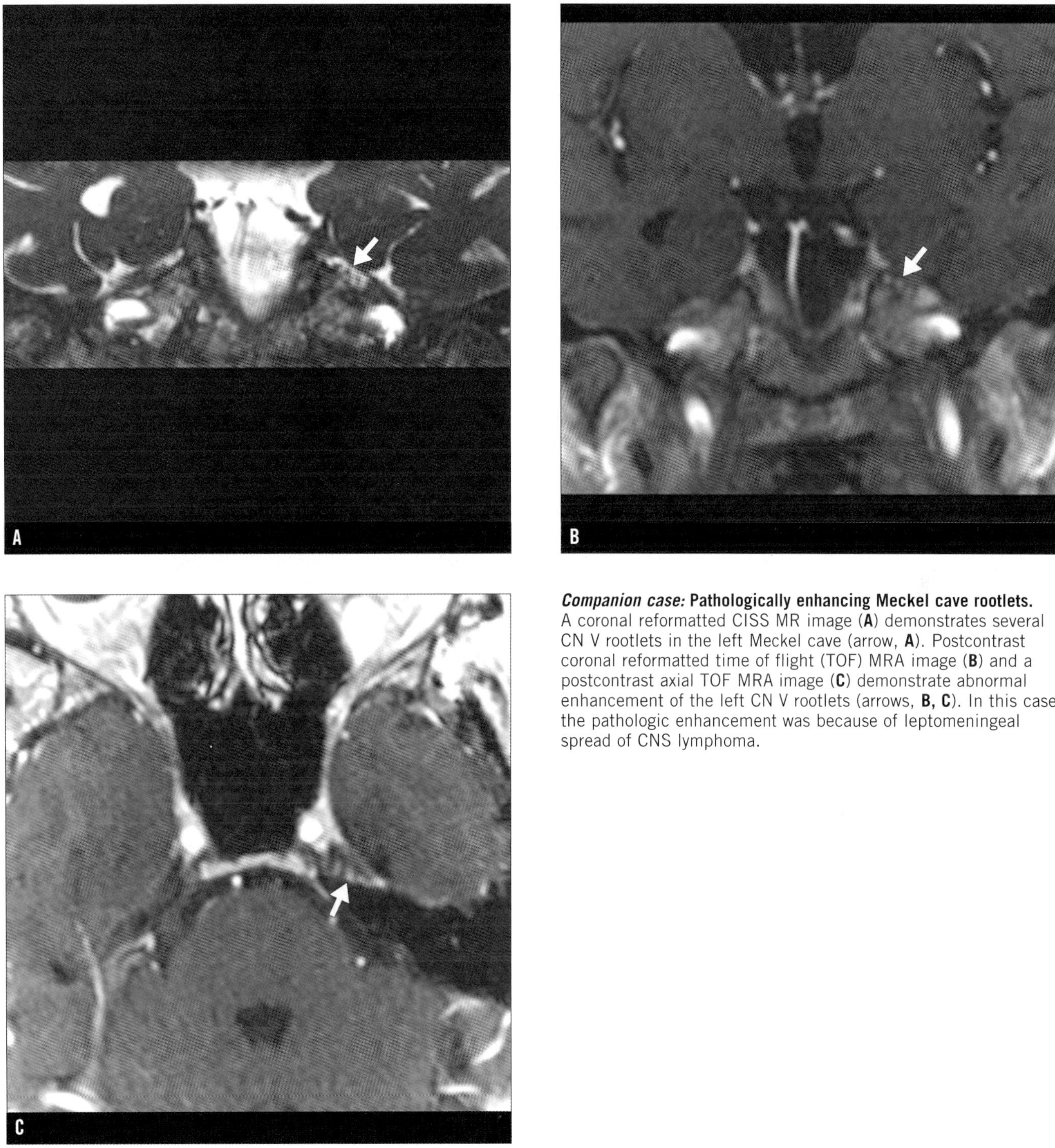

***Companion case:* Pathologically enhancing Meckel cave rootlets.** A coronal reformatted CISS MR image (**A**) demonstrates several CN V rootlets in the left Meckel cave (arrow, **A**). Postcontrast coronal reformatted time of flight (TOF) MRA image (**B**) and a postcontrast axial TOF MRA image (**C**) demonstrate abnormal enhancement of the left CN V rootlets (arrows, **B, C**). In this case, the pathologic enhancement was because of leptomeningeal spread of CNS lymphoma.

REFERENCE

Downs DM, Damiano TR, Rubinstein D. Gasserian ganglion: appearance on contrast-enhanced MR. *AJNR Am J Neuroradiol.* 1996;17(2):237-241.

CASE 32 Normal sensory and motor roots of the CN V cisternal segment

The sensory root of the cisternal segment of CN V is significantly larger and is located inferior relative to the motor root of CN V. The sensory root of CN V travels toward the pons, and is thus afferent, whereas the motor root of CN V travels from the pons and is efferent. Instead of entering the Meckel cave and joining the sensory root in the trigeminal ganglion, the motor root exits the skull base caudally through foramen ovale as a separate root. From there, the motor root then joins the sensory root of CN V to innervate the muscles of mastication.

The motor root of CN V may sometimes be mistaken for the superior cerebellar artery on coronal MR imaging, which is the vessel most commonly implicated in vascular impingement of the CN V cisternal segment and trigeminal neuralgia. Tracing the superior cerebellar artery back to its origin along the basilar artery will resolve any confusion.

Normal sensory and motor roots of the CN V cisternal segment

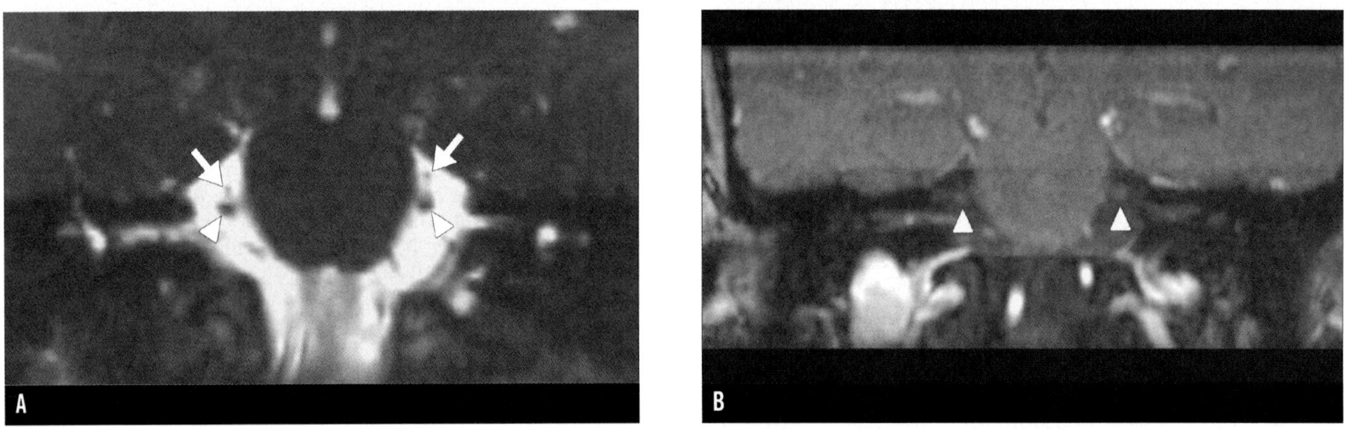

A coronal reformatted constructed interference in the steady state (CISS) MR image (**A**) demonstrates the larger sensory roots of both CN V cisternal segments (arrowheads, **A**) relative to the smaller and more cephalad located motor roots of CN V (arrows, **A**). The lack of enhancement in this area on a coronal postcontrast TOF MRA image (**B**) excludes that the motor roots demonstrated on the CISS sequence represent the superior cerebellar arteries. The bilateral sensory roots of CN V are demonstrated on image **B** (arrowheads, **B**). Several axial CISS images (**C**-**E**) demonstrate the smaller motor roots of the CN V cisternal segments (arrows, **D**, **E**) relative to the larger sensory roots (arrowheads, **C**).

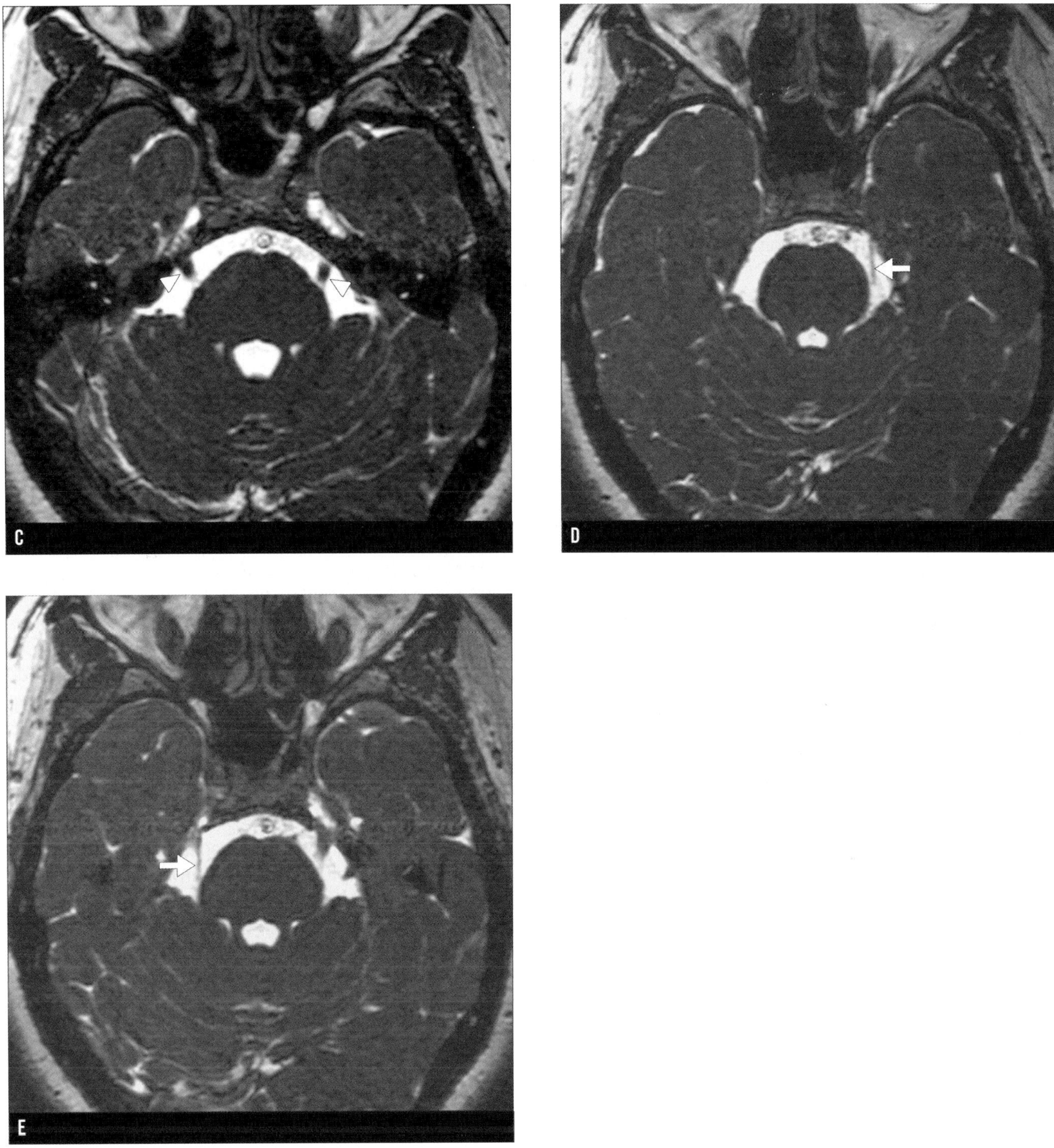

REFERENCE

Williams LS, et al. MR imaging of the trigeminal ganglion, nerve, and the perineural vascular plexus: normal appearance and variants with correlation to cadaver specimens. *AJNR Am J Neuroradiol.* 2003;24(7):1317-1323.

CASE 33 The jugular foramen and pars nervosa

The jugular foramen is an osseous channel at the skull base situated between the temporal and occipital bones, and it serves as a conduit between the posterior fossa and jugular fossa. The anatomy of the jugular foramen is complex, and as a result, there are different anatomic descriptions of this region. The conflicting anatomic descriptions are further complicated by the terms jugular foramen and jugular fossa, which are sometimes erroneously used interchangeably. The jugular fossa, which houses the jugular bulb, resides immediately caudal to the jugular foramen, and its roof is formed by the undersurface of the petrous temporal bone.

According to Rhoton, the jugular foramen is separated into three compartments, two venous and one neural. The neural compartment contains the pars nervosa, representing CN IX-XI, and is situated between the two venous compartments. With high-resolution MR imaging, the CN IX portion of the pars nervosa can be demonstrated as a separate structure from the CNX/XI complex of the pars nervosa.The two venous compartments, termed the sigmoid and the petrosal compartments, house portions of the sigmoid sinus and the inferior petrosal sinus, respectively. The venous compartments are partially separated by dural septa and intrajugular processes arising from the occipital and temporal bones. The sigmoid compartment is the larger of the two venous compartments and is located posterolaterally in the jugular foramen, whereas the petrosal compartment is located anteromedially in the jugular foramen.

As stated above, there are other anatomic descriptions of the jugular foramen. One such description also subdivides the jugular foramen by intrajugular processes and dural septa arising from the temporal and occipital bones, but describes only 2 instead of 3 compartments: an anterior compartment termed the pars nervosa and a posterior compartment termed the pars vascularis. In this anatomic description, the pars nervosa contains the inferior petrosal sinus and CN IX, whereas the pars vascularis contains CN X/XI as well as the jugular bulb. For the remaining text and imaging cases provided herein, the anatomy of the jugular foramen described by Rhoton is used.

COMPANION CASES

- **Nonocclusive distal sigmoid venous sinus and jugular bulb thrombus.** A small nonocclusive thrombus in the distal aspect of the sigmoid venous sinus may simulate the normal pars nervosa, although the former is located within the sigmoid venous compartment of the jugular foramen, whereas the pars nervosa is located adjacent to the sigmoid venous compartment, as discussed above.
- **CN IX-XI complex schwannoma.** Because these nerves are closely positioned to one another, determining the nerve of origin of a schwannoma along the course of these nerves within the cerebellar-medullary cistern is frequently not possible, so they are often referred to as a CN IX-XI complex schwannoma.
- **CT occult glomus jugulare tumor.** A glomus jugulare tumor is a paraganglioma that arises from the adventitia of the jugular bulb. Normally, this tumor results in osseous destruction of the jugular foramen on CT and is an enhancing mass on both CT and MRI. The case provided illustrates how a glomus jugulare tumor can be easily overlooked on CT, particularly when there is only subtle or absent erosion of the jugular foramen. A high index of suspicion, such as with unexplained tinnitus, is often necessary to identify a subtle glomus jugulare tumor. On conventional MRI, contrast-enhanced MPRAGE imaging is frequently helpful. Usually noninvasive imaging with a time-of-flight MRA or contrast-enhanced MRA of the neck will demonstrate flow-related signal and enhancement, respectively, related to vessels within a glomus tumor jugulare. A catheter angiogram can be performed to confirm the presence of the vascular mass as well as for embolization purposes.

The jugular foramen and pars nervosa

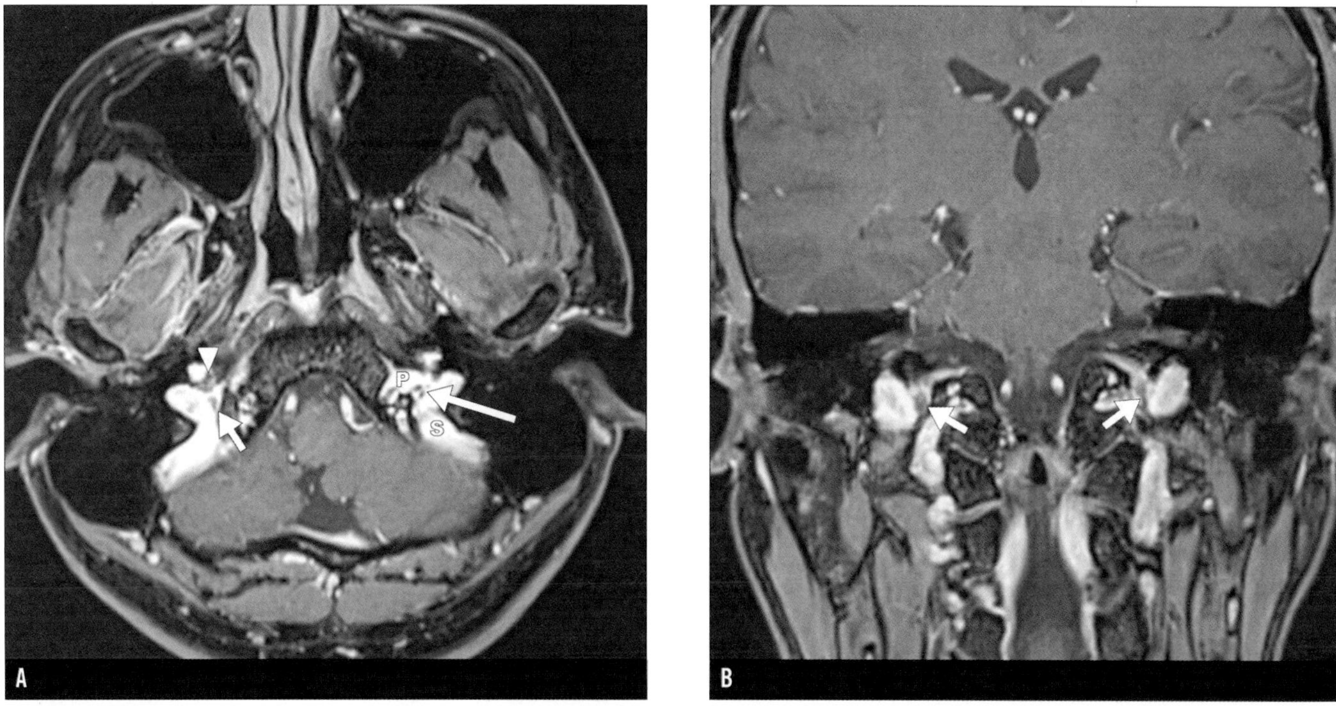

A postcontrast axial T1 VIBE MR image from a 3T magnet (**A**) depicts the right CN IX (arrowhead, **A**) and the right CN X/XI complex (short arrow, **A**) of the pars nervosa as well as the left inferior petrosal sinus (P) and left sigmoid sinus (S). A long arrow on image **A** denotes the intrajugular processes and dural septum which subdivide the inferior petrosal sinus compartment from the sigmoid sinus compartment. A coronal postcontrast T1 VIBE (**B**) MR image of the same patient also demonstrates a portion of each pars nervosa (arrows, **B**).

The jugular foramen and pars nervosa

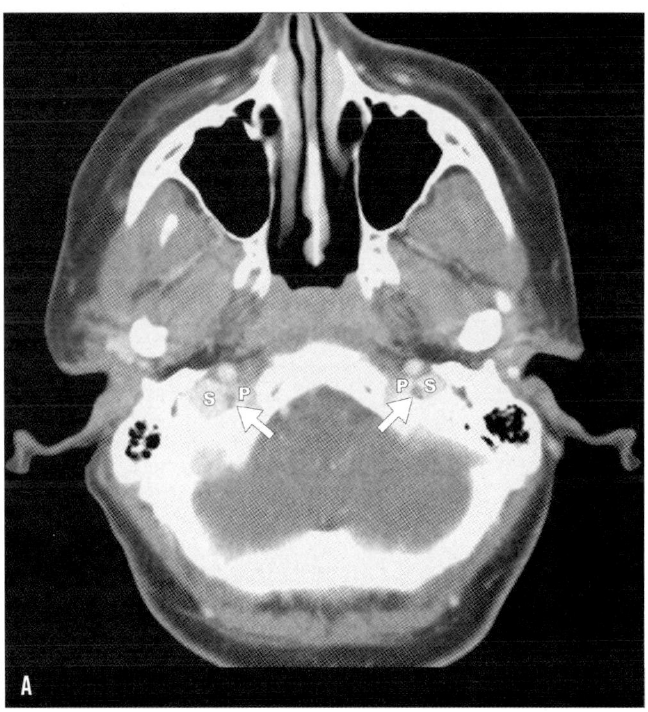

Different patient. A postcontrast axial CT image (**A**) demonstrates the normal jugular foramen on each side. The bilateral pars nervosa (CN IX-XII) (arrows), both sigmoid sinus compartments/ jugular bulb (S), and both inferior petrosal sinus compartments (P) are well-depicted on this image. Care should be taken not to misinterpret the normal pars nervosa for nonocclusive thrombus.

Companion case: Nonocclusive distal sigmoid venous sinus and jugular bulb thrombus

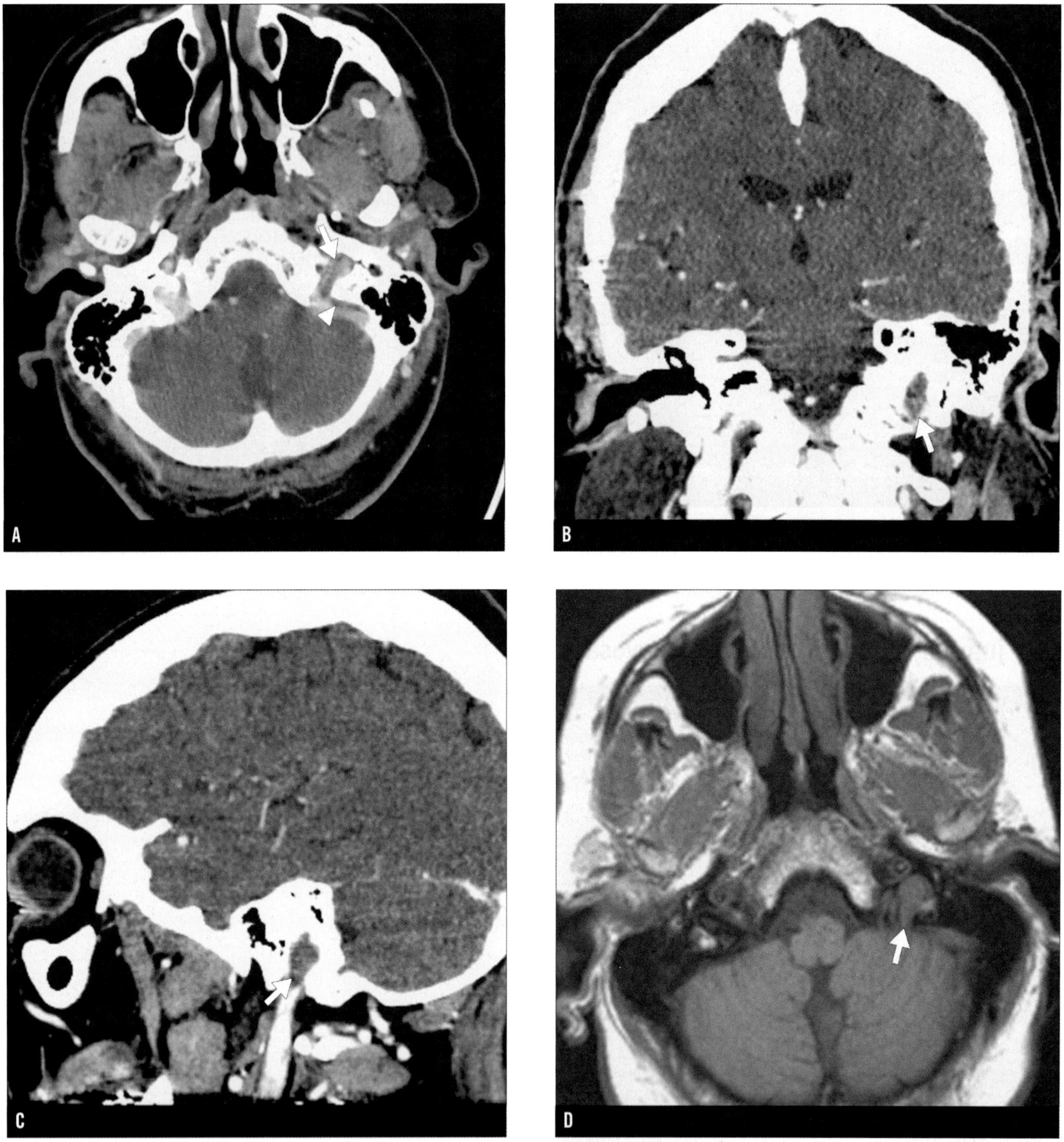

Axial (**A**), coronal reformatted (**B**), and sagittal reformatted (**C**) postcontrast CT images from a CTV demonstrate nonocclusive thrombus within the left jugular bulb (arrows, **A-C**) and distal sigmoid venous sinus (arrowhead, **A**). Unenhanced axial T1 (**D**), axial T2 (**E**), and postcontrast axial T1 (**F**) MR images obtained 1 hour after the CTV. The jugular bulb thrombus is T1 isointense (arrow, **D**) and T2 hyperintense (arrow, **E**). Interestingly, the thrombus enhances in this case (arrow, **F**). While most venous thrombi do not enhance on MRI, a chronic thrombus may enhance, and if it does, may be occult on a postcontrast T1-weighted MR image.

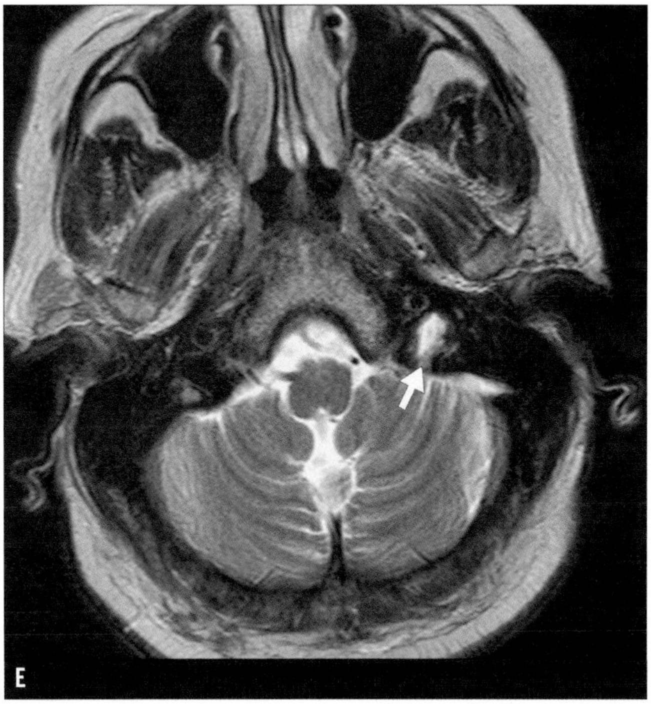

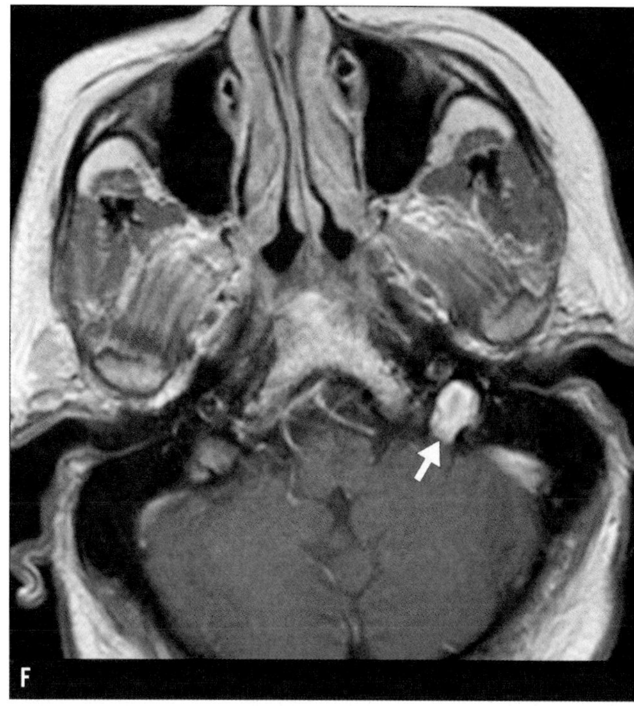

Companion case: Small nonocclusive distal sigmoid sinus thrombus

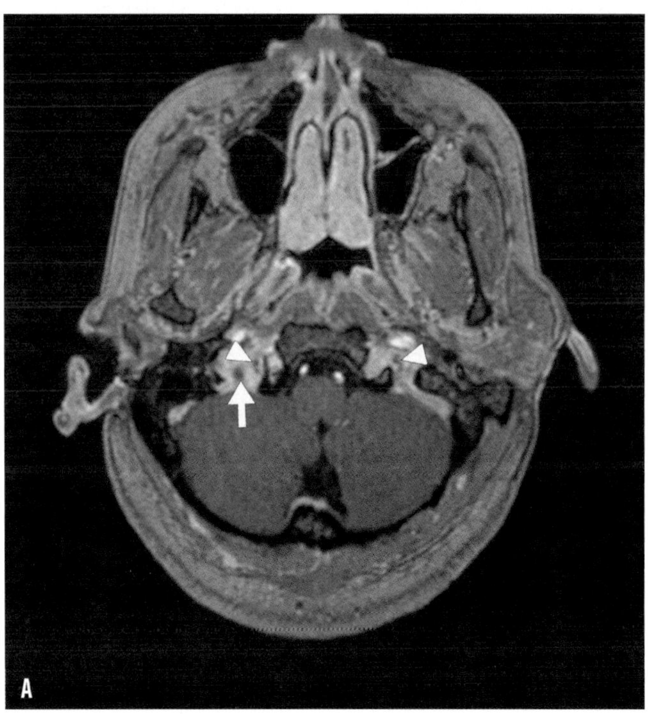

Postcontrast axial MPRAGE MR image (**A**) demonstrates a very small nonocclusive thrombus in the distal sigmoid sinus (arrow). The normal pars nervosa is demonstrated bilaterally (arrowheads).

Companion case: CN IX-XI complex schwannoma

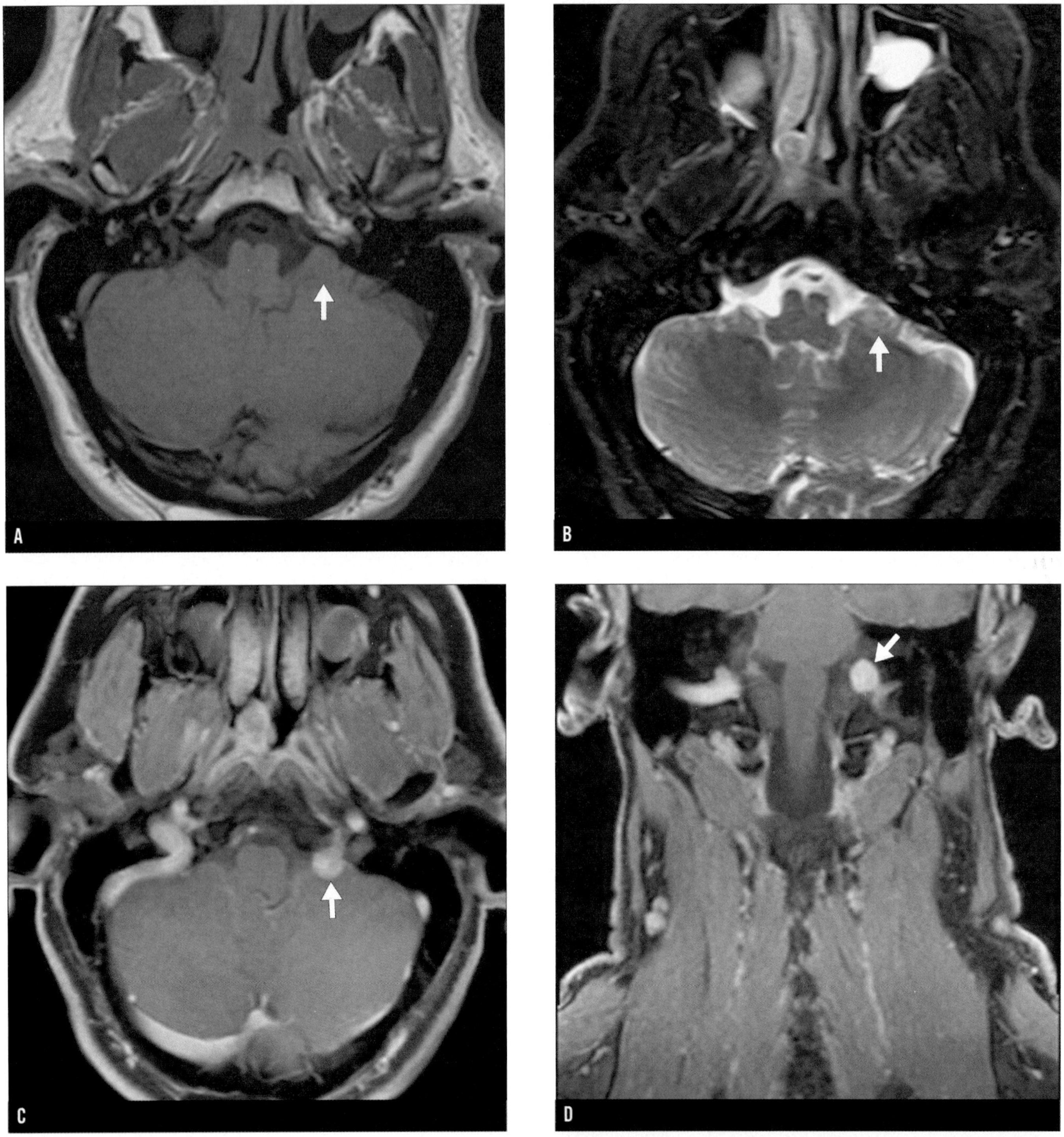

Unenhanced axial T1 (**A**), axial T2 with fat suppression (**B**), and axial (**C**), coronal (**D**), and sagittal (**E**) postcontrast T1 with fat suppression MR images demonstrate a homogeneously enhancing, T2 isointense lesion at the left cerebellar-medullary junction that extends into the left jugular foramen (arrows, **A-E**). The lesion is consistent with a schwannoma along the expected course of CN IX through XI. However, the precise nerve involvement is difficult to determine because of the close proximity of these nerves to one another in this region.

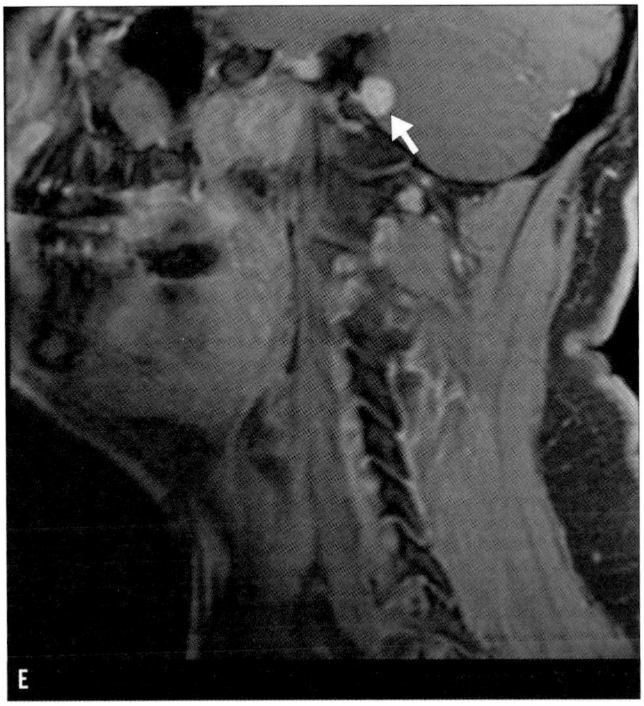

Companion case: CT occult glomus jugulare tumor

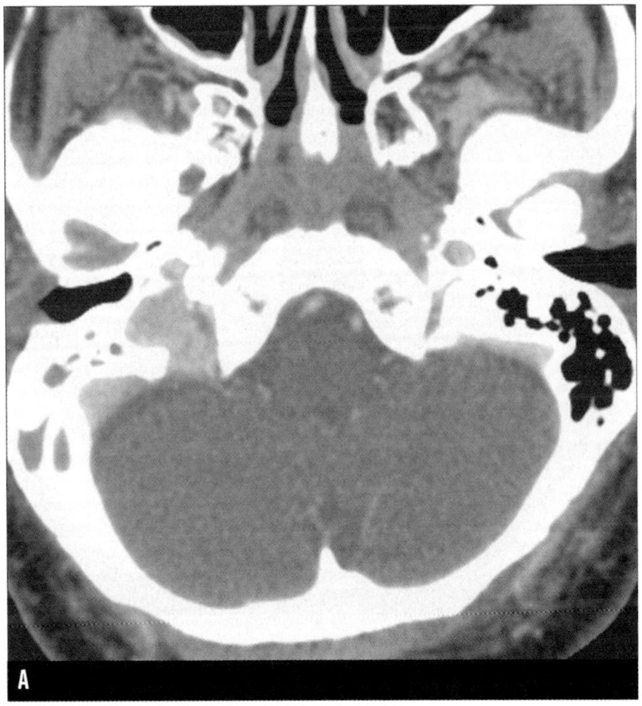

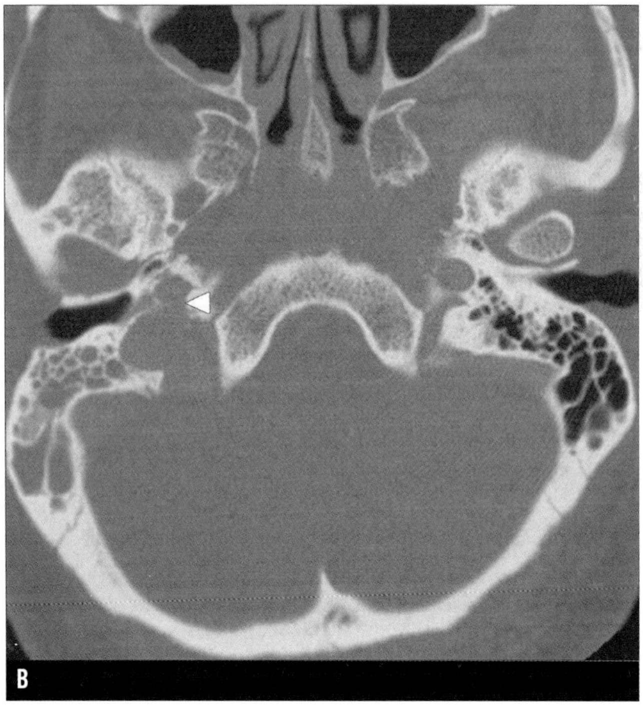

A contrast-enhanced axial CT image viewed with a brain window (**A**) is unremarkable, with apparent normal enhancement of the right jugular bulb. A CT image at the same level as image **A** but viewed with a bone window (**B**) demonstrates possible erosion along the posterior wall of the right petrous carotid canal which was not identified over several studies (arrowhead, **B**). Axial T1 (**C**), axial T2 (**D**), and contrast-enhanced axial T1 with fat suppression (**E**) MR images demonstrate T1 shortening (short arrow, **C**), mild T2 prolongation (short arrow, **D**), and enhancement in the right jugular foramen (short arrow, **E**), nonspecific findings that could simply represent incidental slow flow within normal vein. However, an axial CISS image (**F**) best demonstrates that the distal right sigmoid sinus is displaced medially (long arrow, **F**). A source image from a TOF MRA (**G**) demonstrates several small vessels with flow-related signal traversing the right jugular foramen, suspicious for a glomus jugulare (short arrow, **G**). A lateral image from a catheter angiogram (**H**) confirms a vascular mass consistent with a glomus jugulare (short arrow, **H**). This mass is likely being fed by the jugular branch of the neuromeningeal trunk (arrowhead, **H**), which in turn arises from the ascending pharyngeal artery.

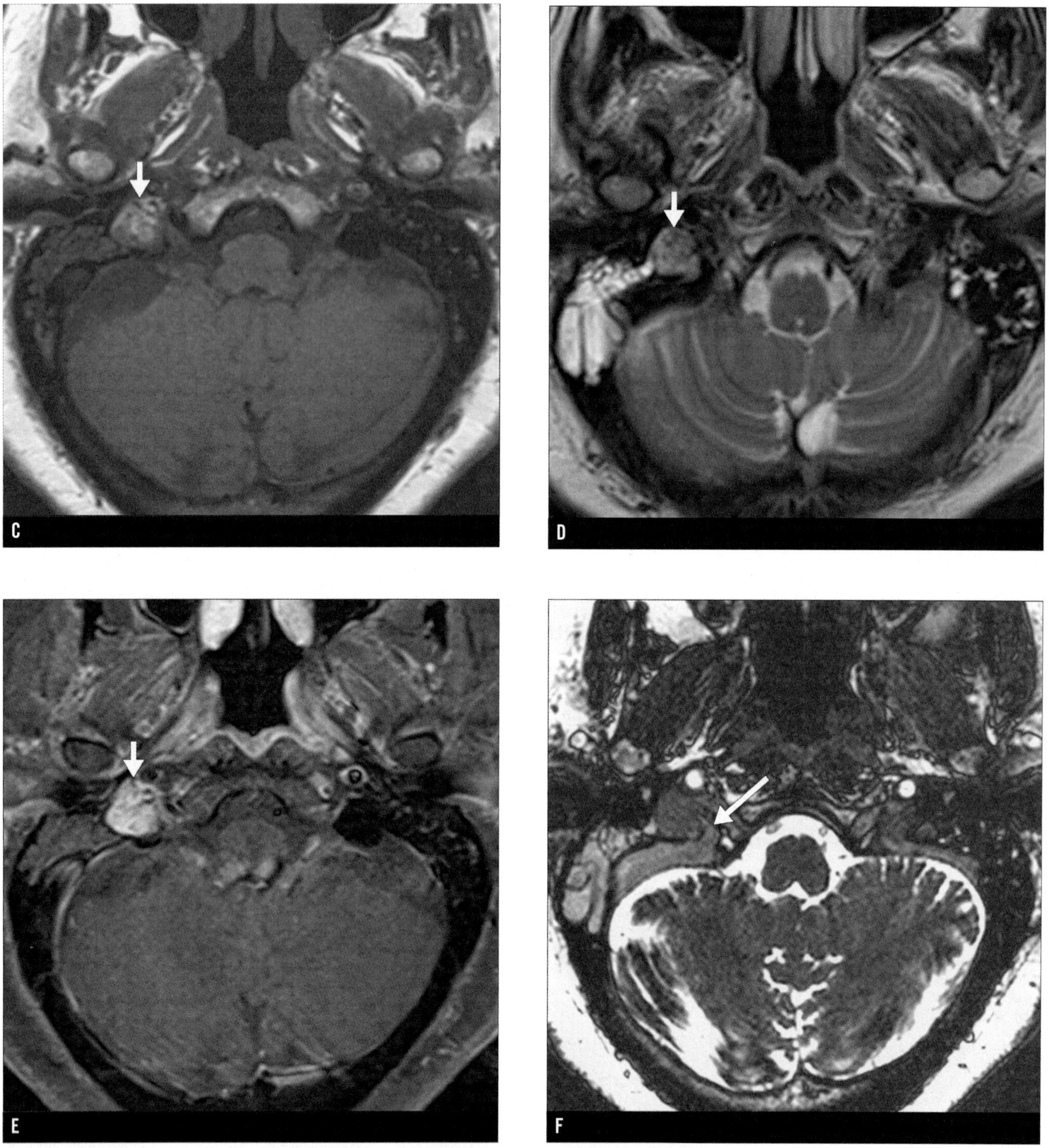
C
D
E
F

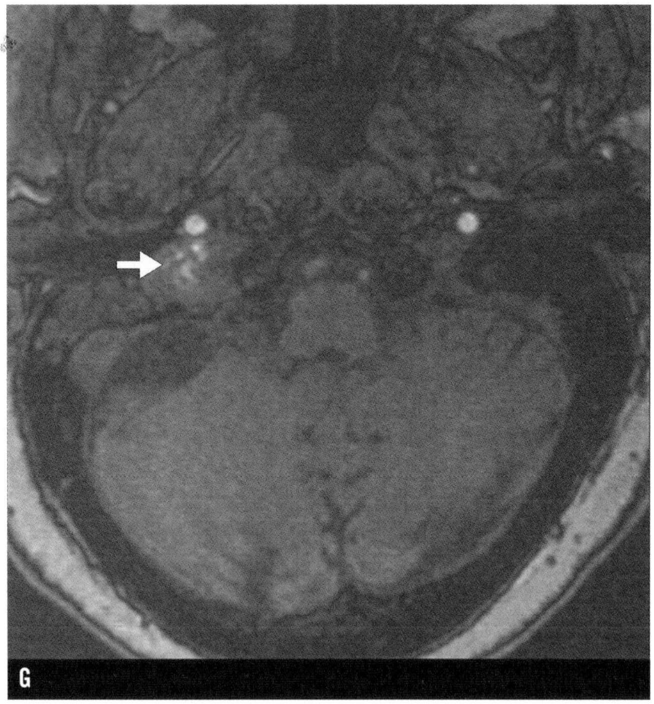

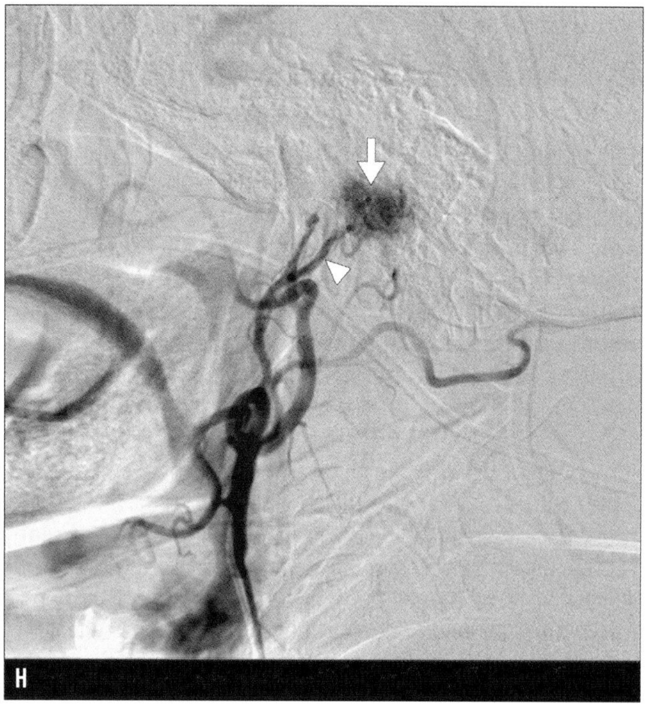

REFERENCES

Rhoton AL. Jugular foramen. *Neurosurgery.* 2000;47(suppl 3):267-285.

Linn J, Peters F, Moriggl B, Naidich TP, Brückmann H, Yousry I. The jugular foramen: imaging strategy and detailed anatomy at 3T. *AJNR Am J Neuroradiol.* 2009;30:34-41.

CASE 34 Normal spinal accessory nerve root

The spinal accessory nerve (CN XI) has traditionally been described as arising from two separate nuclei, a cranial nucleus (nucleus ambiguus) and a spinal nucleus. However, recent literature refuting this conventional teaching maintains that CN XI has only one nucleus, that being the spinal nucleus. If true, then this also raises the question whether the spinal accessory nerve can be considered a cranial nerve, given the lack of a cranial nucleus in this scenario. With that said, there are six or seven rootlets that extend posterolaterally from each spinal cord nucleus to form a single spinal root on each side of the spinal cord, which subsequently travel cephalad. The CN XI spinal roots can occasionally be identified on MRI (particularly MPRAGE) and may appear focally prominent, sometimes simulating a lesion. While pathology (eg, a schwannoma) involving a spinal accessory nerve root can be difficult to exclude, identification of these roots should not routinely be attributed to pathology.

COMPANION CASE

- **Presumed spinal accessory nerve schwannoma.** Suggesting the presence of a spinal accessory nerve schwannoma is best made by MRI, by documenting a change in size of the finding on at least 2 studies, and/or determining that the finding is significantly larger than expected for a normal spinal accessory nerve root. While an exact measurement of the upper limits of normal for a spinal accessory nerve root is likely not known, a measurement of at least 5 mm or greater in axial dimension is probably sufficient to suggest the presence a schwannoma of this nerve.

Normal spinal accessory nerve root

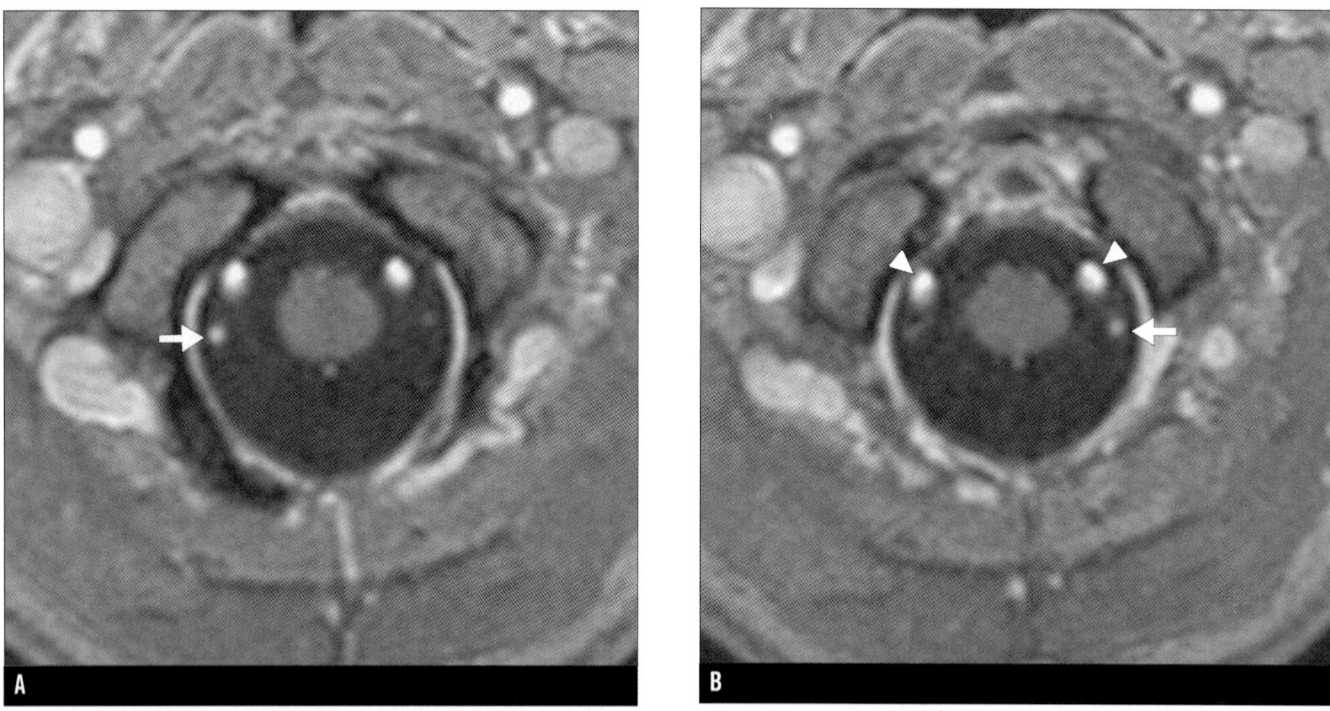

Postcontrast axial MPRAGE MR images through the upper cervical cord (**A**, **B**) demonstrate two symmetric, apparently enhancing rounded foci lateral to the upper cervical spinal cord, compatible with spinal accessory roots (arrows, **A**, **B**). The normal intradural vertebral arteries are present anteriorly (arrowheads, **B**). Similar findings are present on axial MPRAGE MR images from two other patients (**C**, **D**), although the spinal accessory root is asymmetrically larger on the left than the right for Patient **C** and enhancing to a slightly greater degree on the left than the right for Patient **D** (arrows, **C**, **D**). While it can be difficult to exclude a lesion, such as a schwannoma, particularly in asymmetric cases, it is not uncommon to visualize spinal accessory nerve roots on MR imaging. The left spinal accessory nerve root for Patient **D** was stable for 5 years on a follow-up MRI.

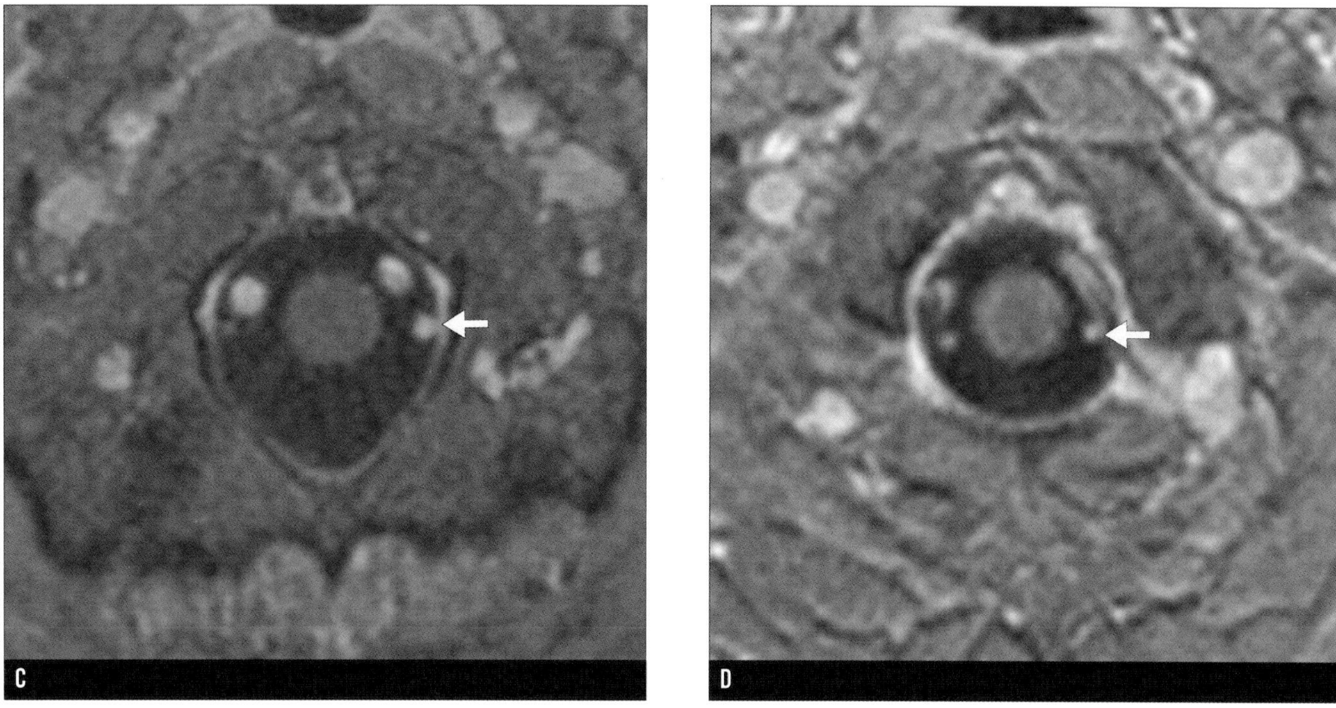

Companion case: Presumed spinal accessory nerve root schwannoma

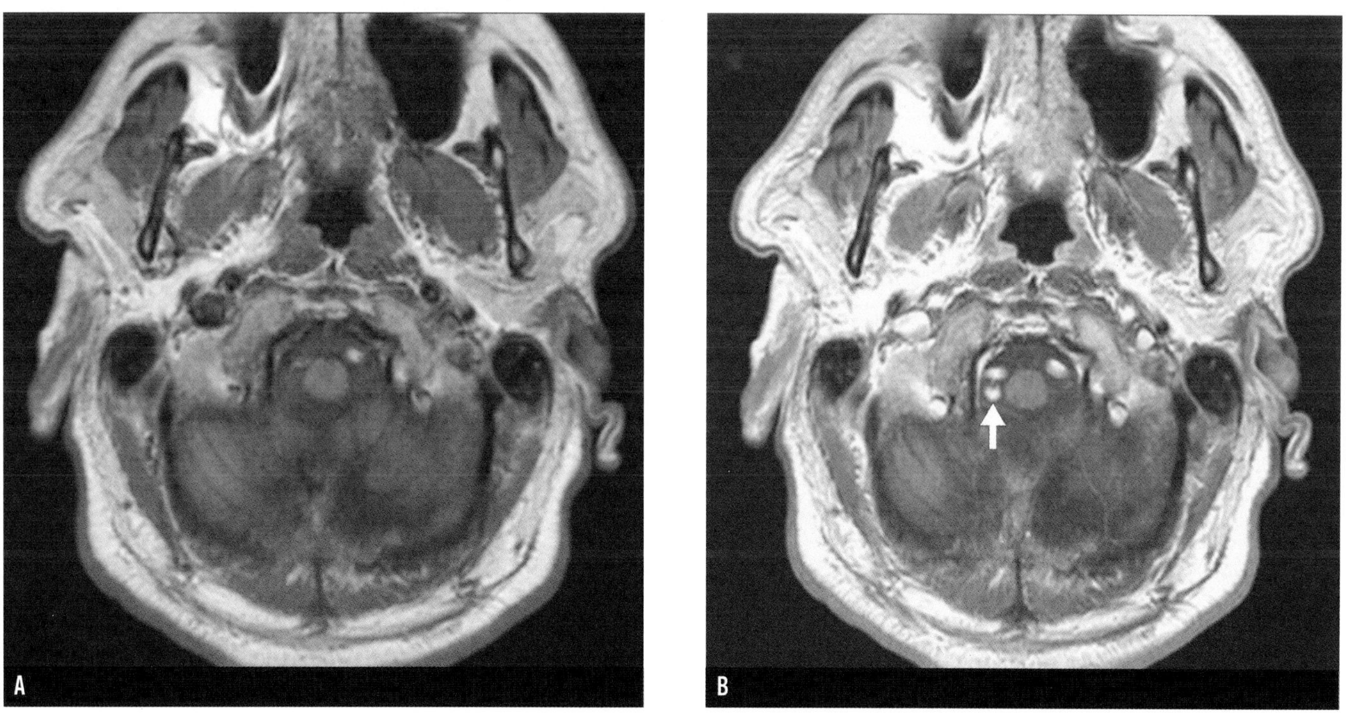

Axial T1 (**A**), postcontrast axial T1 (**B**), postcontrast coronal T1 (**C**), and axial T2 (**D**) MR images demonstrate an enhancing, T2 isointense, oval lesion posterior to the right vertebral artery (arrows, **B-D**). This patient was asymptomatic. However, the finding is larger than expected for a normal CN XI (> 5 mm) and therefore presumed to represent an incidental, small schwannoma.

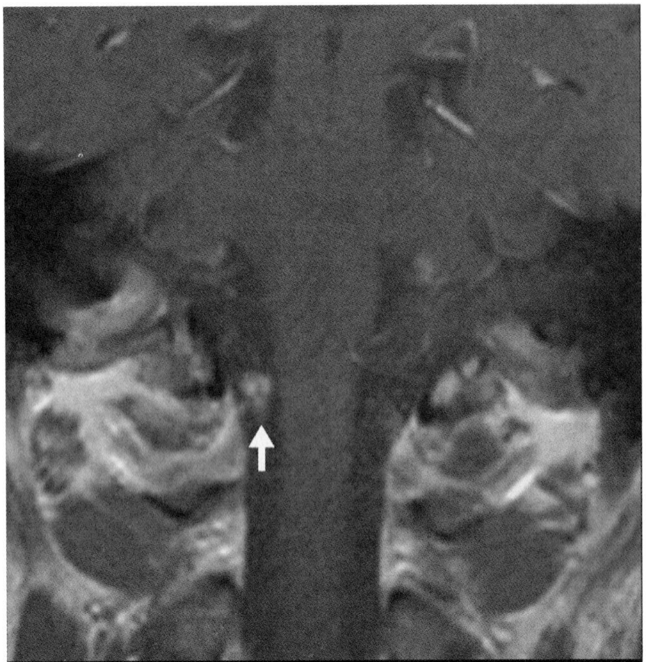

C

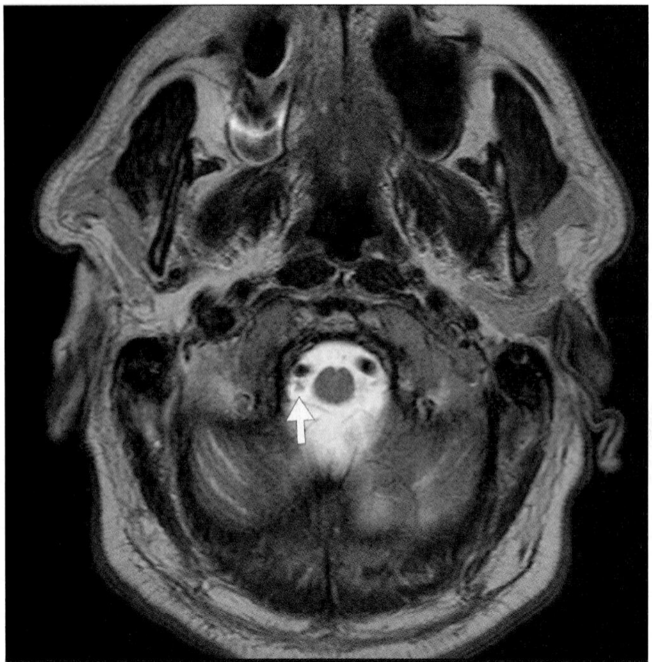

D

REFERENCES

Davagnanam, Chavda SV. Identification of the normal jugular foramen and lower cranial nerve anatomy: contrast-enhanced 3D fast imaging employing steady-state acquisition MR imaging. *AJNR Am J Neuroradiol.* 2008;29:574-576.

Lachman N, Acland RD, Rosse C. Anatomical evidence for the absence of a morphologically distinct cranial root of the accessory nerve in man. *Clin Anat.* 2002;15(1):4-10.

Leblanc, André. *Encephalo-Peripheral Nervous System: Vascularisation, Anatomy, Imaging.* Berlin: Springer, 2001.

Linn J, Peters F, Moriggl B, Naidich TP, Brückmann H, Yousry I. The jugular foramen: imaging strategy and detailed anatomy at 3T. *AJNR Am J Neuroradiol.* 2009;30:34-41.

CASE 35 Normal hypoglossal canal enhancement

There are paired hypoglossal canals which course anterolaterally along the ventral aspect of the basiocciput. The hypoglossal canal (also called anterior condylar canal) consistently enhances on postcontrast imaging studies in part because of a traversing anterior condylar vein. In addition, the hypoglossal artery, which is a neuromeningeal branch of the ascending pharyngeal artery, traverses the hypoglossal canal and contributes to the enhancement within the canal. The hypoglossal nerve can often be identified as a linear focus of hypoenhancement traversing through the hypoglossal canal.

Care should be taken not to misinterpret normal vascular enhancement in the hypoglossal canal as pathology, unless the enhancement pattern is different from the contralateral side, or there are secondary signs of pathology. Conversely, an enhancing mass may be occult on postcontrast CT or postcontrast spin-echo T1-weighted MRI because of the normal vascular enhancement in the hypoglossal canal. Therefore, utilizing a bone window on CT or other sequences on MRI are frequently necessary for accurate imaging interpretation. A bone window on CT is useful to assess for osseous remodeling, destruction, or tumoral mineralization that may be present with a hypoglossal mass. On MRI, T2, unenhanced T1, or contrast-enhanced MPRAGE imaging will often demonstrate a mass in the hypoglossal canal, if present.

COMPANION CASES

- **Asymmetrically enlarged anterior condylar vein.** Like veins elsewhere, one may encounter incidental asymmetry of the anterior condylar vein in the hypoglossal canal compared to its contralateral counterpart. When present, asymmetry of this vein may simulate a hypoglossal canal mass. Identifying similar imaging characteristics with other veins in the vicinity usually helps to correctly differentiate an incidentally enlarged anterior condylar vein from a mass.
- **CN XII meningioma.** While uncommon, occasionally meningiomas of the skull base can track along nerve a nerve, exit the skull base, and extend into the infratemporal fossa. The presence of mineralization within the mass and regional osseous hyperostosis helps differentiate a meningioma tracking along a skull base nerve from a schwannoma arising from a skull base nerve. Meningiomas are usually iso- to hypointense on T2 and diffusely enhance on MRI, although if mineralized, they may heterogeneously enhance.
- **CN XII schwannoma.** A schwannoma arising from a skull base nerve is far more common than a meningioma tracking along a skull base nerve. In contradistinction to a meningioma, a schwannoma usually remodels and smoothly enlarges a skull base foramen, best appreciated by CT. On MRI, a schwannoma is usually T2 hyperintense and enhances, although it may be quite heterogeneous on both T2 and postcontrast imaging, depending on the presence of cystic degeneration as well as the ratio of Antoni A (densely cellular) and Antoni B (loosely organized tissue) content.

Normal hypoglossal canal enhancement

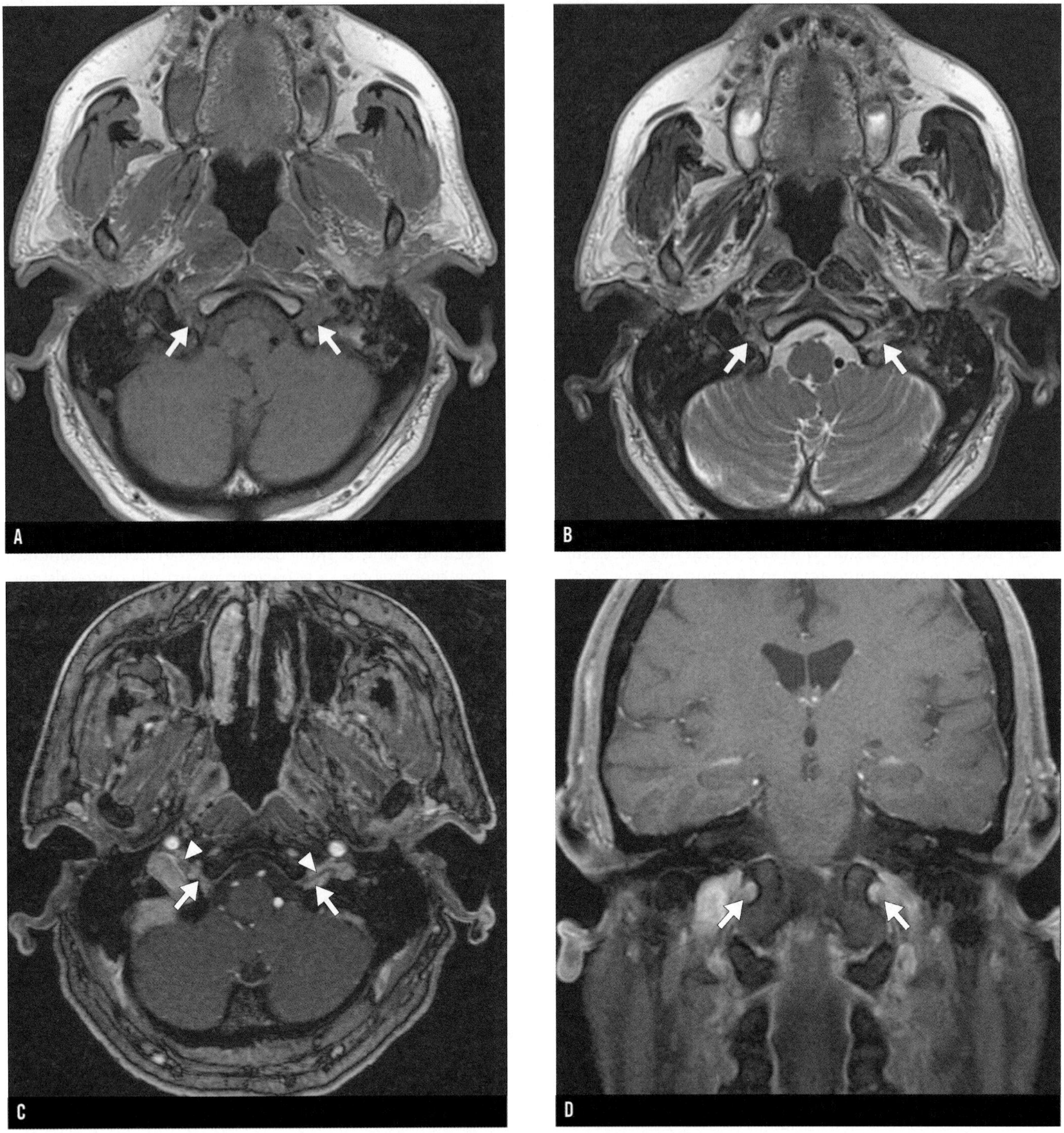

Unenhanced axial T1 (**A**), axial T2 (**B**), postcontrast axial MPRAGE (**C**), and postcontrast coronal T1 with fat suppression (**D**) MR images demonstrate the normal signal characteristics and expected enhancement of the hypoglossal canals (arrows, **A**-**D**). The normal hypoglossal nerves are identified as single, thin, linear foci of hypointense signal traversing through the hypoglossal canals on image **C** (arrowheads, **C**).

Companion case: Asymmetrically enlarged condylar vein

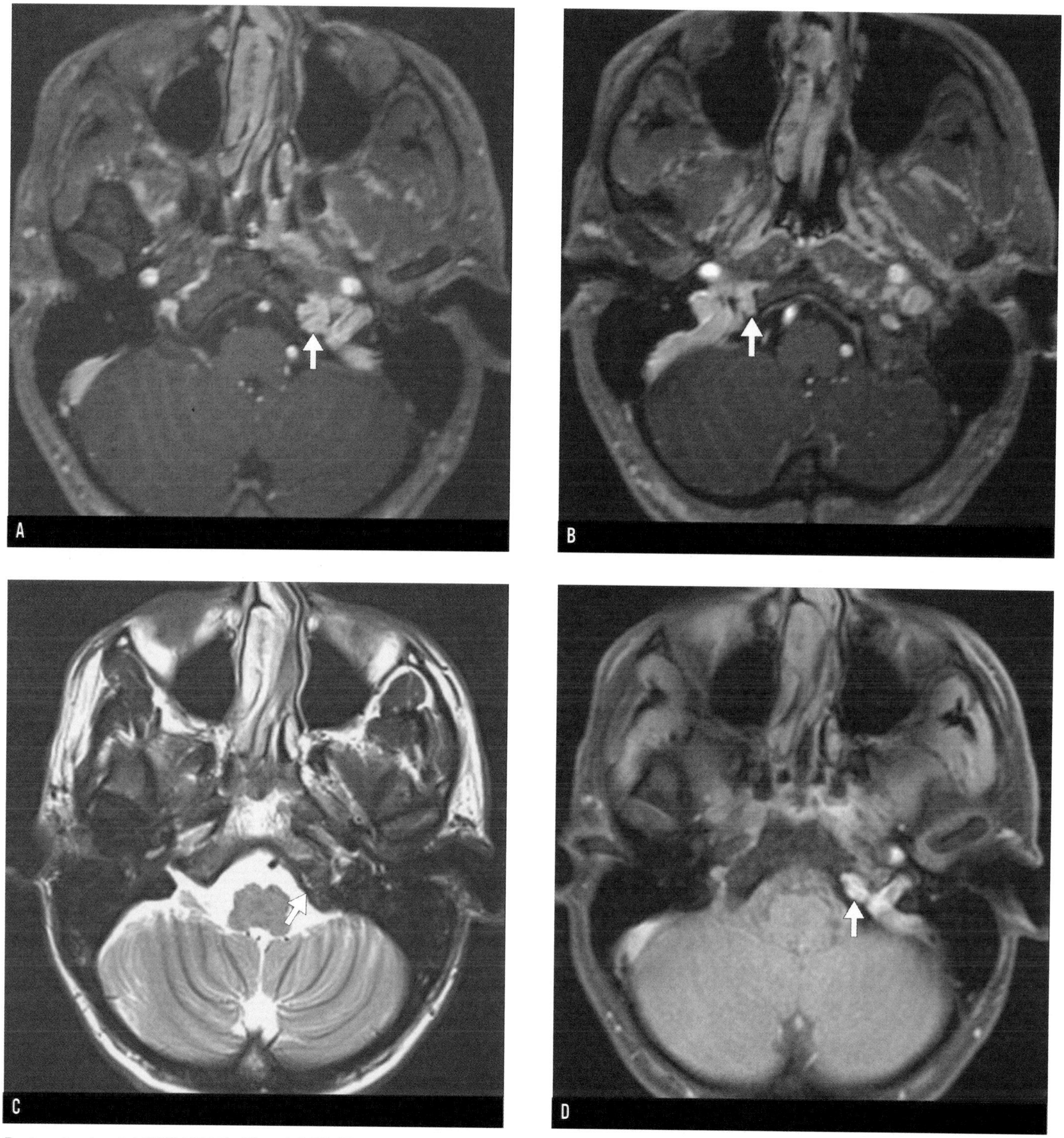

Postcontrast axial MPRAGE (**A, B**), axial T2 (**C**), and unenhanced axial T1 (**D**) MR images performed on a 3T magnet demonstrate asymmetric enhancement within the left hypoglossal canal (arrow, **A**) relative to the right hypoglossal canal (arrow, **B**). Image **C** does not demonstrate a focal abnormality in the left hypoglossal canal (arrow, **C**). Image **D** demonstrates incidental, normal flow-related signal within the anterior condylar vein (arrow, **D**). Normal flow-related signal within arteries and veins is often present with 3T unenhanced T1-weighted imaging, as is present in this case. The asymmetry of the finding did initially raise concern for a focal abnormality in the left hypoglossal canal. However, the enhancement in the hypoglossal canal was contiguous with additional veins anterior and inferior to the hypoglossal canal, known as the anterior condylar confluence (not shown). Coupled with the presence of normal venous flow-related signal in this region on unenhanced T1-weighted imaging, the finding is most compatible with incidental asymmetry of the anterior condylar vein rather than a mass.

Companion case: CN XII meningioma

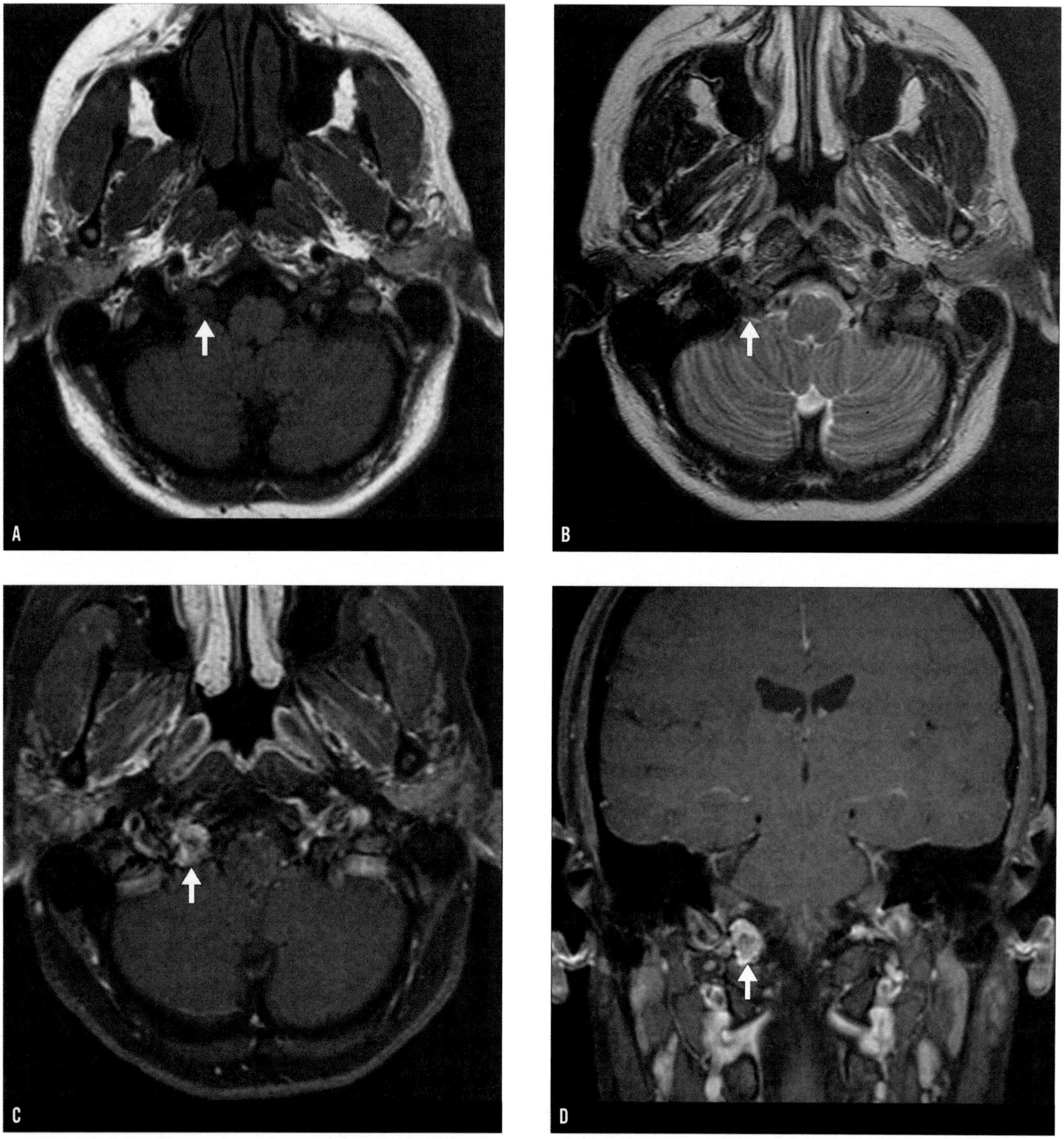

Axial unenhanced T1 (**A**), axial T2 (**B**), postcontrast axial T1 with fat suppression (**C**), and coronal postcontrast T1 with fat suppression (**D**) MR images demonstrate a bulbous, mildly T2 hypointense, enhancing mass extending from the right cerebellar-medullary cistern into right hypoglossal canal (arrows, **A-D**). The enhancing right hypoglossal canal is abnormally expanded on image **D** (arrow). An axial unenhanced T1-weighted MR image through the tongue (**E**) demonstrates abnormal fatty infiltration of the right hemitongue (arrow, **E**). These findings are compatible with a right hypoglossal canal mass with chronic denervation atrophy of the right hemitongue. An axial CT image through the right hypoglossal canal (**F**) demonstrates abnormal expansion and mild wall sclerosis of the right hypoglossal canal related to the mass which is partially calcified (arrow, **F**). The presence of calcium is rare in benign schwannomas but common with meningiomas. The mass was a hypoglossal meningioma at pathology.

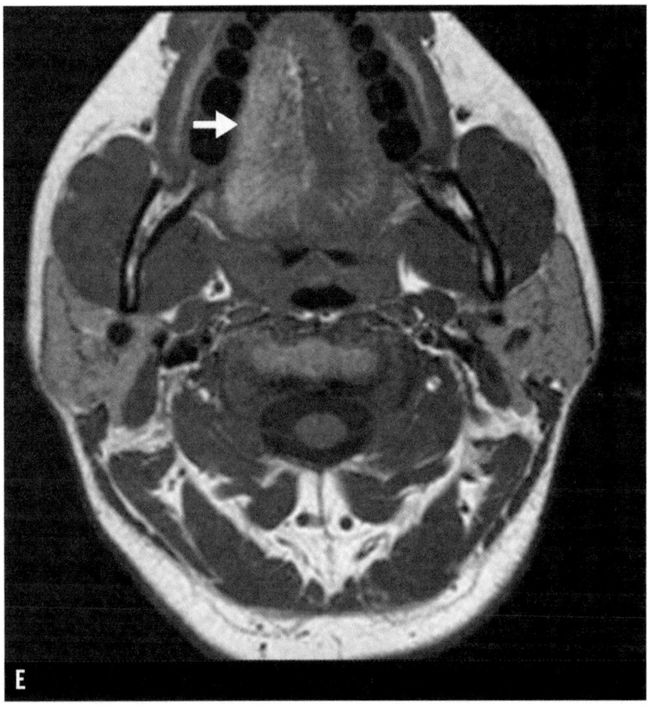

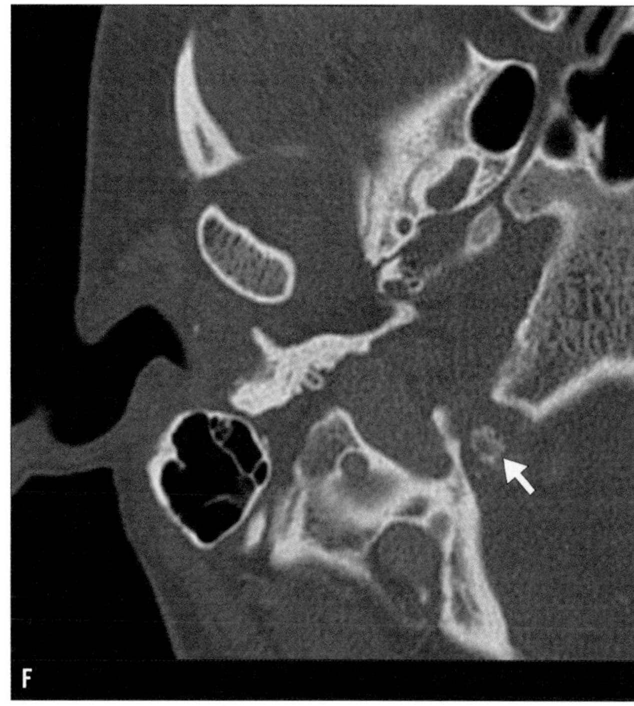

Companion case: CN XII schwannoma

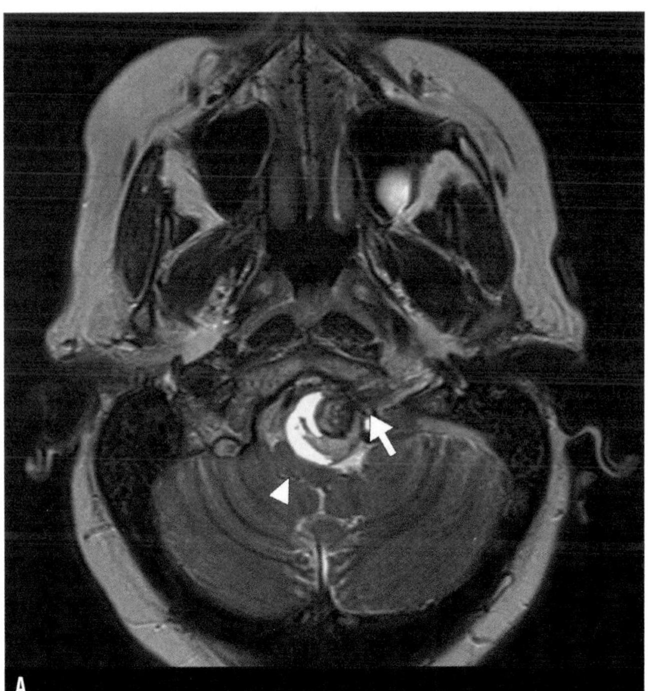

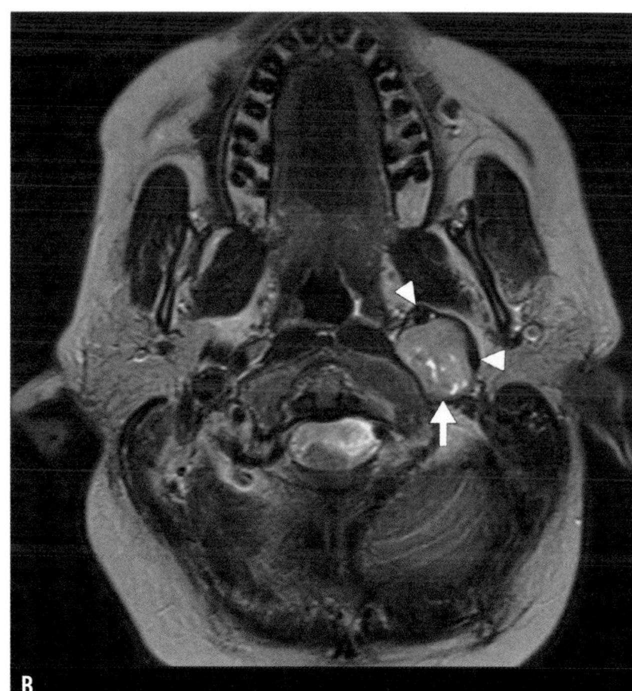

Axial T2 (**A**, **B**) and postcontrast axial MPRAGE (**C**, **D**) MR images demonstrate a T2 heterogeneous and enhancing mass extending from the left premedullary cistern, through the left hypoglossal canal (arrows, **A**, **C**), and into the left poststyloid parapharyngeal space (arrows, **B**, **D**). The lesion markedly deforms the medulla oblongata (arrowheads, **A**, **C**) and displaces the distal left cervical carotid artery and proximal left internal jugular vein (arrowheads, **B**, **D**). The mass was a hypoglossal nerve schwannoma at pathology.

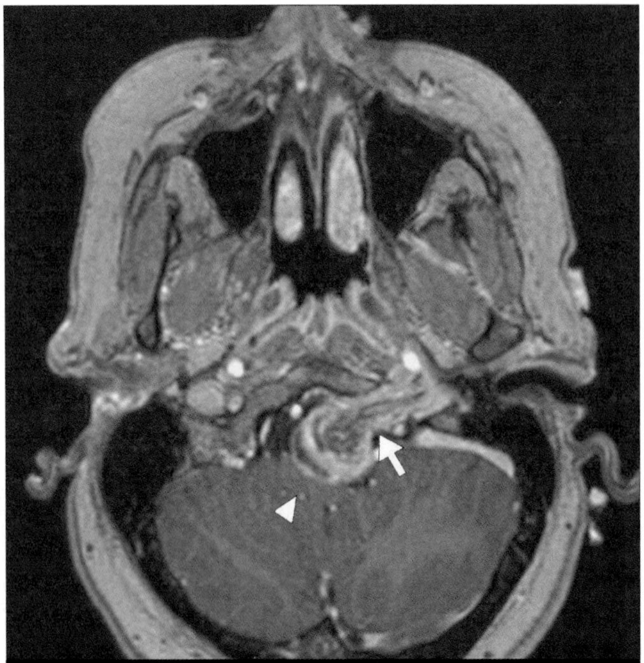

C

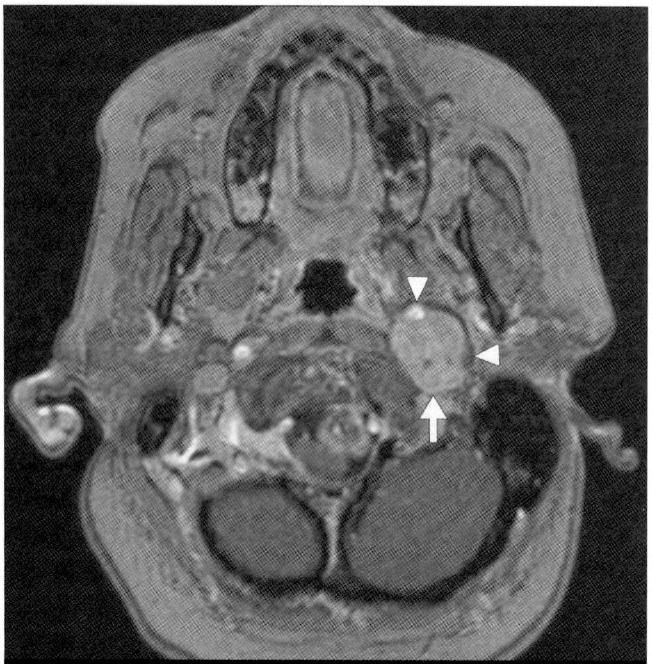

D

REFERENCES

Ernst R, Bulas R, Tomsick T, van Loveren H, Aziz KA. Three cases of dural arteriovenous fistula of the anterior condylar vein within the hypoglossal canal. *AJNR Am J Neuroradiol.* 1999;20:2016-2020.

San Millán Ruíz D, Gailloud P, Rüfenacht DA, Delavelle J, Henry F, Fasel JH. The craniocervical venous system in relation to cerebral venous drainage. *AJNR Am J Neuroradiol.* 2002;23(9):1500-1508.

Tanoue S, Kiyosue H, Sagara Y, Hori Y, Okahara M, Kashiwagi J, Mori H. Venous structures at the craniocervical junction: anatomical variations evaluated by multidetector row CT. *Br J Radiol.* 2010;83(994):831-840. Epub July 2010.

Voyvodic F, Whyte A, Slavotinek J. The hypoglossal canal: normal MR enhancement pattern. *AJNR Am J Neuroradiol.* 1995;16(8):1707-1710.

CASE 36 Mastoid emissary veins

Emissary veins traverse the calvarium and connect the intracranial venous system with the extracranial venous system. Blood in emissary veins typically flows away from the brain, although these veins are valveless and therefore blood may flow in either direction. There are many types of emissary veins and they are described based on their anatomic location. One of the more common emissary veins is the mastoid emissary vein, which anastomoses the suboccipital venous plexus or posterior auricular vein with the sigmoid sinus. In one large study examining skulls from cadavers, the mastoid emissary foramina and veins were present in 98% of skulls on the right and in 72% of skulls on the left. In the same study, the mean diameter at the level of the mastoid foramen measured 3.5 mm with a range of 1.1 to 5.6 mm.

Emissary veins have been shown to represent significant venous outflow pathways, particularly in the upright position. They are also important in the setting of bilateral jugular venous obstruction or idiopathic intracranial hypertension, as they can serve as a "safety valve" for venous drainage.

COMPANION CASES

- **Mildly enlarged mastoid emissary vein in Crouzon syndrome.** In syndromic craniosynostosis cases, such as Crouzon and Apert syndrome, jugular venous outflow stenosis or atresia results in compensatory enlargement of emissary veins. When large, emissary veins that are breached during a rectosigmoid or far lateral approach craniotomy can result in massive hemorrhage. Additionally, large mastoid emissary vein coagulation during surgery has been reported to cause cerebellar infarction. If large emissary veins are encountered at imaging and surgery is being contemplated in that region, then describing these veins and notifying the surgeon to their presence is warranted.
- **Acquired occipital bone vascular channels related to a large arteriovenous fistula.** Emissary veins can enlarge with high-flow vascular lesions, including arteriovenous fistulas. Additionally, if present, arterial feeders supplying a fistula can grow transosseously and anastomose with the affected dural venous sinus, resulting in small osseous channels in the calvarium.

Mastoid emissary veins

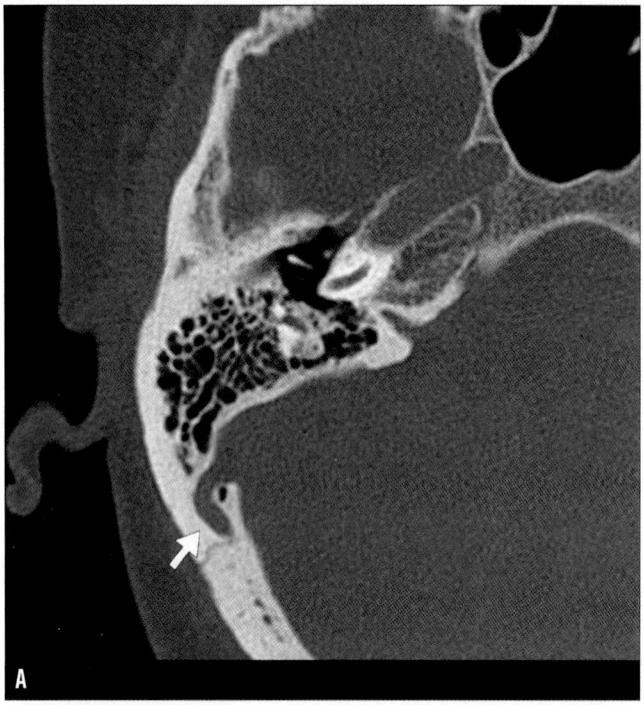

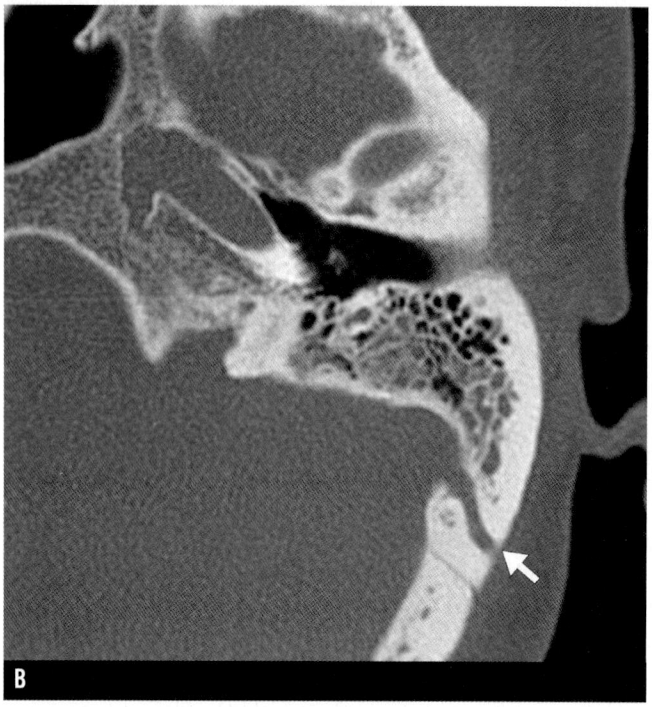

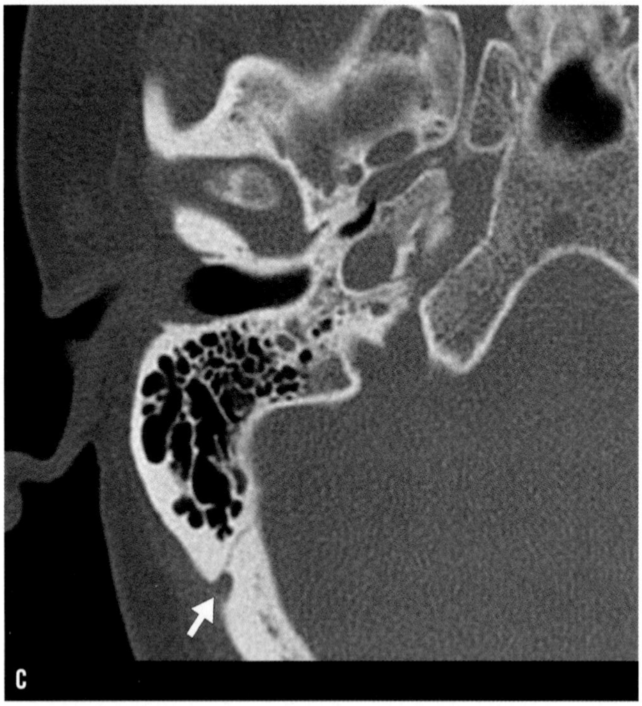

Axial CT images through the mastoid portions of the temporal bones (**A-C**) demonstrate typical bilateral mastoid emissary veins (arrows, **A-C**).

Companion case: Mildly enlarged mastoid emissary vein in Crouzon syndrome

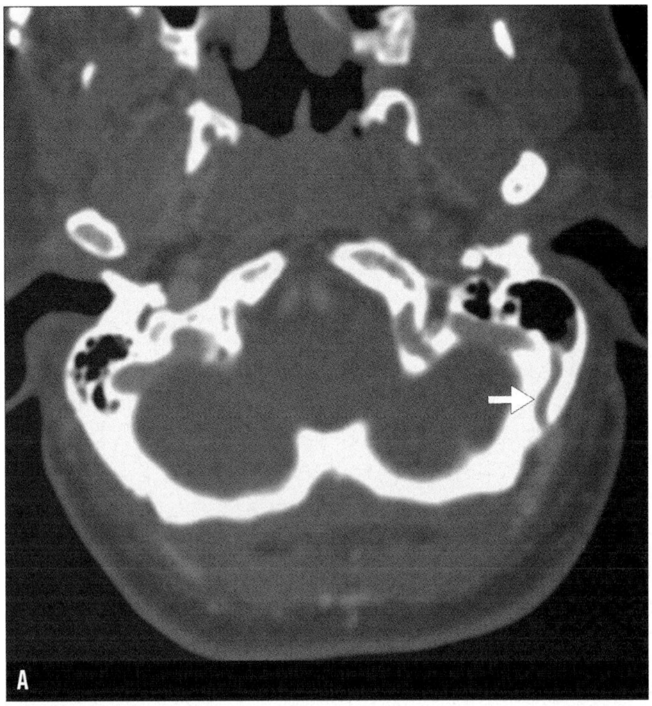

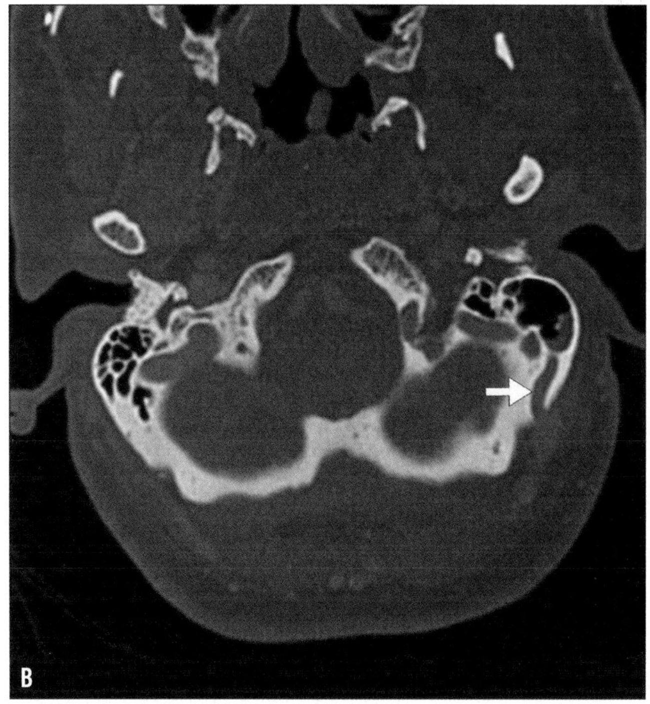

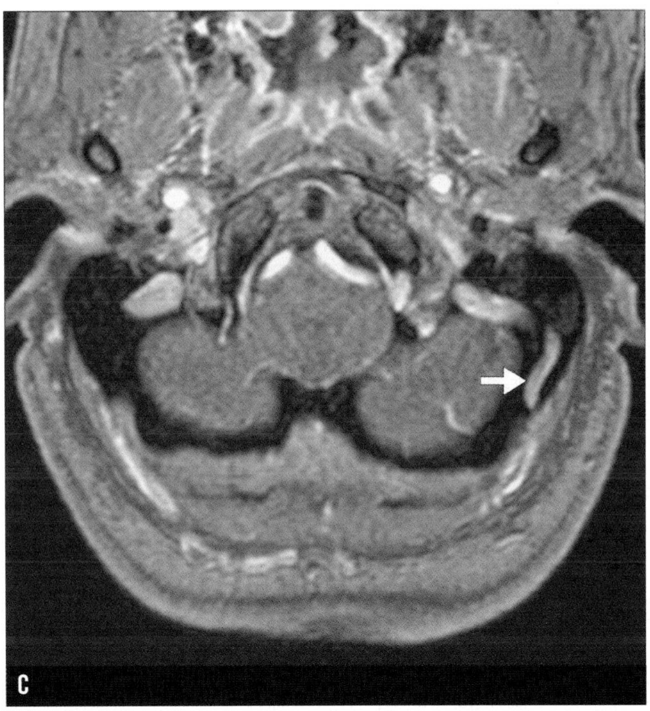

A contrast-enhanced axial CT image through the occipital-mastoid junction viewed with an intermediate window (**A**) and bone window (**B**) demonstrate a mildly enlarged left mastoid emissary vein (arrows, **A, B**). A postcontrast axial MPRAGE MR image through the same level (**C**) demonstrates normal enhancement of the left mastoid emissary vein (arrow, **C**).

Companion case: Acquired occipital bone vascular channels related to a large arterio-venous fistula

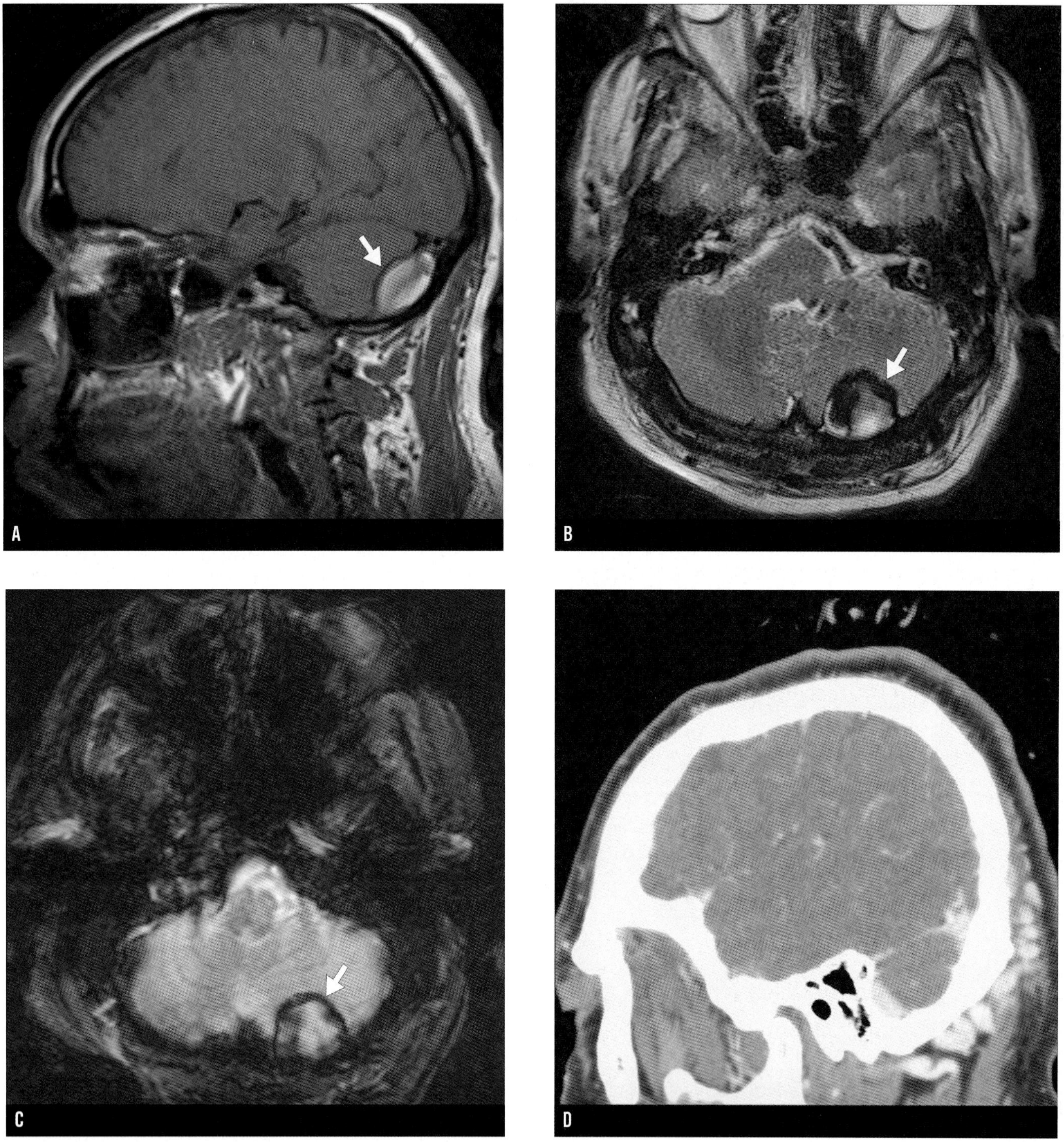

Unenhanced sagittal T1 (**A**), axial T2 BLADE (**B**), and axial GRE (**C**) MR images demonstrate an elliptical lesion that is T1 hyperintense, heterogeneous on T2, and containing peripheral gradient susceptibility located within the left parasagittal posterior aspect of the posterior fossa (arrows, **A**-**C**). This is compatible with a thrombosed varix, most likely of the left occipital sinus. Sagittal reformatted (**D**) and axial (**E**) CT images from a CTA demonstrate innumerable abnormally enlarged suboccipital vessels which represented the occipital arteries. Coronal reformatted (**F**) and axial (**G**) CT images from the same study viewed with a bone window demonstrate innumerable small osseous channels in the occipital calvarium. The findings suggest a dural arterio-venous fistula with multiple abnormal transcalvarial occipital arteries supplying the dural fistula. A right occipital arterial injection during a cerebral angiogram viewed in the AP (**H**) and lateral (**I**) projections confirm an extensive dural arterio-venous fistula with multiple fistulous connections from occipital artery branches.

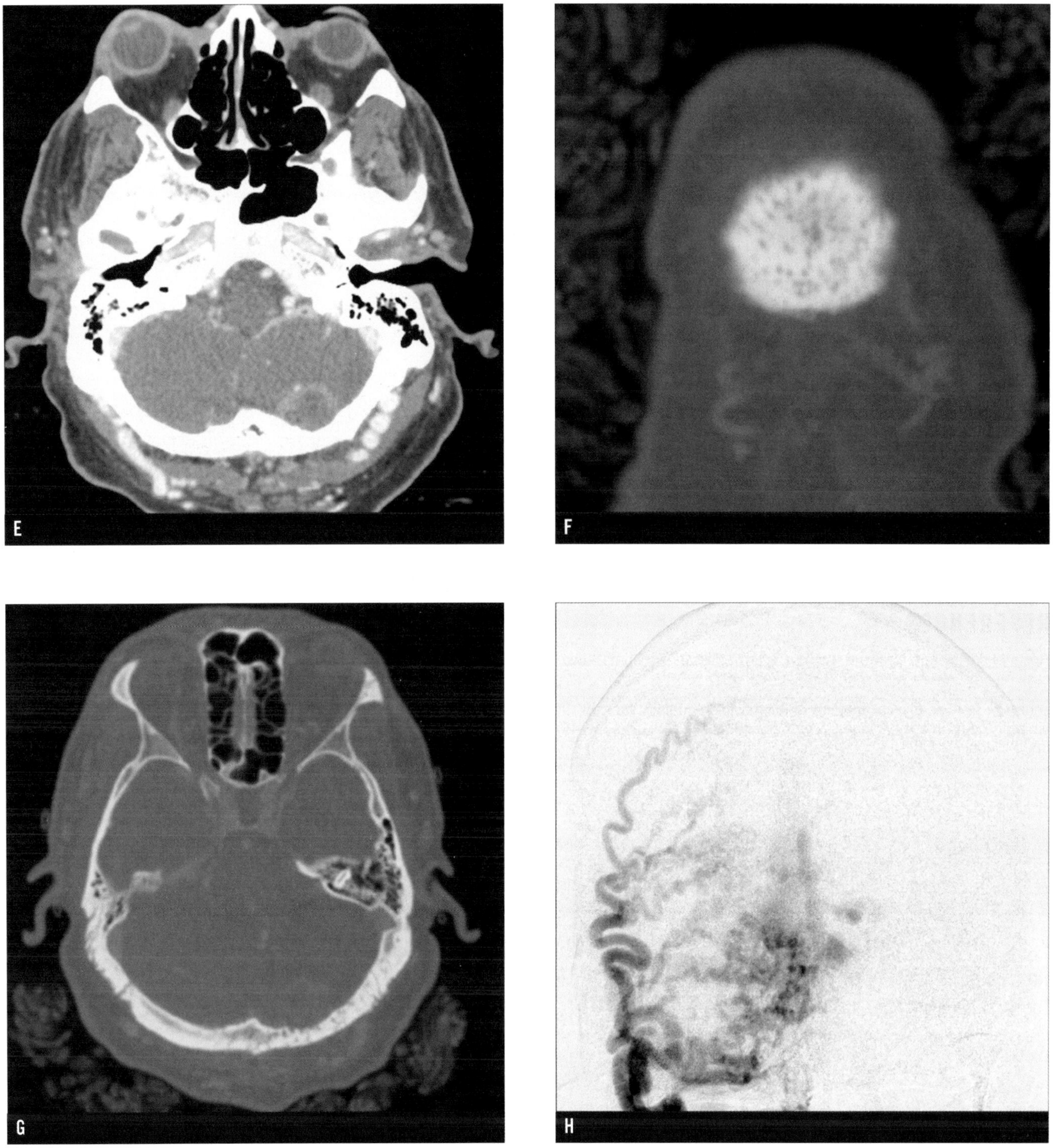

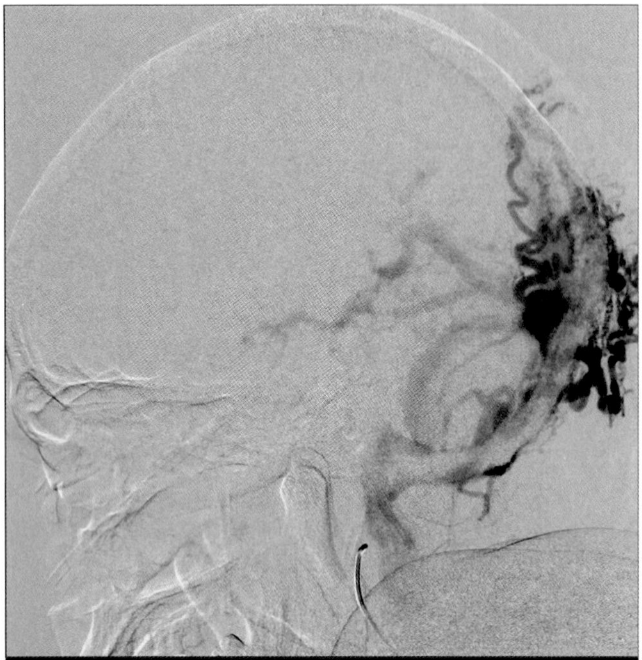

I

REFERENCES

Hoshi M, Yoshida K, Ogawa K, Kawase T. Hypoglossal neurinoma—two case reports. *Neurol Med Chir.* 2000;40:489-493.

Louis RG Jr, et al. Clinical anatomy of the mastoid and occipital emissary veins in a large series. *Surg Radiol Anat.* 2009;31(2):139-144. Epub October 2008.

Reis CV, et al. Anatomy of the mastoid emissary vein and venous system of the posterior neck region: neurosurgical implications. *Neurosurgery.* 2007;61:193-201.

CASE 37 Posterior condylar canal and vein

Similar to other emissary veins, the posterior condylar vein anastomoses the intracranial venous system with the extracranial venous system. The posterior condylar canal contains the posterior condylar vein and the meningeal branch of the occipital artery. The canal is located just medial to the sigmoid sinus and traverses in an anteromedial direction, from posterior to anterior. The posterior condylar vein most commonly arises from the sigmoid sinus, traverses the posterior condylar canal, and drains into the suboccipital cavernous sinus (a venous plexus surrounding the distal horizontal segment of the vertebral artery).

Posterior condylar canal and vein

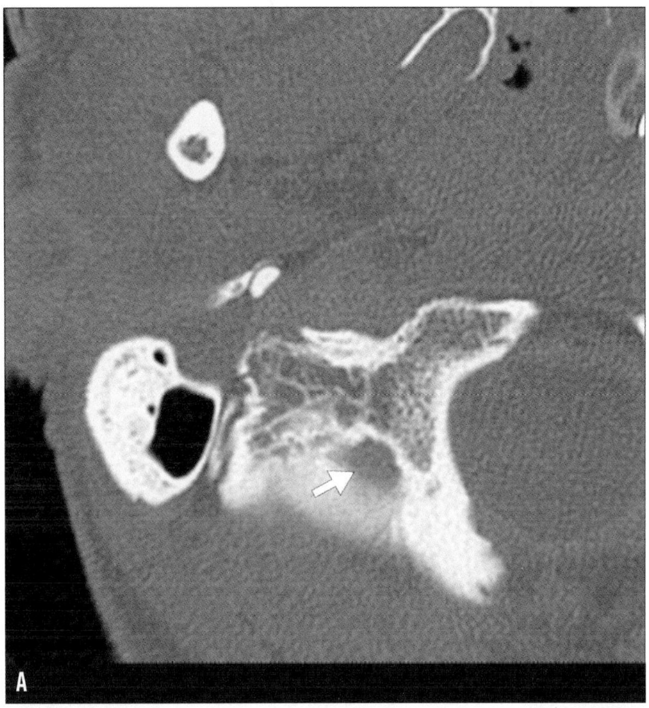

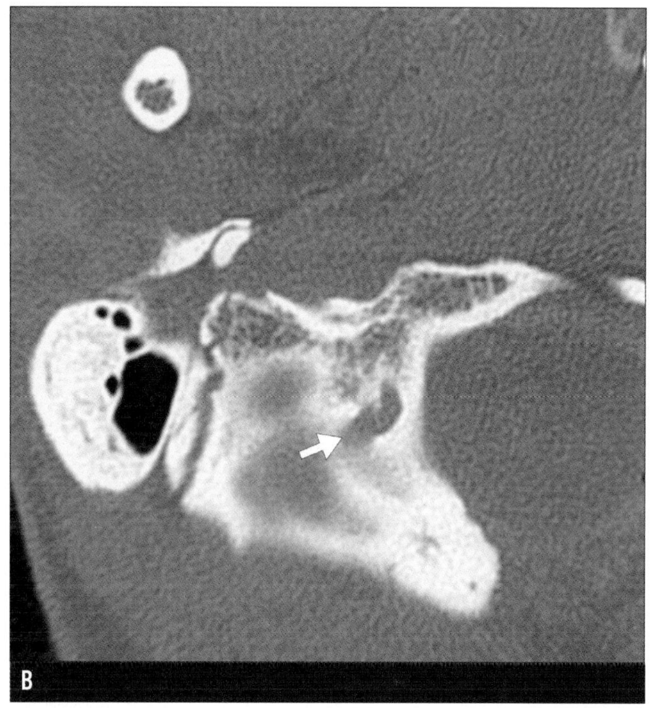

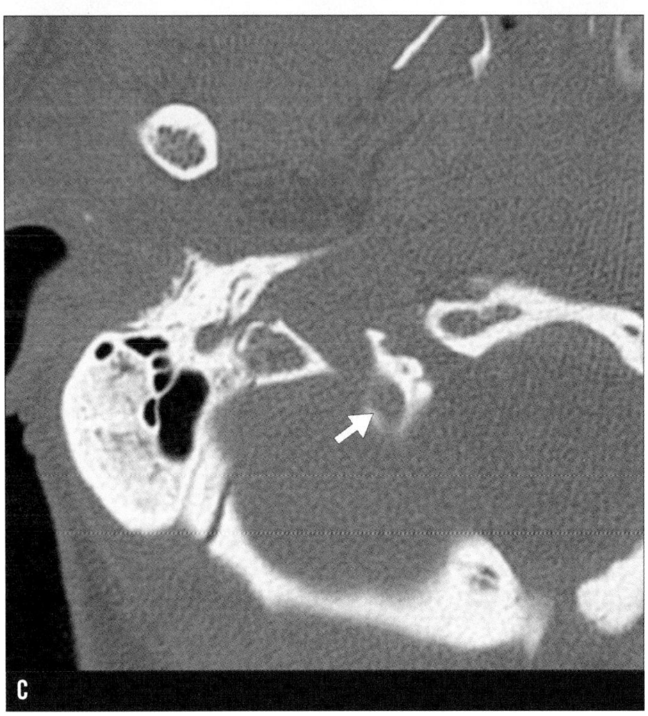

Axial CT images through the bilateral occipital-mastoid junctions viewed with a bone window (**A-E**) demonstrate the normal posterior condylar canals (arrows, **A-E**). Axial images from a CTA viewed with a soft tissue window (**F, G**) demonstrate enhancement occupying the posterior condylar canals related to normal posterior condylar veins (arrows, **F, G**).

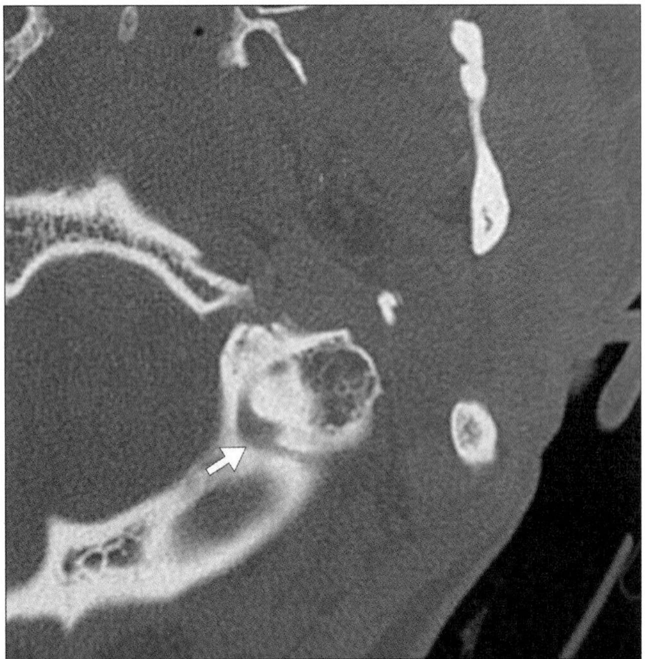
D

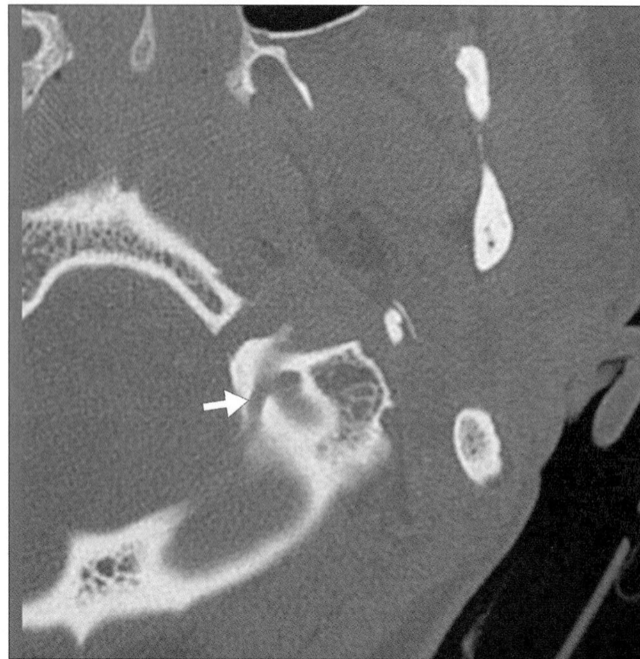
E

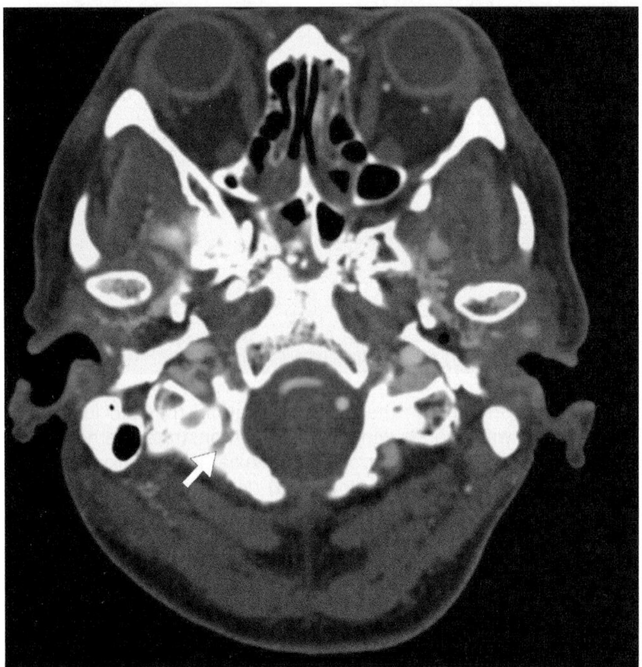
F

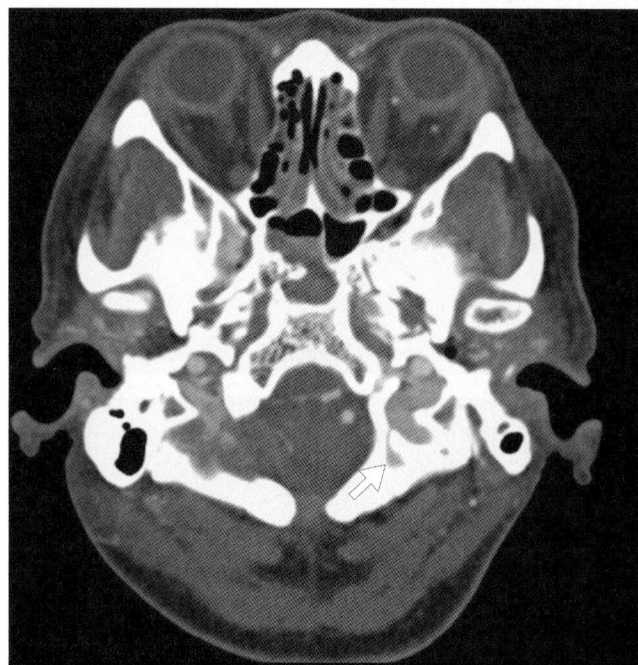
G

REFERENCES

Kiyosue H, et al. Dural arteriovenous fistula involving the posterior condylar canal. *AJNR Am J Neuroradiol.* 2007;28(8):1599-1601.

San Millán Ruíz D, Gailloud P, Rüfenacht DA, Delavelle J, Henry F, Fasel JH. The craniocervical venous system in relation to cerebral venous drainage. *AJNR Am J Neuroradiol.* 2002;23(9):1500-1508.

Tanoue S, et al. Venous structures at the craniocervical junction: anatomical variations evaluated by multidetector row CT. *Br J Radiol.* 2010;83(994):831-840. Epub July 2010.

CASE 38 Petrosquamosal sinus

The petrosquamosal sinus is an uncommon emissary vein that arises from the posterolateral aspect of the transverse sinus and traverses along the superolateral border of the petrous temporal bone. The petrosquamosal sinus can drain via one of two pathways: anteroinferiorly into the retromandibular vein, or anteromedially through the foramen ovale and into the pterygoid venous plexus.

Petrosquamosal sinus

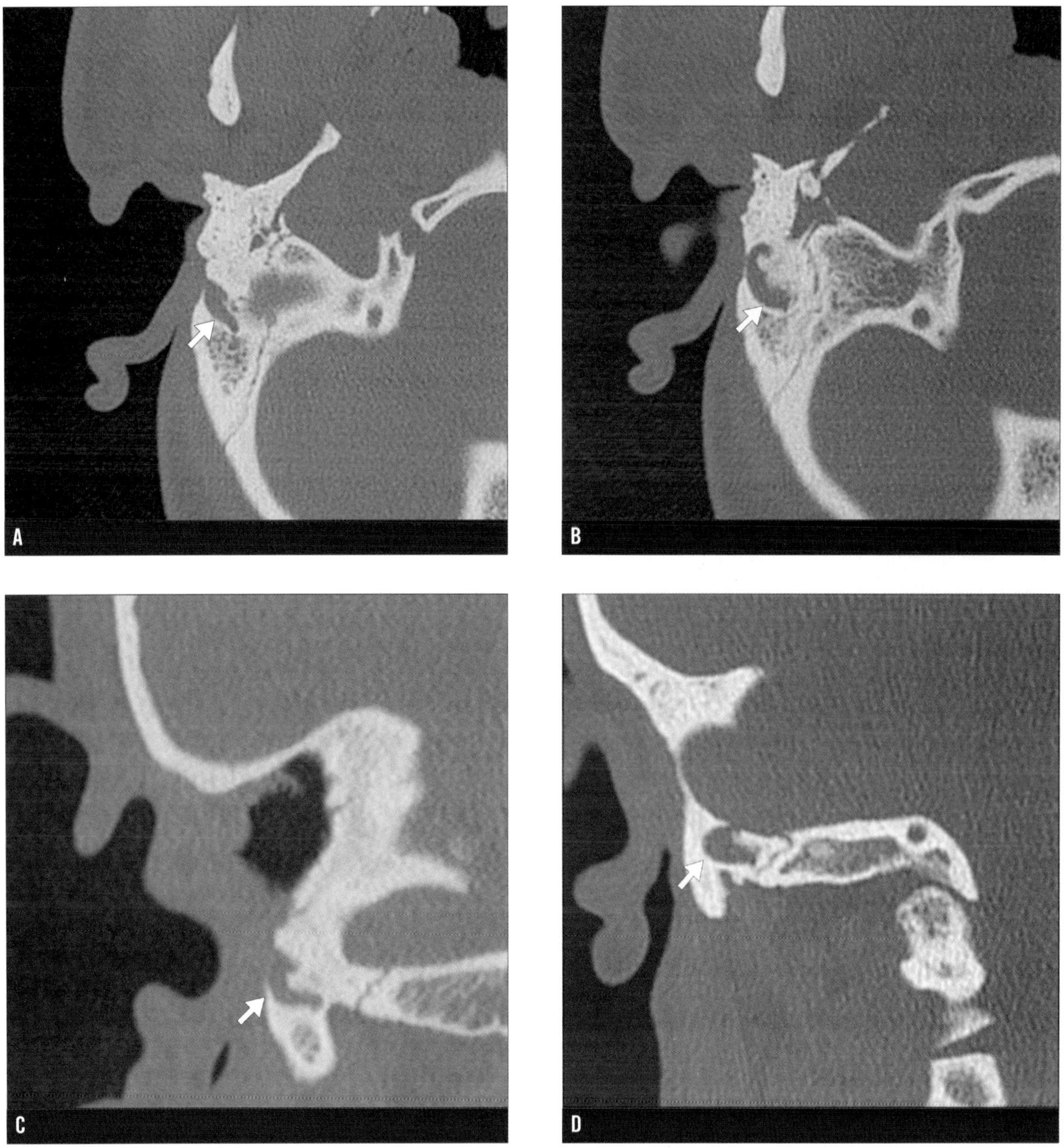

Axial (**A**, **B**) and direct coronal (**C**, **D**) CT images demonstrate a tortuous, circumscribed lucency along the lateral aspect of the right temporal bone, compatible with a petrosquamosal sinus just prior to exiting the skull base (arrows, **A-D**). Axial T1 (**E**), postcontrast axial T1 with fat suppression (**F**), and axial T2 (**G**) MR images of the same patient demonstrate the petrosquamosal sinus as a mildly enhancing, T2 hyperintense structure compatible with slow venous flow (arrows, **E-G**). Given its course, this petrosquamosal sinus likely anastomoses with the right retromandibular vein (not shown).

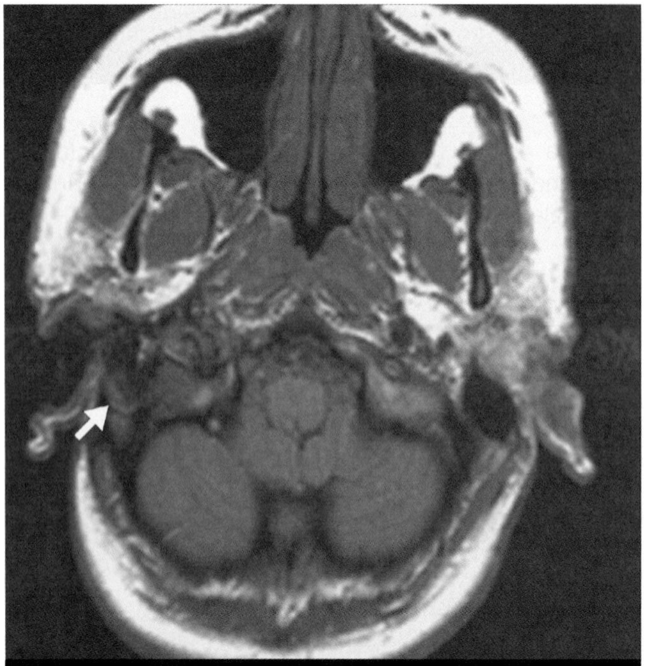

E

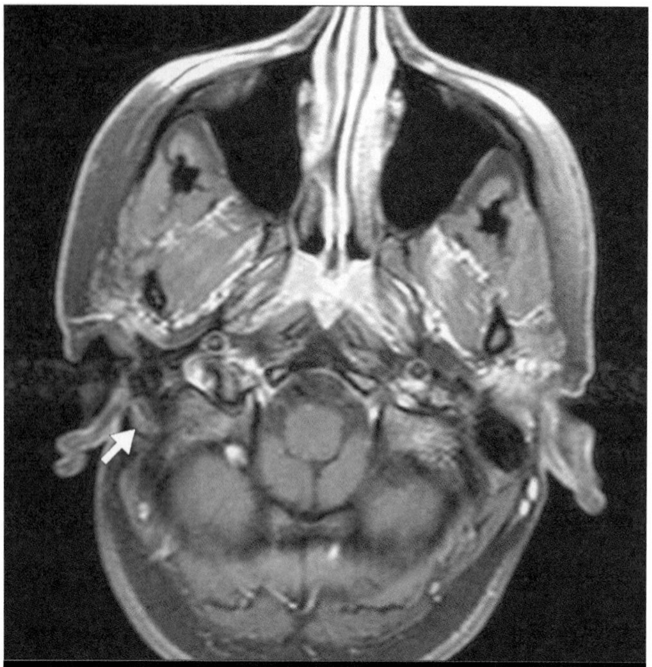

F

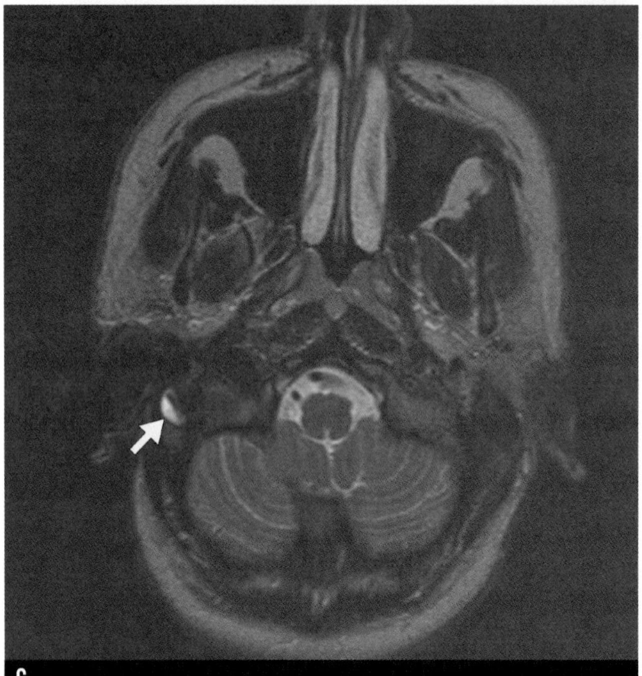

G

REFERENCE

Marsot-Dupuch K, Gayet-Delacroix M, Elmaleh-Bergès M, Bonneville F, Lasjaunias P. The petrosquamosal sinus: CT and MR findings of a rare emissary vein. *AJNR Am J Neuroradiol.* 2001;22(6):1186-1193.

CASE 39 Occipital sinus

The occipital sinus originates from the torcular herophili and traverses along the occipital crest directly inferior the cerebellar hemisphere, most commonly draining into the sigmoid sinus. However, occasionally an occipital sinus may drain into the marginal sinus, which is a sinus located along the lateral aspect of the foramen magnum.

Occipital sinus

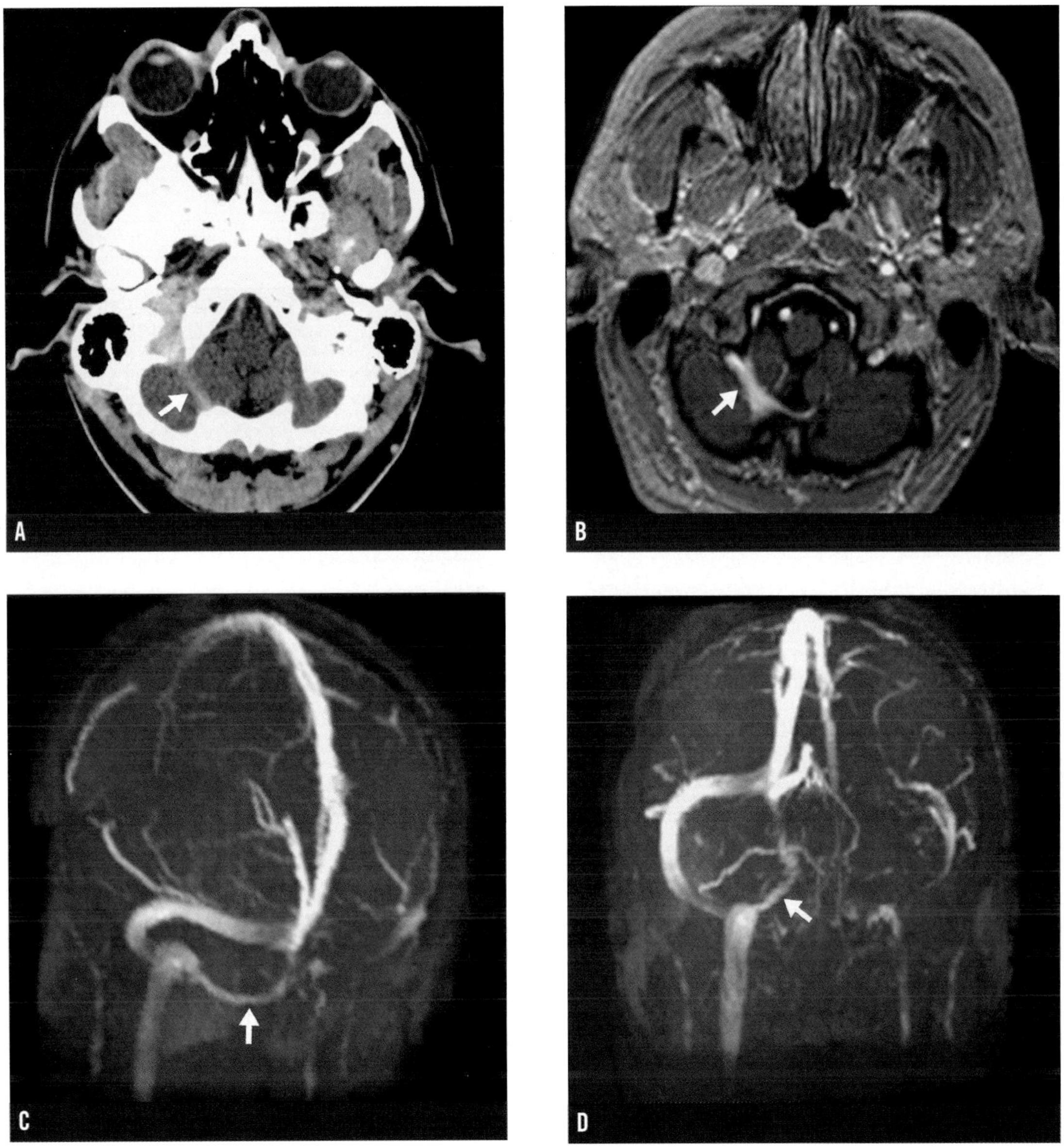

An axial postcontrast CT image from a CTA (**A**), a postcontrast axial MPRAGE MR image (**B**), and two maximum intensity projection images from an MRV (**C**, **D**) demonstrate a normal right occipital sinus (arrows, **A**-**D**).

REFERENCE

Tanoue S, et al. Venous structures at the craniocervical junction: anatomical variations evaluated by multidetector row CT. *Br J Radiol.* 2010;83(994):831-840. Epub July 2010.

CASE 40 Air-tissue interface artifact on 3T MRI

Tissue susceptibility refers to the inherent magnetism of a particular tissue. The greater the degree of tissue susceptibility, the more there is an effect on local resonance frequencies, resulting in increasing spin dephasing, image distortion, and signal loss. In addition, a small local magnetic field gradient and susceptibility artifact arises when two immediately adjacent tissues/structures have a significantly different amount of susceptibility. This susceptibility artifact is often present at the skull base where a significant disparity in the amount of susceptibility exists between the paranasal sinuses and brain. MRI susceptibility artifacts also increase at higher magnetic fields. Susceptibilty artifacts on postcontrast T1-weighted imaging may simulate abnormal enhancement. However, the same artifact is usually also present on unenhanced T1-weighted imaging, aiding in appropriately identifying the finding as artifactual on the postcontrast sequence. These artifacts can be improved by increasing receiver bandwidth, applying parallel imaging techniques, and shortening the TE.

Air-tissue interface artifact on 3T MRI

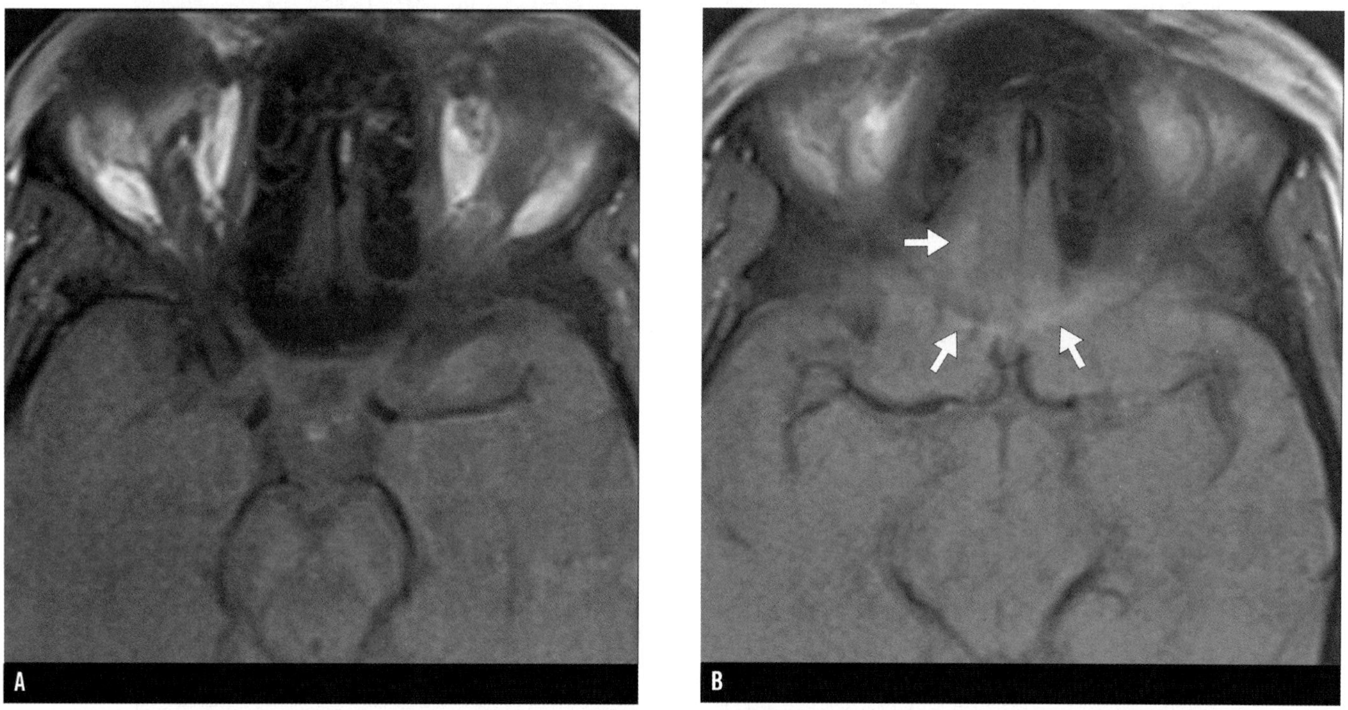

Unenhanced axial T1-weighted and postcontrast axial T1-weighted MR images through the ethmoid air cells (**A, D,** respectively), frontal sinuses and ethmoid air cells (**B, E,** respectively), and the anterior cranial fossa (**C, F,** respectively). This study was performed on a 3 Tesla magnet and demonstrates susceptibility artifact along the anterior skull base related to an air-tissue interface between the paranasal sinuses and the overlying brain. (arrows, **B, C, E, F**). The artifact on the postcontrast T1-weighted images could be mistaken for abnormal enhancement if it is not noticed on the precontrast T1-weighted images.

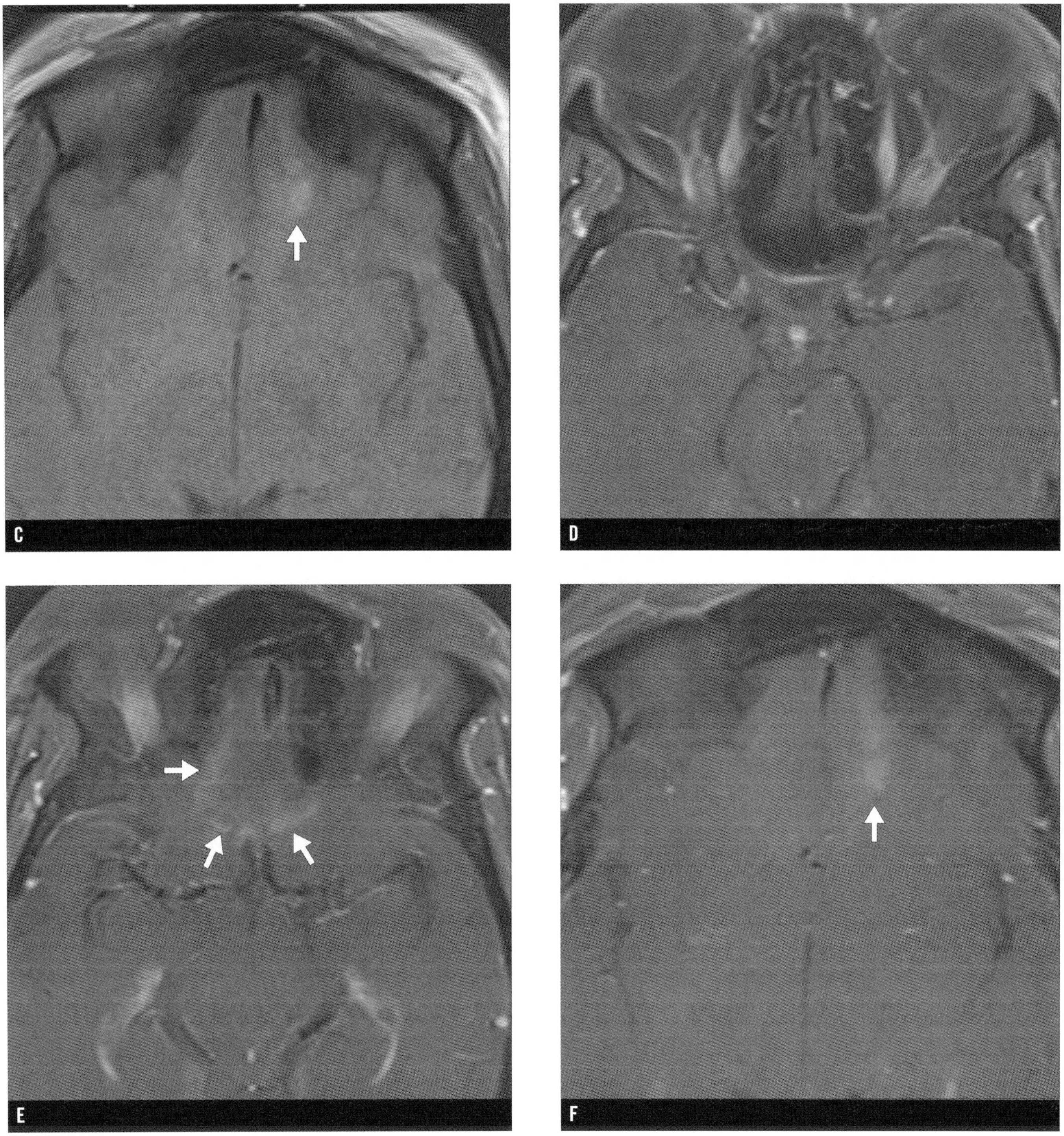

REFERENCES

Frayne R, Goodyear BG, Dickhoff P, Lauzon ML, Sevick RJ. Magnetic resonance imaging at 3.0 Tesla: challenges and advantages in clinical neurological imaging. *Invest Radiol.* 2003;38(7):385-402.

Vargas MI, Delavelle J, Kohler R, Becker CD, Lovblad K. Brain and spine MRI artifacts at 3Tesla. *J Neuroradiol.* 2009;36(2):74-81. Epub October 2008. Review.

CHAPTER 8

TEMPORAL BONE

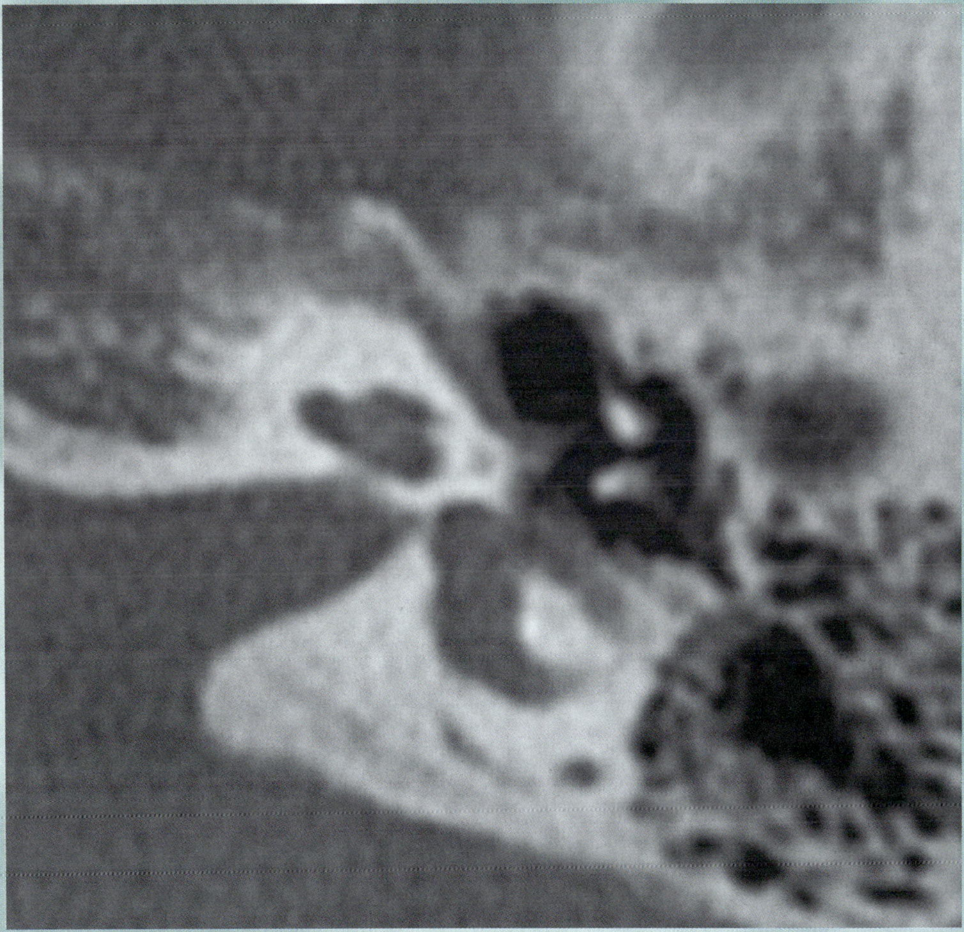

Erin N. McComb, Achilles G. Karagianis

VIII. TEMPORAL BONE

1. Cauliflower or boxer's ear
   i. *Companion case*: Auricular keloid
   ii. *Companion case*: Auricular squamous cell carcinoma
2. Auricular mineralization
3. Auricular reconstruction
4. Partial ossification of the cartilaginous EAC
5. Normal anterior tympanic plate lucencies
   i. *Companion case*: Fractures of the anterior tympanic plates
6. Osseous EAC size variation
   i. *Companion case*: EAC exostoses
   ii. *Companion case*: EAC osteoma
7. EAC cerumen
   i. *Companion case*: EAC squamous cell carcinoma
   ii. *Companion case*: EAC adenoid cystic carcinoma
   iii. *Companion case*: EAC cholesteatoma
   iv. *Companion case*: Keratosis obturans
8. Tympanoplasties
9. Myringotomy tubes
   i. *Companion case*: Displaced myringotomy tube into the EAC
   ii. *Companion case*: Displaced myringotomy tube into the tympanic cavity
   iii. *Companion case*: Displaced earring into the EAC
10. Atticoantrostomy
11. Mastoidectomies
    i. *Companion case*: Automastoidectomy
    ii. *Companion case*: Progressive mastoidectomy fat graft enhancement because of fat necrosis
12. Varying degrees of normal ossicular mineralization
    i. *Companion case*: Tympanosclerosis
    ii. *Companion case*: Ossicular erosion from a cholesteatoma
13. Suspensory ligaments of the ossicles
    i. *Companion case*: Bony bar
14. Tensor tympani muscle and tendon
15. Ossicular prostheses
16. Storage of the incus in the mastoid bowl
17. Deep sinus tympani
18. Persistent stapedial artery
19. Aberrant internal carotid artery
20. Lateralized petrous internal carotid artery
21. High-riding jugular bulb
    i. *Companion case*: Dehiscent high-riding jugular bulb
    ii. *Companion case*: High-riding jugular bulb dehiscent with the posterior semicircular canal
22. Jugular bulb diverticulum
    i. *Companion case*: Jugular bulb diverticulum dehiscent with the mastoid air cells
    ii. *Companion case*: Jugular bulb diverticulum dehiscent with the hypotympanum
23. Aberrant sigmoid sinus with a sigmoid sinus diverticulum
    i. *Companion case*: Aberrant sigmoid sinus with a dehiscent sigmoid sinus diverticulum
24. Cochlear cleft
    i. *Companion case*: Fenestral otosclerosis
    ii. *Companion case*: Retrofenestral otosclerosis
    iii. *Companion case*: Otosyphilis
25. Apparent abnormal inner ear signal on 5-mm T2-weighted MR imaging
    i. *Companion case*: Labyrinthitis ossificans
26. Intratympanic steroid injection
    i. *Companion case*: Intralabyrinthine hemorrhage
    ii. *Companion case*: Acute labyrinthitis
    iii. *Companion case*: Intralabyrinthine schwannoma
27. Cochlear implant
28. Fully implantable hearing system
29. Conventional hearing aids
30. Bone-anchored hearing device
31. False-positive superior semicircular canal dehiscence
    i. *Companion case*: Superior semicircular canal dehiscence
32. Repair of superior semicircular canal dehiscence
33. Singular canal
34. Subarcuate canal
35. Variations of the IAC
    i. *Companion case*: Congenital X-linked hearing loss
36. Petrous temporal bone marrow simulating an IAC lesion on MRI
37. Asymmetry of the petrous apices
    i. *Companion case*: Intraosseous venous malformation (intraosseous hemangioma)
38. Petrous apex effusion
    i. *Companion case*: Cholesterol granuloma
    ii. *Companion case*: Petrous apicitis
39. Petrous apex cephalocele
40. Infracochlear drainage of the petrous apex
41. Variations of temporal bone pneumatization
    i. *Companion case*: Hyperpneumatization of the temporal bone with spontaneous pneumatocele formation
    ii. *Companion case*: Fibrous dysplasia
    iii. *Companion case*: Osteopetrosis
42. Arachnoid granulations
    i. *Companion case*: Spontaneous CSF leaks with idiopathic intracranial hypertension
    ii. *Companion case*: Endolymphatic sac tumor
43. Hyperostosis temporalis interna
    i. *Companion case*: Meningioma-associated calvarial hyperostosis
44. Normal facial nerve enhancement on MRI
    i. *Companion case*: Bell palsy
45. Normal IAC vasculature simulating pathologic CN VII/VIII enhancement on MRI
    i. *Companion case*: Leptomeningeal tumor spread along the CN VII/VIII complexes
46. Dehiscence of the facial nerve canal tympanic segment
    i. *Companion case*: Facial nerve prolapse
    ii. *Companion case*: Aberrant, low-lying facial nerve canal tympanic segment
47. Stapedius and chorda nerves
    i. *Companion case*: Perineural spread along chorda tympani nerve
48. The facial hiatus and greater superficial petrosal nerve
    i. *Companion case*: Longitudinal fracture through the facial nerve canal genu and facial hiatus
    ii. *Companion case*: Perineural spread along the greater superficial petrosal nerve
49. Microvascular decompression of CN VII

CASE 1 Cauliflower or boxer's ear

The auricle has a rich vascular network. Blunt trauma to the ear, which may occur with contact sports such as boxing and wrestling, can result in an auricular hematoma. Because the auricular cartilage receives nutrients from the overlying perichondrium, a hematoma can devitalize the auricular cartilage by disrupting the perichondrium from the auricular cartilage. This devitalized cartilage can result in fibrosis and the formation of neocartilage, ultimately deforming the auricle. The deformed auricle has been termed a "cauliflower ear," since it resembles the cauliflower vegetable, or a "boxer's ear," since it commonly occurs in boxers. A cauliflower or boxer's ear is often mineralized and abnormally thickened relative to a normal auricle.

COMPANION CASES

- **Auricular keloid.** A keloid represents an abnormally exuberant healing response that results from excessive deposition of collagen and glycoprotein. It extends beyond the borders of the original wound and is frequently elevated by more than 4 mm. In addition to being cosmetically unappealing, keloids may be painful and pruritic. A keloid most often occurs in patients younger than 30 years, and those patients with dark pigmented skin are at a 15- to 20-fold increased risk to develop a keloid. A keloid will form in susceptible patients following some form of trauma, such as surgery or burns; in the case of the auricle, a keloid may develop following ear piercing, otoplasty, or skin trauma. Keloids may appear 3 months or years following the insult, do not regress, and have a high recurrence rate, regardless of treatment. Small keloids may be treated with intralesional steroid injection, pressure dressings, and silicone elastomer sheeting. If a large or recurrent keloid is present, then surgery is the primary therapeutic option. CT imaging findings may include a mass-like, irregular, soft tissue density lesion that can enlarge over successive examinations. On MRI, the lesion will be isointense to muscle on T1, hypointense on T2, and may enhance.
- **Auricular squamous cell carcinoma.** While most tumors of the pinna are basal cell carcinomas, squamous cell carcinoma (SCC) accounts for 60% to 80% of all carcinomas of the temporal bone. The local extent of temporal bone SCC is the primary determinant of survival. Other poor prognostic indicators include facial paralysis, dural involvement, lymph node involvement, and positive margins following resection. Surgery and radiotherapy are the treatment of choice for these neoplasms. On CT, an SCC of the auricle will be identified as a soft tissue mass. If large enough, temporal bone erosion or destruction may be identified with CT. On MRI, an SCC is usually isointense to muscle on T1, iso- to hyperintense to muscle on T2, and enhances.

Cauliflower or boxer's ear

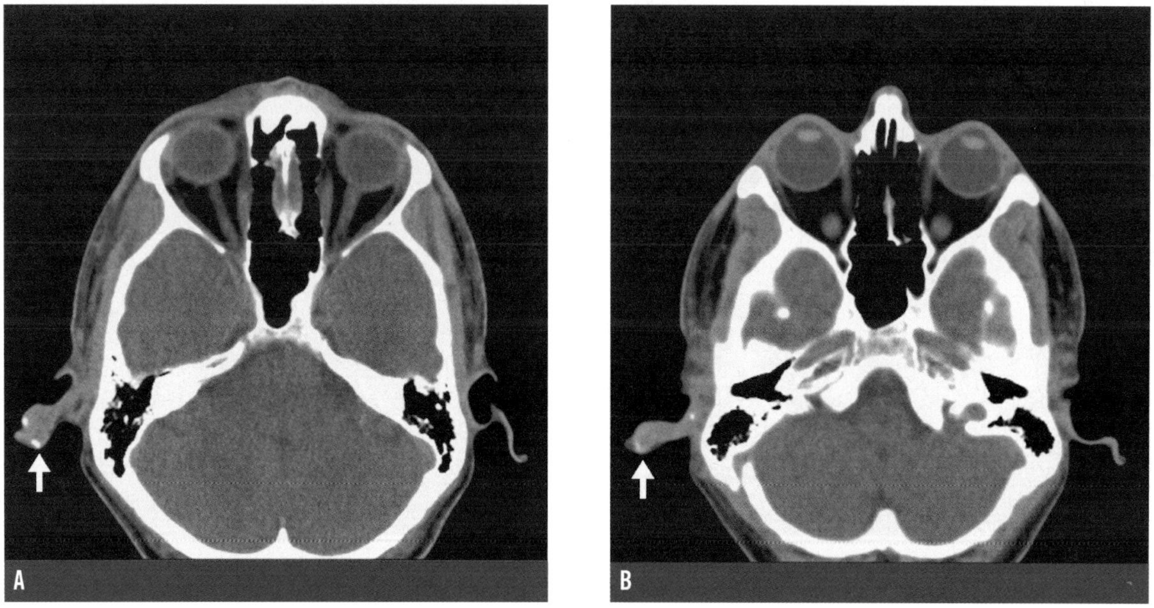

Unenhanced axial CT images (**A**, **B**) demonstrate a deformity of the right auricle with soft tissue thickening and mineralization, compatible with a cauliflower or boxer's ear (arrows, **A**, **B**). The left auricle is normal.

Cauliflower or boxer's ear

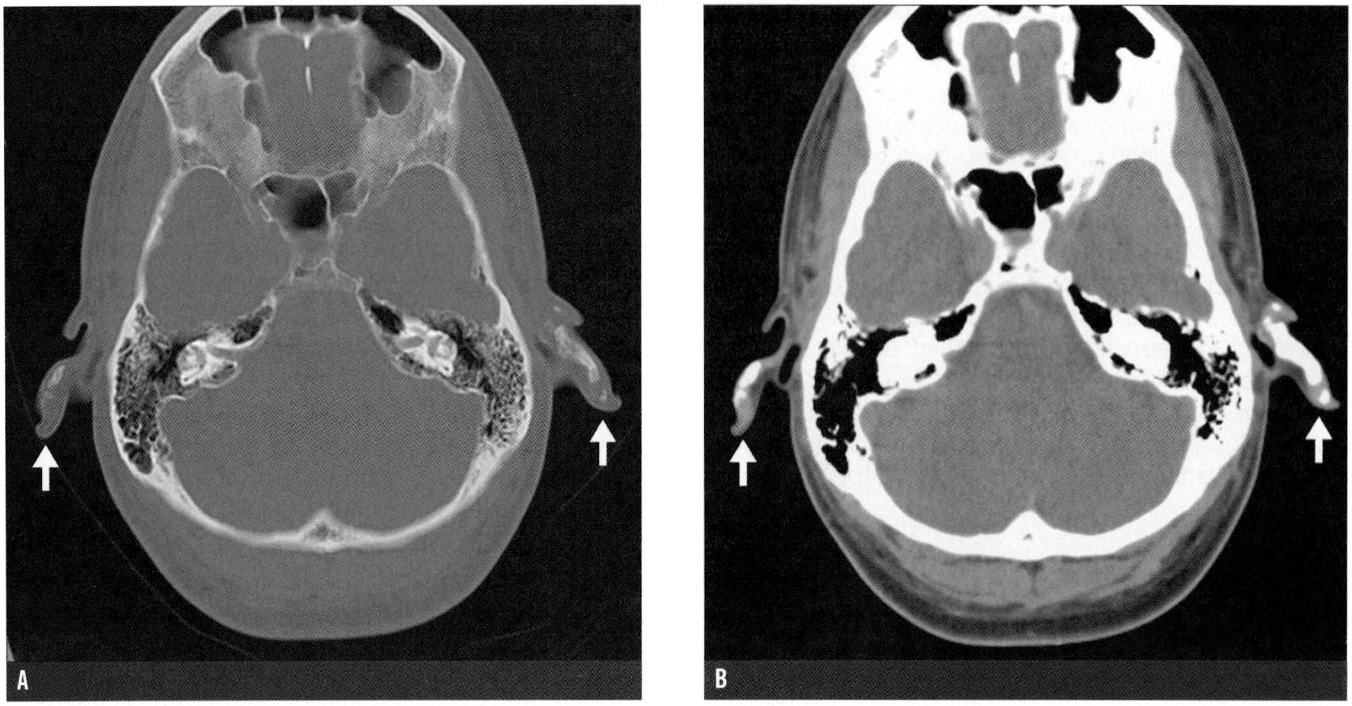

Different patient. An unenhanced axial CT image viewed with a bone window (**A**) and soft tissue window (**B**) demonstrate deformity of the left greater than right auricles associated with soft tissue thickening and mineralization, compatible with bilateral cauliflower or boxer's ears (arrows, **A**, **B**).

Companion case: Auricular keloid

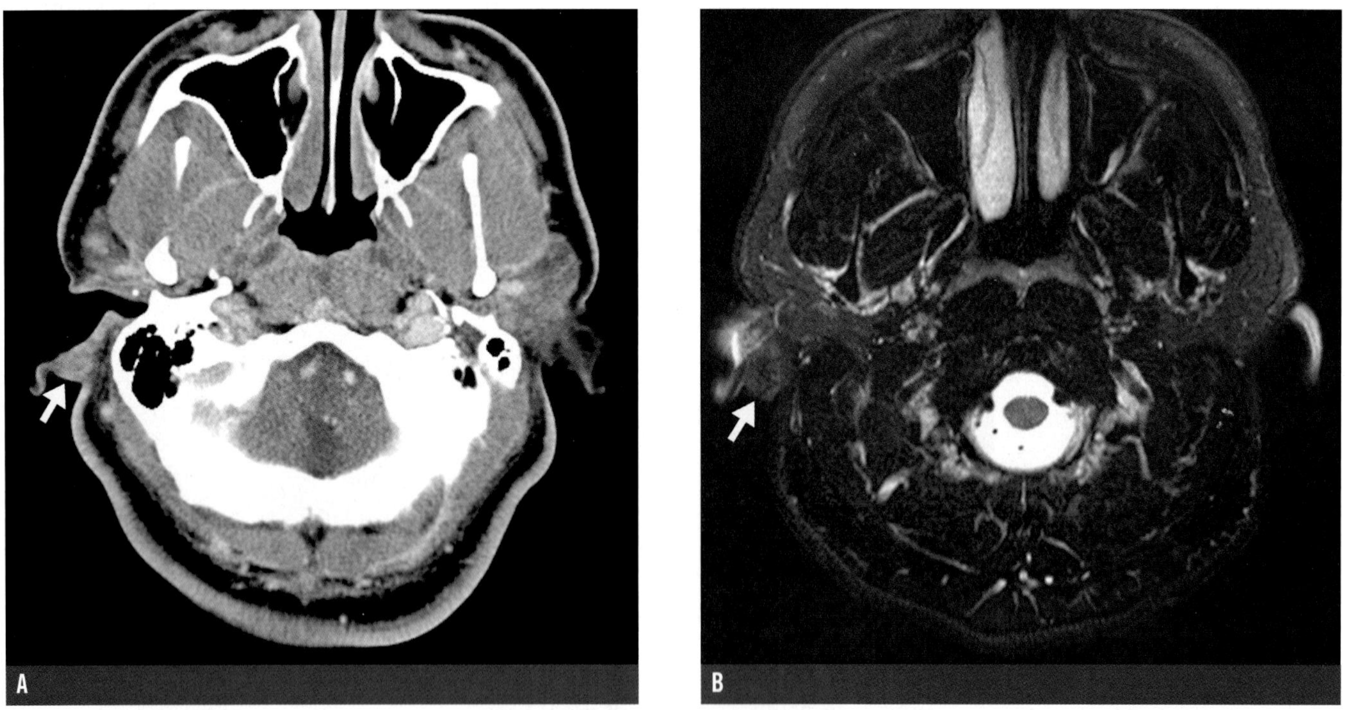

A postcontrast axial CT image through the level of the auricles (**A**) demonstrates a small focal lesion along the posterior aspect of the right pinna (arrow, **A**) that was new from a prior study obtained 6 months earlier (not shown). Fat-suppressed axial T2 (**B**), axial T1 (**C**), and fat-suppressed postcontrast axial T1 (**D**) MR images obtained 2 weeks later demonstrate the same finding to be relatively isointense to muscle on T2 (arrow, **B**) and enhance (arrow, **D**). A fat-suppressed postcontrast axial T1-weighted MR image (**E**) obtained 1 year later demonstrates continued increase in size of the mass. An unenhanced sagittal T1-weighted MR image from the same study (**F**) best demonstrates the lesion conforming to the posterior wall of the pinna (arrows, **F**). Based on these images, the lesion is nonspecific and the differential diagnosis includes several possibilities, including squamous cell carcinoma. However, this represented a keloid on clinical examination.

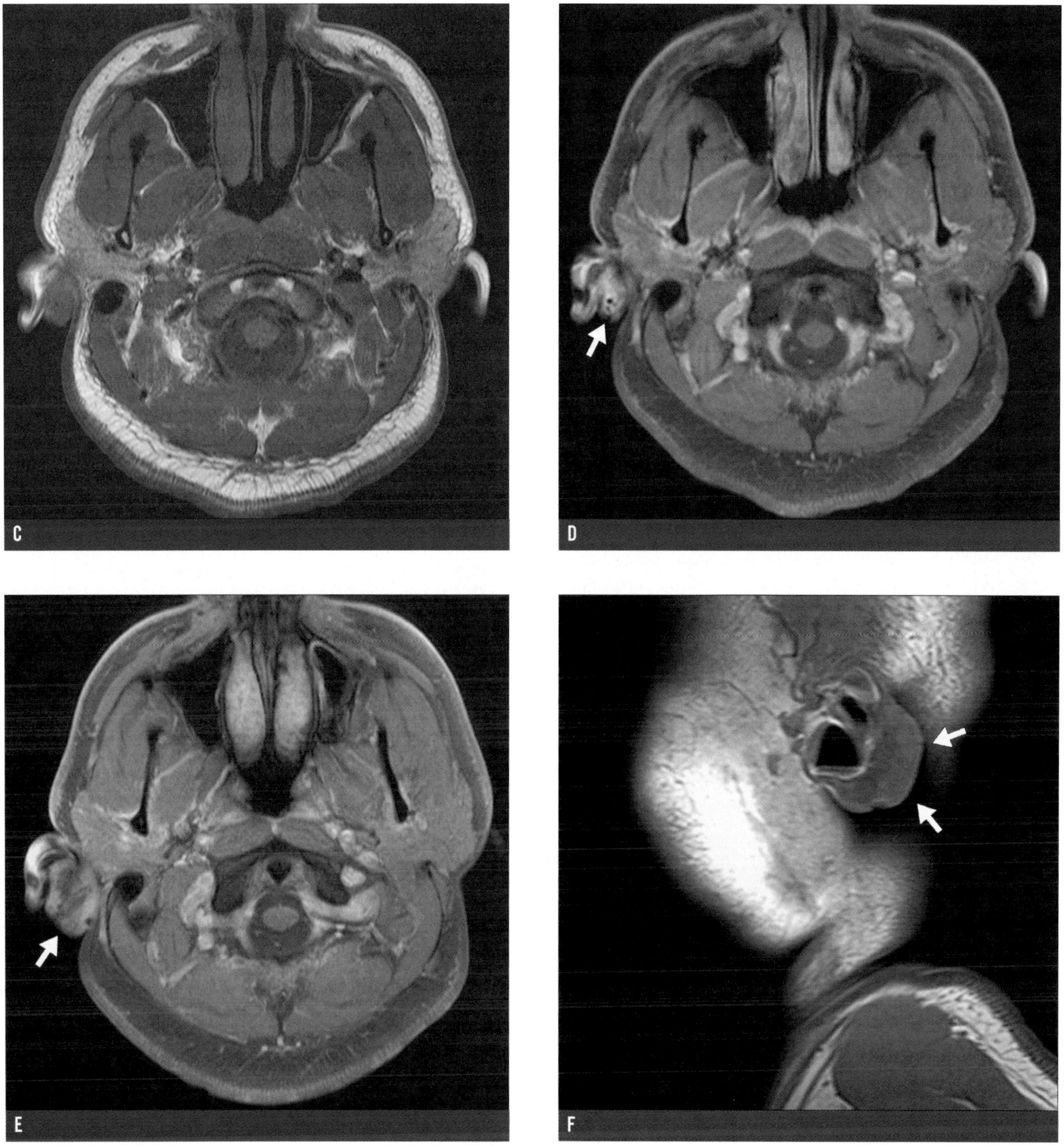
C
D
E
F

Companion case: Auricular squamous cell carcinoma

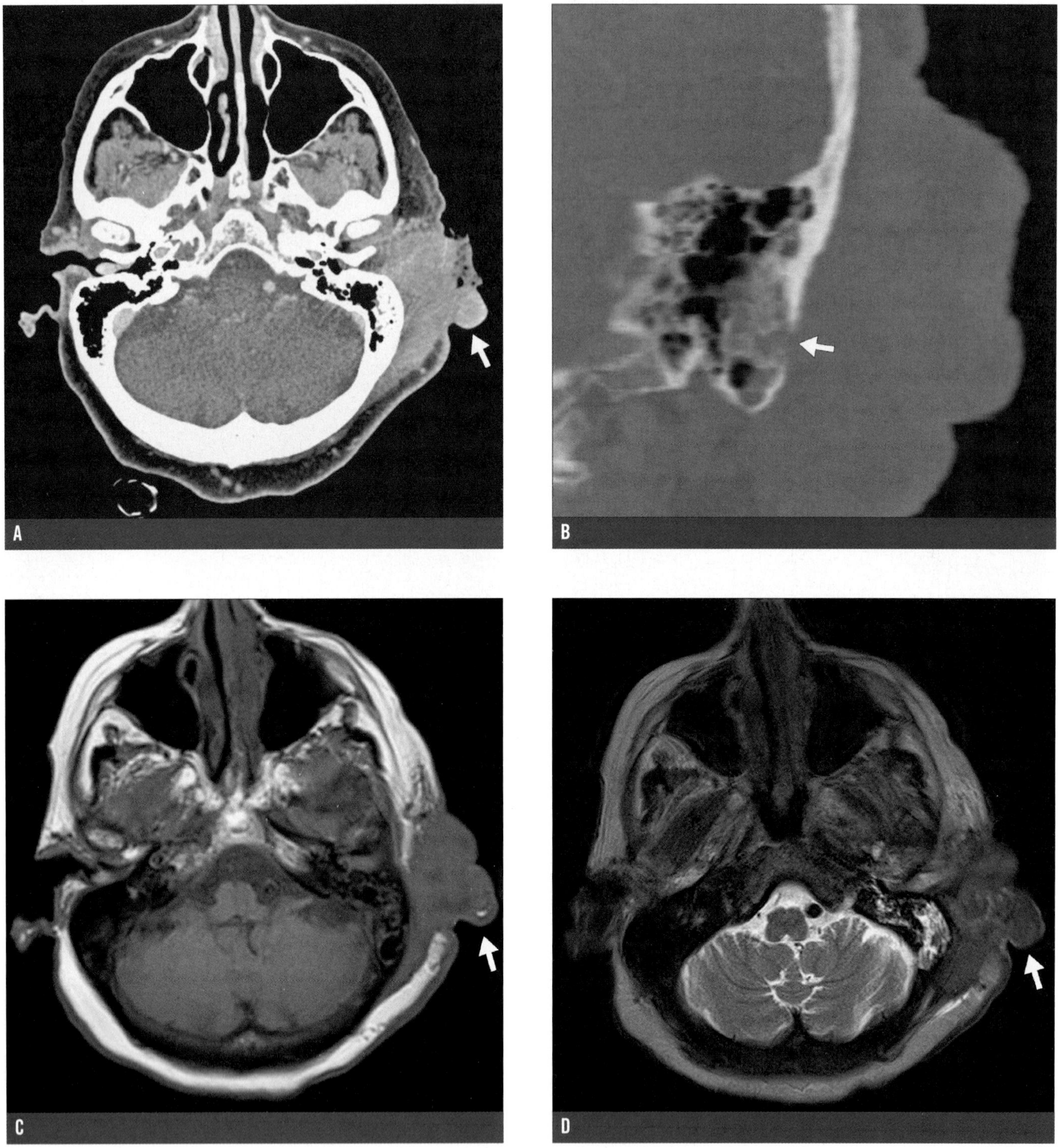

A contrast-enhanced axial CT image (**A**) demonstrates a large left auricular mass (arrow, **A**). A coronal reformatted CT image from the same study (**B**) demonstrates focal osseous erosion of the adjacent mastoid (arrow, **B**). Axial T1 (**C**), axial T2 (**D**), and fat-suppressed contrast-enhanced coronal T1 (**E**) MR images demonstrate the mass to be relatively T1 and T2 isointense to muscle and diffusely enhancing (arrows, **C**-**E**). The large size of the mass and the evidence of erosion favor an aggressive neoplasm. In this case, squamous cell carcinoma was found at pathology.

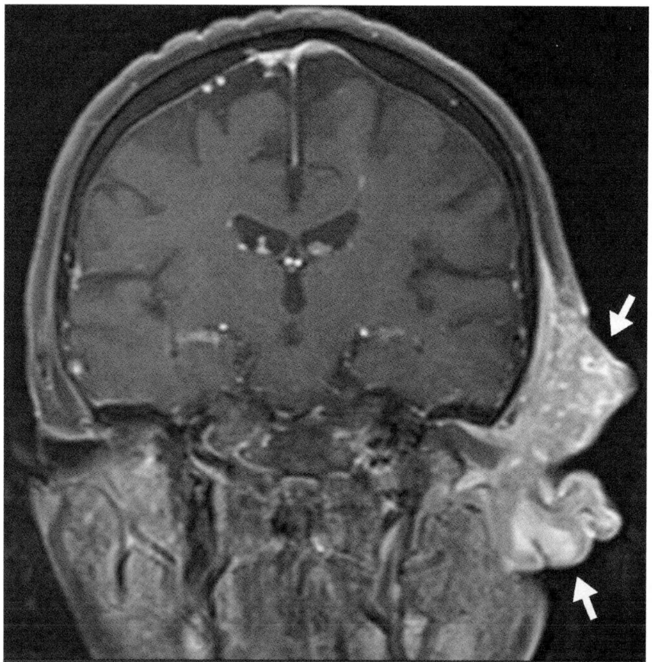

E

REFERENCES

Barrs DM. Temporal bone carcinoma. *Otolaryngol Clin North Am.* 2001;34(6):1197-1218.

Froelich K, Staudenmaier R, Kleinsasser N, Hagen R. Therapy of auricular keloids: review of different treatment modalities and proposal for a therapeutic algorithm. *Eur Arch Otorhinolaryngol.* 2007;264(12):1497-1508.

Greywoode JD, Pribitkin EA, Krein H. Management of auricular hematoma and the cauliflower ear. *Facial Plast Surg.* 2010;26(6):451-455.

Juckett G, Hartman-Adams H. Management of keloids and hypertrophic scars. *Am Fam Physician.* 2009;80(3):253-260.

Mudry A, Wolfgang P. Auricular hematoma and cauliflower deformation of the ear: from art to medicine. *Otol Neurotol.* 2009;30:116-120.

CASE 2 Auricular mineralization

Mineralization of the auricle can result in a partially or totally rigid ear, termed auricular petrification or ossification. This is a common entity and can occur because of ectopic calcification or ossification, although some believe that this entity may represent a continuum from calcification to ossification. The etiology of auricular mineralization is varied and includes severe hypothermia (frostbite), endocrinopathies, and inflammatory conditions such as chondritis/perichondritis, trauma, radiation, and syphilis. Idiopathic cases have also been reported in the literature. Patients are often asymptomatic, although there may be discomfort when pressure is applied to the ear. In contrast to a cauliflower ear, physical examination does not reveal an obvious deformity of the pinna.

Auricular mineralization

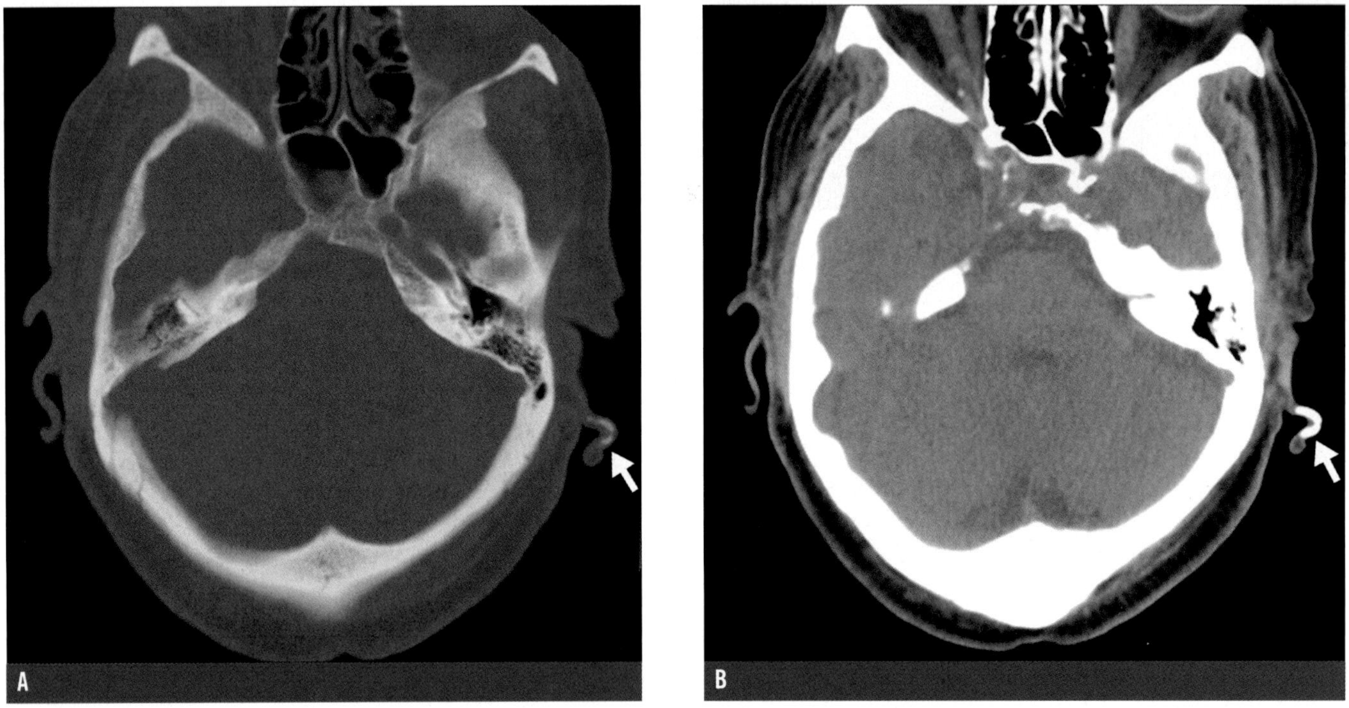

An unenhanced axial CT image viewed with a bone window (**A**) and soft tissue window (**B**) demonstrates mineralization of the left auricle without deformity or soft tissue thickening (arrows, **A**, **B**).

Auricular mineralization

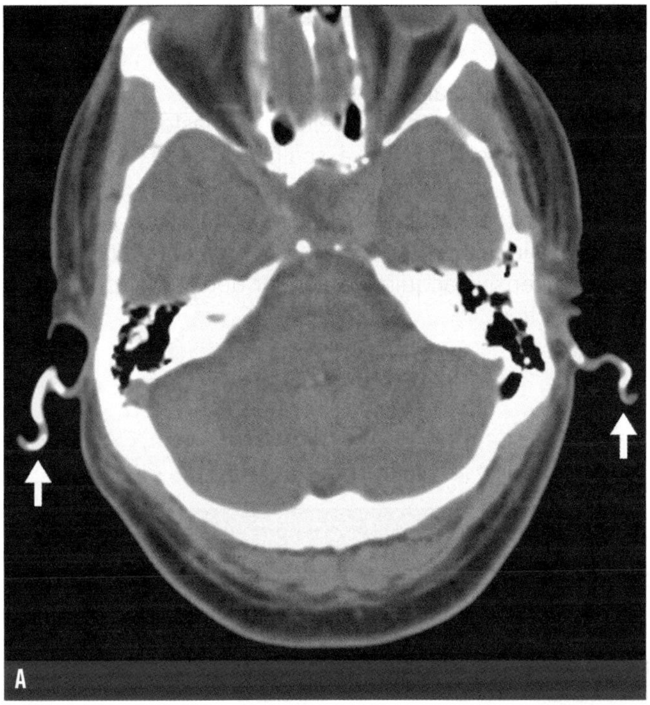

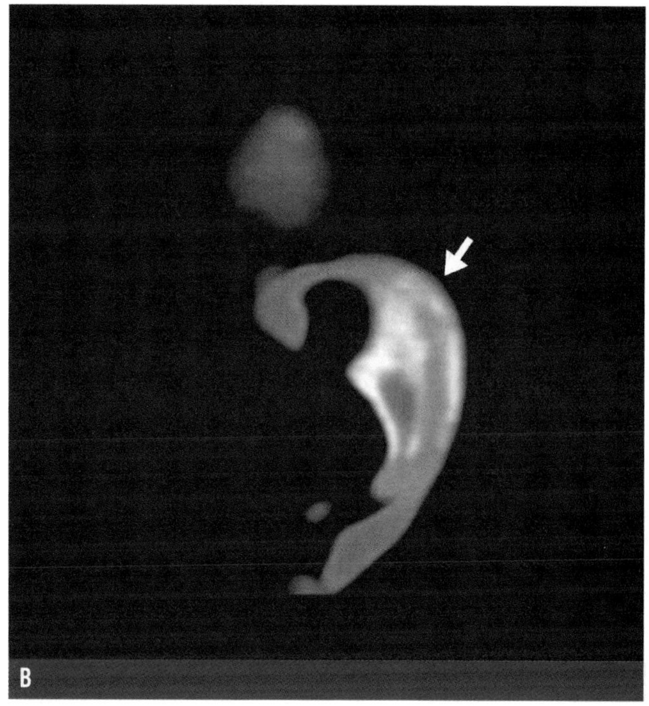

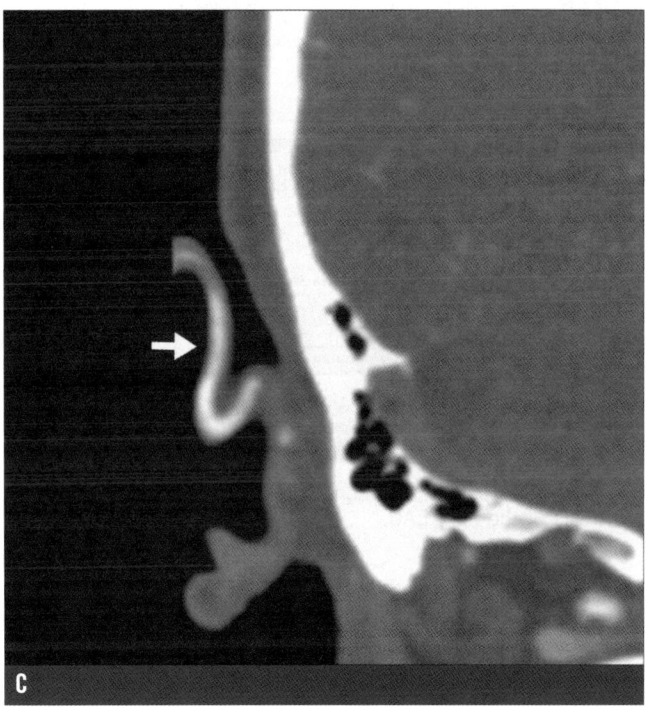

Different patient. An unenhanced axial CT image (**A**) demonstrates mineralization of the auricles without deformity or soft tissue thickening (arrows, **A**). Unenhanced sagittal reformatted (**B**) and coronal reformatted (**C**) CT images of the right auricle from the same patient demonstrate the appearance of auricular mineralization in these planes (arrows, **B**, **C**).

REFERENCES

High WA, Larson MJ, Hoang MP. Idiopathic bilateral auricular ossificans. *Arch Pathol Lab Med.* 2004;128:1432-1434.

Sites PC, Boyd AS, Zic J. Auricular ossificans (ectopic ossification of the auricle). *J Am Acad Dermatol.* 2003;49:142-144.

Gossner J. Prevalence of the petrified ear: a computed tomographic study. *Eur Arch Otorhinolaryngol.* 2014;271(1):195-197.

CASE 4 Partial ossification of the cartilaginous EAC

The external auditory canal (EAC) has a cartilaginous portion and an osseous portion. The cartilaginous portion is a continuation of the conchal and tragal cartilage and comprises approximately the lateral 1/3 of the EAC. The osseous portion comprises the remaining medial 2/3 of the EAC. The cartilaginous EAC has a posterior-superior angulation, whereas the osseous EAC has an anterior-inferior angulation. This configuration results in an "S-shaped" course of the EAC.

The cartilaginous EAC is composed of an incomplete ring of elastic cartilage that is deficient along its superior aspect, termed the incisura terminalis. Fibrous tissue attaches the EAC to the squamosal portion of the temporal bone at the incisura terminalis. The cartilaginous EAC is lined by stratified squamous epithelium, ceruminous glands, and hair follicles. The ceruminous glands contribute to the formation of cerumen which lubricates and cleans the EAC, kills bacteria, and traps foreign particles with the help of EAC hair cells. Two or three variably present small defects, termed the fissures of Santorini, are located along the anterior aspect of the cartilaginous EAC. The fissures of Santorini allow for greater flexibility of the cartilaginous EAC but may also serve as a conduit for infection or malignancy.

Ossification can sometimes develop in the cartilage of the EAC and is a normal variant. When present, it is best visualized by CT imaging and may appear as a single ossified structure or as discontinuous ossified structures paralleling the course of the cartilaginous EACs.

Partial ossification of the cartilaginous EAC

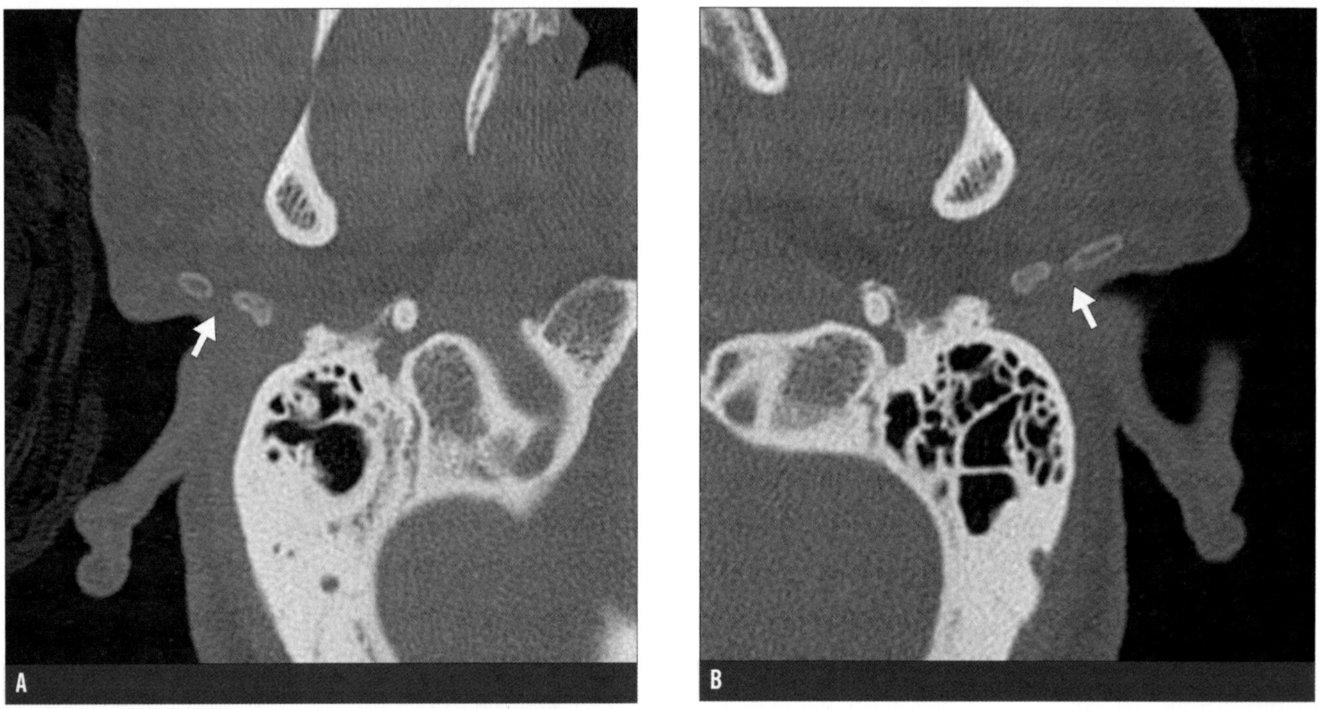

Axial (**A**, **B**) and coronal reformatted (**C**, **D**) CT images of the temporal bones demonstrate incidental partial ossification along the anterior and inferior walls of the cartilaginous EACs. (arrows, **A-D**)

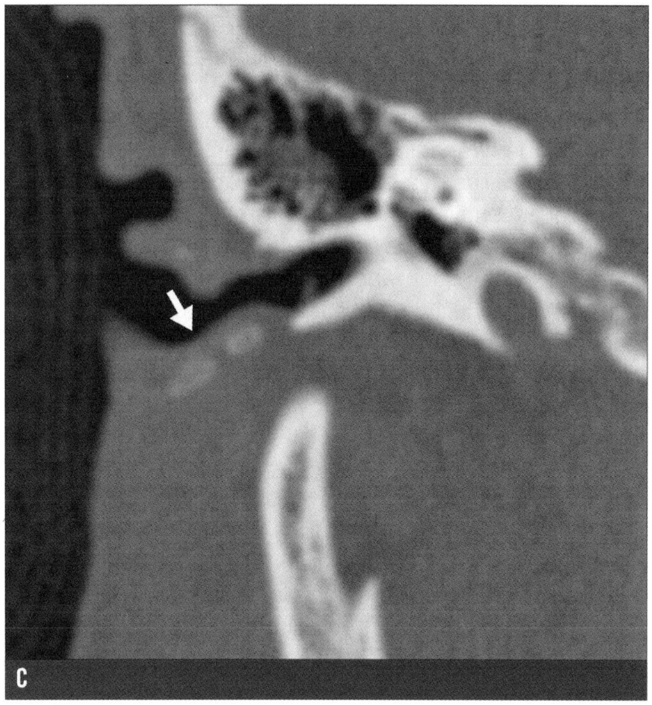

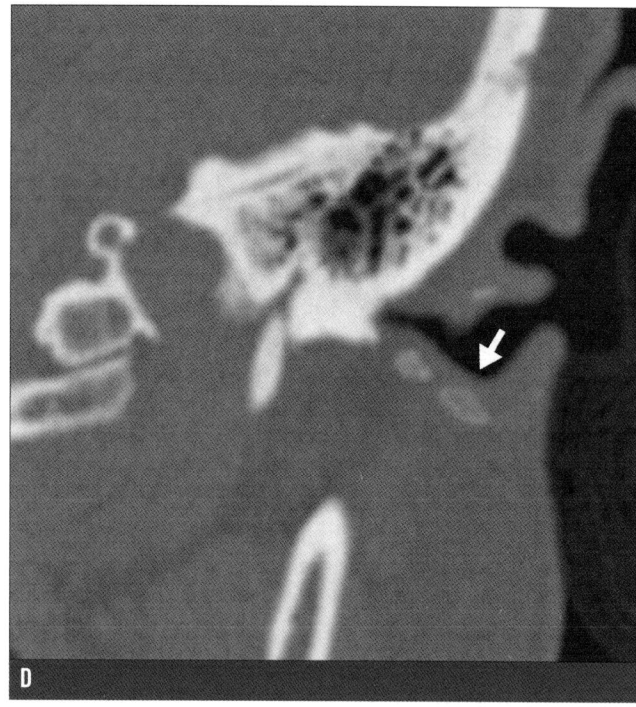

Partial ossification of the cartilaginous EAC

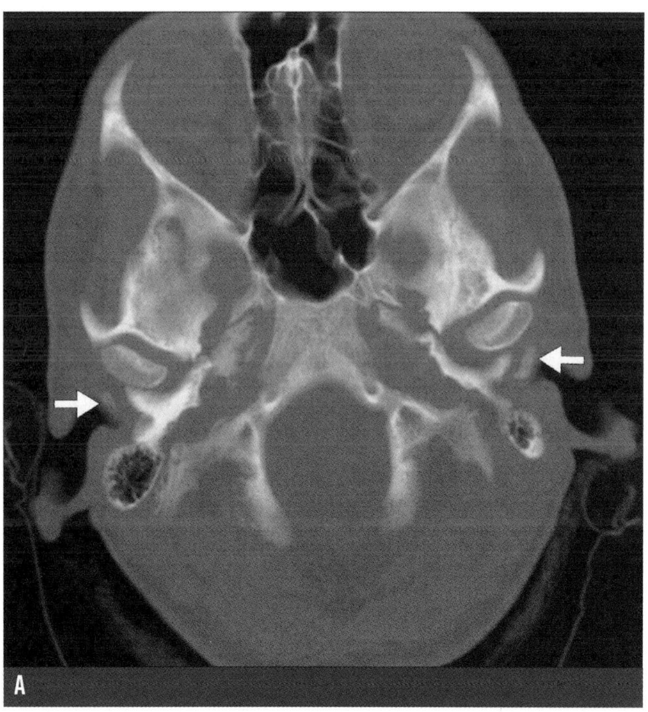

Different patient. An axial CT image (**A**) demonstrates incidental partial ossification of the anterior walls of the cartilaginous EACs (arrows).

REFERENCES

Chakeres DW, Kapila A, LaMasters D. Soft-tissue abnormalities of the external auditory canal: Subject review of CT findings. *Radiology*. 1985;156:105-109.

Kelly KE, Mohs DC. The external auditory canal. Anatomy and physiology. *Otolaryngol Clin North Am*. 1996;5:725-739.

CASE 5 Normal anterior tympanic plate lucencies

The tympanic portion of the temporal bone forms the anterior, inferior, and a portion of the posterior wall of the osseous EAC. The anterior wall of the tympanic portion of the temporal bone is referred to as the anterior tympanic plate. Several anatomic variations within or adjacent to anterior tympanic plate can occur, and it is important to distinguish these variants from an anterior tympanic plate fracture. One of the more commonly described variations is a persistent foramen tympanicum, also known as the foramen of Huschke. This entity represents a developmental focal osseous dehiscence rather than a foramen that contains neural or vascular elements; therefore, the use of the word foramen is a misnomer. The foramen tympanicum is located at the anterior, inferior aspect of the osseous EAC and along the posterior-medial aspect of the temporomandibular joint (TMJ) condylar fossa. Occasionally, a foramen tympanicum may be associated with TMJ pain or dysfunction related to soft tissue herniation from the TMJ into the defect. There have also been reports of salivary gland or TMJ fistulas associated with a persistent foramen tympanicum, with patients usually presenting with otorrhea in these settings.

The tympanosquamous suture is another normal structure in this region that can mimic an anterior tympanic plate fracture. As the name implies, this suture is located between the tympanic and squamous portions of the temporal bone. The tympanosquamous suture is identified as linear lucency on an axial CT image that parallels the anterior tympanic plate. The petrotympanic fissure is also located in this region and is anteromedial to, and is contiguous with, the tympanosquamous suture. Notably, the chorda tympani nerve and the anterior tympanic branch of the maxillary artery pass through the petrotympanic fissure.

COMPANION CASE

- **Fractures of the anterior tympanic plates.** The anterior tympanic plate is commonly injured following direct trauma to the EAC. This structure may also be fractured following injury to the mandible, either from direct injury to the condyle or from an axial force to the mandibular mentum that drives the condyle through the anterior tympanic plate. Differentiating a fracture from a normal variant lucency along the anterior tympanic plate can be difficult, although air adjacent to the lucency frequently aids in identifying the presence of a fracture. Additionally, sagittal reformatted CT imaging through the area of concern is often helpful to further assess equivocal fractures that are present on axial imaging.

Persistent foramina tympanicum (Foramina of Huschke)

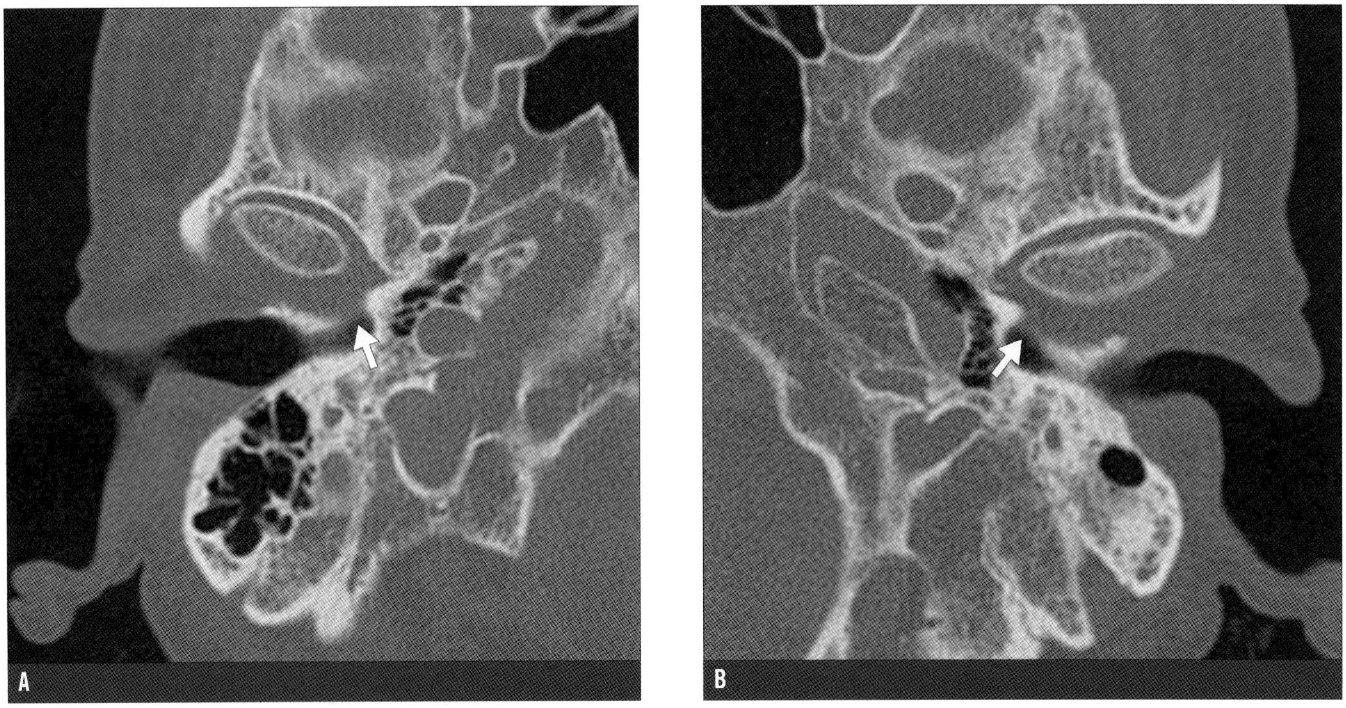

Axial CT images of the right (**A**) and left (**B**) temporal bones demonstrate bilateral persistent foramina tympanicum (arrows, **A**, **B**).

Tympanosquamous suture and petrotympanic fissure

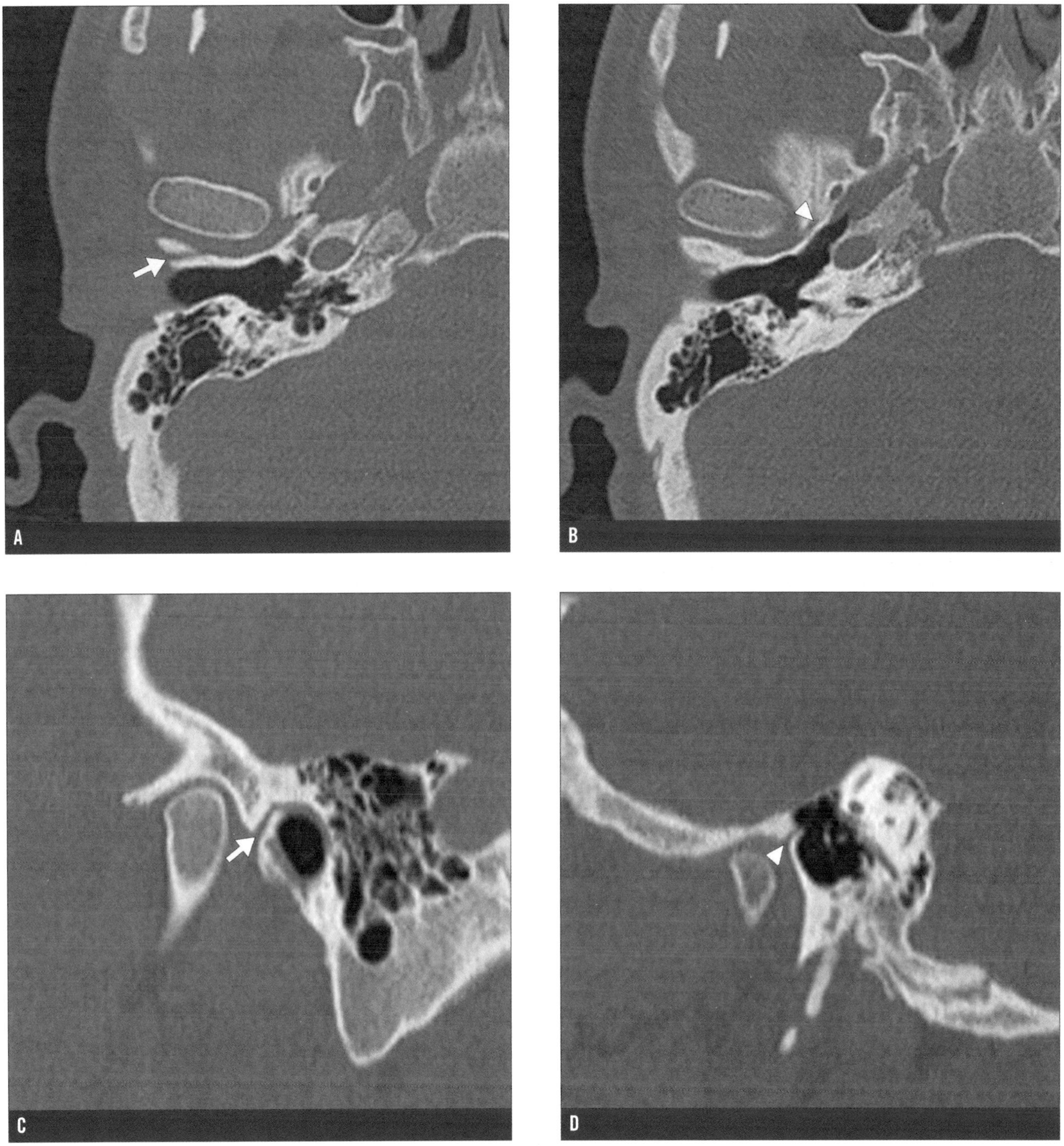

Axial (**A**, **B**) and sagittal reformatted (**C**, **D**) CT images of the right temporal bone demonstrate the normal tympanosquamous suture (arrows, **A**, **C**) and the normal contiguous petrotympanic fissure (arrowheads, **B**, **D**).

Companion case: Fractures of the anterior tympanic plates

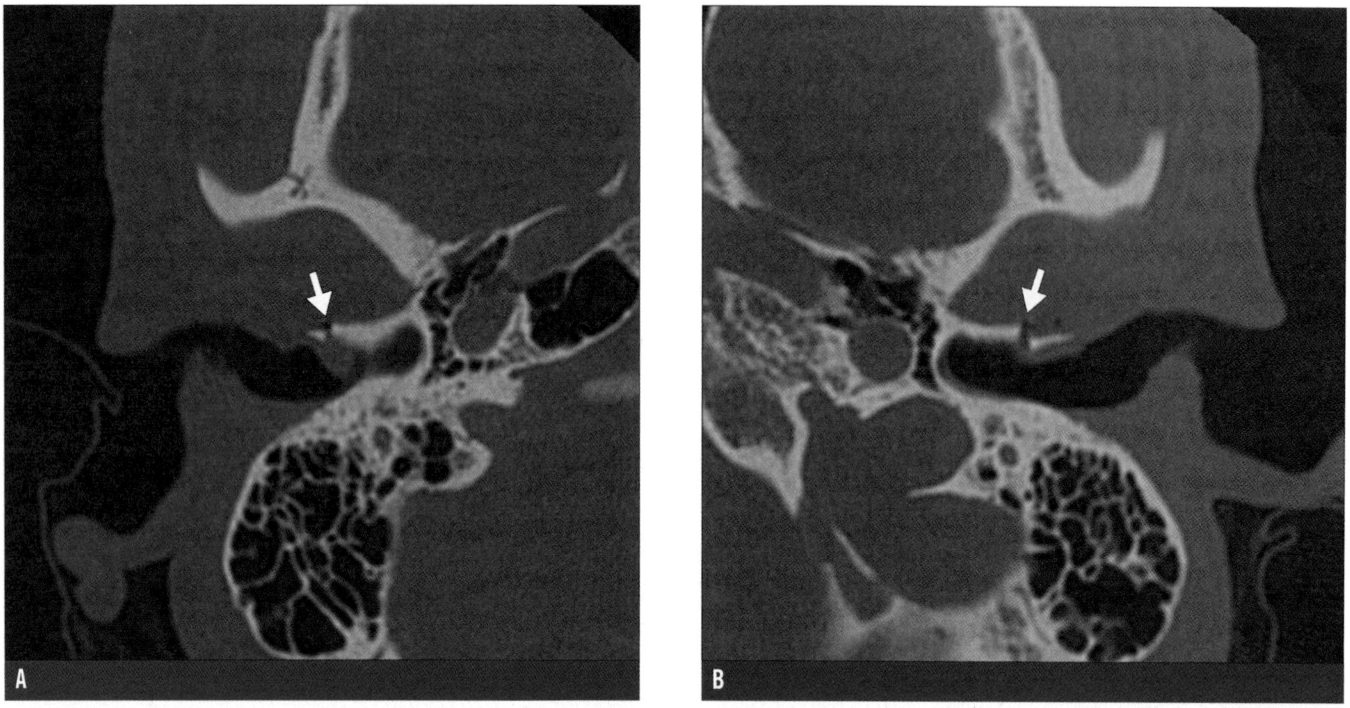

Axial CT images of the right (**A**) and left (**B**) temporal bones demonstrate bilateral anterior tympanic plate fractures following mandibular trauma (arrows, **A**, **B**). Note the presence of air immediately adjacent to these fractures, a finding that is consistent with the presence of acute fractures and not normal suture variation of the anterior tympanic plates.

REFERENCES

Connor SEJ, Tan G, Fernando R, Chaudhury N. Computed tomography pseudofractures of the mid face and skull base. *Clinical Radiology*. 2005;60:1268-1279.

Heffez L, Anderson D, Mafee M. Developmental defects of the tympanic plate: case reports and review of the literature. *J Oral Maxillofac Surg*. 1989;47:1336-1340.

Lacout A, Marsot-Dupuch K, Smoker WRK, Lasjaunias P. Foramen tympanicum, or foramen of Huschke: pathologic cases and anatomic CT study. *Am J Neuroradiol*. 2005;26:1317-1323.

CASE 6 Osseous EAC size variation

The average external auditory canal (EAC) measures approximately 0.6 to 0.7 cm in diameter and 3 cm in length, although the osseous EAC can vary in size, from a capacious EAC to a congenitally atretic EAC that manifests as only a bony plate.

The EAC is formed by the first branchial groove and develops with membraneous ossification, as does the remainder of the temporal bone. The osseous EAC becomes fully canalized by the seventh month of gestation but continues to develop after the first year of life. When viewed from a lateral perspective, the caudal aspect of the osseous EAC is "U" shaped during the first year of life. At the age of 1 year, new bone develops anteriorly and posteriorly along the lower half of the U-shaped EAC and grows toward one another, ultimately obliterating the lower half of U-shape configuration as it continues to transform into the adult EAC. Presumably, an EAC that is markedly capacious in the craniocaudal dimension represents failure of the new bone to develop and fuse at the caudal aspect of the developing EAC.

A developmentally capacious osseous EAC is incidental, though cerumen may accumulate within the deep recesses of a capacious EAC and may be difficult to remove. A developmentally narrow osseous EAC is also frequently incidental, although this may result in obstruction, accumulation of cerumen, and hearing loss.

COMPANION CASES

- **EAC exostoses.** EAC exostoses are also known as "surfer's ear," because of the proclivity of exostoses to develop with cold water exposure. EAC exostoses typically present as multiple, broad-based, and smooth osseous lesions that develop in both osseous EACs. Histopathologically, an exostosis is characterized by concentric, dense layers of subperiosteal bone with abundant osteocytes surrounded by periosteum and covered by squamous epithelium. The lamellar osseous configuration gives rise to a histopathologic "onion-skin" configuration. There is a relative paucity of fibrovascular channels within an exostosis which may help differentiate this entity from an osteoma on histopathology; however, this feature has been refuted as a reliable discriminator by some authors. Exostoses have a reported incidence of 0.6% and are significantly more common than an EAC osteoma. When sizable, EAC exostoses narrow the osseous EAC and predispose the patient to cerumen impaction and conductive hearing loss. Other symptoms that may occur with this entity include vertigo, pain, and tinnitus.
- **EAC osteoma.** An EAC osteoma is a benign osseous tumor that is usually found incidentally and in only one ear. It is a single, often pedunculated mass that is associated with a stalk of bone usually arising from either the tympanosquamous or tymapanomastoid suture of the osseous EAC. Histopathologically, an EAC osteoma consists of lamellated bone, fibrovascular channels, and a small amount of osteocysts surrounded by periosteum and covered by squamous epithelium. However, as alluded to above, histopathology may not reliably discriminate an EAC osteoma from an EAC exostosis, and the diagnosis is often made in conjunction with the clinical and radiological findings. Like exostoses, an osteoma can predispose the patient to cerumen impaction and conductive hearing loss, with symptoms of vertigo, pain, and tinnitus also having been described.

Patulous osseous EACs

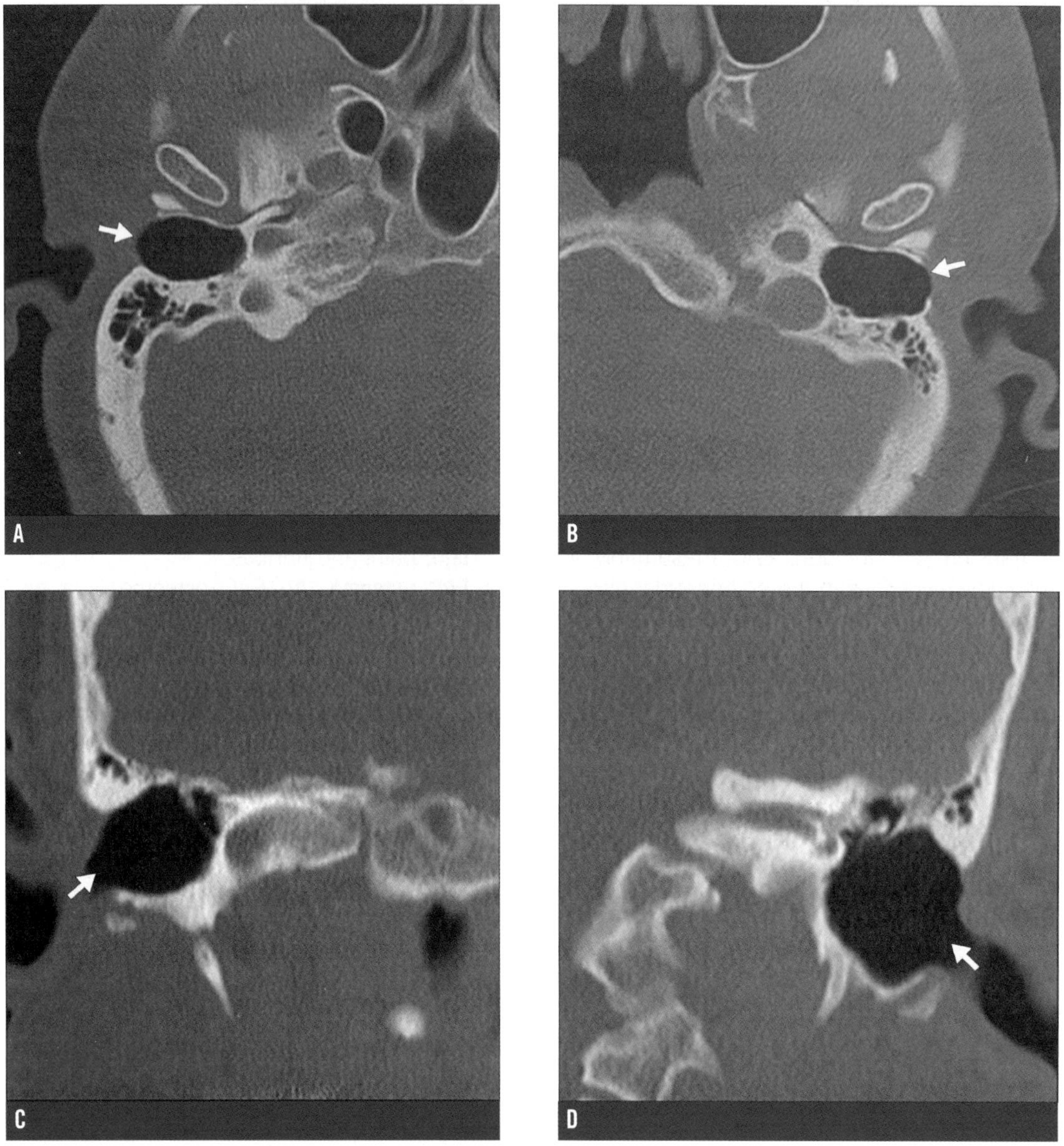

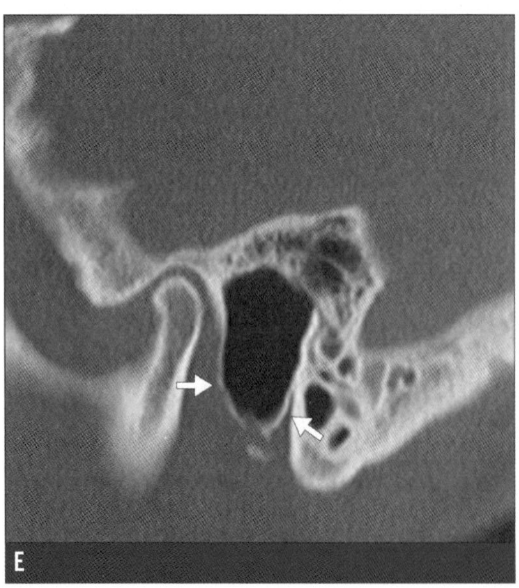

Axial CT images of the right (**A**) and left (**B**) temporal bones as well as coronal reformatted CT images of the right (**C**) and left (**D**) temporal bones demonstrate patulous bilateral osseous EACs, left slightly larger than right (arrows, **A-D**). A sagittal reformatted image of the left temporal bone (**E**) demonstrates a pronounced "U" shape to the caudal aspect of the osseous EAC (arrows, **E**), likely the result of failed developmental closure, as described in the main text. Patulous EACs such as this may predispose the patient to excessive cerumen accumulation, particularly along the inferior recess of the osseous EAC.

Narrowed osseous EACs

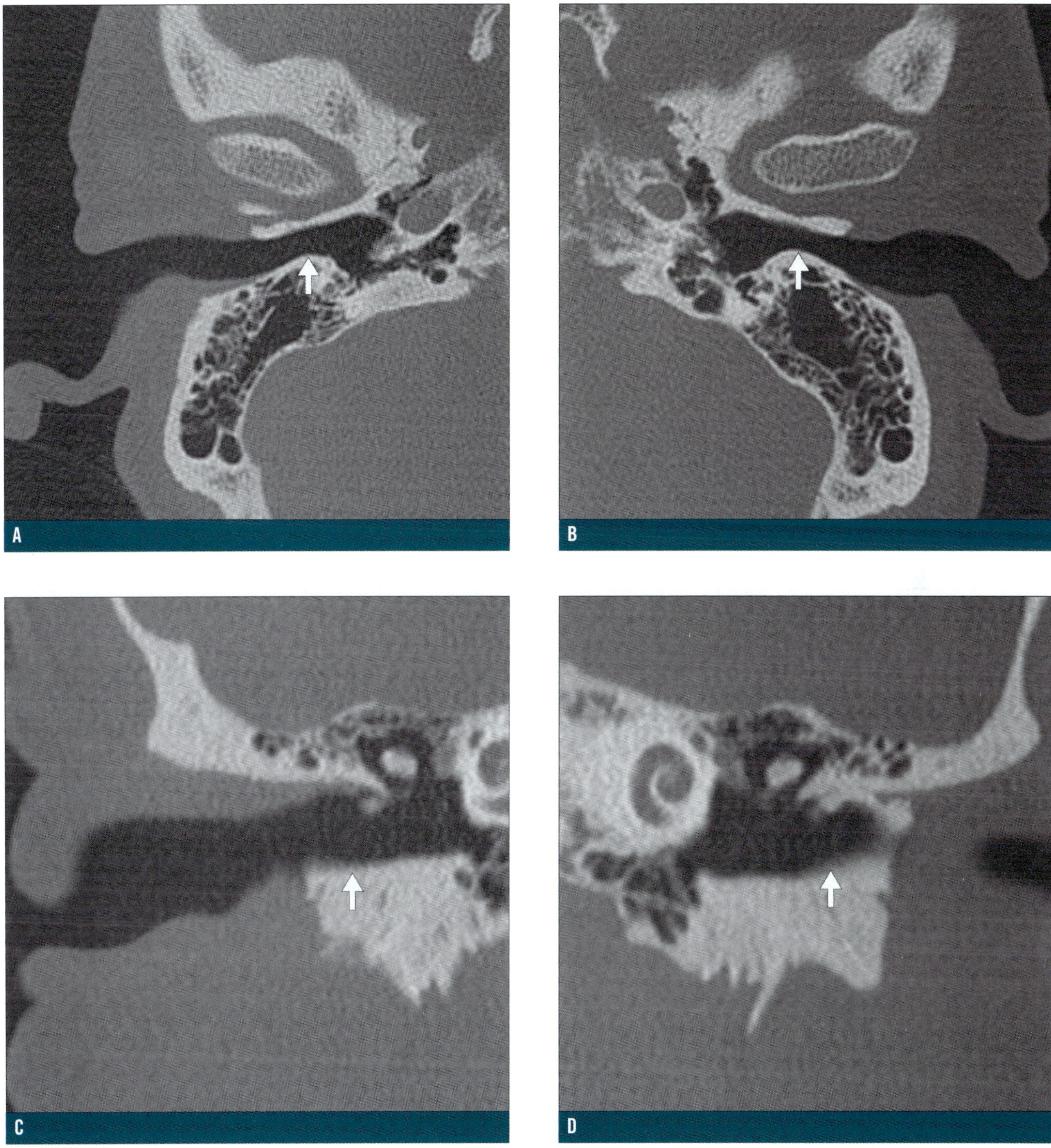

Axial CT images of the right (**A**) and left (**B**) temporal bones and coronal reformatted CT images of the right (**C**) and left (**D**) temporal bones demonstrate narrowed osseous EACs in the AP and CC dimensions, left slightly more pronounced compared to the right (arrows, **A**-**D**).

Companion case: EAC exostoses

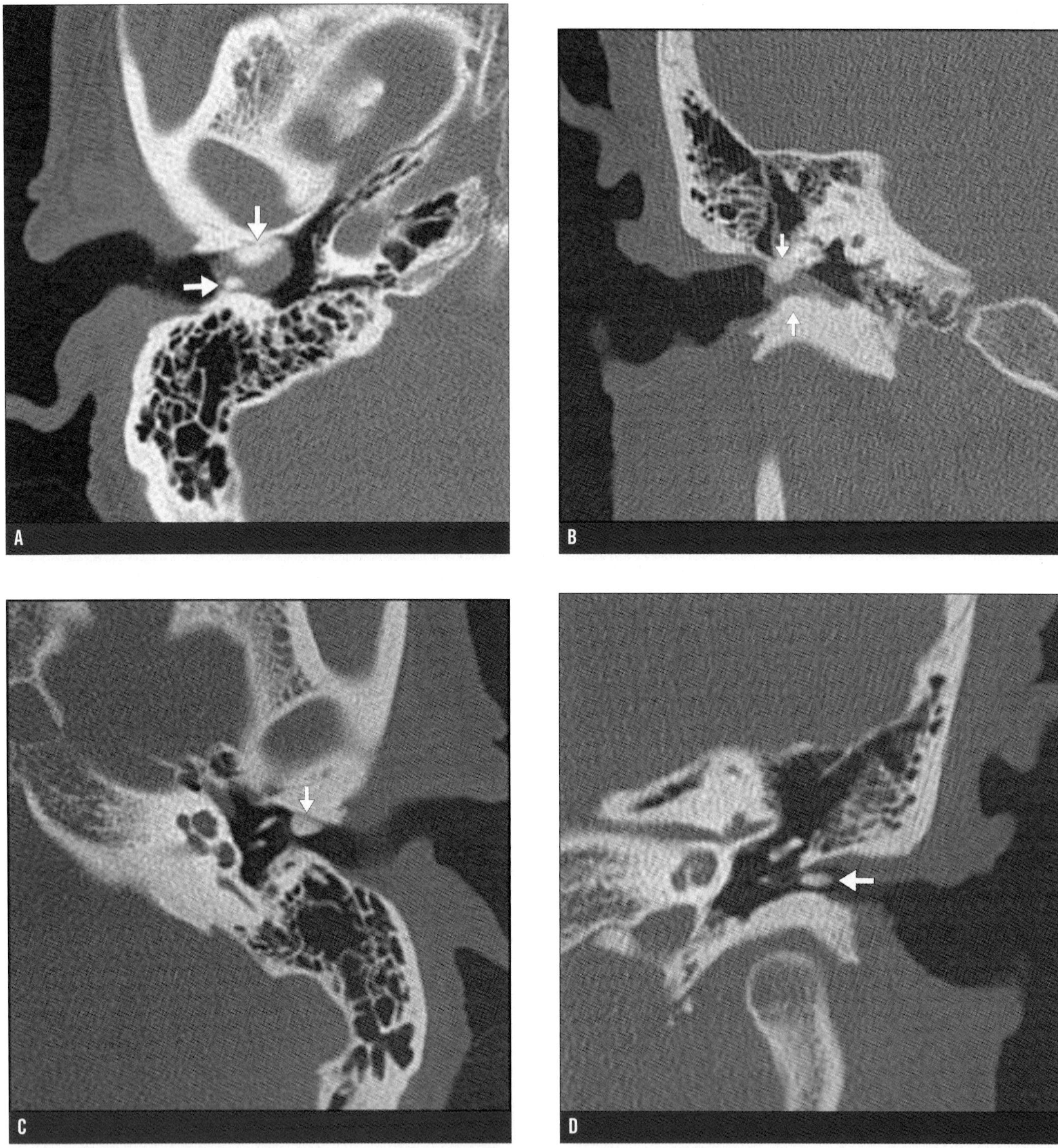

Axial and direct coronal CT images of the right temporal bone (**A**, **B**, respectively) and left temporal bone (**C**, **D**, respectively) demonstrate multiple smooth osseous excrescences arising along the walls of the osseous EACs, compatible with multiple exostoses (arrows, **A**-**D**). There is soft tissue within the right osseous EAC at the level of, and deep to, the exostoses, presumably representing impacted cerumen.

Companion case: EAC osteoma

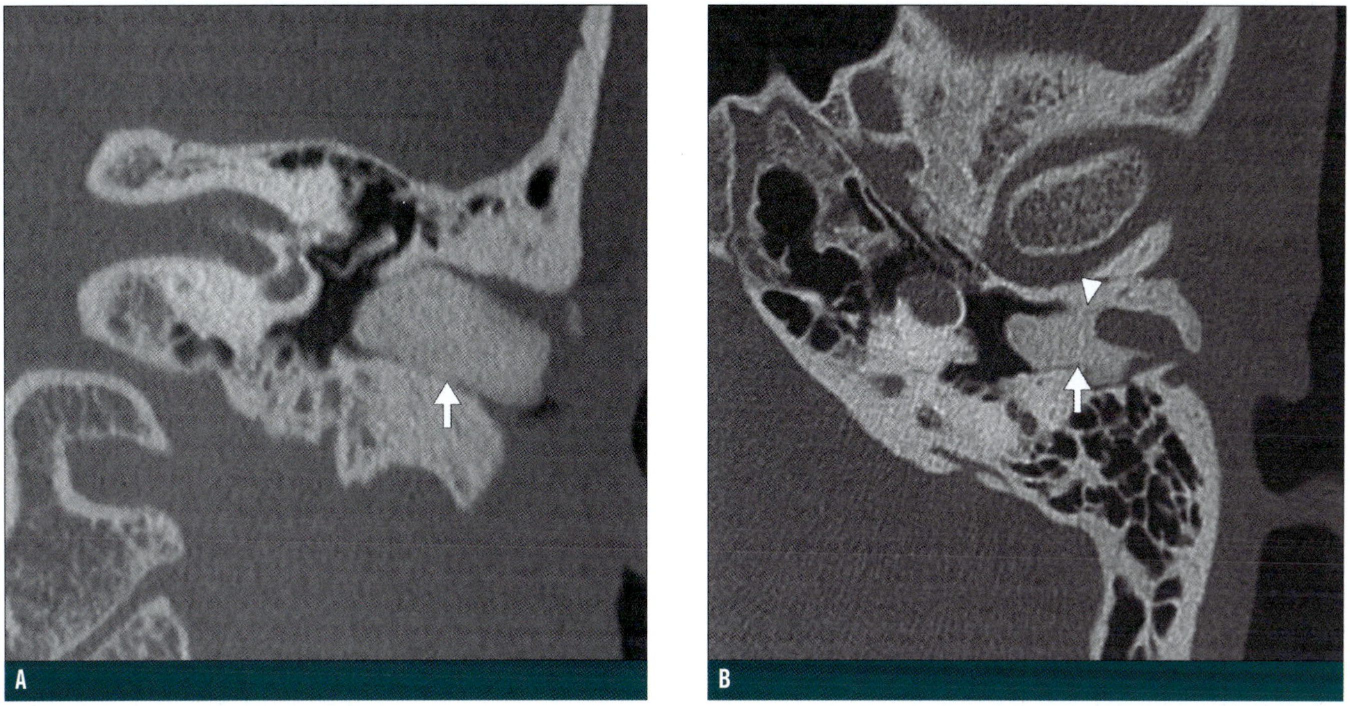

Coronal reformatted (**A**) and axial (**B**) CT images of the left temporal bone demonstrate a large, ossified mass occupying nearly the entire osseous left EAC (arrows, **A**, **B**). There is evidence of a narrow stalk of bone attaching the osseous mass with the anterior tympanic plate, likely arising from the tympanosquamous suture (arrowhead, **B**). The contralateral right EAC was normal (not shown). The pedunculation and unilaterality are compatible with an EAC osteoma.

REFERENCES

Carbone PN, Nelson BL. External auditory osteoma. *Head Neck Pathol.* 2012;6(2):244-246

Fenton JE, Turner J, Fagan PA. A histopathologic review of temporal bone exostosis and osteomata. *Laryngoscope.* 1996;106(5):624-628.

Gulya AJ, Minor LB, Poe DS, eds. *Glasscock- Shambaugh Surgery of the Ear.* 6th ed. Shelton, CT: People's Medical Publishing House; 2010.

Lacout A, Marsot-Dupuch K, Smoker WRK, Lasjaunias P. Foramen tympanicum, or foramen of Huschke: pathologic cases and anatomic CT study. *Am J Neuroradiol.* 2005;26:1317-1323.

CASE 7 EAC cerumen

Cerumen, or ear wax, functions to lubricate and clean the external auditory canal (EAC), kill bacteria, and trap foreign particles with the help of EAC hair cells. Cerumen represents a combination of sloughed epithelial cells and secretions. Epithelial migration originates at the center of the tympanic membrane and extends laterally along the EAC toward the external auditory meatus. Cerumen is considered to be impacted when there are associated symptoms (eg, hearing loss, ear pain, aural fullness) or if the cerumen prevents adequate medical assessment. Certain factors believed to predispose to cerumen impaction include tympanic membrane disorders and atrophy of the EAC apocrine glands, which can result in cerumen being dryer and harder. Cerumen can mimic neoplastic and nonneoplastic lesions of the EAC on imaging, although a small amount of soft tissue in the EAC in an otherwise asymptomatic patient almost always represents incidental cerumen. Cerumen can usually be differentiated from other EAC lesions on CT by a thin rim of air surrounding the cerumen; however, the presence of surrounding air does not exclude significant pathology if there is concern clinically.

COMPANION CASES

- **EAC squamous cell carcinoma.** A primary carcinoma of the EAC is relatively rare. Statistically, it is more common to have a carcinoma arise outside the EAC and subsequently invade the EAC than it is to have a primary EAC carcinoma. The diagnosis of an EAC primary malignancy is often delayed because patients commonly present with nonspecific ear complaints, such as otalgia, that may be incorrectly attributed to chronic otitis externa. The most common primary tumor of the EAC is squamous cell carcinoma (SCC), accounting for approximately 80% of all primary EAC malignancies. Risk factors for SCC of the EAC include chronic inflammation or irritation. SCC can destroy regional bone, undergo perineural spread, and frequently metastasizes to the lymph nodes and lungs. On CT, an SCC of the EAC will be identified as a soft tissue mass that is often associated with osseous erosion. On MRI, SCCs are usually isointense to muscle on T1, iso to hyperintense to muscle on T2, and enhance.
- **EAC adenoid cystic carcinoma.** Adenoid cystic carcinoma (ACC) accounts for only 5% of all malignancies affecting the EAC. Like ACC elsewhere, an ACC of the EAC can be slow-growing but has a high risk of recurrence, a propensity for perineural spread (sometimes with skip lesions), and is associated with a high risk of distant metastasis, particularly to the lungs. While metastatic disease to the lymph nodes can certainly occur with ACC, this is not a predominant feature of ACC compared to other tumors, such as SCC. The MR imaging features of ACC are similar to SCC of the EAC and are usually isointense to muscle on T1, iso to hyperintense to muscle on T2, and they enhance.
- **EAC cholesteatoma.** A cholesteatoma is a lesion that is lined by keratinizing squamous epithelium and is pathologically identical to an epidermoid. Cholesteatoma is a misnomer because it does not contain fat nor does it represent a neoplasm. These lesions most commonly develop in the middle ear, but they can arise elsewhere, including from the EAC. EAC cholesteatomas usually occur spontaneously, although there are reports of EAC cholesteatomas developing following trauma or surgery, presumably because of displaced epidermal tissue. Cholesteatomas can involve multiple EAC walls, although the inferior and posterior walls are most commonly affected. On CT, EAC cholesteatomas appear as a soft tissue lesion often associated with osseous EAC erosion. MRI with diffusion-weighted imaging (DWI) is frequently helpful to distinguish an EAC cholesteatoma from other lesions affecting the EAC. Like epidermoids elsewhere in the head and neck, a cholesteatoma will restrict on diffusion-weighted imaging. Newer non-EPI diffusion-weighted imaging sequences (eg, DWI-HASTE and DWI-BLADE) offer improved resolution, thinner section acquisition, and less artifact compared to EPI diffusion-weighted imaging, although they have longer image acquisition times.
- **Keratosis obturans.** The pathogenesis of keratosis obturans (KO) is not fully understood. KO is characterized by a plug of keratin debris that develops in a lamellar fashion, usually associated with chronic inflammation and hyperplasia of the adjacent epithelium. There is clinical overlap between KO and EAC cholesteatoma. However, KO usually occurs in younger patients, is bilateral, results in acute conductive hearing loss, and is acutely painful, and the patients often have concomitant sinusitis or bronchiectasis. By contrast, patients with EAC cholesteatoma are usually older, only one ear is affected, otorrhea is often present, the pain is chronic and dull in character, there is no hearing loss, and there are no associated sinus or lung findings. KO usually results in diffuse, smooth widening of the EAC, whereas an EAC cholesteatoma results in focal erosions.

EAC cerumen

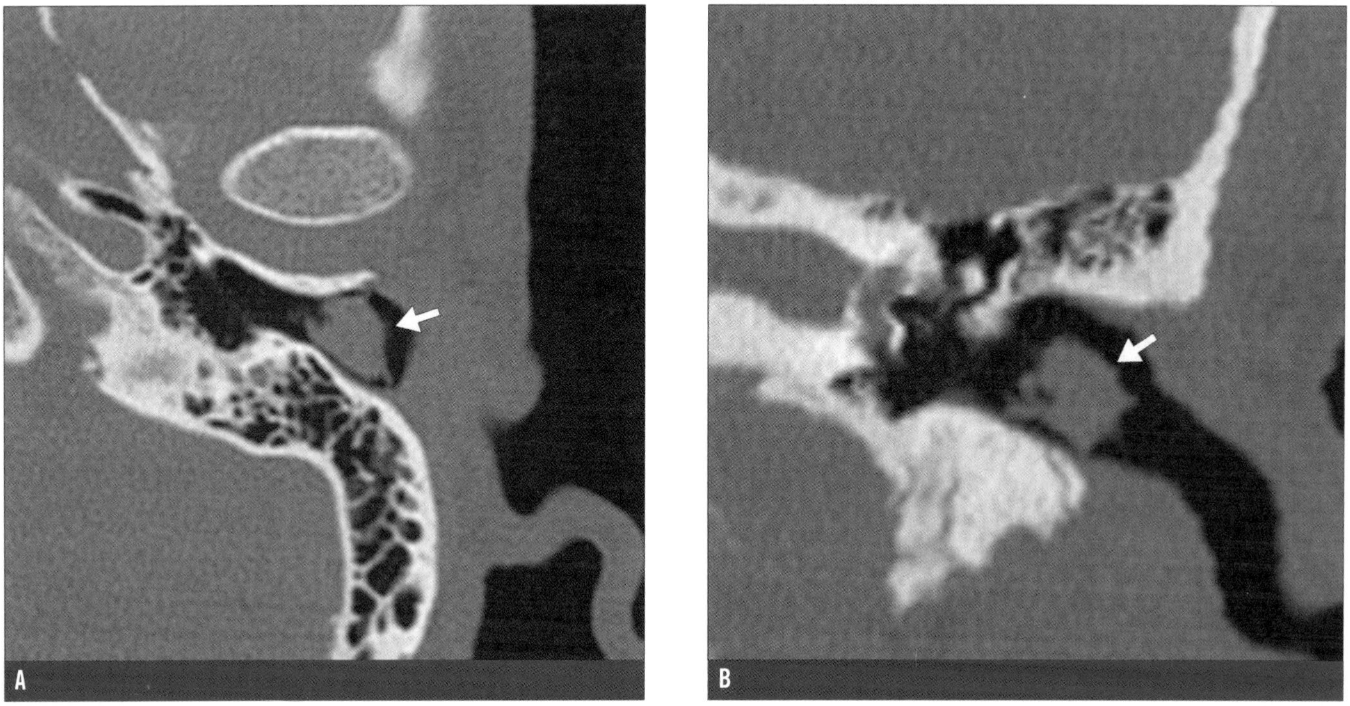

Unenhanced axial (**A**) and coronal reformatted (**B**) CT images of the left temporal bone demonstrate rounded soft tissue in the EAC, compatible with cerumen (arrows, **A**, **B**). There is a thin rim of air surrounding the cerumen, a helpful imaging finding to differentiate cerumen from other entities.

Companion case: EAC squamous cell carcinoma

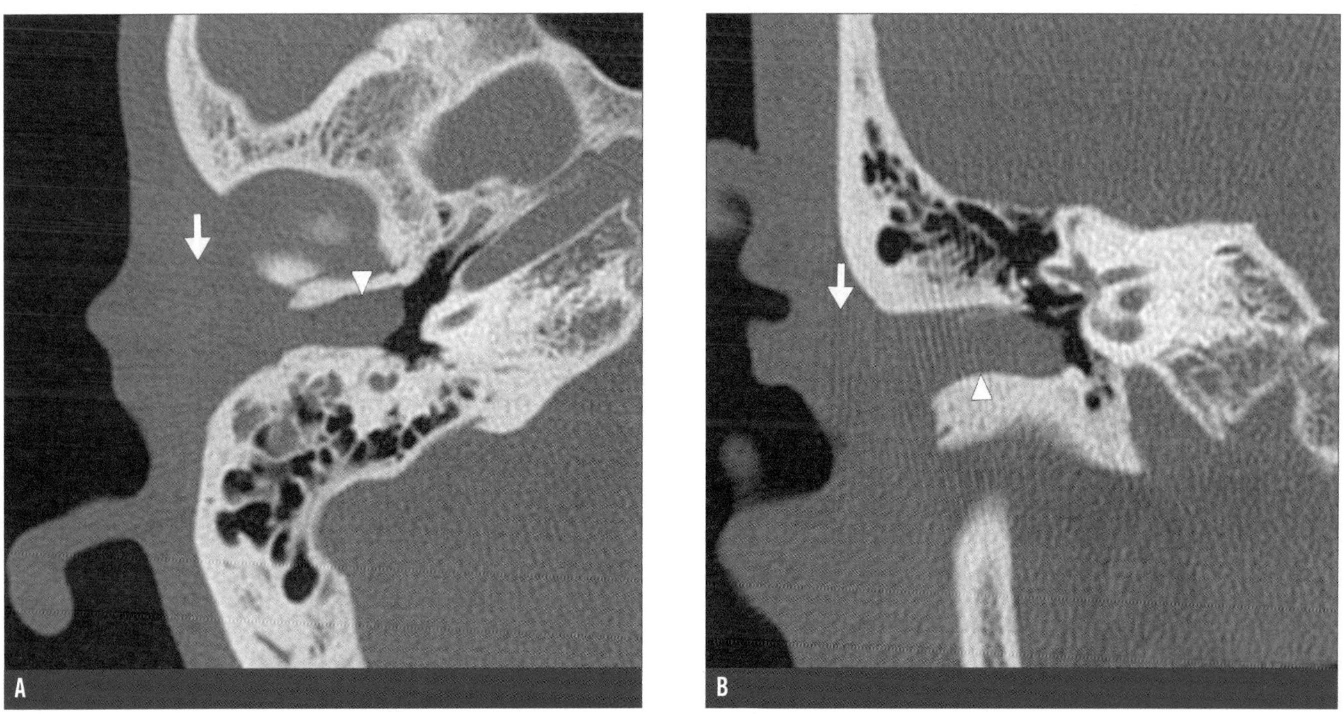

Axial (**A**) and direct coronal (**B**) CT images of the right temporal bone demonstrate abnormal soft tissue completely occupying the entire EAC which could be mistaken for cerumen (arrowheads, **A**, **B**). There is no evidence of osseous erosion, although a soft tissue mass is suggested in the cartilaginous portion of the EAC (arrows, **A**, **B**). An unenhanced coronal reformatted CT image viewed with a soft tissue window (**C**) confirms a soft tissue abnormality occupying the cartilaginous EAC (arrow, **C**). The lesion is nonspecific by CT, although given the abnormal soft tissue, a tumor or infection should be suspected. In this case, squamous cell carcinoma was present at pathology.

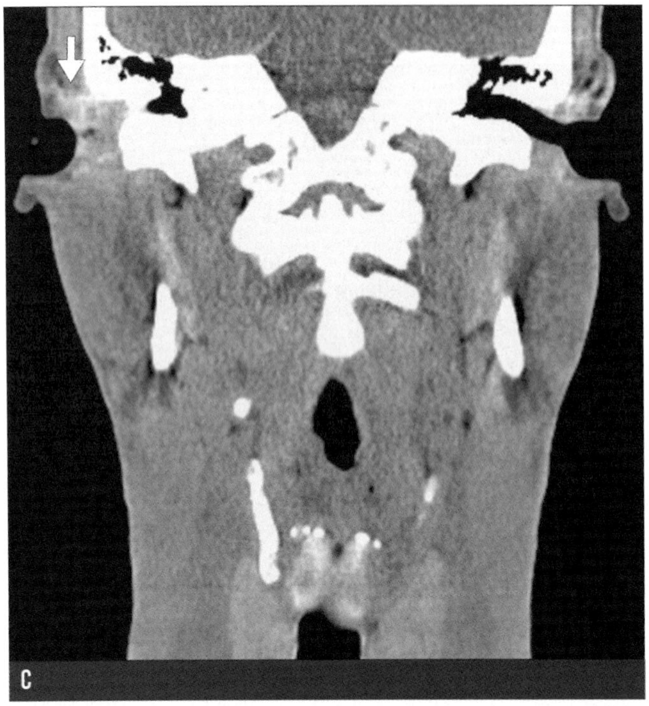

Companion case: EAC adenoid cystic carcinoma

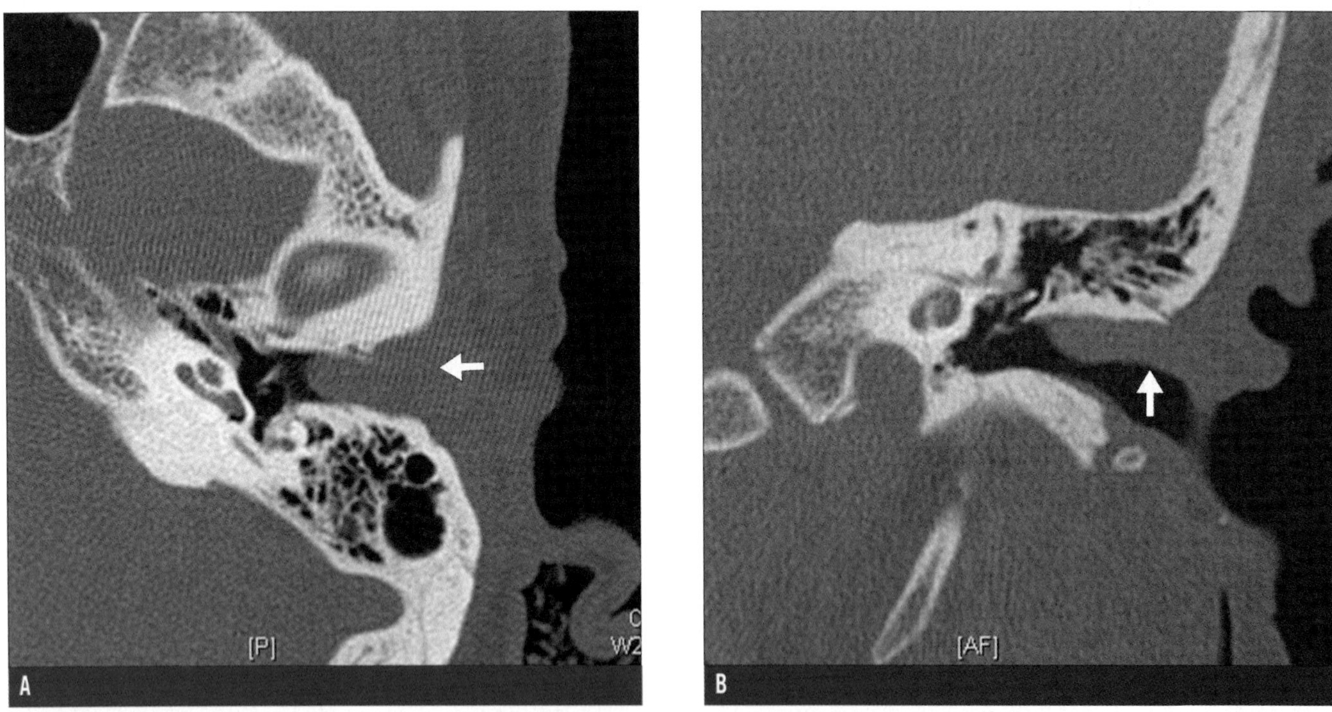

Axial (**A**) and direct coronal (**B**) CT images of the left temporal bone demonstrate abnormal soft tissue occupying the superior aspect of the cartilaginous and osseous portions of the left EAC that could be mistaken for cerumen (arrows, **A**, **B**). However, the finding is isolated to the superior wall of the EAC, rather than centered in the lumen of the EAC, as is typical of cerumen. Furthermore, air does not circumferentially surround the lesion, a finding often identified with cerumen. Axial T1 (**C**), fat-suppressed postcontrast axial T1 (**D**), axial T2 (**E**), and fat-suppressed postcontrast coronal T1 (**F**) MR images of the same patient demonstrate the finding to be T1 and T2 isointense (relative to muscle) as well as enhance (arrows, **C-F**). In this case, this lesion represented an adenoid cystic carcinoma, although any number of tumors, including squamous cell carcinoma, could have this appearance. However, cerumen should not enhance and would not be in the differential, particularly based on the MRI.

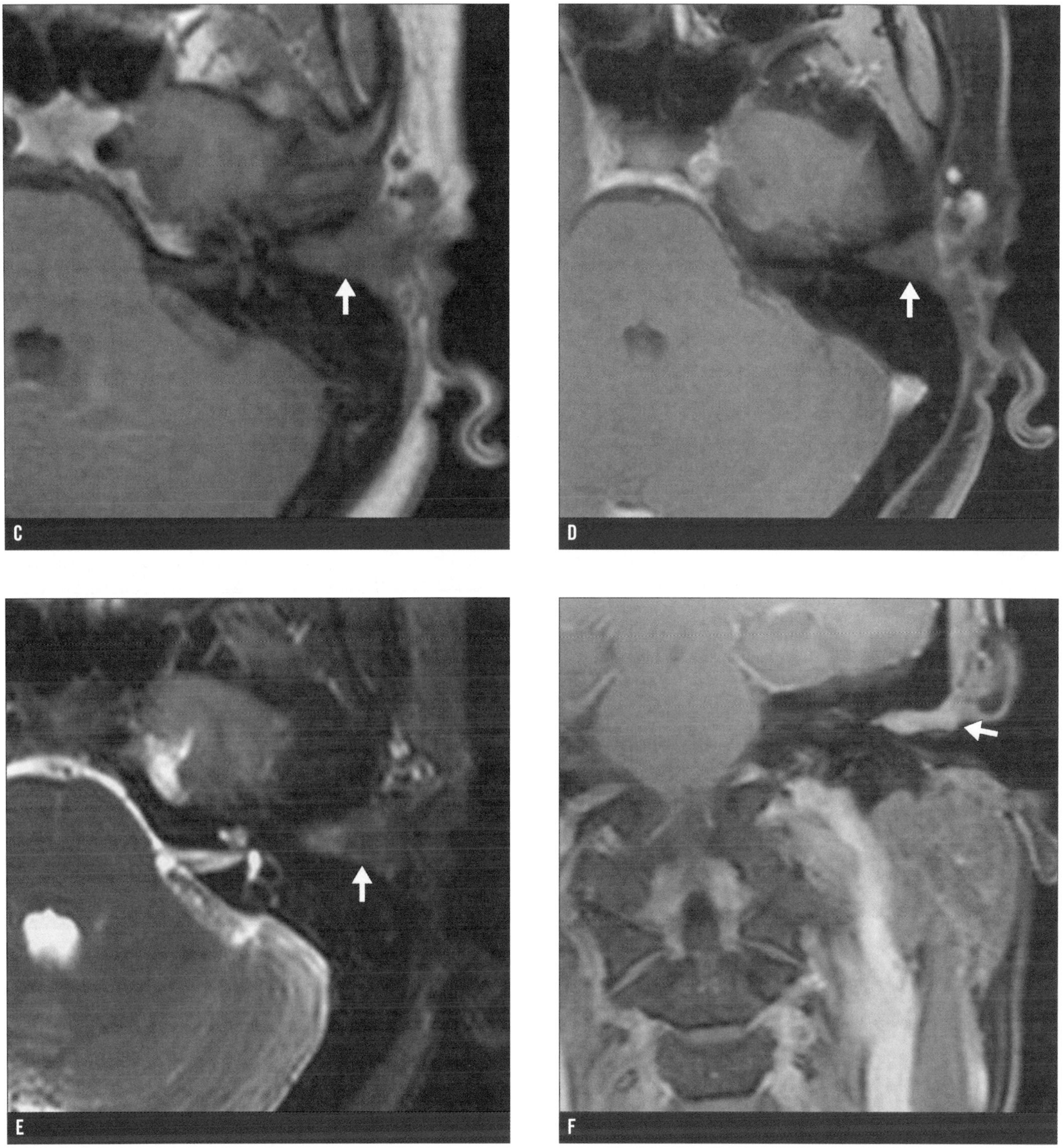
C
D
E
F

Companion case: EAC cholesteatoma

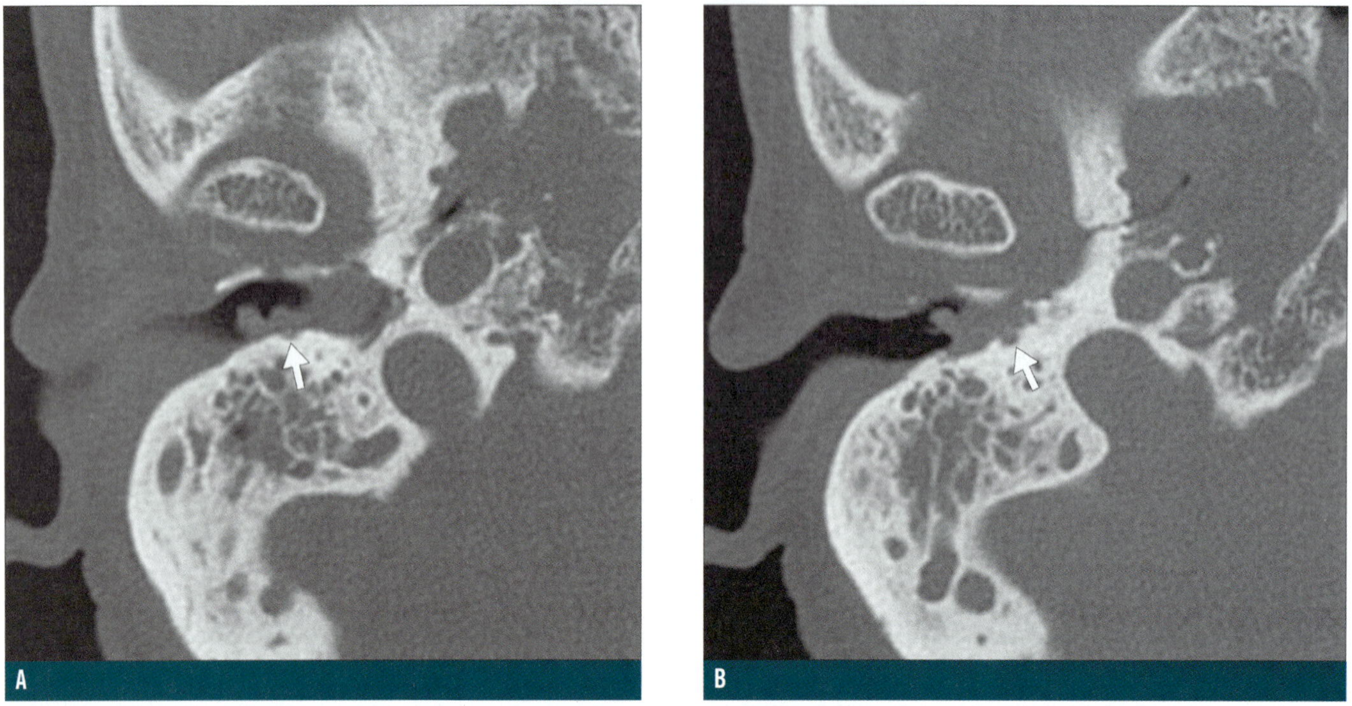

Axial CT images of the right temporal bone (**A**, **B**) demonstrate abnormal soft tissue occupying the posterior-inferior aspect of the EAC. While there is air adjacent to a portion of the lesion, it does not surround the finding, as may be identified with cerumen. Additionally, there is evidence of osseous erosion that suggests an aggressive process (arrows, **A**, **B**), in this case an EAC cholesteatoma.

Companion case: Keratosis obturans

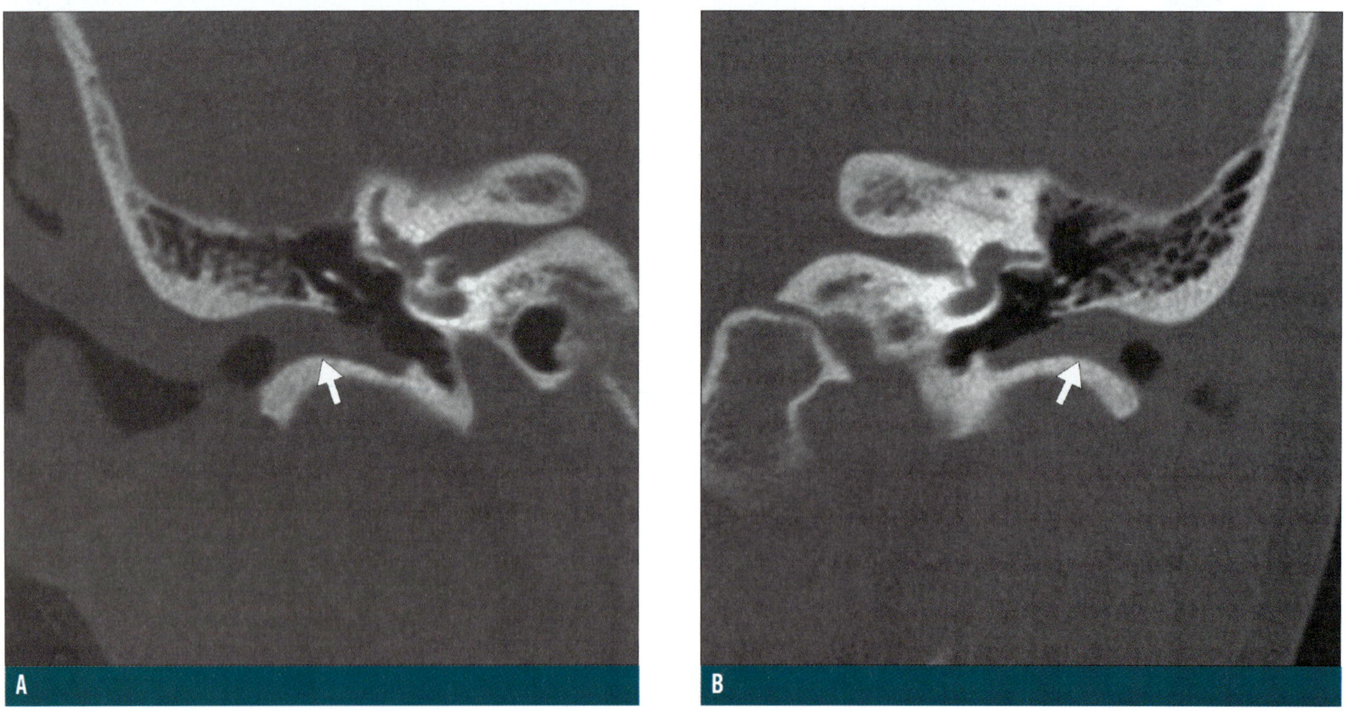

Direct coronal CT images of the right (**A**) and left (**B**) temporal bones demonstrate abnormal soft tissue occupying the bilateral EACs (arrows, **A**, **B**), without a rim of air or evidence of associated osseous erosion. While nonspecific based on imaging, the imaging findings are compatible keratosis obturans in this patient who had a clinical diagnosis of this entity. *Case courtesy of Barbara Zeifer, MD.*

REFERENCES

Beatrice F, Bucolo S, Cavallo R. Earwax, clinical practice. *Acta Otorhinolaryngol Ital.* 2009;29:1-20.

Chakeres DW, Kapila A, LaMasters D. Soft-tissue abnormalities of the external auditory canal: subject review of CT findings. *Radiology.* 1985; 156:105-109.

Chatra PS. Lesions in the external auditory canal. *Indian J Radiol Imaging.* 2011;21(4):274-278.

Dalton SR, Ferringer T, Mowad CM. Obstruction of the external auditory canal by a keratin cast: Keratosis obturans or cholesteatoma? *J Am Acad Dermatol.* 2011;65(3):e88-e89.

Dong F, Gidley PW, Ho T, Luna MA, Ginsberg LE, Sturgis EM. Adenoid cystic carcinoma of the external auditory canal. *Laryngoscope.* 2008;118(9):1591-1596.

Heilbrun ME, Salzman KL, Glastonbury CM, Harnsberger R, Kennedy RJ, Shelton C. External auditory canal cholesteatoma: clinical and imaging spectrum. *Am J Neuroradiol.* 2003;24:751-756.

Ong CK, Pua U, Chong VFH. Imaging of carcinoma of the external auditory canal: a pictorial essay. *Cancer Imaging.* 2008;8:191-198.

Persaud RA, Hajioff D, Thevasagayam MS, Wareing MJ, Wright A. Keratosis obturans and external ear canal cholesteatoma: how and why we should distinguish between these conditions. *Clin Otolaryngol Allied Sci.* 2004;29(6):577-581.

Schwartz KM, Lane JI, Bolster BD Jr, Neff BA. The utility of diffusion-weighted imaging for cholesteatoma evaluation. *AJNR Am J Neuroradiol.* 2011;32(3):430-436.

CASE 8 Tympanoplasties

A tympanoplasty represents a surgical procedure that reconstructs the tympanic membrane (TM). A tympanoplasty is typically performed during surgical treatment of chronic middle ear pathology, such to remove a cholesteatoma, as well as for atelectatic and tympanosclerotic conditions. Historically, temporalis fascia and perichondrium grafts have been used for a tympanoplasty. However, these grafts offer limited resistance to negative middle ear pressure. A cartilage tympanoplasty is not as susceptible to negative ear pressure and therefore has become the preferred technique for some surgeons to reconstruct the TM. A cartilage tympanoplasty can be performed with a single cartilage plate or with several small, overlapping cartilage strips, the latter referred to as the palisade technique. The cartilage graft can be harvested from the tragal cartilage or from the cymbal cartilage of the conchal bowl. A single cartilage plate is preferred for atelectatic TMs because it is more rigid and offers greater resistance to the redevelopment of atelectasis. The palisade technique is preferred for complex cases, such as when the ossicular chain requires reconstruction, because it allows easier closure of various sized defects. On imaging, a tympanoplasty graft will appear as a thickened TM.

In the 1950s, Wullstein and Zollner developed a classification system for the various types of tympanoplasty, in part based on the function and mechanism of the reconstructed ossicular chain. This classification system has been modified since that time to incorporate new surgical techniques and ossicular prostheses.

- **Type I**—This type represents reconstruction of the TM with a normal ossicular chain.
- **Type II**—This type is performed when the ossicular chain has a lever mechanism, meaning that there is one joint in the ossicular chain between the TM and the oval window. Traditionally, the malleus was absent and the tympanoplasty graft was placed directly onto the native incus. However, this type now also includes the instance when a tympanoplasty graft is placed directly onto a partial ossicular replacement prosthesis (PORP) or incus prosthesis.
- **Type III**—This type is performed when the ossicular chain lacks a lever mechanisim, also referred to as a columella configuration (columella is Latin for "little column"). Typically, the malleus and incus are absent, and the tympanoplasty graft is placed directly onto the stapes superstructure. A type III tympanoplasty may also be performed in conjunction with a PORP or total ossicular replacement prosthesis (TORP), the former placed between the tympanoplasty graft and the stapes superstructure, whereas the latter is placed between the tympanoplasty graft and the stapes footplate or oval window.
- **Type IV**—This type is performed when the malleus, incus, and stapes superstructure are absent, but the stapes footplate is intact and mobile. The tympanoplasty graft is placed directly onto the stapes footplate. In order to maintain normal inner ear function, a "sonic shield" is created by positioning the tympanoplasty graft such that a chamber is formed adjacent to the round window. This procedure is uncommonly performed today because of the advances of modern day ossicular prostheses, and it is usually only performed when the ear is unsuitable for an ossicular reconstruction.
- **Type V**—This type is performed when malleus, incus, and stapes superstructure are absent, and the stapes footplate is fixed. In this case, a fenestration is created in the lateral semicircular canal, and the tympanoplasty graft is placed onto that fenestration. This is rarely performed today.

Tympanoplasty—type I

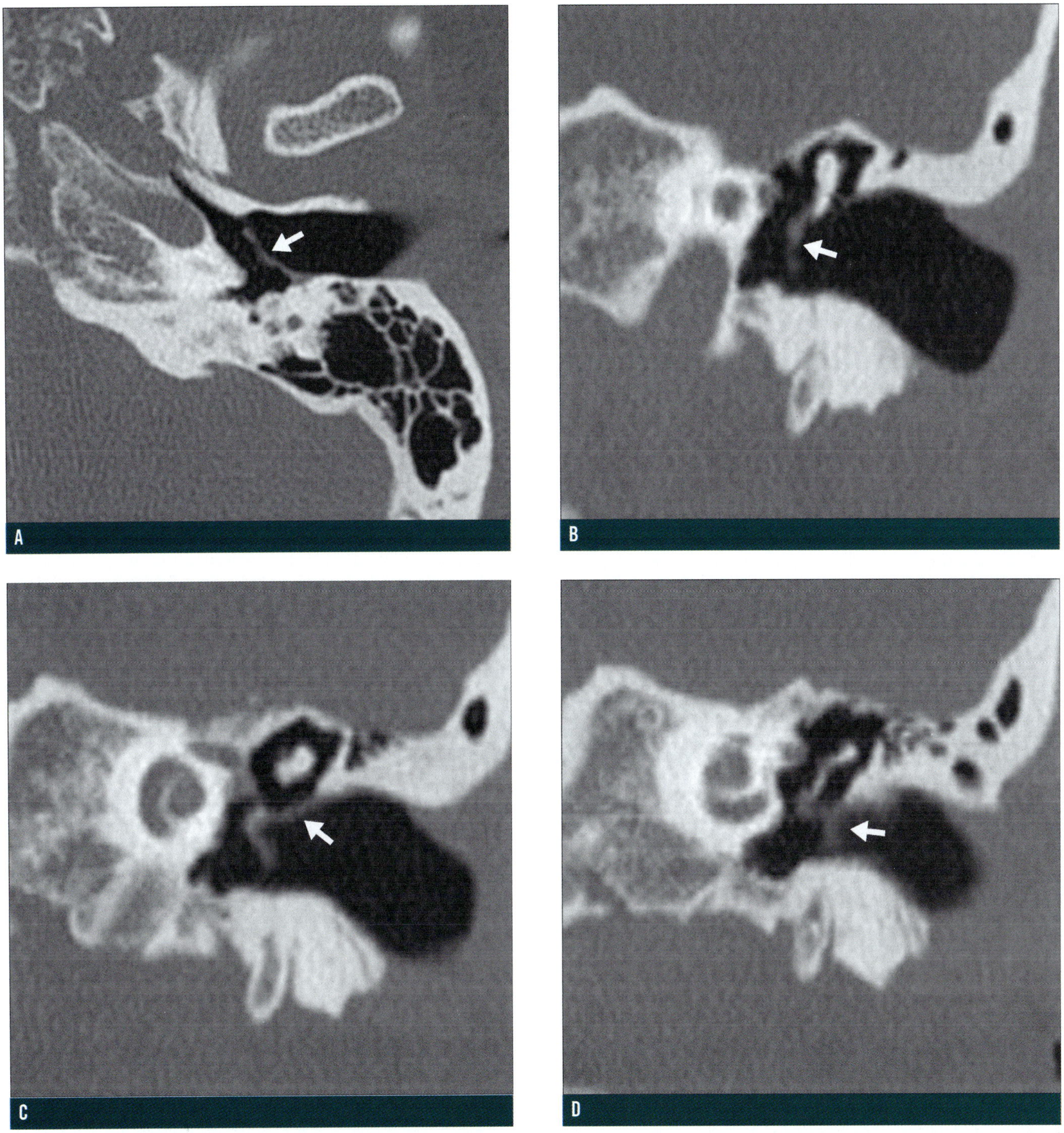

Axial (**A**) and coronal reformatted (**B**-**D**) noncontrast CT images of the left temporal bone demonstrate a thickened TM, compatible with a tympanoplasty graft (arrows, **A**-**D**). The entire ossicular chain was present (not shown in its entirety on the provided images). The findings are compatible with a type I tympanoplasty.

Tympanoplasty—type II

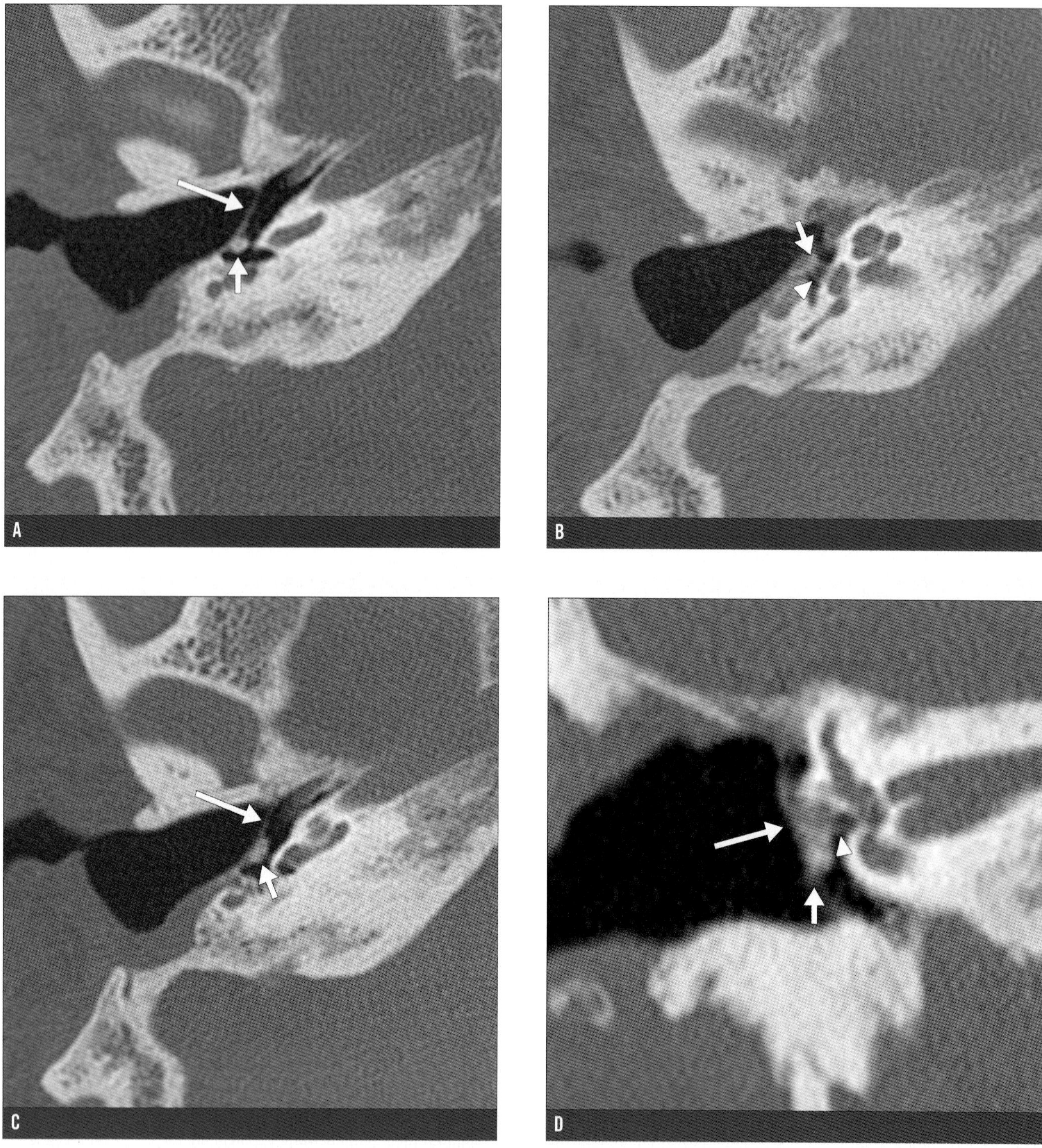

Axial (**A**-**C**) and coronal reformatted (**D**) CT images of the right temporal bone demonstrate a thickened TM, compatible with a tympanoplasty graft (long arrows, **A**, **C**, **D**). The malleus is absent, and there has been placement of an incus interposition graft (short arrows, **A**-**D**) that articulates with the stapes (arrowheads, **B**, **D**). The tympanoplasty graft has been placed onto the incus interposition graft, compatible with a type II tympanoplasty. There are also postoperative changes related to a prior canal wall down mastoidectomy.

Tympanoplasty—type III

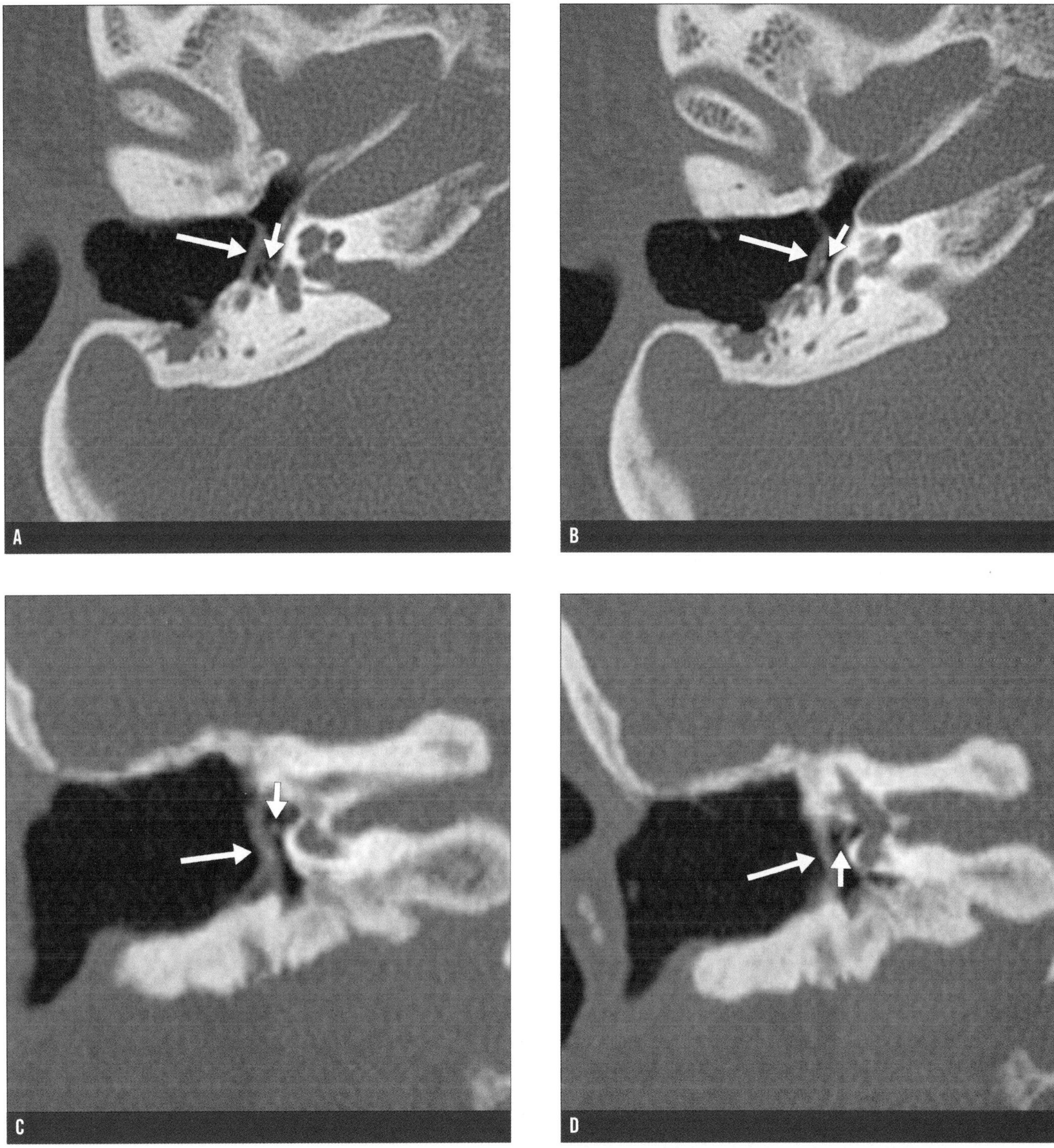

Axial (**A**, **B**) and coronal reformatted (**C**, **D**) CT images of the right temporal bone demonstrate a thickened TM, compatible with a tympanoplasty graft (long arrows, **A-D**). The malleus and incus are absent, and the tympanoplasty graft has been placed directly onto the stapes superstructure (short arrows, **A-D**), compatible with a type III tympanoplasty. There are also postoperative changes related to a prior canal wall down mastoidectomy.

Tympanoplasty—type IV

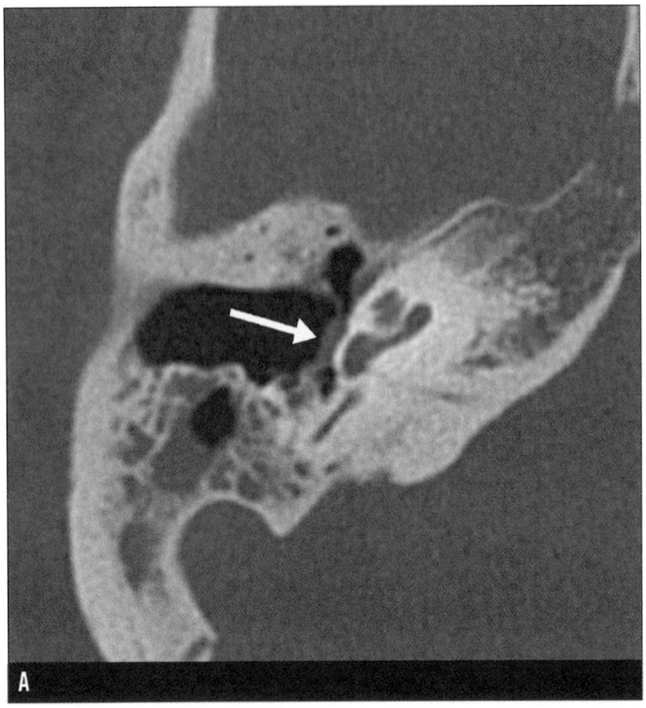

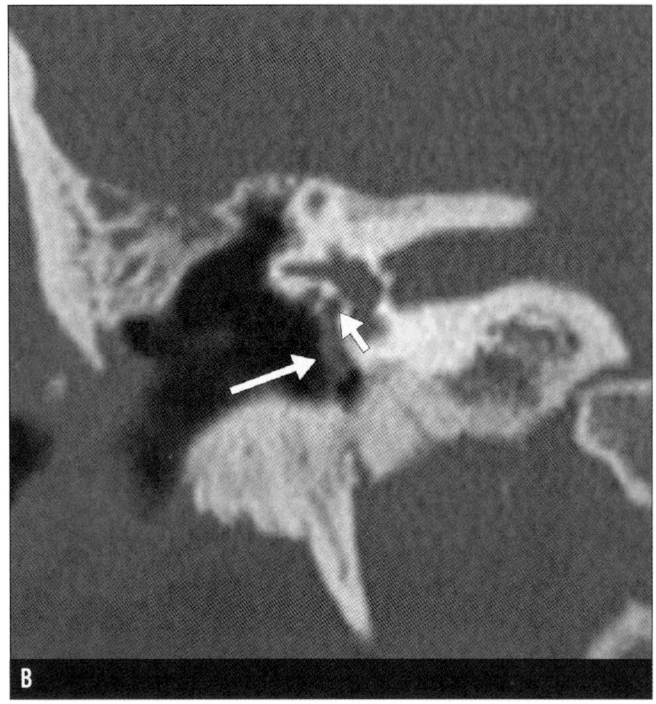

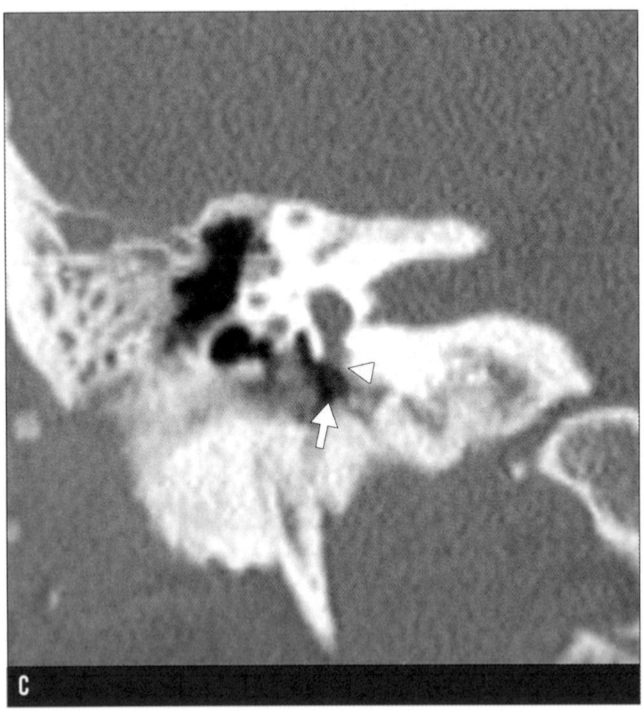

Axial (**A**) and coronal reformatted (**B**) CT images of the right temporal bone demonstrate a thickened TM, compatible with a tympanoplasty graft (long arrows, **A**, **B**). The malleus, incus, and stapes superstructure are absent. At the time of surgery, the stapes footplate was noted to be mobile. The tympanoplasty graft overlies the oval window (short arrow, **B**). An additional coronal reformatted CT image (**C**) demonstrates a "sonic shield" (arrow, **C**) surrounding the round window (arrowhead, **C**). The findings are compatible with a type IV tympanoplasty.

REFERENCES

Alicandri-Ciufelli M, Marchioni D, Grammatica A, Soloperto D, Carpeggiani P, Monzani D, Presutti L. Tympanoplasty: an up-to-date pictorial review. *J Neuroradiol.* 2012;39(3):149-157.

Dornhoffer J. Cartilage tympanoplasty: indications, techniques, and outcomes in a 1,000-patient series. *Laryngoscope.* 2003;113(11):1844-1856.

Dornhoffer JL. Cartilage tympanoplasty. *Otolaryngol Clin North Am.* 2006; 39(6): 1161-1176.

Guneri EA, Ikiz AO, Erdag TK, Sutay S. Cartilage tympanoplasty: indications, techniques, and results. *J Otolaryngol Head Neck Surg.* 2009; 38(3):362-368.

Probst R, Grevers G, Iro H. *Basic Otorhinolaryngology: A step-by-step Learning Guide.* New York, NY: Thieme; 2006.

Yung MW. Type IV tympanoplasty revisited. *Am J Otol.* 1998;19(6):700-703.

CASE 9 Myringotomy tubes

Myringotomy tubes are also known as tympanostomy tubes, pressure-equalizing tubes (PE tubes), or ventilation tubes. Myringotomy tubes are most commonly utilized to treat recurrent episodes of acute otitis media, chronic otitis media, and negative middle ear pressure that results in retraction of the tympanic membrane. A myringotomy or tympanostomy represents a surgical incision in the tympanic membrane through which a myringotomy tube may be placed. The most common site of myringotomy tube placement is the anterior-inferior quadrant of the tympanic membrane. A myringotomy tube straddles the tympanic membrane, with a portion of the tube located in the tympanic cavity and a portion in the external auditory canal. Myringotomy tubes come in a variety of shapes and sizes and can be made of silicone, plastic, or stainless steel. Long-term or "permanent" tubes, such as a Goode T-tube, have a greater longevity than myringotomy tubes, which are considered short-term tubes; however, the majority of these so-called permanent tubes will also eventually extrude. Kalcioglu et al found that T-tubes will stay in an appropriate position for an average of just over 16 months, compared to just over 7 months for a short-term tube. The main complications of a myringotomy tube are tympanic membrane perforation beyond the myringotomy and the formation of granulation tissue, cholesteatoma, or tympanosclerosis. T-tubes have been shown to have a higher rate of tympanic membrane perforation than the short-term tubes.

COMPANION CASES

- **Displaced myringotomy tube into the EAC.**
- **Displaced myringotomy tube into the tympanic cavity.**
- **Displaced earring into the EAC.**

Myringotomy tube

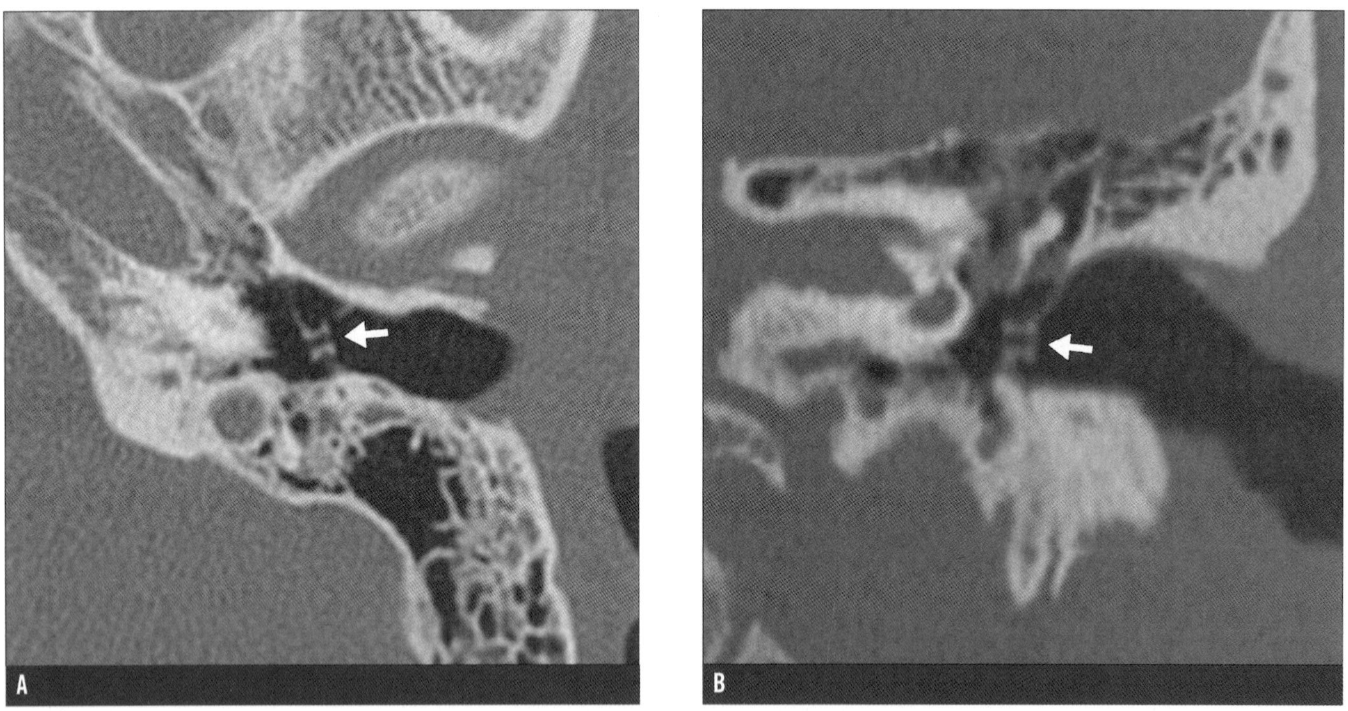

Axial (**A**) and coronal reformatted (**B**) CT images of the left temporal bone demonstrate a myringotomy tube in an appropriate position (arrows, **A**, **B**).

Goode T-tube

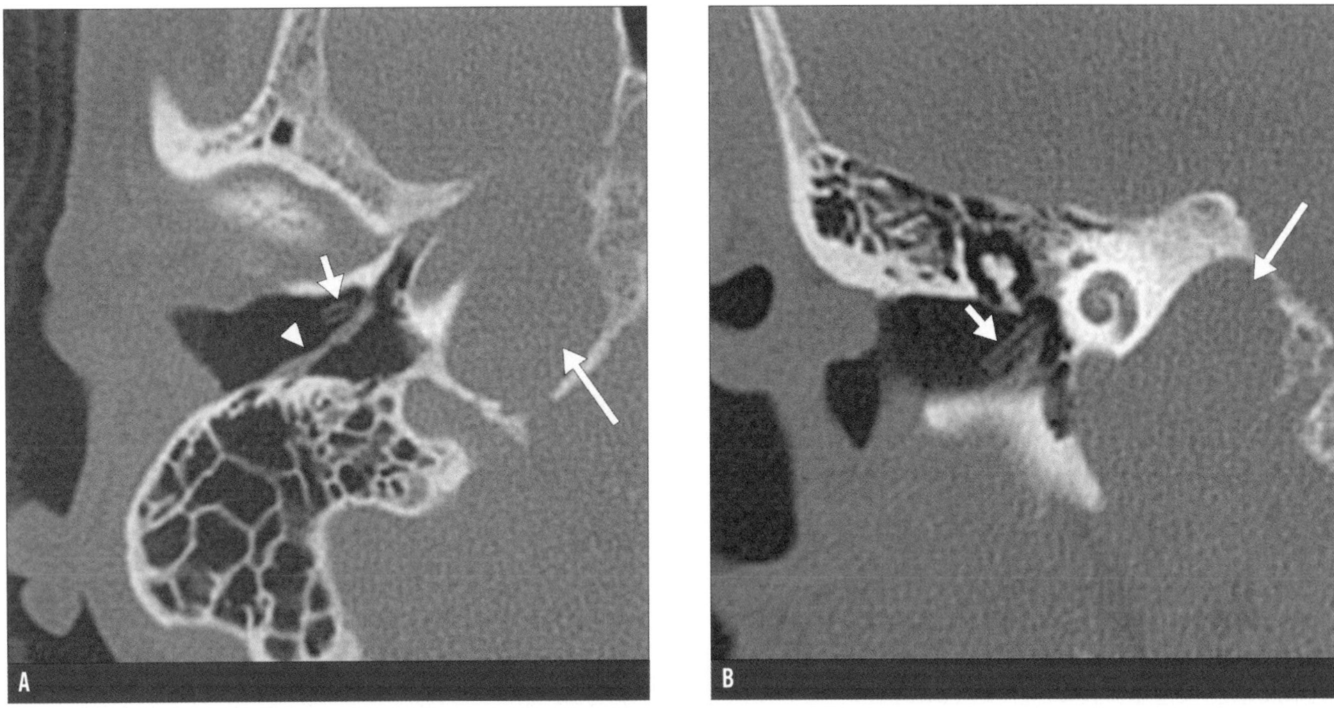

Axial (**A**) and coronal reformatted (**B**) CT images of the right temporal bone demonstrate a Goode T-tube in an appropriate position (short arrows, **A**, **B**), located within the anterior-inferior aspect of a tympanoplasty graft (arrowhead, **A**). There are also findings of a right petrous apex cholesterol granuloma associated with circumscribed, osseous expansion of the petrous apex (long arrows, **A**, **B**).

Companion case: Displaced myringotomy tube into the EAC

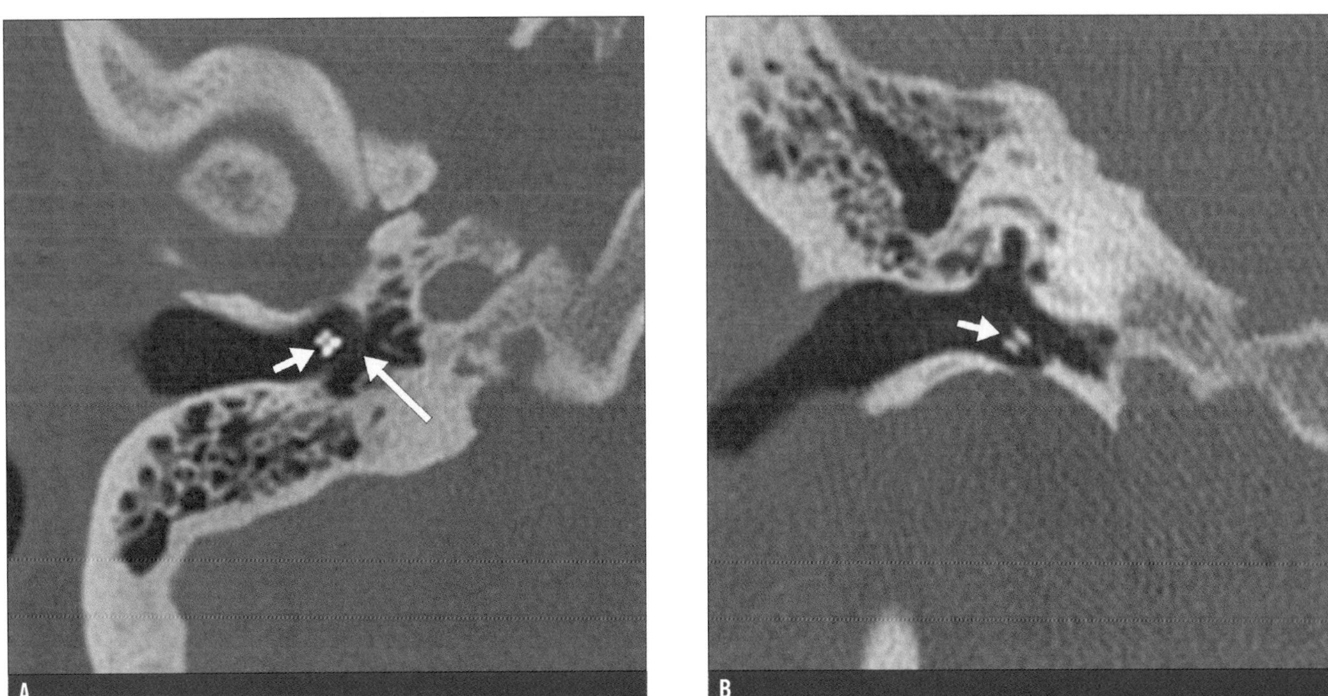

Axial (**A**) and coronal reformatted (**B**) CT images of the right temporal bone demonstrate a displaced myringotomy tube (short arrows, **A**, **B**) located in the EAC and lateral to the tympanic membrane (long arrow, **A**).

Companion case: Displaced myringotomy tube into the tympanic cavity

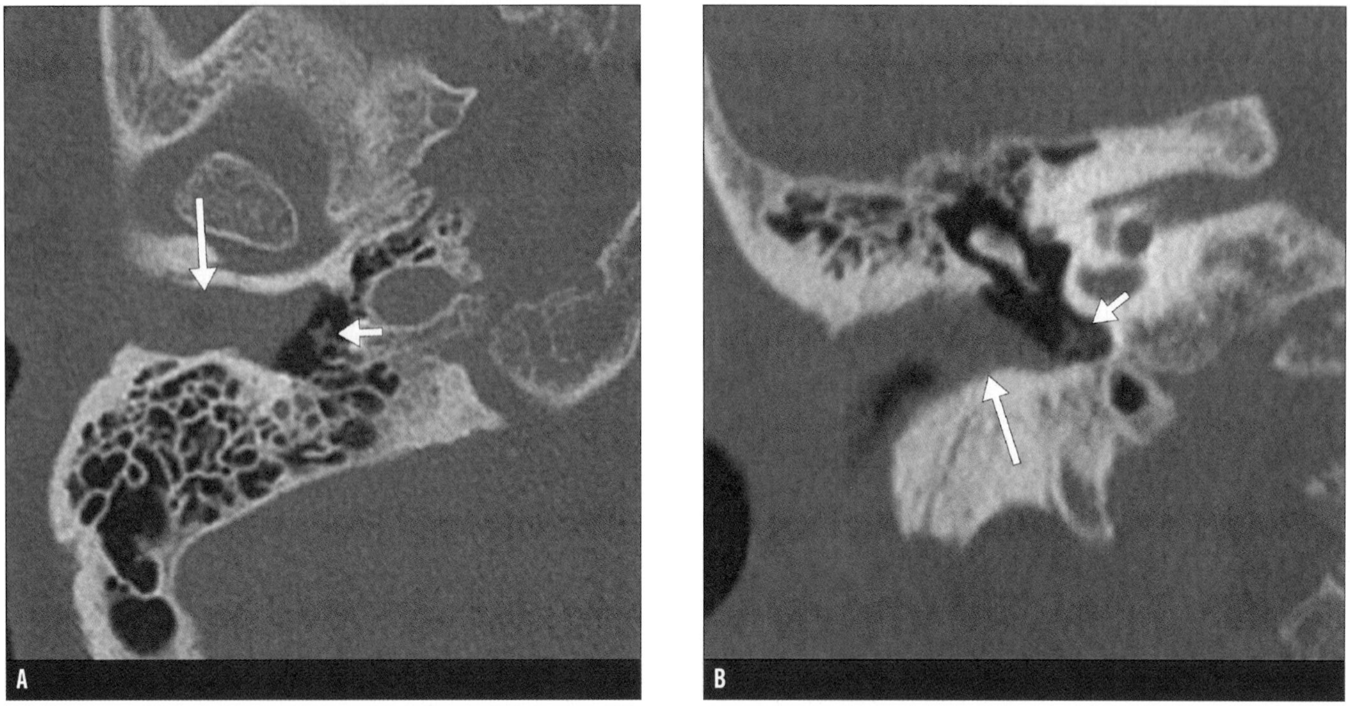

Axial (**A**) and coronal reformatted (**B**) CT images of the right temporal bone demonstrate a displaced myringotomy tube located medial to the tympanic membrane and within the hypotympanum of the tympanic cavity (short arrows, **A**, **B**). The tympanic membrane is not optimally visualized secondary to opacification of the external auditory canal (long arrows, **A**, **B**).

Companion case: Displaced earring into the EAC

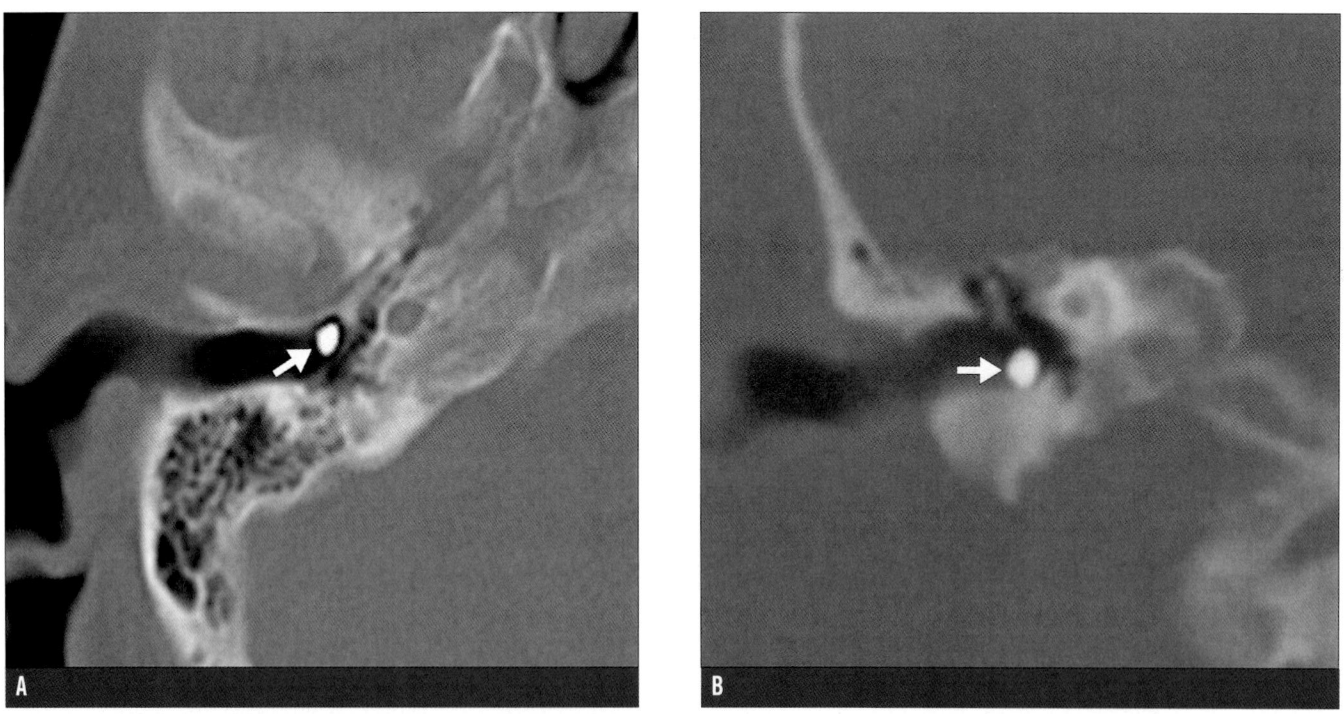

Axial (**A**) and coronal reformatted (**B**) CT images demonstrate a dense metallic structure within the medial-most aspect of the right EAC (arrows, **A**, **B**). The patient lost her right earring for several weeks. The finding represented the lost earring on direct inspection. While a myringotomy tube can be constructed from metal, it should contain a hollow chamber, a finding which is not present in this case.

REFERENCES

Bulkley WJ, Bowes AK, Marlowe JF. Complications following ventilation of the middle ear using Goode T tubes. *Arch Otolaryngol Head Neck Surg.* 1991;117:895-898.

Goode RL. Long-term middle ear ventilation with T tubes: the perforation problem. *Otolaryngol Head Neck Surg.* 1996;115(6):500-501.

Kalcioglu MT, Cokkeser Y, Kizilay A, Ozturan O. Follow-up of 366 ears after tympanostomy tube insertion: why is it draining? *Otolaryngol Head Neck Surg.* 2003;128(4):560-564.

Klein MA, Kelly JK, Eggleston D. Recognizing tympanostomy tubes on temporal bone CT: typical and atypical appearances. *AJR Am J Roentgenol.* 1988;150:1411-1414.

CASE 10 Atticoantrostomy

The attic (also called epitympanum or epitympanic recess) represents the superior aspect of the tympanic cavity cephalad to the level of the superior margin of the tympanic membrane. An atticotomy is a surgical procedure that is performed to gain access to the attic and is commonly utilized to remove a cholesteatoma from the epitympanum. An atticotomy can be performed via a postauricular (ie, posterior to the auricle) or an endaural (ie, through the external auditory canal) incision. The lateral wall of the attic and the scutum are then removed. This is followed by a resection that generally proceeds from an anterior to posterior fashion, with the surgeon removing as much of the native temporal bone as necessary to visualize and completely resect the lesion. Thus, the surgery may entail an atticotomy (ie, isolated to the attic), an attico-antrostomy (ie, involving the attic and aditus ad antrum), or an atticotomy with a limited mastoidectomy. A tympanoplasty and cartilage reconstruction of the scutum can be performed following removal of the lesion. Typically, an atticotomy and its variations are less invasive than a mastoidectomy and are usually associated with fewer long-term complications.

Atticoantrostomy

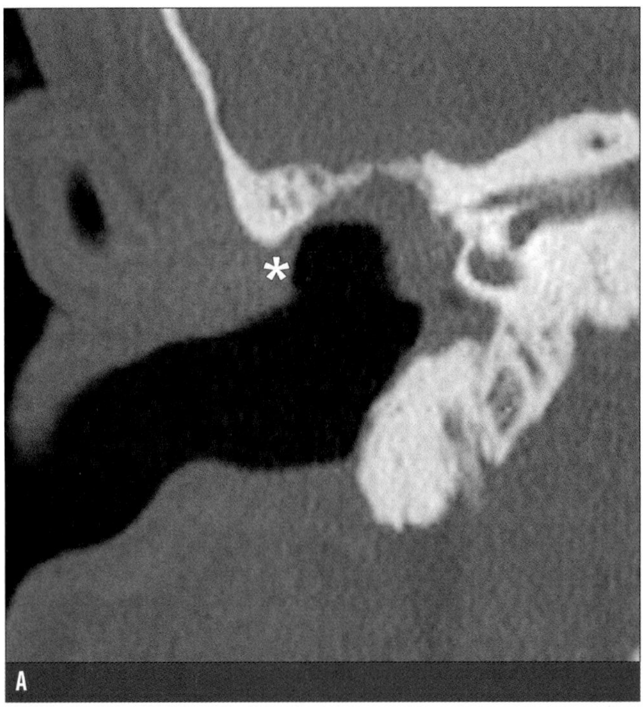

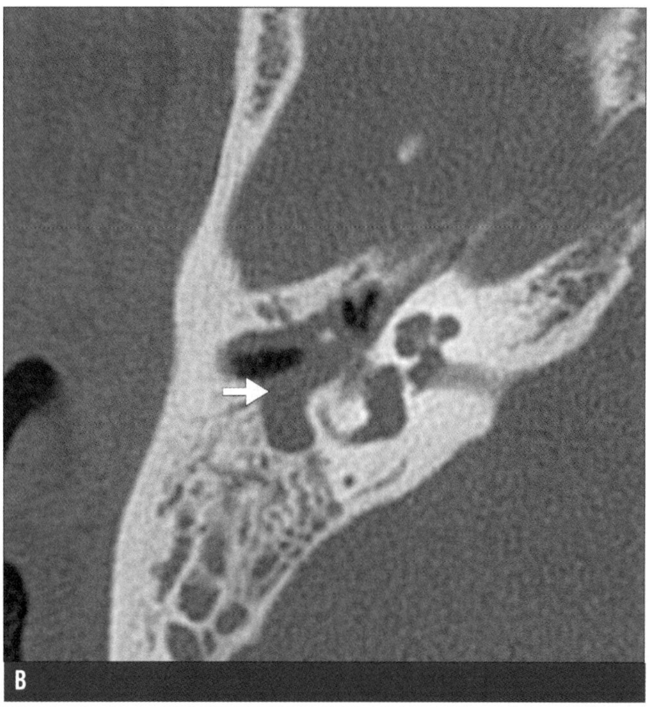

Coronal reformatted (**A**) and axial (**B**) CT images of the right temporal bone of a patient with a history of a cholesteatoma. These images demonstrate postsurgical changes, including removal of the scutum and lateral wall of the attic (asterisk, **A**) as well as widening of the aditus ad antrum (arrow, **B**), compatible with an atticoantrostomy. Soft tissue opacification of the tympanic cavity is nonspecific and may represent granulation tissue or residual/recurrent cholesteatoma.

REFERENCES

Haberman RS. *Middle ear and Mastoid Surgery.* New York, NY: Thieme; 2004.

Nikolopoulos TP, Gerbesiotis P. Surgical management of cholesteatoma: the two main options and the third way – atticotomy/limited mastoidectomy. *Int J Pediatr Otorhinolaryngol.* 2009;73(9):1222-1227.

Pennings RJ, Cremers CW. Postauricular approach atticotomy: a modified closed technique with reconstruction of the scutum with cymbal cartilage. *Ann Otol Rhinol Laryngol.* 2009;118(3):199-204.

CASE 11 Mastoidectomies

A mastoidectomy refers to removal of a portion or all of the mastoid air cells. A mastoidectomy may be performed to remove a cholesteatoma, to treat suppurative otitis media, or to treat mastoiditis that is refractory to medical treatment. There are two main types of mastoidectomy: a canal wall up and a canal wall down mastoidectomy. With a canal wall up mastoidectomy, the posterior wall of the external auditory canal (EAC) is preserved. By contrast, with a canal wall down mastoidectomy, the posterior wall of the EAC is removed. A canal wall up mastoidectomy involves removal of the mastoid air cells as well as the Koerner septum, which is an osseous plate located along the lateral wall of the mastoid antrum. This allows for communication between the mastoid bowl (ie, the surgically formed mastoid bed), the mastoid antrum, and the epitympanum. A canal wall down mastoidectomy encompasses the same surgery as the canal wall up mastoidectomy, with the exception of also removing the posterior wall of the EAC.

A canal wall up mastoidectomy is more often performed than a canal wall down mastoidectomy, in part because it preserves the EAC and thus the normal clearing and lubrication function of the EAC cerumen. Furthermore, patients with a canal wall down mastoidectomy may require frequent debridement of the mastoid bowl because of chronic drainage. A canal wall down mastoidectomy results in a wider exposure than a canal wall up mastoidectomy and is performed when a wider exposure is needed to visualize and completely remove the abnormality.

Techniques to reconstruct the posterior wall of the EAC following a canal wall down mastoidectomy have been developed in an attempt to prevent complications associated with the lack of an EAC. If the native posterior wall of the EAC is diseased and cannot be reconstructed, then mastoid cortical bone, a temporalis fascial graft, and/or mastoid periosteum may be used for the reconstruction.

COMPANION CASES

- **Automastoidectomy.** An automastoidectomy is rare and is most commonly the result of a cholesteatoma. In this setting, a cholesteatoma creates an osseous cavity in the mastoid air cells, often associated with erosion of the posterior wall of the EAC, the outer wall of the attic, and the mastoid antrum. If the cholesteatoma becomes large enough and erodes through the outer mastoid bone cortex, then the cholesteatoma may extrude through the defect, in essence treating itself in the process. The resultant mastoid cavity can mimic the appearance of a surgical mastoidectomy on imaging.
- **Progressive mastoidectomy fat graft enhancement because of fat necrosis.** A fat graft may be utilized during a mastoidectomy to eliminate the dead space created by the surgery. Necrosis of the fat graft may occur within days following surgery, but it often progresses over months to years. When fat necrosis occurs, the graft size will shrink, occasionally leading to ineffective graft closure. On CT, the mastoidectomy fat graft undergoing fat necrosis will progressively diminish in size and may undergo patchy enhancement. On MRI, fat necrosis enhancement can be rather striking and simulate residual or recurrent tumor, in the appropriate clinical setting. Therefore, awareness of the natural progression of fat necrosis is imperative when interpreting postoperative cases that contain fat packing.

Canal wall up mastoidectomy

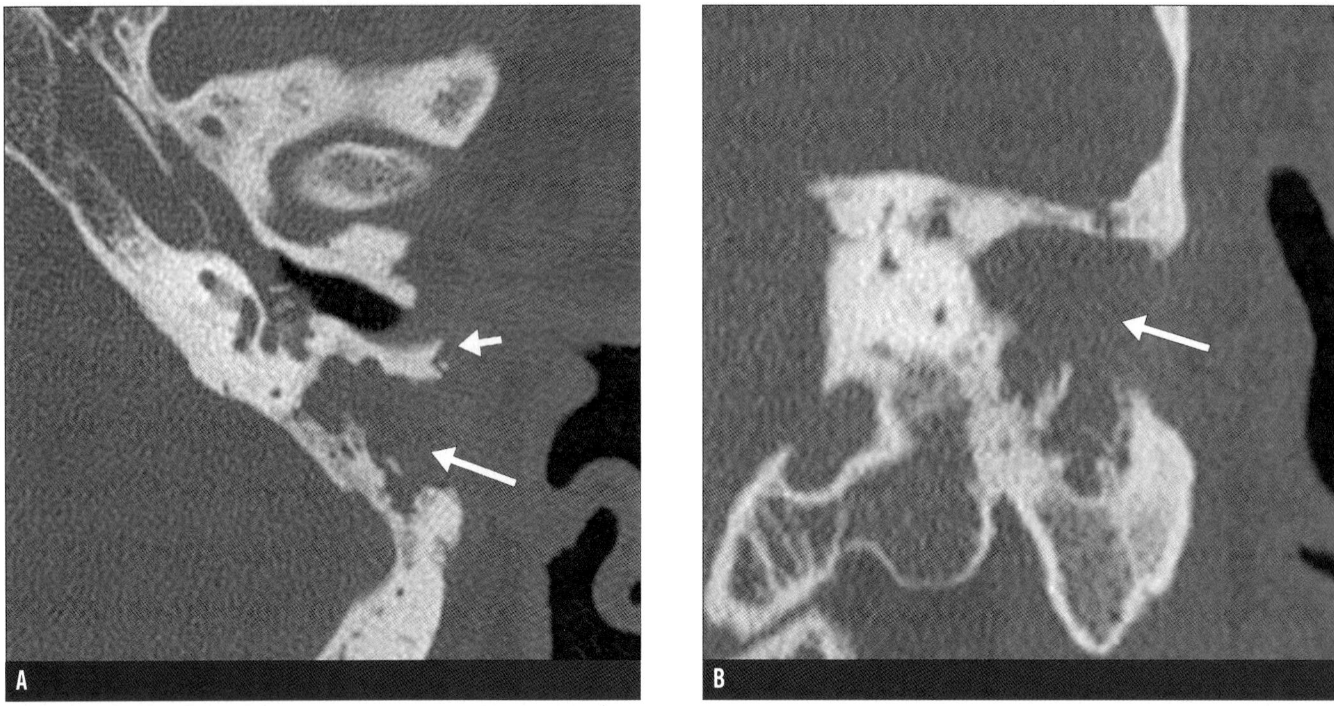

Axial (**A**) and coronal reformatted (**B**) CT images of the left temporal bone demonstrate typical findings of a canal wall up mastoidectomy, including maintenance of the posterior wall of the EAC (short arrow, **A**). There is nonspecific opacification of the left mastoid bowl that may represent incidental granulation tissue or granulation tissue (long arrows, **A**, **B**).

Canal wall down mastoidectomy

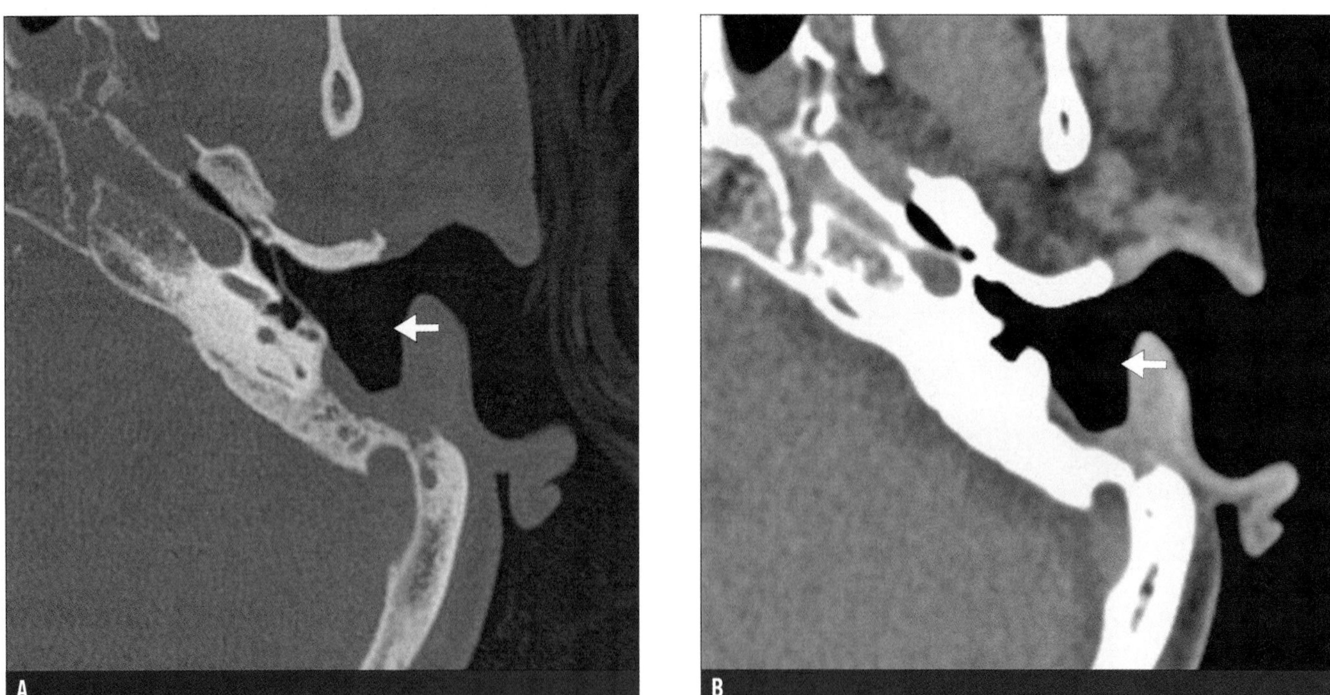

Noncontrast axial CT images of the left temporal bone viewed with a bone window (**A**) and a soft tissue window (**B**). The images demonstrate a typical left canal wall down mastoidectomy with absence of the posterior wall of the EAC (arrows, **A**, **B**). Peripherally located nonspecific soft tissue is present within the mastoid bowl.

Canal wall down mastoidectomy with reconstruction of the posterior wall

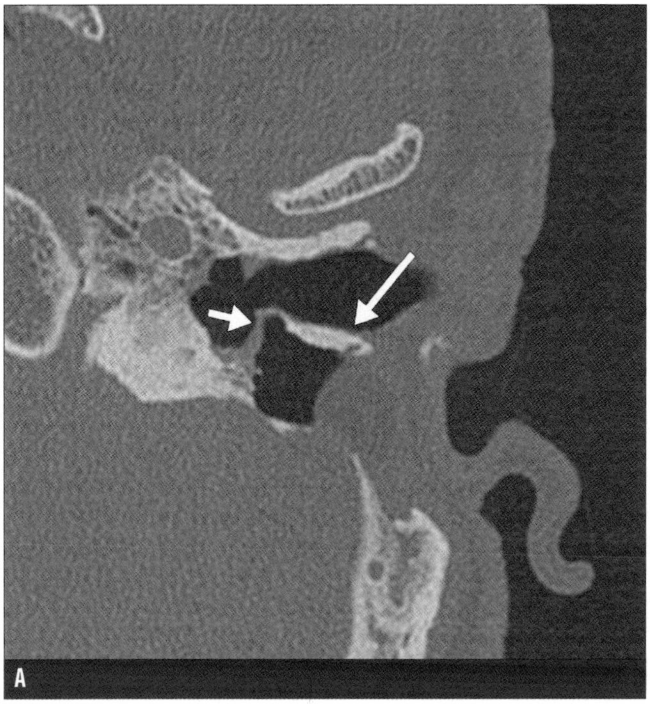

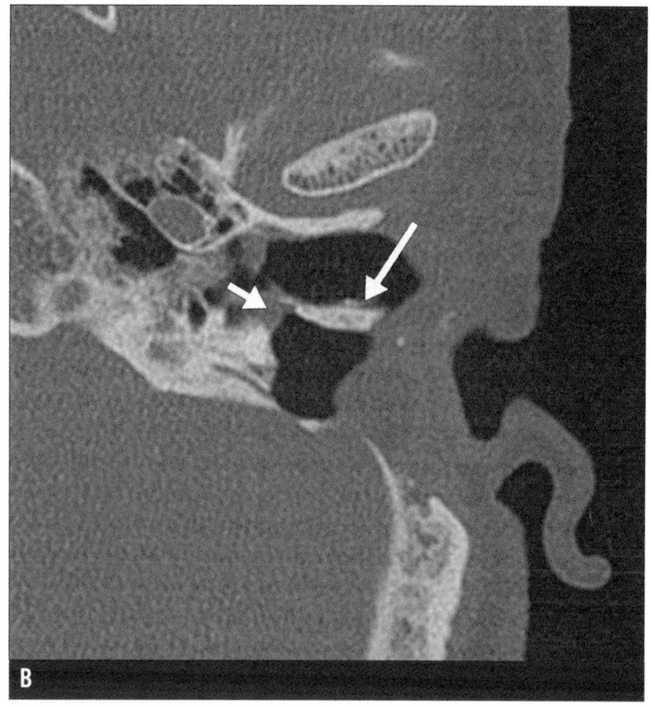

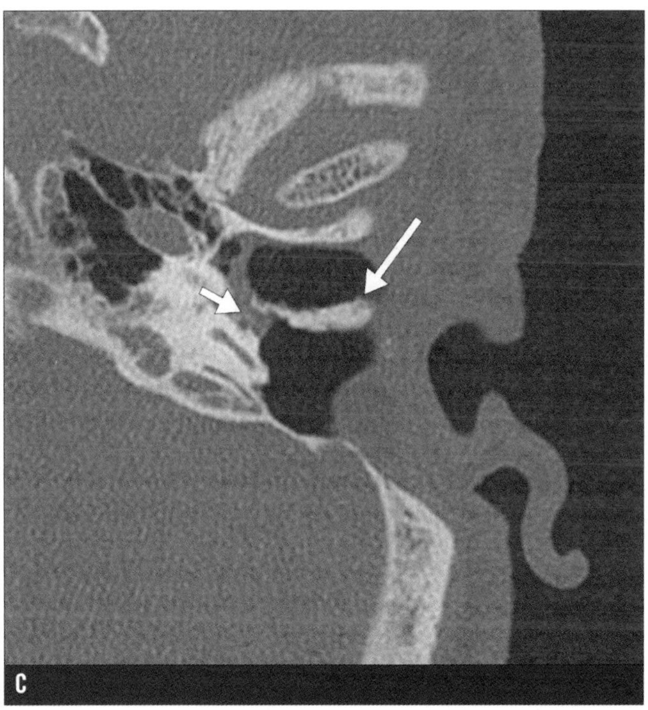

Axial CT images of the left temporal bone (**A**-**C**) demonstrate postsurgical changes from a prior left canal wall down mastoidectomy with reconstruction of the posterior wall of EAC (long arrows, **A**-**C**). The discontinuity along the posterior wall of the EAC (short arrows, **A**-**C**) differentiates a reconstructed posterior wall following a canal wall down mastoidectomy from a canal wall up mastoidectomy with an intact EAC.

Companion case: Automastoidectomy

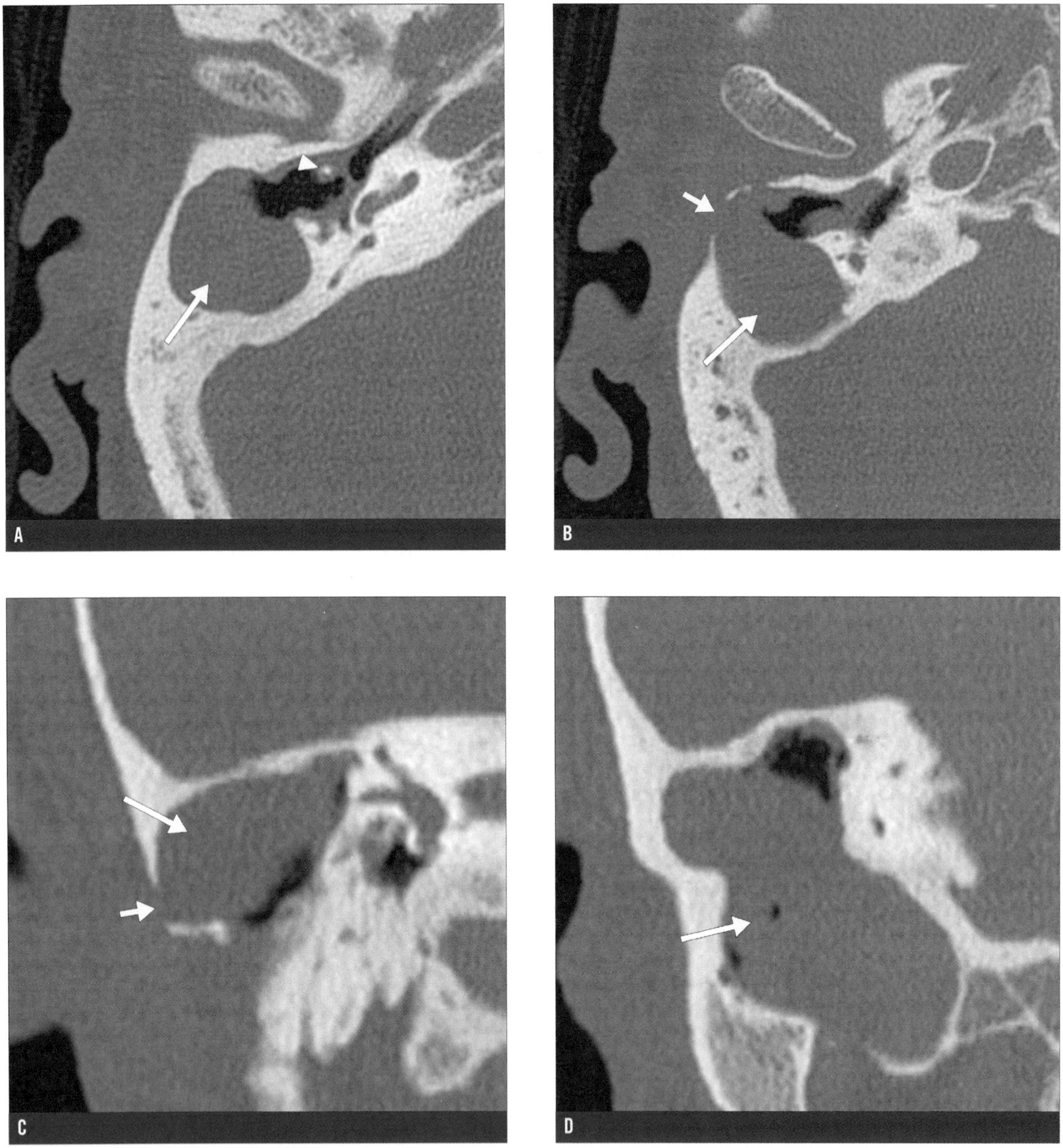

Axial (**A**, **B**) and coronal reformatted (**C**, **D**) CT images of the right temporal bone demonstrate a large osseous lucency centered in the mastoid (long arrows, **A-D**) that communicates with the tympanic cavity. There is near-complete soft tissue opacification of this lucency with a focal area of osseous dehiscence laterally (short arrows, **B**, **C**). There is also erosion of the ossicles, with only a small portion of the malleus remaining (arrowhead, **A**). Axial T2 (**E**), fat-suppressed postcontrast axial T1 (**F**), axial DWI (**G**), and an axial ADC map (**H**) MR images of the right temporal bone demonstrate the mastoid lesion to be heterogeneous on T2 (short arrow, **E**), nonenhancing (short arrow, **F**), and diffusion-restricting (short arrows, **G**, **H**), compatible with an epidermoid/cholesteatoma. This patient did not have a history of right temporal bone surgery. Therefore, the CT and MR imaging characteristics are compatible with an automastoidectomy secondary to an epidermoid/cholesteatoma.

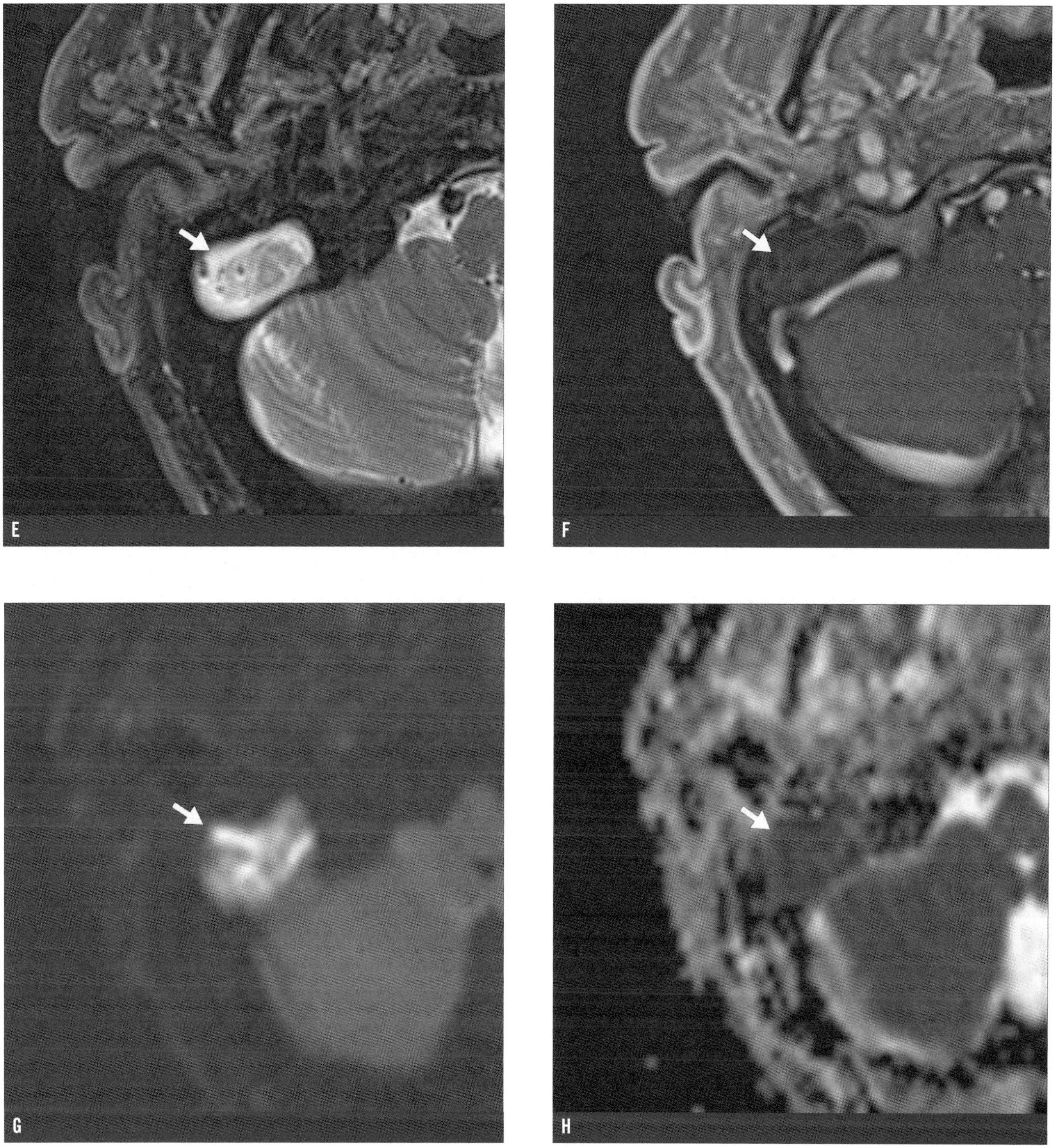
E
F
G
H

Companion case: Progressive mastoidectomy fat graft enhancement because of fat necrosis

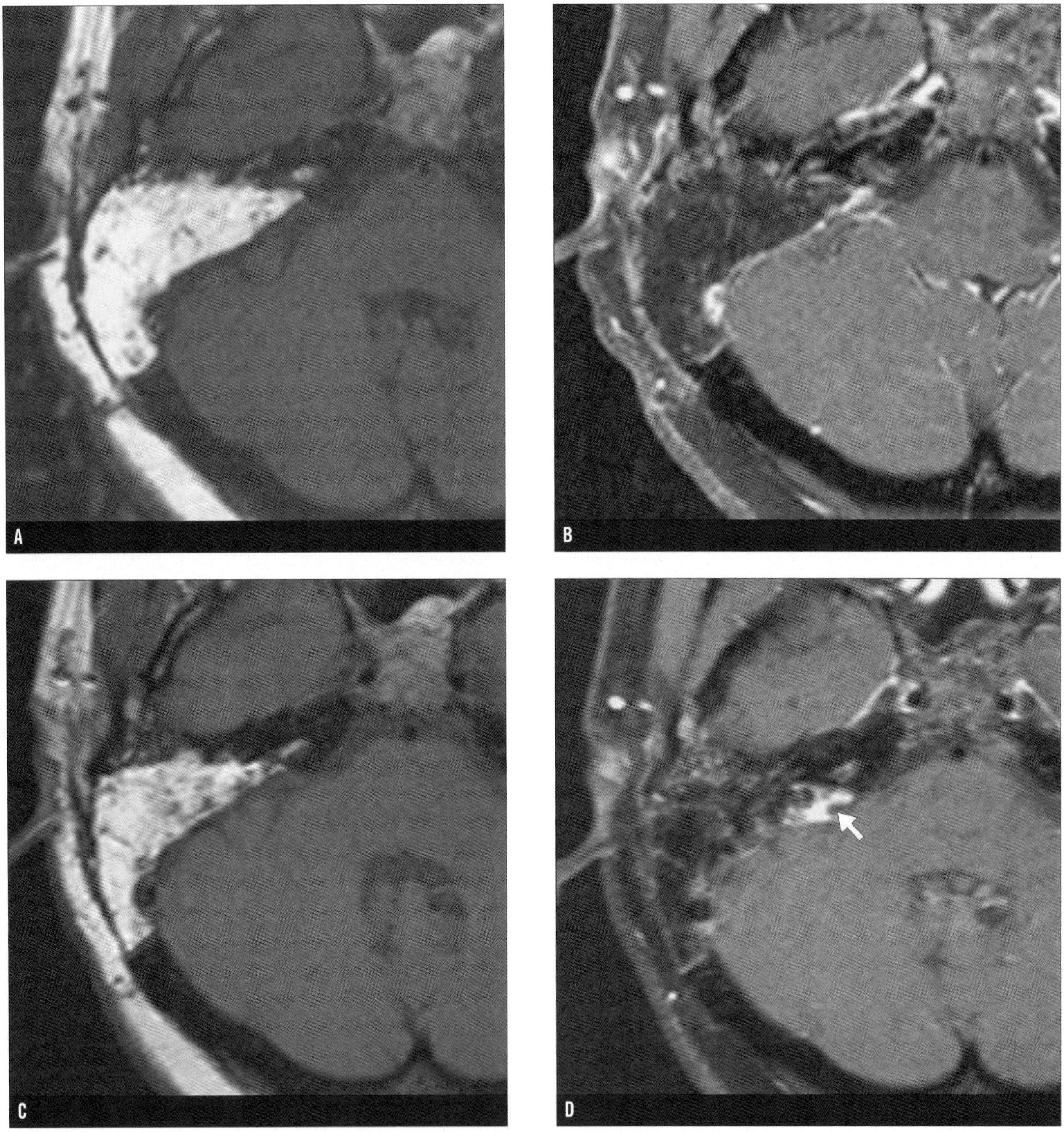

Axial T1 (**A**) and fat-suppressed contrast-enhanced axial T1 (**B**) MR images demonstrate extensive fat packing in a right mastoidectomy following resection of a right cerebellopontine angle schwannoma that extended into the right IAC. The fat completely suppresses at this stage, without evidence of enhancement. The same sequences obtained 6 months later (**C**, **D**) demonstrate a mild decrease in the amount of fat packing and interval development of patchy mild enhancement. A small focal nodular area of enhancement was described as possible recurrent tumor (arrow, **D**). The same sequences obtained 1 year later (**E**, **F**) and approximately 3 years later (**G**, **H**) demonstrate progressive diminution of the right mastoid fat packing, increased enhancement due to progressive fat necrosis, and no evidence of recurrent tumor.

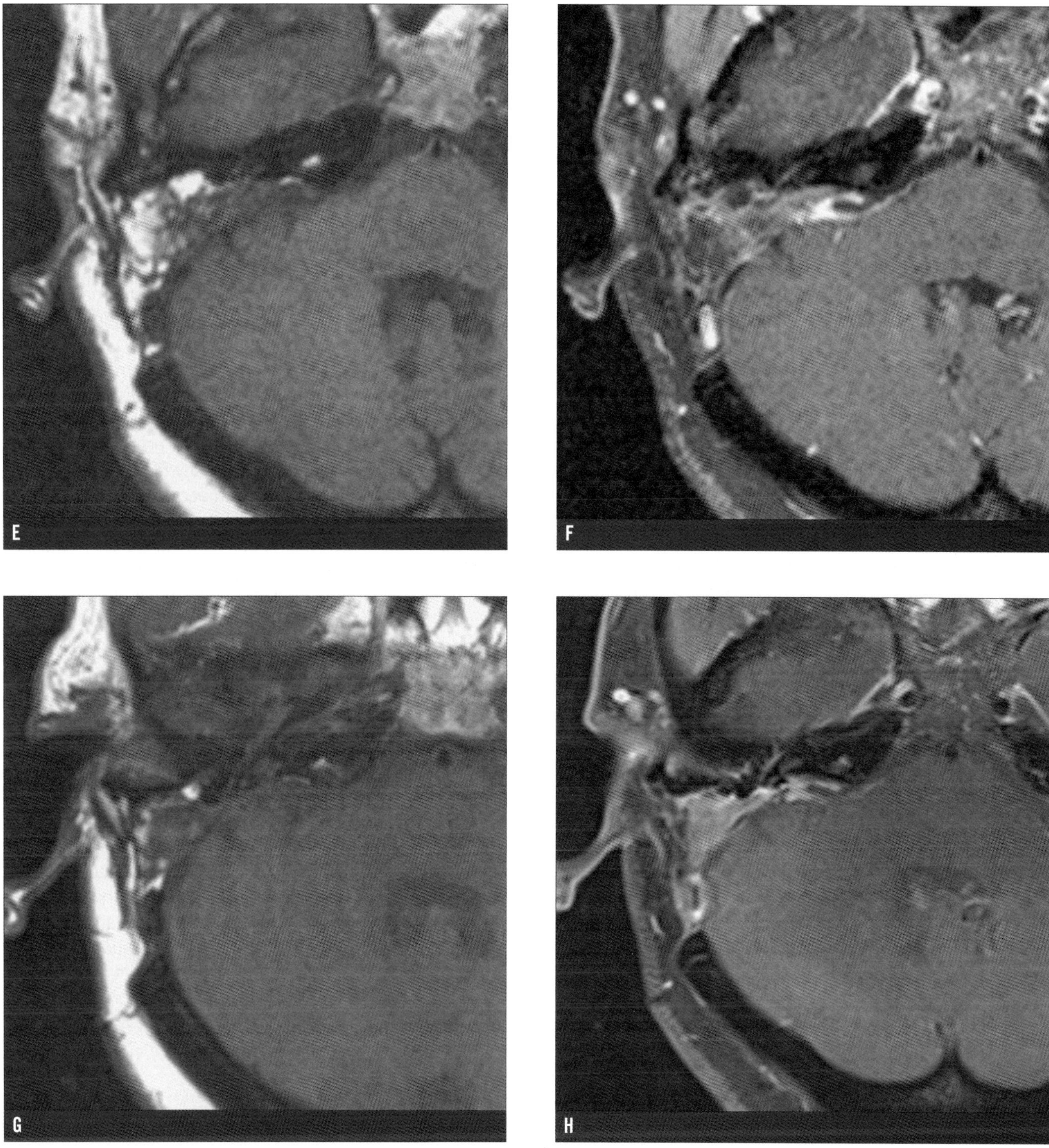

REFERENCES

De Aquino JEAP, Filho NAC, De Aquino JNP. Total reconstruction after canal wall down mastoidectomy with posterior wall of the external auditory canal and allograft ossicular eardrum. *Int Arch Otorhinolaryngol.* 2007;11(2):116-127.

Ginat DT, Martuza RL. Postoperative imaging of vestibular schwannomas. *Neurosurg Focus.* 2012;33(3):E18.

Loh LE. How I do it—post mastoidectomy reconstruction. *Singapore Med J.* 1989;30(6):528-529.

Mukherji SK, et al. CT of the temporal bone: findings after mastoidectomy, ossicular reconstruction, and cochlear implantation. *AJR Am J Roentgenol.* 1994;163:1467-1471.

Nardis PF, Teramo M, Giunta S, Bellelli A. Unusual cholesteatoma shell: CT findings. *J Comput Assist Tomogr.* 1988;12(6):1084-1085.

Offiah CE, Ramsden RT, Gillespie JE. Imaging appearances of unusual conditions of the middle and inner ear. *Br J Radiol.* 2008; 81(966):504-514.

CASE 12 Varying degrees of normal ossicular mineralization

The malleus and incus develop from the first branchial arch and are considered long bones. However, in addition to being much smaller, they are unique from the long bones of the appendicular skeleton in that they develop from a single ossification center. Fully matured ossicles contain both bone and cartilage. The malleus and incus can have varying degrees of mineralization on CT, likely on a developmental basis. Occasionally, the lack of complete mineralization can mimic ossicular erosion or tympanosclerosis.

COMPANION CASES

- **Tympanosclerosis.** Tympanosclerosis results from abnormal deposition of calcified hyalinized connective tissue and represents the end result of a paradoxical healing response to chronic otitis media. Tympanosclerosis is a general term that encompasses any portion of the middle ear and tympanic membrane that may be affected by this process. The calcified hyalinized connective tissue manifests as multifocal calcification involving the tympanic membrane or middle ear on CT. Osteoneogenesis may also occur, with new bone formation involving the tympanic cavity, ossicles, or suspensory ligaments of the ossicles, resulting in ossicular fixation and conductive hearing loss. The affected ossicles may appear enlarged, irregular, and heterogeneous. The degree of hearing loss may be out of proportion to the degree of debris; thus, a small amount of tympanosclerosis may result in a large degree of conductive hearing loss.
- **Ossicular erosion from a cholesteatoma.** A cholesteatoma is a pearly white mass consisting of keratinizing squamous epithelium and may be acquired or congenital. A cholesteatoma is a misnomer because it does not contain fat nor does it represent a neoplasm. An acquired cholesteatoma generally occurs in adults. It is related to a retraction pocket and perforation of the tympanic membrane (usually affecting pars flaccida) that results in the accumulation of keratinized epithelium in the middle ear, most commonly in the Prussak space and epitympanum. An acquired cholesteatoma is often associated with osseous erosions, most commonly ossicular and/or scutal erosion, but it may also erode the tegmen and lateral semicircular canal. If a cholesteatoma erodes the lateral semicircular canal, then it may be necessary to leave a small portion of the cholesteatoma over the erosion during surgery in order to tamponade the defect and prevent a perilymphatic fistula.

  A congenital cholesteatoma differs from an acquired cholesteatoma in several ways. A congenital cholesteatoma is related to ectopic rests of keratinized epithelium and usually occurs in younger patients. The tympanic membrane is intact with this entity, a key clinical finding that differentiates this lesion from an acquired cholesteatoma. Additionally, a congenital cholesteatoma is often located medial to the ossicular chain and displaces it laterally. While osseous erosions do occur with a congenital cholesteatoma, the degree of erosion is relatively mild compared to an acquired cholesteatoma. Both acquired and congenital cholesteatomas are pathologically identical to an epidermoid; therefore, a cholesteatoma will restrict on MR diffusion-weighted imaging. Newer non-EPI diffusion-weighted imaging sequences (eg, DWI-HASTE and DWI-BLADE) offer improved resolution, thinner section acquisition, and less artifact compared to EPI diffusion-weighted imaging, although they have longer image acquisition times. It is important to note that the presence of tympanic cavity soft tissue without associated erosion on CT does not exclude the presence of a cholesteatoma, as it is certainly possible that a cholesteatoma could be present but has not yet caused an erosion at the time of imaging. Thus, most soft tissue findings in the middle ear that are not associated with erosions are nonspecific and could represent granulation tissue, cholesteatoma, or another entity.

Incidental notch in the head of the malleus

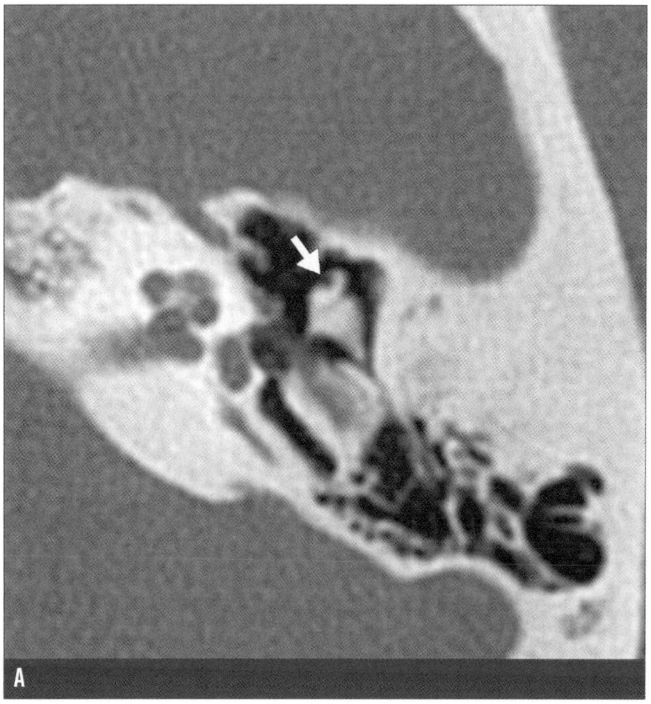

An axial CT image of the left temporal bone (**A**) demonstrates lucency in the head of the malleus (arrow). This is a normal finding and represents an incidental notch in the head of the malleus, possibly in part due to image angulation. This finding can mimic a focal erosion.

Incidental decreased mineralization of the incus

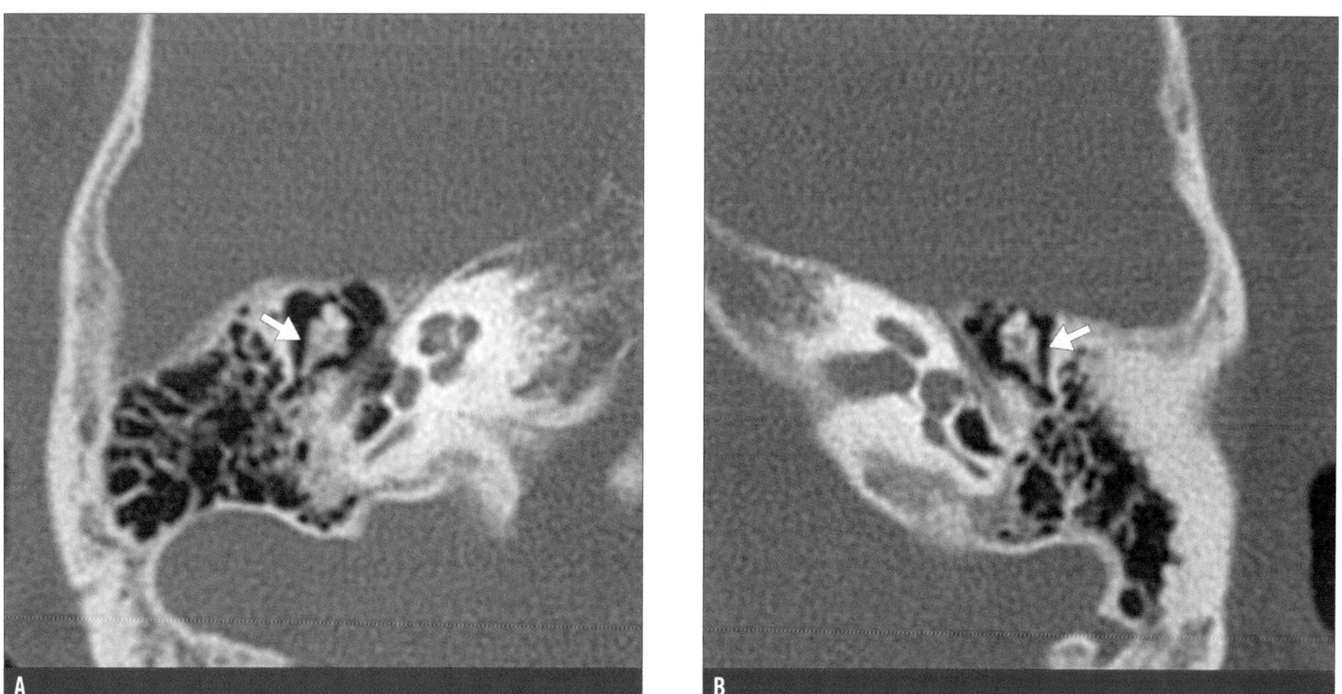

Axial CT images of the right (**A**) and left (**B**) temporal bones demonstrate decreased mineralization centered in the body of the incus bilaterally (arrows, **A**, **B**). Given the symmetric appearance and the lack of middle ear disease, this finding is most likely incidental.

Companion case: Tympanosclerosis

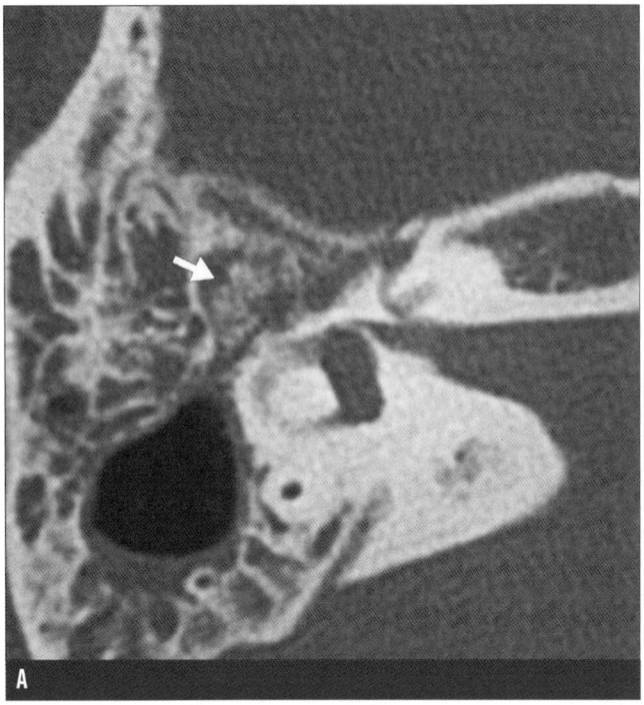

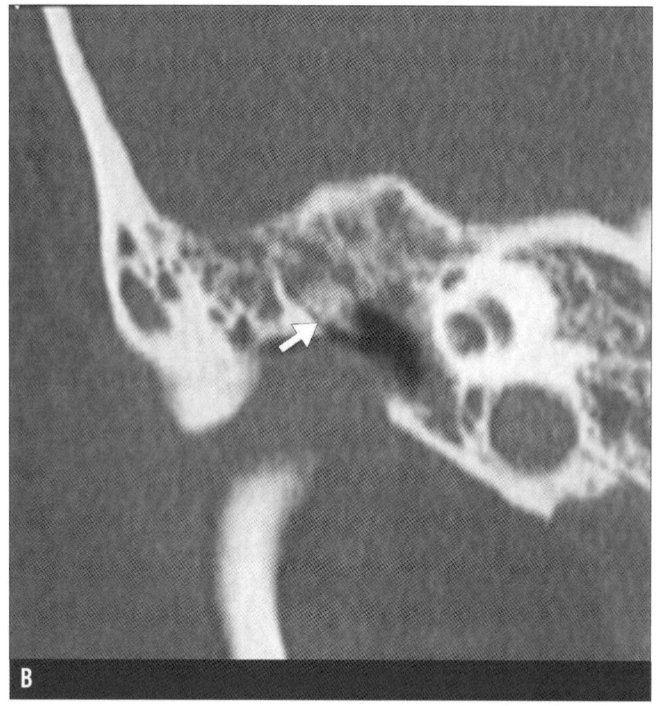

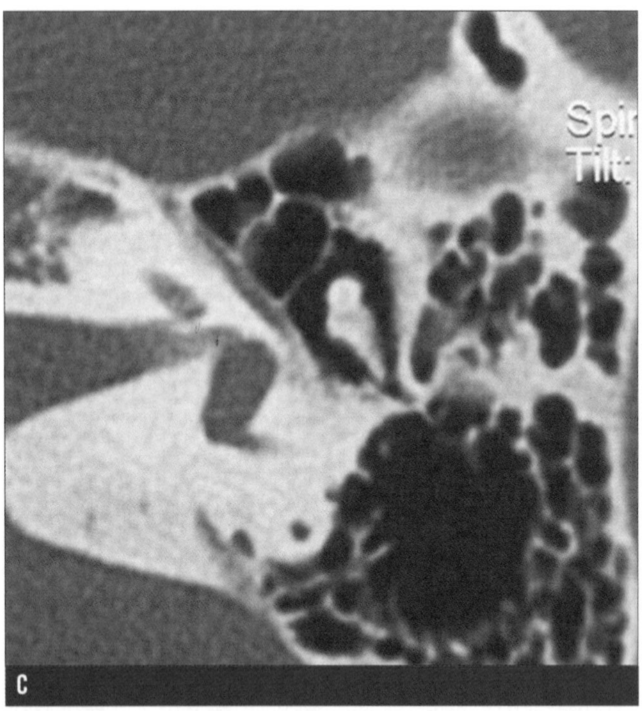

Axial (**A**) and direct coronal (**B**) CT images of the right temporal bone demonstrate partial opacification of the tympanic cavity and mastoid air cells with marked demineralization and enlargement of the malleus and incus (arrows, **A**, **B**). These findings are compatible with chronic otomastoiditis and tympanosclerosis affecting the ossicles. An axial CT image of the left temporal bone from the same patient (**C**) demonstrates normal mineralization of the malleus and incus.

Companion case: Ossicular erosion from a cholesteatoma

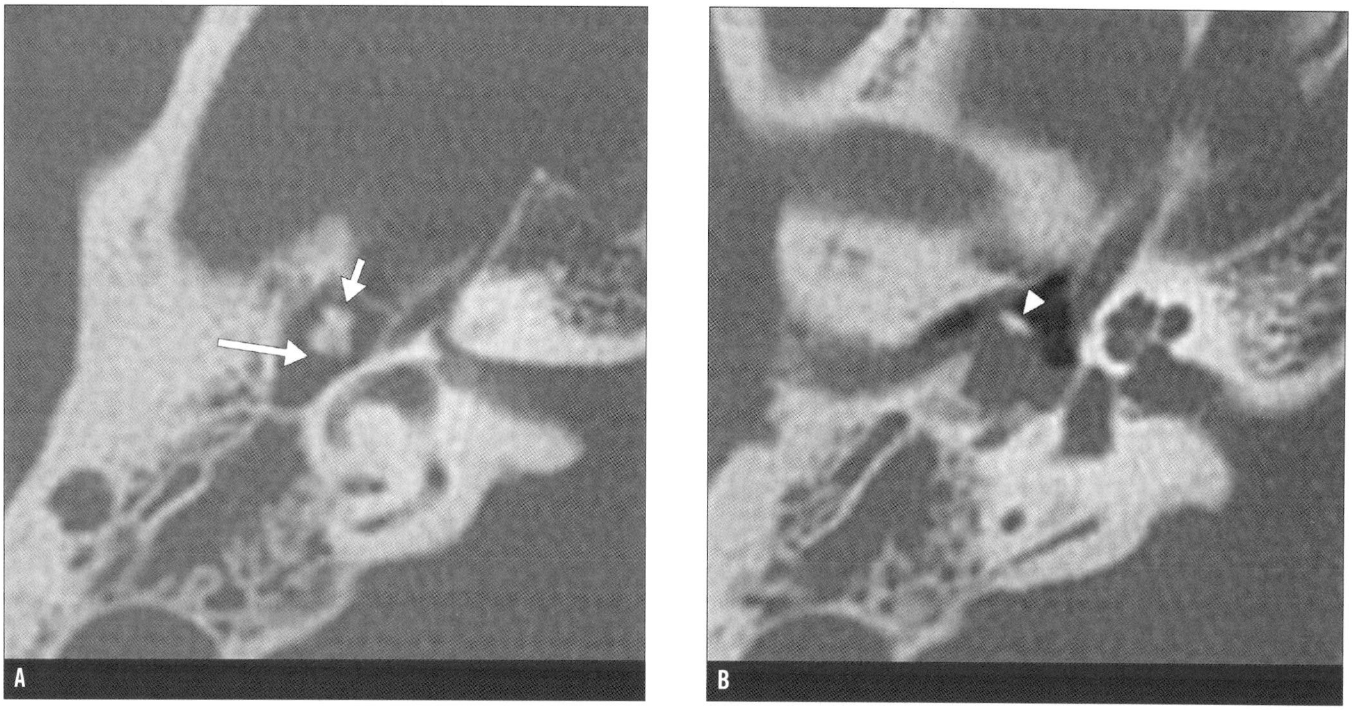

An axial CT image of the right temporal bone (**A**) demonstrates abnormal soft tissue in the tympanic cavity with erosions of the head of the malleus (short arrow, **A**) as well as the body and short process of the incus (long arrow, **A**). An axial CT image of the more caudal aspect of the right tympanic cavity (**B**) demonstrates abnormal soft tissue in the tympanic cavity and only the manubrium of the malleus to be present (arrowhead, **B**). The long process of the incus, which should be parallel and located posterior to the manubrium of the malleus, is absent. These ossicular erosions were the result of an acquired cholesteatoma.

REFERENCES

Mafee MF, Aimi K, Kahen HL, Valvassori GE, Capek V. Chronic otomastoiditis: a conceptual understanding of CT findings. *Radiology.* 1986;160(1):193-200.

Offiah CE, Ramsden RT, Gillespie JE. Imaging appearances of unusual conditions of the middle and inner ear. *Br J Radiol.* 2008;81(966):504-514.

Rodriguez-Vazquez JF. Development of the stapes and associated structures in human embryos. *J Anat.* 2005;207(2):165-173.

Schwartz KM, Lane JI, Bolster BD Jr, Neff BA. The utility of diffusion-weighted imaging for cholesteatoma evaluation. *AJNR Am J Neuroradiol.* 2011;32(3):430-436.

Swartz JD, Wolfson RJ, Marlowe FI, Popky GL. Postinflammatory ossicular fixation: CT analysis with surgical correction. *Radiology.* 1985;154(3):697-700.

Whyte JR, Gonzalez L, Cisneros AI, Yus C, Torres A, Sarrat R. Fetal development of the human tympanic ossicular chain articulations. *Cells Tissues Organs.* 2002;171(4):241-249.

Yates PD, Flood LM, Banerjee A, Clifford K. CT scanning of middle ear cholesteatoma: what does the surgeon want to know? *Br J Radiol.* 2002;75(898):847-852.

CASE 13 Suspensory ligaments of the ossicles

There are four main suspensory ligaments of the middle ear: anterior malleal, lateral malleal, superior malleal, and posterior incudal, with the latter having both medial and lateral portions. The anterior malleal ligament originates from the head of the malleus and inserts onto the anterior epitympanic wall. The lateral malleal ligament originates from the neck of the malleus and inserts onto the osseous margin of the tympanic notch (at the tip of the scutum). Of note, the lateral malleal ligament defines the cephalad margin of the Prussak space. The superior malleal ligament originates from the head of the malleus and inserts onto the epitympanic roof. The medial and lateral portions of the posterior incudal ligament originate from the short process of the incus and insert along the ventral-medial and ventral-lateral aspects of the incudal fossa, which is a fossa located just posterior to the short process of the incus. The malleal ligaments are identified more frequently than the incudal ligament on CT, although all the ligaments are now easier to identify with improvements in CT scanner technology. Occasionally, a relatively normal thickness suspensory ligament may mineralize, although it is unclear whether this is a finding that can contribute to conductive hearing loss or if it is an incidental finding.

Superior malleal ligament

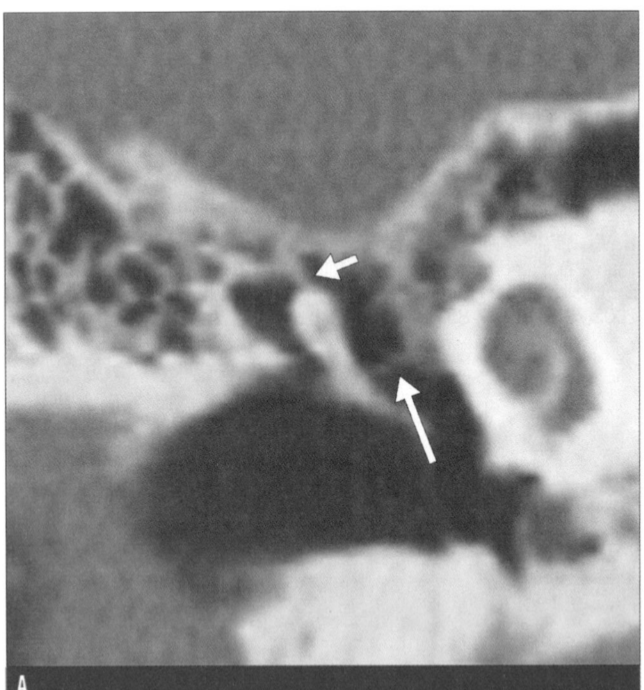

A coronal reformatted CT image of the right temporal bone (**A**) demonstrates a normal superior malleal ligament (short arrow) extending from the head of the malleus to the epitympanic roof. A normal tensor tympani tendon is also identified (long arrow).

COMPANION CASE

- **Bony bar.** A bony bar represents solid osseous fusion of an ossicle with a surrounding osseous wall or rarely the facial nerve canal. The most common location of a bony bar occurs between the head of the malleus and the anterior epitympanic wall. A thick bony bar can be associated with conductive hearing loss. However, subtle abutment of an ossicle with a wall of the tympanic cavity does not necessarily constitute a bony bar, and further investigation is likely needed to determine its relevance in relation to conductive hearing loss. Occasionally, a bony bar can take the form of an abnormally thickened and mineralized suspensory ligament, which can be associated with conductive hearing loss in the appropriate clinical context.

Lateral malleal ligament

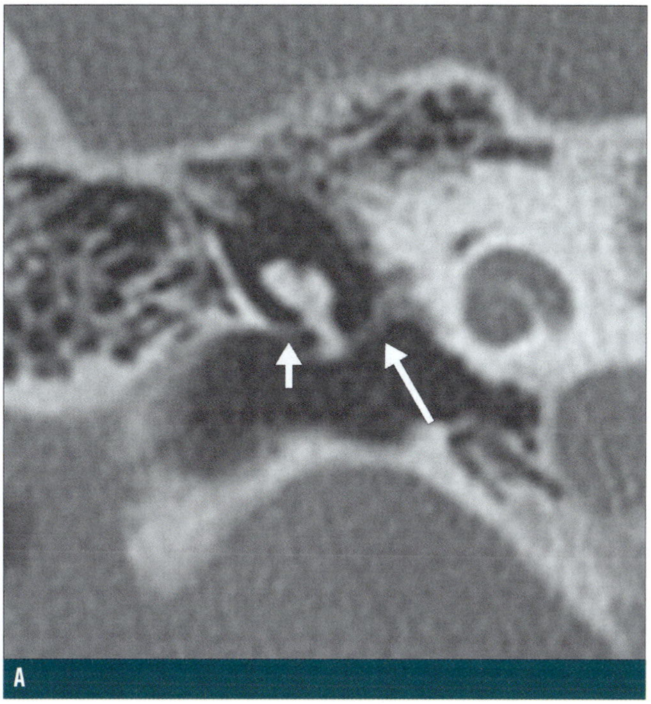

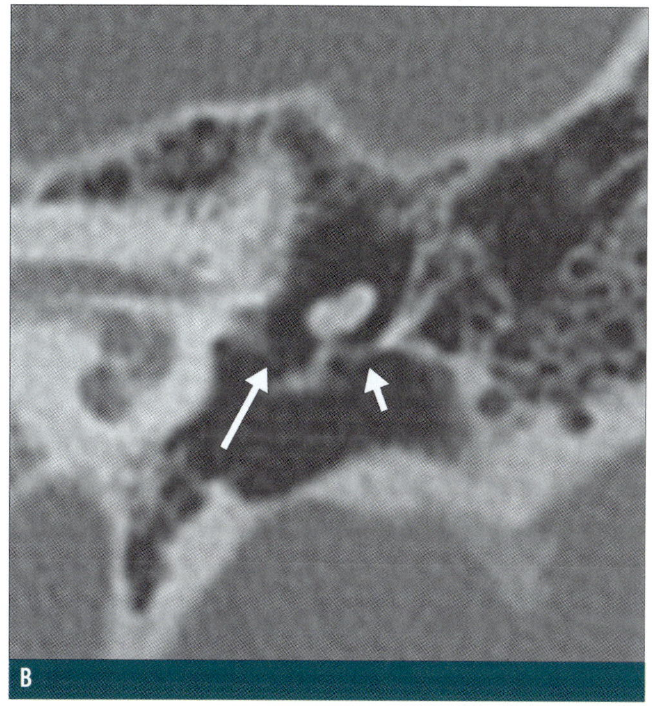

Coronal CT images of the right (**A**) and left (**B**) temporal bones demonstrate the normal lateral malleal ligaments extending from the neck of the mallei to the regions of the scutal tips (short arrows, **A**, **B**). The lateral malleal ligament delinates the cephalad margin of the Prussak space. The normal tensor tympani tendons are also appreciated bilaterally (long arrows, **A**, **B**).

Anterior malleal ligament

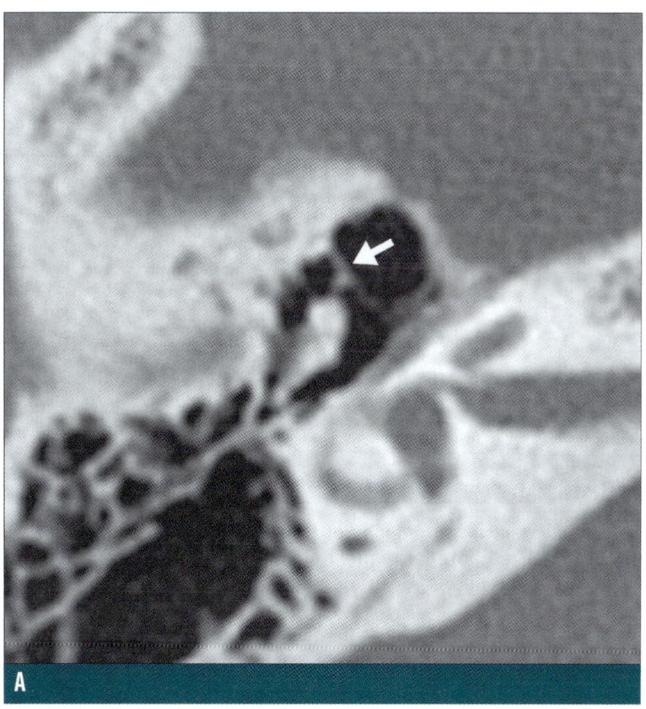

An axial CT image of the right temporal bone (**A**) demonstrates a normal anterior malleal ligament, extending from the head of the malleus to the lateral aspect of the anterior epitympanic wall (arrow).

Posterior incudal ligament

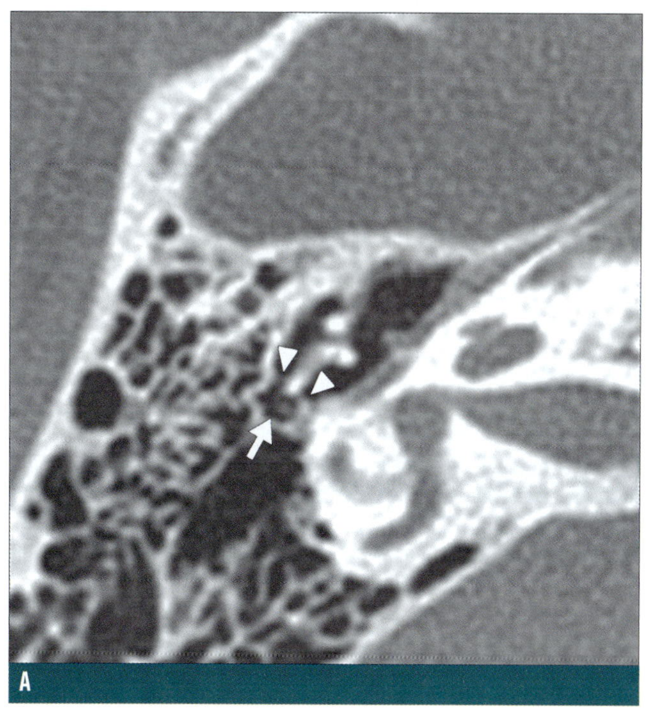

An axial CT image of the right temporal bone (**A**) demonstrates the normal medial and lateral portions of the posterior incudal ligament (arrowheads), extending from the short process of the incus to the ventral-medial and ventral-lateral portions of the incudal fossa (arrow).

Companion case: Bony bars

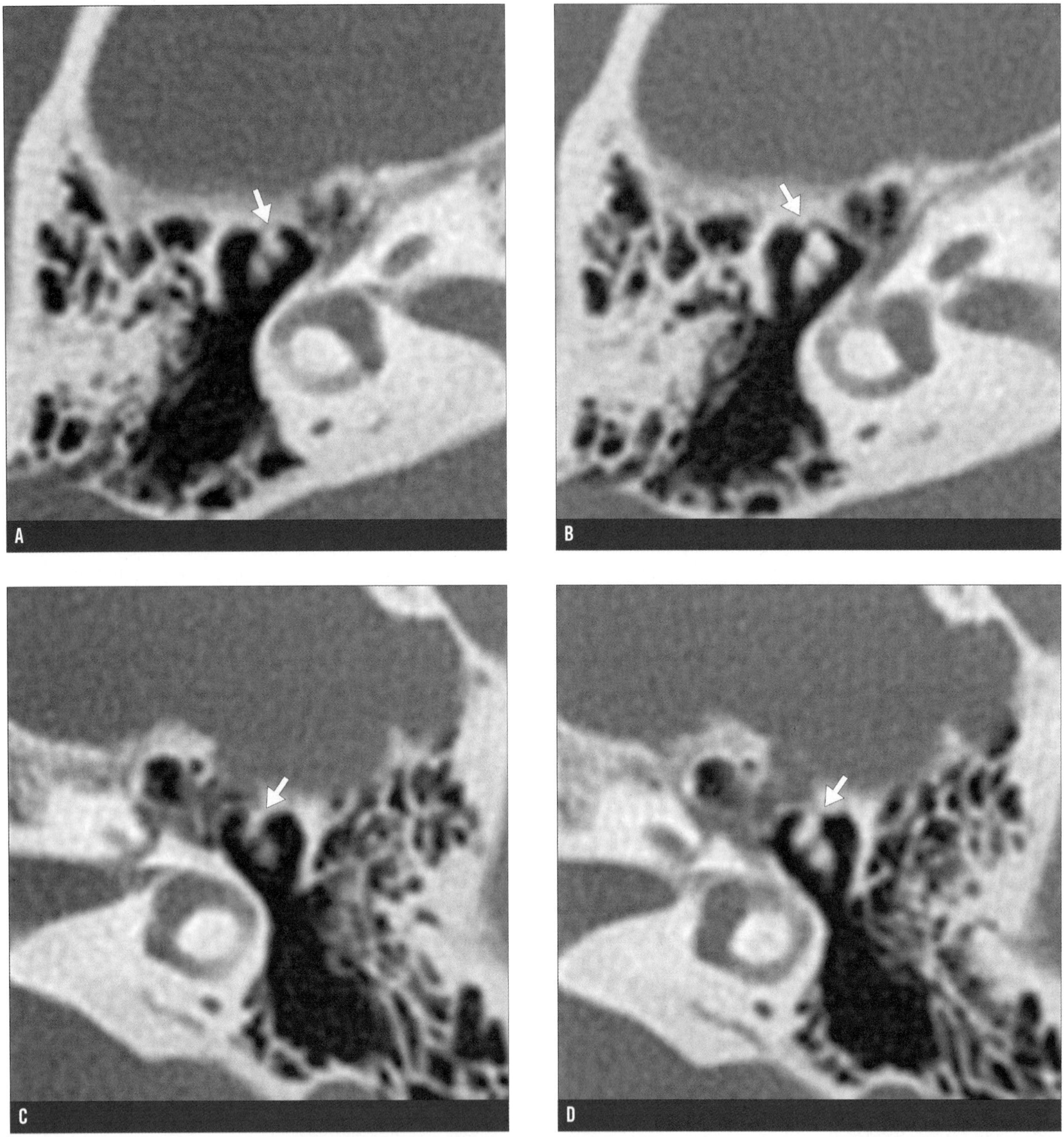

Axial CT images of the right (**A**, **B**) and left (**C**, **D**) temporal bones demonstrate bony bars in the regions of the bilateral anterior malleal ligaments (arrows, **A**-**D**). These bars may represent abnormally thickened and mineralized anterior malleal ligaments or simply osseous fusion in these regions. While a finding such as this can be associated with conductive hearing loss, its significance depends on the clinical context.

Companion case: Bony bar

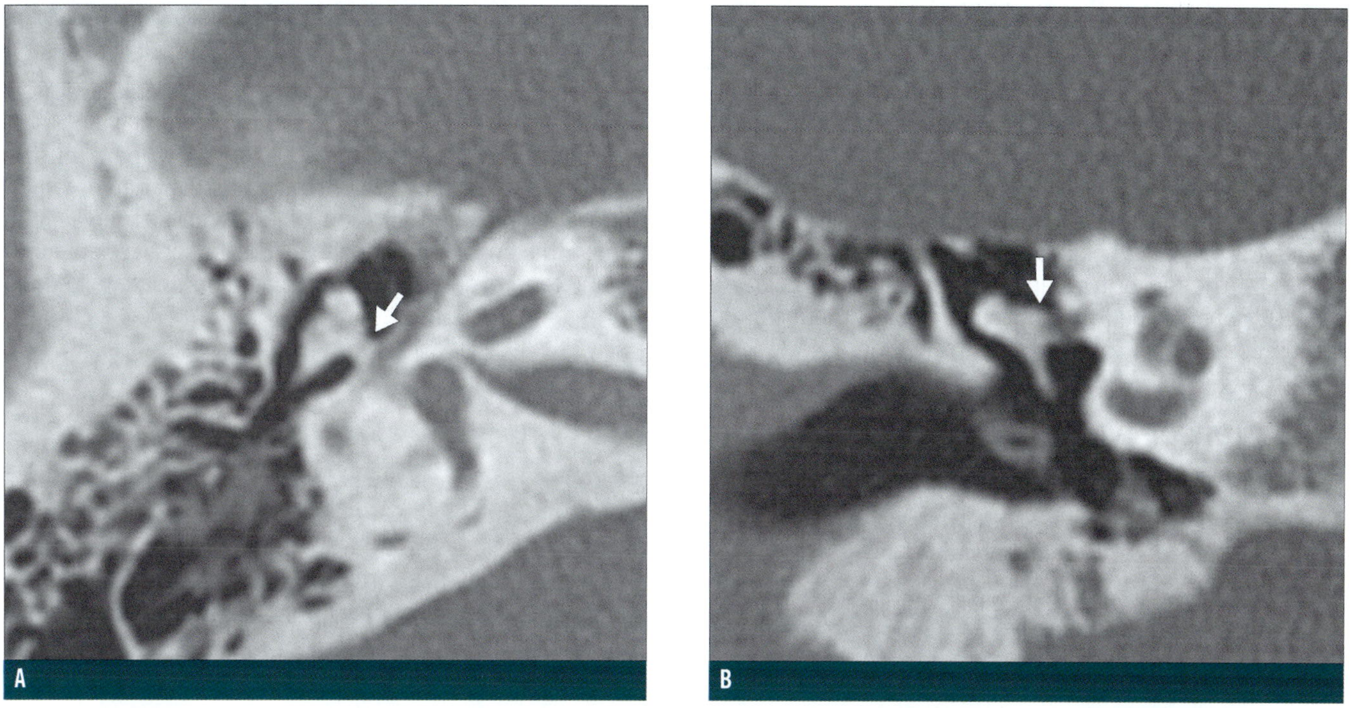

Axial (**A**) and coronal reformatted (**B**) CT images of the right temporal bone demonstrate a bony bar that extends from the incus to the tympanic segment of the facial nerve canal (arrows, **A**, **B**). A bony bar can be associated with conductive hearing loss, in the appropriate clinical context.

REFERENCES

Jager L, et al. CT of the normal temporal bone: comparison of multi-and single detector row CT. *Radiology*. 2005;235:133-141.

Lemmerling MM, Stambuck, HE, Mancuso AA, Antonelli PJ, Kubilis PS. CT of the normal suspensory ligaments of the ossicles in the middle ear. *Am J Neuroradiol*. 1997;18:471-477.

Park K, Choung Y. Isolated congenital ossicular anomalies. *Acta Oto-Laryngologica*. 2009;129:419-422.

CASE 14 Tensor tympani muscle and tendon

The tensor tympani muscle and tendon function to reduce the efficiency of sound conduction by dampening ossicular vibrations. This is achieved by increasing the tension on the tympanic membrane, thereby decreasing the vibratory amplitude of the malleus. The end result is to protect the inner ear against loud noises, most effective at greater than 5000 Hz. The tensor tympani muscle courses through an osseous canal termed the semicanal, located cephalad to the osseous portion of the Eustachian tube. The tendon enters the tympanic cavity and courses laterally with an approximate 90° angle at the level of the cochlea to insert onto the neck of the malleus. The tensor tympani muscle is supplied by a branch of the mandibular nerve, which represents the third division of CN V, by a nerve aptly named the tensor tympani nerve. The tensor tympani muscle and tendon are readily appreciated on CT examinations of the temporal bones.

Tensor tympani muscle and tendon

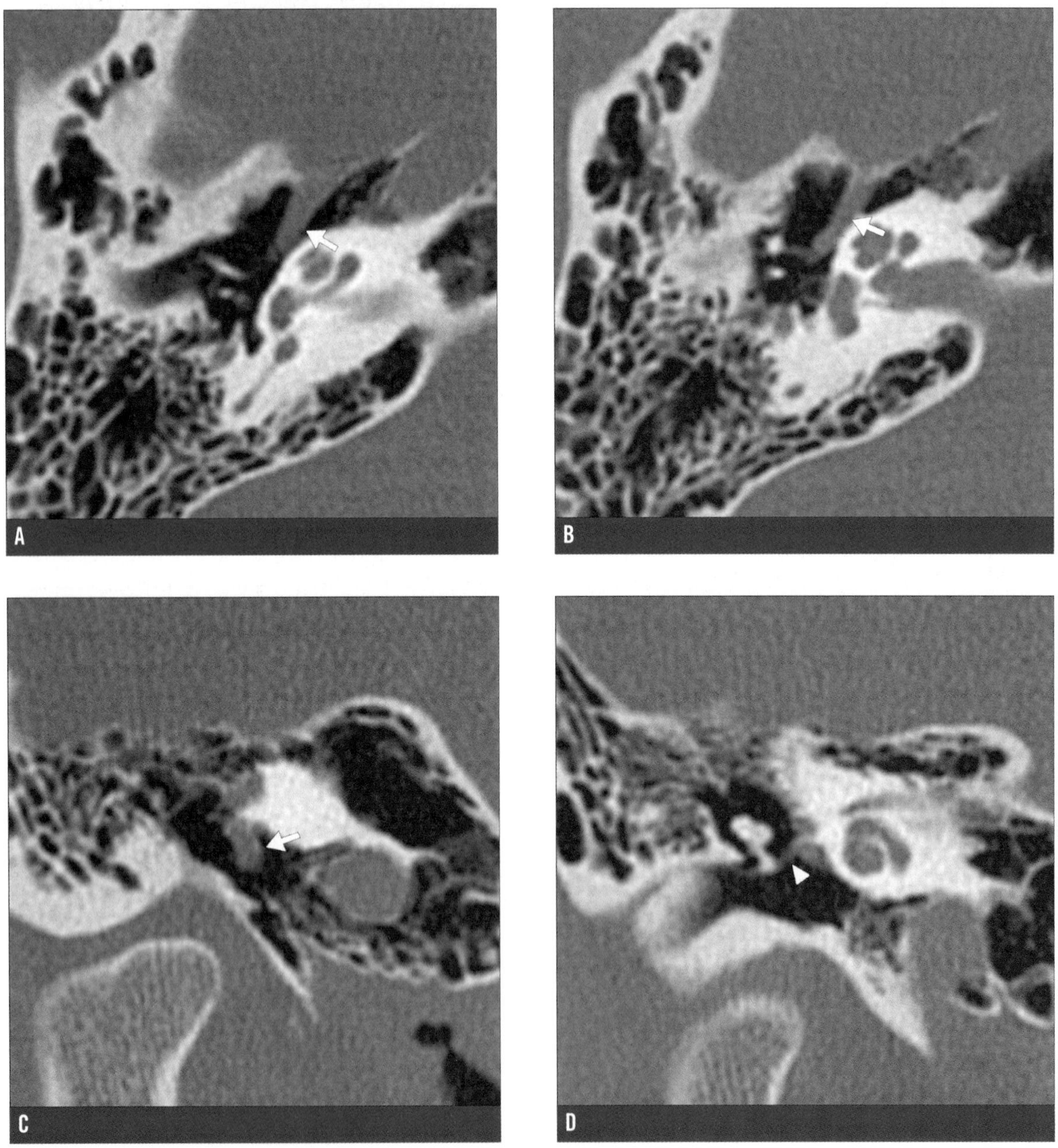

Axial (**A**, **B**) and coronal reformatted (**C**, **D**) CT images of the right temporal bone demonstrate a normal tensor tympani muscle (arrows, **A-C**) and a normal tensor tympani tendon (arrowhead, **D**) inserting onto the neck of the malleus.

Tensor tympani muscle and tendon

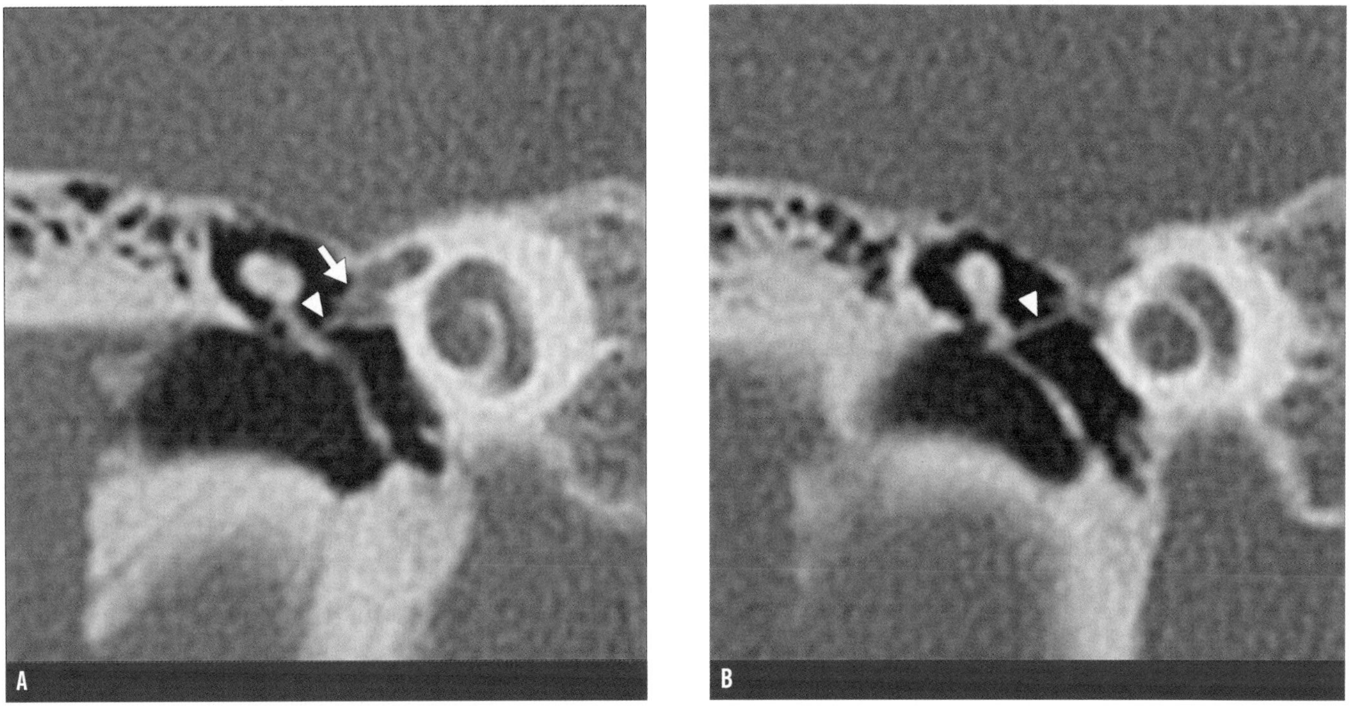

Different patient. Coronal reformatted CT images of the right temporal bone (**A**, **B**) demonstrate the tensor tympani muscle in cross section (arrow, **A**) and the tensor tympani tendon (arrowheads, **A**, **B**) undergoing its normal sharp lateral turn at the level of the cochlea to insert onto the neck of the malleus.

REFERENCE

Jager L, et al. CT of the normal temporal bone: comparison of multi-and single detector row CT. *Radiology*. 2005;235:133-141.

Ossicular prostheses may be of the presculpted synthetic variety or they may be carved from a graft. Grafts can be harvested from the same patient (ie, autograft) or, much less commonly, from a human donor (ie, allograft). An allograft is rarely used today because of the risk of transmittable diseases, such as HIV. An autograft is typically carved from the incus; if the incus is not present, then the head of the malleus is used.

Ossicular autografts may undergo necrosis or granuloma formation. Other complications inherent with all types of ossicular prostheses include subluxation and dislocation of the prosthesis with subsequent conductive hearing loss. There is evidence that there are less complications and improved stability of a prosthesis when the reconstruction uses an intact manubrium of the malleus (if present) as a strut.

The type of ossicular prosthesis that is chosen is based upon which portion of the ossicular chain is damaged.

- If the entire ossicular chain is damaged:
  - TORP (Total ossicular replacement prosthesis)
- If the malleus and incus are damaged, but the stapes is intact:
  - PORP (Partial ossicular replacement prosthesis)
- If the incus or the incus and stapes are damaged:
  - Incus interposition graft
  - Wehrs incus prosthesis or Wehrs incus stapes replacement prosthesis
  - Kartush incus strut prosthesis or Kartush incus-stapes strut prosthesis
- If the incudostapedial joint is damaged:
  - Applebaum incudostapedial joint prosthesis
- If the stapes is damaged:
  - Stapes prosthesis

TOTAL OSSICULAR REPLACEMENT PROSTHESIS

A TORP is placed when the entire ossicular chain is absent or nearly completely absent. A TORP is a synthetic graft that extends from the tympanoplasty graft to the footplate of the stapes or the oval window. Typically, the head of a TORP is constructed from hydroxyapatite and is placed against the tympanoplasty graft, although frequently a thin piece of cartilage is placed between the tympanoplasty graft and the TORP in order to decrease the risk of extrusion. There are several varieties of TORP head shapes which are available, including broad flat tops that are centered or off-centered relative to the shaft of the prosthesis. The off-centered variety has the added benefit of improved visualization of the stapes footplate or oval window during placement, though it may not be as balanced as a TORP that has its head centered. The shaft is most commonly constructed of a polyethylene sponge, fluoroplastic, or a polymer of hydroxyapatite and polyethylene. The distal end of the shaft of a TORP attaches to a surgically formed hole (usually via a laser) that is made at the stapes footplate, termed a stapedotomy. It may also be placed onto graft material that is placed over the oval window following a stapedectomy (ie, removal of the stapes superstructrure and at least a portion of the stapes footplate) and secured into place by Gelfoam.

Multiple different brands, sizes, and shapes of TORPs exist. Some of the more commonly used TORPs include: Black Oval-Top, Grace Medical, Richards, Goldenberg, Haberman, and Dornhoffer. A Grace Medical TORP can be either fixed (Fixed Length Total Ossicular, FLTO) or adjustable (Adjustable Length Total Ossicular, ALTO).

PARTIAL OSSICULAR REPLACEMENT PROSTHESIS

A PORP is a synthetic graft that extends from the tympanoplasty graft to the capitulum (also called head) of the stapes. The stapes superstructure (which includes the capitulum and stapes crura) should be intact in order to insert a PORP. The head and neck of a PORP are constructed from the same materials that can be used for a TORP, as described in the TORP section. As with a TORP, the head of a PORP may be centered or off-centered.

There are several different sizes, shapes, and brands of a PORP. Many of the brands are the same as those found with a TORP and are also discussed in the TORP section.

INCUS INTERPOSITION GRAFT

The incus interposition graft is intended to bypass a diseased incus. If the diseased incus is salvageable and can be used as an autograft, then the incus is removed and reshaped. Knowledge of the incus anatomy is imperative in order to understand the reshaping and placement of an incus interposition graft. In individuals with normal anatomy, the body of the incus articulates with the head of the malleus, the short process is directed posteriorly toward the aditus ad antrum, and the long process extends caudally, immediately posterior to and paralleling the manubrium (ie, handle) of the malleus. A short process, termed the lenticular process, extends at an approximate 90° angle medially from the distal aspect of the long process of the incus to articulate with the stapes capitulum (ie, head). With an incus interposition graft procedure, after the incus is removed from the middle ear, the reshaping of the incus commences. A small notch is formed along the short process of the incus in order to attach the graft to the manubrium of the malleus. If the stapes is still intact, then the lenticular process of the incus is removed and a concavity is carved along the long process of the incus in order to articulate with the head of the stapes. If the stapes is destroyed, then the long process of the incus is maintained for an adequate length that would allow for direct articulation with the oval window.

Incus interposition grafts are particularly prone to subluxation and dislocation because of the precarious nature of these surgically formed articulations. These grafts may also undergo necrosis or granuloma formation.

WEHRS INCUS PROSTHESIS

A Wehrs incus prosthesis is a synthetic prosthesis that is used for ossicular reconstruction when the incus is completely destroyed or when the native incus is too diseased to serve as an adequate autograft. The Wehrs prosthesis is constructed from hydroxyapatite. The head of this prosthesis articulates with the manubrium of the malleus, whereas an opening at the distal shaft of this prosthesis articulates with the stapes capitulum. The head of the Wehrs prosthesis is available in a single notch type (appears like a shoe with the toes bent upward) or a double notch type (simulates a "W"). In the case of the double notch type, either notch can be used, and the notch that is more suitable to affix to the manubrium of the malleus is selected. If the stapes superstructure is absent, a Wehrs incus stapes replacement prosthesis may be used, which extends from the manubrium of the malleus to the stapes footplate.

KARTUSH INCUS STRUT PROSTHESIS

A Kartush incus strut prosthesis is another type of synthetic prosthesis that may be used for ossicular reconstruction when the incus is completely destroyed or too diseased to be utilized as an autograft. This type of prosthesis is an option when when the stapes superstructure is present, in which case a Kartush incus strut prosthesis is used, or when the stapes superstructure is destroyed, in which case a Kartush incus-stapes strut prosthesis is used. The prosthesis is constructed of hydroxyapatite and has the shape of a column, with the addition of a small notch at its proximal end that attaches the manubrium of the malleus. The distal end of the prosthesis attaches to either the stapes superstructure or the stapes footplate, depending on the status of the stapes.

APPLEBAUM PROSTHESIS

An Applebaum prosthesis is a synthetic, L-shaped graft constructed of hydroxyapatite and is used to reconstruct an incudostapedial joint. This prosthesis is most commonly used when there is an erosion of the long process of the incus or a focal erosion at the incudostapedial joint resulting in ossicular chain disruption. Notches at each end of this L-shaped prosthesis articulate with the amputated long process of the incus and the capitulum of the stapes.

STAPES PROSTHESIS

A stapes prosthesis is placed when the ossicular pathology is isolated to the stapes. Common indications include stapes footplate fixation to the oval window as a result of otosclerosis (also called otospongiosis), various congenital abnormalities, prior trauma, and tympanosclerosis. There are numerous types of stapes prostheses, including a Teflon piston, stainless steel piston, wire prosthesis, and polymeric silicone prosthesis. A stapes prosthesis is placed following either a stapedectomy or a stapedotomy. A stapedectomy refers to removal of the stapes superstructure (ie, the crura and capitulum) as well as removal of a portion or the entire stapes footplate. A graft is placed over the exposed oval window and the distal end of the stapes prosthesis is placed onto the graft. A stapedotomy refers to a small hole that is surgically drilled into the stapes footplate in the setting of a destroyed stapes superstructure or following removal of the residual stapes superstructure. The distal end of the stapes prosthesis is placed into the stapedotomy. Proximally, the stapes prosthesis can articulate with the long process of the incus by a wire loop, such as with the Gyrus SMart Piston prosthesis, or by a bucket handle configuration, such as with the Robinson bucket prosthesis. In addition to the complications that may be present with other types of prostheses (namely dislocation and subluxation), a stapes prosthesis may also be complicated by subluxation through the oval window into the vestibule of the inner ear with subsequent formation of a perilymphatic fistula.

Total ossicular replacement prosthesis—Grace Medical ALTO

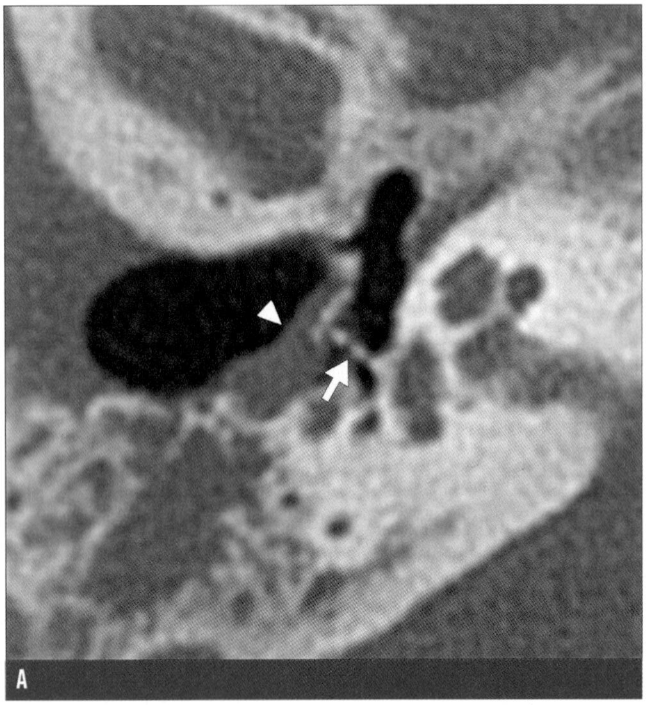

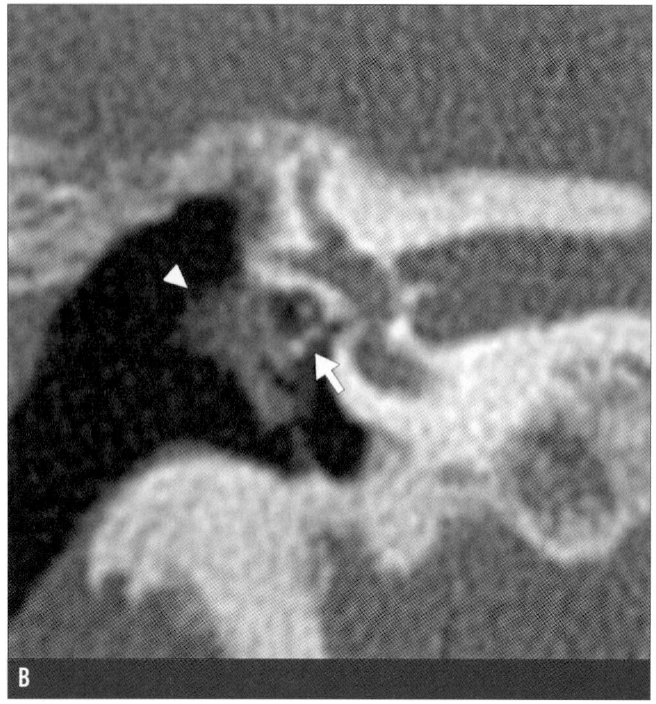

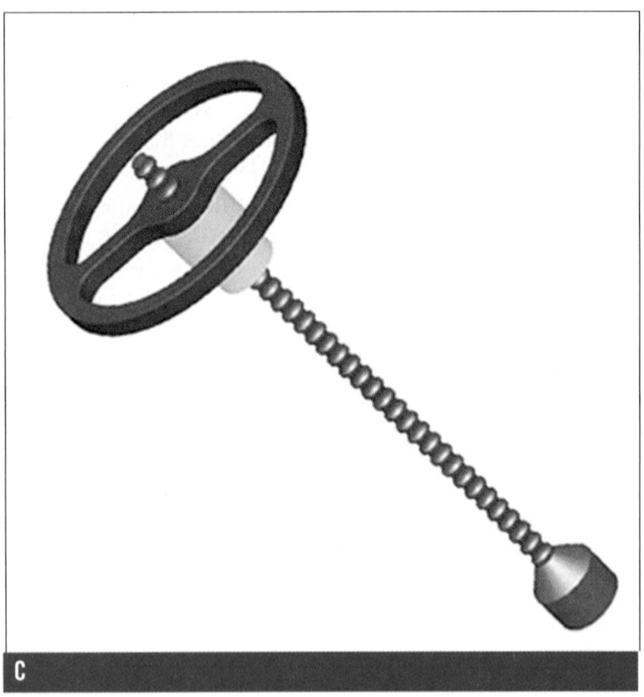

Axial (**A**) and direct coronal (**B**) CT images of the right temporal bone demonstrate a well-positioned Grace Medical TORP (arrows, **A**, **B**) extending from a tympanoplasty graft (arrowheads, **A**, **B**) to the stapes footplate at the oval window. Image **C** is a graphic illustration of a Grace Medical ALTO TORP.

Total ossicular replacement prosthesis—Richards

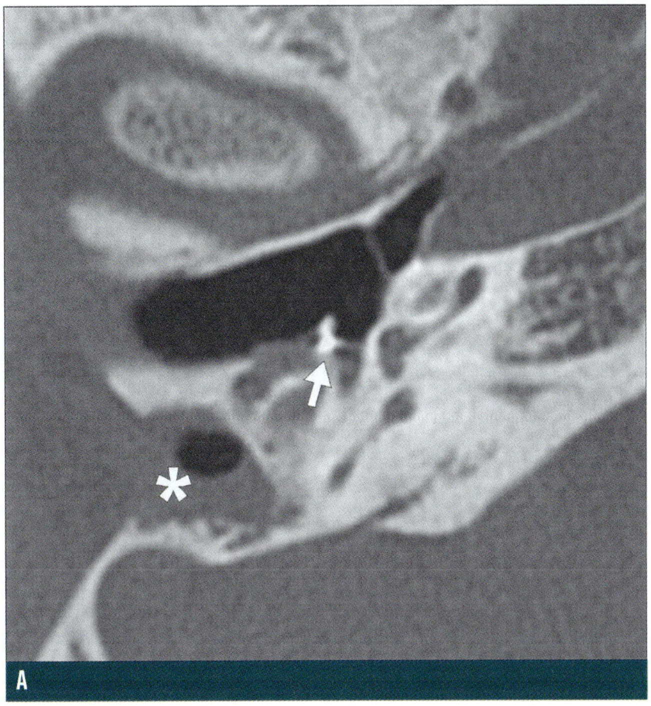

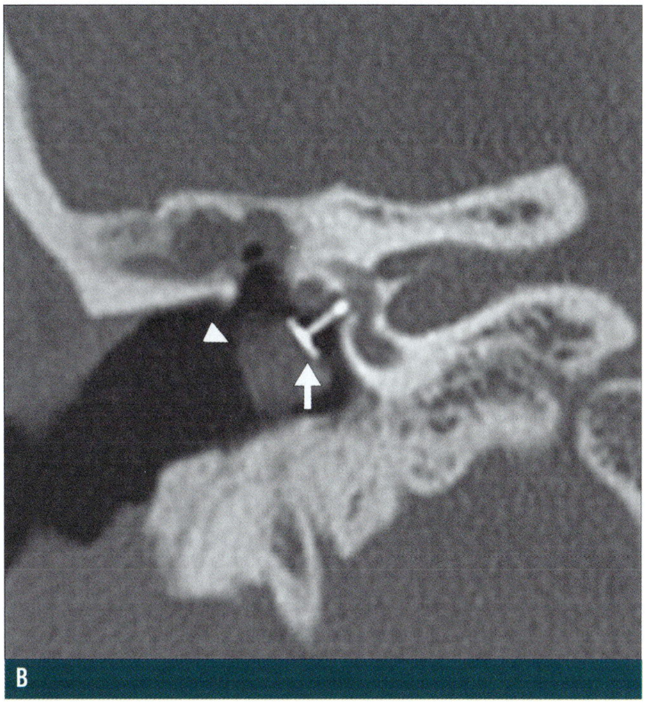

Axial (**A**) and coronal (**B**) CT images of the right temporal bone demonstrate a Richards TORP (arrows, **A**, **B**), with its tip appropriately positioned at the stapes footplate within the oval window. However, the TORP is positioned posteriorly within the tympanic cavity. In addition, while there is soft tissue lateral to the head of the TORP that may represent a portion of a tympanoplasty graft (arrowhead, **B**), there is likely a large tympanoplasty graft perforation on image **A**, possibly accounting for the posterior positioning of the TORP. A prior canal wall up mastoidectomy has been also performed, with partial opacification of the mastoid bowl (asterisk, **A**).

Partial ossicular replacement prosthesis—Grace Medical ALPO

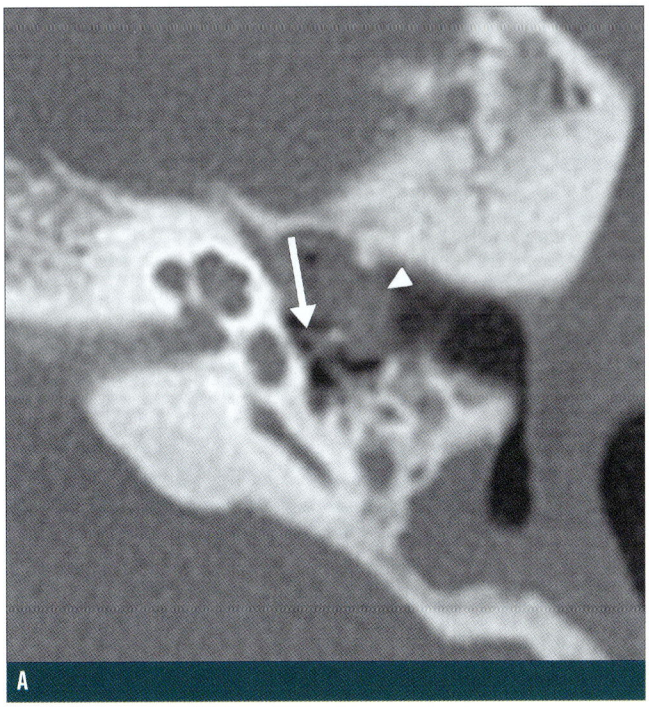

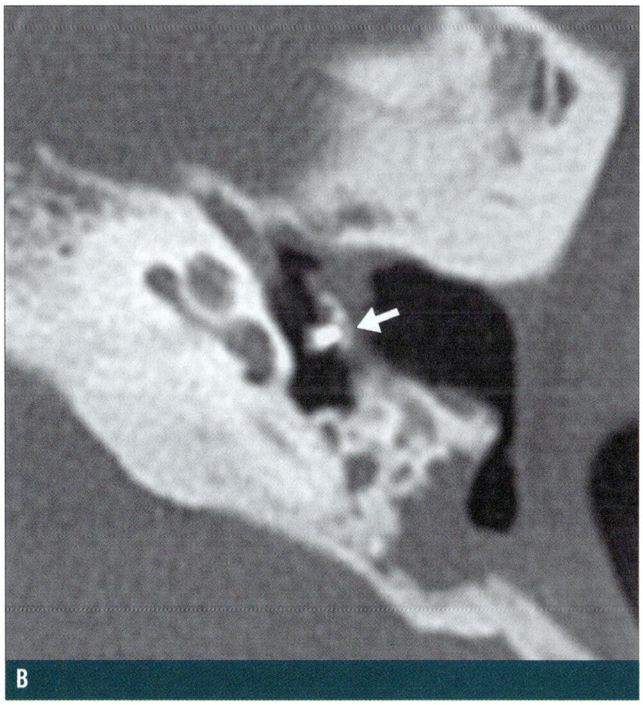

Axial (**A**, **B**) and direct coronal (**C**, **D**) CT images of the left temporal bone demonstrate an appropriately positioned Grace Medical ALPO PORP (short arrows, **B**-**D**). The native stapes crura are visualized (long arrows, **A**, **C**). A prior canal wall up mastoidectomy has been performed. There is nonspecific soft tissue adjacent to the tympanoplasty graft and PORP (arrowhead, **A**).

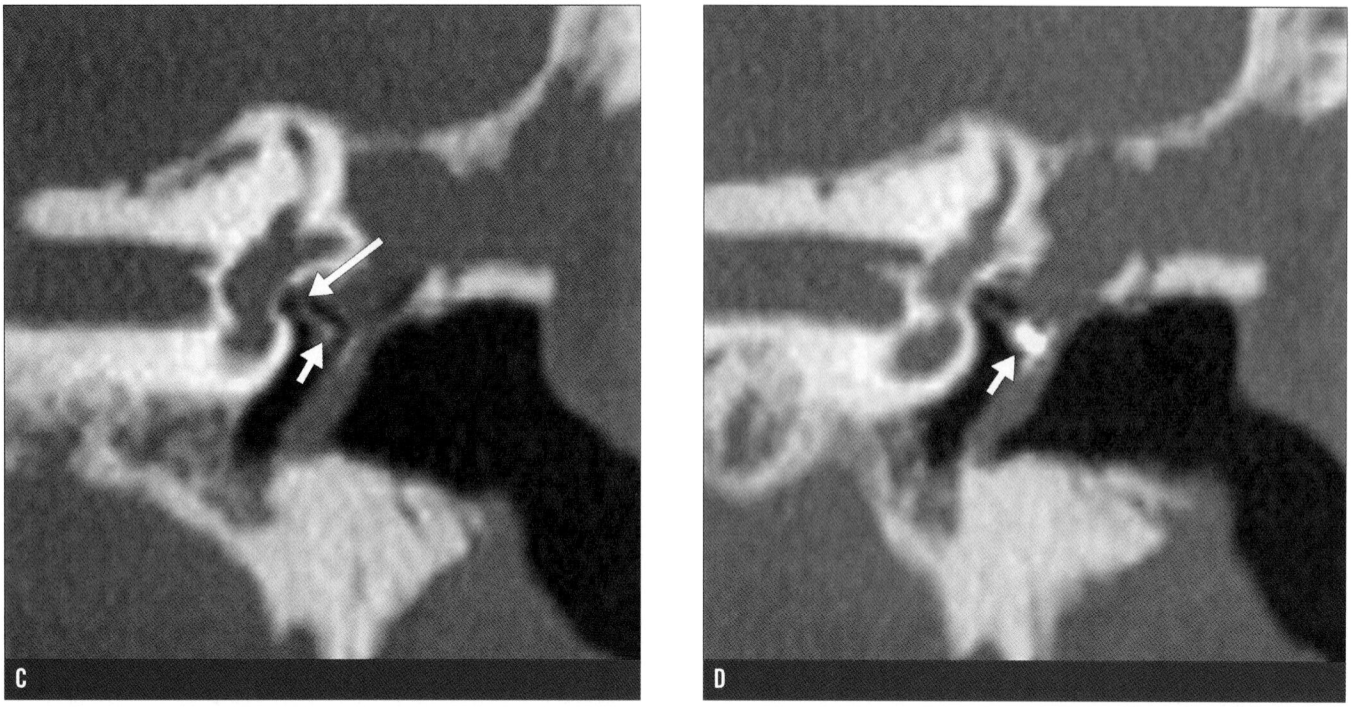

Displaced partial ossicular replacement prosthesis—Haberman

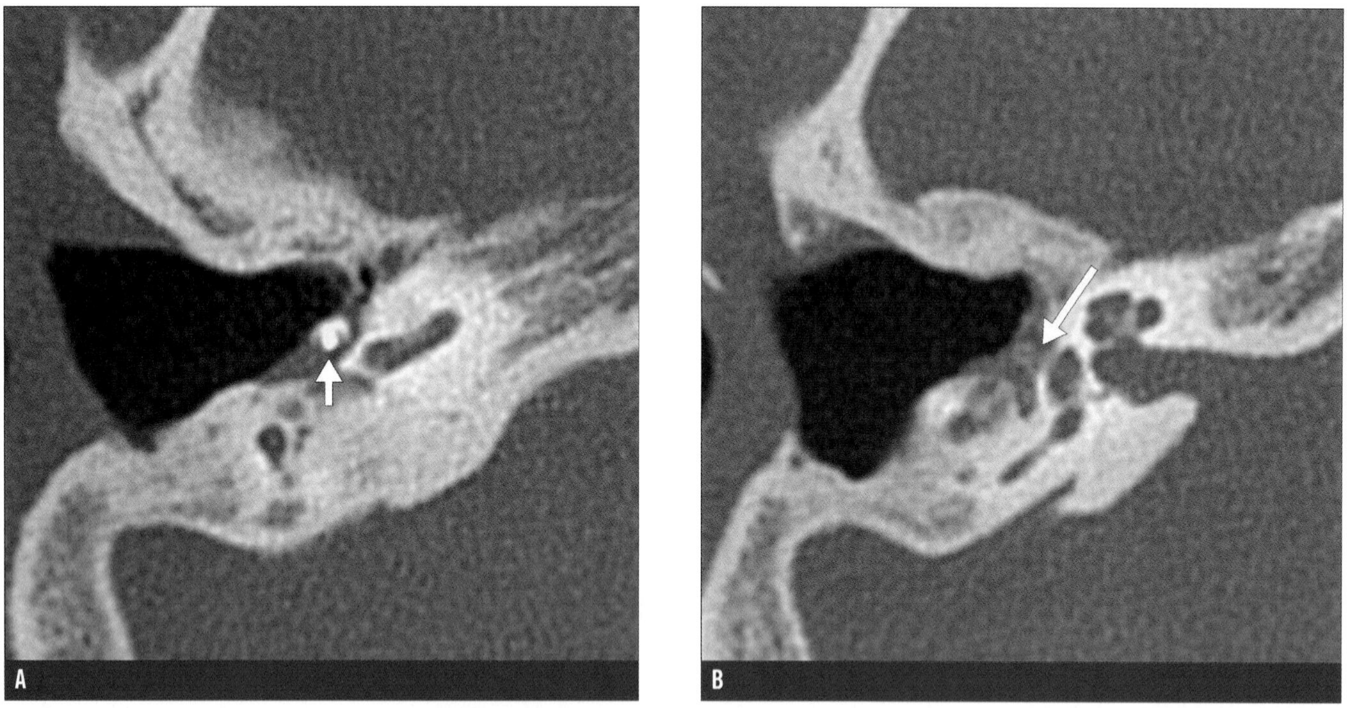

Axial CT images from inferior to superior (**A**, **B**) and a direct coronal CT image (**C**) of the right temporal bone. Images **A** and **B** demonstrate a canal wall down mastoidectomy and a Haberman PORP (short arrows, **A**, **C**) extending from a markedly retracted and/or perforated tympanoplasty graft to the region of the capitulum of the stapes. The stapes superstructure is poorly visualized but present (long arrow, **B**). Image **C** best demonstrates an abnormal vertical orientation of the PORP, rather than the normal perpendicular positioning of the PORP relative to the tympanoplasty graft. In this case, the vertical positioning of the PORP likely reflects displacement and presumably results in poor conductive hearing. Any abnormal positioning of a prosthesis should be conveyed to the clinician in order to determine whether repositioning of the prosthesis is necessary. Image **D** is a graphic illustration of a Haberman PORP.

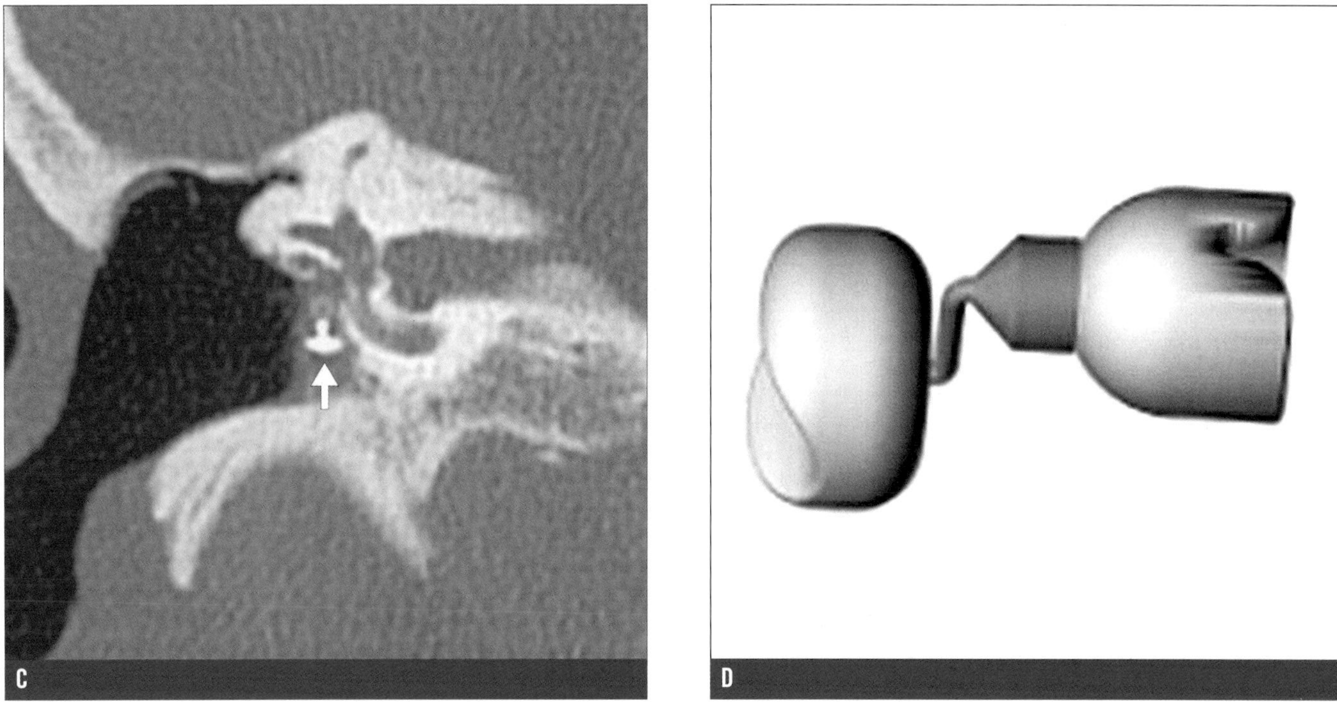

Incus interposition graft

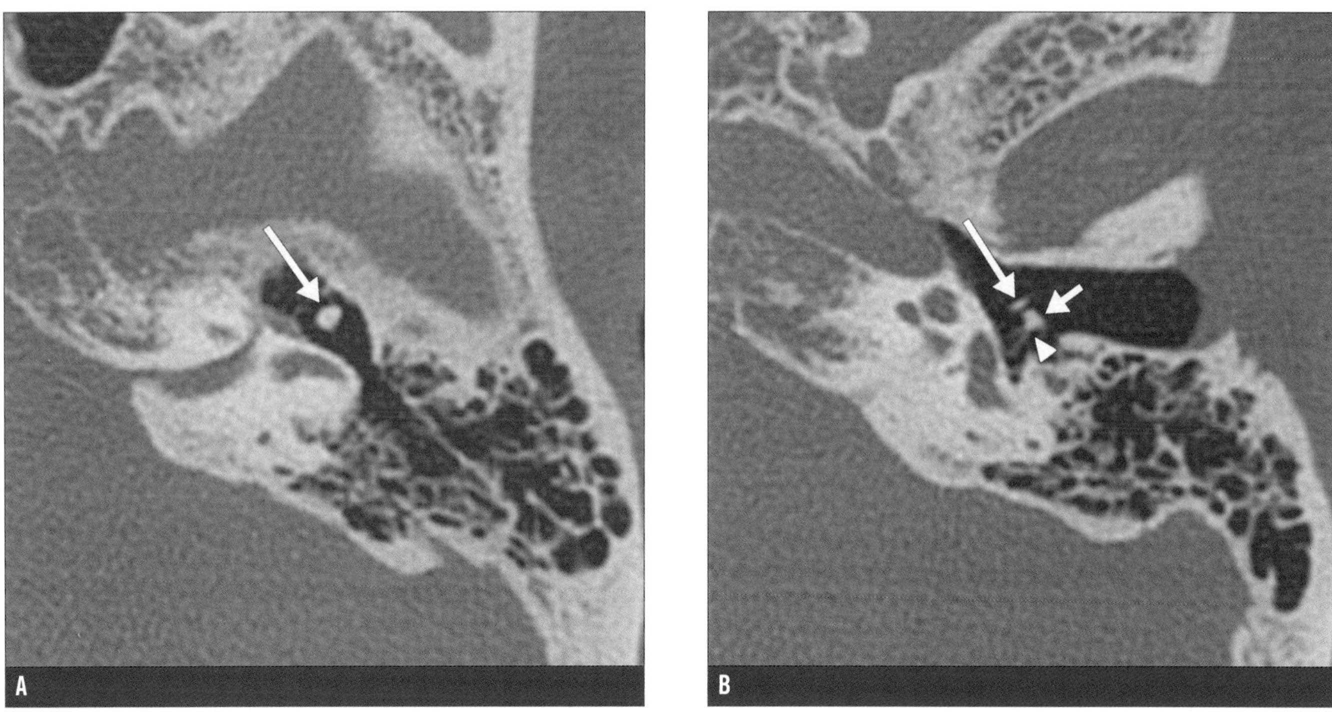

Axial (**A-D**) and coronal reformatted (**E-H**) CT images of the left temporal bone demonstrate an appropriately positioned incus interposition graft. Image **A** demonstrates a normal head of the malleus (long arrow, **A**) and absence of the body and short process of the incus, which normally reside posterolateral to the malleus head. Images **B-D** demonstrate the manubrium of the malleus (long arrows, **B-D**) and the incus interposition graft (short arrows, **B-D**), each abutting one another at the umbo of the malleus (**D**). The incus interposition graft articulates with the capitulum of the stapes on image **B** (arrowhead). A small notch along the medial surface of the incus interposition graft, which was formed to allow articulation with the stapes capitulum, is visualized on images **C** and **D**. Image **E** demonstrates a normal malleus in the coronal plane (long arrow, **E**). Images **F-H** demonstrate the incus interposition graft (short arrows, **F-H**). Image **G** demonstrates the stapes capitulum articulating with the carved notch along the medial margin of the stapes interposition graft (arrowhead, **G**). One of the stapes crura (arrowhead, **H**) is identified extending from the incus interposition graft towards the oval window.

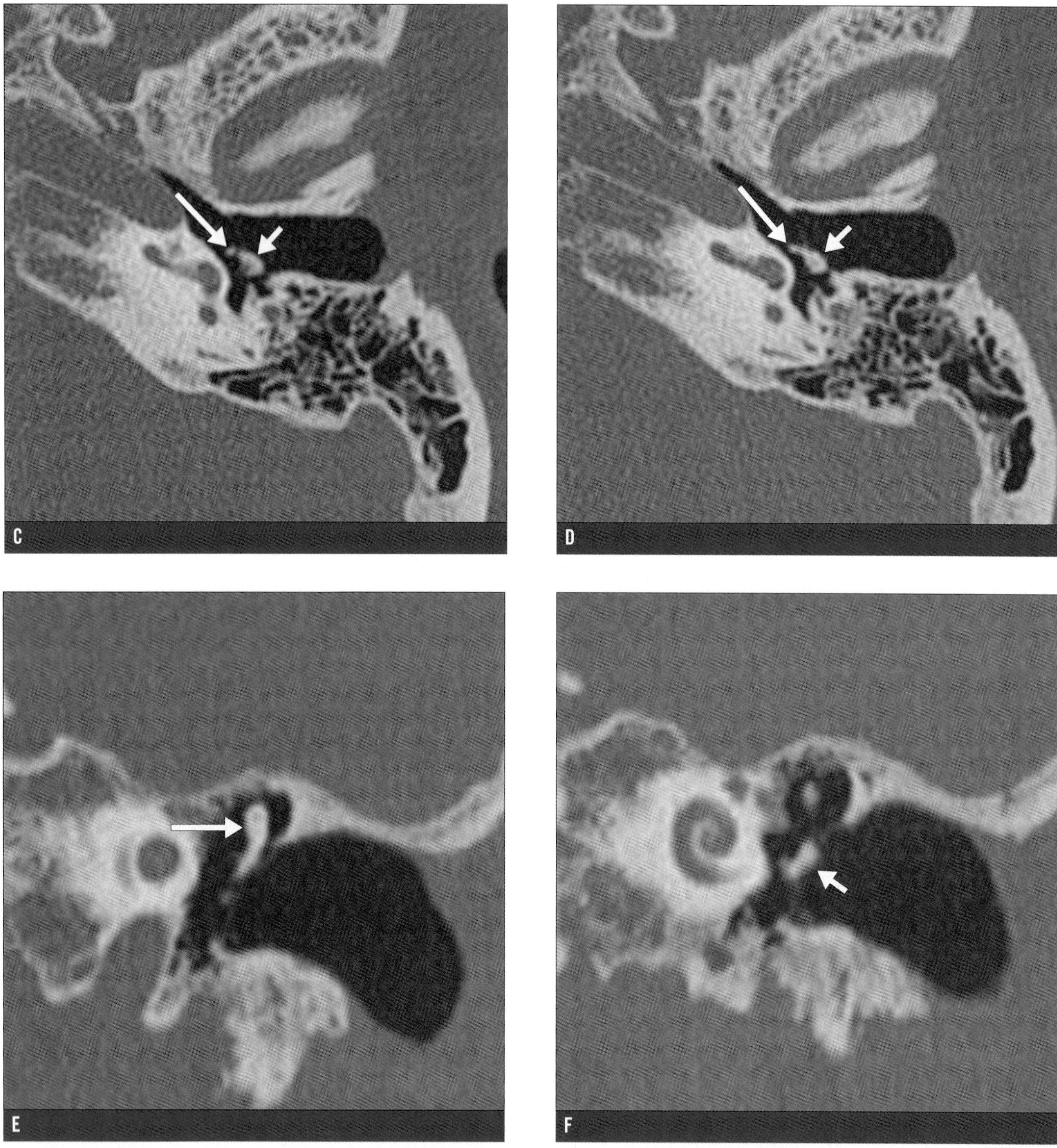
C
D
E
F

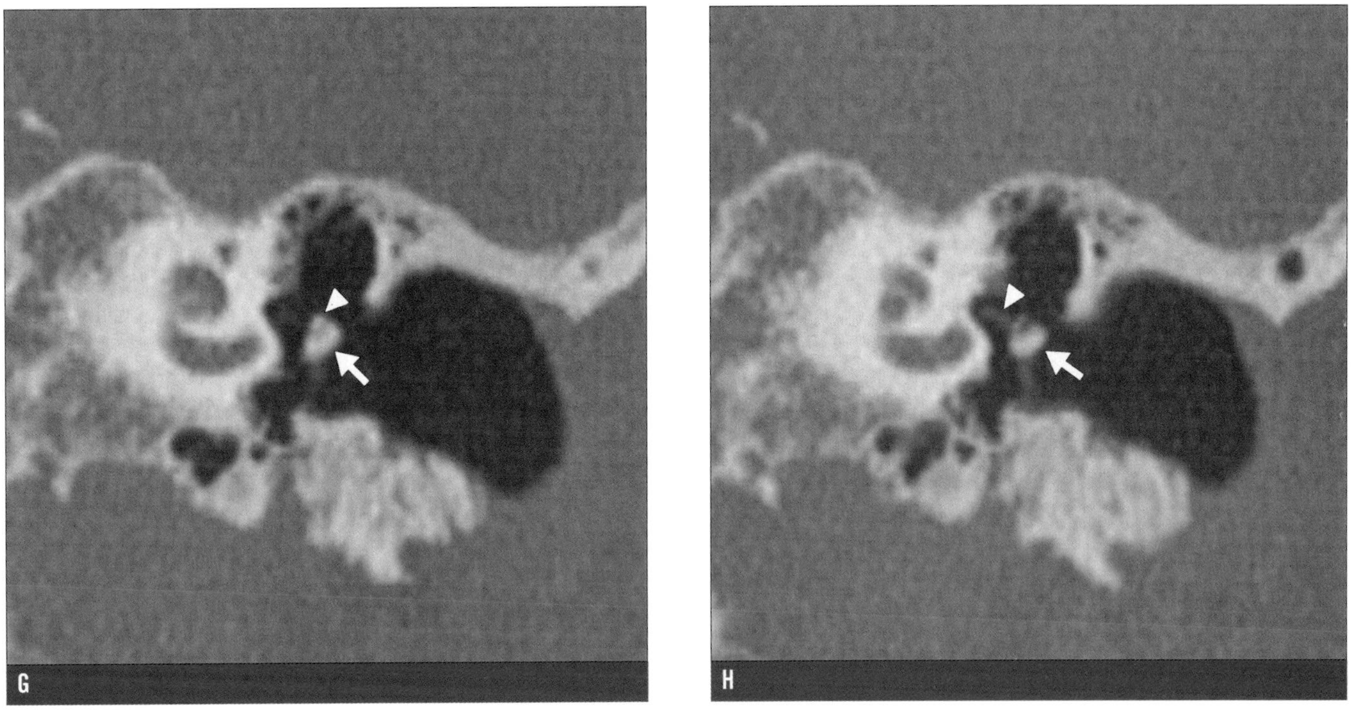

Dislocated double notch Wehrs incus prosthesis

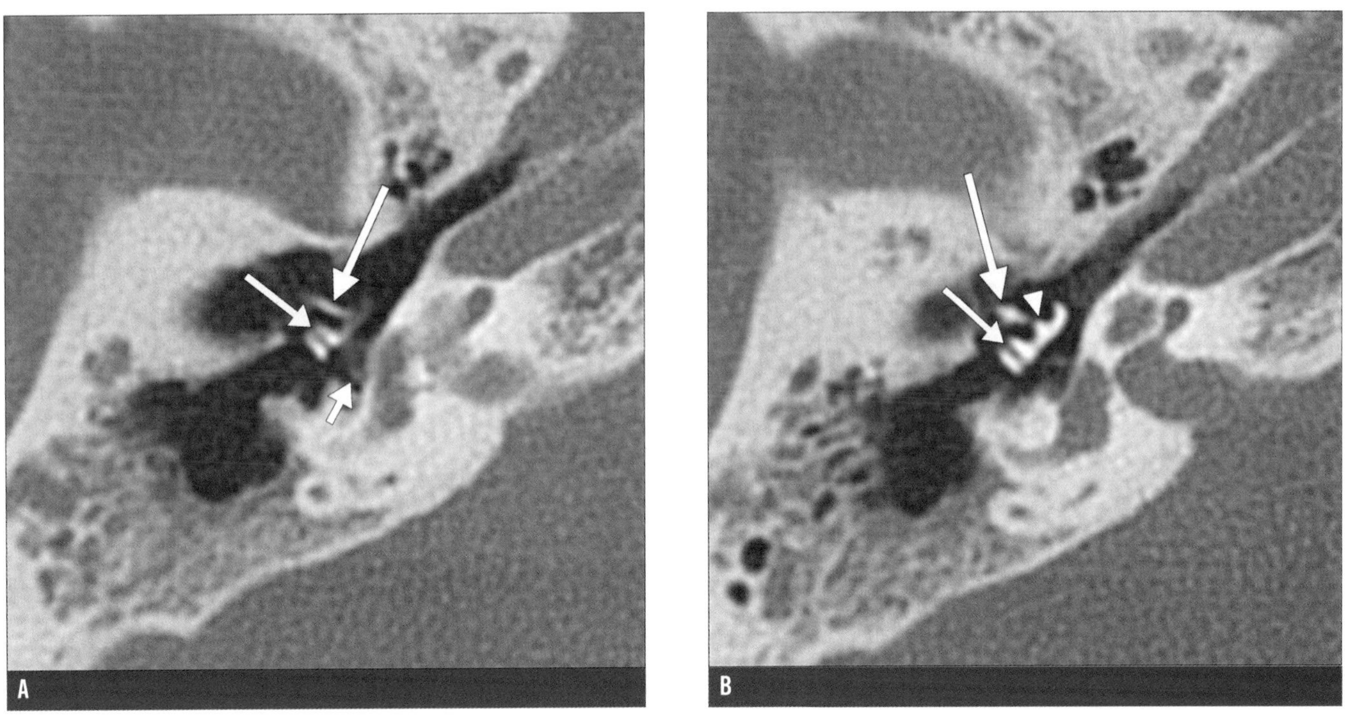

Axial (**A**, **B**) and direct coronal (**C**, **D**) CT images of the right temporal bone. There is a double notch Wehrs incus prosthesis situated between the manubrium of the malleus (long arrows, **A**, **B**) and the stapes superstructure (short arrows, **A**, **C**). On image **B**, the two notches of the Wehrs prosthesis are identified, with an eminence subdividing them (arrowhead, **B**). An apparent third notch on the axial images located along the lateral aspect of the prosthesis represents a hollow core within the proximal aspect of the shaft and not a true notch (medium arrows, **A**, **B**). In this case, the manubrium of the malleus is not positioned within one of the two notches of the prosthesis but is rather perched along the eminence between the notches, best appreciated on image **B**, compatible with a proximal prosthesis dislocation. While a portion of the prosthesis abuts the capitulum of the stapes on image **C** (arrowhead), the distal end of the prosthesis is also dislocated and caudally directed instead of medially directed toward the stapes, best appreciated on image **D** (arrowhead). The hollow core within the proximal aspect of the shaft is also demonstrated on image **D** (medium arrow). Images **E** and **F** are graphic illustrations of a double notch (**E**) and single notch (**F**) Wehrs prosthesis.

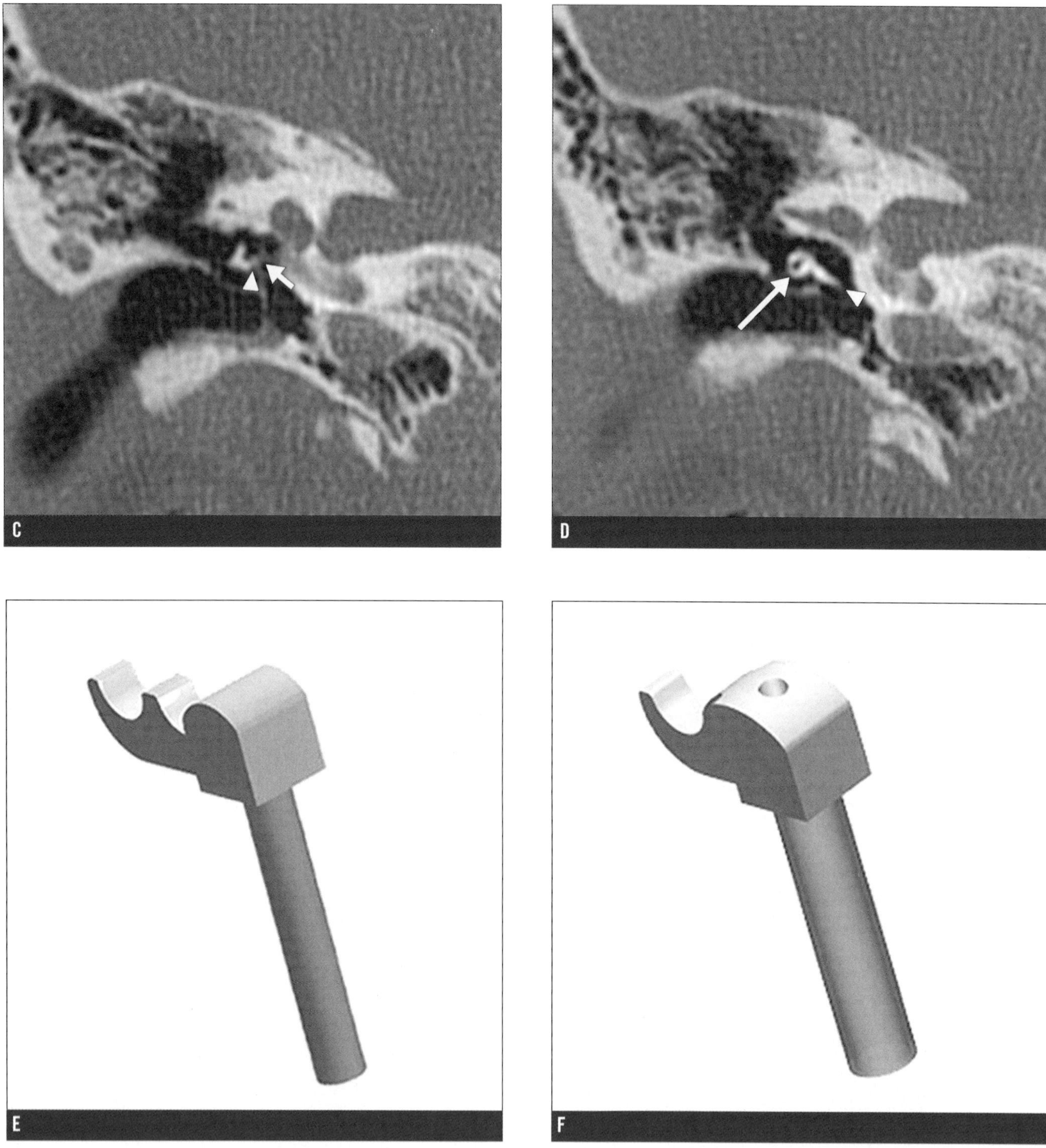
C
D
E
F

Kartush incus-stapes strut prosthesis

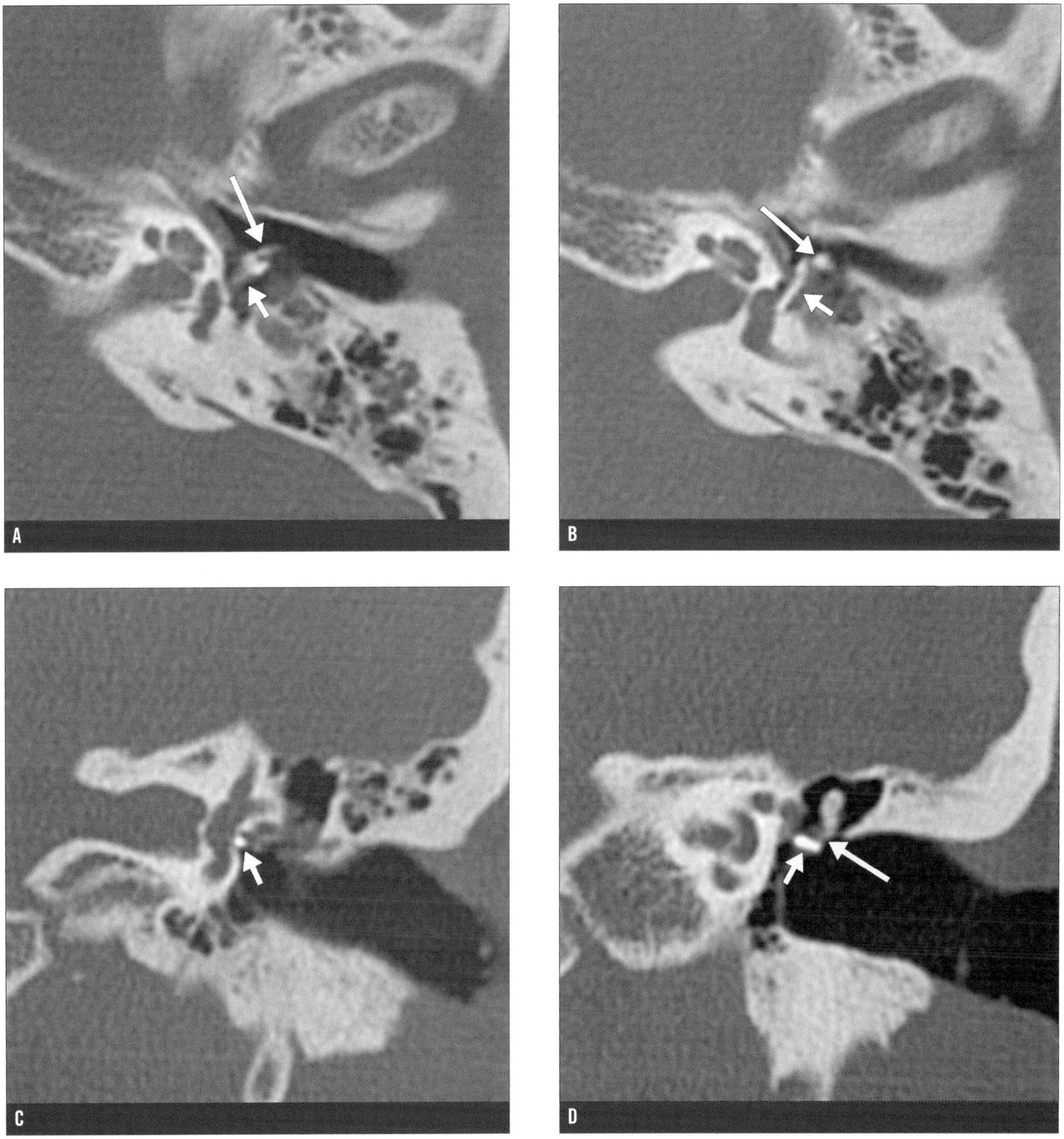

Axial (**A**, **B**) and direct coronal (**C**, **D**) CT images of the left temporal bone demonstrate a Kartush incus-stapes strut prosthesis (short arrows, **A**-**D**) that extends from the manubrium of the malleus (long arrows, **A**, **B**, **D**) to the stapes footplate (**B**, **C**).

Applebaum prosthesis

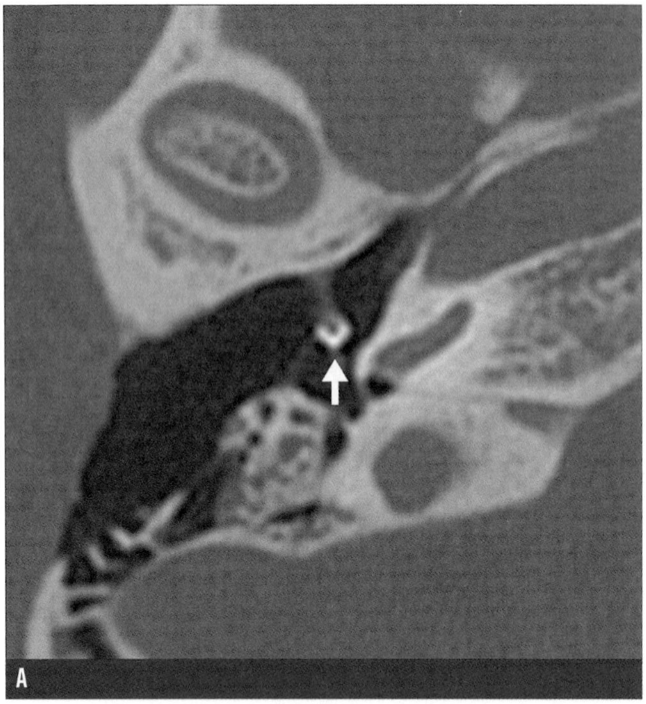

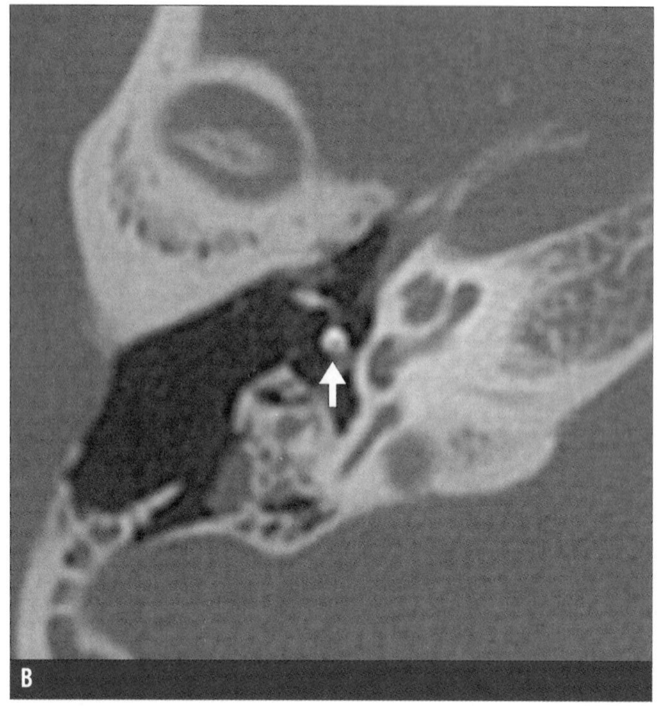

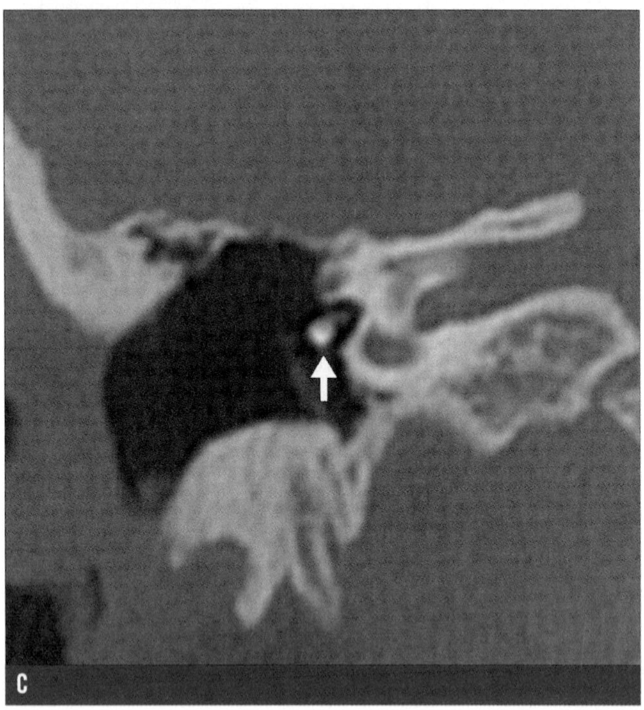

Axial (**A**, **B**) and direct coronal (**C**) CT images of the right temporal bone demonstrate an appropriately positioned Applebaum prosthesis (arrows, **(A-C)**. Normally, an Applebaum prosthesis is placed to bridge the gap between an eroded long process of the incus or focal erosion centered at the incudostapedial joint. However, in this case, the incus was completely destroyed by a cholesteatoma and the residual manubrium of the malleus was attached to the proximal aspect of the prosthesis. The distal end of prosthesis was attached to the capitulum of the stapes, as expected. While this prosthesis has an "L-type" configuration, the L shape is not well demonstrated on these images secondary to the orientation of the prosthesis relative to the plane of imaging. There has also been a prior canal wall down mastoidectomy.

Stapes prosthesis—Gyrus SMart Piston

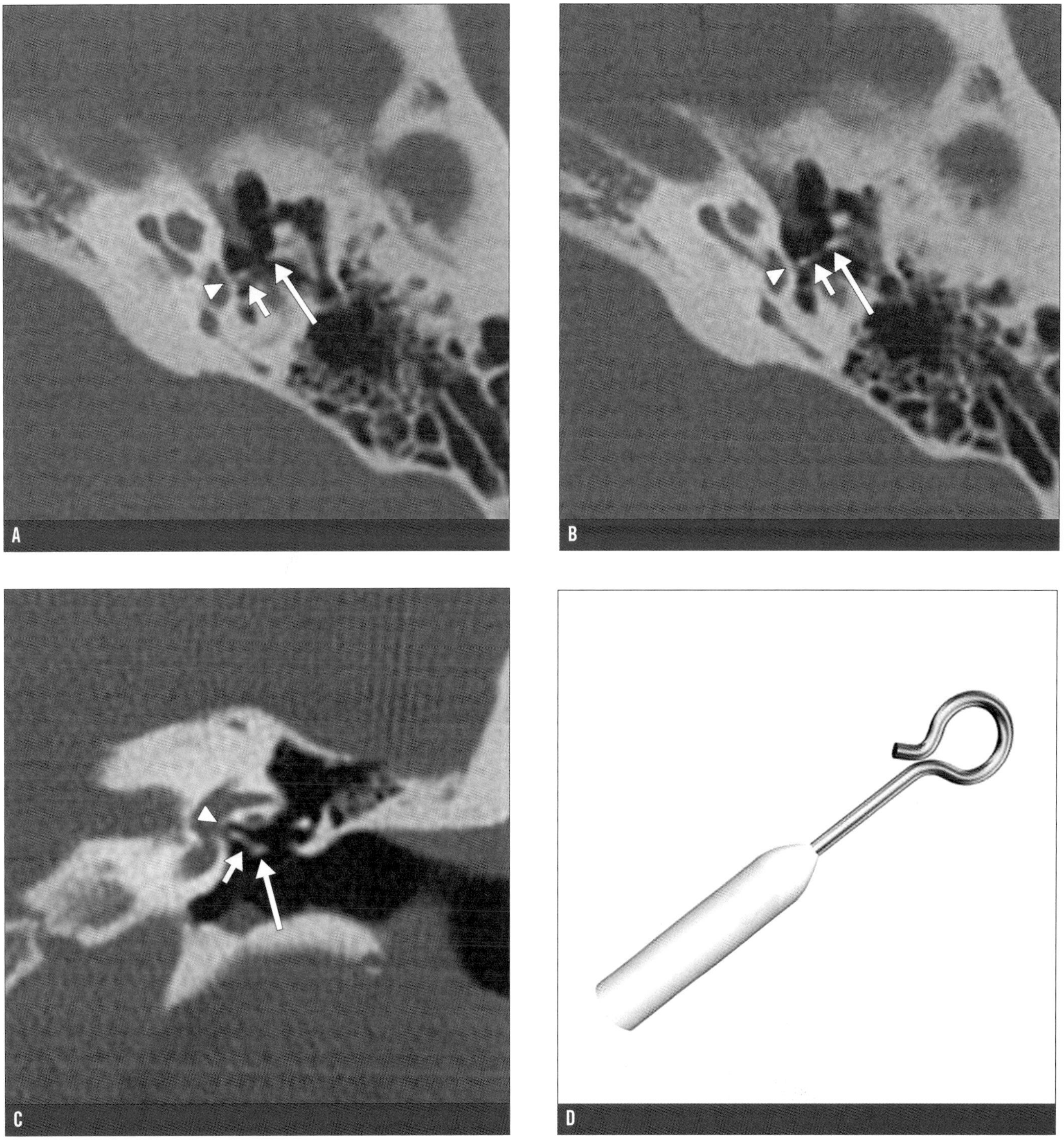

Axial (**A**, **B**) and direct coronal (**C**) CT images of the left temporal bone. There is a Gyrus SMart Piston stapes prosthesis in an appropriate position (short arrows, **A-C**), extending from the long process of the incus (long arrows, **A-C**) to the oval window (arrowheads, **A-C**). Image **D** is a graphic illustration of a Gyrus SMart Piston stapes prosthesis.

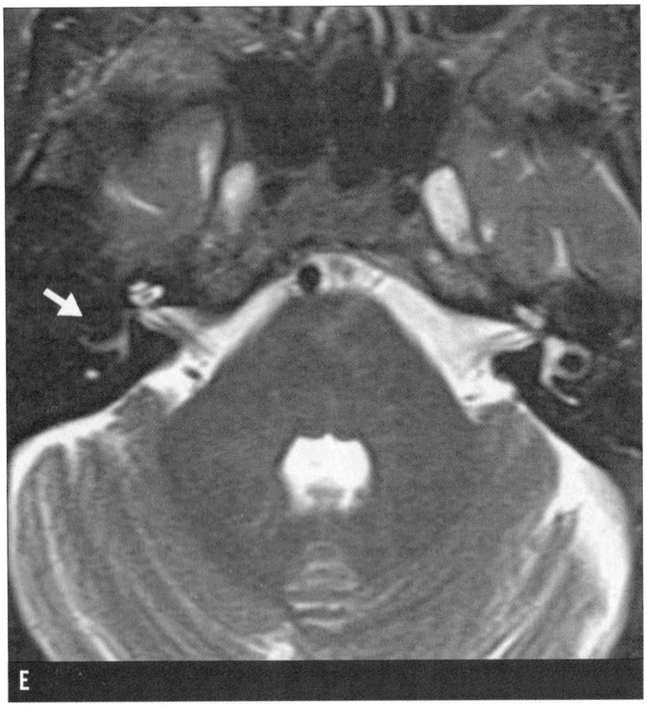

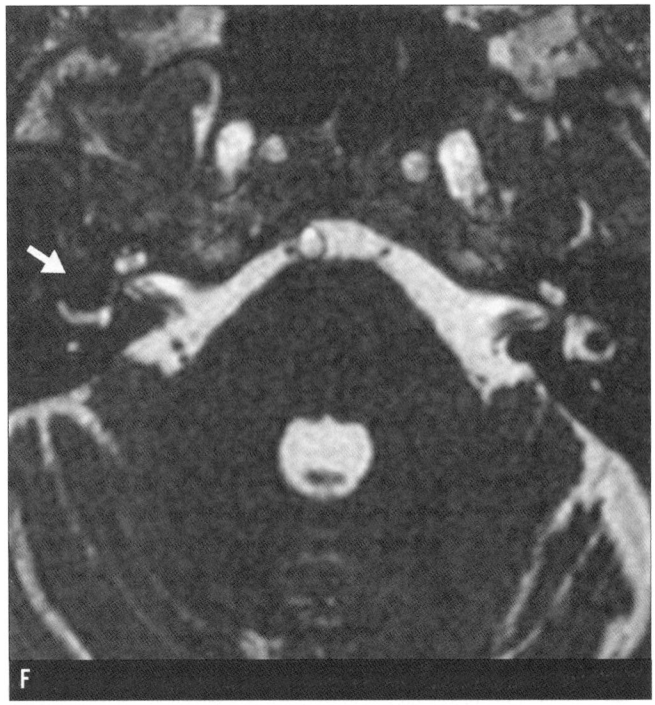

REFERENCES

Al-Qudah M, Dawes PJ. How we do it: modified Wehrs incus ossiculoplasty. *Clin Otolaryngol.* 2005;30(5):461-464.

Al-Qudah M, Dawes PJ. Malleus-stapes assembly: experience with two prostheses. *J Laryngol Otol.* 2006;120(9):736-739.

Mukherji SK, et al. CT of the temporal bone: findings after mastoidectomy, ossicular reconstruction, and cochlear implantation. *AJR Am J Roentgenol.* 1994;163:1467-1471.

Richard Wiet. *Ear and Temporal Bone Surgery: Minimizing Risks and Complications.* Thieme.

Stone JA, Mukherji SK, Jewett BS, Carrasco VN, Castillo M. CT Evaluation of prosthetic ossicular reconstruction procedures: what the otologist needs to know. *Radiographics.* 2000;20:593-605.

CASE 16 Storage of the incus in the mastoid bowl

An ossicular chain autograft (ie, the patient's own ossicle used as a graft) may be harvested to reconstruct a damaged ossicular chain. Occasionally, this procedure may require storage of the harvested ossicle, typically the incus, prior to an ossicular reconstruction (also called ossiculoplasty). Storage of a harvested incus is often performed during a two-stage ossiculoplasty, such as may be performed to treat a middle ear cholesteatoma associated with ossicular destruction. The first stage entails removal of the cholesteatoma and assessment of the native ossicular chain. If the incus is salvageable and can be used as an autograft at the time of the first stage of surgery, it can be stored, usually either in the mastoidectomy bowl or in the tragus. The second stage occurs several months later at which time the harvested incus can be used for the ossiculoplasty. A stored ossicle can simulate unintended ossicular displacement or other osseous abnormality on CT.

Storage of the incus in the mastoid bowl

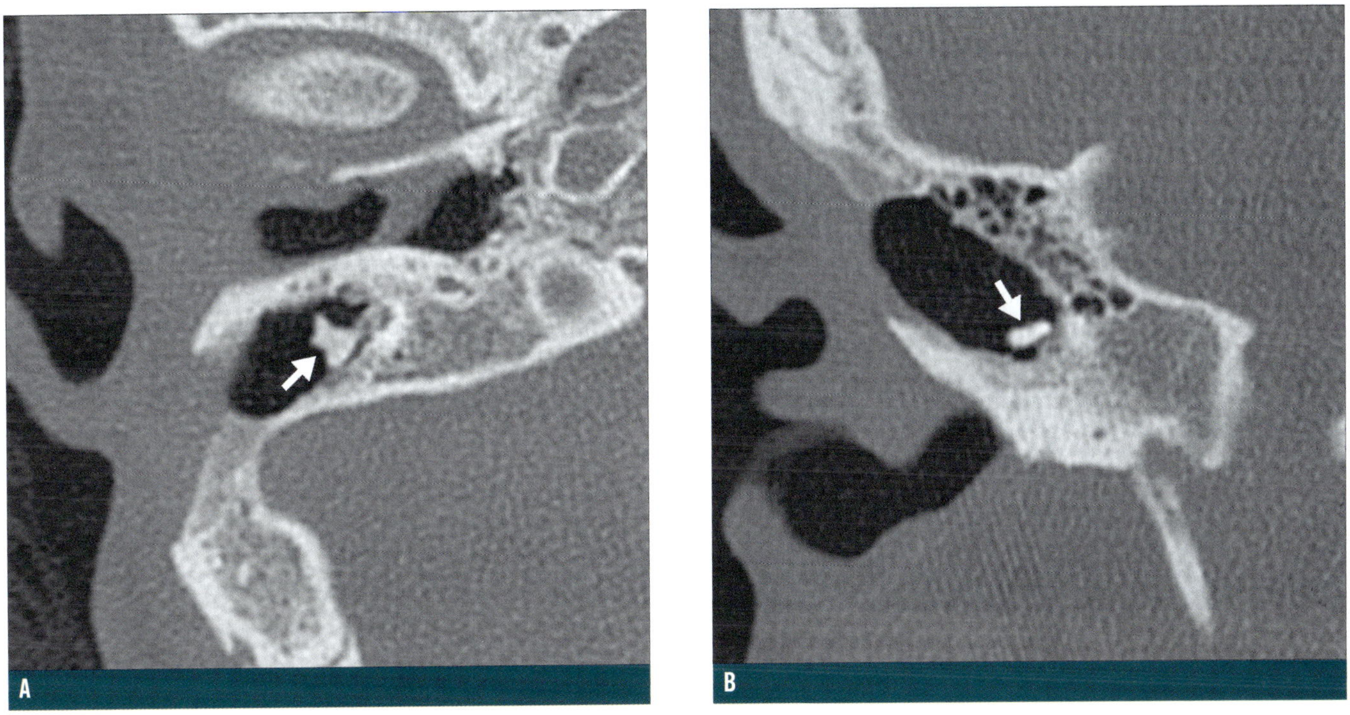

Axial (**A**) and coronal reformatted (**B**) CT images of the right temporal bone demonstrate a canal wall up right mastoidectomy with storage of the incus in the mastoid bowl (arrows, **A**, **B**).

REFERENCE

Gyo K, Hato N, Shinomori Y, Hakuba N. Storage of the incus in the mastoid bowl for use as a columella in staged tympanoplasty. *Auris Nasus Larynx*. 2007;34(1):5-8.

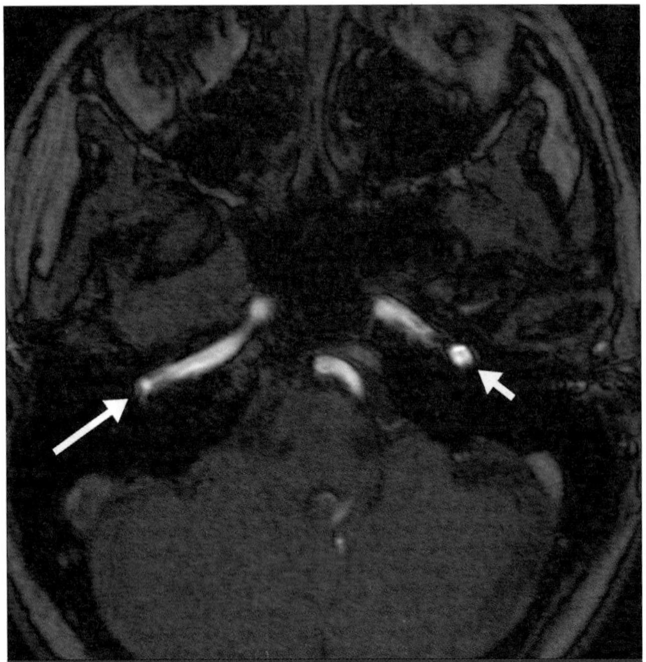
C

REFERENCES

Davis WL, Harnsberger HR. MR angiography of an aberrant internal carotid artery. *Am J Neuroradiol.* 1991;12:1225.

Koesling S, Kunkel P, Schul T. Vascular anomalies, sutures and small canals of the temporal bone on axial CT. *Eur J Radiol.* 2005;54:335-343.

Lasjaunias P, Berenstein A, Ter Brugge KG. *Surgical Neuroangiography, Clinical Vascular Anatomy and Variations.* 2nd ed. New York, NY: Springer-Verlag; 2001.

Lefournier V, Vasdev A, Bessou P, Boubagra K. A persistent pharyngohyostapedial artery: embryologic Implications. *AJNR Am J Neuroradiol.* 1999;20:271-274.

Lo WWM, Solti-Bohman LG, McElveen JT. Aberrant carotid artery: radiologic diagnosis with emphasis on high-resolution computed tomography. *Radiographics.* 1985;5:985-993.

CASE 20 Lateralized petrous internal carotid artery

A lateralized petrous internal carotid artery (ICA) is a rare variation of the ICA as it traverses within the temporal bone. In this variant, the posterior genu, which is located at the junction between the vertical and horizontal portions of the petrous ICA, is located posterolateral to its typical location. On axial CT images of patients with a lateralized petrous ICA, the posterior genu of the petrous ICA extends to, or beyond, an imaginary line drawn perpendicular to the midportion of the basal turn of the cochlea. A lateralized petrous ICA may also partially extend into the anterior aspect of the mesotympanum. Furthermore, the posterior margin of the petrous carotid canal wall with this entity is often thinned or dehiscent. As a result of its lateralized course, the petrous ICA will be elongated in the axial dimension.

Patients with a lateralized petrous ICA are frequently asymptomatic, but they can present with pulsatile tinnitus and vertigo. In cases where there is associated osseous dehiscence, a retrotympanic reddish mass may be seen clinically. It is important for the surgeon to be aware of this variant prior to middle ear surgery in order to avoid vascular injury.

A lateralized petrous ICA should be distinguished from an aberrant ICA, as the latter is an anomaly that enters the tympanic cavity via an enlarged inferior tympanic canaliculus, whereas a lateralized petrous ICA does not. Furthermore, while a lateralized petrous ICA may partially extend into the anterior aspect of the mesotympanum, an aberrant ICA traverses the entire mesotympanum from posterior to anterior. Differentiating a lateralized petrous ICA from an aberrant ICA is readily made by CT and usually by MRA. However, differentiating these two entities on catheter angiography may be difficult because of the lack of adequate osseous landmarks.

Left lateralized petrous internal carotid artery

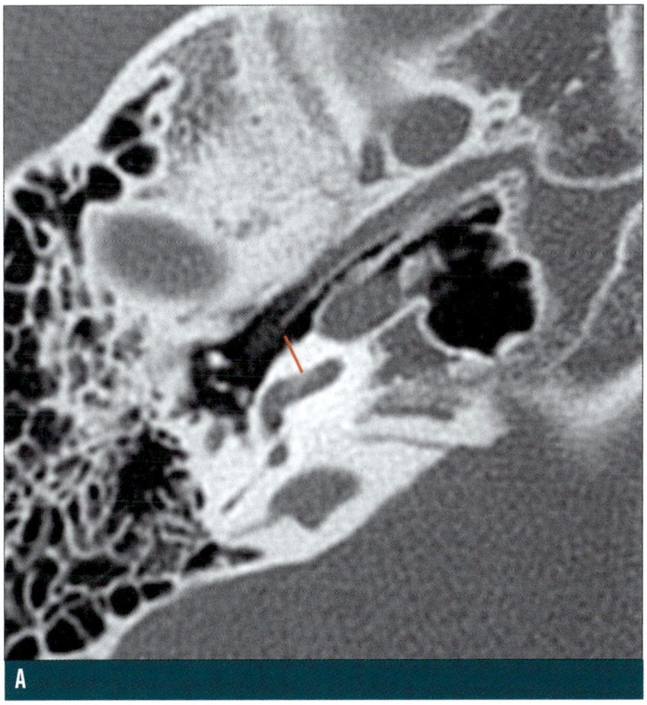

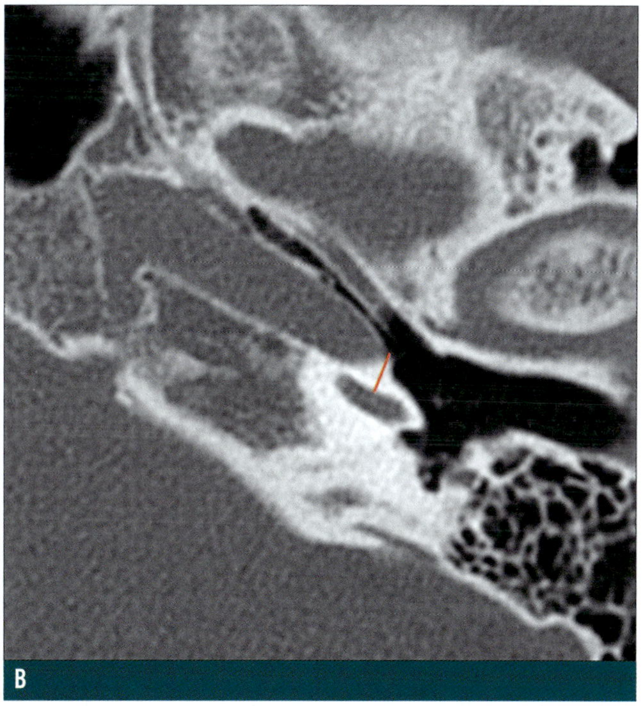

Axial CT images of the right (**A**) and left (**B**) temporal bones demonstrate a lateralized left petrous ICA compared to the normal right side. Specifically, the posterior genu of the left petrous ICA extends to the approximate level of an imaginary line drawn perpendicular to the midportion of the basal turn of the left cochlea (red line, **B**), whereas this is not present on the right (red line, **A**). There is no associated osseous dehiscence of the left lateralized petrous ICA in this case. Coronal reformatted CT images of the right temporal bone (**C**) and left temporal bone (**D**) demonstrate the difference in position of the petrous ICA posterior genus, with the left posterior genu significantly more lateral compared to the right posterior genu with respect to the cochleae (red vertical lines, **C**, **D**). A collapsed maximum intensity projection axial MRA image of the same patient (**E**) also demonstrates the lateral course of the left petrous ICA, which appears as an elongated left petrous ICA (arrow, **E**) relative to the contralateral right petrous ICA.

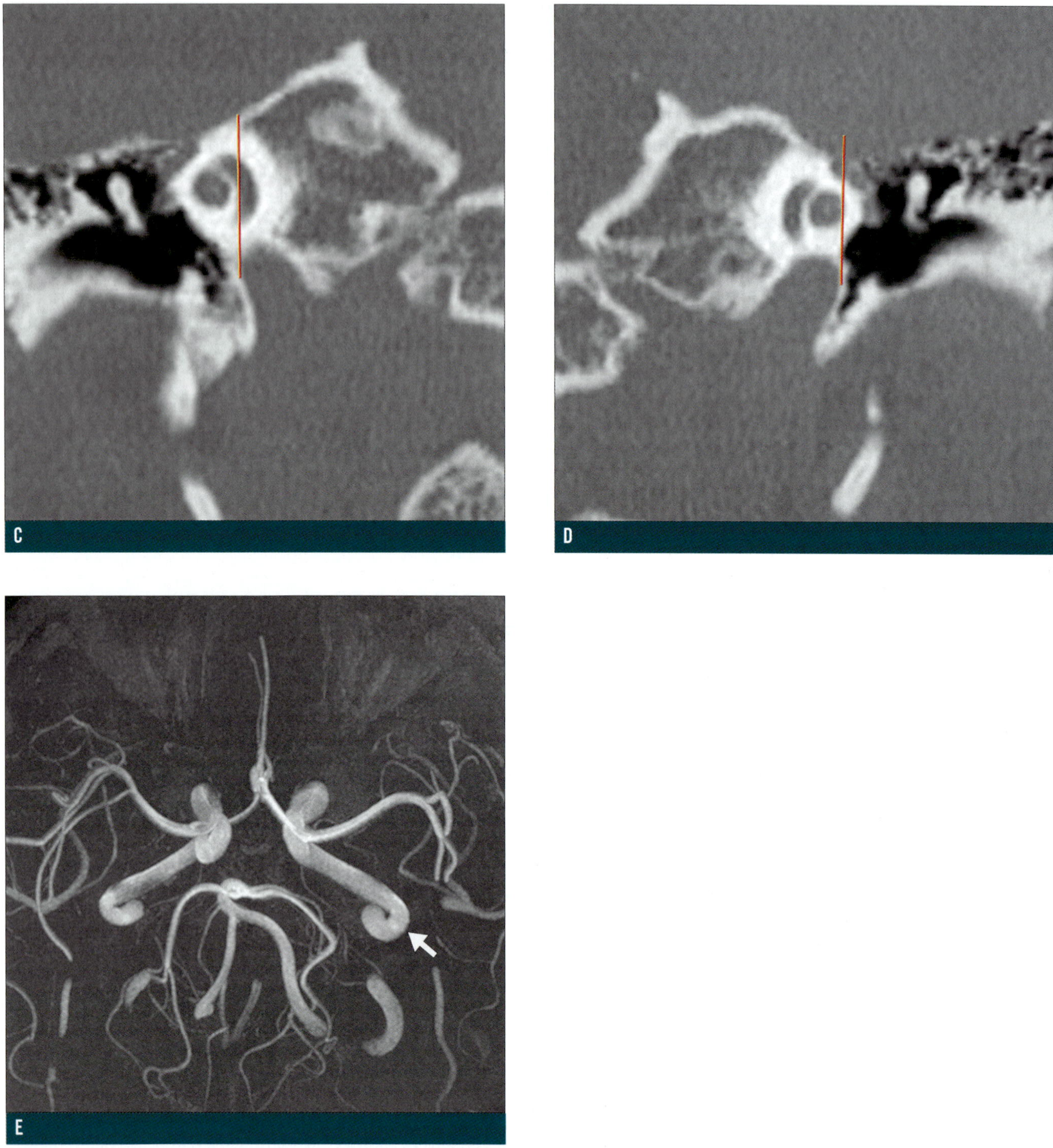

Lateralized petrous internal carotid arteries

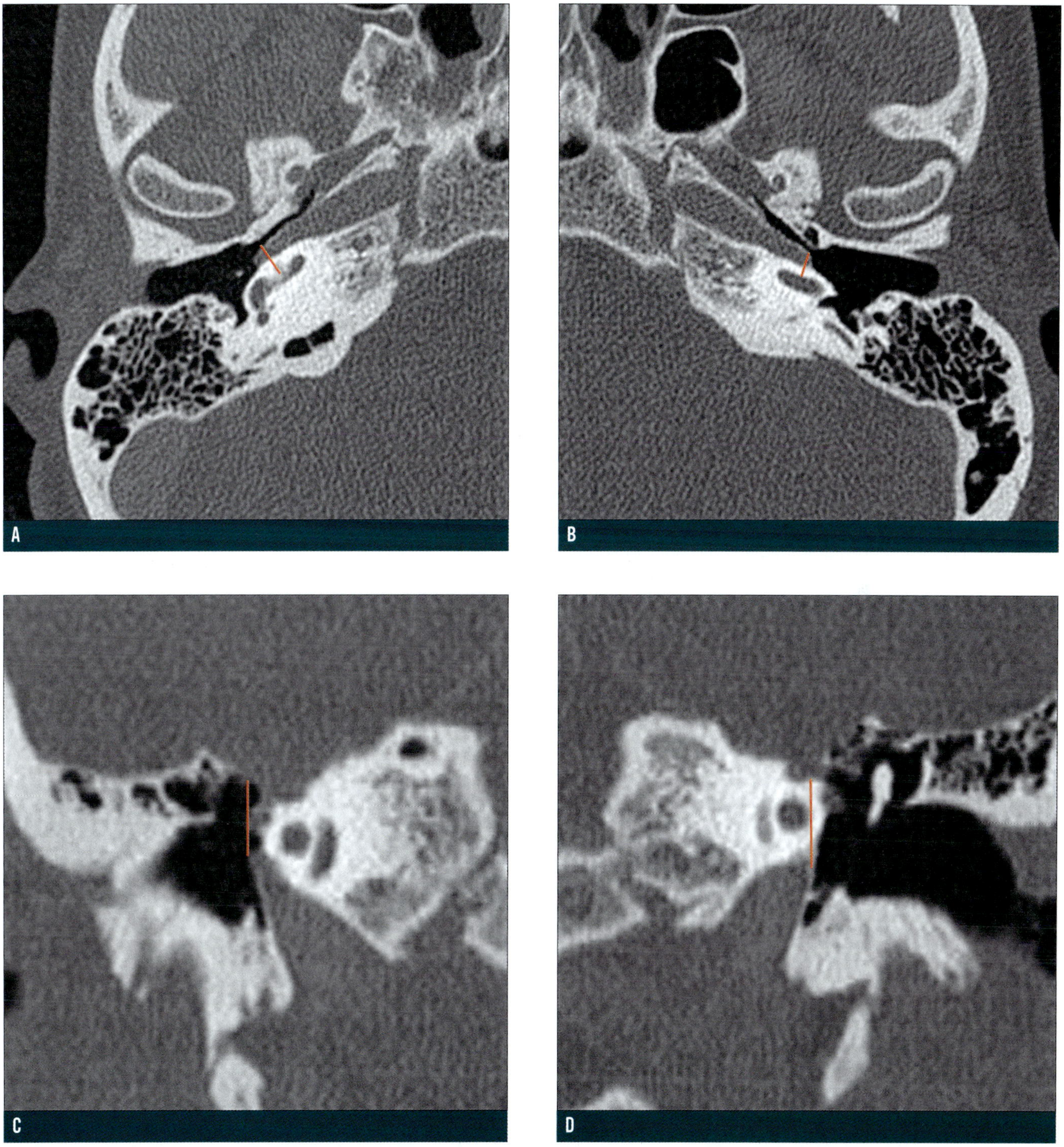

Axial CT images of the right (**A**) and left (**B**) temporal bones and coronal reformatted CT images of the right (**C**) and left (**D**) temporal bones demonstrate lateralized petrous ICAs. The posterior genus of the petrous ICAs extend lateral to imaginary lines drawn perpendicular to the midportions of the basal turns of each cochlea (red lines, **A**, **B**). They are also more lateral than normal relative to each cochlea on the coronal reformatted images, right more so than left (vertical red lines, **C**, **D**). There is apparent osseous dehiscence along the posterior margin of the lateralized right petrous ICA. Furthermore, the posterior margins of the lateralized petrous ICAs bulge into the mesotympanums, right more so than left.

REFERENCE

Glastonbury CM, Harnsberger HR, Hudgins PA, Salzman KL. Lateralized petrous internal carotid artery: imaging features and distinction from the aberrant internal carotid artery. *Neuroradiology*. 2012;54(9):1007-1013.

CASE 21 High-riding jugular bulb

The jugular bulb represents the superior-most portion of the internal jugular vein and is a continuation of the sigmoid sinus. It is focally dilated and located within the jugular foramen of the skull base. It forms after the age of 2 and its size may change during the first 40 years of life, after which its size stabilizes. Normally, the superior margin (dome) of the jugular bulb resides caudal to the hypotympanum of the tympanic cavity. However, occasionally its dome can extend more cephalad than normal (ie, high-riding) and potentially cause symptoms, such as tinnitus. The definition of a high-riding jugular bulb varies among authors. Various definitions that have been proposed include when the jugular bulb dome resides cephalad to the scutum, extends to within 2 mm of the internal auditory canal floor, or when it resides to the level of the round window or basal turn of the cochlea, among other definitions. Despite various opinions on what constitutes a high-riding jugular bulb, the proposed definitions described above are at the same approximate horizontal level. Identifying a high-riding jugular bulb prior to surgery is important as it can be inadvertently breached by the unsuspecting surgeon.

COMPANION CASES

- **Dehiscent high-riding jugular bulb.** The bone adjacent to a high-riding jugular bulb can be dehiscent with the hypotympanum of the tympanic cavity. When present, this may be identified as a smooth, bluish mass at otoscopy. A high-riding jugular bulb can also be dehiscent with the mastoid portion of the facial nerve canal, vestibular aqueduct, and the posterior semicircular canal.
- **High-riding jugular bulb dehiscent with the posterior semicircular canal.** Symptoms that may occur with semicircular canal dehiscence relate to the concept of a third mobile window and include hearing loss, autophony, tinnitus, and aural fullness. As stated above, a high-riding jugular bulb may sometimes be dehiscent with the posterior semicircular canal. While often asymptomatic, a study by Gopen et al demonstrated that 7 of 10 noniatrogenic cases of symptomatic posterior semicircular canal dehiscence were the result of a dehiscent, high-riding jugular bulb. Therefore, clinical correlation is needed when such a finding is encountered by CT imaging.

High-riding jugular bulb

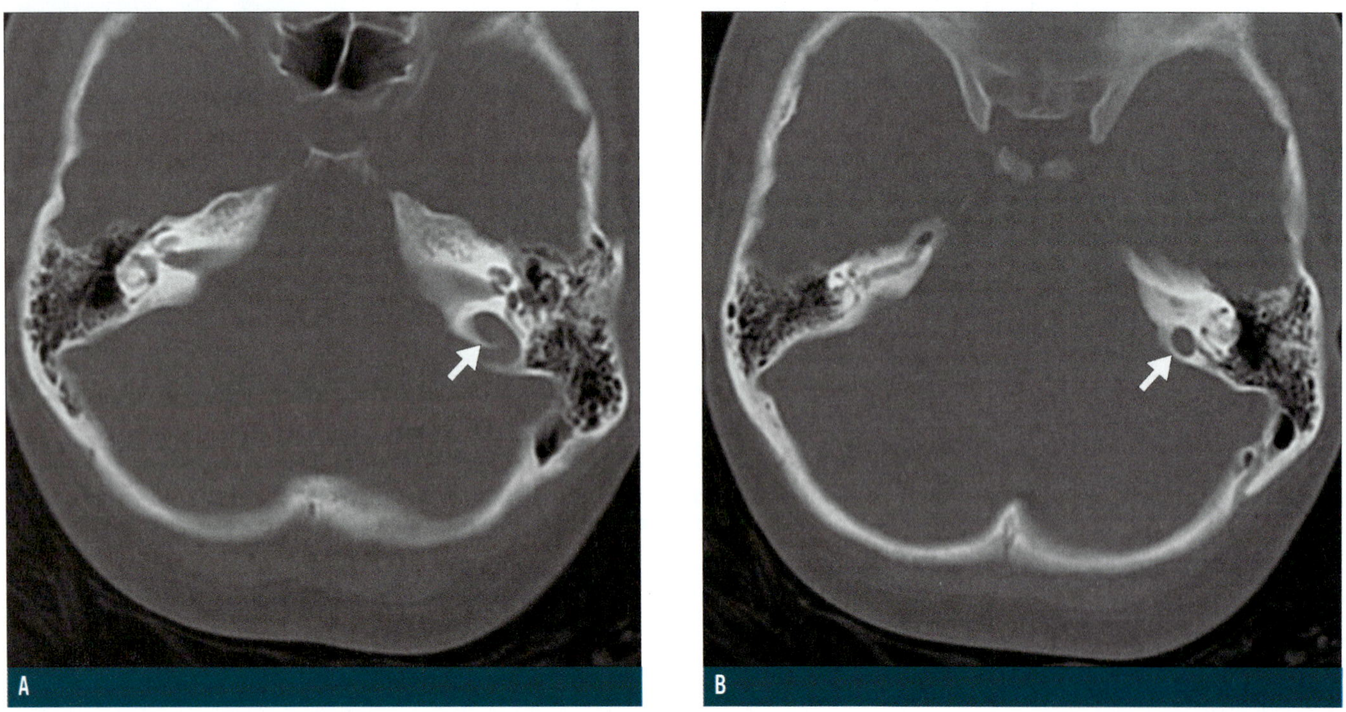

Axial CT images of the temporal bones (**A**, **B**) demonstrate a high-riding left jugular bulb (arrows, **A**, **B**). Its location satisfies various definitions that have been proposed for the diagnosis of a high-riding jugular bulb, including being located above the level of the IAC floor, cephalad to the round window/basal turn of the cochlea, and cephalad to the scutum.

Companion case: Dehiscent high-riding jugular bulb

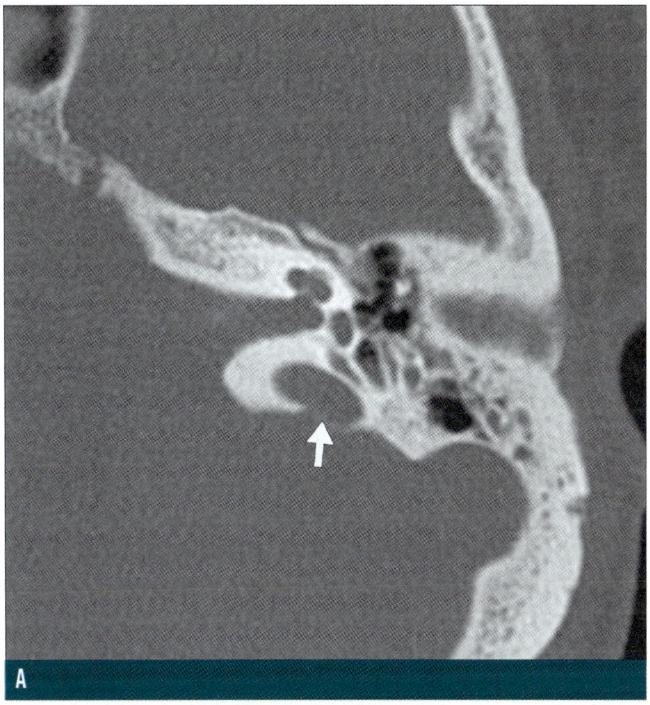

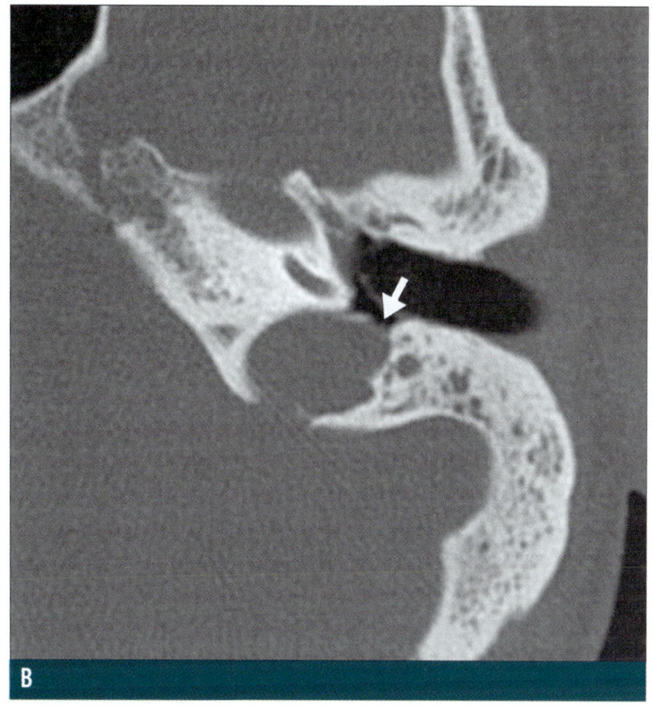

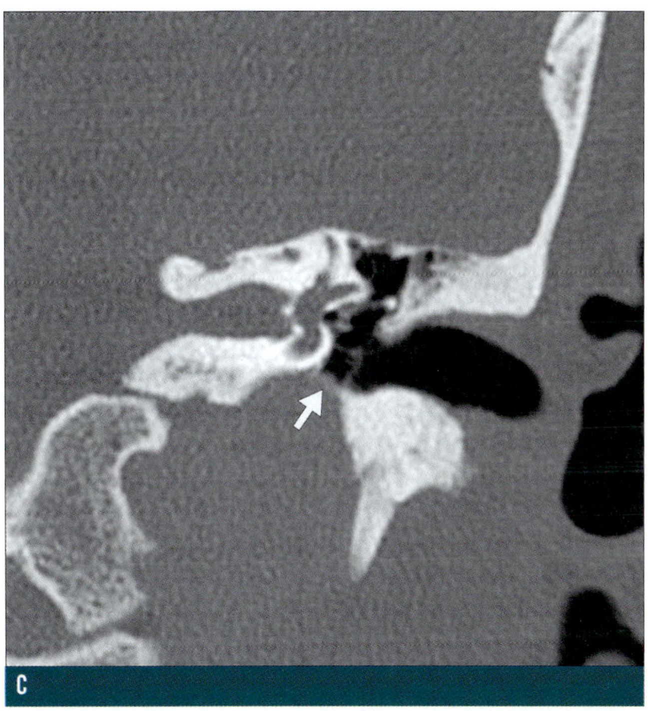

An axial CT image of the left temporal bone (**A**) demonstrates a high-riding left jugular bulb (arrow, **A**). This jugular bulb extends to the level of the IAC and at least up to the level of the middle turn of the cochlea and oval window, clearly meeting the criteria of a high-riding jugular bulb proposed by various authors, as described in the text. Axial (**B**) and coronal reformatted (**C**) CT images of the same patient reveal focal osseous dehiscence of the high-riding jugular bulb with the hypotympanum (arrows, **B**, **C**).

Companion case: High-riding jugular bulb dehiscent with the posterior semicircular canal

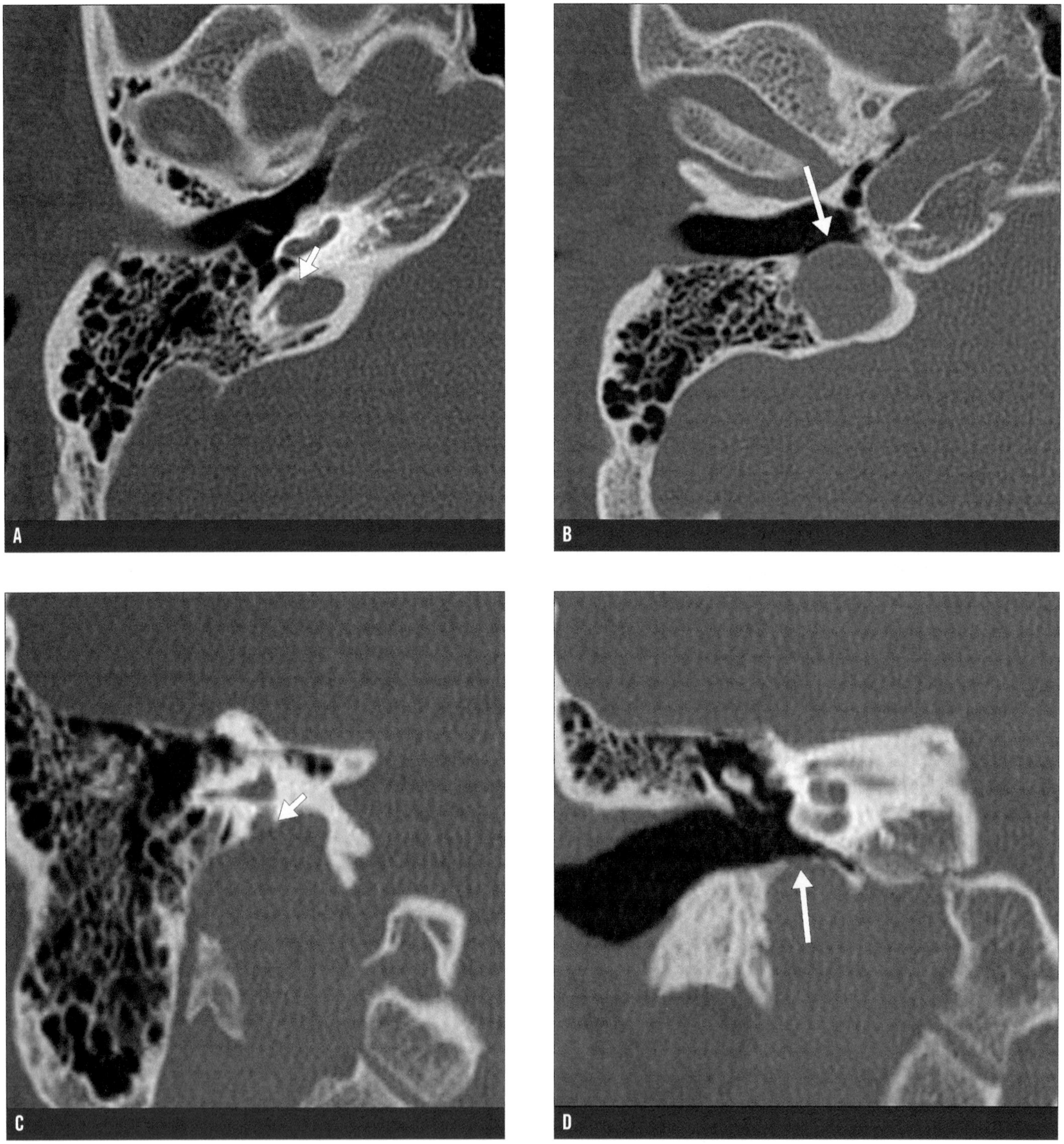

Axial (**A**, **B**) and coronal reformatted (**C**, **D**) CT images of the right temporal bone. There is a high-riding right jugular bulb that communicates with the posterior semicircular canal (short arrows, **A**, **C**). The bone between the jugular bulb and the hypotympanum appears thinned but intact on axial imaging (long arrow, **B**), although it is likely partially dehiscent when viewed on coronal reformatted imaging (long arrow, **D**). While this finding may be incidental and asymptomatic, correlation with clinical symptoms referable to semicircular canal dehiscence is necessary to determine its significance.

REFERENCES

Atilla S, Akpek S, Uslu S, Ilgit E, Isik S. Computed tomographic evaluation of surgically significant vascular variations related with the temporal bone. *Eur J Radiol.* 1995;20:52-56.

Friedmann DR, Eubig J, Winata LS, Pramanik BK, Merchant SN, Lalwani AK. Prevalence of jugular bulb abnormalities and resultant inner ear dehiscence: a histopathologic and radiologic study. *Otolaryngol Head Neck Surg.* 2012;147(4):750-756.

Gopen Q, Zhou G, Poe D, Kenna M, Jones D. Posterior semicircular canal dehiscence: first reported case series. *Otol Neurotol.* 2010;31(2):339-344.

Hourani R, Carey J, Yousem DM. Dehiscence of the jugular bulb and vestibular aqueduct: Findings on 200 consecutive temporal bone computed tomography scans. *J Comput Assist Tomogr.* 2005;29(5):657-662.

Koesling S, Kunkel P, Schul T. Vascular anomalies, sutures and small canals of the temporal bone on axial CT. *Eur J Radiol.* 2005;54:335-343.

Tomura N, Sashi R, Kobayashi M, Hirano H, Hashimoto M, Watarai J. Normal variations of the temporal bone on high-resolution CT: Their incidence and clinical significance. *Clin Radiol.* 1995;50:144-148.

CASE 22 Jugular bulb diverticulum

A jugular bulb diverticulum is a focal vascular outpouching of the jugular bulb that often extends into the temporal bone. There has been debate in the literature as to whether a jugular bulb diverticulum represents a normal variant or a vascular anomaly. It has been postulated that a jugular bulb diverticulum may occur because of regional vascular turbulence at the junction between the internal jugular vein and sigmoid sinus, resulting in a focally weakened venous wall. This finding is considered rare, although there has been speculation that the true prevalence of a jugular bulb diverticulum is greater than reported, presumably because most are not associated with symptoms. Symptoms of a jugular bulb diverticulum may include hearing loss, vertigo, and pulsatile tinnitus.

COMPANION CASES

Like a high-riding jugular bulb, a jugular bulb diverticulum may be dehiscent with adjacent structures, including the mastoid air cells and hypotympanum.

- **Jugular bulb diverticulum dehiscent with the mastoid air cells.**
- **Jugular bulb diverticulum dehiscent with the hypotympanum.**

Jugular bulb diverticulum

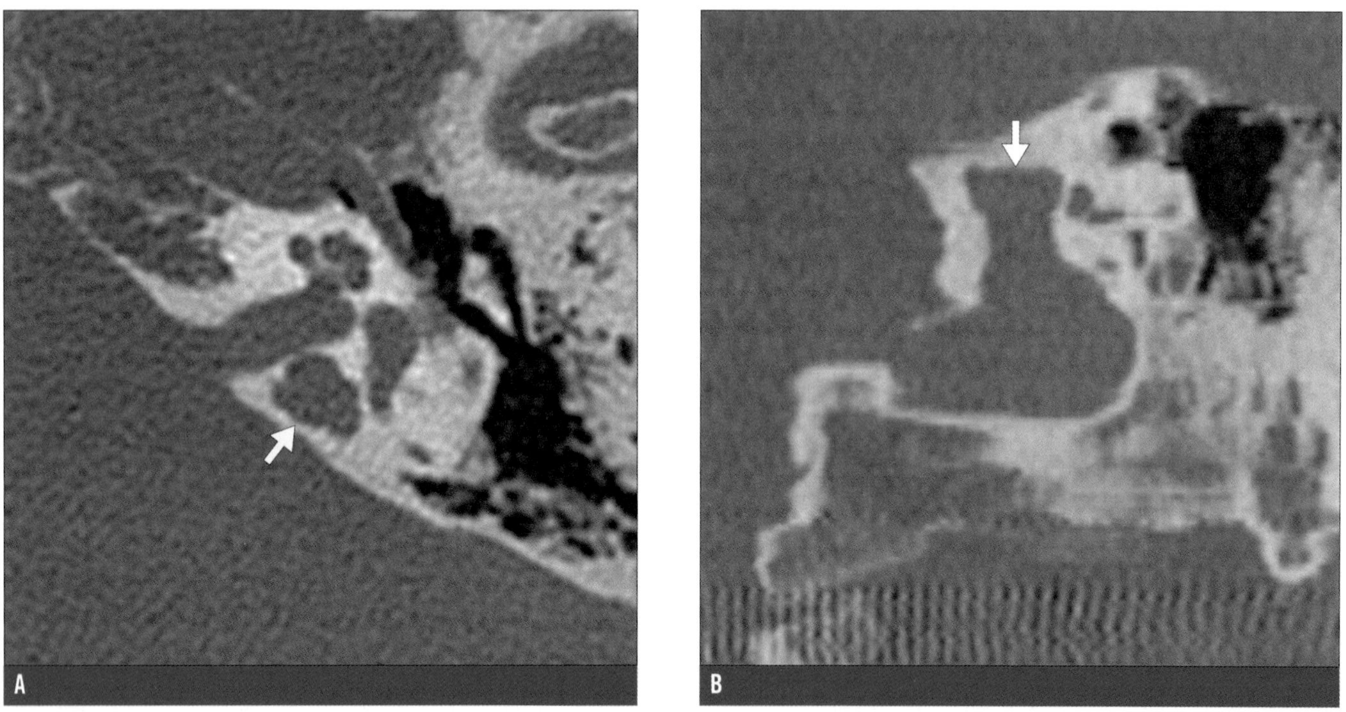

Axial (**A**) and coronal reformatted (**B**) CT images of the left temporal bone demonstrate a focal, cephalad-directed jugular bulb diverticulum (arrows, **A**, **B**).

Companion case: Jugular bulb diverticulum dehiscent with the mastoid air cells

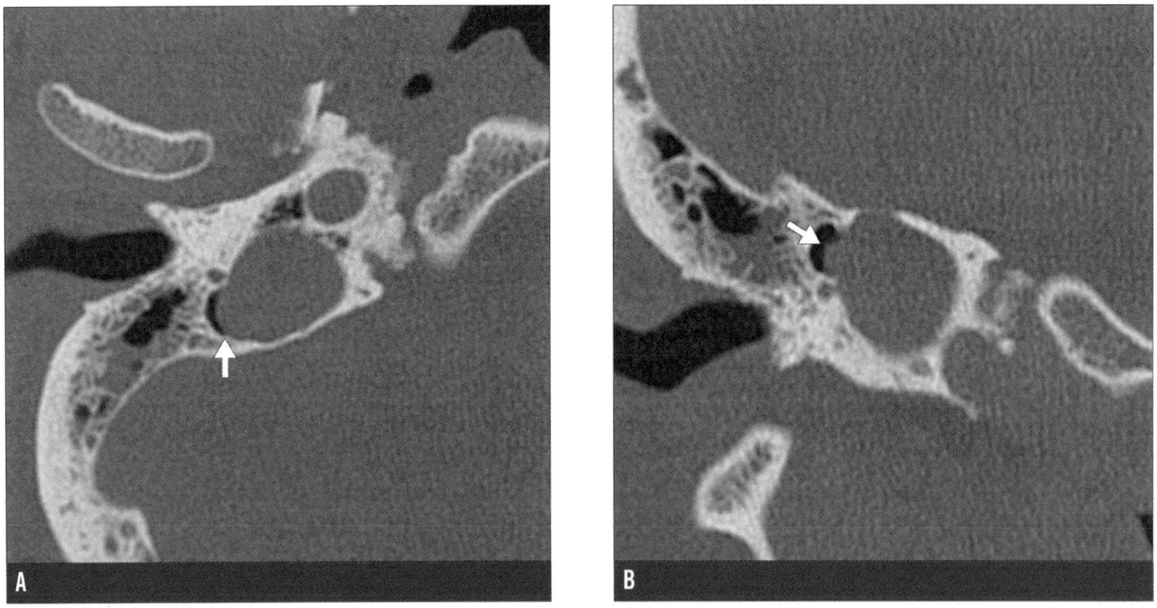

Axial (**A**) and coronal reformatted (**B**) CT images of the right temporal bone demonstrate a focal, posterolaterally directed vascular outpouching of the right jugular bulb, compatible with a jugular bulb diverticulum (arrows, **A**, **B**). The finding is associated with a focal osseous defect of the adjacent mastoid air cells, with a thin rim of residual air immediately adjacent to the jugular bulb diverticulum.

Companion case: Jugular bulb diverticulum dehiscent with the hypotympanum

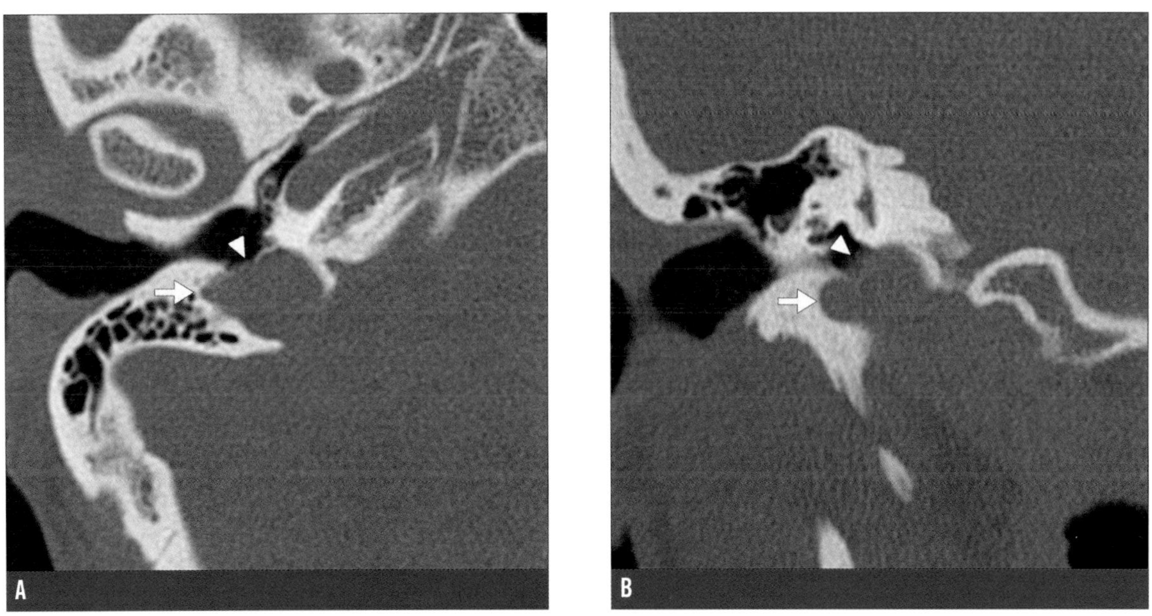

Axial (**A**) and coronal reformatted (**B**) CT images of the right temporal bone demonstrate a vascular outpouching of the right jugular bulb directed laterally, compatible with a jugular bulb diverticulum (arrows, **A**, **B**). There is also associated focal osseous dehiscence of the hypotympanum (arrowheads, **A**, **B**).

REFERENCES

Bilgen C, Kirazli T, Ogut F, Totan S. Jugular bulb diverticula: clinical and radiologic aspects. *Otolaryngol Head Neck Surg.* 2003;128(3): 382-386.

Bush ML, Jones RO, Given C. The value of CT venography in the diagnosis of jugular bulb diverticulum: a series of 3 cases. *Ear Nose Throat J.* 2009;88(4):4-7.

Koesling S, Kunkel P, Schul T. Vascular anomalies, sutures and small canals of the temporal bone on axial CT. *Eur J Radiol.* 2005;54:335-343.

CASE 23 Aberrant sigmoid sinus with a sigmoid sinus diverticulum

An aberrant sigmoid sinus courses more laterally or anteriorly relative to the typical course of the sigmoid sinus. It can also be associated with a superimposed focal vascular outpouching, or diverticulum, of the sigmoid sinus. If a surgeon is unaware of an aberrant course of the sigmoid sinus and/or a sigmoid sinus diverticulum, then inadvertent vascular breach of the sigmoid sinus may occur during surgery. A sigmoid sinus diverticulum can be associated with pulsatile tinnitus, especially if a superimposed osseous dehiscence is present. When symptomatic and not amenable to conservative management, a sigmoid sinus diverticulum can be treated surgically with a transmastoid reconstruction of the sinus.

COMPANION CASE

- **Aberrant sigmoid sinus with a dehiscent sigmoid sinus diverticulum.**

Aberrant sigmoid sinus with a sigmoid sinus diverticulum

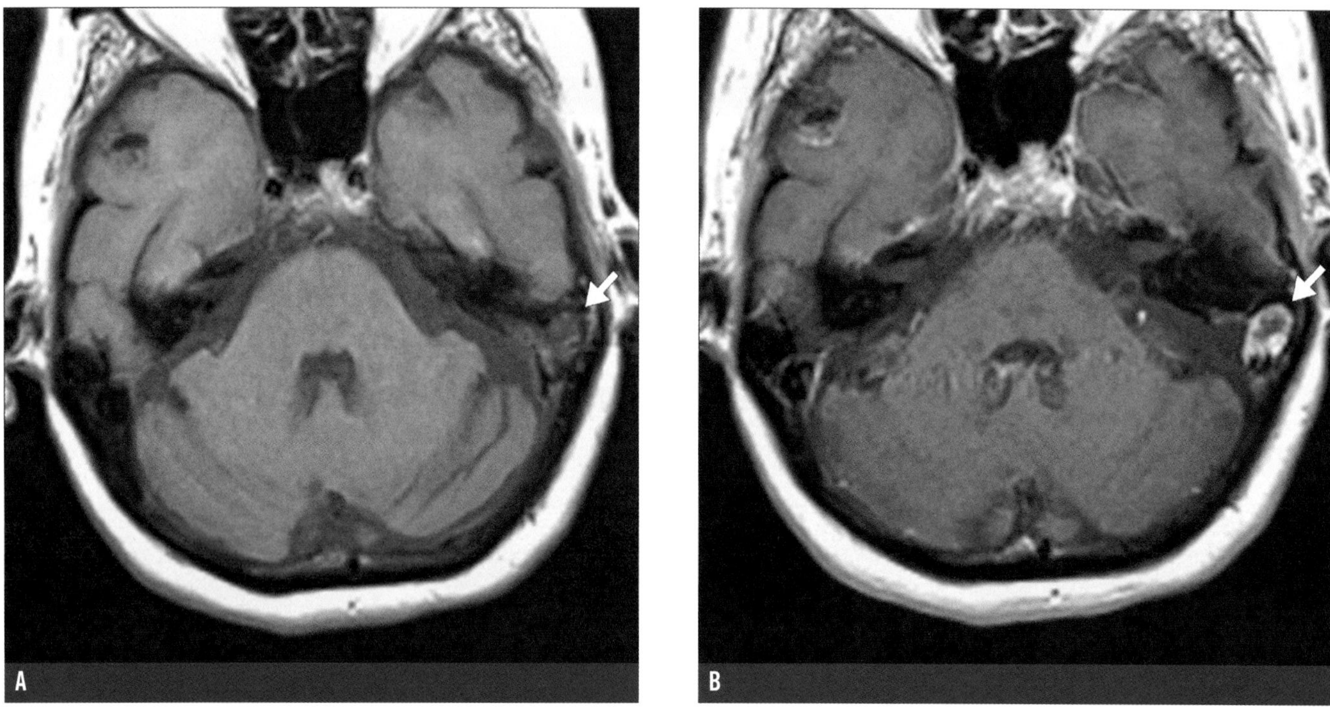

Axial T1 (**A**), postcontrast axial T1 (**B**), axial FLAIR (**C**), and coronal T2 (**D**) MR images demonstrate a lateral, aberrant course of the left sigmoid sinus with an associated left sigmoid sinus diverticulum (arrows, **A-D**). Elevated signal in the left sigmoid sinus on images **C** and **D** relates to flow dynamics, which can sometimes simulate a dural sinus thrombosis on MRI examinations of the brain.

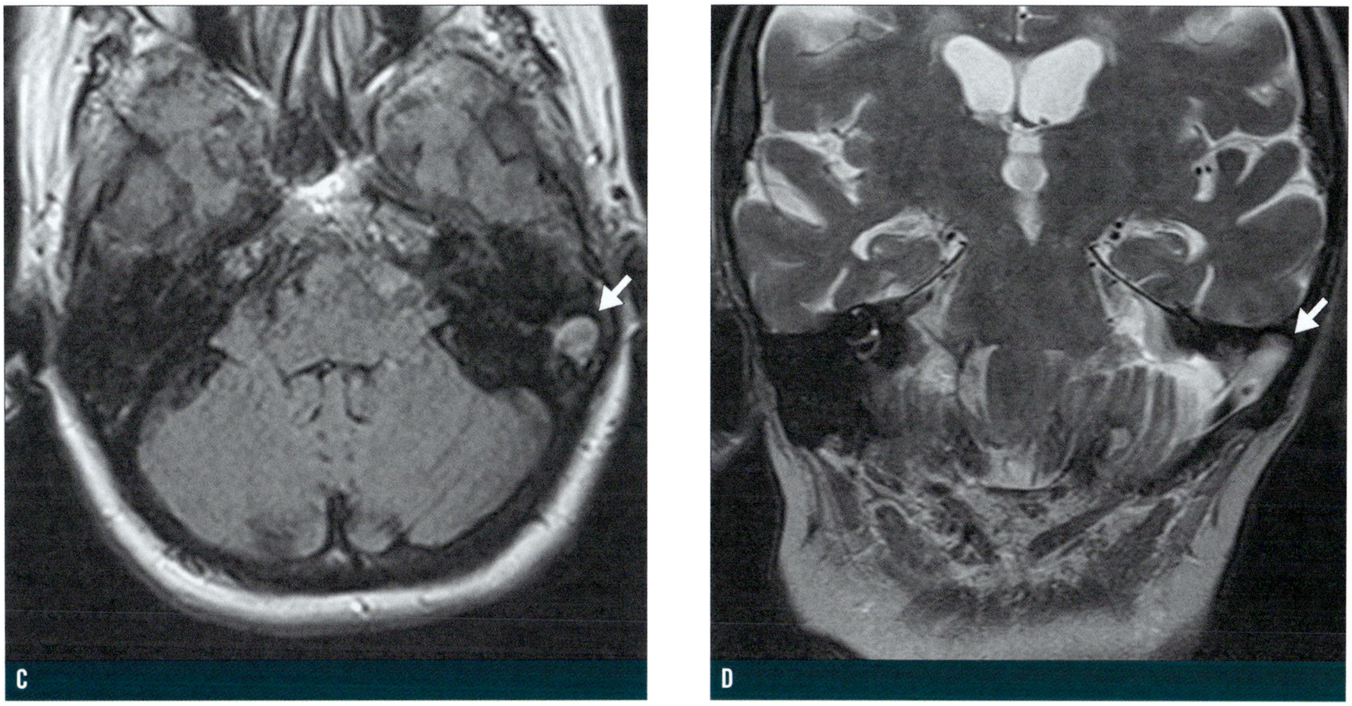

Companion case: Aberrant sigmoid sinus with a dehiscent sigmoid sinus diverticulum

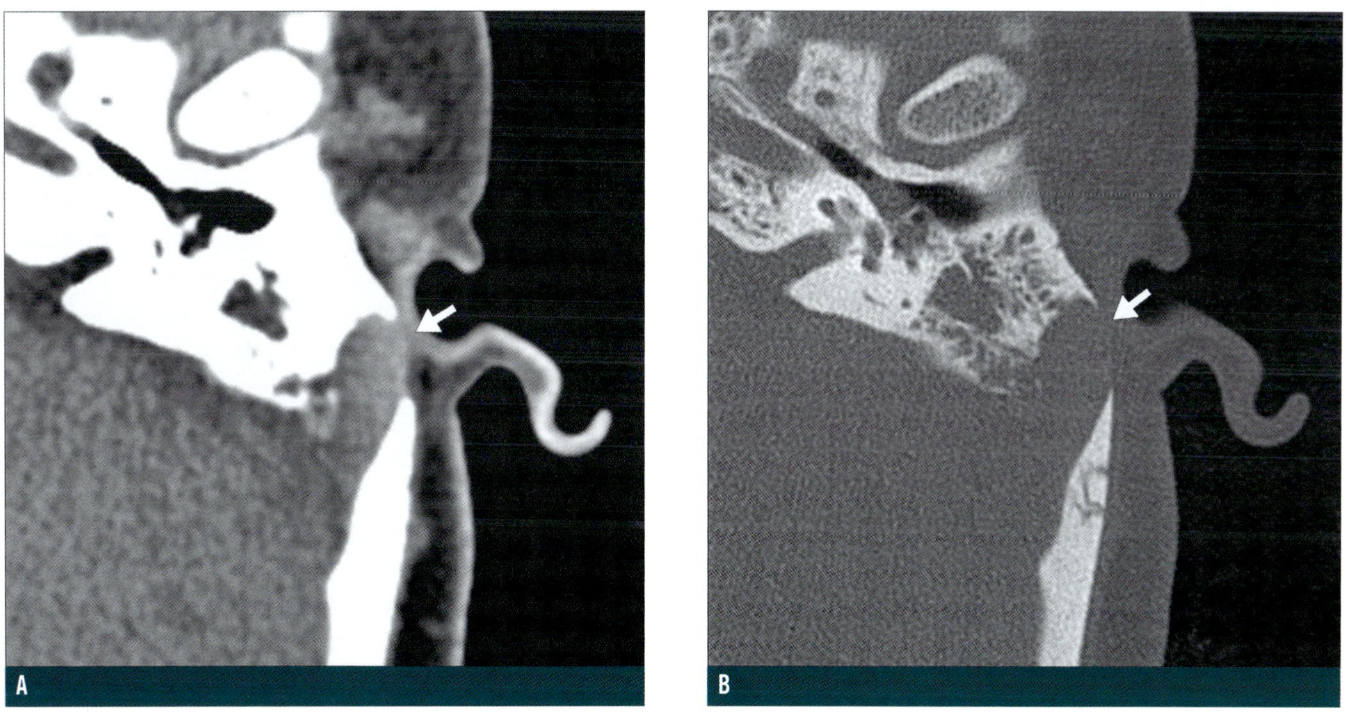

An unenhanced axial CT image viewed with a soft tissue window (**A**), an axial CT image viewed with a bone window (**B**), and an unenhanced coronal reformatted CT image viewed with a soft tissue window (**C**) demonstrate an aberrant, lateral course of the left sigmoid sinus with an associated diverticulum and focal osseous dehiscence (arrows, **A-C**). A coronal 2D TOF MRV source image (**D**) and an axial 3D TOF MRA source image (**E**) of the same patient also demonstrate a lateral course of the left sigmoid sinus associated with a sigmoid diverticulum (arrows, **D**, **E**).

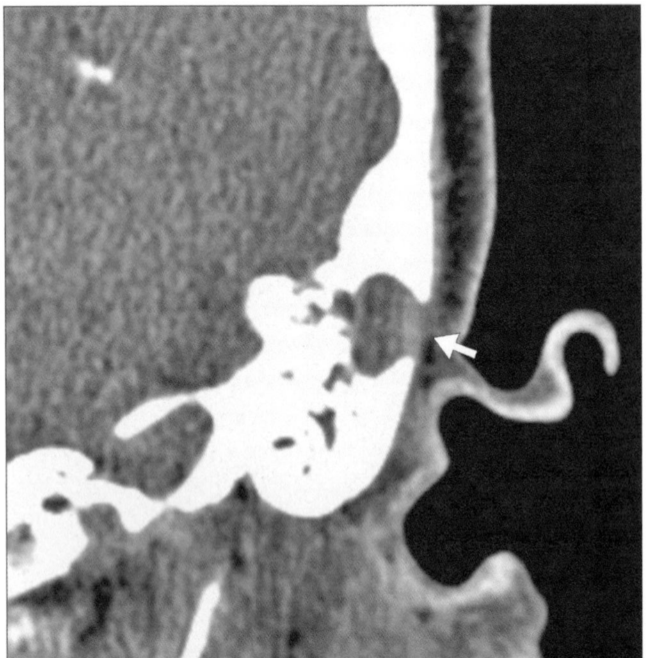

C

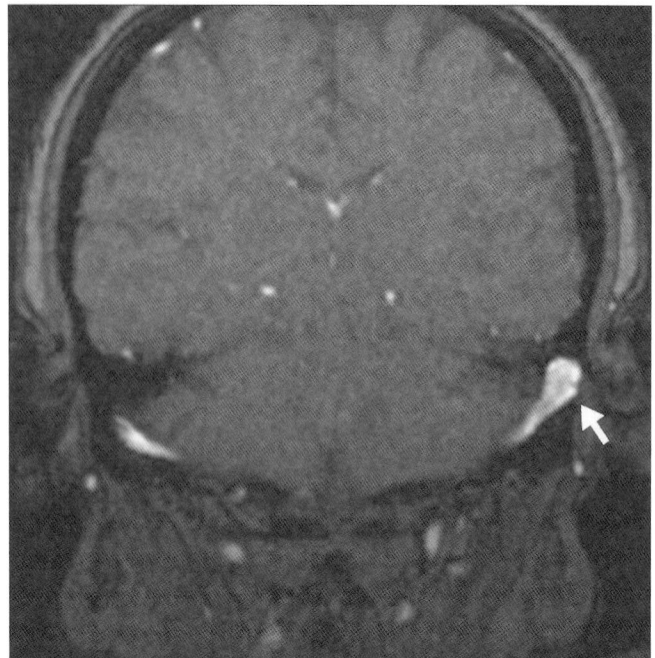

D

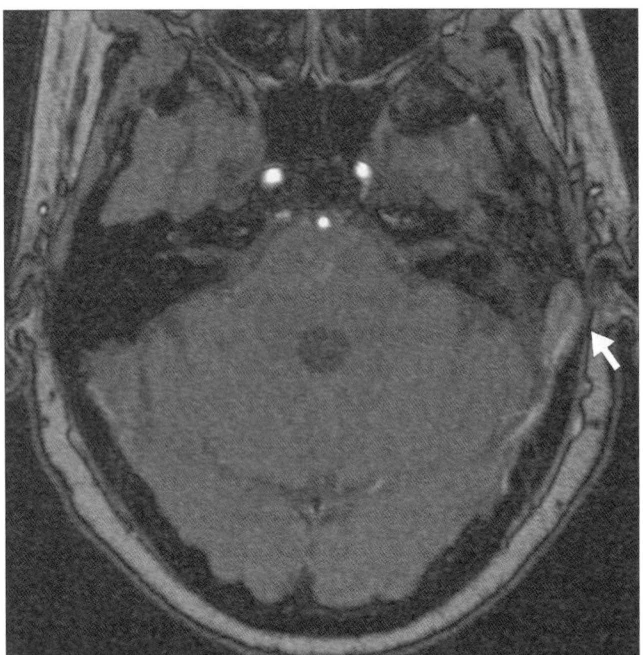

E

REFERENCES

Atilla S, Akpek S, Uslu S, Ilgit E, Isik S. Computed tomographic evaluation of surgically significant vascular variations related with the temporal bone. *Eur J Radiol.*1995;20:52-56.

Eisenman DJ. Sinus wall reconstruction for sigmoid sinus diverticulum and dehiscence: a standardized surgical procedure for a range of radiographic findings. *Otol Neurotol.* 2011;32(7):1116-1119.

Koesling S, Kunkel P, Schul T. Vascular anomalies, sutures and small canals of the temporal bone on axial CT. *Eur J Radiol.* 2005;54:335-343.

Otto KJ, Hudgins PA, Abdelkafy W, Mattox DE. Sigmoid sinus diverticulum: a new surgical approach to the correction of pulsatile tinnitus. *Otol Neurotol.* 2007;28(1):48-53.

CASE 24 Cochlear cleft

A cochlear cleft is identified as a discrete, punctate lucency in the otic capsule located immediately ventral to the oval window, typically best identified on axial CT temporal bone imaging. On coronal CT temporal bone imaging, it may manifest as a curvilinear lucency that parallels the basal turn of the cochlea. Although incidental and benign, the etiology of a cochlear cleft is unclear. The otic capsule has three layers: an outer periosteal layer, a middle or endochondral layer, and an inner endosteal layer. In the normal fetus, the endochondral layer is composed of small cartilaginous islands. Most of these cartilaginous islands undergo endochondral ossification. However, immediately ventral to the oval window, cartilage persists and fibrous tissue develops, resulting in a normal fibrocartilagenous structure termed the fissula ante fenestram. The typical fissula ante fenestram is not identified as a discrete lucency on CT temporal bone imaging. Instead, its location is inferred as a small region of dense osseous bone immediately ventral to the oval window that is of the same osseous density as the remainder of the otic capsule. It is likely that a cochlear cleft lucency represents a normal but lucent fissula ante fenestram or a residual nonossified cleft in the endochondral layer of the otic capsule. A cochlear cleft is more commonly identified in children than adults on CT. It has been reported to be present in up to 41% of children by Chadwell et al.

The significance of a cochlear cleft is not in identifying this benign finding on CT temporal bone imaging, but rather not misinterpreting this finding as fenestral otosclerosis. Indeed, the location of a cochlear cleft is the same as typical fenestral otosclerosis, located immediately ventral to the oval window. However, with a cochlear cleft, the finding on CT temporal bone imaging is discrete and punctate, rather than the ill-defined, usually larger lucency commonly identified with fenestral otosclerosis.

COMPANION CASES

- **Fenestral and retrofenestral otosclerosis.** Otosclerosis, also termed otospongiosis, is a bone disease that affects the endochondral layer of the otic capsule. It is of unknown etiology but there is evidence that it may be hereditary (autosomal dominant). Histologically, there is disordered bone resorption, new otospongiotic bone formation, vascular proliferation, and formation of connective tissue stroma. There are two patterns of otosclerosis, fenestral and retrofenestral (also called cochlear). Fenestral otosclerosis is significantly more common than the retrofenestral pattern. A fenestral component of otosclerosis is almost always present with retrofenestral otosclerosis. Thus, the current belief is that fenestral and retrofenestral otosclerosis represent a disease continuum. Fenestral otosclerosis is bilateral in approximately 80% of cases; therefore, it is imperative to scrutinize the contralateral temporal bone if otosclerosis is identified in one temporal bone. On CT temporal bone imaging, the fenestral form of otosclerosis appears as an ill-defined osseous lucency centered at the fissula ante fenestram, often extending to involve the oval window. Additionally, more advanced cases of fenestral otosclerosis can be associated with focally proliferative otospongiotic bone that encroaches upon the anterior crus of the stapes. This can result in poor visualization along the distal aspect of the anterior crus of the stapes on CT temporal bone imaging. Retrofenestral otosclerosis is typically a more extensive form of otosclerosis that results in a lucent halo surrounding the otic capsule, and again, almost always includes the fissula ante fenestram. Moreover, retrofenestral otosclerosis may involve and narrow the round and oval windows, resulting in significant functional compromise of these structures. With fenestral otosclerosis, patients often have a conductive hearing loss secondary to abnormal fixation of the stapes footplate. A mixed hearing loss (ie, conductive and sensorineural) is usually present with the retrofenestral variety. The sensorineural hearing loss in retrofenestral otosclerosis is believed to be the result of hyaline deposition within the spiral ligament.
- **Otosyphilis.** Otosyphilis can occur from either an acquired or congenital syphilis infection. Histologically, there is an endarteritis and a mononuclear infiltration, which result in diminished blood flow and necrosis. In the otic capsule, these findings manifest as osseous resorption. On CT temporal bone imaging, otosyphilis results in a permeative osseous lucency involving the otic capsule as well as the ossicles. The ossicular involvement helps differentiate otosyphilis from retrofenestral otosclerosis, which does not affect the ossicles. In addition, while the otic capsule lucency associated with otosyphilis can appear similar to retrofenestral otosclerosis, the lucency with syphilis is more ill-defined and permeative. Finally, the otospongiotic bone that accumulates at the fissula ante fenestram and occasionally along the ventral crus of the stapes with otosclerosis is not present with otosyphilis. Symptoms of otosyphilis include bilateral sensorineural hearing loss, tinnitus, and vertigo.

Cochlear cleft

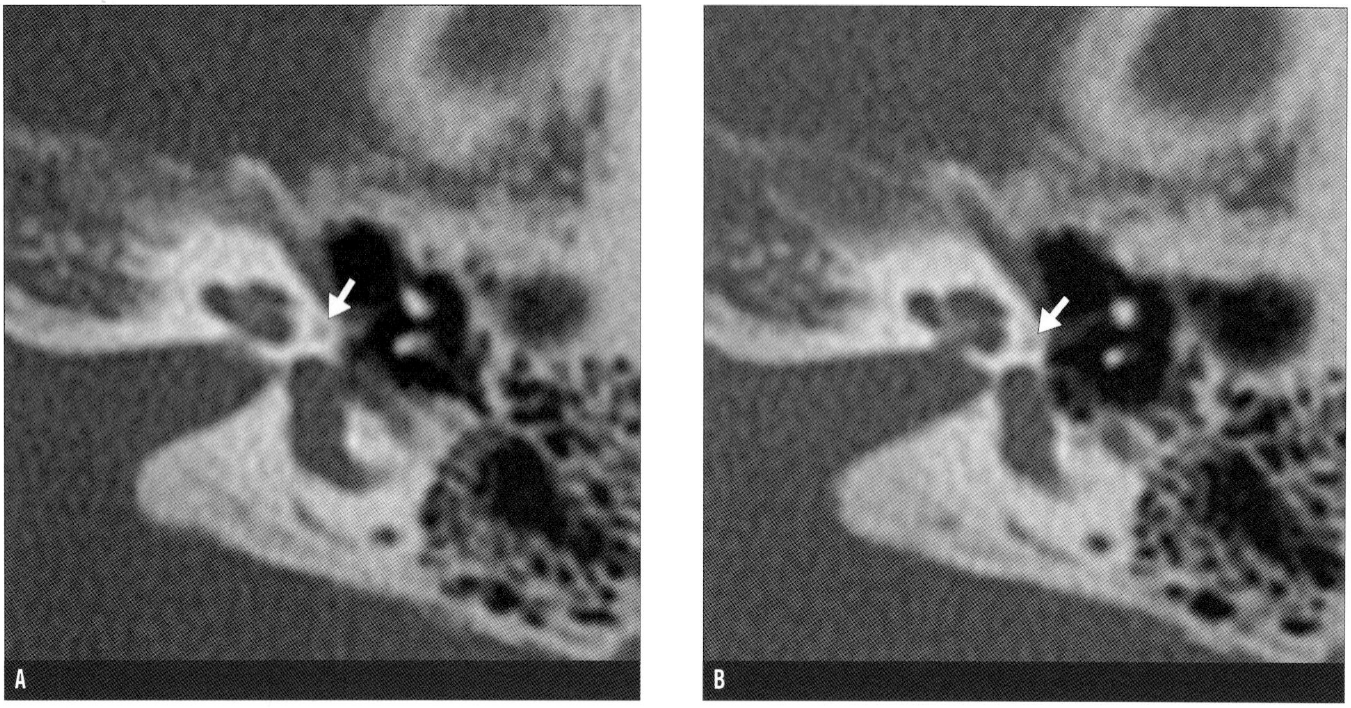

Axial CT images of the left temporal bone (**A**, **B**) demonstrate a discrete, punctate lucency in the fissula ante fenestram (arrows, **A**, **B**). The lucency is more discrete and defined than typically present with fenestral otosclerosis. Additionally, the lucency does not extend to the oval window, a finding that is often present with fenestral otosclerosis.

Companion case: Fenestral otosclerosis

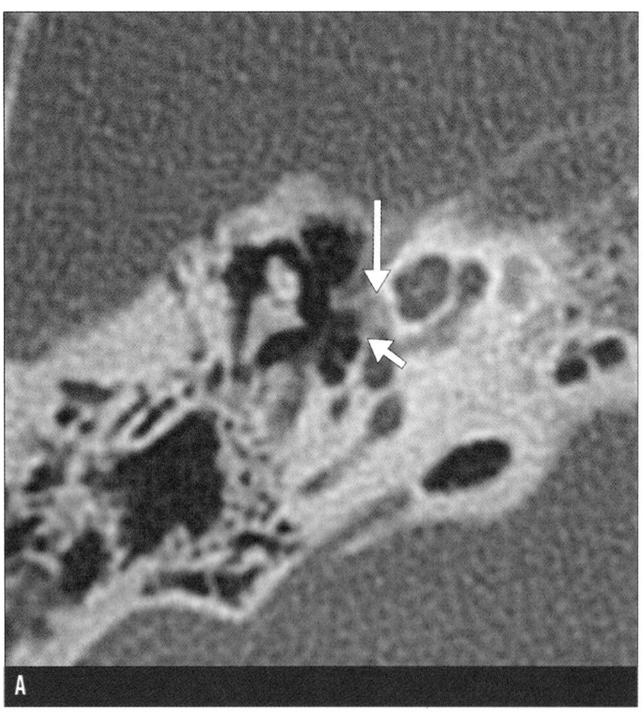

An axial CT image of the right temporal bone (**A**) demonstrates an ill-defined lucency involving the fissula ante fenestram (long arrow), significantly larger and more ill-defined compared to the punctate and discrete lucency identified with a cochlear cleft. A subtle amount of otospongiotic bone is demonstrated along the anterior crus of the stapes (short arrow), further differentiating this entity from a cochlear cleft.

Companion case: Retrofenestral otosclerosis

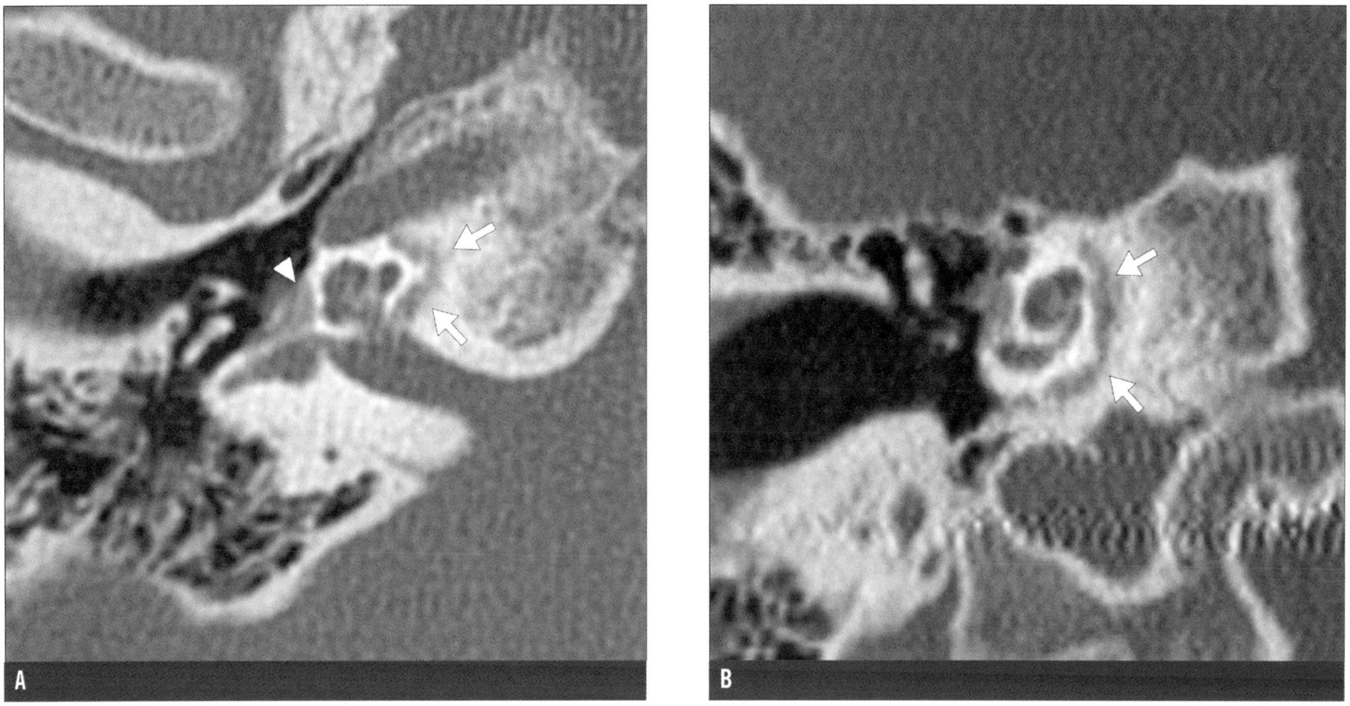

Axial (**A**) and coronal reformatted (**B**) CT images of the right temporal bone demonstrate abnormal osseous lucency involving the otic capsule surrounding the cochlea, compatible with retrofenestral (also called cochlear) otosclerosis (arrows, **A**, **B**). There is also involvement of the fissula ante fenestram (arrowhead, **A**).

Companion case: Otosyphilis

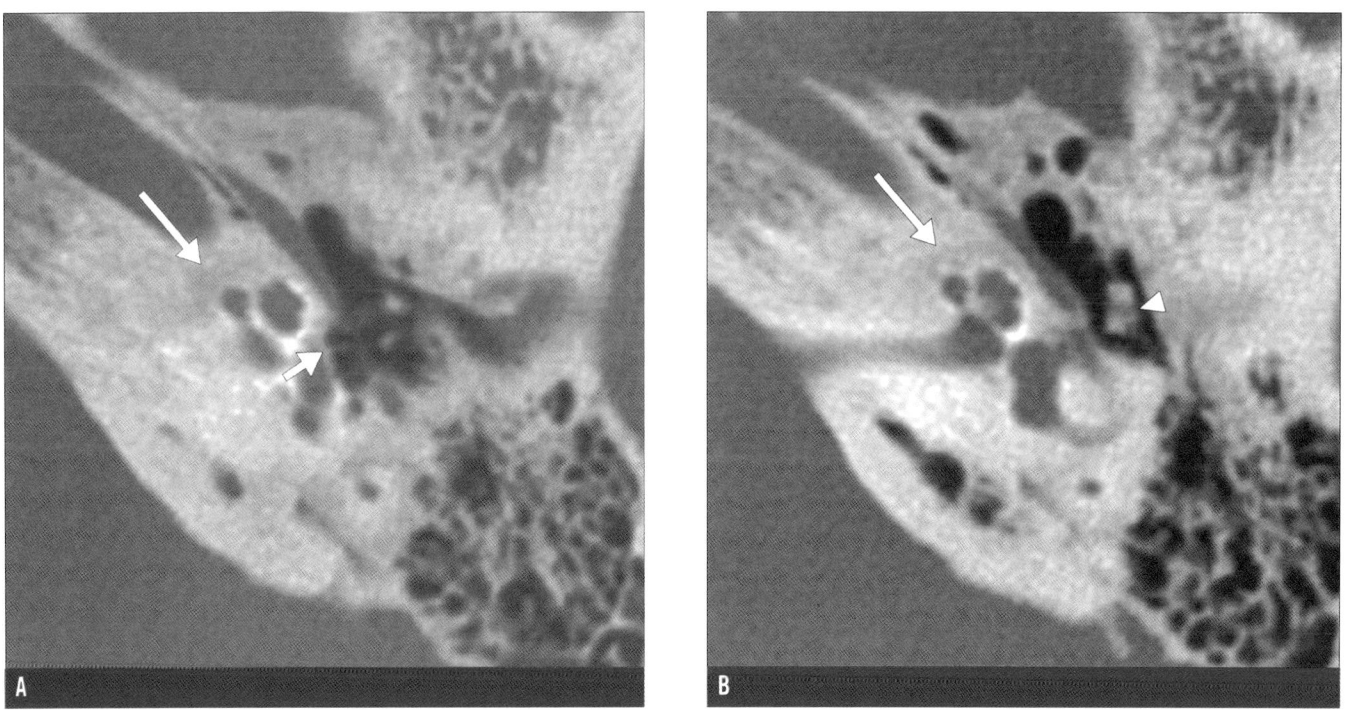

Axial CT images of the left temporal bone (**A**-**C**) demonstrate an abnormal, permeative lucency within the majority of the otic capsule (long arrows, **A**-**C**). While the pattern is similar to retrofenestral otosclerosis, the lucency is more ill-defined, a finding typical of otosyphilis. There is also subtle, abnormal ossicular lucency within the body of the incus (arrowhead, **B**) and the head of the malleus (arrowhead, **C**). Ossicular lucency is often seen with otosyphilis but is not a feature of otosclerosis. Furthermore, while there is lucency at the fissula ante fenestram, there is lack of otospongiotic bone accumulation along the anterior crus of the stapes (short arrow, **A**), a finding that may be present with otosclerosis. *Case courtesy of Barbara Zeifer, MD.*

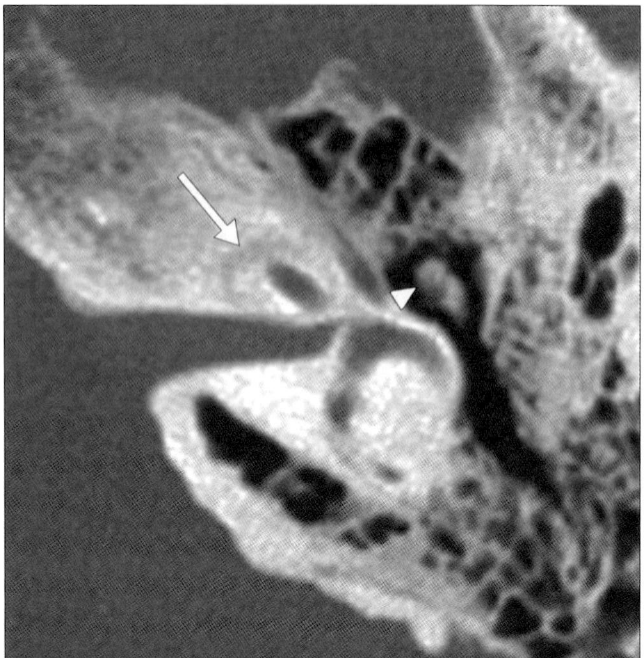

C

REFERENCES

Chadwell JB, Halsted MJ, Choo DI, Greinwald JH, Benton C. The cochlear cleft. *Am J Neuroradio.* 2004;25:21-24.

Lee TC, Aviv RI, Chen JM, Nedzelski JM, Fox AJ, Symons SP. CT grading of otosclerosis. *Am J Neuroradiol.* 2009;30:1435-1439.

Quesnel AM, et al. Correlation of computed tomography with histopathology in otosclerosis. *Otol Neurotol.* 2013;34(1):22-28.

Sonne JE, Zeifer B, Linstrom C. Manifestations of otosyphilis as visualized with computed tomography. *Otol Neurotol.* 2002;23(5):806-807.

Vincente Ade O, Yamashita HK, Albernaz PL, Penido Nde O. Computed tomography in the diagnosis of otosclerosis. *Otolaryngol Head Neck Surg.* 2006;134(40):685-692.

Yimate K, Srirompotong S, Lertsukprasert K. Otosyphilis: a review of 85 cases. *Otolaryngol Head Neck Surg.* 2007;136(1):67-71.

CASE 25 Apparent abnormal inner ear signal on 5-mm T2-weighted MR imaging

The inner ear structures—which include the cochlea, vestibule, and semicircular canals—have both osseous and membranous components. The osseous labyrinth represents the bony portion of the inner ear and is best imaged with CT. The membranous labyrinth resides deep to the osseous labyrinth and contains endolymph. Interposed between the membranous labyrinth and the osseous labyrinth is perilymph. By MRI, the perilymph and endolymph are isointense to CSF on T1- and T2-weighted imaging and are nonenhancing. With dedicated 3-mm T2-weighed MR imaging, the fluid within the cochlea, semicircular canals, and vestibule should be identified in its entirety. However, routine MRI brain examinations are typically performed with 5-mm slice thickness, which can lead to incomplete visualization of the inner ear fluid and volume averaging with the adjacent bone. This volume averaging appears as T2 signal loss within the inner ear and can simulate pathology, such as labyrinthitis ossificans. Thus, an MRI diagnosis of labyrinthitis ossificans should only be made with dedicated 3-mm or thinner T2-weighted imaging or CISS imaging.

COMPANION CASE

- **Labyrinthitis ossificans**. Labyrinthitis (or labyrinthine) ossificans represents an abnormal ossification of the membranous labyrinth. This is the result of a paradoxical healing response that may occur following acute labyrinthitis, inner ear hemorrhage, or because of a tumor. The imaging findings of labyrinthitis ossificans include abnormal bone deposition within the inner ear on CT and loss of the normal inner ear signal on all MRI pulse sequences, best appreciated on thin (3 mm or less) T2-weighted imaging or CISS imaging. The lateral semicircular canal and the basal turn of the cochlea are the two most commonly affected structures with labyrinthitis ossificans. Typically, there is deposition of fibrous tissue prior to ossification of the membranous labyrinth. Studies have demonstrated that MRI may be more sensitive than CT to detect this early fibrotic stage, since fibrous tissue in the membranous labyrinth would be occult on CT but would result in the loss of normal T2 hyperintense signal on MRI. Additionally, MRI may demonstrate patchy enhancement during this fibrotic stage. It is important to determine the location of labyrinthitis ossificans prior to cochlear implantation. Specifically, labyrinthitis ossificans affecting the cochlea may result in difficulty with a traditional cochlear implant approach and require drilling into the cochlea, whereas labyrinthitis ossificans isolated to the vestibule typically does not impair cochlear implant placement.

Apparent abnormal inner ear signal on 5-mm T2-weighted MR imaging

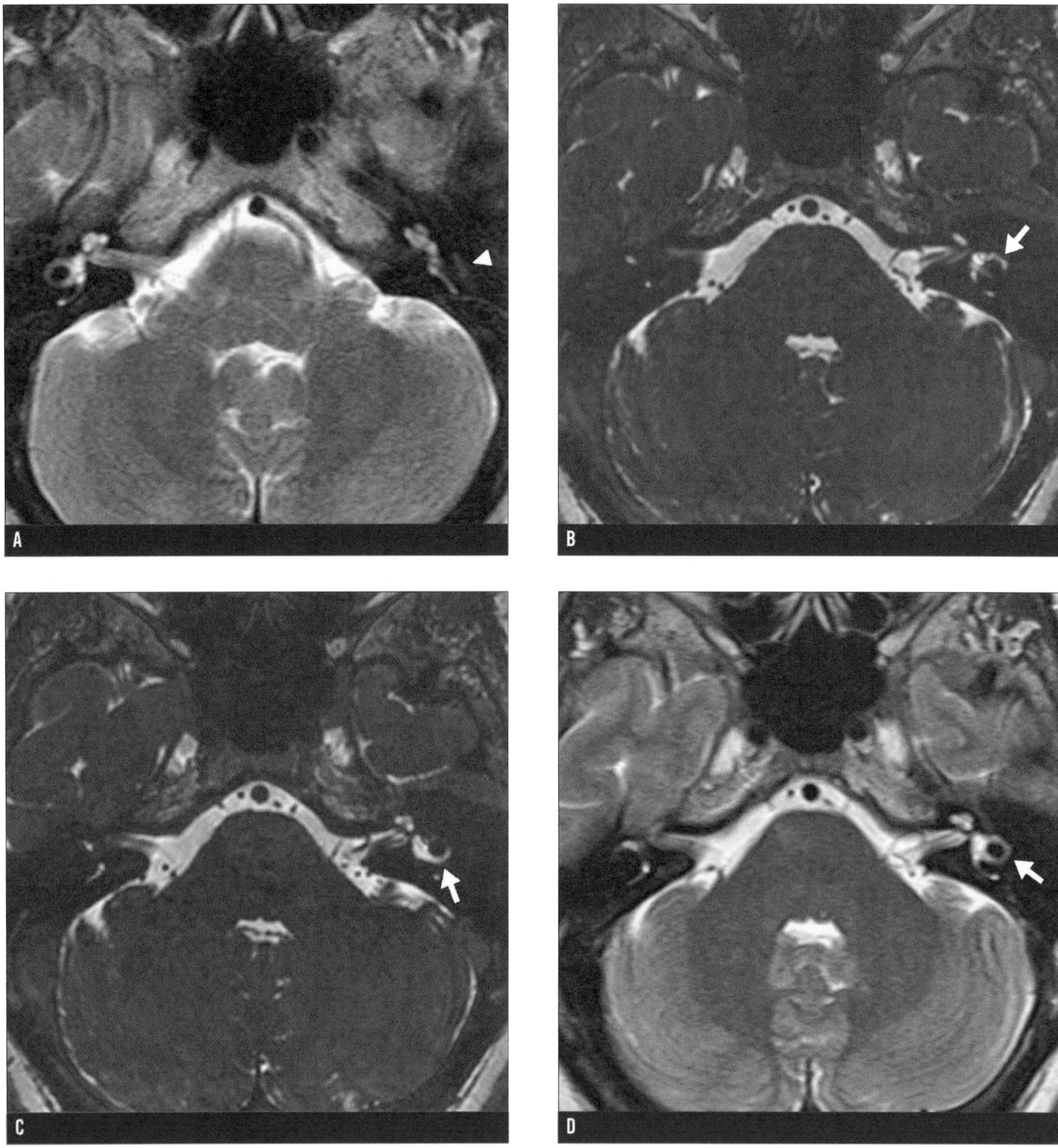

A 5-mm axial T2-weighted MR image of the temporal bones (**A**) demonstrates apparent loss of T2 hyperintense signal in the left lateral semicircular canal (arrowhead, **A**). 1-mm axial CISS (**B**, **C**) and 3-mm axial T2 (**D**) MR images of the left temporal bone from the same patient demonstrate normal T2 hyperintense signal in the left lateral semicircular canal (arrows, **B**-**D**). This case illustrates that the apparent loss of T2 hyperintense signal within the inner ear on 5 mm T2-weighted images can be a technical finding and is related to volume averaging with adjacent bone. It is common to not visualize the entire inner ear fluid signal on T2-weighted MR images obtained with a 5-mm slice thickness, but the entire inner ear fluid signal should be visualized on T2-weighted MR images obtained with 3-mm or thinner slice thickness, assuming the images are free of artifact.

Companion case: Labyrinthitis ossificans

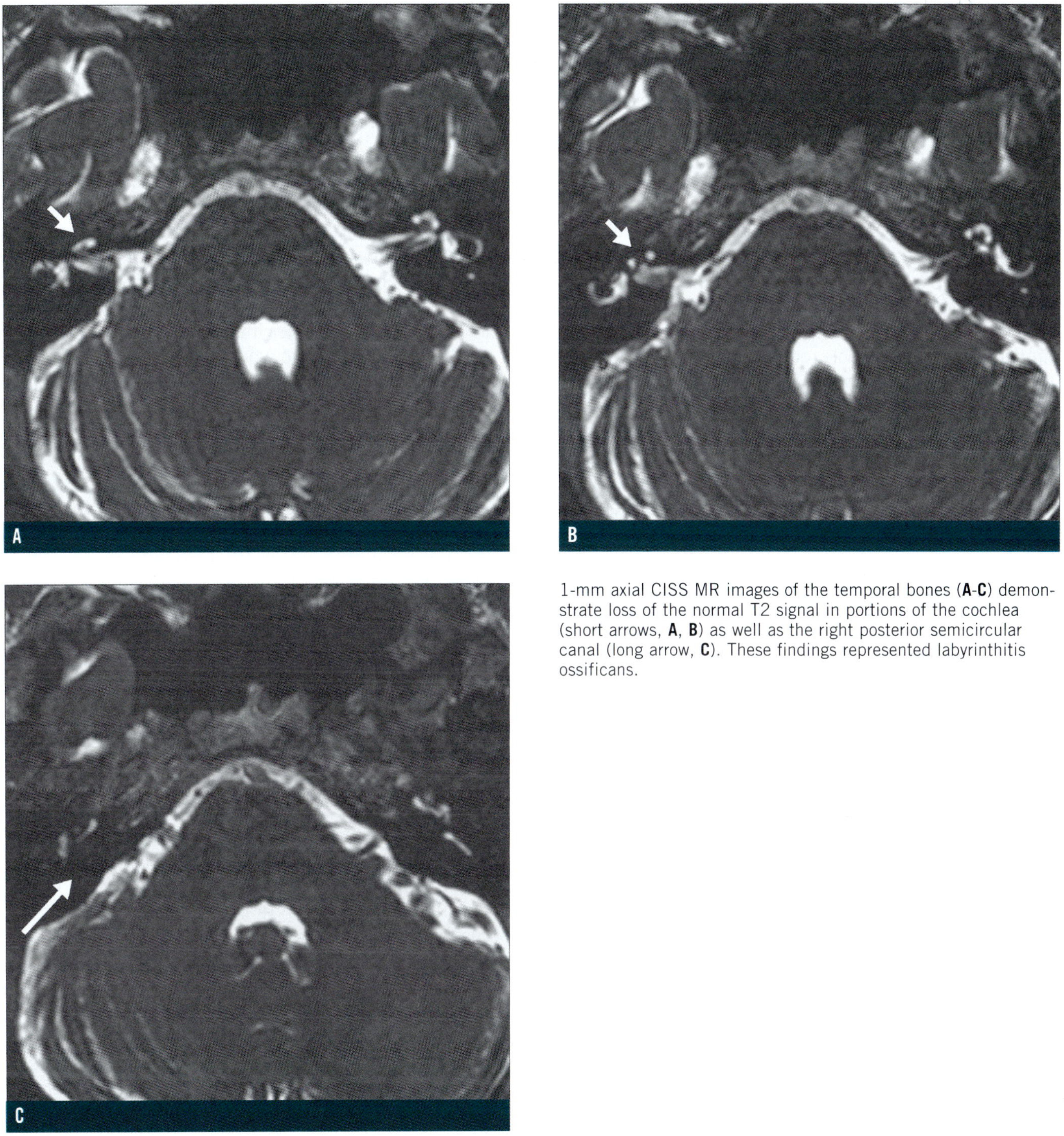

1-mm axial CISS MR images of the temporal bones (**A**-**C**) demonstrate loss of the normal T2 signal in portions of the cochlea (short arrows, **A**, **B**) as well as the right posterior semicircular canal (long arrow, **C**). These findings represented labyrinthitis ossificans.

REFERENCES

Abdullah A, Mahmud MR, Maimunah A, Zulfiqar MA, Saim L, Mazlan R. Preoperative high resolution CT and MR imaging in cochlear implantation. *Ann Acad Med Singapore*. 2003;32(4):442-445.

Chan CC, Saunders DE, Chong WK, Hartley BE, Raglan E, Rajput K. Advancement in post-meningitic lateral semicircular canal labyrinthitis ossificans. *J Laryngol Otol*. 2007;121(2):105-109.

Isaacson B, Booth T, Kurtz JW Jr, Lee KH, Roland PS. Labyrinthitis ossificans: how accurate is MRI in predicting cochlear obstruction? *Otolaryngol Head Neck Surg*. 2009;140(5):692-696.

CASE 26 Intratympanic steroid injection

An intratympanic injection (ie, injection into the middle ear) of dexamethasone may be performed to treat sudden sensorineural hearing loss or Ménière disease. Additionally, intratympanic dexamethasone has been utilized to treat acoustic trauma in an effort to reduce cochlear hair cell loss. The steroid administration can be performed in the office by either a single injection or by a continuous infusion of steroid over several days via a microcatheter placed in the round window niche. During the injection, the patient is asked to tilt their head 45° toward the unaffected ear. The steroid injected into the middle ear diffuses through the semipermeable round window membrane into the scala tympani perilymph. The steroid concentration in the inner ear with this technique is far greater compared to when steroids are administered systemically. Following an intratympanic steroid injection, MR imaging demonstrates abnormally hyperintense signal within the cochlea on precontrast T1-weighted and FLAIR sequences, potentially simulating inner ear pathology such as acute hemorrhage and proteinaceous debris. Therefore, it is imperative for the radiologist to be aware of a recent intratympanic steroid injection in order to avoid misinterpreting the MRI findings. There is usually no significant enhancement or abnormal signal within the inner on T2-weighted MR imaging following an intratympanic steroid injection.

COMPANION CASES

- **Intralabyrinthine hemorrhage.** Inner ear hemorrhage may result from several causes, including leukemia, sickle cell disease, treatment effect, tumor (eg, endolymphatic sac tumor), or trauma. Acute hemorrhage in the inner ear will be occult by CT. By MRI, acute hemorrhage in the inner ear will be intrinsically T1 shortened, elevated in signal on FLAIR, and nonenhancing. A discrete abnormality will usually not be identified on T2-weighted imaging. Profound hearing loss and vertigo are often present with intralabyrinthine hemorrhage.
- **Acute labyrinthitis.** Acute labyrinthitis represents an acute inflammation of the inner ear. There are numerous causes of acute labyrinthitis, including hematogenic (viral), tympanogenic (acute or chronic otomastoiditis), meningogenic, traumatic, or postsurgical. The hematogenic and meningogenic causes usually result in bilateral acute labyrinthitis, whereas the other causes usually result in unilateral acute labyrinthitis. Symptoms of acute labyrinthitis include sudden hearing loss, tinnitus, and vertigo.

  Acute labyrinthitis is occult on CT. On MRI, proteinaceous debris in the inner ear manifests as mildly elevated precontrast T1 signal and pronounced elevated FLAIR signal. Enhancement throughout the inner ear is the hallmark imaging finding of acute labyrinthitis, although this can be isolated to either the cochlea or vestibule, in which case the finding may be more specifically termed an acute cochleitis and vestibulitis, respectively. Importantly, there is no focal abnormality of the inner ear signal on T2-weighted MR imaging with acute labyrinthitis. This is in contradistinction to an intralabyrinthine schwannoma, which is associated with focal hypointense signal on thin section T2-weighted imaging and focal, rather than diffuse, enhancement. If there is still doubt as to whether the finding represents acute labyrinthitis or another entity, such as an intralabyrinthine schwannoma, then a follow-up MRI study is often helpful; the degree of enhancement will decrease with an uncomplicated acute labyrinthitis but will persist with an intralabyrinthine schwannoma.

  Occasionally, an acute labyrinthitis will develop into labyrinthitis ossificans because of a paradoxical healing response that results in fibroosseous deposition within the inner ear. Therefore, follow-up MR imaging in this setting may demonstrate resolved or resolving enhancement on postcontrast T1-weighted imaging as well as focal hypointense signal within the inner ear on T2-weighted or CISS imaging. On CT, labyrinthitis ossificans that progresses from the fibrous phase to the osseous phase will manifest as foci of mineralization within the inner ear structures.
- **Intralabyrinthine schwannoma.** An intralabyrinthine schwannoma (ILS) is a benign nerve sheath tumor of the inner ear. An ILS may occur in various locations within the labyrinth, including intracochlear, intravestibular, transmodiolar (traversing the modiolus of the cochlea), transmacular (traversing the macula of the vestibule), vestibulocochlear (involving the vestibule and cochlea), and transotic (traversing from the internal auditory canal through the inner ear and into the middle ear). The most common symptom of an ILS is hearing loss, although tinnitus, imbalance, and vertigo may also occur. Unless the lesions are large and result in osseous remodeling, an ILS will be occult by CT. On MRI, these lesions are usually focally enhancing and focally hypointense on T2, a combination of findings that are not present with acute labyrinthitis, intralabyrinthine hemorrhage, or following an intratympanic steroid injection. Elevated FLAIR signal and mildly elevated intrinsic T1 signal may also be present with an ILS, presumably because of proteinaceous debris. Hearing preservation surgery is not an option with an ILS. Therefore, most of these lesions are managed conservatively with observation and serial MR imaging.

Intratympanic steroid injection

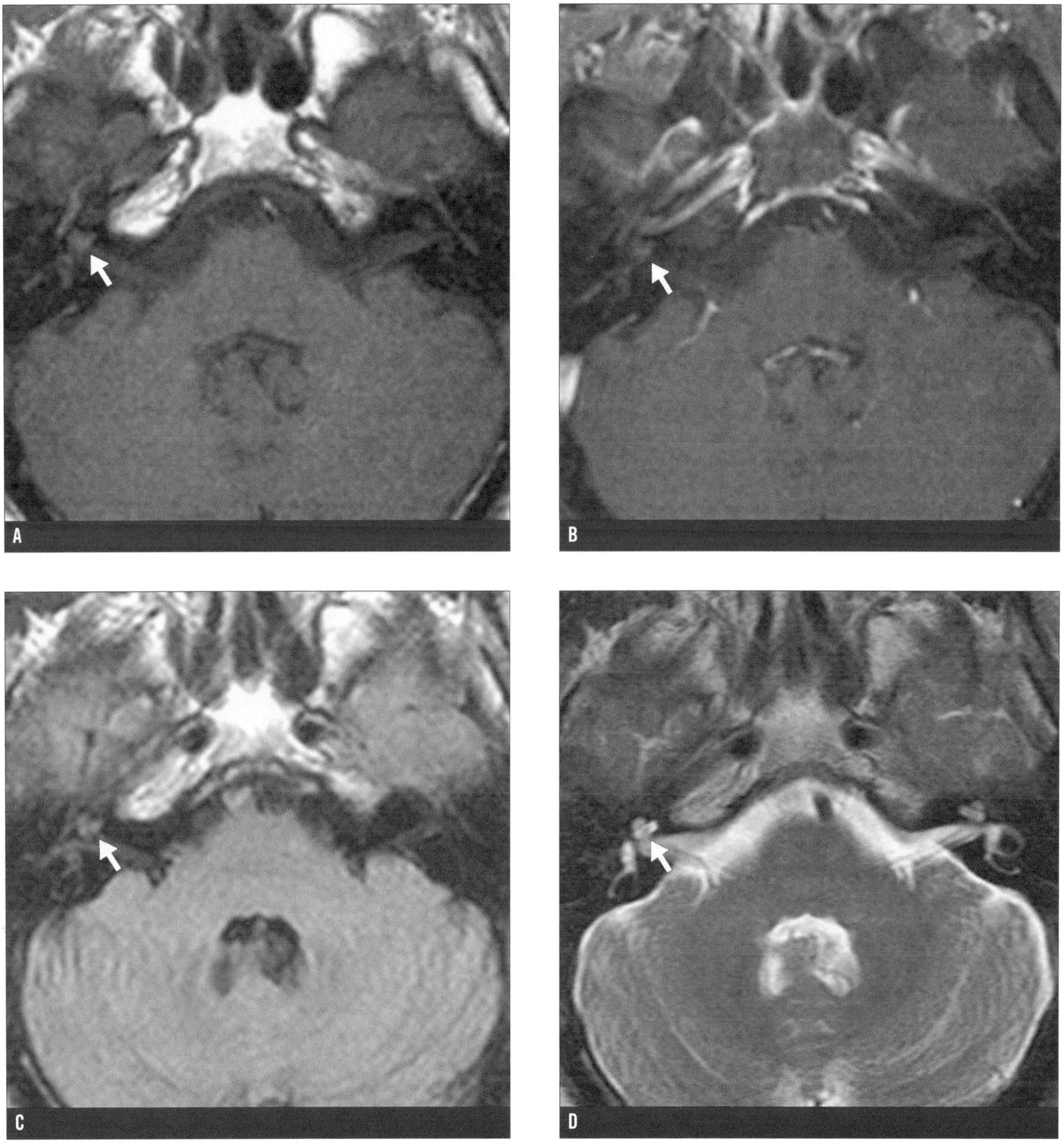

Axial T1 (**A**), fat-suppressed postcontrast axial T1 (**B**), axial FLAIR (**C**), and axial T2 (**D**) MR images of the temporal bones of a patient with a history of sudden sensorineural hearing loss. Image **A** demonstrates subtle intrinsic T1 signal within the right cochlea (arrow, **A**) and image **C** demonstrates elevated FLAIR signal within the right cochlea (arrow, **C**). Relative to precontrast imaging, there is no enhancement within the right cochlea (arrow, **B**) and there is also no abnormal T2 signal within the right cochlea (arrow, **D**). This patient had a history of a right intratympanic steroid injection accounting for the findings. However, acute hemorrhage or abnormal proteinaceous debris in the inner ear can have the same imaging appearance.

Companion case: Intralabyrinthine hemorrhage

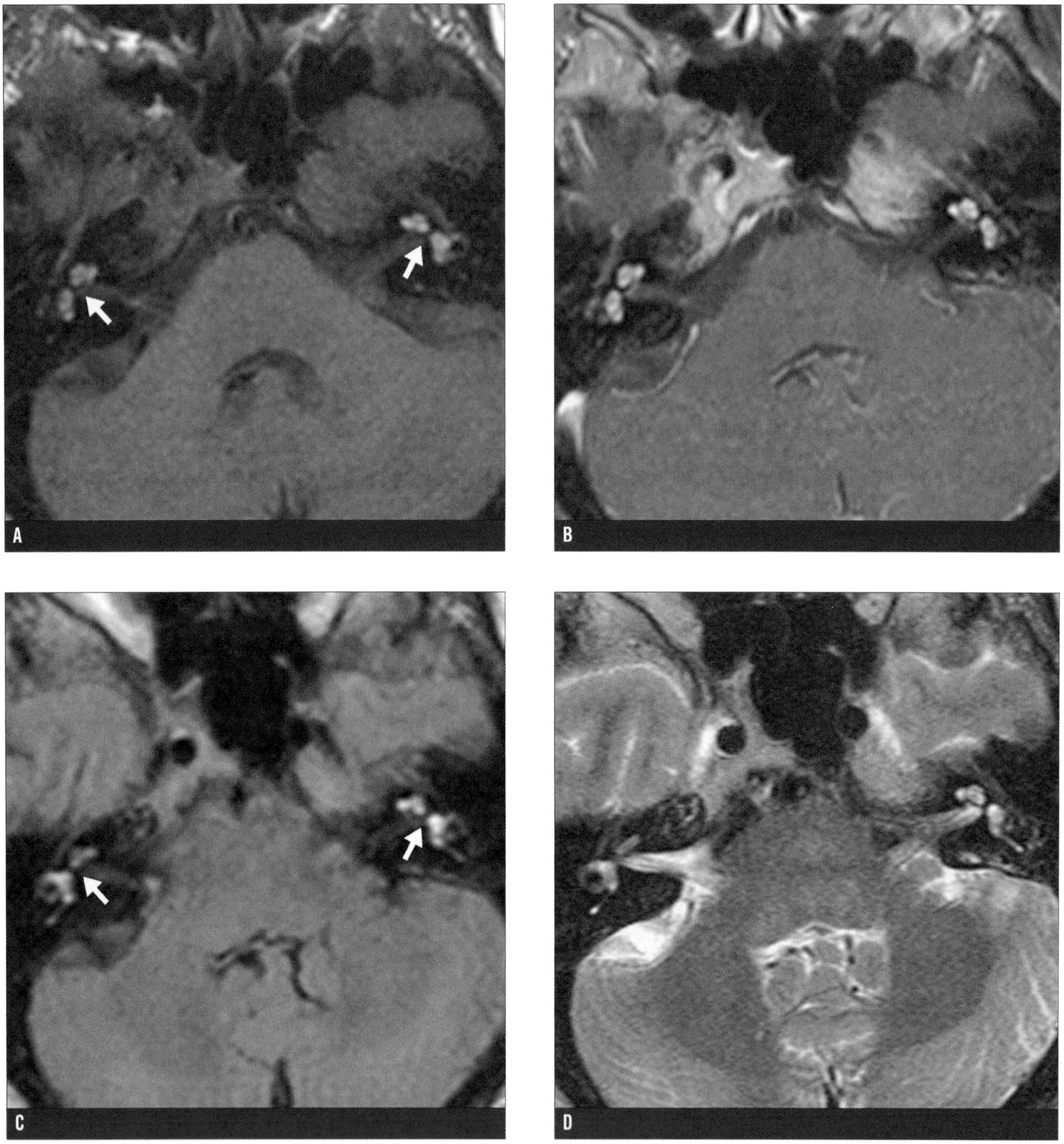

Axial T1 (**A**), fat-suppressed postcontrast axial T1 (**B**), axial FLAIR (**C**), and axial T2 (**D**) MR images of the temporal bones of a patient with a history of sudden sensorineural hearing loss, ataxia, and leukemia demonstrate extensive abnormal intrinsic T1 signal (arrows, **A**) and hyperintense FLAIR signal (arrows, **C**) within the inner ears, compatible with intralabyrinthine hemorrhage. Relative to precontrast imaging, there is no overt enhancement (**B**) and there is no focal abnormal signal on T2-weighted imaging (**D**) within either inner ear. Unenhanced axial T1-weighted images obtained 2 months later (**E, F**) demonstrate near resolution of the intralabyrinthine hemorrhage, with only a small amount of residual hemorrhage within the right inner ear (arrows, **E, F**).

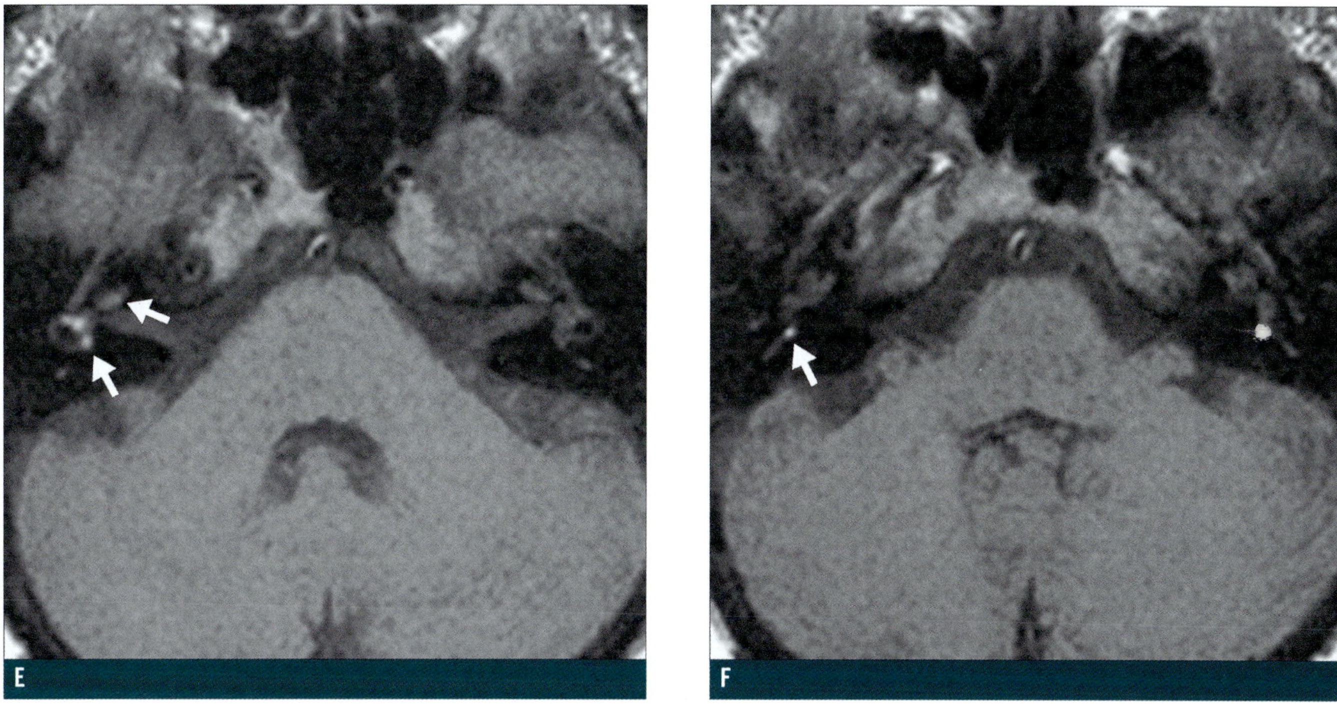

Companion case: Acute labyrinthitis

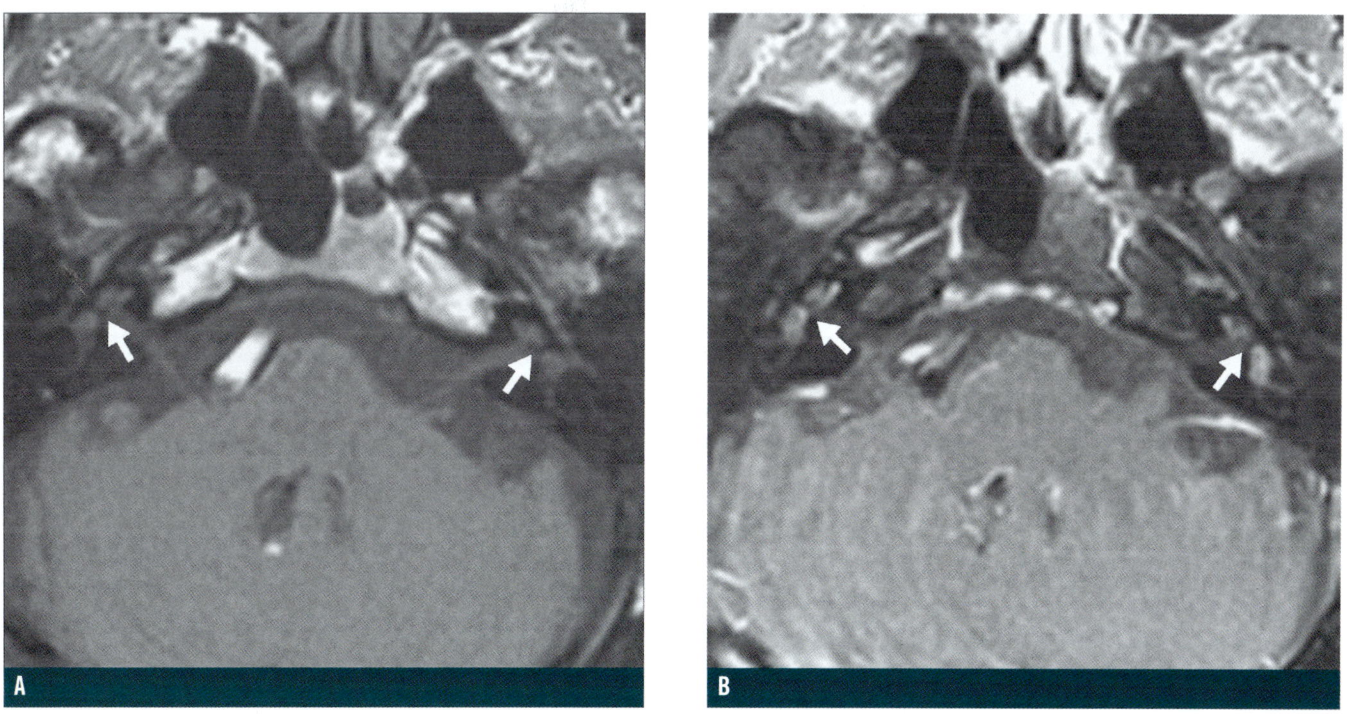

Axial T1 (**A**), fat-suppressed postcontrast axial T1 (**B**), axial FLAIR (**C**), and axial T2 (**D**) MR images of the temporal bones. Image **A** demonstrates only minimal intrinsic T1 signal in the inner ears (arrows, **A**). However, there is enhancement (arrows, **B**) and elevated FLAIR signal (arrows, **C**) in the inner ears. The inner ear T2 signal on image **D** is unremarkable. The findings are compatible with bilateral acute labyrinthitis. The lack of focal hypointense T2 signal in the inner ears aids in differentiating acute labyrinthitis from inner ear schwannomas.

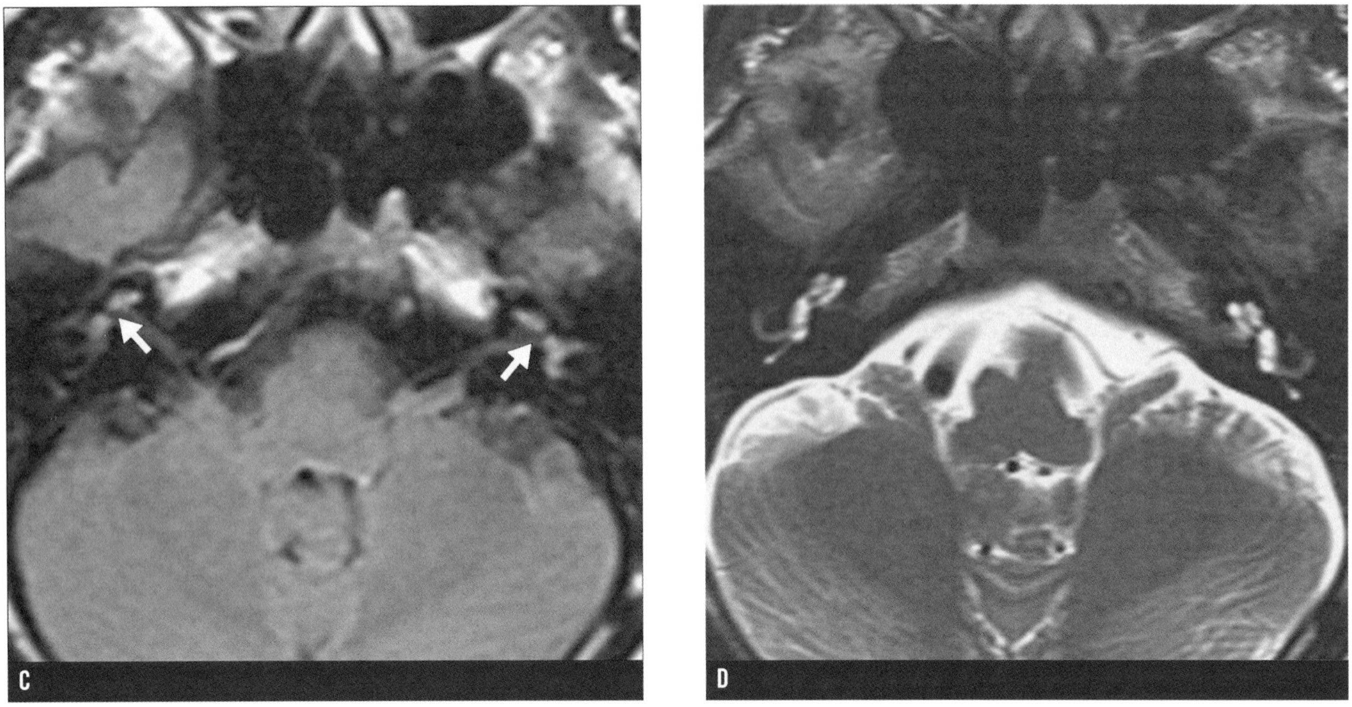

Companion case: Intralabyrinthine schwannoma

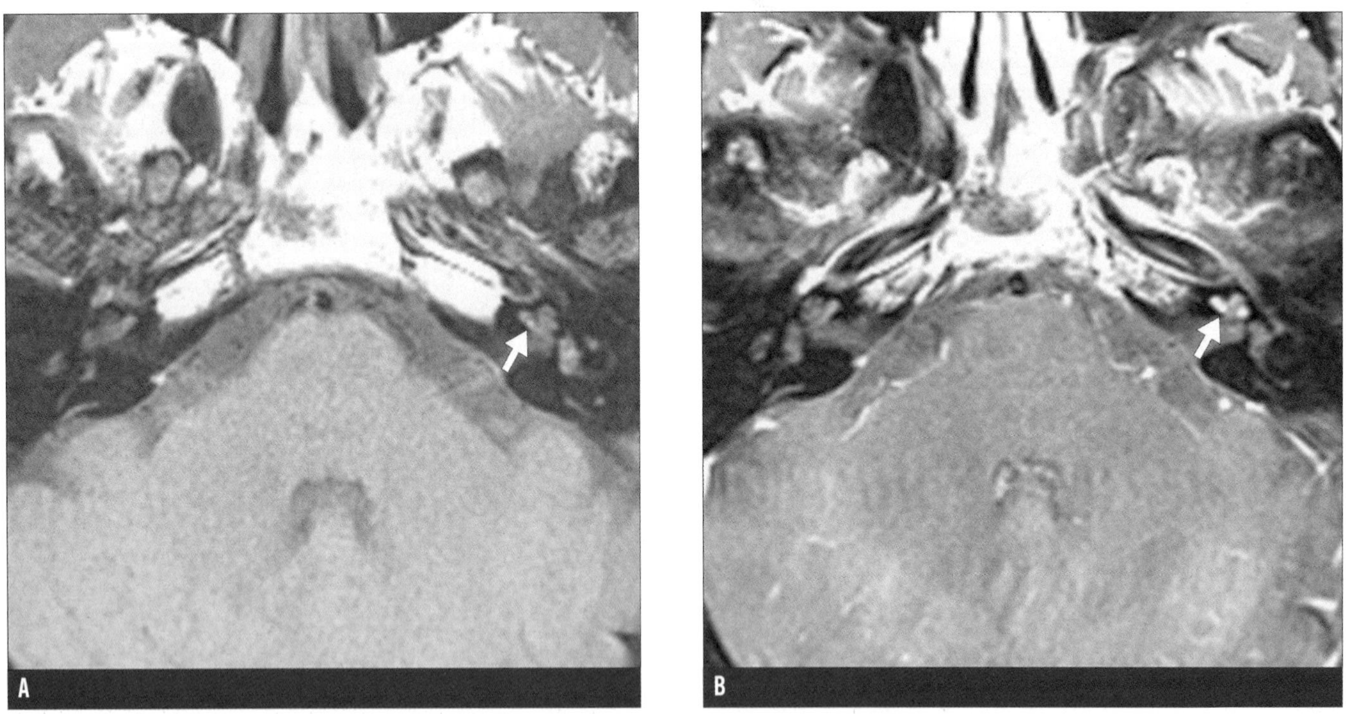

Axial T1 (**A**), fat-suppressed postcontrast axial T1 (**B**), axial FLAIR (**C**), and axial T2 (**D**) MR images of the temporal bones. There is minimal, if any, intrinsic T1 signal in the left cochlea (arrow, **A**) but there is pronounced enhancement (arrow, **B**) and elevated FLAIR signal (arrow, **C**). Additionally, there is focal hypointense T2 signal in the left cochlea (arrow, **D**). These findings are compatible with an intralabyrinthine schwannoma (ILS). The presence of enhancement and focal hypointense T2 signal differentiates an ILS from an intratympanic steroid injection, which does not have these imaging characteristics. Moreover, the focal hypointense T2 signal abnormality helps differentiate an ILS from an acute labyrinthitis, which is not a feature of acute labyrinthitis. However, if there is still doubt as to whether the finding represents an ILS or acute labyrinthitis, then follow-up imaging will reveal persistent enhancement with the former but improved or resolved enhancement with the latter.

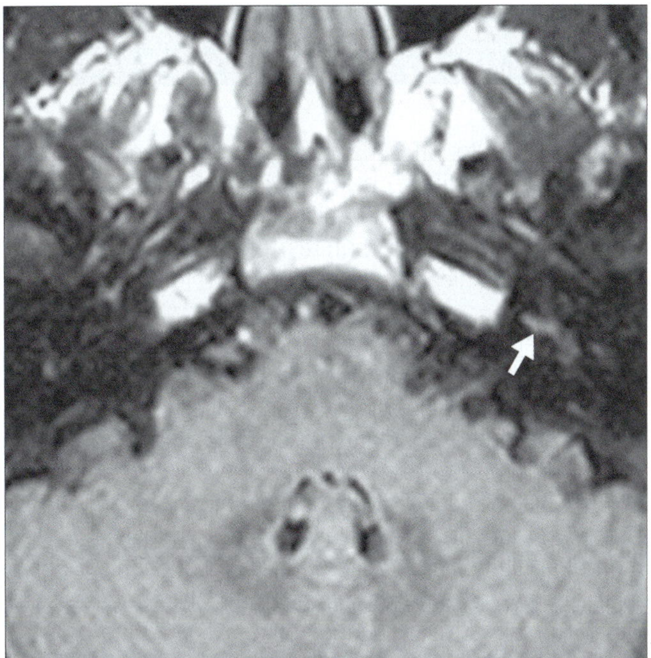

C

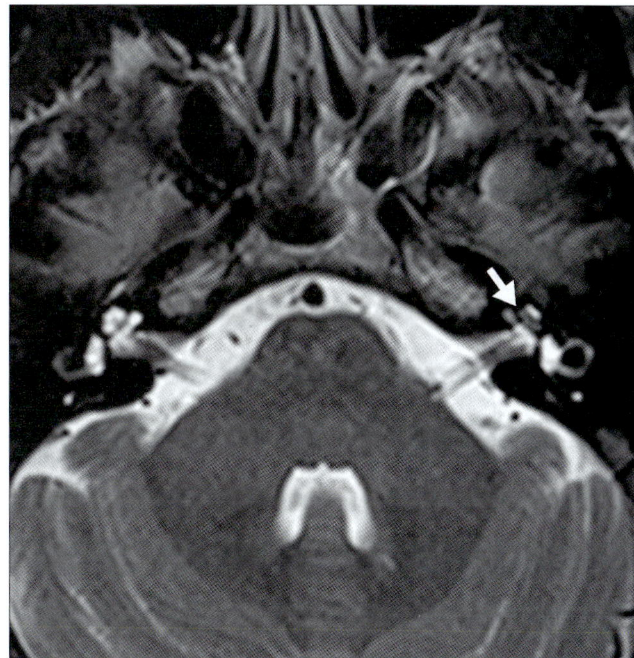

D

REFERENCES

Jagannathan J, et al. Endolymphatic sac tumor demonstrated by intralabyrinthine hemorrhage. Case report. *J Neurosurg*. 2007;107(2):421-425.

Ozdogan F, et al. Investigation of the cochlear effects of intratympanic steroids administered following acoustic trauma. *Laryngoscope*. 2012;122(4):877-882.

Petrovic BD, Futterer SF, Hijaz T, Russell EJ, Karagianis AG. Frequency and diagnostic utility of intralabyrinthine FLAIR hyperintensity in the evaluation of internal auditory canal and inner ear pathology. Acad Radiol. 2010;17(8):992-1000. doi: 10.1016/j.acra.2010.04.002.

Phillips JS, Westerberg B. Intratympanic steroids for Meniere's disease or syndrome. *Cochrane Database Syst Rev*. 2011;7:CD008514.

Poh AC, Tan TY. Sudden deafness due to intralabyrinthine haemorrhage: a possible rare late complication of head and neck irradiation. *Ann Acad Med Singapore*. 2007;36(1):78-82.

Saito N, Nadgir RN, Flower EN, Sakai O. Clinical and radiologic manifestations of sickle cell disease in the head and neck. *Radiographics*. 2010;30(4):1021-1034.

Salzman KL, Childs AM, Davidson HC, Kennedy RJ, Shelton C, Harnsberger HR. Intralabyrinthine schwannomas: imaging diagnosis and classification. *AJNR Am J Neuroradiol*. 2012;33(1):104-109.

Spear SA, Schwartz SR. Intratympanic steroids for sudden sensorineural hearing loss: a systematic review. *Otolaryngol Head Neck Surg*. 2011;145(4):534-543.

Whitehead RE, MacDonald CB, Melhem ER, McMahon L. Spontaneous labyrinthine hemorrhage in sickle cell disease. *AJNR Am J Neuroradiol*. 1998;19(8):1437-1440.

CASE 27 Cochlear implant

A cochlear implant may be placed in those patients who have profound sensorineural hearing loss that does not benefit from either conventional hearing aids or from a fully implantable hearing system (the latter described in Case 28 of this chapter). A cochlear implant functions by providing direct stimulation of the spiral ganglion cells within the cochlea. The implant consists of two main components: an external component, which the patient wears, and an internal component, which is implanted into the patient. The external component consists of an external transmitter as well as a behind-the-ear housing that contains a microphone, battery pack, and speech processor. The internal component consists of a receiver/stimulator device that is implanted into the subcutaneous tissues posterior to the auricle, a ground wire that is usually implanted into the temporalis musculature, and an electrode array that is placed into the cochlea. For placement of the electrode array, a mastoidectomy is performed and the electrode is inserted into the tympanic cavity via a facial recess approach. The electrode array is then placed through the round window, or through a surgically drilled hole in the cochlea (termed a cochleostomy) adjacent to the round window, and advanced into the scala tympani of the cochlea. Optimal placement of the electrode array is achieved when the array traverses the proximal 1.5 turns of the cochlea and when its tip terminates in the middle turn of the cochlea.

MR compatibility varies significantly among cochlear implant brands and manufacturers. The external transmitter and the implanted receiver stimulator appose one another and are held together by magnets. Some types of cochlear implants contain internal magnets that are MRI compatible at 1.5 T, some have internal magnets that can be removed without surgery prior to MR imaging, and others contain internal magnets that must be surgically removed prior to MR imaging. Also, these devices can create marked artifact on MRI, with or without a magnet in place. Ultimately, the ability to safely scan patients with a cochlear implant requires referencing the package insert of the cochlear implant in question to determine MR compatibility.

Preoperative CT imaging is typically performed to assess for the presence of relative or absolute contraindications prior to placement of a cochlear implant. These include advanced cochlear otosclerosis with involvement and compromise of the round window niche, advanced labyrinthitis ossificans, congenital cochlear malformations, (especially labyrinthine aplasia) and hypoplasia of the internal auditory canal (which may suggest cochlear nerve aplasia). Labyrinthitis ossificans may also be assessed with MRI, primarily with thin section T2-weighted or CISS imaging. In fact, MRI may be more sensitive than CT in identifying labyrinthitis ossificans, particularly during the fibroosseous stage (prior to the development of mineralization). If labyrinthitis ossificans is encountered, then localizing which portion of the inner ear affected by the labyrinthitis ossificans is critical. Pronounced labyrinthitis affecting the cochlea may result in a physical obstruction and preclude placement of the electrode. Conversely, if only the vestibule is affected by labyrinthitis ossificans, then placement of the electrode into the cochlea will typically be unimpeded. If cochlear nerve aplasia is suspected, then an MRI of the internal auditory canal may be performed, often including a sagittal oblique CISS/FIESTA sequence. If the cochlear nerve is indeed absent by imaging, then placement of a cochlear implant may not be of benefit. However, there is literature describing that some patients can still benefit from cochlear implantation despite an apparent absence of the cochlear nerve on dedicated MR imaging of the internal auditory canals.

Cochlear implant

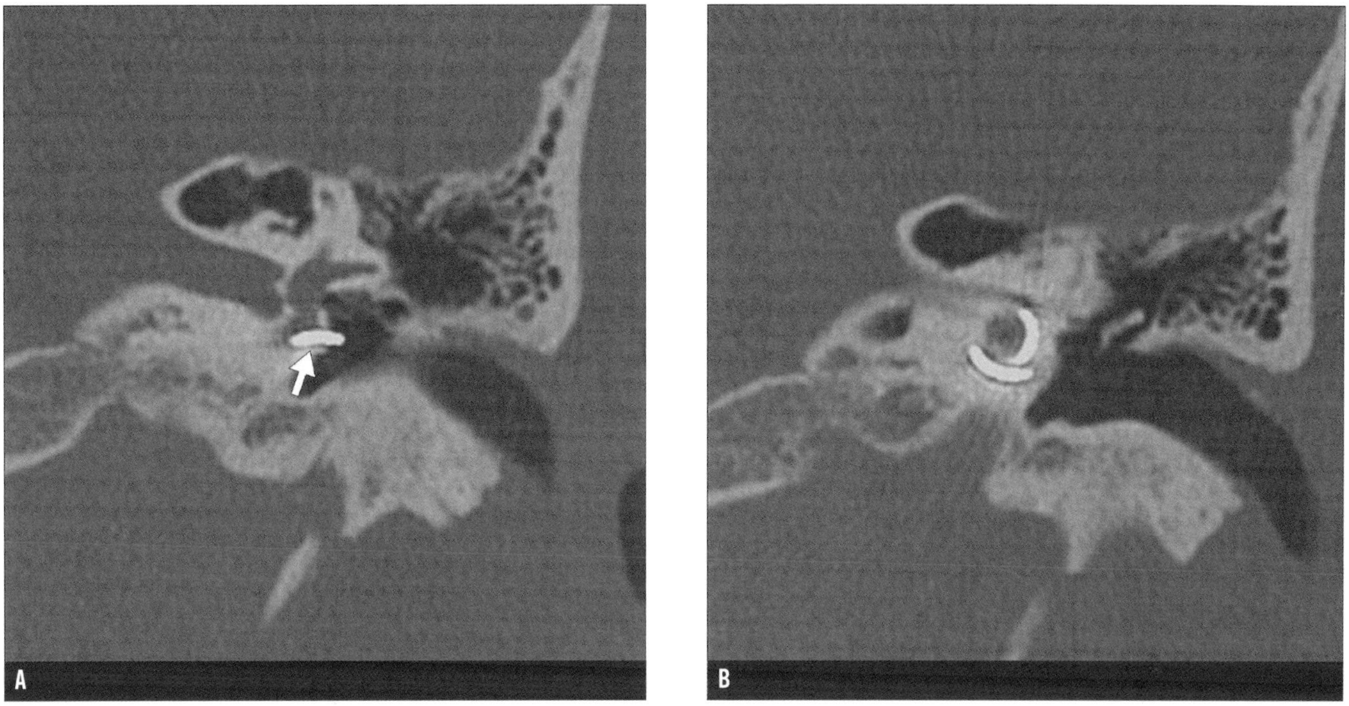

Coronal reformatted (**A**, **B**) and axial (**C**,**D**) CT images of the left temporal bone of a patient with profound bilateral sensorineural hearing loss demonstrate a canal wall up mastoidectomy with the electrode array of a cochlear implant traversing the round window (short arrows, **A**, **C**) and entering the cochlea. The tip of the electrode array terminates within the middle turn of the cochlea (long arrow, **D**).

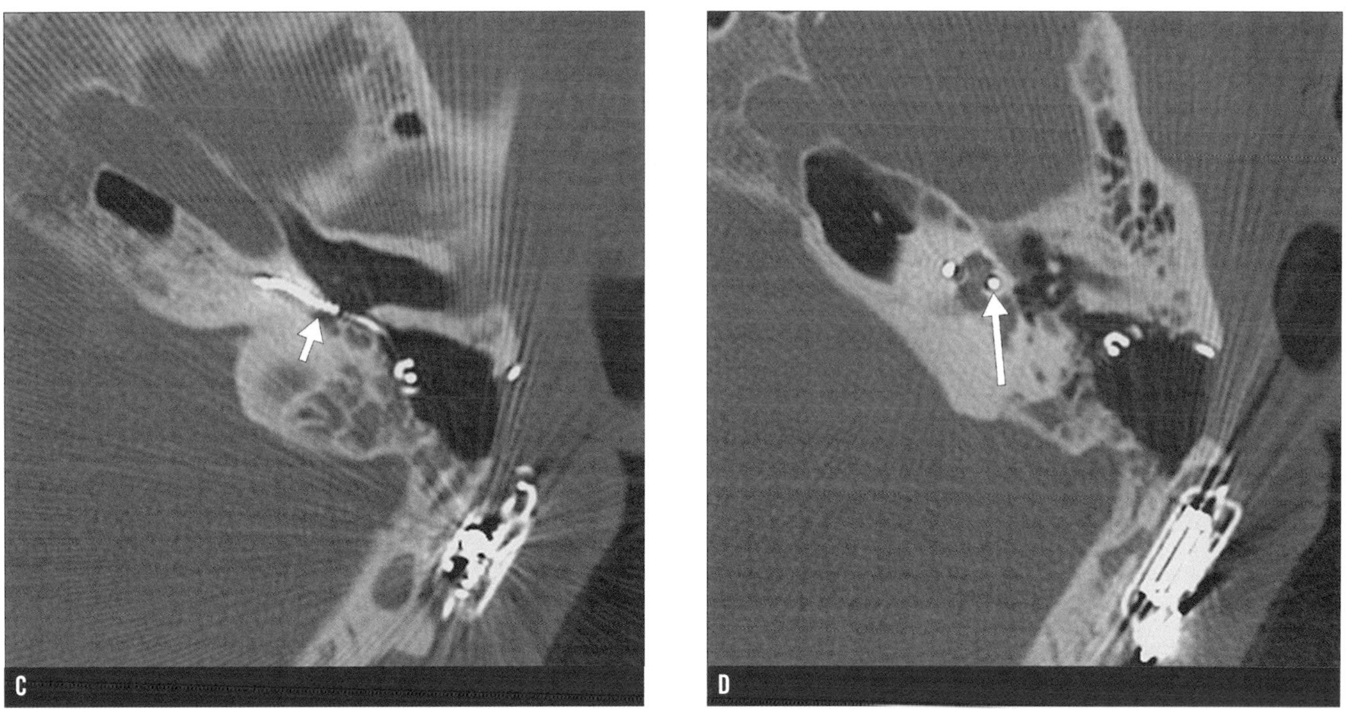

Cochlear implant

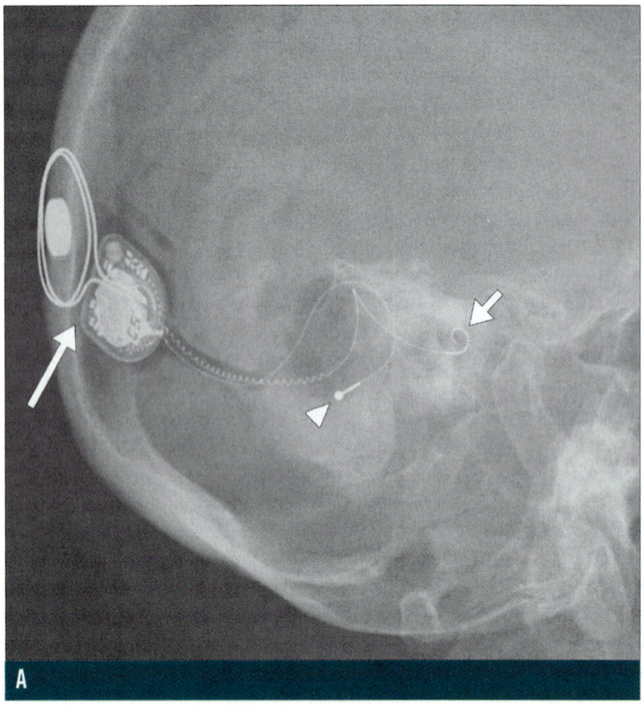

Different patient. An oblique lateral radiograph of the skull (**A**) demonstrates a cochlear implant overlying the posterior calvarium and traversing an inner ear. The receiver/stimulator is located posterior to the auricle (long arrow). The electrode array emanates from the receiver/stimulator toward the temporal bone. A curved appearance at the distal aspect of the electrode array suggests an appropriate intracochlear location of the electrode (short arrow). The ground electrode is located near the mastoid tip (arrowhead) when correlated with other views (not shown).

REFERENCES

Jain R, Mukherji SK. Cochlear implant failure: imaging evaluation of the electrode course. *Clin Radiol.* 2003;58(4):288-293.

Mukherji SK, et al. CT of the temporal bone: findings after mastoidectomy, ossicular reconstruction, and cochlear implantation. *AJR Am J Roentgenol.* 1994;163:1467-1471.

Teymouri J, Hullar TE, Holden TA, Chole RA. Verification of computed tomographic estimates of cochlear implant array position: a micro-CT and histologic analysis. *Otol Neurotol.* 2011;32(6):980-986.

Warren FM 3rd, Wiggins RH 3rd, Pitt C, Harnsberger HR, Shelton. Apparent cochlear nerve aplasia: to implant or not to implant? *Otol Neurotol.* 2010;31(7):1088-1094.

CASE 28 Fully implantable hearing system

A fully implantable hearing system (FIHS) is generally used for patients with less than profound sensorineural hearing loss. An FIHS offers several advantages over conventional hearing aids, including low sound distortion, a wider range of frequency responses, and limited feedback. Additionally, an FIHS can be used in environments that are not appropriate for conventional hearing aids, such as swimming, showering, and certain sports. However, unlike conventional hearing aids, placement of FIHS is invasive and requires an atticotomy or a mastoidectomy.

A FIHS consists of a device to house the electronics (composed of a microphone, electronic amplifier, and a battery source) which is placed posterior to the auricle. An FIHS also has a transducer that is attached to the mastoid bone and a transducer tip that is typically attached to the incus. The device results in direct electromechanical stimulation of the ossicular chain and allows for superior sound fidelity compared to conventional hearing aids, which simply function as a loudspeaker. In cases where there is an abnormal ossicular chain that results in a conductive hearing loss in addition to the sensorineural hearing loss, the transducer tip is fitted with a prosthesis. This prosthesis may be attached to the long process of the incus or stapes head (when present), the stapes footplate (when the stapes superstructure is absent), the round window (in cases of stapes footplate fixation), or the oval window.

An FIHS differs from a cochlear implant in that the electrode used for a cochlear implant extends into the cochlea and directly stimulates the spiral ganglion. A cochlear implant is used in patients with profound sensorineural hearing loss who would not benefit from an FIHS.

Fully implantable hearing system

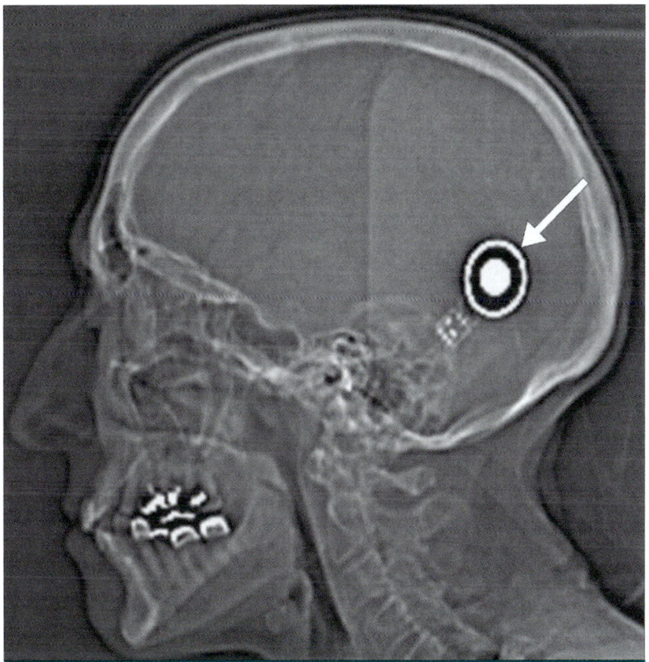

A

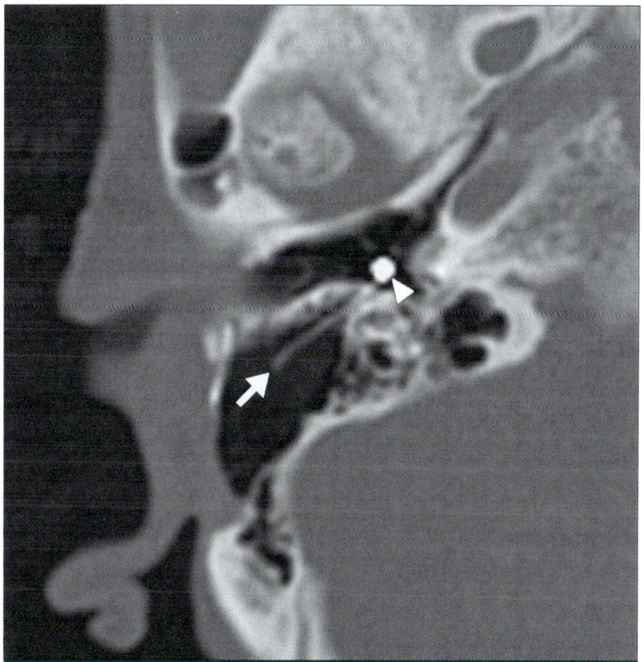

B

A lateral scout view of the calvarium (**A**) and multiple axial CT images (**B-D**) demonstrate a fully implantable hearing system of the right temporal bone. The device that holds the electronics is located posterior-superior to the auricle (long arrows, **A**, **D**). The transducer lead extends through a canal wall up mastoidectomy and enters the tympanic cavity via a facial recess approach (short arrows, **B**, **C**). The tip of the transducer is located at the expected location of the long process of the incus where it is attached to the ossicular chain (arrowheads, **B**, **C**).

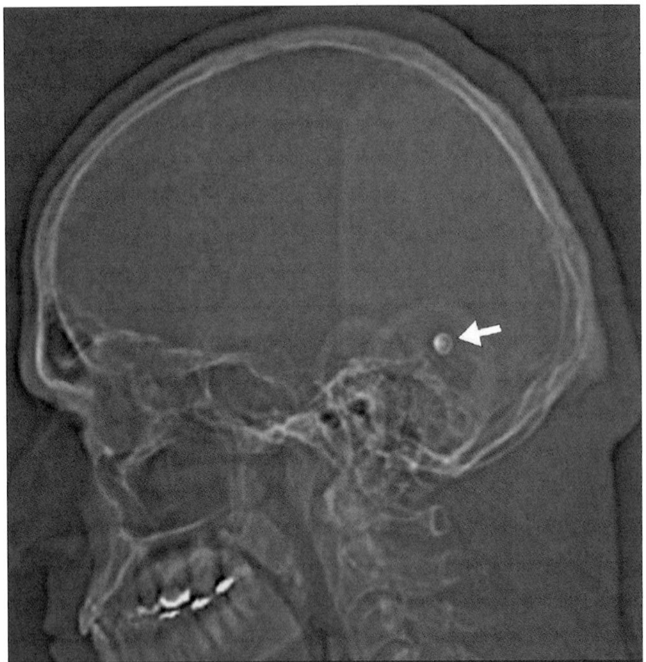

C

REFERENCES

Dun CA, Faber HT, de Wolf MJ, Cremers CW, Hol MK. An overview of different systems: the bone-anchored hearing aid. *Adv Otorhinolaryngol.* 2011;71:22-31.

Janssen RM, Hong P, Chadha NK. Bilateral bone-anchored hearing aids for bilateral permanent conductive hearing loss: a systematic review. *Otolaryngol Head Neck Surg.* 2012;147(3):412-422.

Novakovic D, Meller CJ, Makeham JM, Brazier DH, Forer M, Patel NP. Computed tomographic analysis of outer calvarial thickness for osseointegrated bone-anchored hearing system insertion. *Otol Neurotol.* 2011;32(3):448-452.

CASE 31 False-positive superior semicircular canal dehiscence

Semicircular canal (SCC) dehiscence represents a small defect involving the osseous labyrinth of an SCC. The superior SCC is most commonly affected, usually from an unknown etiology, although a lateral or posterior SCC dehiscence may also occur, with lateral SCC dehiscence most commonly the result of an erosion from a tympanic cavity cholesteatoma. While not all patients with an SCC dehiscence are symptomatic, some patients with SCC dehiscence may present with a clinical scenario termed Tullio phenomenon. Tullio phenomenon is characterized by disequilibrium, vertigo, and oscillopsia (oscillation of the visual field) that is induced by low frequency or loud noises (eg, ambulance siren, jet engines, etc). Other symptoms described with this phenomenon include diplacusis (the perception of a single auditory stimulus as two separate sounds that may differ in time or pitch) and autophony (the perception of a person's own voice, breathing, or other self-generated sounds as unusually loud). These various symptoms are related to the formation of a "third mobile window" at the SCC dehiscence, with the other two windows being the normal round and oval windows.

The mechanisms that result in the varied symptoms of Tullio phenomenon are rather complex. With typical hearing, sound travels via both air conduction (ie, from the tympanic membrane to the ossicles, and then to the inner ear) and bone conduction (which directly stimulates the inner ear). If a third mobile window is present, then bone conduction can oscillate the intracranial meninges at the third mobile window, resulting in standing inner ear fluid waves and subsequent amplification of sound. This mechanism likely accounts for autophony. In addition, because sound conduction travels faster through bone than through air, sound from bone conduction will reach the third mobile window faster than sound entering from the tympanic cavity. This mechanism likely accounts for the symptoms of diplacusis because the same sound is reaching the inner ear at different points in time. Moreover, when loud, low frequency sound energy reaches the inner ear fluid (via air and/or bone conduction), the third mobile window allows for a low resistance pathway toward the third mobile window. This results in stimulation of the SCC afferents and torsional eye movement. By the same token, raising the intracranial pressure, such as with a Valsava maneuver, results in meningeal depression at the third mobile window, generating a torsional eye movement in the opposite direction to the that occurring from loud, low-frequency sounds. These rotational eye movements explain the symptoms of oscillopsia with Tullio phenomenon. Finally, there is evidence that an SCC dehiscence can cause low frequency sensorineural hearing loss. The proposed mechanism is that the low resistance pathway of the third mobile window shunts acoustic energy from the cochlea, resulting in less cochlear stimulation and subsequent sensorineural hearing loss.

In many cases, routine coronal reformatted images are sufficient to confirm or exclude a diagnosis of superior SCC dehiscence. However, in some cases, the bone covering the superior SCC is thin but intact, and partial volume effect on the coronal reformatted images can result in a false-positive interpretation of superior SCC dehiscence. In these cases, Stenver plane (perpendicular to the superior SCC) and Poschl plane (parallel to the superior SCC) reformatted CT images can be performed to better assess the integrity of the osseous superior SSC. In addition, imaging with a slice thickness of less than 1 mm (eg, 0.6 mm) will improve evaluation for SSC dehiscence. As stated above, not all cases of SSC dehiscence are symptomatic; therefore, clinical assessment is necessary to determine the significance of SSC dehiscence.

COMPANION CASE

- **Superior semicircular canal dehiscence.**

False-positive superior semicircular canal dehiscence

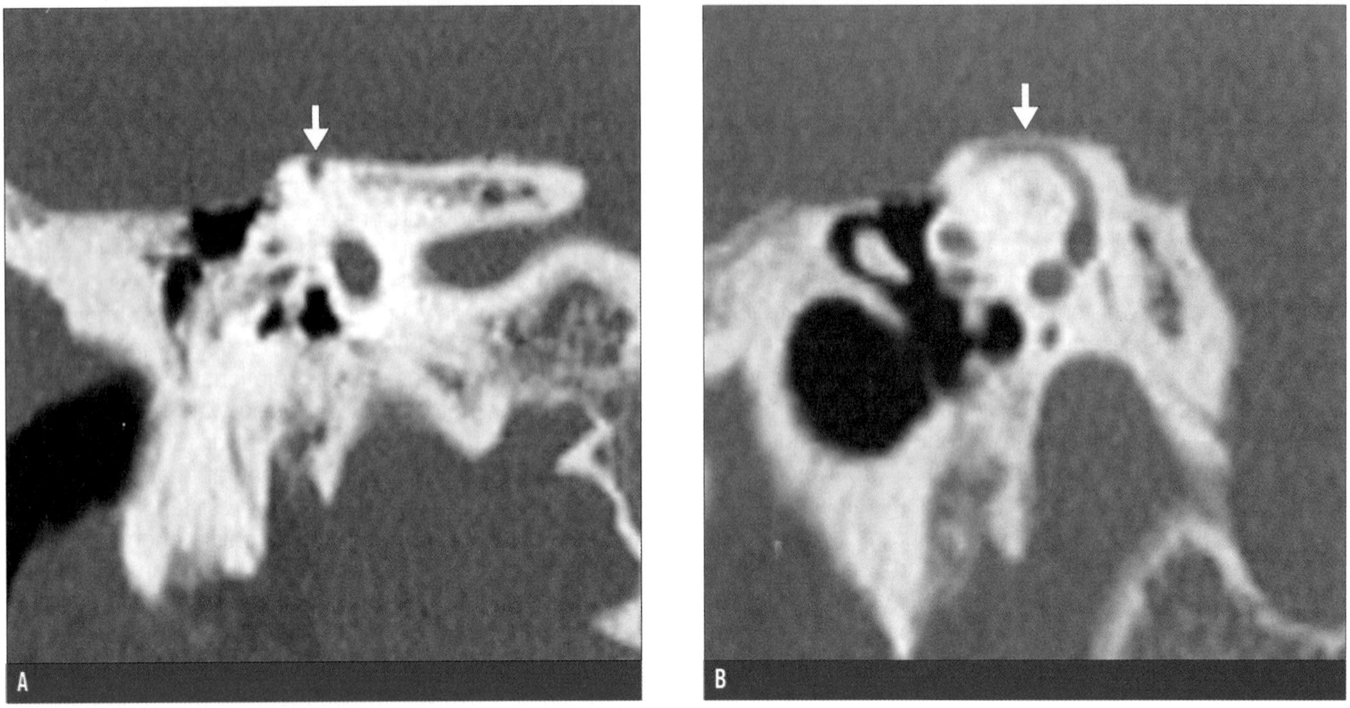

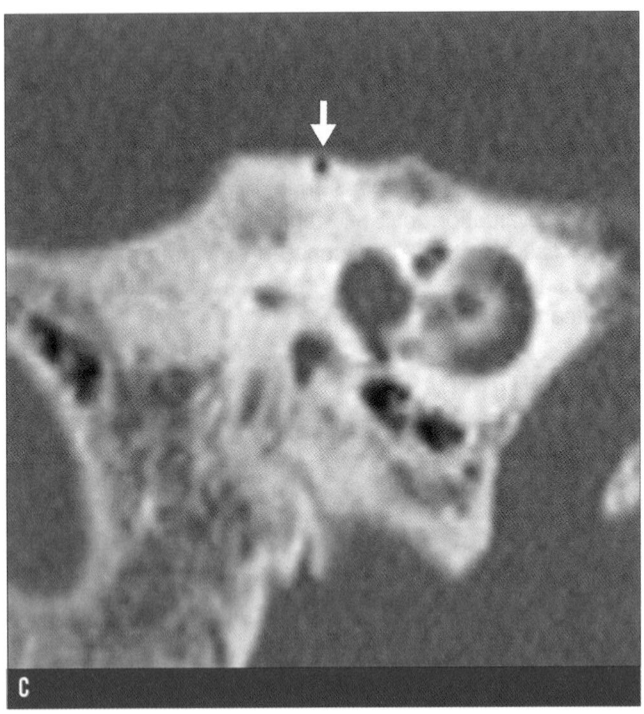

A 1-mm coronal reformatted CT image of the right temporal bone (**A**) demonstrates an apparent osseous defect involving the superior semicircular canal (arrow, **A**). 0.6-mm Poschl plane (**B**) and Stenver plane (**C**) reformatted CT images of the right temporal bone from the same study demonstrate that the osseous covering of the superior semicircular canal is intact (arrows, **B**, **C**). Therefore, the apparent dehiscence on image **A** is related to partial volume effect.

Companion case: Superior semicircular canal dehiscence

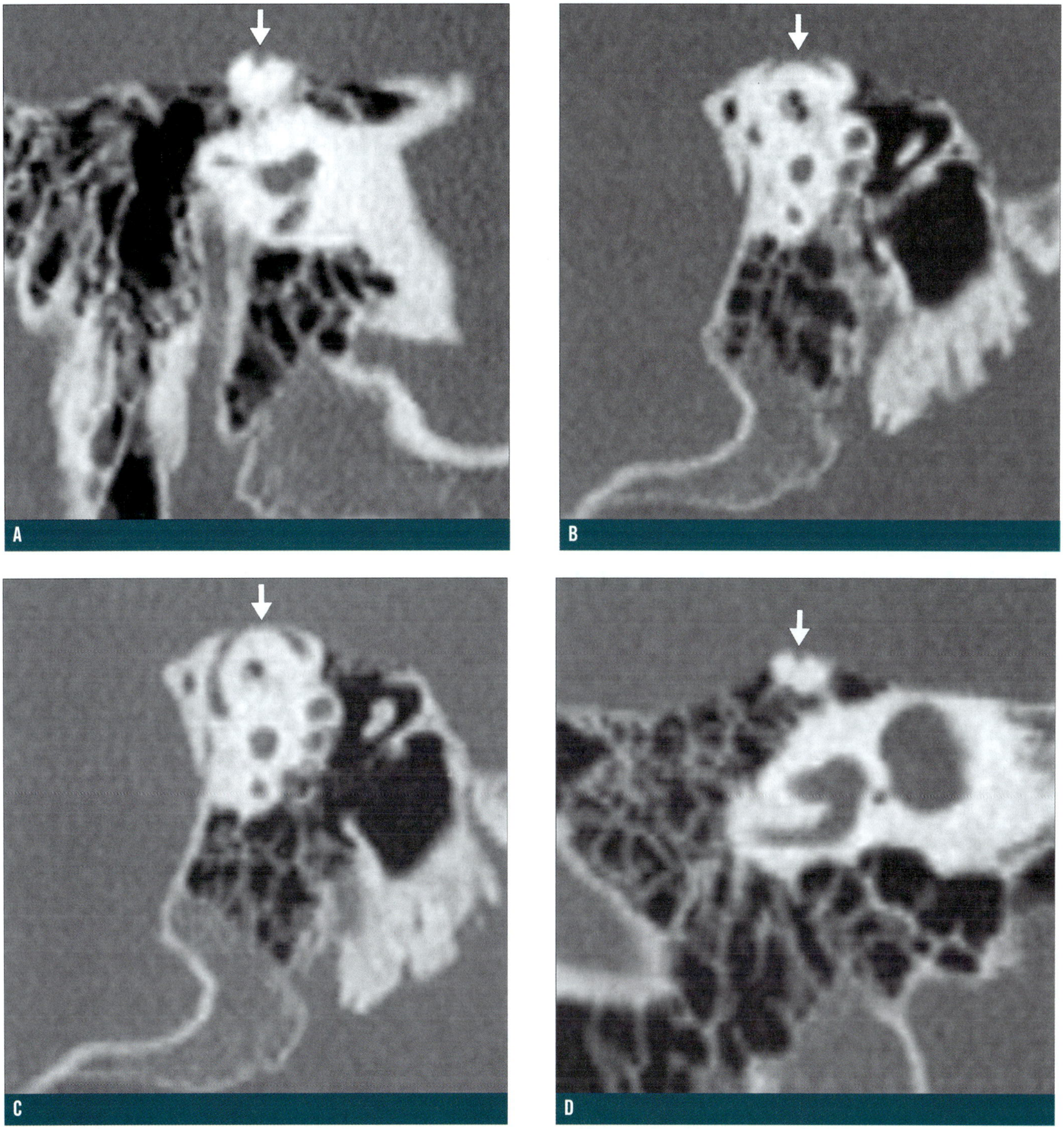

1-mm coronal (**A**), 0.6-mm Poschl plane (**B**, **C**), and 0.6-mm Stenver plane (**D**) reformatted CT images of the right temporal bone demonstrate an osseous defect involving the superior semicircular canal consistent with superior semicircular canal dehiscence (arrows, **A**-**D**). The presence of this finding in the Poschl and Stenver planes confirms that the finding on image **A** is not related to partial volume effect.

REFERENCES

Branstetter BF, Harrigal C, Escott EJ, Hirsch BE. Superior semicircular canal dehiscence: oblique reformatted CT images for diagnosis. *Radiology*. 2006;238(3):938-942.

Curtin HD. Superior semicircular canal dehiscence syndrome and multi-detector row CT. *Radiology*. 2003;226:312-314.

Kaski D, Davies R, Luxon L, Bronstein AM, Rudge P.The Tullio phenomenon: a neurologically neglected presentation. *J Neurol*. 2012;259(1):4-21.

Mikulec AA, et al. Superior semicircular canal dehiscence presenting as conductive hearing loss without vertigo. *Otol Neurotol*. 2004;25(2):121-129.

Exposure to loud or low frequency sound that induces disequilibrium, vertigo, and oscillopsia (oscillation of the visual field) is termed Tullio phenomenon. Most commonly, this entity occurs in the setting of semicircular canal dehiscence, typically affecting the superior semicircular canal. See the preceding case for a more complete discussion of Tullio phenomenon.

Most patients with Tullio phenomenon are treated conservatively with avoidance of precipitants and/or with sound attenuation earmolds. Surgical repair of a semicircular canal defect is reserved for patients with debilitating symptoms, most often vestibular symptoms or those related to marked autophony (defined as the perception of a person's own voice, breathing, or other self-generated sounds as unusually loud). The two main surgical approaches for repair of superior semicircular canal dehiscence are resurfacing and plugging. For the resurfacing technique, a middle fossa craniotomy is typically performed, and the osseous dehiscence is repaired with either a fascial or bone graft. The plugging technique involves packing the semicircular canal with fascia and bone dust to occlude the lumen. The plugging technique can be performed by either a transmastoid approach, or less commonly, via a middle fossa craniotomy. There is a risk of graft migration with the resurfacing technique and a risk of damage to the vestibular and cochlear structures with the plugging technique.

Repair of superior semicircular canal dehiscence

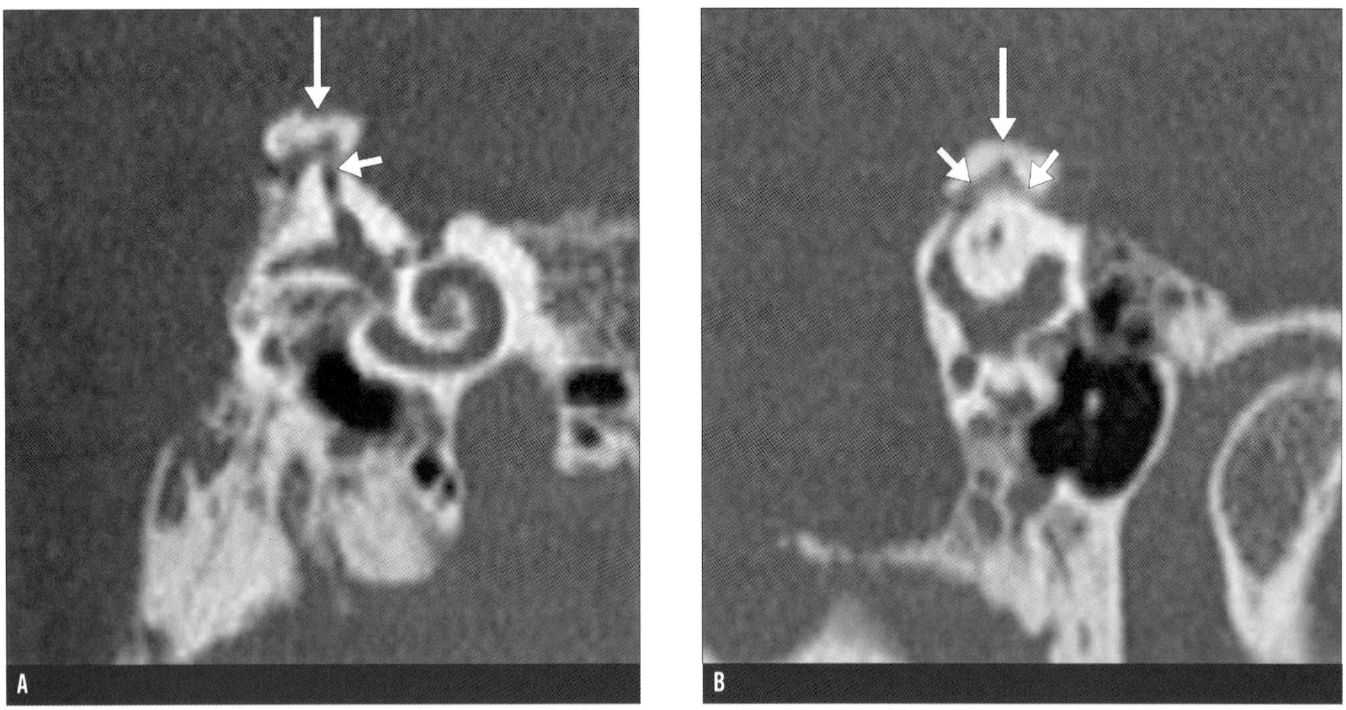

Stenver plane (**A**) and Poschl plane (**B**) reformatted CT images of the right temporal bone demonstrate a bone graft (long arrows, **A**, **B**) overlying a superior semicircular canal osseous dehiscence (short arrows, **A**, **B**), compatible with a resurfacing surgical technique. The bone graft is appropriately positioned, although clinical assessment is needed to determine the efficacy of the graft.

REFERENCES

Amoodi HA, Fawaz MM, McNeil M, Bance M. Transmastoid resurfacing of superior semicircular canal dehiscence. *Laryngoscope*. 2011;121(5):1117-1123.

Kaski D, Davies R, Luxon L, Bronstein AM, Rudge P. The Tullio phenomenon: a neurologically neglected presentation. *J Neurol*. 2012;259(1):4-21.

Lundy L, Zapala D, Moushey J. Cartilage cap occlusion technique for dehiscent superior semicircular canals. *Otol Neurotol*. 2011;32:1281-1284.

Teixido M, Seymour PE, Kung B, Sabra O. Transmastoid middle fossa craniotomy repair of superior semicircular canal dehiscence using a soft tissue graft. *Otol Neurotol*. 2011;32:877-881.

CASE 33 Singular canal

The singular canal is an osseous canal containing the singular nerve (also called posterior ampullary nerve). The singular canal extends from the ampulla of the posterior semicircular canal to the posterior-inferior wall of the internal auditory canal. The singular canal can be identified on most CT temporal bone studies and is a structure that can simulate a fracture.

The singular nerve carries inferior vestibular nerve afferent fibers from the ampulla of the posterior semicircular canal. Rarely, a singular neurectomy can be performed to treat severe benign paroxysmal positional vertigo that is refractory to conservative measures.

Singular canal

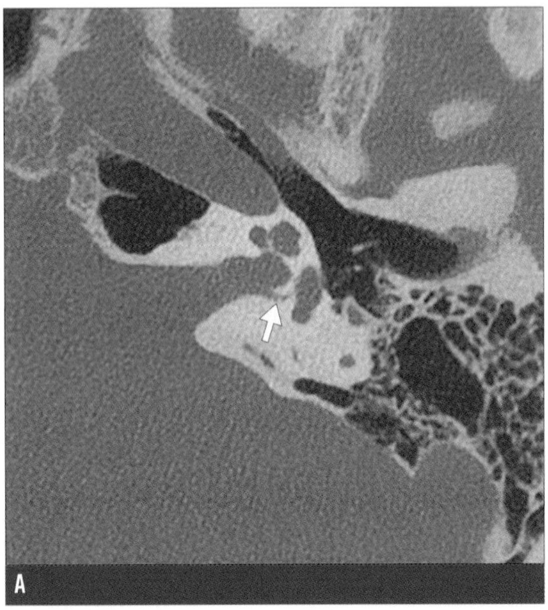

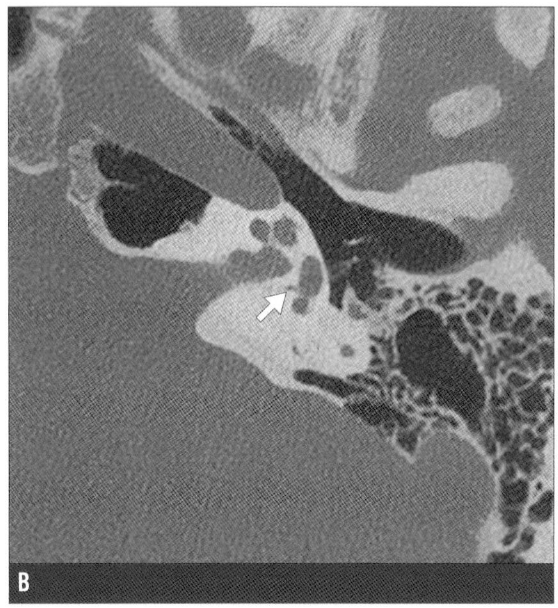

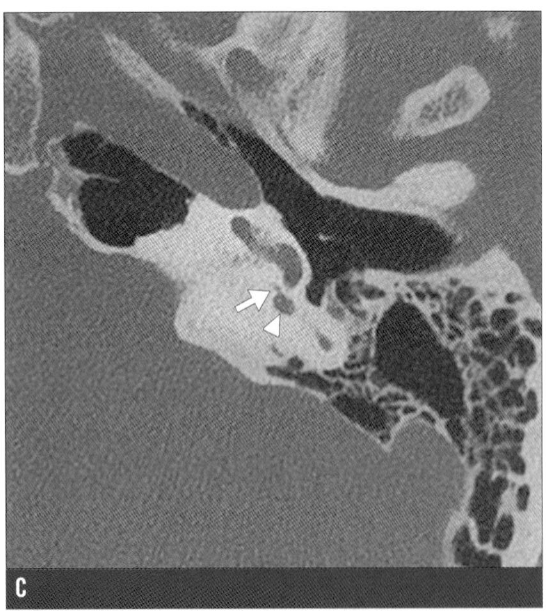

Axial CT images of the left temporal bone (**A-C**) demonstrate a normal singular canal (arrows, **A-C**), extending from the ampulla of the posterior semicircular canal (arrowhead, **C**) to the posterior-inferior wall of the internal auditory canal.

REFERENCE

Connor SEJ, Tan G, Fernando R, Chaudhury N. Computed tomography pseudofractures of the mid face and skull base. *Clin Radiol.* 2005;60:1268-1279.

CASE 34 Subarcuate canal

The subarcuate canal is also referred to as the petromastoid canal. This canal contains the subarcuate artery, which is a branch of the anterior inferior cerebellar artery, and the subarcuate vein. The subarcuate canal is located in the petrous temporal bone and is surrounded by the superior semicircular canal. It traverses between the posterior fossa and the mastoid antrum. Therefore, a subarcuate canal can serve as a conduit for the spread of infection, typically from the mastoid to the posterior fossa.

The subarcuate canal is almost always identified on a temporal bone CT and can simulate a fracture. The subarcuate canal is larger during fetal development and gradually decreases in size during the first few years of life. There are scattered reports of anatomic variations of the subarcuate canal, including unusual enlargement of the canal and an aberrant course.

Subarcuate canal

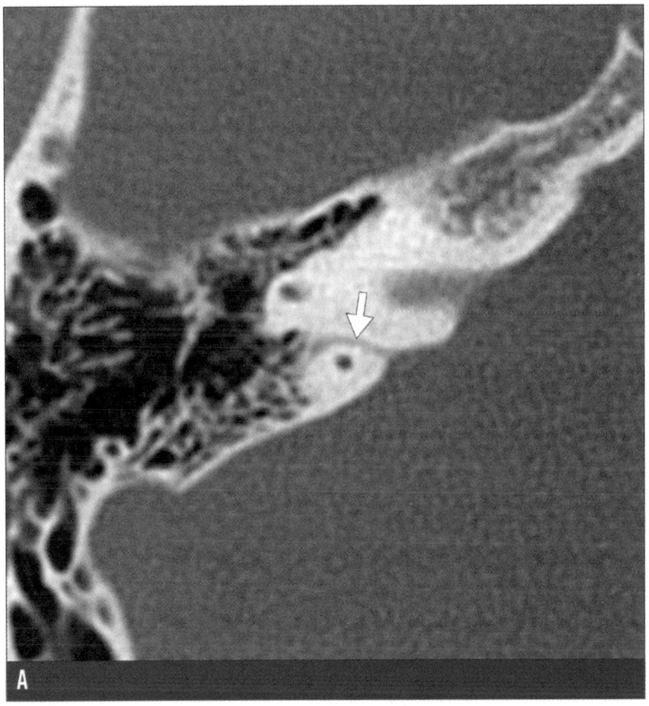

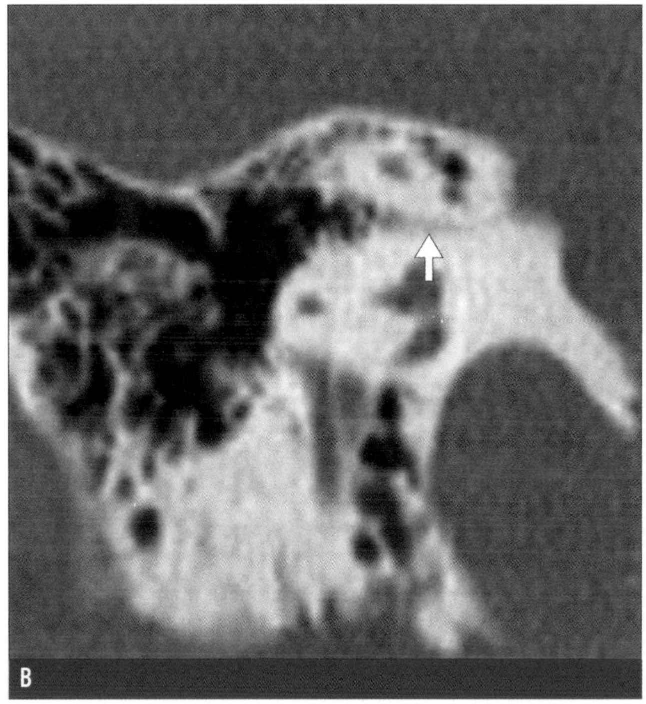

Axial (**A**) and coronal reformatted (**B**) CT images of the right temporal bone demonstrate a normal subarcuate canal (arrows, **A**, **B**) within the petrous temporal bone, traversing between the posterior fossa and mastoid antrum and surrounded by the superior semicircular canal.

Enlarged subarcuate canal

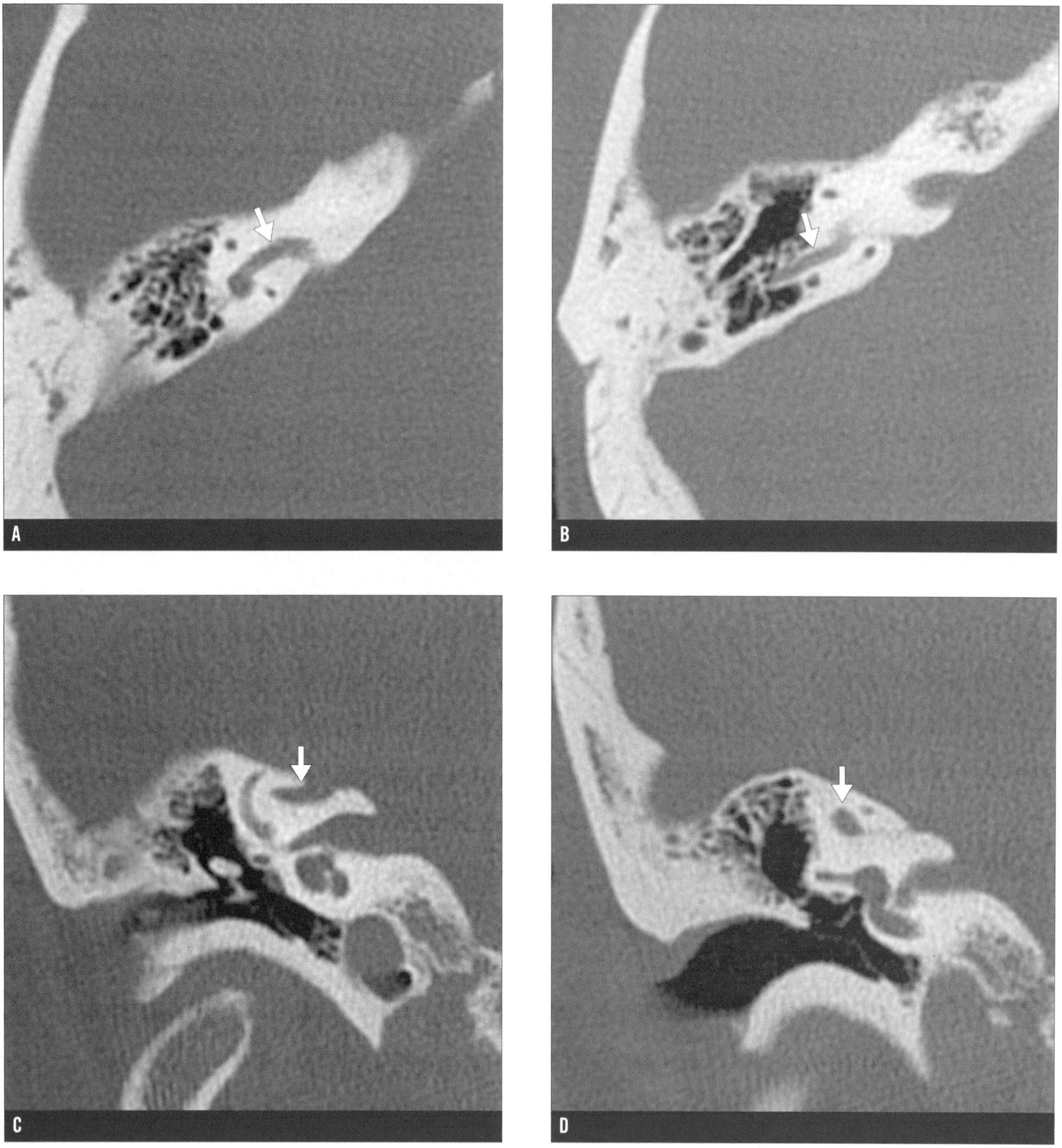

Axial (**A**, **B**) and coronal reformatted (**C**, **D**) CT images of the right temporal bone demonstrate an unusually large subarcuate canal (arrows, **A**-**D**).

Aberrant course of the subarcuate canal

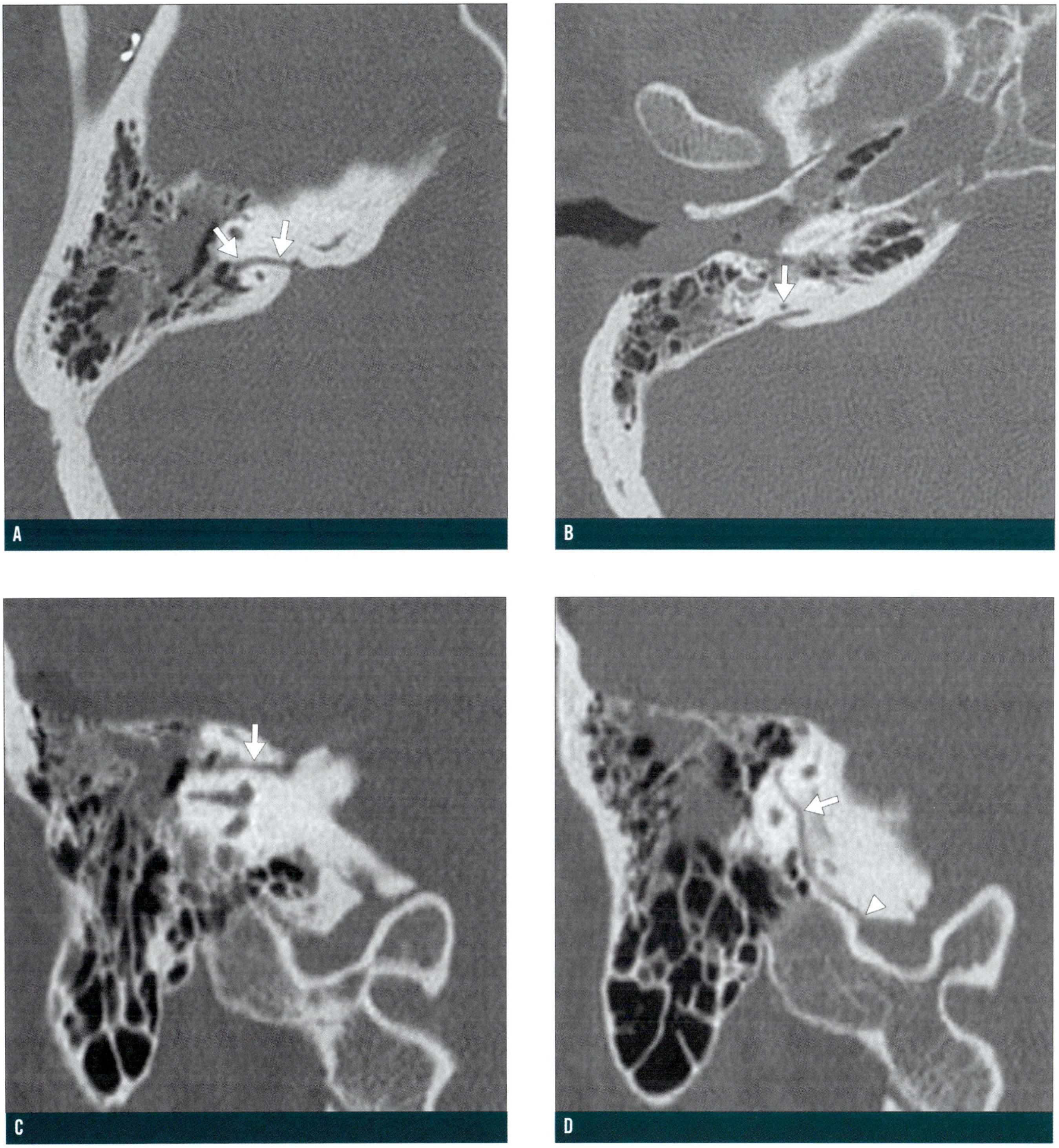

Axial (**A**, **B**) and coronal reformatted (**C**, **D**) CT images of the right temporal bone demonstrate an aberrant course of the subarcuate canal (arrows, **A-D**). It begins traversing normally between the limbs of the superior semicircular canal (**A**, **C**), makes a hairpin turn to extend inferiorly (**B**, **D**), and terminates at the lateral margin of the jugular foramen (arrowhead, **D**)

REFERENCES

Connor SEJ, Tan G, Fernando R, Chaudhury N. Computed tomography pseudofractures of the mid face and skull base. *Clin Radiol.* 2005;60:1268-1279.

Migirov L, Kronenberg J. Radiology of the petromastoid canal. *Otology & Neurotology.* 2006;27:410-413.

CASE 35 Variations of the IAC

The internal auditory canal (IAC) can vary widely in its size and shape, typically ranging from 2 to 8 mm in diameter. Studies of temporal bone development have demonstrated that the inner ear structures are fully developed at birth. Similarly, the fundus of the IAC (the lateral-most portion of the IAC) has fully developed its size and conical shape by birth. However, the middle segment of the IAC and the porus acusticus (entrance to the IAC) continue to develop until adolescence. Some studies have suggested that the shape of the IAC adapts to the cranial growth, likely accounting for its variable appearance among patients.

Patulous IACs are typically asymptomatic and incidental. However, developmental stenosis of the IAC, typically considered less than 2 mm in diameter, may be associated with congenital abnormalities such as aplasia or hypoplasia of the vestibulocochlear nerve. Rarely, the IAC may be duplicated or even triplicated. Acquired stenosis of the IAC is most commonly related to an exostosis or osteoma at the porus acusticus. These acquired lesions are slow growing and are typically diagnosed only when symptoms develop. Symptoms include hearing and vestibular dysfunction related to compression of the vestibulocochlear nerve. The traversing facial nerve is less commonly affected in these settings.

COMPANION CASE

- **Congenital X-linked hearing loss.** This rare entity represents an X-linked chromosomal abnormality that is associated with an abnormal fistulous communication between the IAC and the cochlea. The fistulous communication is usually bilateral and results in a perilymphatic hydrops with progressive and profound sensorineural hearing loss. There is also a component of a conductive hearing loss that is attributable to abnormal stapes fixation. The stapes fixation and superimposed inner ear hydrops predisposes these patients to a so-called "stapes gusher" during a stapedotomy or stapedectomy. The stapes gusher results in marked loss of perilymph that is often catastrophic and can result in total deafness. Congenital X-linked hearing loss is present primarily in males, although female carriers can have a milder form of the disease.

  The imaging hallmarks of this entity represent manifestations of the fistulous communication between the IAC and cochlea. These imaging findings include a deficient lamina cribrosa (bony plate separating the inner ear from the IAC fundus), a deficient cochlear modiolus (central osseous axis of the cochlea which contains the spiral ganglion), and an abnormally enlarged cochlear fossette (osseous opening of the cochlea). The cochlea is also frequently dysmorphic. The IACs are patulous, although as discussed above, this finding in isolation is frequently incidental. Abnormal enlargement of the facial nerve canals has also been described.

Patulous IACs

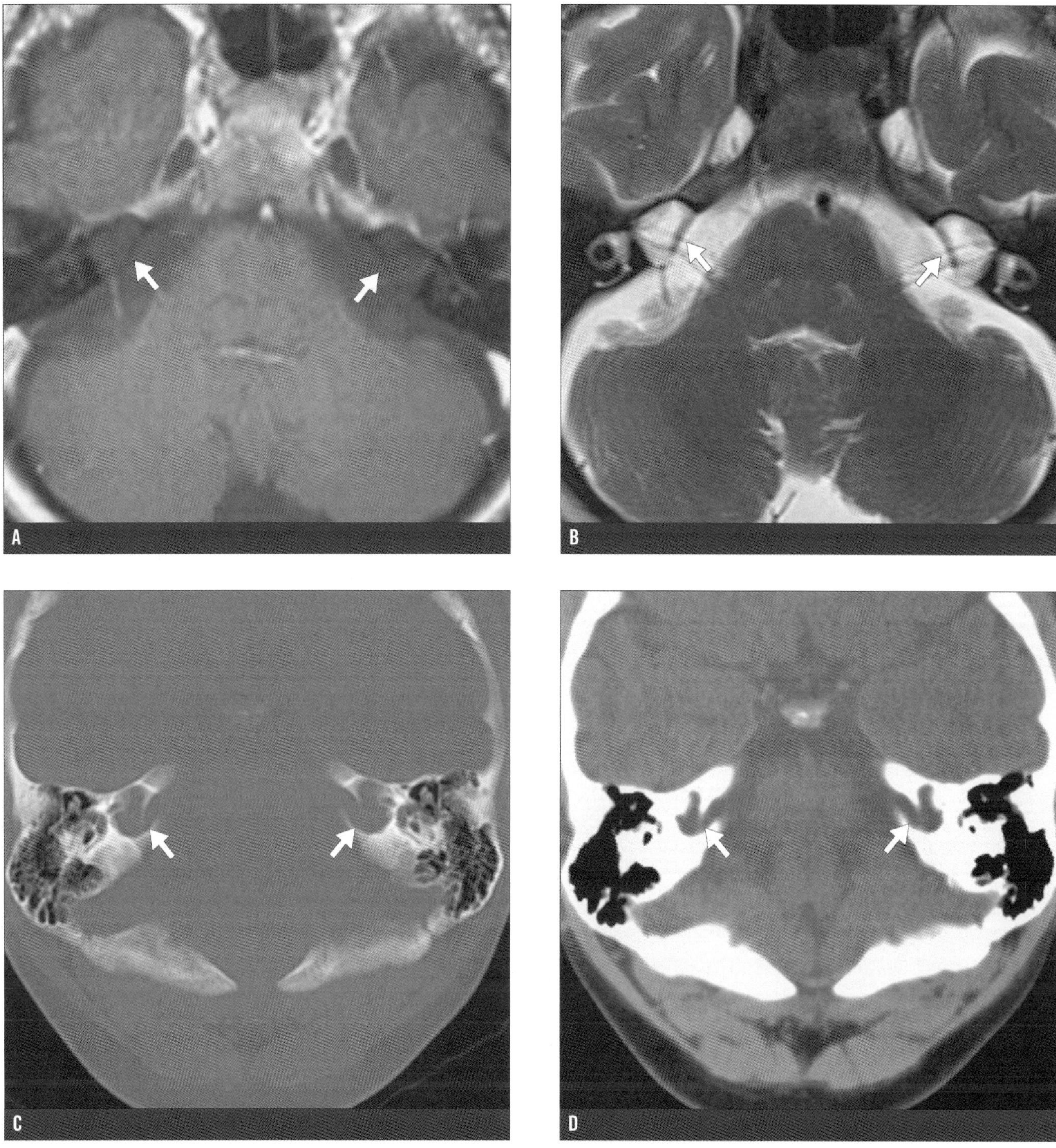

Axial T1 (**A**) and axial T2 (**B**) MR images of the IACs as well as noncontrast axial CT images through the temporal bones of the same patient viewed with a bone window (**C**) and a soft tissue window (**D**) demonstrate patulous bilateral IACs, an incidental finding in this patient (arrows, **A**-**D**).

Developmental stenosis of the IAC

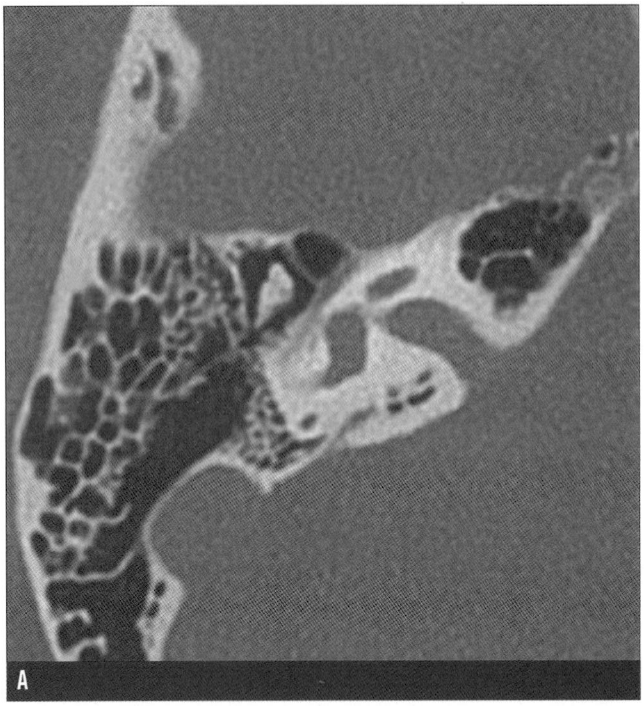

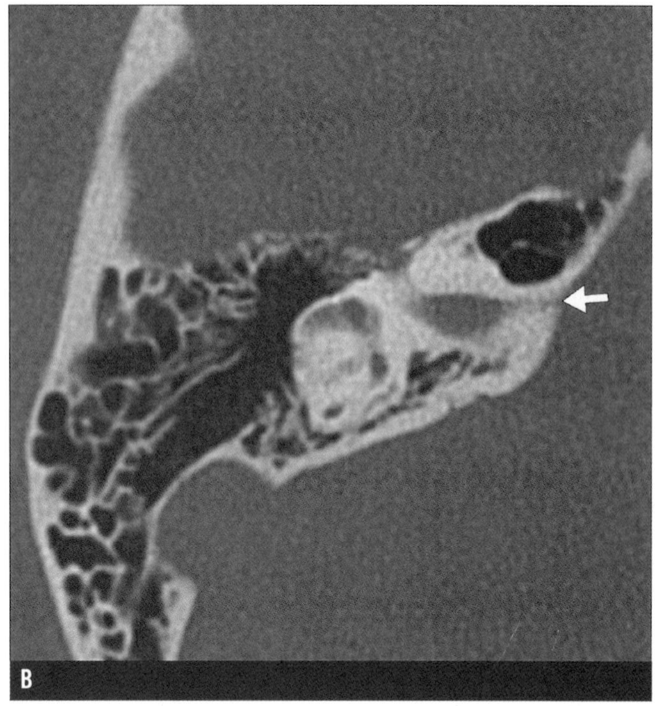

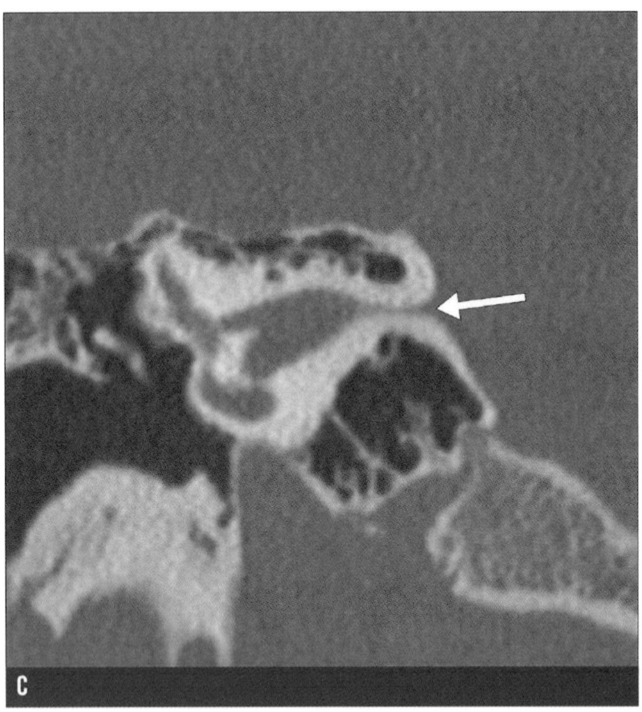

Axial CT images of the right temporal bone (**A**, **B**). On image **B**, there is a focal osseous density in the region of the right IAC porus acusticus that raises the possibility of an exostosis or osteoma (short arrow, **B**). However, a coronal reformatted CT image (**C**) demonstrates symmetric narrowing of the right IAC (long arrow, **C**), compatible with a developmental stenosis. This patient did not have a history of a congenital anomaly or right sensorineural hearing loss. The finding in this case was incidental.

Companion case: Congenital X-linked hearing loss

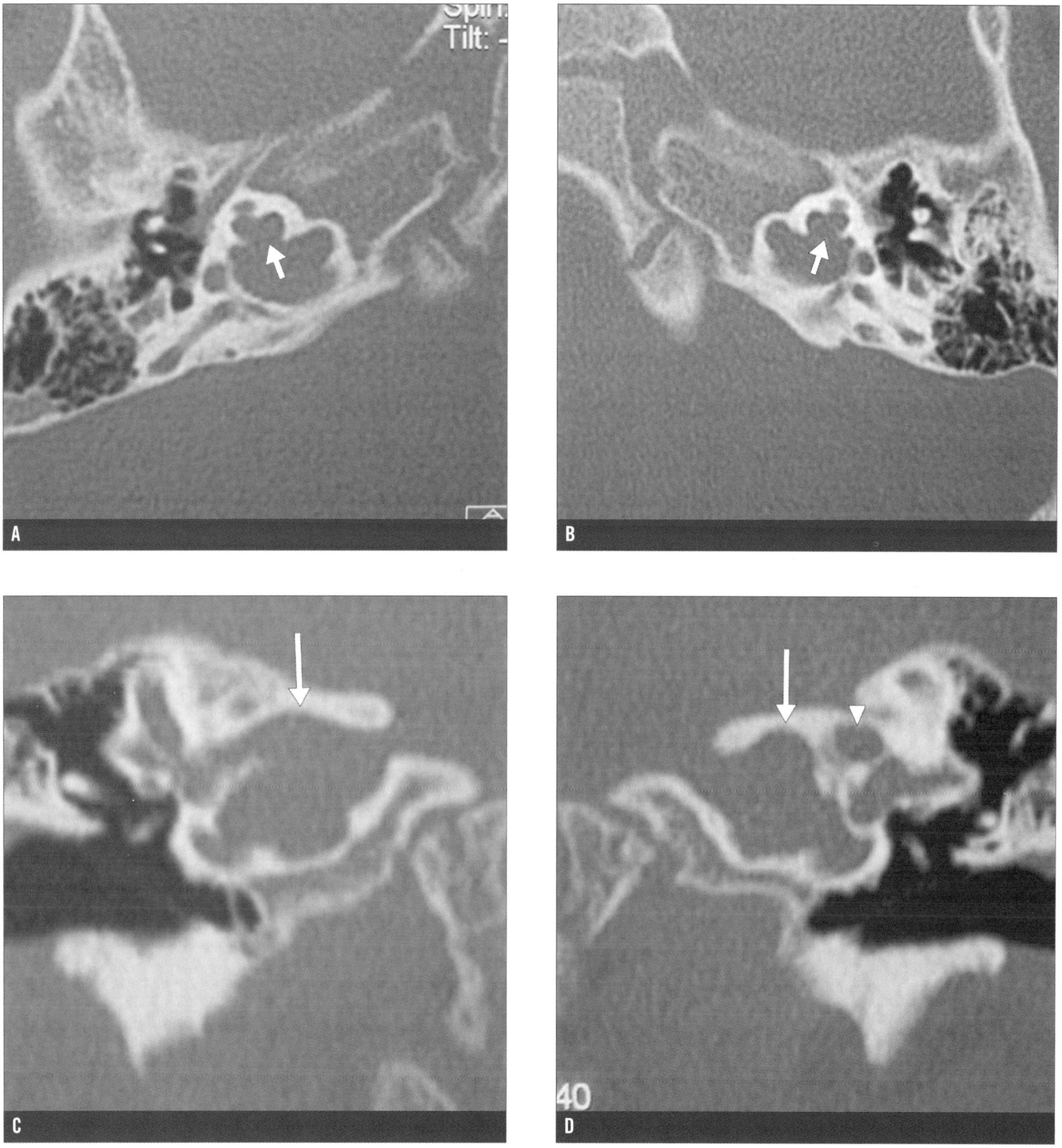

Axial (**A**, **B**) and coronal reformatted (**C**, **D**) CT images of the temporal bones demonstrate classic findings of congenital X-linked hearing loss. There is deficiency of the laminae cribrosae and cochlear modioli as well as enlarged cochlear fossettes (short arrows, **A**, **B**). The cochleae are also dysmorphic. The IACs are patulous, a common manifestation of this entity, but in isolation a frequently incidental finding (long arrows, **C**, **D**). Abnormal enlargement of the labyrinthine segment of the left facial nerve canal is partially imaged (arrowhead, **D**). *Case courtesy of Hugh D. Curtin, MD, FACR.*

REFERENCES

Baik FM, Nguyen L, Doherty JK, Harris JP, Mafee MF, Nguyen QT. Comparative case series of exostoses and osteomas of the internal auditory canal. *Ann Otol Rhinol Laryngol.* 2011;120(4):255-260.

Bonaldi LV, do Lago A, Crema LC, Fukuda Y, Smith RL. Internal auditory canal: pre- and postnatal growth. *J Otolaryngol.* 2004;33(4):243-247.

Kumar G, Castillo M, Buchman CA.X-linked stapes gusher: CT findings in one patient. *AJNR Am J Neuroradiol.* 2003;24(6):1130-1132.

Lowe LH, Vézina LG. Sensorineural hearing loss in children. *Radiographics.* 1997;17(5):1079-1093.

Migirov L. Patulous internal auditory canal. *Arch Otolaryngol Head Neck Surg.* 2003;129(9):992-993.

Lee SY, et al. Narrow duplicated or triplicated internal auditory canal (3 cases and review of literature): can we regard the separated narrow internal auditory canal as the presence of vestibulocochlear nerve fibers? *J Comput Assist Tomogr.* 2009;33(4):565-570.

CASE 36 Petrous temporal bone marrow simulating an IAC lesion on MRI

Occasionally, volume averaging with the petrous temporal bone on an MRI of the brain/IACs may simulate a mass in the IAC, particularly along its medial aspect. If the petrous temporal bone is marrow containing, then the volume averaging will result in intrinsic T1 hyperintense signal that appears to reside in the IAC. Consequently, it follows that a non-fat-suppressed post-contrast T1-weighted sequence will also reveal hyperintensity in the same area, possibly simulating an enhancing lesion such as an IAC schwannoma. Thus, it is critical to evaluate the precontrast T1-weighted sequence in this scenario in order to avoid misinterpretation. Employing a fat suppression technique will result in suppression of the marrow fat and further support volume averaging with the petrous temporal bone. If there is still doubt, then a CT of the temporal bones should clarify the matter. If the volume averaging on MRI is with dense cortical petrous temporal bone, then the volume averaging will be hypointense on all MR pulse sequences, including contrast-enhanced sequences, and will not simulate an enhancing mass on MRI.

Petrous temporal bone marrow simulating an IAC lesion on MRI

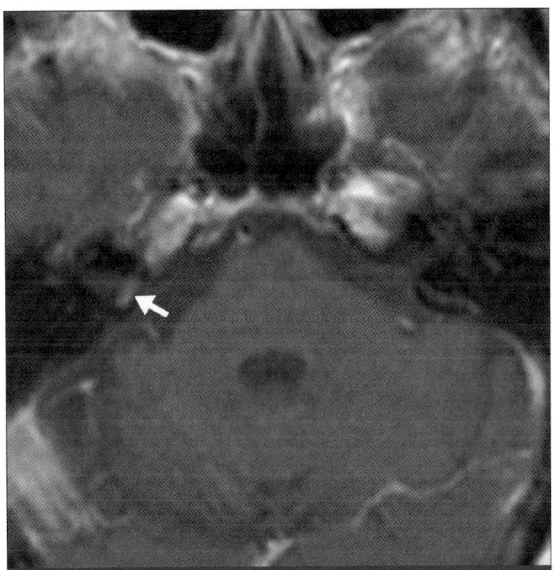

A

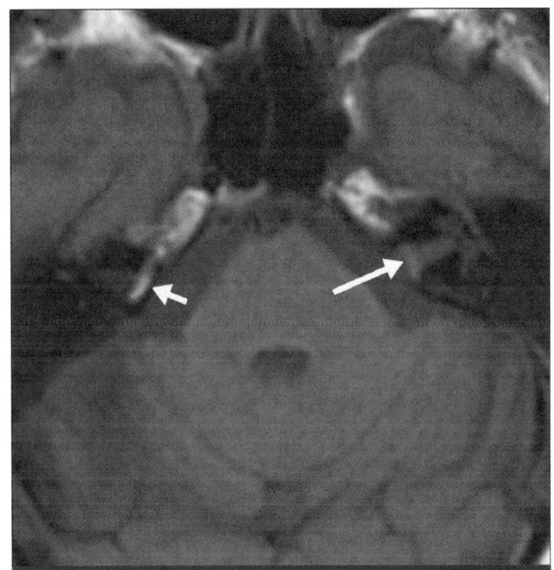

B

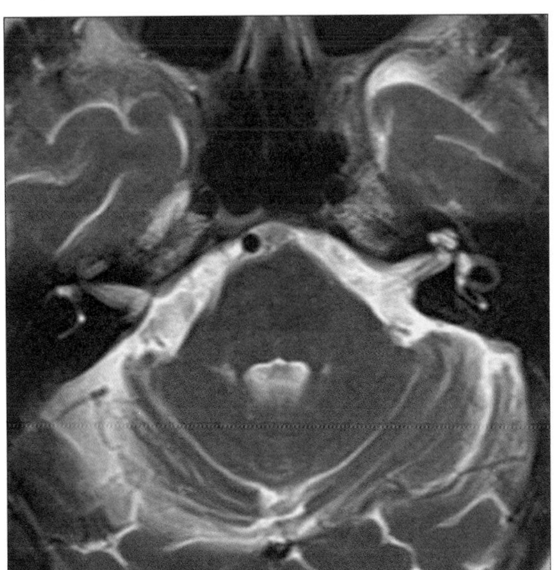

C

Postcontrast axial T1-weighted MR image of the temporal bones (**A**) demonstrates an apparent lesion along the right porus acusticus (short arrow, **A**). However, evaluation of the unenhanced axial T1-weighted MR image (**B**) demonstrates that this finding is intrinsically T1 hyperintense (short arrow, **B**). A similar intrinsically T1 hyperintense finding on the left is also demonstrated on image **B** (long arrow), which is not identified on image **A** because of slice selection. An axial T2-weighted MR image (**C**) does not demonstrate a focal abnormality along either porus acusticus. The findings on the T1-weighted images represent incidental volume averaging of normal petrous marrow and not masses within the IACs.

Petrous temporal bone marrow simulating an IAC lesion on MRI

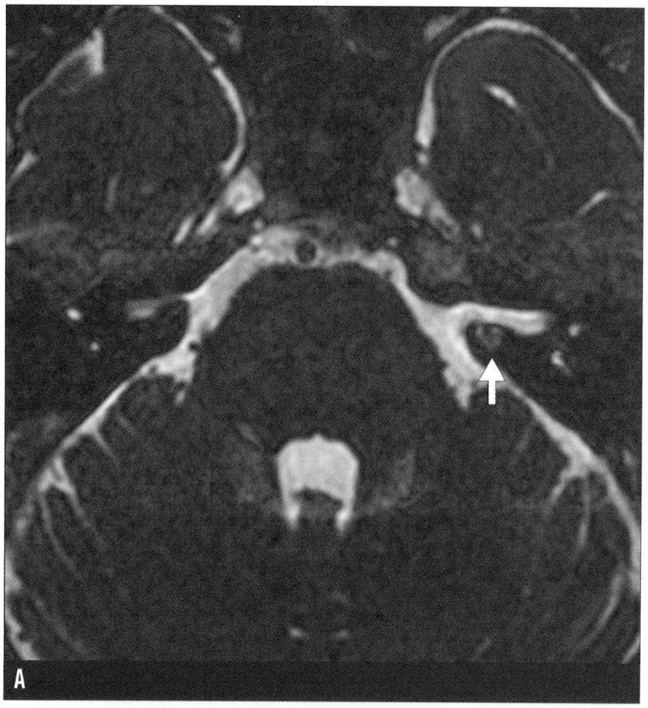

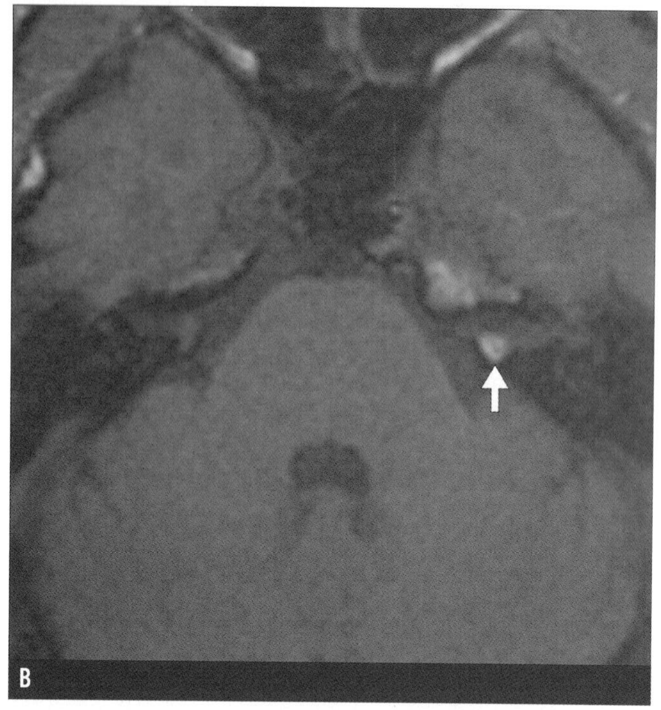

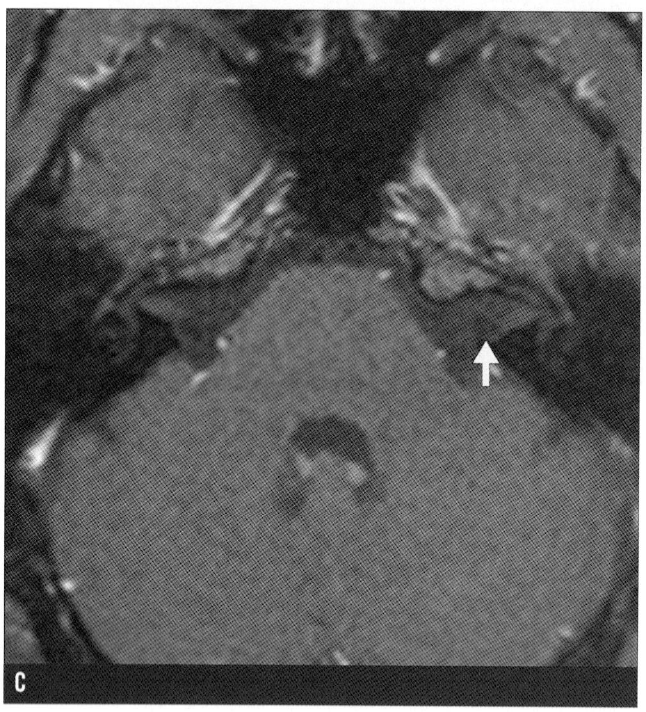

Different patient. Axial CISS (**A**), axial T1 (**B**), and fat-suppressed postcontrast axial T1 (**C**) MR images demonstrate a pseudomass along the posterior wall of the left IAC near the porus acusticus (arrows, **A**-**C**). This finding is intrinsically T1 hyperintense on image **B** and fully suppresses on image **C**, compatible with normal fatty marrow within the adjacent petrous temporal bone.

REFERENCES

Connor SEJ, Leung R, Natas S. Imaging of the petrous apex: a pictorial review. *Br J Radiol.* 2008;81:427-435.

Moore KR, Harnsberger HR, Shelton C, Davidson HC. Leave me alone lesions of the petrous apex. *Am J Neuroradiol.* 1998;19(4):733-738.

Virapongse C, Sarwar M, Bhimani S, Sasaki C, Shapiro R. Computed tomography of temporal bone pneumatization: normal pattern and morphology. *AJR Am J Roentgenol.* 1985;145:473-481.

CASE 37 Asymmetry of the petrous apices

The petrous portion of the temporal bone can be pneumatized, composed of dense cortical bone, or contain a variable amount of marrow fat. With such variability, asymmetry of the petrous apices is a common finding. When present, asymmetry of the petrous apices can mimic a skull base lesion on MRI, particularly when one side contains intrinsically T1 hyperintense marrow fat and the other side is diffusely pneumatized and thus hypointense. However, normal petrous apex marrow fat has the same signal on all MRI pulse sequences as normal fat elsewhere, such as orbital fat. Thus, comparing the petrous marrow fat with orbital fat on various pulse sequences should allow for an appropriate diagnosis of incidental petrous marrow fat. Furthermore, normal petrous apex marrow fat will completely suppress on a fat-suppressed T1-weighted MRI sequence, an imaging technique that can confirm the presence of normal fat if there is still a question regarding the finding. On CT, normal fatty marrow-containing petrous temporal bone will be subtly lucent, sometimes containing regions with Hounsfield units compatible with fat.

COMPANION CASE

- **Intraosseous venous malformation (intraosseous hemangioma).** Historically, a fat-containing lesion in bone that typically enhances has been termed an intraosseous hemangioma. However, more recent histopathologic literature supports that this entity is more appropriately characterized as a venous malformation. On CT, an intraosseous venous malformation is usually lucent and contains coarse osseous trabeculations. Hounsfield units within the lucency may reveal fat attenuation. On MRI, an intraosseous venous malformation is usually T2 hyperintense, enhances, and may contain solid or speckled intrinsic T1 hyperintense signal because of the presence of fat.

Normal asymmetric petrous apex marrow

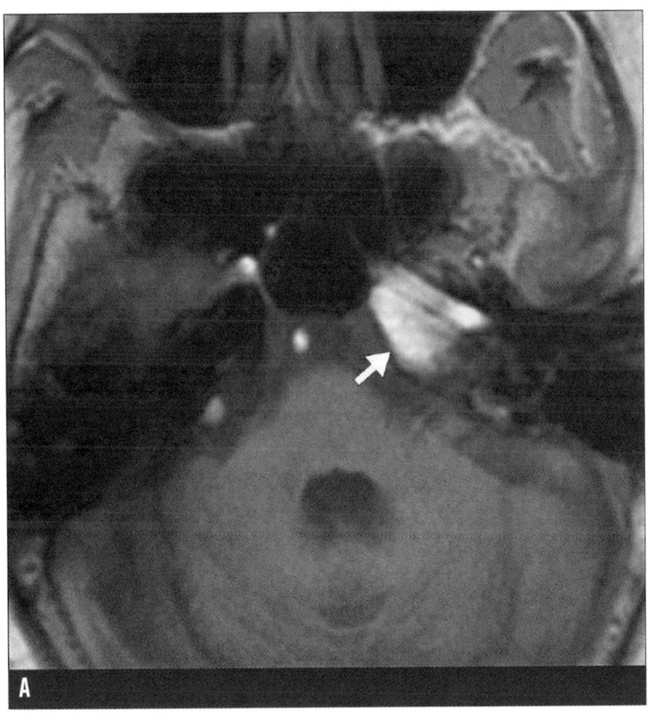

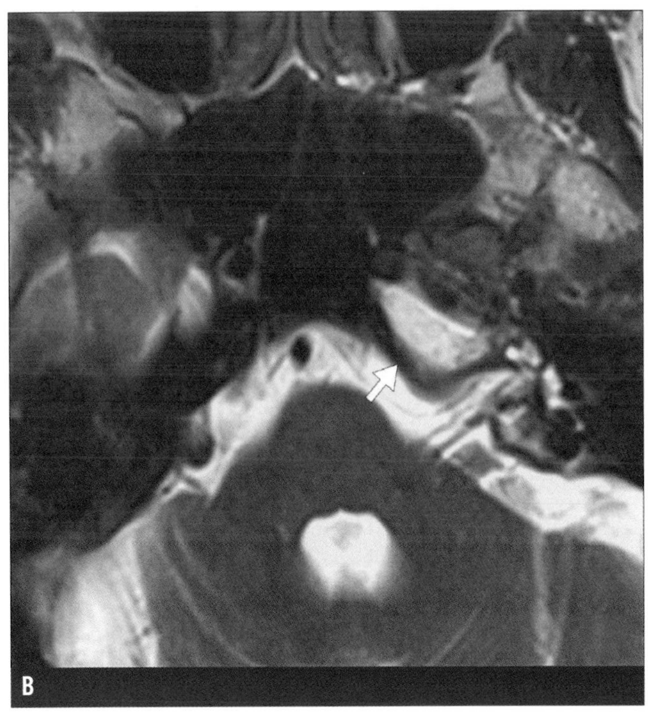

Axial T1 (**A**), axial T2 (**B**), and postcontrast coronal MPRAGE (**C**) MR images through the petrous apices demonstrate hyperintense T1 signal (arrow, **A**), hyperintense T2 signal (arrow, **B**), and no enhancement (arrow, **C**) of the left petrous apex relative to the right. The intrinsically T1 hyperintense signal on image **A** also suppresses on a fat-suppressed postcontrast coronal T1-weighted MR image (arrow, **D**). Furthermore, the left petrous apex signal follows normal fat signal elsewhere on all pulse sequences. Thus, the signal is compatible with normal fat-containing marrow in the left petrous apex and does not represent a skull base mass. Axial CT images of the same patient viewed with a bone window (**E**) and an intermediate window (**F**). Image **E** demonstrates pneumatization of the right petrous apex and nonpneumatization of the left petrous apex (arrow, **E**). Image **F** demonstrates mild lucency within the left petrous apex compatible with fatty marrow (arrow, **F**), corroborating the finding on MRI.

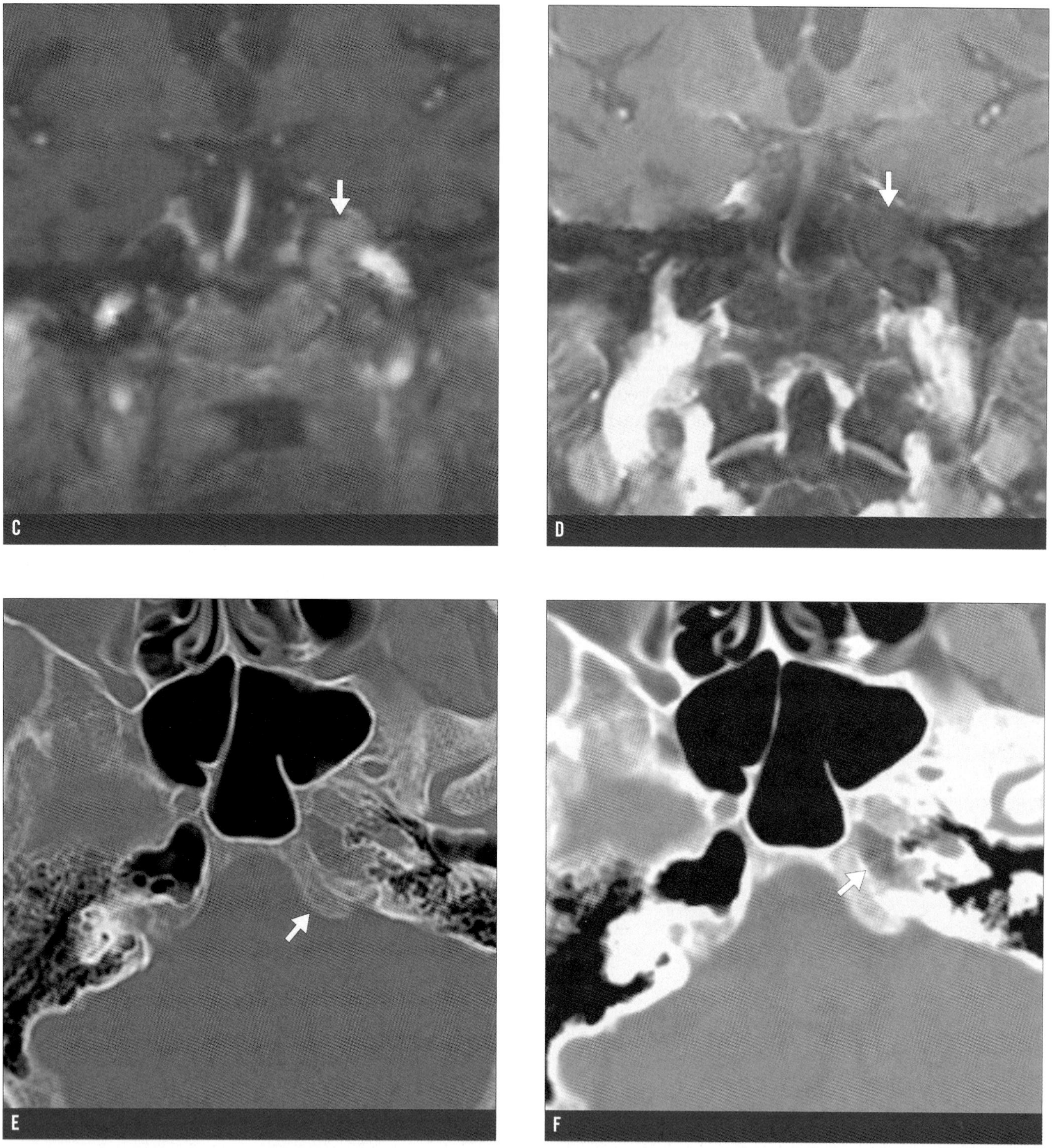
C
D
E
F

Normal island of nonpneumatized petrous apex marrow

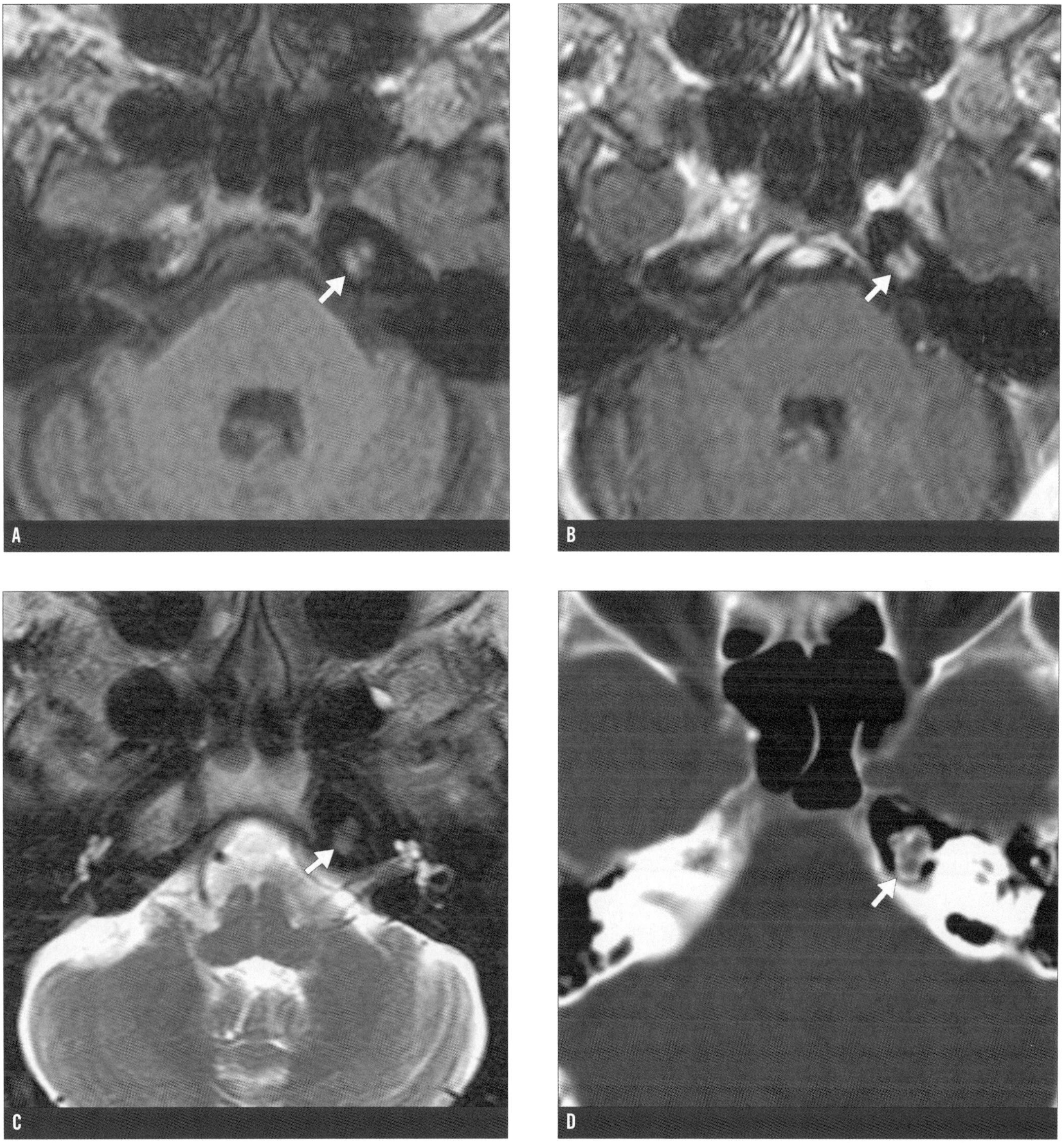

Axial T1 (**A**), postcontrast axial MPRAGE (**B**), and axial T2 (**C**) MR images through the petrous apices demonstrate a nonenhancing, T1 and T2 hyperintense focus in the anterior aspect of the left petrous apex (arrows, **A**-**C**). The possibility of a cholesterol granuloma was raised on this study. An axial CT image viewed with an intermediate window (**D**) demonstrates the finding to contain attenuation compatible with fat (arrow, **D**), which was confirmed with Hounsfield units. Therefore, the finding is compatible with an island of nonpneumatized normal fatty marrow in the petrous apex and not consistent with a cholesterol granuloma.

Companion case: Intraosseous venous malformation (intraosseous hemangioma)

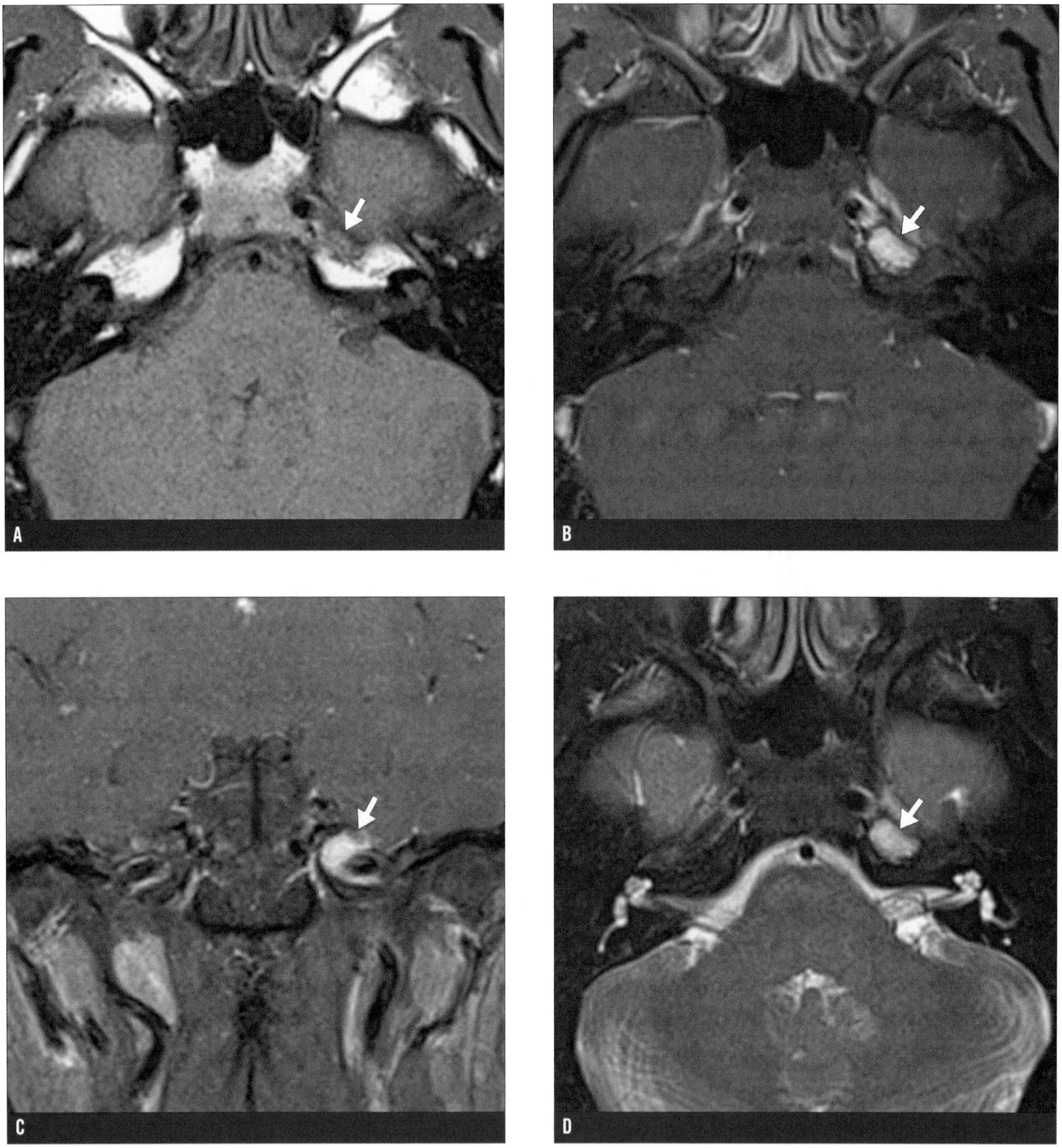

Axial T1 (**A**), fat-suppressed postcontrast axial T1 (**B**), fat-suppressed postcontrast coronal T1 (**C**), and fat-suppressed axial T2 (**D**) MR images demonstrate a focal lesion of the left petrous apex (arrows, **A**-**D**). Image **A** demonstrates the finding to be mostly T1 hypointense with subtle speckled foci of intrinsic T1 shortening. Images **B** and **C** demonstrate diffuse enhancement of the lesion, whereas image **D** reveals the finding to be largely T2 hyperintense. The imaging characteristics are most compatible with an intraosseous venous malformation. However, a follow-up study to document the stability is advisable with this type of finding, as a primary malignancy bone tumor or a metastatic lesion could have a similar appearance. The finding in this patient was entirely stable on a study obtained 2 years later (not shown). While an intraosseous venous malformation frequently contains speckled fat, the fat is usually less pronounced compared to asymmetric petrous apex marrow fat. In this patient, abundant fatty marrow is present elsewhere within the petrous apices, with expected suppression on the fat-saturated sequences.

REFERENCES

Connor SEJ, Leung R, Natas S. Imaging of the petrous apex: a pictorial review. *Br J Radiol.* 2008;81:427-435.

Lowe LH, Marchant TC, Rivard DC, Scherbel AJ. Vascular malformations: classification and terminology the radiologist needs to know. *Semin Roentgenol.* 2012;47(2):106-117.

Moore KR, Harnsberger HR, Shelton C, Davidson HC. Leave me alone lesions of the petrous apex. *Am J Neuroradiol.* 1998;19(4):733-738.

Politi M, et al. Intraosseous hemangioma of the skull with dural tail sign: radiologic features with pathologic correlation. *AJNR Am J Neuroradiol.* 2005;26:2049-2052.

Virapongse C, Sarwar M, Bhimani S, Sasaki C, Shapiro R. Computed tomography of temporal bone pneumatization: Normal pattern and morphology. *AJR Am J Roentgenol.* 1985;145:473-481.

Fluid accumulation in the petrous apex likely occurs because of obstruction of small osseous channels that are located between the petrous apex and middle ear. The MRI appearance of fluid in the petrous apex can vary and depends upon the protein content of the fluid. If the fluid does not contain a significant amount of protein, then petrous apex fluid will generally appear hypointense on T1, hyperintense on T2, and hypointense on FLAIR. If the fluid in the petrous apex is proteinaceous, then it will often appear hyperintense on T1, variable on T2, and hyperintense on FLAIR, potentially simulating a cholesterol granuloma on MRI. In cases where there is difficulty in distinguishing a proteinaceous petrous apex effusion from a cholesterol granuloma on MRI, correlation with CT (preferably thin section temporal bone imaging) is often helpful. If the petrous apex in question contains preserved osseous septa and no evidence of petrous apex expansion on CT imaging, then a diagnosis of a petrous apex effusion can be favored. If there is evidence of expansion of an opacified petrous apex with septal destruction/loss on CT imaging, then a pathologic process should be considered, such as a cholesterol granuloma. Occasionally, one may encounter opacification of a petrous apex air cell that is inherently devoid of osseous septations. In this case, it may be difficult to differentiate a petrous apex effusion from a newly developing cholesterol granuloma. Either correlation with prior CT imaging or follow-up imaging to assess for change would likely be necessary in this setting. Finally, there is literature that describes symptomatic petrous apex effusions, although this should only be considered in the appropriate clinical context and when other etiologies for the patient's symptoms have been excluded.

COMPANION CASES

- **Cholesterol granuloma.** A cholesterol granuloma (CG), also known as a cholesterol cyst, is an expansile lesion that arises in a pneumatized osseous structure and is the result of localized repeated hemorrhage. The most common location of a CG is the petrous apex, although they have also been reported to arise in other areas, including other portions of the temporal bone, the orbit, and the paranasal sinuses. Pathologically, a CG is characterized by an inflammatory reaction to hemorrhagic byproducts and is composed of brown viscous fluid, cholesterol crystals, multinucleated giant cells, hemosiderin-laden macrophages, and granulation tissue. It is often surrounded by a thick capsule that lacks a true epithelial lining. The etiology of a petrous apex CG is not completely understood, although the general consensus is that it forms following occlusion of pneumatized channels located between the petrous apex and middle ear. This is believed to result in negative pressure and extravasation of fluid into the mucosa of the air cells. If the mucosal edema is prolonged, then mucosal breakdown and hemorrhage occurs. The cycle repeats itself and results in an expanding mass in the petrous apex associated with osseous remodeling and air cell erosion. On MRI, a CG does not enhance, is variable in signal on T2-weighted imaging, and at least a portion is intrinsically hyperintense on T1-weighted imaging. However, the signal characteristics depend on the proteinaceous content and/or stage of hemorrhage. On CT, a petrous apex CG is frequently expansile and there is usually clear evidence of petrous apex septal destruction/loss.
- **Petrous apicitis.** Petrous apicitis represents an infection of the petrous temporal bone with formation of a purulent abscess. Petrous apicitis is most commonly secondary to direct spread of a middle ear infection through longitudinal pneumatized channels that connect the middle ear cavity to the petrous apex. This route of infection spread will usually only occur if the petrous apex is pneumatized. However, infection can also spread to the petrous apex via a retrograde thrombophlebitis from the petrous carotid canal venous plexus or direct spread from a malignant otitis externa. Spread of infection from these alternate pathways can also result in a petrous temporal bone infection, even if the petrous temporal bone is nonpneumatized. An infection of a nonpneumatized petrous temporal bone is more appropriately termed an osteomyelitis of the petrous apex.

  The classic clinical triad of a petrous apicitis, termed Gradenigo syndrome, includes an abducens nerve palsy, otorrhea, and pain in the distribution of the trigeminal nerve. However, this triad is not present in all patients with a petrous apicitis. On CT, a petrous apicitis is associated with opacification of the petrous apex air cells and osseous septal destruction. Contrast-enhanced MR imaging can demonstrate enhancing inflammatory soft tissue surrounding and/or within the petrous apex as well as within the infratemporal fossa. There may also be intracranial dural enhancement, enhancement of the affected cranial nerves, and abnormal enhancement/thrombosis of the cavernous sinus. The petrous apex osseous destruction and associated enhancing inflammatory changes distinguish a petrous apicitis from a sterile petrous apex effusion. While both a CG and petrous apicitis are associated with osseous destruction, a CG does not enhance nor is it associated with advanced regional inflammation frequently identified with a petrous apicitis.

Petrous apex effusion

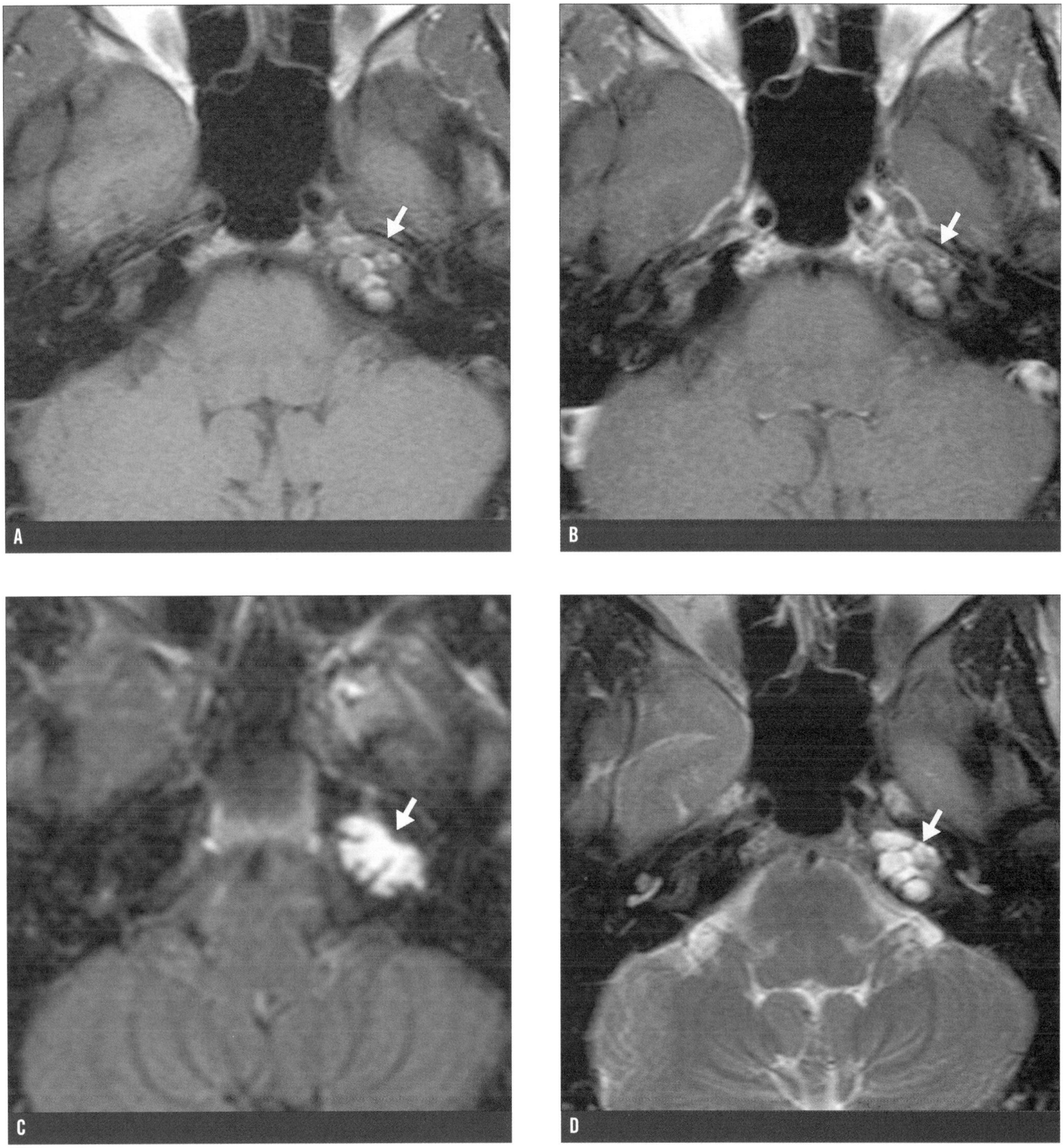

Axial T1 (**A**), postcontrast axial T1 (**B**), axial FLAIR (**C**), and axial T2 (**D**) MR images through the mid skull base demonstrate an intrinsically T1 hyperintense, T2/FLAIR hyperintense, nonenhancing lesion in the left petrous apex (arrows, **A**-**D**). There is thin, curvilinear FLAIR and T2 hypointense signal throughout the lesion, suggesting intact petrous apex septa and favoring a petrous apex effusion. Axial (**E**) and coronal reformatted (**F**) CT images of the left temporal bone from the same patient demonstrate intact petrous apex septa (arrows, **E**, **F**). An axial CT image through the petrous apices (**G**) does not demonstrate evidence of left petrous apex expansion relative to the contralateral, well-aerated petrous apex. These CT findings are consistent with a petrous apex effusion and effectively exclude a cholesterol granuloma.

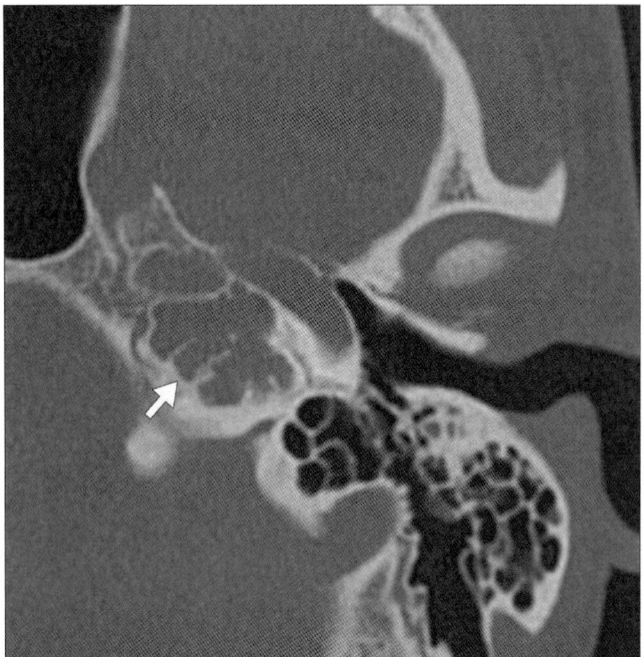
E

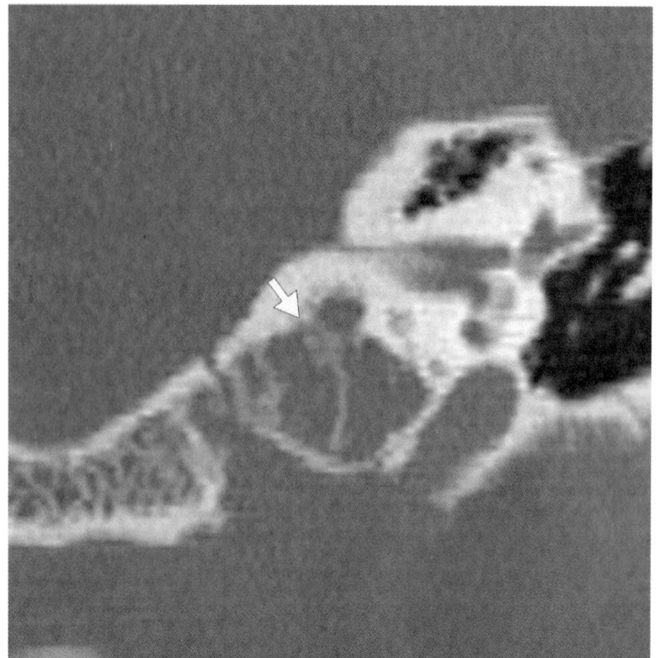
F

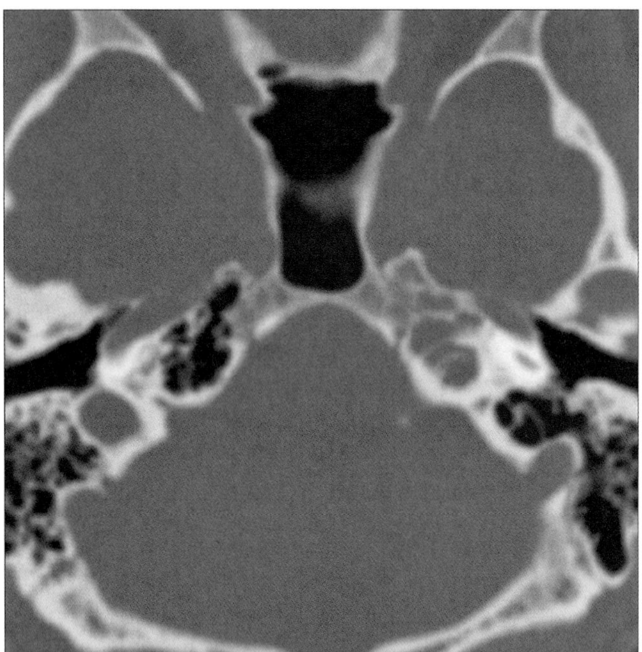
G

Petrous apex effusion

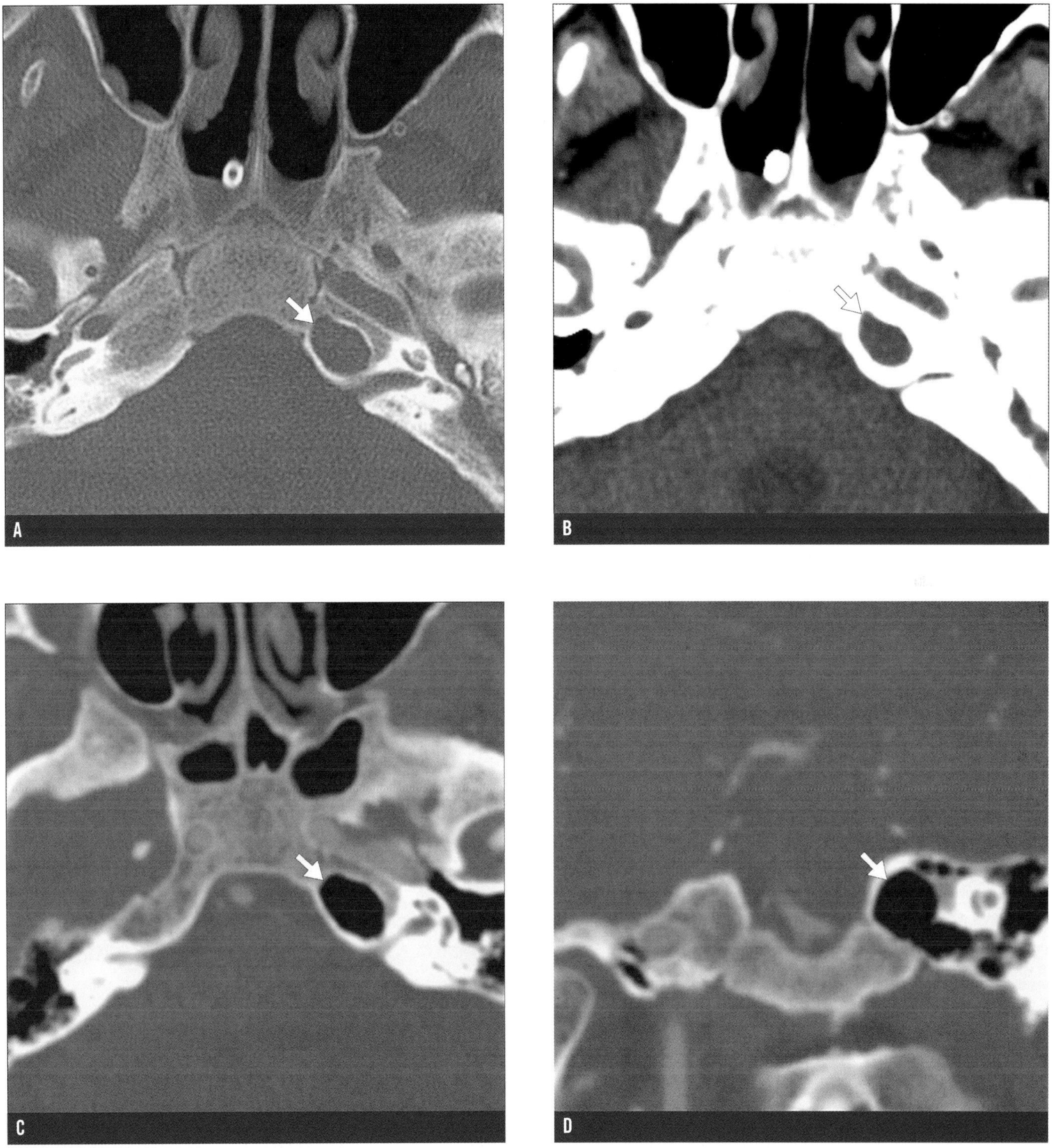

Different patient. Axial CT images viewed with a bone window (**A**) and a soft tissue window (**B**) demonstrate a focal, circumscribed, oval lucency in the left petrous apex that is opacified (arrows, **A**, **B**). The visualized left mastoid air cells and both tympanic cavities are also opacified. The finding in the petrous apex was interpreted as a petrous apex mucocele or a cholesterol granuloma, largely because of its shape. However, axial (**C**) and coronal reformatted (**D**) images from a CTA of the head obtained 1 month earlier demonstrate the left petrous apex to contain an aerated, oval air cell that is exactly the same size as the opacified air cell from the study obtained 1 month later (arrows, **C**, **D**). Thus, the finding on images **A** and **B** simply represents an effusion and not a mucocele or cholesterol granuloma. Axial T1 (**E**) and axial T2 (**F**) MR images obtained on the same day as images **C** and **D** demonstrate lack of signal in this same area of the left petrous apex, also compatible with aeration of this air cell (arrows, **E**, **F**).

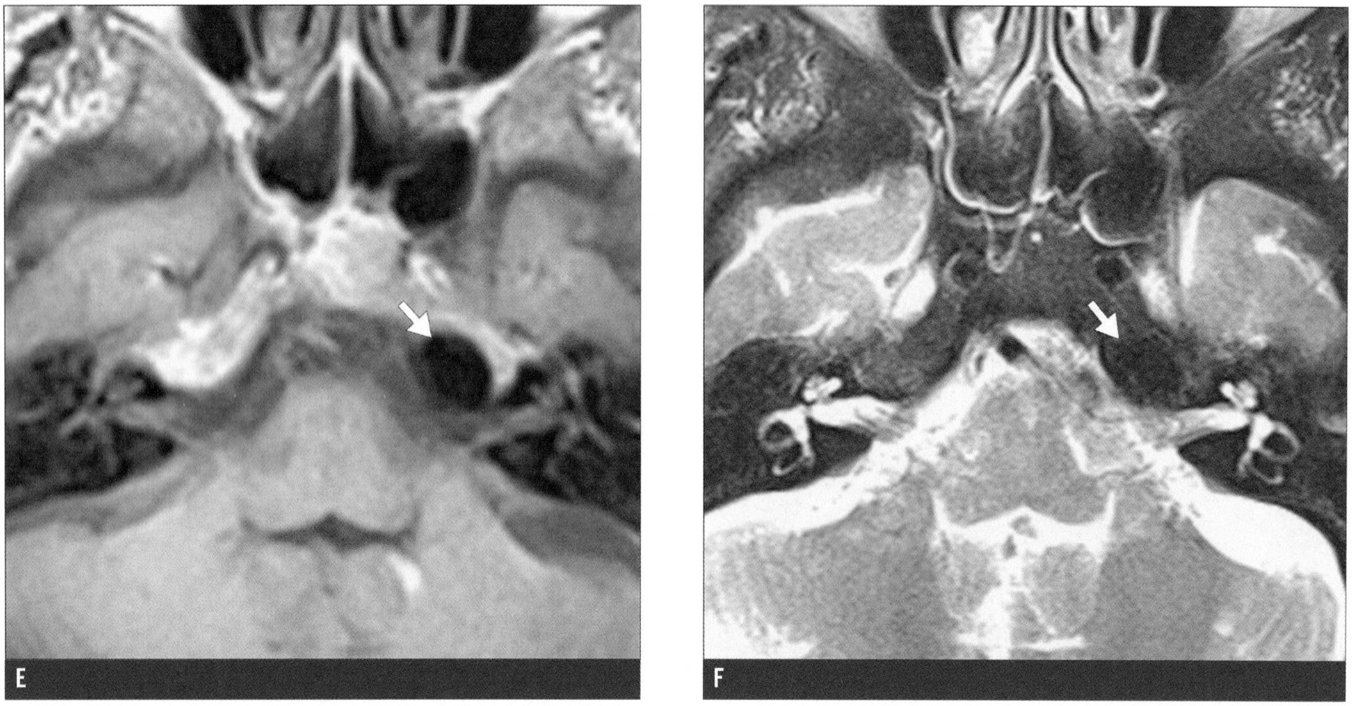

Companion case: Cholesterol granuloma

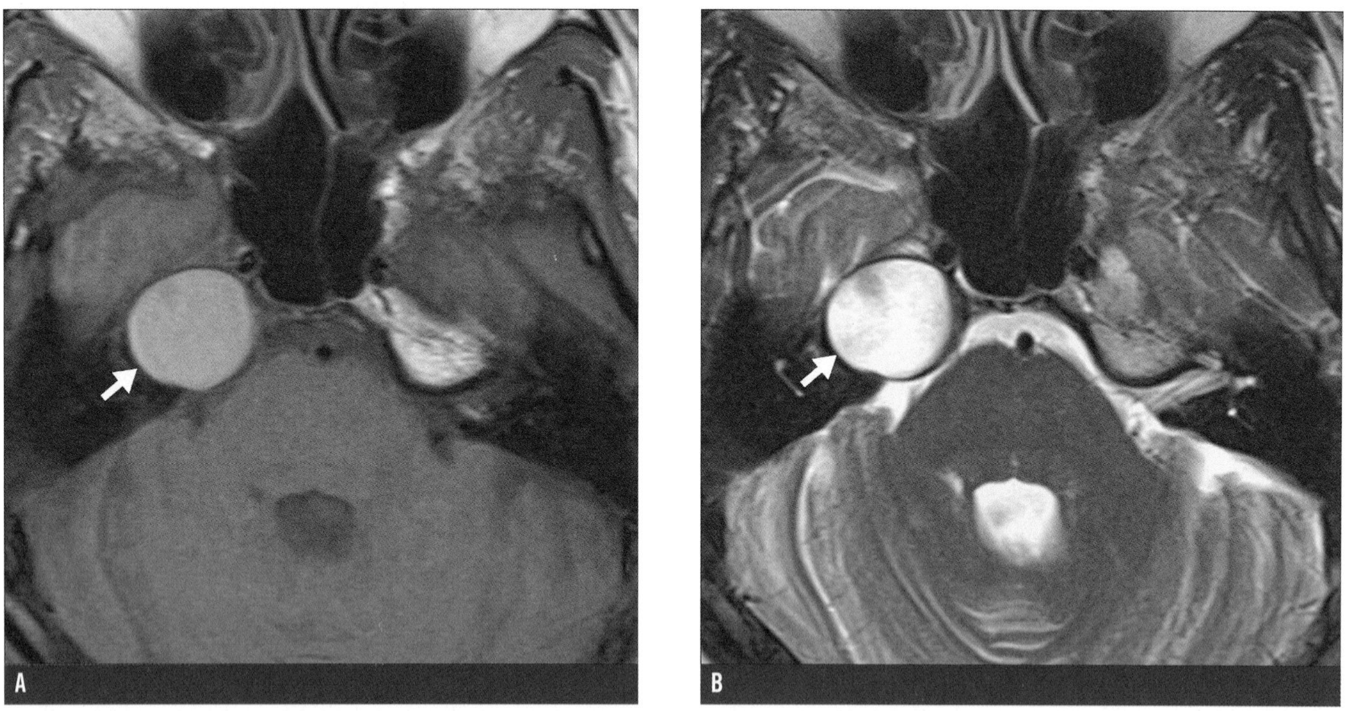

Axial T1 (**A**), axial T2 (**B**), and fat-suppressed postcontrast coronal T1 (**C**) MR images demonstrate a nonenhancing, T1 and T2 hyper-intense, expansile lesion centered in the right petrous apex, compatible with a cholesterol granuloma (arrows, **A**-**C**). An axial CT image through the same region viewed with a bone window (**D**) demonstrates the expansile lesion to contain smooth osseous borders which appear dehiscent (arrow, **D**). Notably, there are no identifiable petrous apex air cell septa. This is in contradistinction to normal petrous apex marrow fat or a sterile petrous apex effusion, neither of which are expansile or associated with petrous apex air cell disruption. A noncontrast axial CT image viewed with a soft tissue window (**E**) demonstrates the lesion to be isodense to brain (arrow, **E**). The density on CT as well as the signal characteristics on MRI can vary with a cholesterol granuloma, depending on the proteinaceous content and/or stage of hemorrhage.

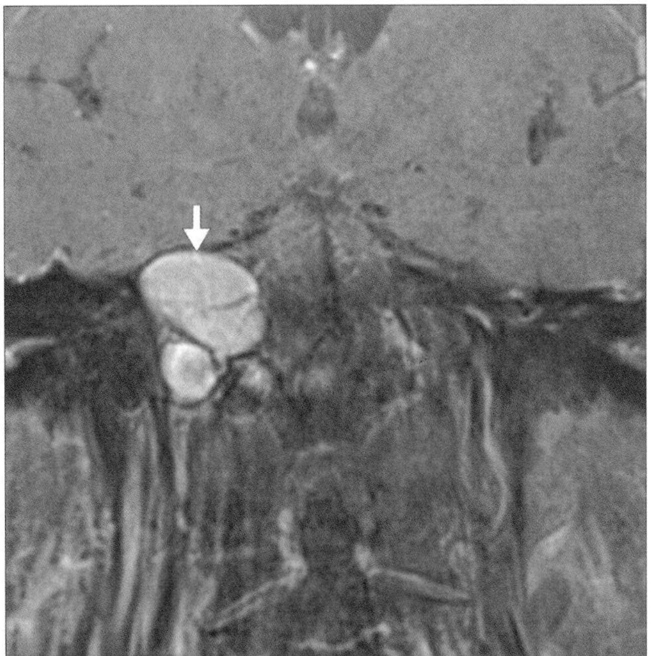
C

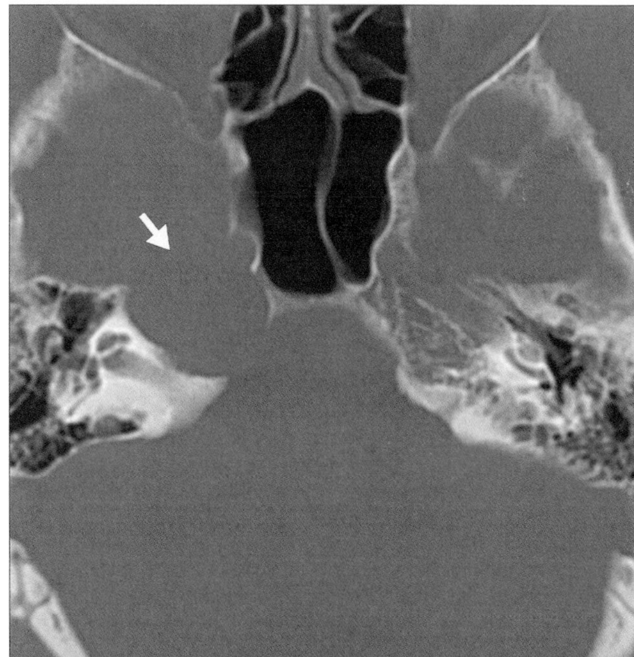
D

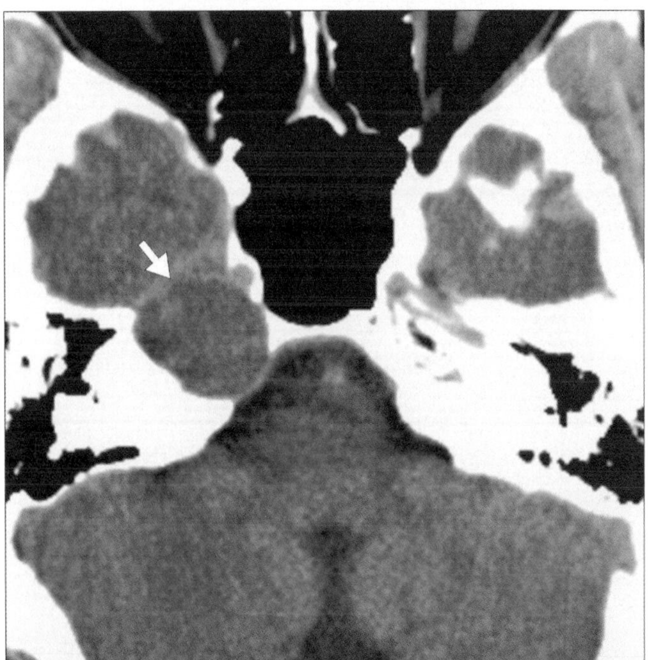
E

Companion case: Petrous apicitis

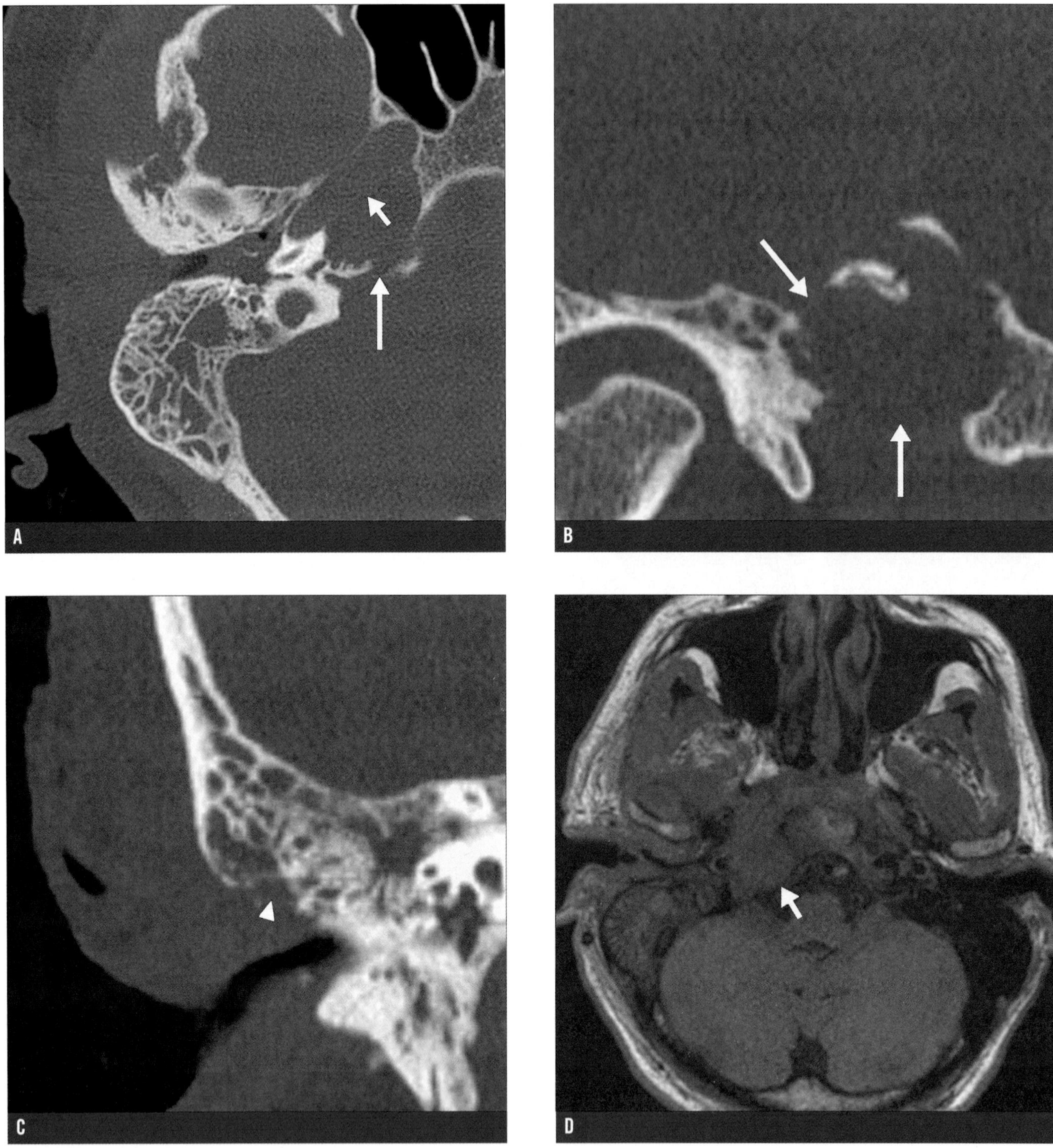

Axial (**A**) and coronal reformatted (**B**, **C**) CT images demonstrate an expansile, erosive lesion involving the right petrous apex (long arrows, **A**, **B**) as well as erosion of a portion of the right mastoid air cells (arrowhead, **C**). The expansile lesion in the right petrous apex has eroded the posteromedial wall of the petrous carotid canal (short arrow, **A**). Axial T1 (**D**) and axial T2 (**E**) MR images through the skull base demonstrate T1 isointense signal (short arrow, **D**) and T2 hyperintense signal (short arrow, **E**) in the right petrous apex. An axial T1-weighted MR image through the suprazygomatic temporal fossa (**F**) demonstrates T1 isointense signal and abnormal thickening of the right temporalis muscle (short arrow, **F**). Fat-suppressed postcontrast axial T1-weighted MR images through the petrous apices (**G**) and the suprazygomatic temporal fossae (**H**) demonstrate marked peripheral enhancement in the right petrous apex (short arrows, **G**) and right suprazygomatic temporal fossa (short arrow, **H**). A small amount of intracranial, extraaxial enhancement in the lateral aspect of the right middle cranial fossa is also present (arrowhead, **H**), compatible with intracranial extension of this process. Axial DWI (**I**) and its corresponding ADC map (**J**) through the petrous apices demonstrate diffusion restriction in the right petrous apex lesion (short arrows, **I**, **J**). The constellation of findings is consistent with a right petrous apicitis with multiple areas of osseous erosion as well as extracranial and intracranial extension of infection.

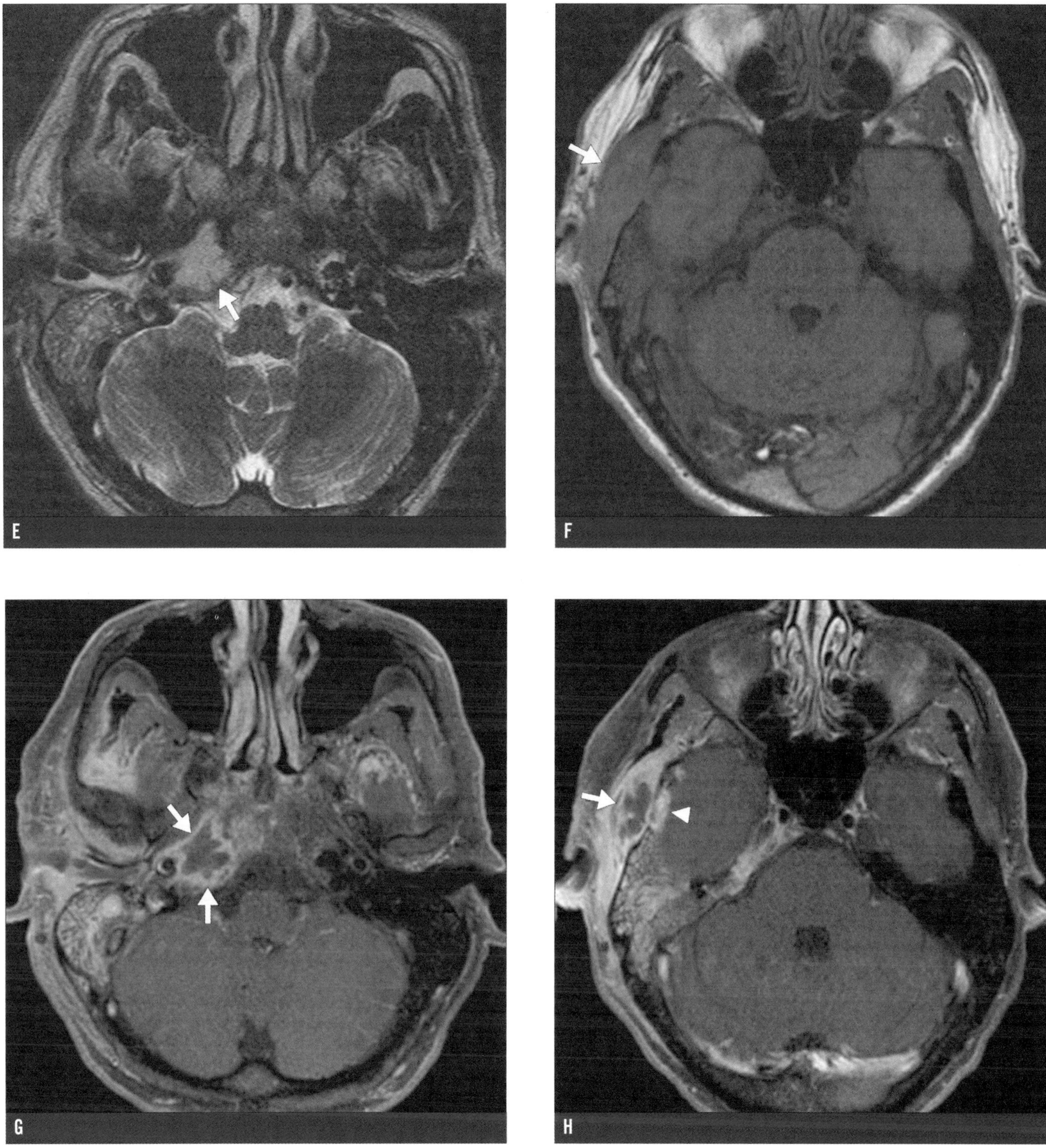
E
F
G
H

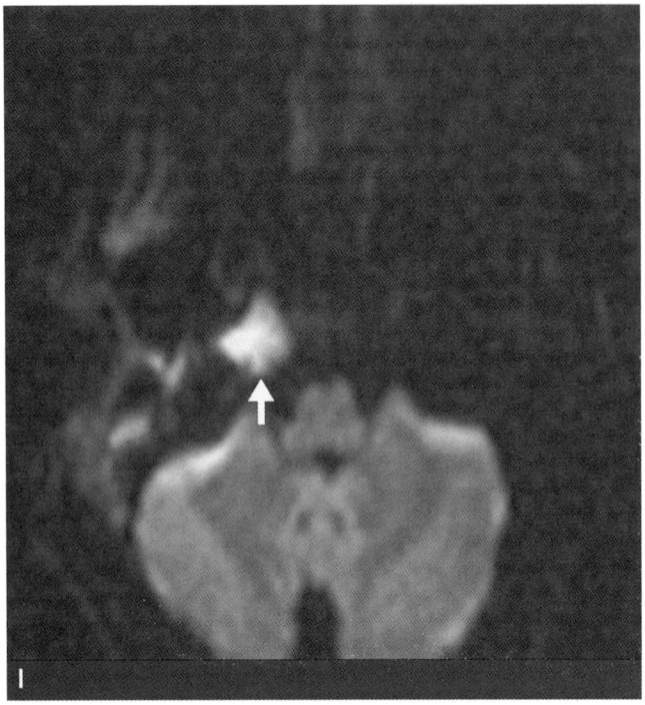

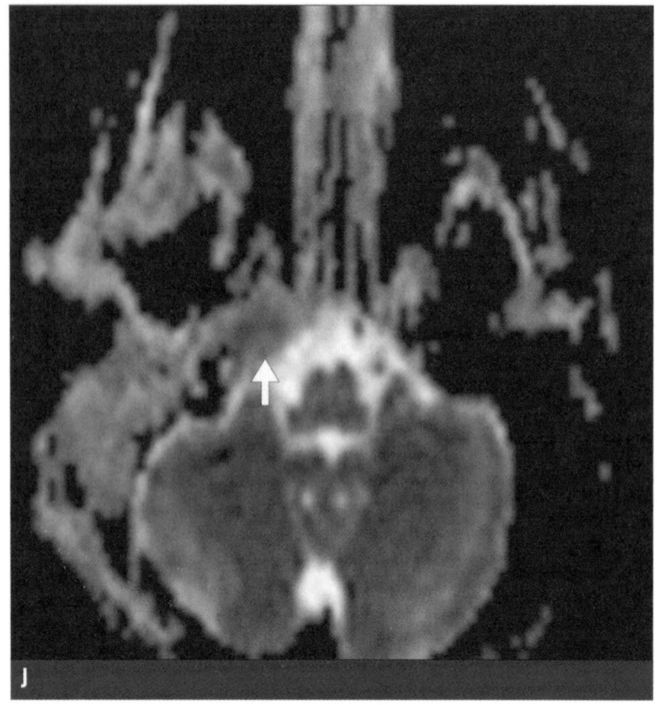

REFERENCES

Connor SEJ, Leung R, Natas S. Imaging of the petrous apex: a pictorial review. *Br J Radiol.* 2008;81:427-435.

Lee YH, Lee NJ, Kim JH, Song JJ. CT, MR and gallium SPECT in the diagnosis and treatment of petrous apicitis presenting as multiple cranial neuropathies. *Br J Radiol.* 2005;78:948-951.

Moises, A. Petrous apex effusion: a clinical disorder. *Laryngoscope.* 2006;116:1349-1356.

Moore KR, et al. Petrous apex cephaloceles. *Am J Neuroradiol.* 2001;22(10):1867-1871.

Murugasu E, Yong TT, Yoon CP. Invasive middle ear cholesterol granuloma involving the basal turn of the cochlea with profound sensorineural hearing loss. *Otol Neurotol.* 2004;25:231-235.

Razek AA, Huang BY. Lesions of the petrous apex: classification and findings at CT and MR imaging. Radiographics. 2012;32(1):151-173.

Royer MC, Pensak ML. Cholesterol granulomas. *Curr Opin Otolaryngol Head Neck Surg.* 2007;15(5):319-322.

A petrous apex cephalocele is a protrusion of meninges and cerebrospinal fluid (CSF) that arises from the ipsilateral Meckel cave and herniates into the adjacent petrous apex. This lesion is contiguous with the posterolateral margin of the Meckel cave. A petrous apex cephalocele may be unilateral or bilateral. Because petrous apex cephaloceles contain CSF, they are CSF equivalent on all MRI pulse sequences as well as on CT. CT will also demonstrate smooth remodeling and occasionally expansion of the petrous apex.

Petrous apex cephaloceles are typically incidental findings and of no clinical significance. Occasionally, they may be associated with meningitis and CSF leaks as well as cranial nerve palsies. However, surgical intervention should only be performed if there is sufficient clinical evidence that the patient's symptoms arise from the finding. Otherwise, these are "leave me alone" findings.

Petrous apex cephaloceles

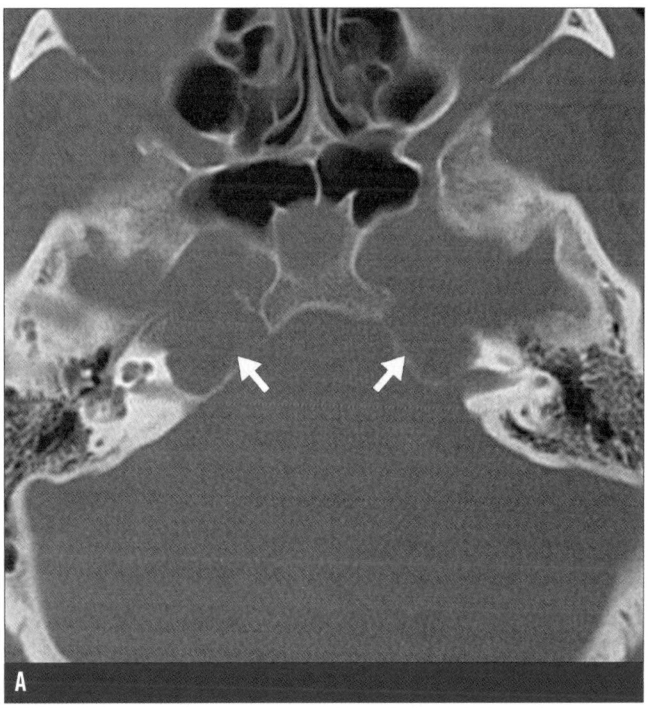

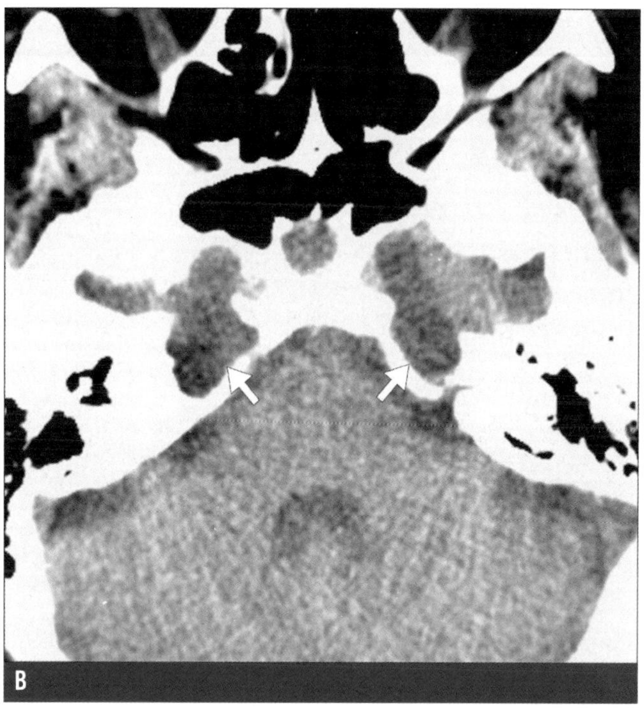

An axial CT image at the level of the petrous apices viewed with a bone window (**A**) demonstrates smooth expansion of the petrous apices (arrows, **A**). A noncontrast axial CT image viewed with a soft tissue window at the same level as image **A** (**B**) demonstrates CSF equivalent density in the petrous apices (arrows, **B**) which are contiguous with the CSF within each Meckel cave. Axial T1 (**C**, **D**), axial T2 (**E**, **F**), axial FLAIR (**G**), and contrast-enhanced coronal reformatted MPRAGE (**H**) MR images of the same patient demonstrate the petrous apex findings to be nonenhancing and CSF equivalent (arrows, **C**-**H**). Images **C**-**F** perhaps best demonstrate the herniation of the CSF and meninges from the Meckel caves into the petrous apices. These imaging findings are consistent with bilateral petrous apex cephaloceles. This patient was asymptomatic from these findings.

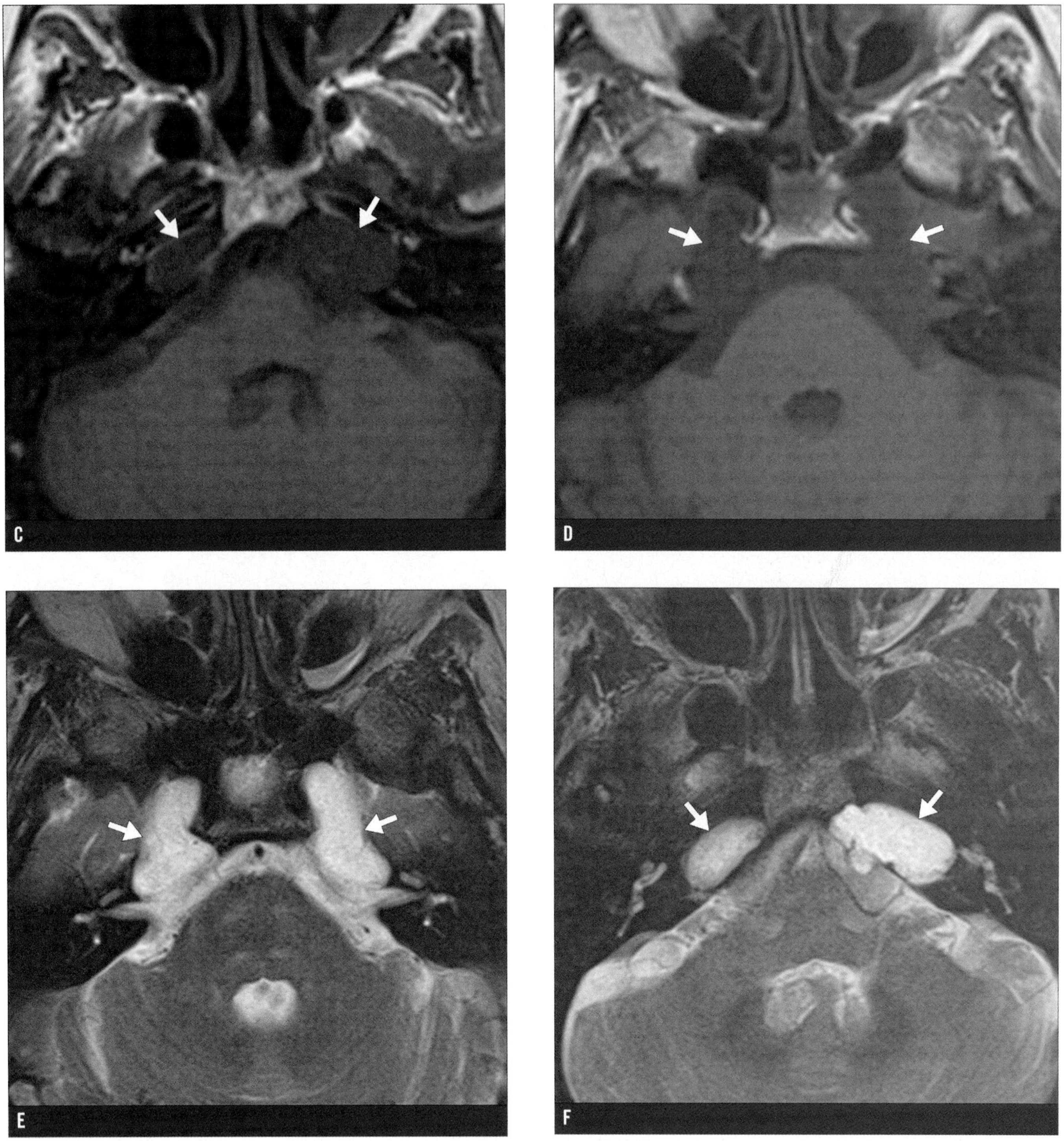
C
D
E
F

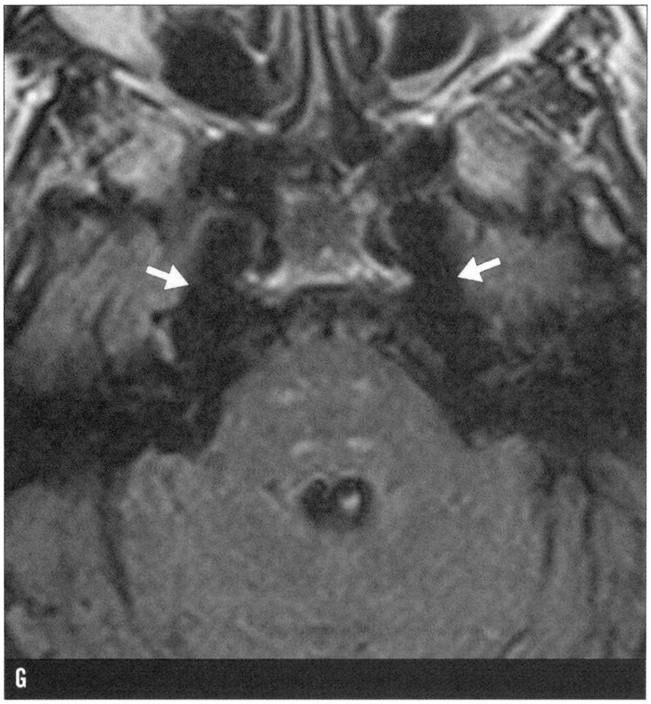

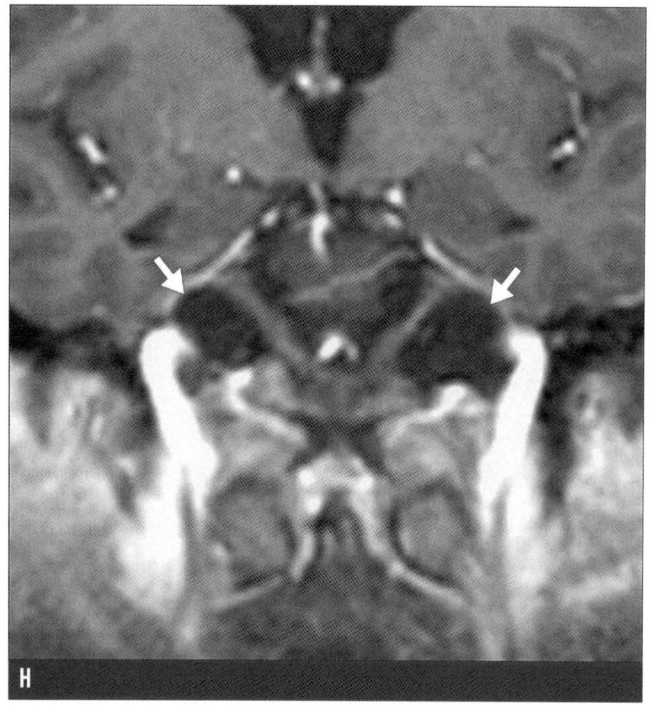

Petrous apex cephalocele

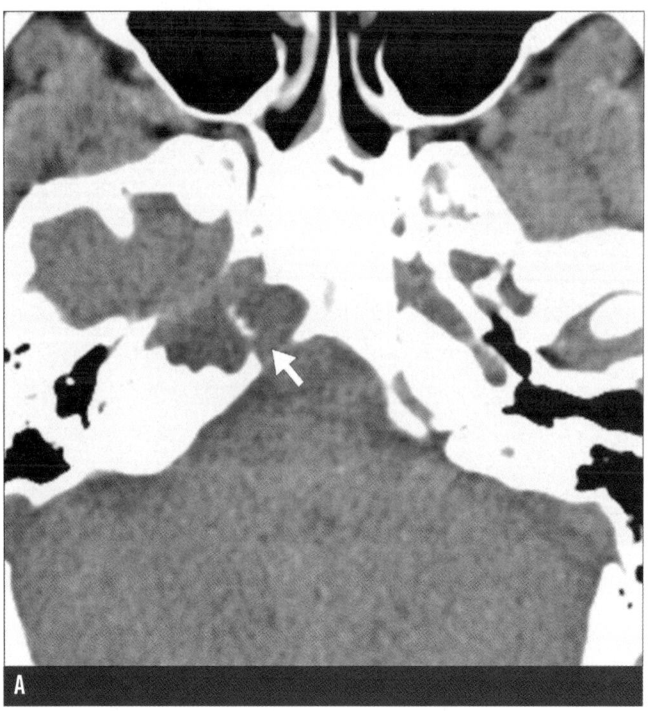

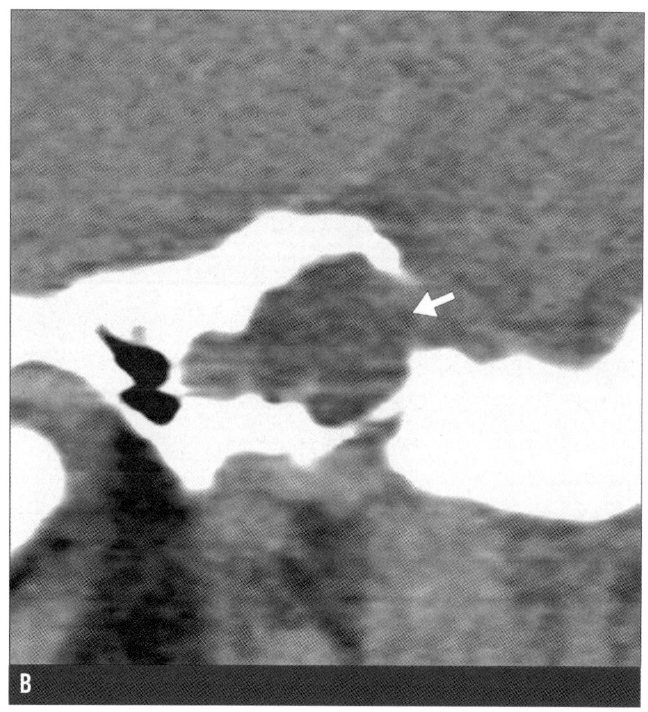

Different patient. Noncontrast axial (**A**) and direct coronal (**B**) CT images through the mid skull base viewed with a soft tissue window demonstrate a CSF equivalent lesion in the right petrous apex (arrows, **A**, **B**). Thin section axial (**C**) and a direct coronal (**D**) CT images through the right mid skull base viewed with a bone window demonstrate smooth osseous expansion of the right petrous apex (arrows, **C**, **D**). There is also erosion of the posteromedial wall of the right petrous carotid canal (arrowheads, **C**). Axial FLAIR (**E**), axial T2 (**F**), postcontrast axial MPRAGE (**G**), and postcontrast coronal MPRAGE (**H**) MR images of the same patient demonstrate the finding to be CSF equivalent and nonenhancing on MRI (arrows, **E**-**H**). The findings based on CT and MRI are compatible with a right petrous apex cephalocele. The clinical implication of the right petrous carotid canal erosion was unclear, although the patient was not symptomatic from these findings at the time of either imaging study.

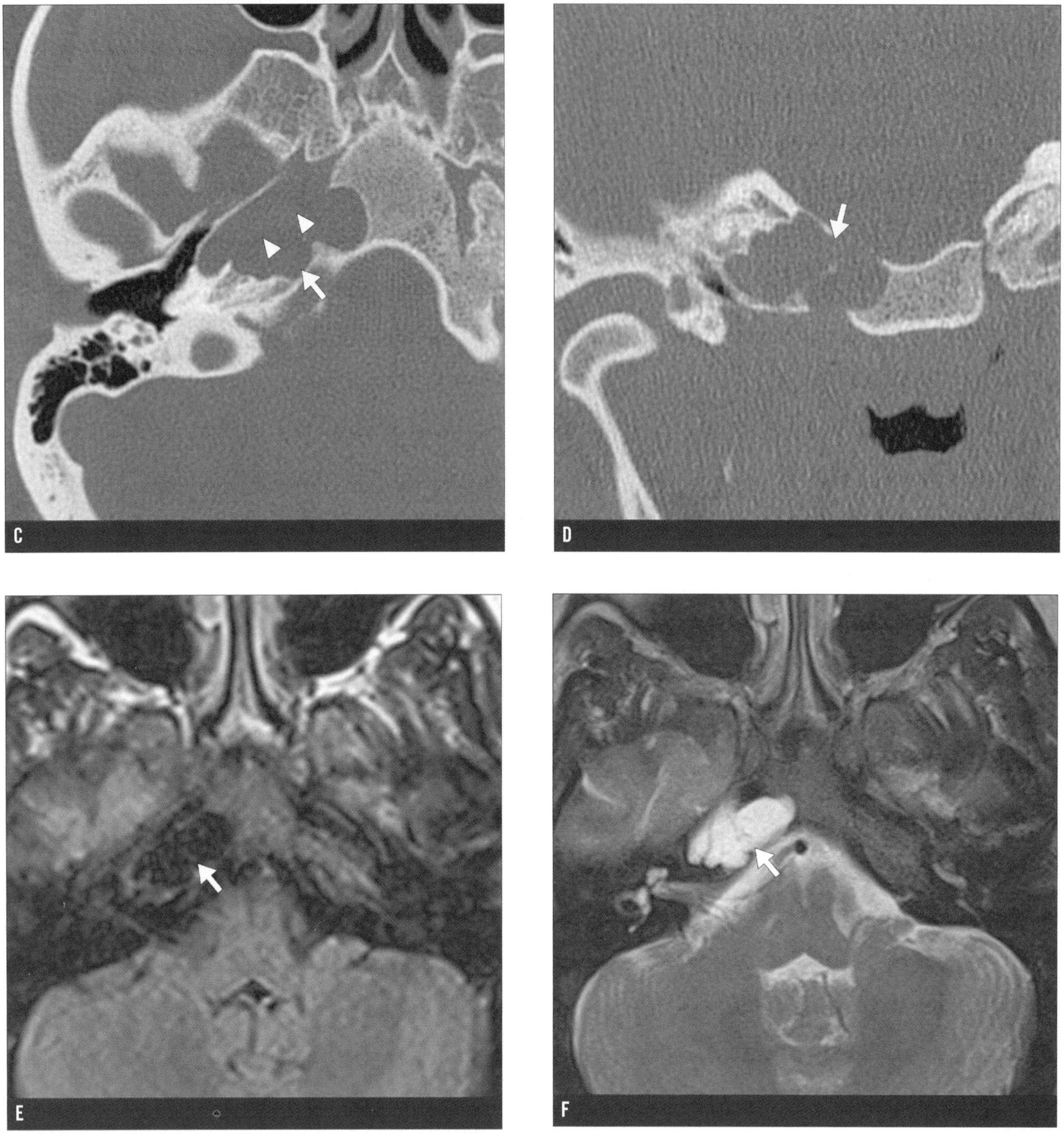

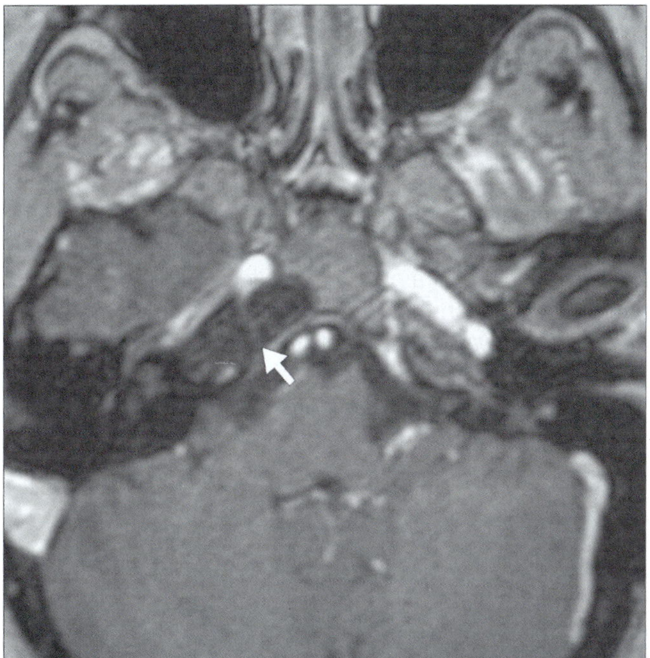

G

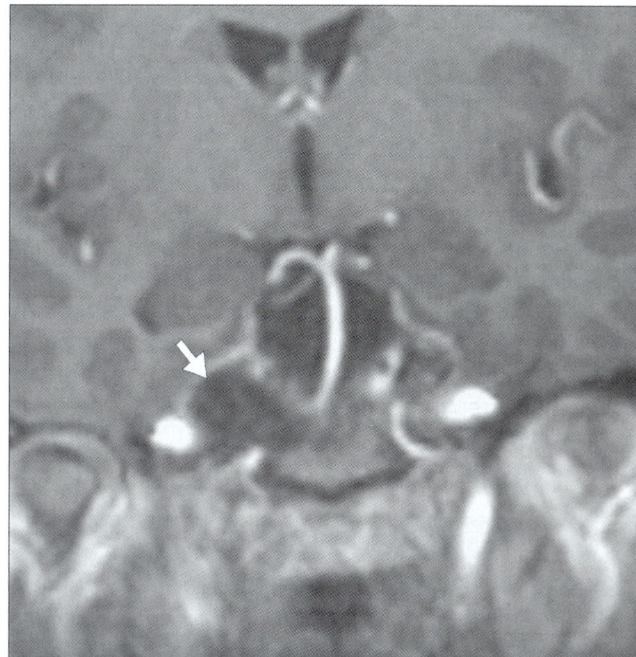

H

REFERENCES

Connor SEJ, Leung R, Natas S. Imaging of the petrous apex: a pictorial review. *Br J Radiol.* 2008;81:427-435.

Jacob M, Gujar S, Trobe J, Gandhi D. Spontaneous resolution of a Meckel cave arachnoid cyst causing sixth cranial nerve palsy. *J Neuroophthalmol.* 2008;28(3):186-191.

Moore KR, et al. Petrous apex cephaloceles. *Am J Neuroradiol.* 2001;22(10):1867-1871.

Schick B, Draf W, Kahle G, Weber R, Wallenfang T. Occult malformations of the skull base. *Arch Otolaryngol Head Neck Surg.* 1997;123(1):77-80.

CASE 40 Infracochlear drainage of the petrous apex

The most common indication for surgical drainage of a petrous apex is to treat a cholesterol granuloma. There are several different surgical approaches to drain a petrous apex. The surgical approach is dependent on the hearing status and the spatial relationship between the petrous apex lesion and the adjacent neurovascular structures. If hearing in the affected ear is preserved, then an infracochlear or infralabyrinthine approach is preferred. If there is profound, irreparable hearing loss in the affected ear, then a translabyrinthine or transotic approach may be performed. Drainage of a petrous apex cholesterol granuloma may or may not include removal of the cyst lining. The most common cause of cholesterol granuloma recurrence following surgical drainage is the development of fibrous and/or granulation tissue leading to obstruction of the drainage pathway. Placement of a silicone-based, Silastic catheter to drain a petrous apex cholesterol granuloma often results in an improved surgical outcome.

Infracochlear drainage of the petrous apex without a Silastic catheter

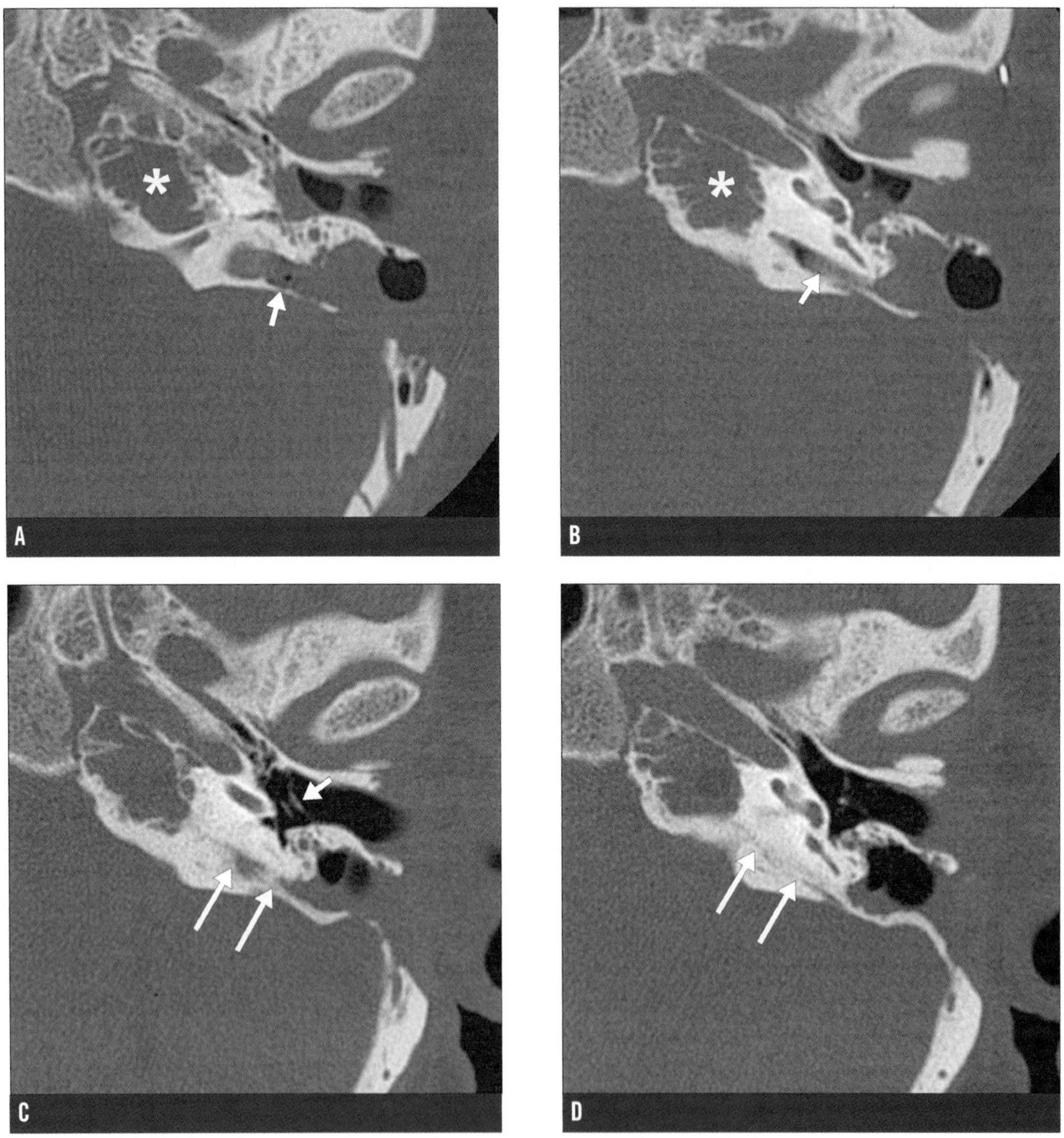

Axial CT images of the left temporal bone (**A**, **B**) demonstrate a cholesterol granuloma (asterisks, **A**, **B**) and postoperative changes related to an infracochlear approach to treat the lesion (short arrows, **A**, **B**). A silicone-based catheter was not placed along the surgical tract in this case. Axial CT images of the left temporal from the same patient 2 years following the surgery (**C**, **D**) demonstrate osseous overgrowth of the majority of the surgical tract (long arrows, **C**, **D**), an undesired but not unexpected finding. A myringotomy tube is also in place (short arrow, **C**).

Infracochlear drainage of the petrous apex with a Silastic catheter

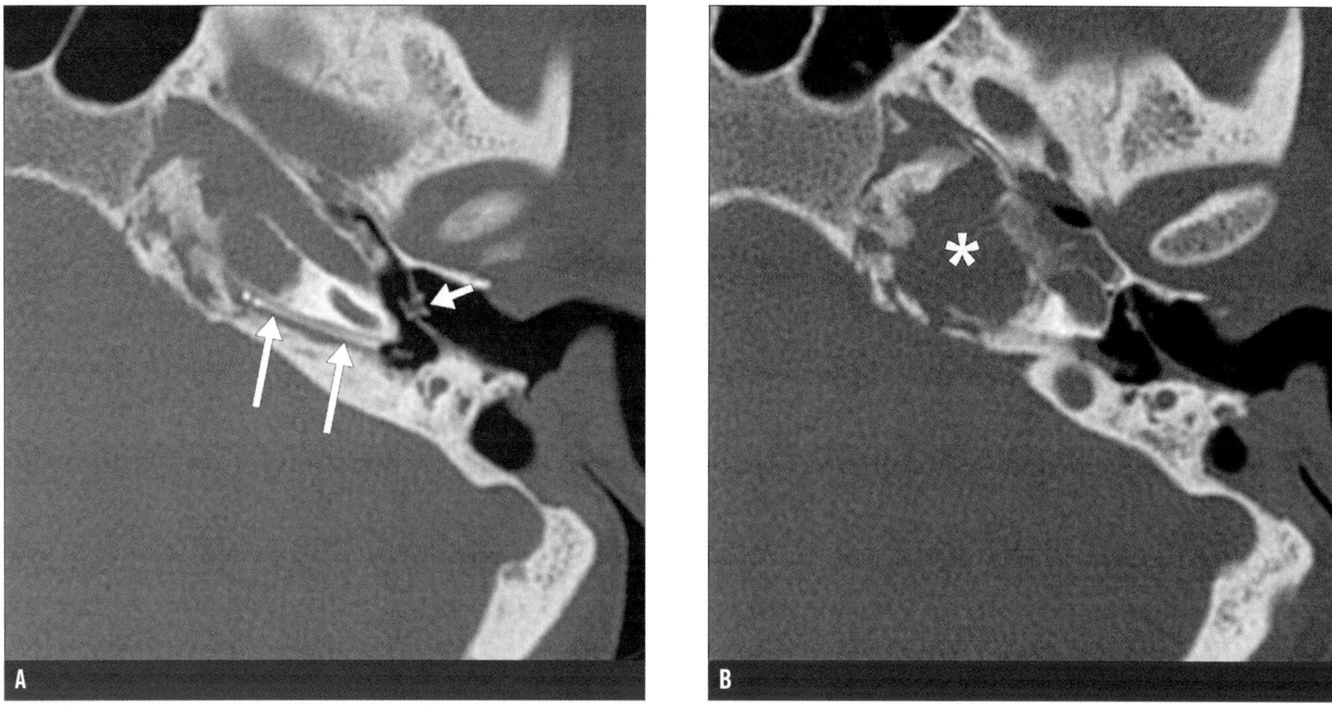

Different patient. Axial CT images of the left temporal bone (**A**, **B**) of a patient with a cholesterol granuloma. The images demonstrate post-operative changes from an infracochlear approach with placement of a silicone-based catheter (long arrows, **A**). The focal osseous expansion of the left petrous apex represents the cholesterol granuloma (asterisk, **B**). A myringotomy tube is incidentally noted (short arrow, **A**).

REFERENCES

Brackmann DE, Toh EH. Surgical management of petrous apex cholesterol granulomas. *Otol Neurotol.* 2002;23:529-533.

Sanna M, Dispenza F, Mathur N, De Stefano A, De Donato G. Otoneurological management of petrous apex cholesterol granuloma. *Am J Otolaryngol.* 2009;30(6):407-414.

Air cells develop from osseous cavities which contain bone marrow. The marrow dedifferentiates into loose connective tissue and eventually becomes a thin-lined membrane attached to the periosteum. There are three stages of mastoid pneumatization. During the infantile stage (from birth to 2 years), the mastoid air cells begin to develop. During the transitional stage (2-5 years), the mastoid enlarges and there is migration of air cells to the periphery. After 5 years of age (the adult stage), mastoid pneumatization ceases.

The spectrum of temporal bone pneumatization can vary from an aplastic/hypoplastic tympanic cavity and mastoid air cells to an extensively pneumatized temporal bone that can include the mastoid air cells, petrous apex, and squamosal portions of the temporal bone. There is some controversy as to whether Eustachian tube dysfunction influences the degree of temporal bone pneumatization; however, it is generally accepted that chronic middle ear disease in a child can result in ipsilateral hypoplasia of the mastoid air cells and tympanic cavity.

COMPANION CASES

- **Hyperpneumatization of the temporal bone with spontaneous pneumatocele formation.** When the amount of pneumatization of the temporal bones or paranasal sinuses is greater than expected, then the term hyperpneumatization is used. There are several different types of hyperpneumatized states that have been described. A hypersinus represents a hyperpneumatized sinus/air cell that is enlarged but its walls do not bulge beyond the expected confines of the mother bone. A pneumocele represents an expanded air cell that bulges outside the confines of the mother bone but it has thin but intact walls. Pneumosinus dilatans is also an expanded air cell that bulges outside the confines of the mother bone but it has a normal osseous wall thickness. However, pneumosinus dilatans has been associated with other entities, such as a meningioma, which can induce a hyperostosis. Finally, a pneumatocele is a separate collection of air that arises from a hyperpneumatized air cell or cells and extends into the adjacent soft tissue. When it extends intracranially, it is typically epidural in location and may be termed an intracranial pneumatocele or simply pneumocephalus.

  While the etiology of hyperpneumatization with pneumatocele formation of the temporal bones has not been fully elucidated, the most likely mechanism relates to a chronic, intermittent, increased intraluminal pressure in the pharynx that is transmitted through the Eustachian tube, presumably with an associated ball-valve mechanism. This increased pressure may be the result of a Valsava maneuver, excessive coughing or sneezing, and scuba or sky diving. Clinical manifestations may include headache, hemiplegia, hemiparesis, aphasia, visual changes, vomiting, and tinnitus. The air likely escapes the hyperpneumatized air cell(s) via a defect along a regional suture. The literature describes improvement symptomatically and radiographically with myringotomy tube placement. There are also reports of spontaneous resolution of the extratemporal air. When epidural air is present, prophylactic antibiotics should be considered in order to prevent meningitis and epidural phlegmon/abscess.
- **Fibrous dysplasia.** With fibrous dysplasia, normal bone is replaced by fibrous tissue consisting of spindle cell bundles and immature woven bone. This process causes expansion of the affected bone. The most common CT appearance of fibrous dysplasia is a ground-glass (sclerotic) pattern. However, fibrous dysplasia can less commonly appear as a heterogeneously lucent and slcerotic lesion (Pagetoid form) or as a cystic lesion (cystic form). On MRI, fibrous dysplasia has a nonspecific appearance and can mimic other osseous lesions, including malignant entities. Thus, any suspicious osseous lesion on MRI should be interpreted in combination with CT, or when appropriate, radiographs. Typically, fibrous dysplasia is low to intermediate in signal on T1 and avidly enhances on MRI. The T2 signal characteristics are variable and depend on the ratio of mineralized matrix to fibrous tissue. In the temporal bone, the external auditory canal is the most common site of involvement; however, the otic capsule can also be affected.
- **Osteopetrosis.** Osteopetrosis is a rare, heritable skeletal disorder that may be autosomal recessive or autosomal dominant and results in defective bone remodeling. The autosomal recessive form is usually diagnosed within the first few months of life; these patients rarely survive childhood. The autosomal dominant form is more common and is typically diagnosed in late childhood or adolescence. Although patients have increased bone density with osteopetrosis, paradoxically, these patients have an increased risk of fracture. The temporal bone manifestations of osteopetrosis include diffusely thickened, extensive sclerosis of the temporal bones resulting in poor temporal bone pneumatization. There are several neuro-otologic complications of osteopetrosis, including a sensorineural and conductive hearing loss, ossicular fixation, and vertigo. Marked sclerotic osseous overgrowth narrows the skull base canals and foramina, often resulting in cranial nerve palsies. Furthermore, pronounced narrowing of the internal auditory canals and petrous carotid canals may occur with this entity.

Temporal bone hyperpneumatization

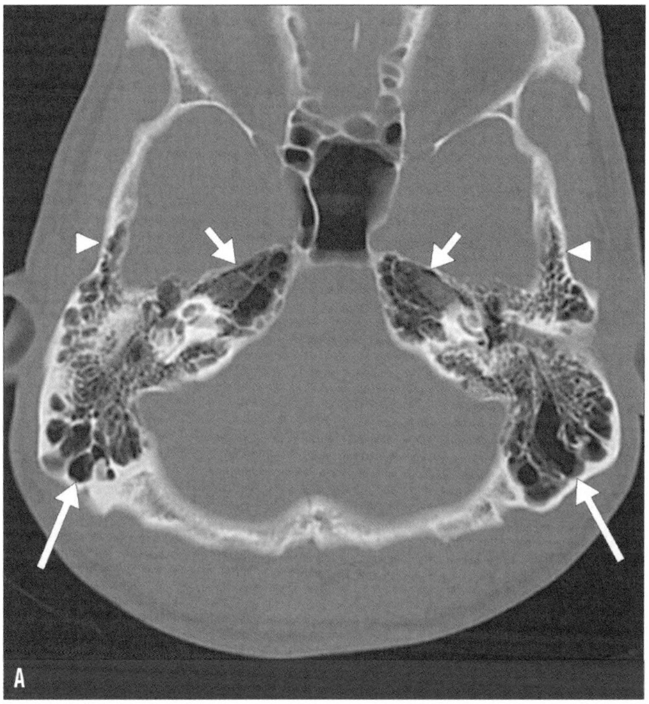

An axial CT of the temporal bones (**A**) demonstrates extensive pneumatization of the petrous apices (short arrows), mastoid air cells (long arrows), and squamosal portions of the temporal bones (arrowheads).

Temporal bone hyperpneumatization

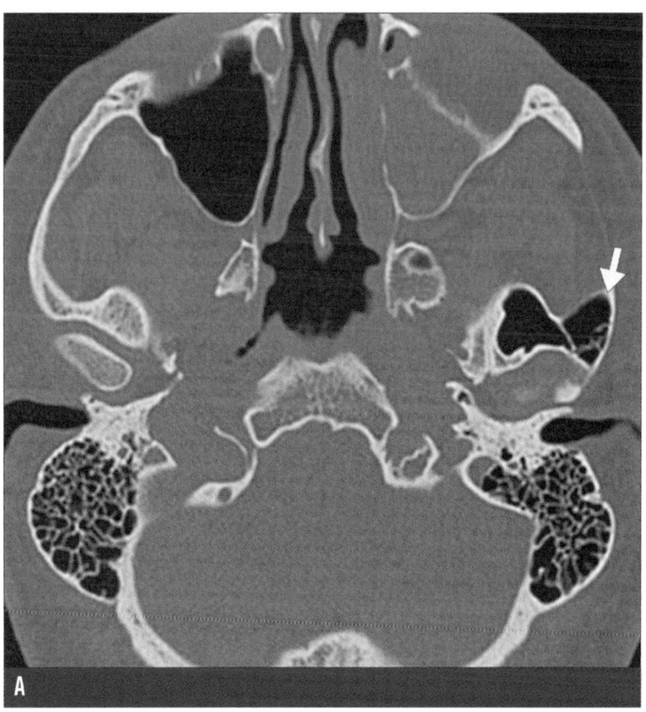

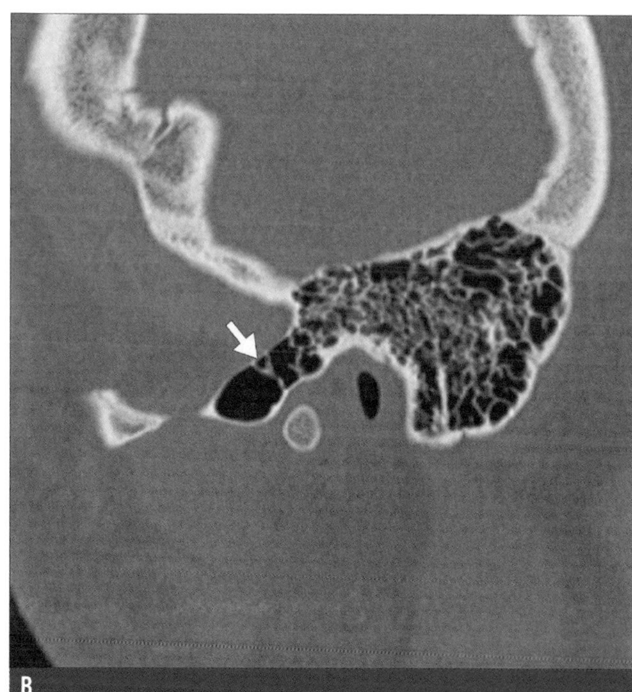

Different patient. Axial (**A**), sagittal reformatted (**B**), and coronal reformatted (**C**) CT images of the temporal bones demonstrate extensive pneumatization of the mastoid portions of the temporal bones as well as the temporal process of the left zygomatic arch (arrows, **A-C**). The hyperpneumatization of the left zygomatic arch enlarges this region of bone beyond its expected confines and there is associated mild thinning of the cortical bone. Therefore, the finding affecting the left zygomatic process can be considered a pneumocele, a type of hyperpneumatization.

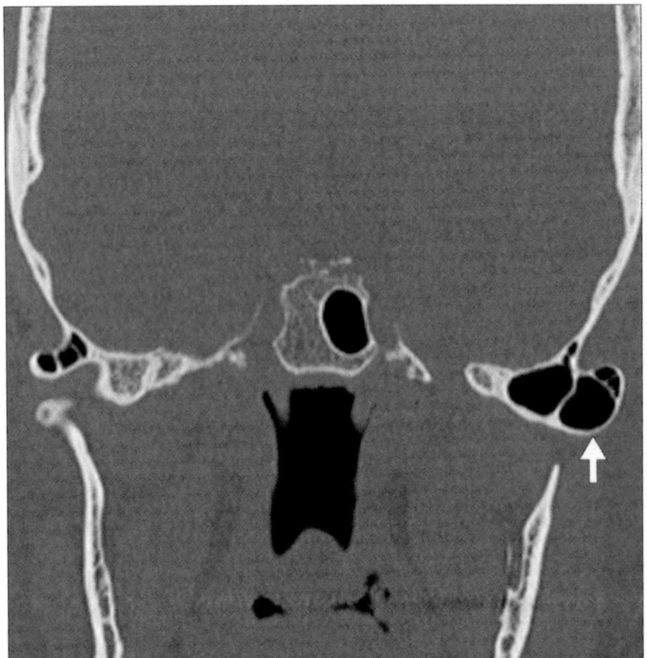

C

Mastoid air cell underpneumatization

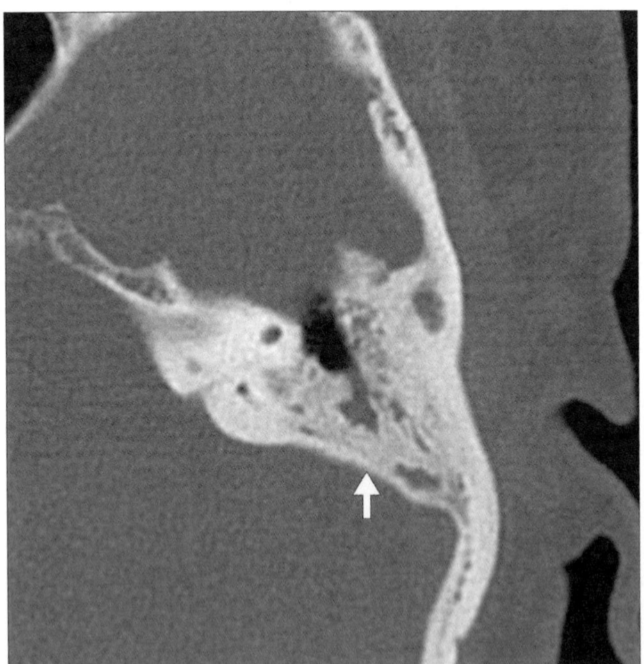

A

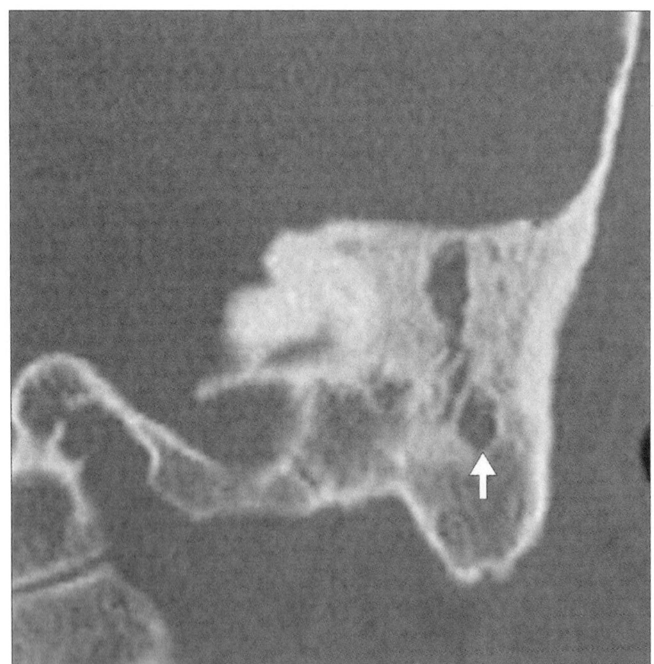

B

Axial (**A**) and coronal reformatted (**B**) CT images through the left temporal bone demonstrate largely opacified, hypoplastic left mastoid air cells (arrows, **A**, **B**). Mastoid air cell underpneumatization can be a manifestation of chronic middle ear disease.

Absent mastoid pneumatization

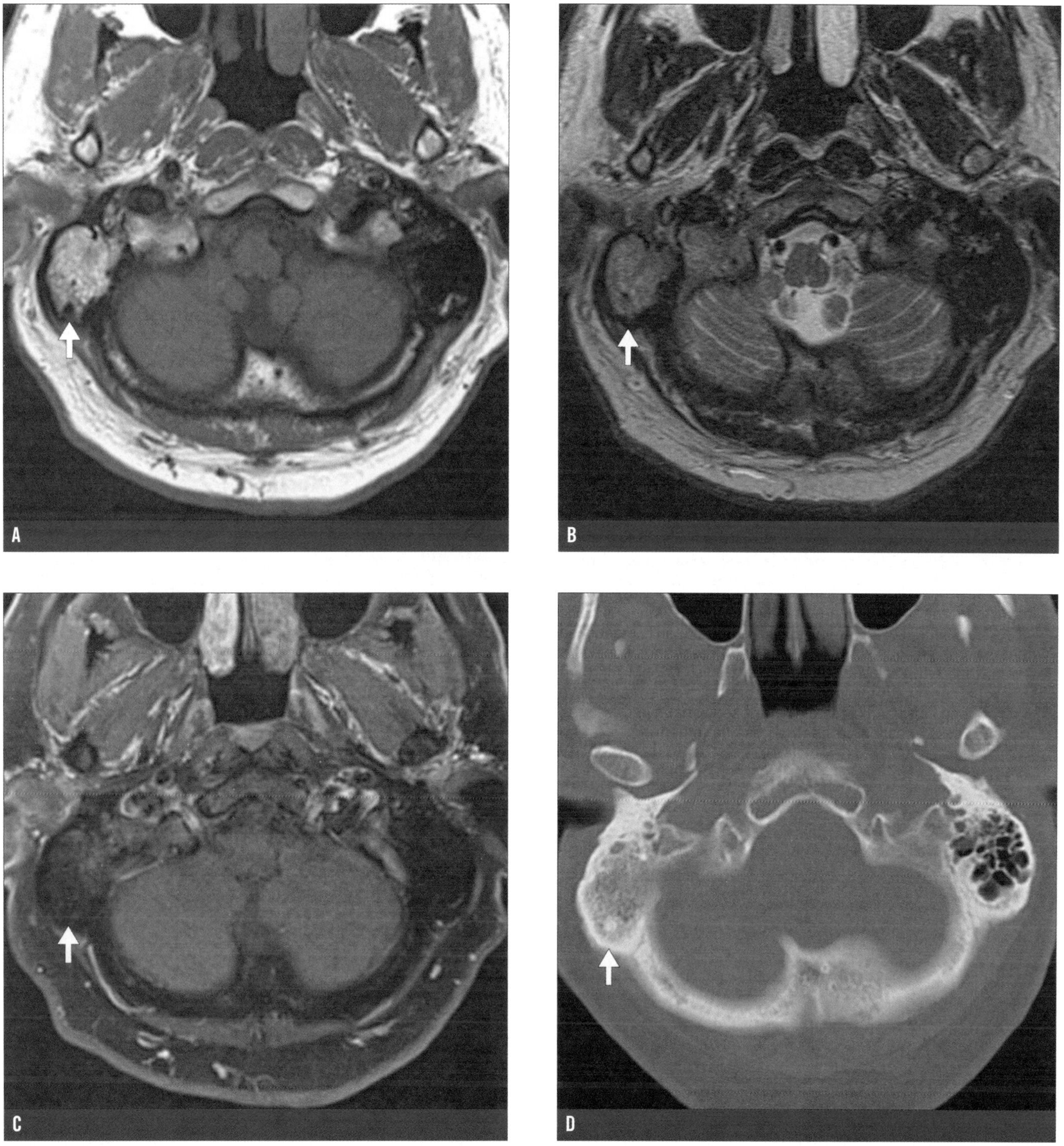

Axial T1 (**A**) and axial T2 (**B**) MR images of the temporal bones demonstrate hyperintense T1 and mildly hyperintense T2 signal in the right mastoid compared to the left (arrows, **A**, **B**). A fat-suppressed postcontrast axial T1-weighted MR image (**C**) demonstrates suppression of the hyperintense T1 signal, compatible with incidental marrow fat (arrow, **C**). An axial CT image of the temporal bones from the same patient (**D**) demonstrates absent pneumatization of the right mastoid air cells compared to the contralateral side, accounting for the asymmetric marrow fat on the right relative to the left (arrow, **D**).

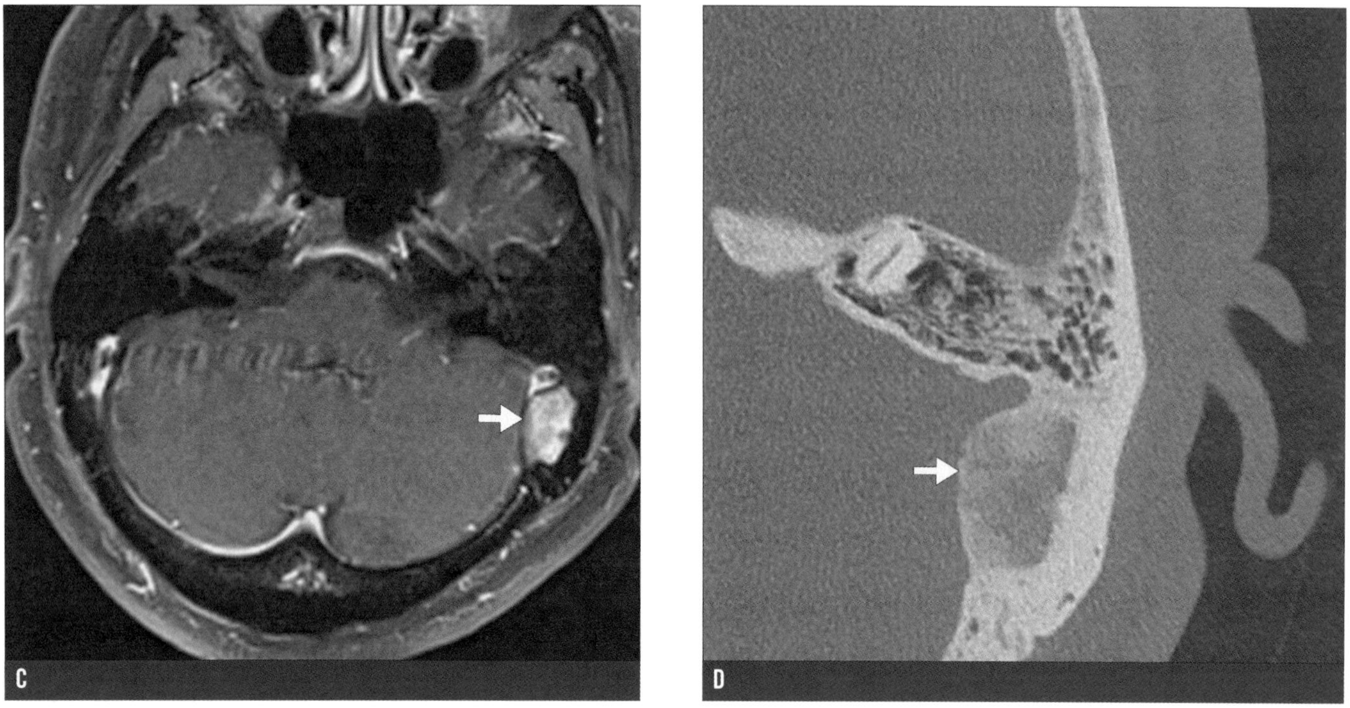

Companion case: Osteopetrosis

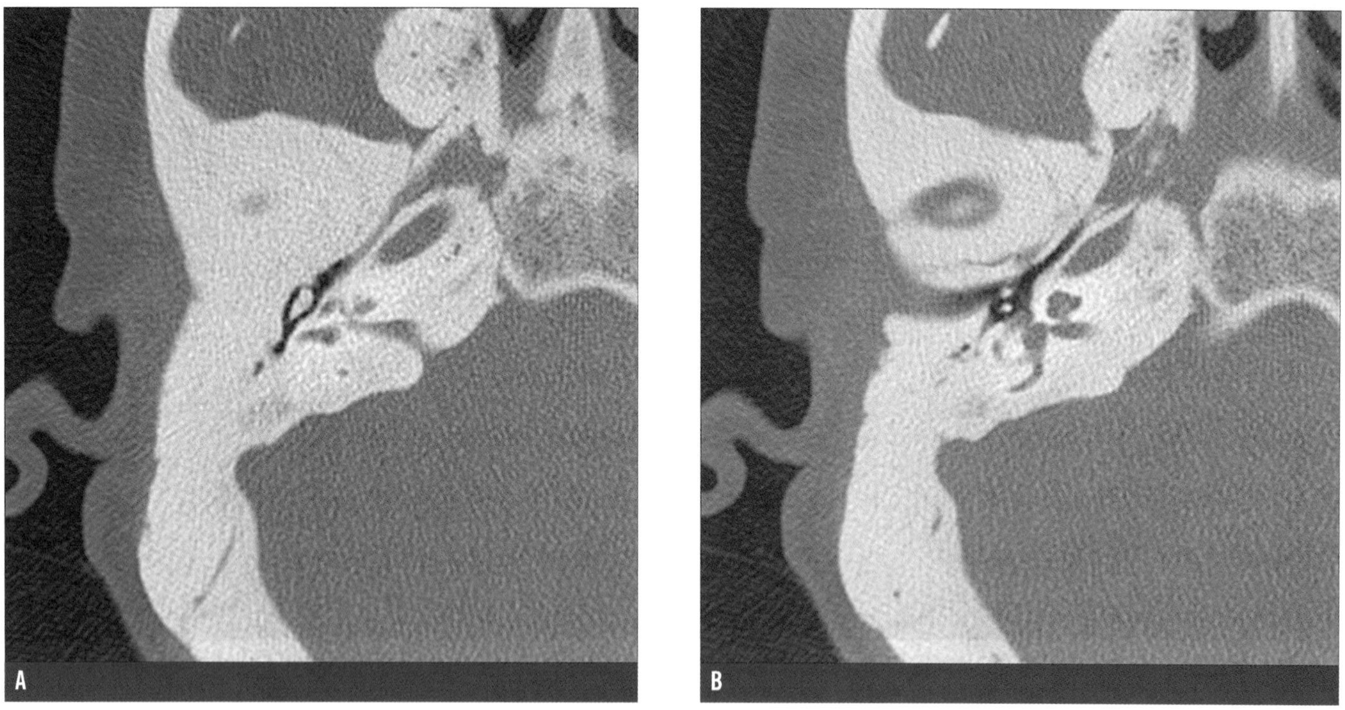

Axial CT images of the right temporal bone (**A**, **B**) and a coronal reformatted CT image of the temporal bones (**C**) demonstrate diffuse increased bone density and bone overgrowth throughout the temporal bones associated with marked paucity of temporal bone aeration, consistent with osteopetrosis. Symmetric narrowing of the IACs is also demonstrated on image **C** (arrows). Narrowing of the skull base canals and foramina is often present with osteopetrosis.

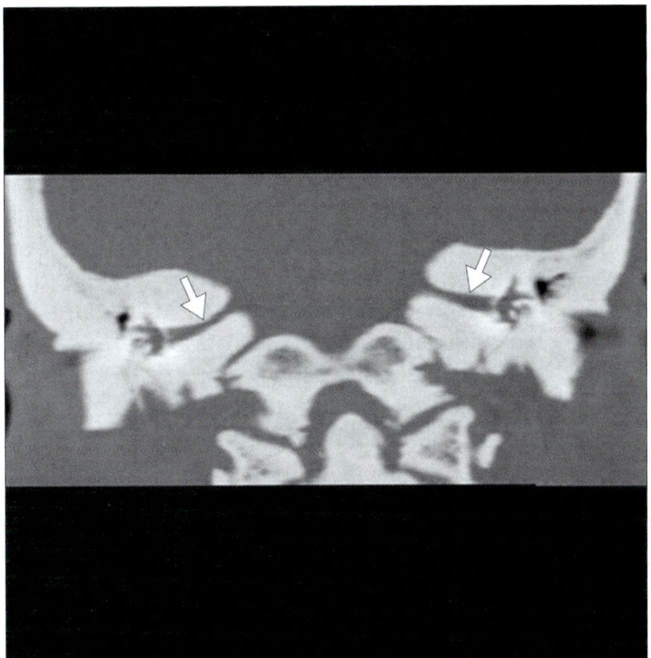
C

REFERENCES

Abdel-Aziz T, Upile T, Scholtz LU, Sudhoff HH. Osteopetrosis of the temporal bone. *Otol Neurotol.* 2012;33(6):e45-e46.

Añorbe E, Aisa P, Saenz de Ormijana J. Spontaneous pneumatocele and pneumocephalus associated with mastoid hyperpneumatization. *Eur J Radiol.* 2000;36(3):158-160.

Brown EW, Megerian CA, McKenna MJ, Weber A. Fibrous dysplasia of the temporal bone: imaging findings. *AJR Am J Roentgenol.* 1995;164:679-682.

Chong VFH, Khoo JBK, Fan YF. Fibrous dysplasia involving the base of the skull. *AJR Am J Roentgenol.* 2002;178:717-720.

Koc A, Ekinci G, Bilgili AM, Akpinar IN, Yakut H, Han T. Evaluation of the mastoid air cell system by high resolution computed tomography: three-dimensional multiplanar volume rendering technique. *J Laryngol Otol.* 2003;117:595-598.

Massmann A, et al. Atypical extensive extratemporal hyper-pneumatization of the skull base including the cervical spine: case report and review of the literature. *Spine (Phila Pa 1976).* 2012;37(3):E199-E202.

Parizel PM, et al. Pneumosinus dilatans in anterior skull base meningiomas. *Neuroradiology.* 2013;55(3):307-311

Virapongse C, Sarwar M, Bhimani S, Sasaki C, Shapiro R. Computed tomography of temporal bone pneumatization: normal pattern and morphology. *AJR Am J Roentgenol.* 1985;145:473-481.

Wemhoff M, Jain R, Rock J. Hyperpneumatization of the skull base: case report. *Neurosurgery.* 2012;70(3):E789-E793

Zhao N, Wang DD, Huang X, Karri SK, Wu H, Zheng M. Sponta-neous otogenic pneumocephalus presenting with occipital subcutaneous emphysema as primary symptom: could tension gas cause the destruction of cranial bones? *J Neurosurg.* 2011;115(4):679-683.

CASE 42 Arachnoid granulations

Arachnoid granulations are normal meningothelial-lined herniations of the arachnoid membrane that protrude through the dura mater into the venous lacunae and venous sinuses along the surface of the brain. They are functionally and histologically similar to arachnoid villi and allow for filtration and resorption of cerebrospinal fluid (CSF) into the venous circulation.

When arachnoid granulations affect the skull base, they often appear as lytic abnormalities on CT, sometimes simulating metastatic disease. The contents of an arachnoid granulation are most often CSF equivalent, unless an arachnoid granulation is large (>1 cm), in which case it may not be CSF equivalent. When a less than 1 cm lucency or fluid signal focus involving the skull base is encountered on CT or MRI, respectively, then it is helpful to determine whether the contents of the finding are CSF equivalent and whether the finding communicates with the adjacent subarachnoid space; if both of these imaging criteria are satisfied, then the finding is most compatible with an arachnoid granulation. An arachnoid granulation that does not overlie a pneumatized air cell is most often incidental. However, if it does overlie a pneumatized air cell, such as the pneumatized portions of the temporal bones, and the intervening bone is sufficiently thinned and/or dehiscent, then the patient is at risk for a CSF leak from an arachnoid granulation rupture.

COMPANION CASES

- **Spontaneous CSF leaks with idiopathic intracranial hypertension.** CSF leaks are considered to be spontaneous if there is no clear etiology for the leak, such as secondary to trauma, neoplasm, or congenital abnormality. Some authors believe that arachnoid villi/granulations enlarge because of increasing CSF volume and intracranial pressure. This is particularly notable in patients with idiopathic intracranial hypertension (IIH), also known as pseudotumor cerebri, who often have several prominent arachnoid granulations. In these patients, if the arachnoid granulations are located over the paranasal sinuses or temporal bones, they can rupture and result in spontaneous CSF leaks. A meningocele, particularly at the genu of the facial nerve canal, may also develop in these patients. Patients with IIH are typically female, obese, and may have numerous symptoms, including headaches, diplopia, and vision loss. Their CSF opening pressure is elevated, and their symptoms improve with drainage of CSF. Imaging findings in patients with IIH may include multiple arachnoid granulations at the skull base, a partially empty sella, and dilated optic nerve sheath complexes. If a CSF leak is present in a patient with IIH, then fluid will be identified in the affected pneumatized air cell and an arachnoid granulation overlying the fluid-filled air cell will often be identified, frequently with a focal osseous defect demonstrated by CT.
- **Endolymphatic sac tumor.** An endolymphatic sac tumor (ELST) represents a papillary cystadenomatous tumor of the endolymphatic sac and is rare. Most ELSTs occur sporadically and are unilateral, although bilateral ELSTs are pathognomonic of von Hippel-Lindau syndrome. CT imaging of ELSTs demonstrates adjacent petrous temporal bone osseous erosion/destruction and intratumoral calcification. On MRI, ELSTs can have heterogeneous, intrinsically hyperintense T1 signal related to subacute hemorrhage or proteinaceous debris and portions of the tumor will usually enhance.

Arachnoid granulations

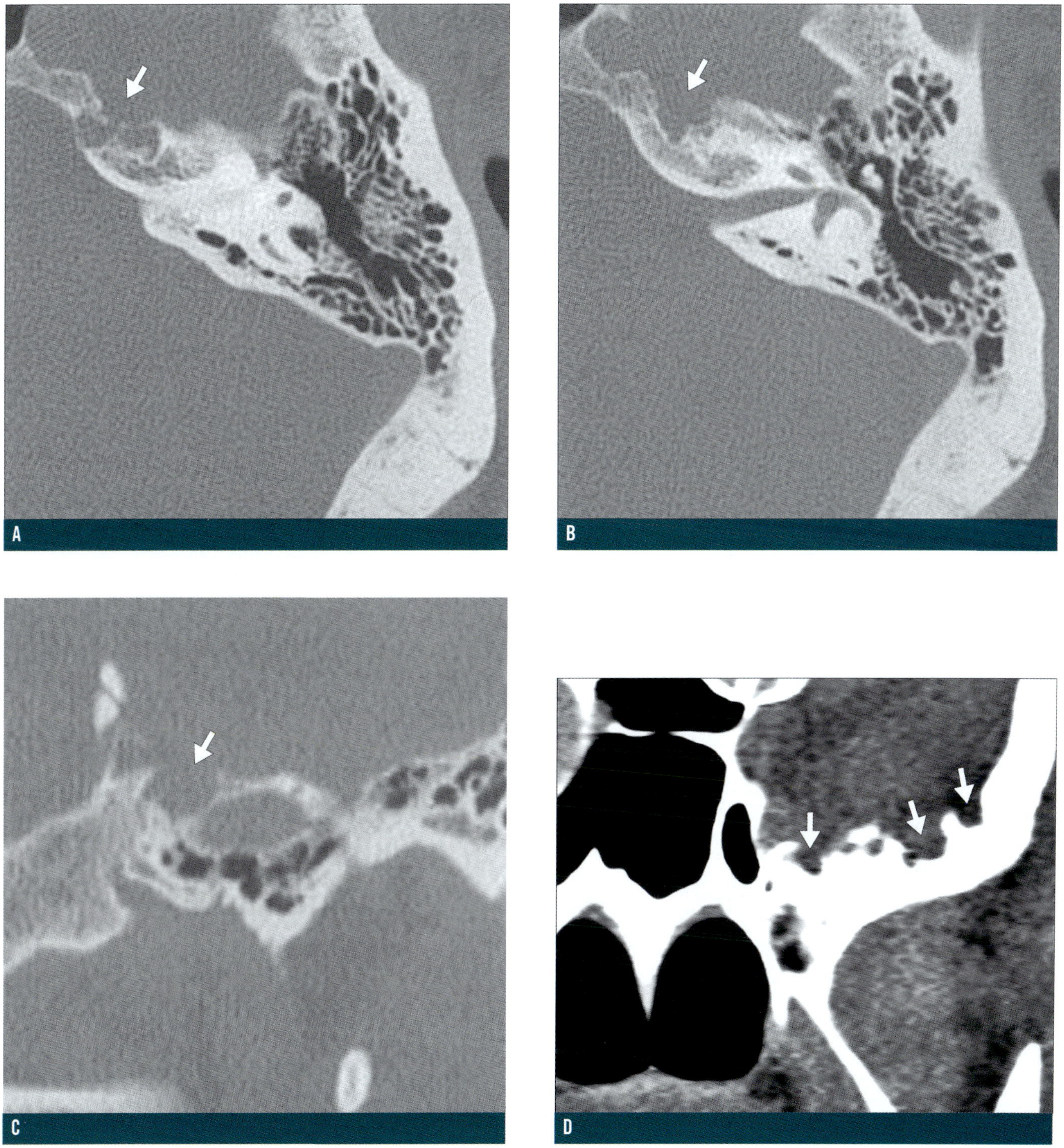

Axial (**A**, **B**) and coronal reformatted (**C**) CT images of the left temporal bone viewed with a bone window demonstrate a clustered area of circumscribed lucencies involving the left petrous apex, raising the possibility of a skull base mass (arrows, **A**-**C**). A noncontrast coronal reformatted CT image of the left temporal bone from the same patient viewed with a soft tissue window (**D**) demonstrates several lucencies along the middle cranial fossa floor (arrows, D) which extended to the petrous apex (not shown). When viewed on the PACS workstation, these lucencies contained CSF equivalent attenuation and communicated with the adjacent CSF, compatible with incidental arachnoid granulations.

Companion case: Spontaneous CSF leaks related to idiopathic intracranial hypertension

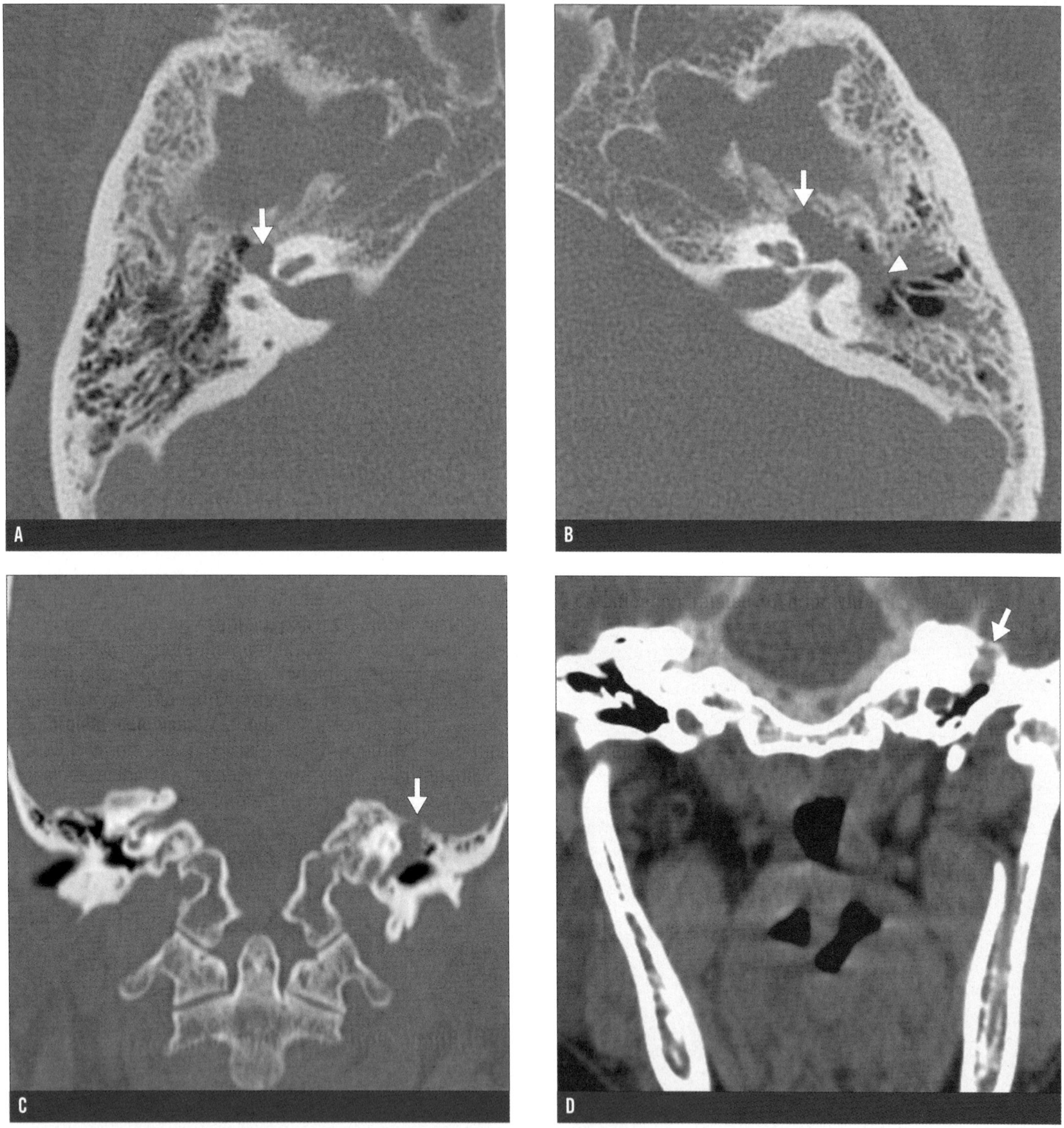

Axial CT images of the temporal bones (**A**, **B**) demonstrate osseous expansion involving the genu of each facial nerve canal (arrows, **A**, **B**), as well as fluid in the left mastoid (arrowhead, **B**). A coronal reformatted CT image from the same study (**C**) demonstrates a subtle focal osseous defect along the cephalad aspect of the left facial nerve genu (arrow, **C**). A coronal reformatted CT image of the same patient following a cisternogram (**D**) demonstrates contrast extending into the left facial nerve canal genu (arrow, **D**). Axial T2-weighted MR imaging of the right (**E**) and left (**F**) temporal bones demonstrates elevated T2 signal within the expanded genu of each facial nerve canal (arrows, **E**, **F**) and fluid in the left mastoid (arrowhead, **F**). A motion-degraded fat-suppressed postcontrast axial T1-weighed MR image of the left temporal bone (**G**) does not demonstrate gross enhancement within the genu of the left facial nerve canal (arrow, **G**), effectively excluding a schwannoma. Lack of enhancement was also demonstrated within the genu of the right facial nerve canal (not shown). The combination of the CT and MRI findings suggests meningoceles within the genu of each facial nerve canal (possibly related to ruptured arachnoid granulations) and an associated CSF leak affecting the left temporal bone. A coronal reformatted CT image from a cisternogram of the same patient viewed with a soft tissue window (**H**) demonstrates contrast extending through an osseous defect into the right olfactory recess (arrow, **H**). These findings are also compatible with a CSF leak. The presence of multiple CSF leaks and meningoceles/arachnoid granulations, particularly in an obese female with headaches, should raise the possibility of idiopathic intracranial hypertension.

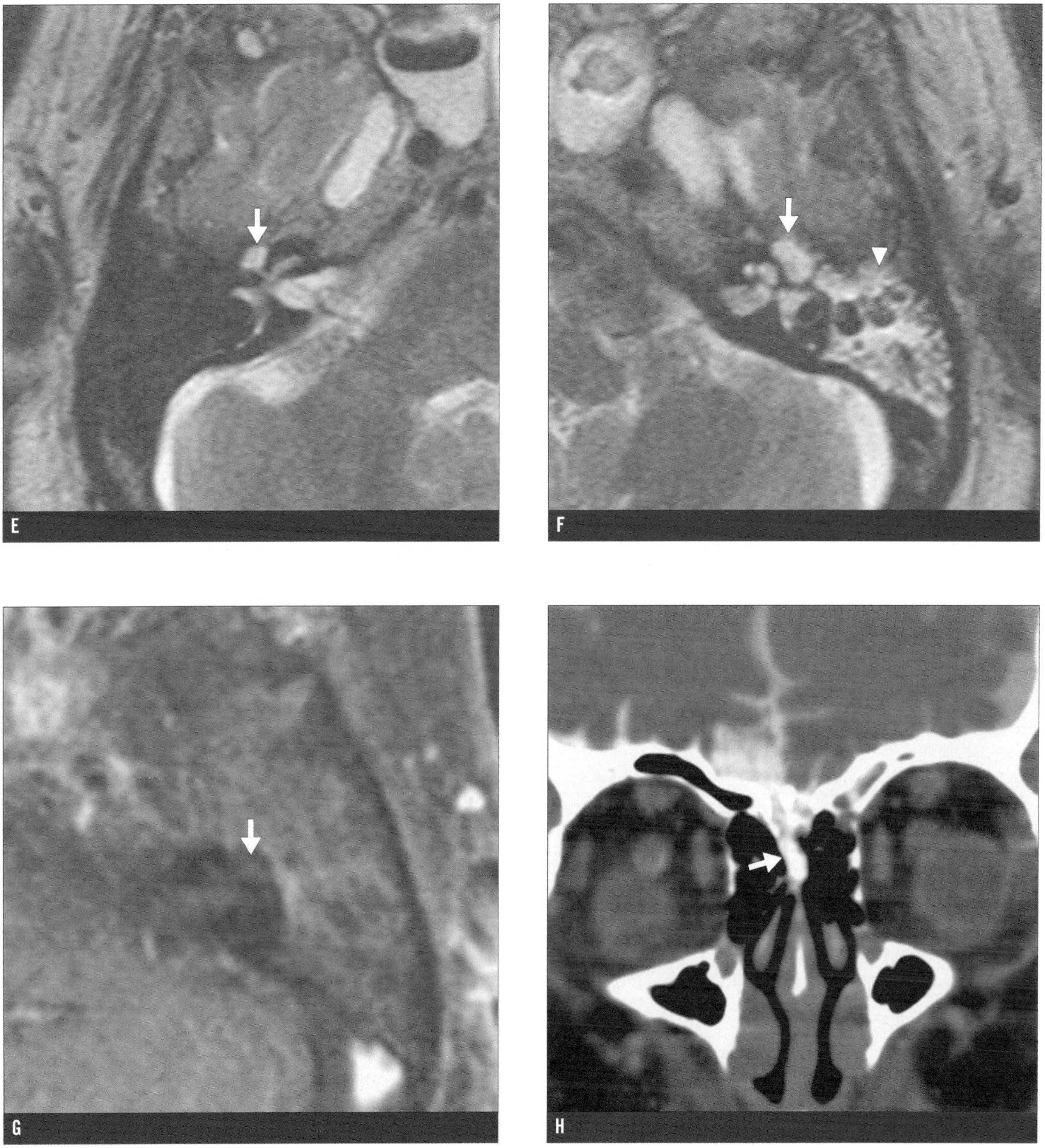
E
F
G
H

Companion case: Endolymphatic sac tumor

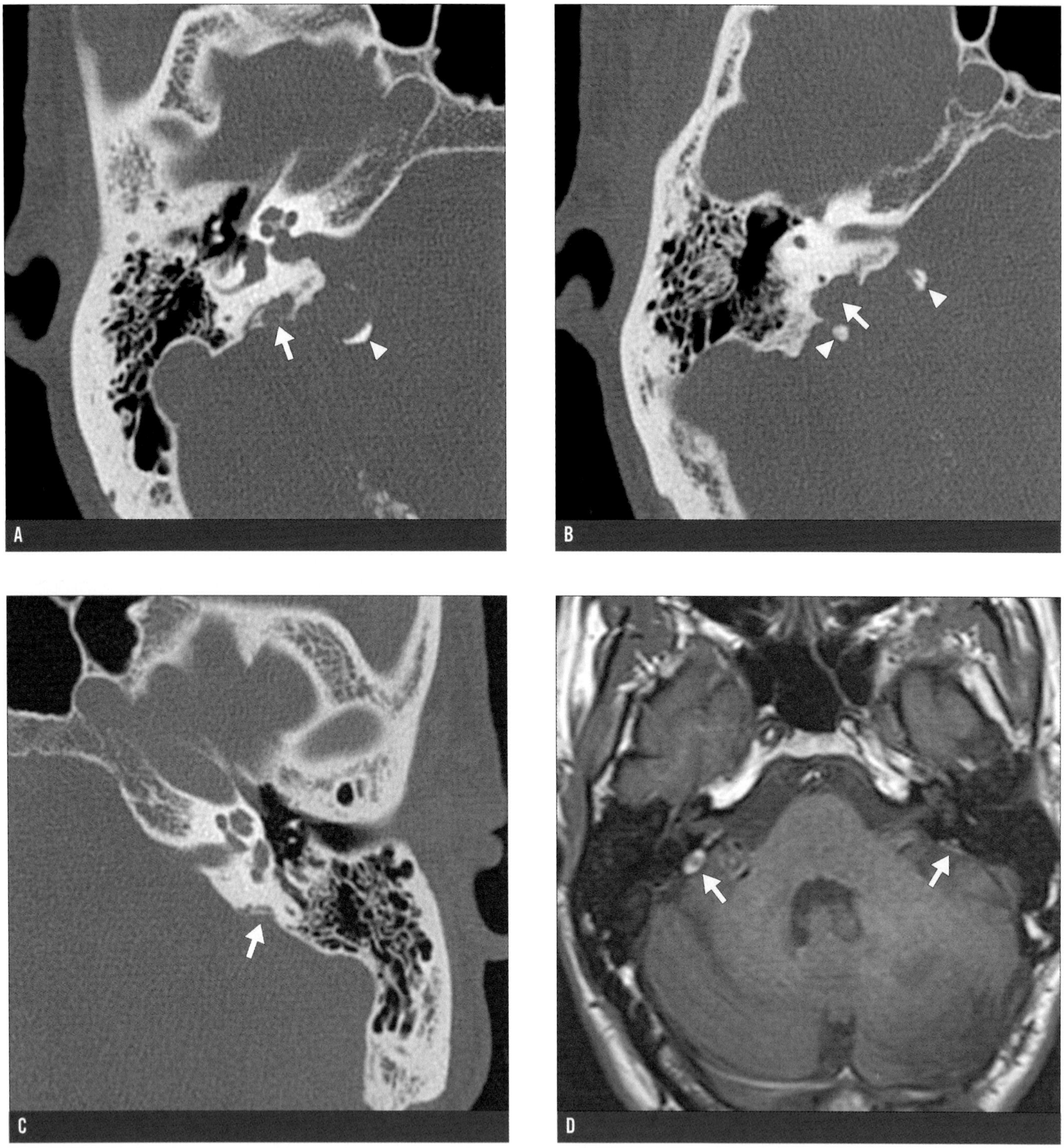

Axial CT images of the right (**A**, **B**) and left (**C**) temporal bones of a patient with Von Hippel Lindau demonstrate areas of osseous irregularity along the dorsal aspects of the petrous temporal bones in the region of the vestibular aqueducts, right worse than left (arrows, **A-C**), similar to what can be identified with arachnoid granulations. However, focal coarse calcifications are also identified adjacent to the right petrous temporal bone erosion, raising the possibility of intratumoral calcifications (arrowheads, **A**, **B**). Axial T1 (**D**), axial T2 (**E**), and fat-suppressed postcontrast axial T1 (**F**) MR images of the temporal bones from the same patient demonstrate focal abnormalities in the regions of the endolymphatic sacs, corresponding to the areas of osseous lucency demonstrated on the CT. A portion of each lesion is intrinsically hyperintense on T1 (right more so than left) (arrows, **D**), and each lesion is heterogeneously hypointense on T2 (arrows, **E**). While there is no appreciable enhancement of the lesion on the right, the lesion on the left minimally enhances (arrow, **F**). The findings are compatible with bilateral endolymphatic sac tumors in this patient with von Hippel-Lindau.

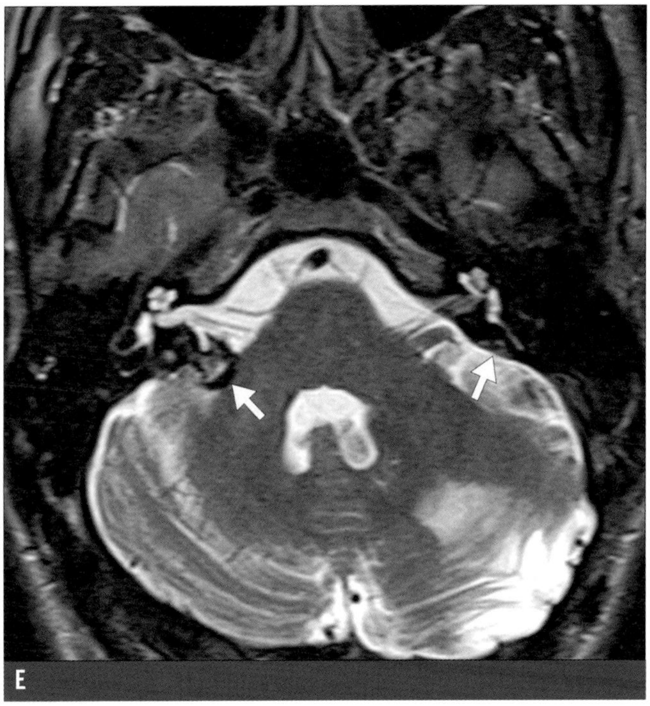

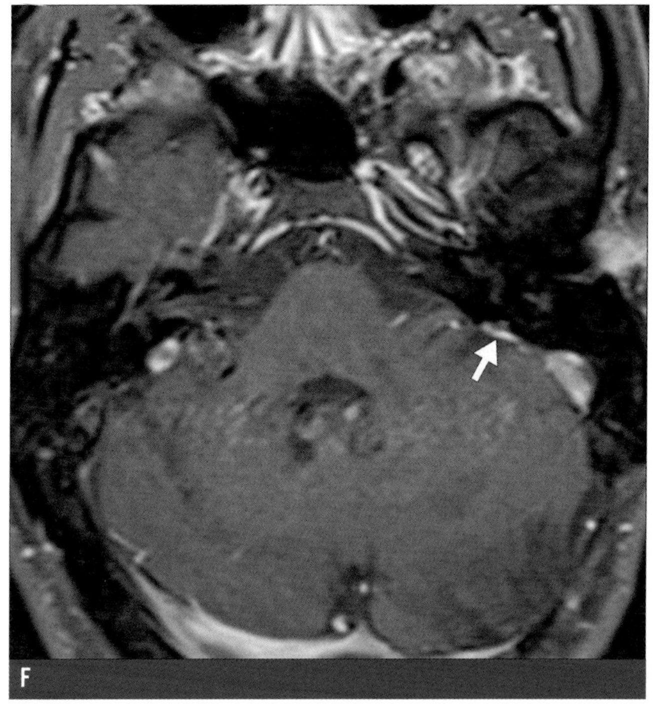

REFERENCES

Chen F, Deng XF, Liu B, Zou LN, Wang DB, Han H. Arachnoid granulations of middle cranial fossa: a population study between cadaveric dissection and in vivo computed tomography examination. *Surg Radiol Anat.* 2011;33(3):215-221. Epub October 2010.

Goddard JC, Meyer T, Nguyen S, Lambert PR. New considerations in the cause of spontaneous cerebrospinal fluid otorrhea. *Otol Neurotol.* 2010;31(6):940-945.

Lloyd KM, DelGaudio JM, Hudgins PA. Imaging of skull base cerebrospinal fluid leaks in adults. *Radiology.* 2008;248:725-736.

Lo WW et al., Endolymphatic sac tumors: radiologic appearance. *Radiology.* 1993;189(1):199-204.

Patel NP, Wiggins RH, Shelton C. The radiologic diagnosis of endolymphatic sac tumors. *Laryngoscope.* 2006;116:40-46.

Schuknecht B, Simmen D, Briner HR, Holzmann D. Nontraumatic skull base defects with spontaneous CSF rhinorrhea and arachnoid herniation: imaging findings and correlation with endoscopic sinus surgery in 27 patients. *Am J Neuroradiol.* 2008;29:542-549.

Trimble CR, Harnsberger HR, Castillo M, Brant-Zawadzki M, Osborn AG. "Giant" arachnoid granulations just like CSF?: NOT!! *AJNR Am J Neuroradiol.* 2010;31(9):1724-1728. Epub June 2010.

Yew M, et al. Arachnoid granulations of the temporal bone: a histologic study of dural and osseous penetration. *Otol Neurotol.* 2011;32:602-609.

Calvarial hyperostosis interna is a benign entity manifested by cancellous new bone formation that arises along the inner table of the calvarium. It is frequently identified incidentally and is present predominately in middle-aged or elderly women. Hyperostosis can occur along a focal portion of the calvarium or it can diffusely involve the calvarium. It is often bilateral and described by location (eg, hyperostosis frontalis, hyperostosis parietalis, hyperostosis temporalis, diffuse calvarial hyperostosis, etc), with frontal bone involvement being the most common. Despite being originally described in 1765, the etiology of calvarial hyperostosis interna remains unproven. While it is most likely a hormonally driven process, other hypotheses, including genetic, viral, and dietary have also been proposed. The prevalence is estimated to be between 5% to 12% of the general population, although this percentage increases among older age groups.

Radiographically, there is wavy or nodular new bone formation along the inner calvarial table, with the bone formation sometimes described as "pearls on a string" or "bullets" that project into the calvarial vault. Hyperostosis tends to be less dense than normal cortical bone. On CT and MRI, the cancellous bone will also have a thickened, nodular contour and may contain normal marrow fat. The presence of normal marrow can aid in differentiating this entity from other processes, such as malignancy or Paget disease.

Hyperostosis frontalis interna usually has no significant clinical implications. However, advanced cases of skull base hyperostosis (such as may occur with a hereditary form of hyperostosis termed hyperostosis cranialis interna) can result in calvarial foraminal stenoses and impingement of the traversing cranial nerves. Also, there are rare reports of calvarial hyperostosis interna resulting in mass effect upon the subjacent brain necessitating surgical intervention.

COMPANION CASE

- **Meningioma-associated calvarial hyperostosis.** Meningiomas are the most common nonglial primary central nervous system tumor. Meningiomas arise from meningothelial cells and are therefore extraaxial tumors that may occur anywhere along the dura. Other locations where meningiomas arise include the orbits (from the optic nerve sheath), ventricles, paranasal sinuses, and the diploic space of bone. On noncontrast CT, an intracranial meningioma will be an extraaxial, hyperdense tumor that may contain mineralization and is frequently associated with hyperostosis of the adjacent calvarium. On MRI, an intracranial meningioma will usually be isointense to brain on T1- and T2-weighted imaging and will diffusely enhance on postcontrast T1-weighted imaging. However, when mineralized, the mineralized portions of a meningioma will be hypointense on T1- and T2-weighted imaging and will not enhance following contrast. When arising from the intracranial dura, a meningioma will often have a dural tail emanating from a broad-based dural attachment on MRI. A meningioma on MRI will also be frequently surrounded by a CSF cleft, except along its broad-based dural attachment.

Hyperostosis temporalis interna

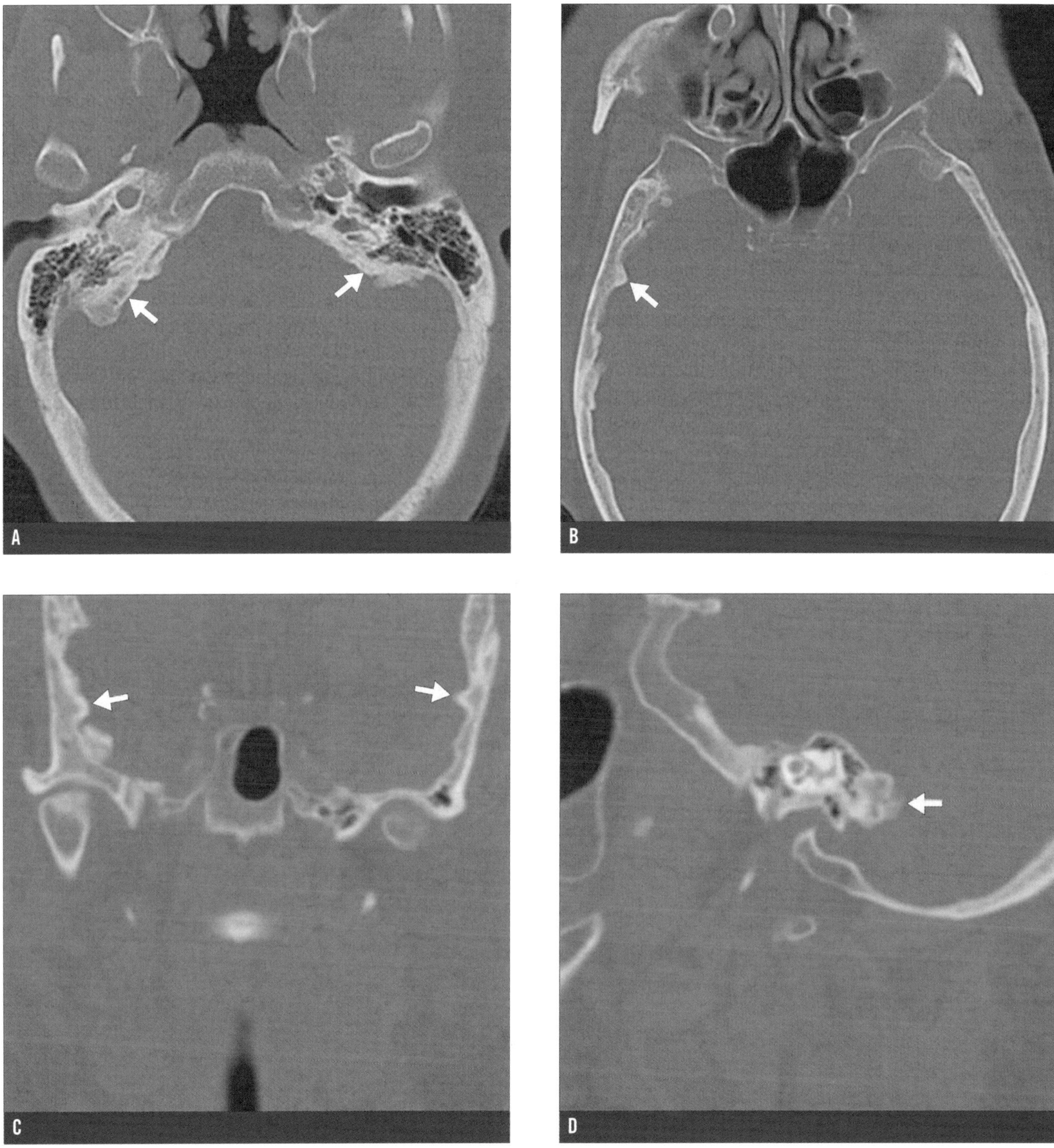

An axial CT image through the petrous temporal bones (**A**) and squamosal temporal bones (**B**) as well as a coronal reformatted CT image through the middle cranial fossae (**C**) demonstrate hyperostotic, lobulated, marrow-containing bone along the right greater than left dorsal aspects of the petrous temporal bones (arrows, **A**) as well as along the inner table of the squamosal portions of the temporal bones (arrows, **B**, **C**). A sagittal reformatted CT image through the right petrous temporal bone (**D**) demonstrates the petrous temporal bone hyperostosis in the sagittal plane (arrow, **D**).

Companion case: Meningioma-associated calvarial hyperostosis

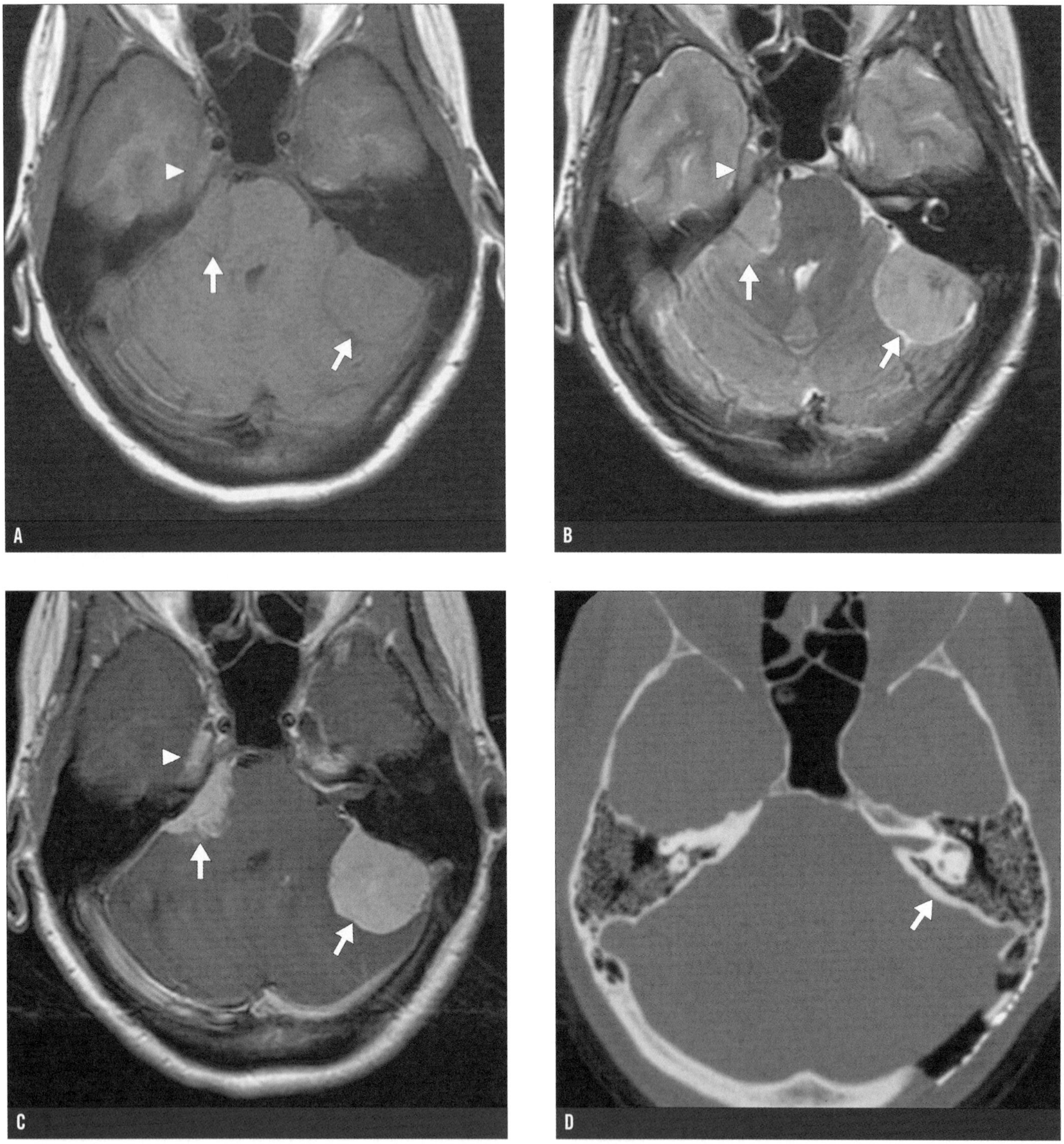

Axial T1 (**A**), axial T2 (**B**), and postcontrast axial T1 (**C**) MR images through the posterior fossa demonstrate meningiomas in the bilateral aspects of the posterior fossa (arrows, **A-C**) and a similar but smaller mass in the right Meckel cave that either represents an additional meningioma or a schwannoma (arrowheads, **A-C**). An axial CT image through the temporal bones (**D**) and a sagittal reformatted CT image through the left temporal bone (**E**) demonstrate meningioma-associated hyperostosis along the dorsal aspect of the left petrous temporal bone (arrows, **D**, **E**). A sagittal reformatted CT image through the right petrous temporal bone (**F**) demonstrates the normal right petrous temporal bone for comparison purposes (arrow, **F**). Whenever hyperostosis involving the calvarium is identified, evaluation for an intracranial mass as a cause of the hyperostosis, particularly a meningioma, should be performed.

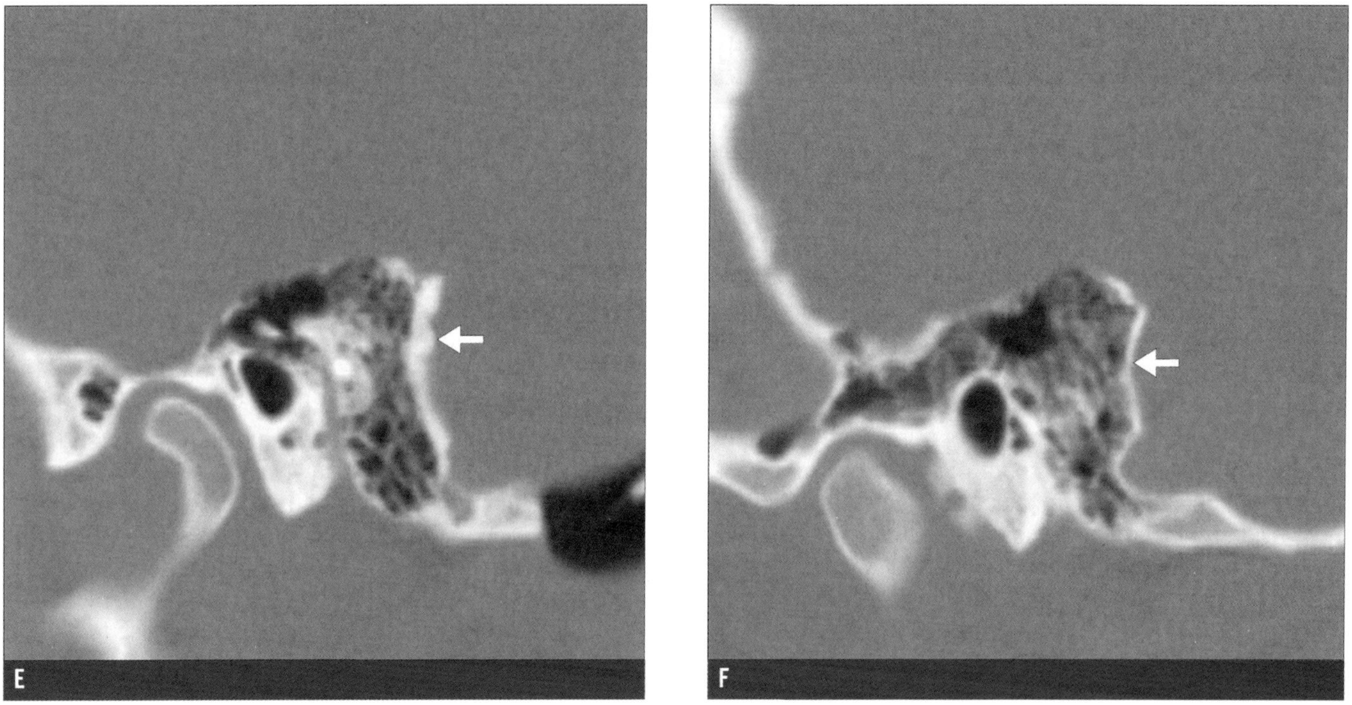

REFERENCES

Buetow MP, Buetow PC, Smirniotopoulos JG. Typical, atypical, and misleading features in meningioma. *Radiographics.* 1991;11(6):1087-1106.

Chaljub G, Johnson RF 3rd, Johnson RF Jr, Sitton CW. Unusually exuberant hyperostosis frontalis interna: MRI. *Neuroradiology.* 1999;41:44-45.

She S, Szakacs J. Hyperostosis frontalis interna: case report and review of literature. *Ann Clin Lab Sci. 2004.* 34(2).206-208.

Waterval JJ, van Dongen TM, Stokroos RJ, De Bondt BJ, Chenault MN, Manni JJ. Imaging features and progression of hyperostosis cranialis interna. *AJNR Am J Neuroradiol.* 2012;33(3):453-461.

Normal enhancement of the facial nerve will frequently be identified within the facial canal on 1.5T MRI. The portions of the facial nerve that normally enhance include the geniculate, tympanic, and mastoid segments and to a lesser, variable degree, the labyrinthine segment. This normal enhancement is related to a circumneural arteriovenous plexus that extends from the labyrinthine segment to the stylomastoid foramen. The amount of arteriovenous plexus varies along these portions of the facial nerve, with relatively less plexus along the labyrinthine segment. Conversely there is a greater amount of arteriovenous plexus at the geniculate and tympanic segments, resulting in more avid enhancement of these segments on MRI. While the intracanalicular (ie, within the internal auditory canal) and cisternal segments of a normal facial nerve should not enhance on 1.5T imaging, one retrospective study demonstrated that on a 3T magnet, the normal facial nerve can also enhance at the distal intracanalicular segment. In addition, there is more robust facial nerve enhancement with 3T MR imaging. The greater extent and degree of facial nerve enhancement on a 3T study relates to the higher field strength and should be accounted for when evaluating the facial nerve on a 3T study. However, any significant asymmetric enhancement of the facial nerve on a fat-suppressed spin-echo T1-weighted sequence, regardless of the site of enhancement or magnet strength, should be viewed with suspicion.

COMPANION CASE

- **Bell palsy.** Bell palsy is the most common cause of acute unilateral facial nerve palsy. It is the result of an acute inflammatory reaction that causes facial nerve edema and predominantly occurs at the geniculate ganglion. While it has been proposed that it is the result of a latent herpetic infection that is reactivated by various stressors, Bell palsy is still considered idiopathic. Bell palsy occurs abruptly, typically over 1 to 3 days, sometimes afflicting the patient overnight and first noticed upon waking from sleep. It is self-limiting in 70% to 80%, with symptoms peaking in the first week and gradually improving over 3 weeks to 3 months. Symptoms of Bell palsy include a unilateral facial palsy that involves the entire face and includes the forehead. The forehead involvement in Bell palsy is a helpful clinical feature to differentiate this lower motor neuron entity from a facial paralysis that is the result of an upper motor neuron abnormality, such as from a cerebral infarction or multiple sclerosis. Because there is crossed neural supply to the forehead from both cerebral hemispheres, patients with a unilateral upper motor neuron lesion will be able to wrinkle their forehead, whereas those with a lower motor neuron lesion, such as Bell palsy, will not. The facial nerve pathology with Bell palsy will be occult by CT. On MRI, there is asymmetric enhancement of the facial nerve, most often affecting the genu and labyrinthine segments, but the distal intracanalicular, proximal tympanic and mastoid segments may also be affected. The MRI enhancement pattern is uniform and there is no abnormal enlargement of the facial nerve on MRI or the facial nerve canal on CT. This is in contradistinction to perineural spread of tumor, which also enhances but often thickens the facial nerve on MRI and may enlarge portions of the facial nerve canal on CT. Nevertheless, when asymmetric facial nerve enhancement is encountered on MRI, regardless of whether the facial nerve is thickened, then inspection of the adjacent structures (eg, the parotid gland) should be performed to exclude other causes of abnormal facial nerve enhancement, such as perineural spread of tumor.

Normal facial nerve enhancement with a 1.5T magnet

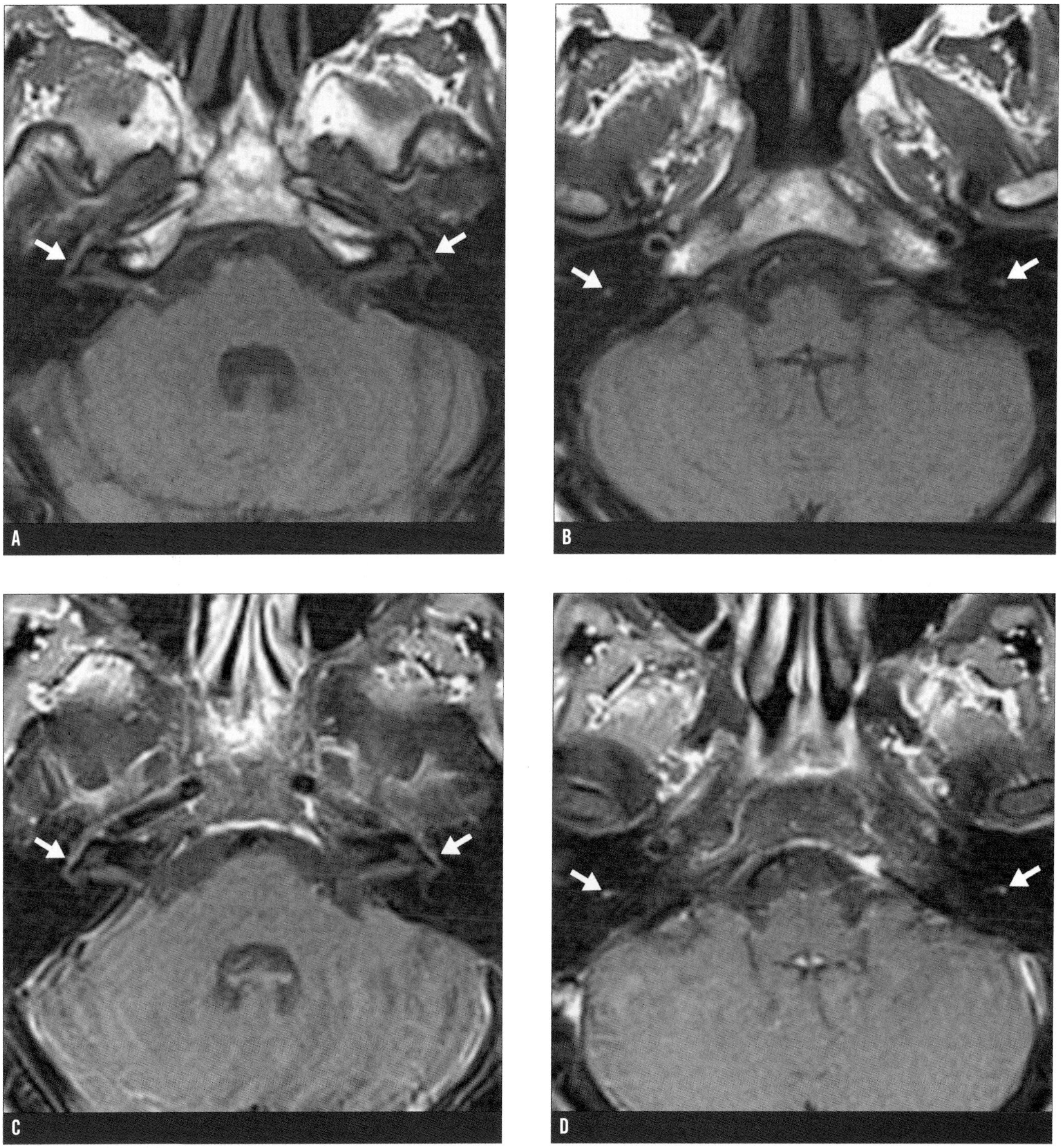

Axial T1 (**A**, **B**) and fat-suppressed postcontrast axial T1 (**C**, **D**) MR images through the temporal bones obtained on a 1.5T magnet. Images **A** and **B** demonstrate mild incidental T1 shortening along the tympanic segments (arrows, **A**) and mastoid segments (arrows, **B**) of the facial nerves that is likely technical. Images **C** and **D** demonstrate mild symmetric enhancement of the tympanic segments (arrows, **C**) and mastoid segments (arrows, **D**). Symmetric mild enhancement of these portions of the facial nerves is a normal, expected finding and relates to a normal circumneural arteriovenous plexus.

Normal facial nerve enhancement with a 1.5T versus 3.0T magnet

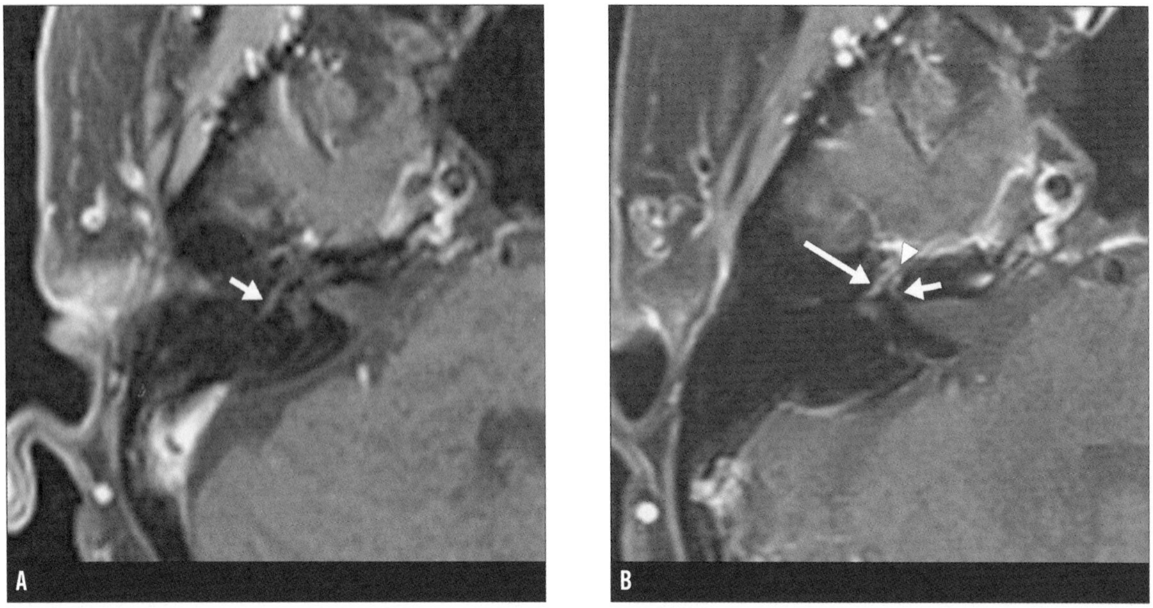

Fat-suppressed postcontrast axial T1-weighted MR images of the right temporal bone on a 1.5T magnet (**A**) and a 3.0T magnet 8 months later (**B**). On image **A**, there is normal expected enhancement of the tympanic segment of the right facial nerve (short arrow, **A**). On image **B**, there is an overall greater degree and more diffuse enhancement of the right facial nerve, with enhancement of the labyrinthine (short arrow, **B**), geniculate (arrowhead, **B**), and tympanic segments (long arrow, **B**). While there is more enhancement of the right facial nerve on the 3T image, this enhancement is still normal and relates to the greater field strength of the 3T scanner. The patient did not have symptoms related to the right facial nerve on either study.

Companion case: Bell palsy

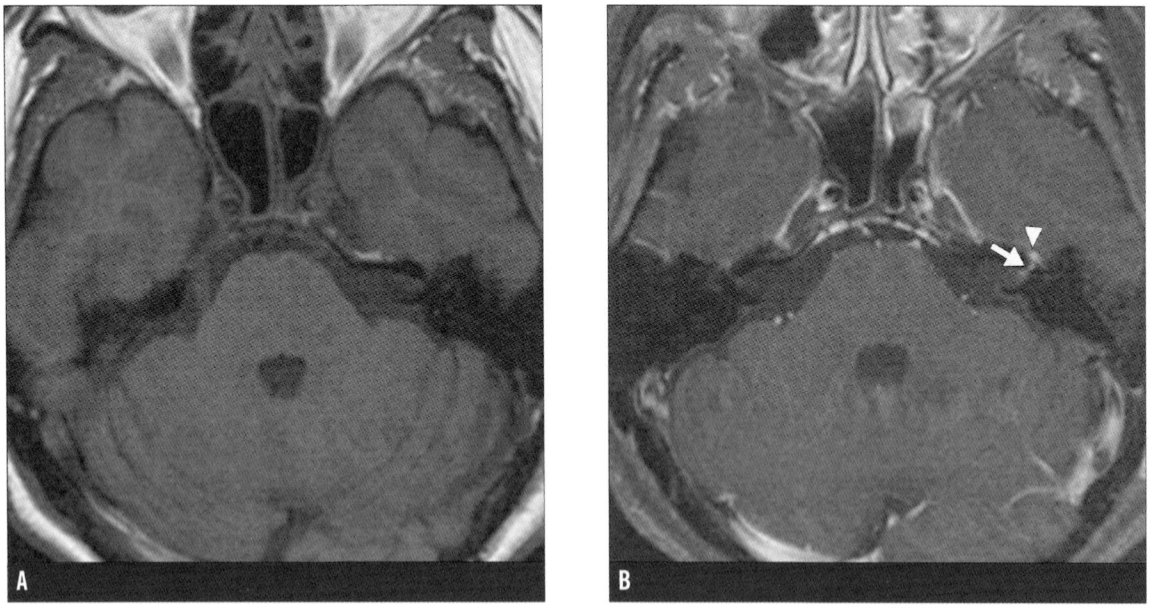

Axial T1 (**A**) and fat-suppressed postcontrast axial T1 (**B-D**) MR images through the temporal bones demonstrate typical findings of Bell palsy. Image **B** demonstrates asymmetric enhancement of the left labyrinthine segment (arrow, **B**) and left genu (arrowhead, **B**). Image **C** demonstrates asymmetric enhancement of the left tympanic segment (arrow, **C**), whereas image **D** demonstrates asymmetric enhancement of the left mastoid segment (arrow, **D**). The asymmetric nature of the findings is abnormal. While other causes of facial nerve enhancement exist, such as perineural spread of tumor, the enhancement in this case is thin and uniform, compatible with Bell palsy. There was no abnormal enhancement of the surrounding structures, such as the parotid gland (not shown). Furthermore, this patient had a clinical history and symptoms compatible with Bell palsy.

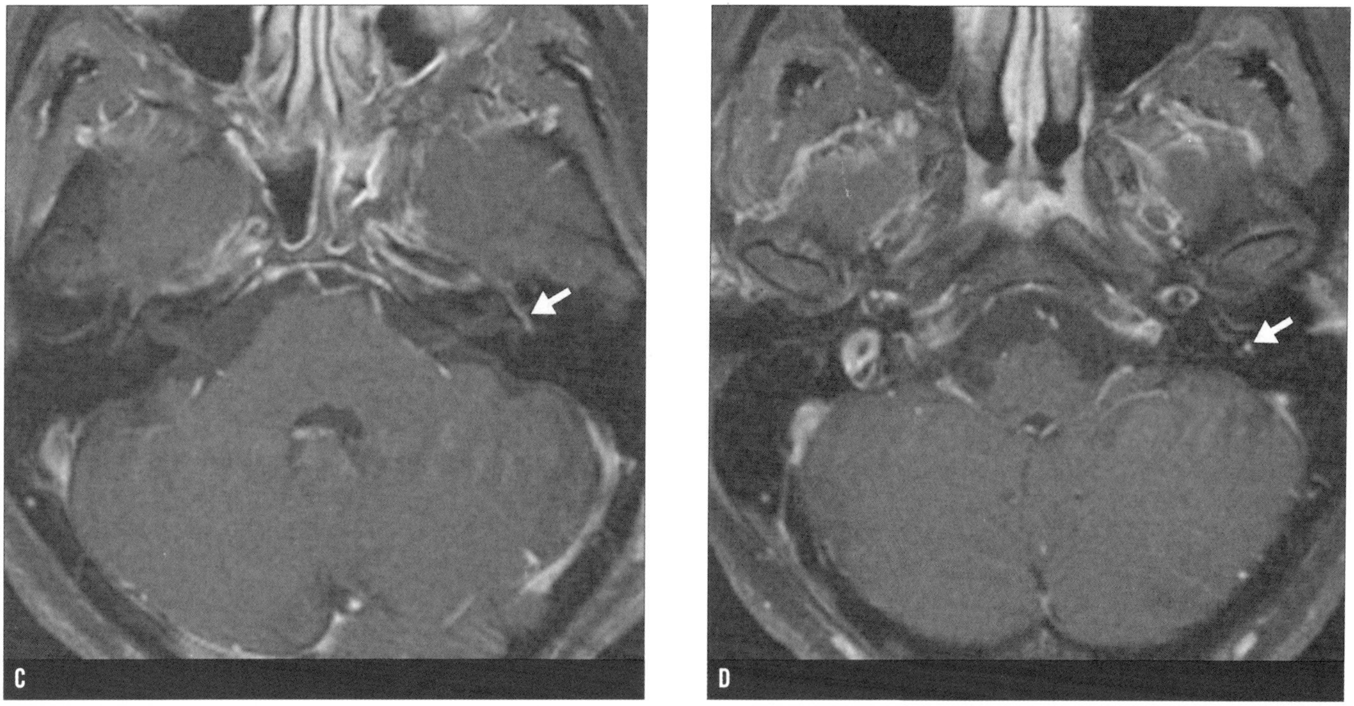

REFERENCES

Gebarski SS, Telian SA, Niparko JK. Enhancement along the normal facial nerve in the facial canal: MR imaging and anatomic correlation. *Radiology.* 1992;183:391-394.

Hong HS, et al. Enhancement pattern of the normal facial nerve at 3.0 T temporal MRI. *Br J Radiol.* 2010;83(986):118-121.

Martin-Duverneuil N, et al. Contrast enhancement of the facial nerve on MRI, normal or pathological? *Neuroradiology.* 1997;39:207-212.

Tiemstra JD, Khatkhate N. Bell's palsy: diagnosis and management. *Am Fam Physician.* 2007;76(7):997-1002.

CASE 45 Normal IAC vasculature simulating pathologic CN VII/VIII enhancement on MRI

Normal MRI vascular enhancement may occur in the internal auditory canal (IAC) as a result of normal traversing arteries and veins. The most common arteries to traverse the IAC include the anterior inferior cerebellar artery (AICA) as well as the labyrinthine and subarcuate arteries, which are typically branches of the AICA. The venous drainage in the IAC is complex, but includes the labyrinthine vein, which drains into the superior petrosal sinus. These vessels traversing the IAC may simulate pathologic cranial nerve (CN) VII/VIII enhancement on MRI, such as from leptomeningeal spread of tumor. This pitfall is particularly true when viewing the IAC with high-resolution 3D MR imaging, such as with an MPRAGE sequence. However, if there is true abnormal enhancement of the nerves on MRI, then the pathology should also be evident with spin-echo T1-weighted postcontrast imaging, preferably obtained with fat suppression.

COMPANION CASE

- **Leptomeningeal tumor spread along the CN VII/VIII complexes**

Normal IAC vasculature simulating pathologic CN VII/VIII enhancement on MRI

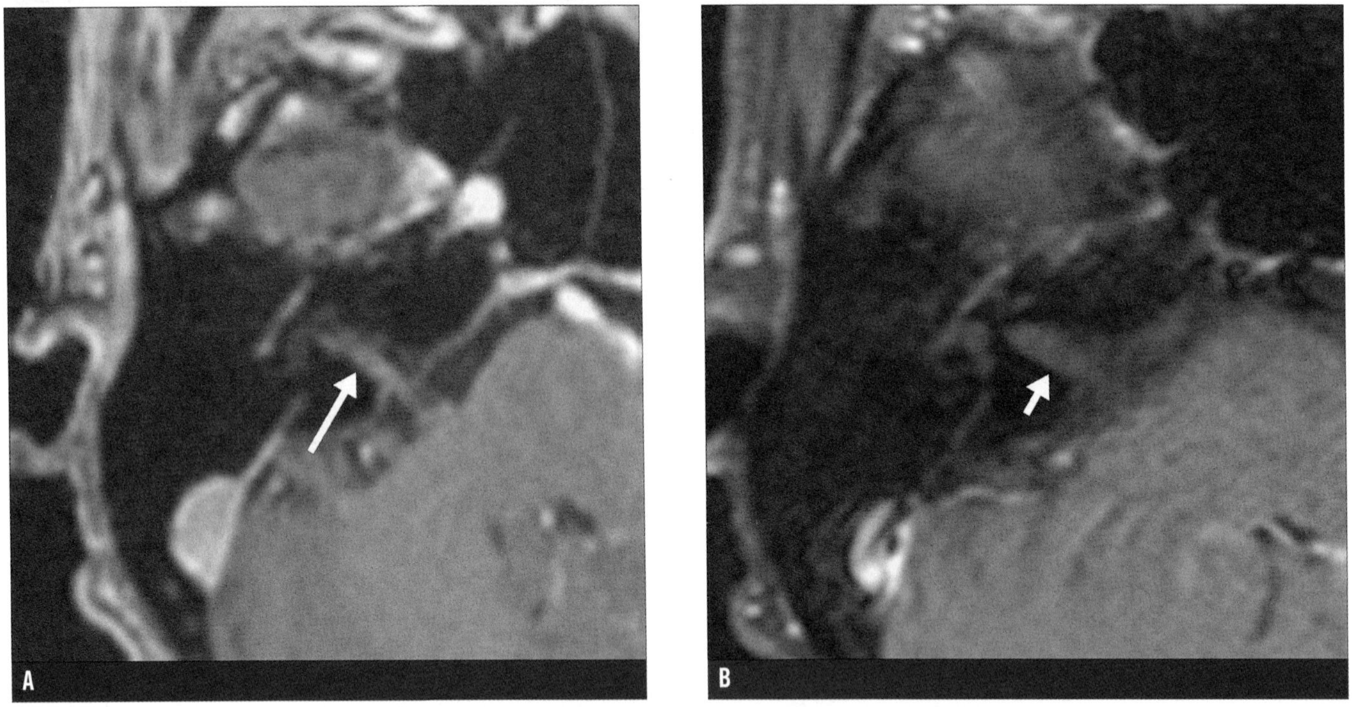

Postcontrast axial MPRAGE (**A**) and fat-suppressed postcontrast axial T1 (**B**) MR images of the right temporal bone from the same study. There is apparent abnormal enhancement of the right CN VII/VIII complex on image **A** (long arrow). However, there is no abnormal enhancement of the right CN VII/VIII complex on image **B** (short arrow). The patient did not have right facial or vestibulocochlear nerve symptoms. This spurious CN VII/VIII complex enhancement is particularly common on MPRAGE imaging. Thus, determining pathologic IAC nerve enhancement solely on the basis of a contrast-enhanced MPRAGE sequence should only be made when it is clearly pathologic and/or if it is confirmed with other sequences, such as with a postcontrast spin-echo T1-weighted sequence.

Companion case: Leptomeningeal tumor spread along the CN VII/VIII complexes

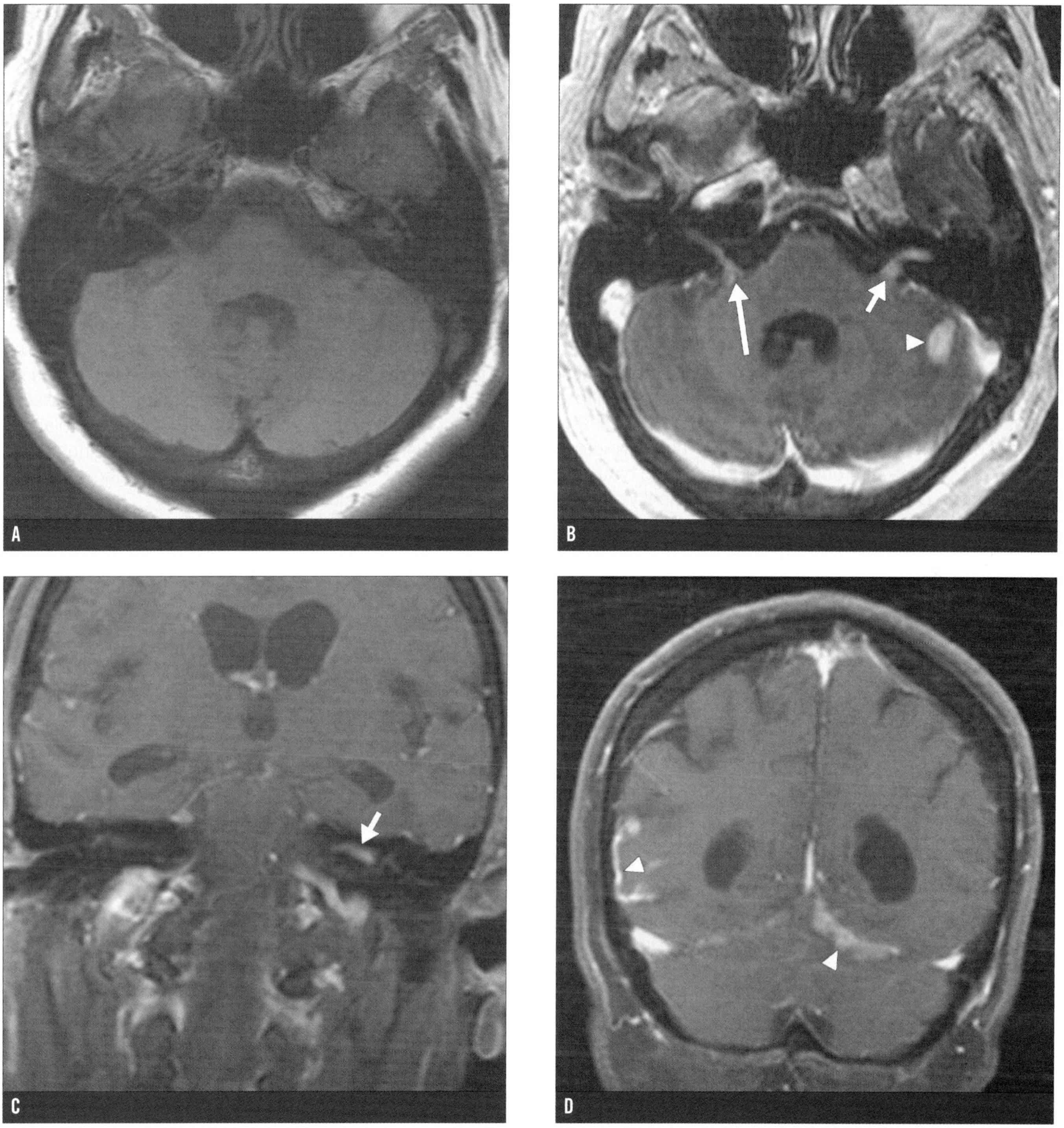

Axial T1 (**A**), postcontrast axial MPRAGE (**B**), and fat-suppressed postcontrast coronal T1 (**C**) MR images of a patient with breast cancer demonstrate abnormal enhancement in the left IAC (short arrows, **B**, **C**) and to a lesser degree the right IAC (long arrow, **B**). The enhancement within the right IAC on image **B** was confirmed on another fat-suppressed postcontrast image (not shown). Image **B** as well as a fat-suppressed postcontrast coronal T1-weighted MR image of the brain (**D**) demonstrate parenchymal, pachymeningeal, and leptomeningeal tumor spread elsewhere (arrowheads, **B**, **D**). The bilateral IAC enhancement is compatible with leptomeningeal spread of tumor along the CN VII/VIII complexes.

REFERENCE

Lescanne E, Velut S, Lefrancq T, Destrieux C. The internal acoustic meatus and its meningeal layers: a microanatomical study. *J Neurosurg.* 2002;97:1191-1197.

Microdissection studies have demonstrated that portions of the facial nerve canal can be dehiscent, usually involving the tympanic segment. The incidence of dehiscence ranges from 12% to 55% in various studies. However, an intact osseous covering of the facial nerve tympanic segment may be too thin to be visualized by CT. Therefore, it can be difficult to definitively diagnose facial nerve canal dehiscence on CT unless it is associated with prolapse of the facial nerve through the dehiscence.

COMPANION CASES

- **Dehiscence of the facial nerve canal tympanic segment with prolapse.** Facial nerve tympanic segment prolapse has been reported to occur in up to 25% of cases of facial nerve dehiscence. When the facial nerve tympanic segment prolapses through a dehiscence, the tympanic segment is caudally positioned and frequently overlies the oval window, typically resting upon the superior aspect of the stapes crural arch. If present, this stapes crural abutment by the facial nerve may result in a conductive hearing loss. A facial nerve tympanic segment prolapse is also important to identify prior to stapes/oval window-related surgeries, as the unsuspecting surgeon could damage the facial nerve in this setting.
- **Aberrant, low-lying facial nerve canal tympanic segment.** Occasionally, there can be an abnormally low-lying facial nerve canal tympanic segment without an associated osseous dehiscence, with a reported incidence of approximately 4%. This would more appropriately be termed an aberrant facial nerve, rather than a prolapsed facial nerve. This is because with an aberrant facial nerve, the course of both the facial nerve and osseous canal is abnormal, whereas in the case of a prolapsed facial nerve, the osseous canal course is normal in position but, by virtue of the prolapse, the facial nerve is abnormal in position.

Dehiscence of the facial nerve canal tympanic segment

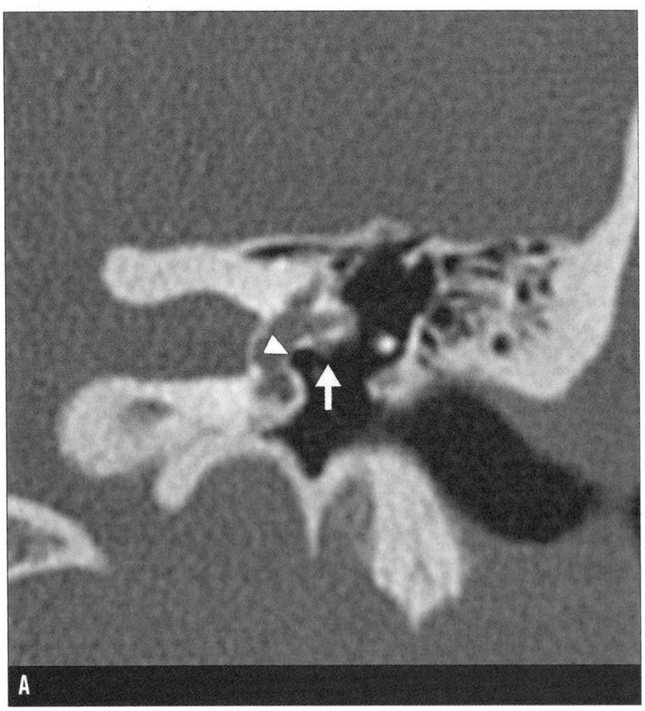

A coronal reformatted CT image of the left temporal bone (**A**) demonstrates a lack of discrete bone surrounding the tympanic portion of the facial nerve, suggesting osseous dehiscence of this portion of the facial nerve canal (arrow). However, despite the apparent dehiscence, the facial nerve tympanic segment is in a normal position and does not overlie the oval window (arrowhead), a finding which would be important to identify if it were present.

Companion case: Facial nerve prolapse

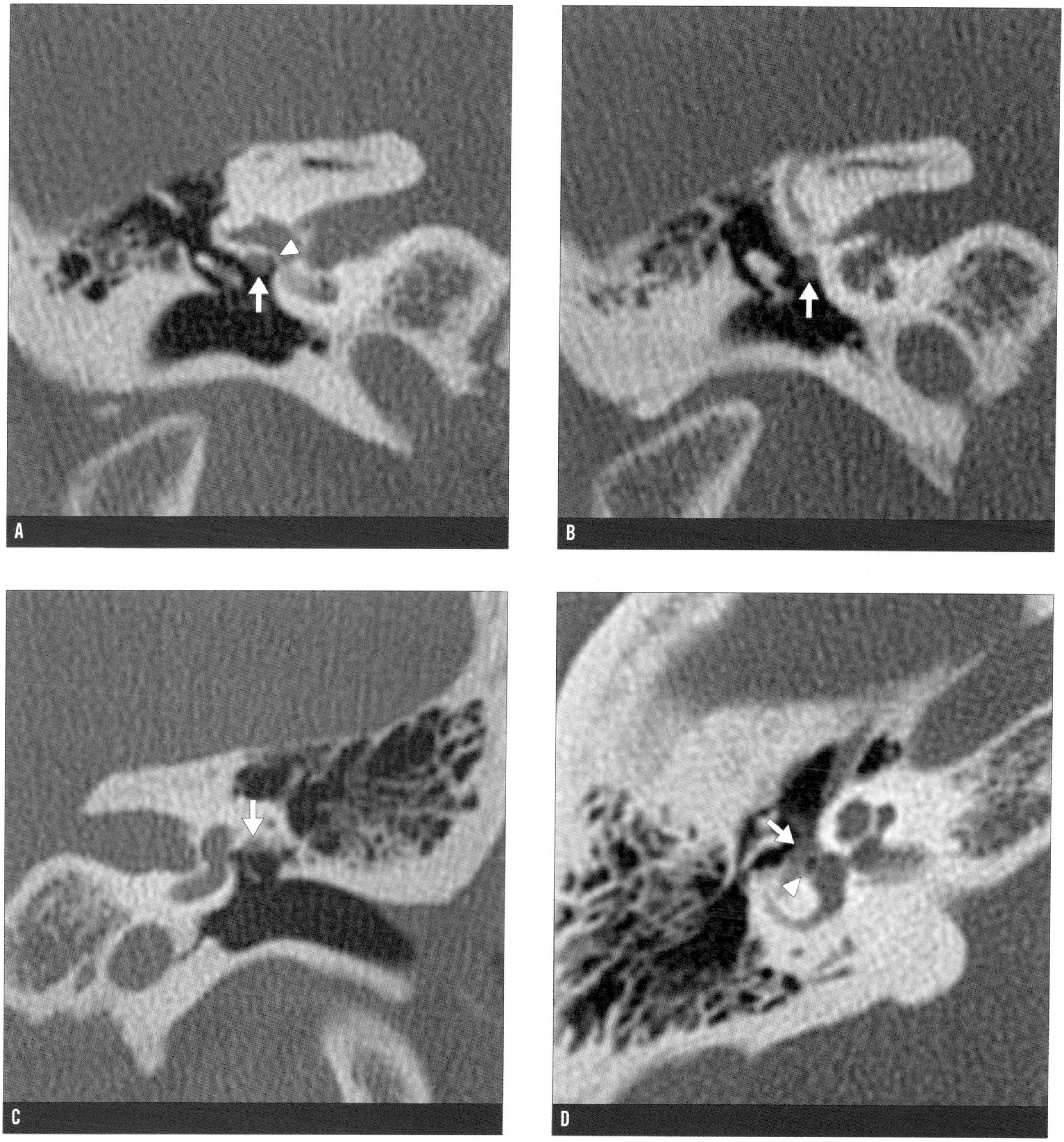

Contiguous coronal reformatted CT images of the right temporal bone (**A**, **B**) demonstrate osseous dehiscence along the right facial nerve canal tympanic segment associated with caudal prolapse of the nerve (arrows, **A**, **B**). The tympanic segment overlies the oval window (arrowhead, **A**) and predisposes the nerve to a greater chance of injury during surgery that involves the stapes and/or oval window. A coronal reformatted CT image of the left temporal bone from the same patient (**C**) demonstrates the normal relationship of the facial nerve tympanic segment (arrow, **C**) relative to the oval window. An axial CT image of the right temporal bone from the same patient (**D**) demonstrates the facial nerve tympanic segment prolapse in the axial plane (arrow, **D**), residing at the same level as the oval window and lying upon the stapes crural arch (arrowhead, **D**).

Companion case: Aberrant, low-lying facial nerve canal tympanic segment

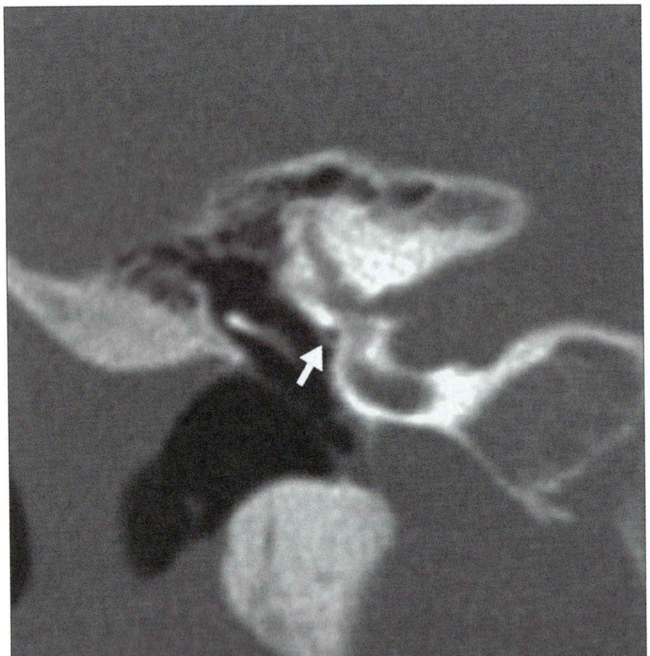

A

A coronal CT image of the right temporal bone (**A**) demonstrates the facial nerve tympanic segment to be abnormally caudal in position and to reside within the oval window (arrow). However, a subtle amount of intact facial nerve canal wall bone is identified surrounding this portion of the facial nerve. Therefore, this is compatible with an aberrant course of the facial nerve, rather than a facial nerve prolapse.

REFERENCES

Kharat RD, Golhar SV, Patil CY. Study of intratemporal course of facial nerve and its variations – 25 temporal bones dissection. *Indian J Otolaryngol Head Neck Surg*. 2009;61:39-42.

Swartz J. The facial nerve canal: CT analysis of the protruding tympanic segment. *Radiology*. 1984;153:443-447.

CASE 47 Stapedius and chorda nerves

There are two branches along the mastoid segment of the facial nerve that may be identified by CT imaging, the stapedius nerve, and the chorda tympani nerve. The stapedius nerve arises from the proximal mastoid segment of the facial nerve and extends anteriorly. The nerve supplies the stapedius muscle which is housed within the pyramidal eminence, a pyramid-shaped structure interposed between the more medially located sinus tympani and the more laterally located facial recess. Because of their extremely small size, the stapedial nerve and muscle may not be identified as separate structures. The stapedial tendon may sometimes be identified on CT as it extends into the tympanic cavity and inserts upon the stapes neck. The function of the stapedius tendon and muscle is to protect the inner ear from loud noise. When the stapedius muscle contracts, it decreases stapes superstructure movement, thereby decreasing inner ear stimulation.

The chorda tympani nerve is the second branch of the facial nerve mastoid segment and is usually best identified on CT when the images are obtained with a 0.6-mm or less slice thickness. The chorda tympani nerve arises from the lateral aspect of the distal facial nerve mastoid segment and ascends (ie, in the opposite direction of the facial nerve) for a short distance within the facial nerve canal. The chorda tympani nerve then exits the distal aspect of the facial nerve canal mastoid segment (a variable distance but usually approx. 4-5 mm superior to the stylomastoid foramen) and ascends within its own bony canal of the mastoid termed the posterior canaliculus, a very small canal measuring only 0.3 to 0.5 mm in diameter. The chorda tympani nerve then exits the posterior canaliculus and enters the posterolateral aspect of the tympanic cavity. Within the tympanic cavity, the chorda tympani nerve arches anterosuperiorly and traverses between the neck or manubrium of the malleus and the long process of the incus. The nerve then exits along the medial aspect of the petrotympanic fissure and descends anteriorly. Approximately 1 to 2 cm after exiting the skull base, the chorda tympani nerve joins the lingual nerve (a branch of the trigeminal nerve V3 segment) on its way toward the oral cavity. There are preganglionic parasympathetic fibers of the chorda tympani nerve which synapse in the submandibular ganglion. The postganglionic fibers then pass directly to the submandibular gland and duct as well as rejoin the lingual nerve to innervate the sublingual gland. The lingual nerve, as well as fibers of the chorda tympani nerve, then enter the tongue.

While there is likely a complex interplay among nerves in and around the oral cavity, the function of the chorda tympani nerve is primarily twofold. One function is to provide secretomotor innervation to the submandibular and sublingual glands (via efferent parasympathetics from the superior salivatory nucleus) allowing for salivary secretion from these glands. The other function is to convey afferent taste fibers from the anterior two-thirds of the tongue to the nucleus solitarius in the brainstem.

COMPANION CASE

- **Perineural spread along the chorda tympani nerve**

Stapedius muscle and nerve

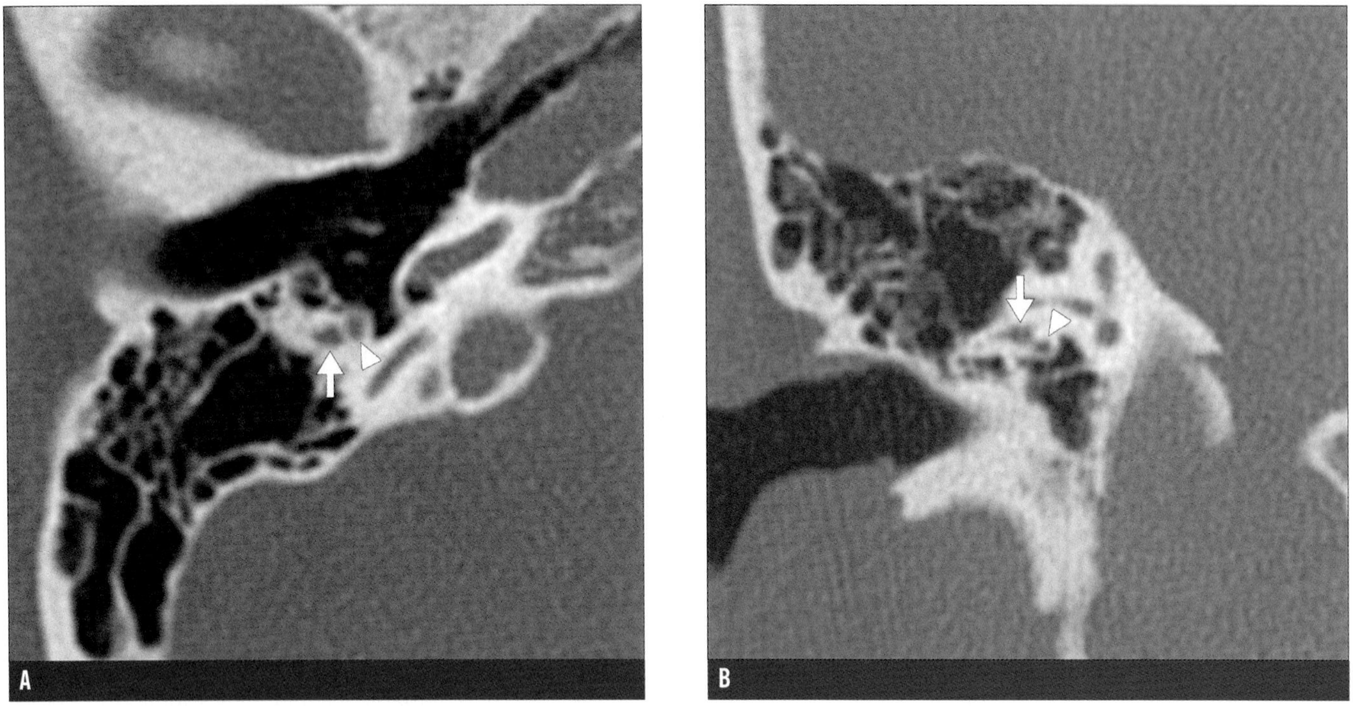

Axial (**A**) and coronal reformatted (**B**) CT images of the right temporal bone demonstrate two distinct osseous canals. One osseous canal contains the stapedius muscle and nerve (arrowheads, **A**, **B**). The other represents the proximal facial nerve mastoid segment (arrows, **A**, **B**), which contains the facial nerve and gives rise to the stapedius nerve.

Stapedius muscle and tendon

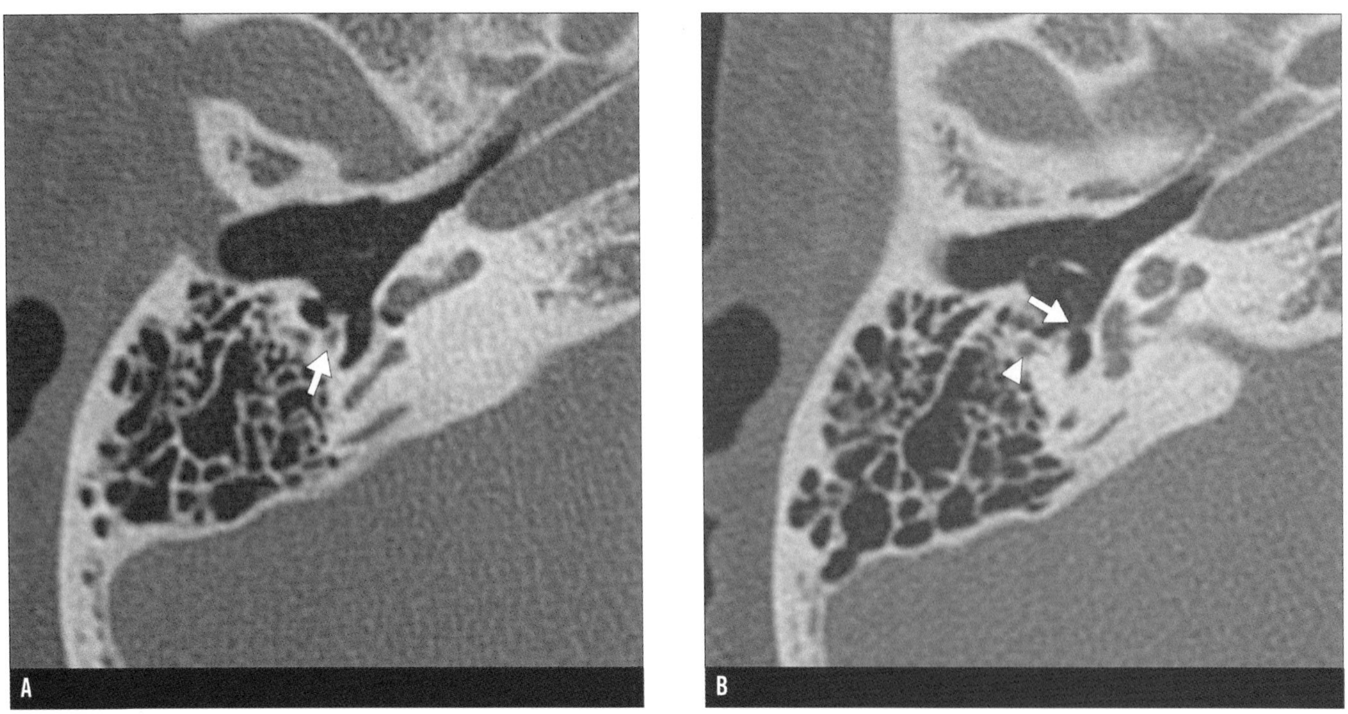

Axial CT images of the right temporal bone (**A**-**C**) demonstrate the normal stapedius muscle/nerve (arrow, **A**) and the stapedius tendon (arrows, **B**, **C**) inserting onto the neck of the stapes. The proximal aspect of the facial nerve canal mastoid segment is also demonstrated on these images (arrowheads, **B**, **C**).

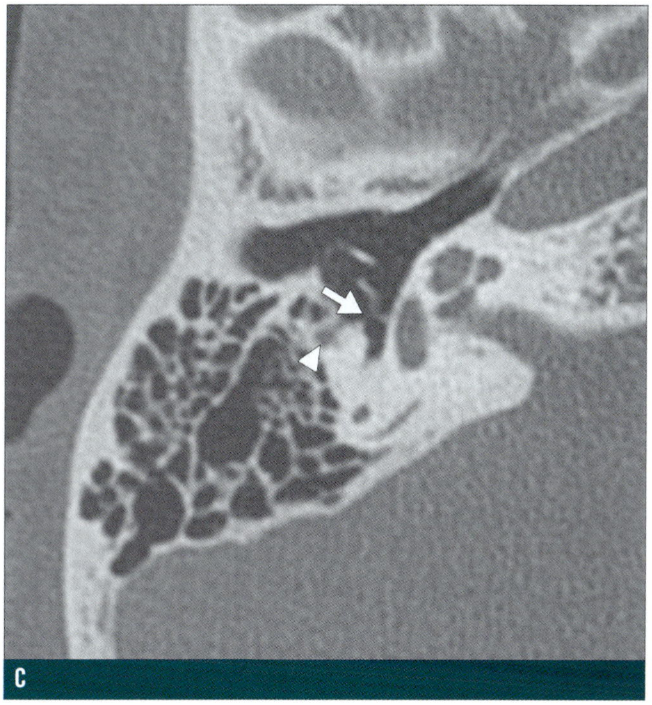

Chorda tympani nerve within the posterior canaliculus

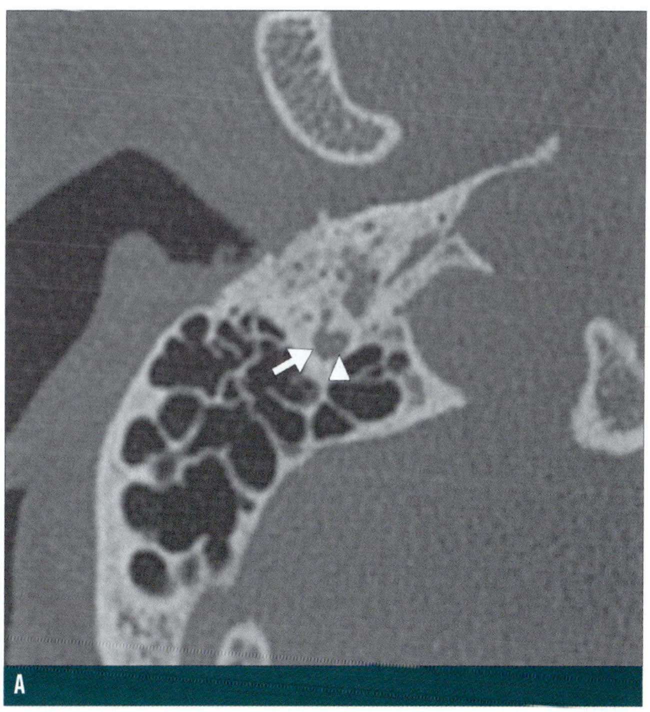

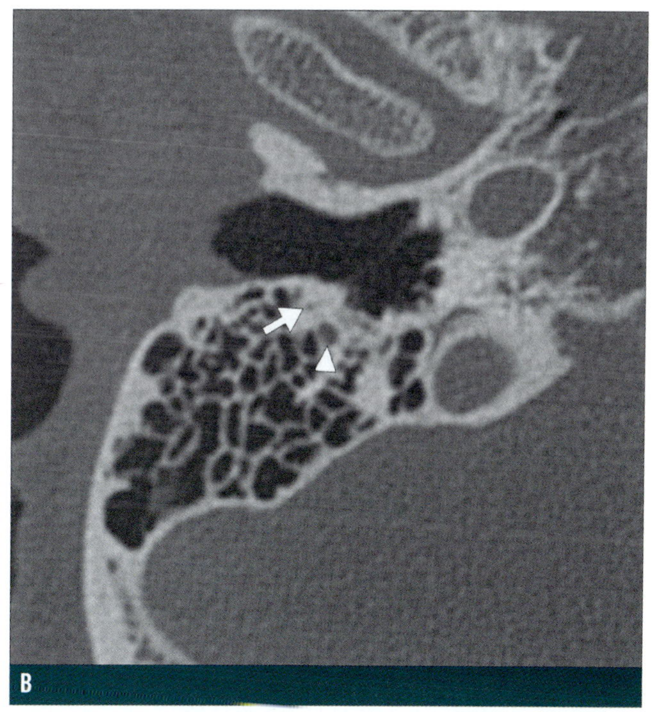

Axial CT images obtained through the mastoid portion of the right temporal bone from inferior to superior (**A**-**C**) demonstrate the normal chorda tympani nerve ascending through mastoid within the posterior canaliculus (arrows, **A**-**C**) and its relationship relative to the facial nerve canal mastoid segment (arrowheads, **A**-**C**). The typical origin of the posterior canaliculus as it arises from the distal aspect of the facial nerve canal mastoid segment is demonstrated on image **A**. A Pöschl plane reformatted CT view of a different patient (**D**) perhaps best demonstrates the relationship between the chorda tympani nerve within the posterior canaliculus (arrow, **D**) and the facial nerve (arrowhead, **D**).

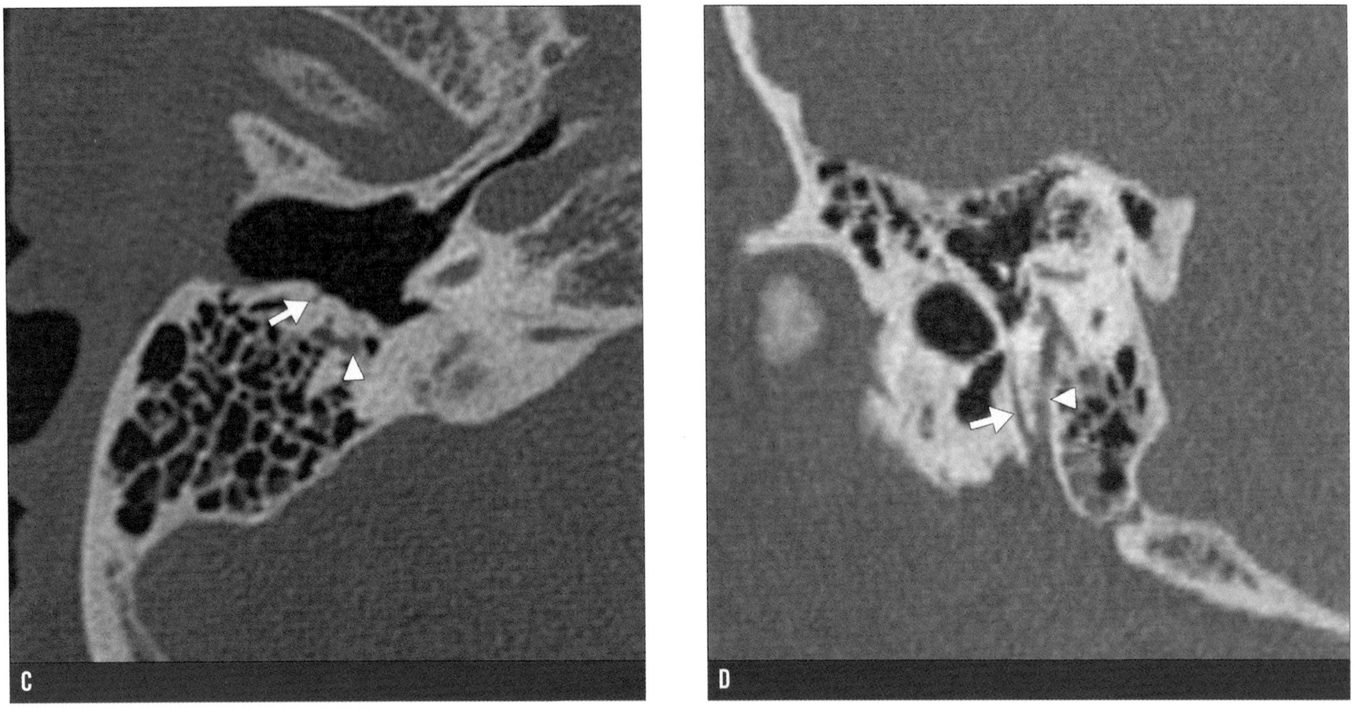

Chorda tympani nerve traversing the tympanic cavity

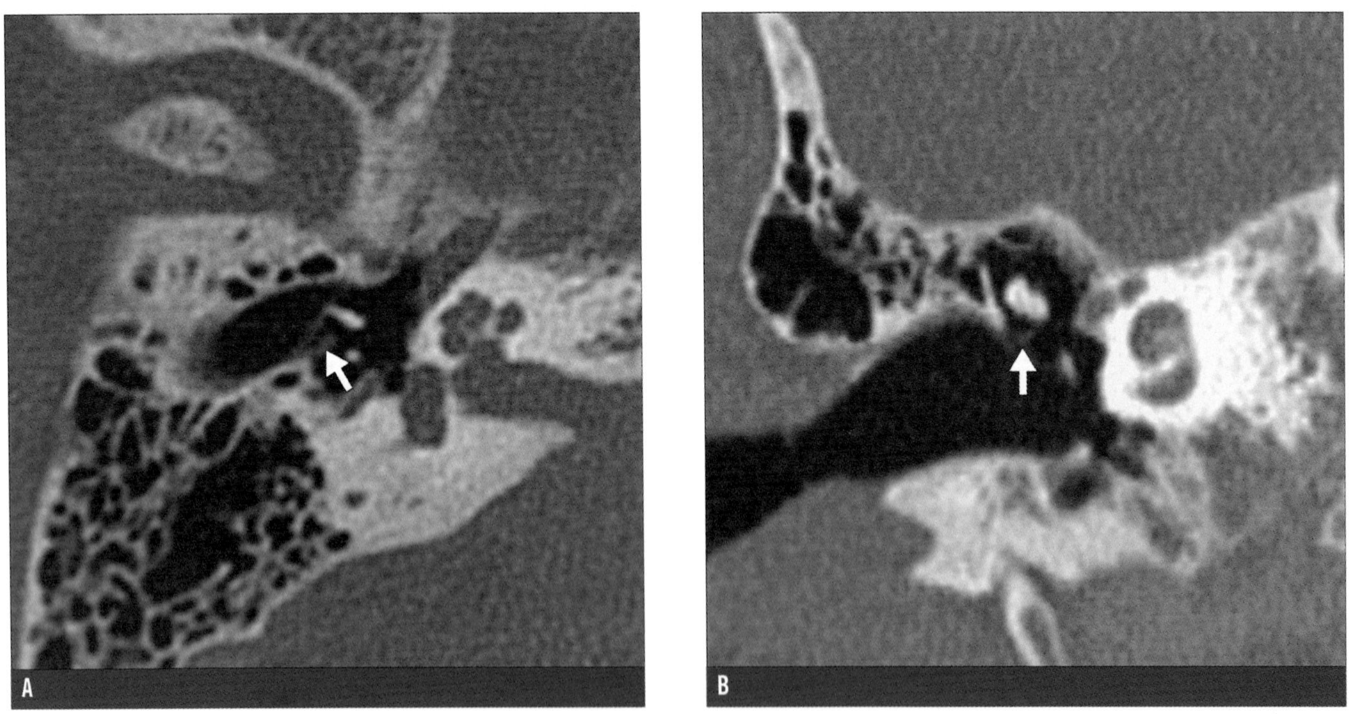

Axial (**A**) and coronal reformatted (**B**) CT images of the right temporal bone demonstrate a subtle linear density traversing the right tympanic cavity (arrows, **A**, **B**), representing the normal chorda tympani nerve as it traverses between the neck/manubrium of the malleus and the long process of the incus.

Companion case: Perineural spread along the chorda tympani nerve

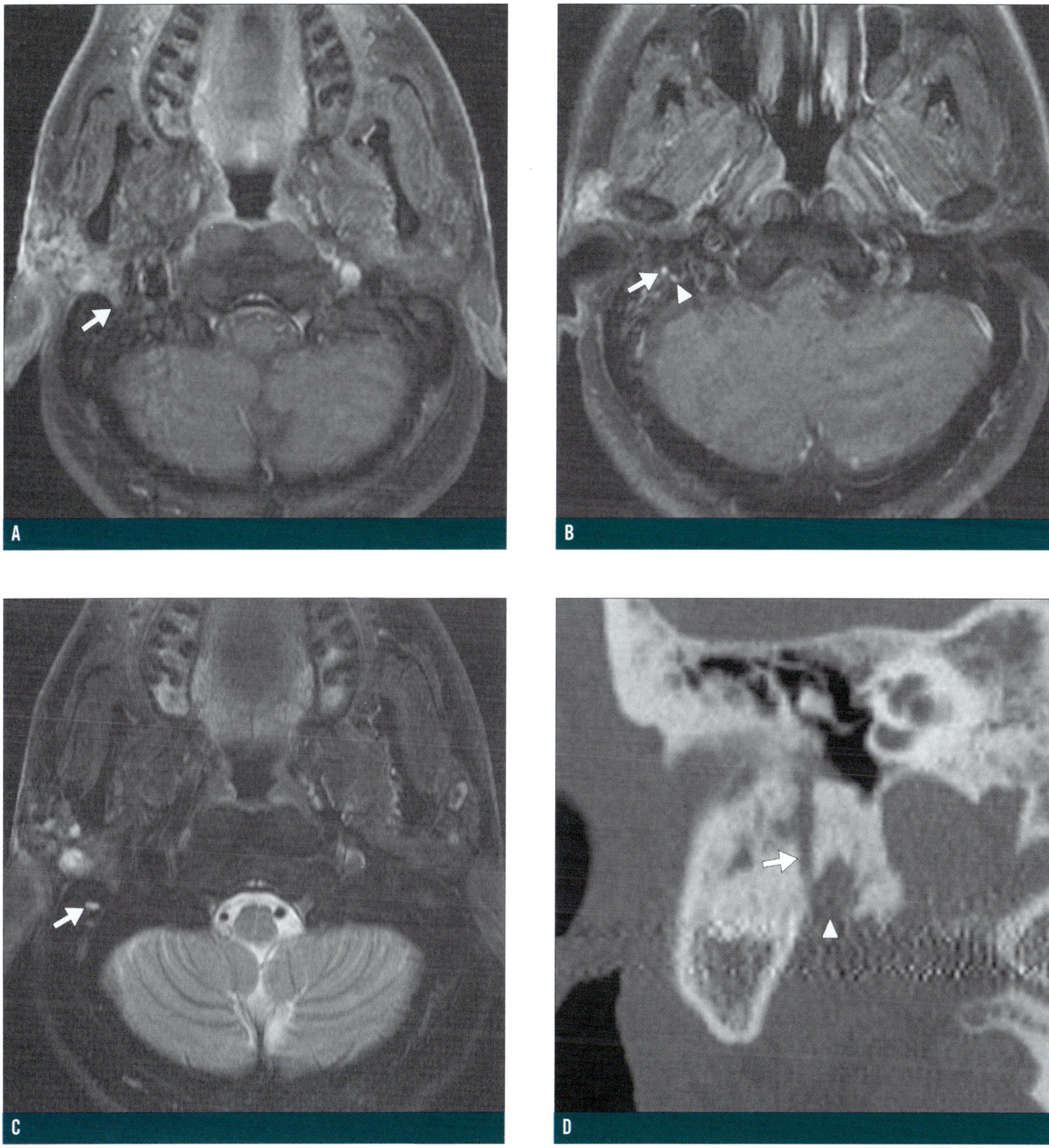

Fat-suppressed postcontrast axial T1-weighted MR images (**A**, **B**) demonstrate a mass of the right parotid gland extending into the right stylomastoid foramen (arrow, **A**) and two discrete foci of enhancement in the inferior right mastoid representing the chorda tympani nerve (arrow, **B**) and mastoid segment of the facial nerve (arrowhead, **B**). A fat-suppressed axial T2-weighted MR image (**C**) demonstrates a discrete focus of hyperintense signal representing the right chorda tympani nerve (arrow, **C**), clearly asymmetric when compared to the contralateral left mastoid. A coronal reformatted CT image of the right temporal bone (**D**) demonstrates the posterior canaliculus (which contains the chorda tympani nerve) (arrow, **D**) to extend to the level of the stylomastoid foramen (arrowhead, **D**). Axial CT images of the right (**E**) and left (**F**) temporal bones demonstrate marked enlargement of the right posterior canaliculus (arrow, **E**) compared to the left (arrow, **F**) but fairly symmetric mastoid segment facial nerve canals (arrowheads, **E**, **F**). The chorda tympani nerve and its posterior canaliculus usually arise from the facial nerve mastoid segment approximately 4-5 mm superior to the stylomastoid foramen, although their origin is variable among patients.. In this case, their origin near the right stylomastoid foramen allowed direct access of the tumor into the posterior canaliculus. This tumor represented carcinoma ex pleomorphic adenoma and perineural tumor spread along the chorda tympani nerve was confirmed at pathology.

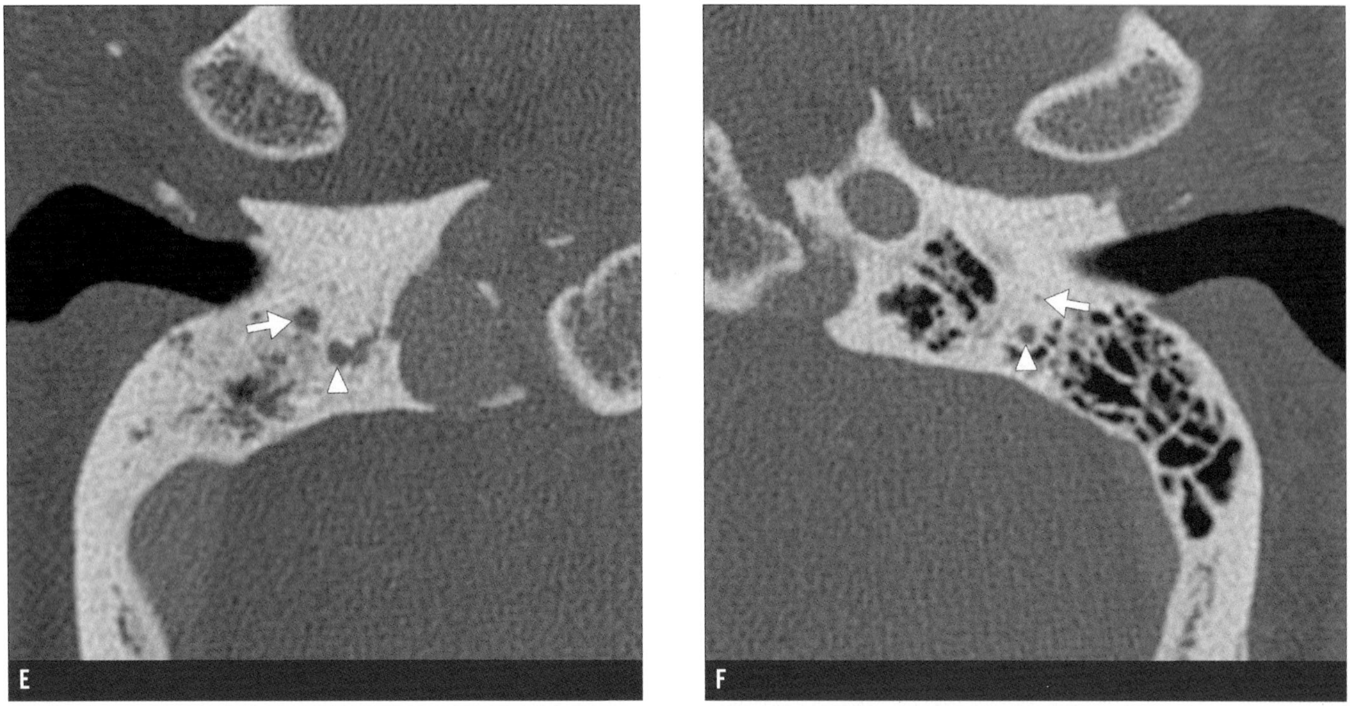

REFERENCES

McManus LJ, Dawes PJ, Stringer MD. Clinical anatomy of the chorda tympani: a systematic review. *J Laryngol Otol.* 2011;125(11): 1101-1108.

McManus LJ, Dawes PJ, Stringer MD. Surgical anatomy of the chorda tympani: a micro-CT study. *Surg Radiol Anat.* 2012;34(6):513-518.

Rodríguez-Vázquez JF. Development of the stapedius muscle and pyramidal eminence in humans. *J Anat.* 2009;215(3):292-299.

CASE 48 The facial hiatus and greater superficial petrosal nerve

The greater superficial petrosal nerve (GSPN) is a branch of the facial nerve that carries both efferent parasympathetic fibers and afferent sensory fibers. The GSPN arises at the level of the geniculate ganglion of cranial nerve (CN) VII. It exits anteromedially via an osseous opening termed the facial hiatus, which is located along the ventral margin of the facial nerve canal anterior genu. The GSPN then traverses along the cephalad margin of the petrous temporal bone and subsequently inferior to the Meckel cave. From here, the GSPN joins the deep petrosal nerve to give rise to the vidian nerve (also called nerve of the pterygoid canal). This nerve traverses anteriorly toward the pterygopalatine fossa, where preganglionic parasympathetic fibers synapse at the sphenopalatine (also called pterygopalatine) ganglion. The postganglionic parasympathetic fibers supply the lacrimal glands to provide lacrimation as well as the palate and nasal mucosa to provide secretory and vasomotor innervation. Sensation fibers arising from the palate and nasopharynx traverse afferently within the GSPN on their way to the brainstem.

When viewed on axial CT imaging utilizing a bone algorithm, the facial hiatus is characterized as a linear, discrete, lucency arising anteromedially from the apex of the facial nerve canal anterior genu. It is important not to mistake the normal facial hiatus for a fracture in the setting of trauma.

COMPANION CASES

- **Longitudinal fracture through the facial nerve canal genu and facial hiatus.**
- **Perineural spread along the GSPN**. As discussed above, the GSPN arises from the facial nerve and extends to the pterygopalatine fossa via the vidian nerve. Because the V2 division of CN V also extends into the pterygopalatine fossa, the GSPN can serve as a conduit for perineural spread of tumor between CN VII and CN V. As an aside, other potential routes of perineural spread between CN VII and CN V exist via the auriculotemporal nerve and between the chorda tympani nerve (a branch of CN VII) with the lingual nerve (a branch of CN V).

The facial hiatus and greater superficial petrosal nerve

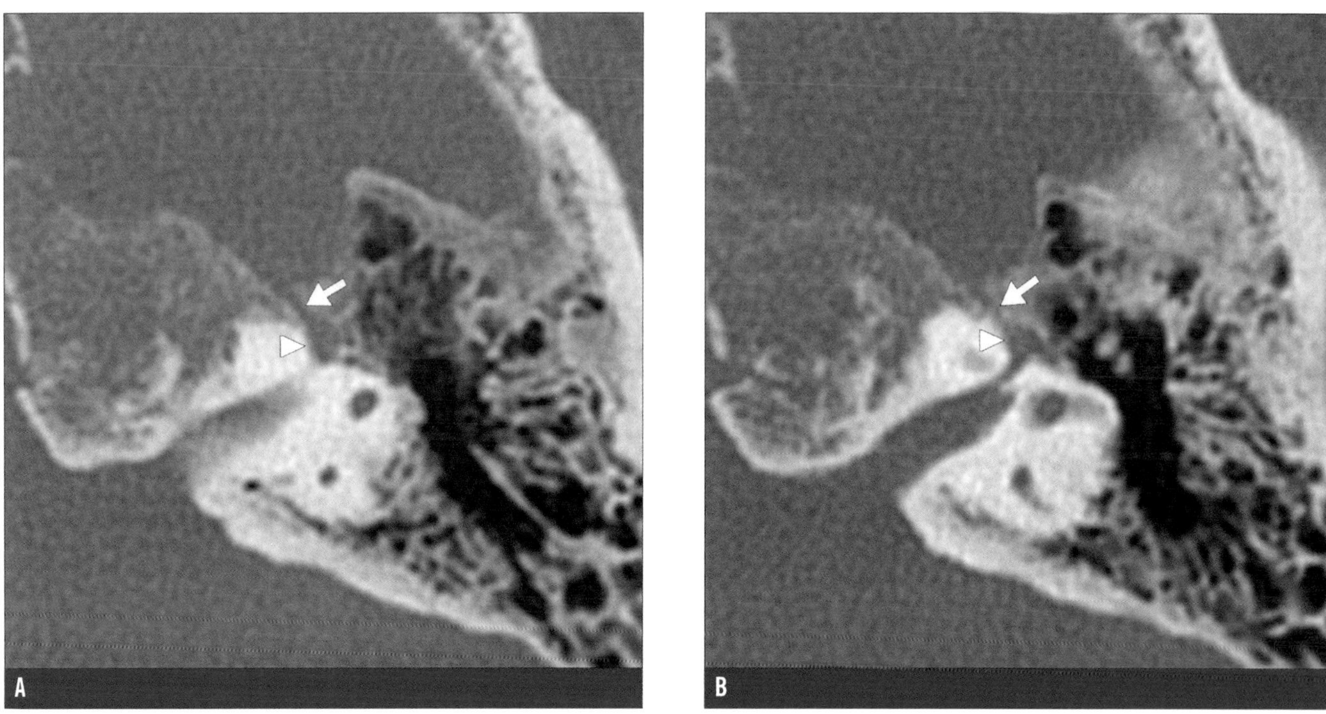

Axial CT images of the left temporal bone (**A**, **B**) demonstrate the normal facial nerve canal anterior genu, which houses the geniculate ganglion (arrowheads, **A**, **B**). The facial hiatus is located at the apex of the anterior genu and represents the location where the greater superficial petrosal nerve exits the temporal bone (arrows, **A**, **B**). It is important not to mistake the normal facial hiatus for a fracture in the setting of trauma.

Companion case: Longitudinal fracture though the facial nerve canal genu and facial hiatus

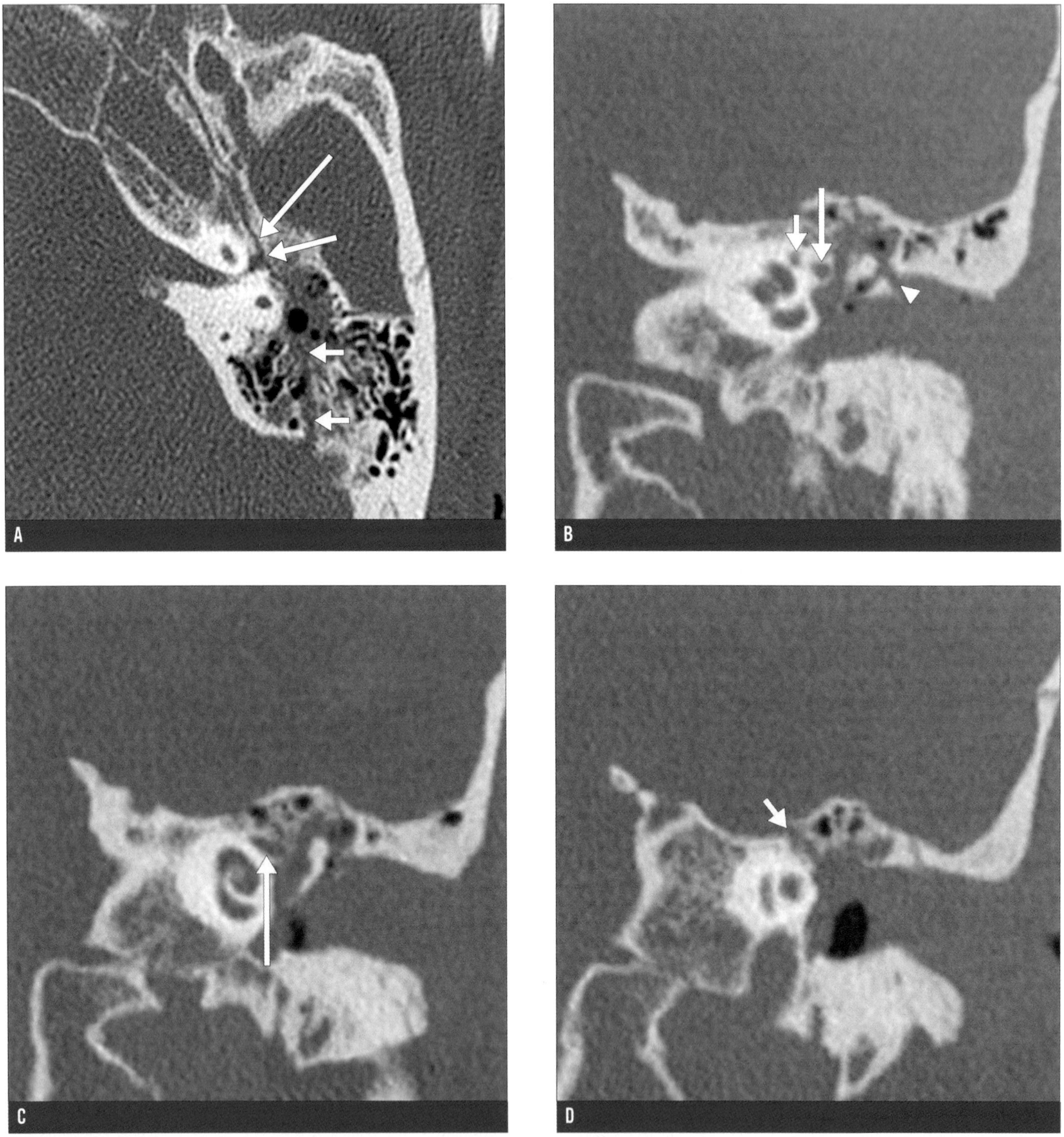

An axial CT image through the left temporal bone (**A**) demonstrates a longitudinal fracture through the temporal bone (short arrows, **A**). This fracture involves the genu of the facial nerve canal (medium arrow, **A**) as well as likely the facial hiatus and extending anteriorly (long arrow, **A**), although involvement of the facial hiatus is difficult to verify by axial imaging alone. Coronal reformatted images of the left temporal bone (**B-D**). Image **B** demonstrates the osseous canals of the facial nerve labyrinthine segment (also called fallopian canal) (short arrow, **B**) and the proximal aspect of the facial nerve tympanic segment (medium arrow, **B**). A fracture involving the scutum is also demonstrated (arrowhead, **B**). Image **C** demonstrates the genu of the facial nerve canal (long arrow, **C**) which houses the geniculate ganglion and is located at the union of the labyrinthine and tympanic segments of the facial canal. Immediately anterior to image **C** (**D**), a fracture line is clearly identified extending through the region of the facial hiatus, corroborating the finding on image **A**.

Companion case: Perineural spread along the greater superficial petrosal nerve

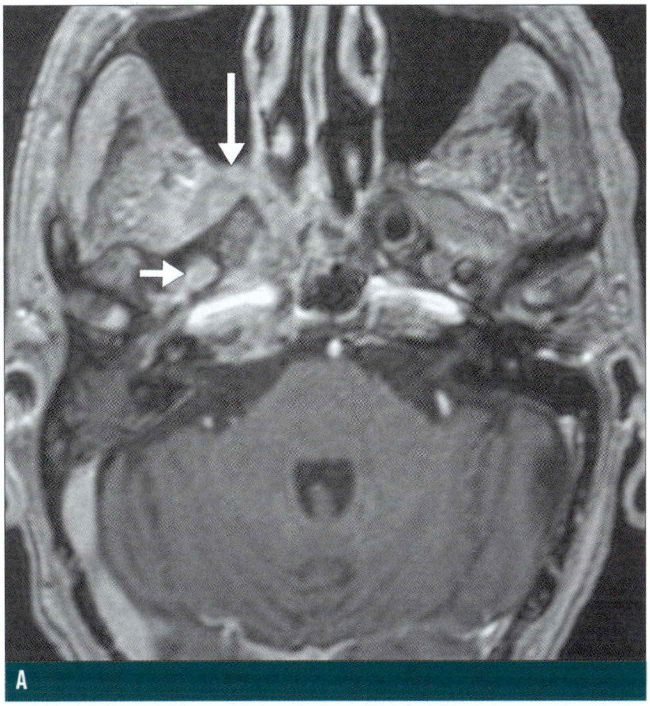

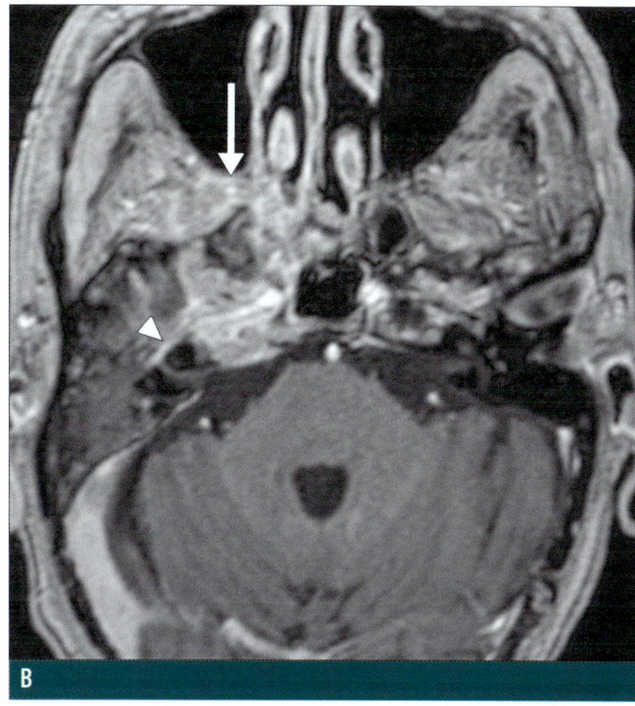

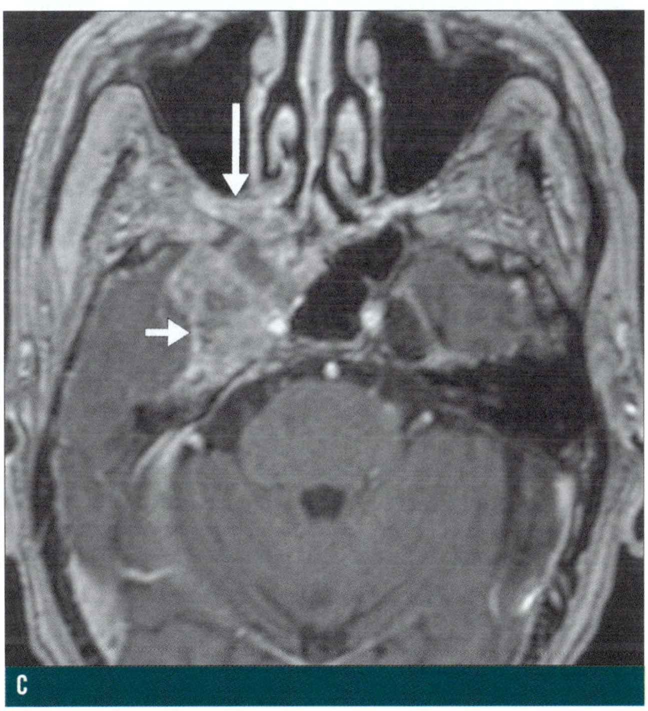

Postcontrast axial MPRAGE MR images (**A**-**C**) demonstrate extensive perineural spread of tumor in a patient with nasopharyngeal carcinoma. There is tumor occupying and expanding the right pterygopalatine fossa (long arrows, **A**-**C**), occupying and expanding the right Meckel cave (short arrow, **C**), involving the right foramen ovale (short arrow, **A**), and extending along the greater superficial petrosal nerve (arrowhead, **B**). This case illustrates one of the routes of perineural spread between branches of CN V and CN VII.

REFERENCES

Alfieri A, Strauss C, Prell J, Peschke E. History of the nervus intermedius of Wrisberg. *Ann Anat.* 2010 20;192(3):139-144.

Ginsberg LE, De Monte F, Gillenwater AM. Greater superficial petrosal nerve: anatomy and MR findings in perineural tumor spread. *Am J Neuroradiol.* 1996;17:389-393.

Jager L, et al. CT of the normal temporal bone: comparison of multi-and single detector row CT. *Radiology.* 2005;235:133-141.

Jordan, D. The Nervus Intermedius. *Arch Ophthalmol.* 1993;111(12): 1691-1692.

Shao YX, Xie X, Liang HS, Zhou J, Jing M, Liu EZ. Microsurgical anatomy of the greater superficial petrosal nerve. *World Neurosurg.* 2012;77(1):172-182.

Surgical microvascular decompression of CN VII is most commonly performed to treat symptoms of hemifacial spasm caused by vascular compression of the nerve. Typically, the decompression is performed by separating the offending vessel from CN VII with synthetic material, usually in the form of a small felt pledget composed of polytetrafluoroethylene (PTFE). If the vascular compression is caused by the vertebral artery, the vertebral artery may be surgically separated from the nerve and stabilized in position by suturing the artery to a suitable adjacent structure. In cases when a pledget is used for microvascular decompression, CT imaging will demonstrate an iso- to hyperdense structure at the cerebellopontine angle on the side of surgery. On MRI, a pledget will manifest as a small geographic area of isointense T1 and hypointense T2 signal.

Microvascular decompression of CN VII

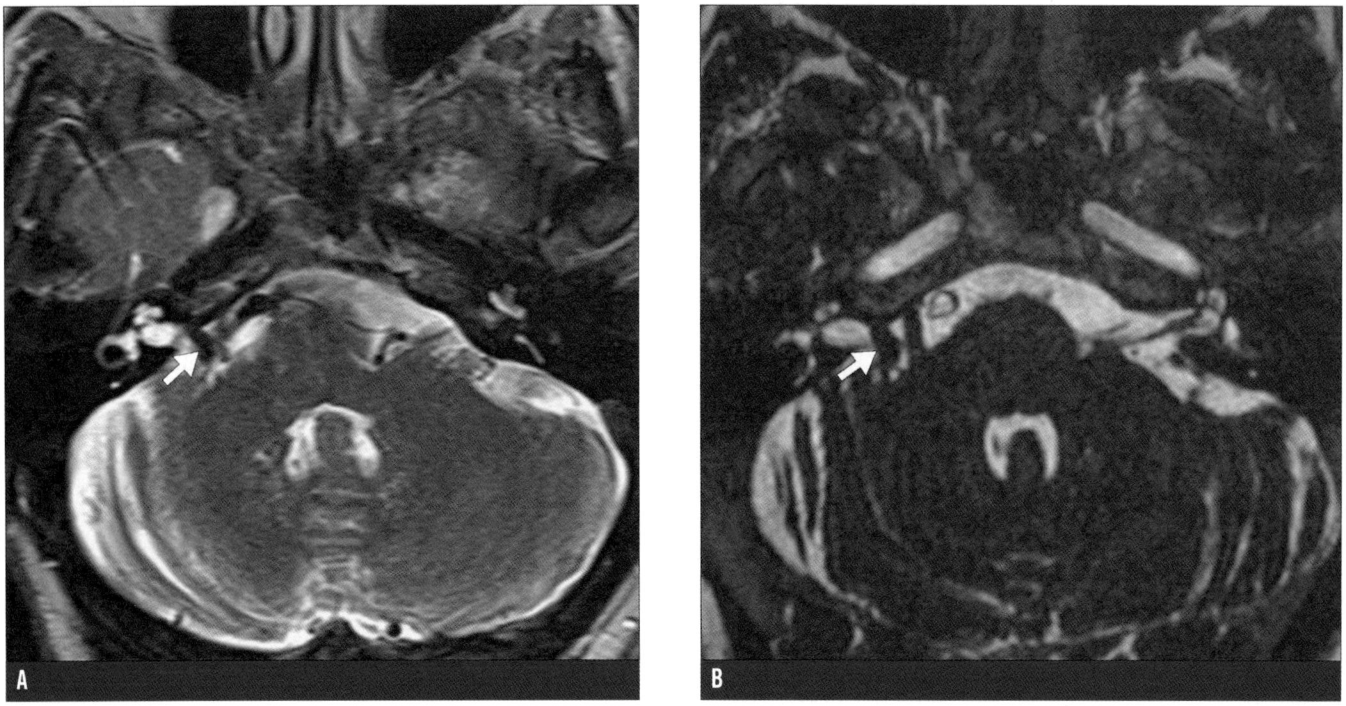

Axial T2 (**A**), axial CISS (**B**), axial T1 (**C**), and fat-suppressed postcontrast axial T1 (**D**) MR images of a patient with a prior history of right hemifacial spasm demonstrate a geographic area in the right cerebellopontine angle that is low in signal on T2 (arrows, **A**, **B**), isointense on T1 (arrow, **C**), and mildly enhancing (arrow, **D**), compatible with a PTFE pledget used for microvascular decompression of CN VII. The mild enhancement in this region presumably reflects granulation tissue.

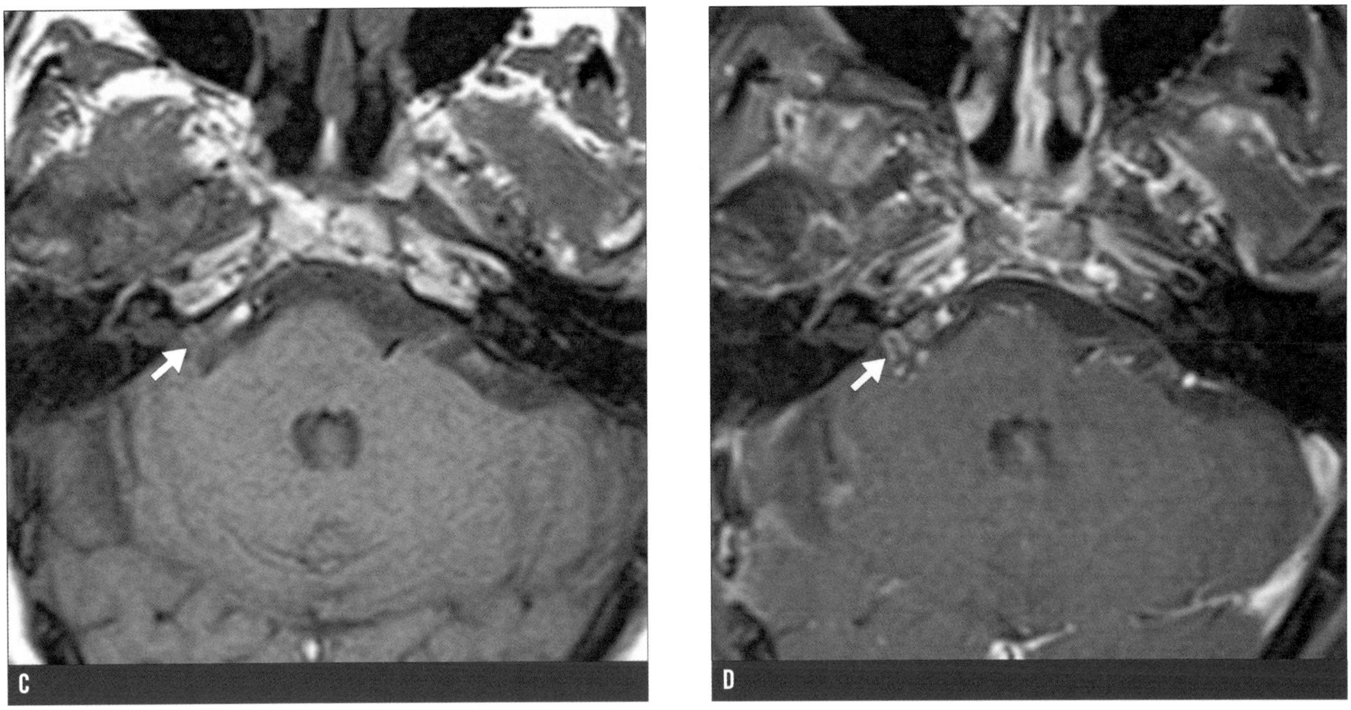

Microvascular decompression of CN VII

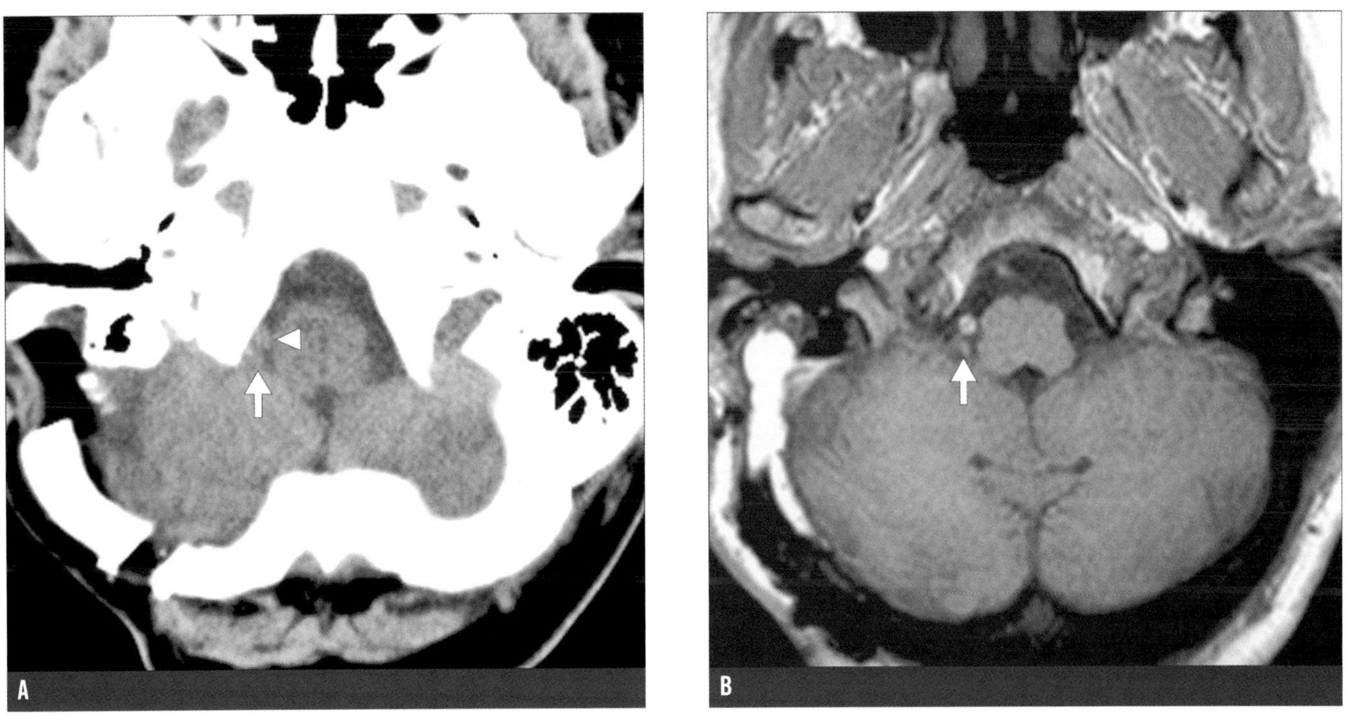

Different patient. An axial CT image (**A**) of a patient with a prior history of right hemifacial spasm demonstrates a barely perceptible isodense structure at the right cerebellopontine angle (arrow, **A**) representing a PTFE pledget used for microvascular decompression of the right facial nerve. The intracranial right vertebral artery is identified immediately anterior to the pledget (arrowhead, **A**). A right retrosigmoid craniotomy was used to gain access to the right cerebellopontine angle. Axial T1 (**B**) and axial T2 (**C**) MR images of the same patient demonstrate the pledget to be isointense on T1 (arrow, **B**) and hypointense on T2 (arrow, **C**). Note that placement of the pledget is somewhat caudal to the expected location of the CN VII cisternal segment because the offending vessel was profoundly tortuous.

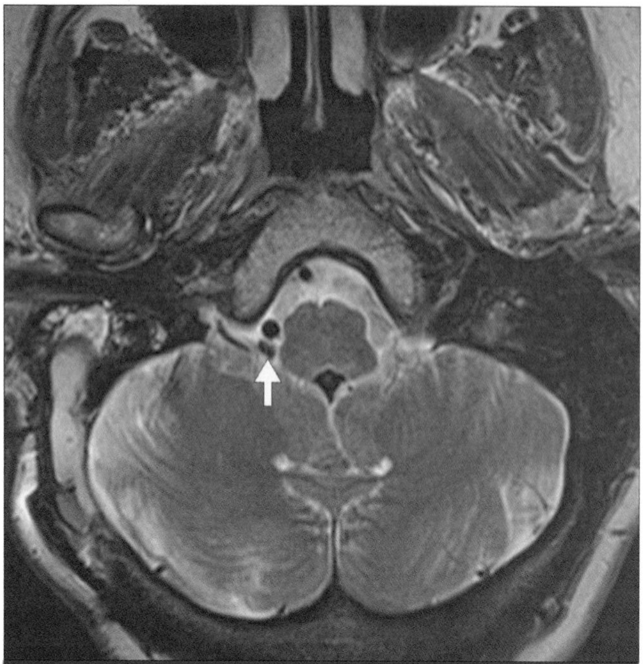

C

REFERENCES

Ferreira M, Walcott BP, Nahed BV, Sekhar LN. Vertebral artery pexy for microvascular decompression of the facial nerve in the treatment of hemifacial spasm. *J Neurosurg.* 2011;114:1800-1804.

Mitsuoka H, Tsunoda A, Okuda O, Sato K, Makita J. Delineation of small nerves and blood vessels with three-dimensional fast spin-echo MR imaging: comparison of presurgical and surgical findings in patients with hemifacial spasm. *Am J Neuroradiol.* 1998;19:1823-1829.

Nagaseki Y, et al. Postoperative oblique sagittal MR imaging of microvascular decompression for hemifacial spasm. *Acta Neurochir.* 1999;141(7):737-742.

CHAPTER 9

ORBIT

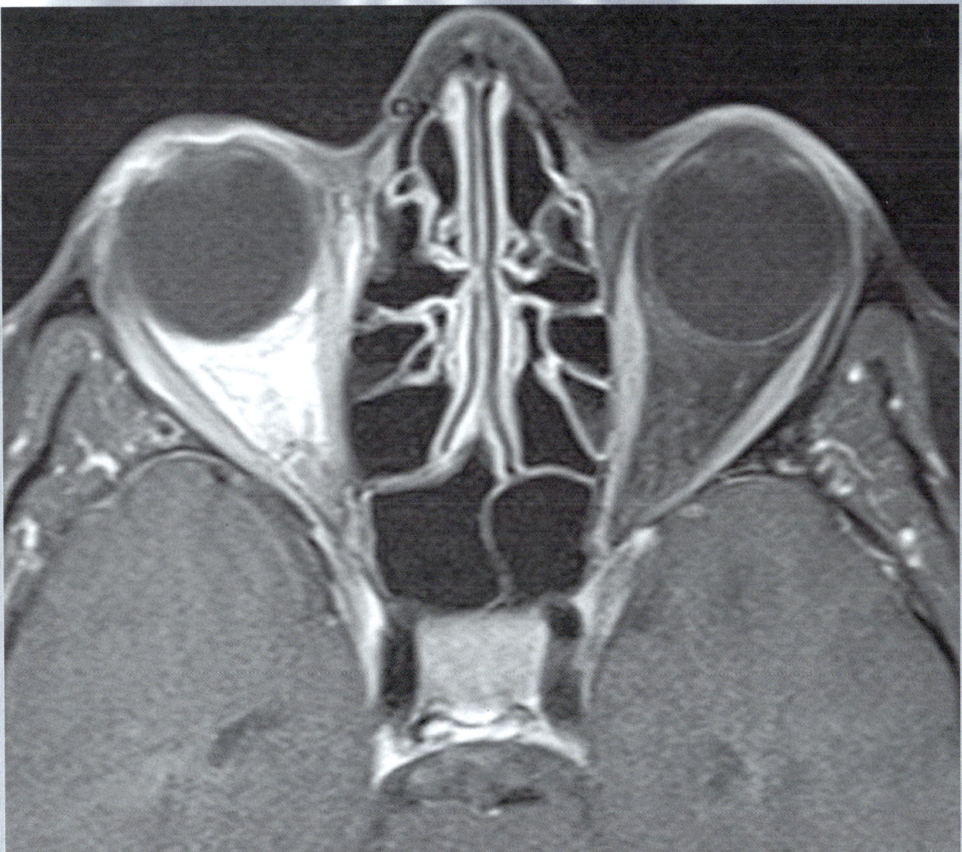

Kamran A. Shah, Achilles G. Karagianis,
Tarek A. Hijaz

IX. ORBIT

1. Senile scleral calcification
    i. *Companion case*: Glass foreign bodies
    ii. *Companion case*: Sclerochoroidal calcifications due to renal failure
    iii. *Companion case*: Choroidal osteoma
    iv. *Companion case*: Calcification related to prior vitreous hemorrhage
2. Optic disc drusen
    i. *Companion case*: Calcified retinal drusen
3. Trochlear calcification
    i. *Companion case*: Small metallic foreign body simulating the trochlea
    ii. *Companion case*: Ophthalmic artery atherosclerosis
    iii. *Companion case*: Brown syndrome
4. Axial myopia
    i. *Companion case*: Buphthalmos
    ii. *Companion case*: Coloboma
    iii. *Companion case*: Staphyloma
5. Axial hyperopia
    i. *Companion case*: Microphthalmia
    ii. *Companion case*: Ocular hypotony
6. Phthisis bulbi
    i. *Companion case*: Retinoblastoma
    ii. *Companion case*: Persistent hypertrophic primary vitreous
7. Apparent globe proptosis
    i. *Companion case*: Thyroid ophthalmopathy
    ii. *Companion case*: Traumatic proptosis
    iii. *Companion case*: Spontaneous subperiosteal orbital hematoma
    iv. *Companion case*: Encapsulated venous malformation (cavernous hemangioma)
    v. *Companion case*: CN V, V1 division orbital schwannoma
    vi. *Companion case*: Orbital extension of an intracranial meningioma
    vii. *Companion case*: Silent sinus syndrome
8. Inferior oblique muscle insertion simulating an epibulbar mass
    i. *Companion case*: Conjunctival epithelial inclusion cyst
    ii. *Companion case*: Conjunctival dermoid (epibulbar dermoid)
9. Extraocular muscle contraction simulating thyroid ophthalmopathy
    i. *Companion case*: Thyroid ophthalmopathy
    ii. *Companion case*: Treatment of metastatic melanoma with a CTLA-4 receptor monoclonal antibody (ipilimumab)
    iii. *Companion case*: Orbital pseudotumor
    iv. *Companion case*: Extraocular muscle denervation atrophy from CN III avulsion
10. Enlarged optic nerve sheath
    i. *Companion case*: Idiopathic intracranial hypertension (pseudotumor cerebri)
    ii. *Companion case*: Optic nerve sheath meningocele
    iii. *Companion case*: Optic nerve sheath enlargement due to a mass
    iv. *Companion case*: Optic nerve atrophy
    v. *Companion case*: Optic nerve sheath meningioma
    vi. *Companion case*: Optic nerve sheath hemorrhage
11. Optic nerve sheath tortuosity
    i. *Companion case*: Marked optic nerve sheath complex tortuosity and distortion due to birth trauma
    ii. *Companion case*: Optic pathway glioma
12. Pseudofractures of the orbit
    a. Supraorbital foramen
    b. Infraorbital canal and foramen
        i. *Companion case*: Infraorbital canal fracture
    c. Sphenofrontal (also called frontosphenoid) suture
    d. Sphenozygomatic (also called zygomaticosphe-noid) suture
        i. *Companion case*: Sphenozygomatic suture buckle fracture and sutural diastasis
    e. Zygomaticofrontal (also called frontozygomatic) suture
        i. *Companion case*: Zygomaticofrontal suture diastasis
    f. Zygomaticofacial foramen
    g. Duplicated zygomaticofacial foramen
    h. Zygomaticotemporal foramen
    i. Anterior and posterior ethmoidal canals
        i. *Companion case*: Inadvertent anterior ethmoidal artery surgical laceration
13. Incidental thinning of the orbital walls
    i. *Companion case*: Cocaine abuse
    ii. *Companion case*: Allergic fungal sinusitis
    iii. *Companion case*: Mucocele
14. Medialization of the lamina papyracea
    i. *Companion case*: Lamina papyracea fracture
    ii. *Companion case*: Orbital decompression for thyroid ophthalmopathy
15. Orbital roof sclerotic focus
    i. *Companion case*: Fibrous dysplasia
16. Normal and pathologic appearances of the lacrimal glands
    i. *Companion case*: Lacrimal gland prolapse
    ii. *Companion case*: Subconjunctival orbital fat prolapse
    iii. *Companion case*: Symmetric lacrimal gland enlargement due to a chronic disease state
    iv. *Companion case*: Sjögren syndrome
    v. *Companion case*: Lymphoma
    vi. *Companion case*: Pleomorphic adenoma
    vii. *Companion case*: Adenoid cystic carcinoma
    viii. *Companion case*: Adenocarcinoma
    xi. *Companion case*: Metastatic disease to the lacrimal gland
17. Normal variation in size of the superior ophthalmic vein
    i. *Companion case*: Orbital venous varix
    ii. *Companion case*: Superior ophthalmic vein thrombosis
    iii. *Companion case*: Carotid-cavernous fistula
18. Globe motion artifact
19. Cosmetic MRI artifact
    i. *Companion case*: Chemosis
20. Incomplete suppression of orbital fat on MRI
    i. *Companion case*: Postseptal orbital cellulitis

CASE 1 Senile scleral calcification

Senile scleral calcifications are a common, incidental CT finding in the elderly. These occur at sites of senescent thinning of the sclera, classically immediately anterior to the insertion points of the medial and lateral rectus muscles, although they can occur adjacent to other extraocular muscles. From a clinical perspective, these are asymptomatic, circumscribed, gray lesions situated approximately 3 mm posterior to the limbus. Senile scleral calcifications are rarely present before the seventh decade, and their incidence increases with advancing age.

COMPANION CASES

- **Glass foreign bodies.** Depending on the type of glass of which they are composed, glass fragments as small as 0.5 mm can be detected by CT. However, certain types of glass may be entirely missed by CT, and direct inspection is always necessary if there is a high clinical suspicion of a glass foreign body in the globe or periorbital soft tissues.
- **Sclerochoroidal calcifications due to renal failure.** More diffuse, plaque-like calcifications of the sclera and choroid may be present in patients with a history of an underlying derangement of calcium or phosphorus metabolism (eg, hyperparathyroidism, chronic renal insufficiency, vitamin D toxicity).
- **Choroidal osteoma.** A choroidal osteoma is a benign, slow-growing lesion composed of mature bone that resides along the posterior choroid in a juxtapapillary location (ie, adjacent to the optic disc). This lesion is of unknown etiology, most often unilateral, and classically presents in healthy, young women in their 20s and 30s. Patients may be initially asymptomatic, but they often have gradual visual blurring or visual loss. Fundoscopy is suggested to assess for neovascularization, the presence of which may lead to the potential loss of visual acuity related to hemorrhage and scarring. Because of their commonly small size and osseous composition, most lesions are not evident on MRI. The lack of significant enhancement on contrast-enhanced T1-weighted images is useful in differentiating a choroidal osteoma from other lesions, such as a retinoblastoma, choroidal melanoma, metastasis, and choroidal hemangioma; however, there are numerous other nonenhancing causes of calcification along the retina, choroid, and sclera that can simulate a choroidal osteoma, including calcified prior retinal/choroidal hemorrhage, idiopathic dystrophic calcification, and sclerochoroidal calcification, to name a few. The juxtapapillary location of a choroidal osteoma may help differentiate this entity from the other causes of calcification affecting the globe.
- **Calcification related to prior vitreous hemorrhage.** Vitreous hemorrhage may occur from numerous causes, including retinal detachment, choroidal detachment, trauma, diabetic retinopathy, and age-related macular degeneration. As with hemorrhage elsewhere in the body, old vitreous hemorrhage may calcify. The calcification may occur focally in the center of the vitreous chamber or along its periphery.

Senile scleral calcifications

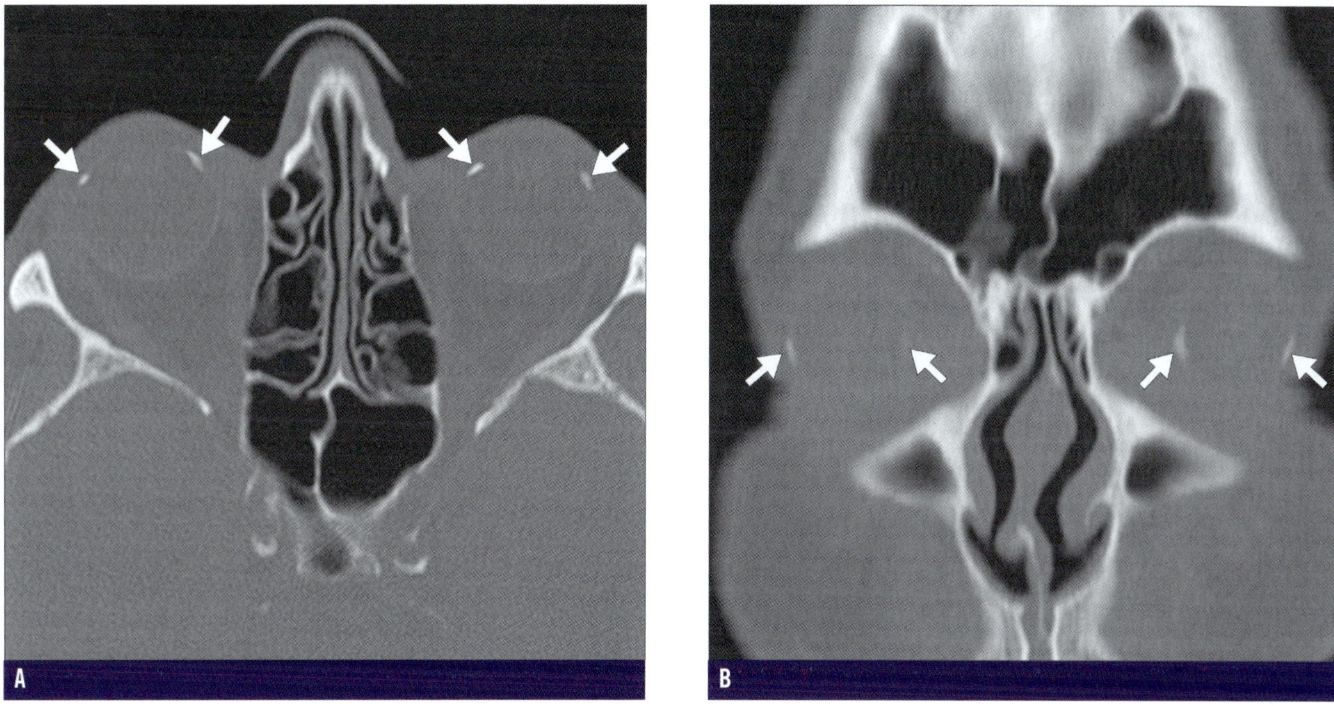

Axial and coronal reformatted CT images (**A**, **B**) demonstrate calcifications at the insertion points of the medial and lateral rectus muscles, compatible with senile scleral calcifications (arrows, **A**, **B**).

Companion case: Glass foreign bodies

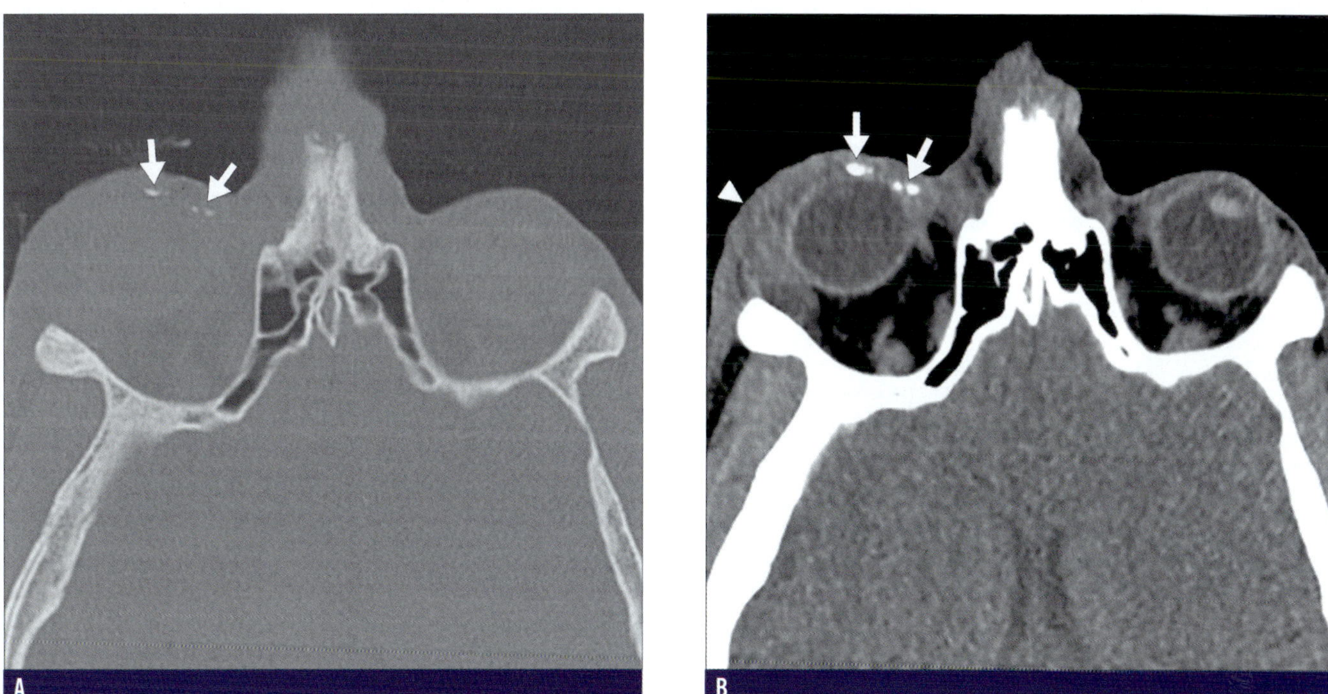

Axial CT images viewed with a bone window (**A**) and soft tissue window (**B**), as well a coronal reformatted CT image viewed in a bone window (**C**), demonstrate several hyperdense foci overlying the right globe (arrows, **A-C**). These foci might be mistaken for scleral or senile calcifications at the extraocular muscle insertions. However, image **B** also demonstrates right periorbital soft tissue swelling (arrowhead), whereas image **C** demonstrates a minimally displaced acute fracture of the nasal septum (arrowhead), consistent with a history of recent trauma. On ophthalmologic examination, the hyperdense foci were found to represent pieces of glass.

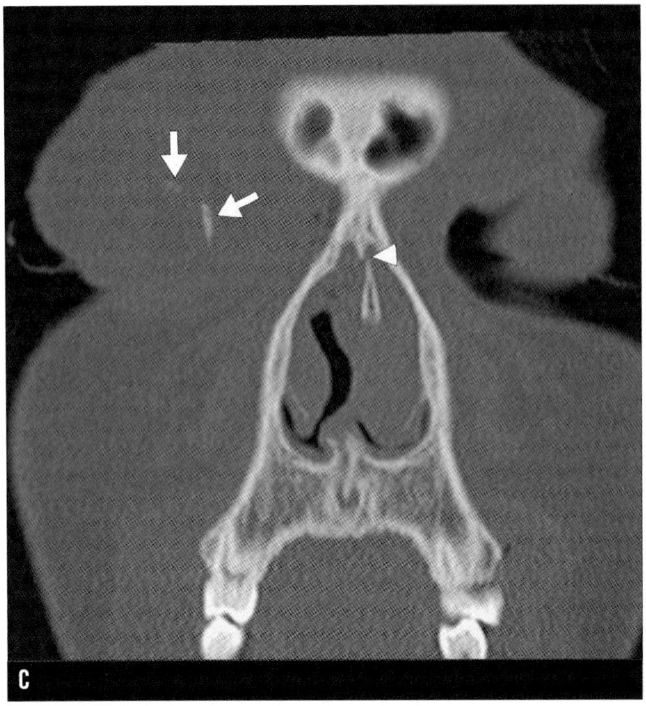

C

Companion case: Sclerochoroidal calcifications due to renal failure

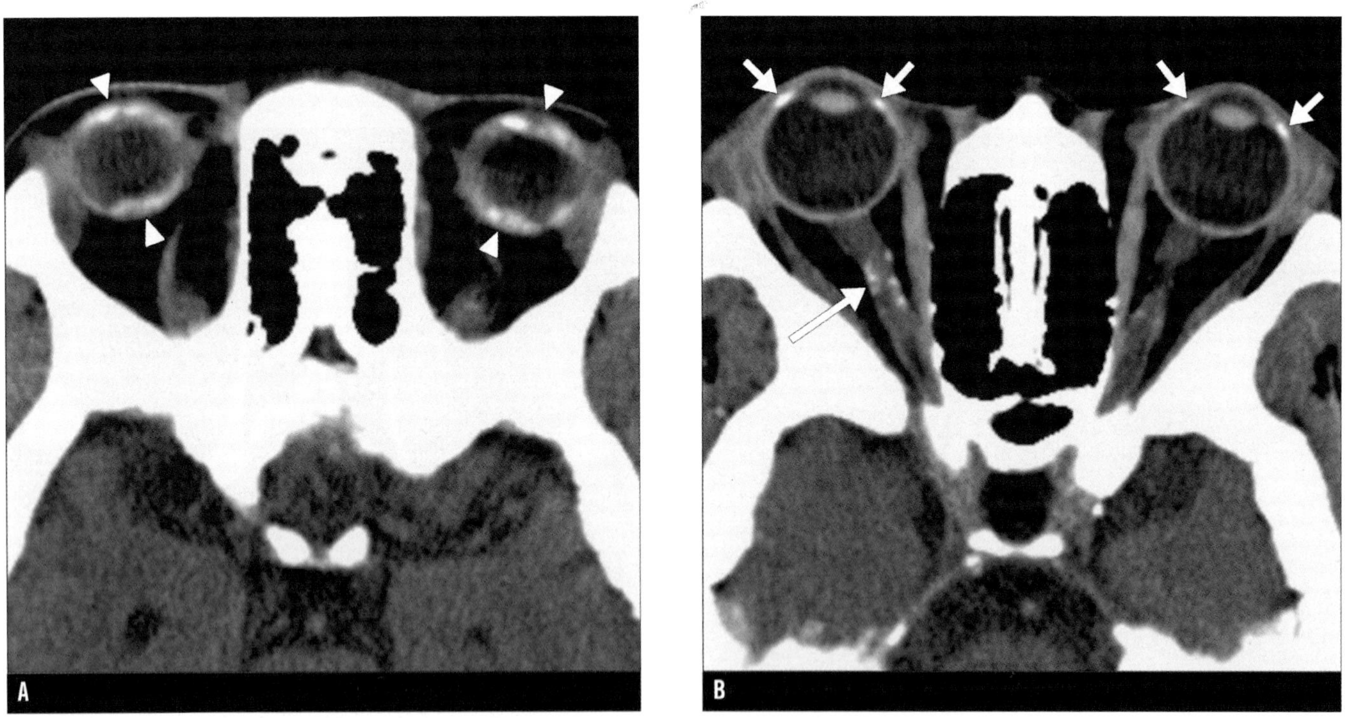

A B

An axial CT image through the orbits (**A**) demonstrates diffuse scleral calcifications along the anterior and posterior scleral margins of the upper aspects of the globes (arrowheads, **A**). An axial CT image through the mid aspect of the globes (**B**) demonstrates punctate calcifications along the right optic nerve sheath (long arrow, **B**). These findings can be seen with an abnormality of calcium or phosphorus metabolism, in this case chronic renal failure. Senile type calcifications at the insertion sites of the medial and lateral rectus muscles are also present (short arrows, **B**).

Companion case: Choroidal osteoma

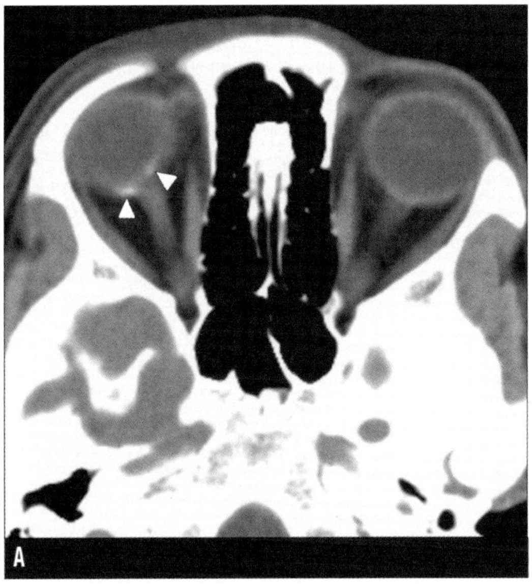

An axial CT image (**A**) demonstrates curvilinear, peripapillary calcifications abutting the margins of the right optic disc in a 35-year-old woman without visual complaints (arrowheads). The findings were presumed to represent choroidal osteomas given their peripapillary location, the lack of vision loss, and the age of the patient. However, several other causes of mineralization are in the differential diagnosis, including old calcified retinal/choroidal hemorrhage, idiopathic dystrophic calcification, or sclerochoroidal calcification, the latter typically present in patients with a history of disordered calcium and phosphate metabolism.

Companion case: Calcification related to prior vitreous hemorrhage

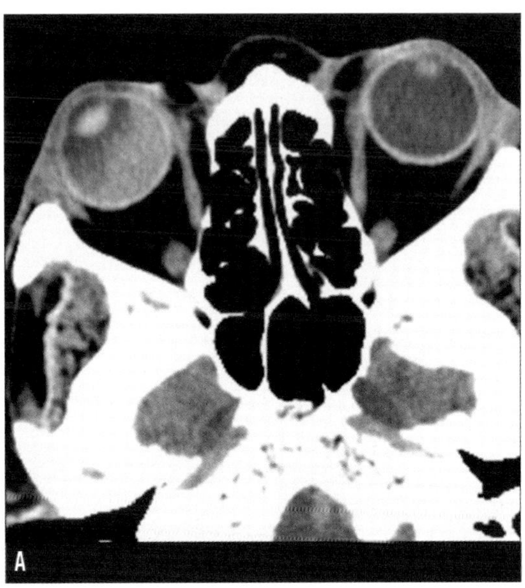

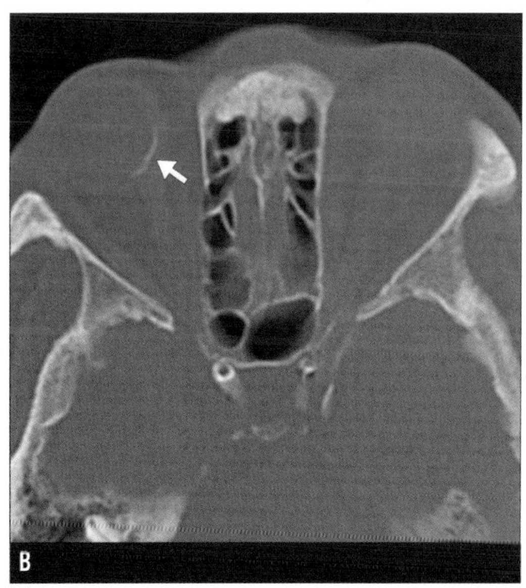

An unenhanced axial CT image viewed with a soft tissue window (**A**) demonstrates diffuse right globe vitreous hemorrhage in a patient with a history of elevated INR and retinal artery occlusion. Because of the diffuse nature of the hemorrhage, it cannot be accurately determined if this was caused by a retinal detachment, choroidal detachment, or other causes. Several years later, an unenhanced axial CT image viewed with a bone window (**B**) demonstrates curvilinear calcification along the left aspect of the globe retina and/or choroid compatible with dystrophic calcification from the prior vitreous hemorrhage.

REFERENCES

Alorainy I. Senile scleral plaques: CT. *Neuroradiology.* 2000;42(2):145-148.

Browning DJ. Choroidal osteoma: observations from a community setting. *Ophthalmology.* 2003;110(7):1327-1334.

Bryan RN, Lewis RA, Miller SL. Choroidal osteoma. *AJNR Am J Neuroradiol.* 1983;4(3):491-494.

DePotter P, Shields JA, Shields CL, Rao VM. Magnetic resonance imaging in choroidal osteoma. *Retina.* 1991;11(2):221-223.

Gordon RN, Slamovits TL, Rosenbaum PS, and Bellos J. Calcified scleral plaques imaged on orbital computed tomography. *Am J Ophthalmol.* 1999;127:461-463.

Kadrmas EF, Weiter JJ. Choroidal osteoma. *Int Ophthalmol Clin.* 1997;37(4):171-182.

Kubal WS. Imaging of orbital trauma. *Radiographics.* 2008;28(6):1729-1739. doi: 10.1148/rg.286085523.

Mafee MF, Karimi A, Shah J, Rapoport M, Ansari SA. Anatomy and pathology of the eye: role of MR imaging and CT. *Neuroimaging Clin N Am.* 2005;15(1):23-47.

Murray JL, Hayman LA, Tang RA and Schiffman JS. Incidental Asymptomatic Orbital Calcifications. *J Neuroophthalmol.* 15(4);1995:203-208.

Shields CL, Shields JA, Augsburger JJ. Choroidal osteoma. *Surv Ophthalmol.* 1988;33(1):17-27.

CASE 2 Optic disc drusen

Optic disc drusen (ODD) are calcific deposits that occur at the optic disc. The cause of ODD is unknown, though axonal degeneration of the optic nerve resulting in calcium deposition has been proposed. ODDs are common findings occurring in approximately 1% of the general population and in up to 3% of patients with a family history of ODD. ODD are usually bilateral when present. On CT, ODD manifests as a punctate focus of mineralization at the optic nerve head.

ODD are most often asymptomatic without loss of visual acuity, although some degree of visual field loss may occur and can be progressive. ODD can result in an elevation of the optic nerve head observed during ophthalmoscopy, resulting in "pseudopapilledema."

COMPANION CASE

- **Calcified retinal drusen.** Drusen of the retina is a different clinical entity than ODD. Drusen of the retina are soft or hard excrescences that may calcify and form outside the confines of the disc, between the retinal pigment epithelium and Bruch membrane. For orientation, the retinal pigment epithelium is the outermost cell layer of the retina and resides just outside the confines of the photoreceptive layer (ie. rods and cones). Bruch membrane represents the innermost portion of the choroid and resides immediately posterior to the retinal pigment epithelium. This form of drusen is associated with age-related macular degeneration, which is not the case with ODD.

Optic disc drusen

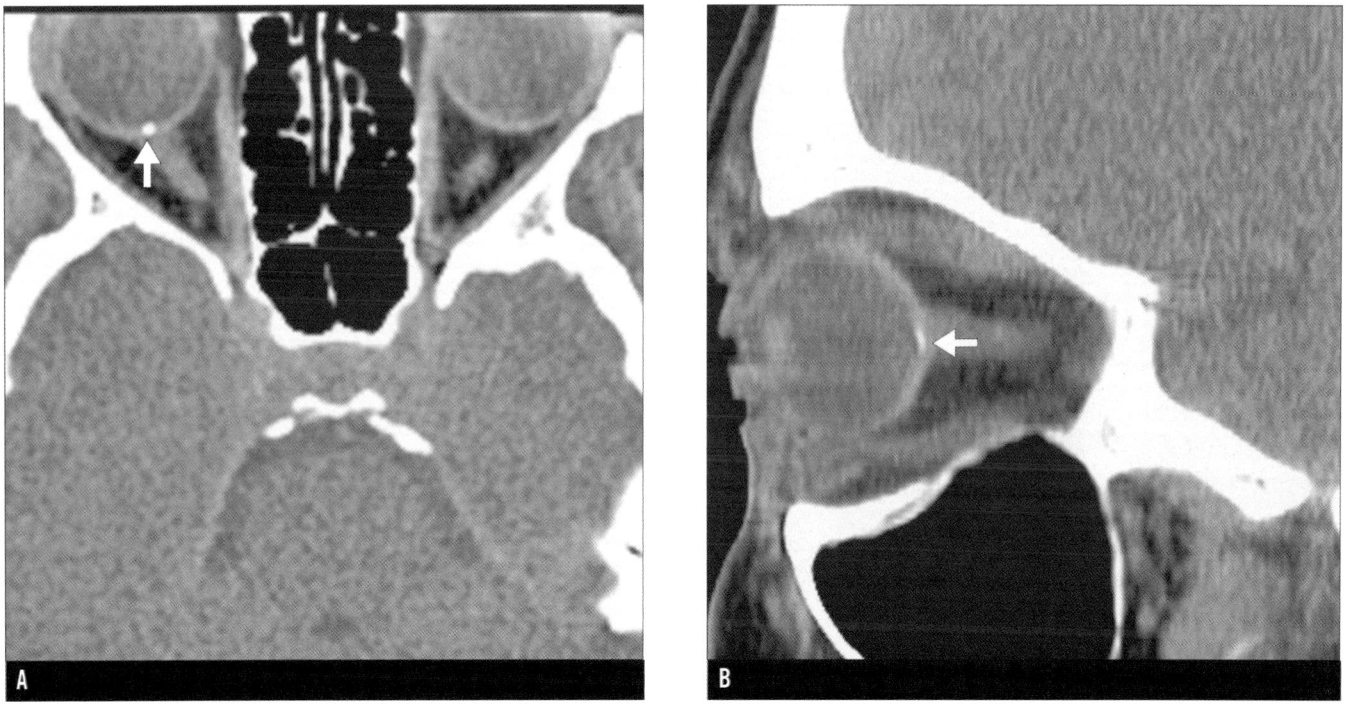

Axial (**A**) and sagittal reformatted (**B**) unenhanced CT images demonstrate a punctate calcification at the right optic nerve head, compatible with drusen (arrows, **A**, **B**).

Companion case: Calcified retinal drusen

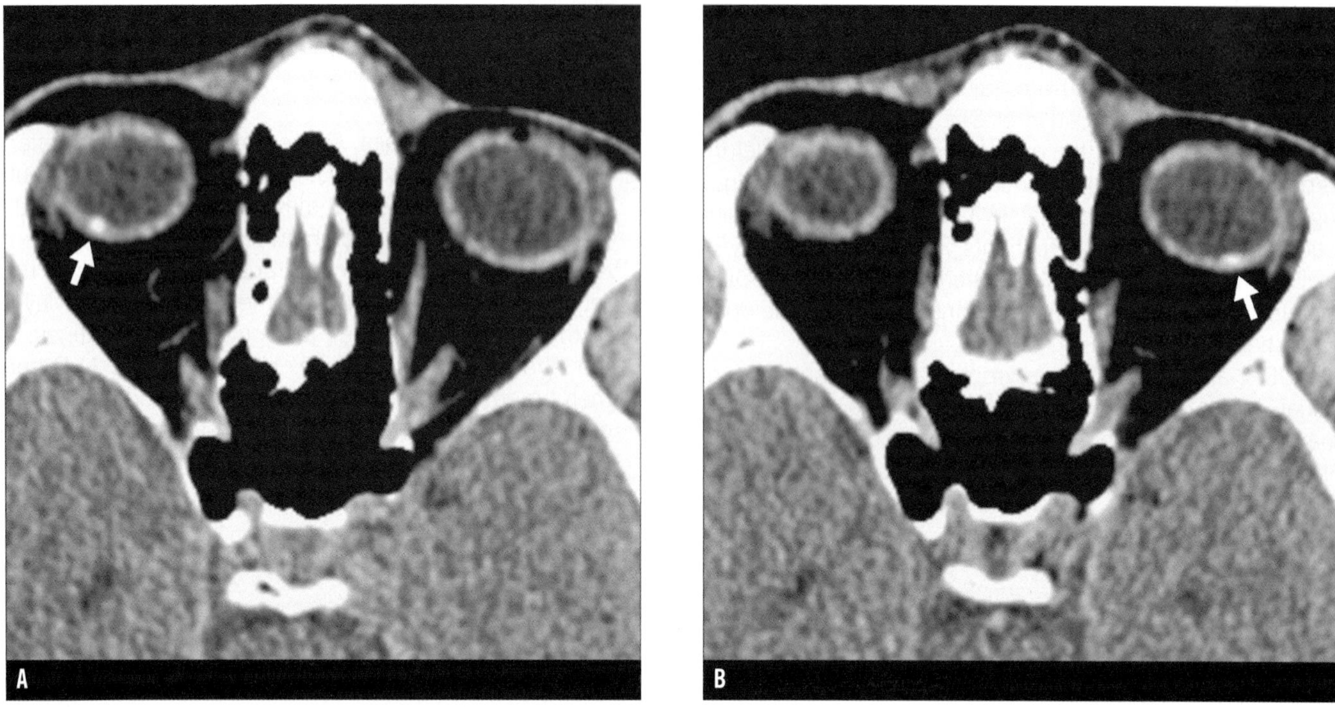

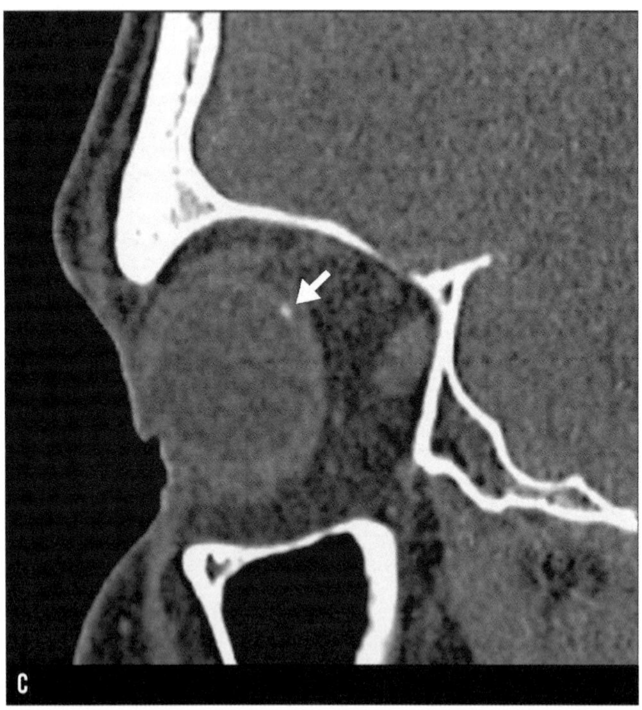

Unenhanced axial (**A**, **B**) and sagittal reformatted (**C**) CT images demonstrate a punctate focus of mineralization along the retinal surface of the globes that resides outside the confines of the optic nerve heads, compatible with calcified retinal drusen (arrows, **A**-**C**).

REFERENCES

Davis PL, Jay WM. Optic nerve head drusen. *Semin Ophthalmol.* 2003;18(4):222-242.

Lam BL, Morais CG Jr, Pasol J. Drusen of the optic disc. *Curr Neurol Neurosci Rep.* 2008;8(5):404-408.

Williams MA, Craig D, Passmore P, Silvestri G. Retinal drusen: harbingers of age, safe havens for trouble. *Age Ageing.* 2009;38(6):648-654. doi: 10.1093/ageing/afp136. Epub September 2009.

CASE 3 Trochlear calcification

Latin for pulley, the trochlea of the orbit is a normal cartilaginous structure located in the superomedial aspect of the orbit through which the tendon and sheath of the superior oblique muscle pass. The trochlea often calcifies and can mimic a foreign body. These asymptomatic calcifications can be unilateral or bilateral, and they occur in approximately 25% to 30% of patients older than 50. In patients younger than 40, there is an association with diabetes mellitus.

COMPANION CASES

- **Small metallic foreign body simulating the trochlea.** CT is extremely sensitive for detection of metallic foreign bodies and is able to determine their presence even when they are smaller than 1 mm. Any unexplained metallic foreign body in the orbit is a contraindication to imaging with MRI, since if placed in a powerful magnetic field, such a foreign body could result in blindness.
- **Ophthalmic artery atherosclerosis.** Atherosclerotic calcifications within the orbit are typically present in patients with advanced atherosclerotic disease elsewhere, especially in the setting of severe hypertension, diabetes mellitus, or renal failure.
- **Brown syndrome.** The function of the superior oblique muscle and tendon is complex and includes internally rotating, abducting, and depressing the eye into a "down and out" position when it contracts. First described by an ophthalmologist named Harold Whaley Brown in 1946, Brown syndrome (also called superior oblique tendon sheath syndrome) is a rare entity that occurs when the superior oblique muscle/tendon, for a variety of reasons, is unable to lengthen. Clinically, it is primarily characterized by restricted elevation of the affected globe above the horizontal during adduction. In essence, the affected eye is functionally tethered by the tight superior oblique muscle/tendon.

  Both congenital and acquired forms of Brown syndrome exist. Among the causes of congenital Brown syndrome is a short or taut superior oblique tendon sheath complex. The acquired form is often inflammatory and results in thickening of the sheath and swelling of the tendon. It can be seen in several settings, including trauma, sinusitis, rheumatoid arthritis, and systemic lupus erythematosus. Brown syndrome is usually unilateral, affecting only one globe 90% of the time.

  Imaging of the acquired form with MRI, which is more sensitive than CT, may reveal thickening of the superior oblique tendon on a T1-weighted sequence and hyperintense signal with enhancement on T2-weighted and post-gadolinium fat-saturated sequences, respectively. While Brown syndrome can resolve spontaneously after many years, a variety of surgeries, including tenotomy, tenectomy, and split-tendon lengthening, the latter a tendon weakening and slackening procedure, have been utilized for treatment.

Trochlear calcifications

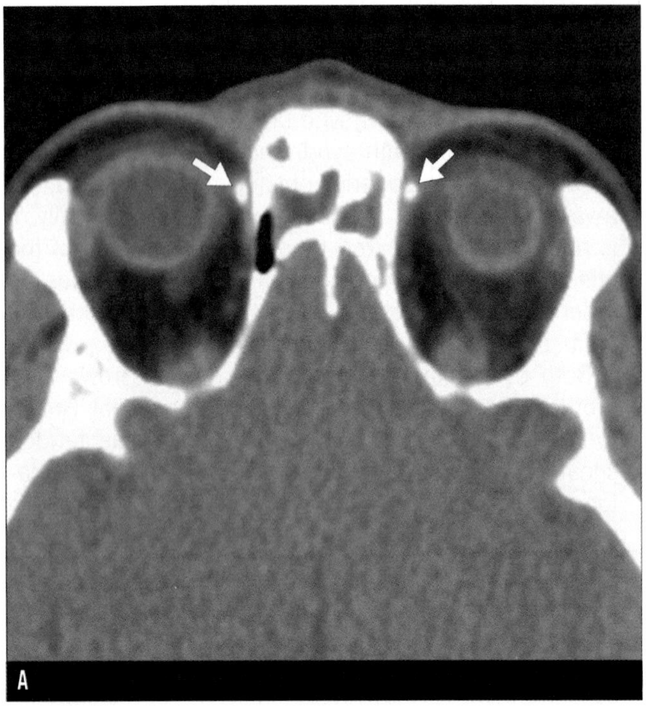

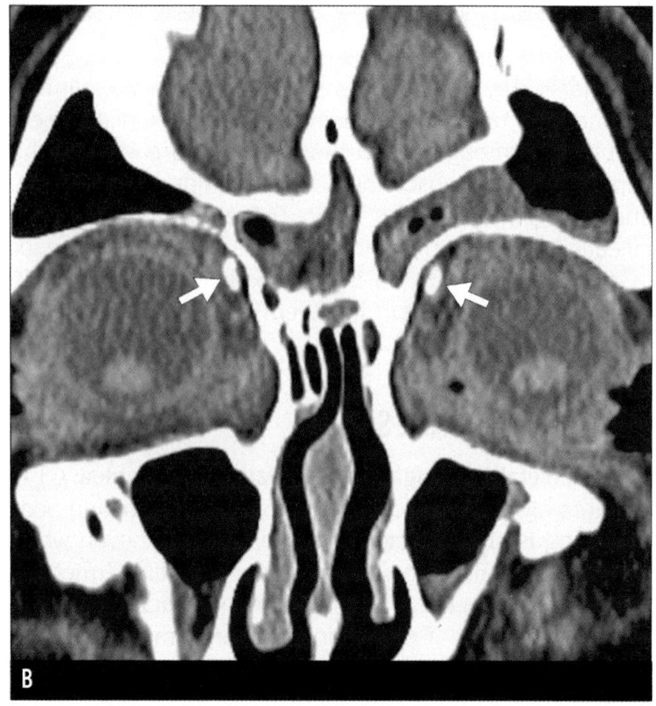

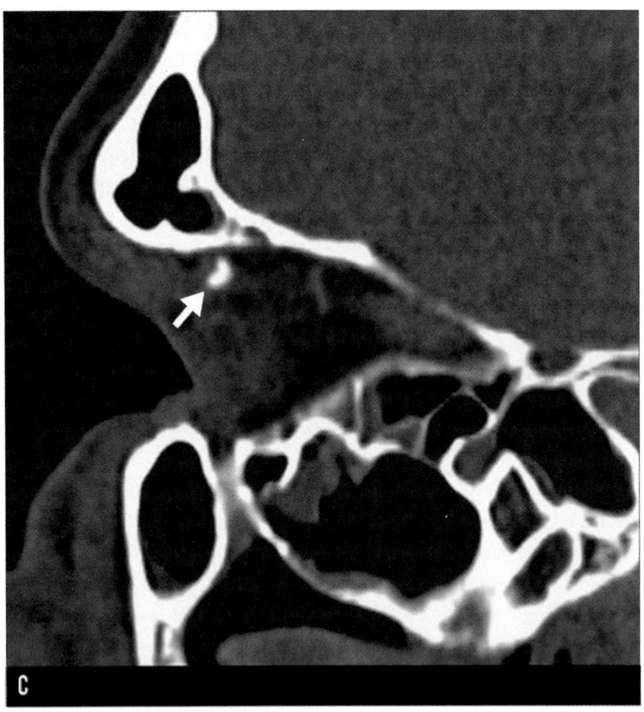

Axial (**A**), coronal reformatted (**B**), and sagittal reformatted (**C**) CT images demonstrate incidental calcification of the trochlear apparatus of the orbits (arrows, **A**-**C**).

Companion case: Small metallic foreign body simulating the trochlea

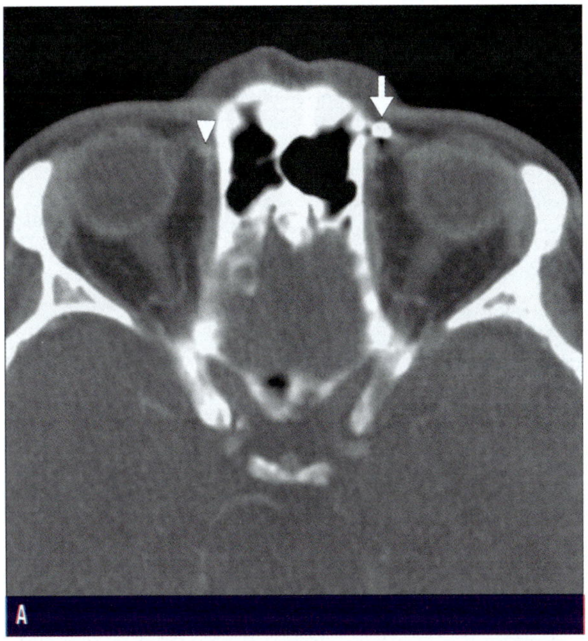

An unenhanced axial CT image of the orbits (**A**) demonstrates a foreign body in the superior nasal quadrant of the left orbit (arrow), which could be confused with calcification of the trochlea. However, this finding is denser than would be expected for a calcified trochlea and is most consistent with metal. In addition, the foreign body is located more anterior than expected for the trochlea. As a reference, the right trochlea is subtly identified (arrowhead).

Companion case: Ophthalmic artery atherosclerosis

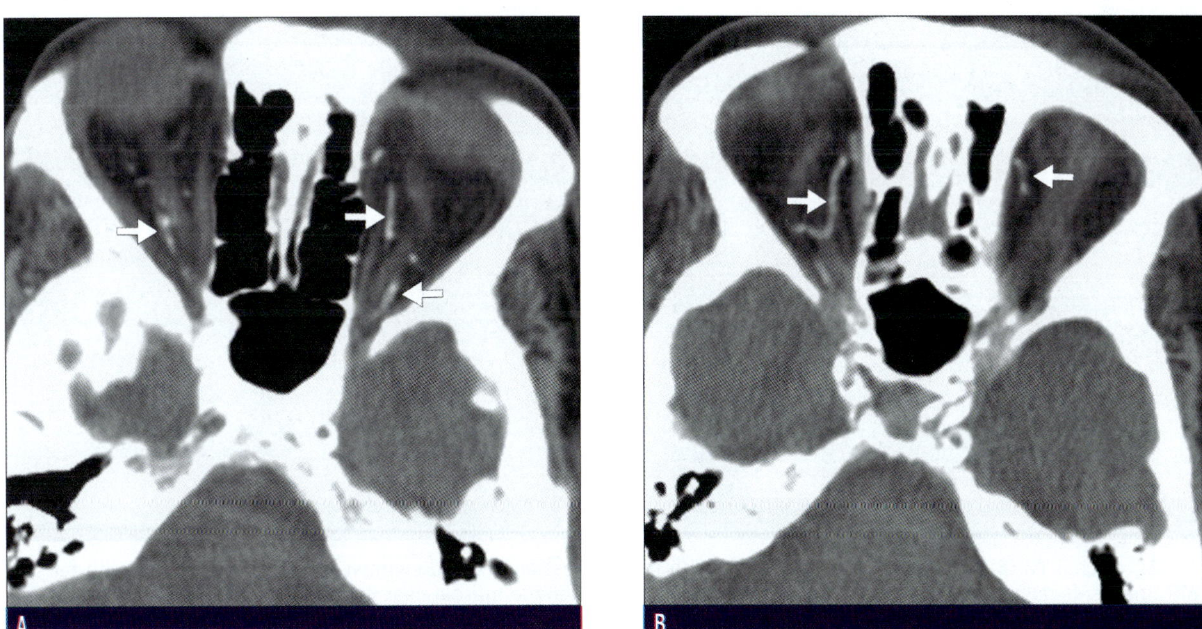

Axial CT images (**A**, **B**) demonstrate atherosclerotic calcifications involving the bilateral ophthalmic arteries in a patient with a history of chronic renal failure (arrows, **A**, **B**).

Companion case: Brown syndrome (CT)

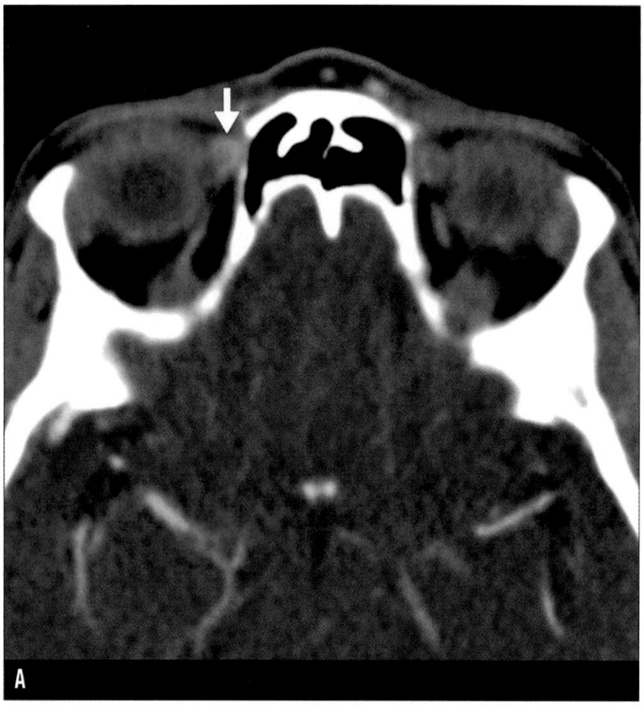

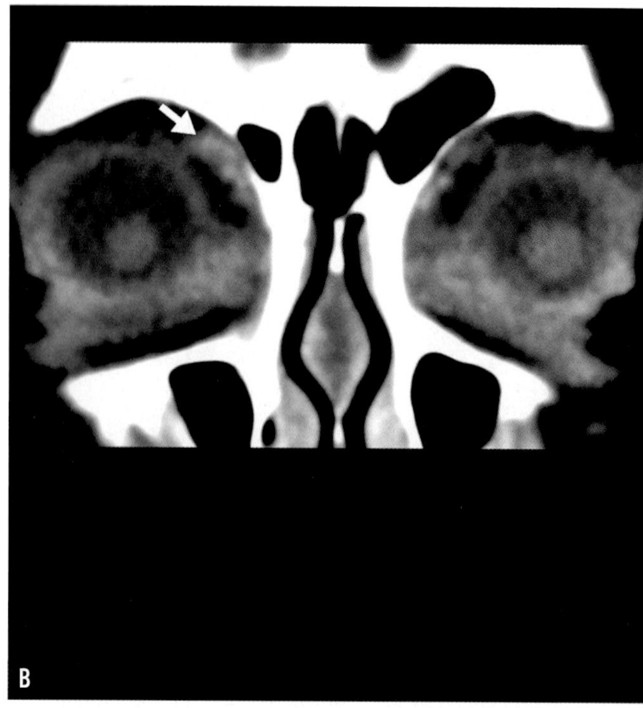

Axial (**A**) and coronal reformatted (**B**) contrast-enhanced axial CT images demonstrate asymmetric apparent enhancement of the right superior oblique tendon sheath (arrows, **A**, **B**). This patient had numerous clinical episodes of superior oblique tendon dysfunction. The imaging findings and clinical scenario are consistent with Brown syndrome.

Companion case: Brown syndrome (MRI)

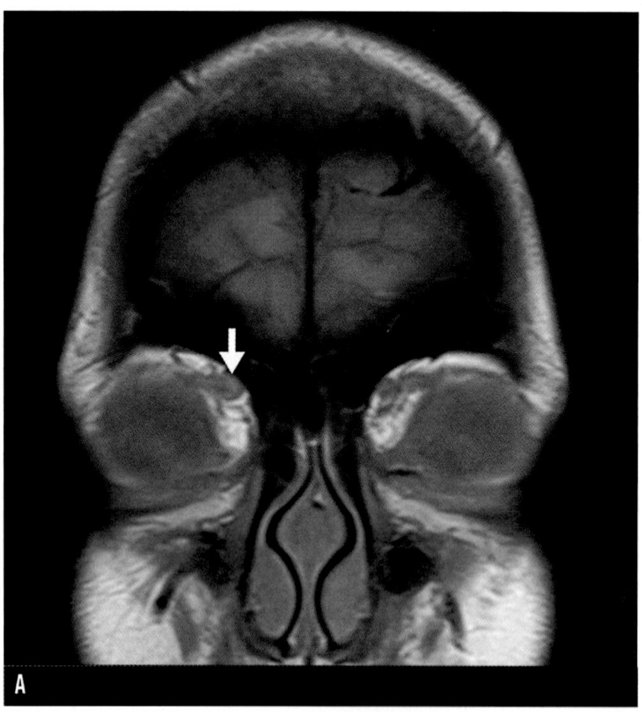

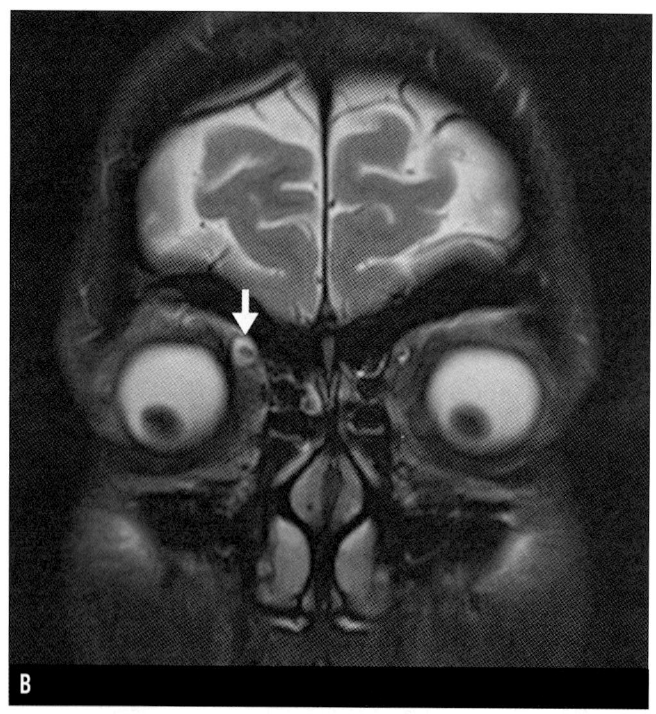

Coronal T1 (**A**), coronal T2 (**B**), contrast-enhanced axial T1 with fat suppression (**C**), and contrast-enhanced coronal T1 with fat suppression (**D**) MR images demonstrate a T2 hyperintense, enhancing superior oblique muscle near its tendon sheath, compatible with inflammation and edema (arrows, **A-D**). This patient presented with double vision and tenderness over superomedial aspect of right orbit with restricted elevation and adduction of the right globe. The imaging findings and clinical presentation are consistent with Brown syndrome.

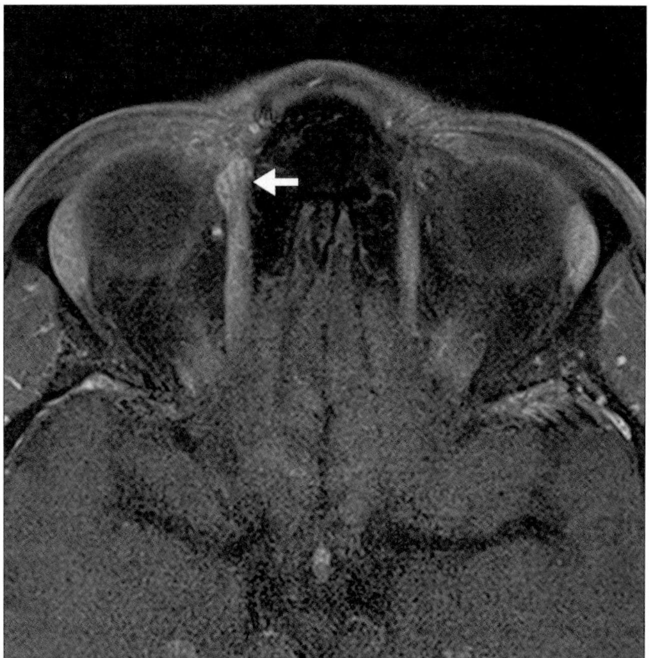

C

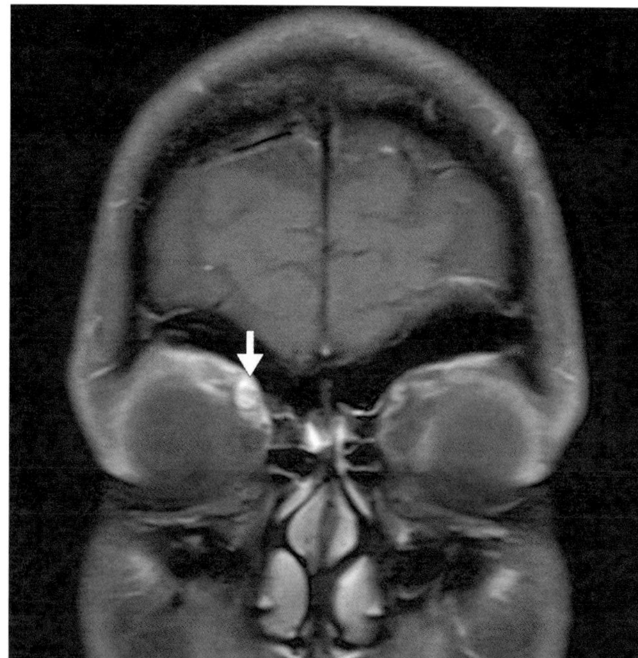

D

REFERENCES

Currie S, Goddard T. MR Imaging Features of Acquired Brown Syndrome. *Am J Neuroradiol.* 2009;30:1778-1779.

Hart BL, Spar JA, Orrison Jr, WW. Calcification of the trochlear apparatus of the orbit: appearance and association with diabetes and age. *AJR Am J Roentgenol.* 1992;159:1291-1294.

Kim JH, Hwang JM. Magnetic resonance imaging in congenital Brown syndrome. *Graefes Arch Clin Exp Ophthalmol.* 2015.

Manley DR, Alvi RA. Brown's syndrome. *Current Opinion in Ophthalmology.* 2011; 22:432-440.

CASE 4 Axial myopia

Axial myopia is idiopathic enlargement of the globe in its anteroposterior dimension. It is the most common cause of macrophthalmia, may be unilateral or bilateral, and may be associated with painless proptosis. Because of the ocular elongation, light is focused anterior to the retina, and as a result, patients often have impaired vision. On imaging, the enlarged eye may be associated with scleral thinning.

COMPANION CASES

- **Buphthalmos.** Buphthalmos refers to an abnormally enlarged globe which has uniform or irregular walls due to elevated intraocular pressure (glaucoma). It is usually the result of a congenital or infantile glaucoma, and only rarely secondary to an acquired glaucoma. This entity almost exclusively arises in children, likely because their sclera is soft and malleable. Buphthalmos may be sporadic or it may occur in patients with neurofibromatosis type I or Sturge-Weber syndrome, among other entities.
- **Coloboma.** A coloboma is the result of an embryologic failure of fusion affecting any portion of the eye, including the eyelid, cornea, iris, lens, choroid, retina, or optic nerve. Posterior colobomata are smooth, focal outpouchings of the vitreous humor through a gap or defect of ocular tissue. The posterior colobomata typically occur at or near the optic nerve head.
- **Staphyloma.** A staphyloma is an acquired outpouching of the vitreous humor secondary to ectasia of the sclera-uveal coat. It is associated with age-related myopia. The combination of anteroposterior elongation and thinning of the posterior aspect of the globe is characteristic of the posterior subtype of this entity. As opposed to a coloboma of the posterior aspect of the globe, a staphyloma does not involve the optic nerve head but is rather most commonly located along the posterior-temporal aspect of the globe. An anterior form of staphyloma also exists.

Axial myopia

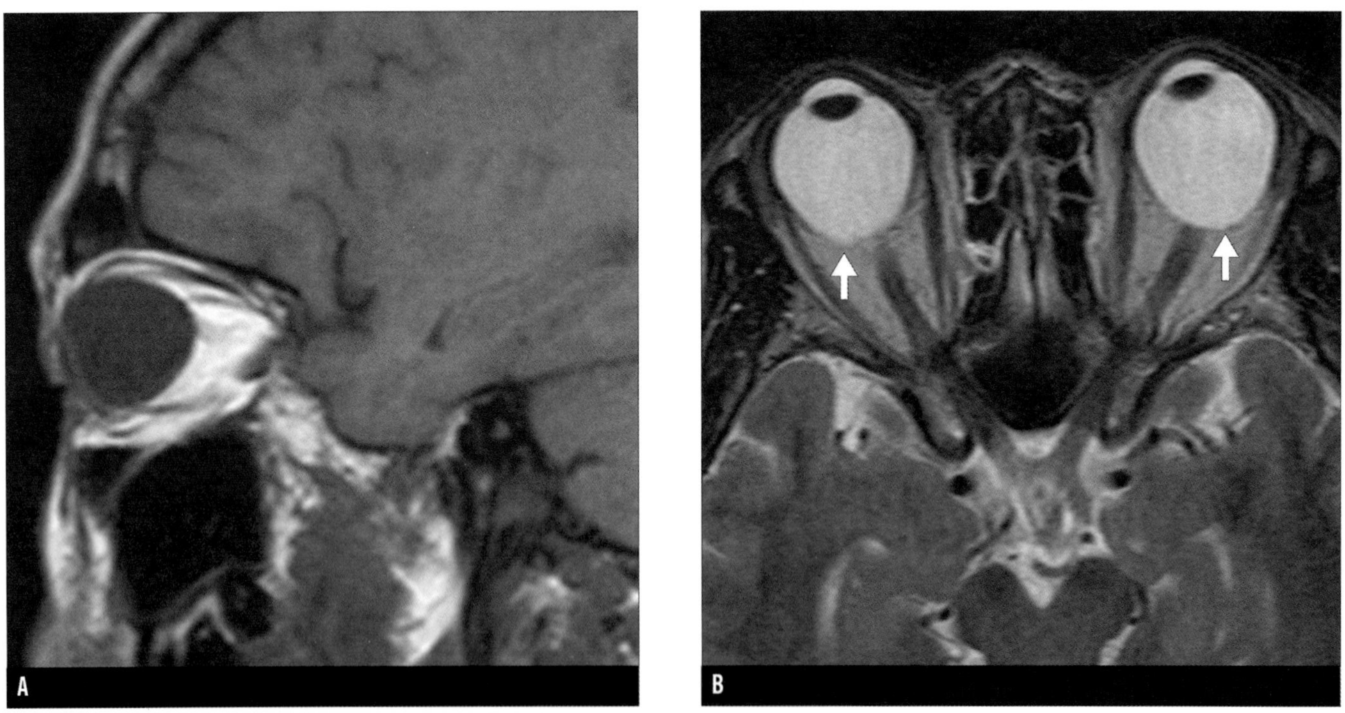

Sagittal T1 (**A**) and axial T2 (**B**) MR images demonstrate anterior to posterior elongation of the globes, consistent with axial myopia. Posterior scleral thinning is best demonstrated on image **B** (arrows), a finding often present with axial myopia.

Companion case: Unilateral buphthalmos

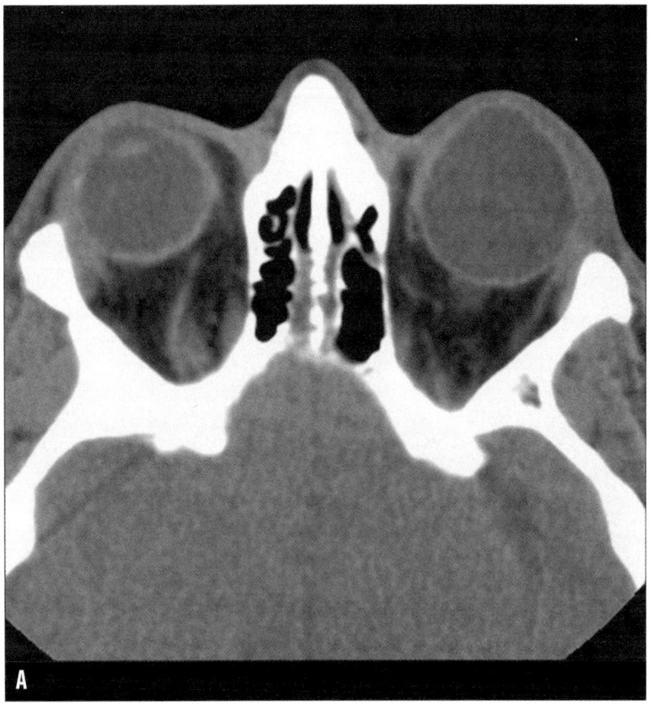

An unenhanced axial CT image of the orbits in a patient with congenital left eye blindness (**A**) demonstrates diffuse left globe enlargement and absence of the left globe intraocular lens, compatible with buphthalmos and congenital aphakia, respectively.

Companion case: Bilateral buphthalmos

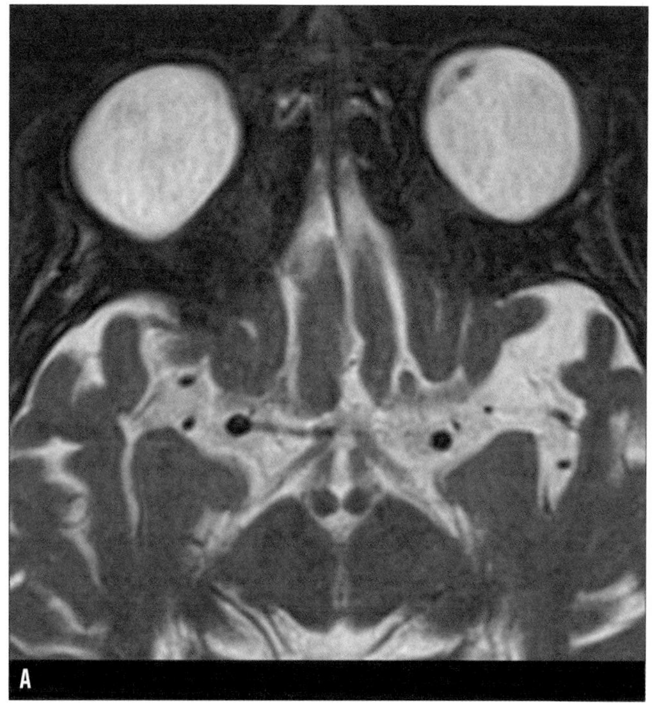

An axial T2 MR image through the orbits demonstrates enlargement and contour irregularity of the globes, consistent with buphthalmos. The globes are directed medially, either representing a bilateral esotropia or transiently present during the scan.

Companion case: Coloboma

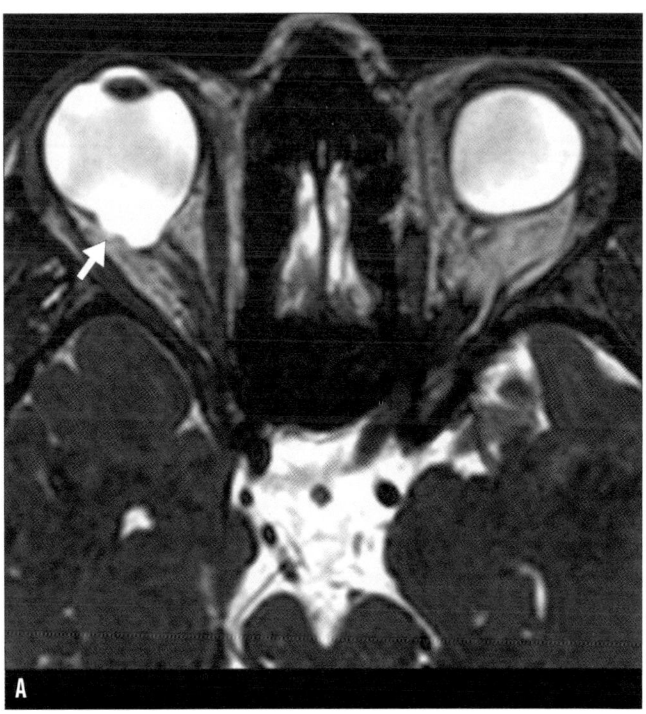

An axial CISS MR image (**A**) demonstrates smooth-shaped, dome-like, focal posterior outpouchings through a gap along the posterior scleral margin of the right globe at and adjacent to the optic nerve head insertion, compatible with a coloboma (arrow).

Companion case: Staphyloma

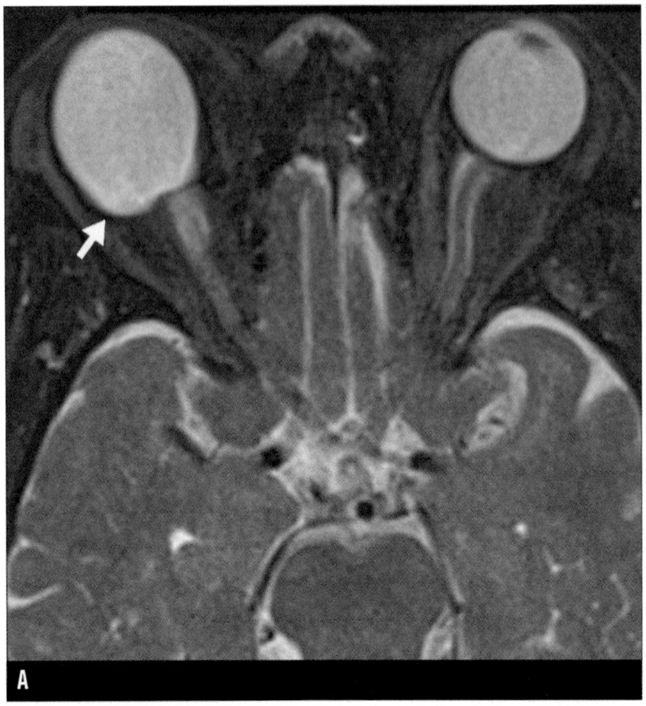

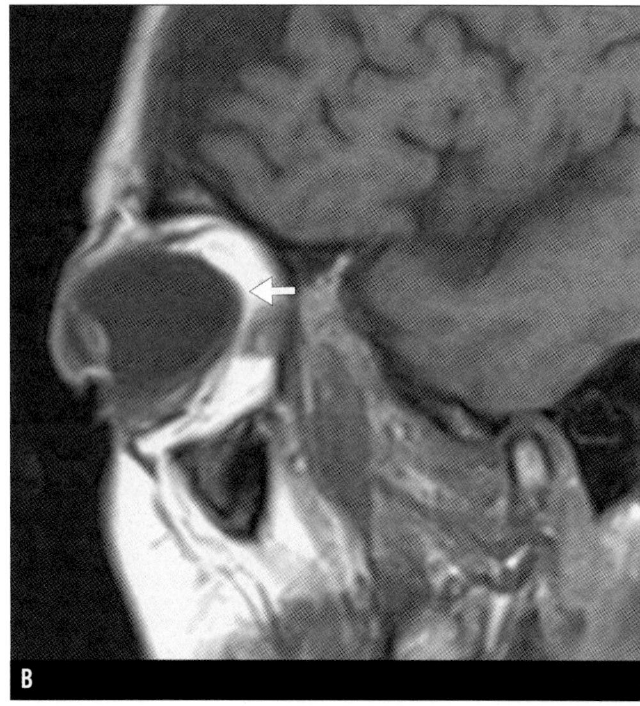

Axial T2 (**A**) and sagittal T1-weighted (**B**) MR images demonstrate smooth outpouchings of vitreous humor at the posterolateral aspect of an intact right globe compatible with a staphyloma (arrows, **A**, **B**). This is in contradistinction to a posterior coloboma, which is associated with a focal defect in the globe and typically occurs at or adjacent to the optic nerve head. There is also anteroposterior enlargement of the right globe, consistent with axial myopia, a finding often present with a staphyloma.

REFERENCES

Hsiang HW, et al. Clinical characteristics of posterior staphyloma in eyes with pathologic myopia. *Am J Ophthalmol.* 2008;146(1):102-110.

Onwochei BC, et al. Ocular colobomata. *Surv Ophthalmol.* 2000;45(3):175-194.

Smith M, Castillo M. Imaging and differential diagnosis of the large eye. *Radiographics.* 1994;14:721-728.

Som PM, Curtin HD. Head and Neck Imaging. Vol 5. St. Louis, MO: Mosby Elsevier; 2011.

CASE 5 Axial hyperopia

Axial hyperopia is present when the anteroposterior (AP) dimension of the globe is shorter than the transverse dimension. In a normal-sized globe, a normal cornea and lens can generate enough optical power to focus light directly upon the retina. However, with axial hyperopia, as an object moves closer to the eye, the optical power of a normal cornea and lens is often insufficient to accommodate the shortened AP dimension of the globe, resulting in the light being focused posterior to the retina. This results in farsightedness, which is defined as the ability to retain focus on faraway objects but the inability to focus on objects that are near.

COMPANION CASES

- **Microphthalmia.** Microphthalmia is defined as a globe that has an AP length that is two standard deviations below normal; this corresponds to less than 21 mm in an adult and less than 19 mm in a 1-year-old child. Simple microphthalmia is a term used when the globe is small but otherwise structurally normal, whereas the term complex microphthalmia is used when other abnormalities of the globe are also present. Microphthalmia may be unilateral or bilateral. It may also be sporadic or associated with congenital infections or genetic abnormalities. While the finding may be incidental in some patients, in most cases a microphthalmic eye is abnormal and the patient is blind in the affected eye.
- **Ocular hypotony.** The normal intraocular pressure is typically between 10 and 20 mmHg, with a mean of approximately 15.5 mmHg. The intraocular pressure in normal individuals varies throughout the day, with intraocular pressure usually lower at night because of a decrease in aqueous humor production. Abnormally low intraocular pressure is termed ocular hypotony. While sources vary in their reported thresholds, ocular hypotony may be considered to be present when the intraocular pressure is less than 6.5 mm Hg, or when the intraocular pressure is low enough to cause symptoms. There are numerous causes of ocular hypotony, including a scleral leak following surgery, an overfiltering bleb related to a glaucoma drainage device, trauma to the globe, and iridocyclitis (inflammation of the iris and ciliary body), the latter resulting in ocular hypotony because of poor aqueous production. Ocular hypotony can result in cataract formation, choroidal effusion, inflammation, and hypotony maculopathy. Hypotony maculopathy occurs when ocular hypotony results in an inward collapse of the sclera. The choroidal and retinal folds that occur because of the inward collapse of the sclera affect the macula, resulting in vision loss.

Axial hyperopia

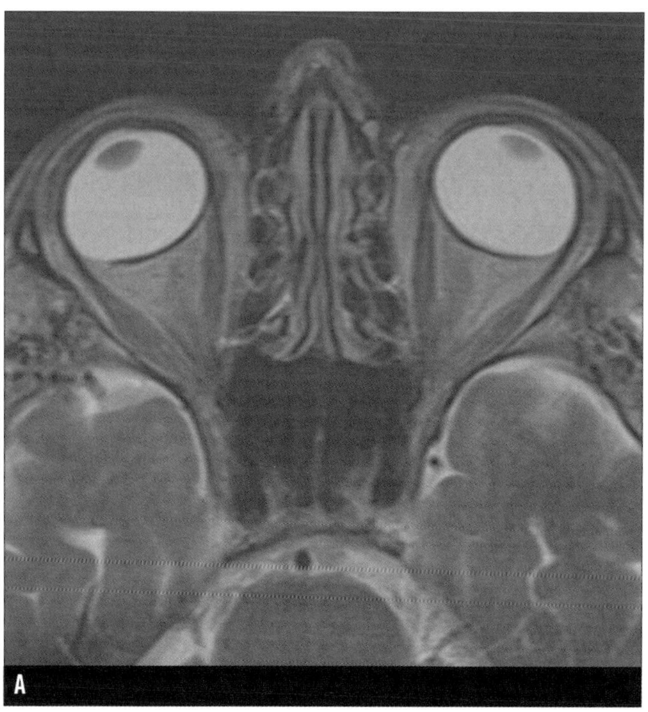

An axial T2-weighted MR image (**A**) demonstrates a decreased anteroposterior dimension of the globes, compatible with hyperopic globes.

Companion case: Microphthalmia

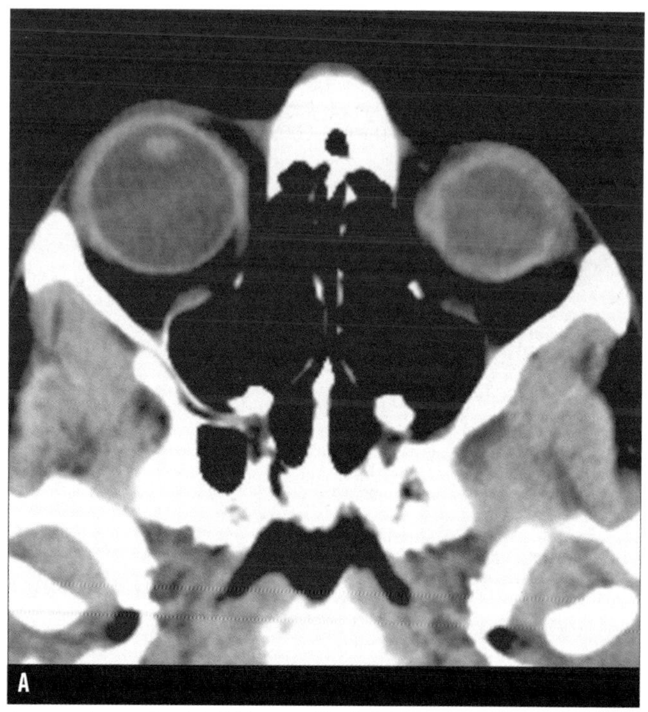

An unenhanced axial CT image (**A**) demonstrates left globe microphthalmia with absence of a left ocular lens (ie, aphakia).

Companion case: Ocular hypotony

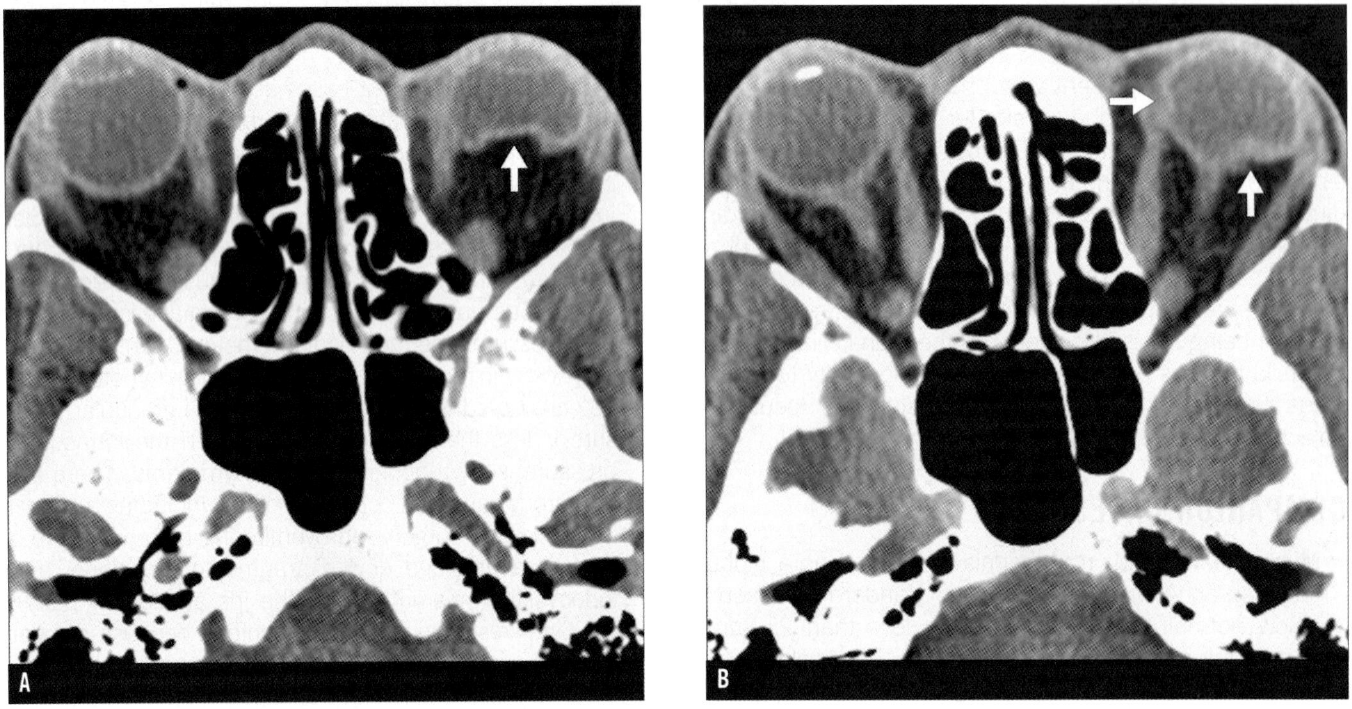

Unenhanced axial CT images (**A**, **B**) demonstrate the left globe to be significantly smaller than its contralateral counterpart and to have irregular contours, findings, which are compatible with left globe hypotony (arrows, **A**, **B**). This was presumably secondary to a vitreous leak.

REFERENCES

Cheng HM, Singh OS, Kwong KK, Xiong J, Woods BT, Brady TJ. Shape of the myopic eye as seen with high-resolution magnetic resonance imaging. *Optom Vis Sci.* 1992;69(9):698-701.

Costa VP, Arcieri ES. Hypotony maculopathy. *Acta Ophthalmol Scand.* 2007;85(6):586-597. Epub June 2007.

Mafee MF, Valvassori GE, Becker M. *Imaging of the Head and Neck. Textbook.* 2nd ed. New York: Thieme; 2005.

Rahman A, Mendonca M, Simmons RB, Simmons RJ. Hypotony after glaucoma filtration surgery. *Int Ophthalmol Clin.* 2000 Winter;40(1):127-136.

Verma AS, Fitzpatrick DR. Anophthalmia and microphthalmia. *Orphanet J Rare Dis.* 2007;2:47.

CASE 6 Phthisis bulbi

Phthisis bulbi refers to a shrunken, irregularly shaped, end-stage appearance of a globe, which is the result of a variety of congenital or acquired insults. Congenital infections such as syphilis, rubella, and toxoplasmosis may result in phthisis bulbi. Acquired causes of phthisis bulbi include trauma, infection, and radiation exposure. This entity is frequently associated with dystrophic calcification and sometimes ossification. The patient is blind in the affected eye.

COMPANION CASES

- **Retinoblastoma.** Retinoblastoma (Rb) is a primitive neuroectodermal tumor arising from the retina and is the most common cause of leukocoria in a child. Rb may be sporadic or inherited, with a mean age at presentation of 18 months. About two-thirds of cases are unilateral. Trilateral and quadrilateral forms, in which bilateral Rb occurs in concert with lesions in the pineal and/or suprasellar regions, have also been described. On CT, Rb is characterized by a hyperattenuating mass usually associated with calcifications arising from the retina of a normal-sized globe. On MRI, it is often mildly intrinsically T1 hyperintense and T2 hypointense relative to the vitreous humor. Rb enhances following contrast administration.
- **Persistent hypertrophic primary vitreous.** During normal fetal development, the primary vitreous provides nourishment to the developing lens and retina. The hyaloid artery traverses the primary vitreous and is the main arterial supply for these structures. During the second month of gestation, the normal primary vitreous regresses and is replaced by the secondary vitreous, which ultimately forms the definitive vitreous body. As the primary vitreous regresses, it is reduced in volume and is displaced centrally, forming the hyaloid canal (also called Cloquet canal) which contains the hyaloid artery. The hyaloid canal traverses the center of the globe from the lens to the optic disc. In persistent hypertrophic primary vitreous (PHPV), the primary vitreous fails to regress and instead proliferates, forming a retrolental mass. The centrally located hyaloid canal often persists with this entity as well. PHPV is classified as anterior or posterior PHPV, depending on which structures of the globe are affected, although the most common form of PHPV is a combination of both. On imaging, the retrolental mass is of variable thickness and the globe is typically microphthalmic. Occasionally, one may encounter an upright wine glass configuration, in which the retrolental mass represents the bowl of the glass and the hyaloid canal represents the stem. On MRI, the globe vitreous in PHPV is usually T1 and T2 hyperintense, the retrolental mass often enhances following contrast administration, and a funnel-shaped retinal detachment with the posterior form of this entity may be present. Unlike Rb, calcification is not a characteristic finding with PHPV. PHPV is most often unilateral and is the second most common cause of leukocoria in the pediatric population, after retinoblastoma.

Apparent globe proptosis

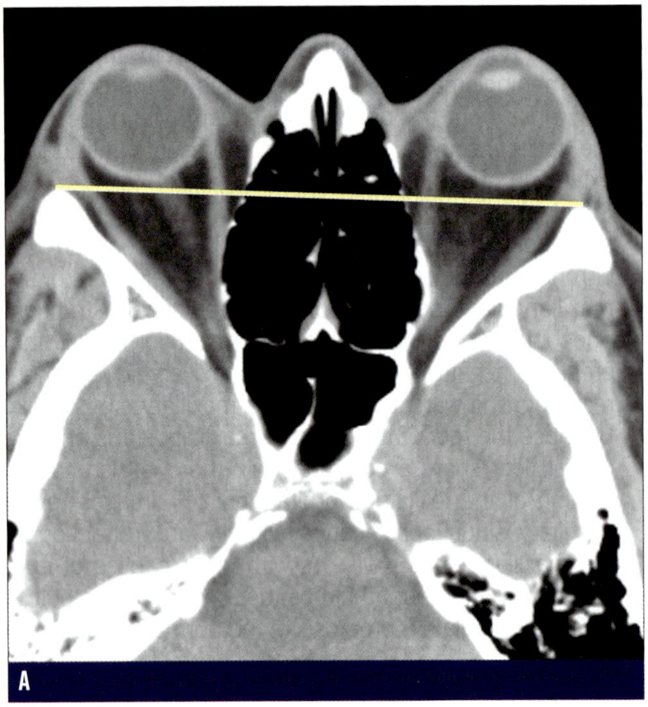

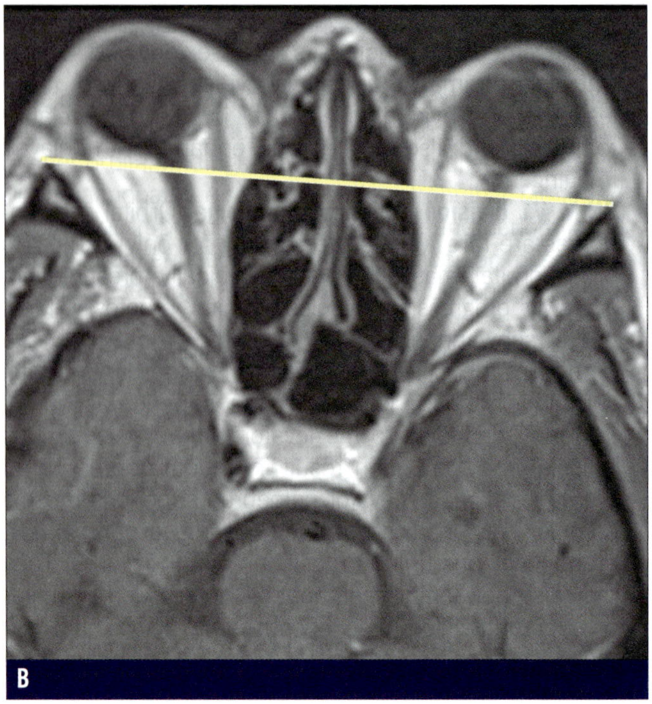

An axial CT image (**A**) and an axial T1-weighted MR image (**B**) demonstrate symmetric apparent proptosis of the globes, which protrude beyond the interzygomatic line. These findings are nonspecific and need to be correlated with the patient's history, laboratory values, and physical examination to determine significance. In this patient, there was no clinical history of proptosis and therefore the findings were presumably due to demographic variation in globe position rather than related to a pathologic proptosis.

Companion case: Thyroid ophthalmopathy

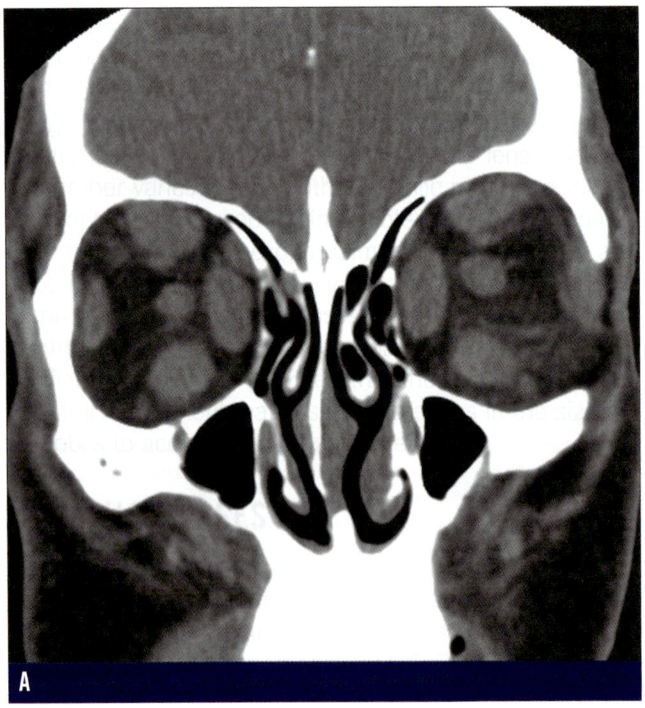

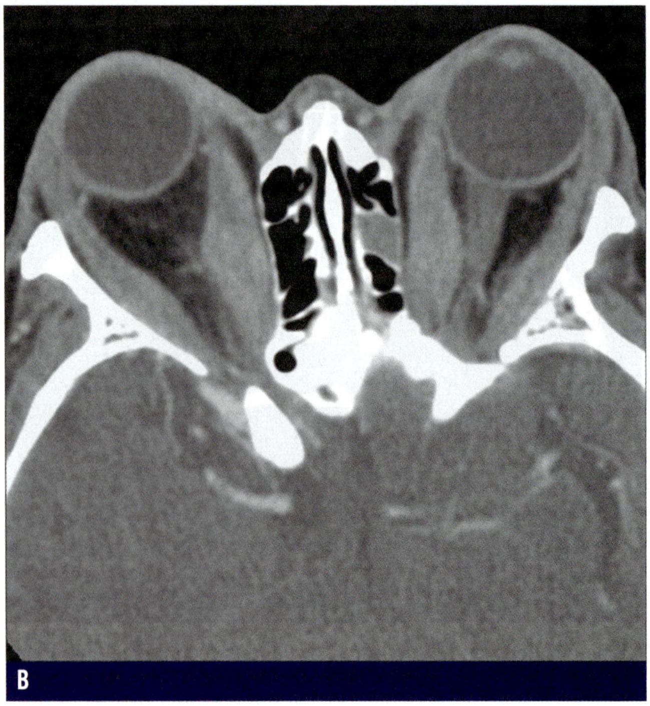

Unenhanced coronal reformatted (**A**) and postcontrast axial (**B**) CT images demonstrate marked bilateral proptosis associated with extensive enlargement of all of the extraocular muscles and retrobulbar stranding, consistent with thyroid ophthalmopathy.

Companion case: Traumatic proptosis

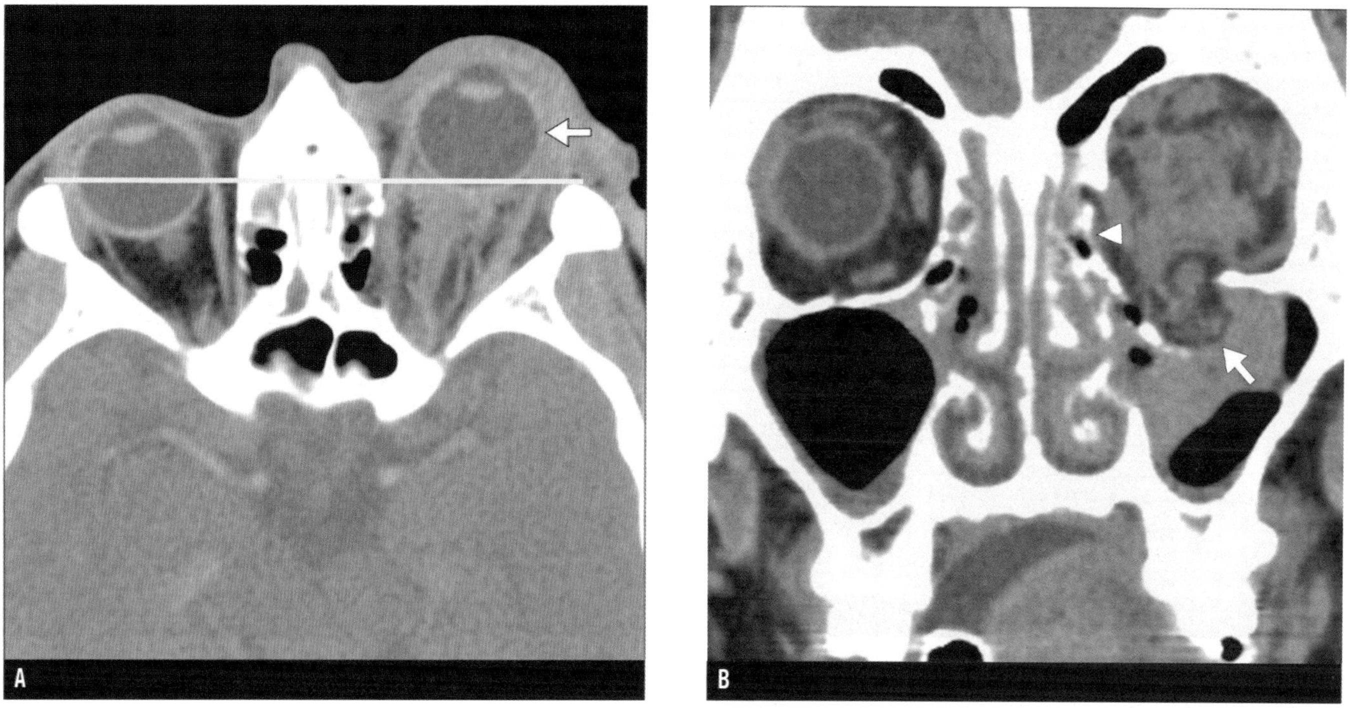

Postcontrast axial (**A**) and coronal reformatted (**B**) CT images demonstrate marked left globe proptosis (arrow, **A**) following trauma. There is extensive left intraconal hemorrhage as well as left periorbital soft tissue swelling. Also present are fractures of the left lamina papyracea (arrowhead, **B**) and a depressed fracture of the left orbital floor, the latter associated with downward herniation of the orbital fat and the left inferior rectus muscle (arrow, **B**).

Companion case: Spontaneous subperiosteal orbital hematoma

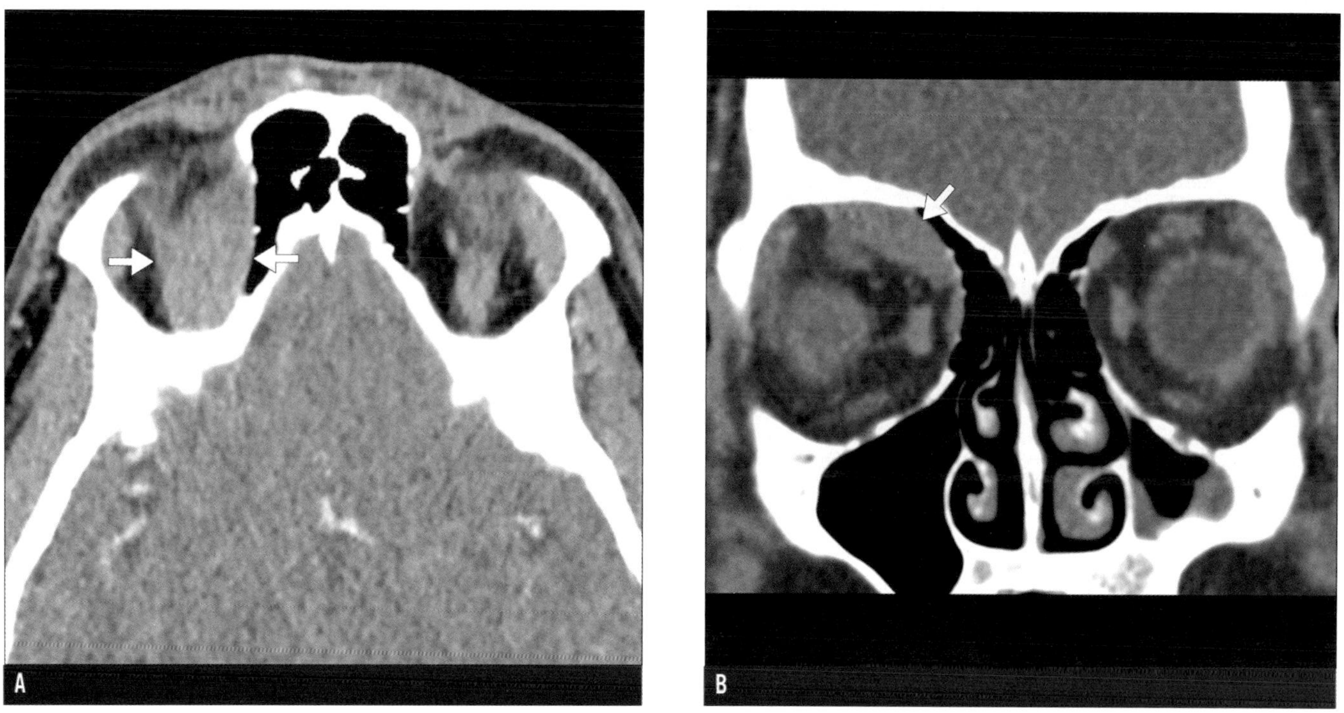

Axial (**A**) and coronal reformatted (**B**) contrast-enhanced CT images demonstrate a soft tissue density lesion in the superomedial aspect of the extraconal right orbit in this patient with 6 days of progressive right globe proptosis, clinical restriction of the superior rectus/levator palpebrae superioris complex and superior oblique muscle, and no history of trauma (arrows, **A**, **B**). Sagittal T1 (**C**), coronal T2 with fat suppression (**D**), and contrast-enhanced coronal T1 with fat suppression (**E**) MR images demonstrate the finding to be intrinsically T1 hyperintense (arrow, **C**), hypointense on T2 (arrow, **D**), and to not undergo fat suppression (arrow, **E**). The clinical history and imaging findings are compatible with a spontaneous subperiosteal orbital hematoma.

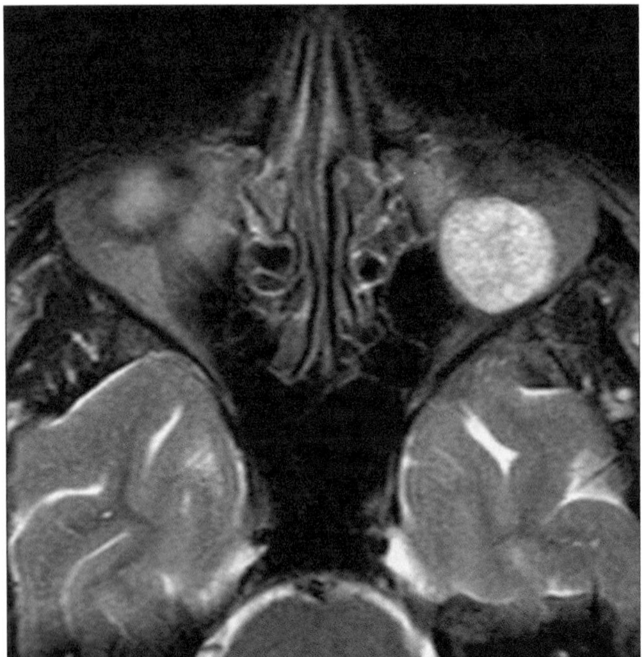

E

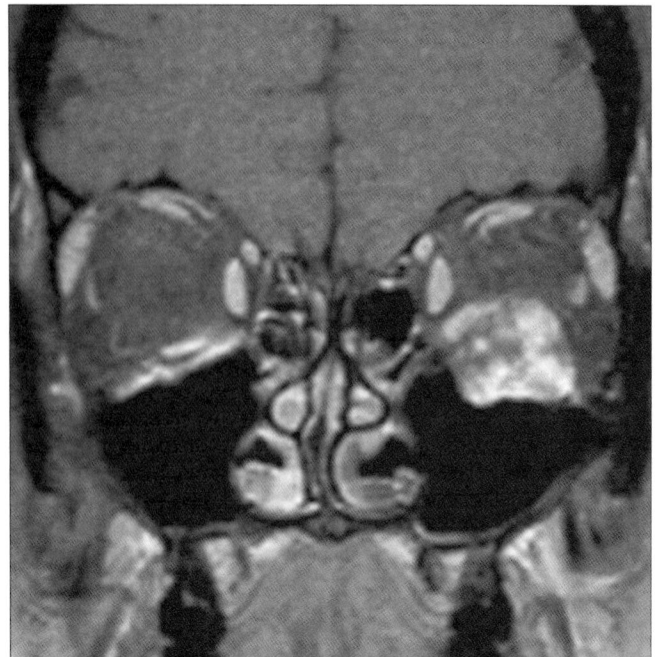

F

Companion case: CN V, V1 division orbital schwannoma

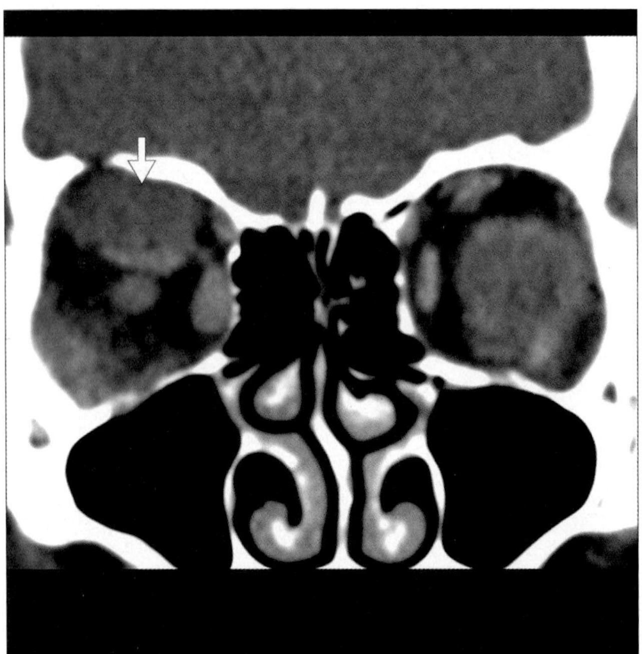

A

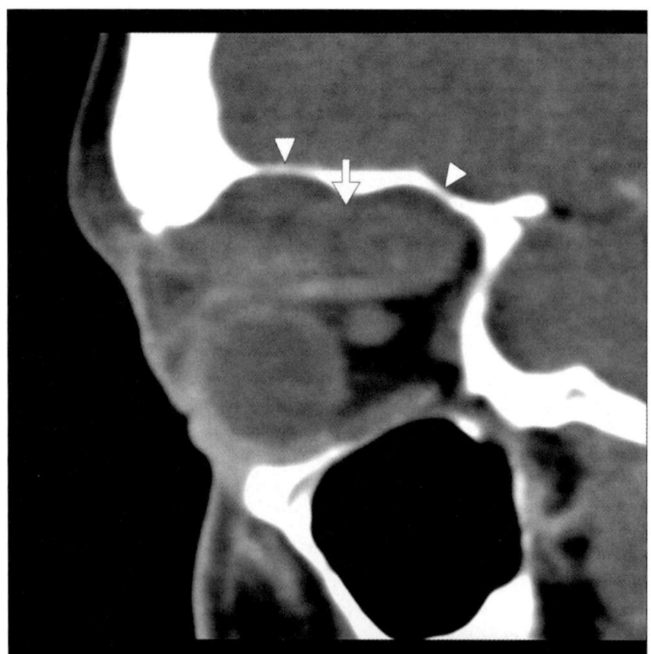

B

Coronal reformatted (**A**) and sagittal reformatted (**B**) contrast-enhanced CT images demonstrate a large, minimally presumably enhancing extraconal mass in the superior aspect of the right orbit (arrows, **A**, **B**) caudally displacing the right superior rectus/levator palpebrae superioris complex and remodeling the right orbital roof (arrowheads, **B**). There is also caudal displacement of the right globe (hypoglobus), and other images demonstrated mild right globe proptosis (not shown). Coronal T2 with fat suppression (**C**), sagittal T2 with fat suppression (**D**), axial T1 (**E**), contrast-enhanced axial T1 with fat suppression (**F**), and contrast-enhanced coronal T1 with fat suppression (**G**) MR images demonstrate the mass to be heterogeneous on both T2 and following contrast (arrows, **C**-**G**) with a characteristic T2 hyperintense, nonenhancing target sign sometimes identified with nerve sheath tumors (asterisks, **C**, **D**, **F**, **G**). This was pathologically proven to represent a schwannoma of the frontal nerve, a branch of the CN V, V1 division.

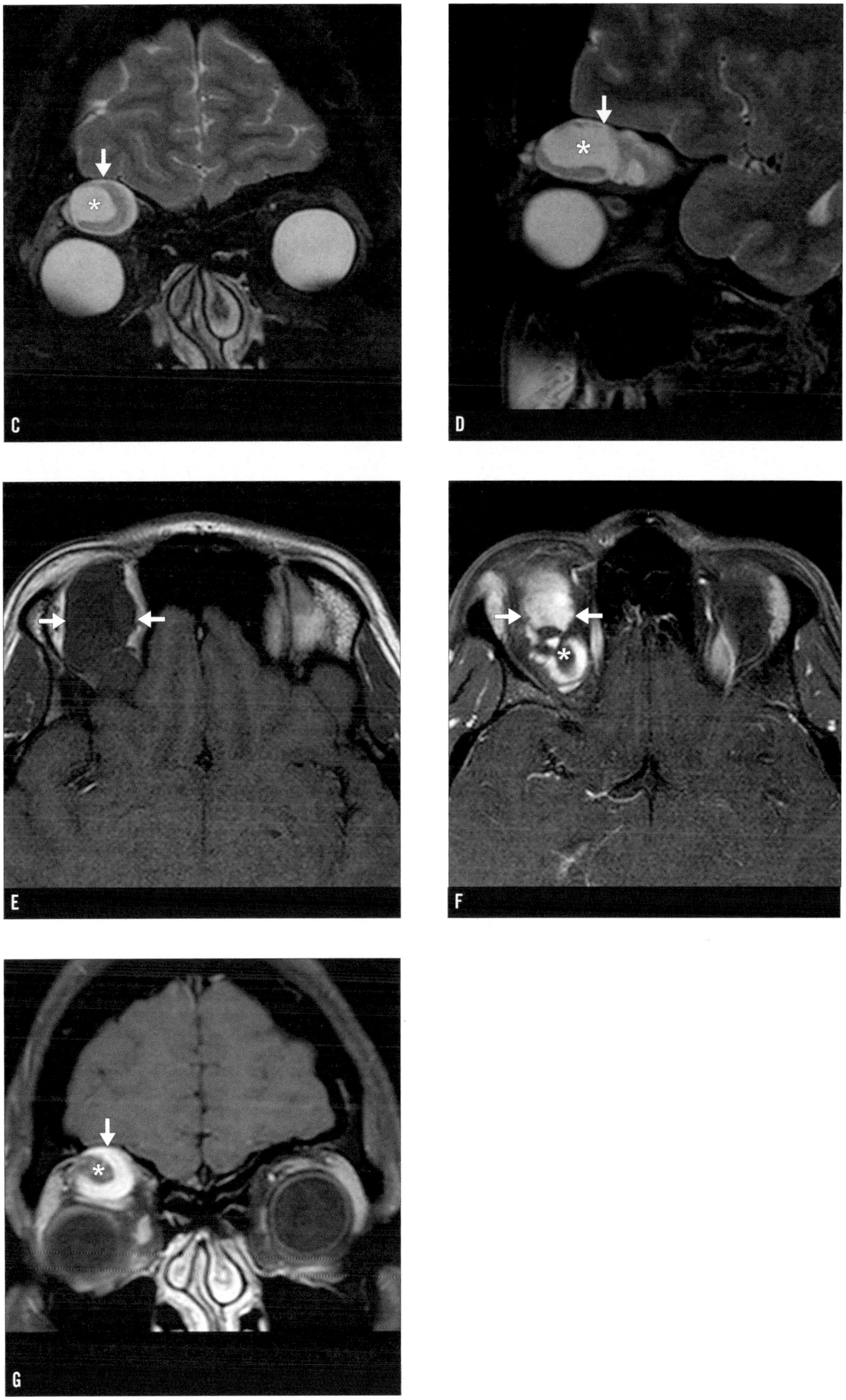
C
D
E
F
G

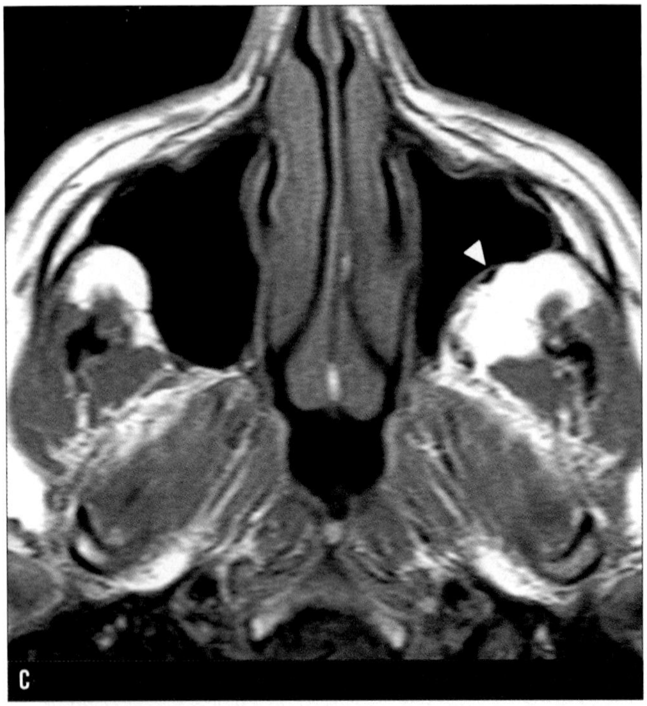

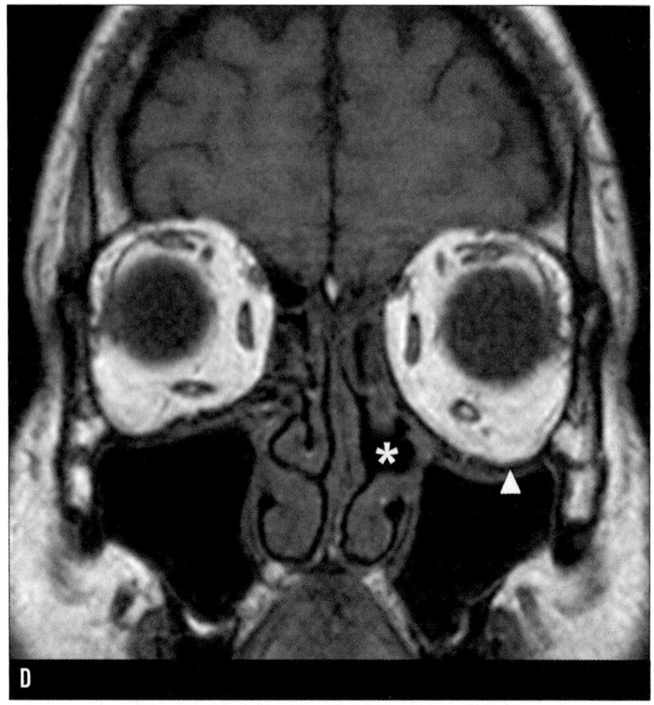

REFERENCES

B. Devenney-Cakir, R. Selouan, B.F. Branstetter IV, E. Melhem, and L.A. Loevner Spontaneous Bilateral Subperiosteal Orbital Hematomas in the Setting of Increased Transvenous Pressure. Neurographics 2015 March/ April; 5(2):64– 67.

Bingham CM, et al. Axial Globe Position Measurement: A Prospective Multicenter Study by the International Thyroid Eye Disease Society. *Ophthal Plast Reconstr Surgl.* 2015;20(20):1-7.

Comprehensive manual of ophthalmology, E. Ahmed. JP Medical. 2001, Pg 130.

de Juan, Jr E, Hurley DP, Sapira JD. Racial differences in normal values of proptosis. *Arch Intern Med.* 1980;140:1230-1231.

Dollfus H, Verloes A. Dysmorphology and the orbital region: A practical clinical approach. *Surv Ophthalmol.* November-December 2004;49 (6);547-561.

Fidor-Mikita E, Krupski W. Computed tomography imaging of orbits in thyroid orbitopathy. *JPCCR.* 2008;2(1):59-63.

Hayashi Y, Watanabe T, Kita D, Hayashi Y, Takahira M, Hamada J. Orbital cystic schwannoma originating from the frontal nerve. Case Rep Ophthalmol Med. 2012;2012:604574.

Hilal SK, Trokel SL. Computerized tomography of the orbit using thin sections. *Semin Roentgenol.* 1977;12:137-147.

Hira NK, Lipham WJ, Marciniak MM. Silent sinus syndrome. *Optometry.* September 2004;75(9):589-594.

Jayaram A, Lissner GS, Cohen LM, Karagianis AG. Potential Correlation Between Menopausal Status and the Clinical Course of Orbital Cavernous Hemangiomas. Ophthal Plast Reconstr Surg. 2014 Aug 26.

Lam DS, NG JS, To KF, Abdulah V, Liew CT, Tso MO. Cystic schwannoma of the orbit. Eye (Lond). 1997;11 (Pt 6):798-800.

Lee JS, Lim DW, Lee SH, Oum BS, Kim HJ, Lee HJ. Normative measurements of Korean orbital structures revealed by computerized tomography. *Acta Ophthalmol Scand.* 2001;79:197-200.

Lloyd GA. The radiological investigation of proptosis. *Br J Radiol.* 1970;43:1-18.

Ozgen A, Ariyurek M. Normative measurements of orbital structures using CT. *AJR Am J Roentgenol.* April 1998;170:1093-1096.

Sheikh M, Abalkhail S, Doi SA, Al-Shoumer KA. Normal measurement of orbital structures: implications for the assessment of Graves' ophthalmopathy. *Australas Radiol.* June 2007;51(3):253-256.

Smoker WR, Gentry LR, Yee NK, Reede DL, Nerad JA. Vascular lesions of the orbit: more than meets the eye. *Radiographics.* January-February 2008;28(1):185-204

CASE 8 Inferior oblique muscle insertion simulating an epibulbar mass

The inferior oblique muscle is located just cephalad to the orbital floor, originating a few millimeters posterior to the medial aspect of the inferior orbital rim and immediately lateral to the lacrimal sac fossa. The origin of this muscle is in contrast to the remaining extraocular muscles, which originate from the annulus of Zinn. Occasionally, the scleral insertion of the inferior oblique muscle at the inferolateral margin of the globe can appear thickened on axial imaging (particularly on CT), simulating the appearance of an epibulbar or conjunctival mass. This appearance may in part be due to the lack of a defined musculotendinous junction associated with the inferior oblique muscle, a unique anatomic characteristic of this muscle relative to the other extraocular muscles.

COMPANION CASES

- **Conjunctival epithelial inclusion cyst.** Conjunctival epithelial inclusion cysts are benign lesions lined by non-keratinizing squamous epithelium, sometimes accompanied by mucin-producing goblet cells. Primary conjunctival cysts are the result of sequestration of conjunctival epithelium during embryologic development. However, approximately two-thirds of conjunctival cysts are secondary, either the result of traumatic or iatrogenic displacement of the conjunctival epithelium into the orbit. On CT, these lesions are like uncomplicated cysts elsewhere in the body, and they are either uni- or multilocular in morphology. Conjunctival epithelial inclusion cysts on MRI are thin-walled, T2 hyperintense, T1 hypointense, and nonenhancing lesions.
- **Conjunctival dermoid (epibulbar dermoid).** Conjunctival dermoids are lined by stratified squamous epithelium and contain fat, pilosebaceous units, and collagen. They are exophytic lesions that arise along the conjunctiva, usually in the superior nasal quadrant of the orbit. These lesions may be uniformly fatty or heterogeneous on CT and MRI, depending on their contents, and only their walls may enhance.

Inferior oblique muscle insertion simulating an epibulbar mass

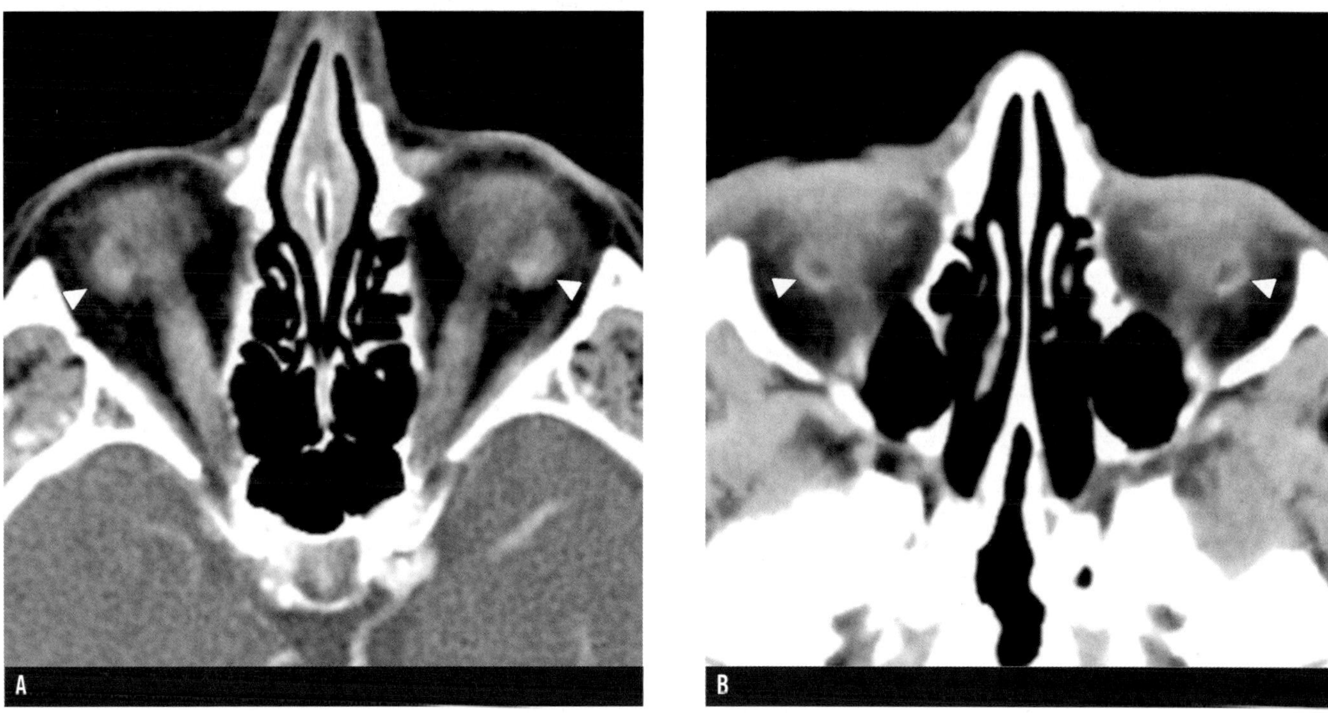

Contrast-enhanced axial CT images (**A**, **B**) demonstrate symmetric apparent lesions along the inferior margins of each globe (arrowheads, **A**, **B**). On a coronal reformatted CT image from the same study (**C**), the apparent abnormalities correspond to the normal insertion sites of the inferior oblique muscles (arrows, **C**).

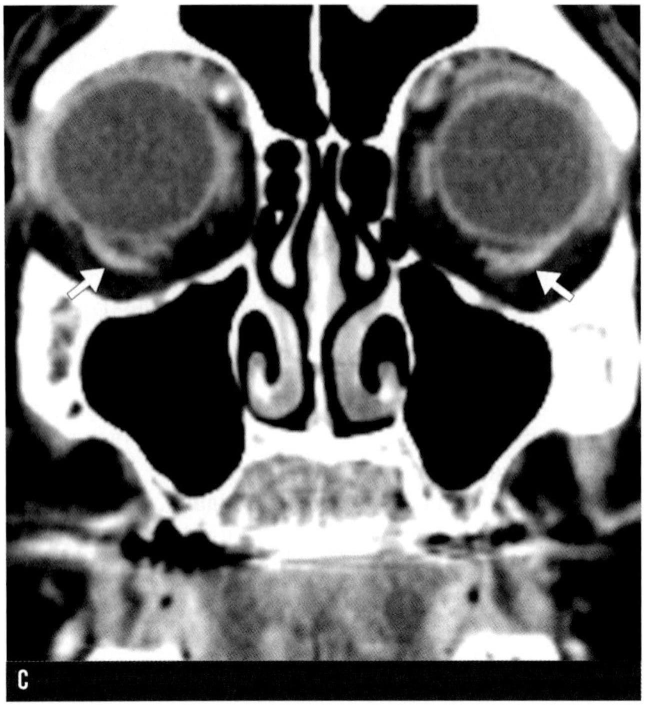

Companion case: Conjunctival epithelial inclusion cyst associated with a scleral buckle

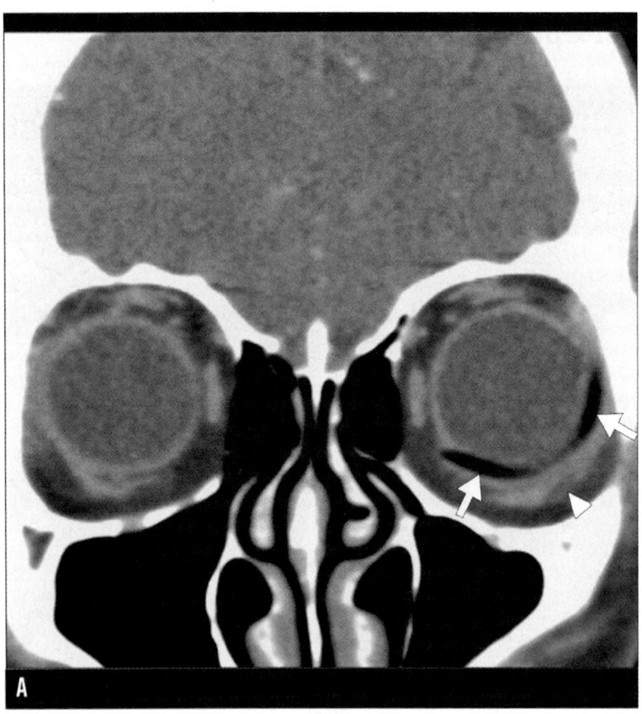

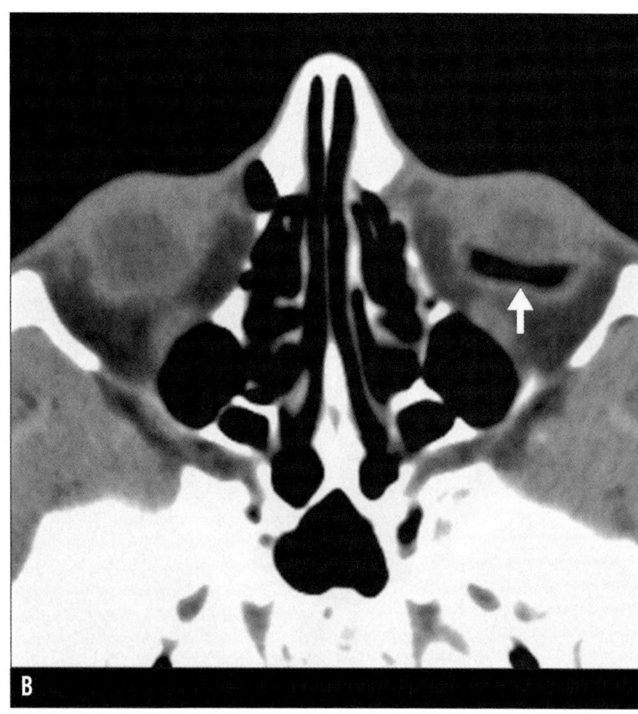

Contrast-enhanced coronal reformatted (**A**, **C**) and axial (**B**, **D**) CT images demonstrate segmental scleral buckling, characterized by a silicone sponge located along the lateral and inferior margins of the left globe (arrows, **A, B**). A small, low-density, cystic-appearing lesion is present adjacent to the sponge and conjunctiva, consistent with a conjunctival epithelial inclusion cyst (arrowheads, **A**, **C**, **D**).

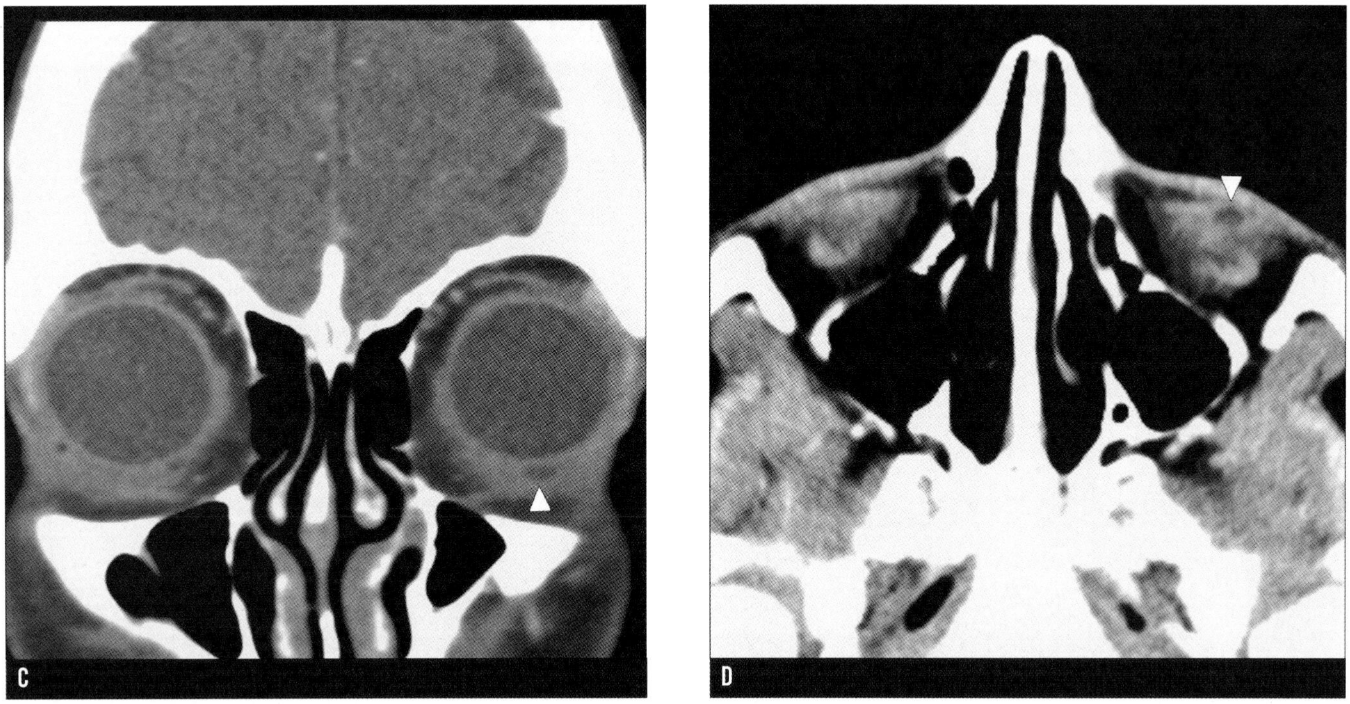

Companion case: Conjunctival epithelial inclusion cyst following strabismus surgery

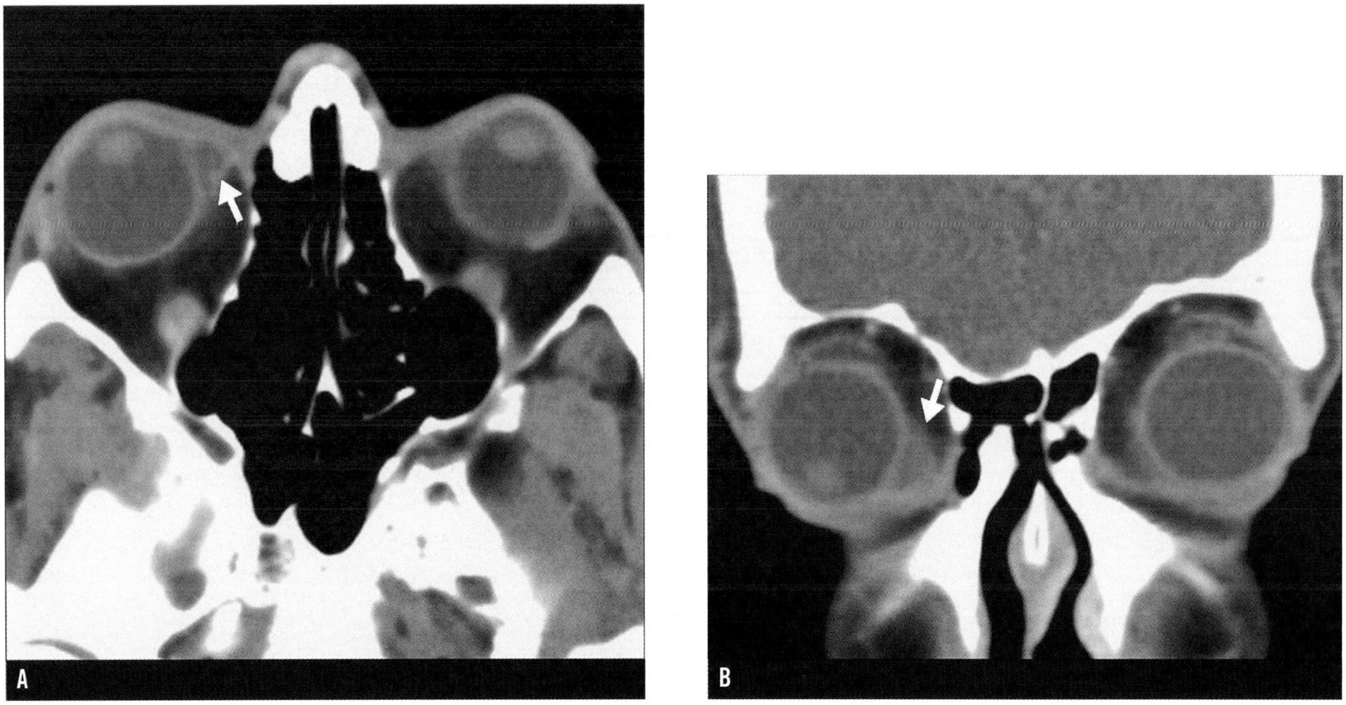

Axial (**A**) and coronal reformatted (**B**) unenhanced CT images demonstrate a hypoattenuating lesion intimately associated with the insertion site of the right medial rectus muscle (arrows, **A**, **B**). In this patient who had just undergone strabismus surgery, the finding is most compatible with a conjunctival epithelial inclusion cyst. However, in the absence of a history of surgery, a conjunctival (epibulbar) dermoid could have a similar appearance.

Companion case: Conjunctival epithelial inclusion cyst

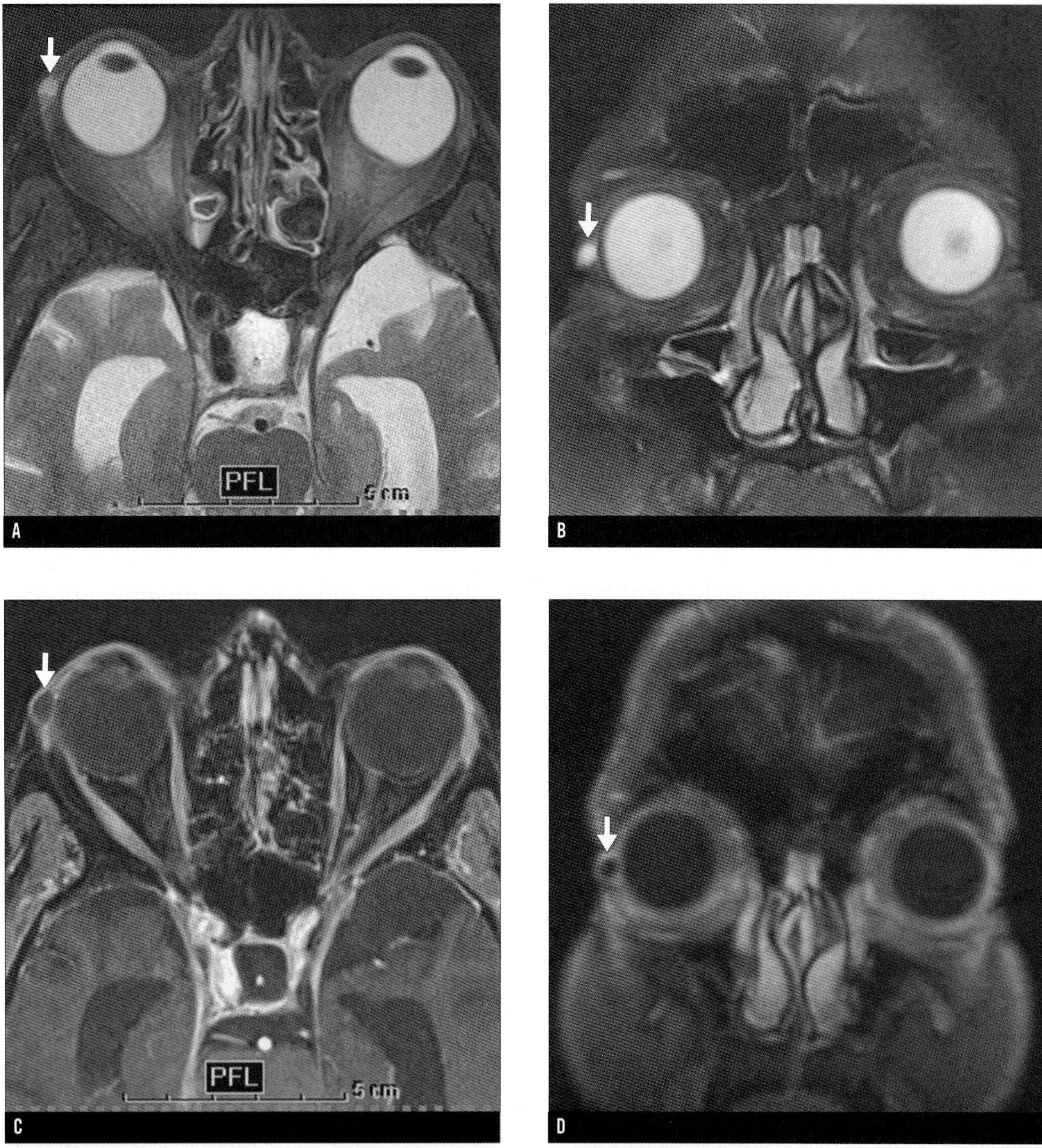

Fat-suppressed axial T2 (**A**), fat-suppressed coronal T2 (**B**), fat-suppressed contrast-enhanced axial T1 (**C**), and contrast-enhanced coronal MPRAGE (**D**) MR images. These images demonstrate a mildly T2 heterogeneous and peripherally enhancing lesion (relative to noncontrast imaging, not shown) located along the lateral conjunctival surface of the right globe, compatible with a conjunctival epithelial inclusion cyst (arrows, **A**-**D**). This finding was entirely stable for 7 years.

Companion case: Conjunctival dermoid (epibulbar dermoid)

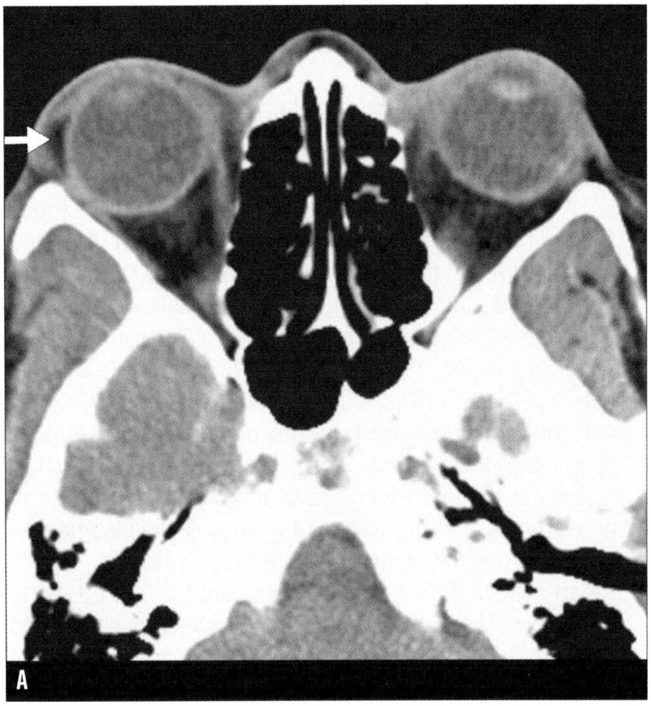

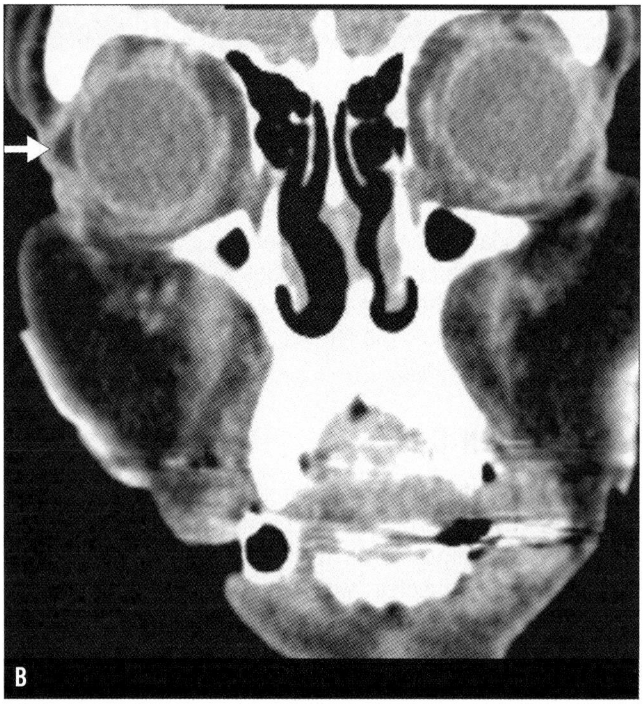

Unenhanced axial (**A**) and coronal reformatted (**B**) CT images demonstrate a circumscribed, elliptical, fat-attenuation lesion along the lateral aspect of the right globe, compatible with a conjunctival dermoid (arrows, **A**, **B**).

REFERENCES

Miller TM, Mafee MF. Computed tomography scanning in the evaluation of ocular motility disorders. *Radiol Clin North Am.* 1987;25:733-752.

Som PM and Curtin HD. *Head and Neck Imaging.* 4th ed. St. Louis, MO: Mosby Inc; 2003.

Yalçin B, Ozan H. Insertional pattern of the inferior oblique muscle. *Am J Ophthalmol.* 2005;139(3):504-508.

CASE 9 Extraocular muscle contraction simulating thyroid ophthalmopathy

The extraocular muscles will appear thickened when they contract during imaging and may occasionally simulate pathology, such as thyroid ophthalmopathy. This is particularly true when a pronounced directional gaze is present during the scan. For example, when the globes are directed inferiorly, the inferior rectus muscles will be contracted and thickened, and when the gaze is directed to the right, the right lateral and left medial rectus muscles will be contracted and thickened.

COMPANION CASES

- **Thyroid ophthalmopathy.** Thyroid ophthalmopathy (also called thyroid orbitopathy) most frequently manifests as exophthalmos and fusiform enlargement of the extraocular muscles with sparing of the musculotendinous junctions. The process is typically bilateral (90%) and asymmetric (70%). About 90% of cases are associated with Graves disease. Less frequent causes include Hashimoto thyroiditis, thyroid carcinoma, primary hyperthyroidism, and neck irradiation. The most commonly involved muscles (in order from most to least frequent) are the inferior, medial, superior recti, and lateral recti followed by the superior and inferior oblique muscles.
- **Treatment of metastatic melanoma with a CTLA-4 receptor monoclonal antibody (ipilimumab)**. Treatment with ipilimumab may result in a Graves ophthalmopathy-like syndrome and may be accompanied by manifestations of thyroiditis. The imaging findings are identical to typical thyroid orbitopathy, with the onset of abnormalities occurring as soon as 6 to 12 weeks after the start of ipilimumab therapy.
- **Orbital pseudotumor.** Orbital pseudotumor is a painful, nongranulomatous inflammatory process that can affect almost any portion of the orbit. It is believed to part of a recently described IgG4-related disease spectrum, which includes several other head and neck entities, such as Mikulicz disease, Hashimoto thyroiditis, Riedel thyroiditis, and lymphocytic hypophysitis of the pituitary gland. Entities elsewhere in the body that are also considered part of the IgG4-related disease spectrum includes autoimmune pancreatitis, sclerosing cholangitis, and retroperitoneal fibrosis, to name a few. Multiorgan involvement or elevated serum levels of IgG4 are very helpful in establishing the diagnosis, although not required. Histopathologically, the appearance of these lesions is similar, regardless of the organ, and are characterized by an abundance of IgG4-positive plasma cells and lymphocytes with associated organ fibrosis. On CT, it can manifest as ill-defined infiltration of the orbital fat or be tumefactive in appearance. On MRI, pseudotumor is most frequently iso- to hypointense on T1-weighted imaging and iso- to hypointense on T2-weighted imaging. Unlike thyroid orbitopathy, pseudotumor affecting the extraocular muscles usually does not spare the musculotendinous junction.
- **Extraocular muscle denervation atrophy from CN III avulsion.** Denervation atrophy may be identified on imaging as early as 4 to 6 weeks after the inciting injury. Acute muscle denervation atrophy manifests as increased T2 signal and enhancement, with volume loss and fatty atrophy of the muscle occurring over time. Head trauma, even when relatively mild, can result in cranial nerve injury. In the case of CN III, one theory implicates the petroclival ligament as a contributing factor to injury of this nerve. With this proposed mechanism, the petroclival ligament acts as a fulcrum during downward herniation of the brainstem as a result of the trauma injuring and rarely severing the nerve.

Inferior gaze simulating thyroid ophthalmopathy

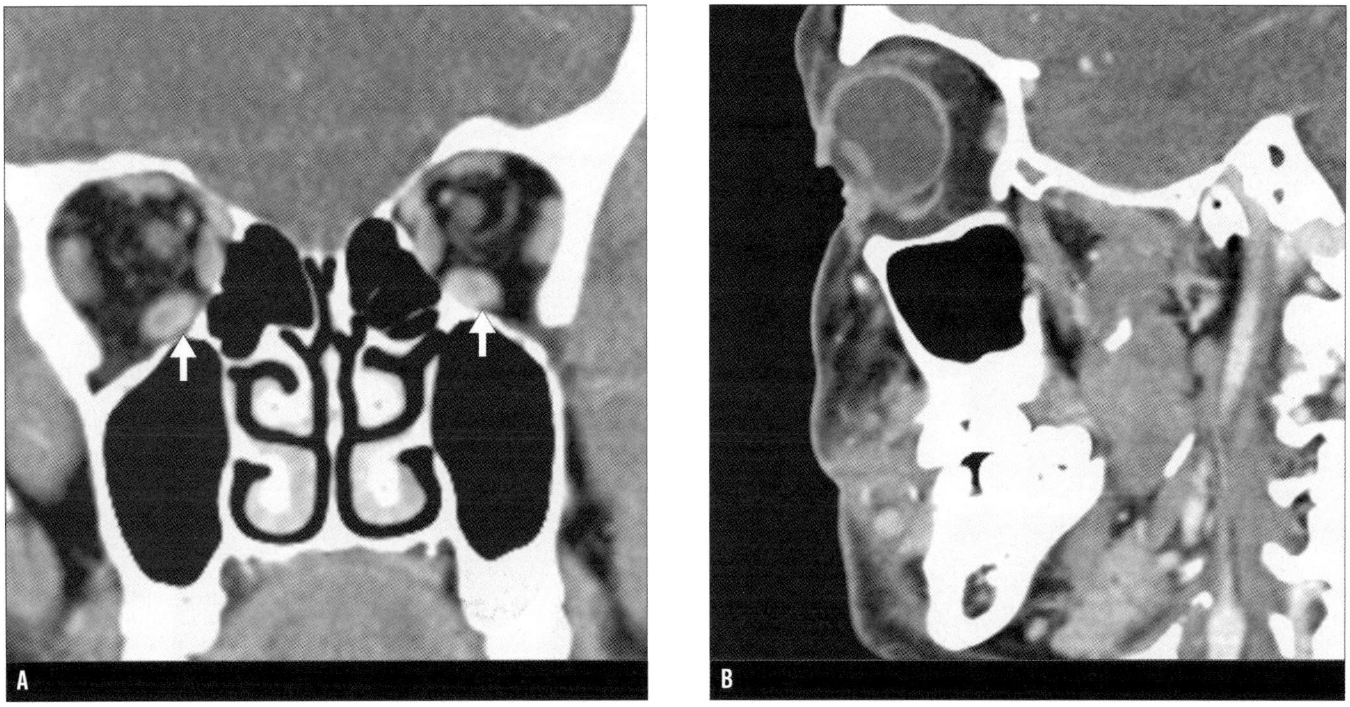

A coronal reformatted CT image (**A**) demonstrates thickening of the inferior rectus muscles (arrows, **A**), often the first extraocular muscle affected with thyroid ophthalmopathy. However, a sagittal reformatted CT image (**B**) demonstrates an inferior gaze during the scan. The contraction of the inferior rectus muscles during the inferior gaze explains their appearance on the coronal reformatted image.

Superior gaze simulating thyroid ophthalmopathy

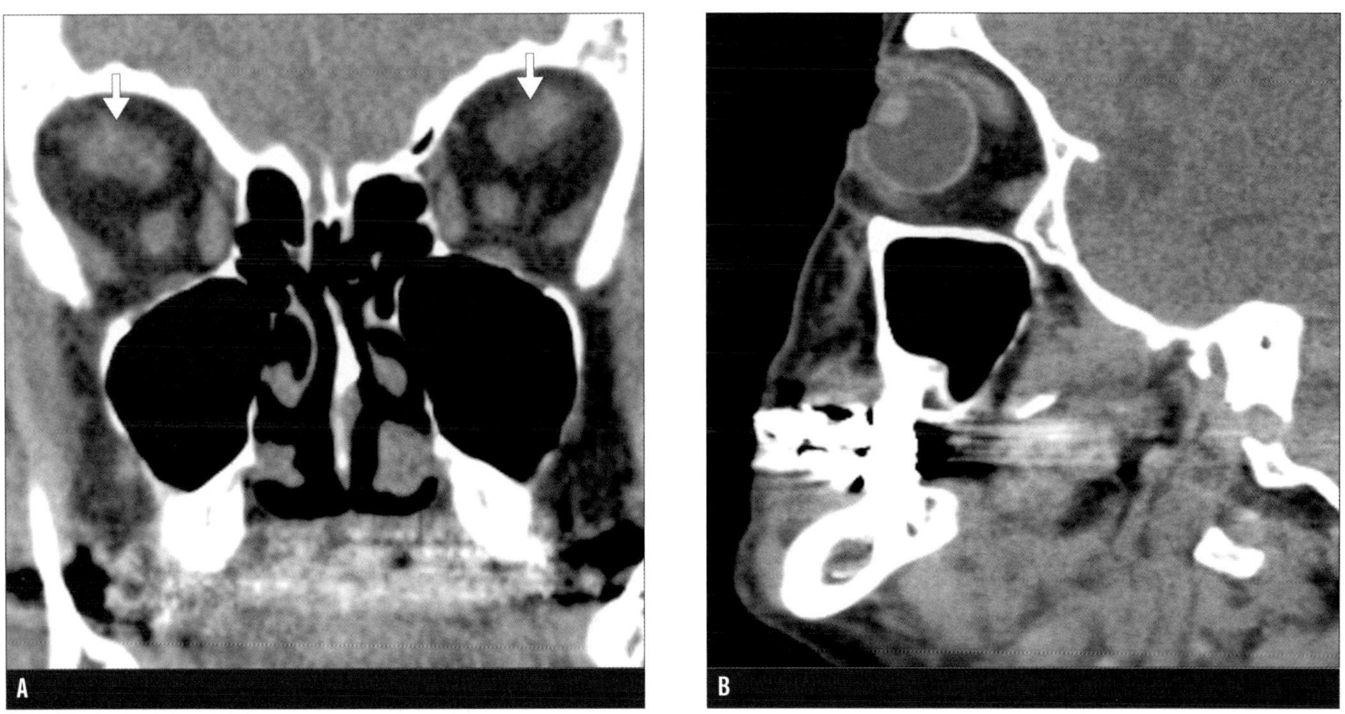

A coronal reformatted CT image (**A**) demonstrates thickening of the bilateral superior rectus/levator palpebrae superioris muscle complexes (arrows, **A**). A sagittal reformatted image (**B**) demonstrates a superior gaze. The contraction of the superior rectus/levator palpebrae superioris muscle complexes during the superior muscle gaze explains their appearance on the coronal reformatted image.

Horizontal gaze simulating thyroid ophthalmopathy

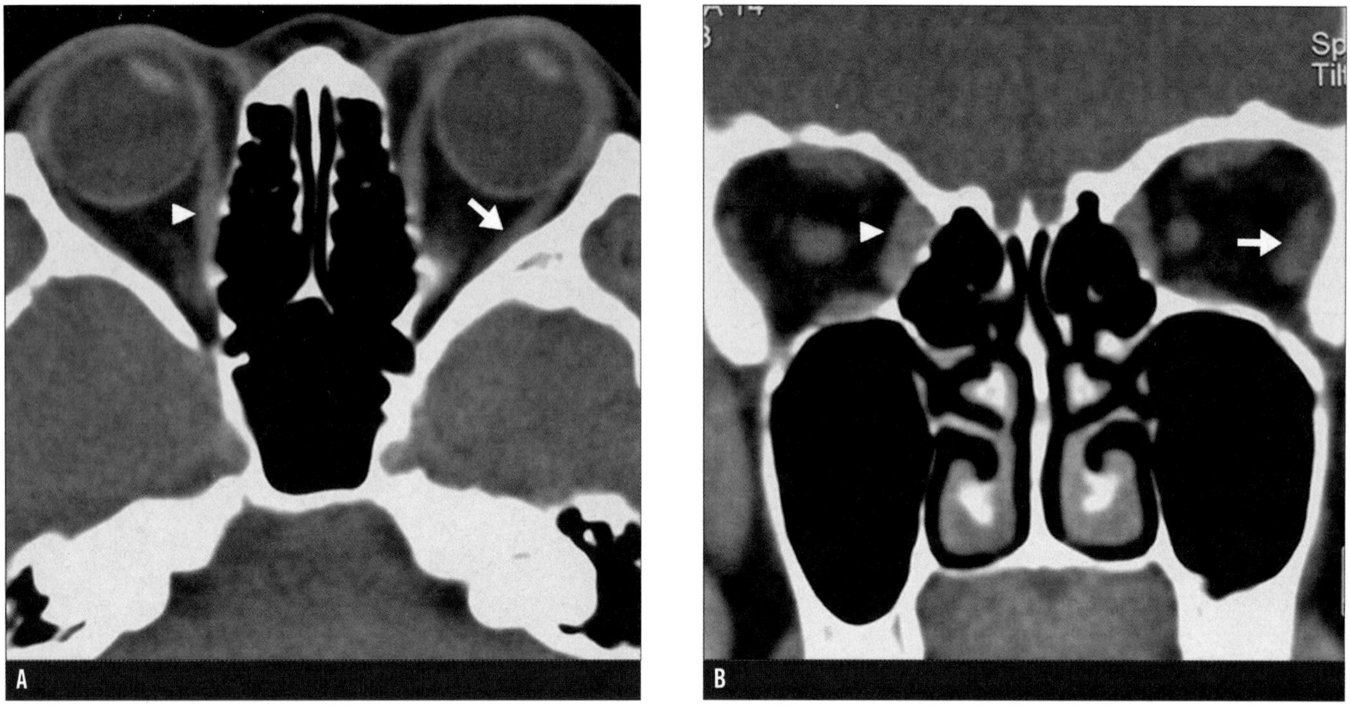

Axial (**A**) and coronal reformatted (**B**) CT images demonstrate asymmetric thickening of the right medial rectus (arrowheads, **A**, **B**) and left lateral rectus (arrows, **A**, **B**) muscles when compared to their contralateral counterparts. Leftward-directed gaze is clearly demonstrated on the axial image. The muscular contraction of the right medial rectus muscle and the left lateral rectus muscle account for their thickening on the images.

Companion case: Thyroid ophthalmopathy

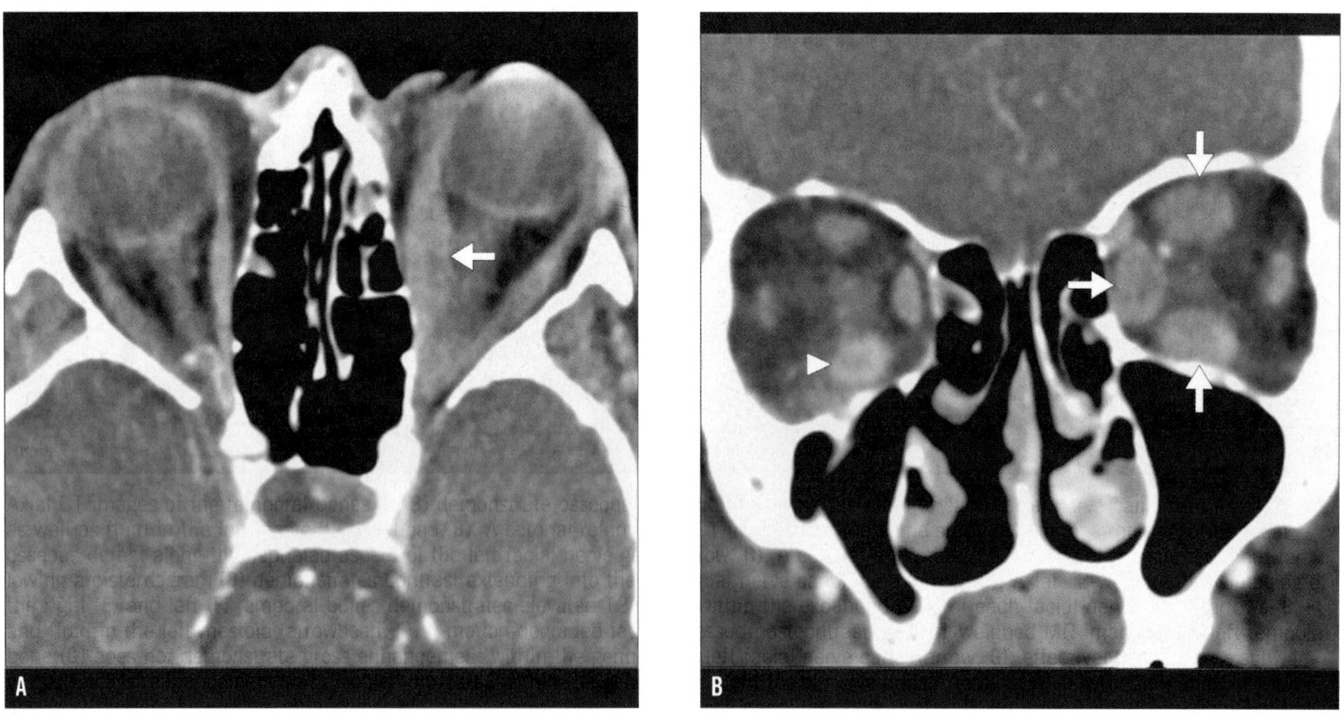

Contrast-enhanced axial (**A**) and coronal reformatted (**B**) CT images demonstrate marked enlargement of several left extraocular muscles (arrows, **A**, **B**) as well as the right inferior rectus muscle (arrowhead, **B**). There is also pronounced stranding of the retrobulbar fat, right greater than left. The findings are compatible with thyroid ophthalmopathy.

Companion case: Treatment of metastatic melanoma with a CTLA-4 receptor monoclonal antibody (ipilimumab)

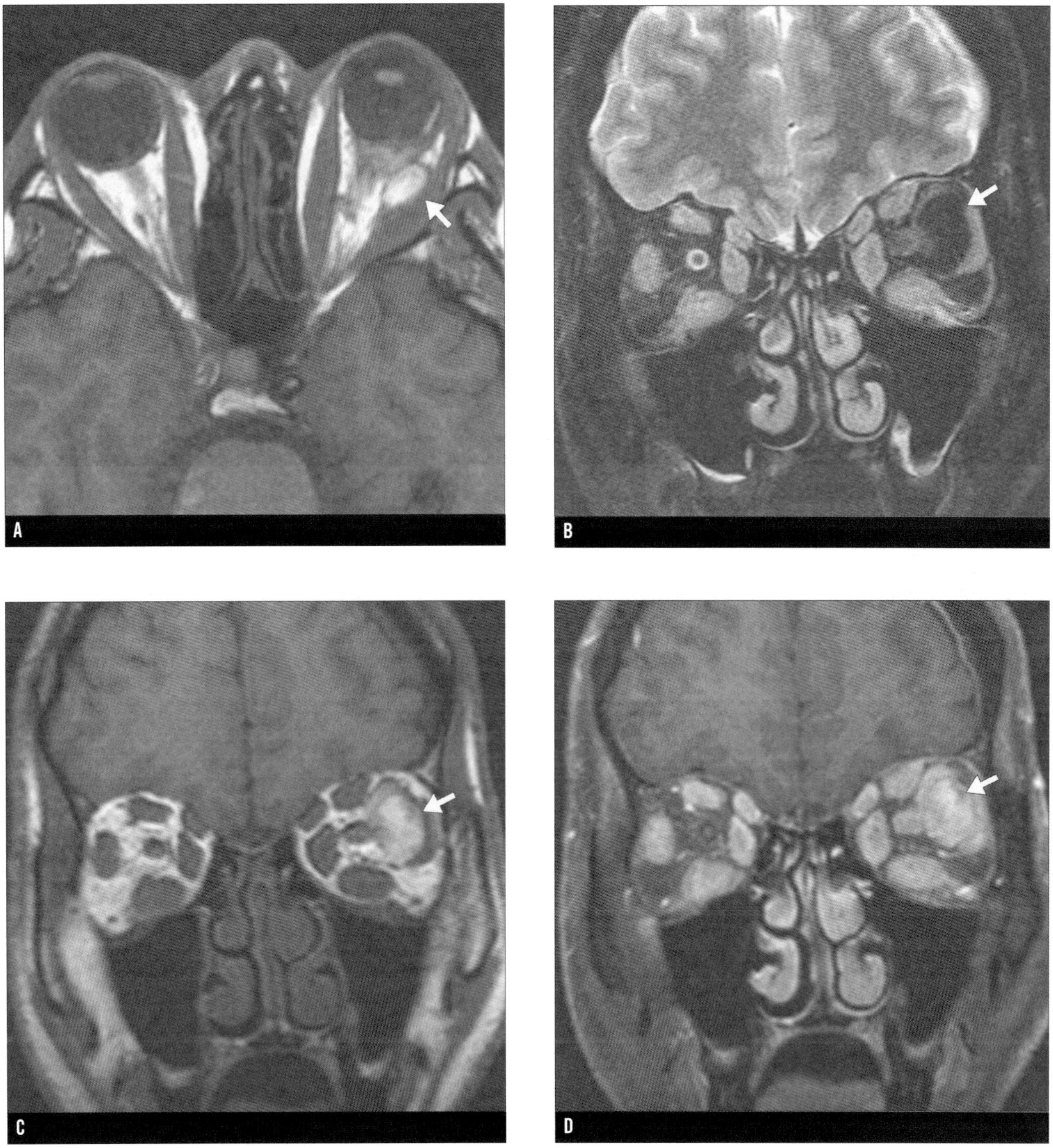

Axial T1 (**A**), coronal T2 with fat suppression (**B**), coronal T1 (**C**), and fat-suppressed postcontrast coronal T1 (**D**) MR images demonstrate marked, diffuse enlargement of the extraocular muscles of the orbits. A heterogeneously enhancing mass in the superolateral aspect of the left orbit represents a choroidal melanoma that has spread into the retrobulbar fat (arrows, **A-D**). Axial T1 (**E**) and postcontrast coronal T1 with fat suppression (**F**) MR images performed 2 months prior demonstrate the extraocular muscles to be normal in size. The melanoma mass in the left orbit is grossly stable between the two studies (arrows, **E, F**). In the interim between the two studies, the patient was treated with ipilimumab. Given this history, the marked extraocular muscle enlargement on images **A-D** is consistent with an ipilimumab-induced thyroid ophthalmopathy-like syndrome.

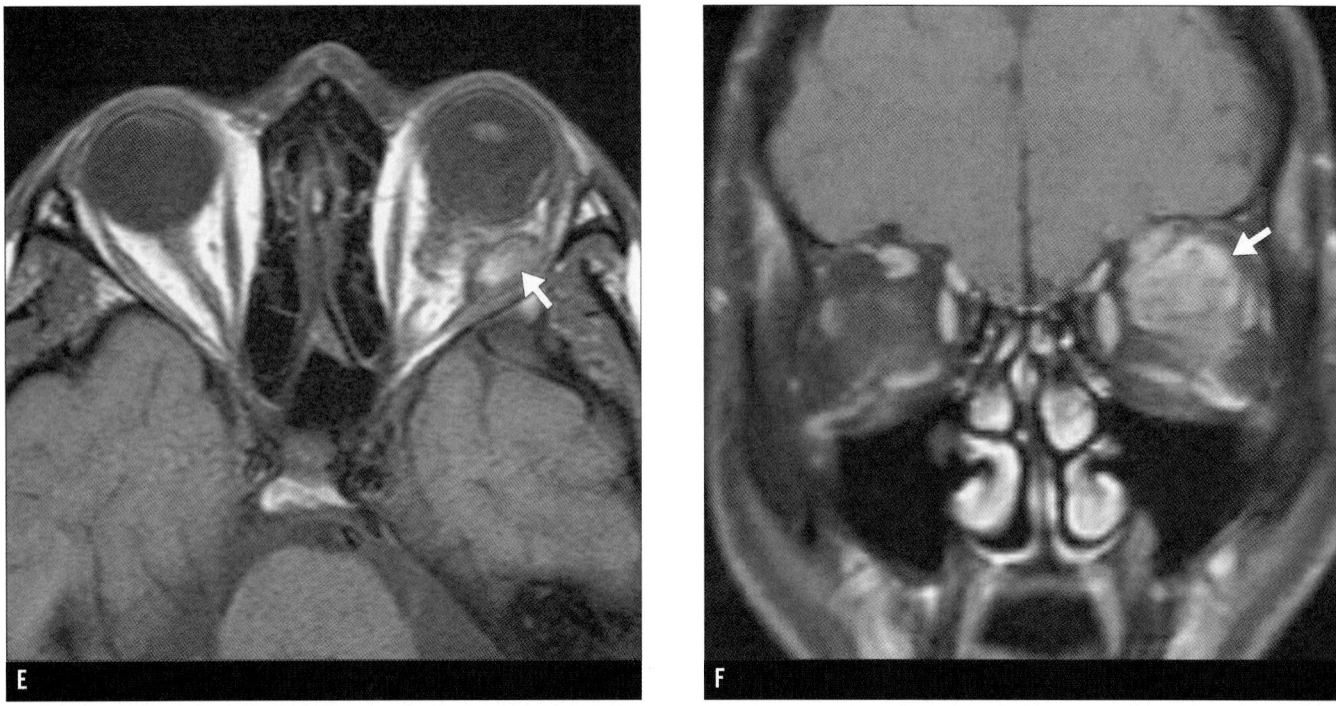

Companion case: Orbital pseudotumor

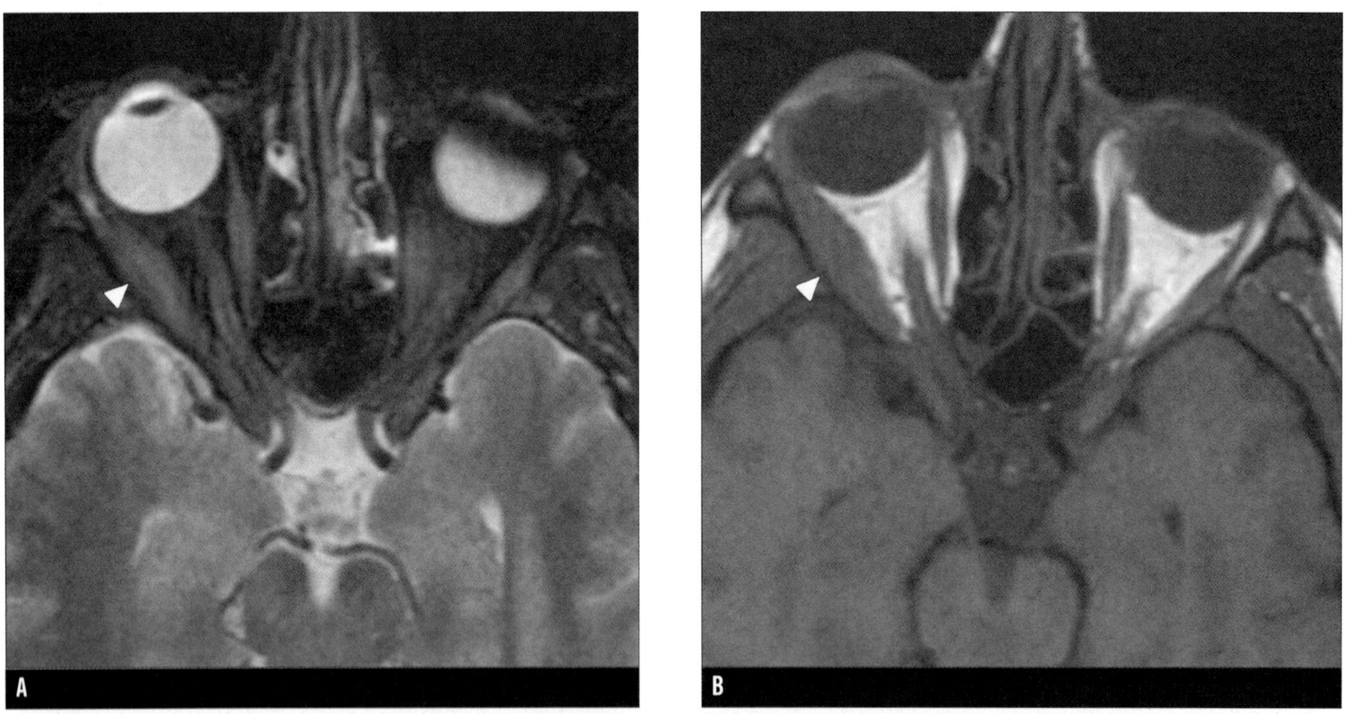

MR imaging through the orbits with fat-suppressed axial T2 (**A**), axial T1 (**B**, **C**), coronal T1 (**D**) and fat-suppressed postcontrast T1 in the axial (**E**, **F**), and coronal (**G**) planes demonstrate abnormal extraconal soft tissue in the lateral and inferior aspects of the right orbit which infiltrates the lateral and inferior rectus muscles and extends lateral to the confines of the orbit (arrowheads, **A**, **B**, **D**, **E**, **G**). The lesion is isointense on T1 and T2 relative to the extraocular muscles and enhances diffusely. Contiguous abnormal soft tissue also extends into the right pterygopalatine fossa and retromaxillary fat (arrows, **C**, **F**). The findings result in proptosis of the right globe. The imaging findings are nonspecific and include numerous etiologies, including inflammatory pseudotumor and lymphoma. On biopsy, this patient was found to have orbital pseudotumor.

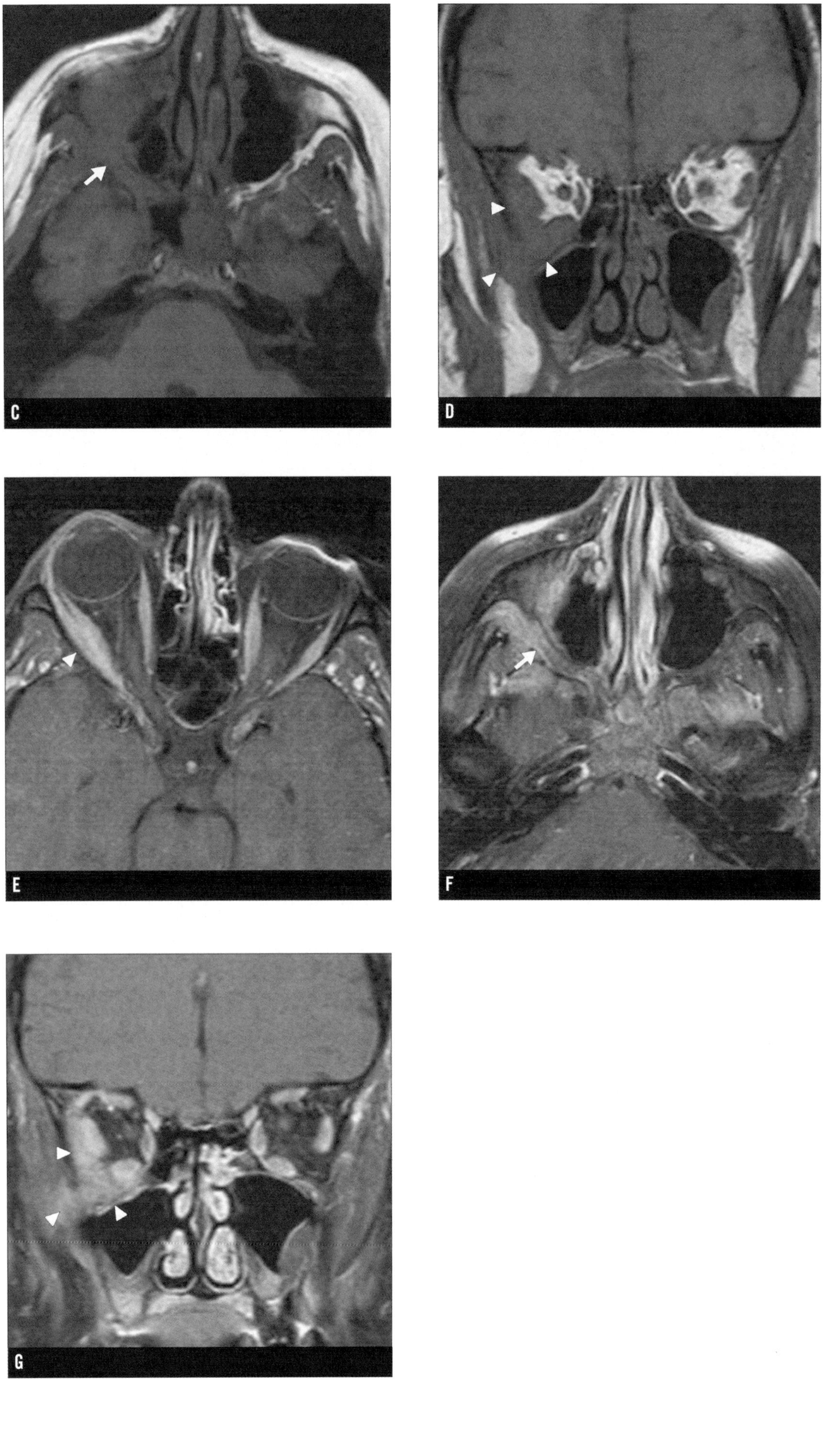
C
D
E
F
G

Companion case: Extraocular muscle denervation atrophy from CN III avulsion

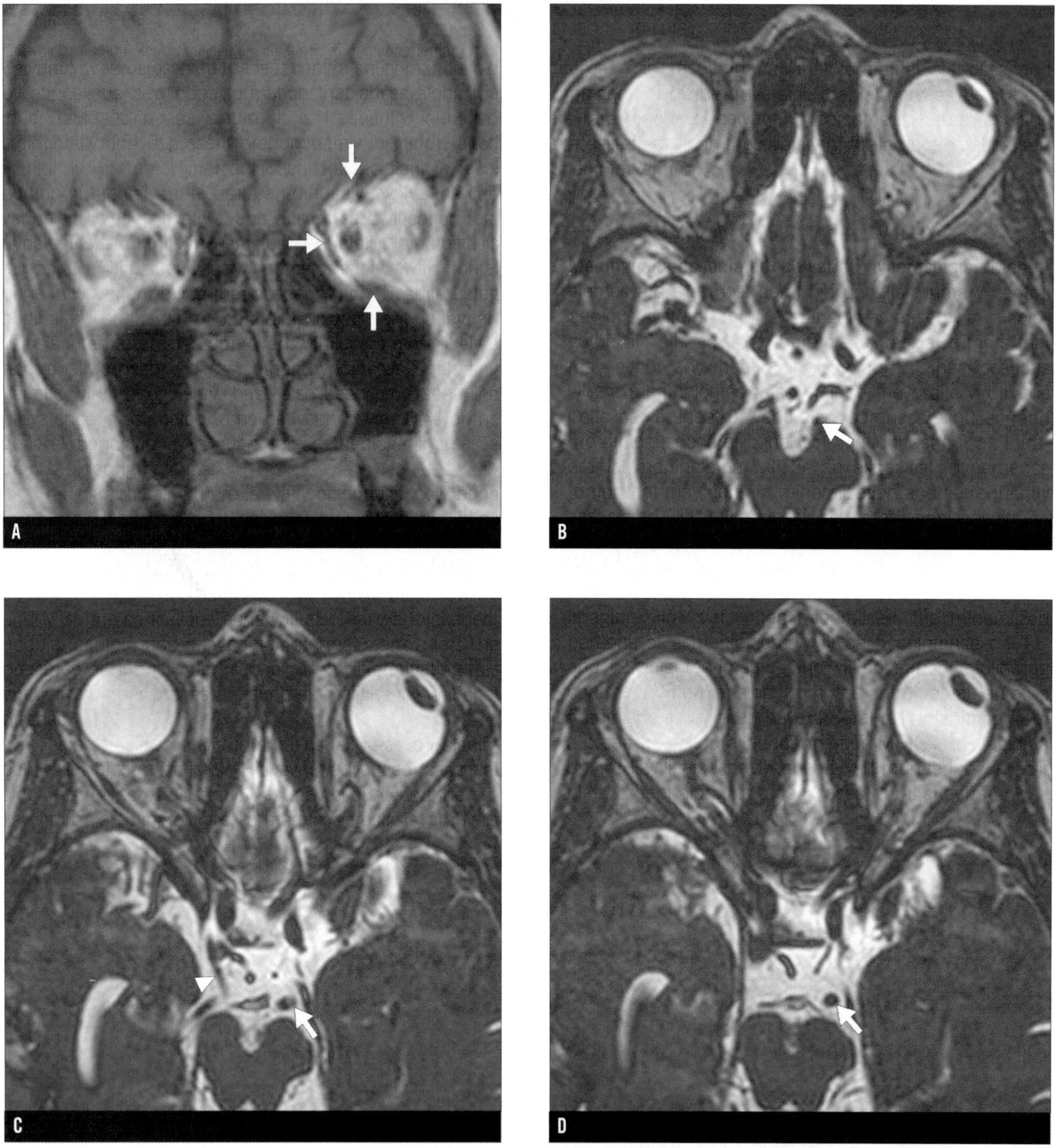

A coronal T1-weighted MR image (**A**) demonstrates atrophy of the left medial rectus muscle, inferior rectus muscle, and superior rectus/levator palpebrae superioris complex (arrows, **A**) when compared to the right. A series of CISS MR images beginning at the level of the interpeduncular cistern and extending cephalad (**B-D**) demonstrate a left globe exotropia and an abrupt termination of the mid-cisternal segment of the left oculomotor nerve (arrows, **B-D**), compatible with a nerve avulsion. The proximal portion of the avulsed left oculomotor nerve is asymmetrically thicker than the normal right oculomotor nerve (arrowhead, **C**), likely because of nerve retraction following the avulsion. This patient was involved in a motor vehicle collision 9 months prior to this imaging and had a clinically dense left oculomotor nerve palsy. The left oculomotor nerve avulsion explains the left extraocular muscle denervation atrophy present on image **A** as well as the left globe exotropia, the latter due to unopposed contraction of the left lateral rectus muscle.

REFERENCES

Borodic G, Hinkle DM, Cia Y. Drug-induced graves disease from CTLA-4 receptor suppression. *Ophthal Plast Reconstr Surg.* 2011;27(4):e87-e88.

Coello AF, Canals AG, Gonzalez JM, Martín JJ. Cranial nerve injury after minor head trauma. *J Neurosurg.* 2010;113(3):547-555.

Dhaliwal A, West AL, Trobe JD, Musch DC. Third, fourth, and sixth cranial nerve palsies following closed head injury. *J Neuroophthalmol.* 2006;26(1):4-10.

Fidor-Mikita E, Krupski W. Computed tomography imaging of orbits in thyroid orbitopathy. *J Preclin Clin Res.* 2008; 2(1):59-63.

Kato K, Tomura N, Takahashi S, Watarai J. Motor denervation of tumors of the head and neck: changes in MR appearance. *Magn Reson Med Sci.* 2002;1(3):157-164.

Katsuno M, Kobayashi S, Yokota H, Teramoto A. [Primary oculomotor nerve palsy due to mild head injury–report of two cases]. *Brain Nerve.* 2008;60(1):89-91.

Min L, Vaidya A, Becker C. Thyroid autoimmunity and ophthalmopathy related to melanoma biological therapy. *Eur J Endocrinol.* 2011;164(2): 303-307. Epub November 2010.

Narla LD, Newman B, Spottswood SS, Narla S, Kolli R. Inflammatory pseudotumor. *Radiographics.* 2003;23(3):719-729. Review. Erratum in: Radiographics. 2003;23(6):1702.

Nugent RA, et al. Graves orbitopathy: correlation of CT and clinical findings. *Radiology.* 1990;177:675-682.

Pemberton JD, Fay A. Idiopathic sclerosing orbital inflammation: a review of demographics, clinical presentation, imaging, pathology, treatment, and outcome. *Ophthal Plast Reconstr Surg.* 2012;28(1):79-83.

Weber AL, Romo LV, Sabates NR. Pseudotumor of the orbit. Clinical, pathologic, and radiologic evaluation. *Radiol Clin North Am.* 1999;37(1):151-168, xi.

Just as the optic nerves are direct extensions of the brain, the optic nerve sheaths are direct extension of the intracranial dura mater. In addition to surrounding the optic nerves, the optic nerve sheaths enclose the same cerebrospinal fluid (CSF) that bathes the brain. The volume of CSF enclosed by the optic nerve sheath may vary widely among normal individuals and reflect the intracranial pressure. A number of studies have examined the relationship between the optic nerve sheath diameter in both intracranial hypertension and hypotension. In patients with hydrocephalus or idiopathic intracranial hypertension, previously enlarged optic nerve sheath diameters may decrease in response to therapeutic shunting. Conversely, a decreased optic nerve sheath diameter may reflect intracranial hypotension.

COMPANION CASES

- **Idiopathic intracranial hypertension (pseudotumor cerebri).** While an optic nerve sheath diameter of >6 mm may be present with idiopathic intracranial hypertension, this is not a specific finding and can be present normally. Nevertheless, optic nerve sheaths of this diameter should prompt an assessment for other imaging findings of idiopathic intracranial hypertension, the most significant of which is posterior globe flattening, and when pronounced clinically, papilledema. Nonspecific imaging findings that may also be associated with this entity include a concave deformity of the superior aspect of the pituitary gland, an "empty" sella turcica appearance, and superior ophthalmic vein dilation. Ultimately, the diagnosis of idiopathic intracranial hypertension is based on the clinical assessment of the patient, abnormal elevated opening CSF pressure (>25-28 cm CSF), and/or alleviation of symptoms following a lumbar puncture with drainage of a large volume of CSF.
- **Optic nerve sheath meningocele.** Primary dilation of the optic nerve sheath, which cannot be attributed to an underlying cause such as idiopathic intracranial hypertension or a mass, is referred to as an optic nerve sheath meningocele. While optic nerve sheath meningoceles may have a benign course, there have been reports linking them to progressive visual changes, headaches (particularly retrobulbar), ophthalmologic findings (such as choroidal folds), and neurofibromatosis type I.
- **Optic nerve sheath enlargement due to a mass.** A mass within the orbit, such as at the orbital apex, may compress the optic nerve and impede CSF flow within the sheath. In these cases, the sheath may become distended in between the lesion and the globe.
- **Optic nerve atrophy.** Depending on the literature cited, a normal optic nerve measures approximately 3 to 4 mm in diameter. Studies have also demonstrated that a normal optic nerve progressively decreases in overall diameter as it courses from the globe toward the orbital apex. Optic nerve atrophy is generally considered to be present with a diameter of less than 2.5 mm. MRI is the preferred modality for radiological evaluation of the optic nerve. CT is inadequate for this task because the optic sheath cannot be reliably differentiated from the nerve, unless intrathecal contrast is administered and the patient is positioned to allow the flow of contrast into the optic sheath. On MRI, the presence of optic nerve atrophy can simulate an increased amount of CSF within the optic sheath. Optic atrophy can result from a myriad of causes, including ischemia, glaucoma, tumor compression, infection, demyelinating disease, and radiation. Clinically, there is optic nerve pallor when evaluated with ophthalmoscopy, and the patient has vision loss.
- **Optic nerve sheath meningioma.** Meningiomas of the optic nerve sheath are benign, slow-growing tumors which arise from arachnoid cap cells. Findings on CT include thickening of the optic nerve sheath and occasionally tram-track calcifications. On MRI, the lesions are isointense on T1-weighted images and isointense to hypointense on T2-weighted images, depending to some extent on the amount of associated calcification, if present.
- **Optic nerve sheath hemorrhage.** Retinal and/or vitreous hemorrhage that occurs in the setting of extensive subarachnoid hemorrhage, such as secondary to an intracranial aneurysm rupture or severe head trauma, is termed Terson syndrome. Occasionally with this entity, hemorrhage may also be identified within the optic nerve sheath. Retrobulbar anesthetic injection prior to ocular surgery has been associated with inadvertent injection into the optic nerve sheath, resulting in optic nerve sheath hemorrhage and marked visual loss.

Enlarged optic nerve sheath

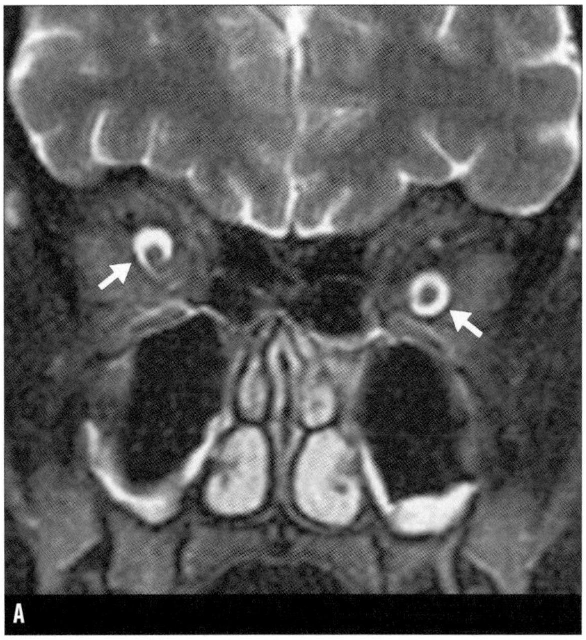

A coronal T2-weighted MR image with fat suppression (**A**) demonstrates an increased amount of CSF within the optic nerve sheaths (arrows). This patient did not have other imaging or clinical findings of intracranial hypertension, and the enlarged optic nerve sheaths were incidental findings. However, given that there are reports of visual issues in the setting of enlarged optic nerve sheaths (ie, optic nerve sheath meningoceles), an ophthalmologic examination may be warranted if this finding is encountered.

Companion case: Idiopathic intracranial hypertension (pseudotumor cerebri)

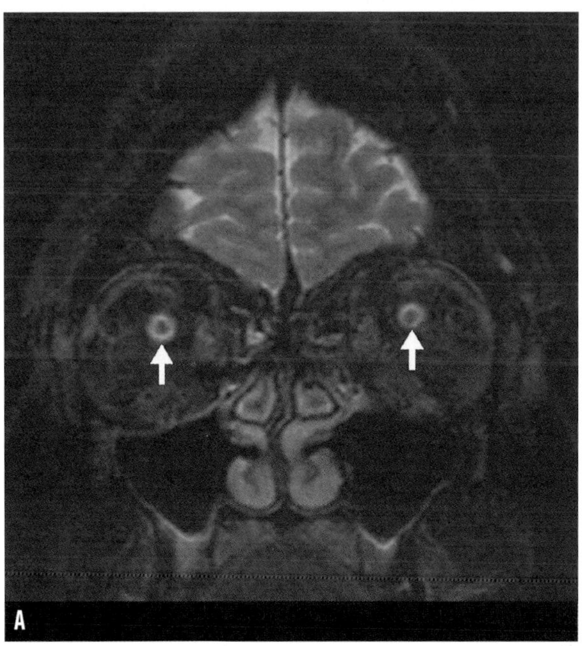

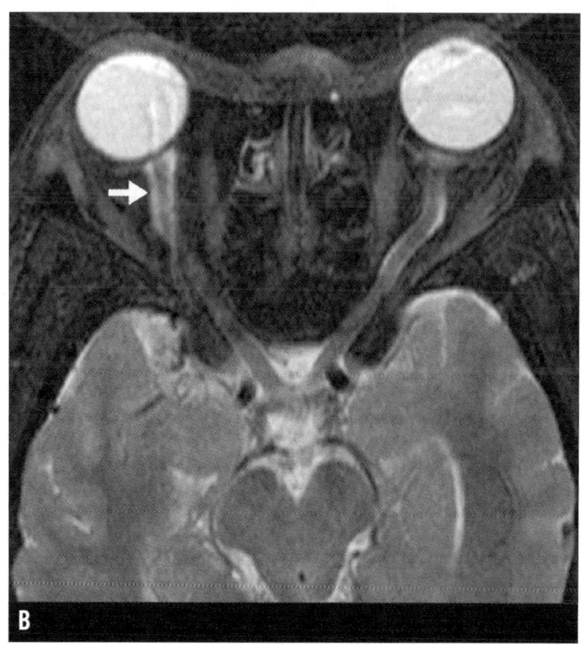

Coronal (**A**) and axial (**B**, **C**) fat-suppressed T2-weighted MR images demonstrate prominent CSF within the optic nerve sheath complexes (arrows, **A**-**C**). A sagittal T1-weighted MR image of the same patient (**D**) demonstrates a partially empty sella (arrow, **D**). While these findings are nonspecific, this patient had an elevated CSF opening pressure of 30 cm H_2O and clinical symptoms compatible with idiopathic intracranial hypertension.

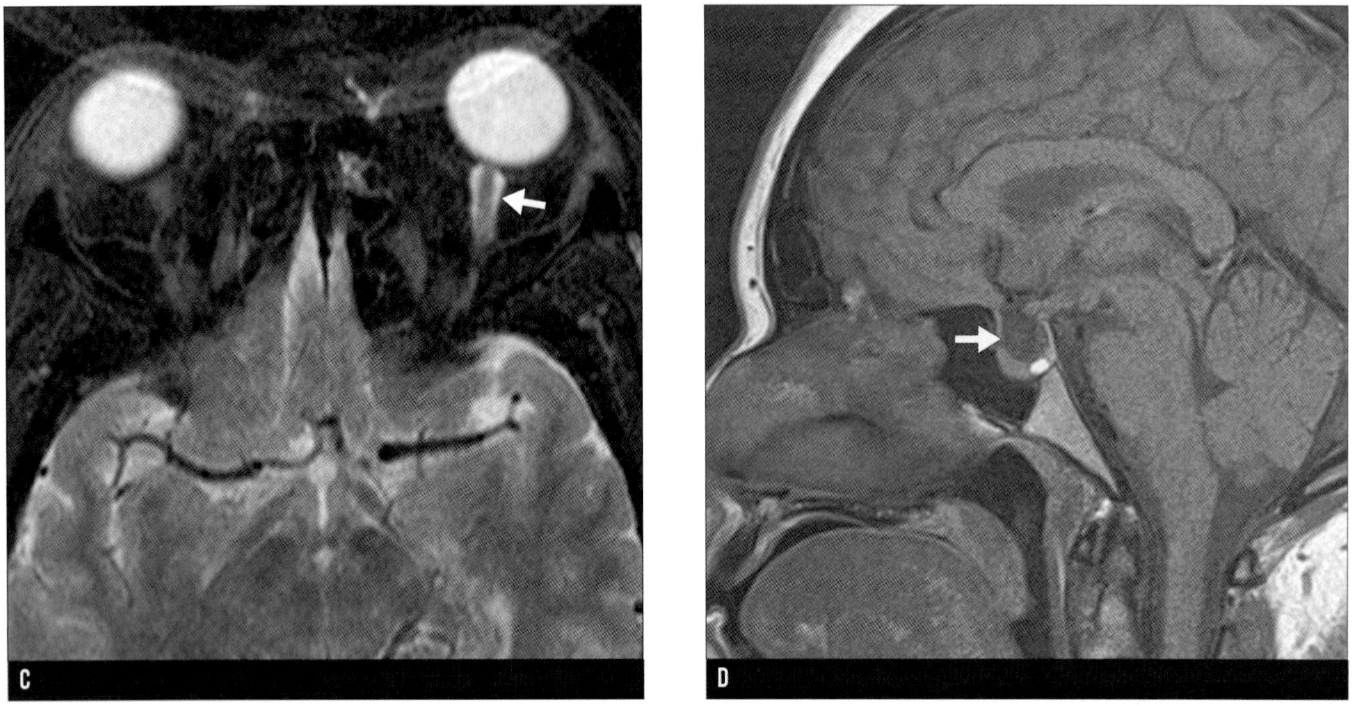

Companion case: Optic nerve sheath meningocele

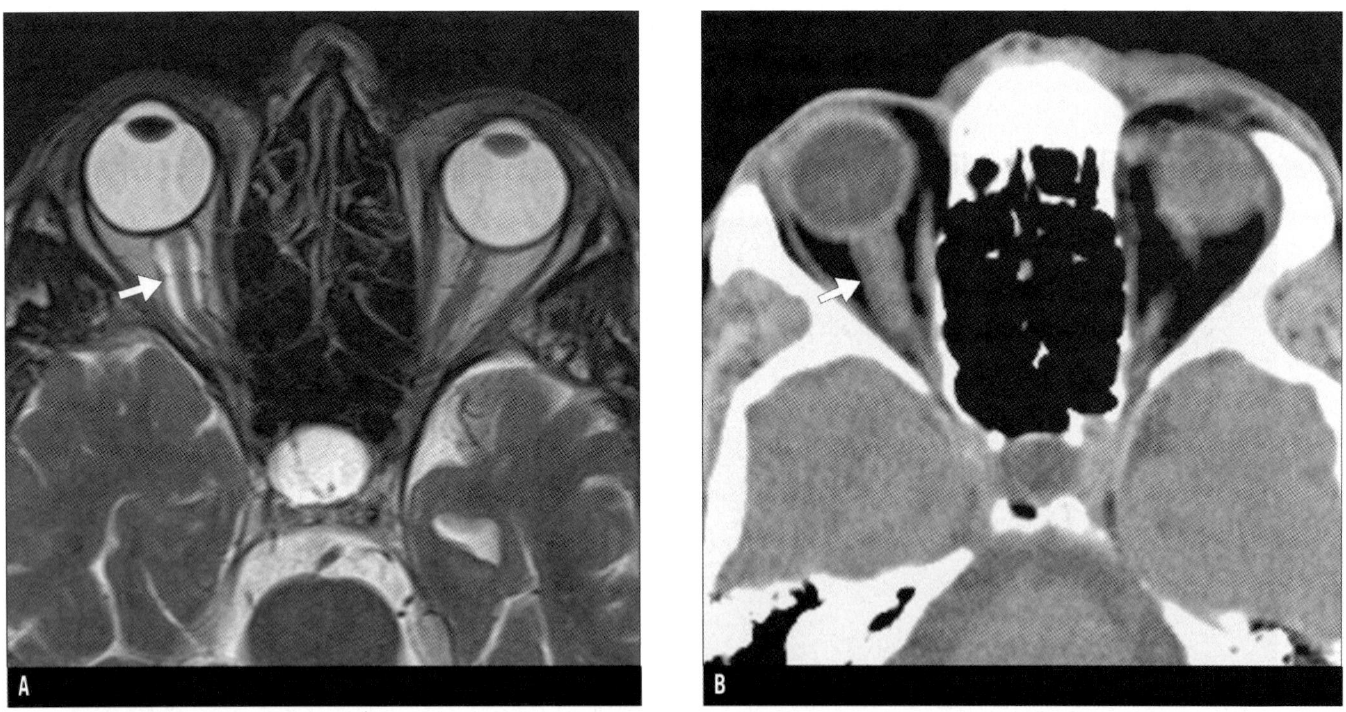

An axial T2-weighted MR image (**A**) demonstrates asymmetric enlargement of the right optic nerve sheath (arrow, **A**) with a larger amount of CSF within the sheath relative to the left optic nerve sheath. Unenhanced axial CT images obtained 3 years earlier (**B**, **C**) demonstrate stable enlargement of the right optic nerve sheath complex (arrow, **B**) relative to the left. The findings are compatible with a right optic nerve sheath meningocele. There was no provided history of visual loss for this patient. However, an ophthalmologic examination may be warranted if confronted with such a finding, given reports in the literature of visual issues with this entity.

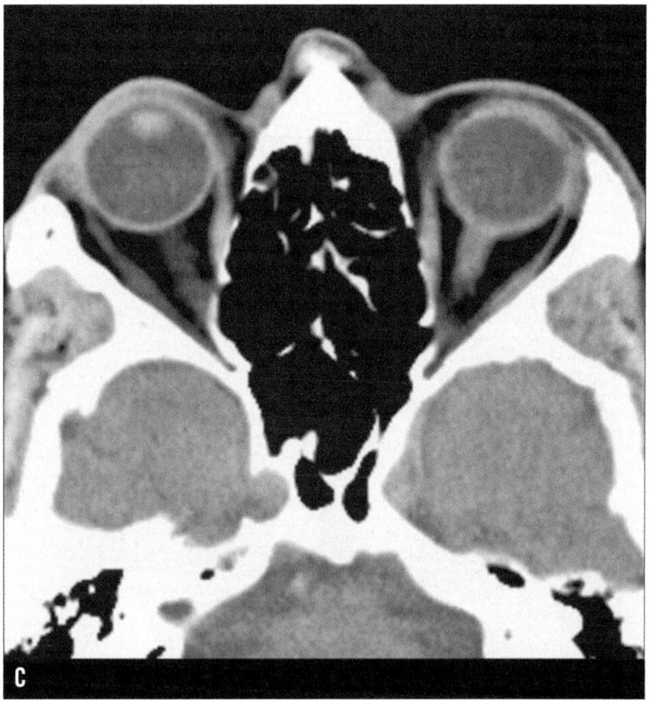

Companion case: Optic nerve sheath enlargement due to a mass

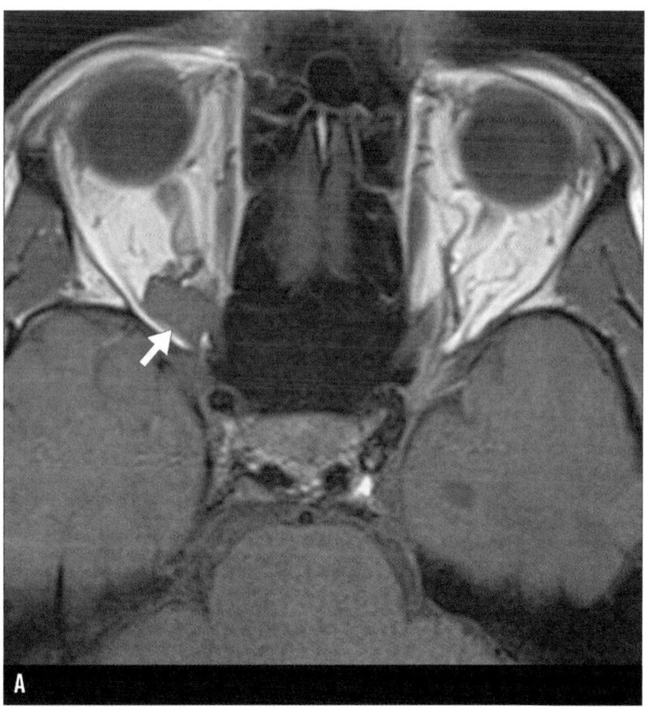

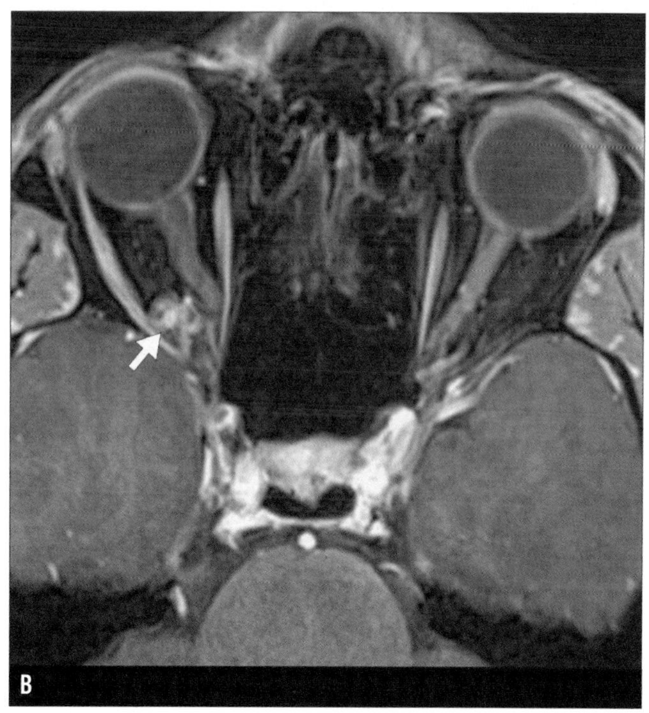

Precontrast axial T1 (**A**), postcontrast axial T1 with fat suppression (**B**), axial T2 with fat suppression (**C**), coronal T2 with fat suppression (**D**), and axial CISS (**F**) MR images demonstrate a T1 isointense, T2 hyperintense, CISS isointense, heterogeneously enhancing mass at the right orbital apex, likely representing an encapsulated venous malformation (arrows, **A C**, **E**). This mass medially displaces and impinges the posterior aspect of the right optic nerve sheath complex, likely resulting in obstruction of the right optic nerve sheath CSF and dilation of the majority of the sheath anterior to the mass (arrowheads, **D**, **E**).

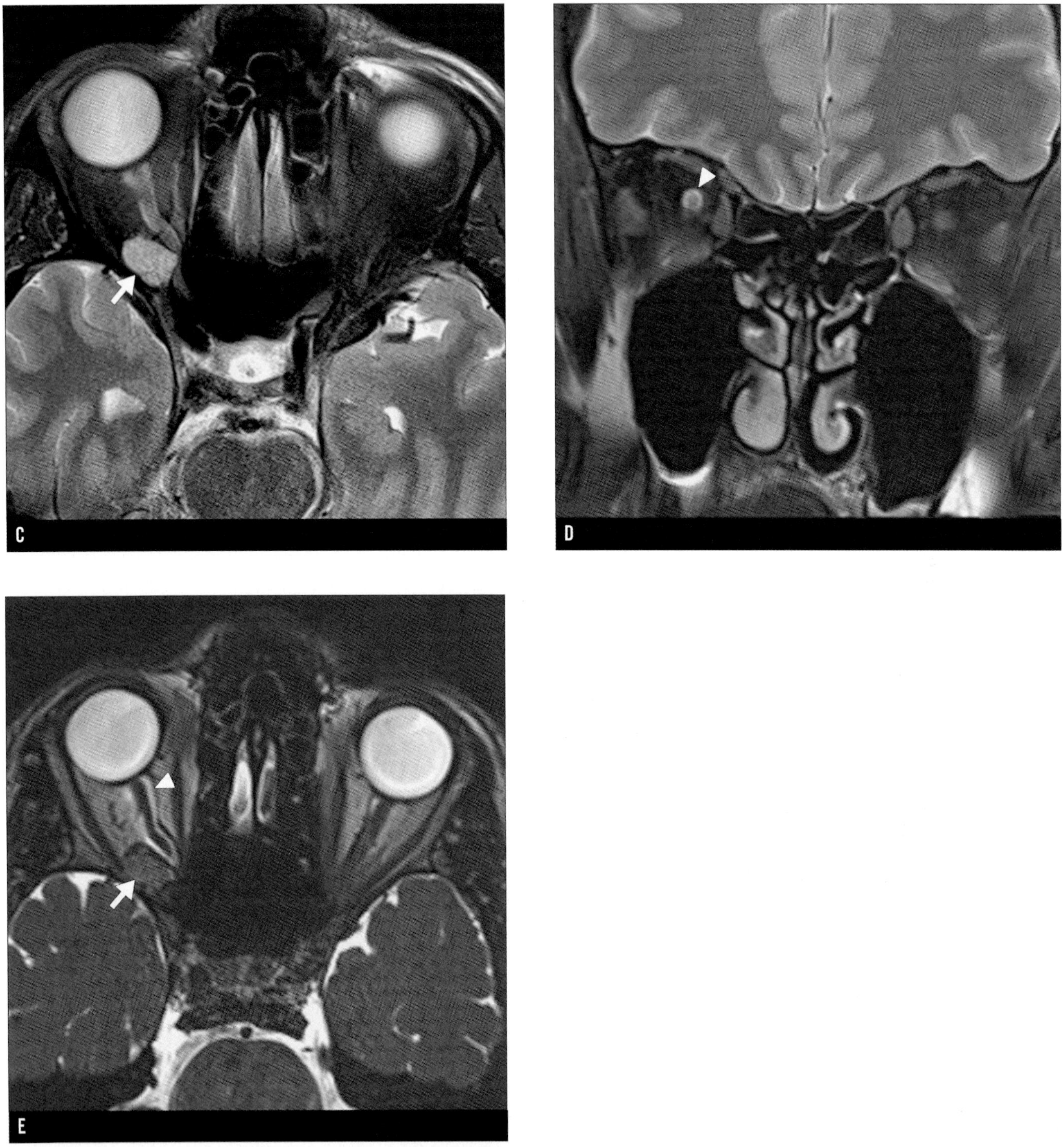
C
D
E

Companion case: Optic nerve atrophy

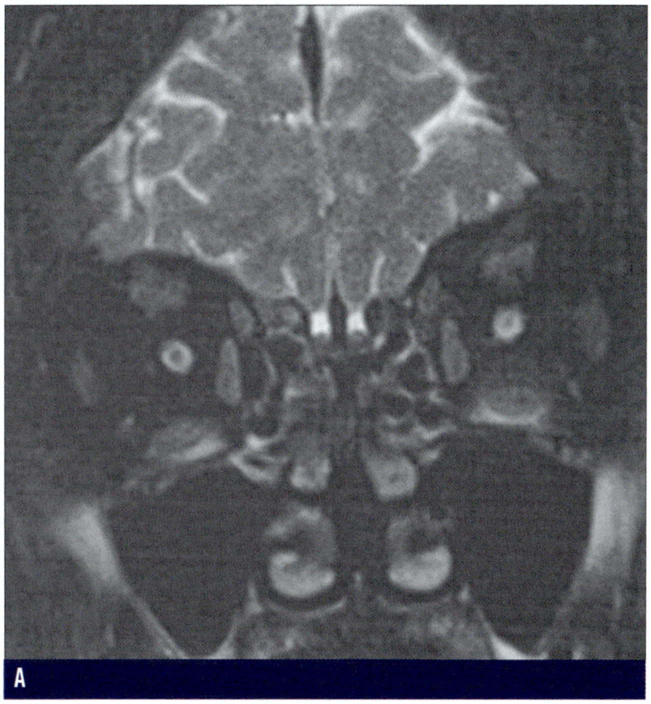

A coronal T2 fat-suppressed MR image (**A**) demonstrates left optic nerve atrophy, measuring significantly less than 3 mm in diameter. There is also likely mild right optic nerve atrophy. While the optic nerve sheaths appear enlarged, this is related to optic nerve atrophy rather than an overabundance of CSF within the optic nerve sheaths.

Companion case: Optic nerve sheath meningioma

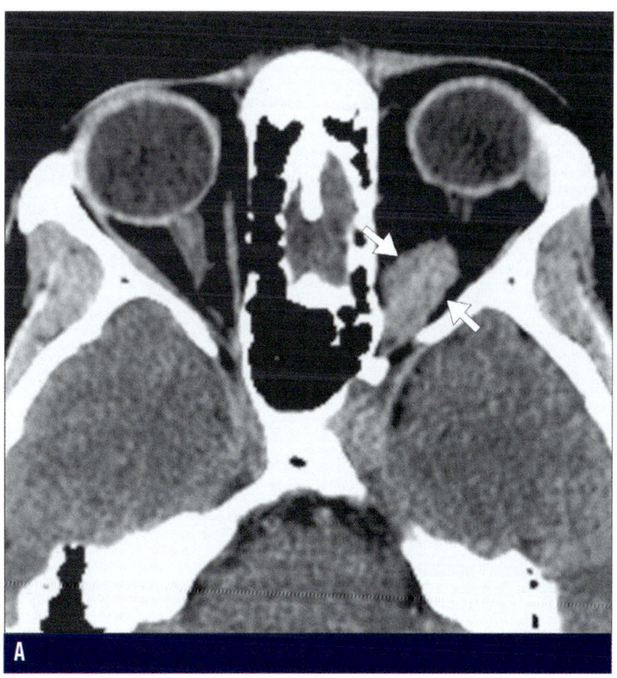

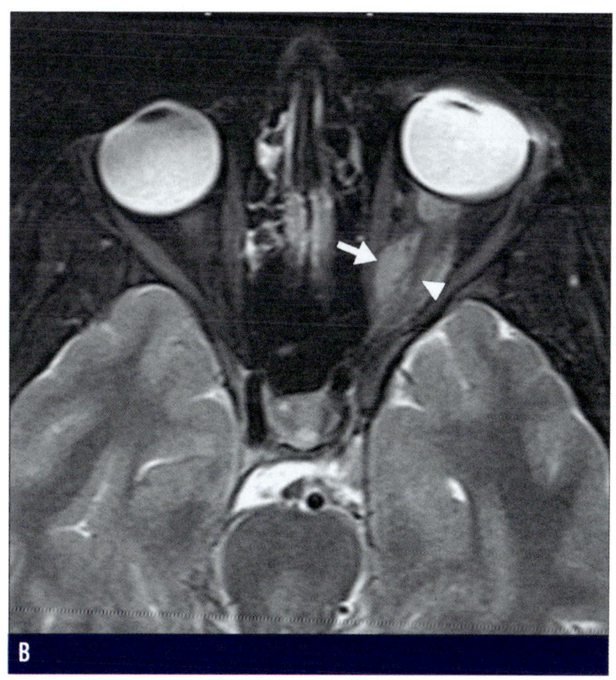

An axial CT image (**A**) demonstrate a relatively isodense mass along the posterior two-thirds of the intraconal left orbital nerve, extending toward the orbital apex (arrows, **A**). Axial T2 with fat suppression (**B**), axial T1 (**C**), and postcontrast axial and coronal T1 with fat suppression (**D**, **E**, respectively) MR images demonstrate the same mass (arrows, **B-E**) which circumferentially surrounds the left optic nerve (arrowheads, **B**, **D**, **E**). The mass is T1 isointense and T2 hyperintense when compared to the extraocular muscles, and it enhances avidly. The imaging findings are consistent with an optic nerve sheath meningioma.

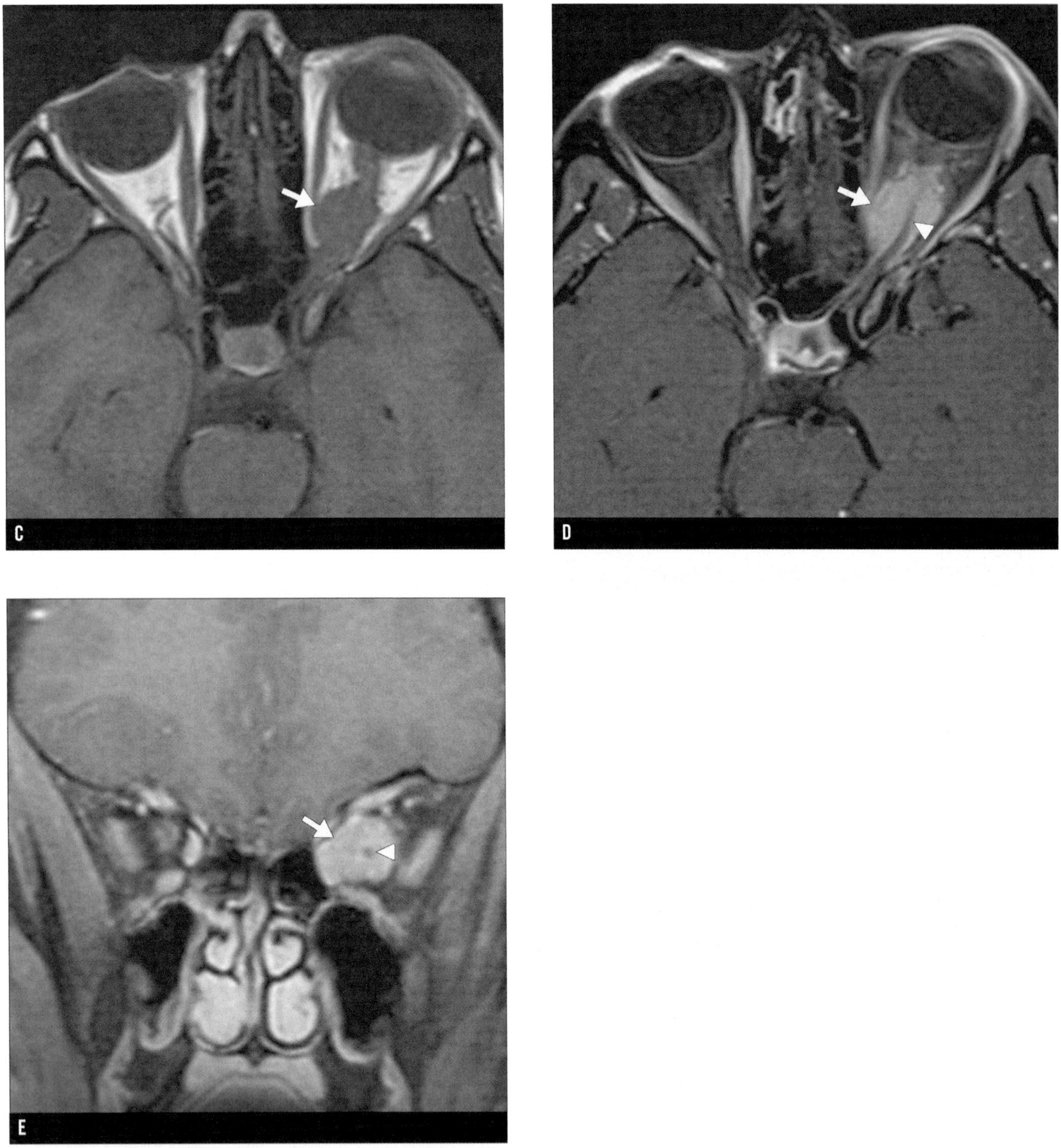
C
D
E

Companion case: Optic nerve sheath hemorrhage

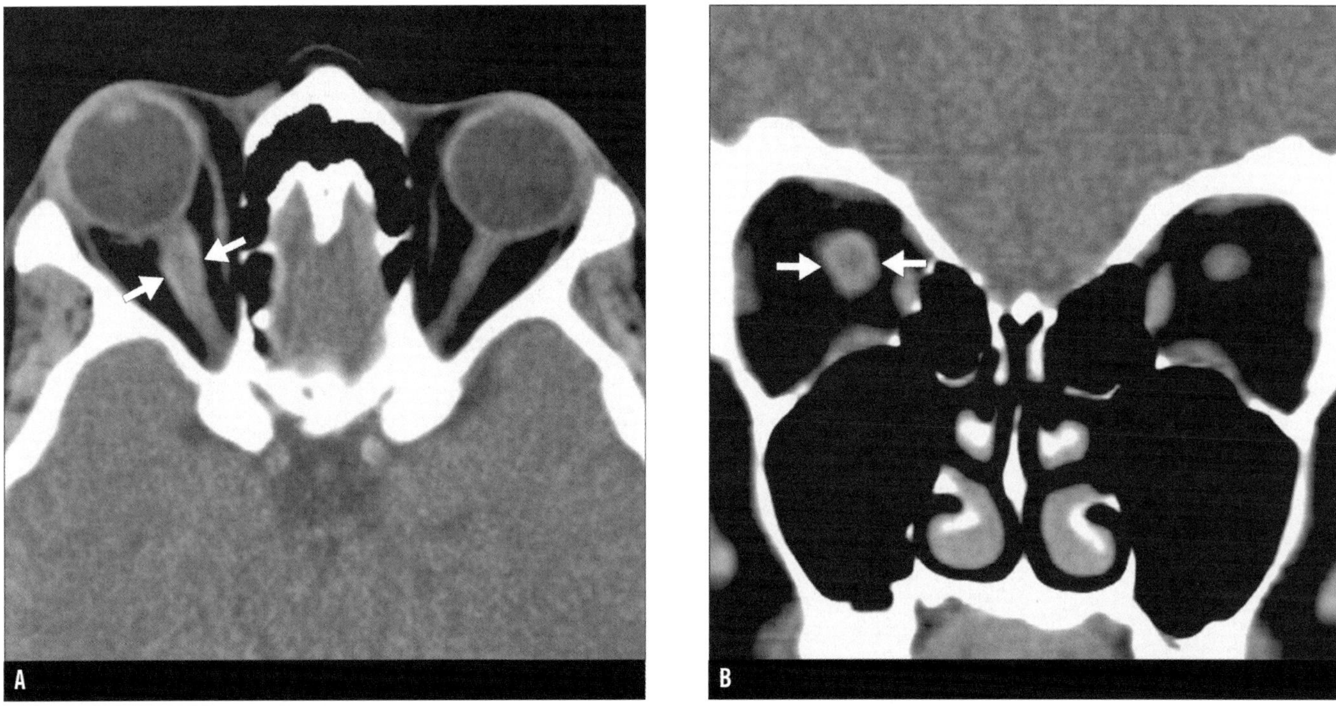

Axial (**A**) and coronal reformatted (**B**) unenhanced CT images demonstrate abnormal circumferential hyperdensity within an expanded right optic nerve sheath and surrounding the intraorbital portion of the right optic nerve (arrows, **A**, **B**). The findings are consistent with blood products within the right optic nerve sheath. Mild right proptosis is also present. One day prior to this study, the patient had undergone a right trabeculectomy with retrobulbar anesthetic injection for treatment of glaucoma. The anesthetic was presumably inadvertently injected into the right optic nerve sheath resulting in the hemorrhage.

REFERENCES

Agid R, Farb RI, Willinsky RA, Mikulis DJ, Tomlinson G. Idiopathic intracranial hypertension: the validity of cross-sectional neuroimaging signs. *Neuroradiology.* 2006;48(8):521-527. Epub May 2006.

Dural Jungkim S, Khurshid SG, Fenton S. Ectasia of the optic nerve sheath. *Acta Ophthalmol Scand.* 2005;83(2):266-267.

Garrity JA, Trautman JC, Bartley GB, et al. Optic nerve sheath meningoceles: Clinical and radiographic features in 13 cases with a review of the literature. *Ophthalmology.* 1990;97:1519-1531.

Gauntt CD, Sherry RG, Kannan C. Terson syndrome with bilateral optic nerve sheath hemorrhage. *J Neuroophthalmol.* 2007;27(3):193-194.

Geeraerts T, et al. Use of T2-weighted magnetic resonance imaging of the optic nerve sheath to detect raised intracranial pressure. *Crit Care.* 2008;12(5):R114. Epub September 2008.

Karim S, Clark RA, Poukens V, Demer JL. Demonstration of systematic variation in human intraorbital optic nerve size by quantitative magnetic resonance imaging and histology. *Invest Ophthalmol Vis Sci.* 2004;45(4):1047-1051.

Lagrèze WA, et al. Retrobulbar optic nerve diameter measured by high-speed magnetic resonance imaging as a biomarker for axonal loss in glaucomatous optic atrophy. *Invest Ophthalmol Vis Sci.* 2009;50(9):4223-4228. doi: 10.1167/iovs.08-2683. Epub April 2009.

Mesa-Gutiérrez JC, Quiñones SM, Ginebreda JA. Optic nerve sheath meningocele. *Clin Ophthalmol.* 2008;2(3):661-668.

Mashima Y, Oshitari K, Imamura Y, Momoshima S, Shiga H, Oguchi Y. High-resolution magnetic resonance imaging of the intraorbital optic nerve and subarachnoid space in patients with papilledema and optic atrophy. *Arch Ophthalmol.* 1996;114(10):1197-1203.

Muller PJ, Deck JH. Intraocular and optic nerve sheath hemorrhage in cases of sudden intracranial hypertension. *J Neurosurg.* 1974;41(2):160-166.

Ortiz O, Schochet SS, Kotzan JM, Kostick D. Radiologic-pathologic correlation: meningioma of the optic nerve sheath. *AJNR Am J Neuroradiol.* 1996;17(5):901-906.

Parravano JG, Toledo A, Kucharczyk W. Dimensions of the optic nerves, chiasm, and tracts: MR quantitative comparison between patients with optic atrophy and normals. *J Comput Assist Tomogr.* 1993;17(5):688-690.

Pautler SE, Grizzard WS, Thompson LN, Wing GL.Blindness from retrobulbar injection into the optic nerve. *Ophthalmic Surg.* 1986;17(6):334-337.

Saeed P, Rootman J, Nugent RA, White VA, Mackenzie IR, Koornneef L. Optic nerve sheath meningiomas. *Ophthalmology.* 2003;110(10):2019-2030.

Shoftya B, Ben-Sirab L, Constantinia S, Freedmana S, Keslerc A. Optic nerve sheath diameter on MR imaging: establishment of norms and comparison of pediatric patients with idiopathic intracranial hypertension with healthy controls. *AJNR Am J Neuroradiol.* 2012;33:366-369.

Som PM and Curtin HD. *Head and Neck Imaging.* 4th ed. St. Louis, MO: Mosby Inc; 2003.

Watanabe A, Kinouchi H, Horikoshi T, Uchida M, Ishigame K. Effect of intracranial pressure on the diameter of the optic nerve sheath. *J Neurosurg.* 2008;109(2):255-258.

Whiteley W, Al-Shahi R, Warlow CP, Zeidler M, Lueck CJ.CSF opening pressure: reference interval and the effect of body mass index. *Neurology.* 2006;67(9):1690-1691.

Wolf AL, Alexander L, Matthias W, Hans-Christian H , Jürgen H, Thorsten AB. Morphometry of the retrobulbar human optic nerve: comparison between conventional sonography and ultrafast magnetic resonance sequences invest. Ophthalmol Vis Sci. 2007;48(5):1913-1917.

CASE 11 Optic nerve sheath tortuosity

The intraorbital segment of the optic nerve is approximately 25 mm in length, whereas the distance from the posterior margin of the globe to the orbital apex is less than 20 mm. The excess length of the optic nerve allows the globe to move freely and accounts for its sometimes sinuous appearance on imaging. It is thought that up to 9 mm of globe proptosis can occur before the optic nerve begins to cause traction on the globe.

It is worth noting that in children with neurofibromatosis type 1, marked optic nerve tortuosity without enhancement may presage the eventual development of an optic glioma. Consequently, close follow-up of these patients is warranted.

COMPANION CASES

- **Marked optic nerve sheath complex tortuosity and distortion due to birth trauma.** Several traumatic orbital complications may occur during a forceps delivery including corneal edema, lid edema, seventh cranial nerve palsy, hyphema, choroidal rupture, and optic nerve damage. These complications often coexist with orbital fractures. In the absence of an orbital fracture, these complications likely occur because of sudden traumatic rotation of the globe during a forceps delivery.
- **Optic pathway glioma.** An optic pathway glioma (OPG) in childhood is a WHO grade I juvenile pilocytic astrocytoma that often occurs in the setting of neurofibromatosis type I. The adult form of an OPG are often more aggressive clinically and by imaging than the juvenile form. When it affects the optic nerve, the juvenile form of an OPG is characterized by fusiform enlargement of the nerve, sometimes with exaggerated tortuosity. On MRI, the tumor is iso- to slightly hypointense on T1-weighted images and slightly hyperintense on T2-weighted images. Enhancement is variable and depends on tumor histology.

Optic nerve sheath tortuosity

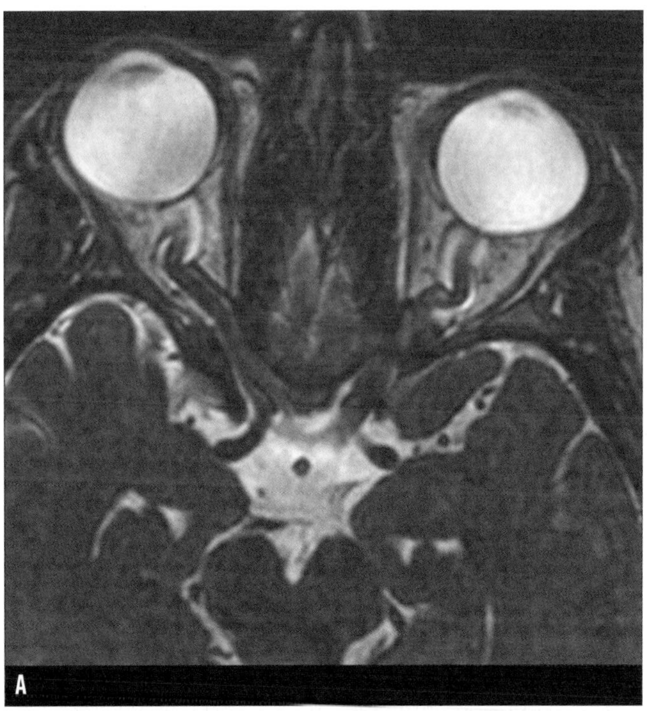

An axial CISS MR image (**A**) demonstrates a pronounced sinuous appearance of the optic nerve sheath complexes. This tortuosity is a normal finding.

Optic nerve sheath tortuosity

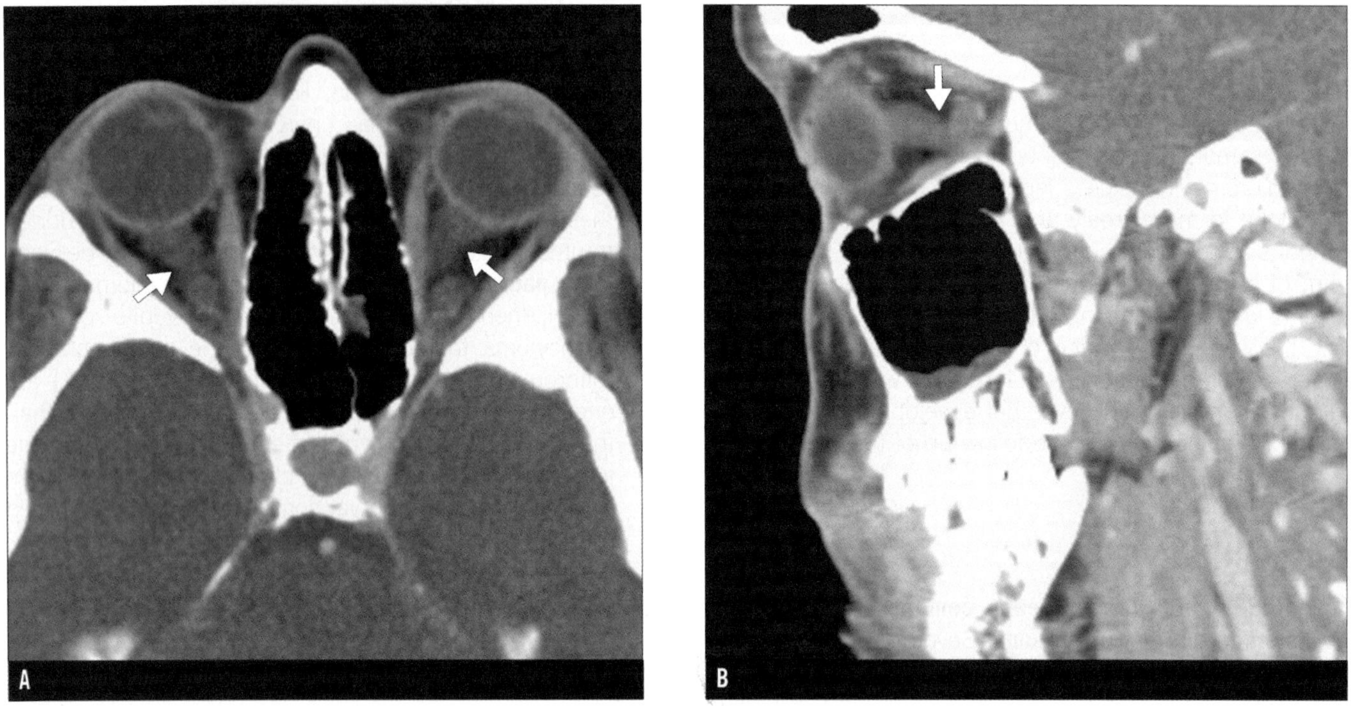

Different patient. Axial (**A**) and reformatted (**B**) contrast-enhanced CT images demonstrate normal redundancy of the optic nerve sheath complexes (arrows, **A**, **B**).

Companion case: Marked optic nerve sheath complex tortuosity and distortion due to birth trauma

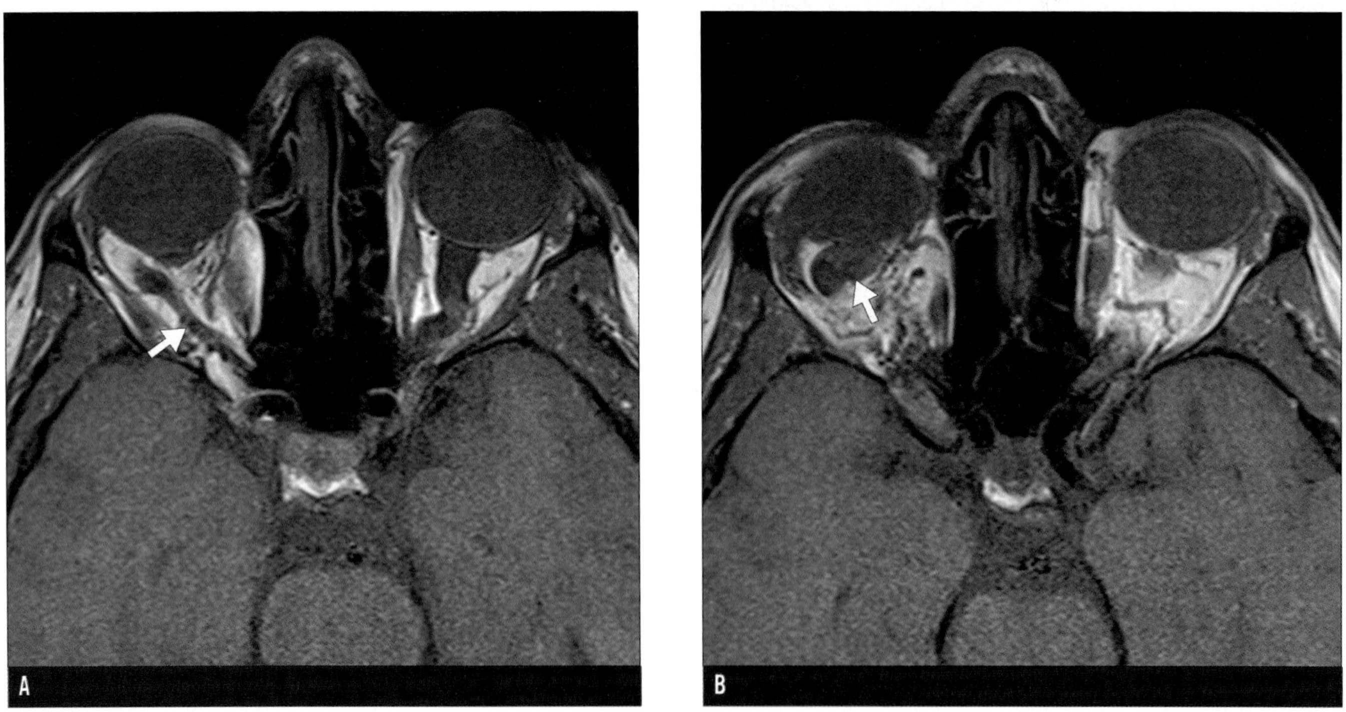

Axial T1 (**A**, **B**), coronal T1 (**C**), and coronal T2 with fat suppression (**D**) MR images demonstrate marked tortuosity and distortion of the right optic nerve and its surrounding sheath (arrows, **A-D**). There is also pronounced distortion of several right extraocular muscles in this patient with right orbit birth trauma.

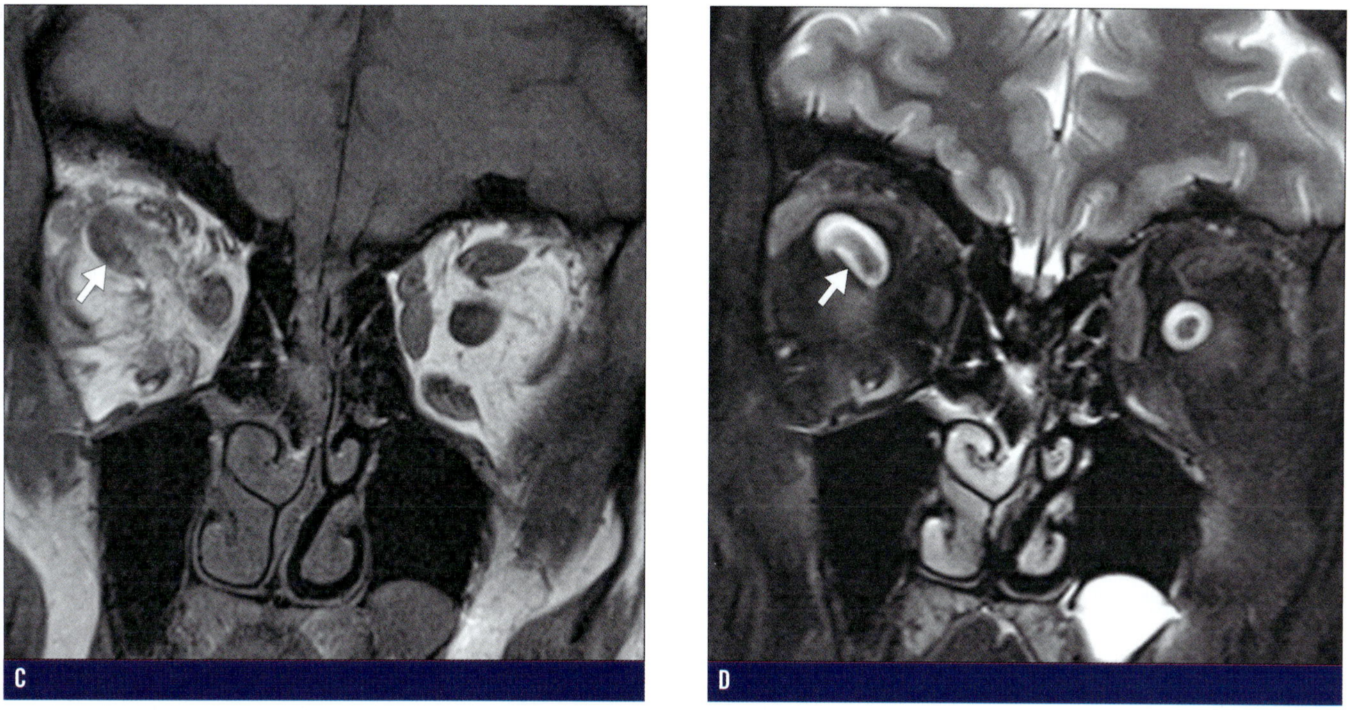

Companion case: Optic pathway glioma

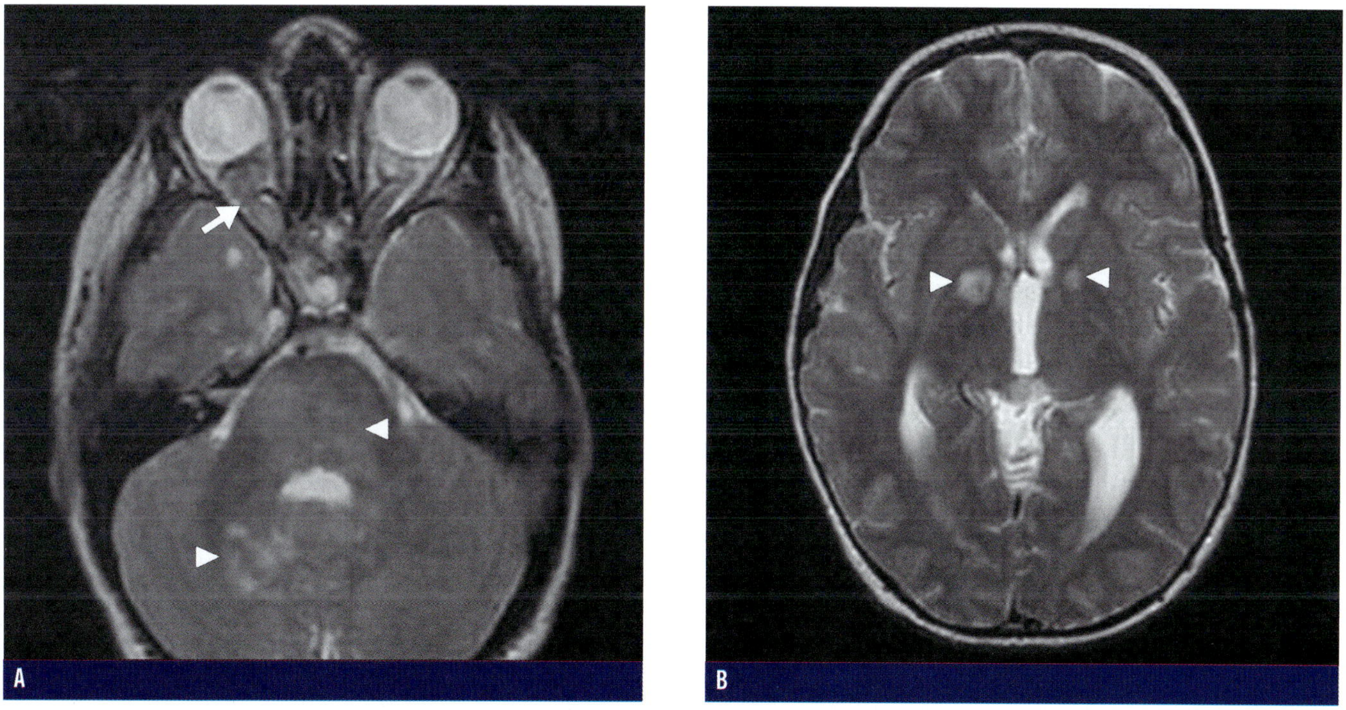

An axial T2-weighted MR image (**A**) demonstrates redundancy of the optic nerves and thickening of the right optic nerve (arrow, **A**). Several scattered focal areas of T2 prolongation are present in the posterior fossa (arrowheads, **A**). Another axial T2-weighted image (**B**) more cephalad (**B**) demonstrates foci of T2 prolongation in the bilateral basal ganglia (arrowheads, **B**). The foci of T2 prolongation are compatible with neurofibromatosis "spots." Given the clinical scenario, the right optic nerve finding likely represents an optic glioma.

REFERENCES

Armstrong GT, et al. Defining optic nerve tortuosity. *AJNR Am J Neuroradiol.* 2007;28(4):666-671.

Chung EM, Smirniotopoulos JG, Specht CS, Schroeder JW, Cube R. From the archives of the AFIP: pediatric orbit tumors and tumorlike lesions: nonosseous lesions of the extraocular orbit. *Radiographics.* 2007;27(6):1777-1799.

Glazer JS. *Neuro-Ophthalmology.* 3rd ed. Philadelphia, PA: Lippincott Williams & Wilkins; 1999: 77-79.

Khalil SK, Urso RG, Mintz-Hittner HA. Traumatic optic nerve injury occurring after forceps delivery of a term newborn. *J AAPOS.* 2003;7(2):146-147.

Millar WS, Tartaglino LM, Sergott RC, Friedman DP, Flanders AE. MR of malignant optic glioma of adulthood. *AJNR Am J Neuroradiol.* 1995;16(8):1673-1676.

Miller NR, Newman NJ, Biousse V, Kerrison JB. *Walsh & Hoyt's Clinical Neuro-Ophthalmology: The Essentials.* 6th ed. Philadelphia, PA: Lippincott Williams & Wilkins; 2005: 27-28.

Unsöld R, DeGroot J, Newton TH. Images of the optic nerve: anatomic-CT correlation. *AJR Am J Roentgenol.* 1980;135:767-773.

CASE 12 Pseudofractures of the orbit

Normal structures of the osseous orbit occasionally can be mistaken for acute fractures in the setting of trauma. Familiarity with these normal structures can prevent misdiagnosis.

- **Supraorbital foramen**. This foramen is located at or near the midline of the superior orbital rim and transmits the supraorbital artery and nerve (V1 division of CN V).
- **Infraorbital canal and foramen**. The canal typically traverses the floor of the orbit, although variations exist, including the distal portion traversing within the anterosuperior aspect of the maxillary sinus lumen or traversing along the posterolateral wall of the maxillary sinus (further discussed in Chapter 6). The infraorbital foramen is located near the midline of the inferior orbital rim. Both structures transmit the infraorbital artery and nerve (V2 division of CN V). A fracture of the orbital floor and/or rim often results in disruption of the infraorbital canal and/or foramen and paresthesias of the midface.

Companion case: **Infraorbital canal fracture.**

- **Sphenofrontal (also called frontosphenoid) suture**. Often demonstrated on CT along the superolateral aspect of osseous orbit, this suture attaches the posterior margin of the frontal bone orbital plates with the ventral margin of the lesser wings of the sphenoid bone.
- **Sphenozygomatic (also called zygomaticosphenoid) suture**. This suture is located along the mid-lateral wall of osseous orbit and attaches the lateral portion of the greater wing of the sphenoid bone to the posteromedial margin of the zygomatic bone. Buckling of this suture may occur following trauma.

Companion case: **Sphenozygomatic suture buckle fracture and sutural diastasis.**

- **Zygomaticofrontal (also called frontozygomatic) suture**. This suture is located along the superolateral wall of the osseous orbit and attaches the frontal process of the zygoma with the zygomatic process of the frontal bone. This suture may become diastatic following trauma. Comparison with the contralateral counterpart is often necessary to identify a subtle diastasis of this suture.

Companion case: **Zygomaticofrontal suture diastasis.**

- **Zygomaticofacial foramen**. This foramen is a small aperture located along the mid malar aspect of the zygomatic body and transmits the zygomaticofacial vessels and nerve. The zygomaticofacial nerve is one of two branches that arise from the zygomatic nerve (itself a branch of the V2 division of CN V), with the other branch being the zygomaticotemporal nerve. The zygomaticofacial nerve supplies sensory innervation to the ipsilateral cheek.
- **Duplicated zygomaticofacial foramen.** Occasionally, there are duplicated foramen visualized along the mid zygomatic body, one transmitting the vessels and the other transmitting the nerve.
- **Zygomaticotemporal foramen**. This foramen resides within the frontal process of the zygomatic bone, approximately 1 cm caudal to the frontozygomatic suture. The zygomaticotemporal nerve courses through this foramen and supplies a patch of skin measuring approximately 3 cm in diameter along the ipsilateral forehead and temple region. As stated above, the zygomaticotemporal nerve is one of the two branches that arise from the zygomatic nerve.
- **Anterior and posterior ethmoidal canals**. The anterior ethmoidal artery (AEA) typically arises from the distal one-third of the intraorbital ophthalmic artery. The AEA exits the orbit via the anterior ethmoidal foramen and then the anterior ethmoidal canal, the latter representing medially directed, pyramidal-shaped notch located along the superior aspect of the lamina papyracea. The anterior ethmoidal canal serves as a surgical landmark and demarcates the posterior edge of the frontal recess. An anterior ethmoidal canal may sometimes simulate a lamina papyracea fracture, although this can usually be differentiated from a fracture by its typical morphology and location. From the anterior ethmoidal canal, the AEA may directly enter the skull base, or it may first traverse the ethmoid labyrinth prior to entering the skull base. The AEA may or may not be surrounded by bone if it traverses the ethmoid labyrinth, with the latter scenario rendering it more vulnerable to surgical injury.

  The posterior ethmoidal artery (PEA) has a more variable origin. While the PEA typically arises from the proximal one-third of the intraorbital ophthalmic artery, it may also arise from the anterior ethmoidal artery or from the middle meningeal artery. The PEA exits the orbit via the posterior ethmoidal foramen and continues into the posterior ethmoidal canal, both of which are located posterior to the anterior ethmoidal foramen/canal and a few millimeters anterior to the sphenoid sinus. From there, the PEA enters the skull base. The PEA is encased by bone and is therefore less prone to surgical trauma.

Companion case: **Inadvertent anterior ethmoidal artery surgical laceration.**

The AEA and the anterior ethmoidal canal are avoided during functional endoscopic sinus surgery (FESS) in order to prevent injury to the AEA. However, identification of the AEA and/or anterior ethmoidal canal may be difficult during FESS if they are obscured by polyps or a mass. If breached near its exit from the anterior ethoidal canal, the AEA can retract intraorbitally and result in uncontrolled superomedial extraconal orbital hemorrhage with associated proptosis, elevated intraorbital pressure, lid edema, and vision loss. In addition, injury to the AEA may occur following trauma to the lamina papyracea as well as during orbital surgery, including to repair a lamina papyracea fracture, as in the case provided.

Supraorbital foramen

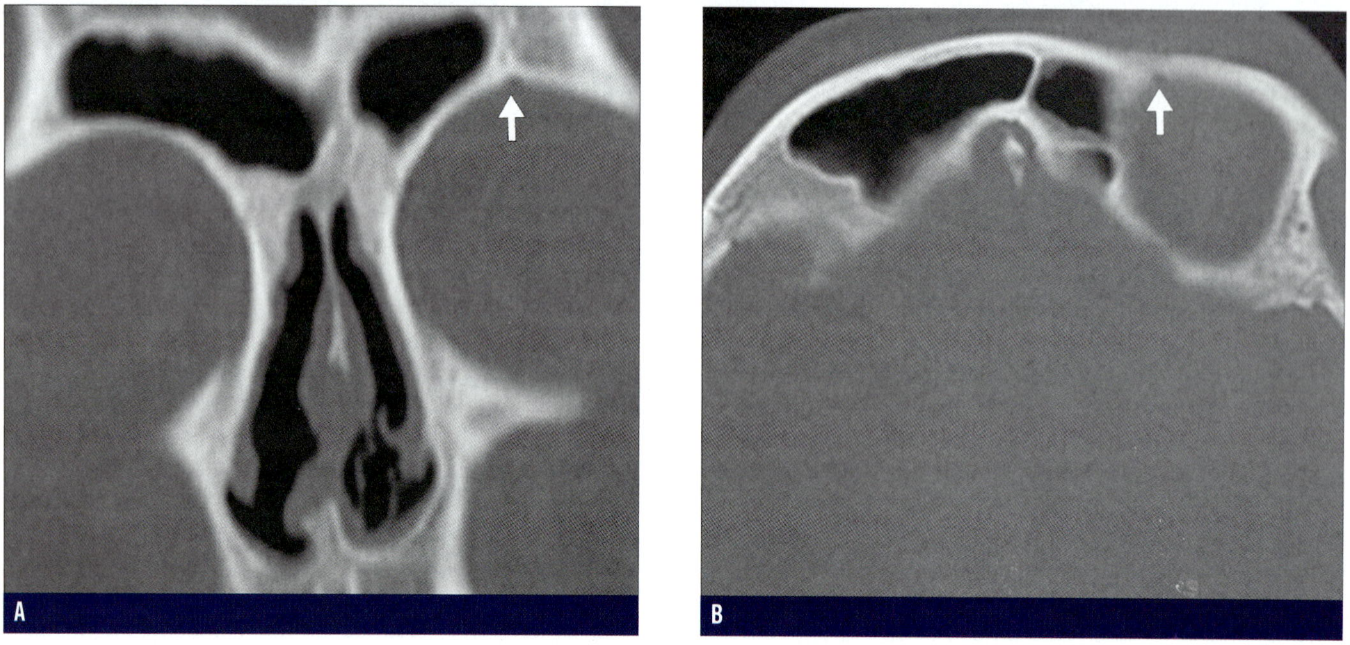

Coronal reformatted (**A**) and axial (**B**) CT images demonstrate a normal left supraorbital foramen (arrows, **A**, **B**).

Infraorbital canal and foramen

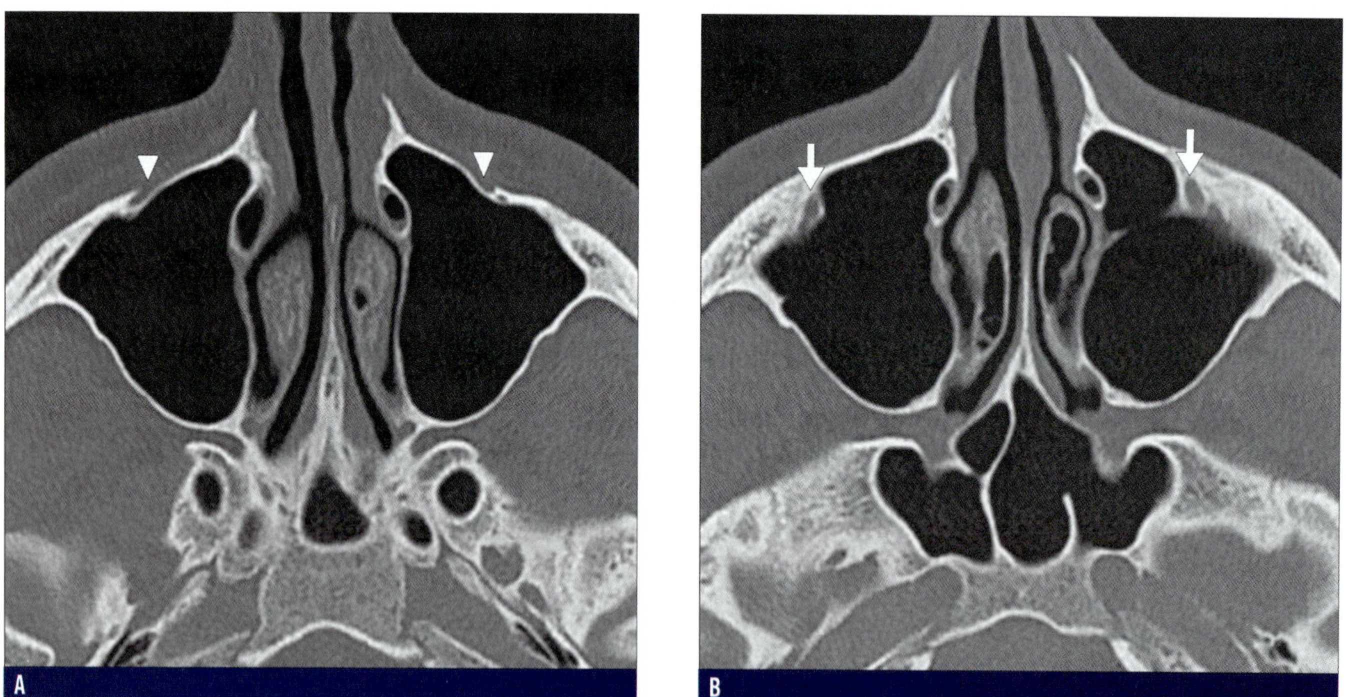

Axial (**A**, **B**), coronal reformatted (**C**, **D**), and sagittal reformatted (**E**, **F**) CT images demonstrate the normal infraorbital foramina (arrowheads, **A**, **C**, **E**) and the normal infraorbital canals (arrows, **B**, **D**, **F**).

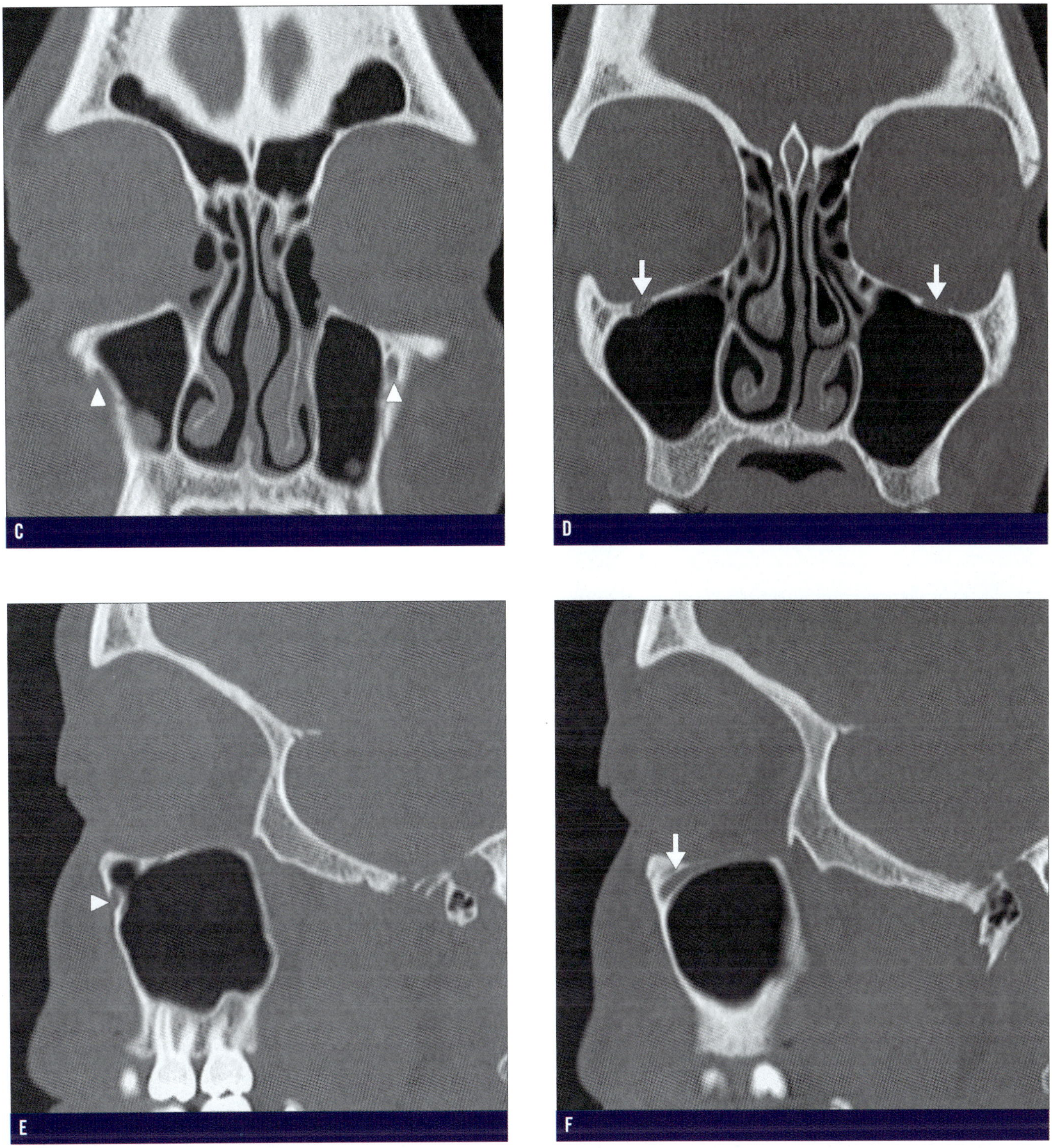
C
D
E
F

Companion case: Infraorbital canal fracture

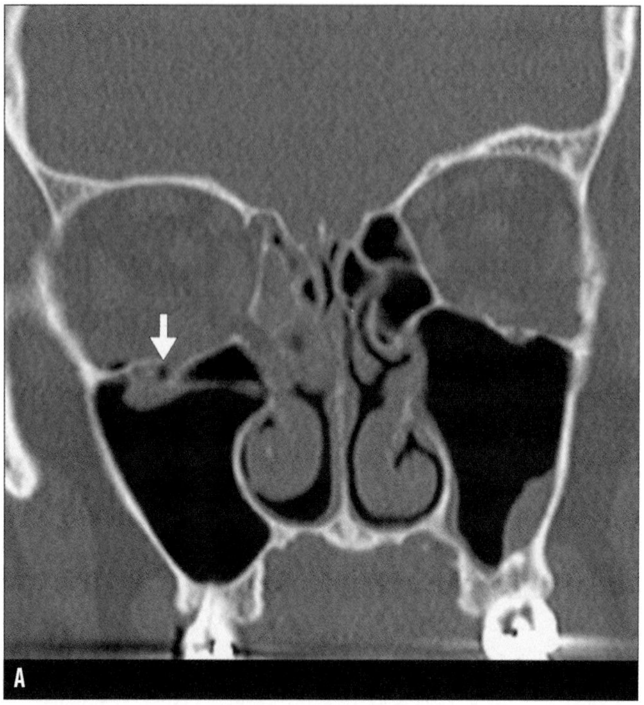

A coronal reformatted CT image (**A**) demonstrates a fracture through the right infraorbital canal associated with a small focus of air (arrow). Air within or adjacent to the infraorbital canal is often a helpful clue alerting one to the presence of a fracture. Correlation for V2 symptomatology is indicated when a fracture involving the infraorbital canal or foramen is encountered.

Sphenofrontal (also called frontosphenoid) suture

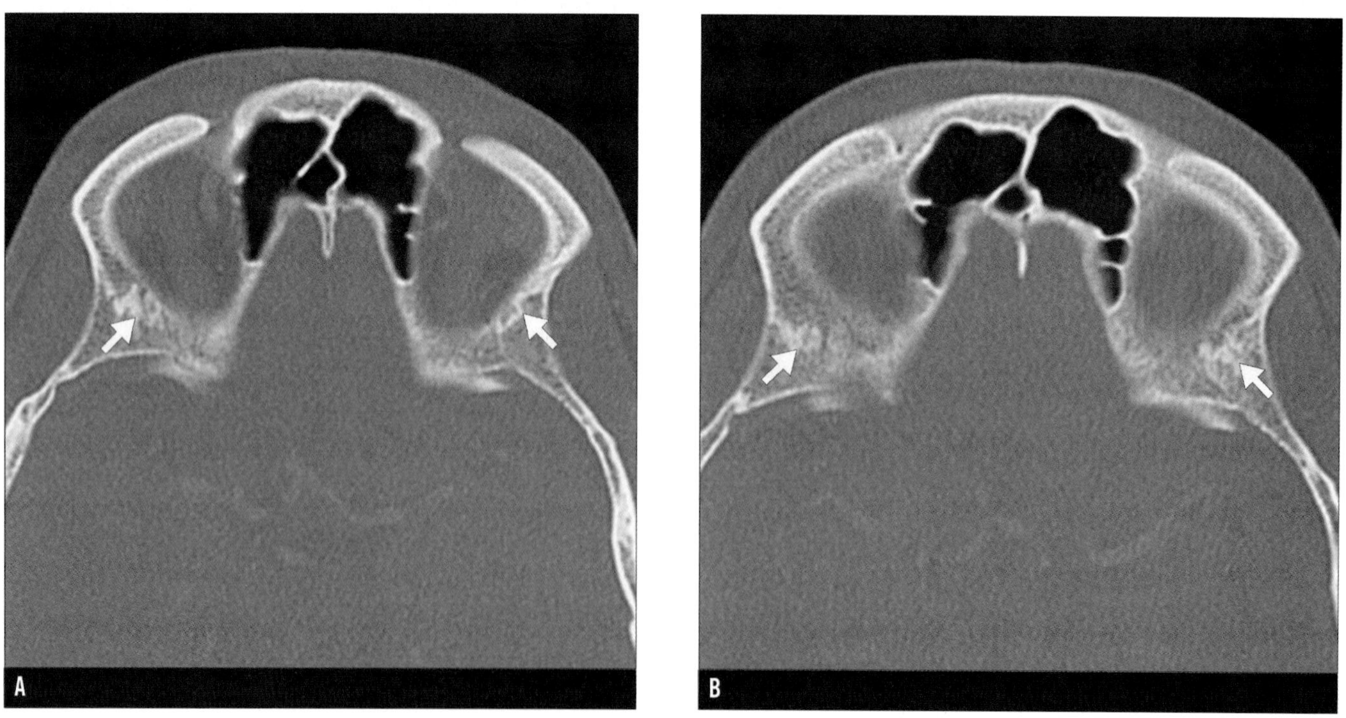

Axial CT images (**A**, **B**) demonstrate normal sphenofrontal sutures (arrows, **A**, **B**).

Sphenozygomatic (also called zygomaticosphenoid) suture

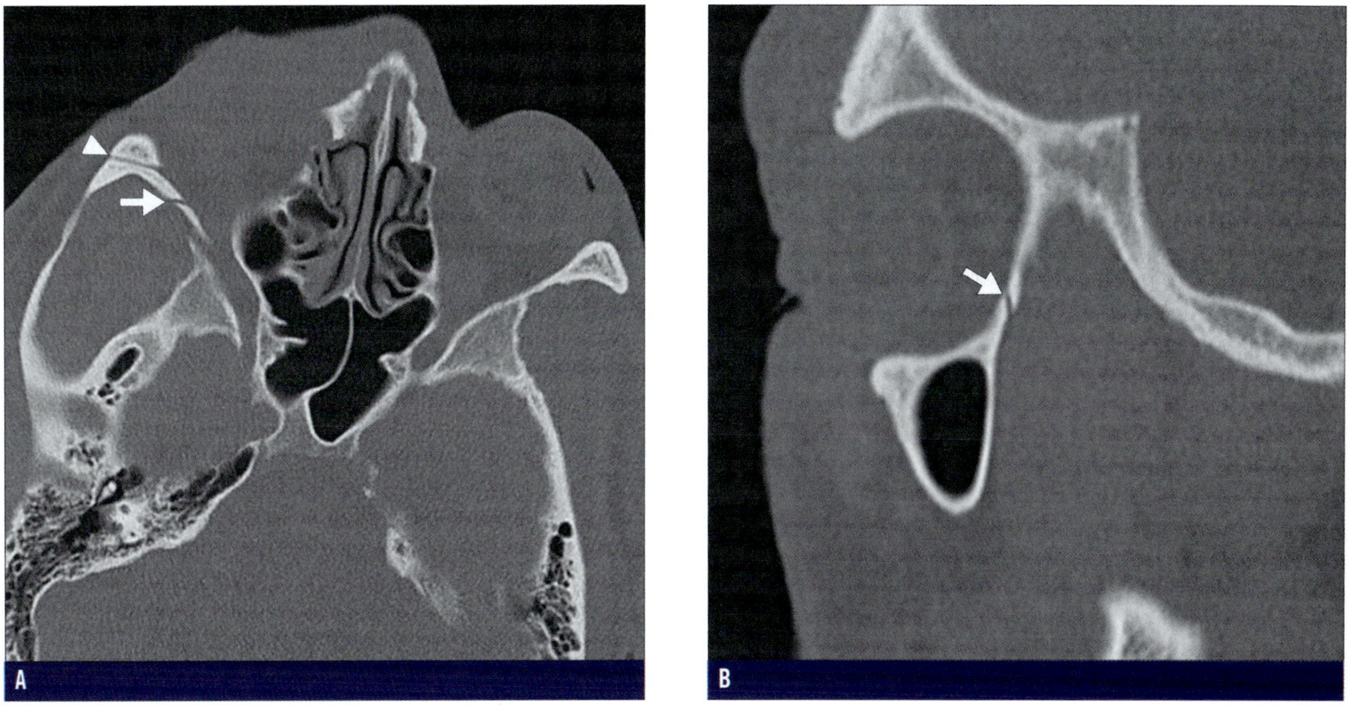

Axial (**A**) and sagittal reformatted (**B**) CT images demonstrate a normal right sphenozygomatic suture (arrows, **A**, **B**). This particular sphenozygomatic suture has distinct, nonsclerotic margins, simulating a fracture. A normal right zygomaticofacial foramen is also identified (arrowhead, **A**).

Sphenozygomatic (also called zygomaticosphenoid) suture

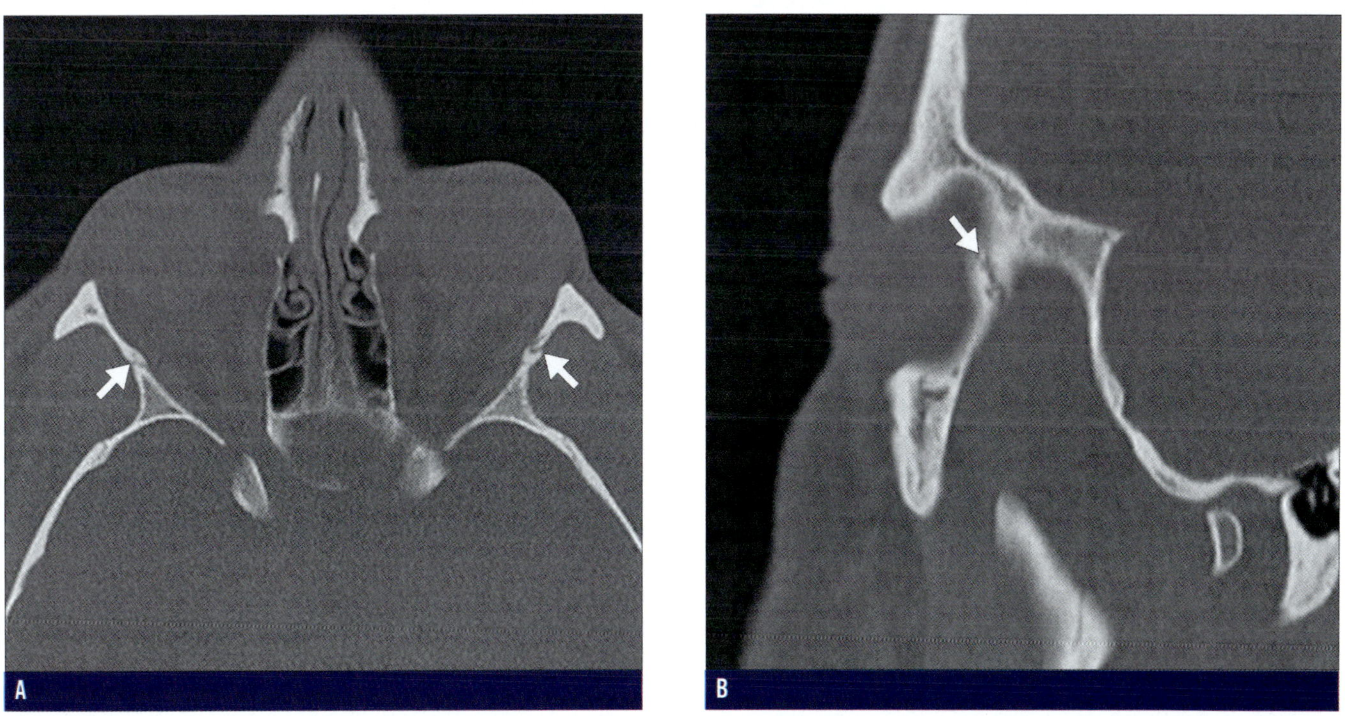

Different patient. Axial (**A**) and sagittal reformatted (**B**) CT images demonstrate normal sphenozygomatic sutures (arrows, **A**, **B**). In this patient, these sutures have sclerotic margins, typical of a suture.

Companion case: Sphenozygomatic suture buckle fracture and sutural diastasis

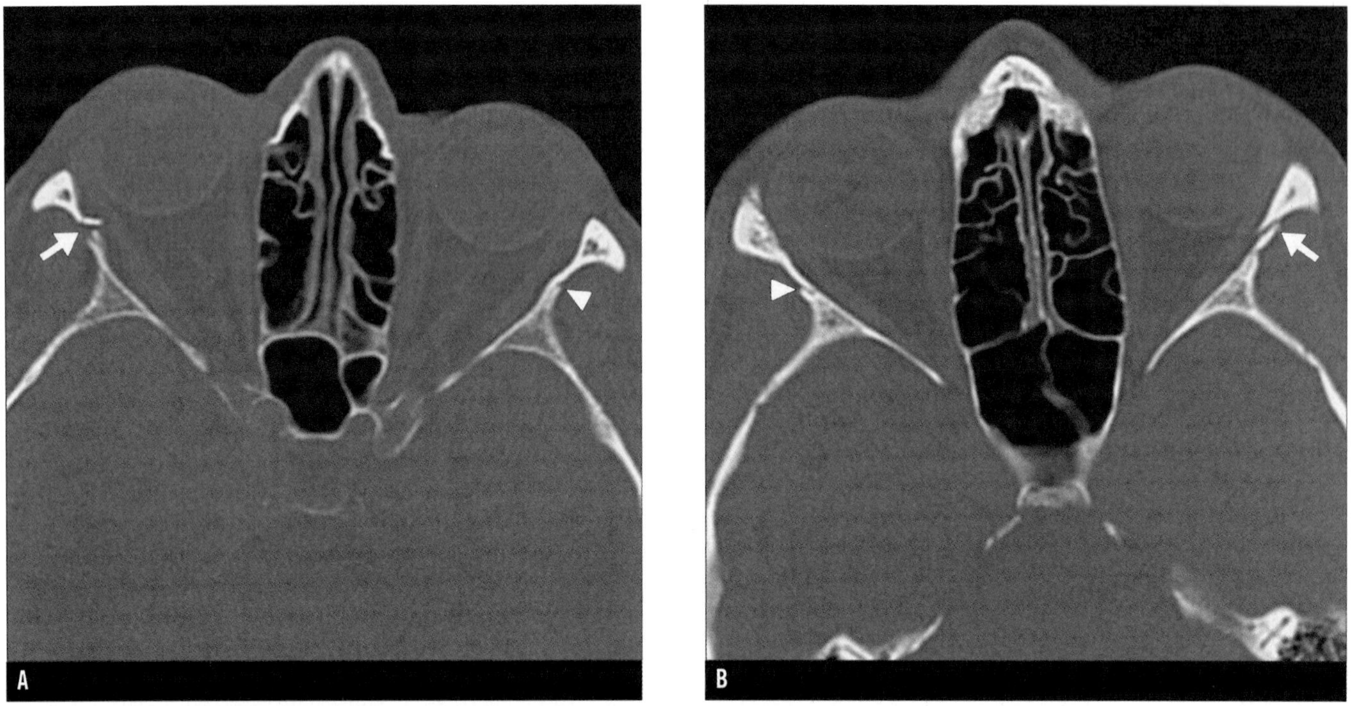

An axial CT image (**A**) demonstrates an acute fracture with buckling of the right sphenozygomatic suture (arrow, **A**). A normal left sphenozygomatic suture is present (arrowhead, **A**). An axial CT image of a different patient (**B**) demonstrates subtle diastasis of the left sphenozygomatic suture (arrow, **B**). A normal right sphenozygomatic suture is denoted for reference (arrowhead, **B**).

Zygomaticofrontal (also called frontozygomatic) suture

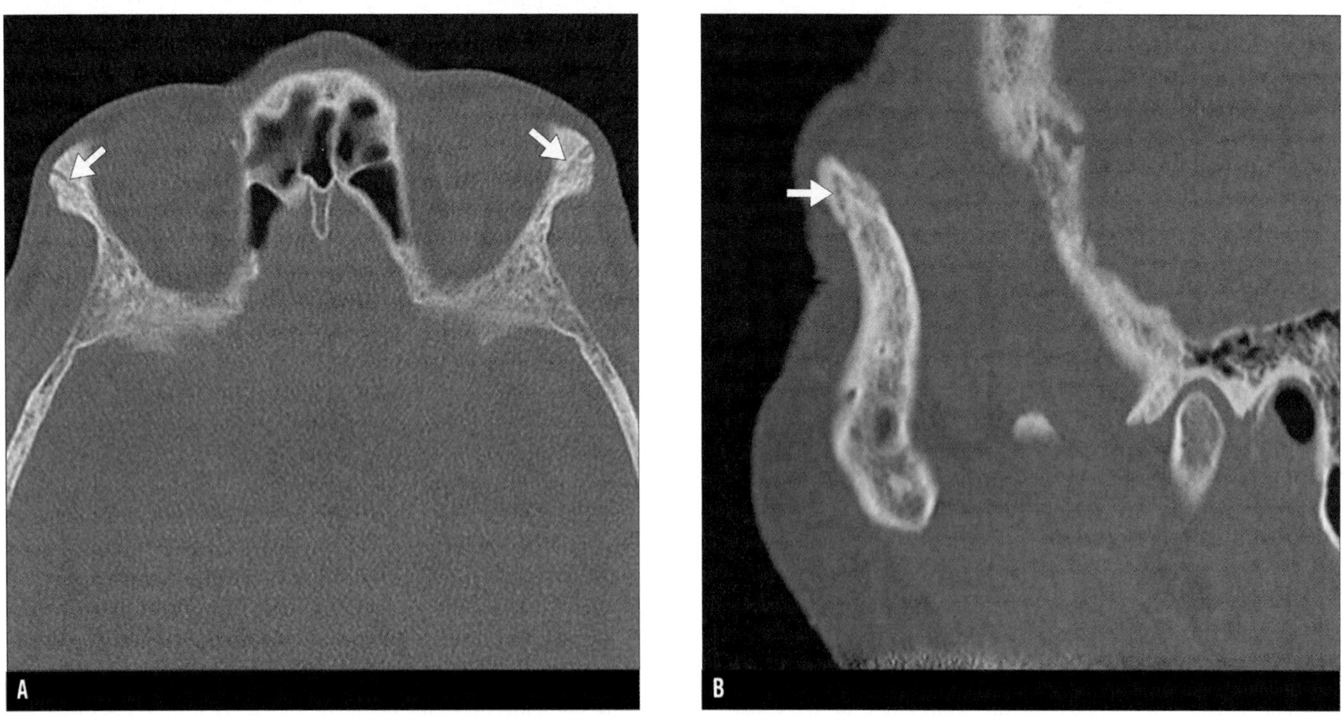

Axial (**A**), sagittal reformatted (**B**), and coronal reformatted (**C**, **D**) CT images demonstrate normal zygomaticofrontal sutures (arrows, **A**-**D**).

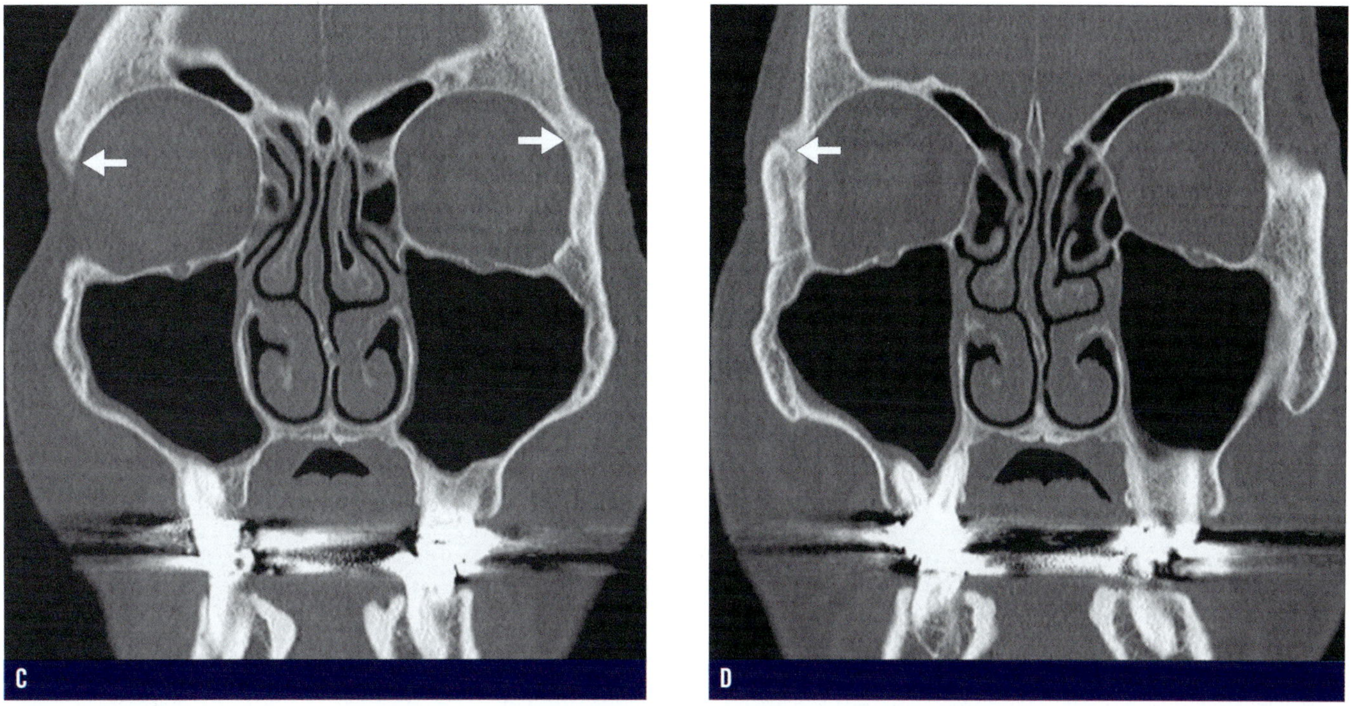

Companion case: Zygomaticofrontal suture diastasis

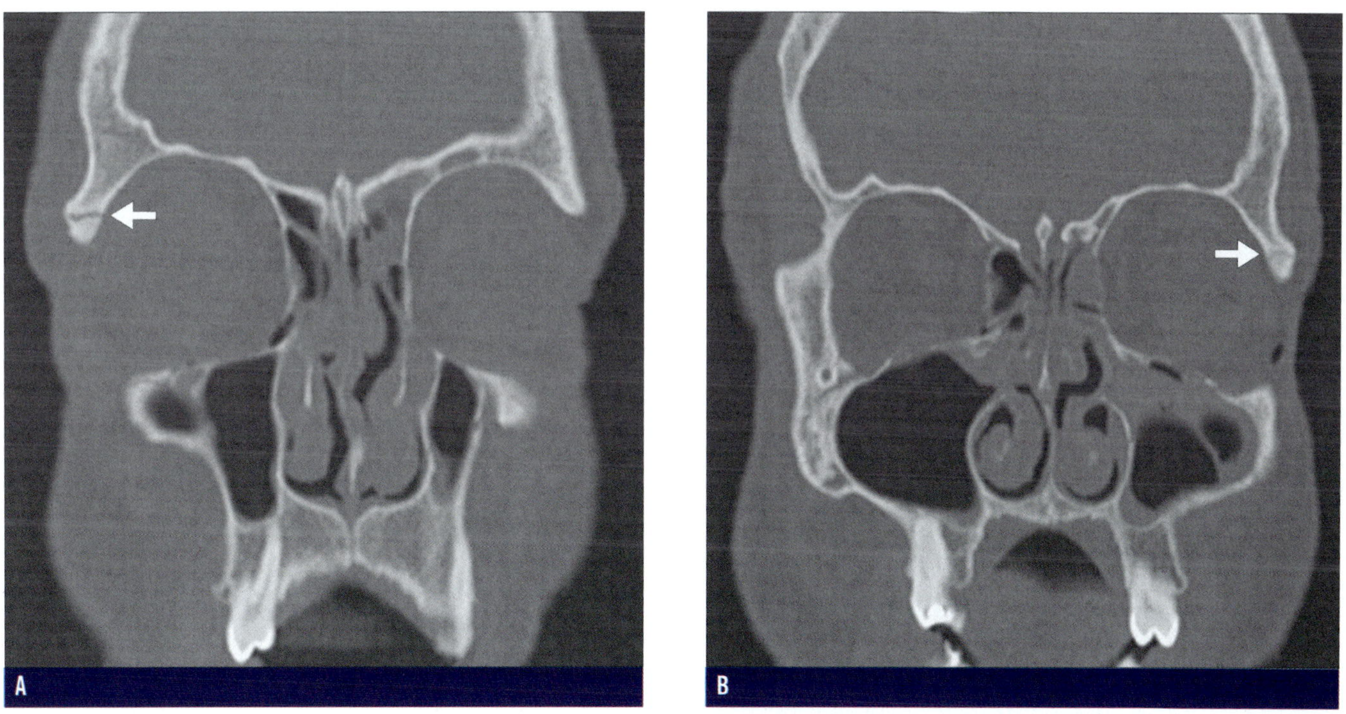

Coronal reformatted CT images through the right zygomaticofrontal suture (**A**) and left zygomaticofrontal suture (**B**) demonstrate a mild diastasis of the right zygomaticofrontal suture (arrow, **A**) and a normal left zygomaticofrontal suture (arrow, **B**). This patient had extensive right facial fractures (most of which are not shown). The presence of a mild diastasis of this suture may only be noticed if it is compared with the contralateral suture and when viewed with coronal or sagittal reformatted imaging.

Zygomaticofacial foramen

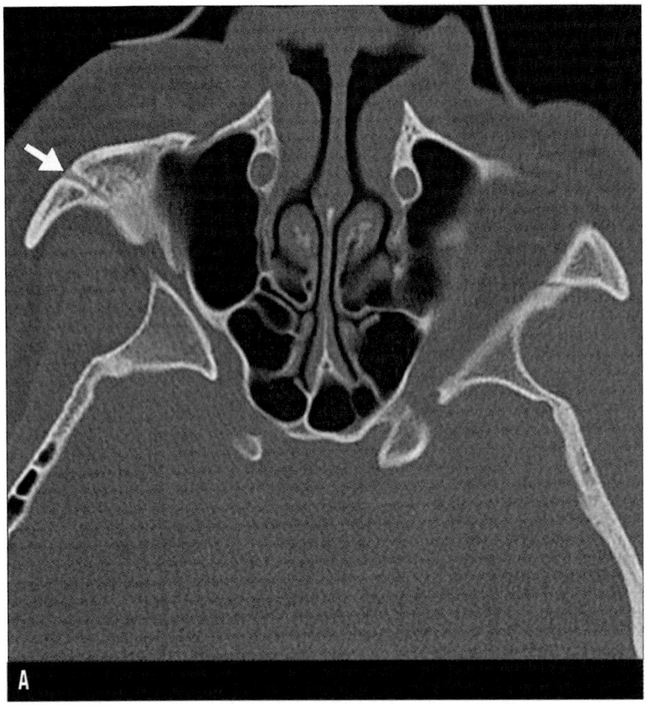

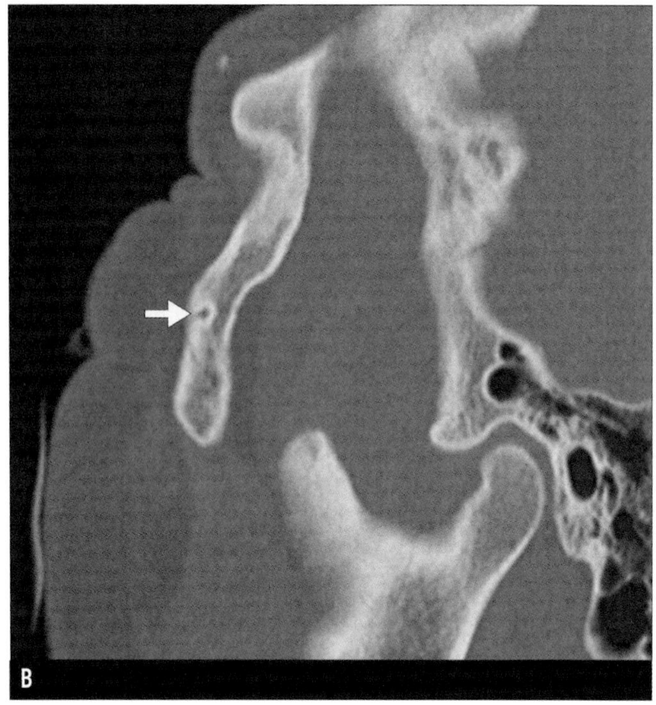

Axial (**A**) and sagittal reformatted (**B**) CT images demonstrate a normal right zygomaticofacial foramen (arrows, **A**, **B**).

Duplicated zygomaticofacial foramen

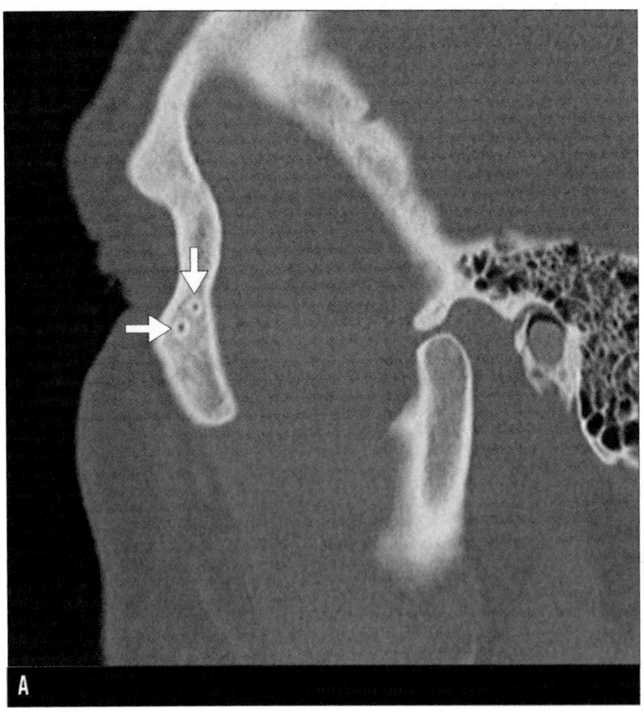

A sagittal reformatted CT image (**A**) demonstrates a duplicated zygomaticofacial foramen (arrows), one for the zygomaticofacial vessels and the other for the zygomaticofacial nerve.

Zygomaticotemporal foramen

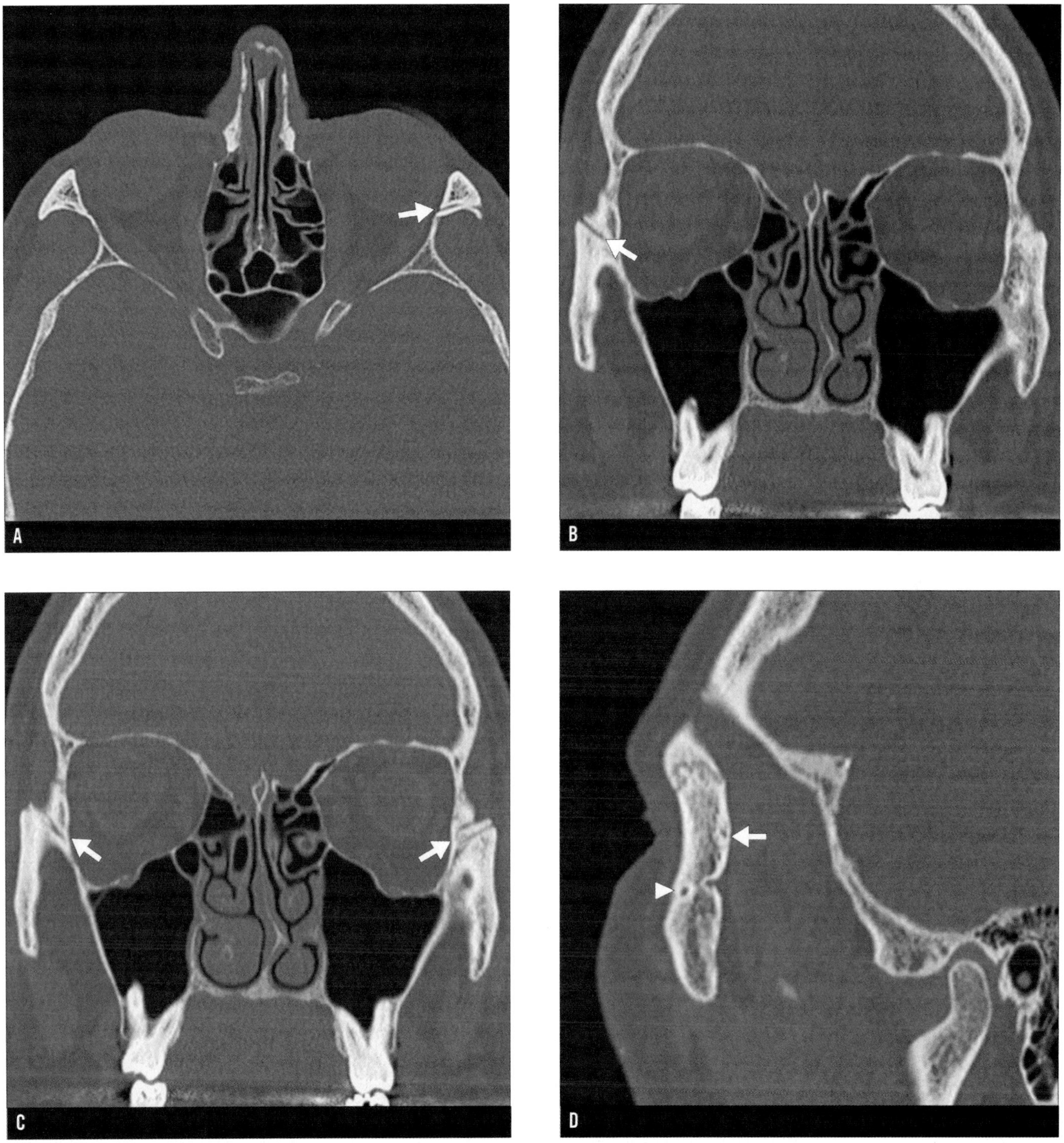

Axial (**A**), coronal reformatted (**B**, **C**), and sagittal reformatted (**D**) CT images demonstrate normal zygomaticotemporal foramina (arrows, **A**-**D**). Image **D** demonstrates the normal relationship of the zygomaticofacial foramen (arrowhead) relative to the zygomaticotemporal foramen.

Anterior and posterior ethmoidal canals

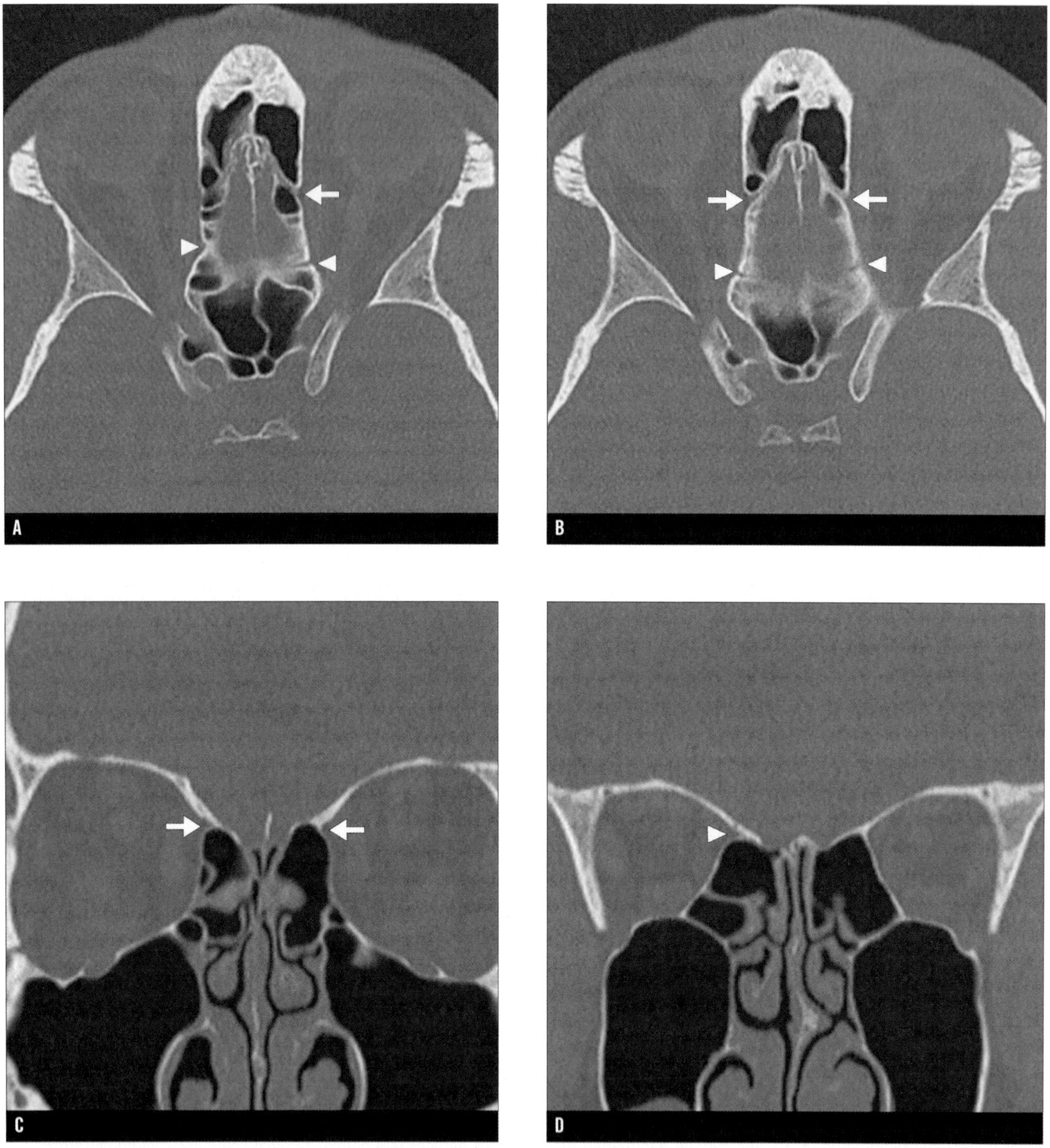

Axial (**A**, **B**) and coronal reformatted (**C**, **D**) CT images demonstrate the normal anterior ethmoidal canals (arrows, **A**-**C**) and the normal posterior ethmoidal canals (arrowheads, **A**, **B**, **D**). The anterior and posterior foramina are located at the entrance site of each canal.

Companion case: Inadvertent anterior ethmoidal artery surgical laceration

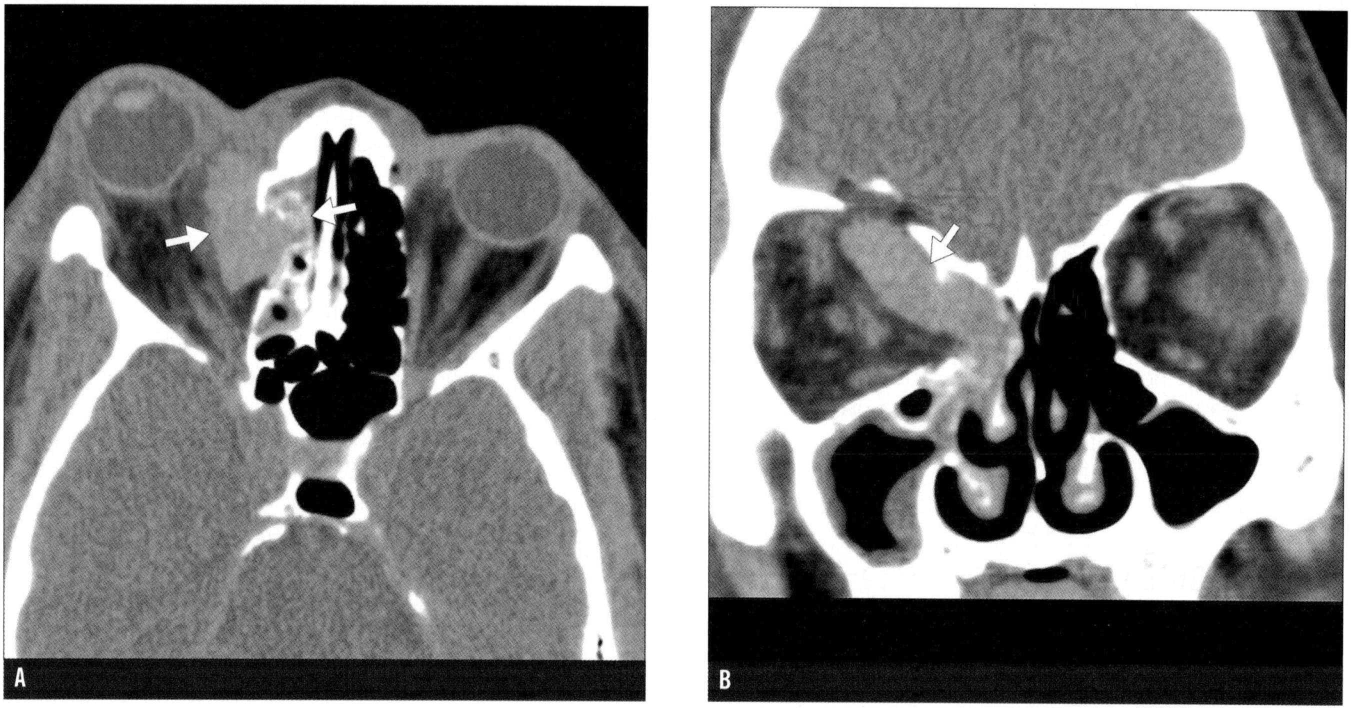

Axial (**A**) and coronal reformatted (**B**) unenhanced CT images demonstrate right globe proptosis and a large hyperattenuating lesion located within the superomedial aspect of the extraconal right orbit (arrows, **A**, **B**). These images were obtained immediately following surgery to repair a large right lamina papyracea fracture. The finding in the superomedial right orbit was not present preoperatively. Given the location and sequence of events, the finding is most consistent with surgical laceration of the right anterior ethmoidal artery.

REFERENCES

Cankal F. et al. Evaluation of the anterior and posterior ethmoidal canal by computed tomography. *Clinl radiol.* Nov 2004 59(11);1034-1040.

Connor SEJ, et al. Computed tomography pseudofractures of the mid face and skull base. *Clini Radiol.* 2005;60:1268-1279.

Meloni F et al. Anatomic variations of surgical importance in ethmoid labyrinth and sphenoid sinus. A study of radiological anatomy. *Surg Radiol Anat.* 1992;14:65-70.

Moon HJ et al. Surgical anatomy of the anterior ethmoidal canal in ethmoid roof. *Laryngoscope.* 2001;111:900-904.

Pigadas N, Lloyd RE. Haematoma of anterior ethmoidal artery after reduction of fracture of zygomatic complex. *Br J Oral Maxillofac Surg.* 2005;43(5):417-419.

Stankiewicz JA, Chow JM. Two faces of orbital hematoma in intranasal (endoscopic) sinus surgery. *Otolaryngol Head Neck Surg.* 1999;120(6):841-847.

Calvarial thickness can vary widely among individuals. The thickness of the calvarium is primarily dependent on the width of the diploic space, and it may range from a few millimeters to over a centimeter. In some individuals, the bone may be so thin as to appear dehiscent on CT.

Any part of the orbital walls may be thinned, particularly the orbital roofs, which can be fragile and even dehiscent, frequently best identified in the coronal plane on CT. Orbital roof dehiscence is most often identified in older patients, likely the result of osseous absorption, resulting in direct contact of the periorbita with the overlying dura. This finding is most often a normal variant, although care should be taken to exclude an underlying lesion, such as an arachnoid cyst, mucocele, or cephalocele.

COMPANION CASES

- **Cocaine abuse.** Inhaled cocaine results in a vasoconstriction that may lead to nasal mucosa inflammation, ulceration, or nasal septal perforation. Superinfection and progressive osteocartilaginous necrosis may cause eventual destruction of the nasal turbinates, paranasal sinuses, and rarely, the hard palate.
- **Allergic fungal sinusitis.** Allergic fungal sinusitis (AFS) is the most common form of fungal sinusitis. It is immune-mediated and affects immunocompetent individuals. One hallmark of AFS on imaging is multifocal expansion and remodeling of the sinuses, often with bulging into adjacent structures, such as the orbits. On CT, hyperdense, inspissated secretions (known as allergic mucin), and/or fungal colonization are characteristically present. On MRI, the sinus contents do not enhance and are of variable T1 signal, with characteristic, markedly hypointense T2 signal, which can mimic the appearance of normally aerated sinuses (also called pseudoaeration).
- **Mucocele.** Mucoceles are the most common expansile lesion of the paranasal sinuses. The inciting incident is obstruction of the sinus ostium, with subsequent complete mucous opacification of the affected sinus. With time, this mucous opacification enlarges and forms a mucocele, often causing smooth remodeling and thinning of the sinus walls. The density and signal characteristics of mucoceles on CT and MRI, respectively, will vary depending upon their viscosity and protein content. However, on CT they are iso- to mildly hyperdense, whereas on MRI, they are most often T1 isointense and T2 hyperintense.

Incidental thinning and apparent dehiscence of the orbital walls

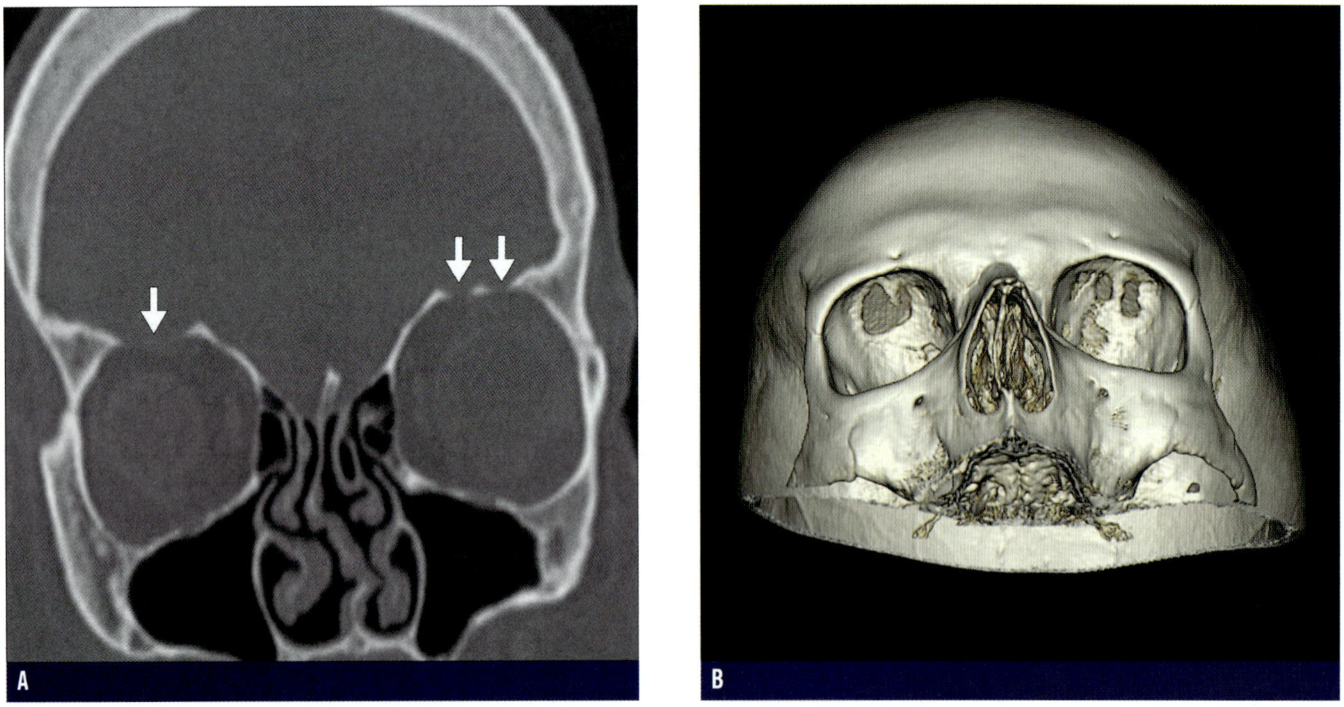

A coronal reformatted CT image (**A**) demonstrates incidental apparent dehiscence of the orbital roofs (arrows, **A**). A 3D reconstruction image from the same study (**B**) demonstrates the bilateral orbital roof apparent dehiscence to a better advantage. Axial (**C**) and coronal reformatted (**D**) CT images from another patient demonstrate normal incidental thinning of the lateral orbital walls (arrows, **C**, **D**).

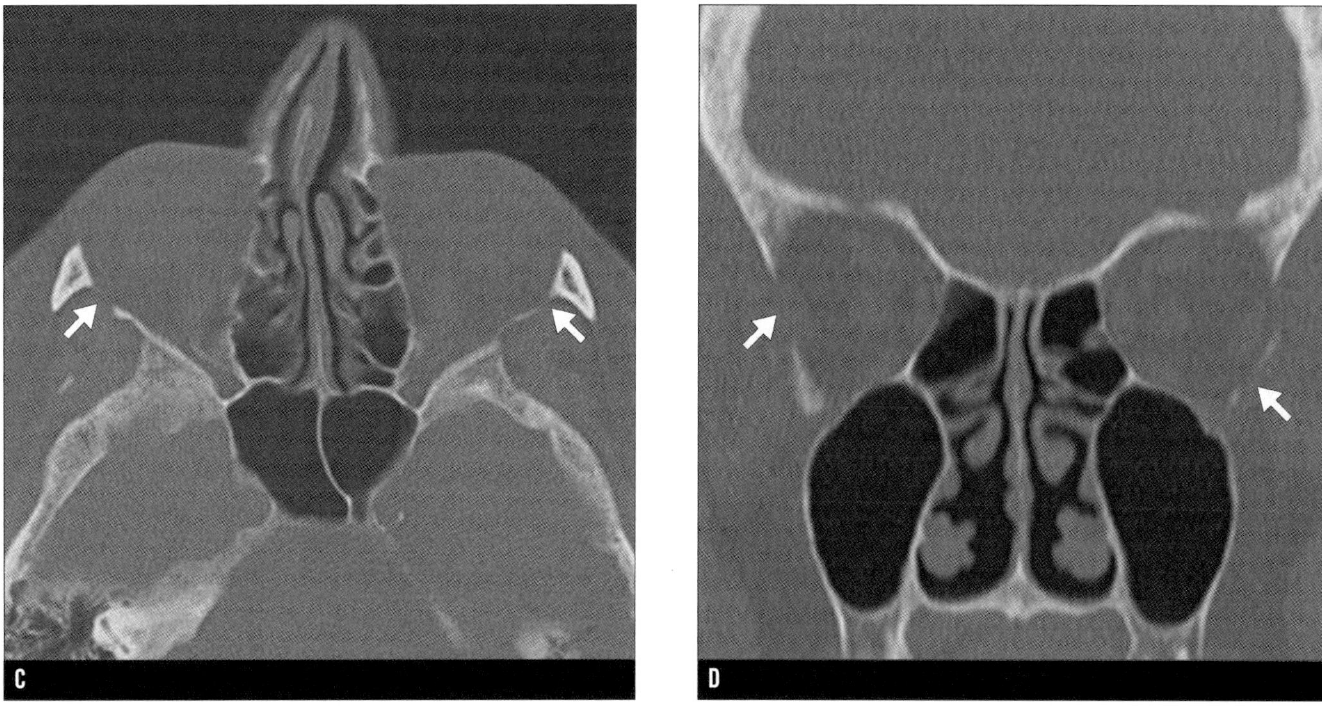

Companion case: Cocaine abuse

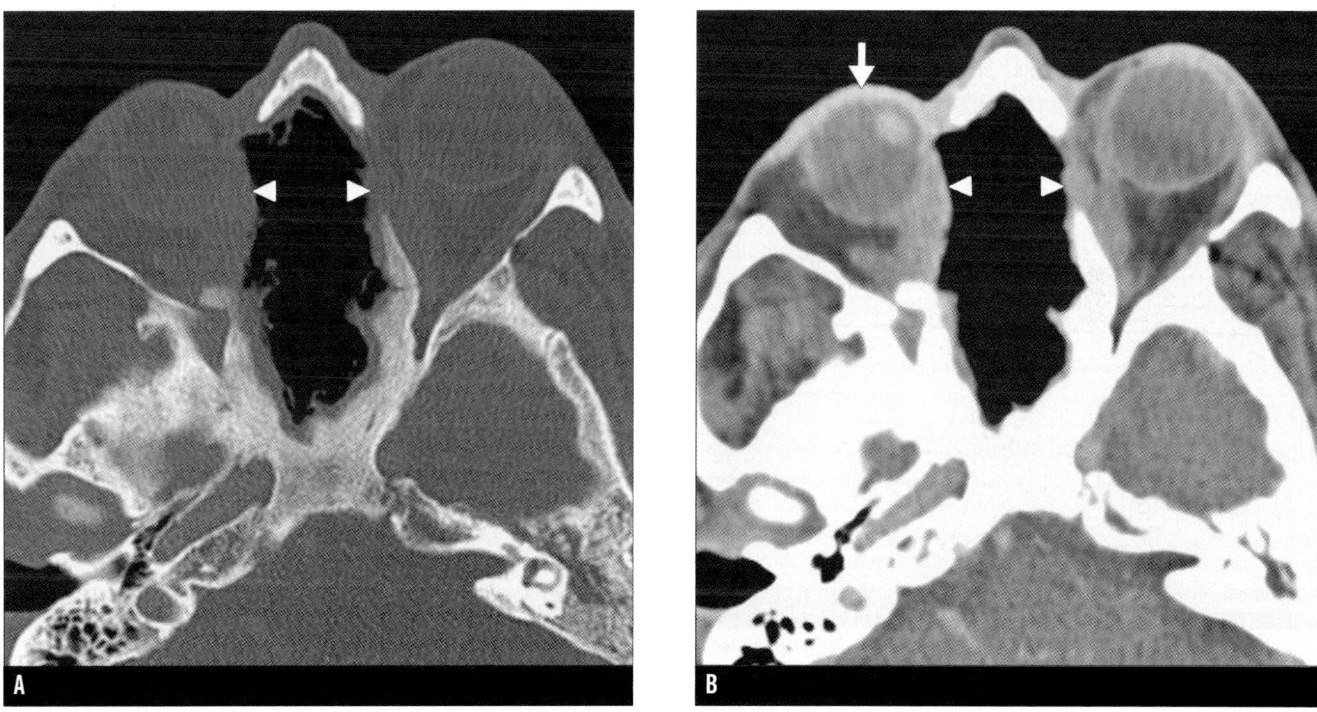

Axial (**A**, **B**) and coronal reformatted (**C**, **D**) CT images viewed with a bone window (**A**, **C**) and soft tissue window (**B**, **D**) demonstrate extensive osseous destruction, including complete absence of the nasal septum, nasal turbinates, ethmoid labyrinth, ostiomeatal complexes, ventral wall of the sphenoid sinus, and medial walls of the maxillary sinuses. There is also marked osseous loss with frank dehiscence of the bilateral lamina papyracea (arrowheads, **A**, **C**) and cribriform plate (arrows, **C**, **D**). A large right oral antral fistula is present (asterisk, **D**). Abnormal soft tissue is present within the medial extraconal space of the orbits (arrowheads, **B**, **D**). Marked right globe esotropia is also present (arrow, **B**). Axial T1 (**E**) and postcontrast axial T1 with fat suppression (**F**) MR images from an MRI performed 2 years later demonstrate similar findings as the above described CT, including a thick rind of nonspecific enhancing tissue in the medial extraconal space of the orbits (arrowheads, **E**, **F**). While these findings could be secondary to a variety of causes (including infectious, neoplastic, and granulomatous etiologies), in this case, extensive cocaine abuse was the culprit.

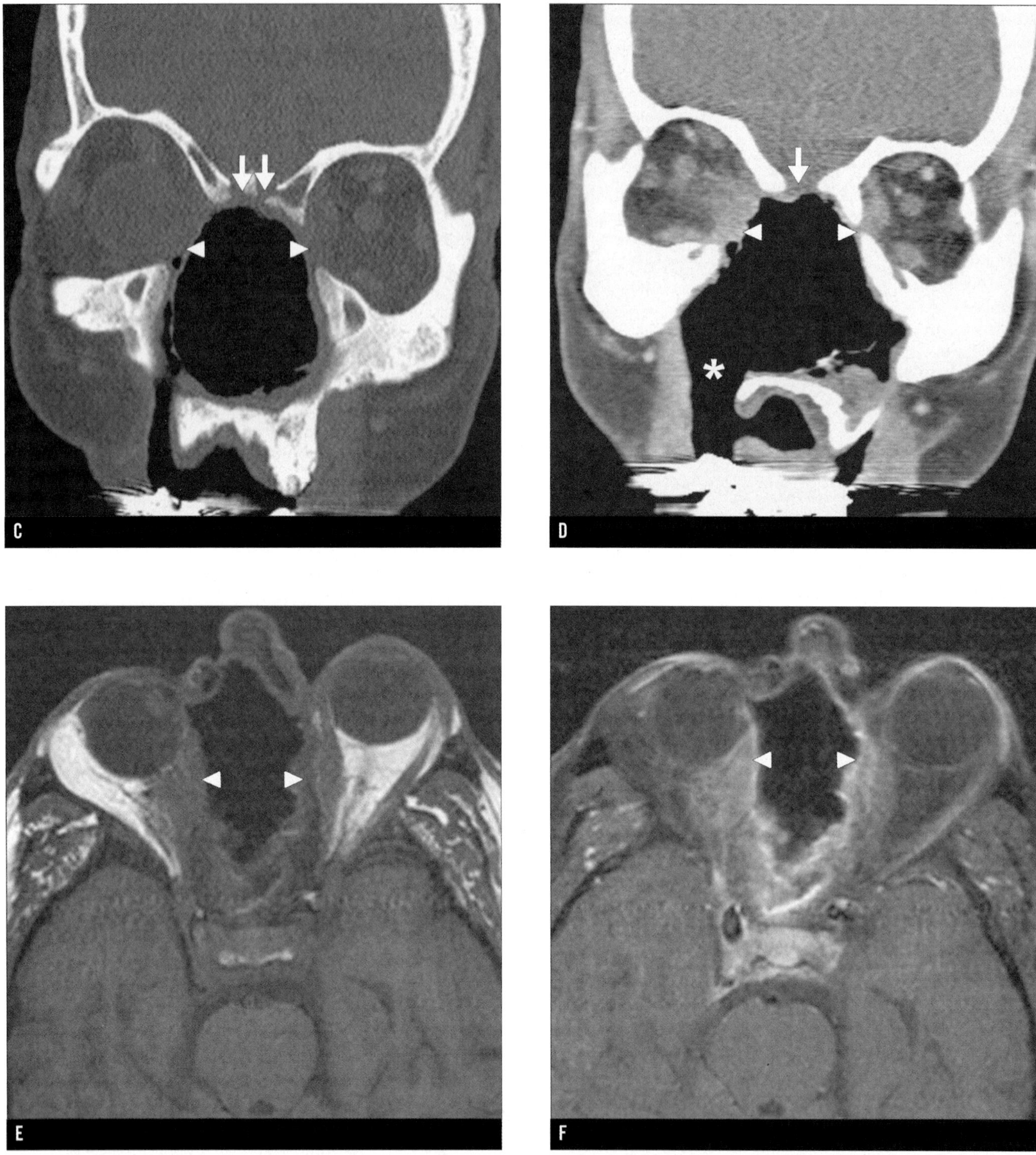
C
D
E
F

Companion case: Allergic fungal sinusitis

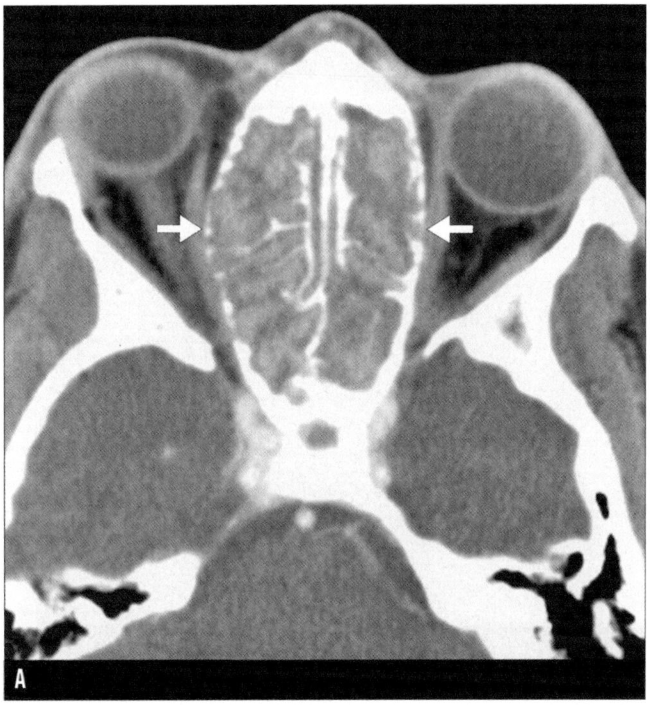

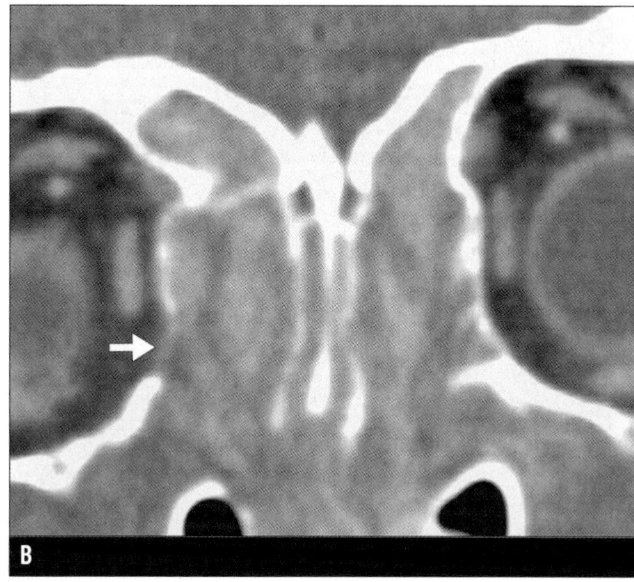

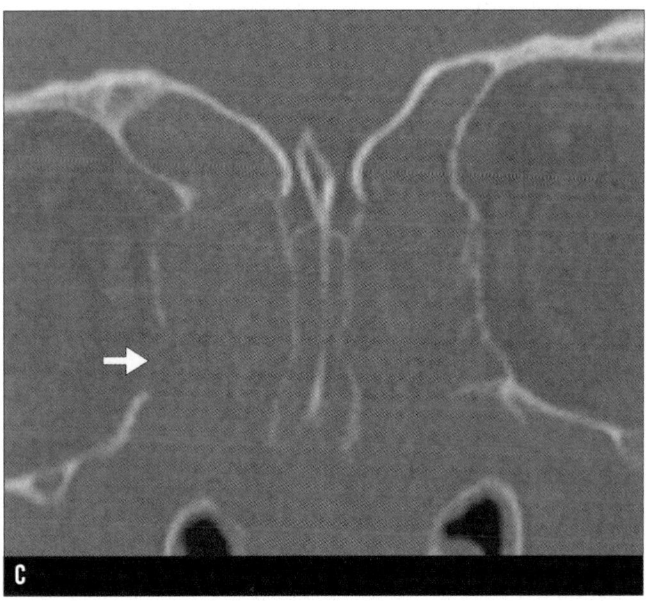

An unenhanced axial CT image viewed with a soft tissue window (**A**) demonstrates extensive high-density sinus opacification within an expanded ethmoid labyrinth and sphenoid sinus, associated with lateral bowing of the lamina papyracea (arrows, **A**). Coronal reformatted CT images viewed in a soft tissue window (**B**) and bone window (**C**) demonstrate demineralization and remodeling of the lamina papyracea, with evidence of focal dehiscence involving the right lamina papyracea (arrows, **B**, **C**). The multiple sinus opacification, increased sinus disease attenuation, and sinus expansion associated with remodeling, thinning, and dehiscence of the osseous walls are consistent with allergic fungal sinusitis.

Companion case: Mucocele

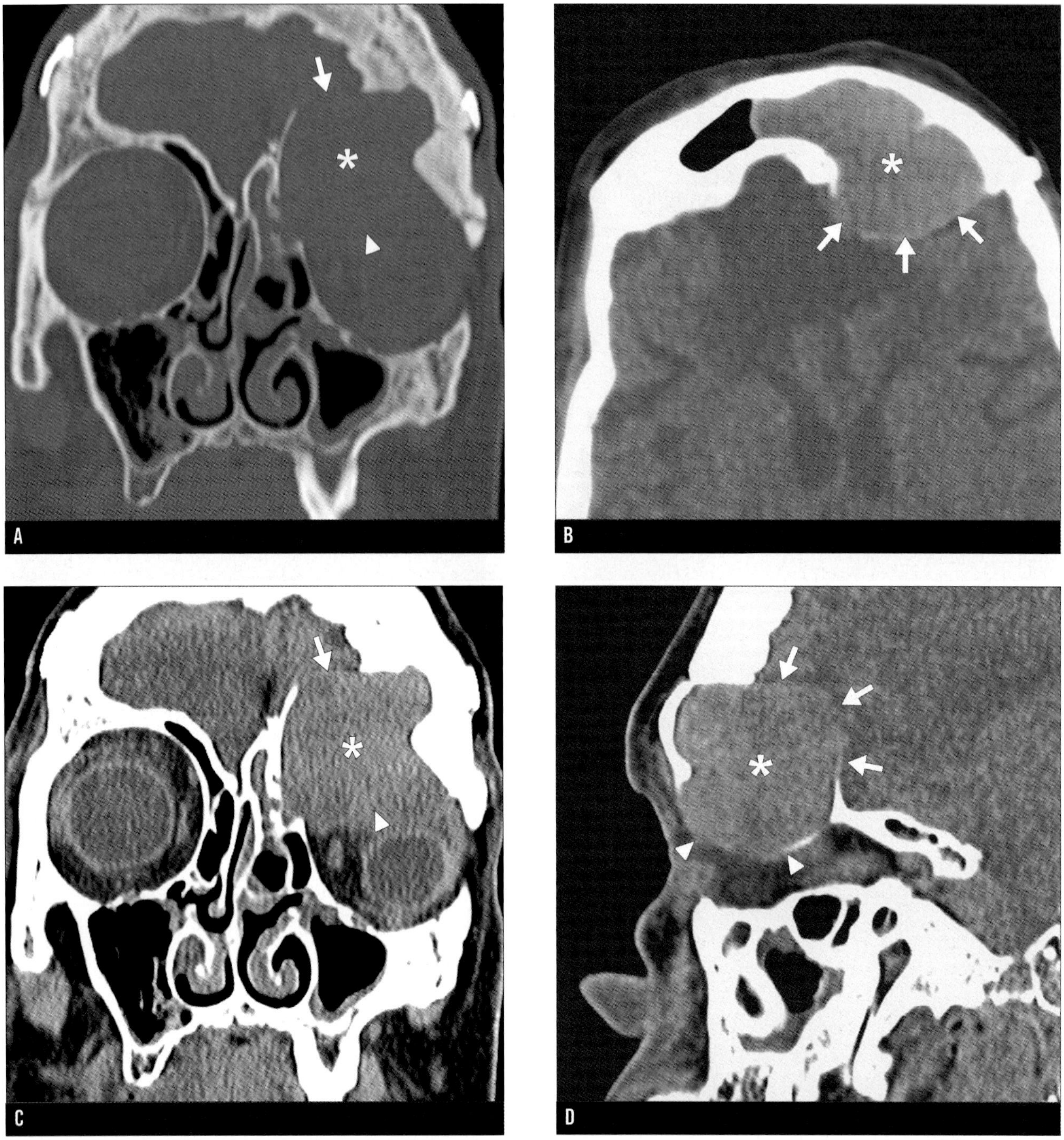

A coronal reformatted CT image viewed with a bone window (**A**) and axial (**B**), coronal reformatted (**C**), and sagittal reformatted (**D**) CT images viewed with a soft tissue window demonstrate a mildly hyperdense, markedly expanded, left frontal sinus compatible with a large mucocele (asterisks, **A-D**). The mucocele is associated with marked demineralization and dehiscence involving portions of the posterosuperior wall of the left frontal sinus (arrows, **A-D**) and left orbital roof/floor of the left frontal sinus (arrowheads, **A, C, D**). The large mucocele results in significant mass effect upon the left orbital contents.

REFERENCES

Aribandi M, McCoy VA, Bazan C 3rd. Imaging features of invasive and noninvasive fungal sinusitis: a review. *Radiographics*. 2007;27(5):1283-1296.

Barkovich AJ, Vandermarck P, Edwards MS, Cogen PH. Congenital nasal masses: CT and MR imaging features in 16 cases. *AJNR Am J Neuroradiol*. 1991;12(1):105-116.

Freyschmidt J, Alban K, Zimmer EA, Schmidt H. *Freyschmidt's "Koehler/Zimmer" Borderlands of Normal and Early Pathologic Findings in Skeletal Radiography*. 5th ed. Stuttgart: Thieme; New York; 2003.

Gupta A, Hawrych A, Wilson WR. Cocaine-induced sinonasal destruction. *Otolaryngol Head Neck Surg*. 2001;124(4):480.

Han MH, Chang KH, Min YG, Choi WS, Yeon KM, Han MC. Nontraumatic prolapse of the orbital contents into the ethmoid sinus: evaluation with screening sinus CT. *Am J Otolaryngol.* 1996;17(3):184-189.

Jordan DR, Mawn L, Anderson RL. Surgical anatomy of the ocular adnexa: a clinical approach. 2nd ed. New York: Oxford University Press; 2012.

Lowe LH, Booth TN, Joglar JM, Rollins NK. Midface anomalies in children. *Radiographics.* 2000;20(4):907-922.

Meloni F, Mini R, Rovasio S, Stomeo F, Teatini GP. Anatomic variations of surgical importance in ethmoid labyrinth and sphenoid sinus. A study of radiological anatomy. *Surg Radiol Anat.* 1992;14(1):65-70.

Meyers RM, Valvassori G. Interpretation of anatomic variations of computed tomography scans of the sinuses: a surgeon's perspective. *Laryngoscope.* 1998;108(3):422-425.

Morón FE, Morriss MC, Jones JJ, Hunter JV. Lumps and bumps on the head in children: use of CT and MR imaging in solving the clinical diagnostic dilemma. *Radiographics.* 2004;24(6):1655-1674.

Moulin G, et al. Dehiscence of the lamina papyracea of the ethmoid bone: CT findings. *AJNR Am J Neuroradiol.* 1994;15(1):151-153.

Seeley MJ, Waterhouse DR, Shetty S, Gathercole JS, Seeley CJ. Boundary issues: a case of nontraumatic bilateral dehiscence of the lamina papyracea. *Arch Otolaryngol Head Neck Surg.* 2010;136(1):88-89.

Seyer BA, Grist W, Muller S. Aggressive destructive midfacial lesion from cocaine abuse. *Oral Surg Oral Med Oral Pathol Oral Radiol Endod.* 2002;94(4):465-470.

CASE 14 Medialization of the lamina papyracea

The ethmoid septa are thought to act as a supporting lattice that help to maintain the normal position of the medial orbital walls. Internal ethmoidectomies involve resection of many or all of these septa and can lead to medial bowing of the lamina papyracea. The resultant expansion in orbital volume may cause mild posterior displacement of the globe and mild enophthalmos.

COMPANION CASES

- **Lamina papyracea fracture.** Lamina papyracea fractures occur most commonly in conjunction with fractures of the orbital floor, with the latter the most common site of orbital blow-out fractures. Lamina papyracea fractures are less frequently identified in isolation, given the reinforcing strut characteristics of the ethmoid septa. When assessing orbital floor fractures, it is important to assess for imaging evidence of extraocular muscle entrapment within the osseous defect, although clinical evidence of muscle entrapment can be occult on imaging. With chronic fractures, enophthalmos may result when there is sufficient herniation of the orbital contents into the osseous defect.
- **Orbital decompression for thyroid ophthalmopathy.** Surgical decompression of the orbits in patients with thyroid ophthalmopathy may be performed to treat advanced proptosis, compressive optic neuropathy, and exposure keratitis. There is currently no single accepted technique for optimal orbital decompression. There are a variety of surgical approaches that have been employed, including removal of one or more of the osseous orbital walls, orbital fat, or a combination of both. Endoscopic, external, and combined approaches have been utilized to perform orbital surgical decompression, with minimally invasive forms of the procedure becoming more commonplace. A combined approach with excellent outcomes described by Kingdom et al includes an endoscopic approach that removes the lamina papyracea as well as a transconjunctival approach via a lateral canthotomy and cantholysis in order to achieve inferior and lateral orbital wall decompression. Importantly, the inferomedial aspect of the orbit (also called inferomedial orbital strut) is preserved during this procedure to prevent inferomedial displacement of the globe and new or worsening diplopia. The infraorbital neurovascular bundle is also left intact. The amount of bone and fat removed depends on the degree of proptosis and the extent of desired decompression.

Medialization of the lamina papyracea

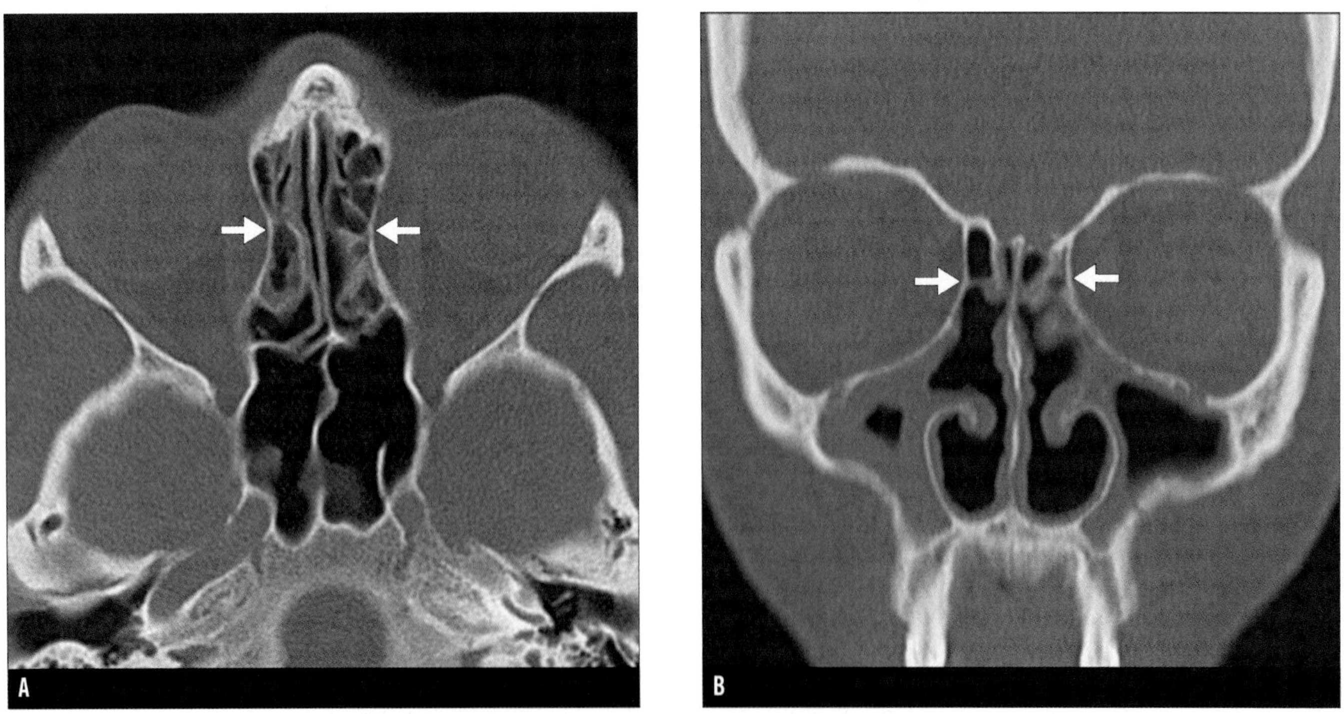

Axial (**A**) and coronal reformatted (**B**) CT images demonstrate smooth and symmetric medialization of the lamina papyracea in this patient who underwent bilateral partial internal ethmoidectomies and uncinectomies (arrows, **A, B**).

Companion case: Lamina papyracea fracture

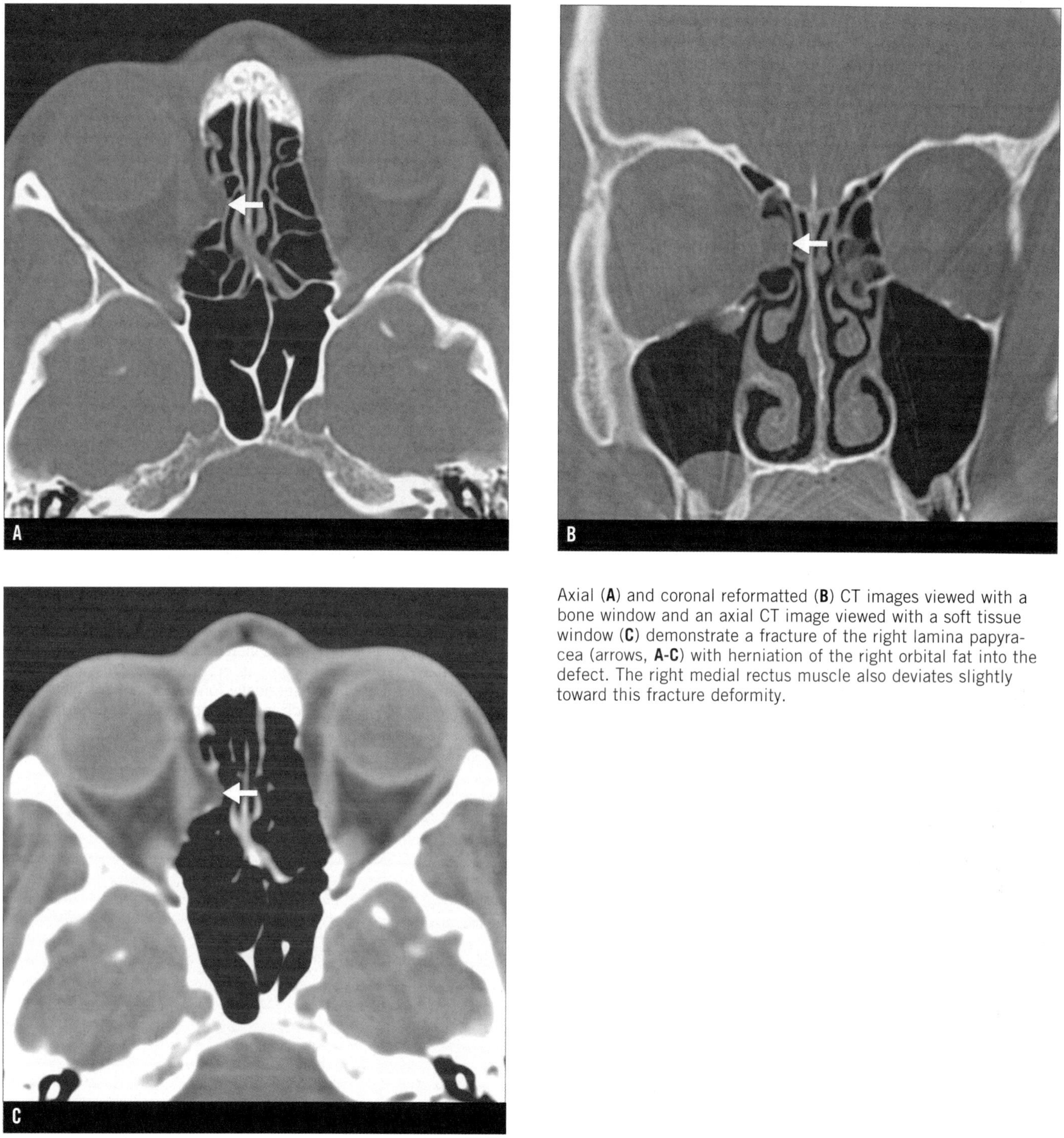

Axial (**A**) and coronal reformatted (**B**) CT images viewed with a bone window and an axial CT image viewed with a soft tissue window (**C**) demonstrate a fracture of the right lamina papyracea (arrows, **A-C**) with herniation of the right orbital fat into the defect. The right medial rectus muscle also deviates slightly toward this fracture deformity.

Companion case: Orbital decompression for thyroid ophthalmopathy

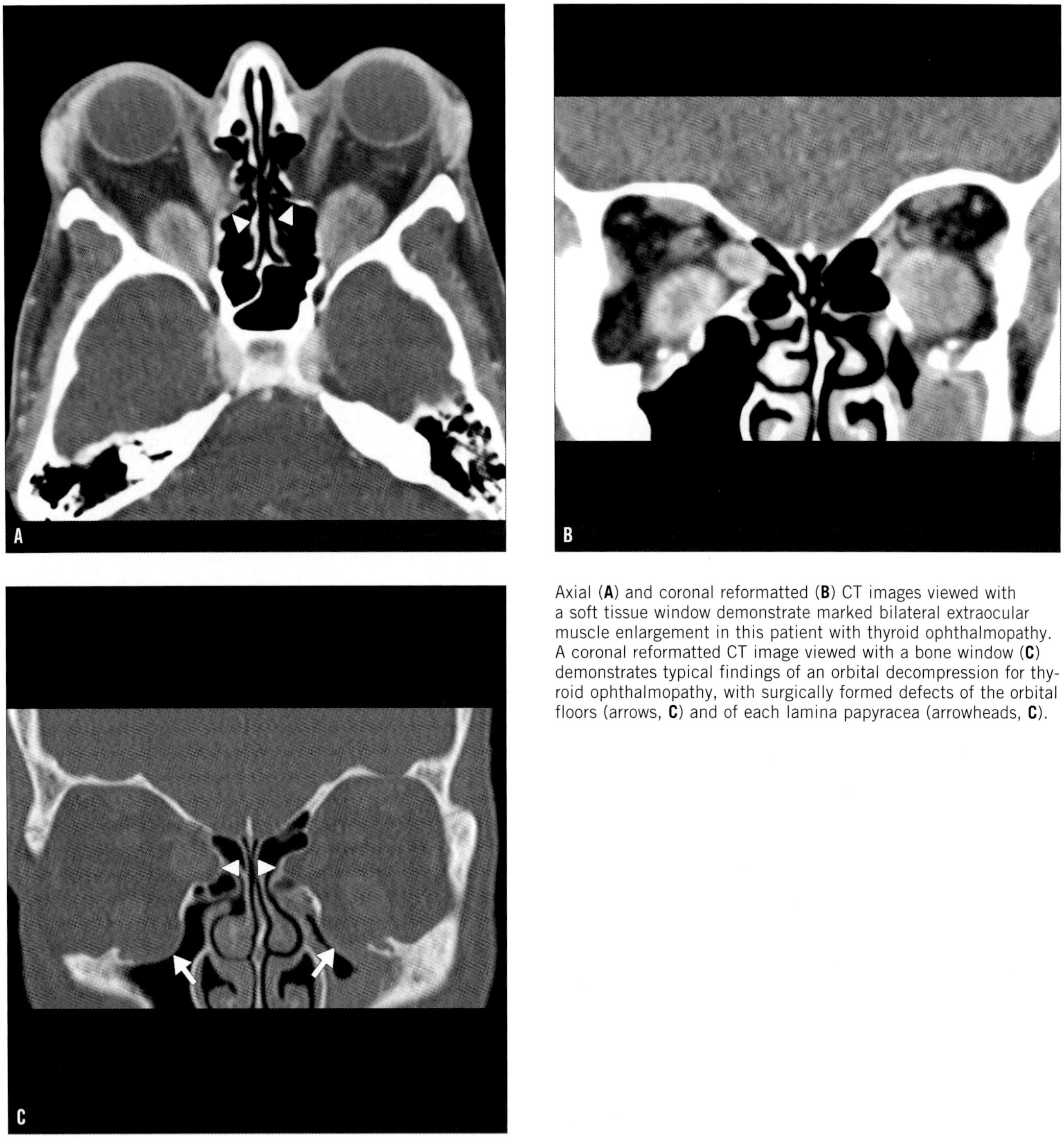

Axial (**A**) and coronal reformatted (**B**) CT images viewed with a soft tissue window demonstrate marked bilateral extraocular muscle enlargement in this patient with thyroid ophthalmopathy. A coronal reformatted CT image viewed with a bone window (**C**) demonstrates typical findings of an orbital decompression for thyroid ophthalmopathy, with surgically formed defects of the orbital floors (arrows, **C**) and of each lamina papyracea (arrowheads, **C**).

REFERENCES

Cunnane ME, Platt M, Caruso PA, Metson R, Curtin HD. Medialization of the lamina papyracea after endoscopic ethmoidectomy: comparison of preprocedure and postprocedure computed tomographic scans. *J Comput Assist Tomogr.* 2009;33(1):79-81.

Kingdom TT, Davies BW, Durairaj VD. Orbital decompression for the management of thyroid eye disease: An analysis of outcomes and complications. *Laryngoscope.* 2015 Apr 17 [Epub ahead of print].

Mirvis SE, Shanmuganathan K. *Imaging in Trauma and Critical Care.* 2nd ed. Philadelphia, PA: Saunders; 2003.

Wu W, et al. Endoscopic Medial Orbital Fat Decompression for Proptosis in Type 1 Graves Orbitopathy. *Am J Ophthalmol.* 2015;159:277-284.

CASE 15 Orbital roof sclerotic focus

A single sclerotic focus with nonaggressive features is sometimes identified on CT imaging within the orbital process of the frontal bone along superolateral aspect of the orbital roof. Occasionally, a lucent center may be present within the area of sclerosis on CT. The finding is often bilateral. On MRI, these foci are usually T1 and T2 hypointense and they do not enhance. In many cases, these findings are bilateral and symmetric. In our experience, they are stable on multiyear follow-up examinations performed for other reasons. The etiology of this sclerotic focus is unclear, although one hypothesis is that it may represent a remnant of a frontal bone primary ossification center.

COMPANION CASE

- **Fibrous dysplasia.** Fibrous dysplasia is a developmental abnormality in which benign fibro-osseous tissue proliferates within the medullary cavity of bone. Fibrous dysplasia may be an isolated lesion (monostotic) or involve multiple sites (polyostotic), the latter a characteristic finding in patients with McCune-Albright syndrome. Seventy-five percent of patients with fibrous dysplasia present before the age of 30. On pathologic examination, fibrous dysplasia consists of trabecular bone surrounded by fibrous tissue.

  While these lesions frequently have a characteristic "ground glass" appearance, the quantity of trabecular bone within them, as well as the extent to which this bone is mineralized, accounts for the variability in density observed when they are imaged with radiography. Therefore, these lesions can also appear lytic or have mixed patterns (so-called pagetoid). As these lesions slowly increase in size, endosteal scalloping and osseous expansion can occur. These lesions typically have sharp borders and can be surrounded by a sclerotic rim, which can vary in thickness.

  On MRI, fibrous dysplasia has a variable appearance on T1- and T2-weighted sequences, depending on whether the lesion is primarily of the ground-glass, lytic, or mixed type. Fibrous dysplasia may enhance on postcontrast sequences, with the degree of enhancement ranging from mild to avid. The enhancement on MRI associated with fibrous dysplasia can mimic a malignancy. Therefore, one should always interpret any suspicious osseous lesion on MRI in conjunction with either radiographs or CT.

Orbital roof sclerotic focus

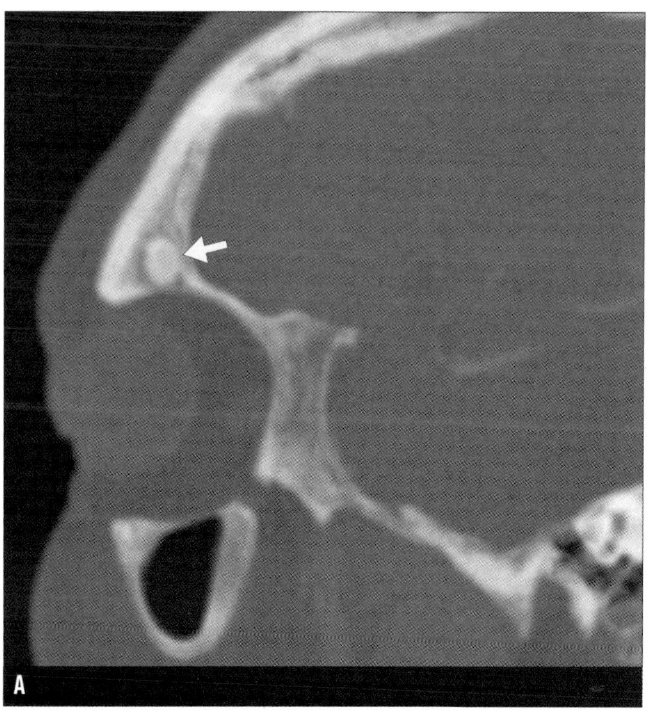

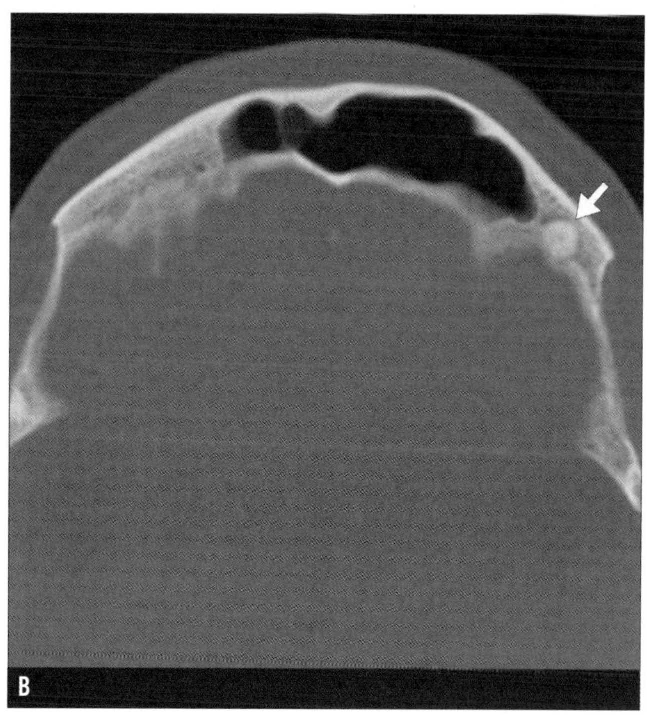

Sagittal reformatted (**A**) and axial (**B**) CT images as well as axial T2 with fat suppression (**C**) and postcontrast axial T1 (**D**) MR images demonstrate a sclerotic, nonenhancing lesion located within the lateral aspect of the left orbital roof (arrows, **A-D**). This lesion was unchanged for over 7 years on follow-up imaging.

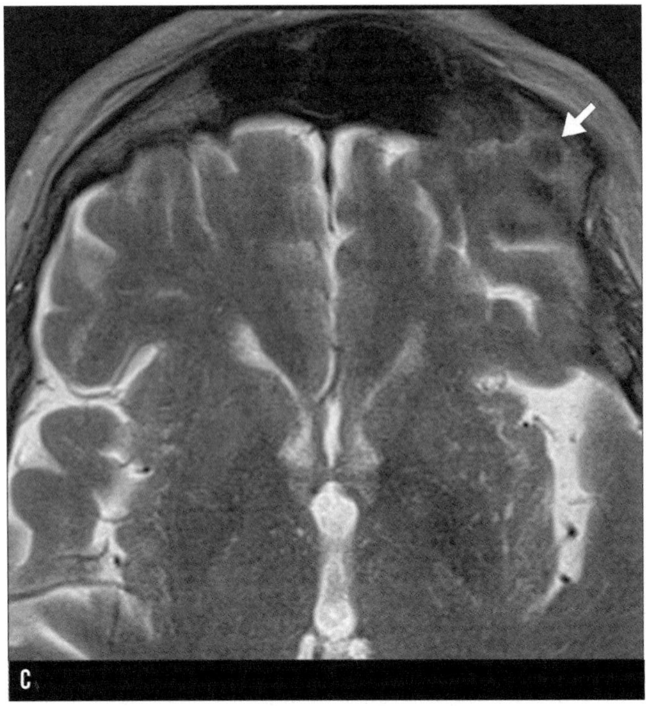

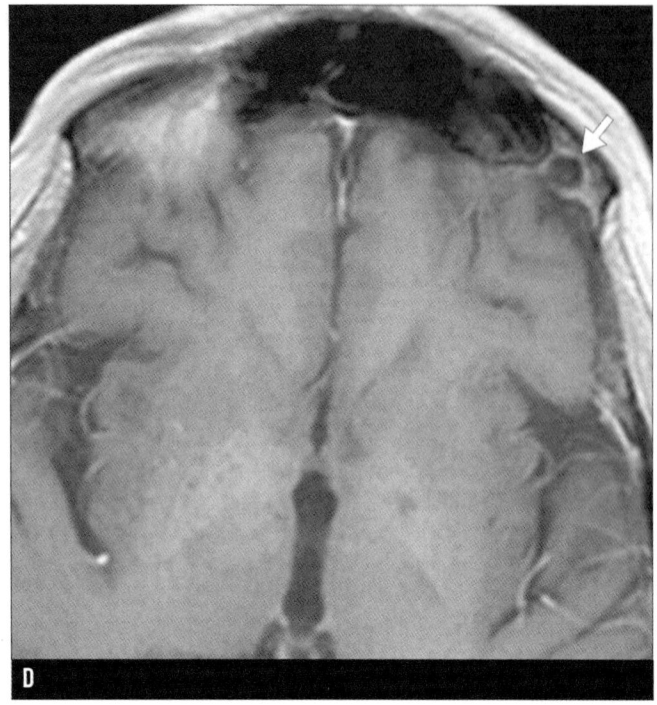

Companion case: Fibrous dysplasia

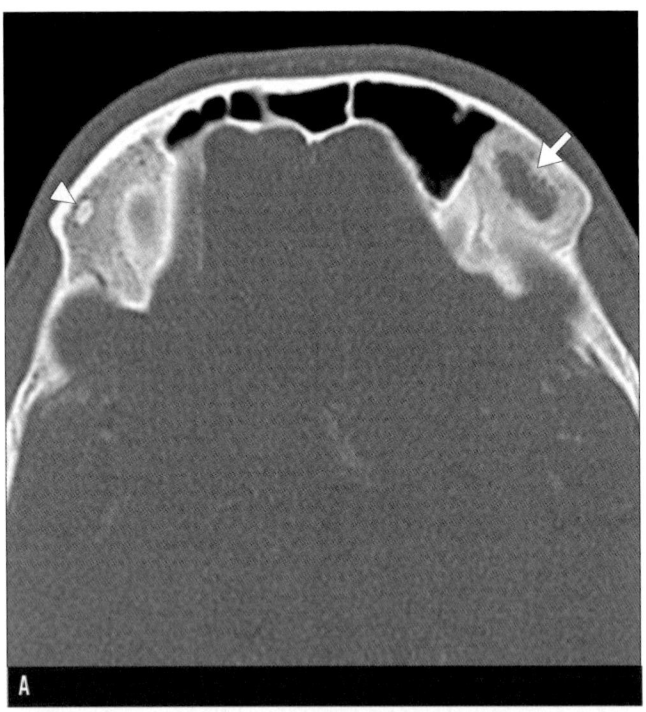

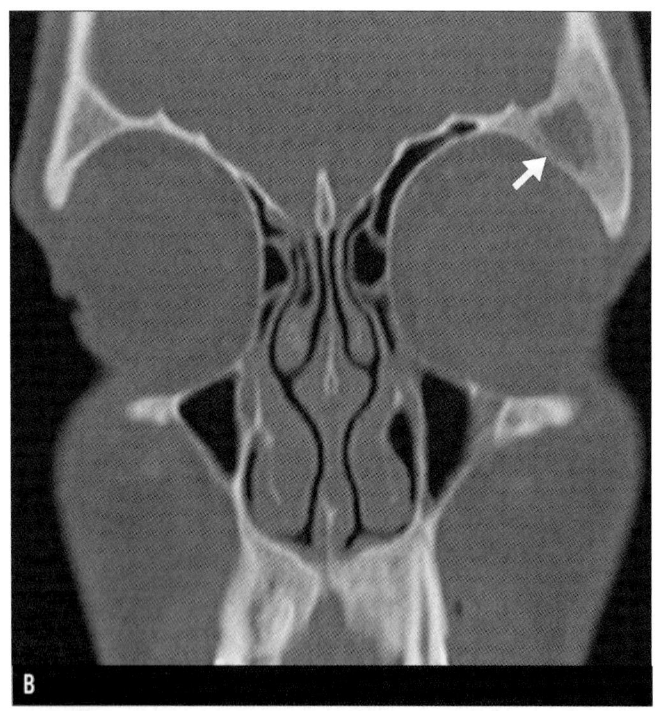

Axial (**A**) and coronal reformatted (**B**) CT images demonstrate an expansile lesion of the left orbital roof (arrows, **A, B**) characterized by a central lucent area that is surrounded by ground-glass attenuation. A normal variant sclerotic focus within the lateral aspect of the right orbital roof is also present (arrowhead, **A**). Axial T2 with fat suppression (**C**), axial T1 (**D**), and postcontrast axial T1 (**E**) MR images of the same patient demonstrates the same left orbital roof intraosseous lesion to be centrally T2 hyperintense (corresponding to the lucent component on CT), whereas the periphery of the lesion is T2 hypointense (corresponding to the ground-glass portion of the lesion on CT). The central component of the lesion is T1 isointense and enhances following contrast administration. The patient had no history of malignancy. The CT and MR findings, in addition to the lack of a history of malignancy, are most compatible with a mixed form of fibrous dysplasia.

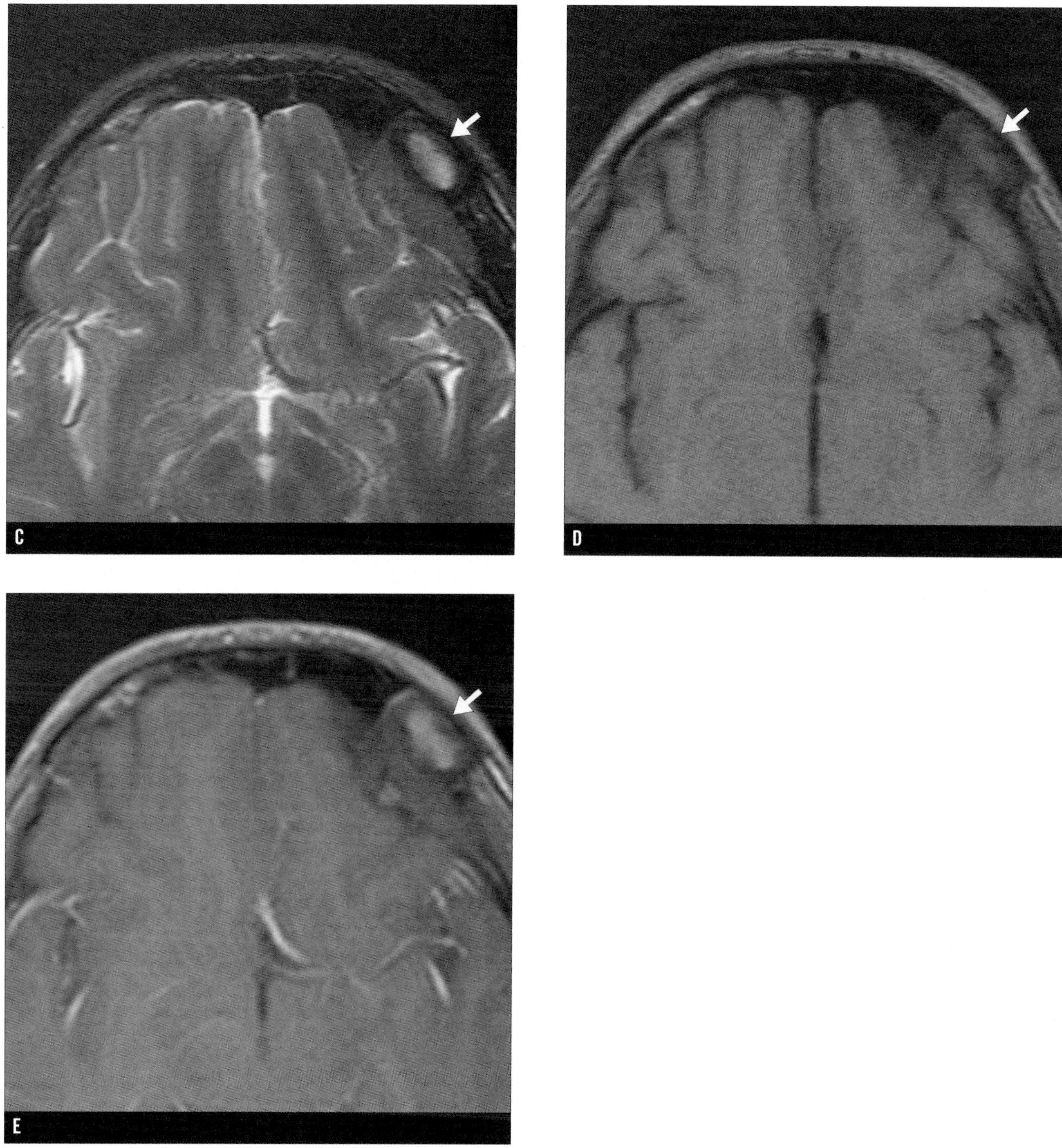

REFERENCES

Cerase A, Priolo F. Skeletal benign bone-forming lesions. *Eur J Radiol.* 1998;27:(Suppl 1):S91-S97.

Eversole R, Su L, ElMofty S. Benign fibro-osseous lesions of the craniofacial complex. A Review. *Head Neck Pathol.* 2008;2(3):177-202.

Gould CF, et al. Bone tumor mimics: avoiding misdiagnosis. *Curr Probl Diagn Radiol.* 2007;36(3):124-141.

Inman VT, Saunders JBCM. The ossification of the human frontal bone with special reference to its presumed pre- and post-frontal elements. *J Anat.* 1937;71(Pt 3):383-394.

Kransdorf MJ, Moser RP, Gilkey FW. Fibrous dysplasia. *Radiographics.* 1990;10(3):519-537.

CASE 16 Normal and pathologic appearances of the lacrimal glands

The lacrimal glands are located anteriorly within the superolateral aspect of each orbit. While there is no true anatomical division, the lacrimal glands can be subdivided into a palpebral portion (under the eyelid) and an orbital portion (within the osseous orbit). These glands can vary in size among individuals, with mild, symmetrically enlarged but otherwise normal glands sometimes noted on imaging. Unilateral enlargement should always be viewed with suspicion, whereas bilateral enlargement will often need to be correlated with the patient's clinical history to determine significance. The lacrimal glands, like the salivary glands, are subject to senescent involution (ie, atrophy).

COMPANION CASES

- **Lacrimal gland prolapse.** Lacrimal gland prolapse is an acquired condition in which the palpebral portion of the gland herniates and causes bulging of the lateral upper eyelid. There are a variety of causes of lacrimal gland prolapse, including diffuse enlargement or displacement of the lacrimal gland, laxity of lacrimal gland suspensory ligaments due to aging, and trauma.

  Lacrimal gland prolapse has been reported in 15% of patients presenting for blepharoplasty, and it is important to identify this entity before surgery to avoid inadvertent injury to the gland. Surgical repair of lacrimal gland prolapse has been achieved by suture suspension to the orbital rim periosteum. Another approach involves suturing the Whitnall ligament (superior transverse ligament within the upper eyelid) to the superior orbital rim periosteum anterior to the lacrimal gland fossa and over the gland. Resection of the palpebral portion of the lacrimal gland has been performed in the past but has since been abandoned due to resultant impaired tear production.

  On imaging, the prolapsed palpebral portion of the lacrimal gland is identical to the remainder of the gland as visualized on CT and on all MRI sequences. If not, then other possibilities to explain the finding enter the differential.
- **Subconjunctival orbital fat prolapse.** Subconjunctival fat prolapse is an acquired lesion typically characterized by herniation of intraconal fat in the superotemporal quadrant, although cases of superonasal prolapse have also been reported. It is presumed that the prolapse occurs because of weakness of the Tenon capsule due to aging, trauma, or surgery.

  Typically, subconjunctival fat prolapse occurs in elderly obese male individuals. Occasionally, subconjunctival fat prolapse is misdiagnosed as a dermolipoma, although the latter is more common in younger females. The key feature distinguishing these two entities on imaging is that prolapsed subconjunctival fat is continuous with the intraconal fat. In dermolipoma, the lesion is separate from the intraconal fat. Surgical excision of the prolapsed fat may be performed to relieve discomfort or for cosmesis.

  Subconjunctival fat prolapse follows fat attenuation and signal on CT and MRI, respectively.
- **Symmetric lacrimal gland enlargement due to a chronic disease state.** Individuals with a history of chronic alcohol abuse, especially those with resultant cirrhosis, sometimes exhibit asymptomatic diffuse enlargement of the bilateral salivary glands and lacrimal glands, termed sialadenosis (or sialosis). These changes are presumed to be secondary to a neuropathic process affecting the autonomic innervation of these glands. Similar asymptomatic, symmetrically enlarged lacrimal glands may be present with other chronic disease states, including malnourished patients, diabetes mellitus, obesity, and after chronic exposure to certain medications or chemicals. Asymptomatic symmetric enlargement of the lacrimal glands has also been described in pregnancy.
- **Sjögren syndrome.** Sjögren syndrome is an autoimmune disorder characterized by keratoconjunctivitis sicca (dry eyes) and xerostomia (dry mouth). Sjögren syndrome is associated with lymphocytic infiltration of the salivary and lacrimal glands, initially producing glandular enlargement but ultimately resulting in glandular atrophy. This syndrome commonly occurs in conjunction with an underlying connective tissue disorder, most commonly rheumatoid arthritis. On MRI, the lacrimal glands may be heterogeneous on T1- and T2-weighted sequences. Characteristic punctate T2 hyperintense foci, intrinsically T1 hyperintense fatty deposits, and areas of speckled enhancement may be identified. Sjögren syndrome is associated with lymphoma; therefore, lymphoma should be suspected in a patient with Sjögren syndrome when an enlarging solid lesion in the lacrimal gland is present.
- **Lymphoma.** Lymphoproliferative disease is a subcategory of nonepithelial lesions of the lacrimal gland and includes both lymphoid hyperplasia and lymphoma. The lacrimal gland is the sole orbital structure with native lymphocytes and plasma cells. Both primary and secondary (ie, systemic) forms of lacrimal gland lymphoma occur, with a median age of diagnosis near 60. Interestingly, there has been an increase over time in the proportion lacrimal gland lymphoma relative to other malignant tumors of the lacrimal gland.

  The imaging findings of lymphoma include circumscribed, diffuse enlargement of the lacrimal gland with an oblong shape conforming to the adjacent bone. While epithelial tumors (eg pleomorphic adenoma, etc) may also diffusely involve the lacrimal gland, they are often focal, a finding not typically identified with lacrimal gland lymphoma. Orbital lymphoma is typically isointense to muscle on T1- and T2-weighted MR images, enhance homogeneously following gadolinium administration, and restrict on diffusion weighted imaging.

- **Pleomorphic adenoma.** Pleomorphic adenoma (also called benign mixed tumor) is the most common tumor of the lacrimal gland. These tumors most often present in middle-aged patients as a slow growing, painless lacrimal gland mass. Pleomorphic adenomas (like other tumors containing epithelial cells) are usually focal tumors, unlike lymphoma, which generally involves the entire lacrimal gland. However, if large, a minor salivary gland tumor of the lacrimal gland may also involve the entire gland. On CT, pleomorphic adenomas are usually cicrumscribed, smoothly contoured tumors. While most often noncalcified, of the minor salivary gland tumors, pleomorphic adenomas are the type that most often calcify. On occasion, these tumors remodel the adjacent osseous orbit. On MRI, pleomorphic adenomas are T1 isointense and often markedly homogeneously T2 hyperintense. They can enhance homogeneously or heterogeneously on CT and MR, and delayed imaging may be necessary to visualize the enhancement, particularly on CT.
- **Adenoid cystic carcinoma.** Adenoid cystic carcinoma (ACC) is the most common malignant epithelial tumor of the lacrimal gland. The median age at diagnosis is 50, and pain, facial asymmetry, and a firm mass in the lacrimal fossa are common at presentation. Pain associated with ACC has been attributed to its tendency for early peripheral nerve, vascular, and extraocular muscle invasion. On imaging, ACC typically has irregular margins, infiltrates surrounding tissues, and results in osseous destruction. When metastatic, ACC has a proclivity to spread to lungs (sometimes with large "cannonball" lung metastases) and may also metastasize to the bone and dura. While it may metastasize to lymph nodes, it does so significantly less frequently than other tumors of this region. MRI is the preferred imaging modality for ACC, as it is particularly helpful in identifying perineural tumor spread. The lesion is usually isointense to muscle on T1- and T2-weighted imaging, and it enhances moderately. On CT, ACC may contain calcification.

  The current standard of care for local treatment of ACC is surgery and postoperative radiotherapy. In cases in which the tumor is extensive and infiltrative, subtotal or total orbital exenteration may be necessary. In unresectable cases and/or with metastatic disease, chemotherapy may be administered. Recurrence rates for ACC are reported to be as high as 75%, and death is usually a result of distant metastases and intracranial spread.
- **Adenocarcinoma.** Primary adenocarcinoma of the lacrimal gland is an aggressive neoplasm, prone to both recurrence and early lymphatic as well as distant metastatic spread. Like ACC, but unlike benign tumors such as pleomorphic adenoma, pain is a common presenting symptom with this neoplasm. On imaging, aggressive features such as extraorbital extension, nodal metastatic disease, an infiltrative appearance, calcification, and osseous destruction may be present.
- **Metastatic disease to the lacrimal gland.** Breast cancer is the most common source of metastases to the orbit and may involve essentially any part of the orbit. Scirrhous metastatic breast cancer to the orbit may result in orbital fibrosis and enophthalmos. Other malignancies known to metastasize to the orbit in adults include prostate cancer, gastrointestinal malignancies, lung cancer, and sarcomas. Neuroblastoma accounts for most orbital metastases in children. On imaging, metastatic tumors may be infiltrative, although encapsulated tumors are not uncommon. Metastases are often T1 hypointense and T2 hyperintense when compared to orbital fat, and they almost always enhance.

Normal lacrimal glands (CT)

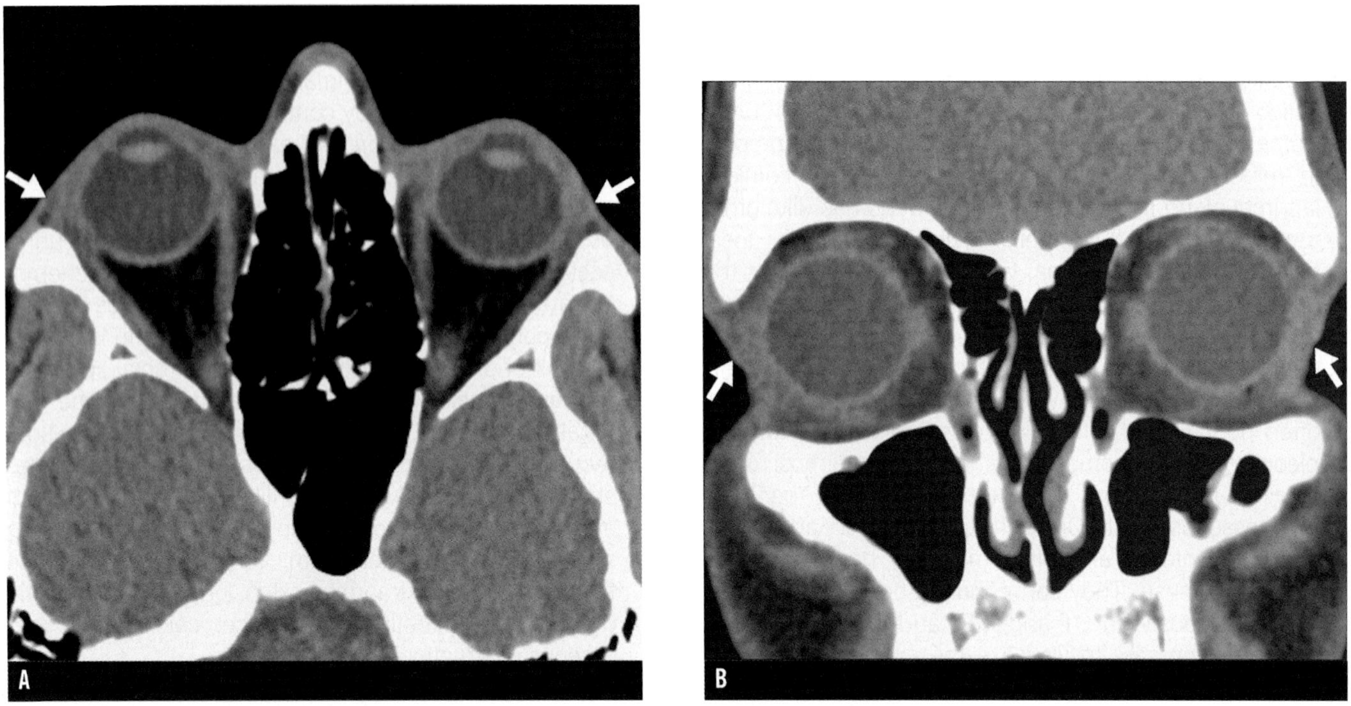

Axial (**A**) and coronal reformatted (**B**) CT images demonstrate normal lacrimal glands (arrows, **A**, **B**).

Normal lacrimal glands (MRI)

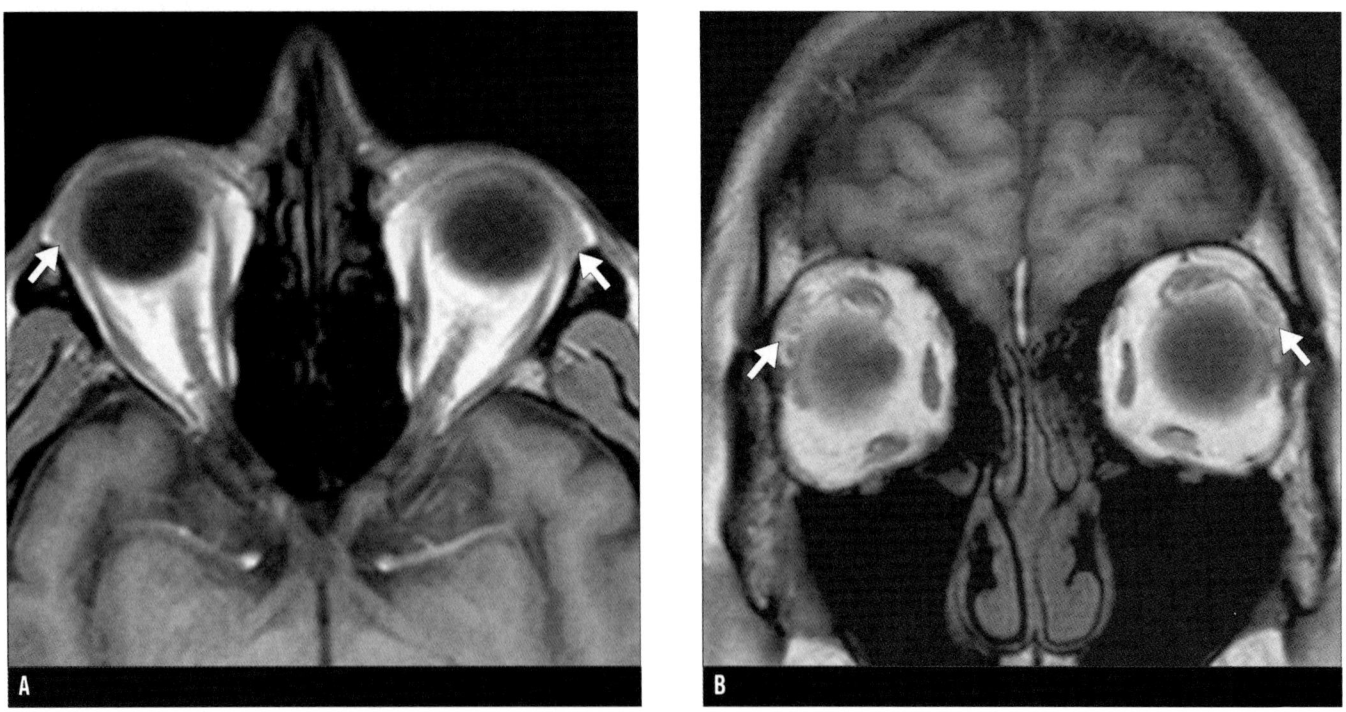

Axial T1 (**A**), coronal T1 (**B**), fat-suppressed coronal T2 (**C**), and postcontrast fat-suppressed coronal T1 (**D**) MR images demonstrate the MRI appearance of normal lacrimal glands (arrows, **A**-**D**).

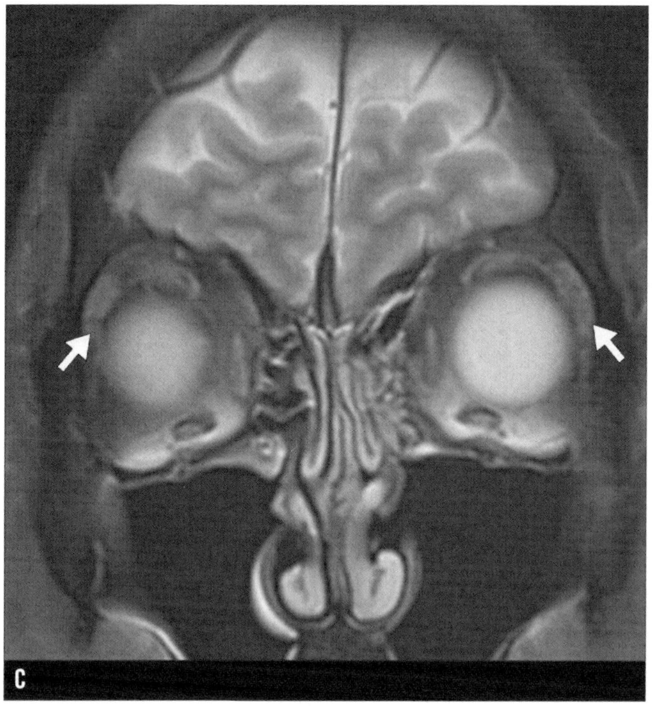

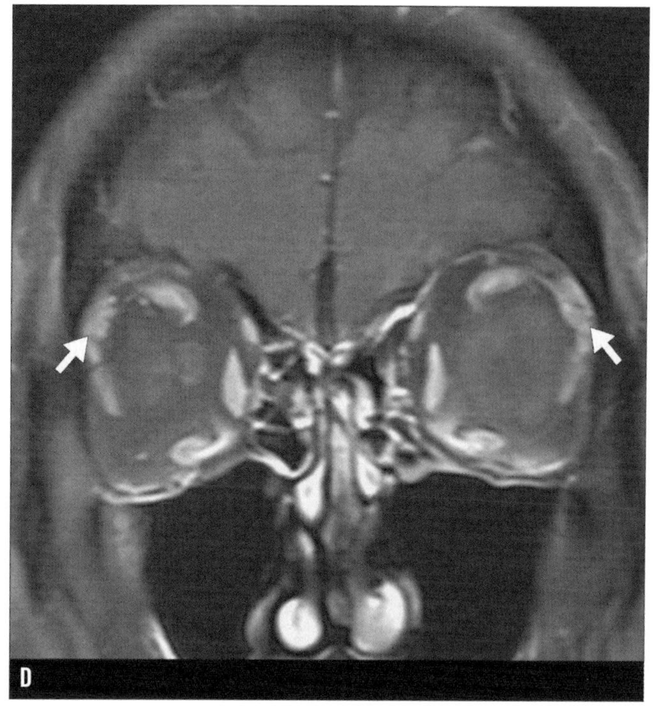

Companion case: Lacrimal gland prolapse

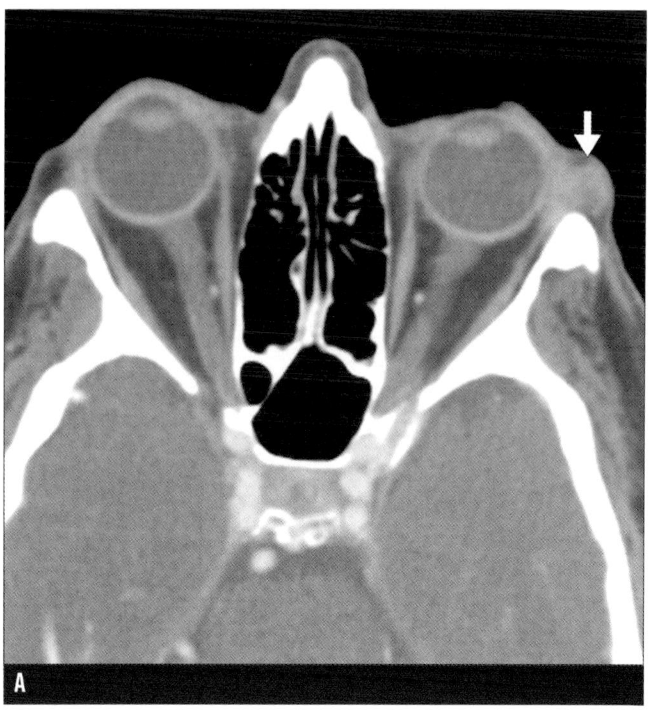

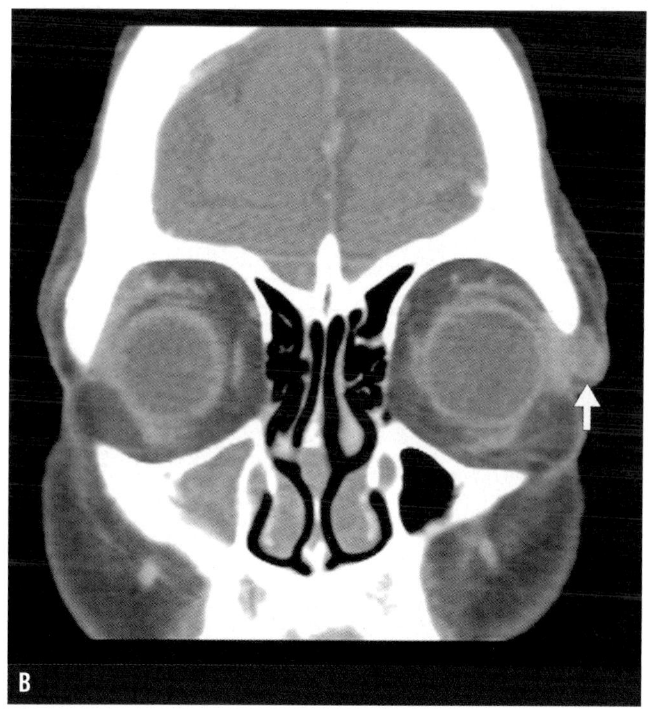

Axial (**A**) and coronal reformatted (**B**) contrast-enhanced CT images demonstrate asymmetric soft tissue in the left upper eyelid which was palpable (arrows, **A**, **B**). Coronal T1 (**C**) and contrast-enhanced coronal T1 with fat suppression (**D**) MR images demonstrate the same soft tissue asymmetry to enhance on MRI (arrows, **C**, **D**). A contrast-enhanced coronal T1-weighed MR image with fat suppression located more posteriorly than image **D** (**E**) demonstrates the normal position of the right lacrimal gland (arrow, **E**). The finding in the left upper eyelid was isodense and isointense compared to the contralateral lacrimal gland on CT and all MR sequences, respectively. The finding is compatible with incidental left lacrimal gland prolapse.

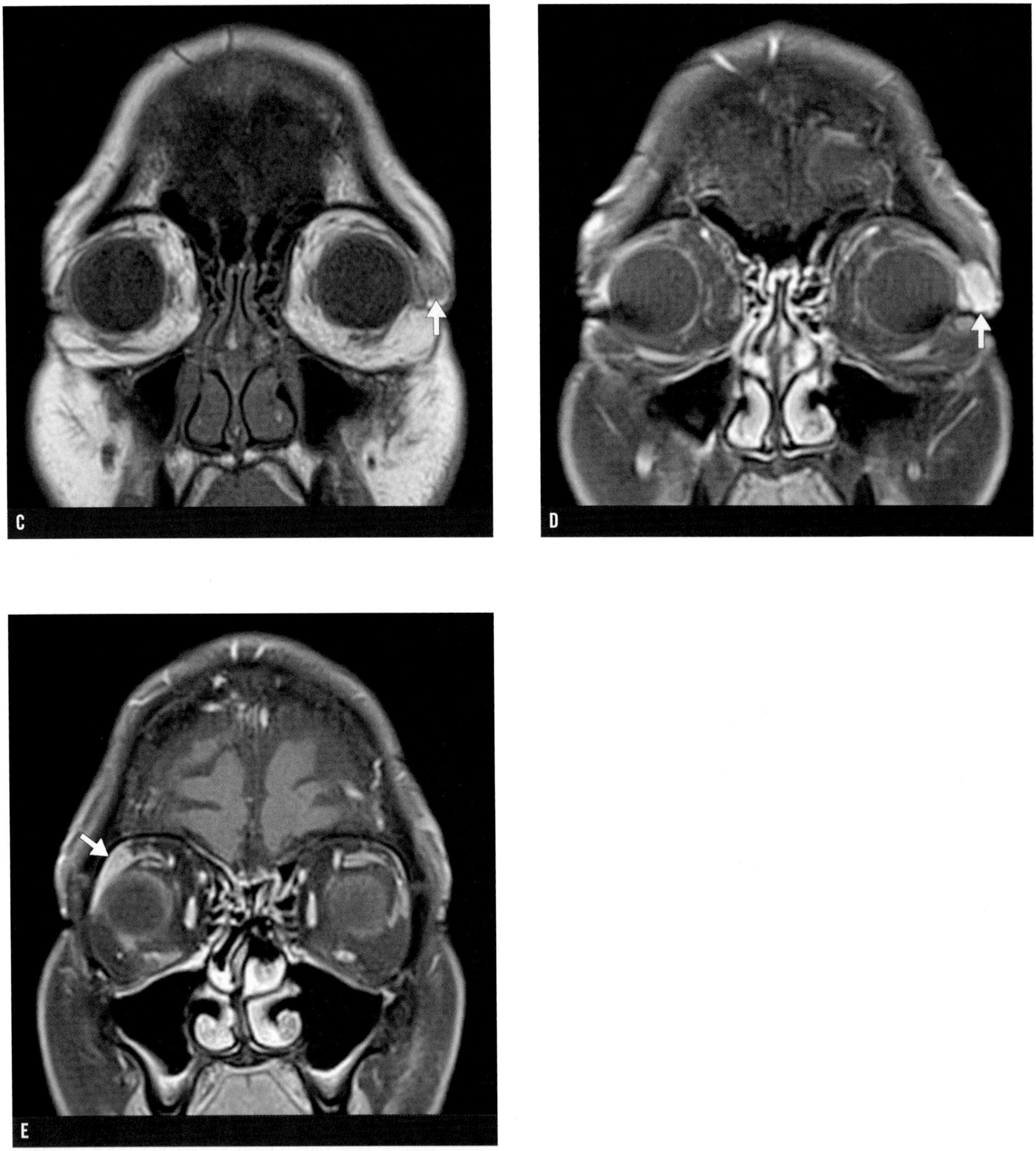
C
D
E

Companion case: Subconjunctival orbital fat prolapse

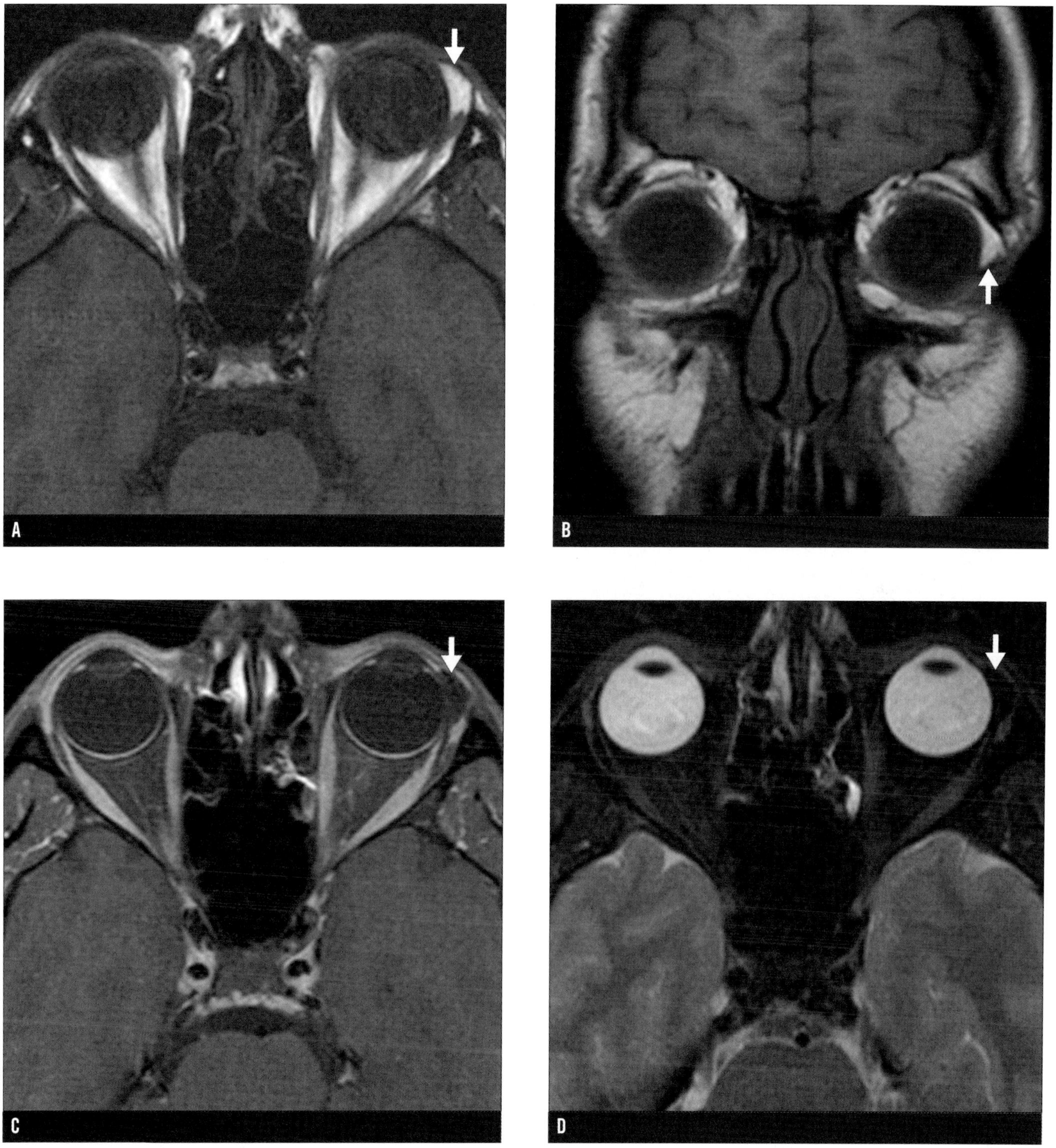

Axial T1 (**A**), coronal T1 (**B**), contrast-enhanced axial T1 with fat suppression (**C**), and axial T2 with fat suppression (**D**) MR images of a patient who presents with a "mass of the left lacrimal gland." There is a T1 hyperintense, circumscribed lesion along the temporal and superotemporal aspect of the left globe (arrows, **A**, **B**). This finding fully suppresses on fat suppressed imaging, in keeping with normal fat that has prolapsed into the subconjunctiva of the globe (arrows, **C**, **D**).

Companion case: Symmetric lacrimal gland enlargement due to a chronic disease state: chronic alcohol abuse

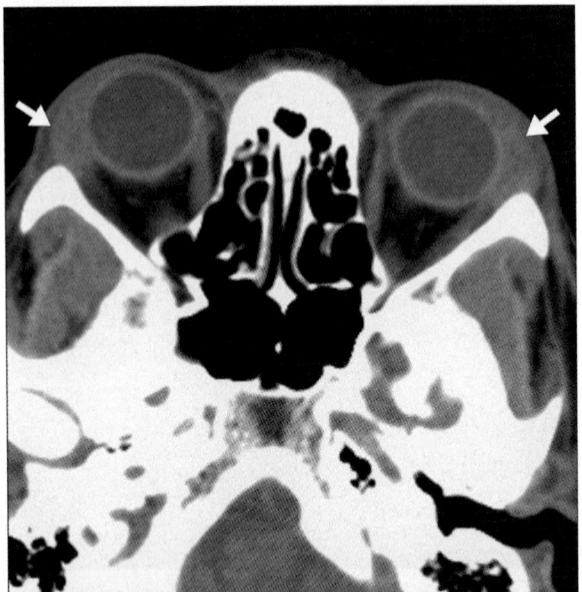

A

An axial CT image (**A**) demonstrates symmetrically enlarged, homogenous lacrimal glands in a patient who has a history of alcohol abuse. While nonspecific, symmetrically enlarged lacrimal glands are often present in patients who have a history of a chronic disease state, such as chronic alcohol abuse.

Companion case: Symmetric lacrimal gland enlargement due to a chronic disease state: diabetes mellitus

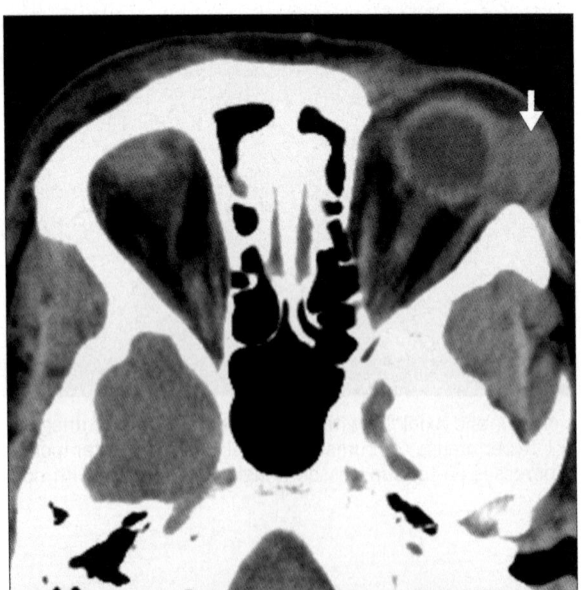

A

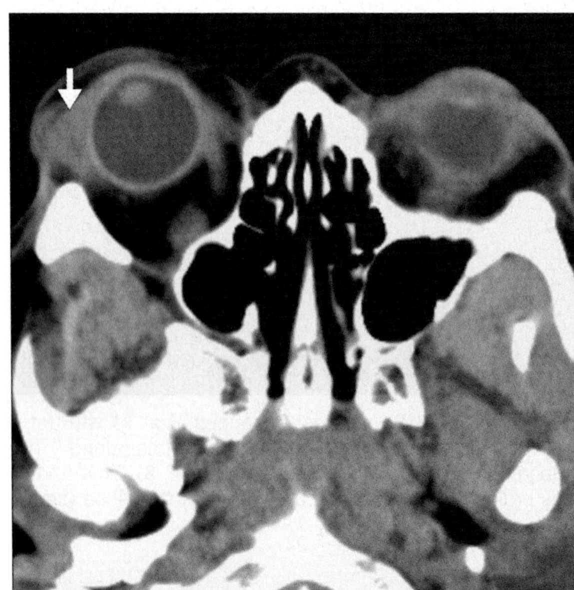

B

Axial CT images (**A**, **B**) demonstrate enlarged lacrimal glands in a patient with diabetes mellitus (arrows, **A**, **B**). These findings were stable on a CT scan performed 5 years earlier (not shown).

Companion case: Sjögren syndrome

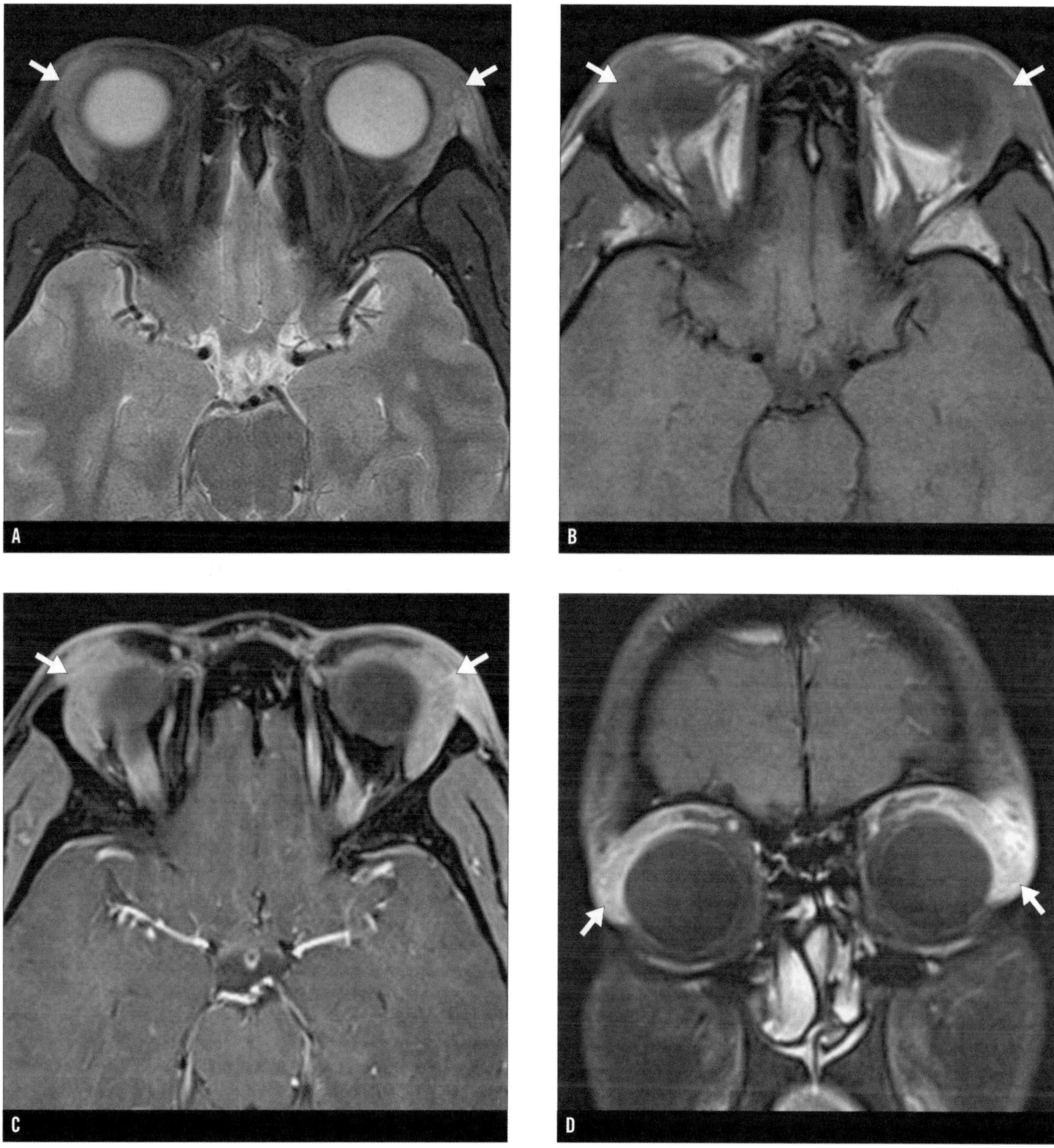

Axial T2 with fat suppression (**A**), axial T1 (**B**), postcontrast fat-suppressed axial T1 (**C**), and postcontrast fat-suppressed coronal T1 (**D**) MR images demonstrate symmetric enlargement of the lacrimal glands (arrows, **A**-**D**). These findings are nonspecific and can be present in several entities. One of the lacrimal glands from this patient was biopsied and demonstrated pathologic findings consistent with Sjögren syndrome.

Companion case: Lymphoma

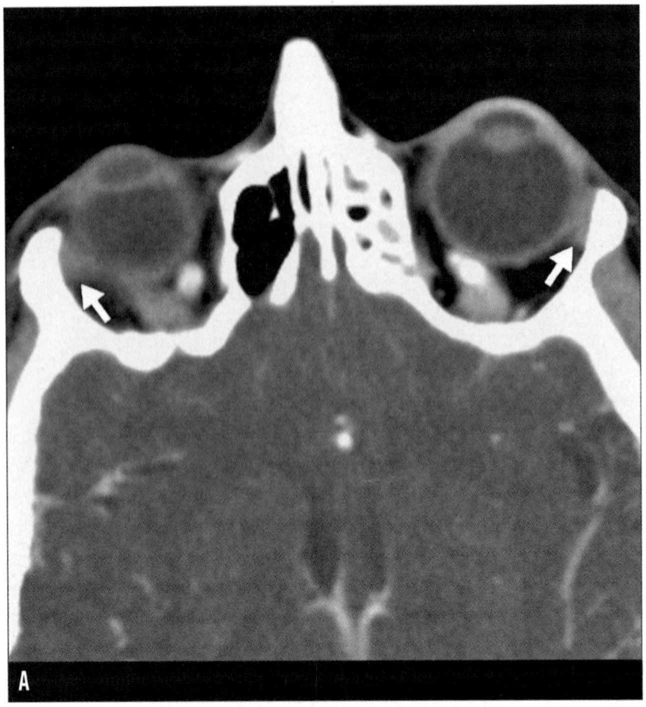

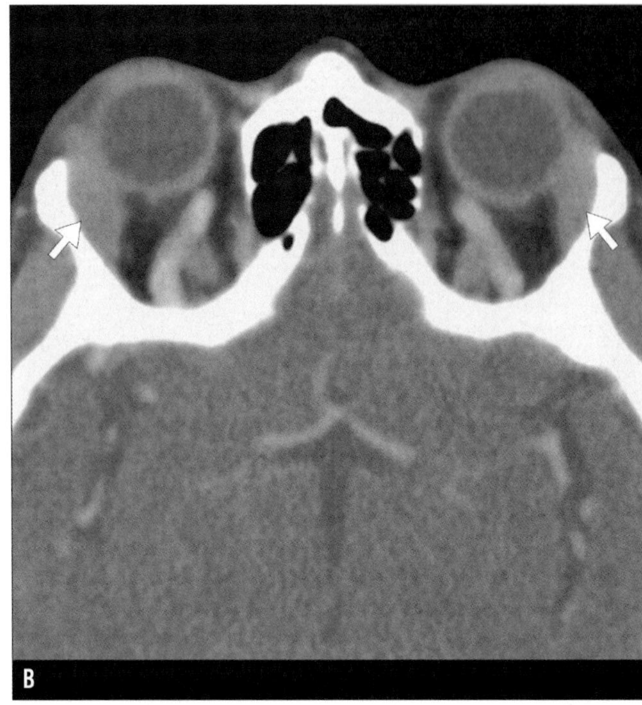

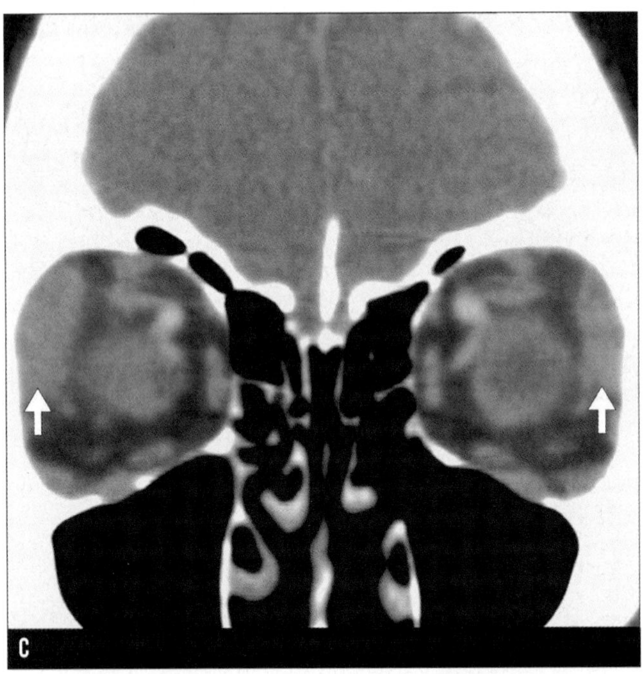

A contrast-enhanced axial CT image (**A**) demonstrates normal-sized lacrimal glands (arrows, **A**). Five years later, contrast-enhanced axial (**B**) and coronal reformatted (**C**) CT images demonstrate marked, diffuse enlargement of the lacrimal glands (arrows, **B**, **C**). This patient had extensive systemic lymphoma. The findings on images **B** and **C** are concordant with lymphomatous infiltration of the lacrimal glands.

Companion case: Pleomorphic adenoma

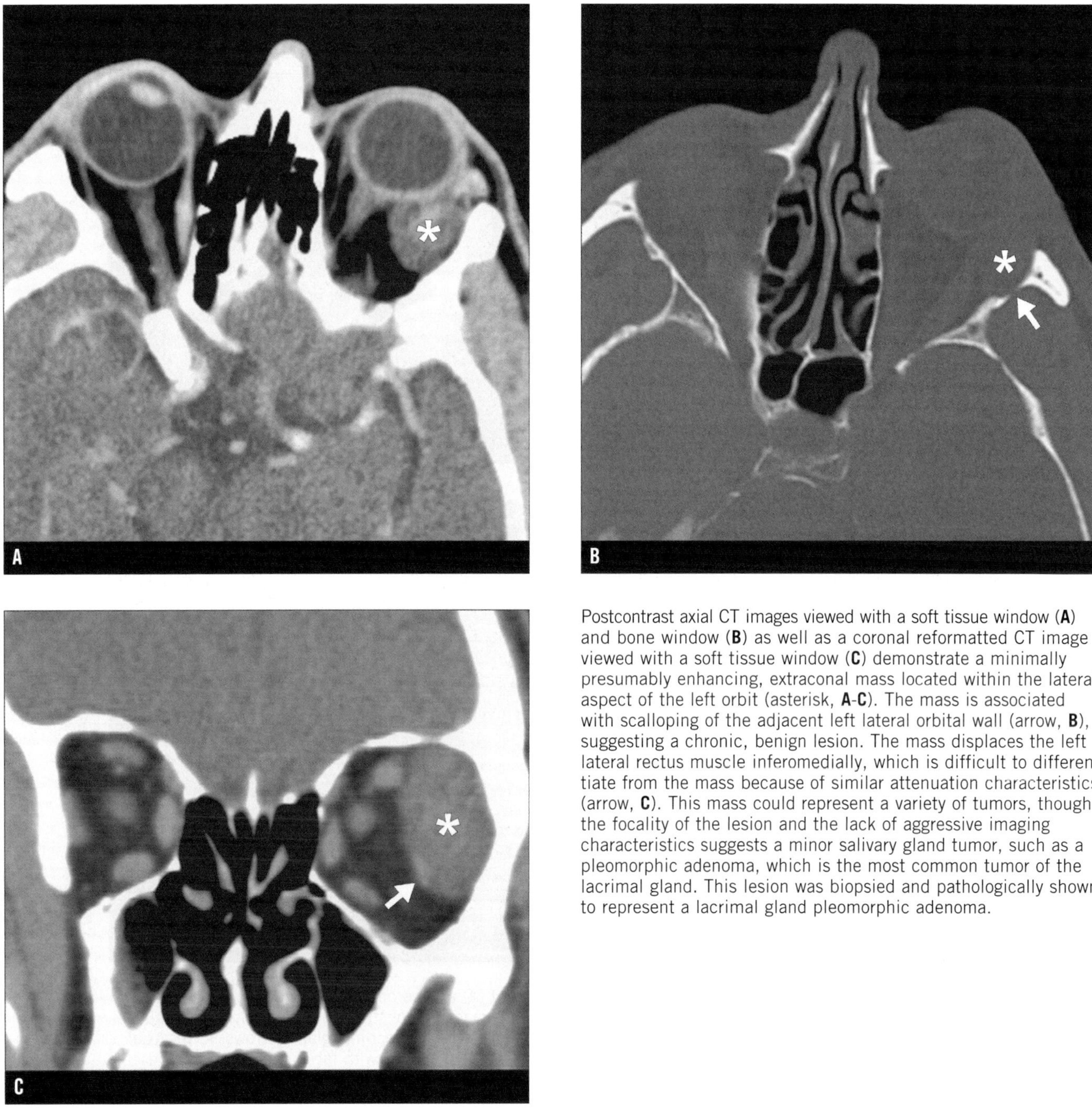

Postcontrast axial CT images viewed with a soft tissue window (**A**) and bone window (**B**) as well as a coronal reformatted CT image viewed with a soft tissue window (**C**) demonstrate a minimally presumably enhancing, extraconal mass located within the lateral aspect of the left orbit (asterisk, **A**-**C**). The mass is associated with scalloping of the adjacent left lateral orbital wall (arrow, **B**), suggesting a chronic, benign lesion. The mass displaces the left lateral rectus muscle inferomedially, which is difficult to differentiate from the mass because of similar attenuation characteristics (arrow, **C**). This mass could represent a variety of tumors, though the focality of the lesion and the lack of aggressive imaging characteristics suggests a minor salivary gland tumor, such as a pleomorphic adenoma, which is the most common tumor of the lacrimal gland. This lesion was biopsied and pathologically shown to represent a lacrimal gland pleomorphic adenoma.

Companion case: Adenoid cystic carcinoma

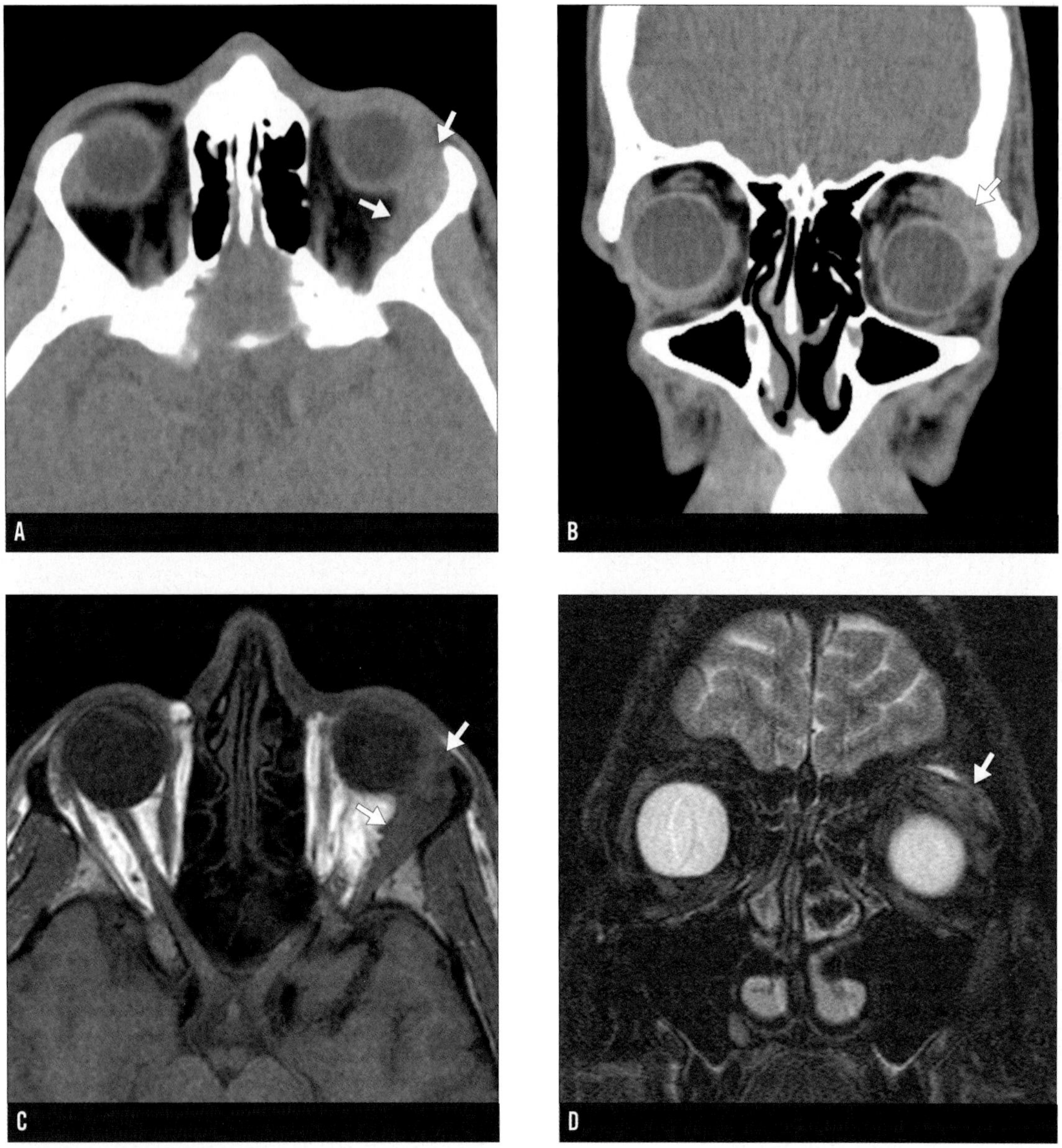

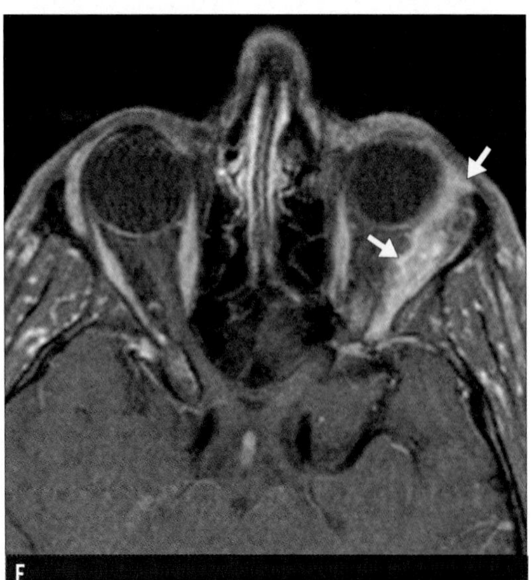

Axial (**A**) and coronal reformatted (**B**) unenhanced CT images demonstrate diffuse, asymmetric enlargement of the left lacrimal gland (arrows, **A**, **B**). Axial T1 (**C**), coronal T2 with fat suppression (**D**), and contrast-enhanced axial T1 with fat suppression (**E**) MR images demonstrate diffuse, abnormal enhancement of the left lacrimal gland with irregular, ill-defined margins, in this case representing left lacrimal gland adenoid cystic carcinoma (arrows, **C**-**D**).

Companion case: Adenocarcinoma

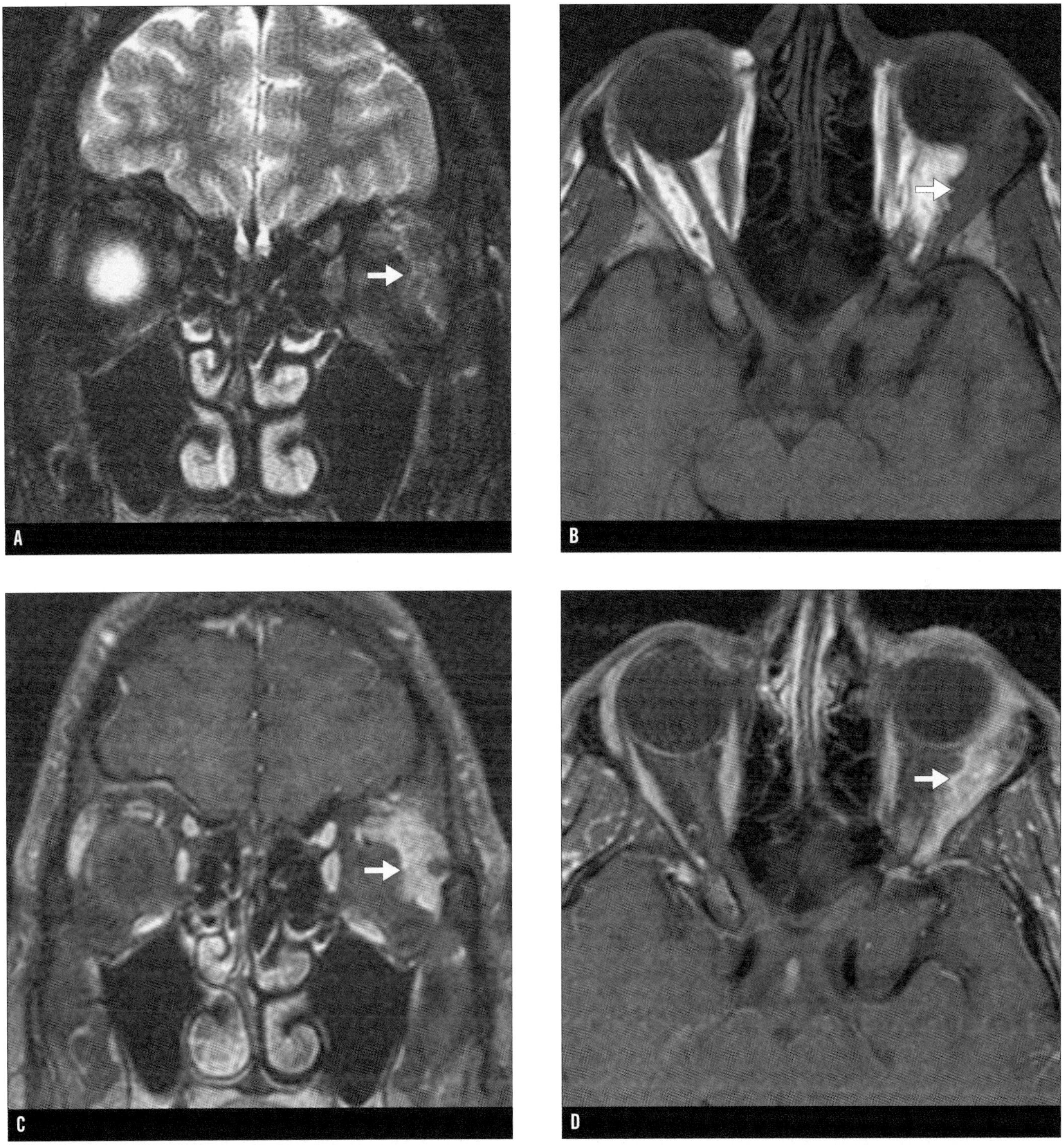

Coronal T2 with fat suppression (**A**), axial T1 (**B**), and postcontrast coronal T1 with fat suppression (**C**) and postcontrast axial T1 with fat suppression (**D**) MR images demonstrate an irregularly marginated, extraconal mass located in the superolateral aspect of the left orbit that arises from the left lacrimal gland. Relative to the extraocular muscles, the mass is T1 isointense (arrow, **B**), heterogeneous but primarily hypointense on T2 (arrow, **A**), and avidly enhances following contrast administration (arrows, **C**, **D**). The left lateral rectus muscle is inseparable from the mass. The patient underwent an orbital exenteration, and pathology demonstrated primary lacrimal gland invasive adenocarcinoma. The irregular margins and the heterogeneous T2 signal characteristics help differentiate this aggressive neoplasm from a benign minor salivary gland tumor of the lacrimal gland.

Companion case: Metastatic disease to the lacrimal gland

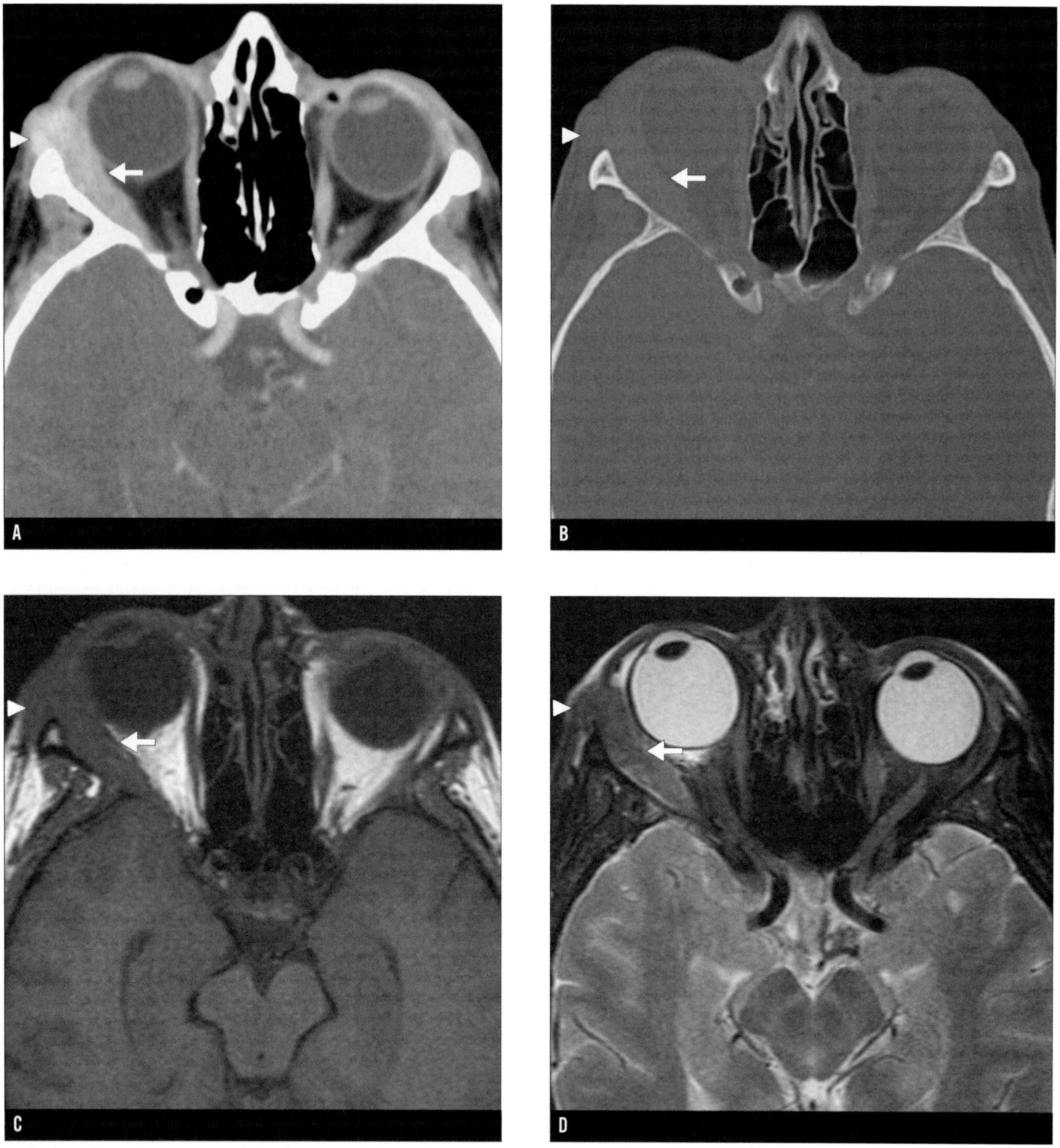

Postcontrast axial CT images viewed with a soft tissue window (**A**) and bone window (**B**) as well as axial T1 (**C**), fat-suppressed axial T2 (**D**), postcontrast fat-suppressed axial T1 (**E**), and postcontrast fat-suppressed coronal T1 (**F**) MR images were obtained on a 57-year-old woman with a history of breast cancer complaining of new onset right orbital pain and proptosis. Imaging demonstrates mild right globe proptosis resulting from an irregularly marginated, enhancing mass involving the right lacrimal gland (arrows, **A-F**) and extending anterolateral relative to the lateral right orbital wall (arrowheads, **A-F**). The mass is inseparable from the right lateral rectus muscle. Numerous intracranial and osseous metastases were also present (not shown). Given the imaging findings and clinical context, the findings are consistent with a metastases to the right lacrimal gland.

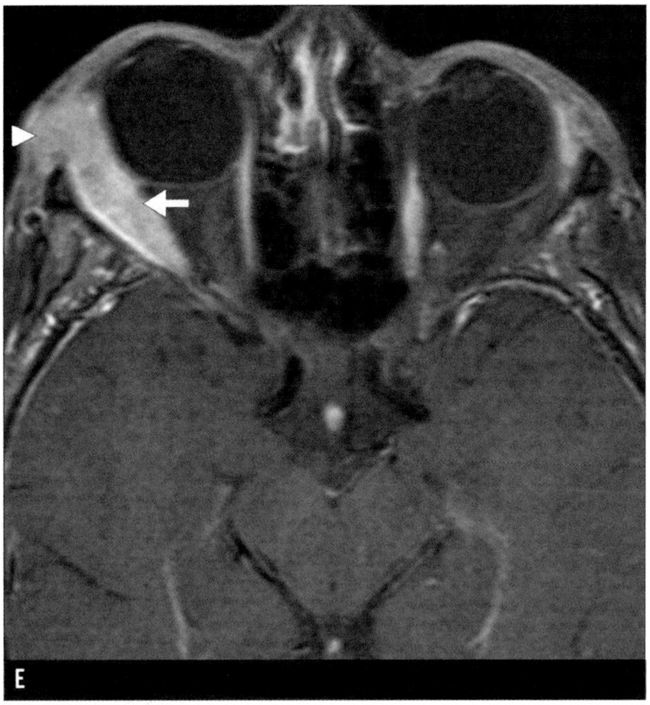

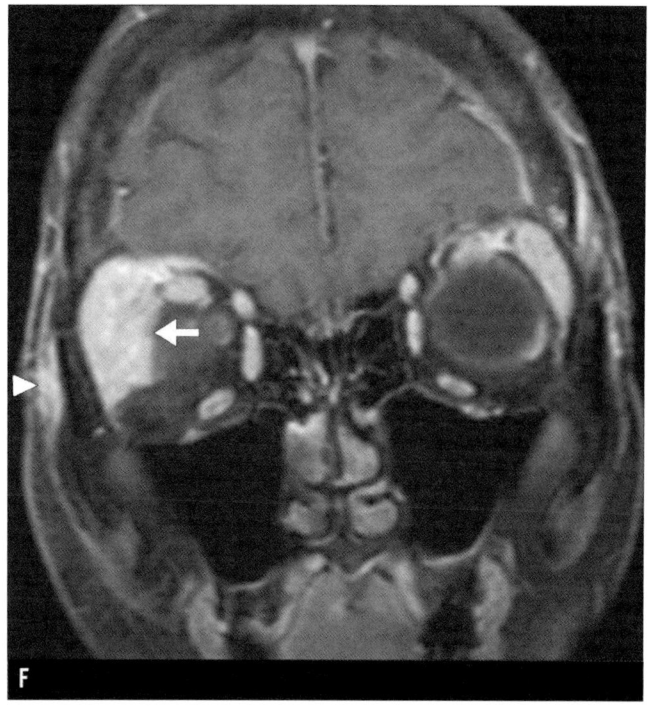

REFERENCES

Andreoli MT, Aakalu V, Setabutr. Epidemiological Trends in Malignant Lacrimal Gland Tumors. *Otolaryng Head Neck.* 2015;152(2):279-283.

Friedhofer H, et al. Lacrimal Gland Prolapse: Management During Aesthetic Blepharoplasty: review of the Literature and Case Reports. *Aesth Plast Surg.* 2009;33:647-653.

Guggenheimer J, Close JM, Eghtesad B. Sialadenosis in patients with advanced liver disease. *Head Neck Pathol.* 2009;3(2):100-105. Epub March 2009.

Gündüz K, Shields CL, Günalp I, Shields JA. Magnetic resonance imaging of unilateral lacrimal gland lesions. *Graefes Arch Clin Exp Ophthalmol.* 2003;241(11):907-913. Epub October 2003.

Heaps RS, Miller NR, Albert DM, Green WR, Vitale S. Primary adenocarcinoma of the lacrimal gland. A retrospective study. *Ophthalmology.* 1993;100(12):1856-1860.

Izumi M, et al. MR features of the lacrimal gland in Sjögren's syndrome. *AJR Am J Roentgenol.* 1998;170(6):1661-1666.

Kim E, et al. Subconjunctival fat prolapse and dermolipoma of the orbit: differentiation on CT and MRI imaging. *Am J Neuroradiol.* 2011;32:465-467.

Mafee MF, Edward DP, Koeller KK, Dorodi S. Lacrimal gland tumors and simulating lesions. Clinicopathologic and MR imaging features. *Radiol Clin North Am.* 1999;37(1):219-239, xii.

Mallen-St. Clair, J, et al. Epidemiology and treatment of lacrimal gland tumors: a population-based cohort analysis. *JAMA Otolaryngol Head Neck Surg.* 2014;140(12):1110-1116.

Mandel L, Vakkas J, Saqi A. Alcoholic (beer) sialosis. *J Oral Maxillofac Surg.* 2005;63(3):402-405.

Massry GG. Prevalence of lacrimal gland prolapse in the functional blepharoplasty population. *Ophthal Plast Reconstr Surg.* 2011;27(6):410-413.

McNab AA. Subconjunctival fat prolapse. *Aust Nz J Ophthal.* 1999;27:33-36.

Morley AMS, Malhotra R. Subconjunctival prolapse of the palpebral lobe of the lacrimal gland occurring in association with occult orbital fat herniation. *Orbit.* 2009;28(6):430-432.

Prabhakaran VC, et al. Lesions mimicking lacrimal gland pleomorphic adenoma. *Br J Ophthalmol.* 2010;94(11):1509-1512.

Shields JA, Shields CL, Brotman HK, Carvalho C, Perez N, Eagle RC Jr. Cancer metastatic to the orbit: the 2000 Robert M. Curts Lecture. *Ophthal Plast Reconstr Surg.* 2001;17(5):346-354.

Shields JA, Shields CL, Epstein JA, Scartozzi R, Eagle RC Jr. Review: primary epithelial malignancies of the lacrimal gland: the 2003 Ramon L. Font lecture. *Ophthal Plast Reconstr Surg.* 2004;20(1):10-21.

Tamboli DA, Harris MA, Hogg JP, Realini T, Sivak-Callcott JA. Computed tomography dimensions of the lacrimal gland in normal Caucasian orbits. *Ophthal Plast Reconstr Surg.* 2011;27(6):453-456.

Tonami H, Matoba M, Yokota H, Higashi K, Yamamoto I, Sugai S. CT and MR findings of bilateral lacrimal gland enlargement in Sjögren syndrome. *Clin Imaging.* 2002;26(6):392-396.

Ueno H, Ariji E, Izumi M, Uetani M, Hayashi K, Nakamura T. MR imaging of the lacrimal gland. Age-related and gender-dependent changes in size and structure. *Acta Radiol.* 1996;37(5):714-719.

Vaidhyanath R, et al. Lacrimal fossa lesions: pictorial review of CT and MRI features. *Orbit.* 2008;27:410-418.

Viana GAP, et al. Prolapsed orbital fat: 15 consecutive cases. *Scan J Plast Reconstr Surg Hand Surg.* 2009;43:330-334.

Vlachostergios PJ, Voutsadakis IA, Papandreou CN. Orbital metastasis of breast carcinoma. *Breast Cancer (Auckl).* 2009;3:91-97.

Von Holstein SL, et al. Epithelial tumors of the lacrimal gland: a clinical, histopathological, surgical and oncological survey. *Acta Ophthalmol.* 2013;91:195-206.

Wright JE, Rose GE, and Garner A. Primary malignant neoplasms of the lacrimal gland. *Br J Ophthalmol.* 1992;76(7):401-407.

CASE 17 Normal variation in size of the superior ophthalmic vein

The superior ophthalmic vein (SOV) is a valveless vein responsible for the majority of the orbital venous drainage. The course of the SOV is remarkably constant. It arises from the confluence of the supraorbital and angular veins, extends posteriorly within the superior aspect of the orbit, through the superior orbital fissure, and ultimately terminates in the cavernous sinus. While its course is predictable, the normal SOV can exhibit great variability in diameter, ranging from 2 mm up to 1 cm in some literature.

The Monroe-Kellie doctrine states that the sum of the brain, CSF, and intracranial blood volume is constant. Therefore, if the brain volume is not altered, a decrease in CSF volume will result in an increase in the amount of intracranial blood volume. This is readily observed in the setting of intracranial hypotension which results in a decrease in CSF volume but engorgement of intracranial venous structures. Thus, one would logically conclude that the SOV, being valveless, would enlarge in the setting of intracranial hypotension and decrease in caliber with intracranial hypertension. However, there is discrepant literature describing the effects of intracranial pressure as they relate to the caliber of the SOV. A study by Chen CC et al studied the size of the SOV with ultrasound in patients with intracranial hypotension and did find an increase in the caliber of the SOV in this setting. Conversely, a study by Chen WT et al found a decrease in SOV caliber in patients with intracranial hypotension and a study by Rohr et al found an increase in SOV caliber with secondary intracranial hypertension. Clearly, further investigation is needed and other factors may account for the discrepant conclusions of these studies. Nevertheless, one must always consider an underlying pathologic process when confronted with abnormally enlarged SOVs (particularly when asymmetric), including a venous varix, cavernous sinus thrombosis, carotid-cavernous fistula, and cavernous sinus meningioma/schwannoma.

COMPANION CASES

- **Orbital venous varix.** An orbital venous varix refers to venous enlargement which is believed to arise from congenital weakness of the orbital vein wall. Because of free communication with the venous system, an orbital varix may enlarge with increases in venous pressure secondary to coughing, bending forward, or breath holding, sometimes resulting in a "stress proptosis" when large. Varices may also thrombose and undergo hemorrhage, sometimes leading to a rapid onset of painful, sustained proptosis. Often, a venous varix will enlarge and enhance more intensely on postcontrast CT imaging if the patient is placed in a prone position and performs a Valsalva maneuver during the imaging.
- **Superior ophthalmic vein thrombosis.** SOV thrombosis is most commonly secondary to an infectious process, such as sinusitis or a facial infection. The thrombosis within the SOV may extend posteriorly and result in cavernous sinus thrombosis. Patients may present with a multitude of symptoms, such as orbital pain, proptosis, visual changes, periorbital edema, chemosis (conjunctival edema), cranial nerve palsies, and headache. On CT and MRI, thrombosis of the SOV and cavernous sinus often result in enlargement of these structures and accompanied by vascular engorgement of the extraocular muscles, exophthalmos, and periorbital edema. On contrast-enhanced studies, filling defects may be apparent in the SOV and/or cavernous sinus.
- **Carotid-cavernous fistula.** A carotid-cavernous (CC) fistula may occur spontaneously or be the result of trauma, surgery, or atherosclerosis. The gradient of flow occurs from the high-flow internal carotid artery to the low-flow cavernous sinus. The increased venous pressure is transmitted to the orbital venous system, in particular the SOV. The elevated venous pressure results in ipsilateral orbital inflammation/chemosis, pulsatile proptosis, and frequently an audible bruit by auscultation. On imaging, typically unilateral SOV and ipsilateral cavernous sinus enlargement is identified by CT or MRI. On CT, the arterialized veins may be more hyperattenuating with contrast than the veins unaffected by the fistula, a helpful imaging finding if present. Time-resolved MR imaging will usually reveal arteriovenous shunting, which can be confirmed with catheter angiography, if necessary. Catheter angiography has the added benefit of providing a means for lesion embolization.

Normal variation in size of the superior ophthalmic vein

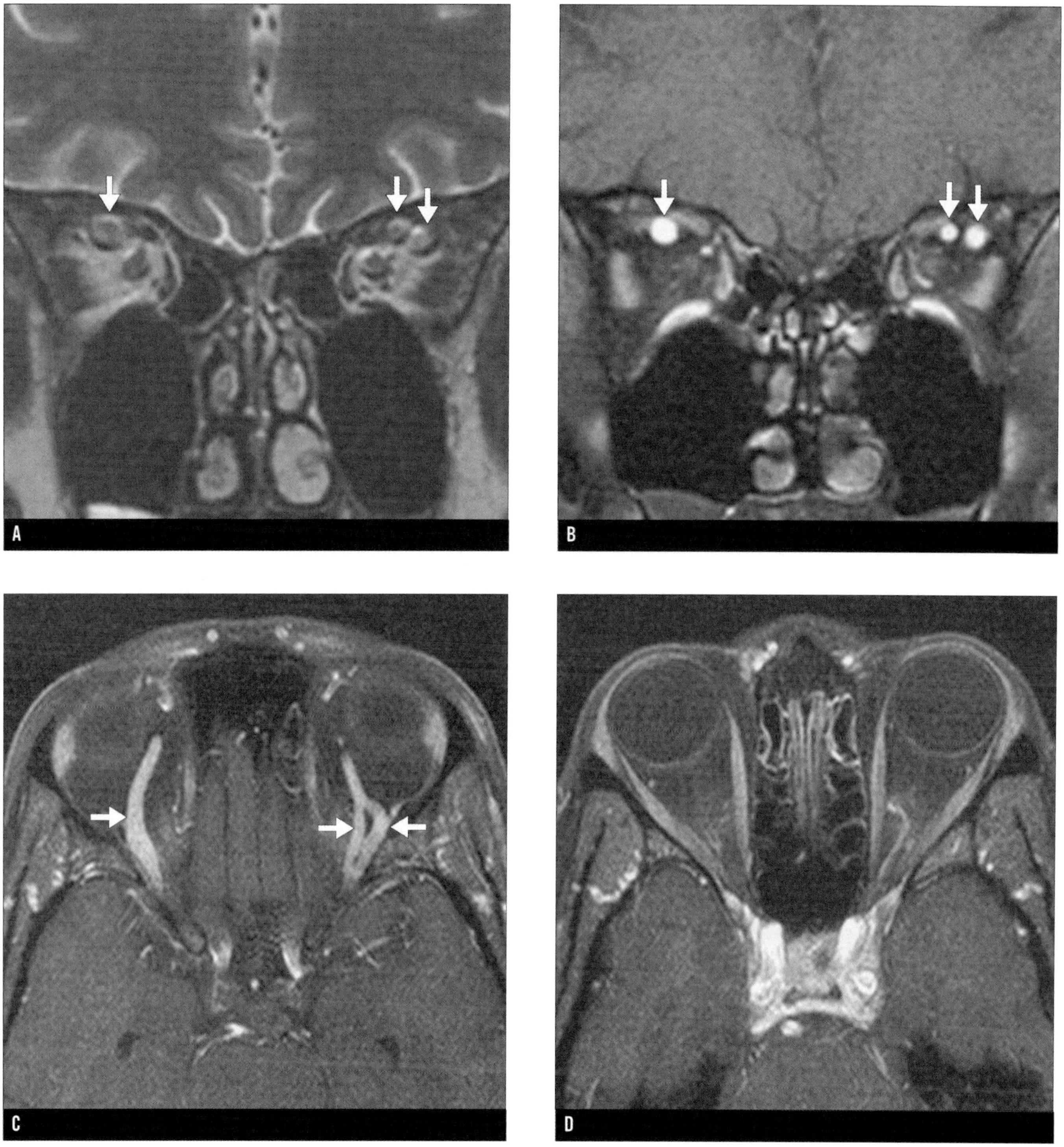

Coronal T2 (**A**) as well as coronal (**B**) and axial (**C**, **D**) fat-suppressed postcontrast T1-weighted MR images demonstrate enlargement of the bilateral SOVs (arrows, **A**-**C**), with the right SOV larger than the left and an incidental fenestration of the left SOV (arrows, **C**). The cavernous sinus is symmetric, there is no abnormal tangle of vessels in the region of the cavernous sinus or adjacent brain, no imaging evidence of proptosis, and the patient did not have a clinical history of a painful, red eye or an orbital bruit. The normal SOV can be variable in size. Furthermore, an asymmetrically enlarged SOV can be a normal finding; however, when encountered, findings to explain the finding (ie, carotid-cavernous fistula, cavernous sinus thrombosis, etc) should be excluded.

Companion case: Small orbital venous varix

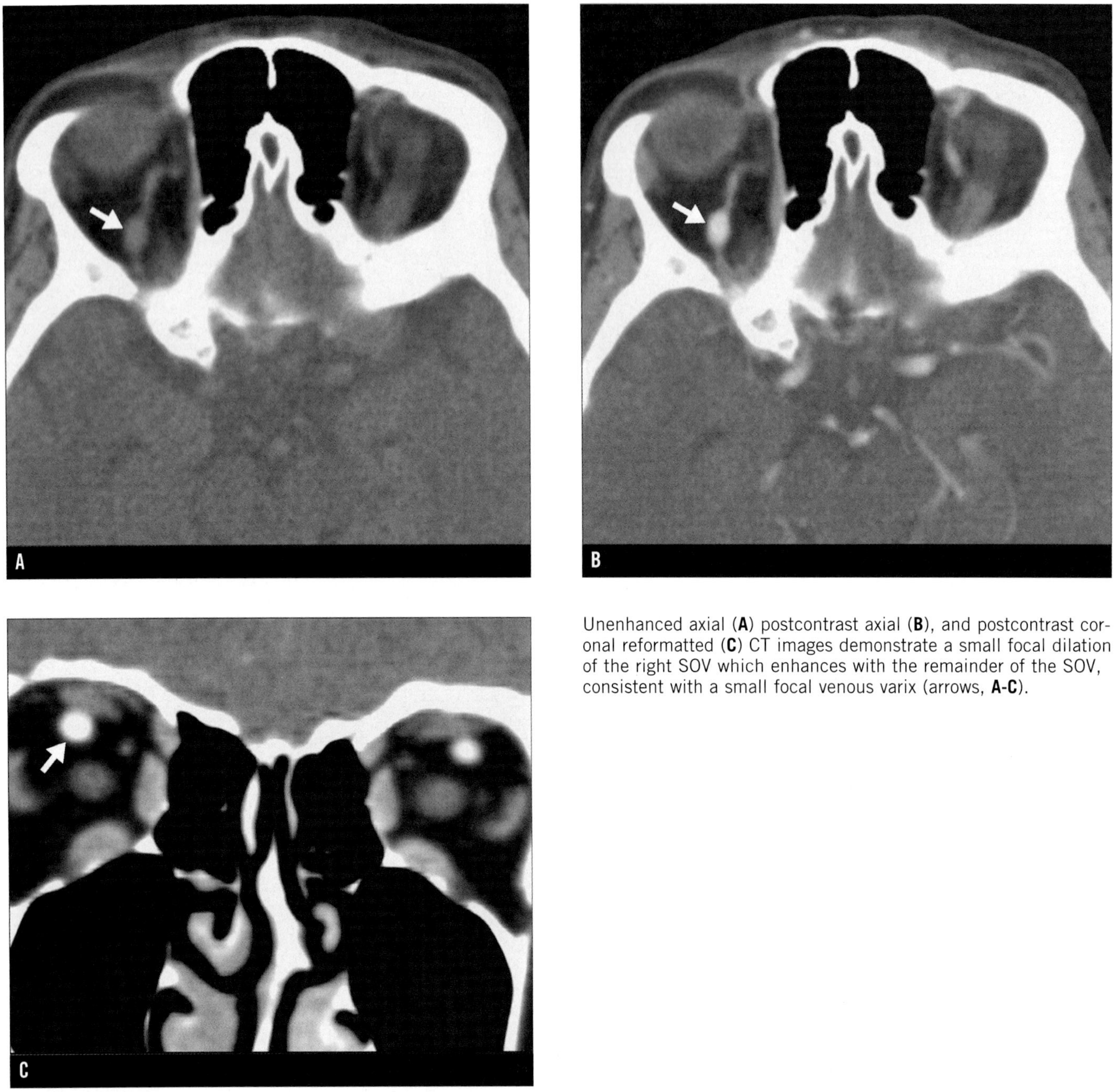

Unenhanced axial (**A**) postcontrast axial (**B**), and postcontrast coronal reformatted (**C**) CT images demonstrate a small focal dilation of the right SOV which enhances with the remainder of the SOV, consistent with a small focal venous varix (arrows, **A-C**).

Companion case: Large orbital venous varix

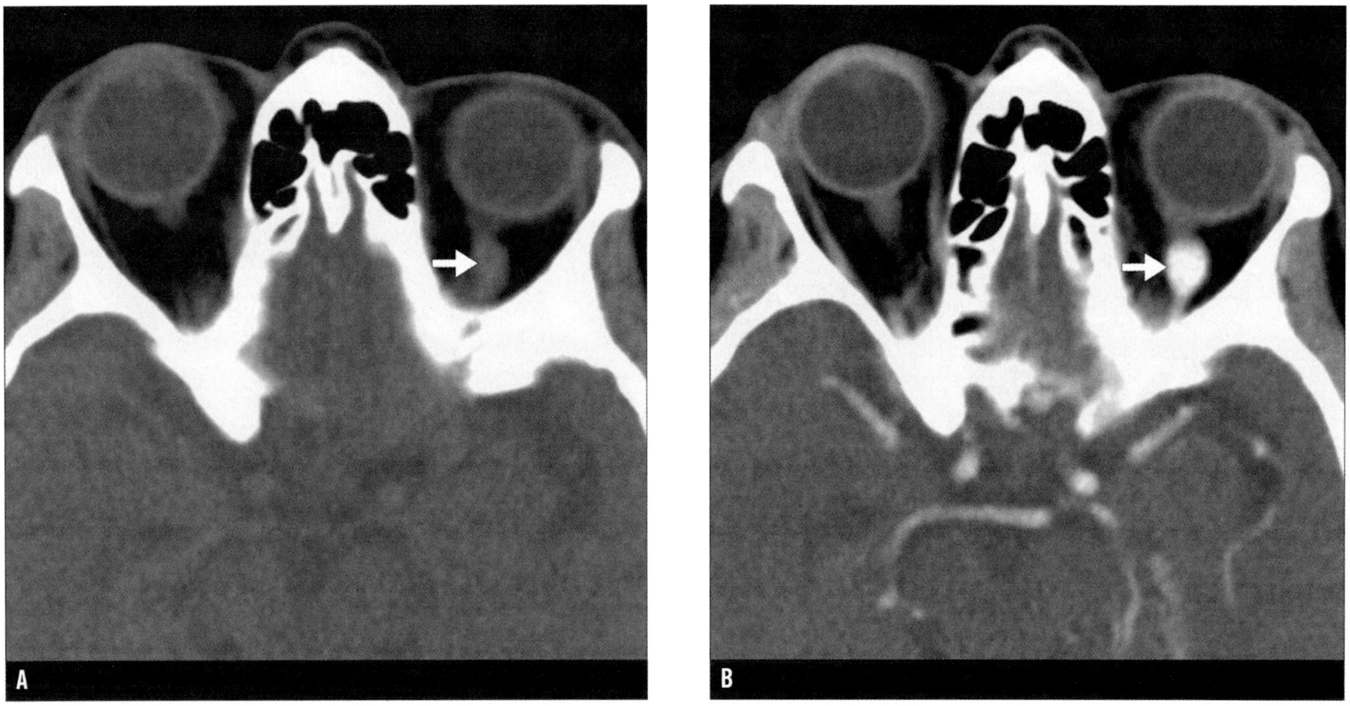

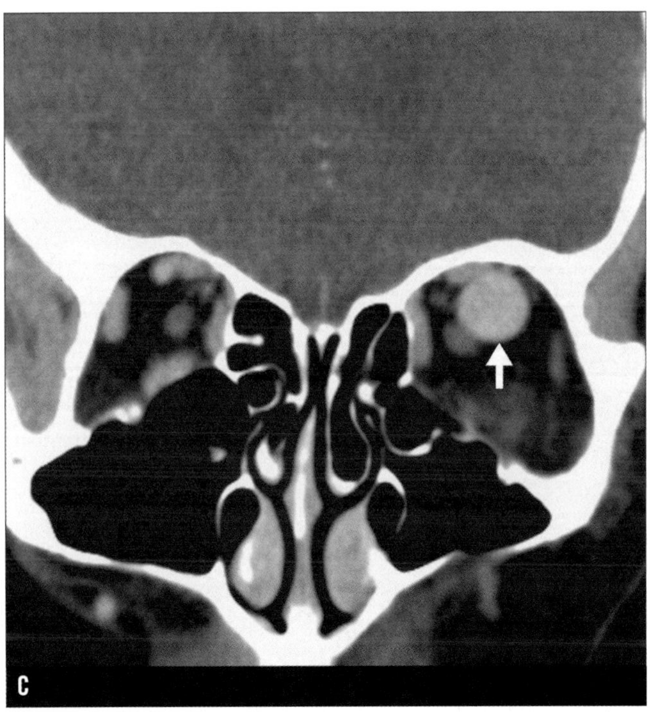

Unenhanced axial (**A**) and contrast-enhanced axial (**B**) CT images performed while the patient was in the supine position demonstrate mild enlargement with enhancement of the left SOV (arrows, **A**, **B**). A contrast-enhanced direct coronal CT image from the same study obtained while the patient was in the prone position (**C**) demonstrates significant enlargement of the left SOV, compatible with an orbital varix (arrow, **C**). Typically, placing the patient in a prone position and/or imaging during a Valsalva maneuver will enlarge an orbital varix.

Companion case: Superior ophthalmic vein thrombosis

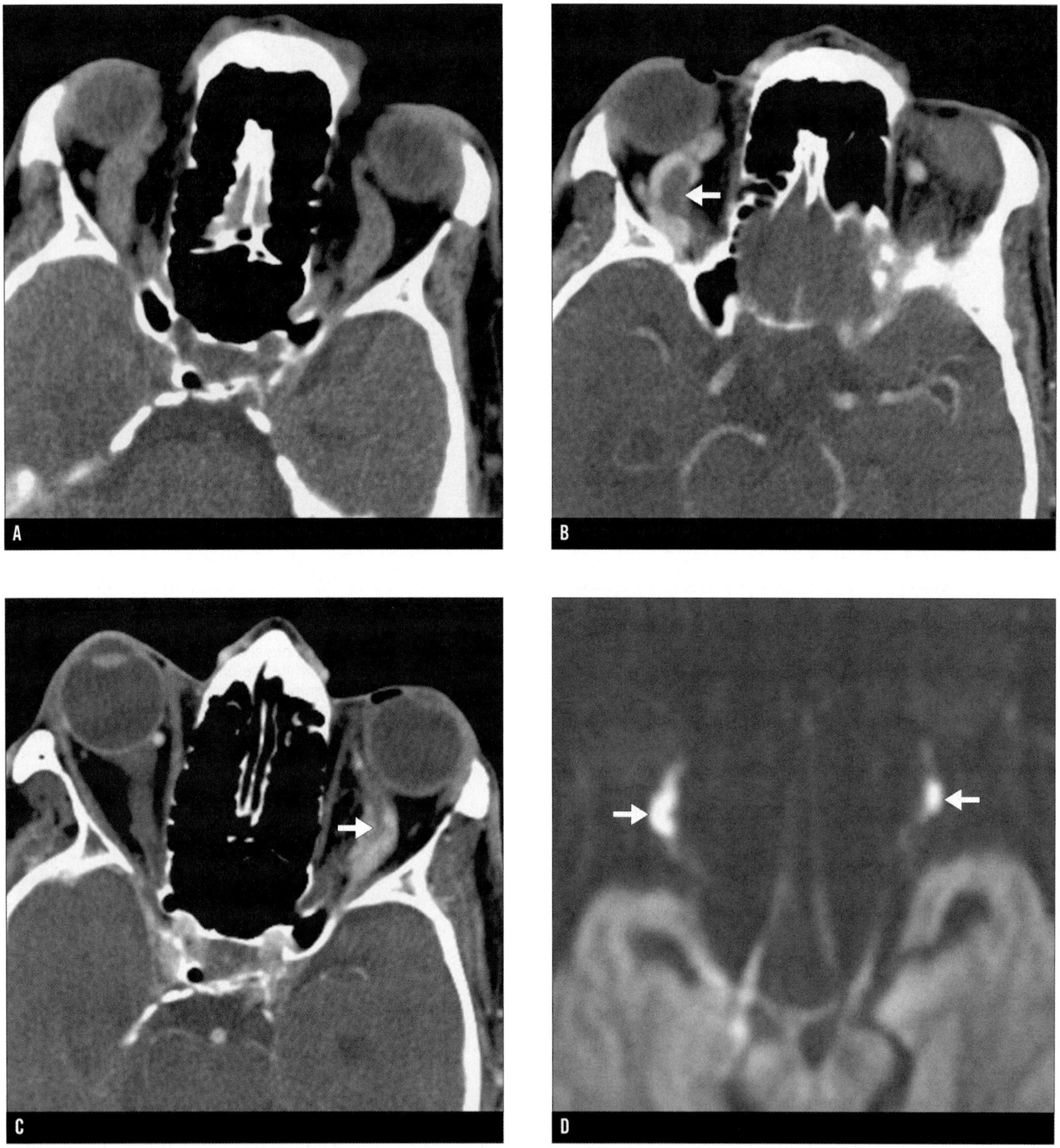

Unenhanced axial (**A**) as well as postcontrast axial (**B**, **C**) CT images demonstrate enlarged bilateral SOVs which contain a large amount of nonenhancing, nonocclusive thrombus centrally (arrows, **B**, **C**). Axial diffusion (**D**), axial ADC (**E**), axial T1 (**F**), axial T2 (**G**), and postcontrast axial MPRAGE (**H**) MR images of the same patient demonstrate the MR appearance of partial SOV thrombosis. Restricted diffusion within a thrombus may sometimes be evident, as is present in this case (arrows, **D**, **E**). The thrombus is intrinsically hyperintense on T1 (**F**) and heterogeneously hyperintense on T2 (**G**), compatible with the presence of late subacute methemoglobin. The thrombus does not enhance on the postcontrast images in this particular case (arrows, **H**), although thrombus may enhance on MR imaging. With any case of SOV thrombosis, one should evaluate for any extension of the thrombus into the cavernous sinus, which is unremarkable in this patient on an axial MPRAGE MR image (**I**).

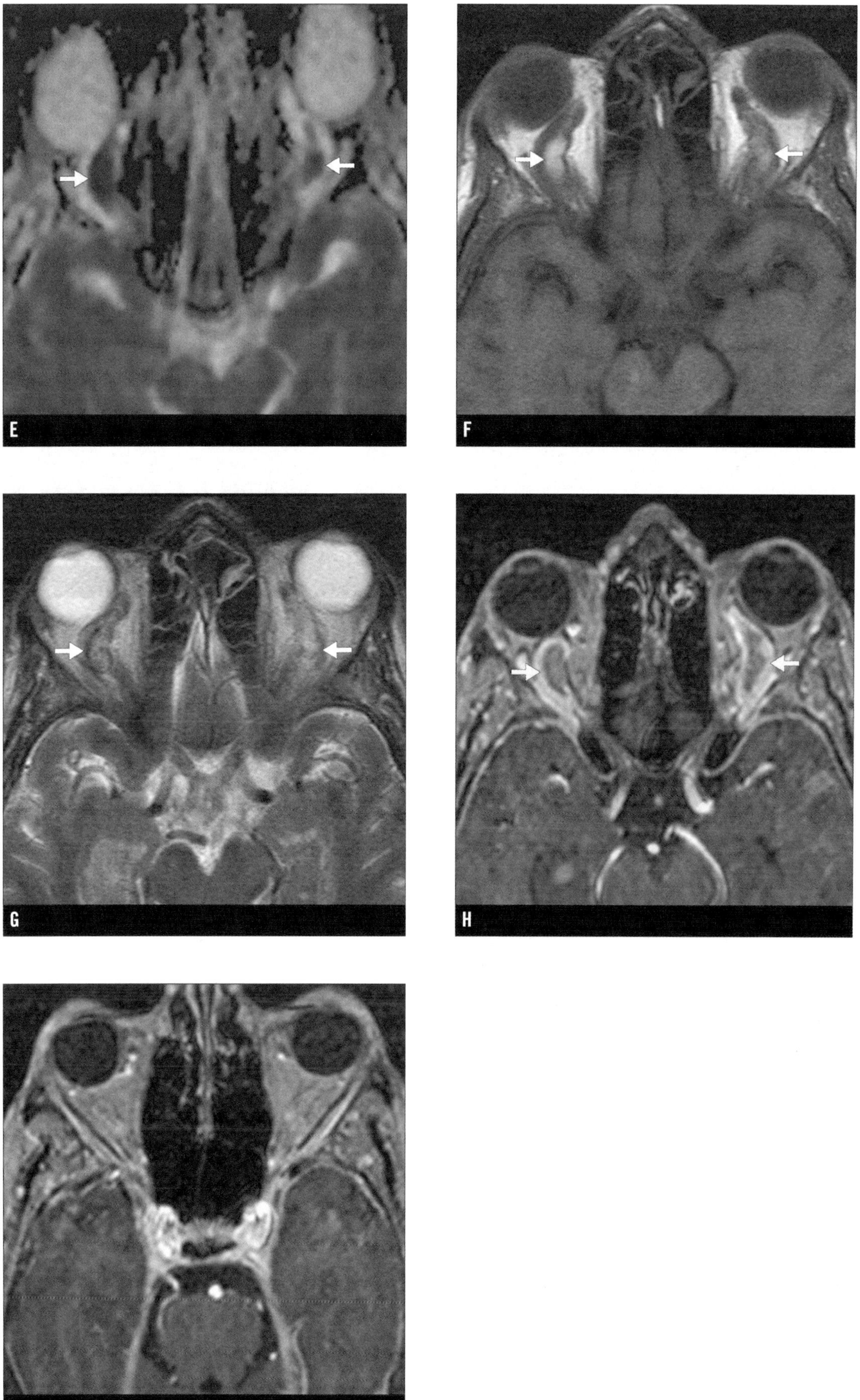
E
F
G
H
I

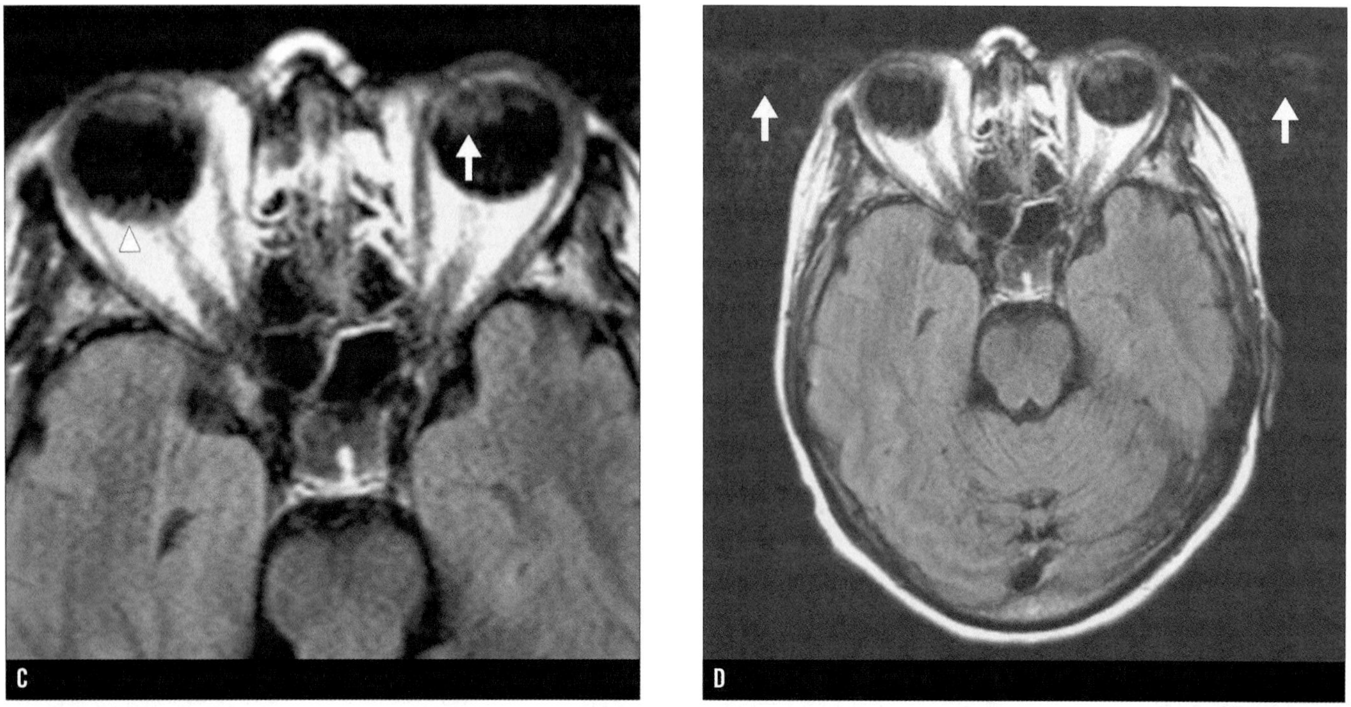

Globe and optic nerve sheath motion: Artifactual duplication of the optic nerve sheath

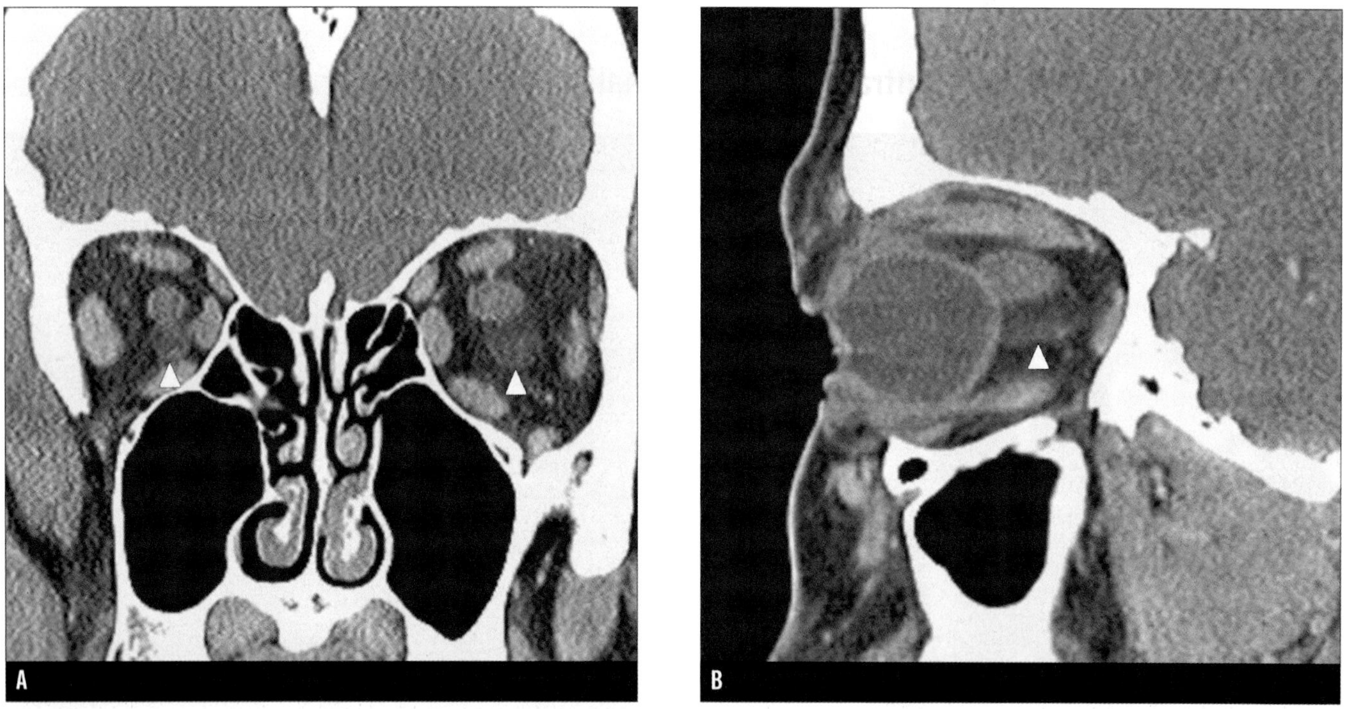

Unenhanced coronal reformatted (**A**) and reformatted (**B**) CT images demonstrate linear, apparent soft tissue density located inferior to and paralleling both optic nerve sheath complexes, simulating bilateral optic nerve sheath duplication (arrowheads, **A**, **B**). A T1-weighted MR image of the same patient (**C**) demonstrates a normal, single optic nerve sheath complex and normal retrobulbar fat (the other orbit is not shown but was also normal). The finding on CT was completely artifactual.

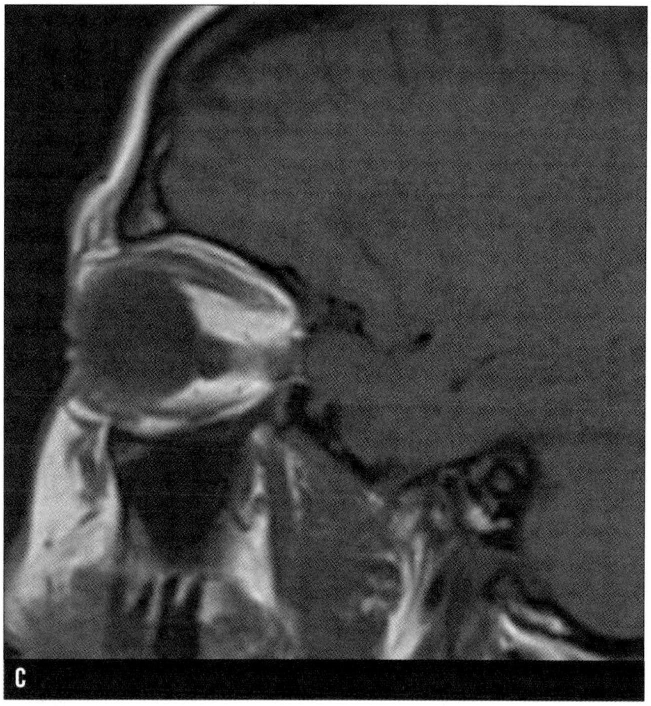

REFERENCES

Barrett JF, Keat N. Artifacts in CT: recognition and avoidance. *Radiographics.* 2004;24:1679-1691.

Herrick RC, et al. Artifacts and pitfalls in MR Imaging of the orbit: a clinical review. *Radiographics.* 1997;17:707-724.

Malhotra A, et al. Ocular anatomy and cross-sectional imaging of the eye. *Semin Ultrasound CT MR.* 2011;32(1):2-13.

CASE 19 Cosmetic MRI artifact

Mascara, eyeliner, and eye shadow cosmetics can be a source of artifact on MRI. This is the result of iron oxide pigments that are used in these products. These ferromagnetic substances cause local magnetic field heterogeneity, which results in image distortion and obscuration of regional structures, particularly at the anterior aspects of the orbits. The MR artifact of the ferromagnetic substances increases with increasing field strength.

In the setting of brain imaging, such artifact is usually of no consequence, although if an MRI is being performed specifically to evaluate for orbital pathology, it is worthwhile to advise the patient to forgo wearing makeup, particularly when an MRI is performed with a 3T magnet.

COMPANION CASE

- **Chemosis.** Chemosis (conjunctival edema) can be due to infection, such as conjunctivitis or episcleritis, and can result in both edema and enhancement on imaging. Inflammation secondary to allergy or chemical irritation is another common cause of chemosis. Rarer causes include inflammatory processes such as orbital pseudotumor or sarcoidosis, systemic processes such as thyroid ophthalmopathy, and vascular pathology such as a carotid-cavernous fistula or cavernous sinus thrombosis.

Cosmetic MRI artifact

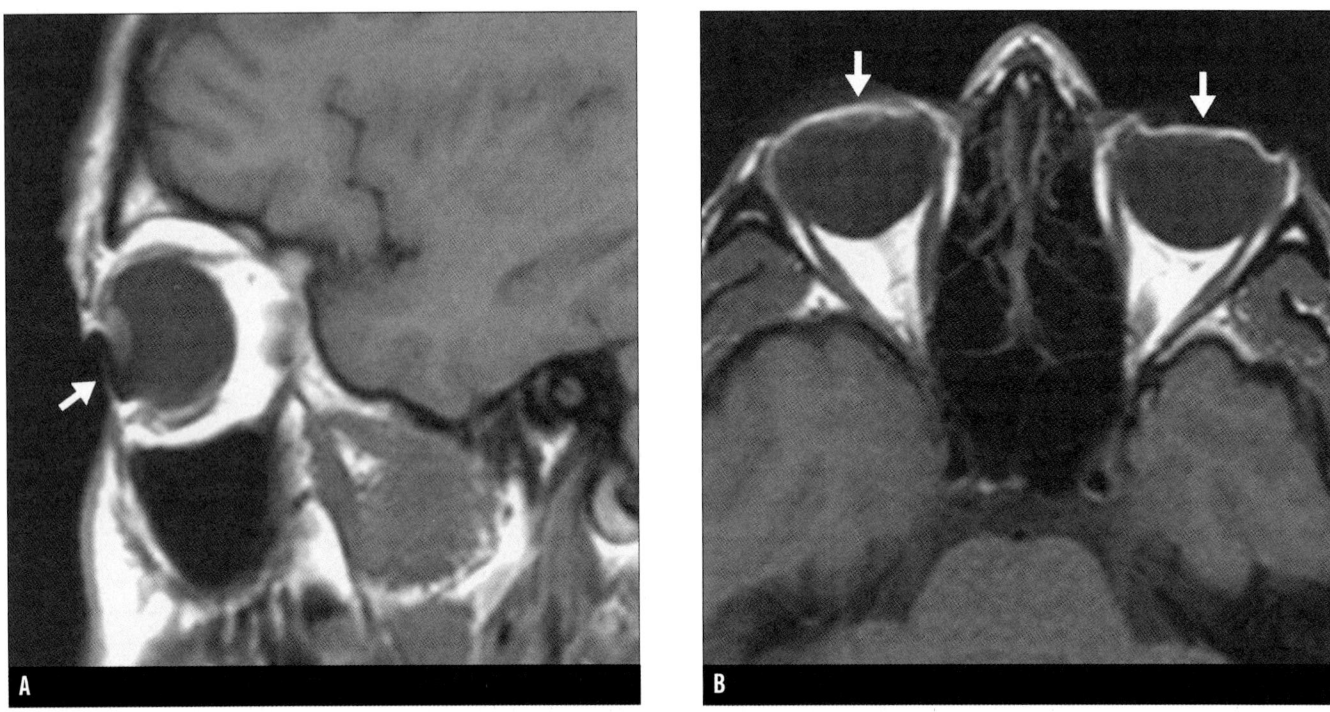

Sagittal T1 (**A**), axial T1 (**B**), and contrast-enhanced axial T1 with fat suppression (**C**) MR images demonstrate symmetric, wavy, horizontally oriented signal abnormality along the anterior aspects of the globes resulting in an apparent globe contour abnormality. This represented artifact from eye makeup.

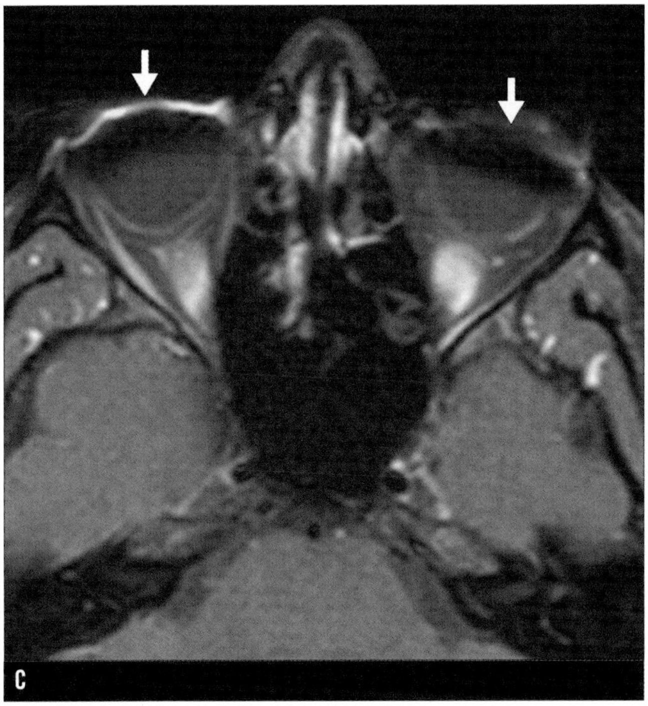

Companion case: Chemosis

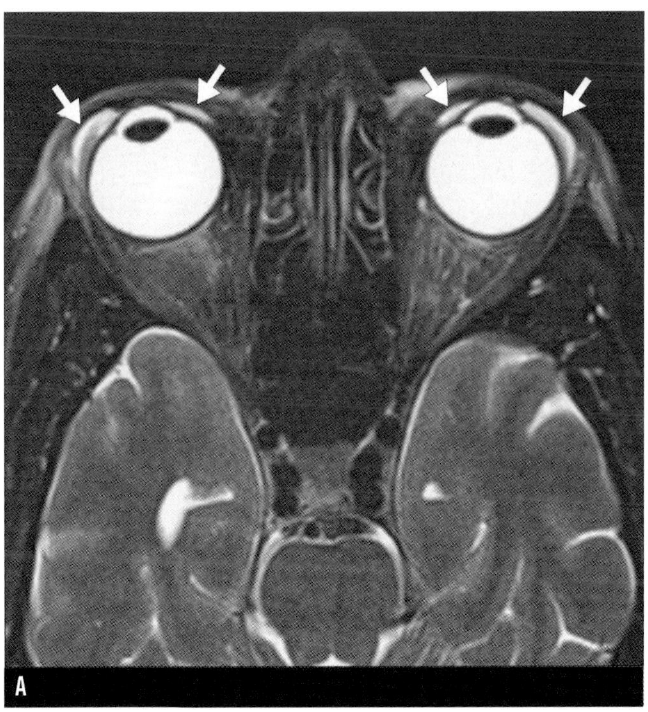

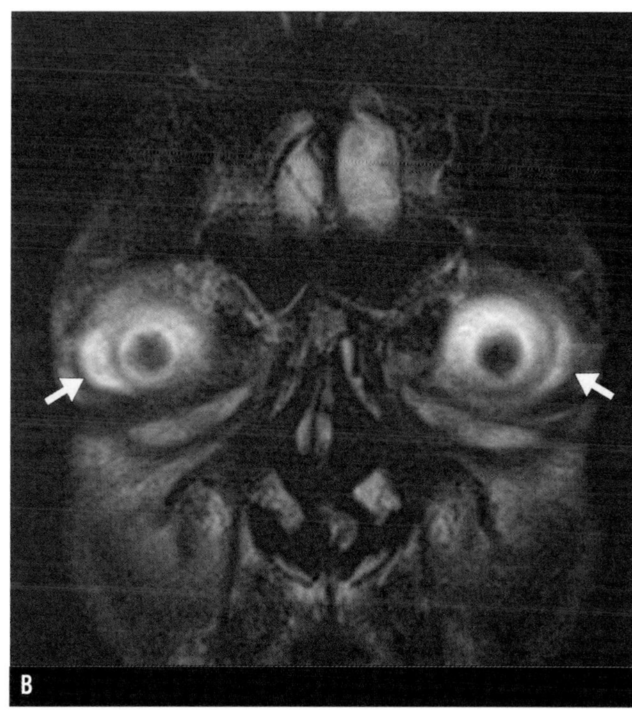

Axial T2 (**A**), coronal T2 (**B**), postcontrast axial T1 (**C**), and postcontrast coronal T1 (**D**) MR images with fat suppression were obtained in this patient with a history of Sweet syndrome, a febrile neutrophilic dermatosis. There is increased T2 signal and heterogeneous enhancement of the bilateral conjunctiva consistent with chemosis (arrows, **A**-**C**). In addition, there is edema and heterogeneous enhancement of the retrobulbar fat (**A**, **C**, **D**), including enhancement along the optic nerve sheaths (**C**, **D**). The findings are consistent with an inflammatory/infectious process, in keeping with Sweet syndrome.

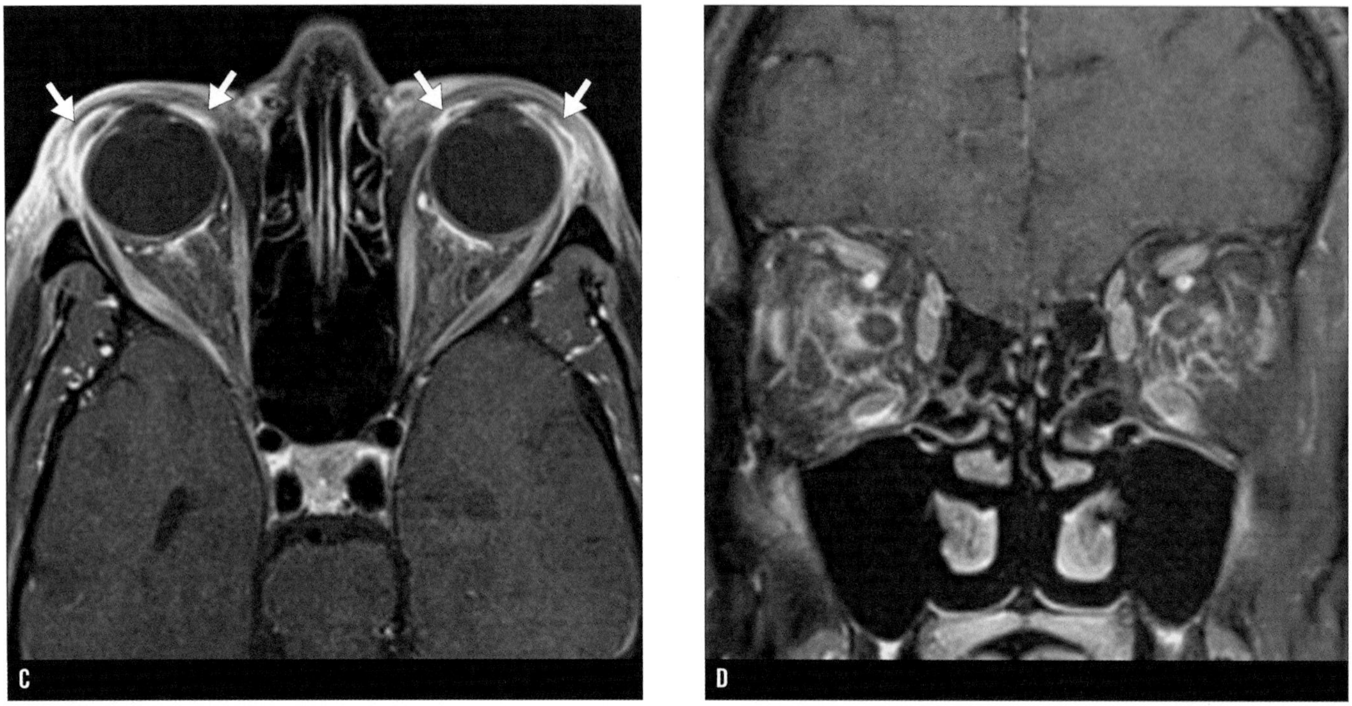

Companion case: Chemosis

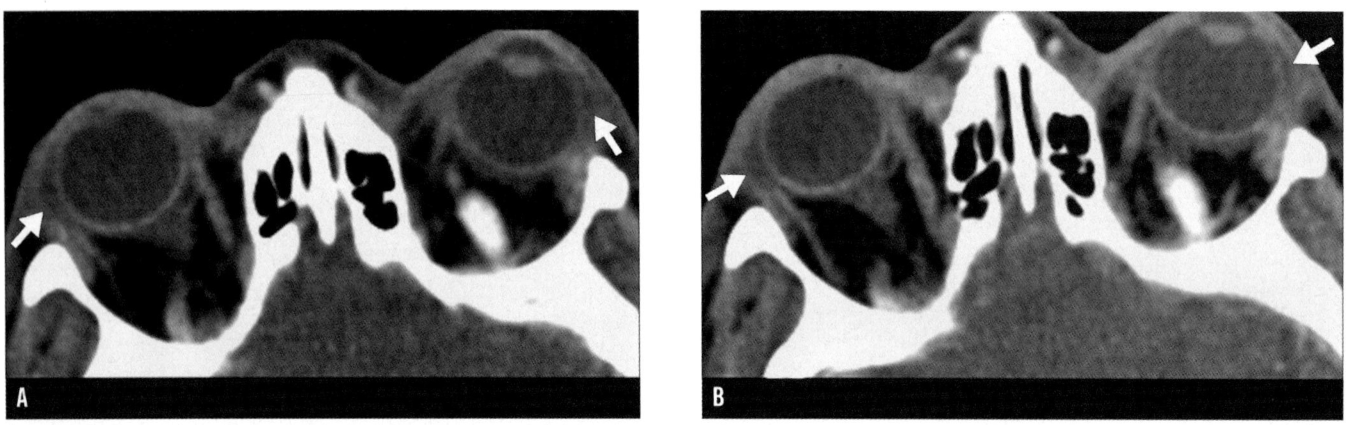

Different patient. Postcontrast axial CT images (**A**, **B**) demonstrate fluid attenuation along the anterolateral aspects of the globes (arrows, **A**, **B**). The patient had acute angioedema and clinical findings of bilateral chemosis.

REFERENCES

Karesh JW, On AV, Hirschbein MJ. Noninfectious orbital inflammatory disease. In: Tansman W, Jaeger EA, eds. *Duane's Foundations of Clinical Ophthalmology.* 15th ed. Philadelphia, PA: Lippincott Williams & Wilkins; 2009:chap 35.

Rubenstein JB, Virasch V. Conjunctivitis: infections and noninfections. In: Yanoff M, Duker JS, eds. *Ophthalmology.* 3rd ed. St. Louis, MO: Mosby Elsevier; 2008:chap 4.6.

Sacco DC, et al. Artifacts caused by cosmetics in MR imaging of the head. *AJR Am J Roentgenol.* 1987;148:1001-1004.

CASE 20 Incomplete suppression of orbital fat on MRI

Incomplete suppression of the orbital fat occurs commonly and usually results from nonuniformity of the local magnetic field. One of the most frequent causes of this artifact is related to the presence of dental hardware. This can be particularly misleading if the dental hardware is more pronounced on one side of the oral cavity. In this setting, there is often increased signal throughout the orbital fat on both fat-suppressed T1- and T2-weighted sequences ipsilateral to the greater amount of dental hardware, often simulating an inflammatory process or an infiltrating lesion in that orbit. This type of artifact can also be the result of facial reconstructive metallic hardware or, to a lesser degree, because of air-tissue interfaces (ie, the paranasal sinuses). In addition, this artifact is more pronounced with increasing field strength. If incomplete suppression of the orbital fat is suspected as a cause of intraorbital signal abnormality, then evaluating the nonfat-suppressed spin-echo T1-weighted sequence is helpful; if there is no focal abnormality on the spin-echo T1-weighted sequence without fat saturation, then the finding is likely artifactual.

COMPANION CASE

- **Postseptal orbital cellulitis.** Postseptal cellulitis is an infectious process which extends posterior to the orbital septum. MR imaging findings include T2 prolongation and abnormal enhancement in the postseptal orbital fat. Some degree of fat stranding should be present on spin-echo T1-weighted imaging without fat suppression if there is true postseptal cellulitis (particularly in advanced cases) as opposed to MR artifact, as discussed above.

Incomplete suppression of orbital fat on MRI

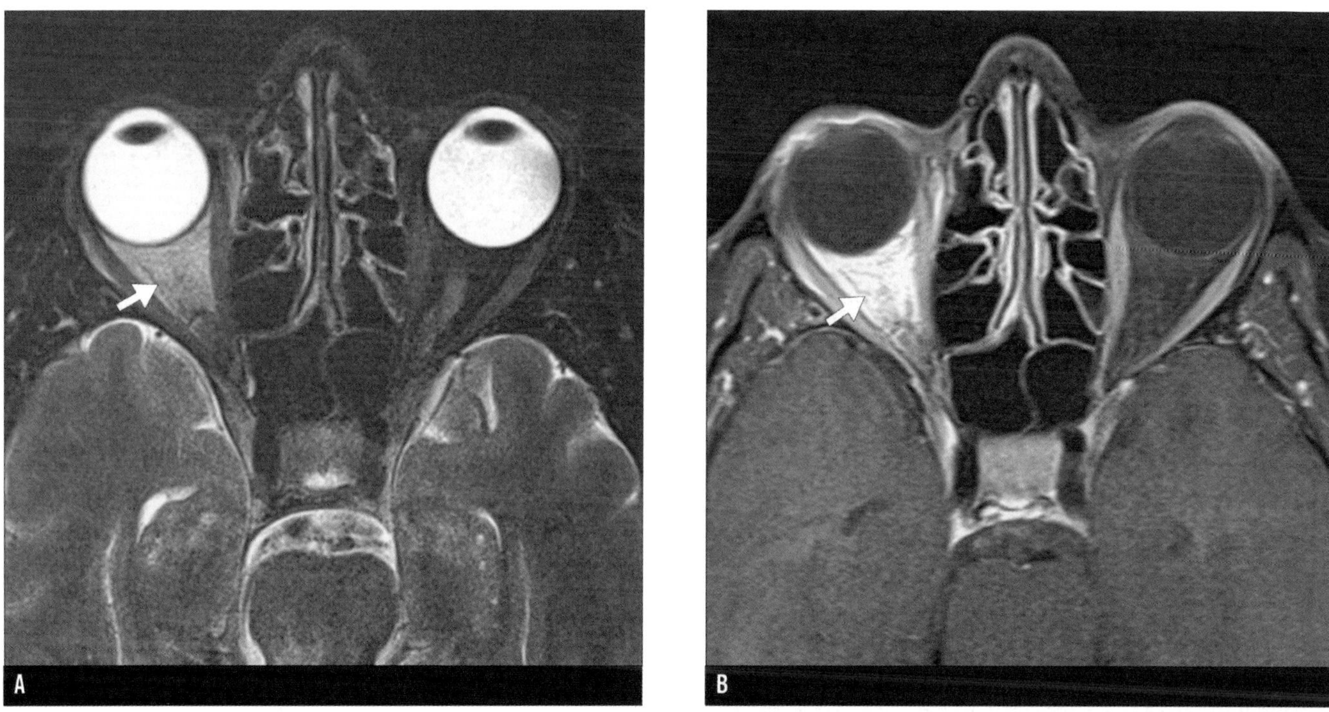

Axial T2 (**A**), contrast-enhanced axial T1 (**B**), and contrast-enhanced coronal T1 (**C**) MR images with fat suppression demonstrate asymmetrically elevated T2 signal and apparent enhancement in the right retrobulbar fat, suggesting an infiltrating right orbital abnormality (arrows, **A-C**). However, unenhanced axial T1 (**D**) and coronal T1 (**E**) MR images without fat suppression from the same study demonstrate normal and symmetric right retrobulbar fat compared to the left. The apparent asymmetric abnormality localized to the right orbit on images **A-C** were entirely artifactual and related to incomplete fat suppression from an asymmetrically larger amount of dental amalgam on the right (arrows, **E**).

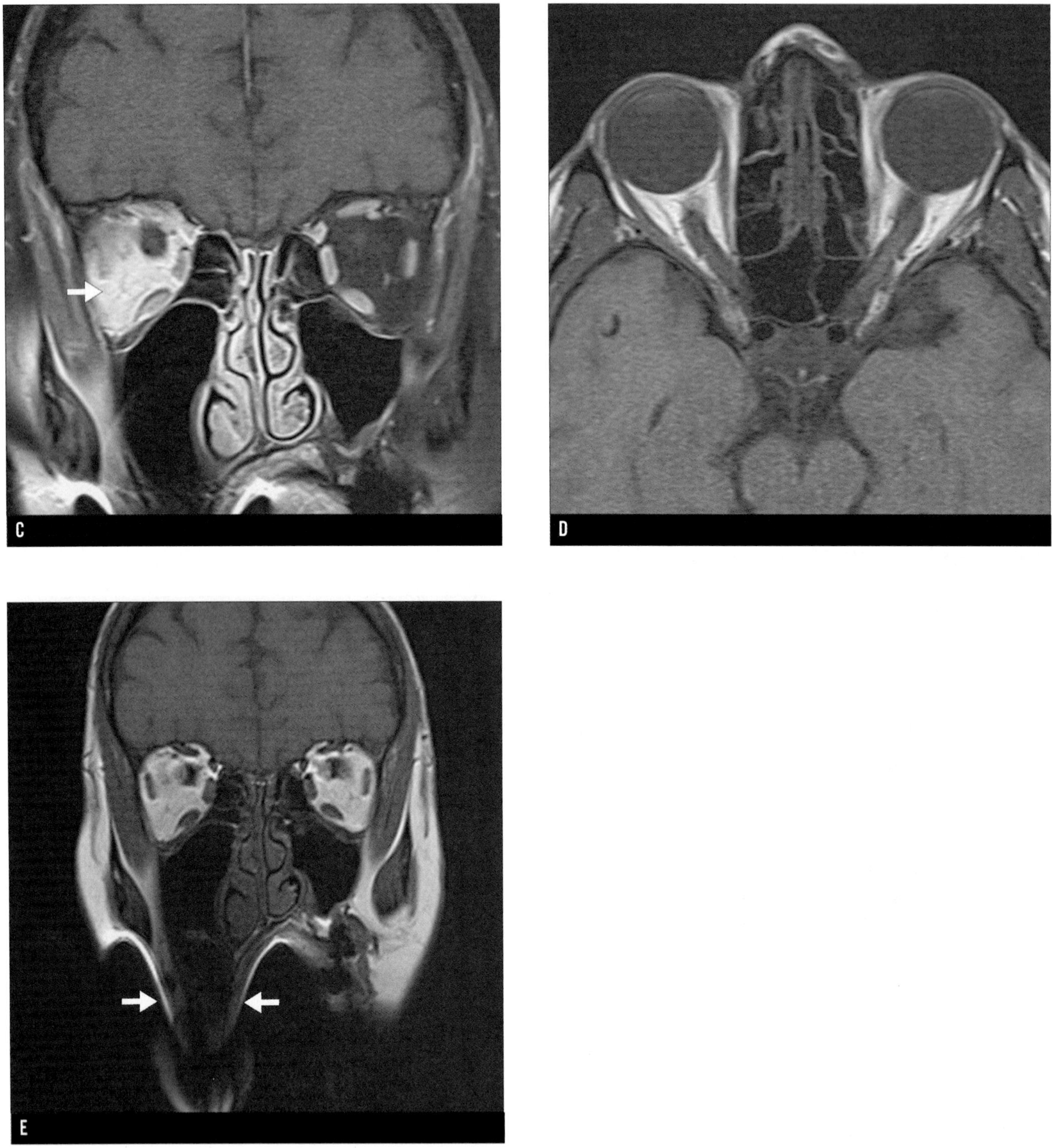
C
D
E

Incomplete suppression of orbital fat on MRI

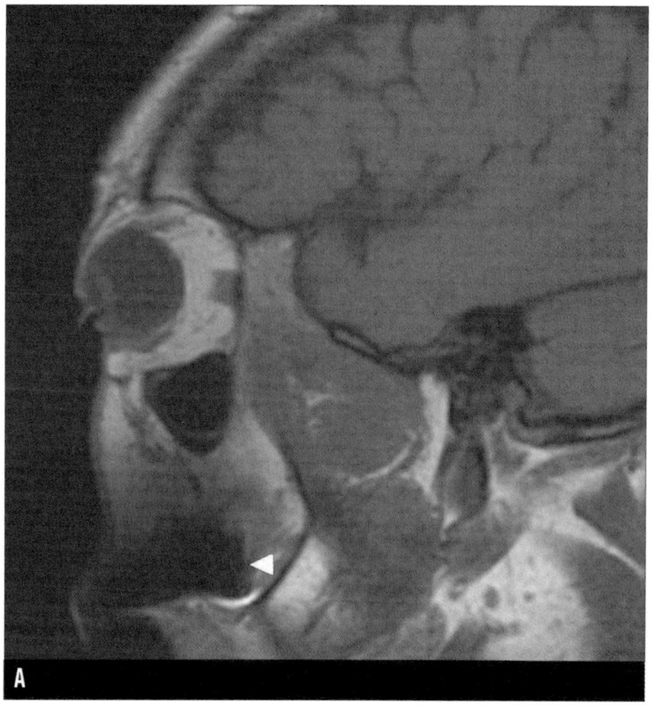

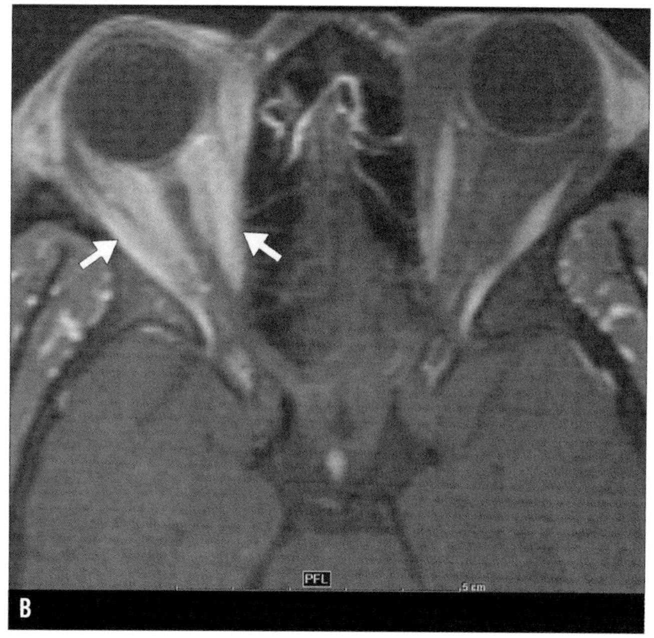

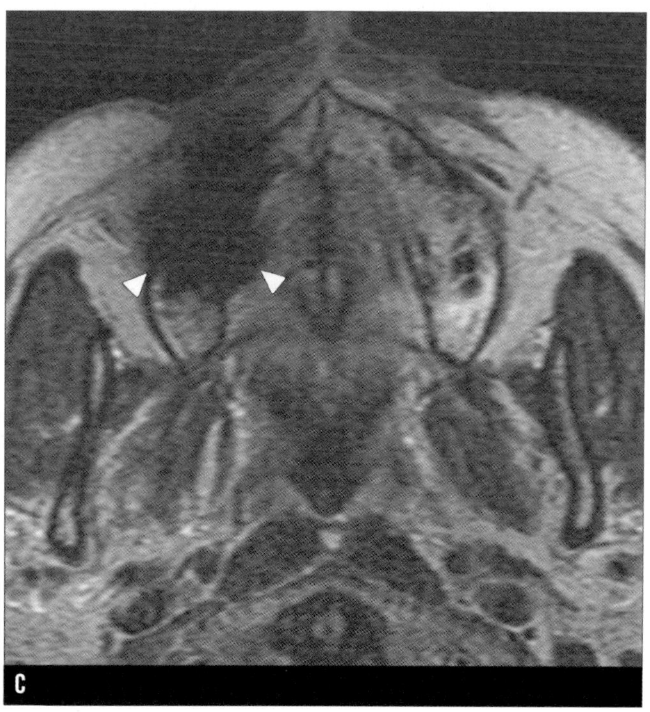

Different patient. Unenhanced sagittal T1 (**A**), postcontrast axial T1 with fat suppression (**B**), and axial T2 (**C**) MR images. There is extensive increased T1 signal localized to the right orbital fat (arrows, **B**). This apparent asymmetric orbital abnormality is artifactual and due to incomplete fat suppression from susceptibility effects related to dental hardware on the right (arrowheads, **A**, **C**). This is confirmed by the normal retrobulbar fat on the image **A**, which would be expected to be stranded if this were a true inflammatory/infiltrative process.

Incomplete suppression of orbital fat on MRI

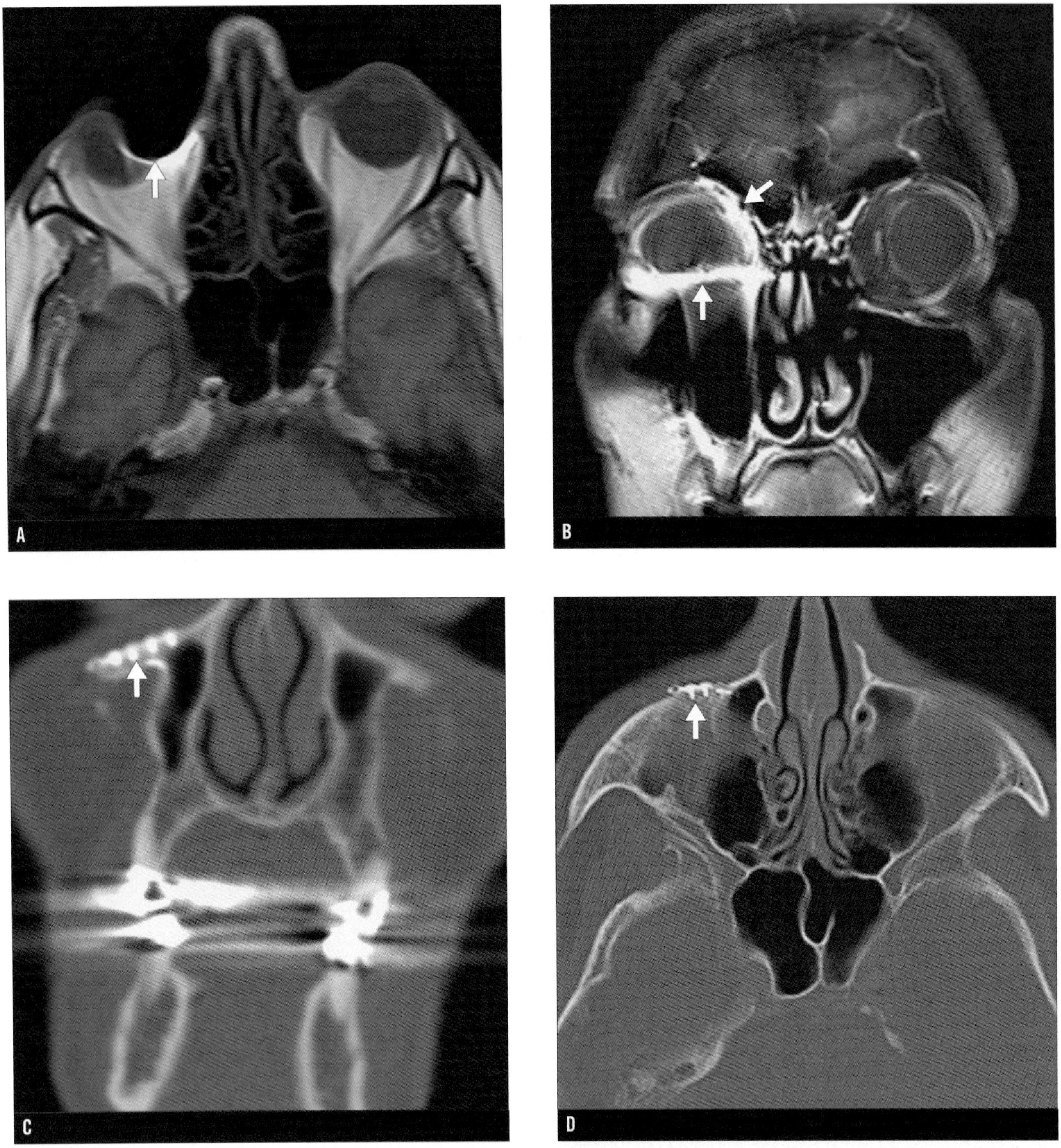

Different patient. An unenhanced axial T1-weighted MR image (**A**) demonstrates an apparent contour abnormality and signal void along the medial aspect of the right globe (arrow, **A**). A fat-suppressed postcontrast coronal T1-weighted MR image (**B**) demonstrates apparent linear and curvilinear enhancement along the inferior and superomedial aspects of the right orbit, respectively (arrows, **B**). These findings result from susceptibility effects related to fracture fixation hardware demonstrated on coronal reformatted (**C**) and axial (**D**) CT images of the same patient (arrows, **C**, **D**).

Companion case: Postseptal orbital cellulitis

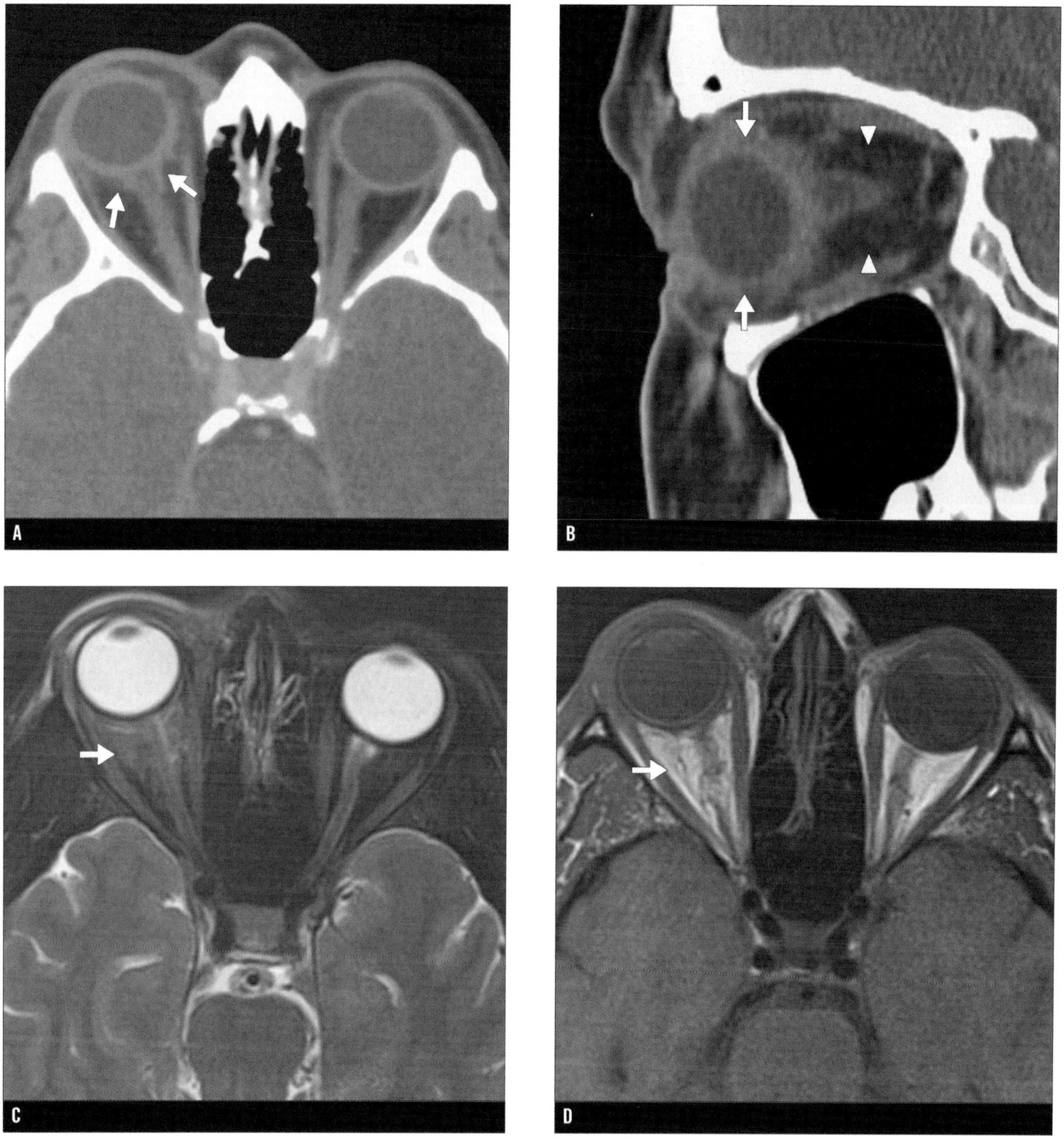

Contrast-enhanced axial (**A**) and sagittal reformatted (**B**) CT images demonstrate right globe scleral thickening (arrows, **A**, **B**) and stranding of the intraconal fat (arrowheads, **B**) consistent with postseptal orbital cellulitis. Fat-suppressed axial T2 (**C**), axial T1 (**D**), and fat-suppressed postcontrast axial T1 (**E**) MR images of the same patient demonstrate changes of right postseptal cellulitis on MRI. The retrobulbar fat is edematous on T2 (arrow, **C**) and enhances following contrast (arrow, **E**). In addition, there is fat stranding on image **D** (arrow), verifying that there is true inflammation rather than artifact on the fat-suppressed sequences. There is also right globe proptosis, in keeping with posteptal orbital cellulitis.

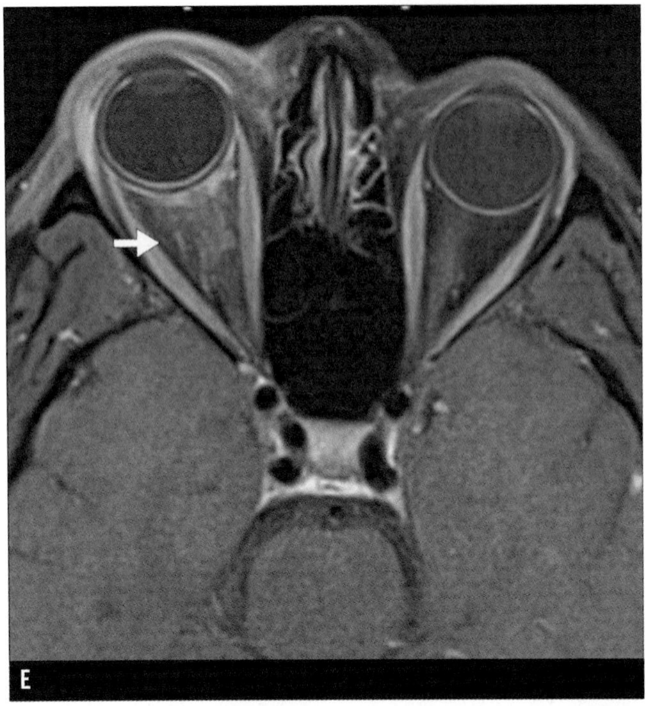

REFERENCE

Herrick RC, et al. Artifacts and Pitfalls in MR Imaging of the orbit: a clinical review. *Radiographics*. 1997;17:707-724.

CASE 21 Ocular prostheses and orbital implants

An ocular prosthesis is an artificial eye that is used when the globe has been damaged, enucleated, or congenitally abnormal (eg, microphthalmia). These prostheses are fabricated and fitted by an ocularist and usually constructed from plastic acrylic, although occasionally they are made from cryolite glass. Plastic acrylic is far more commonly utilized for a variety of reasons, including superior durability relative to glass. The pupil, iris, and conjunctiva are custom painted by the ocularist with the intent of simulating a real eye. There are multiple different types of ocular prostheses, ranging from a prosthetic contact lens used for a scarred cornea to a scleral shell fitted over a residual shrunken globe (ie, phthisis bulbi).

If a globe is not present, then an orbital implant is placed within the orbit, and the ocular prosthesis is custom-fitted over it. Orbital implants are usually round or oval in shape and may be nonintegrated (nonporous) or integrated (porous). Nonintegrated implants are usually solid and typically made of plastic acrylic. Another type of nonintegrated orbital implant is the hollow glass spherical orbital implant; this low-cost implant is rarely used today in the United States but is still used successfully in other parts of the world and has a similar safety profile of plastic acrylic. A mesh is placed over a nonintegrated orbital implant, and the extraocular muscles are attached to the mesh to allow for movement of the implant. Integrated implants are typically constructed of hydroxyapatite or polyethelene and offer several advantages over nonintegrated implants. Because of their porous nature, integrated implants allow for fibrovascular ingrowth directly into the implant, thereby decreasing the incidence of implant migration. Integrated implants also allow direct attachment of the extraocular muscles onto the implant, resulting in improved implant mobility. In addition, an ocular prosthesis can be attached directly to an integrated implant via a peg, which is typically constructed of titanium. One end of the peg is fitted into the ocular prosthesis whereas the other end is fitted into the orbital implant. While peg fixation often results in a more natural movement of the ocular prosthesis, placement of a peg can be technically challenging for the surgeon and can be associated with long-term complications.

Enhancement of the extraocular muscles on MRI in the setting of an orbital implant suggests an intact vascular supply to the muscles. Additionally, enhancement extending toward the center of a porous implant suggests fibrovascular ingrowth and a healthy implant.

Orbital implant

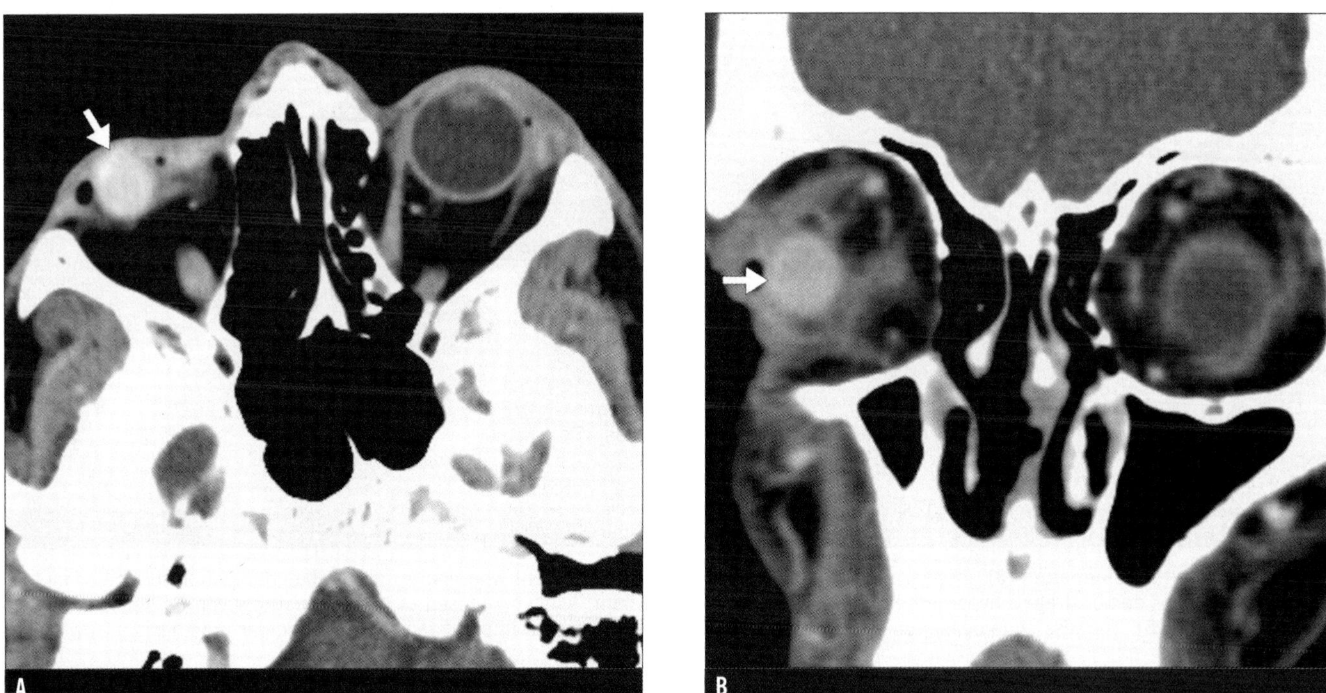

Axial (**A**), coronal reformatted (**B**), and sagittal reformatted (**C**) contrast-enhanced CT images demonstrate a hyperdense, spherical right orbital implant in this patient who is status post enucleation following a stab wound to the right eye (arrows, **A-C**). The orbital implant is likely composed of hydroxyapatite, given its high density. Expected, normal granulation tissue is appreciated surrounding the surface of the orbital implant.

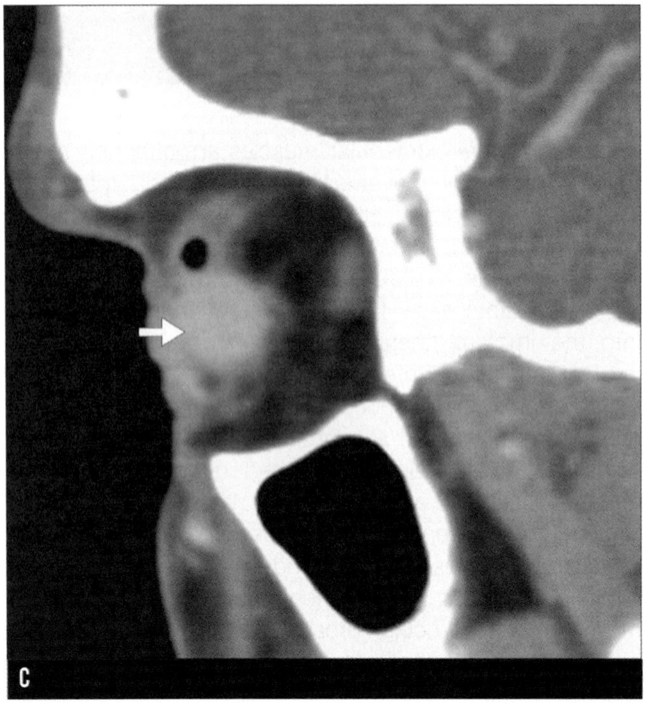

Ocular prosthesis and an orbital implant

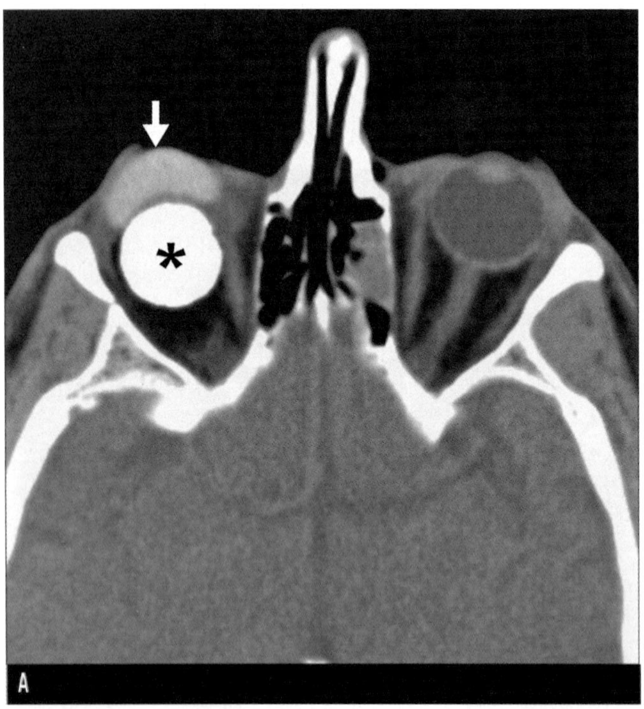

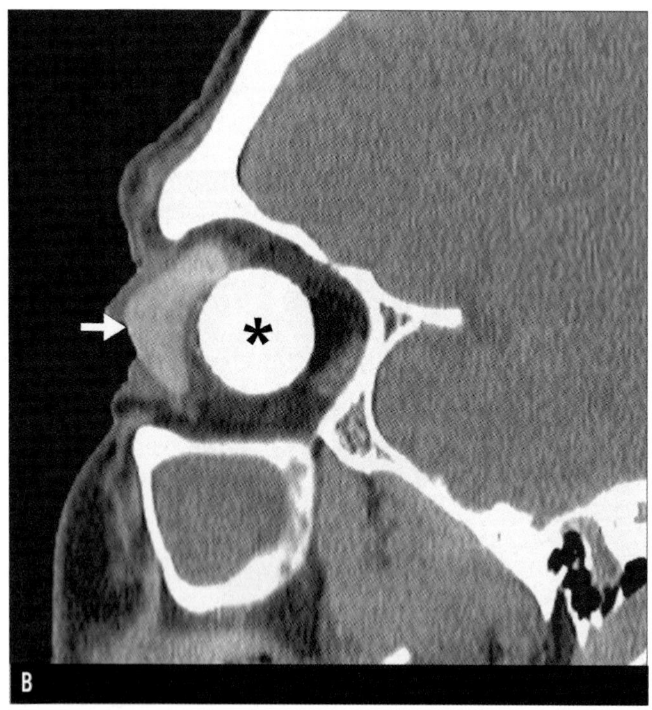

Axial (**A**) and sagittal reformatted (**B**) unenhanced CT images of the orbits in a patient who had a right globe enucleation for ocular melanoma. The images demonstrate a hyperdense, spherical right orbital implant, likely composed of hydroxyapatite given its dense appearance (asterisks, **A**, **B**). The less hyperdense, curvilinear structure overlying the orbital implant represents an ocular prosthesis (arrows, **A**, **B**).

Ocular prosthesis and an orbital implant with fibrovascular ingrowth on MRI

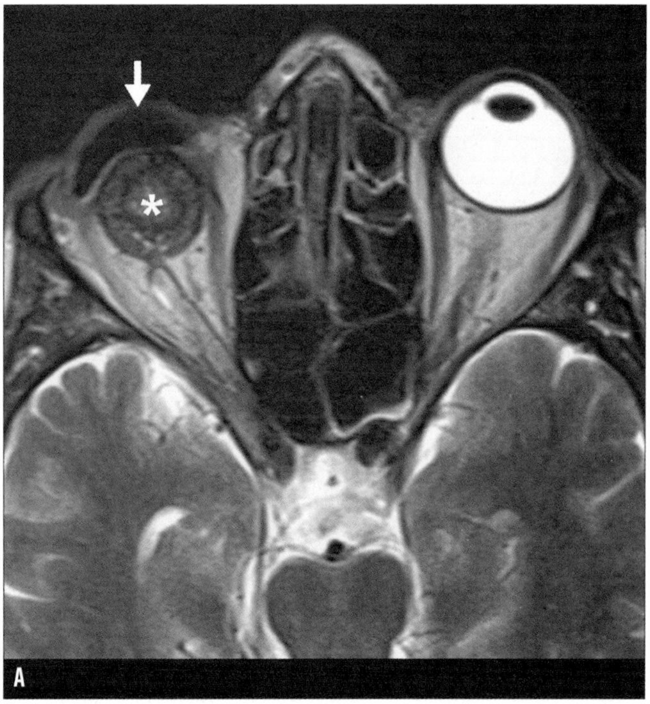

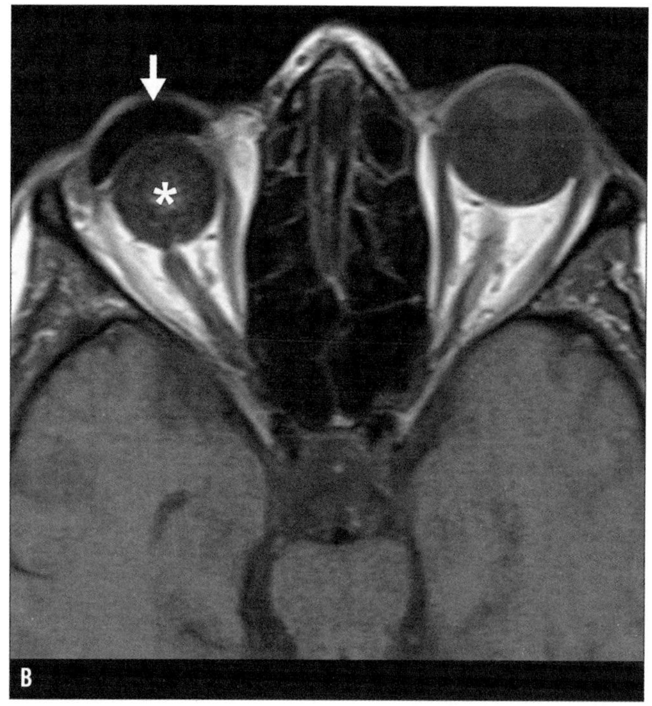

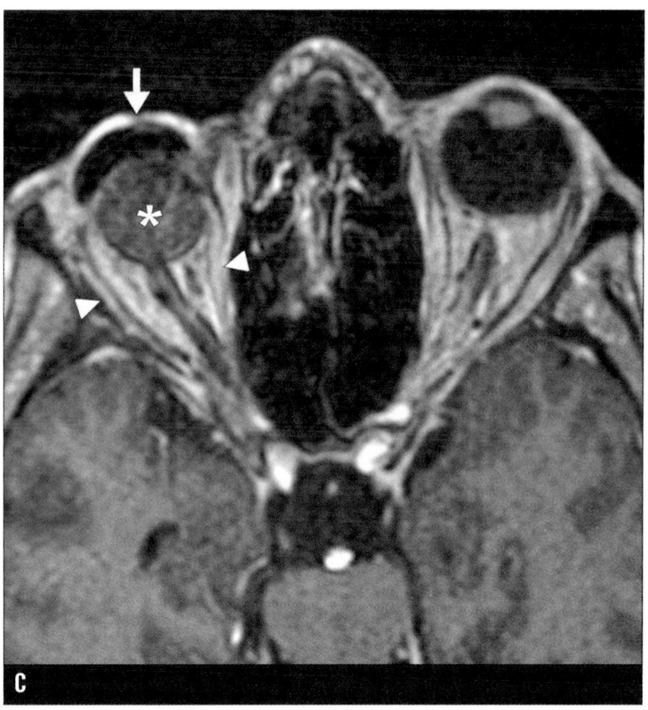

Axial T2 (**A**), axial T1 (**B**), and postcontrast axial MPRAGE (**C**) MR images demonstrate appropriate positioning of an orbital implant (asterisks, **A**-**C**) and an overlying ocular prosthesis (arrows, **A**-**C**) in this patient who had a right globe enucleation because of recurrent globe infection following trauma. Enhancement of the orbital implant is compatible with fibrovascular ingrowth (**C**). This fibrovascular ingrowth is compatible with a healthy integrated orbital implant, with the implant likely composed of either hydroxyapatite or polyethylene. Enhancement of the extraocular musculature suggests an intact vascular supply to the musculature (arrowheads, **C**).

Orbital implant with a pegged ocular prosthesis

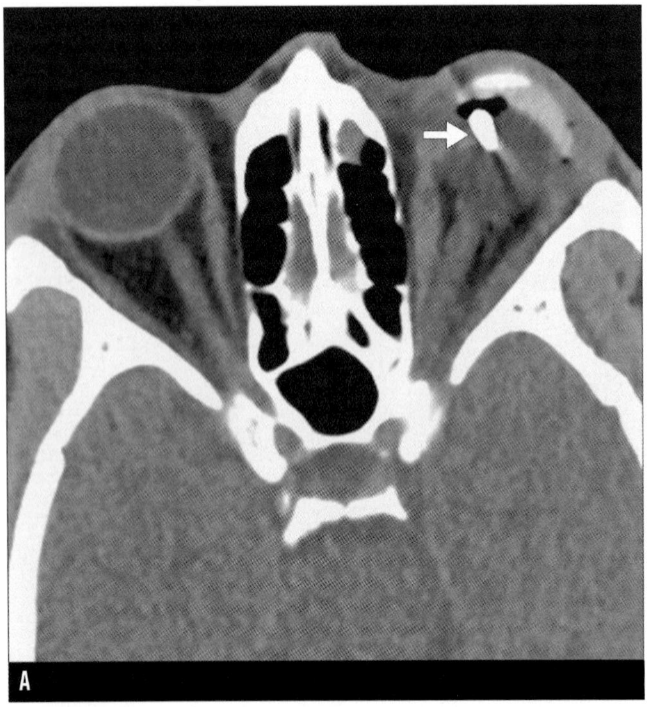

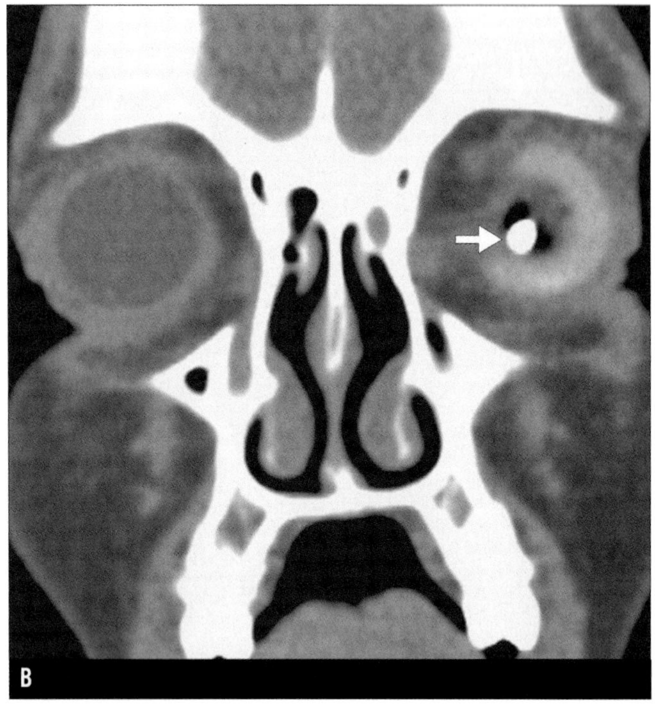

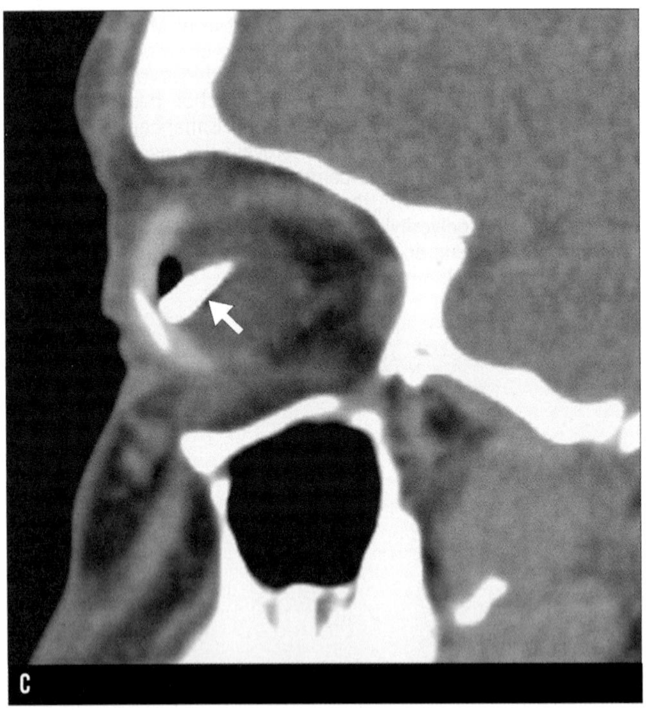

Axial (**A**), coronal reformatted (**B**), and sagittal reformatted (**C**) unenhanced CT images demonstrate the normal appearance of an integrated left orbital implant pegged to an overlying ocular prosthesis. The orbital implant is likely constructed of polyethylene, given its hypoattenuating appearance. The metallic peg (arrows, **A**-**C**) anchors the overlying ocular prosthesis to the orbital implant, allowing for a more natural movement of the ocular prosthesis.

Hollow glass spherical orbital implant

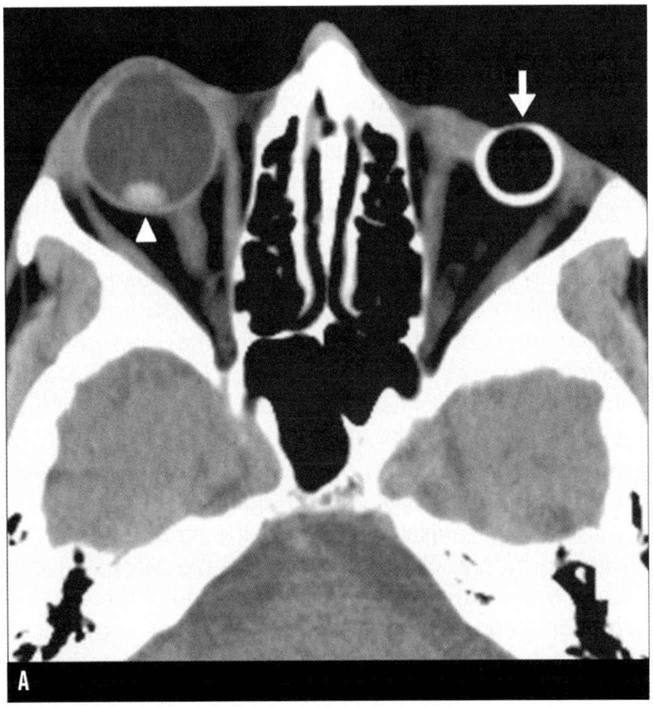

An axial CT image (**A**) demonstrates a hollow glass left orbital implant (arrow). Incidentally, a native right globe lens is dislocated and lies dependently in the vitreous chamber of the right globe (arrowhead).

REFERENCES

Ainbinder DJ, Haik BG, Mazzoli RA. Anophthalmic socket and orbital implants: role of CT and MR imaging. *Radiol Clin North Am.* 1998;36(6):1133-1147.

Custer PL. Enucleation: past, present, and future. Ophthal Plast *Reconstr Surg.* 16(5):316-321.

Custer PL, et al. Orbital implants in enucleation surgery. *Ophthalmology.* 2003;110(10):2054-2061.

De Potter P, Duprez T, Cosnard G. Postcontrast magnetic resonance imaging assessment of porous polyethylene orbital implant (Medpor). *Ophthalmology.* 2000;107(9):1656-1660.

Hunter T, et al. Medical devices of the head, neck, and spine. *RadioGraphics.* 2004;24:257-285.

Patil SB, Meshramkar R, Naveen BH, Patil NP. Ocular prosthesis: a brief review and fabrication of an ocular prosthesis for a geriatric patient. *Gerodontology.* 2008;25(1):57-62.

Raizada K, Rani D. Ocular prosthesis. *Cont Lens Anterior Eye.* 2007;30:152-162.

CASE 22 Intraocular lens implant

Intraocular lens (IOL) implants are used to replace a diseased lens and are most commonly performed for the treatment of senile cataract formation. The normal human crystalline lens is made up of three concentric components. From peripheral to central, these layers are the outer capsule (hard outer layer), the cortex (soft intermediate layer), and the nucleus (hard center). IOL implant surgery begins with dilating the pupil, anesthetizing the eye, and performing an incision into the sclera or cornea. This is followed by formation of a hole in the anterior outer capsule of the lens (termed capsulorhexis), removal of the anterior portion of the lens cortex, and phacoemulsification of the lens nucleus. Phacoemulsification allows for removal of the lens nucleus and is accomplished with an ultrasonic tool that uses vibrations to break the nucleus of the diseased lens into several pieces, after which these pieces are emulsified and aspirated. During this procedure, aspirated fluids from the globe are replaced with a balanced salt solution via an irrigation system, which serves to maintain pressure in the eye and prevent ocular hypotonia. The posterior cortical portion of the lens that remains is then aspirated. The preserved posterior outer capsule and the remaining anterior outer capsule are referred to as the capsular bag and serve as a lattice for placement of the IOL implant. The lens is inserted through the incision and carefully placed into the capsular bag.

If the capsular bag is damaged during surgery, or if it is inherently weak (eg, following infection, patients with Marfan syndrome, etc) then IOL implantation into the capsular bag may not be an option. Several other locations for IOL implant placement exist, including situating the implant in the ciliary sulcus posterior to the iris, or placing the IOL in the anterior chamber and fixing it along the superficial aspect of iris, the latter termed an anterior chamber IOL. Anterior chamber IOLs may also be placed in the presence of an intact native crystalline lens in order to improve refractive power.

The IOL implant consists of a central optical lens component and typically two footplates, termed haptics, which serve to stabilize the device. Today, the central optic lens component may be made from polymethylmethacrylate, silicone, or acrylic, and some IOLs are foldable. An IOL implant is significantly thinner than a native lens because of the relatively high refractive index of the material used in the implant. On CT, an optical lens component of the implant will appear thin and hyperdense, whereas the haptics may be visible as punctate foci along the lateral margins of the IOL implant. On MRI, the optical lens component of the implant will appear as a linear area of signal void on both T1- and T2-weighted sequences. The haptics may be visible as punctate foci of hypointense signal along the lateral margins of the implant on MRI.

COMPANION CASES

- **Native lens and intraocular lens implant subluxation and dislocation.** There are several peripherally located zonules that attach the native crystalline lens to the ciliary body. The zonules serve to hold the lens in place and play an important role in accommodation. A lens subluxation or dislocation (termed ectopia lentis) most commonly occurs following blunt trauma, in which globe deformation results in tearing of the zonular attachments. By virtue of its position, the iris impedes anterior subluxation or anterior dislocation of the lens. Therefore, a posterior subluxation or posterior dislocation is more common. With partial zonular ligament tears, the lens may become angled posteriorly and subluxed into the vitreous humor. With complete tears, the dislocated lens usually lies within the dependent portion of the vitreous humor. Lens subluxations or dislocations may occur with native lenses or IOL implants. Nontraumatic lens subluxations or dislocations may be associated with connective tissue disorders, such as Marfan syndrome or homocystinuria.
- **Subluxation of a calcified cataract.** Most cataracts develop a cloudy appearance on ophthalmologic examinations and do not calcify. However, calcification of a native crystalline lens cataract may sometimes be identified by CT or US. Calcification of a cataract may also occur following inadequate removal of the lens cortex during the phacoemulsification stage of IOL implant surgery. In this setting, the epithelial cells that remain may migrate along the posterior aspect of the capsular bag and result in "after cataract" (also called posterior capsular opacification), which is a potential complication of this procedure. It is this posterior capsular opacification that can calcify and may be identified on imaging. Finally, some hydrophilic acrylic IOL implants have a predilection to calcify.
- **Aphakia.** Aphakia is the term used to describe absence of the lens, either the native lens or an IOL implant. This most commonly occurs following surgical removal of the lens, although aphakia may also occur as a result of trauma or be associated with congenital anomalies. The lens is responsible for accommodation and accounts for 20 diopters of refraction, whereas the cornea accounts for an additional 40 diopters of refraction. While the lens contributes less than the cornea to overall refraction, the combined effect of loss of refractive power due to absence of the lens coupled with loss of accommodation results in hyperopia (farsightedness).
- **Displaced Soemmering ring and a dislocated intraocular lens implant.** A Soemmering ring is circumferential, proliferated epithelial tissue and fibrosis that occurs when residual lens debris following IOL surgery becomes

trapped along the periphery between the posterior capsule and the remaining anterior capsule of the capsular bag. Because the central portion of the ring is usually clear, there is typically no visual disturbance as a result of a Soemmering ring. However, a Soemmering ring may represent a precursor of posterior capsular opacity, which as described above, represents a secondary cataract of the posterior capsule following cataract surgery. Rarely, a Soemmering ring and the capsular bag, including the IOL implant, may dislocate.

Posterior chamber intraocular lens implant

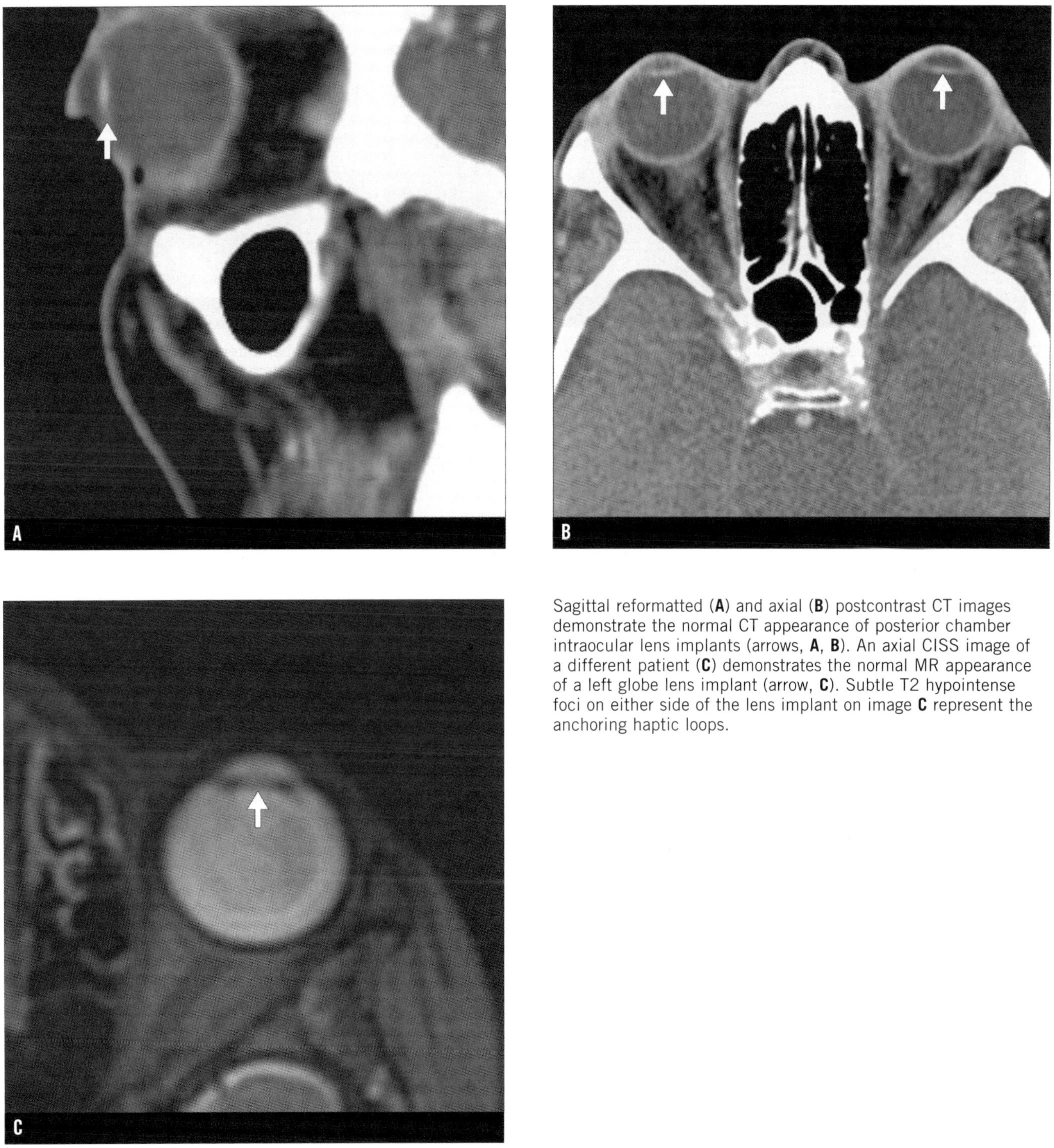

Sagittal reformatted (**A**) and axial (**B**) postcontrast CT images demonstrate the normal CT appearance of posterior chamber intraocular lens implants (arrows, **A**, **B**). An axial CISS image of a different patient (**C**) demonstrates the normal MR appearance of a left globe lens implant (arrow, **C**). Subtle T2 hypointense foci on either side of the lens implant on image **C** represent the anchoring haptic loops.

Anterior chamber intraocular lens implant

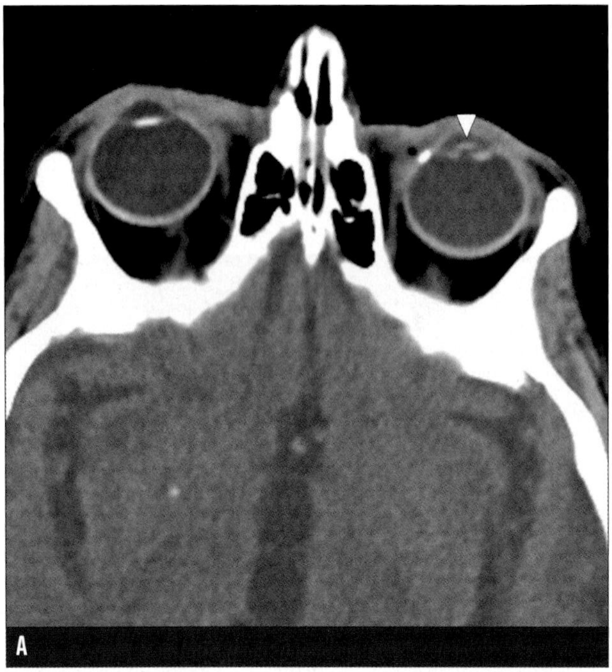

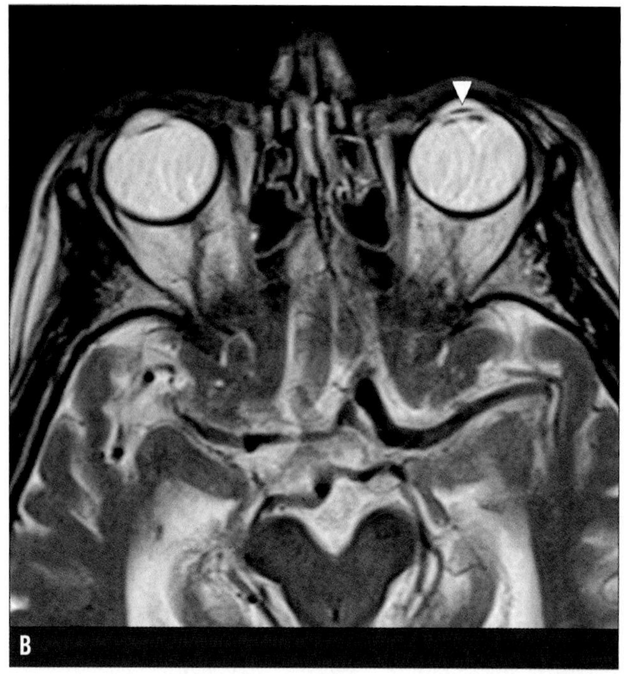

An axial CT image (**A**) demonstrates an intraocular lens implant that resides in the anterior chamber anterior to the ciliary body and iris (arrowhead, **A**). An axial T2-weighted MR image of the same patient (**B**) demonstrates the same finding (arrowhead, **B**). While this appears to be an abnormally subluxed lens implant, it is appropriately positioned and represents an anterior chamber intraocular lens implant.

Companion case: Intraocular lens implant subluxation

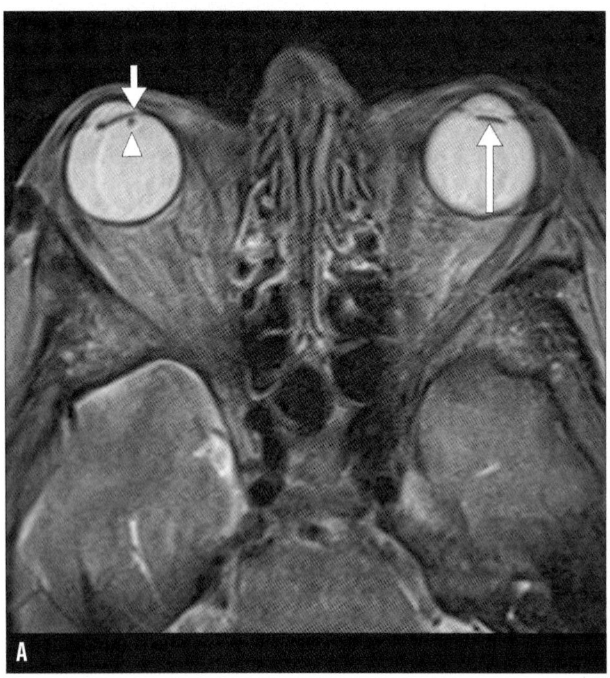

An axial T2-weighted MR image (**A**) demonstrates the normal appearance of a left intraocular lens implant situated appropriately in the posterior chamber of the globe (long arrow). However, the right lens implant has subluxed, with the medial edge of the lens implant anteriorly positioned (short arrow). A T2 hypointense focus along the medial posterior margin of the right lens implant presumably represents a displaced haptic loop (arrowhead).

Companion case: Intraocular lens implant dislocation

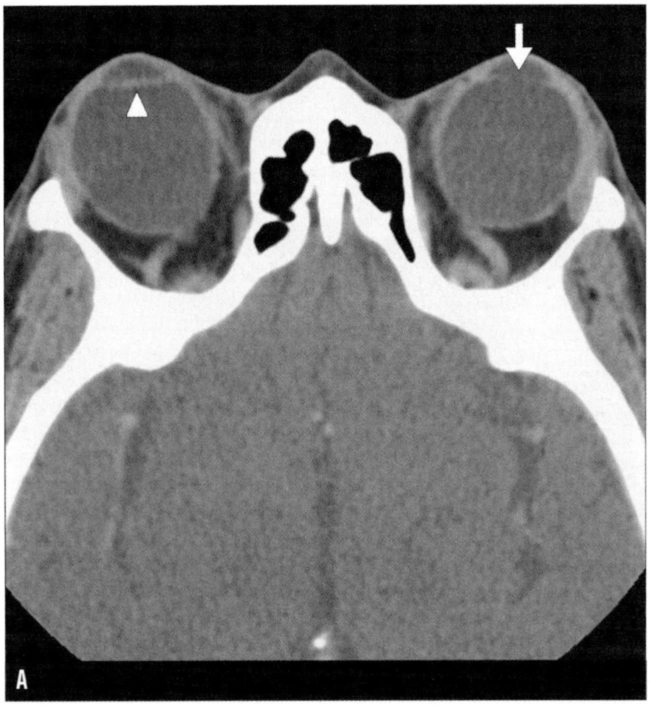

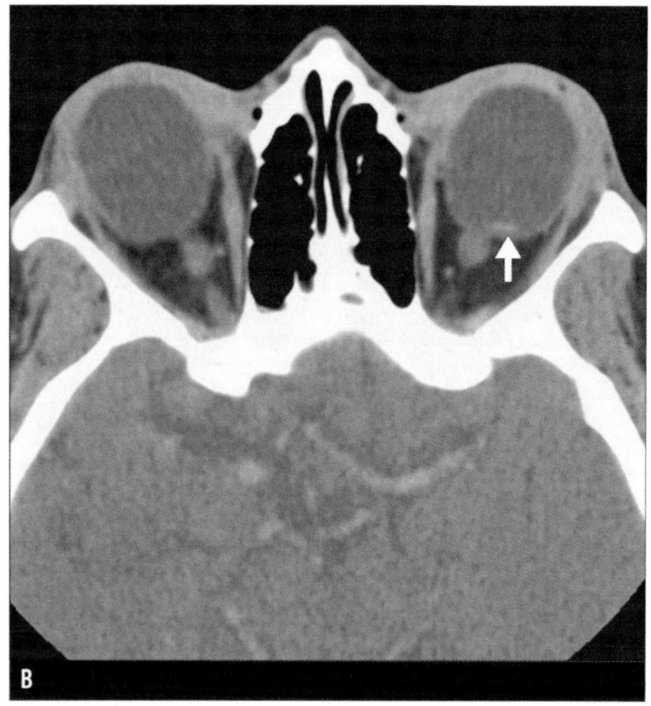

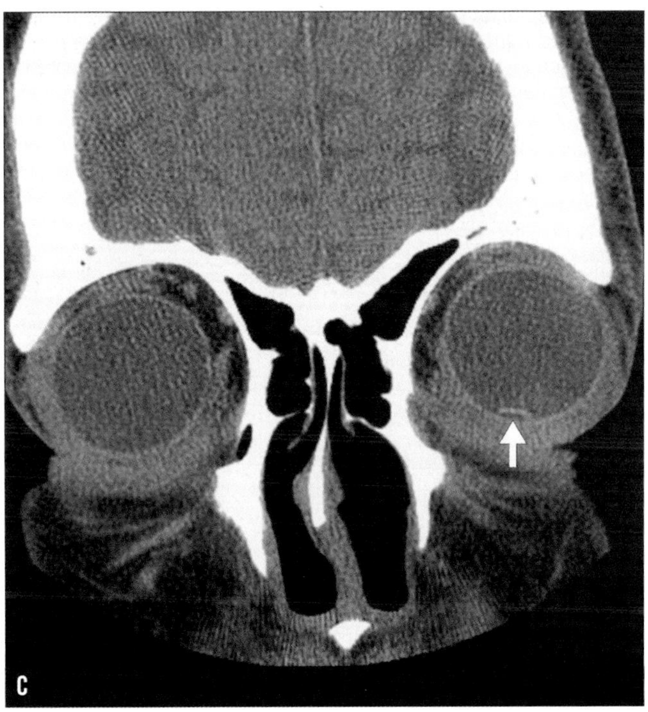

Supine axial (**A**, **B**) and prone direct coronal (**C**) unenhanced CT images of the orbits. Image **A** demonstrates left globe aphakia (arrow, **A**). However, images **B** and **C** demonstrate a dislocated lens implant lying dependently in the left vitreous chamber (arrows, **B**, **C**). An appropriately positioned right lens implant is present (arrowhead, **A**). The globes are elongated in anteroposterior dimension, compatible with axial myopia.

Companion case: Native lens subluxation

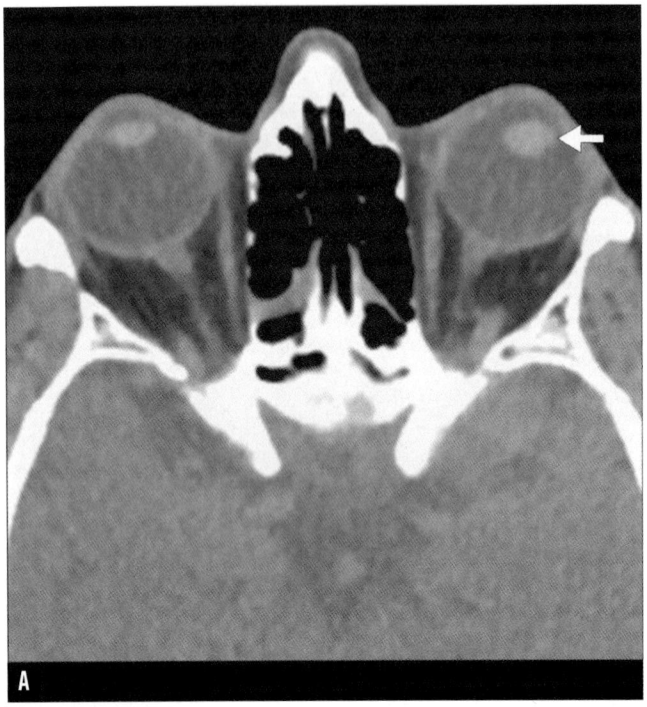

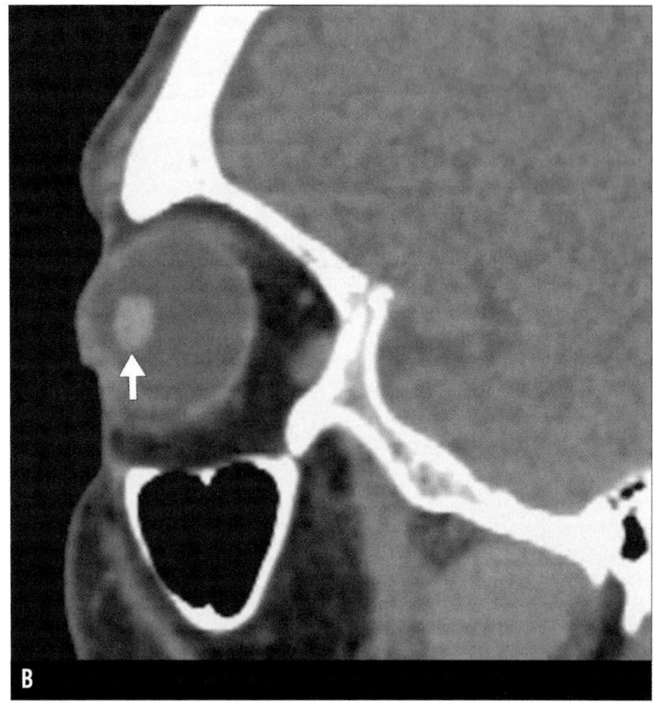

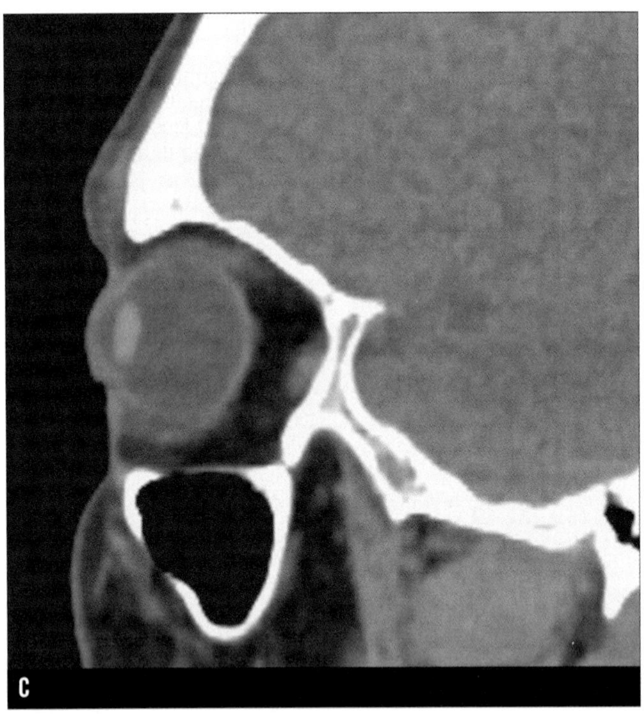

Unenhanced axial (**A**) and sagittal reformatted CT images of the left (**B**) and right (**C**) globes demonstrate posterior and lateral subluxation of the native left lens (arrows, **A**, **B**) when compared to the normally positioned native right lens.

Companion case: Native lens dislocation

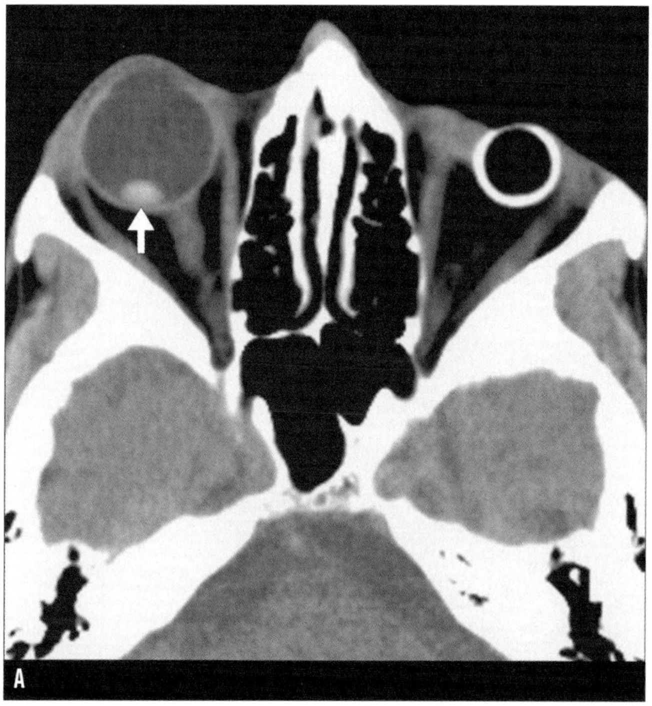

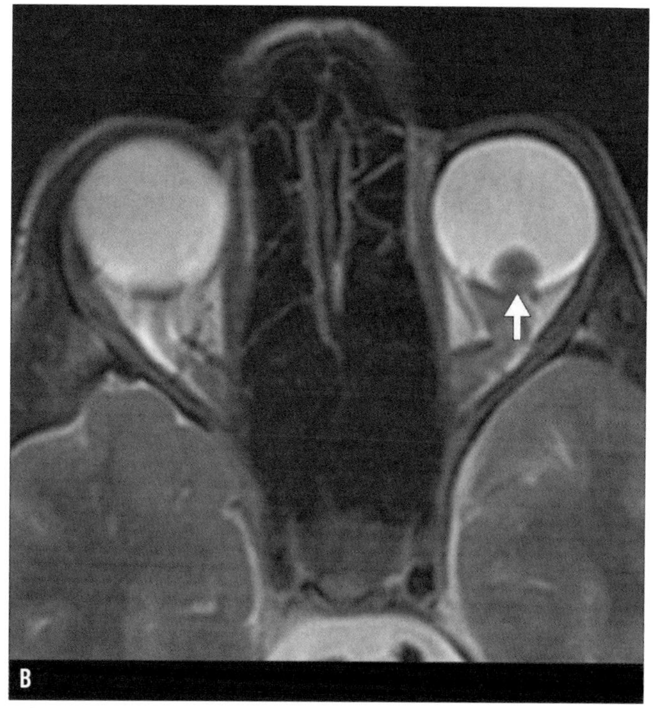

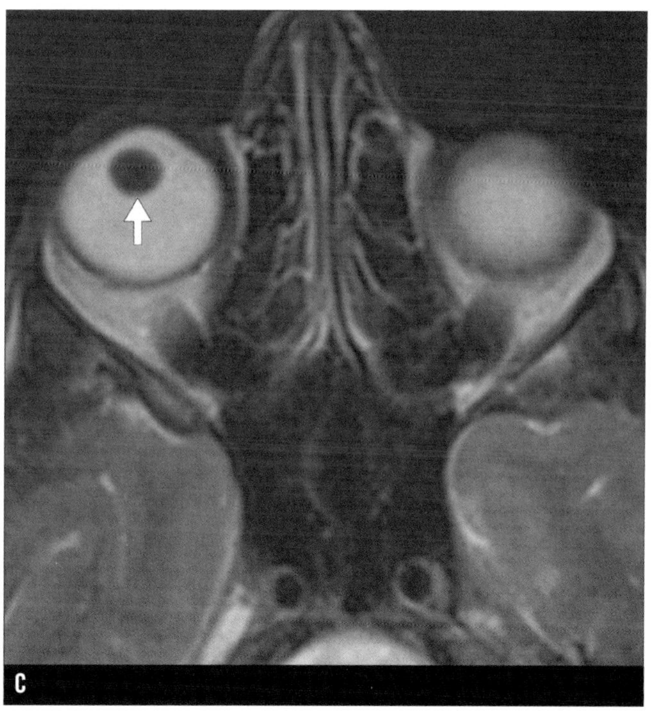

An axial CT image (**A**) demonstrates the native right lens lying dependently in the vitreous chamber of the right globe, compatible with a native right lens dislocation (arrow, **A**). A hollow glass left orbital implant is also present on image **A**. Axial T2-weighted images of a different patient (**B**, **C**) demonstrate frank dislocation of the left lens (arrow, **B**) and at least subluxation of the right lens (arrow, **C**). Images **B** and **C** are from a patient with Marfan syndrome.

Companion case: Subluxation of a calcified cataract

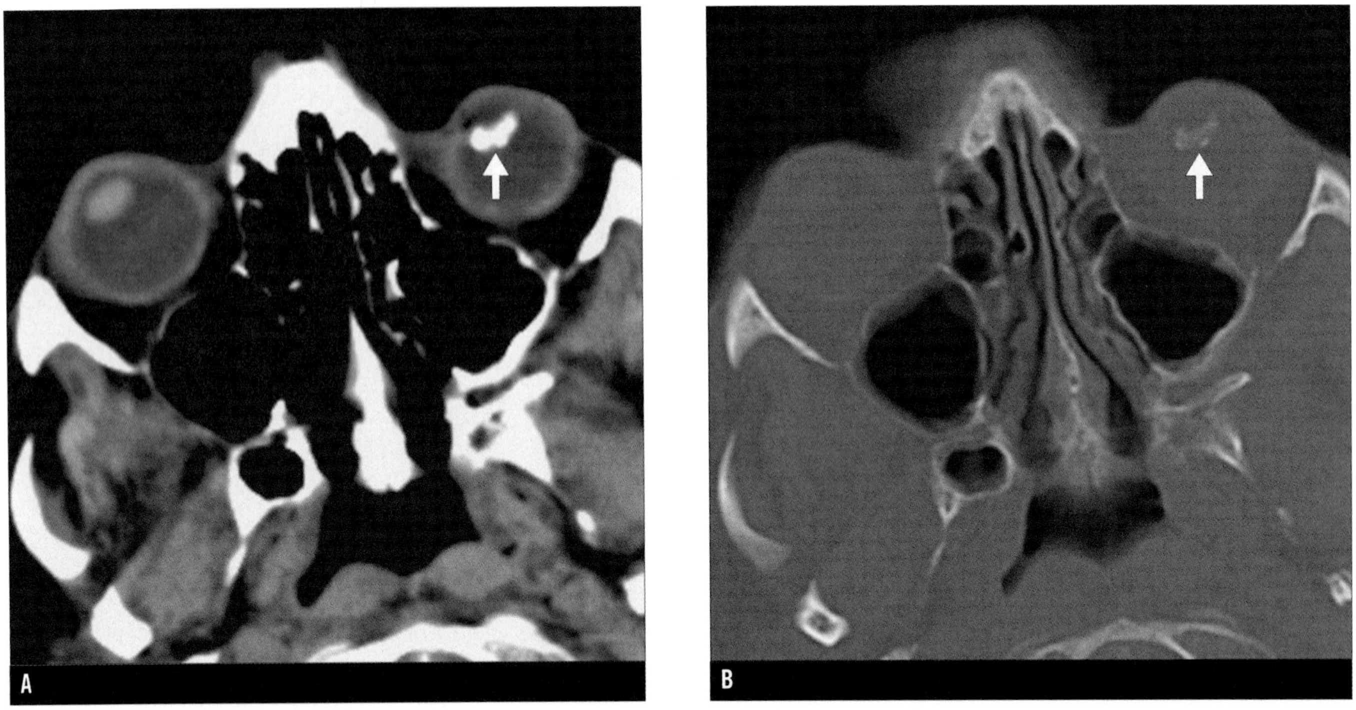

Unenhanced axial CT images viewed with a soft tissue window (**A**) and bone window (**B**) demonstrate mild posterior subluxation of a heavily calcified left globe cataract (arrows, **A**, **B**).

Companion case: Congenital aphakia

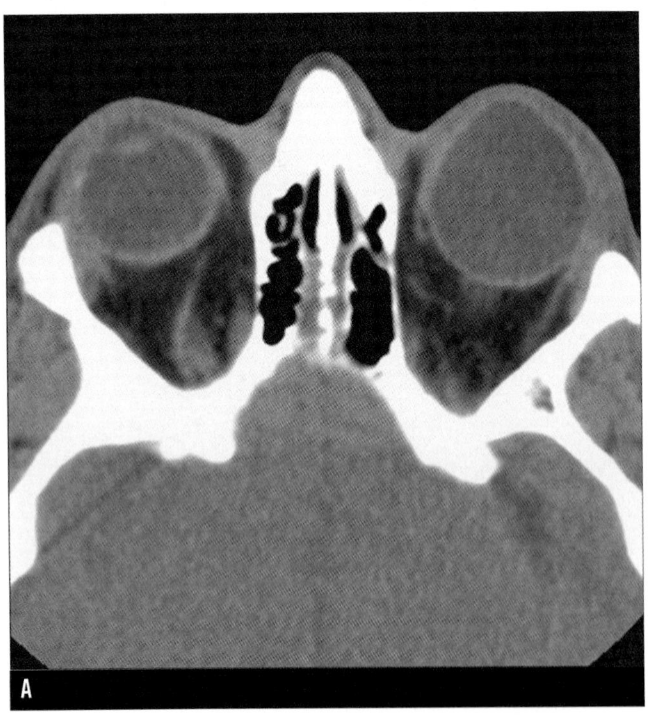

An unenhanced axial CT image of the orbits of a patient with congenital left eye blindness (**A**) does not demonstrate an identifiable left globe lens, consistent with congenital aphakia. The left globe is diffusely enlarged, likely due to congenital glaucoma (buphthalmos).

Companion case: Displaced Soemmering ring and a dislocated intraocular lens implant

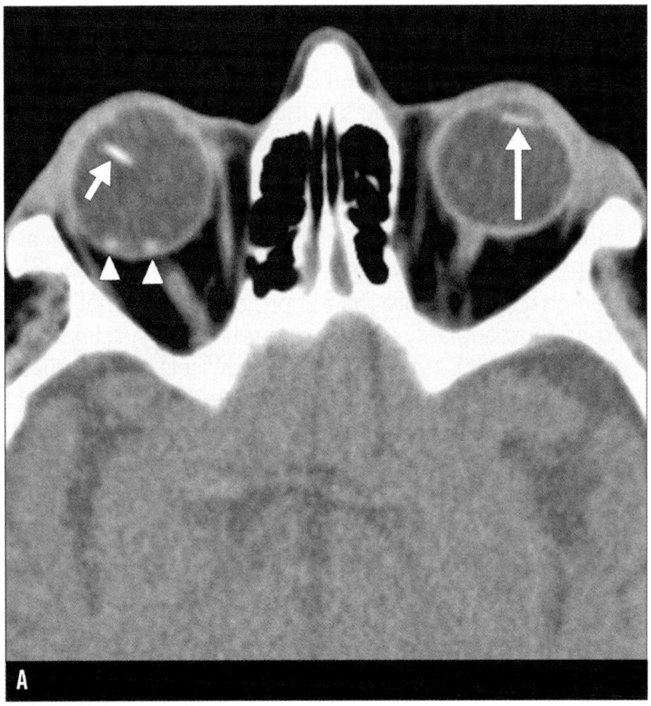

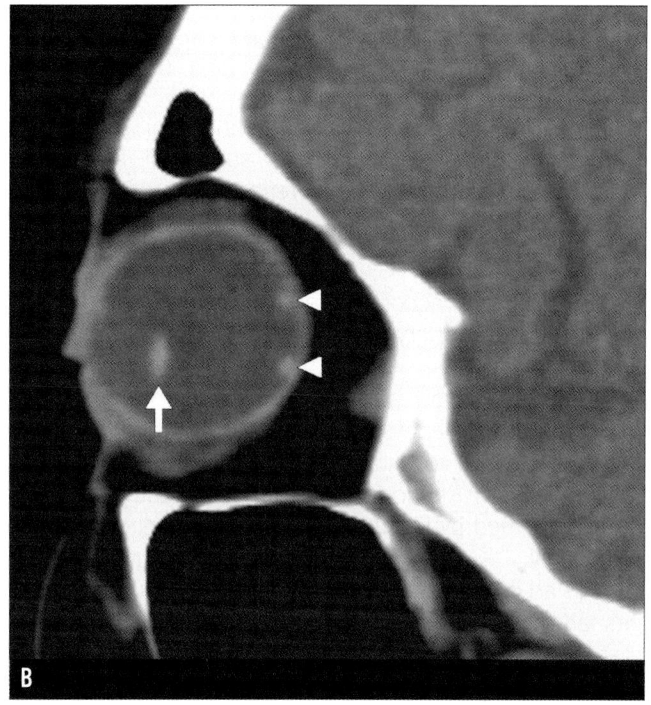

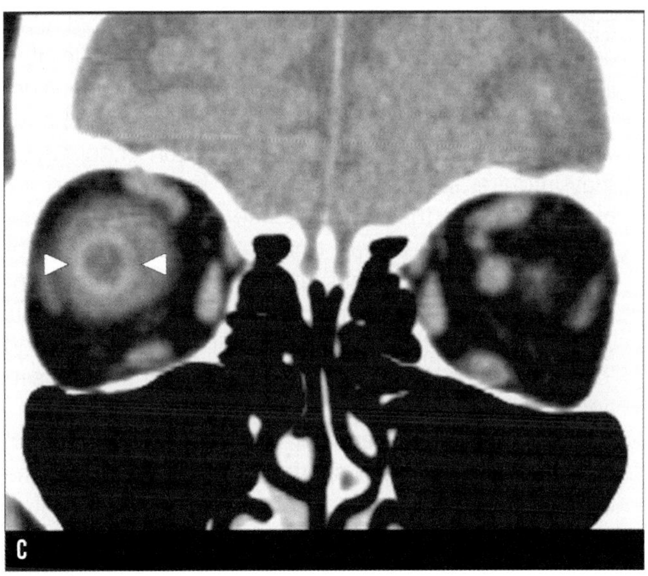

Axial (**A**), sagittal reformatted (**B**), and coronal reformatted (**C**) unenhanced CT images of the orbits, with image **C** obtained through the posterior aspect of the right globe. Images **A** and **B** demonstrate posterior and lateral dislocation of a right lens implant (arrows, **A, B**). This patient had a clinical history of a right lens capsular bag displacement. In the dependent portion of the right vitreous chamber, there is a hyperdense, ring-shaped structure representing a peripherally calcified displaced Soemmering ring (arrowheads, **A**, **B**, **C**). A nondisplaced left lens implant is also present (long arrow, **A**).

REFERENCES

Eleftheriadis H, Amoros S, Bilbao R, Teijeiro MA. Spontaneous dislocation of a phakic refractive lens into the vitreous cavity. *J Cataract Refract Surg*. 2004;30(9):2013-2016.

Guha GS. Soemmering's ring and its dislocations. *Brit J Ophthal*. 1951;35:226.

Kubal WS. Imaging of orbital trauma. *Radiographics*. 2008;28:1729-1739.

Kuo MD, et al. In Vivo CT and MR appearance of prosthetic intraocular lens. *Am J Neuroradiol*. 1998;19:749-753.

Root, T. Anatomy of the Eye. *The Free Online Ophthalmology Book!*. N.p., n.d. Web. 5 Apr 2015.

Syam P, et al. Hydroview lens implant calcification: 186 exchanges at a district general hospital. Eye (Lond). 2008;22(3):325-331. Epub 2006 Oct 20.

Surgical repair of retinal detachment is based upon two fundamental concepts:

1. Mechanical apposition of the retinal tear that allows vitreous humor to enter the subretinal space (ie, space between the sensory retina and retinal pigment epithelium).
2. Preventing retears

These goals are accomplished through vitrectomy and retinopexy, laser or cryotherapy fusion of retinal tears, and scleral buckling.

Vitrectomy involves surgical removal of the vitreous gel to enable direct access and repair of the retinal detachment as well as to allow for drainage of the subretinal fluid collection. Retinopexy, or intraocular tamponade, is then performed by filling the vitreous chamber with gas or silicone oil.

An advantage that pneumatic retinopexy (also called gas tamponade) has compared to silicone oil retinopexy is that the gas used with pneumatic retinopexy is naturally resorbed, generally within 3 days to 8 weeks, depending on the specific gas utilized. However, many agents require prolonged prone head positioning postoperatively and temporarily leave the patient without vision, limiting its tolerance. Gas tamponade results in an expected air-fluid level in the vitreous cavity which can simulate a complication, such as an infection.

The advantage of silicone oil retinopexy relative to pneumatic retinopexy is that it does not require prone head positioning postoperatively. Furthermore, because silicone oils are transparent, the patient retains vision during the convalescent period. Silicone oils may be surgically removed after at least 8 weeks of tamponade, or the silicone oil may be left permanently. On CT, silicone oil is hyperattenuating relative to the normal vitreous humor. On MRI, silicone oil is generally hyperintense to normal vitreous on T1-weighted images and of variable signal on T2-weighted images. Silicone oils will decrease in signal intensity with fat suppression techniques. On MRI, chemical shift artifact may also be identified on nonfat-suppressed MR images at the interface between the silicone oil and vitreous fluid. These imaging characteristics can be of value in differentiating silicone oil from vitreous hemorrhage. Because silicone oils have a lower specific gravity than normal vitreous fluid, reaccumulation of normal vitreous fluid will reside dependent to the silicone oil and result in a silicone oil-vitreous fluid level.

COMPANION CASES

- **Vitreous hemorrhage.** The vitreous chamber has a volume of approximately 4 cc and occupies the majority of the globe. Anatomically, it is bound anteriorly by the posterior lens capsule and the posterior margin of the lens zonular fibers, anterolaterally by the ciliary body, and posterolaterally by the internal limiting membrane layer of the retina. Hyaluronic acid and collagen constitutes only 1 percent of the vitreous but gives the vitreous its gelatinous consistency. Water comprises the remaining 99 percent of the vitreous. There are three basic mechanisms that may result in vitreous hemorrhage: rupture of abnormal vessels that result from neovascularity (ie, diabetic retinopathy, retinal vein occlusion, etc), rupture of normal vessels (ie, traumatic vitreous traction tearing vessels, perforating or blunt trauma, Terson syndrome, etc), or hemorrhage from regional pathology (hemorrhagic tumors, etc). On imaging, vitreous hemorrhage will occupy a portion or all of the vitreous chamber and is not confined by anatomic boundaries that are frequently identified with retinal or choroidal detachments described below.
- **Terson syndrome.** This entity represents retinal and/or vitreous hemorrhage that occurs in the setting of intracranial subarachnoid hemorrhage, most often when the hemorrhage is severe. The globe hemorrhage usually manifests within the first few days of subarachnoid hemorrhage and is the result of sudden, severe, elevated intracranial pressure and retinal venous hypertension. While some patients with Terson syndrome do not have vision loss, significant visual deficits often occur which may require surgical intervention. In addition, some have suggested that the presence of Terson syndrome may portend an overall poorer clinical morbidity or mortality compared to those patients without Terson syndrome. The most common imaging finding in patients with Terson syndrome is a crescent or nodule-shaped focus of hemorrhage located along the retina in the setting of subarachnoid hemorrhage.
- **Retinal hemorrhage, papillitis with marked papilledema, and optic nerve sheath surgical fenestration.** First-line treatments for papilledema secondary to increased intracranial pressure, such may be present with idiopathic intracranial hypertension (also called pseudotumor cerebri), include medical management with carbonic anhydrase inhibitors and corticosteroids as well as cerebrospinal fluid diversion via a lumbar drain. However, in some cases, an optic nerve sheath fenestration and ventriculoperitoneal shunting may be performed to halt and ultimately reverse optic neuropathy, if present. Early detection of papilledema and its attendant clinical manifestations is important to prevent permanent vision loss.

  Optic nerve sheath fenestration is achieved by surgical creation of a rectangular window in the sheath. Generally, the surgery is performed unilaterally on the more affected side, and it tends to be very effective. On imaging, one may identify ill-defined stranding (CT or MRI) and enhancement (MRI) adjacent to the optic nerve sheath related to the egress of fluid, as is present in the case provided.

- **Retinal detachment.** Understanding the pathophysiology of retinal detachment requires knowledge of retinal anatomy. The human retina contains several layers of neurons that are interconnected by layers of synapses. Retinal detachment occurs when fluid, such as hemorrhage, extends into a potential space known as the subretinal space. The subretinal space is located between the photoreceptive layer, which is the outer-most neuronal layer of the retina, and the retinal pigment epithelium (RPE). The RPE is a pigmented cell layer of the retina that is interposed between the photoreceptive layer and the underlying choroid and serves numerous functions, including light absorption.

  The ophthalmic artery gives rise to the arterial supply of the retina, namely the central retinal artery and short posterior ciliary arteries. The central retinal artery supplies the inner layers of the retina and the short posterior ciliary arteries merge to form the choroid, which supplies the outer layers of the retina, including the photoreceptive layer. The photoreceptive layer contains rods and cones which are vital for vision and is dependent on the underlying choroid not only for its blood supply but also for nutrients. Thus, when retinal detachment occurs, the photoreceptive layer becomes separated from the choroid and ischemia with vision loss ensues.

  Retinal detachment occurs via three main mechanisms: a rhegmatogenous tear (ie, retinal tear) that results in vitreous fluid entering the subretinal space, a subretinal serous/exudative fluid accumulation resulting from a lesion of the RPE or choroid (eg, choroidal melanoma, uveitis, etc), or vitreoretinal adhesions (eg, diabetic retinopathy or vitreous liquefaction) which can retract and detach the photoreceptive layer from the RPE.

  On CT or MRI, a retinal detachment will spare the optic nerve head (also called optic disc) because the subretinal space surrounds but does not overlie the optic nerve head; however, it is worth noting that the ganglion layer of the retina (an inner retinal layer) merges at the optic nerve head and gives rise to the optic nerve. The ora serrata represents the junction between the anterior margin of the photoreceptive layer of the retina and the ciliary body. Therefore, a retinal detachment does not extend anterior to the ora serrata. Because of this anatomy, a retinal detachment may have a V-shaped configuration, with the apex of the "V" representing the spared optic nerve head and the most anterior aspects of the "V" terminating at the ora serrata.
- **Choroidal detachment.** Choroidal detachment occurs when fluid or hemorrhage (such as may occur from uveitis or trauma) accumulates in the suprachoroidal space. The suprachoroidal space represents a potential space located between the choroid and sclera. Accumulated fluid in the suprachoroidal space is not bounded by the ora serrata anteriorly as is fluid in the subretinal space. Also, the choroid is mechanically tethered to the sclera via short posterior ciliary arteries, vortex veins, and short ciliary nerves posterolaterally along the globe at a considerable distance from the optic nerve head. Thus, a choroidal detachment not only spares the optic nerve head, but also spares a more sizeable portion of the posterior globe compared to a retinal detachment. Nevertheless, even with the aforementioned anatomical constraints defining the characteristic appearance of a retinal and choroidal detachments, sometimes these two forms of detachment cannot be differentiated from one another by imaging alone. This is particularly true when there is diffuse hemorrhage within the vitreous chamber, which may occur from numerous causes, including from retinal and/or choroidal detachments.
- **Circumscribed choroidal hemangioma.** A circumscribed choroidal hemangioma (CCH) is a rare, benign vascular hamartoma which is believed to be congenital. While CCH is an isolated finding, the diffuse variant of choroidal hemangioma can be associated with Sturge-Weber syndrome.

  Clinically, CCH presents as a unilateral, red-orange or grayish lesion in the posterior choroid, typically near and temporal to the optic disc. It can mimic a variety of other lesions, including melanoma, metastatic disease, choroidal osteoma, central serous chorioretinopathy, or retinal detachment.

  Typically, CCH is diagnosed with ophthalmoscopy and ultrasonography, the latter demonstrating high internal acoustic reflectivity. On MRI, CCH has a lentiform shape, and most are T1 hyperintense relative to the vitreous, although they can be T1 isointense. A CCH tends to be isointense relative to the vitreous on T2-weighted imaging. On gadolinium-enhanced images, CCH undergoes centrifugal or homogenous enhancement. Melanoma can appear similar to CCH, although melanoma is most often T2 hypointense and may have a more irregular enhancement pattern.

  While individuals with CCH may be asymptomatic, the lesion can impair vision via accumulation of subretinal fluid. Potential treatment options include photocoagulation, radiotherapy, transthermotherapy, and photodynamic therapy.
- **Uveitis.** The uvea is a contiguous structure that is formed by a combination of the choroid, ciliary body, and iris of the globe; thus, infection/inflammation of any of these structures constitutes a uveitis. An anterior uveitis, often referred to as iritis, is the most common form of uveitis. A posterior uveitis may affect the choroid or choroid and retina, and is referred to as choroiditis and chorioretinitis, respectively. If the inflammation/infection affects the ciliary body, then the term cyclitis is used. A panuveitis is present when all layers of the uvea are affected. There are numerous causes of uveitis, including a frank orbital infection, autoimmune disorders (eg, ankylosing spondylitis, rheumatoid arthritis, etc), and toxin exposure. Imaging findings of uveitis can be identified on MRI but are often absent on CT. On MR imaging, enhancement

of the affected portions of the uvea will often be identified. Hyperintense FLAIR signal along the affected uvea and within the vitreous may also be identified, the latter reflecting proteinaceous debris in the vitreous chamber.

- **Endophthalmitis.** Acute endophthalmitis refers to a pyogenic globe infection and is an ophthalmologic emergency requiring a prompt diagnosis to effectively treat. Two subcategories of endophthalmitis exist, exogenous and endogenous. Exogenous is the more common type and usually occurs following surgery (eg, cataract surgery), corneal ulcers, or penetrating injury. The endogenous form results from hematogenous spread of an infection and usually occurs in immunocompromised patients. On MRI, there will be hyperintense FLAIR signal and enhancement along the periphery or throughout the globe. Hemorrhage and/or proteinaceous debris in the globe with or without retinal detachment may be present. Restricted diffusion involving affected portions of the globe has also been reported. The infection may spread to other portions of the orbit, including the retrobulbar fat and extraocular muscles, as well as to the periorbital regions.

Vitrectomy and pneumatic retinopexy (CT)

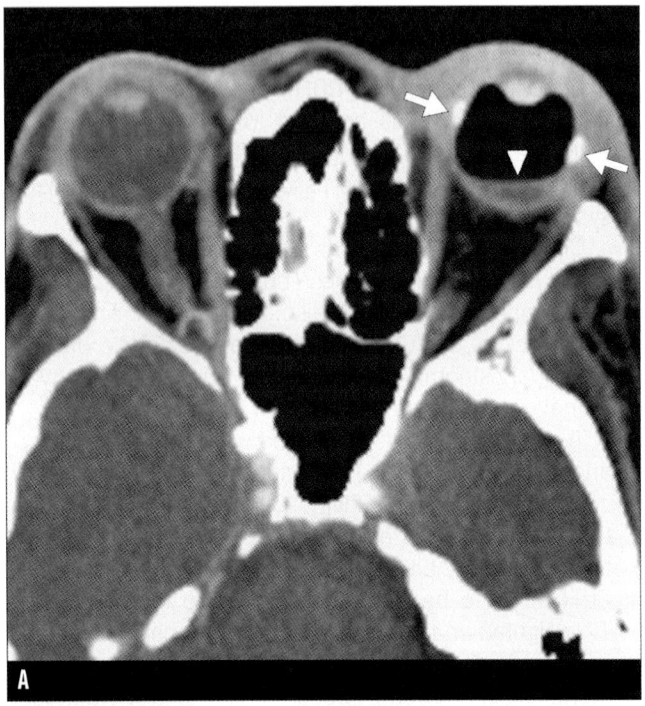

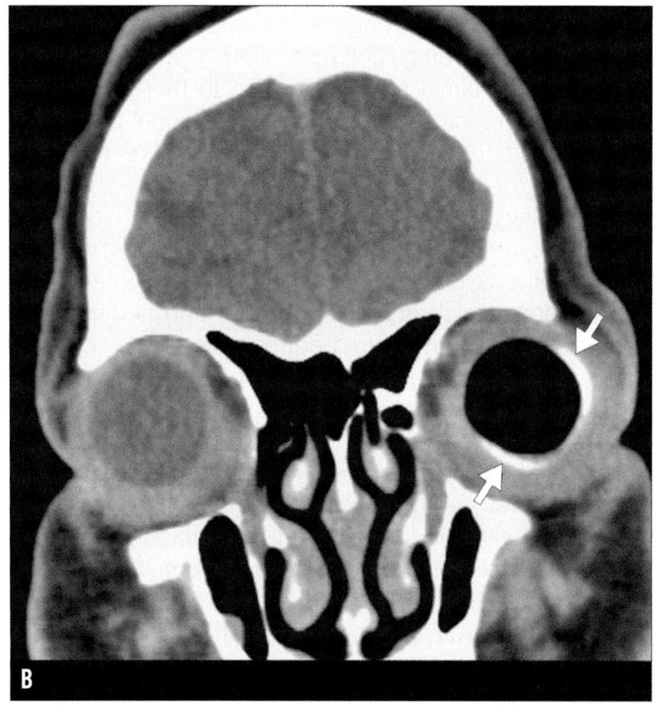

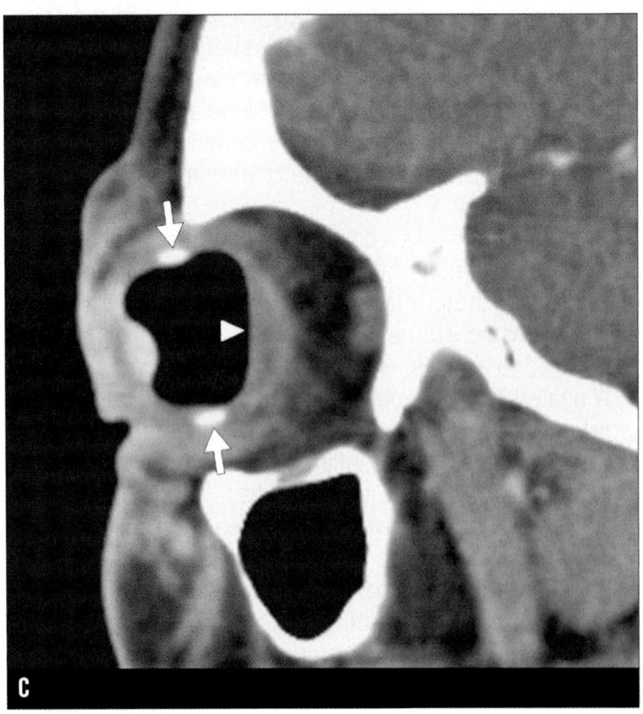

Axial (**A**), coronal reformatted (**B**), and sagittal reformatted (**C**) contrast-enhanced CT images demonstrate changes of a hyperdense silicone scleral buckle (arrows, **A-C**), vitrectomy, and pneumatic retinopexy (gaseous tamponade) of the left globe, with an associated air-fluid level (arrowheads, **A**, **C**). Gas tamponade will often contain air-fluid levels because of the expected reaccumulation of normal vitreous fluid.

Vitrectomy and pneumatic retinopexy (MRI)

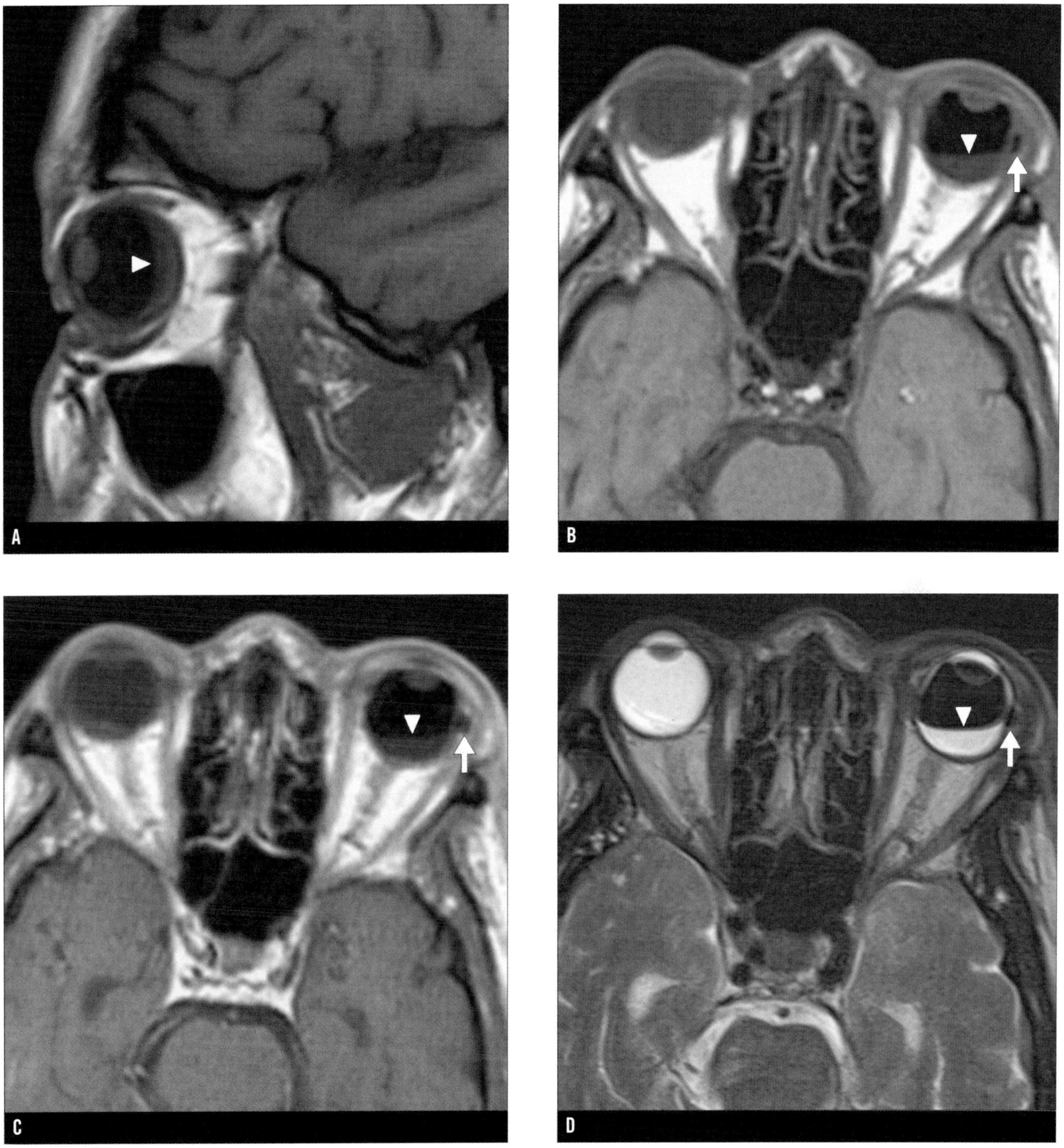

Same patient. Sagittal T1 (**A**), axial T1 (**B**), postcontrast axial T1 (**C**), and axial T2 (**D**) MR images demonstrate lack of signal within the anterior three-fourths of the left globe vitreous chamber, suggestive of gas. An associated fluid level is present within the dependent one-fourth of the vitreous chamber (arrowheads, **A-D**). The dependent fluid represents expected reaccumulation of the normal vitreous fluid. T1 and T2 hypointense signal corresponding to a left silicone scleral buckle is also identified (arrows, **B-D**).

Vitrectomy and silicone oil retinopexy (CT)

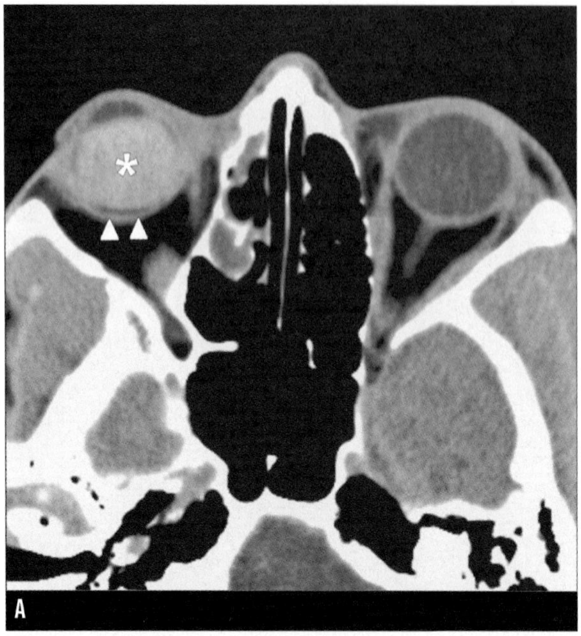

An unenhanced axial CT image (**A**) demonstrates high-density material in the right globe vitreous chamber compatible with vitreous silicone oil placed after a vitrectomy (asterisk). Because silicone oils have a lower specific gravity than vitreous fluid, it is normal to identify normal vitreous fluid layering dependently to the instilled silicone (arrowheads).

Vitrectomy and silicone oil retinopexy (CT and MRI)

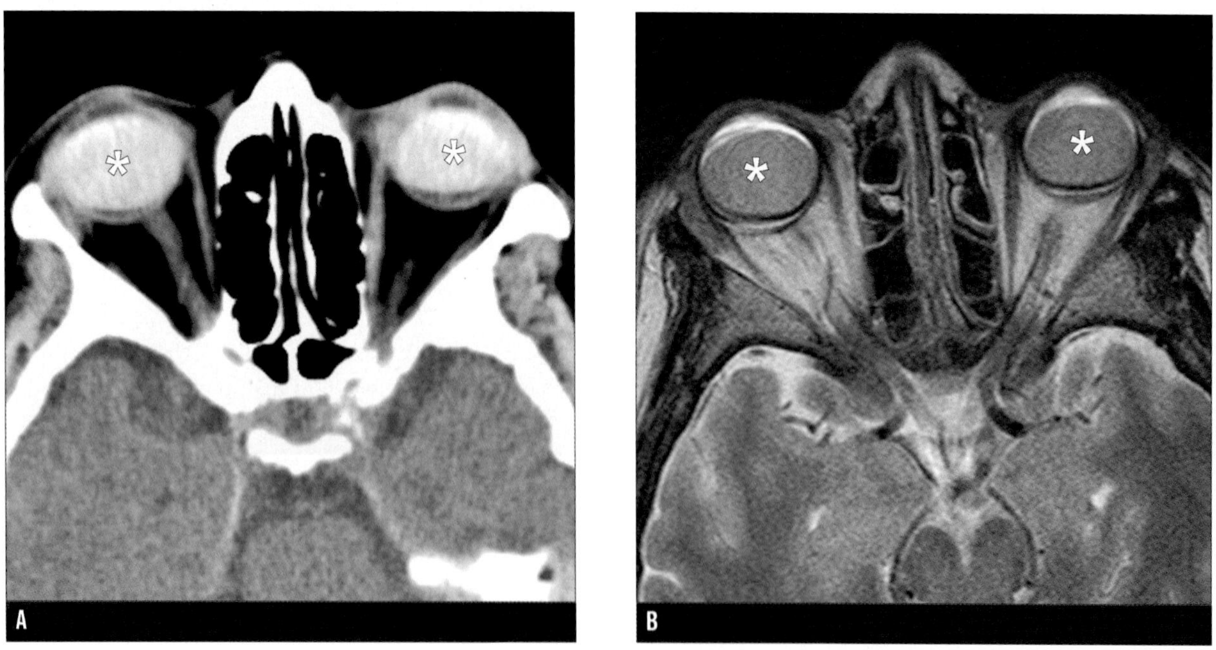

Different patient. An unenhanced axial CT image (**A**) demonstrates hyperdense material in the vitreous chambers of the globes, consistent with the presence of silicone oil (asterisks). Axial T2 (**B**), axial T1 (**C**), and postcontrast axial T1 with fat suppression (**D**) MR images demonstrate the silicone oil to be T2 hypointense, T1 isointense, and nonenhancing relative to normal vitreous fluid (asterisks, **B**-**D**). On image **D**, the signal of the silicone oil is more hypointense relative to image **C** because of suppression of the silicone oil lipids.

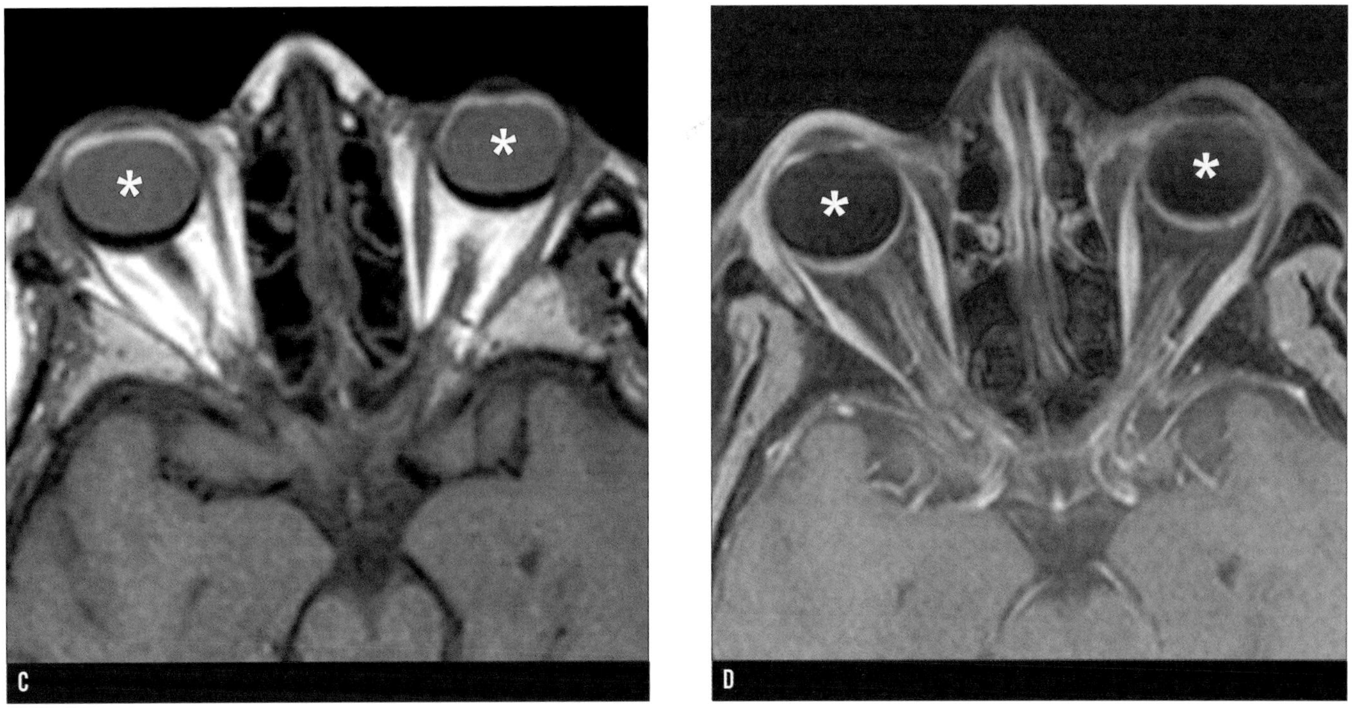

Companion case: Vitreous hemorrhage

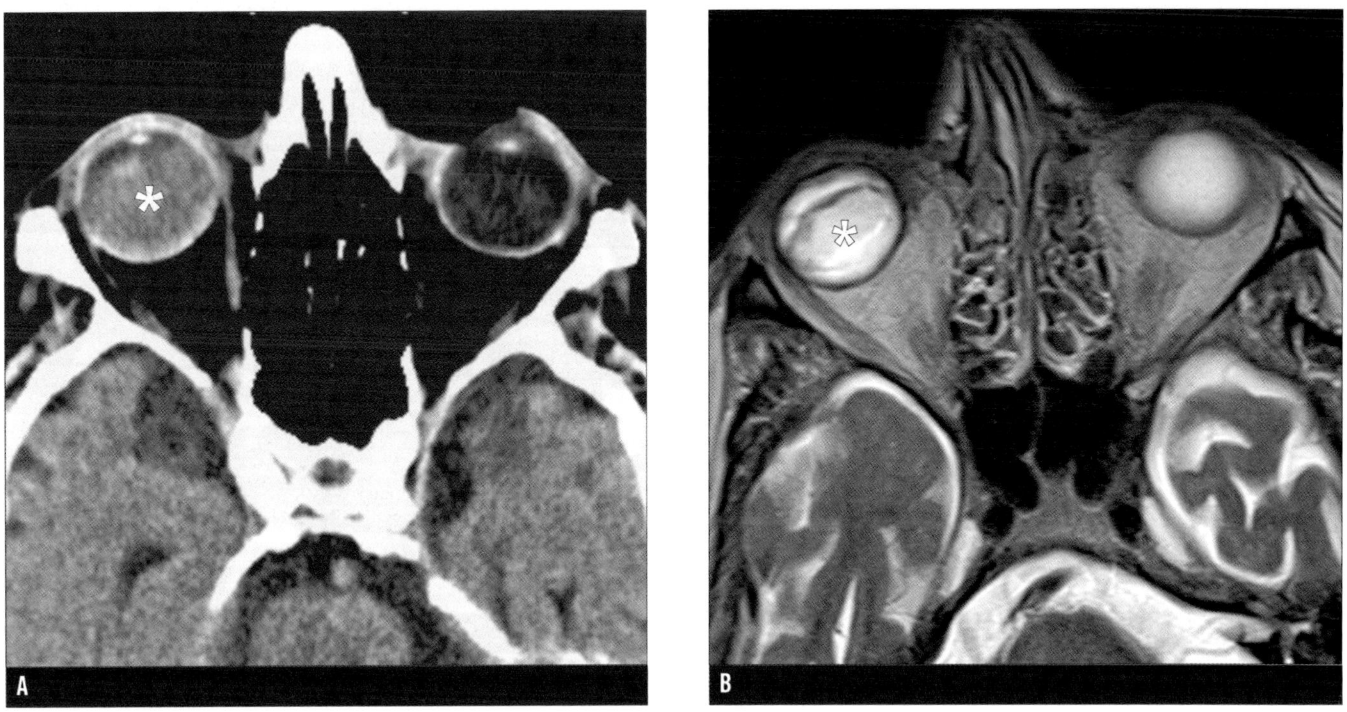

An unenhanced axial CT image (**A**) demonstrates hyperattenuation within the right globe vitreous chamber (asterisk, **A**). However, the density of the finding is not as elevated as would be expected with a silicone oil retinopexy and more concordant with the density of hemorrhage. Axial T2 (**B**), axial T1 (**C**), and postcontrast axial T1 (**D**) MR images of the same patient demonstrate primarily elevated T2 signal, elevated T1 signal, and no enhancement within the right vitreous chamber (asterisks, **B**-**D**). These MRI imaging characteristics are also more consistent with vitreous hemorrhage rather than silicone oil retinopexy.

REFERENCES

Berdahl, John P., Prithvi Mruthyunjaya, Ingrid U. Scott, and Sharon Fekrat. "Vitreous Hemorrhage: Diagnosis and Treatment." *Vitreous Hemorrhage: Diagnosis and Treatment.* American Academy of Ophthalmology, Mar. 2007. Web. 05 Apr. 2015.

Fonseca PF, et al. Visual outcomes of surgical intervention for pseudotumor cerebri: optic nerve sheath fenestration versus cerebrospinal fluid diversion. *Br J Opthalmol.* 2014;98:1360-1363.

Heimann H, Damato B. Congenital vascular malformations of the retina and choroid. *Eye.* 2010;24:459-467.

Heimann H, Jmor F, Damato B. Imaging of retinal and choroidal vascular tumours. *Eye.* 2013;27:208-216.

Khuu T, Hoffman DJ. Circumscribed choroidal hemangioma: A case report and review of the literature. *Optometry.* 2006;77:384-391.

Kiel JW. *The Ocular Circulation.* San Rafael, CA: Morgan & Claypool Life Sciences; 2010.

Killer HE, Jaggi GP, Miller NR. Progressive Optic Neuropathy in Idiopathic Intracranial Hypertension After Optic Nerve Sheath Fenestration. *J Neuro-Ophthalmol.* 2010;30:205.

Lane JI, Watson RE, Witte JF, McCannel CA. Retinal detachment: imaging of surgical treatments and complications. *Radiographics.* 2003;23(4):983-994.

Lane JI, Watson RE Jr, Witte RJ, McCannel CA. Retinal detachment: imaging of surgical treatments and complications. *Radiographics.* 2003;23(4):983-994.

LeBedis CA, Sakai O. Nontraumatic orbital conditions: diagnosis with CT and MR imaging in the emergent setting. *Radiographics.* 2008;28(6):1741-1753. doi: 10.1148/rg.286085515.

Li Yim J, et al. Treatment review of sight threatening circumscribed choroidal haemangioma. *Int J Ophthalmol.* 2010;3(2):168-171.

Mafee MF, Peyman GA. Retinal and choroidal detachments: role of magnetic resonance imaging and computed tomography. *Radiol Clin North Am.* 1987;25(3):487-507.

Root, Tim. Anatomy of the Eye. *The Free Online Ophthalmology Book! (Ophthobook.com).* N.p., n.d. Web. 5 Apr. 2015.

Rumboldt Z, Moses C, Wieczerzynski U, Saini R. Diffusion-weighted imaging, apparent diffusion coefficients, and fluid-attenuated inversion recovery MR imaging in endophthalmitis. *AJNR Am J Neuroradiol.* 2005;26:1869-1872.

Stroszczynski C, et al. Choroidal Hemangioma. MR Findings and Differentiation from Uveal Melanoma. *Am J Neuroradiol.* 1998;19:1441-1447.

Swallow CE, Tsuruda JS, Digre KB, Glaser MJ, Davidson HC, Harnsberger HR. Terson syndrome: CT evaluation in 12 patients. *AJNR Am J Neuroradiol.* 1998;19:743-747.

Yu E, Laughlin S, Kassel EE, Messner HA, Yucel YH. Nocardial endophthalmitis and subretinal abscess: CT and MR imaging features with pathologic correlation: a case report. *AJNR Am J Neuroradiol.* 2005;26:1220-1222.

CASE 24 Scleral buckling

Scleral buckling (also called scleral banding) is a mainstay of retinal detachment surgical repair. A scleral buckle is a device that may be placed radially (parallel to the rectus muscles) or circumferentially, completely encircling the globe. Moreover, it may be segmental and placed only over the region of retinal tear. The purpose of a buckle is to indent the globe and thus relieve vitreous traction on the retina. This promotes reapposition of the detached retina wall and helps prevent vitreous humor from entering the subretinal space via retinal tears.

Currently, the most commonly used buckling elements are composed of solid silicone. Silicone-based scleral buckles are hyperdense on CT and hypointense on MRI. However, because of their lack of signal, silicone scleral buckles may be difficult to detect on MRI, and their presence may only be inferred by the contour abnormality of the globe caused by the buckle. Solid silicone buckles may be separated from the sclera by interposed porous silicone sponges, which have air density on CT. On occasion, silicone sponges have also been utilized without an accompanying hard silicone buckle. All scleral buckles are sutured in place and are permanent devices, unless a complication necessitates their removal. In the past, the free edges of silicone scleral buckles were secured by MR-compatible small tantalum metallic clips, although these are no longer used.

COMPANION CASE

- **Hydrogel segmental scleral buckle with fragmentation and expansion.** In the 1970s and 1980s, hydrogels, such as Miragel, were frequently employed as buckling elements. These hydrogels were used because of two perceived advantages: their apparent ability to absorb and slowly release water-soluble antibiotics, and because of the lack of a potential dead space that existed between these scleral buckles and the globe, thereby theoretically limiting the risks of infection. However, hydrogel buckles were prone to expansion, fragmentation, and fibrosis, and they were discontinued in 1995.

Circumferential silicone scleral buckling

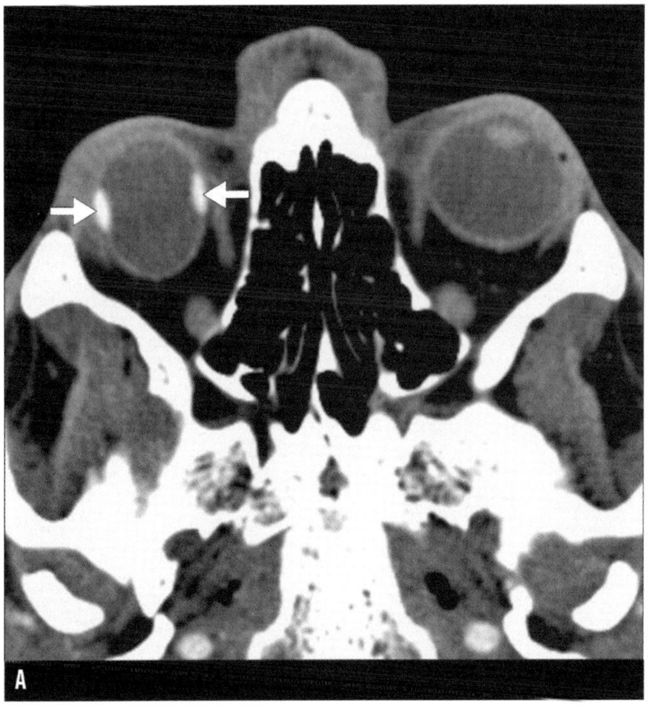

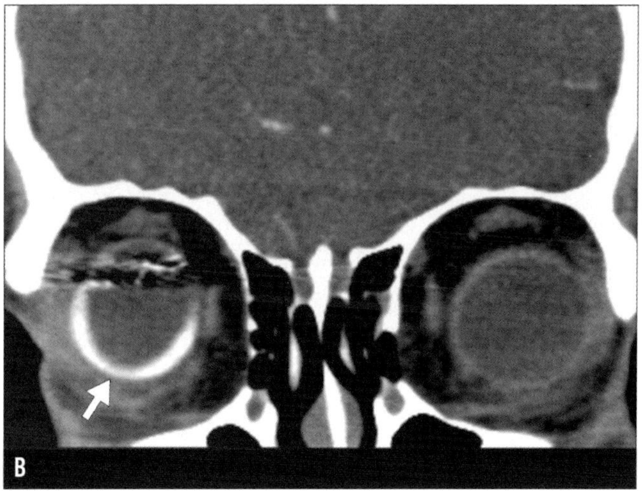

Axial (**A**), coronal reformatted (**B**), and sagittal reformatted (**C**) unenhanced CT images demonstrate a circumferential silicone scleral buckle encircling the right globe (arrows, **A-C**). The scleral buckle in this case results in pronounced narrowing of the right globe diameter, more so than is typically present. By indenting the globe, a scleral buckle decreases vitreous traction and promotes reapposition of a retinal detachment. Incidental note is made of a metallic foreign body posterior to the right globe (arrowhead, **C**), unrelated to the scleral buckle. Postcontrast axial T1 (**D**) and axial T2 (**E**) MR images of a different patient demonstrate how relatively occult a scleral buckle may be on MRI. The scleral buckle is only faintly apparent and is perhaps best appreciated by the mild contour deformity of the right globe as a result of the scleral buckle (arrows, **E**).

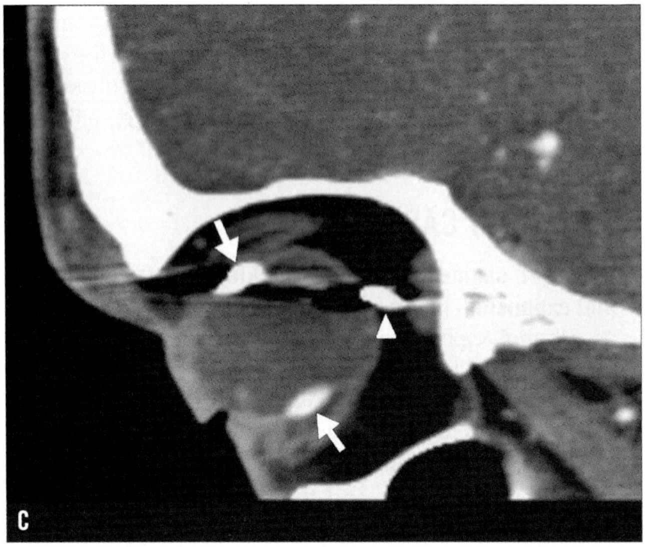
C

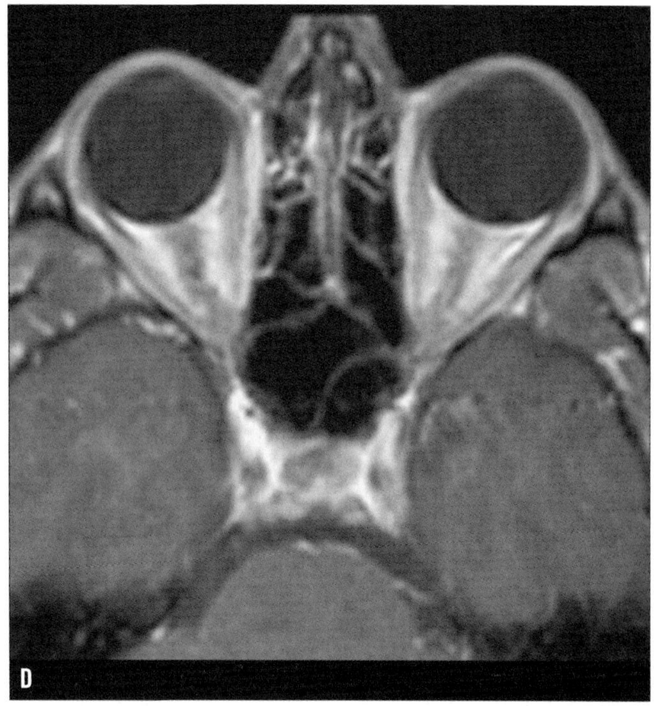
D

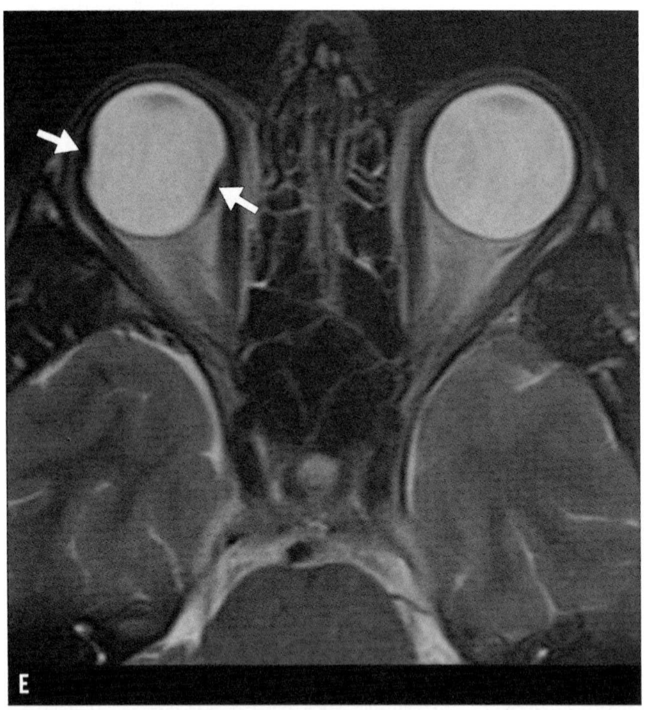
E

Circumferential silicone scleral buckling secured with a metallic clip

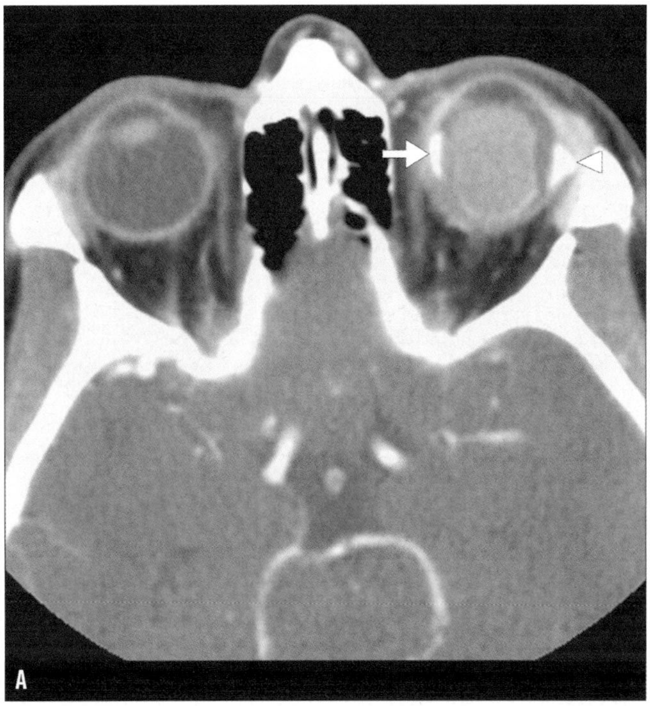

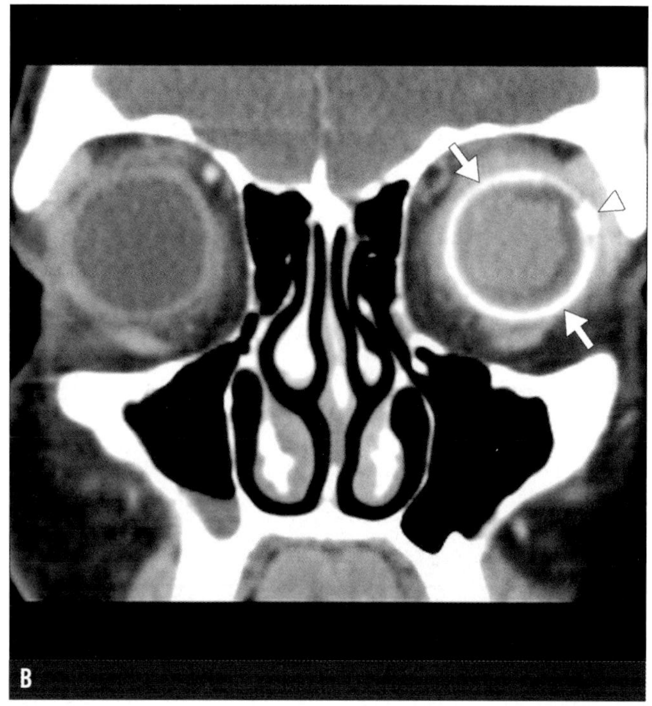

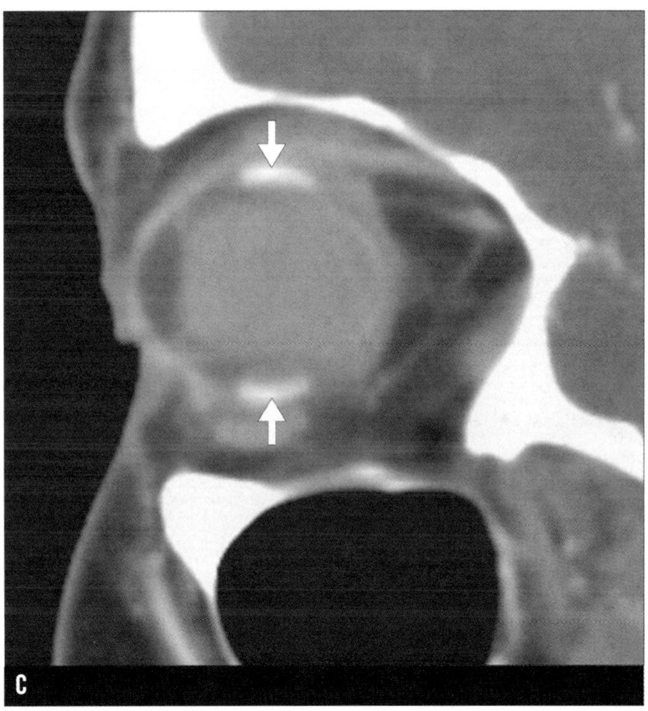

Axial (**A**), coronal reformatted (**B**), and sagittal reformatted (**C**) contrast-enhanced CT images demonstrate postprocedural changes of a left vitrectomy with hyperdense silicone oil tamponade. There is a circumferential hyperdensity outlining the left scleral margin, consistent with a silicone scleral buckle (arrows, **A**-**C**). The free edges of the silicone buckle are secured by a slightly more hyperdense clip (arrowheads, **A**, **B**), typically composed of tantalum, an MRI-compatible material.

Circumferential silicone sponge scleral buckling

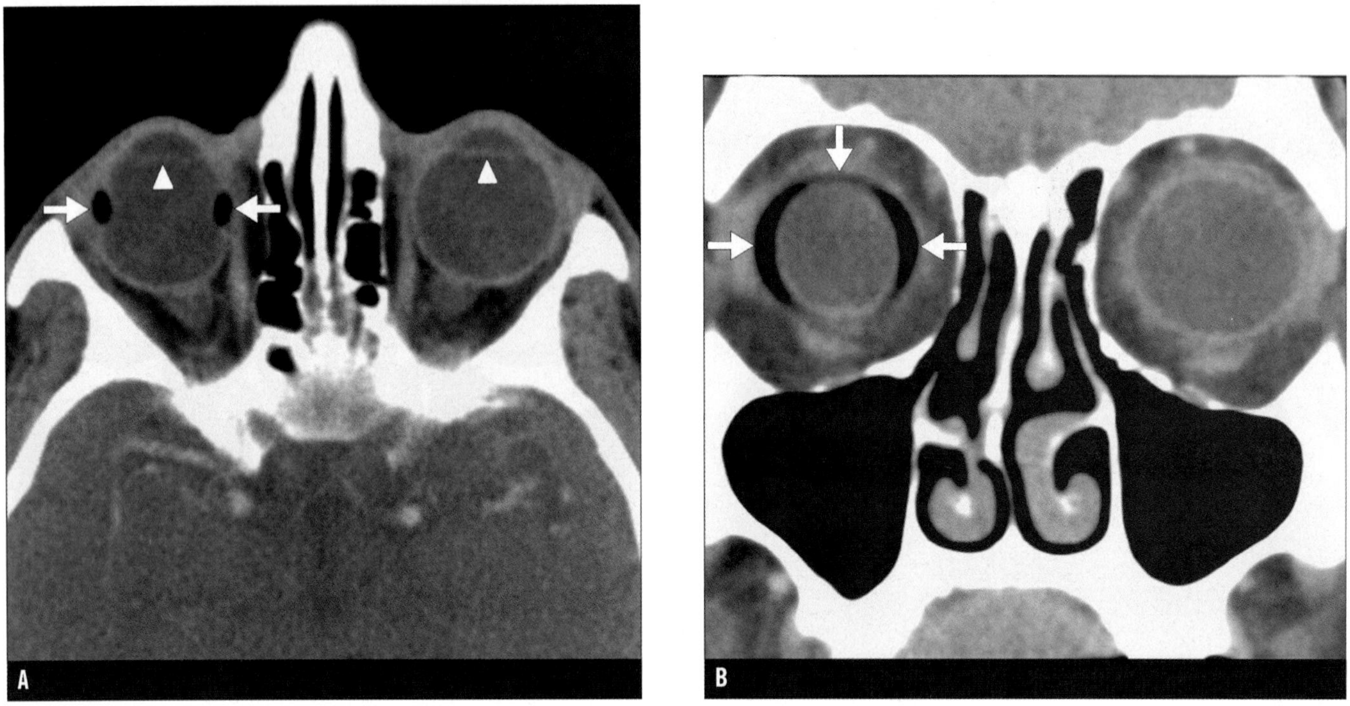

Axial (**A**) and coronal reformatted (**B**) unenhanced CT images demonstrate an air-attenuation ring encircling and deforming the right globe, consistent with circumferential silicone sponge (arrows, **A**, **B**). Bilateral intraocular lens replacements are also present (arrowheads, **A**).

Segmental silicone sponge scleral buckling

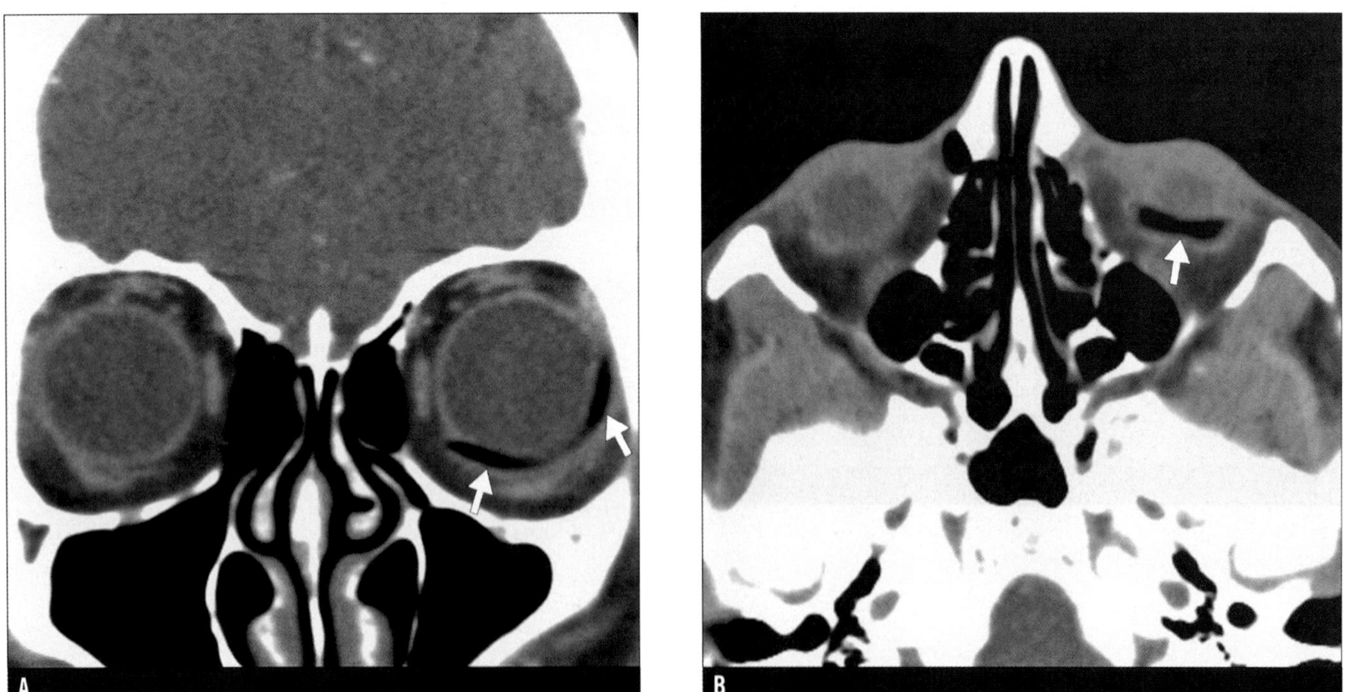

Coronal reformatted (**A**) and axial (**B**, **C**) unenhanced CT images demonstrate segmental scleral buckling with placement of a silicone sponge only along the lateral and inferior margins of the left globe (arrows, **A**-**C**).

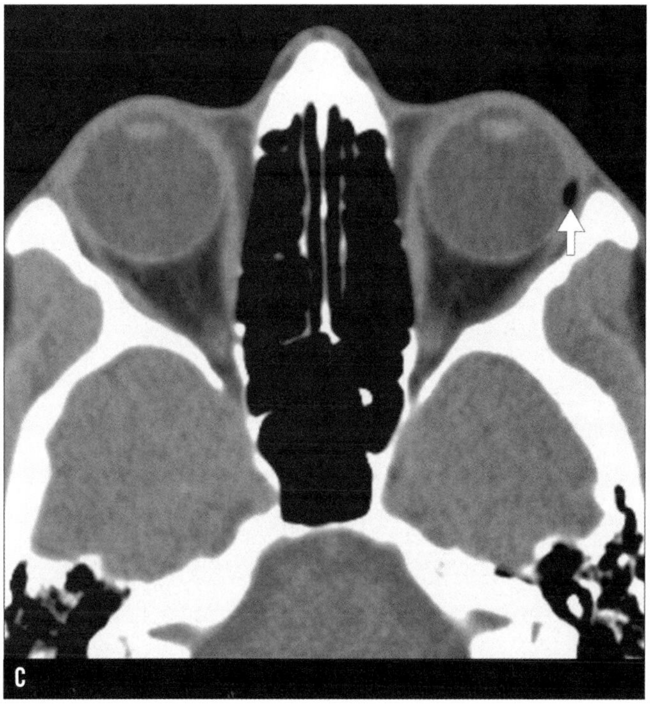

Hydrogel segmental scleral buckle

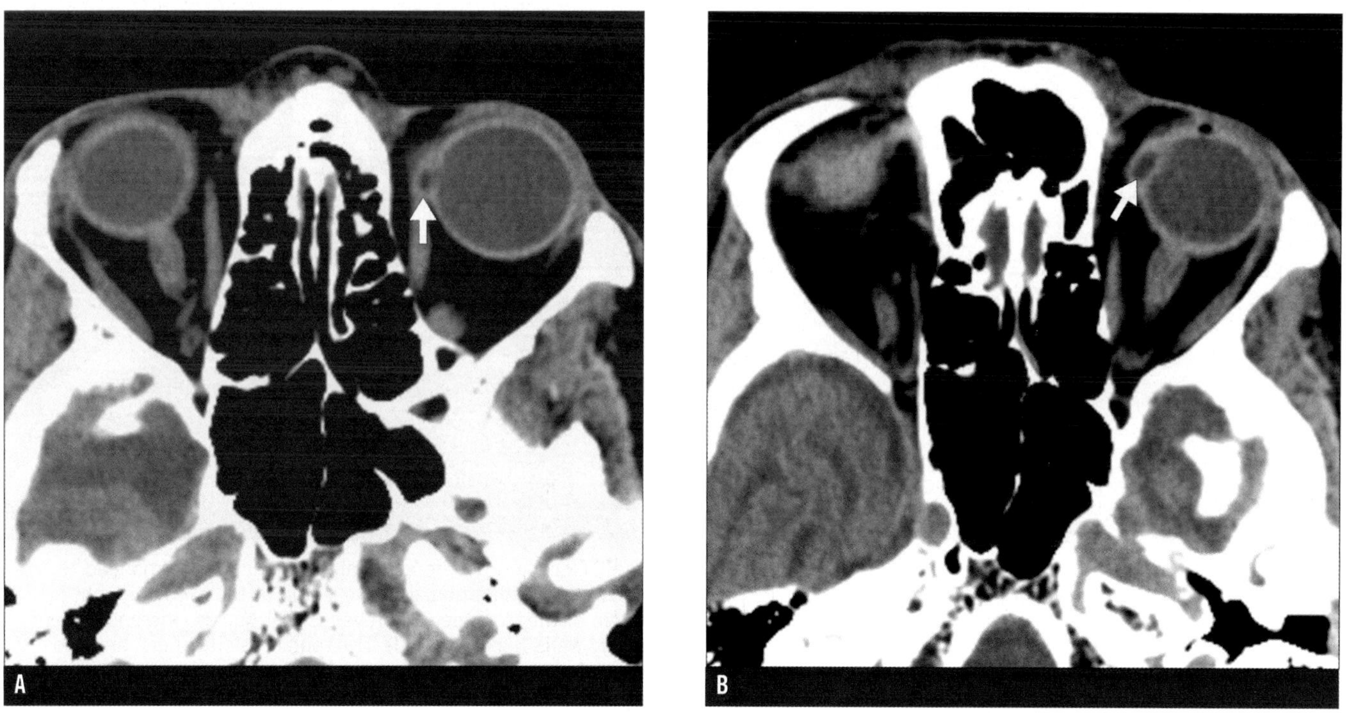

Unenhanced axial CT images (**A**-**C**) demonstrate a fluid density segmental scleral buckle along the medial and superior aspects of the left globe (arrows, **A**-**C**). Given the density, this likely represents a hydrogel scleral buckle.

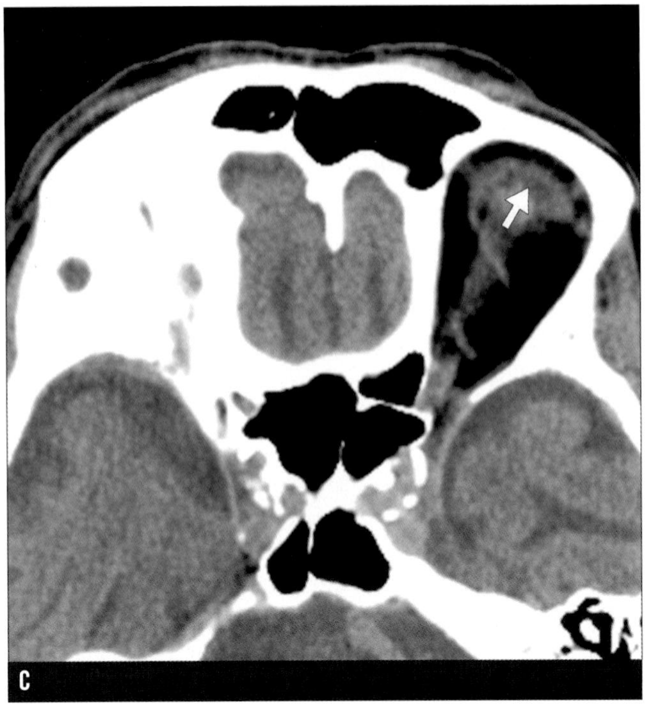

Companion case: Hydrogel segmental scleral buckle with fragmentation and expansion

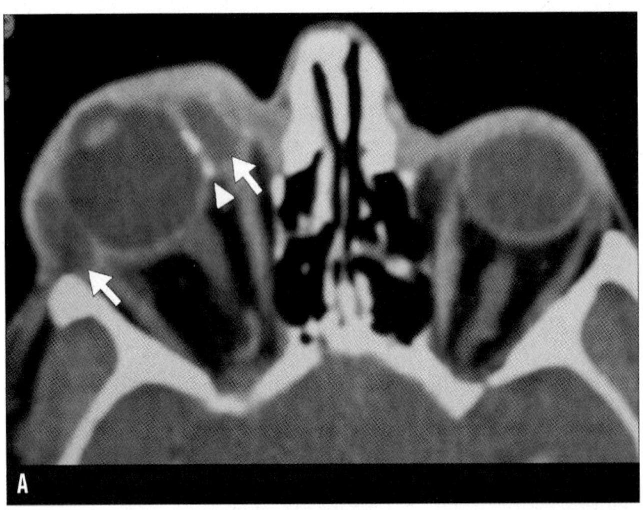

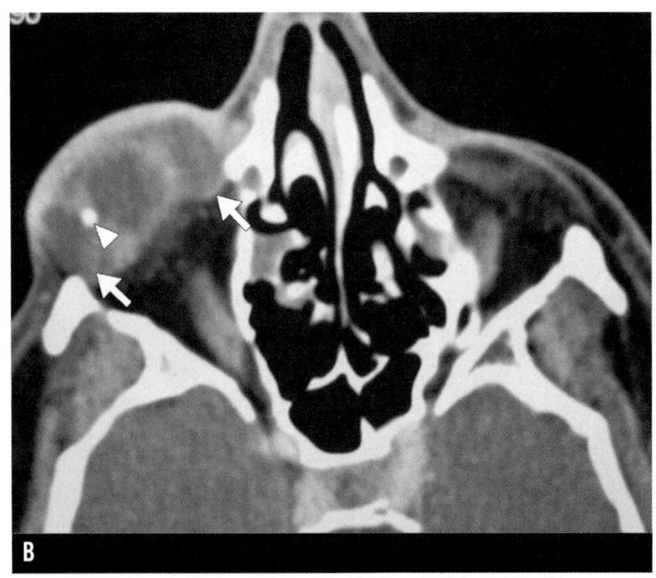

Axial (**A**-**C**) and coronal reformatted (**D**, **E**) images from a contrast-enhanced CT of the orbits demonstrate a dramatically expanded Hydrogel scleral buckle (short arrows, **A**-**E**). There is associated right globe proptosis with induration and thickening of the overlying right lid soft tissues, suggestive of an accompanying cellulitis. Along the nasal margin of the expanded Hydrogel scleral buckle, there is a seemingly unconnected fluid collection with thickening and presumably enhancing walls (long arrow, **C**). Dystrophic calcifications are also noted (arrowheads, **A**-**E**). The constellation of findings are compatible with Hydrogel scleral buckle expansion and fragmentation with an accompanying cellulitis. The apparently separate fluid collection on image **C** could represent additional buckle fragmentation or an abscess. Regardless, surgical exploration and scleral buckle removal is warranted in this setting. *Case courtesy of Hugh D. Curtin, MD, FACR*

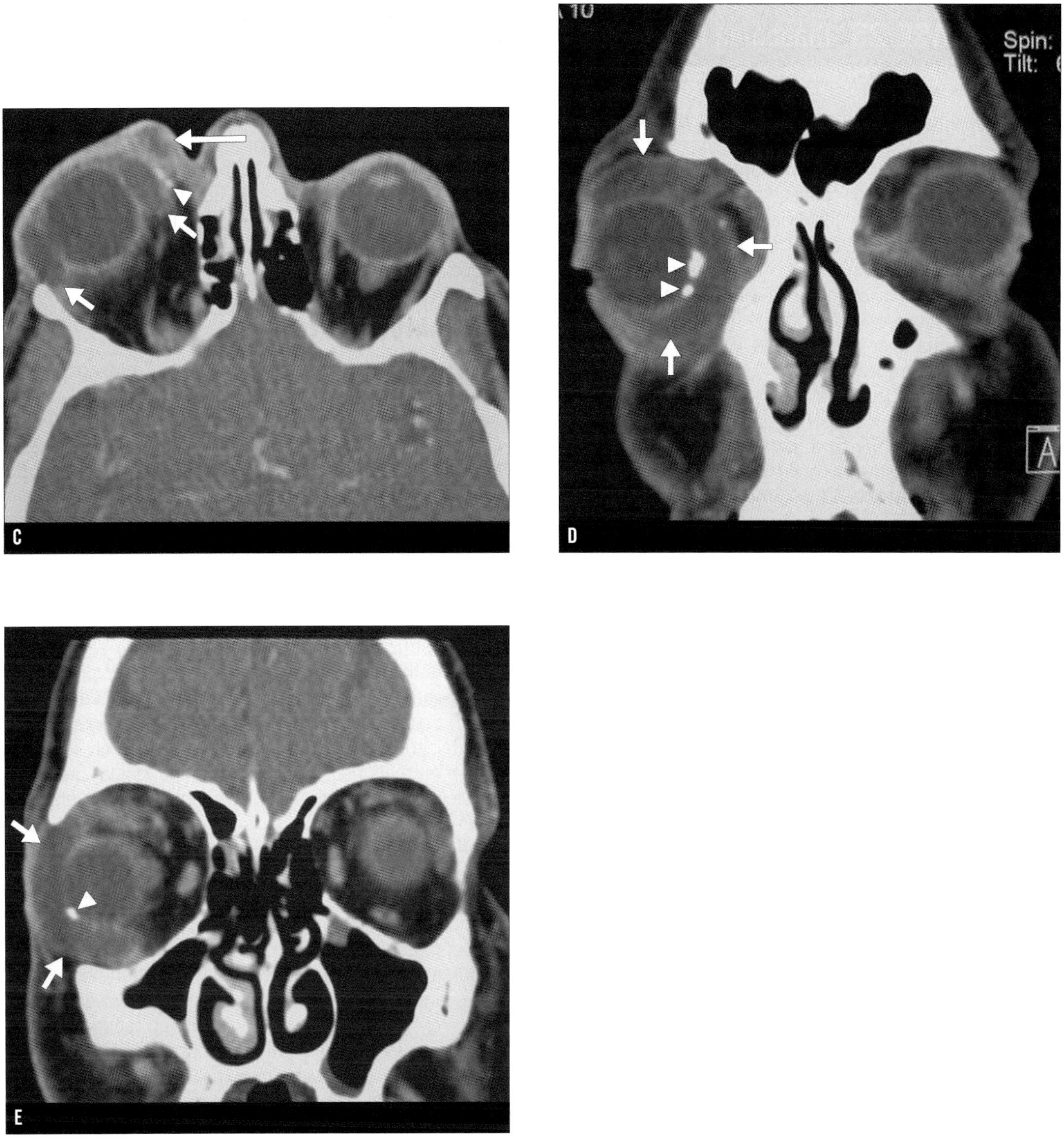

REFERENCES

Baino F. Scleral buckling biomaterials and implants for retinal detachment surgery. *Med Eng Phys.* 2010;32:945-956.

Lane JI, Randall JG, Campeau NG, Overland PK, McCannel CA, Thomas A. Matskolmaging of hydrogel episcleral buckle fragmentation as a late complication after retinal reattachment surgery. *AJNR Am J Neuroradiol.* 2001;22:1199-1202.

Lane JI, Watson RE, Witte JF, McCannel CA. Retinal detachment: imaging of surgical treatments and complications. *Radiographics.* 2003;23(4):983-994.

CASE 25 Glaucoma drainage devices

Glaucoma is one of the leading causes of preventable blindness in the United States and is the result of abnormally elevated intraocular pressure. Aqueous humor, which serves to provide nourishment for the lens and cornea, is produced by the ciliary body and enters the posterior chamber of the eye (not to be confused with the vitreous chamber, which is much larger and resides posterior to the posterior chamber). From here, the aqueous humor traverses anteriorly through the pupil and exits the anterior chamber of the globe laterally at the iridocorneal angle. A trabecular meshwork filters the aqueous humor, and the aqueous humor ultimately drains into the blood stream via the canal of Schlemm. If there is loss of this homeostasis, either by a dysfunctional and/or debris-filled trabecular meshwork (open-angle glaucoma) or from a narrowed angle between the cornea and iris (closed-angle glaucoma), then elevated intraocular pressure ensues. The elevated intraocular pressure results in degeneration of the ganglion cells within the retina at the optic nerve head and culminates in vision loss.

Traditionally, a trabeculectomy was the gold standard for the treatment of glaucoma. However, glaucoma drainage devices are currently being used with increasing frequency because of their significantly improved effectiveness and safety profile. Glaucoma drainage devices are surgically implanted devices that may be used as the primary surgical option in patients with medically refractory glaucoma, following a failed trabeculectomy, or if a trabeculectomy is not an option. These devices consist of two main components, an outflow device (endplate) and a tube to drain the aqueous humor. The tube is placed either in the anterior or posterior chamber, and the endplate is most often placed in the superior temporal quadrant of the orbit adjacent to the globe.

Currently, there are two types of glaucoma drainage devices: valved and nonvalved types. Valved glaucoma drainage devices, such as the Ahmed (New World Medical, Inc., Rancho Cucamonga, CA) and Krupin (Hood Laboratories, Pembroke, MA), utilize a pressure-sensitive, unidirectional valve that regulates aqueous egress. The aqueous egress only occurs at a level above a certain pressure, thus reducing the risk of globe hypotony. A fibrous bleb forms around the drained aqueous humor along the endplate. This fibrous bleb, in addition to the surface area of the endplate, provides additional resistance to the system. Nonvalved glaucoma drainage devices, such as the Baerveldt glaucoma drainage device (Abbott medical optics, Abbott Park, IL), do not contain a pressure-sensitive valve but rather rely on the fibrous bleb to prevent globe hypotony. The drained aqueous humor in both the valved and nonvalved systems is resorbed through the fibrous bleb via the venous and lymphatic system of the adjacent tissues.

COMPANION CASE

- **Large glaucoma drainage device bleb.** There are several complications related to a glaucoma drainage device which may be identified on imaging studies, including implant extrusion, tube malposition, or intraocular hemorrhage. While it is normal for fluid to accumulate around an implanted valve, abnormal progressive enlargement of a bleb, termed a giant reservoir, may occur. A giant reservoir is most commonly identified with an Ahmed glaucoma valve device. On imaging, a giant reservoir is characterized as an oval, fluid equivalent, nonenhancing lesion that is subdivided by a T1 and T2 hypointense linear structure representing the silicone-based endplate of the drainage device. The giant reservoir is often surrounded by a dense fibrous capsule (termed a Tenon cyst) that is impervious to the egress of aqueous humor contained by the giant reservoir, subsequently resulting in shunt malfunction and elevated intraocular pressure. A vicious cycle may ensue, resulting in further enlargement of the giant reservoir and progressive proptosis.
- **Solitary fibrous tumor.** A solitary fibrous tumor (SFT) is a rare tumor that most often occurs in the pleura, pericardium, or peritoneum, but can occur in extrapleural sites, including the meninges and head and neck, amongst others. Orbital SFTs typically have a more indolent course than those identified elsewhere in the body, and they are cured by complete excision. However, incomplete excision is associated with a high recurrence rate and the risk of malignant transformation. The lesion is typically a slow-growing, circumscribed, highly vascular mass that can be found anywhere in the orbit. Relative to muscle, an SFT is generally T1 isointense and T2 iso- to hypointense, the latter reflecting its fibrous content. Internal areas of T2 hyperintensity can sometimes be identified and are related to cystic degeneration or internal hemorrhage. Adjacent osseous remodeling may also be present.

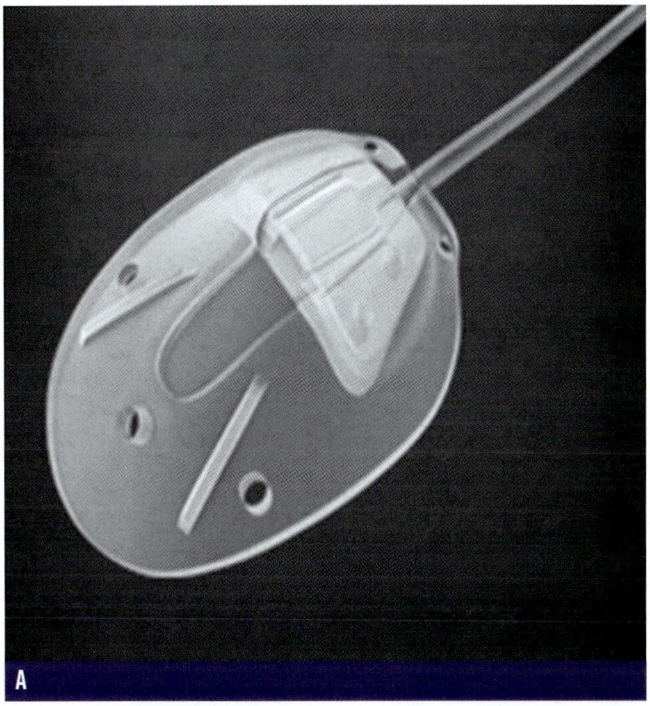

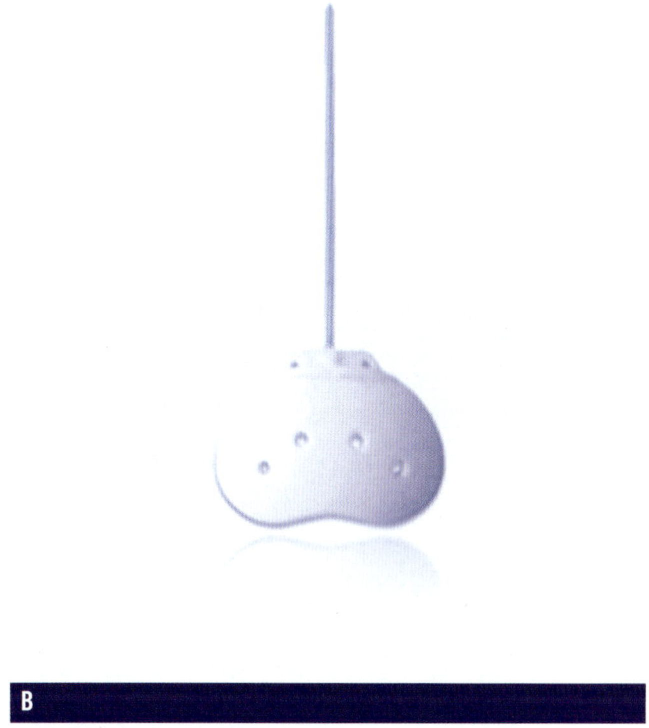

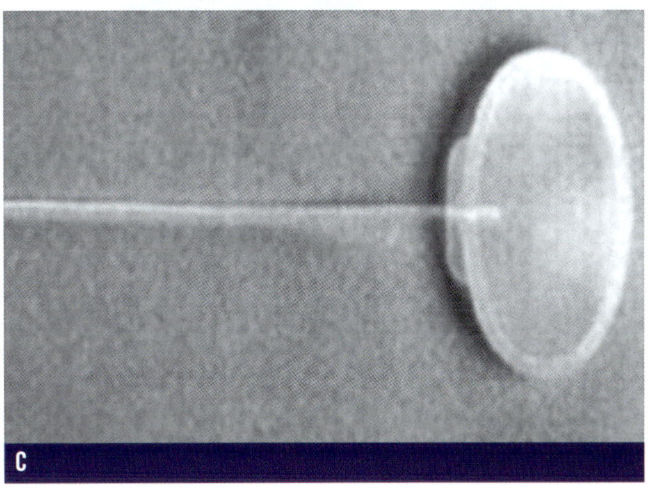

A Ahmed glaucoma drainage device
B Baerveldt glaucoma drainage device
C Krupin glaucoma drainage device

Krupin glaucoma drainage device

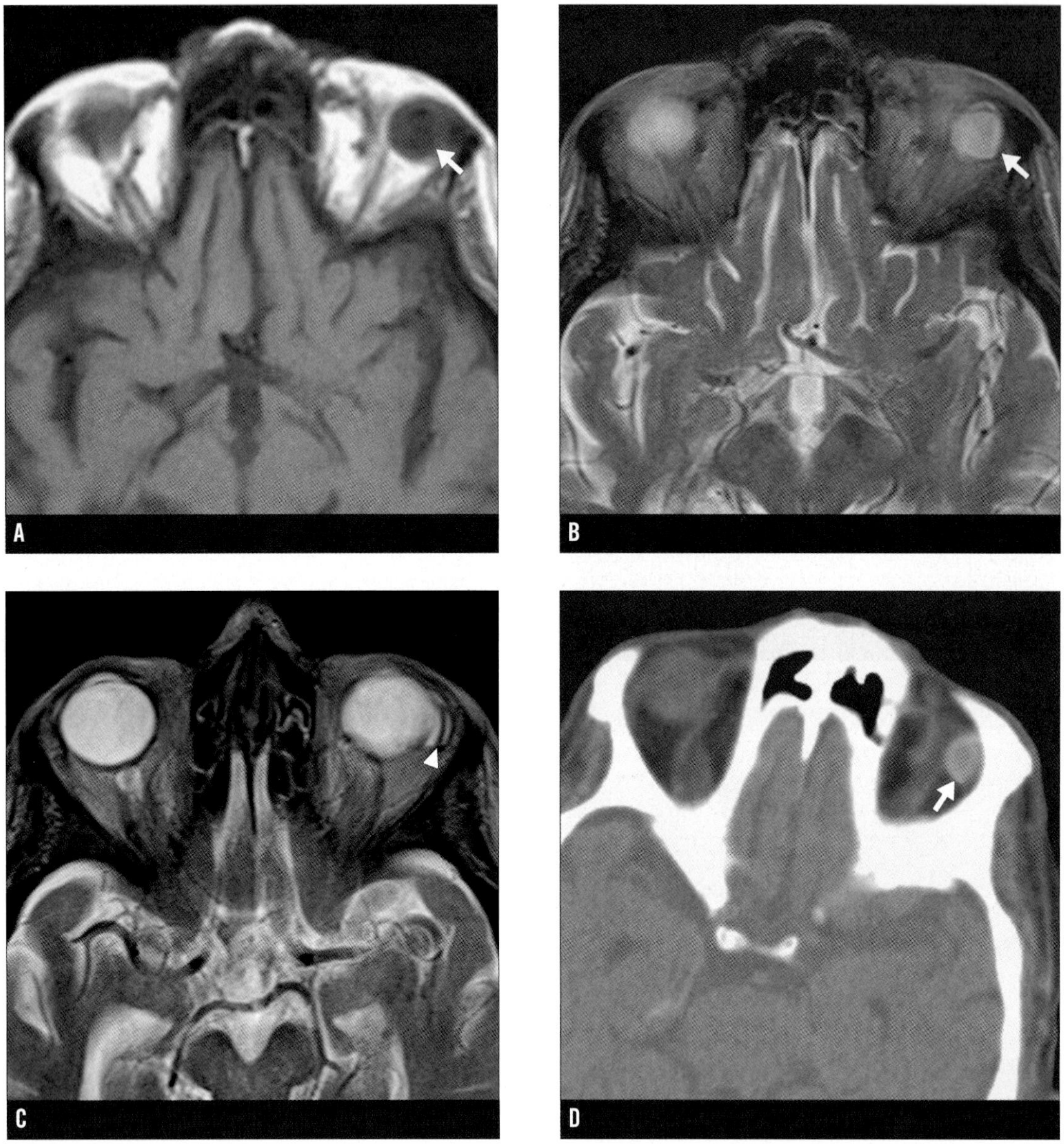

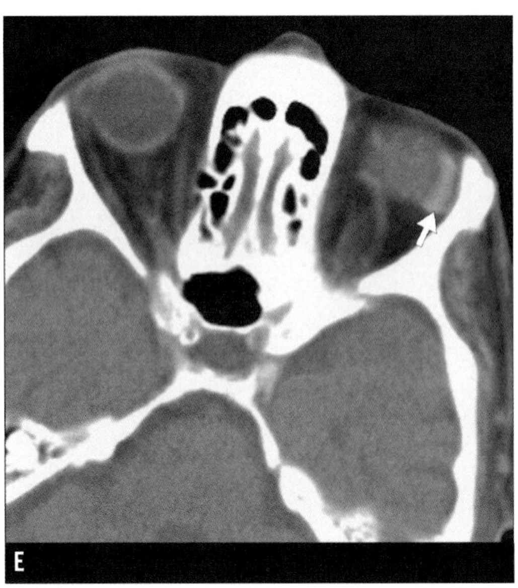

Unenhanced axial T1 (**A**) and axial T2 (**B**, **C**) MR images as well as unenhanced axial CT images (**D**, **E**) demonstrate a Krupin glaucoma drainage device implanted in the superotemporal quadrant of the left orbit. The oval decreased T1 signal (arrow, **A**) and increased T2 signal (arrow, **B**) represent the fluid contained by a fibrous capsule adjacent to the endplate of the drainage device. A curvilinear focus of decreased T2 signal (arrowhead, **C**) represents a portion of the endplate, which is surrounded by fluid. The increased attenuation on CT represents the endplate of the device (arrows, **D**, **E**).

Baerveldt glaucoma drainage device

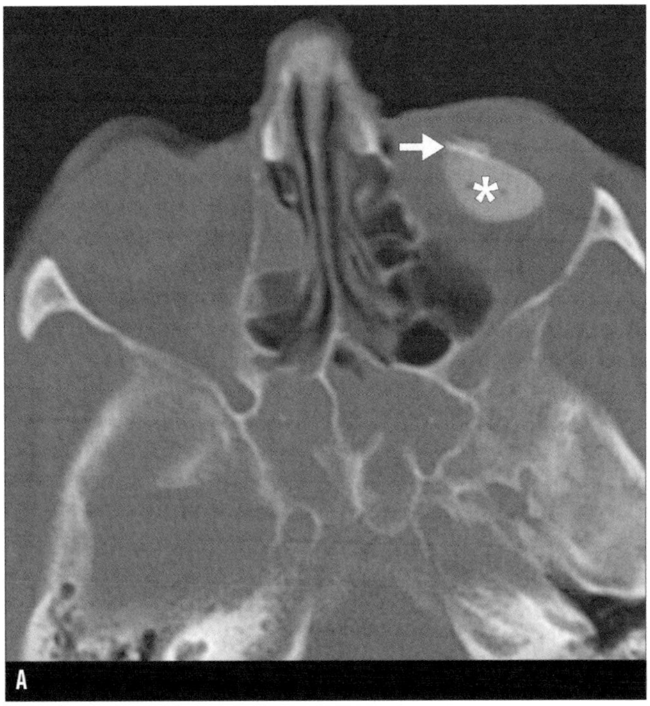

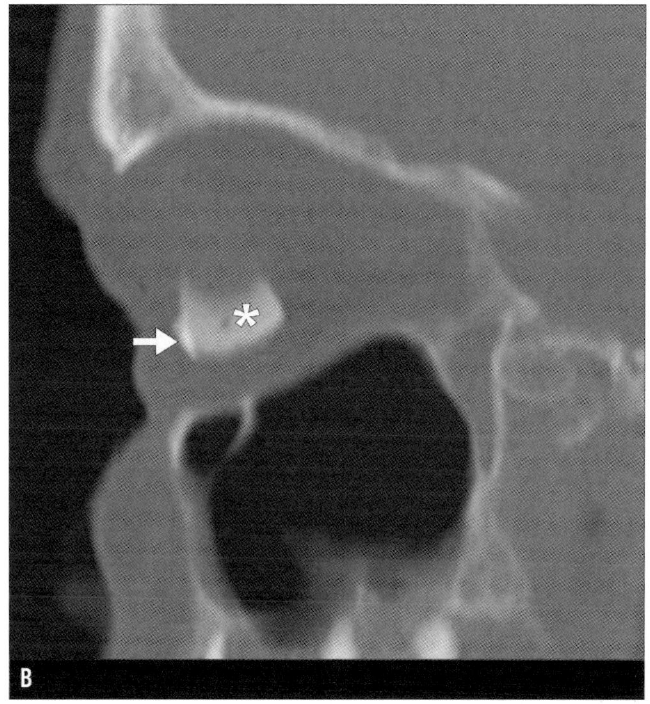

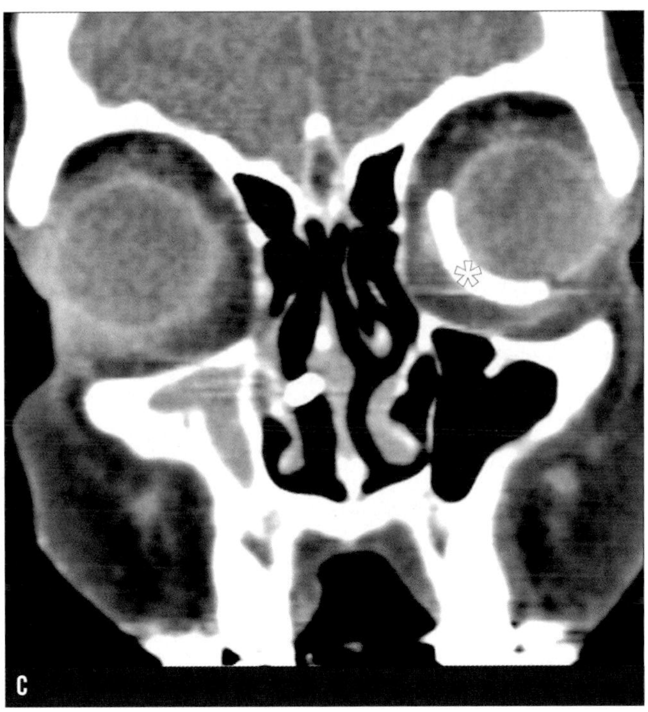

Axial (**A**) and sagittal reformatted (**B**) CT images viewed with a bone window as well as a coronal reformatted CT image viewed with a soft tissue window (**C**) demonstrate the endplate of the Baerveldt glaucoma drainage device (asterisks, **A**-**C**) and its tubing (arrows, **A**, **B**) placed in the inferonasal quadrant of the left orbit. The silicone used in a Baerveldt glaucoma drainage device is impregnated with barium, allowing easy visualization of this device by plain film and CT.

Glaucoma drainage device (unknown type)

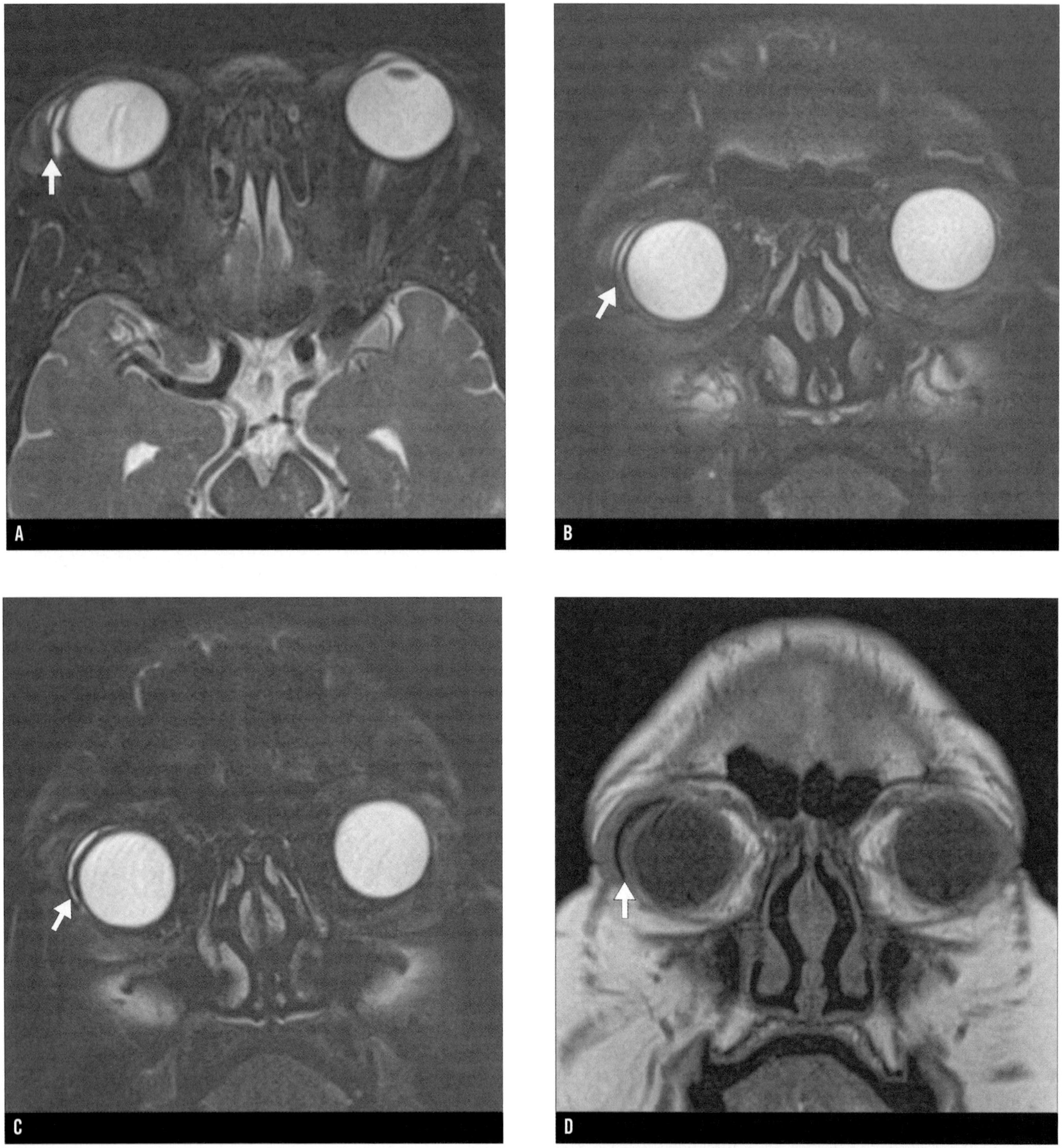

Fat-suppressed axial T2 (**A**), fat-suppressed coronal T2 (**B**, **C**), and coronal T1 (**D**) MR images demonstrate a glaucoma drainage device within the superior temporal quadrant of the right orbit. The type of glaucoma device was not detailed in the history, though typical findings are present, with thin, curvilinear T1 and T2 hypointense signal representing the endplate of the device (arrows, **A**-**D**) and aqueous fluid accumulating on both sides of the endplate.

Companion case: Large glaucoma drainage device bleb

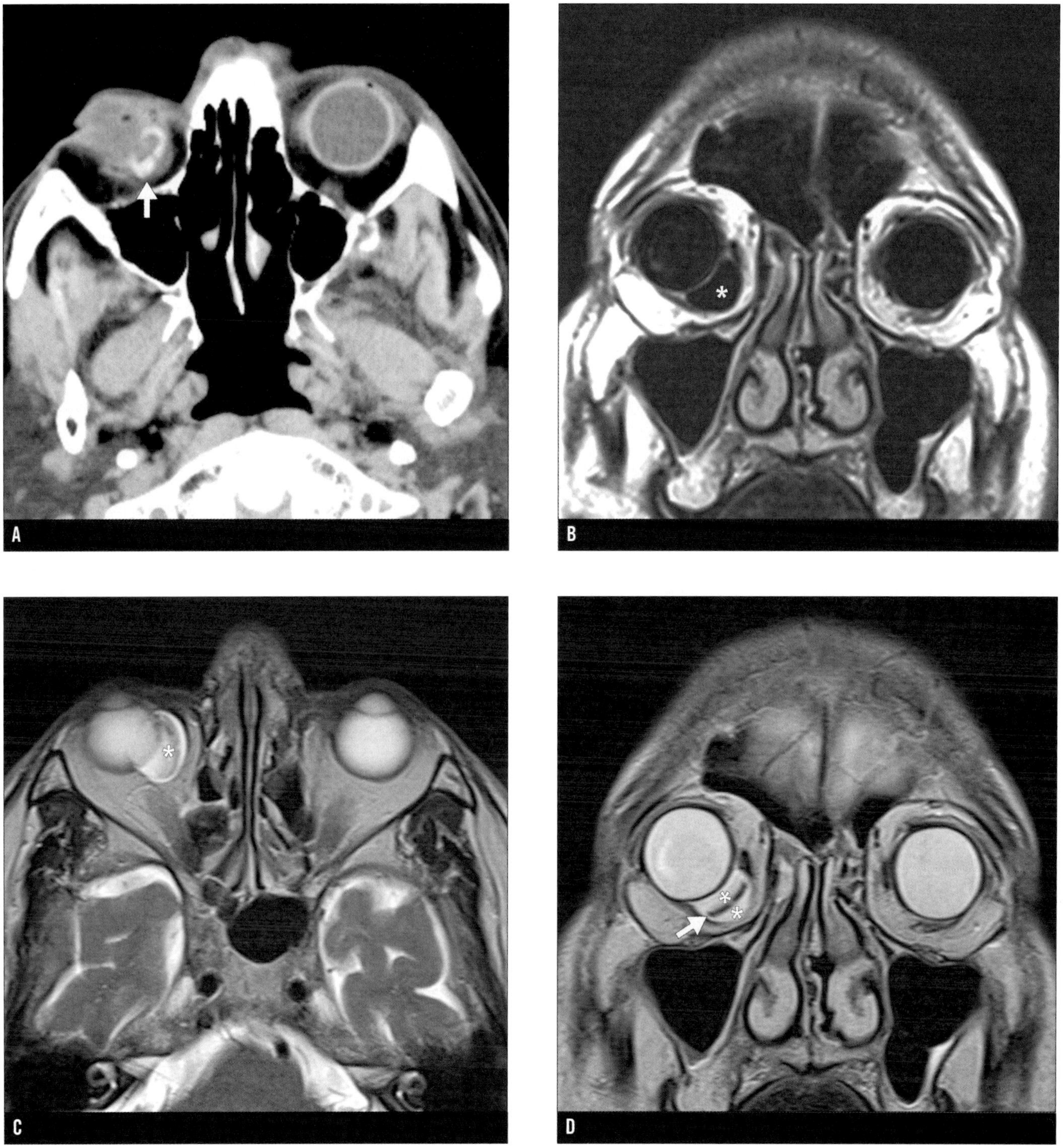

An unenhanced axial CT image (**A**) demonstrate a curvilinear high-density foreign body surrounded by fluid attenuation (arrow, **A**). Coronal T1 (**B**) and axial T2 (**C**) MR images demonstrate a large oval fluid collection abutting the inferior nasal quadrant of the right globe (asterisks, **B**, **C**). A coronal T2-weighted MR image (**D**) more clearly demonstrates that the curvilinear structure on image **A** represents a glaucoma drainage device (arrow, **D**), which is surrounded by a large bleb (asterisks, **D**). The large bleb results in unintended displacement of the right globe, best appreciated on image **D**.

Companion case: Solitary fibrous tumor

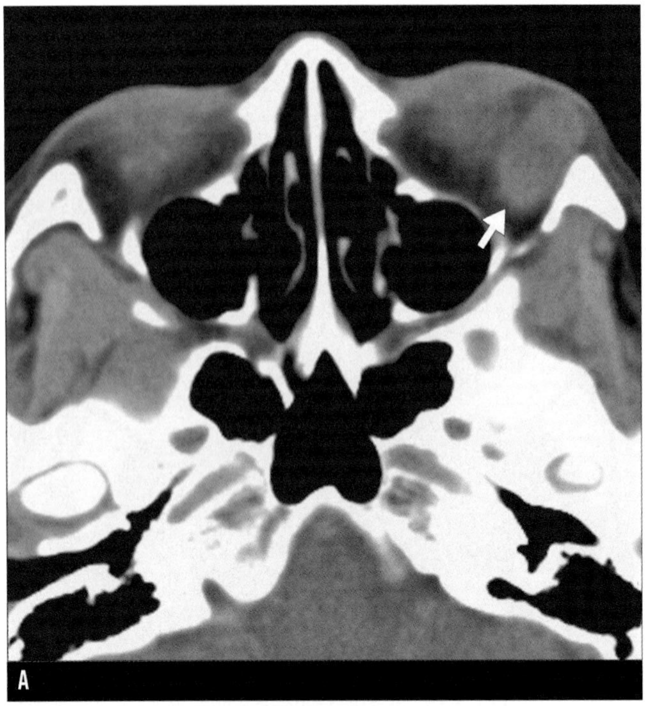

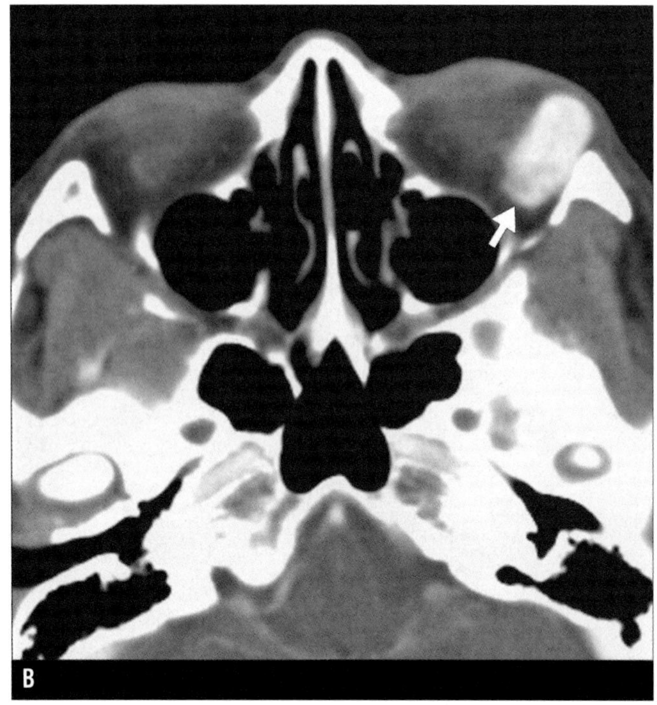

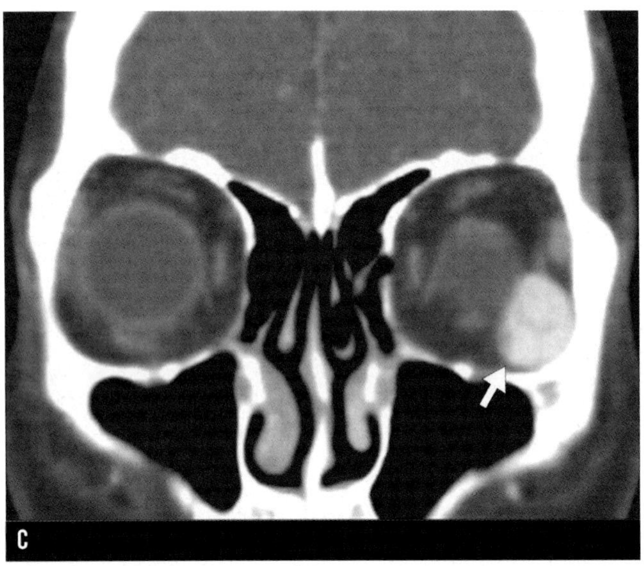

Unenhanced axial (**A**) as well as contrast-enhanced axial (**B**) and coronal reformatted (**C**) CT images demonstrate a circumscribed, extraconal mass in the inferolateral aspect of the left orbit (arrows, **A-C**). The mass avidly and uniformly enhances following contrast. While nonspecific, this mass represented a solitary fibrous tumor at pathology. In addition to the frank enhancement, this lesion is differentiated from a glaucoma drainage device by its shape; a glaucoma device endplate is thin and curvilinear, whereas the finding in this case is clearly a solid, oval mass.

REFERENCES

Bernardini FP, de Conciliis C, Schneider S, Kersten RC, Kulwin DR. Solitary fibrous tumor of the orbit: is it rare? Report of a case series and review of the literature. *Ophthalmology.* 2003;110(7):1442-1448.

Ceballos EM, Parrish RK 2nd. Plain film imaging of Baerveldt glaucoma drainage implants. *AJNR Am J Neuroradiol.* 2002;23(6):935-937.

Festa S, Lee HJ, Langer P, Klein KM. Solitary fibrous tumor of the orbit: CT and pathologic correlation. *Neuroradiology.* 1999;41(1):52-54.

Jeon TY, Kim HJ, Kim ST, Chung TY, Kee C. MR imaging features of giant reservoir formation in the orbit: an unusual complication of Ahmed glaucoma valve implantation. *AJNR Am J Neuroradiol.* 2007;28(8):1565-1566.

Kim HJ, et al. Solitary fibrous tumor of the orbit: CT and MR imaging findings. *AJNR Am J Neuroradiol.* 2008;29(5):857-862.

Lim K, et al. Glaucoma drainage devices; past, present, and future. *Br J Ophthalmol.* 1998;82(9):1083-1089.

Patel S, Pasquale LR. Glaucoma drainage devices: a review of the past, present, and future. *Semin Ophthalmol.* 2010;25(5-6):265-270.

Root T. "Anatomy of the Eye (Ophthobook.com)." *The Free Online Ophthalmology* Book! (*Ophthobook.com*). N.p., n.d. Web. 5 Apr. 2015.

CASE 26 Eyelid weight implant

The muscles of facial expression are innervated by the facial nerve. One of these muscles of facial expression, the orbicularis oculi, functions to close the eye. This muscle function is counteracted by the levator palpebrae muscle, which functions to elevate the upper eyelid. Instead of the facial nerve, the levator palpebrae muscle is innervated by the oculomotor nerve. Thus, with a facial paralysis - as may occur following trauma to the facial nerve, Bell palsy, or a brain lesion affecting the facial nerve motor nucleus - the orbicularis oculi muscle is unable to function and the levator palpebrae muscle is unopposed. This results in eyelid retraction and the patient's inability to completely close their eyes, a condition termed lagophthalmos. In addition to cosmetic issues and dry eyes, lagophthalmos can result in serious complications from corneal exposure, including keratitis, ulceration, and sometimes blindness.

Eyelid weight implants are used to treat lagophthalmos in the setting of a complete facial nerve paralysis. These eyelid weights are placed in the superior eyelid of the affected eye and counteract the unopposed contraction of the levator palpebrae superioris muscle, thereby allowing for improved corneal protection. Eyelid weight implants can be made of gold, platinum, or platinum/viridium, but gold is favored because of its density, malleability, and low reactivity. Eyelid weight implants are MRI-compatible and are hypointense on both T1- and T2-weighted imaging. On CT, extensive streak artifact related to eyelid weight implants is typically present. If eyelid weight implantation is identified by imaging, then it can be safely assumed that the patient has an ipsilateral facial nerve paralysis.

Eyelid weight implant (CT)

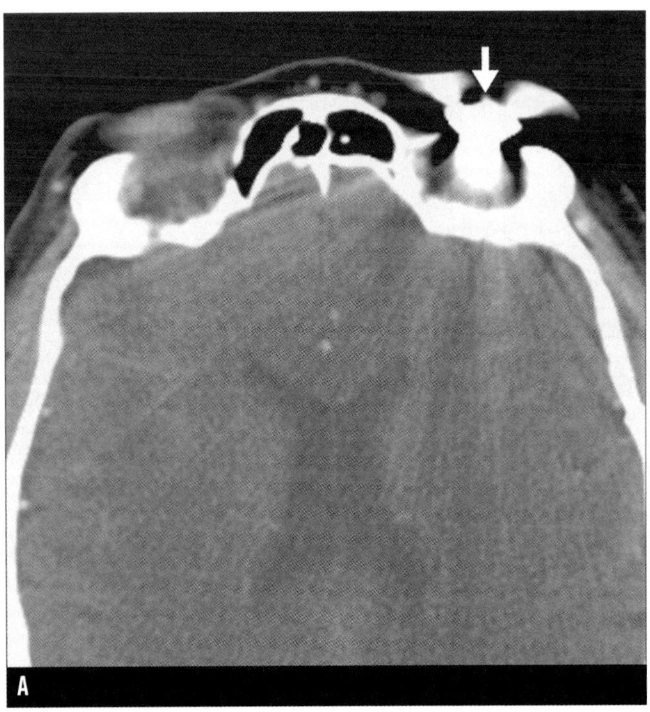

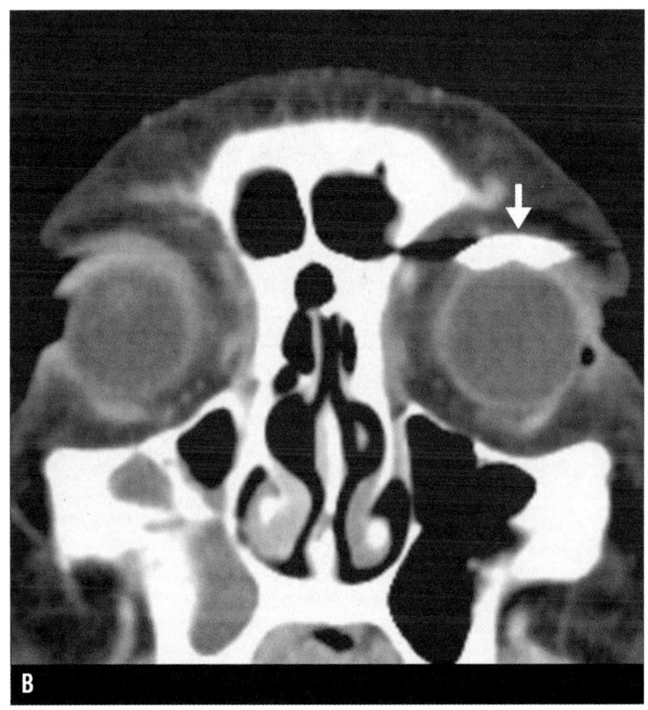

Axial (**A**), coronal reformatted (**B**), and sagittal reformatted (**C**) unenhanced CT images demonstrate a metallic prosthesis implanted in the left upper eye lid, compatible with an eyelid weight (arrows, **A**-**C**). If an eyelid weight is identified by imaging, then it can be safely assumed that the patient has an ipsilateral facial nerve paralysis. An axial CT image was obtained following the left facial nerve paralysis (**D**). This patient developed a left facial nerve injury during a canal wall up mastoidectomy (arrowhead, **D**) to drain a left petrous apex collection (arrow, **D**).

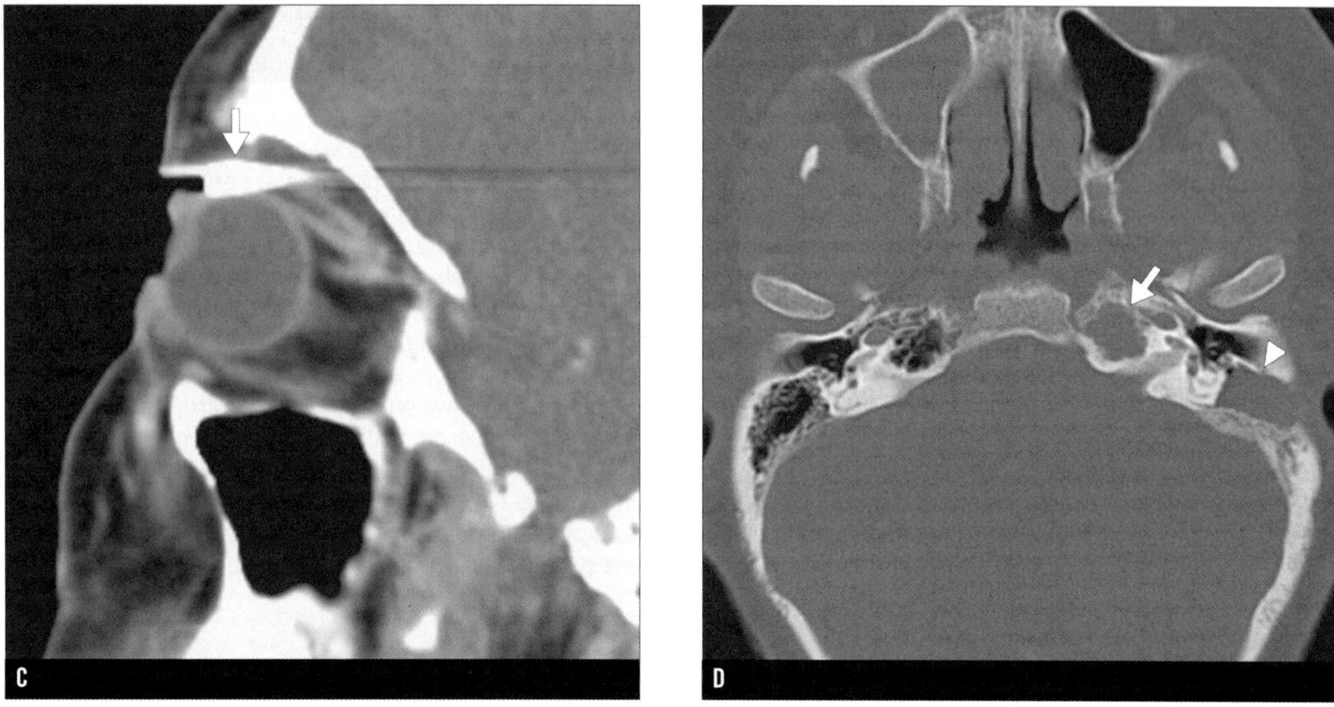

Eyelid weight implant (CT and MRI)

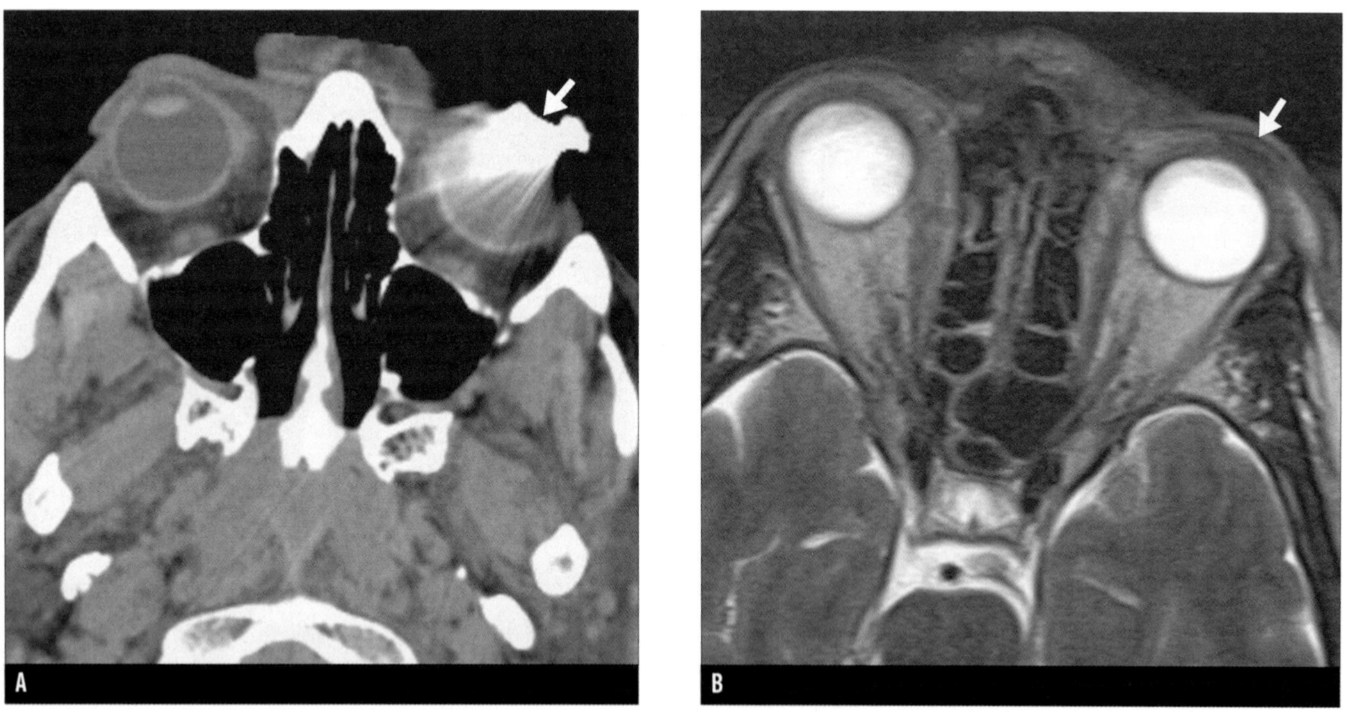

Different patient. An unenhanced axial CT image (**A**) demonstrates a left upper eyelid weight prosthesis (arrow, **A**). Extensive streak artifact is present, a common occurrence with these metallic eyelid implants. Axial T2 (**B**), unenhanced axial T1 (**C**), contrast-enhanced axial T1 (**D**), and unenhanced T1 (**E**) MR images demonstrate the typical MRI appearance of an eyelid weight prosthesis, which is hypointense on both T1- and T2-weighted images (arrows, **B**-**E**). This patient developed a left facial nerve paralysis following a left suboccipital craniotomy and partial mastoidectomy for resection of a large left cerebellopontine angle vestibular schwannoma. A small amount of residual tumor at the left cerebellopontine angle is present on image **D** (arrowhead).

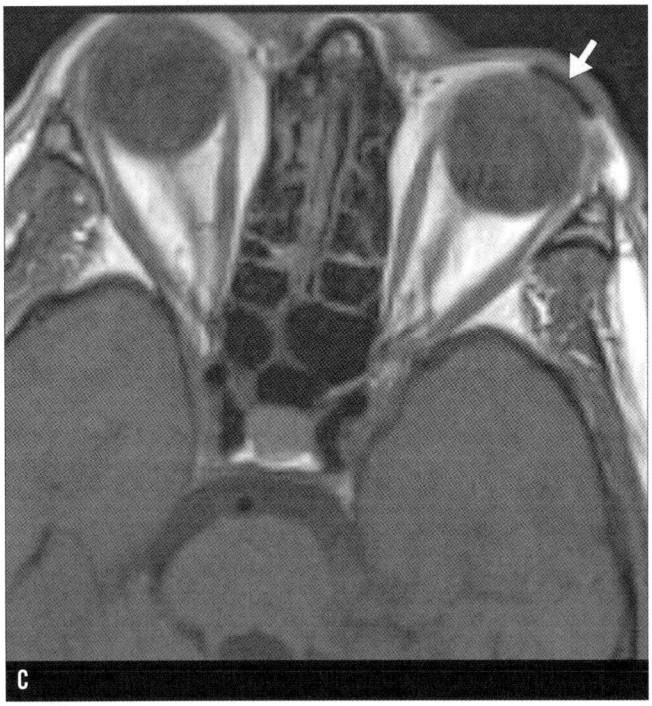

C

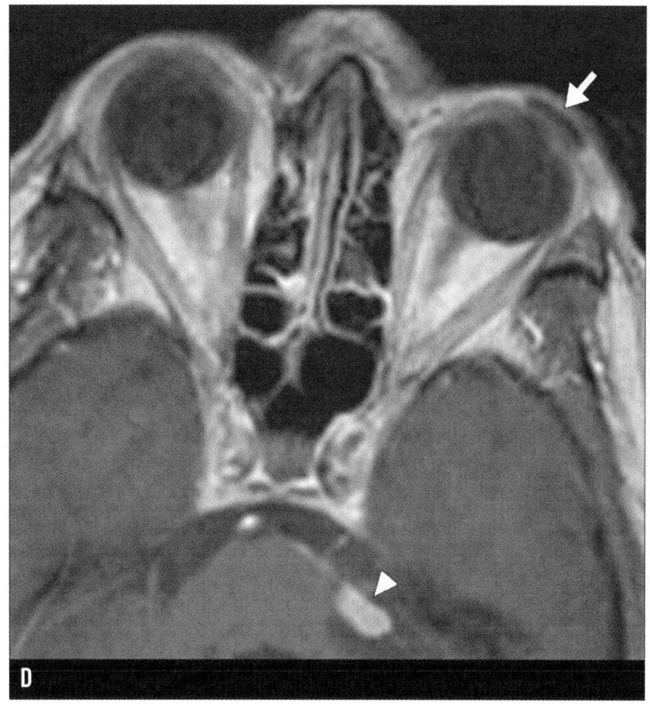

D

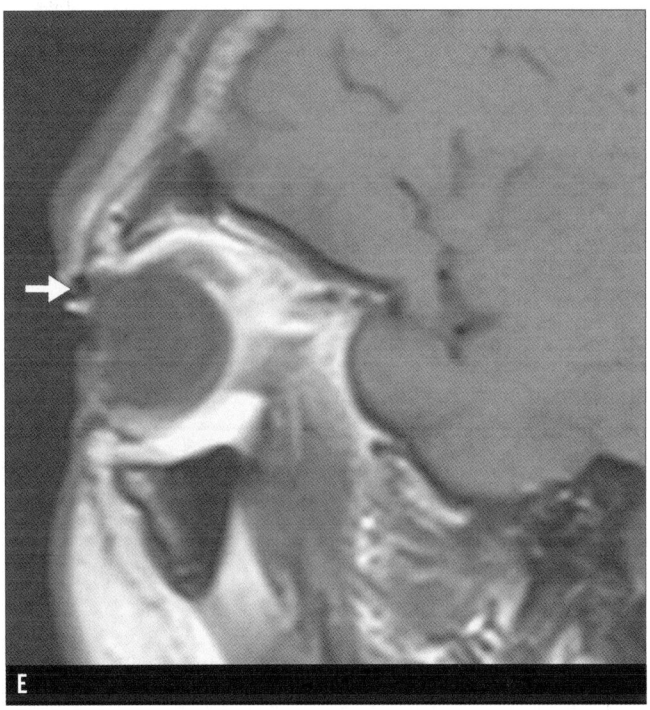

E

REFERENCES

Dalkiz M, et al. Gold weight implantation for rehabilitation of the paralysed eyelid. *Int J Oral Maxillofac Surg*. 2007;36:522-526.

Swanger RS, et al. Postsurgical imaging of the globe. *Semin Ultrasound CT MRI*. 2011:32(1):57-63.

CASE 27 Air beneath eyelid (Pneumofornix)

The conjunctival fornices represent potential spaces between the globe and each eyelid. They are subdivided into four quadrants (superior, inferior, medial, and lateral), and can be thought of as a *cul-de-sac* created by the reflections of the palpebral and bulbar conjunctiva. Air may accumulate in the conjunctival fornices (also called pneumofornix) and is usually best identified on CT, although on occasion, it may also be identified on MRI. Air pockets in the superior or inferior fornices tend to be larger than those found in the medial or lateral fornices. Typically, these incidental collections of air beneath the eyelids are identified in the elderly, presumably due to redundancy of the eyelid skin (dermatochalasis). Air collections beneath the eyelids are incidental findings.

COMPANION CASES

- **Orbital emphysema following trauma.** Orbital emphysema is most commonly secondary to fractures of one or more of the orbital walls that results in a direct communication between the orbit and the adjacent paranasal sinuses. Gas will often be identified in the postseptal space in this setting, sometimes accompanied by palpebral and subcutaneous emphysema. Other causes of orbital emphysema include foreign bodies, conjunctival laceration, infection, and following surgery.
- **Wooden foreign body in the orbit.** On CT, a wooden foreign body may be hypoattenuating or hyperattenuating, depending on the amount of air or radiopaque substances that are contained within the cellulose matrix of the wood. In addition, an aerated wooden foreign body may become more attenuating over time as water content in the wood increases. Generally, a wooden foreign body in the orbit on CT will have a linear, discrete margin that has air or near-air Hounsfield attenuation and does not substantially change in location between CT studies.

Air beneath eyelids (CT)

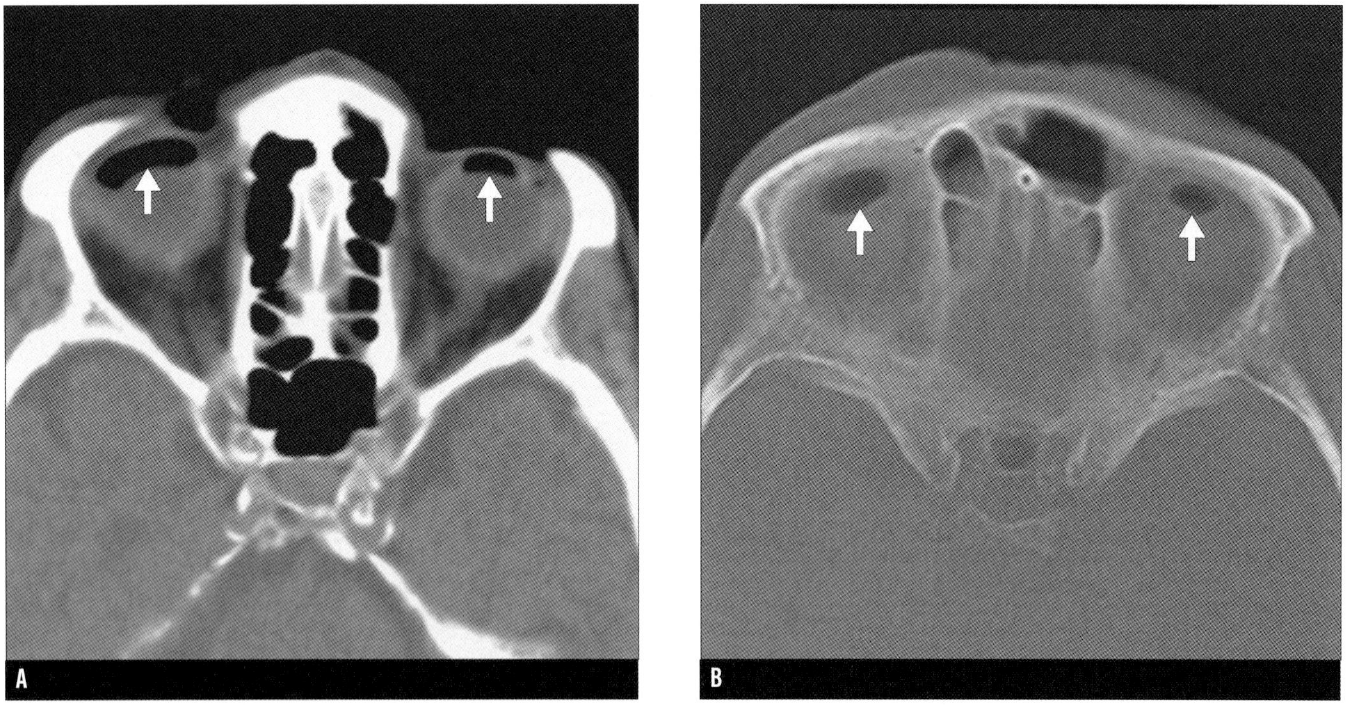

Unenhanced axial CT images viewed with a soft tissue window (**A**) and bone window (**B**) as well as a sagittal reformatted CT image viewed with an intermediate window (**C**) demonstrate the typical CT appearance of air in the bilateral superior conjunctival fornices (ie, under the superior eyelids) (arrows, **A**-**C**).

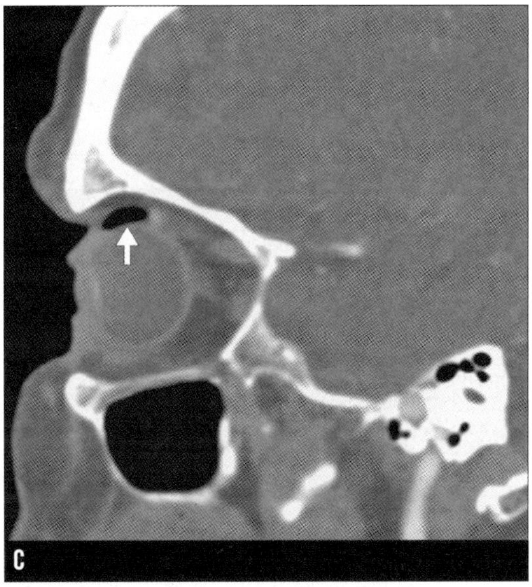

Air beneath eyelid (MRI)

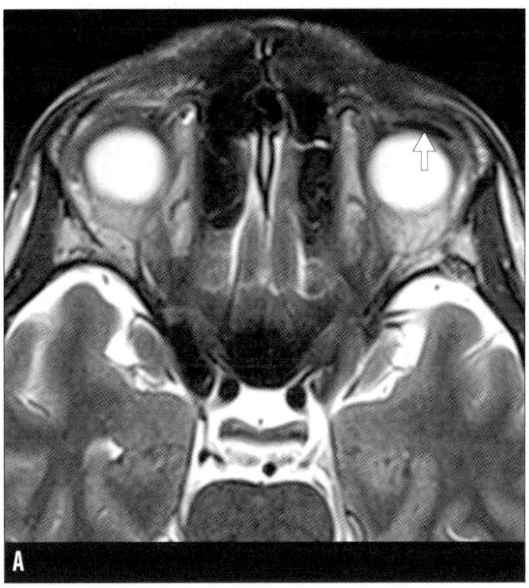

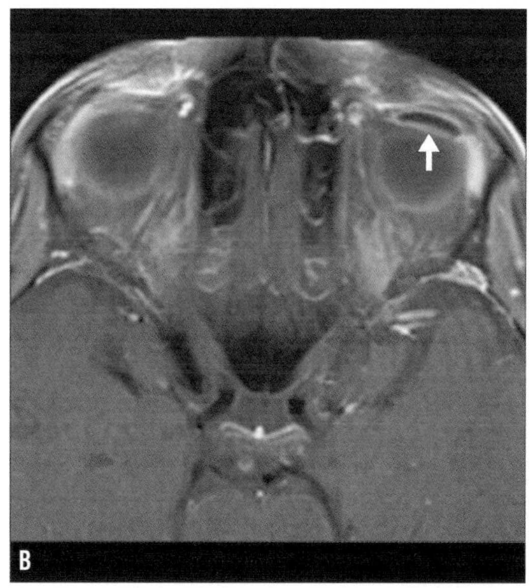

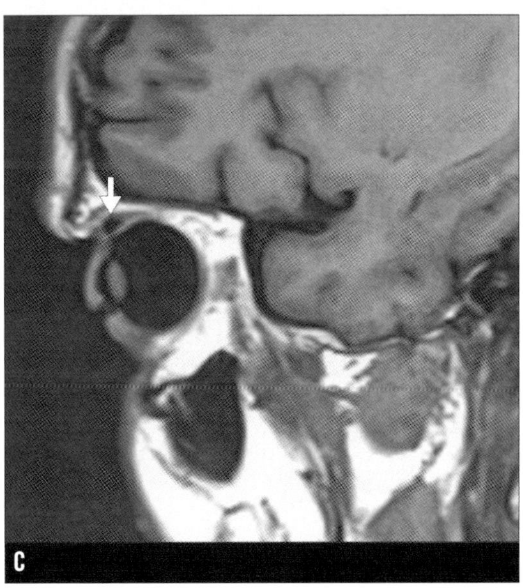

Different patient. Axial T2 (**A**), contrast-enhanced fat-suppressed axial T1 (**B**), and unenhanced T1 (**C**) MR images demonstrate a curvilinear focus of hypointense signal situated in the superior aspect of the left orbit, beneath the left upper eyelid (arrows, **A**-**C**). While nearly identical in appearance, this is differentiated from a metallic eyelid weight used for lagophthalmos, which is located within the substance of the eyelid rather than deep to the eyelid. This was confirmed as air on CT imaging (not shown).

Companion case: Orbital emphysema following trauma

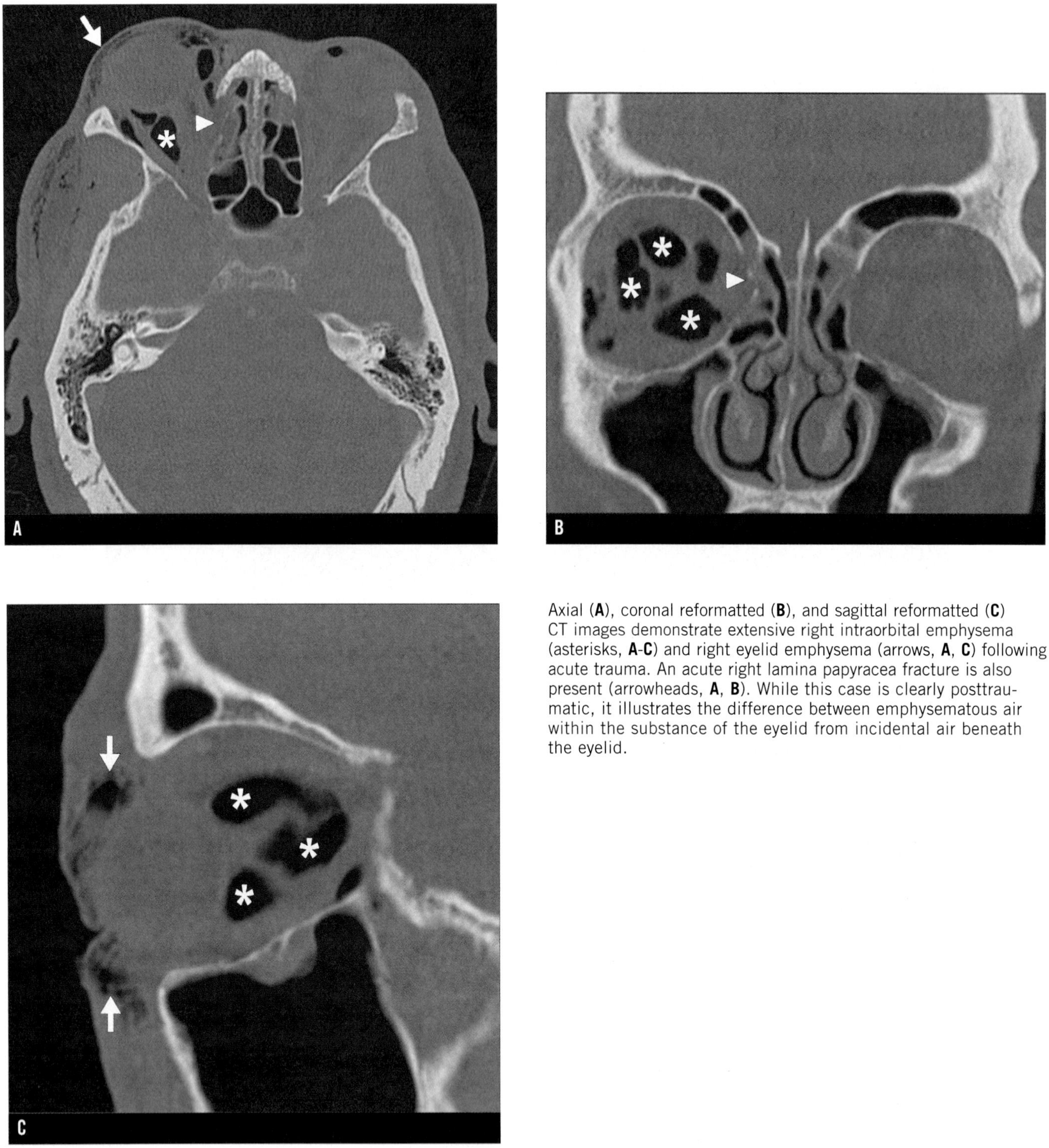

Axial (**A**), coronal reformatted (**B**), and sagittal reformatted (**C**) CT images demonstrate extensive right intraorbital emphysema (asterisks, **A-C**) and right eyelid emphysema (arrows, **A**, **C**) following acute trauma. An acute right lamina papyracea fracture is also present (arrowheads, **A**, **B**). While this case is clearly posttraumatic, it illustrates the difference between emphysematous air within the substance of the eyelid from incidental air beneath the eyelid.

Companion case: Wooden foreign body in the orbit

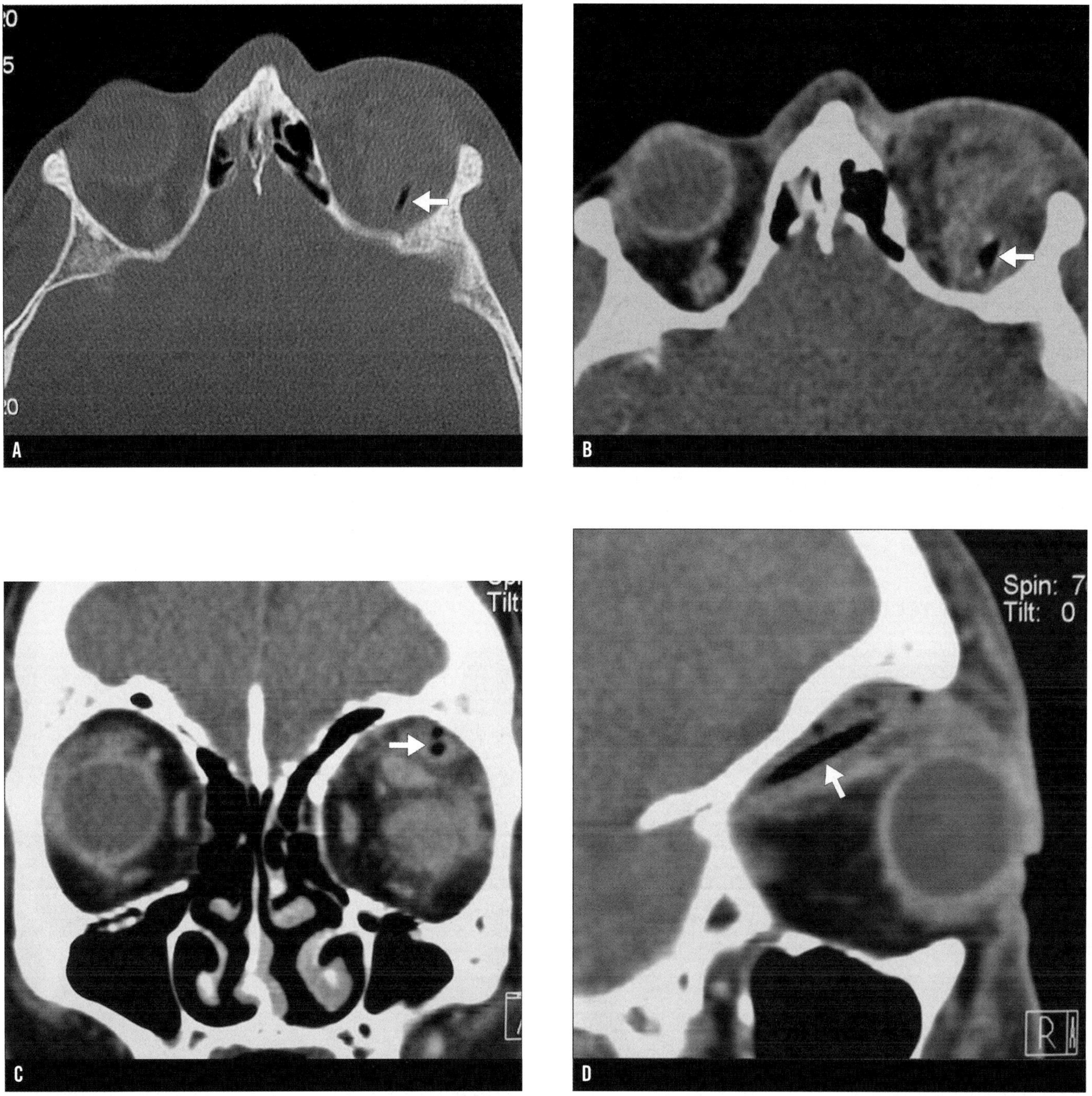

An axial CT image viewed with a bone window (**A**) and axial (**B**), coronal reformatted (**C**), and sagittal reformatted (**D**) CT images viewed with a soft tissue window demonstrate a linear focus of air within the superior extraconal space of the left orbit (arrows, **A**-**D**). This finding represents air within a wood branch that traumatically penetrated the left orbit.

REFERENCES

Ho VT, McGuckin JF Jr, Smergel EM. Intraorbital wooden foreign body: CT and MR appearance. *AJNR Am J Neuroradiol.* 1996;17:134-136.

Kubal WS. Imaging of orbital trauma. *Radiographics.* 2008;28(6):1729-1739. doi: 10.1148/rg.286085523.

Patcl BC, ct al. "Pncumofornix" (air under the eyelid): a normal finding. *Ophthalmic surg Lasers.* 1997;28(6):520.

Zimmer-Galler IE, Bartley GB. Orbital emphysema: case reports and review of the literature. *Mayo Clin Proc.* 1994;69(2):115-121.

CASE 28 Orbital wall reconstruction

A variety of materials have been used to reconstruct orbital blowout fractures. Titanium mesh has been the most widely used alloplastic material because of its nonreactivity and malleability. Although the incidence of infection is rare, the presence of a long-term, indwelling foreign body predisposes to this complication. As a result, there has been interest in the utilization of resorbable mesh materials, particularly for the pediatric population. Currently commercially available resorbable mesh implants retain their structural integrity for approximately 2 months, providing sufficient time to form fibrous tissue as the fracture begins to heal and they are nearly completely resorbed within 9 months, thereby minimizing the long-term risk of infection.

COMPANION CASE

- **Malpositioned titanium mesh placed for orbital wall reconstruction.** The purpose of orbital blowout reconstruction is to provide support for the orbital contents, prevent enophthalmos, release entrapped soft tissues, and to restore or preserve normal ocular motility. A malpositioned mesh implant, regardless of type, may result in deleterious consequences, such as an intraorbital hematoma, optic nerve injury/impingement, extraocular muscle dysfunction, vascular compromise, and a poorly positioned globe. The position of the mesh implant, which should ideally appose the fractured orbital wall, as well as any complications that may result from the implant should be assessed on every postoperative imaging study that has a mesh reconstruction.

Orbital floor reconstruction

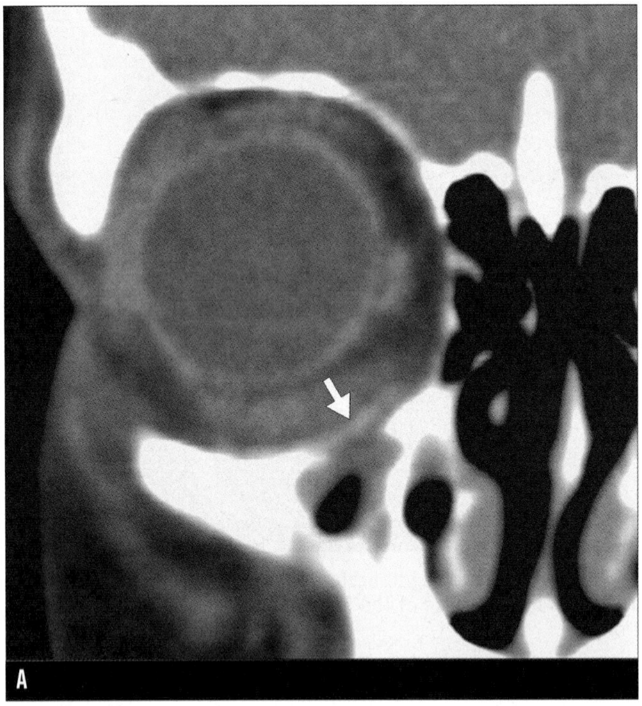

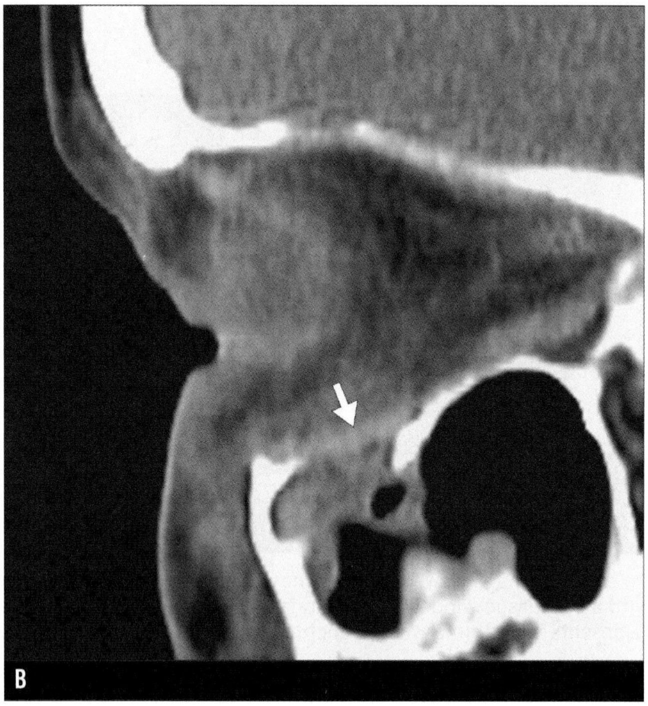

Coronal reformatted (**A**) and sagittal reformatted (**B**) unenhanced CT images viewed with a soft tissue window demonstrate subtle, linear hyperdensity along the right orbital floor overlying a fracture deformity (arrows, **A**, **B**). The linear hyperdensity represents a resorbable mesh that is sometimes used for orbital floor reconstructions. However, following surgery, the patient exhibited worsening diplopia on upward gaze for unclear reasons. A repeat surgery was performed and the resorbable material was replaced with a titanium mesh. Coronal reformatted (**C**) and reformatted (**D**) unenhanced CT images viewed with an intermediate window following the repeat surgery demonstrates the newly placed titanium mesh along the right orbital floor (arrows, **C**, **D**).

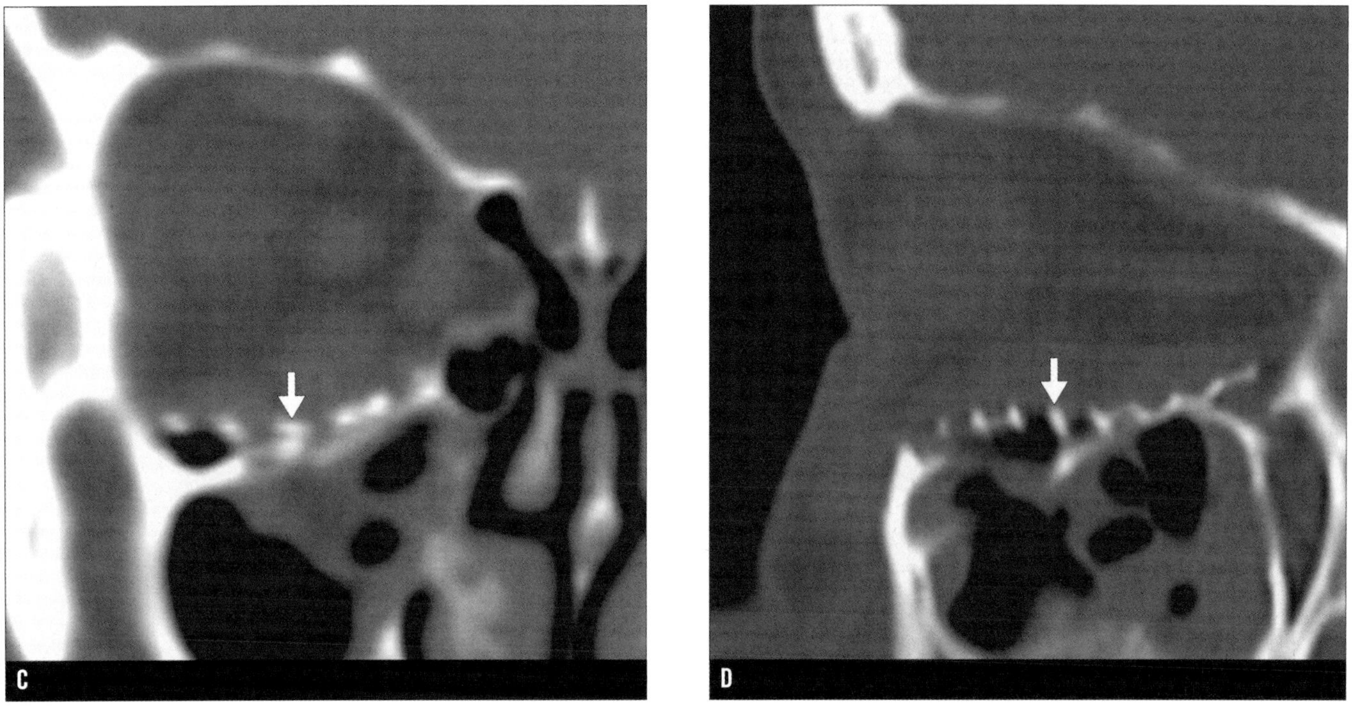

Orbital floor reconstruction

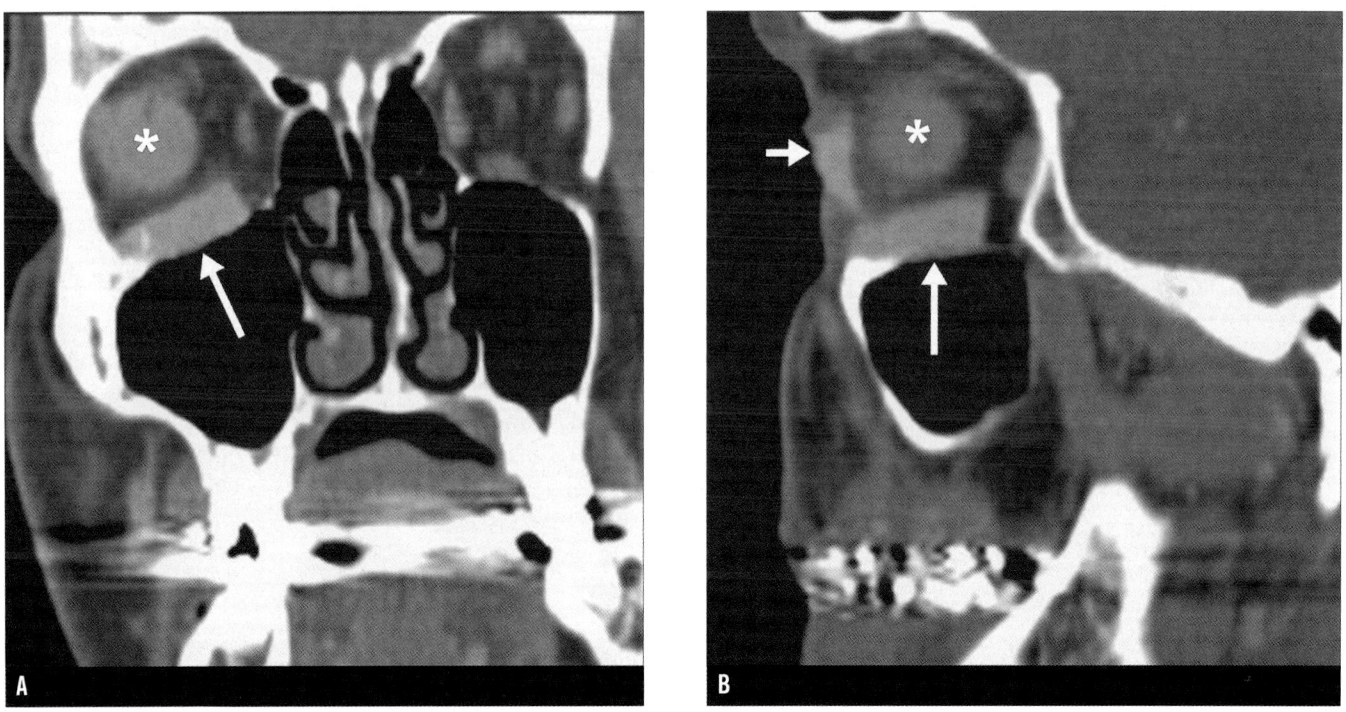

Different patient. Coronal reformatted (**A**), reformatted (**B**), and axial (**C**) postcontrast CT images demonstrate an unusually thick orbital floor prosthesis (long arrows, **A-C**). The increased thickness of the floor prosthesis was likely utilized to elevate an orbital implant (asterisks, **A**, **B**) and ocular prosthesis (short arrow, **B**) into a more anatomically appropriate position. A small circlage wire (arrowhead, **C**) was used to affix the prosthesis.

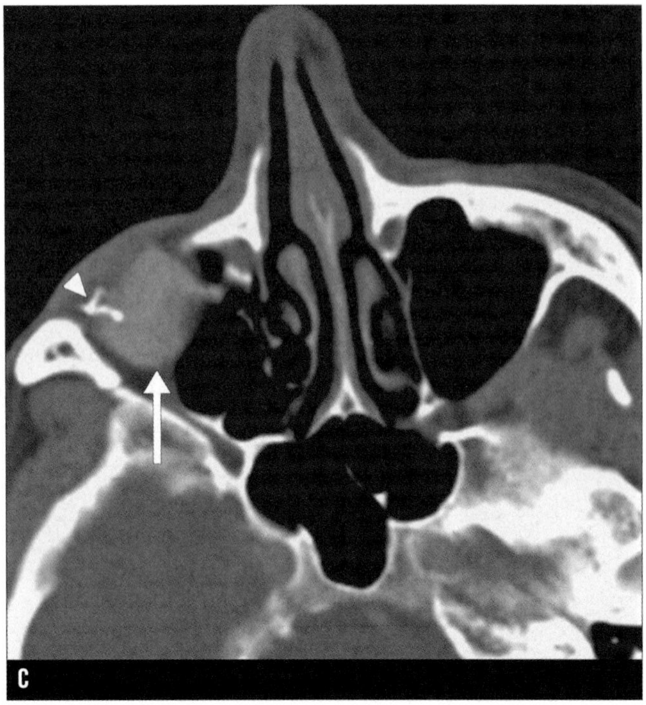

Companion case: Malpositioned titanium mesh placed for orbital wall reconstruction

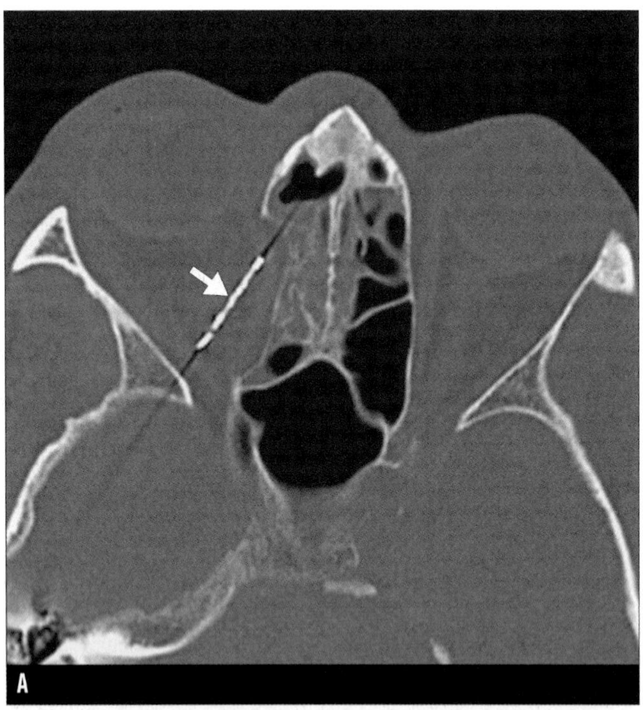

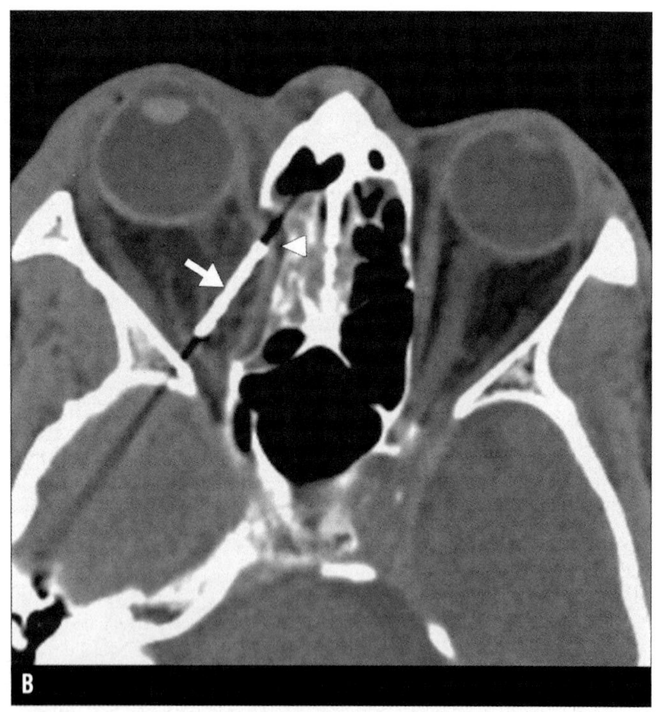

Axial CT images viewed with a bone window (**A**) and soft tissue window (**B**) demonstrate a poorly positioned, obliquely oriented titanium mesh that was placed to treat an orbital blowout fracture (arrows, **A**, **B**). The titanium mesh impinges upon the mid right medial rectus muscle (arrowhead, **B**), and this muscle unintentionally resides outside the confines of the titanium mesh. Coronal reformatted images viewed with a bone window (**C**) and soft tissue window (**D**) also demonstrate the right medial rectus muscle to inappropriately reside outside the confines of the titanium mesh (arrow, **D**).

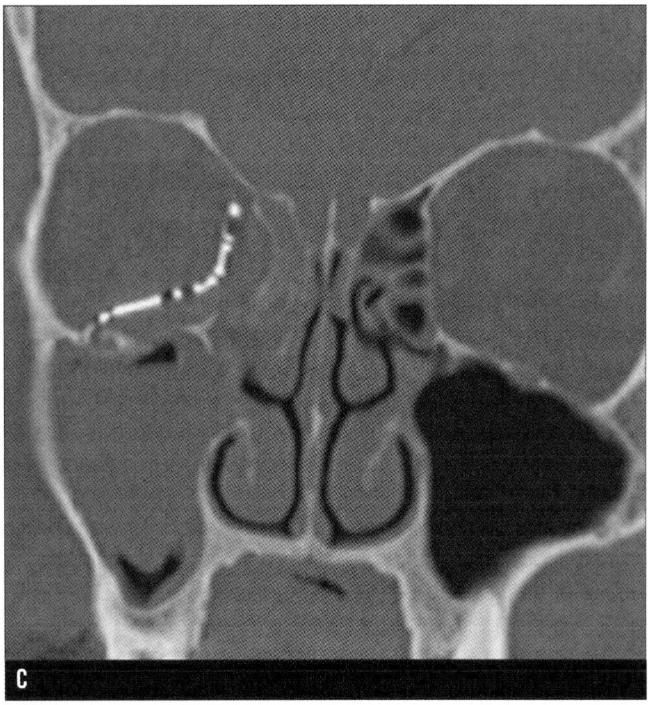

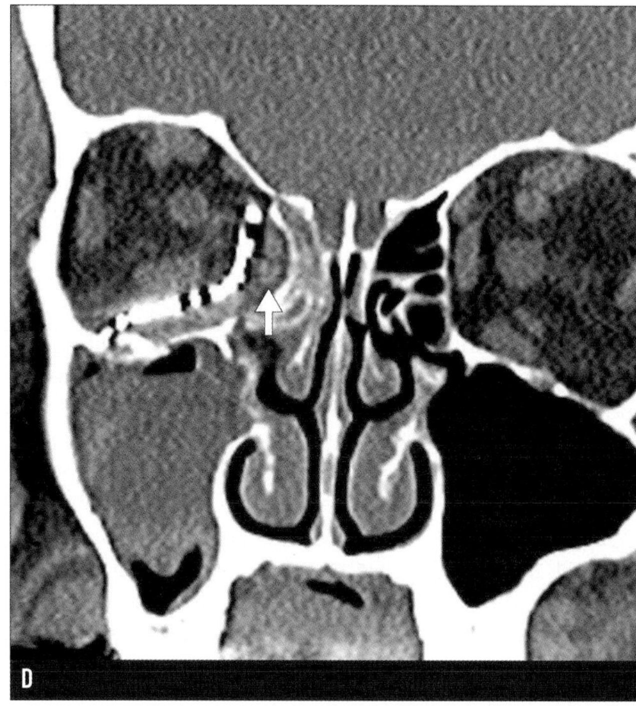

REFERENCES

Hollier LH, Rogers N, Berzin E, Stal S. Resorbable mesh in the treatment of orbital floor fractures. *J Craniofac Surg.* 2001;12(3):242-246.

O'Connell JE, Hartnett C, Hickey-Dwyer M, Kearns GJ. Reconstruction of orbital floor blow-out fractures with autogenous iliac crest bone: a retrospective study including maxillofacial and ophthalmology perspectives. *J Craniomaxillofac Surg.* 2015;43(2):192-198

CASE 29 Treatment-related effects involving the orbit

The effects of radiation therapy can be identified within soft tissues as early as 2 to 12 days after the initiation of therapy. Initially, there is detachment of the endothelial lining of small arteries, veins, and lymphatic vessels leading to increased permeability and interstitial edema. Within 1 to 4 months, there is progressive fibrosis and soft tissue thickening. Radiation-induced endothelial proliferation results in the complete obstruction of small arteries, veins, and lymphatics, causing progression of the interstitial edema. This process can continue for up to 8 months, after which collateral vessels develop and the interstitial fluid is resorbed. Irreparable damage to the orbits and optic pathway may occur when they are in the radiotherapy field; therefore, every attempt is made to exclude these structures from the radiotherapy field when they are not involved with tumor. Chemotherapy, alone or in combination with radiation, may also result in tissue damage and interstitial edema.

These deleterious effects to the orbits from radiation and chemotherapy can sometimes be visualized on imaging, and when present, may simulate an infectious process or tumor infiltration of the orbits.

COMPANION CASES

- **Retrobulbar metastatic breast carcinoma.** Breast cancer is the most common neoplasm to metastasize to the orbit. Metastases from breast cancer may involve any portion of the orbit and often have an infiltrative appearance. Scirrhous breast cancer may result in an enophthalmos from associated orbital fibrosis.
- **Orbital sarcoid.** Sarcoidosis is a disease characterized by the presence of noncaseating granulomas, usually occurring in adults between the third and fifth decades of life. Almost any organ can be affected, and approximately 25% of individuals have ophthalmologic involvement. Some of the more common ophthalmologic presentations include keratoconjunctivitis and uveitis. The optic nerve, optic chiasm, eyelid, retrobulbar fat, extraocular muscles and osseous orbit are other potential targets of sarcoidosis, either individually or in combination with one another. Sarcoidosis confined to the orbits is uncommon, although when it occurs, it usually manifests as lacrimal gland pathology. Affected orbital structures characteristically enhance and are relatively hypointense on T2-weighted MR images.

Treatment-related effects involving the orbit

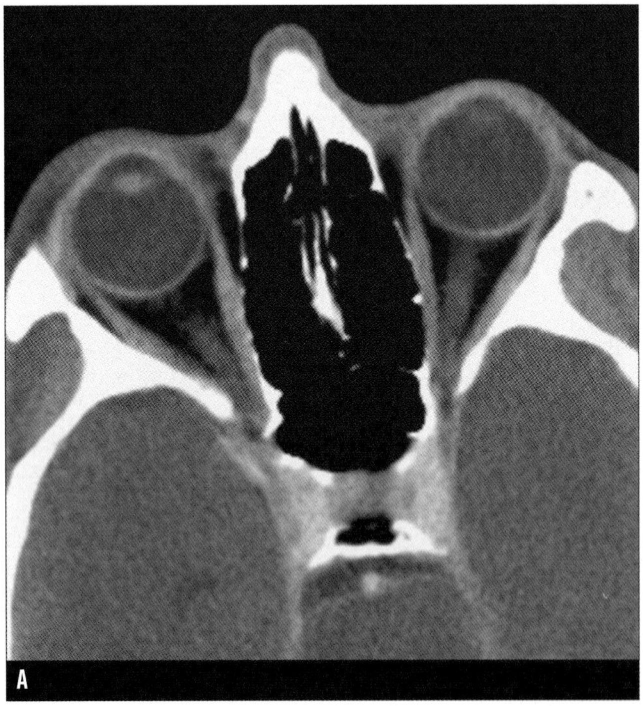

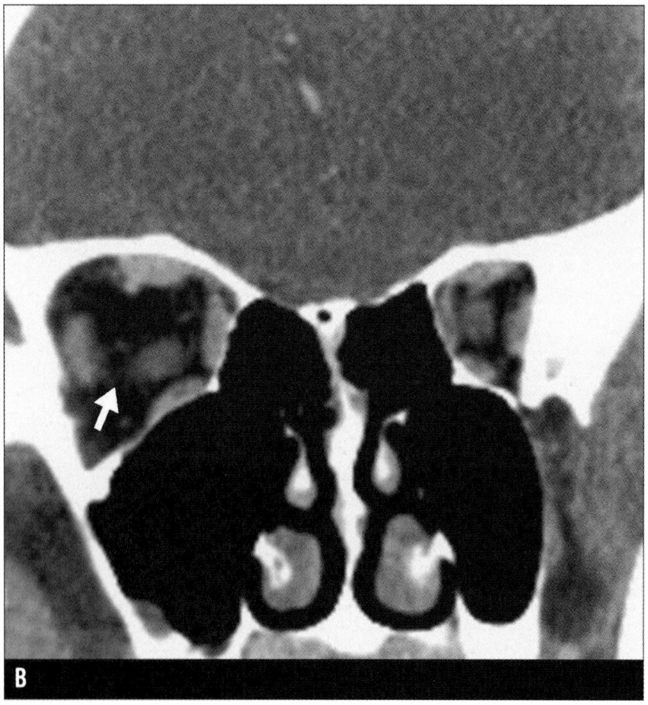

Axial (**A**) and coronal reformatted (**B**) contrast-enhanced CT images 2 months following completion of chemotherapy and radiation therapy for squamous cell carcinoma of the tongue in a 27-year-old patient. Images **A** and **B** demonstrate a relatively unremarkable appearance of the orbits, except for perhaps a trace amount of fat stranding in the right orbit (arrow, **B**). Axial (**C**) and coronal reformatted (**D**) contrast-enhanced CT images of the same patient 4 months following completion of chemotherapy and radiation demonstrate extensive infiltration of the intraorbital and periorbital fat. The findings likely represent a combination of tissue damage from chemotherapy/radiation as well as treatment related anasarca, as similar imaging findings were present in the chest, abdomen, and pelvis (not shown).

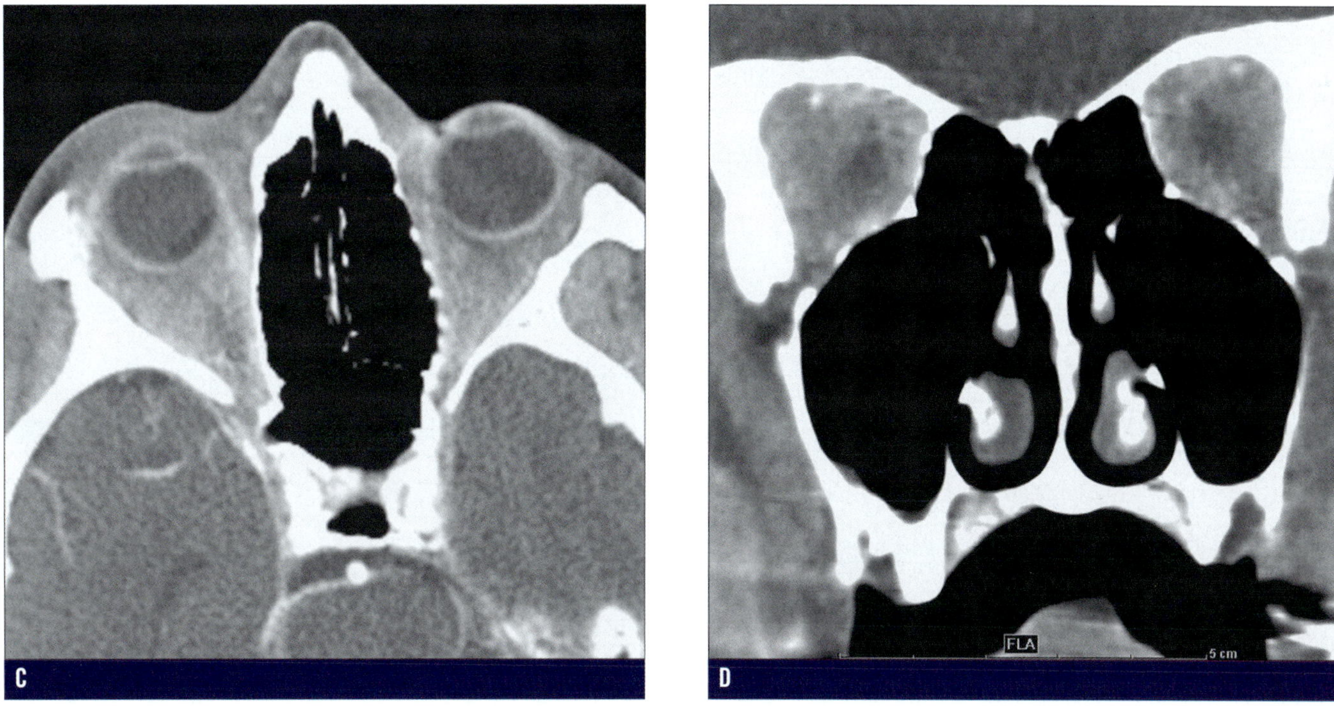

Companion case: Bilateral retrobulbar metastatic breast carcinoma

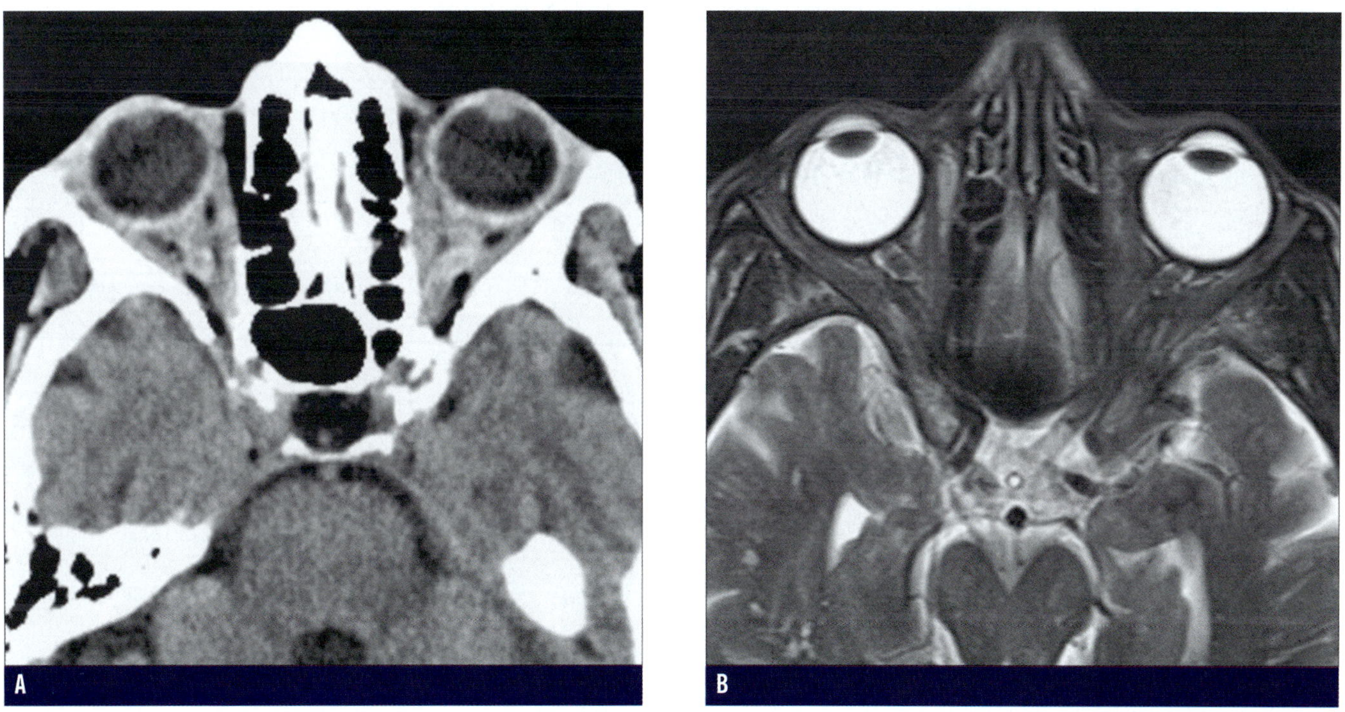

An unenhanced axial CT image (**A**) as well as axial T2 (**B**), unenhanced axial T1 (**C**), and contrast-enhanced coronal T1 with fat suppression (**D**) MR images demonstrate bilateral enophthalmos with heterogeneity and diffuse enhancement of the bilateral retrobulbar fat. In this patient with a history of breast carcinoma, the findings are consistent with diffuse bilateral retrobulbar metastatic infiltration.

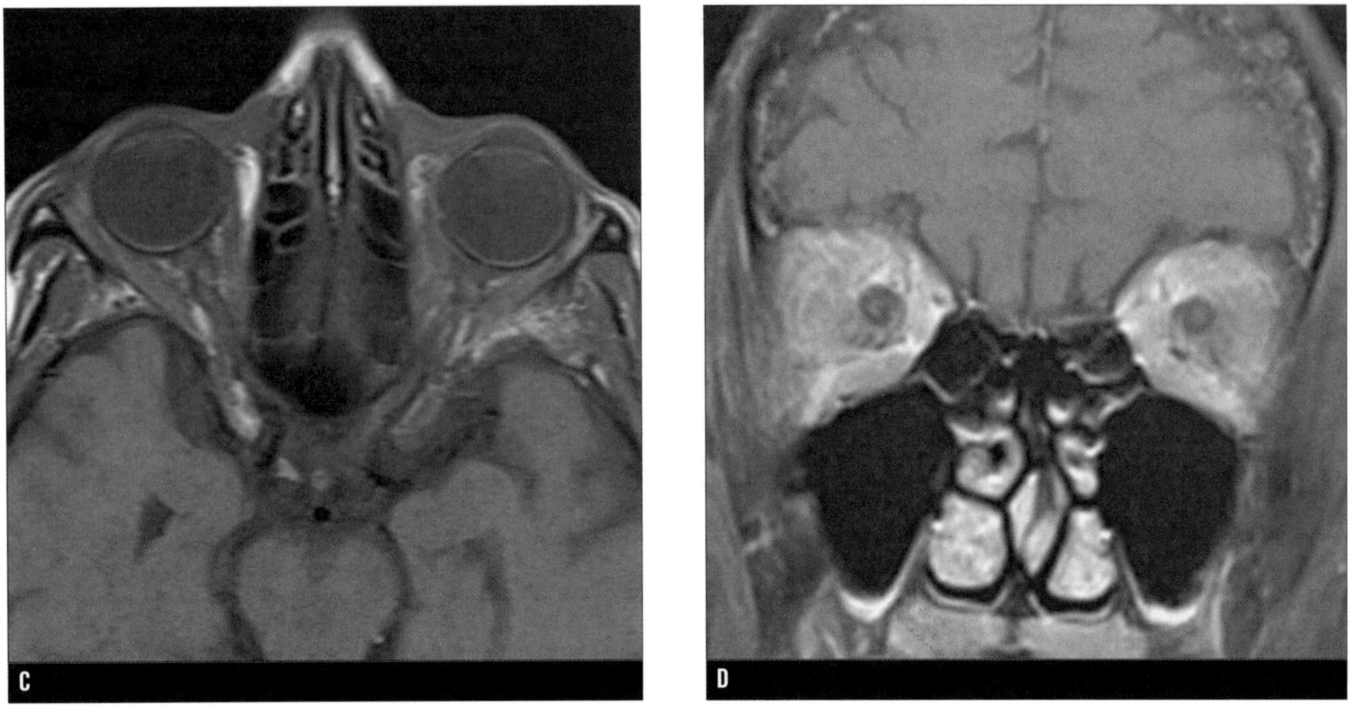

Companion case: Unilateral retrobulbar metastatic breast carcinoma

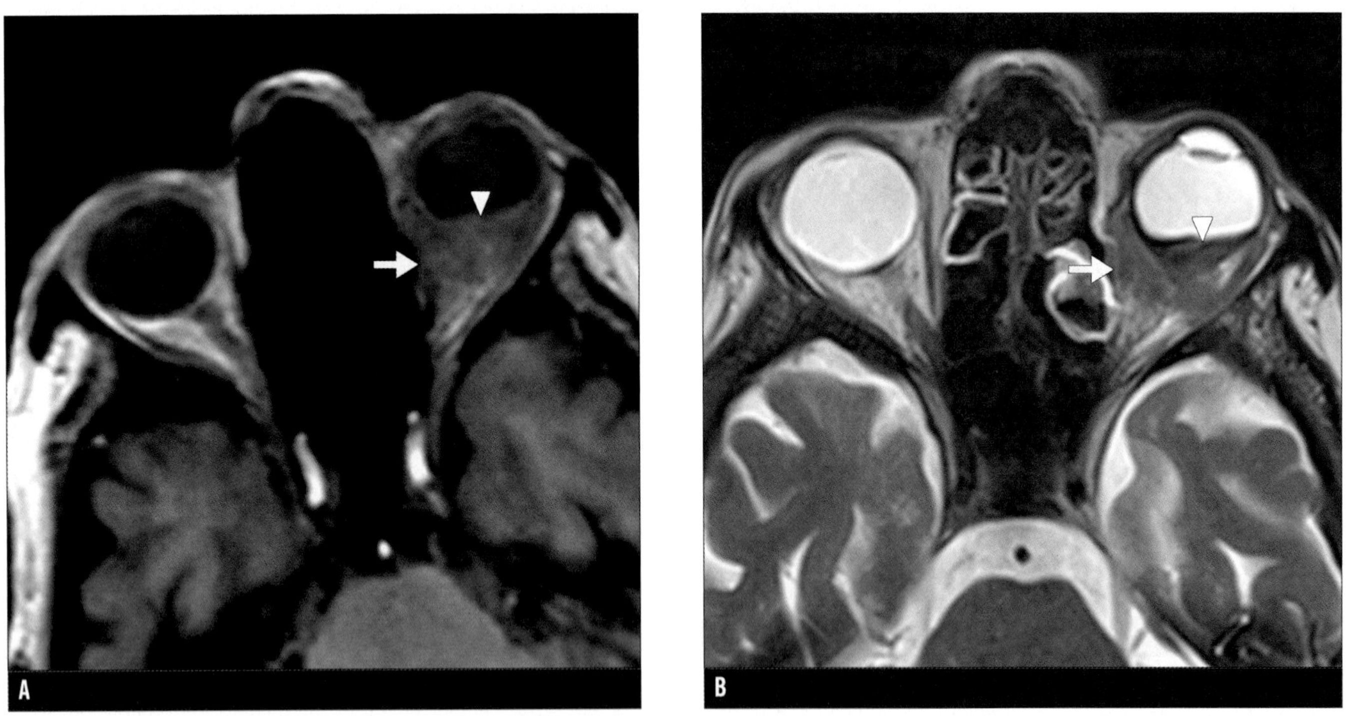

Different patient. Axial T1 (**A**), axial T2 (**B**), axial MPRAGE (**C**), and contrast-enhanced coronal T1 with fat suppression (**D**) MR images demonstrate an infiltrating left retrobulbar lesion that is, T1 hypointense (arrow, **A**), T2 hypointense (arrow, **B**), and diffusely enhancing (arrows, **C**, **D**) which invades the posterior aspect of the left globe (arrowheads, **A**-**C**). This represented a metastatic lesion from breast carcinoma.

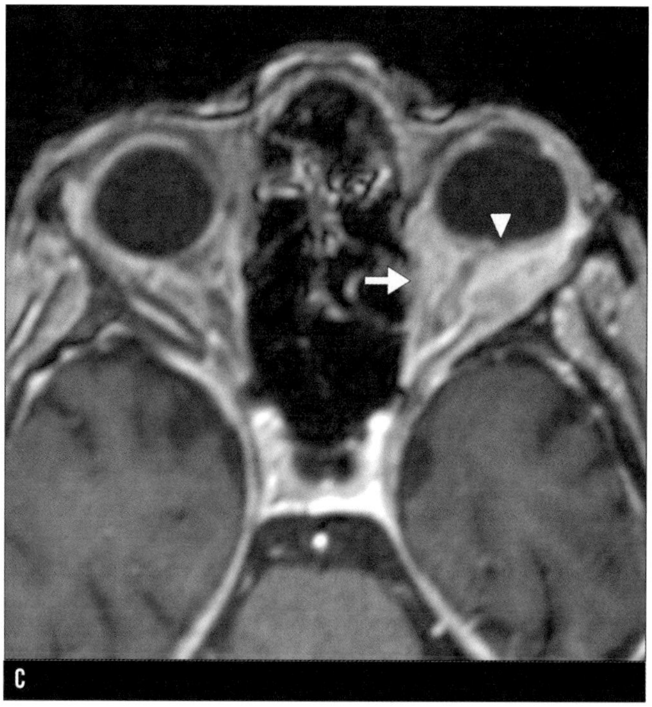

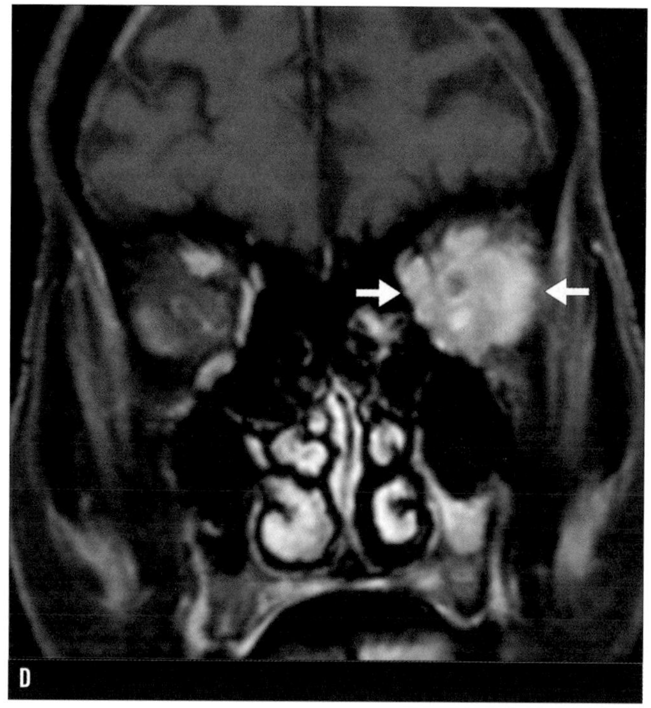

Companion case: Orbital sarcoid

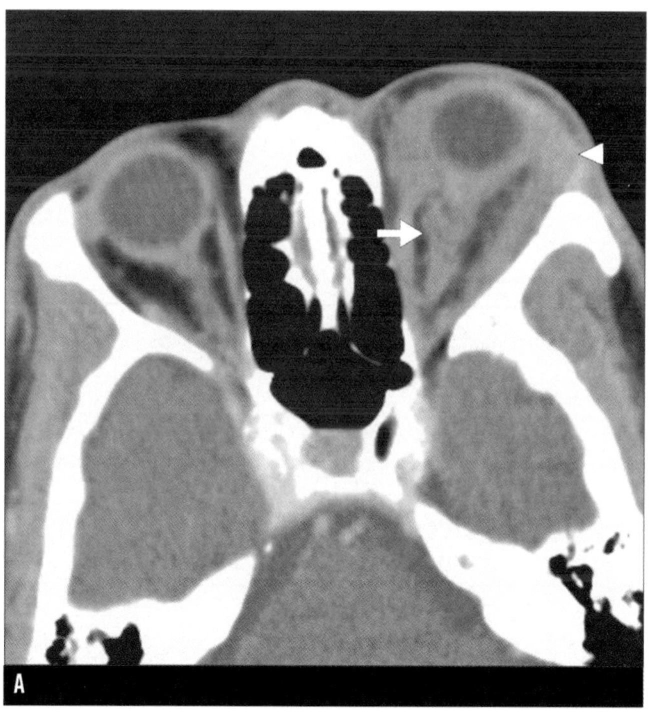

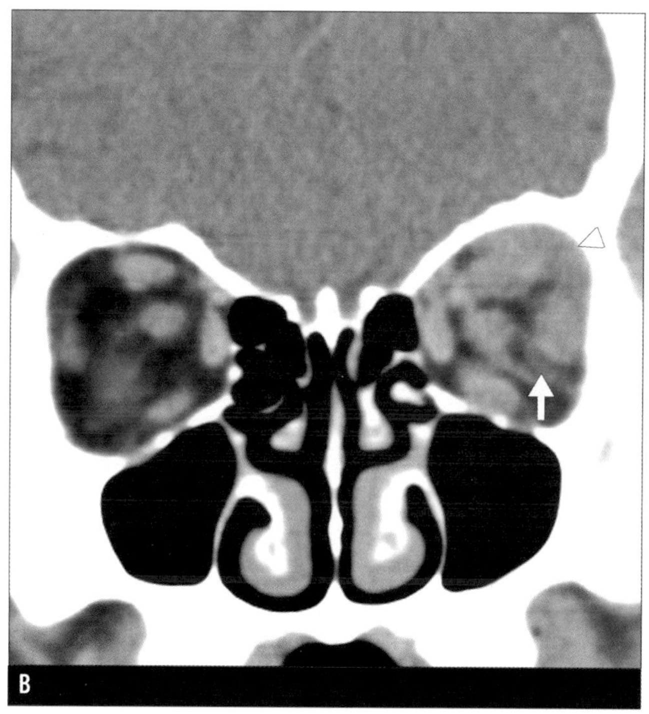

Axial (**A**) and coronal reformatted (**B**) contrast-enhanced CT images demonstrate heterogeneous infiltration of the left retrobulbar fat (arrows, **A**, **B**), diffuse enlargement of the left lacrimal gland (arrowheads, **A**, **B**), and diffuse enlargement of the left extraocular muscles. There is moderate left globe proptosis. Mild stranding of the right retrobulbar fat is also present. While the findings are nonspecific, in this case the findings represented orbital sarcoidosis.

REFERENCES

Mafee MF. Orbit: embryology, anatomy, and pathology. In: Som PM, Curtin HD, eds. *Head and Neck Imaging.* 4th ed. St. Louis, MO: Mosby; 2003:529-654.

Mavrikakis I, Rootman J. Diverse clinical presentations of orbital sarcoid. *Am J Ophthal.* November 2007;144(5):769-775.

Mukherji SK, Mancuso AA, Kotzur IM, Mendenhall WM, Kubilis PS, Tart RP, Lee WR, Freeman D. Radiologic appearance of the irradiated larynx. Part I. Expected changes. *Radiology.* October 1994;193(1):141-148.

Nömayr A, Lell M, Sweeney R, Bautz W, Lukas P. MRI appearance of radiation-induced changes of normal cervical tissues. *Eur Radiol.* 2001;11(9):1807-1817.

Simon EM, et al. Systemic sarcoidosis with bilateral orbital involvement: MR findings. *Am J Neuroradiol.* 1998;19:336-337.

Som PM, Lawson W, Urken ML. The posttreatment neck: clinical and imaging considerations. *Head and Neck Imaging.* St. Louis, MO: Mosby; 2003.

There are various types of surgical procedures that may be employed to treat the diseased orbit. For example, during an orbital evisceration, the majority of the globe is removed, although its scleral coating is left in place. This procedure, followed by placement of an orbital implant, may be performed to treat a variety of disorders, including the nonfunctioning or painful eye, phthisis bulbi, microphthalmia, endophthalmitis, and cosmetic deformity.

Enucleation entails removal of the entire globe, including the sclera. Enucleation, followed by placement of an orbital implant, may be performed for treatment of all of the conditions for which evisceration may be considered. In addition, it may be performed to treat intraocular tumors or in patients in whom definitive treatment is needed to prevent sympathetic ophthalmia, an autoimmune granulomatous uveitis of both eyes that may result in complete blindness following trauma to one eye.

An orbital exenteration is the most radical of the orbital surgeries. It involves removal of the entire orbit, including the globe, eyelids, and remaining orbital contents. This procedure is reserved for malignant tumors, invasive mucormycosis, chronic and unrelenting orbital pain, or severe orbital deformity. A partial orbital exenteration may also be performed, which is a surgical procedure that preserves a portion of the orbit. As one might expect, a partial orbital exenteration is more cosmetically appealing than a complete exenteration. Occasionally, the muscular component of a myocutaneous flap placed into an orbital exenteration defect may undergo enhancement on MRI, particularly with delayed imaging. This can simulate recurrent tumor. One helpful imaging finding to differentiate normal myocutaneous flap enhancement from recurrent tumor may be identified on the precontrast, nonfat-suppressed T1-weighted images. If fat is interspersed within the finding on this sequence, then the enhancement most likely relates to incidental enhancement of the myocutaneous flap rather than recurrent tumor.

Orbital exenteration

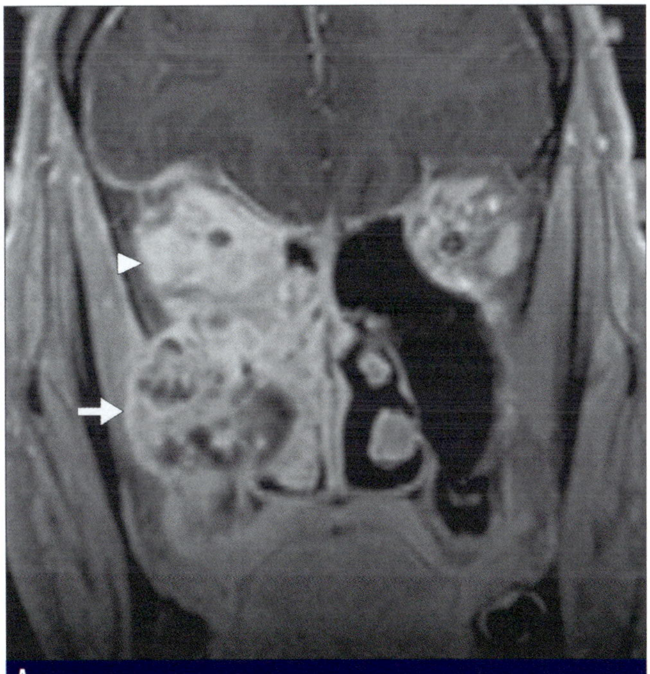

A

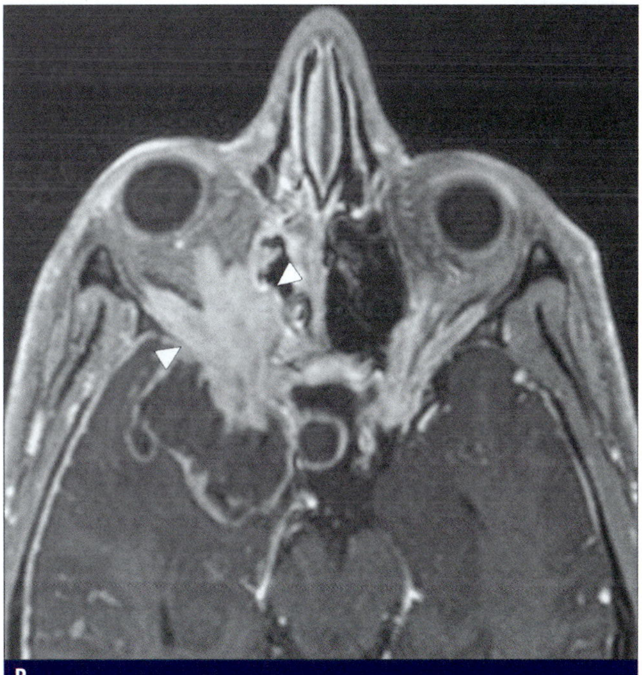

B

Coronal reformatted MPRAGE (**A**) and axial MPRAGE (**B**) contrast-enhanced MR images of a patient with a right maxillary sinus adenoid cystic carcinoma. Image **A** demonstrates a lobulated, heterogeneously enhancing mass occupying the right maxillary sinus (arrow, **A**). This tumor infiltrates multiple structures, including the right orbit (arrowheads, **A**, **B**). The mass results in right globe proptosis. Unenhanced axial (**C**, **D**) as well as enhanced coronal reformatted (**E**, **F**) CT images of the same patient viewed with a bone window (**C**, **E**) and soft window (**D**, **F**) demonstrate the immediate postsurgical changes of a right orbital exenteration and maxillectomy with a myocutaneous flap reconstruction placed along the right face and into the orbital exenteration (arrows, **D**, **F**). Embolic coils were placed to iatrogenically sacrifice the right internal carotid artery prior to surgery (arrow, **C**). Expected postoperative pneumocephalus and subcutaneous emphysema are also identified. Unenhanced axial T1 (**G**), unenhanced coronal T1 (**H**), and fat-suppressed contrast-enhanced axial T1 (**I**) MR images demonstrate the MRI appearance of the myocutaneous flap (arrows, **G-I**). The enhancing tissue along the posterior aspect of the orbital exenteration represents the enhancing muscular component of the myocutaneous flap and not residual/recurrent tumor (arrow, **I**). While poorly visualized on image **G**, a subtle amount of fat interspersed within this area was identified, helping to identify that the enhancement was related to the myocutaneous flap.

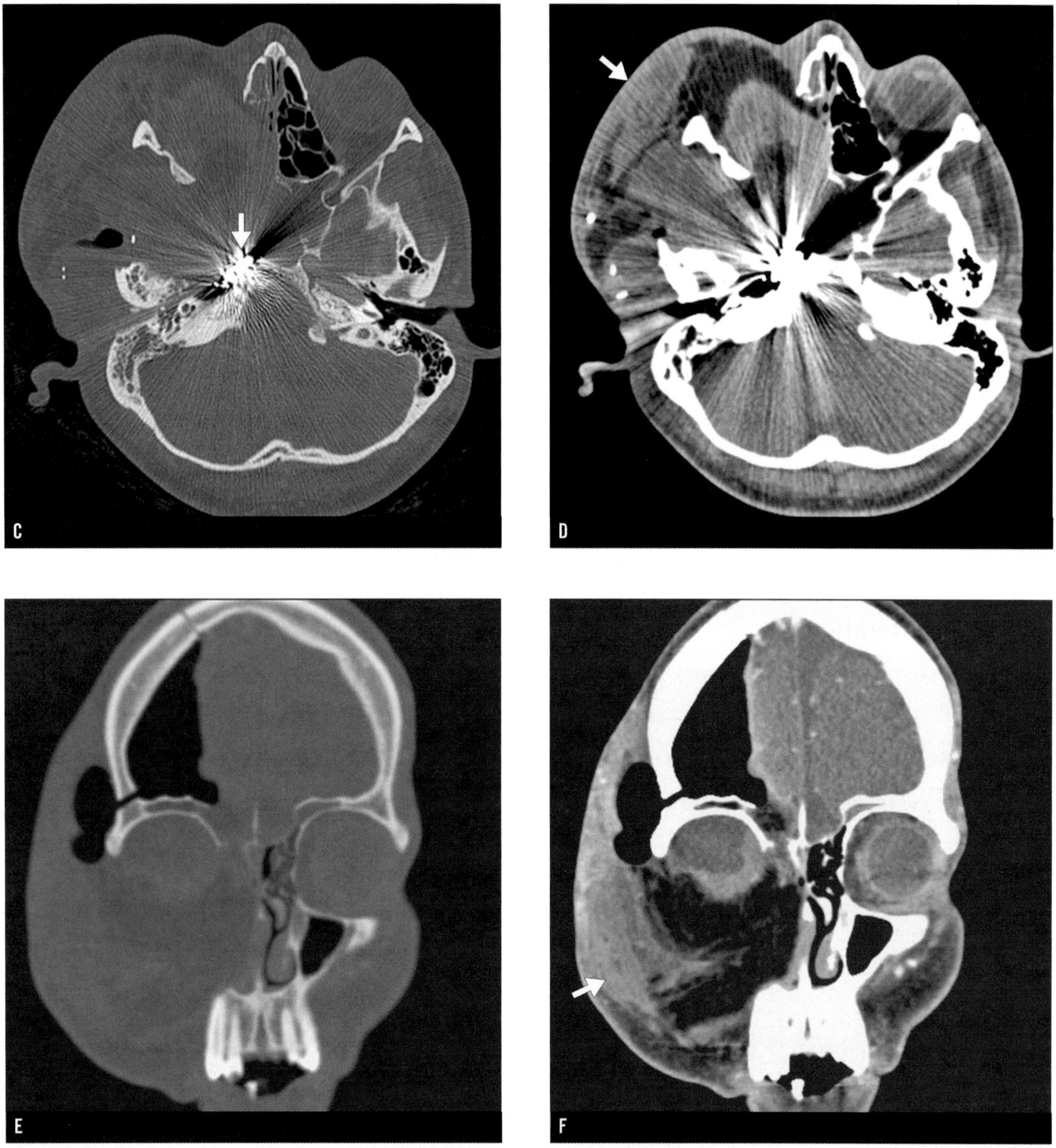
C
D
E
F

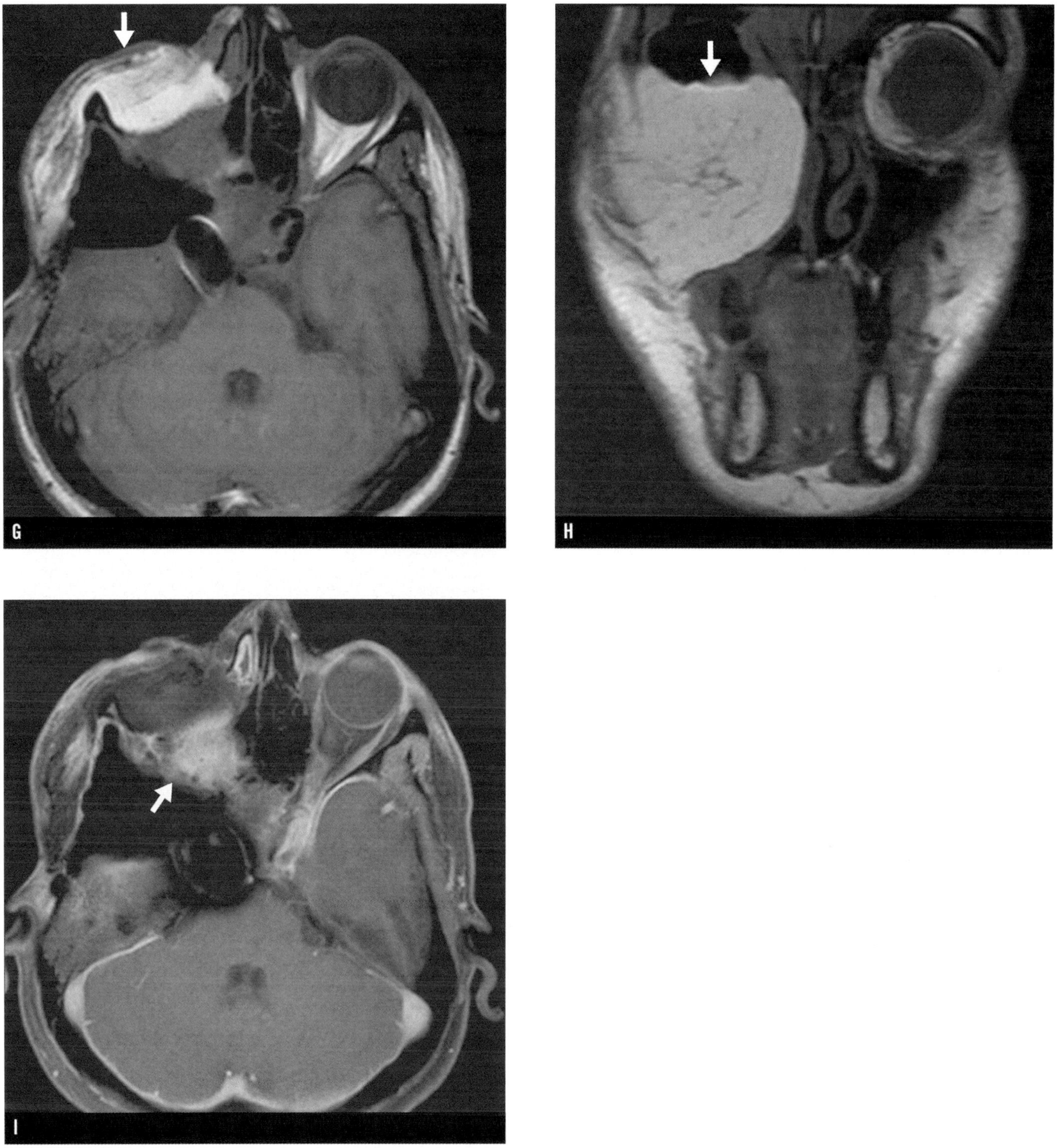
G
H
I

Orbital exenteration

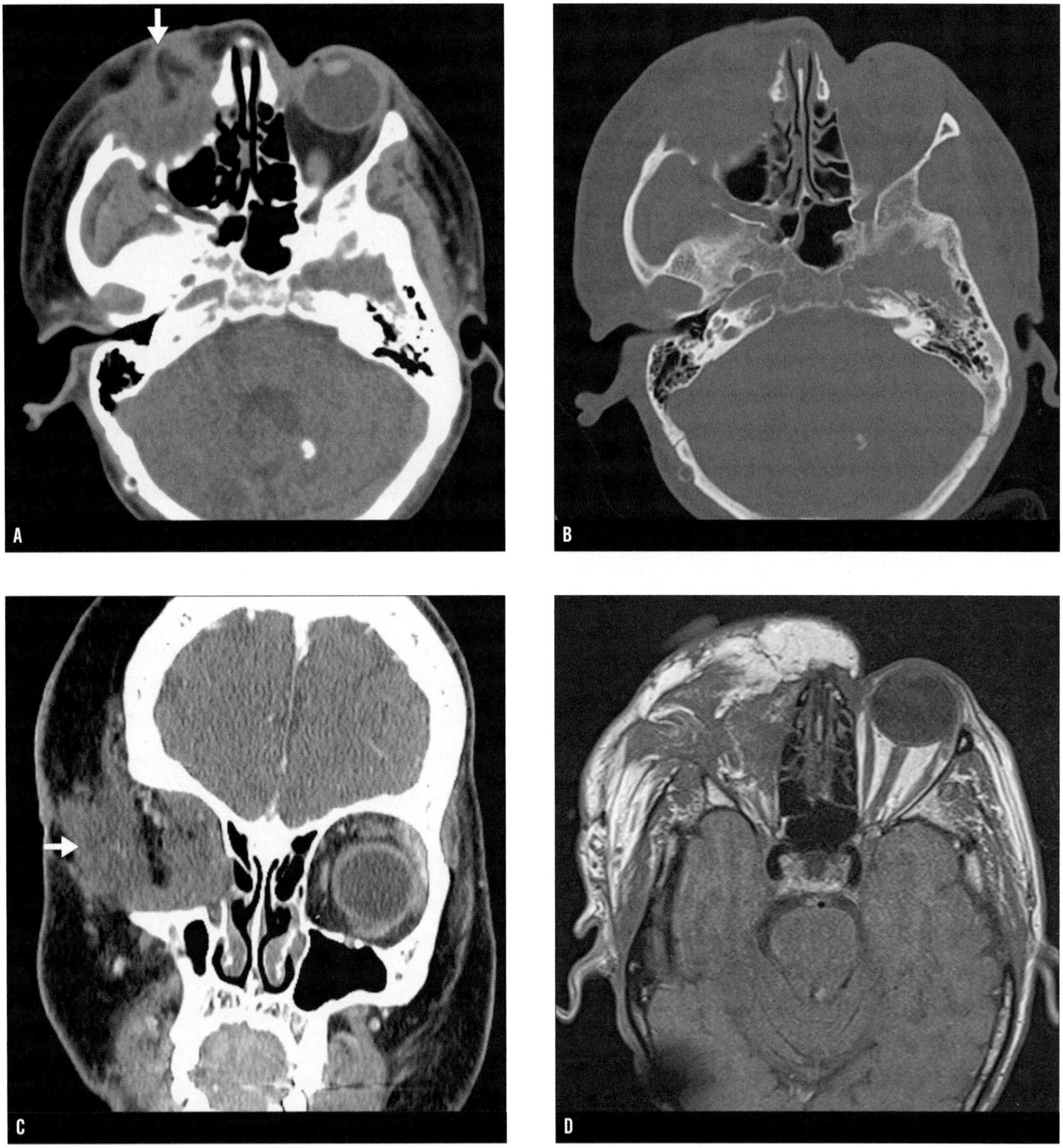

Different patient. Unenhanced axial CT images viewed in a soft tissue window (**A**) and bone window (**B**) as well as a contrast-enhanced coronal reformatted CT image viewed with a soft tissue window (**C**) demonstrate a right orbital exenteration with a myocutaneous flap placed into the exenteration defect (arrows, **A**, **C**). Axial T1 (**D**), coronal T1 (**E**), sagittal T1 (**F**), fat-suppressed contrast-enhanced axial T1 (**G**), and fat-suppressed contrast-enhanced coronal T1 (**H**) MR images of the same patient demonstrate the MRI appearance of a right orbital exenteration and myocutaneous flap placement. Image **H** was acquired after image **G** and delayed enhancement of the soft tissue in the right orbital exenteration is identified, simulating tumor (arrow, **H**). However, this simply represents expected delayed enhancement of the myocutaneous flap and not recurrent tumor. This is supported by the presence of scattered fat within the orbital exenteration on precontrast T1-weighted imaging, which would not be expected if this were recurrent tumor.

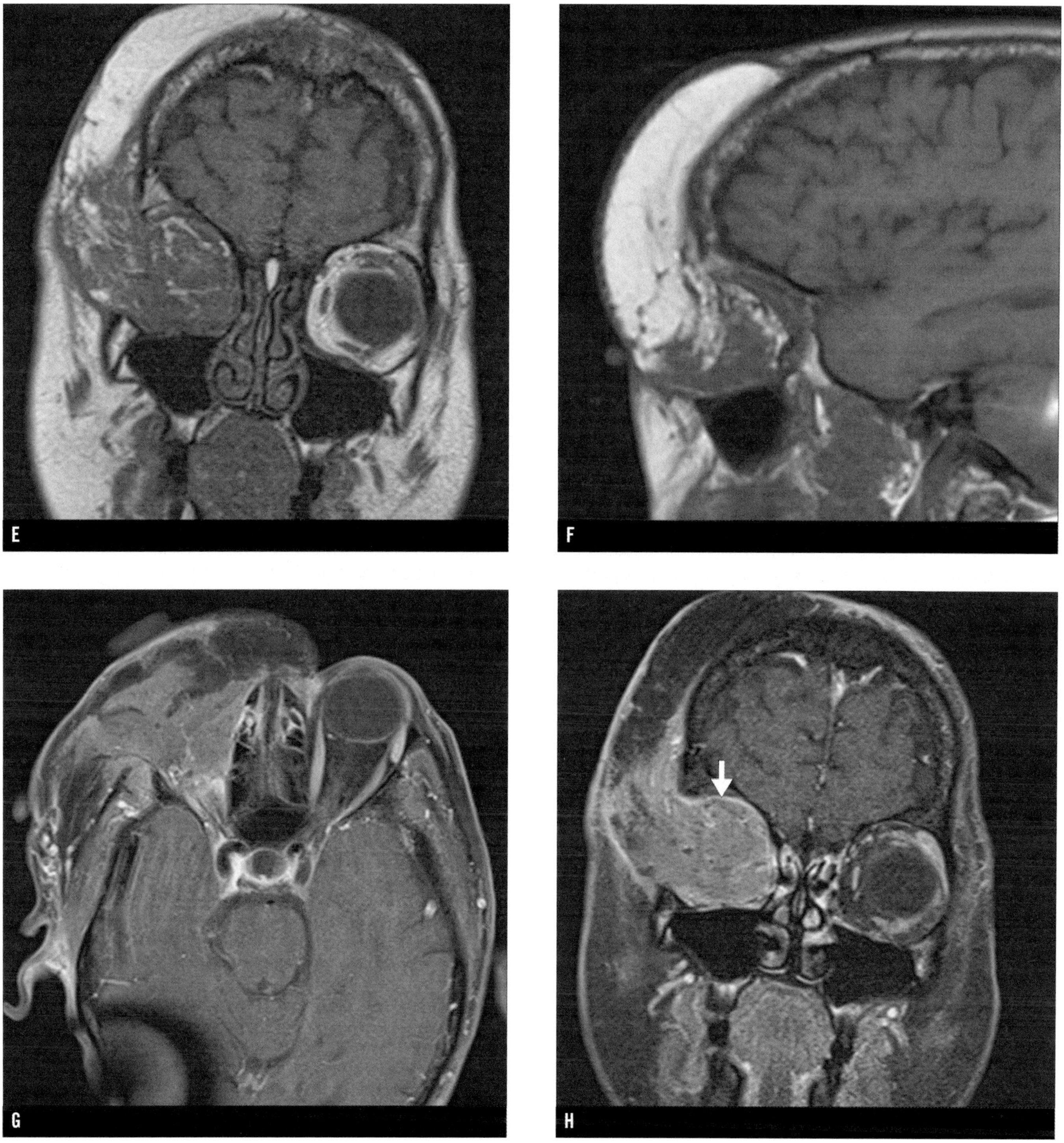

REFERENCE

Yanoff M, Jay SD, James JA. *Ophthalmology*. Edinburgh, Scotland: Mosby Elsevier; 2009.

CASE 31 Incidental tears and air in the nasolacrimal duct

Tears, which are produced by the lacrimal gland, accessory glands, and meibomian glands, bathe and lubricate the globe. Tears, unless excessive, normally traverse medially and collect at the medial canthus of the orbit. Blinking, muscular contraction, and capillary action promote drainage of tears into the superior and inferior puncta. These puncta are small openings for the superior and inferior canaliculi, which are small, horizontally oriented ducts embedded within the superior and inferior eyelids, respectively. These canaliculi merge to form a short common canaliculus, which then drains into a vertically oriented lacrimal sac. The lacrimal sac, which is bulbous at its superior aspect and tapers inferiorly, serves as a temporary reservoir for tears. The lacrimal sac resides within the lacrimal fossa, which is located anterior to the orbital septum. Thus, a lesion isolated to the lacrimal fossa is preseptal in location. Tears then drain caudally into the nasolacrimal duct, which is an inferior extension of the lacrimal sac. The nasolacrimal duct has a long proximal intraosseous portion and a short distal membranous portion, the latter embedded within the nasal mucosa. The lacrimal sac and nasolacrimal duct contain several valves, the most significant and distal-most valve termed the valve of Hasner. A small, slit-like opening allows tears to exit into the inferior meatus, and the tears are then either swallowed or exit via the nasal vestibule. Obstruction of the nasolacrimal system can occur at any level of the nasolacrimal duct system. When obstructed, excessive tearing typically ensues, which is an entity termed epiphora. Some of the more common causes of obstruction include congenital stenosis, trauma, inflammation, dacryoliths (calculi), surgery, tumor, and radiation.

The bone surrounding the nasolacrimal duct, named the nasolacrimal canal, is consistently symmetric to its contralateral counterpart in the normal state. However, air within one nasolacrimal duct and tears in the other will result in asymmetry of the nasolacrimal ducts within the canals. Air and/or tear opacification of the nasolacrimal ducts is normal and should not be confused with pathology when the nasolacrimal canals are symmetric and have normal osseous margins. However, an asymmetrically enlarged or irregular nasolacrimal canal margin on CT associated with soft tissue and/or abnormal enhancement should be viewed with suspicion. An MRI is often indicated in this scenario. In addition, a dacryocystogram, a procedure which entails contrast instillation into the nasolacrimal duct after accessing the punctum of either the superior or inferior canaliculus, may also be of benefit to evaluate the integrity of the nasolacrimal system.

COMPANION CASES

- **Fibrous dysplasia of the frontal process of the maxilla.** With fibrous dysplasia, normal bone is replaced by fibrous tissue consisting of spindle cell bundles and immature woven bone. This process results in expansion of the affected bone. It may affect a single site (monostotic) or multiple sites (polyostotic). The most common CT appearance of fibrous dysplasia is a ground-glass (sclerotic) pattern. However, fibrous dysplasia can less commonly appear as a heterogeneously sclerotic and lucent lesion (Pagetoid form) or as a cystic lesion (cystic form). On MRI, fibrous dysplasia has a nonspecific appearance and can mimic other osseous lesions, including malignant entities. Thus, any suspicious osseous lesion on MRI should be interpreted in combination with CT, or when appropriate, radiographs. Typically, fibrous dysplasia is low to intermediate in T1 signal and enhances on MRI. The T2 characteristics are variable and depend on the ratio of mineralized matrix to fibrous tissue. Due to its expansile nature, strategically located fibrous dysplasia may result in compromise of the nasolacrimal canal and result in epiphora.
- **Dacryocystocele.** A dacryocystocele is a mucocele that typically forms near the medial canthus of the orbit. These are secondary to obstruction of the nasolacrimal drainage apparatus. The most common etiology of a dacryocystocele in an infant is secondary to congenital persistence of a membrane involving the valve of Hasner, which is located at the distal aspect of the nasolacrimal duct. Causes of a dacryocystocele in the adult include trauma or tumors that result in scarring and obstruction of the nasolacrimal apparatus. Dacryocystoceles can peripherally enhance, particularly if acutely inflamed, but they do not centrally enhance. The precontrast T1 and T2 signal characteristics of a dacryocystocele depend on its protein contents, although most often it is isointense on T1 and hyperintense on T2.
- **Nasolacrimal duct squamous cell carcinoma.** Malignancies of the lacrimal sac and nasolacrimal duct are rare and include transitional cell carcinoma, squamous cell carcinoma, adenoid cystic carcinoma, mucoepidermoid carcinoma, and adenocarcinoma. Symptoms of these malignancies include epiphora, a palpable mass (either of the primary tumor or from a postobstructive dacryocystocele), epistaxis, and blood-tinged tears. On CT, most tumors are solid, and bone destruction or erosion is often identified with aggressive malignancies. On MRI, a squamous cell carcinoma affecting these structures will typically be isointense on T1, iso- to hypointense on T2, and enhance. Abnormal bone marrow signal on MRI may also be identified with aggressive tumors, such as squamous cell carcinoma.

Normal tears and air in the nasolacrimal duct

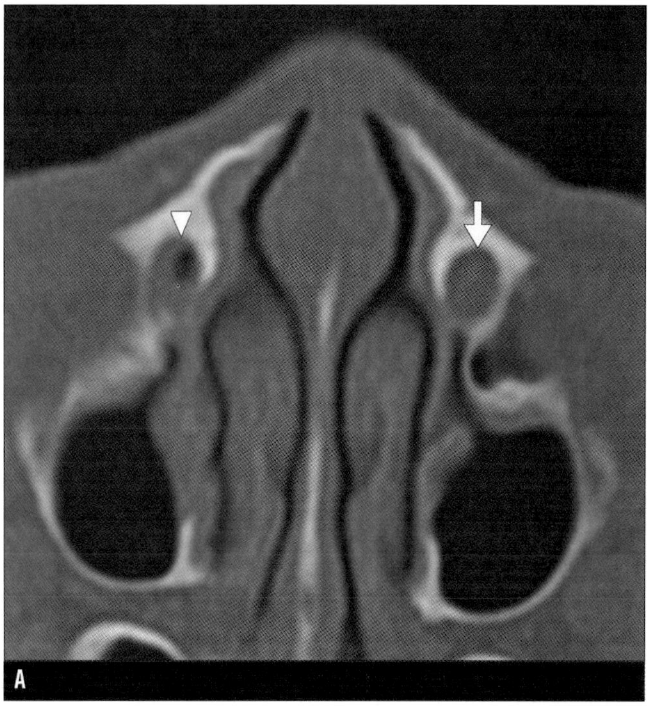

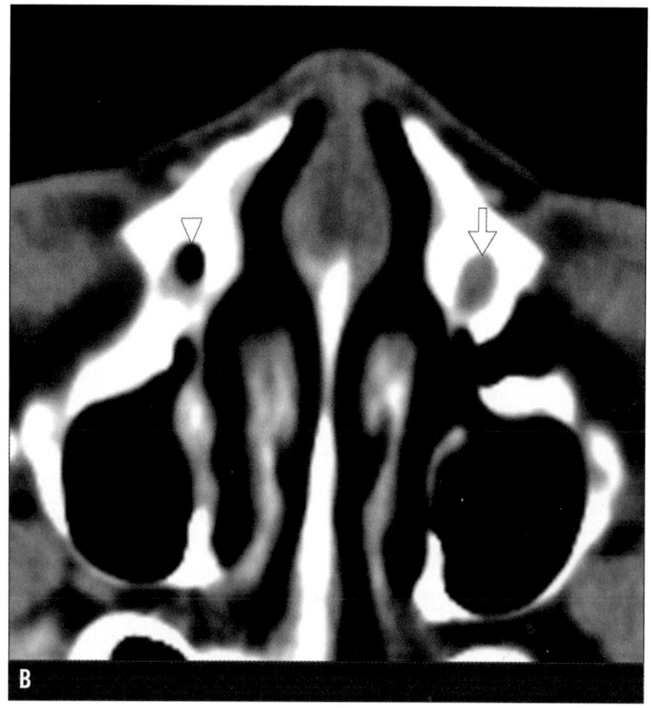

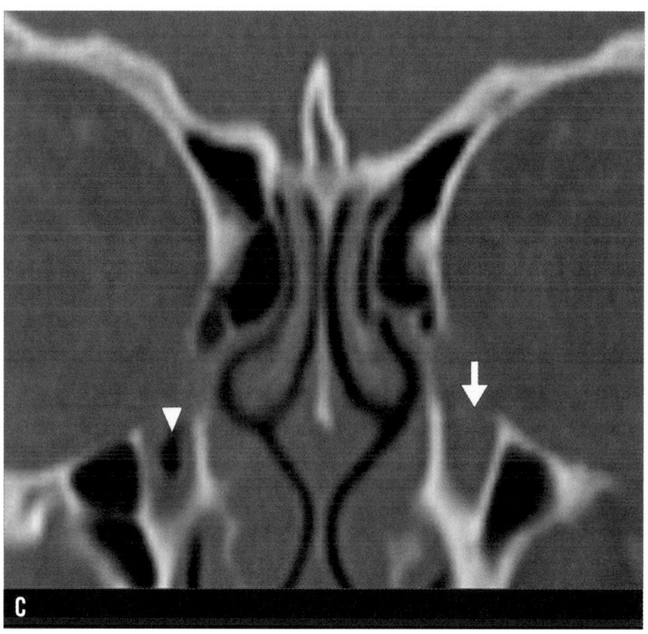

Unenhanced axial CT images viewed with a bone window (**A**) and soft tissue window (**B**) as well as a coronal reformatted CT image viewed with a bone window (**C**) demonstrate complete opacification of the left nasolacrimal duct (arrows, **A**-**C**) and a partially air-filled right nasolacrimal duct (arrowheads, **A**-**C**). The nasolacrimal canals are symmetric and there were no symptoms referable to the nasolacrimal system. This appearance is very common and normal.

Companion case: Fibrous dysplasia of the frontal process of the maxilla

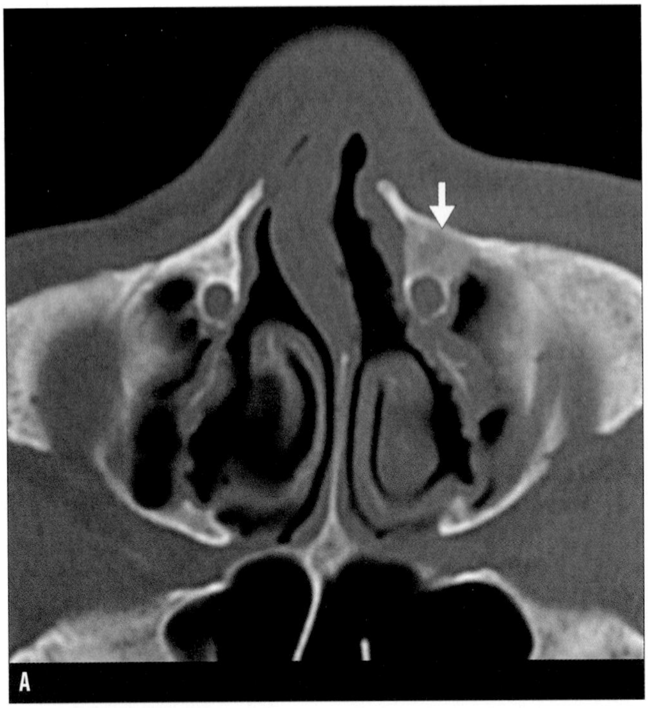

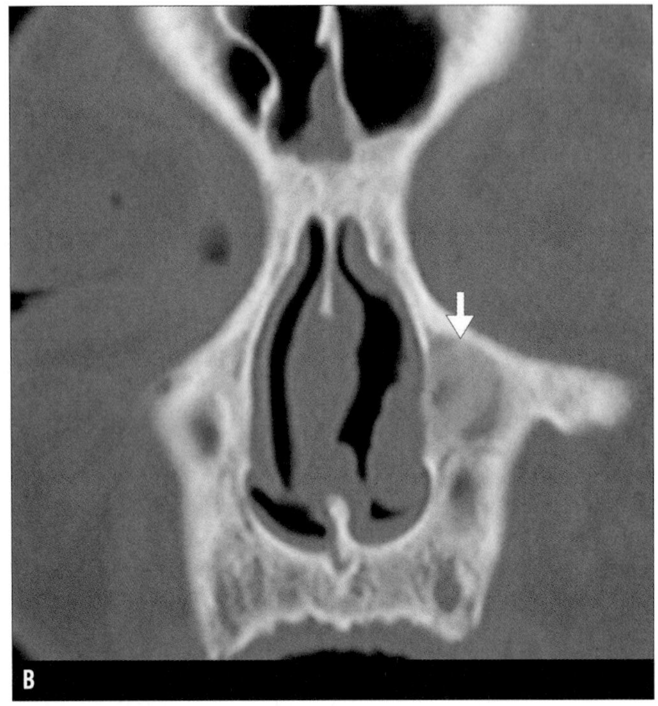

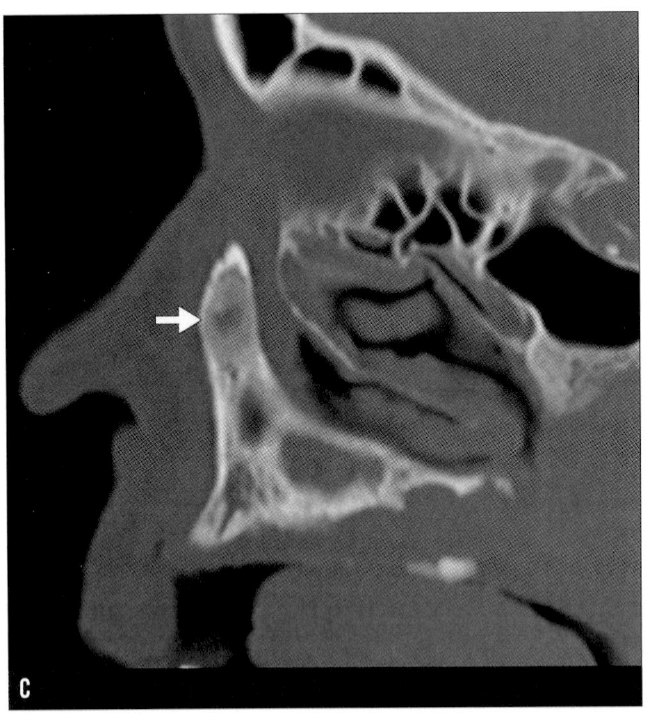

Axial (**A**), coronal reformatted (**B**), and sagittal reformatted (**C**) CT images demonstrate a slightly expansile, ground-glass lesion involving the left frontal process of the maxilla, compatible with fibrous dysplasia (arrows, **A**-**C**).

Companion case: Fibrous dysplasia of the frontal process of the maxilla with nasolacrimal canal narrowing

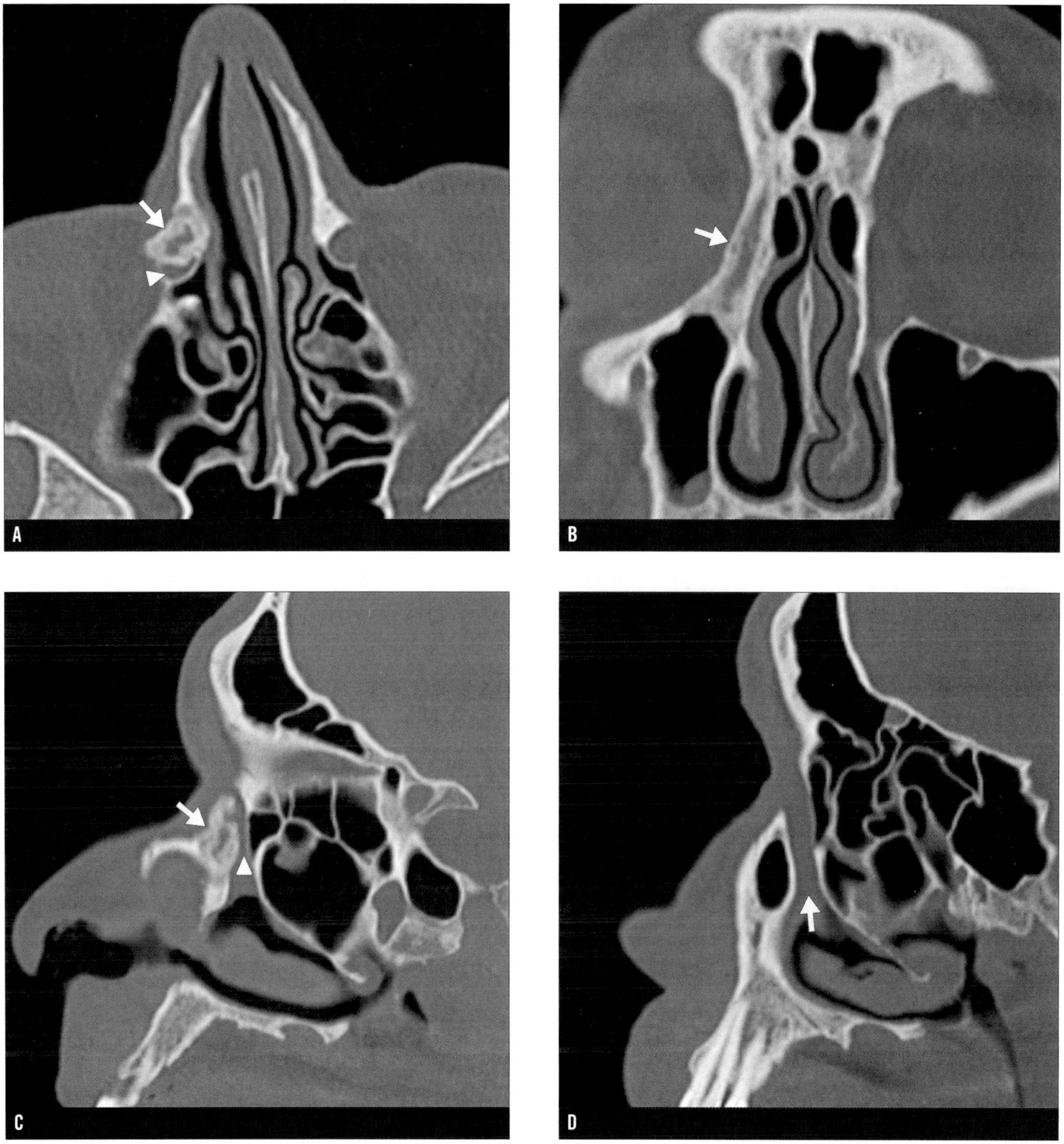

Axial (**A**) and coronal reformatted (**B**) CT images performed on a patient with right eye epiphora (excessive tearing) demonstrate an expansile, ground-glass lesion involving the right frontal process of the maxilla compatible with fibrous dysplasia (arrows, **A**, **B**). This area of fibrous dysplasia results in focal narrowing of the right nasolacrimal canal (arrowhead, **A**). Sagittal reformatted CT images obtained through the right nasolacrimal canal (**C**) and left nasolacrimal canal (**D**) also illustrate the fibrous dysplasia (arrow, **C**) to result in marked asymmetric narrowing of the right nasolacrimal canal (arrowhead, **C**) compared to left (arrow, **D**). This finding was likely the cause of the patient's right eye epiphora.

Companion case: Dacryocystocele

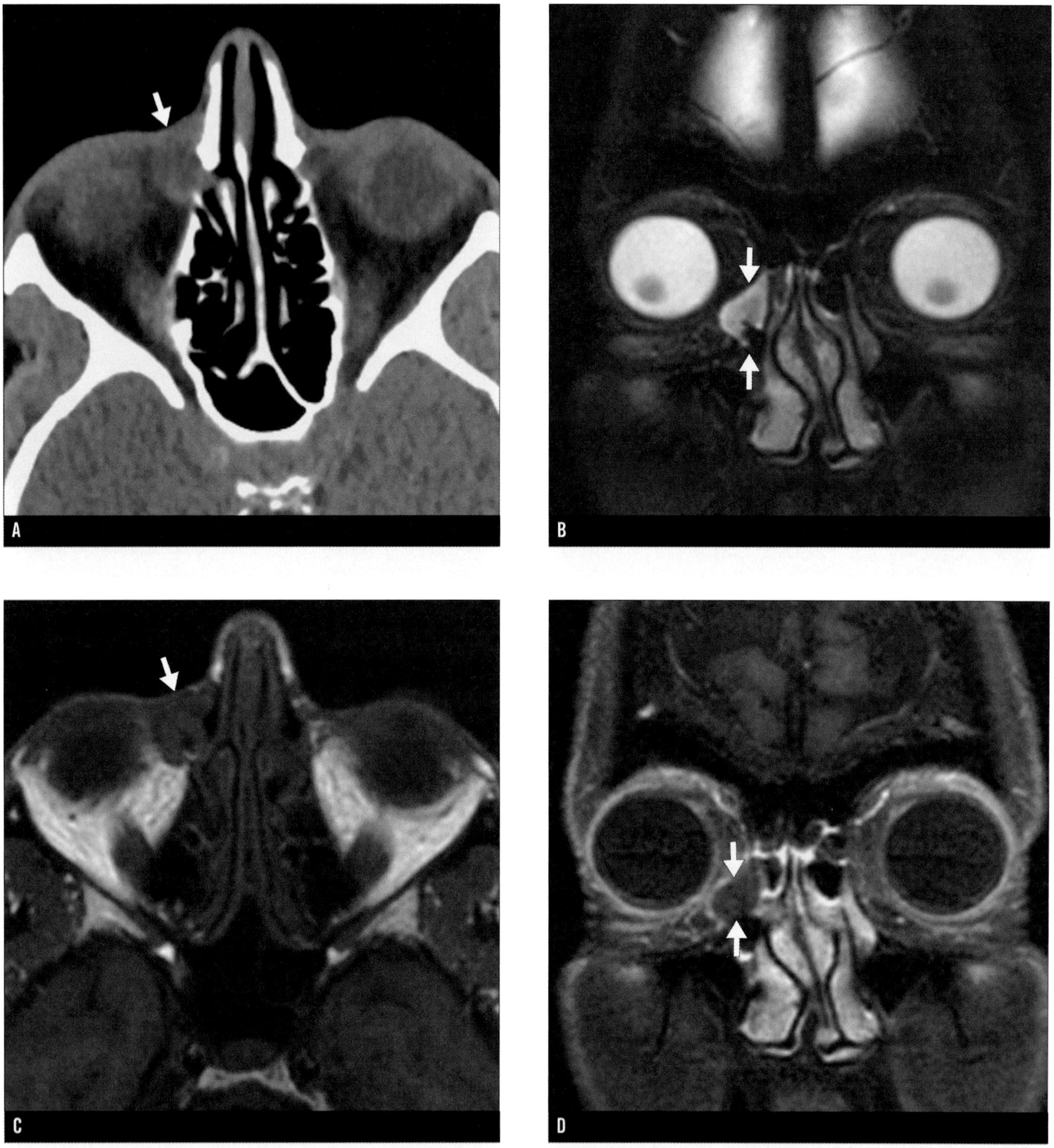

An axial noncontrast CT image (**A**) demonstrates a relatively isodense lesion in the region of the right medial canthus (arrow, **A**). Coronal T2 with fat suppression (**B**), axial T1 (**C**) and contrast-enhanced coronal T1 with fat suppression (**D**) MR images demonstrate a T1 hypointense, T2 hyperintense, rim-enhancing lesion in the region of the right medial canthus and extending into the right lacrimal sac fossa, most compatible with a dacryocystocele (arrows, **B**-**D**).

Companion case: Nasolacrimal duct squamous cell carcinoma

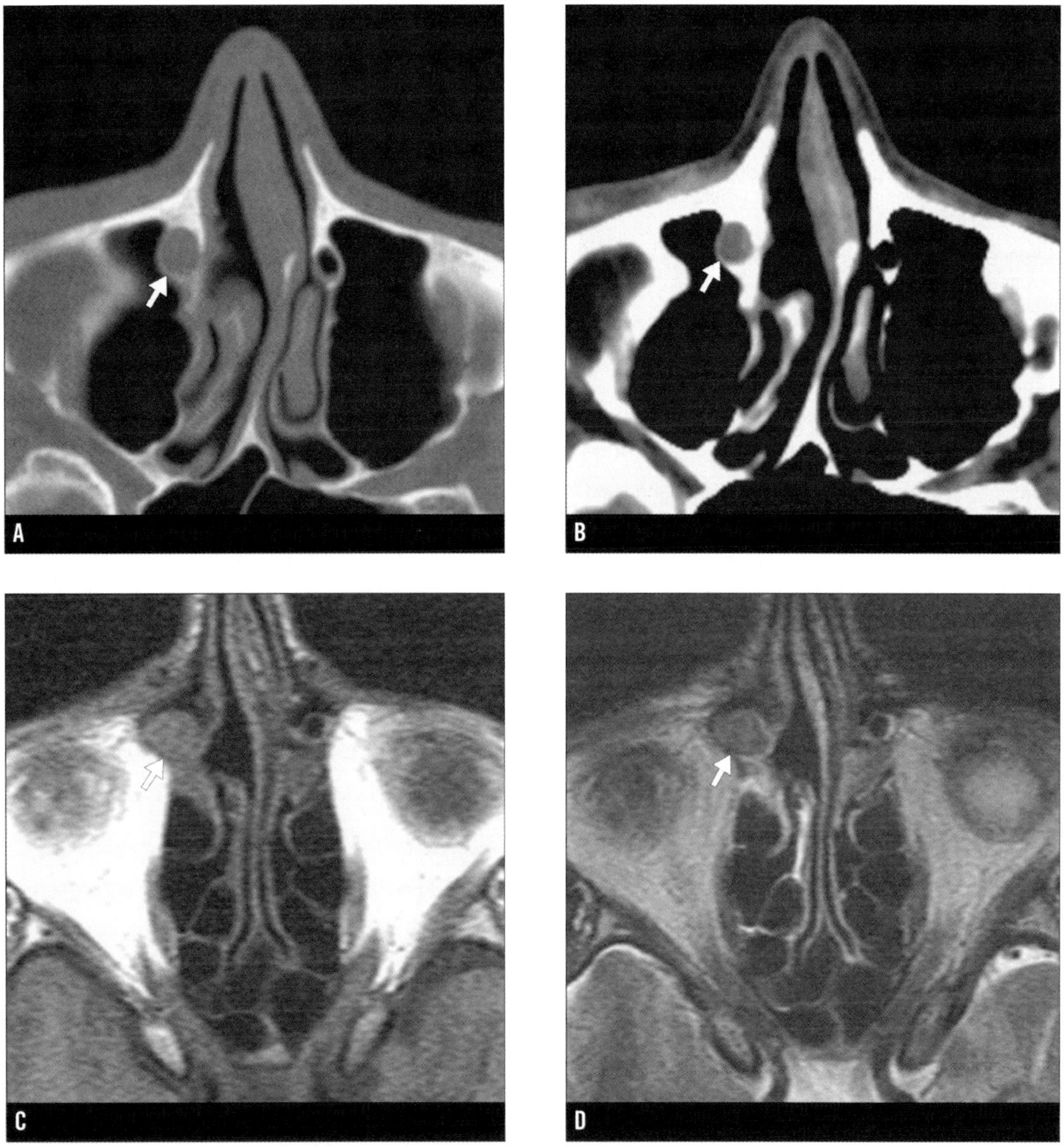

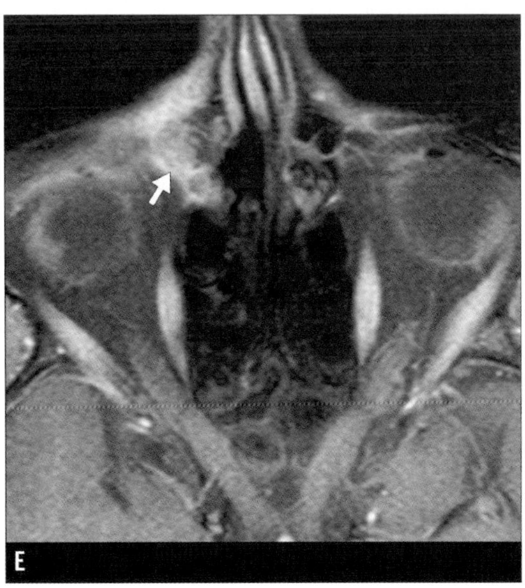

An unenhanced axial CT image viewed with a bone window (**A**) and soft tissue window (**B**) demonstrates opacification and asymmetric enlargement of the right nasolacrimal canal (arrows, **A**, **B**). Axial T1 (**C**), axial T2 (**D**), and contrast-enhanced axial T1 with fat suppression (**E**) MR images demonstrate the contents of the right nasolacrimal duct finding to be T2 hypointense and to enhance, in this case shown to represent a squamous cell carcinoma of the nasolacrimal duct at pathology (arrows, **C**-**E**).

REFERENCES

Camilleri AE. Craniofacial fibrous dysplasia. *J Laryngol Otol* 1991;105:662-66.

Clauser L, Marchetti C, Piccione M, Bertoni F. Craniofacial fibrous dysplasia and Ollier's disease: combined transfrontal and transfacial resection using the nasal-cheek flap. *J Craniofac Surg* 1996;7(2):140-44.

Cruz AAV, Constanzi M, Attie de Castro FA, Carlos dos Santos AC. Apical involvement with fibrous dysplasia: implications for vision. *Ophthal Plast Reconstr Surg.* 2007;23(6):450-454.

Debnam JM, Esmaeli B, Ginsberg LE. Imaging characteristics of dacryocystocele diagnosed after surgery for sinonasal cancer. *AJNR Am J Neuroradiol.* 2007;28(10):1872-1875. Epub October 2007.

Demirdover C, Sahin B, Ozkan HS, Durmus EU, Oztan HY. Isolated fibrous dysplasia of the zygomatic bone. *J Craniofac Surg* 2010;21:1583-1584.

Farrer RS, Mohammed TL, Hahn FJ. MRI of childhood dacryocystocele. *Neuroradiology.* 2003;45(4):259-261.

MacDonald-Jankowski DS. Fibro-osseous lesions of the face and jaws. *Clin Radiol.* 2004;59:11-25.

Manfre L, de Maria M, TTodaro E, Mangiameli A, Ponte F, Lagalla R. MR dacrocystography: comparison with dacrocystography and CT dacrocystography. *AM J Neuroradiol.* 2000;21(6):1145-1150.

McCluskey P, Wingae R, Benger R, McCarthy S. Monostotic fibrous dysplasia of the orbit: an unusual lacrimal fossa mass. *Br J Opthalmol* 1993;77:54-56.

Rahangdale SR, Castillo M, Shockley W. MR in squamous cell carcinoma of the lacrimal sac. *AJNR Am J Neuroradiol.* 1995;16(6):1262-1264.

Russell EJ, Czervionke L, Huckman M, Daniels D, McLachlan D. CT of the inferomedial orbit and the lacrimal drainage apparatus: normal and pathologic anatomy. *AJR Am J Roentgenol.* 1985;145(6):1147-1154.

Shah ZK, Peh WCG, Koh WL, Shek TWH. Magnetic resonance imaging appearances of fibrous dysplasia. *Br J Radiol.* 2005;78:1104-1115

Yang BT, Wang YZ, Wang XY, Wang ZC, Xian JF, Li J. Fibrous dysplasia-like appearance of the frontal process of the maxilla on CT: prevalence in North China. AJNR *Am J Neuroradiol.* 2011;32(3):471-473.

CASE 32 Dacryocystorhinostomy

A dacryocystorhinostomy is a surgical procedure which creates a direct communication between the lacrimal sac and nasal cavity. It is typically performed to treat epiphora (excessive tearing) when the epiphora is the result of a nasolacrimal duct obstruction that cannot be treated by other means (such as probing). A dacryocystorhinostomy can be performed from either an endoscopic or external approach. An endoscopic dacryocystorhinostomy has some advantages over the external approach, including lack of external scarring and maintenance of the pumping action of the orbicularis oculi muscle on the lacrimal sac. Following an endoscopic or external dacryocystorhinostomy, a temporary silicone stent is placed to maintain patency of the newly created passage and is subsequently removed several days later.

Dacryocystorhinostomy

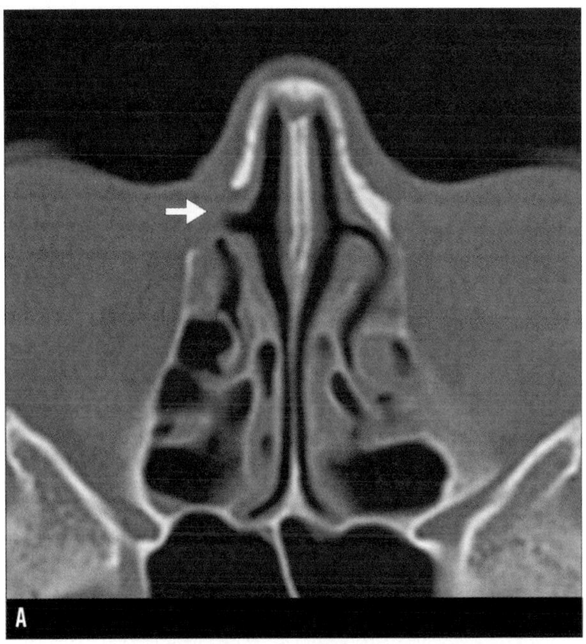

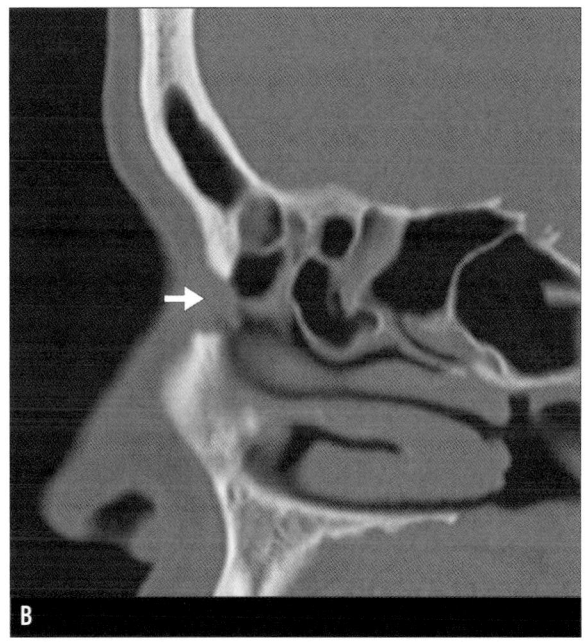

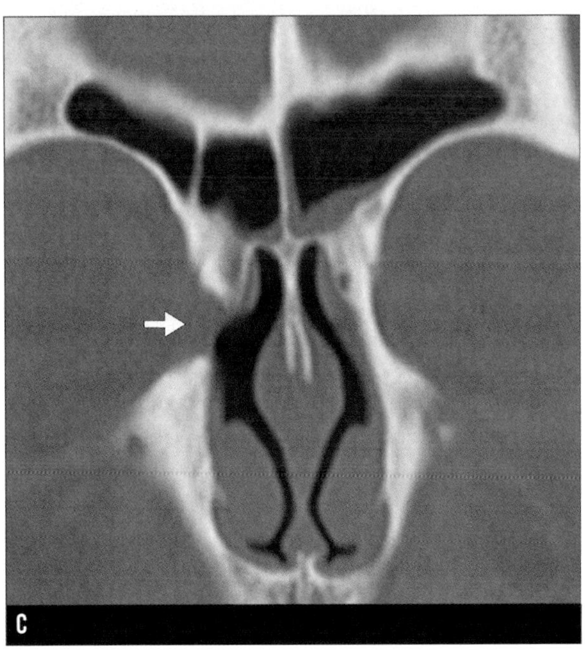

Axial (**A**), sagittal reformatted (**B**), and coronal reformatted (**C**) CT images demonstrate postsurgical changes of right dacryocystorhinostomy, which allows drainage of the lacrimal sac directly into the nasal cavity (arrows, **A**-**C**).

Dacryocystorhinostomy

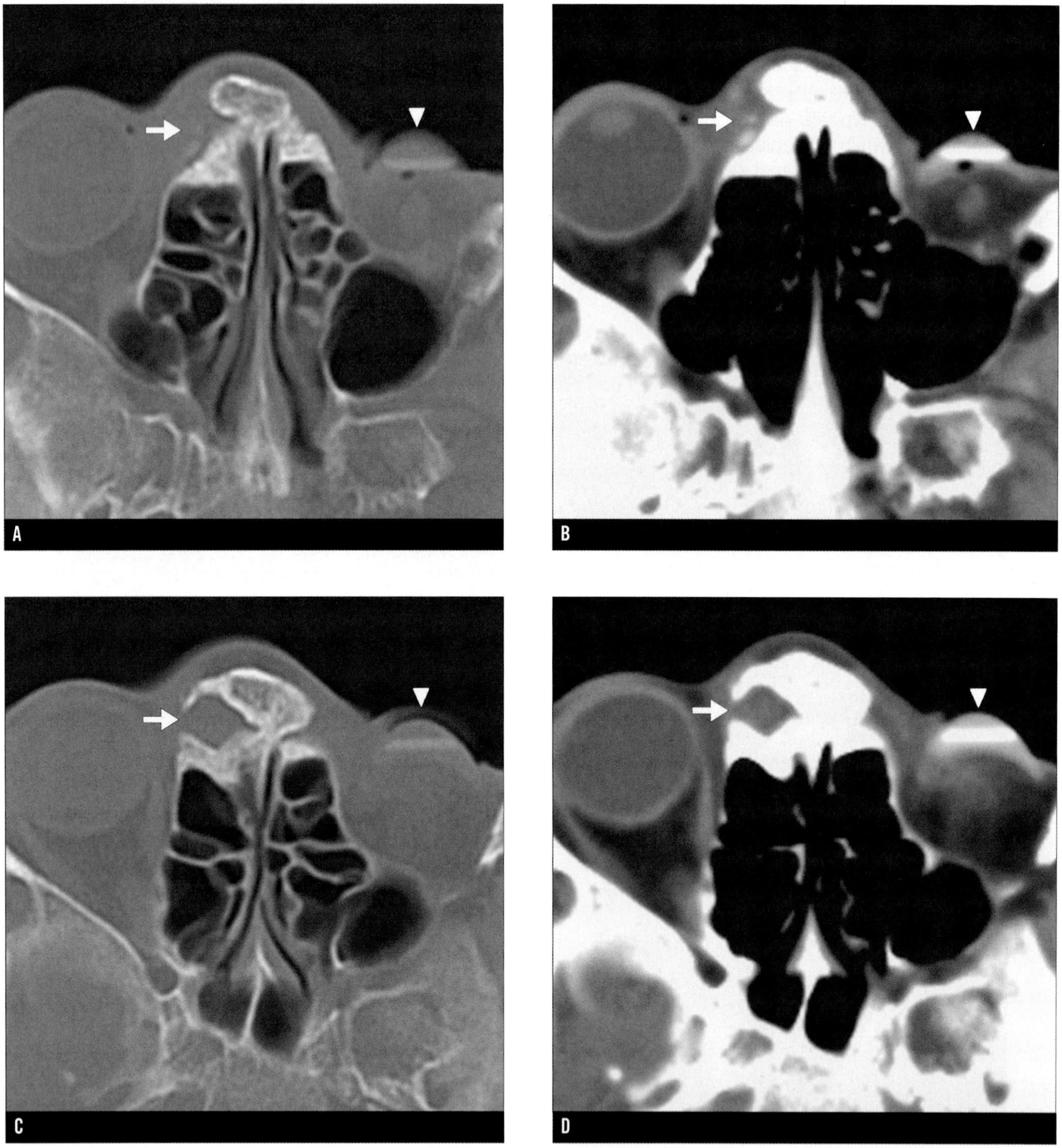

Different patient. Unenhanced axial CT images viewed with a bone window (**A**, **C**) and soft tissue window (**B**, **D**) demonstrate postsurgical changes of a prior right dacryocystorhinostomy (arrows, **A**-**D**). Incidentally, the left globe has been surgically removed and there is an overlying ocular prosthesis (arrowheads, **A**-**D**).

Dacryocystorhinostomy tube

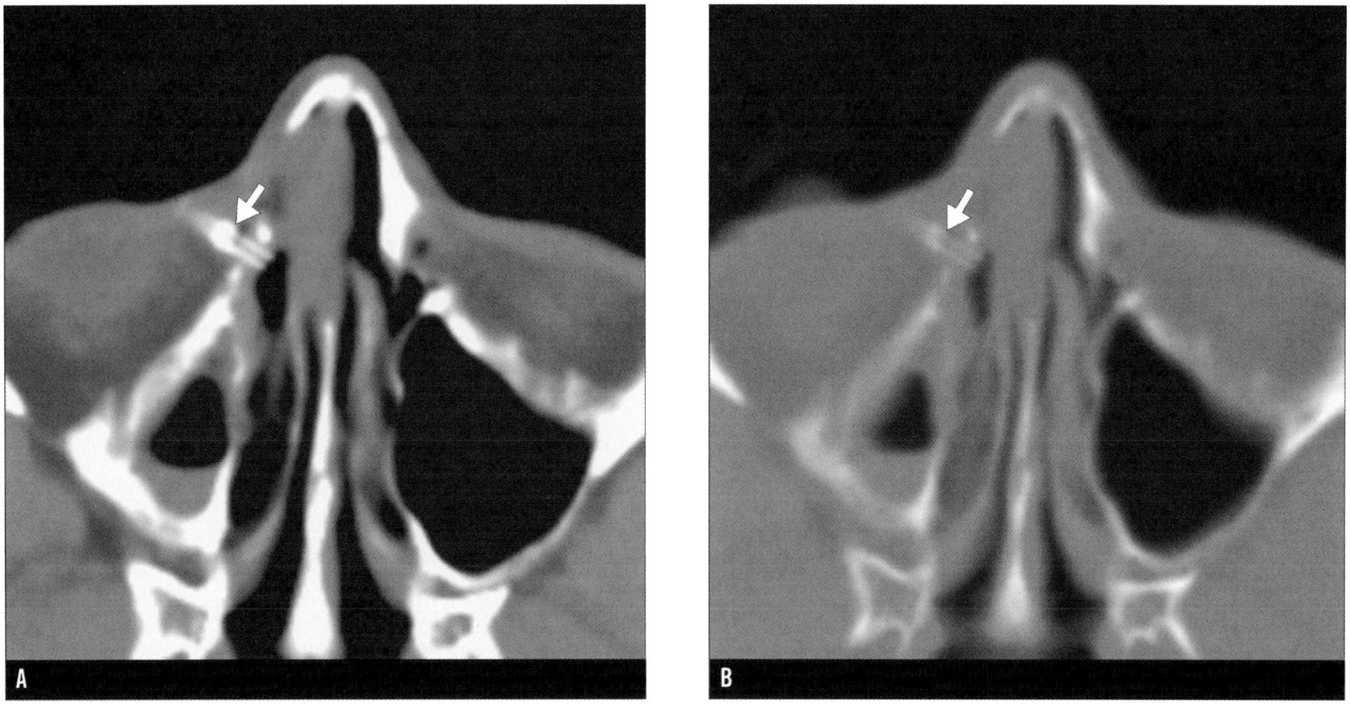

Axial CT images viewed with a soft tissue window (**A**) and bone window (**B**) demonstrate postsurgical changes of a right dacryocystorhinostomy with placement of a silicone tube (arrows, **A**, **B**).

REFERENCES

Dailey RA, Tower, RN. Frosted jones pyrex tubes. *Ophthal Plast Reconstr Surg*. 2005;21(3):185-187.

Dolman PJ. Comparison of external dacryocystorhinostomy with nonlaser endonasal dacryocystorhinostomy. *Ophthalmology*. 2003;110;78-84.

Sonkhya N, Mishra P. Endoscopic transnasal dacryocystorhinostomy with nasal mucosal and posterior lacrimal sac flap. *J Laryngol Otol*. 2009;123(3):320-326.

Trotter WL, Meyer DR. Endoscopic conjunctivodacryocystorhinostomy with Jones tube placement. *Ophthalmology*. 2000;107(6);1206-1209.

CHAPTER 10

FACE

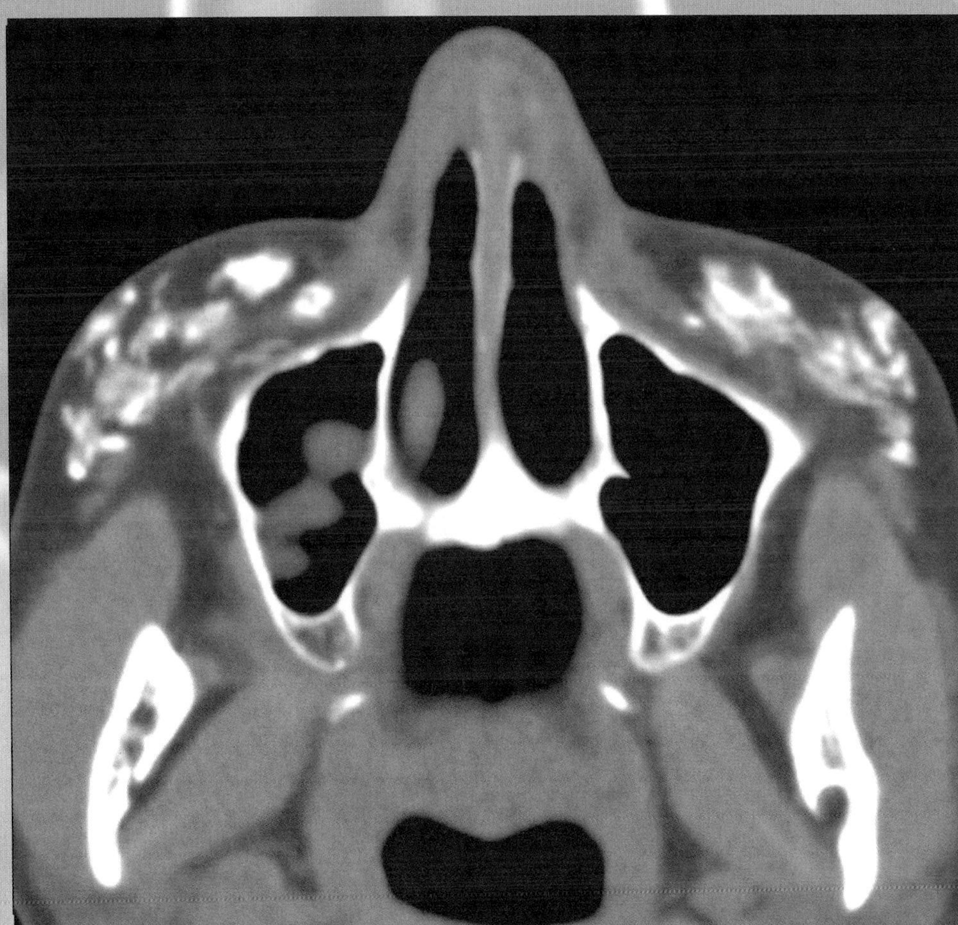

Vanessa A. Lewis, Achilles G. Karagianis, Benjamin P. Liu

X. FACE

1. Nasolabial fold cyst
2. Epidermal inclusion cyst
3. Dermal calcifications
    i. *Companion case*: Glass fragments in the face following trauma
    ii. *Companion case*: Shotgun injury to the face
4. Incomplete MRI fat suppression simulating a facial cellulitis
    i. *Companion case*: Facial cellulitis
    ii. *Companion case*: Port-wine stain
5. Mimetic muscle atrophy
    i. *Companion case*: Parry-Romberg syndrome
    ii. *Companion case*: CN V, V3 denervation atrophy
6. Rhytidectomy (facelift) and forehead lift
7. Cosmetic injectable filler
    i. *Companion case*: Hypermetabolic cosmetic injectable filler on PET imaging
    ii. *Companion case*: Inadvertent cosmetic injection into a Stensen duct
    iii. *Companion case*: Rapidly hardening hydroxyapatite cement for fracture stabilization
8. Malar implant prostheses
9. Reduction rhinoplasty
    i. *Companion case*: Valvular collapse
    ii. *Companion case*: Saddle-nose deformity
10. Augmentation and reconstruction rhinoplasty
    i. *Companion case*: Nasal ala cartilage mineralization
11. Facial piercings and rings
12. Pseudofractures of the facial bones
    i. *Companion case*: Nasomaxillary suture diastasis
    ii. *Companion case*: Nondisplaced zygomatic arch fracture
13. Reanimation for facial paralysis
    i. *Companion case*: Zygomaticus major muscle full-thickness tear
14. Facial reconstruction flap
    i. *Companion case*: Necrotizing fasciitis
    ii. *Companion case*: Venous malformation
    iii. *Companion case*: Natural killer/T-cell lymphoma, nasal type with facial involvement
15. Diseases affecting the face that simulate malignancy
    a. Fibrous dysplasia
    b. Venous malformation of bone (osseous hemangioma)
    c. Renal osteodystrophy
    d. Paget disease
    e. Osteopetrosis

Nasolabial fold cysts (also called nasoalveolar cysts or Klestadt cysts) are rare cysts that lie deep to the nasolabial folds or nasal ala. They are nonodontogenic, extraosseous cysts that overlie, but do not arise from, the maxillary alveolus. Initially, nasolabial cysts were believed to arise from retained epithelium trapped between the lateral nasal and maxillary processes of the developing embryo. An alternative theory, and generally more accepted, suggests that these originate from remnants of nasolacrimal duct epithelium. Histologically, nasolabial fold cysts are lined with pseudostratified columnar epithelium and mucin-producing cells, the same cells that form the nasolacrimal duct.

A nasolabial fold cyst is usually occult and is most often painless. It typically presents clinically if there is effacement of the nasolabial fold or if it becomes infected. They are up to three times more common in women and are most often identified in the fourth or fifth decades. Bilateral cysts are less common than unilateral cysts, the former accounting for up to 11% of all cases.

Radiographs are often negative, although occasionally they may reveal erosions of the adjacent maxillary alveolus. CT will usually demonstrate an oval, cystic lesion deep to the nasal ala or nasolabial fold. On MRI, the T1 and T2 signal characteristics of the cyst are variable and depend on the proteinaceous content of the cyst. The cyst wall rarely enhances unless it is infected. The treatment is surgical enucleation via a sublabial incision. At surgery, the cysts are usually composed of a thick fibrous capsule containing yellow serous fluid or mucoid material.

Nasolabial fold cyst

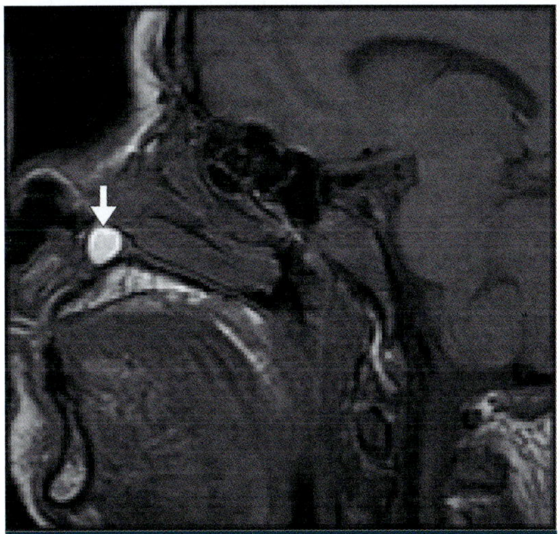
A

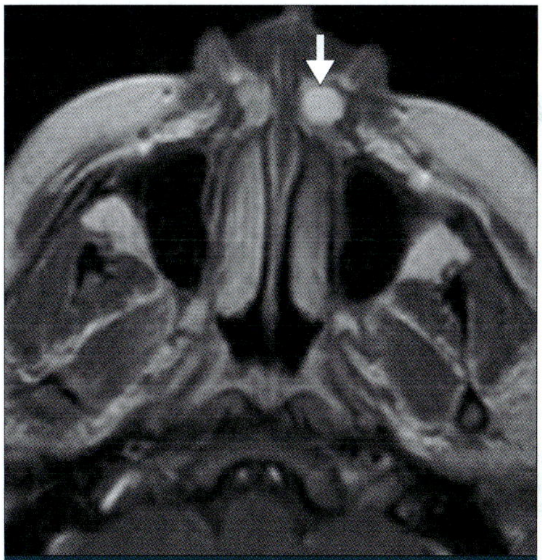
B

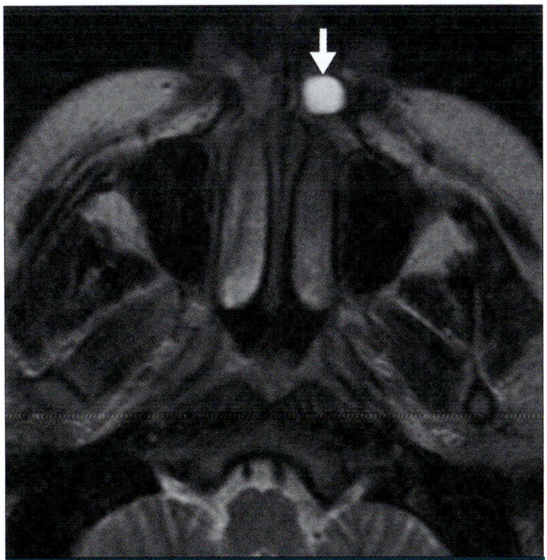
C

Sagittal T1 (**A**), contrast-enhanced axial T1 (**B**), and axial T2 (**C**) MR images demonstrate a round, intrinsically T1 hyperintense, T2 hyperintense, and nonenhancing lesion deep to the left nasal ala, consistent with an incidental nasolabial fold cyst (arrows, **A**-**C**). The intrinsic T1 hyperintense signal is representative of elevated protein content within the cyst.

Nasolabial fold cyst

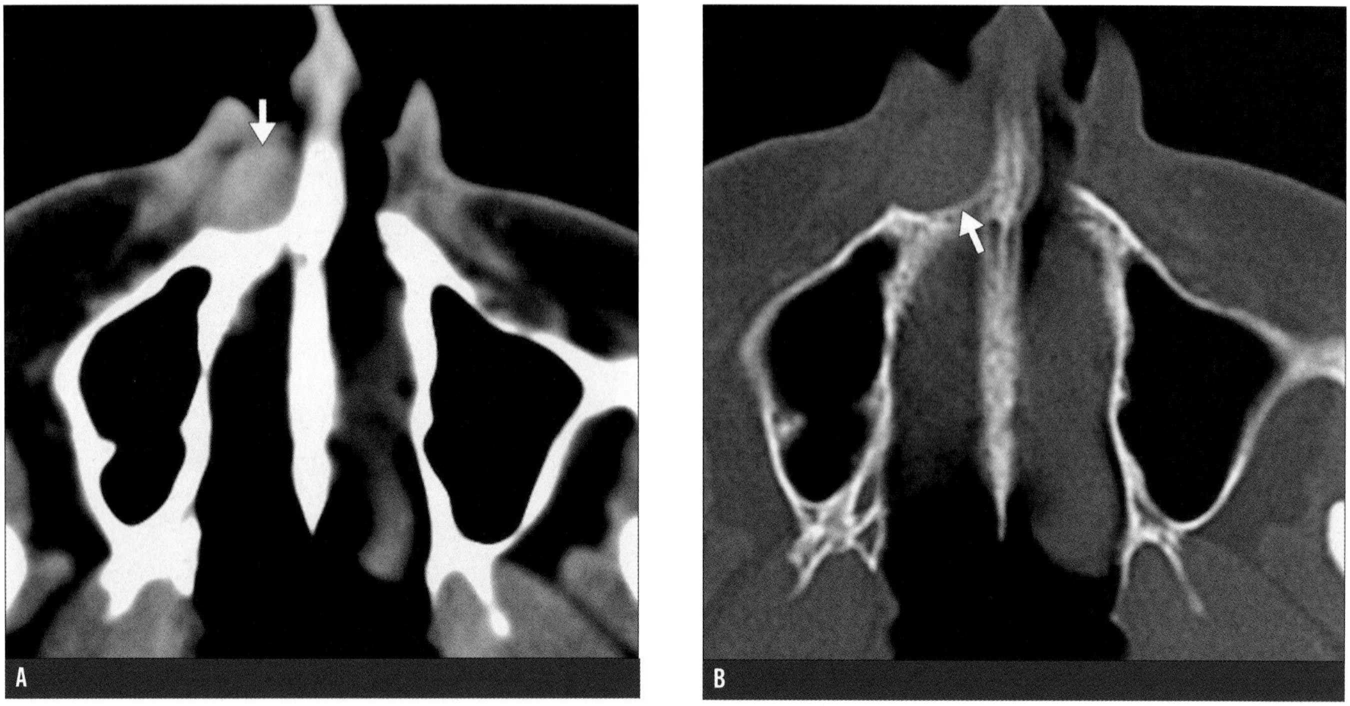

Unenhanced axial CT images viewed with a soft tissue window (**A**) and bone window (**B**) demonstrate an oval soft tissue lesion deep to the right nasolabial fold and nasal ala (arrow, **A**) associated with smooth osseous scalloping of the paramedian right aspect of the maxillary alveolus (arrow, **B**), consistent with an incidental right nasolabial fold cyst.

REFERENCES

Boffano P, Gallesio C, Campisi P, Roccia FJ. Diagnosis and surgical treatment of a nasolabial cyst. *Craniofac Surg.* 2011;22(5):1946-1948.

Kato H, et al. Nasoalveolar cyst: imaging findings in three cases. *Clin Imaging.* 2007;31:206-209.

Marcoviceanu M, et al. Report of rare bilateral nasolabial cysts. J *Craniomaxillofac Surg.* 2009;37:83-86.

Tanimoto K, Kakimoto N, Nishiyama H, Murakami S, Kishino M. MRI of nasoalveolar cyst: case report. *Oral Surg.* 2005;99:221-224.

Yuen H, Julian CL, Samuel CY. Nasolabial cysts: clinical features, diagnosis, and treatment. *Brit J Oral Maxillofac Surg.* 2007;45:293-297.

CASE 2 Epidermal inclusion cyst

Epidermal inclusion cysts are the most common cutaneous cysts and result from implantation or rests of the epidermal elements in the dermis and subcutaneous soft tissues. These cysts are pathologically identical to epidermoid cysts located elsewhere in the body and are composed of keratin, protein, cholesterol, and cell membrane lipids. The term sebaceous cyst should be avoided to describe this entity because an epidermal inclusion cyst does not arise from the sebaceous glands. Moreover, while sebaceous cysts do occur in the same locations as epidermal inclusion cysts, they are significantly less common. Epidermal inclusion cysts are benign, slow-growing lesions; however, there are rare reports of associated malignancies.

Epidermal inclusion cysts are unilocular, circumscribed, round to oval lesions that reside in the subcutaneous tissue and usually abut the dermis. They are fluid attenuating on CT. On MRI, they are primarily iso- to hypointense on T1 relative to muscle (although they may contain small foci of mildly intrinsic T1 hyperintense signal), hyperintense on T2, and often restrict on diffusion-weighted imaging, similar to epidermoids elsewhere. Epidermal inclusion cysts do not centrally enhance on CT or MRI. A thin capsule surrounding these lesions is often appreciated on imaging. Epidermal inclusion cysts may also mineralize, particularly in the elderly.

Epidermal inclusion cyst

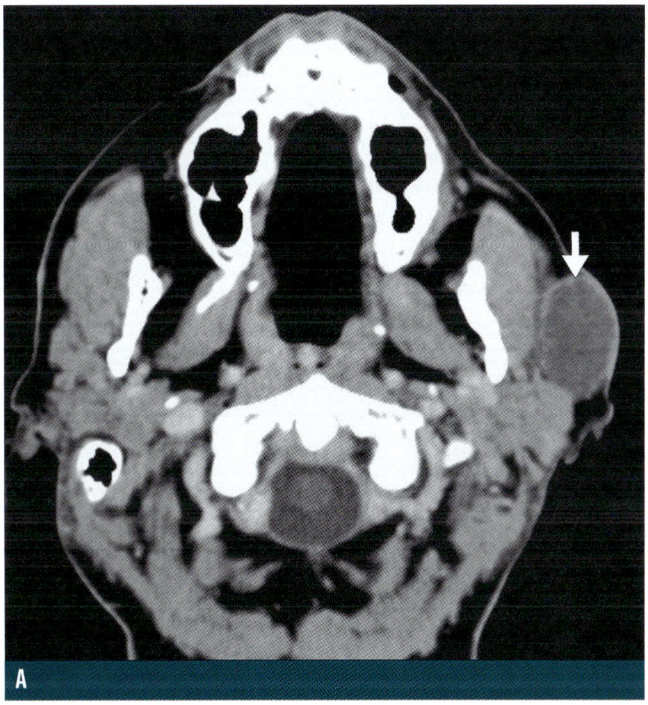

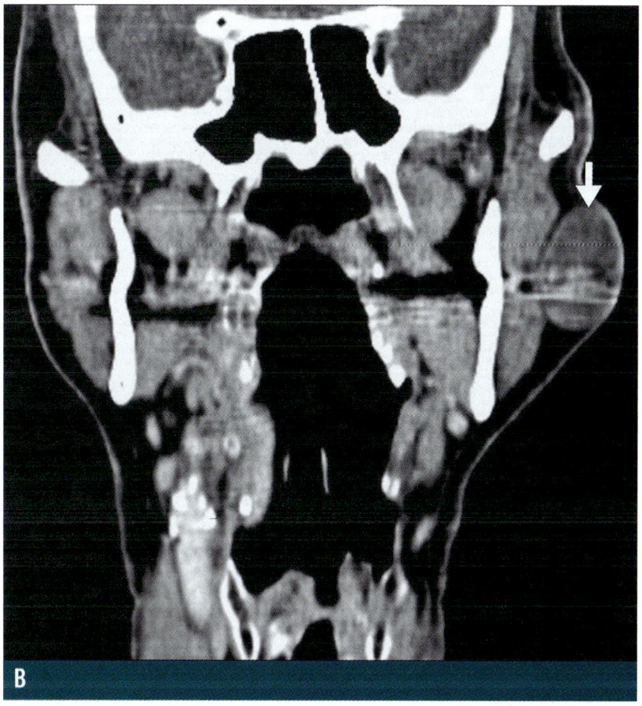

Axial (**A**) and coronal reformatted (**B**) contrast-enhanced CT images demonstrate an oval, circumscribed, hypoattenuating, and nonenhancing lesion in the subcutaneous soft tissues of the left lateral face (arrows, **A**, **B**). This finding was present for many years. Its stability, circumscribed appearance, subcutaneous location, and abutment of the overlying dermis suggests that the lesion represents an epidermal inclusion cyst. Sagittal T1 (**C**), axial DWI (**D**), and axial ADC map (**E**) MR images demonstrate the lesion to be hypointense on T1 (arrow, **C**) and restrict on DWI (arrows, **D**, **E**), also in keeping with the diagnosis of an epidermal inclusion cyst.

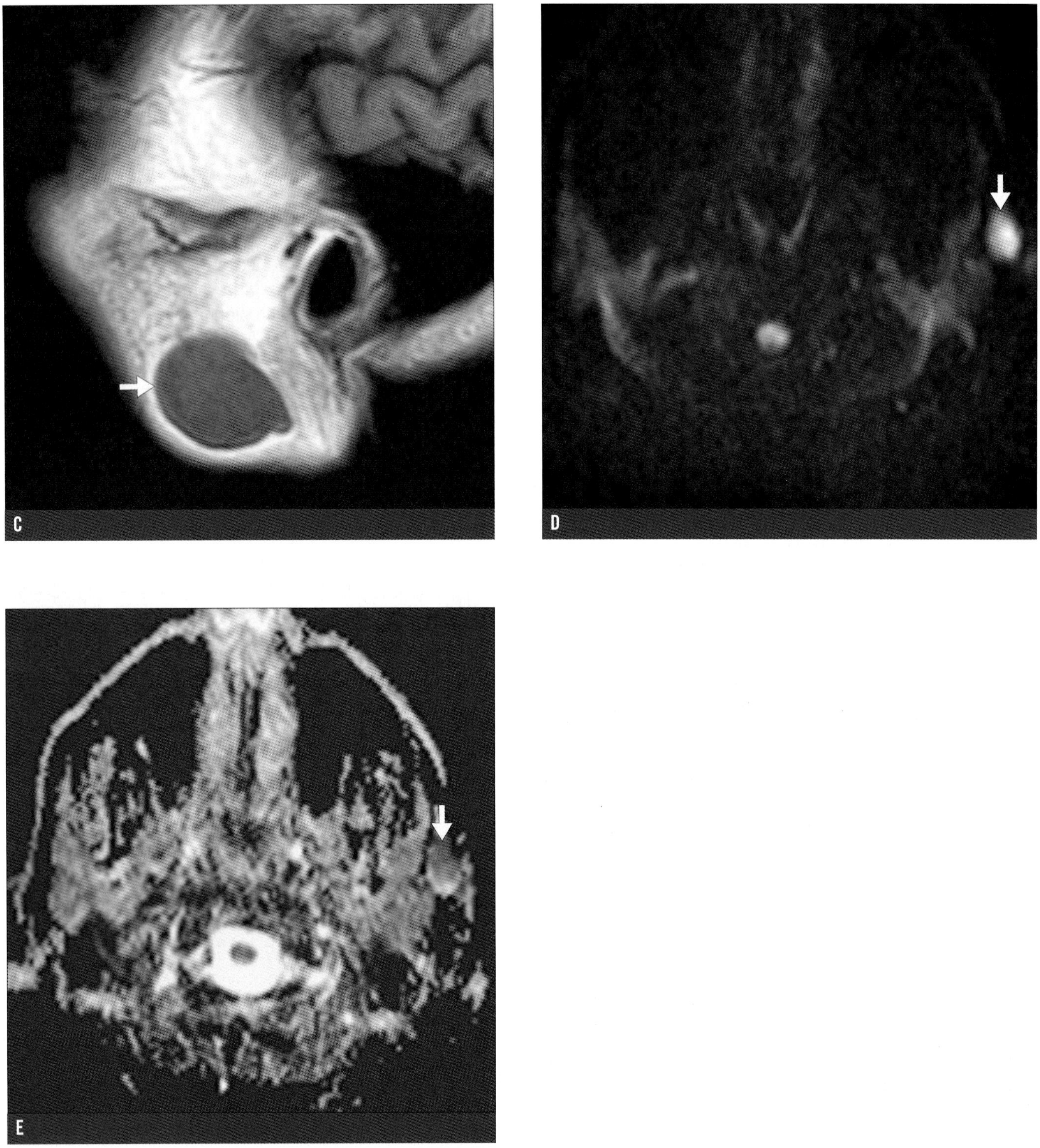

C
D
E

Spontaneous rupture of an epidermal inclusion cyst

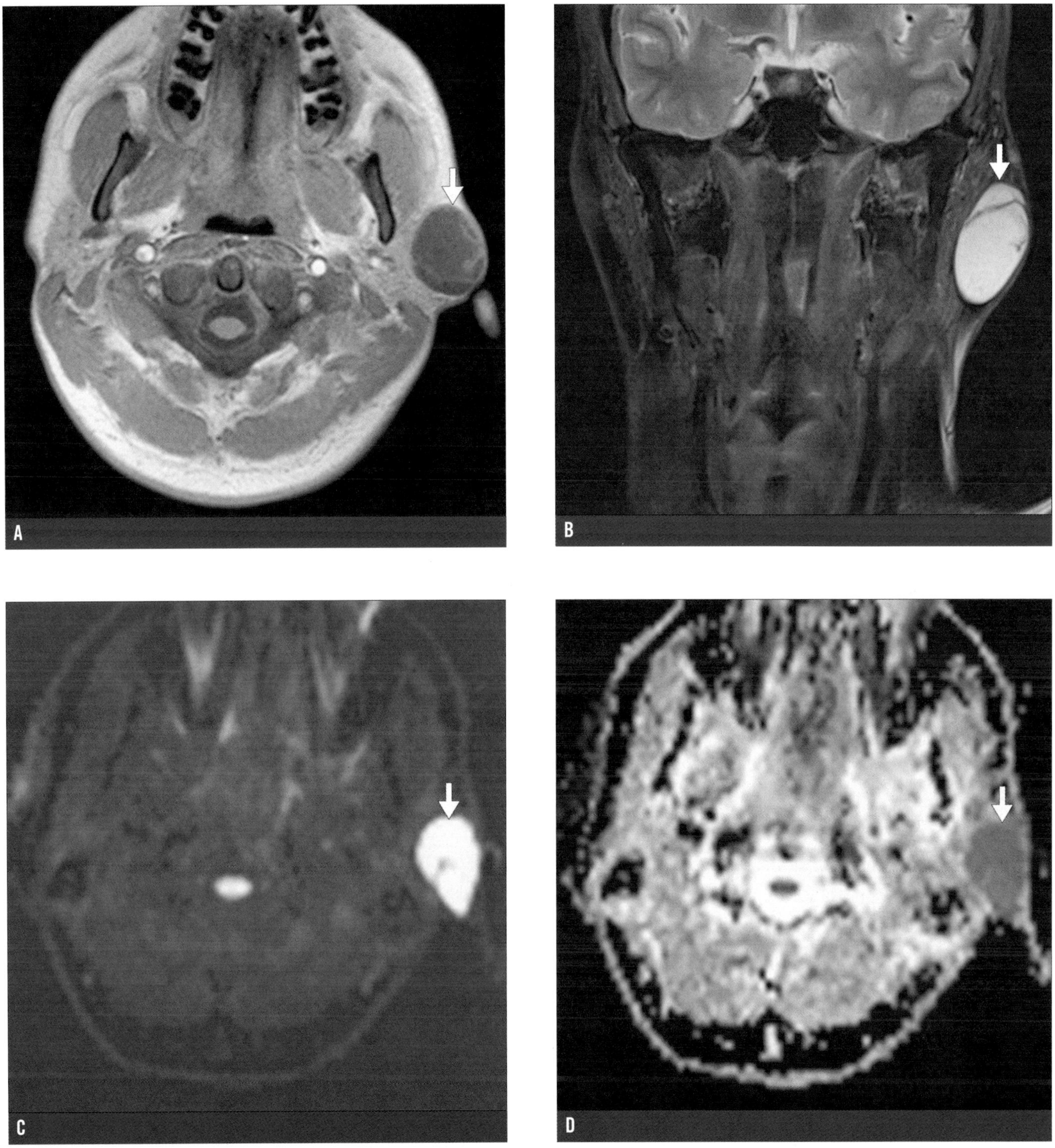

Different patient. Axial T1 (**A**), fat-suppressed coronal T2 (**B**), axial DWI (**C**), and axial ADC map (**D**) MR images demonstrate a T1 hypointense, T2 hyperintense, circumscribed lesion that contains mildly T1 hyperintense and discrete T2 hypointense internal septations as well as diffusely restricts on DWI (arrows, **A**-**D**). The lesion is located immediately deep to the dermis as well as overlies and results in mass effect upon the subjacent left parotid gland. The findings are most compatible with an epidermal inclusion cyst. Several months later, and without a history of interval surgical intervention or trauma, axial T1 (**E**) and fat-suppressed axial T2 (**F**) MR images of the same patient demonstrate a marked decrease in size of the lesion with less mass effect upon the subjacent left parotid gland. Otherwise, the lesion is unchanged in its imaging appearance, including the previously demonstrated internal septations. These findings represent spontaneous rupture of an epidermal inclusion cyst.

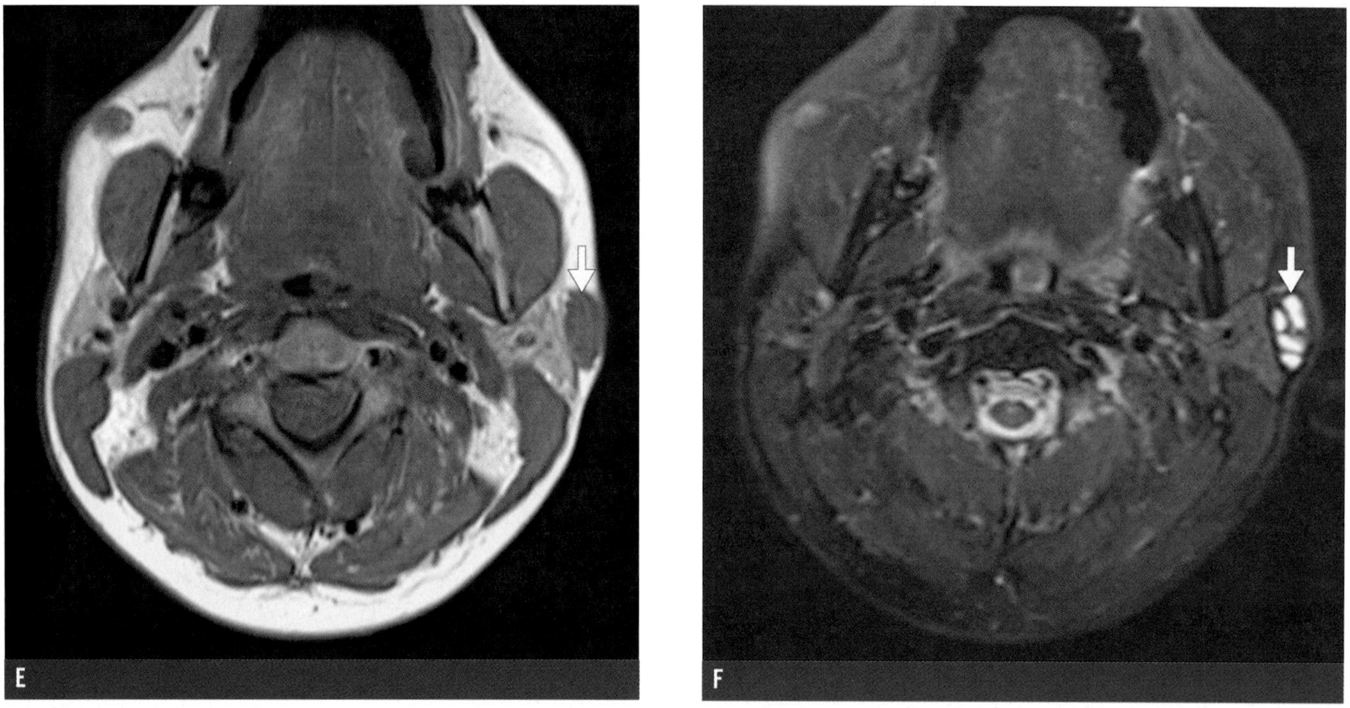

Calcified epidermal inclusion cyst

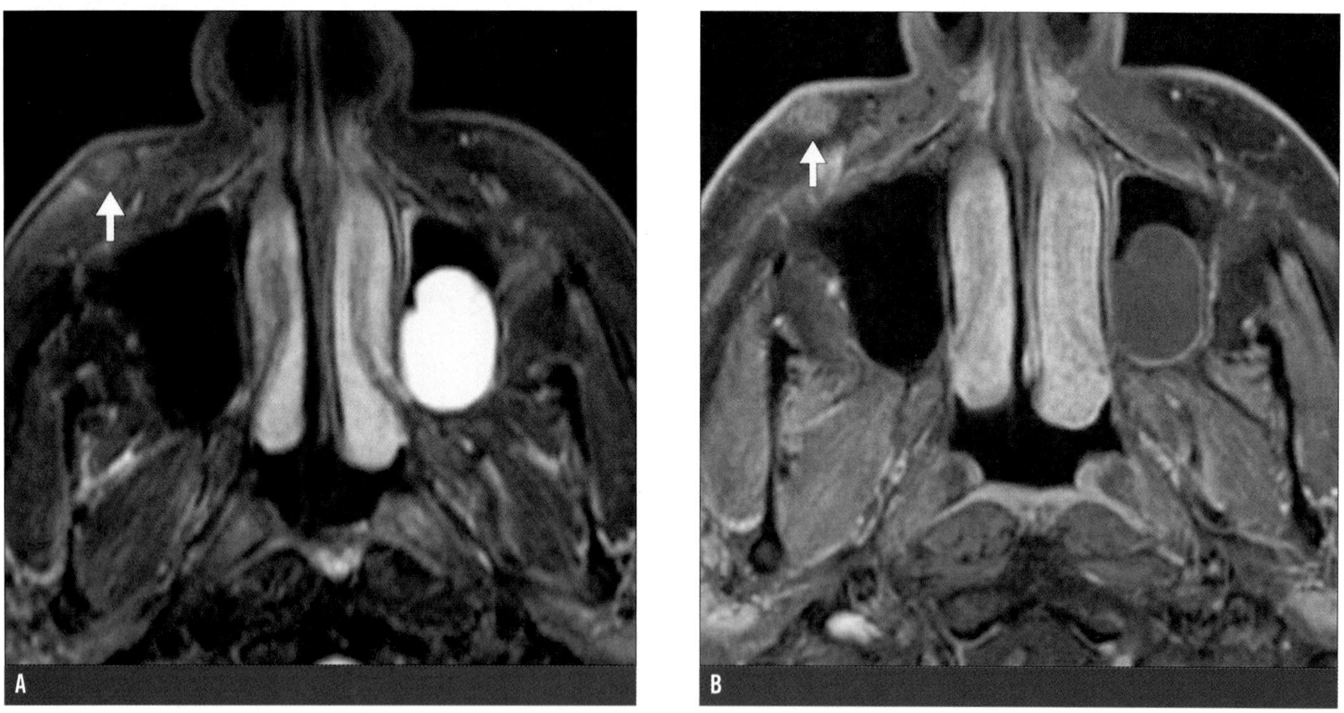

Fat-suppressed axial T2 (**A**) and fat-suppressed contrast-enhanced axial T1 (**B**) MR images demonstrate a T2 hypointense, nonenhancing (relative to unenhanced T1-weighted imaging, not shown) oval lesion in the subcutaneous soft tissues of the right cheek (arrows, **A**, **B**). An unenhanced axial CT image viewed with a bone window (**C**) and a sagittal reformatted CT image viewed with a soft tissue window (**D**) demonstrate the same finding to be diffusely calcified (arrows, **C**, **D**). The imaging characteristics are compatible with a calcified epidermal inclusion cyst.

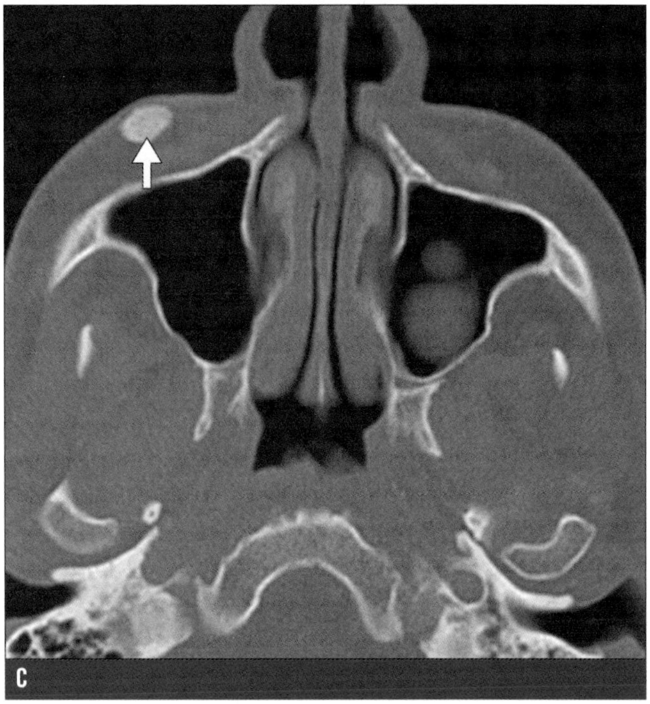

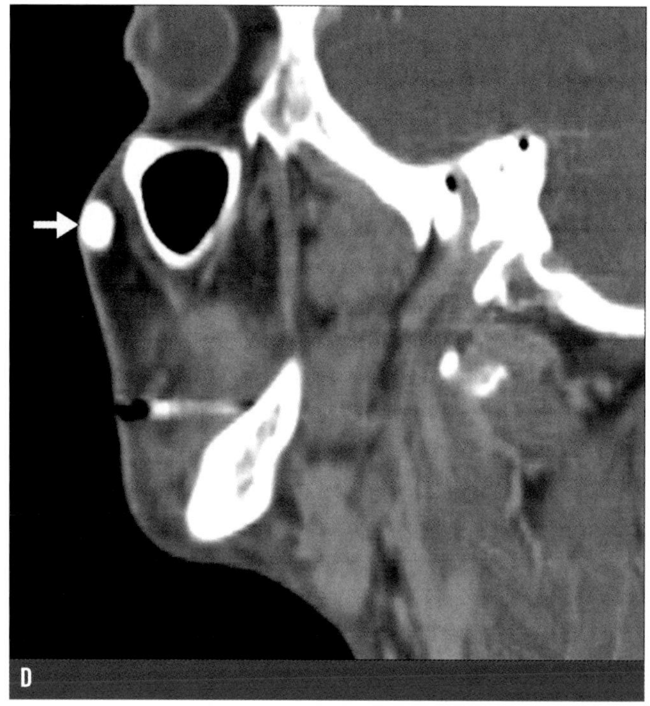

REFERENCE

Kim HK, Kim SM, Lee SH, Racadio JM, Shin MJ. Subcutaneous epidermal inclusion cysts: ultrasound (US) and MR imaging findings. *Skeletal Radiol.* 2011;40(11):1415-1419.

CASE 3 Dermal calcifications

There is scant radiologic literature pertaining to benign skin calcifications apart from the mammography literature, although many of the conclusions made in the mammography literature can be extrapolated to imaging of the skin elsewhere. Incidentally detected small foci (less than 5 mm) of calcium density at the skin surface of the scalp and face are common. Sebaceous glands are abundant in the scalp and face, and dermal calcifications most likely result from calcium formation within obstructed sebaceous glands. The term pseudocalcification is used to describe foreign substances on the skin surface that may mimic calcifications, such as powders, creams, adhesives, or high-density environmental particles.

On CT, dermal calcifications of the face related to obstructed sebaceous glands are identified as punctate, hyperdense foci isolated to the dermis. They may occur anywhere on the face, although they are most commonly located within the dermis of the forehead and cheeks. Unless dermal calcifications are extensive, they are typically occult by MRI.

COMPANION CASES

- **Glass fragments in the face following trauma.** Glass foreign bodies involving the face are common following motor vehicle collisions and industrial accidents. Glass is radiopaque and can be detected on radiography, if large enough in size. However, helical CT is superior to radiographs in its ability to detect glass fragments. Detection of these fragments is dependent on the size as well as the type of glass. As small as 0.5 mm glass fragments can be detected by helical CT. Interestingly, the glass from green and brown beer bottles is often higher in density on CT relative to other types of glass, such as glass from spectacles. With respect to the globe, the detection of foreign bodies can be dependent on location, with one study demonstrating a significantly greater sensitivity in detecting glass in the anterior chamber relative to other portions of the globe, such as along the corneal surface. The detection of glass foreign bodies is significantly less sensitive with MRI when compared to CT or radiography.
- **Shotgun injury to the face.** Bullet injuries to the face often lead to complex facial fractures and extensive soft tissue damage. A shotgun shell contains numerous pellets that can be made from various substances, including lead or composites from steel, tungsten, or bismuth. On CT or radiography, these metallic pellets will appear as numerous, round, metallic foci scattered diffusely in the injured area, with some pellets often fairly remote from the site of impact. Bullets, pellets, and shrapnel frequently contain ferromagnetic materials; therefore, caution should be exercised if an MRI is performed in patients injured with these metals, especially if they are located adjacent to vital structures. MRI is contraindicated if these metallic objects are located on or within the globe.

Dermal calcifications

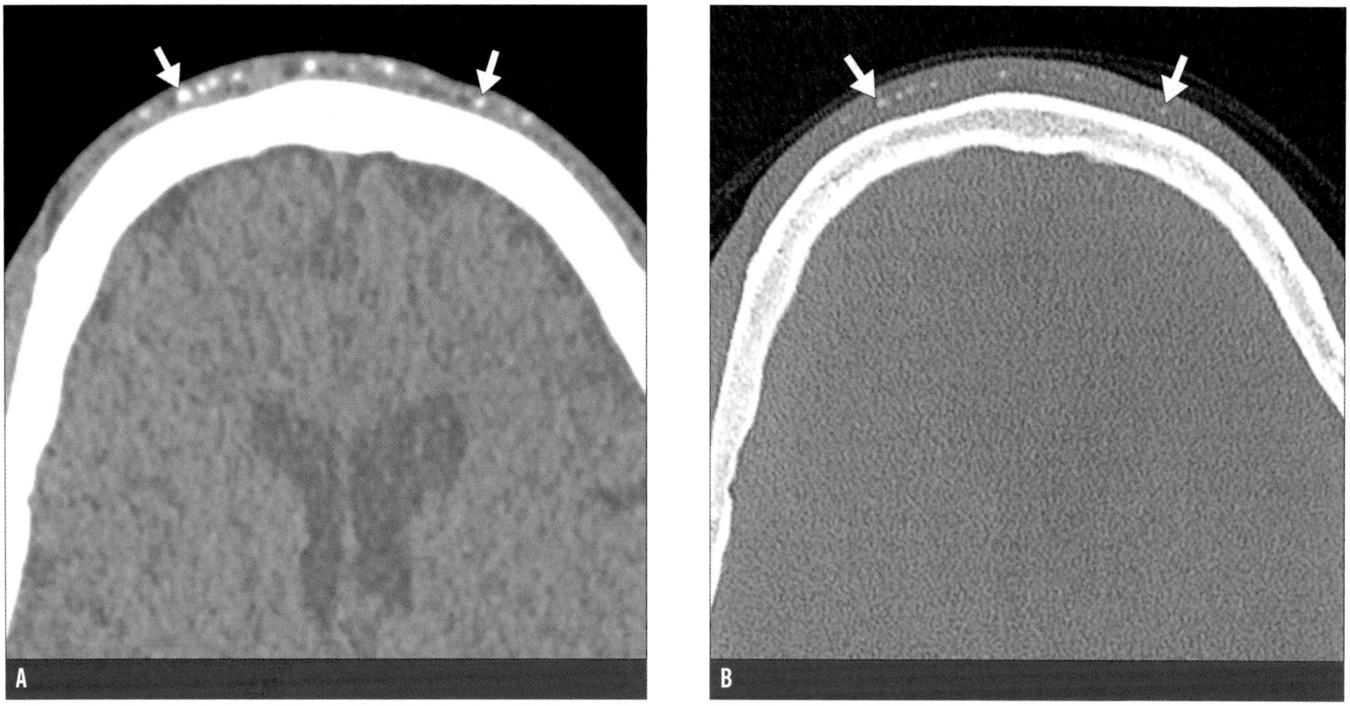

Axial CT images viewed with a soft tissue window (**A**) and bone window (**B**) demonstrate numerous punctate foci of mineralization within the dermis of the forehead, compatible with dermal calcifications. The lack of soft tissue swelling and the location of the calcified foci isolated to the dermis help differentiate this incidental finding from foreign bodies.

Dermal calcifications

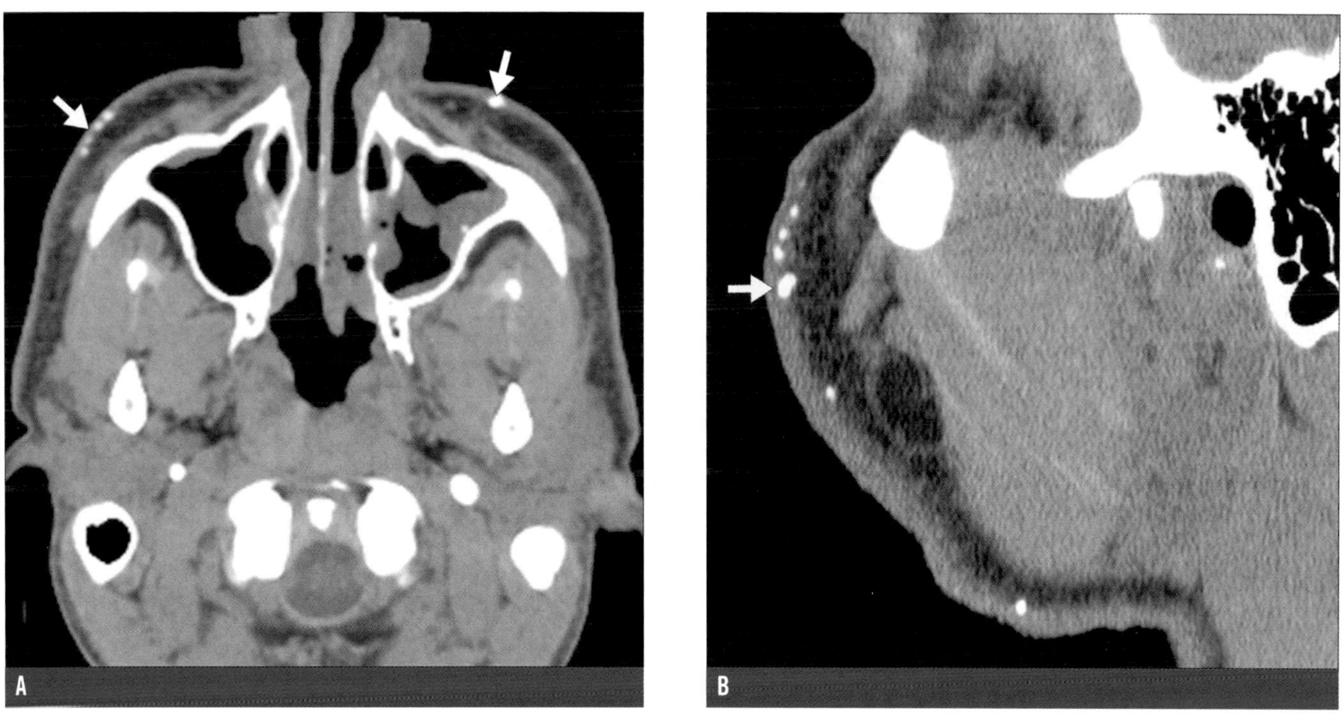

Different patient. Axial (**A**) and sagittal reformatted (**B**) CT images viewed with soft tissue window demonstrate numerous punctate hyperdense foci within the dermis of the cheeks, compatible with incidental dermal calcifications (arrows, **A**, **B**).

Companion case: Glass fragments in the face following trauma

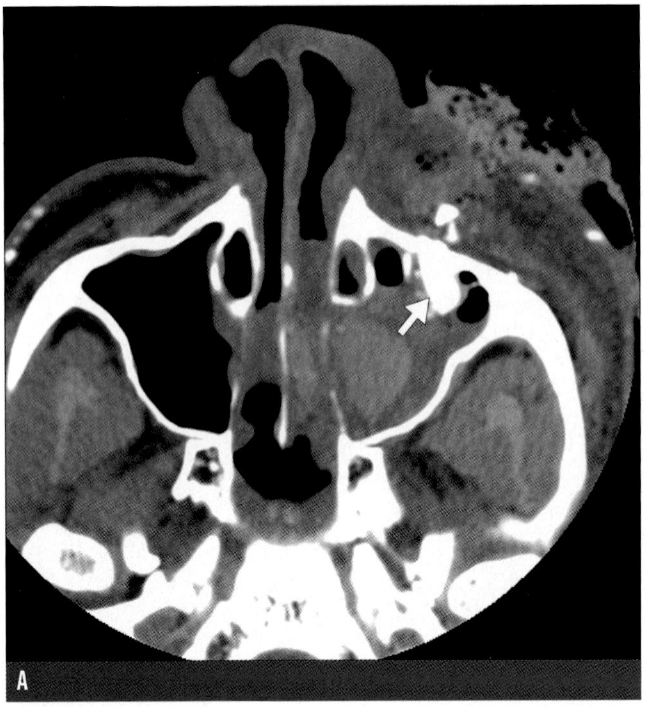

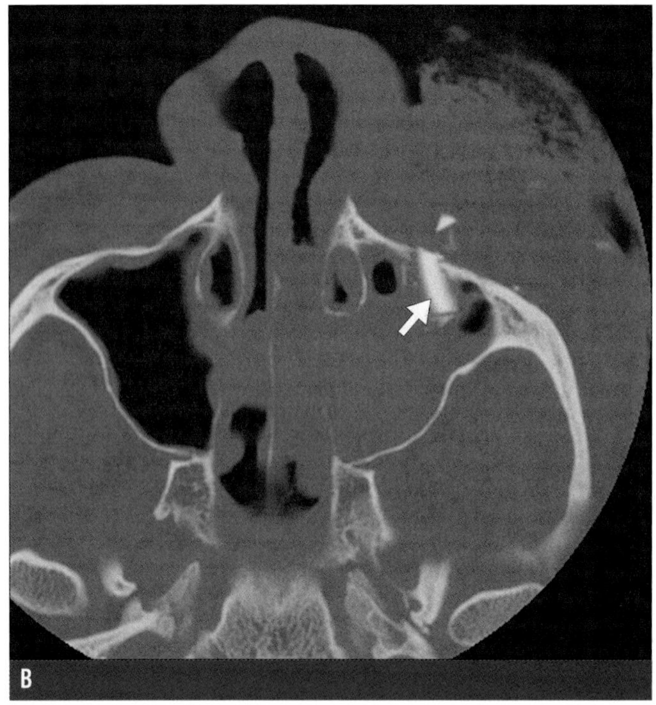

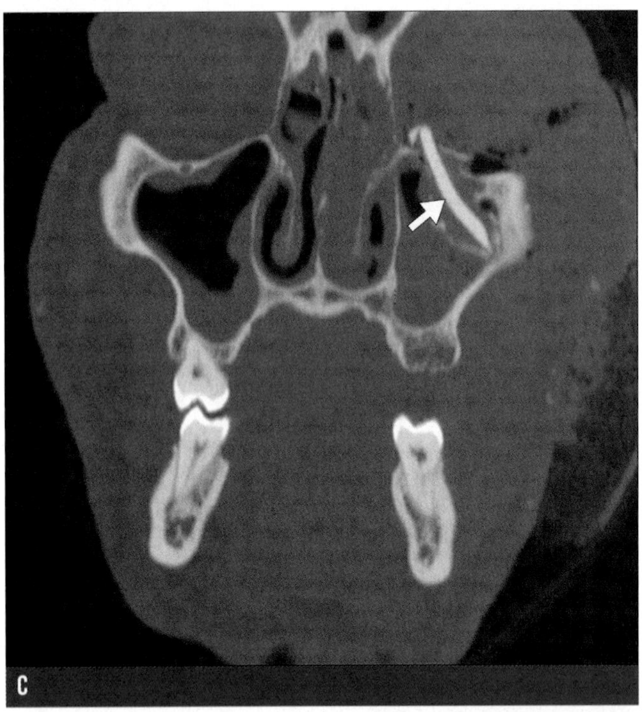

The same patient as in the preceding case immediately following trauma. Axial CT images of the face viewed with a soft tissue window (**A**) and bone window (**B**) as well as a coronal reformatted CT image viewed with a bone window (**C**). These CT images demonstrate extensive left facial swelling and lacerations with several foreign bodies embedded within the left face (glass by history), including a large fragment of glass embedded within the left maxillary sinus and extending into the left orbit (arrows, **A**-**C**). The previously present dermal calcifications in the cheeks are also identified.

Companion case: Glass fragments in the face following trauma

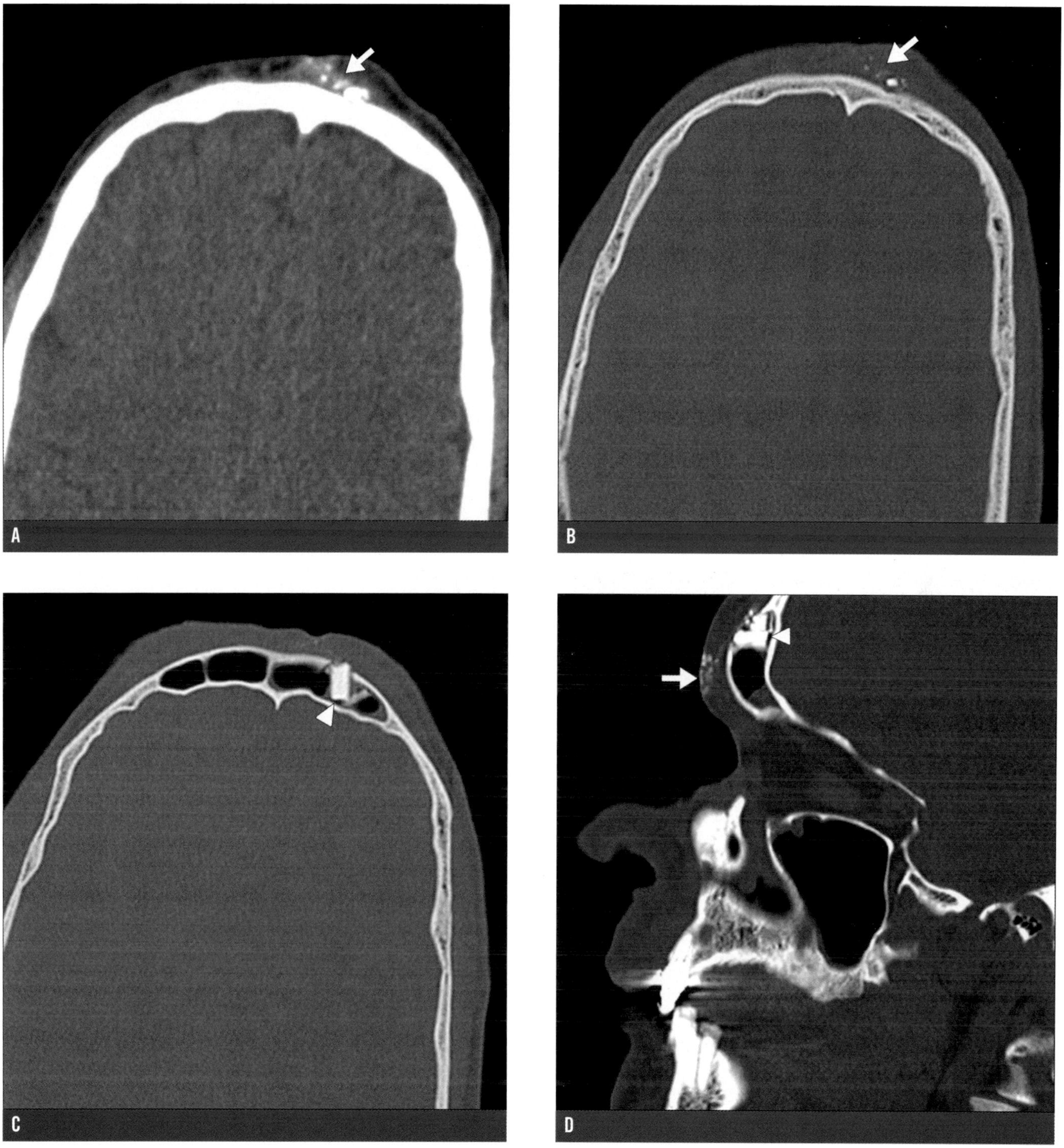

Different patient. Axial CT images viewed with a soft tissue window (**A**) and bone window (**B**, **C**) as well as a sagittal reformatted CT image viewed with a bone window (**D**) obtained from a patient immediately following a motor vehicle collision. The images demonstrate several linearly oriented and punctate foci of increased attenuation that extend into the deep subcutaneous soft tissues of the forehead and are associated with forehead edema (arrows, **A, B, D**). A larger focus of increased attenuation extends through a left frontal sinus outer table fracture and resides within the left frontal sinus lumen (arrowheads, **C**, **D**). These foci of increased attenuation represented glass foreign bodies.

Companion case: Shotgun injury to the face

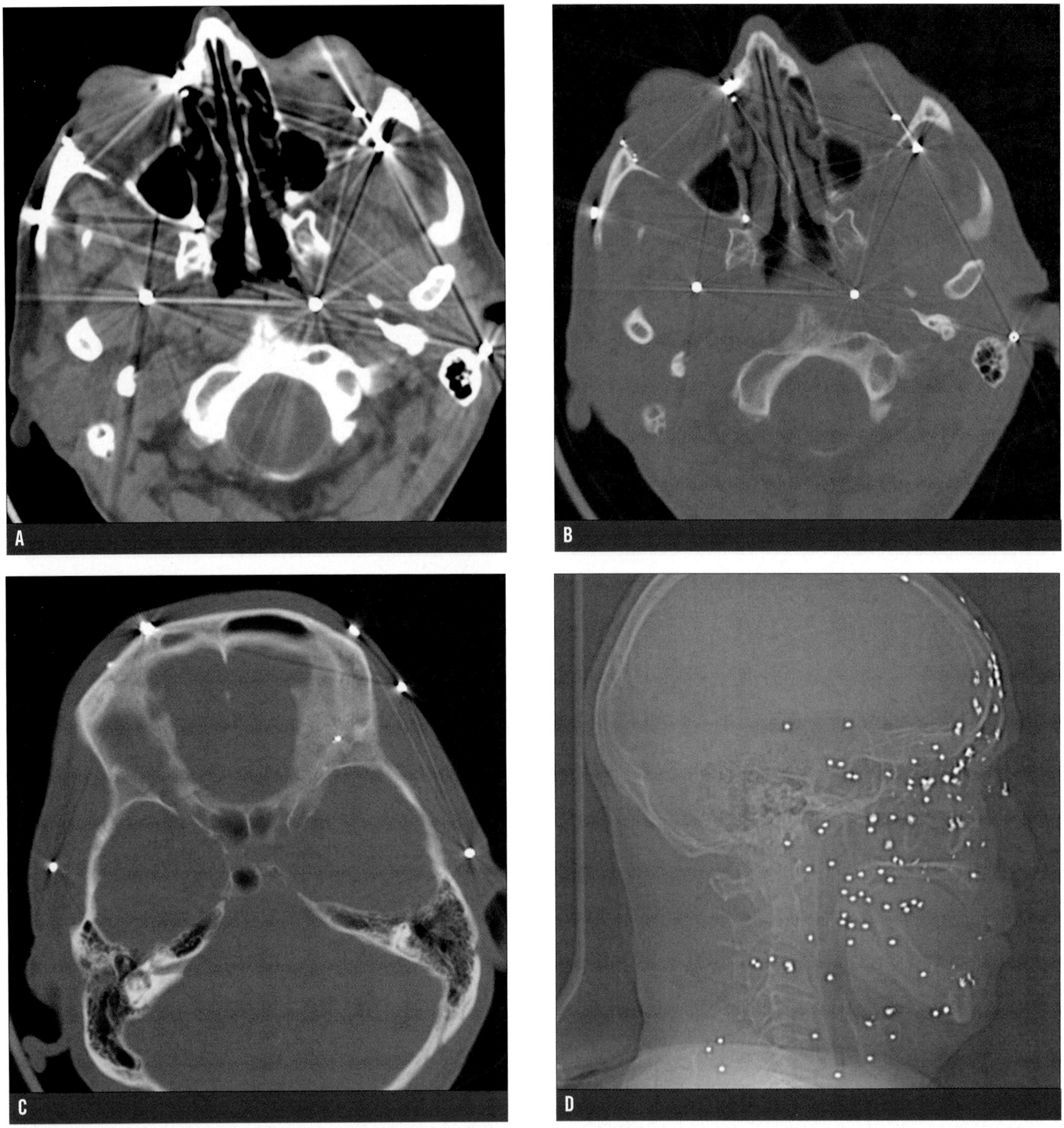

Axial CT images viewed with a soft tissue window (**A**) and bone window (**B**, **C**) demonstrate numerous small metallic fragments associated with streak artifact located within the superficial and deep soft tissues of the face and infratemporal fossa, compatible with a shotgun injury to the face. A sagittal scout image from the same study (**D**) best demonstrates the extensive nature of the injury.

REFERENCES

Ayaviri NAM, et al. Isolated primary osteoma cutis of the head: case report. *Can J Plast Surg.* 2006;14(1):33-36.

Basler RSW, Watters JH, Taylor WB. Calcifying acne lesions. *Int J Dermatol.* 1977;16(9):755-758.

Gor DM, Kirsch CF, Leen J, Turbin R, Von Hagen S. Radiologic differentiation of intraocular glass: evaluation of imaging techniques, glass types, size, and effect of intraocular hemorrhage. *AJR Am J Roentgenol.* 2001;177:1199-1203.

Hunter TB, Talijanovic MS. Foreign bodies. *Radiographics.* 2003;23:731-757.

Picca DA, Shaw de Paredes E. Calcification in the breast: A radiologic perspective. *Appl Radiol.* 2003;32(9):29-37.

CASE 4 Incomplete MRI fat suppression simulating a facial cellulitis

Fat, along with water and gadolinium, is an essential source of signal on MR imaging. Fat is hyperintense on both T1- and T2-weighted sequences, unless fat suppression (FS) techniques are applied. T2-weighted FS sequences are extremely useful for highlighting edema in bones and soft tissues. Contrast-enhanced T1-weighted imaging with FS is ideal for identifying enhancing lesions while suppressing potentially confounding soft tissue fat and marrow fat.

Multiple techniques to subtract fat signal are available. Traditional spin-echo-based FS sequences utilize a presaturation pulse at a frequency specific to fat. This technique allows only signal from fat to be eliminated. It can be applied to T1- and T2-weighted sequences with excellent signal preservation of nonfat-containing tissues. The major disadvantage of this technique is that large areas of fat may not suppress if their precessional frequency is shifted by a heterogeneous magnetic field. Metal, such as from prior spinal surgery or dental amalgam, will cause pronounced field heterogeneity and will often result in incomplete FS. Other causes of poor FS include poor MR magnet shimming and disparate interfaces such as bone-air. In some instances, a large enough frequency shift may occur such that water, instead of fat, is suppressed in some areas.

Short T1 (or short tau) inversion recovery (STIR) is an alternative technique that allows for subtraction of fat signal. This inversion recovery sequence is timed so that the rephasing pulse occurs when fat signal returns to baseline (ie, its null point). In addition to fat, water signal within the fat is suppressed, often resulting in improved tumor conspicuity. However, if fat is intermixed within tumor such that its relaxation time shifts, it will not fully suppress, potentially resulting in underestimation of tumoral fat. Furthermore, because of the timing of the pulse, some signal is lost from all tissues. This results in decreased signal-to-noise relative to spin-echo-based FS sequences. However, STIR is not as affected by field heterogeneities compared to conventional spin-echo-based FS sequences. Thus, STIR is more efficient at suppressing fat than conventional spin-echo-based FS sequences in the presence of metal or other causes of field heterogeneity.

Knowledge of the causes of incomplete fat suppression and their appearance on MRI is essential in order to avoid image misinterpretation. Incomplete fat suppression should be suspected when there are geographic areas of increased signal that cross tissue planes. Importantly, if there is a true lesion on a contrast enhanced T1-weighted or on a T2-weighted FS sequence, then the lesion will usually be identified on the precontrast T1-weighted non-FS sequence. Conversely, if a finding is not identified on the precontrast T1-weighted non-FS sequence, then artifact accounting for the finding on a FS sequence should be considered.

COMPANION CASES

- **Facial cellulitis.** Cellulitis is a superficial soft tissue infection caused by bacteria invading the skin, often occurring via a skin defect. A patient with cellulitis will present with erythema, pain, and swelling of the affected area. On CT, the skin will be frequently thickened and the subjacent subcutaneous fat will be inflamed. MRI may delineate the extent of the infection to a better advantage relative to CT, but MRI is usually reserved to exclude complications, such as abscess formation. On MRI, the skin will be also be thickened and the inflamed tissue will be T1 hypointense, T2 hyperintense, and enhance.
- **Port-wine stain.** A port-wine stain (PWS) is considered by some authors to be one of the vascular malformations of the head and neck, the others being arteriovenous malformation (AVM), venous malformation, and lymphatic malformation. A PWS is a congenital abnormal ectasia of the superficial cutaneous vascular plexus and is a lesion which has slow vascular flow. This lesion is characterized by a geographic, reddish skin lesion (hence the term "port wine") and most commonly affects the head and neck. More than 40% of PWSs are confined to the cutaneous distribution of the cranial nerve V. Sturge-Weber and Klippel-Trenaunay-Weber syndrome are commonly associated with a PWS. In contrast to capillary hemangiomas, a PWS does not involute with time but may in fact progress and develop nodularity, increasing the risk of spontaneous bleeding. While there are many treatment options which have varying success, the current treatment of choice for a PWS is laser photocoagulation.

  There is a paucity of literature describing the MRI appearance of a PWS. However, it stands to reason that the increased vascularity of the lesion may be detectable by MRI. In the case presented, the patient's known PWS was characterized by skin thickening, T2 hyperintense signal, and enhancement.

Incomplete MRI fat suppression simulating a facial cellulitis

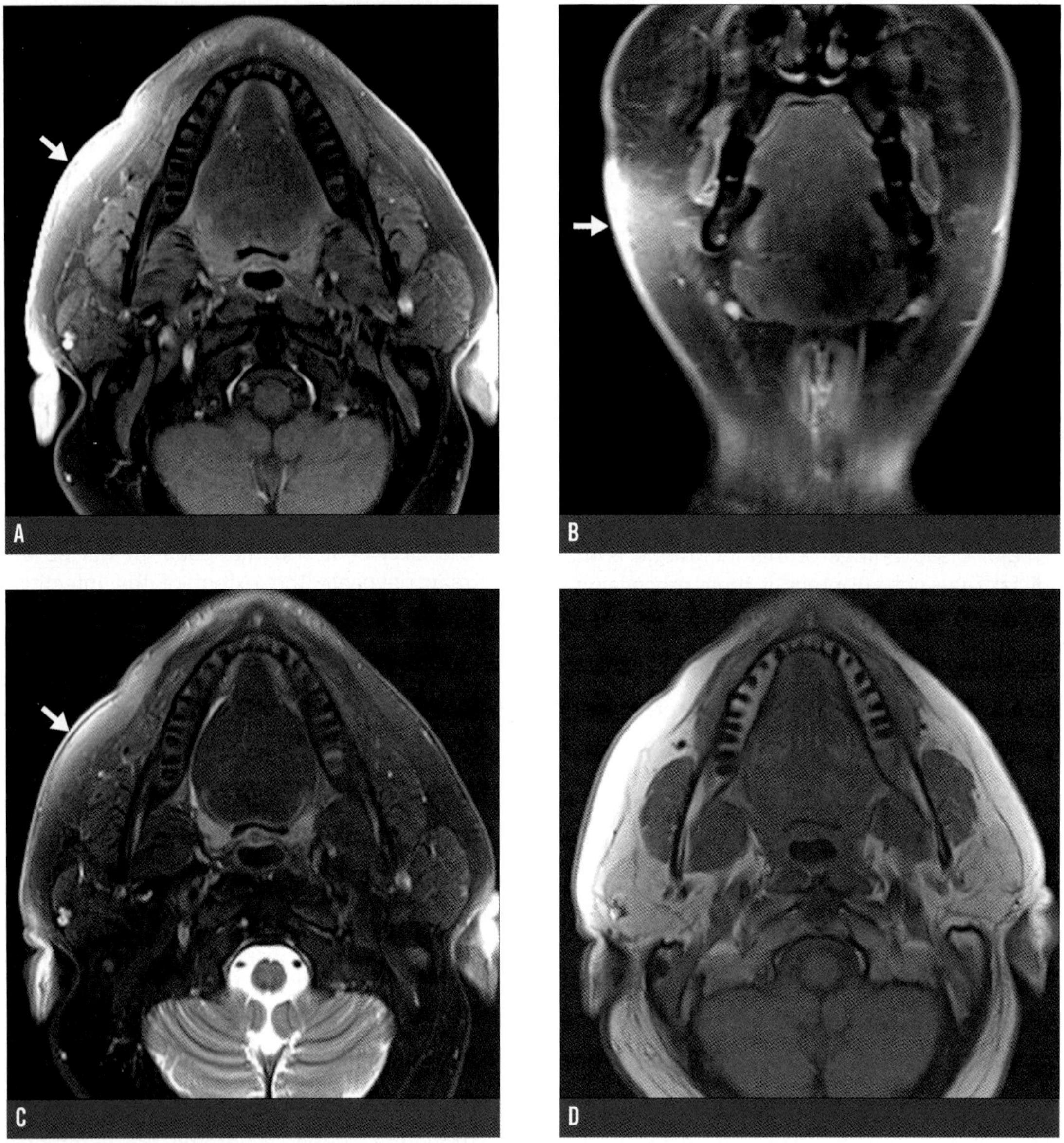

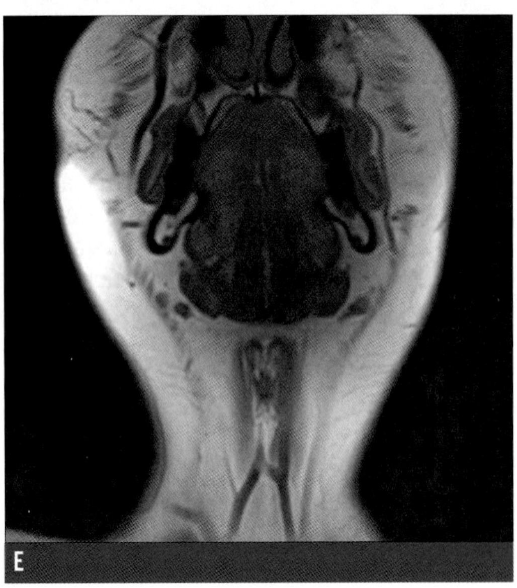

Postcontrast fat-suppressed axial T1 (**A**), postcontrast fat-suppressed coronal T1 (**B**), and fat-suppressed axial T2 (**C**) MR images demonstrate elevated signal along the right face soft tissues simulating abnormal enhancement (arrows, **A**, **B**) and edema (arrow, **C**). Axial T1 (**D**) and coronal T1 (**E**) MR images from the same study do not demonstrate evidence of a lesion or edema of the right face soft tissues. The findings on images **A-C** represent MRI field heterogeneity resulting in incomplete fat suppression. If abnormal signal is detected on the fat-suppressed sequences, then a true abnormality is usually identified on the nonfat-suppressed T1-weighted images.

Incomplete MRI fat suppression simulating a facial cellulitis

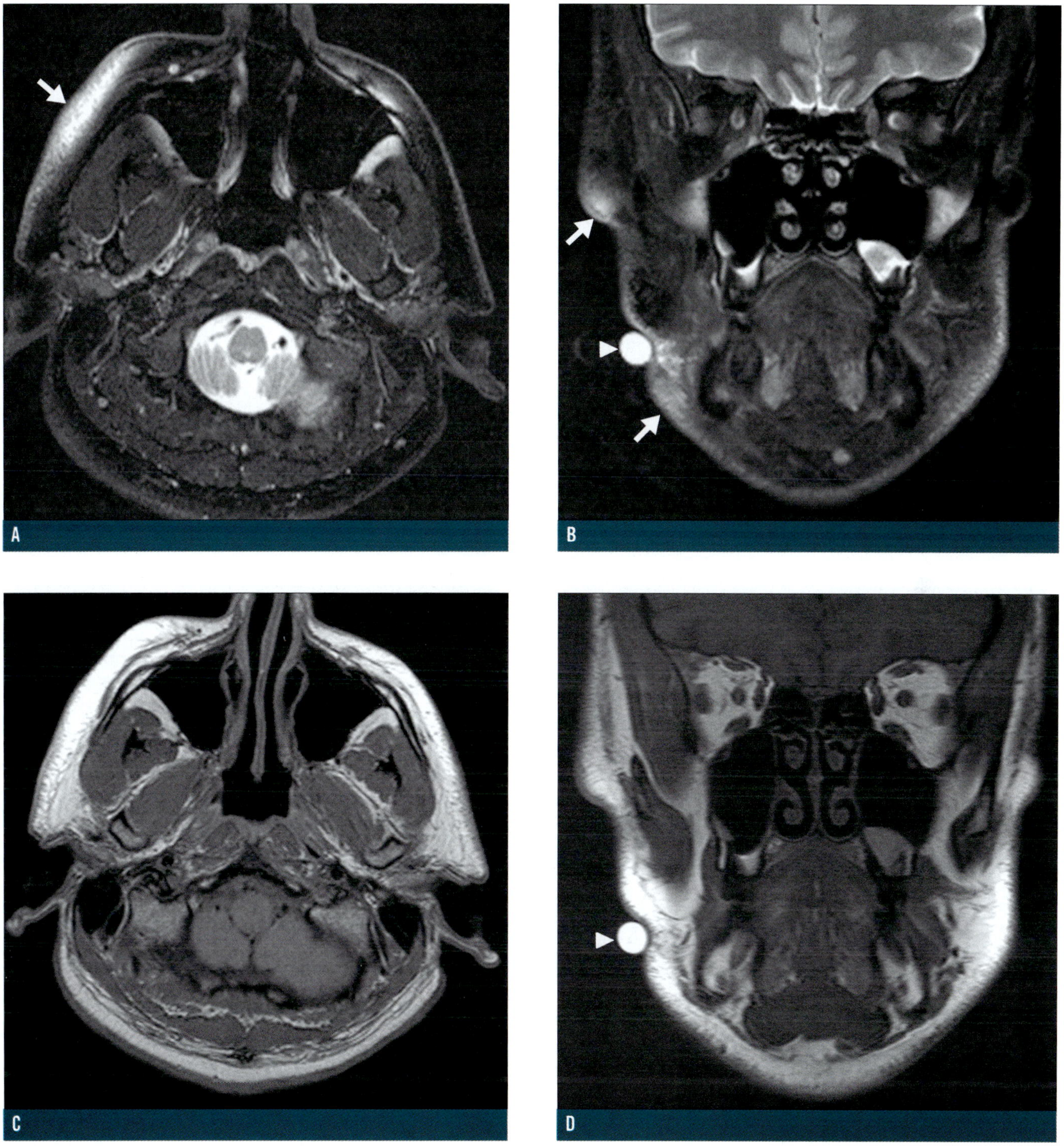

Different patient. Fat-suppressed axial T2 (**A**) and fat-suppressed coronal T2 (**B**) MR images demonstrate elevated T2 signal along the right aspect of the face (arrows, **A, B**). Axial T1 (**C**) and coronal T1 (**D**) MR images do not demonstrate signal abnormality or evidence of soft tissue edema, effectively excluding a significant abnormality along the right aspect of the face. A vitamin E capsule denotes the clinical area of concern (arrowheads, **B, D**).

Companion case: Facial cellulitis

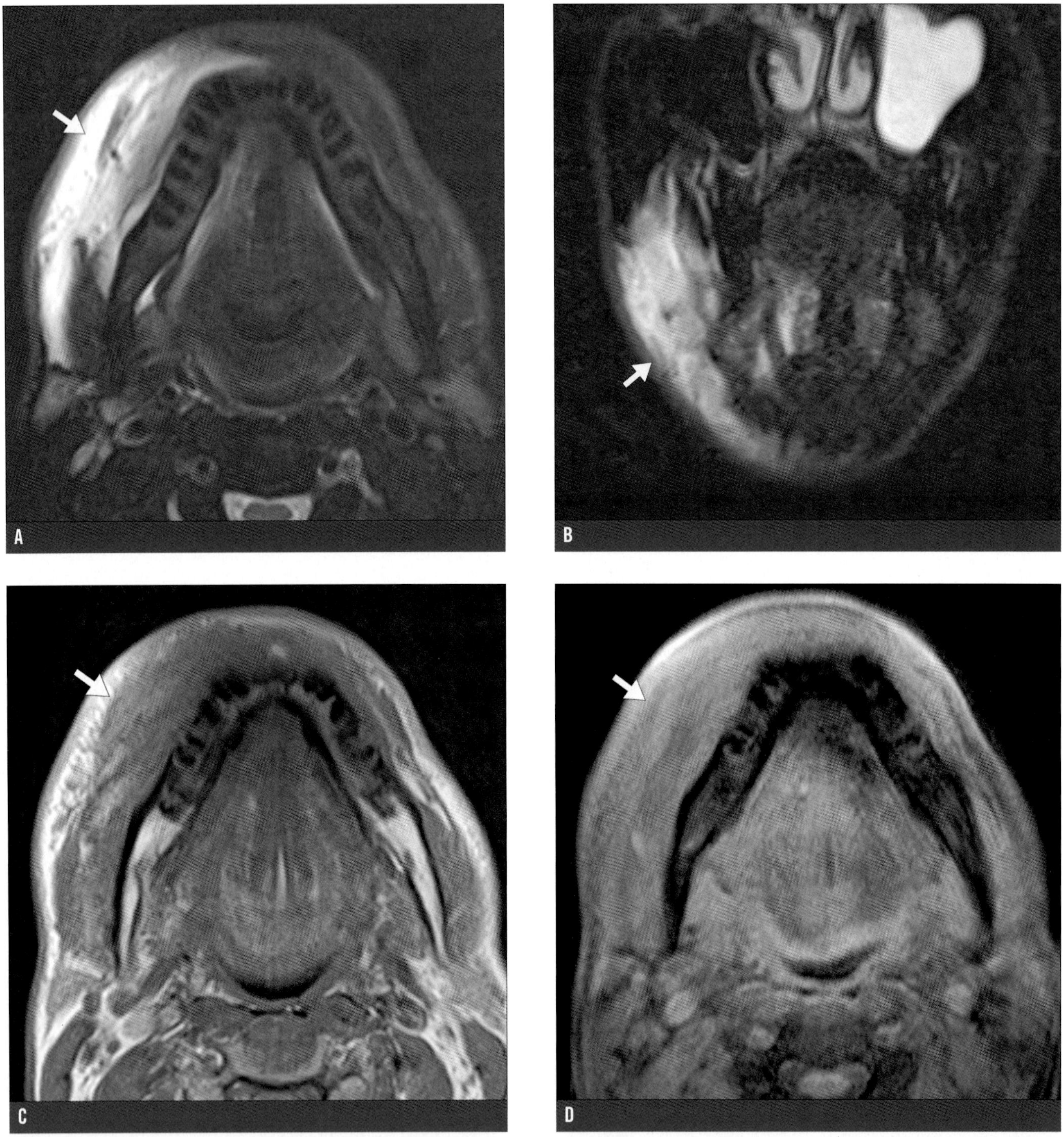

Fat-suppressed axial T2 (**A**) and fat-suppressed coronal T2 (**B**) MR images demonstrate elevated T2 signal with asymmetric thickening of the right facial soft tissues relative to the left (arrows, **A**, **B**). An axial T1-weighted MR image (**C**) demonstrates abnormal, heterogeneous T1 signal and soft tissue thickening corresponding to the abnormalities on images **A** and **B** (arrow, **C**). A fat-suppressed contrast-enhanced axial T1-weighted MR image (**D**) demonstrates abnormal enhancement and also asymmetric soft tissue thickening of the right facial soft tissues (arrow, **D**). This patient had a dental abscess (not shown) that resulted in these findings.

Companion case: Port-wine stain

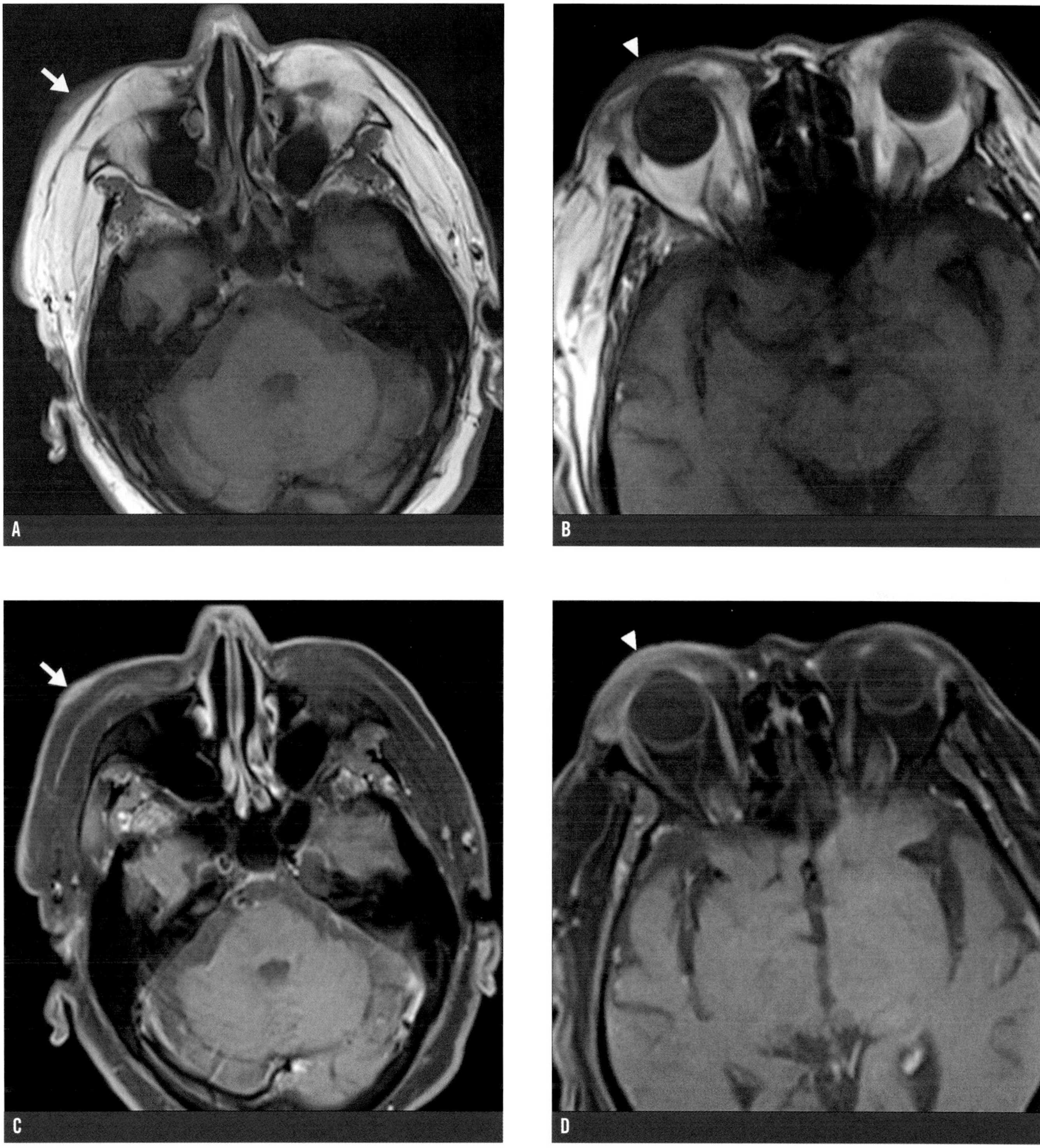

Axial T1 (**A**, **B**), contrast-enhanced axial T1 with fat suppression (**C**, **D**), and coronal T2 with fat suppression (**E**, **F**) MR images demonstrate subtle enhancement and T2 prolongation involving the right cheek (arrows, **A**, **C**, **E**, **F**) and right periorbital soft tissues (arrowheads, **B**, **D**, **E**) in this patient with a known right face port-wine stain.

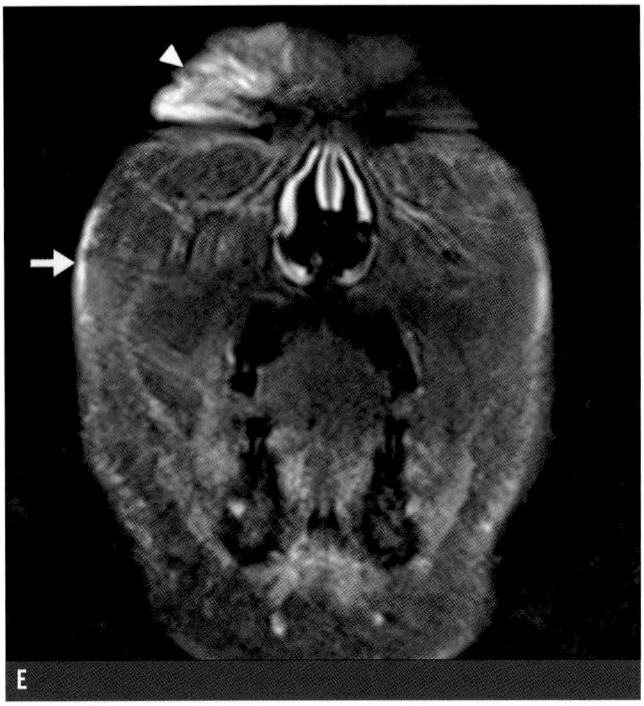

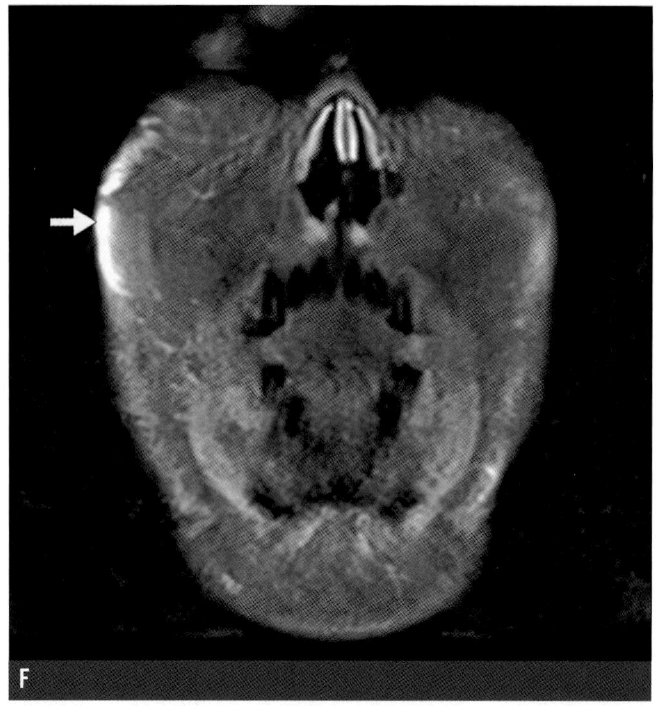

REFERENCES

Delfaut EM, et al. Fat suppression in MR imaging: techniques and pitfalls. *Radiographics.* 1999;19:373-382.

Bitar R, et al. MR pulse sequences: what every radiologist wants to know but is afraid to ask. *Radiographics.* 2006;26(2):513–537.

Minkis K, Geronemus RG, Hale EK. Port wine stain progression: a potential consequence of delayed and inadequate treatment? *Lasers Surg Med.* 2009;41(6):423-426.

Taber KH, et al. Pitfalls and artifacts encountered in clinical MR imaging of the spine. *Radiographics.* 1998;18(6):1499-1521.

Turecki MB, et al. Imaging of musculoskeletal soft tissue infections. *Skeletal Radiol.* 2010;39:957-971.

CASE 5 Mimetic muscle atrophy

The muscles of facial expression, also termed the mimetic muscles, are innervated by CN VII. There are multiple muscles of facial expression and include: the frontal belly of the occipitofrontalis, procerus, depressor supercilii, corrugator supercilii, orbicularis oculi, nasalis, levator labii superioris alaeque nasi, depressor septi nasi, nasalis, zygomaticus major and minor, levator labii superioris, buccinator, risorius, orbicularis oris, levator anguli oris, depressor anguli oris, depressor labii inferioris, mentalis, and the platysma.

The majority of the facial muscles have an osseous origin and a dermal or subcutaneous insertion. The SMAS, or superficial muscular aponeurotic system, is contiguous with the temporoparietal as well as the parotid fascia and connects the facial muscles to the overlying dermis and subcutaneous soft tissues. It is this facial muscle attachment to the SMAS that allows for facial expressions. This anatomic arrangement is unique compared to the rest of the body. Elsewhere in the body, the subcutaneous tissues and skin are not attached to the underlying musculature but instead are separated from the musculature by an investing layer of fascia. On imaging, the SMAS appears as a thin curvilinear structure in the subcutaneous fat of the face.

Many of the facial muscles lie in close proximity and are difficult to delineate on imaging. In addition, they are often oriented oblique to the plane of imaging and are small in caliber. However, many muscles of facial expression can be identified by CT and MR imaging, including the frontal belly of the occipitofrontalis, orbicularis oculi, zygomaticus major, buccinator, orbicularis oris, and the platysma muscle, to name a few.

After exiting the stylomastoid foramen, the facial nerve divides into multiple branches to innervate the muscles of facial expression. Some of the major facial nerve branches include the temporal, zygomatic, buccal, mandibular, cervical, and posterior auricular nerves.

Denervation atrophy of the mimetic muscles usually occurs following permanent facial nerve injury, such as following trauma or surgery that transects the nerve. An atypical Bell palsy or perineural spread of tumor can also result in chronic facial nerve injury and subsequent mimetic muscle denervation atrophy. Both CT and MRI are able to demonstrate chronic mimetic muscle denervation atrophy, which manifests as asymmetric volume loss of the affected muscles.

COMPANION CASES

- **Parry-Romberg syndrome.** Also known as progressive hemifacial atrophy, Parry-Romberg syndrome (PRS) is a rare disorder of unknown etiology that is characterized by progressive, unilateral facial atrophy that affects the skin, subcutaneous tissues, muscles, and occasionally the underlying bone and cartilage. There is unilateral facial deformity and shrinkage, with deviation of the nose and mouth toward the affected side. There are numerous systemic manifestations that have been associated with PRS, including neurologic (seizures, migraines, trigeminal neuralgia, ipsilateral brain atrophy, ipsilateral white matter abnormality on MRI), ophthalmologic (ipsilateral enophthalmos, glaucoma, uveitis), and oral abnormalities (ipsilateral hemitongue atrophy, orthodontic abnormalities). PRS typically begins in the first decade of life and slowly progresses for 2 to 20 years before stabilizing. While there is no consensus with respect to the etiology of PRS, some consider it in the spectrum of localized scleroderma.

  PRS shares similar features with hemifacial microsomia, although the latter is a congenital abnormality and essentially nonprogressive. PRS can simulate CN V, V3 denervation atrophy, although with CN V, V3 denervation atrophy, all the muscles of mastication on the affected side are typically abnormal, whereas PRS is generally a more localized phenomenon. In addition, the skin and subcutaneous tissues are atrophic with PRS, a finding that is not usually present with CN V, V3 denervation atrophy.
- **CN V, V3 denervation atrophy.** The V3 (mandibular) division of CN V innervates the muscles of mastication. V3 denervation atrophy occurs when there is injury along the course of the V3 division of CN V, involving the Meckel cave, or when a lesion involves the brainstem at the level of the CN V nuclei.

  While CT can detect chronic denervation, MRI is superior at demonstrating the evolutionary changes of denervation atrophy, from acute to chronic. See Chapter 7 for further description of CN V, V3 denervation atrophy.

Mimetic muscle atrophy

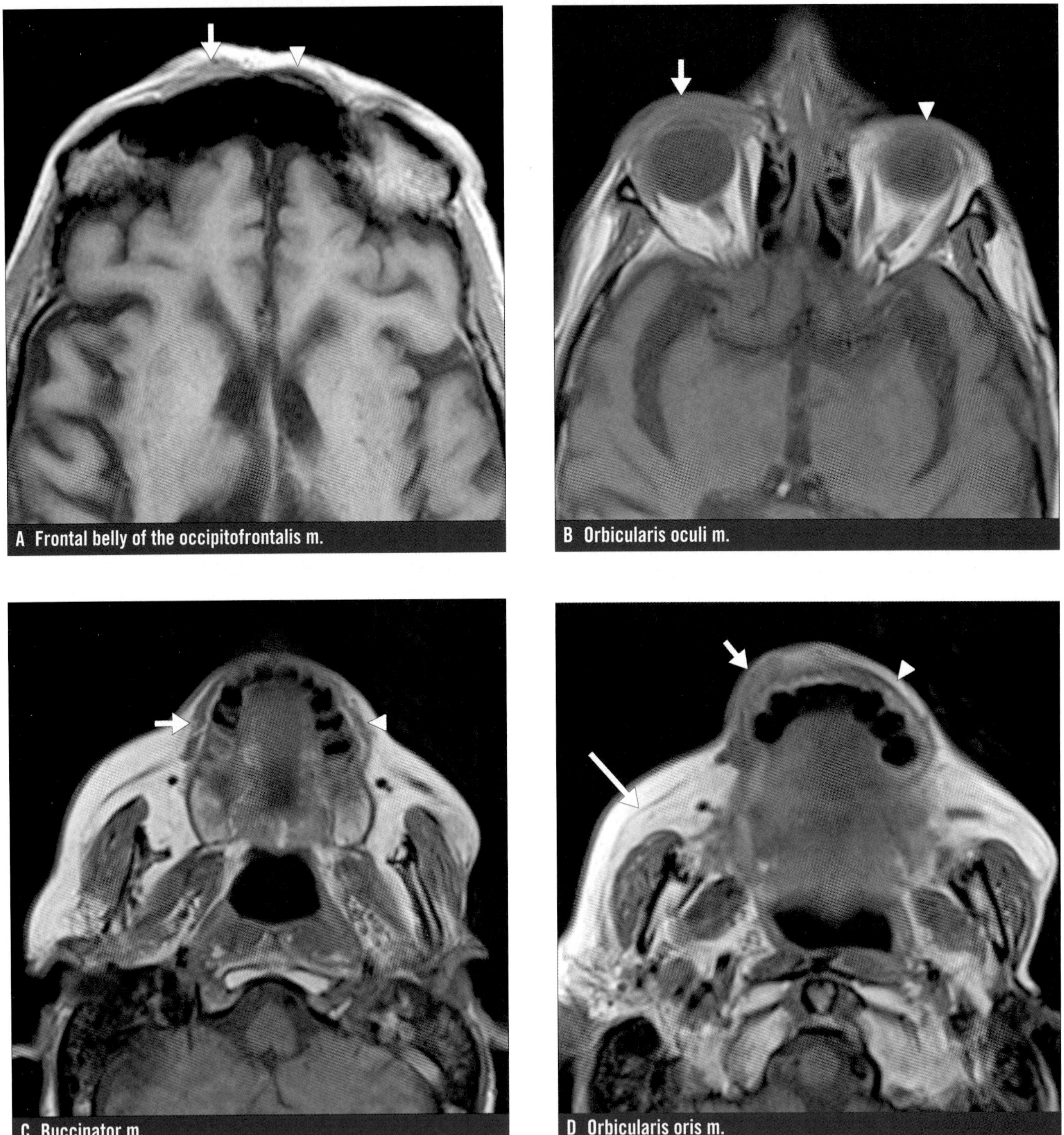

Several axial T1 (**A**-**F**) and coronal T1 (**G**-**I**) MR images through the face demonstrate left mimetic muscle atrophy in a patient with chronic left facial nerve injury. The arrowheads denote the atrophic left mimetic muscle and the short arrows denote their normal-sized counterpart on the right. The long arrow on image **D** denotes a portion of the SMAS.

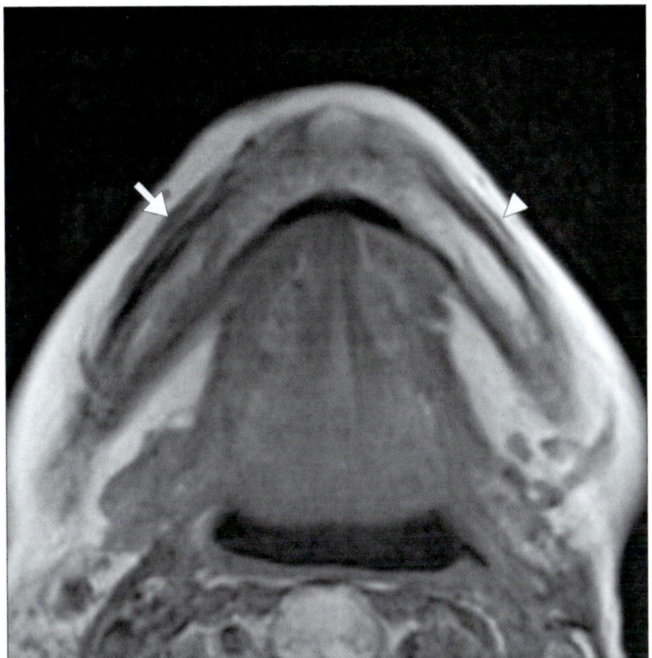

E Depressor anguli oris m.

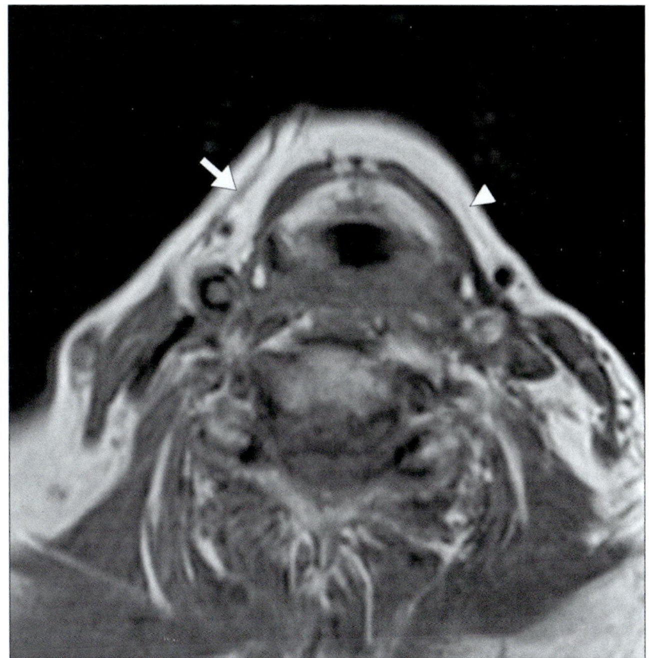

F Platysma m.

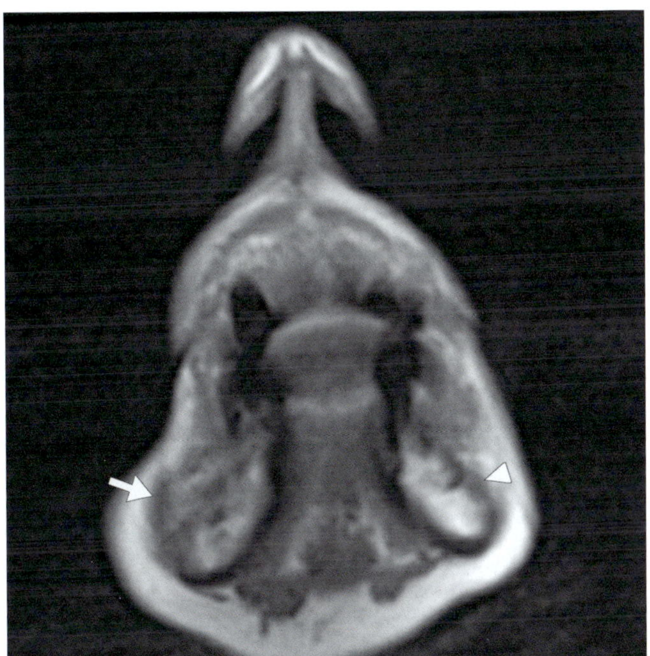

G Depressor anguli oris m.

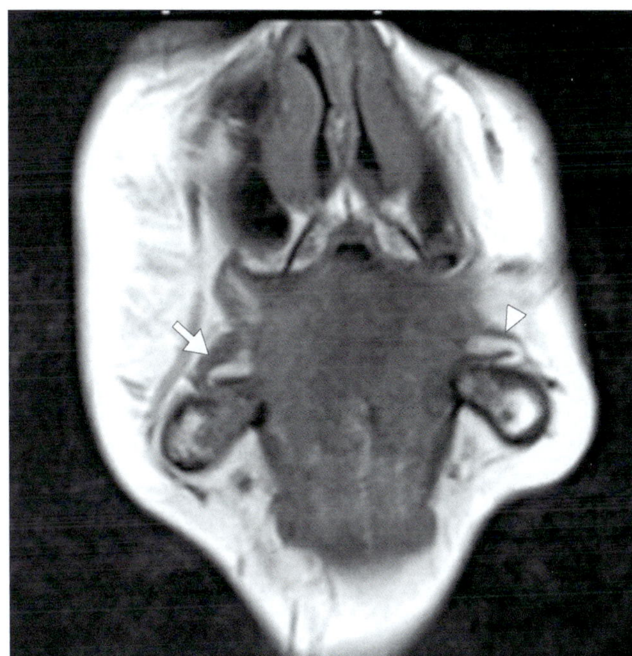

H Buccinator m.

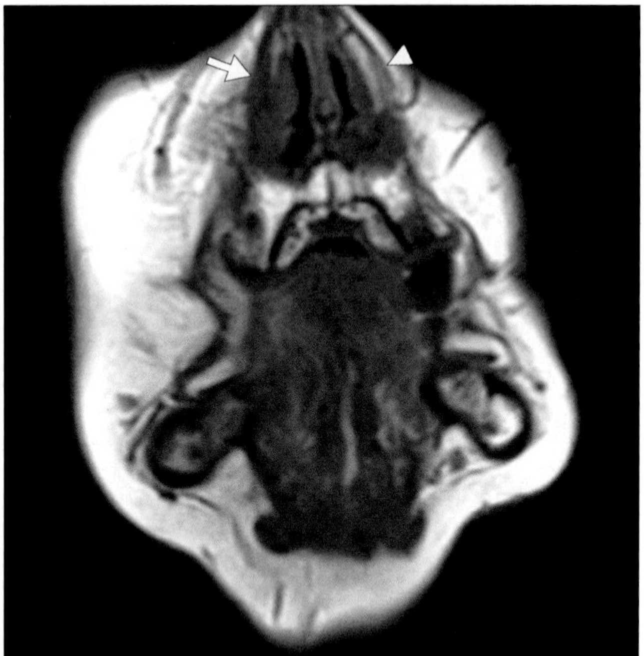

I Levator labii superioris alaeque nasi m.

Companion case: Parry-Romberg syndrome

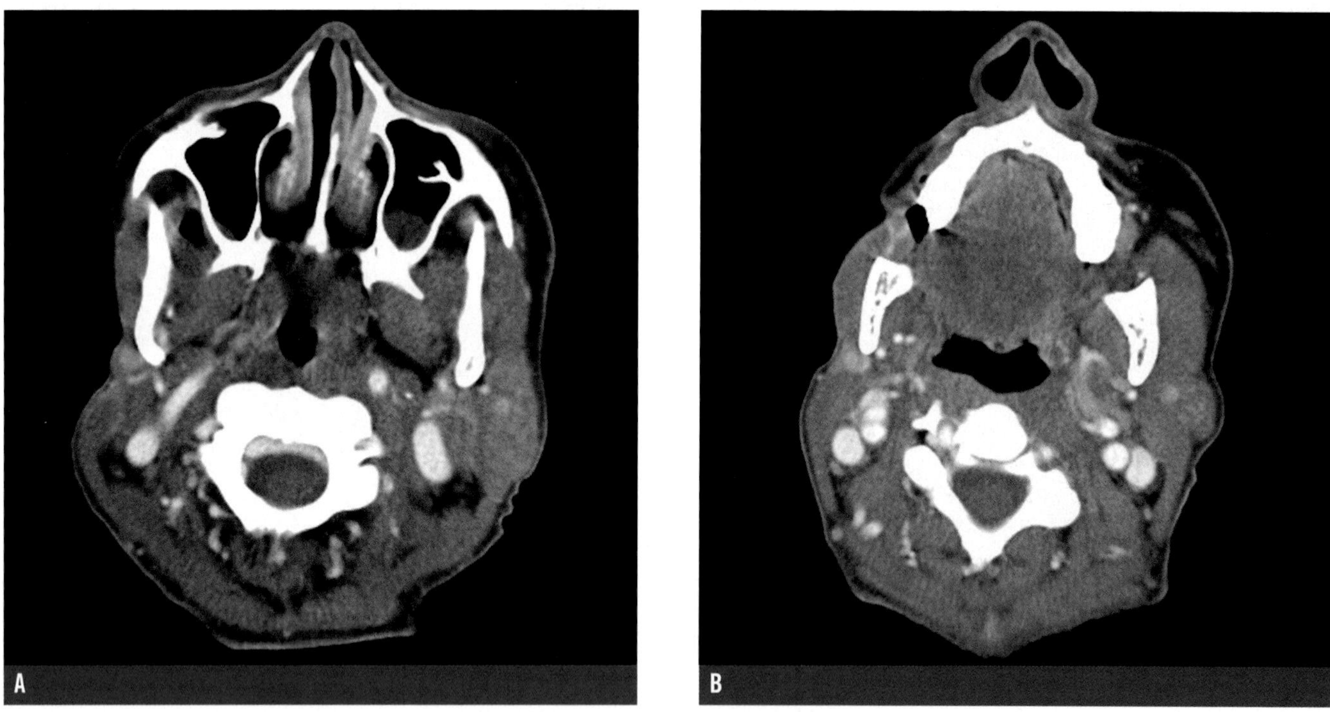

Axial (**A**, **B**) and coronal reformatted (**C**) contrast-enhanced CT images demonstrate pronounced atrophy of the right face, in particular the skin, subcutaneous tissues, and masseter muscle. This patient was diagnosed with Parry-Romberg syndrome approximately 20 years prior to this study.

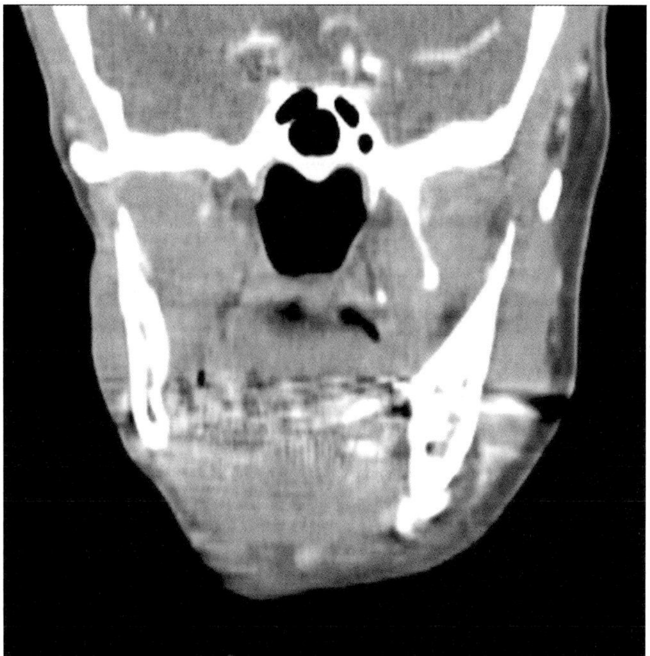

C

Companion case: CN V, V3 denervation atrophy

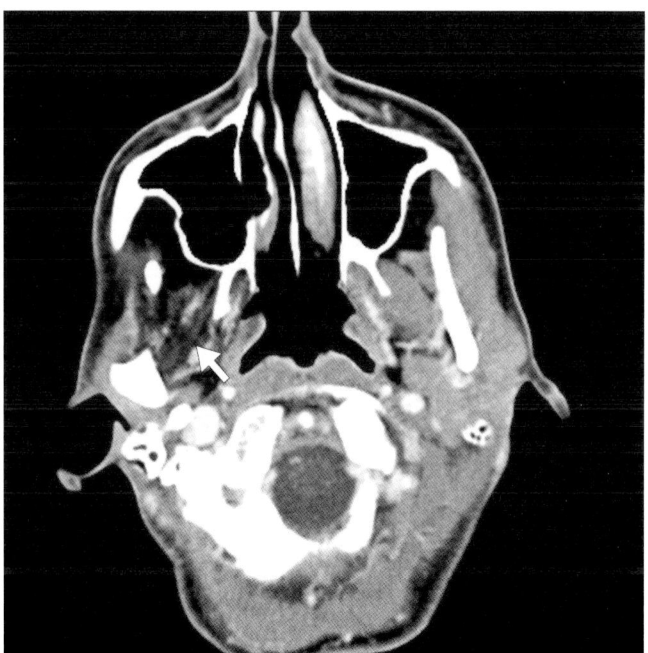

A

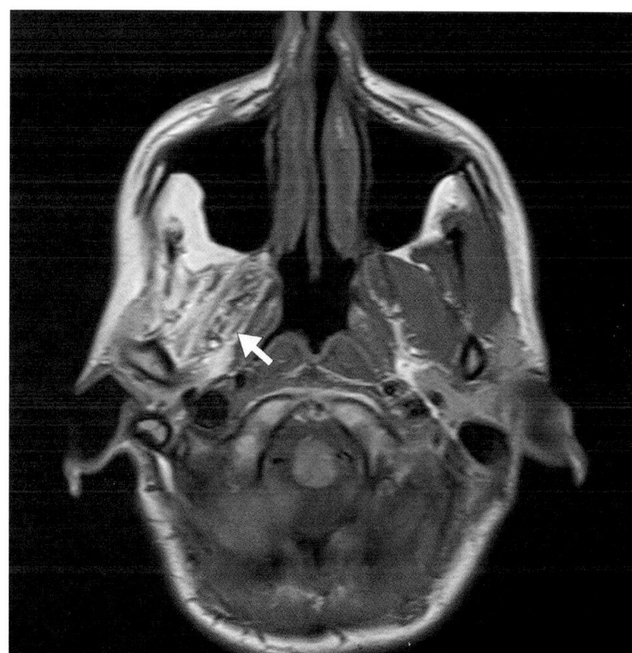

B

A postcontrast axial CT image (**A**) and an axial unenhanced T1-weighted MR image (**B**) demonstrate marked atrophy of the right muscles of mastication, compatible with CN V, V3 denervation atrophy (arrows, **A**, **B**).

REFERENCES

Agur AMR, Lee MJ, Grant JCB. *Grant's Atlas of Anatomy.* Philadelphia, PA: Lippincott Williams & Wilkins; 1999.

Deshingkar SA , Barpande SR, Bhavthankar J D, Humbe JG. Progressive hemifacial atrophy (Parry-Romberg Syndrome). *Contemp Clin Dent.* 2012;3(suppl 1): S78-S81.

El-Kehdy J, Abbas O, Rubeiz N. A review of Parry-Romberg syndrome. *J Am Acad Dermatol.* 2012;67(4):769-784.

Fischbein NJ, Kaplan MJ, Jackler RK, Dillon WP. MR imaging in two cases of subacute denervation change in the muscles of facial expression. *AJNR Am J Neuroradiol.* 2001;22:880-884.

Harnsberger HR, Dillon WP. Major motor atrophic patterns in the face and neck: CT evaluation. *Radiology.* 1985;155:665-670.

Hutto JR, Vattoth S. A practical review of the muscles of facial mimicry with special emphasis on the superficial musculoaponeurotic system. *AJR Am J Roentgenol.* 2015;204(1):W19-W26.

CASE 6 Rhytidectomy (facelift) and forehead lift

Over the past 30 years, the number of cosmetic surgeries that are performed worldwide has soared. There are several surgical techniques that may be employed for facial rejuvenation of the midface (termed rhytidectomy or facelift) and of the forehead (termed forehead lift).

Rhytidectomies improve the aging effects of the midface and lower eyelid. Various different incisions may be used, although they typically extend caudal from behind the hairline of the temple to the pretragal region, continue immediately caudal and posterior to the pinna, and terminate at the occipital scalp hairline. Dissection begins superficial to the investing fascia of the zygomaticus major. The tissue is released from the underlying bones and sutures, microscrews, or tissue adhesives are used to secure the tissues to the periosteum after the lift procedure. Some of these materials used to secure the rhytidectomy may be identified on imaging. Malar implants, if desired, may also be placed at the time of the rhytidectomy.

A forehead lift (also called browlift) is performed to raise the eyebrows as well as to minimize expression lines along the forehead, bridge of nose, and between the eyes in an effort to gain a more youthful appearance. Forehead lift procedures can be performed with a variety of different surgical techniques, including an endoscopic approach, a wide coronal incision, or with limited incisions directly over the brow or mid forehead.

The endoscopic approach of a forehead lift entails the use of an endoscope that is placed through several strategically placed small incisions which are made behind the hairline. The goal of the procedure is to elevate and release the skin as well as supporting tissues from the underlying bone. Each brow is then lifted in a superolateral vector and fixed in position. Various surgical materials may be used to fix the brow in position and the type used depends on the surgeon's preference. Some of these materials are the same as those used during a rhytidectomy and include: sutures, microscrews, fixation posts, absorbable wires/tines, tissue adhesives, and mini plates.

The coronal incision used for a forehead lift is an older and more invasive technique that entails making a pretragal incision which extends cephalad and behind the hairline to the contralateral pretragal region. Some techniques extend this incision immediately caudal and posterior to the pinna into the immediately adjacent occipital hairline. The coronal incision allows the surgeon to reflect the entire forehead anteriorly in order to release the scalp from the underlying periosteum. A portion of the forehead is frequently removed during the coronal incision. The forehead is then retracted and sutured into place. The coronal incision may be identified on cross-sectional imaging, particularly on MRI.

Both the endoscopic and coronal surgical techniques of a forehead lift may involve resecting portions of the corrugator and procerus muscles which are responsible for frown lines. The coronal incision, while offering greater exposure, usually results in greater morbidity relative to the endoscopic technique, including a greater incidence of numbness, larger scars, and alopecia.

Rhytidectomy with preauricular postsurgical changes

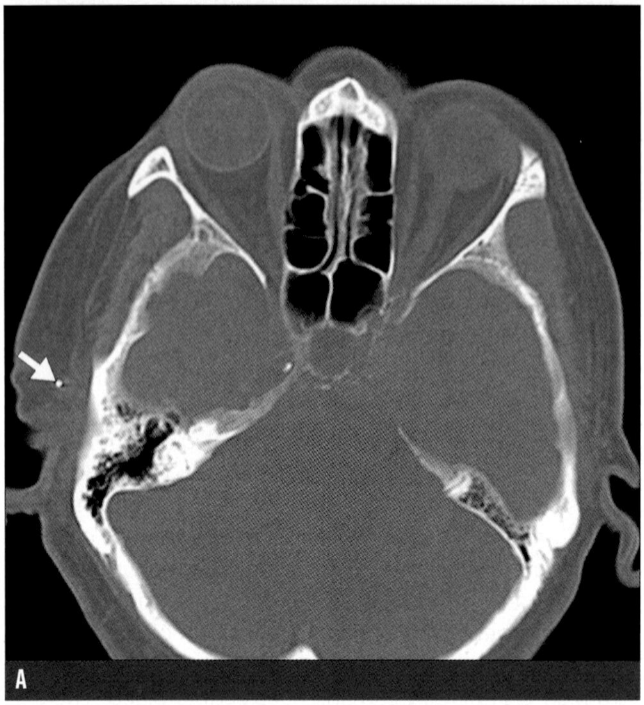

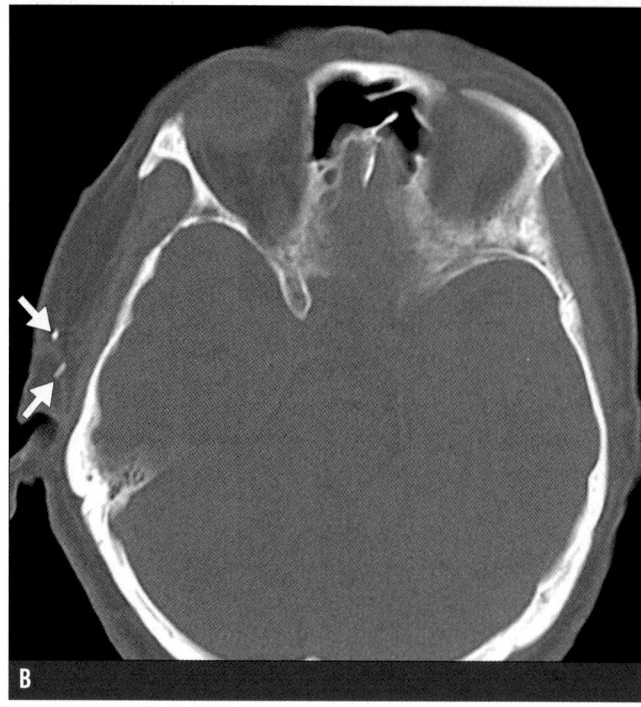

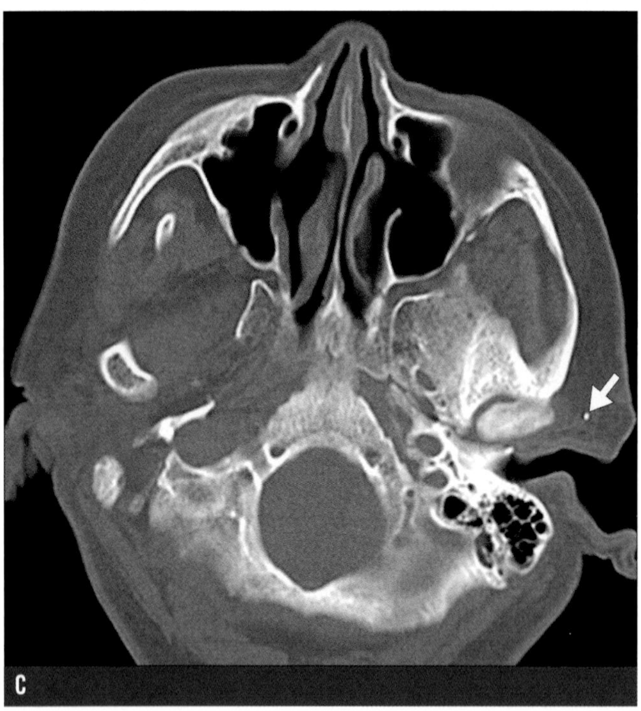

Axial unenhanced CT images (**A**-**C**) demonstrate surgical clips in the bilateral preauricular regions, compatible with postsurgical changes related to a prior rhytidectomy (arrows, **A**-**C**).

Rhytidectomy utilizing microscrew fixation

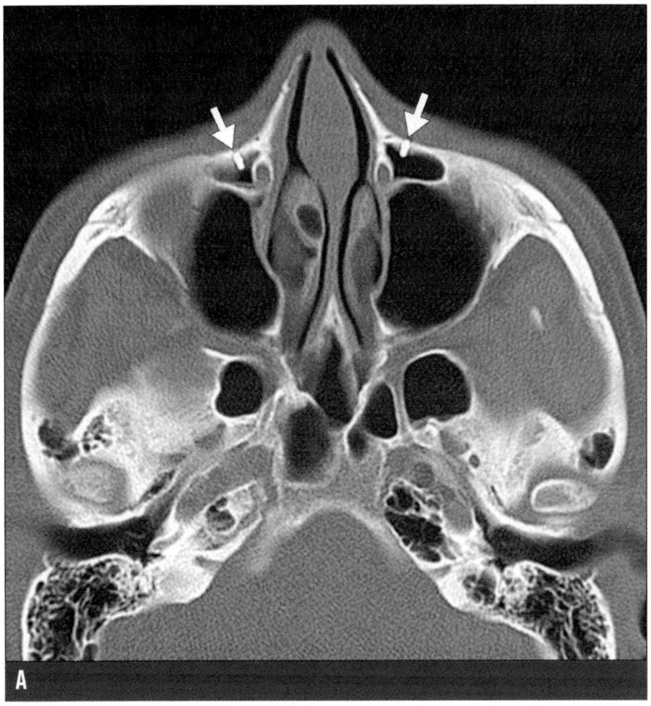

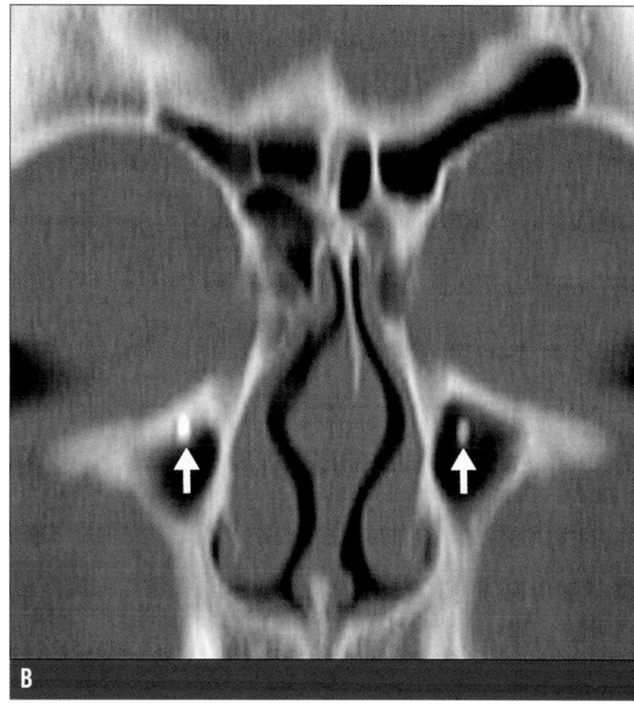

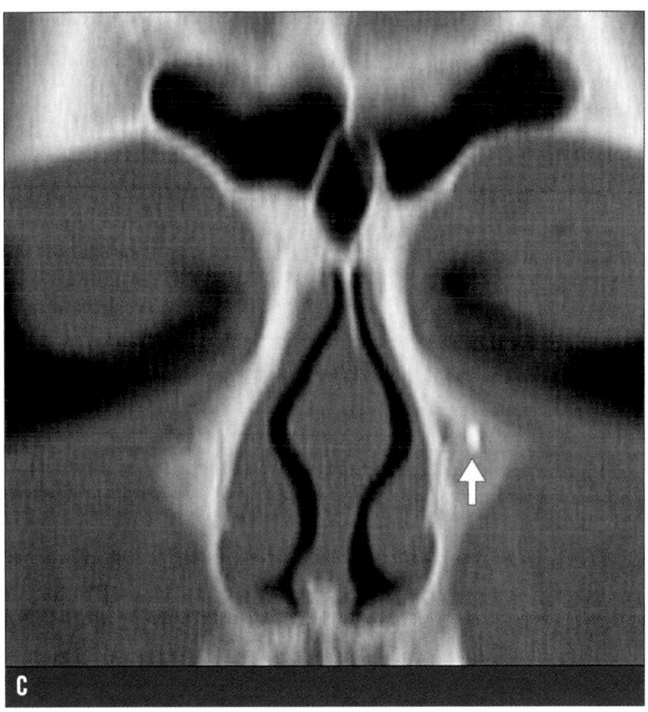

Axial (**A**) and coronal reformatted (**B**, **C**) CT images demonstrate paired screws deep to the nasolabial folds that represent microscrews utilized during a rhytidectomy procedure (arrows, **A**-**C**).

Forehead lift utilizing a coronal incision

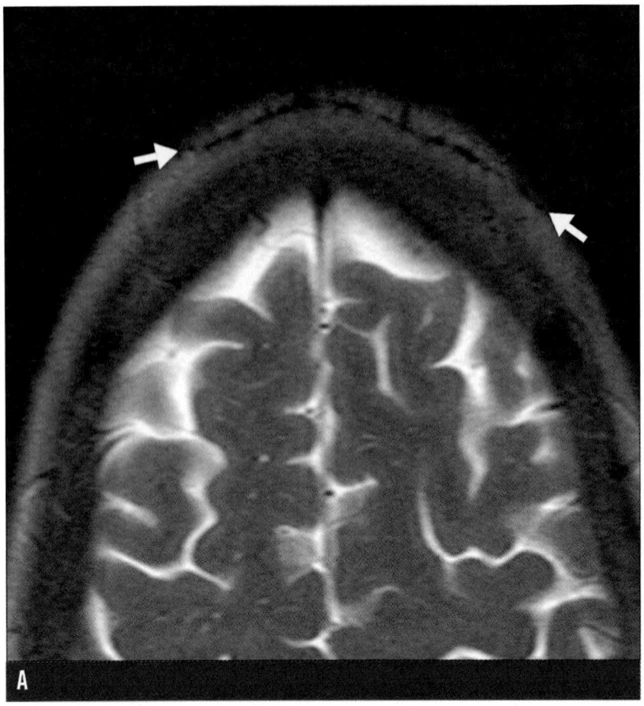

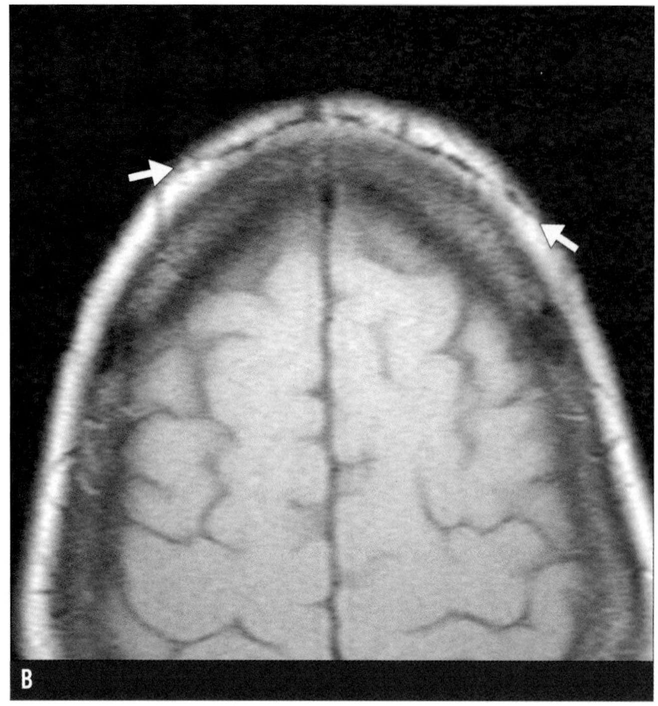

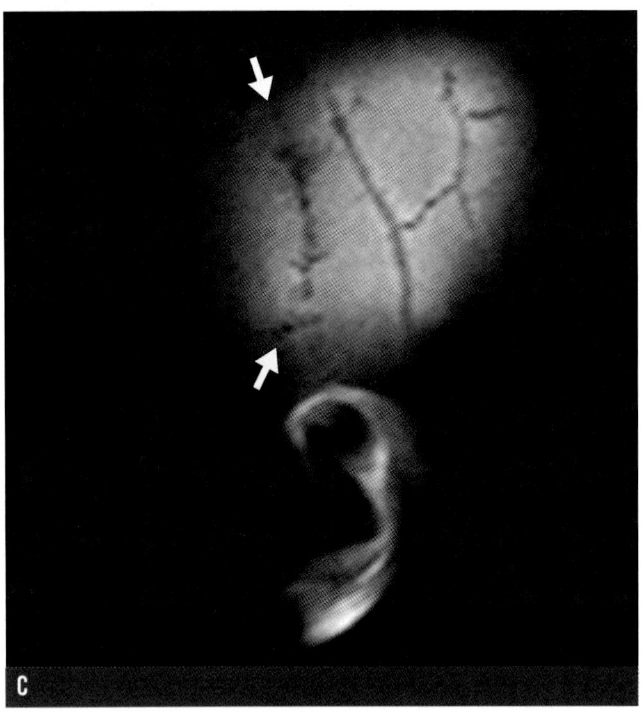

Axial T2 (**A**), axial T1 (**B**), and sagittal T1 (**C**) MR images demonstrate a coronal type incision performed for a forehead lift (arrows, **A**-**C**). The coronal incision was placed above the hairline so that the scar is not visible.

Forehead lift utilizing microscrew fixation

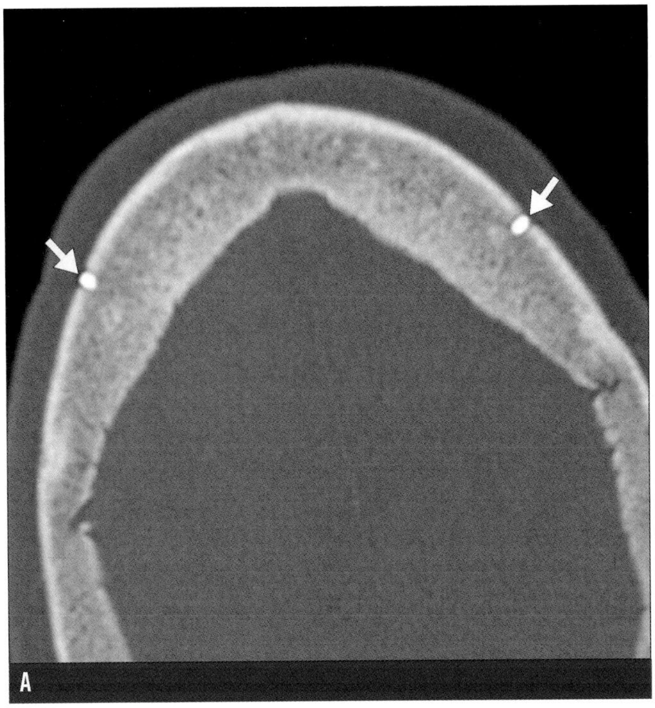

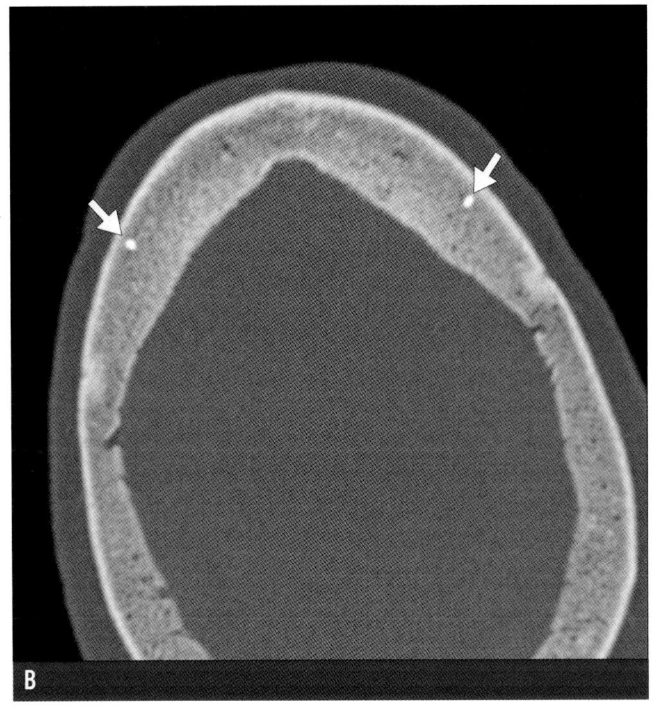

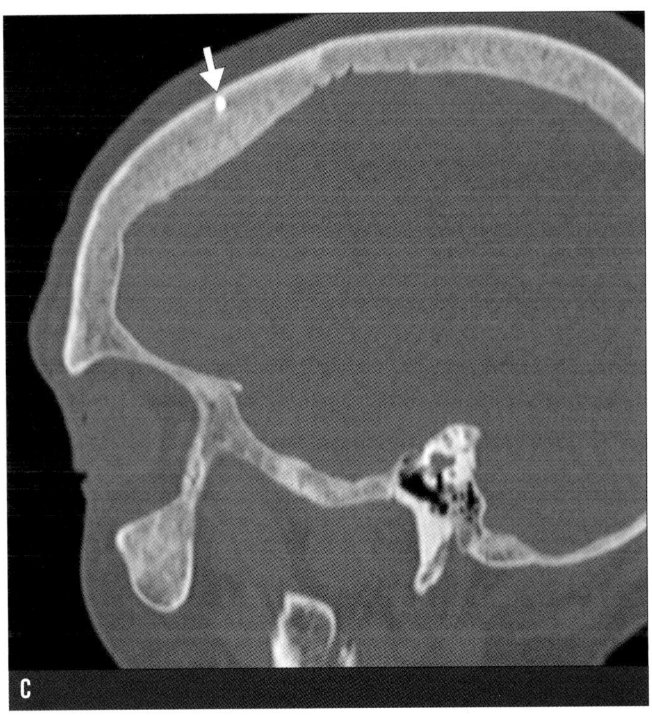

Axial (**A**, **B**) and sagittal reformatted (**C**) CT images demonstrate small metallic densities embedded within the bilateral aspects of the frontal calvarium (arrows, **A**-**C**). These metallic densities represent microscrews that are sometimes used to secure a forehead lift.

Forehead lift with screw tracts from prior microscrew fixation

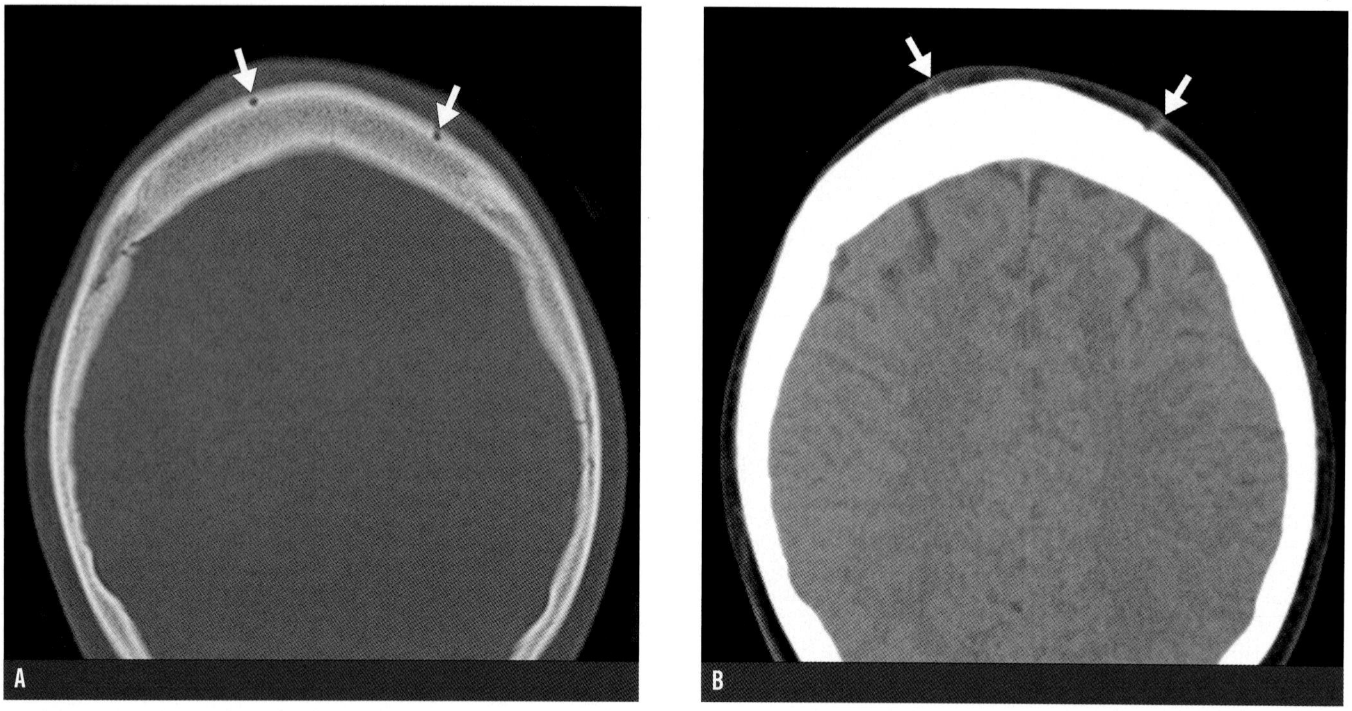

Axial CT images viewed with a bone window (**A**) and soft tissue window (**B**). Image **A** demonstrates paired small tracts within the bilateral aspects of the frontal calvarium (arrows, **A**). Image **B** demonstrates subtle small hyperdensities in the subcutaneous tissues of the scalp immediately overlying these osseous tracts (arrows, **B**). The findings are consistent with remnant tracts following removal of microscrews that were placed during a forehead lift procedure.

REFERENCES

Finn JC. An overview of techniques, indications, and approaches to the mid face lift. *Dermatol Clin.* 2005;23(3):505-514.

Gladstone GJ, Myint S, Black EH, Brazzo BG, Nesi FA. Fundamentals of facelift surgery. *Ophthalmol Clin North Am.* 2005;18(2):311-317.

Guyuron B. An evidence based approach to face lift. *Plast Reconstr Surg.* 2010;126(6):2230-2233.

Knize D. Anatomic concepts for brow lift procedures. *Plast Reconstr Surg.* 2009;124(6):2118-2126.

Patrocinio LG. Forehead lift: a 10-year review. *Arch Facial Plast Surg.* 2008;10(6):391-394.

CASE 7 Cosmetic injectable filler

Cosmetic injectable fillers have become increasingly popular for facial rejuvenation. They are approved for use in HIV lipoatrophy and for soft tissue augmentation to treat unwanted moderate-to-severe facial wrinkles and folds. Commonly injected locations include the cheeks, malar eminence, nasolabial folds, lips, philtrum, marionette lines (lines that extend caudal from the corner of the mouth), chin, tear trough (sunken area caudal to the inner canthus), and glabellar folds.

There are various types of cosmetic fillers that may be utilized and include: calcium hydroxylapatite (CaHA), collagen, hyaluronic acid, polytetrafluoroethylene, liquid silicone, poly-L-lactic acid, and polyacrylamide gel.

- CaHA fillers (eg, Radiesse) are used to treat wrinkles and facial lipoatrophy. CaHA fillers are composed of CaHA microspheres suspended in a methylcellulose gel matrix. These fillers are hyperattenuating (approximately 300-700 Hounsfield units) and appear infiltrative on CT. On MRI, CaHA fillers are heterogeneous hypo- to isointense on T1- and T2-weighted imaging and may mildly enhance on MRI. In addition, CaHA will be FDG-PET avid. The literature differs as to the etiology of this PET avidity, some stating that it is related to attenuation correction artifacts whereas others stating that it is likely due to a mild foreign body granulomatous reaction. These fillers will gradually resorb and last 2 or more years.
- Collagen fillers are naturally occurring proteins and can be obtained from various sources, including bovine, porcine, and human tissue. They are utilized to treat scars as well as wrinkles and can last up to 12 months. Collagen fillers follow fluid attenuation and signal on CT and MRI, respectively, and they can be associated with subcutaneous fat stranding. Minimal enhancement on MRI may last up to 2 months.
- Hyaluronic acid filler (eg, Restylane, Juvéderm) is nonpermanent, biodegradable material used for facial augmentation and to treat HIV-related lipoatrophy. Hyaluronic acid fillers follow fluid density and signal on CT and MRI, respectively. Minimal peripheral enhancement can be visualized for up to 2 months following injection. Because it is nonpermanent, loss of filler volume can be observed over serial imaging studies. If needed, this filler can be reversed by the injection of hyaluronidase.
- Polytetrafluoroethylene filler (eg, Gore-Tex) is a permanent, inert material that is used to treat the lips, nasolabial folds, and glabellar folds. GoreTex is high in attenuation on CT, measuring approximately 300 to 400 Hounsfield units. On MRI, GoreTex is low in signal relative to fat on both T1 and T2 sequences.
- Poly-L-lactic acid filler (eg, Sculptra) is used for facial cosmesis as well as to treat HIV-related lipoatrophy. This filler is synthetic (made from corn starch) and is reported to promote collagen formation. It has soft tissue attenuation on CT and is associated with fat stranding.
- Polyacrylamide gel fillers are high in water content and follow fluid density and signal on CT and MRI, respectively. On MRI, a low T2 rim of signal can be identified, likely reflective of fibrous capsule formation.
- Liquid silicone filler is a permanent agent that has been used for several decades to treat acne scars and for facial cosmesis. On CT, liquid silicone is iso- to slightly hyperattenuating compared to soft tissue. The signal on MRI depends on the viscosity of the liquid silicone used; however, liquid silicone is usually T1 hyperintense and T2 iso- to hypointense relative to water. Liquid silicone injections can result in severe and irreparable damage to the face, particularly with nonmedical grade formulas. Its use for facial cosmesis is controversial, and with the exception of approved clinical trials, it is no longer FDA-approved for facial cosmesis.

Although most cosmetic injectable fillers have a favorable safety profile and are a cornerstone of many dermatological practices, multiple complications have been reported in the literature. Early complications include skin discoloration, skin necrosis, immediate hypersensitivity reactions, or overcorrection. Late complications include infection, granulomatous reactions, delayed hypersensitivity reactions, filler migration, and scarring (particularly with liquid silicone).

COMPANION CASES

- **Hypermetabolic cosmetic injectable filler on PET imaging.** While the literature has described CaHA fillers as being PET avid, it is likely that other cosmetic fillers may also be PET avid. In the case provided herein, the lack of increased density of the filler on CT clearly indicates that it does not represent CaHA. Instead, the cosmetic filler used for this patient, who is a patient afflicted with HIV, is isodense relative to soft tissue and thus likely represents either poly-L-lactic acid or hyaluronic acid. Regardless of the filler, the clinical history of a prior cosmetic facial injection is important in order to avoid misinterpreting a PET examination.
- **Inadvertent cosmetic injection into a Stensen duct.** There is at least one case report of sialadenitis and infiltration of the Stensen duct following injection of a cosmetic filler. Inadvertent injection of a cosmetic filler into a Stensen duct may result in duct obstruction and acute parotitis as well as sialodochitis.
- **Rapidly hardening hydroxyapatite cement for fracture stabilization.** Several alloplastic materials have been used to correct craniofacial deformities, including methylmethacrylate, high-density polyethylene, silicone, and hydroxyapatite cement. These materials have various advantages and disadvantages. A disadvantage of

methylmethacrylate is that it generates a thermogenic reaction and potential local tissue damage. Silicone and high-density polyethylene are manufactured as solid materials and require molding or cutting prior to their use. However, with rapidly hardening hydroxyapatite cement, placement of this material generates an isothermic reaction with less tissue damage, and it can be molded by hand. Hydroxyapatite cement is eventually replaced by normal bone and bonds by osteogenesis. Possible complications of hydroxyapatite cement used in this setting include seroma, implant displacement, and infection, although these complications are uncommon.

Cosmetic injectable filler: Cheeks

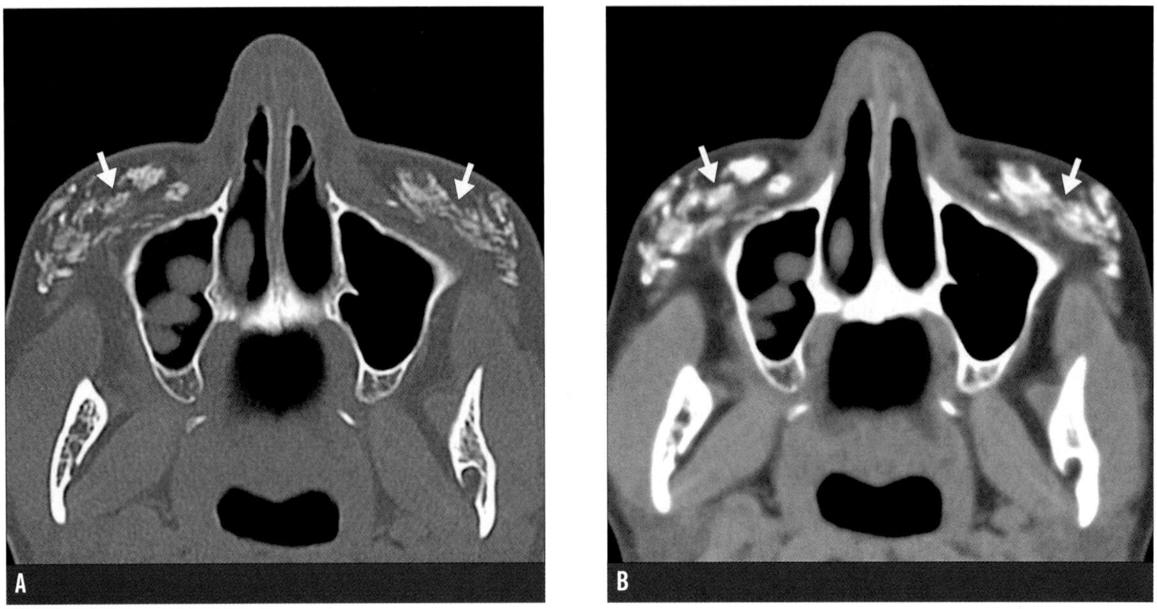

Unenhanced axial CT images viewed with a bone window (**A**) and soft tissue window (**B**) demonstrate heterogeneous hyperdense material within the cheeks, compatible with cosmetic injectable filler, in this case CaHA (arrows, **A**, **B**).

Cosmetic injectable filler: Cheeks

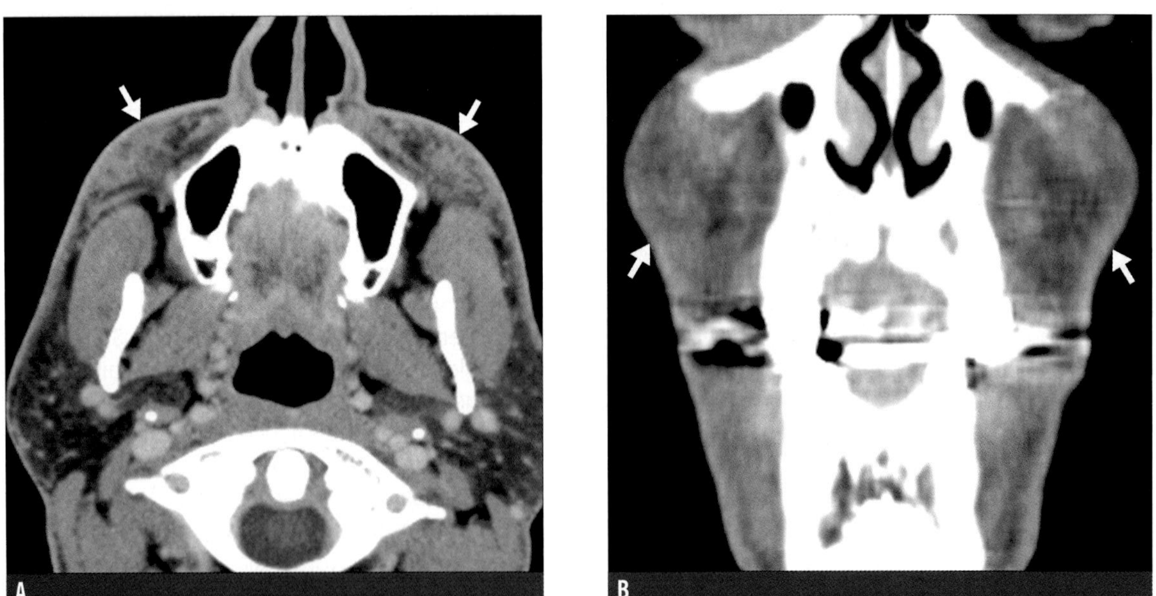

Different patient. Axial (**A**) and coronal reformatted (**B**) unenhanced CT images of a patient with HIV demonstrate heterogeneous soft tissue density within the cheeks, compatible with cosmetic injectable filler (arrows, **A**-**B**). Given the density, the cosmetic injectable filler most likely represents either hyaluronic acid or poly-L-lactic acid.

Cosmetic injectable filler: Cheeks

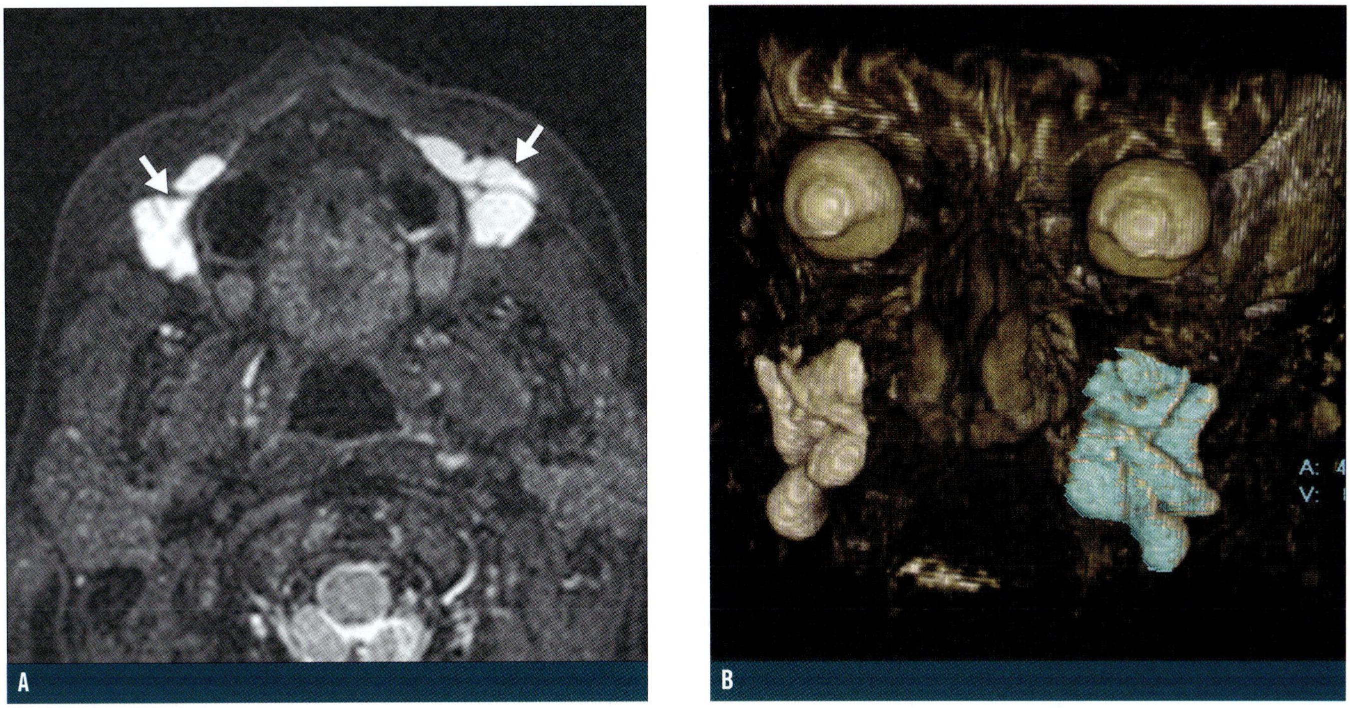

Different patient. A fat-suppressed axial T2-weighted MR image (**A**) demonstrates multilobulated T2 hyperintense signal in the cheeks compatible with cosmetic injectable filler, in this case Restylane. A volumetric T2-weighted reconstructed image (**B**) illustrates the cosmetic injectable filler volume to a better advantage.

Cosmetic injectable filler: Nasolabial fold

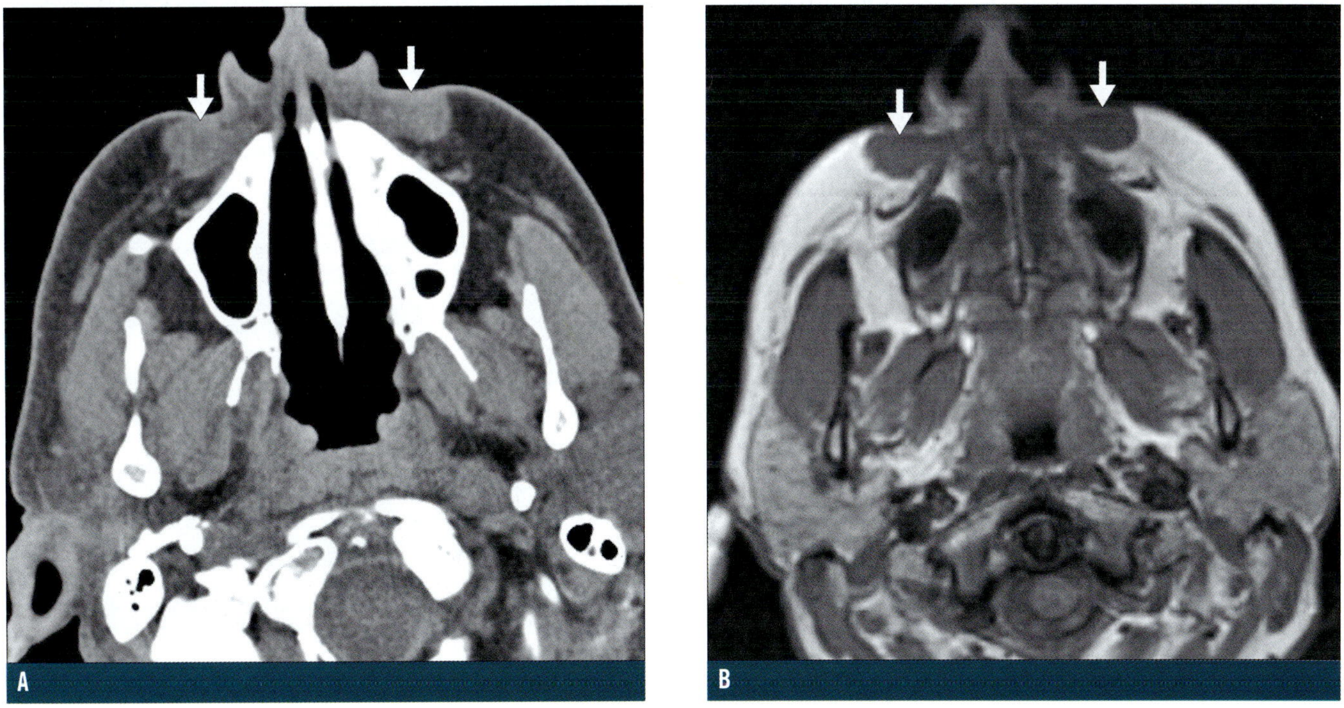

An unenhanced axial CT image (**A**) demonstrates confluent soft tissue density deep to the nasolabial folds (arrows, **A**). Unenhanced axial T1 (**B**), axial T2 (**C**), and contrast-enhanced axial T1 (**D**) MR images of the same patient demonstrate the findings to be isointense on T1 relative to muscle (arrows, **B**) and hyperintense on T2 relative to muscle (arrows, **C**) and undergoes minimal, if any, enhancement (arrows, **D**). The findings are consistent with cosmetic injectable filler. The exact type of filler used in this case is not known, although given its overall appearance, it likely represents either hyaluronic acid or polyacrylamide gel.

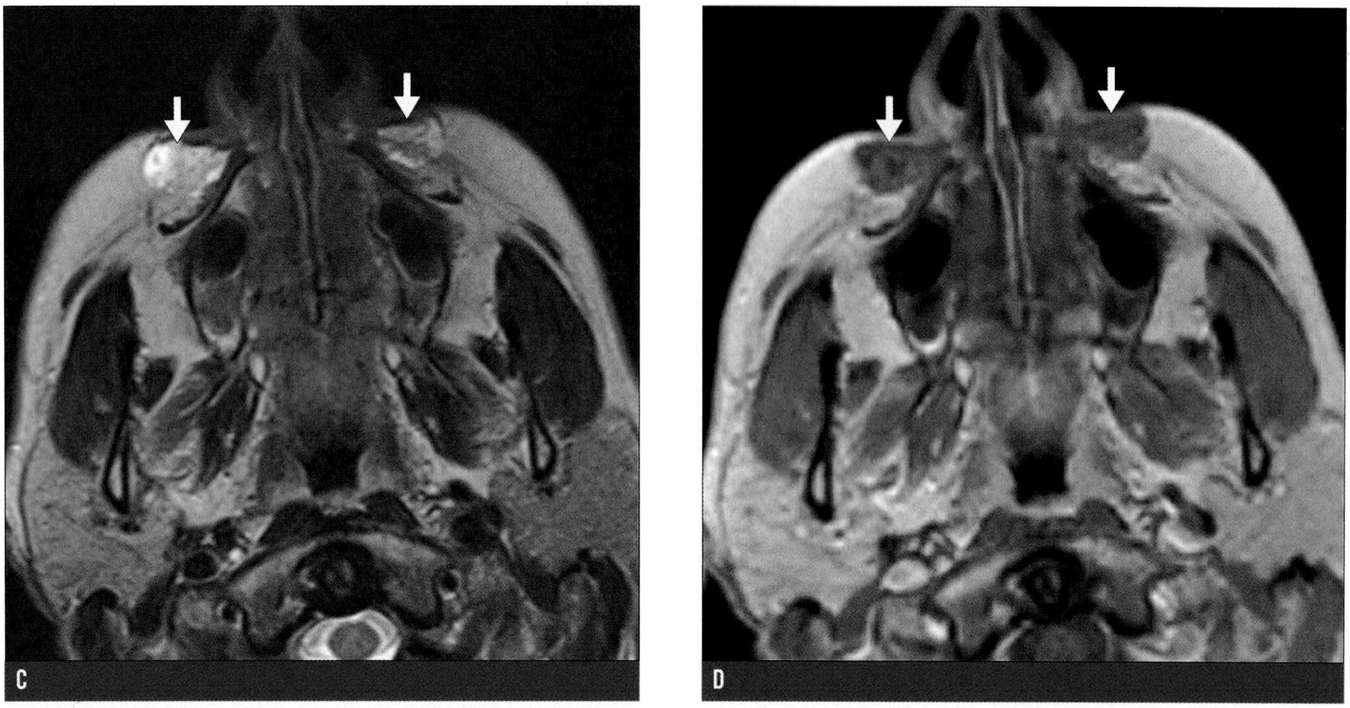

Cosmetic injectable filler: Nasolabial fold

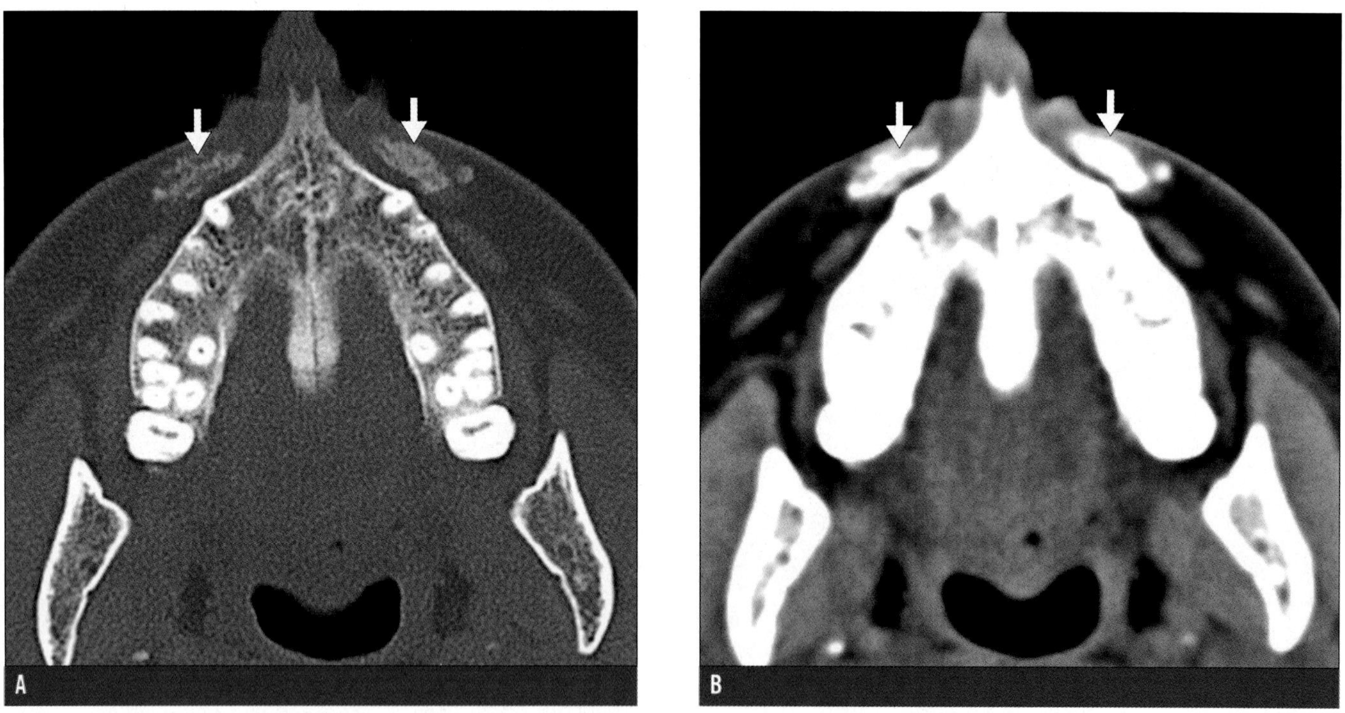

Different patient. Unenhanced axial CT images viewed with a bone window (**A**) and soft tissue window (**B**) demonstrate heterogeneous increased attenuation within the subcutaneous fat of the nasolabial folds, compatible with cosmetic injectable filler, either CaHA or polytetrafluoroethylene (Gore-Tex) (arrows, **A**, **B**).

Cosmetic injectable filler: Malar eminence

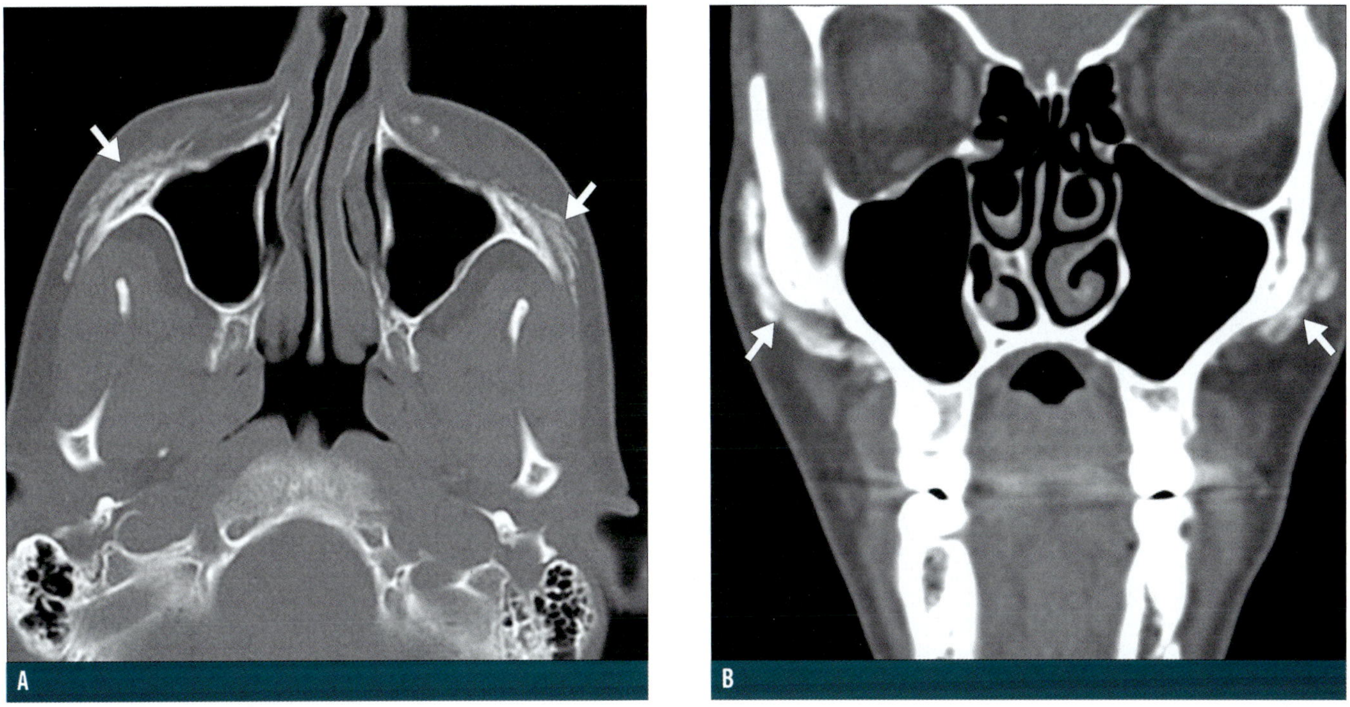

An unenhanced axial CT image viewed with a bone window (**A**) as well as an unenhanced coronal reformatted CT image viewed with a soft tissue window (**B**) demonstrate heterogeneous increased attenuation overlying the malar eminences, compatible with cosmetic injectable filler (arrows, **A**, **B**). The density of this filler measured between 300 and 400 Hounsfield units and thus represents either CaHA or polytetrafluoroethylene (Gore-Tex).

Cosmetic injectable filler: Malar eminence

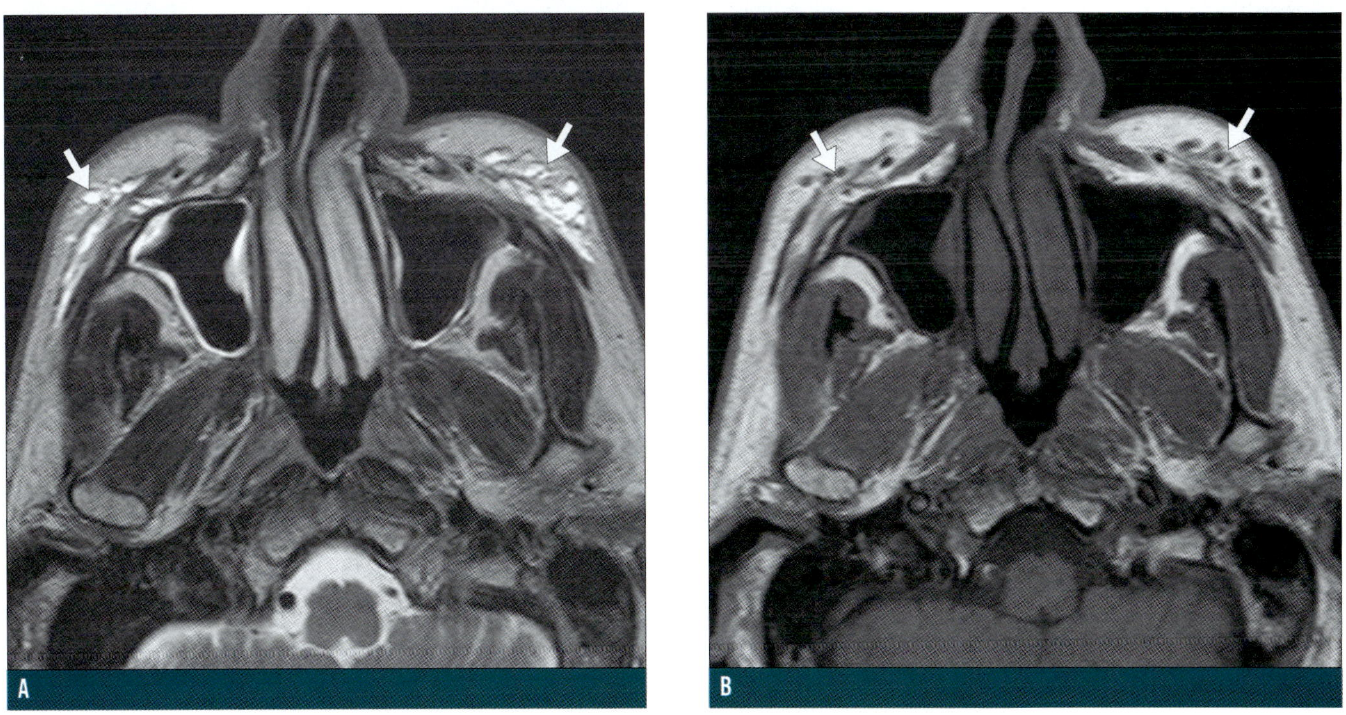

Different patient. Axial T2 (**A**), axial T1 (**B**), and contrast-enhanced axial T1 (**C**) MR images demonstrate multilobulated T2 hyperintense, T1 isointense, and nonenhancing foci over the malar eminences, compatible with cosmetic injectable filler (arrows, **A**-**C**). Given the fluid signal and infiltrative nature, this filler probably represents collagen.

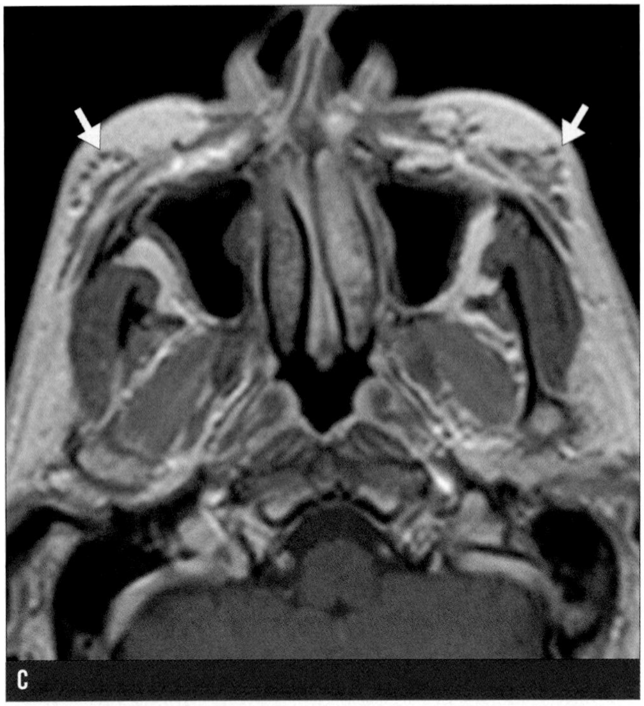

C

Cosmetic injectable filler: Chin

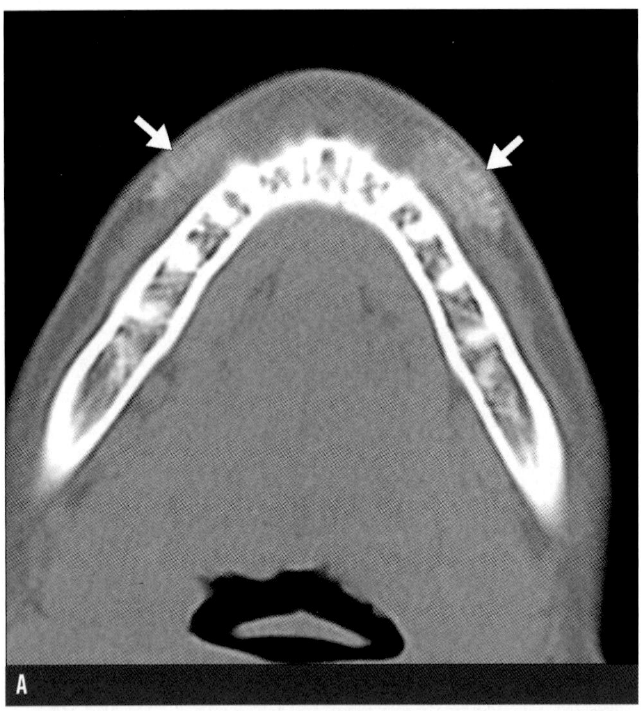

A

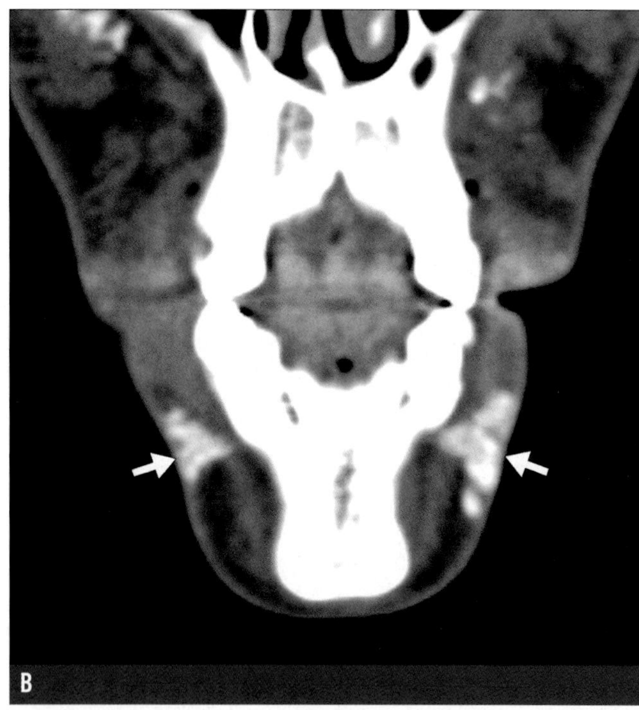

B

An unenhanced axial CT image viewed with a bone window (**A**) as well as an unenhanced coronal reformatted CT image viewed with a soft tissue window (**B**) demonstrate focal increased attenuation within the subcutaneous soft tissues on both sides of the chin, compatible with cosmetic injectable filler (arrows, **A**, **B**). The density of this filler measured between 300 and 400 Hounsfield units and thus likely represents either CaHA or polytetrafluoroethylene (Gore-Tex).

Cosmetic injectable filler: Philtrum

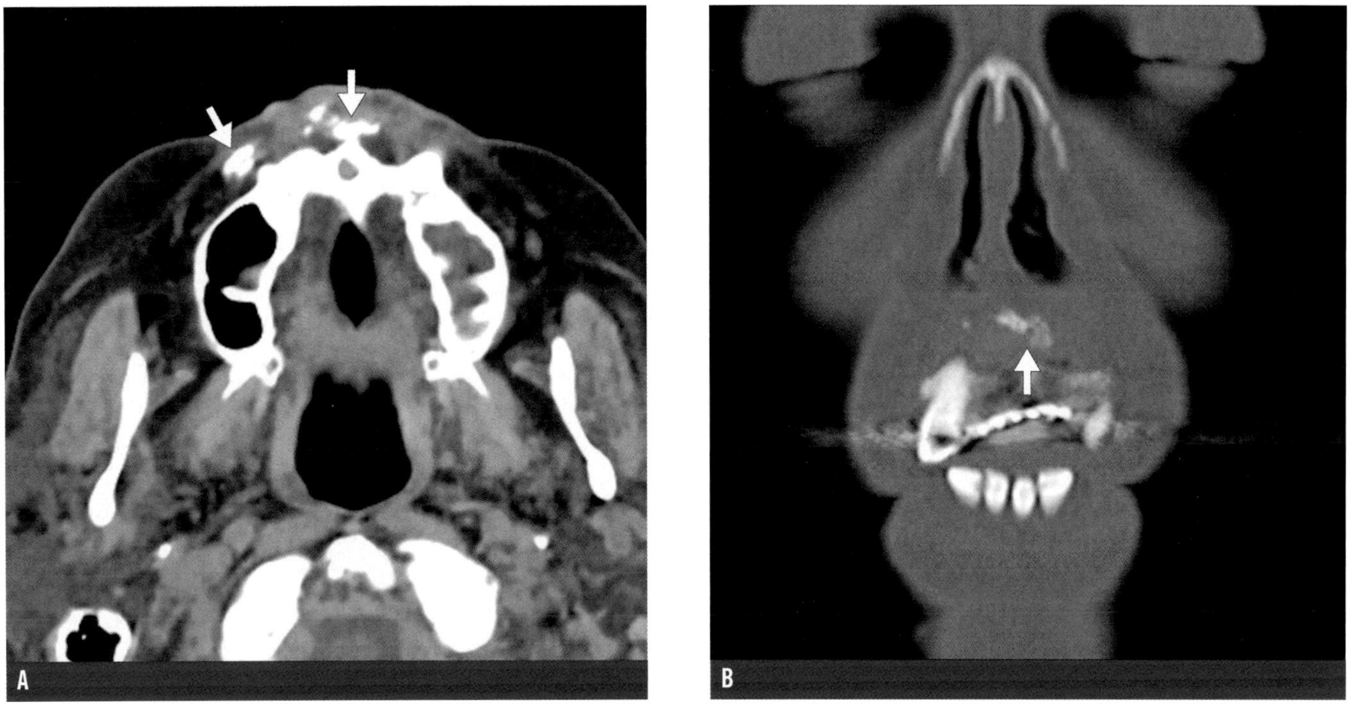

An unenhanced axial CT image viewed with a soft tissue window (**A**) and an unenhanced coronal reformatted CT image viewed with a bone window (**B**) demonstrate patchy foci of increased attenuation in the subcutaneous soft tissues of the philtrum, compatible with cosmetic injectable filler (arrows, **A**, **B**). The density of this filler measured greater than 700 Hounsfield units and is therefore most compatible with CaHA.

Cosmetic injectable filler: Glabella

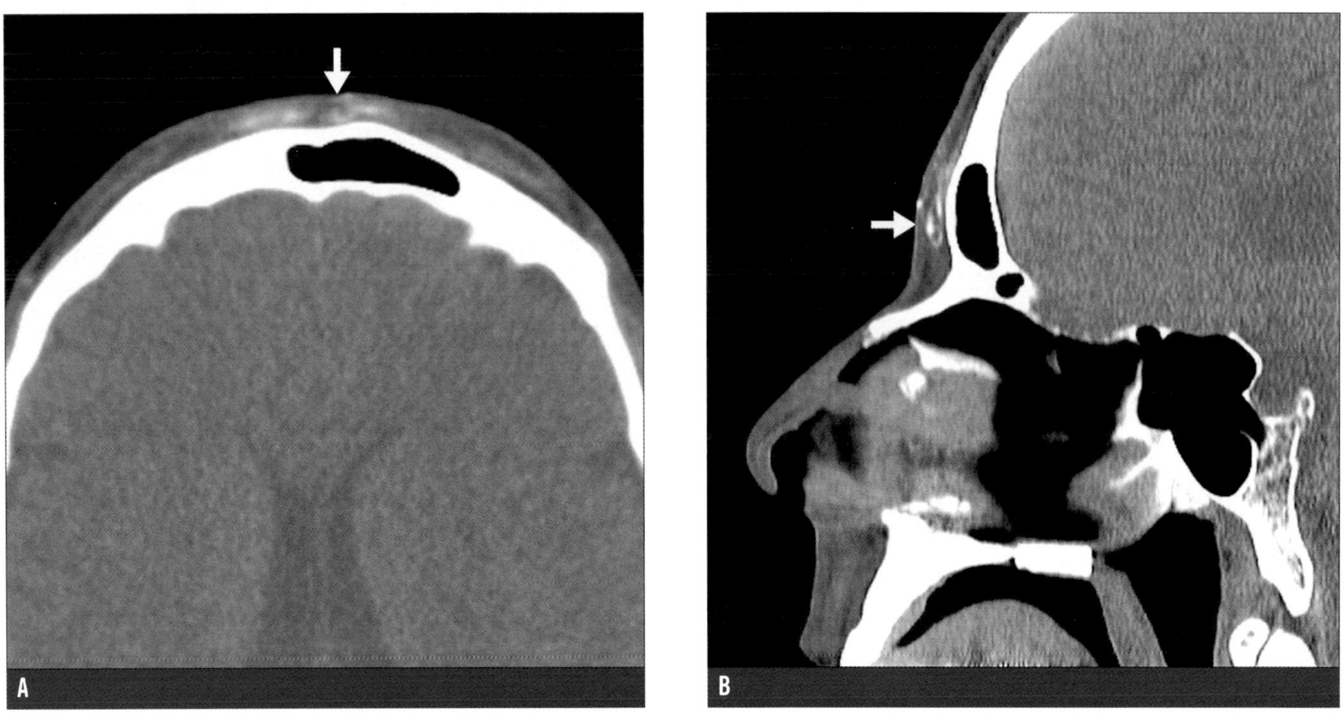

Axial (**A**) and sagittal reformatted (**B**) unenhanced CT images viewed with an intermediate window demonstrate hyperattenuating material in the subcutaneous soft tissues of the glabella, compatible with cosmetic injectable filler (arrows, **A**, **B**). This density of this filler measured up to 300 Hounsfield units and is thus compatible with either CaHA or polytetrafluoroethylene (Gore-Tex).

Cosmetic injectable filler: Lips

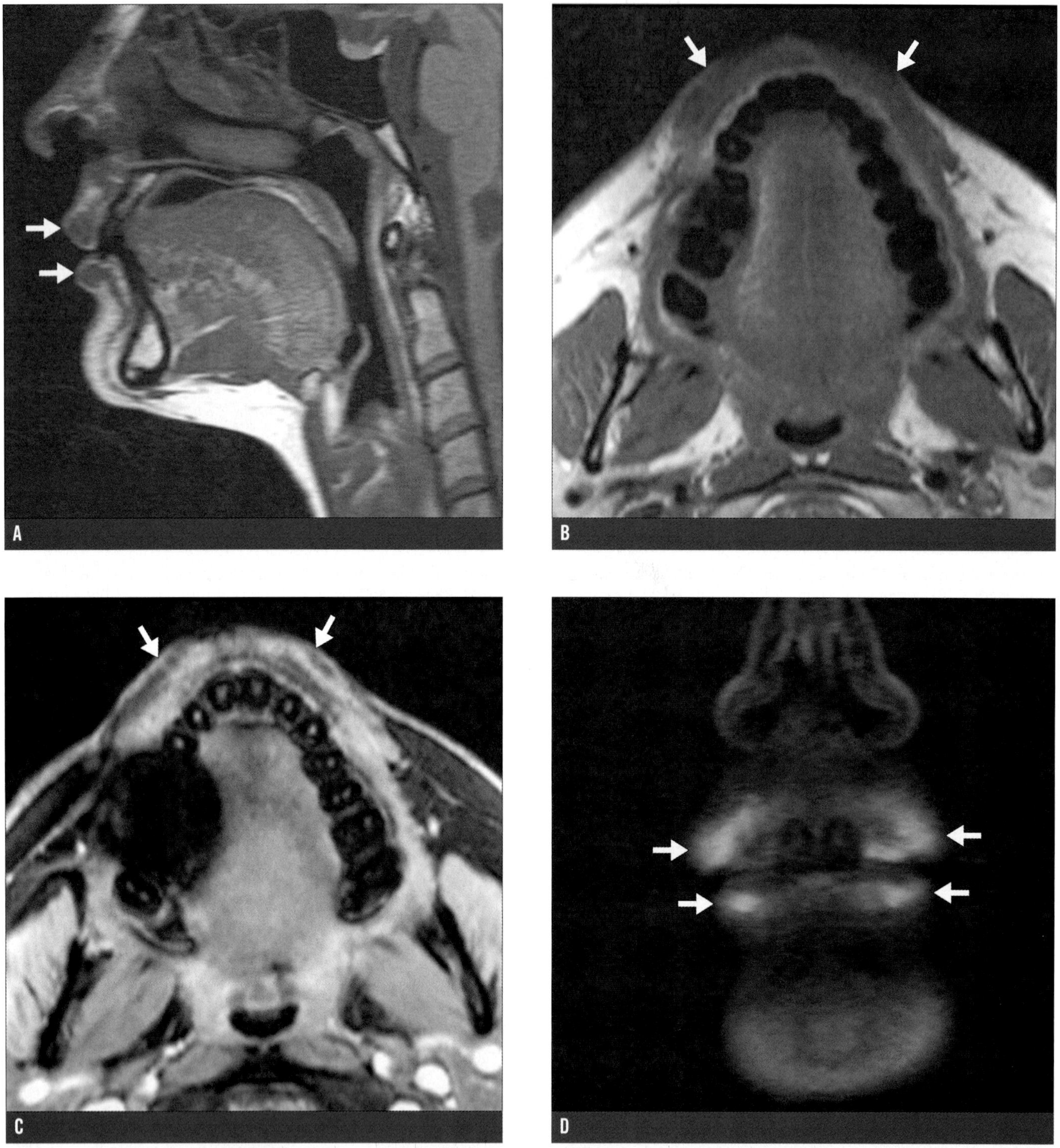

Sagittal T1 (**A**), axial T1 (**B**), fat-suppressed contrast-enhanced axial T1 (**C**), and fat-suppressed coronal T2 (**D**) MR images demonstrate mildly enlarged upper and lower lips which are T1 isointense (arrows, **A**, **B**), minimally enhancing (arrows, **C**), and T2 hyperintense (arrows, **D**), compatible with cosmetic augmentation of the lips. Given the signal and location of the filler, the filler used likely represents hyaluronic acid.

Companion case: Hypermetabolic cosmetic injectable filler on PET imaging

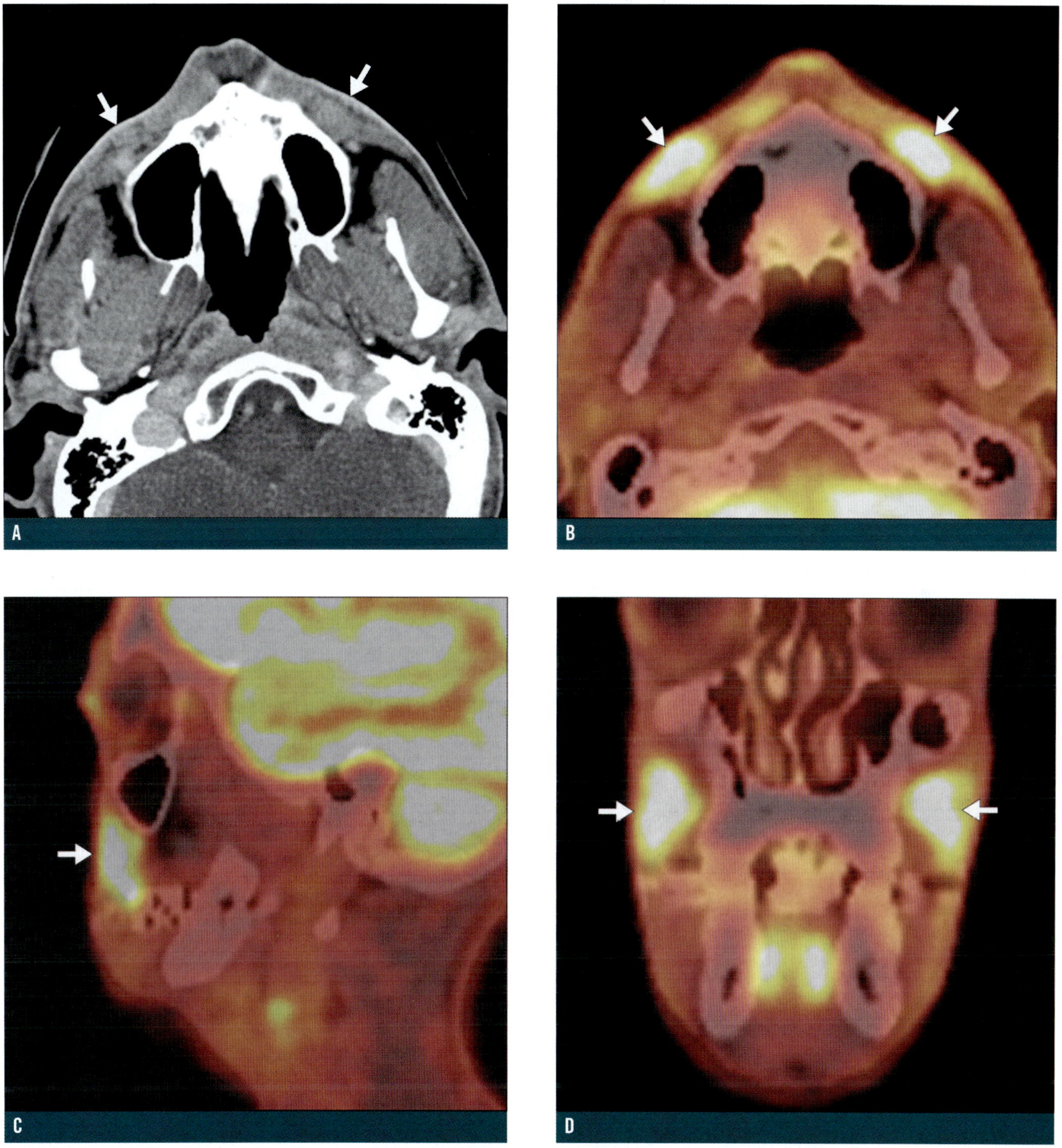

A contrast-enhanced axial CT image (**A**) demonstrates soft tissue density infiltrating the premalar fat, compatible with cosmetic injectable filler (arrows, **A**). The exact type of cosmetic injectable filler used for this patient is not known. However, this patient has HIV, and given its overall appearance, the cosmetic injectable filler likely represents either poly-L-lactic acid or hyaluronic acid. Axial (**B**), sagittal reformatted (**C**), and coronal reformatted (**D**) PET images of the same patient demonstrate the cosmetic injectable filler to be PET avid, an incidental finding.

Companion case: Inadvertent cosmetic injection into a Stensen duct

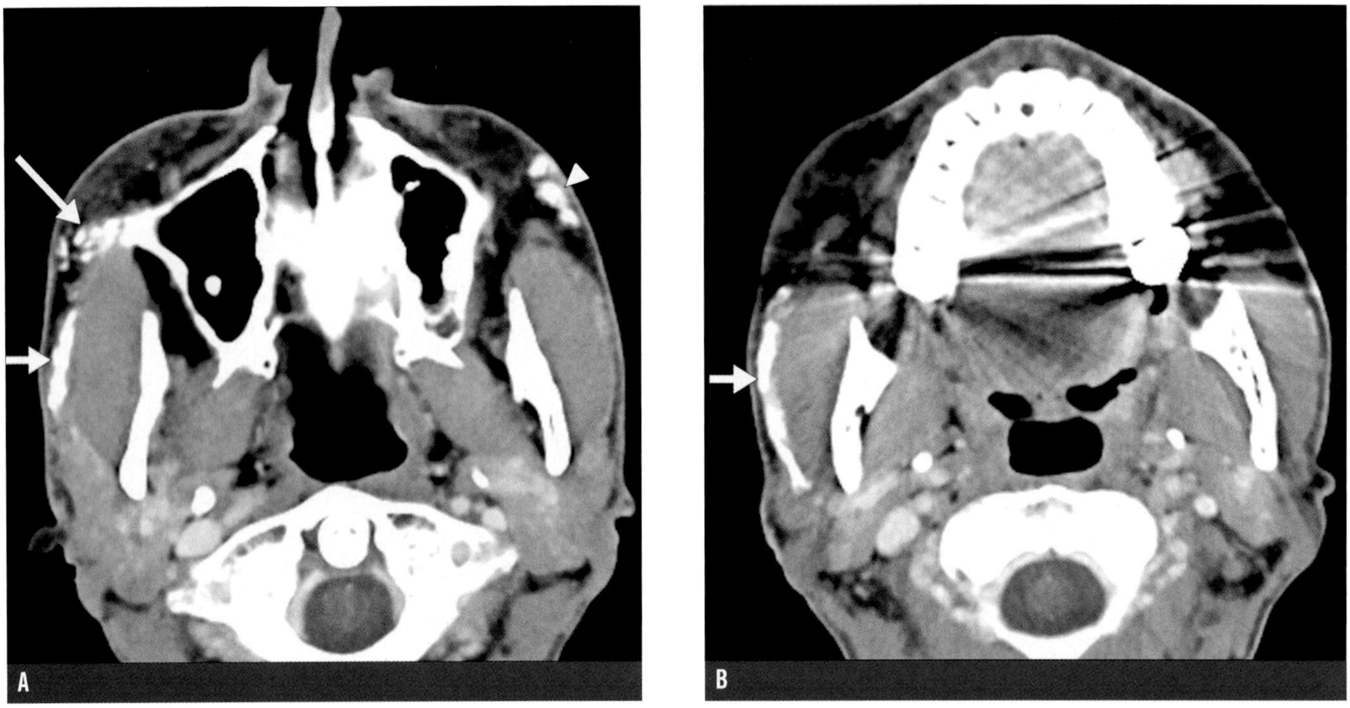

Contrast-enhanced axial CT images (**A**, **B**) demonstrate abnormal increased attenuation within the right Stensen duct (arrows, **A**, **B**) related to inadvertent injection during placement of CaHA cosmetic filler into the right cheek (long arrow, **A**). Cosmetic injectable filler was also placed into the left cheek (arrowhead, **A**).

Companion case: Rapidly hardening hydroxyapatite cement for fracture stabilization

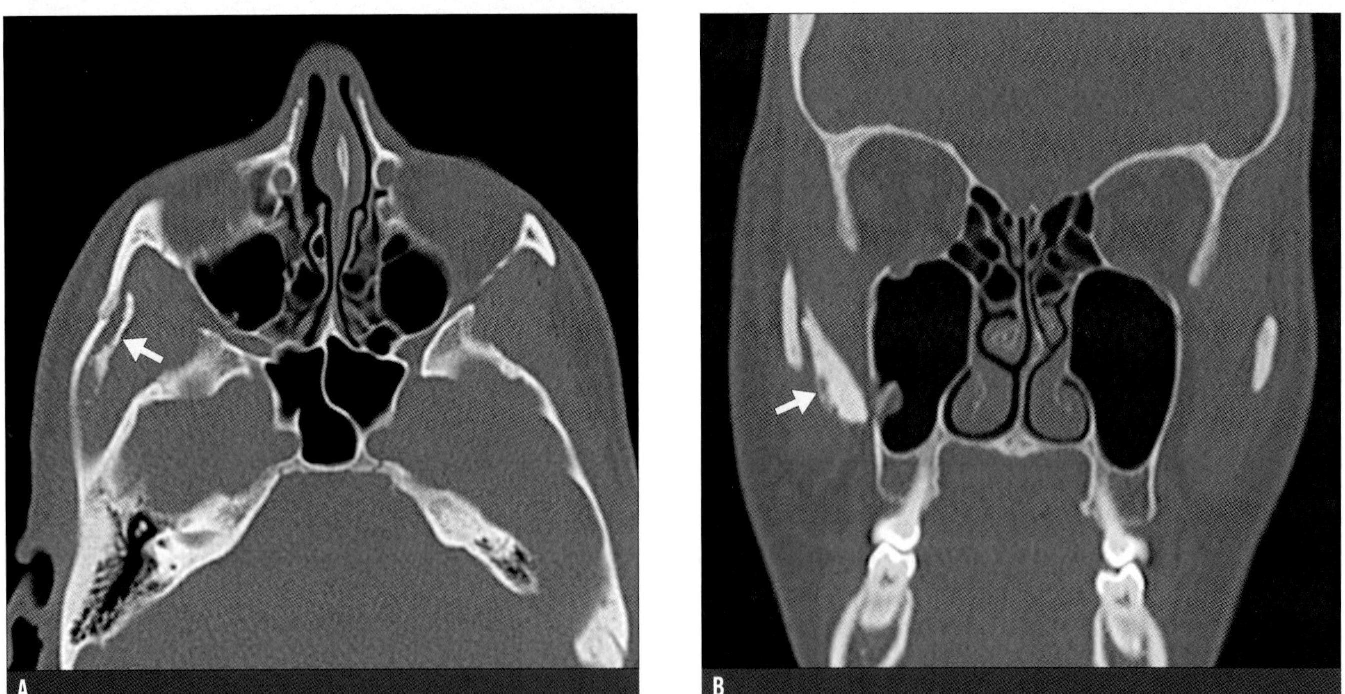

Axial (**A**) and coronal reformatted (**B**) CT images demonstrate a high density material deep to a right zygomatic arch fracture representing rapidly hardening hydroxyapatite cement (arrows, **A**, **B**). Following reduction of the right zygomatic arch fracture under ultrasound guidance, this cement was molded by hand and placed via ultrasound guidance through an incision in the right suprazygomatic soft tissues. The hydroxyapatite cement was placed to stabilize the right zygomatic arch fracture.

REFERENCES

Caruthers A, Liebskind M, Carruthers J, Forster BB. Radiographic and computed tomographic studies of calcium hydroxylapatite for treatment of HIV-associated facial lipoatrophy and correction of nasolabial folds. *Dermatol Surg.* 2008;34:S78-S84.

Feeney JN, Fox JJ, Akhurst T. Radiological impact of the use of calcium hydroxylapatite dermal fillers. *Clin Radiol.* 2009;64:897-902.

Ginat DT, Schatz CJ. Imaging features of midface injectable fillers and associated complications. *AJNR Am J Neuroradiol.* 2012;34:1488-1495.

Lee DW, Kim JY, Lew DH. Use of rapidly hardening hydroxyapatite cement for facial contouring surgery. *J Craniofac Surg.* 2010;21(4):1084-1088

Nichols BJ, Carpenter J, Hribar KP, Go J, Rice DH. Acute parotitis after injection of poly-L-lactic acid for malar augmentation: a case report and review of relevant anatomy. *Dermatol Surg.* 2011;37(3):381-386.

Vasquez J, Rosenthal DI. Bilateral, symmetrical soft tissue calcifications in the face. *Skeletal Radiol.* 2010;39:387-389.

CASE 8 Malar implant prostheses

Malarplasty, which includes augmentation of the malar and/or submalar (premaxillary) space, is often used to restore cheek volume loss. Options for malarplasty include synthetic injectable fillers, autologous fat grafts, or prosthetic implants. Prosthetic implants are increasingly becoming more common, given their ease of implantation and low rate of complications. Malar implants are placed over the malar eminences (zygomatic processes of the maxilla) and zygomatic bones, whereas submalar implants are placed over the anterior walls of the maxillary sinuses. The implants are secured with either sutures or screws. Malar implants may be placed in conjunction with a rhytidectomy (facelift).

Prosthetic malar implants can be synthesized from various materials including: silicone rubber, porous polytetrafluoroethylene (Medpor), expanded polytetrafluoroethylene (Gore-Tex), and polymethylmethacrylate (PMMA). Silicone rubber implants, which are the most commonly used malar implants, are denser than soft tissue on CT and are best visualized with bone windows. On MRI, silicone rubber implants are hypointense on T1- and T2-weighted sequences. Medpor is hypoattenuating on CT whereas on MRI it is hypointense relative to fat on T1- and T2-weighted sequences. Gore-Tex and PMMA are dense on CT while on MRI they are hypointense to fat on T1- and T2-weighted sequences.

Infection of an implant within 2 weeks after implantation occurs at a rate of 3.8%. Other rarer complications include implant migration, implant displacement, foreign body reaction, heterotopic bone formation, and osseous erosion.

Malar implant prostheses

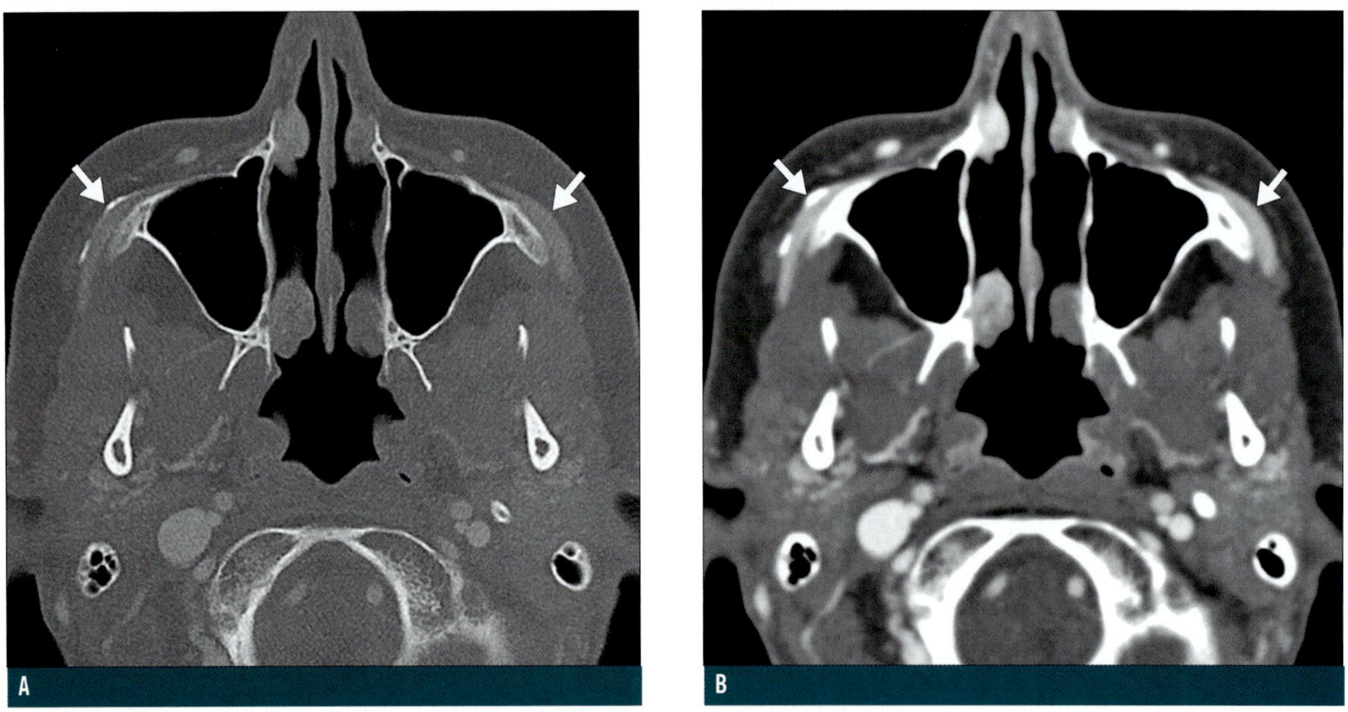

A contrast-enhanced axial CT image viewed with a bone window (**A**) as well as axial (**B**), coronal reformatted (**C**), and sagittal reformatted (**D**) contrast-enhanced CT images viewed with a soft tissue window demonstrate smooth, curvilinear, high-density prosthetics overlying the malar eminences, compatible with malar implant prostheses (arrows, **A-D**). Images **B** and **D** demonstrate a small amount of dystrophic mineralization associated with the malar implants.

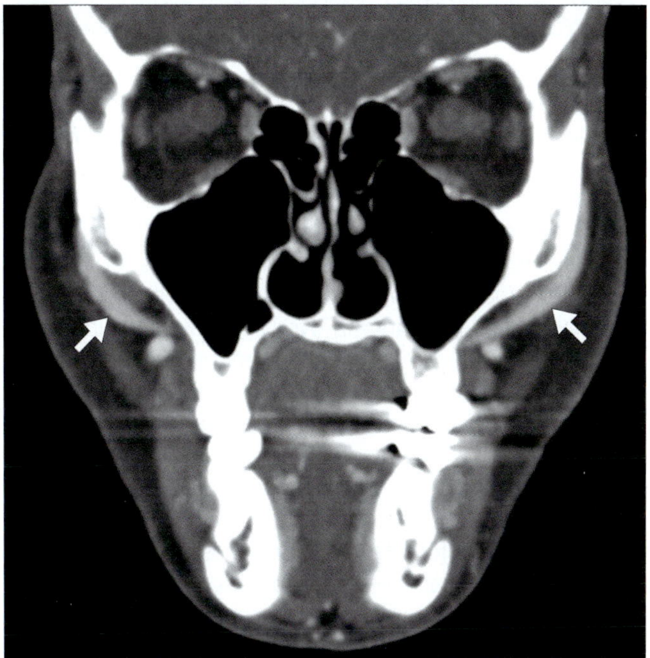

C

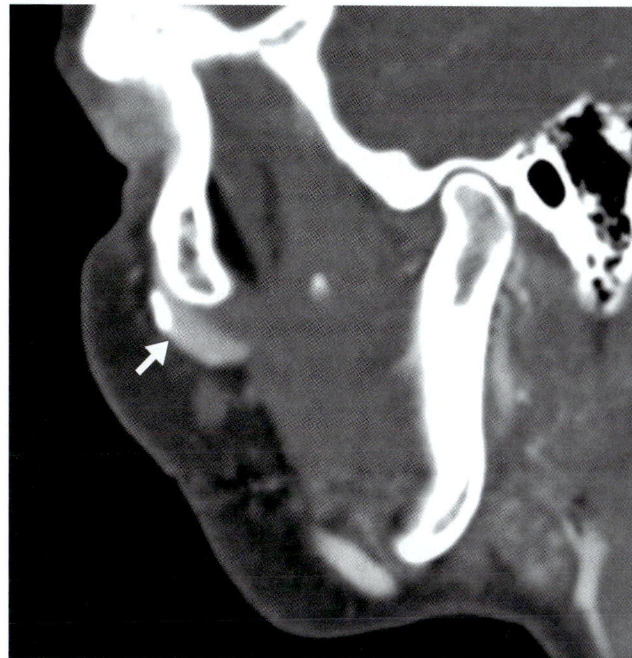

D

REFERENCES

Binder WJ, Azizzadeh B. Malar and submalar augmentation. *Facial Plast Surg Clin North Am.* 2008;16:11-32.

Coskun U, et al. Imaging of porous polyethylene implant by using multidetector spiral computed tomography. *J Craniofac Surg.* 2008;19:156-158.

Niamtu J 3rd. Essentials of cheek and midface implants. *J Oral Maxillofac Surg.* 2010;68:1420-1429.

Schatz CJ, Ginat DT. Imaging of cosmetic facial implants and grafts. *AJNR Am J Neuroradiol.* 2012;34:1674-1681.

CASE 9 Reduction rhinoplasty

A reduction rhinoplasty is a cosmetic surgical procedure that is performed to reduce the size of a large nose or to correct a congenital or acquired nasal deformity in an effort to render the nose more aesthetically pleasing. Bilateral reduction osteotomies (also called lateral osteotomies) are performed along the frontal (also called nasal) processes of the maxilla to reduce the size of the nose, realign deviated nasal bones or a nasal bridge deformity, or alter the width of the osseous nasal vault. On CT, a reduction rhinoplasty is characterized by symmetric defects located at the base of the frontal processes of the maxilla, sometimes with overriding of the fractured segments as a result of the reduction. A reduction rhinoplasty may be difficult to identify by MRI; however, typically the nasal bridge will be unusually straight following a reduction rhinoplasty on sagittal imaging with CT and MRI.

COMPANION CASES

- **Valvular collapse.** The nasal valve is the narrowest portion of the nasal airway. The term valvular collapse is used when this region is overly narrowed. Valvular collapse can be external (ie, anterior) or internal (ie, posterior). An external collapse occurs at the nasal ala level, whereas an internal collapse occurs at the mid aspect of the nose at the level of the lateral nasal cartilages. While there are various causes of valvular collapse, including aging, valvular collapse most commonly occurs following an overly aggressive rhinoplasty or the lack of cartilage reattachment during a rhinoplasty. In both instances, there is subsequent loss of cartilage support. Valvular collapse results in an overly pinched or a depressed appearance of the nose and a reduction of inspired air (particularly during maximal inspiration) because of the cartilage collapse.
- **Saddle-nose deformity.** A saddle-nose deformity represents a focal nasal bridge depression that results from underlying nasal cartilage and osseous destruction. This most often occurs in the setting of granulomatosis with polyangiitis (also called Wegener granulomatosis), sarcoidosis, cocaine use, trauma, or the result of a surgical complication.

Reduction rhinoplasty

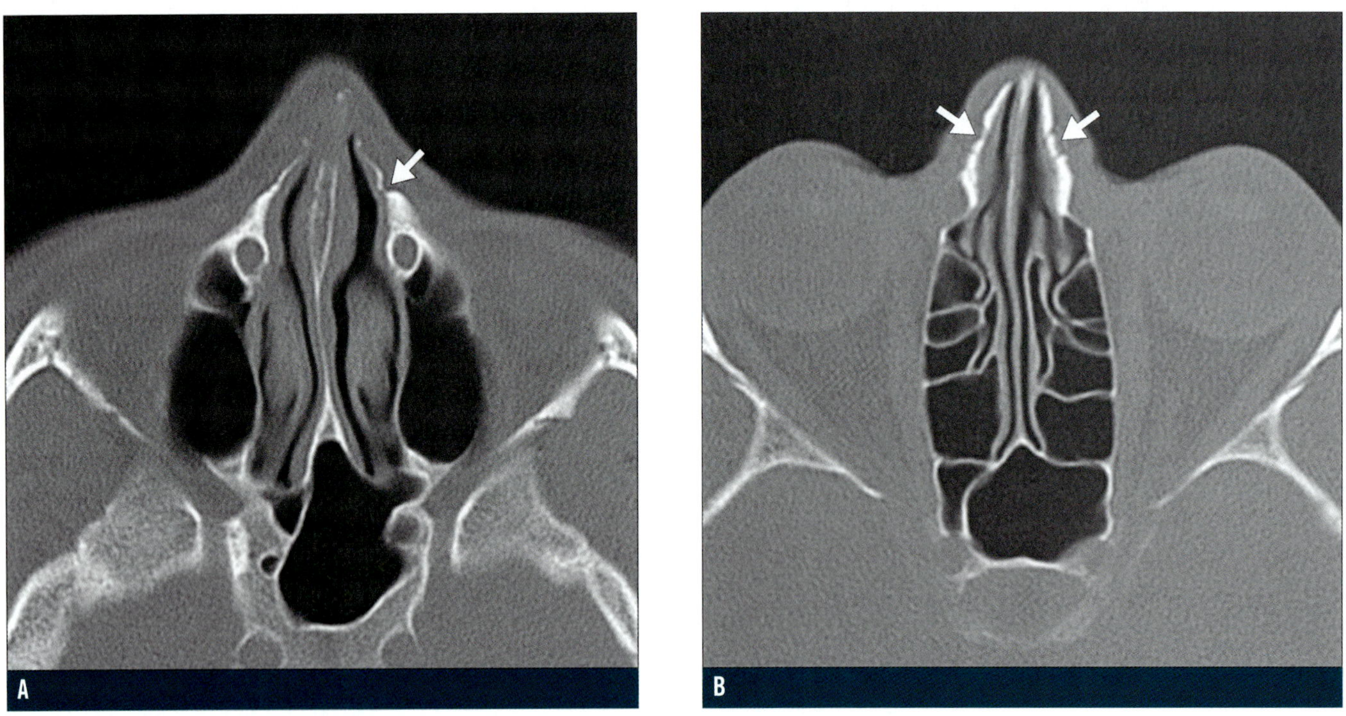

Axial CT images through the nasal bones (**A**, **B**) demonstrate chronic fractures through the frontal processes of the maxilla, compatible with a reduction rhinoplasty (arrows, **A**, **B**). A midline sagittal reformatted CT image through the nose (**C**) demonstrates the reduction rhinoplasty in the sagittal plane with a pronounced upturn of the nasal columella, a complication that may occur if an inordinate amount of nasal tip cartilage is removed during surgery (arrowhead, **C**).

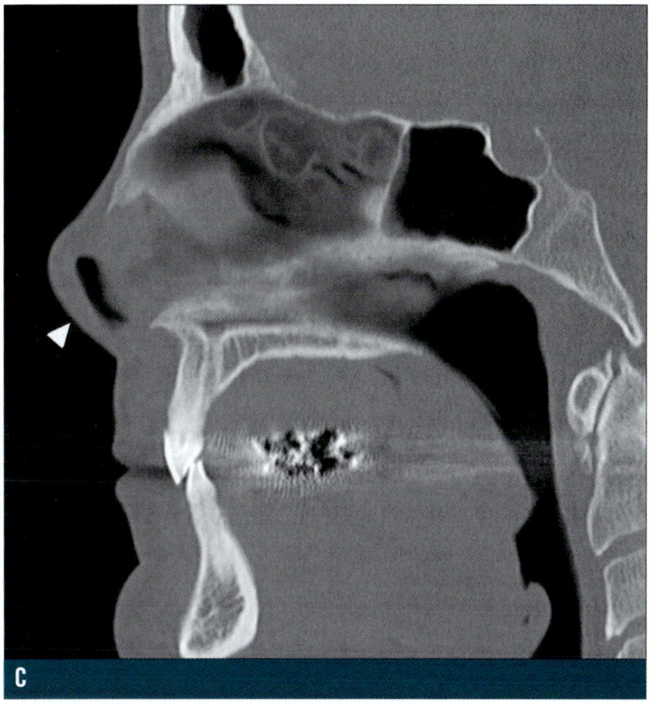

Reduction rhinoplasty

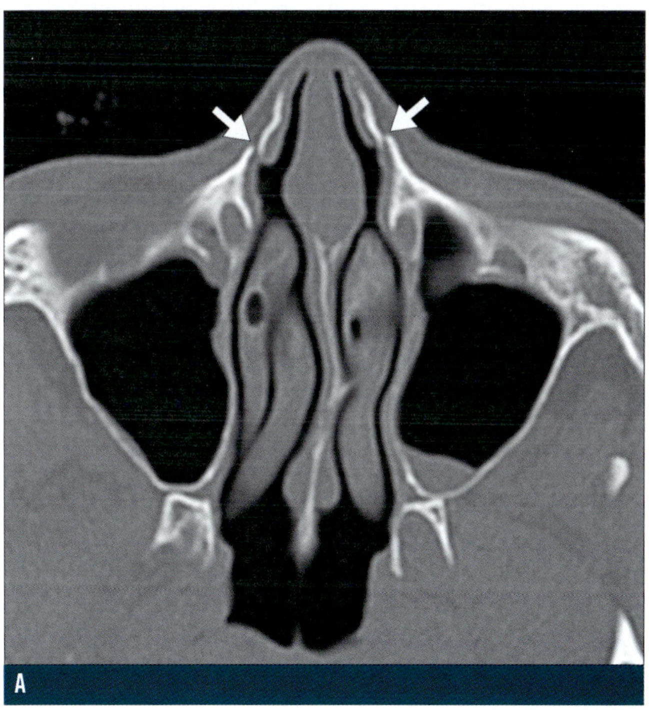

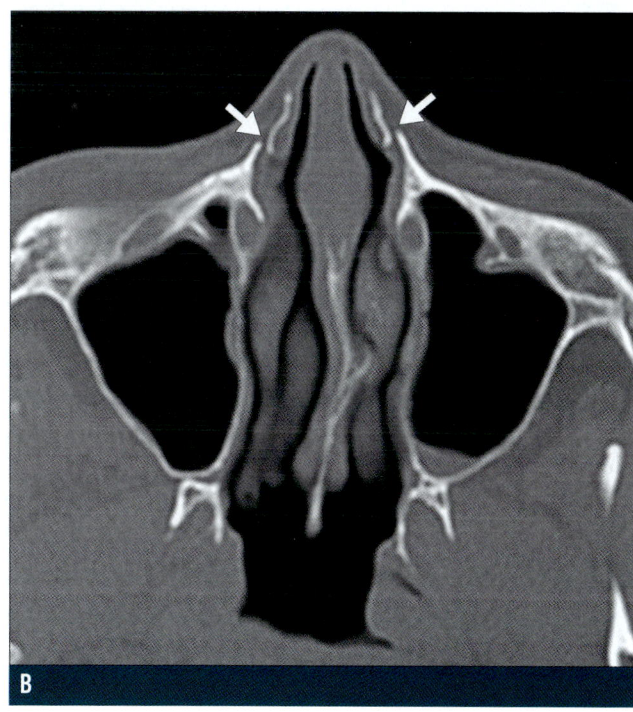

Different patient. Axial CT images through the nose demonstrate chronic osseous defects within the frontal processes of the maxilla (arrows, **A**, **B**). The distal fractured segments of the maxillary frontal processes are reduced medially relative to the proximal fractured segments of the maxillary frontal processes, resulting in a more desirable smaller nasal profile.

Companion case: Valvular collapse

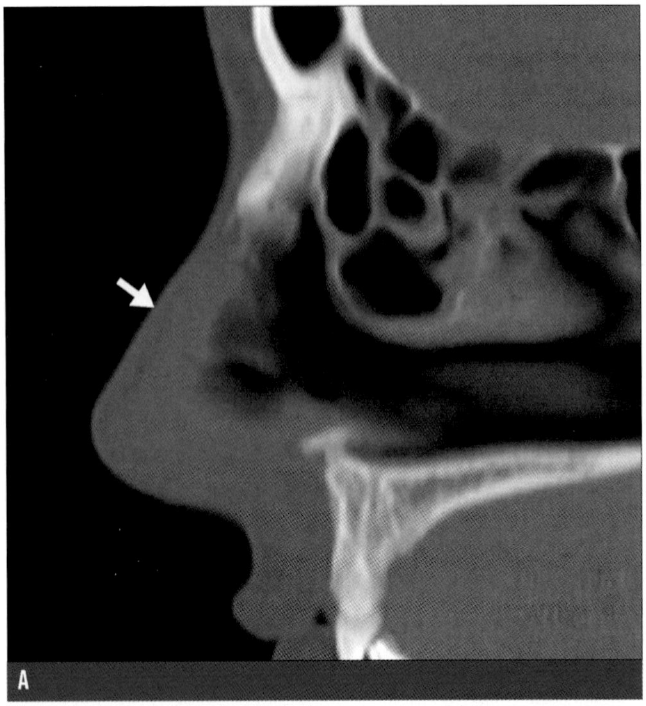

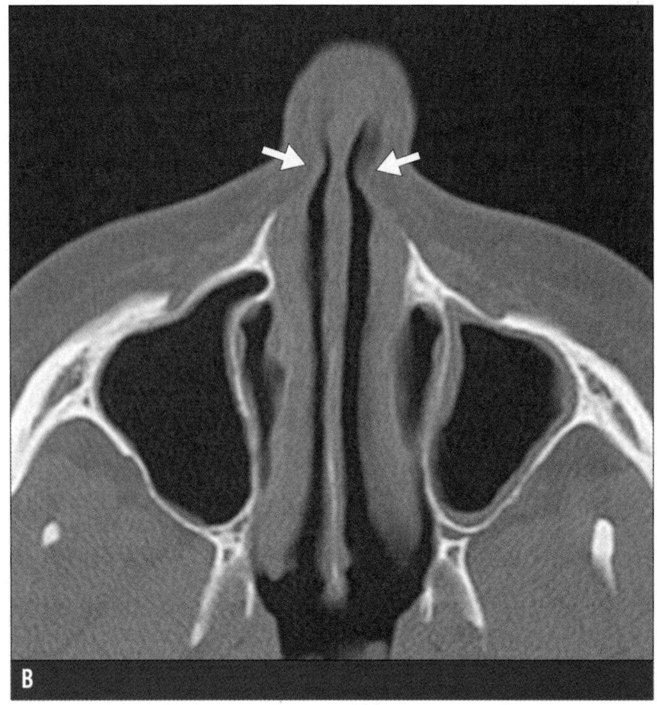

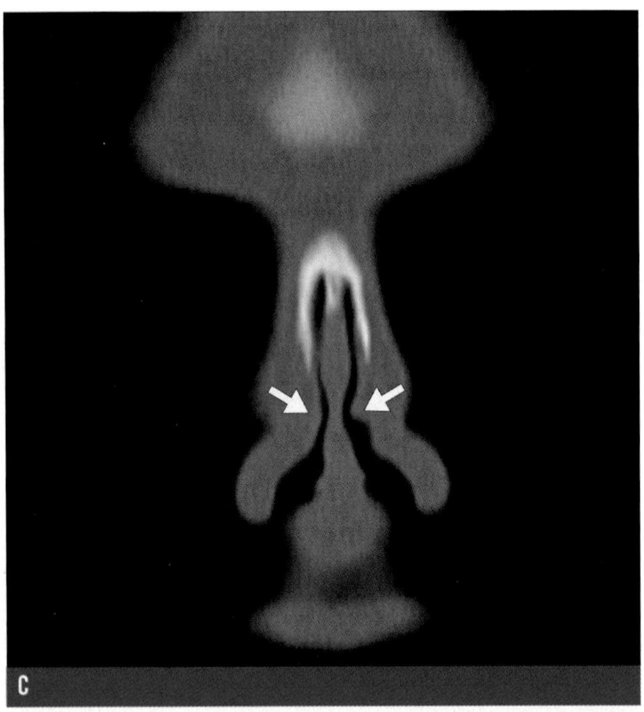

Sagittal reformatted (**A**), axial (**B**), and coronal reformatted (**C**) CT images through nose. Image **A** demonstrates a straightened nasal bridge suggestive of a prior nasal rhinoplasty (arrow, **A**). Images **B** and **C** demonstrate a "pinched" nasal airway appearance compatible with valvular collapse (arrows, **B**, **C**). This valvular collapse was located at the mid aspect of the nose at the level of the lateral nasal cartilages (when cross referencing), compatible with an internal (ie, posterior) valvular collapse.

Companion case: Saddle-nose deformity

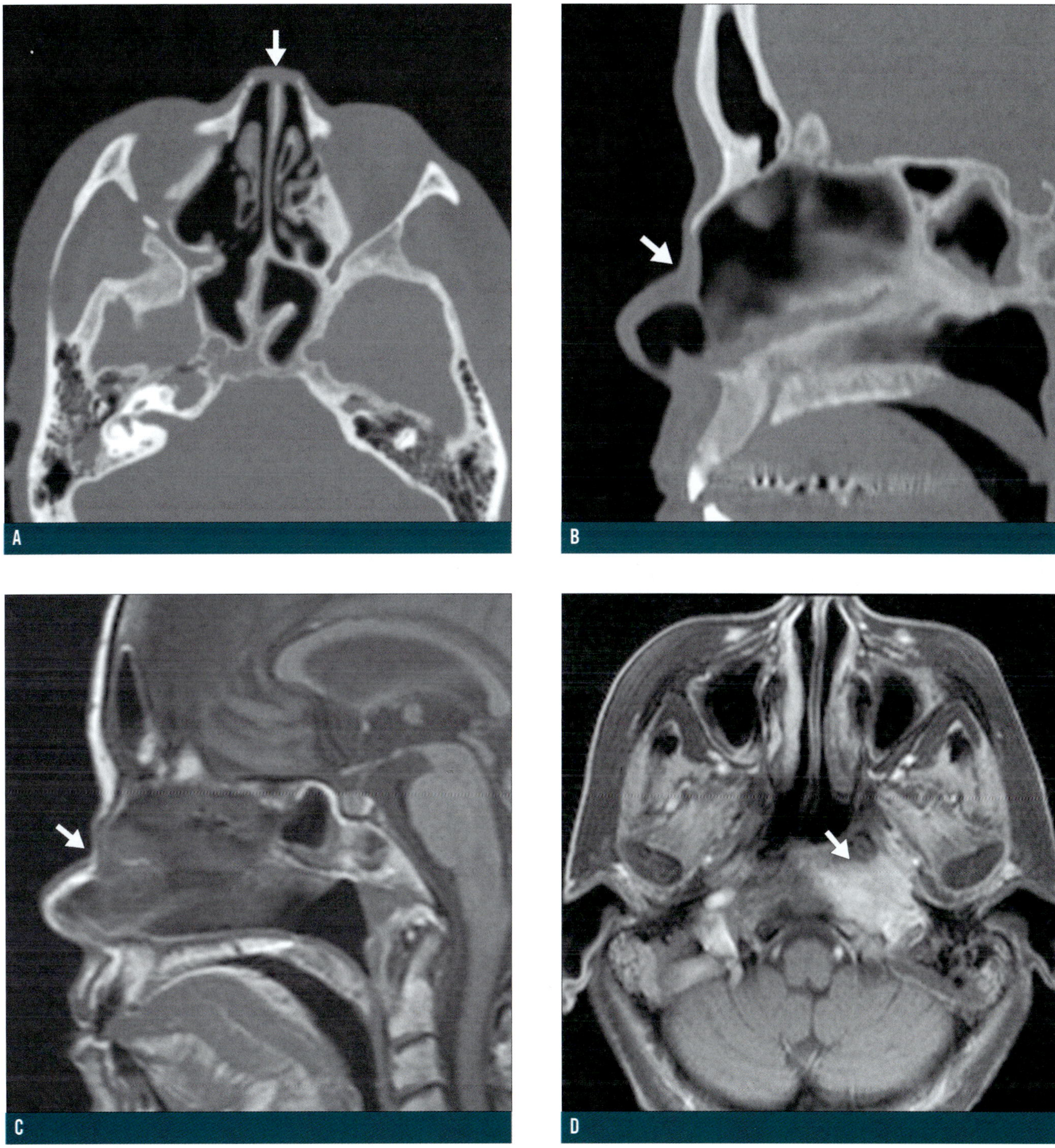

Axial (**A**) and sagittal reformatted (**B**) CT images demonstrate a focal depression along the bridge of the nose in this patient with granulomatosis with polyangiitis (also called Wegener granulomatosis), compatible with a saddle-nose deformity (arrows, **A**, **B**). A sagittal T1-weighted MR image (**C**) demonstrates the same finding (arrow, **C**). A contrast-enhanced axial T1-weighted MR image with fat suppression (**D**) demonstrates a mass at the left aspect of the mid skull base representing an additional area involved by granulomatosis with polyangiitis Wegener granulomatosis (arrow, **D**).

REFERENCES

Conrad K, et al. Applications of GORE-TEX implants in rhinoplasty reexamined after 17 years. *Arch Facial Plast Surg.* 2008;10(4):224-231.

Grammer L. Greenberger, P. Patterson's allergic diseases. *Allergic diseases: Diagnosis and Management.* 7th ed. Philadelphia, PA: Lippincott Williams & Wilkins; 2009.

Park SS. Fundamental principles in aesthetic rhinoplasty. *Clin Exp Otorhinolaryngol.* 2011;4(2):55-66.

Rohrich RJ, Ahmad J. Rhinoplasty. *Plastic Reconstr Surg.* 2011;128(2):49e-73e.

Thomsen J, Balle V, Tos M. Rhinology: A State of the Art : Proceedings of the Xvth Congress of the European Rhinologic Society and the Xiiith International Symposium on European Rhinologic Society Congress, 1994.

Schatz CJ, Ginat DT. Imaging features of rhinoplasty. *AJNR Am J Neuroradiol.* 2014;35(2):216-222.

CASE 10 Augmentation and reconstruction rhinoplasty

An augmentation rhinoplasty is a form of rhinoplasty whereby autogenous and/or alloplastic material is surgically implanted along the nose, such as the dorsum (nasal bridge) or the radix (root), in order to alter the nasal contour and improve nasal aesthetics. Materials that may be used for nasal augmentation include autologous bone and/or cartilage harvested from septal, otic, or intercostal cartilages as well as alloplastic materials composed of silicone, polytetrafluoroethylene, porous polyacrylamide gel, and calcium hydroxylapatite. Complications of nasal augmentation include infection, implant extrusion, and implant deformity.

Nasal tip reconstruction is a type of rhinoplasty that is performed for cosmesis as well as for maintenance of function. The shape of the normal nasal tip is determined by the shape and location of the alar cartilages as well as by the overlying skin. In the case of a large nasal tip, cartilage trimming and/or contouring may be performed to reduce the size of the nasal tip. For diminutive nasal tips, a columellar strut (discussed below) or a prosthetic tip graft may be placed to augment the nasal tip. Occasionally, a bone graft obtained from the nasal dorsum during a dorsal hump resection may be utilized for nasal tip augmentation.

The columella, Latin for "little column," represents the skin covered soft tissue that separates the nostrils at the inferior aspect of the nose. The columella is critical for nasal tip support. Columella reconstruction may be used to correct congenital, infectious, posttraumatic, or postsurgical defects affecting the columella. An abnormally widened columella may be narrowed by excision. Columellar augmentation may be performed in conjunction with nasal bridge augmentation via L-strut implants, where the long portion of the "L" is placed along the nasal dorsum and the short portion is placed along the columella.

COMPANION CASE

- **Nasal ala cartilage mineralization.** Just like cartilages elsewhere in the body, incidental mineralization of the nasal ala cartilages may occur. Nasal ala cartilage mineralization may result from benign senescence, related to implants placed for nasal augmentation, or a sequela of prior trauma/hemorrhage. Mineralization of a cartilage implant performed for nasal augmentation may develop 5 to 10 years following cartilage implantation, usually without deformation. However, of the various implants that may mineralize, a silicone implant that mineralizes is the type that is most likely to result in soft tissue deformation.

Nasal augmentation

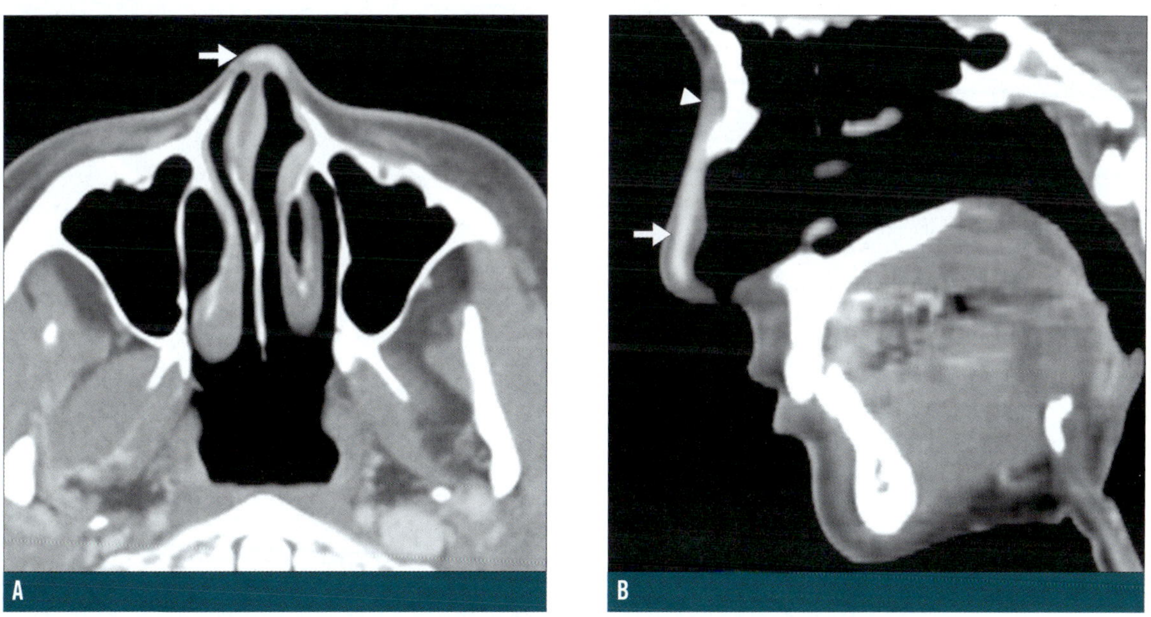

Axial (**A**) and sagittal reformatted (**B**) noncontrast CT images demonstrate a thin, hyperdense surgical prosthesis extending along the nasal dorsum (arrows, **A**, **B**) and nasal radix (arrowhead, **B**), compatible with a nasal augmentation procedure. The implant used in this case was likely constructed of polytetrafluoroethylene.

Nasal augmentation

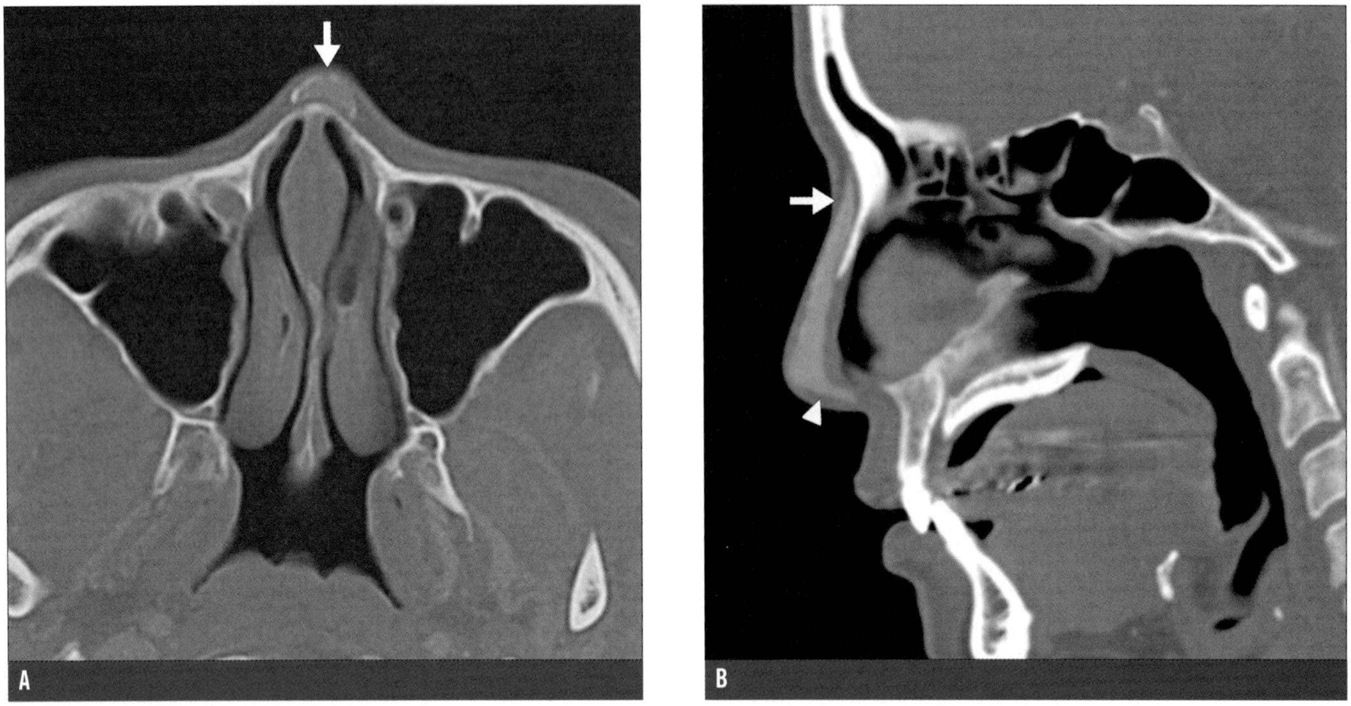

Different patient. Axial (**A**) and sagittal reformatted (**B**) CT images demonstrate a surgical prosthesis extending from the radix of the nose (arrow, **A, B**) to the columella (arrowhead, **B**), consistent with nasal augmentation. The implant used in this case was likely constructed from silicone.

Nasal augmentation

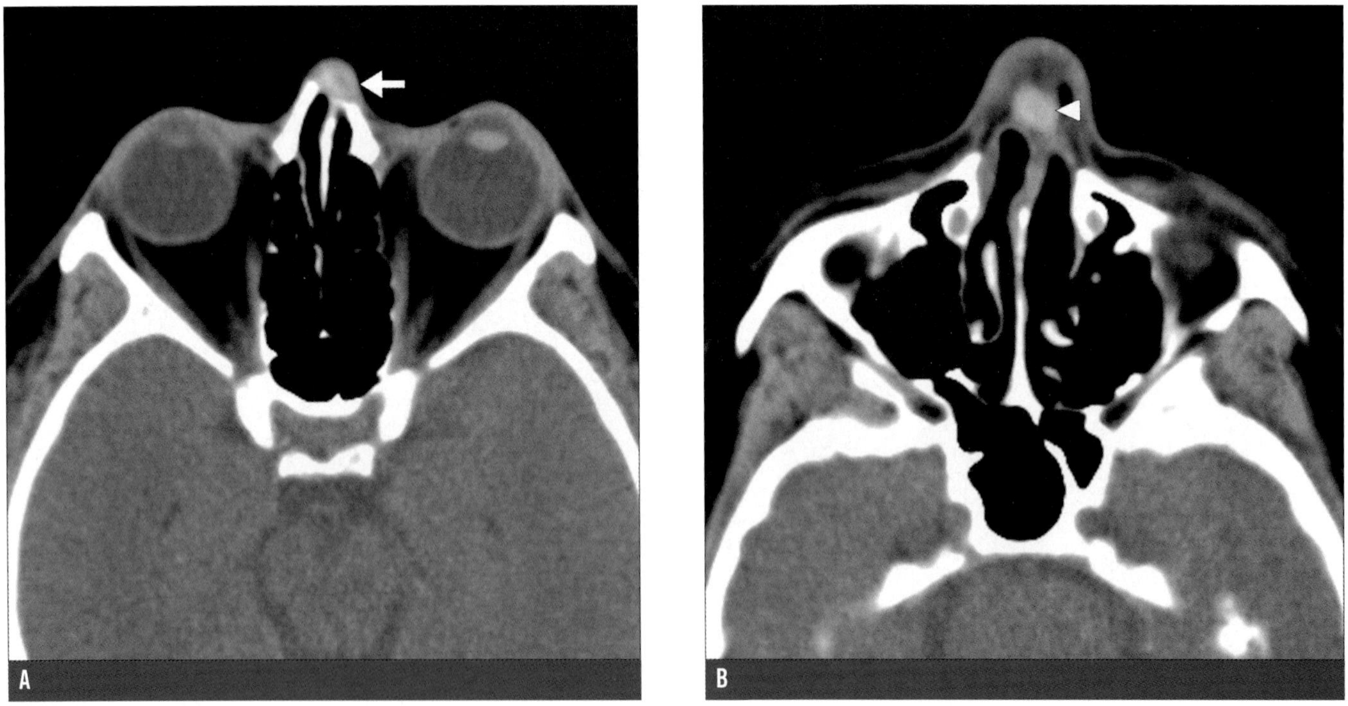

Different patient. Axial (**A**, **B**) and sagittal reformatted (**C**, **D**) unenhanced CT images. There is a surgical prosthesis placed along the nasal radix (long arrow, **C**) and a portion of the nasal dorsum (short arrows, **A**, **D**). This prosthesis was incorporated into the nasal septum (arrowheads, **B**, **D**).

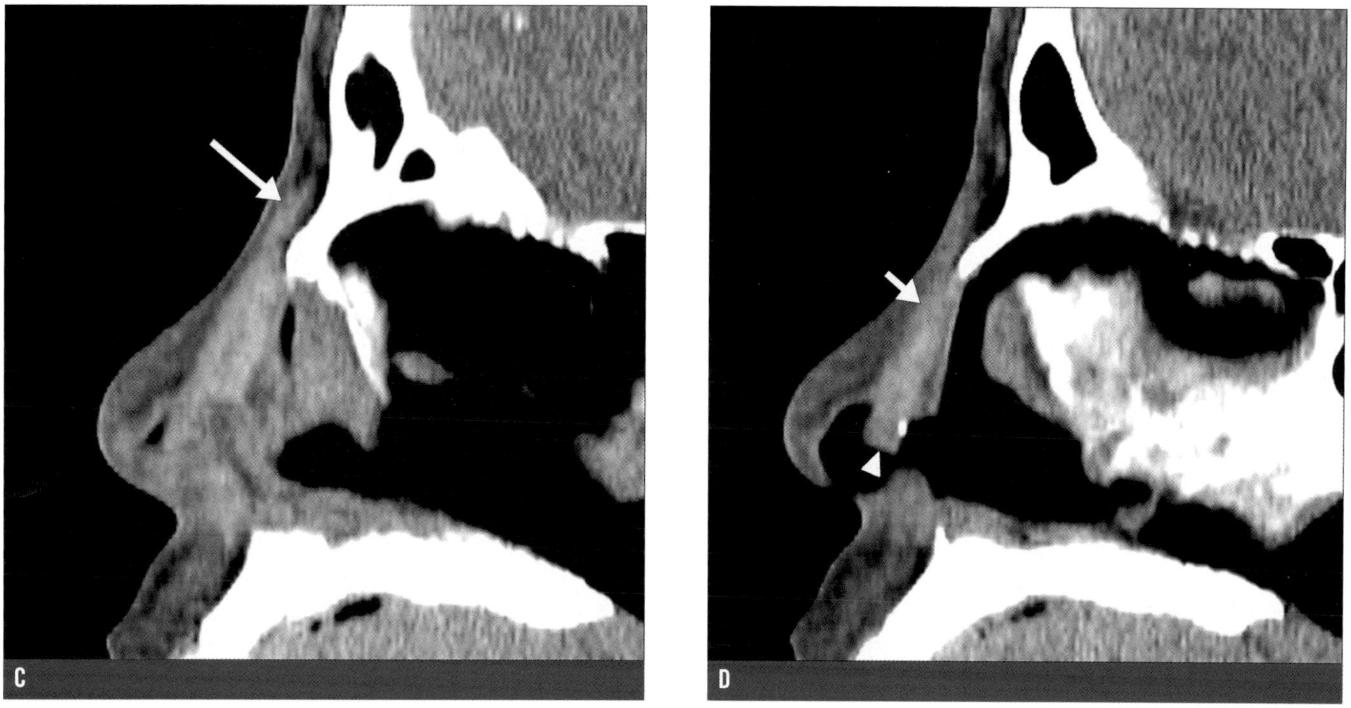

Nasal augmentation and reduction rhinoplasty

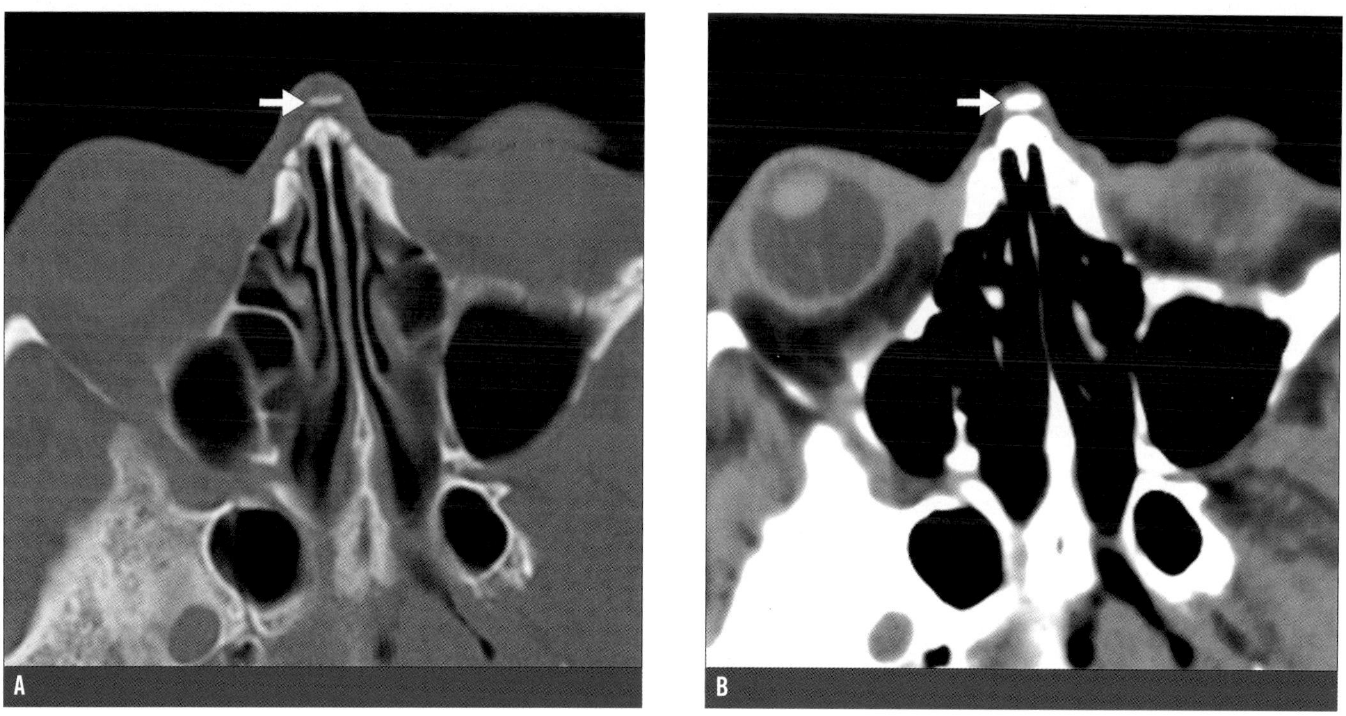

Unenhanced axial CT images viewed with a bone window (**A**) and soft tissue window (**B**) demonstrate thin bone graft along the radix of the nose (arrows, **A, B**). A sagittal reformatted image viewed with a bone window (**C**) demonstrates the finding to augment and parallel the nasal radix (arrow, **C**). A more caudal CT image relative to images **A** and **B** viewed with a bone window (**D**) demonstrates concomitant reduction rhinoplasty changes (arrows, **D**).

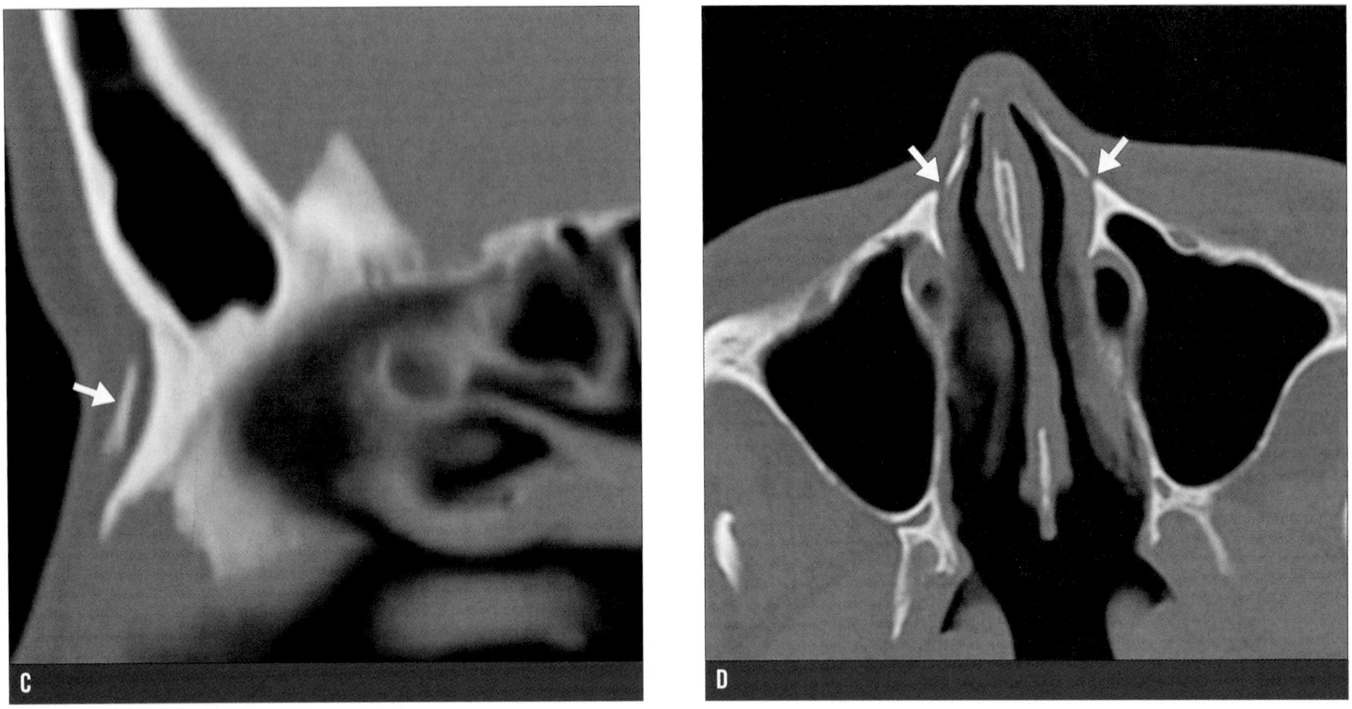

Nasal augmentation

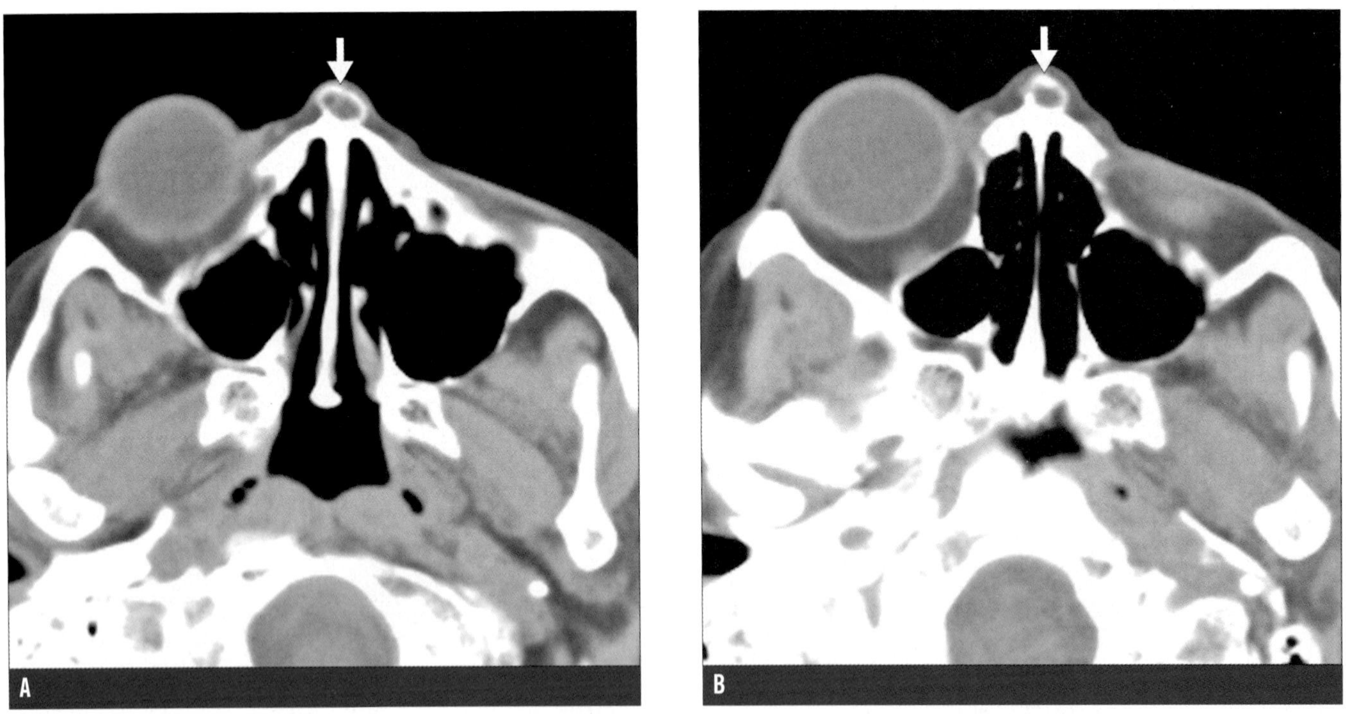

Unenhanced axial CT images viewed with an intermediate window (**A**, **B**) demonstrate an oval, peripherally hyperdense structure located in the subcutaneous soft tissues at the dorsum of the nose, compatible with a prior nasal augmentation procedure (arrows, **A**, **B**).

Nasal augmentation

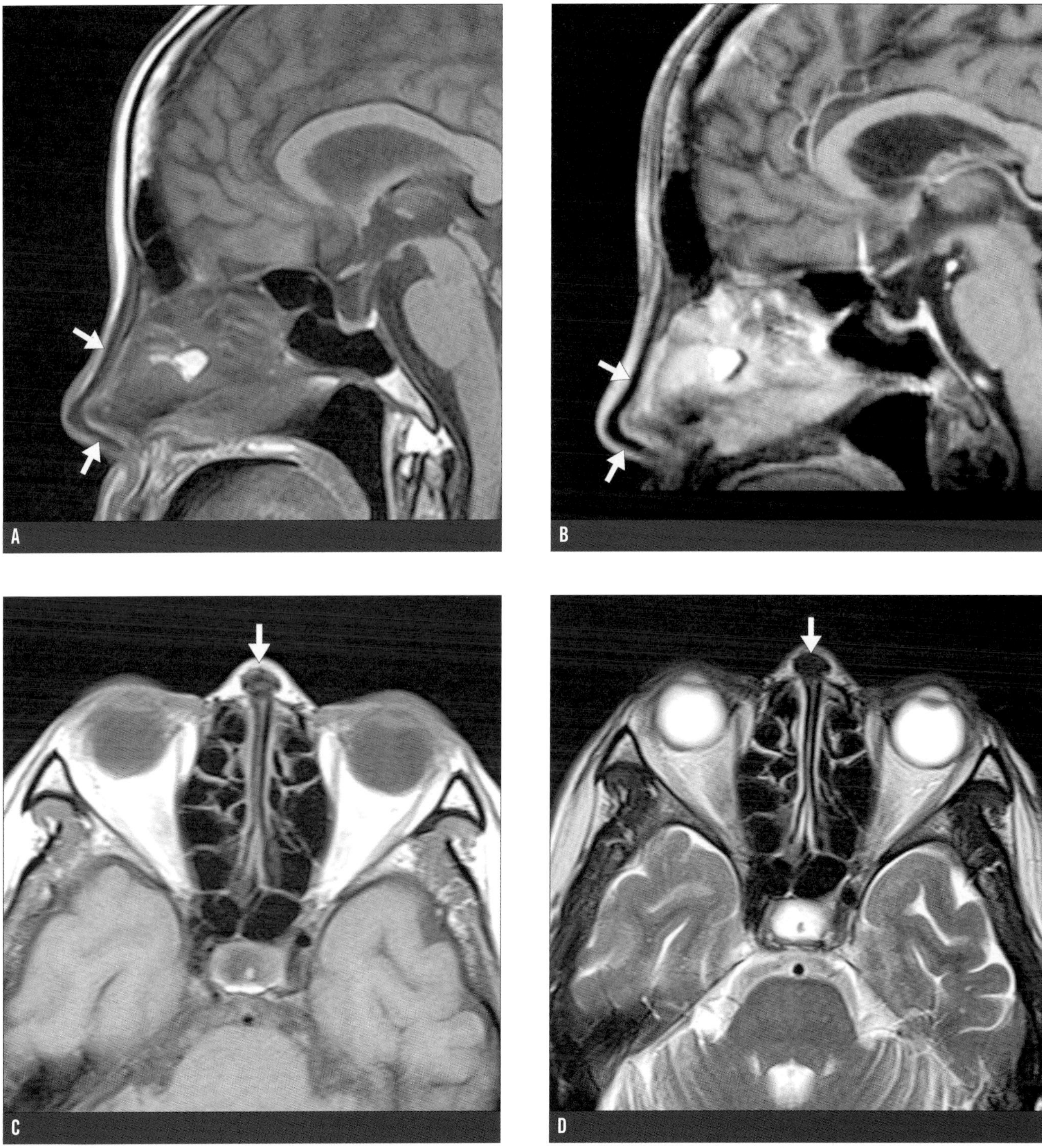

Different patient. Precontrast sagittal T1 (**A**), postcontrast sagittal T1 with fat suppression (**B**), precontrast axial T1 (**C**), and axial T2 (**D**) MR images demonstrate a linear nose prosthesis extending along the nasal bridge and along the columella, compatible with a prior nasal augmentation procedure utilizing an L-strut implant (arrows, **A**-**D**).

Nasal tip reconstruction

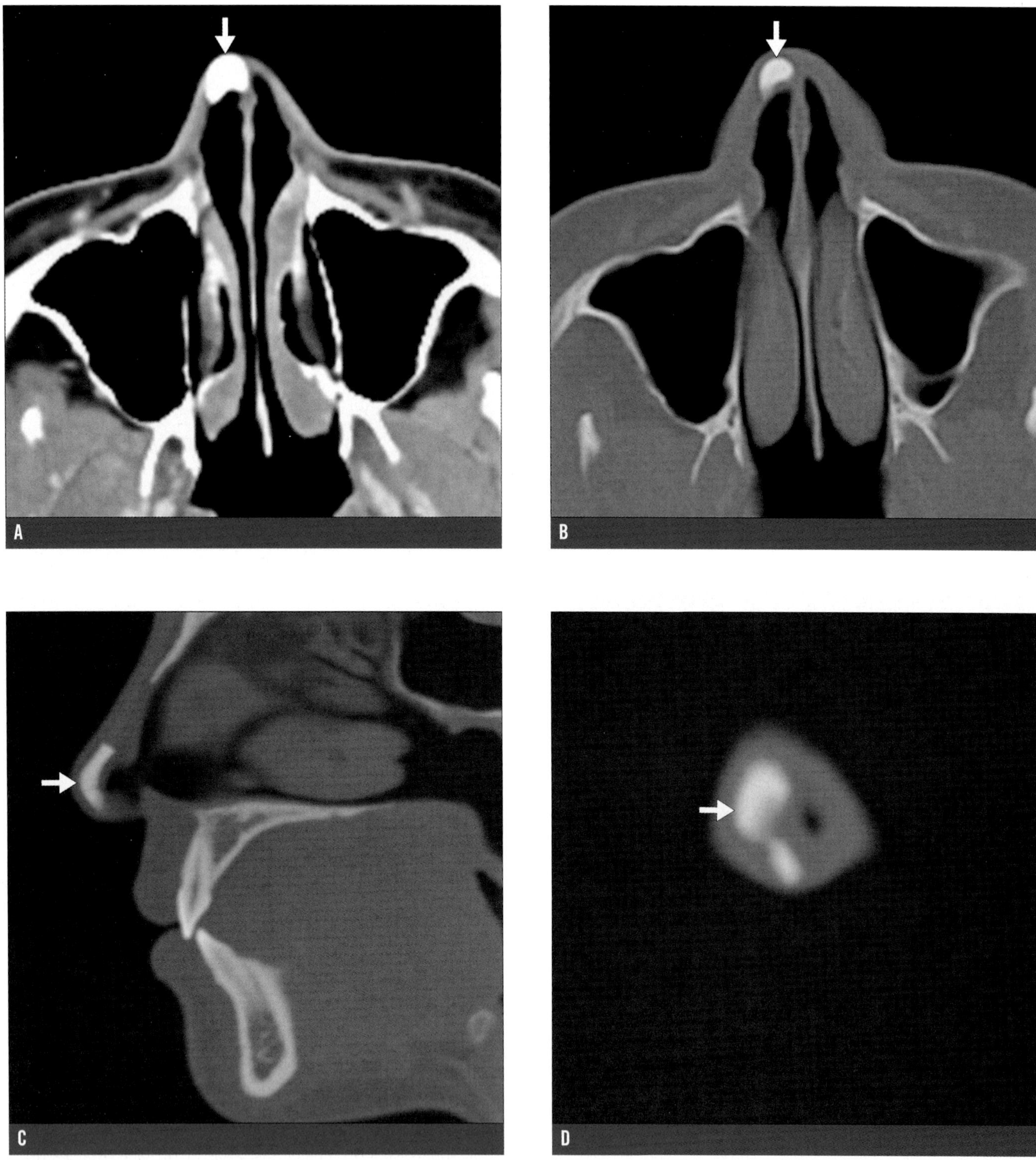

Unenhanced axial CT images viewed a soft tissue window (**A**) and bone window (**B**) as well as sagittal reformatted (**C**) and coronal reformatted (**D**) CT images viewed with a bone window demonstrate an ossific density over the right aspect of the nasal tip, compatible with nasal tip reconstruction (arrows, **A-D**).

Columella reconstruction

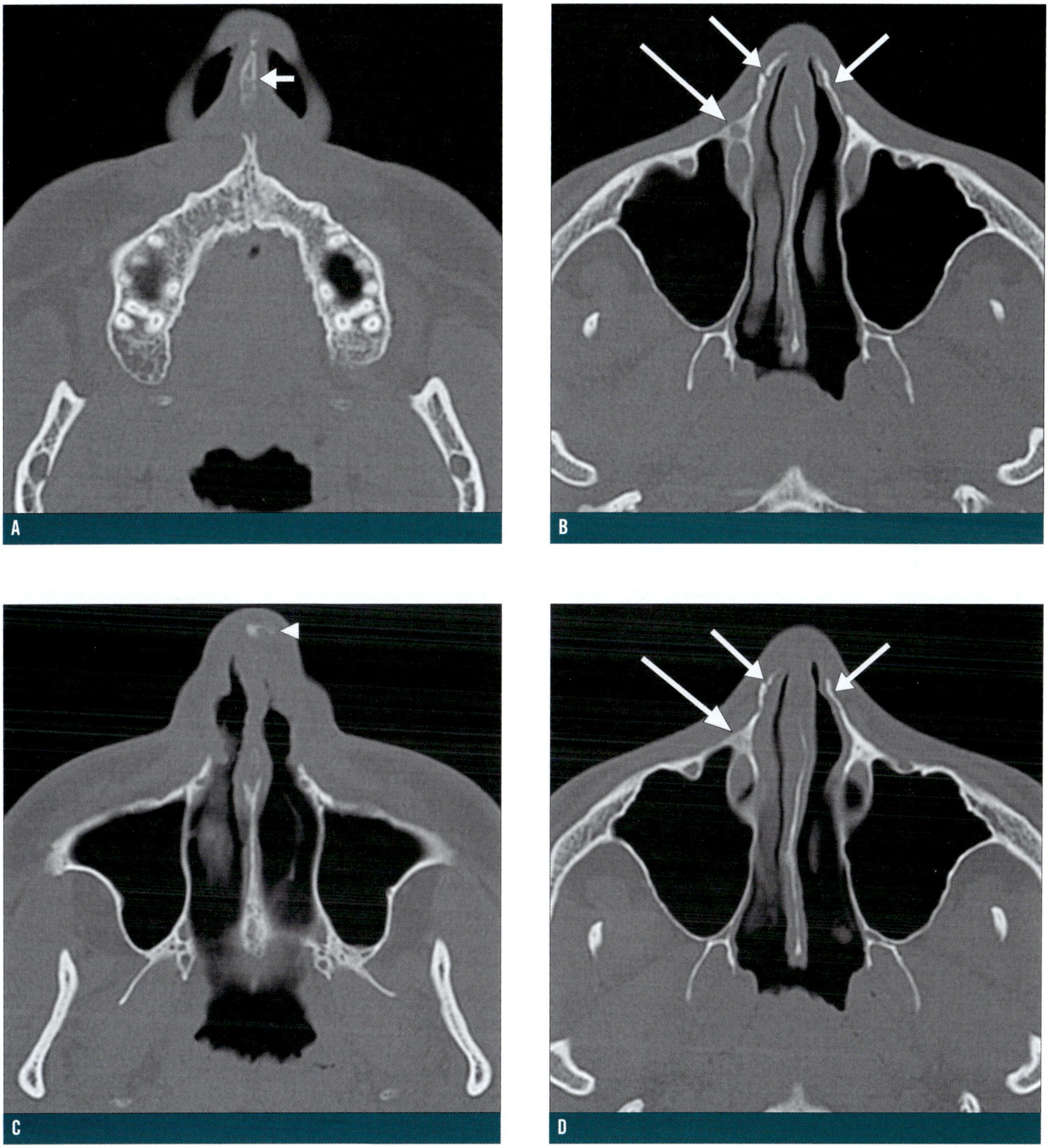

Axial (**A-D**), coronal reformatted (**E**), and sagittal reformatted (**F**) CT images through the nose. There is ossification along the columella (short arrows, **A, E, F**) as well as near the tip of the nose (arrowheads, **C, F**), compatible with bone placed for nasal reconstructive purposes. Multiple old fractures involving the nasal arch likely represent postoperative changes related to a reduction rhinoplasty (medium arrows, **B, D**). Image **F** demonstrates pronounced straightening of the nasal bridge, also compatible with prior nasal reconstructive surgery. Incidental note is also made of fibrous dysplasia involving the right frontal process of the maxilla (long arrows, **B, D**).

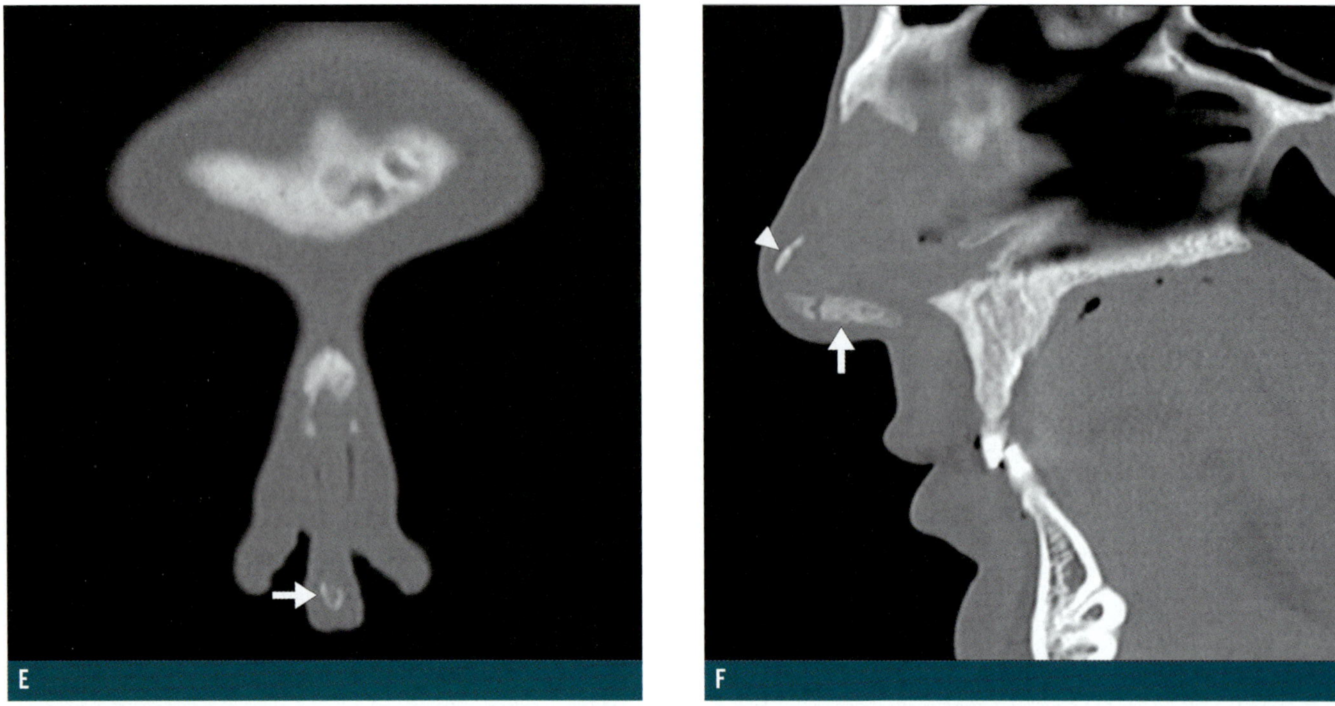

Companion case: Nasal ala cartilage mineralization

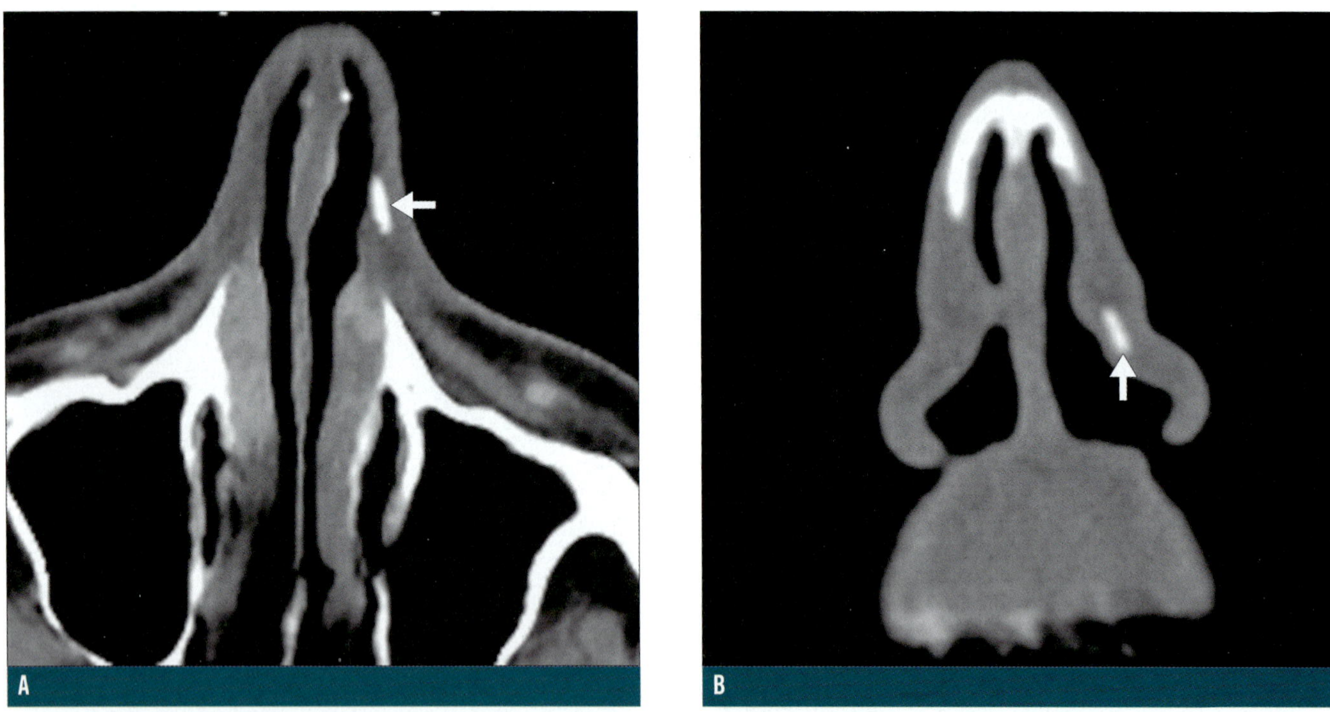

Axial (**A**) and coronal reformatted (**B**) CT images demonstrate linear mineralization within the left nasal ala, compatible with incidental mineralization of the left nasal ala cartilage.

REFERENCES

Becker DG, Park SS. *Revision Rhinoplasty*. New York: Thieme, New York and Stuttgart; 2008.

Faris C, Vuyk HD. Reconstruction of nasal tip and columella. *Facial Plast Surg Clin North Am*. 2011;19:25-62.

Huizing EH, De Groot JAM. *Functional Reconstructive Nasal Surgery*. New York: Thieme, New York and Stuttgart; 2003.

Pak MW, et al. Late complications of nasal augmentation using silicone implants. *J Laryngol Otol*. 1998;112:1074-1077.

Schatz CJ, Ginat DT. Imaging features of rhinoplasty. *AJNR Am J Neuroradiol*. 2014;35(2):216-222.

Thomsen J, Balle V, Tos M. Rhinology: A State of the Art: Proceedings of the Xvth Congress of the European Rhinologic Society and the Xiiith International Symposium on European Rhinologic Society Congress, 1994. New York: Kugler publications, NY; 1995.

CASE 11 Facial piercings and rings

While ear piercing has been around for thousands of years, facial piercing has become increasingly prevalent in the last 40 years. Common sites of facial piercing include the eyebrows, nose, cheeks, lips, tongue frenulum, and oral tongue. There are multiple complications that have been described with body piercing, with infection being the most common. Other reported complications include granulomatous reaction, scarring or keloids, perichondritis, gingival damage, and dental fractures. Serious complications, such as sepsis or airway obstruction, are rare but have been reported.

Nose ring and right nose piercing

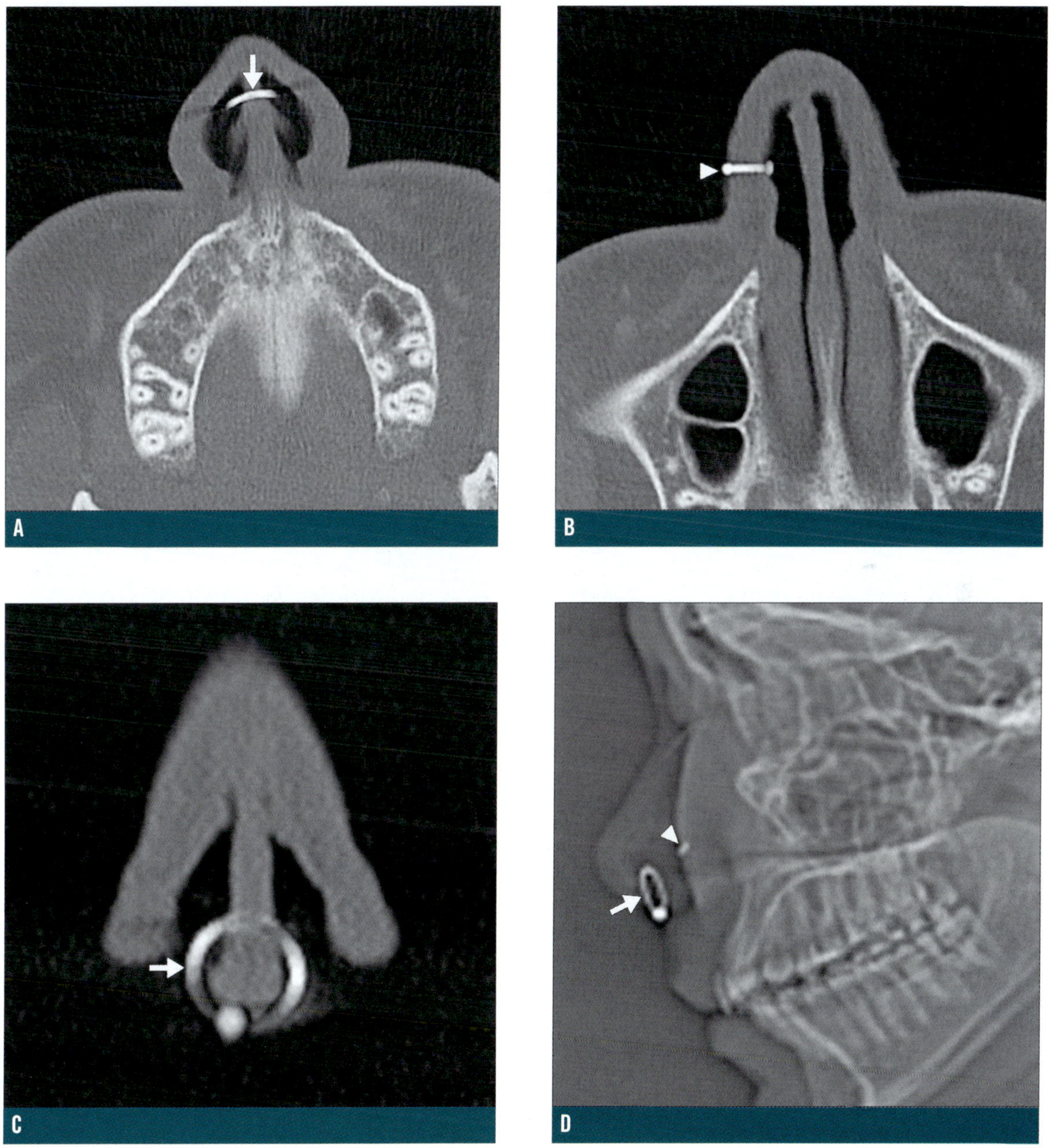

Axial (**A**, **B**) and coronal reformatted (**C**) CT images demonstrate a metallic nose ring through the columella (arrows, **A**, **C**) and a metallic nose piercing in the right nasal ala (arrowhead, **B**). A sagittal scout image from the same CT study (**D**) also demonstrates the nose ring (arrow, **D**) and nasal ala piercing (arrowhead, **D**).

Eyebrow ring

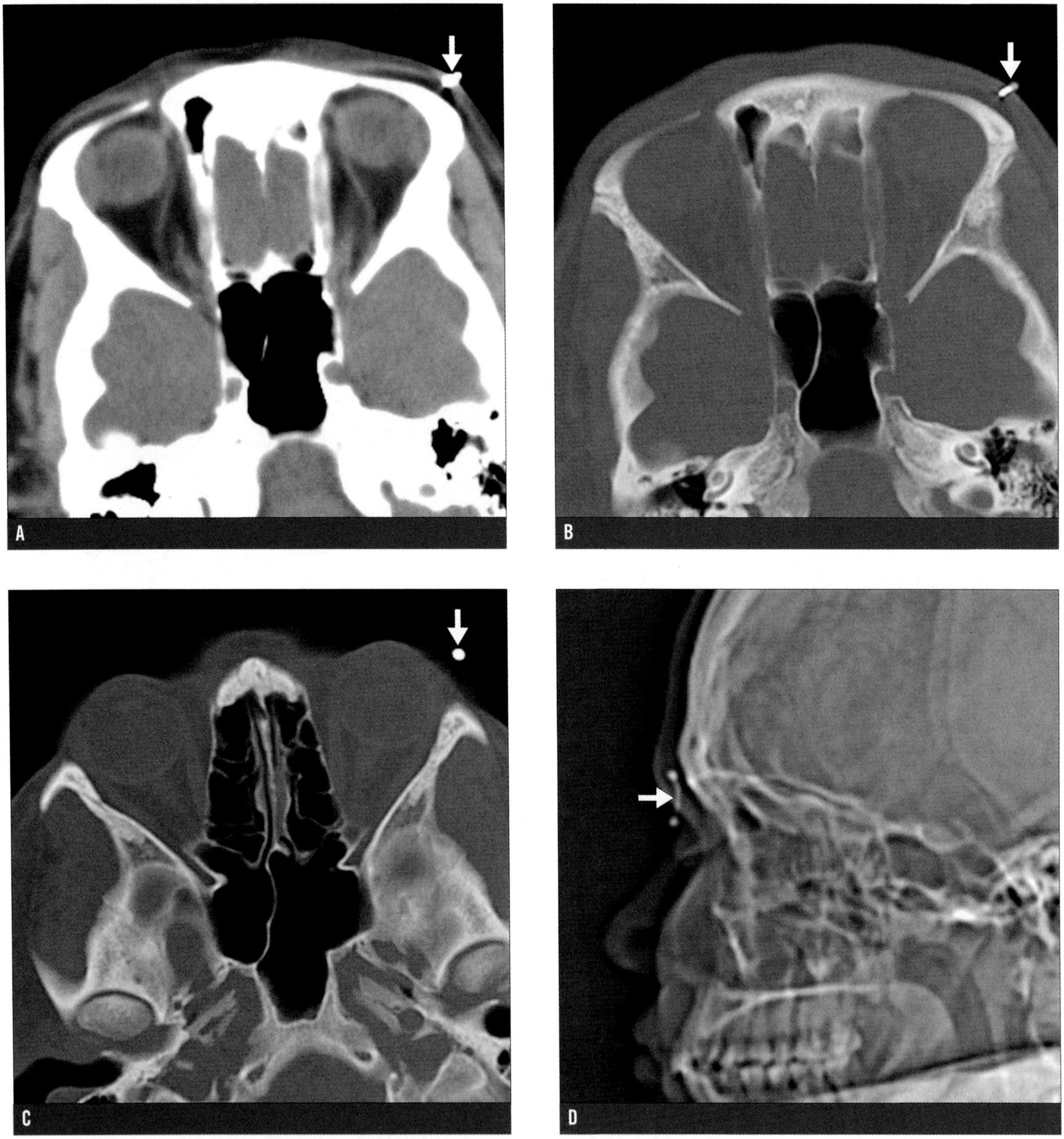

Unenhanced axial CT images viewed with a soft tissue window (**A**) and bone window (**B**, **C**) as well as a sagittal scout image (**D**) demonstrate a curvilinear metallic structure along the left supraorbital soft tissues, compatible with an eyebrow ring (arrows, **A-D**).

Lip piercing

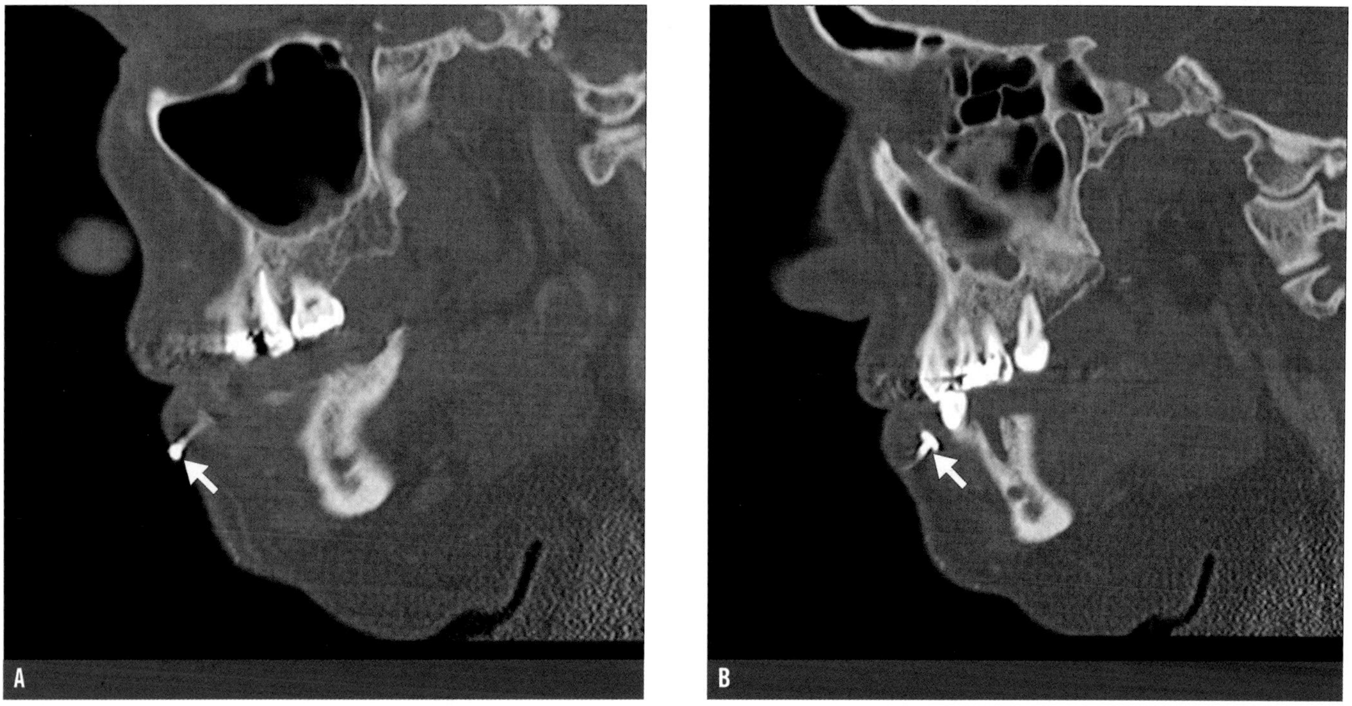

Sagittal reformatted CT images (**A**, **B**) demonstrate a metallic piercing along the lower lip (arrows, **A**, **B**).

REFERENCES

Lopez-Jornet P, Navarro-Guardiola C, Camacho-Alonso F, Vincente-Ortega V, Yanez-Gascon J. Oral and facial piercings: a case series and review of the literature. *Inter J Dermatol.* 2006;45:805-809.

Stirn A. Body piercing: medical consequences and psychological motivations. *Lancet.* 2003;361:1205-1215.

Waugh M. Body piercing: where and how. *Clin Dermatol.* 2007;25:407-411.

Vascular channel in the diploic space of the maxillary frontal process

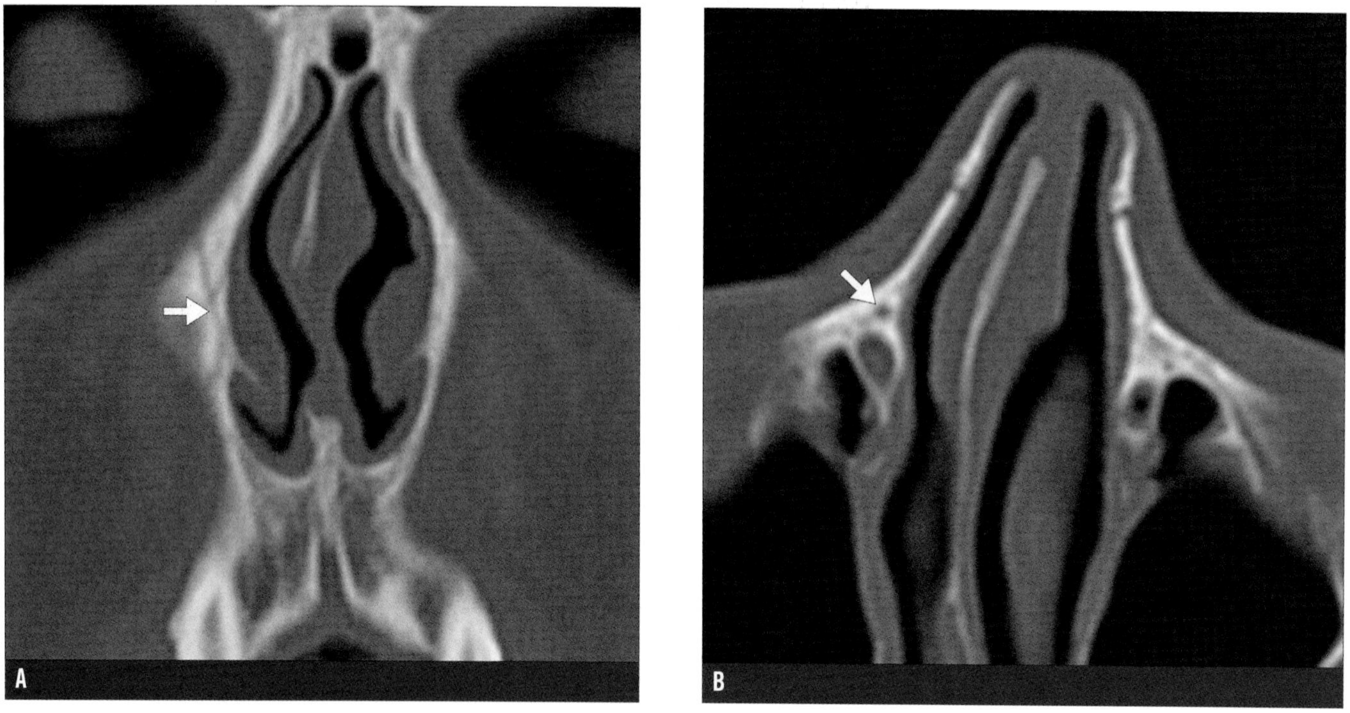

A coronal reformatted CT image (**A**) demonstrates a vertically oriented lucency that could be mistaken for a fracture (arrow, **A**). However, an axial CT image (**B**) demonstrates that this finding corresponds to a round lucency isolated within the diploic space of the frontal process of the maxilla, compatible with an incidental vascular channel and not a fracture (arrow, **B**).

Zygomaticotemporal suture

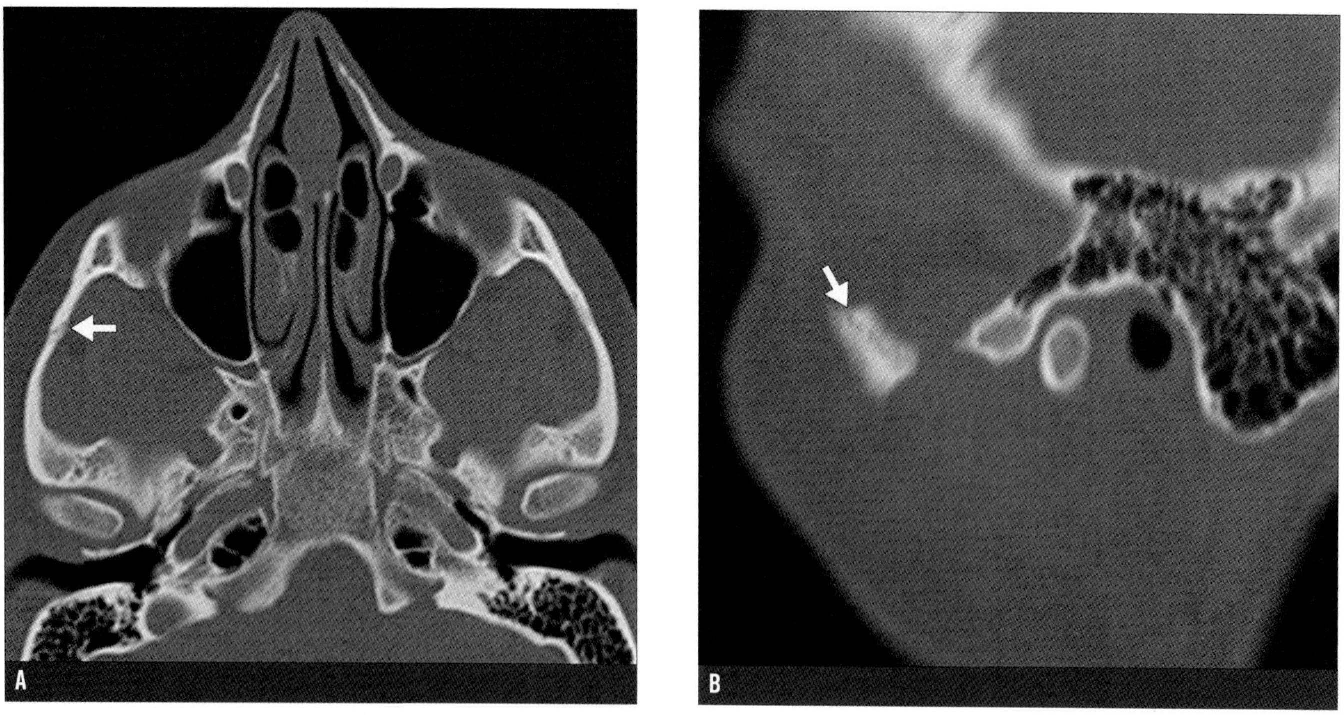

An axial CT image (**A**) and a sagittal reformatted CT image through the right zygomatic arch (**B**) demonstrate a finely serrated lucency through the mid aspect of the right zygomatic arch, compatible with a normal zygomaticotemporal suture (arrows, **A**, **B**). This suture joins the temporal process of the zygomatic bone with the zygomatic process of the temporal bone.

Companion case: Nondisplaced zygomatic arch fracture

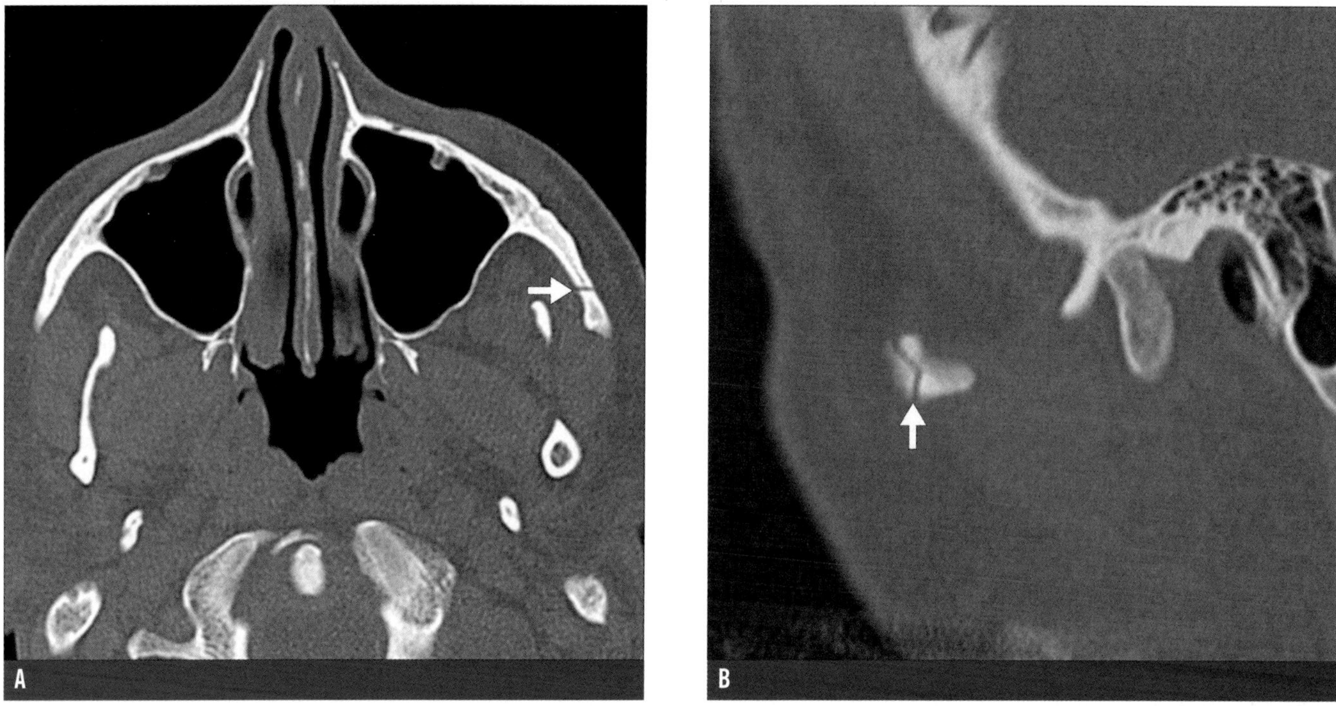

An axial CT image (**A**) and a sagittal reformatted CT image through the left zygomatic arch (**B**) demonstrate a discrete lucency through the left zygomatic arch (arrows, **A, B**) which is not identified involving the visualized right zygomatic arch on image **A** (nor was it identified on the remaining images through the right zygomatic arch that are not shown). Moreover, the lucency through the left zygomatic arch has margins that are not sclerotic and lacks a fine serrated margin typically identified with a suture. The patient had trauma to the left zygomatic bone and the finding is compatible with a nondisplaced acute left zygomatic arch fracture.

REFERENCES

Aviv RI, Casselman J. Orbital imaging: part 1. Normal anatomy. *Clin Radiol*. 2005;60:279-287.

Connor SEJ, Tan G, Fernando R, Chaudhury N. Computed tomography pseudofractures of the mid face and skull base. *Clin Radiol*. 2005;60:1268-1279.

Hopper RA, Salemy S, Sze RW. Diagnosis of midface fractures with CT: what the surgeon needs to know. *Radiographics*. 2006;26:783-793.

Facial reanimation surgical techniques are performed to treat facial paralysis. There are several different types of facial reanimation techniques which are broadly characterized into neural, musculofascial transpositions, facial plastic surgeries, and facial prostheses. The neural and musculofascial transpositions will be discussed here, whereas facial plastic surgery and facial prostheses are discussed elsewhere in this chapter.

The type of neural technique employed depends on several factors. If the facial nerve is transected but can be reapproximated, then a primary nerve repair may be performed. However, if the nerve cannot be reapproximated, then a nerve interposition graft from a donor nerve, such as the sural nerve, may be utilized. If the proximal end of the facial nerve is not accessible, a crossover nerve anastomosis technique could be considered. A crossover nerve technique utilizes a portion of a regional nerve (typically the hypoglossal nerve) and attaches it to the transected facial nerve. This is achieved by splitting a portion of the donor nerve in a longitudinal fashion (while maintaining the integrity of the remaining donor nerve), reflecting the split portion of the donor nerve superiorly toward the transected facial nerve, and attaching this portion of the donor nerve via an end-to-end neurorrhaphy to the transected facial nerve. However, using this technique entails risk to the donor nerve end organ; in the case of the hypoglossal nerve, there is a risk of developing ipsilateral tongue atrophy.

Occasionally, a facial nerve repair is not an option, either due to technical limitations or because of prohibitive surgical risks with the crossover technique. Additionally, an inadequate or failed treatment response with reinnervation techniques can occur. In these settings, other facial reanimation techniques, such as musculofascial transposition, are an option. Musculofascial transposition techniques may be performed with regional muscles and/or their tendons, such as the masseter or temporalis muscles/tendons, or with distal muscle free flaps such as with the palmaris longus or gracilis muscles. One of the more common musculofascial reanimation surgical techniques is the temporalis tendon transfer, which entails performing an osteotomy through the coronoid process of the mandible and mobilizing the temporalis tendon. The tendon is then attached to the muscles at the corner of the mouth, a region which is referred to as the modiolus. If the tendon is not long enough to attach to the modiolus, then a fascia lata interposition graft may be utilized.

COMPANION CASE

- **Zygomaticus major muscle full-thickness tear.** The zygomaticus major muscle is a paired muscle of facial expression that extends from the zygomatic bone to the modiolus. The function of the zygomaticus major muscle is to allow one to smile by drawing the modiolus superiorly and posteriorly. Therefore, a deep laceration of the zygomaticus major muscle severely impairs the ability to smile on the side of injury. On axial imaging, the zygomaticus major muscle is located immediately anterior to the facial vein and parallels the anteromedial aspect of the Stensen duct, the latter traversing immediately posterior to the facial vein.

Reanimation for facial paralysis

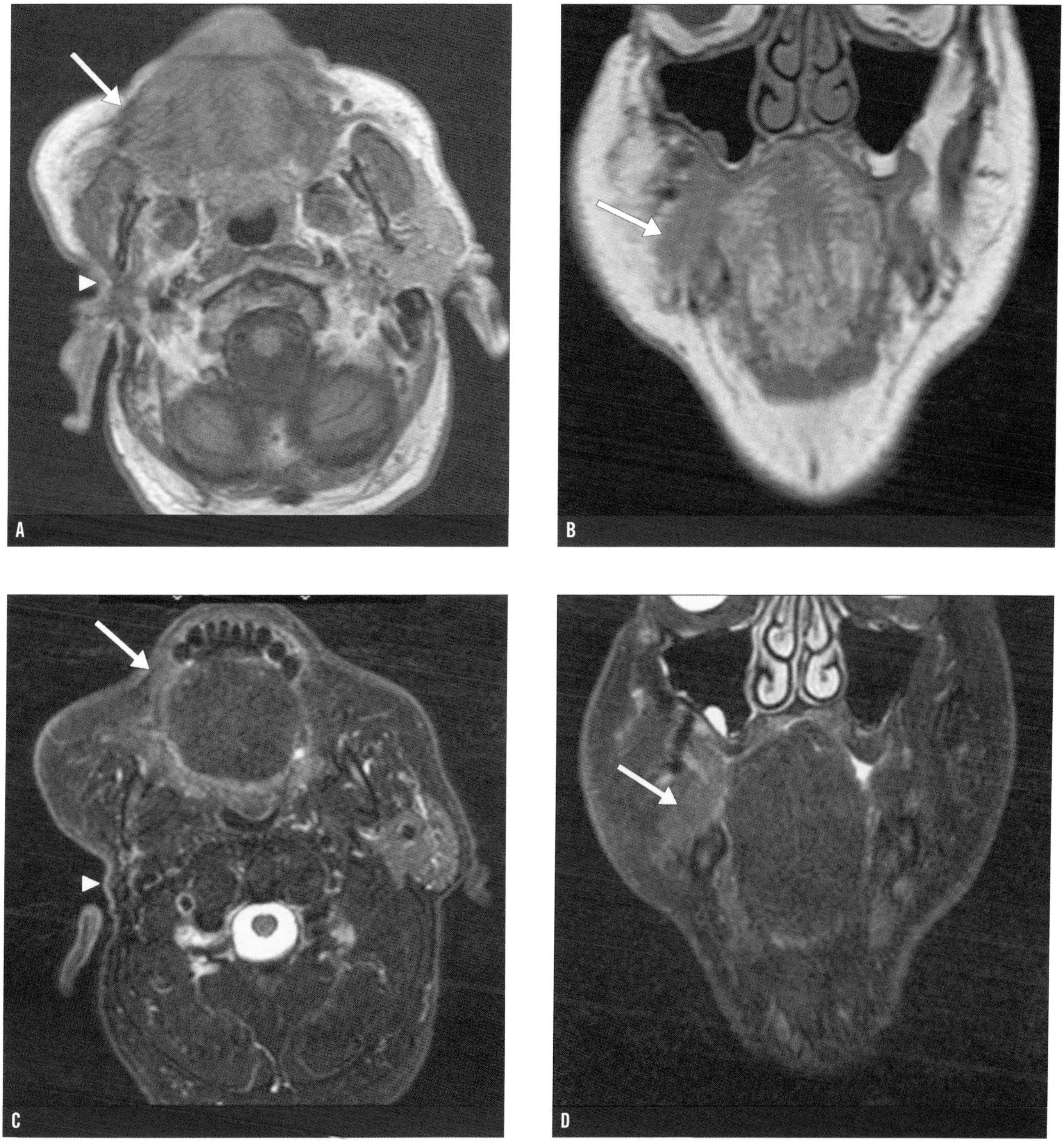

Axial and coronal T1 (**A**, **B**, respectively) and axial and coronal T2 with fat suppression (**C**, **D**, respectively) MR images of a patient with a history of high-grade right parotid adenocarcinoma. There are postsurgical changes of a prior right parotidectomy (arrowheads, **A**, **C**). In addition, there are findings of a right facial reanimation surgery with a temporalis tendon transfer and fascia lata interposition graft attached to the lateral aspect of the mouth, a region which is referred to as the modiolus (long arrows, **A**-**D**). Axial (**E**, **F**) and coronal reformatted (**G**) contrast-enhanced CT images of the same patient. There is asymmetric soft tissue in the right buccal space at the level of the modiolus, again representing facial reanimation surgery with a temporalis tendon transfer and fascia lata interposition graft (long arrows, **F**, **G**). There is a metallic weight in the right upper eyelid (short arrows, **E**, **G**), which was placed to treat the patient's inability to close their eyes (lagophthalmos) as a result of the previous right facial paralysis. A right parotidectomy is also identified on image **F** (arrowhead).

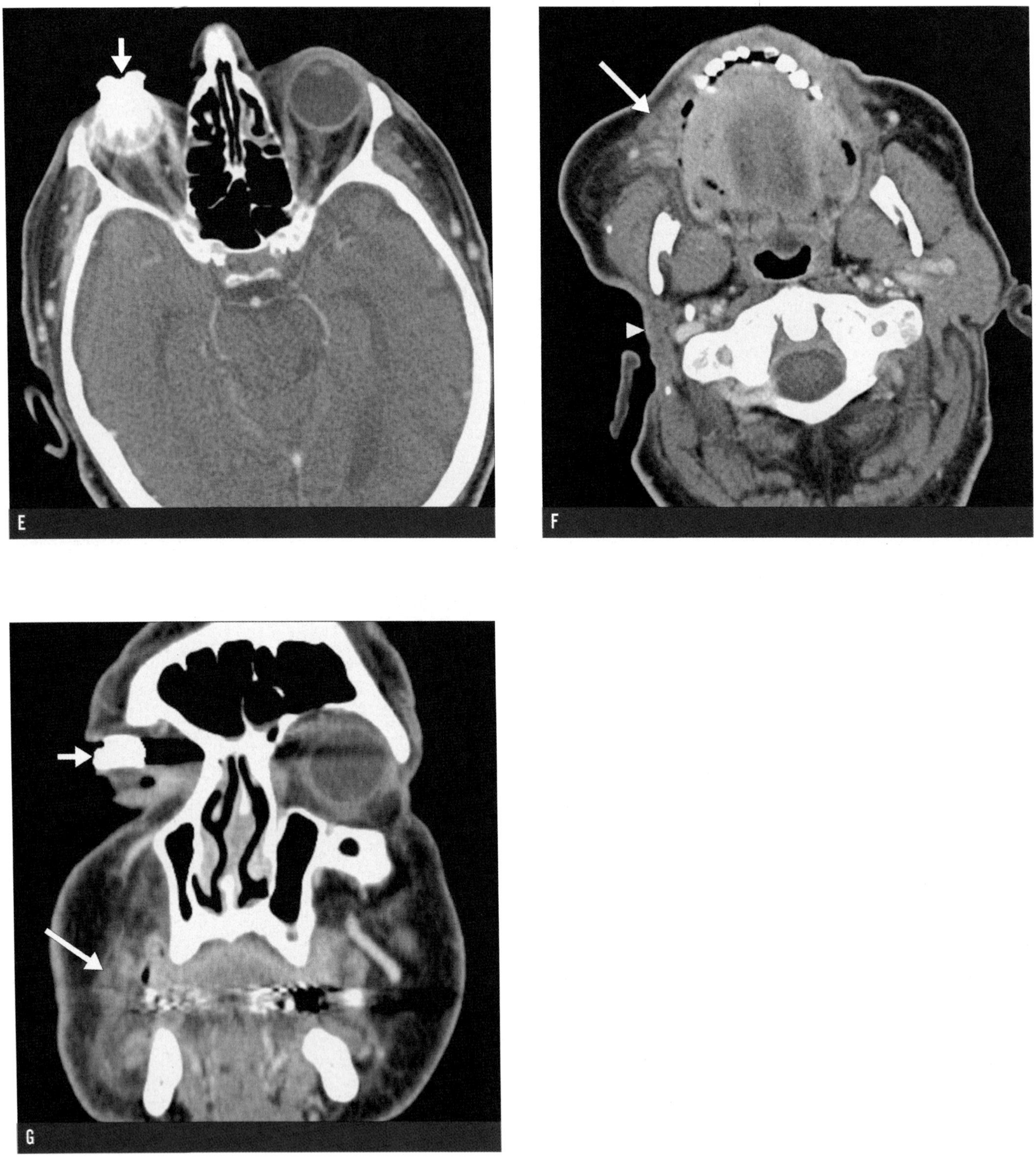
E
F
G

Companion case: Zygomaticus major muscle full-thickness tear

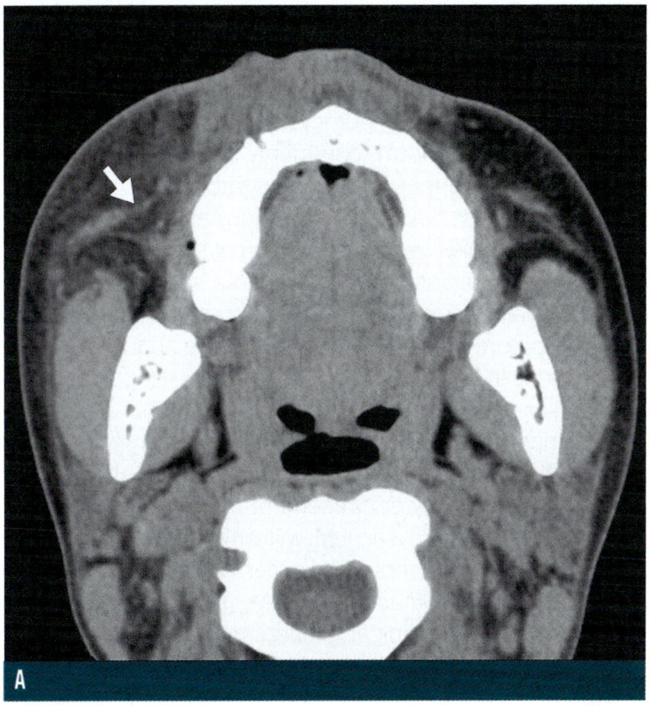

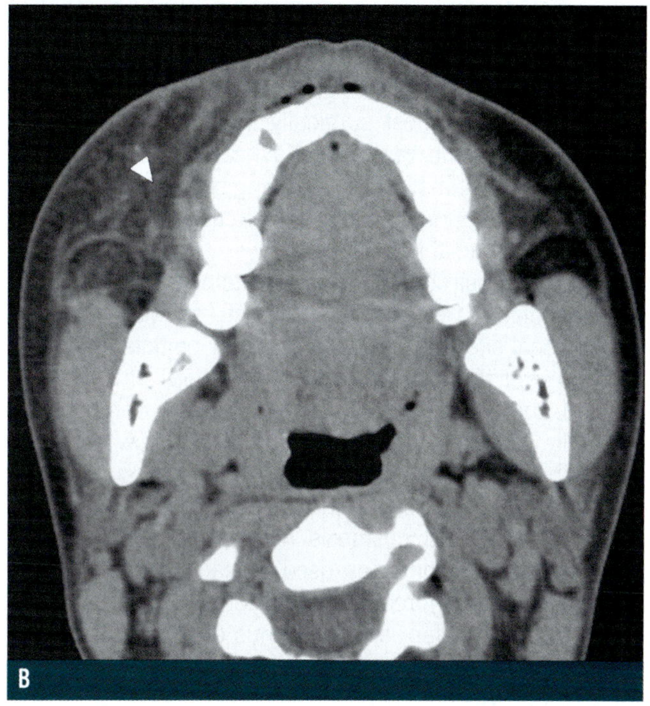

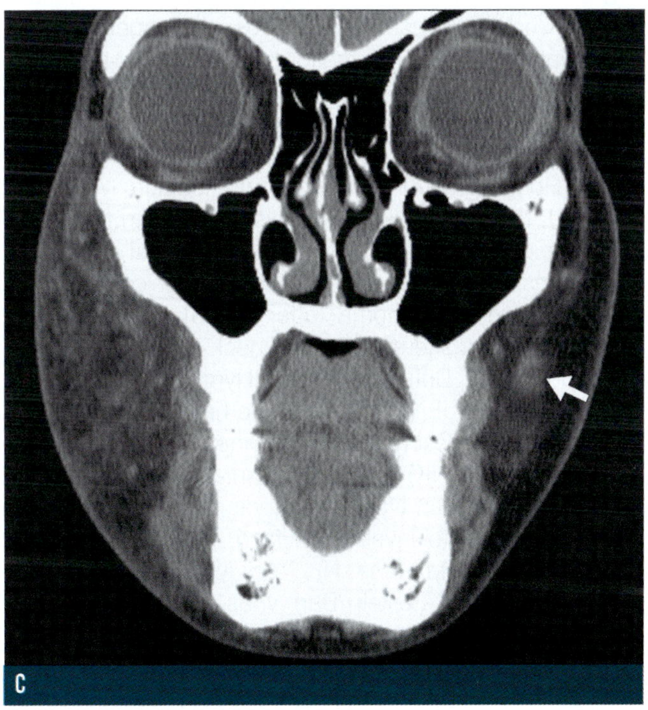

An unenhanced axial CT image (**A**) and an unenhanced axial CT image slightly more caudal (**B**) obtained on a patient following a deep right face laceration. Images **A** and **B** demonstrate extensive right face edema. Image **A** demonstrates the right zygomaticus major muscle (arrow, **A**) but image **B** demonstrates absence of this muscle (arrowhead, **B**). An unenhanced coronal reformatted image (**C**) demonstrates the normal left zygomaticus major muscle (arrow, **C**) and the lack of a normal right zygomaticus major muscle at this level. These findings are compatible with a right zygomaticus major muscle full-thickness tear.

REFERENCES

Byrne PJ, Kim M, Boahene K, Millar J, Moe K. Temporalis tendon transfer as part of a comprehensive approach to facial reanimation. *Arch Facial Plast Surg*. 2007;9(4):234-241.

Hoffman WY. Reanimation of the paralyzed face. *Otolaryngol Clin North Am*. 1992;25(3):649-667.

Revenaugh PC, Knott PD, Scharpf J, Fritz MA. Simultaneous anterolateral thigh flap and temporalis tendon transfer to optimize facial form and function after radical parotidectomy. *Arch Facial Plast Surg*. 2012;14(2):104-109.

Facial defects may be congenital, posttraumatic, or the result of surgery. Most surgically induced facial defects occur following the removal of a head and neck malignancy. Facial reconstruction following surgery is frequently necessary for wound closure, oral function, orbital support, or to improve facial aesthetics.

Flap reconstructions may be obtained from a remote site and placed over the facial defect (free flap) or taken from a local site with an intact vascular pedicle and repositioned over the facial defect (pedicle flap). If a free flap is used, then an adequate vascular pedicle from the flap (typically 10-12 cm) is usually required to allow for a vascular anastomosis to the native vessels and subsequent flap viability. The size of the defect, desired functional result, and desired cosmesis help determine the muscle choice. Common flaps used for facial reconstruction include a radial forearm flap, rectus abdominis flap, temporal muscle flap, and latissimus dorsi flap. On imaging, reconstruction flaps are initially edematous and of increased T2 signal on MRI. Subacutely, the flap muscle may enhance and mimic a tumor recurrence in patients who have malignancy. In addition to muscle, fat and bone may also be identified within the flap.

COMPANION CASES

- **Necrotizing fasciitis.** Necrotizing fasciitis is a rapidly progressive soft tissue infection that can be fatal without immediate and appropriate medical and surgical treatment. Less than 10% of cases occur in the cervical and/or facial region. A dental infection is usually the culprit when necrotizing fasciitis involves the face. Clinically, patients present with progressive erythema and swelling with eventual soft tissue crepitus and necrosis. On imaging, necrotizing fasciitis may initially appear as relatively minor inflammation. However, this may quickly progress and spread over hours to days with affected areas containing marked fat stranding, gas dissecting along fascial planes, and peripherally enhancing fluid collections.
- **Venous malformation.** Vascular malformations of the head and neck are a diverse group of lesions and include arteriovenous malformation (AVM), venous malformation (VM), and lymphatic malformation (LM). Vascular malformations may be high-flow lesions (AVM), low-flow lesions (VM, LM), or mixed (a combination of VM and LM). Properly categorizing these lesions is important in order to determine appropriate treatment. Most vascular malformations are present at birth, although trauma can result in an AVM.

  VMs are an abnormal collection of venous channels, fat, and degenerated muscle matrix. The veins in a VM can thrombose and form phleboliths, the latter considered pathognomonic of this entity. LMs represent an abnormal collection of lymphatic vessels. LMs are subcategorized into macrocystic and microcystic forms. The macrocystic form, commonly referred to as a cystic hygroma, is composed of large cystic spaces containing proteinaceous fluid and lymphocytes that are interspersed around septa. The microcystic form contains 2 mm or smaller-sized cysts within a solid matrix.

  The hallmark of a vascular malformation is its transpatial nature (ie, often involving more than one compartment in the neck) and its softness to palpation. A vascular malformation may or may not be associated with mass effect. On MRI, both a VM and a macrocystic LM will be hyperintense on T2. Following contrast, a VM will contain patchy enhancement throughout the lesion, whereas a macrocystic LM will only enhance along its periphery and/or septa. A hemorrhagic fluid level may be identified in a macrocystic LM, frequently associated with an abrupt clinical enlargement, and is strongly suggestive of a macrocystic LM when present. However, VMs and LMs frequently coexist in a lesion, and when a lesion contains both entities, the term venolymphatic malformation is used. MRI is usually superior to CT in evaluating vascular malformations of the head and neck.
- **Natural killer/T-cell lymphoma, nasal type with facial involvement.** Lymphoma is broadly subdivided into Hodgkin lymphoma and non-Hodgkin lymphoma (NHL), the former almost always confined to the lymph nodes, whereas the latter may be extranodal in location. The head and neck is the second most common site of extranodal lymphoma (after the GI tract), and the most frequent site of head and neck involvement is the Waldeyer ring. Diffuse large B cell lymphoma is the most common type of NHL to affect the head and neck.

  Previously described as midline lethal granuloma, natural killer (NK)/T-cell lymphoma, nasal type is an extranodal form of NHL that affects the nasal cavity and often spreads to involve the face, nasopharynx, orbit, and infratemporal fossa. NK/T-cell lymphoma is strongly associated with Epstein-Barr virus and it is the most common cellular subtype of nasal lymphoma. While rare in the Western population, it is relatively more common in patients who reside in Asia, Mexico, and South America. Clinical symptoms include nasal obstruction, nasal discharge, epistaxis, and nasal pain. On CT, a NK/T-cell lymphoma of the nasal cavity will be heterogeneously enhancing and frequently destroys adjacent bone (eg, the bones of the nasal cavity, maxillary sinus, and lamina papyracea). On MRI, the tumor is usually isointense to muscle on T1-weighted imaging, hypo- to isointense on T2-weighted imaging, and heterogeneously enhances. As with lymphoma elsewhere, restricted diffusion may be evident within the lesion on DWI.

Facial reconstruction flap

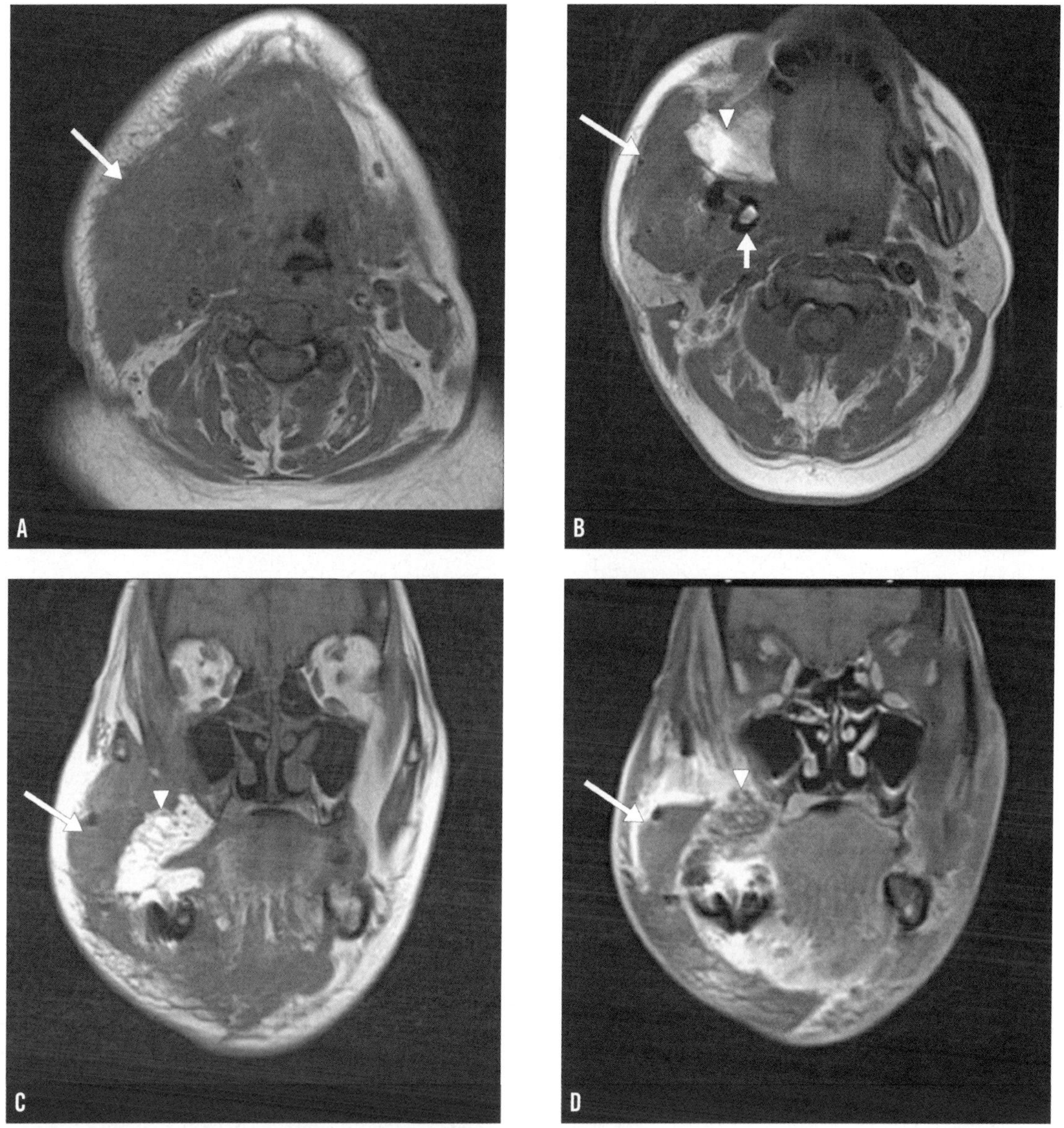

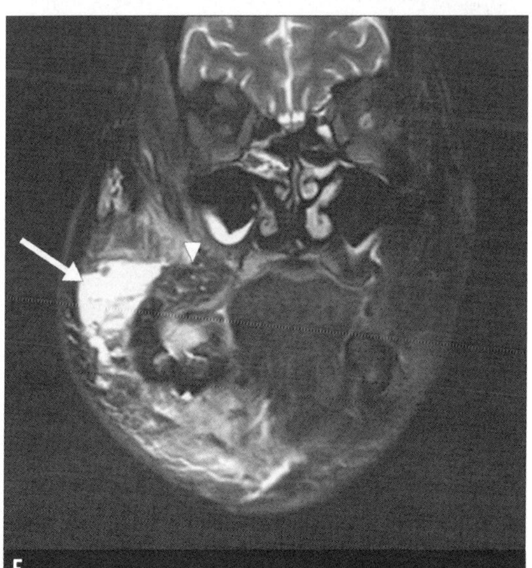

Axial T1 (**A**, **B**), coronal T1 (**C**), contrast-enhanced fat-suppressed coronal T1 (**D**), and fat-suppressed coronal T2 (**E**) MR images demonstrate a large amount of heterogeneous soft tissue over the right aspect of the face. Without appropriate history, the lesion could be misinterpreted as a large soft tissue mass. However, this patient did have a large osteomyocutaneous fibula free flap that was placed following resection of a mucoepidermoid carcinoma. There is an edematous muscular component (long arrows, **A**-**E**) and a fat component (arrowheads, **B**-**E**), the latter suppressing on the fat-suppressed images. The presence of focal, nonanatomic fat within the finding is a clue that this is a surgical flap rather than a tumor. A portion of the fibula is also identified (short arrow, **B**).

Companion case: Necrotizing fasciitis

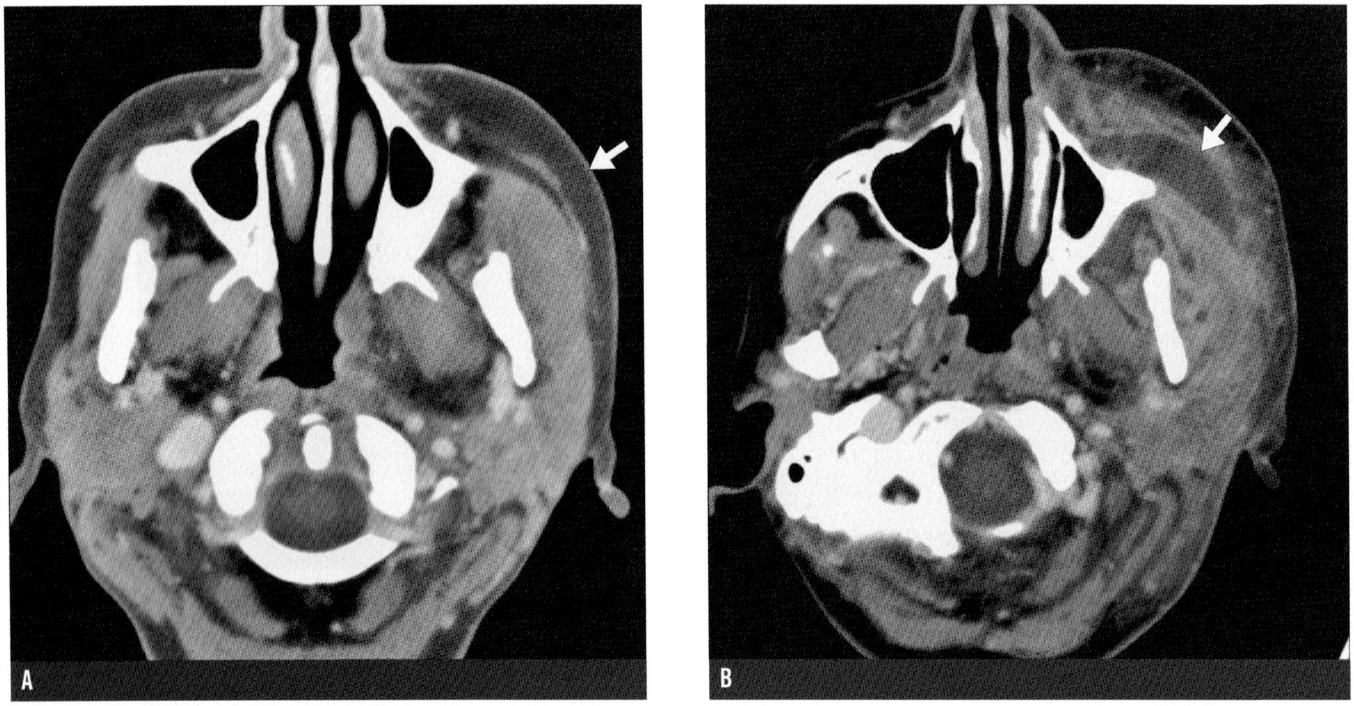

A contrast-enhanced axial CT image of a patient with acute left face pain on admission (**A**) demonstrates asymmetric enlargement of the left masseter muscle with overlying mild subcutaneous inflammatory stranding (arrow, **A**). Three days later, a contrast-enhanced axial CT image (**B**) demonstrates marked worsening of the left face inflammatory change, with a new large fluid collection developing in the anterior left face (arrow, **B**). This patient had necrotizing fasciitis of unknown etiology that required multiple surgical debridements, although the patient did eventually recover.

Companion case: Venous malformation

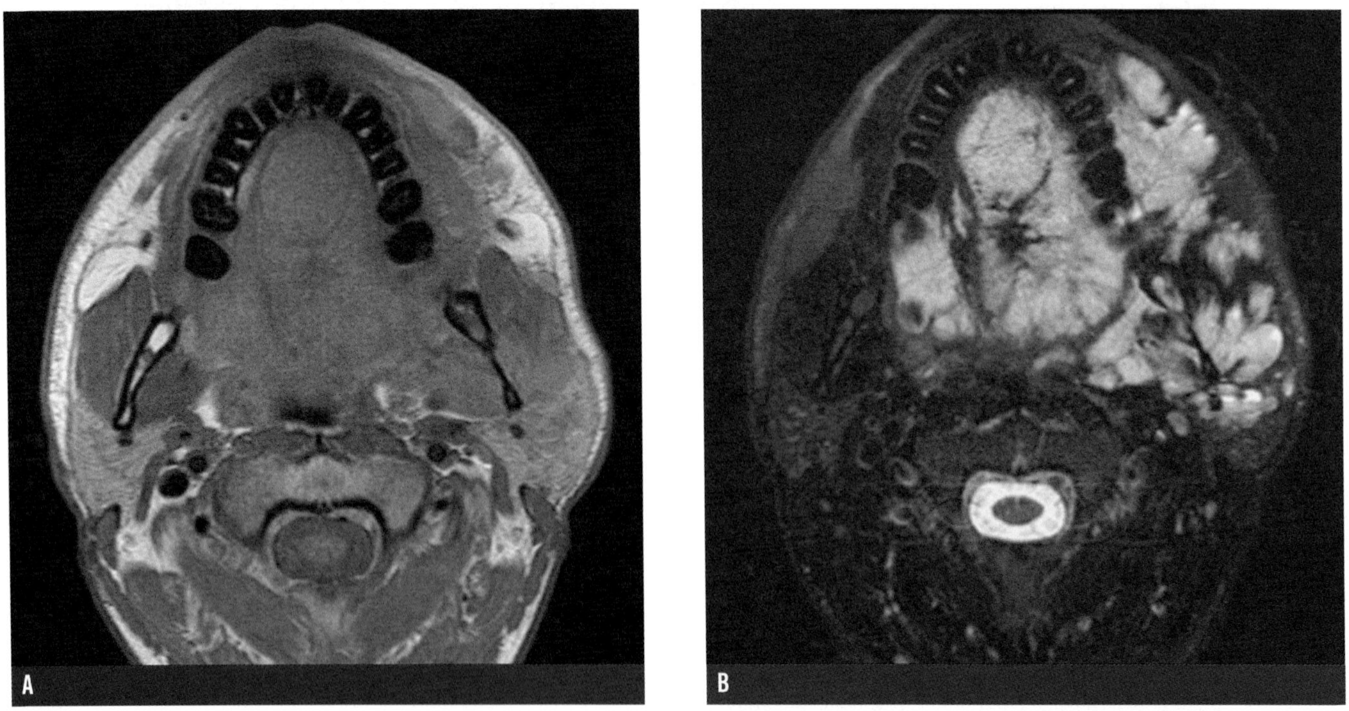

Axial T1 (**A**), fat-suppressed axial T2 (**B**), fat-suppressed contrast-enhanced axial T1 (**C**) and fat-suppressed contrast-enhanced coronal T1 (**D**) MR images demonstrate a large, T2 hyperintense, and diffusely enhancing transpatial abnormality affecting multiple facial compartments including the left masticator space, parapharyngeal space, and oral cavity. The elevated T2 signal, diffuse enhancement, and transpatial involvement are consistent with a large venous malformation.

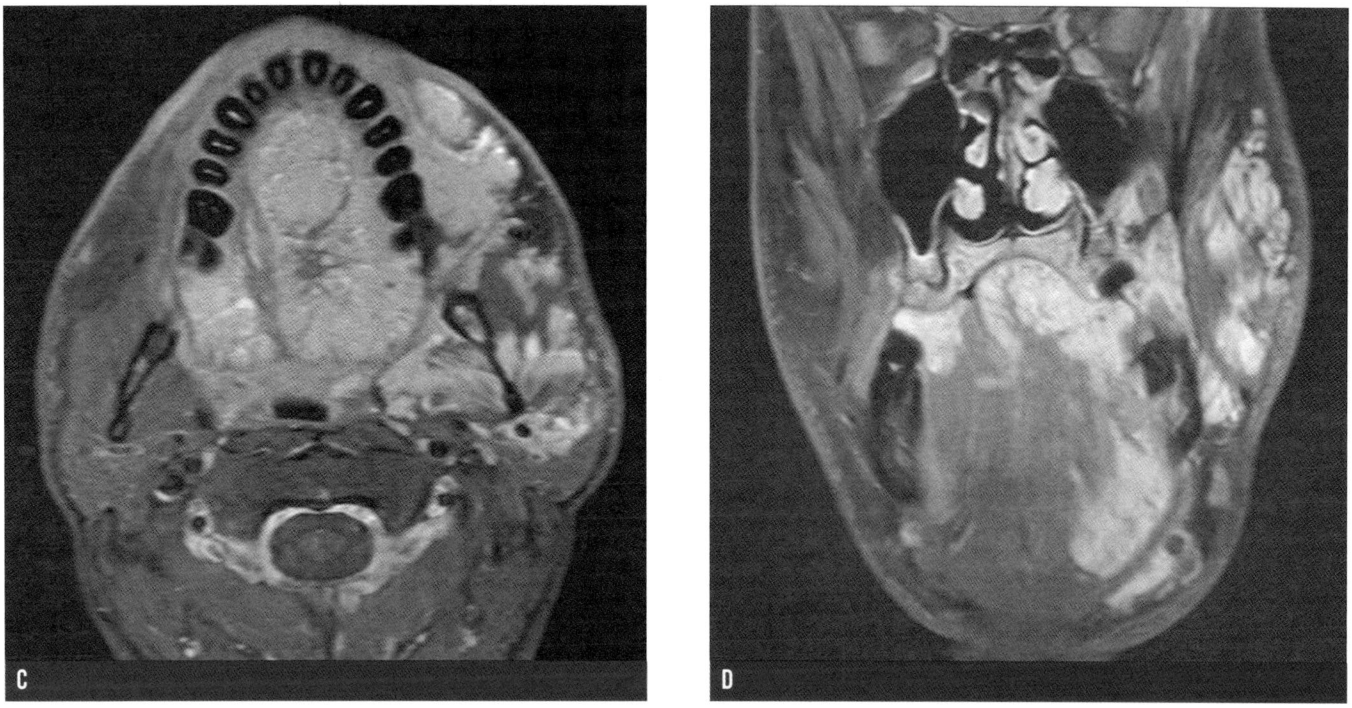

Companion case: Natural killer/T-cell lymphoma, nasal type with facial involvement

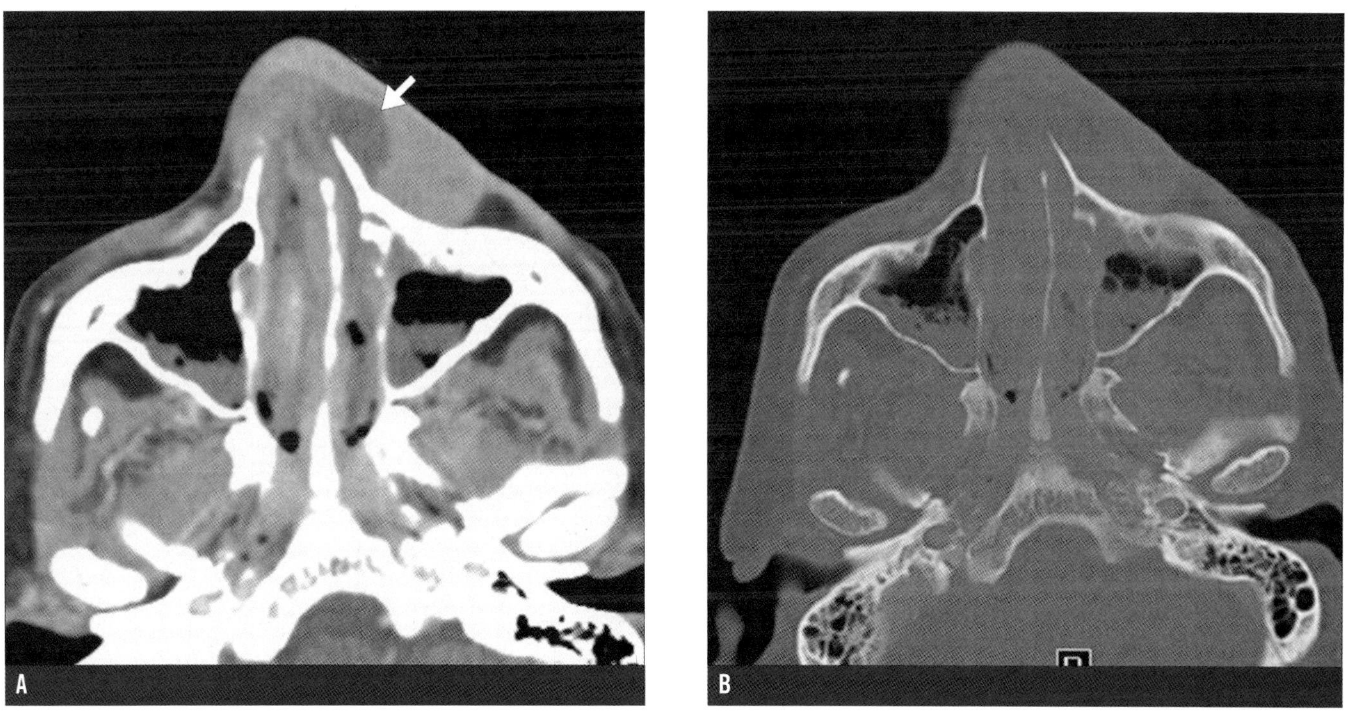

Contrast-enhanced axial CT images viewed with a soft tissue window (**A**) and bone window (**B**) as well as a contrast-enhanced coronal reformatted CT image viewed with a soft tissue window (**C**) obtained through the face. These images demonstrate a large, heterogeneous lesion involving the left face and nose. The mass does not result in underlying osseous destruction but contains a necrotic component (arrows, **A**, **C**). There is a paucity of surrounding inflammatory stranding, suggesting that the lesion represents a tumor rather than an infection. This lesion is nonspecific and the differential diagnosis includes several different types of tumors; in this case, the lesion was diagnosed as natural killer/T-cell lymphoma, nasal type at pathology. While there is no evidence of bone destruction in this case, natural killer/T-cell lymphoma, nasal type does have a propensity to destroy regional bone. The patient was of Mexican descent, a potential clue to the diagnosis given the greater risk to develop this tumor in those who originate from Mexico (along with those from Asia and South America) compared to the general population.

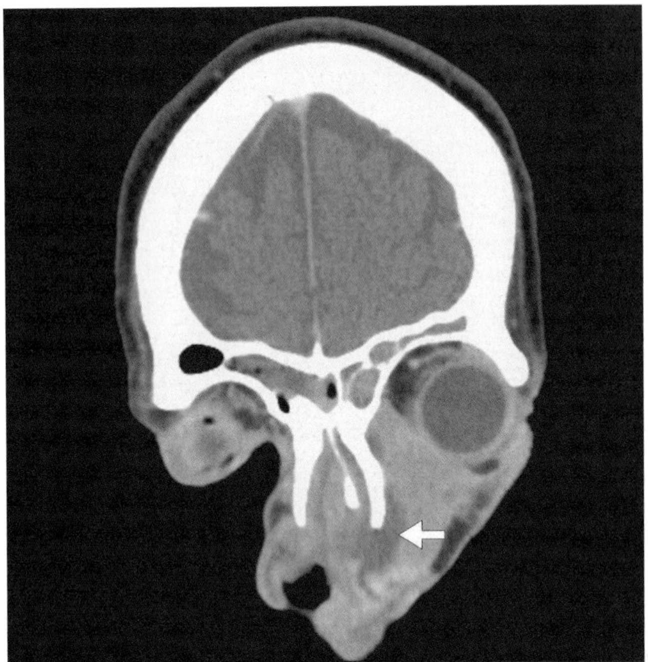

C

REFERENCES

Baker SR. Regional flaps in facial reconstruction. *Otolaryngol Clin North Am.* 1990;23:925-946.

Kim EY, et al. Primary peripheral T cell lymphoma of the face other than mycosis fungoides: computed tomography and magnetic resonance findings. *J Comp Assist Tomogr.* 2004;28(5):670-675.

McCarthy CM, Cordeiro PG. Microvascular reconstruction of oncologic defects of the midface. *Plast Reconstr Surg.* 2010;126(6):1947-1959.

McCafferty IJ, Jones RG. Imaging and management of vascular malformations. *Clin Radiol.* 2011;66(12):1208-1218.

Naidich MJ, Weissman JL. Reconstructive myofascial skull-base flaps: normal appearance on CT and MR imaging studies. *Am J Radiol.* 1996;167:611-614.

Ord R, Coletti D. Cervico-facial necrotizing fasciitis. *Oral Dis.* 2009;15:133-141.

Ou CH, et al. Nasal NK/T-cell lymphoma: computed tomography and magnetic resonance imaging findings. *J Chin Med Assoc.* 2007;70(5):207-212.

Thomas AG, Vaidhyanath R, Kirke R, Rajesh A. Extranodal lymphoma from head to toe: part 1, the head and spine. *Am J Roentgenol.* 2011;197(2):350-356.

Fibrous dysplasia. With fibrous dysplasia, normal bone is replaced by fibrous tissue consisting of spindle cell bundles and immature woven bone. This process results in expansion of the affected bone. It may affect a single site (monostotic) or multiple sites (polyostotic). The most common CT appearance of fibrous dysplasia is a ground-glass (sclerotic) pattern. However, fibrous dysplasia can less commonly appear as a heterogeneously lucent and sclerotic lesion (Pagetoid) or as a cystic lesion. On MRI, fibrous dysplasia has a nonspecific appearance and can mimic other osseous lesions, including malignant entities. Thus, any suspicious osseous lesion on MRI should be interpreted in combination with CT, or when appropriate, radiographs. Typically, fibrous dysplasia demonstrates low-to-intermediate T1 signal and avid enhancement on MRI. The T2 characteristics are variable and depend on the ratio of mineralized matrix to fibrous tissue.

Venous malformation of bone (hemangioma). Historically, an at least partially intrinsic T1 hyperintense osseous lesion in bone that typically enhances on MRI has been termed an intraosseous hemangioma. However, more recent literature describing its histopathology supports that this entity is more appropriately termed a venous malformation of bone. On CT, an intraosseous venous malformation of the face contains some lucency and frequently contains coarse osseous trabeculations. Hounsfield units within the lucency may reveal fat attenuation, a finding that usually confirms this benign entity.

Renal osteodystrophy. Renal osteodystrophy is a disorder of calcium and phosphate metabolism. With chronic renal failure, phosphate retention and decreased synthesis of vitamin D leads to hypocalcemia and subsequent secondary hyperparathyroidism. These metabolic abnormalities result in either elevated bone turnover osteodystrophy (ie, increased bone resorption and bone formation) or depressed bone turnover/aplastic osteodystrophy (ie, osteomalacia).

There are multiple imaging features involving the body that may be associated with renal osteodystrophy. Classic features include generalized osteopenia, subperiosteal bone resorption, subchondral bone resorption, "rugger jersey" spine appearance, Brown tumors, and vascular as well as periarticular soft tissue calcifications. In addition, patients with renal osteodystrophy often have findings consistent with osteomalacia that can result in pathologic fractures.

Manifestations of renal osteodystrophy involving the face are less common. Three main radiographic appearances of renal osteodystrophy affecting the face have been described. In osteitis fibrosa cystica, the most common radiographic appearance, there is diffuse cortical thinning of multiple bones, coarsened trabeculae, and lytic lesions, often with a superimposed "salt and pepper" skull related to mixed sclerotic and lytic lesions affecting the calvarium. A second radiographic manifestation of renal osteodystrophy may have a fibrous dysplasia-like appearance with loss of corticomedullary junction differentiation. The third appearance, and most rare, is termed uremic leontiasis ossea, a profound facial abnormality characterized by marked maxillary and mandibular enlargement, channeling within bone, and cortical bone loss.

Paget disease. Paget disease is a metabolic bone disorder of unknown etiology that typically affects the elderly and is characterized by extensive bone remodeling, sclerosis, and thickening. Clinically, patients with Paget disease may be asymptomatic although they will have an elevated serum alkaline phosphatase and they can be disfigured from the disease. There is facial involvement in approximately 11% of patients afflicted with Paget disease, and if the face and/or calvarium are involved, the expanded bone may narrow foramina and canals, sometimes resulting in cranial neuropathies. Paget disease is associated with giant cell tumor formation and there is a risk of malignant sarcomatous transformation.

Paget disease is often readily diagnosed with radiographs. However, CT may allow for a diagnosis as well as provide additional information regarding the extent of disease affecting the face. There are three characteristic phases of Paget disease that are observed with radiographs and CT imaging: osteolytic, mixed lytic-sclerotic, and blastic (also called sclerotic). In the initial phase, Paget disease presents as a lucent lesion with a leading edge of resorption. The mixed lytic-sclerotic phase is the most commonly diagnosed phase of Paget disease by radiographs or CT. Imaging features at this stage includes cortical thickening, osseous expansion, and coarse trabeculae, classically resulting in a "cotton-wool" appearance when it affects the skull. The final stage, the blastic stage, manifests as progressive new bone formation with increased osseous density, medullary sclerosis, and markedly increased bone volume.

MRI is significantly less useful than CT or plain films to diagnose Paget disease. On MRI, the visualized osseous cortices will be thickened and any osteolytic areas that may be present will be hyperintense on T2-weighted imaging and enhance. Any sclerotic areas that are present will be hypointense on all pulse sequences. While MRI is not the preferred imaging modality to diagnose Paget disease, MRI as well as CT are useful to evaluate for the presence of sacromatous degeneration. Paget disease may also be assessed with a whole body bone scan with Tc-99m labeled MDP. With this imaging study, the affected bone with undergo increase uptake.

Osteopetrosis. Osteopetrosis, derived from the Greek words for bone (osteo) and stone (petra), is a rare, heritable skeletal disorder that results in defective bone remodeling and extensive diffuse osseous sclerosis. The autosomal recessive form is usually diagnosed within the first few months of life; these patients rarely survive childhood. The autosomal dominant form is more common and is typically diagnosed in late childhood or adolescence. Although patients have increased bone density with osteopetrosis, paradoxically, these patients have an increased risk of fracture. Complications of osteopetrosis affecting the face or skull base include cranial nerve palsies and optic atrophy secondary to narrowing of the neural and vascular foramina. On CT, there is extensive increased attenuation and thickening of the skull as well as lack of a definable diploic space. On MRI, the skull is diffusely expanded, hypointense on all pulse sequences, and does not enhance following contrast.

Fibrous dysplasia of the zygomatic bone

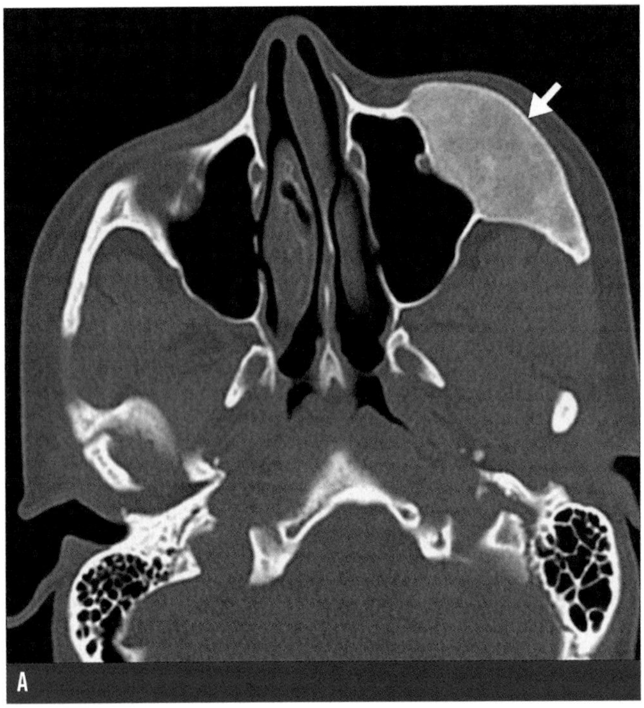

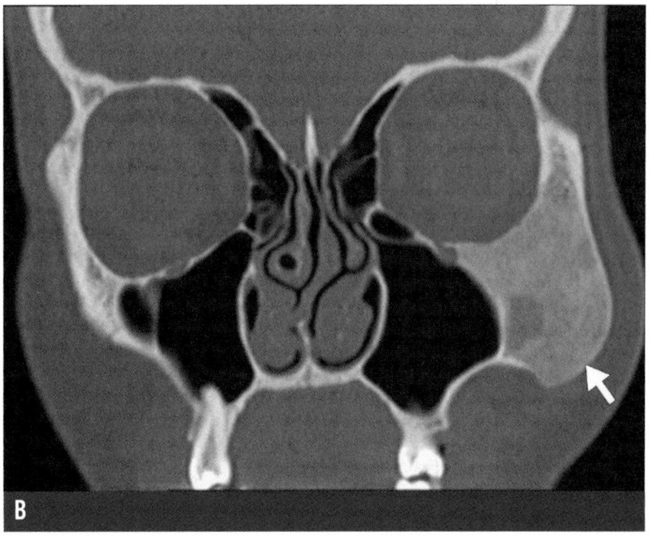

Axial (**A**) and coronal reformatted (**B**) CT images demonstrate a large, expansile, ground-glass abnormality involving the left zygomatic bone, compatible with fibrous dysplasia (arrows, **A**, **B**).

Fibrous dysplasia of the right maxillary sinus

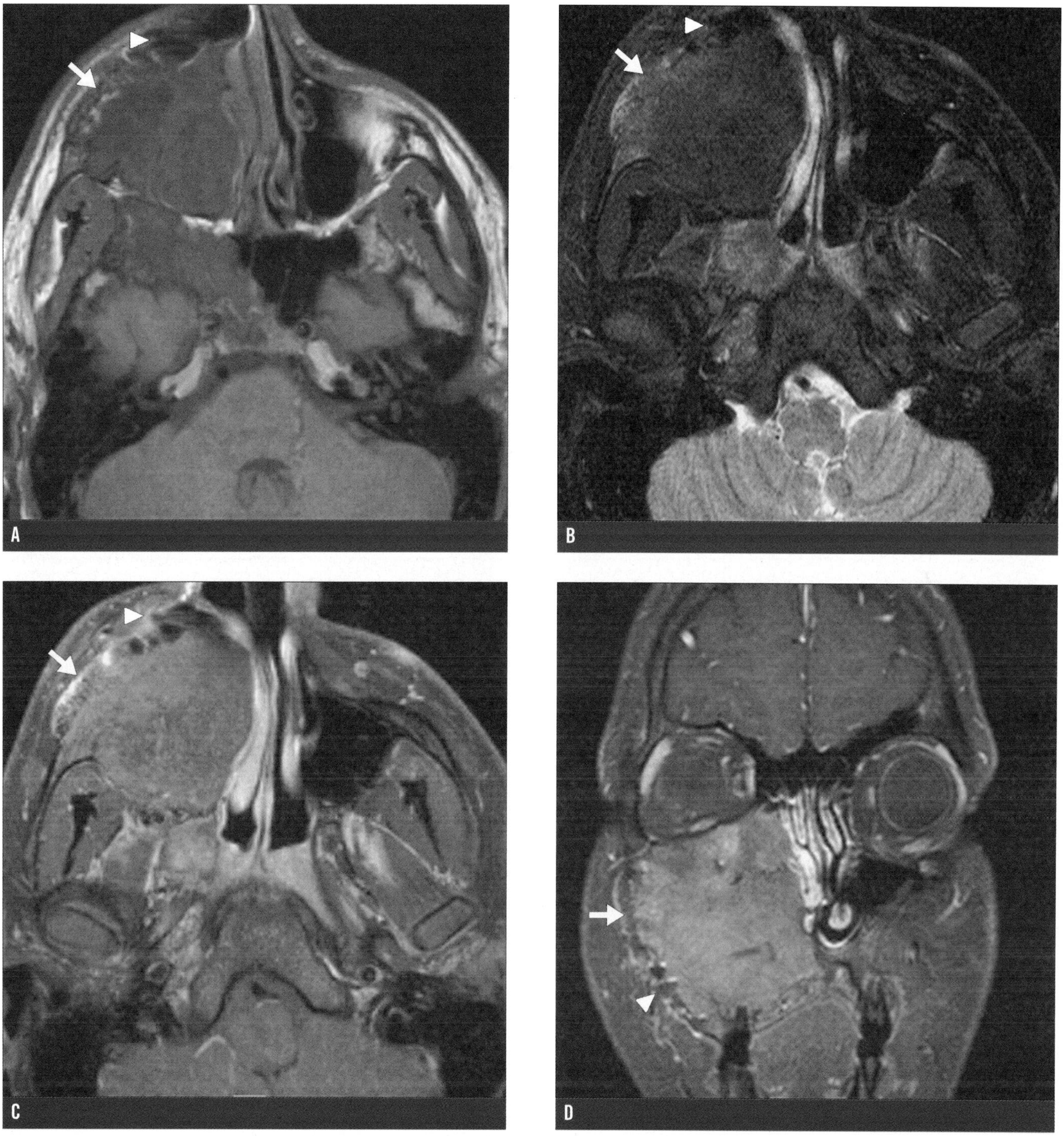

Axial T1 (**A**), fat-suppressed axial T2 (**B**), fat-suppressed contrast-enhanced axial T1 (**C**) and fat-suppressed contrast-enhanced coronal T1 (**D**) MR images demonstrate a large, expansile, T2 hypointense, mildly enhancing lesion occupying the entire right maxillary sinus (arrows, **A-D**). This lesion is nonspecific by MRI and could represent a malignancy based on the MR imaging findings. However, this lesion represented pathologically proven benign fibrous dysplasia. This case emphasizes that a bone lesion demonstrated on MRI should be correlated with plain films, or preferably CT, which would have likely been diagnostic of this entity. Incidentally noted is metallic artifact from prior surgery (arrowheads, **A-D**).

Fibro-osseous lesion of the zygomatic bone and/or arrested pneumatization of the maxillary sinus

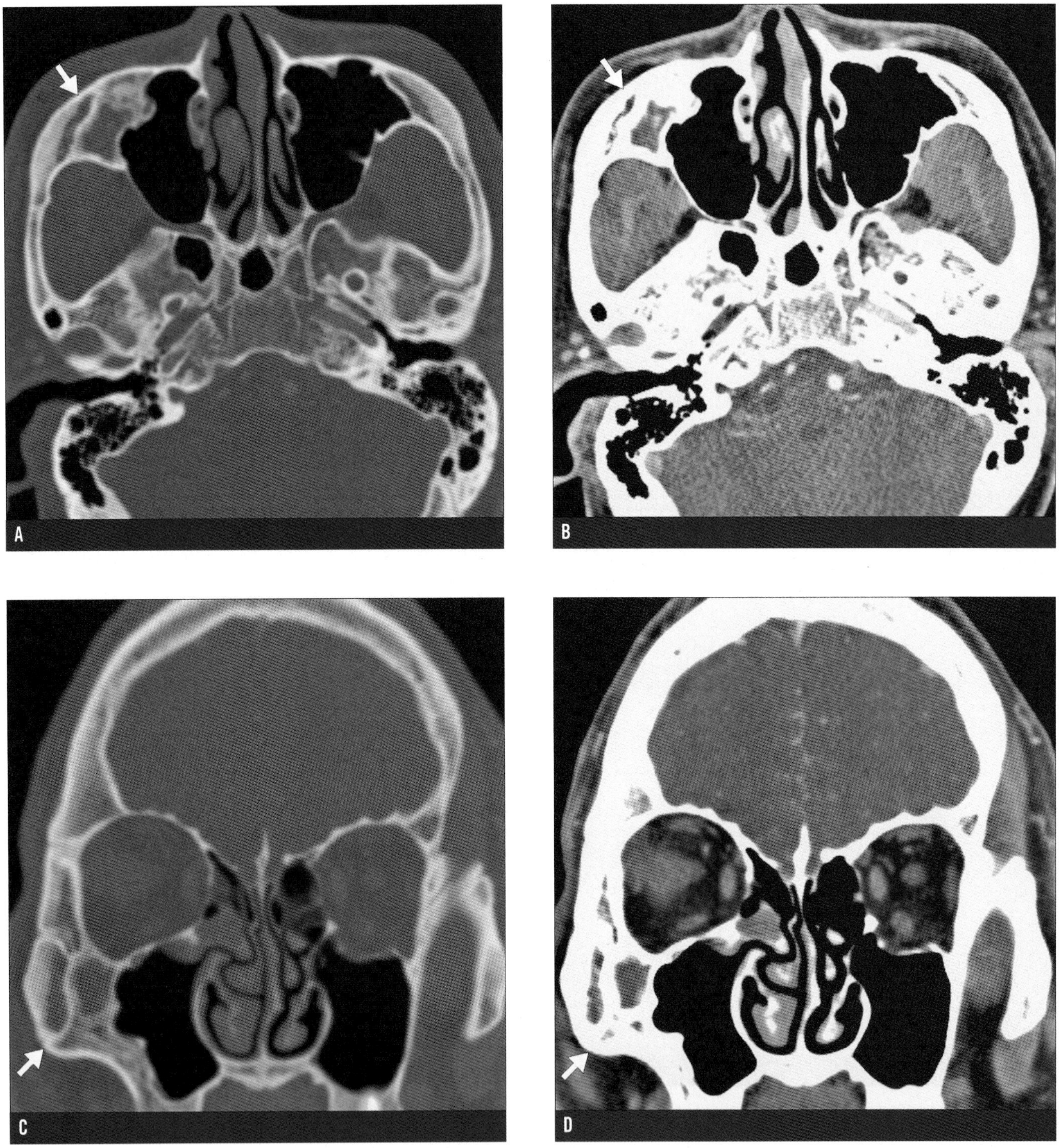

Contrast-enhanced axial CT images viewed with a bone window (**A**) and soft tissue window (**B**) as well as contrast-enhanced coronal reformatted CT images viewed with a bone window (**C**) and soft tissue window (**D**) demonstrate an expansile, partially ground-glass, partially lucent lesion involving the right zygomatic bone and extending into the right maxillary sinus (arrows, **A**-**D**). The finding contains soft tissue attenuation on images **B** and **D** suggestive of normal marrow. While nonspecific, this is a benign entity and likely represents a fibro-osseous lesion (eg, fibrous dysplasia) of the right zygomatic bone, arrested pneumatization of the maxillary sinus, or a combination of both.

Zygomatic bone venous malformation (osseous hemangioma)

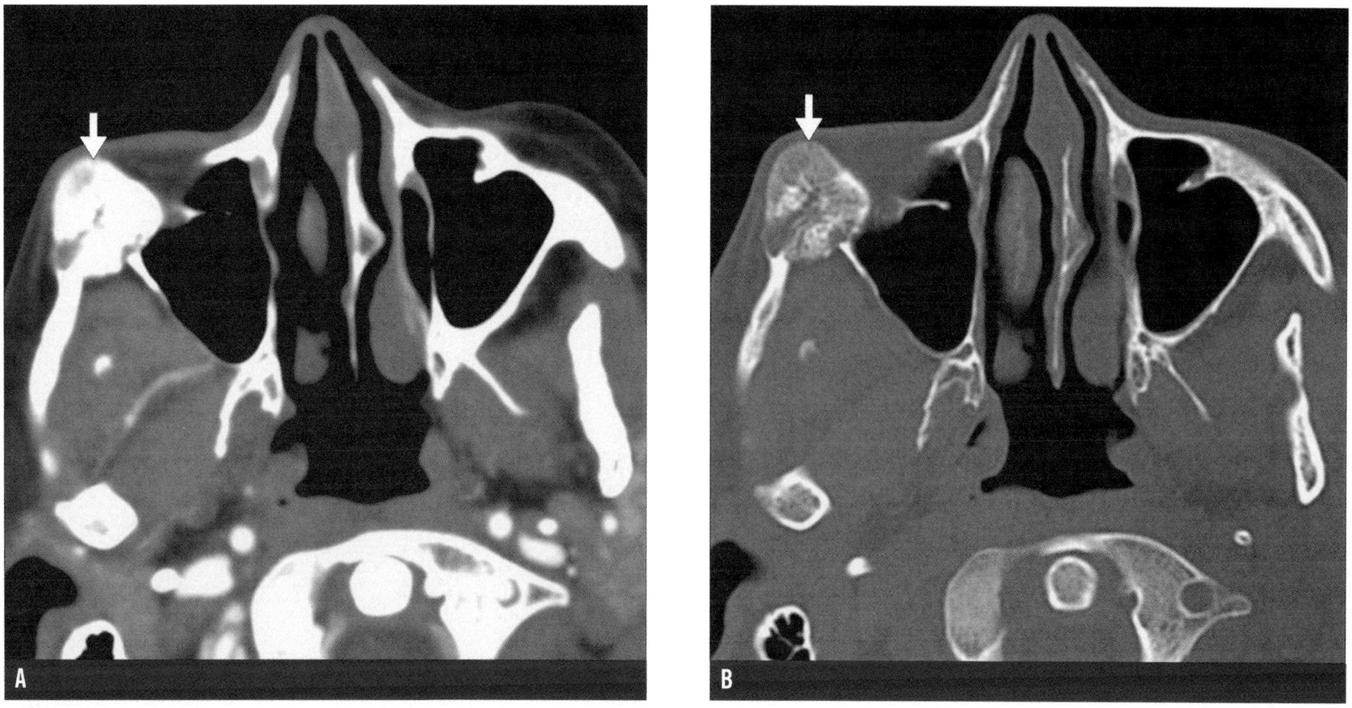

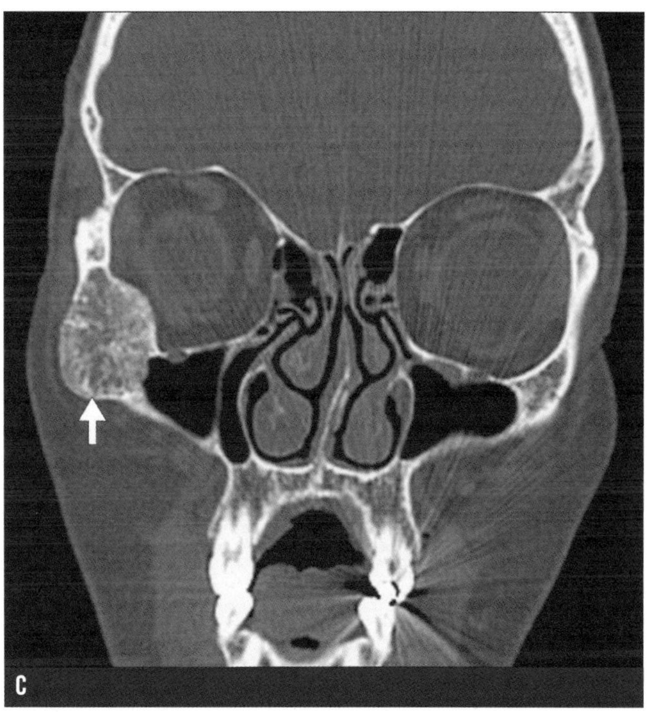

Contrast-enhanced axial CT images viewed with a soft tissue window (**A**) and bone window (**B**) as well as a coronal CT image viewed with a bone window (**C**) demonstrate a round, expansile lesion involving the right zygomatic body associated with radially directed course trabeculations, compatible with a zygomatic bone venous malformation (also called osseous hemangioma) (arrows, **A**-**C**). This finding was stable for many years.

Renal osteodystrophy

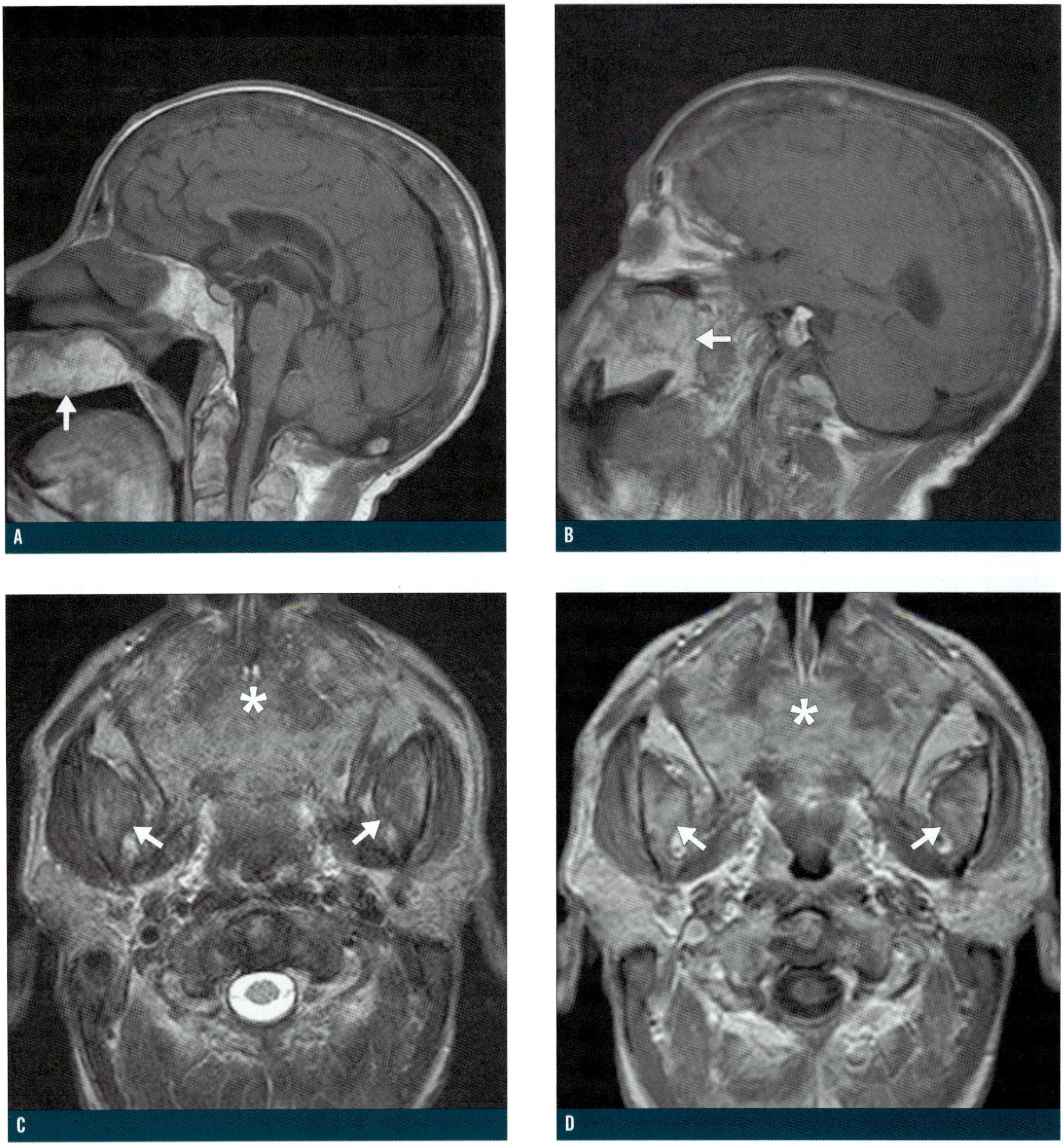

Sagittal T1 (**A**, **B**), axial T2 (**C**), and contrast-enhanced axial T1 (**D**) MR images demonstrate numerous osseous abnormalities in this patient with end-stage renal disease. Image **A** demonstrates marked enlargement of the hard palate (arrow, **A**), whereas image **B** demonstrates marked enlargement of the maxillary alveolus (arrow, **B**) resulting in a pronounced decreased volume of the maxillary sinus lumen. Images **A** and **B** also demonstrate diploic space enlargement and heterogeneity of the calvarium. Images **C** and **D** demonstrate diffuse enlargement and diffuse heterogeneous marrow signal of the hard palate (asterisks, **C**, **D**) and mandibular rami (arrows, **C**, **D**). Axial CT images of the same patient viewed with a bone window (**E**, **F**) demonstrate the CT correlate, with expansion and heterogeneous attenuation of the hard palate (asterisk, **E**), mandibular rami (arrows, **E**, **F**), and maxillary alveolus (asterisks, **F**). A sagittal scout image from the same study (**G**) perhaps best demonstrates the diffuse osseous abnormality, including the marked enlargement of the maxilla and mandible.

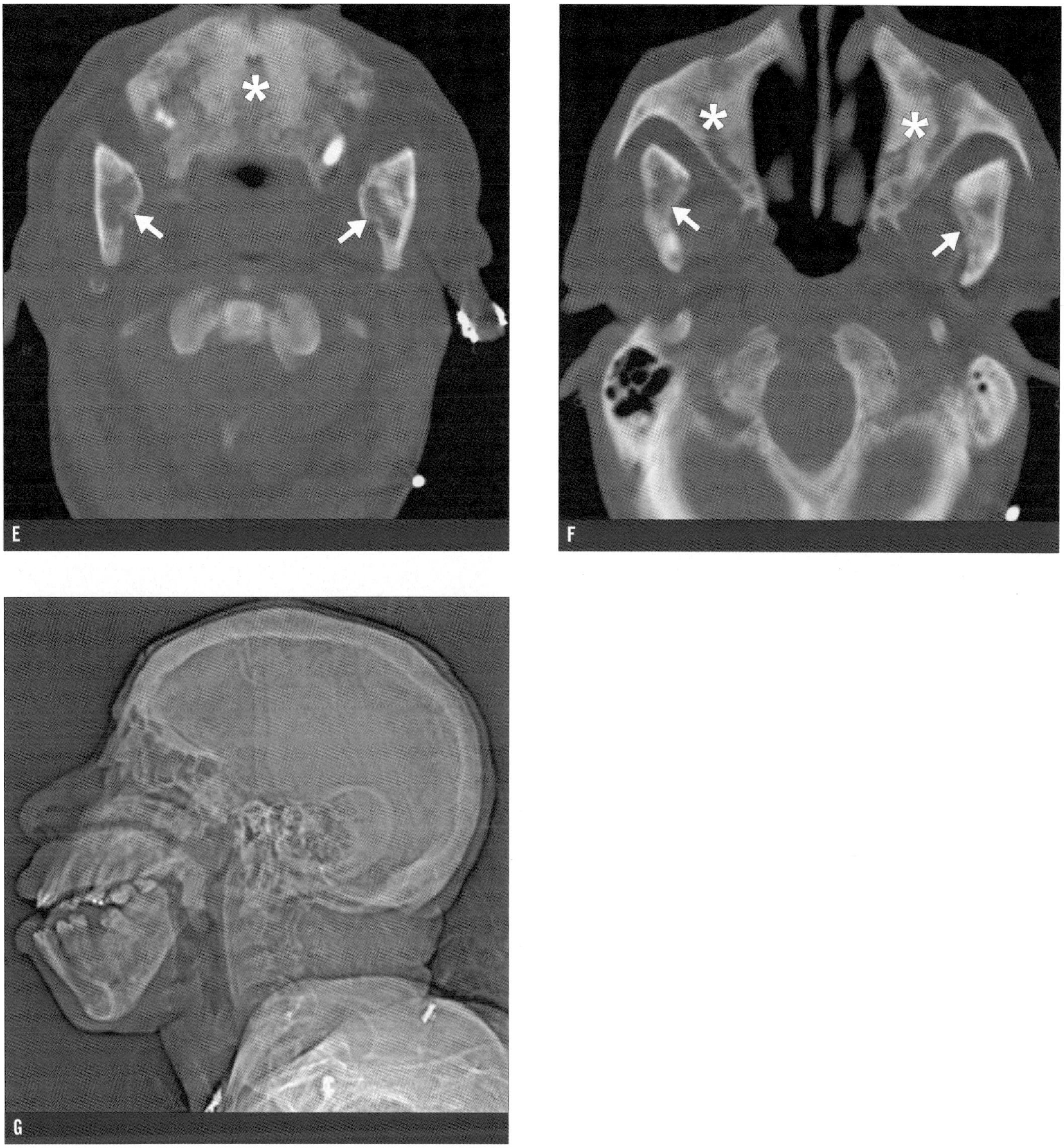
E
F
G

Paget Disease

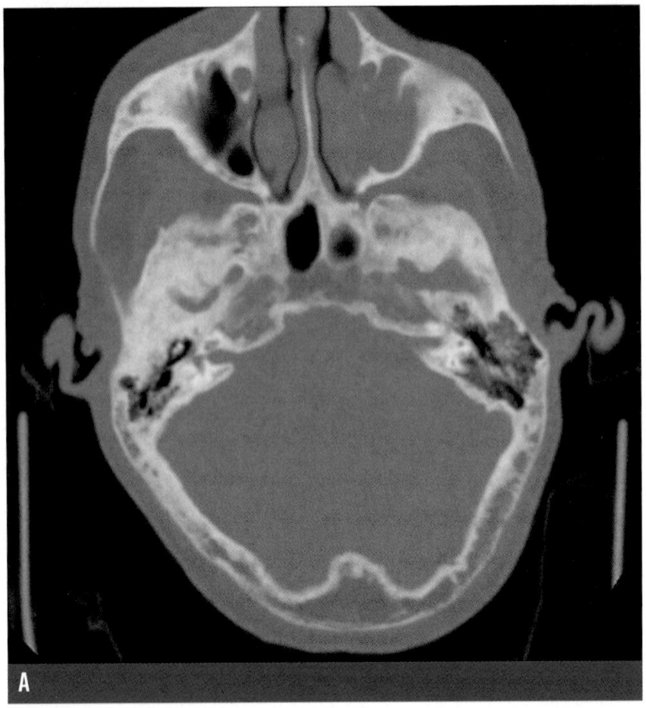

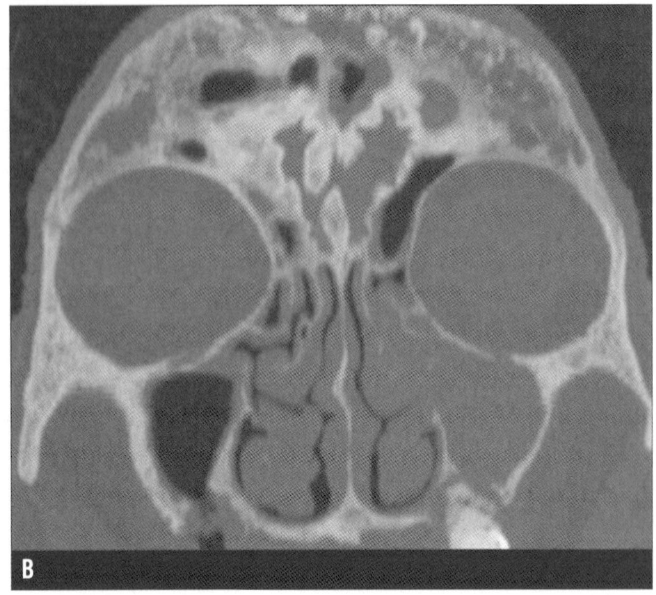

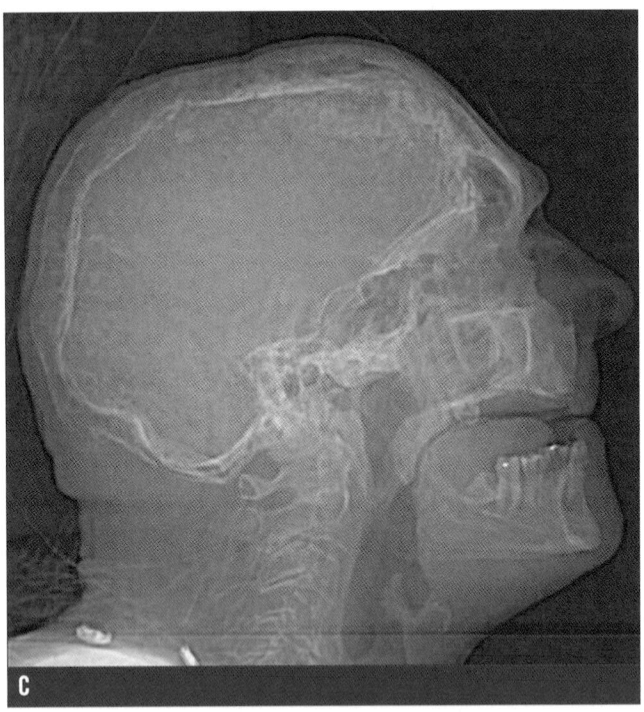

Axial (**A**) and coronal reformatted (**B**) CT images as well as a sagittal scout image from the same study (**C**) demonstrate diffuse cortical thickening, osseous expansion, and patchy sclerosis of the visualized osseous structures, compatible with Paget disease.

Osteopetrosis

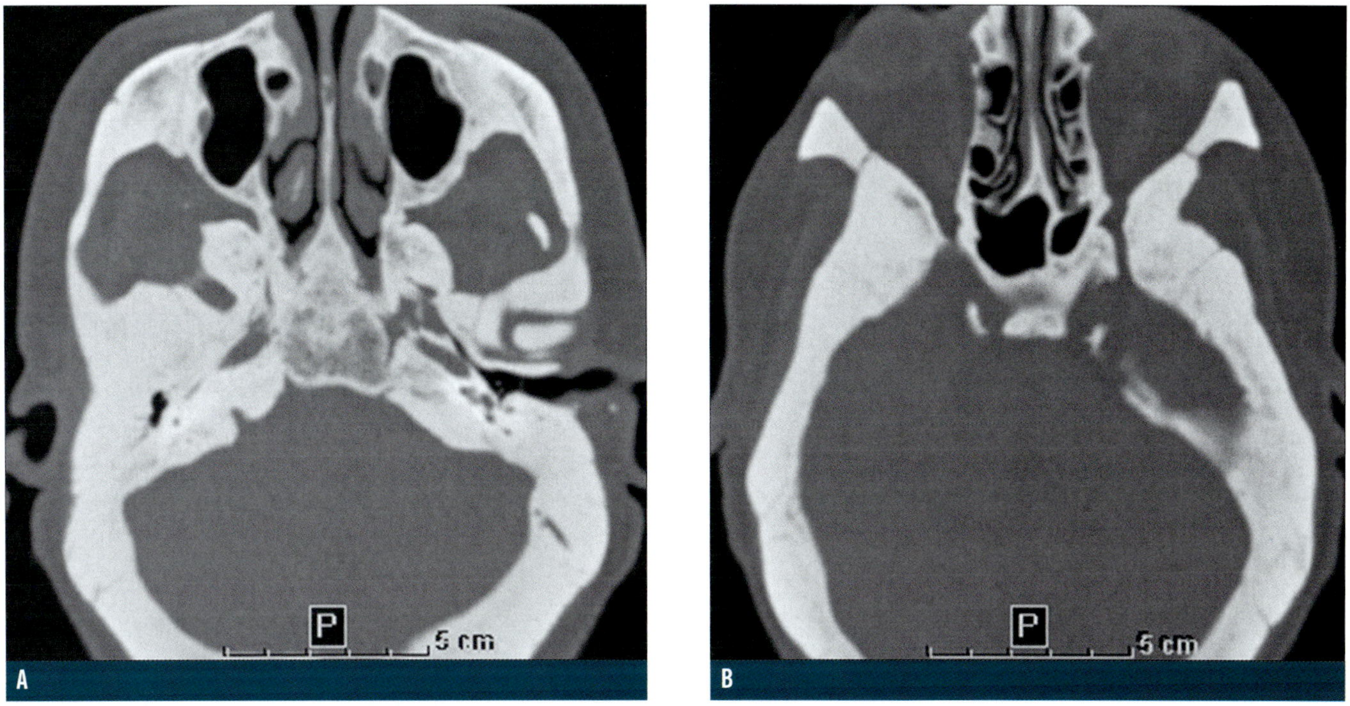

Axial CT images (**A**, **B**) demonstrate diffuse sclerosis of the visualized face and skull in this patient with a history of osteopetrosis.

REFERENCES

Camilleri AE. Craniofacial fibrous dysplasia. *J Laryngol Otol.* 1991;105:662-666.

Chang JI, Som PM, Lawson W. Unique imaging findings in the facial bones of renal osteodystrophy. *AJNR Am J Neuroradiol.* 2007;26:608-609.

Clauser L, Marchetti C, Piccione M, Bertoni F. Craniofacial fibrous dysplasia and Ollier's disease: combined transfrontal and transfacial resection using the nasal-cheek flap. *J Craniofac Surg.* 1996;7(2):140-144.

Cortis K, Micallef K, Mizzi A. Imaging Paget's disease of bone—from head to toe. *Clin Radiol.* 2011;66(7):662-672.

Cruz AAV, Constanzi M, Attie de Castro FA, Carlos dos Santos AC. Apical involvement with fibrous dysplasia: implications for vision. *Ophthal Plast Reconstr Surg.* 2007;23(6):450-454.

Cure JK, Key, LL, Goltra DD, VanTassel P. Cranial MR imaging of osteopetrosis. *AJNR Am J Neuroradiol.* 2000;21:1110-1115.

Demirdover C, Sahin B, Ozkan HS, Durmus EU, Oztan HY. Isolated fibrous dysplasia of the zygomatic bone. *J Craniofac Surg.* 2010;21:1583-1584.

Elster AD, Theros EG, Key LL, Chen MY. Cranial imaging in autosomal recessive osteopetrosis: part I. Facial bones and calvarium. *Radiology.* 1992;183(1):129-135.

Eversole R, Su L, El Mofty S. Benign fibro-osseous lesions of the craniofacial complex: a review. *Head Neck Pathol.* 2008;2(3):177-202.

Ihde LL, et al. Sclerosing bone dysplasias: review and differentiation from other causes of osteosclerosis. *Radiographics.* 2011;31:1865-1882.

Jevtic V. Imaging of renal osteodystrophy. *Eur J Radiol.* 2003;46(2):85-95.

Lowe LH, Marchant TC, Rivard DC, Scherbel AJ. Vascular malformations: classification and terminology the radiologist needs to know. *Semin Roentgenol.* 2012;47(2):106-117.

MacDonald-Jankowski DS. Fibro-osseous lesions of the face and jaws. *Clin Radiol.* 2004;59:11-25.

Martin D, Chapman T. Infantile osteopetrosis on head CT. *Pediatr Radiol.* 2009;39:308.

Shah ZK, Peh WCG, Koh WL, Shek TWH. Magnetic resonance imaging appearances of fibrous dysplasia. *Br J Radiol.* 2005;78:1104-1115.

CHAPTER 11

CALVARIUM, SCALP, AND THE TEMPORALIS MUSCULATURE

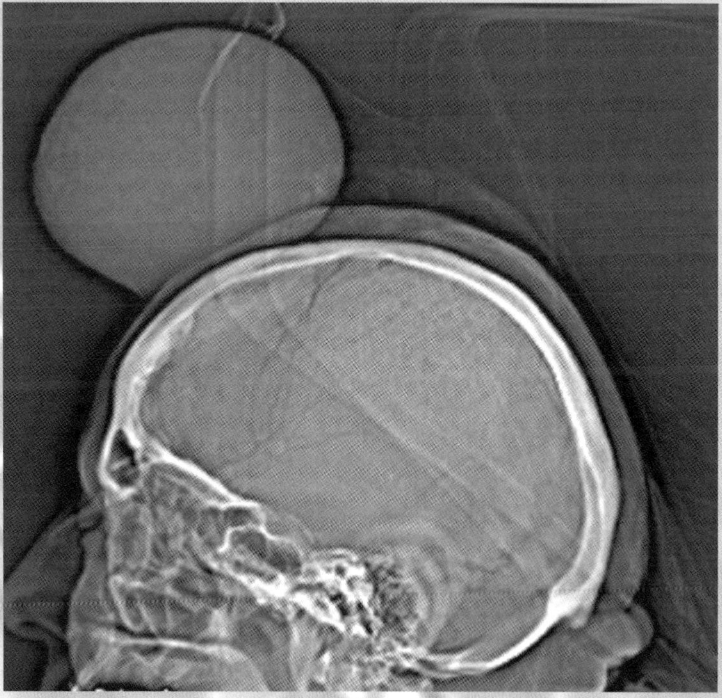

Noah Schwind, Achilles G. Karagianis

XI. CALVARIUM, SCALP, AND THE TEMPORALIS MUSCULATURE

1. Calvarial arachnoid granulations
   i. *Companion case*: Calvarial meningocele
   ii. *Companion case*: Arachnoid cyst
   iii. *Companion case*: Cerebellar herniation into the calvarium

2. Calvarial diploic veins and venous lakes
   i. *Companion case*: Venous malformation of bone (osseous hemangioma)
   ii. *Companion case*: Multiple myeloma
   iii. *Companion case*: Sinus pericranii

3. Parietal foramina
   i. *Companion case*: Incidental parietal calvarial thinning
   ii. *Companion case*: Burr hole

4. Calvarial hyperostosis interna
   a. *Companion case*: Dyke-Davidoff-Mason

5. Various nonmalignant entities that may diffusely affect the calvarium
   a. Red marrow
   b. Osteopetrosis
   c. β-Thalassemia
   d. Renal osteodystrophy
   e. Paget disease
      i. *Companion case*: Myelofibrosis
      ii. *Companion case*: Metastatic disease

6. Various nonmalignant entities that may focally affect the calvarium
   a. Osteoma
   b. Enostosis
   c. Venous malformation of the calvarium (osseous hemangioma)
   d. Calvarial epidermoid
   e. Benign fibro-osseous calvarial lesion
   f. Calvarial meningioma
      i. *Companion case*: Sclerotic metastatic disease
      ii. *Companion case*: Metastatic melanoma to the calvarium
      iii. *Companion case*: Radiation-induced calvarial osteosarcoma

7. External occipital protuberance
   i. *Companion case*: Calvarial osteoma of the outer table

8. Cranial suture variants

9. Craniosynostoses

10. Wormian bones

11. Middle meningeal artery calvarial groove or canal
   i. *Companion case*: Nondisplaced squamosal temporal bone fracture

12. Temporalis muscle hypertrophy
   i. *Companion case*: Temporalis muscle venous malformation
   ii. *Companion case*: Temporalis muscle/fascia insertion hyperostosis

13. Folliculitis keloidalis nuchae
   i. *Companion case:* Cutaneous acute myeloid leukemia
   ii. *Companion case:* Chronic scalp trauma

14. Scalp inclusion cysts
   i. *Companion case*: Hidradenitis suppuritiva
   ii. *Companion case*: Keloids
   iii. *Companion case*: Neurofibromas of the scalp
   iv. *Companion case*: Metastatic disease to the scalp
   v. *Companion case*: Skin clip artifact simulating a scalp lesion on MRI

15. Scalp lipoma
   i. *Companion case*: Pectoralis muscle flap to repair a scalp defect

16. Scalp dermal calcifications
   i. *Companion case*: Foreign bodies in the scalp following trauma

17. Hair transplantation

18. Scalp soft tissue expander
   i. *Companion case*: Ommaya reservoir

19. Cranioplasties

CASE 1 Calvarial arachnoid granulations

Arachnoid granulations are normal meningothelial-lined herniations of the arachnoid membrane that protrude through the dura mater and into the venous lacunae and dural venous sinuses along the surface of the brain. They are functionally and histologically similar to arachnoid villi and allow for filtration and resorption of cerebrospinal fluid (CSF) into the venous circulation. Most often, arachnoid granulations are CSF equivalent in their signal intensity and attenuation on MRI and CT, respectively, although occasionally they may deviate from CSF on MRI, particularly when large or "giant" (>1 cm). On MRI and CT, arachnoid granulations can usually be identified communicating with the adjacent subarachnoid space CSF. This is particularly important when an arachnoid granulation extends into a dural venous sinus. When this occurs, identifying its communication with the CSF helps differentiate this often incidental finding from a focal dural venous sinus thrombosis. Occasionally, a vessel, typically a vein, may be identified extending into a suspected calvarial arachnoid granulation, effectively confirming that the finding represents this entity.

Arachnoid granulations are most often incidental and completely asymptomatic. However, some authors believe that arachnoid villi will enlarge because of increasing CSF volume and intracranial pressure, resulting in giant arachnoid granulations. Similarly, some have shown that a strategically located arachnoid granulation of sufficient size within a dural venous sinus may result in abnormally elevated intracranial venous pressure and intracranial hypertension. Thus, it currently remains unclear if some giant arachnoid granulations may cause, or are the result of, intracranial hypertension. In addition, the larger the arachnoid granulation, the more often it may cause osseous irregularities, remodeling, and erosion. Patients with idiopathic intracranial hypertension (also called pseudotumor cerebri) often have several prominent arachnoid granulations. In these patients, arachnoid granulations that are located over the paranasal sinuses or temporal bones can rupture and result in spontaneous CSF leaks.

COMPANION CASES

- **Calvarial meningocele.** A cephalocele is a generic term that is used when the intracranial meninges and/or brain herniate outside the expected confines of the cranium. The term cranial meningocele is used when meninges and CSF, but not brain, herniate outside the cranium, whereas the term encephalocele is used when brain also herniates through the defect. The more specific terms calvarial meningocele or calvarial encephalocele may be used when the finding involves the cranial vault (ie, upper skull). As expected, a meningocele will follow CSF attenuation and signal on CT and MRI, respectively. A giant arachnoid granulation and a focal meningocele involving the calvarium are likely within the same imaging spectrum, although histologically the former herniates through the dura.
- **Arachnoid cyst.** An arachnoid cyst represents a benign, CSF-containing, congenital lesion located within the arachnoid. Arachnoid cysts are smooth lesions that are most often unilocular, do not communicate with the ventricular system, and frequently have mass effect. The calvarium and brain are often molded by the cyst, and removal of the cyst does not result in reversal of the molded calvarial or brain contour. Most arachnoid cysts are supratentorial, and of those, most are located in the middle cranial fossa. While the etiology of an arachnoid cyst is unknown, one theory suggests that there is arachnoid separation and/or a diverticulum during development that fills with CSF. These lesions do not enhance and almost always follow CSF attenuation and signal on CT and MRI, respectively. Uncommonly, proteinaceous debris or hemorrhage may develop in an arachnoid cyst, particularly following trauma. Differentiating an arachnoid cyst from a giant arachnoid granulation (>1 cm) can be difficult. When large, arachnoid cysts will be associated with mass effect upon the adjacent brain, whereas a giant arachnoid granulation is typically not associated with mass effect upon the brain. Additionally, veins do not traverse an arachnoid cyst because it represents a contained cyst, whereas veins may traverse an arachnoid granulation.
- **Cerebellar herniation into the calvarium.** A true cephalocele that involves the cranial vault (either a meningocele or encephalocele) is present when meninges and/or brain herniate through both the inner as well as the outer tables of the calvarium. Otherwise, the finding is more appropriately characterized as a cephalocele herniating into the calvarium. This distinction is made because a true cephalocele is more likely to be associated with symptoms, such as a CSF leak, as opposed to a herniation of intracranial contents that is contained by the outer table of the calvarium, which is typically asymptomatic. Other instances where a true cephalocele may be identified include those that extend completely through skull base, including those that extend through the skull base foramina, into the paranasal sinuses, or into pneumatized portions of the temporal bones.

Calvarial arachnoid granulation

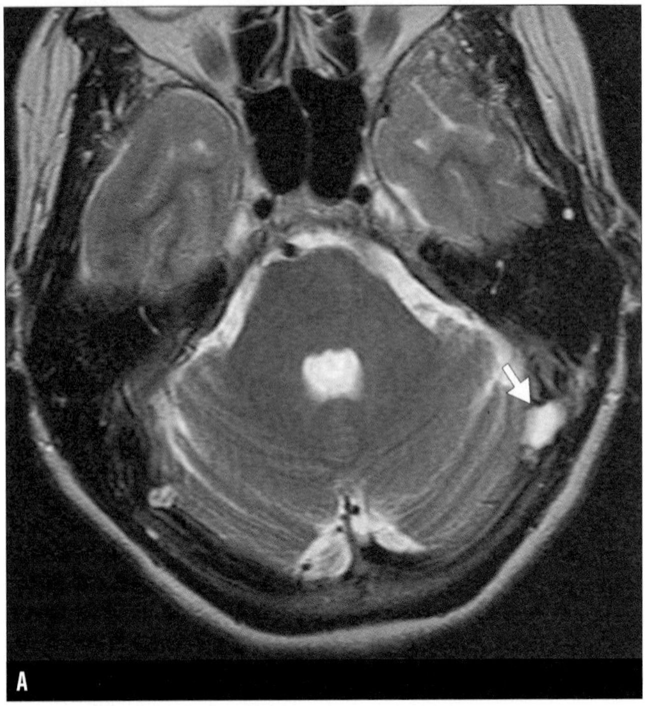

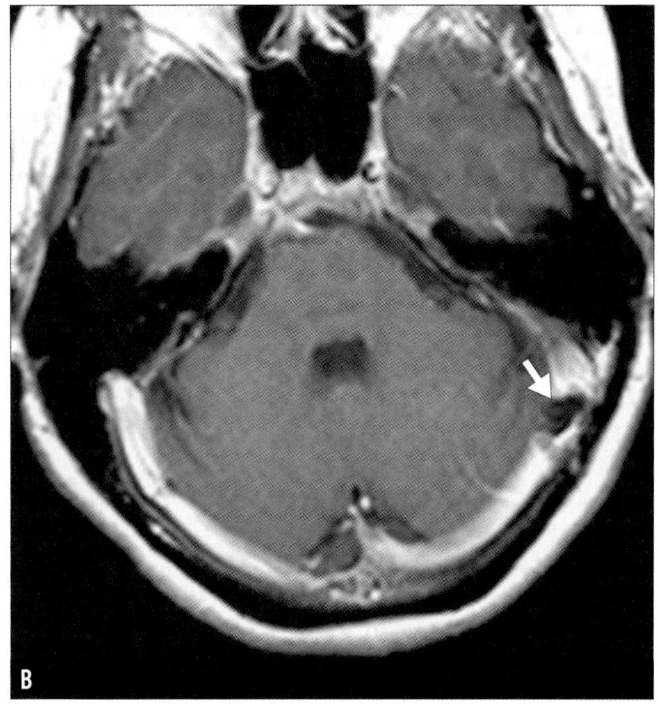

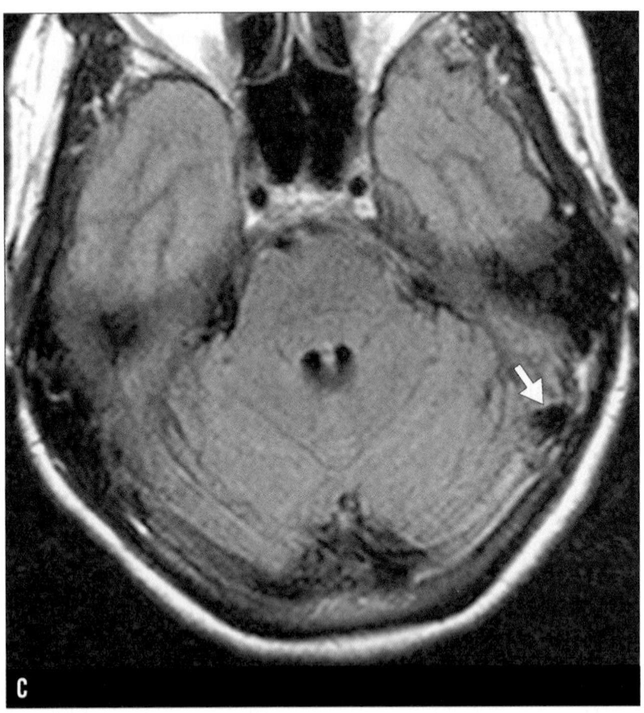

Axial T2 (**A**), contrast-enhanced axial T1 (**B**), and axial FLAIR (**C**) MR images demonstrate a CSF-equivalent focus projecting into the distal left transverse sinus (arrows, **A**-**C**). Given its morphology and location, this finding simulates a focal dural venous sinus thrombosis. However, when evaluating all the pertinent images from several sequences, this finding communicated with the adjacent CSF. The communication with the adjacent CSF as well as the CSF-equivalent signal of the finding is consistent with an arachnoid granulation, rather than a dural venous sinus thrombosis.

Calvarial arachnoid granulation

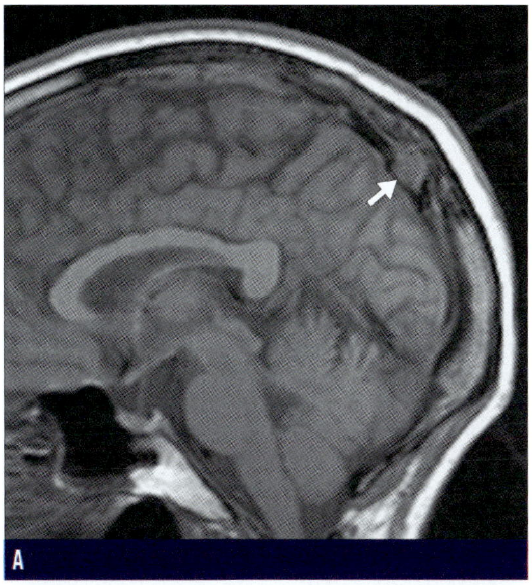

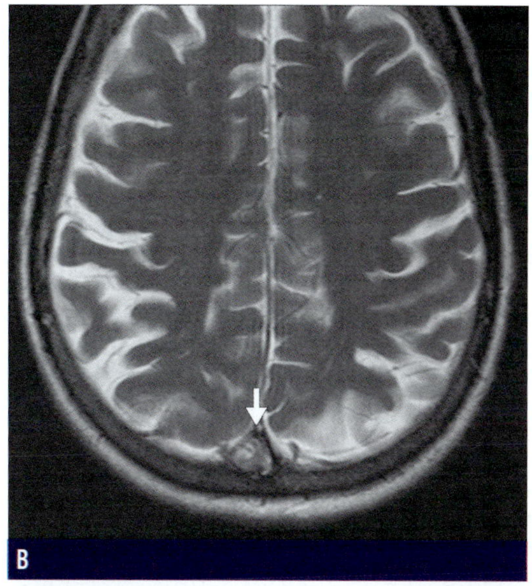

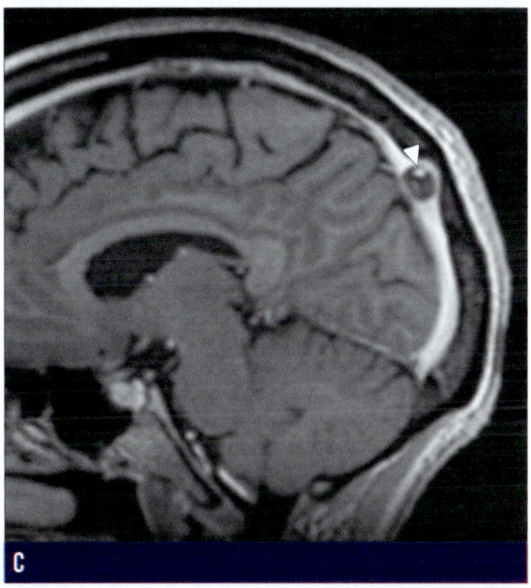

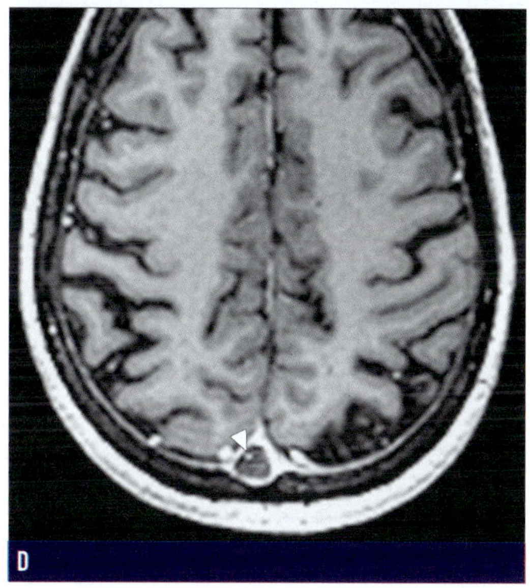

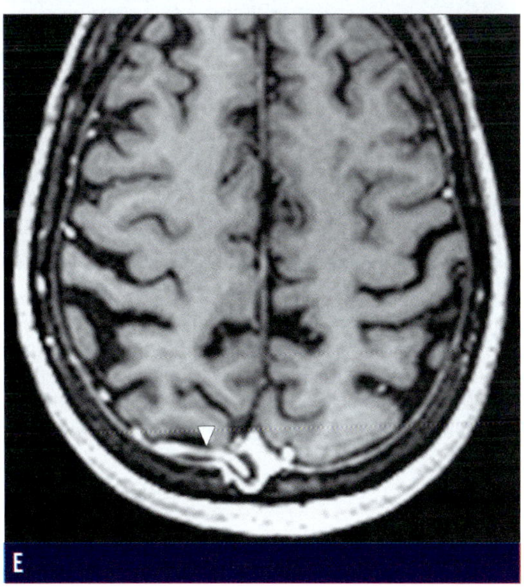

Different patient. Sagittal T1 (**A**) and axial T2 (**B**) MR images demonstrate a T1 isointense, heterogeneously T2 hyperintense focus in the region of the superior sagittal sinus, raising the possibility of a focal dural venous sinus thrombosis or other lesion (arrows, **A**, **B**). Sagittal (**C**) and axial (**D**, **E**) postcontrast MPRAGE MR images demonstrate the finding to be situated within the superior sagittal sinus. A punctate-enhancing focus identified within the finding on images **C** and **D** (arrowheads, **C**, **D**) is clearly identified as a vein entering the finding on image **E** (arrowhead, **E**). The findings are compatible with an arachnoid granulation and not a focal dural venous sinus thrombosis.

Giant calvarial arachnoid granulation

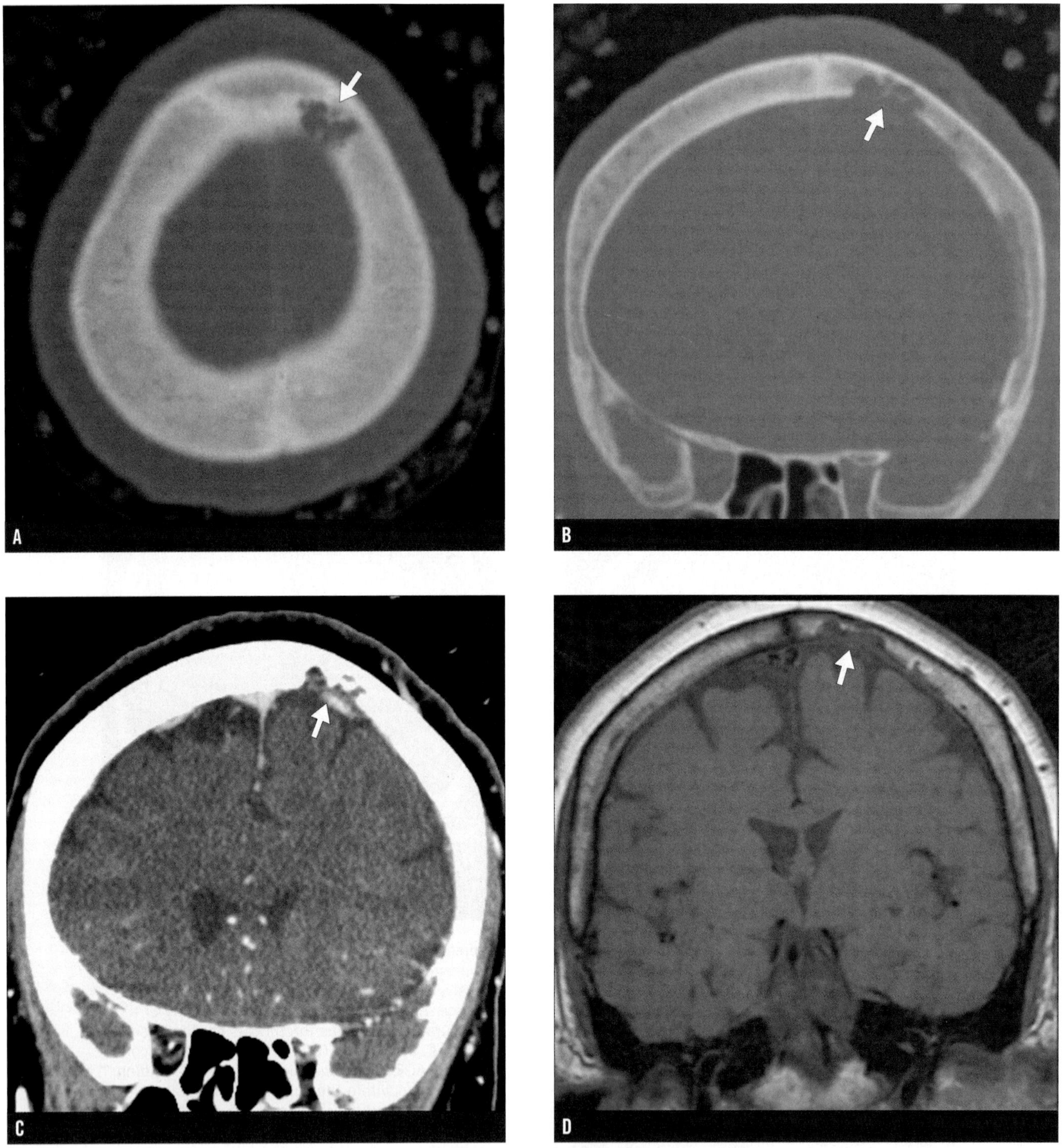

Contrast-enhanced axial (**A**) and coronal reformatted (**B**) CT images viewed with a bone window and the same image as **B** viewed with a soft tissue window (**C**). Images **A** and **B** demonstrate a focal lucency significantly larger than 1 cm located in the anterior aspect of the left parietal bone (arrows, **A**, **B**). Image **C** demonstrates a vessel that traverses the calvarial lucency and which communicates with the subarachnoid space (arrow, **C**). These findings are in keeping with a giant arachnoid granulation. Coronal T1 (**D**), contrast-enhanced coronal T1 with fat suppression (**E**), and coronal T2 with fat suppression (**F**) MR images of the same patient demonstrate the calvarial lesion to be mildly lobulated, T1 hypointense (arrow, **D**), peripherally enhancing (arrow, **E**), and to contain CSF-equivalent T2 signal (arrow, **F**), again compatible with a giant arachnoid granulation.

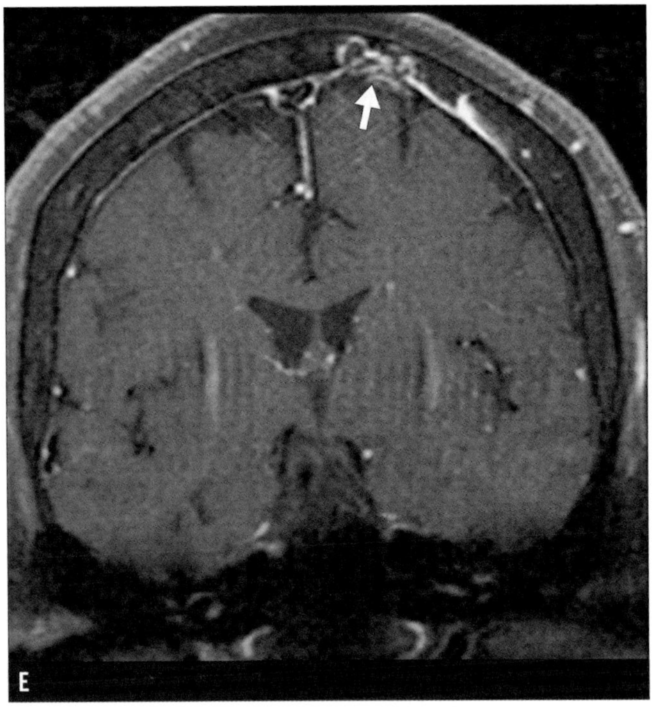

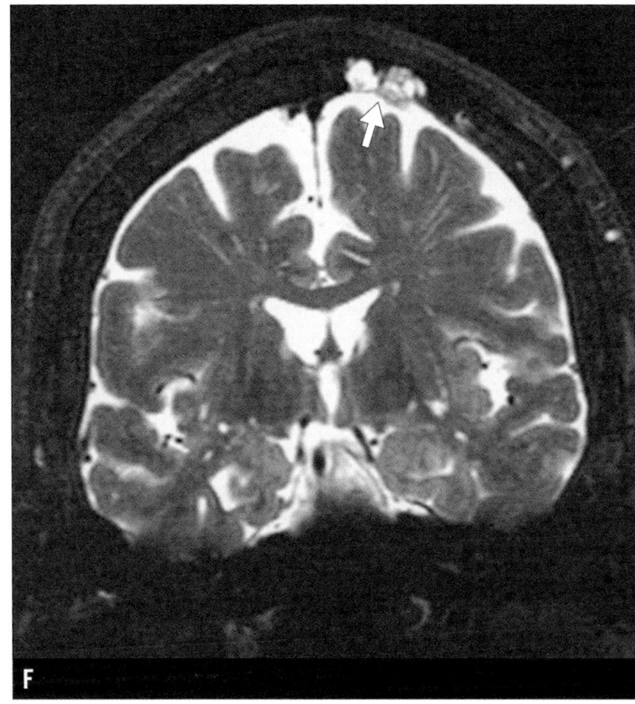

Companion case: Calvarial meningocele

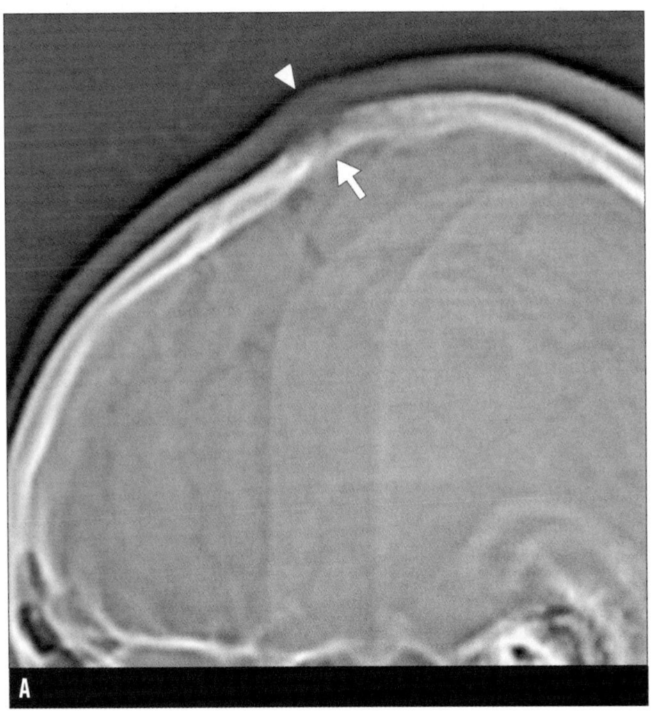

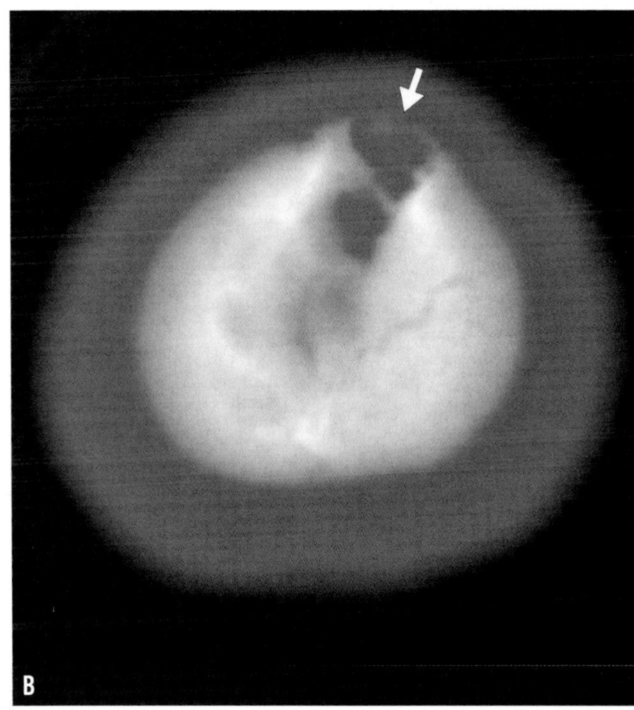

A sagittal scout image from a CT brain examination (**A**) demonstrates a focal lytic lucency at the calvarial vertex (arrow, **A**) associated with slight bulging of the overlying scalp (arrowhead, **A**). Axial CT images from the same study viewed with a bone window (**B**) and soft tissue window (**C**) demonstrate the lytic finding to extend through the inner and outer tables of the calvarium and to contain hypoattenuation, although it is difficult to determine whether it is a benign or malignant finding based on this CT study. Contrast-enhanced coronal T1 with fat suppression (**D**) and sagittal T2 (**E**) MR images of the brain from the same patient demonstrate the finding to be located to the left of the superior sagittal sinus, to contain CSF-equivalent fluid, and to be devoid of herniated brain tissue (arrows, **D**, **E**). A contrast-enhanced sagittal MPRAGE MR image (**F**) demonstrates a small vein (arrowhead, **F**) traversing this protruding CSF collection, indicating that the finding is contiguous with the subarachnoid space and effectively excluding an arachnoid cyst. Given that the finding extends through both the inner and outer tables of the calvarium, best demonstrated on CT, the finding is most consistent with a calvarial meningocele rather than a giant arachnoid granulation.

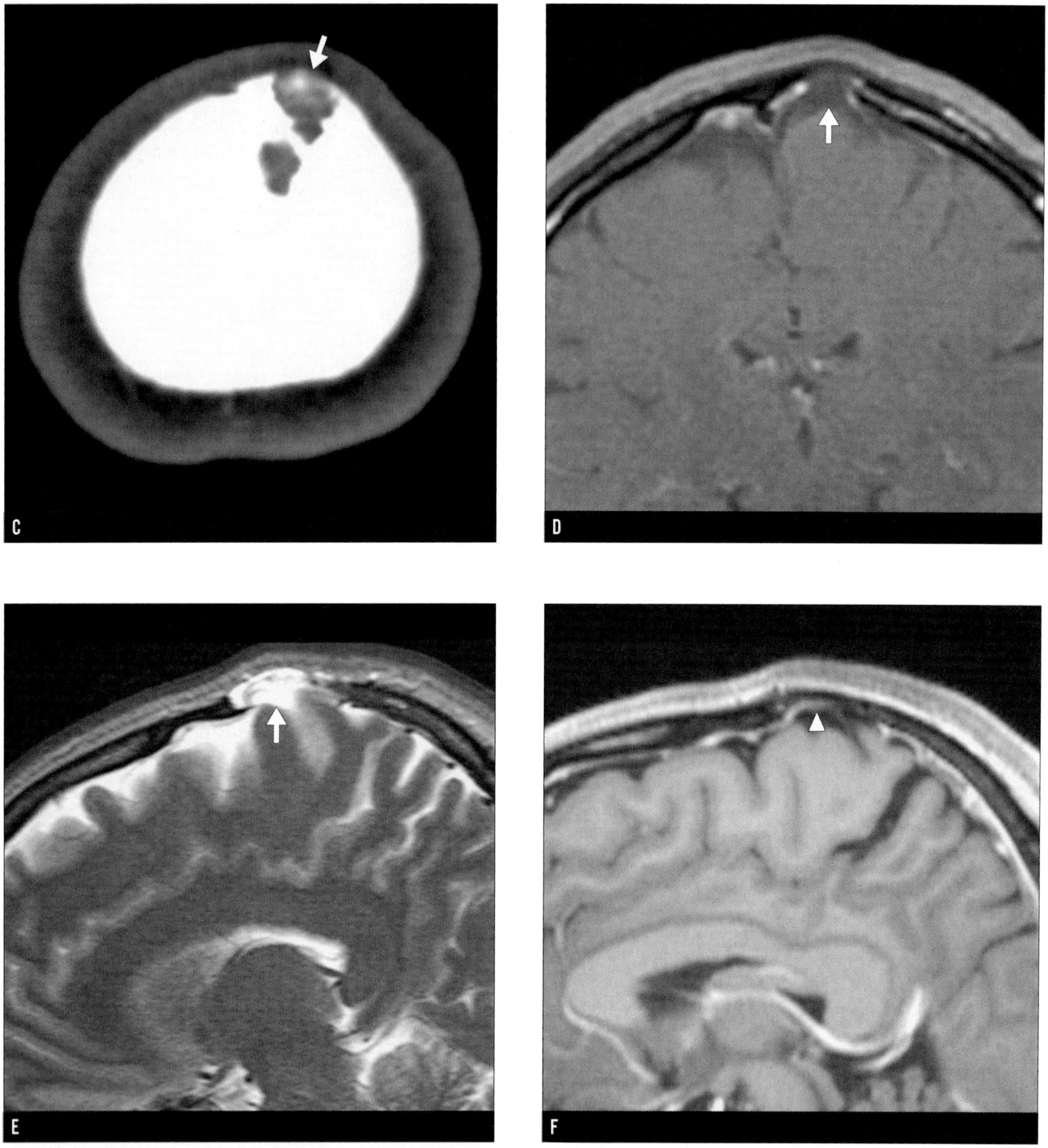
C
D
E
F

Companion case: Arachnoid cyst

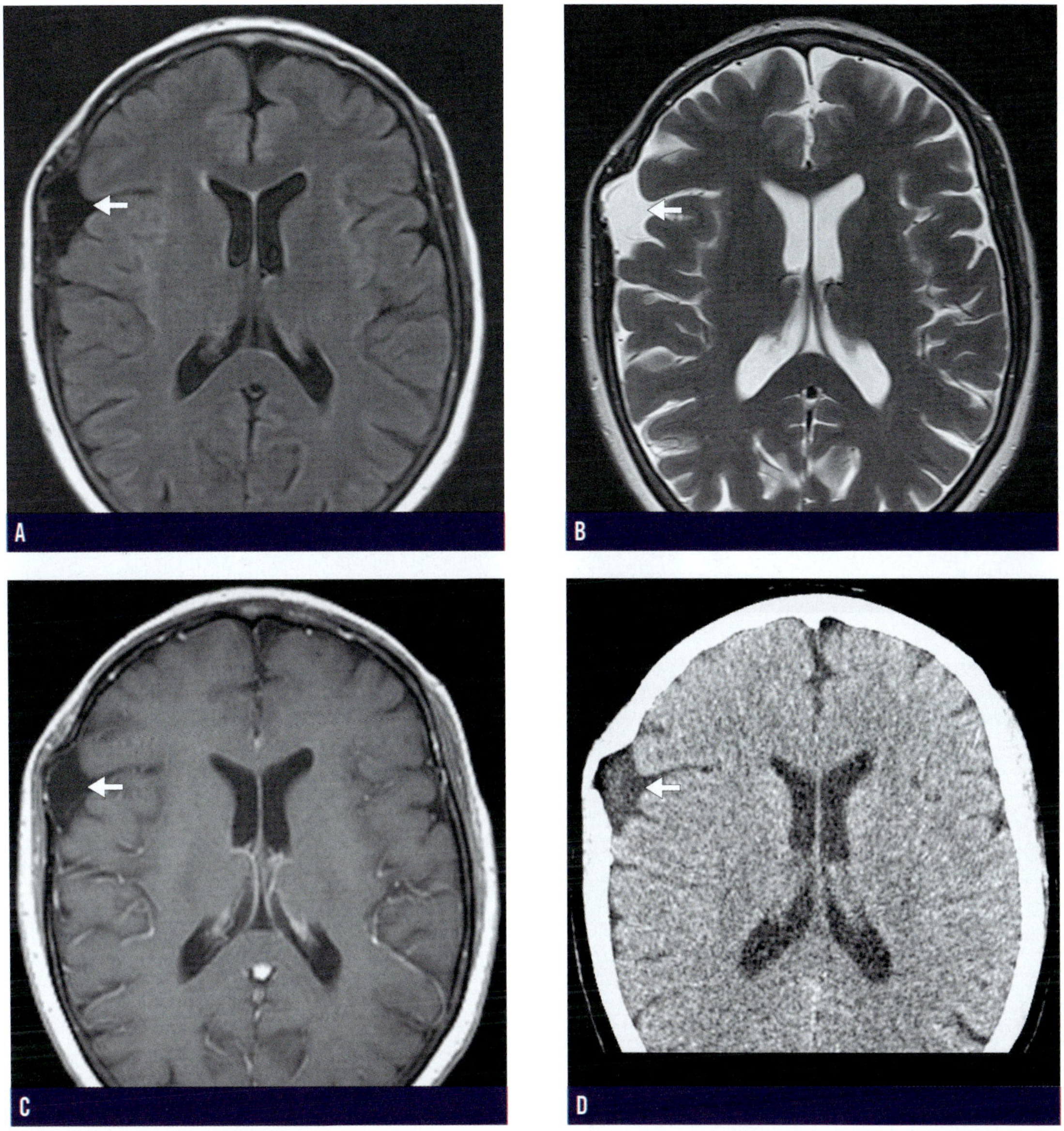

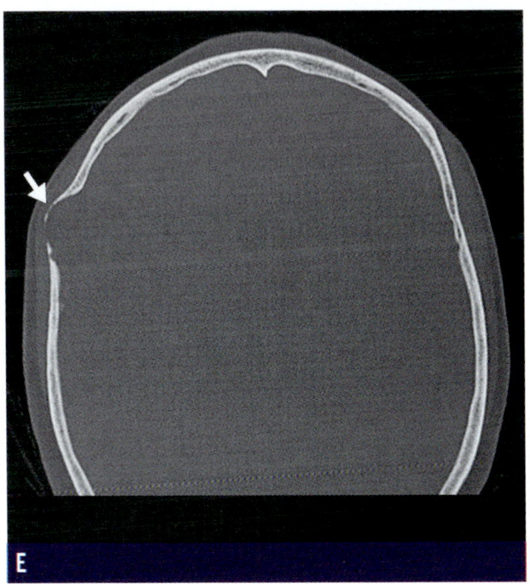

Axial FLAIR (**A**), axial T2 (**B**), and contrast-enhanced axial T1 (**C**) MR images demonstrate focal lateral bulging of the calvarium that is occupied by CSF-equivalent fluid (arrows, **A-C**). There is no sizeable vein traversing this focal CSF collection to suggest that the finding directly communicates with the subarachnoid space, an imaging characteristic that would be compatible with a large arachnoid granulation. Furthermore, there is mass effect upon the subjacent brain, a finding that is not associated with a large arachnoid granulation. An axial CT image of the same patient viewed with a brain window (**D**) also demonstrates CSF-equivalent fluid within the finding (arrow, **D**). An axial CT image viewed with a bone window (**E**) better demonstrates the lateral bulging of the calvarium and associated calvarial thinning, although the outer table of the calvarium remains intact (arrow, **E**). The findings are most compatible with an arachnoid cyst.

Companion case: Cerebellar herniation into the calvarium

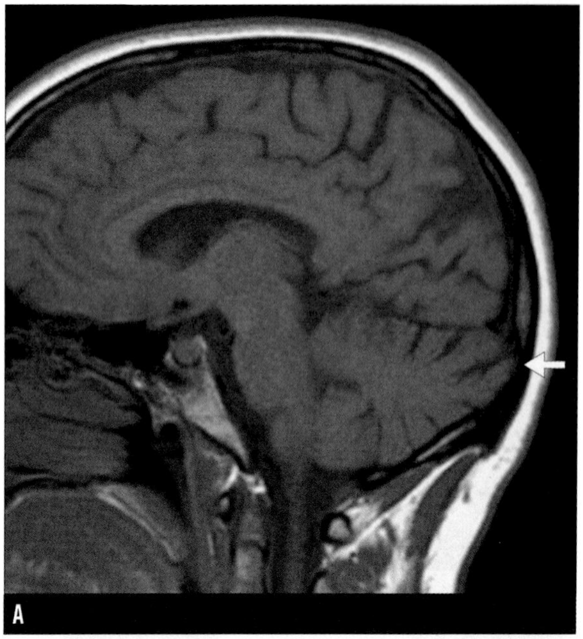

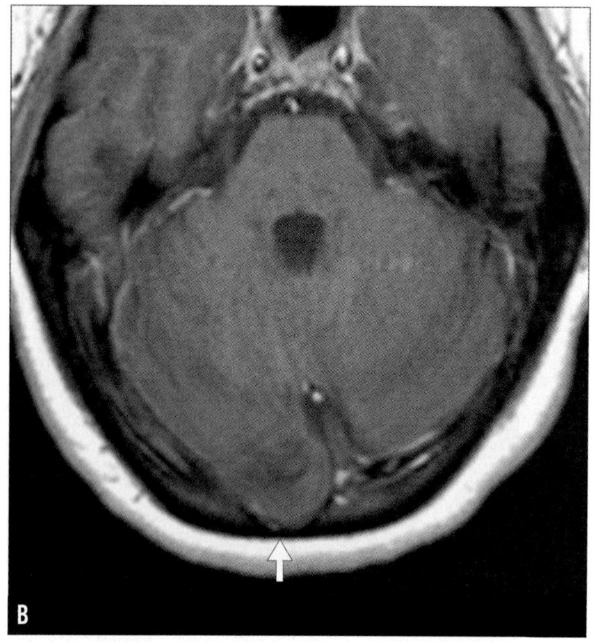

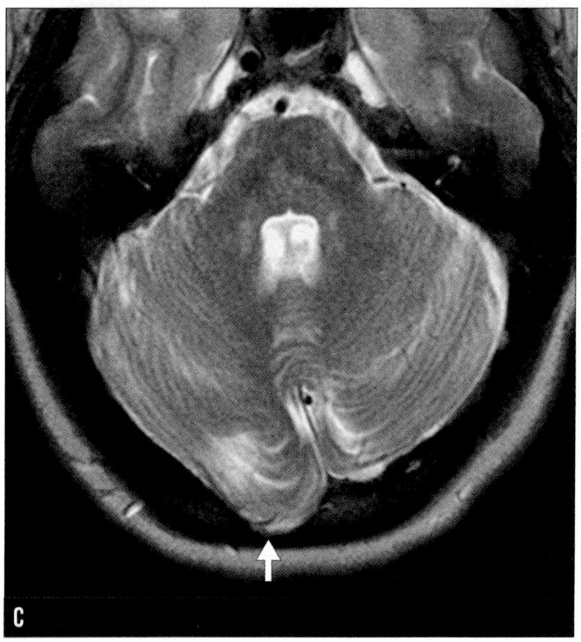

Sagittal T1 (**A**), contrast-enhanced axial T1 (**B**), and axial T2 (**C**) MR images demonstrate distortion and herniation of the posterior right cerebellar folia into a smooth inner table deficiency along the parasagittal right aspect of the occipital bone (arrows, **A**-**C**). However, the outer table of the occipital calvarium is intact and therefore the finding does not fit strict criteria for an encephalocele. Therefore, the finding is more appropriately characterized as cerebellar herniation into the calvarium rather than a true encephalocele.

REFERENCES

Battal B, Castillo M. Brain herniations into the dural venous sinuses or calvarium: MRI of a recently recognized entity. *Neuroradiol J.* 2014;27(1):55-62.

Battal B, Hamcan S, Akgun V, Sari S, Karaman B. Brain herniation with surrounding CSF into the skull or encepholecele? *J Neuroradiol.* 2015.

Chan WC, et al. Focal brain herniation into giant arachnoid granulation: a rare occurrence. *Eur J Radiol* 2011;78:e111-e113.

Chen F, Deng XF, Liu B, Zou LN, Wang DB, Han H. Arachnoid granulations of middle cranial fossa: a population study between cadaveric dissection and in vivo computed tomography examination. *Surg Radiol Anat.* 2011;33(3):215-221. Epub October 12, 2010.

Goddard JC, Meyer T, Nguyen S, Lambert PR. New considerations in the cause of spontaneous cerebrospinal fluid otorrhea. *Otol Neurotol.* 2010;31(6):940-945.

Osborn AG, Preece MT. Intracranial cysts: radiologic-pathologic correlation and imaging approach. *Radiology.* 2006;239(3):650-664.

Trimble CR, Harnsberger HR, Castillo M, Brant-Zawadzki M, Osborn AG. "Giant" arachnoid granulations just like CSF?: NOT!! *AJNR Am J Neuroradiol.* 2010;31(9):1724-1728. Epub June 25, 2010.

Zheng H, Zhou M, Zhao B, Zhou D, He L. Pseudotumor cerebri syndrome and giant arachnoid granulation: treatment with venous sinus stenting. *J Vasc Interv Radiol.* 2010;21(6):927-929.

CASE 2 Calvarial diploic veins and venous lakes

The calvarial diploic venous system is a large network of valveless veins located between the inner and outer tables of the calvarial cortex. The calvarial diploic venous system communicates with the intracranial venous system as well as the venous system that drains soft tissues of the scalp, the latter via transosseous connections termed emissary veins. Diploic veins appear by approximately the eighth week of development and continue to develop in size and distribution into early childhood, undergoing minimal change after the age of five. Venous lakes (also called venous lacunae) represent focally dilated diploic veins and aid in resorbing cerebrospinal fluid from arachnoid granulations, much like dural venous sinuses.

There is no correlation between the size of the skull and the size of diploic venous system. Several studies have identified different diploic vein and venous lake patterns in the calvarium. Specifically, seven different patterns have been described using radiography, including "serpentine" and "thousand lakes" subtypes. There tends to be symmetry in the size and pattern of diploic veins between the two sides of the calvarium, a characteristic that may help differentiate this normal anatomy from pathology.

On radiography or CT, diploic veins are identified as discrete venous channels. Venous lakes are typically are typically round or oval lucent areas that contain distinct corticated margins, with or without regional thinning of the cortex. On MRI, diploic veins enhance like other surrounding venous structures and may have flow voids on T2-weighted imaging. Venous lakes will also enhance on MRI but may be T2 hyperintense, likely secondary to slow venous flow.

COMPANION CASES

- **Venous malformation of bone (osseous hemangioma).** A focal, nonaggressive, at least partially intrinsic T1 hyperintense osseous lesion that enhances on MRI has historically been termed a benign intraosseous hemangioma. However, more recent literature evaluating the histopathology of this lesion supports that this entity is more appropriately termed a venous malformation of bone. On CT, an intraosseous venous malformation of the calvarium is largely lucent and frequently contains coarse osseous trabeculations. Hounsfield units within the lucency often reveals fat attenuation, a finding that usually confirms this benign entity.
- **Multiple myeloma.** Multiple myeloma (MM) is disease of malignant plasma cells that generally affects older patients. A patient with MM typically presents with fatigue and bone pain as well as fractures, hypercalcemia, and renal insufficiency. MM is often diagnosed following the detection of a blood and/or urine monoclonal protein, known as the M protein. The amount of M protein and other paraproteins combined with the serum hemoglobin level, calcium level, renal function, and the number of lytic lesions on a skeletal survey aid in determining the staging and prognosis of the disease. Four distinct patterns of the MM disease spectrum have been described with plain film radiography, including plasmacytoma (a solitary bone lesion that may progress to MM), diffuse skeletal involvement (also called myelomatosis), diffuse skeletal osteopenia, and sclerosing myeloma. On CT, discrete lytic lesions, expansile osseous lesions associated with soft tissue masses, diffuse osteopenia, fractures, and rarely osteosclerosis may be identified. MRI likely best depicts the extent and location of disease burden, with tumor foci usually identified as hypointense on T1, hyperintense on STIR, and enhancing on postcontrast T1-weighted imaging with fat suppression. Because MM is a metabolically active disease, PET imaging is also useful. While nuclear medicine bone scan imaging may reveal uptake in areas of bone reaction, it tends to underestimate the degree of MM disease burden.
- **Sinus pericranii.** Sinus pericranii (SP) is a venous anomaly characterized by tightly packed varicosities located within the scalp that directly communicate with the dural venous sinuses via diploic veins. SP is most commonly located in the frontal region of the calvarium at or near the midline. SP is typically congenital, and it may be associated with an intracranial developmental venous anomaly. SP is most often an incidental lesion. Treatment is usually reserved for cosmetic purposes or if there are persistent symptoms, such as headaches or localized pain, which may be the result of acute thrombosis of the lesion. CT and MR angiography/venography are excellent modalities to delineate the epicranial varicosities as well as their connection with the intracranial dural venous sinuses. They may also reveal associated intracranial developmental venous anomalies, the presence of a skull defect, a venous malformation of the calvarium (osseous hemangioma), or thrombus within the SP. A T2-weighted sequence may reveal flow voids and/or increased T2 signal within the SP, the latter related to slow vascular flow. Intraluminal intrinsic T1 shortening may be identified on T1-weighted MRI if an acute thrombus in the SP is present. Direct catheter angiography is typically not required unless treatment is planned.

Calvarial diploic veins and venous lakes

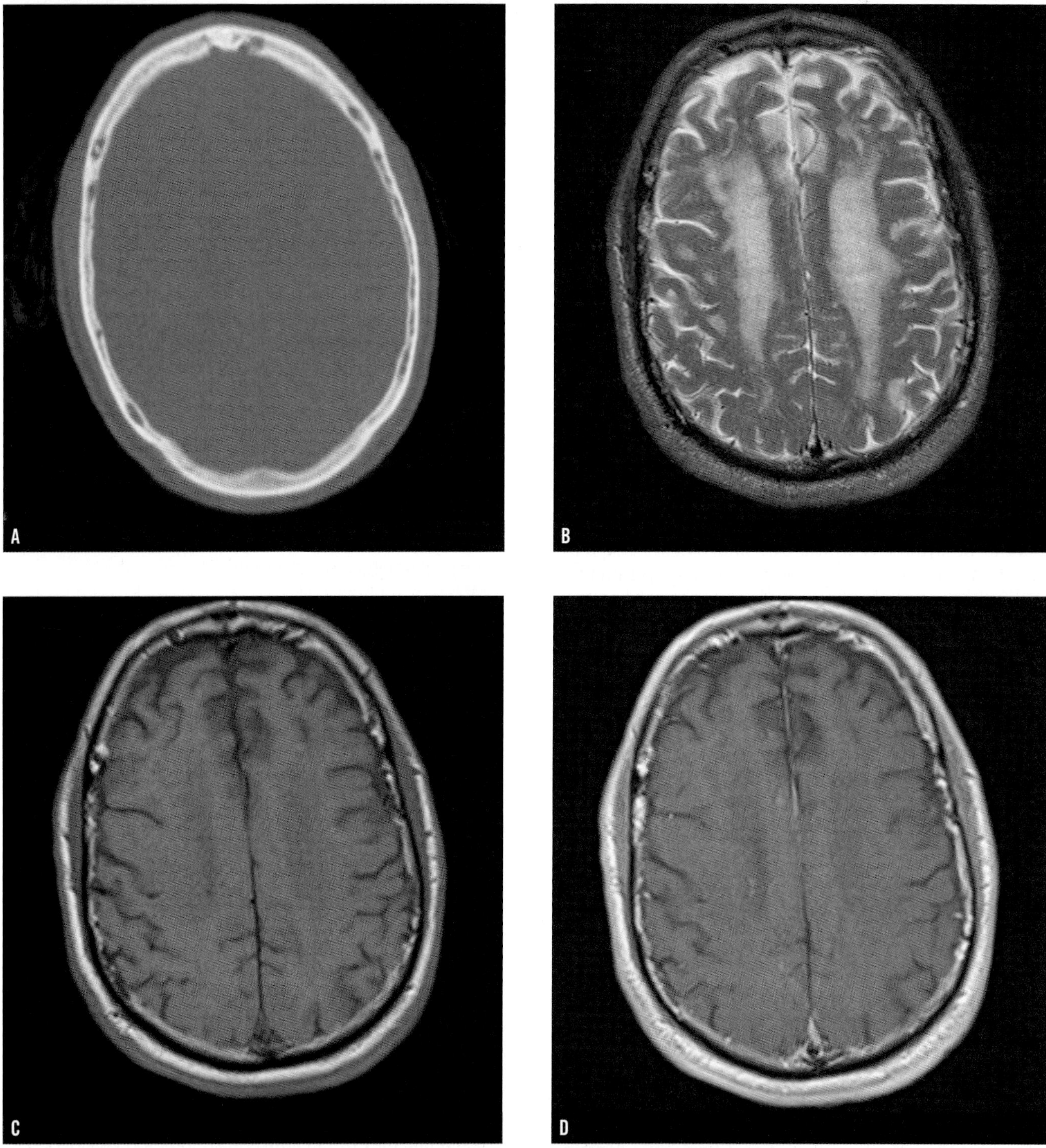

An axial CT image (**A**) demonstrates multiple lucencies within the diploic space of the calvarium. Many of these lucencies were identified on multiple other images and were linear in morphology. Axial T2 with fat suppression (**B**), axial T1 (**C**), and contrast-enhanced axial T1 (**D**) MR images demonstrate these lucencies to correspond to small foci of hyperintense T2 signal, hypointense T1 signal, and enhancement. The findings are related to incidentally enlarged calvarial diploic veins and venous lakes.

Calvarial diploic veins and venous lakes

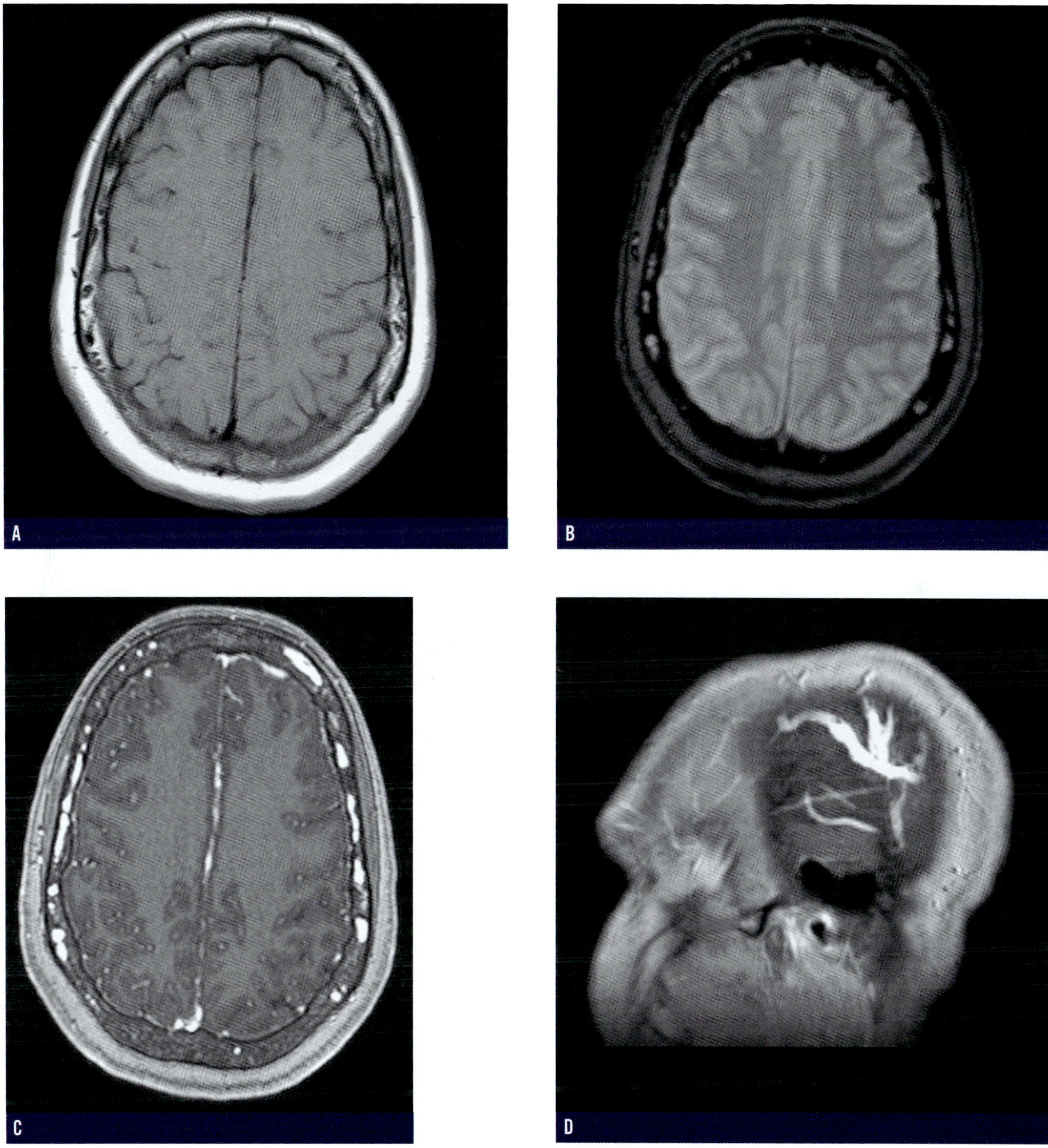

Different patient. Axial T1 (**A**), axial GRE (**B**), contrast-enhanced axial MPRAGE (**C**), and contrast-enhanced sagittal reformatted MPRAGE (**D**) MR images demonstrate multiple contiguous enhancing areas within the diploic space of the calvarium, compatible with large diploic veins. Some of these findings are not contiguous and are therefore consistent with venous lakes.

Companion case: Venous malformation of bone (osseous hemangioma)

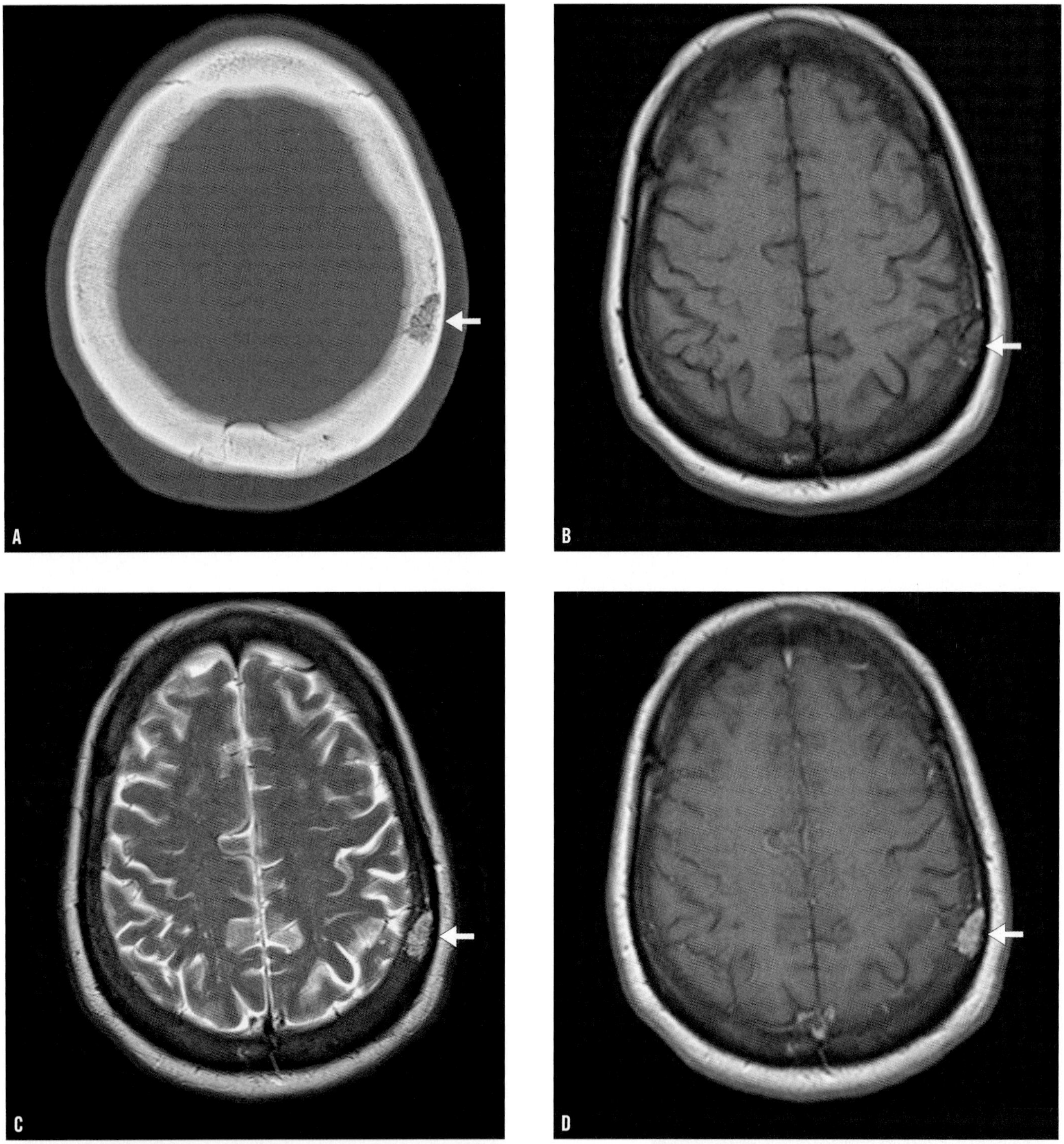

An axial CT image (**A**) demonstrates a discrete, lucent lesion in the left parietal calvarium that contains speckled foci of increased attenuation, compatible with a "honeycomb" pattern (arrow, **A**). Axial T1 (**B**), axial T2 (**C**), and contrast-enhanced axial T1 (**D**) MR images of the same patient demonstrate the finding to be mostly precontrast T1 isointense with speckled T1 hyperintense foci (arrow, **B**), hyperintense on T2 (arrow, **C**), and enhance (arrow, **D**). The imaging findings are most consistent with a benign calvarial venous malformation, historically referred to as a calvarial osseous hemangioma.

Companion case: Multiple myeloma

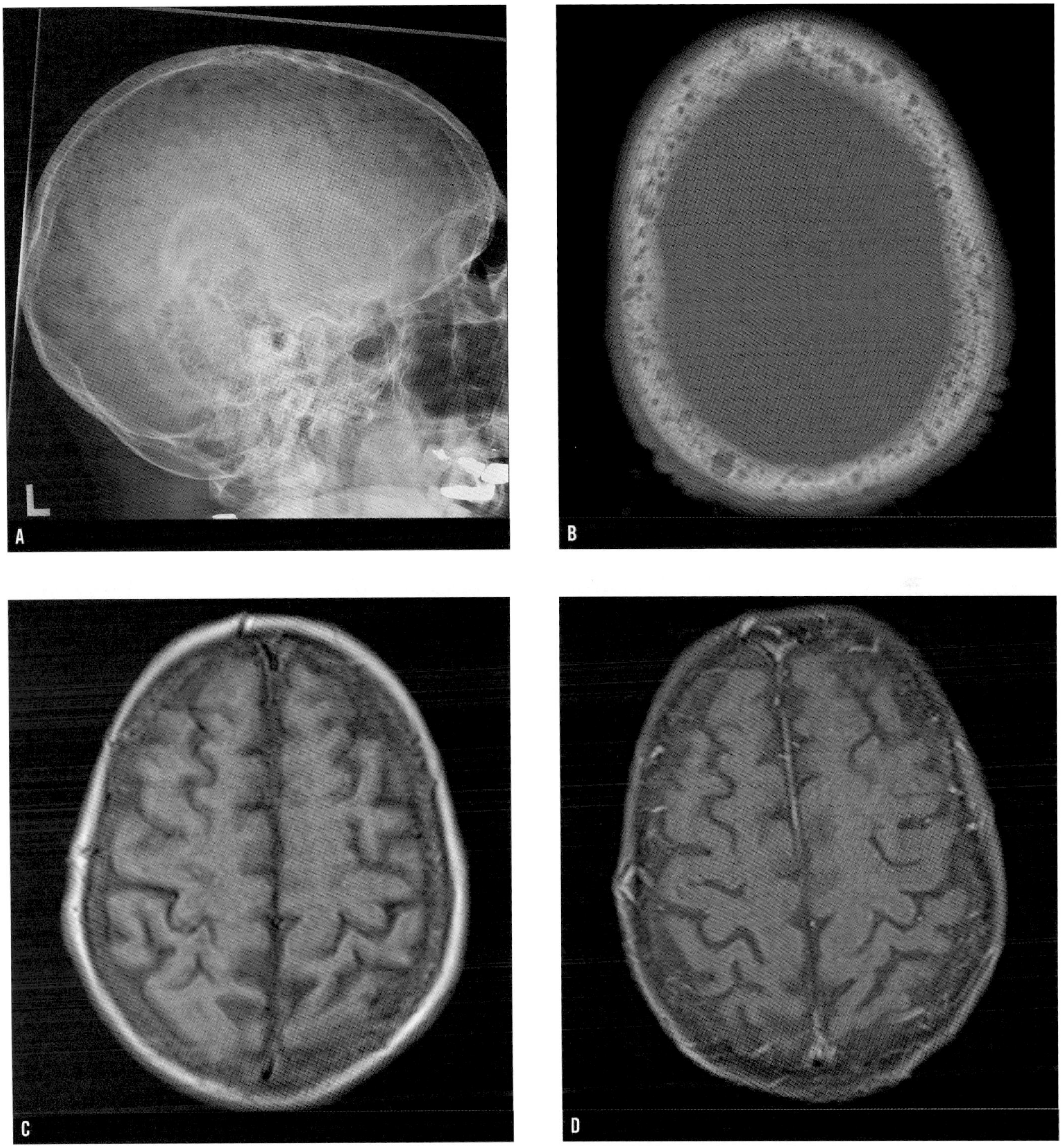

A lateral skull radiograph (**A**) and an axial CT image (**B**) of the same patient demonstrate innumerable lytic foci throughout the calvarium. Axial T1 (**C**) and contrast-enhanced fat-suppressed axial T1 (**D**) MR images of the same patient demonstrate subtle patchy enhancement of the calvarium interspersed among normal venous enhancement within the calvarium. These findings represented diffuse multiple myeloma. Multiple myeloma is most often strikingly STIR hyperintense (not shown).

Companion case: Sinus pericranii

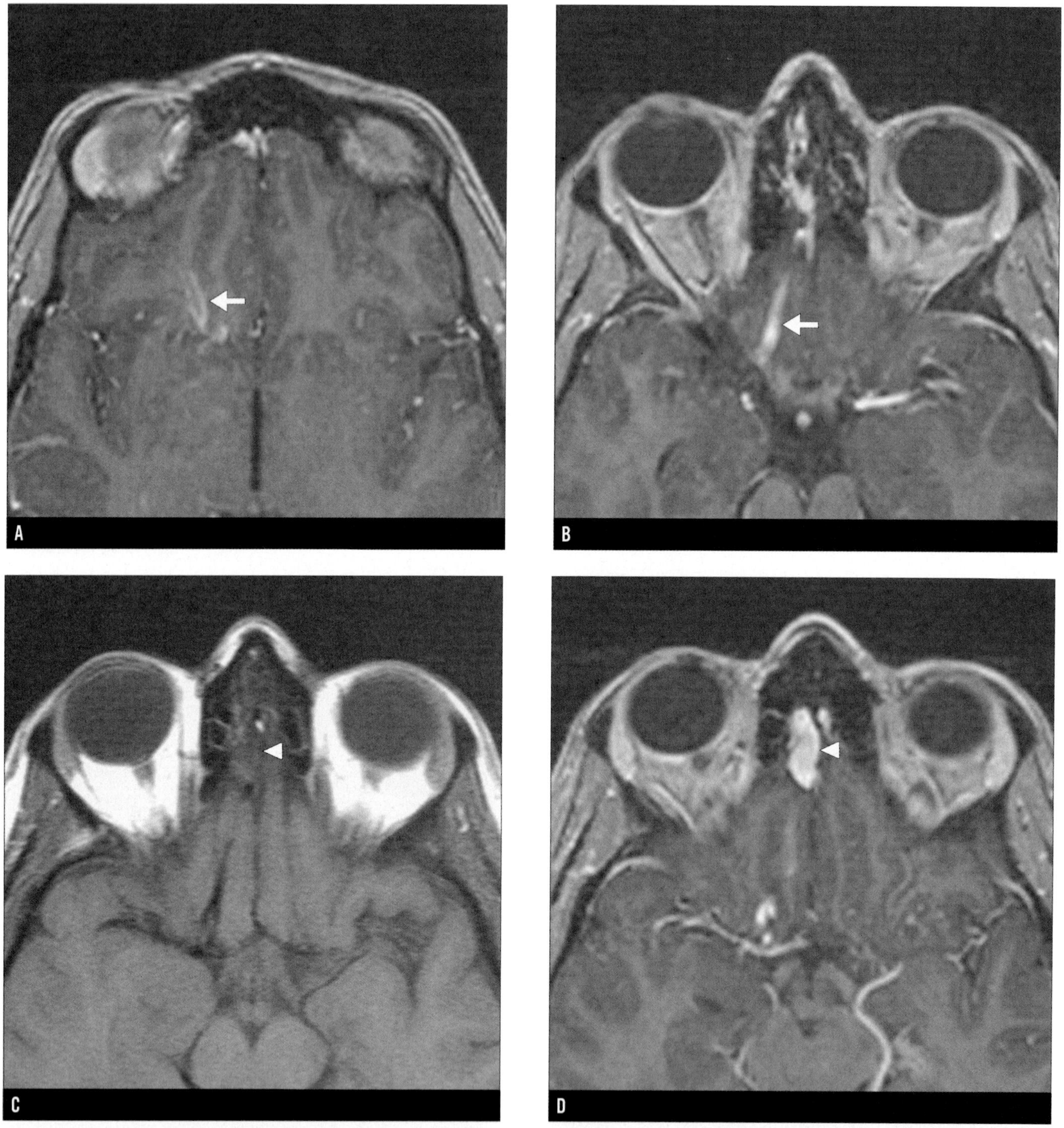

Contrast-enhanced axial MPRAGE MR images (**A**, **B**) demonstrate a prominent developmental venous anomaly (DVA) in the inferior aspect of the right frontal lobe (short arrows, **A**, **B**). Unenhanced axial MPRAGE (**C**) and contrast-enhanced axial MPRAGE (**D**) MR images demonstrate an oval-enhancing focus in the region of the right olfactory groove (arrowheads, **C**, **D**) which communicated with the DVA (not shown). Axial T1 (**E**), axial T2 (**F**), and contrast-enhanced fat-suppressed axial T1 (**G**) MR images demonstrate hypointense T1 and T2 signal with corresponding enhancement in the diploic space of the parasagittal right frontal calvarium (short arrows, **E**-**G**) associated with subtle similar signal characteristics within the overlying subgaleal soft tissues along the right aspect of the forehead (arrowheads, **E**-**G**). An axial CT image of the same patient (**H**) demonstrates subtle lucency within the diploic space of the right parasagittal aspect of the frontal bone (short arrow, **H**), corresponding to the signal abnormality in the calvarium on MRI. Frontal (**I**) and lateral (**J**) images from a catheter angiogram of the same patient demonstrate the DVA (short arrows, **I**, **J**) communicating with a venous pouch (arrowheads, **I**, **J**), the latter corresponding to the oval-enhancing focus in the right olfactory groove on MRI. The enhancing abnormality extends anterior to the calvarium and into the right frontal scalp soft tissues (long arrow, **J**). The constellation of findings is compatible with sinus pericranii. The finding in the frontal bone is consistent with an associated venous malformation of bone (also called osseous hemangioma). This patient complained of stress-related fullness behind the eyes.

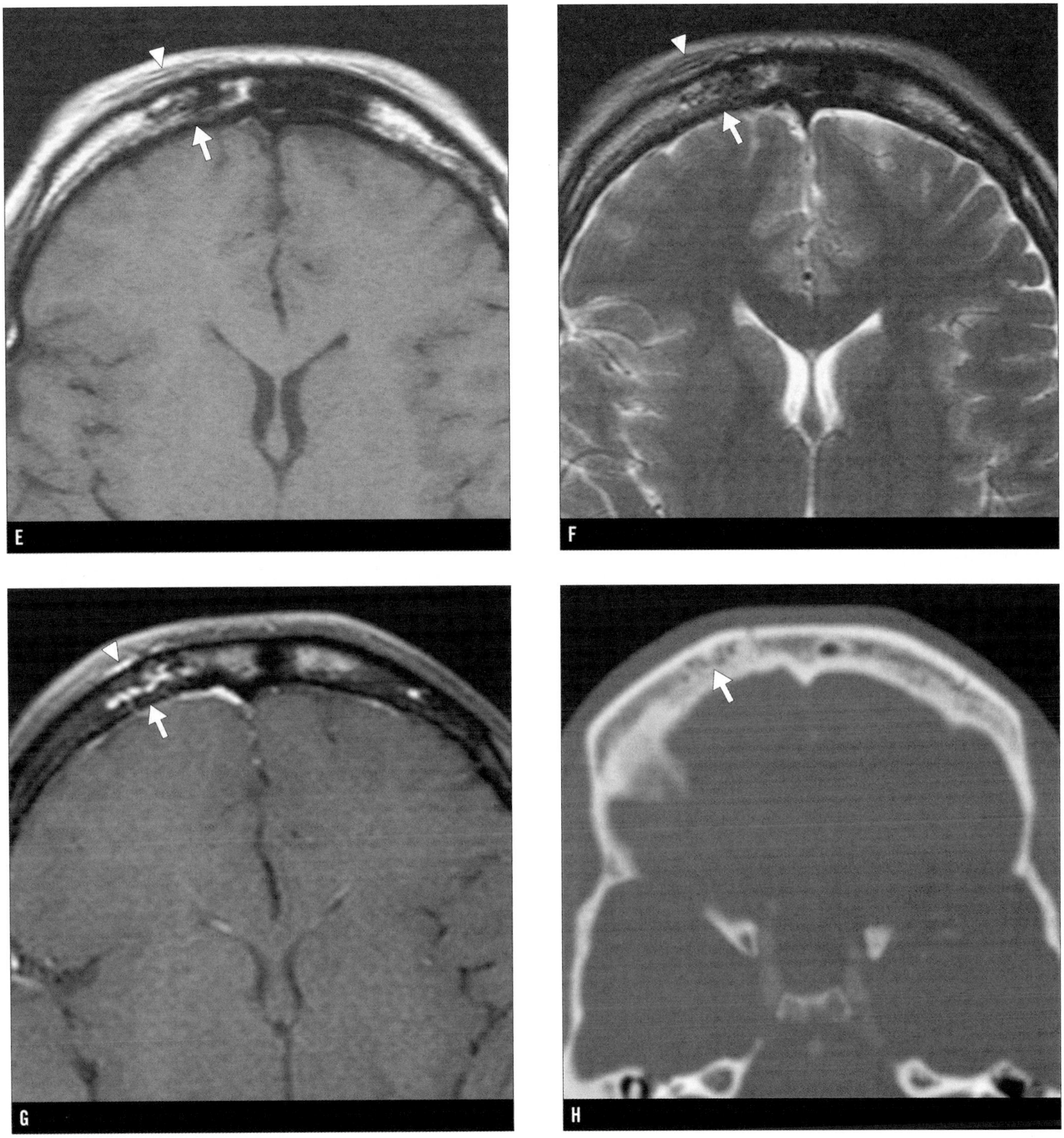
E
F
G
H

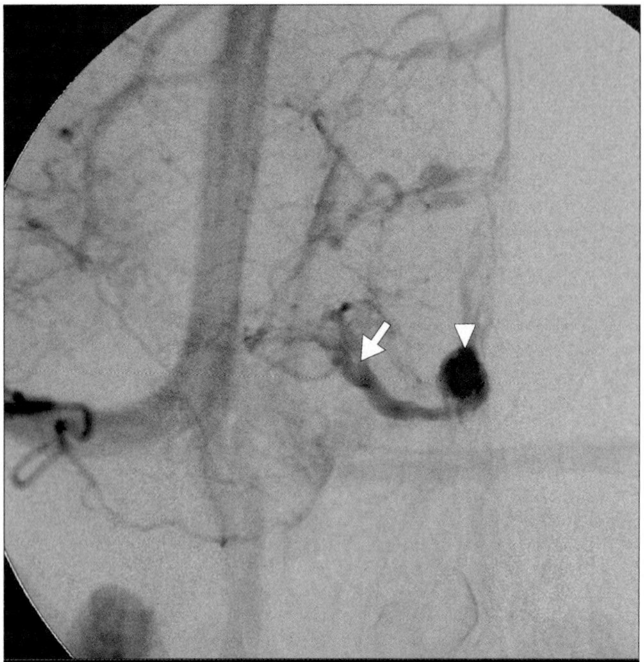

I

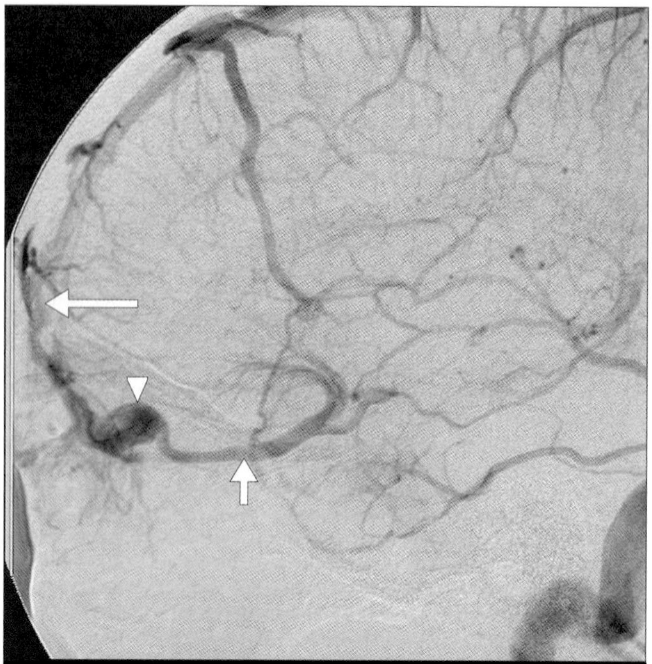

J

REFERENCES

Amaral L, et al. MR Imaging for the evaluation of lesions of the cranial vault. *Arq Neuropsiquiatr.* 2003;61(3-A): 521-532.

Angtuaco EJ, et al. Multiple myeloma: clinical review and diagnostic imaging. *Radiology.* 2004;231(1):11-23.

Carpenter JS, et al. Sinus pericranni: clinical and imaging findings in two cases of spontaneous partial thrombosis. *AJNR Am J Neuroradiol.* 2004;25:121-125.

Gandolfo C, et al. Sinus pericranii: diagnostic and therapeutic considerations in 15 patients. *Neuroradiology.* 2007;49(6):505-514.

Garcia-Gonzalez U, et al. The diploic venous system: surgical anatomy and neurosurgical implications. *Neurosurg Focus.* 2009;27(5):E2.

Hershkovitz I, et al. The elusive diploic vein: anthropological and anatomical perspective. *Am J Phys Anthropol.* 1999;108:345-358.

Jivraj K, et al. Diploic venous anatomy studied in-vivo by MRI. *Clin Anat.* 2009;22(3):296-301.

Lowe LH, Marchant TC, Rivard DC, Scherbel AJ. Vascular malformations: classification and terminology the radiologist needs to know. *Semin Roentgenol.*2012;47(2):106-117.

CASE 3 Parietal foramina

Parietal foramina represent well-corticated developmental foramina that are located within the paramedian parietal bones near the parietal eminence. These are considered normal variants and have an estimated prevalence of approximately 60% to 70%. Parietal foramina are believed to represent remnants of the primitive parietal notch, an area of relative slow bone development that typically disappears by the fifth month of fetal development.

Parietal foramina are most often small, usually only 1 to 2 mm in diameter, although a size of up to 5 mm still considered normal. Parietal foramina larger than 5 mm, termed enlarged parietal foramina, among other names, are also typically benign but rarely can be associated with intracranial anomalies. Parietal foramina are typically located within a few centimeters of midline and a few centimeters superior to the lambdoidal suture. Although these foramina are typically paired, a unilateral parietal foramen can also occur. Parietal foramina are covered by the scalp. In many cases, parietal foramina permit the passage of small emissary veins, termed the veins of Santorini, which anastomose the occipital vein to the superior sagittal sinus.

COMPANION CASES

- **Incidental parietal calvarial thinning.** Parietal bone thinning is believed to be an acquired, progressive thinning of both parietal bones, though there are a few reports of unilateral involvement. It appears radiographically as either flat or grooved thinning of the parietal bones, typically between the sagittal suture and the parietal prominence. Parietal thinning is uncommon and is usually identified in osteoporotic female patients who are older than 50 years. It is typically of no clinical significance, though there are reports of patients presenting with fractures of the thinned parietal bone. Parietal thinning is relatively diffuse in its extent, unlike parietal foramina which represent focal osseous lucencies.
- **Burr hole.** A burr hole is a surgically drilled calvarial defect utilized for device placement or for various surgical procedures that necessitate access to the intracranial compartment. On CT, these defects extend through entire thickness of the calvarium and can be associated with air as well as fluid superficial, within, or deep to the defect shortly after surgical creation. On MRI, elevated T2 signal may occupy the defect, and there may be enhancement along the margin of the defect on contrast-enhanced T1-weighted imaging. Displaced calvarial bone fragments may be identified within the brain following drilling of a burr hole. Burr holes are usually easily differentiated from parietal foramina by their location, history of prior intervention, and the lack of well-corticated bone along the margin of the defect.

Parietal foramina

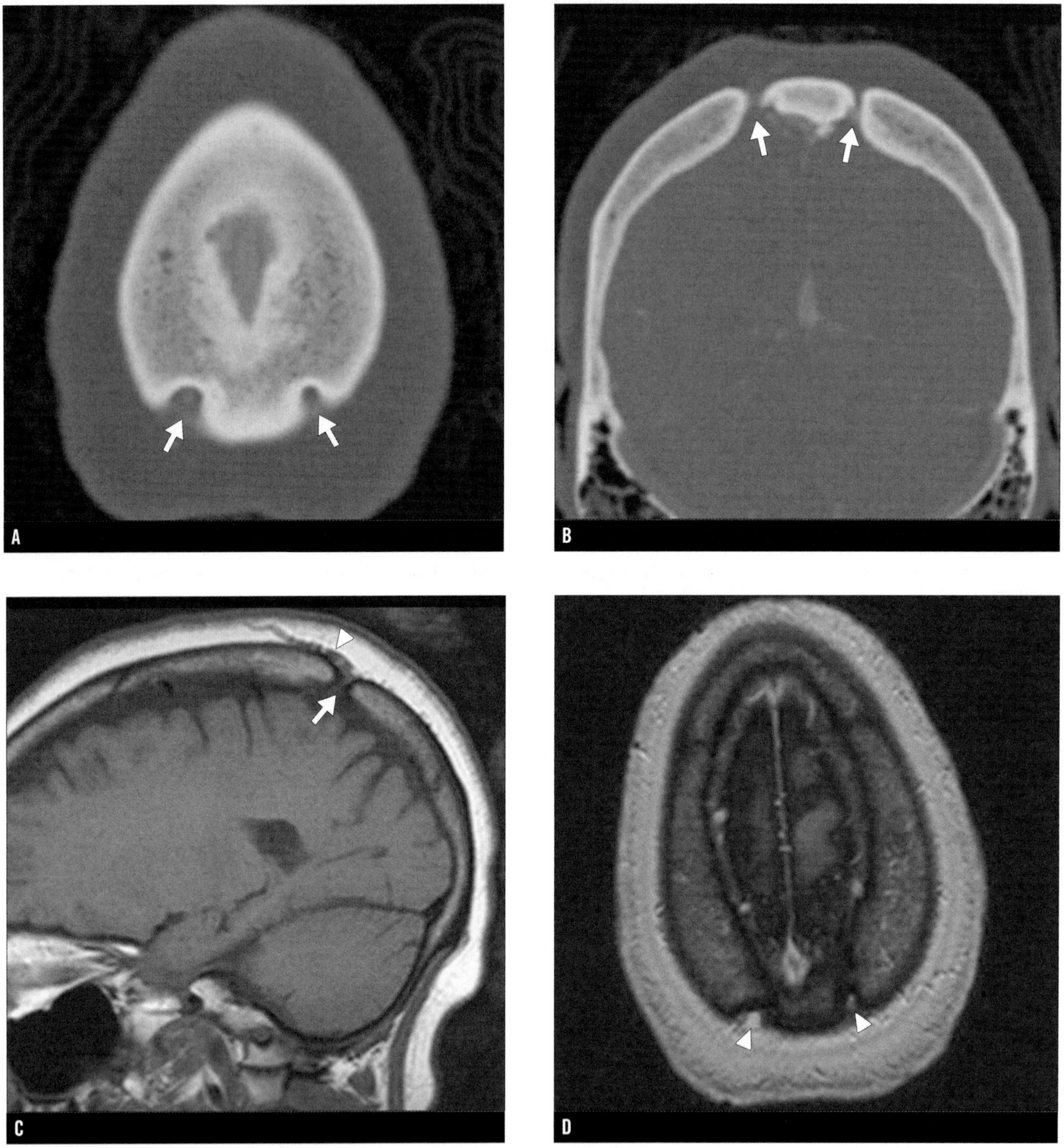

Axial (**A**) and coronal reformatted (**B**) CT images demonstrate paired, corticated lucencies at the vertex of the parietal bones (arrows, **A**, **B**). A sagittal T1-weighted MR image of the same patient (**C**) demonstrates one of the osseous defects in the sagittal plane (arrow, **C**). A contrast-enhanced axial MPRAGE MR image of the same patient (**D**) demonstrates that the foramina contain small enhancing vessels (arrowheads, **D**). One of these vessels is also identified traversing the scalp on image **C** (arrowhead). The findings are compatible with incidental parietal foramina which contain normal traversing veins (veins of Santorini).

Large parietal foramina

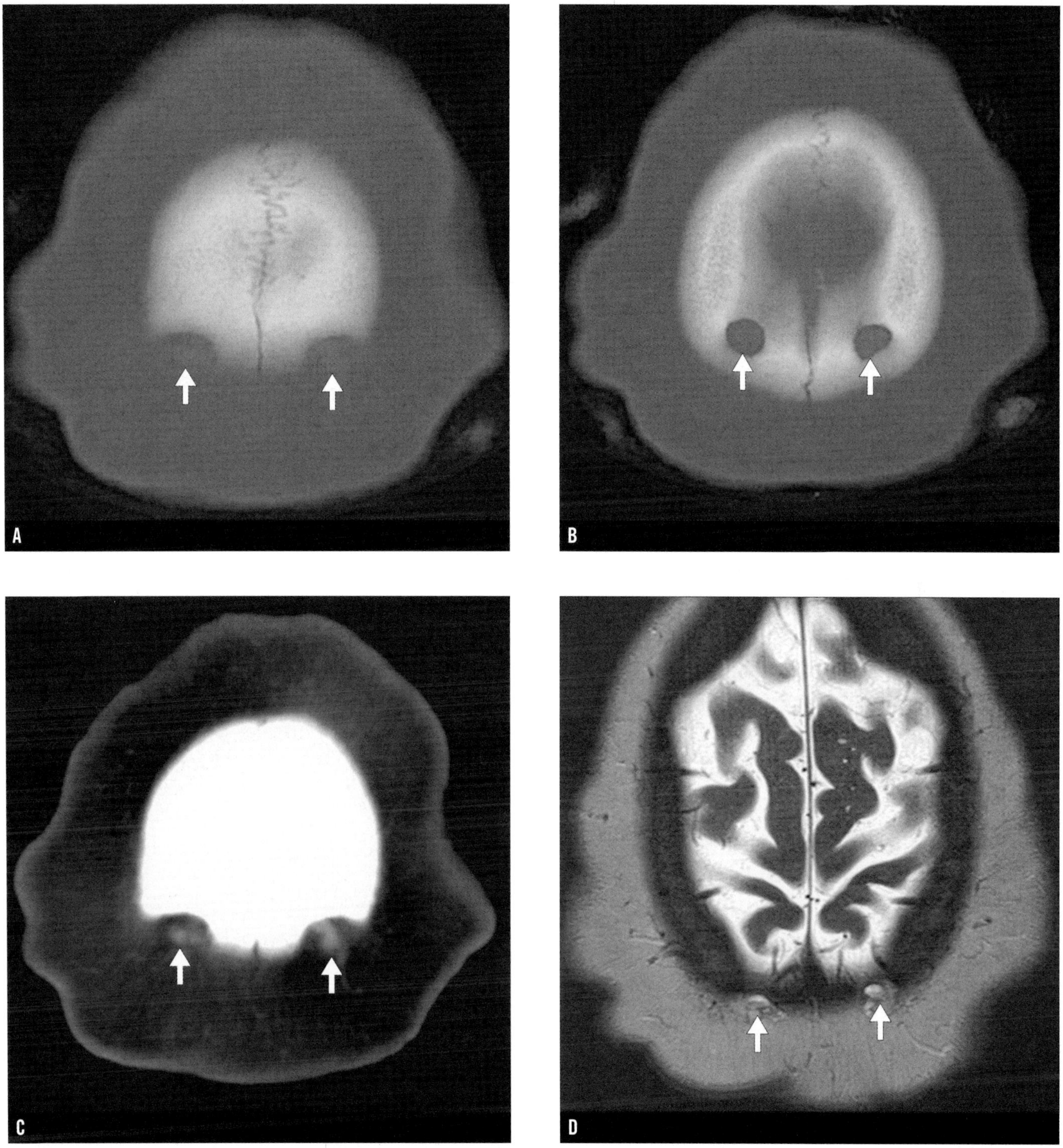

Axial CT images through the vertex of the calvarium viewed with a bone window (**A**, **B**) and soft tissue window (**C**) demonstrate large, circumscribed, paired lucencies within the parietal bones (arrows, **A**-**C**). Image **C** also demonstrates focal soft tissue density within these lucencies. Axial T2 (**D**), axial T1 (**E**), and contrast-enhanced axial T1 (**F**) MR images of the same patient demonstrate the MR correlate (arrows, **D**-**F**). Image **F** demonstrates subtle enhancement traversing the defects. The findings are compatible with incidentally enlarged parietal foramina that contain normal traversing veins (veins of Santorini).

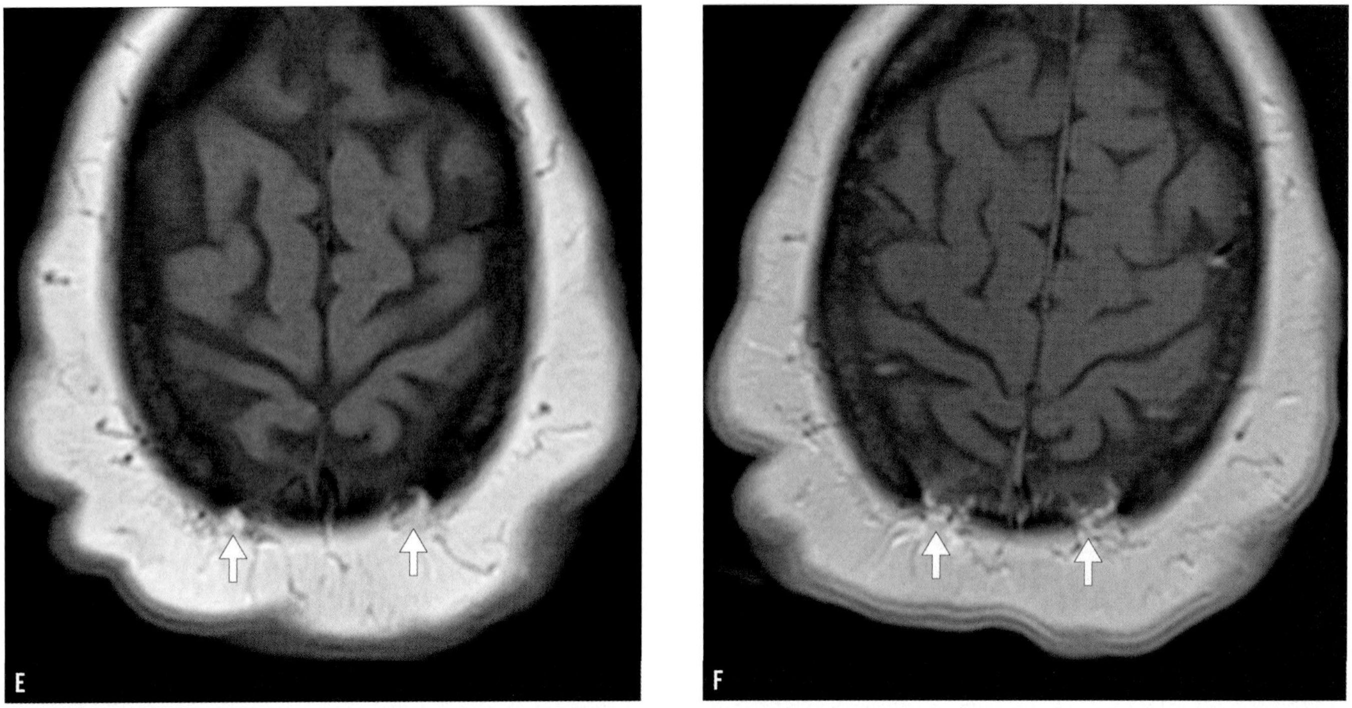

Parietal foramen

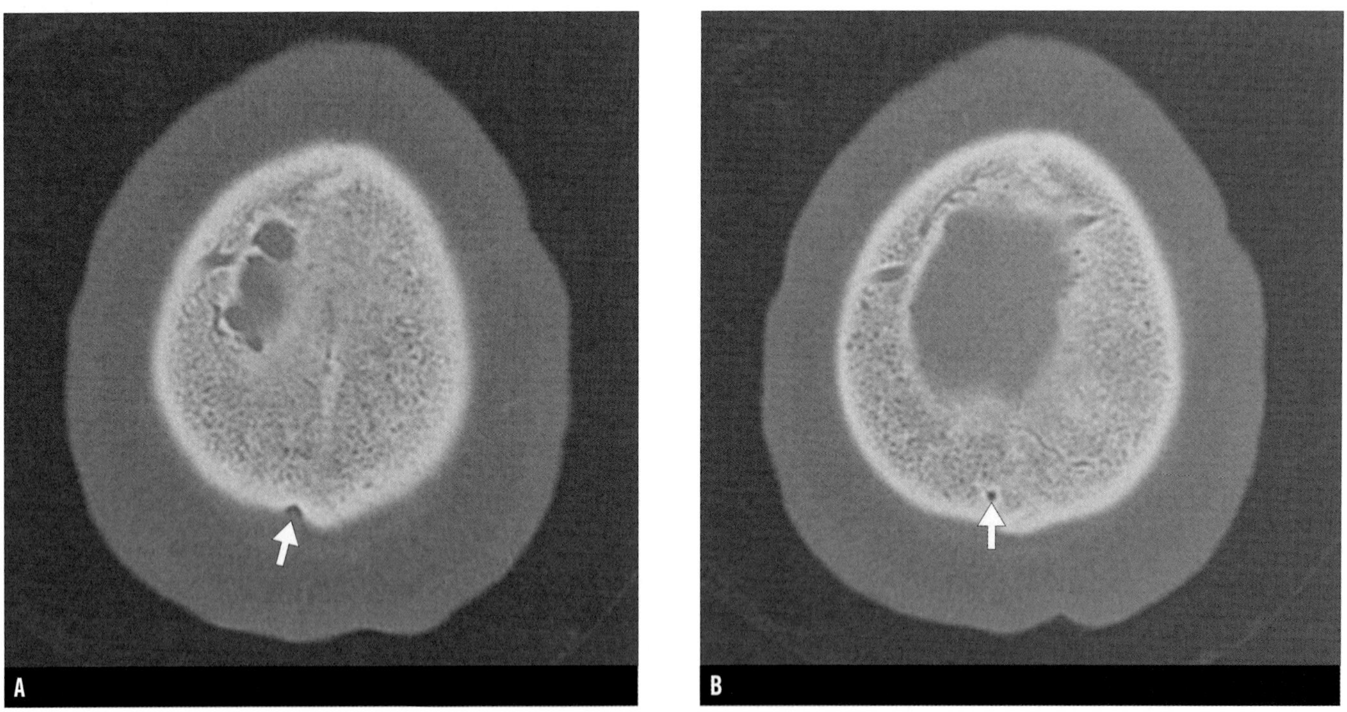

Axial (**A**, **B**), sagittal reformatted (**C**), and coronal reformatted (**D**) CT images demonstrate a unilateral right parietal foramen (arrows, **A**-**D**), a normal finding.

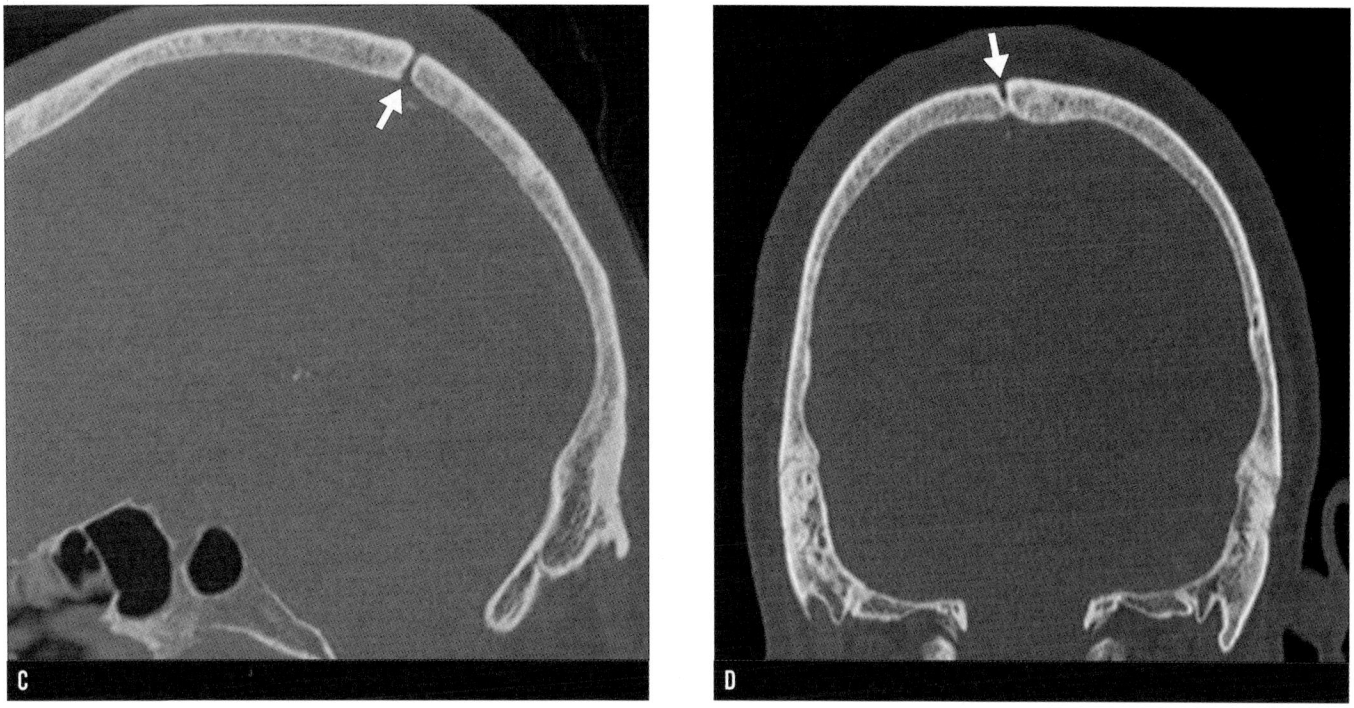

Companion case: Incidental parietal calvarial thinning

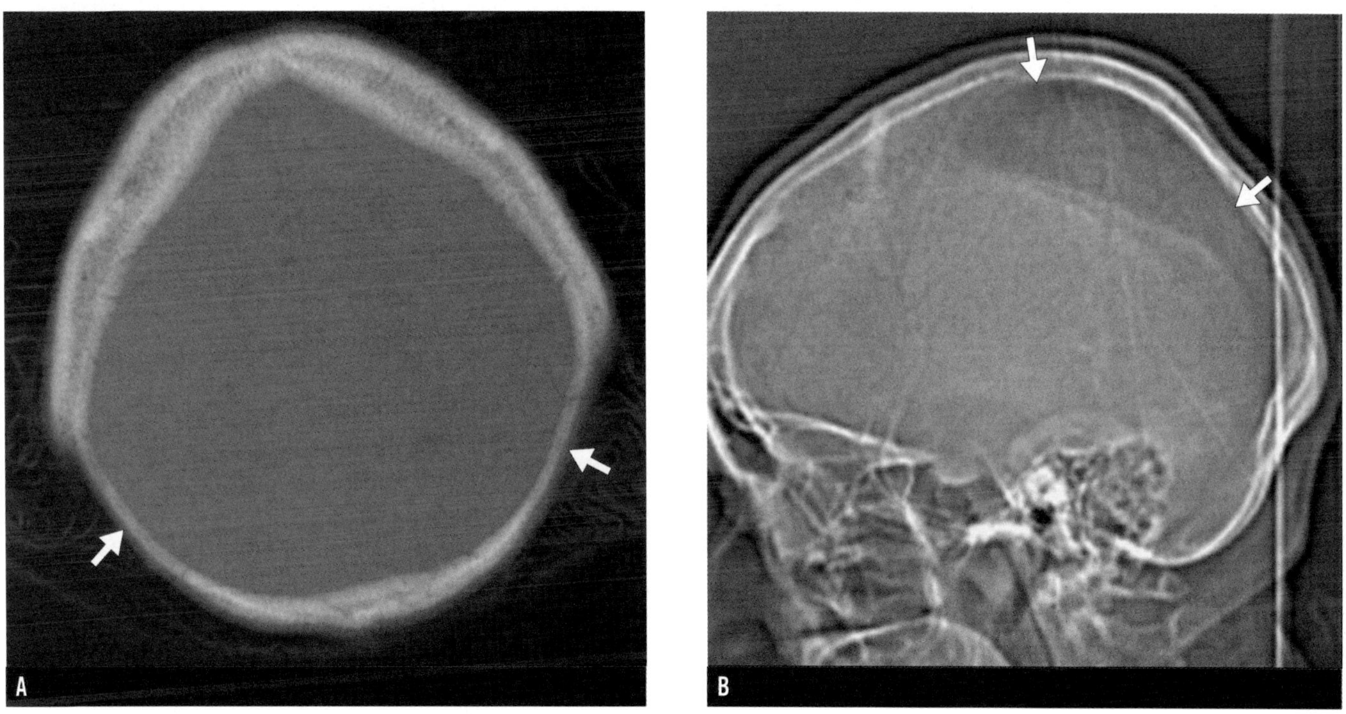

An axial CT image (**A**) and a lateral scout image from the same CT study (**B**) demonstrate pronounced bilateral parietal calvarial thinning, an incidental finding (arrows, **A**, **B**). Axial T2 (**C**) and coronal MPRAGE (**D**) MR images demonstrate the same incidental finding on MRI (arrows, **C**, **D**).

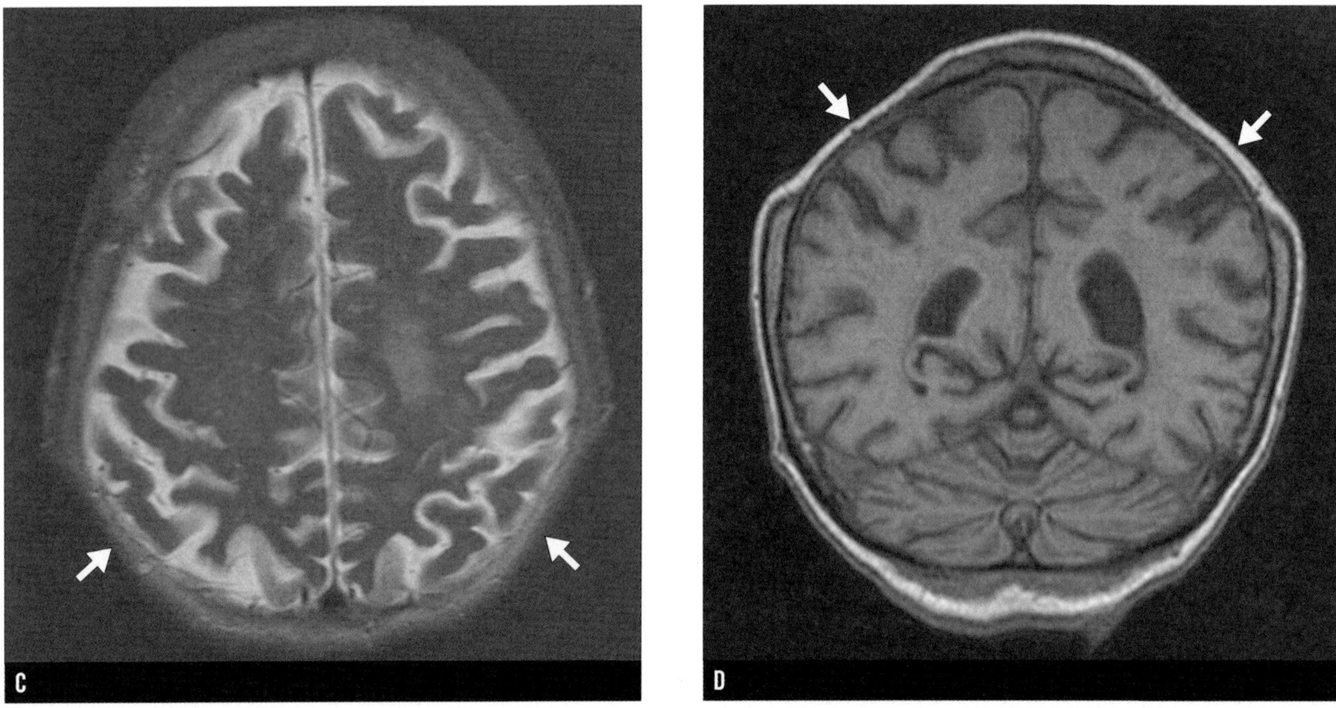

Companion case: Burr hole

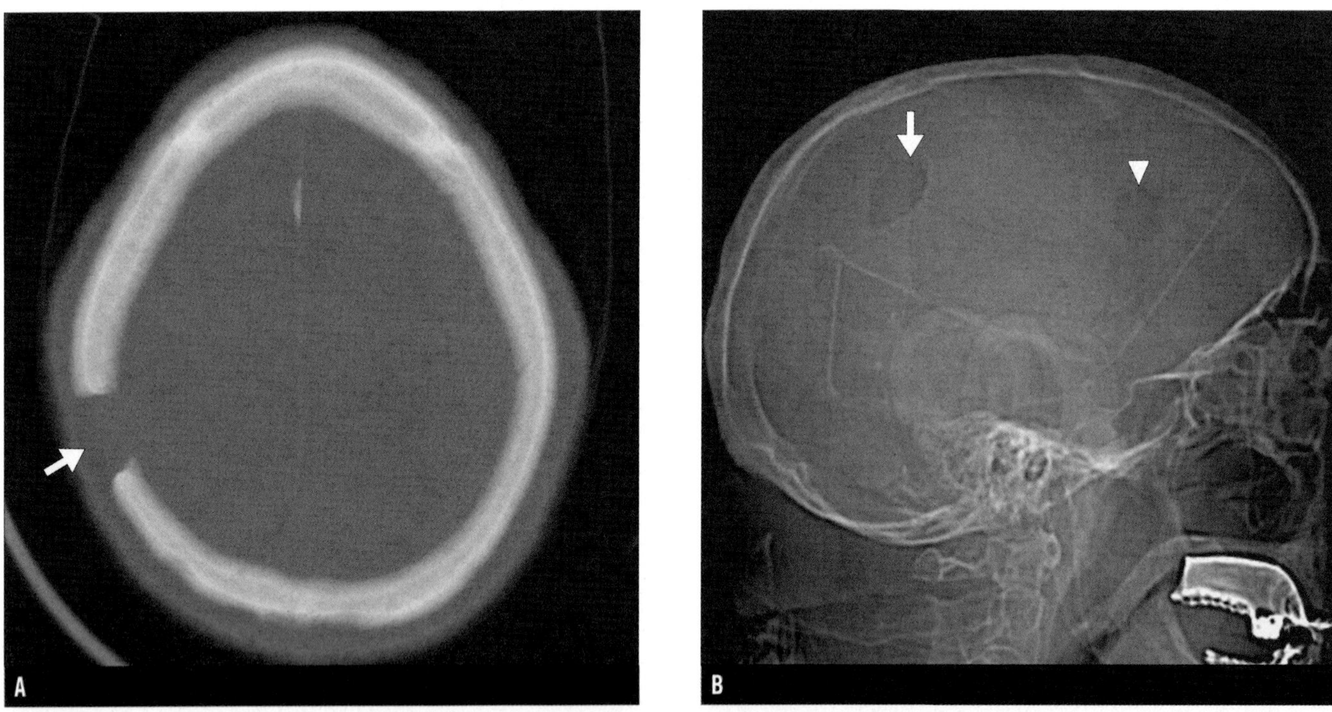

An axial CT image (**A**) and a sagittal scout image from the same study (**B**) demonstrate a right parietal burr hole (arrows, **A**, **B**), which is located more anterior and inferior to the expected location of a parietal foramen. This patient also had a frontal burr hole, as demonstrated on image **B** (arrowhead).

REFERENCES

Cederlung CG, Andren L, Olivercrona H. Progressive bilateral thinning of the parietal bones. *Skeletal Radiol.* 1982;8:29-33.

Kortesis B, et al. Surgical management of foramina parietalia permagna. *J Craniofac Surg.* 2003;14(4):538-544.

Reddy AT, Hedlund GL, Percy AK. Enlarged parietal foramina; association with cerebral venous and cortical anomalies. *Neurology.* 2000;54:1175-1178.

Sinclair AG, Scoffings DF. Imaging of the post-operative cranium. *Radiographics.* 2010;30:461-482.

CASE 4 Calvarial hyperostosis interna

Calvarial hyperostosis interna represents benign cancellous new bone formation that arises along the inner table of the calvarium. It is frequently identified incidentally and is present predominately in middle-aged or elderly women. Hyperostosis can occur along a focal portion of the calvarium or it can diffusely involve the calvarium. It is often described by location (eg, hyperostosis frontalis, hyperostosis parietalis, hyperostosis temporalis, diffuse calvarial hyperostosis, etc), with frontal bone involvement being the most common. Despite being originally described in 1765, the etiology of calvarial hyperostosis interna remains unproven. While it is most likely a hormonally driven process, other hypotheses, including genetic, viral, and dietary, have been proposed. The prevalence is estimated to be between 5% to 12% of the general population, although this percentage increases among older age groups.

Radiographically, there is wavy or nodular new bone formation along the inner calvarial table, with the bone formation sometimes described as "pearls on a string" or "bullets" that project into the calvarial vault. On CT and MRI, the cancellous bone will also have a thickened, nodular contour and may contain marrow, a finding that can aid in differentiating this benign entity from other processes, such as malignancy or Paget disease.

Calvarial hyperostosis interna usually has no significant clinical implications, although there are rare reports of calvarial hyperostosis interna that resulted in mass effect upon the subjacent brain and which necessitated surgical intervention.

COMPANION CASE

- **Dyke-Davidoff-Mason.** First described in 1933, Dyke-Davidoff-Masson (DDM) syndrome is characterized by hemicalvarial thickening associated with ipsilateral cerebral hemiatrophy and ex vacuo dilation. There is often associated ipsilateral hyperpneumatization of the paranasal sinuses and mastoid air cells. DDM can be either congenital or acquired and may be clinically associated with hemiplegia, hemiparesis, mental impairment, and epilepsy. The diagnosis of the congenital form is often made clinically in the prenatal or neonatal period, whereas the acquired type usually occurs following a severe brain insult at a young age, such as secondary to advanced infection, trauma, or hemorrhage.

Calvarial hyperostosis temporalis and frontalis interna

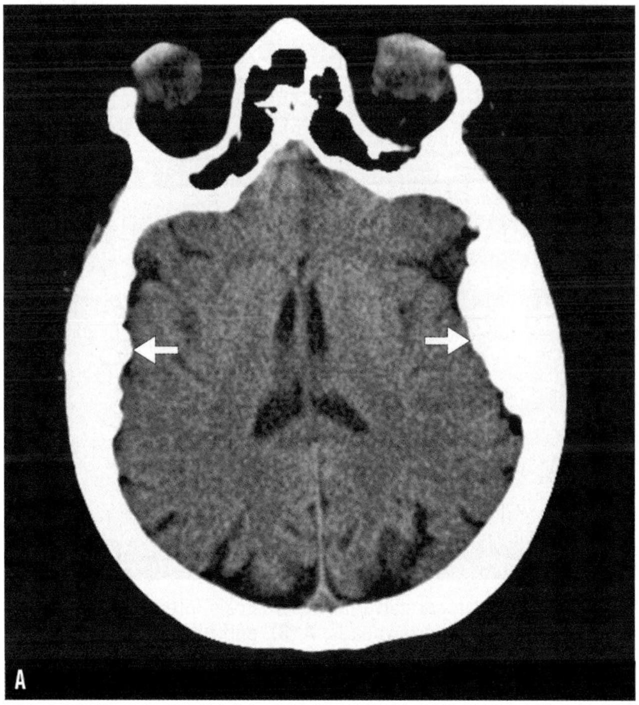

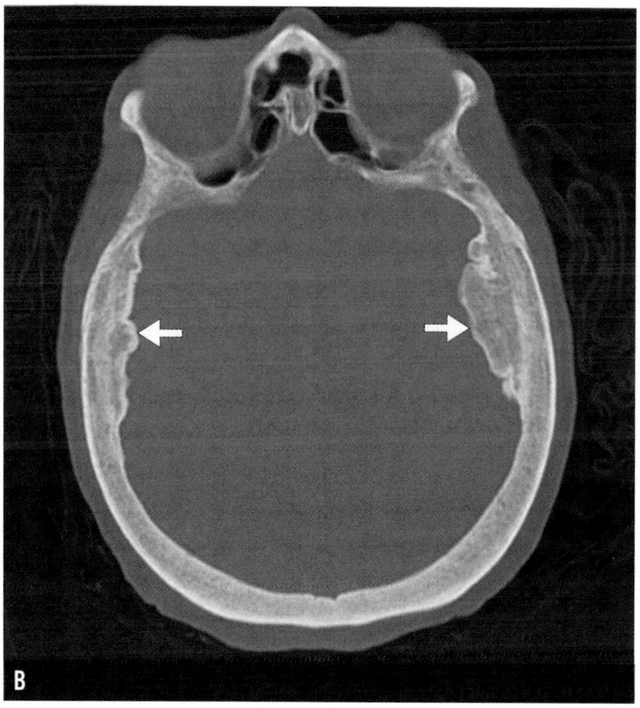

Unenhanced axial CT images viewed with a brain window (**A**) and bone window (**B**, **C**) demonstrate lobulated, marrow-containing, hyperostotic bone along the inner table of the squamosal portions of the temporal bones (short arrows, **A**, **B**) and the inner table of the frontal bone bilaterally (long arrows, **C**), compatible with hyperostosis temporalis interna and hyperostosis frontalis interna, respectively. There is subtle preservation of the CSF surrounding the crowded temporal lobes on image **A**, suggesting that there is no significant mass effect from the hyperostosis temporalis interna.

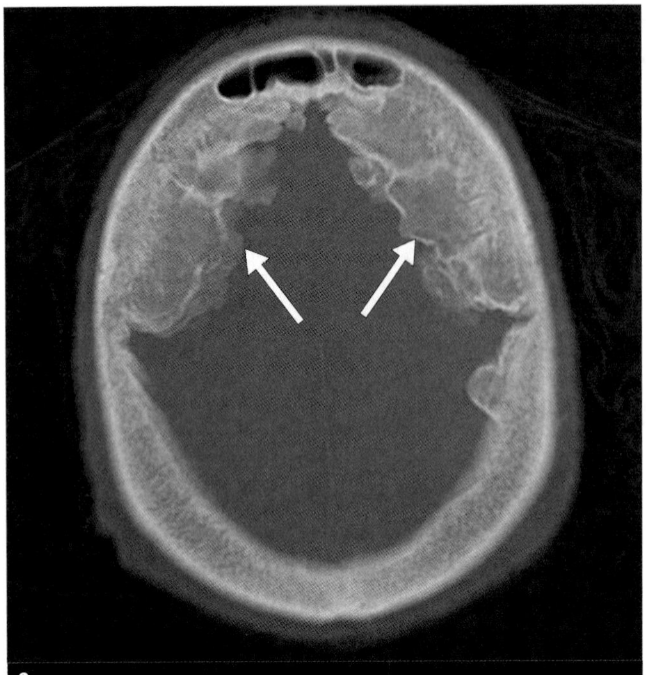

C

Calvarial hyperostosis frontalis, parietalis, and temporalis interna

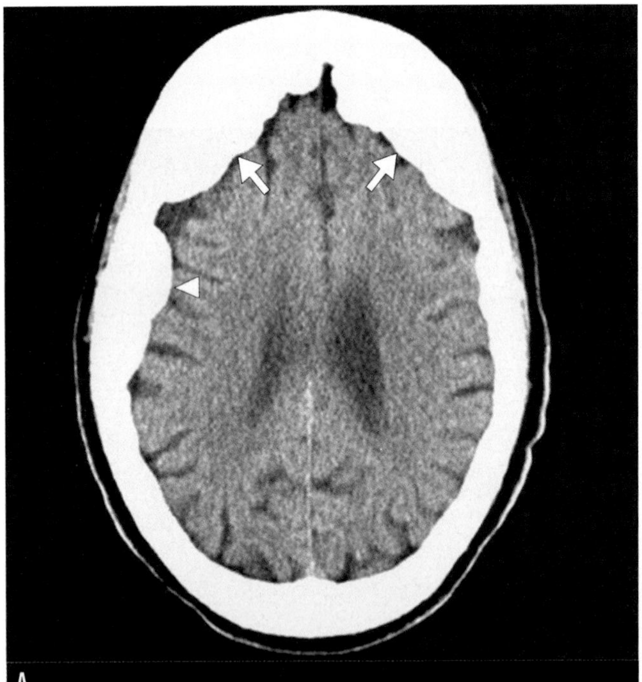

A

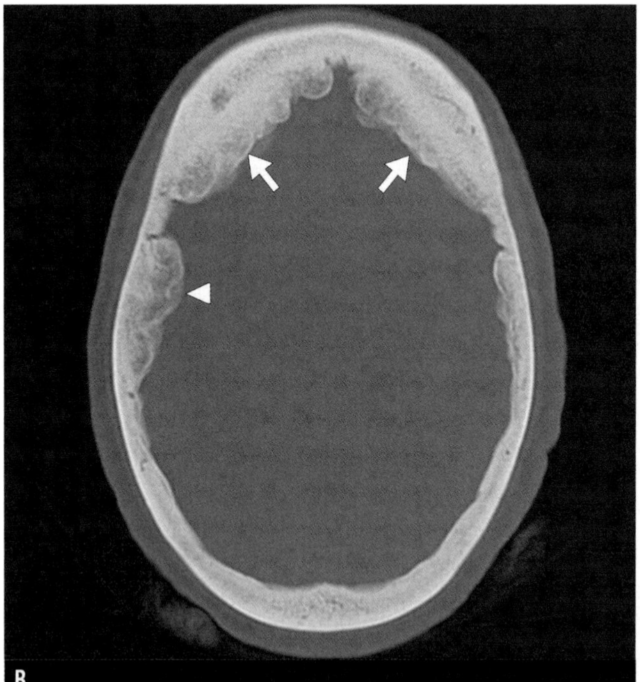

B

Axial CT images viewed with a brain window (**A**) and bone window (**B**, **C**) demonstrate multifocal calvarial hyperostosis interna, including bilateral hyperostosis frontalis interna (short arrows, **A**, **B**), right hyperostosis parietalis interna (arrowheads, **A**, **B**), and bilateral hyperostosis temporalis interna (long arrows, **C**).

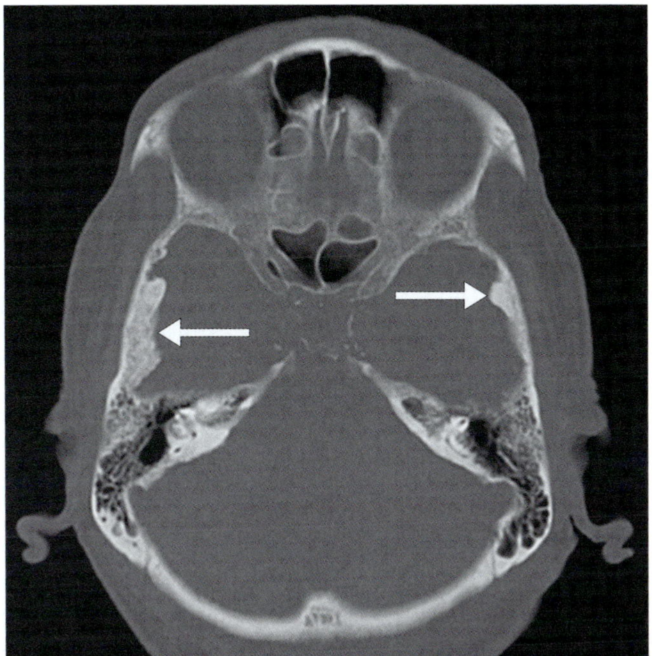

C

Calvarial hyperostosis frontalis interna

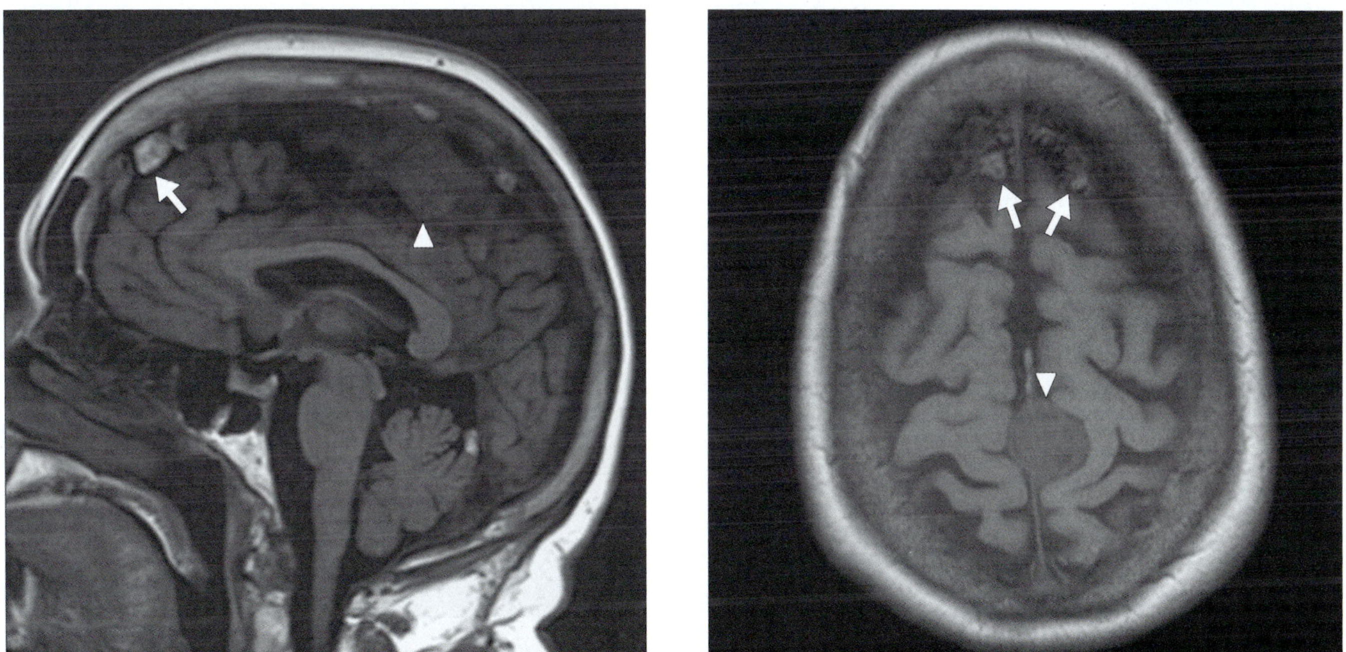

A B

Unenhanced sagittal T1 (**A**) and axial T1 (**B**) MR images demonstrate several hyperintense and hypointense T1 foci located deep to the frontal calvarium, possibly representing an extra-axial abnormality, such as hemorrhage (arrows, **A**, **B**). These foci are hypointense on a T2-weighted MR image (arrows, **C**). A contrast-enhanced coronal T1-weighted MR image with fat suppression (**D**) demonstrates the findings to be diffusely hypointense (arrows, **D**), including the precontrast T1 hyperintense portion of the findings. An unrelated meningioma is also present on images **A** through **C** (arrowheads). An axial CT image (**E**) and a sagittal scout image (**F**) of the same patient demonstrate that the findings along the inner table of the frontal bone relate to hyperostosis frontalis interna, a normal variant (arrows, **E**, **F**). The precontrast T1 hyperintense signal on images **A** and **B** which suppressed on image **D** represents fatty marrow within the hyperostosis frontalis interna.

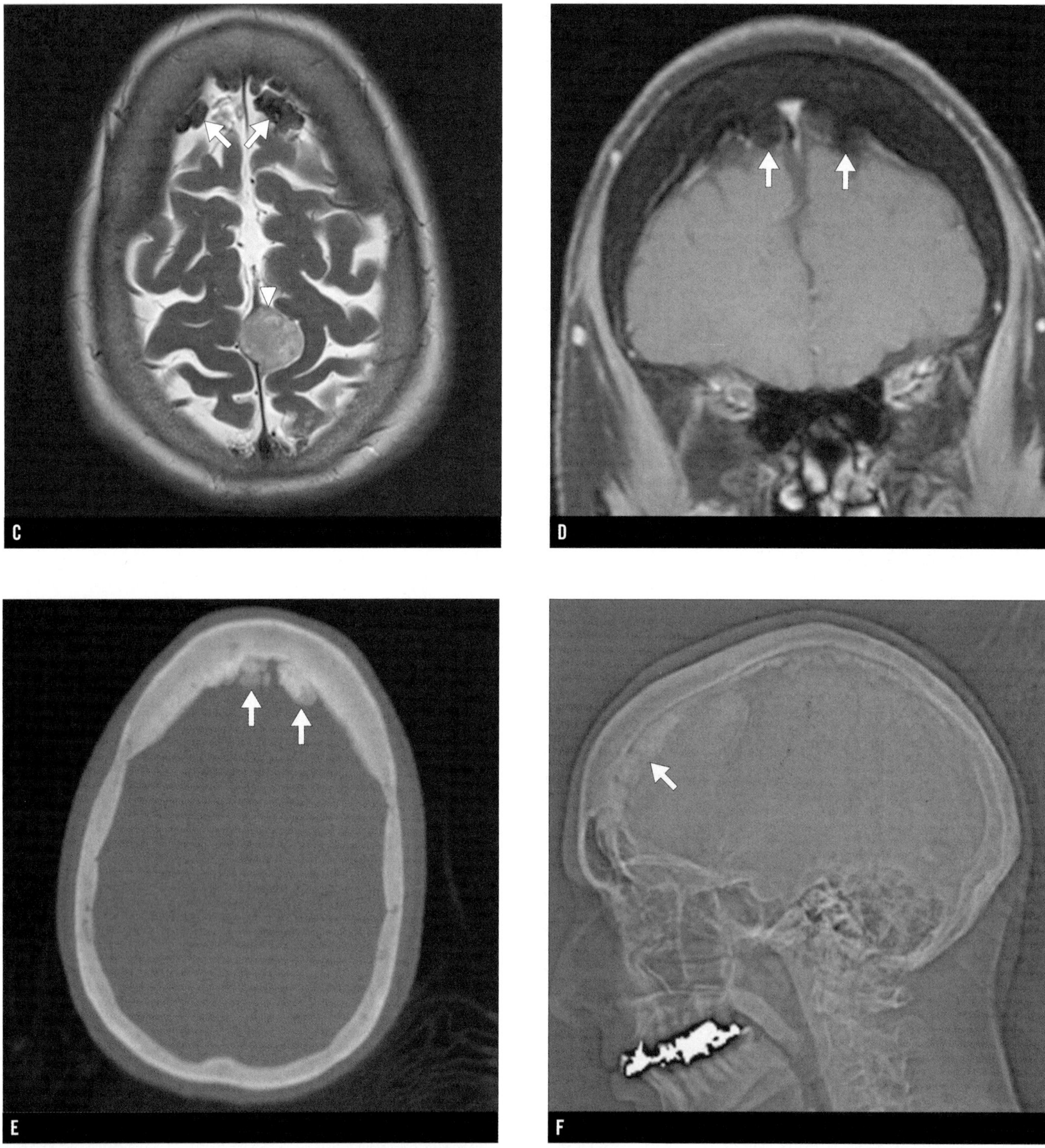
C
D
E
F

Calvarial hyperostosis occipitalis interna

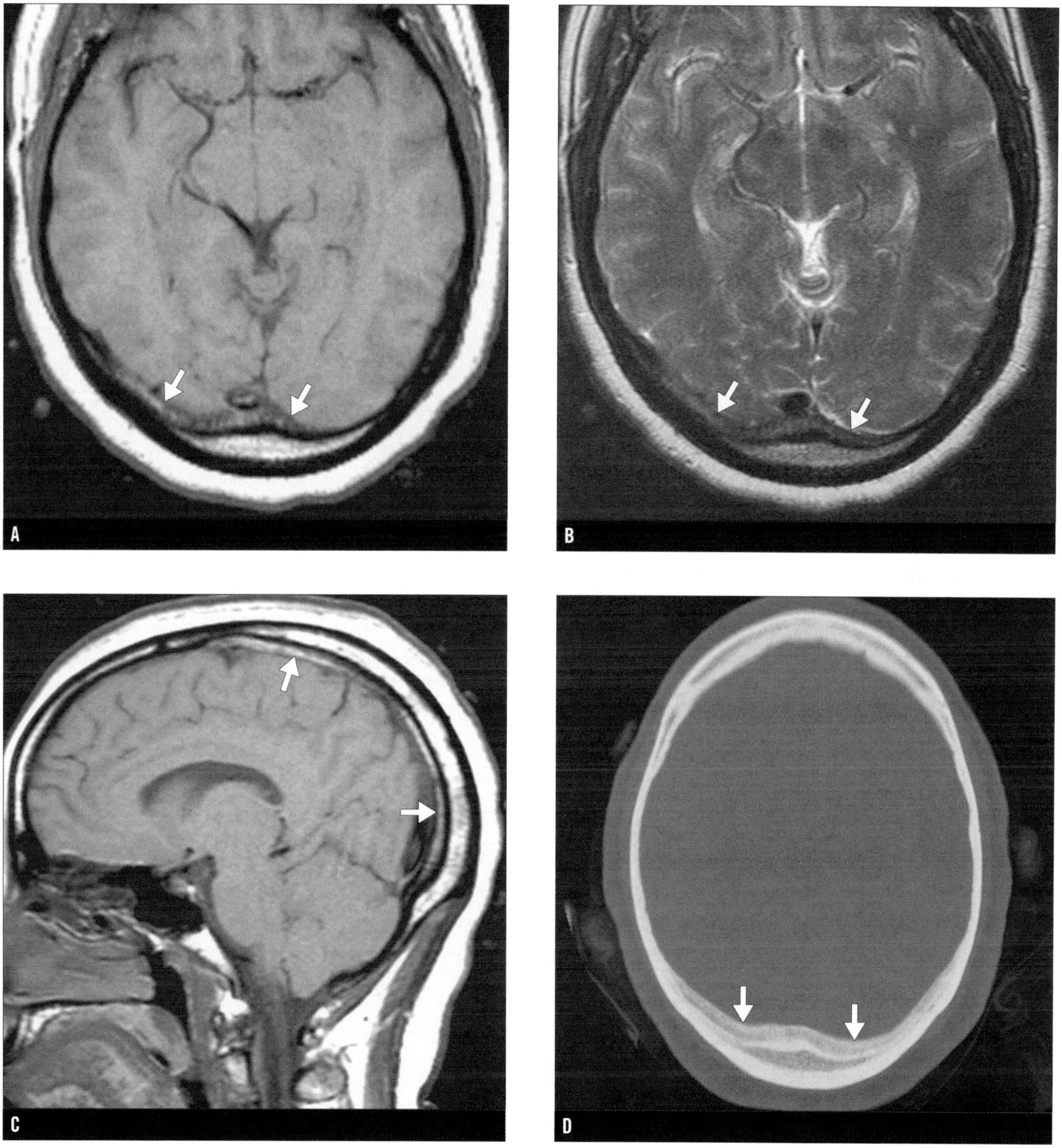

Axial T1 (**A**) and axial T2 (**B**) MR images demonstrate mildly T1 hyperintense and T2 hypointense signal relative to brain along the inner margin of the occipital bone, raising the possibility of an extra-axial abnormality such as hemorrhage (arrows, **A, B**). A sagittal T1-weighted MR image from the same study (**C**) demonstrates the continuous T1 shortening to reside deep to the occipital and parietal bones (arrows, **C**). An axial CT image of the same patient (**D**) demonstrates the finding to simply represent incidental hyperostosis along the inner table of the occipital calvarium (arrows, **D**).

Companion case: Dyke-Davidoff-Mason

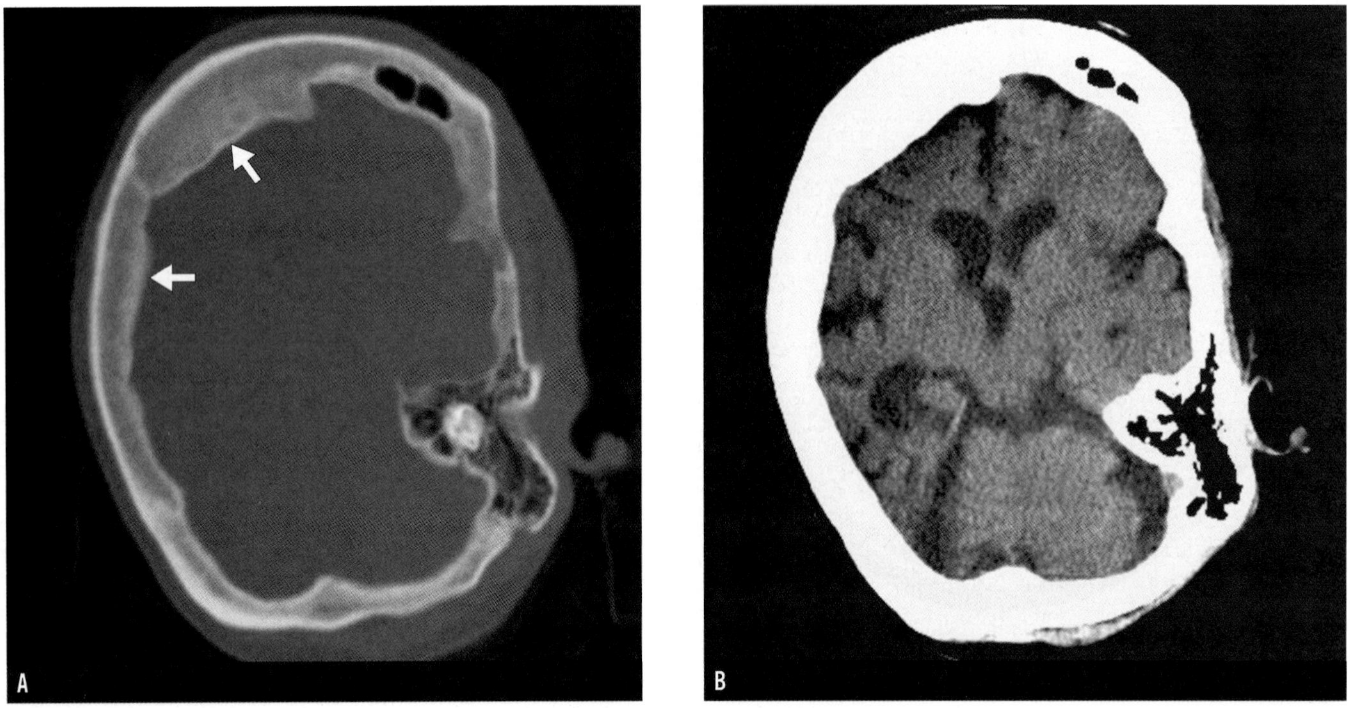

Axial CT images viewed with a bone window (**A**) and brain window (**B**) demonstrate marked unilateral right calvarial thickening (arrows, **A**) associated with pronounced ipsilateral brain volume loss, compatible with Dyke-Davidoff-Mason.

REFERENCES

Chaljub G, et al. Unusually exuberant hyperostosis frontalis interna: MRI. *Neuroradiology*. 1999;41:44-45.

Devriendt W, et al. Hyperostosis frontalis interna: forensic Issues. *J Forensic Sci*. 2005.50(1):143-146.

She R, Szakacs J. Hyperostosis frontalis interna: case report and review of literature. *Ann Clin Lab Sci*. 2004;34(2):206-208.

Tasdemir HA, et al. Dyke-Davidoff-Masson syndrome. *Clin Imag*. 2002;26(1):13-17.

CASE 5 Various nonmalignant entities that may diffusely affect the calvarium

There are numerous nonmalignant entities that may diffusely affect the calvarium. Some of the more common entities are described below.

- **Red marrow.** Normal red marrow is responsible for hematopoiesis and is composed of 40% fat, 40% water, and 20% protein, whereas yellow marrow is predominately composed of fat (80%). By the age of 15, there is complete conversion from red to yellow marrow in the calvarial diploic space in the majority of patients. However, obese patients (particularly women), as well as smokers, can have red marrow in the calvarial diploic space well into their adult life.

  Red marrow cannot be differentiated from yellow marrow on CT. On MRI, normal red marrow is either T1 isointense or slightly T1 hyperintense to muscle, whereas normal yellow marrow is T1 hyperintense relative to muscle. Differentiating normal red marrow from pathologic entities can be difficult. Some helpful imaging findings that support normal red marrow include homogeneously mild hypointense T1 signal, lack of osseous expansion, and lack of osseous erosion/destruction.
- **Osteopetrosis.** Osteopetrosis, derived from the Greek words for bone (osteo) and stone (petra), is a rare, heritable skeletal disorder characterized by diffuse osseous sclerosis. The osseous sclerosis occurs as a result of defective osteoclast activity and the inability to resorb bone. The autosomal recessive form is usually diagnosed within the first few months of life; these patients rarely survive childhood. The autosomal dominant form is more common and is typically diagnosed in late childhood or adolescence. Although the bone density is increased with osteopetrosis, the affected bones are associated with an increased risk of fracture. Other complications of osteopetrosis that may affect the face and skull base include cranial nerve palsies and optic atrophy secondary to narrowing of the neural and vascular foramina. On CT, there is extensive increased attenuation and thickening of the skull as well as a lack of a definable diploic space. On MRI, the skull is diffusely expanded, hypointense on all pulse sequences, and does not enhance following contrast.
- **β–Thalassemia.** First described in 1927, β-thalassemia is a hereditary anemia that results in deficient synthesis of β-globin, a polypeptide that is necessary for the normal formation and function of hemoglobin within red blood cells. The abnormal function of the red blood cells results in shorter cellular lifespan which, in turn, requires increased erythropoiesis. As a result, the skull in β-thalassemia is characterized by widening of the diploic space, thinning of the outer cortex, and a "hair-on-end" appearance along the surface of the skull related to vertically oriented trabeculations. The marrow signal within the diploic space can vary depending on patient's age or treatment; however, it is often T1 and T2 hypointense because of red marrow erythropoiesis. Marrow overgrowth from erythropoiesis can also result in underpneumatization of the paranasal sinuses, lateralization of the orbits, and inferior displacement of the central incisors, an appearance historically referred to as a "rodent facies." Extramedullary hematopoiesis can manifest as masses which reside outside the calvarial diploic space.
- **Renal osteodystrophy.** Renal osteodystrophy is a disorder of calcium and phosphate metabolism that occurs secondary to chronic renal failure. Patients with renal osteodystrophy often have osteomalacia that can result in pathologic fractures. Renal osteodystrophy can have a myriad of appearances on CT and MRI. On CT, the skull will often be thickened, may have a salt-and-pepper appearance due to trabecular resorption, or may be diffusely sclerotic with a paucity of a definable diploic space. On MRI, the skull may be thickened, heterogeneously hypointense on T1 and T2, and heterogeneously enhance.
- **Paget disease.** Paget disease (also called osteitis deformans) is a metabolic bone disorder of genetic etiology that typically affects the elderly and is characterized by rapid bone turnover, remodeling, sclerosis, and osseous expansion. Clinically, patients may be asymptomatic but will have an elevated serum alkaline phosphatase and can be disfigured from the disease. Paget disease usually diffusely affects the calvarium, but it may also be focal disease, particularly in the early phase. When Paget disease affects the skull base, the thickened bone may narrow foramina and canals, sometimes resulting in cranial neuropathies.

  There are three characteristic phases of Paget disease that are observed with radiographs and CT imaging: osteolytic, mixed lytic-sclerotic, and blastic (also called sclerotic). During the osteolytic phase, the skull is characterized by osteoporosis circumscripta, a well-defined lucent lesion that can progressively increase in size, involve the inner and outer cortices, cross sutures, and may even involve the entire calvarium. On MRI, this lytic phase is heterogeneous on T1 and T2 and will typically heterogeneously enhance. Also during the mixed phase, mixed osteolytic and osteoblastic activity results in a "cotton-wool" appearance, manifested by cortical thickening and foci of sclerosis with surrounding areas of lucency. Also during the mixed phase, the marrow signal becomes more homogenous on MRI compared to the lytic phase, with hyperintense fatty marrow signal predominating. Speckled intramedullary enhancement on MRI may also be identified during the mixed phase. In the final phase, osteoblastic activity predominates and results in more diffuse sclerosis and trabecular coarsening, with an overall decrease in T1 and T2 signal on MRI. Paget disease may be identified with a whole body bone scan labeled with Tc-99m MDP, which will demonstrate increased uptake during all three phases of Paget disease, although it is generally least active in the final phase.

COMPANION CASES

- **Myelofibrosis.** Myelofibrosis is a rare form of chronic leukemia that results in fibrosis of the bone marrow. It may be primary (idiopathic) or the result of other disease entities, such as polycythemia vera or essential thrombocytopenia. While it usually develops slowly and patients may be symptom free for years, the median survival is poor and only between 3.5 and 5.5 years. On CT, there may be focal or diffuse sclerosis of the skull and a resultant paucity of the diploic space. On MRI, myelofibrosis will be hypointense on T1 and T2 but hyperintense on STIR. Enhancement of myelofibrosis has been described in the literature, although in the companion case provided, no enhancement is evident. Other findings that may be identified on imaging with myelofibrosis include extramedullary hematopoiesis, lymphadenopathy, splenomegaly, and portal venous hypertension.
- **Metastatic disease.** Diffuse metastatic disease involving the calvarium can simulate some of the entities discussed above, in particular renal osteodystrophy and Paget disease. Cortical breakthrough, an adjacent soft tissue mass, focal expansion, and of course clinical history are all helpful in distinguishing metastatic disease from these other entities, although some imaging overlap does exist. On CT, patchy lucent and sclerotic areas may be present, largely dependent on the osteolytic or osteoblastic nature of the metastatic disease, respectively. Similarly, on MRI, the imaging features are varied and depend on the type of metastatic disease. Usually, the most problematic metastatic lesions to diagnose on CT and MRI tend to be of the osteoblastic variety. Osteoblastic metastatic lesions may not enhance on MRI and can simulate benign osseous lesions on both CT and MRI, such as enostoses. History in these cases is paramount.

Red marrow

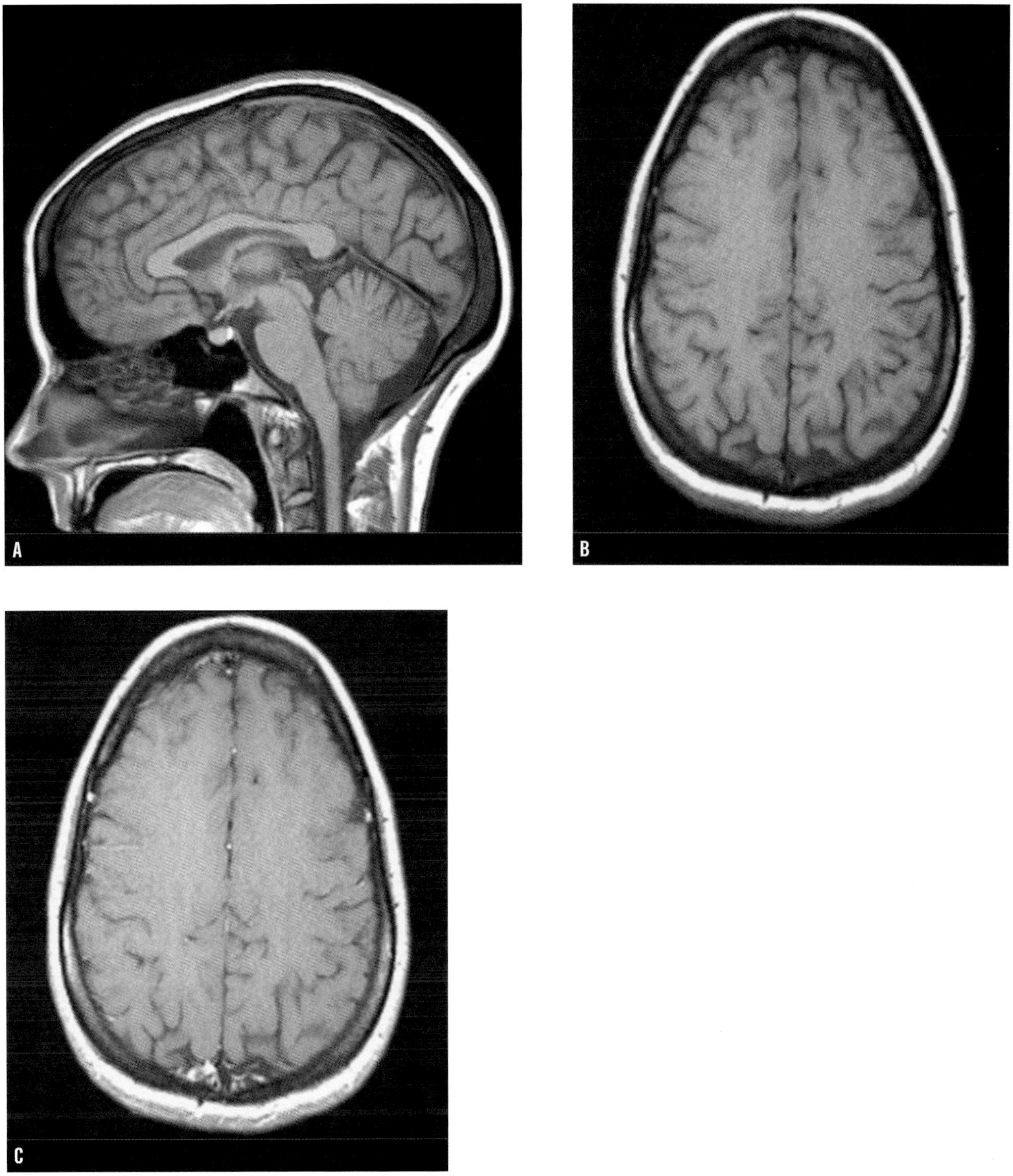

Sagittal T1 (**A**), axial T1 (**B**), and postcontrast axial T1 (**C**) MR images demonstrate mildly diffuse hypointense T1 signal throughout the calvarial marrow without enhancement, compatible with normal red marrow in this 37-year-old female patient.

Osteopetrosis

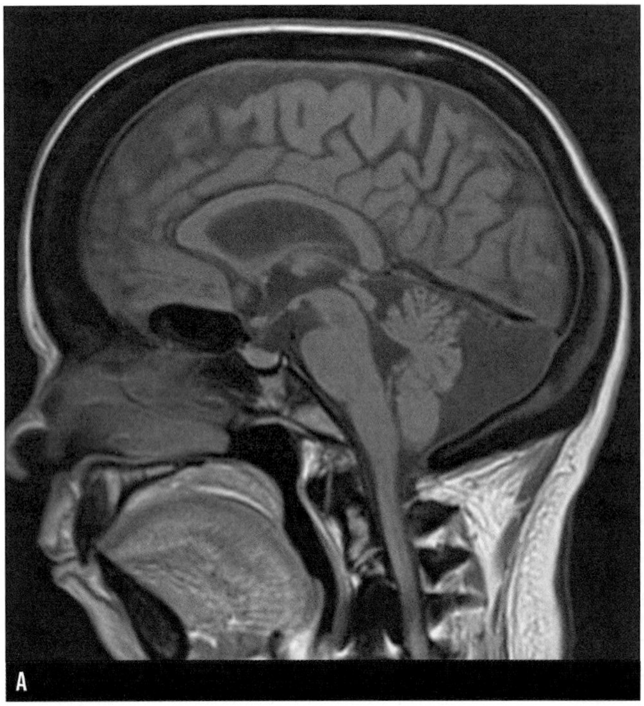

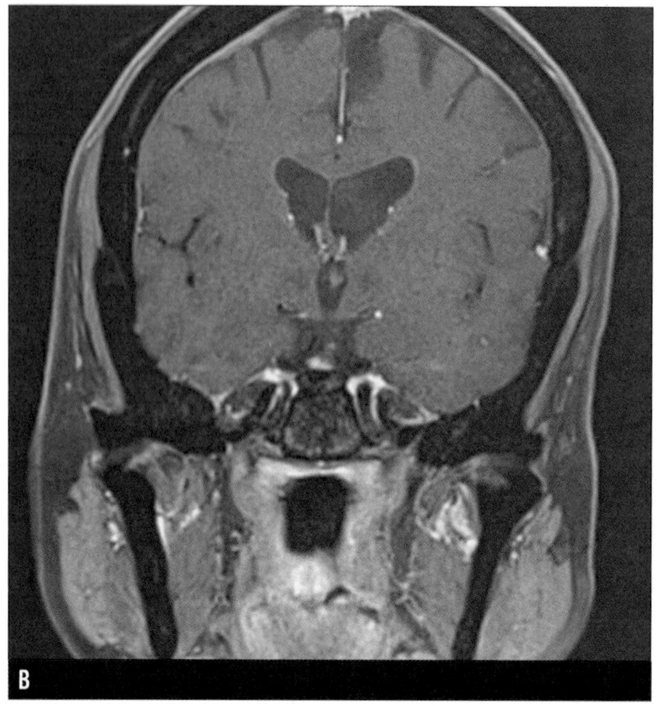

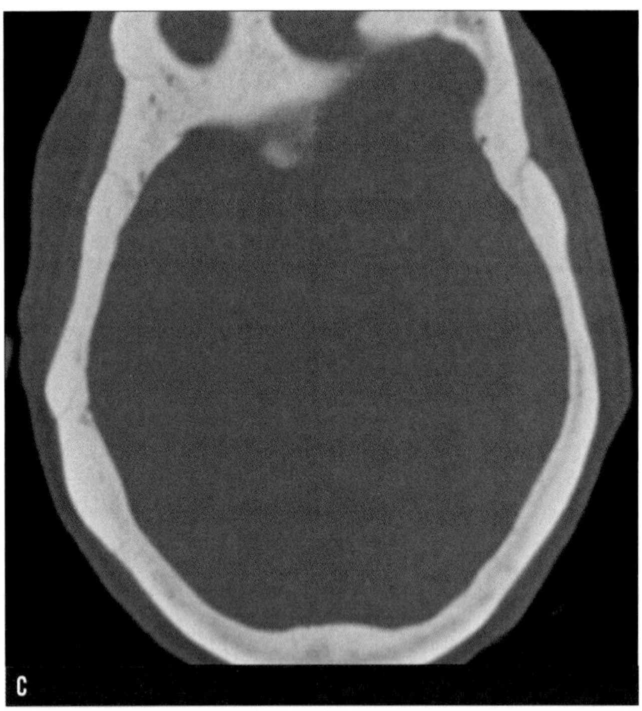

Sagittal T1 (**A**) and contrast-enhanced coronal T1 with fat suppression (**B**) MR images demonstrate diffuse, markedly hypointense calvarial marrow associated with osseous expansion in this patient with osteopetrosis. An axial CT image of the same patient (**C**) demonstrates the CT correlate with marked diffuse sclerosis and osseous expansion.

β–Thalassemia

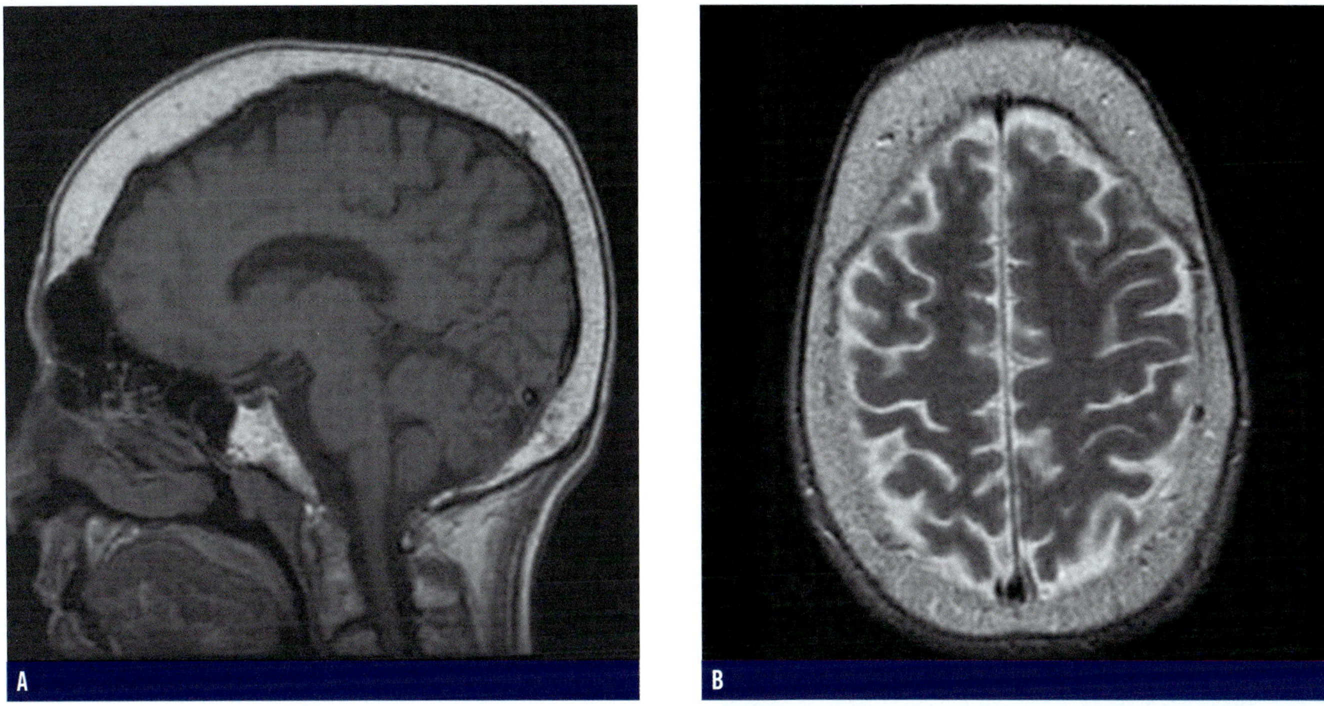

Sagittal T1 (**A**) and axial T2 (**B**) MR images demonstrate marked calvarial expansion with extensive increased T1 and T2 signal throughout the calvarium in this patient with a history of β-thalassemia. While not present in this case, most commonly, the marrow signal is depressed on T1- and T2-weighted imaging with β-thalassemia because of red marrow erythropoiesis.

Renal osteodystrophy

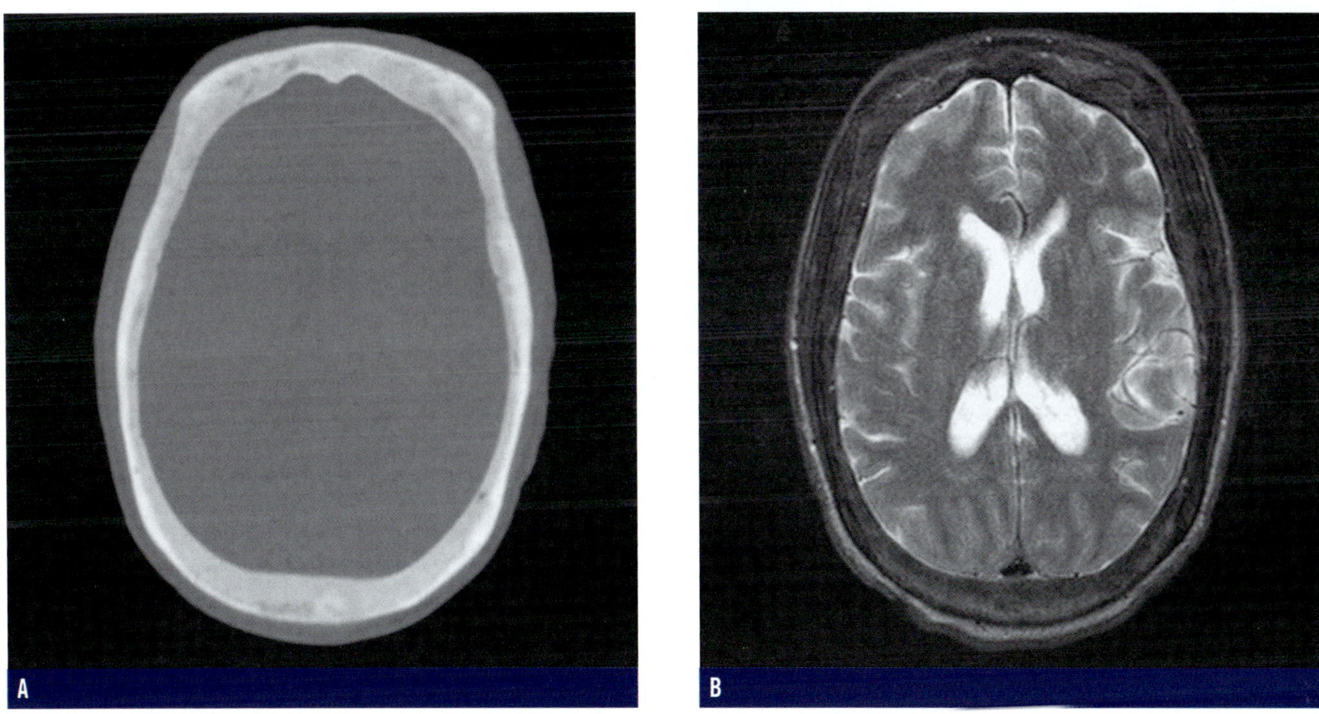

An axial CT image (**A**) demonstrates diffuse calvarial expansion, sclerosis, and paucity of a diploic space. Axial T2 (**B**), axial T1 (**C**), sagittal T1 (**D**), and contrast-enhanced axial T1 (**E**) MR images of the same patient demonstrate diffusely heterogeneous marrow signal with patchy enhancement and diffuse calvarial expansion in this patient with renal osteodystrophy. The findings on CT are relatively specific for renal osteodystrophy, whereas the findings on MRI could easily be mistaken for metastatic disease. Thus, when confronted with similar MR imaging findings, correlation should be made with CT, and of course, clinical history.

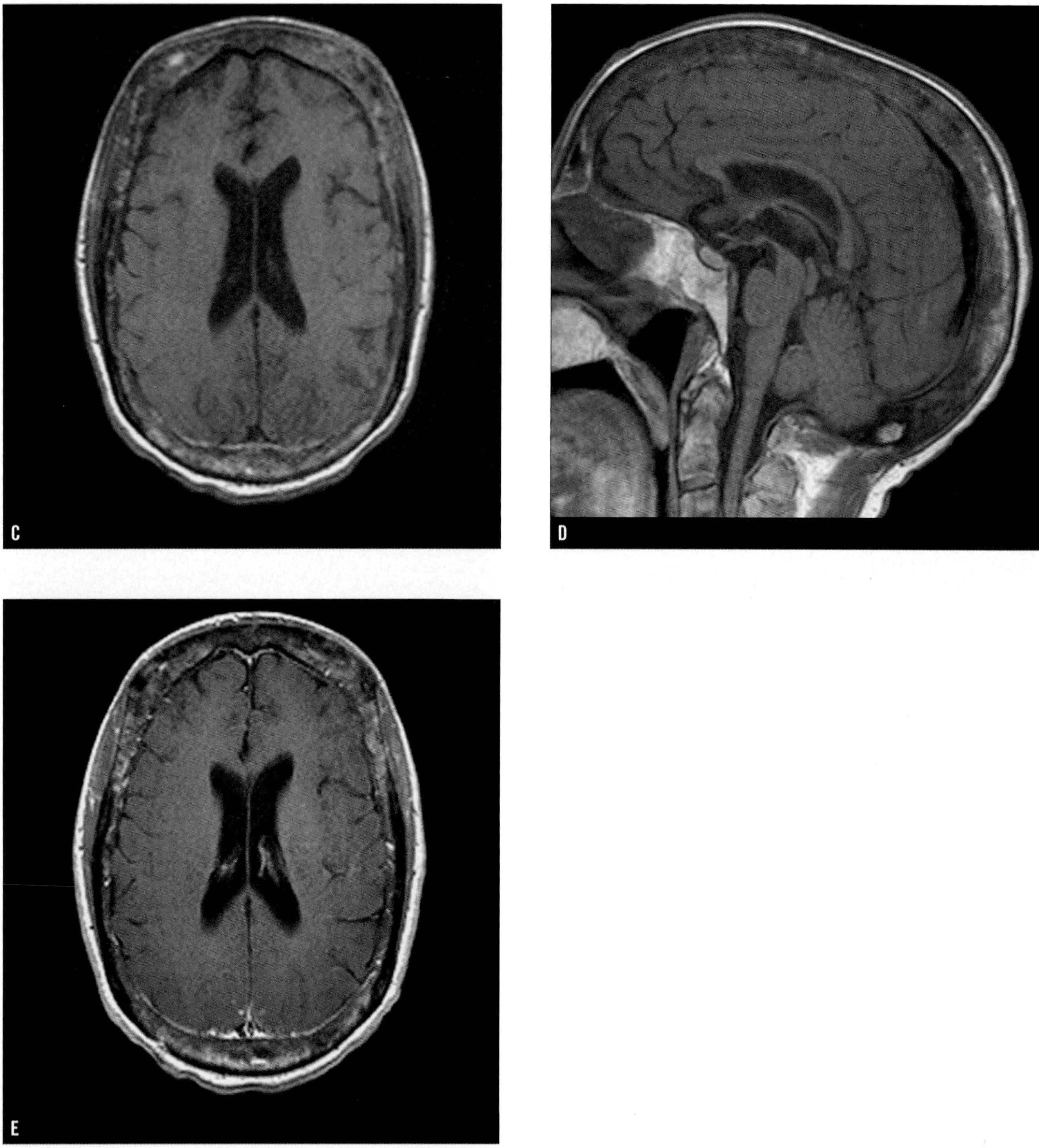
C
D
E

Renal osteodystrophy

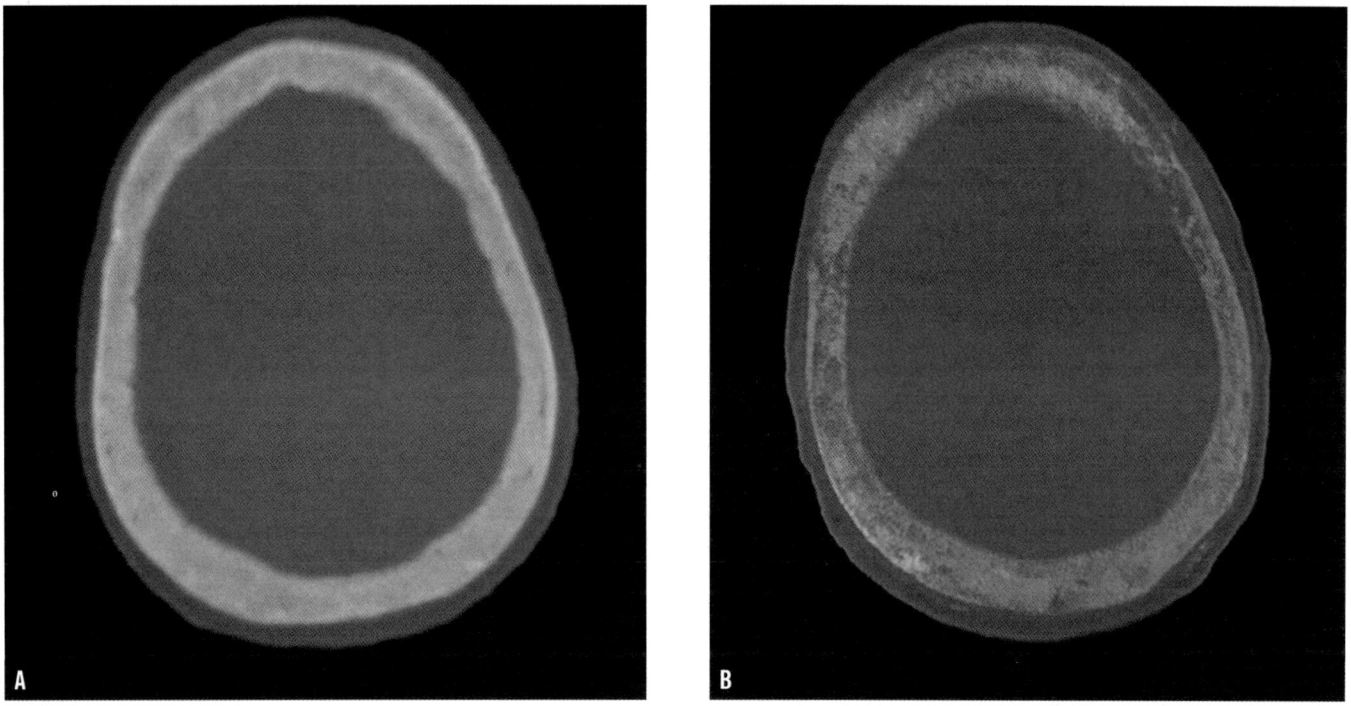

Different patient. An axial CT image (**A**) and a CT image at the same approximate level 3 years later (**B**) of a patient with end-stage renal disease. Image **A** demonstrates diffuse, abnormal increased attenuation of the calvarium with paucity of a diploic space, but with only minimal heterogeneity. Image **B** demonstrates marked loss of bone density which is now markedly heterogeneous and has a "salt and pepper" appearance. This case illustrates the varying osseous appearances that may occur with renal osteodystrophy.

Paget disease

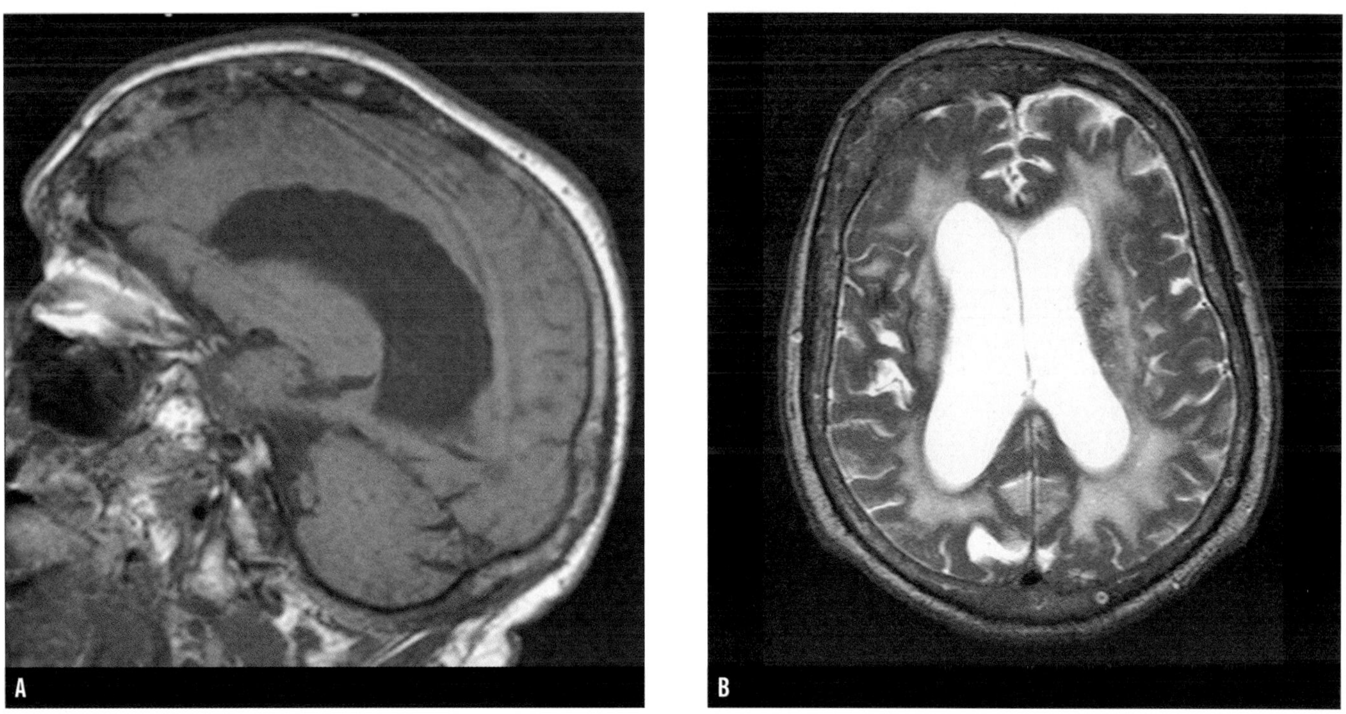

Sagittal T1 (**A**), axial T2 (**B**), axial T1 (**C**), and contrast-enhanced axial T1 (**D**) MR images demonstrate diffusely heterogeneous marrow signal with patchy enhancement and focal expansion along the right aspect of the frontal calvarium. An axial CT image of the same patient (**E**) demonstrates diffuse patchy sclerosis as well as focal calvarial expansion along the right aspect of the frontal calvarium. This type of patchy sclerosis is often referred to as a "cotton-wool" appearance. The imaging pattern is most consistent with Paget disease. Paget disease may focally or diffusely involve the calvarium.

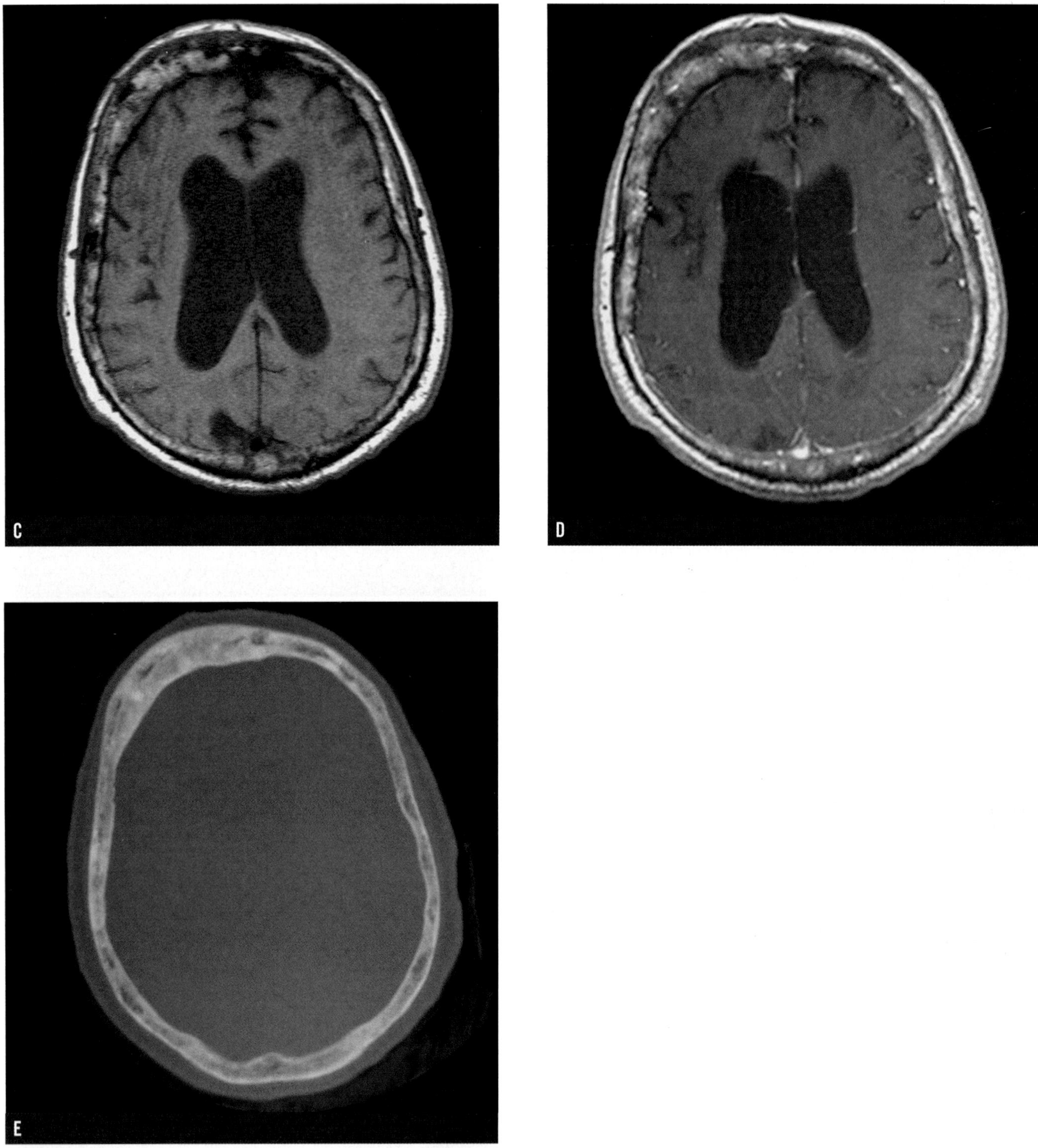
C
D
E

Companion case: Myelofibrosis

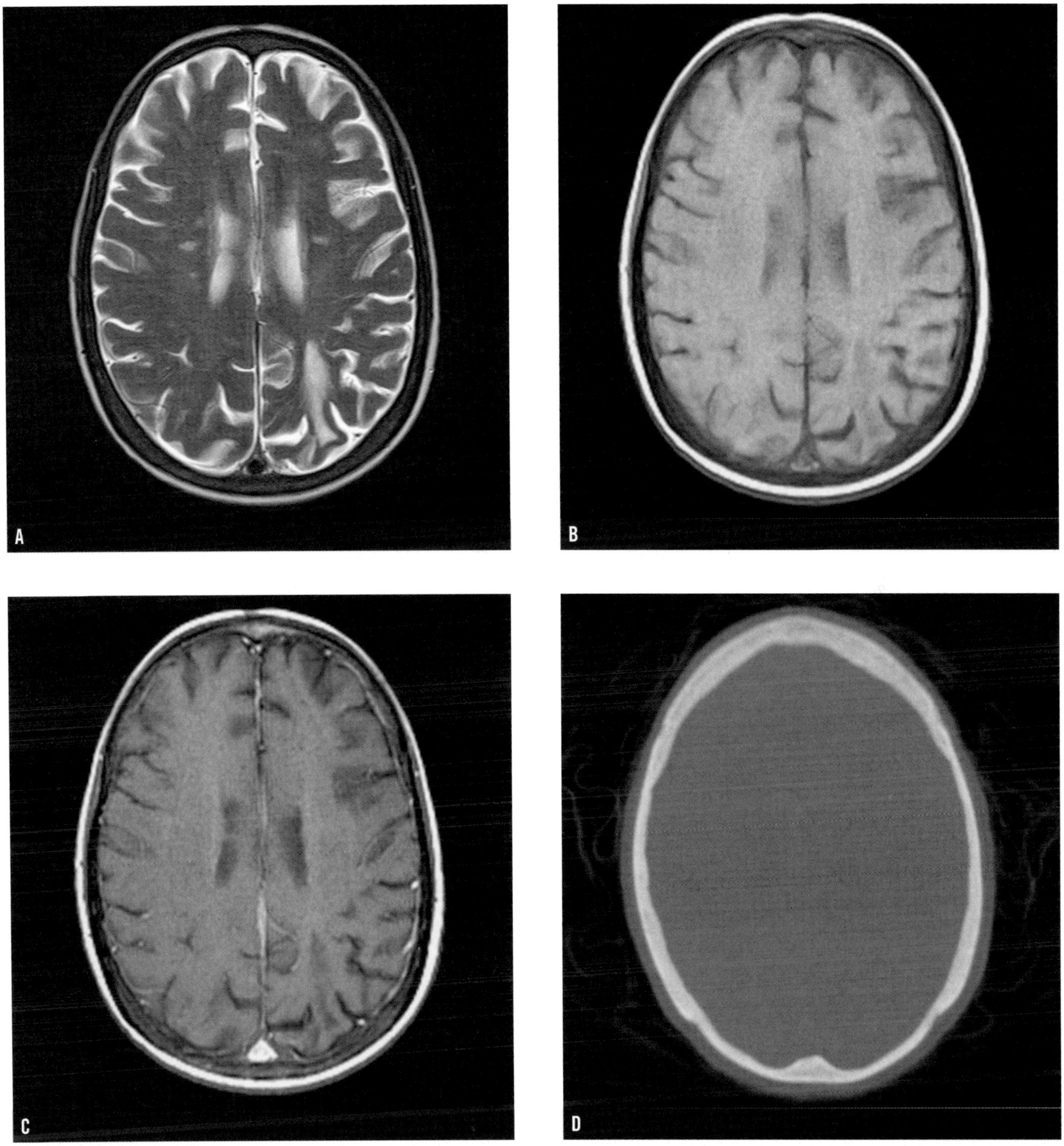

Axial T2 (**A**), axial T1 (**B**), and contrast-enhanced axial T1 (**C**) MR images demonstrate diffuse hypointense signal in the calvarial marrow on images **A** and **B** that does not enhance on image **C**. The marrow space is not expanded. While the signal is abnormal, these MR findings can be seen in any number of diffuse marrow processes, including pronounced benign red marrow conversion. An axial CT image of the same patient (**D**) demonstrates a diffuse osseous sclerosis with a relative paucity of the calvarial diploic space, although this can be identified in normal patients as well. This patient had known myelofibrosis, and the imaging findings, while nonspecific, are compatible with this entity.

Companion case: Metastatic disease

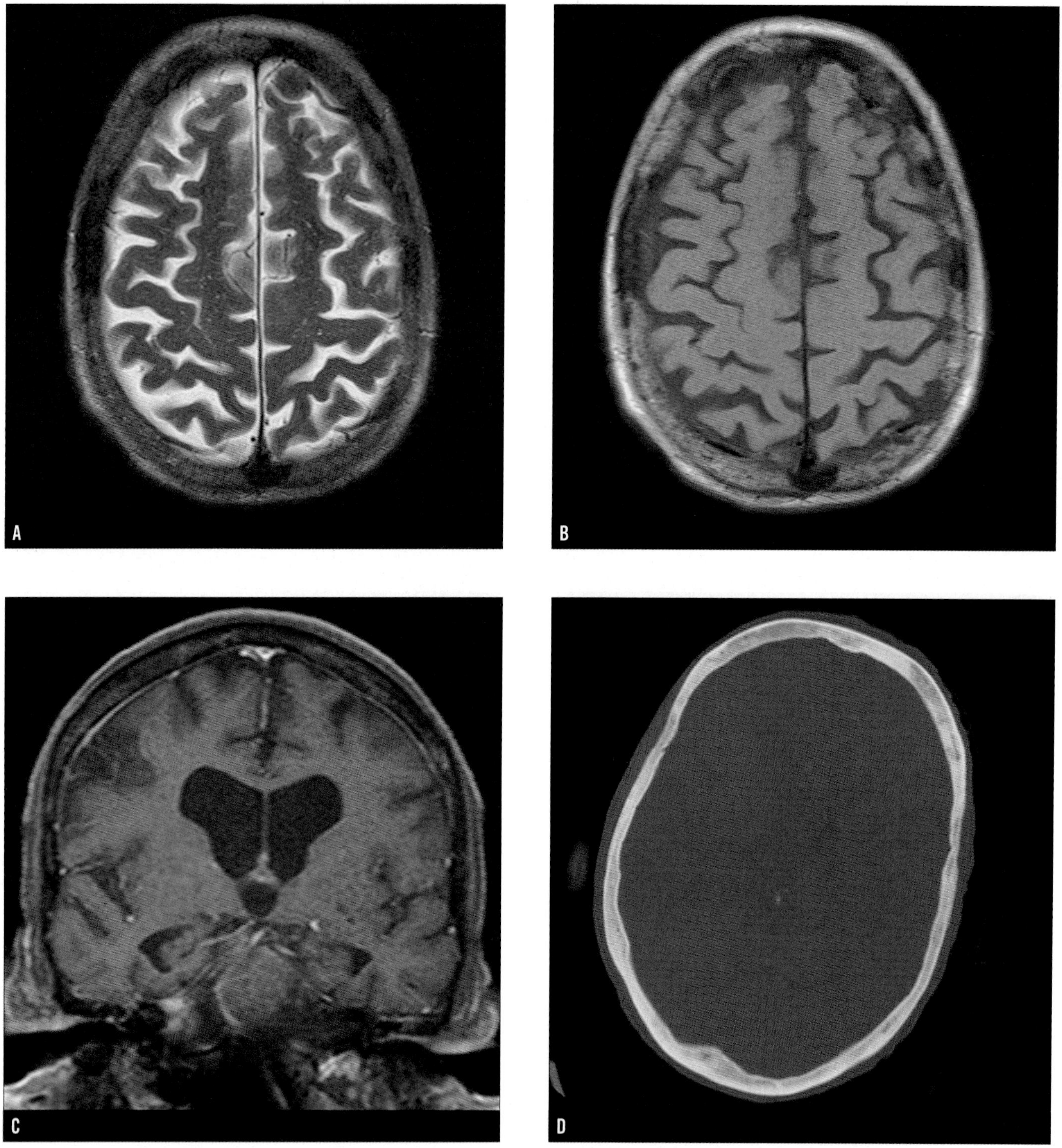

Axial T2 (**A**), axial T1 (**B**), and contrast-enhanced coronal T1 with fat suppression (**C**) MR images demonstrate focal areas of T1 and T2 hypointense signal in the calvarium with minimal, if any, enhancement. An axial CT image of the same patient (**D**) demonstrates patchy areas of sclerosis without calvarial expansion. These findings were related to metastatic breast carcinoma.

REFERENCES

Amano Y, Onda M, Amano M, Kumazaki T. Magnetic resonance imaging of myelofibrosis. STIR and gadolinium-enhanced MR images. *Clin Imag.* 1997;21(4):264-268.

Brouard R, et al. The lucent rim: a radiographic and computed tomography sign of Paget's disease of the skull. *Eur Radiol.* 2006;16(6):1308-1311.

Cai M, et al. Clinical and radiological observation in a surgical series of 36 cases of fibrous dysplasia of the skull. *Clin Neurol Neurosurg.* 2012;114(3):254-259.

Curé JK, et al. Cranial MR imaging of osteopetrosis. *AJNR Am J Neuroradiol.* 2000;21(6):1110-1115.

Eversole R, Su L, ElMofty S. Benign fibro-osseous lesions of the craniofacial complex. A review. *Head Neck Pathol.* 2008;2(3):177-202.

Foster K, et al. MRI of the marrow in the paediatric skeleton. *Clin Radiol.* 2004;59(8):651-673.

Guermazi A, de Kerviler E, Cazals-Hatem D, Zagdanski AM, Frija J. Imaging findings in patients with myelofibrosis. *Eur Radiol.* 1999;9(7): 1366-1375.

Lacativa, PG, et al. Prevalence of radiological findings among cases of severe secondary hyperparathyroidism. *Sao Paulo Med J.* 2009;127(2): 71-77.

Lymphoma and leukemia society. Myelofibrosis facts. http://www.lls.org/. Lymphoma and Leukemia Society, 1 Apr. 2012. Web. 26 Apr. 2015.

Smith SE, et al. From the archives of the AFIP. radiological spectrum of Paget's disease of the bone and its complications with pathological correlation. *Radiographics.* 2002;22:1191–1216.

Tunaci M, et al. Imaging features of thalassemia. *Eur Radiol.* 1999;9:1804-1809.

Yildirim T, et al. MRI evaluation of cranial bone marrow signal intensity and thickness in chronic anemia. *Eur J Radiol.* 2005;53(1):125-130.

CASE 6 Various nonmalignant entities that may focally affect the calvarium

There are numerous nonmalignant entities that may focally affect the calvarium. Some of the more common entities are described below.

- **Osteoma.** Osteomas are osseous hamartomas of unknown etiology. Calvarial osteomas are sclerotic, round to oval osseous densities that arise from either the inner or outer calvarial cortex. Osteomas are usually asymptomatic lesions, unless they result in mass effect on adjacent structures, and they are typically identified incidentally on imaging studies or by direct palpation. Osteomas of the mandible or multiple osteomas, while often identified sporadically, are associated with Gardner syndrome.

  On radiographs or CT, calvarial osteomas are smoothly marginated, densely sclerotic juxtacortical lesions. On MRI, they are usually diffusely hypointense on all pulse sequences because of tightly packed lamellar bone. However, osteomas may have small areas of internal heterogeneous signal that represent small amounts of cancellous bone marrow. Enhancement of osteomas is rare and , when present, likely represents vascularity within cancellous bone.

  Multiple terms for osteomas exist, including bone hamartoma, surface or ivory osteoma, as well as exostosis. The later term should be avoided, as an exostosis is synonymous with an osteochondroma arising from the peripheral tubular bones and has distinctly different imaging and pathological findings.
- **Enostosis.** An enostosis, or bone island, represents a hamartomatous deposit of cortical bone located within the medullary space. Enostoses are common, found incidentally in up to 14% of cadavers, and are likely developmental in nature. Enostoses can be solitary or multifocal.

  On imaging, enostoses are homogenously sclerotic foci that are round or ovoid in shape and range from 1 to 20 mm, with the term giant bone island typically reserved for lesions greater than 2 cm. The borders may be smooth, spiculated, or feathered. The spiculated or feathered appearance is attributed to cortical bone that is interspersed within the surrounding medullary bone. On MRI, enostoses are hypointense on all pulse sequences. Osteopoikilosis is an autosomal dominant bone dysplasia characterized by innumerable enostoses scattered throughout the skeleton and is most often identified in patients younger than 20 years of age.
- **Venous malformation of the calvarium (osseous hemangioma).** A focal, nonaggressive, at least partially intrinsic T1 hyperintense osseous lesion that enhances on MRI has historically been termed a benign intraosseous hemangioma. However, more recent literature evaluating the histopathology of this lesion supports that this entity is more appropriately termed a venous malformation of bone. On CT, an intraosseous venous malformation of the calvarium is largely lucent and frequently contains coarse osseous trabeculations. Hounsfield units within the lucency often reveals fat attenuation, a finding that usually confirms this benign entity.
- **Calvarial epidermoid.** An epidermoid represents an ectodermal inclusion cyst. An epidermoid cyst contains debris, water, cholesterol, and keratin that accumulates from progressive desquamation of the cyst wall, often resulting in a lamellated pattern at pathology. A calvarial epidermoid usually resides within the diploic space. When large, a calvarial epidermoid may result in a bulging contour along the surface of the calvarium and/or subjacent mass effect upon the underlying brain. On CT, the majority of calvarial epidermoids are hypoattenuating diploic space masses which may focally expand the calvarium as well as result in cortical thinning and/or erosion. On MRI, they are near CSF signal on T1- and T2-weighted imaging, although they frequently will contain mild, sometimes swirling T1 shortening. Most epidermoids do not enhance, but if they do, they will usually only enhance peripherally to a mild degree. A classic epidermoid is hyperintense on FLAIR and will restrict on diffusion-weighted imaging (DWI).
- **Benign fibro-osseous calvarial lesion.** Benign fibro-osseous lesions of the calvarium and face represent a collection of lesions that contain variable amounts of fibrous and osseous dysplasia.

  They may be classified as follows:
  - Bone dysplasias (eg, fibrous dysplasia and Paget disease
  - Cemento-osseous dysplasia (most frequently present in the tooth-bearing regions of the jaw)
  - Inflammatory/reactive processes (eg, osteomyelitis)
  - Metabolic disease (eg, hyperparathyroidism)
  - Neoplastic lesions (eg, ossifying fibroma)

  With fibrous dysplasia, the normal bone is replaced by fibrous tissue consisting of spindle cell bundles and immature woven bone. This process causes expansion of the affected bone. The most common CT appearance of fibrous dysplasia is a ground-glass (sclerotic) pattern, although fibrous dysplasia can less commonly appear as a heterogeneously sclerotic and lucent lesion (Pagetoid form) or as a cystic lesion (cystic form). On MRI, fibrous dysplasia is most often low-to-intermediate in signal on T1, variable in signal on T2, and may enhance. However, the MR imaging appearance of fibrous dysplasia depends on the ratio of mineralized matrix and fibrous tissue, and it may sometimes mimic an aggressive tumor. Thus, any suspicious osseous lesion on MRI should be interpreted in combination with CT, or when appropriate, radiographs. Fibrous dysplasia may be monostotic or polyostotic. There are multiple conditions that are associated with fibrous dysplasia, including McCune-Albright syndrome, Mazabraud syndrome, and tuberous sclerosis. Craniofacial involvement is seen in almost all cases of polyostotic fibrous dysplasia.

Differentiating fibrous dysplasia from Paget disease can be difficult. Unlike Paget disease, fibrous dysplasia more commonly affects the calvarium in a focal manner, often arises in young patients, is stable later in adult life, commonly affects the face, and does not have a "cotton-wool" appearance that is classically associated with Paget disease. While fibrous dysplasia can have an elevated alkaline phosphatase level during the proliferative phase, alkaline phosphatase is not elevated after the lesion becomes quiescent. This is in contradistinction to Paget disease in which the alkaline phosphatase level is consistently elevated.

- **Calvarial meningioma.** Meningiomas that originate directly from the calvarium or skull base are uncommon tumors. Calvarial meningiomas often arise near the sutures and develop from arachnoid rests or cap cells that have presumably undergone abnormal migration during embryogenesis. Most calvarial meningiomas are osteoblastic and induce hyperostosis, although occasionally lytic calvarial meningiomas may occur, which tend to be more aggressive. On CT, most calvarial meningiomas will result in thickening and sclerosis of the diploic space as well as of the inner and outer calvarial tables. Regions of osteolysis and periosteal reaction may also be identified. On MRI, calvarial meningiomas tend to be T1 hypointense, T2 hyperintense, and heterogeneously enhance. MRI may be slightly more sensitive in detecting an extraosseous soft tissue component, a finding which is usually more homogeneously enhancing relative to the calvarial component.

COMPANION CASES

- **Sclerotic metastatic disease.** Osteoblastic metastasis occurs via hematogenous spread of tumor and is a complex process driven by cytokines and hormones which allow for tumor invasion into bone. Differentiating an enostosis from a sclerotic metastasis (such as may occur with prostate cancer, breast cancer, and thyroid cancer, among others) is often difficult by CT or MRI, particularly without adequate clinical history.

  Osteoblastic metastasis should be considered in cases where the lesion is symptomatic or has increased in size by more than 25% in 6 months, as an enostosis is typically asymptomatic and usually increases in size at much slower rate, if at all. Bone scintigraphy is a frequently helpful imaging modality to distinguish enostoses from osteoblastic metastases. Osteoblastic metastases are typically active lesions on bone scintigraphy. Conversely, enostoses are typically inactive lesions on bone scintigraphy, although rare cases of radioisotope uptake by an enostosis have been reported.
- **Metastatic melanoma to the calvarium.** The lifetime risk of developing melanoma has increased over the last century, and sun exposure, particularly when intermittent, is the leading environmental risk factor. In the year 2000, it was estimated that 1 in 75 individuals will develop melanoma, and the risk of development increases with age. Because most melanocytes in the body are present in the skin, and since the skin is readily exposed to the sun, melanoma overwhelmingly arises from the skin. However, melanocytes are also present in the eyes, mucosa, and internal organs, and thus melanoma may arise from these structures as well. Melanomas frequently contain melanin, a substance that is intrinsically T1 hyperintense on MRI; therefore, enhancement of a metastatic melanoma lesion may be relatively occult on MRI. However, amelanotic melanomas also exist and will not contain intrinsic T1 hyperintensity signal. Melanomas will commonly metastasize to organs and lymph nodes, sometimes several years after an apparent cure. Melanoma that is metastatic to bone will most frequently result in an osteolytic lesion centered within the medullary cavity. Melanoma is typically FDG-18 avid on PET, although up to 13% of melanomas will have only minimal PET avidity.
- **Radiation-induced calvarial osteosarcoma.** There has been an increase in the prevalence of radiation-induced tumors because of an increase in survival rates among cancer patients. In the setting of radiation to the head, the radiation-induced tumor type and grade is believed to be proportional to the radiation dose. A lower dose of radiation to the head (<15 Gy) usually results in lower-grade tumors, such as a meningioma. Conversely, a higher radiation dose (usually 55-60 Gy) typically results in higher-grade tumors, such as a calvarial osteosarcoma, although radiation-induced osteosarcoma (RIO) of the calvarium with radiation doses as low as 16 Gy have been reported. RIOs constitute approximately 3% to 5% of all osteosarcomas, and the risk of developing an osteosarcoma among those irradiated is believed to be less than 1%. RIOs usually occur at the margin of the irradiated field; this has been postulated to be due to only partial cell death at the margin of the irradiated field, with viable cells maintaining their ability to proliferate into a sarcoma. RIOs are clinically suspected when there is pain or swelling at the site of radiation. A RIO is often more locally aggressive and of a higher grade than a sporadic calvarial osteosarcoma, although the rate of metastatic disease is much less with an RIO than with a sporadic osteosarcoma.

  In order to meet the diagnostic criteria of a RIO, a sarcoma must occur within the field of radiation, should not be present prior to radiation, is histologically different from the primary tumor, and has an asymptomatic latency period following radiation. A sufficient latency period is generally regarded to be at least 3 to 4 years, although latency periods up to 50 years after radiation have been reported.

On CT, the imaging findings of RIO most often include a soft tissue mass, osseous destruction, tumor matrix mineralization, and a periosteal reaction. On MRI, a RIO is iso- to hypointense on T1, heterogeneous on T2, and moderately to avidly enhances following contrast administration. Complete surgical excision is the treatment of choice. Nevertheless, the 5-year survival of RIO is dismal and is generally less than 20% to 30%. This is considerably worse compared to sporadic osteosarcomas, which are estimated to have a 5-year survival of approximately 70%.

Calvarial osteoma of the outer table

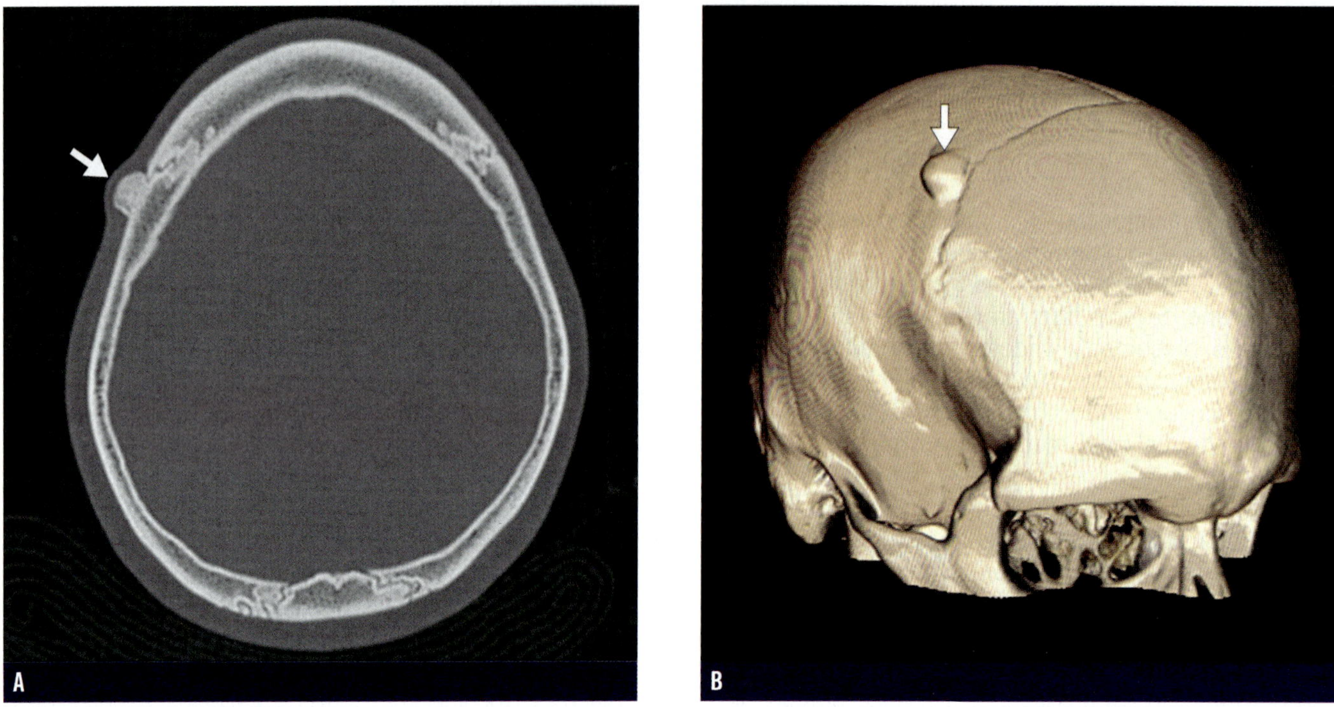

Axial (**A**) and 3D reconstructed (**B**) CT images demonstrate a focal, exophytic, round osseous excrescence arising from the anterior aspect of the right parietal bone outer table, compatible with a calvarial osteoma (arrows, **A**, **B**).

Pedunculated calvarial osteoma of the outer table

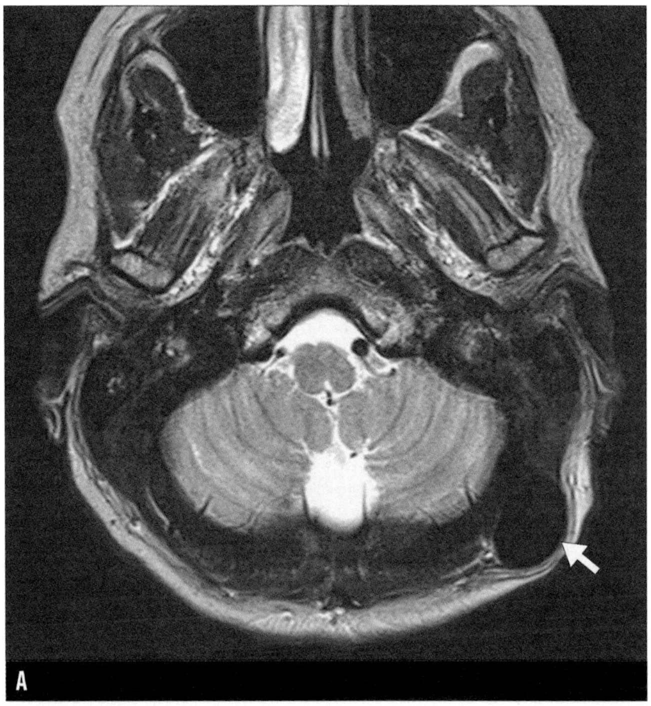

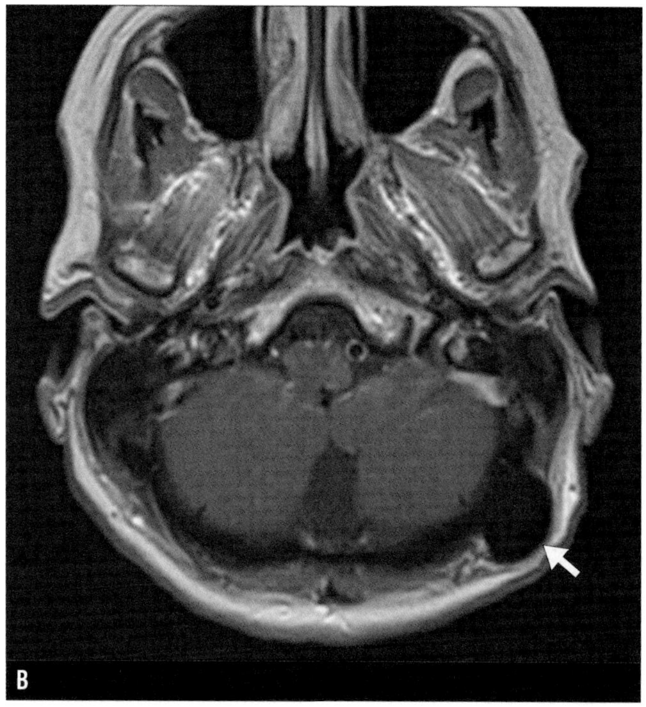

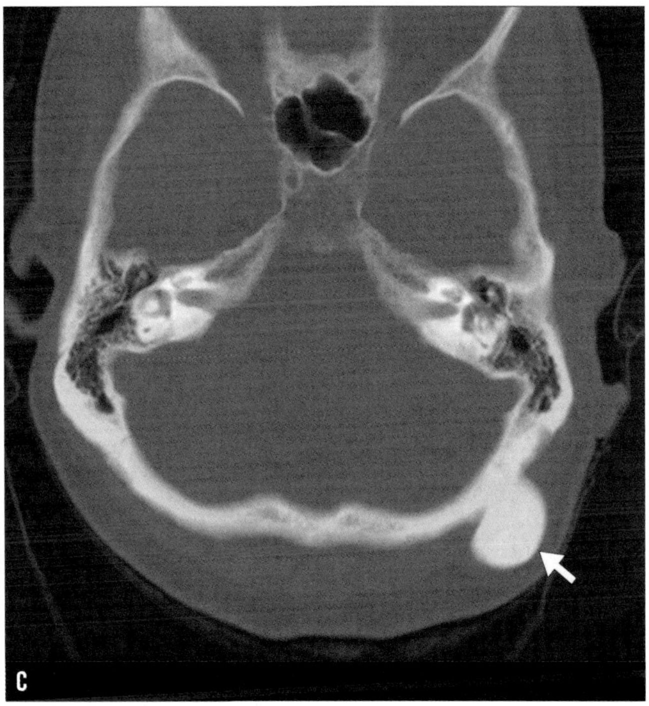

Axial T2 (**A**) and contrast-enhanced axial T1 (**B**) MR images demonstrate an oval, diffusely T1 and T2 hypointense, nonenhancing lesion along the left aspect of the occipital bone outer table (arrows, **A**, **B**). An axial CT image (**C**) demonstrates the finding on MRI to be a densely ossified lesion arising from the occipital bone outer table and projecting into the subgaleal soft tissues, compatible with a large osteoma (arrow, **C**).

Enostosis

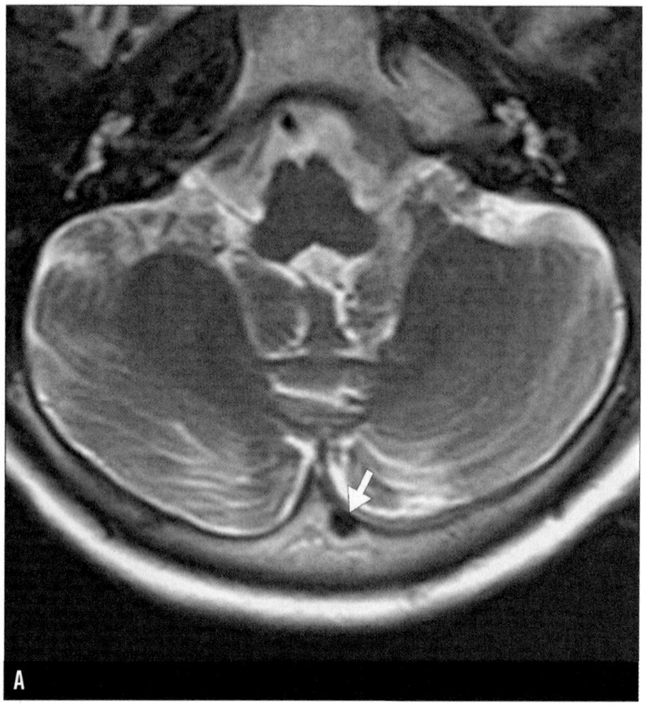

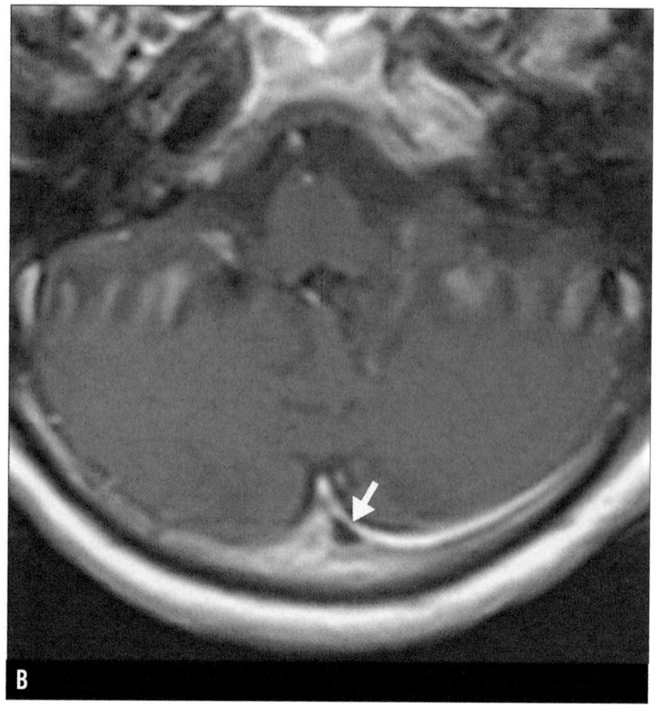

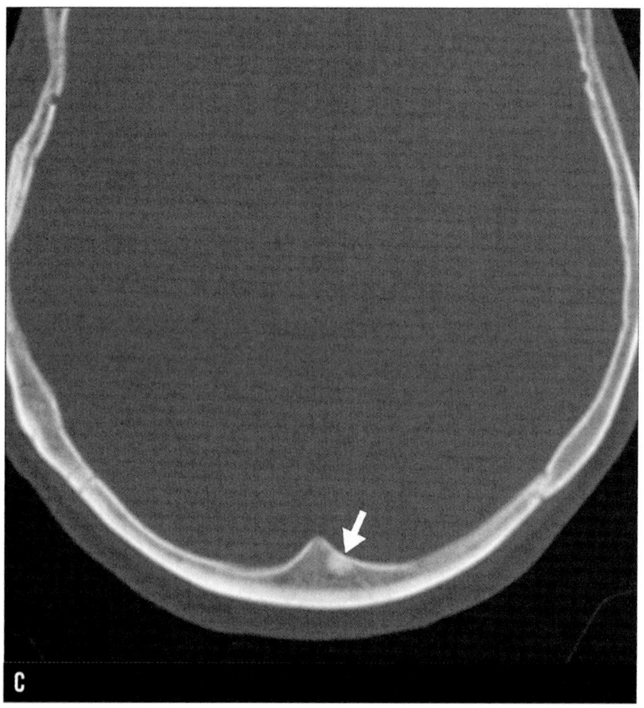

Axial T2 (**A**) and contrast-enhanced axial T1 (**B**) MR images demonstrate a small, nonenhancing focus of T1 and T2 hypointense signal located near the midline of the occipital calvarium (arrows, **A**, **B**). An axial CT image of the same patient (**C**) demonstrates the finding to represent a small focus of sclerosis (arrow, **C**). There were no other similar findings involving the remainder of the visualized osseous structures, and the patient did not have a history of malignancy. The finding is most consistent with a small calvarial enostosis.

Venous malformation of the calvarium (osseous hemangioma)

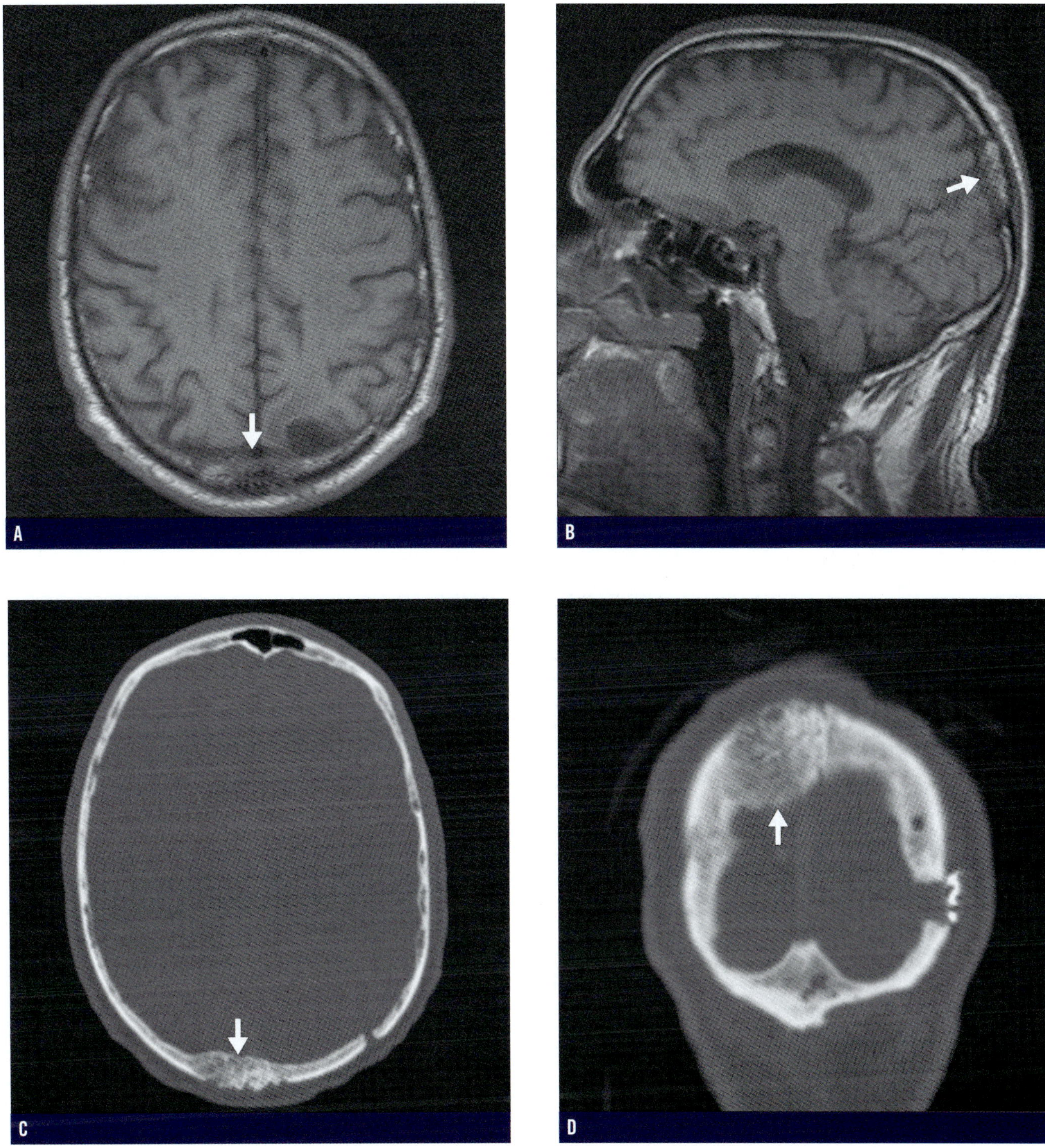

Axial T1 (**A**) and sagittal T1 (**B**) MR images demonstrate a focal, heterogeneous T1 lesion with speckled intrinsic T1 hyperintensity involving the posterior paramedian right parietal calvarium (arrows, **A**, **B**). Axial (**C**) and coronal reformatted (**D**) CT images of the same patient demonstrate the lesion to be mildly expansile and contain a "honeycomb" pattern (arrows, **C, D**). The imaging findings are most consistent with a benign calvarial venous malformation, traditionally termed an osseous hemangioma.

Calvarial epidermoid

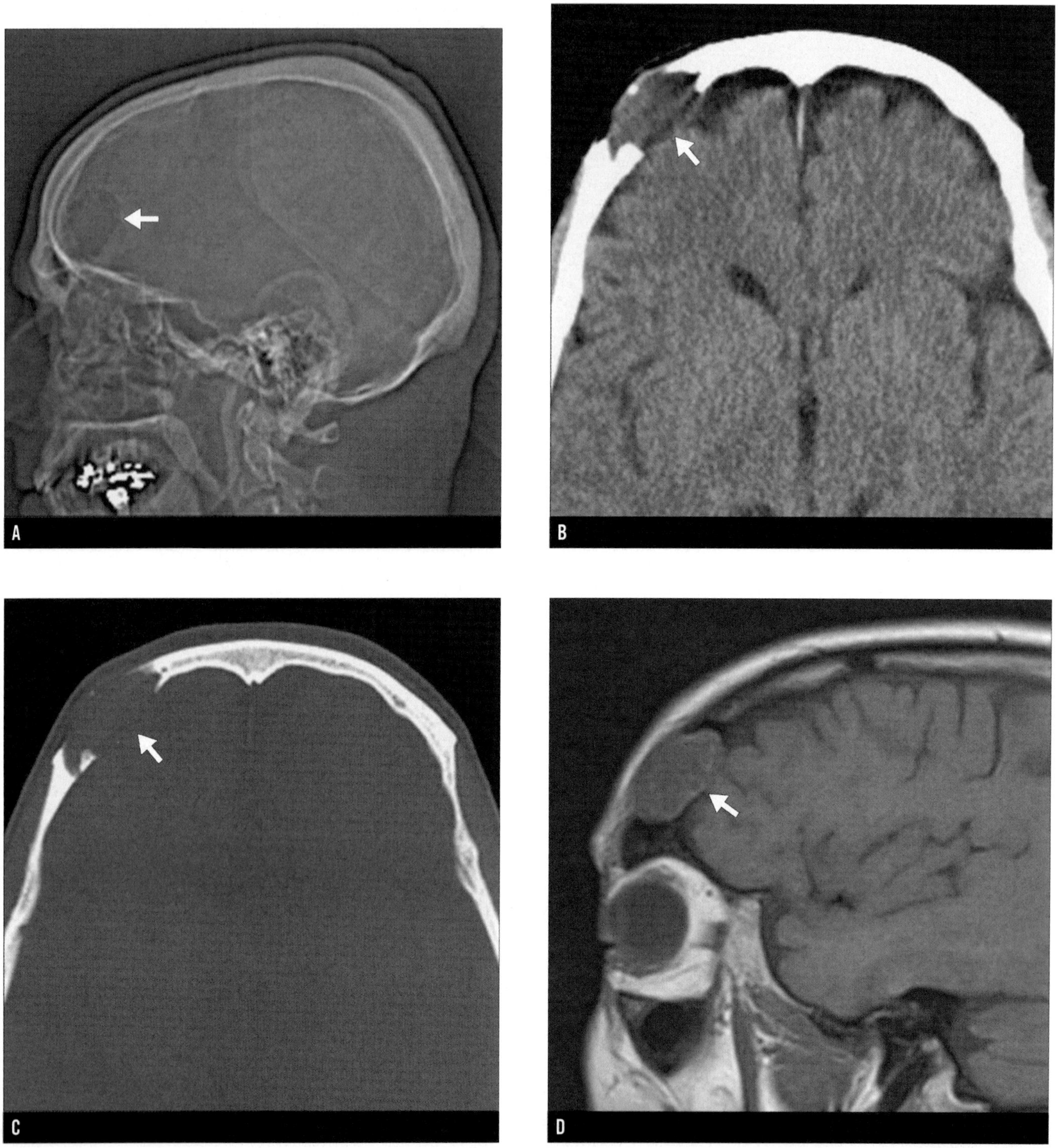

A sagittal scout image from a CT (**A**) demonstrates a discrete lucency involving the frontal calvarium (arrow, **A**). Axial CT images from the same study viewed with a brain window (**B**) and bone window (**C**) demonstrate the finding to be a hypoattenuating mass centered in the diploic space of the frontal calvarium associated with osseous expansion and marked thinning of the inner and outer cortices (arrows, **B**, **C**). Sagittal T1 (**D**), axial T2 (**E**), axial FLAIR (**F**), axial DWI (**G**), and axial ADC map (**H**) MR images of the same patient demonstrate the finding to be mostly T1 hypointense with scattered swirls of minimal T1 shortening, T2 hyperintense, mildly FLAIR hyperintense, and to restrict on DWI (arrows, **D**-**H**). The imaging findings are consistent with a calvarial epidermoid.

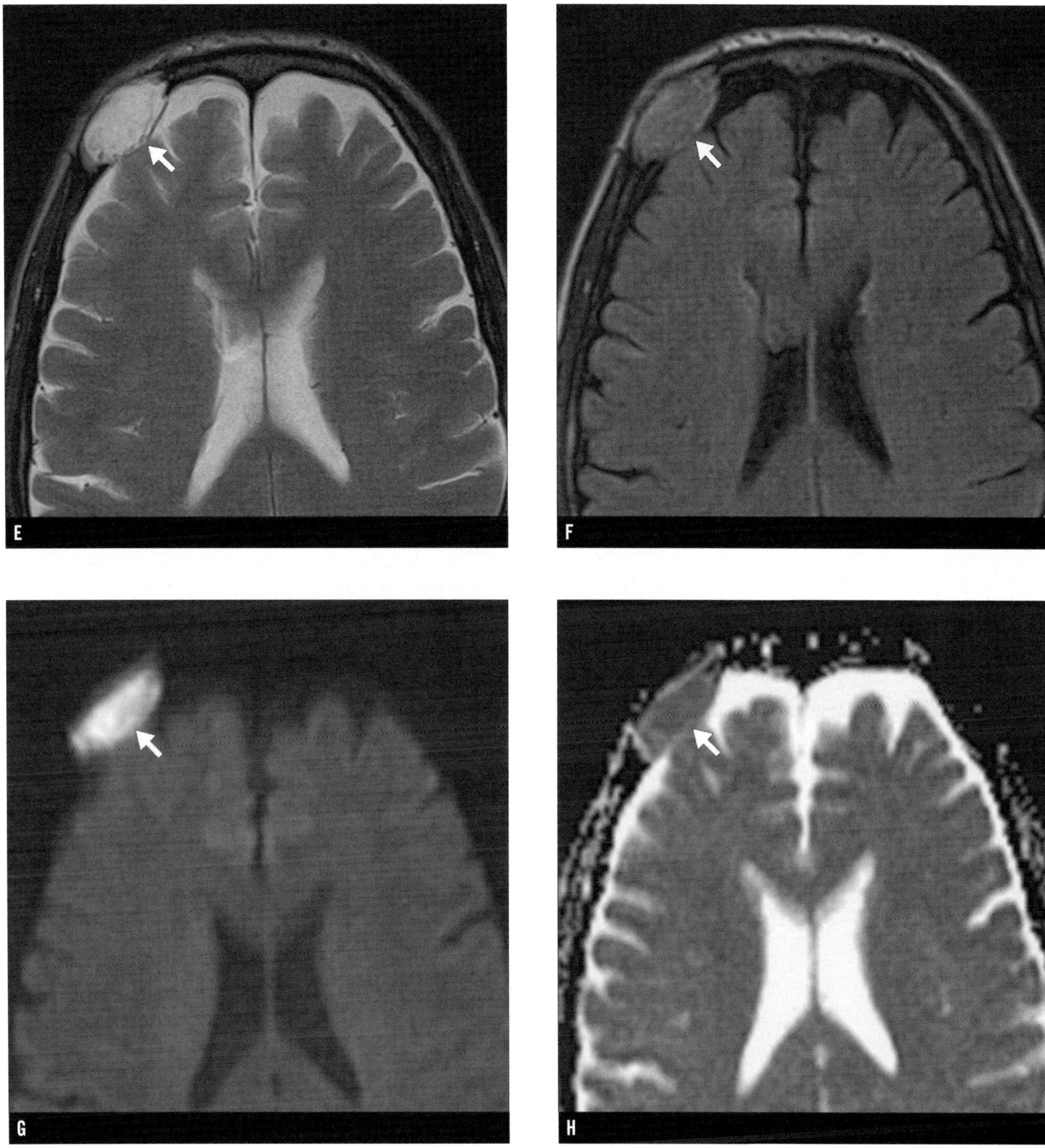
E
F
G
H

Benign fibro-osseous calvarial lesion: Ground-glass (sclerotic) form of fibrous dysplasia

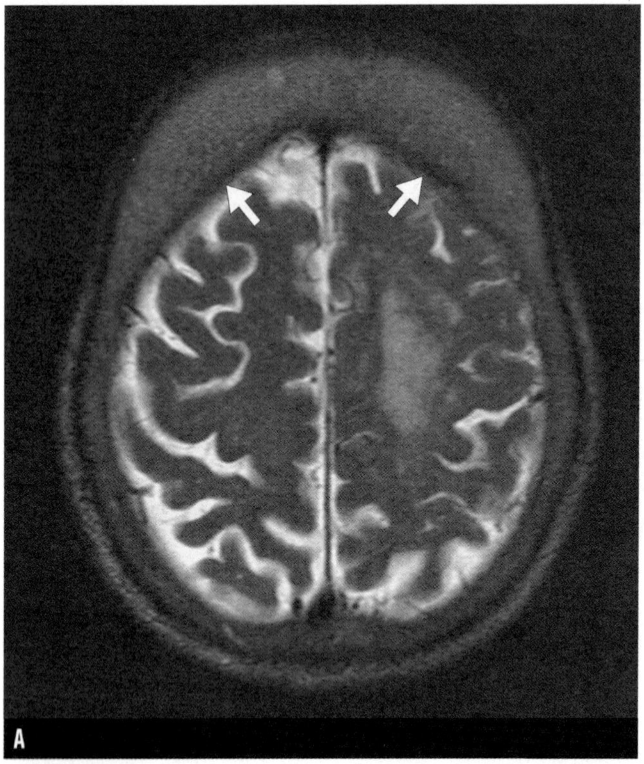

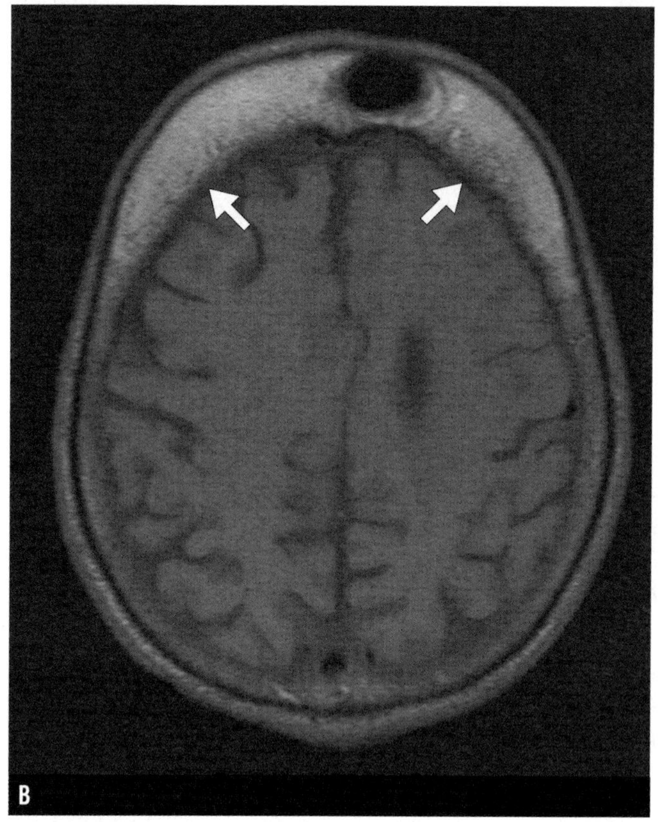

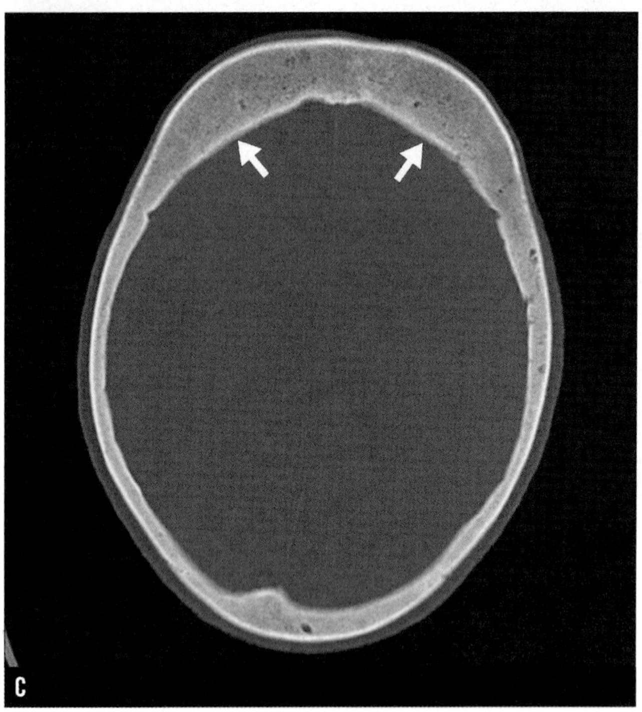

Axial T2 (**A**) and axial T1 (**B**) MR images demonstrate diffuse expansion of the frontal calvarium with mildly hyperintense T2 signal and pronounced T1 shortening in the marrow (arrows, **A**, **B**). An axial CT image of the same patient (**C**) demonstrates pronounced expansion and a "ground-glass" appearance of the frontal calvarium, most compatible with fibrous dysplasia. (arrows, **C**) The ground-glass appearance and the lack of irregular lobulation along the inner table of the frontal bone differentiate this entity from hyperostosis frontalis interna.

Benign fibro-osseous calvarial lesion: Fibrous dysplasia

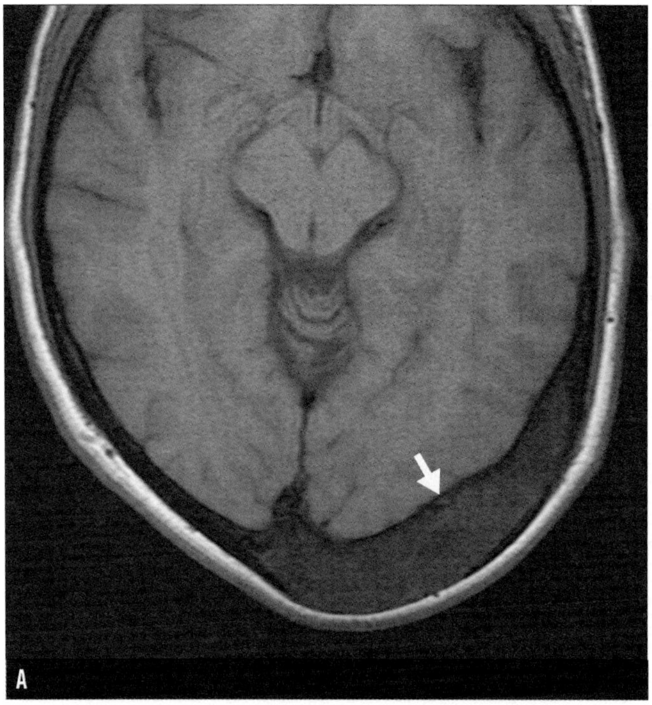

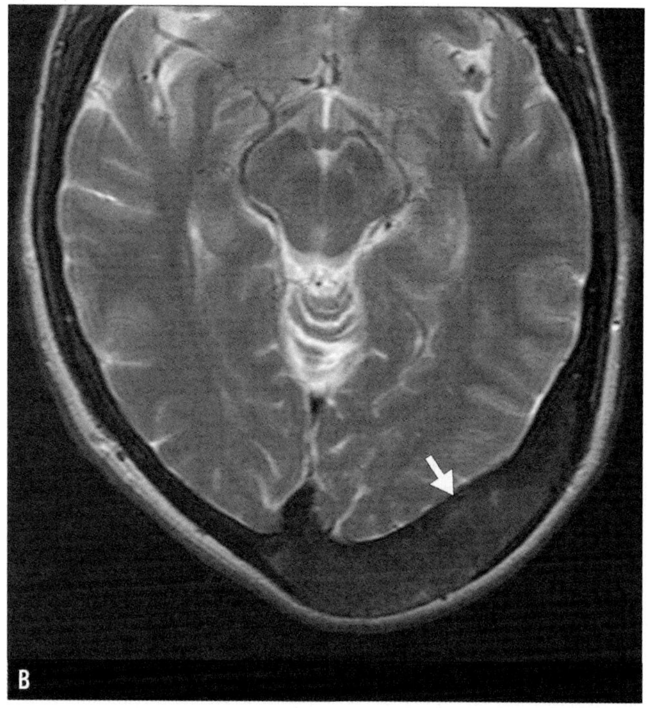

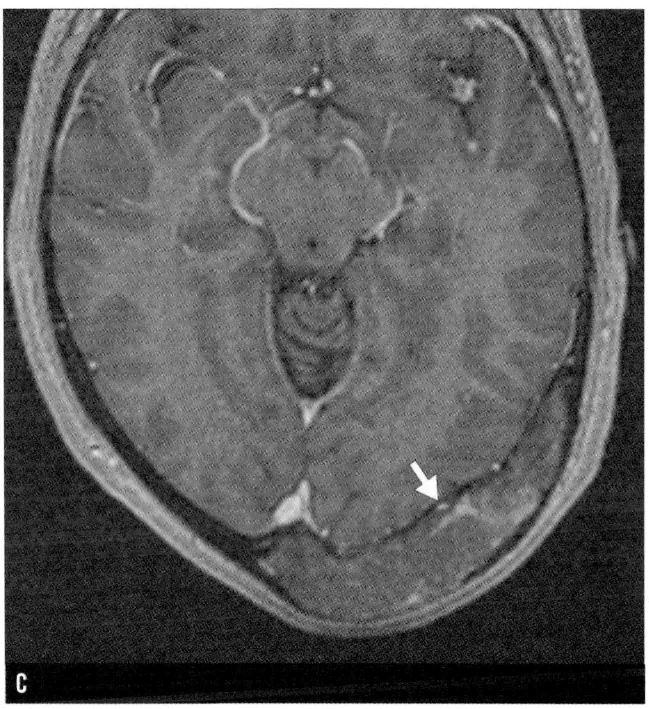

Axial T1 (**A**), axial T2 (**B**), and postcontrast axial MPRAGE (**C**) MR images demonstrate an expansile lesion of the left parietal and occipital bones that is heterogeneous on T1 and T2 and heterogeneously enhances (arrows, **A**-**C**). The imaging findings are most compatible with fibrous dysplasia, although correlation with CT imaging in cases such as these is usually prudent for confirmation.

Benign fibro-osseous calvarial lesion: Cystic form of fibrous dysplasia

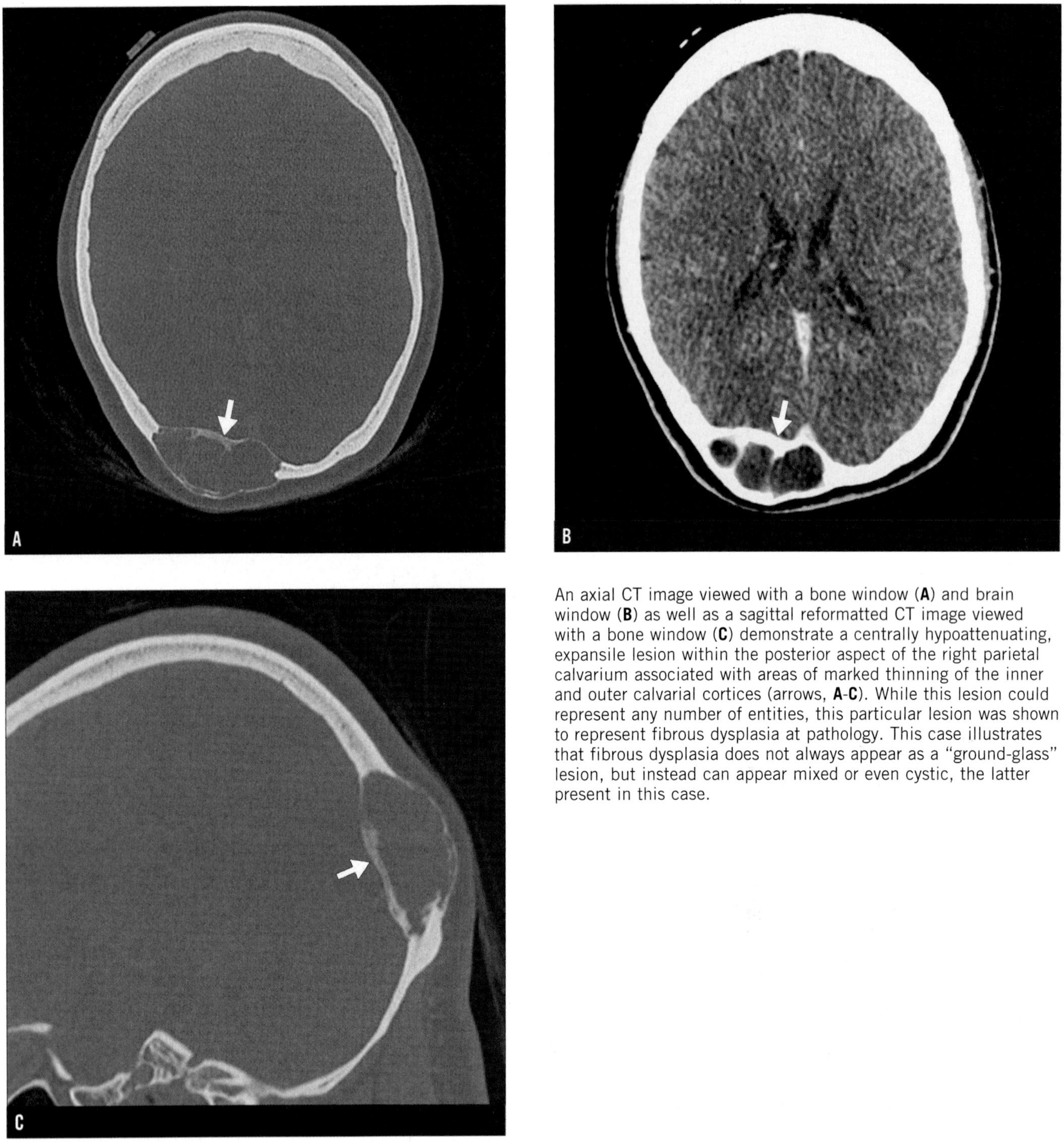

An axial CT image viewed with a bone window (**A**) and brain window (**B**) as well as a sagittal reformatted CT image viewed with a bone window (**C**) demonstrate a centrally hypoattenuating, expansile lesion within the posterior aspect of the right parietal calvarium associated with areas of marked thinning of the inner and outer calvarial cortices (arrows, **A**-**C**). While this lesion could represent any number of entities, this particular lesion was shown to represent fibrous dysplasia at pathology. This case illustrates that fibrous dysplasia does not always appear as a "ground-glass" lesion, but instead can appear mixed or even cystic, the latter present in this case.

Partially cystic benign fibro-osseous calvarial lesion

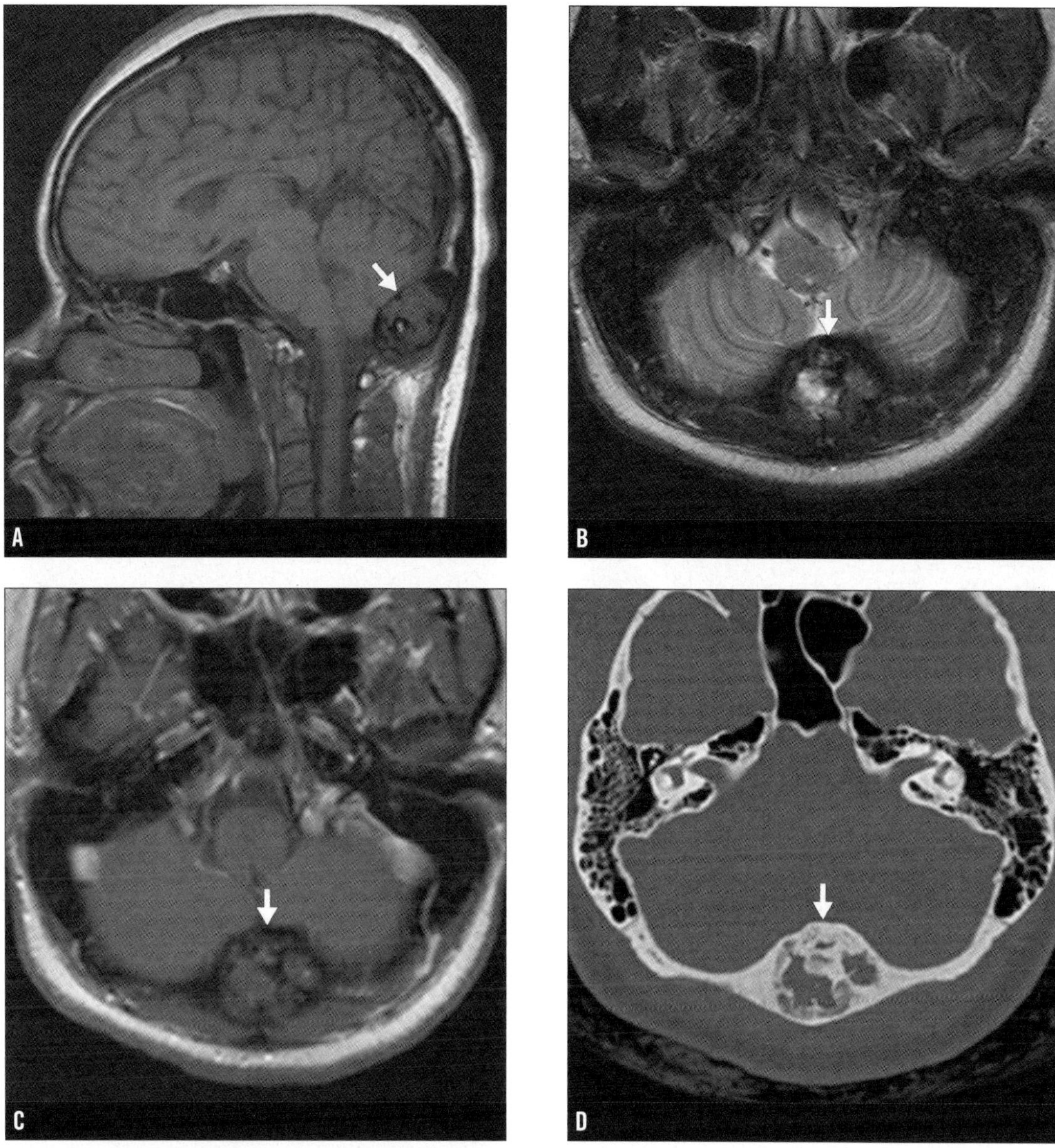

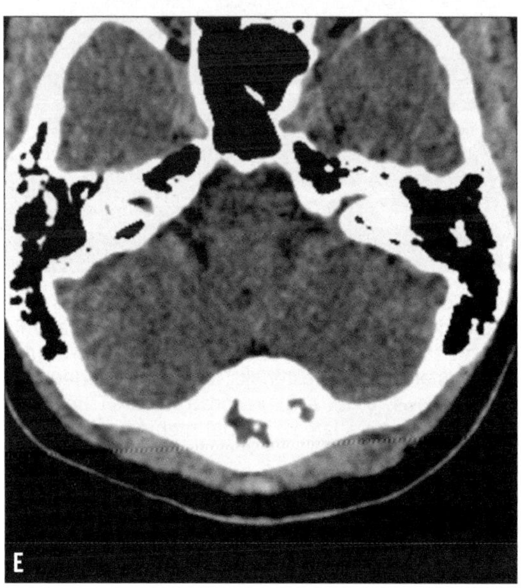

Sagittal T1 (**A**), axial T2 (**B**), and contrast-enhanced axial T1 (**C**) MR images demonstrate an expansile, centrally T1 isointense and T2 hyperintense, minimally enhancing lesion centered in the inferior midline aspect of the occipital bone (arrows, **A-C**). An axial CT image of the same patient viewed with a bone window (**D**) demonstrates the lesion to have thickened peripheral sclerosis and to contain coarse osseous trabeculations (arrow, **D**). The same axial CT image viewed with a soft tissue window (**E**) does not demonstrate an adjacent soft tissue abnormality, and the central lucent area approximates marrow attenuation. This finding was stable for several years. The overall imaging characteristics are compatible with a fibro-osseous lesion, most likely the cystic form of fibrous dysplasia.

Calvarial meningioma

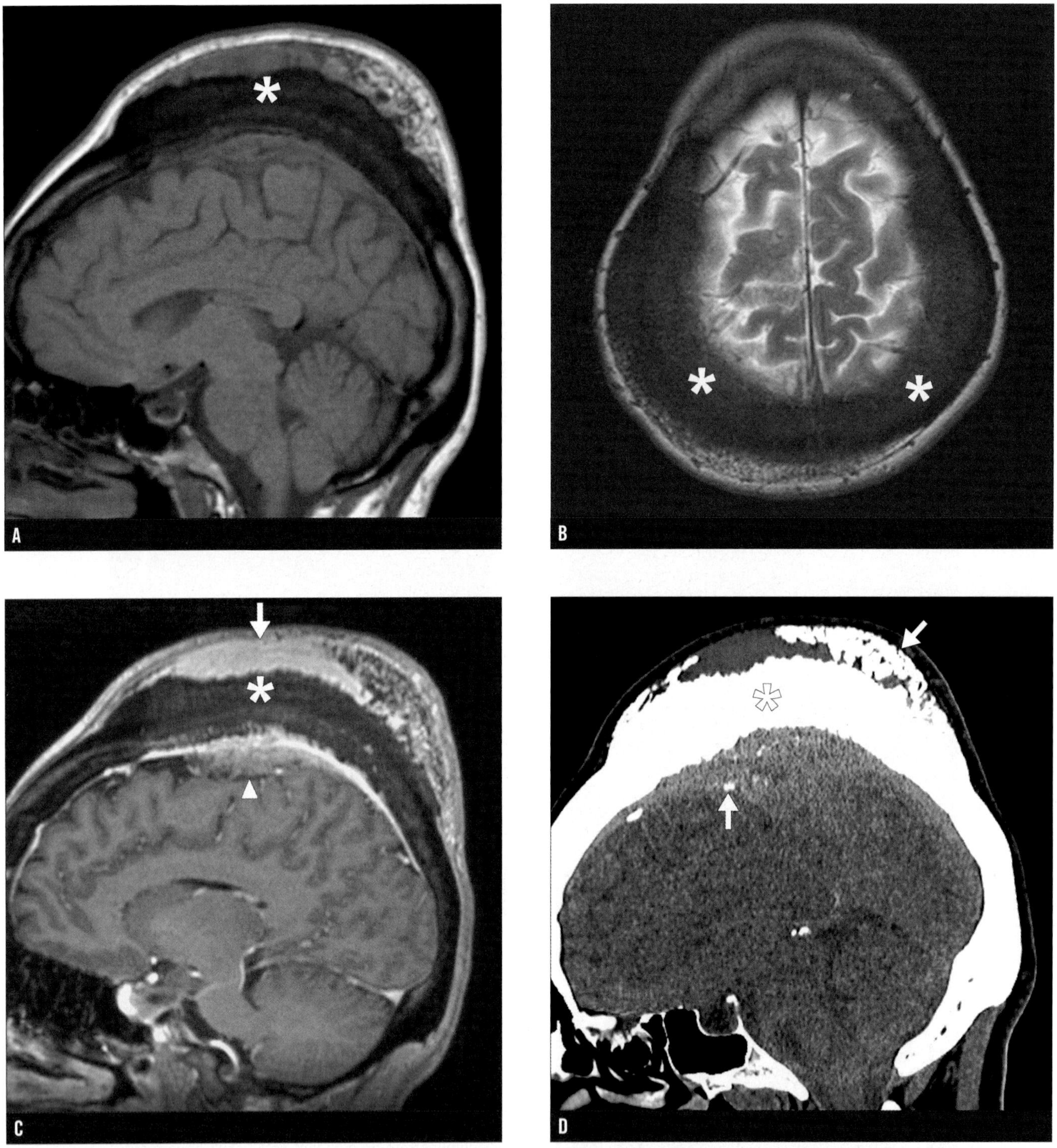

Sagittal T1 (**A**), axial T2 (**B**), and sagittal postcontrast MPRAGE (**C**) MR images demonstrate a large calvarial vertex mass that is associated with pronounced calvarial thickening (asterisks, **A-C**), subgaleal enhancement (arrow, **C**), and underlying dural enhancement (arrowhead, **C**). Unenhanced sagittal reformatted CT images viewed with a soft tissue window (**D**) and bone window (**E**) of the same patient demonstrate marked osseous thickening of the calvarial vertex with irregular margins (asterisks, **D**, **E**) and scattered mineralization of the subgaleal component, and to a lesser degree, the dural component (arrows, **D**, **E**). A 3D reconstructed CT image viewed in the lateral projection (**F**) demonstrates the 3D correlate of the finding. This lesion represents a large calvarial meningioma.

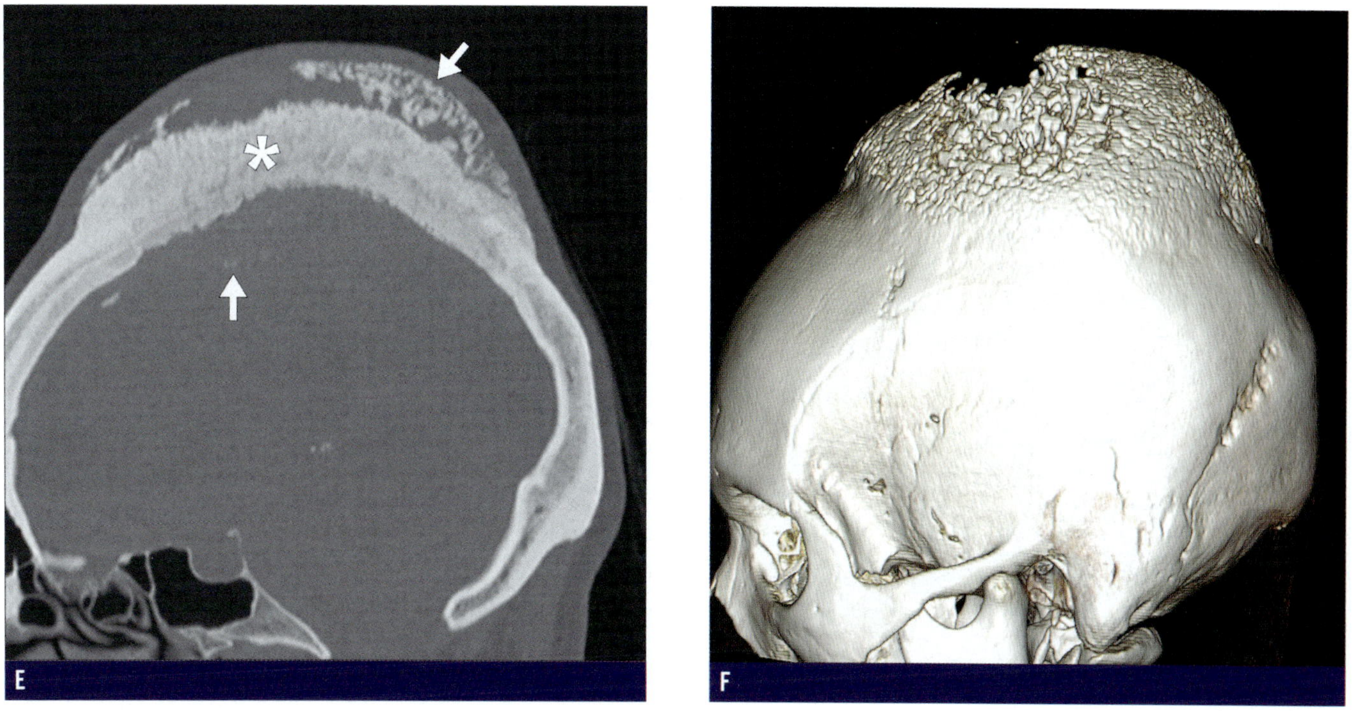

Companion case: Sclerotic metastatic disease

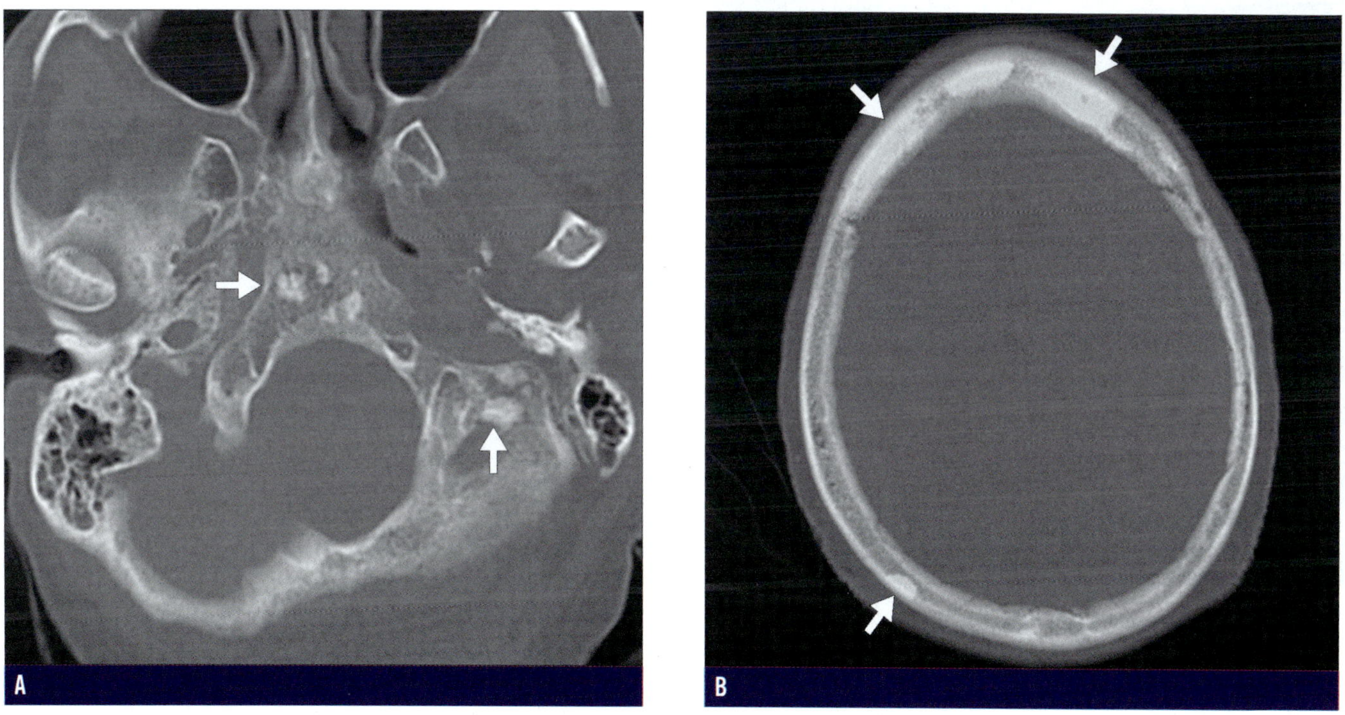

An axial CT image through the skull base (**A**) demonstrates several sclerotic foci involving the basiocciput, a nonspecific finding that could represent several enostoses or other entities, such as sclerotic metastases (arrows, **A**). An axial CT image more cephalad (**B**) demonstrates several additional small and large sclerotic lesions affecting the calvarium (arrows, **B**). Axial T1 (**C**), axial T2 (**D**), and contrast-enhanced axial T1 (**E**) MR images of the same patient demonstrate the same foci from image **B** to be T1 hypointense, T2 hypointense, and nonenhancing (arrows, **C**-**E**). This patient has metastatic breast cancer, and the findings are most consistent with sclerotic, nonenhancing metastases.

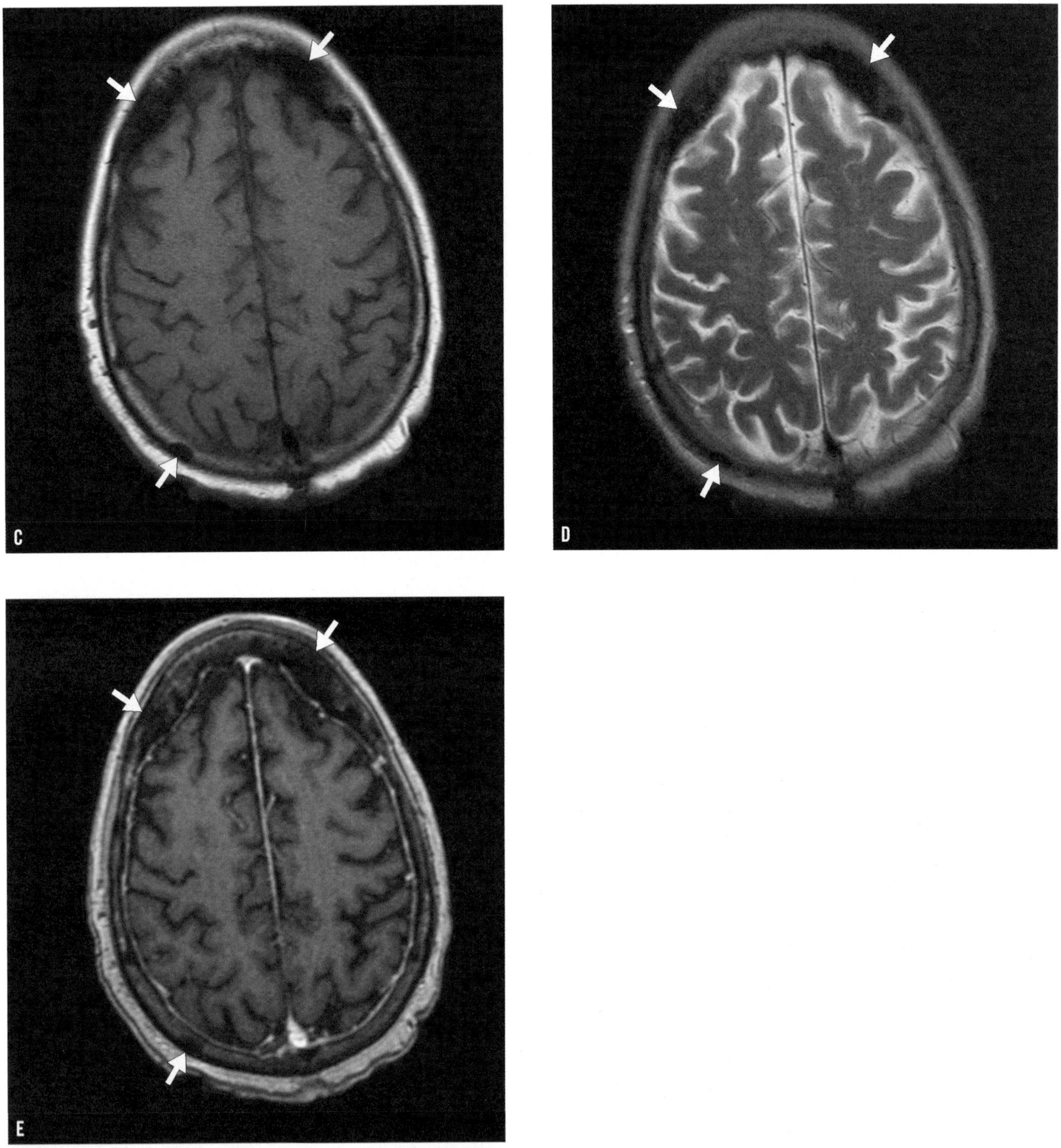
C
D
E

Companion case: Metastatic melanoma to the calvarium

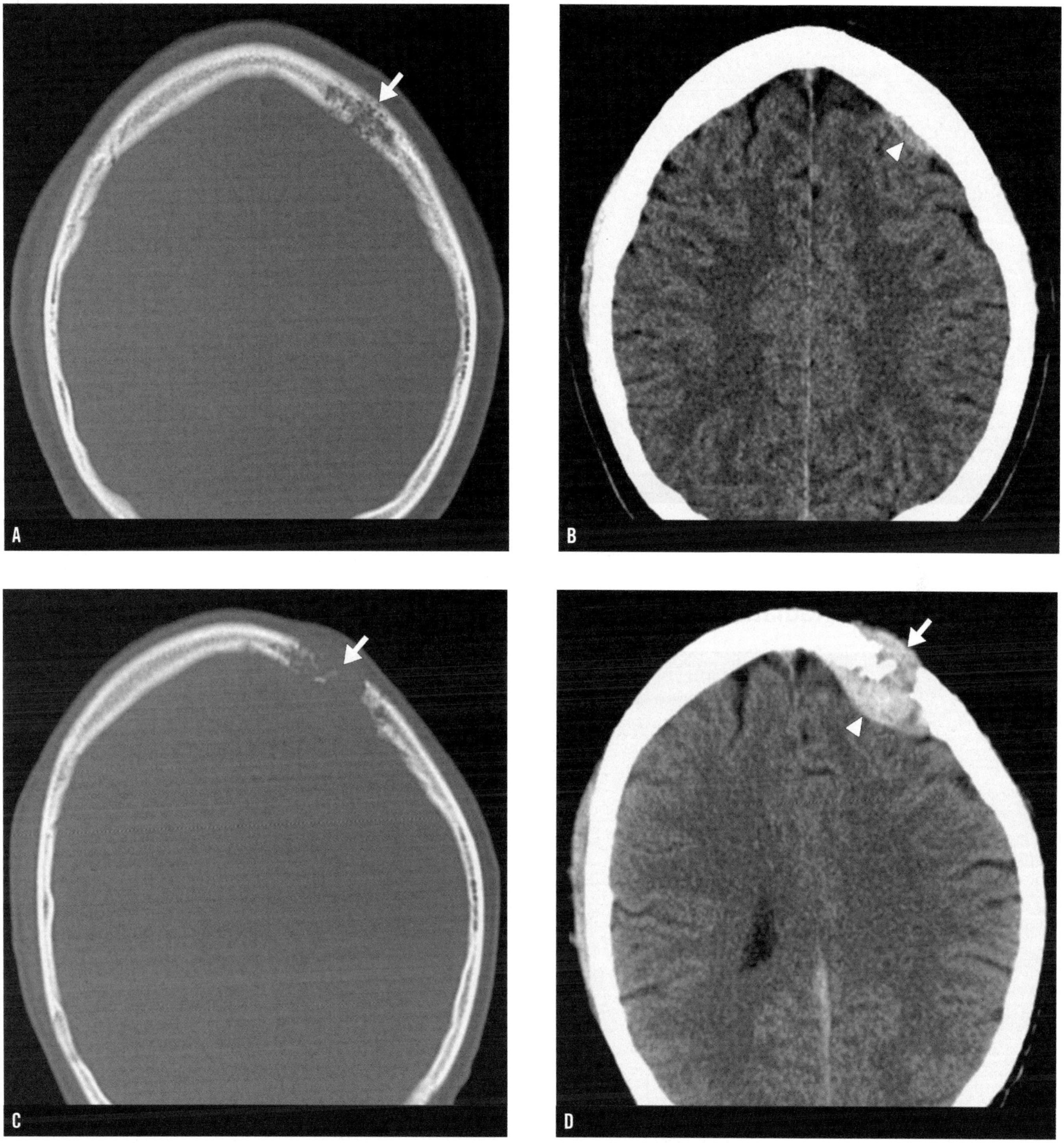

Unenhanced axial CT images viewed with a bone window (**A**) and brain window (**B**) demonstrate a permeative lesion involving the diploic space and inner table along the left aspect of the frontal calvarium (arrow, **A**) associated with a small, intracranial, extra-axial soft tissue component (arrowhead, **B**). Five months later, unenhanced axial CT images viewed with a bone window (**C**) and brain window (**D**) demonstrate a significant increase in size of the lesion. There is greater destruction of the frontal calvarium (arrow, **C**) with a larger intracranial, extra-axial component (arrowhead, **D**) and a new subgaleal component (arrow, **D**). Unenhanced sagittal T1 (**E**) and contrast-enhanced coronal T1 with fat suppression (**F**) MR images of the same patient obtained on the same date as images **C** and **D**. These MR images demonstrate the lesion to be diffusely precontrast T1 hyperintense (arrow, **E**) and also reveal a large amount of intracranial extension with dural enhancement (arrows, **F**). This case represented a melanoma metastasis, with the T1 shortening on image **E** related to the presence of melanin.

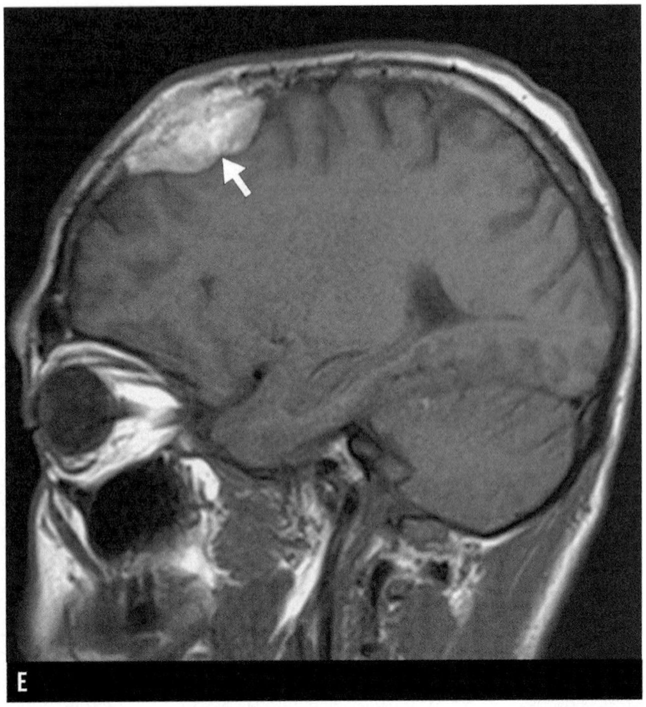

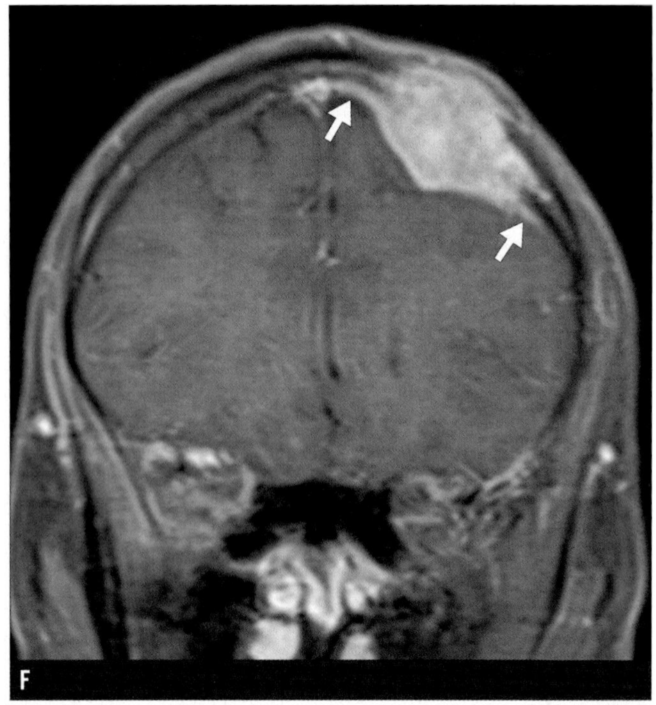

Companion case: Radiation-induced calvarial osteosarcoma

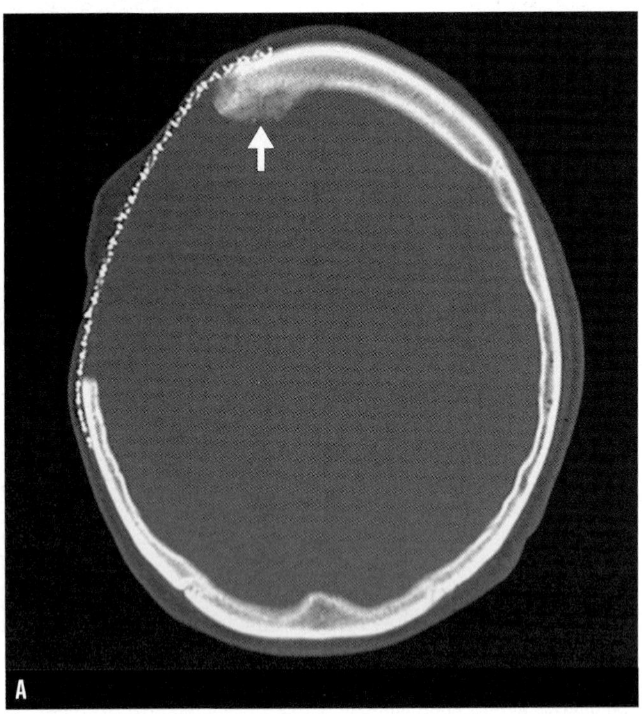

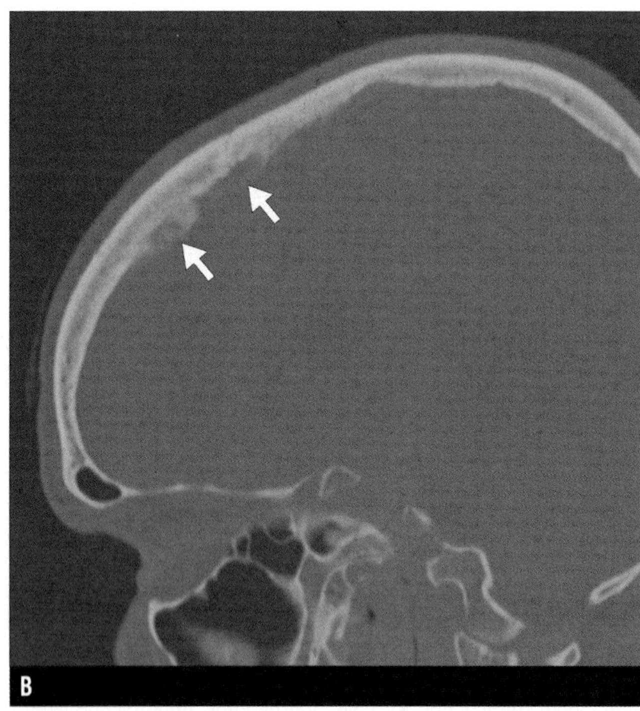

Axial (**A**) and right parasagittal reformatted (**B**) CT images viewed with a bone window demonstrate a mildly spiculated, irregular osseous overgrowth along the anterior margin of a titanium mesh cranioplasty, pathologically shown to represent osteosarcoma (arrows, **A**, **B**). This patient had previous surgery and radiation to the brain several years prior to this examination for treatment of a right frontal lobe anaplastic astrocytoma . This osseous abnormality was pathologically shown to represent a calvarial osteosarcoma, and given the clinical scenario, it was compatible with the radiation-induced type.

REFERENCES

Amaral L, et al. MR imaging for evaluation of lesions of the cranial vault: a pictorial essay. *Arq Neuropsiquiatr.* 200361(3-A): 521-532.

Baik FM, et al. Comparative case series of exostoses and osteoma of the internal auditory canal. *Ann Oto Rhinol Laryngol.* 2011;120(4):255-260.

Cai PQ, et al. CT and MRI of radiation-induced sarcomas of the head and neck following radiotherapy for nasopharyngeal carcinoma. *Clin Radiol.* 2013;68(7):683-689.

Camels V, et al. Osteoblastic and mixed spinal metastases: evaluation of the analgesic efficacy of percutaneous vertebroplasty. *Am J Neuroradiol.* 2007;28:570-574.

Chalain T, Tan B. Ivory osteoma of the craniofacial skeleton. *J Craniofac Surg.* 2003;14(5):729-735.

Eversole R, Su L, ElMofty S. Benign fibro-osseous lesions of the craniofacial complex. A review. *Head Neck Pathol.* 2008;2(3):177-202.

Goltzman D. (). Mechanisms of the development of osteoblastic metastases. *Cancer.* 1997;80:1581-1587.

Greenspan A, Steiner G., Knutzon R. Bone island (enostosis): clinical significance and radiologic and pathologic correlations. *Skeletal Radiol.* 1991;20:85-90.

Ito T, et al. Radiation-induced osteosarcomas after treatment for frontal gliomas: a report of two cases. *Brain Tumor Pathol.* 2010;27(2):103-109.

Lee HY, et al. Intraosseous meningioma: CT and MR Appearance. *J Comput Assist Tomogr.* 1992;16(6):1000-1001.

Lowe LH, Marchant TC, Rivard DC, Scherbel AJ. Vascular malformations: classification and terminology the radiologist needs to know. *Semin Roentgenol.* 2012;47(2):106-117.

O'Regan K, et al. Imaging of radiation-associated sarcoma. *AJR Am J Roentgenol.* 2011;197(1):W30-W36.

Osborn AG, Preece MT. Intracranial cysts: radiologic-pathologic correlation and imaging approach. *Radiology.* 2006;239(3):650-664.

Patel AJ, et al. Radiation-induced osteosarcomas of the calvarium and skull base. *Cancer.* 2011;117(10):2120-2126.

Patnana M, et al. Multimethod imaging, staging, and spectrum of manifestations of metastatic melanoma. *Clin Radiol.* 2011;66(3): 224-236.

Puranik A, Sankhe S, Goel N, Mahore A. Cerebral shading sign in a giant intraparenchymal white epidermoid. *Neurol India.* 2012;60(2):265-266.

Zanetti R, et al. Comparison of risk patterns in carcinoma and melanoma of the skin in men: a multi-centre case-case-control study. *Br J Cancer.* 2006;94(5):743-751.

CASE 7 External occipital protuberance

The external occipital protuberance (EOP) is a midline osseous projection arising from the external surface of the occipital bone squama and represents the insertion site of the nuchal ligament. Identification of the EOP is clinically relevant as a landmark for the treatment of greater and lesser occipital nerve neuropathy in patients with chronic occipital headaches (eg, during therapeutic injections) as well as for surgical planning (eg, during craniocervical fixation).

There is a variable appearance of the EOP among individuals, and a classification scheme of three distinct appearances exists: smooth, crest (ie, pointed posteriorly), and spine (ie, caudally beaked appearance). The EOP is generally larger in males compared to females. Interestingly, the size of the EOP is used by forensic investigators and anthropological researchers to discriminate the gender of skeletal remains. An EOP represents the second most reliable anatomic structure for this purpose, second only to the shape of the pelvic anatomy.

The EOP rarely results in a diagnostic imaging dilemma, aided mainly by its characteristic location. It has been speculated that increased physical activity involving the neck muscles leads to progressive enlargement. Occasionally, a patient may complain of discomfort or cosmetic deformity when an EOP is unusually large. An abnormally enlarged EOP may occur sporadically or can be identified in patients afflicted by acromegaly.

COMPANION CASE

- **Calvarial osteoma of the outer table.** Calvarial osteomas are osseous hamartomas of unknown etiology. They are sclerotic, round to oval osseous densities that arise from either the inner or outer calvarial cortex. Osteomas are usually asymptomatic lesions, unless they result in mass effect on adjacent structures, and they are typically identified incidentally on imaging studies or by direct palpation. Osteomas of the mandible or multiple osteomas, while often identified sporadically, are associated with Gardner syndrome.

  On radiographs or CT, calvarial osteomas are smoothly marginated, densely sclerotic juxtacortical lesions. On MRI, they are usually diffusely hypointense on all pulse sequences because of tightly packed lamellar bone. However, osteomas may have small areas of internal heterogeneous fat signal that represent small amounts of cancellous bone marrow. Enhancement of osteomas is rare and, when present, likely represents vascularity within cancellous bone.

  Multiple terms for osteomas exist, including bone hamartoma, surface or ivory osteoma, as well as exostosis. The latter term should be avoided, as an exostosis is synonymous with an osteochondroma arising from the peripheral tubular bones and has distinctly different imaging and pathological findings.

External occipital protuberance

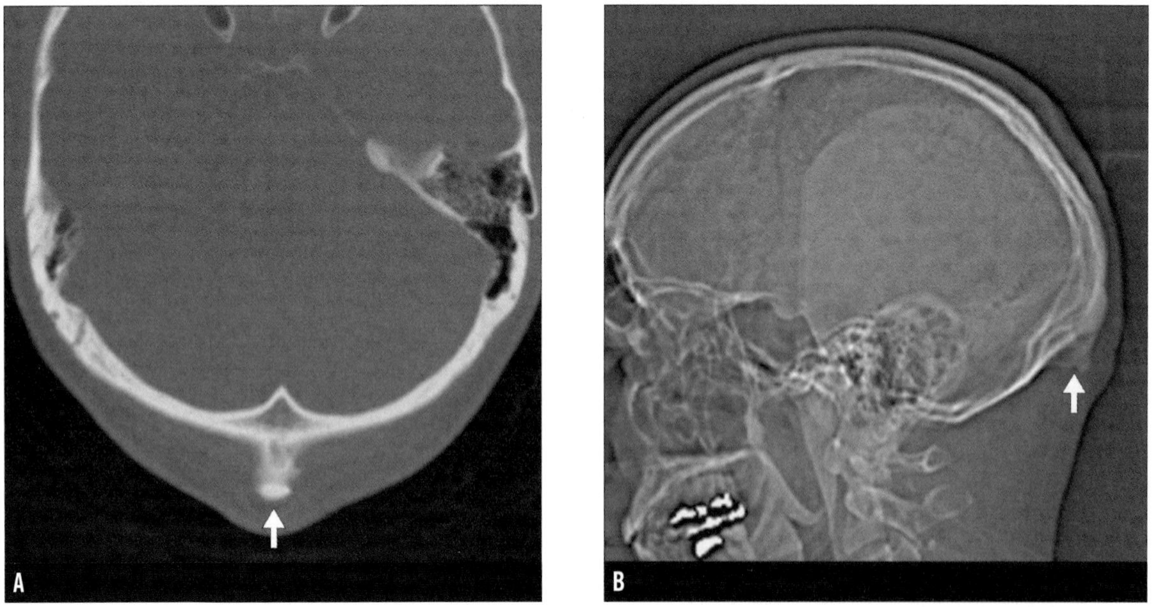

An axial CT image (**A**) and a sagittal scout image from the same study (**B**) demonstrate a large-sized, but normal external occipital protuberance (arrows, **A**, **B**). This type of external occipital protuberance would be classified as a "spine" type, because of its slightly caudal directed morphology. This patient presented to his physician for surgical removal of this finding, which was clinically suspected to represent an osteoma.

External occipital protuberance

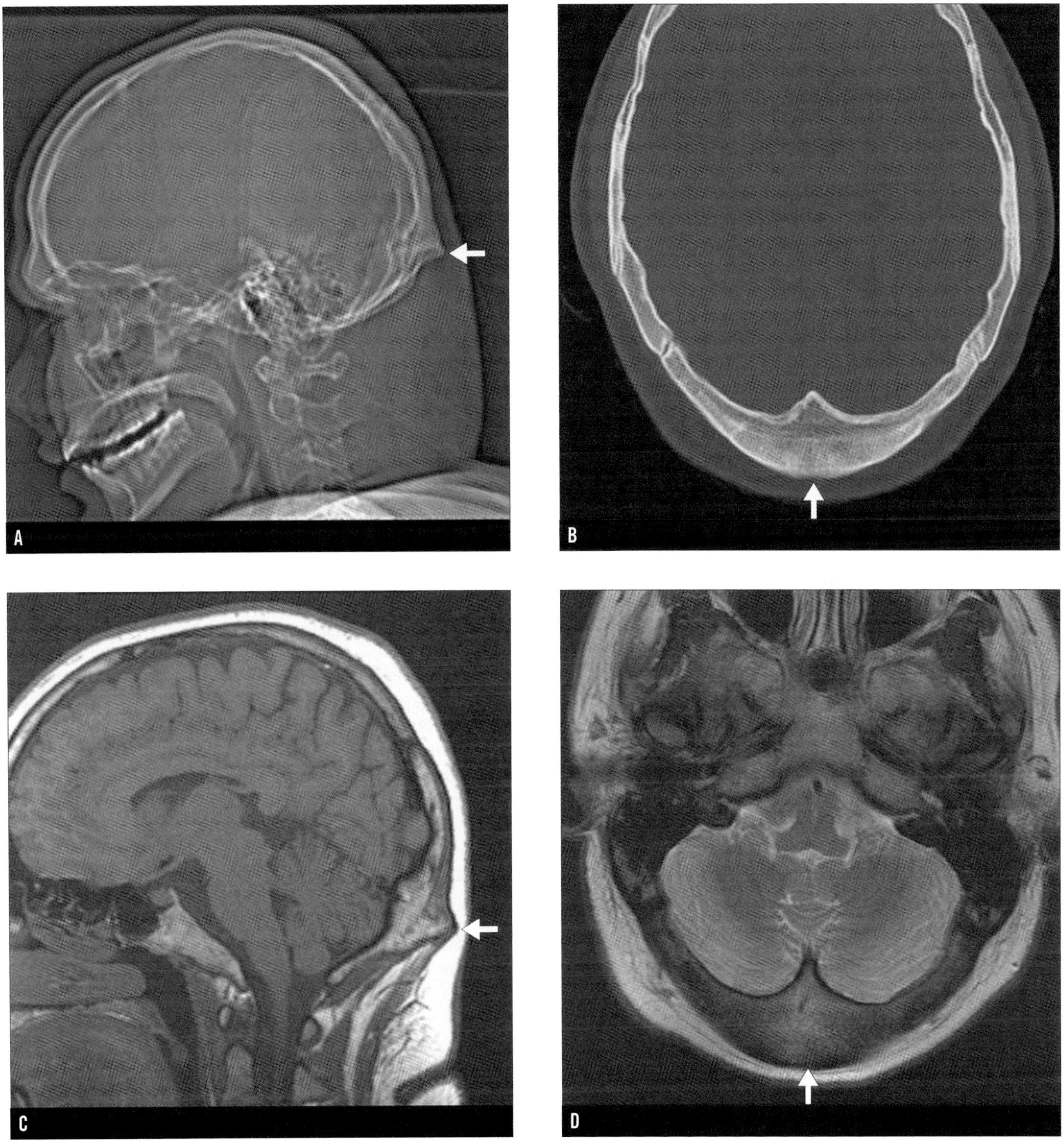

Different patient. A sagittal scout (**A**) and an axial CT image from the same study (**B**) demonstrate a large, broad-based external occipital protuberance (arrows, **A**, **B**). Sagittal T1 (**C**) and axial T2 (**D**) MR images demonstrate the MRI correlate (arrows, **C**, **D**). This external occipital protuberance would be classified as a "crest" type of morphology because its apex is directed posteriorly.

Companion case: Calvarial osteoma of the outer table

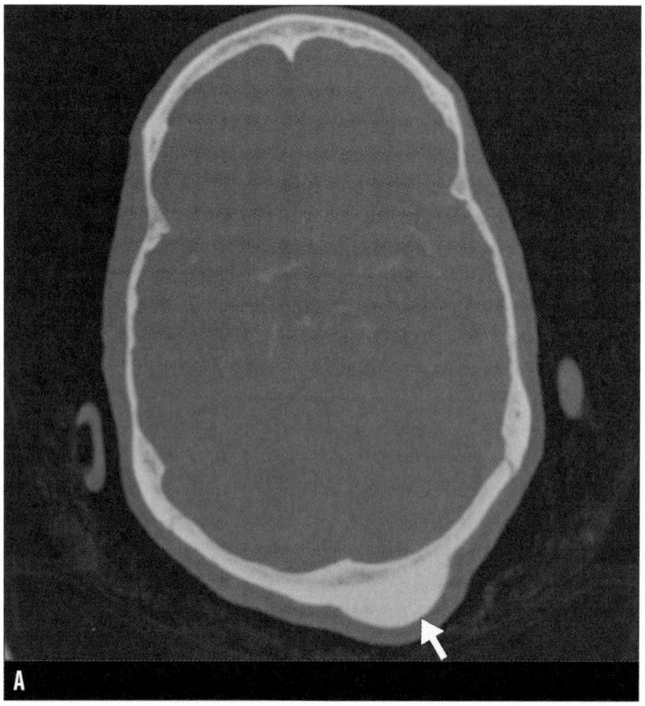

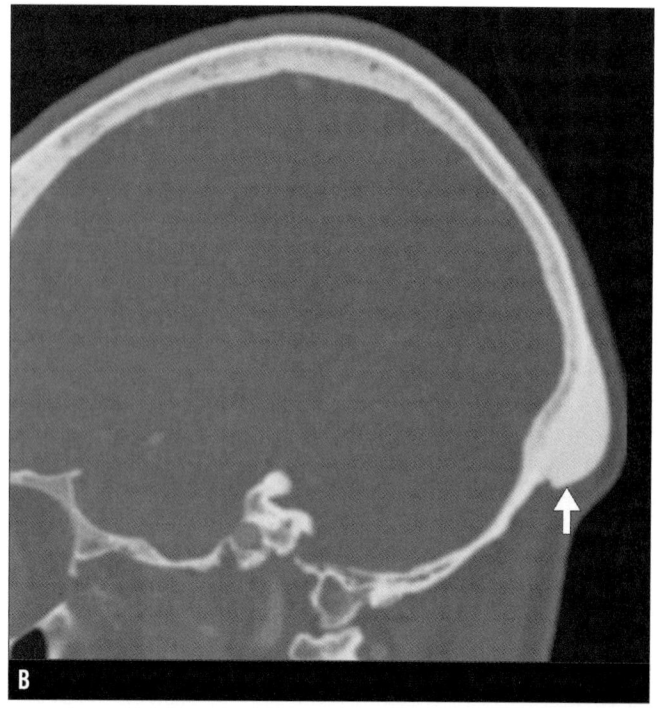

Contrast-enhanced axial (**A**) and sagittal reformatted (**B**) CT images demonstrate a large, broad-based lesion arising from the outer table of the occipital bone (arrows, **A**, **B**). This lesion is located to the left of midline, a finding that is not present with a typical external occipital protuberance. In addition, the posterior margin of the finding is smooth rather than posteriorly angulated as is often identified with an external occipital protuberance. Therefore, the lesion is most compatible with a large outer table calvarial osteoma.

REFERENCES

Bonakdarpour A, Reinus WR, Khurana JS. *Diagnostic Imaging of Musculoskeletal Diseases: A Systematic Approach*. Totowa, NJ: Humana Press, Inc.; 2009.

Gülekon IN, Turgut HB. The external occipital protuberance: can it be used as a criterion in the determination of sex? *J Forensic Sci*. 2003;48(3):1-4.

Hertel G, Hirschfelder H. In vivo and in vitro CT analysis of the occiput. *Eur Spine J*. 1999;8:27-33.

Tubbs RS, et al. Anatomical study of the third occipital nerve and its potential role in occipital headache/neck pain following midline dissections of the craniocervical junction. *J Neurosurg Spine*. 2011;15(1):71-75.

CASE 8 Cranial suture variants

In the normal newborn, there are typically five main calvarial vault sutures. These sutures allow the calvarium to mold during passage through the birth canal and allow the brain adequate room to grow later in life.

The calvarial vault sutures are as follows:

- One AP directed sagittal suture, located between the two parietal bones
- One transversely directed coronal suture, located between the parietal and frontal bones
- One AP directed metopic suture, located between the two frontal bones
- Two obliquely oriented lambdoidal sutures, located between the parietal and occipital bones

The metopic suture is the first to close by 9 months of age, although a normal metopic suture may persist throughout adult life. The remaining sutures progressively narrow to less than 2 mm during the first 1 to 2 years of life. However, these remaining sutures do not fuse until the third decade of life. When sutures do begin to fuse, the general progression of fusion is from posterior to anterior and from lateral to medial, depending on the direction of the suture. The exception to this rule is the metopic suture, which fuses from anterior to posterior.

Additional normal sutures can be identified incidentally in the pediatric patient and are not uncommon. These are related to the presence of several calvarial ossification centers which do not always fuse to one another antenatally. These additional sutures can be broadly categorized as accessory sutures, but most have specific names based on a historic or anatomic basis. Accessory sutures tend to be bilateral and symmetric, but they may also be unilateral and complex. Accessory sutures may be confused with fractures in the pediatric patient, particularly following trauma. The lack of overlying soft tissue swelling or hematoma formation, identifying the expected interdigitating and sclerotic margins of normal sutures, and knowledge of the normal ossification centers as well as the expected location of accessory sutures are helpful in differentiating an accessory suture from a fracture.

The occipital region has the greatest variation of accessory sutures because it contains six different ossification centers. The six ossification centers include (from superior to inferior): two interparietal centers, a single supraoccipital center, two exoccipital centers, and a single basioccipital center. Several distinct accessory sutures have been described and are named based on their location relative to the adjacent ossification centers. In the example given, the two interparietal centers have yet to fuse with one another, resulting in what is known as the superior median fissure (or suture) of the occiput.

Metopic suture

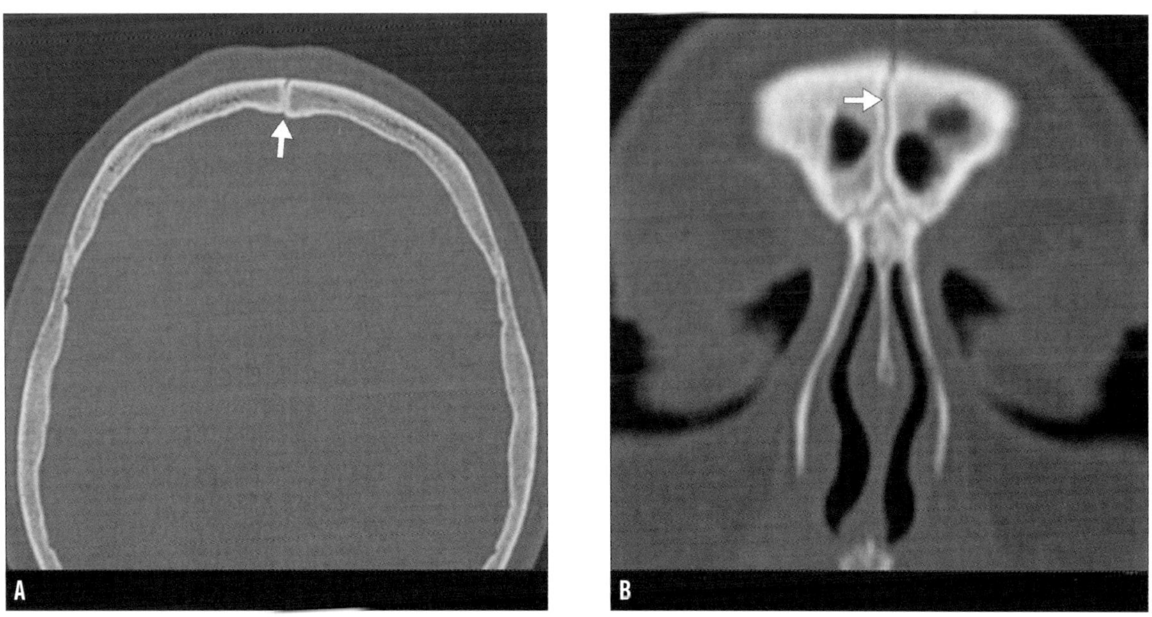

Axial (**A**) and coronal reformatted (**B**) CT images demonstrate a midline frontal calvarial linear lucency compatible with a normal persistent metopic suture (arrows, **A**, **B**).

Superior median fissure (suture) of the occiput

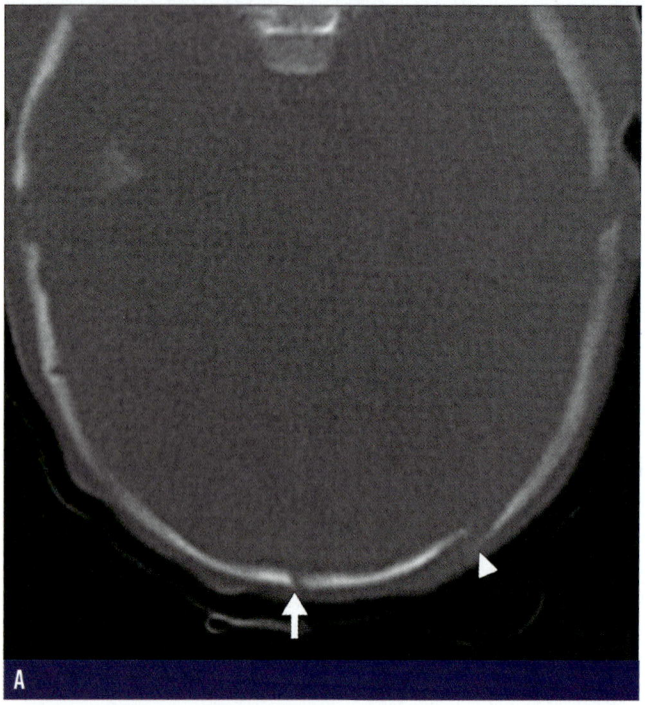

A

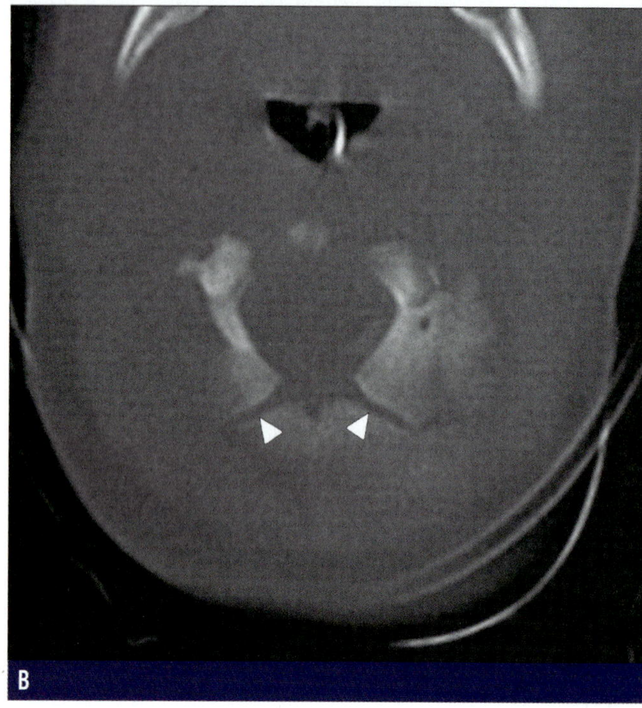

B

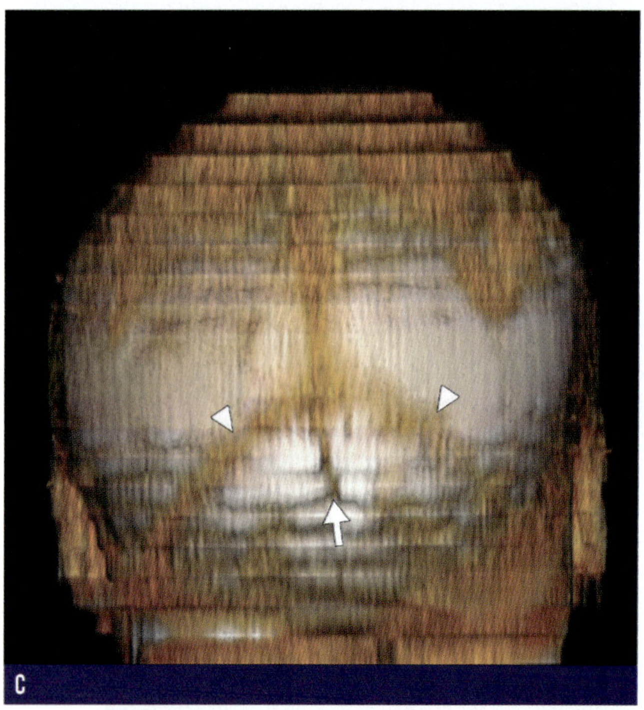

C

Axial CT images (**A**, **B**) demonstrate a normal superior median fissure of the occiput in a newborn (arrow, **A**), a finding that could be confused with a calvarial fracture. The normal lambdoid sutures are shown as a reference (arrowheads, **A**, **B**), with the left lambdoid suture associated with normal overriding because of molding during childbirth (arrowhead, **A**). A 3D reconstructed image from the same study (**C**) demonstrates the normal superior median fissure (arrow, **C**) and the normal lambdoid sutures (arrowheads, **C**).

REFERENCES

Choudhary AK, et al. Occipital sutures and its variations: the value of 3D-CT and how to differentiate it from fractures using 3D-CT? *Surg Radiol Anat.* 2010;32(9):807-816.

Mitchell LA, et al. Normal sagittal and coronal suture widths by using CT imaging. *AJNR Am J Neuroradiol.* 2011;32(10):1801-1805.

Sanchez T, et al. Skull fracture vs. accessory sutures: how can we tell the difference? *Emerg Radiol.* 2010;17(5):413-418.

Tubbs RS, et al. Does the mendosal suture exist in the adult? *Clin Anat.* 2007;20(2):124-125.

CASE 9 Craniosynostoses

Craniosynostosis is the abnormal, premature complete or partial closure of one or more cranial sutures, occurring in 1 in 2100 to 2500 live births. Craniosynostosis is usually not part of a syndrome, with only 15% of all cases related to syndromic or other developmental abnormalities. However, craniosynostosis is one of the features in over 180 syndromes. Furthermore, syndromic cases of craniosynostosis are more likely to involve more than one suture. Craniosynostosis is often clinically evident early in life because it can restrict normal brain development and results in an abnormally shaped head. The pathophysiology is not completely understood, although environmental and genetic factors likely play a role in its development.

Radiographic studies are typically used to confirm the clinical suspicion of a craniosynostosis as well as to describe any associated abnormalities, such as a Chiari malformation, hydrocephalus, or venous outflow obstruction. The imaging spectrum of craniosynostosis includes perisutural sclerosis, osseous bridging across the affected suture, and complete absence of the sutures. There is restricted growth perpendicular to the fused suture as well as compensatory overgrowth of other regions of the skull. Assessment of the cranial vault with 3D CT is superior compared to plain films. MRI is most often utilized to assess for underlying brain anomalies, if any, rather than to assess for a subtle craniosynostosis, although the skull shape on MRI usually allows for an accurate determination of the type of craniosynostosis.

- **Scaphocephaly (dolichocephaly).** Scaphocephaly (Greek, meaning boat-shaped head) and dolichocephaly (Greek, meaning elongated head) are used interchangeably and represent premature closure of the sagittal suture. Scaphocephaly is the most common isolated craniosynostosis, accounting for approximately 40% to 50% of all cases. It is four times more common in males than females, and it can be associated with neurological symptoms in up to one-third of cases. The restricted growth perpendicular to the sagittal suture results in an elongated calvarial shape characterized by frontal bossing, occipital bulging, and hypertelorism.
- **Brachycephaly.** Brachycephaly (Greek, meaning short head) occurs because of bicoronal and skull base synostosis. Bicoronal suture closure results in a short AP and a widened transverse dimension of the skull. Brachycephaly is the craniosynostosis which is most often associated with syndromes.
- **Trigonocephaly.** The metopic suture normally closes by 9 months of age, although normal metopic suture closure as early as 3 months of age has been described. Premature closure of the metopic suture can result in trigonocephaly (Greek, meaning triangle-shaped head). Up to one-third of trigonocephaly cases may be syndromic. Trigonocephaly is usually easily diagnosed clinically as it results in a characteristic triangular-shaped, underdeveloped forehead with a prominent metopic ridge and hypotelorism.
- **Plagiocephaly.** Plagiocephaly (Greek, meaning oblique-shaped head) is a descriptive term used to characterize the skull shape and may or may not be due to a craniosynostosis. Anterior plagiocephaly is most often the result of a unicoronal synostosis, yielding fusion and flattening of the ipsilateral frontal and parietal bones with normal contralateral skull growth. Posterior plagiocephaly is usually not the result of a craniosynostosis but rather due to prolonged positioning of the infants head in a supine position, often termed positional or deformation occipital plagiocephaly. This type of plagiocephaly has increased over the last two decades because of the "back to sleep" campaign which has been promoted to reduce the risk of sudden infant death syndrome. Posterior plagiocephaly can also be caused by unilateral lambdoidal synostosis, which adopts more of a trapezoid skull shape, often best assessed with 3D CT imaging.

Scaphocephaly (dolichocephaly)

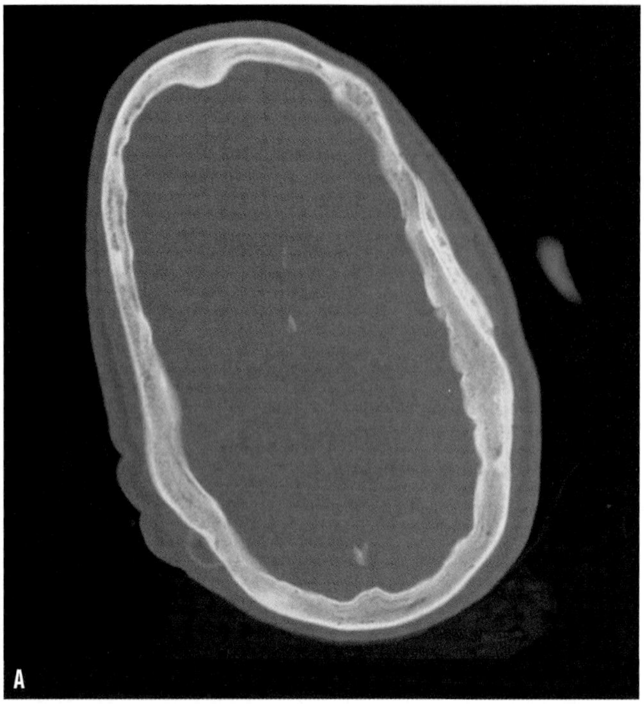

An axial CT image (**A**) demonstrates an anterior-to-posterior elongated calvarial shape, compatible with scaphocephaly.

Scaphocephaly (dolichocephaly)

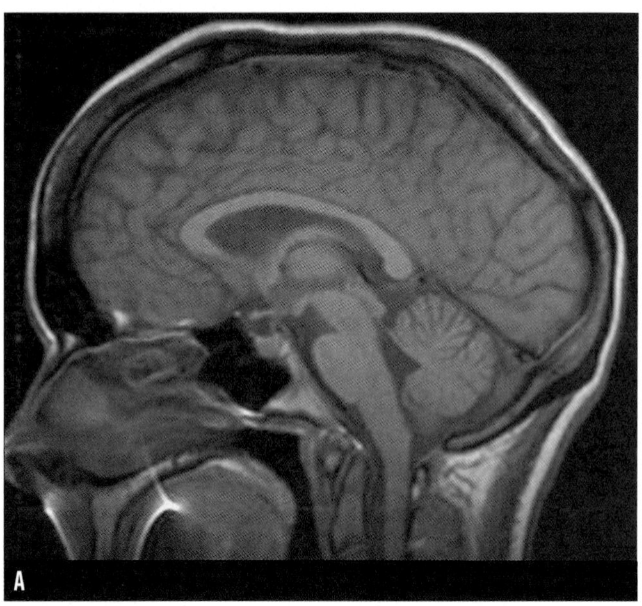

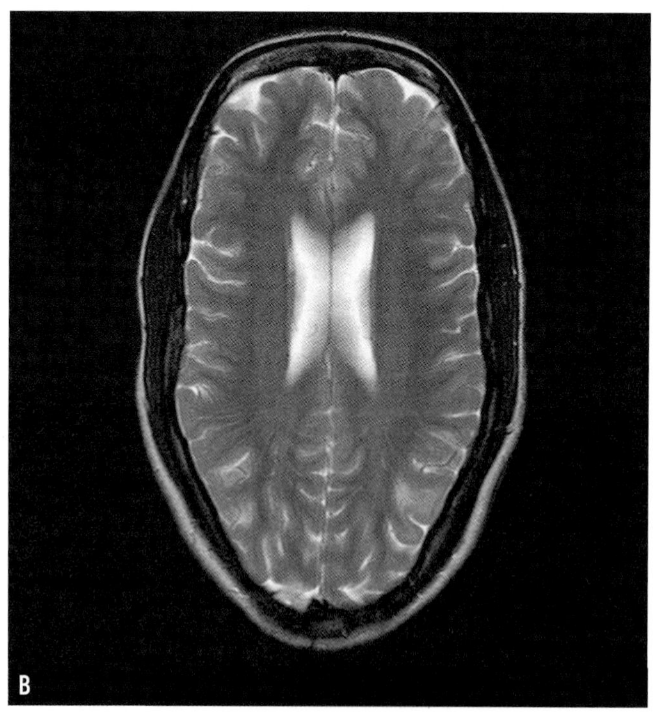

Different patient. Sagittal T1 (**A**) and axial T2 (**B**) MR images demonstrate an anterior-to-posterior elongated calvarial shape, compatible with scaphocephaly.

Brachycephaly

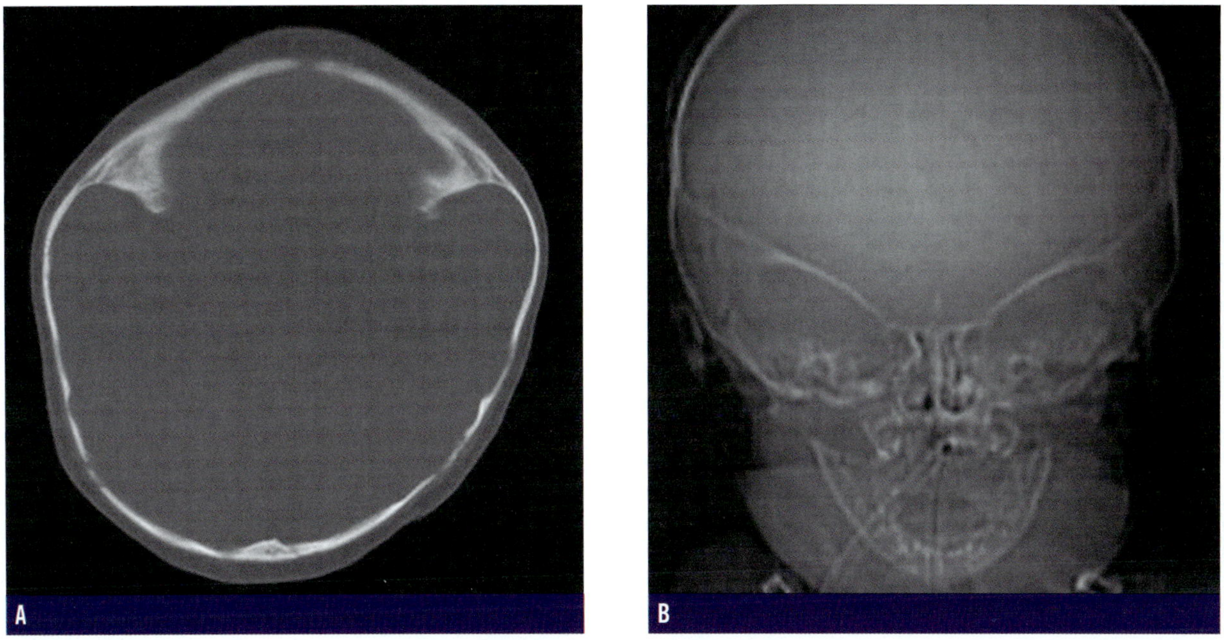

An axial CT image of a newborn with Apert syndrome (**A**) demonstrates a widened transverse dimension relative to the anterior-posterior dimension of the calvarium, consistent with brachycephaly. A frontal scout image from the same study (**B**) also demonstrates the enlarged transverse dimension of the calvarium.

Trigonocephaly

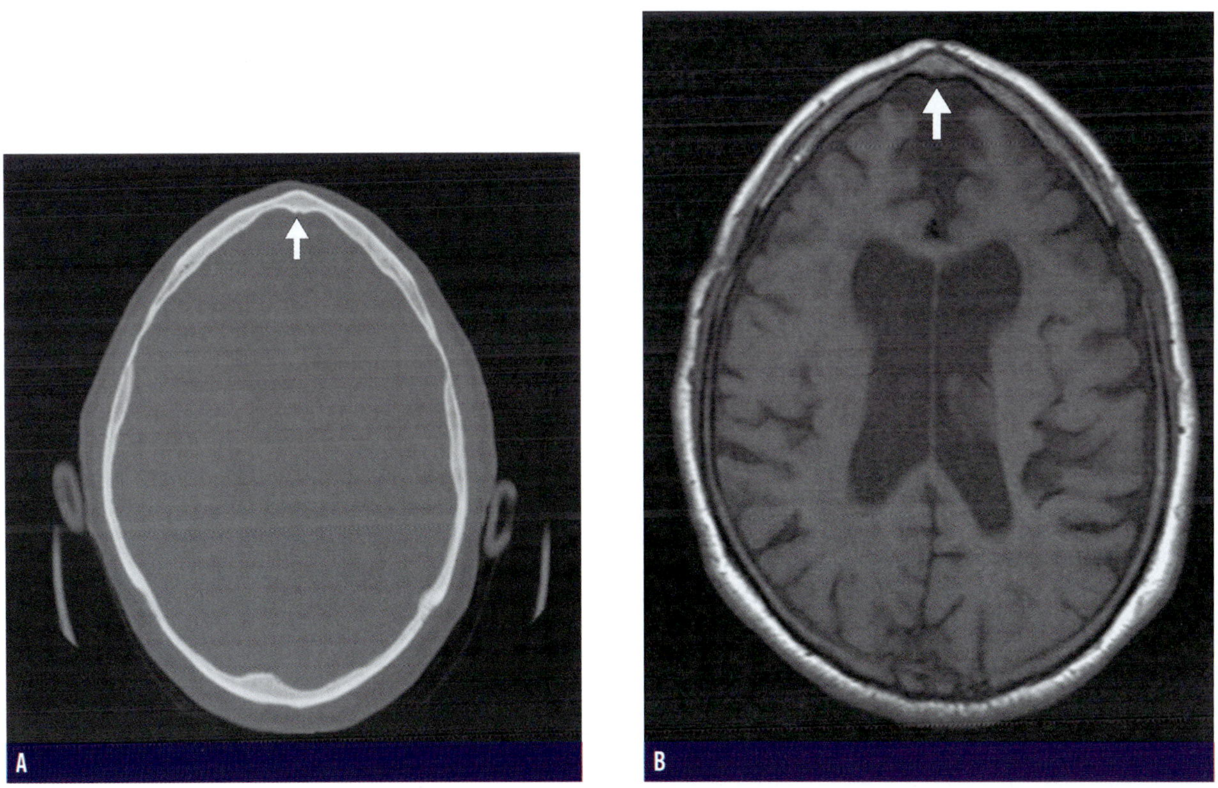

An axial CT image (**A**) and an axial T1-weighted MR image (**B**) of an adult patient demonstrate a ventrally angulated forehead at the midline, compatible with trigonocephaly (arrows, **A**, **B**).

Unilateral synostosis (anterior plagiocephaly)

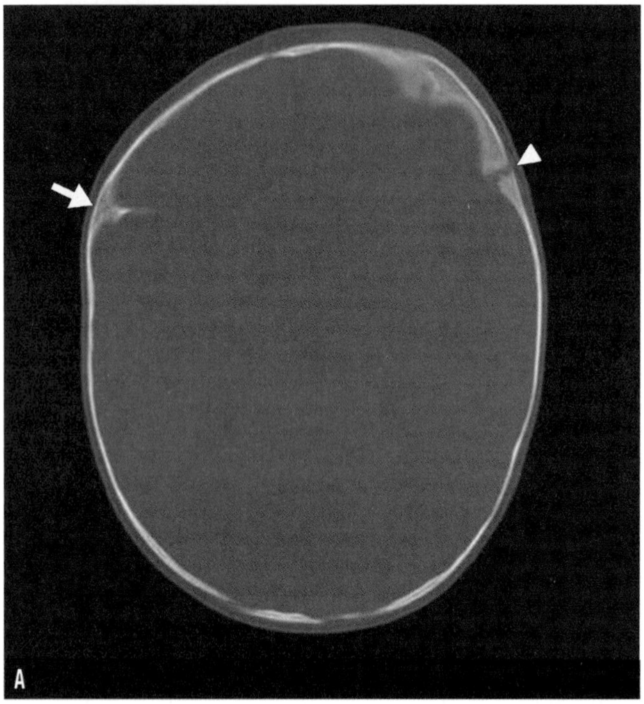

An axial CT image of a newborn (**A**) demonstrates unilateral synostosis of the right aspect of the coronal suture (arrow) and a normal, unfused left aspect of the coronal suture (arrowhead).

Posterior plagiocephaly

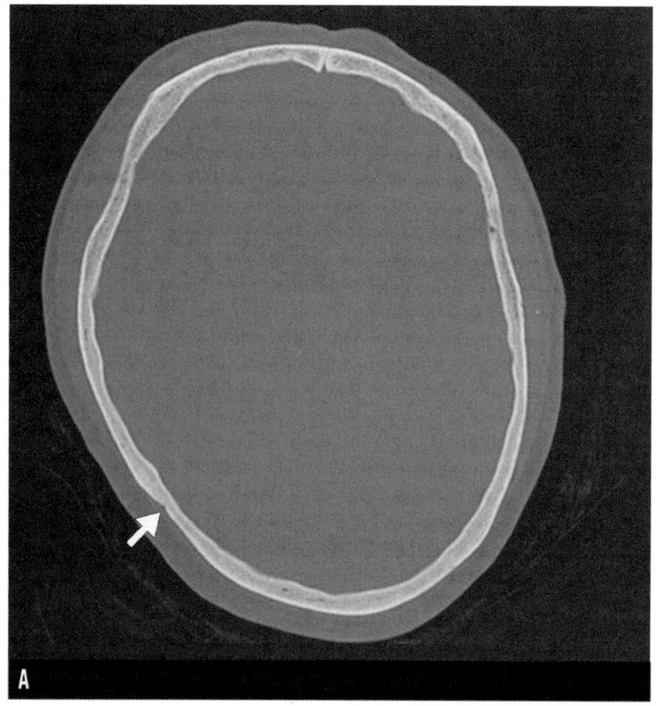

An axial CT image (**A**) demonstrates asymmetric flattening of the calvarium involving the right parietal and temporal bones, consistent with posterior plagiocephaly (arrow).

Posterior plagiocephaly

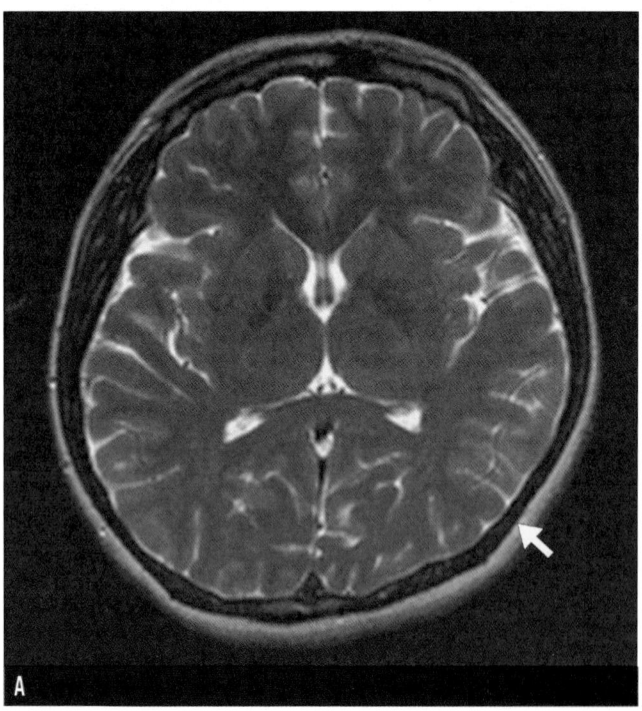

Different patient. An axial T2-weighted MR image (**A**) demonstrates flattening along the left posterior aspect of the calvarium, consistent with posterior plagiocephaly (arrow). The underlying brain is unremarkable.

REFERENCES

Kirmi O, et al. Craniosynostosis: A radiological and surgical perspective. *Semin Ultrasound CT MRI.* 2009;30:492-512.

Levi B, et al. Cranial suture biology: from pathways to patient care. *J Craniofac Surg.* 2012;23:13-19.

Nagaraja S, et al. Craniosynostosis. *Clin Radiol.* 2013;68:284-292.

Vu HL, Panchal J, Parker EE, Levine NS, Francel P. The timing of physiologic closure of the metopic suture: a review of 159 patients using reconstructed 3D CT scans of the craniofacial region. *J Craniofac Surg.* 2001;12(6):527-532.

CASE 10 Wormian bones

Wormian bones, also termed supernumerary ossicles or intrasutural bones, were first described by Dr. Olaus Worm. These represent small, irregular-shaped bones of varying sizes that occur between sutures. They have sclerotic borders and interdigitating margins, identical to the sutures of the calvarium. The etiology of Wormian bones has not been fully elucidated.

There is a large range of the reported prevalence of Wormian bones in the general population, from as low as 8% to more than 50%. The majority of Wormian bones are completely idiopathic and clinically insignificant. Some authors have described a greater prevalence of Wormian bones in cases of craniosynostosis, positional plagiocephaly, and in patients with hydrocephalus. Moreover, many diseases associated with Wormian bones have been described in the literature, including osteogenesis imperfecta, Menke syndrome, and cleidocranial dysostosis, to name a few. More than 10 Wormian bones may suggest the presence of osteogenesis imperfecta, and further evaluation for this disease should be considered in such cases.

Wormian bones are often named for the adjacent suture or fontanelle that it occupies, such as Wormian bones (or ossicles) at the bregma (representing the junction of the coronal and sagittal sutures), lambdoid Wormian bones, or sagittal Wormian bones.

Wormian bone

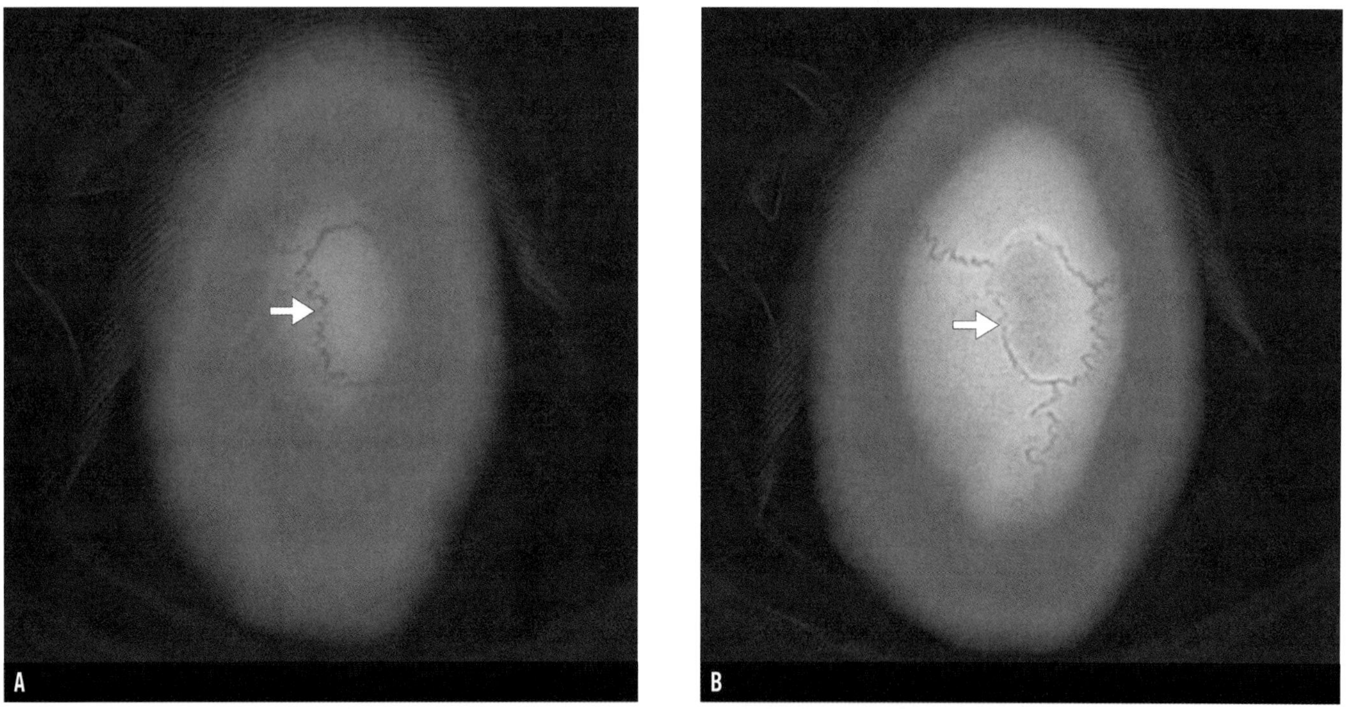

Axial CT images of a 46-year-old patient (**A**, **B**) demonstrate a single Wormian bone (arrows, **A**, **B**) located at the bregma, which represents the junction between the sagittal suture and the coronal suture.

Wormian bones

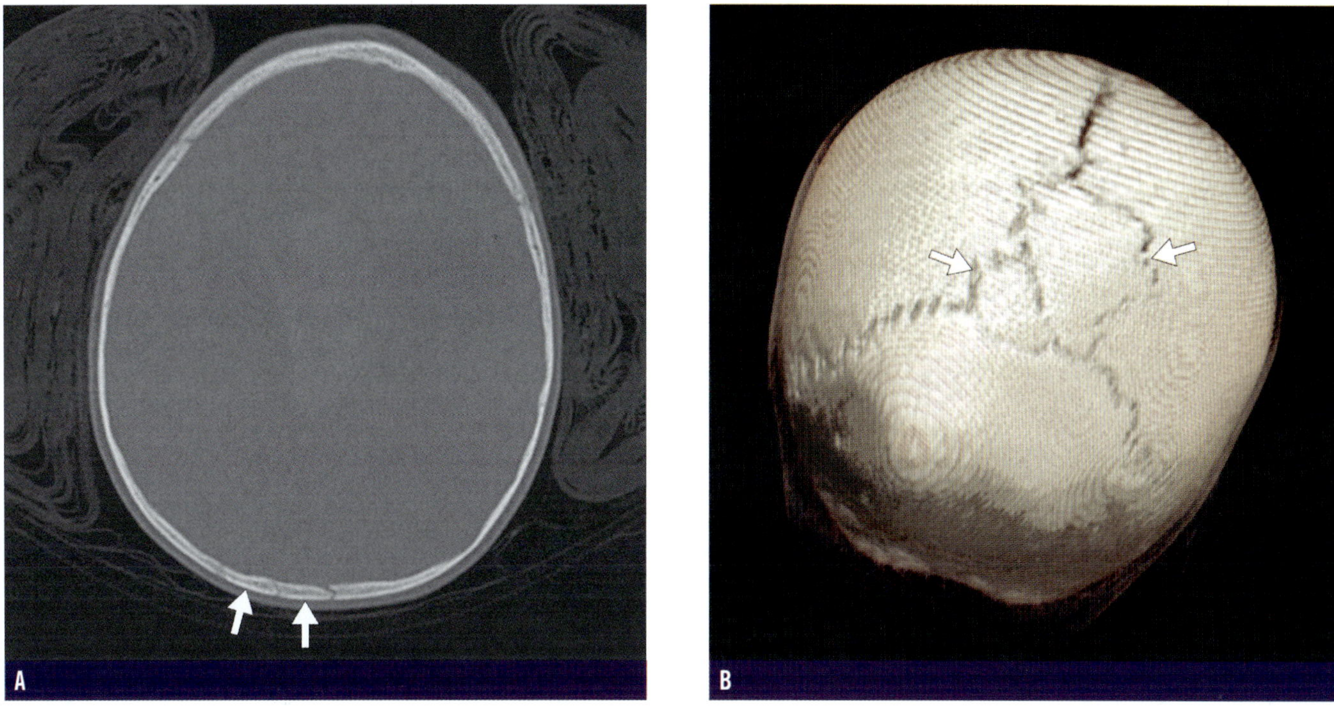

An axial CT image (**A**) and a 3D reconstructed CT image from the same study (**B**) of a 19-month-old patient demonstrate two small bones at the junction between the sagittal and lambdoid sutures, compatible with two Wormian bones (arrows, **A**, **B**).

Wormian bones

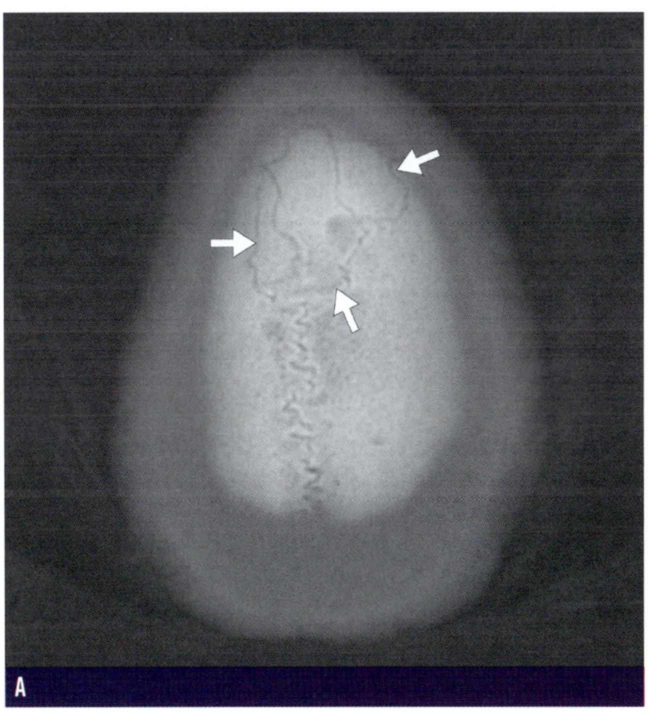

An axial CT image of a 39-year-old patient (**A**) demonstrates three Wormian bones along the anterior aspect of the sagittal suture (arrows).

REFERENCES

Barberini F, et al. An unusually-wide human bregmatic Wormian bone: anatomy, tomographic description, and possible significance. *Surg Radiol Anat.* 2008;30(8):683-687.

Marti B, et al. Wormian bones in a general paediatric population. *Diagn Interv Imaging.* 2013;94:428-432.

O'Loughlin VD. Effects of different kinds of cranial deformation on the incidence of wormian bones. *Am J Phys Anthropol.* 2004;123(2):146-155.

Samson TD, Beals SP, Rekate HL. Massive Wormian bone at the cranial apex: identification, correction, and outcome. *J Craniofac Surg.* 2008;19(1):96-100.

CASE 11 Middle meningeal artery calvarial groove or canal

The internal maxillary artery, a branch of the external carotid artery, gives rise to several of its own branches. One of its branches, the middle meningeal artery, enters the skull via the foramen spinosum and then divides into anterior and posterior branches. The anterior branch traverses anterolaterally through the middle cranial fossa and ascends along the anterior aspect of the parietal bone, whereas the posterior branch traverses posteriorly along the squamosal portion of the temporal bone. Both branches subdivide further distally. Although there is a wide variation of the middle meningeal artery branching pattern among individuals, the pattern of branching tends to be symmetric in each individual. A study by Ma et al of the middle meningeal arterial anatomy as it relates to the pterion of the calvarium demonstrated that the anterior branch of this artery may run along the inner skull surface in a groove or within the diploic space in a canal, with canals more commonly identified in women.

COMPANION CASE

- **Nondisplaced squamosal temporal bone fracture.** The calvarial groove or canal of the middle meningeal artery could be mistaken for a calvarial fracture, particularly on skull radiographs. However, several imaging findings aid in differentiating a normal middle meningeal artery groove or canal from a calvarial fracture on CT. A normal middle meningeal artery groove or canal may be favored by identifying its typical location along the anterior to mid aspect of the cranial vault, the presence of corticated/sclerotic margins, an intact outer table, and the lack of overlying scalp edema or underlying acute brain injury.

Middle meningeal artery calvarial groove

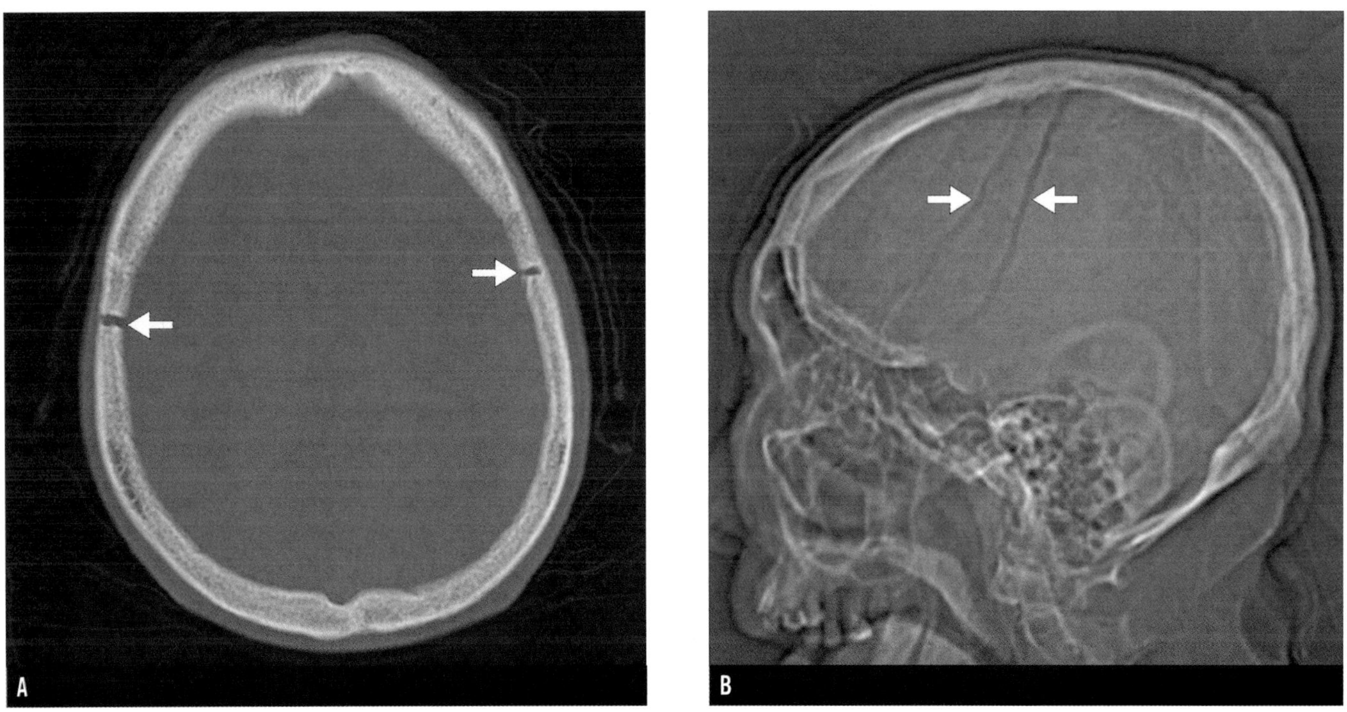

An axial CT image (**A**) demonstrates large, symmetric lucencies involving the inner table and diploic space of the parietal bones, with sparing the outer table, compatible with large middle meningeal artery calvarial grooves (arrows, **A**). These are also identified on a lateral scout image from the same CT study (**B**) (arrows).

Companion case: Nondisplaced squamosal temporal bone fracture

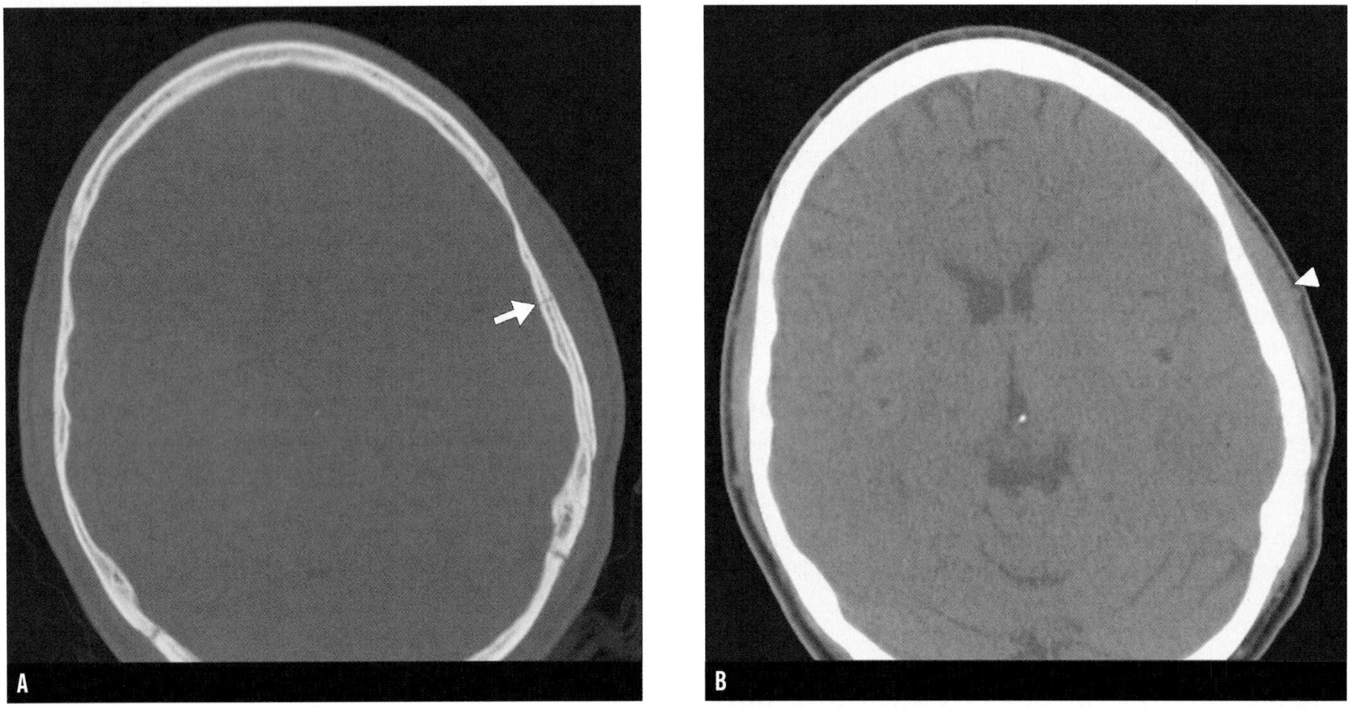

An axial CT image viewed with a bone window (**A**) demonstrates a subtle asymmetric lucency along the squamosal portion of the left temporal bone (arrow, **A**). This lucency traverses the inner and outer tables of the affected calvarium, unlike a middle meningeal artery groove or canal which spares the outer table. The same axial image viewed with an intermediate window (**B**) demonstrates mild overlying muscular edema in this patient who sustained an injury to this area (arrowhead, **B**). The finding in the calvarium is compatible with a nondisplaced fracture.

REFERENCES

Bruner E, Averini M, Manzi G. Endocranial traits. Prevalence and distribution in a recent human population. *Eur J Anat.* 2003;7(1):23-33.

Ellis JA, et al. Pre-operative intracranial meningioma embolization. *Expert Rev Neurother.* 2011;11(4):545-556.

Hu KTP, Lam WMW, Chau MT. Why does the fracture not heal? Vascular channel mimicking skull fracture. *HK J Paediatr.* 2011;16:184-187.

Ma S, et al. Reappraising the surface anatomy of the pterion and its relationship to the middle meningeal artery. *Clin Anat.* 2012;25(3):330-339.

Muro K, et al. True aneurysm on the posterior meningeal artery associated with a dural arteriovenous fistula: case report. *Neurosurgery.* 2010;67(3):E876-E877.

CASE 12 Temporalis muscle hypertrophy

The muscles of mastication include the masseter, the medial and lateral pterygoids, and the temporalis muscles. Masticatory muscle hypertrophy, first described in 1880, may be congenital or acquired, with the acquired types sometimes attributed to nervous behavior leading to bruxism or secondary to temporomandibular joint dysfunction.

Masticatory muscle hypertrophy may involve any of the muscles of mastication, although it most commonly affects the masseter muscle, and it may be unilateral or bilateral. Isolated unilateral or bilateral temporalis muscle hypertrophy usually presents as asymptomatic temple swelling. However, unilateral headaches related to ipsilateral temporalis muscle hypertrophy have been described. Moreover, bilateral temporalis muscle hypertrophy can result in a harsh facial appearance, sometimes referred to as Minotaur syndrome.

There are no set size imaging criteria for masticatory muscle hypertrophy, although in unilateral cases comparison with the contralateral side is usually sufficient for diagnosis. Radiographs are typically unremarkable, but they may demonstrate soft tissue fullness, hyperostotic bone formation at the tendinous insertion sites, temporomandibular joint degeneration, or dental malocclusion. Asymmetric FDG-18 uptake on positron emission tomography (PET) scans may be identified in cases of unilateral masticatory muscle hypertrophy. While CT or MRI can confirm a clinical suspicion of masticatory muscle hypertrophy, the main role of these imaging modalities is to exclude an underlying pathologic process that could account for unilateral masticatory muscle enlargement, such as a vascular malformation, myositis, lipomatous lesion, or lymphoma. CT is helpful in diagnosing a lipoma or revealing phleboliths associated with a venous malformation as a cause of masticatory muscle enlargement. However, subtle isodense tumor or other abnormalities accounting for muscle enlargement could be occult on CT, particularly on unenhanced imaging. MRI with contrast is usually more sensitive to evaluate for an underlying solid soft tissue mass that may cause unilateral masticatory muscle enlargement.

Treatment of masticatory muscle hypertrophy is typically performed for cosmetic purposes and depends on the degree of severity. Conservative treatment in mild cases includes nocturnal bite plates or cognitive behavior modification to decrease bruxism. More severe cases are treated with botulism toxin injection, radiofrequency ablation, or surgical resection of muscle and bone.

COMPANION CASES

- **Temporalis muscle venous malformation.** Vascular malformations are generally subdivided into low-flow lesions (ie, venous malformations, lymphatic malformations, or mixed malformations) and high-flow lesions, such as an arteriovenous malformation (AVM). Properly categorizing these lesions is important in order to determine appropriate treatment. Most vascular malformations are present at birth, although some lesions, such as an AVM, may result from trauma.

  Venous malformations (VM) represent an abnormal collection of venous channels, fat, and degenerated muscle matrix. The venous components of a VM can thrombose and form phleboliths, the latter considered pathognomonic of this entity. Lymphatic malformations (LM) represent an abnormal collection of lymphatic vessels. LMs are subcategorized into macrocystic and microcystic forms. The macrocystic form, commonly referred to as a cystic hygroma, is composed of large cystic spaces containing proteinaceous fluid and lymphocytes that are interspersed around septa. The microcystic form contains 2 mm or smaller sized cysts within a solid matrix. Mixed lesions refer to low flow vascular lesions which contain both venous and lymphatic components (so-called venolymphatic malformations).

  The hallmark of a vascular malformation is its transspatial nature (ie, often involving more than one compartment in the neck) and softness to palpation. A vascular malformation may or may not be associated with mass effect. On MRI, both a VM and a macrocystic LM will be hyperintense on T2. Following contrast, a VM will contain patchy enhancement throughout the lesion, whereas a macrocystic LM will only enhance along its periphery and/or along its septa. When a hemorrhagic fluid level within a loculated fluid collection is associated with abrupt clinical enlargement, then the diagnosis of a macrocystic LM should be suspected. MRI is usually superior to CT at evaluating vascular malformations of the head and neck.
- **Temporalis muscle/fascia insertion hyperostosis.** There are two arched, slightly elevated, adjacent osseous ridges running in parallel along outer table of the mid parietal bones, termed the superior and inferior temporal lines. The superior temporal line represents the origin of the temporalis fascia, whereas the inferior temporal line represents the origin of the temporalis muscle. Rarely, focal hyperostosis of the temporal lines (ie, enthesophyte formation) may occur and be identified on CT imaging.

Unilateral temporalis muscle hypertrophy

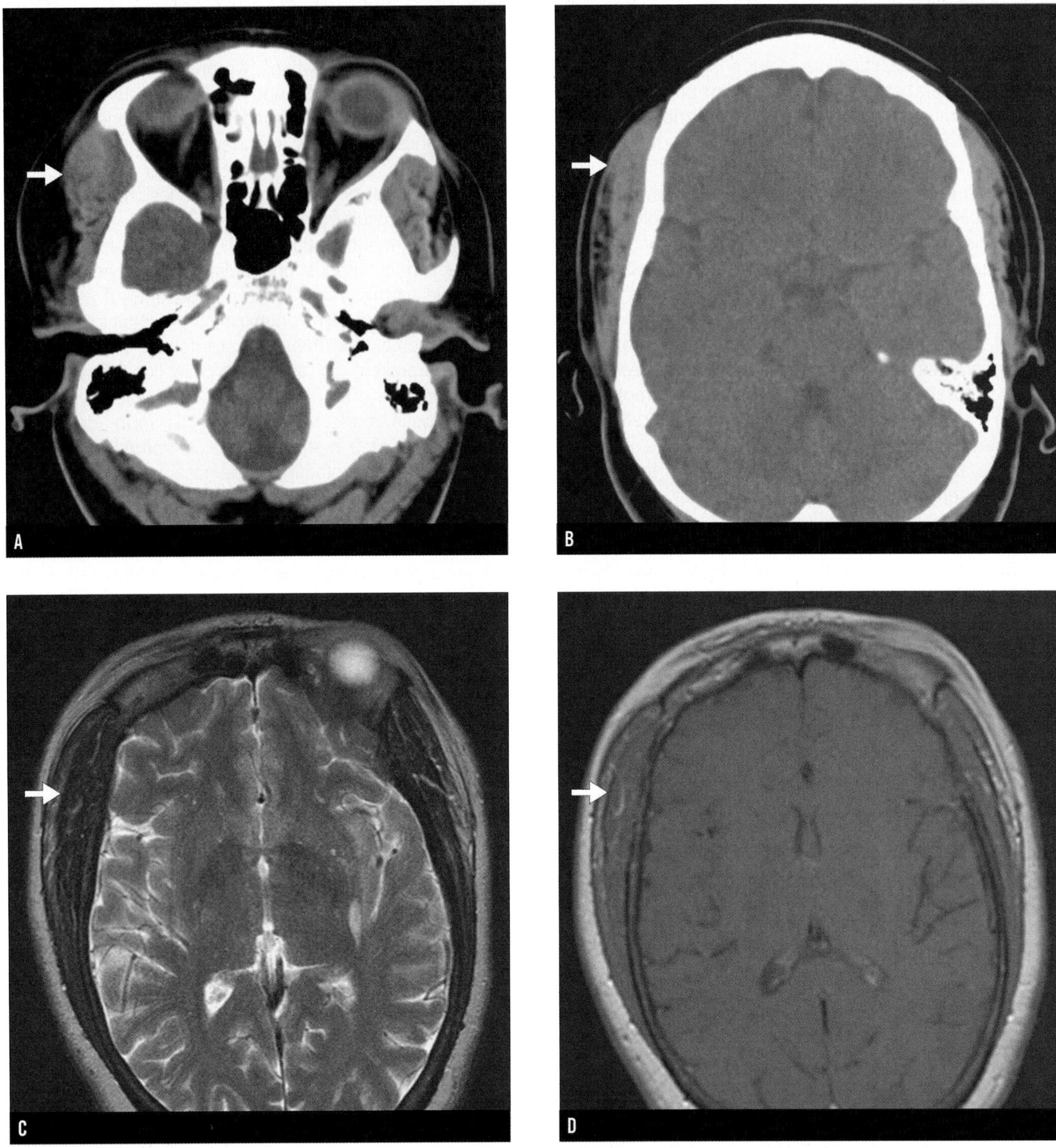

Axial CT images (**A**, **B**) demonstrate asymmetric enlargement of the right temporalis muscle (arrows, **A**, **B**). Axial T2 (**C**) and contrast-enhanced axial T1 (**D**) MR images of the same patient also demonstrate asymmetric enlargement of the right temporalis muscle (arrows, **C**, **D**) without evidence of a focal tumor to account for the enlargement. The finding is consistent with unilateral right temporalis muscle hypertrophy.

Bilateral temporalis muscle hypertrophy

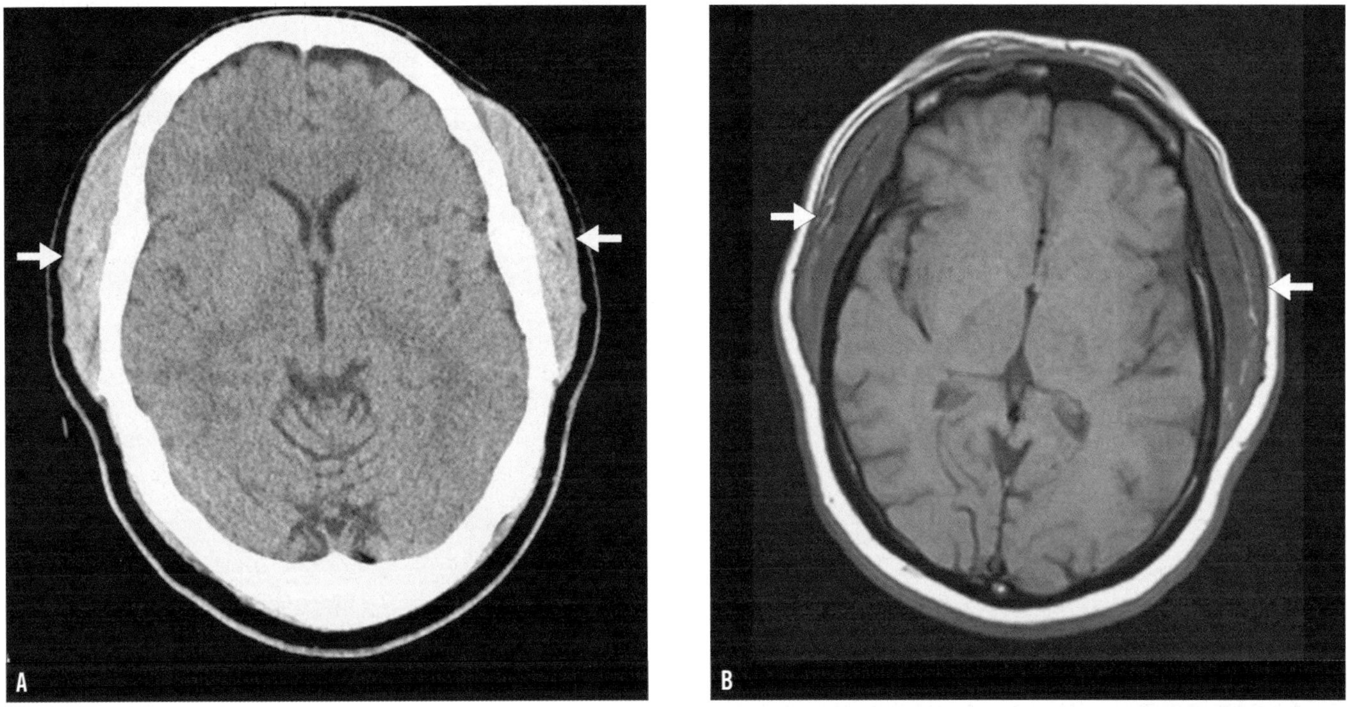

An unenhanced axial CT image (**A**) and an axial T1-weighted MR image of the same patient (**B**) demonstrate pronounced symmetric hypertrophy of the suprazygomatic portions of the temporalis muscles (arrows, **A**, **B**).

Companion case: Temporalis muscle venous malformation

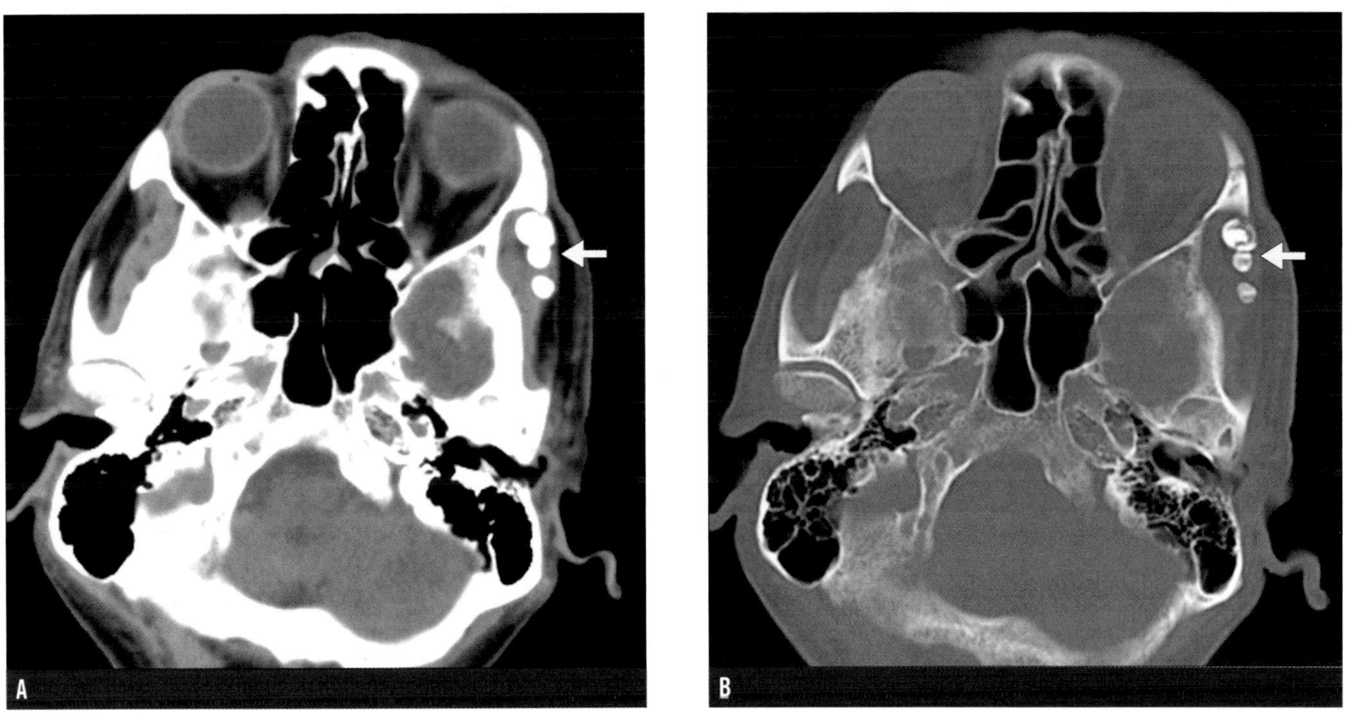

Unenhanced axial CT images viewed with a brain window (**A**) and bone window (**B**) demonstrate asymmetric enlargement of the suprazygomatic portion of the left temporalis muscle which contains several circumscribed mineralized structures, compatible with phleboliths (arrows, **A**, **B**). Axial T1 (**C**), axial T2 with fat suppression (**D**), and contrast-enhanced axial T1 with fat suppression (**E**) MR images of the same patient demonstrate expected signal loss of the phleboliths on all three pulse sequences (arrows, **C-E**), which are surrounded by T2 hyperintensity on image **D** and enhancement on image **E**. These findings are consistent with a venous malformation resulting in the left temporalis muscle enlargement.

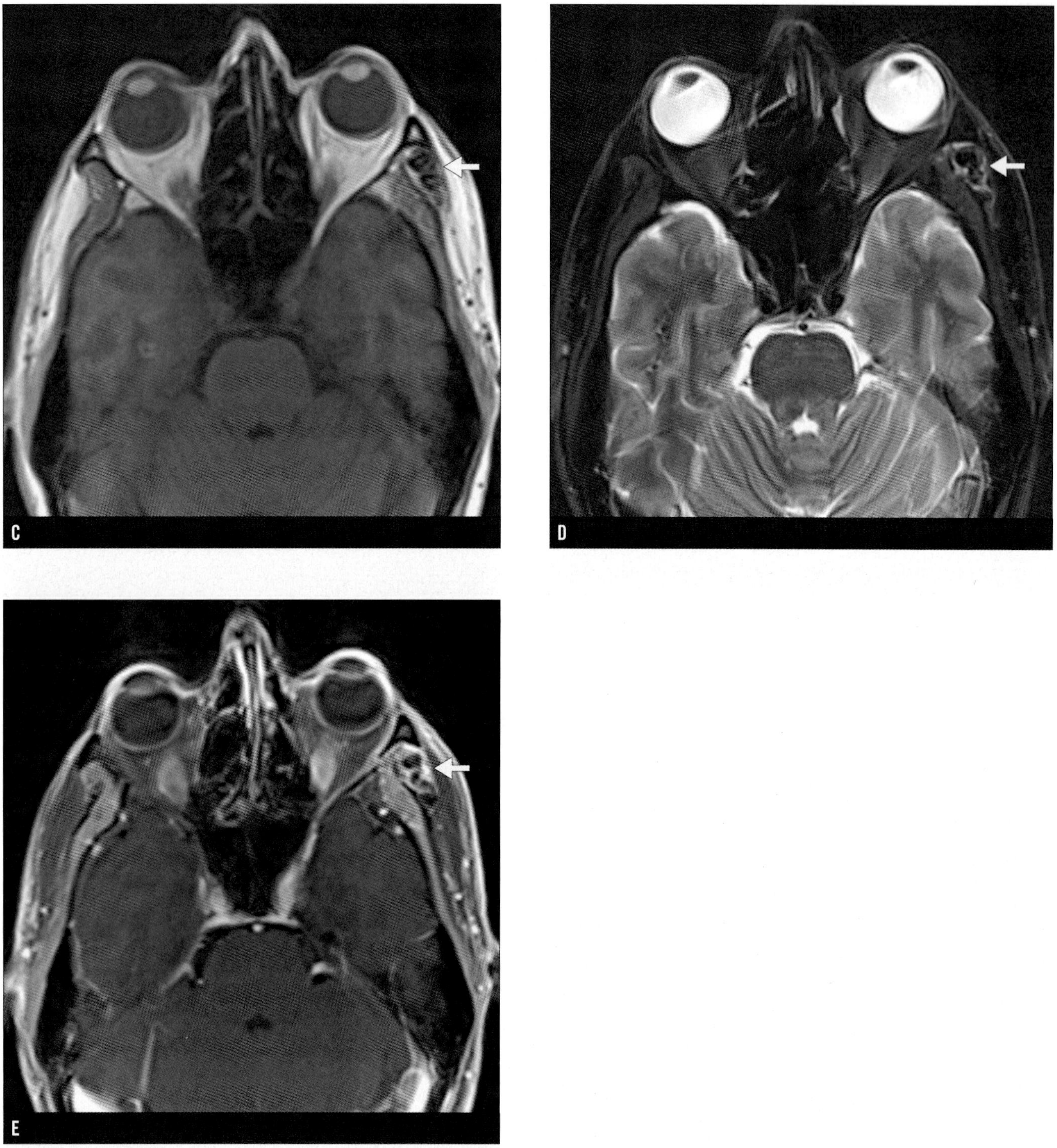
C
D
E

Companion case: Temporalis muscle/fascia insertion hyperostosis

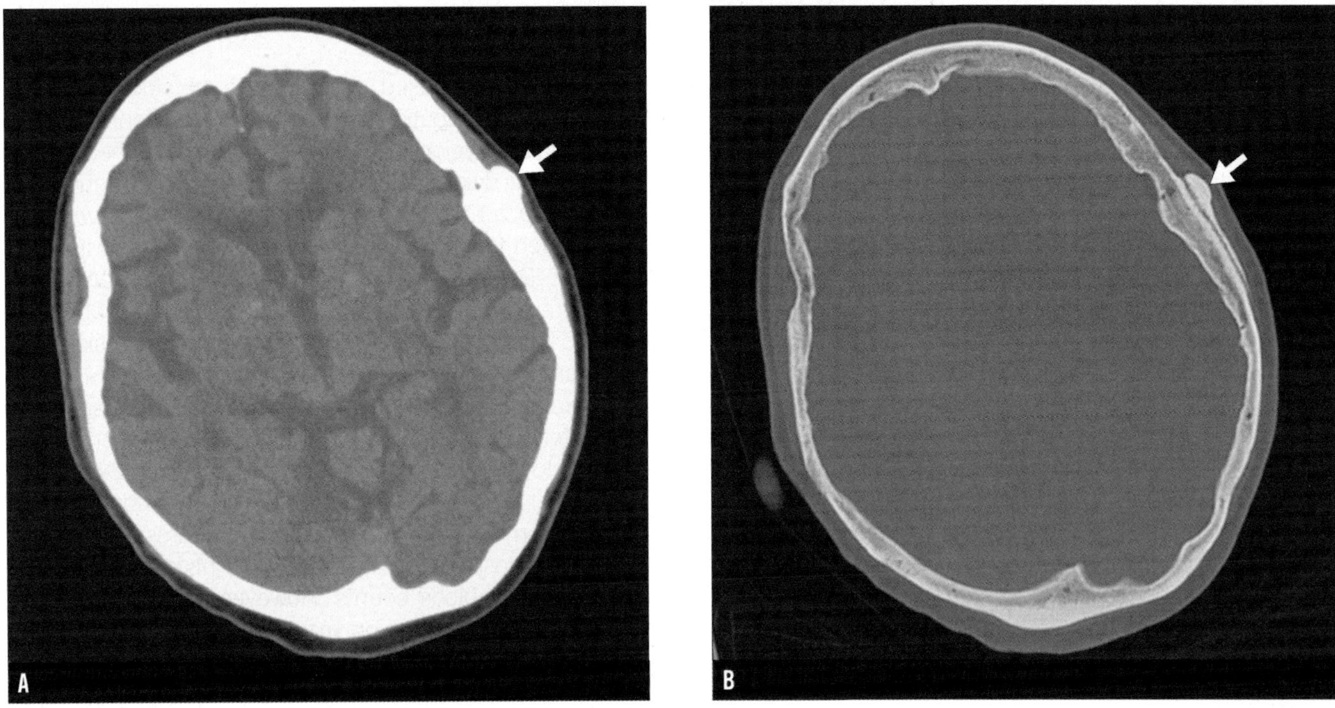

Axial CT images viewed with an intermediate window (**A**) and a bone window (**B**) demonstrate pronounced focal hyperostosis along the one or both left temporal lines (arrows, **A**, **B**). The temporal lines represent the origins of the temporalis muscle and fascia.

REFERENCES

Ihn YK, Park YH, Chung SK. FDG uptake in benign asymmetric hypertrophy of the masticator muscles. *Clin Nucl Med* 2006;31(4):221-222.

Lo JL, Chen YR. The volume of muscles of mastication in patients receiving mandibular contouring surgery: a comparative study. *J Plastic Reconstr Aesthet Surg.* 2007;60(2):125-129.

Morselli PG. Temporalis muscle hypertrophy: a new plastic surgery procedure. *Plast Reconstr Surg.* 2000;106(5):1156-1161.

Ozturk E, et al. Unilateral temporalis muscle hypertrophy with contralateral masseteric hypertrophy. *Dentomaxillofac Radiol.* 2007;36(5):296-297.

Prantl L, et al. Recurrence of isolated unilateral temporalis muscle hypertrophy: case report. *Aesthetic Plast Surg.* 2005;29(6): 574-575.

Vordenbaumen S, Grois SJ, Dihne M. Isolated unilateral temporal muscle hypertrophy: a rare cause of hemicranial headache. *Headache.* 2009;49(5):779-782.

CASE 13 Folliculitis keloidalis nuchae

Folliculitis keloidalis nuchae (FKN), also termed acne keloidalis nuchae, represents a scarring alopecia and keloid formation that occurs along the occipital soft tissues in patients of African descent. FKN is the result of a hair folliculitis, typically beginning as fibrotic papules or nodules that progress to keloid formation. The etiology is unclear, although close razor shaving along the nape of the neck has been implicated in some cases.

Given the multifocal and infiltrative nature of the folliculitis, keloid formation with FKN can be multifocal, residing deep or exophytically along the occipital soft tissues. Wortsman et al evaluated FKN with ultrasound and found full thickness cutaneous inflammation with dilated, anechoic or hypoechoic, fluid-filled fistulous tracts between enlarged hair follicles. The CT appearance of FKN is typically of an infiltrative, heterogeneous subcutaneous lesion in the suboccipital subcutaneous fat that is isoattenuating to muscle. On MRI, the abnormality is iso- to hypointense to muscle on T1- and T2-weighted imaging and may enhance.

COMPANION CASES

- **Cutaneous acute myeloid leukemia.** Cutaneous acute myeloid leukemia (also called chloroma, myeloid sarcoma, or granulocytic sarcoma) is a localized extramedullary neoplasm composed of immature myeloid precursor cells found in patients with acute or chronic myeloid leukemia, myeloproliferative disorder, or other myelodysplastic disorders. The term chloroma is derived by its characteristic gross pathologic green tint which is attributed to the presence of myeloperoxidase within the tumor. These tumors can be found in almost any organ but are particularly common in the soft tissues and skin. On CT, cutaneous acute myeloid leukemia lesions are enhancing soft tissue abnormalities, either en plaque or exophytic in morphology. On MRI, these lesions are isointense to muscle on T1-weighted images and isointense to slightly hyperintense to muscle on T2-weighted images. Generally, these lesions will enhance homogenously on CT or MRI unless central necrosis is present. The diagnosis is usually aided by a history of leukemia or abnormal blood counts. However, a cutaneous acute myeloid leukemia lesion may precede the diagnosis of leukemia or myelodysplastic syndrome.
- **Chronic scalp trauma.** Repetitive scalp injury, such as may occur with alcoholic patients, can result in chronic scalp thickening, presumably because of an old, organized hematoma with subsequent scar formation. When present, this finding will simulate an acute localized injury. Misinterpreting this finding as acute trauma can be avoided by recognizing its on prior imaging, if available.

Folliculitis keloidalis nuchae

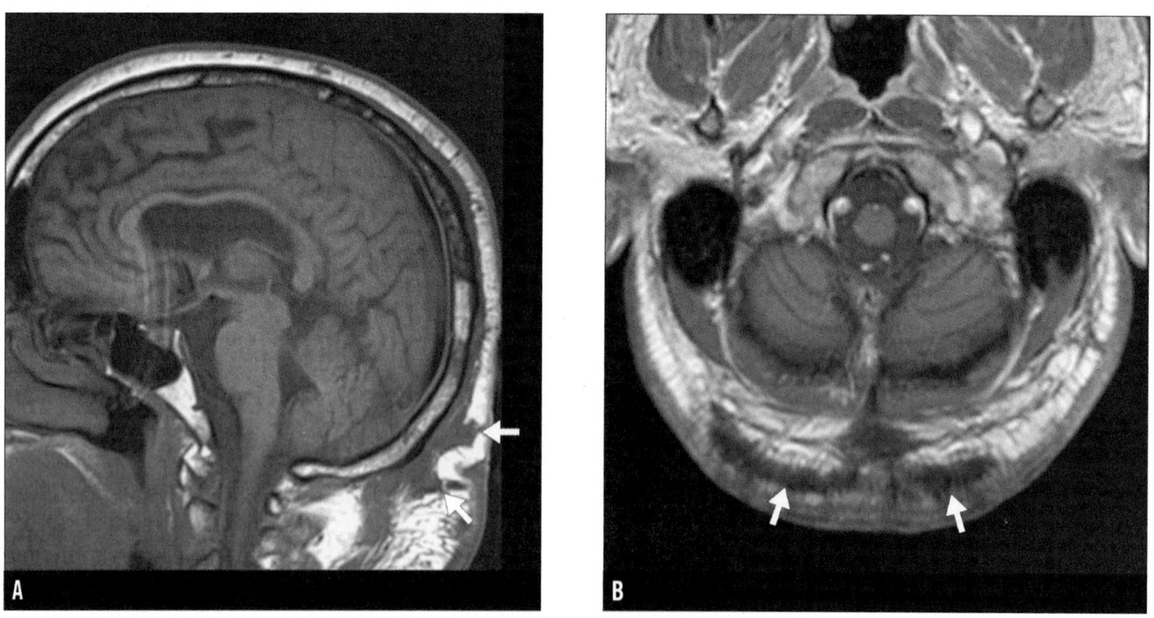

Sagittal T1 (**A**), contrast-enhanced axial T1 (**B**), and axial T2 (**C**) MR images demonstrate pronounced linear and nodular areas of abnormal signal located in the suboccipital soft tissues. Relative to muscle, these findings are which are T1 iso- to hypointense, essentially T2 isointense, and do not enhance (arrows, **A-C**). An unenhanced axial CT image of the same patient (**D**) demonstrates the CT correlate (arrows, **D**). A couple punctate calcifications in the soft tissue abnormality on image D are likely related to the finding. These findings represent keloid formation secondary to prior folliculitis. This patient was an asymptomatic African American patient.

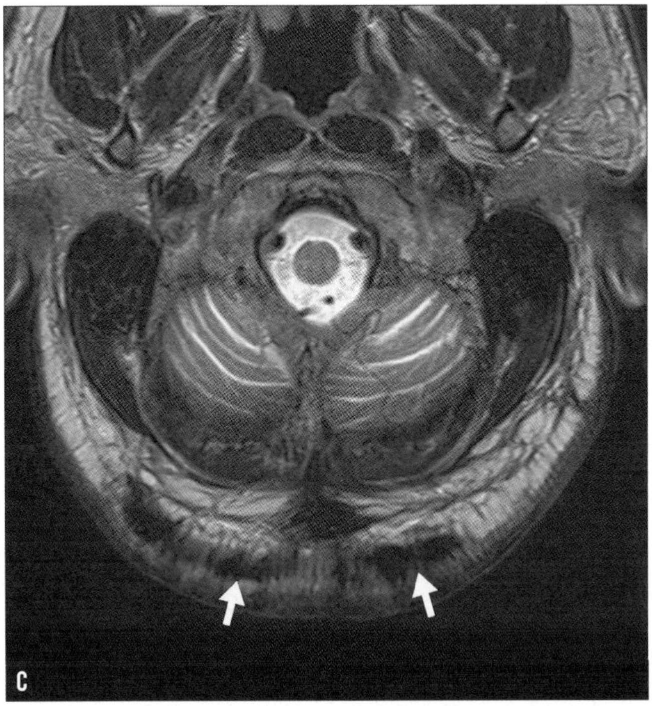

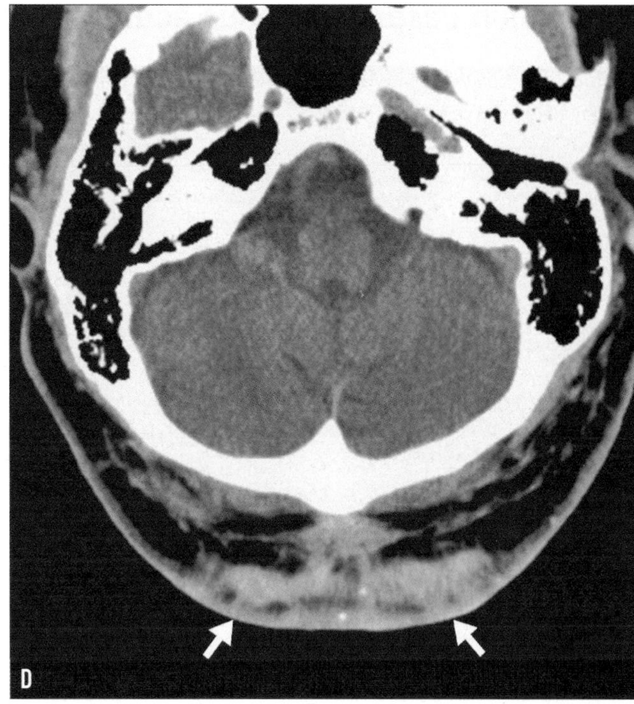

Folliculitis keloidalis nuchae

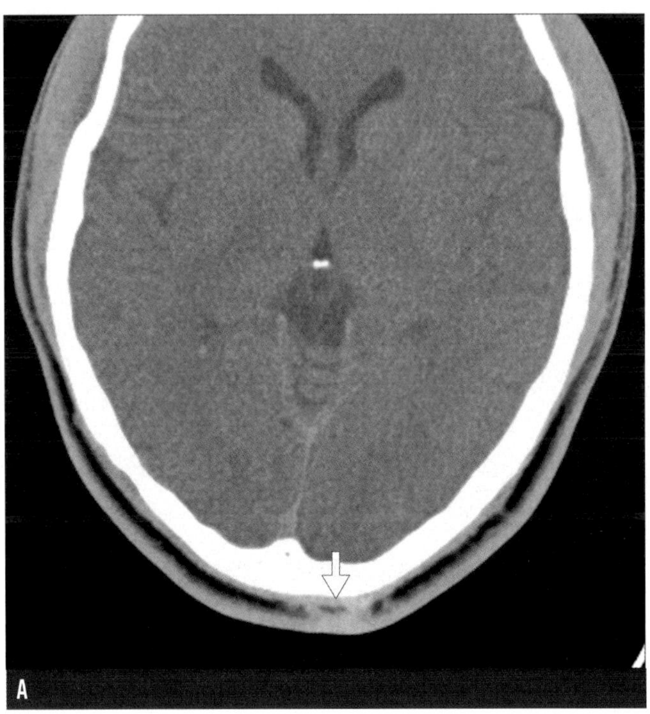

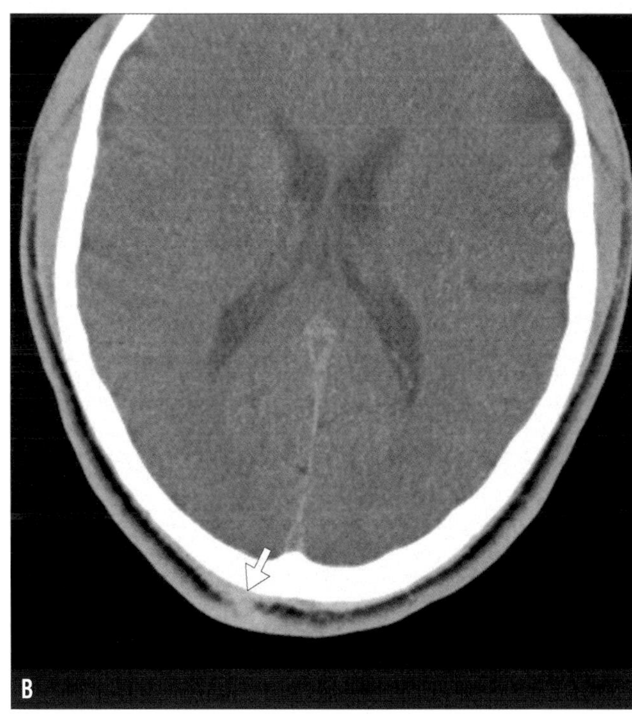

Different patient. Unenhanced axial CT images of a patient who is of African American descent (**A**, **B**) demonstrate linear and nodular areas of soft tissue density within the subcutaneous soft tissues of the occipital scalp (arrows, **A**, **B**), without a history of trauma to this area. The findings are most compatible with small areas folliculitis keloidalis nuchae.

Companion case: Cutaneous acute myeloid leukemia

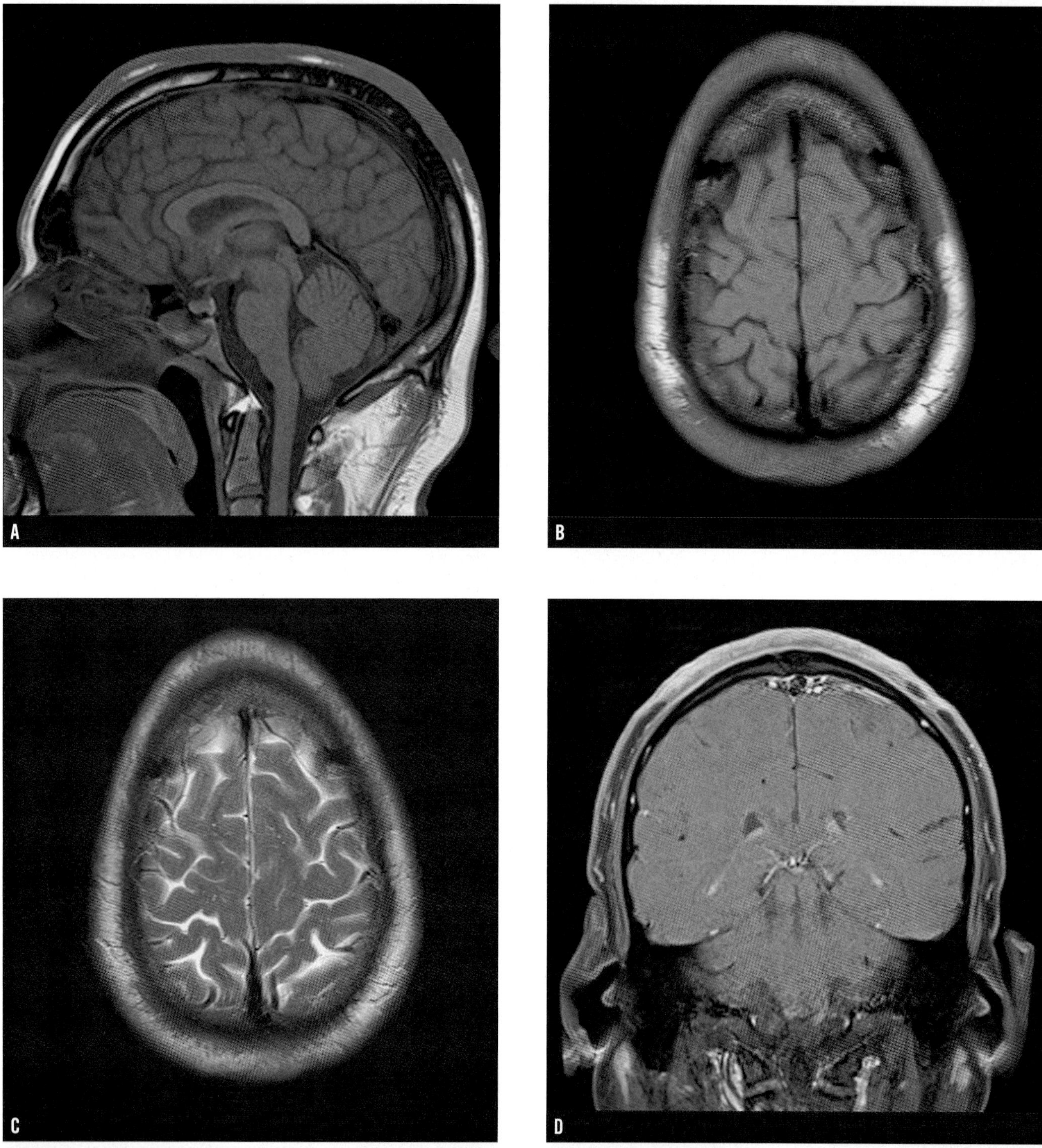

Sagittal T1 (**A**), axial T1 (**B**), axial T2 (**C**), and contrast-enhanced coronal T1 with fat suppression (**D**) MR images demonstrate a T1 iso-intense, mildly T2 hyperintense, diffusely enhancing infiltrating scalp lesion, pathologically proven to represent cutaneous acute myeloid leukemia.

Companion case: Chronic scalp trauma

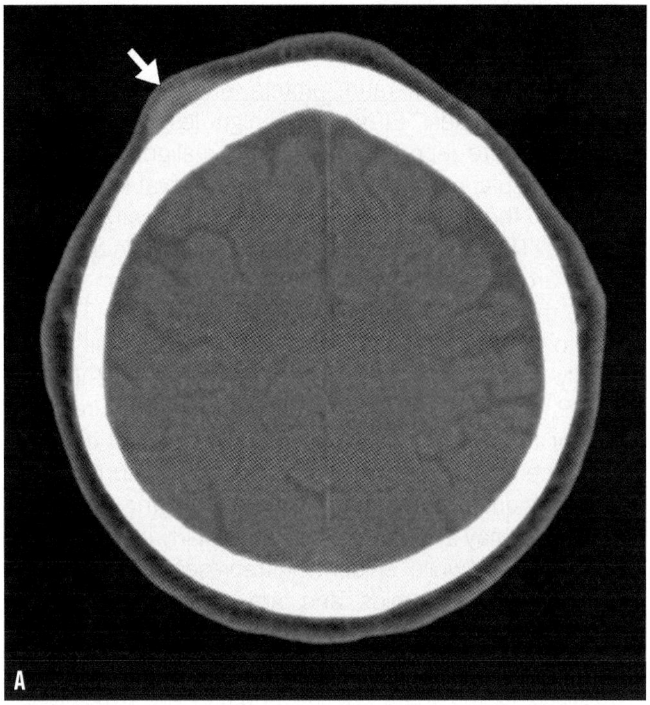

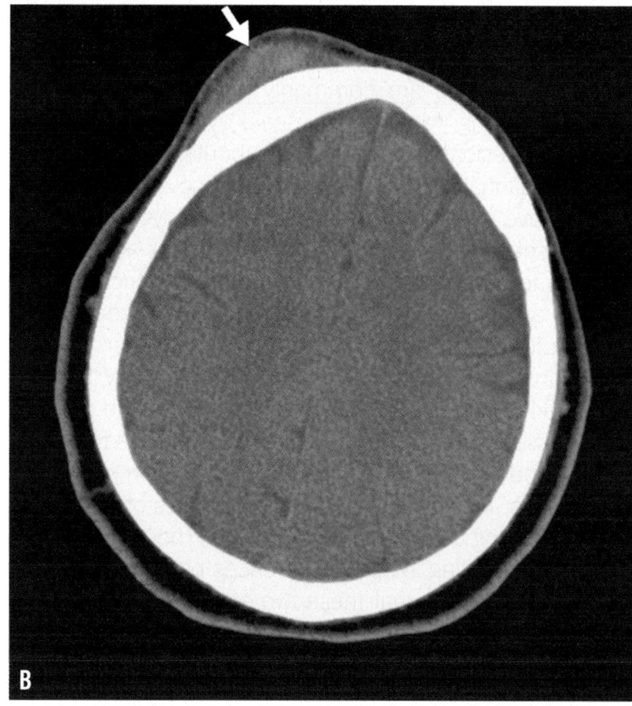

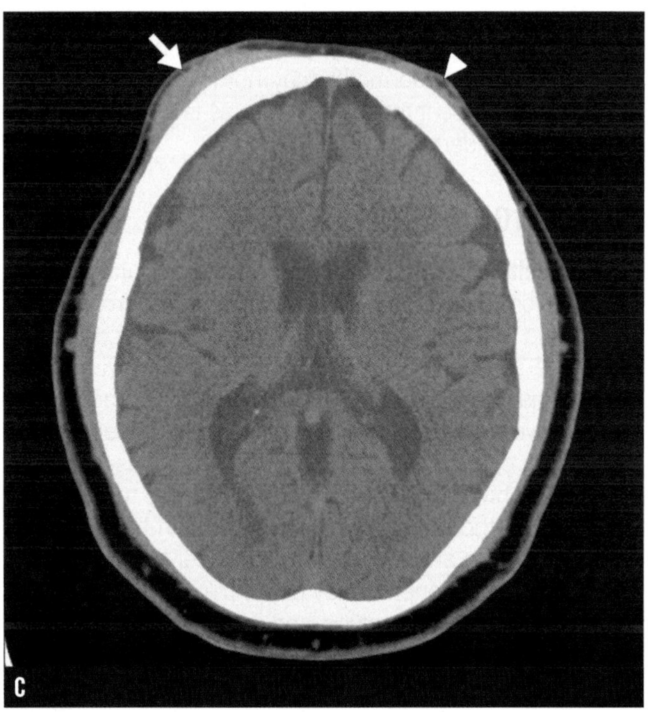

An axial unenhanced CT image (**A**) demonstrates an apparent focal subgaleal hematoma along the right frontal scalp in a chronic alcoholic patient following trauma (arrow, **A**). A follow-up unenhanced CT image of the head obtained 4 years later (**B**) demonstrates the same finding but larger (arrow, **B**). A follow-up CT of the head 8 years after image **B** (**C**) demonstrates the same right frontal scalp subgaleal finding (arrow, **C**) as well as new mild scalp thickening along the left frontal scalp (arrowhead, **C**). There were numerous intervening studies that demonstrated the same right frontal scalp finding, many of which were misread as an "acute subgaleal hematoma." Repetitive scalp injury, such as may be occur with alcoholic patients, can result in chronic scalp thickening, presumably because of an old, organized hematoma and scar.

REFERENCES

Khumalo NP, Gumedze F, Lehloenya R.Folliculitis keloidalis nuchae is associated with the risk for bleeding from haircuts. *Int J Dermatol.* 2011;50(10):1212-1216.

Ko SW, et al. Granulocytic sarcoma manifested as a parametrial mass mimicking a haemorrhagic abscess: a case report with CT and MR findings. *Br J Radiol.* 2007;80(955):e128-e130.

Ogunbiyi A, George A. Acne keloidalis in females: case report and review of literature. *J Natl Med Assoc.* 2005;97(5):736-738.

Shinagare AB, et al. MRI for evaluation of myeloid sarcoma in adults: a single-institution 10-year experience. *AJR Am J Roentgenol.* 2012;199(6):1193-1198.

Wortsman X, et al. Sonography in pathologies of scalp and hair. *Br J Radiol.* 2012;85:647-655.

Benign scalp cysts are commonly encountered clinically and with imaging. Most benign scalp cysts are round, circumscribed lesions located in the subcutaneous fat of the scalp. Traditionally, most benign-appearing scalp cysts on imaging have been described as sebaceous cysts. However, the term sebaceous cyst should be avoided as an all-inclusive term to describe these lesions because a trichilemmal cyst (TC) and an epidermal inclusion cyst (EIC) are far more common lesions to involve the scalp, and neither a TC or an EIC arise from a sebaceous gland. In a study by Türk et al, of 345 patients undergoing resections of one or more scalp masses, approximately 41% were TCs, 15% EICs, 8% lipomas, and only 5% were sebaceous cysts, with numerous other lesions, including several different types of malignancies, comprising the remaining pathology. There is a paucity of literature detailing imaging differences between a TC and EIC, but it is unlikely that these two entities can be reliably differentiated by CT or MRI.

- **Trichilemmal cyst.** A TC is estimated to be present in 5% to 10% of the general population and is the most common scalp mass. A TC, also referred to as a pilar cyst, arises from the outer root sheath of the hair follicle, termed the trichilemma. Clinically, TCs are firm, mobile lesions, and some are associated with overlying alopecia. The vast majority of TCs are found in women older than 60 years, greater than 90% are found in the scalp, and they are often multiple. Some TCs have an autosomal dominant inheritance pattern. Histologically, the contents of a TC consist of keratinous debris and breakdown products, and its walls resemble the normal trichilemma. On CT, these lesions are circumscribed, round, subcutaneous scalp masses that may contain calcification. On MRI, they are most often isointense on T1-weighted imaging, hyperintense on T2-weighted imaging, and do not enhance. There is a paucity of literature describing the MR diffusion-weighted imaging characteristics of a TC, but it is well known that most epidermoid cysts will restrict on this sequence. More aggressive lesions may also arise from a TC or arise de novo. These are the proliferating trichilemmal tumor (PTT) (generally considered benign but can be locally aggressive and can progressively enlarge) and the rare malignant trichilemmal tumor (MTT). A PTT and MTT have similar T1 and T2 signal characteristics as a TC, but these more aggressive lesions enhance on MRI and a MTT may have irregular margins.
- **Epidermal inclusion cyst.** While an EIC is the second most common benign scalp cyst after a TC, it is the most common subcutaneous cyst of the head and neck. An EIC results from rests or implantation of the epidermal elements into the dermis and subcutaneous soft tissues. These cysts are pathologically identical to epidermoid cysts located elsewhere in the body and are composed of keratin, protein, cholesterol, and cell membrane lipids. EICs are benign lesions; however, there are rare reports of associated malignancies. EICs are unilocular, circumscribed, round to oval lesions that reside in the subcutaneous tissue and typically abut the dermis. They usually grow slowly over years to decades. They are fluid attenuating or isoattenuating on CT. On MRI, they are primarily iso- to hypointense on T1 relative to muscle (although they may contain small foci of mildly intrinsic T1 hyperintense signal), hyperintense on T2, and often restrict on diffusion-weighted imaging, similar to epidermoids elsewhere. EICs do not centrally enhance on CT or MRI. A thin capsule surrounding these lesions is often appreciated on imaging. Similar to TCs, EICs may also mineralize, particularly in the elderly.

  So-called "white" epidermoids represent proteinaceous-containing epidermoids and are rare. These epidermoids are termed "white" because their protein content results in intrinsically hyperintense T1 signal on MRI, as opposed to the more typical, primarily T1 hypointense signal identified for the vast majority of epidermoids. They are usually hypointense on T2 and may be hyperattenuating on CT. Additionally, depending on their protein content, white epidermoids may not restrict on DWI and may not be hyperintense on FLAIR, as is typically present with most epidermoids.

COMPANION CASES

- **Hidradenitis suppuritiva.** Hidradenitis suppurativa (HS) is a chronic, disfiguring disease that results from occlusion and subsequent rupture of the pilosebaceous unit into the surrounding dermis. This, in turn, gives rise to inflammation, abscess, and sometimes sinus tract formation. Severe cases of HS may even result in septicemia. HS most commonly develops along skin folds, although uncommonly it may also occur along the neck, ears, and face without developing along the skin folds of these areas. Women are three times more likely to develop HS than men, and genetics may play a role in developing the disease. Cigarette smoking and obesity are believed to increase the risk and severity of HS.

  Imaging is not used to diagnose HS, although HS may be utilized to evaluate for complications of HS. On CT, HS may appear as focal, hypoattenuating fluid collections in the subcutaneous soft tissues, sometimes simulating scalp inclusion cysts. On MRI, HS typically manifests as a T1 hypointense, T2 hyperintense, rim-enhancing collection(s) with associated edema and overlying skin thickening. HS may be avid on positron emission tomography. However, the findings of HS on any given imaging study are often indistinguishable from other inflammatory or infectious skin conditions.

- **Keloids.** A keloid is composed of abnormally excessive collagen and glycoproteins that occurs as a result of an exuberant healing response. It extends beyond the borders of the original wound and is frequently elevated by more than 4 mm. In addition to being cosmetically unappealing, keloids may be painful and pruritic. A keloid most often occurs in individuals younger than 30 years, and those patients with dark pigmented skin have a 15- to 20-fold increased risk of developing a keloid. A keloid will form in susceptible patients following some form of trauma, including surgery or burns. Keloids may appear in as little as 3 months or years later following the insult, do not regress without treatment, and have a high recurrence rate regardless of treatment. Small keloids may be treated with intralesional steroid injection, cryotherapy, pressure dressings, and silicone elastomer sheeting. If a large or recurrent keloid is present, then surgery is the primary therapeutic option. CT imaging findings may include a mass-like, irregular, soft tissue density lesion that can enlarge over successive examinations. On MRI, the lesion will be iso- to hypointense to muscle on T1- and T2-weighted imaging and may enhance.
- **Neurofibromas of the scalp.** Neurofibromas are the result of an abnormal proliferation of Schwann cells, perineural cells, and endoneurial fibroblasts within the skin and subcutaneous soft tissues. In the setting of neurofibromatosis Type I (NF-I), innumerable neurofibromas involving the scalp may be identified. On CT, scalp neurofibromas in patients with NF-I are usually small, variable-sized, iso- to hypoattenuating soft tissue polypoid lesions that are localized within the scalp subcutaneous tissues and/or protrude from the scalp. On MRI, scalp neurofibromas in patients with NF-I are isointense to soft tissue on T1 and T2, and usually enhance following contrast. Most scalp neurofibromas in patients with NF-I are stable or undergo slow growth over several years.
- **Metastatic disease to the scalp.** Up to 5% to 10% of all cancer patients may develop a metastasis to the dermis. While any malignancy may metastasize to the soft tissues, breast carcinoma is the most common culprit in women. In men, melanoma followed by lung carcinoma are the most frequently identified causes of metastasis to the soft tissues. Clinically, these metastatic lesions are usually multifocal, small, rubbery, or hard lesions. On imaging, the lesions are typically isointense relative to muscle on T1, iso- to mildly hyperintense to relative to muscle on T2, may restrict on DWI (particularly melanoma), and will usually enhance.
- **Skin clip artifact simulating a scalp lesion on MRI.** Metal can result in image distortion, signal loss, and signal "pile-up." Signal loss can result from two principal mechanisms. The first mechanism is when the metal object results in local differences in atomic spins which leads to spin-spin dephasing and loss of the MR signal. The second occurs when the metal object alters the frequency of atomic spins within a voxel such that those protons localize to a different voxel. The voxel which loses the protons loses signal, whereas the voxel which acquires the additional protons will have increased signal, otherwise known as signal "pile-up." In the scalp, a metallic clip often results in a signal pile and may simulate a scalp lesion, such as a scalp inclusion cyst.

Scalp inclusion cysts

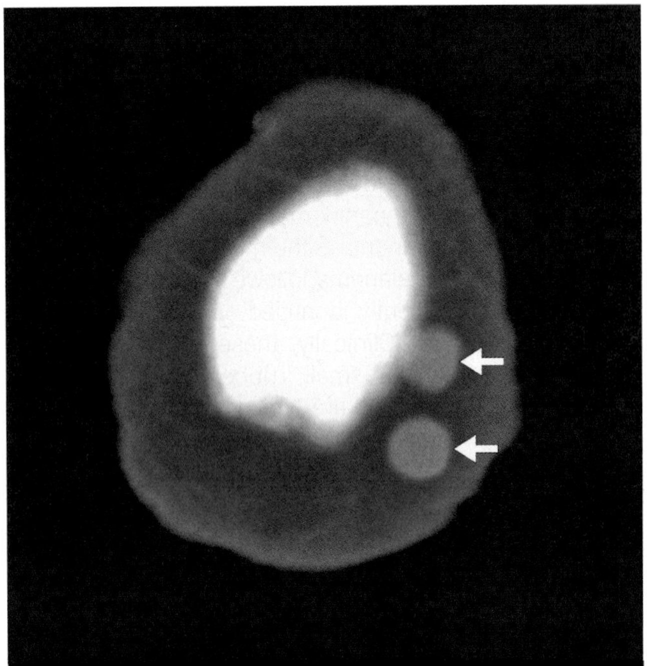

A

An axial noncontrast CT image at the vertex (**A**) demonstrates several round, circumscribed soft tissue density lesions embedded within the subcutaneous soft tissue of the scalp (arrows, **A**). These findings are statistically most compatible with either trichilemmal cysts or epidermal inclusion cysts.

Scalp inclusion cyst containing mineralization

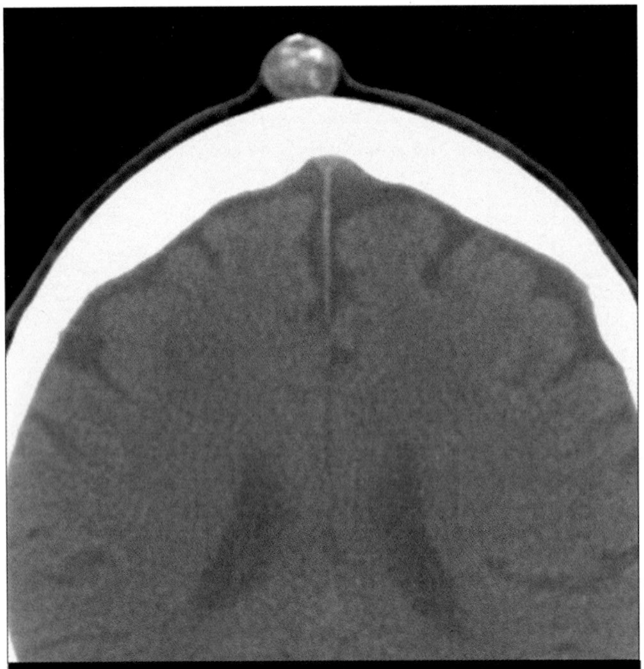

A

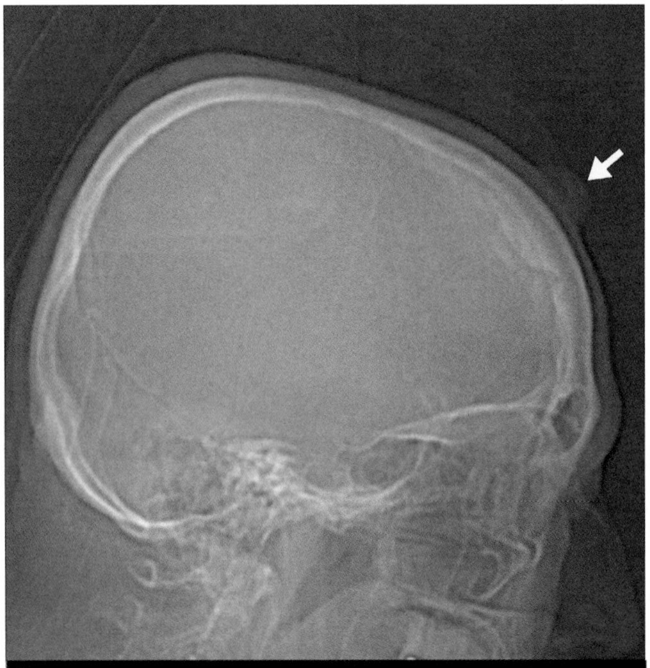

B

An unenhanced axial CT image (**A**) demonstrates a round, partially calcified lesion within the frontal scalp subcutaneous soft tissues. A lateral scout image from the same CT study (**B**) also demonstrates the finding (arrow, **B**). Statistically, this finding is most compatible with either a trichilemmal cyst or an epidermal inclusion cyst.

Enlarging presumed scalp epidermal inclusion cyst

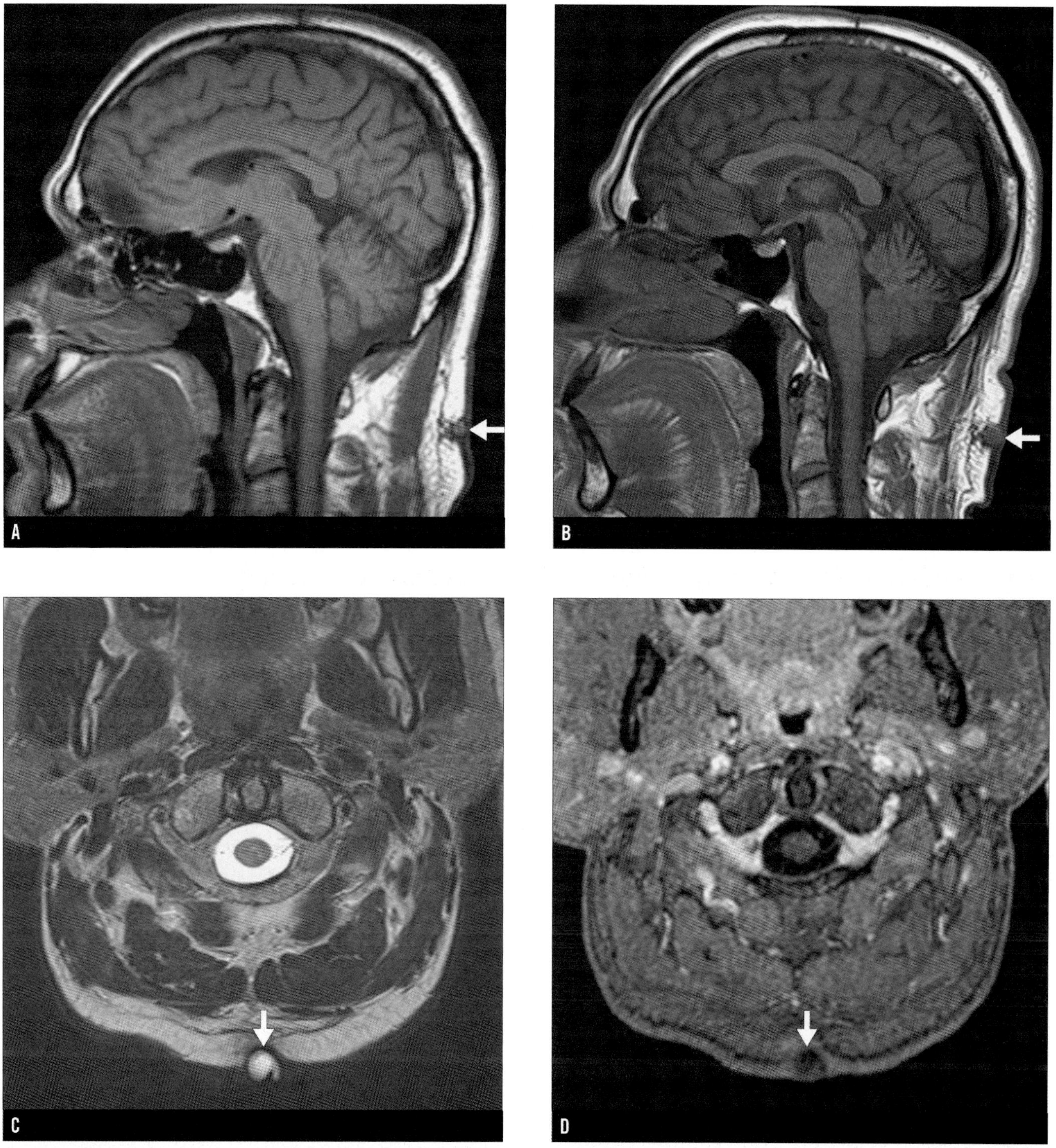

A sagittal T1-weighted MR image (**A**) demonstrates a small, round focus of T1 isointense signal (relative to muscle) in the upper posterior neck subcutaneous soft tissues (arrow, **A**). A follow-up MRI 1 year later with sagittal T1 (**B**), axial T2 (**C**), postcontrast axial MPRAGE (**D**), axial DWI (**E**), and axial ADC map (**F**) MR images. The lesion has mildly increased in size and remains T1 isointense (arrow, **B**). It is also T2 hyperintense (**C**), nonenhancing (**D**), and restricts on DWI (arrows, **E**, **F**) . Given the diffusion restriction, the finding most likely represents an enlarging epidermal inclusion cyst.

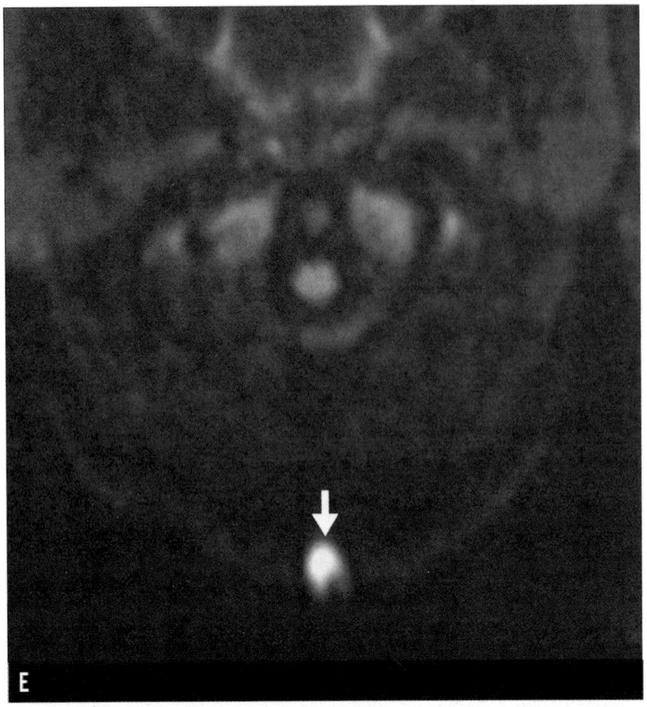

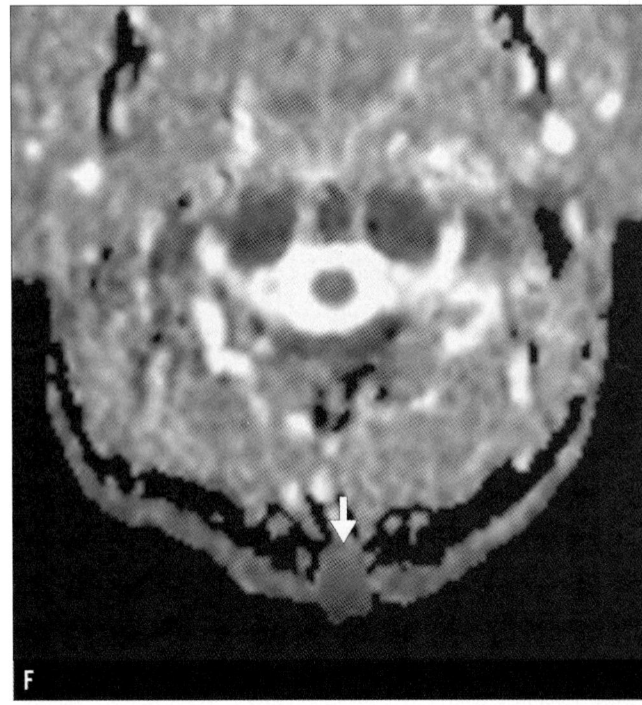

Scalp epidermal inclusion cyst with adjacent osseous remodeling

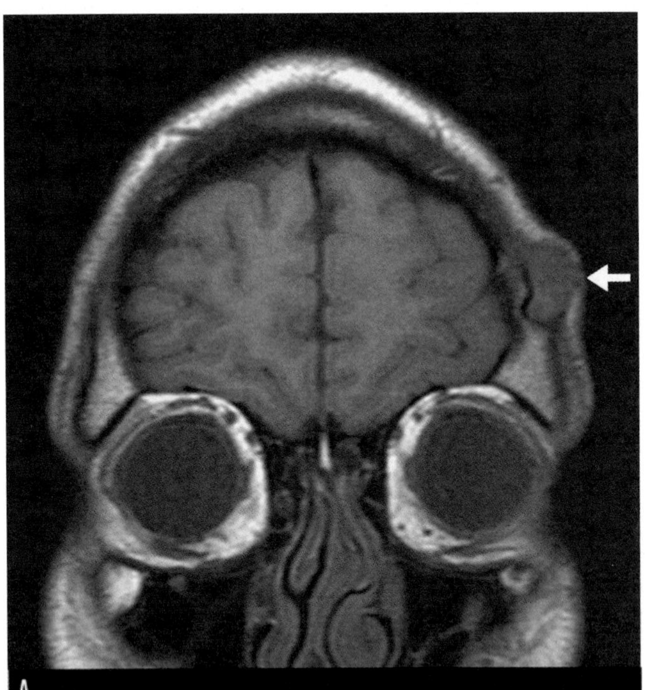

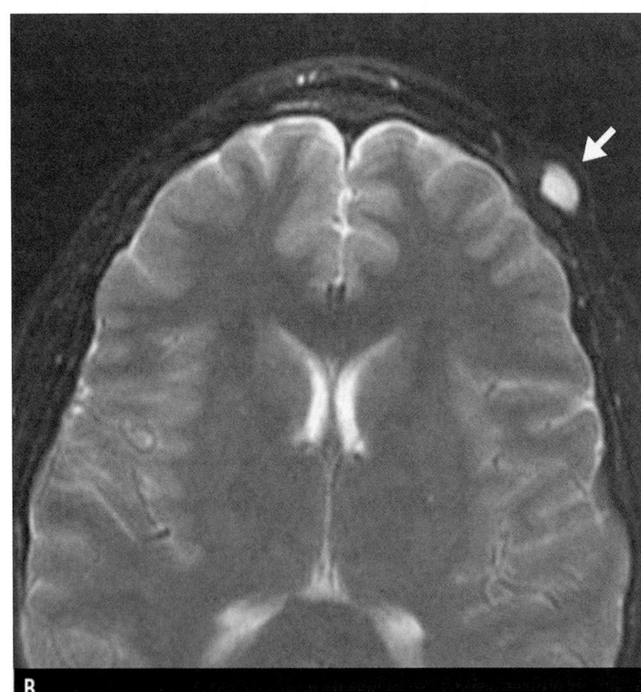

Coronal T1 (**A**), fat-suppressed axial T2 (**B**), and fat-suppressed contrast-enhanced axial T1 (**C**) MR images demonstrate an oval lesion in the left frontal scalp tissues that is largely T1 isointense with small foci of T1 shortening (arrow, **A**), hyperintense on T2 (arrow, **B**), and nonenhancing (arrow, **C**). Image **A** best demonstrates smooth osseous remodeling of the subjacent calvarium. Unenhanced axial CT images viewed with a brain window (**D**) and bone window (**E**) demonstrate the same finding to be hypoattenuating (arrow, **D**) and result in smooth osseous remodeling (arrow, **E**). This lesion was removed and pathologically proven to represent an epidermal inclusion cyst.

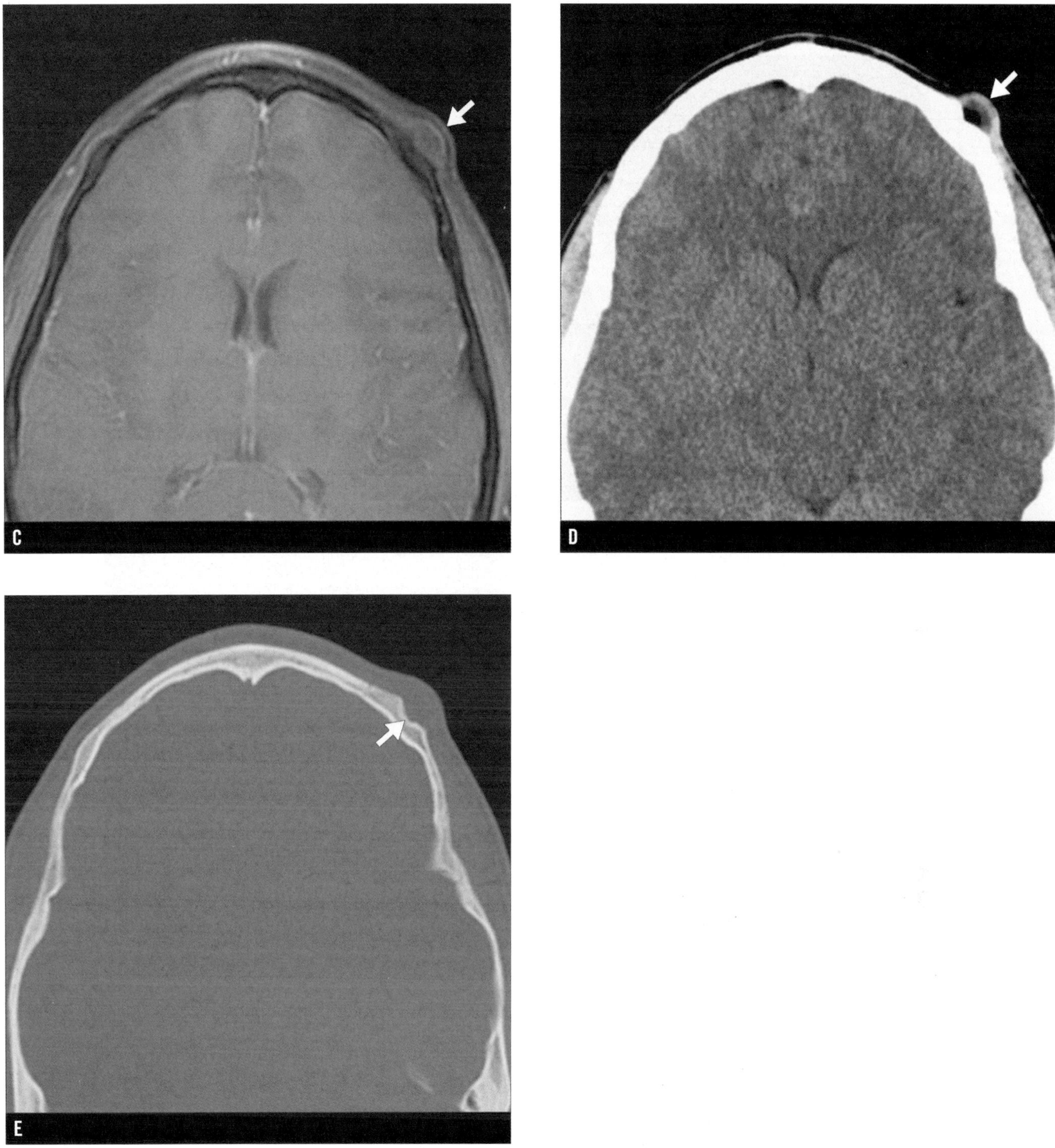
C
D
E

"White" epidermal inclusion cyst

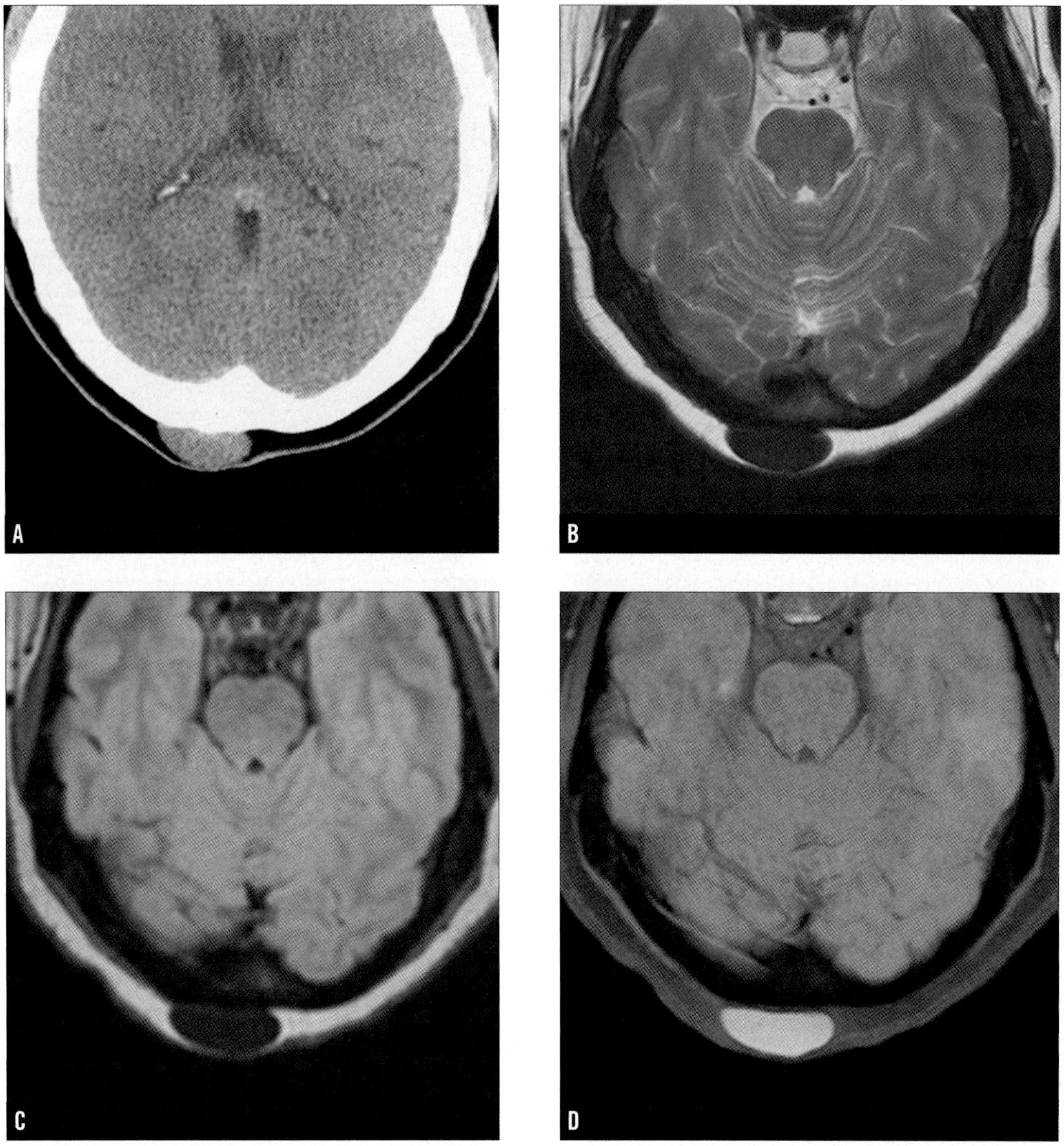

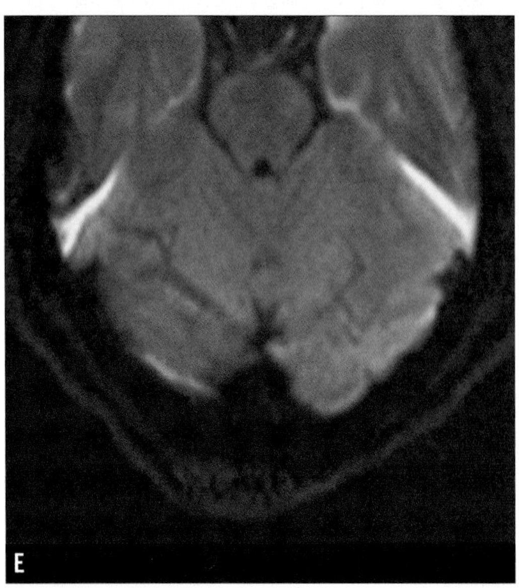

An unenhanced axial CT image (**A**) demonstrates an isoattenuating, circumscribed, oval lesion within the subcutaneous soft tissues of the right paramedian occipital scalp. This finding was stable for over 12 years. Axial T2 (**B**), axial FLAIR (**C**), unenhanced axial T1 with fat suppression (**D**), and axial diffusion (**E**) MR images demonstrate the finding to be T2 and FLAIR hypointense, T1 hyperintense, and non-restricting. Given the stability and benign appearance, this finding was not removed. However, the lesion is most compatible with a so-called "white" epidermal inclusion cyst because of its characteristic intrinsic T1 signal on MRI.

Trichilemmal cyst

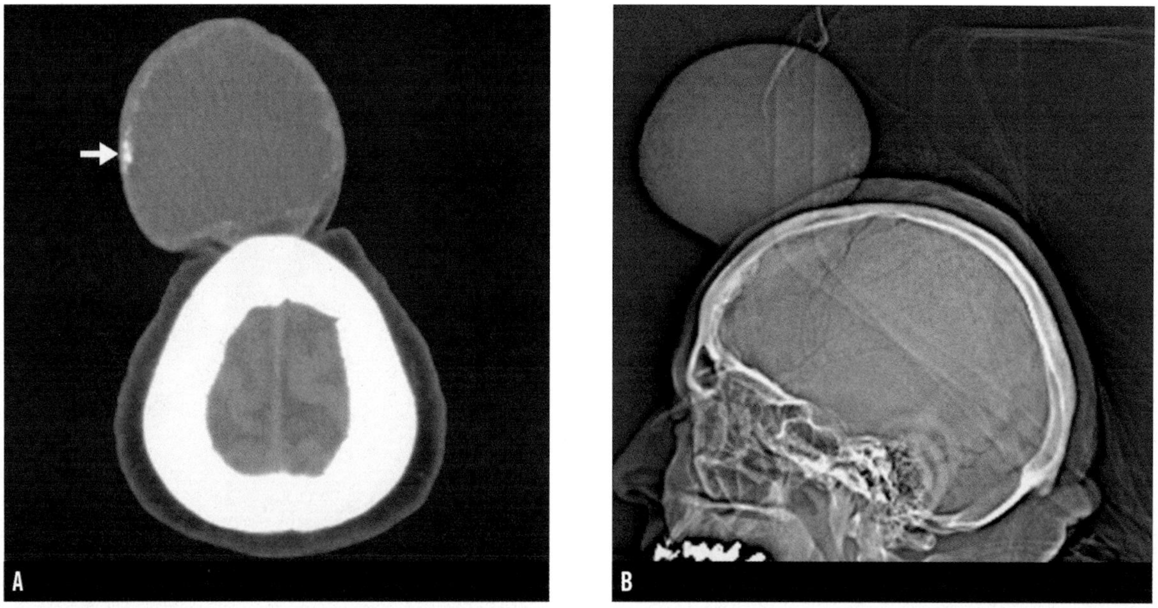

An unenhanced axial CT image (**A**) and a lateral scout image from the same CT study (**B**) demonstrate an extremely large, exophytic, intermediate density mass that is contiguous with the right frontal scalp at the vertex. A small amount of mineralization is present along the periphery (arrow, **A**). This was removed and pathologically proven to represent a massive trichilemmal cyst with surrounding areas of fibrosis, foreign body giant cell reaction, calcifications and chronic inflammation.

Companion case: Hidradenitis suppuritiva

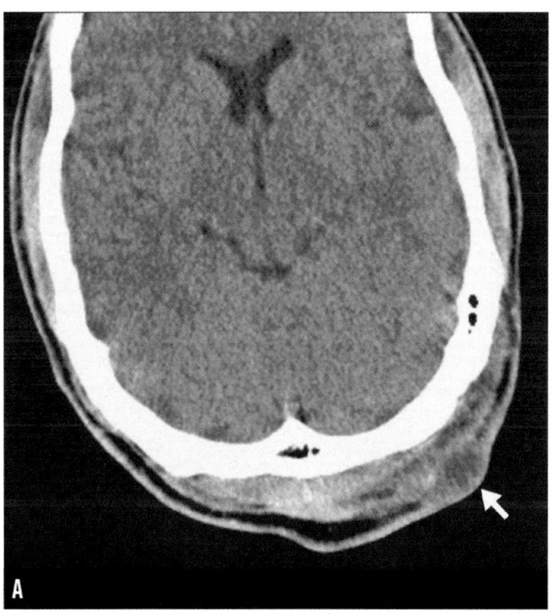

An unenhanced axial CT image (**A**) demonstrates a fluid-attenuating, circumscribed lesion in the subcutaneous tissues of the left suboccipital scalp (arrow). Several similar appearing lesions were present adjacent to this finding on other images (not shown). By imaging alone, the finding is nonspecific and could represent any number of entities that may affect the scalp. However, this finding represented hidradenitis suppurativa, a diagnosis that this patient had for many years. The lesions in this case were actively draining pus and the patient had similar draining lesions in the axilla and groin that were also compatible with this entity.

Companion case: Keloids

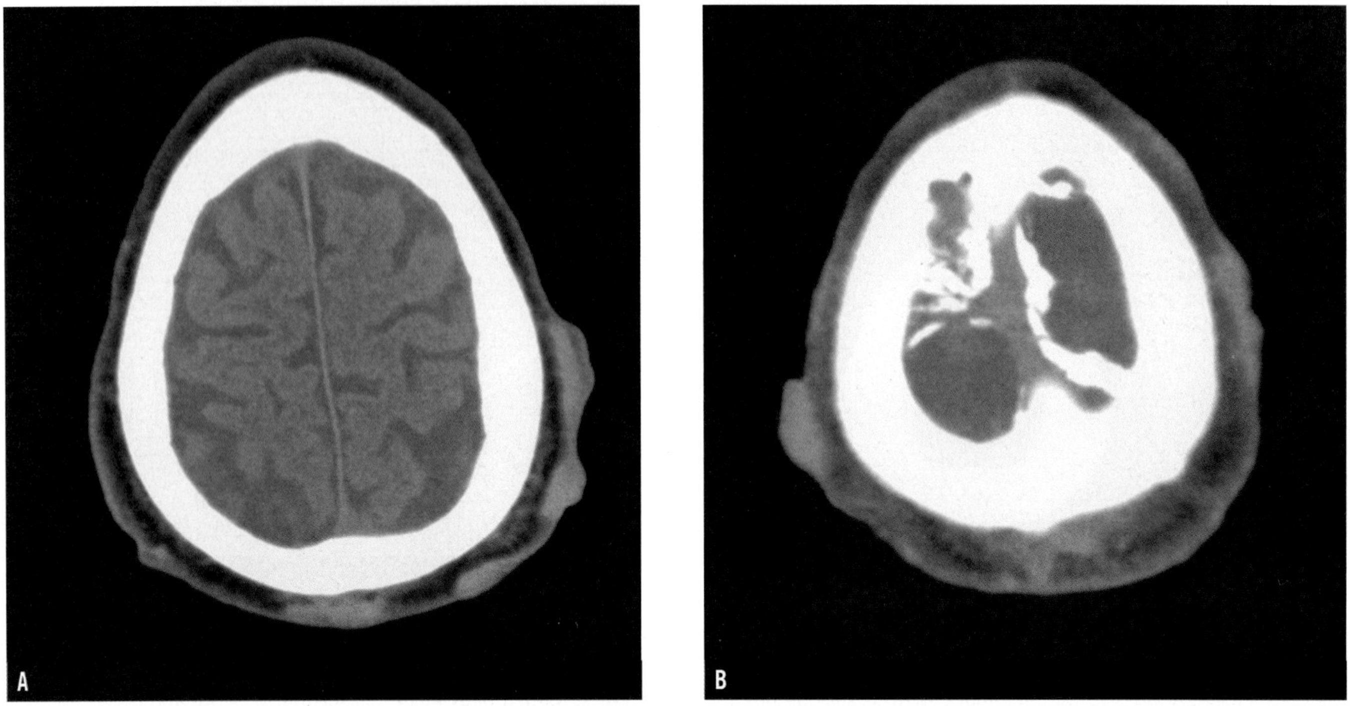

Unenhanced axial CT images (**A**, **B**) demonstrate lobulated, soft tissue masses involving the dermis and subcutaneous soft tissues of the scalp, many of which protrude from the dermal surface. The appearance of these lesions is nonspecific and the findings could represent any number of entities. In this case, these were clinically compatible with multiple keloids.

Companion case: Keloids

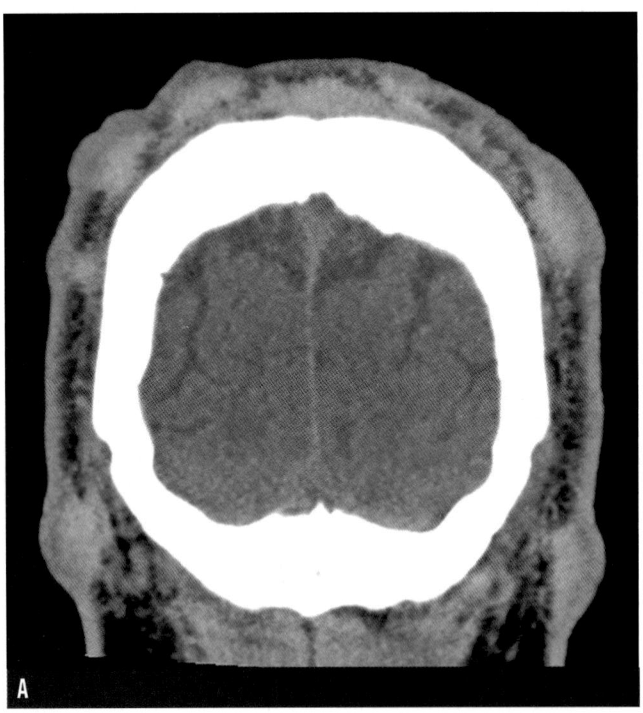

Different patient. An unenhanced coronal reformatted CT image (**A**) demonstrates numerous exophytic scalp keloids which were confirmed clinically.

Companion case: Neurofibromas of the scalp

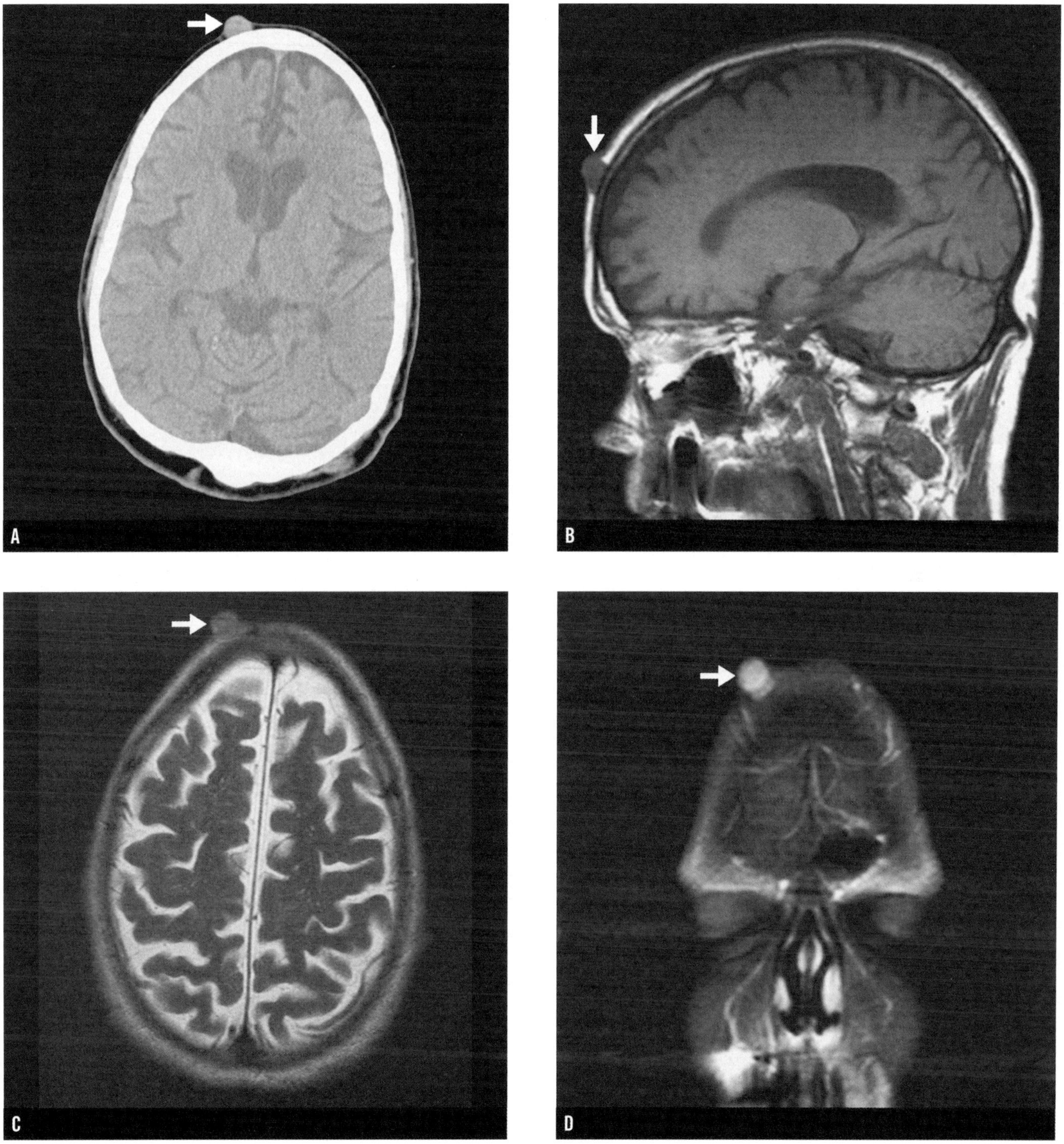

An unenhanced axial CT image (**A**) demonstrate a few of the innumerable small soft tissue nodular foci that were present scattered throughout this patient's scalp, one of which is shown to be protruding outside the confines of the dermis (arrow, **A**). Sagittal T1 (**B**), axial T2 (**C**), and contrast-enhanced fat-suppressed coronal T1 (**D**) MR images demonstrate the protruding lesion to be T1 isointense to muscle, T2 isointense to brain, and enhancing (arrows, **B**-**D**). These findings represented neurofibromas in this patient with a known diagnosis of neurofibromatosis Type I.

Companion case: Metastatic disease to the scalp

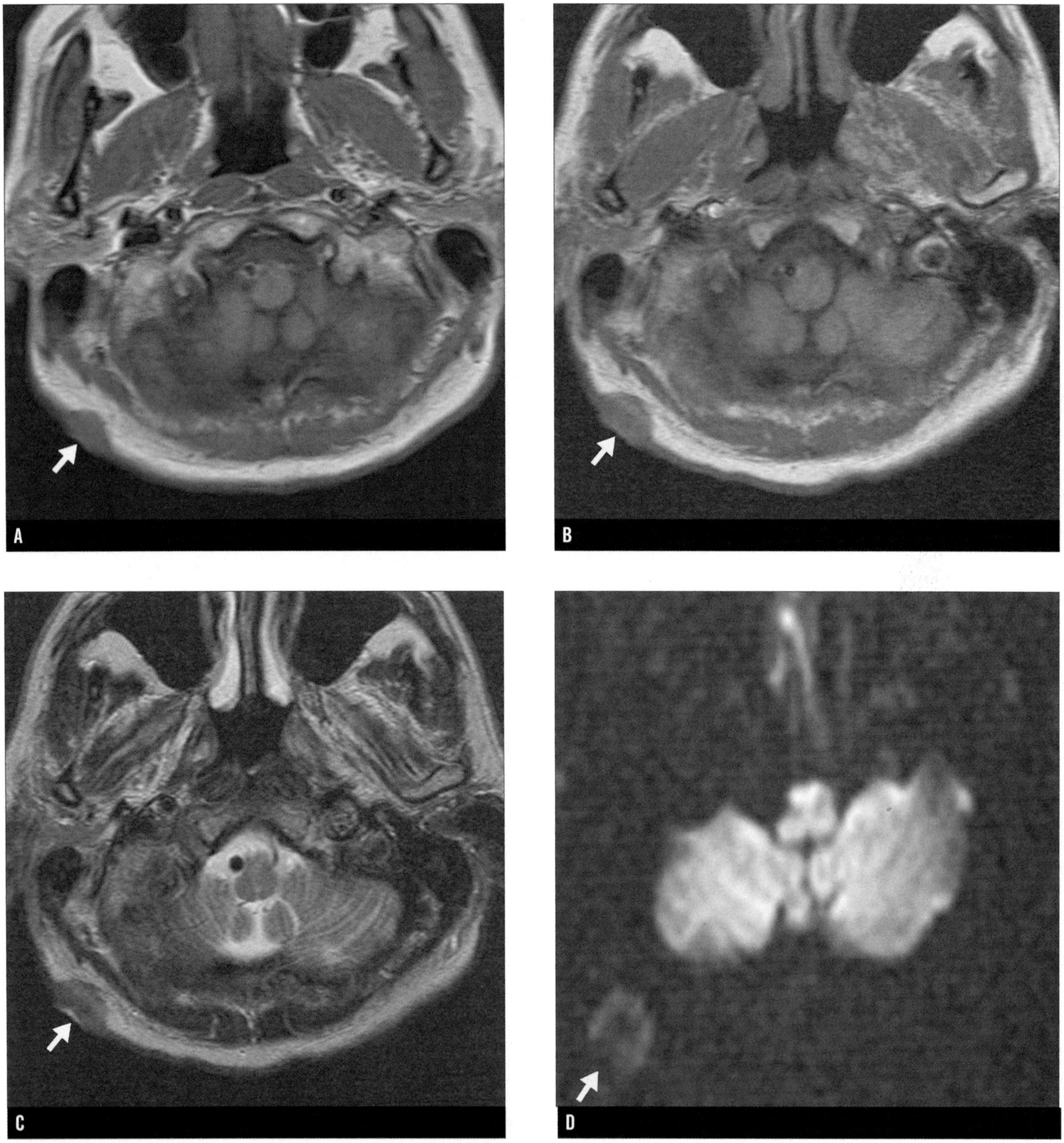

An axial T1-weighted MR image (**A**) demonstrates a focal oval lesion involving the dermis and subcutaneous tissues of the right suboccipital scalp that is isointense to muscle in this patient with metastatic lung cancer (arrow, **A**). Approximately 1 month later, axial T1 (**B**), axial T2 (**C**), axial DWI (**D**), and contrast-enhanced fat-suppressed coronal T1 (**E**) MR images demonstrate the same lesion to have significantly increased its size. It remains similarly isointense on T1 (arrow, **B**), mildly hyperintense to muscle on T2 (arrow, **C**), does not appreciably restrict on DWI (arrow, **D**), and heterogeneously enhances (arrow, **E**). While the findings on T1 and T2 are similar to a benign scalp inclusion cyst, the presence of enhancement does not occur with this entity. In addition, at least with an epidermal inclusion cyst, restricted diffusion is often evident. While scalp inclusion cysts do enlarge, they typically do not significantly enlarge within 1 month, as occurred in this case. Given the history of metastatic lung cancer, the findings are most consistent with metastatic disease to the scalp. An unenhanced axial CT obtained at the same time as the second MRI (**F**) demonstrates the striking similarity between this metastatic lesion and a scalp inclusion cyst. History is paramount when evaluating these findings, particularly on CT.

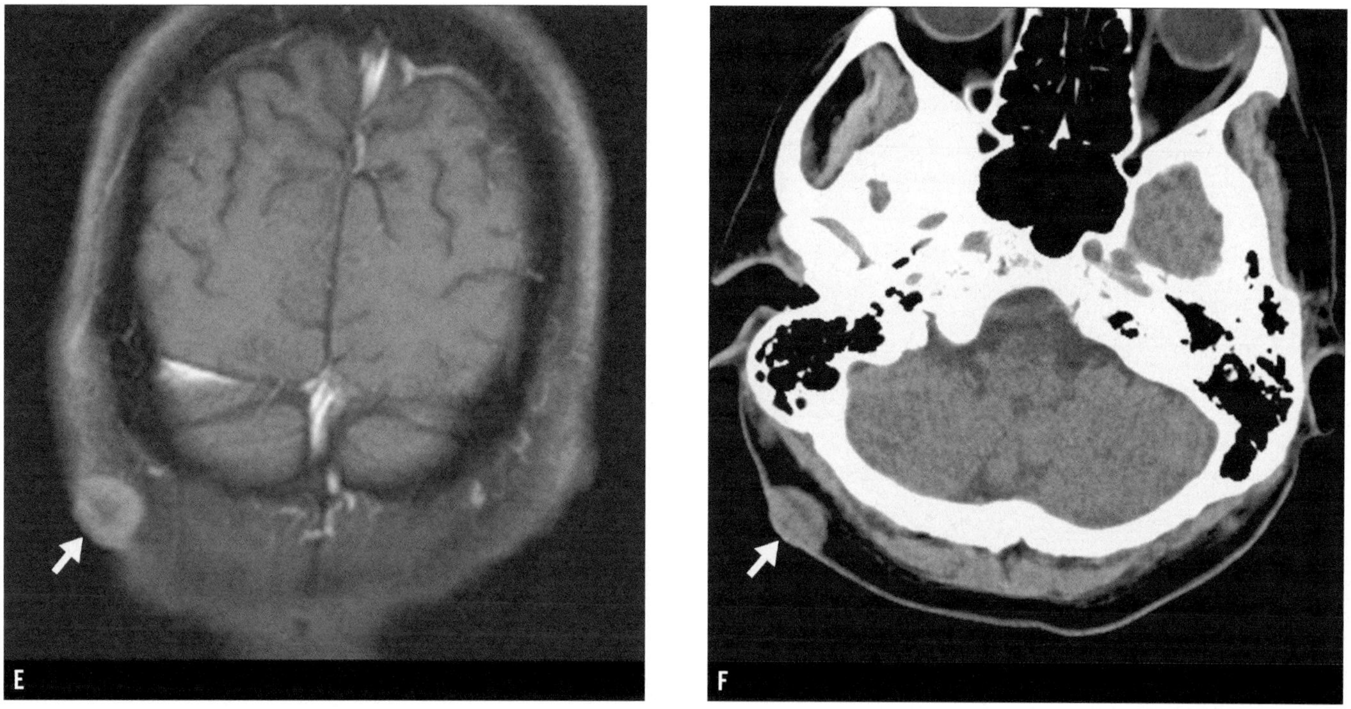

Companion case: Skin clip artifact simulating a scalp lesion on MRI

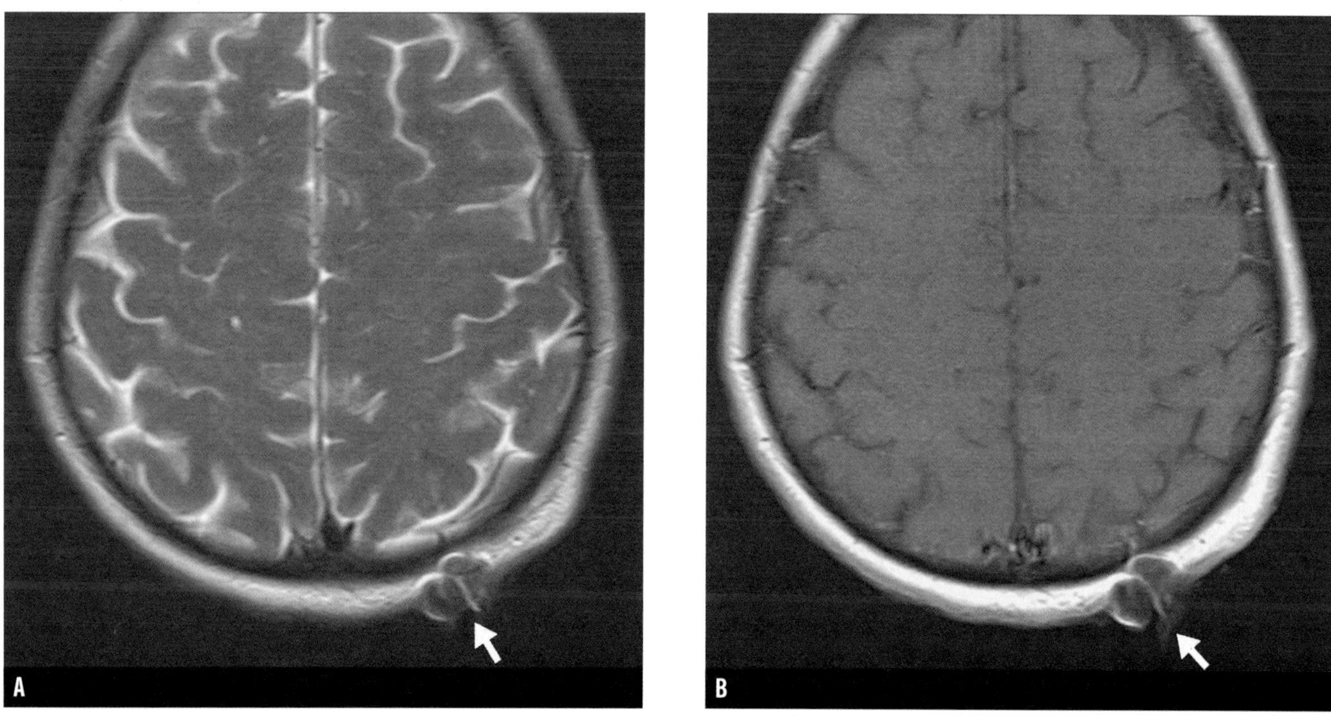

Axial T2 (**A**) and contrast-enhanced axial T1 (**B**) MR images demonstrate an apparent lesion in the left parietal scalp soft tissue (arrows, **A**, **B**). An axial CT image (**C**) and a lateral scout image from the same CT study (**D**) demonstrate the finding on MRI to merely represent artifact associated with skin staples (arrows, **C**, **D**).

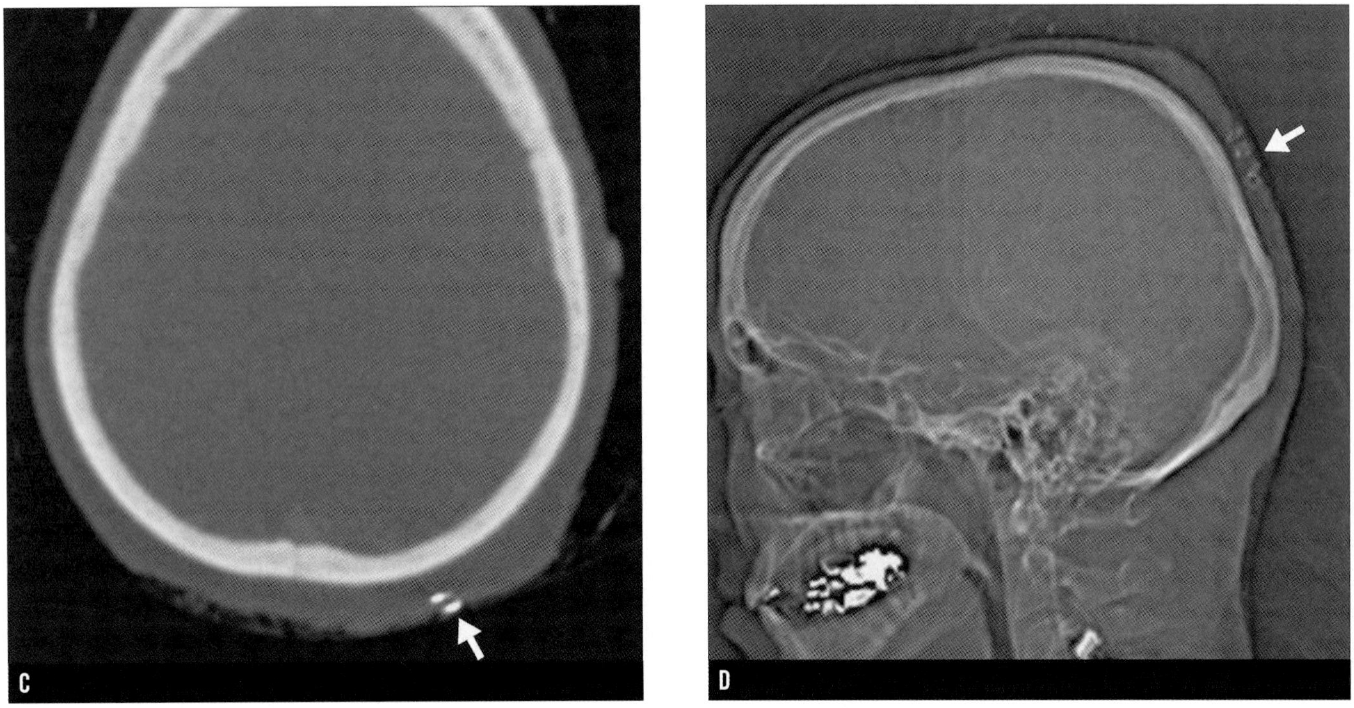

REFERENCES

Beaman FD, Kransdorf MJ, Andrews TR, Murphey MD, Arcara LK, Keeling JH. Superficial soft-tissue masses: analysis, diagnosis, and differential considerations. *Radiographics.* 2007;27(2):509-523.

Fortman BJ, et al. Neurofibromatosis type 1: a diagnostic mimicker at CT. *Radiographics.* 2001;21(3):601-612.

Ibrahim AE, Barikian A, Janom H, Kaddoura I. Numerous recurrent trichilemmal cysts of the scalp: differential diagnosis and surgical management. *J Craniofac Surg.* 2012;23(2):e164-e168.

Ikegami T, Kameyama M, Orikasa H, Yamazaki K. Trichilemmal cyst in the pulp of the index finger: a case report. *Hand Surg.* 2003;8(2):253-255.

Kelly AM, Cronin P. MRI features of hidradenitis suppurativa and review of the literature. *AJR Am J Roentgenol.* 2005;185(5):1201-1204.

Kim HK, Kim SM, Lee SH, Racadio JM, Shin MJ. Subcutaneous epidermal inclusion cysts: ultrasound (US) and MR imaging findings. *Skeletal Radiol.* 2011;40(11):1415-1419. Epub December 4, 2010.

Kitajima K, Imanaka K, Hashimoto K, Hayashi M, Kuwata Y, Sugimura K. Magnetic resonance imaging findings of proliferating trichilemmal tumor. *Neuroradiology.* 2005;47(6):406-410.

Koshelev MV, et al. Concurrent hidradenitis suppurativa, inflammatory acne, dissecting cellulitis of the scalp, and pyoderma gangrenosum in a 16-year-old boy. *Pediatr Dermatol.* 2014;31(1):e20-e21.

Madu P, Kundu RV. Follicular and scarring disorders in skin of color: presentation and management. *Am J Clin Dermatol.* 2014;15(4):307-321.

Puranik A, Sankhe S, Goel N, Mahore A. Cerebral shading sign in a giant intraparenchymal white epidermoid. *Neurol India.* 2012;60(2):265-266.

Satyaprakash AK, Sheehan DJ, Sangüeza OP.Proliferating trichilemmal tumors: a review of the literature. Dermatol Surg. 2007;33(9):1102-1108.

Syed ZU, Hamzavi IH. Atypical hidradenitis suppurativa involving the posterior neck and occiput. *Arch Dermatol.* 2011;147(11):1343-1344.

Türk CÇ, Bacanlı A, Kara NN. Incidence and clinical significance of lesions presenting as a scalp mass in adult patients. *Acta Neurochir* (Wien). 2015;157(2):217-223.

CASE 15 Scalp lipoma

Lipomas are common lesions which represent fatty tissue that is surrounded by a fibrous capsule. Lipomas may contain thin septa and typically measure less than 5 cm, although there are cases of lipomas larger than 10 cm. Lipomas cannot be used for energy stores. As a result, while they can enlarge with weight gain, they do not decrease in size with weight loss. There is no gender predilection, but lipomas are more common in older patients and can be multiple in up to 15% of cases.

Clinically, superficial benign lipomas are almost always soft, mobile, asymptomatic masses that are stable for years. Imaging of a lipoma is usually performed only as a confirmatory examination. On CT, benign lipomas appear as homogenous, circumscribed lesions that measure fat density. On MRI, benign lipomas will follow fat signal on all pulse sequences and, as expected, will suppress on fat-suppressed imaging. Contrast enhancement is not observed within the fatty tissue, but can sometimes be identified along the fibrous capsule or septa. Rarely, foci of mineralization may be associated with a lipoma. Larger lesions with thick septa, nodular areas, or associated enhancing soft tissue should evoke the possibility of a liposarcoma, although this is uncommon in the head and neck region.

Resection of a benign lipoma is typically reserved for the rare symptomatic lesion or for cosmetic reasons. Underlying osseous abnormalities are uncommon; however, scalp lipomas can cause pressure on the outer table of the calvarium and result in calvarial remodeling.

COMPANION CASE

- **Pectoralis muscle flap to repair a scalp defect.** Flap reconstructions may be obtained from a remote site and placed over a scalp defect (free flap) or taken from a local site with an intact vascular pedicle and repositioned over the scalp defect (pedicle flap). The flap used to repair a scalp defect may contain a variety of different tissues, including muscle, fascial tissue, galeal tissue, subcutaneous tissue, and skin. One of the more widely used musculocutaneous flaps is the pectoralis major flap. The pectoralis major flap carries minimal morbidity or functional loss and helps protect against complications, such as cerebrospinal fluid leak. However, disadvantages of the pectoralis muscle flap include excessive tissue bulk over the calvarium and breast/chest distortion.

Scalp lipoma

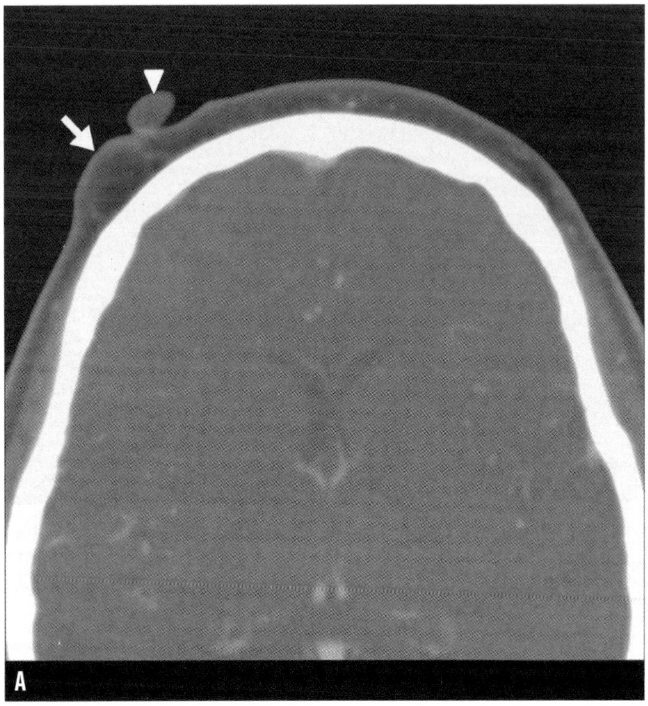

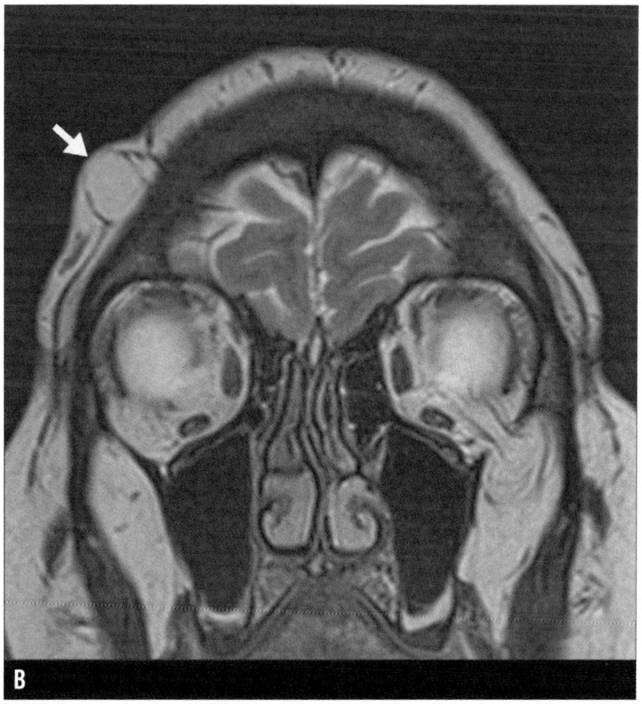

A contrast-enhanced axial CT image (**A**) demonstrates a fat-density lesion within the right frontal scalp subcutaneous soft tissues (arrow, **A**). A vitamin E capsule (arrowhead, **A**) denotes this palpable abnormality. The finding followed fat signal on all MRI pulse sequences on a subsequently performed MRI study, compatible with a benign lipoma. A representative coronal T2-weighted MR image from that study (**B**) demonstrating the lipoma is shown (arrow, **B**).

Scalp lipoma

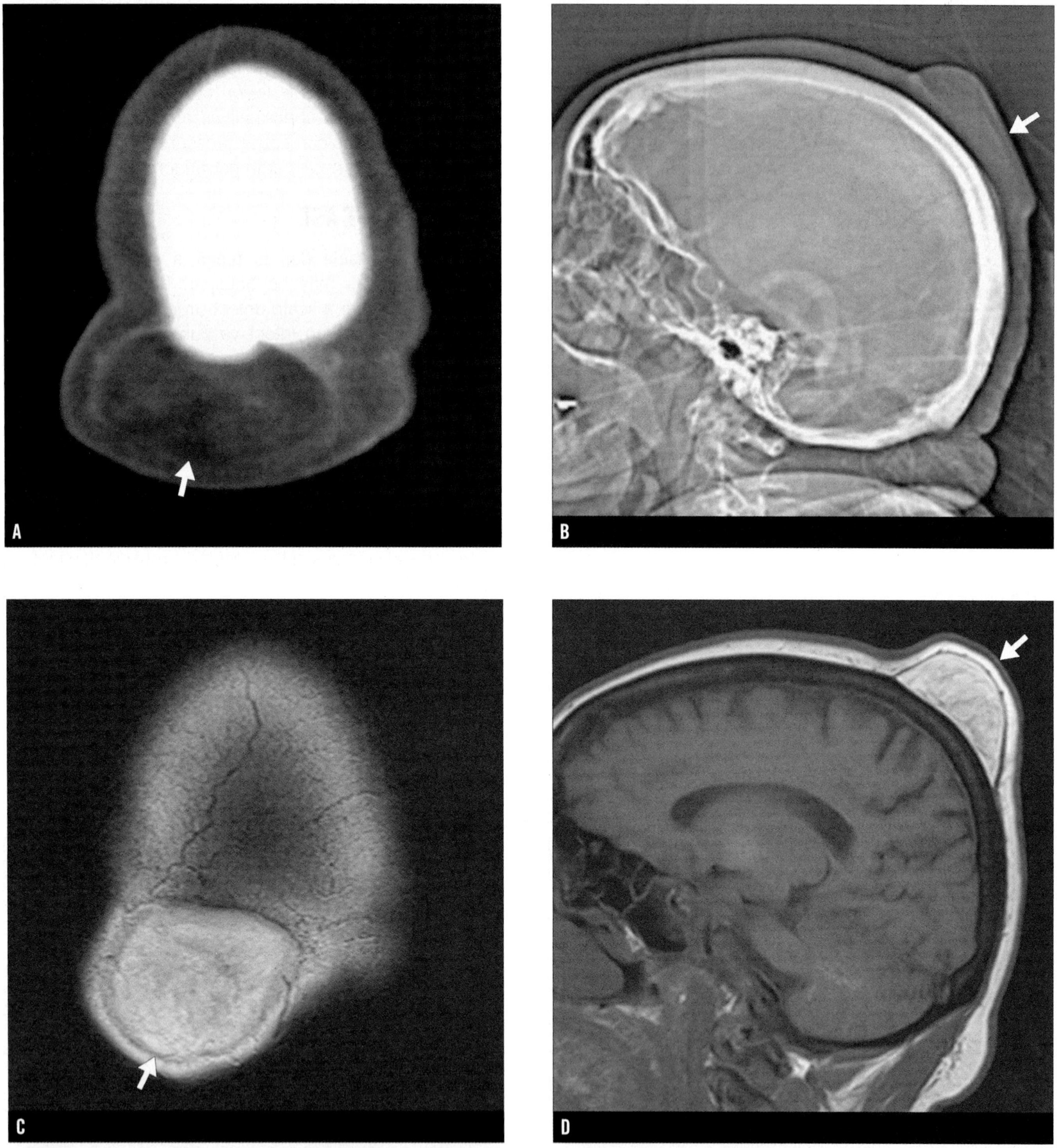

Different patient. An axial CT image (**A**) demonstrates a fat-equivalent lesion at the scalp vertex (arrow, **A**). A lateral scout image from the same CT (**B**) demonstrates flattening of the lesion against the gantry, suggesting that the lesion is soft (arrow, **B**). Axial T2 (**C**) and sagittal T1 (**D**) MR images demonstrate the same finding to be fat equivalent on both sequences (arrows, **C**, **D**). These findings are compatible with a benign scalp lipoma.

Companion case: Pectoralis muscle flap to repair a scalp defect

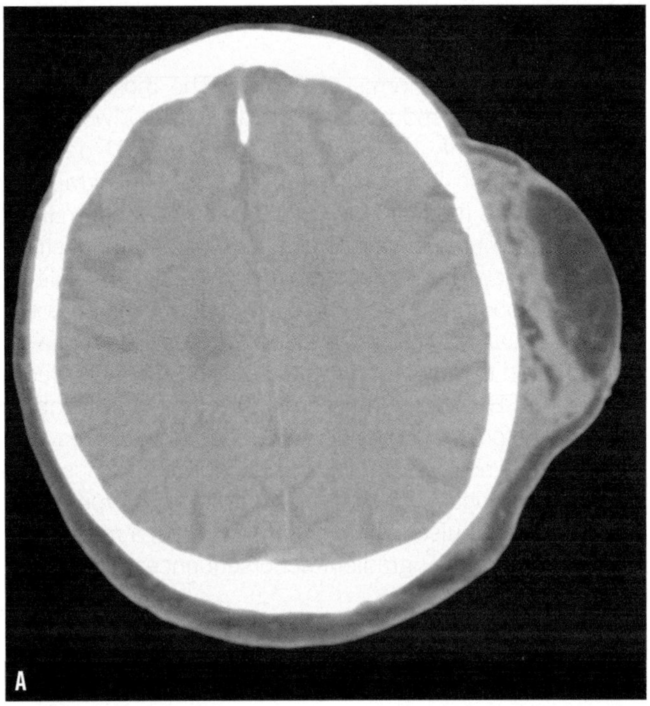

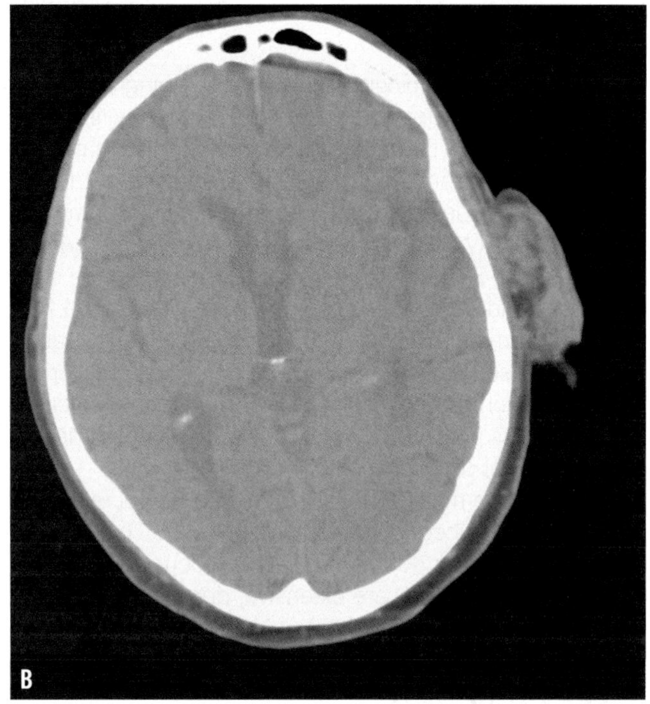

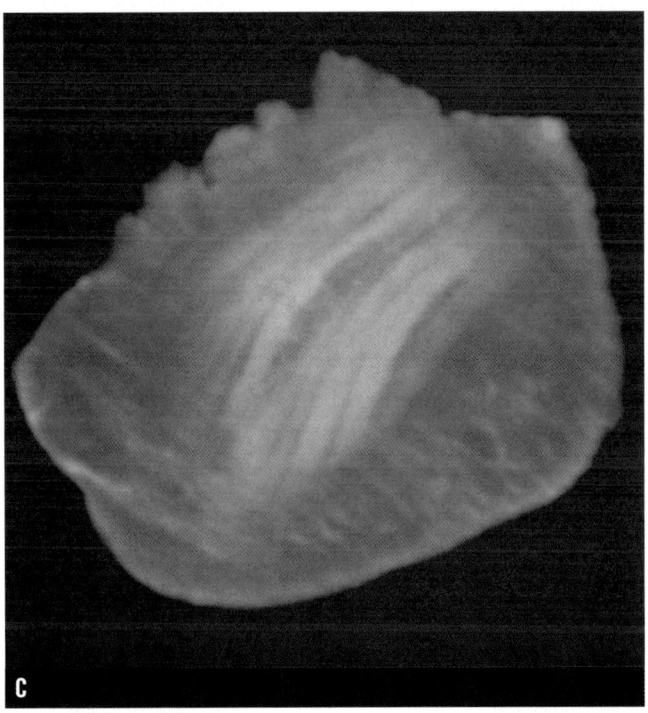

Unenhanced axial CT images (**A**, **B**) demonstrate a large amount of asymmetric fat and muscle along the scalp overlying the left temporal and parietal bones. This represents a pectoralis flap that was placed to repair a scalp defect following resection of a melanoma metastasis. An unenhanced axial CT image at the vertex of the scalp (**C**) best demonstrates muscle fibers intermixed with fat comprising the pectoralis major flap.

REFERENCES

Given CA, et al. Interhemispheric lipoma connected to subcutaneous lipoma via lipomatous stalk. *Pediatr Radiol.* 2005;35(11):1110-1112.

Kato K, et al. Intracranial epidermoid tumor after subcutaneous lipoma excision. *Neurol Med Chir (Tokyo).* 2008;48:262-265.

Kransdorf MJ, et al. Imaging of fatty tumors: distinction of lipoma and well-differentiated liposarcoma. *Radiology.* 2002;224:99-104.

Mustoe TA, Corral CJ. Soft tissue reconstructive choices for craniofacial reconstruction. *Clin Plast Surg.* 1995;22(3):543-554.

CASE 16 Scalp dermal calcifications

There is scant radiologic literature pertaining to benign skin calcifications apart from the mammography literature, although many of the conclusions made in the mammography literature can be extrapolated to imaging of the skin elsewhere. Incidentally detected small foci (<5 mm) of calcium density at the skin surface of the scalp and face are common. Sebaceous glands are abundant in the scalp and face, and dermal calcifications most likely result from calcium formation within obstructed sebaceous glands. The term pseudocalcification is used to describe foreign substances on the skin surface that may mimic calcifications, such as powders, creams, adhesives, or high-density environmental particles.

On CT, dermal calcifications of the scalp related to obstructed sebaceous glands are punctate, hyperdense foci isolated to the dermis. They may occur anywhere on the scalp. Unless they are extensive, dermal calcifications are typically occult on MRI.

COMPANION CASE

- **Foreign bodies in the scalp following trauma.** A foreign body (FB) is often encountered on radiologic studies following various forms of trauma. The most common FBs are composed of glass, metal, stone, or wood. The ability to identify a FB with radiographs or CT depends on the composition and size of the FB. Radiography is the first-line modality for FB detection as it can reliably detect radiopaque glass, stone, and metal without streak artifact. However, radiography usually lacks the ability to detect wood or acrylic FBs. CT is similar in its detection rate but can often improve upon the localization of a FB compared to radiography. Ultrasonography may detect a wooden FB within soft tissues but is limited in its ability to detect foreign bodies located deep within tissues. MRI is typically not used for FB detection, but if a FB is present, it will usually be identified as focally hypointense signal on all pulse sequences. In addition, a metallic FB will bloom on MR gradient echo sequences.

Scalp dermal calcifications

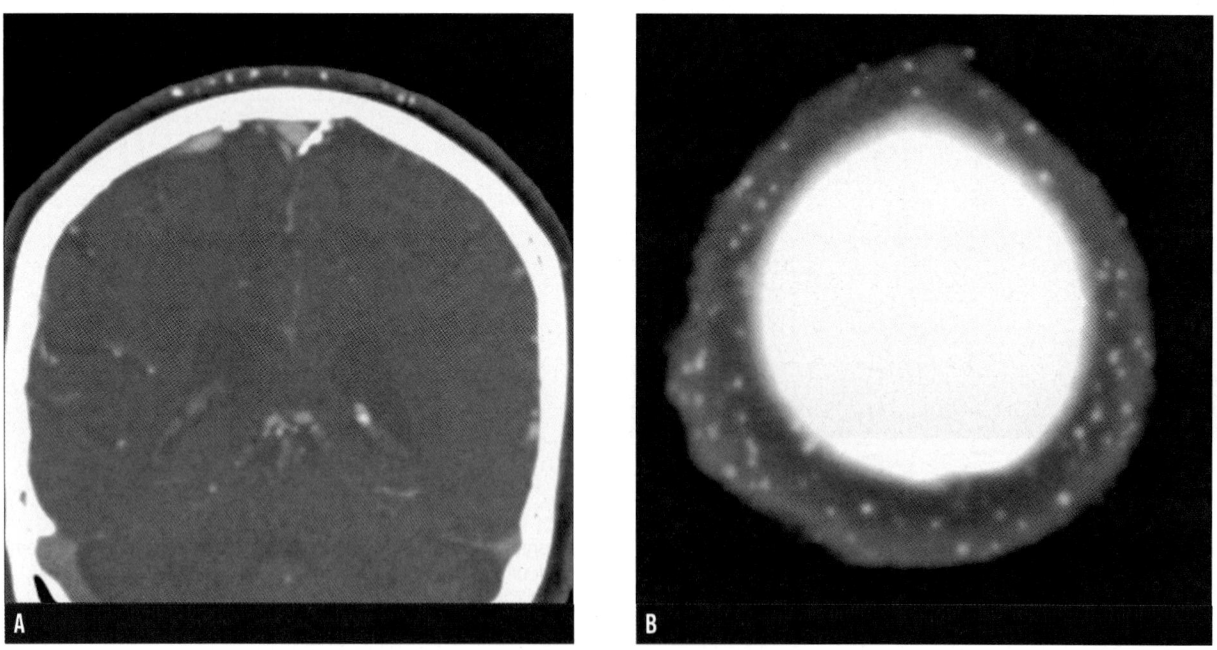

Contrast-enhanced coronal reformatted (**A**) and axial (**B**) CT images demonstrate innumerable punctate foci of mineralization within the dermis of the scalp at the vertex, compatible with dermal scalp calcifications.

Companion case: Foreign bodies in the scalp following trauma

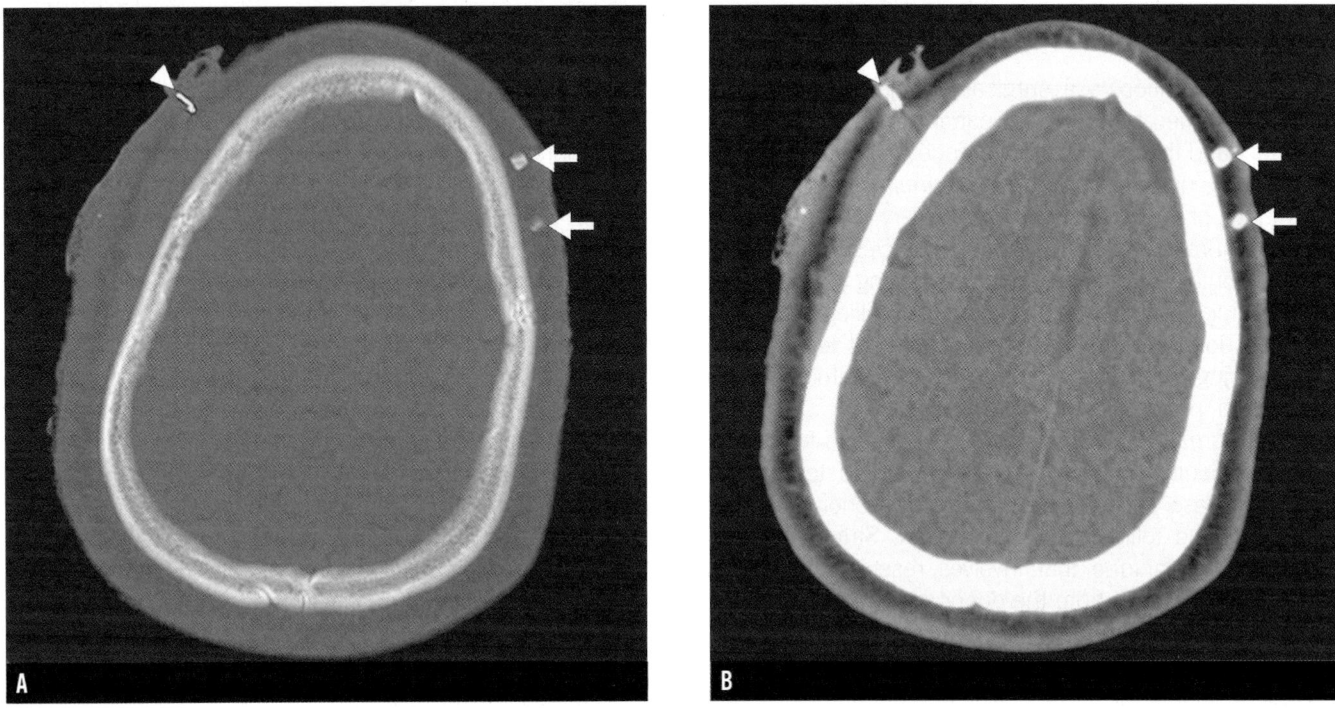

Axial CT images viewed with a bone window (**A**) and brain window (**B**) of a patient who presented to the emergency department following acute trauma. These images demonstrate several foreign bodies in the left frontal scalp that represent glass (arrows, **A**, **B**). A linear metallic foreign body in the right frontal scalp likely represents a metallic staple used to repair a laceration (arrowheads, **A**, **B**).

REFERENCES

Aras MH, et al. Comparison of the sensitivity for detecting foreign bodies among conventional plain radiography, computed tomography and ultrasonography. *Dentomaxillofac Radiol.* 2010;39(2):72-78.

Ayaviri NAM, et al. Isolated primary osteoma cutis of the head: case report. *Can J Plast Surg.* 2006;14(1):33-36.

Basler RS, Watters JH, Taylor WB. Calcifying acne lesions. *Int J Dermatol.* 1977;16(9):755-758.

Picca DA, Shaw de Paredes E. Calcification in the breast: a radiologic perspective. *Appl Radiol.* 2003;32(9):29-37.

CASE 17 Hair transplantation

Hair transplantation is a surgical procedure most commonly performed to treat male pattern baldness. In order to understand the imaging appearance of hair transplantation, a basic understanding of the principles and surgical techniques of this procedure is necessary. At its essence, the procedure involves removing hair follicles from a donor site that contains ample hair and transposing those follicles to the recipient site (ie, balding site). Hair follicles obtained from the donor site are genetically resistant to hair loss; thus, placing them in the balding scalp eventually allows hair growth in the balding areas.

Hair normally grows in groupings of one to four hairs, termed follicular units. There are two main techniques to obtain these follicular units from the donor site: strip harvesting and follicular unit extraction. Strip harvesting is an older technique that involves resecting a strip of hair-containing scalp from the donor site (usually from the occipital area). The hair follicular units are then carefully dissected from the strip. A major disadvantage of the strip harvesting technique is a horizontally oriented scar that results along the occipital scalp, although it can usually be obscured by adjacent native hair. The follicular unit extraction technique is significantly more time consuming and more expensive than the strip harvesting technique, as each follicular unit is meticulously extracted by a fine punch needle as small as 0.6 mm. Only punctate scars remain with this technique and the postoperative discomfort is minimized. With either the strip or follicular unit extraction technique, the balding area is prepared by using a microblade or punch needle to form small recipient sites that allow for placement of the follicular units.

The imaging appearance of the donor site in cases of hair transplantation will depend on whether the strip harvesting or follicular unit extraction technique is used. For strip harvesting, horizontally oriented linear scars in the suboccipital region may be identified. With the follicular unit extraction technique, numerous punctate oval to linear foci will be identified in the suboccipital region. Similar punctate foci will be identified at the recipient site with either technique. Because of the superior soft tissue resolution of MRI relative to CT, these findings will be more easily identified by MRI.

Donor site using the follicular unit extraction technique

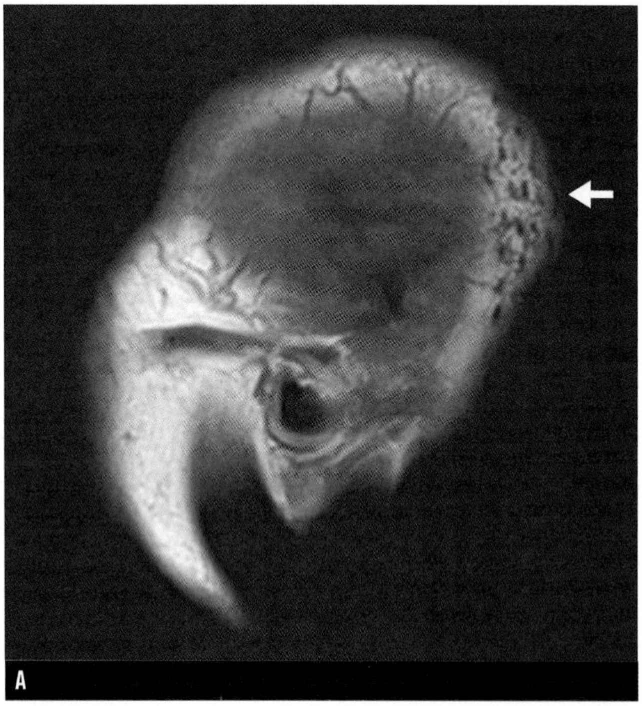

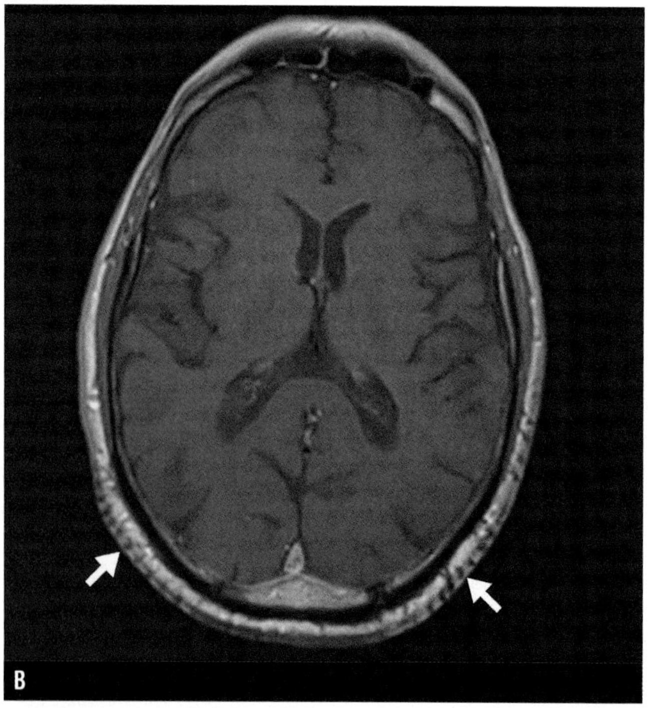

Sagittal T1 (**A**), axial T1 (**B**), and axial T2 (**C**) MR images demonstrate multiple punctate, oval to linear foci within the posterior scalp (arrows, **A-C**). These foci represent the sequela of a follicular extraction technique performed at the donor site during a hair transplantation procedure.

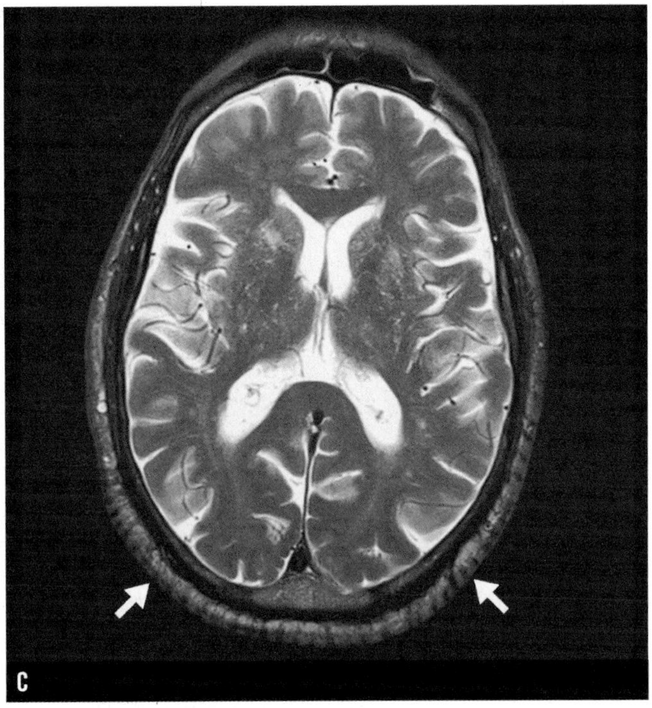

Donor site using the follicular unit extraction technique and recipient site

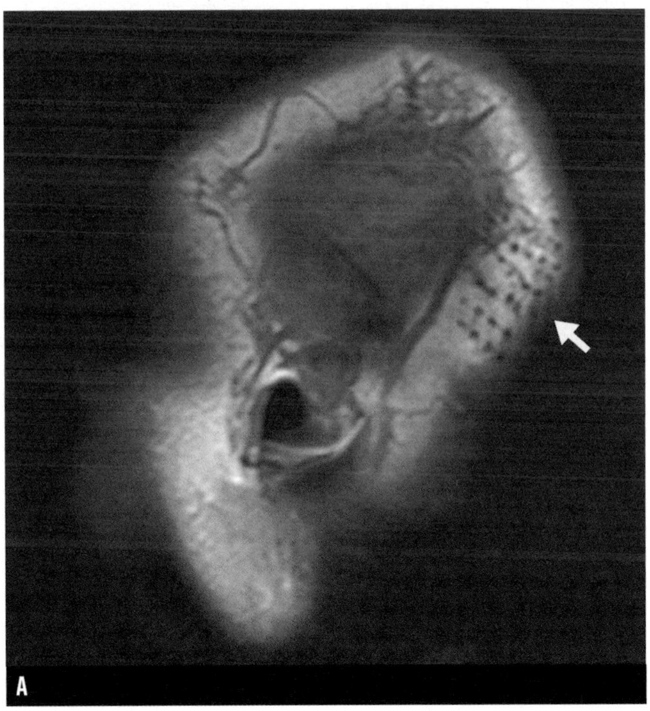

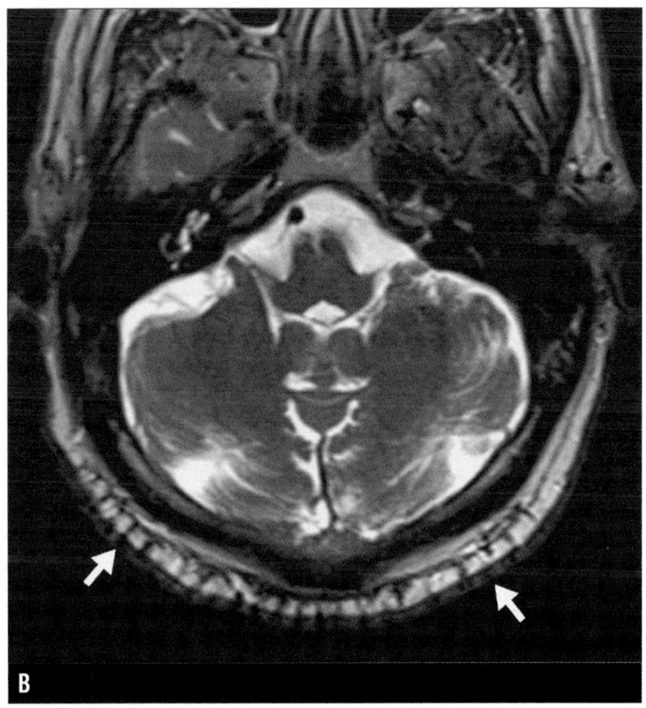

Different patient. Sagittal T1 (**A**), axial T2 (**B**), and contrast-enhanced axial T1 with fat suppression (**C**) MR images demonstrate numerous punctate, linear foci within the occipital scalp (arrows, **A-C**). These foci represent the sequela of the follicular extraction technique performed at the donor site during hair transplantation. Sagittal T1 (**D**), axial T2 (**E**), and axial FLAIR (**F**) MR images from the same study demonstrate numerous oval foci at the location of the recipient site (ie, balding site) for the hair follicles (arrowheads, **D-F**) as well as a portion of the donor site (arrows, **D-F**). An unenhanced axial CT image of the same patient (**G**) demonstrates the CT correlate of the follicular extraction technique sequela (arrows, **G**).

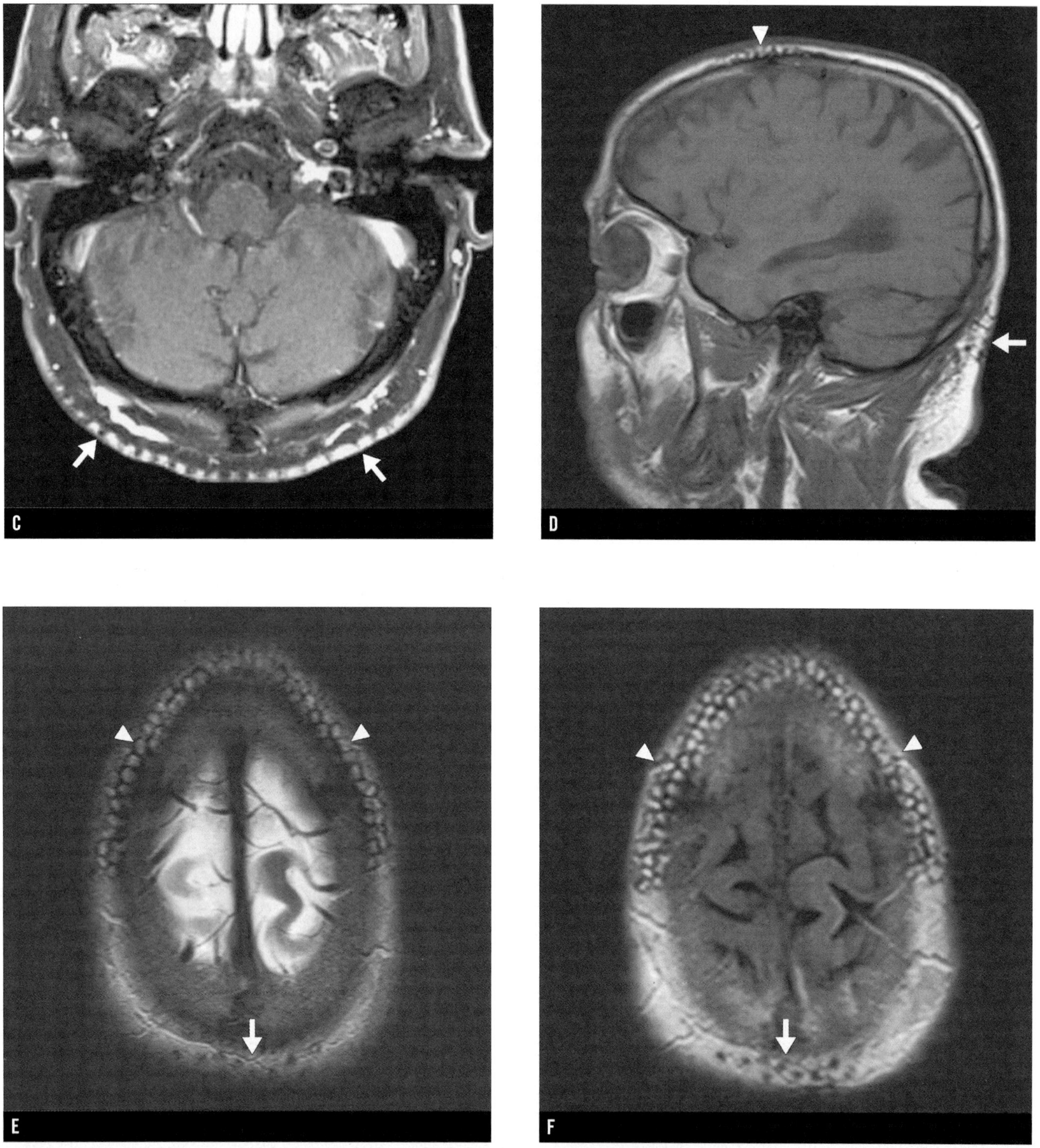
C
D
E
F

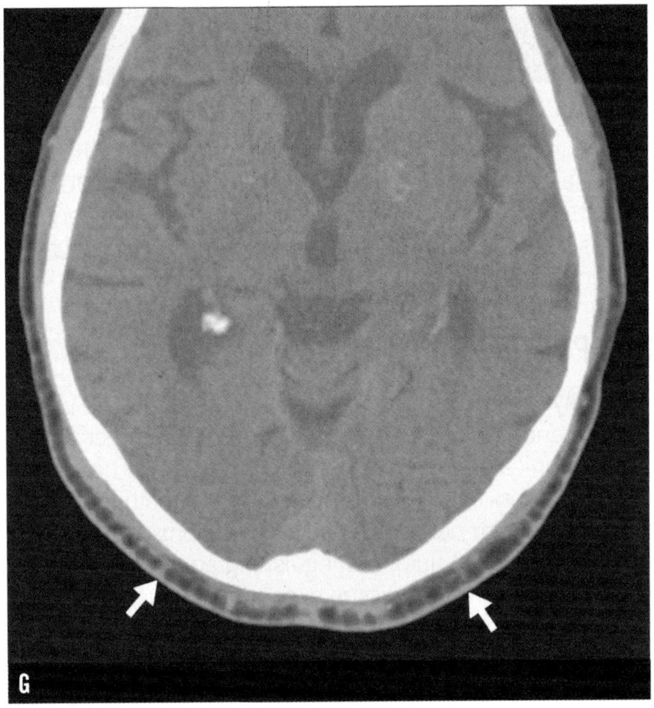

REFERENCES

Avram M, Rogers N. Contemporary hair transplantation. *Dermatol Surg.* November 2009;35(11):1705-1719.

Dua A, Dua K. Follicular unit extraction hair transplant. *J Cutan Aesthet Surg.* 2010;3(2):76-81.

Lee TS, Minton TJ. An update on hair restoration therapy. *Curr Opin Otolaryngol Head Neck Surg.* 2009;17(4):287-294.

As the name implies, soft tissue expanders are surgically placed materials that are used to stretch skin. In regard to the scalp and calvarium, the stretched skin formed by soft tissue expanders is utilized to repair large scalp defects or an underlying calvarial abnormality that requires a large amount of tissue for optimal repair. Examples of scalp or calvarial abnormalities that may require such a repair include those that occur following severe burns, large posttraumatic defects, congenital deformities, or following some craniectomies and cranioplasties. Soft tissue expanders are most commonly utilized during a staged repair, often slowly increasing the volume of the tissue expander over a period of several weeks to months. This allows the skin/scalp to slowly stretch until the desired amount is able to be harvested for the repair.

Tissue expanders come in various shapes and sizes, and their shape can be customized. Typical soft tissue expanders are filled with normal saline, and the expander ports can be located either internally or externally.

On imaging, soft tissue expanders contain fluid attenuation and signal on CT and MRI, respectively. Metallic artifact may be present if a metallic valve is present. A fibrous capsule surrounding the expander may develop and enhance on imaging.

COMPANION CASE

- **Ommaya reservoir.** Ommaya reservoirs are placed in the scalp and are attached to an intracranial catheter which communicates with the ventricular system. These reservoirs allow for direct installation of chemotherapy into the ventricular cerebrospinal fluid and long-term access of cerebrospinal fluid. Distinguishing an Ommaya reservoir from a scalp soft tissue expander is usually obvious, as tissue expanders are typically much larger, may have a distinctly different shape, and are not connected to an intracranial catheter.

Scalp soft tissue expanders

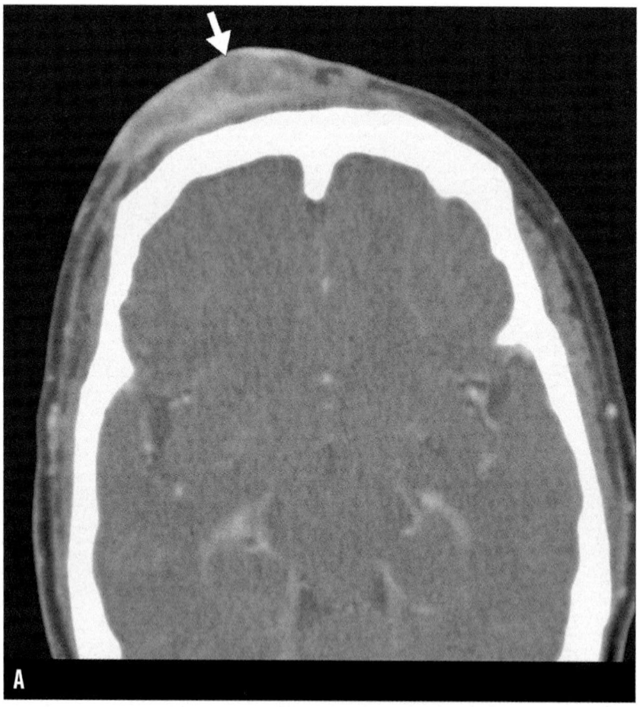

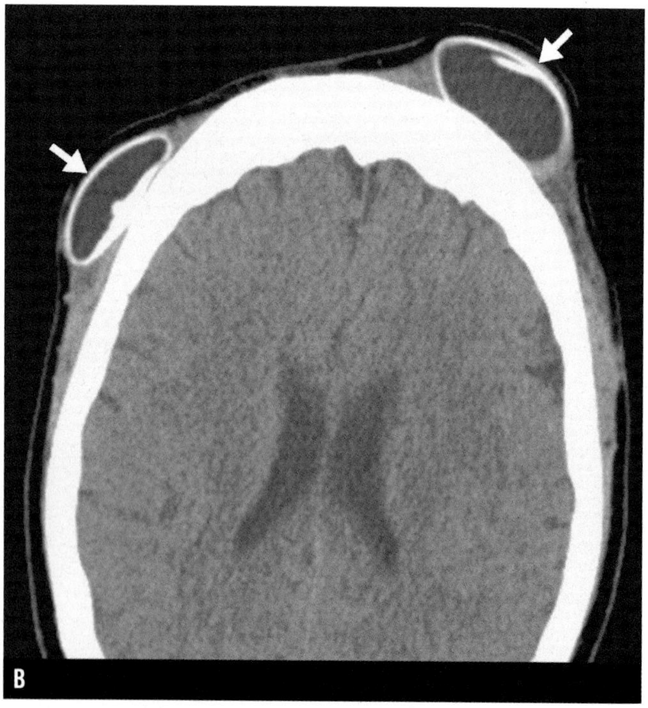

A contrast-enhanced axial CT image (**A**) demonstrates a focal soft tissue inflammatory process involving the right forehead soft tissues (arrow, **A**). This was related to silicone injections that became infected and resulted in granulomatous formation with skin necrosis. Unenhanced axial (**B**) and coronal reformatted (**C**) CT images demonstrate oval soft tissue expanders within the scalp (arrows, **B**, **C**). These soft tissue expanders were placed to stretch the scalp in order to perform future skin grafting. An unenhanced axial CT image following scalp repair (**D**) demonstrates only mild focal soft tissue thickening along the right aspect of the forehead (arrow, **D**).

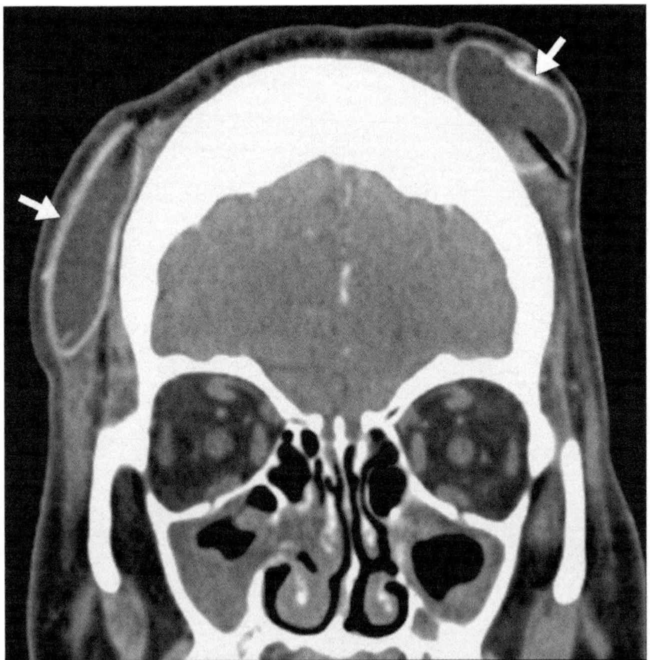
C

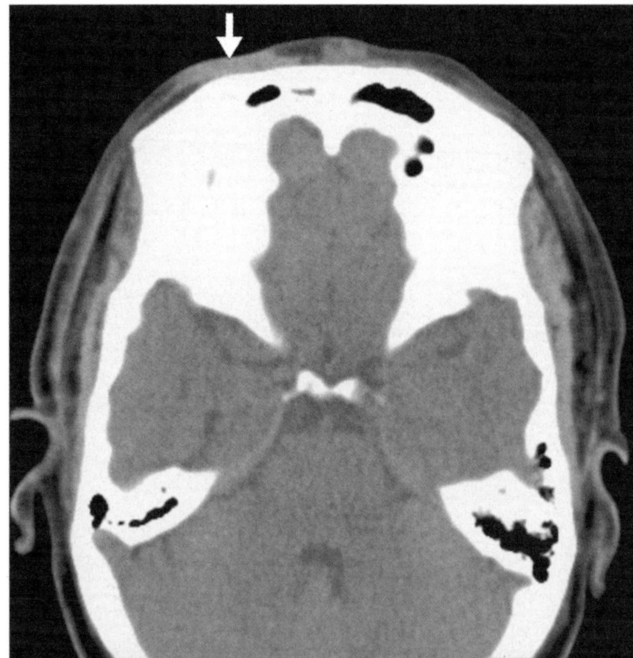
D

Companion case: Ommaya reservoir

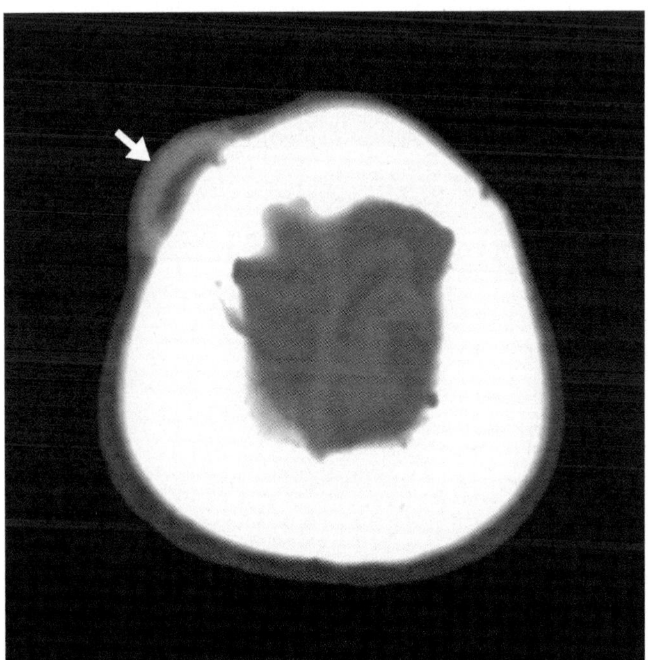
A

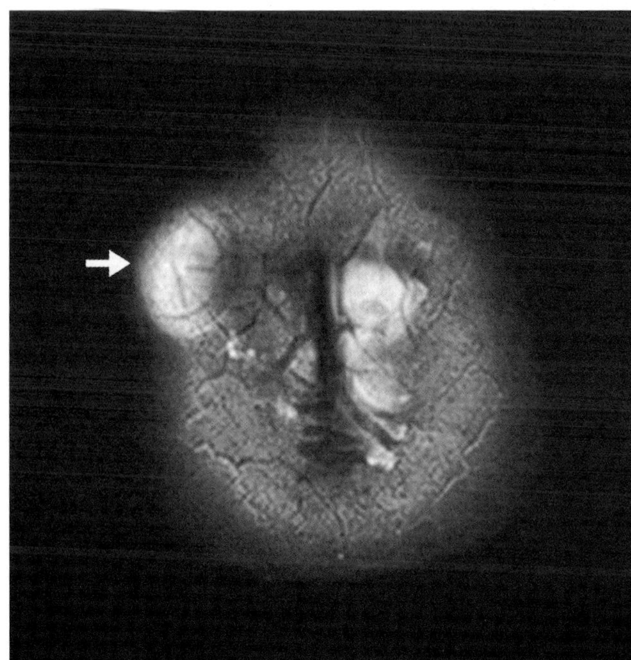
B

An unenhanced axial CT image (**A**) as well as axial T2 (**B**), axial T1 (**C**), and contrast-enhanced fat-suppressed coronal T1 (**D**) MR images demonstrate an Ommaya reservoir within the right vertex scalp soft tissues (arrows, **A**-**D**). This was attached to an intracranial catheter which terminated in the ventricular system (not shown).

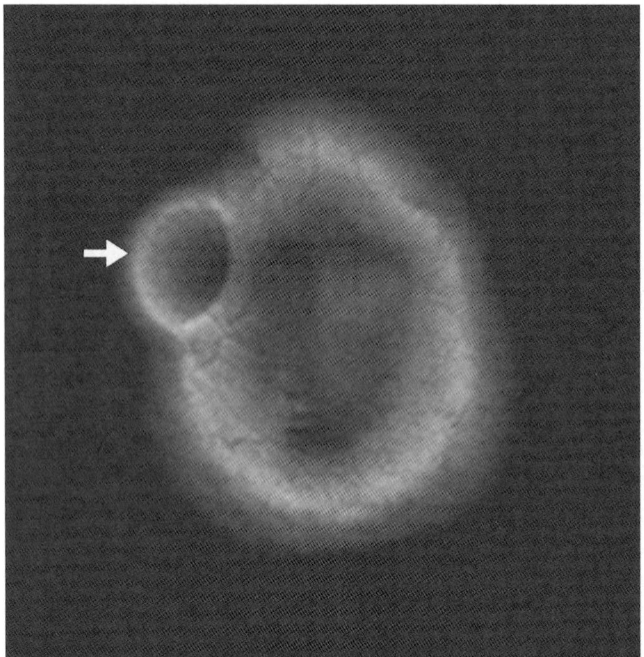

C

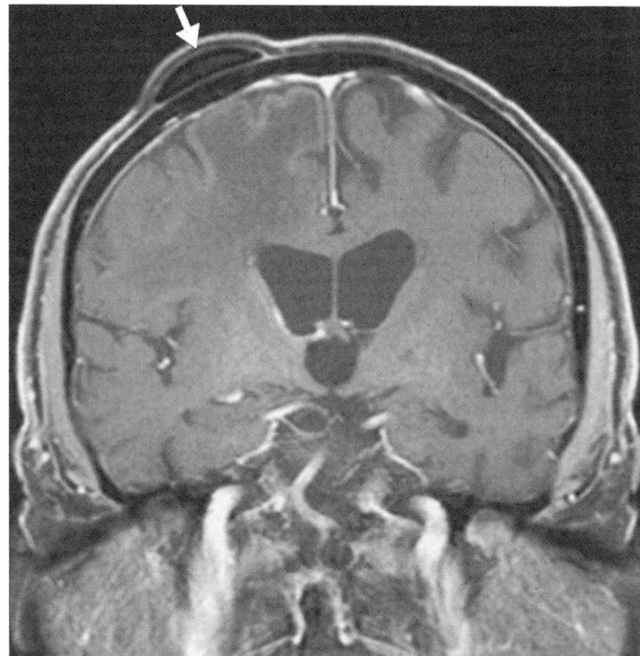

D

REFERENCES

Awad MM. The effect of tissue expanders on the growing craniofacial skeleton. *Indian J Plast Surg.* 2006;39:22-28.

Dickerman RD, Eisenberg MB. Preassembled method for insertion of Ommaya reservoir. *J Surg Oncol.* 2005;89(1):36-38.

Duffy FJ, May JM. Tissue expanders and magnetic resonance imaging: the "hot" breast implant. *Ann Plast Surg.* 1995;35(6):647-649.

Saunders A, Davies AM, Grimer RJ. Magnetic resonance imaging of soft tissue expanders used in the management of musculoskeletal sarcomas. *Br J Radiol.* 1998;7(849):926-929.

Wollina U, Bayyoud Y. Reconstruction of a large scalp defect by the sequential use of dermal substitute, self-filling osmotic tissue expander and rotation flap. *J Cutan Aesthet Surg.* 2010;3:106-110.

CASE 19 Cranioplasties

A cranioplasty is performed to repair a calvarial defect. This procedure has been performed as early as the Renaissance period, and various materials have been used since that time, including gold, silver, and even coconuts. The procedure most often follows removal of a portion of the skull (ie, craniectomy), but it may also be performed in conjunction with a craniotomy to repair congenital skull defects or a posttraumatic calvarial injury. A craniectomy may sometimes be associated with a "sinking skin flap syndrome," also referred to as trephine syndrome. This phenomenon occurs because the pressure of the exposed intracranial compartment is exceeded by the atmospheric pressure. Occasionally, this phenomenon may result in decreased cerebral perfusion, and the degree of retraction may result in significant brain herniation which may require immediate surgical attention. Fortunately, this complication can be readily reversed with a cranioplasty which effectively removes the pressure gradient that causes the sunken brain morphology.

Today, several materials may be used during a cranioplasty, and the imaging characteristics will vary depending on the substance used. Autologous bone is the preferred material used for a cranioplasty, as several studies have demonstrated a lower complication rate when using autologous bone. When autologous bone is not an option, calcium phosphate cement, methyl methacrylate cement, alumina ceramics, bioplastics, bioresorbable scaffolds, titanium, and acrylic resins may be used. Some of these materials may be molded at the time of surgery or may be prefabricated. Calcium phosphate cements will be the same density as bone, although the morphology and thickness of the cement generally differs from the native calvarium and is usually readily discriminated. Acrylic cranioplasty is lucent relative to normal bone and may contain air bubbles that are incorporated during mixing of the resin. On MRI, acrylic will be devoid of signal. Titanium may be utilized in the form of a plate or mesh. As expected, titanium will be hyperattenuating on CT and lack signal on MRI.

Utilizing ribs as construct for a cranioplasty is rarely performed today, particularly because there are numerous other materials currently available the are well tolerated and incur less morbidity. However, rib grafts utilized for a cranioplasty have some positive attributes. They are bendable, have low infection rates, have high fusion rates, and represent an autologous bone source, the latter eliminating the risk of a foreign body reaction. In addition, at least when performed in children, there is almost complete regeneration of the resected rib at the harvest site. On the other hand, a scar and pain may occur at the rib harvest site, the overall procedure time is longer, and the cranioplasty may have an irregular contour. In most cases, the seventh and/or eighth ribs are harvested and an osteotome is used to section the rib(s) in half length-wise; thus, this procedure is often termed a "split-rib" cranioplasty. The ribs are purposefully harvested slightly longer than expected for the size of the craniectomy site. The ribs are bent with a bone bender and then wedged into place within the craniectomy site. Because they are harvested slightly long, the ribs are under mild tension within the craniectomy site which allows for a mild convex bowing and conformation with the remainder of the skull. The ribs are then affixed into place.

Trephine syndrome treated with an autologous cranioplasty flap

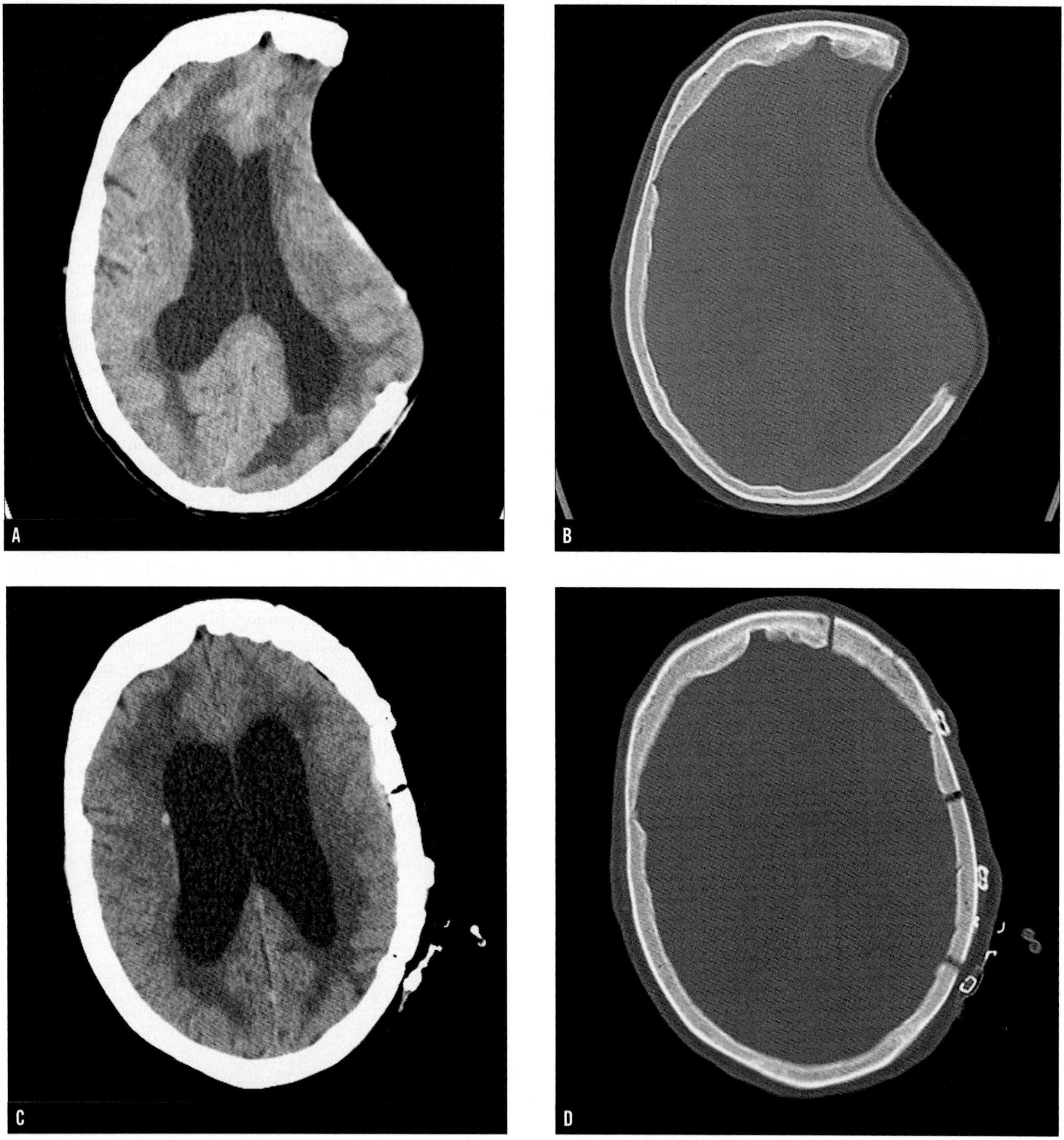

Axial CT images viewed with a brain window (**A**) and bone window (**B**) demonstrate a large left craniectomy defect with a sunken appearance of the brain and left-to-right subfalcine brain herniation, compatible with trephine syndrome. The following day, the patient underwent a cranioplasty. Axial CT images viewed with a brain window (**C**) and bone window (**D**) obtained immediately after the cranioplasty procedure demonstrate the bone flap to be composed of two pieces, but is otherwise of the same density and configuration as the remainder of the calvarium, compatible with an autologous bone flap. The trephine syndrome and associated left-to-right subfalcine brain herniation are completely resolved following the procedure, an expected benefit of the cranioplasty.

Cranioplasty utilizing methyl methacrylate cement

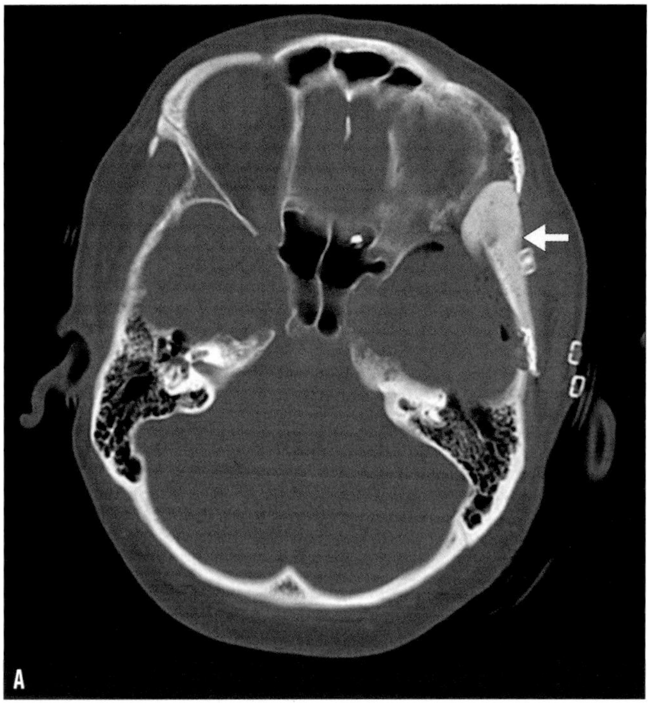

An axial CT image (**A**) demonstrates a left pterional cranioplasty, in this case utilizing methyl methacrylate bone cement (arrow).

Cranioplasty utilizing prefabricated acrylic resin

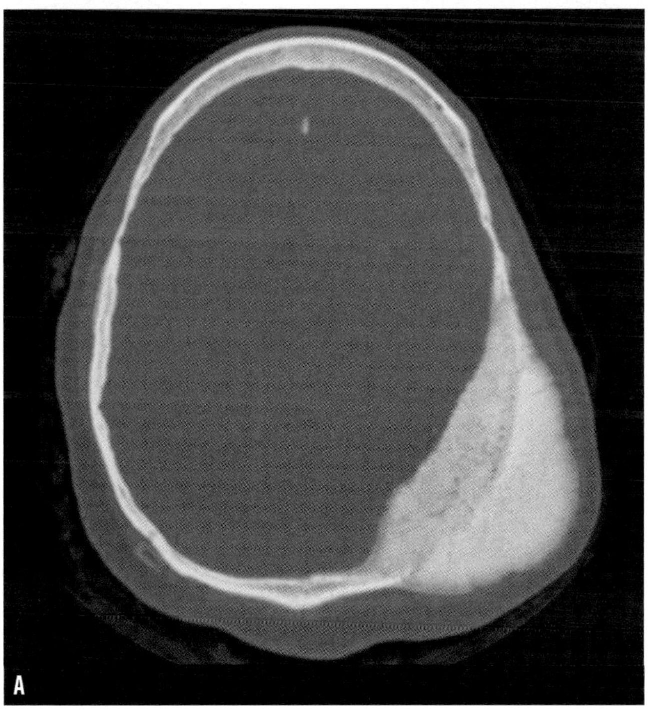

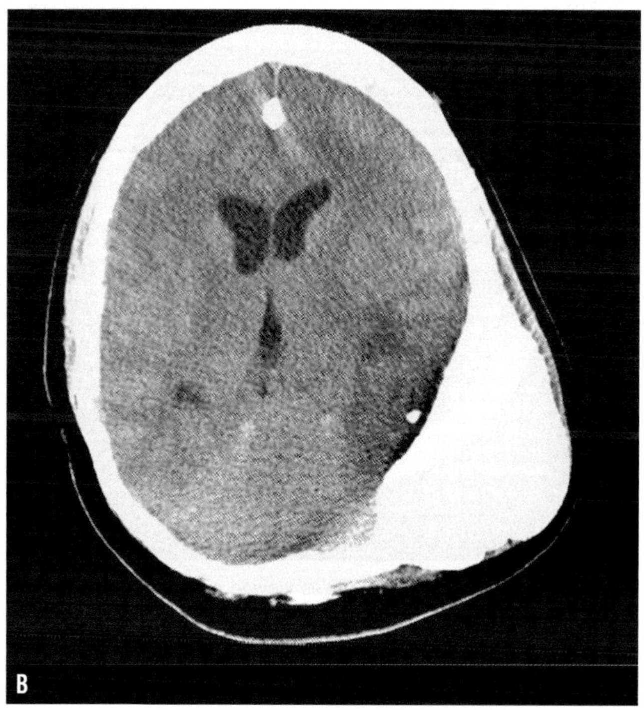

Axial CT images viewed with a bone window (**A**) and brain window (**B**) demonstrate a large ossified mass involving the left parietal calvarium which represents a large intraosseous meningioma. An axial CT image viewed with a bone window following tumor resection and a cranioplasty (**C**) demonstrates a prefabricated acrylic resin flap that was used to close the osseous defect (arrow, **C**).

Cranioplasty performed during the Vietnam War

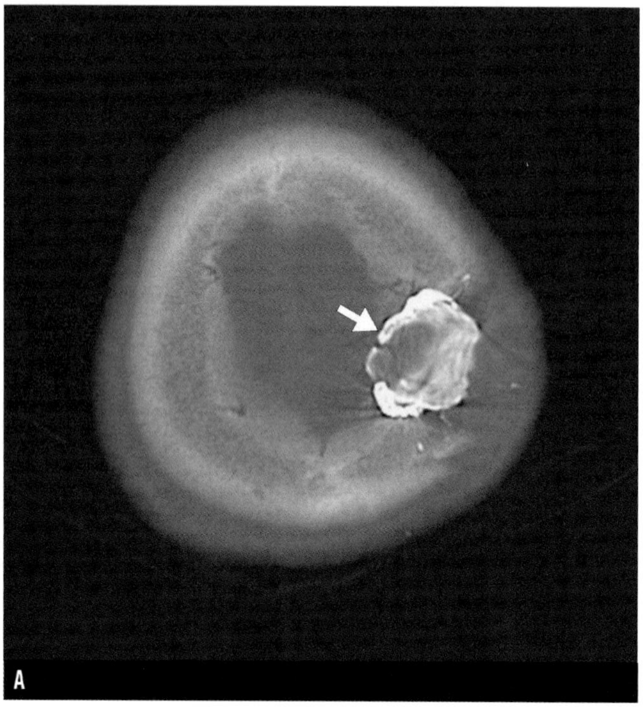

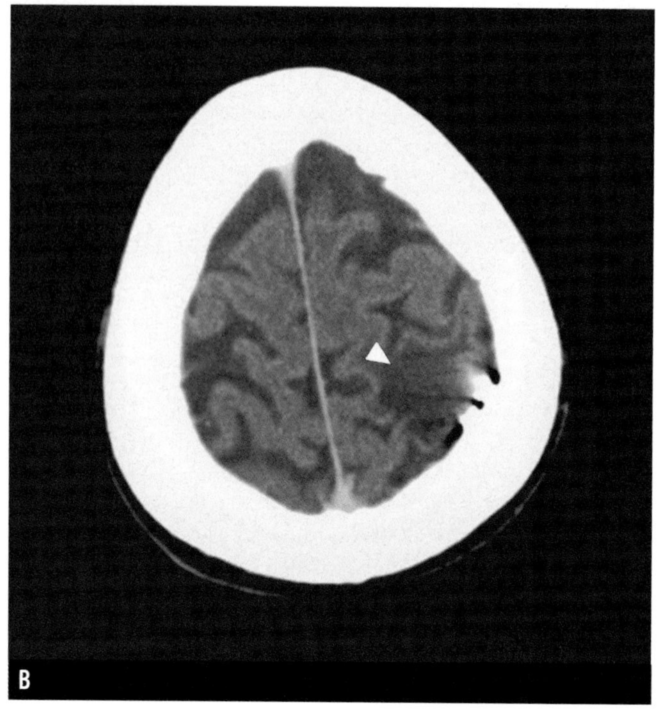

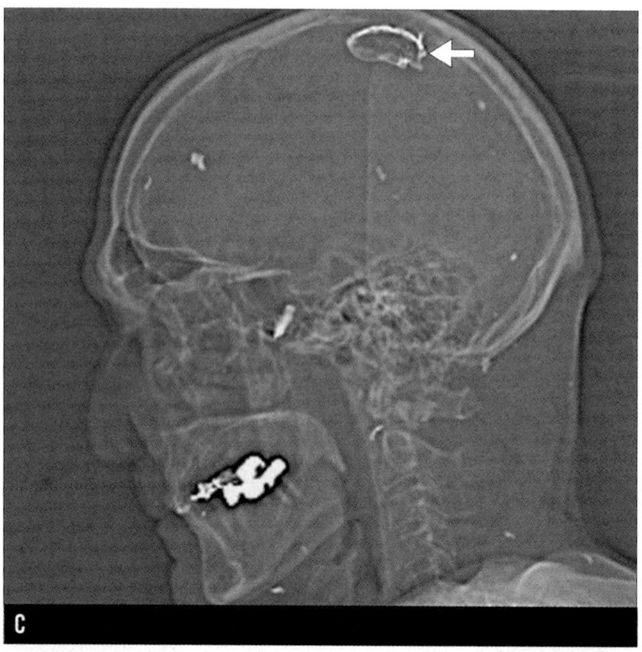

An axial CT image viewed with a bone window (**A**) demonstrates a round hyperattenuating prosthesis within a left vertex craniotomy (arrow, **A**). This represents cranioplasty material that was placed during the Vietnam War after a patient sustained a calvarial injury during combat. An axial CT image viewed with a brain window (**B**) demonstrates underlying encephalomalacia (arrowhead, **B**). Image **C** demonstrates the cranioplasty material (arrow, **C**) as well as numerous other small metallic objects that represent shrapnel. The type of material used for a cranioplasty during the Vietnam War depended on the surgeon's preference, defect size, and topography of the defect. However, the most common material used during that time was acrylic. Other materials used included vitallium, tantalum, stainless steel, silastic, and autologous bone.

Split rib cranioplasty

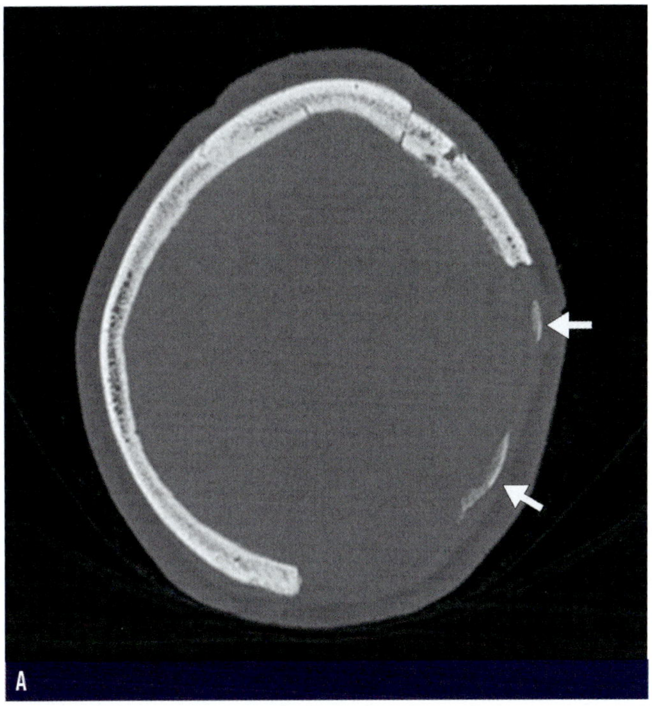

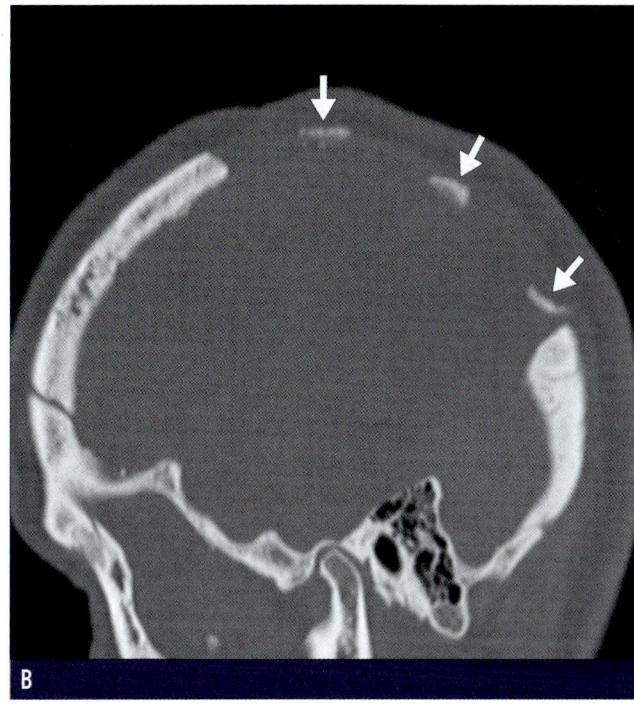

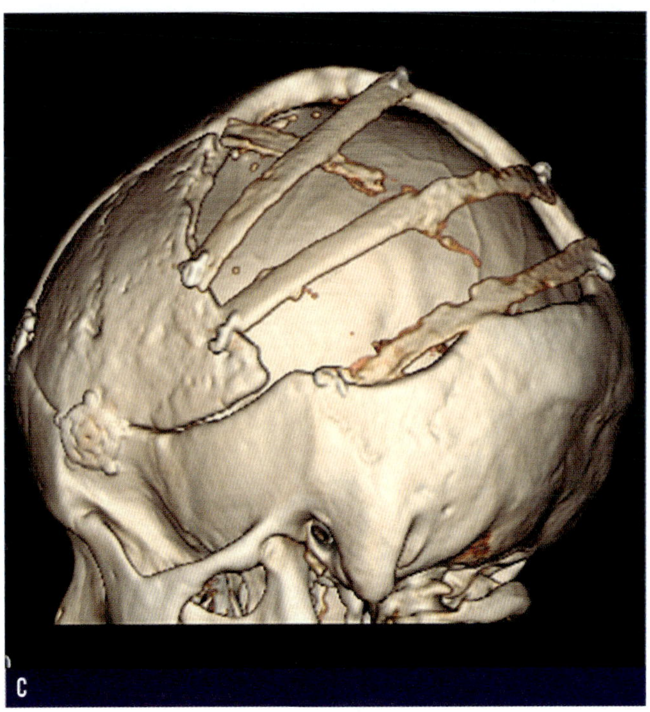

Axial (**A**) and sagittal reformatted (**B**) CT images demonstrate linear strips of bone traversing a large left craniectomy defect, representing a split rib cranioplasty (arrows, **A**, **B**). A 3D reconstruction of these images (**C**) demonstrates the findings to a better advantage.

REFERENCES

Beekmans SJ, Don Griot JP, Mulder JW. Split rib cranioplasty for aplasia cutis congenita and traumatic skull defects: more than 30 years of follow-up. *J Craniofac Surg.* 2007;18(3):594-597.

Chiang HY, et al. Clinical significance of positive cranial bone flap cultures and associated risk of surgical site infection after craniotomies or craniectomies. *J Neurosurg.* 2011;114(6):1746-1754.

Munro IR, Guyuron B. Split-rib cranioplasty. *Ann Plast Surg.* 1981;7(5):341-346.

Rish BL, et al. Cranioplasty: a review of 1030 cases of penetrating head injury. *Neurosurgery.* 1979;4(5):381-385.

Sinclair AG, Scoffings DJ. Imaging of the post-operative cranium. *Radiographics.* 2010;30(2): 461-482.

Spetzger U, et al. Materials and techniques for osseous skull reconstruction. *Minim Invasive Ther Allied Technol.* 2010;19(2):110-121.

Taggard DA, Menezes AH. Successful use of rib grafts for cranioplasty in children. *Pediatr Neurosurg.* 2001;34(3):149-155.

CHAPTER 12

VASCULAR

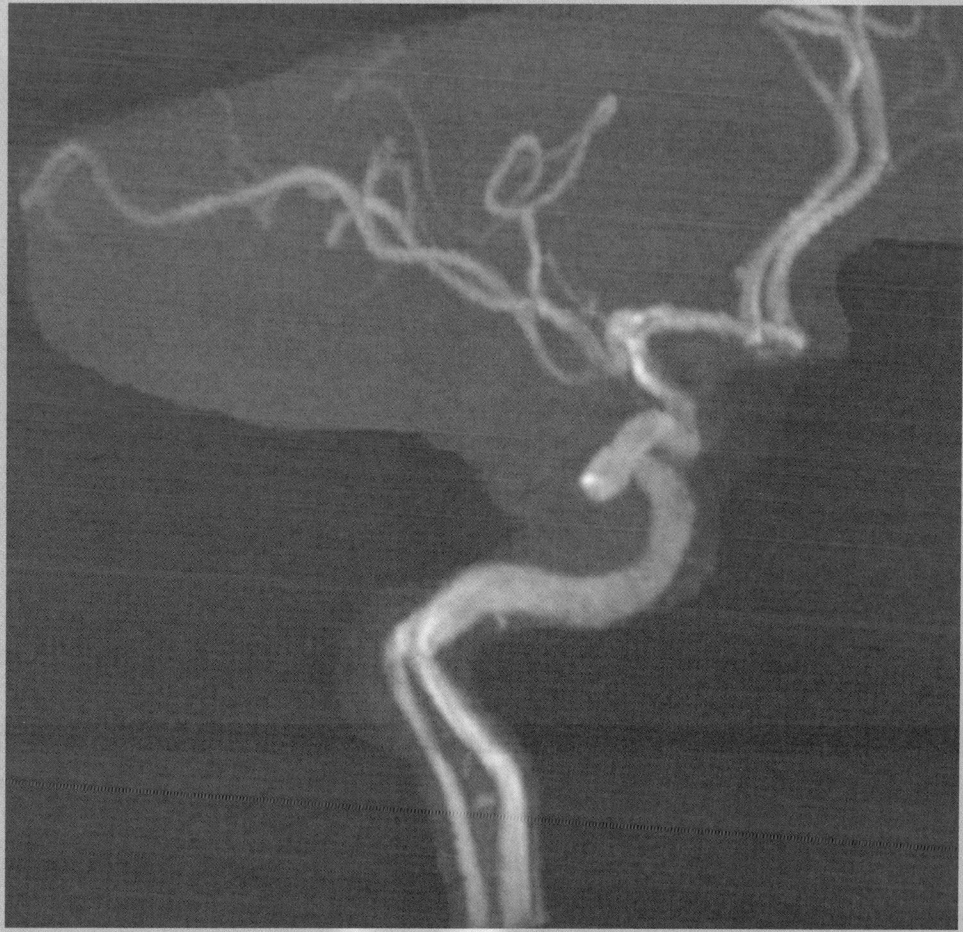

Rishi Seth, Achilles G. Karagianis,
Matthew T. Walker

XII. VASCULAR

1. Common origin of the innominate and left common carotid arteries
   i. *Companion case*: Left common carotid artery originating from the innominate artery
   ii. *Companion case*: Left ECA and left ICA originating from the aortic arch
   iii. *Companion case*: Left ECA originating from the aortic arch and the left ICA originating from the left subclavian artery
2. Right aortic arch and its various branching patterns
3. Left aortic arch with an aberrant right subclavian artery
4. Variations of vertebral artery origin
5. Extraforaminal course of the cervical vertebral artery
6. Hypoplastic vertebral artery
7. Vertebral artery fenestration
8. Cervical vertebral artery tortuosity, kinks, and loops
   i. *Companion case*: Acute cervical vertebral artery dissection
   ii. *Companion case*: Cervical vertebral artery dissection with pseudoaneurysm formation
   iii. *Companion case*: Fibromuscular dysplasia with cervical vertebral artery pseudoaneurysm formation
   iv. *Companion case*: Cervical vertebral artery venous plexus on MRI
9. Retropharyngeal course of the cervical carotid arteries
10. Variation in the location of a carotid artery bifurcation
11. Carotid web
12. Cervical carotid artery tortuosity, kinks, and loops
   i. *Companion case*: Fibromuscular dysplasia
13. Absence of the ICA
14. Persistent pharyngohyoid artery with a normal ipsilateral cervical ICA ("duplicated internal carotid artery")
   i. *Companion case*: Aberrant ICA
15. Carotid endarterectomy
   i. *Companion case*: Chronic cervical ICA dissection with pseudoaneurysm formation and a contralateral acute cervical ICA dissection
   ii. *Companion case*: Carotid endarterectomy with residual thrombosis and a superimposed cervical carotid dissection
   iii. *Companion case*: Carotid endarterectomy with a patch angioplasty and contralateral cervical carotid stent placement
16. Surgical arterial bypass grafts, transpositions, and interposition grafts
17. Persistent embryonic carotid-basilar anastomoses (persistent fetal circulation variants)
18. MRI and CT artifacts of neck vessels

CASE 1 Common origin of the innominate and left common carotid arteries

More than 20 different aortic arch configurations have been described in humans. Of these, the most common aortic branching pattern has separate origins for the innominate, left common carotid, and left subclavian arteries. The second most common branching pattern is a common origin of the innominate and left common carotid arteries, often described as a "common trunk" or a "bovine arch." However, in reality, the aortic arch in bovine gives rise to a single large trunk. Each subclavian artery arises from this large trunk as does a bicarotid trunk, which in turn gives rise to each common carotid artery. This true bovine configuration is rare in humans. Some authors suggest that the term "bovine arch" may have arisen from its cattle horn appearance demonstrated on conventional angiography.

COMPANION CASES

- **Left common carotid artery originating from the innominate artery.** A similar, but less common variation compared to the common origin of the innominate and left common carotid arteries occurs when the left common carotid artery originates as a branch of the proximal innominate artery, rather than as a common trunk.
- **Left ECA and left ICA originating from the aortic arch.** This is an extremely rare variation with only a few case reports described in the literature. In this case, the left common carotid artery never develops. The embryology of this variant is complex and beyond the scope of this text.
- **Left ECA originating from the aortic arch and the left ICA originating from the left subclavian artery.** This variant is similar to the immediately preceding case, except that the left ICA originates from the left subclavian artery instead of the aortic arch. The left common carotid artery also never develops in this setting.

Common origin of the innominate and left common carotid arteries

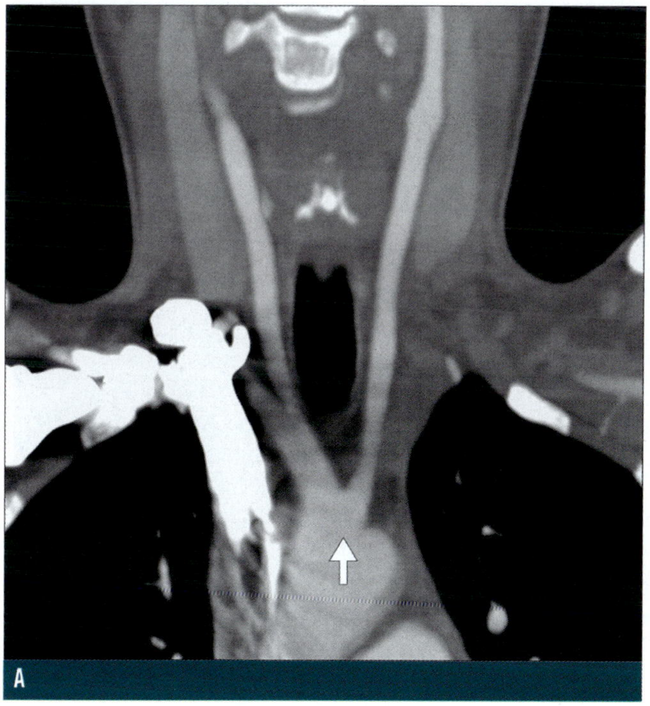

A coronal reformatted image from a CT angiogram of the neck (**A**) demonstrates a short common trunk originating from the aortic arch that gives rise to the innominate and left common carotid arteries (arrow).

Companion case: Left common carotid artery originating from the innominate artery

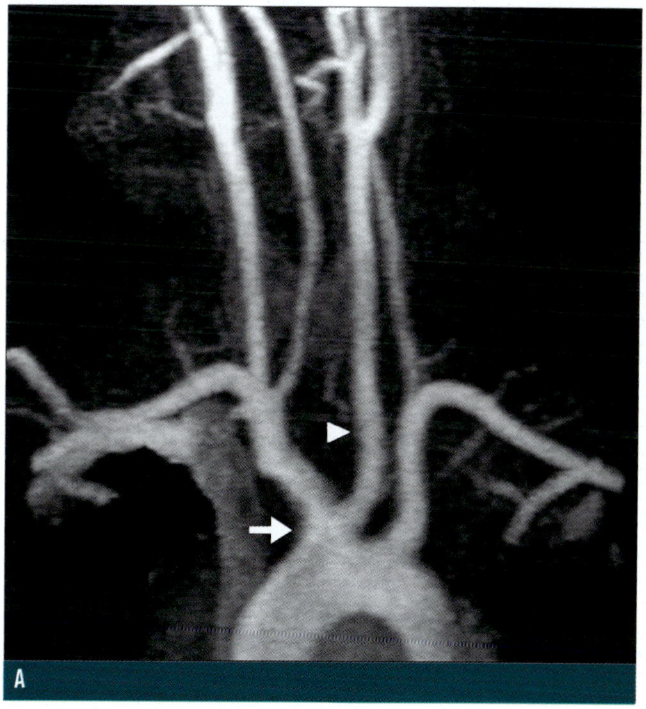

An oblique MIP image from a contrast-enhanced MR angiogram of the neck (**A**) demonstrates a "two-vessel" aortic arch in which the left common carotid artery (arrowhead) originates as a branch along the proximal aspect of the innominate artery (arrow).

Companion case: Left ECA and left ICA originating from the aortic arch

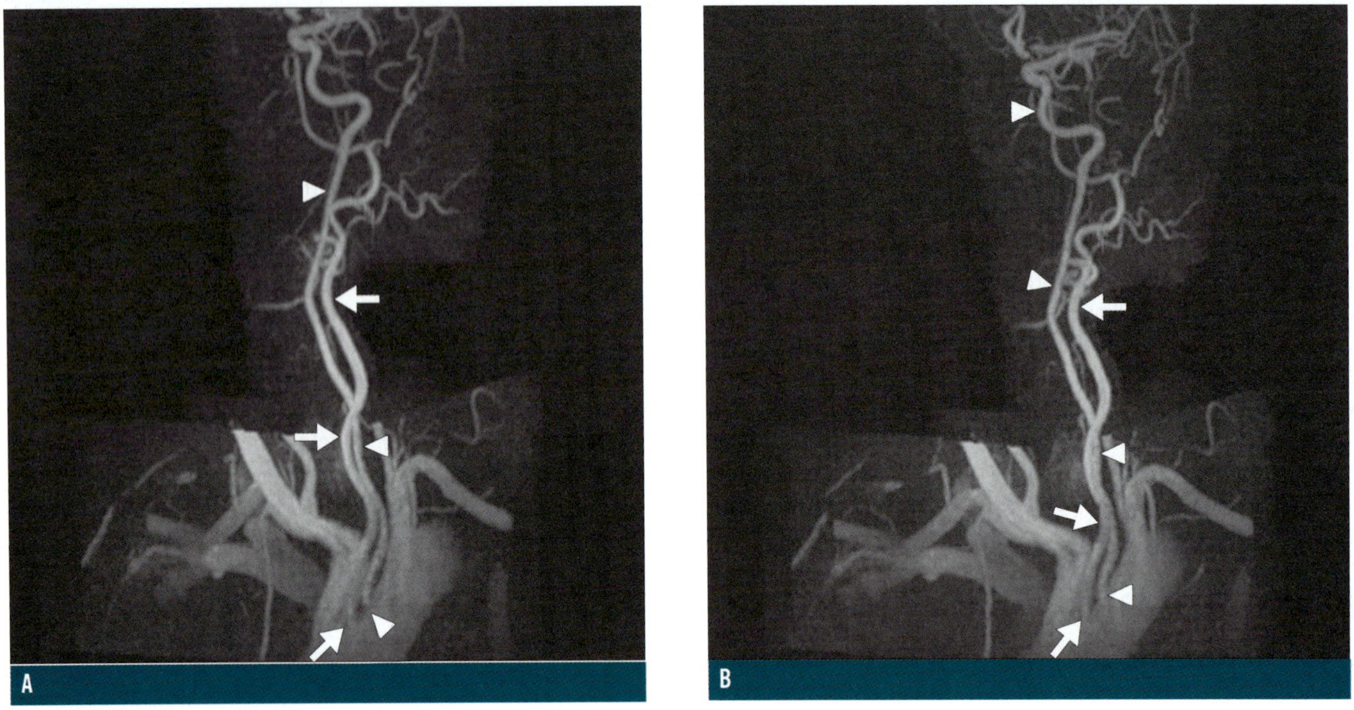

MIP images from a gadolinium-enhanced MRA of the neck (**A, B**) demonstrate both the left ECA (arrows, **A**, **B**) and the left ICA (arrowheads, **A**, **B**) originating directly from the aortic arch. The left common carotid artery never formed.

Companion case: Left ECA originating from the aortic arch and the left ICA originating from the left subclavian artery

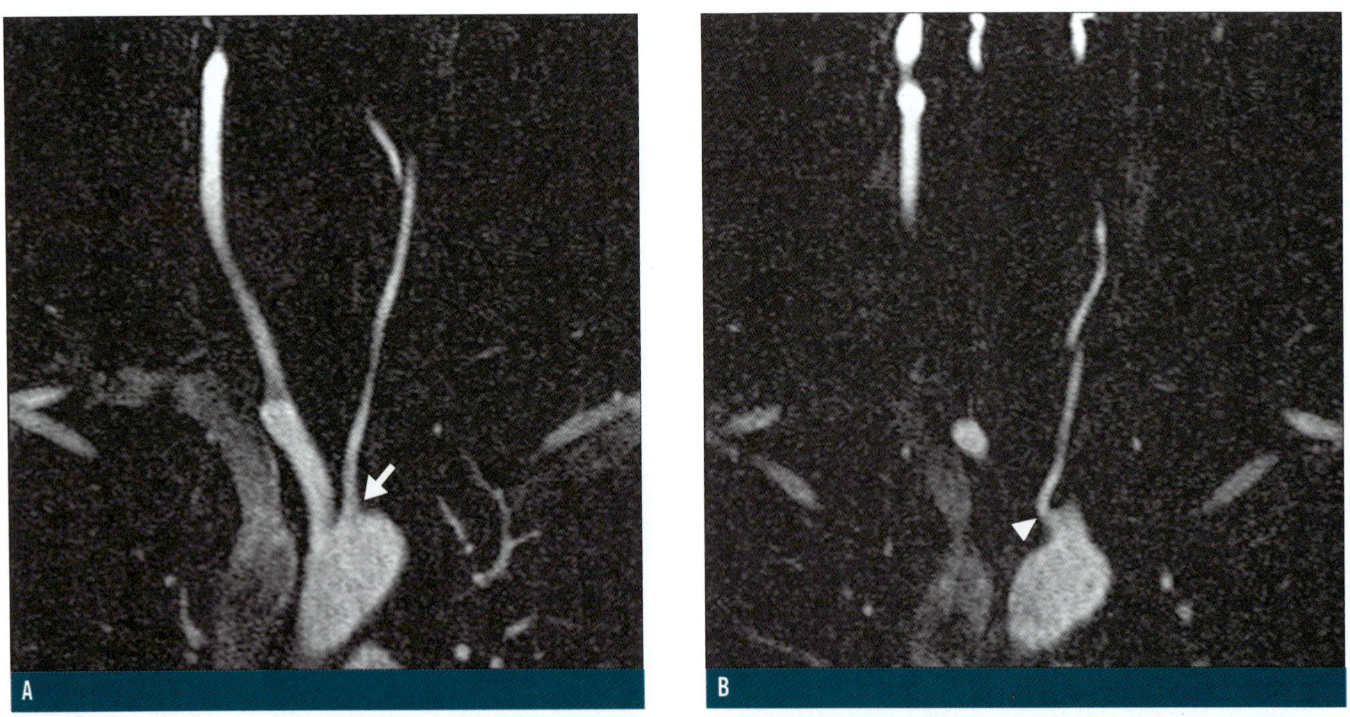

Coronal source images from a gadolinium-infused MRA of the neck (**A**, **B**) demonstrate unusual origins of the left ECA arising from the aortic arch (arrow, **A**) and the left ICA arising from the proximal left subclavian artery (arrowhead, **B**). A MIP image of the left carotid artery (**C**) demonstrates the left ECA (arrows, **C**) and the left ICA (arrowheads, **C**) along their entire course within the neck. The left common carotid artery never developed.

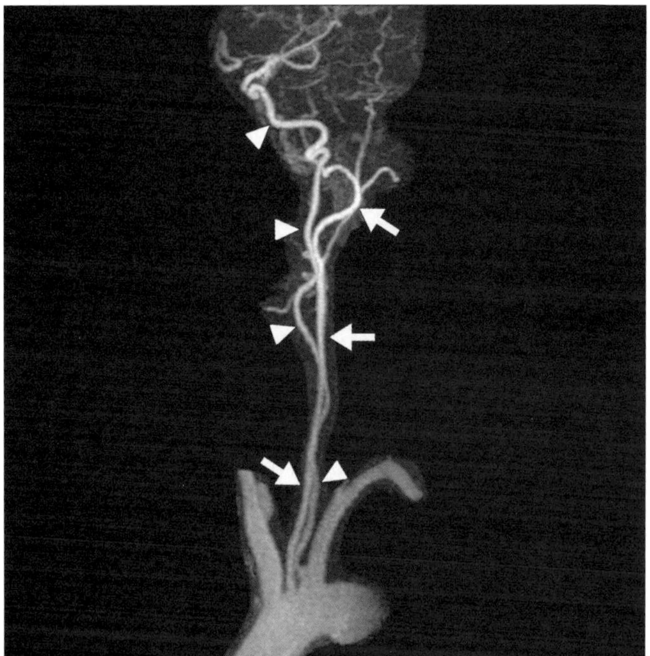

C

REFERENCES

Cakirer S, Karaarslan E, Kayabali M, Rozanes I. Separate origins of the left internal and external carotid arteries from the aortic arch: MR angiographic findings. *AJNR Am J Neuroradiol.* 2002;23(9):1600-1602.

Layton KF, Kallmes DF, Cloft HJ, Lindell EP, Cox VS. Bovine aortic arch variant in humans: clarification of a common misnomer. *AJNR Am J Neuroradiol.* 2006;27(7):1541-1542.

Vitek JJ. Bovine aortic arch. *AJNR Am J Neuroradiol.* 2007;2487:1205.

CASE 2 Right aortic arch and its various branching patterns

A right aortic arch is present when the aortic arch crosses cephalad to the right main stem bronchus. This variant represents persistence of the right fourth embryonic arch and regression of the left fourth arch. Although the aortic arch is absent on the left side, the descending segment of a right aortic arch may be on either side of the spine. There are three primary subgroups of a right aortic arch. They include a right aortic arch with: an aberrant left subclavian artery, an isolated left subclavian artery, and mirror image branching. When a right arch is present, the organs may be in a normal position or completely reversed, termed normal situs (or situs solitus) and situs inversus, respectively. A right arch variant is commonly identified in patients with congenital anomalies of the cardiovascular system, such as truncus arteriosis, tetralogy of Fallot, and pulmonary atresia with a ventricular septal defect.

- **Right aortic arch with an aberrant left subclavian artery.** The right aortic arch with an aberrant left subclavian artery is the most common right arch configuration and results from an interruption of the left fourth aortic arch between the left common carotid and left subclavian arteries. It also represents the most common cause of a symptom-producing vascular ring, with most cases forming a complete vascular ring because of persistence of the ligamentum arteriosum. While a persistent ligamentum arteriosum is typically not visualized by cross-sectional imaging, its presence can be inferred by a left dorsal aortic root remnant termed the "diverticulum of Kommerell". If a ligamentum arteriosum were visualized, it would be identified extending from the diverticulum of Kommerell to the proximal aspect of the left pulmonary artery. Because the vascular ring with this aortic arch branching pattern completely encircles the trachea and esophagus, it can compress these structures and result in airway symptoms and dysphagia, the latter in this setting referred to as dysphagia lusoria. With a right aortic arch and an aberrant left subclavian artery, the left common carotid artery arises from the arch first, followed by the right common carotid and right subclavian arteries, or alternatively, by the innominate artery. The aberrant left subclavian artery is the last branch to arise from the arch. It courses posterior to the esophagus and originates from the diverticulum of Kommerell. This aortic arch pattern is associated with intracardiac defects in approximately 5% to 10% of patients.
- **Right aortic arch with an isolated left subclavian artery.** Of the three primary subgroups of a right aortic arch, the isolated left subclavian artery variety is the least common. In this case, instead of the subclavian artery arising from the aortic arch or left common carotid artery, it joins the pulmonary artery via a left ductus arteriosis, which may or may not be patent. A right aortic arch with an isolated left subclavian artery may be an incidental finding or it may be identified with congenital heart disease, the most common being tetralogy of Fallot. The primary arterial flow to the isolated left subclavian artery is via retrograde arterial flow through the ipsilateral left vertebral artery, which in turn, receives its blood from the contralateral right vertebral artery. This may or may not result in a symptomatic subclavian steal phenomenon. A portion of the retrograde arterial flow to an isolated left subclavian artery may also occur from ECA collaterals. If there is a patent left ductus arteriosis, then flow from an isolated left subclavian artery will be directed into the pulmonary artery, resulting in a so-called "pulmonary steal", increasing the risk of symptoms.
- **Right aortic arch with mirror image branching.** A right aortic arch with mirror image branching occurs when there is an interruption of the dorsal segment of the left arch between the left subclavian artery and the descending aorta. In this pattern, the normal branching pattern is reversed, with the innominate artery on the left and representing the most proximal branch of the arch, followed in succession by the right common carotid artery and right subclavian artery. This pattern is almost always associated with intracardiac defects (98%).

Right aortic arch with situs inversus

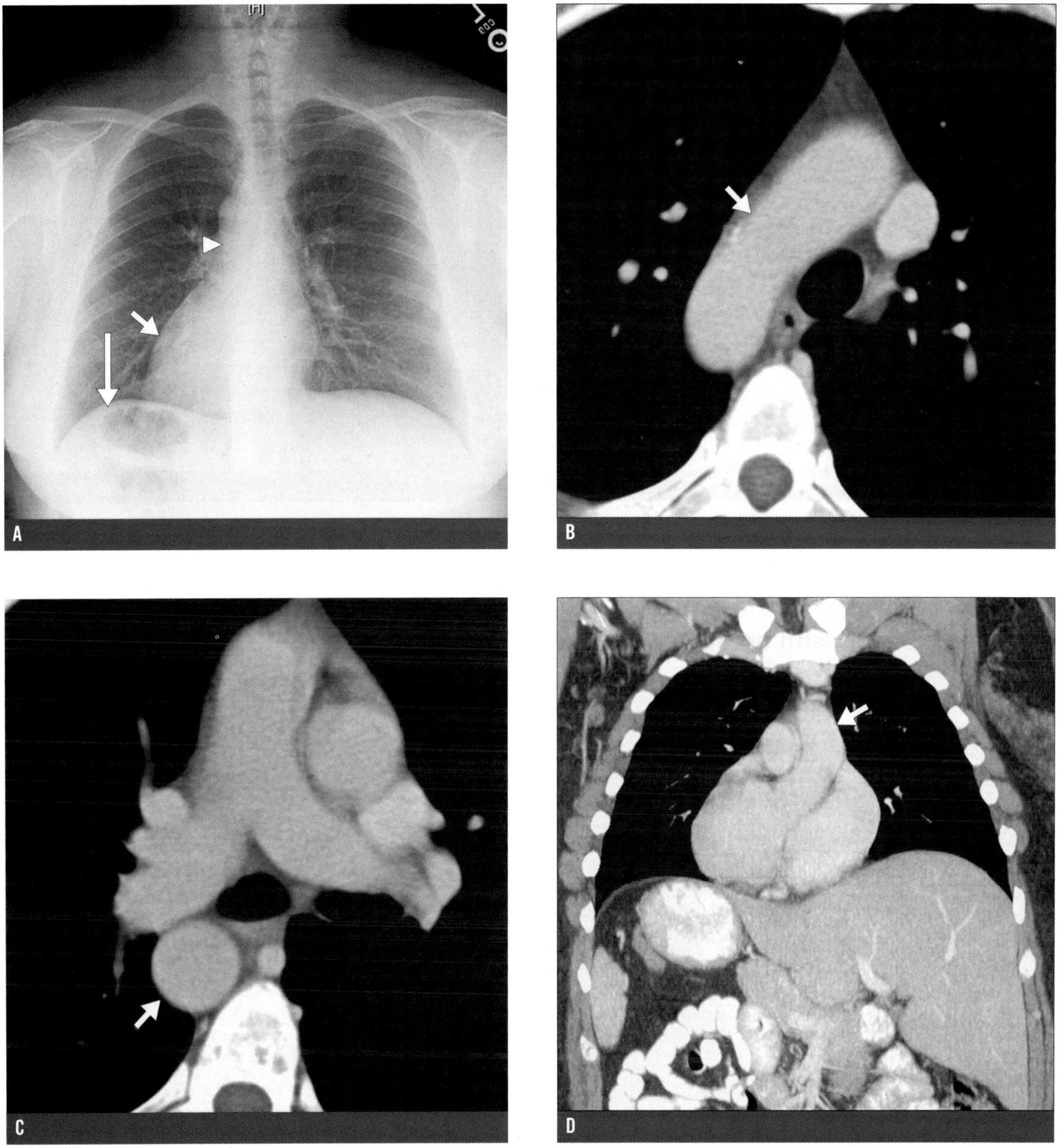

A frontal chest radiograph (**A**) demonstrates a density in the right paratracheal region with loss of the paratracheal stripe, compatible with a right aortic arch (arrowhead, **A**). There is also absence of the aortic knob on the left. The presence of dextrocardia (short arrow, **A**) and right-sided gastric bubble (long arrow, **A**) indicates a situs inversus. Axial postcontrast CT images of the same patient through the aortic arch (**B**) as well as the descending aorta and aortic root (**C**) demonstrate a right-sided aortic arch (short arrow, **B**) and a descending aorta located to the right of midline (short arrow, **C**). Coronal reformatted contrast-enhanced CT images of the same patient (**D-F**) demonstrate the right aortic arch (short arrows, **D, E**) and the right descending aorta (short arrow, **F**). Situs inversus is also demonstrated on images **D-F**.

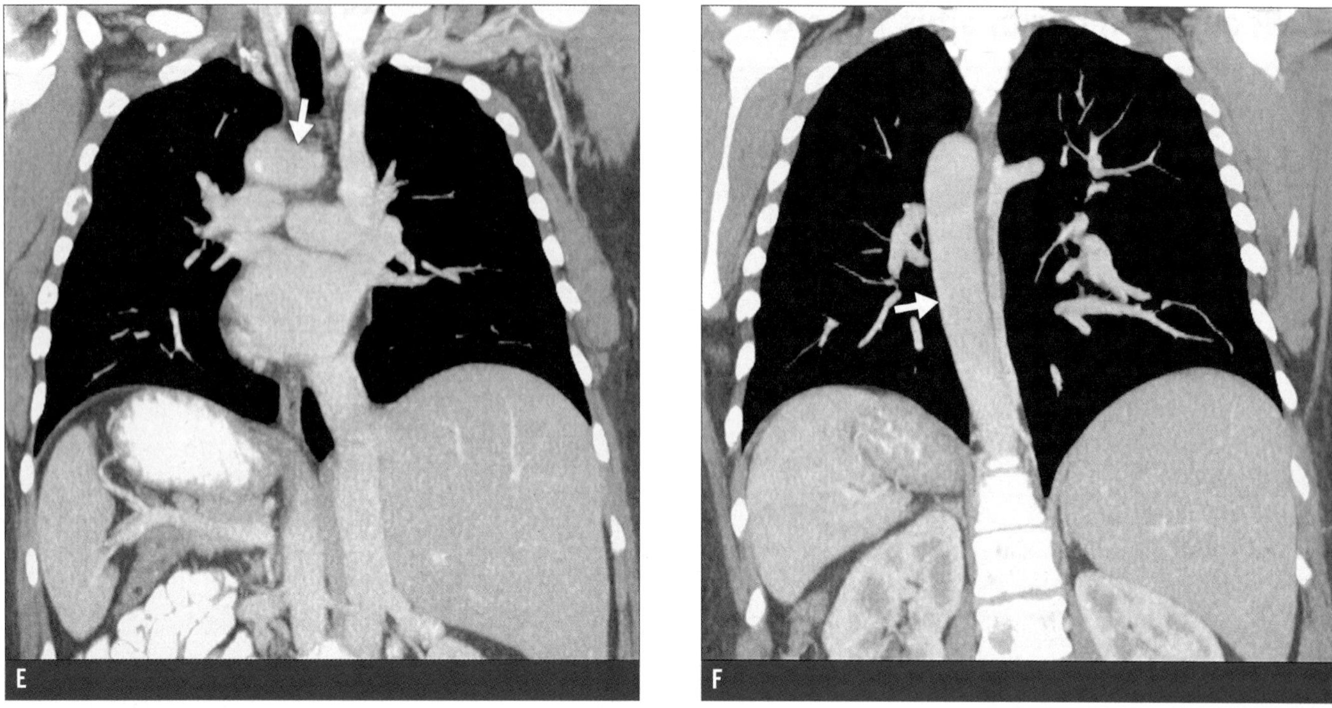

Right aortic arch with an aberrant left subclavian artery

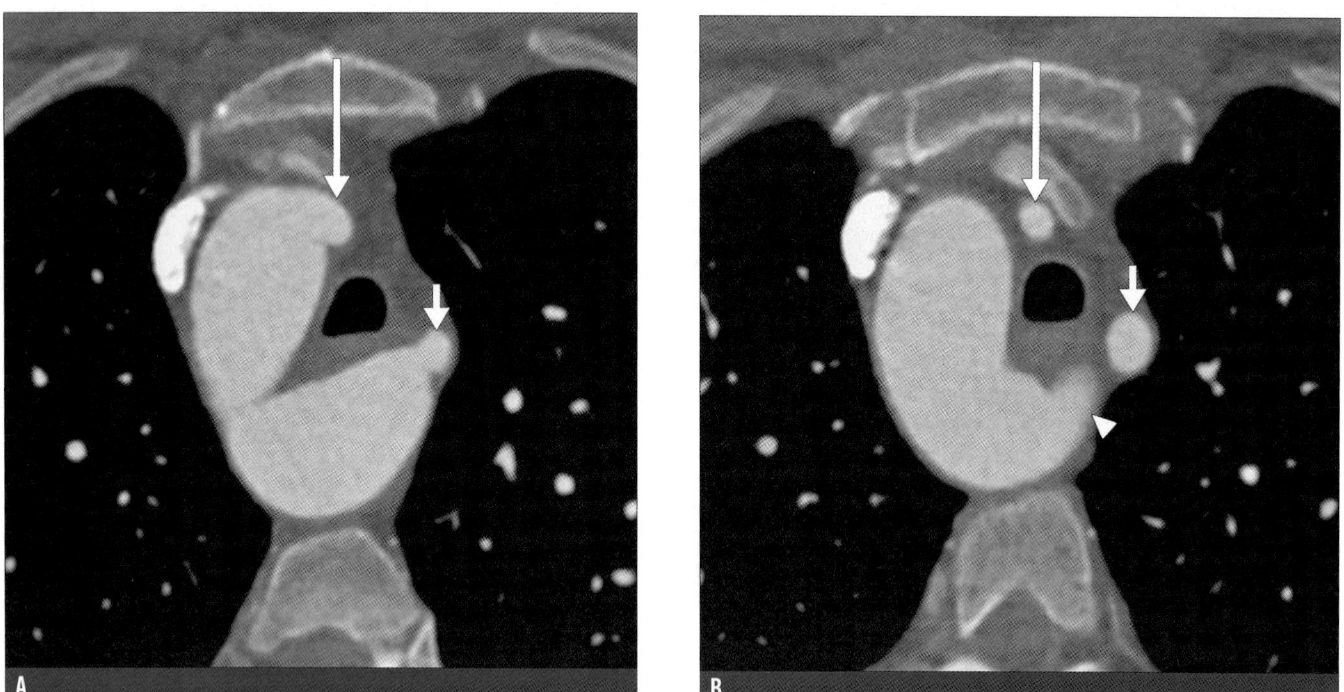

Axial images from a CTA of the chest shown from inferior to superior (**A**-**D**) demonstrate a right aortic arch first giving rise to the left common carotid artery (long arrows, **A**-**D**), followed by the innominate artery (medium arrow, **C**), and lastly an aberrant left subclavian artery (short arrows, **A**-**D**). A diverticulum of Kommerell giving rise to the aberrant left subclavian artery is also present (arrowhead, **B**). This right aortic arch configuration results in mass effect upon the esophagus, as demonstrated on image **A**. The innominate artery gives rise to the typical right subclavian artery (medium arrow, **D**) and the right common carotid artery (arrowhead, **D**). 3D volumetric images generated from the same study shown with an frontal view (**E**) and a lateral view (**F**) demonstrate the left common carotid artery (long arrows, **E**, **F**), the innominate artery (medium arrows, **E**, **F**), and the aberrant left subclavian artery (short arrows, **E**, **F**) associated with a diverticulum of Kommerell (arrowheads, **E**, **F**).

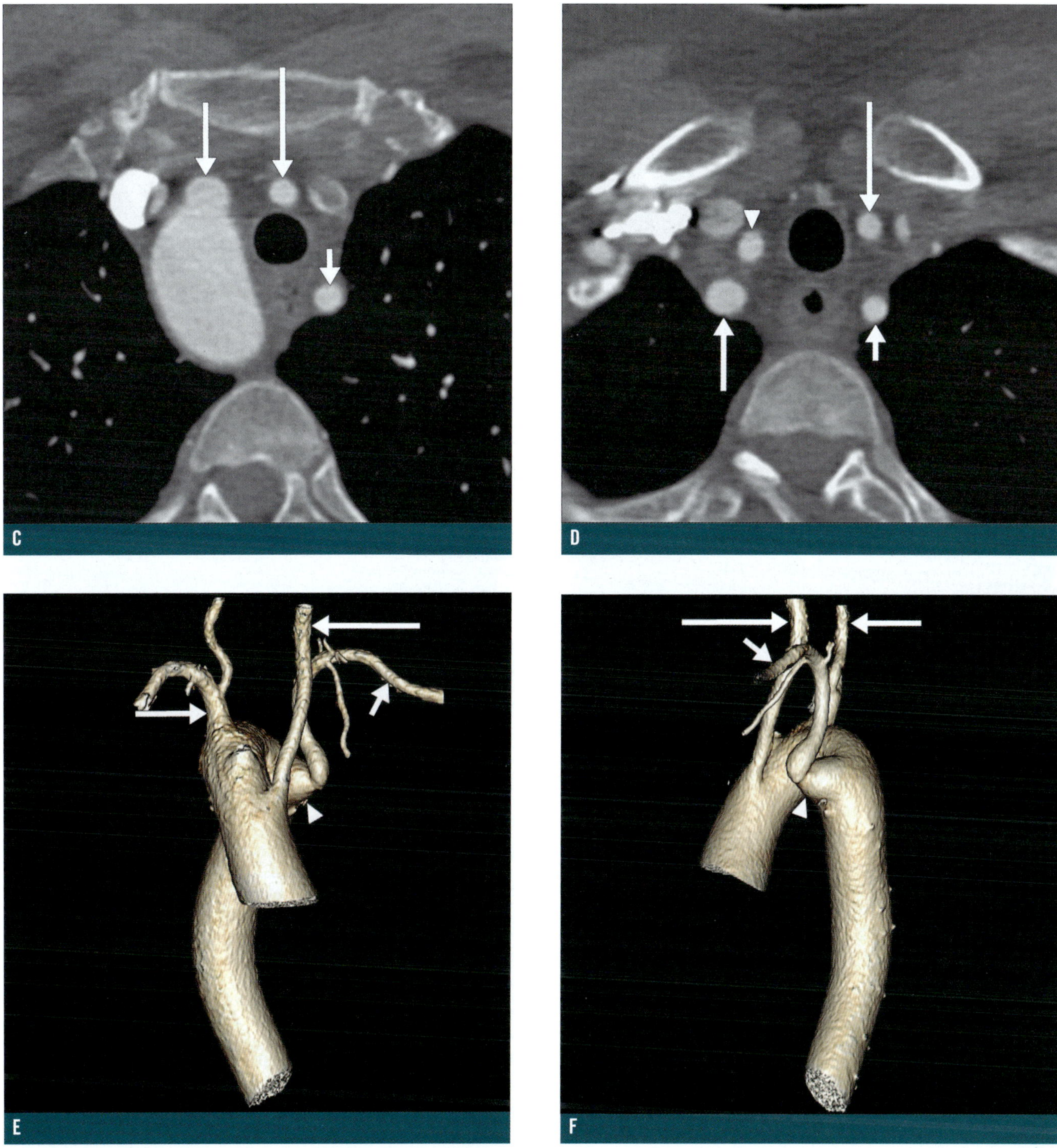
C
D
E
F

Right aortic arch with an isolated left subclavian artery

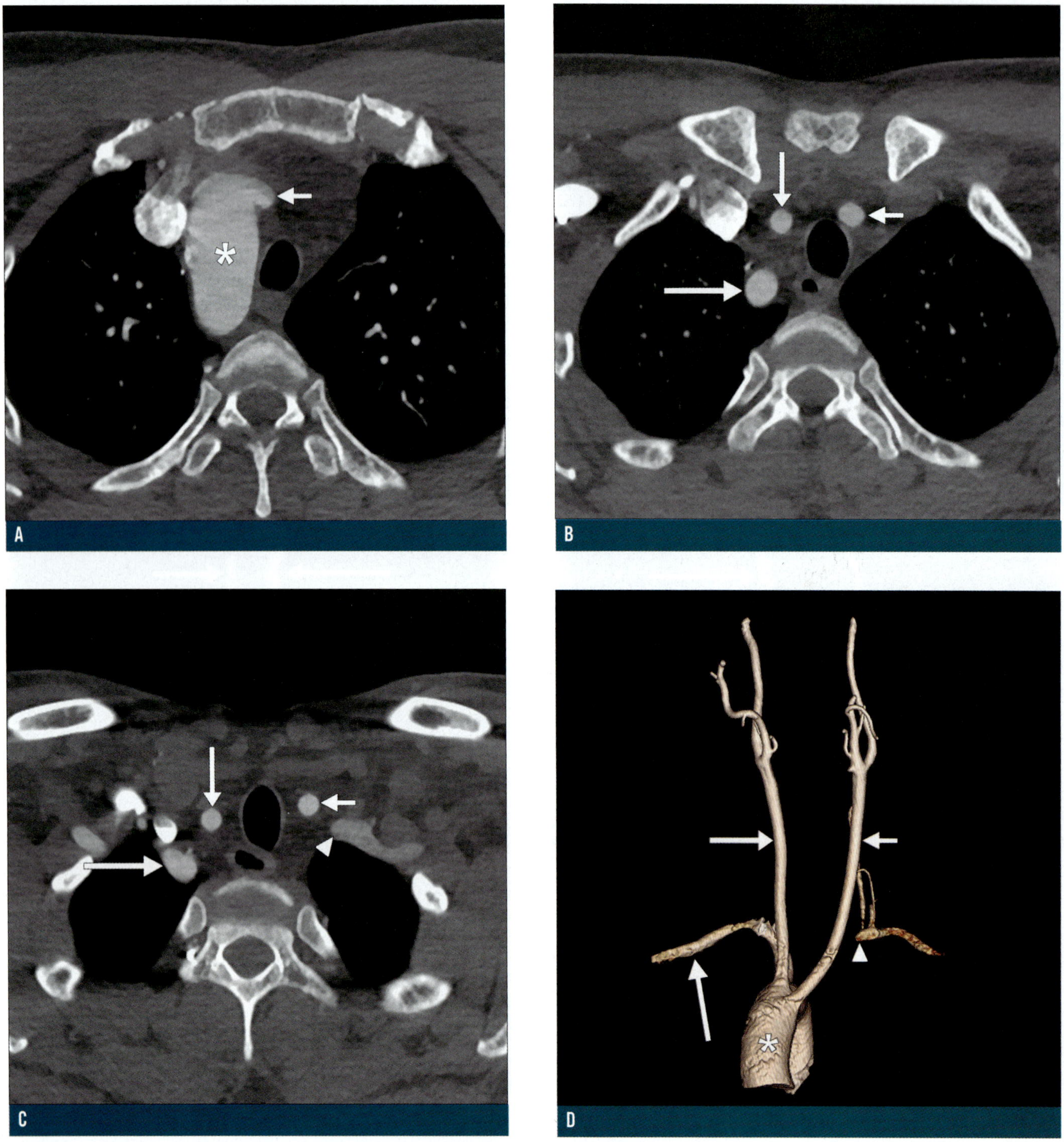

Axial CTA images (**A**-**C**) demonstrate a right aortic arch (asterisk, **A**) and the left common carotid artery (short arrows, **A**-**C**), right common carotid artery (medium arrows, **B**, **C**), and right subclavian artery (long arrows, **B**, **C**) arising in that order from the aortic arch. An isolated left subclavian artery is present (arrowhead, **C**). A 3D volumetric image from the same study (**D**) demonstrates the findings more clearly with the same annotations listed above. A coronal reformatted image (**E**) demonstrates the isolated left subclavian artery (arrowhead, **E**) and the right aortic arch (asterisk, **E**). The left vertebral artery origin arose from the proximal aspect of the isolated left subclavian artery (not shown). Image E demonstrates more robust contrast enhancement of the right vertebral artery (long arrow, **E**) compared to the left vertebral artery (short arrow, **E**). This suggests that there is retrograde arterial flow in the left vertebral artery from the right vertebral artery and likely at least contributes to flow in the isolated left subclavian artery.

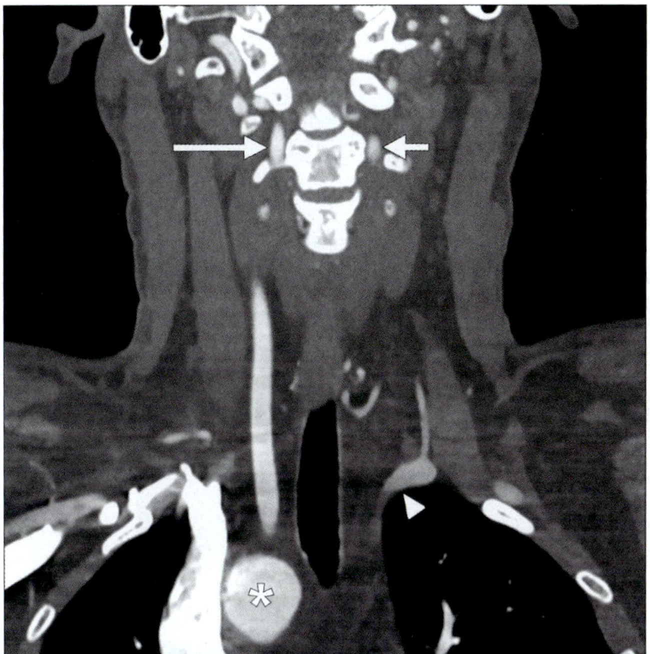

E

Right aortic arch with mirror image branching

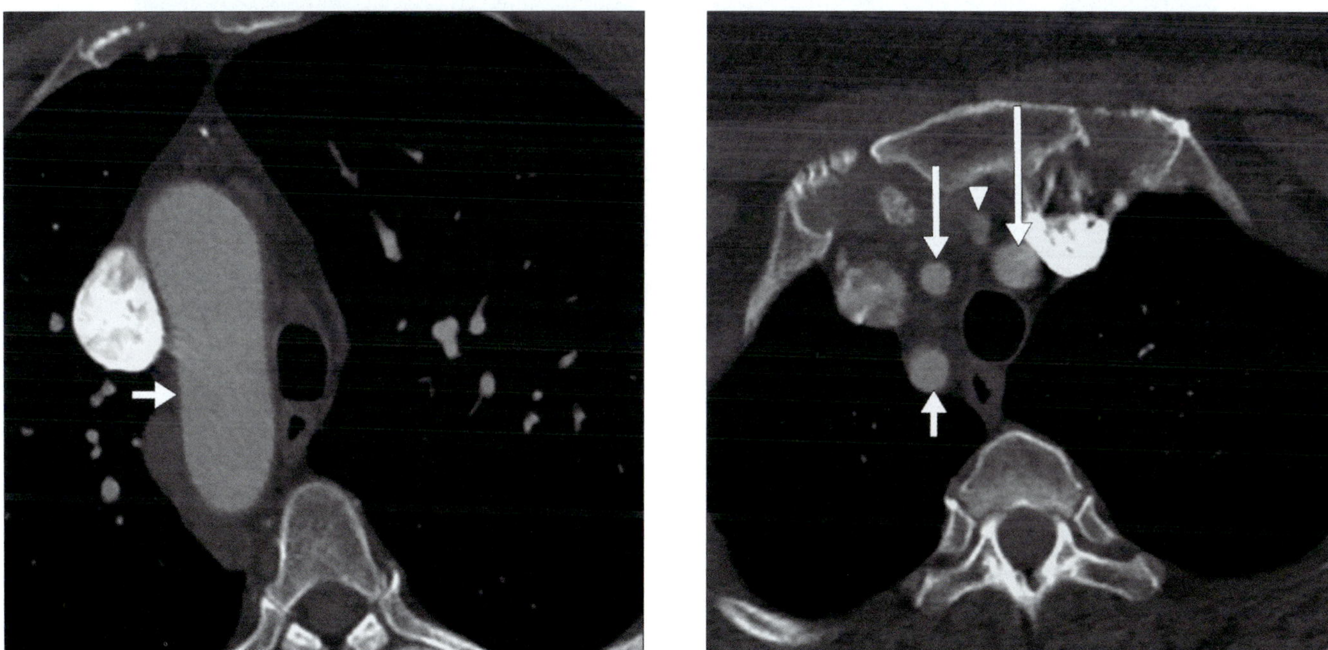

A B

Axial images from a CTA of the chest (**A, B**) demonstrate a right aortic arch (short arrow, **A**) that has mirror image branching with an innominate artery on the left (long arrow, **B**), a separate origin of the right common carotid artery (medium arrow, **B**), and a right subclavian artery (short arrow, **B**) arising in that order from the right aortic arch. A small mediastinal vein is incidentally noted on image **B** (arrowhead, **B**). Coronal reformatted imaging obtained from the same study with images viewed from anterior to posterior (**C-F**) demonstrate the innominate artery on the left (short arrow, **C**), right common carotid artery (short arrow, **D**), right subclavian artery (short arrow, **E**), and a right arch (short arrow, **F**). A 3D volumetric reconstruction from this same study (**G**) demonstrates the right subclavian artery (short arrow), right common carotid artery (medium arrow), and innominate artery (long arrow), the latter bifurcating into the left subclavian and left common carotid arteries.

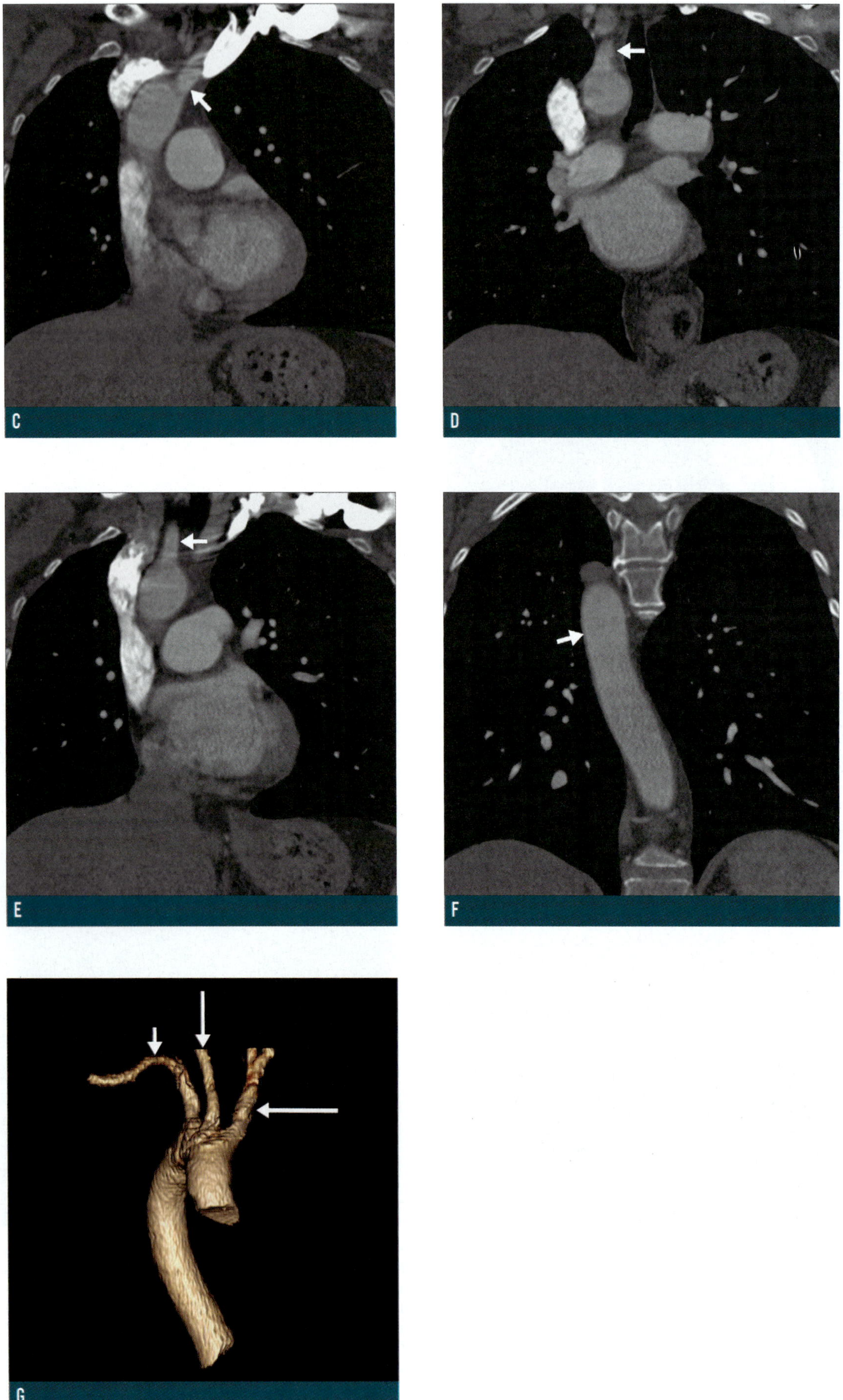
C
D
E
F
G

REFERENCES

Carano N, Piazza P, Agnetti A, Squarcia U. Congenital pulmonary steal phenomenon associated with tetralogy of Fallot, right aortic arch, and isolation of the left subclavian artery. *Pediatr Cardiol.* 1997;18(1):57-60.

Donnelly LF, Fleck RJ, Pacharn P et-al. Aberrant subclavian arteries: cross-sectional imaging findings in infants and children referred for evaluation of extrinsic airway compression. *AJR Am J Roentgenol.* 2002;178 (5): 1269-1274.

McElhinney DB, et al. Congenital obstructive lesions of the right aortic arch. *Ann Thorac Surg.* 1999;67:1194-1202.

Ramos-Duran L, et al. Developmental aortic arch anomalies in infants and children assessed with CT angiography. *AJR Am J Roentgenol.* 2012;198:W466-W474.

Türkvatan A, Büyükbayraktar FG, Ölçer T, Cumhur T. Congenital anomalies of the aortic arch: evaluation with the use of multidetector computed tomography. *Korean J Radiol.* 2009;10(2):176-184.

Whitten CR, et al. A diagnostic approach to mediastinal abnormalities. *Radiographics.* 2007;27:657-671.

CASE 3 Left aortic arch with an aberrant right subclavian artery

An aberrant right subclavian artery arising from a left aortic arch is a common congenital arch anomaly and has a reported prevalence ranging from 0.4% to 2%. This anomaly results from interruption of the dorsal segment of the right arch between the right carotid artery and right subclavian artery. With this anomaly, the first branch arising from the arch is the right common carotid artery, followed in succession by the left common carotid artery and the left subclavian artery. The last branch arising from the arch is the aberrant right subclavian artery, which has a retroesophageal course and may arise from a dilated remnant of the right aortic arch (diverticulum of Kommerell). While this anomaly does not result in a complete vascular ring, such as is typically present with a right aortic and an aberrant left subclavian artery, it can nevertheless result in extrinsic compression of the trachea and/or esophagus. It has been estimated that approximately 10% of patients with a left aortic arch and an aberrant right subclavian artery can have dysphagia, an entity termed dysphagia lusoria in this setting.

Left aortic arch with an aberrant right subclavian artery

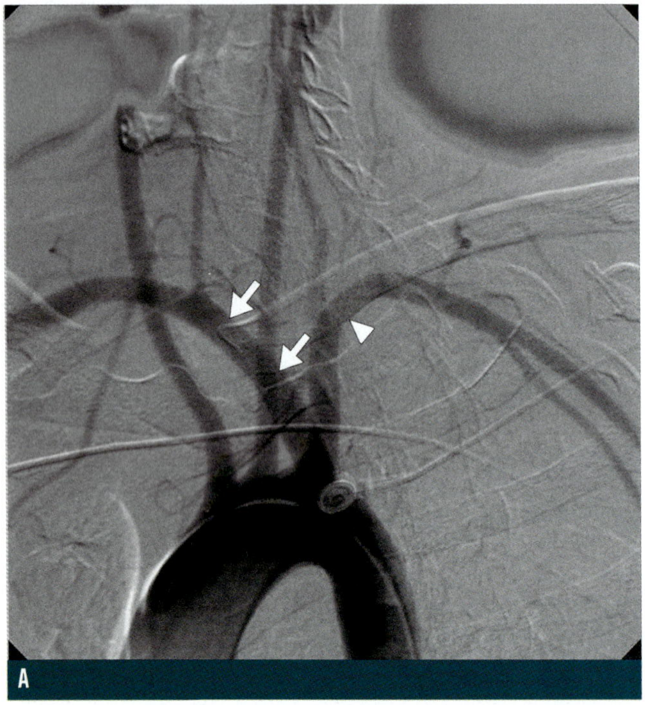

A digitally subtracted frontal angiographic image (**A**) demonstrates an aberrant right subclavian artery (arrows). The right subclavian artery arose distal to the left subclavian artery (arrowhead) on oblique imaging (not shown).

Left aortic arch with an aberrant right subclavian artery

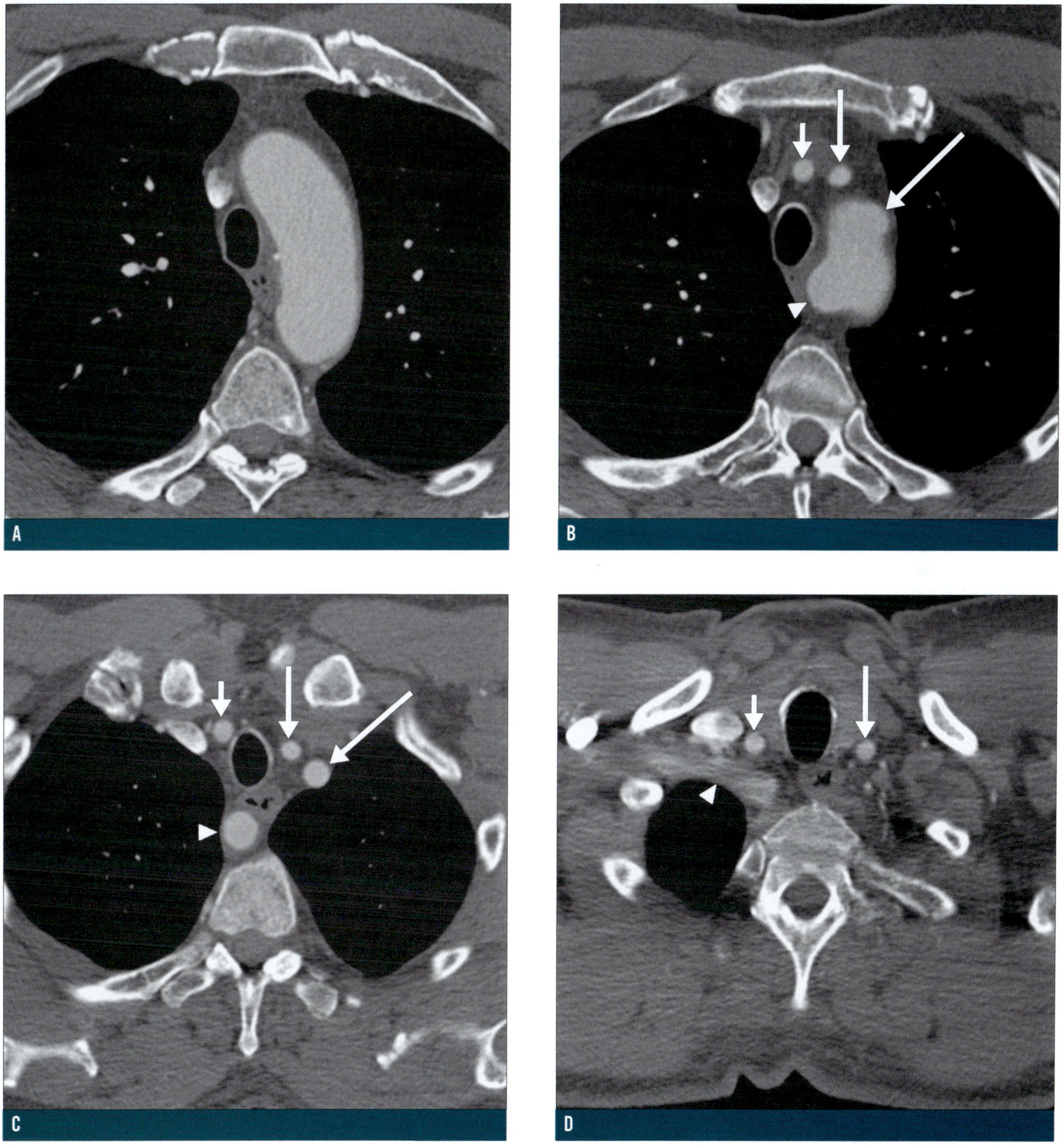

Different patient. Axial CTA images of the chest from inferior to superior (**A-D**). Image **A** demonstrates a left aortic arch. Images **B** through **D** demonstrate the right common carotid artery (short arrows, **B-D**), the left common carotid artery (medium arrows, **B-D**), and the left subclavian artery (long arrows, **B**, **C**) arising from the aortic arch in that order. An aberrant right subclavian artery (arrowheads, **B-D**) arises last from the aortic arch and traverses posterior to esophagus. 3D volumetric images from the same study viewed in a lateral projection (**E**) and frontal projection (**F**) demonstrate the same findings and utilize the same annotation that is listed above.

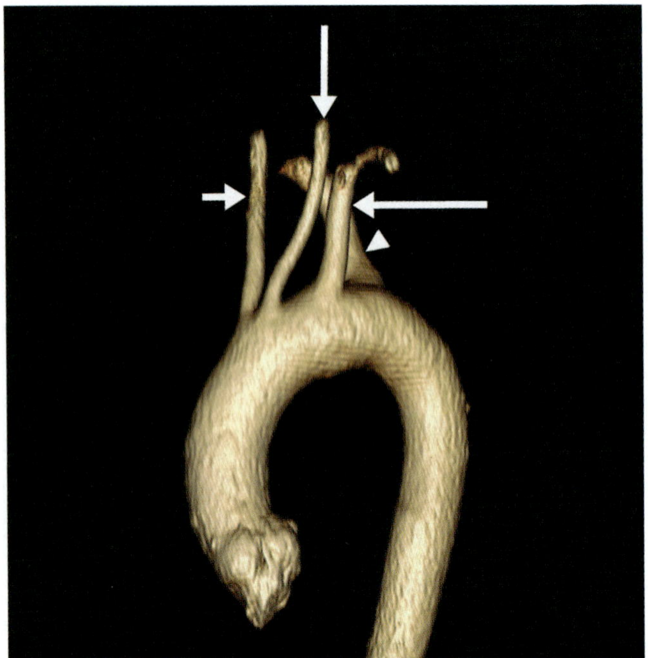
E

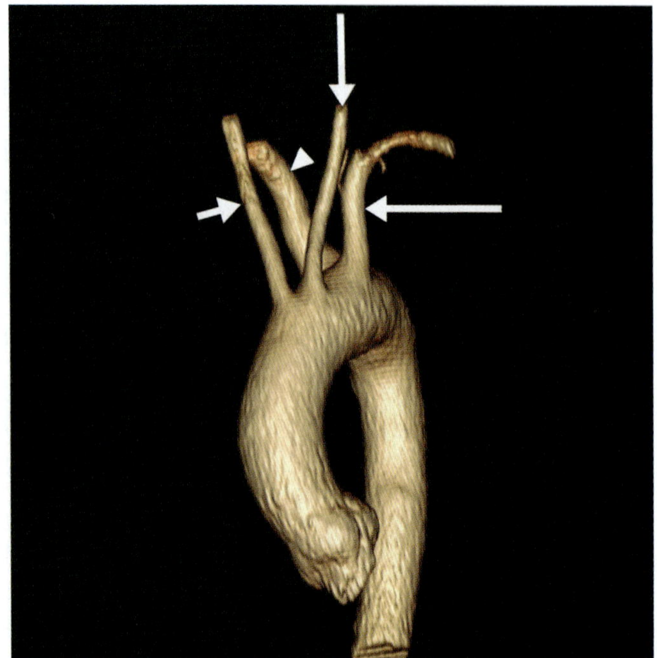
F

REFERENCES

Ka-tak W, Lam WW, Yu SC. MDCT of an aberrant right subclavian artery and of bilateral vertebral arteries with anomalous origins. *AJR Am J Roentgenol.* 2007;188 (3): W274-W275.

Osborn AG. *Diagnostic Cerebral Angiography.* 2nd ed. Philadelphia, PA: LWW; 1999.

Ramos-Duran L, et al. Developmental aortic arch anomalies in infants and children assessed with CT angiography. *AJR Am J Roentgenol.* 2012;198:W466-W474.

Türkvatan A, Büyükbayraktar FG, Ölçer T, Cumhur T. Congenital anomalies of the aortic arch: evaluation with the use of multidetector computed tomography. *Korean J Radiol.* 2009;10(2):176-184.

Whitten CR, et al. A diagnostic approach to mediastinal abnormalities. Radiographics. 2007;27:657-671.

CASE 4 Variations of vertebral artery origin

The vertebral artery is typically the first branch that arises the ipsilateral subclavian artery. However, multiple vertebral artery origin variations have been reported, including arising directly from the aortic arch, common carotid artery, and cervical internal carotid artery. The most frequent variation is a left vertebral artery arising directly from the aortic arch (2.4%-5.8%), usually located between the left common carotid artery and left subclavian artery. In these cases, the vertebral artery typically enters the foramen transversarium at C4 or C5, rather than at the more common C6 level. A right vertebral artery arising directly from the aortic arch is rare; if present, the right vertebral artery most commonly originates on the contralateral side, distal to the left subclavian artery origin. A cervical vertebral artery may also have duplicate origins before forming a single vertebral artery.

Left cervical vertebral artery origin arising directly from the aortic arch

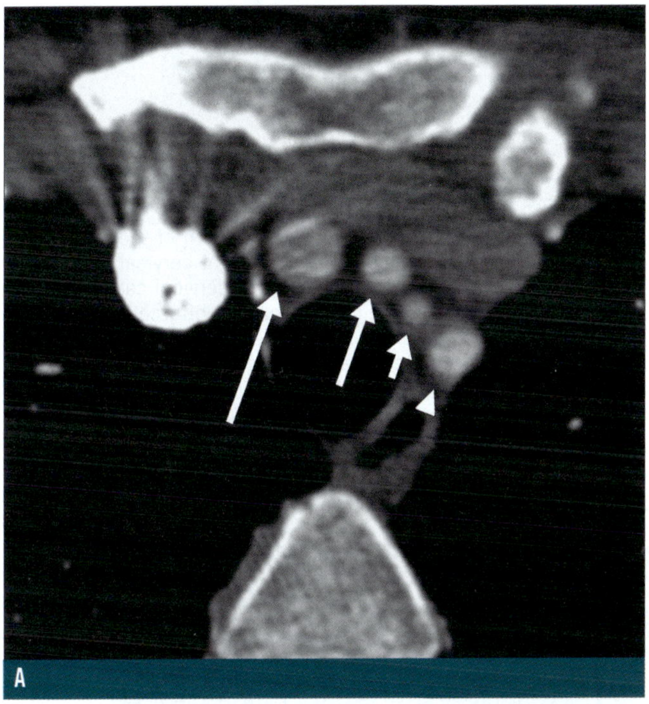

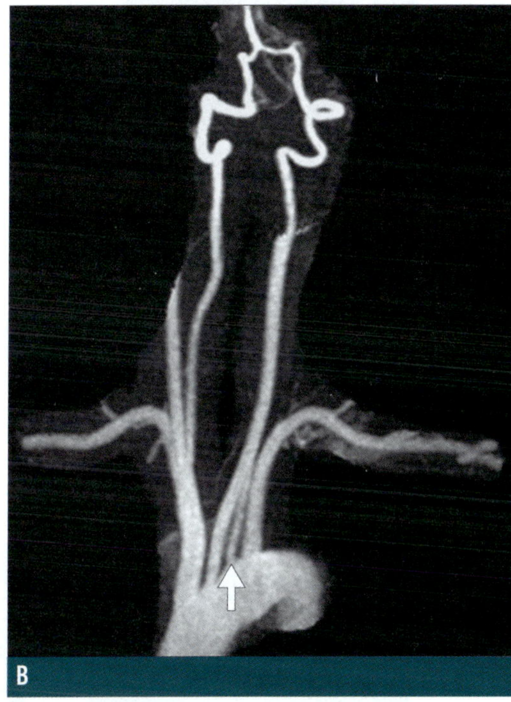

An axial CTA image (**A**) demonstrates the typical configuration of a "four-vessel arch" with the innominate artery (long arrow, **A**), left common carotid (medium arrow, **A**), left cervical vertebral artery (short arrow, **A**), and the left subclavian artery (arrowhead, **A**) arising in succession from the aortic arch. A MIP image from a contrast-enhanced MRA of the same patient (**B**) also demonstrates the four-vessel arch with an aortic arch origin of the left cervical vertebral artery (short arrow, **B**).

Right cervical vertebral artery origin arising directly from the aortic arch distal to the left subclavian artery

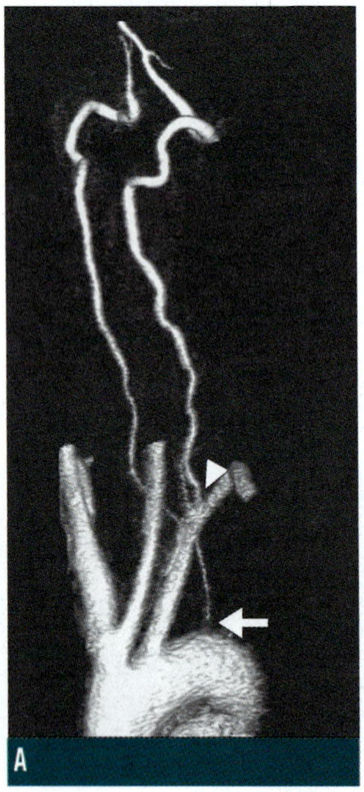

An oblique MIP image from a gadolinium-infused MRA of the neck (**A**) demonstrates the right cervical vertebral artery origin (arrow) to arise from the aortic arch distal to the left subclavian artery. The left cervical vertebral artery origin is conventional, arising from the left subclavian artery (arrowhead).

Right cervical vertebral artery origin arising from the right cervical carotid artery

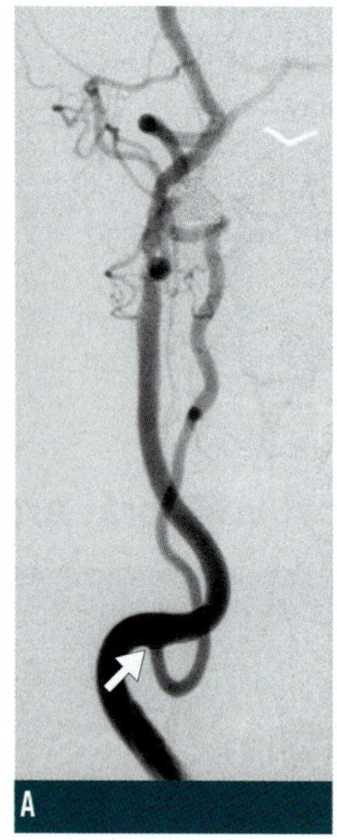

A single image from a catheter angiogram of the right cervical carotid artery (**A**) demonstrates the right cervical vertebral artery origin to arise directly from the right cervical carotid artery (arrow). A normal right cervical carotid bifurcation (ie, a bifurcation with an ECA and ICA) is not evident in this case. Therefore, it is difficult to determine if the right vertebral artery arises from the proximal right ICA or the distal right CCA. However, if it is the former, then one could consider this variant a persistent proatlantal intersegmental artery type I, which is described in Case 17 of this chapter.

Duplicate origin of the left cervical vertebral artery

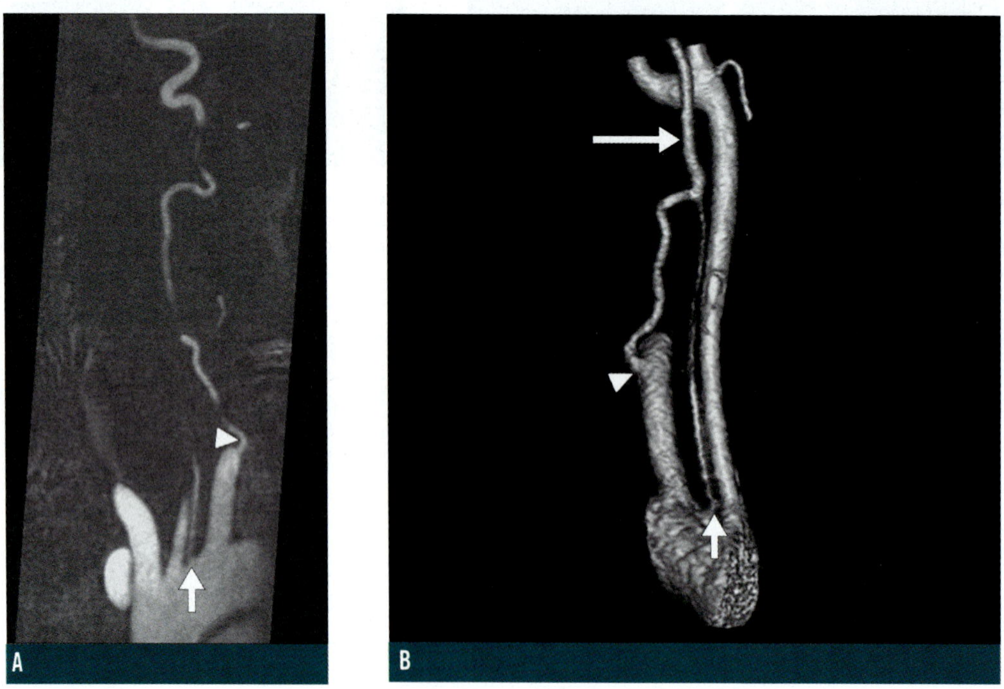

A source image from a gadolinium-infused MRA of the neck (**A**) and 3D volumetric MRA images from the same study (**B**, **C**) demonstrate a duplicate origin of the left cervical vertebral artery, with one origin arising from the aortic arch (short arrows, **A**-**C**) and the other origin arising from the left subclavian artery (arrowheads, **A**-**C**). These vessels unite more cephalad to form a single left cervical vertebral artery (long arrows, **B**, **C**).

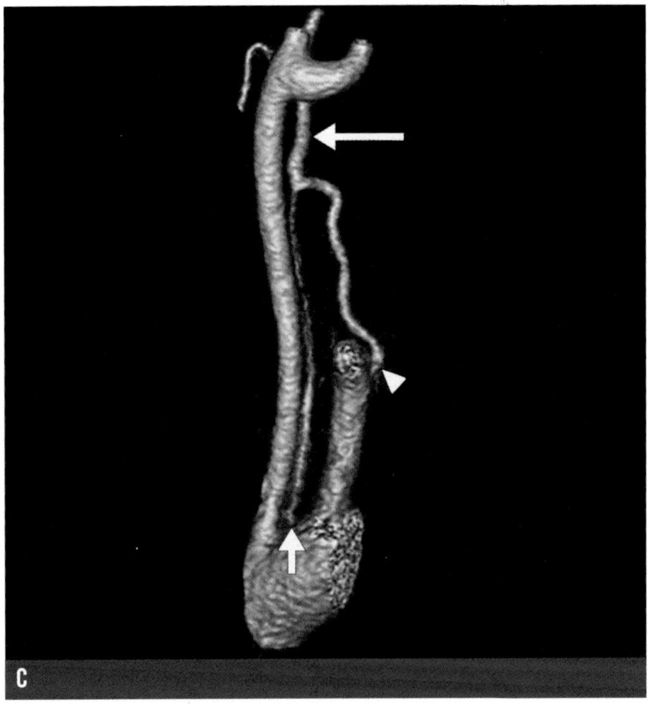

Duplicate origin of the left cervical vertebral artery

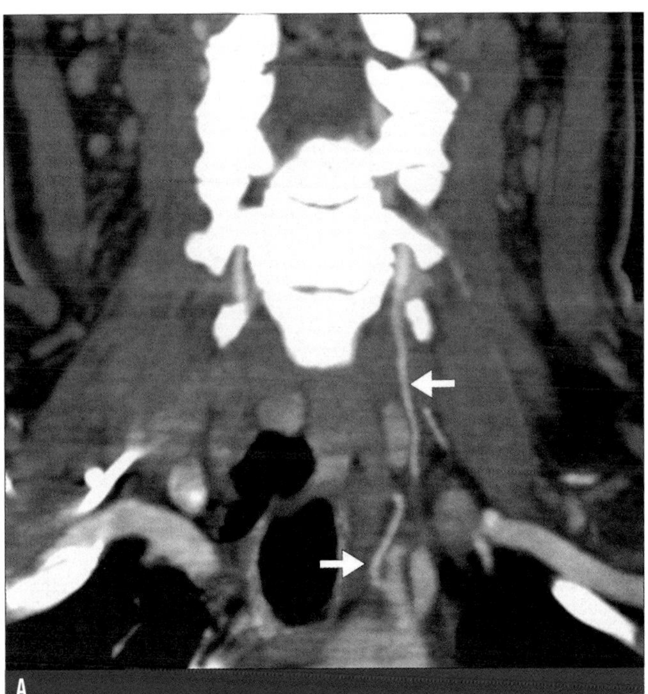

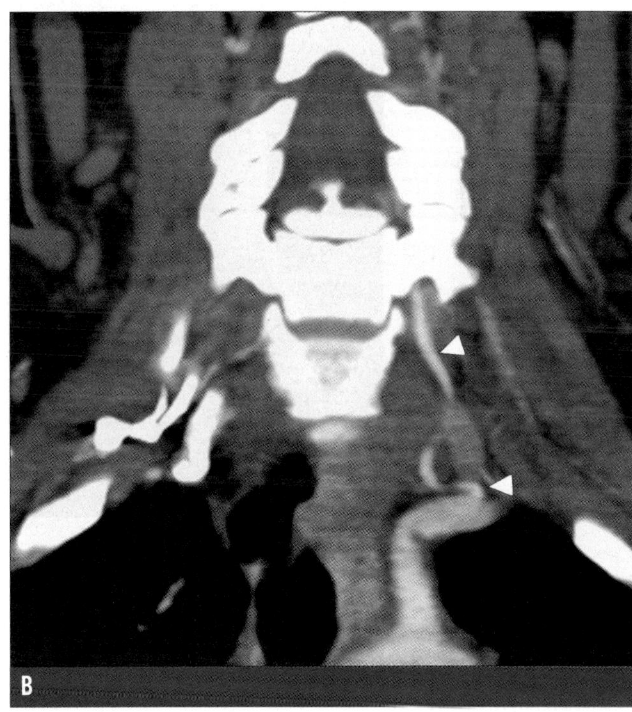

Different patient. Coronal reformatted images from a CTA (**A**, **B**) demonstrate a duplicate origin of the left cervical vertebral artery, with a smaller ventral component arising from the proximal left subclavian artery (arrows, **A**) and a larger dorsal component arising from the more distal left subclavian artery (arrowheads, **B**). The ventral component appears discontinuous on image **A**, but was intact when viewing other images from the study. An axial CT image from the same study (**C**) demonstrates the smaller ventral component (arrow, **C**) and the larger dorsal component (arrowhead, **C**). A left parasagittal reformatted image from the same study (**D**) demonstrates the two vessels uniting at the C5 foramen transversarium (arrow, **D**). A 3D volumetric reconstruction (**E**) best demonstrates the duplication anomaly (arrows, **E**).

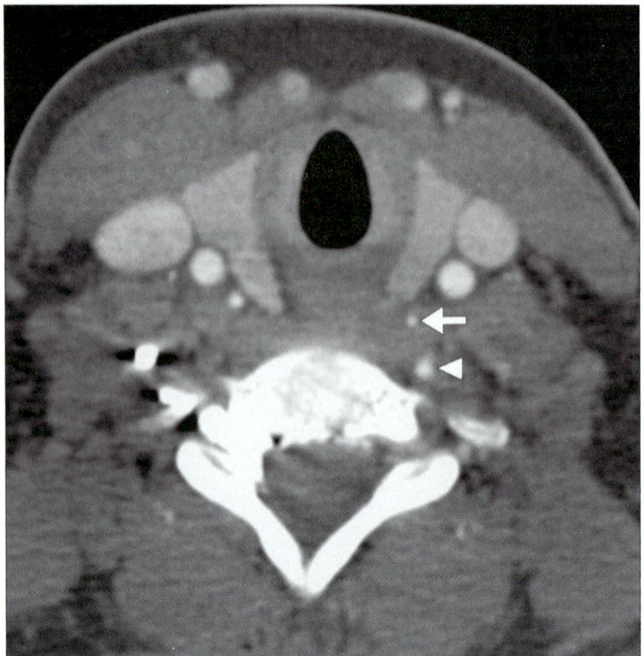

C

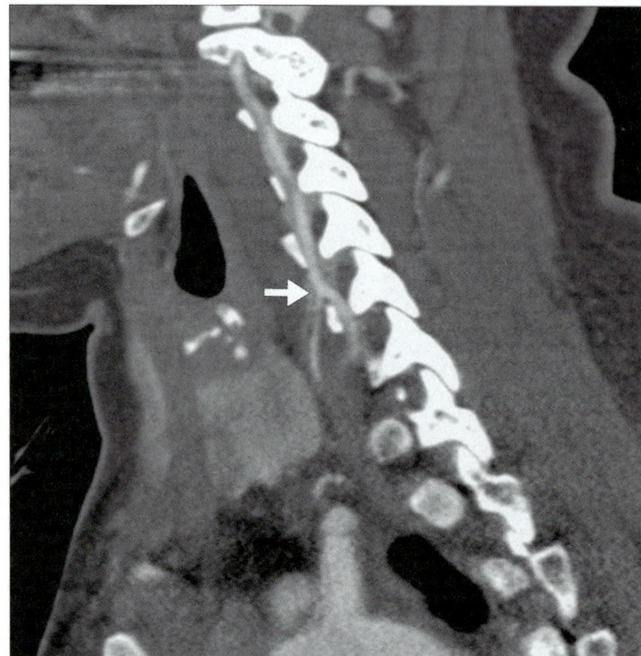

D

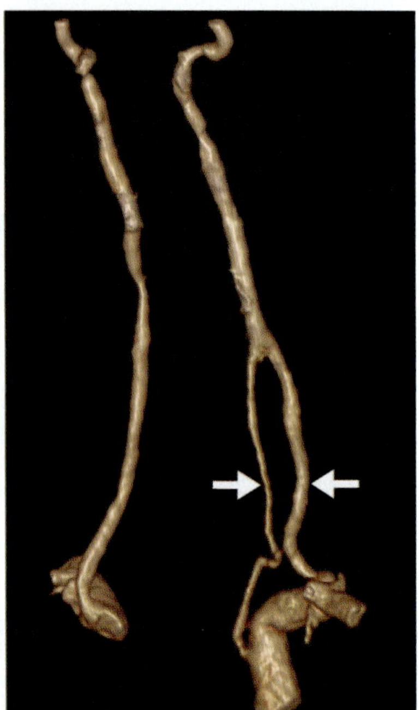

E

REFERENCES

Goray VB, Joshi AR, Garg A, Merchant S, Yadav B, Maheshwari P. Aortic arch variation: a unique case with anomalous origin of both vertebral arteries as additional branches of the aortic arch distal to left subclavian artery. *AJNR Am J Neuroradiol.* 2005;26(1):93-95.

Strub WM, Leach JL, Tomsick TA. Left vertebral artery origin from the thyrocervical trunk: a unique vascular variant. *AJNR Am J Neuroradiol.* 2006;27:1155-1156.

CASE 5 Extraforaminal course of the cervical vertebral artery

Beyond its origin, the cervical vertebral artery typically ascends anterior to the C7 foramen transversarium to enter the C6 foramen transversarium in 92% to 95% of cases. The vertebral artery ascends within the remaining cervical foramina transversaria to the base of the C2 vertebra, at which point it extends posteriorly and cephalad to enter the C1 foramen transversarium. The cervical vertebral artery then traverses superomedially to pierce the cranial dura to become the intracranial (ie, intradural) portion of the vertebral artery. Occasionally, the cervical vertebral artery may have a longer extraforaminal course and enter the foramen transversarium of C5 (5%), C4 (1%-2%), or C3 (0.2%-1%). The longer the extraforaminal course of a cervical vertebral artery, the more prone to injury the artery may become during surgery (eg, anterior cervical discectomy and fusion) or blunt trauma because of the lack of protection normally afforded by the foramina transverseria.

Extraforaminal course of the left cervical vertebral artery

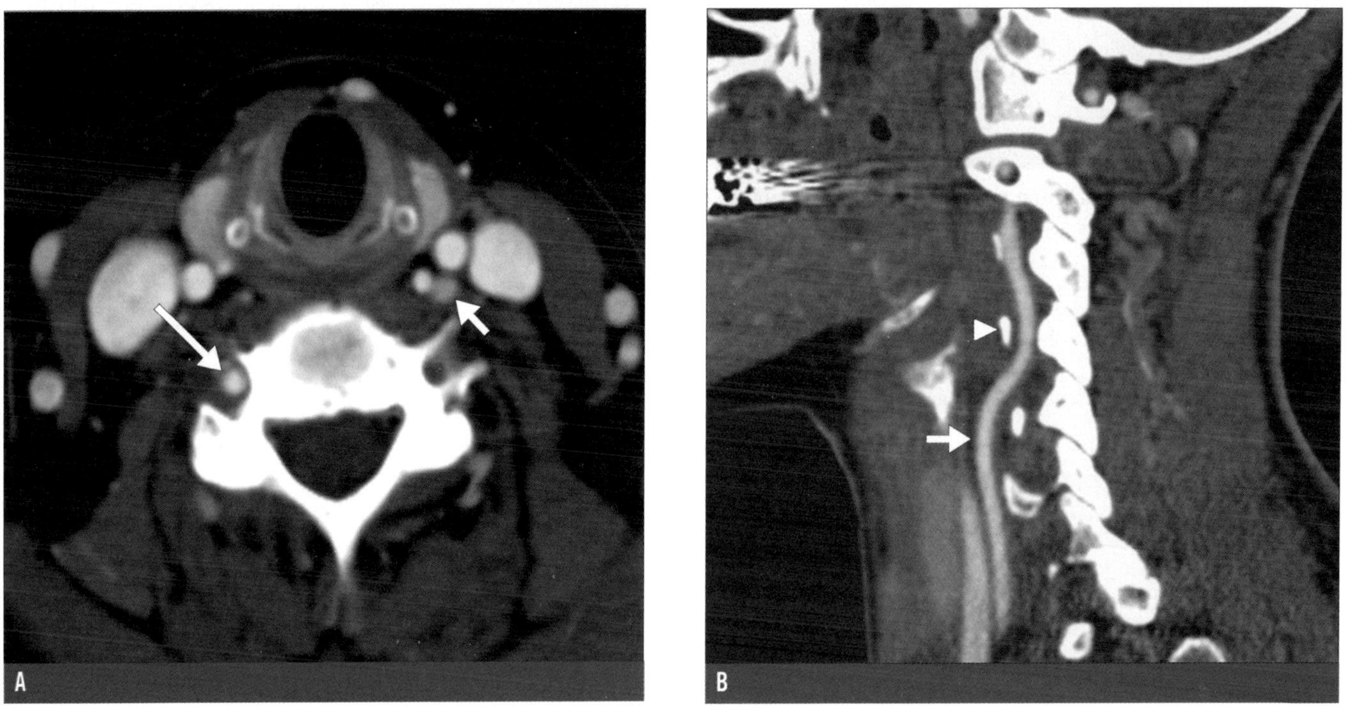

Axial (**A**) and left parasagittal reformatted (**B**) CTA images through the neck demonstrate an extraforaminal course of the left cervical vertebral artery (short arrows, **A, B**), in this case entering the C4 foramen transversarium (arrowhead, **B**). The right vertebral artery enters a more caudal foramen transversarium (long arrow, **A**).

Extraforaminal course of the right cervical vertebral artery

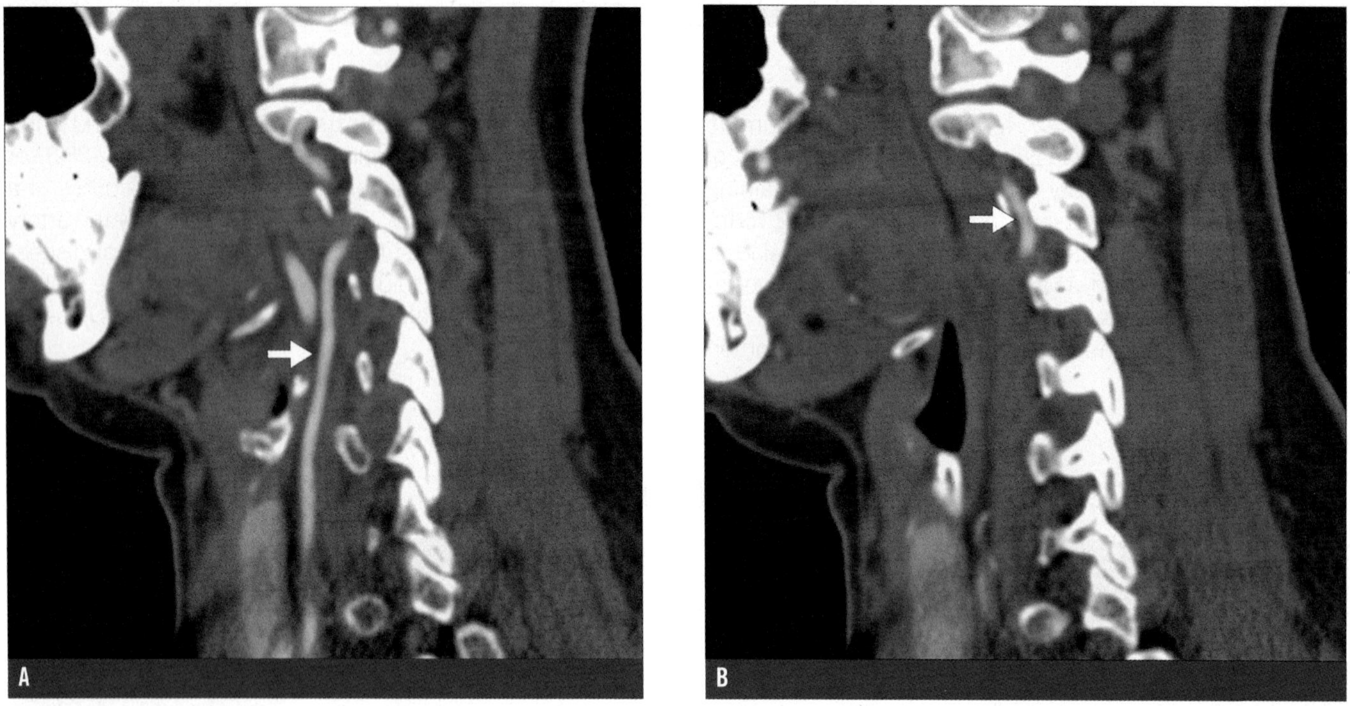

Different patient. Right parasagittal reformatted CTA images (**A, B**) demonstrate the right cervical vertebral artery to be extraforaminal (arrow, **A**) until it enters the C3 foramen transversarium (arrow, **B**).

REFERENCES

Eskander MS, et al. Vertebral artery anatomy: a review of two hundred fifty magnetic resonance imaging scans. *Spine.* 2010;35(23):2035-2040.

Rawal, Jadav H. Anatomical study of variation of vertebral artery entering the foramen transversarium of cervical vertebrae. *Natl J Med Res.* 2012;2(2): 199-201.

CASE 6 Hypoplastic vertebral artery

There is significant variability of the vertebral artery caliber among patients. The left vertebral artery is dominant in approximately 42% of patients, the right vertebral artery is dominant in 25% to 32% of patients, and there is a codominance of the vertebral arteries in approximately 26% of patients. A nondominant vertebral artery may be slightly hypoplastic to markedly hypoplastic (ie, threadlike) compared to the dominant vertebral artery. The foramen transversarium is usually proportional to the size of the ipsilateral vertebral artery. Therefore, a hypoplastic vertebral artery will often be associated with a small caliber foramen transversium compared to the dominant vertebral artery. This observation can be helpful in cases when it is unclear whether the smaller vertebral artery is incidentally hypoplastic or abnormal, such as because of atherosclerosis or arterial dissection.

Occasionally, a hypoplastic intracranial vertebral artery may not anastomose with the basilar artery but instead may terminate as the ipsilateral posterior inferior cerebellar artery (PICA); when this occurs, the contralateral vertebral artery represents the primary antegrade flow to the basilar artery. If the vertebral artery primarily terminates as PICA, but an ipsilateral markedly hypoplastic post-PICA vertebral artery is still present, then the term "functionally terminating in PICA" may be used. If a catheter angiogram is performed on a patient with a vertebral artery that terminates or functionally terminates in PICA, then a hand injection, rather than a power injection, should be performed in order to minimize the risk of arterial rupture.

Hypoplastic right cervical vertebral artery

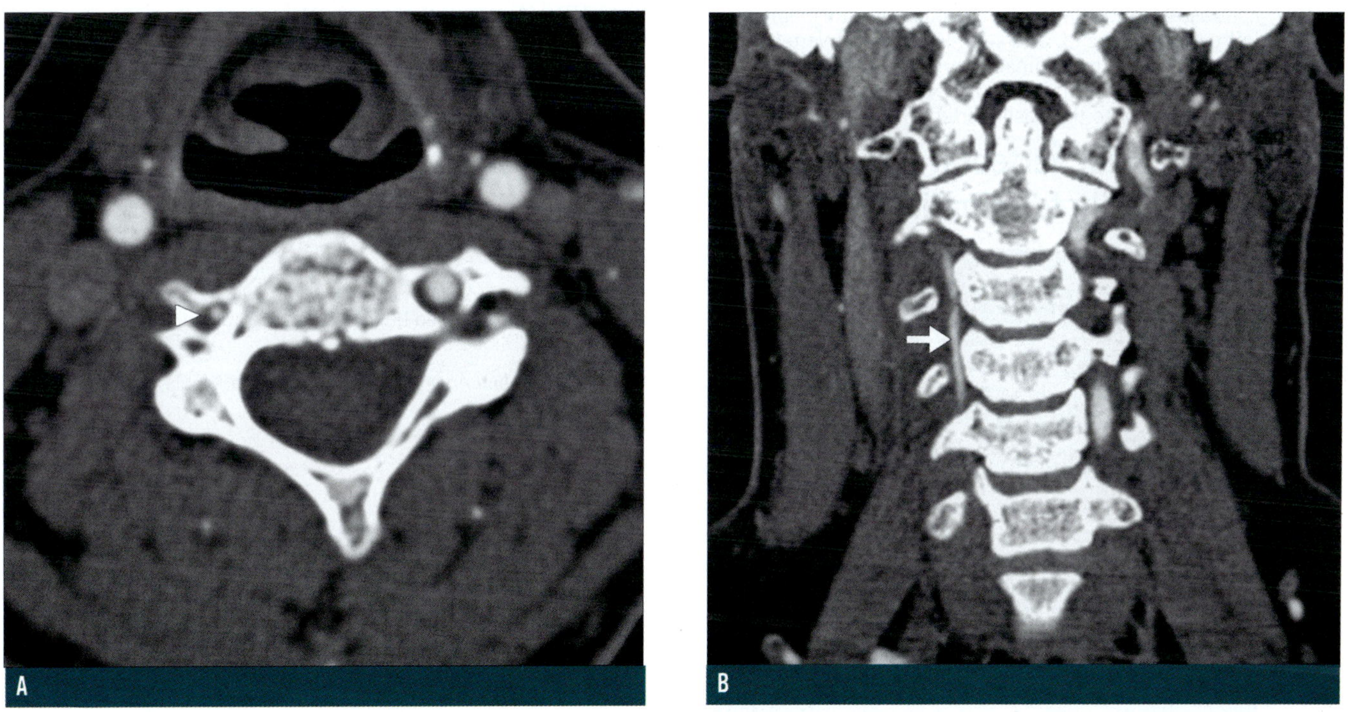

Axial (**A**) and coronal reformatted (**B**) CTA images demonstrate a hypoplastic right cervical vertebral artery within an asymmetrically small right foramen transversarium (arrows, **A, B**).

Hypoplastic left cervical vertebral artery

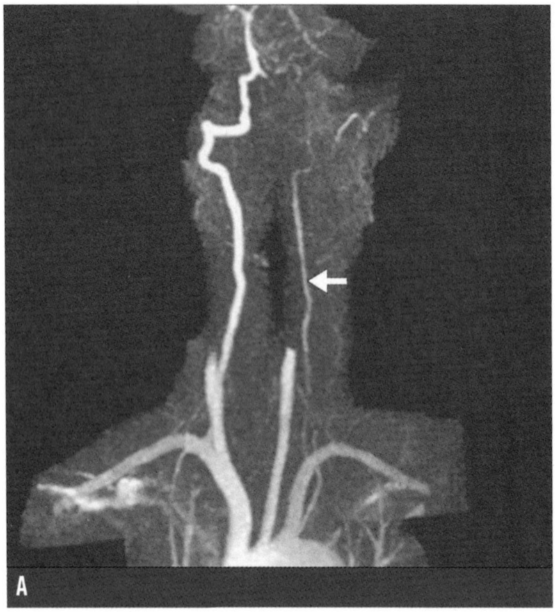

Different patient. A slightly oblique MIP image from a contrast-enhanced MRA (**A**) demonstrates a hypoplastic left cervical vertebral artery (arrow). The left vertebral artery functionally terminated in PICA (not shown), and the right cervical vertebral artery represents the primary antegrade flow to the basilar artery.

Intracranial vertebral artery functionally terminating in PICA

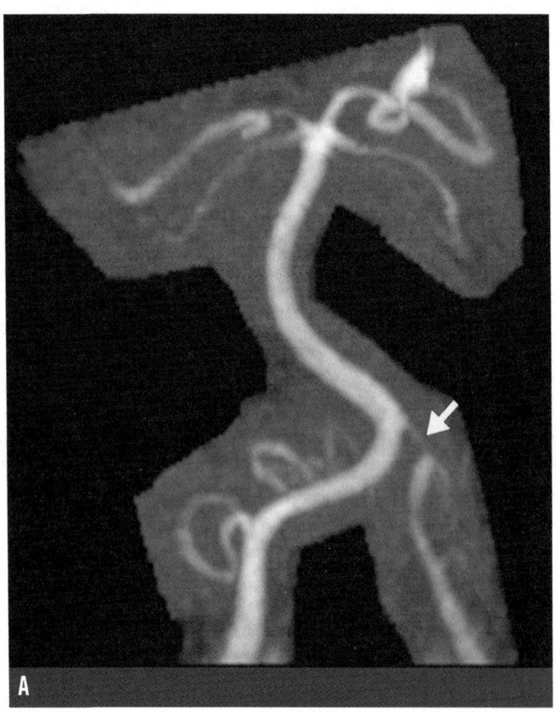

A MIP image of the posterior circulation from a time-of-flight MRA (**A**) demonstrates a markedly hypoplastic intracranial left vertebral artery (arrow) located immediately distal to the origin of the left PICA, compatible with a left vertebral artery that functionally terminates in PICA.

Intracranial vertebral artery terminating in PICA

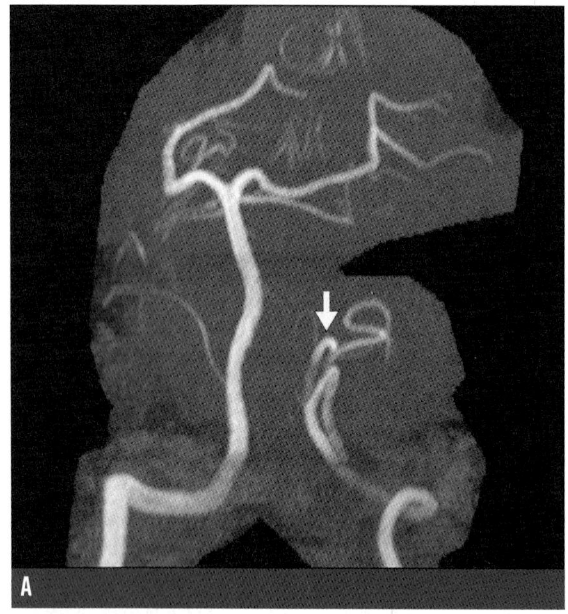

A MIP image of the posterior circulation from a time-of-flight MRA (**A**) demonstrates the intracranial left vertebral artery to completely terminate in PICA (arrow).

REFERENCES

Eskander MS, et al. Vertebral artery anatomy: a review of two hundred fifty magnetic resonance imaging scans. *Spine (Phila Pa 1976).* 2010;35(23):2035-2040.

Jeng JS, Yip PK. Evaluation of vertebral artery hypoplasia and asymmetry by color-coded duplex ultrasonography. *Ultrasound Med Biol.* 2004;30(5):605-609.

Osborn A. *Cerebral Angiography.* 2nd ed. Philadelphia, PA: LWW; 1999.

A fenestration refers to a vessel with a single origin that divides into two parallel segments and reunites anywhere along its more distal course. Fenestrations are a well-known variant of the vertebral artery. In the neck, vertebral artery fenestrations are most frequently present at the C1 to C2 level where the prevalence of unilateral fenestration is approximately 1%. The prevalence of bilateral extracranial vertebral artery fenestrations is rare, estimated to only be approximately 0.01%. Similarly, multiple fenestrations along a single extracranial vertebral artery have only been rarely reported. Intracranial vertebrobasilar system fenestrations are significantly more commonplace. A series by Uchino et al retrospectively reviewed more than 3300 MRA examinations performed on a 1.5T magnet and found intracranial fenestrations with a prevalence of approximately 0.5% involving the intracranial vertebral arteries and approximately 0.2% at the vertebrobasilar junction.

An arterial fenestration is a normal variant that can simulate an arterial dissection. However, patients with fenestrations are at a higher risk for aneurysm formation because of altered normal laminar flow and resultant vessel wall shear stress.

Cervical vertebral artery fenestration

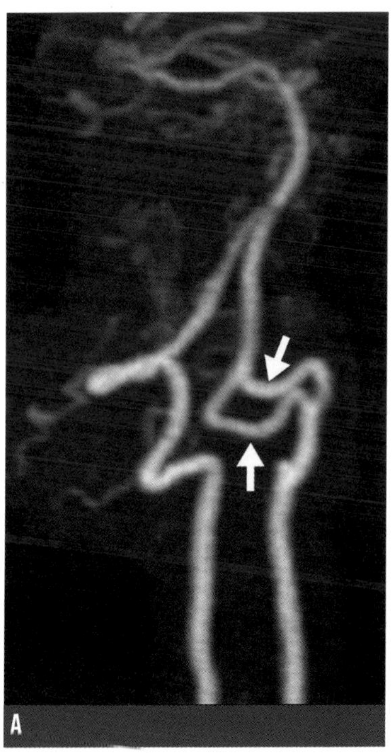

A MIP image from a contrast-enhanced MRA of the neck (**A**) demonstrates a long segment fenestration of the left cervical vertebral artery V3 segment (arrows).

Cervical vertebral artery fenestration

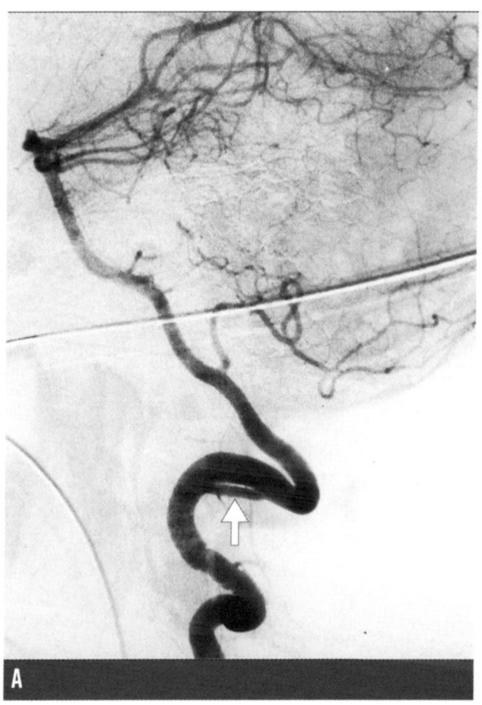

Different patient. A lateral image from a catheter angiogram of the right vertebral artery (**A**) demonstrates a fenestration of the right cervical vertebral artery V3 segment (arrow).

Intracranial vertebral artery fenestration

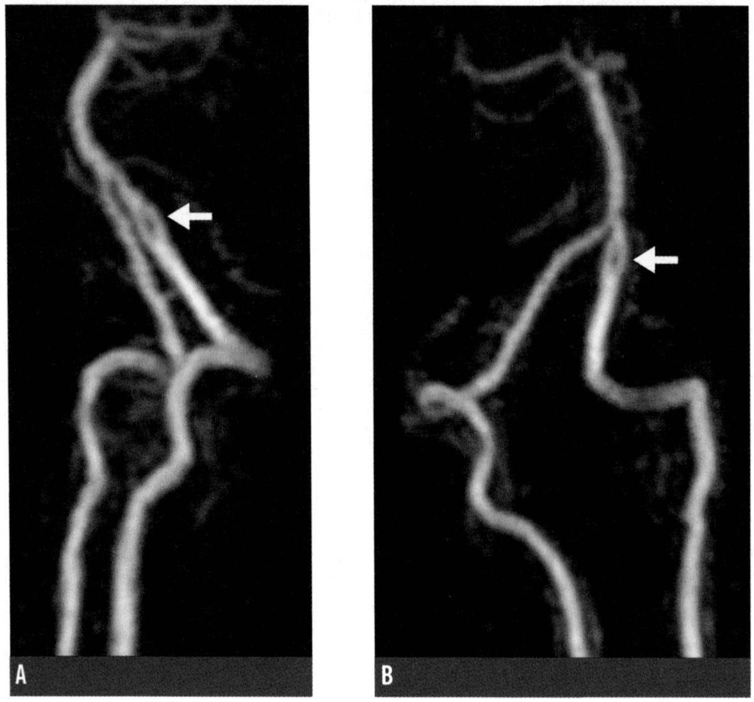

Oblique MIP images from a contrast-enhanced MRA of the neck (**A, B**) demonstrate a short-segment fenestration involving the distal left vertebral artery V4 segment (arrows, **A**, **B**).

REFERENCES

Ionete C, Omojola MF. MR angiographic demonstration of bilateral duplication of the extracanial vertebral artery: unusual course and review of the literature. *AJNR Am J Neuroradiol.* 2006;27(6):1304-1306.

Sim E, Vaccaro A, Berzianovich A, Thaler H, Ullrich CG. Fenestration of the extracranial vertebral artery: review of the literature. *Spine.* 2001;26:139-142.

Uchino A, et al. Fenestrations of the intracranial vertebrobasilar system diagnosed by MR angiography. *Neuroradiology.* 2012;54(5):445-450.

Uchino A, et al. Vertebral artery variations at the C1-2 level diagnosed by magnetic resonance angiography. *Neuroradiology.* 2011;54:19-23.

CASE 8 Cervical vertebral artery tortuosity, kinks, and loops

Tortuosity of the cervical vertebral arteries is a common finding and has been reported to be present in 22% to 47% of individuals. Vertebral artery tortuosity is usually an incidental finding and related to chronic hypertension and/or atherosclerosis. However, some studies have suggested that additional factors, such as cystic medial necrosis (with or without hypertension), may lead to the development of vascular tortuosity. Focal vertebral artery tortuosity typically does not result in arterial flow limitation. However, there are rare reports of a tortuous vertebral artery segment extending into a foramen and resulting in an ipsilateral radiculopathy. Focal tortuosity may also result in erosion of an adjacent vertebral body and/or widening of the surrounding foramen transversarium. Recognizing vertebral artery tortuosity may be important during preoperative planning in order to minimize the risk of iatrogenic injury.

In addition to tortuosity, a cervical vertebral artery may have a focal kink. A focal cervical vertebral artery kink has been described as a cause of vertebrobasilar insufficiency. In some patients, this phenomenon may be exaggerated by head/neck turning, an entity termed "bow hunter syndrome" (also called rotational vertebral artery occlusion). This entity has been termed bow hunter syndrome because when the patient turns their head/neck, such as in a position a bow hunter would assume when shooting an arrow, there is dynamic compromise of a vertebral artery (typically the dominant vertebral artery) that results in vertebrobasilar insufficiency. The vertebral artery compromise in bow hunter syndrome is usually the result of impingement by an uncovertebral or facet joint osteophyte although numerous other causes have been implicated. While the vertebrobasilar insufficiency is usually transient with bow hunter syndrome, lateral medullary infarcts have been described. Bow hunter syndrome is best assessed by conventional angiography which should include head and neck positioning that elicits the symptoms. A CTA examination, again with patient positioning that triggers the symptoms, may also prove useful.

There is literature describing surgical correction of vertebral artery kinks that are responsible for medically refractory vertebrobasilar insufficiency. However, it is likely that the majority of cervical vertebral artery kinks are incidental findings; this is particularly true if a cervical vertebral artery kink is not associated with flow limitation distal to the kink and the contralateral vertebral artery is normal in caliber and course.

Cervical vertebral artery vascular loops are also usually incidental findings, although altered flow dynamics can result in aneurysm formation along the loop.

COMPANION CASES

- **Acute cervical vertebral artery dissection.** Vertebral artery dissections may be spontaneous or related to a traumatic etiology. Traumatic etiologies may occur from accidental and nonaccidental trauma as well as secondary to iatrogenic injury in the setting of vessel catheterization, percutaneous needle placement, or chiropractic manipulation. Spontaneous dissections are most commonly identified in middle-aged women and are sometimes associated with fibromuscular dysplasia.

  Occasionally, an acute vertebral artery dissection may be difficult to diagnose on CTA or MRA, particularly if there is superimposed atherosclerosis. A vascular flap along the vertebral artery is often not identified with an acute vertebral artery dissection. However, a focal abrupt caliber change associated with irregularity of the vertebral artery should raise suspicion of an acute dissection, particularly if there are embolic posterior fossa acute infarcts. Other imaging findings of an acute vertebral artery dissection include intramural hematoma formation (best demonstrated by MRI) and vertebral artery occlusion.
- **Cervical vertebral artery dissection with pseudoaneurysm formation.** An arterial dissection, particularly when chronic, results in a weakened vessel wall and may result in a pseudoaneurysm.
- **Fibromuscular dysplasia with cervical vertebral artery pseudoaneurysm formation.** Fibromuscular dysplasia (FMD) is an arteriopathy of medium- and large-sized vessels. It is most commonly identified in women aged 30 to 50 who have a history of hypertension. The disease most commonly affects the renal arteries, followed by the carotid and vertebral arteries. The exact etiology of this arteriopathy is unknown, but the leading hypothesis suggests an association with α_1-antitrypsin deficiency. Three histologic subtypes of FMD are recognized which are differentiated by the layer of the arterial wall affected. The medial subtype of FMD is by far the most common and represents 90% to 95% of cases, with vascular imaging typically demonstrating thickened concentric rings associated with a "string-of-beads" appearance. The intimal subtype accounts for 5% to 10% of cases and results in intimal thickening, destruction of the internal elastic lamina, and a long tubular vascular stenosis. The adventitial subtype is rare and results in fibrosis of the adventitia as well as of the periarterial tissue, creating asymmetric vascular outpouchings. Continued screening of FMD patients should be considered because of the increased risk of arterial dissection, aneurysm, and arteriovenous fistula formation.
- **Cervical vertebral artery venous plexus on MRI.** An unenhanced fat-saturated axial T1-weighted MRI sequence through the neck is often helpful to diagnose an acute arterial dissection by demonstrating T1 shortening associated within an intramural thrombus, particularly

when evaluating the carotid arteries. However, incidental T1 shortening may occur from flow within the venous plexus that surrounds the cervical vertebral arteries and thus can simulate cervical vertebral artery intramural thrombus. It is important to compare the T1 shortening on the fat-saturated T1-weighted sequence with an MRA of the neck. If a focal vascular contour abnormality is not identified on the accompanying MRA of the neck to correspond with the T1 shortening on the fat-saturated sequence, then the finding on the fat-saturated sequence likely relates to the normal venous plexus that surrounds the vertebral arteries and not an acute vertebral artery dissection. In addition, a poorly timed bolus during a contrast-enhanced MRA of the neck may result in venous contamination of the vertebral artery venous plexus and poor visualization of the vertebral arteries.

Cervical vertebral artery tortuosity and kinking

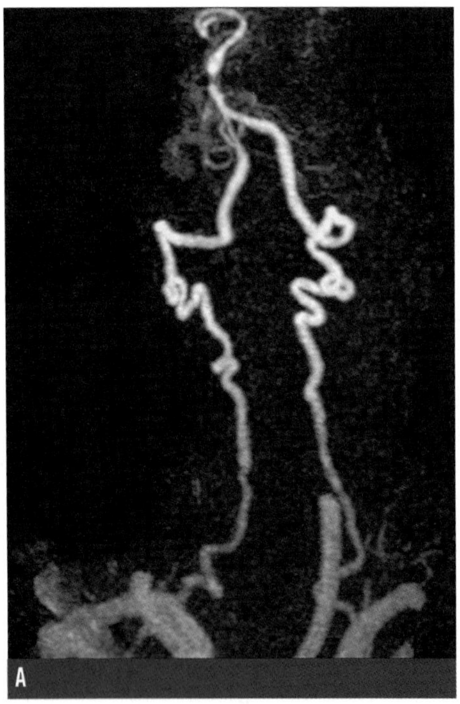

A slightly obliqued MIP image of the cervical vertebral arteries from a gadolinium-enhanced MRA (**A**) demonstrates marked tortuosity of the cervical vertebral arteries. There is no evidence of flow limitation because of the cervical vertebral artery tortuosity and kinking. Therefore, the findings are likely incidental.

Cervical vertebral artery tortuosity and kinking

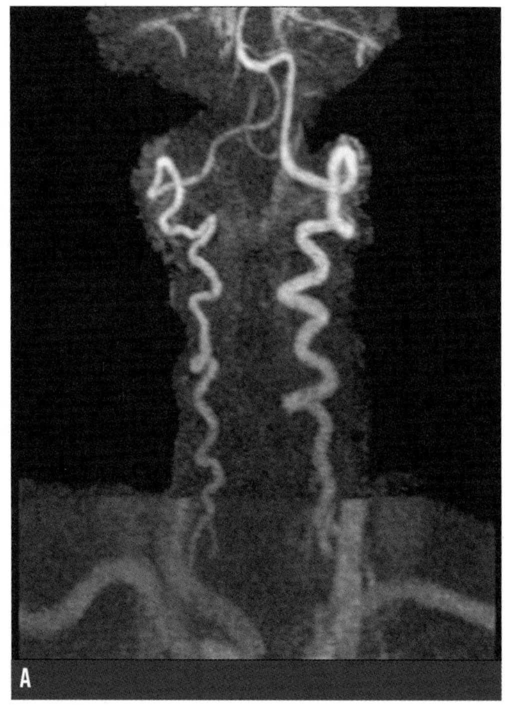

Different patient. A MIP image of the cervical vertebral arteries from a gadolinium-enhanced MRA (**A**) demonstrates marked tortuosity and kinking of both cervical vertebral arteries. These findings are likely incidental as there is no evidence of flow limitation, when allowing for a developmentally smaller right cervical vertebral artery.

Cervical vertebral artery loop

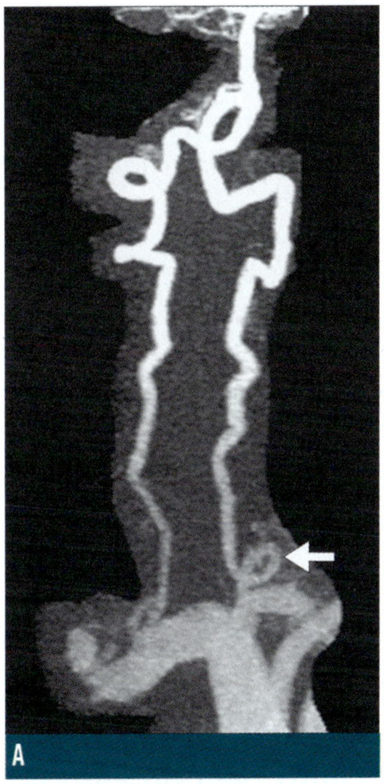

A slightly obliqued MIP image of the cervical vertebral arteries from a gadolinium-enhanced MRA (**A**) demonstrates a 360° loop involving the left cervical vertebral artery V1 segment (arrow).

Companion case: Acute cervical vertebral artery dissection

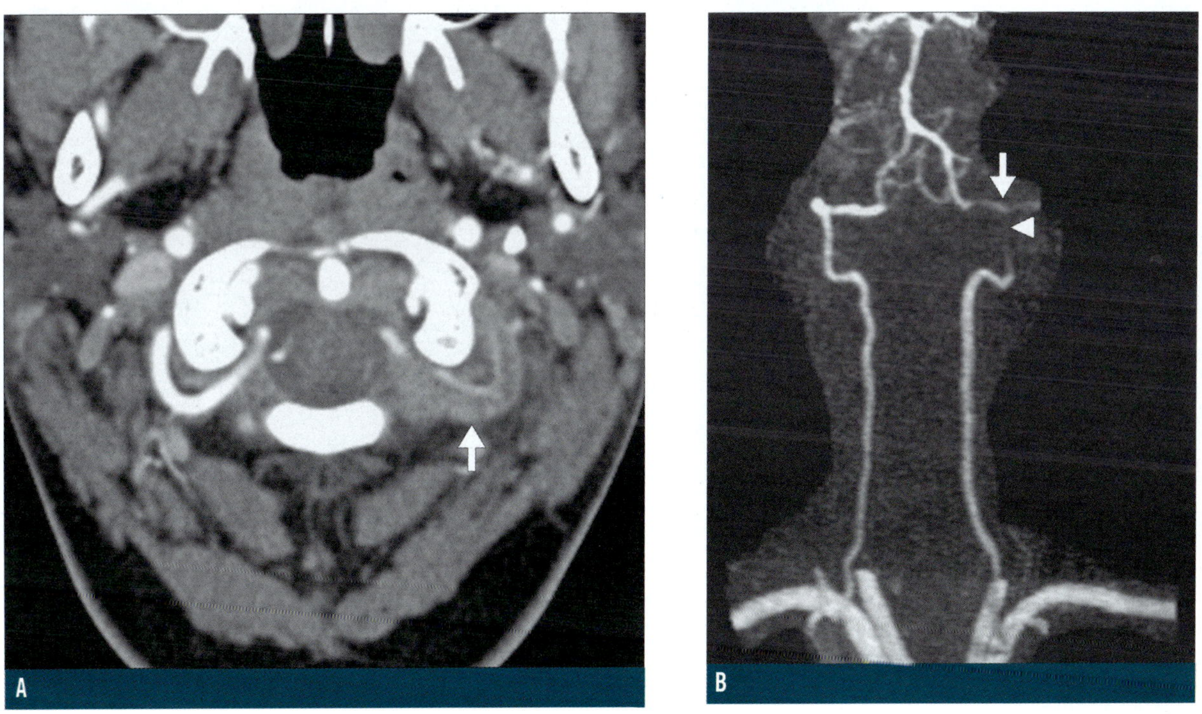

An axial image from a CTA of the head (**A**) demonstrates marked narrowing of the left cervical vertebral artery V3 segment likely because of intramural clot related to an acute arterial dissection (arrow, **A**). This particular finding has been termed the "suboccipital rind sign." A MIP image from a gadolinium-enhanced MRA of the same patient (**B**) demonstrates focal narrowing of the vertical portion (arrowhead, **B**) and horizontal portion (arrow, **B**) of the left cervical vertebral artery V3 segment. An axial fat-suppressed T1-weighted MRI sequence without contrast (**C**) demonstrates a large amount of T1 shortening within the distal portion of the left cervical vertebral artery V3 segment, compatible with an acute vertebral artery dissection (arrow, **C**).

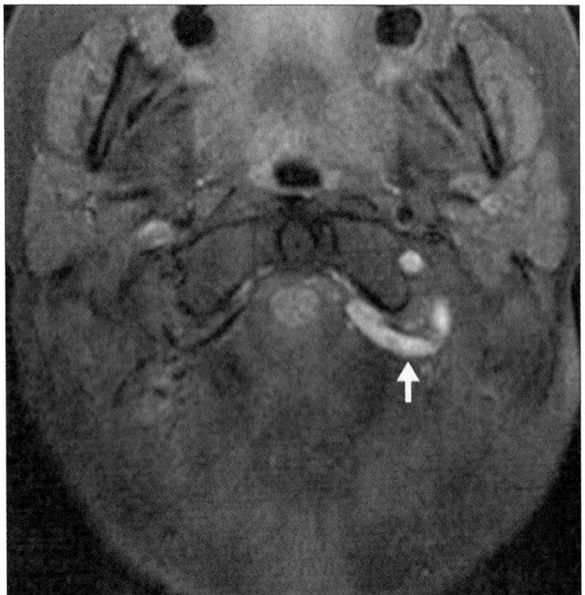
C

Companion case: Cervical vertebral artery dissection with pseudoaneurysm formation

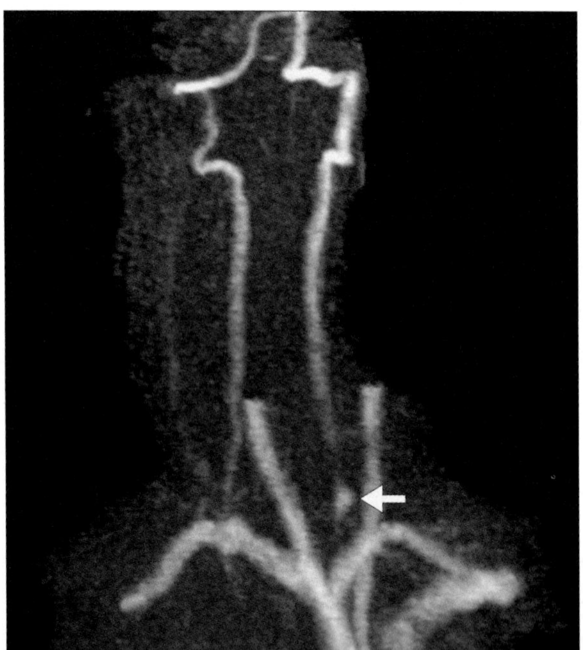
A

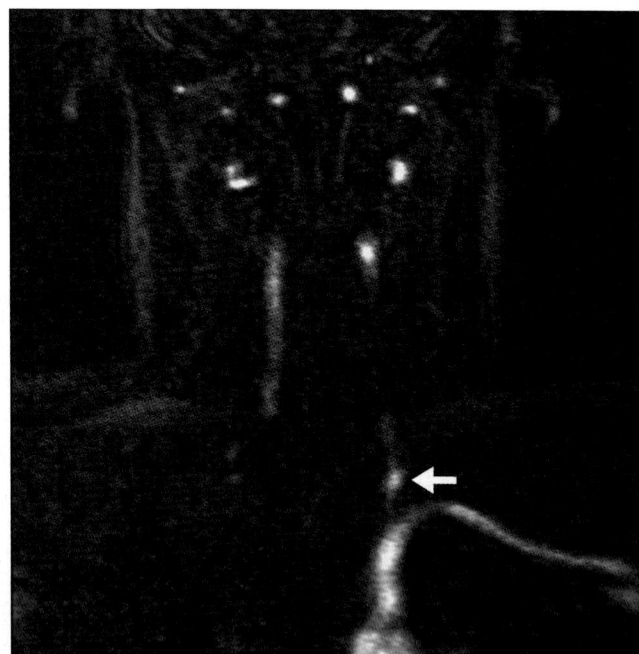
B

A MIP (**A**) and a source image (**B**) from a gadolinium-enhanced MRA demonstrate a small, focal pseudoaneurysm (arrows, **A, B**) involving the left cervical vertebral artery V1 segment with stenosis both proximal and distal to the pseudoaneurysm. An axial unenhanced fat-saturated T1-weighted MR image of the same patient obtained through one of the left cervical vertebral artery V1 segment stenoses (**C**) demonstrates abnormal intramural T1 shortening, compatible with a vertebral artery dissection (arrow, **C**). A MIP image from a gadolinium-enhanced MRA of the same patient following treatment (**D**) demonstrates resolution of the dissection and pseudoaneurysm.

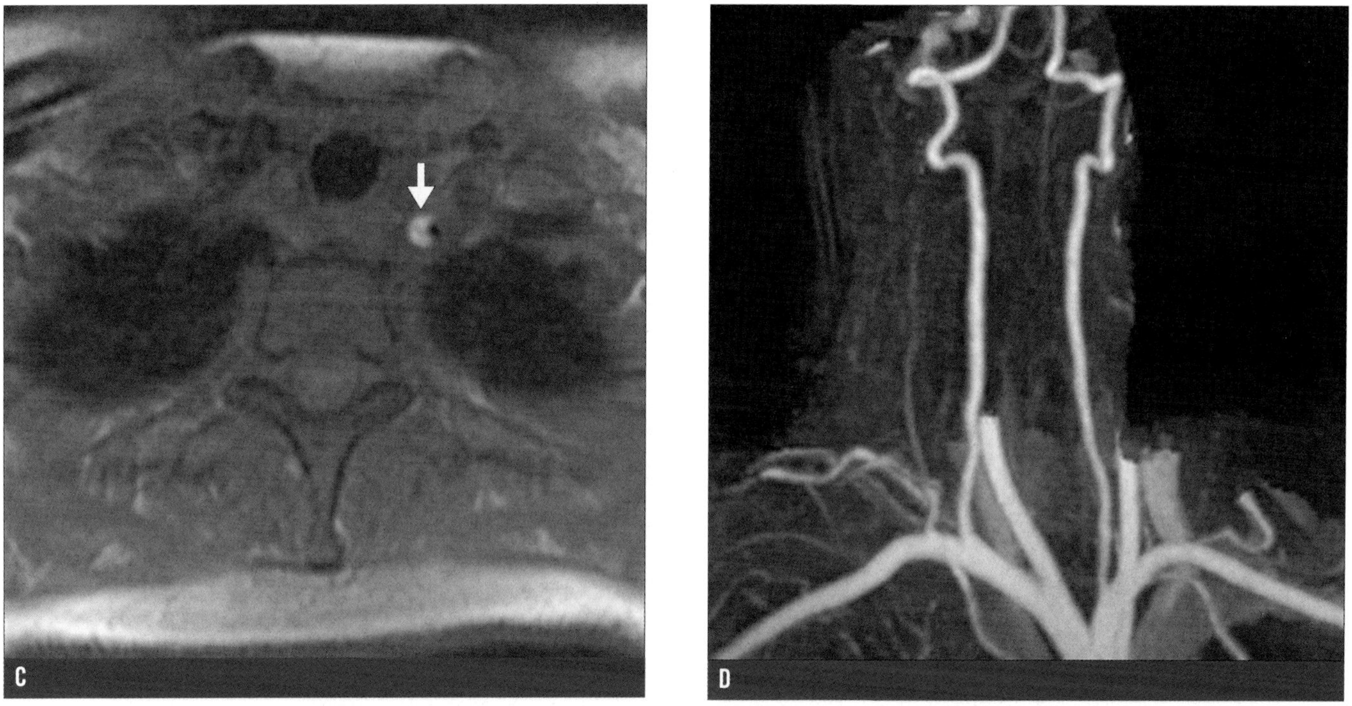

Companion case: Fibromuscular dysplasia with cervical vertebral artery pseudoaneurysm formation

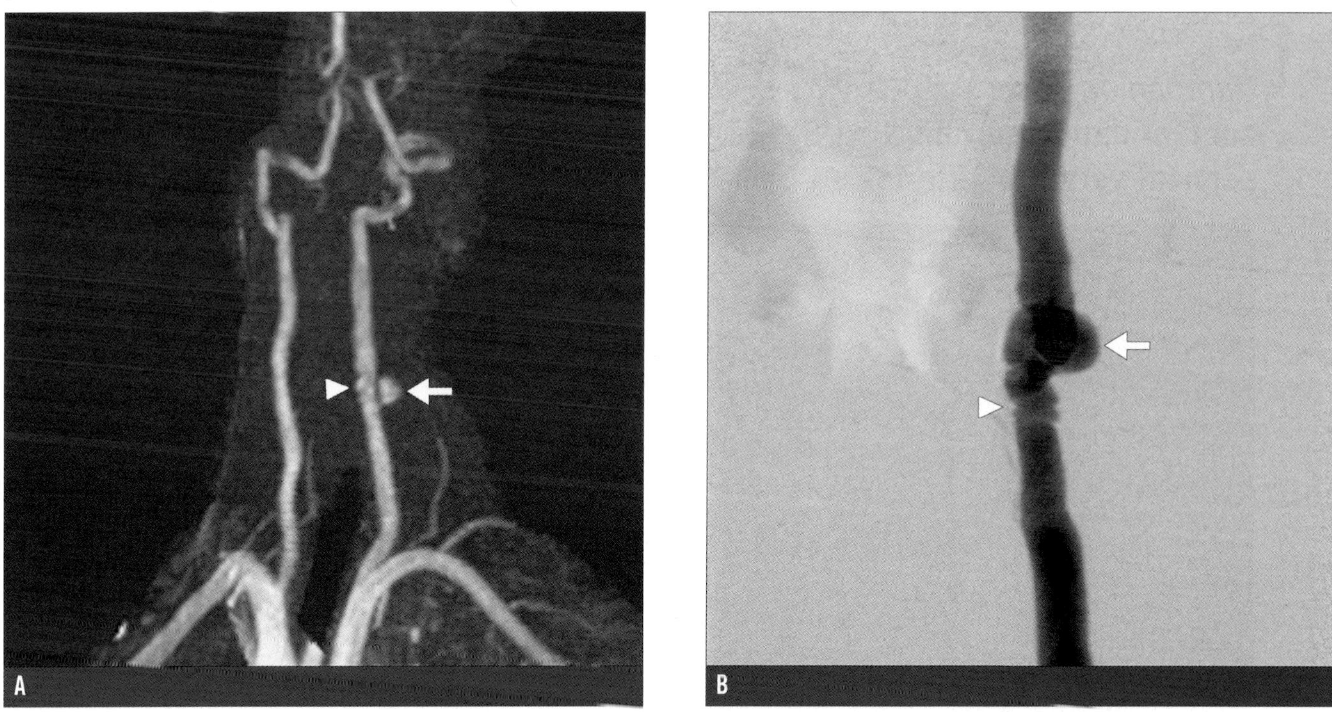

A MIP image obtained from a gadolinium-enhanced MRA (**A**) demonstrates a focal pseudoaneurysm (arrow, **A**) associated with a "beaded" appearance of the immediately adjacent left cervical vertebral artery V2 segment (arrowhead, **A**), the latter finding suggestive of fibromuscular dysplasia. An image from a catheter angiogram of the left cervical vertebral artery performed on the same patient (**B**) demonstrates the same pseudoaneurysm (arrow, **B**) and the immediately adjacent beaded irregularity (arrowhead, **B**). This patient had known fibromuscular dysplasia and widespread beaded arterial irregularity elsewhere.

Companion case: Vertebral artery venous plexuses simulating vertebral artery dissections on MRI

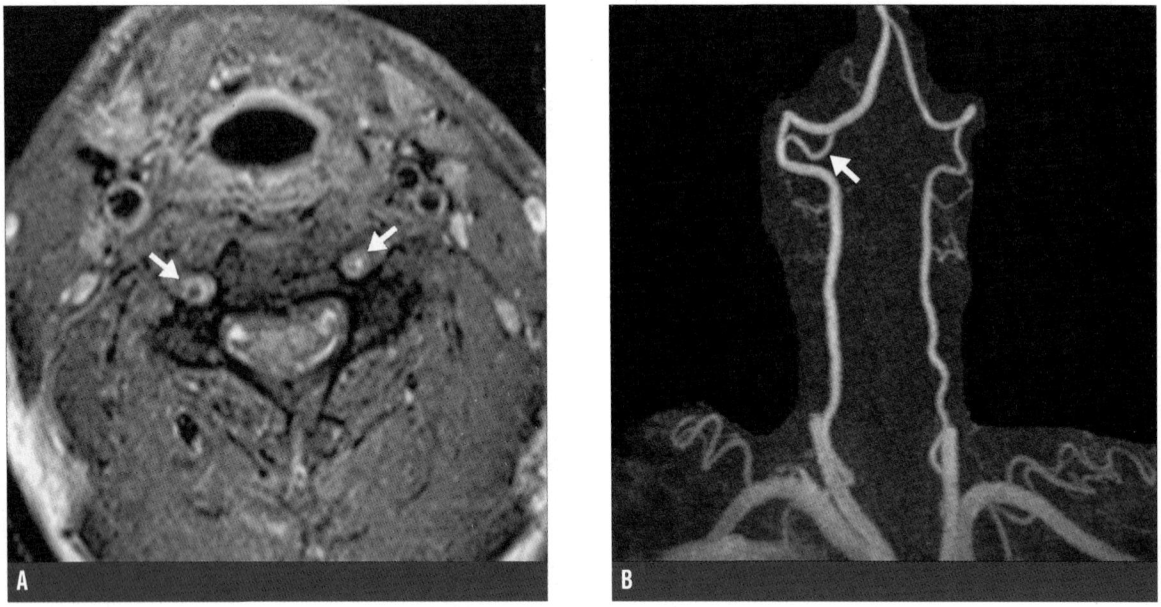

An unenhanced fat-suppressed axial T1-weighted image obtained through the neck at the level of the distal cervical vertebral artery V2 segments (**A**) demonstrates T1 shortening surrounding both cervical vertebral arteries (arrows, **A**), worrisome for possible bilateral vertebral artery dissections. However, a MIP image of the vertebral arteries from a gadolinium-enhanced MRA performed during the same study (**B**) does not demonstrate any stenosis or focal irregularity involving either cervical vertebral artery. The finding on image **A** simply represents normal venous plexuses surrounding the cervical vertebral arteries and not vertebral artery dissections. Incidental note is made of a right vertebral artery V3 segment fenestration (arrow, **B**).

Companion case: Venous contamination surrounding the cervical vertebral arteries on MRI

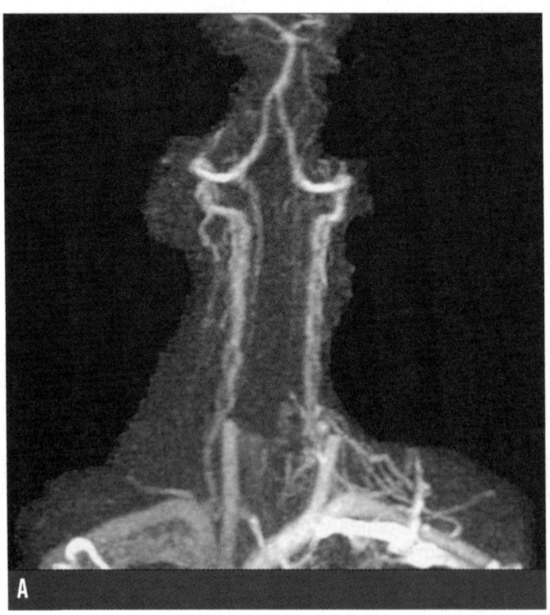

A MIP image from a gadolinium-enhanced MRA (**A**) demonstrates marked venous contamination of the venous plexuses surrounding the cervical vertebral arteries. This was due to poor timing of the contrast bolus.

REFERENCES

Benes V, Netuka D. Surgical correction of symptomatic vertebral artery kinking. *Br J Neurosurg.* 2003;17(2):174-178.

Lum, et al. Vertebral artery dissection with a normal-appearing lumen at multisection CT angiography: the importance of identifying wall hematoma. *AJNR Am J Neuroradiol.* 2009;30:787-792.

Naggara O, et al. Added value of high-resolution MR imaging in the diagnosis of vertebral artery dissection. *AJNR Am J Neuroradiol.* 2010;31(9):1707-1712.

Poonam RS, Rathore NJ. Tortuous vertebral arteries-incidence and clinical implications. *J Clin Diagn Res.* 2011;5(4):780-782.

Taylor WB 3rd, Vandergriff CL, Opatowsky MJ, Layton KF. Bowhunter's syndrome diagnosed with provocative digital subtraction cerebral angiography. *Proc (Bayl Univ Med Cent).* 2012;25(1):26-27.

Zimmerman HB, Farrell WJ. Cervical vertebral erosion caused by vertebral artery tortuosity. *Am J Roentgenol Radium Ther Nucl Med.* 1970;108(4):767-770.

CASE 9 Retropharyngeal course of the cervical carotid arteries

The cervical internal carotid artery (ICA) may have a tortuous course, sometimes projecting medially toward the retropharyngeal space. However, while medialized cervical ICAs may appear to freely reside within the retropharyngeal space on cross-sectional imaging, they are normally anatomically separated medially from the retropharyngeal space by the deep layer of the deep cervical fascia. Thus a cervical ICA with a "retropharyngeal course" likely continues to reside within the carotid space and bows the deep layer of the deep cervical fascia toward the retropharyngeal space. The etiology of a retropharyngeal course of the cervical ICAs has been debated, although some possible etiologies include degenerative laxity of the supporting structures or obesity with resultant medial displacement of the cervical ICAs. Although less common, the carotid bifurcations or common carotid arteries may also bulge toward the retropharyngeal space. If both carotid arteries extend medial enough to appear to contact one another in the retropharyngeal space, then the term "kissing carotid arteries" has been used. A retropharyngeal course of the cervical ICAs often results in apparent abnormal thickening of the prevertebral soft tissues on plain film radiography. This apparent finding may lead the radiologist to believe that an occult fracture or an acute retropharyngeal inflammatory process is present. CT imaging of the neck readily resolves this plain film imaging pitfall.

Uncommonly, a retropharyngeal course of the carotid arteries may be a transient phenomenon, identified on one cross-sectional study only to be absent on a follow-up examination. The etiology of this transient retropharyngeal course has not yet been determined in the literature.

It is important to identify a retropharyngeal course of the cervical carotid arteries on imaging as this may result in asymmetry of the posterior pharyngeal wall which could be mistaken for a submucosal mass during direct inspection of the pharynx. Furthermore, placement of a laryngoscope and/or endotracheal tube in a patient with retropharyngeal course of the cervical carotid arteries may result in carotid injury, such as carotid dissection. A retropharyngeal course of a cervical carotid artery is also a contraindication to robotic surgical removal of an ipsilateral pharyngeal mass.

Retropharyngeal course of the cervical internal carotid arteries

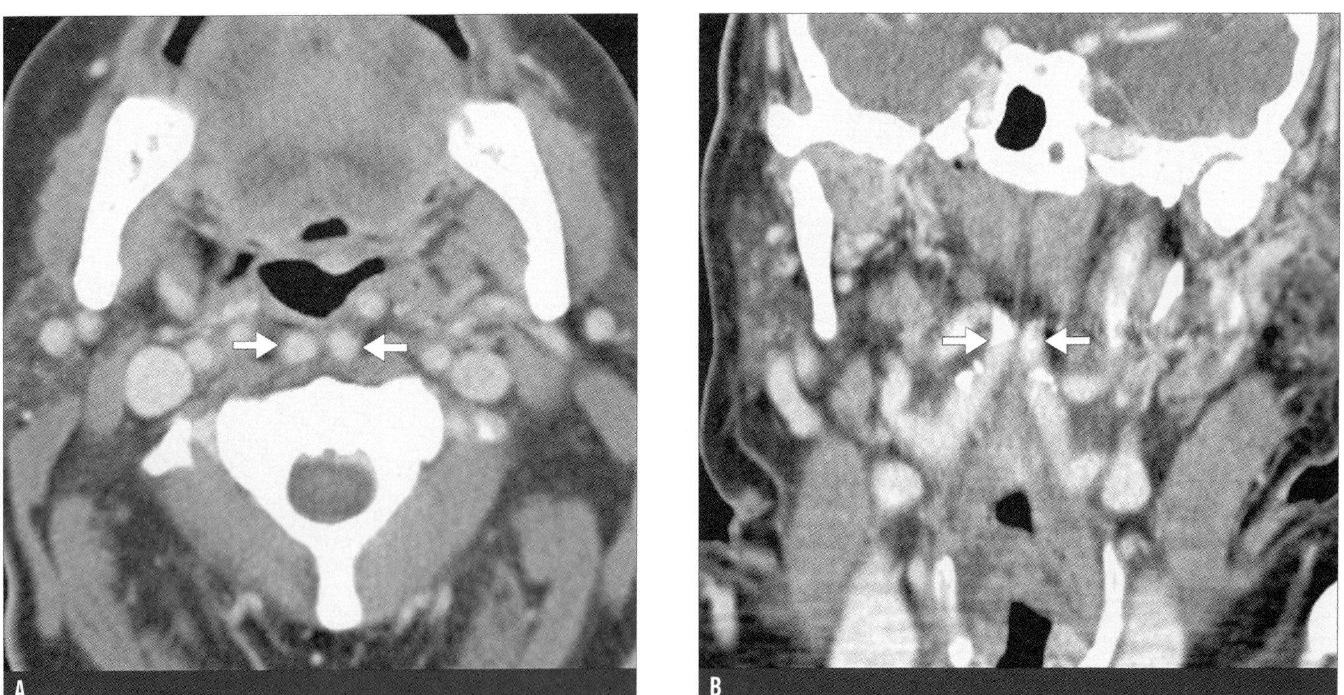

Axial (**A**) and coronal reformatted (**B**) contrast-enhanced CT images of the neck demonstrate a retropharyngeal course of the cervical internal carotid arteries at the level of the oropharynx, which nearly contact each other at the midline, resulting in a near "kissing carotid artery" configuration (arrows, **A**, **B**).

Retropharyngeal course of the carotid bifurcations

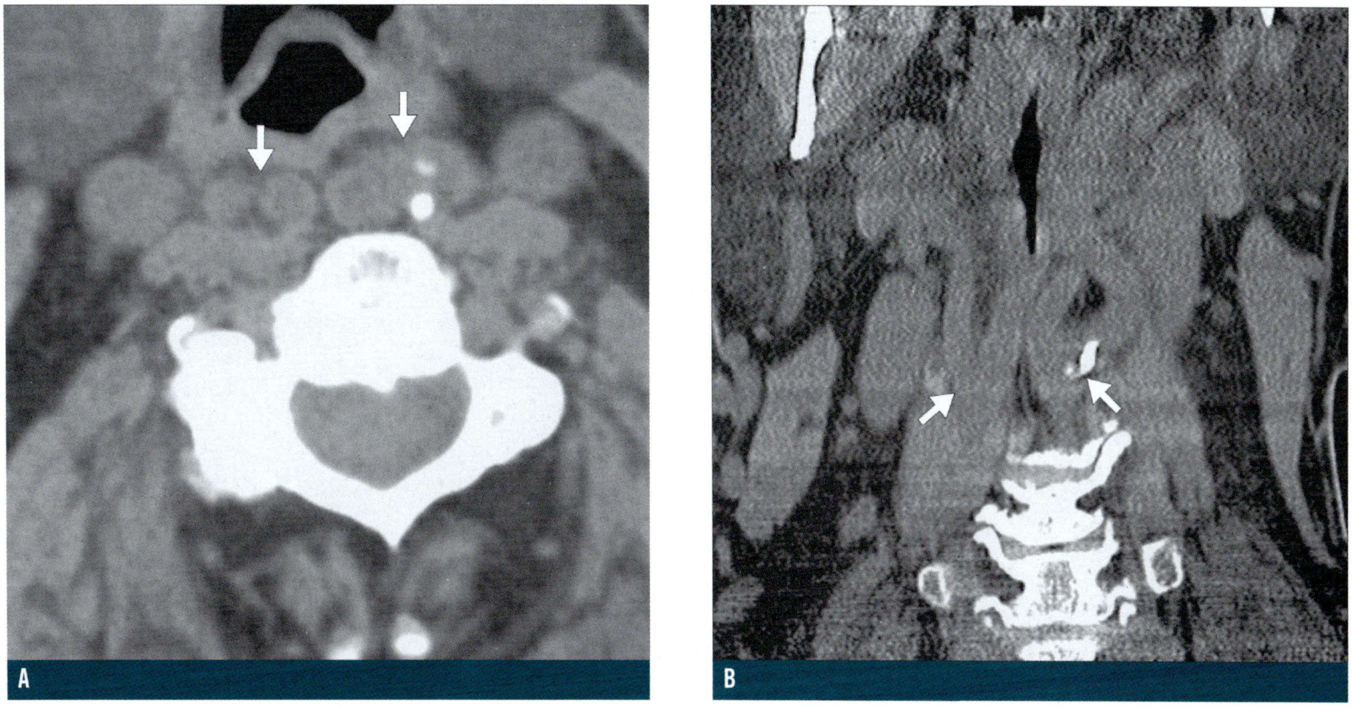

Axial (**A**) and coronal reformatted (**B**) unenhanced CT images from a CT of the cervical spine demonstrate a retropharyngeal course and "kissing" configuration of the carotids bifurcations at the level of the lower oropharynx (arrows, **A**, **B**).

Retropharyngeal course of the common carotid arteries

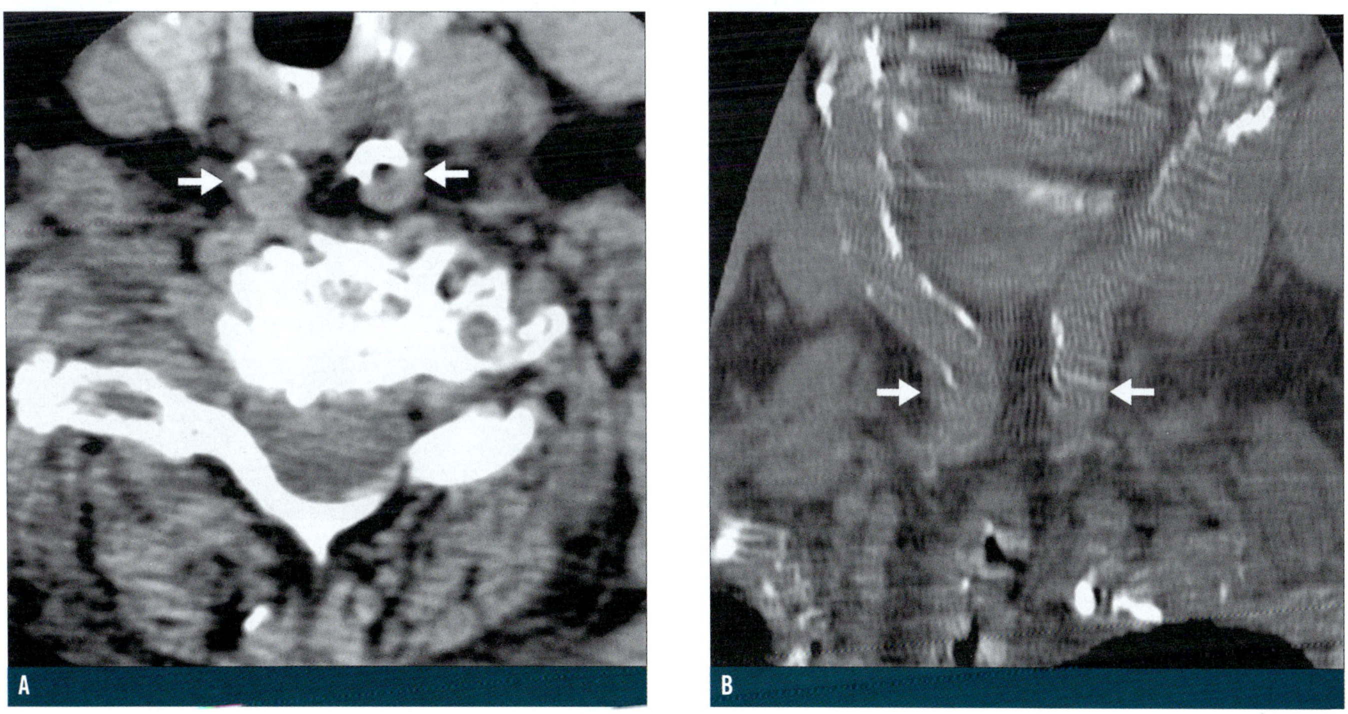

Axial (**A**) and coronal reformatted (**B**) unenhanced CT images from a CT of the cervical spine demonstrate a retropharyngeal course of the common carotid arteries at the level of the hypopharynx (arrows, **A**, **B**).

Transient retropharyngeal course of the cervical internal carotid arteries

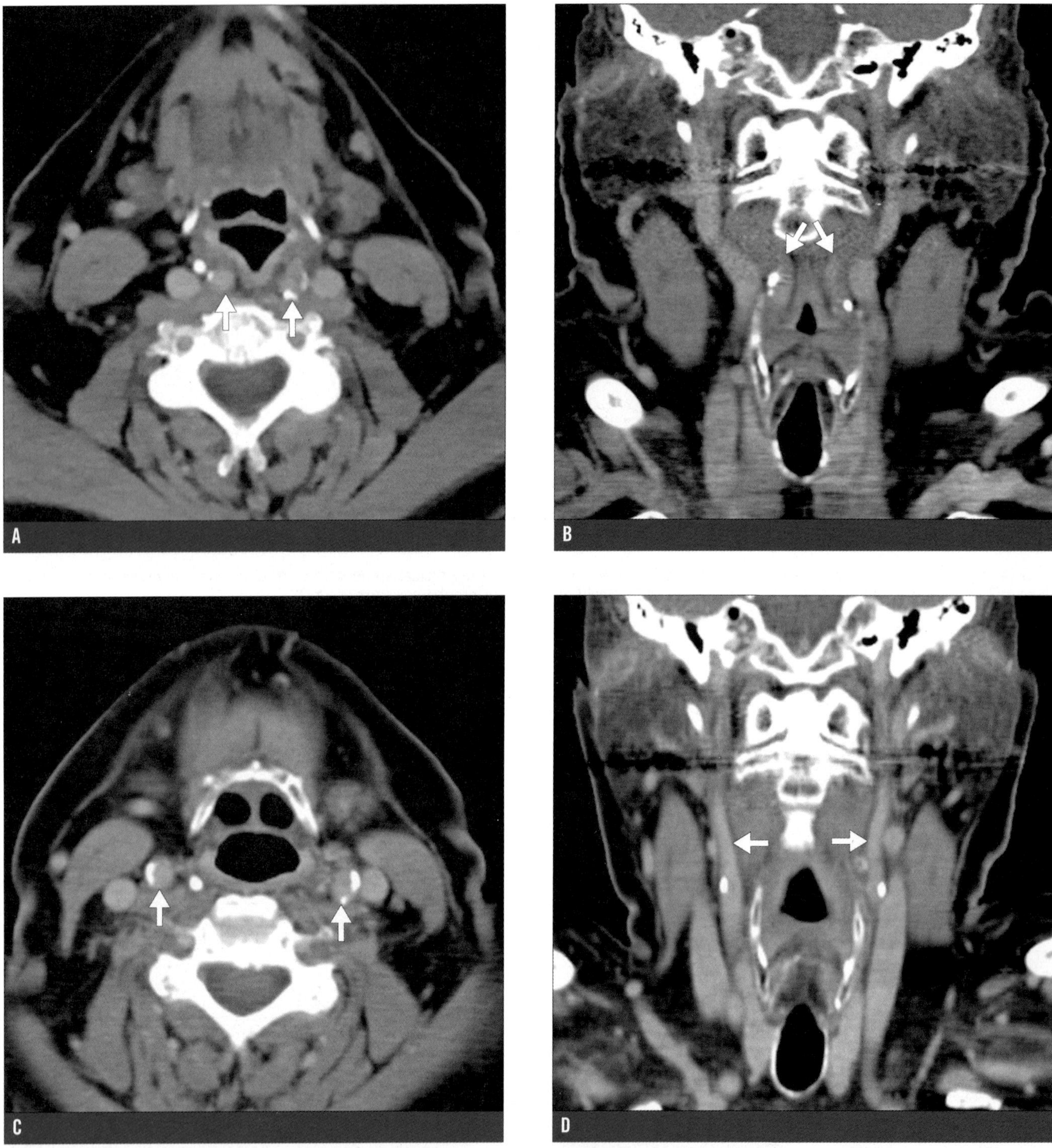

Axial (**A**) and coronal reformatted (**B**) contrast-enhanced CT images demonstrate a retropharyngeal course of the cervical internal carotid arteries (arrows, **A**, **B**). Six months later, axial (**C**) and coronal reformatted (**D**) contrast-enhanced CT images of the same patient demonstrate that the cervical internal carotid arteries no longer have a retropharyngeal course but instead are located in a more typical position (arrows, **C**, **D**). This case illustrates that a retropharyngeal course of the cervical internal carotid arteries may be a transient finding in some patients.

REFERENCES

Fix TJ, Daffner RH, Deeb, ZL. Carotid transposition: Another cause of wide retropharyngeal soft tissues. *AJR Am J Roentgenol.* 1996;167:1305-1307.

Gupta A, Shah AD, Zhang Z, Phillips CD, Young RJ. Variability in the position of the retropharyngeal internal carotid artery. *Laryngoscope.* 2013;123(2):401-403.

Marcucci C, Thomas P, Sewell DA. Retropharyngeal carotid artery: An important anatomic variation for the anesthesiologist. *Anesthesiology.* 2009;111(2):454-455.

Palacios E, Kirsch D, Rojas R. Anomalous course of the carotid arteries in the retropharyngeal space poses a surgical risk. *Ear Nose Throat J.* 2005;84:336-337.

CASE 10 Variation in the location of a carotid artery bifurcation

The common carotid artery typically bifurcates at the level of the C4 vertebral body, which is usually at the superior margin of the thyroid lamina. However, a carotid artery bifurcation may occur as cephalad as C1 or as caudal as T2. An abnormally high bifurcation is important to recognize as it introduces additional surgical challenges that may require a mandibular split osteotomy to gain access to the artery.

Asymmetric location of the carotid bifurcations

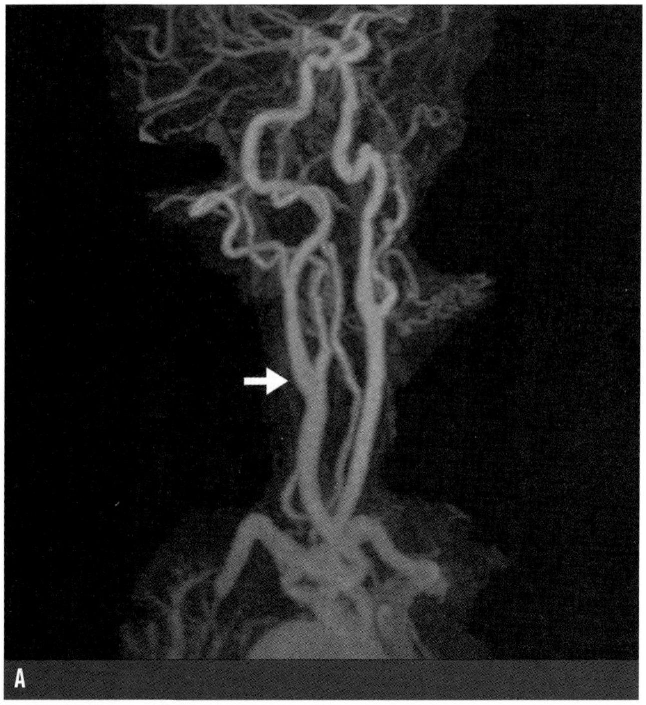

An oblique MIP image from a contrast-enhanced MRA of the neck (**A**) demonstrate an asymmetrically lower right carotid bifurcation (arrow) compared to the left.

High carotid artery bifurcation

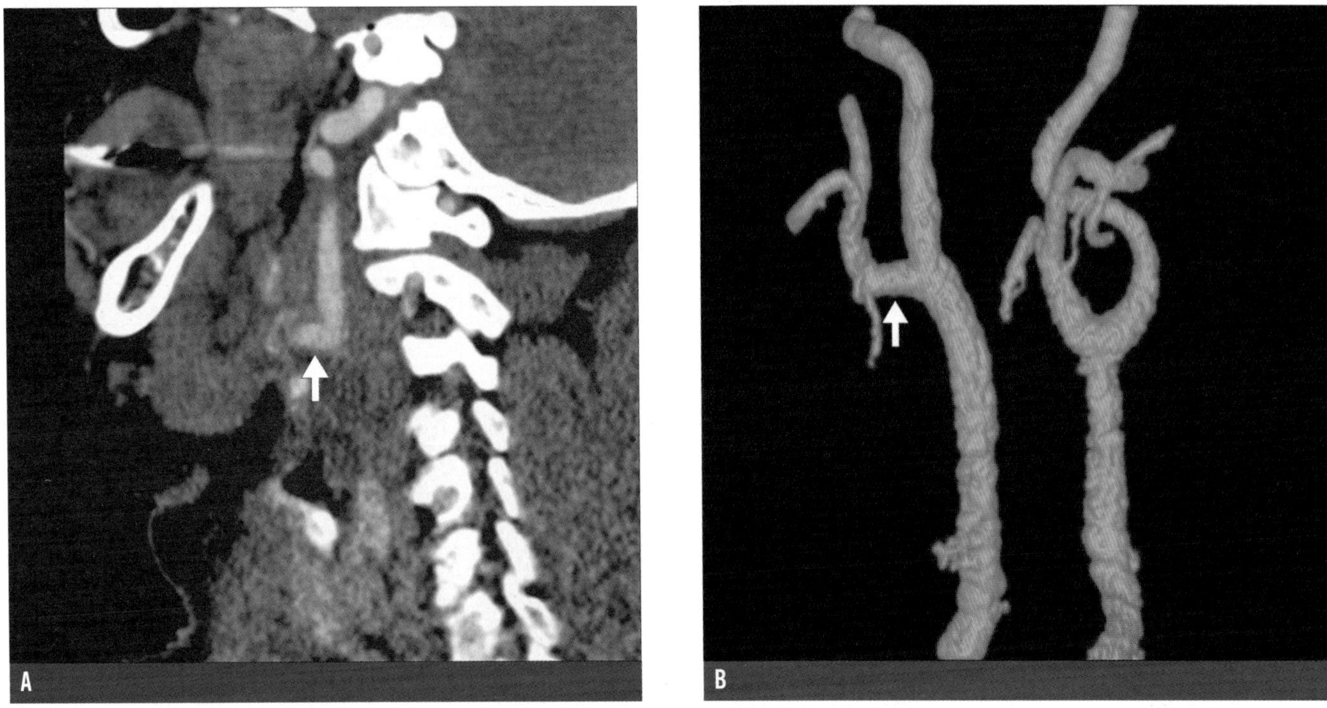

A right parasagittal reformatted image from a CTA of the neck (**A**) demonstrates a high right carotid bifurcation at the approximate C2 to C3 level and the level of the mandible (arrow, **A**). A 3D volumetric image from the same CTA (**B**) demonstrates the relationship of the high right carotid bifurcation (arrow) relative to the left carotid bifurcation.

REFERENCES

Ooigawa H, et al. Non-bifurcating cervical carotid artery. *J Clin Neurosci.* 2006;13(9):944-947.

Osborn A. *Diagnostic Cerebral Angiography.* 2nd ed. Philadelphia, PA: LWW; 1999.

CASE 11 Carotid web

Carotid webs can sometimes be mistaken for intimal flaps that are sometimes identified with an arterial dissection or atherosclerotic disease. Carotid webs are characterized by focal, horizontally oriented intima, often located along the posterior aspect of the carotid bulb. The cause of a carotid web is unknown, although one theory proposes a relationship between carotid web formation and atypical fibromuscular dysplasia. While carotid webs are often incidental findings, altered hemodynamic flow along a carotid web can result in thrombus formation and thromboembolic complications, necessitating anticoagulation or endovascular therapy in this setting.

Carotid web

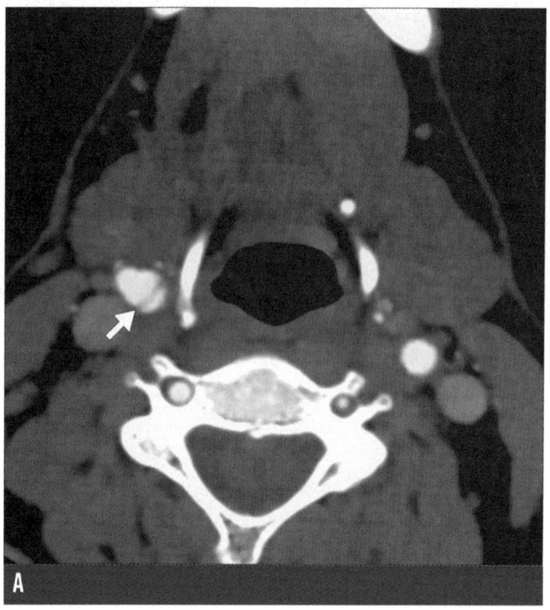

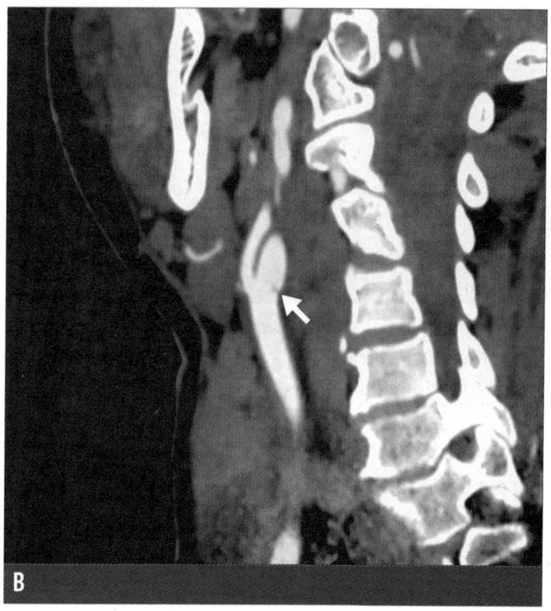

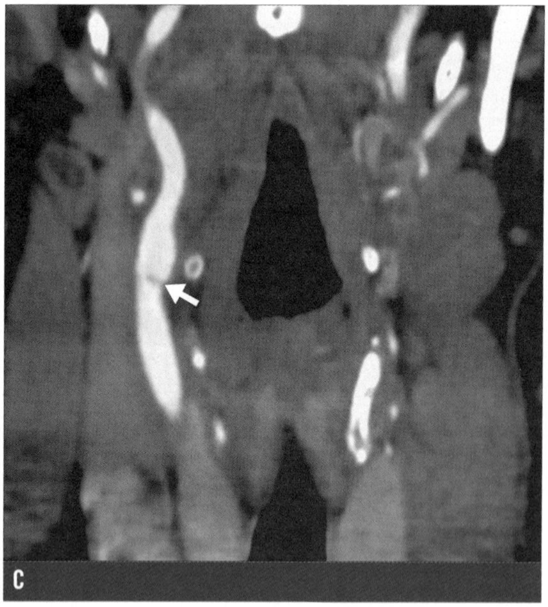

Axial (**A**), sagittal reformatted (**B**), and coronal reformatted (**C**) images from a CTA demonstrate a discrete, horizontally oriented, linear filling defect within the posteromedial aspect of the right carotid bulb, compatible with a carotid web (arrows, **A**-**C**).

Carotid web

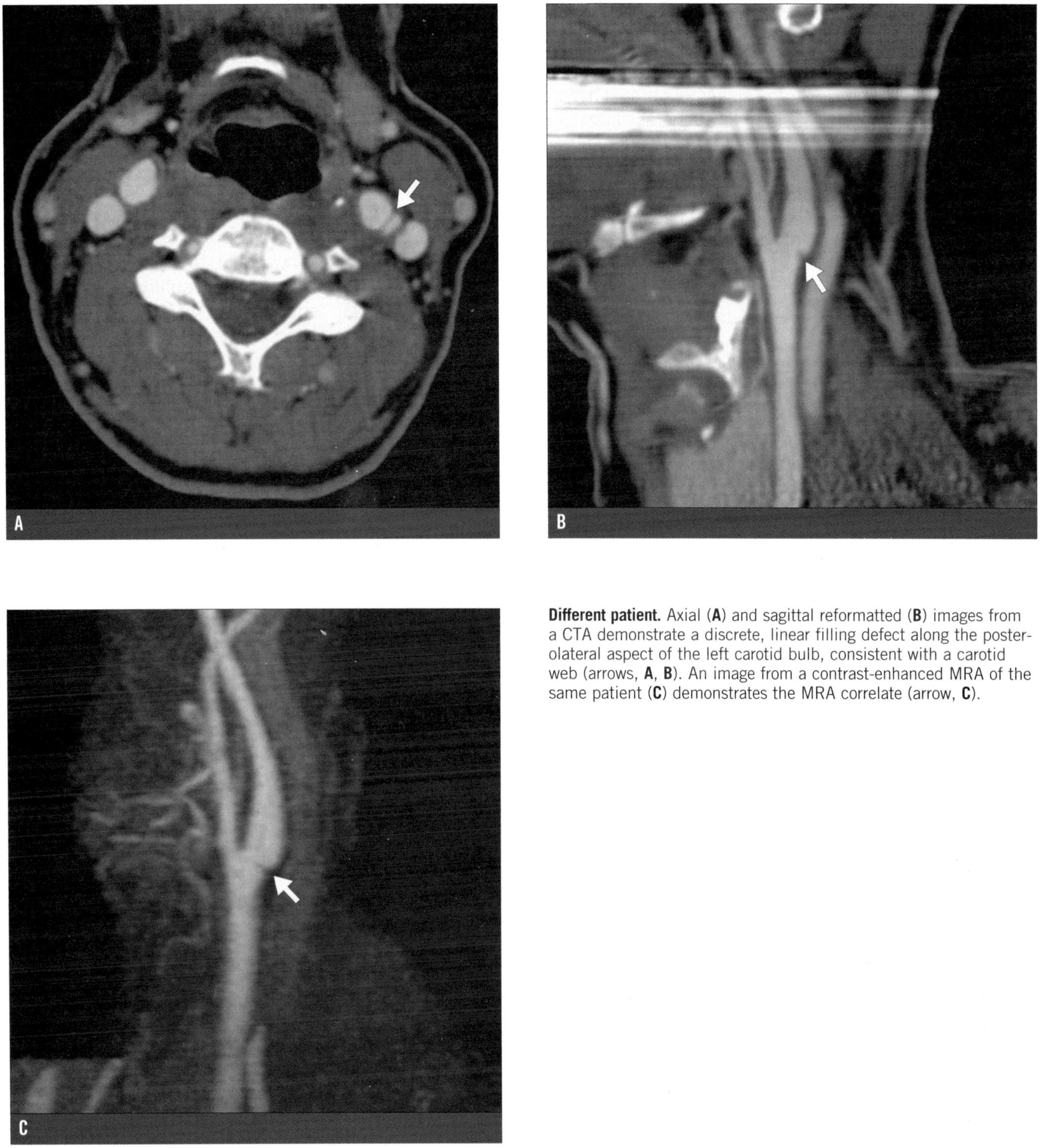

Different patient. Axial (**A**) and sagittal reformatted (**B**) images from a CTA demonstrate a discrete, linear filling defect along the posterolateral aspect of the left carotid bulb, consistent with a carotid web (arrows, **A**, **B**). An image from a contrast-enhanced MRA of the same patient (**C**) demonstrates the MRA correlate (arrow, **C**).

REFERENCES

Kliewer MA, Carroll BA. Ultrasound case of the day. Internal carotid artery web (atypical fibromuscular dysplasia). *Radiographics.* 1991;11(3):504-505.

Morgenlander JC, Goldstein LB. Recurrent transient ischemic attacks and stroke in association with and internal carotid artery web. *Stroke.* 1991;22:94-98.

Cervical carotid artery tortuosity is a relatively common finding and usually occurs in the setting of chronic hypertension and/or atherosclerosis. However, there is literature that describes some cases of cervical carotid artery tortuosity to contain typical or atypical features of fibromuscular dysplasia at pathology. Moreover, although rare, cervical carotid tortuosity has also been observed in children, suggesting some are congenital in nature. While most often incidental findings, a tortuous cervical carotid artery may be inadvertently injured during a surgical procedure, such as during a tonsillectomy, adenoidectomy, or peritonsillar abscess drainage.

Focal cervical carotid artery kinks and loops may also be identified on imaging. These are most likely related to the same etiologies responsible for cervical carotid tortuosity. Cervical carotid kinks may be a source of cerebral emboli or may be temporarily occluded by head/neck rotation resulting in cerebral ischemia. In addition, surgical correction of a cervical carotid kink has been performed in selected cases of cerebral ischemia when other etiologies have been ruled out, although surgical correction for this entity remains controversial. Most cases of a carotid kink are incidental, particularly if there is no flow limitation distal to the kink or focal thrombus associated with the kink on MRA, CTA, or catheter angiography. Finally, because of altered hemodynamics, aneurysms may form along a cervical carotid vascular loop.

Tortuous cervical ICA

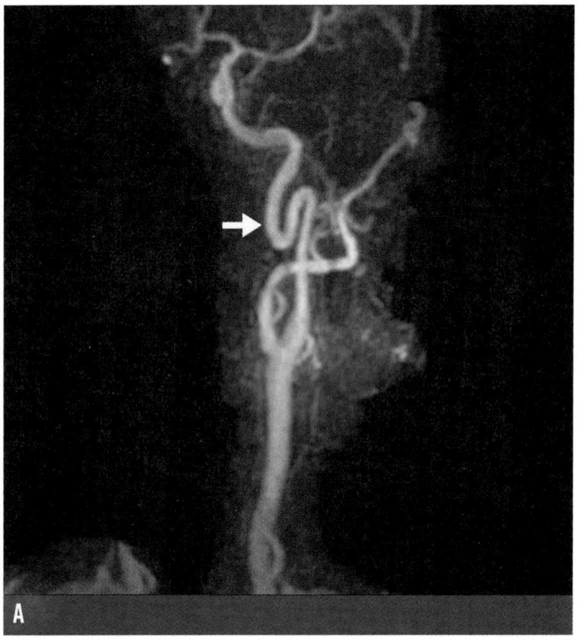

A MIP image from a contrast-enhanced MRA of the left carotid artery (**A**) demonstrates a typical appearance of a tortuous cervical ICA (arrow).

COMPANION CASE

- **Fibromuscular dysplasia.** Fibromuscular dysplasia (FMD) is an arteriopathy of medium- and large-sized vessels. It is most commonly identified in women aged 30 to 50 who have a history of hypertension. The disease most commonly affects the renal arteries, followed by the carotid and vertebral arteries. The exact etiology of this arteriopathy is unknown, but the leading hypothesis suggests an association with α_1-antitrypsin deficiency. Three histologic subtypes of FMD are recognized which are differentiated by the layer of the arterial wall affected. The medial subtype of FMD is by far the most common and represents 90% to 95% of cases, with vascular imaging typically demonstrating thickened concentric rings associated with a "string-of-beads" appearance. The intimal subtype accounts for 5% to 10% of cases and results in intimal thickening, destruction of the internal elastic lamina, and a long tubular vascular stenosis. The adventitial subtype is rare and results in fibrosis of the adventitia as well as of the periarterial tissue, creating asymmetric vascular outpouchings. Continued screening of FMD patients should be considered because of the increased risk of arterial dissection, aneurysm, and arteriovenous fistula formation.

Cervical ICA kink

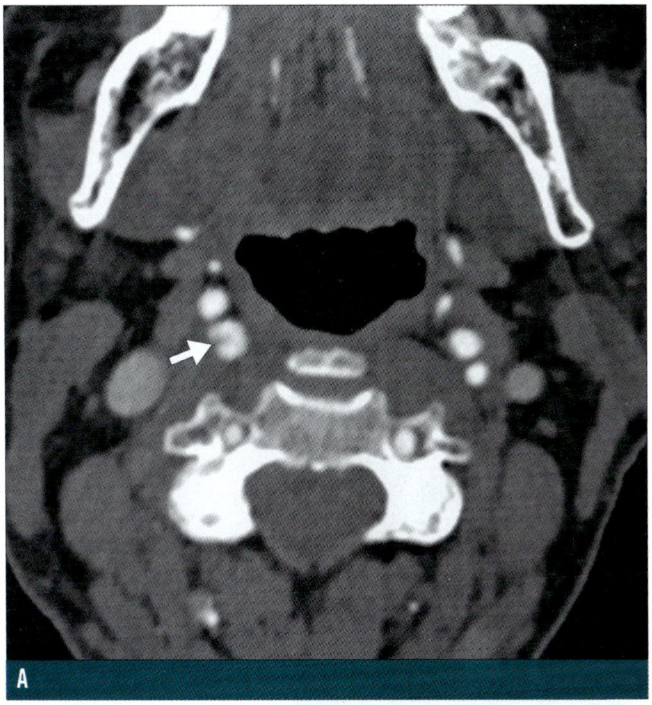

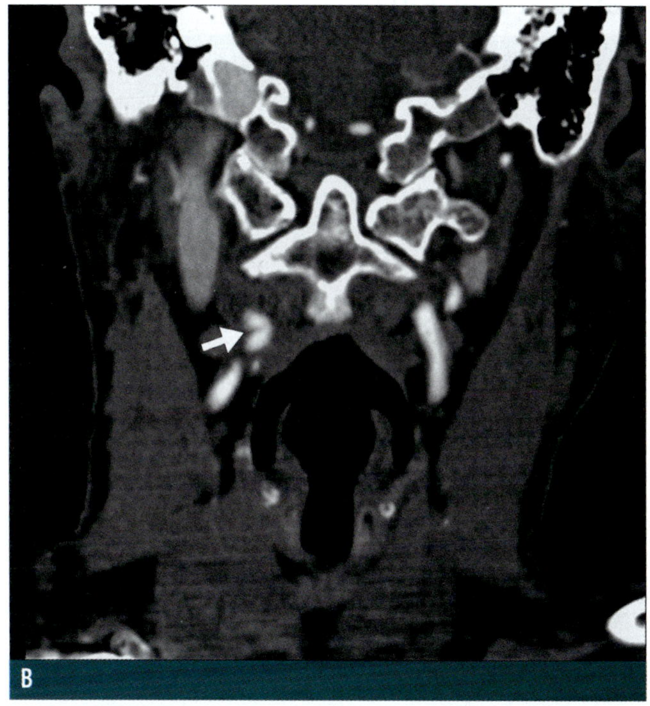

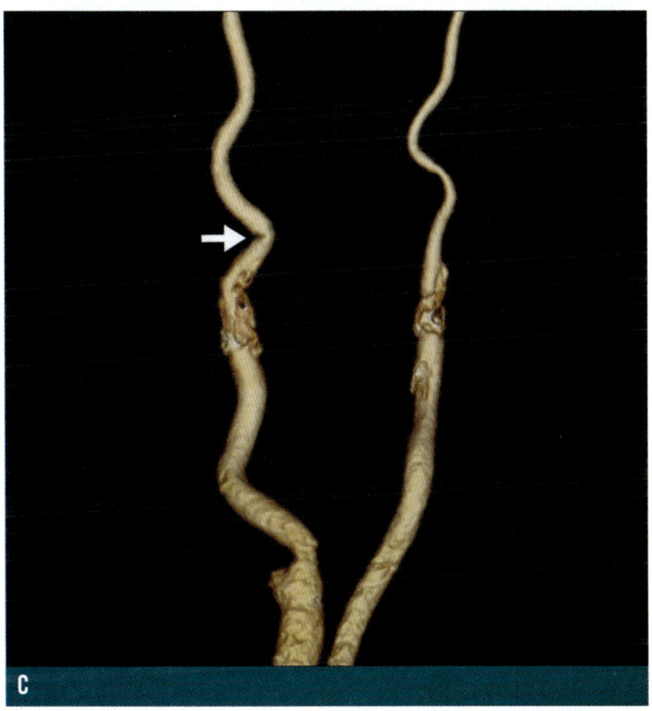

Axial (**A**) and coronal reformatted (**B**) images from a CTA demonstrate a focal kink in the mid right cervical ICA (arrows, **A**, **B**). A 3D volumetric image from the same CTA (**C**) also demonstrates the kink (arrow, **C**). There is no evidence of flow limitation distal to the kink and the finding is therefore likely incidental.

Cervical ICA kink

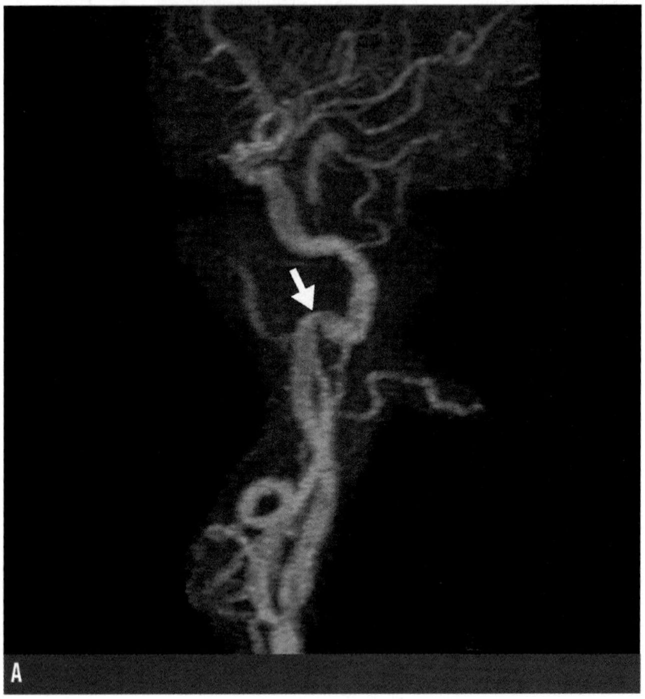

Different patient. A MIP image of the left cervical ICA from a gadolinium-enhanced MRA of the neck (**A**) demonstrates a focal kink in the mid to distal left cervical ICA (arrow).

Cervical ICA loop with aneurysm formation

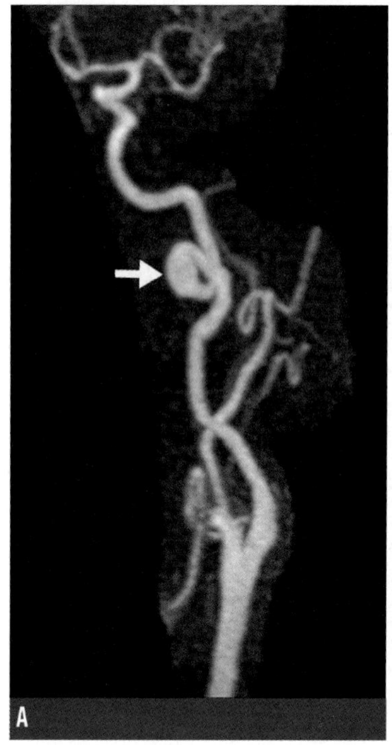

A MIP image from a contrast-enhanced MRA of the left cervical ICA (**A**) demonstrates a 360° loop with fusiform aneurysm formation along the ventral aspect of the loop (arrow).

Companion case: Fibromuscular dysplasia of the cervical ICA

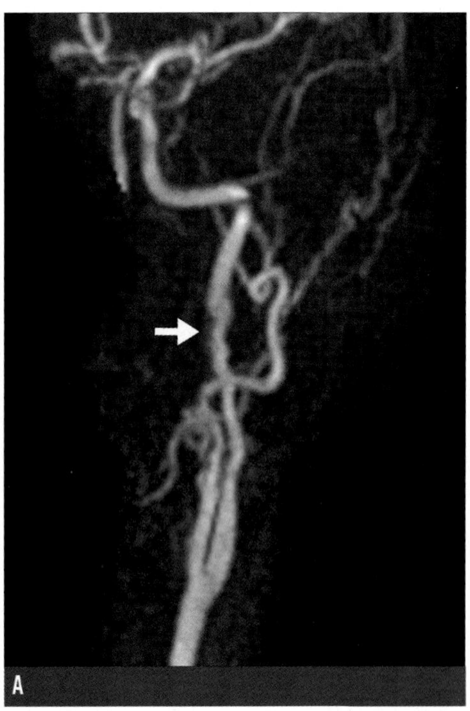

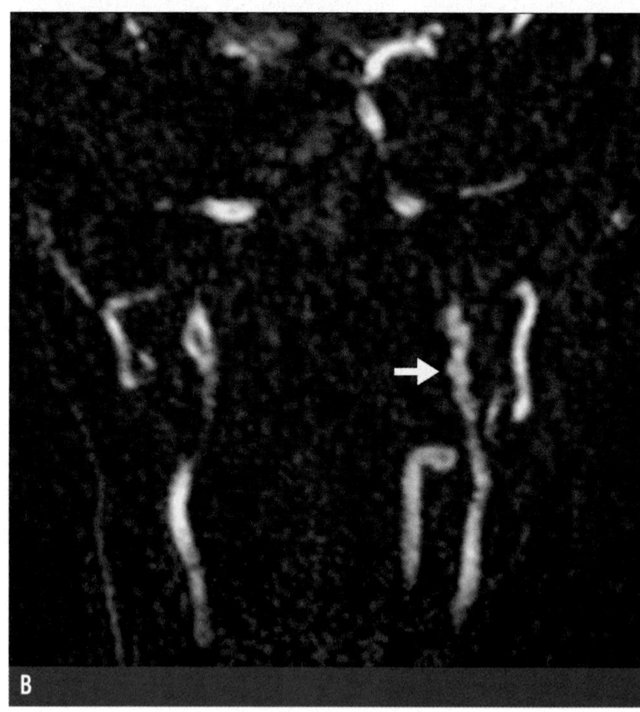

A MIP image from a gadolinium-enhanced MRA (**A**) and a source image from the same study (**B**) demonstrate an irregular, markedly beaded appearance of the mid left cervical ICA (arrows, **A**, **B**). A lateral image of the left carotid artery obtained during a catheter angiogram of the same patient (**C**) also demonstrates a markedly beaded appearance of the left cervical ICA (arrows, **C**). These findings are characteristic of fibromuscular dysplasia.

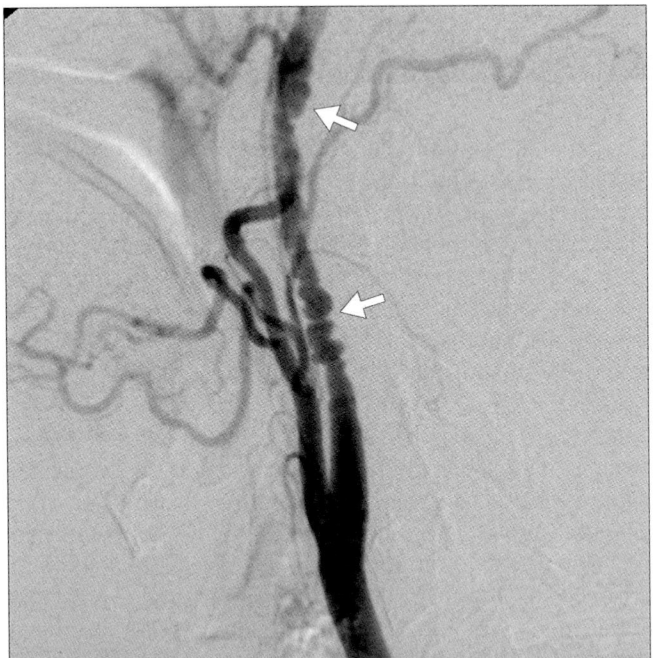

C

REFERENCES

Ballotta E, et al. Surgical vs medical treatment for isolated internal carotid artery elongation with coiling or kinking in symptomatic patients: a prospective randomized clinical study. *J Vasc Surg*. November 2005;42(5):838-846; discussion 846.

Barbour PJ, et al. Internal carotid artery redundancy is significantly associated with dissection. *Stroke*. 1994;25(6):1201-1206.

Benes V, Mohapl M. Alternative surgery for the kinked internal carotid artery. *Acta Neurochir (Wien)*. 2001;143(12):1267-1271; discussion 1271-1272.

Furie DM, Tien RD. Fibromuscular dysplasia of arteries of the head and neck: imaging findings. *AJR Am J Roentgenol*. 1994;162:1205-1209.

Grego F, Lepidi S, Cognolato D, Frigatti P, Morelli I, Deriu GP. Rationale of the surgical treatment of carotid kinking. *J Cardiovasc Surg (Torino)*. 2003;44(1):79-85.

CASE 13 Absence of the ICA

Absence of the ICA is of unknown etiology and represents a rare group of congenital anomalies described by some authors to encompass agenesis, aplasia, and hypoplasia of the ICA. Absence of the ICA occurs in less than 0.01% of the population with only 100 cases having been described in the literature. There is a 3:1 left-to-right predominance of absence of the ICA.

Hypoplasia, aplasia, and agenesis of the ICA are believed to be part of a spectrum. Hypoplasia refers to a small caliber of the ICA associated with a small intracranial ICA canal. Aplasia is present when there is a lack of ICA development characterized by a vascular remnant or fibrous band as well as the presence of a small residual intracranial ICA canal. Agenesis is complete failure of the ICA to develop and includes complete absence of the intracranial ICA canal. Therefore, CT assessment of the skull base to evaluate for the presence of an intracranial ICA canal is helpful to differentiate aplasia from agenesis. Similarly, assessment of the skull base is useful to differentiate diffuse narrowing of the ICA secondary to acquired etiologies (eg, arterial dissection, fibromuscular dysplasia, or severe atherosclerosis) from ICA hypoplasia, as these acquired pathologic processes would be expected to have a normal intracranial ICA canal, whereas the ICA canal would be small in caliber in the setting of a hypoplastic ICA.

If there is absence of the ICA, collateral flow to the remainder of the intracranial territory is typically via the circle of Willis, any persistent fetal circulations, or from external carotid artery collaterals. There is an increased prevalence of intracranial aneurysms associated with absence of the ICA (24%-34%); therefore, radiologic assessment for aneurysms is recommended in these patients.

Aplastic and contralateral hypoplastic intracranial ICAs

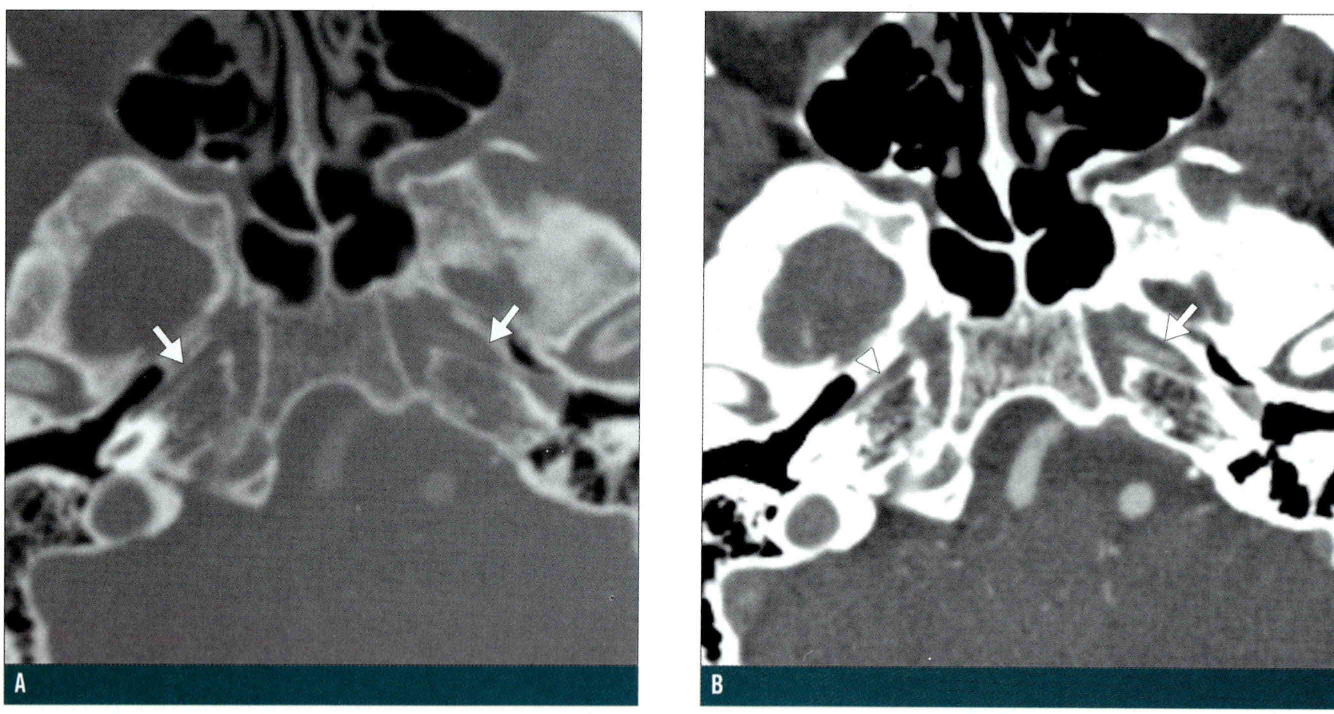

Axial CT images of the skull base from a CTA viewed with a bone window (**A**) and a soft tissue window (**B**) demonstrate bilateral hypoplastic petrous carotid canals (arrows, **A**). On the left, an enhancing hypoplastic ICA is present (arrow, **B**), whereas on the right, an enhancing ICA is not identified, consistent with right ICA aplasia (arrowhead, **B**). Axial images through the upper neck (**C**) and cavernous ICA (**D**) from the same CTA also demonstrate a hypoplastic left cervical ICA (arrow, **C**) and left cavernous ICA (arrow, **D**) as well as a markedly hypoplastic right cervical ICA (arrowhead, **C**). A convincing right cavernous ICA is not identified on image **D**, compatible with intracranial ICA aplasia. Thus, the right ICA is hypoplastic in the neck and aplastic intracranially. A 3D volumetric image from the same study (**E**) demonstrates marked hypoplasia and distal tapering of the right cervical ICA (arrow, **E**).

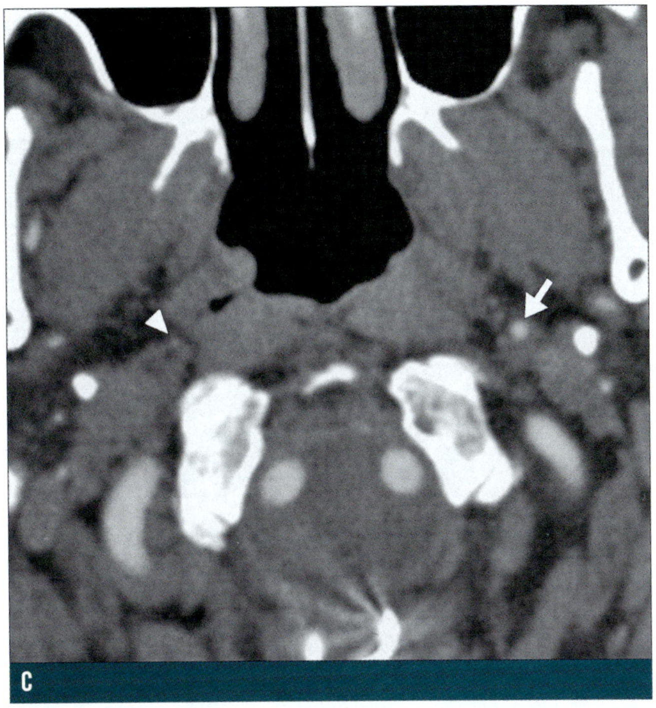
C

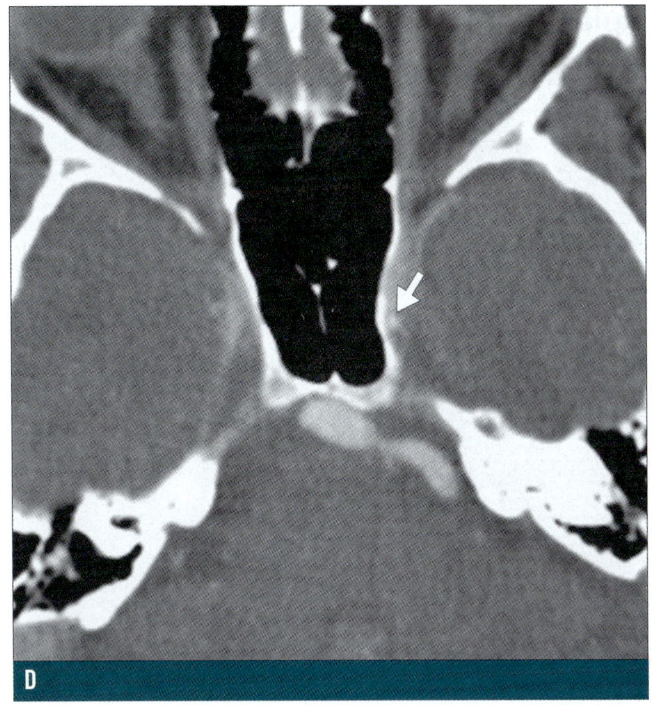
D

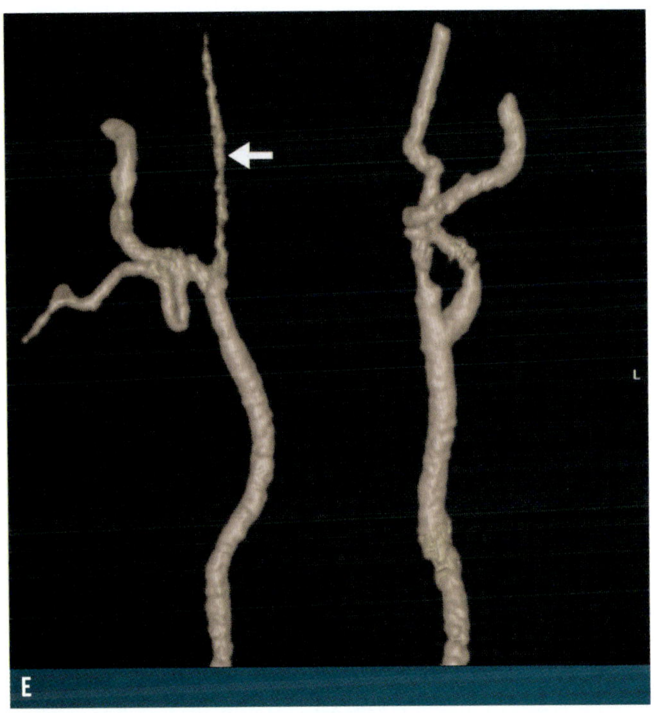
L
E

Aplastic intracranial ICA

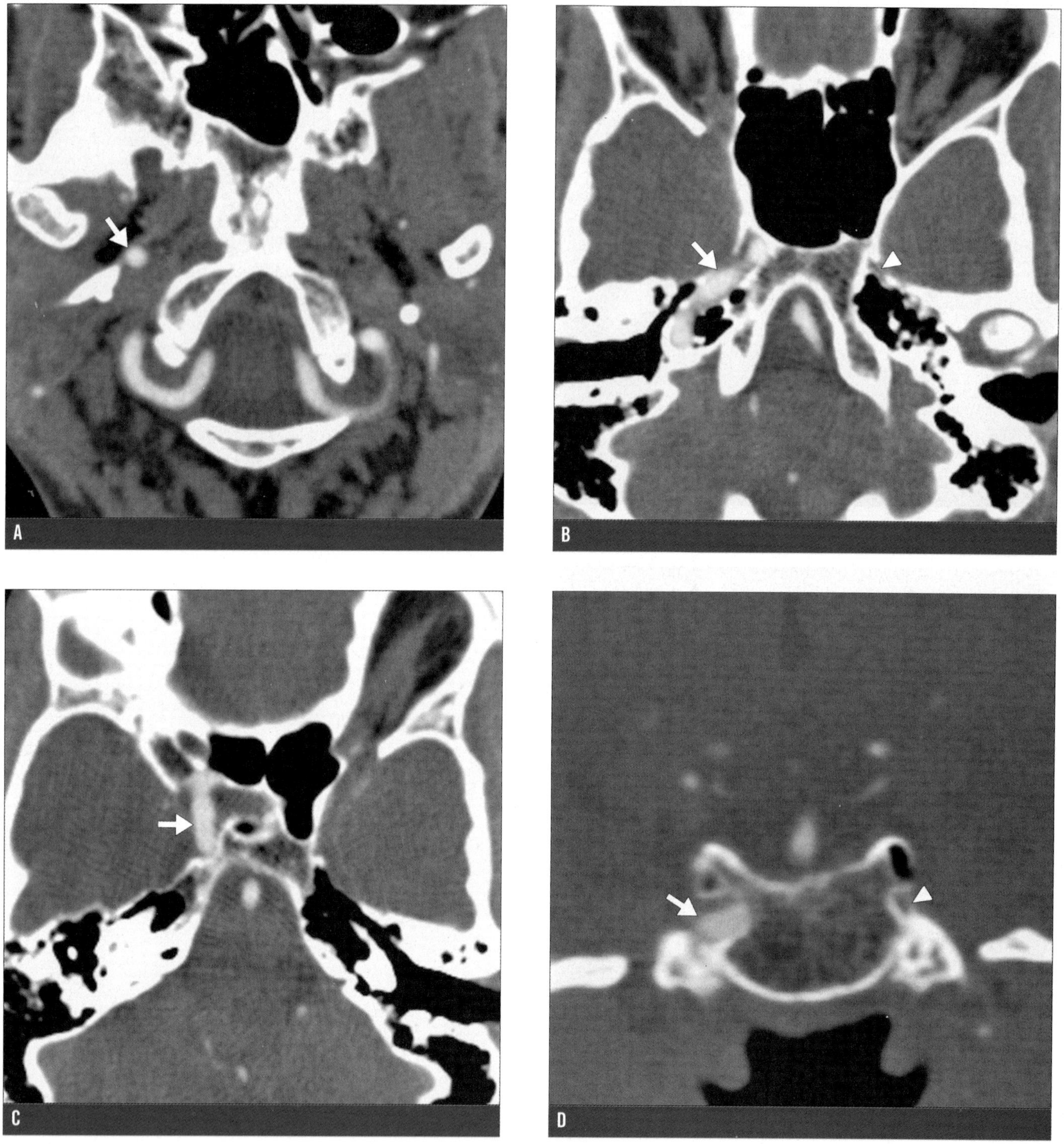

Axial images (**A-C**) and a coronal reformatted image (**D**) from a CTA of the brain. There is lack of an enhancing left ICA and a diminutive intracranial left ICA canal (arrowheads, **B, D**), compatible with left ICA aplasia. A normal-sized right ICA is present (arrows, **A-D**). A 3D volumetric image from the same CTA (**E**) demonstrates the presence of a hypoplastic left cervical ICA (arrow, **E**) which ultimately becomes the aplastic left intracranial ICA. The left common carotid artery (arrowhead, **E**) is also relatively hypoplastic compared to the right. An axial T2-weighted MR image of the same patient (**F**) demonstrates a normal right ICA flow void (arrow, **F**) and lack of a left ICA flow void.

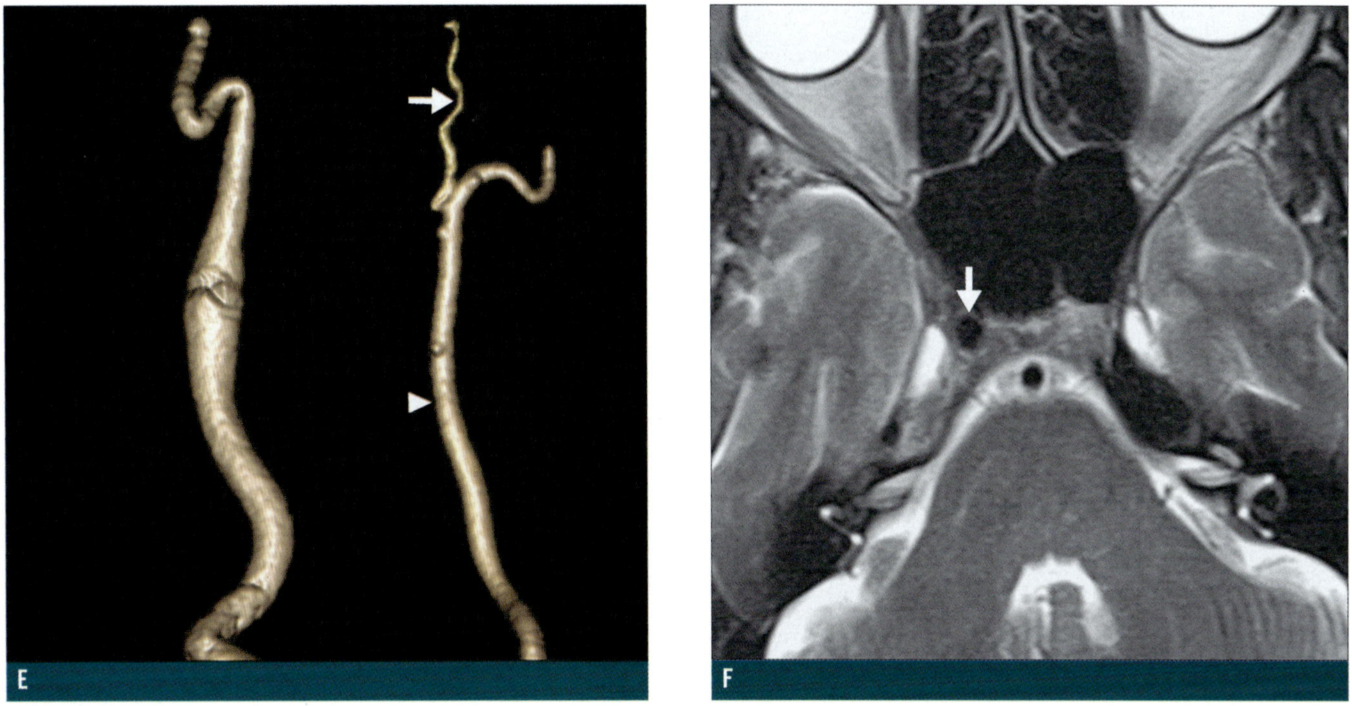

Aplasia versus agenesis of the intracranial ICA

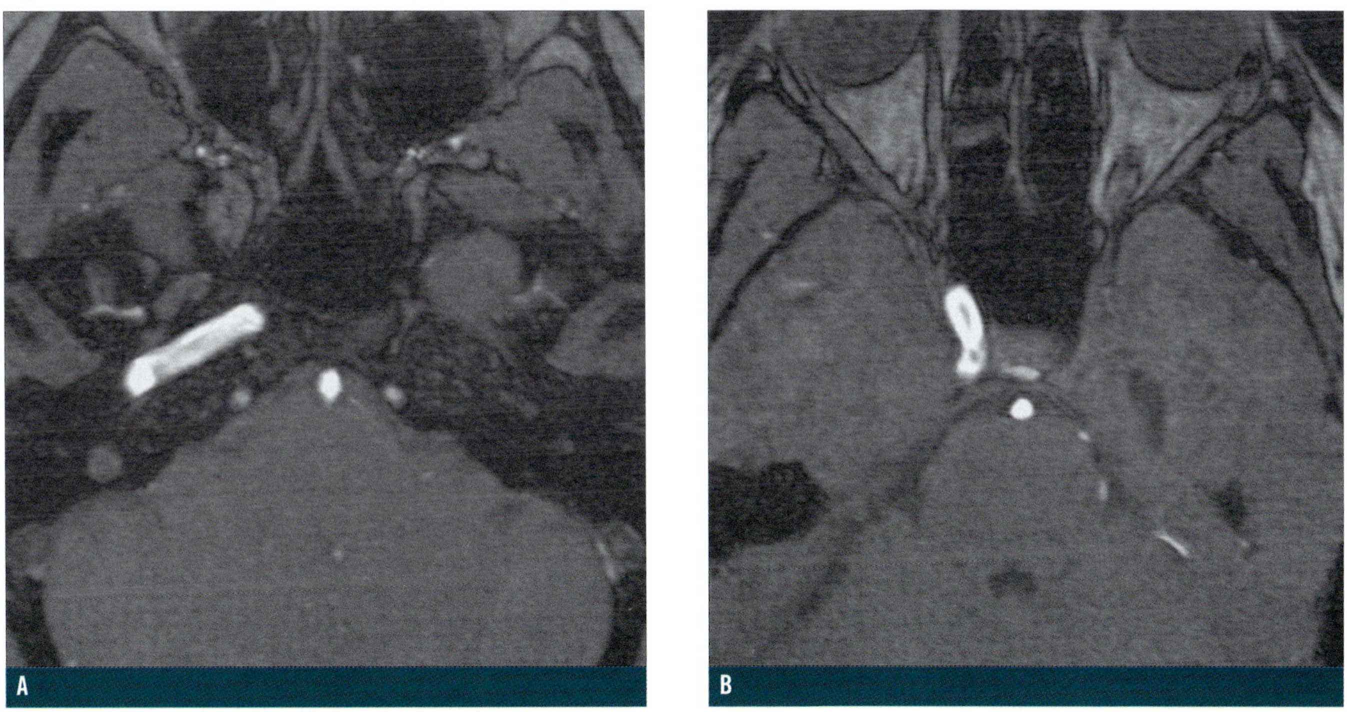

Axial source images from a time-of-flight MRA of the head (**A-C**) demonstrate absence of the intracranial left ICA from the petrous segment to the ophthalmic segment. Supply to the left middle cerebral artery arises from the left posterior communicating artery (arrowhead, **C**). An axial collapsed maximum intensity projection image best demonstrates the variant (**D**). This variant represents either aplasia or agenesis, and differentiating between these two entities is dependent on whether the osseous carotid canal is present. A small osseous carotid canal is present with aplasia, whereas a discernible osseous canal is not present with agenesis. The presence or absence of the osseous carotid canal would be best assessed by CT, which was not available for this patient.

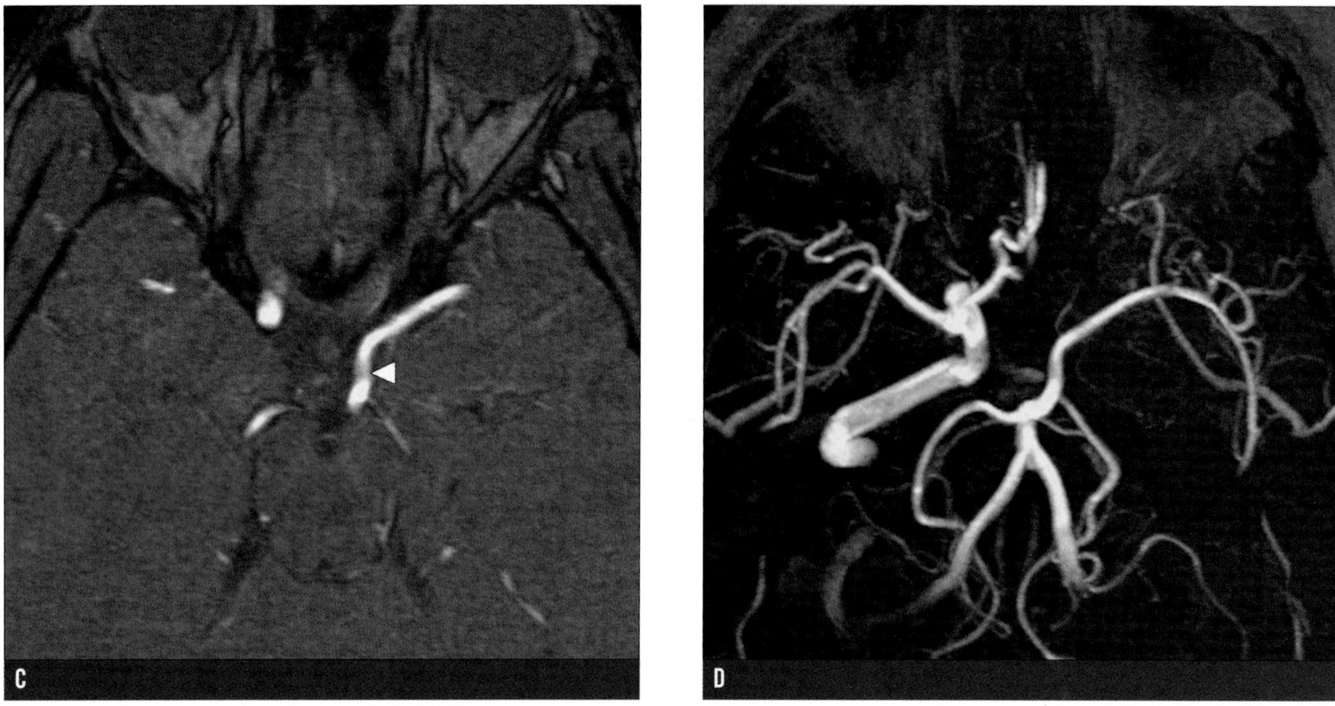

REFERENCES

Given CA, Huang-Hellinger F, Baker MD, Chepuri NB, Morris PP. Congenital absence of the internal carotid artery: case reports and review of the collateral circulation. *AJNR Am J Neuroradiol.* 2001;22:1953-1959.

Midkiff RB, Boykin MW, McFarland DR, Bauman JA. Agenesis of the internal carotid artery with intercavernous anastomosis. *AJNR Am J Neuroradiol.* 1995;16(6):1356-1359.

Sliwka U, Schmidt P, Ruel J, Noth J. Agenesis of the internal carotid artery: color Doppler, CT, and MR angiography findings. *J Clin Ultrasound.* 1998;26(4):213-216.

Taşar M, Yetişer S, Taşar A, Uğurel S, Gönül E, Sağlam M. Congenital absence or hypoplasia of the carotid artery: radioclinical issues. *Am J Otolaryngol.* 2004;25(5):339-349.

CASE 14 Persistent pharyngohyoid artery with a normal ipsilateral cervical ICA ("duplicated internal carotid artery ")

A persistent pharyngohyoid artery with a normal ipsilateral cervical ICA is a rare anomaly that has only been described in a few case reports. During the fourth and fifth weeks of fetal life, a total of six aortic arches develop which give rise to the arterial vasculature in the neck and chest. Of the six aortic arches, the first three arches give rise to the carotid arterial system in the neck. Pertinent to this discussion, the second aortic arch forms the primitive hyoid artery and the third aortic arch forms the cervical ICA. The primitive hyoid artery normally regresses during fetal development and becomes the caroticotympanic artery, which is a diminutive branch of the developed petrous carotid artery. When fully developed, the normal, diminutive caroticotympanic artery anastomoses with the inferior tympanic artery. The inferior tympanic artery is a normal branch of the ascending pharyngeal artery, which, in turn, is typically a branch of the external carotid artery (ECA). Incidentally, because of this normal anastomosis, the caroticotympanic artery can serve as an ECA to ICA collateral pathway in patients with severe internal carotid stenosis proximal to the skull base.

When there is a developmental, abnormally enlarged inferior tympanic artery, and the normal cervical ICA does not regress (as occurs with an aberrant ICA, discussed in the accompanying Companion Case), then the result is an apparent "duplication" of the cervical ICA. In this setting, the abnormally enlarged inferior tympanic artery arises from ascending pharyngeal artery, as expected; however, instead of the ascending pharyngeal artery arising from its typical ECA origin, it may arise from the proximal cervical ICA. The enlarged inferior tympanic artery traverses posterolateral to the cervical ICA as it ascends the neck and enters an abnormally enlarged inferior tympanic canaliculus at the skull base (also called Jacobson canal). Normally, the inferior tympanic canaliculus is a very small foramen located posterolateral to the petrous carotid canal through which a diminutive inferior tympanic artery and the tympanic branch of the glossopharyngeal nerve (also called Jacobson nerve) traverse. After entering the inferior tympanic canaliculus, the abnormally enlarged inferior tympanic artery anastomosis with a persistent primitive hyoid artery. This artery then traverses the tympanic cavity and anastomoses at the junction between the vertical and horizontal portions of the petrous ICA. Collectively, the abnormally enlarged inferior tympanic artery and persistent primitive hyoid artery/enlarged caroticotympanic artery are termed a pharyngohyoid artery (or inferior tympano-caroticotympanic artery). If there is a persistent stapedial artery in conjunction with this anomaly, then the term pharyngohyostapedial artery is used.

A persistent pharyngohyoid artery with a normal ipsilateral cervical ICA is a normal variant. Care should be taken to not mistake this rare developmental variant for pathology, such as a carotid dissection. Conversely, a cervical ICA dissection, most often when focally involving the cervical ICA, can simulate a duplication/fenestration. In these cases, evaluation for vascular irregularity, other areas of arterial dissection, pseudoaneurysm formation, and fibromuscular dysplasia will aid in appropriately diagnosing a cervical ICA dissection.

COMPANION CASE

- **Aberrant ICA.** The term "aberrant ICA" is a misnomer. In actuality, an aberrant ICA represents a persistent pharyngohyoid artery anomaly described above except that there is also complete absence of the normal cervical ICA and the vertical portion of the petrous ICA either secondary to lack of development or regression during fetal life. With an aberrant ICA, the enlarged inferior tympanic artery traverses the tympanic cavity and anastomoses with a persistent primitive hyoid artery. This artery then joins with the horizontal portion of the petrous ICA. The result is the appearance of an ICA that traverses the tympanic cavity—thus the phrase "aberrant carotid artery."

  With an aberrant ICA, there is often a focal arterial stenosis between the inferior tympanic artery and the petrous carotid artery at the level of the enlarged inferior tympanic canaliculus. Additionally, there is a fairly acute angle at the site of the anastomosis on imaging, resulting in a characteristic "seven" or "reverse-seven" imaging appearance, depending on the side affected and whether the finding is viewed from an anterior-to-posterior or posterior-to-anterior direction.

  Symptoms of an aberrant ICA may include tinnitus, hearing loss, vertigo, and rarely otalgia. A retrotympanic reddish-blue mass is often visualized during an otoscopic evaluation.

Persistent pharyngohyoid artery with a normal ipsilateral cervical ICA

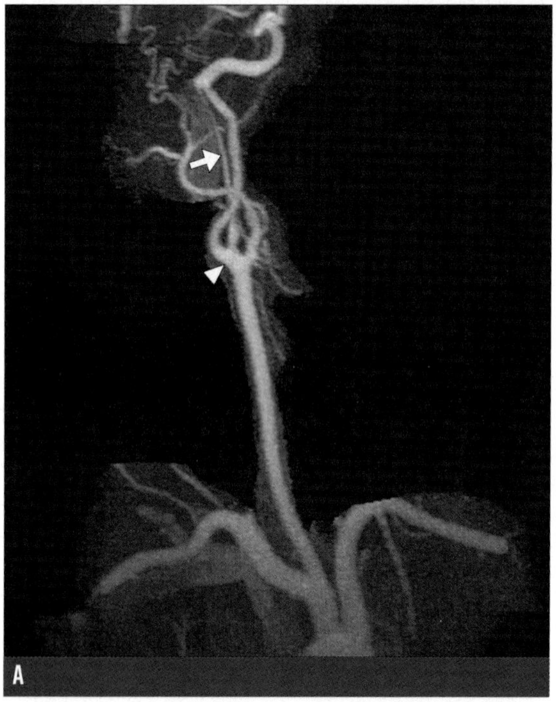

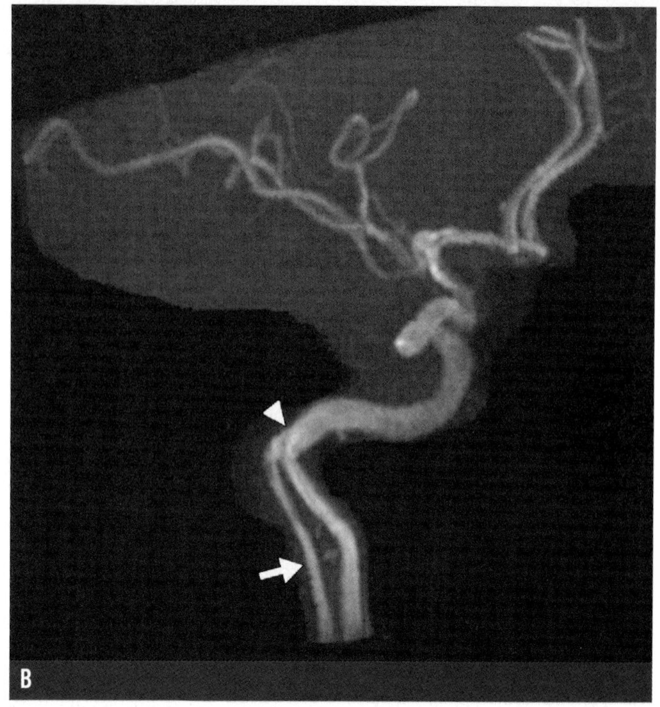

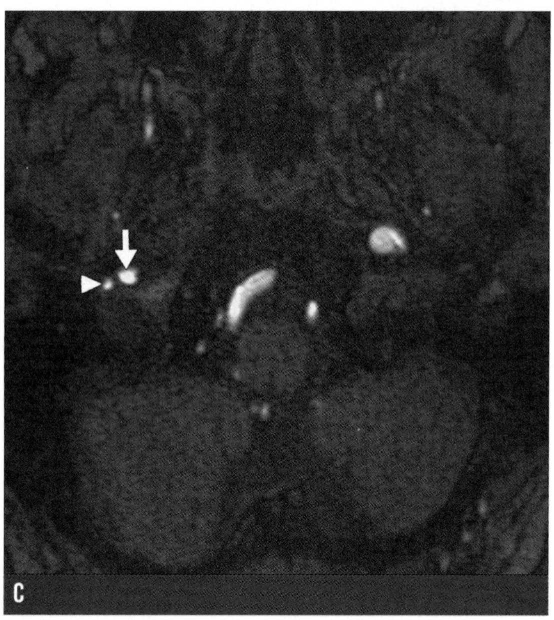

MIP images from a contrast-enhanced MRA of the neck (**A**) and a time-of-flight MRA of the head (**B**) demonstrate a persistent pharyngohyoid artery (arrows, **A**, **B**) arising from the proximal aspect of the right cervical ICA just distal to the bifurcation (arrowhead, **A**). This persistent pharyngohyoid artery parallels the course of the normal cervical right ICA and simulates a "duplicated ICA". A persistent hyoid artery (arrowhead, **B**), which represents a portion of this anomaly, anastomoses the abnormally enlarged inferior tympanic artery portion of the anomaly to the junction of the vertical and horizontal portions of the petrous ICA. Axial source images from the time-of-flight MRA (**C, D**) demonstrate the inferior tympanic artery (arrowhead, **C**), the vertical portion of the petrous ICA (arrow, **C**), and the fusion of both vessels (arrow, **D**). An axial CT image of the skull base viewed with a bone window (**E**) demonstrates the abnormally enlarged right inferior tympanic canaliculus (arrow, **E**).

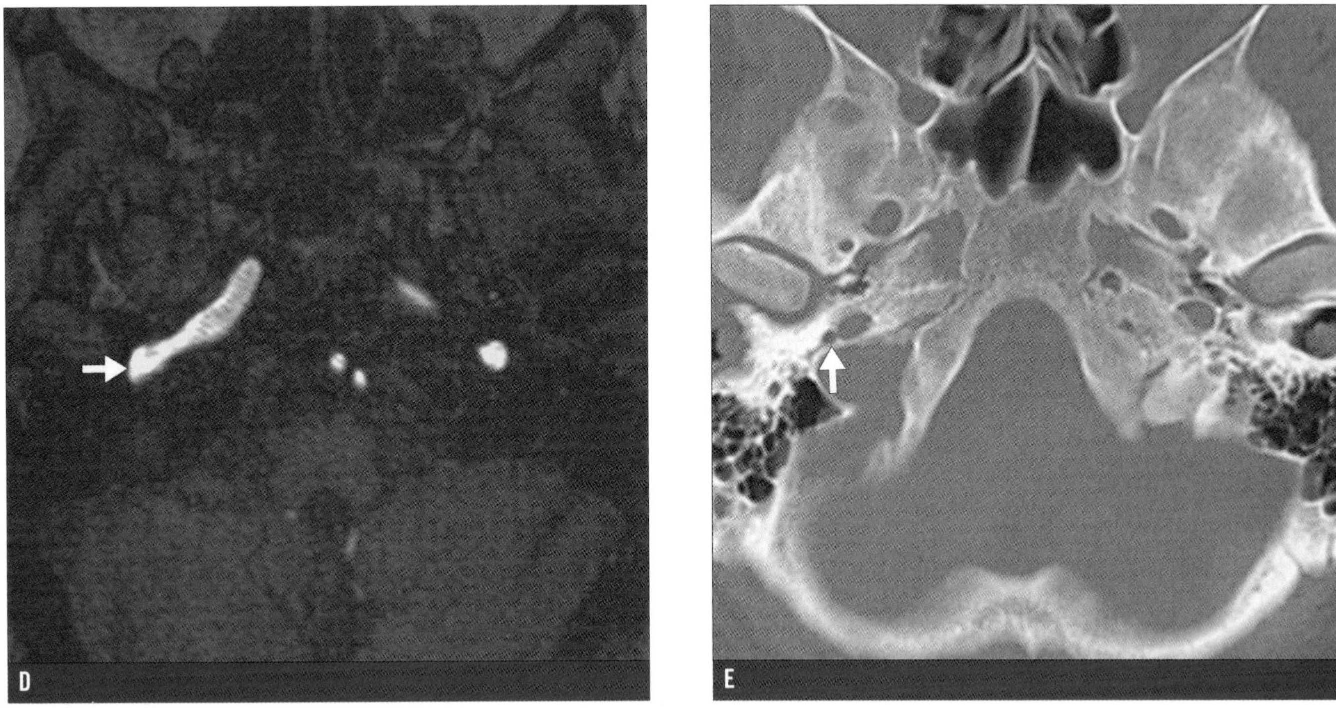

Companion case: Aberrant ICA

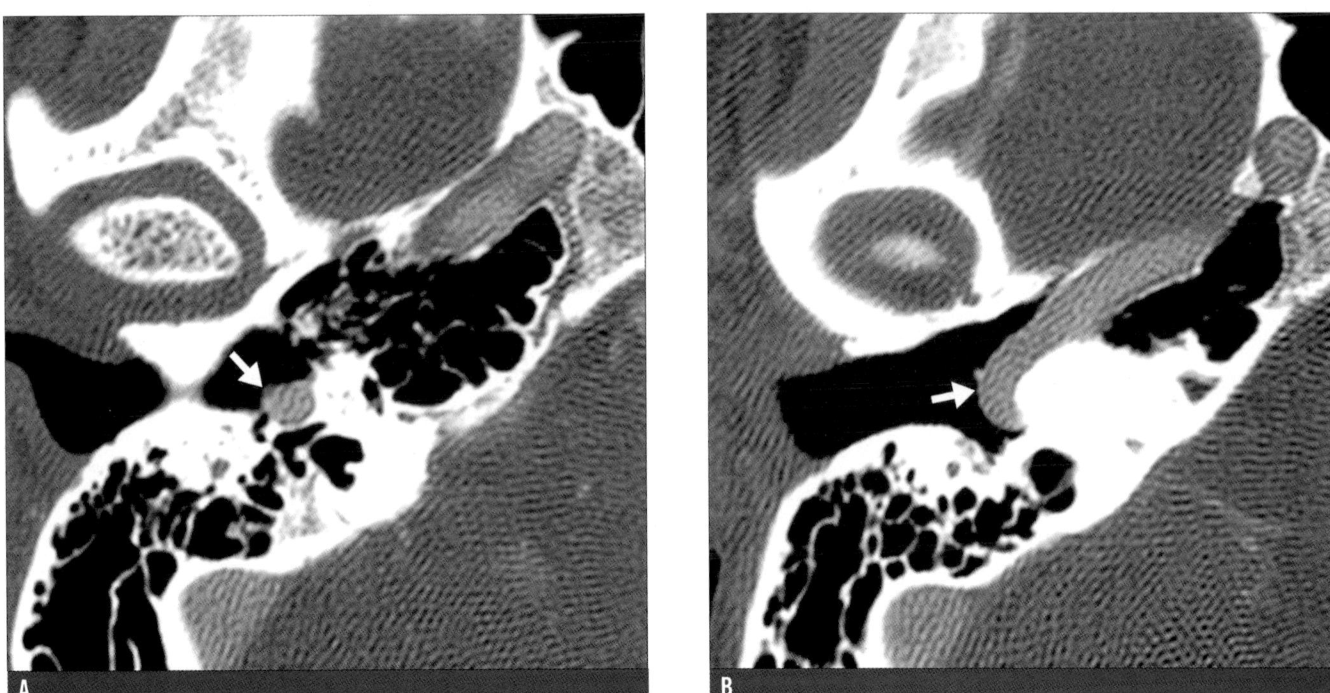

Postcontrast axial CT images of the right temporal bone (**A**, **B**) demonstrate an aberrant right ICA coursing through the right tympanic cavity (short arrows, **A**, **B**). Postcontrast coronal reformatted (**C**) and axial (**D**) CT images of the right temporal bone demonstrate the typical course of an aberrant ICA at this level as it enters the tympanic cavity via an enlarged inferior tympanic canaliculus (long arrows, **C**, **D**).

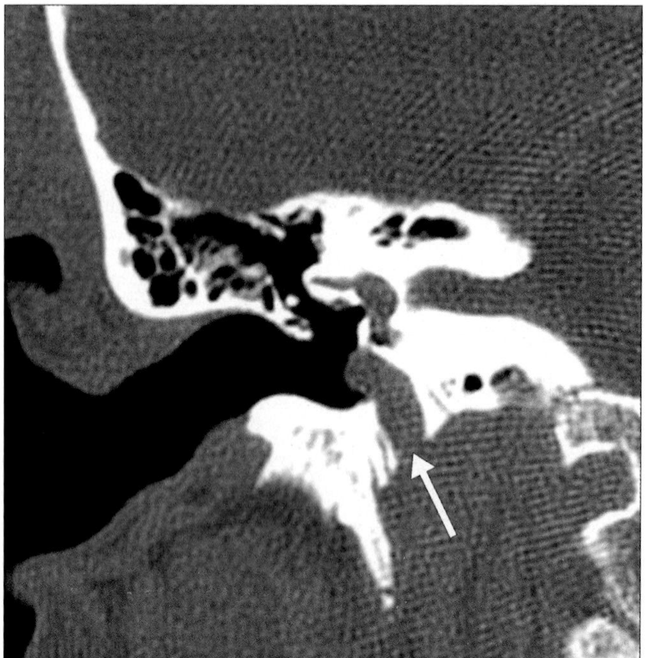

C

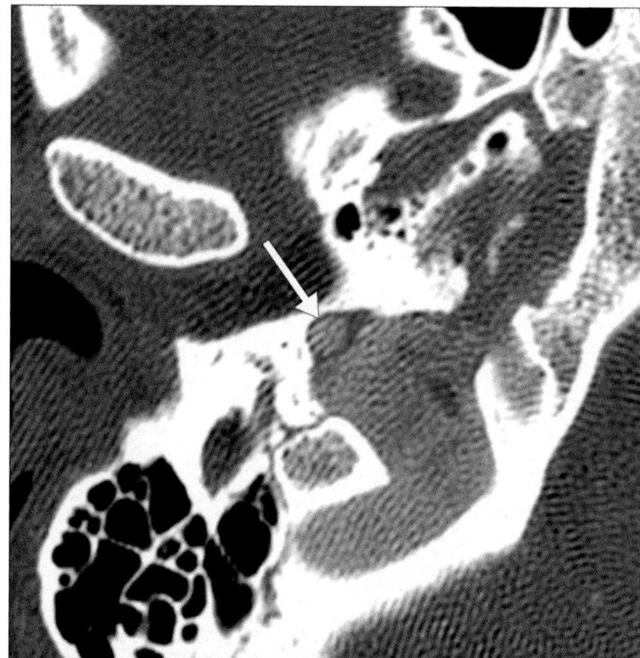

D

REFERENCES

Chess MA, Barsotti JB, Chang JK, Ketonen LM, Westesson PL. Duplication of the extracranial internal carotid artery. *AJNR Am J Neuroradiol.* 1996;16:1545-1547.

Chng SM, Alvarez H, Marsot-Dupuch K, Mercier P, Lasjaunias P. "Duplicated" or "multiple" cervical internal carotid and vertebral arteries from fenestration, duplication and vasa vasorum to segmental rete. *Interv Neuroradiol.* 2004;10:301-307.

Davis WL, Harnsberger HR. MR angiography of an aberrant internal carotid artery. *Am J Neuroradiol.* 1991;12:1225.

Gailloud P, Carpenter J, Heck DV, Murphy KJ. Pseudofenestration of the cervical internal carotid artery: a pathologic process that simulates an anatomic variant. *AJNR Am J Neuroradiol.* 2004;25:421-424.

Killien FC, Wyler AR, Cromwell LD. Duplication of the internal carotid artery. *Neuroradiology.* 1980;19:101-102.

Koesling S, Kunkel P, Schul T. Vascular anomalies, sutures and small canals of the temporal bone on axial CT. *Eur J Radiol.* 2005;54:335-343.

Lasjaunias P, Berenstein A, Ter Brugge KG. *Surgical Neuroangiography, Clinical Vascular Anatomy and Variations.* 2nd ed. New York, NY: Springer-Verlag; 2001.

Lefournier V, Vasdev A, Bessou P, Boubagra K. A persistent pharyngohyostapedial artery: embryologic implications. *AJNR Am J Neuroradiol.* 1999;20:271-274.

Lo WWM, Solti-Bohman LG, McElveen JT. Aberrant carotid artery: radiologic diagnosis with emphasis on high-resolution computed tomography. *Radiographics.* 1985;5:985-993.

Intracranial infarction represents one of the most common causes of morbidity and mortality in the world, with severe carotid artery stenosis accounting for approximately 20% of all ischemic infarcts. Treatment options include medical management, endovascular stenting (with or without angioplasty), and surgery. Among the surgical options, a carotid endarterectomy (CEA), with or without a patch angioplasty, is the mainstay of treatment. The carotid bulb is by far the most common location of a significant cervical carotid atherosclerotic stenosis, and it is the location where the vast majority of CEAs are performed. Multicenter trials have demonstrated a significant decreased incidence of intracranial infarction following a CEA in patients with a cervical internal carotid artery luminal diameter narrowing of 70% or more.

Patch angioplasties are commonly used to supplement a CEA. Patch angioplasties restore the size and often enlarge the carotid artery, thereby improving the hemodynamics compared to a primary CEA closure. Furthermore, when compared with primary closure, the use of a patch angioplasty is associated with a decreased risk of restenosis, occlusion, and cerebral infarction. Patch angioplasties can be performed with either an autogenous vein or synthetic graft. Vein patches may be harvested from the saphenous or jugular veins. Synthetic grafts may be constructed from Dacron, polytetrafluoroethylene (PTFE), or bovine pericardium. Studies have demonstrated durability, long-term efficacy, and low infection rates for these venous patches and synthetic grafts.

On vascular imaging, the site of a CEA is typically patulous, particularly when performed with a patch angioplasty.

COMPANION CASES

- **Chronic cervical ICA dissection with pseudoaneurysm formation and a contralateral acute cervical ICA dissection.** A chronic carotid artery dissection causes vessel wall weakening and sometimes results in pseudoaneursym formation. On vascular imaging, a cervical carotid artery pseudoaneurysm can have a similar appearance to a CEA, particularly when compared to a CEA performed with a patch angioplasty.
- **Carotid endarterectomy with residual thrombosis and a superimposed cervical carotid dissection.** Potential complications of a CEA include residual thrombus, residual or recurrent stenosis, and cervical carotid dissection. These complications most often occur at the margins of the endarterectomy.
- **Carotid endarterectomy with a patch angioplasty and contralateral cervical carotid stent placement.** Approximately 25% of patients with severe cervical carotid artery stenosis have significant comorbidities, often placing these patients at a greater risk for complications during a CEA. Deploying a stent across the stenosis via an endovascular approach is often a preferred option for this cohort of patients. Endovascular stent placement has been demonstrated to be an effective method of treating carotid artery stenosis and has a relatively low complication rate. Typically, a self-expanding endovascular stent is placed across the stenosis and usually performed in conjunction with pre- and post-stenting angioplasty. A distal protection device is often utilized during the procedure to minimize the risk of cerebral embolization.

Carotid endarterectomy

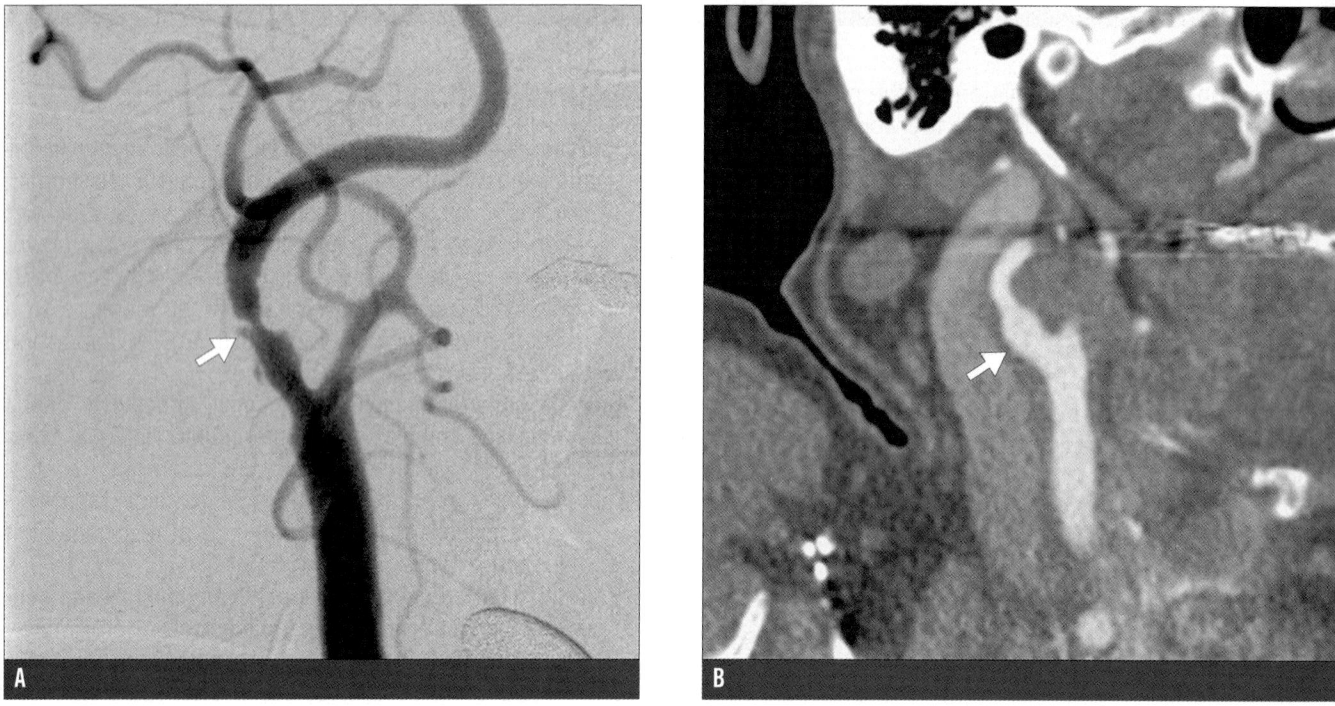

A preoperative digitally subtracted right carotid angiogram (**A**) demonstrates a high-grade ICA stenosis (arrow, **A**). Following a right carotid endarterectomy, a sagittal oblique reformatted image of the right cervical carotid artery from a CTA neck (**B**) demonstrates resolution of the carotid stenosis (arrow, **B**). The carotid bulb is now patulous, a normal finding following an endarterectomy. Despite its patulous appearance, a patch angioplasty was not performed in this case.

Carotid endarterectomy with patch angioplasty

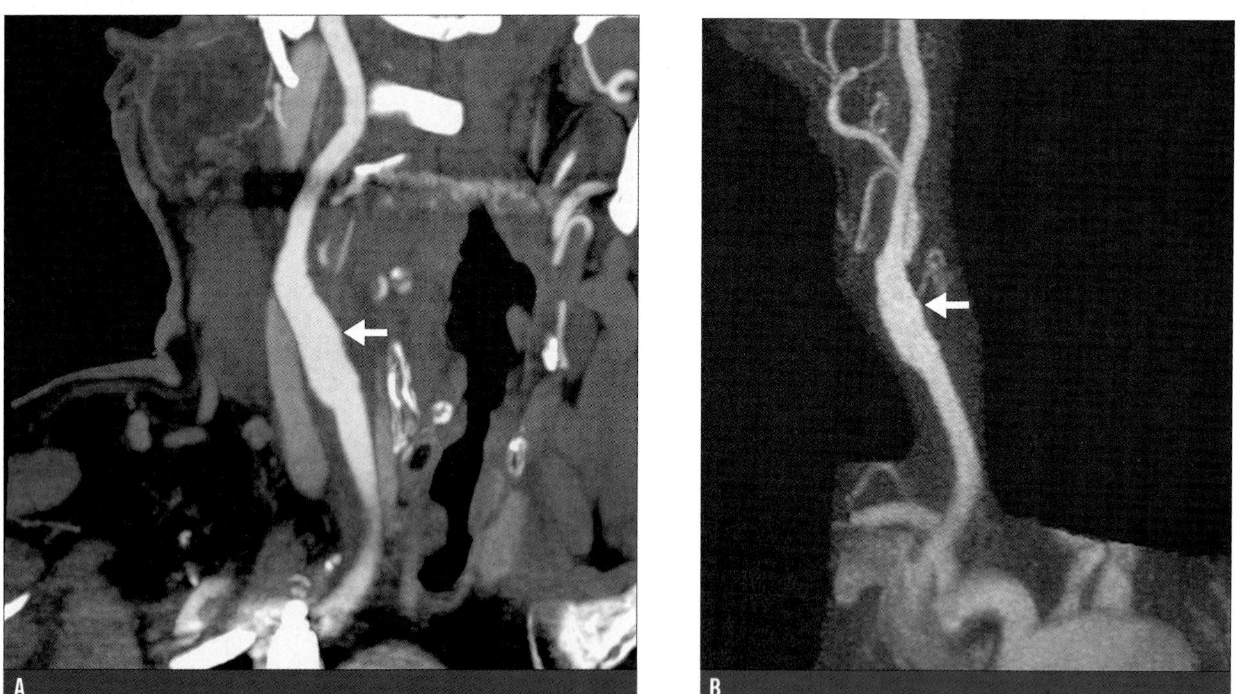

A sagittal reformatted image of the right carotid artery from a CTA of the neck (**A**) demonstrate a bulbous appearance of the distal right common carotid artery and carotid bulb following a carotid endarterectomy and patch angioplasty (arrow, **A**). A MIP image from a gadolinium-enhanced neck MRA of the same patient (**B**) demonstrates the MRI correlate (arrow, **B**).

Companion case: Chronic cervical ICA dissection with pseudoaneurysm formation and a contralateral acute cervical ICA dissection

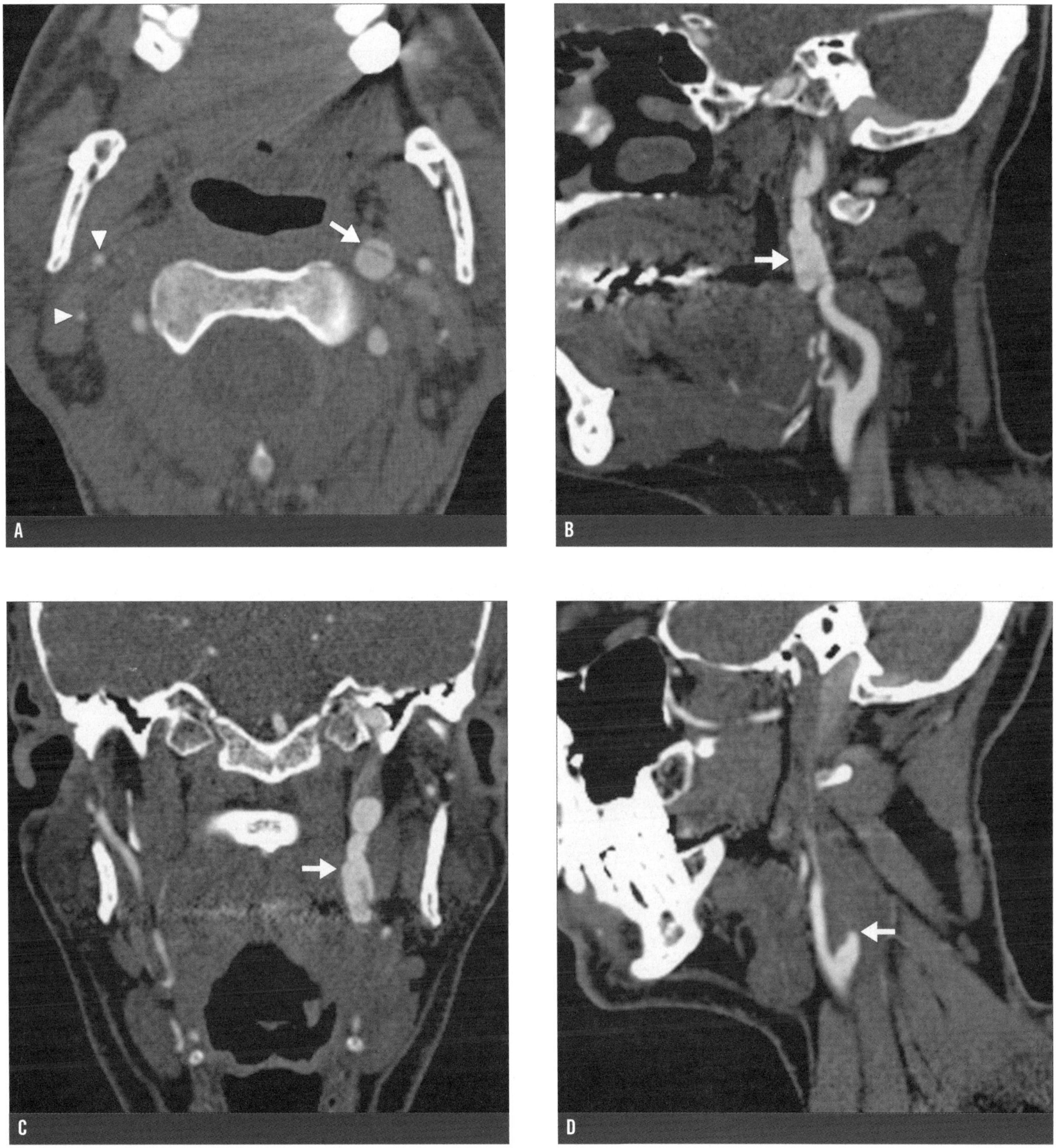

An axial image from a CTA (**A**) demonstrates a focal dissection flap within the left cervical ICA (arrow, **A**) and the presence of several right ECA branches (arrowheads, **A**), but no evidence of a patent right cervical ICA. A sagittal reformatted CTA image through the left cervical ICA (**B**) and a coronal reformatted CTA image (**C**) demonstrate marked pseudoaneurysm formation related to a chronic dissection of the left cervical ICA (arrows, **B**, **C**). A pseudoaneurysm related to a chronic ICA dissection can appear similar to a CEA with a patch angioplasty. A sagittal reformatted CTA image through the right ICA (**D**) demonstrates focal marked tapering of the right cervical ICA related to an acute arterial dissection (arrow, **D**).

Companion case: Carotid endarterectomy with residual thrombus and a superimposed cervical carotid dissection

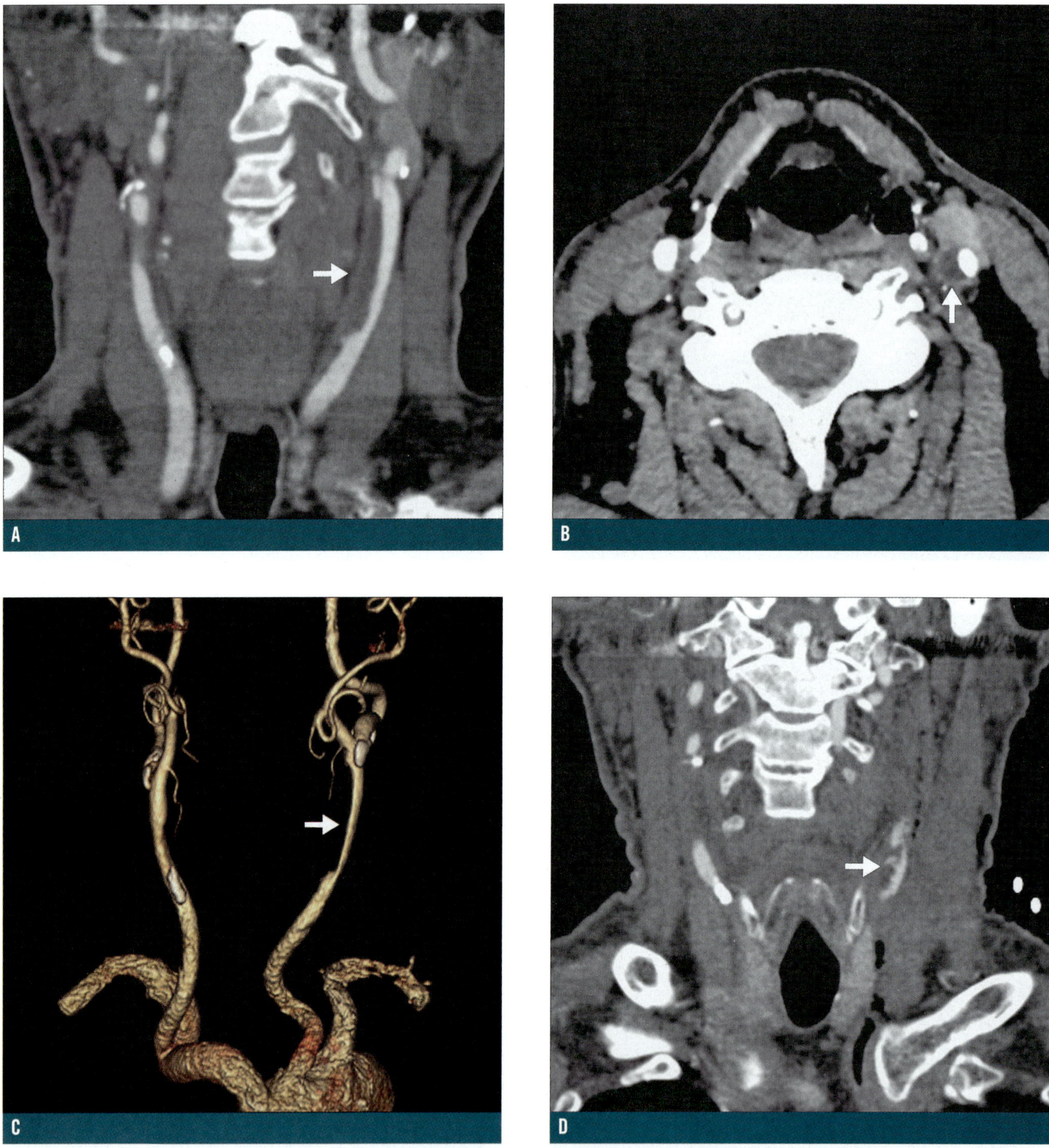

Coronal reformatted (**A**) and axial (**B**) CT images from a neck CTA demonstrate a long segment of noncalcified plaque involving the mid to distal left common carotid artery (arrows, **A**, **B**). A 3D volumetric reconstruction of the carotid arteries (**C**) also demonstrates the finding (arrow, **C**). Coronal reformatted (**D**) and axial (**E**) CT images from a neck CTA of the same patient following a left carotid endarterectomy demonstrate marked irregularity, intraluminal thrombus, and a carotid dissection (arrows, **D**, **E**). A 3D volumetric reconstruction of the carotid arteries (**F**) also demonstrates these findings (arrow, **F**).

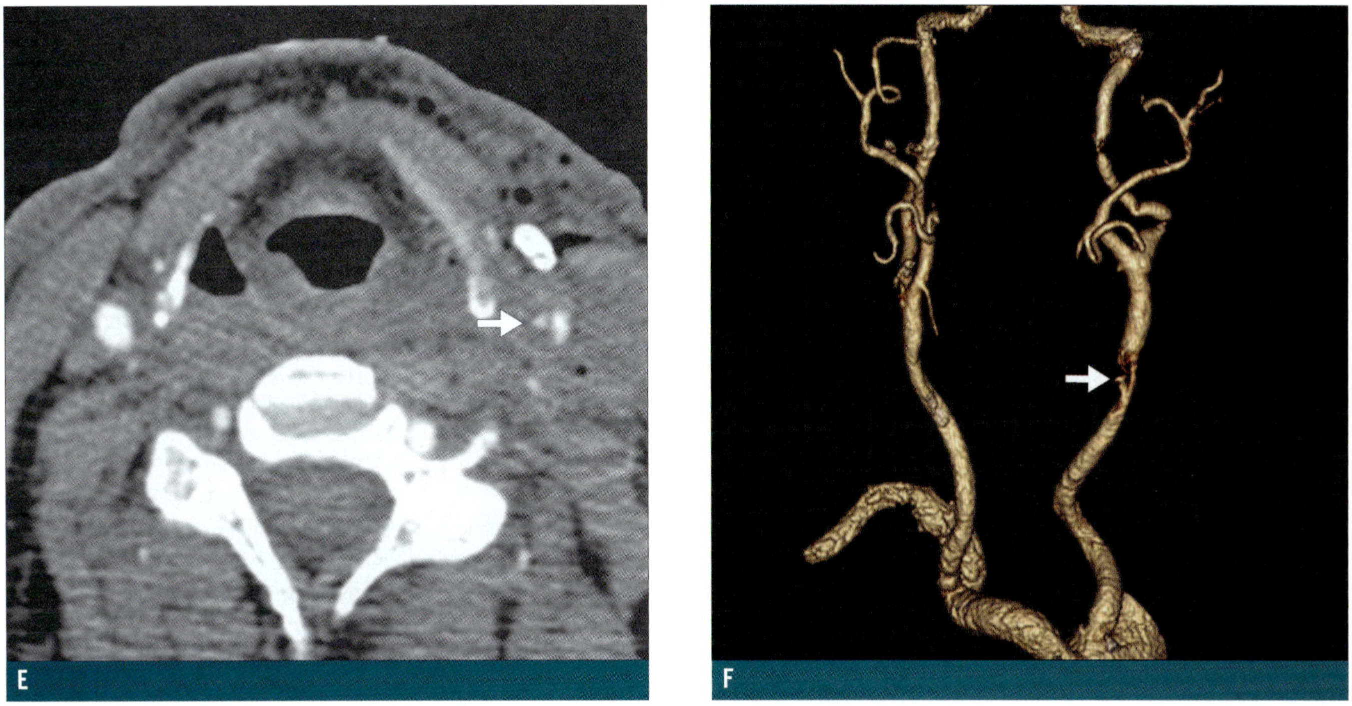

Companion case: Carotid endarterectomy with a patch angioplasty and contralateral cervical carotid stent placement

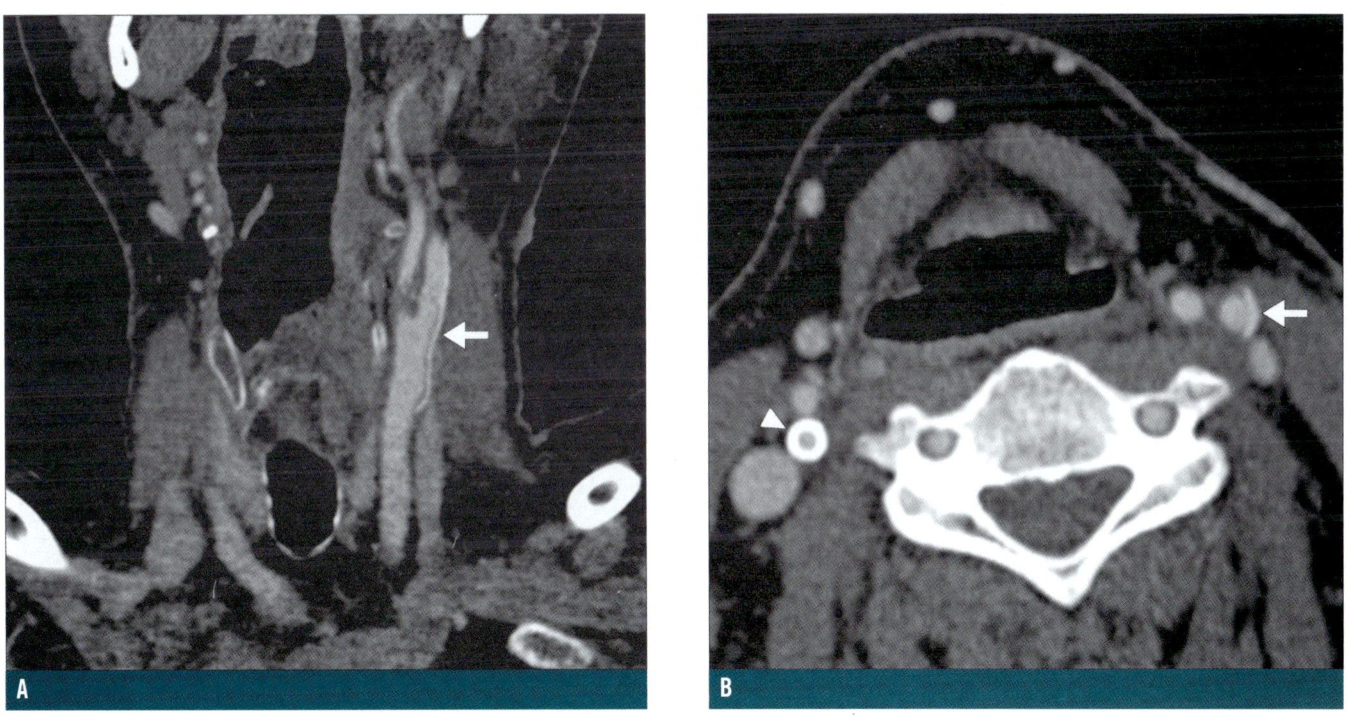

Coronal reformatted (**A**) and axial (**B**) CTA images following a left carotid endarterectomy demonstrate a patulous distal left common carotid artery and left carotid bulb associated with a linear high-density structure along its lateral aspect representing a patch graft (arrows, **A**, **B**). Image (**B**) as well as well as a right parasagittal reformatted CT image viewed with a bone window (**C**) demonstrate the typical appearance of a carotid stent on the right (arrowheads, **B**, **C**).

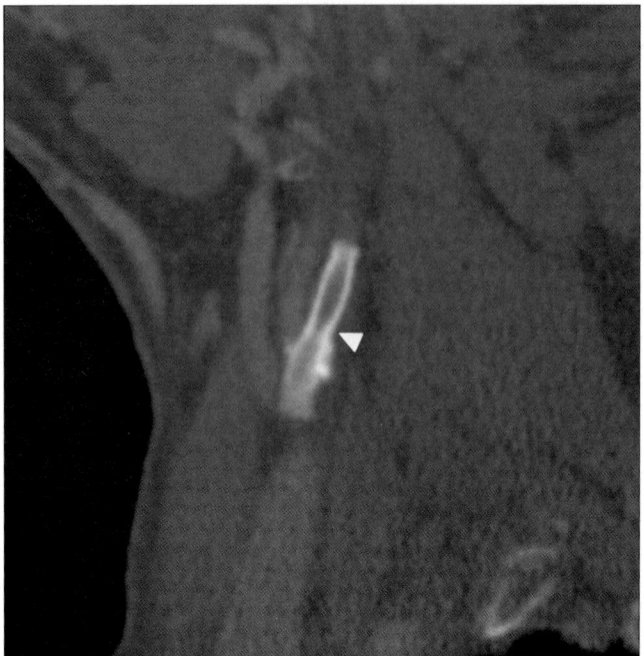

C

REFERENCES

Béatrice Marro, et al. Computerized tomographic angiography scan following carotid endarterectomy. Annals of vascular surgery. 1998;12(5):451-456.

Kim JH, Cho YP, Kwon TW, Kim H, Kim GE. Ten-year comparative analysis of bovine pericardium and autogenous vein for patch angioplasty in patients undergoing carotid endarterectomy. *Ann Vasc Surg.* 2012;26(3):353-358.

Litwinski RA, Wright K, Pons P. Pseudoaneurysm formation following carotid endarterectomy: two case reports and a literature review. *Ann Vasc Surg.* 2006;20:678-680.

North American Symptomatic Carotid Endarterectomy Trial Collaborators. Beneficial effect of carotid endarterectomy in symptomatic patients with high-grade carotid stenosis. *N Engl J Med.* 1991;325:445-453.

Osborn AG. *Diagnostic Cerebral Angiography.* 2nd ed. Philadelphia, PA: LWW; 1999.

Safian RD. Treatment strategies for carotid stenosis in patients at increased risk for surgery. Prog Cardiovasc Dis. 2011;54(1):22-28.

Vitek JJ, Roubin GS, Al-Mubarek N, New G, Iyer SS. Carotid artery stenting: technical considerations. *ANJR Am J Neuroradiol.* 2000;21:1736-1743.

CASE 16 Surgical arterial bypass grafts, transpositions, and interposition grafts

There are a variety of open surgical options available to treat patients with symptomatic lesions of the subclavian, carotid, and vertebral arteries that are not amenable to endovascular therapy or carotid endarterectomy (CEA). These open surgical options include arterial bypass grafting, transposition, or interposition grafting. A bypass graft refers to a venous or synthetic graft used to "bypass" a stenosis or other pathologic finding. The first named vessel in a bypass graft procedure represents the donor vessel, whereas the second named vessel represents the recipient vessel that is being treated. For example, a subclavian to carotid artery bypass is a bypass that utilizes a graft from the subclavian artery to the carotid artery in order to treat a carotid artery lesion. A transposition refers to surgically ligating a diseased vessel distal to a stenosis and anastomosing the distal stump of that vessel to a patent native vessel in order to improve blood flow. The first named vessel of a transposition refers to the vessel that is being treated and manipulated (ie, "transposed"), and the second named vessel represents the recipient vessel. For instance, to treat a proximal subclavian artery stenosis, a subclavian to carotid artery transposition entails ligating and transecting the subclavian artery distal to the level of stenosis and implanting the distal stump end-to-side onto the carotid artery in order to reestablish flow to the subclavian artery. Interposition grafting circumvents an abnormal portion of the same vessel via a venous or synthetic graft. Arterial bypass grafting, transposition, and interposition grafting procedures are performed for a variety of abnormalities, including symptomatic high-grade stenosis (not amenable to CEA or stenting), arterial occlusion, aneurysm formation, and recurrent stenosis following CEA.

CASES

- **Subclavian to carotid artery bypass graft.** See above.
- **Carotid to subclavian artery bypass graft.** A carotid to subclavian artery bypass graft is typically performed in the setting of a subclavian artery stenosis that results in subclavian steal, arm claudication, rest pain, ischemic changes of the hand or digits, or vertebrobasilar symptoms. A carotid to subclavian bypass utilizes a synthetic graft to create a communication between the carotid artery and the subclavian artery that is distal to the level of subclavian artery stenosis/occlusion.
- **Largely thrombosed carotid to subclavian artery bypass graft.**
- **Aorto-bicarotid and left subclavian artery bypass graft.** This type of bypass is typically performed when there are extensive arterial stenoses that need to be bypassed, such as may be seen with vasculitides that affect large vessels.
- **Carotid-to-carotid artery bypass graft.** In a carotid-to-carotid artery bypass procedure, a bypass graft anastomoses the right and left carotid arteries. The graft for this procedure is typically placed low in the midline, extends posterior to the pharynx, and resides ventral to the prevertebral fascia.
- **Vertebral to carotid artery transposition.** This is typically performed to revascularize a stenotic or occluded vertebral artery. For a proximal lesion, the V1 segment of the vertebral artery is ligated distal to the stenosis or occlusion and transposed onto the common carotid artery. Less commonly, a transposition to revascularize the vertebral artery may also be performed to the cervical internal carotid, subclavian, or thyrocervical trunk arteries.
- **Carotid artery interposition graft.** In this case, a graft is utilized to circumvent a diseased portion of the carotid artery by anastomosing the graft proximal and distal to the native carotid artery.

Subclavian to carotid artery bypass graft

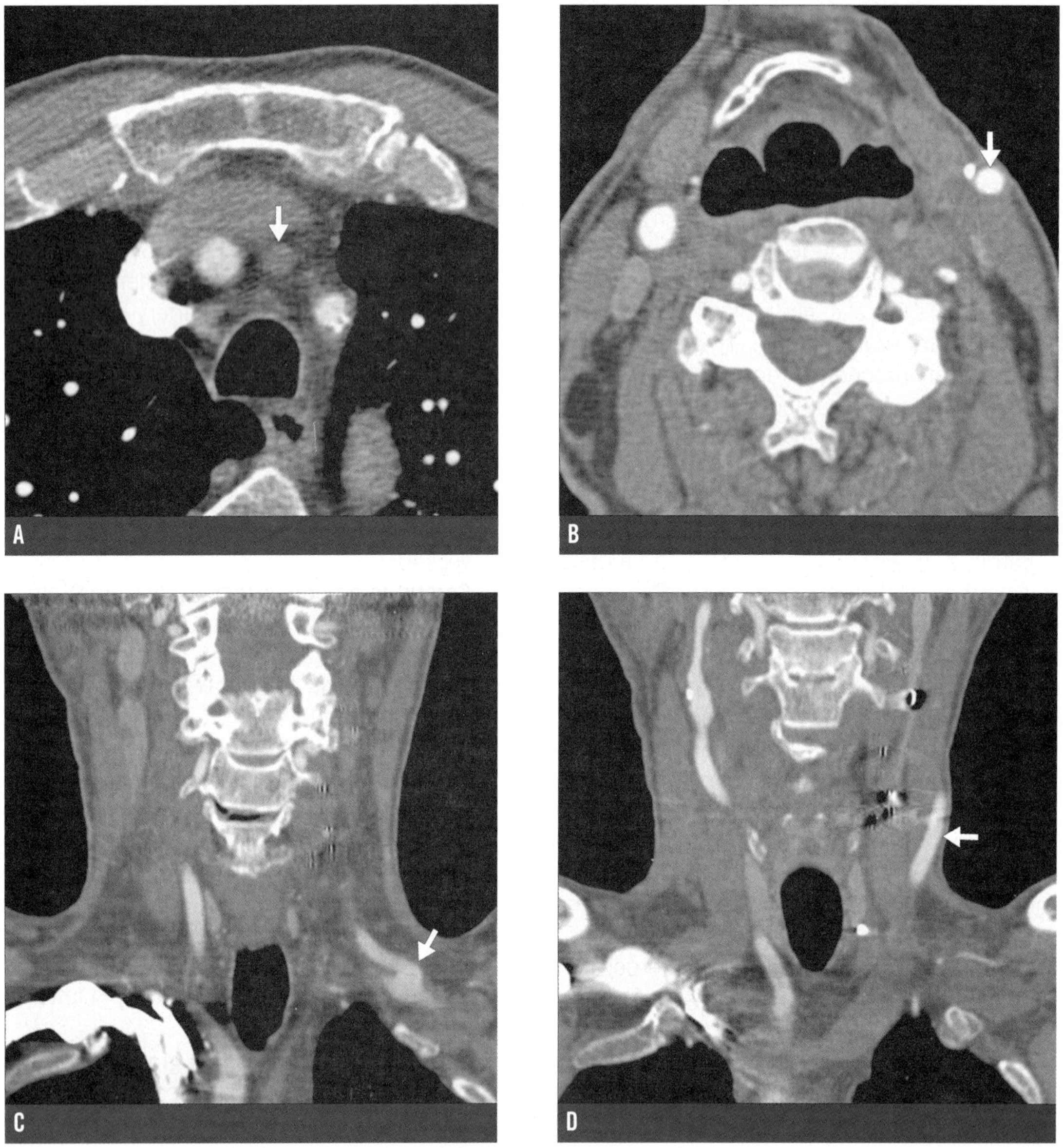

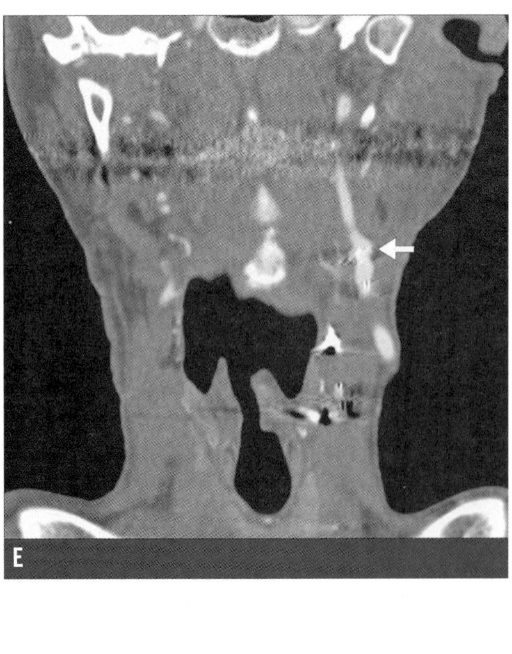

An axial CTA image (**A**) demonstrates absent flow in the proximal left common carotid artery (arrow, **A**). An axial CTA image more superior in the neck (**B**) as well as coronal reformatted CTA images (**C**-**E**) demonstrate a saphenous vein that was utilized to bypass the left subclavian artery to the left cervical internal carotid artery (arrows, **B**-**E**). The flow of blood is from the left subclavian artery to the left carotid artery. This left subclavian to carotid artery bypass was performed after a left carotid endarterectomy patch graft became infected and resulted in a carotid artery perforation (not shown).

Carotid to subclavian artery bypass graft

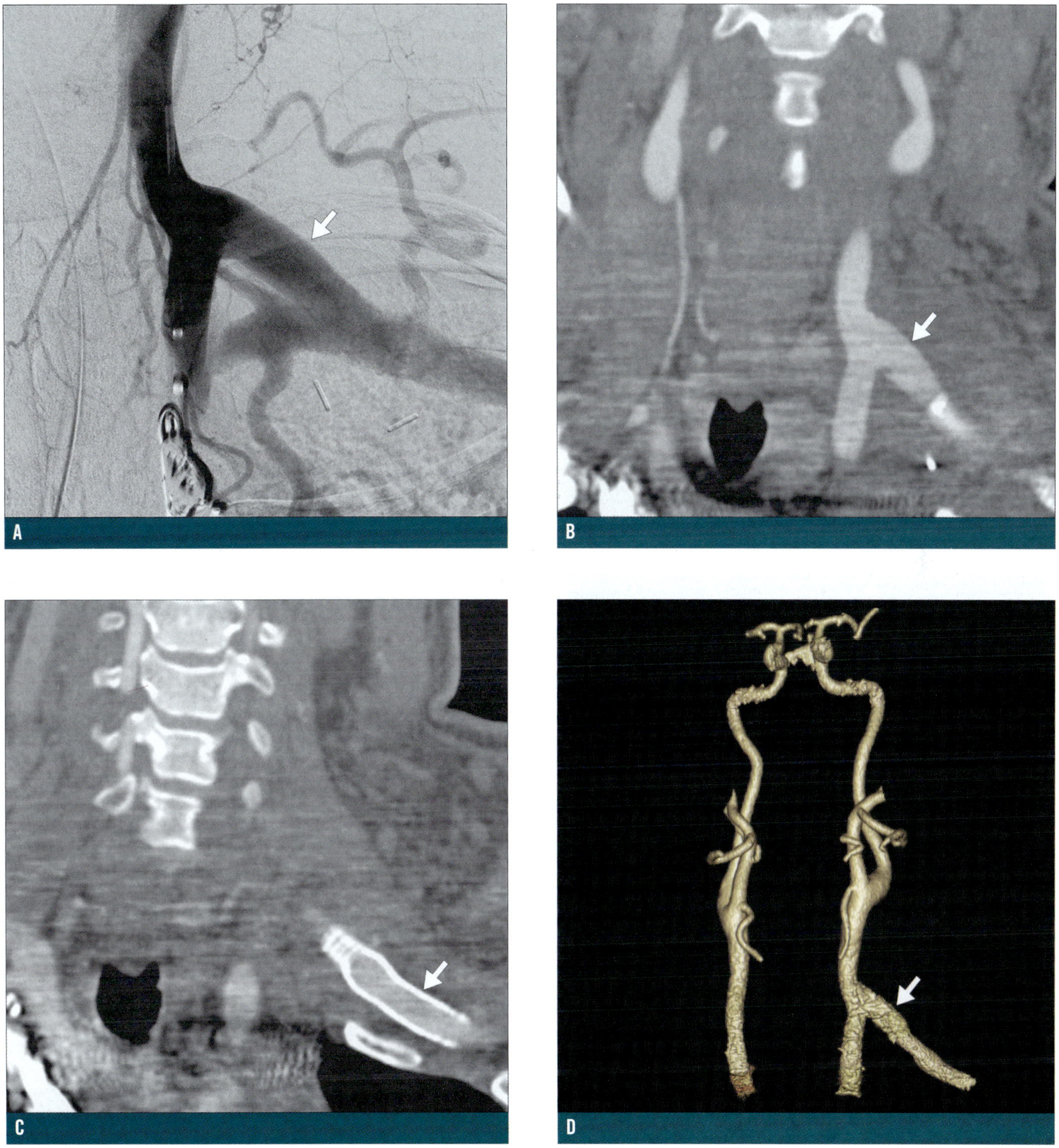

A frontal catheter angiogram image (**A**) demonstrates a patent left carotid artery to subclavian bypass that utilized a polytetrafluoroethylene (PTFE) graft (arrow, **A**). Coronal reformatted images from a follow-up CTA of the neck (**B**, **C**) demonstrate a patent graft (arrow, **B**) as well as a stent that was placed within the graft (arrow, **C**) which was utilized for hemostasis purposes. A 3D volumetric image from the CTA (**D**) also demonstrates the patent bypass graft (arrow, **D**). Prior to the bypass, this patient experienced a type A aortic dissection and was treated with placement of an aortic stent (not shown). The stent did not allow adequate flow of blood into the left subclavian artery, necessitating this carotid to subclavian artery bypass graft. The flow of blood is from the left carotid artery to the left subclavian artery.

Largely thrombosed carotid to subclavian artery bypass graft

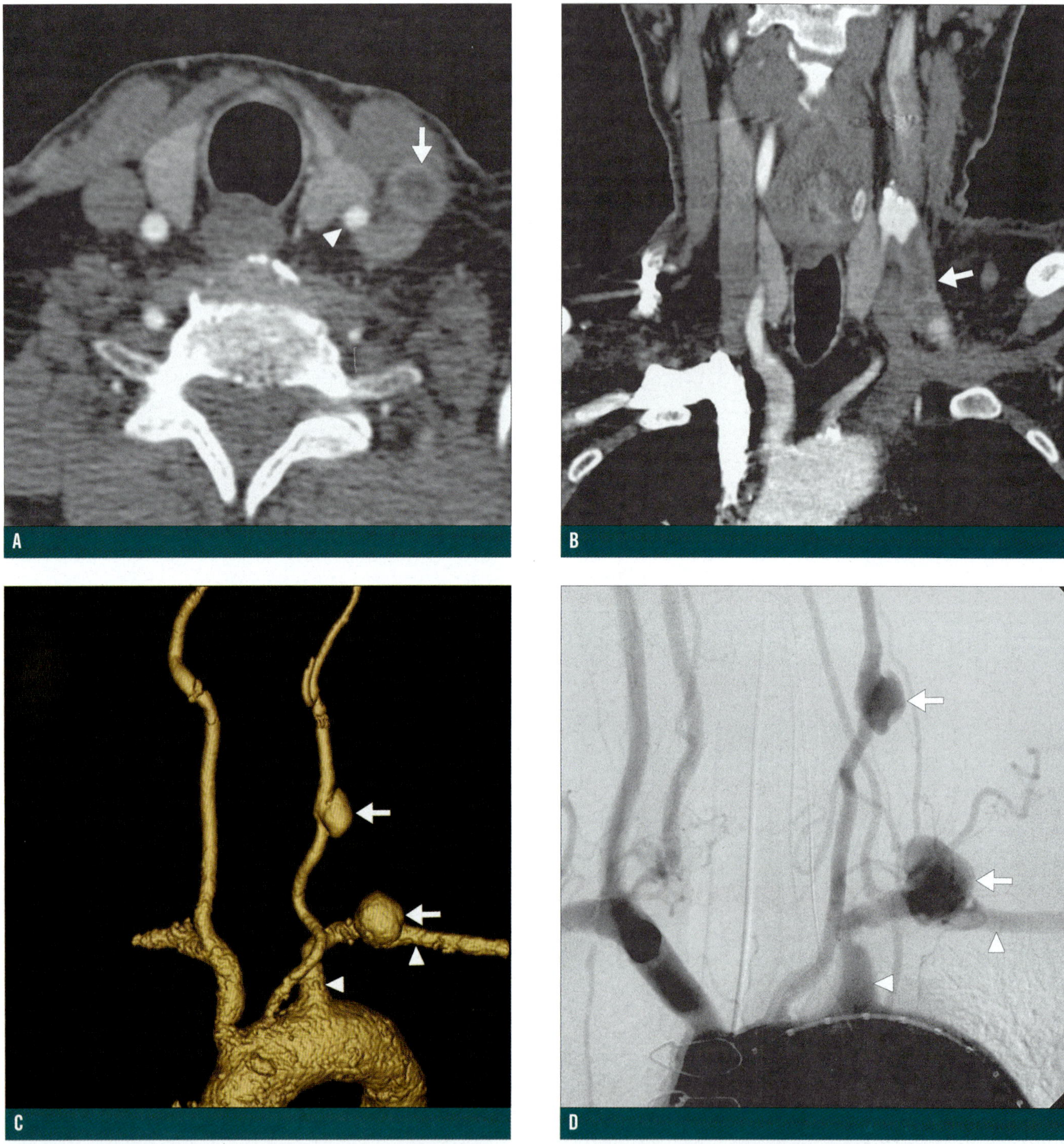

Axial (**A**) and coronal reformatted (**B**) images from a CTA neck demonstrate a largely thrombosed bypass graft that extends from the left common carotid artery to the left subclavian artery (arrows, **A**, **B**). The patent left common carotid artery is shown on image **A** (arrowhead). A 3D volumetric image from the CTA (**C**) and a frontal image from a catheter angiogram (**D**) demonstrate opacification of the proximal and distal ends of the graft (arrows, **C**, **D**) but lack of flow within the intervening portion of the graft. Despite the largely thrombosed graft, the left subclavian artery remains patent (arrowheads, **C**, **D**).

Aorto-bicarotid and left subclavian artery bypass graft

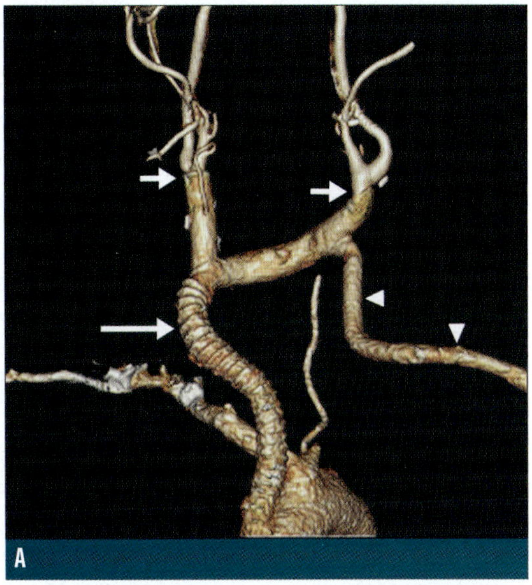

A 3D volumetric image generated from a CTA of the neck (**A**) demonstrates a large graft arising from the aorta (long arrow) that anastomoses with both common carotid arteries (short arrows). There is also additional graft material that bypasses the left subclavian artery (arrowheads). The native left subclavian artery is not visualized on this image. This extensive graft was utilized to treat large vessel occlusion related to Takayasu disease.

Carotid-to-carotid artery bypass graft

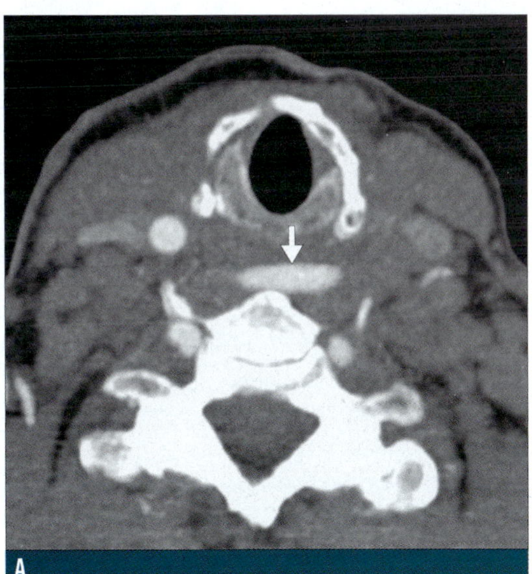

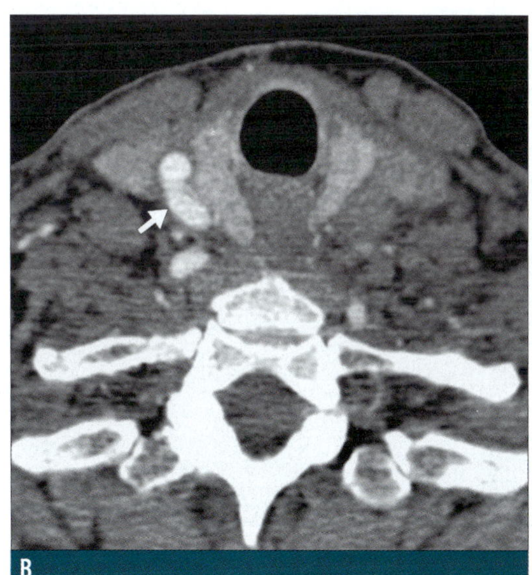

Axial (**A**, **B**) and coronal reformatted (**C**) images from a CTA of the neck demonstrate a bypass graft (Gore-Tex) extending from the proximal right common carotid artery to the distal left common carotid artery. The anastomosis with the right common carotid artery is shown on image **B** (arrow). This graft crosses the midline posterior to the pharynx (arrows, **A**, **C**). A 3D volumetric image (**D**) best demonstrates the proximal anastomosis with the right common carotid artery (arrow, **D**) and the distal anastomosis with the left common carotid artery (arrowhead, **D**). Prior to this surgical bypass, the patient experienced a type A aortic dissection that resulted in thrombosis of the proximal left common carotid artery. This right to left carotid-to-carotid retropharyngeal bypass was then performed to allow blood to travel from the right common carotid artery to the left common carotid artery in order to bypass the thrombosis.

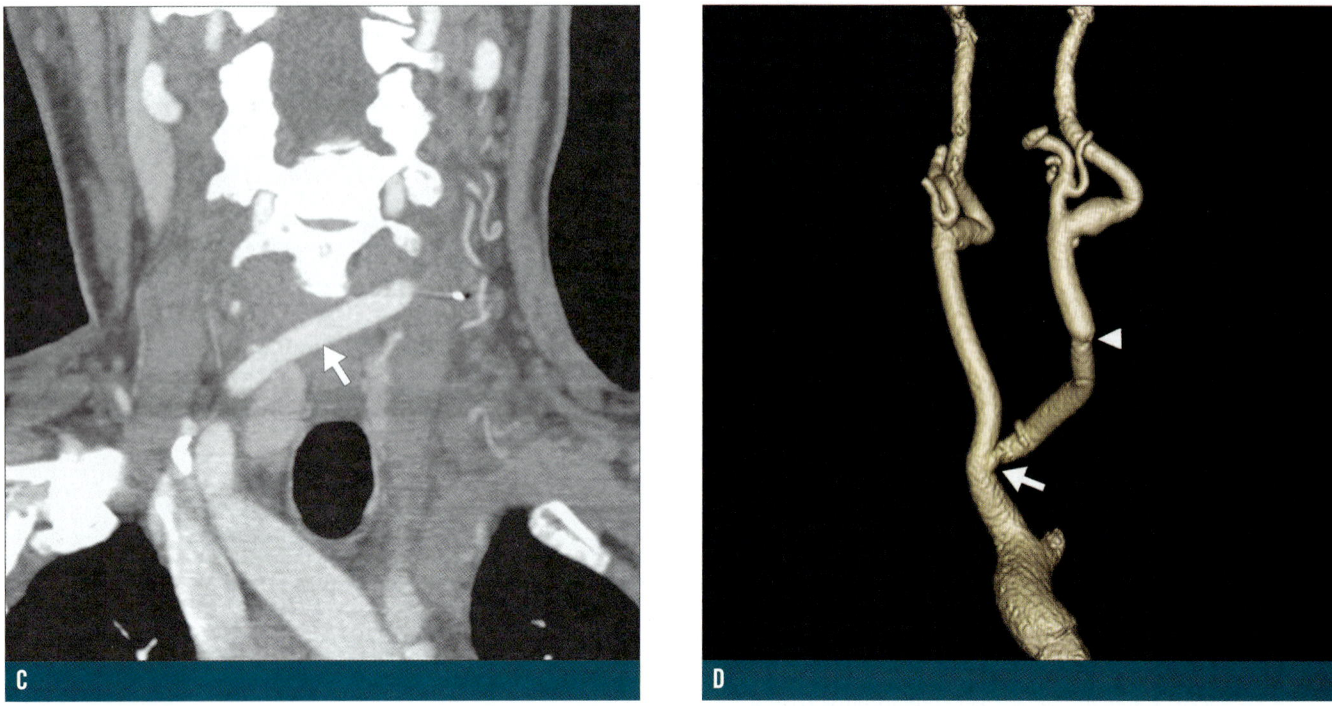

Vertebral to carotid artery transposition

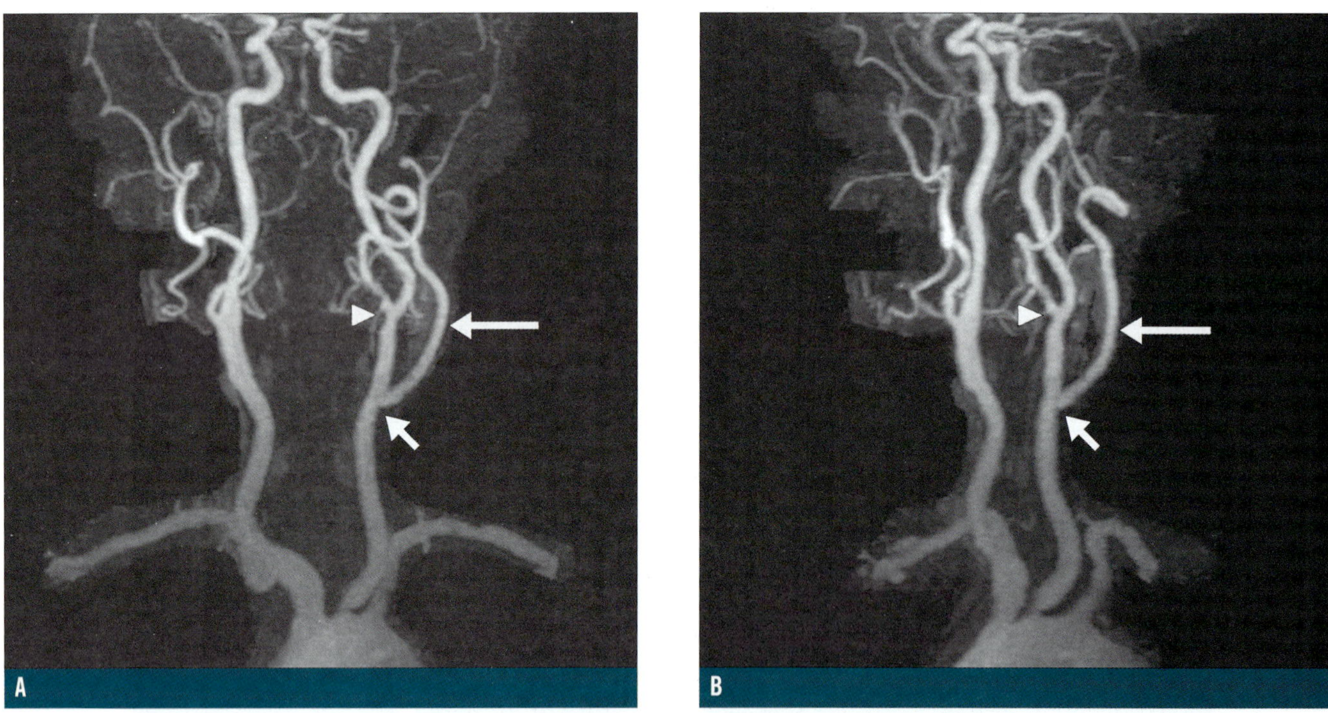

AP (**A**) and oblique (**B**) MIP images from a contrast-enhanced MRA of the neck demonstrate a surgical transposition of the left cervical vertebral artery (long arrows, **A**, **B**) to the mid to distal left common carotid artery (short arrows, **A**, **B**). In this case, the left vertebral artery was ligated distal to the stenosis/occlusion and the distal stump was then transposed end-to-side onto the left common carotid artery. This procedure was performed to allow blood flow to travel from the left common carotid artery to the left vertebral artery. The normal left carotid bifurcation is located more cephalad (arrowheads, **A**, **B**).

Carotid artery interposition graft

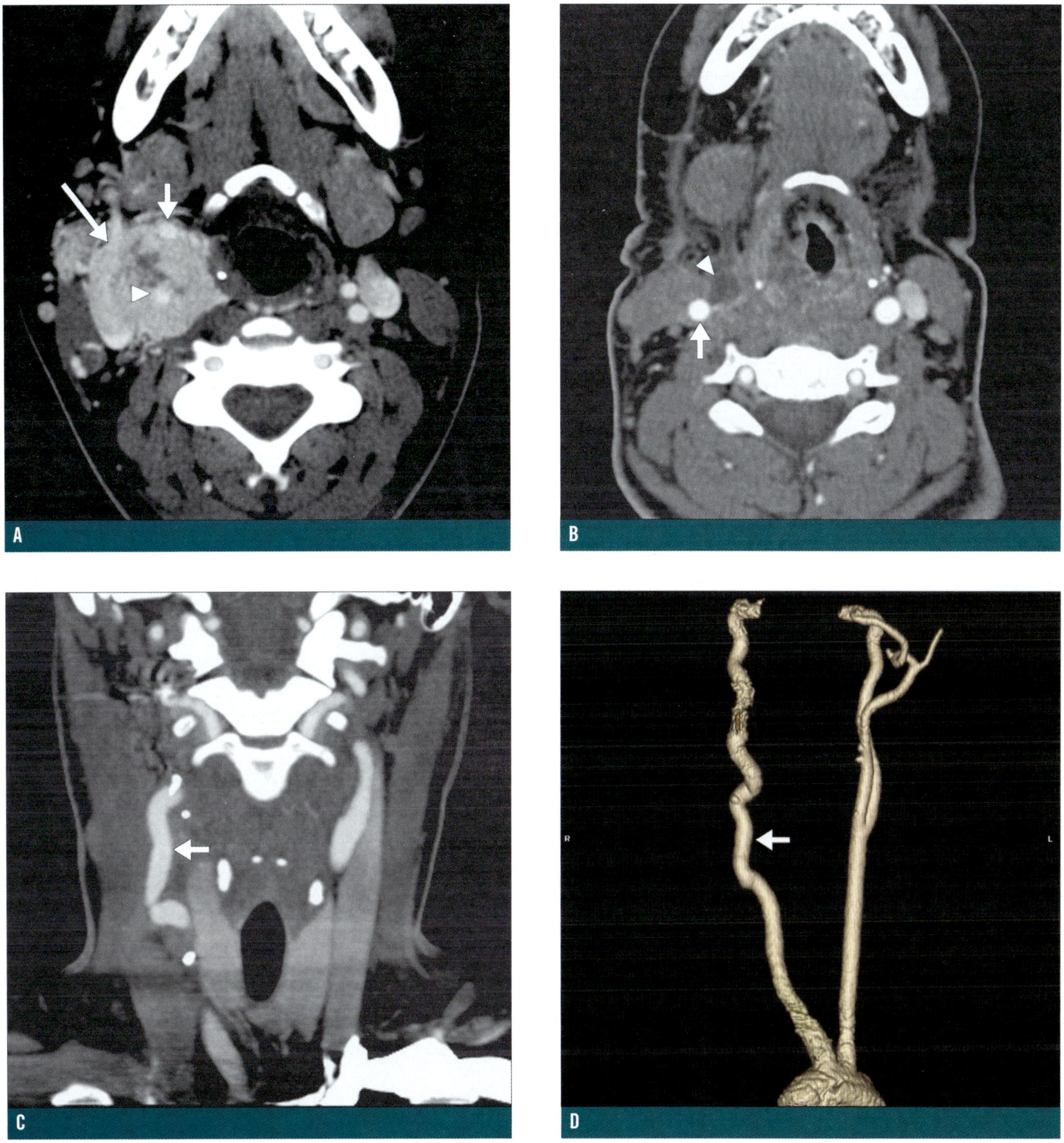

An axial CTA image (**A**) demonstrates a large, heterogeneous mass that was shown to represent a glomus tumor at pathology (long arrow, **A**). This mass completely encased the right cervical internal carotid artery (arrowhead, **A**) and largely encased the right external carotid artery (short arrow, **A**). In order to preserve blood flow to the carotid artery during removal of the glomus tumor, the patient concurrently underwent a carotid artery interposition bypass using a saphenous vein graft. Axial (**B**) and coronal reformatted (**C**) images from a CTA of the neck following removal of the glomus tumor and placement of the bypass graft demonstrate thrombosis of the native right cervical internal carotid artery (arrowhead, **B**) and a patent saphenous vein bypass graft (short arrows, **B**, **C**). A 3D volumetric image obtained from the CTA following surgery (**D**) also demonstrates the patent right saphenous vein bypass graft (short arrow, **D**).

REFERENCES

Abou-Zamzam AM, et al. Extrathoracic arterial grafts performed for carotid artery occlusive disease not amenable to endarterectomy. *Arch Surg*. 1999;134:952-957.

Aiello F, Morrissey NJ. Open and endovascular management of subclavian and innominate arterial pathology. *Semin Vasc Surg*. 2011;24(1):31-35.

Cina CS, et al. Subclavian carotid transposition and bypass grafting: consecutive cohort study and systematic review. *J Vasc Surg*. 2002;35(3):422-429.

Dorafshar AH, Reil TD, Ahn SS, Quinones-Baldrich WJ, Moore WS. Interposition grafts for difficult carotid artery reconstruction: a 17-year experience. *Ann Vasc Surg*. 2008;22:63-69.

Morasch MD. Technique for subclavian to carotid transposition, tips, and tricks. *J Vasc Surg*. 2009;49(1):251-254.

Schardey HM, Meye G, Rau HG, Gradi G, Jaunch KW, Lauterjung L. Subclavian carotid transposition: An analysis of a clinical series and a review of the literature. *Eur J Vasc Endovasc Surg*. 1996;12:431-436.

CASE 17 Persistent embryonic carotid-basilar anastomoses (persistent fetal circulation variants)

There are multiple transient segmental anastomoses between the anterior and posterior circulation that are present during fetal development of the brain. Typically, these primitive anastomoses remain functional for approximately 7 to 10 days and obliterate as the posterior communicating arteries develop. However, one or more of these connections can persist into adulthood and are referred to as persistent embryonic carotid-basilar anastomoses or persistent fetal circulation variants. The majority of these persistent fetal arteries are named for the cranial nerves that they parallel. From superior to inferior, they are: persistent trigeminal, otic, hypoglossal, and proatlantal intersegmental arteries.

While these persistent fetal anastomoses are typically incidental, they may become important in certain situations. For instance, if there is significant cervical internal carotid artery (ICA) atherosclerotic disease, the more distal ipsilateral carotid artery may "steal" blood flow from the posterior circulation via a persistent fetal anastomosis, which tend to be relatively large vessels. Also, particles used during an embolization procedure may inadvertently traverse these anastomoses. Furthermore, evaluation for the presence of these persistent fetal anastomoses should be performed prior to the administration of sodium amobarbital used during a Wada test to prevent inadvertent anesthesia of the brainstem.

- **Persistent trigeminal artery (PTA).** The PTA is the most common persistent embryonic carotid-basilar anastomosis and is present in approximately 0.1% to 0.2% of cerebral angiograms. It is typically identified below the level of the posterior communicating arteries at the approximate level of the sella turcica. It extends posteriorly and medially from the ICA cavernous segment to join the distal one-third of the basilar artery, between the origins of the superior cerebellar artery and the anterior inferior cerebellar artery. Flow within the anastomosis is typically from the ICA toward the basilar artery.
- **Persistent otic artery.** The existence of this persistent fetal circulation anastamosis has been debated in the literature, some arguing that there are no true cases reported and that those which have been reported simply represent a low-lying PTA. This purported persistent anastomotic vessel courses from the lateral aspect of the petrous ICA through the internal auditory canal and joins the caudal aspect of the basilar artery.
- **Persistent hypoglossal artery (PHA).** The PHA is the second most common persistent embryonic carotid-basilar anastomosis, with a prevalence of 0.03% to 0.26%. This persistent embryonic vessel arises from the cervical ICA and parallels CN XII at the skull base. The vessel courses posteromedially through an enlarged hypoglossal canal to join the basilar artery. If a PHA is present, then the posterior communicating arteries are typically absent. Additionally, if the PHA is large, it may replace the intracranial vertebral artery and there may be concomitant hypoplasia or absence of the ipsilateral or bilateral cervical vertebral arteries.
- **Persistent proatlantal intersegmental artery (PPIA).** The PPIA is the most caudal and the last to involute of the persistent embryonic carotid-basilar anastomoses. During fetal development, this artery accompanies the C1 nerve and traverses between the occipital somites and the cervical somites; this artery is termed proatlantal because it resides above C1. Similar to the PHA, if the proatlantal intersegmental artery persists, the ipsilateral or bilateral vertebral arteries may be hypoplastic or even absent.

There are two variants of a PPIA. In the PPIA type I variant, the persistent anastomotic vessel arises from the anteromedial aspect of the cervical ICA and extends cephalad along the ventral aspect of the vertebral bodies. From there, the artery extends horizontally over the atlas to enter the calvarial vault through the foramen magnum, ultimately anastomosing with, or giving rise to, the ipsilateral vertebral artery. The type II variant of the PPIA is less common and is characterized by the PPIA arising from the external carotid artery rather than the cervical ICA.

The PPIA and PHA can be difficult to differentiate, as both arise from the extracranial carotid artery. However, the PHA arises more cephalad in the neck (at the skull base level) and traverses the hypoglossal canal, whereas the PPIA does not.

Persistent trigeminal artery (PTA)

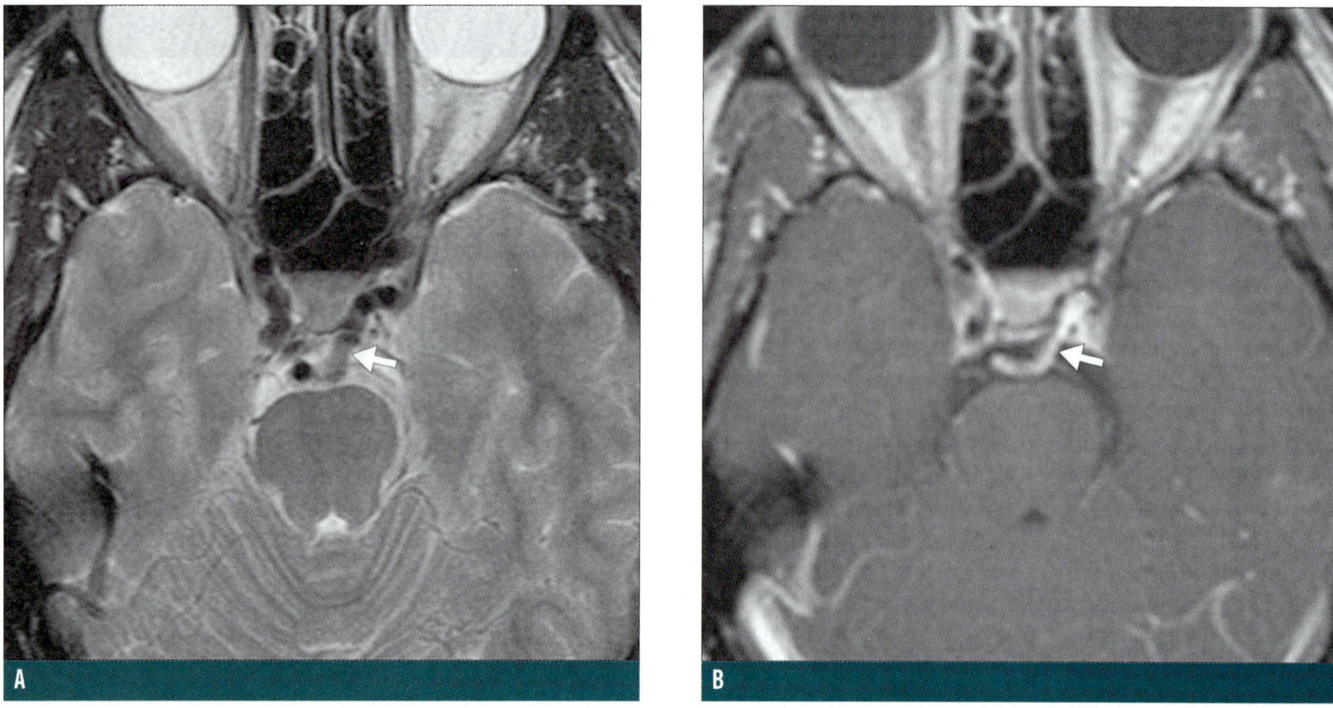

Axial T2 (**A**) and postcontrast axial T1 (**B**) MR images at the level of the cavernous carotid arteries demonstrate a flow void (arrow, **A**) and corresponding vessel enhancement (arrow, **B**) that arises from the cavernous left ICA and joins the distal basilar artery, consistent with a PTA.

Persistent trigeminal artery (PTA)

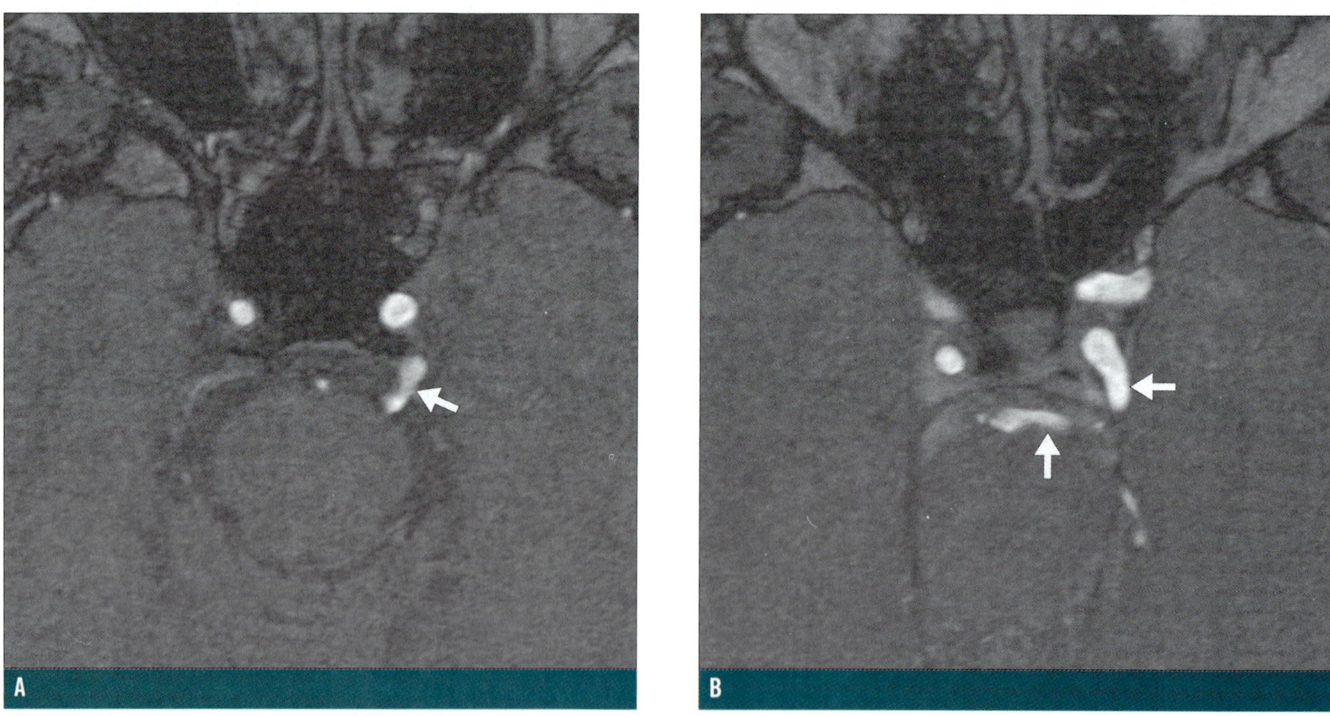

Different patient. Two axial source images from a time-of-flight MRA through the level of the cavernous ICA (**A**, **B**) demonstrate a moderate-sized vessel communicating between the left cavernous ICA and the basilar artery, compatible with a PTA (arrows, **A**, **B**). This is vessel arises too proximal to represent the normal posterior communicating artery, which arises from the supraclinoid carotid artery. An axial collapsed MIP image (**C**) and a lateral MIP image (**D**) from the same MRA also demonstrate the PTA (arrows, **C**, **D**) communicating with the basilar artery (arrowhead, **D**).

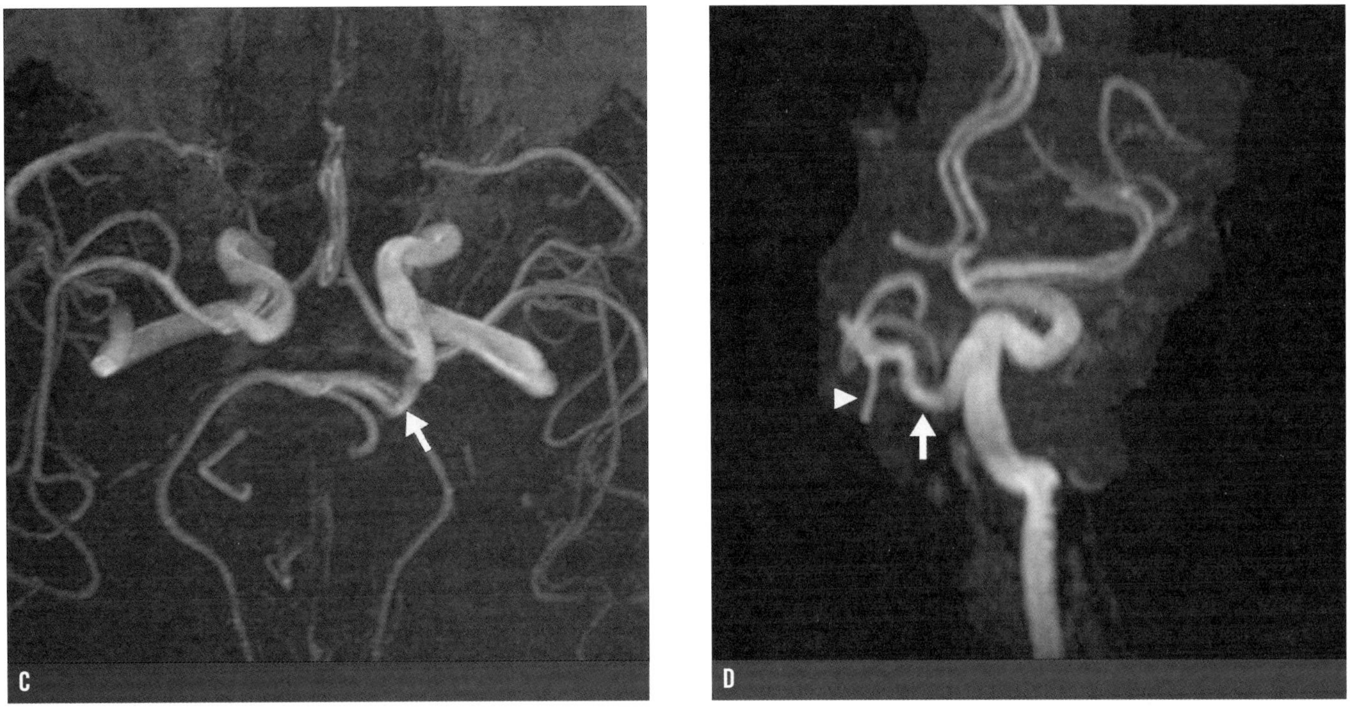

Persistent hypoglossal artery (PHA)

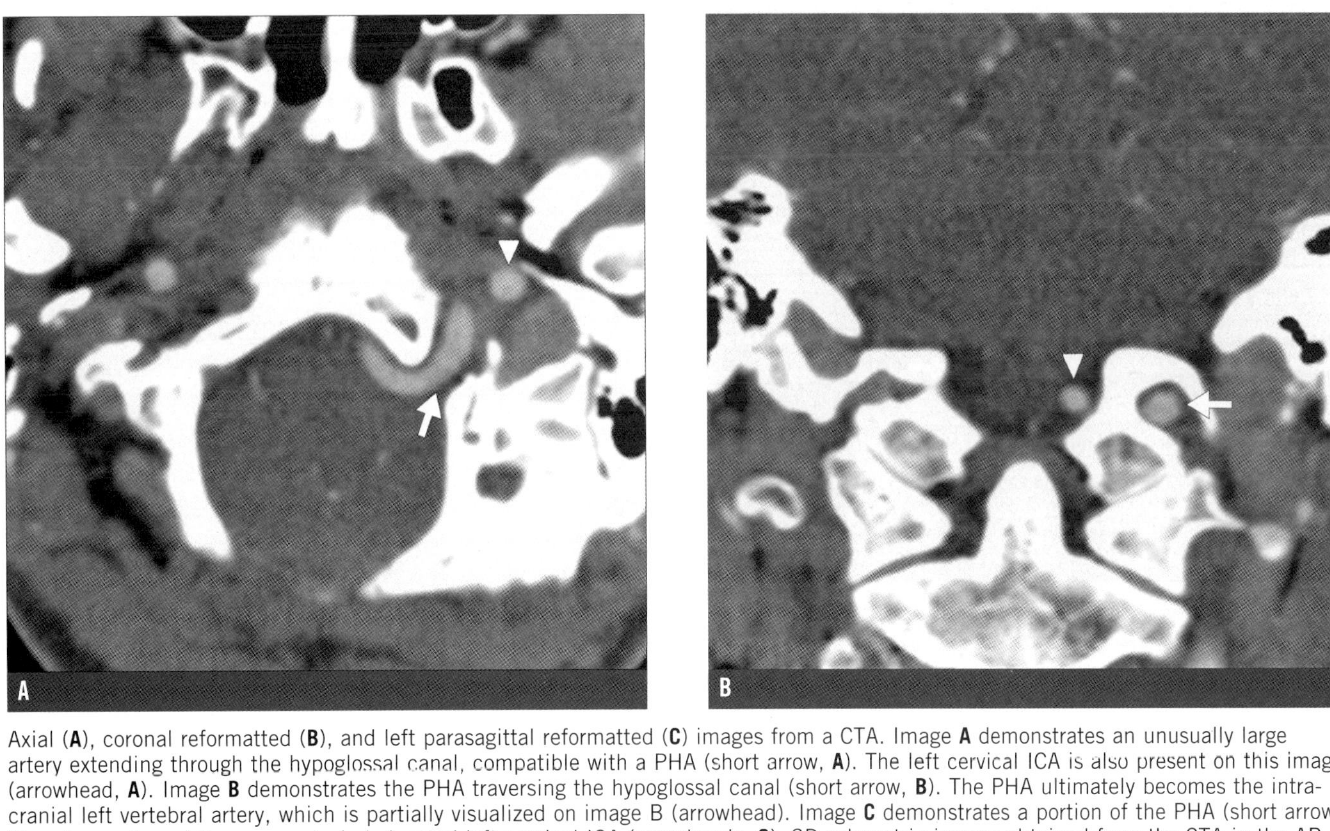

Axial (**A**), coronal reformatted (**B**), and left parasagittal reformatted (**C**) images from a CTA. Image **A** demonstrates an unusually large artery extending through the hypoglossal canal, compatible with a PHA (short arrow, **A**). The left cervical ICA is also present on this image (arrowhead, **A**). Image **B** demonstrates the PHA traversing the hypoglossal canal (short arrow, **B**). The PHA ultimately becomes the intracranial left vertebral artery, which is partially visualized on image B (arrowhead). Image **C** demonstrates a portion of the PHA (short arrow, **C**) and a portion of the more anteriorly located left cervical ICA (arrowheads, **C**). 3D volumetric images obtained from the CTA in the AP plane (**D**) and the lateral plane (**E**) best demonstrate the relationship of the PHA (short arrows, **D**, **E**) and the left cervical ICA (arrowheads, **D**, **E**). The PHA's origin from the left cervical ICA is also demonstrated on image E (long arrow).

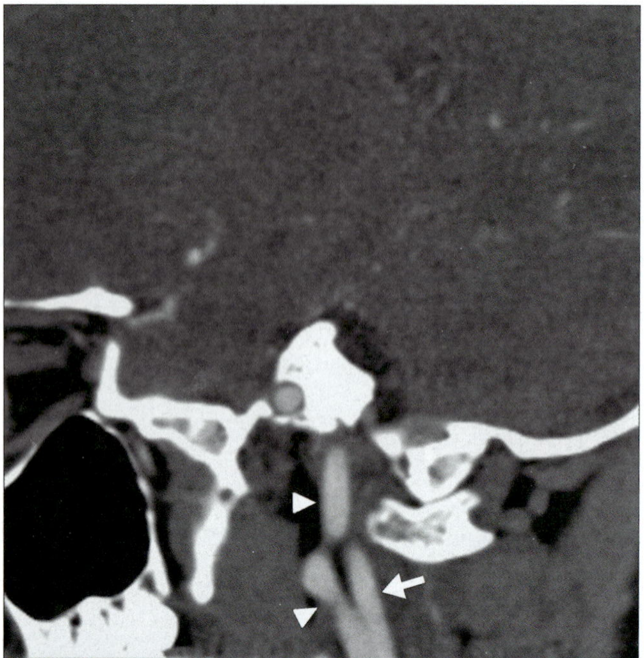
C

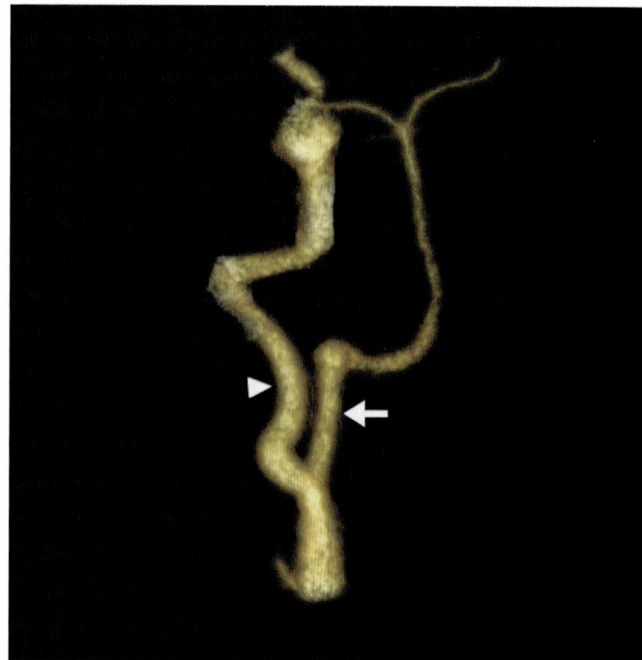
D

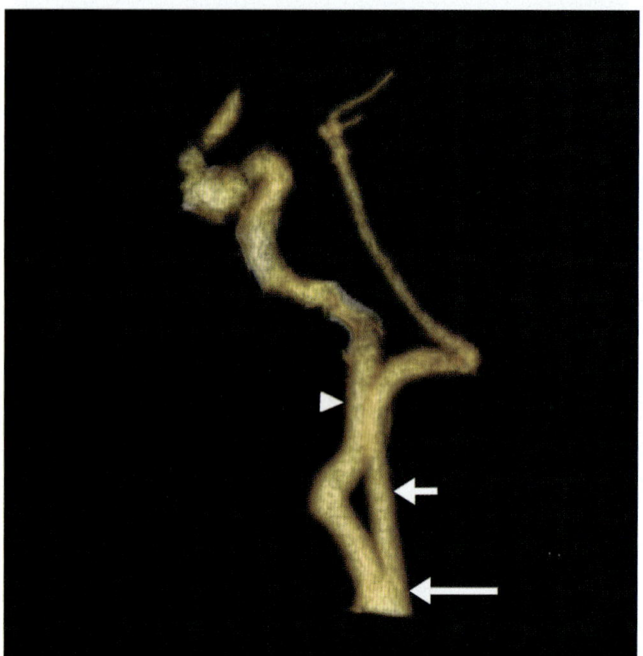
E

Persistent hypoglossal artery (PHA)

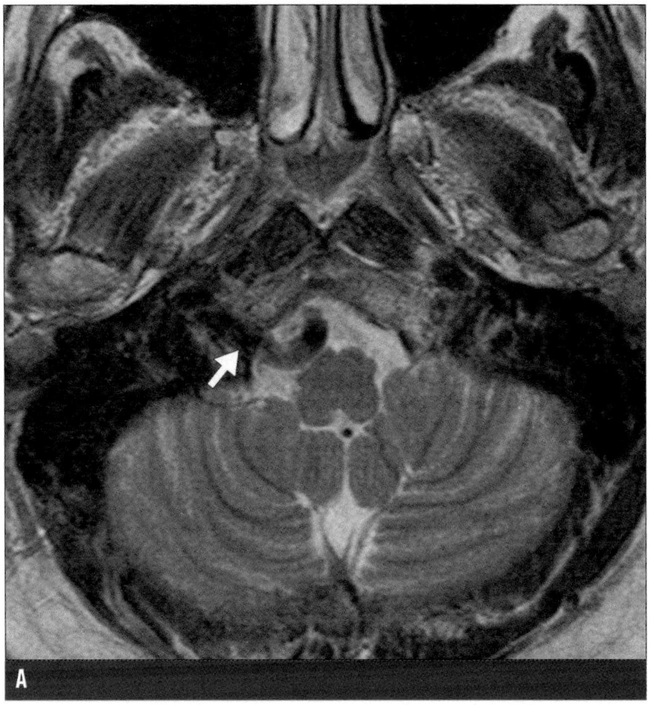

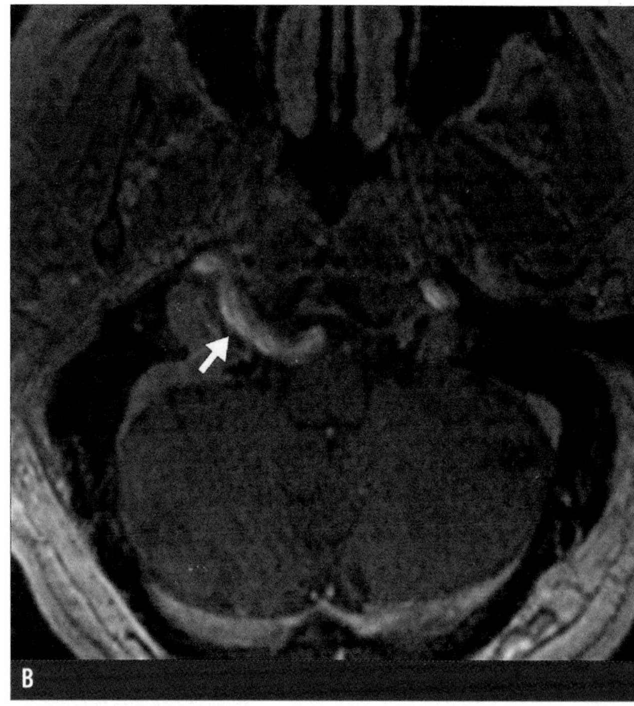

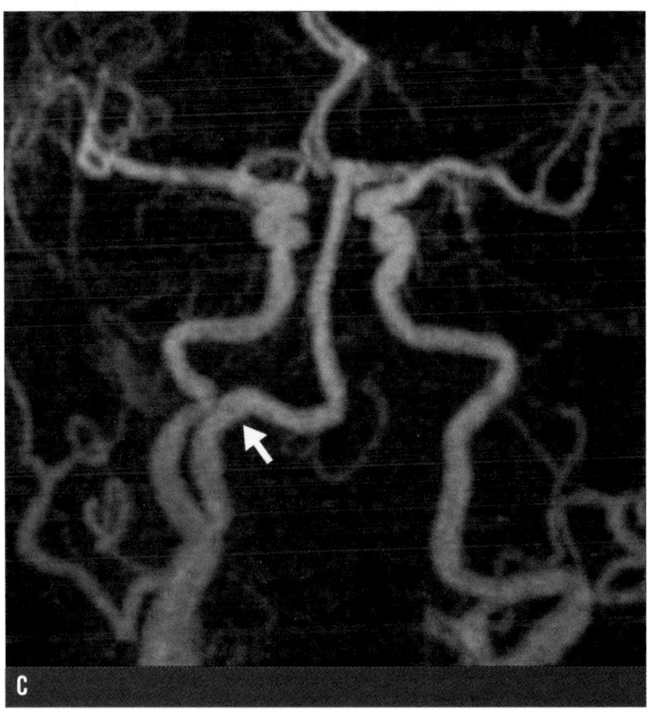

Different patient. Axial T2 (**A**) and an axial source image from a time-of-flight MRA (**B**) demonstrate a PHA traversing the right hypoglossal canal (arrows, **A**, **B**). A MIP image from the MRA (**C**) demonstrates the right PHA (arrow, **C**) communicating between the right cervical ICA and the basilar artery.

Persistent proatlantal intersegmental artery (PPIA)

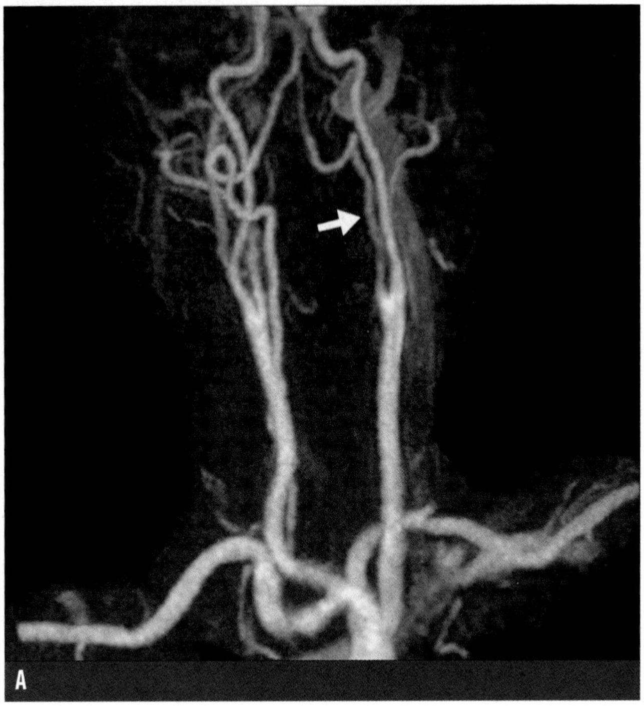

A MIP image from a gadolinium-infused MRA (**A**) demonstrates the distal cervical left vertebral artery (arrow) to originate from the left external carotid artery compatible with a type II PPIA.

REFERENCES

Bhattacharya JJ, Lamin S, Thammaroj J. Otic or mythic? *AJNR Am J Neuroradiol.* 2004;25:160-162.

Gumusa T, Onal B, Ilgita EG. Bilateral persistence of type 1 proatlantal arteries: report of a case and review of the literature. *AJNR Am J Neuroradiol.* 2004;25:1622-1624.

Osborn AG. *Cerebral Angiography.* 2nd ed. Philadelphia, PA: LWW; 1999.

Patel AB, Gandhi CD, Bederson JB. Angiographic documentation of a persistent otic artery. *AJNR Am J Neuroradiol.* 2003;24:124-126.

Uchino A, Sawada A, Takase Y, Kudo S. MR angiography of anomalous branches of the internal carotid artery. *AJR Am J Roentgenol.* 2003;181:1409-1414.

Woodcock R, Cloft H, Dion J. Bilateral type 1 proatlantal arteries with absence of vertebral arteries. *AJNR Am J Neuroradiol.* 2001;22:418-420.

There are a variety of artifacts that may be identified on vascular imaging of the head and neck. Artifact on CT often results from metallic beam hardening. MRI artifacts may be the result of magnetic susceptibility (air-tissue interface, dental amalgam, metallic vascular clips/foreign bodies, orthopedic implants, etc.), CSF pulsation, and truncation artifact. Causes of artifact that may affect CT as well as MR vascular imaging include those related to patient motion and vessel pulsation. Although some imaging artifacts may be obvious, others may simulate disease or obscure disease. In all vascular imaging studies, it is critical to review the vascular source data and reformatted imaging, depending on the type of imaging modality, to help differentiate artifact from true pathology.

On CTA imaging of the neck, vessel tortuosity and pulsation can simulate an intimal flap with a false lumen. This is particularly more common at the caudal aspects of the common carotid arteries where there tends to be a greater degree of vessel tortuosity and the heartbeat is more forceful. Arterial or venous pulsation artifact on MRI may simulate the presence of an intraaxial lesion. This often occurs at the level of the temporal lobe (due to cavernous carotid artery pulsation) and cerebellum (due to the dural venous sinuses) because of "ghosting". Ghosting occurs in the phase encoding direction. In order to minimize this artifact over the area of interest, the short axis of the area imaged is typically chosen for the phase encoding direction. Thus, for the brain, the phase encoding directions is typically set to traverse from right to left, whereas for the neck, it is set to traverse from anterior to posterior. In problematic cases, it is helpful to switch the phase and frequency encoding directions in order to determine whether the finding is pathologic or a true finding. If artifactual, switching the phase and frequency encoding directions will eliminate the artifact. Another helpful technique to assess whether a finding is a true lesion or related to pulsation artifact on MRI is to increase the window width and lower the window level of the image (ie, "widen the window"). This may reveal that the finding extends outside the confines of the calvarium. If the finding does reside outside the confines of the calvarium, and it is located at the same horizontal level as the finding overlying the brain, then the finding is likely artifactual, assuming that the phase encoding direction was performed along the short axis.

Beam hardening on CT or metallic susceptibility artifact on MRI that is located adjacent to the carotid or vertebral arteries may simulate occlusion or dissection of the artery as well as obscure significant portions of the artery on both imaging modalities, precluding the evaluation of a potentially significant finding.

Tortuosity/pulsation artifact simulating a carotid artery dissection on CTA

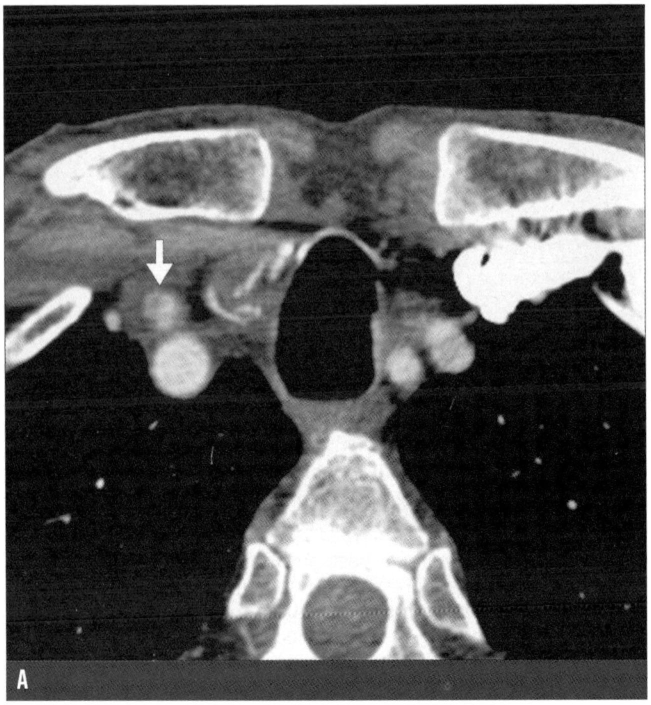

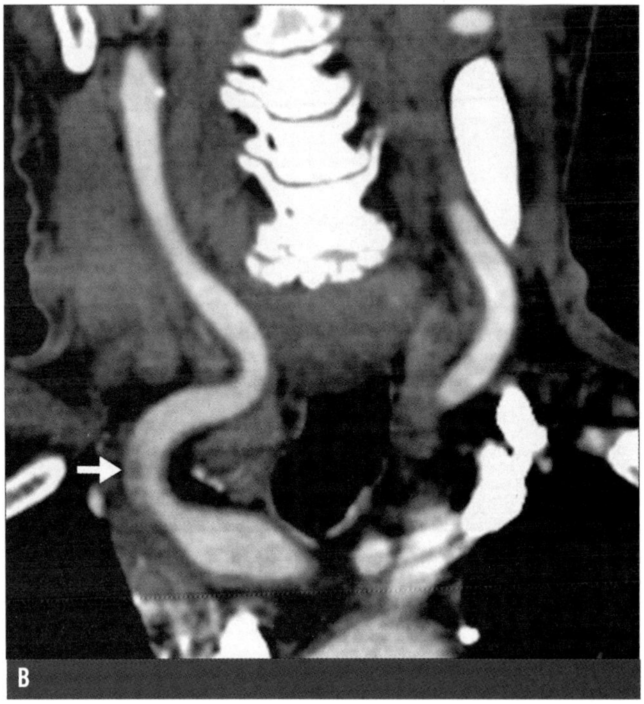

Axial (**A**) and coronal reformatted (**B**) CTA images of the neck demonstrate a possible proximal right common carotid artery dissection (arrows, **A**, **B**). Two MIP images from a gadolinium-infused MRA performed the next day (**C**, **D**) demonstrate a normal proximal right common carotid artery. The apparent finding on the CTA was merely artifactual, possibly related to vessel tortuosity (resulting in turbulent arterial flow and incomplete mixing of contrast with blood) or prominent pulsation of the vessel at this location.

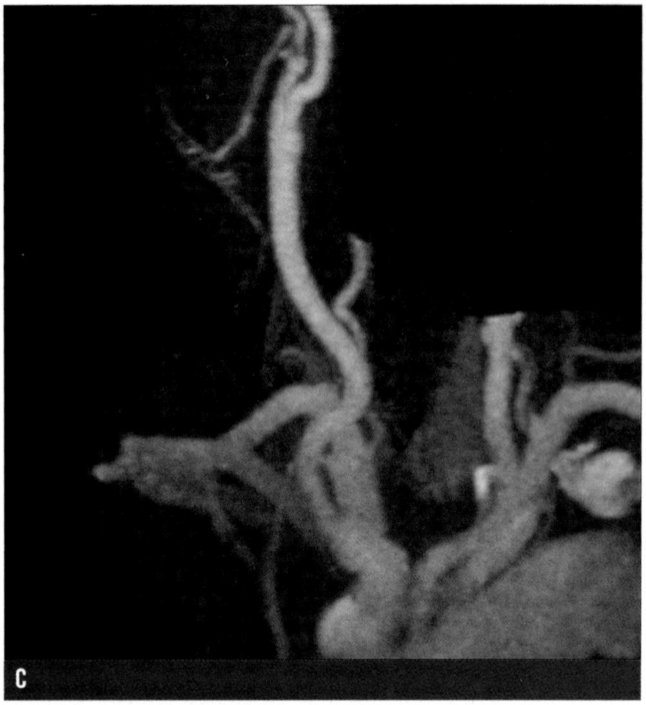

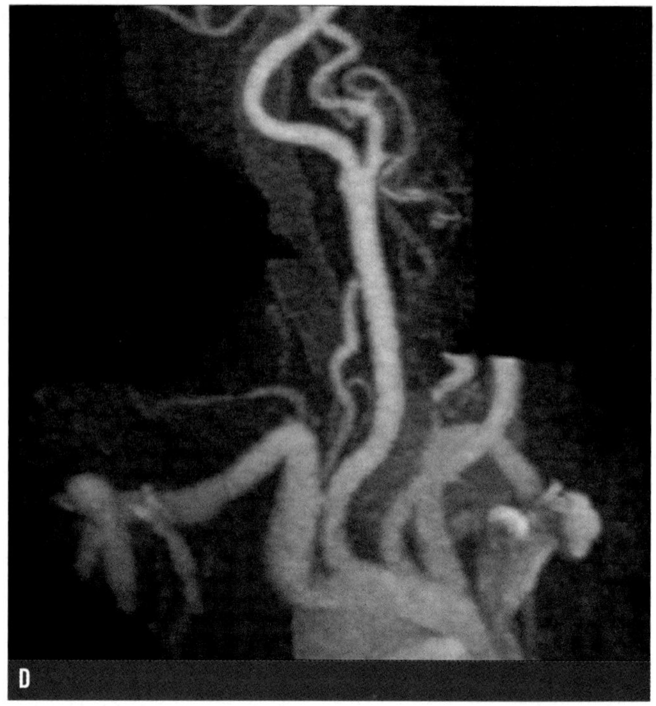

MRI pulsation artifact from the sigmoid sinuses

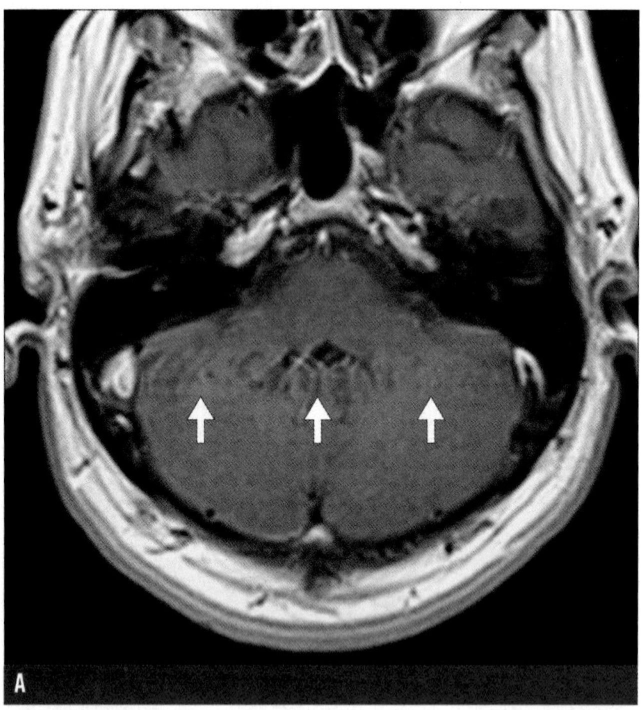

A postcontrast axial T1-weighted MR image (**A**) demonstrates a linear band of pulsation artifact extending across the cerebellum related to the sigmoid sinuses (arrows).

MRI pulsation artifact from the sigmoid sinuses

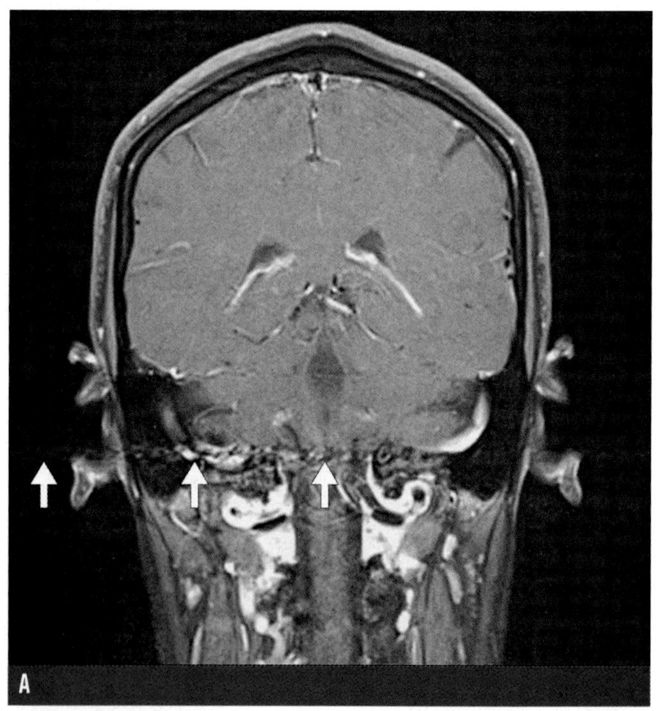

Different patient. A coronal postcontrast T1-weighted MR image performed with fat suppression (**A**) demonstrates a large amount of horizontally oriented pulsation artifact related to the sigmoid sinuses extending through the craniocervical junction and outside the confines of the calvarium (arrows).

MRI pulsation artifact from the cavernous carotid arteries

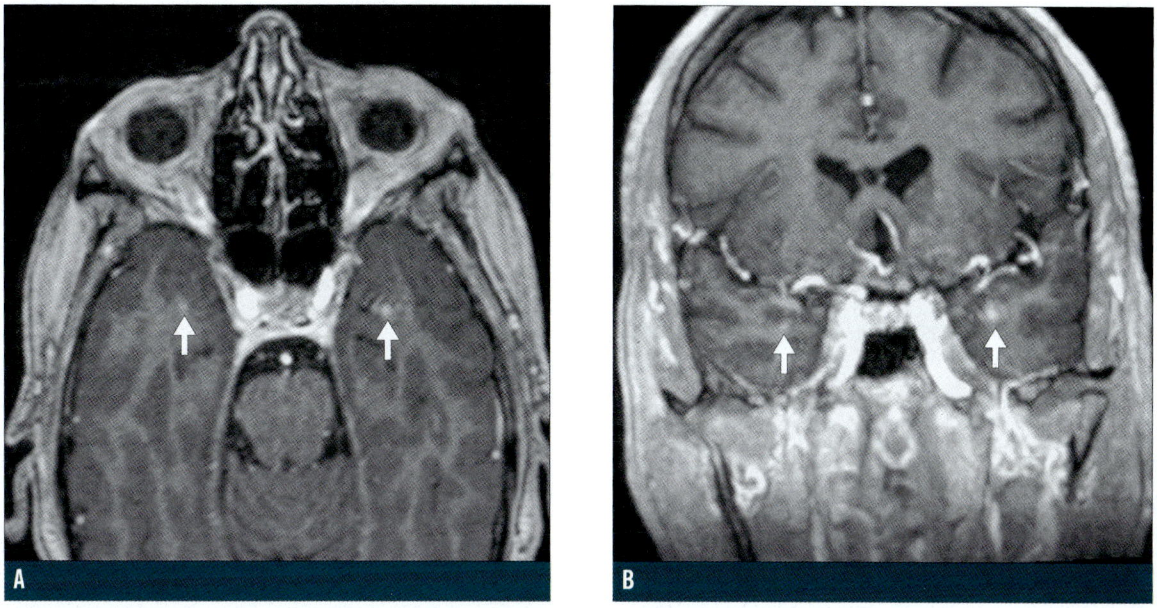

Axial (**A**) and coronal reformatted (**B**) postcontrast MPRAGE MR images demonstrate symmetric punctate foci of apparent enhancement in the medial aspects of both temporal lobes (arrows, **A**, **B**) in a patient being evaluated for intracranial metastatic disease. These foci simply relate to pulsation artifact from the cavernous carotid arteries. This type of artifact often parallels the arteries on multiple consecutive images.

MRI pulsation artifact from the internal jugular veins

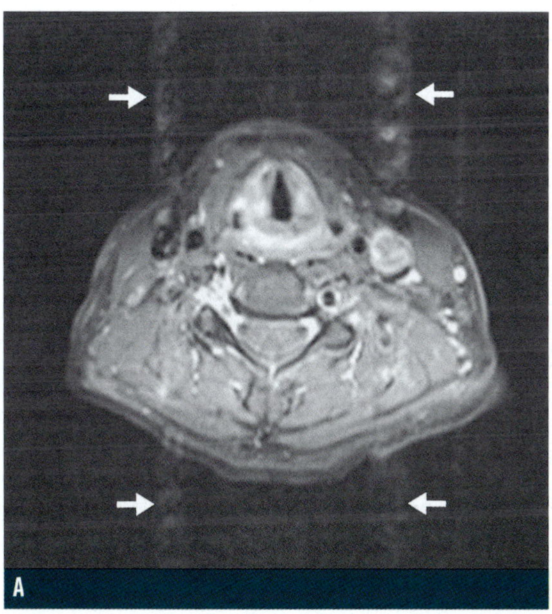

An axial postcontrast T1-weighted MR image with fat saturation (**A**) demonstrates pronounced vertically oriented pulsation artifact related to bilateral internal jugular vein pulsation which extends outside the confines of the neck (arrows). This artifact traverses vertically along the neck, rather than horizontally (as is typically identified on brain imaging). This is because pulsation artifact occurs in the phase encoding direction. In order to minimize this artifact over the area of interest, the short axis of the body part image is chosen for the phase encoding direction. Thus, for the neck, an anterior to posterior direction is typically chosen for the phase encoding direction.

MRA pseudostenosis related to susceptibility artifact

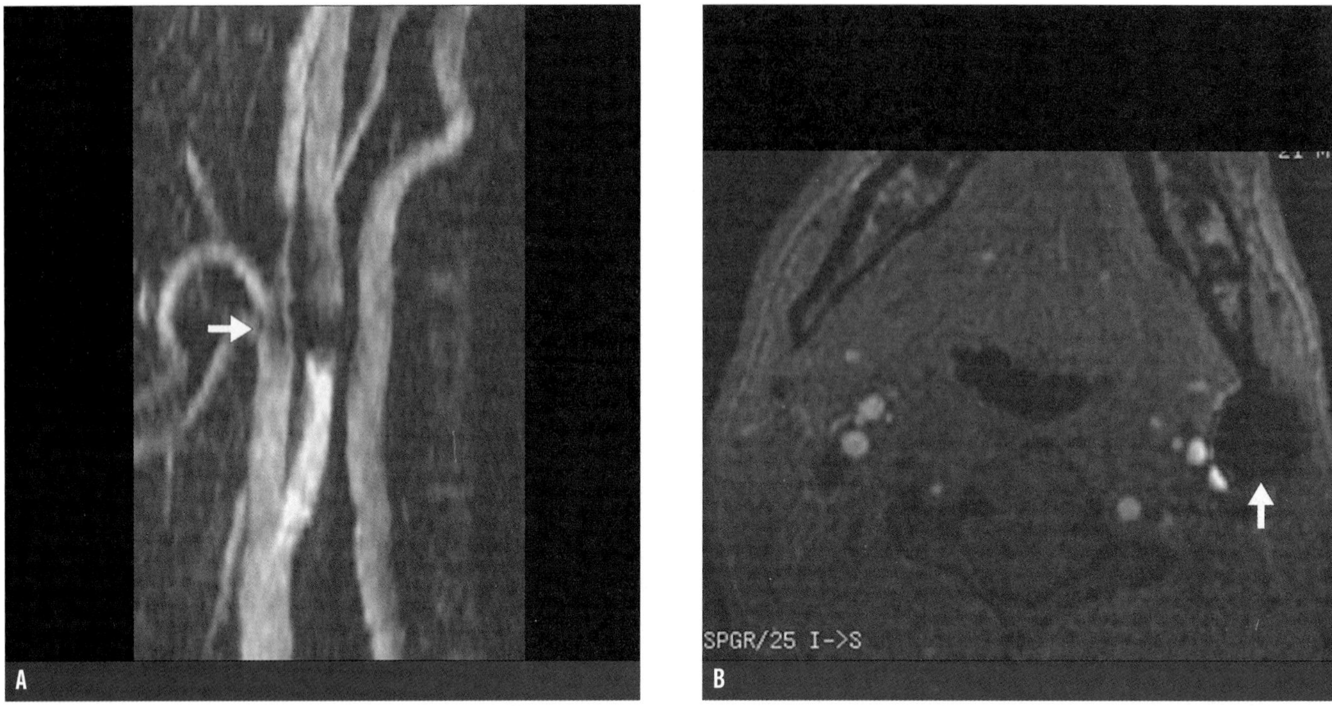

A lateral 2D MIP reconstruction (**A**) and a 2D TOF source image from the same study (**B**). Image **A** demonstrates horizontally oriented signal loss of the proximal left cervical internal and external carotid arteries (arrow, **A**). The morphology of the signal loss suggests that this is artifactual. Review of the source data clearly demonstrates susceptibility artifact (arrow, **B**) resulting in the focally diminished signal of the left cervical internal and external carotid arteries on image **A.**

Artifactual flow gap on MRA because of dental amalgam susceptibility artifact

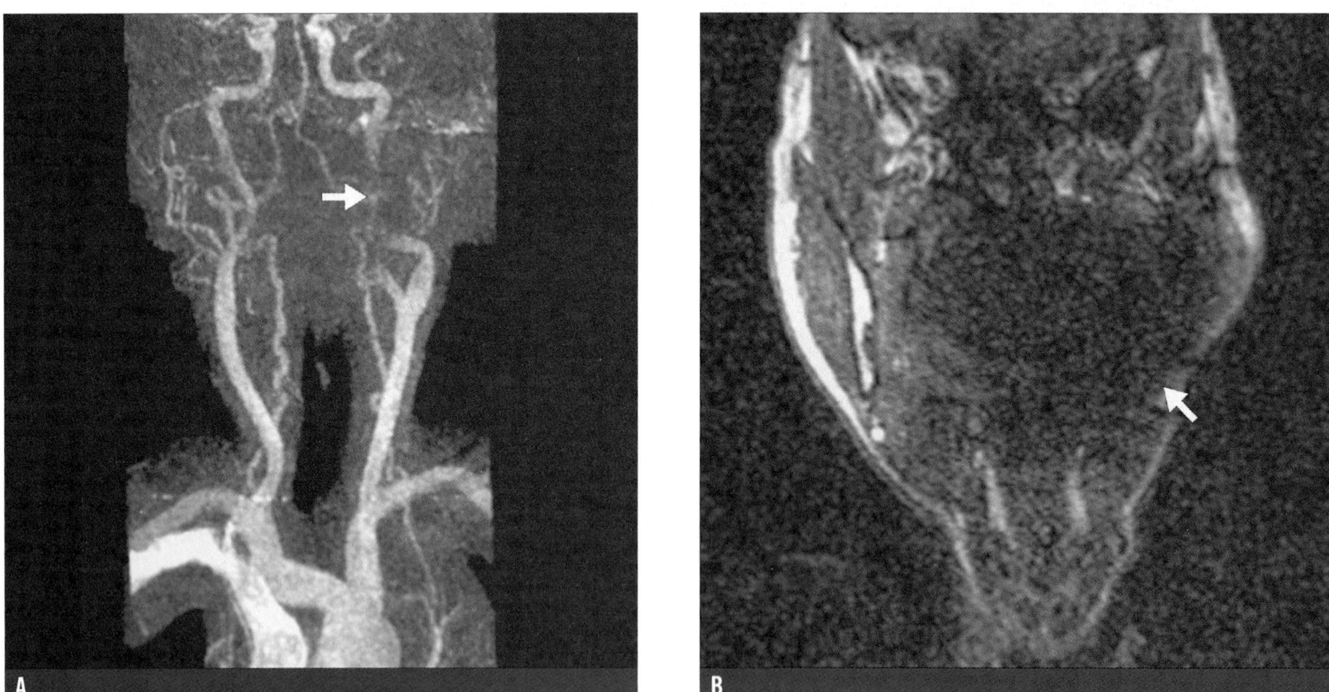

A frontal MIP image from a contrast-enhanced MRA of the neck (**A**) demonstrates an apparent flow gap within the high left cervical ICA (arrow, **A**). A source image from the same study (**B**) demonstrates a large region of susceptibility artifact (arrow, **B**). A sagittal reconstructed image from a CTA of the neck performed on the same patient (**C**) demonstrates horizontally oriented beam-hardening artifact (arrow, **C**) at level of the distal cervical ICA because of metallic dental amalgam. There is normal contrast enhancement and contour of the left cervical ICA on image **C** at the same level as the apparent left ICA flow gap on the accompanying MRA, confirming the artifactual nature of the finding on the MRA.

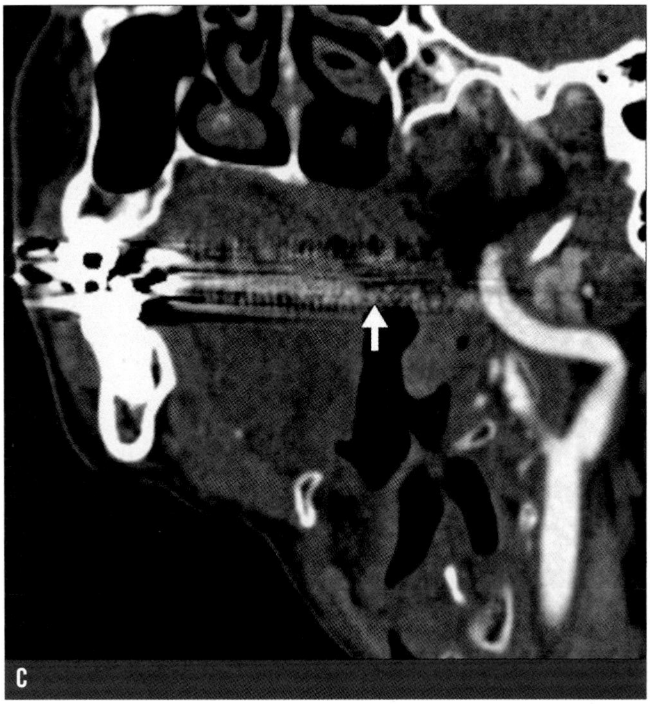

REFERENCES

Provenzale JM, Sarikaya B, Hacein-Bey L, Wintermark M. Causes of misinterpretation of cross-sectional imaging studies for dissection of the craniocervical arteries. *AJR Am J Roentgenol.* 2011:196:45-52.

Vargas MI, Delavelle J, Kohler R, Becker CD, Lovblad K. Brain and spine MRI artifacts at 3 Tesla. *J Neuroradiol.* 2009:36:74-81.

INDEX

Page numbers followed by an *f* indicate figures; page numbers in **boldface** indicate major discussions.

A

B

C

D

E

F

G

H

J

K

L

M

O

T

U

V

W

Z